KU-467-492

Kendig's

Disorders *of the* Respiratory Tract *in* Children

Kendig's

Disorders *of the* Respiratory Tract *in* Children

Seventh Edition

Victor Chernick, MD, FRCPC

Professor Emeritus
Department of Pediatrics, University of Manitoba
Active Staff, Children's Hospital of Winnipeg
Winnipeg, Manitoba, Canada

Thomas F. Boat, MD

Professor and Chair
Department of Pediatrics, University of Cincinnati College of Medicine
Director, Cincinnati Children's Research Foundation
Physician-in-Chief, Department of Pediatrics
Cincinnati Children's Hospital Medical Center
Cincinnati, Ohio

Robert W. Wilmott, BSc (Hons), MD, FRCP (UK)

IMMUNO Professor and Chair
Department of Pediatrics, St. Louis University
Pediatrician-in-Chief, SSM Cardinal Glennon Children's Hospital
St. Louis, Missouri

Andrew Bush, MB, BS (Hons), MA, MD, FRCP, FRCPCH

Professor of Paediatric Respirology
Department of Paediatric Respiratory Medicine
Imperial College at National Heart and Lung Institute
Consultant Paediatric Chest Physician
Department of Paediatrics, Royal Brompton Hospital
London, United Kingdom

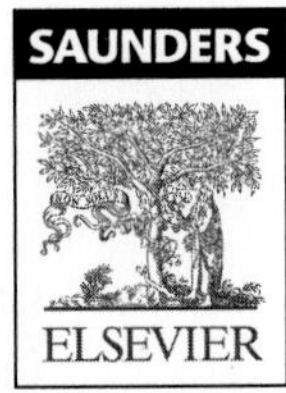

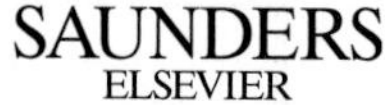

1600 John F. Kennedy Boulevard
Suite 1800
Philadelphia, PA 19103-2899

KENDIG'S DISORDERS OF THE RESPIRATORY TRACT IN CHILDREN
ISBN-13: 978-0-7216-3695-5
ISBN-10: 0-7216-3695-0

Copyright © 2006, Elsevier Inc. All rights reserved.

No part of this publication may be reproduced or transmitted in any form or by any means, electronic or mechanical, including photocopying, recording, or any information storage and retrieval system, without permission in writing from the publisher. Permissions may be sought directly from Elsevier's Health Sciences Rights Department in Philadelphia, PA, USA: phone: (+1) 215-239-3804, fax: (+1) 215-239-3805, e-mail: healthpermissions@elsevier.com. You may also complete your request on-line via the Elsevier homepage (http://www.elsevier.com), by selecting "Customer Support" and then "Obtaining Permissions."

Notice

Knowledge and best practice in this field are constantly changing. As new research and experience broaden our knowledge, changes in practice, treatment, and drug therapy may become necessary or appropriate. Readers are advised to check the most current information provided (i) on procedures featured or (ii) by the manufacturer of each product to be administered, to verify the recommended dose or formula, the method and duration of administration and contraindications. It is the responsibility of the practitioner, relying on his or her own experience and knowledge of the patient, to make diagnoses, to determine dosages and the best treatment for each individual patient, and to take all appropriate safety precautions. To the fullest extent of the law, neither the Publisher nor the Editors assume any liability for any injury and/or damage to persons or property arising out of or related to any use of the material contained in this book.

The Publisher

First Edition 1967. Second Edition 1972. Third Edition 1977. Fourth Edition 1983.
Fifth Edition 1990. Sixth Edition 1998.

Library of Congress Cataloging-in-Publication Data

Kendig's disorders of the respiratory tract in children/[edited by] Victor Chernick ...
[et al.].—7th ed.
p. ; cm.
Includes bibliographical references and index.
ISBN 0-7216-3695-0
1. Pediatric respiratory diseases. I. Title: Disorders of the respiratory tract in children.
II. Chernick, Victor. III. Kendig, Edwin L., 1911–2003
[DNLM: 1. Respiratory Tract Diseases—Child. 2. Respiratory Tract Diseases—Infant.
WS 280 K331 2006]
RJ431.K42 2006
618.92′2—dc22 2005056103

Acquisitions Editor: *Todd Hummel*
Senior Developmental Editor: *Kim J. Davis*
Senior Project Manager: *Joan Sinclair*
Design Direction: *Ellen Zanolle*

Printed in the United States of America.

Last digit is the print number: 9 8 7 6 5 4 3 2 1

Working together to grow
libraries in developing countries
www.elsevier.com | www.bookaid.org | www.sabre.org
ELSEVIER BOOK AID International Sabre Foundation

Dedication

The seventh edition of this book is dedicated to Dr. Edwin Lawrence Kendig, Jr., who died suddenly on February 18, 2003. It was his vision that resulted in the publication of the first edition nearly 40 years ago.

Born in 1911 in Victoria, Virginia, he graduated from the Hampden-Sydney College in 1932, where he was awarded the Gammon Cup for character, scholarship, and athletics. In 1936 he graduated from the University of Virginia School of Medicine, after which he trained in pediatrics at Bellevue Hospital (New York), Johns Hopkins Hospital (Baltimore), and Babies Hospital (Wrightsville Beach, North Carolina).

Dr. Kendig then settled in Richmond, Virginia, where he enjoyed a long and distinguished academic career with a special interest in childhood tuberculosis and sarcoidosis. He had the foresight to realize the unique nature of, and the need for research in, the field of pulmonary disease in children. In addition to his work on this book, renamed *Kendig's Disorders of the Respiratory Tract in Children* beginning with the fifth edition, Dr. Kendig contributed to academic pediatrics at the local, national, and international levels. Indeed, his name became synonymous with the subspecialty of pediatric pulmonology.

A retired professor of pediatrics at the Virginia Commonwealth University's Medical College of Virginia Hospitals, Dr. Kendig was also past president of the Virginia State Board of Medicine, the Virginia Pediatric Society, the Richmond Academy of Medicine, and the American Academy of Pediatrics. For two decades, he served as an official examiner for the American Board of Pediatrics, where he spent 13 years lobbying for the creation of a sub-board of pediatric pulmonology finally instituted in 1986.

Internationally, Dr. Kendig was well known not only for his work on this text but also for his many years of service as a member of the standing committee of the International Pediatric Association. During his career, Dr. Kendig was honored with many tributes, including the Abraham Jacobi Award from the American Academy of Pediatrics and the Distinguished Service Award from the American Medical Association. In 2003 the Medical College of Virginia created the Edwin Lawrence Kendig, Jr., Professorship for Pediatric Pulmonary Diseases.

This textbook is Dr. Kendig's legacy to the subspecialty of pediatric pulmonology. We will miss his wise counsel and his dedication to excellence.

Victor Chernick

Thomas F. Boat

Robert W. Wilmott

Andrew Bush

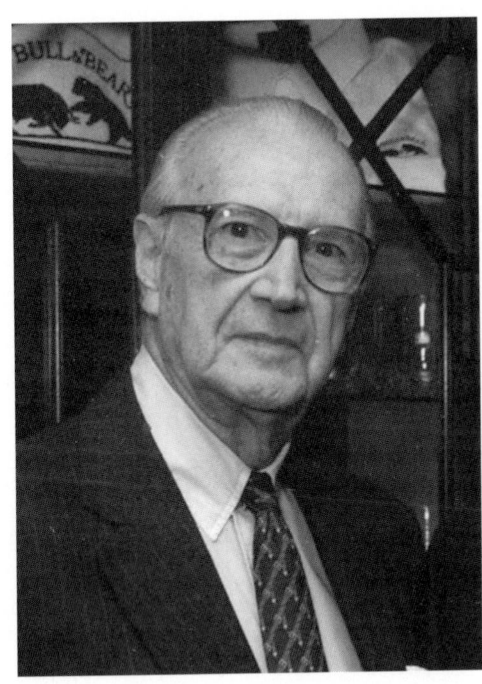

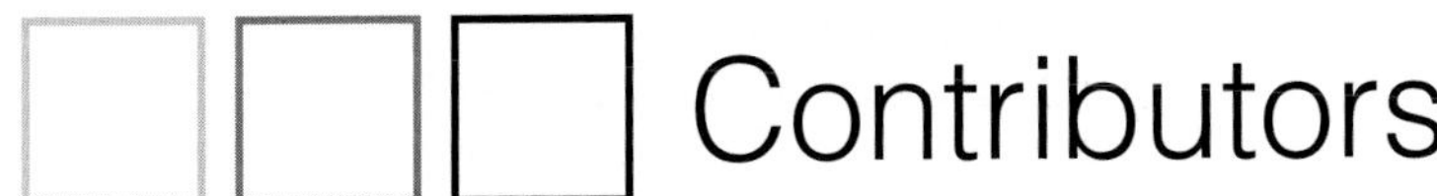

Contributors

Robin Michael Abel, BSc, MBBS, PhD, FRCS (Eng Paeds)
Consultant Paediatric and Neonatal Surgeon, Hammersmith Hospital, London, United Kingdom
Congenital Lung Disease

Steven H. Abman, MD
Professor, Department of Pediatrics, University of Colorado School of Medicine; Director, Pediatric Lung Center, The Children's Hospital, Denver, Colorado
Bronchopulmonary Dysplasia

Mutasim N. Abu-Hasan, MD
Assistant Professor of Clinical Pediatrics, Pediatric Allergy and Pulmonary Division, Pediatrics, University of Iowa College of Medicine, Iowa City, Iowa
Asthma in the Preschool Child

Najma N. Ahmed, MD, MSc, FRCPC
Assistant Professor, Department of Pediatrics, IWK Health Centre, Halifax, Nova Scotia, Canada
Nonpulmonary Manifestations of Cystic Fibrosis

Daniel R. Ambruso, MD
Professor, Department of Pediatrics, University of Colorado School of Medicine; Pediatric Hematologist, Departments of Pediatric Hematology, Oncology, and Bone Marrow Transplantation, The Children's Hospital; Associate Medical Director and Director of Research, Bonfils Blood Center, Denver, Colorado
Chronic Granulomatous Disease of Childhood

Raouf S. Amin, MD
Professor of Pediatrics, Department of Pediatrics, University of Cincinnati College of Medicine; Professor of Pediatrics, Department of Pulmonary Medicine, Cincinnati Children's Hospital Medical Center, Cincinnati, Ohio
Chronic Respiratory Failure; Hypersensitivity Pneumonitis and Eosinophilic Pulmonary Diseases

Robert J. Arceci, MD, PhD
Director and King Fahd Professor of Pediatric Oncology, Department of Oncology, Johns Hopkins University, Baltimore, Maryland
Histiocytic Disorders of the Lung

M. Innes Asher, MD, ONZM, BSc, MBChB, FRACP
Chair in Pediatrics and Head of Department, Department of Pediatrics, Faculty of Medical and Health Sciences, University of Auckland; Paediatric Respiratory Specialist, Respiratory Department, Starship Children's Health, Auckland District Health Board, Auckland, New Zealand
Epidemiology of Asthma

Ian M. Balfour-Lynn, BSc, MD, MBBS, FRCP, FRCPCH, FRCS (Ed), DHMSA
Consultant in Paediatric Respiratory Medicine, Department of Paediatrics, Royal Brompton Hospital, London, United Kingdom
Acute Infections Producing Upper Airway Obstruction

Peter J. Barnes, DM, DSc, FRCP
Professor and Head of Respiratory Medicine, National Heart and Lung Institute, Imperial College; Honorary Consultant Physician, Royal Brompton Hospital, London, United Kingdom
Biology and Assessment of Airway Inflammation

Robyn J. Barst, MD
Professor of Pediatrics, Department of Pediatric Cardiology, Columbia University College of Physicians and Surgeons; Attending Pediatrician, Department of Pediatric Cardiology, Morgan Stanley Children's Hospital of New York Presbyterian Medical Center; Director, Pulmonary Hypertension Center, New York Presbyterian Medical Center, New York, New York
Childhood Pulmonary Arterial Hypertension

Leslie L. Barton, MD
Professor of Pediatrics and Director of Pediatric Residency Program, Department of Pediatrics, University of Arizona School of Medicine; University of Arizona Health Sciences Center; Department of Pediatrics, Tuscon, Arizona
Atypical Pneumonias in Children

Pierre-Yves Berclaz, MD, PhD
Assistant Professor, Division of Pulmonary Medicine, Cincinnati Children's Hospital Medical Center, Cincinnati, Ohio
Rare Childhood Lung Disorders: α_1-Antitrypsin Deficiency, Pulmonary Alveolar Proteinosis, and Pulmonary Alveolar Microlithiasis

Thomas F. Boat, MD
Professor and Chair, Department of Pediatrics, University of Cincinnati College of Medicine; Director, Cincinnati Children's Research Foundation; Physician-in-Chief, Department of Pediatrics, Cincinnati Children's Hospital Medical Center, Cincinnati, Ohio
Pulmonary Hemorrhage and Hemoptysis

Itzhak Brook, MD, MSc
Professor of Pediatrics, Georgetown University School of Medicine, Washington, D.C.
Lung Abscess and Pulmonary Infections Due to Anaerobic Bacteria

James W. Brooks, MD
Emeritus Professor of Surgery, Cardiothoracic Division, Virginia Commonwealth University Health System/Medical College of Virginia; Medical College of Virginia Hospital, Richmond, Virginia
Tumors of the Chest; Disorders of the Respiratory Tract Due to Trauma

Andrew Bush, MB, BS (Hons), MA, MD, FRCP, FRCPCH
Professor of Paediatric Respirology, Department of Paediatric Respiratory Medicine, Imperial College at National Heart and Lung Institute; Consultant Paediatric Chest Physician, Department of Paediatrics, Royal Brompton Hospital, London, United Kingdom
Congenital Lung Disease

Michael R. Bye, MD
Professor of Clinical Pediatrics, Department of Pediatrics, Columbia University; Acting Director, Pediatric Pulmonary Medicine, Department of Pediatrics, Pulmonary Medicine Section, Morgan Stanley Children's Hospital of New York Presbyterian, New York, New York
Lung Injury from Hydrocarbon Aspiration and Smoke Inhalation

Emmanuel Canet, MD, PhD
Director, Research Institute, Servier, Suresnes, France
Chest Wall Function and Dysfunction

Todd C. Carpenter, MD
Associate Professor of Pediatrics, Division of Pediatric Critical Care Medicine, University of Colorado Health Sciences Center; The Children's Hospital, Department of Pediatrics, Denver, Colorado
Acute Respiratory Failure

Robert G. Castile, MD, MS
Professor of Pediatrics, College of Medicine and Public Health, The Ohio State University; Staff Physician, Department of Pediatrics, Children's Hospital, Columbus, Ohio
Pulmonary Function Testing in Children

Anne B. Chang, MBBS, FRACP, MPHTM, PhD
Associate Professor, Department of Paediatrics and Child Health, University of Queensland; Doctor of Respiratory Medicine, Royal Children's Hospital, Brisbane, Queensland, Australia
Bronchiectasis

Victor Chernick, MD, FRCPC
Professor Emeritus, Department of Pediatrics, University of Manitoba; Active Staff, Children's Hospital of Winnipeg, Winnipeg, Manitoba, Canada
The Functional Basis of Respiratory Disease; Pneumonia Secondary to Varicella and Measles

Lyn S. Chitty, PhD, MRCOG
Senior Lecturer, Department of Clinical and Molecular Genetics, Institute of Child Health; Fetal Medicine Unit, Elizabeth Garrett Anderson and Obstetric Hospital, UCLH, London, United Kingdom
Congenital Lung Disease

Allan L. Coates, MDCM
Professor, Departments of Paediatrics and Physiology, University of Toronto; Division of Respiratory Medicine, Department of Paediatrics, Hospital for Sick Children, Toronto, Ontario, Canada
Drug Administration by Aerosol in Children

Giuseppe N. Colasurdo, MD
Associate Professor and Head, Division of Pediatric Pulmonary and Critical Care Medicine, The University of Texas Health Science Center; Director, Respiratory Science Center, Memorial Hermann Children's Hospital, Houston, Texas
Lung Defenses: Intrinsic, Innate, and Adaptive

Misty Colvin, MD, FAAP
Clinical Lecturer of General Pediatrics, Department of Pediatrics, University of Arizona; Director, Pediatric Urgent Care, Department of Urgent Care, Northwest Hospital, Tuscon, Arizona
Atypical Pneumonias in Children

Dan M. Cooper, MD
Professor, Departments of Pediatrics and Bioengineering; GCRC Satellite Director, University of California, Irvine; Professor, Department of Pediatrics, UCI Medical Center; Professor, Department of Pediatrics, Children's Hospital of Orange County, Orange, California; Professor, Department of Pediatrics, Miller's Children's Hospital, Long Beach, California
Pulmonary Function Assessment in the Laboratory during Exercise

Jonathan Corren, MD
Associate Clinical Professor of Medicine, University of California, Los Angeles; Medical Director, Allergy Research Foundation, Los Angeles, California
The Influence of Upper Airway Disease on the Lower Airway

Robin T. Cotton, MD
Professor, Department of Otolaryngology, University of Cincinnati College of Medicine; Director, Department of Pediatric Oncology–Head and Neck Surgery, Cincinnati Children's Hospital Medical Center, Cincinnati, Ohio
Foreign Body Aspiration

James E. Crowe, Jr., MD
Professor, Departments of Pediatrics and Microbiology and Immunology; Director, Vanderbilt Vaccine Center, Vanderbilt University Medical Center, Nashville, Tennessee
Viral Pneumonia

Garry R. Cutting, MD
Professor of Pediatrics and Medicine, Institute of Genetic Medicine, Johns Hopkins University School of Medicine, Baltimore, Maryland
Genetics and Pathophysiology of Cystic Fibrosis

Cori Daines, MD
Assistant Professor of Pediatrics, University of Cincinnati College of Medicine; Assistant Professor of Pediatrics, Department of Pediatric Pulmonary Medicine, Cincinnati Children's Hospital Medical Center, Cincinnati, Ohio
Bronchoscopy and Bronchoalveolar Lavage in Pediatric Patients

Jane C. Davies, MD, MBChB, MRCPCH
Senior Lecturer, Department of Gene Therapy, Imperial College; Honorary Consultant in Paediatric Respiratory Medicine, Royal Brompton Hospital, London, United Kingdom
Acute Infections Producing Upper Airway Obstruction

Jonathan M. Davis, MD
Professor of Pediatrics, Department of Pediatrics, SUNY Stony Brook School of Medicine, Stony Brook, New York; Director of Neonatology; Director, CardioPulmonary Research Institute, Winthrop University Hospital, Mineola, New York
Bronchopulmonary Dysplasia

Pamela B. Davis, MD, PhD
Arline H. and Curtis L. Garvin Research Professor, Department of Pediatrics, Case Western Reserve University School of Medicine; Director, Pediatric Pulmonary Division, Department of Pediatrics, Rainbow Babies and Children's Hospital, Cleveland, Ohio
Pulmonary Disease in Cystic Fibrosis

Robert Dinwiddie, FRCPCH
Honorary Senior Lecturer, Portex Unit, The Institute of Child Health, University of London; Honorary Consultant Paediatrician, Respiratory Unit, Great Ormond Street Hospital for Children, London, United Kingdom
Familial Dysautonomia

Emily L. Dobyns, MD
Associate Professor, Department of Pediatrics, Section of Critical Care Medicine, University of Colorado; Medical Director, PICU, The Children's Hospital/University of Colorado, Denver, Colorado
Acute Respiratory Failure

Michelle Duggan, MB, FFARCSI
Clinical Fellow, Department of Anesthesia, The Hospital for Sick Children, Toronto, Ontario, Canada
Atelectasis

Peter R. Durie, MD, FRCP(C), BSc
Professor, Department of Pediatrics, Faculty of Medicine, University of Toronto; Senior Scientist, Department of Integrative Biology, Research Institute, The Hospital for Sick Children; Staff Physician, Division of Gastroenterology, Hepatology and Nutrition, The Hospital for Sick Children, Toronto, Ontario, Canada
Nonpulmonary Manifestations of Cystic Fibrosis

Anthony G. Durmowicz, MD
Medical Officer, Division of Pulmonary and Allergy Products, Center for Drug Evaluation and Research, Federal Drug Administration, Silver Spring, Maryland
Acute Respiratory Failure

Joanne Embree, MD, FRCPC
Professor and Head, Department of Medical Microbiology, University of Manitoba; Professor and Section Head, Department of Pediatric Infectious Disease, Children's Hospital/Health Sciences Centre, Winnipeg, Manitoba, Canada
Pneumonia Secondary to Varicella and Measles

Leland L. Fan, MD
Professor of Pediatrics, Pulmonary Section, Department of Pediatrics, Baylor College of Medicine; Texas Children's Hospital, Houston, Texas
Interstitial Lung Disease

Philip M. Farrell, MD, PhD
Dean and Vice Chancellor for Medical Affairs, University of Wisconsin Medical School; Robert Turell Professor in Medical Leadership, Department of Pediatrics, University of Wisconsin Hospital and Clinics, Madison, Wisconsin
Neonatal Screening for Cystic Fibrosis

David Gozal, MD
Children's Foundation Chair of Pediatric Research, Professor of Pediatrics, Pharmacology and Toxicology, Psychology and Brain Sciences, Kosair Children's Hospital Research Institute, Department of Pediatrics, University of Louisville; Director, Sleep Medicine and Apnea Center, Kosair Children's Hospital, Louisville, Kentucky
Disorders of Breathing during Sleep

Cameron Grant, MBChB, FRACP, PhD
Associate Professor, Department of Pediatrics, University of Auckland; Consultant Pediatrician, Department of General Pediatrics, Starship Children's Hospital, Auckland District Health Board, Auckland, New Zealand
Epidemiology of Asthma

Anne Greenough, MD, FRCP, FRCPCH
Professor, Division of Asthma, Allergy, and Lung Biology, King's College; Honorary Consultant Paediatrician, Department of Child Health, King's College Hospital, London, United Kingdom
Respiratory Disorders in the Newborn

Jürg Hammer, MD
Associate Professor of Pediatrics, Division of Intensive Care and Pulmonology, University Children's Hospital Basel, Basel, Switzerland
Near-Drowning and Drowning

Jonny Harcourt, FRCS
Consultant ENT Surgeon, Department of Paediatric ENT, Chelsea and Westminster Hospital; Consultant ENT Surgeon, ENT Department, Royal Brompton Hospital, London, United Kingdom
Congenital Lung Disease

Ulrich Heininger, MD
Professor and Doctor of Medicine, Medical School, University of Basel; Professor and Doctor of Medicine, Department of Pediatric Infectious Diseases and Vaccinology, University Children's Hospital, Basel, Switzerland
Pertussis and Other Bordetella *Infections of the Respiratory Tract*

Marianna M. Henry, MD, MPH
Associate Professor of Pediatrics, Department of Pediatrics, University of North Carolina at Chapel Hill; North Carolina Children's Hospital, University of North Carolina Hospitals, Chapel Hill, North Carolina
Sarcoidosis; Lung Injury Caused by Pharmacologic Agents

Peter W. Heymann, MD
Professor of Pediatrics; Head, Division of Pediatric Respiratory Medicine, Department of Pediatrics, University of Virginia, Charlottesville, Virginia
Immunopathogenesis of Asthma

Ellis K.L. Hon, MBBS, FAAP, FHKCP, FHKAM (Paed)
Associate Professor, Department of Pediatrics, The Chinese University of Hong Kong; Honorary Associate Consultant, Department of Pediatrics, NTEC, Prince of Wales Hospital, Hong Kong
Pediatric Severe Acute Respiratory Syndrome

Alan H. Jobe, MD, PhD
Professor of Pediatrics, University of Cincinnati College of Medicine; Professor of Pediatrics, Department of Neonatology/Pulmonary Biology, Cincinnati Children's Hospital Medical Center, Cincinnati, Ohio
The Surfactant System

Richard B. Johnston, Jr., MD
Professor of Pediatrics and Associate Dean for Research Development, University of Colorado School of Medicine; Executive Vice President for Academic Affairs, National Jewish Medical and Research Center, Denver, Colorado
Chronic Granulomatous Disease of Childhood

Sebastian L. Johnston, MD, PhD, FRCP
Professor of Respiratory Medicine, Department of Respiratory Medicine, National Heart and Lung Institute, Imperial College London; Honorary Consultant Physician, Chest and Allergy Clinic, St. Mary's NHS Trust, London, United Kingdom
Diagnosis of Viral Respiratory Illness: Practical Applications

Meyer Kattan, MD, CM
Professor, Department of Pediatrics, Mount Sinai School of Medicine; Chief, Pediatric Pulmonary and Critical Care, Department of Pediatrics, Mount Sinai Medical Center, New York, New York
Respiratory Disorders in Pediatric HIV Infection

Brian P. Kavanagh, MB, BSc, MRCP(I), FRCP(C)
Associate Professor, Departments of Anesthesia, Medicine, and Physiology, University of Toronto; Dr. Geoffrey Barker Chair in Critical Care Medicine, Staff Physician, and Director of Research, Department of Critical Care Medicine, Scientist, Research Institute, Hospital for Sick Children, Toronto, Ontario, Canada
Atelectasis

James S. Kemp, MD
Associate Professor, Pulmonary Division, Department of Pediatrics, St. Louis University School of Medicine; Medical Director, Respiratory Care and Sleep Clinic, Cardinal Glennon Children's Hospital, St. Louis, Missouri
Sudden Infant Death Syndrome and Acute Life-Threatening Events

Carolyn M. Kercsmar, MD
Professor, Department of Pediatrics, Case Western Reserve Medical School; Director, Asthma Center, Department of Pediatrics, Rainbow Babies and Children's Hospital, Cleveland, Ohio
Wheezing in Older Children: Asthma

Leila Kheirandish, MD
Senior Clinical and Research Post-doctoral Fellow, Division of Pediatric Sleep Medicine, Department of Pediatrics, University of Louisville, Louisville, Kentucky
Disorders of Breathing during Sleep

Jennifer Knight-Madden, MBBS, FRCP(C)
Lecturer, Sickle Cell Unit, Tropical Medicine Research Institute, University of the West Indies; Honorary Consultant, Department of Obstetrics, Gynaecology, and Child Health, University Hospital of the West Indies, Kingston, Jamaica
The Lung in Sickle Cell Disease

Alan P. Knutsen, MD
Professor and Director of Pediatric Allergy and Immunology, Department of Pediatrics, Division of Allergy and Immunology, St. Louis University, St. Louis, Missouri
Hypersensitivity Pneumonitis and Eosinophilic Pulmonary Diseases

Thomas M. Krummel, MD, FACS, FAAP
Emile Holman Professor and Chair, Department of Surgery, Stanford University School of Medicine; Professor of Surgery, Department of Surgery, Stanford Hospital and Clinics; Susan B. Ford Surgeon-in-Chief, Department of Pediatric Surgery, Lucile Packard Children's Hospital, Palo Alto, California
Tumors of the Chest; Disorders of the Respiratory Tract Due to Trauma

Claire Langston, MD
Professor, Departments of Pathology and Pediatrics, Baylor College of Medicine; Department of Pathology, Texas Children's Hospital, Houston, Texas
Interstitial Lung Disease

Ada S. Lee, MD
Assistant Professor of Pediatrics, Department of Pediatrics, Columbia University College of Physicians and Surgeons; Assistant Attending Physician, Department of Pediatrics, The Morgan Stanley Children's Hospital of New York–Presbyterian, New York, New York; Consulting Staff, Pediatric Pulmonology, Department of Pediatrics, Northern Westchester Hospital, Mount Kisco, New York
Lung Injury from Hydrocarbon Aspiration and Smoke Inhalation

Margaret W. Leigh, MD
Professor, Department of Pediatrics, University of North Carolina; Attending Physician, UNC Hospitals, Chapel Hill, North Carolina
Influenza; Primary Ciliary Dyskinesia

Ann Marie LeVine, MD
Associate Professor, Department of Pediatrics, University of Florida, Gainesville, Florida
The Surfactant System

Albert Martin Li, MBBch, MRCP (UK), MRCPCH, FHKCP, FHKAM (Paed)
Associate Professor, Department of Paediatrics, Chinese University of Hong Kong; Honorary Associate Consultant, Department of Paediatrics, Prince of Wales Hospital, Shatin, Hong Kong
Pediatric Severe Acute Respiratory Syndrome

Gerald M. Loughlin, MD
Nancy C. Paduano Professor and Chairman, Department of Pediatrics, Weill Medical College of Cornell University; Pediatrician-in-Chief, Phyllis and David Komansky Center for Child Health, New York–Presbyterian Hospital, New York, New York
Bronchitis

Anna M. Mandalakas, MD
Assistant Professor of Pediatrics and Global Health, Department of Pediatrics, Case Western Reserve University; Assistant Professor, Department of Clinical Epidemiology, Rainbow Babies and Children's Hospital, Cleveland, Ohio
Tuberculosis and Nontuberculous Mycobacterial Disease

Paulo J.C. Marostica, MD
Professor of Pediatrics, Department of Pediatrics, Universidade Federal do Rio Grande do Sul; Professor, Department of Emergency Medicine, Hospital de Clinicas de Porto Alegre, Porto Alegre–Rio Grande do Sul (RS), Brazil
Community-Acquired Bacterial Pneumonia

Robert B. Mellins, MD
Professor of Pediatrics, Columbia University; Morgan Stanley Children's Hospital of New York–Presbyterian, New York, New York
Lung Injury from Hydrocarbon Aspiration and Smoke Inhalation

Mark Montgomery, MD, FRCP(C)
Clinical Associate Professor, Department of Child Health, University of Calgary; Consultant, Division of Pediatric Respiratory Medicine, Alberta Children's Hospital, Calgary, Alberta, Canada
Air and Liquid in the Pleural Space

Samira Mubareka, MD, FRCPC
Fellow in Infectious Diseases and Medical Microbiology, Department of Medical Microbiology and Infectious Diseases, University of Manitoba, Winnipeg, Manitoba, Canada
Pneumonia Secondary to Varicella and Measles

Thomas M. Murphy, MD
Associate Professor and Chief, Division of Pulmonary Medicine, Department of Pediatrics, Duke University School of Medicine; Chief, Division of Pulmonary Medicine, Department of Pediatrics, Duke Children's Hospital and Health Center, Durham, North Carolina
The Lung in Sickle Cell Disease

Joseph J. Nania, MD
Assistant Professor of Pediatrics, Department of Pediatrics, Division of Pediatric Infectious Diseases, Vanderbilt University School of Medicine; Vanderbilt Children's Hospital, Department of Pediatrics, Vanderbilt University School of Medicine, Nashville, Tennessee
The Mycoses

Christopher J.L. Newth, MB, ChB, FRCPC
Professor of Pediatrics, Departments of Anesthesiology and Critical Care Medicine, Keck School of Medicine, University of Southern California, Los Angeles, California
Acute Respiratory Distress Syndrome in the Pediatric Patient; Near-Drowning and Drowning

Andrew G. Nicholson, DM, FRCPath
Professor of Respiratory Pathology, National Heart and Lung Institute Division, Imperial College School of Medicine; Consultant Histopathologist, Royal Brompton and Harefield NHS Trust, London, United Kingdom
Congenital Lung Disease

Terry L. Noah, MD
Associate Professor, Department of Pediatrics; Investigator, Center for Environmental Medicine, Asthma, and Lung Biology, University of North Carolina at Chapel Hill; University of North Carolina Hospitals, University of North Carolina, Chapel Hill, North Carolina
Sarcoidosis; Lung Injury Caused by Pharmacologic Agents

Lawrence M. Nogee, MD
Associate Professor of Pediatrics, Department of Pediatrics, Johns Hopkins University School of Medicine; Attending Neonatologist, Division of Neonatology, Johns Hopkins Hospital, Baltimore, Maryland
Genetic Causes of Surfactant Deficiency

Blakeslee E. Noyes, MD
Associate Professor of Pediatrics, Department of Pediatrics, St. Louis University School of Medicine; Division of Pulmonary Medicine, Cardinal Glennon Children's Hospital, St. Louis, Missouri
Pediatric Lung Transplantation

Andrew H. Numa, MBBS, FRACP, FJFICM
Senior Lecturer, Department of Pediatrics, University of New South Wales; Senior Consultant, Department of Intensive Care, Sydney Children's Hospital; Senior Consultant, Department of Respiratory Medicine, Sydney Children's Hospital, Sydney, Australia
Acute Respiratory Distress Syndrome in the Pediatric Patient; Near-Drowning and Drowning

Hugh O'Brodovich, MD, FRCP(C)
Professor and Chair of Paediatrics, R.S. McLaughlin Foundation Chair in Paediatrics at The Hospital for Sick Children, Department of Paediatrics, University of Toronto; Paediatrician-in-Chief and Paediatric Pulmonologist, Department of Paediatrics, The Hospital for Sick Children, Toronto, Ontario, Canada
Pulmonary Edema

Christopher O'Callaghan, FRCP, FRCPCH, PhD, DM
Professor of Paediatrics, Department of Infection, Immunity and Inflammation, University of Leicester, Leicester, United Kingdom
Drug Administration by Aerosol in Children

Øystein E. Olsen, PhD
Consultant Radiologist, Department of Radiology, Great Ormond Street Hospital for Children NHS Trust, London, United Kingdom
Diagnostic Imaging of the Respiratory Tract

Catherine M. Owens, BSc, MBBS, MRCP, FRCR
Consultant Paediatric Radiologist and Clinical Director, Department of Radiology, Great Ormond Street Hospital for Children NHS Trust, London, United Kingdom
Diagnostic Imaging of the Respiratory Tract

Nikolaos G. Papadopoulos, MD, PhD
Lecturer in Pediatric Allergy and Head of Research, Allergy Department, Second Pediatric Clinic, University of Athens, Athens, Greece
Diagnosis of Viral Respiratory Illness: Practical Applications

Hans Pasterkamp, MD, FRCPC
Professor, Department of Pediatrics and Child Health, University of Manitoba; Head, Department of Pediatric Respirology, Winnipeg Children's Hospital, Winnipeg, Manitoba, Canada
The History and Physical Examination

Thomas A.E. Platts-Mills, MD, PhD
Professor of Medicine, Division Chief, Asthma and Allergic Diseases, Asthma and Allergic Diseases Center, University of Virginia, Charlottesville, Virginia
Immunopathogenesis of Asthma

Arnold C.G. Platzker, MD
Professor of Pediatrics, Department of Pediatrics, USC/Keck School of Medicine; Director, Cystic Fibrosis Center, Division of Pediatric Pulmonology, Department of Pediatrics, Children's Hospital of Los Angeles; Attending Physician, Department of Pediatrics, UCLA/Matel Children's Hospital; Adjunct Professor, Department of Pediatrics, UCLA/Mattel Children's Hospital, Los Angeles, California
Gastroesophageal Reflux and Aspiration Syndromes; Pulmonary Involvement in Rheumatoid Disorders of Childhood

Jean-Paul Praud, MD, PhD
Professor, Departments of Pediatrics and Physiology, Université de Sherbrooke, Quebec, Canada; Director, Research Institute, Servier, Suresnes, France
Chest Wall Function and Dysfunction

Stelios Psarras, PhD
Allergy Department, University of Athens, Goudi, Athens, Greece
Diagnosis of Viral Respiratory Illness: Practical Applications

Mobeen H. Rathore, MD
Professor and Chief, Department of Pediatric Infectious Diseases and Immunology, University of Florida; Chief, Section of Infectious Diseases and Hospital Epidemiologist, Wolfson Children's Hospital; Chief, Pediatric Infectious Diseases, Shands Jacksonville Medical Center; Director, Rainbow Center for Women, Adolescent Children and Families, University of Florida, Jacksonville, Florida
Toxocariasis, Hydatid Disease of the Lung, Strongyloidiasis, and Pulmonary Paragonimiasis

Gregory J. Redding, MD
Professor of Pediatrics, University of Washington School of Medicine; Chief, Department of Pulmonary Medicine, Children's Hospital and Regional Medical Center, Seattle, Washington
Bronchiectasis

Michael J. Rock, MD
Professor of Pediatrics, Department of Pediatrics, University of Wisconsin; Department of Pediatrics, American Family Children's Hospital, Madison, Wisconsin
Neonatal Screening for Cystic Fibrosis

Erika Berman Rosenzweig, MD
Assistant Professor of Pediatrics (in Medicine), Department of Pediatric Cardiology, Columbia University College of Physicians and Surgeons; Assistant Attending Pediatrician, Department of Pediatric Cardiology, Morgan Stanley Children's Hospital of New York Presbyterian Medical Center; Pulmonary Hypertension Center, New York Presbyterian Medical Center, New York, New York
Childhood Pulmonary Arterial Hypertension

Michael J. Rutter, MD
Associate Professor of Clinical Otolaryngology-Affiliated, Department of Otolaryngology, University of Cincinnati College of Medicine; Associate Professor, Pediatric Otolaryngology, Department of Otolaryngology, Cincinnati Children's Hospital Medical Center, Cincinnati, Ohio
Foreign Body Aspiration

L. Barry Seltz, MD
Clinical Associate Professor, Department of Pediatrics, University of Arizona, Tuscon, Arizona
Atypical Pneumonias in Children

Amir H. Shahlaee, MD
Assistant Professor of Pediatrics, Division of Pediatric Hematology and Oncology, University of Florida Health Science Center, Gainesville, Florida
Histiocytic Disorders of the Lung

David Sigalet, MD, PhD, FRCSC, FACS
Professor, Department of Surgery, University of Calgary; Regional Division Head, Division of Pediatric General Surgery, Alberta Children's Hospital, Calgary, Alberta, Canada
Air and Liquid in the Pleural Space

Samatha Sonnappa, MD, DCH, MRCP, FRCPCH
Fellow in Paediatric Respiratory Medicine, Department of Paediatric Respiratory Medicine, Great Ormond Street Hospital, London, United Kingdom
Familial Dysautonomia

Chaim Springer, MD
Associate Professor of Pediatrics, Hadassah Medical School, The Hebrew University; Institute of Pulmonology, Hadassah University Hospital, Ein Kerem, Jerusalem, Israel
Pulmonary Function Assessment in the Laboratory during Exercise

James M. Stark, MD, PhD
Associate Professor, Division of Pediatric Pulmonary and Critical Care Medicine, Department of Pediatrics, University of Texas Health Science Center at Houston; Co-director, Respiratory Sciences Center, Memorial Hermann Children's Hospital, Houston, Texas
Lung Defenses: Intrinsic, Innate, and Adaptive

Jeffrey R. Starke, MD
Professor and Vice Chairman, Department of Pediatrics, Baylor College of Medicine; Chief of Pediatrics, Ben Taub General Hospital, Houston, Texas
Tuberculosis and Nontuberculous Mycobacterial Disease

Renato T. Stein, MD
Professor, Department of Pediatrics, Pontificia Universidade Catolica RGS; Head, Pediatric Pulmonary Section, Hospital São Lucas Purcs, Porto Alegre, RS, Brazil
Community-Acquired Bacterial Pneumonia

Kurt R. Stenmark, MD
Professor and Head of Division of Pediatric Critical Care, Department of Pediatrics, University of Colorado, Denver, Colorado
Acute Respiratory Failure

Janet Stocks, PhD
Professor of Respiratory Physiology, Portex Anaesthesia, Intensive Therapy and Respiratory Unit, Institute of Child Health, University College London, London, United Kingdom
Pulmonary Function Tests in Infants and Preschool Children

Dennis C. Stokes, MD
Professor of Pediatrics, Dartmouth Medical School, Hanover, New Hampshire; Section of Pediatric Pulmonology, Department of Pediatrics, Children's Hospital of Dartmouth, Dartmouth-Hitchcock Medical Center, Lebanon, New Hampshire
Pulmonary Infections in the Immunocompromised Pediatric Host

James Temprano, MD
Clinical Fellow, Department of Pediatrics, Division of Allergy and Immunology, St. Louis University Health Sciences Center, St. Louis, Missouri
Hypersensitivity Pneumonitis and Eosinophilic Pulmonary Diseases

Bradley T. Thach, MD
Professor of Pediatrics, Newborn Medicine Division, Washington University School of Medicine and St. Louis Children's Hospital, St. Louis, Missouri
Sudden Infant Death Syndrome and Acute Life-Threatening Events

Bruce C. Trapnell, MD
Professor, Departments of Medicine and Pediatrics, University of Cincinnati College of Medicine; Attending Physician, Department of Pediatrics, Cincinnati Children's Hospital Medical Center; Attending Physician, Department of Medicine, University of Cincinnati College of Medicine, Cincinnati, Ohio
Rare Childhood Lung Disorders: α_1-Antitrypsin Deficiency, Pulmonary Alveolar Proteinosis, and Pulmonary Alveolar Microlithiasis

Colin Wallis, MD, FRCPCH, DCH
Institute Senior Lecturer, Department of Respiratory Paediatrics, The Institute of Child Health; Consultant Paediatrician, Respiratory Unit, Great Ormond Street Hospital for Children, London, United Kingdom
Diagnosis and Presentation of Cystic Fibrosis

Miles Weinberger, MD
Professor and Director, Pediatric Allergy and Pulmonary Division, Department of Pediatrics, University of Iowa, Iowa City, Iowa
Asthma in the Preschool Child

Susan E. Wert, PhD
Associate Professor, Department of Pediatrics, University of Cincinnati College of Medicine; Associate Professor, Division of Pulmonary Biology, Cincinnati Children's Hospital and Medical Center, Cincinnati, Ohio
Molecular Determinants of Lung Morphogenesis

John B. West, MD, PhD, DSc, FRCP, FRACP
Professor of Medicine and Physiology, Department of Medicine, University of California, San Diego, La Jolla, California
The Functional Basis of Respiratory Disease

Jeffrey A. Whitsett, MD
Professor, Department of Pediatrics, University of Cincinnati College of Medicine; Chief, Divisions of Neonatology, Perinatal and Pulmonary Biology, Department of Pediatrics, Cincinnati Children's Hospital Medical Center, Cincinnati, Ohio
Molecular Determinants of Lung Morphogenesis

Robert W. Wilmott, BSc (Hons), MD, FRCP (UK)
IMMUNO Professor and Chair, Department of Pediatrics, St. Louis University; Pediatrician-in-Chief, SSM Cardinal Glennon Children's Hospital, St. Louis, Missouri
Hypersensitivity Pneumonitis and Eosinophilic Pulmonary Diseases

Mary Ellen B. Wohl, MD
Professor of Pediatrics, Harvard Medical School; Division Chief Emeritus, Division of Respiratory Diseases, Children's Hospital of Boston, Boston, Massachusetts
Developmental Physiology of the Respiratory System; Bronchiolitis

Robert E. Wood, MD, PhD
Cincinnati Children's Hospital Medical Center, Division of Pulmonary Medicine, Cincinnati, Ohio
Bronchoscopy and Bronchoalveolar Lavage in Pediatric Patients

Peter F. Wright, MD
Professor of Pediatrics, Pathology and Immunology and Microbiology, Department of Pediatrics, Division of Pediatric Infectious Diseases, Vanderbilt University School of Medicine; Vanderbilt Children's Hospital, Department of Pediatrics, Vanderbilt University School of Medicine, Nashville, Tennessee
The Mycoses

Pamela L. Zeitlin, MD, PhD
Professor of Pediatrics, Department of Pediatrics, Johns Hopkins University School of Medicine, Baltimore, Maryland
Genetics and Pathophysiology of Cystic Fibrosis

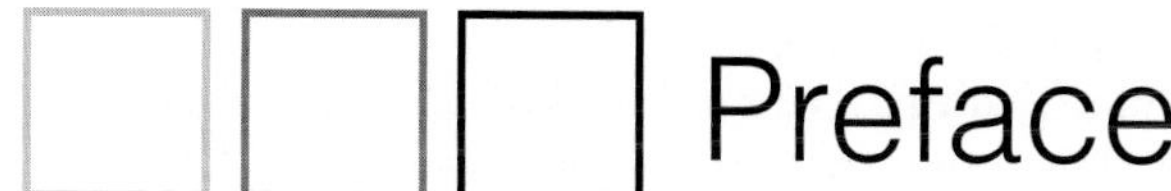

Preface

Since the publication of the sixth edition in 1998, there have been tremendous changes in the subspecialty of pediatric pulmonology. We continue to be amazed by the pace of change and the accumulation of new knowledge. There are now four editors, who have shared the task of assembling chapters, cajoling authors, and ensuring that the book is up-to-date and comprehensive. The general organization of the book remains the same, but because of the complexity of the topics of asthma and cystic fibrosis, they have now graduated to sections of their own. The seventh edition includes 21 new chapters and more than 80 new authors; we thank them all for their hard work and diligence.

Our objective has expanded from that of the first edition. It is our goal to provide a comprehensive textbook of pediatric respiratory disease for the established pediatric respirologist and intensivist; for those who are in training in these subspecialties; and for pediatric practitioners, residents, and interns. In addition, the book is an important resource for roentgenologists, pediatric allergists, thoracic surgeons, and students in allied specialties with a particular interest in pediatric chest disease. Included are both common and rare childhood disorders of the lungs, as well as basic scientific considerations necessary for an understanding of pulmonary disease processes and their effect on pulmonary function. Edwin Kendig's book has become the bible of pediatric pulmonology, and we have strived to continue his tradition in this edition, which is dedicated to his memory.

Once again, the members of the staff at Elsevier (Saunders) have provided superb support, and we are grateful for their sound advice, patience, and attention to detail. In particular, we thank Kim J. Davis, senior developmental editor, who has been extremely diligent and patient with us, and Todd Hummel, who has provided encouragement and sage advice.

Not least, we acknowledge the tremendous support, tolerance, and forbearance of our partners and families, which have made this volume possible.

Victor Chernick, MD

Thomas F. Boat, MD

Robert W. Wilmott, MD

Andrew Bush, MD

Color Plates

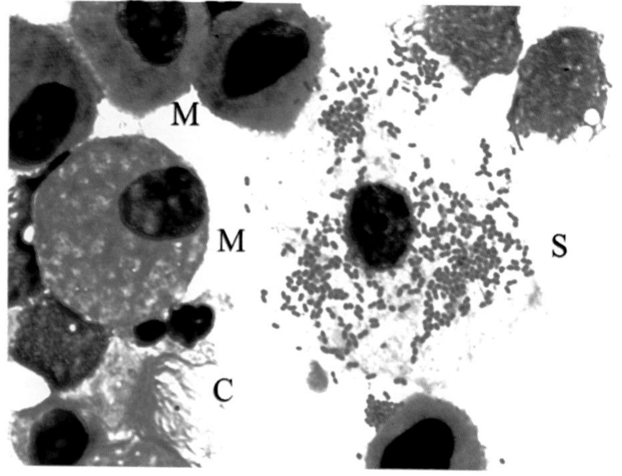

■ **COLOR PLATE 1.** Alveolar macrophages (*M*). Squamous epithelial cell (*S*) with adherent bacteria. Such cells usually represent contamination of the specimen with oral secretions. Ciliated epithelial cell (*C*); these cells are often seen in normal BAL specimens and are of little diagnostic significance. (See Fig. 7-2.)

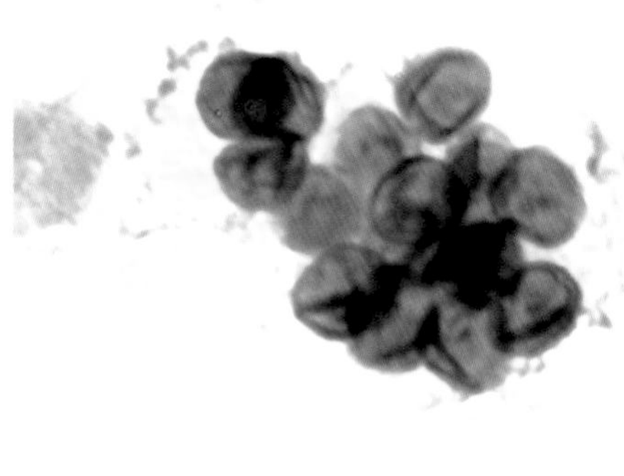

■ **COLOR PLATE 3.** Pneumocysts (methenamine silver stain). (See Fig. 7-4.)

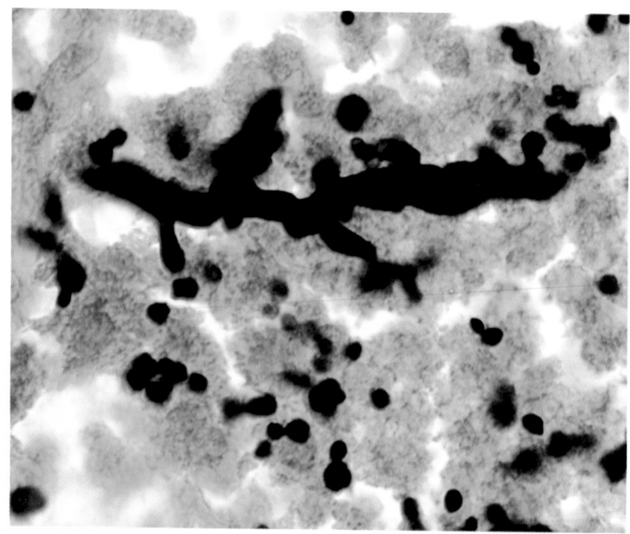

■ **COLOR PLATE 2.** Budding yeast on methenamine silver stain. (See Fig. 7-3.)

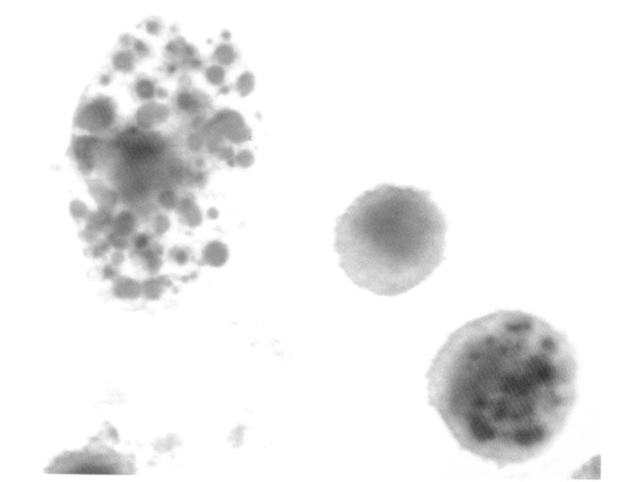

■ **COLOR PLATE 4.** Lipid-laden macrophages (Oil Red O stain). (See Fig. 7-5.)

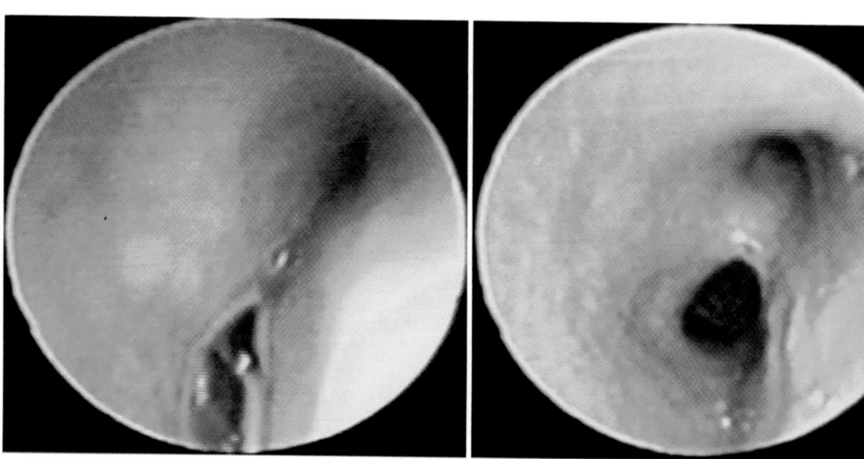

■ **COLOR PLATE 5.** Bronchomalacia, right main bronchus. *Left:* During expiration. *Right:* During inspiration. (See Fig. 7-6.)

■ COLOR PLATE 6. Tracheomalacia. *Left:* During expiration. *Right:* During inspiration. (See Fig. 7-7.)

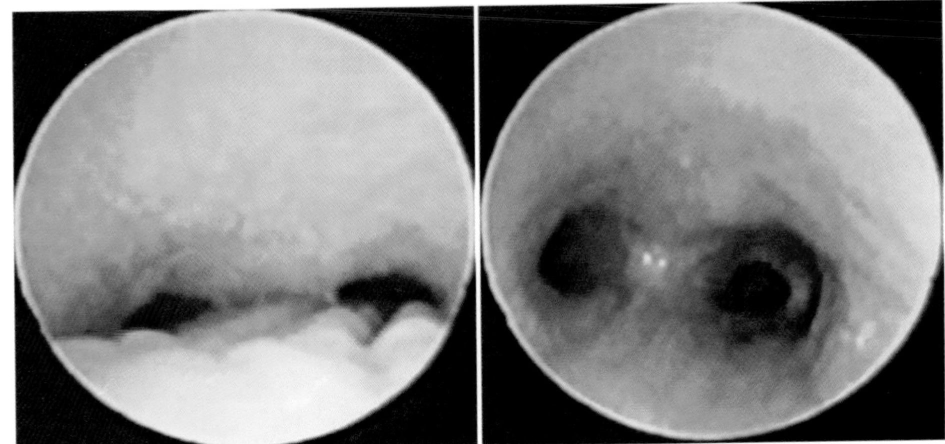

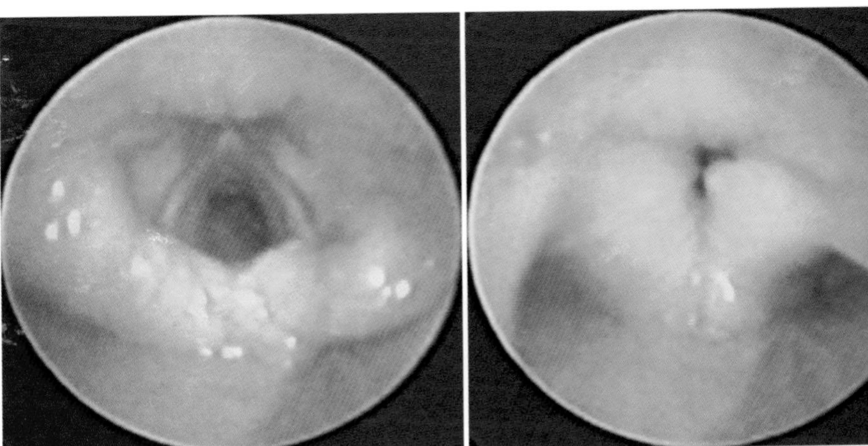

■ COLOR PLATE 7. Laryngomalacia. *Left:* During expiration. *Right:* During inspiration, the arytenoids prolapse into the glottis. (See Fig. 7-8.)

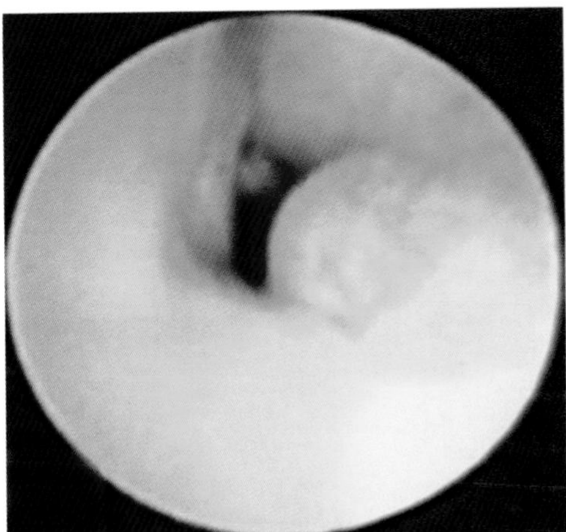

■ COLOR PLATE 8. Infant with persistent stridor, beginning 3 months after intubation. Large subglottic cyst arises from the right side of the subglottic space. (See Fig. 7-9.)

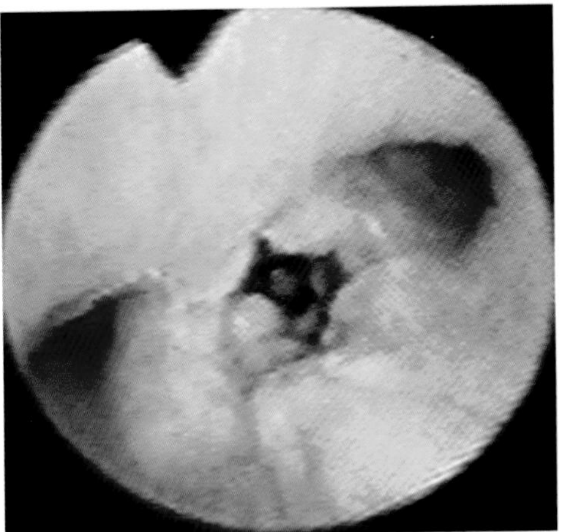

■ COLOR PLATE 9. Endobronchial damage (granulation tissue) resulting from deep endotracheal suctioning. The right middle lobe (*on left*) and the superior segment of the right lower lobe (*on right*) are relatively unaffected; the orifice leading to the basal segments (the direct path of the catheter) is nearly occluded. Continued injury may lead to atelectasis or even complete bronchial stenosis. (See Fig. 7-10.)

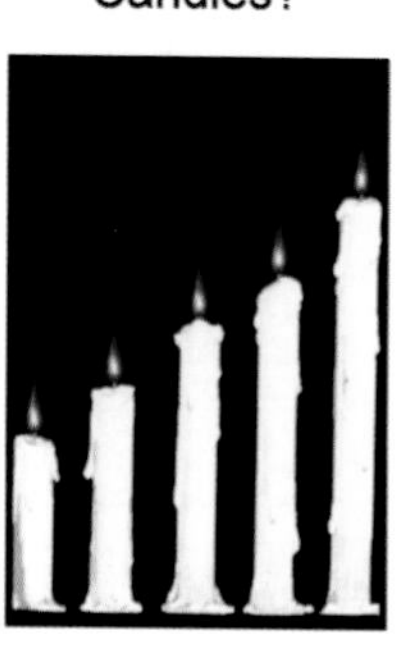

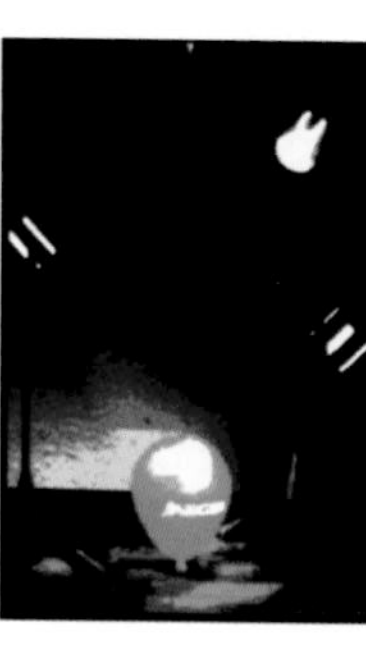

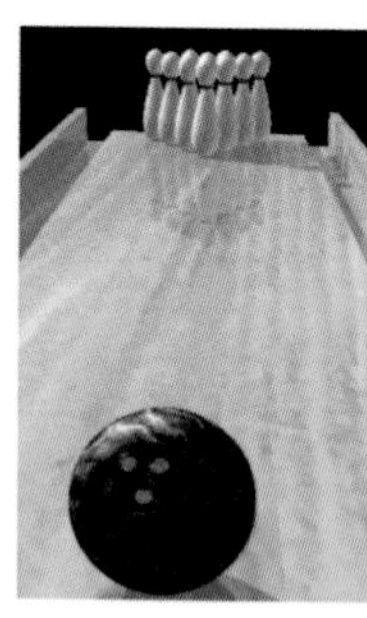

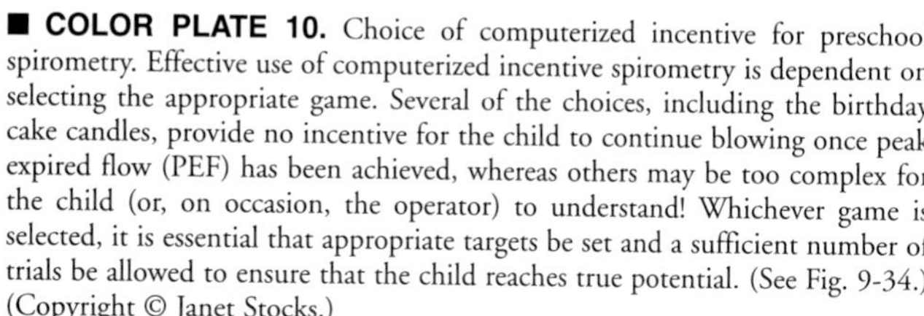

■ **COLOR PLATE 10.** Choice of computerized incentive for preschool spirometry. Effective use of computerized incentive spirometry is dependent on selecting the appropriate game. Several of the choices, including the birthday cake candles, provide no incentive for the child to continue blowing once peak expired flow (PEF) has been achieved, whereas others may be too complex for the child (or, on occasion, the operator) to understand! Whichever game is selected, it is essential that appropriate targets be set and a sufficient number of trials be allowed to ensure that the child reaches true potential. (See Fig. 9-34.) (Copyright © Janet Stocks.)

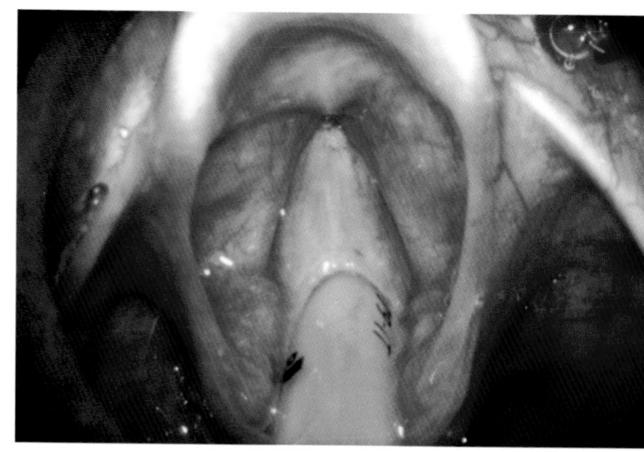

■ **COLOR PLATE 13.** Congenital laryngeal web associated with anterior subglottic stenosis. (See Fig. 17-9.) (Picture reproduced courtesy of Mr. C.M. Bailey.)

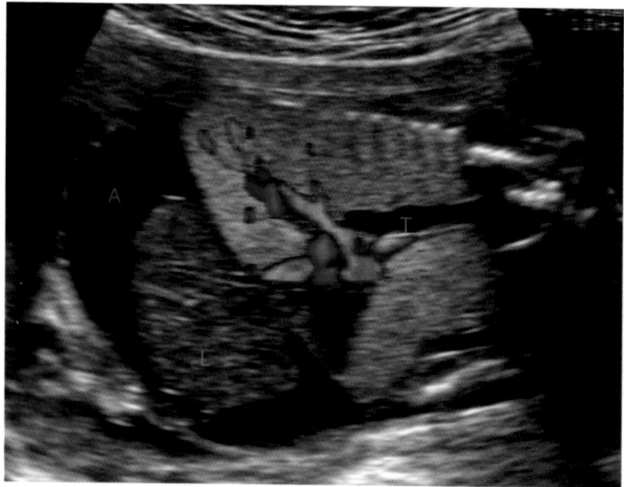

■ **COLOR PLATE 11.** Longitudinal view of a fetus with tracheal agenesis. The heart can be seen highlighted by the color Doppler, with the abnormally dilated trachea (*T*) seen as a fluid-filled structure in the mediastinum. The lungs bulge downward into the ascites (*A*) in the abdominal cavity, in which the liver (*L*) can be seen. (See Fig. 17-7.)

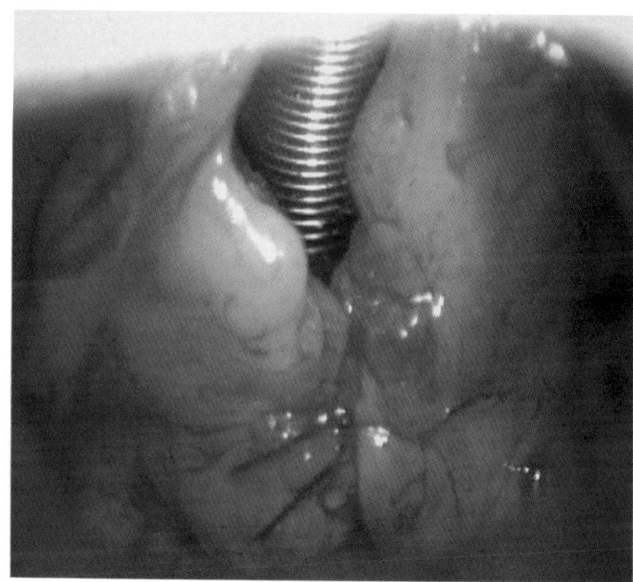

■ **COLOR PLATE 14.** Endoscopic repair of laryngeal cleft type 1. (See Fig. 17-10.)

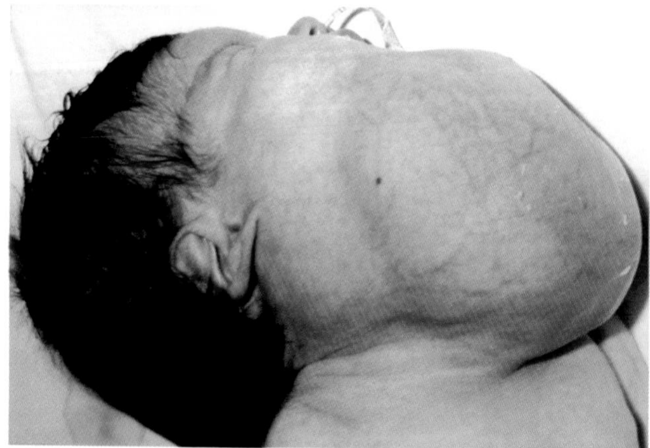

■ **COLOR PLATE 12.** Severe neonatal upper airway obstruction due to cystic hygroma. (See Fig. 17-8.) (Picture reproduced courtesy of Mr. C.M. Bailey.)

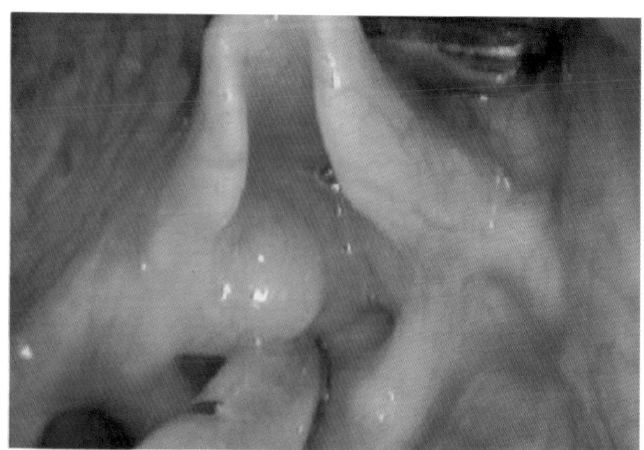

■ **COLOR PLATE 15.** Congenital saccular cyst of aryepiglottic fold. (See Fig. 17-11.)

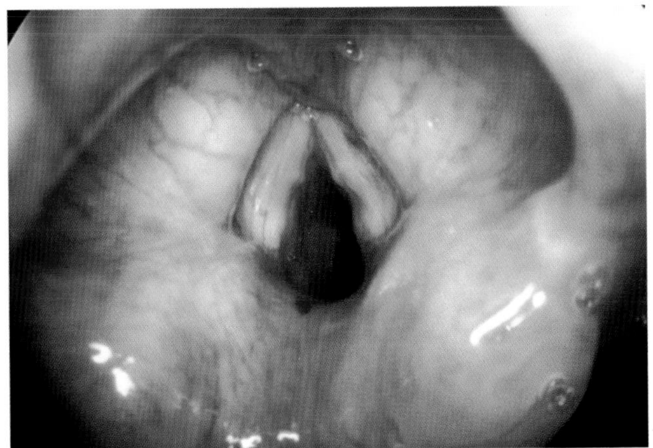

■ **COLOR PLATE 16.** Subglottic hemangioma. (See Fig. 17-12.) (Picture reproduced courtesy of Mr. C.M. Bailey.)

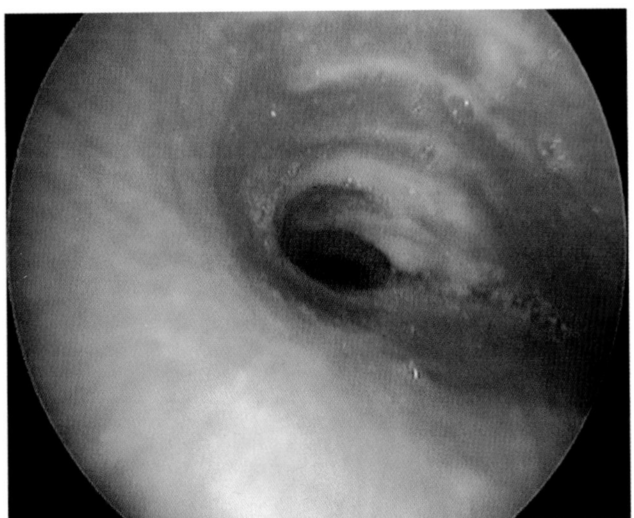

■ **COLOR PLATE 17.** Tracheomalacia, acquired secondary to cardiac surgery. (See Fig. 17-13.)

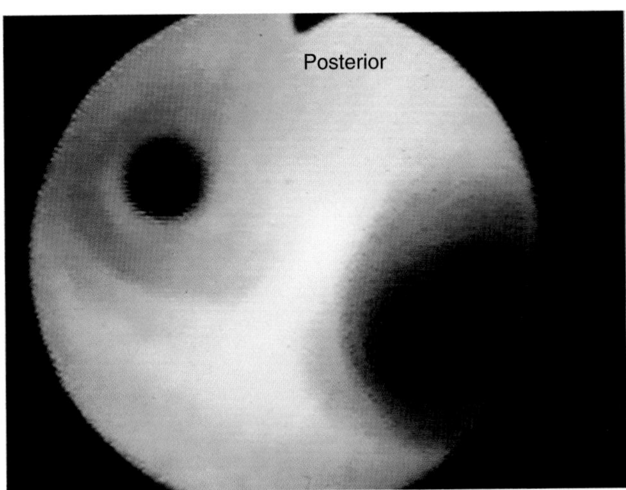

■ **COLOR PLATE 18.** Bronchoscopic view of a single complete cartilage ring at the origin of the right main bronchus. (See Fig. 17-14.)

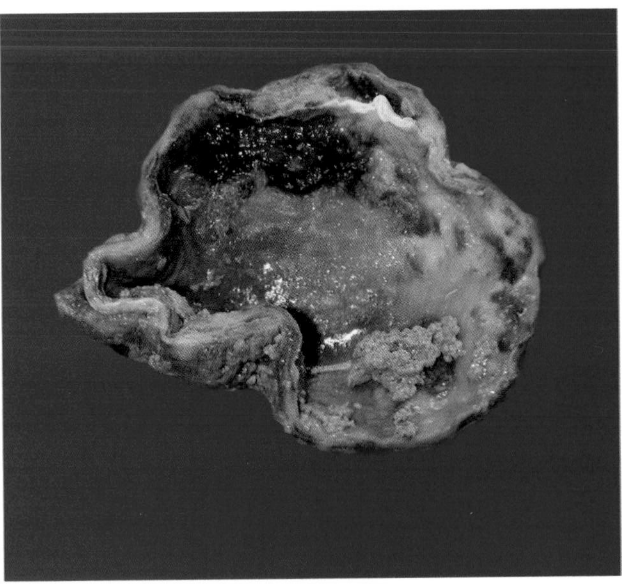

■ **COLOR PLATE 19.** Mediastinal bronchogenic cyst. The inner surface of this unilocular cyst is partly hemorrhagic and partly covered by purulent debris, indicative of recurrent infection. (See Fig. 17-16.)

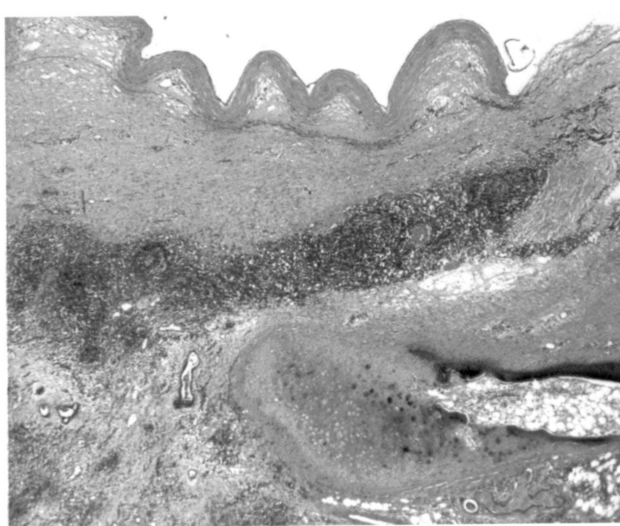

■ **COLOR PLATE 20.** Mediastinal bronchogenic cyst. The lining of the cyst is mainly denuded, while the wall is chronically inflamed. Note the cartilage plate that indicates bronchogenic origin. (See Fig. 17-17.)

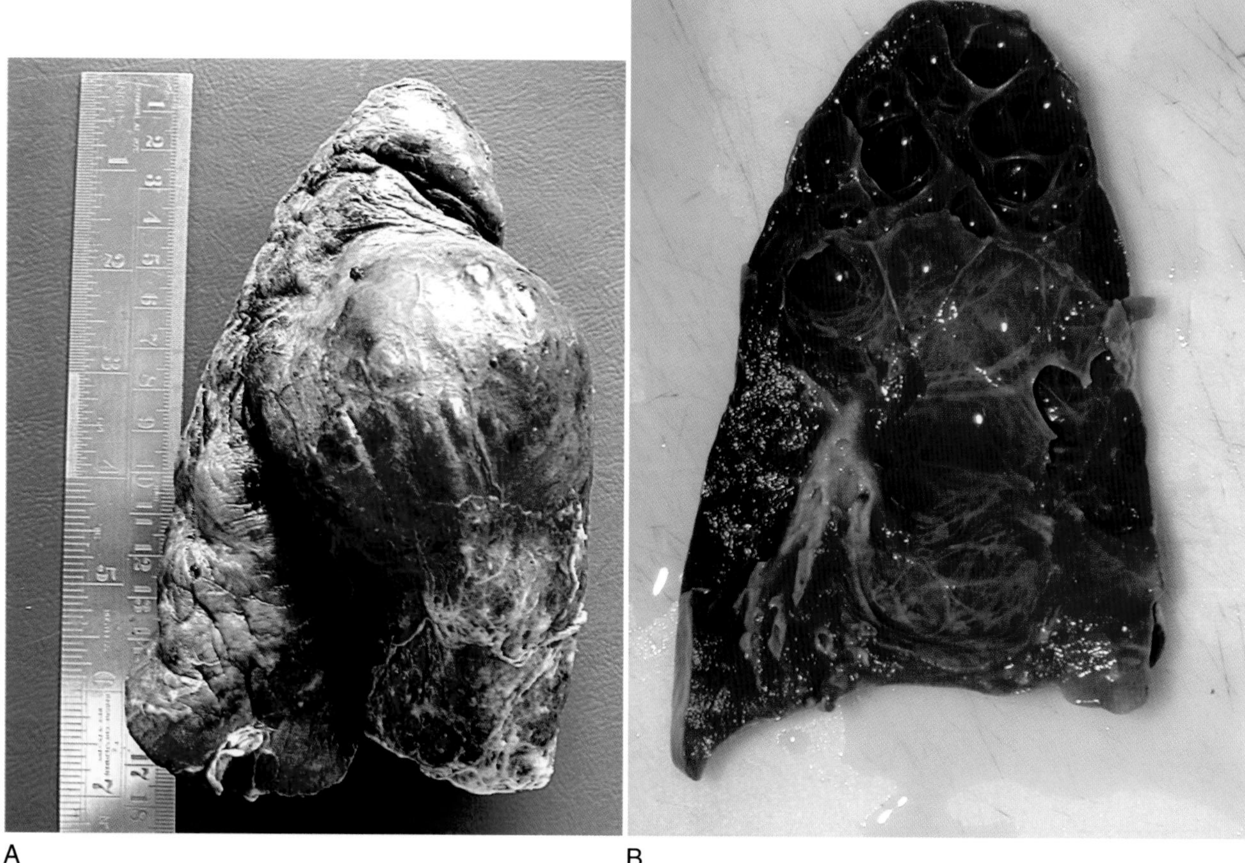

■ **COLOR PLATE 21.** Type 1 CCAM. **A,** A cystic lesion bulges to fill most of the lower lobe. **B,** The cut surface shows a multiloculated cyst replacing most of the parenchyma. (See Fig. 17-18.)

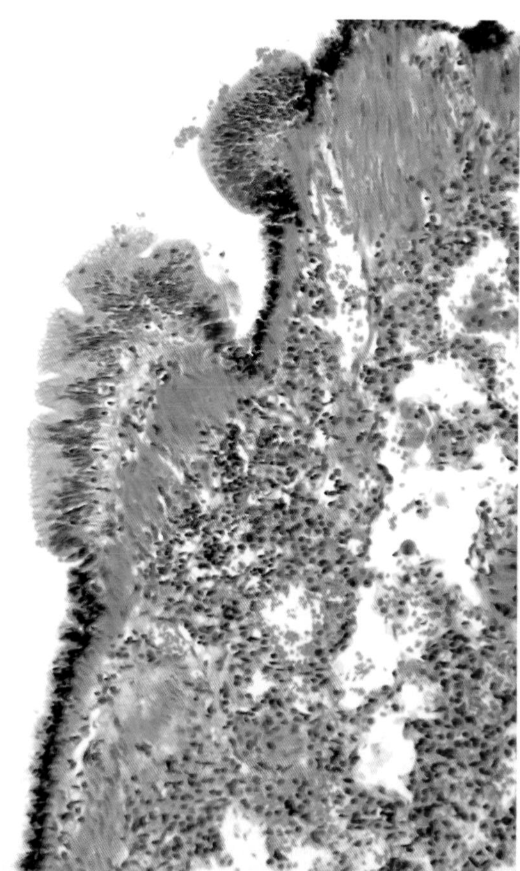

■ **COLOR PLATE 22.** Type 1 CCAM. The cyst lining is mainly of respiratory type, although mucous cell hyperplasia is not infrequently seen. (See Fig. 17-19.)

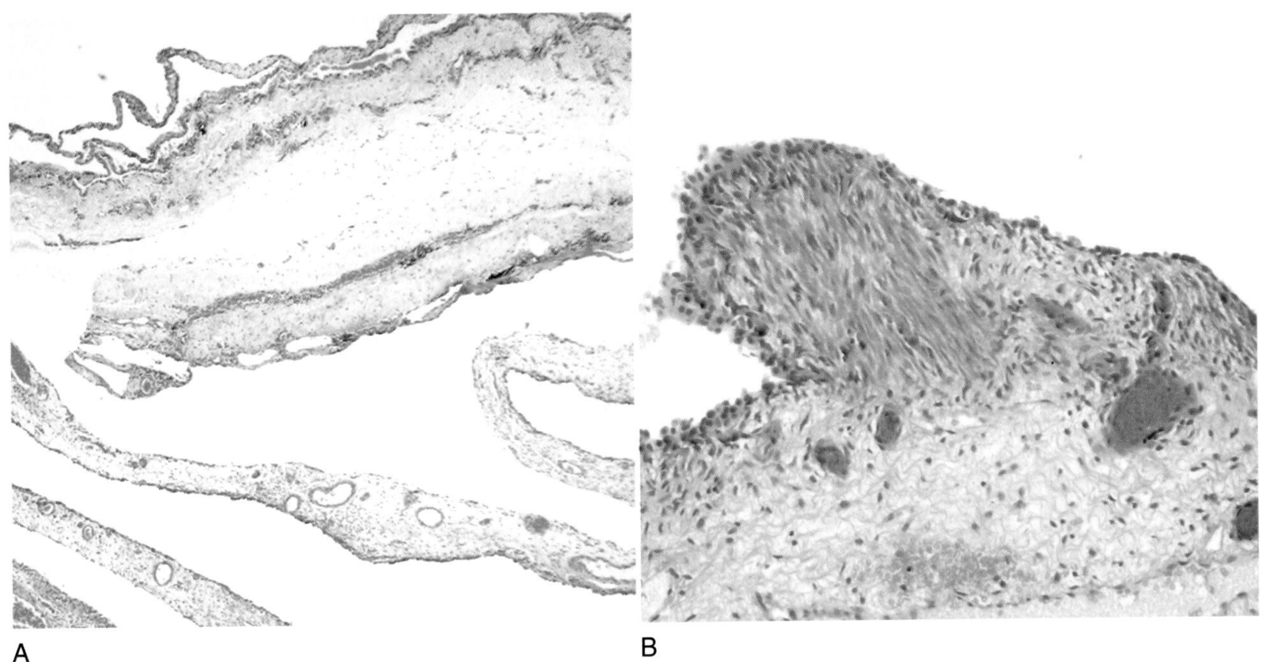

■ **COLOR PLATE 23.** Type 4 CCAM. **A,** These cysts are lined typically by pneumocytes with loose and myxoid fibrous stroma comprising the walls of variably sized thin-walled cysts. **B,** Care must be taken to ensure that no blastematous elements are present, which would then indicate a diagnosis of pleuropulmonary blastoma. (See Fig. 17-20.)

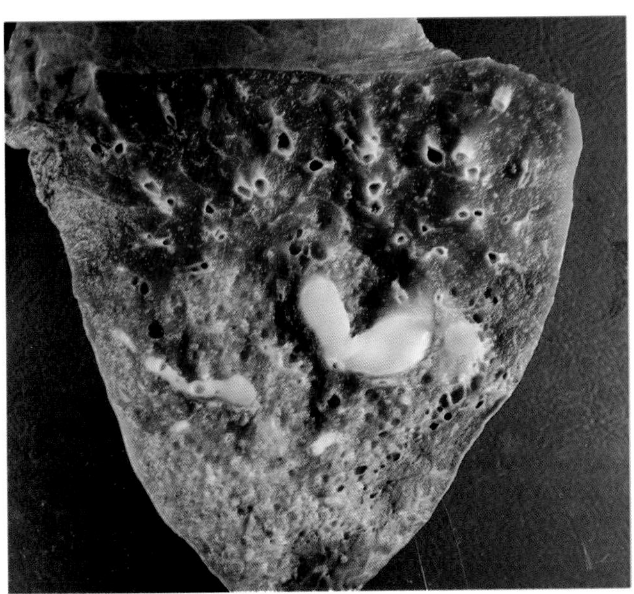

■ **COLOR PLATE 24.** Bronchial atresia. The cut surface of the lung shows dilated airways plugged with mucus with surrounding microcystic changes. Dissection showed atresia at the origin of the apical segmental bronchus. (See Fig. 17-23.)

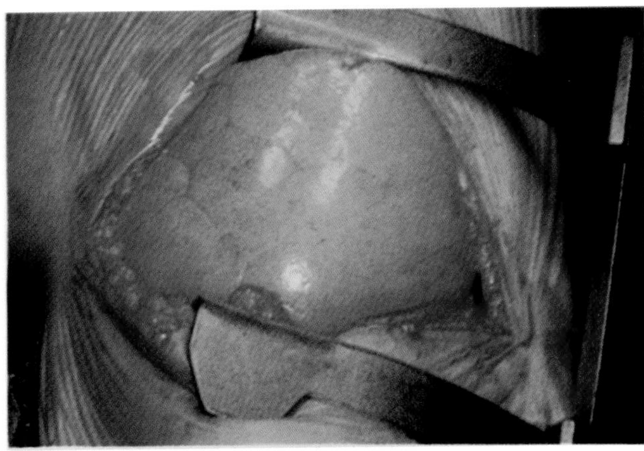

■ **COLOR PLATE 25.** Surgery for congenital large hyperlucent lobe (congenital lobar emphysema). The hyperexpanded lobe protrudes out of the thoracotomy incision. (See Fig. 17-24.)

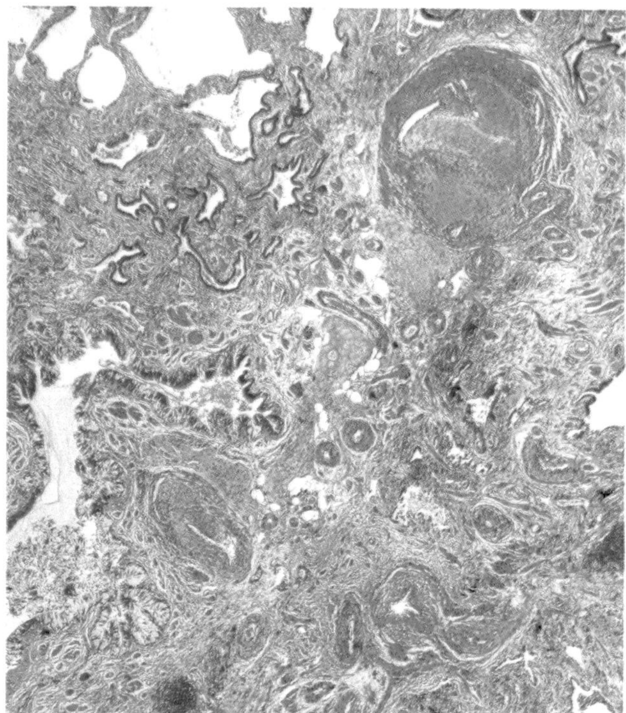

■ **COLOR PLATE 26.** Absence of the pulmonary artery. The parenchyma lacks pulmonary arteries but instead shows very prominent bronchial arteries. (See Fig. 17-27.)

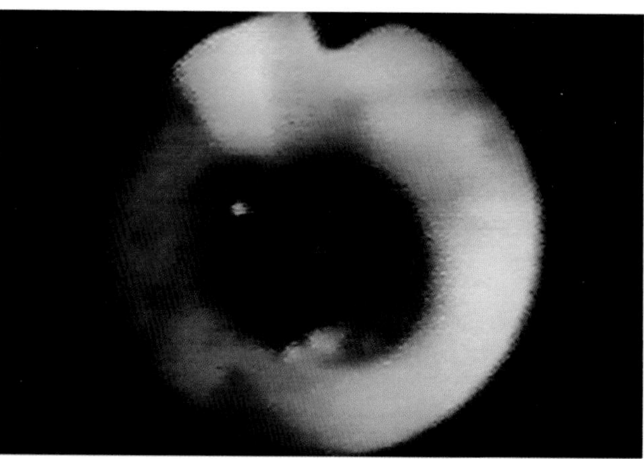

■ **COLOR PLATE 27.** Iatrogenic complete infarction of the trachea, which is black and necrotic. The child had undergone a unifocalization procedure, in which the bronchial arteries had been stripped from the airways and anastomosed to create a pulmonary trunk. The child is intubated, and the blue line marks the endotracheal tube. (See Fig. 17-28.)

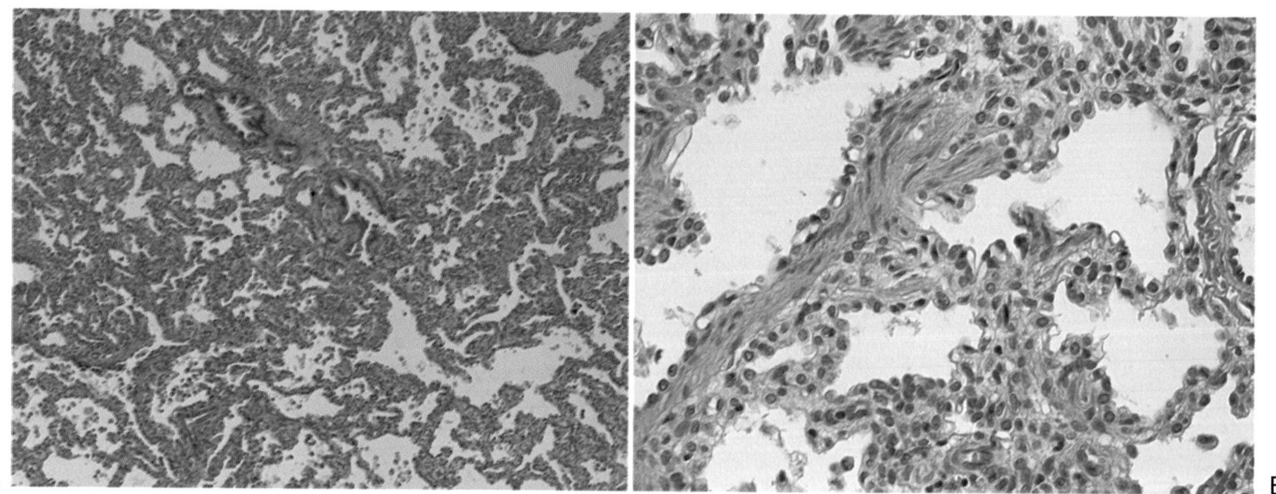

■ **COLOR PLATE 28.** Lung histology from an infant who died with severe bronchopulmonary dysplasia (BPD) following prolonged mechanical ventilation. **A,** Classic features of thickened interstitium, increased cellularity, and fibroproliferative changes. **B,** A higher-powered view that illustrates distal fibroproliferative changes in severe BPD. (See Fig. 19-2.)

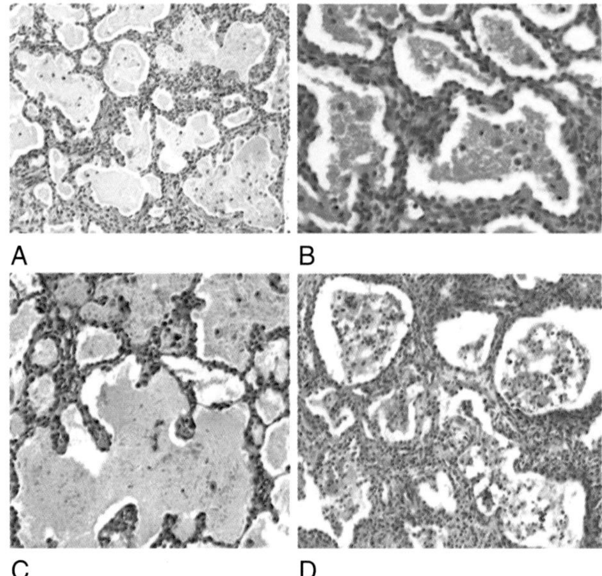

■ **COLOR PLATE 29.** Variable and overlapping histology associated with mutations in genes important in surfactant metabolism. **A,** Results from an SP-B-deficient infant, demonstrating marked accumulation of granular proteinaceous material with entrapped macrophages filling distal airspaces. **B,** Similar pathology from a patient with ABCA3 deficiency (**B**) and from a patient with an SP-C mutation (**C**), although with better preservation of the alveolar architecture in **C**. **D**, Results from a patient with a different SP-C mutation, demonstrating interstitial thickening and accumulations of foamy macrophages in the airspaces, but with scant amounts of proteinaceous material. (See Fig. 20-2.)

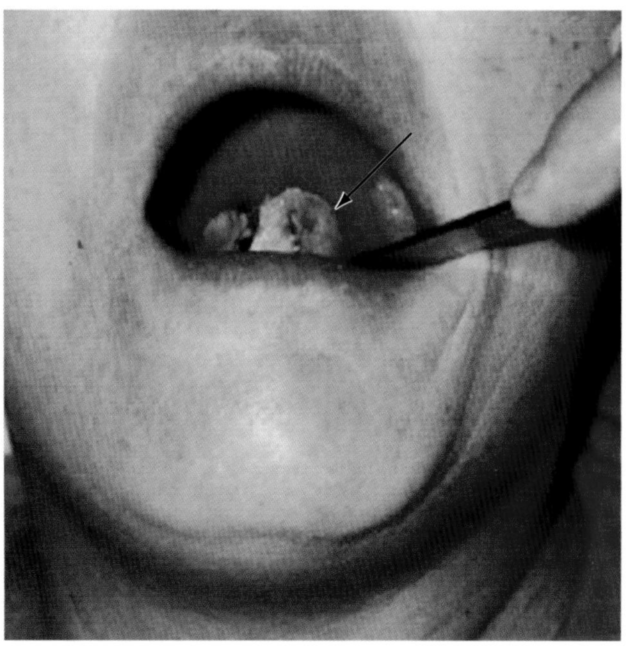

■ **COLOR PLATE 31.** Diphtheritic membrane (*arrow*) extending from the uvula to the pharyngeal wall in an adult. (See Fig. 23-4.) (From Kadirova R, Kartoglu HÜ, Strebel PM: Clinical characteristics and management of 676 hospitalized diphtheria cases. Kyrgyz Republic 1995. J Infect Dis 2000;181[Suppl 1]:S110–S115. Photograph by P. Strebel.)

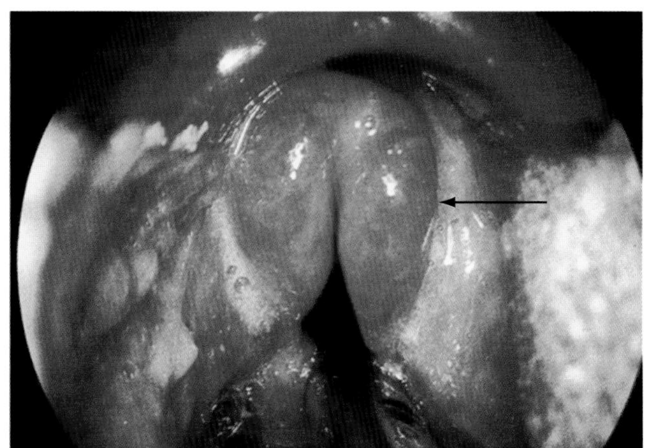

■ **COLOR PLATE 30.** Swollen epiglottis (*arrow*) due to acute epiglottitis in an intubated child. (See Fig. 23-2.) (From Benjamin B, Bingham B, Hawke M, Stammberger H: A Colour Atlas of Otorhinolaryngology. London: Taylor & Francis, 1995, p 292, with permission.)

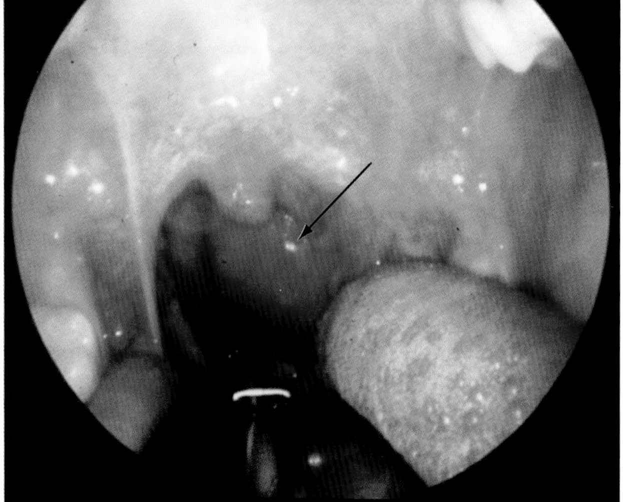

■ **COLOR PLATE 32.** Retropharyngeal abscess behind and to the left of the uvula (*arrow*). The tongue is pressed down and to the left with a tongue depressor. (See Fig. 23-5.) (Photograph courtesy of the Otolaryngology Teaching Set, Department of Ear, Nose & Throat, Great Ormond Street Hospital for Children NHS Trust, London.)

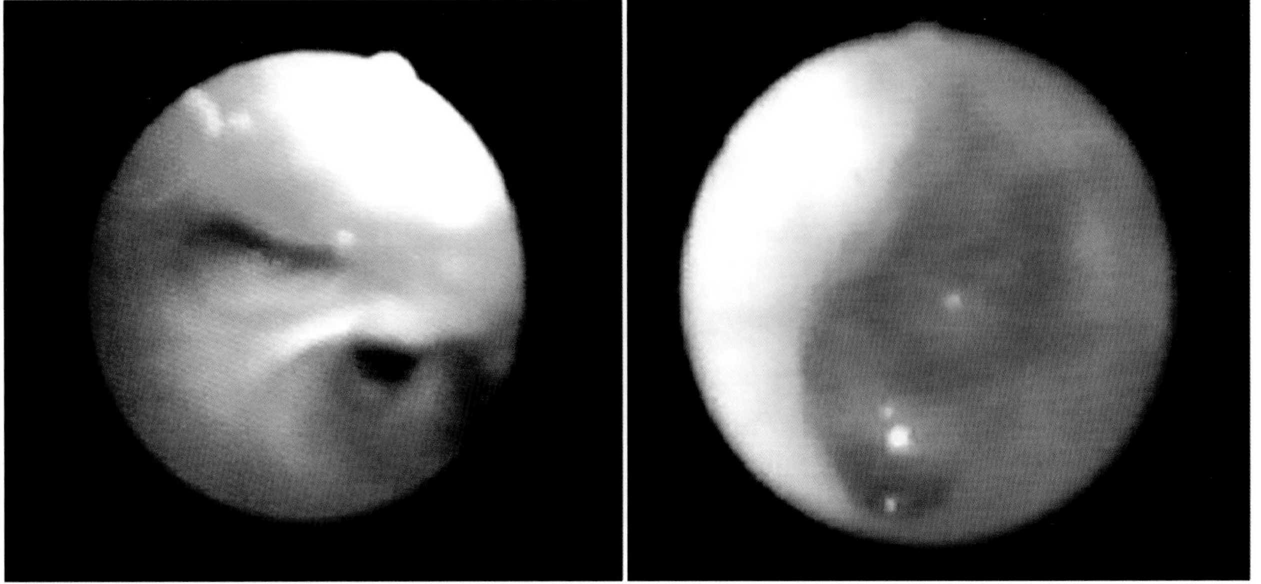

■ **COLOR PLATE 33.** Major airway bronchoscopic findings where bronchiectasis is not present. **A,** Bronchomalacia (airway type II) of the right middle lobe. **B,** Obliterative-like lesion (airway type III) seen in the segmental bronchi (middle of picture) while the adjacent bronchi is widely patent and more inflamed. (See Fig. 29-4.) (Reproduced from Chang AB, Boyce NC, Masters IB, Torzillo PJ, Masel JP: Bronchoscopic findings in children with non–cystic fibrosis chronic suppurative lung disease. Thorax 2002;57:935–938, with permission from the BMJ Publishing Group.)

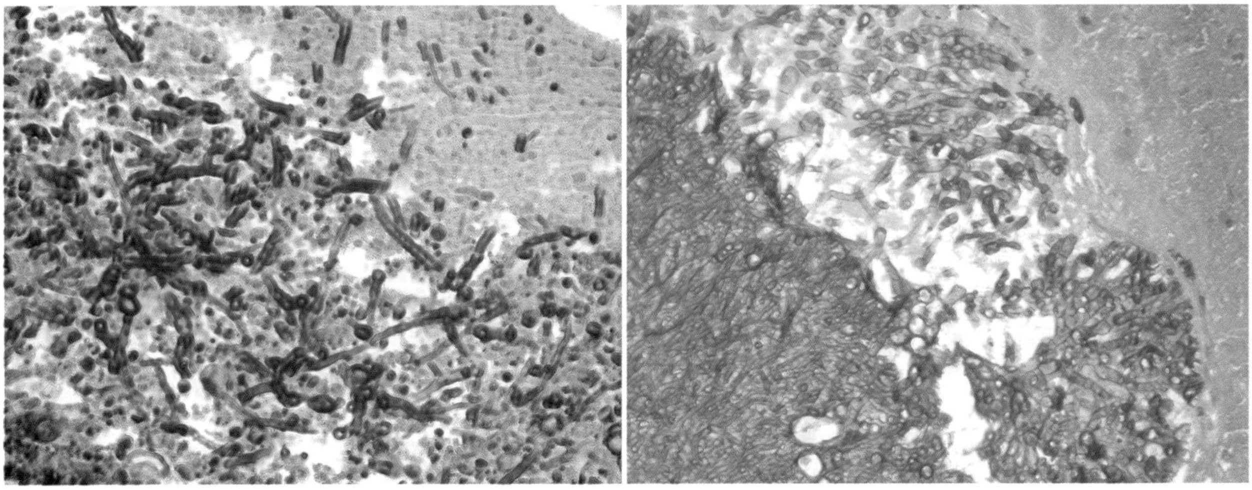

A

B

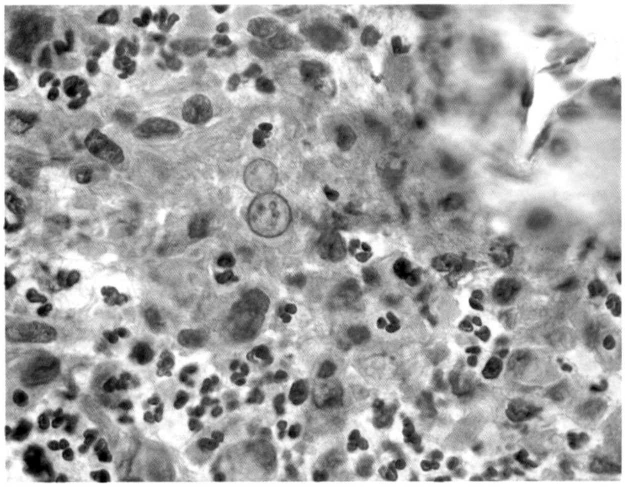

C

Continued

■ **COLOR PLATE 34.** Panels showing the typical morphology of invasive aspergillosis (**A** and **B**), blastomycosis (**C** and **D**), and histoplasmosis (**E** and **F**). **A, C,** and **E,** Hematoxolyn and eosin. **B, D,** and **F,** Gomori's methenamine silver stain. (See Fig. 35-1.)

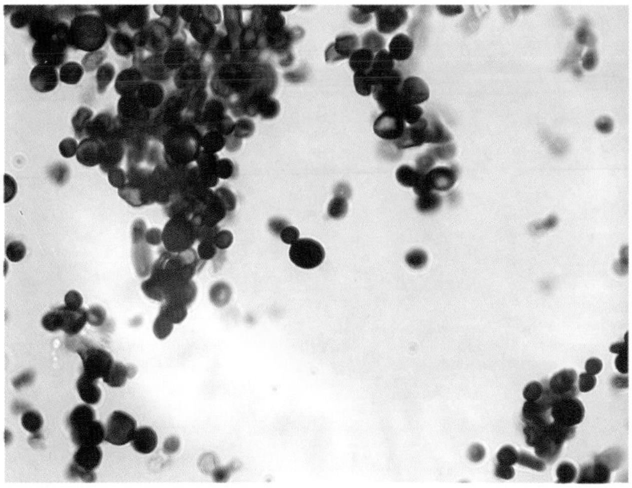

D

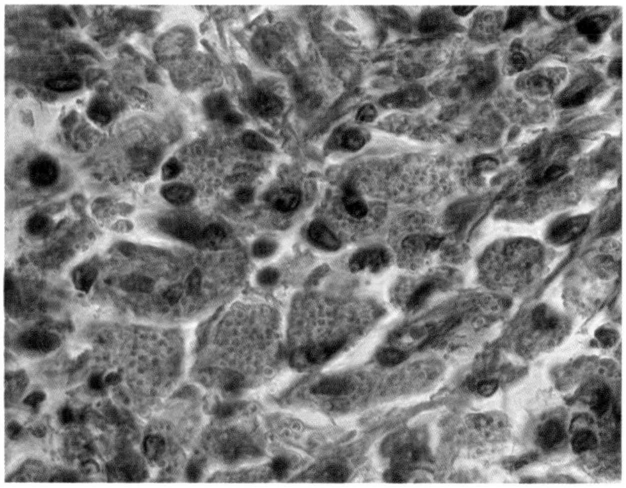

E

■ **COLOR PLATE 34, cont'd**

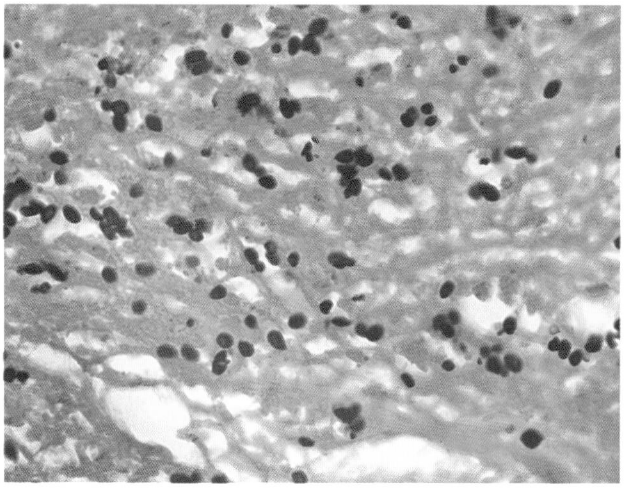

F

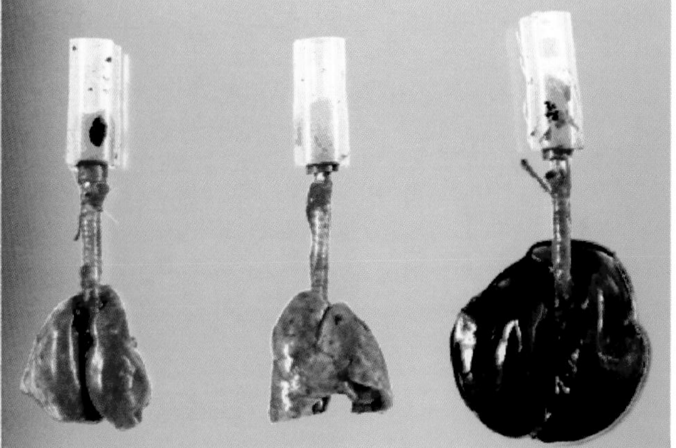

■ **COLOR PLATE 35.** Macroscopic aspect of rat lungs after mechanical ventilation at 45 cm H_2O peak airway pressure. *Left,* Normal lungs. *Middle,* After 5 minutes of high airway pressure mechanical ventilation. Note the focal zones of atelectasis (in particular at the left lung apex). *Right,* After 20 minutes, the lungs were markedly enlarged and congested; edema fluid fills the tracheal cannula. (See Fig. 44-2.) (From Dreyfuss D, Saumon G: Ventilator-induced lung injury. Lessons from experimental studies. Am Rev Respir Crit Care Med 1998; 157:294–323.)

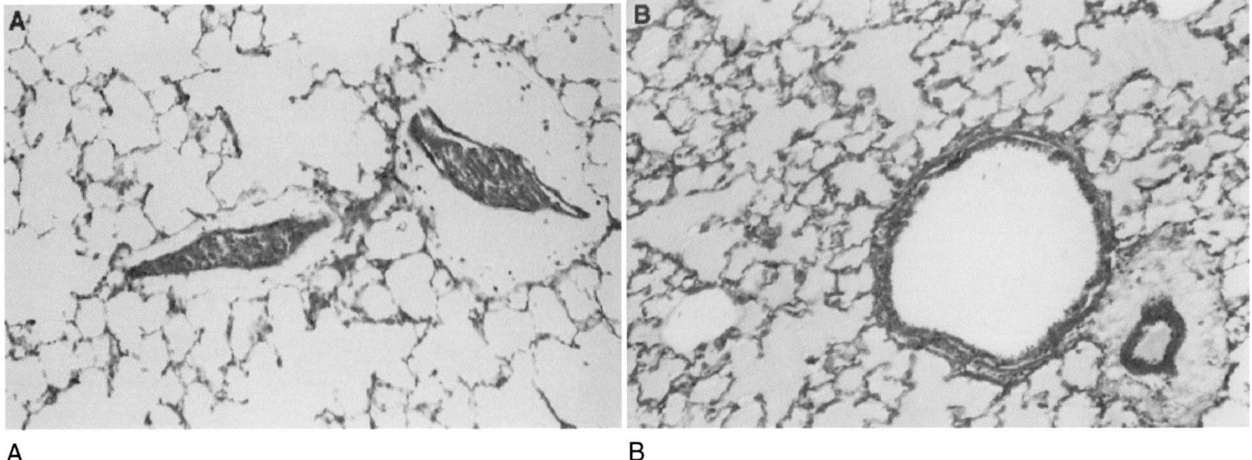

■ **COLOR PLATE 36.** Light microscopic appearance of rat lungs after mechanical ventilation at 45 cm H_2O peak airway pressure. **A,** After 5 minutes of ventilation, interstitial edema is found in large perivascular cuffs. **B,** After 20 minutes of ventilation, there is widespread alveolar edema that fills nearly all the alveoli on this slide. (See Fig. 44-3.) (From Dreyfuss D, Saumon G: Ventilator-induced lung injury. Lessons from experimental studies. Am Rev Respir Crit Care Med 1998;157:294–323.)

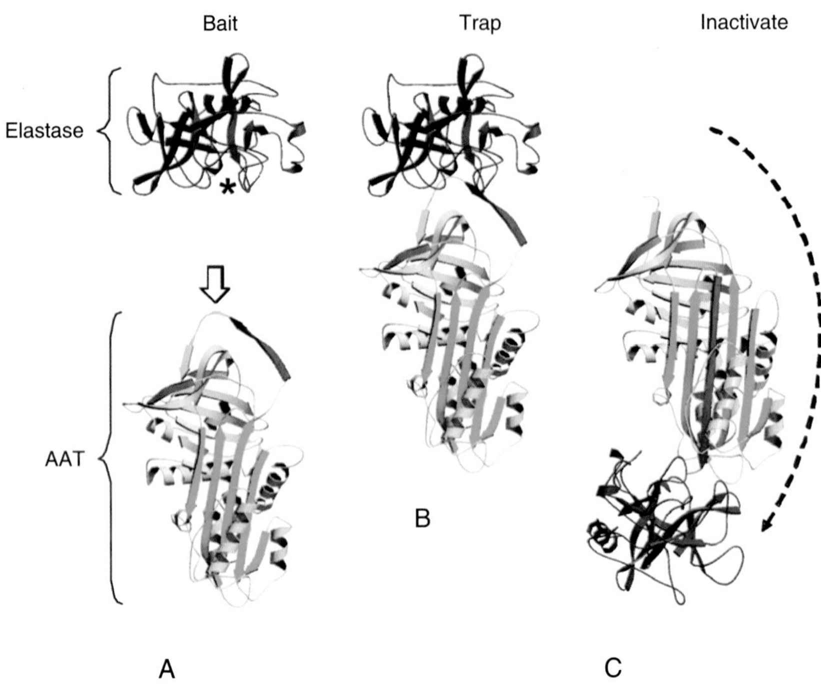

■ **COLOR PLATE 37.** Alpha-1 antitrypsin "baits," traps, and irreversibly inactivates neutrophil elastase using a mousetrap-like action. AAT is a globular protein with a reactive external loop (*open arrow*) (the loop is shown in *red*) that acts as bait for neutrophil elastase by virtue of its ability to bind the active site of the protease (*asterisk*) (**A**). Docking of neutrophil elastase on the reactive external loop of AAT (*red*) (**B**) is associated with movement of the reactive external loop from the upper pole to the lower pole of AAT, its insertion into β-sheet A (*green*) of AAT, and inactivation of the protease (**C**). (See Fig. 52-1.) (From Lomas DA, Parfrey H: Alpha1-antitrypsin deficiency. 4: Molecular pathophysiology. Thorax 2004;59[6]: 529–535.)

■ COLOR PLATE 38. Abnormal folding of Z-type α1-antitrypsin molecules creates a cleft that leads to polymerization into long chains. The structure of AAT is centered on β-sheet A (*green*) and the mobile reactive external loop (*red*). Polymer formation results from the Z variant of AAT (*arrow*) or the S_{iiyama}, M_{malton}, S, or I mutations in the shutter domain (*blue circle*) that open β-sheet A to favor partial insertion (step 1) and the formation of an unstable intermediate (*M**). The patent β-sheet A can either accept the loop of another molecule (step 2) to form dimer (*D*) which then extends into polymers (*P*) or its own loop (step 3) to form a latent conformation (*L*). The individual molecules of AAT within the polymer are shown in various colors. (See Fig. 52-2.) (From Lomas DA, Parfrey H: Alpha1-antitrypsin deficiency. 4: Molecular pathophysiology. Thorax 2004;59[6]: 529–535.)

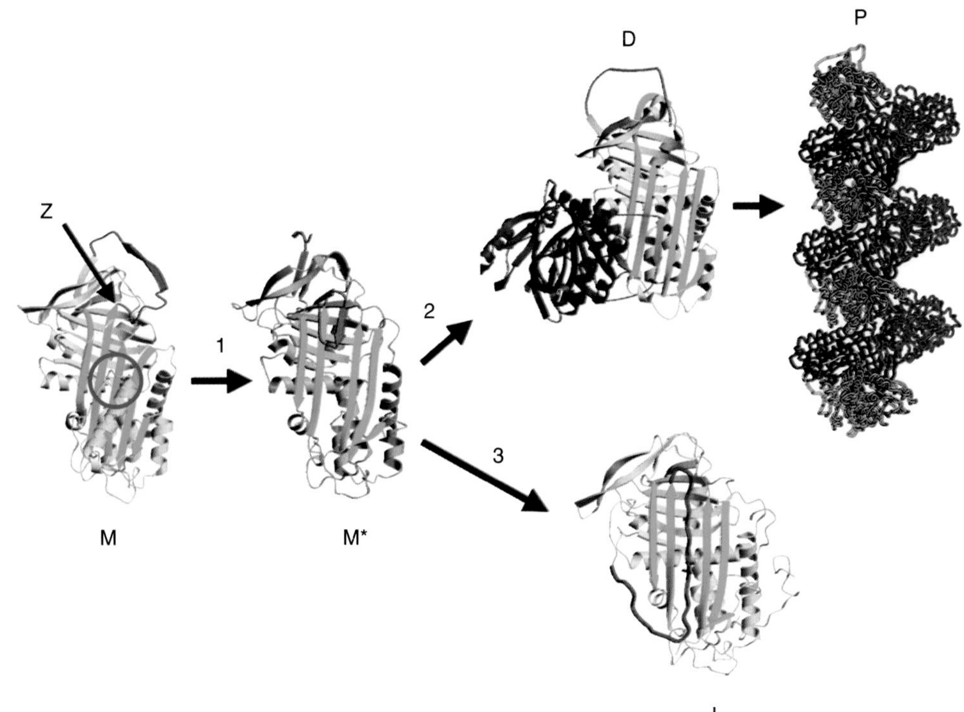

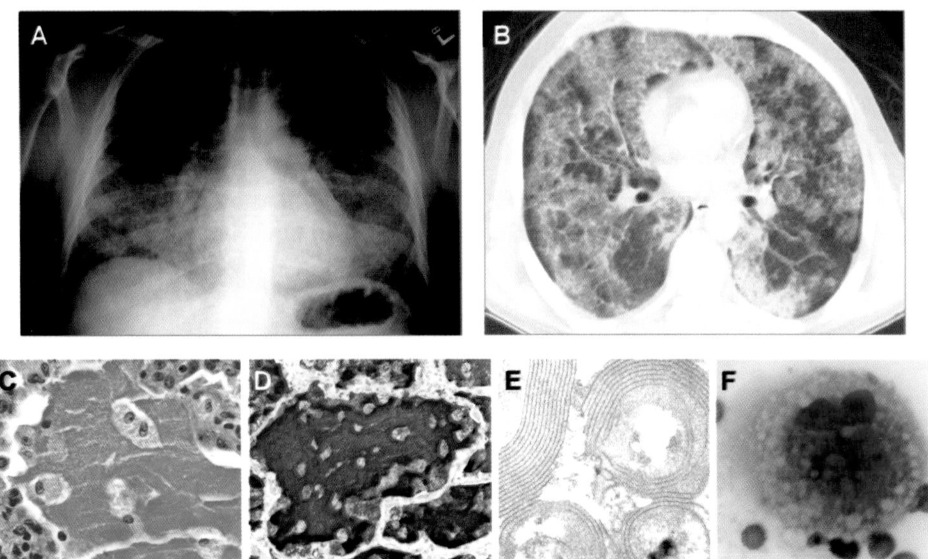

■ COLOR PLATE 39. Radiographic, histologic, and ultrastructural features of pulmonary alveolar proteinosis. **A,** Posteroanterior chest radiograph showing the typical features of pulmonary alveolar proteinosis, including diffuse, patchy, bilateral airspace disease unaccompanied by evidence of cardiac failure, adenopathy, or effusion. **B,** High-resolution computed tomographic scan of the chest showing patchy ground-glass opacification and interlobular septal thickening. This pattern, commonly referred to as "crazy paving," is characteristic, but not diagnostic, of the disease. **C,** Lung biopsy specimen showing intra-alveolar material that stains positively with periodic acid-Schiff reagent. **D,** Immunohistochemical staining of a lung biopsy specimen showing abundant intra-alveolar accumulation of surfactant protein A. **E,** Ultrastructural examination of the bronchoalveolar lavage sediment showing the characteristic features of pulmonary surfactant including laminated membrane structures and amorphous debris. **F,** Cytologic appearance of a "foamy" alveolar macrophage present in bronchoalveolar fluid. (See Fig. 52-3.) (From Ben-Dov I, Kishinevski Y, Roznman J, et al: Pulmonary alveolar proteinosis in Israel. Ethnic clustering. Isr Med Assoc J 1999;1[2]:75–78.)

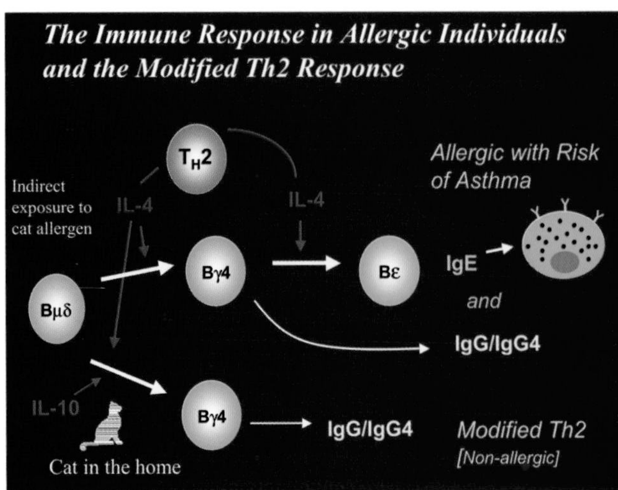

■ **COLOR PLATE 40.** The immune response to cat allergens may take a traditional T-helper 2 (Th2) response with immunoglobulin G4 (IgG4) and IgE antibodies. Alternatively, among children living with a cat a significant number produce IgG1 and IgG4 antibodies to Fel d 1 without IgE (modified Th2 response). The T cells are thought to control IgE production both in nonallergic and allergic children. (See Fig. 54-3.)

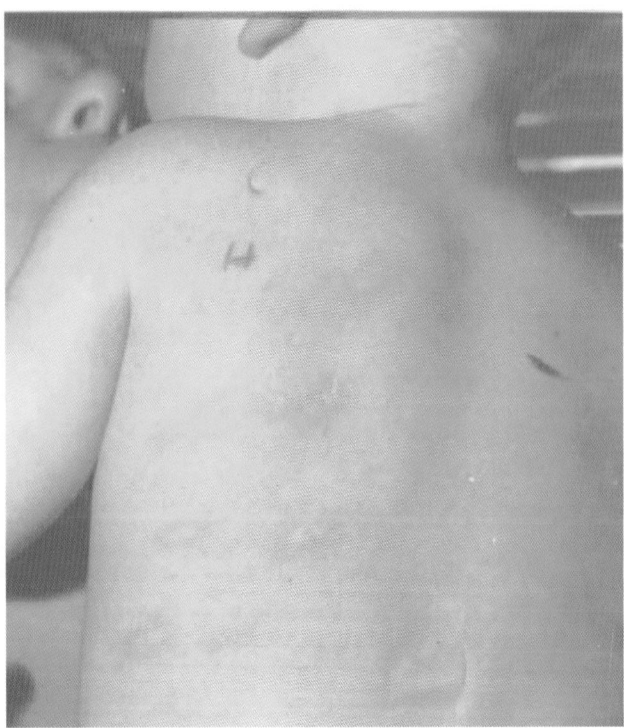

■ **COLOR PLATE 41.** This 11-month-old infant was hospitalized at 9 months of age with severe acute asthma preceded by rhinoconjunctivitis during the peak of the grass pollen season in a northern California valley area. The typical wheal and flare of the multiple related species of grass pollen native to that area are seen on the left side of the infant's back. They are much larger than the histamine control (*H*) with no reactivity to the diluent control (*C*). Skin tests on the right side of the back to other common inhalant allergens were all negative. While immunotherapy using injections of allergenic extracts is rarely indicated at this age, this infant illustrates a striking exception where benefit could reasonably be expected. (See Fig. 55-7.)

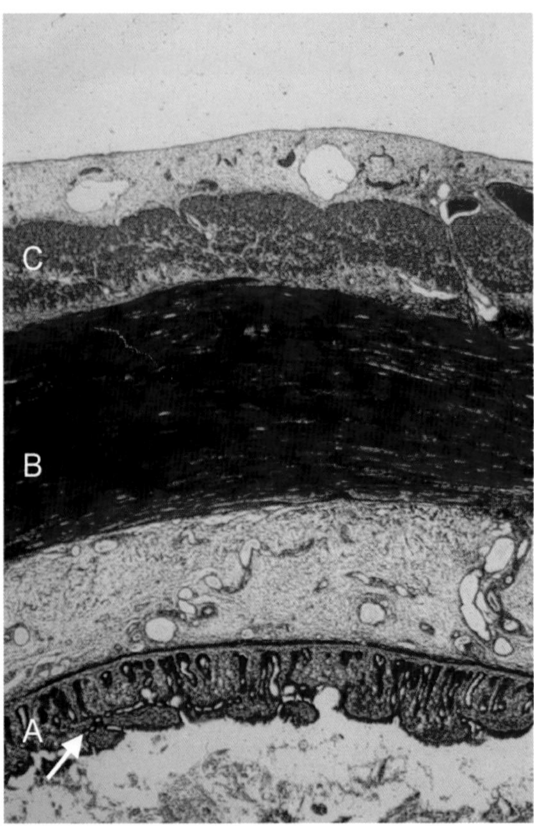

■ **COLOR PLATE 42.** Histologic findings in fibrosing colonopathy. Classification system for CFTR mutations (see the text for details). Intestinal cross-section from a patient with fibrosing colonopathy illustrating nonspecific acute and chronic inflammation in the mucosa (*A* [*arrow*]), hypertrophy of the muscularis mucosa (*B*), and a ring of fibrous tissue (*C*). (See Fig. 62-2.)

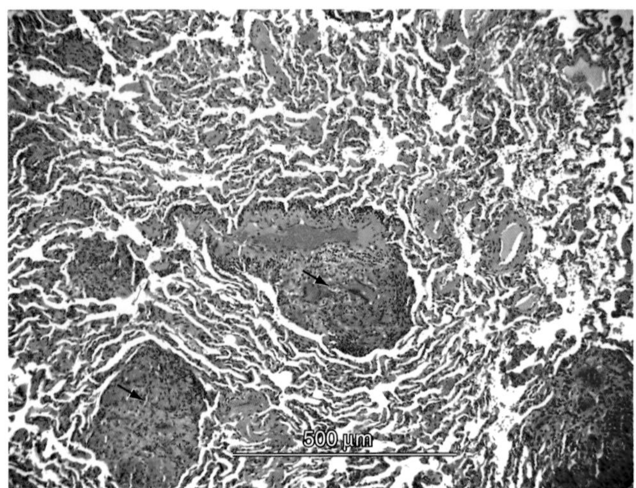

■ **COLOR PLATE 43.** Biopsy of the apex of the left lung from a 15-year-old African American boy with a history of skin lesions, bilateral ankle swelling, a painful red eye, and lung infiltrate (see Fig. 65-2). Biopsy showed non-necrotizing interstitial granulomas (*arrows*). Special stains for acid-fast bacillus and fungi were negative, as were stains for vasculitis. Similar results were found on biopsy of axillary lymph nodes. (See Fig. 65-1.)

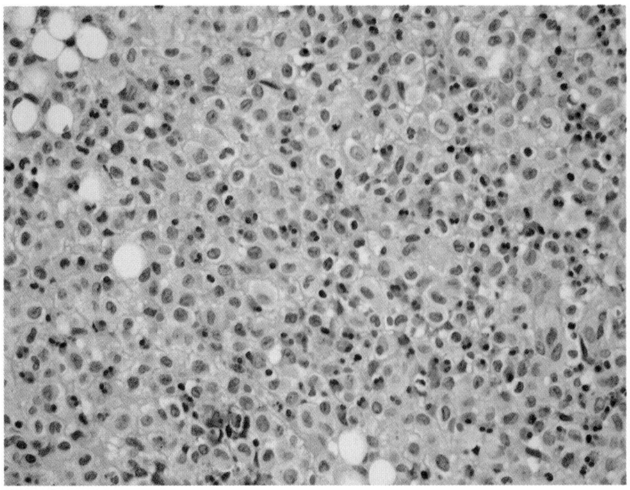

A

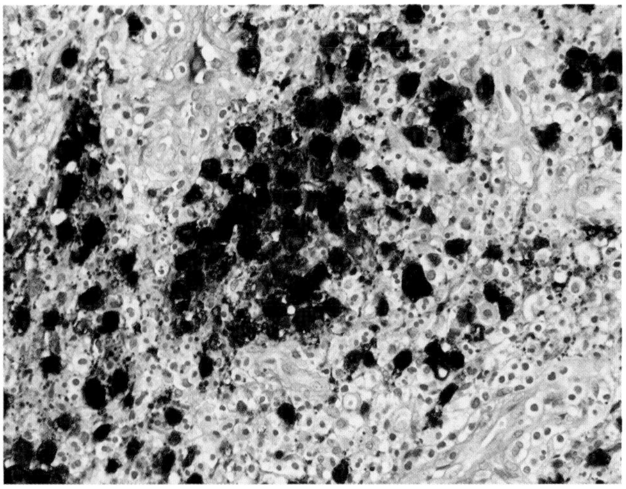

B

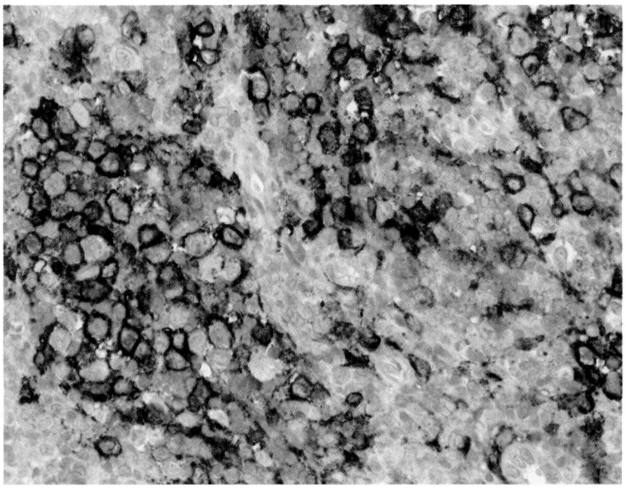

C

■ **COLOR PLATE 44.** **A,** Langerhans cell histiocytosis in bone, showing an admixture of eosinophils and Langerhans cells. The eosinophils contain bilobed nuclei and prominent eosinophilic, granular cytoplasm. The Langerhans cells are the larger cells with variable eosinophilic to clear cytoplasm and indented, cerebriform-like nuclei (hematoxylin and eosin stain, original magnification ×400). Immunostains for S-100 protein (**B**) and CD1a (**C**) highlight Langerhans cells. (See Fig. 66-1.) (Courtesy of Dr. John D. Reith, Department of Orthopaedic Pathology, University of Florida School of Medicine.)

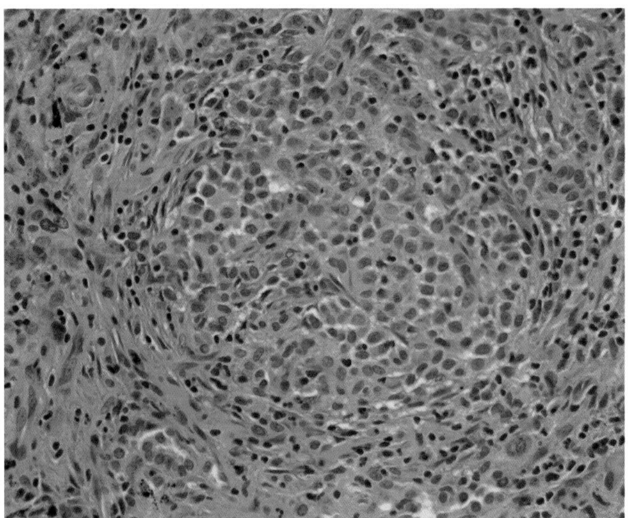

■ **COLOR PLATE 45.** The typical low-power appearance of pulmonary Langerhans cell histiocytosis is of a multiple nodular interstitial infiltrate with a stellate border. At high magnification the cellular infiltrate consists of sheets of Langerhans cells characterized by abundant eosinophilic cytoplasm and prominent nuclear indentation (grooves). Scattered eosinophils are often present. Lymphocytes, macrophages, and fibroblasts may also be present. (See Fig. 66-3.) (Courtesy of Dr. Li Lu, Department of Pathology, University of Florida School of Medicine.)

Contents

SECTION VIII ■ Cystic Fibrosis, 848

SECTION IX ■ Other Diseases with a Prominent Respiratory Component, 902

General Considerations

1 Molecular Determinants of Lung Morphogenesis

Jeffrey A. Whitsett, MD • Susan E. Wert, PhD

OVERVIEW

The adult human lung consists of a gas exchange area of approximately 100 m^2 that provides oxygen delivery and carbon dioxide excretion required for cellular metabolism. In evolutionary terms, the lung represents a relatively late phylogenetic solution for the efficient gas exchange needed for terrestrial survival of organisms of increasing size, an observation that may account for the similarity of lung structure in vertebrates. The respiratory system consists of mechanical bellows and conducting tubules that bring inhaled gases to a larger gas exchange surface that is highly vascularized. Alveolar epithelial cells come into close apposition to pulmonary capillaries, providing efficient transport of gases from the alveolar space to the pulmonary circulation. The delivery of external gases to pulmonary tissue necessitates a complex organ system that (1) keeps the airway free of pathogens and debris, (2) maintains humidification of alveolar gases and precise hydration of the epithelial cell surface, (3) reduces collapsing forces inherent at air-liquid interfaces within the air spaces of the lung, and (4) supplies and regulates pulmonary blood flow to exchange oxygen and carbon dioxide efficiently. The present chapter will provide a framework for understanding the molecular mechanisms that lead to the formation of the mammalian lung, focusing attention to processes contributing to cell proliferation and differentiation involved in organogenesis and postnatal respiratory adaptation. Where possible, the pathogenesis of congenital or postnatal lung disease will be considered in the context of the molecular determinants of pulmonary morphogenesis and function.

ORGANOGENESIS OF THE LUNG

BODY PLAN

Events critical to organogenesis of the lung begin with formation of anteroposterior and proximodistal axes in the early embryo. The body plan is determined by genes that control cellular proliferation and differentiation and depends on complex interactions among many cell types. The fundamental principles determining embryonic organization are currently and rapidly being elucidated in more simple organisms (e.g., *Drosophila melanogaster* and *Caenorhabditis elegans*) and applied to increasingly complex organisms (e.g., mouse and human) as the genes determining axial segmentation, organ formation, cellular proliferation, and differentiation are identified. Segmentation and organ formation in the embryo are profoundly influenced by sets of master control genes that include various classes of transcription factors. Critical to formation of axial body plan are the homeotic, or Hox, genes.[1–7] Hox genes are arrayed in clearly defined spatial patterns within clusters on several chromosomes. Hox gene expression in the developing embryo is determined in part by the position of the individual genes within these gene clusters, which are aligned along the chromosome in the same order as they are expressed along the anteroposterior axis. Complex organisms have more individual Hox genes within each locus and have more Hox gene loci than in simpler organisms. Hox genes encode nuclear proteins that bind to DNA via a conserved homeodomain motif that modulates the transcription of specific sets of target genes. The temporal and spatial expression of these nuclear transcription factors, in turn, control the expression of other Hox genes and their transcriptional targets during morphogenesis and cytodifferentiation.[8–15] Expression of Hox genes influences many downstream genes, such as transcription factors, growth factors, and cell adhesion molecules (CAMs), which are critical to the formation of the primitive endoderm from which the respiratory epithelium is derived. Specification of endoderm requires the activity of a number of transcription factors, including Foxa2,[16–18] β-catenin,[19,20] Sox-17,[21,22] and GATA-6.[23] These transcription factors are also expressed in respiratory epithelial cells of the lung later in development when they play roles in cell differentiation and organ function.

LUNG MORPHOGENESIS

Lung morphogenesis begins during the embryonic period of fetal development as an outpouching of epithelial cells lining the laryngotracheal sulcus at the caudal end of the medial pharyngeal groove of the foregut endoderm.[24] In the mouse, the lung bud forms on day 9 of gestation, comparable with 3 to 4 weeks of gestation in the human. The endoderm develops earlier in embryogenesis with formation of the dorsal plate and primitive notochord, which requires the expression of the transcription factor forkhead homologue Foxa2, previously termed hepatocyte nuclear factor-3β (HNF-3β), a protein also involved in differentiation and gene expression in the respiratory epithelium later in development.[16–18,25–31]

Lung morphogenesis can be subdivided into distinct periods on the basis of the morphologic characteristics of the tissue (Table 1-1 and Figs. 1-1 and 1-2). While the timing of the process is highly species specific, the anatomic events underlying lung morphogenesis are shared by all mammalian species. The reader is referred to several reviews that detail anatomic development of the human lung.[32–36]

The Embryonic Period (3–6 Weeks Postconception)

Relatively undifferentiated epithelial cells of the primitive foregut endoderm form tubules that invade the splanchnic mesoderm and undergo branching morphogenesis. This process requires highly controlled cell proliferation and migration to direct dichotomous branching of the tubules to form the main stem, lobar, and segmental bronchi of the primitive lung (see Fig. 1-1*A*; Fig. 1-2, *E10, E11*). The respiratory epithelium remains relatively undifferentiated and is lined predominantly by columnar epithelium in the embryonic period. Experimental removal of mesenchymal tissue from the embryonic endoderm arrests branching morphogenesis, demonstrating the critical role of mesenchyme in formation of the respiratory tract.[37,38] Interactions between epithelial and mesenchymal cells are mediated by a variety of growth factors and associated receptors that regulate gene transcription in differentiating lung cells. Epithelial-mesenchymal interactions involve both autocrine and paracrine signaling, which are critical to lung morphogenesis.[39,40]

Formation of the larger, more proximal conducting airways, including segmental and subsegmental bronchi, is completed by the 6th week postconception; however, both epithelial and mesenchymal cells of the embryonic lung remain relatively undifferentiated. At this stage, tracheobronchial tubules lack underlying cartilage, smooth muscle, or nerves, and the pulmonary and bronchial vessels are not well developed. Vascular connections with the right and left atria are established at the end of the embryonic period (6–7 weeks), creating the primitive pulmonary vascular bed. Developmental anomalies occurring during this period of development may include tracheal, laryngeal, and esophageal atresia, tracheal stenosis, pulmonary agenesis, tracheoesophageal fistulas, and bronchial malformations.

TABLE 1-1. Morphogenetic periods of human lung development

Period	Age (Weeks)	Structural Events
Embryonic	3–6	Lung buds, trachea, main stem, lobar, and segmental bronchi
Pseudoglandular	6–16	Subsegmental bronchi, terminal bronchioles, acinar tubules, mucous glands, cartilage, smooth muscle
Canicular	16–26	Respiratory bronchioles, acinus formation and vascularization, type I and II cell differentiation
Saccular	26–36	Dilation and subdivision of alveolar
Alveolar	36–maturity	saccules, increase of gas-exchange surface area, further growth and alveolarization of lung, maturation of alveolar capillary network

Pseudoglandular Period (6–16 Weeks Postconception)

The pseudoglandular stage is so named because of the distinct glandular appearance of the lung from 6 to 16 weeks of gestation. During this period, the lung consists primarily of epithelial tubules surrounded by a relatively thick mesenchyme. Branching of the airways continues, and formation of the terminal bronchioles and primitive acinar structures is completed by the end of this period (see Fig. 1-1*A*; Fig. 1-2, *E13, E15*). During the pseudoglandular period, epithelial cell differentiation is increasingly apparent; deposition of cellular glycogen and expression of a number of genes expressed selectively in the distal respiratory epithelium is initiated. Surfactant proteins A, B, and C are first detected at 12 to 14 weeks of human gestation.[41,42] Tracheobronchial glands begin to form in the proximal conducting airways. The airway epithelium is increasingly complex, with basal, mucous, ciliated, and nonciliated secretory cells being detected.[32,33] Neuroepithelial cells, often forming clumps of cells termed neuroepithelial bodies and expressing a variety of neuropeptides and transmitters (e.g., bombesin, calcitonin-related peptide, serotonin, and others), are increasingly apparent along the bronchial/bronchiolar epithelium during this stage of development. Smooth muscle and cartilage are now observed adjacent to the conducting airways. The pulmonary vascular system develops in close relationship to the bronchial and bronchiolar tubules between the 9th and 12th weeks of gestation. Bronchial arteries arise from the aorta and form along the epithelial tubules. Smooth muscle actin and myosin are found in the vascular structures during this period of development.[43–45] A variety of congenital defects may arise during the pseudoglandular stage of lung development, including tracheal-bronchiomalacia, pulmonary sequestration, cystadenomatoid malformation, ectopic lobes, cyst formation, and congenital pulmonary lymphangiectasia. The pleuroperitoneal cavity also closes early in the pseudoglandular period. Failure to close the pleural cavity, often accompanied by herniation of the abdominal contents into the chest (congenital diaphragmatic hernia), leads to lung hypoplasia.

Canalicular Period (16–26 Weeks)

The canalicular period is characterized by luminal expansion, the formation of acinar structures in the distal tubules, thinning of the mesenchyme, and formation of the capillary bed, which comes into close apposition to the dilating acinar tubules (see Fig. 1-1*B*; Fig. 1-2, *E17*). By the end of this period, the terminal bronchioles have divided to form two or more respiratory bronchioles, and each of these have divided into multiple acinar tubules, forming the primitive alveolar ducts and pulmonary acini. Epithelial cell differentiation becomes increasingly complex and is especially apparent in the distal regions of the lung parenchyma. Bronchiolar cells express differentiated features and synthesize Clara cell secretory protein (CCSP).[29,46–48] Cells lining the distal tubules assume cuboidal shapes and express increasing amounts of surfactant proteins (SP-A, SP-B, and SP-C)[29,41,49–52] and phospholipids.[53] Lamellar bodies, composed of surfactant phospholipids and protein, are seen in association with rich glycogen stores in the cuboidal pre–type II cells lining the distal lung tubules.[49,54–57] Some cells of the acinus become squamous, acquiring features of typical type I alveolar epithelial cells. Thinning of the pulmonary mesenchyme continues; the basal lamina of the epithelium and mesenchyme fuse. Capillaries surround the distal acinar tubules, which together will ultimately form the gas exchange region of the lung. By the end of the canalicular period in the human infant (26–28 weeks), gas exchange can be supported after birth, especially when surfactant is provided by administration of exogenous surfactants. Surfactant synthesis and mesenchymal thinning

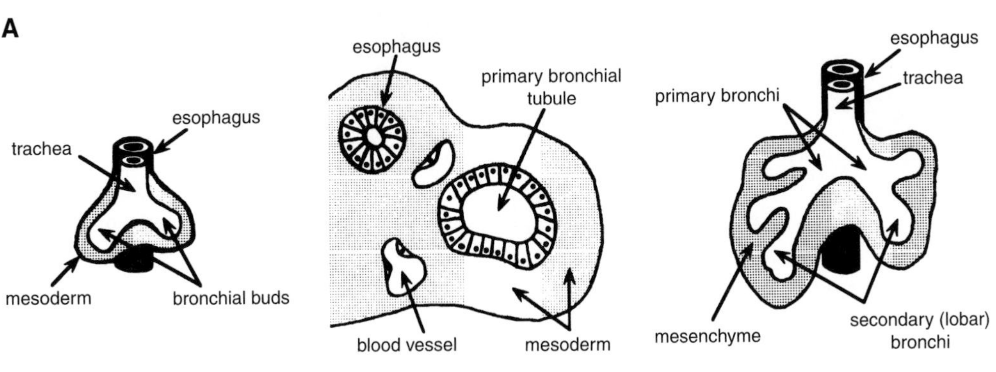

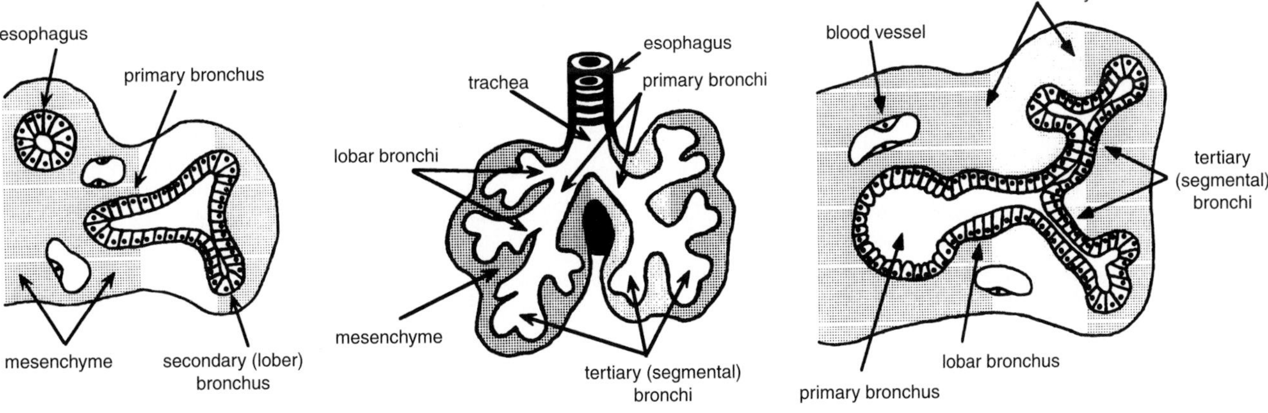

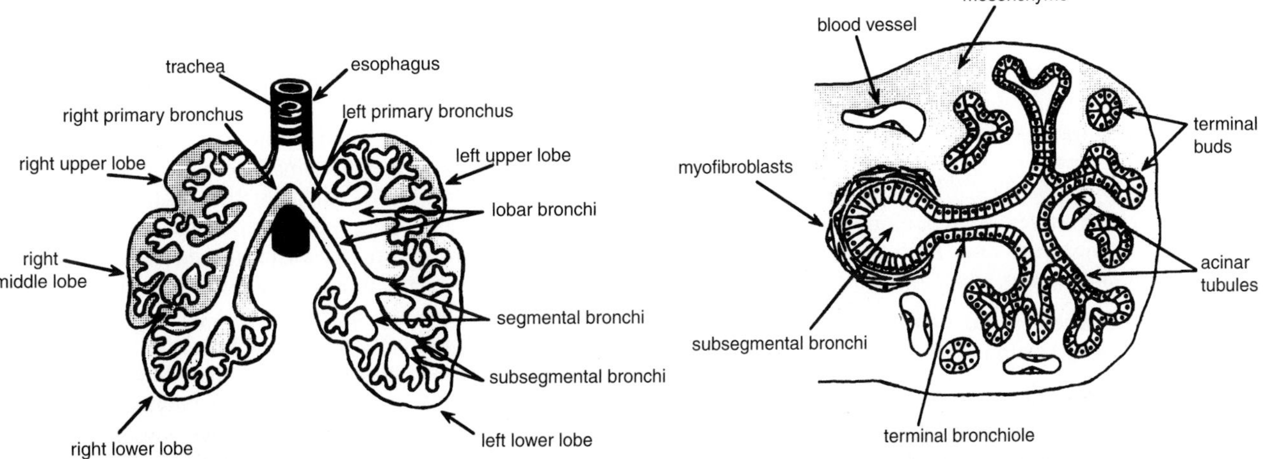

■ **FIGURE 1-1.** **A,** Lung morphogenesis is initiated by the evagination of the lung bud into the surrounding splanchnic mesenchyme during the embryonic stage. Bronchi, bronchioles, and acinar tubules are formed by the process of branching morphogenesis during the pseudoglandular stage.

Continued

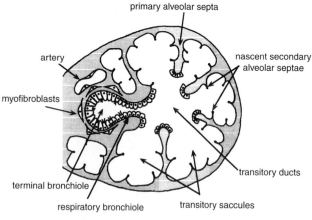

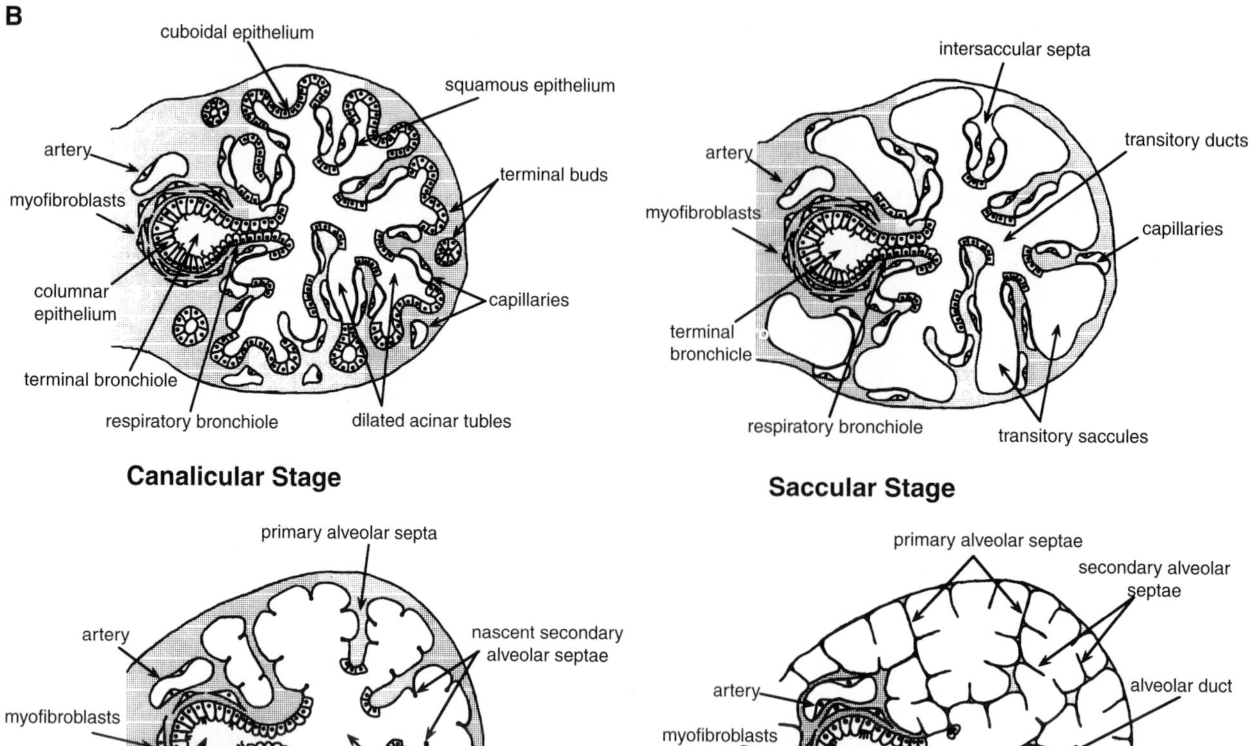

■ **FIGURE 1-1, cont'd. B,** Formation of the capillary bed and expansion of acinar structures is initiated during the canalicular stage. Growth and subdivision of terminal saccules and alveoli continue until early adolescence by septation of the distal respiratory structures to form additional alveoli.

are influenced by glucocorticoids,[58–60] which are administered to mothers to prevent respiratory distress syndrome (RDS) after premature birth.[61,62] Abnormalities of lung development occurring during the canalicular period include pulmonary hypoplasia (caused by diaphragmatic hernia or compression by thoracic or abdominal masses and prolonged rupture of membranes causing oligohydramnios) and renal agenesis, in which amniotic fluid production is impaired. While postnatal gas exchange can be supported late in the canalicular stage, infants born during this period generally suffer severe complications related to decreased pulmonary surfactant, which cause RDS and bronchopulmonary dysplasia, a complication secondary to the therapy for RDS.[63]

Saccular (26–36 weeks) and Alveolar Periods (36 Weeks through Adolescence)

These periods of lung development are characterized by increased thinning of the respiratory epithelium and pulmonary mesenchyme, further growth of lung acini, and development of the distal capillary network (see Fig. 1-1*B*; Fig. 1-2, *E18, P1, A*). In the periphery of the acinus, maturation of type II epithelial cells occurs in association with increasing numbers of lamellar bodies and increased synthesis of surfactant phospholipids[52,53,64] and SP-A, -B, -C, and -D.[29,41,42,49,50,65] The acinar regions of the lung increase in surface area, and proliferation of type II cells continues.[33] Type I cells, derived from differentiation of type II epithelial cells, line an ever-increasing proportion of the surface area of the distal lung. Capillaries become closely associated with the squamous type I cells, decreasing the diffusion distance between the alveolar gas and pulmonary capillaries. Basal laminae of the epithelium and stroma fuse, and the stroma contains increasing amounts of acellular matrix, including elastin and collagen. The abundance of smooth muscle in the pulmonary vasculature increases prior to birth. In human lung, the alveolar period begins near the time of birth and continues through the first decade of life, during which the lung grows primarily by septation and proliferation of the alveoli,[33,34,66] and by elongation and luminal enlargement of the conducting airways. Pulmonary arteries enlarge and elongate in close relationship to the increased growth of the lung.[35] Pulmonary vascular resistance decreases, and considerable remodeling of the pulmonary vasculature and capillary bed continues during the postnatal period.[34] Lung growth remains active until early adolescence, when the entire complement of more than 200 million alveoli has been formed.

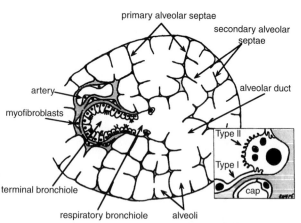

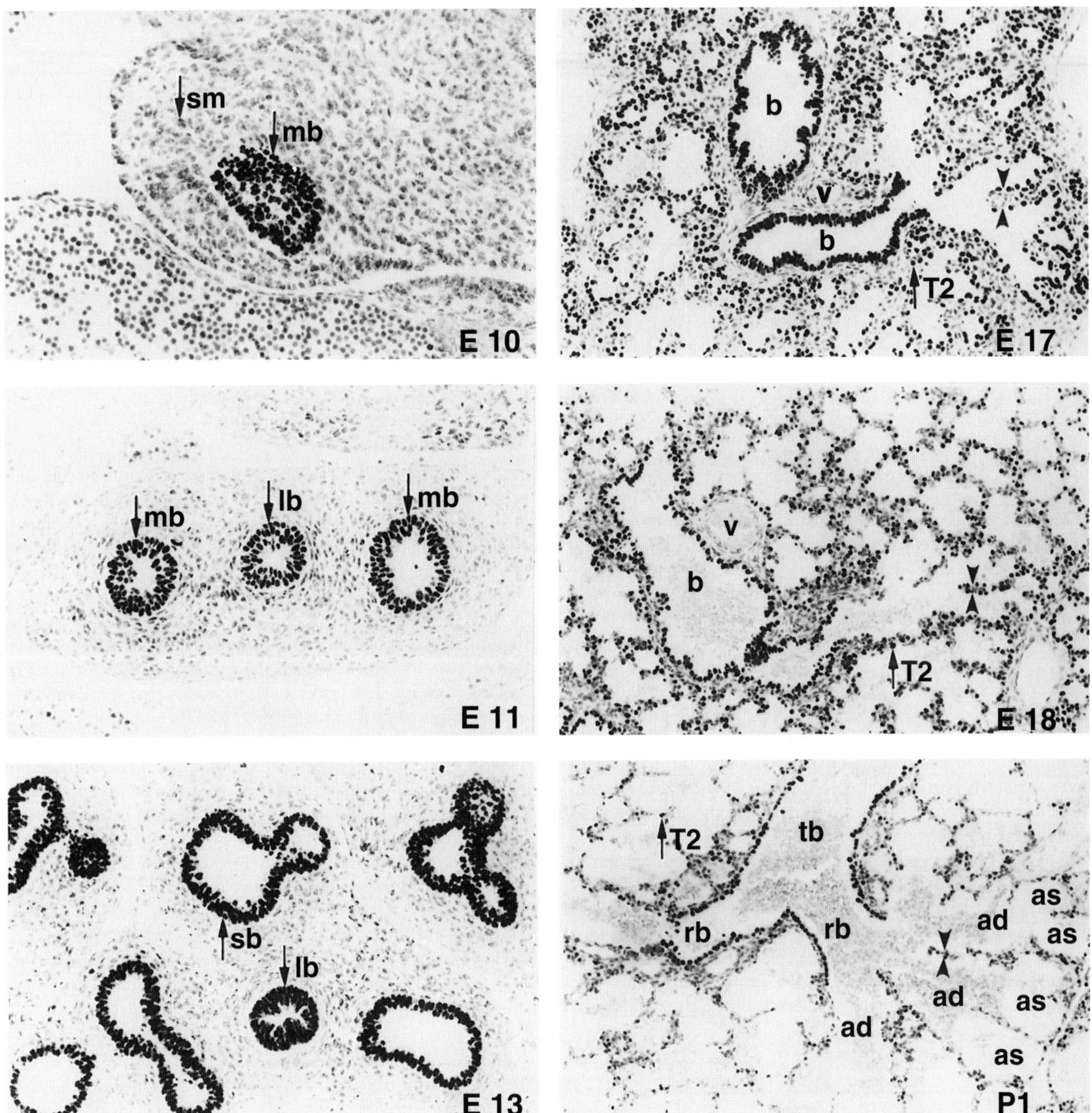

Continued

■ **FIGURE 1-2.** Mouse lung morphogenesis. Lung sections obtained from mice on embryonic days 10 *(E10),* 11 *(E11),* 13 *(E13),* 15 *(E15),* 17 *(E17),* and 18 *(E18),* postnatal day 1 *(P1),* and in adulthood *(A)* were stained for thyroid transcription factor-1, a marker for embryonic respiratory epithelial cells and differentiated type II cells. Mouse lung morphogenesis begins at E9.5 with outgrowth of paired lung buds from the foregut. Epithelium of the main stem bronchus (*E10,* mb) is surrounded by splanchnic mesenchyme (*E10,* sm). During the pseudoglandular stage (E12–E16), two main stem bronchi undergo extensive branching morphogenesis to form the conducting airways, including lobar bronchi (*E11 and E13,* lb), segmental bronchi (*E13,* sb), bronchioles (*E15,* b), and terminal lung buds (*E15,* tlb). Terminal lung buds dilate to form canal-like structures during the canalicular stage *(E17)* and further dilate to form saclike structures during the saccular stage *(E18),* near the end of gestation. After birth, the distal airways expand further and subdivide to form true alveolar structures *(P1, A).* Terminal bronchiole (tb), respiratory bronchiole (rb), alveolar duct (ad), and alveolar sac (as) are illustrated in *P1.* Distal airway remodeling during the canalicular, saccular, and alveolar stages is accompanied by thinning of the mesenchyme (notice the distance between the two arrowheads in *E17, E18, and P1*), differentiation of type I and type II cells (T2 in *E17, E18, P1, and A*), and evagination of blood vessels. A complicated alveolar network is observed in adult lung *(A).* Bar = 64 μm. v, vessel. (Courtesy of Dr. Lan Zhou.)

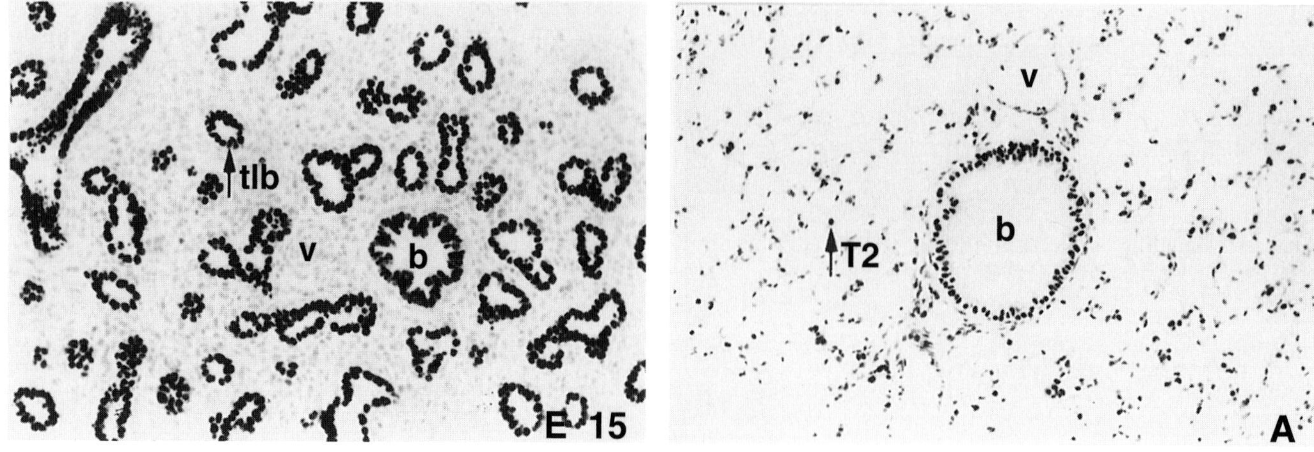

■ **FIGURE 1-2, cont'd**

CONTROL OF GENE TRANSCRIPTION DURING LUNG MORPHOGENESIS

Numerous regulatory mechanisms influence cell commitment, proliferation, and terminal differentiation required for formation of the mammalian lung (Fig. 1-3). These events must be precisely controlled in all organs to produce the complex body plan characteristic of higher organisms. In the mature lung, approximately 40 distinct cell types can be distinguished on the basis of morphologic and biochemical criteria.[67] Distinct pulmonary cell types arise primarily from subsets of endodermal and mesodermal progenitor cells (see Fig. 1-3). Pleuripotent or multipotent cells receive precise temporal and spatial signals that commit them to differentiated pathways, which ultimately generate the heterogeneous cell types present in the mature organ. The information directing cell proliferation and differentiation during organogenesis is derived from the genetic code contained within the DNA of each cell in the organism. Unique subsets of messenger RNAs (mRNAs), directing the synthesis of a variety of polypeptides, are expressed in each cell type, ultimately determining cell proliferation, structure, and behavior. Unique features of differentiating cells are controlled by the relative abundance of these mRNAs, which, in turn, determine the relative abundance of proteins synthesized by each cell. Cellular proteins influence morphologic, metabolic, and proliferative behaviors of cells, characteristics that traditionally have been used to assign cell phenotype by using morphologic and cytologic criteria. Gene expression in each cell is also determined by the structure of DNA-protein complexes that comprise the chromatin within the nucleus of each cell. Chromatin structure, in turn, influences the accessibility of individual genes to the transcriptional machinery. Diverse extracellular and intracellular signals also influence gene transcription, mRNA processing, mRNA stability, and translation, processes that determine the relative abundance of proteins produced by each cell.

Only a small fraction of the genetic material present in the nucleus represents regions of DNA that direct the synthesis of mRNAs encoding proteins. There is an increasing awareness that sequences in the noncoding regions of genes influence DNA structure and contain promoter and enhancer elements (usually in flanking and intronic regions of each gene) that determine levels of transcription. The ongoing nucleotide sequencing and identification of expressed complementary DNA (cDNA) sequences encoded within the human genome provide increasing insight into the amount of the genetic code used to synthesize the cellular proteins produced by each organ. At present, nearly all of the expressed cDNAs have been identified and

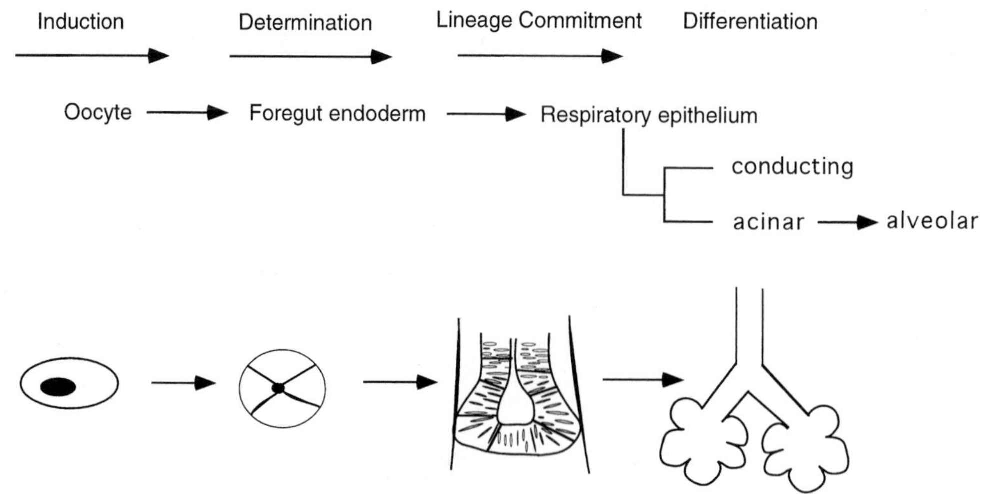

■ **FIGURE 1-3.** Pulmonary morphogenesis is determined by the genetic code in the oocyte and involves the precise control of cell proliferation, differentiation, or death of subsequent cells that ultimately form a complex organ containing more than 40 diverse cell types.

partially sequenced for most human organs.[68] Analysis of these mRNAs reveals distinct, and often unique, subsets of genes that are expressed in each organ, as well as the relative abundance and types of polypeptides encoded by these mRNAs. Of interest, proteins bearing signaling and transcriptional regulatory information are among the most abundant of various classes of proteins in human cells. Organ complexity in higher organisms is derived, at least in part, by the increasingly complex array of signaling molecules that govern cell behavior. Regulatory mechanisms controlling transcription are listed in Figure 1-4.

TRANSCRIPTIONAL CASCADES/HIERARCHIES

Gene transcription is modulated primarily by the binding of transcriptional factors (or transacting factors), which are nuclear proteins that bind to regulatory motifs consisting of ordered nucleotides (specific nucleotide sequences). The order of these specific nucleotide sequences determines recognition sites within the DNA (*cis*-acting elements) that are bound by these nuclear proteins. The binding of transcriptional factors to the *cis*-acting elements influences the activity of RNA polymerase II, which binds, in turn, to sequences near the transcription start site of target genes, initiating mRNA synthesis. Numerous families of transcription factors have been identified, and their activities are regulated by a variety of mechanisms, including post-translational modification and interactions with other proteins or DNA, as well as by their ability to translocate or remain in the nucleus.[69,70] Transcription factors also activate the transcription of other downstream nuclear factors, which, in turn, influence the expression of additional transacting factors. The number and cell specificity of transcriptional factors have proven to be large and are represented by diverse families of proteins categorized on the basis of structural motifs of their DNA binding or *trans* activating domains.[71–73] These interacting cascades of factors comprise a network with vast capabilities to influence target gene expression. The family of transcription factors (homeodomain, helix-turn-helix-containing family of DNA-binding proteins) represents an example of such a regulatory motif. A series of *HOX* genes are located in arrays containing large numbers of distinct genes arranged 3′ to 5′ in distinct loci within human chromosomes. Hox genes bind to and activate other downstream Hox gene family members that, in turn, bind to and activate the transcription of additional related and unrelated transcription factors, altering the activity of paired-homeodomain-containing genes (Pax), winged helix genes (Fox), zinc finger genes, such as retinoic acid receptors (RARs) or leucine-zipper transcription factors, that may also interact at the transcriptional level. Such cascades are now well characterized in organisms such as in *D. melanogaster*[74] and *C. elegans*.[75–77] Mammalian homologues exist in many of these genes, and their involvement in similar regulatory cascades influences gene expression and organogenesis in more complex organisms.[7,8,10,12,15] In the lung, thyroid transcription factor-1 (TTF-1) and Fox family members are involved in regulatory cascades that determine organogenesis and lung epithelial specific gene expression, and it is highly likely that many other nuclear transcription factors influence lung growth and development. Stat-3, β-catenin, GATA-6, POD-1, Foxa2, nuclear factor-1 (NF-1), Foxf1, Gli family members, Ets family members, N-*myc*, CCAAT/enhancer binding protein (C/EBP) family members, retinoic acid receptors, and glucocorticoid receptors, all nuclear transcription factors, influencing lung growth, cytodifferentiation, and function.[30,39,78,79]

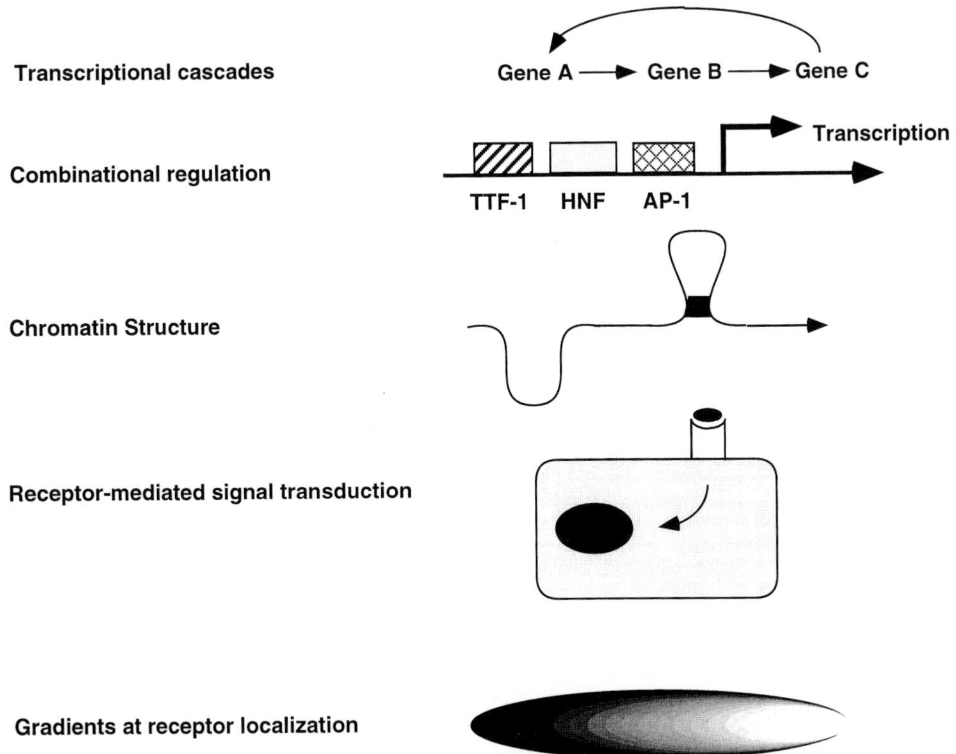

FIGURE 1-4. Diverse cellular mechanisms regulate varying levels of gene transcription that, in turn, control messenger RNA and protein synthesis governing cell differentiation and function during lung development.

COMBINATORIAL REGULATION OF GENE TRANSCRIPTION

The regulatory regions of target genes in eukaryotes are highly complex, usually containing numerous *cis*-acting elements that bind various nuclear transcription proteins. Nuclear proteins may bind DNA as monomers or oligomers, or form homo- or hetero-oligomers with other transcriptional proteins. Furthermore, many transcriptional proteins are modified by posttranslational modifications that are induced by receptor occupancy or phosphorylation/dephosphorylation events. Binding of transcription factors, or groups of transcription factors, may also perturb the structural organization of DNA (chromatin), making sites in the promoter regions more or less accessible to other nuclear proteins. Numerous *cis*-acting elements and their cognate *trans*-acting proteins interact with the basal transcriptional apparatus to regulate mRNA synthesis. The precise stoichiometry and specificity of the occupancy of the various DNA-binding sites influence either positively or negatively the transcription of specific target genes. This mode of regulation is characteristic of most eukaryotic cells, including those of the lung. For example, in pulmonary epithelial cells, a distinct set of transcription factors including TTF-1, activator protein-1 (AP-1), Fox family members, RARs, Stat-3, NF-1, and SP-1 regulate expression of surfactant protein genes that influence postnatal respiratory adaptation.[30]

INFLUENCE OF CHROMATIN STRUCTURE ON GENE EXPRESSION

The structure of chromatin is a critical determinant of the ability of target genes to respond to regulatory information influencing gene transcription. The abundance and organization of histones and other chromatin-associated proteins, including nuclear transcriptional proteins, influence the structure of DNA at genetic loci. The accessibility of regulatory regions within genes or groups of genes for binding and regulation by transcription factors is often dependent on chromatin structure. Changes in chromatin structure are likely determined by the process of cell differentiation during which target genes are made available or unavailable to the regulatory influences of transcription factors. Thus, the activity of a transcription factor at one time in development may be entirely distinct from that at another time. Chemical modification of DNA (e.g., methylation of cytosine) is also known to modify the ability of *cis*-active elements to bind and respond to regulatory influences. cytosine-guanine (CG)– rich islands are found in transcriptionally active genes, and methylation of these regions may vary developmentally or in response to signals that may influence gene transcription.[69] Chromatin structure, in turn, is influenced by post-transcriptional modification of histones and other DNA-associated proteins by acetylation, methylation, and phosphorylation, which is regulated by transcriptional complex and coactivator proteins that interact with the basal transcriptional machinery via polymerase II to alter gene transcription.[69]

RECEPTOR-MEDIATED SIGNAL TRANSDUCTION

Receptor-mediated signaling is well recognized as a fundamental mechanism for transducing extracellular information. Such signals are initiated by the occupancy of membrane-associated receptors capable of initiating additional signals (known as secondary messengers), such as cyclic adenosine monophosphate, calcium, and inositide phosphates, which influence the activity and function of intracellular polypeptides (kinases, phosphatases, proteases, etc.). These polypeptides, in turn, may alter the abundance of transcription factors, the activity of ion channels, or changes in membrane permeability, which subsequently modify cellular behaviors. Receptor-mediated signal transduction, induced by ligand-receptor binding, mediates endocrine, paracrine, and autocrine interactions on which cell differentiation and organogenesis depend. For example, fibroblast growth factor (FGF), Wnt, bone morphogenic protein (BMP), vascular endothelial growth factor (VEGF), ephrins, Notch/Delta, and sonic hedge hog (SHH) signaling have been implicated in organogenesis in many organs, including the lung.[40,80]

GRADIENTS OF SIGNALING MOLECULES AND LOCALIZATION OF RECEPTOR MOLECULES

Chemical gradients within tissues, and their interactions with membrane receptors located at distinct sites within the organ, can provide critical information during organogenesis. Polarized cells have basal, lateral, and apical surfaces with distinct subsets of signaling molecules (receptors) that allow the cell to respond in unique ways to focal concentrations of regulatory molecules. Secreted ligands (e.g., Wnts and SHH) function in gradients that are further influenced by binding of the ligand to basement membranes or proteoglycans. Spatial information is established by gradients of the signaling molecules and the presence and abundance of receptors at specific cellular sites. Such systems provide positional information to the cell that influences its behavior (e.g., shape, movement, proliferation, differentiation, polarized transport, etc.).

NONTRANSCRIPTIONAL MECHANISMS

While regulation of gene transcription is an important factor in organogenesis, numerous regulatory mechanisms, including control of transcriptional RNA expression, mRNA stability, protein translation, and degradation, are also known to provide further refinement in the abundance of mRNAs and proteins synthesized by a specific cell, which ultimately determine its structure and function.[69]

TRANSCRIPTIONAL MECHANISMS CONTROLLING GENE EXPRESSION DURING PULMONARY DEVELOPMENT

While knowledge of the determinants of gene regulation in lung development is rudimentary at present, a number of transcription factors and signaling networks that play critical roles in lung morphogenesis have been identified.[30,39,78,79,81] Lung morphogenesis depends on formation of definitive endoderm, which, in turn, signals from the splanchnic mesenchyme to initiate organogenesis along the foregut, forming thyroid, liver, pancreas, lung, and portions of the gastrointestinal tract.[82] The ventral plate of the endoderm in mammals forms under the direction of Foxa2, a transcription factor that is known to play a critical role in committing progenitor cells of the endoderm to form the primitive foregut.[16,25] Foxa2 is member of a large family of nuclear transcription factors, termed the winged helix family of transcription factors, that are involved in cell commitment, differentiation, and gene transcription in a variety of organs, such as the central nervous system and derivatives of the foregut endoderm, including the gastrointestinal tract, lung, and liver.[83] Foxa2 plays a critical role in organogenesis of the lung. Foxa2 is required for the formation of foregut endoderm, from which the lung bud is derived by evagination of a subset of endodermal cells into the splanchnic mesenchyme at approximately 3 to 4 weeks of gestation in the human. While Foxa2 plays a critical role in formation and commitment of progenitor cells to form the foregut endoderm, Foxa2 also influences the expression of specific genes in the respiratory epithelium later in development.[29,84–88] Conditional deletion of Foxa2 in respiratory epithelial cells of the developing lung caused respiratory distress at birth, Foxa2 regulating surfactant protein and phospholipid production, as well as morphologic maturation of the lung at birth.[89] Deletion of Foxa2 after birth caused goblet cell metaplasia, airspace enlargement, and inflammation during the postnatal period.[31] Deletion of mouse Foxa2 prior to birth resulted in delayed pulmonary maturation associated with decreased surfactant lipid and protein expression and the development of a respiratory distress–like syndrome.[89] Thus, Foxa2 plays a critical role in specification of foregut endoderm in the early embryo, and is used again in the perinatal and postnatal period to direct alveolarization, postnatal lung function, and homeostasis.

TTF-1 (or Nkx2.1) is a 38-kd nuclear protein, containing a homeodomain DNA-binding motif, that is critical for formation of the lung and for regulation of a number of highly specific gene products produced only in the respiratory epithelium. TTF-1 is also expressed in the thyroid and in specific regions of the developing central nervous system. In the lung, TTF-1 is expressed in the respiratory epithelium of the primitive lung bud[29,90–92] (see Fig. 1-2). Ablation of the mouse *Titf-1* gene impairs lung morphogenesis, resulting in hypoplastic lungs lined by a poorly differentiated respiratory epithelium and lacking gas exchange areas.[90] Substitution of a mutant *Titf-1* gene that lacks phosphorylation sites substantially rescues lung function in the *Titf-1* knockout mouse.[93] Expression of a number of genes, including those regulating surfactant homeostasis, fluid and electrolyte transport, host defense, and vasculogenesis, was regulated by TTF-1 phosphorylation prior to birth. TTF-1 regulates the expression of a number of genes in a highly specific manner in the respiratory epithelium, including surfactant proteins A, B, C, and CCSP.[85,94–98] TTF-1 functions in concert with other transcription factors, including GATA-6, NF-1, Stat-3, nuclear factor of activated T cells (NFAT), Foxa1 and Foxa2, and RARs to regulate lung-specific gene transcription. *Titf-1* gene transcription itself is modulated by the activity of Foxa2, which binds to the promoter enhancer region of the *Titf-1* gene, thus creating a transcriptional network.[88,99] A combinatorial mode of regulation is evidenced by the apposition of clustered TTF-1 *cis*-active elements and Foxa2-binding sites in target genes, such as the *SP-B* and *CCSP* genes.[84–87,100] The stoichiometry, timing, and distinct combinations of transcription factors, as well as posttranscriptional modification of TTF-1 by phosphorylation, are involved in differential, lung epithelial cell, gene expression throughout lung development. TTF-1 and other transcription factors are recruited to complexes at regulatory sites of target genes that influence respiratory epithelial cell differentiation, providing and translating spatial information required for the formation of the highly diverse epithelial cell types lining distinct regions of the respiratory tract. In the mature human lung, more than a dozen distinct epithelial cell types are readily distinguished, yet all are derived from progenitor cells originating in the foregut endoderm.

EPITHELIAL-MESENCHYMAL INTERACTIONS AND LUNG MORPHOGENESIS

In vivo and in vitro experiments support the concept that branching morphogenesis and differentiation of the respiratory tract depends on reciprocal signaling between endodermally derived cells of the lung buds and the pulmonary mesenchyme/stroma. This interdependency depends on autocrine and paracrine interactions that are mediated by the various signaling mechanisms governing cellular behavior[40,80] (Fig. 1-5). Similarly, autocrine/paracrine interactions are known to be involved in cellular responses of the postnatal lung, generating signals that regulate cell proliferation and differentiation necessary for its repair and remodeling following injury. The splanchnic mesenchyme produces a number of growth factors critical for migration and proliferation of cells in the lung buds, including FGF-10, FGF-7, FGF-9, and Wnt family members. In a complementary manner, epithelial cells of the lung tubules produce Wnt7b, Wnt5a, SHH, BMP-4, FGF-9, VEGF, and platelet-derived growth factor (PDGF) that activate receptors on target cells in the mesenchyme.[79,80]

BRANCHING MORPHOGENESIS, VASCULARIZATION, AND SACCULATION

Two distinct processes, branching and sacculation, are critical to morphogenesis of the mammalian lung. The major branches of the conducting airways of the human lung are completed by week 16 by a process of dichotomous branching, initiated by the bifurcation of the main stem bronchi early in the embryonic period of lung development. Epithelial-lined tubules of ever-decreasing diameter are formed from the proximal to distal region of the developing lung. Pulmonary arteries and veins form along

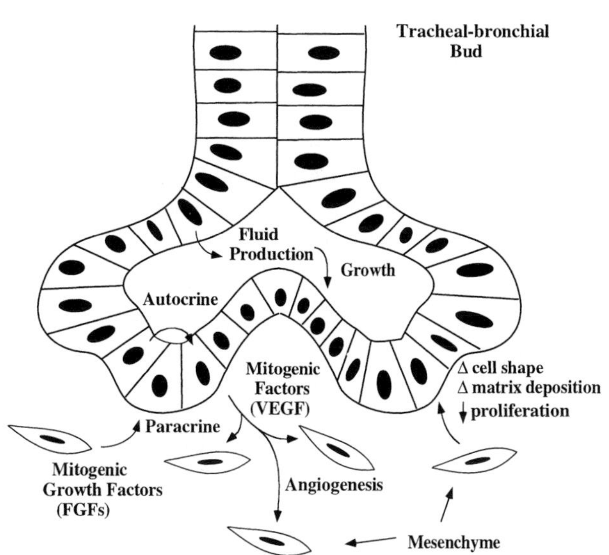

FIGURE 1-5. Branching morphogenesis is initiated by the evagination of the foregut endoderm into the splanchnic mesenchyme. Bronchi and bronchioles are formed by dichotomous branching, which depends on the precise regulation of cell proliferation and differentiation. Autocrine-paracrine interactions among various pulmonary cells are mediated by growth factors and receptors that influence cellular behaviors that are critical to lung formation.

the tubules and ultimately invade the acinar regions, where capillaries form between the arteries and veins, completing the pulmonary circulation. The bronchial vasculature arises from the aorta, providing nutrient supply predominantly to bronchial and bronchiolar regions of the lung. In contrast, the acinus (composed of bronchiolar portal and alveolar regions) is supplied by the pulmonary arterial system. Lymphatics and nerves form along the conducting airways, the latter being prominent in hilar, stromal, and vascular tissues, but lacking in the alveolar regions of the lung. A distinct period of lung sacculation and alveolarization begins in the late canalicular period (16 weeks and thereafter), forming the acinus that ultimately consists of the respiratory bronchiole, alveolar duct, and alveoli. During sacculation, a unique pattern of vascular supply forms the capillary network surrounding each saccule, providing an ever-expanding gas exchange area that is completed in adolescence. Both vasculogenesis and angiogenesis contribute to formation of the pulmonary vascular system.[36] Signaling via SHH, VEGF-A, Foxf1, Notch/Delta, ephrins, and PDGF plays important roles in pulmonary vascular development. VEGF-A is a critical factor in vasculogenesis in many tissues. However, overexpression of the VEGF-A 164 isoform disrupts pulmonary vascular endothelium in newborn conditional transgenic mice, causing pulmonary hemorrhage.[101]

CONTROL OF LUNG PROLIFERATION DURING BRANCHING MORPHOGENESIS

Dissection of the splanchnic mesenchyme from the lung buds arrests cell proliferation, branching, and differentiation of the pulmonary tubules in vitro.[37,38,40] Both in vitro and in vivo experiments strongly support the concept that the mesenchyme produces growth factors critical to the formation of respiratory tubules. In addition, lung growth is influenced by mechanical factors, including the size of the thoracic cavity and by stretch. For example, complete occlusion of the fetal trachea in utero enhances lung growth, while drainage of lung liquid or amniotic fluid causes lung hypoplasia. Regional control of proliferation is required for the process of dichotomous branching: division is enhanced at the lateral edges of the growing bud and inhibited at branch points.[102] Precise positional control of cell division is determined by polypeptides derived from the mesenchyme (e.g., growth factors or matrix molecules) that selectively decrease proliferation at clefts and increase cell proliferation at the edges of the bud (see Fig. 1-5). Proliferation in the respiratory tubule is dependent on a number of growth factors, including the FGF family of polypeptides. In vitro, FGF-1 and FGF-7 (keratinocyte growth factor, KGF) partially replace the requirement of pulmonary mesenchyme for continued epithelial cell proliferation and budding.[103,104] FGF polypeptides are produced by the mesenchyme during lung development and bind to and activate a splice variant of FGF receptor II (FGF-R2) that is present on respiratory epithelial cells, completing a paracrine loop.[105,106] Blockade of FGF-R2 signaling in the epithelium of the developing lung bud in vivo, using a dominant-negative FGF receptor mutant, completely blocked dichotomous branching of all conducting airway segments except the primary bronchi.[107] FGF-10 produced at localized regions of mesenchyme near the tips of the lung buds creates a chemoattractant gradient that activates the FGF-R2IIIb receptor in epithelial cells of the lung buds, which influences cell migration, differentiation, and proliferation required for branching morphogenesis.[108] Deletion of FGF-10 or FGF-R2IIIb blocked lung bud formation, resulting in lung agenesis.[109,110] Increased expression of FGF-10 or FGF-7 in the fetal mouse lung caused severe pulmonary lesions with all of the histologic features of cystadenomatoid malformations.[111,112] FGF-7 is also mitogenic for mature respiratory epithelial cells in vivo, enhancing proliferation of bronchiolar and alveolar cells when administered intratracheally to the lungs of adult rats.[113] Since FGF-7 is produced during lung injury, it is likely that FGF signaling molecules mediate cell proliferation or migration to influence repair.[114] FGF-7 and FGF-1 increase expression of surfactant proteins in vitro and in vivo, suggesting that these factors enhance type II cell differentiation.[111,115,116] Signaling polypeptides known to influence branching morphogenesis and differentiation of the respiratory tract are listed in Box 1-1.

ROLE OF EXTRACELLULAR MATRIX, CELL ADHESION, AND CELL SHAPE

The pulmonary mesenchyme is relatively loosely packed, and there is little evidence that cell type is specified during the early embryonic period of lung development. However, with advancing gestation, increasing abundance of extracellular matrix molecules, including laminin, fibronectin, collagens, elastin, and proteoglycans, is readily detected surrounding the developing epithelial tubules. Variability in the presence and abundance of various matrix molecules surrounding the tubules may influence differentiation and cell interactions.[117–123] Mesenchymal cells differentiate to form distinct vascular elements, endothelium, and smooth muscle and distinct fibroblastic cells that arise from the relatively undifferentiated progenitor cells of the splanchnic mesenchyme. While little is known regarding the factors influencing the differentiation of the pulmonary mesenchyme, the development of pulmonary vasculature is dependent on VEGFs.[124] VEGF-A is expressed by respiratory epithelial cells, stimulating pulmonary vasculogenesis mediated via paracrine signaling to receptors that are expressed by progenitor cells in the mesenchyme.[125–129] PDGF-α chain secreted by the respiratory epithelium influences proliferation and differentiation of myofibroblasts in the developing lung; deletion of PDGF-α causes pulmonary malformation in transgenic mice.[130] The organization of both mesenchyme and epithelium is further

BOX 1-1 Secreted Polypeptides Influencing Lung Morphogenesis and Differentiation

- Transforming growth factor-β (TGF-β)
- Bone morphogenic proteins (BMP-4)
- Fibroblast growth factors (FGF-1, FGF-7, FGF-9, FGF-10)
- Platelet-derived growth factor (PDGF)
- Epidermal/transforming growth factors (EGF/TGF-α)
- Sonic hedge hog (SHH)
- Vascular endothelial growth factor (VEGF-A)
- Hepatocyte growth factor (HGF)
- Insulin-like growth factors (IGFs)
- Granulocyte-macrophage colony-stimulating factor (GM-CSF)
- Wnt family members

modulated by CAMs of various classes, including the cadherins, integrins, and polypeptides, forming tight and gap junctions that contribute to cellular organization and polarity of various tissues during pulmonary organogenesis.[118,120,131] In vitro, inhibitors of collagen, elastin, and glycosaminoglycan (GAG) synthesis, and antibodies to various extracellular and cell attachment molecules, alter cell proliferation and branching morphogenesis of the embryonic lung.[119] Furthermore, the surrounding acellular matrix contains adhesion molecules that interact with attachment sites within cell membranes that in turn influence cell shape. Cell shape is determined, at least in part, by the organization of these cell attachment molecules to the cytoskeleton. Cell shape influences intracellular routing of cellular proteins and secretory products, determining the sites of secretion. Cell shape, polarity, and mobility are further influenced by the cytoskeletal proteins that interact with extracellular matrix, as well as neighboring cells. The organization of cell shape, via the cytoskeleton and its attachments, in turn, modifies cell differentiation in the lung.[132–134] For example, epithelial cells grown on intracellular matrix gels at an air-liquid interface form a highly polarized cuboidal epithelium that maintains cell differentiation and polarity of secretions in vitro. Loss of cell shape is associated with the loss of differentiated features such as surfactant protein and lipid synthesis, demonstrating the profound influence of cell shape on gene expression and cell behavior.

AUTOCRINE-PARACRINE INTERACTIONS IN LUNG INJURY AND REPAIR

As in lung morphogenesis, autocrine-paracrine signaling plays a critical role in the process of repair following lung injury. The repair processes in the postnatal lung, as in lung morphogenesis, require the precise control of cell proliferation and differentiation and, as such, are likely influenced by many of the signaling molecules and transcriptional mechanisms that mediate lung development. Events involved in lung repair may recapitulate events occurring during development in which progenitor cells undergo proliferation and terminal differentiation following lung injury. While many of the mechanisms involved in lung repair and development may be shared, it is also clear that the fetal and postnatal lung respond in distinct ways to autocrine-paracrine signals. Cells of the postnatal lung have undergone distinct phases of differentiation and may have different proliferative potentials or respond in unique ways to the signals evoked by lung injury. For example, after acute or chronic injury, increased production of polypeptide growth factors or cytokines may cause pulmonary fibrosis or pulmonary vascular remodeling in neonatal life, mediated by processes distinct from those occurring during normal lung morphogenesis.[135–140] The role of inflammation and the increasing activity of the immune system that accompanies postnatal development also distinguishes the pathogenesis of disease in the fetal and postnatal lungs.

HOST DEFENSE SYSTEMS

Distinct innate and adaptive defense systems mediate various aspects of host responses in the lung. During the postnatal period, the numbers and types of immune cells present in the lung expand markedly.[141] Alveolar macrophages, dendritic cells, lymphocytes of various subtypes, polymorphonuclear cells, eosinophils, and mast cells each have distinct roles in host defense. Immune cells mediate acute and chronic inflammatory responses accompanying lung injury or infection. Both the respiratory epithelium and inflammatory cells are capable of releasing and responding to a variety of polypeptides that initiate the expression of genes that are involved in (1) cytoprotection (e.g., antioxidants, heat shock proteins); (2) adhesion, influencing the attraction and binding of inflammatory cells to epithelial and endothelial cells of the lung; (3) cell proliferation, apoptosis, and differentiation that occur following injury or infection; and (4) innate host defense. An increasing array of cytokines and chemokines have now been identified that contribute to host defense following injury of the lung.[142–148]

The adaptive immune system includes both antibody and cell-mediated responses to antigenic stimuli. Adaptive immunity depends on the presentation of antigens by macrophages, dendritic cells, or the respiratory epithelium to mononuclear cells, triggering the expansion of immune lymphocytes and initiating antibody production and cytotoxic activity needed to remove infected cells from the lung. The lung contains active lymphocytes (natural killer cells, helper and cytotoxic T cells) that are present within the parenchyma and alveolus. Organized populations of mononuclear cells are also found in the lymphatic system along the conducting airways, termed the bronchiolar-associated lymphocytes (BALT). Cytokines and chemokines (interleukin-1 [IL-1], IL-8, tumor necrosis factor-α, RANTES [regulated on activation, normal T-expressed and secreted], granulocyte-macrophage colony-stimulating factor [GM-CSF], macrophage inflammatory protein-1α [MIP-1α], etc.) are produced by respiratory epithelial and other pulmonary cells, providing proliferative and/or differentiative signals to inflammatory cells that, in turn, amplify these signals by releasing cytokines or other inflammatory mediators within the lung.[149] Receptors for some of these signaling molecules have been identified in pulmonary epithelial cells.[150] For example, GM-CSF plays a critical role in surfactant homeostasis. Genetic ablation of GM-CSF or GM-CSF-IL-3/5β chain receptor causes alveolar proteinosis associated with macrophage dysfunction and surfactant accumulation.[151–155] Pulmonary alveolar proteinosis in adults is associated with high-affinity autoantibodies against GM-CSF that block receptor activation required for surfactant catabolism by alveolar macrophages.[156] However, GM-CSF stimulates both differentiation and proliferation of Type II epithelial cells, as well as activating alveolar macrophages to increase surfactant catabolism. Thus, GM-CSF acts in an autocrine-paracrine fashion as a growth factor for the respiratory epithelium. A number of growth factors, including GM-CSF, FGFs, EGF, TGF-α, PDGF, insulin-like growth factor-1 (IGF-1), TGF-β, and others, are released by lung cells following injury (see Box 1-1). These polypeptide growth factors likely play a critical role in stimulating proliferation of the respiratory epithelial cells required to repair the injured respiratory epithelium.[140,157] For example, intratracheal administration of FGF-7 causes marked proliferation of the adult respiratory epithelium and protects the lung from various injuries.[113]

INNATE DEFENSES

The lung also has innate defense systems that function independently of those provided by the mesodermally derived immune system. The respiratory epithelium and other lung cells secrete a variety of polypeptides that serve defense functions, including bacteriocidal polypeptides (lysozyme and defensins), collectins (surfactant proteins A and D), and other polypeptides that enhance macrophage activity involved in the clearance of bacteria and other pathogens. SP-A and SP-D, both members of the collectin family of mammalian lectins,[158] are secreted by the respiratory epithelium and bind to and enhance the phagocytosis of pathogenic organisms by alveolar macrophages.[159–170] Polypeptide factors with bacteriocidal activity, such as the defensins, are produced by various cells in response to inflammation within the lung, and are likely to play roles in host defense.[171–177] Thus, the immune system and accompanying production of chemokines and cytokines serve in an autocrine-paracrine fashion to modulate expression of genes mediating innate and immune-dependent defenses, as well as cell growth, critical to the repair of the parenchyma after injury. Uncontrolled proliferation of stromal cells leads to pulmonary fibrosis, just as uncontrolled growth of the respiratory epithelium produces pulmonary adenocarcinoma. Chronic inflammation, whether through inhaled particles, infection, or immune responses, may therefore establish ongoing proliferative cascades that lead to fibrosis and abnormal alveolar remodeling associated with chronic lung disease.[139]

GENE MUTATIONS IN LUNG DEVELOPMENT AND FUNCTION

Knowledge of the role of specific genes in lung development and function is expanding rapidly, extending our understanding of the role of genetic mutations that cause lung malformation and disease. Mutations in the DNA code may alter the abundance and function of encoded polypeptides, causing changes in cell behavior that lead to lung malformation and dysfunction. While poorly understood at present, a congenital malformation, termed acinar dysplasia, is associated with decreased or absent levels of TTF-1, Foxa2, and surfactant proteins; lungs from these infants are severely hypoplastic and lack peripheral airways at birth.[178] Such findings implicate the transcription factors TTF-1 and Foxa2, or their upstream regulators, in acinar dysplasia. Mutations in *TTF-1* cause lung hypoplasia and hypothyroidism.[179] Mutations in *SOX-9* influence the growth of the chest wall and cause lung hypoplasia in campomelic dwarfism.[180–184] Similarly, defects in SHH and FGF receptor signaling have been associated with lung and tracheobronchial malformation in human infants.[185,186] Thus, it is increasingly apparent that mutations in genes influencing transcriptional and signaling networks that control lung morphogenesis cause pulmonary malformations in infants.

Postnatally, mutations in various genes critical to lung function, host defense, and inflammation are associated with genetic disease in humans. Hereditary disorders affecting lung function include cystic fibrosis (cystic fibrosis transmembrane conductance regulator protein [CFTR]), hereditary surfactant protein B deficiency,[187,188] alveolar proteinosis (GM-CSF or receptors),[189] emphysema (α_1-antitrypsin deficiency), pulmonary fibrosis, interstitial lung disease, and respiratory distress (SP-C and ATP-binding cassette transporter 3 [ABCA3]),[190–192] and lymphangiomyomatosis (tuberous sclerosis complex [Tbc]). Mutations in polypeptides controlling neutrophil oxidant production lead to bacterial infections as seen in chronic granulomatous disease. The severity of disease associated with these monogenetic disorders is often strongly influenced by other inherited genes or environmental factors (e.g., smoking) that ameliorate or exacerbate underlying lung disease. The identification of "modifier genes" and the role of gene dosage in disease susceptibility will be critical in understanding the pathogenesis and clinical course of pulmonary disease in the future.

SUMMARY

The molecular and cellular mechanisms controlling lung morphogenesis and function provide a fundamental basis for understanding the pathogenesis and therapy of pulmonary diseases in children and adults. Future advances in pulmonary medicine will depend on the identification of new genes, and their encoded polypeptides, that play critical roles in lung formation and function. Knowledge regarding the complex signaling pathways that govern lung cell behaviors during development and after injury will provide the basis for new diagnostic and therapeutic approaches that will influence clinical outcomes. Diagnosis of pulmonary disease will be facilitated by the identification of new gene mutations that cause abnormalities in lung development and function. Since many of the events underlying lung morphogenesis may also be involved in the pathogenesis of lung disease postnatally, elucidation of molecular pathways governing lung development will provide the knowledge needed to understand the cellular and molecular basis of lung diseases. Advances in recombinant DNA technology and the ability to synthesize bioactive polypeptides and to add or to delete genes via DNA transfer are also likely to influence the therapy of pulmonary disease in the future.

REFERENCES

1. Favier B, Dolle P: Developmental functions of mammalian Hox genes. Mol Hum Reprod 1997;3:115–131.
2. Mark M, Rijli FM, Chambon P: Homeobox genes in embryogenesis and pathogenesis. Pediatr Res 1997;42:421–429.
3. Gellon G, McGinnis W: Shaping animal body plans in development and evolution by modulation of the Hox expression patterns. Bioessays 1998;20:116–125.
4. Veraksa A, del Campo M, McGinnis W: Developmental patterning genes and their conserved functions. From model organisms to humans. Mol Genet Metab 2000;69:85–100.
5. Goodman FR, Scambler PJ: Human HOX gene mutations. Clin Genet 2001;59:1–11.
6. Goodman FR: Congenital abnormalities of body patterning; embryology revisited. Lancet 2003;362:651–662.
7. Hombria JC, Lovegrove B: Beyond homeosis—HOX function in morphogenesis and organogenesis. Differentiation 2003;71:461–476.
8. Botas J: Control of morphogenesis and differentiation by HOM/Hox. Curr Opin Cell Biol 1993;5:1015–1022.
9. Bogue CW, Gross I, Vasavada H, et al: Identification of *Hox* genes in newborn lung and effects of gestational age and retinoic acid on their expression. Am J Physiol 1994;266:L448–L454.
10. Lufkin T: Transcriptional regulation of vertebrate Hox genes during embryogenesis. Crit Rev Eukaryot Gene Expr 1997;7:195–213.
11. Mann RS, Affolter M: Hox proteins meet more partners. Curr Opin Genet Dev 1998;8:423–429.
12. Pradel J, White RA: From selectors to realizators. Int J Dev Biol 1998; 42:417–421.
13. Chariot A, Gielen J, Merville MP, et al: The homeodomain-containing proteins. An update on their interacting partners. Biochem Pharmacol 1999;58:1851–1857.
14. Deschamps J, van den Akker E, Forlani S, et al: Initiation, establishment and maintenance of Hox gene expression patterns in the mouse. Int J Dev Biol 1999;43:635–650.
15. Lohmann I, McGinnis W: Hox genes: It's all a matter of context. Curr Biol 2002;12:R514–R516.
16. Ang SL, Wierda A, Wong D, et al: The formation and maintenance of the definitive endoderm lineage in the mouse. Involvement of HNF3/forkhead proteins. Development 1993;119:1301–1315.
17. Ang SL, Rossant J: HNF-3β is essential for node and notochord formation in mouse development. Cell 1994;78:561–574.

18. Weinstein DC, Ruiz I, Altaba A, et al: The winged-helix transcription factor HNF-3 beta is required for notochord development in the mouse embryo. Cell 1994;78:575–588.
19. Wodarz A, Nusse R: Mechanisms of Wnt signaling in development. Annu Rev Cell Dev Biol 1998;14:59–88.
20. Huelsken J, Behmers J: The Wnt signaling pathway. J Cell Sci 2002; 115:3977–3978.
21. Kanai-Azuma M, Kanai Y, Gad JM, et al: Depletion of definitive gut endoderm in Sox17-null mutant mice. Development 2002;129:2367–2379.
22. Sinner D, Rankin S, Lee M, et al: Sox17 and β-catenin cooperate to regulate the transcription of endodermal genes. Development 2004;131:3069–3080.
23. Morrisey EE, Tang Z, Sigrist K, et al: GATA-6 regulates HNF4 and is required for differentiation of visceral endoderm in the mouse embryo. Genes Dev 1998;12:3579–3590.
24. Moore KL: The respiratory system. In: Moore KL, ed: The Developing Human—Clinically Oriented Embryology, 5th ed. Philadelphia: WB Saunders, 1993, pp 226–236.
25. Monaghan AP, Kaestner KH, Grau E, et al: Postimplantation expression patterns indicate a role for the mouse forkhead/HNF-3 alpha, beta and gamma genes in determination of the definitive endoderm, chordamesoderm and neuroectoderm. Development 1993;119:567–578.
26. Sasaki H, Hogan BL: Differential expression of multiple fork head related genes during gastrulation and axial pattern formation in the mouse embryo. Development 1993;118:47–59.
27. Sasaki H, Hogan BLM: HNF 3β as a regulator of fetal plate development. Cell 1994;70:103–115.
28. Hackett BP, Bingle CD, Gitlin JD: Mechanisms of gene expression and cell fate determination in the developing pulmonary epithelium. Annu Rev Physiol 1996;58:51–71.
29. Zhou L, Lim L, Costa RH, et al: Thyroid transcription factor-1, hepatocyte nuclear factor 3, surfactant protein B, C, and Clara cell secretory protein in developing mouse lung. J Histochem Cytochem 1996;44:1183–1193.
30. Costa RH, Kalinichenko VV, Lim L: Transcription factors in mouse lung development and function. Am J Physiol 2001;280:L823–L838.
31. Wan H, Kaestner KH, Ang S-L, et al: Foxa2 regulates alveolarization and goblet cell hyperplasia. Development 2004;131:953–964.
32. Scarpelli EM: Lung cells from embryo to maturity. In: Scarpelli EM, ed: Pulmonary Physiology. Fetus, Newborn, Child, and Adolescent, 2nd ed. Philadelphia: Lea & Febiger, 1990, pp 42–82.
33. Thurlbeck WM: Pre- and postnatal organ development. In: Chernick V, Mellins RB, eds: Basic Mechanisms of Pediatric Respiratory Disease. Cellular and Integrative. Philadelphia: BC Decker, 1991, pp 23–35.
34. Burri PH: Structural aspects of prenatal and postnatal development and growth of the lung. In: McDonald JA, ed: Lung Growth and Development, 1st ed. New York: Marcel Dekker, 1997, p 1.
35. deMello DE, Reid LM: Pre- and postnatal development of the pulmonary circulation. In: Chernick J, Mellins RB, eds: Basic Mechanisms of Pediatric Respiratory Disease. Cellular and Integrative. Philadelphia: BC Decker, 1991, pp 36–54.
36. deMello DE, Reid LM: Embryonic and early fetal development of human lung vasculature and its functional implications. Pediatr Dev Pathol 2000;3:439–449.
37. Spooner BS, Wessells NK: Mammalian lung development. Interactions in primordium formation and bronchial morphogenesis. J Exp Zool 1970;175:445–454.
38. Masters JRW: Epithelial-mesenchymal interaction during lung development. The effect of mesenchymal mass. Dev Biol 1976;51:98–108.
39. Cardoso WV: Molecular regulation of lung development. Annu Rev Physiol 2001;63:471–494.
40. Shannon JM, Hyatt BA: Epithelial-mesenchymal interactions in the developing lung. Annu Rev Physiol 2004;66:625–645.
41. Khoor A, Gray ME, Hull WM, et al: Developmental expression of SP-A and SP-A mRNA in the proximal and distal respiratory epithelium in the human fetus and newborn. J Histochem Cytochem 1993;41:1311–1319.
42. Khoor A, Stahlman MT, Gray ME, et al: Temporal-spatial distribution of SP-B and SP-C proteins and mRNAs in the developing respiratory epithelium of the human lung. J Histochem Cytochem 1994;42:1187–1199.
43. Leslie KO, Mitchell JJ, Woodcock-Mitchell JL, et al: Alpha smooth muscle actin expression in developing and adult human lung. Differentiation 1990;44:143–149.
44. Woodcock-Mitchell J, White S, Stirewalt W, et al: Myosin isoform expression in developing and remodeling rat lung. Am J Respir Cell Mol Biol 1993;8:617–625.
45. Miano JM, Cserjesi P, Ligon KL, et al: Smooth muscle myosin heavy chain exclusively marks the smooth muscle lineage during mouse embryogenesis. Circ Res 1994;75:803–812.
46. Singh G, Singh J, Katyal SL, et al: Identification, cellular localization, isolation, and characterization of human Clara cell-specific 10 kd protein. J Histochem Cytochem 1988;36:73–80.
47. Strum JM, Singh G, Katyal S, et al: Immunochemical localization of Clara cell protein by light and electron microscopy in conducting airways of fetal and neonatal hamster lung. Anat Rec 1990;227:77–86.
48. Ten Have-Opbroek AAW, DeVries ECP: Clara cell differentiation in the mouse. Ultrastructural morphology and cytochemistry for surfactant protein A and Clara cell 10 kD protein. Microsc Res Tech 1993;26:400–411.
49. Schellhase DE, Emrie PA, Fisher JH, et al: Ontogeny of surfactant proteins in the rat. Pediatr Res 1989;26:167–174.
50. Endo H, Oka T: An immunohistochemical study of bronchial cells producing surfactant protein A in the developing human fetal lung. Early Hum Dev 1991;25:149–156.
51. Otto-Verberne CJM, Ten Have-Opbroek AAW, DeVries ECP: Expression of the major surfactant-associated protein, SP-A, in Type II cells of human lung before 20 weeks of gestation. Eur J Cell Biol 1990;53: 13–19.
52. Weaver TE, Whitsett JA: Function and regulation of expression of pulmonary surfactant-associated proteins. Biochem J 1991;273:249–264.
53. Batenburg JJ, Hallman M: Developmental biochemistry of alveoli. In: Scarpelli EM, ed: Pulmonary Physiology. Fetus, Newborn, Child, and Adolescent. Philadelphia: Lea & Febiger, 1991, pp 106–139.
54. Williams MC, Mason R: Development of the type II cell in the fetal rat lung. Am Rev Respir Dis 1977;115:37–47.
55. Hilfer SR: Development of terminal buds in the fetal mouse lung. Scanning Electron Microsc 1983;111:1378–1401.
56. Chi EY: The ultrastructural study of glycogen and lamellar bodies in the development of fetal monkey lung. Exp Lung Res 1985;8:275–289.
57. Ten Have-Opbroek AAW, Otto-Verberne CJM, Dubbeldam JA: Ultrastructural characteristics of inclusion bodies of type II cells in late embryonic mouse lung. Anat Embryol 1990;181:317–323.
58. Whitsett JA, Weaver TE, Clark JC, et al: Glucocorticoid enhances surfactant proteolipid Phe and pVal synthesis and RNA in fetal lung. J Biol Chem 1987;262:15618–15623.
59. Ballard PL: Hormonal regulation of pulmonary surfactant. Endocr Rev 1989;10:165–181.
60. Mendelson CR, Boggaram V: Hormonal control of the surfactant system in fetal lung. Annu Rev Physiol 1991;53:415–440.
61. Jobe AH, Soll RF: Choice and dose of corticosteroid for antenatal treatments. Am J Obstet Gynecol 2004;190:878–881.
62. Yeomans ER: Prenatal corticosteroid therapy to prevent respiratory distress syndrome. Semin Perinatol 1993;17:253–259.
63. Jobe AH: Antenatal factors and the development of bronchopulmonary dysplasia. Semin Neonatol 2003;8:9–17.
64. Rooney SA, Young SL, Mendelson CR: Molecular and cellular processing of lung surfactant. FASEB J 1994;8:957–967.
65. Crouch E, Rust K, Marienchek W, et al: Developmental expression of pulmonary surfactant protein D (SP-D). Am J Respir Cell Mol Biol 1991; 5:13–18.
66. Langston C, Kida K, Reed M, et al: Human lung growth in late gestation and in the neonate. Am Rev Respir Dis 1984;129:607–613.
67. Gail DB, Lenfant CJM: Cells of the lung. Biology and clinical implications. Am Rev Respir Dis 1983;127:366–387.
68. Adams MD, Kerlavage AR, Fleischman RD, et al: Initial assessment of human gene diversity and expression patterns based upon 83 million nucleotides of cDNA sequence. Nature 1995;377:3–174.
69. Lewin B: Genes VIII. New York: Prentice-Hall, 2003.
70. Latchman DS: Eukaryotic Transcription Factors. San Diego, CA: Academic, 2003.
71. Mitchell DJ, Tjian R: Transcriptional regulation in mammalian cells by sequence specific DNA binding proteins. Science 1989;245:371–378.
72. Pabo CO, Sauer RT: Transcription factors: Structural families and principles of DNA recognition. Ann Rev Biochem 1992;61:1053–1095.
73. Vellanoweth RL, Supakar PC, Arun KR: Transcription factors in development growth and aging. Lab Invest 1994;70:784–799.
74. Davis GK, Patel NH: Short, long, and beyond. Molecular and embryological approaches to insect segmentation. Annu Rev Entomol 2002;47: 669–699.
75. Salser SJ, Kenyon C: Patterning *C. elegans*. Homeotic cluster genes, cell fates and cell migrations. Trends Genet 1994;10:159–164.
76. Kenyon CJ, Austin J, Costa M, et al: The dance of the Hox genes. Patterning the anteroposterior body axis of *Caenorhabditis elegans*. Cold Spring Harb Symp Quant Biol 1997;62:293–305.
77. Aboobaker AA, Blaxter ML: Hox gene loss during dynamic evolution of the nematode cluster. Curr Biol 2003;13:37–40.

78. Cardoso WV: Transcription factors and pattern formation in the developing lung. Am J Physiol 1995;269:L429–L442.
79. Warburton D, Schwarz M, Tefft D, et al: The molecular basis of lung morphogenesis. Mech Dev 2000;92:55–81.
80. Kaplan F: Molecular determinants of fetal lung organogenesis. Mol Genet Metab 2000;71:321–341.
81. Whitsett JA, Korfhagen TR: Regulation of gene transcription in respiratory epithelial cells. Am J Respir Cell Mol Biol 1996;14:118–120.
82. Wells JM, Melton DA: Vertebrate endoderm development. Annu Rev Cell Dev Biol 1999;15:393–410.
83. Clevidence DE, Overdier DG, Tao W, et al: Identification of nine tissue-specific transcription factors of the hepatocyte nuclear factor3/forkhead DNA-binding-domain family. Proc Natl Acad Sci U S A 1993;90:3948–3952.
84. Sawaya PL, Stripp BR, Whitsett JA, et al: The lung-specific CC10 gene is regulated by transcription factors from the AP-1, octamer, and hepatocyte nuclear factor-3 families. Mol Cel Biol 1993;13:3860–3871.
85. Bohinski RJ, DiLauro R, Whitsett JA: The lung-specific surfactant protein B gene promoter is a target for thyroid transcription factor 1 and hepatocyte nuclear factor 3, indicating common factors for organ-specific gene expression along the foregut axis. Mol Cell Biol 1994;14:5671–5681.
86. Clevidence DE, Overdier DG, Peterson RS, et al: Members of the HNF-3/forkhead family of transcription factors exhibit distinct cellular expression patterns in lung and regulate the surfactant protein B promoter. Dev Biol 1994;166:195–209.
87. Sawaya PL, Luse DS: Two members of the HNF-3 family have opposite effects on a lung transcriptional element; HNF-3α stimulates and HNF-3β inhibits activity of region I from the Clara cell secretory protein (CCSP) promoter. J Biol Chem 1994;269:22211–22216.
88. Ikeda K, Shaw-White JR, Wert SE, et al: Hepatocyte nuclear factor 3 activates transcription of TTF-1 in respiratory epithelial cells. Mol Cell Biol 1996;16:3626–3636.
89. Wan H, Xu Y, Ikegami M, et al: Foxa2 is required for transition to air breathing at birth. Proc Natl Acad Sci U S A 2004;101:14449–14454.
90. Kimura S, Hura Y, Pinlau T, et al: The T/ebp null mouse. Thyroid specific enhancer binding protein is essential for organogenesis of the thyroid, lung ventral forebrain, and pituitary. Genes Dev 1996;10:60–69.
91. Lazzaro D, Price M, de Felice M, et al: The transcription factor TTF-1 is expressed at the onset of thyroid and lung morphogenesis and in restricted regions of the foetal brain. Development 1991;113:1093–1104.
92. Stahlman MT, Gray ME, Whitsett JA: Expression of thyroid transcription factor-1 (TTF-1) in fetal and neonatal human lung. J Histochem Cytochem 1996;44:673–678.
93. DeFelice M, Silberschmidt D, DiLauro R, et al: TTF-1 phosphorylation is required for peripheral lung morphogenesis, perinatal survival, and tissue-specific gene expression. J Biol Chem 2003;278:35574–35583.
94. Bruno MD, Bohinski RJ, Huelsman KM, et al: Lung cell specific expression of the murine surfactant protein A gene is mediated by interactions between the SP-A promoter and thyroid transcription factor-1. J Biol Chem 1995;270:6531–6536.
95. Kelly SE, Bachurski CJ, Burhans MS, et al: Transcription of the lung-specific surfactant protein C gene is mediated by thyroid transcription factor-1. J Biol Chem 1996;271:6881–6888.
96. Yan C, Sever Z, Whitsett JA: Upstream enhancer activity in the human surfactant protein B gene is mediated by thyroid transcription factor 1. J Biol Chem 1995;270:24852–24857.
97. Ray MK, Chen C-Y, Schwartz RJ, et al: Transcriptional regulation of a mouse Clara cell specific protein (mCC10) gene by the NKx transcription factor family member thyroid transcription factor 1 and cardiac muscle-specific homeobox protein (CSx). Mol Cell Biol 1996;16:2056–2064.
98. Zhang L, Whitsett JA, Stripp BR: Regulation of Clara cell secretory protein gene transcription by thyroid transcription factor-1. Biochim Biophys Acta 1997;1350:359–367.
99. Ikeda K, Clark JC, Shaw-White JR, et al: Gene structure and expression of human thyroid transcription factor-1 in respiratory epithelial cells. J Biol Chem 1995;270:8108–8114.
100. Bingle CD, Gitlin JD: Identification of hepatocyte nuclear factor-3 binding sites in the Clara cell secretory protein gene. Biochem J 1993;295:227–232.
101. Le Cras TD, Spitzmiller RE, Albertine KH, et al: VEGF causes pulmonary hemorrhage, hemosiderosis, and air space enlargement in neonatal mice. Am J Physiol 2004;287:L134–L142.
102. Kauffman SL: Cell proliferation in the mammalian lung. Int Rev Exp Pathol 1980;22:131–191.
103. Nogawa H, Ito T: Branching morphogenesis of embryonic mouse lung epithelium in mesenchyme-free culture. Development 1995;121:1015–1022.
104. Deterding, RR, Jacoby CR, Shannon JM: Acidic fibroblast growth factor and keratinocyte growth factor stimulated fetal rat pulmonary epithelial growth. Am J Physiol 1996;271:L495–L505.
105. Han RN, Liu J, Tanswell AK, et al: Expression of basic fibroblast growth factor and receptor—Immunolocalization studies in developing rat fetal lung. Pediatr Res 1992;31:435–440.
106. Peters KG, Werner S, Chen G, et al: Two FGF receptor genes are differentially expressed in epithelial and mesenchymal tissues during limb formation and organogenesis in the mouse. Development 1992;114:233–243.
107. Peters K, Werner S, Liao X, et al: Targeted expression of a dominant negative FGF receptor blocks branching morphogenesis and epithelial differentiation of the mouse lung. EMBO J 1994;13:3296–3301.
108. Sekine K, Ohuchi H, Fujiwara M, et al: FGF10 is essential for limb and lung formation. Nat Genet 1999;21:138–141.
109. Min H, Danilenko DM, Scully SA, et al: *Fgf-10* is required for both limb and lung development and exhibits striking functional similarity to *Drosophila branchless*. Genes Dev 1998;12:3156–3161.
110. Arman E, Haffner-Krausz R, Chen Y, et al: Targeted disruption of fibroblast growth factor (FGF) receptor 2 suggests a role for FGF signaling in pregastrulation mammalian development. Proc Natl Acad Sci U S A 1998;95:5082–5087.
111. Tichelaar JW, Lu W, Whitsett JA: Conditional expression of fibroblast growth factor-7 in the developing and mature lung. J Biol Chem 2000;275:11858–11864.
112. Clark JC, Tichelaar JW, Wert SE, et al: FGF-10 disrupts lung morphogenesis and causes pulmonary adenomas in vivo. Am J Physiol 2001;280:L705–L715.
113. Ulich TR, Yi ES, Longmuir K, et al: Keratinocyte growth factor is a growth factor for type II pneumocytes in vivo. J Clin Invest 1994;93:1298–1306.
114. Charafeddine L, D'Angio CT, Richards JL, et al: Hyperoxia increases keratinocyte growth factor mRNA expression in neonatal rabbit lung. Am J Physiol 1999;276:L105–L113.
115. Sugahara K, Rubin JS, Mason RJ: Keratinocyte growth factor increases mRNAs for SP-A and SP-B in adult rat alveolar type II cells in culture. Am J Physiol 1995;269:L344–L350.
116. Cardoso WV, Itoh A, Nogawa H, et al: FGF-1 and FGF-7 induce distinct patterns of growth and differentiation in embryonic lung epithelium. Dev Dyn 1997;208:398–405.
117. Guzowski DE, Blau H, Bienkowski RS: Extracellular matrix in developing lung. In: Scarpelli EM, ed: Pulmonary Physiology: Fetus, Newborn, Child, and Adolescent. Philadelphia: Lea & Febiger, 1990, pp 83–105.
118. Pilewski JM, Albelda SM: Adhesion molecules in the lung. An overview. Am Rev Respir Dis 1993;148(6; Suppl):31–37.
119. Hilfer SR: Morphogenesis of the lung. Control of embryonic and fetal branching. Annu Rev Physiol 1996;58:93–113.
120. Kampman KA, McDonald JA: Adhesion molecules in lung morphogenesis. In: Ward PA, Fantone JC, eds: Lung Biology in Health and Disease, Vol 89. New York: Marcel Dekker, 1996, pp 99–126.
121. Spurzem JR, Rennard SI, Romberger DJ: Interactions between pulmonary epithelial cells and extracellular matrix. In: Ward PA, Fantone JC, eds: Lung Biology in Health and Disease, Vol 89. New York: Marcel Dekker, 1996, pp 127–146.
122. Crouch E, Mecham RP, Davila RM, et al: Collagen and elastic fiber proteins in lung development. In: McDonald JA, ed: Lung Development, 1st ed. New York: Marcel Dekker, 1997, p 327.
123. Shannon JM, Deterding RR: Epithelial-mesenchymal interactions in lung development. In: McDonald JA, ed: Lung Growth and Development, 1st ed. New York: Marcel Dekker, 1997, p 81.
124. Ferrara N, Houch KA, Jakeman LB, et al: The vascular endothelial growth factor family of polypeptides. J Cell Biochem 1991;47:211–218.
125. Peters KG, DeVries C, Williams LT: Vascular endothelial growth factor receptor expression during embryogenesis and tissue repair suggests a role in endothelial differentiation and blood vessel growth. Proc Natl Acad Sci U S A 1993;90:8915–8919.
126. Monacci WT, Merrill MJ, Oldfield EH: Expression of vascular permeability factor/vascular endothelial growth factor in normal rat tissues. Am J Physiol 1993;264:C995–C1002.
127. Breier G, Albrecht U, Sterrer S, et al: Expression of vascular endothelial growth factor during embryonic angiogenesis and endothelial cell differentiation. Development 1992;114:521–532.

128. Breier G, Clauss M, Risau W: Coordinate expression of vascular endothelial growth factor receptor-1 (flt-1) and its ligand suggests a paracrine regulation of murine vascular development. Dev Dyn 1995;20:228–239.
129. Millauer B, Wizigmann-Voos S, Schnürch H, et al: High affinity VEGF binding and developmental expression suggest flk-1 as a major regulator of vasculogenesis and angiogenesis. Cell 1993;72:835–846.
130. Boström H, Willetts K, Pekny M, et al: PDGF-A signalling is a critical event in lung alveolar myofibroblast development and alveogenesis. Cell 1996;85:863-873.
131. Liley H, Bernfield M: Mechanisms of development and repair of the lung. In: Chernick V, Mellins RB, eds: Basic Mechanisms of Pediatric Respiratory Disease. Cellular and Integrative. Philadelphia: BC Decker, 1991, pp 11–22.
132. Shannon JM, Mason RJ, Jennings SD: Functional differentiation of alveolar type II epithelial cells in vitro. Effects of cell shape, cell-matrix interactions and cell-cell interactions. Biochim Biophys Acta 1987;931: 143–156.
133. Sanchez-Esteban J, Tsai SW, Sang J, et al: Effects of mechanical forces on lung-specific gene expression. Am J Med Sci 1998;316:200–204.
134. Sanchez-Esteban J, Cicchiello LA, Wang Y, et al: Mechanical stretch promotes alveolar epithelial type II cell differentiation. J Appl Physiol 2001;91:589–595.
135. Finkelstein JN, Horowitz S, Sirkin R, Ryan RM: Cellular and molecular responses to lung injury in relation to induction of tissue repair and fibrosis. Clin Perinatol 1992;19:603–620.
136. Valliant P, Menard O, Vignaud JM, et al: The role of cytokines in human lung fibrosis. Monaldi Arch Chest Dis 1996;51:145–152.
137. O'Reilly MA, Stripp BR, Pryhuber GS: Epithelial-mesenchymal interactions in the alteration of gene expression and morphology following lung injury. Microsc Res Tech 1997;38:473–479.
138. DeMayo F, Minoo P, Plopper CG, et al: Mesenchymal-epithelial interactions in lung development and repair. Are modeling and remodeling the same process? Am J Physiol 2002;283:L510–L517.
139. Chapman HA: Disorders of lung matrix remodeling. J Clin Invest 2004; 113:148–157.
140. Warburton D, Bellusci S: The molecular genetics of lung morphogenesis and injury repair. Paediatr Respir Rev 2004;5(Suppl A):283–287.
141. Kamani NR, Bonagura VR: Developmental immunology of the lung. In: Scarpelli EM, ed: Pulmonary Physiology. Fetus, Newborn, Child, and Adolescent, 2nd ed. Philadelphia: Lea & Febiger, 1990, pp 140–160.
142. Elias JA, Freundlich B, Kern JA, et al: Cytokine networks in the regulation of inflammation and fibrosis in the lung. Chest 1990;97:1439–1445.
143. Kelley J: Cytokines of the Lung. New York: Marcel Dekker, 1992.
144. Lukas NW, Ward PA: Inflammatory mediators, cytokines, and adhesion molecules in pulmonary inflammation and injury. Advan Immunol 1996; 62:257–304.
145. Standiford TJ: Cytokines and pulmonary host defenses. Curr Opin Pulm Med 1997;3:81–88.
146. Zhang P, Summer WR, Bagby GJ, et al: Innate immunity and pulmonary host defense. Immunol Rev 2000;173:39–51.
147. Strieter RM, Belperio JA, Keane MP: Cytokines in innate host defense in the lung. J Clin Invest 2002;109:699–705.
148. Strieter RM, Belperio JA, Keane MP: Host innate defenses in the lung. The role of cytokines. Curr Opin Infect Dis 2003;16:193–198.
149. Adler KB, Fischer BM, Wright DT, et al: Interactions between respiratory epithelial cells and cytokines. Relationships to lung inflammation. Ann NY Acad Sci 1994;725:120–145.
150. Sheperd VL: Cytokine receptors of the lung. Am J Respir Cell Mol Biol 1991;5:403–410.
151. Dranoff G, Crawford AD, Sadelain M, et al: Involvement of granulocyte-macrophage colony stimulating factor in pulmonary homeostasis. Science 1994;264:713–716.
152. Lieschke GJ, Stanley E, Grail D, et al: Mice lacking both macrophage- and granulocyte-macrophage colony-stimulating factor have macrophages and coexistent osteoporosis and severe lung disease. Blood 1994;84:27–35.
153. Stanley E, Lieshke GJ, Grail D, et al: Granulocyte/macrophage colony stimulating factor-deficient mice show no major perturbation of hematopoiesis but develop a characteristic pulmonary pathology. Proc Natl Acad Sci U S A 1994;91:5592–5594.
154. Huffman JA, Hull WM, Dranoff G, et al: Pulmonary epithelial cell expression of GM-CSF corrects the alveolar proteinosis in GM-CSF-deficient mice. J Clin Invest 1996;97:649–655.
155. Ikegami M, Ueda T, Hull W, et al: Surfactant metabolism in transgenic mice after granulocyte macrophage-colony stimulating factor ablation. Am J Physiol 1996;270:L650–L658.
156. Trapnell BC, Whitsett JA: GM-CSF regulates pulmonary surfactant homeostasis and alveolar macrophage-mediated innate host defense. Annu Rev Physiol 2002;64:775–802.
157. Perkett EA: Role of growth factors in lung repair and diseases. Curr Opin Pediatr 1995;7:242–249.
158. Sastry K, Ezekowitz RA: Collectins. Pattern recognition molecules involved in first line host defense. Curr Opin Immunol 1993;5:59–66.
159. Van Iwaarden JF, Pikaar JC, Storm J, et al: Binding of surfactant protein A to the lipid A moiety of bacterial lipopolysaccharides. Biochem J 1994; 303:407–411.
160. McNeely TB, Coonrod JD: Aggregation and opsonization of type A but not type B *Hemophilus influenzae* by surfactant protein A. Am J Respir Cell Mol Biol 1994;11:114–122.
161. Limper AH, Crouch EC, O'Riordan DM, et al: Surfactant protein-D modulates interaction of *Pneumocystis carinii* with alveolar macrophages. J Lab Clin Med 1995;126:416–422.
162. Geertsma MF, Nibbering PH, Haagsman HP, et al: Binding of surfactant protein A to C1q receptors mediates phagocytosis of *Staphylococcus aureus* by monocytes. Am J Physiol 1994;267:L578–L584.
163. Downing JF, Pasula R, Wright JR, et al: Surfactant protein A promotes attachment of *Mycobacterium tuberculosis* to alveolar macrophages during infection with human immunodeficiency virus. Proc Natl Acad Sci U S A 1995;92:4848–4852.
164. Benne CA, Kraaijeveld CA, van Strijp JAG, et al: Interactions of surfactant protein A with influenza A viruses. Binding and neutralization. J Infect Dis 1995;171:335–341.
165. Wright JR: Immunomodulatory functions of surfactant. Semin Respir Crit Care Med 1995;16:61–68.
166. Tino MJ, Wright JR: Surfactant protein A stimulates phagocytosis of specific pulmonary pathogens by alveolar macrophages. Am J Physiol 1996;270:L677–L688.
167. Williams MD, Wright JR, March KL, et al: Human surfactant protein A enhances attachment of *Pneumocystis carinii* to rat alveolar macrophages. Am J Respir Cell Mol Biol 1996;14:232–238.
168. LeVine AM, Whitsett JA: Pulmonary collectins and innate host defense of the lung. Microbes Infect 2001;3:161–166.
169. Crouch E, Wright JR: Surfactant proteins A and D and pulmonary host defense. Annu Rev Physiol 2001;63:521–554.
170. McCormack FX, Whitsett JA: The pulmonary collectins, SP-A and SP-D, orchestrate innate immunity in the lung. J Clin Invest 2002;109: 707–712.
171. Bevins CL: Antimicrobial peptides as agents of mucosal immunity. Ciba Found Symp 1994;186:250–260.
172. Ganz T: Biosynthesis of defensins and other microbial peptides. Ciba Found Symp 1994;186:62–71.
173. Ganz T, Lehrer RI: Defensins. Curr Opin Immunol 1994;6:584–589.
174. Kagan BL, Ganz T, Lehrer RI: Defensins. A family of antimicrobial and cytotoxic peptides. Toxicology 1994;87:131–149.
175. van Wetering S, Sterk PJ, Rabe KF, et al: Defensins. Key players or bystanders in infection, injury, and repair in the lung? J Allergy Clin Immunol 1999;104:1131–1138.
176. Cole AM, Waring AJ: The role of defensins in lung biology and therapy. Am J Respir Med 2002;1:249–259.
177. Schutte BC, McCray PB Jr: β-Defensins in lung host defense. Ann Rev Physiol 2002;64:709–748.
178. Wert SE, Profitt SA, Kirwin KL, et al: Acinar dysplasia is associated with the absence of TTF-1 and HNF-3β expression during human lung development. Pediatr Res 1996;39:355A.
179. Devriendt K, Vanhole C, Matthijs G, et al: Deletion of thyroid transcription factor-1 gene in an infant with neonatal thyroid dysfunction and respiratory failure. N Engl J Med 1998;338:1317–1318.
180. Houston CS, Opitz JM, Spranger JW, et al: The campomelic syndrome. Review, 17 cases, and follow up on the currently 17-year-old boy first reported by Maroteaux et al in 1971. Am J Med Genet 1983;15: 3–28.
181. Foster JW, Dominguez-Steglich MA, Guioli S, et al: Campomelic dysplasia and autosomal sex reversal caused by mutations in an SRY-related gene. Nature 1994;372:525–530.
182. Wagner T, Wirth J, Meyer J, et al: Autosomal sex reversal and campomelic dysplasia are caused by mutations in and around the SRY-related gene SOX9. Cell 1994;79:1111–1120.
183. Mansour S, Hall CM, Pembrey ME, et al: A clinical and genetic study of campomelic dysplasia. J Med Genet 1995;32:415–420.
184. Mansour S, Offiah AC, McDowall S, et al: The phenotype of survivors of campomelic dysplasia. J Med Genet 2002;39:597–602.

185. Pepicelli CV, Lewis PM, McMahon AP: Sonic hedgehog regulates branching morphogenesis in the mammalian lung. Curr Biol 1998;8: 1083–1086.
186. Kan SH, Elanko N, Johnson D, et al: Genomic screening of fibroblast growth-factor receptor 2 reveals a wide spectrum of mutations in patients with syndromic craniosynostosis. Am J Hum Genet 2002;70:472–486.
187. Nogee LM: Alterations in SP-B and SP-C expression in neonatal lung disease. Annu Rev Physiol 2004;66:601–623.
188. Nogee LM: Genetic mechanisms of surfactant deficiency. Biol Neonate 2004;85:314–318.
189. Trapnell BC, Whitsett JA, Nakata K: Pulmonary alveolar proteinosis. N Engl J Med 2003;349:2527–2539.
190. Nogee LM, Dunbar AE 3rd, Wert SE, et al: A mutation in the surfactant protein C gene associated with familial interstitial lung disease. N Engl J Med 2001;344:573–579.
191. Nogee LM: Abnormal expression of surfactant protein C and lung disease. Am J Respir Cell Mol Biol 2002;26:641–644.
192. Shulenin S, Nogee LM, Annilo T, et al: ABCA3 gene mutations in newborns with fatal surfactant deficiency. N Engl J Med 2004;350: 1296–1303.

2 The Surfactant System

Ann Marie LeVine, MD • Alan H. Jobe, MD

Pulmonary surfactant is a complex substance with multiple functions in the microenvironments of the alveoli and small airways. The traditional functions of surfactant are the biophysical activities to keep the lungs open, to decrease the work of breathing, and to prevent alveolar flooding. More recently, most of the components of surfactant were found to contribute to innate host defenses and injury responses in the lung. Surfactant deficiency states occur with prematurity and with severe lung injury syndromes. Recent studies in humans and in mice are defining an expanding number of genetic and metabolic abnormalities that disrupt surfactant and cause lung diseases that range from lethal respiratory failure at birth to chronic interstitial lung disease in later life. Our goal is to summarize those aspects of surfactant biology that are relevant to children.

SURFACTANT COMPOSITION AND METABOLISM

COMPOSITION

Surfactant recovered from lungs by bronchoalveolar lavage contains about 80% phospholipids, about 8% protein, and about 8% neutral lipids, primarily cholesterol (Fig. 2-1). The phosphatidylcholine species of the phospholipids contribute about 70% by weight to surfactant. The phospholipids in surfactant are unique relative to the lipid composition of lung tissue or other organs. About 50% of the phosphatidylcholine species have two palmitic acids or other saturated fatty acids esterified to the glycerol-phosphorylcholine backbone, resulting in "saturated" phosphatidylcholine, which is the principal surface-active component of surfactant. About 8% of surfactant is the acidic phospholipid phosphatidylglycerol. Surfactant from the immature fetus contains relatively large amounts of phosphatidylinositol, which then decreases as phosphatidylglycerol appears with lung maturity.

Four surfactant-specific proteins have been identified and their functions in part elucidated.[1,2] Surfactant protein A (SP-A) is a water-soluble collectin coded on human chromosome 10. The 24-kd protein is heavily glycosylated in the carboxy-terminal region to yield a reduced protein of about 36 kd. SP-A forms a collagen-like triple helix that then aggregates to form a multimeric protein with a molecular size of 650 kd. SP-A contributes to the biophysical properties of surfactant primarily by decreasing protein-mediated inhibition of surfactant function. The major functions of SP-A are an innate host defense protein and as a regulator of inflammation in the lung.[1] SP-A levels are low in surfactant from preterm lungs and increase with corticosteroid exposure. SP-A is not a component of surfactants used for treatment of respiratory distress syndrome (RDS).

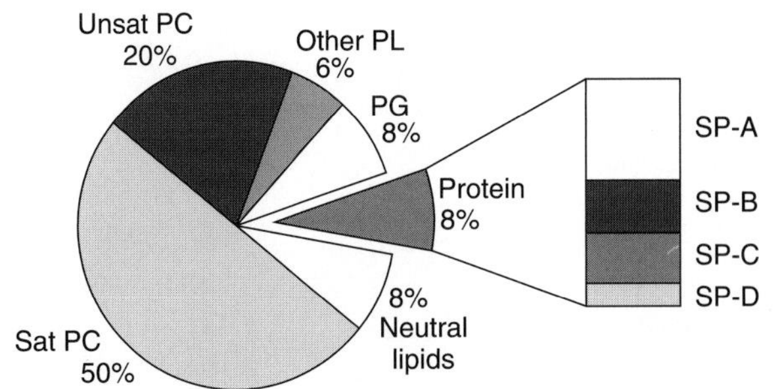

FIGURE 2-1. Composition of surfactant. Saturated phosphatidylcholines are the major components of alveolar surfactant. The proteins contribute about 8% to the weight of surfactant.

SP-B is a small hydrophobic protein that contributes about 2% to the surfactant mass.[2] The SP-B gene is on human chromosome 2, and the primary translation product is 40 kd. The protein is clipped in the type II cell to become an 8-kd protein prior to associating with phospholipids to form lamellar bodies. SP-B facilitates surface absorption of lipids and the development of low surface tensions on surface area compression. A genetic lack of SP-B causes a loss of normal lamellar bodies in type II cells, a lack of mature SP-C, and the appearance of incompletely processed SP-C in the airspaces.[3]

The SP-C gene is on chromosome 8, and its primary translation product is a 22-kd protein that is processed to an extremely hydrophobic 4-kd protein that is associated with lipids in lamellar bodies.[4] The messenger RNA (mRNA) for SP-C appears in cells lining the developing airways from early gestation. With advancing lung maturation, the mRNA for SP-C becomes localized only to type II cells. The sequence and cellular localization of SP-C have been remarkably conserved across species. SP-B and SP-C function cooperatively to optimize rapid adsorption and spreading of phospholipids on a surface and to facilitate the development of low surface tensions on surface area compression. Surfactants prepared by organic solvent extraction of natural surfactants or from lung tissue contain SP-B and SP-C. Such surfactants are similar to natural surfactants when evaluated for in vitro surface properties or for function in vivo.

SP-D is a 43-kd hydrophilic collectin with structural similarities to SP-A with a collagen-like domain and a glycosylated head group that gives it lectin-like functions.[5] SP-D is synthesized by type II cells and by Clara cells, as well as in other epithelial sites. Like the other SPs, its expression is developmentally regulated and induced by glucocorticoids and inflammation. SP-D is soluble and not associated with the surfactant lipids or other surfactant proteins.

SURFACTANT METABOLISM AND SECRETION

The synthesis and secretion of surfactant by the type II cell is a complex sequence of biochemical events that results in the release by exocytosis of lamellar bodies to the alveolus.[6] Enzymes within the endoplasmic reticulum use glucose, phosphate, and fatty acids as substrates for phospholipid synthesis. The details of how the surfactant components condense with SP-B and SP-C to form the surfactant lipoprotein complex within lamellar bodies remain obscure. Ultrastructural abnormalities of type II cells with SP-B deficiency and ABCA3 deficiency in full-term infants indicate that these gene products are essential for lamellar body formation.[4,7] A basal rate of surfactant secretion occurs continuously, and surfactant secretion can be stimulated by a number of mechanisms. Type II cells increase surfactant secretion in response to β agonists and purines. Surfactant secretion also is stimulated by mechanical stretch such as with lung distention and hyperventilation.

The alveolar pool size of saturated phosphatidylcholine of about 2 μmol/kg in the adult human is equivalent to about 4 mg/kg surfactant.[8] The lung tissue of the adult human contains about 28 μmol/kg. Thus, about 7% of the lung saturated phosphatidylcholine is in the secreted pool. The surfactant pool size per kilogram probably changes little with age after the newborn period. While no estimates exist for the full-term human, full-term animals have alveolar pool sizes of about 100 mg/kg, and this large pool decreases to adult values by 1 week of age in rabbits, for example. The alveolar surfactant pool size in the adult (and presumably young child) is small relative to other mammalian species (e.g., about 30 mg/kg in adult sheep), which may make the human lung more susceptible to surfactant deficiency with lung injury. Infants with RDS have alveolar surfactant pool sizes of less than 5 mg/kg.

The metabolic activity of surfactant was measured in animals using radioisotopes to pulse label surfactant components, which then were tracked from synthesis to secretion and catabolism or recycling.[9] Surfactant components are synthesized rapidly from precursors and then packaged in lamellar bodies for storage and secretion. The time from synthesis to peak alveolar secretion of the newly synthesized surfactant is about 6 hours in adult rabbits. The turnover time for surfactant lipids is about 5 hours, with about 50% of the lipids being recycled from the airspaces back into lamellar bodies for resecretion. No measurements of surfactant metabolism have been reported in older children or adult humans. The few measurements in large juvenile or adult animals indicate that surfactant is dynamically metabolized by efficient recycling from secretion to uptake for resecretion. The surfactant proteins also are recycled to variable extents.

More extensive measurements of surfactant metabolism have been made in developing animals and in preterm and full-term infants. In general, alveolar pool sizes are larger per kilogram body weight, secretion rates may be lower, and turnover times longer at full term. Recycling is very efficient in the newborn. Stable isotopically labeled precursors of surfactant lipids were used for studies in newborn humans.[10] These studies will be extended to children and adults in the near future.

ALVEOLAR LIFE CYCLE OF SURFACTANT

After secretion, surfactant goes through a series of form transitions in the airspace (Fig. 2-2). The lamellar bodies unravel to form the elegant structure called tubular myelin. This lipoprotein array has SP-A at the corners of the lattice and requires at least SP-A, SP-B, and the phospholipids for its unique structure.[11] Tubular myelin and other large surfactant lipoprotein structures are the reservoir in the fluid hypophase for the formation of the surface film within the alveolus and small airways. The hypophase is a very thin fluid layer covering the distal epithelium with a volume of about 0.5 mL/kg body weight that has a surfactant concentration of perhaps 10 mg/mL. New surfactant enters the surface film, and "used" surfactant leaves in the form of small vesicles. The surface-active tubular myelin forms contain SP-A, SP-B, and SP-C while the biophysically inactive small vesicular forms that are recycled and catabolized contain very little protein. The total surfactant pool size is less than the amount of active surfactant because 30% to 50% of the alveolar phospholipids are in catabolic forms in the normal lung.

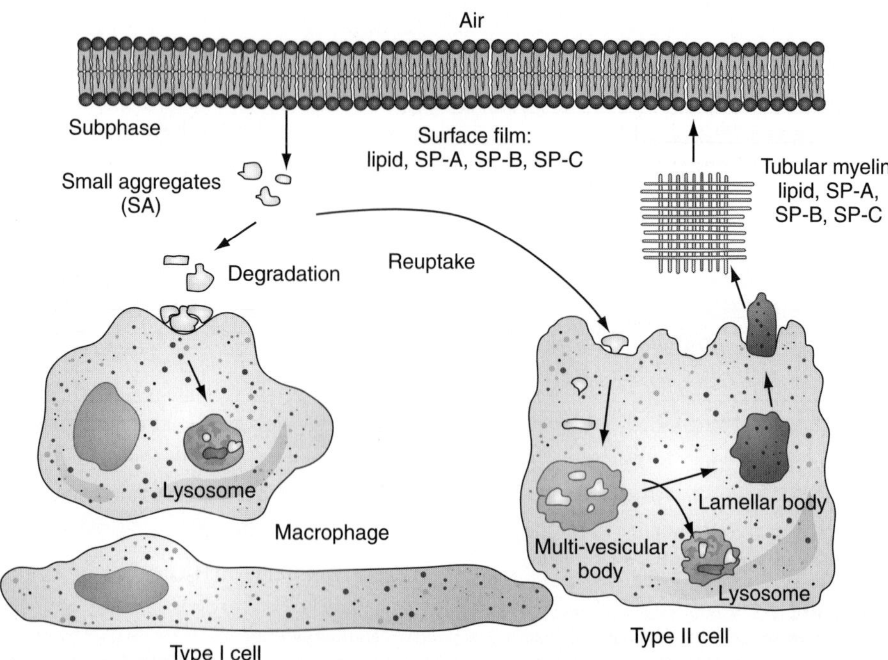

FIGURE 2-2. Alveolar life cycle of surfactant. Surfactant is secreted from lamellar bodies in type II cells. In the alveolar fluid lining layer, the surfactant transforms into tubular myelin and other surfactant protein–rich forms that facilitate surface adsorption. The lipids are catabolized as small vesicular forms by macrophages and type II cells and recycled by type II cells.

In the preterm infant, conversion from surface active to inactive forms occurs more rapidly, probably because less surfactant proteins are present. Pulmonary edema and products of lung injury can accelerate form conversion and cause a depletion of the surface active fraction of surfactant despite normal or high total surfactant pool sizes.[12]

Surfactant is catabolized primarily by type II cells and alveolar macrophages. Granulocyte-macrophage colony-stimulating factor deficiency prevents alveolar macrophages from catabolizing surfactant and results in the clinical syndrome of alveolar proteinosis. The important concept is that the alveolar pool of functional surfactant is maintained by dynamic metabolic processes that include secretion, reuptake, and resecretion balanced by catabolism.

SURFACTANT FUNCTION

ALVEOLAR STABILITY

Alveoli are polygonal with flat surfaces and curvatures where the walls of adjacent alveoli intersect. Alveoli are interdependent in that their structure is determined by the shape and elasticity of neighboring alveolar walls. The forces acting on the pulmonary microstructure are chest wall elasticity, lung tissue elasticity, and surface tensions of the air-fluid interfaces of the small airways and alveoli. Although the surface tension of surfactant decreases with surface area compression and increases with surface area expansion, the surface area of an alveolus changes little with tidal breathing. The low surface tensions resulting from surfactant help to prevent alveolar collapse and keep interstitial fluid from flooding the alveoli. Surfactant also keeps small airways from filling with fluid and thus prevents the potentially ensuing luminal obstruction.[13] If alveoli collapse or fill with fluid, the shape of adjacent alveoli will change, which can result in distortion, overdistention, or collapse. When positive pressure is applied to a surfactant-deficient lung, the more normal alveoli will tend to overexpand and the alveoli with inadequate surfactant will collapse, generating a nonhomogeneously inflated lung.

PRESSURE-VOLUME CURVES

The static effects of surfactant on a surfactant-deficient lung are evident from the pressure-volume curve of the preterm lung (Fig. 2-3). Preterm surfactant-deficient rabbit lungs do not begin to inflate until pressures exceed 20 cm H_2O.[14] The pressure needed to open a lung unit is related to the radius of curvature and surface tension of the meniscus of fluid in the airspace leading to the lung unit. The units with larger radii and lower surface tensions will "pop" open first because, with partial expansion, the radius increases and the forces needed to finish opening the unit decrease. Surfactant decreases the opening pressure from greater than 20 to 15 cm H_2O in this example with preterm rabbit lungs. Because surfactant does not alter airway diameter, the decreased opening pressure results from surface adsorption of the surfactant to the fluid in the airways. The inflation is more uniform as more units open at lower pressures, resulting in less overdistention of the open units.

A particularly important effect of surfactant on the surfactant-deficient lung is the increase in maximal volume at maximal pressure. In this example, maximal volume at 30 cm H_2O is increased over two times with surfactant treatment. Surfactant also stabilizes the lung on deflation. The surfactant-deficient lung collapses at low transpulmonary pressures, whereas the surfactant-treated lung retains about 30% of the lung volume on deflation. This retained volume is similar to the total volume of the surfactant-deficient lung at 30 cm H_2O and demonstrates how surfactant treatments increase the functional residual capacity of the lung.

HOST DEFENSE FUNCTIONS OF SURFACTANT

SP-A enhances microbial phagocytosis by macrophages because it acts as opsonin, can directly stimulate macrophage activity, and is chemotactic for alveolar macrophages and peritoneal macrophages.[15] SP-A binds a variety of microorganisms, including bacteria, viruses, and fungi, and stimulates the release of oxygen radicals from alveolar macrophages. SP-A also regulates cytokine production by macrophages, granulocytes,

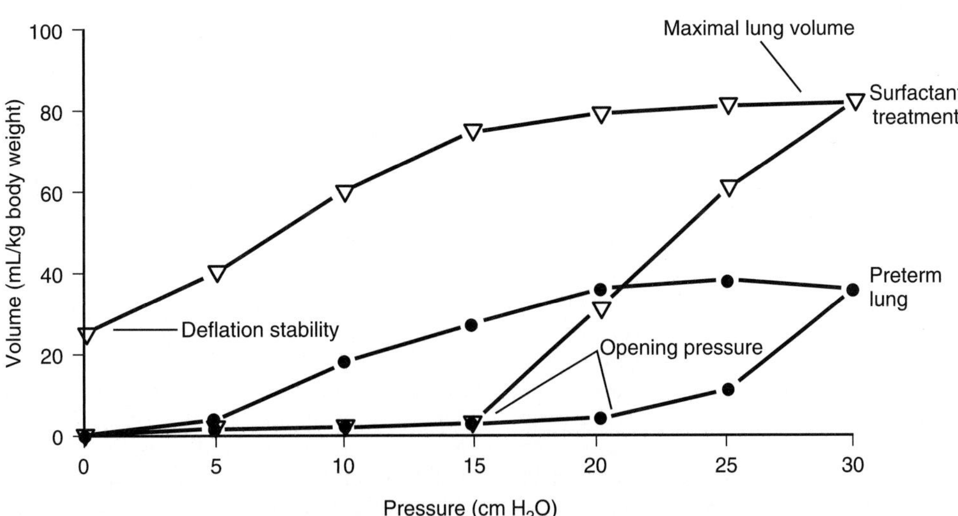

■ **FIGURE 2-3.** Effect of surfactant treatment on surfactant deficient lungs. These idealized pressure-volume curves illustrate the effect of surfactant treatment with natural sheep surfactant on the opening pressure, the maximal lung volume, and the deflation stability of lungs from preterm rabbits. (Curves based on data from Rider ED, Jobe AH, Ikegami M, Sun B: Different ventilation strategies alter surfactant responses in preterm rabbits. J Appl Physiol 1992;73:2089–2096.)

and lymphocytes. SP-A has multiple roles in regulating innate immune and inflammatory responses in the lung during acute lung injury.[16] SP-A also may contribute to adaptive immune responses. SP-A inhibits the maturation of dendritic cells in response to potent T-cell stimulators and enhances the endocytic ability of dendritic cells. In addition, SP-A down-regulates lymphocyte activity and proliferation. Thus, SP-A may have a complex role in adaptive immune responses.[17]

The hydrophobic surfactant proteins SP-B and SP-C may also have host defense functions. Although SP-B can inhibit bacterial growth in vitro, overexpression of SP-B or reduced expression of SP-B in the lungs of mice did not alter bacterial clearance, suggesting that the SP-B is not involved in innate host defense.[18] However, elevated levels of SP-B in the lungs of endotoxin-exposed mice decreased pulmonary inflammation.[19] Thus, SP-B may contribute to modulation of inflammation in the injured lung. SP-C binds lipopolysaccharide and blocks the production of tumor necrosis factor-α by macrophages.[20] However, possible roles for SP-C in bacterial clearance or lung inflammation in vivo have not been evaluated.

SP-D increases phagocytosis of gram-negative and gram-positive bacteria, viruses, fungi, and parasites by alveolar macrophages in a calcium-dependent manner.[1] SP-D also enhances calcium-dependent uptake of *Escherichia coli, Streptococcus pneumoniae,* and *Staphylococcus aureus* by neutrophils. In addition to binding microorganisms, SP-D is more chemotactic than SP-A for monocytes and neutrophils. Both SP-A and SP-D increase the production of oxygen radicals by alveolar macrophages, down-regulate lymphocyte activity and proliferation, and inhibit allergen-induced proliferation of lymphocytes.[16,17] SP-D has an important role in regulating innate and adaptive immune responses in the lung.

SURFACTANT DEFICIENCY

THE PRETERM INFANT WITH RESPIRATORY DISTRESS SYNDROME

RDS in preterm infants is a surfactant deficiency that initially does not include lung injury. The surfactant system normally is mature by about 35 weeks' gestation, but early appearance of surfactant and lung maturation is frequent for infants delivered prematurely. Early maturation is thought to occur in response to fetal stress resulting in increased fetal cortisol levels, or by exposure of the fetal lung to inflammation as a result of chorioamnionitis. Maternal treatments with corticosteroids to decrease the risk of RDS are routinely given if preterm delivery before 32 to 34 weeks' gestation is anticipated.[21] Induced lung maturation includes not only an induction of surfactant but also thinning of the mesenchyme, which increases lung gas volumes. Unless preterm infants have early lung maturation, they develop progressive respiratory distress from birth characterized by tachypnea, grunting, an increased work of breathing, and cyanosis. Infants who have died of RDS have alveolar pool sizes of surfactant of less than 5 mg/kg. Although this amount is similar in amount to the surfactant recovered from healthy adult humans, surfactant from the preterm infant has decreased function, probably because it contains less of the surfactant proteins that are critical for biophysical function.[22] The surfactant from the preterm infant also is more susceptible to inactivation by edema fluid, and the preterm lung is easily injured if a stable functional residual capacity (FRC) is not maintained or if the lung is overstretched.

THE INJURED MATURE LUNG

Acute respiratory distress syndrome (ARDS) describes an overwhelming inflammatory reaction within the pulmonary parenchyma leading to global lung dysfunction. ARDS is defined by acute onset, an oxygenation index less than 200 mm Hg, bilateral infiltrates on chest x-ray, and a pulmonary capillary wedge pressure of less than 18 mm Hg or absence of clinical evidence for left-sided heart failure. The etiology of ARDS is multifactorial and can occur in association with lung injury secondary to trauma, sepsis, aspiration, pneumonia, massive blood transfusions, or near drowning to name some associations. It is a common disease, affecting roughly 15% to 20% of all patients ventilated in the adult intensive care unit (ICU) and 1% to 4.5% of patients in the pediatric ICU. ARDS has a high mortality rate of 40% to 50%.

Impairment of surfactant with ARDS can result from inhibition, degradation, or decreased production.[12] The proteinaceous pulmonary edema characteristic of ARDS can inactivate surfactant by dilution and by competition for the interface. Plasma proteins known to inhibit surfactant function include serum albumin, globulin, fibrinogen, and C-reactive protein. In addition to proteins, phospholipases A2 and C, along with their products, fatty acids, and dipalmitin inhibit surface activity. Epithelial cell injury by inflammatory mediators can decrease surfactant production and contribute to surfactant deficiency.

Surfactant is present in the alveoli as tubular myelin and lipoprotein aggregates that are biophysically active and as small vesicles that are not bioactive. Normally in the lung, about 50% of surfactant is present in the bioactive form that has a high SP-B and SP-C content. In ARDS, small vesicular forms increase and deplete the pool of active surfactant.

The composition of surfactant is altered in ARDS. In bronchoalveolar lavage fluid (BALF) from patients with ARDS, there is a reduced phospholipid content and abnormal phospholipid composition.[23] SP-A, SP-B, and SP-C also are decreased in BALF from patients with ARDS. The surfactant protein levels can remain low for at least 14 days after the onset of ARDS. Changes in surfactant composition including phospholipids, fatty acids, and proteins likely represent alveolar type II cell injury with altered metabolism, secretion, or recycling of components. SP-A and SP-B concentrations are also reduced in the lungs of patients at risk for ARDS, even before the onset of lung injury clinically. In contrast, SP-D levels in BALF remain normal, except in a subgroup of patients who later died. Decreased SP-D levels in BALF were 85.7% sensitive and 74% specific in predicting death with ARDS.[24]

GENETIC DEFICIENCIES OF SURFACTANT IN MICE AND HUMANS

SP-A-deficient mice have normal survival without changes in surfactant composition, function, secretion, and reuptake; however, there is no tubular myelin.[25] SP-A-deficient mice are highly susceptible to various bacterial (group B *Streptococcus, Haemophilus influenza, Pseudomonas aeruginosa*) and viral (respiratory syncytial virus [RSV], influenza A virus) pathogens in vivo.[16] There are currently no documented genetic deficiencies of SP-A in humans. However, polymorphisms in the human genes for SP-A affecting their function have been identified, and humans with these polymorphisms have increased susceptibility to infections with respiratory syncytial virus and *Mycobacterium tuberculosis.*[26]

Gene-targeted mice lacking SP-B and infants with hereditary SP-B deficiency demonstrate the critical role of SP-B in surfactant function, homeostasis, and lung function.[27] Targeted disruption of the mouse SP-B gene caused respiratory failure at birth. Despite normal lung structure, the mice failed to inflate their lungs postnatally. Type II cells of SP-B-deficient mice had large multivesicular bodies but did not have lamellar bodies, and the proteolytic processing of pro-SP-C (the preprocessed form of SP-C) was disrupted.[2] Infants with SP-B deficiency die from respiratory distress in the early neonatal period with the same anatomic findings.[28] Mutations leading to partial SP-B function have been associated with chronic lung disease in infants. Mice and infants without the adenosine triphosphate–binding cassette transporter A3 (ABCA3) have type II cells without lamellar bodies and the same lethal respiratory failure phenotype.[7]

SP-C-deficient mice survive and have normal surfactant composition and amounts. However, surfactant isolated from the SP-C-deficient mice forms less stable bubbles, demonstrating a role for SP-C in developing and maintaining lipid films.[29] SP-C mutations recently were identified in families with familial interstitial lung disease that can present in childhood or in adulthood.[30] These individuals have lungs with a thickened interstitium, infiltration with inflammatory cells and macrophages, fibrosis, and abnormalities of the respiratory epithelium.

SP-D-deficient mice develop increased surfactant lipid pools in the lung, indicating that SP-D plays a critical role in the regulation of surfactant homeostasis. SP-D also regulates alveolar macrophage function because SP-D-deficient mice accumulate foamy activated macrophages in the lung and develop emphysema due to increased oxidant and metalloproteinase expression by these macrophages.[1] SP-D-deficient mice are also highly susceptible to infection by influenza A virus and RSV.[16] SP-D deficiency has not been described in humans.

SURFACTANT TREATMENT OF SURFACTANT DEFICIENCY

RESPIRATORY DISTRESS SYNDROME

The respiratory morbidities of preterm infants with RDS have decreased strikingly in recent years because of the combined effects of antenatal corticosteroid treatments and more gentle approaches to mechanical ventilation. The original randomized trials of surfactant for RDS evaluated treatments given after the disease was established, generally after 6 hours of age. Other trials evaluated treatment of all high-risk infants soon after birth to prevent RDS. Subsequent trials demonstrated that treatments of the highest-risk infants (generally infants with birth weights less than 1 kg) as soon after birth as convenient and before significant mechanical ventilation will minimize lung injury. However, many very low birth weight infants can be transitioned to air breathing successfully using continuous positive airway pressure (CPAP), and the decision to treat with surfactant can be made after the initial stabilization at birth. An advantage of allowing the infant to breathe spontaneously with CPAP used to recruit and maintain FRC is that hyperventilation and overdistention of the delicate preterm lung can be avoided. Larger infants who develop RDS generally are treated with oxygen and nasal CPAP until the oxygen concentration approaches 40%. They then are treated with surfactant. Preterm infants will respond to surfactant treatments even if the treatment is delayed for several days.

Full-term infants with severe meconium aspiration or pneumonia also will respond to surfactant treatments with improved oxygenation. Surfactant also can improve lung function in infants with the group B streptococcal sepsis/pneumonia syndrome. Current practice is to treat most any infant with severe respiratory failure with surfactant because there seems to be no contraindications.

The surfactants that are commercially available for clinical use in infants are made from organic solvent extracts of animal lungs or alveolar lavages of animal lungs. While there are differences in composition, the clinical results do not demonstrate any compelling differences in clinical responses. All of the commercial surfactants lack SP-A, contain SP-C, and have variable amounts of SP-B. Surfactants that contain synthetic peptides or surfactant proteins are being developed for clinical use.

ACUTE RESPIRATORY DISTRESS SYNDROME

ARDS is a significant therapeutic challenge for intensivists despite recent advances in understanding pathophysiology and new treatment modalities. Surfactant content and composition are altered in ARDS, resulting in decreased surface activity, atelectasis, and decreased lung compliance.[12] Surfactant treatment for ARDS can improve gas exchange, but to a lesser degree than that seen with RDS. ARDS results in primarily surfactant inactivation rather than deficiency, and surfactant inhibitors such as plasma proteins and inflammatory mediators decrease the efficacy of treatment. Several recent pilot studies in adults and children have examined surfactant therapy in ARDS.

Adults with ARDS treated with a natural bovine surfactant had significant improvements in gas exchange and a trend toward decreased mortality.[31] Walmrath and colleagues examined the efficacy of bronchoscopic administration of a bovine surfactant preparation in adult patients with ARDS. Patients demonstrated improved gas exchange, recruitment of collapsed alveoli, and improved ventilation-perfusion mismatch.[32] A phase II study in Europe recently evaluated the efficacy of intratracheal administration of a recombinant SP-C in ARDS patients.[33] Patients were randomized to receive either standard therapy alone or standard therapy plus recombinant SP-C surfactant, given as either 200 mg/kg in four doses or 500 mg/kg in four doses. The lower-dose group had significant improvement in oxygenation index, and patients were weaned more rapidly from the ventilator compared with the standard therapy group. Results in the high-dose group were not different from those of the standard therapy group.

In a large trial, full-term infants with severe respiratory failure treated with surfactant had improved oxygenation and required less extracorporeal membrane oxygenation (ECMO) than did controls.[34] Children with ARDS or acute lung injury (ALI) have been treated with a number of different surfactants in small trials. No large or definitive trials of surfactant for respiratory failure in children have been performed. Representative responses have improved oxygenation and decreased ventilator days,[35] results that are consistent with the larger trials in adults with ARDS.

There is strong experimental evidence that alterations in the pulmonary surfactant system play an important role in the pathophysiology of ARDS.[36] While it is still unclear whether mortality and morbidity from ARDS will be reduced, surfactant treatments can improve oxygenation, improve lung compliance, and decrease the need for ventilatory support.

REFERENCES

1. McCormack FX, Whitsett JA: The pulmonary collectins, SP-A and SP-D, orchestrate innate immunity in the lung. J Clin Invest 2002;109:707–712.
2. Whitsett JA, Weaver TE: Hydrophobic surfactant proteins in lung function and disease. N Engl J Med 2002;347:2141–2148.
3. Nogee LM: Genetics of the hydrophobic surfactant proteins. Biochim Biophys Acta 1998;1408:323–333.
4. Weaver TE, Conkright JJ: Function of surfactant proteins B and C. Annu Rev Physiol 2001;63:555–578.
5. Crouch E, Wright JR: Surfactant proteins a and d and pulmonary host defense. Annu Rev Physiol 2001;63:521–554.
6. Mason RJ, Voelker DR: Regulatory mechanisms of surfactant secretion. Biochim Biophys Acta 1998;1408:226–240.
7. Shulenin S, Nogee LM, Annilo T, et al: ABCA3 gene mutations in newborns with fatal surfactant deficiency. N Engl J Med 2004;350: 1296–1303.
8. Rebello CM, Jobe AH, Eisele JW, Ikegami M: Alveolar and tissue surfactant pool sizes in humans. Am J Respir Crit Care Med 1996;154:625–628.
9. Jobe AH, Rider ED: Catabolism and recycling of surfactant. In: Robertson B, van Golde LMG, Batenburg JJ, eds: Pulmonary surfactant. From molecular biology to clinical practice. Amsterdam: Elsevier, 1992.
10. Torresin M, Zimmermann LJ, Cogo PE, et al: Exogenous surfactant kinetics in infant respiratory distress syndrome. A novel method with stable isotopes. Am J Respir Crit Care Med 2000;161:1584–1589.
11. Schurch S, Green FHY, Bachofen H: Formation and structure of surface films. Captive bubble surfactometry. Biochim Biophys Acta 1998;1408: 180–202.
12. Lewis JF, Jobe AH: Surfactant and the adult respiratory distress syndrome. Am Rev Respir Dis 1993;147:218–233.
13. Enhorning G, Duffy LC, Welliver RC: Pulmonary surfactant maintains patency of conducting airways in the rat. Am J Respir Crit Care Med 1995; 151:554–556.
14. Rider ED, Jobe AH, Ikegami M, Sun B: Different ventilation strategies alter surfactant responses in preterm rabbits. J Appl Physiol 1992;73: 2089–2096.
15. Wright JR, Youmans DC: Pulmonary surfactant protein A stimulates chemotaxis of alveolar macrophage. Am J Physiol 1993;264:L338–L344.
16. LeVine AM, Whitsett JA: Pulmonary collectins and innate host defense of the lung. Microbes Infect 2001;3:161–166.
17. Hohlfeld JM, Erpenbeck VJ, Krug N: Surfactant proteins SP-A and SP-D as modulators of the allergic inflammation in asthma. Pathobiology 2002; 70:287–292.
18. Akinbi HT, Bhatt H, Hull WM, Weaver TE: Altered surfactant protein B levels in transgenic mice do not affect clearance of bacteria from the lungs. Pediatr Res 1999;46:530–534.
19. Epaud R, Ikegami M, Whitsett JA, et al: Surfactant protein B inhibits endotoxin-induced lung inflammation. Am J Respir Cell Mol Biol 2003;28:373–378.
20. Augusto LA, Synguelakis M, Johansson J, et al: Interaction of pulmonary surfactant protein C with CD14 and lipopolysaccharide. Infect Immun 2003;71:61–67.
21. Crowley P: Prophylactic Corticosteroids for Preterm Birth. The Cochrane Library, Issue 2. Oxford, UK: Update Software, 2001.
22. Ueda T, Ikegami M, Jobe AH: Developmental changes of sheep surfactant: In vivo function and in vitro subtype conversion. J Appl Physiol 1994;76: 2701–2706.
23. Gunther A, Siebert C, Schmidt R, et al: Surfactant alterations in severe pneumonia acute respiratory distress syndrome, and cardiogenic lung edema. Am J Respir Crit Care Med 1996;153:176–184.
24. Greene KE, Wright JR, Steinberg KP: Serial changes in surfactant-associated proteins in lung and serum before and after onset of ARDS. Am J Respir Crit Care Med 1999;160:1843–1850.
25. Ikegami M, Korfhagen TR, Bruno MD, et al: Surfactant metabolism in surfactant protein A-deficient mice. Am J Physiol 1997;272: L479–L485.
26. Lofgren J, Ramet M, Renko M, et al: Association between surfactant protein A gene locus and severe respiratory syncytial virus infection in infants. J Infect Dis 2002;185:283–289.
27. Clark JC, Wert SE, Bachurski CJ, et al: Targeted disruption of the surfactant protein B gene disrupts surfactant homeostasis, causing respiratory failure in newborn mice. Proc Natl Acad Sci U S A 1995;92: 7794–7798.
28. Nogee LM, Wert SE, Profitt SA, et al: Allelic heterogeneity in hereditary SP-B deficiency. Am J Respir Crit Care Med 2000;161:973–981.
29. Glasser SW, Burhans MS, Korfhagen TR, et al: Altered stability of pulmonary surfactant in SP-C deficient mice. Proc Natl Acad Sci U S A 2001;98:6366–6371.
30. Thomas AQ, Lane K, Phillips J III, et al: Heterozygosity for a surfactant protein C gene mutation associated with usual interstitial pneumonitis and cellular nonspecific interstitial pneumonitis in one kindred. Am J Respir Crit Care Med 2002;165:1322–1328.
31. Gregory TJ, Steinberg KP, Spragg R, et al: Bovine surfactant therapy for patients with acute respiratory distress syndrome. Am J Respir Crit Care Med 1997;155:1309–1315.
32. Walmrath D, Gunter A, Ghofrani HA, et al: Bronchoscopic surfactant administration in patients with severe ARDS and sepsis. Am J Respir Crit Care Med 1996;154:57–62.
33. Spragg RG, Lewis JF, Wurst W, et al: Treatment of acute respiratory distress syndrome with recombinant surfactant protein C surfactant. Am J Respir Crit Care Med 2003;167:1562–1566.
34. Lotze A, Mitchell BR, Bulas DI, et al: Multicenter study of surfactant (beractant) use in the treatment of term infants with severe respiratory failure. Survanta in Term Infants Study Group. J Pediatr 1998; 132:40–47.
35. Moller JC, Schaible T, Roll C, et al: Treatment with bovine surfactant in severe acute respiratory distress syndrome in children. A randomized multicenter study. Intens Care Med 2003;29:437–446.
36. Poynter SE, Levine AM: Surfactant biology and clinical application. Crit Care Clin 2003;19:459–472.

3 Developmental Physiology of the Respiratory System

Mary Ellen B. Wohl, MD

Respiratory diseases are among the four leading causes of death in the United States.[1] Immaturity of the lung has been a major contributing factor to infant mortality, although in recent years this has been reduced by the antenatal administration of corticosteroids and the postnatal administration of surfactants. However, respiratory distress of the newborn still ranks fifth as a contributor to infant mortality. After infancy, mortality rates related to respiratory causes are low but are still included in the 10 most frequent causes of death. Respiratory morbidity rates, on the other hand, are high, and respiratory diseases continue to be one of the most common causes of hospital admissions and absence from school.

AGE SPECIFICITY OF RESPIRATORY PATHOGENS

Certain respiratory pathogens are age specific: they produce disease of consequence at certain ages and not at other ages. Some respiratory infections, such as cytomegalovirus pneumonia, depend on exposure in utero. With the exception of infections in the immunocompromised host, cytomegalovirus rarely causes disease beyond the perinatal period. Other infectious agents, such as chlamydia and group B streptococci, cause pneumonia after exposure of the host during birth. Respiratory syncytial virus produces bronchiolitis in infants but usually only upper respiratory symptoms in school-aged children and adults. Parainfluenza virus causes croup in the child between 2 and 3 years old. Acute epiglottitis, rarely seen since *Hemophilus influenzae* B vaccination became commonplace, is usually, but not always, seen in children 2 to 7 years of age. *Mycoplasma* rarely produces disease in preschool children but is a common cause of bronchopneumonia in school-aged children and young adults.

Part of the age specificity of respiratory pathogens is related to development of the immune system, of defenses within the lung itself,[2,3] and to age-related exposure. The influence of age on respiratory structure and function, however, may contribute to this age specificity and is the subject of this chapter.

AGE AND RESPIRATORY STRUCTURE

The respiratory system continues to develop from birth to young adulthood. Some of the steps in the development of the lung have a strong influence on lung function during childhood and on the pattern of respiratory disease. There have been a number of reviews of lung development in recent years elucidating the mechanisms underlying morphogenesis, molecular regulation, maturation, and vascular development.[4–7] This chapter considers the structural factors of lung development.

AIRWAYS

The airways are derived from an outpouching of the ventral groove of the embryo. During the embryonal period of lung development, the proximal branches are formed. Further branching of the airways, which is more or less dichotomous, occurs during the pseudoglandular period, so named because of the appearance of the lung on microscopic section. By the 17th week of gestation, the full number of generations of conducting airways has been established.[7,8] Thereafter, no new conducting airways develop, but there is continuing growth (increase in length and diameter) of the existing airways, remodeling of the peripheral airways,[9] and thinning of the respiratory epithelium.

The airway wall and the respiratory epithelium change during gestation and postnatal life. During fetal life, the thick, columnar, glycogen-rich epithelium develops cilia and thins, particularly in the periphery of the airway. The thinning of the epithelium continues postnatally in the human. Although the epithelium of the infant's airway, like the adult's, is a ciliated pseudostratified columnar type in the trachea and gradually thins to a columnar type in the bronchioles, there are substantial differences. The infant's airway epithelium contains a higher ratio of mucous glands than the adult's, and the constituents of the secretions may change throughout childhood.[10] The respiratory epithelium is substantially thicker, approaching (at a given generation of airways) the thickness found in asthmatics.[11] The rate of tracheal mucociliary clearance, studied in animals, is greater in the young adult than in the infant.[12] Smooth muscle is present in the airways of the fetus early in development and extends from the trachea to the alveolar ducts in both newborns and adults.[13] Between 5 and 17 weeks of gestation airway wall cells differentiate to form cartilage, submucosal glands, smooth muscle, and types of epithelial cells. In the rabbit, the amount of smooth muscle is increased and the amount of cartilage is decreased in the immature compared with the mature animal.[14] In contrast to the work of James,[11] airway wall thickness is similar in both mature and immature rabbits.[14] The amount of cartilage increase in the first years of life, contributing to the stiffening of the airways observed in the first months of an infant's postnatal life.[15]

Postnatal growth of the airway has been investigated by only a limited number of anatomic studies in humans, and the data are conflicting.[16,17] Hislop and associates[16] show the infant's airway to be a miniature of the adult's. The limited anatomic and more extensive physiologic studies on excised human lung performed by Hogg and co-workers[17] suggest that peripheral airways, those distal to the 10th or 12th generation, increase in size relative to the central airways until age 5 years (Fig. 3-1).

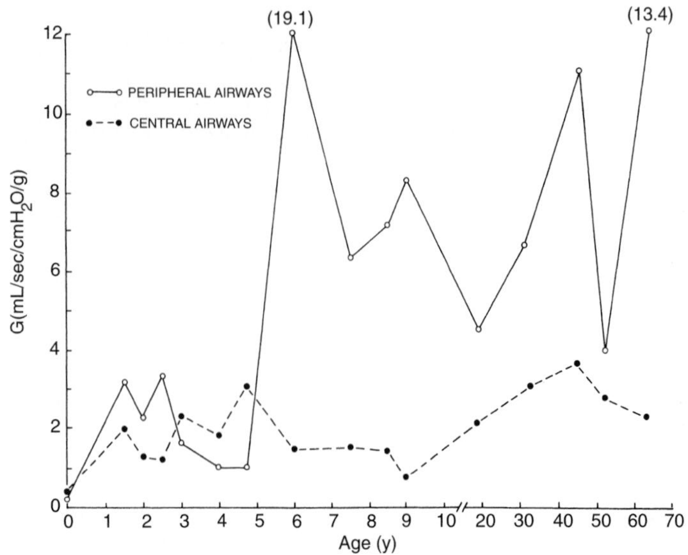

■ FIGURE 3-1. Comparison of peripheral and central airway conductance as a function of age in normal human lungs. The data are corrected for size by expressing the conductance as mL/sec/g of lung and for lung inflation by expressing all data at a transpulmonary pressure of 5 cm H_2O. (Replotted from Hogg JC, Williams J, Richardson JB, et al: Age as a factor in the distribution of lower-airway conductance and in the pathologic anatomy of obstructive lung disease. N Engl J Med 1970;282:1283.)

■ ALVEOLI AND LUNG PARENCHYMA

Whereas the airways are established in early gestational life and grow by enlargement, the alveoli develop in late gestational life and early childhood by forming new structures (i.e., alveolar ducts and alveoli). Only later do they grow by enlargement[9] (Fig. 3-2). The development of alveoli is preceded by the formation of saccules at the end of the budding airway. These structures—larger, thicker walled, and more irregular than alveoli—are probably capable of sustaining gas exchange. From 28 to 32 weeks of gestation, some of the subdivisions of the saccules have the cupped shape and single capillary layer characteristic of alveoli, but infants born at less than 28 weeks have virtually no alveoli.

Approximately 150 million alveoli are present at birth in the full-term infant. The number is likely to be extremely variable. Pulmonary hypoplasia is diagnosed when a baby has an associated abnormality (i.e., a congenital renal abnormality or a diaphragmatic hernia), and may be considered when a newborn develops a spontaneous pneumothorax. In all likelihood, considerable variability in lung size as expressed by the number of terminal units may go undetected by the pediatrician but may influence the child's respiratory reserve. Dunhill[18] carried out morphometric studies on lungs obtained at autopsy. His data suggest that most of the 300 million alveoli present in the adult lung are formed by the age of 2 years. Current data suggest that this is an underestimation of the number or alveoli present in the adult lung[19] and that mean data have a wide range. The variability in the number of alveoli present at a given age[20] makes the age at which the increase in alveolar number ceases less certain. Nonetheless, a substantial fraction of the total number of alveoli is formed in the first few months and years of life. Thereafter, growth of alveoli takes place for the most part by enlargement.

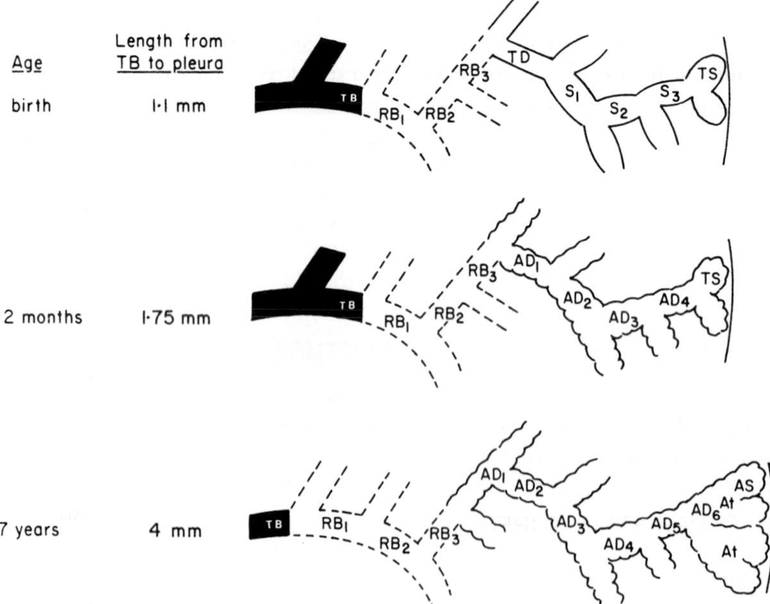

■ FIGURE 3-2. Diagram showing that the lung grows initially by increasing the number of alveoli by the ingrowth of septa and formation of the alveolar ducts. AD, alveolar duct; RB, respiratory bronchiole; TB, terminal bronchiole. (Modified from Hislop A, Reid L: Development of the acinus in the human lung. Thorax 1974;29:90.)

It seems reasonable to assume that factors that influence growth of the fetus during the last trimester and during the first year of life would be of particular importance to lung development. Some of these factors are under active investigation. Nutrition,[21] vitamin A,[22] administration of corticosteroids,[23] hyperoxia,[24] and maternal smoking[25] play important roles in lung development. Although both collagen and elastin are important in airway morphogenesis and branching, the interstitium of the lung contains little collagen and elastin during late gestation and at birth. This near absence of collagen and elastin may contribute to the relative ease of rupture of air spaces in the premature lung. Elastin, which appears to be closely related to the development of alveoli, increases during early postnatal life. Lung collagen also increases during postnatal life. The formation and changing ratio of elastin and collagen probably contribute to the change in volume-pressure relationships of the lung and to the increased stiffness of the lung with increasing age until young adulthood.

■ PULMONARY VESSELS

The pulmonary arterial system develops by vasculogenesis, the production of vessels from endothelial cells differentiating from mesenchymal precursors, and angiogenesis, the sprouting of new vessels from preexisting vessels. It appears that until about 17 weeks of gestation new vessels are produced by vasculogenesis and the airway acts as a template. Postnatally there is a marked increase in the number of arteries in the acinus that seem to be formed by angiogenesis.[7] To some extent, the postnatal development of acinar arteries and capillaries parallels the postnatal development of alveoli. The pulmonary veins originate as proliferating endothelial cells that migrate away from the artery, are surrounded by lymphatic channels, and never develop any smooth muscle.

The origins of smooth muscle cells include cells that migrate from the airway into the vessel wall at the penultimate generation of the airway and form the innermost layer of the vessel wall. Later, fibroblasts differentiate and express both alpha and gamma actin. Finally, endothelial cells, later in development, express alpha actin and form smooth muscle cells.[7] Muscular arteries extend only to the level of the terminal bronchioles in the fetus and young child, and during childhood, muscle extends out to the alveolar duct, and in the adult out to the alveoli. A number of studies of the pulmonary vascular system relating structure to function have been carried out, and these reveal differences between infants and adults. The extension of muscle out into the acinus and the rise in the ratio of arteries to alveoli that occurs during childhood is consistent with an increasing responsiveness to acute hypoxia with increasing age. However, the development of the fetal and infant lung is strongly influenced by chronic hypoxia with decreased airway, vascular, and alveolar development.

Although structural features of the infant's pulmonary vasculature may influence the infant's response to a variety of vasoconstrictors and vasodilators, there may be substantial differences in response governed at the cellular level between infants and adults. This is an active area of investigation and beyond the scope of this chapter.

■ OTHER STRUCTURES

In the adult, collateral ventilation—the movement of gas from one acinus to another—occurs through holes in the alveoli (the pores of Kohn) and epithelium-lined channels between terminal bronchioles and adjacent alveoli (the canals of Lambert). These structures may be present in the infant lung, but they are probably not of sufficient size to allow for air drift. Although collateral pathways in the adult are probably not of great significance for ventilation, they do help to prevent absorption of gas in regions distal to airway obstruction. The relative absence of functional collateral pathways probably contributes to the patchy atelectasis so common in airway disease of infants and young children.

■ CHEST WALL

Considerable structural changes occur in the chest wall, particularly during early postnatal life. In infancy the ribs are oriented in a horizontal plane. As growth occurs, they slant in a progressively caudal direction. By 10 years of age they have the downward slope of adults.[26] Ossification of the rib cage sternum and vertebrae begins in utero and continues until about age 25. Calcification of costal cartilage can continue into old age. Muscle mass develops progressively throughout childhood and adolescence and in some into adulthood.

In adults, lung volume at end-expiration or functional residual capacity (FRC) is mainly set passively by the balance between the inward recoil of the lung and outward recoil of the chest wall. Newborns have compliant chest walls that would allow nearly complete collapse of lungs if it were not for the activity of muscles. Expiratory braking occurs by active glottic narrowing and by the interruption of expiration by the onset of inspiration, or by both mechanisms. Indeed, the major function of the active Hering-Breuer reflex in infants may be to terminate expirations before lung volume gets too small. This response may disappear once the chest wall has become stiff enough to prevent collapse. End-expiratory lung volume is actively maintained by infants until about 6 to 12 months of age, when the passive characteristics of the lung and chest wall appear to determine resting end-expiratory lung volume.[27]

The easy collapsibility of the rib cage is probably advantageous during birth, when it allows for deformation of the chest as it passes through the birth canal and for easier expulsion of liquid from the lungs before the first breath. Thereafter the collapsibility is probably disadvantageous but affordable in a healthy infant because of relatively small metabolic demands. The parenchyma of the lungs develops during the postnatal period, and the rib cage may be thought of as doing the same. The infant rib cage "caves in" during obstructed inspiration, whereas the adult rib cage does not.

■ AGE AND RESPIRATORY FUNCTION

Respiratory structures change remarkably during growth. What are the functional implications of such changes? Lung volume and volume-pressure relationships (e.g., pulmonary compliance) should reflect parenchymal (alveolar) development, and airflows and pressure-flow relationships (resistances and conductances) should reflect airway development. But the relationships are not as direct as they might seem.

Pulmonary compliance depends on the number of air spaces expanded, the size and geometry of the air spaces, the characteristics of their surface lining layer, and the properties of the lung parenchyma that change with growth and maturation.

Changes in the shape, magnitude, or curvilinearity of volume-pressure curves do point to maturational changes in growing lungs.

The lung volume at which airways close is higher in younger children (7 years) and in elderly adults than in older children and young adults.[28] Airway closure in infants is graphically illustrated by the atelectasis observed in dependent portions of the lung in computed tomography scans. Lung recoil is reduced in younger lungs[29–31] and increases as the lungs mature in early adulthood to decline again in the elderly[32] (Fig. 3-3).

Measurements of chest wall compliance in the tidal range in children younger than 4 years[33] further confirm the marked stiffening of the chest wall in early childhood suggested by the measurements of Thorsteinsson and co-workers[34] and the earlier measurements of Sharp and co-workers.[35] Chest wall compliance corrected for body and therefore lung size was about 50% greater in infants younger than 1 year compared to children older than 1 year. Furthermore, the relationship between chest wall and lung compliance changes. In infants chest wall compliance is threefold greater than lung compliance, but in children and adults these values are virtually equal. These marked physiologic changes in mechanical properties of both the lung and the chest wall parallel the remarkable growth of these structures.

Pressure-volume curves of the total respiratory system[34] mimic those of the lung in young children in that they are more curvilinear and at a given pressure the respiratory system is at a higher fraction of its total volume. However, for individuals 2 to 16 months of age, curves are very similar, probably reflecting increasing inward recoil of the lung balanced by increasing outward recoil of the chest wall. Overall, the total respiratory system becomes increasingly stiff with increasing age, and these changes are particularly remarkable in the child younger than 5.

Changes in airways and pulmonary and total respiratory system resistance with age are difficult to interpret, since they involve a substantial and often variable contribution from the upper airway, notably the glottis. This upper airway resistance can comprise more than 50% of measured resistance, making measurements of resistance less useful for inferring growth patterns in normal subjects or changes associated with diseased lungs. The available measurements of resistance, despite the limitations noted above, suggest that resistance declines through infancy and compliance increases, but the increase in compliance is greater than the reduction in resistance during the first years of life.[36] These observations and the observation that specific conductance in infant lungs is greater than in older lungs is entirely consistent with the sequence of airway and parenchymal development.[37] The airways in the newborn lung are large compared with the relatively scanty parenchyma they serve.

Maximal expiratory flow (MEF) does not depend on any manipulation of the glottis and reflects only the intrathoracic properties of the lung and airway. It is another measure of airway properties, depending on the physical properties of the gas, the physical properties of the airway wall, the elastic recoil of the lung, the degree of lung inflation, and the resistive pressure losses along the airway. Nevertheless, MEF-volume curves can be interpreted in terms of the relative size of airways and parenchyma. The average slope of a flow-volume curve (i.e., the best straight line fit to the descending portion of the curve) expresses the mean maximum rate of emptying. This rate depends on the relative sizes of the airways and lung parenchyma. The smaller the lung, the more rapidly it empties through an airway of a given size and resistance. Similarly, the greater the size of the airways, and hence the lower their resistance, the more rapidly a lung of a given size empties. Estimates of rates of lung emptying can be made for infants, children, and adults. The lung of the infant empties four times faster than the lung of an adult, with rate constants of 7.8 compared to 1.7 (rate constant is flow/volume, which is 1/time, i.e., rate).[38] Data collected in children 3 weeks to 15 years of age supports the relative greater increase in lung parenchyma growth relative to airway growth throughout childhood.[36]

The available measurements from infancy to adolescence reflect and parallel structural changes in the lungs. Compliance in

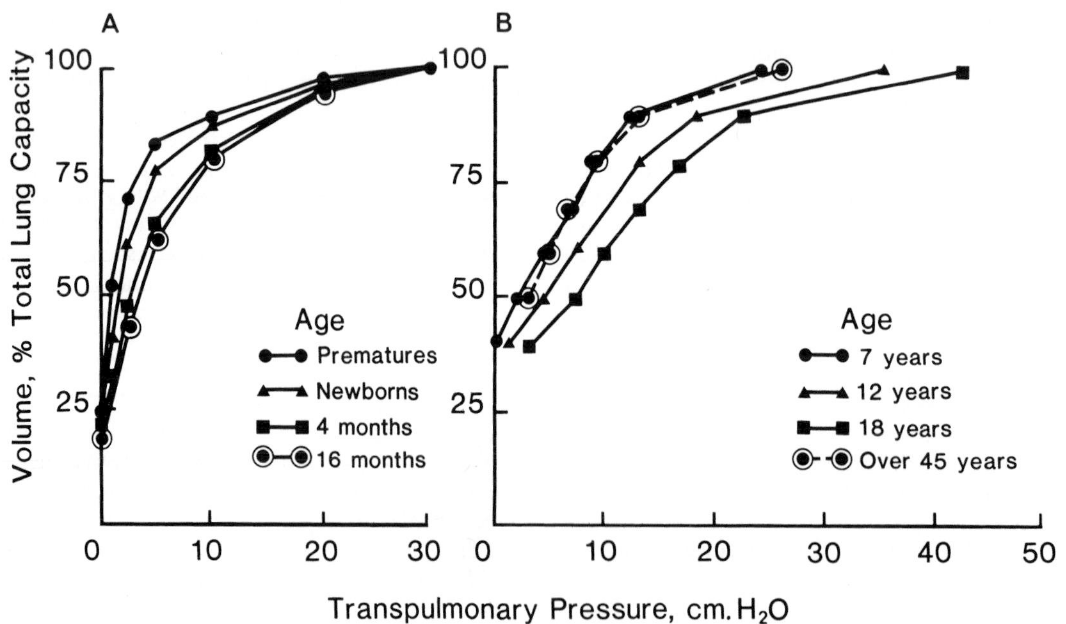

■ **FIGURE 3-3.** Deflation volume-pressure curves of the lung. **A,** Data plotted from curves on excised lungs obtained by Fagan.[29,30] The lung volume at a transpulmonary pressure of 30 cm H_2O is taken as 100% of total lung capacity. **B,** Data taken from the work of Zapletal and co-workers[31] are plotted in solid lines. Age is estimated from height. For comparison, the curve for subjects older than 45 years is shown with dashed lines.[32] With increasing age up to young adulthood the curves become straighter, and at a given lung volume elastic recoil is greater. The curve from elderly subjects (*dashed line*) resembles that from a 7-year-old.

absolute terms increases as new alveoli develop, but the changes in shape of the volume-pressure curve suggest that to some extent maturation makes the lung relatively stiffer. As the volume of the lung parenchyma enlarges relative to airway volume, specific conductance and indices of rates of emptying fall. However, these broad developmental changes may not be as important to the occurrence of lung disease as individual variability. In adults, considerable variability in indices of airway and lung size exists. Some individuals apparently have relatively large airways and small lungs, and vice versa. Some data indicate substantial tracking of lung volumes and of indices of airway size that have been documented from age 6 years through adolescence.[39] These observations suggest that this dysanapsis between airway and lung parenchyma growth begins in early life and presumably is genetically determined. Whether it bears on disease susceptibility remains to be seen, but there is increasing epidemiologic evidence that disease in childhood, at least the occurrence of wheezing with lower respiratory infections, is linked to physiologic indicators of lung and airway size established during early infancy.[40–42]

AGE, STRUCTURE, FUNCTION, AND AIRWAY REACTIVITY

Data from a number of investigators suggest that infants' and children's airways are more reactive to methylcholine and histamine than are the airways of adults.[42] Under static conditions the amount, location, and length-tension relationship determine the contractile response of smooth muscle. However, airway reactivity may be modulated by cyclic changes in tidal volume and cyclic changes in force applied to the smooth muscle.[43,44] This force may be altered by the number of attachments to the airway wall, elastic recoil of the lung, airway wall thickness both inside and outside the airway, and presence of fluid within the airway.[45] A number of these factors, for example, the thickness of the airway wall and the number of parenchymal attachments, are altered by growth of the lung.

Edema of the outer airway wall, which occurs in viral illnesses, pulmonary overcirculation, and inflammation of the airway wall, uncouples the attachments of the parenchyma to the airway wall. This results in increased airway reactivity to inhaled bronchoconstrictors.

To evaluate airway reactivity, usually increasing concentrations of a bronchoconstrictor, methacholine or histamine, are nebulized and inhaled. The dose required to produce a decrease in a measured parameter of some fixed percentage of baseline value is used as the expression of reactivity, for example, a 20% decline in forced expiratory volume in 1 second (FEV_1).

Infants and young children have lower inspiratory flow rates than do adults and will entrain less air to dilute the nebulizer output. Normal children 6 months to 1 year of age have inspiratory flow rates that approximate nebulizer output and will deliver a higher dose of the bronchoconstricting agent to the airways.[46] On the other hand, adjusting the concentration of the bronchoconstrictor on a mg/kg basis results in very little drug or bronchoconstrictor delivered to the child, since the dose is further "size corrected" by the lower minute ventilation of smaller subjects. In studies where "dose" appears to be adequately controlled, younger human subjects appear to be more reactive than older ones.

The younger lung thus has many of the features of the asthmatic lung. These structural features may be important determinants of the frequency of wheezing in young children and the increased response to bronchoconstricting agents. It does not require a greater inflammatory response, cytokine release, or smooth muscle response, although these may or may not be present.

AGE STRUCTURE, FUNCTION, AND MANIFESTATION OF DISEASE

When the structure and mechanical behavior of the young infant's and child's respiratory system are compared to those of the mature adult (but not the elderly), important differences emerge that are likely to influence the pattern of disease. Some of these differences, such as the reduced lung recoil, are shared by the elderly and likely influence the pattern of respiratory disease in that population as well.

1. The young lung lacks elastic recoil; as a result, airways are less well supported. This will be particularly true if there are fewer parenchymal attachments.[16] Greater airway closure favors inhomogeneity of gas exchange and the development of patchy atelectasis frequently observed in the child under school age.
2. Airway walls of young lungs may be thicker.[10,16] This, combined with reduced elastic recoil, favors greater airway narrowing for any degree of smooth muscle contraction.
3. The chest wall is relatively more compliant in the young child and stiffens with increasing age. As a result, the infant can develop paradoxical respiration. Respiratory muscle activation during inspiration can produce inward displacement of the rib cage, contributing to increased respiratory work for a given level of ventilation, particularly during rapid eye movement (REM) sleep. The apparent fatigue resistance of the infant's respiratory muscles may offset the increased demand for respiratory work. The deformability of the chest wall influences findings on physical examination. Chest wall–abdominal paradox may be normal in the premature infant during REM sleep but not in the older child or adult.
4. Finally, infants and children have frequent respiratory tract infections, particularly if they attend daycare, school, or come from large families. It may be that the profuse secretions are aspirated and with a shorter path length to peripheral airways, the epithelium lining these structures becomes infected. Airway cell sloughing, loss of ciliated epithelial cells, injury to epithelial cells with cytokine release, and possible increased bronchovascular permeability contribute to airway wall thickening, edema of the airway wall, and attenuation of the tethering effects of parenchymal–airway wall attachments. The effects of any degree of airway smooth muscle contraction will be exaggerated and contribute to the uneven ventilation and perfusion and modest hypoxemia observed in so many children with respiratory tract infections.

REFERENCES

1. Arias E, Smith BL: Deaths. Preliminary data for 2001. Natl Vital Stat Rep 2003;51:1.
2. Whitsett JA: Intrinsic and innate defenses in the lung. Intersection of pathways regulating lung morphogenesis, host defense, and repair. J Clin Invest 2002;109:565.

3. McCormack FX, Whitsett JA: The pulmonary collectins, SP-A and SP-D, orchestrate innate immunity in the lung. J Clin Invest 2002;109:707.
4. Hilfer SR: Morphogenesis of the lung. Control of embryonic and fetal branching. Ann Rev Physiol 1996;58:93.
5. Cardoso WV: Molecular regulation of lung development. Annu Rev Physiol 2001;63:471.
6. McMurtry IF: Introduction. Pre- and postnatal lung development, maturation, and plasticity. Am J Physiol Lung Cell Mol Physiol 2002;282:L341.
7. Hislop AA: Airway and blood vessel interaction during lung development. J Anat 2002;201:325.
8. Bucher U, Reid L: Development of the intrasegmental bronchial tree. The pattern of branching and development of cartilage at various stages of intra-uterine life. Thorax 1961;16:207.
9. Hislop A, Reid L: Development of the acinus in the human lung. Thorax 1974;29:90.
10. Matsuba K, Thurlbeck WM: A morphometric study of bronchial and bronchiolar walls in children. Am Rev Respir Dis 1972;105:908.
11. James A, Christmas T: Mechanisms of bronchial hyperresponsiveness in infants. Am Rev Respir Dis 1989;139:A106.
12. Wanner A, Salathé M, O'Riordan TG: Mucociliary clearance in the airways. Am J Respir Crit Care Med 1996;154:1868.
13. Leslie K, Mitchell J, Woodcock-Mitchell J, Low R: Alpha smooth muscle actin expression in developing and adult human lung. Differentiation 1990; 44:143.
14. McCray P, Nakamura K: Development of airway smooth muscle. Lung Growth and Development. New York: Marcel Dekker, 1997.
15. Croteau JR, Cook CD: Volume-pressure and length-tension measurements in human tracheal and bronchial segments. J Appl Physiol 1961;16:170.
16. Hislop A, Muir DCF, Jacobsen M, et al: Postnatal growth and function of the pre-acinar airways. Thorax 1972;27:265.
17. Hogg JC, Williams J, Richardson JB, et al: Age as a factor in the distribution of lower-airway conductance and in the pathologic anatomy of obstructive lung disease. N Engl J Med 1970;282:1283.
18. Dunhill MS: Postnatal growth of the lung. Thorax 1962;17:329.
19. Ochs M, Nyengaard JR, Jung A, et al: The number of alveoli in the human lung. Am J Respir Crit Care Med 2004;169:120.
20. Brody JS, Thurlbeck WM: Development, growth, and aging of the lung. In: Fishman AP, ed: Handbook of Physiology. Vol III. Mechanics of Breathing. Part 1. The Respiratory System. Bethesda, Md: American Physiological Society, 1986, p 355.
21. Sosenko IRS, Frank L: Nutritional influences on lung development and protection against chronic lung disease. Semin Perinatol 1991;15:462.
22. Massaro D, Massaro GDC: Retinoids, alveolus formation, and alveolar deficiency. Clinical implications. Am J Respir Cell Mol Biol 2003;28:271.
23. Tschanz SA, Makanya AN, Haenni B, Burri PH: Effects of neonatal high-dose short-term glucocorticoid treatment on the lung. A morphologic and morphometric study in the rat. Pediatr Res 2003;53:72.
24. Haworth SG, Hislop AA: Lung development—The effects of chronic hypoxia. Semin Neonatol 2003;8:1.
25. Hanrahan JP, Tager IB, Segal MR, et al: The effect of maternal smoking during pregnancy on early infant lung function. Am Rev Respir Dis 1992; 145:1129.
26. Openshaw P, Edwards S, Helms P: Changes in rib cage geometry during childhood. Thorax 1984;39:624.
27. Colin AA, Wohl MEB, Mead J, et al: Transition from dynamically maintained to relaxed end-expiratory volume in human infants. J Appl Physiol 1989; 67:2107.
28. Mansell AL, Bryan C, Levison H: Airway closure in children. J Appl Physiol 1972;33:711.
29. Fagan DG: Post-mortem studies of the semistatic volume-pressure characteristics of infants' lungs. Thorax 1976;31:534.
30. Fagan DG: Shape changes in static V-P loops from children's lungs related to growth. Thorax 1977;32:198.
31. Zapletal A, Paul T, Samanek M: Pulmonary elasticity in children and adolescents. J Appl Physiol 1976;40:953.
32. Turner JM, Mead J, Wohl MEB: Elasticity of human lungs in relation to age. J Appl Physiol 1968;25:664.
33. Papastamelos C, Panitch HB, England SE, Allen JL: Developmental changes in chest wall compliance in infancy and early childhood. J Appl Physiol 1995;78:179.
34. Thorsteinsson A, Larsson A, Jonmarker C, Werner O: Pressure-volume relations of the respiratory system in healthy children. Am J Respir Crit Care Med 1994;150:421.
35. Sharp JT, Druz WS, Balagot RC, et al: Total respiratory compliance in infants and children. J Appl Physiol 1970;29:775.
36. Lanteri CJ, Sly PD: Changes in respiratory mechanics with age. J Appl Physiol 1993;74:369.
37. Stocks J, Godfrey S: Specific airway conductance in relation to postconceptional age during infancy. J Appl Physiol 1977;43:144.
38. Bryan AC, Wohl MEB: Respiratory mechanics in children. In: Fishman AP, ed: Handbook of Physiology. Vol. III, Part 1. Mechanics of Breathing. The Respiratory System. Bethesda, Md: American Physiological Society, 1986, p 179.
39. Martin TR, Feldman HA, Fredberg JJ, et al: The relationship between maximal expiratory flows and lung volumes in growing humans. J Appl Physiol 1988;65:822.
40. Martinez F, Morgan W, Wright A, et al: Diminished lung function as a predisposing factor for wheezing respiratory illness in infants. N Engl J Med 1988;319:1112.
41. Martinez F, Morgan W, Wright A, et al: Initial airway function is a risk factor for recurrent wheezing respiratory illnesses during the first three years of life. Am Rev Respir Dis 1991;143:312.
42. Martinez FD, Wright AL, Taussig LM, et al: Asthma and wheezing in the first six years of life. N Engl J Med 1995;332:133.
43. Fredberg JJ: Frozen objects. Small airways, big breaths, and asthma. J Allergy Clin Immunol 2000;106:615.
44. Seow CY, Fredberg JJ: Historical perspective on airway smooth muscle. The saga of a frustrated cell. J Appl Physiol 2001;91:938.
45. Moreno R, Hogg J, Paré PD: Mechanics of airway narrowing. Am Rev Respir Dis 1986;133:1171.
46. Le Souëf PN: Validity of methods used to test airway responsiveness in children. Lancet 1992;339:1282.

4 The Functional Basis of Respiratory Disease

Victor Chernick, MD • John B. West, MD

Knowledge of the normal development and physiologic function of the lungs is required to understand the pathophysiology that is seen in disease. Historically, our understanding of lung function was derived solely from clinical observation and postmortem histologic examination. The development of invasive and noninvasive techniques that were capable of assessing lung function in living subjects greatly improved our understanding of lung physiology on an "organ basis." There has been an explosion of knowledge in cellular and molecular biology, which are covered in detail in other chapters in this section. This chapter will concentrate on organ physiology.

NORMAL LUNG ANATOMY AND CELL FUNCTION

A knowledge of normal lung anatomy is one of the basic requirements for understanding lung function in health and disease. Because detailed descriptions of lung anatomy are available elsewhere, this section will focus on selected aspects of gross and microscopic anatomy to enable the reader to understand the physiologic changes that occur in congenital and acquired lung disease.

AIRWAYS

The basic structure of the airways is already present at birth, and thus neonates and adults share a common bronchopulmonary anatomy (Fig. 4-1). When airways divide, they do so by dichotomous branching, but the number of times that branching occurs varies. For example, there may be anywhere from 10 (hilar region) to 25 (basal region) airway divisions before the gas-exchanging units are reached. This airway variability has physiologic implications; different pathways will have different resistances to airflow, and a heterogeneous distribution of gases or inhaled particles may occur. As the bronchi branch and decrease in size, they lose their cartilage and become bronchioles. Ultimately, a terminal bronchiole opens up into the gas-exchanging area of the lung (Fig. 4-2).

The airways are lined with an epithelial membrane that gradually changes from ciliated pseudostratified columnar epithelium in the bronchi to a ciliated cuboidal epithelium near the gas-exchanging units. Ciliated cells predominate throughout this epithelium and are responsible for propelling mucus from the peripheral airways to the pharynx. This mucociliary transport system is an important defense mechanism of the lungs. The mucous layer has two parts, a superficial gel layer and a deeper sol layer. The cilia form a dense, long carpet on top of the epithelial cells, and their coordinated to-and-fro action propels the gel mucous layer toward the oropharynx. Cilia are a derivative of the centrioles, and there are approximately 200 of them on the apex of each ciliated cell. The cilia are anchored within the cell with a basal body that is oriented in the direction of mucous movement. The shaft of the cilium has a central pair of single tubules that are connected via radial spokes to nine peripheral pairs of tubules. The tip of the cilium has tiny hooklets that probably help grab the gel component of the mucous layer and propel it forward. The cilium has a beat frequency of 12 ± 1 SD Hz and is coordinated both with other cilia on that cell and concurrently with the cilia on adjacent cells to yield a synchronized wave flowing up the airway. Primary ciliary dyskinesia (PCD) is a group of disorders that includes Kartagener's syndrome and the erroneously named immotile cilia syndrome. In PCD there are defects within the tubules, in their inner or outer dynein arms, or in the radial arms that result in a disorganized movement of the cilia that precludes normal mucociliary transport and results in chronic bronchitis and repeated pneumonias (see Chapter 63).

Mucous glands, which are present in large and small bronchi, are the chief source of airway secretions, and contain both serous and mucus-producing cells. Goblet cells are seen in the trachea and bronchi. They produce mucin within their rough endoplasmic reticulum and Golgi apparatus. Mucin is a viscous mixture of acid glycoproteins that contributes to the mucous layer. Mucous glands and goblet cells can increase in number in disorders such as chronic bronchitis, the result being mucous hypersecretion and increased sputum production. There are several other cell types found within the airways; however, their functional significance is less well understood. The basis cell, commonly seen within the pseudostratified columnar epithelium, is undifferentiated and may be a precursor of ciliated or secretory cells. The brush cell has a dense tuft of broad, short microvilli and is only rarely seen within the conducting airways and alveolar space. Clara cells are seen exclusively within the bronchiolar region of the lung. Their physiologic role has been uncertain, but data suggest that they may play two important roles. First, because they contain but do not synthesize surfactant apoproteins, they may recycle surfactant within the distal lung unit. Second, they are capable of actively transporting sodium from their apical to their basal side and thus may be involved in the reabsorption of fluid from the distal lung unit.

There are curious cells found within the airways that are believed to possess neuroendocrine properties. They are known under a variety of names, including Feyrter or Kulchitsky cells. Histochemical staining indicates that they contain a variety of vasoactive peptides, including serotonin and kinins, so these cells may belong to the class of amine precursor uptake and decarboxylation (APUD) cells. These neuroendocrine cells are innervated and are found more frequently, and in groups (neuroepithelial bodies), within the fetal airways or in pediatric disorders characterized by chronic hypoxemia (e.g., bronchopulmonary dysplasia).

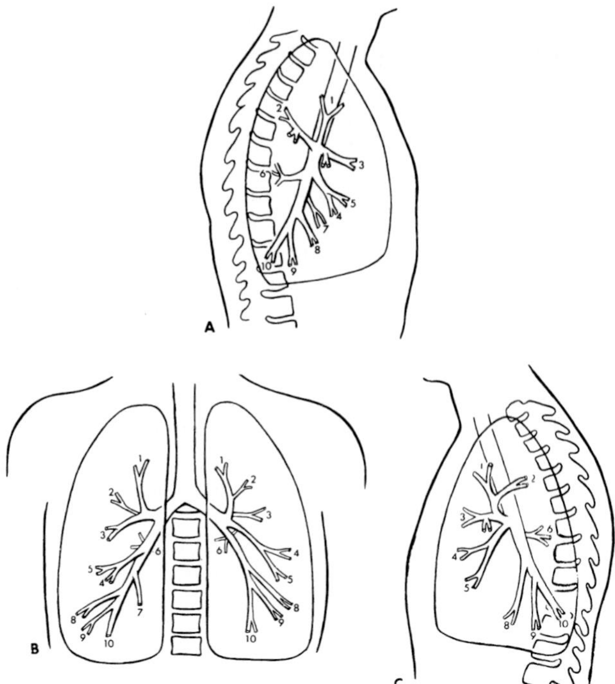

■ **FIGURE 4-1.** The nomenclature of bronchopulmonary anatomy, from a report by the Thoracic Society in 1950. **A,** Right lateral view. **B,** Anterior view. **C,** Left lateral view. (Adapted from Negus V: The Biology of Respiration. Baltimore: Williams & Wilkins, 1955.)

Histologically, the remainder of the airway consists of the submucosa, with its network of blood vessels and nerves, and a variable amount of smooth muscle and cartilage. Within the submucosa are found mast cells containing vasoactive peptides and amines, cells of the immune system (plasma cells, lymphocytes, and phagocytes), and mucous glands. In the main stem bronchi, cartilage is present in C-shaped rings. However, as further branching occurs, progressively less cartilage is present, so that bronchi 2 mm in diameter have cartilage only at the origins of the bronchioles. Cartilage adds structural rigidity to the airway and thus plays an important role in maintaining airway patency, especially during expiration. Congenital deficiency of airway cartilage and hence airway instability has been associated with bronchiectasis (Williams-Campbell syndrome) and congenital lobar emphysema.

The smooth muscle content of the airway also varies with its anatomic location. In the largest airways a muscle bundle connects the two ends of the C-shaped cartilage. As the amount of cartilage decreases, the smooth muscle assumes a helical orientation and gradually becomes thinner, ultimately reaching the alveolar ducts. Muscle contraction increases airway rigidity in all airways and terminal respiratory units.

Although it has been widely assumed that the airway muscles of newborn infants are inadequate for bronchoconstriction, this assumption is not correct. Even premature infants have smooth muscle, and although the amount may be statistically less than that seen in adults, it is likely enough to constrict the infant's much more compliant airways. Indeed, pulmonary function test results have demonstrated that airway resistance can be altered with bronchodilating drugs. The belief that infants have little or no smooth muscle in their airways is even less tenable in such disorders as bronchopulmonary dysplasia and left-to-right congenital heart disease, in which hypertrophy of the airway smooth muscle has been demonstrated by morphometric measurement. Congenital deficiency of large-airway smooth muscle and elastic fibers is associated with marked dilatation of the trachea and bronchi, which promotes retention of airway secretions and ultimately leads to recurrent pulmonary sepsis (Mounier-Kuhn syndrome).

■ TERMINAL RESPIRATORY UNIT

The terminal respiratory (gas-exchanging) unit consists of the structures distal to the terminal bronchiole: the respiratory bronchioles (bronchioles with alveoli budding from their walls), alveolar ducts, and alveoli. This unit is also known as an acinus

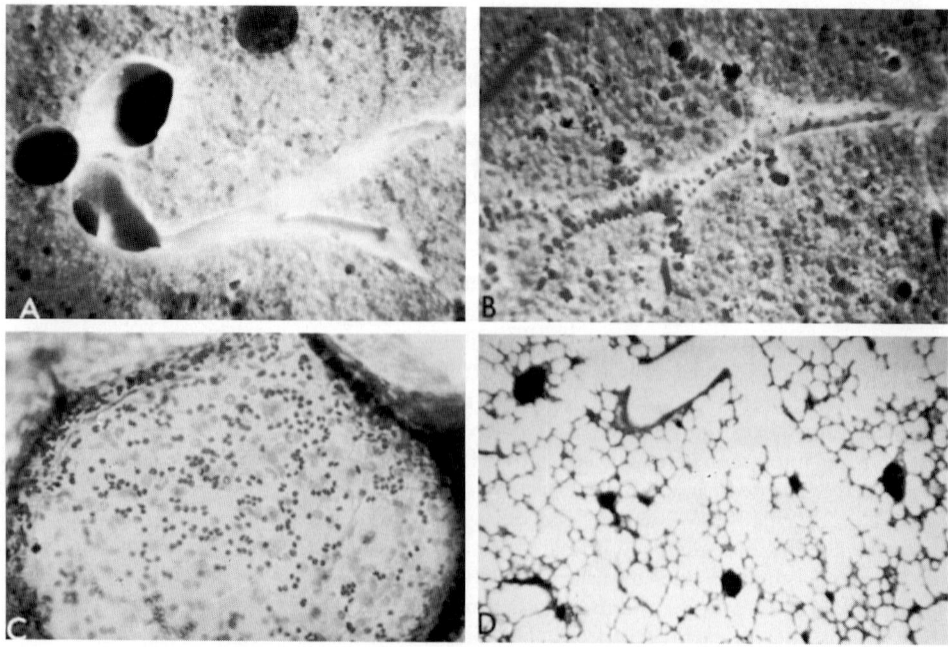

■ **FIGURE 4-2.** The architecture of the lung. **A,** Fresh frozen cat lung. Segmental cartilaginous bronchus and branches. The pulmonary artery is close to the airway; the pulmonary vein is in a more peripheral location (original magnification ×4). **B,** Fresh frozen cat lung (original magnification ×4). Terminal bronchiole with many alveolar ducts arising from it. **C,** Thick section of cat lung. A single alveolar wall is in the plane of focus. Individual red blood cells in alveolar capillaries are clearly seen (original magnification ×100). **D,** Guinea pig, fixed thin section. The terminal respiratory unit, with alveoli shown as outpouchings of the alveolar duct, arises from the terminal bronchiole at the top of the picture. Note that three vessels, probably pulmonary veins, mark the distal boundaries of the unit (original magnification ×15). (From Dr. Norman Staub [All but **A** appeared in color in]: The interdependence of pulmonary structure and function. Anesthesiology 1963;24:831–834.)

and may be considered the basic functional unit of the lung. Terminal respiratory units are well suited for gas exchange. In the adult lung these units have a total gas volume of 2500 mL and a surface area of about 80 m^2, yet all alveoli are within 5 mm of the closest terminal bronchiole. True alveoli are not spherical but more closely resemble hexagons with flat, sheet-like surfaces. The average alveolar diameter ranges from 250 to 300 μm. Within the terminal respiratory units, two types of intercommunicating channels provide collateral ventilation for the gas-exchanging units. The alveolar pores of Kohn are holes in the alveolar wall 3 to 13 μm in diameter that perhaps provide channels for gas movement between contiguous alveoli. These pores are not present in newborn lungs. The canals of Lambert are accessory channels that connect a small airway to an airspace normally supplied by a different airway.

The alveoli are lined by two types of epithelial cells (Fig. 4-3). The type I epithelial cell is an extremely broad, thin (0.1 to 0.5 μm) cell that covers 95% of the alveolar surface. It is a markedly differentiated cell possessing few organelles. The type II epithelial cells are more numerous than type I cells, but owing to their cuboidal shape, type II cells occupy only 5% of the alveolar surface area (Table 4-1). They are characterized histologically by microvilli and osmophilic inclusion bodies.

The type II epithelial cell maintains homeostasis within the alveolar space in several ways. First, it is the source of pulmonary surfactant and as such indicates maturity of the lung; it decreases the surface tension at the alveolar air-liquid interface. Second, this cell is likely the precursor of the alveolar type I cell and thus plays a key role in the repair process following lung injury. Third, it is capable of actively transporting ions against an electrochemical gradient and likely is involved in both fetal lung liquid secretion and, postnatally, the reabsorption of fluid from the airspace following the development of alveolar pulmonary edema (see the later section on Fetal Lung Liquid Secretion).

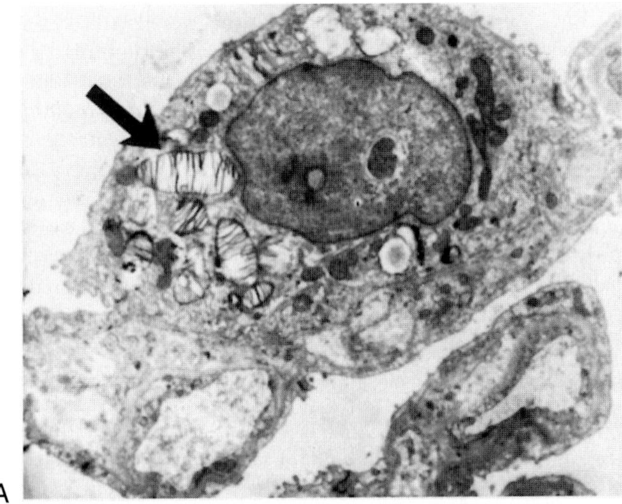

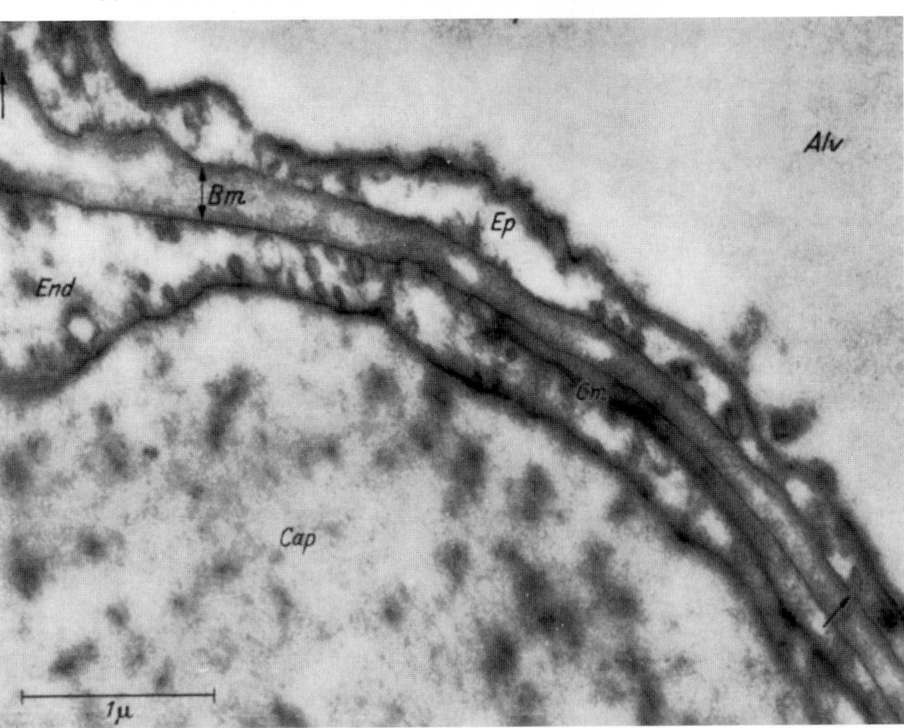

■ **FIGURE 4-3.** **A,** Electron micrograph of a type II epithelial cell. This particular cell is from a dog's lung but is similar to those found in all mammalian lungs. The airspace is in the upper portion of the figure. The *arrow* points to the osmophilic inclusions that are thought to be associated with the alveolar lining substance. The cell rests on a basement membrane that separates it from the capillary endothelium in the lower part of the picture. **B,** Normal human lung showing the attenuated alveolar cytoplasm of a type I epithelial cell. Alv, alveolus; Bm, basement membrane; Cap, capillary; Cm, erythrocyte cell membrane; End, capillary endothelium; Ep, cytoplasmic layer of an epithelial cell. (**A,** Courtesy of E.S. Boatman and H.B. Martin. **B,** From Schultz H: The Submicroscopic Anatomy and Pathology of the Lung. Berlin: Springer-Verlag, 1959.)

■ **TABLE 4-1.** Cellular characteristics of the human lung

Cell Type	Total Cells (%)	Apical Surface Area (μm²)
Epithelium		
Alveolar type I	8.3	5098
Alveolar type II	15.9	183
Endothelium	30.2	1353
Interstitial	36.1	
Alveolar macrophages	9.4	

Data from Crapo JD, Barry BE, Gehr P, et al: Cell number and cell characteristics of the normal human lung. Am Rev Respir Dis 1982;125:740–745.

Two pediatric disorders associated with the type II epithelial cell are (1) its lack of maturity and surfactant secretion in respiratory distress syndrome and (2) its excessive and disordered secretion of surfactant in alveolar proteinosis.

The cell junctions (zonulae occludentes) between alveolar type I and type II epithelial cells are very tight and restrict the movement of both macromolecules and small ions such as sodium and chloride. This tightness is an essential characteristic of the cells lining the alveolar space; it enables the active transport of ions. Also these tight junctions provide a margin of safety for patients susceptible to pulmonary edema: significant interstitial pulmonary edema can be present without alveolar flooding occurring, thus preserving gas exchange.

There is a thick side and a thin side to the alveolar capillary membrane. Gas exchange is thought to occur predominantly on the thin side, where there are only the alveolar epithelial cell, fused basement membranes, and capillary endothelial cell (see Fig. 4-3). Capillaries undergo considerable stress (e.g., during exercise or lung hyperinflation) and must have great tensile strength. This strength is mainly imparted by type IV collagen located in the basement membrane. The thick side of the barrier consists of connective tissue, amorphous ground substance, and scattered fibroblasts. The thick side, in addition to providing structural support, acts as a site of fluid and solute exchange.

■ PULMONARY VASCULAR SYSTEM

The lung receives blood from both ventricles. The entire right ventricular output enters the lung via the pulmonary arteries, and blood ultimately reaches the gas-exchanging units by one of the pulmonary arterial branching systems. Conventional arteries accompany the bronchial tree and divide with it, each branch accompanying the appropriate bronchial division. Supernumerary arteries do not travel with the airways but directly supply the gas-exchanging units. These extra arteries actually outnumber the conventional ones and supply approximately one third of the pulmonary capillary bed. Their specific physiologic role is unclear. The pulmonary capillary bed is the largest vascular bed in the body and covers a surface area of 70 to 80 m². The network of capillaries is so dense that it may be thought of as a sheet of blood interrupted by small vertical supporting posts. The pulmonary veins return blood to the left atrium via conventional and supernumerary branches. By virtue of their larger numbers and thinner walls, the pulmonary veins provide a large reservoir for blood and help maintain a constant left ventricular output in the face of a variable pulmonary arterial flow.

The bronchial arteries, usually three in number, provide a source of well-oxygenated systemic blood to the lungs. This blood supply nourishes the walls of the bronchi, bronchioles, blood vessels, and nerves in addition to perfusing the lymph nodes and most of the visceral pleura. There are numerous communications between the bronchial arterial system and the remainder of the pulmonary vascular bed: a portion of the blood returns to the right atrium via bronchial veins, and a portion drains into the left atrium via pulmonary veins. Although normally the bronchial arteries receive only 1% to 2% of the cardiac output, they hypertrophy in chronically infected lungs, and blood flow may easily increase by more than 10-fold. This is clinically important because virtually all hemoptysis originates from the bronchial vessels in such disorders as cystic fibrosis or bronchiectasis.

Histologically, the pulmonary arteries can be classified as elastic, muscular, partially muscular, or nonmuscular. The elastic pulmonary arteries are characterized by elastic fibers embedded in their muscular coat, whereas the smaller muscular arteries have a circular layer of smooth muscle bounded by internal and external elastic laminae. As arteries decrease further in size, only a spiral of muscle remains (partially muscular arteries), which ultimately disappears so that vessels still larger than capillaries have no muscle in their walls (nonmuscular arteries). In the adult lung, elastic arteries are greater than 1000 μm in diameter, and muscular arteries range from 150 to 100 μm. In the pediatric age group, histologic structure is not as easily determined from vessel size. Reid and co-workers have demonstrated that during growth of the lung a remodeling of the pulmonary vasculature occurs. Muscularization of the arteries lags behind multiplication of alveoli and appearance of new arteries. Therefore, the patient's age must be considered before histologic structure can be assumed from vessel size within the pulmonary acinus (Fig. 4-4). Notably, in the fetus and newborn the amount of pulmonary arterial smooth muscle is increased and regresses after birth. This is functionally important since a high pulmonary arterial resistance is a feature of the fetal circulation in association with a large right to left shunt via the ductus arteriosus.

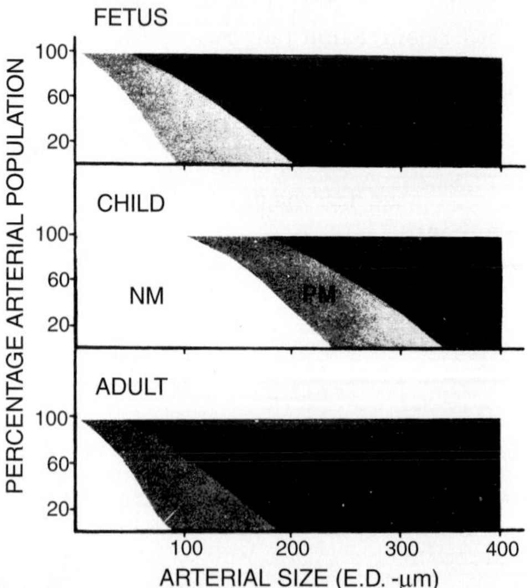

■ **FIGURE 4-4.** The populations of the three arterial types: muscular (M), partially muscular (PM), and nonmuscular (NM), in fetus, child, and adult. The distribution of structure in size is similar in fetus and adult, whereas during childhood NM and PM structures are found in much larger arteries. E.D., external diameter. (From Reid LM: The pulmonary circulation. Remodelling in growth and disease. Am Rev Respir Dis 1979;119:531.)

The endothelium of the pulmonary vascular system is continuous and nonfenestrated. It is an intensely active cell layer and is not just serving a passive barrier function. The endothelial cell produces a glycocalyx that interacts with blood-borne substances and blood cellular elements, thereby influencing such homeostatic functions as hemostasis. The endothelium produces von Willebrand factor, which is part of the factor VIII complex and is necessary for normal platelet function. Similarly, there are enzymes located on the surface and within the cell itself that are capable of synthesizing, altering, or degrading blood-borne vasoactive products. The individual cells are separated by gaps of approximately 35 Å in radius, which allow the free movement of water and small ions but restrict the movement of proteins. The cells and the basement membrane on which they sit carry different net surface charges, which affect the movement of anionic macromolecules such as proteins and thus affect lung water and solute exchange (see Chapter 43). The capacity of the pulmonary endothelium and its basement membrane to restrict fluid and protein movement is impressive. It has been estimated that the amount of lung lymph flow is only 10 to 20 mL/hr despite a total blood flow of 300,000 mL/hr.

LYMPHATIC SYSTEM

There is an extensive interconnecting network of lymphatic vessels throughout the lung. The major function of this network is to collect the protein and water that has moved out of the pulmonary vascular space and to return it to the circulation, thus maintaining the lung at an appropriate degree of hydration. The lymphatic vessels travel alongside the blood vessels in the loose connective tissue of the pleura and bronchovascular spaces. It is likely that there are no lymphatics within the alveolar wall itself and that juxta-alveolar lymphatics represent the beginning of the pulmonary lymphatic system. Histologically, the lymphatic capillaries consist of thin, irregular endothelial cells lacking a basement membrane. Occasionally, there are large gaps between endothelial cells that allow direct communication with the interstitial space. Larger lymphatic vessels contain smooth muscle in their walls that undergoes rhythmic contraction. This muscular contraction plus the presence of funnel-shaped, monocuspid valves ensures an efficient unidirectional flow of lymph. In addition to helping maintain lung water balance, the lymphatic system is one of the pulmonary defense mechanisms. It aids in removal of particulate matter from the lung, and aggregates of lymph tissue near major airways contribute to the host's immune response.

INNERVATION OF THE LUNG

The lung is innervated by both components of the autonomic nervous system. Parasympathetic nerves arise from the vagus nerve, and sympathetic nerves are derived from the upper thoracic sympathetic ganglia. These branches congregate around the hila of the lung to form the pulmonary plexus. Myelinated and nonmyelinated fibers then enter the lung tissues and travel along with and innervate the airways and blood vessels. Although the anatomic location of pulmonary nerves has been elucidated, their physiologic role in health and disease is incompletely understood. In general, the airways constrict in response to vagal stimulation and dilate in response to adrenergic stimulation. The pulmonary vasculature appears to be maximally dilated under normal conditions, and it is difficult to demonstrate any significant physiologic effect of either parasympathetic or sympathetic stimulation. The vascular response, however, is influenced by age and initial vascular tone. For example, in fetal lungs where there is an abundance of pulmonary vascular smooth muscle, vagal stimulation results in significant vasodilatation, and sympathetic stimulation results in marked vasoconstriction.

Sensory nerves from the lungs are vagal in origin and arise from slowly and rapidly adapting receptors and from C-fiber receptors. The slowly adapting (stretch) receptors, located in the smooth muscle of the airway, are stimulated by an increase in lung volume or transpulmonary pressure. They induce several physiologic responses including inhibition of inspiration (Hering-Breuer reflex), bronchodilatation, increased heart rate, and decreased systemic vascular resistance. The rapidly adapting vagal (irritant) receptors are activated by a wide variety of noxious stimuli, ranging from mechanical stimulation of the airways to anaphylactic reactions within the lung parenchyma. The rapidly adapting receptors induce hyperpnea, cough, and constriction of the airways and larynx. C-fiber receptors are the terminus of nonmyelinated vagal afferents. They include the J receptors that are located near the pulmonary capillaries and are stimulated by pulmonary congestion and edema; they evoke a sensation of dyspnea and induce rapid shallow breathing along with laryngeal constriction during expiration.

In addition to the sympathetic and parasympathetic nervous systems, humans and several other species have a third nervous system within their lungs. The noncommittal name *nonadrenergic noncholinergic nervous system* has been chosen because its function and properties are not understood. Purines, substance P, and vasoactive intestinal polypeptide have been suggested as possible neurotransmitters for this system.

INTERSTITIUM

The interstitium plays several roles in lung function in addition to providing a structural framework that consists of insoluble proteins. The ground substance influences cell growth and differentiation and lung water and solute movement. The cells contained within the interstitial region of the lung not only play individual roles that result from their contractile or synthetic properties but they also interact with other cells, such as the endothelium and epithelium, to alter the basic structure and function of the lung.

Most of the interstitial matrix of the lung is composed of type I collagen. Type I collagen, along with the less common types II, III, IV, and V, forms a structural, fibrous framework within the lung. The three principal components of this framework, which include the axial, peripheral, and septal fiber systems, are illustrated in Figure 4-5. Elastin, a contractile insoluble protein, provides elasticity and support to the structures. Both elastin and collagen turn over very slowly under normal conditions. However, rapid remodeling with changes in these proteins sometimes occurs. In diseases such as α_1-antitrypsin deficiency (affecting elastin) and pulmonary fibrosis (affecting collagen), there are marked qualitative and quantitative changes in these proteins. The remainder of the matrix is made up of proteoglycans and glycosaminoglycans. These carbohydrate-protein complexes can affect cell proliferation and differentiation in addition to their known effect on cell adhesion and attachment (e.g., laminin) and ability to diminish fluid movement (glycosaminoglycans).

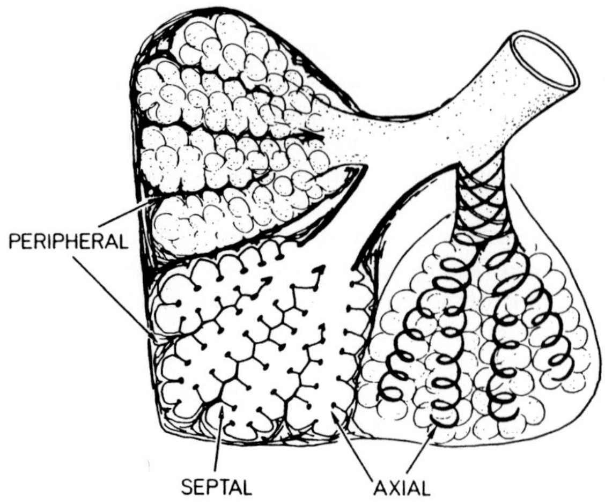

■ **FIGURE 4-5.** Schematic diagram of the fibrous support of the lung. See text for detail. (From Weibel ER, Bachofen H: How to stabilize the alveoli. Surfactant or fibers. News Physiol Sci 1987;2:72–75.)

Fibroblasts are capable of synthesizing collagen, elastin, and glycosaminoglycans and hence contribute significantly to the composition of the lung's interstitial space. They can be found within all of the interstitial regions of the lung, although their apparent structure may change. For example, because "myofibroblasts" contain obvious contractile elements, they may represent fibroblasts that are capable of contraction, or they may be cells that are intermediate between fibroblasts that are capable of contraction, or they may be cells that are intermediate between fibroblasts and smooth muscle cells. Similarly, it is likely that morphologically similar fibroblasts are not similar in terms of proliferative capacity and ability to synthesize various types of collagen. Data suggest that fibrotic lung diseases are characterized by the loss of the normal heterogeneous fibroblast population and that there may be a selection for certain clones that promote inappropriate collagen deposition within the lung parenchyma.

Smooth muscle cells are contractile interstitial cells that influence the bronchomotor and vasomotor tone within the conducting airways and blood vessels. They are also seen within the free edge of the alveolar septa, and they form an alveolar entrance ring that is capable of constricting or dilating. The smooth muscle cells form bundles connected by nexus or gap junctions that enable electrical coupling and synchronous contraction. The pericyte is another interstitial cell that is found between the basement membrane and the endothelium. It is believed to be a precursor cell that can differentiate into a mature vascular smooth muscle cell.

There are a variety of interstitial cells that are concerned with immune and nonimmune defense of the lung. The interstitial macrophage and the alveolar macrophage are predominantly responsible for nonimmune defense, which they manage by ingesting particulate matter and removing it from the lung. These macrophages are capable of secreting many compounds, including proteases and cytokines (substances capable of modulating the growth and function of other cells). B and T lymphocytes are present in the lung and especially within the bronchus-associated lymphoid tissue, where they contribute to the humoral and cellular-mediated immune response.

Although not within the interstitium per se, there are large numbers of intravascular granulocytes that adhere to the pulmonary endothelium. Indeed, next to the bone marrow and spleen, there are more granulocytes within the lung than in any other organ. These granulocytes can be released into the systemic circulation during such stimuli as exercise or the infusion of adrenalin, and this demargination is responsible for the concomitant blood leukocytosis. These leukocytes are also in a prime location for movement into the lung should an infection or inflammatory stimulus occur. There is much evidence to suggest that the pulmonary granulocyte contributes to the pulmonary dysfunction seen in acute lung injury or acute respiratory distress syndrome. Leukocytes also contain proteases that are thought to play a role in the development of emphysema and in the lung destruction that occurs in cystic fibrosis.

■ GROWTH AND DEVELOPMENT OF THE LUNG

■ PRENATAL LUNG GROWTH

Intrauterine growth and development of the lung have been divided into various stages with names that reflect the respective histologic appearance of the lung, the region of the lung that is most obviously developing, or both. Obviously, all the regions of the lung are developing during the various stages; in addition, there are variations in growth rates among individual fetuses. Thus, there is no exact differentiation between the various stages. However, the major reason for identifying these stages of development is to improve our understanding of how and why specific congenital lesions occur. Obviously, the child with unilateral lung agenesis must have had defective lung development much earlier than another child with a peripheral congenital lung cyst.

The five stages of lung development are (1) embryonic (days 26 to 52), (2) pseudoglandular (day 52 to week 16), (3) canalicular (weeks 16 to 28), (4) saccular (weeks 28 to 36), and (5) alveolar (week 36 to term). This classification recognizes that there are true alveoli present in the human lung before birth, with the first being seen at 29 to 32 weeks of gestation. This example illustrates the inexact nature of staging lung development, since the alveolar period does not "begin" until 36 weeks (Fig. 4-6).

The lung first appears in the embryonic period as a ventral outpouching of the primitive gut. The primary bronchi elongate into the mesenchyme and divide into the two main bronchi. In the pseudoglandular period, the branching continues by means of a higher mitotic rate in the epithelium relative to the mesenchyme. The mesenchyme differentiates into cartilage, smooth muscle, and connective tissue around the epithelial tubes. By the end of the pseudoglandular period (16 weeks) all the major conducting airways, including the terminal bronchioles, have formed. The canalicular period is characterized by the development of respiratory bronchioles, each of which ends in two or three thin-walled dilatations called terminal sacs or primitive alveoli. Vascularization of the lung interstitium intensifies, and the glandular appearance is lost as there is a decrease in the relative amount of connective tissue. Further differentiation of the respiratory portion of the lung takes place during the saccular period. During this period, there is for the first time close contact between the airspace and the bloodstream, as the pulmonary capillaries rapidly proliferate and the epithelium thins. Gas exchange is now possible, although obviously it is not optimal. Elastic fibers, which will be important in

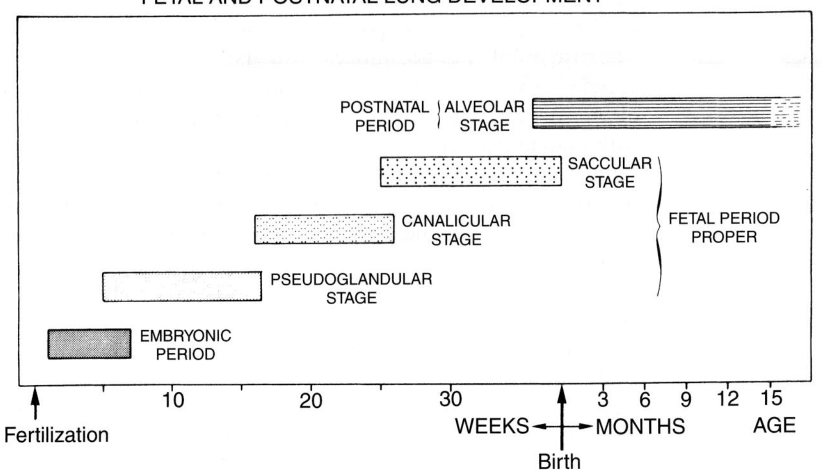

■ **FIGURE 4-6.** Various stages of lung development. The actual separation of individual stages is not discrete, and it overlaps. Note that the alveolar stage commences before birth. (From Burri PH: Fetal and postnatal development of the lung. Annu Rev Physiol 1984;46:617–628. © 1984 by Annual Reviews, Inc.)

subsequent true alveolar development, are beginning to be laid down. At this time, cuboidal (type II) and thin (type I) epithelial cells line the airspace. During the alveolar period, further refinement takes place as tiny secondary septa form on the walls of the larger saccules. These outpouchings grow into the lumen and form the walls of true alveoli, thus further increasing the surface area available for gas exchange.

The development of the pulmonary vasculature coincides with the development of the airways. During the embryonic period, the main pulmonary artery arises from the sixth branchial arch and nourishes the developing lung bud. Throughout the pseudoglandular period, arteries are evident alongside the conducting airways. In addition to the conventional arteries that branch and travel with the airways, supernumerary arteries are evident by 12 weeks of gestation. By 16 weeks of gestation, all preacinar arterial branches have formed; although these will increase in size and length, no new preacinar branches will appear. During the canalicular period, the lung develops a rich vascular supply that is closely associated with the respiratory bronchioles. As saccules begin to develop during the saccular period, capillaries can be found within the walls of the airspaces in close contact with the epithelium. Gas exchange can now occur.

The maturation of surfactant production has been studied intensively since the discovery that prematurely born infants with hyaline membrane disease had abnormal surface tension at the air-liquid interface. It is now known that the source of pulmonary surfactant is the mature type II epithelial cell. When the type II epithelial cell first appears within the lung during the saccular stage, however, it is immature and contains much intracellular glycogen. Many drugs and hormones, including steroids and thyroid and peptide hormones, can influence surfactant biosynthesis and accelerate lung maturation. The surfactant system is discussed in detail in Chapter 2.

The control of lung development is complex and is now known to be strongly influenced by interactions between the pulmonary epithelium and mesenchyme. A family of about 28 fibroblast growth factors are important in regulating cell proliferation, migration, and differentiation during lung development. Epithelium isolated in vitro does not undergo morphogenesis; when it is recombined with pulmonary mesenchyme, development resumes. In a similar manner, it has been demonstrated that the mesenchymal signals can be organ specific. For example, submandibular mesenchyme can induce mammary gland epithelium to express submandibular epithelium gene products. Thus, defects in lung epithelial development could conceivably result from abnormalities within the mesenchymal rather than the epithelial structures.

The mesenchyme's influence on lung development can be classified as instructive (directive) or permissive. The former influence instructs the epithelium to take a specific developmental pathway (e.g., to differentiate into a type II versus a ciliated epithelial cell). In contrast, permissive inductions allow an already committed cell to express its capabilities (e.g., a type II cell to start secreting surfactant).

■ FETAL LUNG LIQUID SECRETION

Fetal lung liquid secretion is essential for normal lung development. Exactly when the lung begins to secrete fluid is unknown, but the secretion is well established by the second half of gestation and is produced at a rate of 4 to 5 mL/kg/hr. Analysis of fetal lung liquid has demonstrated that it is neither a mere ultrafiltrate of plasma nor aspirated amniotic fluid. The lung fluid relative to plasma has higher concentrations of chloride (155 mM) and potassium (6 mM), similar sodium concentration, and markedly lower bicarbonate (3 mM) concentration. The lung liquid protein concentration is so low that it is comparable with cerebrospinal fluid (0.03 g/dL). Fetal lung liquid secretion is dependent on the active transport of electrolytes into the airspace.

There are two requirements for the active secretion of fluid into the developing airspaces (Fig. 4-7). First, there must be an electrochemical gradient for ion movement that will carry water with it. The source of energy for the active transport is the sodium-potassium adenosine triphosphatase (ATPase) located on the basolateral epithelial cell membrane. As the pump extrudes sodium out of the cell, there is a linked reentry of this sodium along with chloride (and perhaps potassium) back into the cell down sodium's electrochemical gradient. The intracellular chloride concentration rises, and it exits out into the airspace through chloride channels in the apical membrane, driven out by the electrical gradient (the inside of the cell membrane is negative relative to the lumen). The second requirement for ion transport is a very tight epithelial membrane, which is necessary to establish these gradients and to prevent rapid backward flow

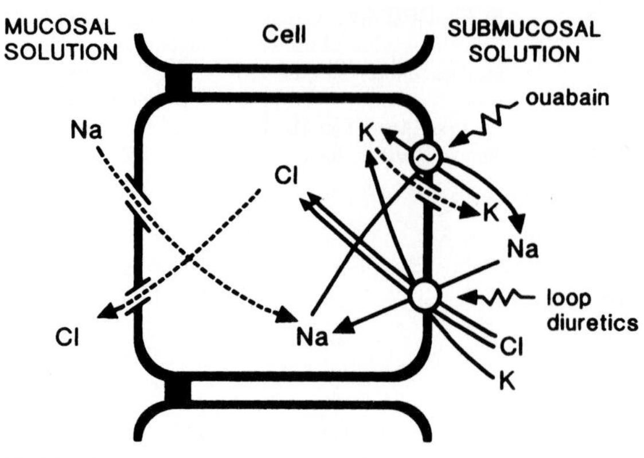

■ **FIGURE 4-7.** A model of pathways for active transport of electrolytes by a pulmonary epithelial cell. In fetal life, chloride (Cl) secretion predominates and presumably occurs via the apical Cl channel. After birth, sodium (Na) absorption is dominant. Ouabain inhibits the Na-K ATPase pump, whereas loop diuretics can inhibit the Na:K:2Cl cotransporter, thus impeding Cl secretion. See text for details. (From Welsh M: Electrolyte transport by airway epithelia. Physiol Rev 1987;67:1143–1184.)

of ions and water between the cells. This requirement is met by the extremely tight interepithelial junctions that restrict the movement of these small ions. Data from fetal sheep suggest that the airspace's epithelium is tight and remarkably constant between 50% of gestation and term. Interference with fetal lung liquid secretion or fetal lung distention by liquid results in a maldeveloped lung with a reduced number of terminal airspaces.

THE LUNG AT BIRTH

Many dramatic changes must occur in the lungs during the transition from intrauterine to extrauterine life. The lung's epithelium must change from fluid secretion to fluid absorption, the distal lung units must fill with and retain the inhaled air, and blood flow must increase approximately 20-fold.

Just before birth the lungs contain approximately 30 mL/kg of fetal lung liquid. At the time of birth it is essential that fetal lung liquid secretion decrease so that the lung liquid can be cleared to allow for normal gas exchange. The control mechanisms for this decrease in secretion are incompletely understood, but evidence suggests that catecholamines released before or during the birth process will decrease secretion, possibly by inhibiting chloride ion transport, opening sodium channels in the apex of the epithelial cell, thereby converting it into a sodium reabsorbing membrane, or both. It has also been demonstrated that this effect of catecholamines is dependent on gestational age. In the more immature fetus, β agonists have little effect on lung liquid secretion, and thus the immature fetus may have greater difficulty clearing the airspace fluid when making the transition to breathing air. The process of labor itself will increase the amount of sodium-potassium ATPase activity in the type II epithelial cells; which aspect of labor is important is unknown. Fetal lung liquid is cleared at birth by several mechanisms; approximately one third is squeezed out during the birth process, and the remainder is absorbed by the epithelium; the fluid is then taken up by pulmonary vessels or cleared by the lymphatics. Failure of normal lung water clearance at birth is simply one type of pulmonary edema, and it results in respiratory distress (wet lung syndrome or transient tachypnea of the newborn).

The assessment of lung function in early stages of development is based chiefly on measurement in lambs, which provides insight into the direction of changes that occur with time, although exact analogies to the human subject are speculative. The distensibility of the lung early in gestation is much less than at term. When peak volumes are expressed as milliliters per gram of lung tissue, it is evident that the potential airspace is small with respect to lung mass. The ability to retain air at end-expiration, which depends on the presence of the pulmonary surfactant, does not appear until later in the canalicular stage of development. In the lamb it appears between days 120 and 130 of a 147-day gestation. In the human it appears probably between the 20th and the 24th weeks of gestation, with a wide distribution over this period.

In utero, little blood flows through the lung despite a relatively high perfusion pressure, because of the abundance of pulmonary vascular smooth muscle and the vasoconstrictor effect of the low fetal partial pressure of oxygen (PO_2) (<30 mm Hg). Although during the last trimester, concomitant with surfactant production, blood flow increases to 7% of the cardiac output, it is only at birth that marked increases in the capacity and distensibility of the pulmonary vasculature occur. Several mechanisms are responsible for the changes in circulation. Inflation of the lung with air results in mechanical distention of the vessels, and improvement in oxygenation removes hypoxic vasoconstriction. In addition, the rise in partial pressure of oxygen in arterial blood (PaO_2) induces granulocytes in the lung to release massive quantities of kinin. This kinin alters the tissue concentrations of prostaglandins and helps to mediate the vasoconstriction of the ductus arteriosus and umbilical vessels and to dilate the pulmonary vascular bed. Both prostacyclin and nitric oxide have a significant regulatory role on pulmonary vascular tone in the perinatal period. The concentration of both prostaglandin 1-synthase and nitric oxide synthase (NOS) increase with development, especially near term. Neonatal lung NOS expression is decreased in persistent pulmonary hypertension of the newborn. With increasing postnatal age, vascular muscle regresses so that the wall/lumen ratio decreases. After about 10 days of extrauterine life, the lumina are wider, regardless of the gestational age of the baby. The events of birth have little effect on other aspects of lung development, including histochemical maturation.

POSTNATAL LUNG GROWTH

The postnatal growth of the lung continues into the adolescent years and perhaps beyond. It is important to remember that the lung of the newborn is not a miniature of the lung of the adult; during growth, tracheal diameter approximately triples, alveolar dimensions increase about fourfold, and alveolar numbers increase about 10-fold while body mass increases about 20-fold. Other anatomic relationships of the infant's and child's lungs are similar to those in the adult's lung (see Figs. 4-1 and 4-2). The internal surface area of the lung maintains a close relationship to body mass (approximately 1 m^2/kg of body weight), and the proportion of total lung weight represented by each lobe is remarkably constant from infancy to adulthood. Average values of lung lobe weight expressed as a percentage of total lung weight are as follows: right upper lobe 19.5%, right middle lobe 8.3%, right lower lobe 25.3%, left upper lobe 22.5%, and left lower lobe 24.6%.

The preacinar blood vessels and airways have developed by 16 weeks' gestation, and although they do increase in size after birth, the majority of postnatal lung growth involves the terminal respiratory unit.

New secondary septa continue to appear on the walls of the saccules and grow into the airspace, thus creating more true alveoli. Alveoli continue to increase in number through segmentation of these primitive alveoli and through transformation of terminal bronchioles into respiratory bronchioles, a process known as alveolarization. The number of alveoli rapidly increases from 20 million to 200 million by the third year of life, but then alveolar multiplication slows.

There is no agreement about when alveolar multiplication ceases (2 vs. 8 years), but few if any new alveoli develop after 8 years of age. Further growth of the airspace then occurs through increases in alveolar dimensions. In the mature adult lung, the number of alveoli varies from 200 million to 600 million, and an individual alveolus is 250 to 350 μm in diameter. The reason for the variable number of alveoli in the adult lung is unknown but seems to be related to total lung volume. Indeed, in the adult there are about 170 alveoli per mm^3 of lung parenchyma.

As alveolar multiplication occurs, new blood vessels appear within the acinus, so the ratio between the numbers of alveoli and arteries remains relatively constant throughout childhood. Branching of conventional arteries continues until 18 months of age, whereas supernumerary arteries continue to appear until 8 years of age.

Throughout childhood there is an increase in the concentration of arteries to alveoli. The alveolar/arterial ratio is 20:1 in the newborn, 12:1 in a 2-year-old child, and 8 to 10:1 in the older child. The muscularization of the arteries lags behind during childhood, with a return to muscularization of more peripheral arteries by adult life (see Fig. 4-7).

VENTILATION AND MECHANICS OF BREATHING

The principal function of the lung is to perform gas exchange, that is, to enrich the blood with oxygen and cleanse it of carbon dioxide. An essential feature of normal gas exchange is that the volume and distribution of ventilation are appropriate. Ventilation of the lung depends on the adequacy of the respiratory pump (muscles and chest wall) and the mechanical properties of the airways and gas-exchanging units.

It is traditional and useful to consider mechanical events as belonging to two main categories: the static-elastic properties of the lungs and chest wall and the flow-resistive or dynamic aspects of moving air. Changes in one category may be associated with compensatory changes in the other. Thus, many diseases affect both static and dynamic behavior of the lungs. Often the principal derangement is in the elastic properties of the tissues or in the dimensions of the airways, and the treatment or alleviation of symptoms depends on distinguishing between them.

Before we discuss the mechanical aspects of lung function and gas exchange, it is important to review several basic physical laws concerning the behavior of gases and also the related abbreviations and symbols that will be used.

DEFINITIONS AND SYMBOLS

The principal variables for gases are as follows:

V = gas volume
$\dot{V}$ = volume of gas per unit time
P = pressure
F = fractional concentration in dry gas
R = respiratory exchange ratio, carbon dioxide/oxygen
f = frequency
D_L = diffusing capacity of lung

The designation of which volume or pressure is cited requires a small capital letter after the principal variable. Thus, VO_2 = volume of oxygen; P_B = barometric pressure.

I = inspired gas
E = expired gas
A = alveolar gas
T = tidal gas
D = dead space gas
B = barometric pressure

When both location of the gas and its species are to be indicated, the order is V_IO_2, which means the volume of inspired oxygen.

STPD = standard temperature, pressure, dry (0°C, 760 mm Hg)
BTPS = body temperature, pressure, saturated with water vapor
ATPS = ambient temperature, pressure, saturated with water vapor

The principal designations for blood are as follows:

S = percentage saturation of gas in blood
C = concentration of gas per 100 mL of blood
Q = volume of blood
$\dot{Q}$ = blood flow per minute
a = arterial
$\bar{v}$ = mixed venous
c = capillary

All sites of blood determinations are indicated by lowercase initials. Thus, $PaCO_2$ = partial pressure of carbon dioxide in arterial blood; PO_2 = partial pressure of oxygen in mixed venous blood; and PaO_2 = partial pressure of oxygen in a capillary.

Properties of Gases

Gases behave as an enormous number of tiny particles in constant motion. Their behavior is governed by the gas laws, which are essential to the understanding of pulmonary physiology.

Dalton's law states that the total pressure exerted by a gas mixture is equal to the sum of the pressures of the individual gases. The pressure exerted by each component is independent of the other gases in the mixture. For instance, at sea level, air saturated with water vapor at a temperature of 37°C has a total pressure equal to the atmospheric or barometric pressure (P_B = 101.3 kilopascals or 30 inches of mercury or 760 mm Hg), with the partial pressures of the components as shown in:

$$P_B = 760 \text{ mm Hg} = P_{H_2O} \text{ (47 mm Hg)} + P_{O_2} \text{ (149.2 mm Hg)} + P_{N_2} \text{ (563.5 mm Hg)} + P_{CO_2} \text{ (0.3 mm Hg)}$$

The gas in alveoli contains 5.6% carbon dioxide, BTPS. If P_B = 760 mm Hg, then,

$$P_{ACO_2} = 0.056(760 - 47) = 40 \text{ mm Hg}$$

Boyle's law states that at a constant temperature, the volume of any gas varies inversely as the pressure to which the gas is subjected: PV = k. Because respiratory volume measurements may be made at different barometric pressures, it is important to know the barometric pressure and to convert to standard pressure, which is considered to be 760 mm Hg.

Charles' law states that if the pressure is constant, the volume of a gas increases in direct proportion to the absolute temperature. At absolute zero (−273°C), molecular motion ceases. With increasing temperature, molecular collisions increase, so that at constant pressure, volume must increase.

In all respiratory calculations, water vapor pressure must be taken into account. The partial pressure of water vapor increases with temperature but is independent of atmospheric pressure. At body temperature (37°C), fully saturated gas has a PH_2O of 47 mm Hg.

Gases may exist in physical solution in a liquid, escape from the liquid, or return to it. At equilibrium, the partial pressure of a gas in a liquid medium exposed to a gas phase is equal in the two phases. Note that in blood the sum of the partial pressures of all the gases does not necessarily equal atmospheric pressure. For example, in venous blood, PO_2 has fallen from the 100 mm Hg of the arterial blood to 40 mm Hg, while PCO_2 has changed from 40 to 46 mm Hg. Thus, the sum of the partial pressures of O_2, CO_2, and N_2 in venous blood equals 655 mm Hg.

ELASTIC RECOIL OF THE LUNG

The lung is an elastic structure that tends to decrease its size at all volumes. The elasticity of the lung depends on the structural components (although elastic fibers are not essential for normal performance), the geometry of the terminal airspaces, and the presence of an air-liquid interface. When a lung is made airless and is then inflated with liquid, the elastic recoil pressure at large volumes is less than half that of a lung inflated to the same volume with air. Thus, the most significant determinant of the elastic properties of the lung is the presence of an air-liquid interface.

The increase of elastic recoil in the presence of an air-liquid interface results from the forces of surface tension. What is surface tension? When molecules are aligned at an air-liquid interface, they lack opposing molecules on one side. The intermolecular attractive forces are then unbalanced, and the resultant force tends to move molecules away from the interface. The effect is to reduce the area of the surface to a minimum. In the lungs the forces at the air-liquid interface operate to reduce the internal surface area of the lung, and thus they augment elastic recoil. A remarkable property of the material at the alveolar interface, the alveolar lining layer or pulmonary surfactant, is its ability to achieve a high surface tension at large lung volumes and a low surface tension at low volumes. Surfactant is a phospholipid-protein complex that when compressed forms insoluble, folded-surface films of low surface tension. The ability to achieve a low surface tension at low lung volumes tends to stabilize the airspaces and prevent their closure.

The exact method of lung stabilization and the concomitant role of surfactant in this stabilization can be debated. The classic interpretation is that without surfactant the smaller alveoli would tend to empty into the larger alveoli in accordance with the Laplace relationship, which relates the pressure across a surface (P) to surface tension (T) and radius (r) of curvature. For a spherical surface, P = 2T/r. The smaller the radius, the greater is the tendency to collapse.

The difficulty with this hypothesis is that the individual lung units are drawn as independent but communicating bubbles or spheres (Fig. 4-8). This is not representative of structure of the lung because the alveolar walls are planar, not spherical. In addition, the inside wall of one alveolus is the outside wall of the adjacent alveolus. This last explanation has been utilized to develop the interdependence model of lung stability, which indicates that surface and tissue forces interact to maintain the lungs' inherent structure, with the fibrous components playing an important role (see Fig. 4-8).

The elastic recoil of the lung is responsible for the lung's tendency to pull away from the chest wall with the resultant subatmospheric pressure in the pleural space. Lung recoil can therefore be derived from measurement of the pleural pressure when no airflow is occurring and alveolar pressure is zero. (The pressure measurement is taken with the patient holding his breath for a brief period with the glottis open.)

The pressure within the esophagus can be used as an index for mean pleural pressure. This is a reasonable assumption as long as there is no paradoxical rib cage movement. However, it is not a reasonable assumption for premature infants, term infants in rapid eye movement (REM) sleep, and older infants with severe lung disease. For these infants, no average pleural pressure exists, and calculations of resistance and compliance will not be accurate using this method. When pleural pressure is estimated with an esophageal balloon, one must be careful to avoid artifacts resulting from the gravitational pressure of the mediastinum. For this reason, these measurements are best performed with the patient in the upright or lateral rather than the supine position. Once a series of pressure measurements has been made during brief breath-holds at different lung volumes, a pressure-volume curve of the lung can be constructed (Fig. 4-9).

COMPLIANCE OF THE LUNG

The pressure-volume curve of the lung describes two measurements of the elastic properties of the lung: elastic recoil pressure and lung compliance. Elastic recoil pressure is the pressure generated at a given lung volume, whereas compliance is the slope of the pressure-volume curve, or the volume change per unit of pressure:

$$\text{Compliance} = \frac{\Delta\text{volume}}{\Delta\text{pressure}} = \frac{\text{L}}{\text{cm H}_2\text{O}}$$

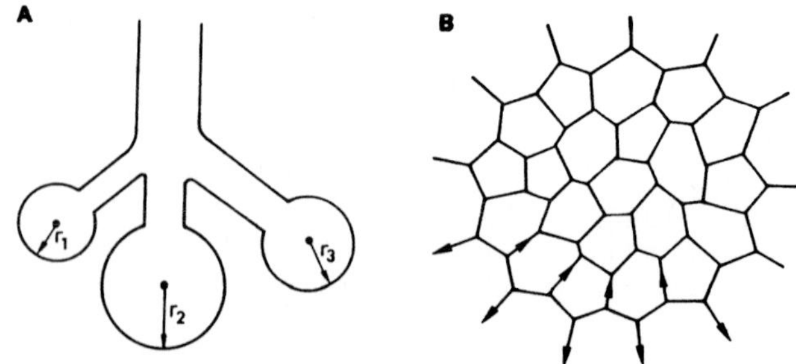

FIGURE 4-8. **A,** Classic model of the distal lung, in which individual alveoli would be controlled by Laplace's law: $P = 2\gamma/r$. Small alveoli would empty into large alveoli. **B,** Interdependence model of the lung, in which alveoli share common planar and not spherical walls. Any decrease in the size of one alveolus would be stabilized by the adjacent alveoli. (From Weibel ER, Bachofen H: How to stabilize the alveoli. Surfactant or fibers. News Physiol Sci 1987;2:72–75.)

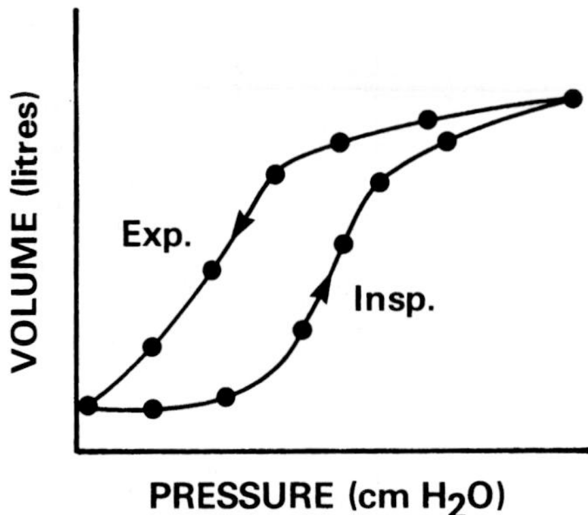

FIGURE 4-9. Pressure-volume curve of a normal lung. Pleural pressure and lung volume are simultaneously determined during brief breath-holds. Lung compliance is calculated from data obtained on the expiratory portion of the pressure-volume curve.

Compliance depends on the initial lung volume from which the change in volume is measured and the ventilatory events immediately preceding the measurement as well as the properties of the lung itself. At large lung volumes, compliance is lower, because the lung is nearer its elastic limit. If the subject has breathed with a fixed tidal volume for some minutes, portions of the lung are not participating in ventilation, and compliance may be reduced. A few deep breaths, with return to the initial volume, will increase compliance. Thus, a careful description of associated events is required for correct interpretation of the measurement.

Changes in lung compliance occur with age (Table 4-2). Of course, the smaller the subject, the smaller is the change in volume, so that $\Delta V/\Delta P$ is close to 6 mL/cm H_2O in infants, and is 125 to 190 mL/cm H_2O in adults. It is more relevant to a description of the elastic properties of the lung to express the compliance in relation to a unit of lung volume such as the functional residual capacity (FRC). Note that with age, as shown in Table 4-2, the compliance of the lung/FRC, or the specific compliance, changes much less.

It is worth reemphasizing that total lung compliance is a function not only of the lung's tissue and surface tension characteristics but also of its volume. This is especially important to remember when compliance has been measured in newborn infants with respiratory distress syndrome (RDS). The total compliance is a composite of the lung's elastic properties and the number of open lung units. In RDS, sudden changes in total measured compliance (if uncorrected for simultaneously measured lung gas volume) will predominantly, if not exclusively, reflect the opening and closing of individual lung units.

TABLE 4-2. Lung compliance (C_L) with age

	mL/cm H_2O	C_L/FRC
Newborns		
3 hr	4.75 ± 1.67	0.041 ± 0.01
24 hr	6.24 ± 1.45	0.055 ± 0.01
Infants		
1 mo–2 yr	7.9	0.038
Children		
Average age 9 yr	77	0.063
Young adult males	184	0.050
Young adult females	125	0.053
Adults over 60 yr	191	0.041

FRC, functional residual capacity.

Lung compliance may also be measured during quiet breathing with pressure and volume being recorded at end-inspiration and end-expiration. The resultant value is the dynamic lung compliance. Although dynamic lung compliance does reflect the elastic properties of the normal lung, it is also influenced by the pressure required to move air within the airways. Therefore, dynamic lung compliance increases with increased respiratory rate and with increased airway resistance. Airflow is still occurring within the lung after it has ceased at the mouth, and pleural pressure reflects both the elastic recoil of the lung and the pressure required to overcome the increased airway resistance. Indeed, dynamic lung compliance can be used as a sensitive test of obstructive airway disease.

ELASTIC PROPERTIES OF THE CHEST WALL

The chest wall is also an elastic structure, but in contrast to the lung, it tends to push outward at low volumes and inward at high volumes. These phenomena are illustrated when air is introduced into the pleural space: the lung collapses and the chest wall springs outward.

Compliance of the chest wall can be measured by considering the pressure difference between the pleural space or esophagus and the atmosphere, per change in volume. Significant changes in thoracic compliance occur with age (Fig. 4-10). In the range of normal breathing, the thorax of the infant is nearly infinitely compliant. The pressures measured at different lung volumes are about the same across the lung as those measured across lung and thorax together. The functional significance of the high compliance of the neonatal thorax is observed when there is lung disease. The necessarily greater inspiratory effort and more negative pleural pressure can "suck" in the chest wall, resulting in less effective gas exchange and a higher work of breathing.

With advancing age the thorax becomes relatively stiffer. Changes in volume-pressure relations are profitably considered only if referred to a reliable unit, such as a unit of lung volume or a percentage of total lung capacity. Considered on a percentage basis, compliance of the thorax decreases with age. How much of this change is contributed by changes in tissue properties, such as increasing calcification of ribs and connective tissue changes, and how much is a disproportionate growth of the chest wall relative to the lung remains unclear.

LUNG VOLUMES

Definition

The partition of commonly used lung volumes can be understood by studying Figure 4-11. The spirogram on the left represents the volume of air breathed in and out by a normal subject. The first portion of the tracing illustrates normal breathing and is called the tidal volume (V_T). The subject then makes a maximal inspiration followed by a maximum expiration: the volume of expired air is the vital capacity (VC). The volume of air that still remains in the lung after a maximal expiration is the residual volume (RV), whereas the volume of air remaining in the lung after a normal passive expiration is the FRC. The maximum amount of air that a subject can have in the lungs is called the total lung capacity (TLC). In healthy young subjects, TLC correlates best with the subject's sitting height.

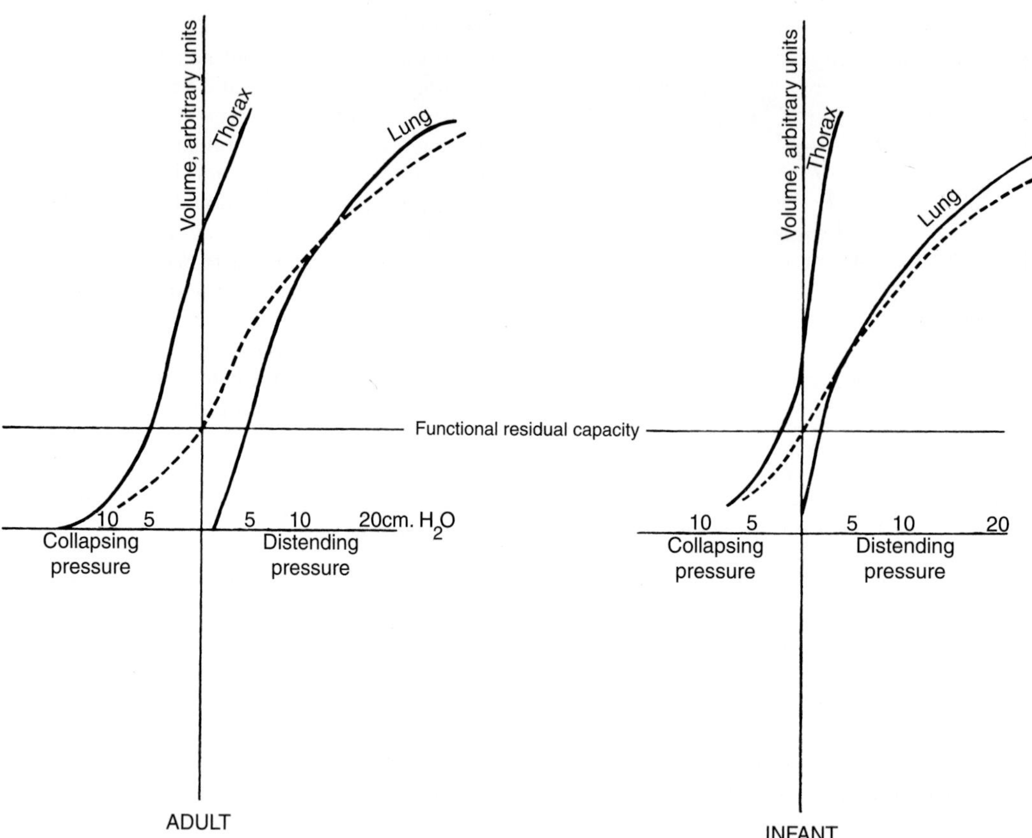

■ **FIGURE 4-10.** Pressure-volume relations of lungs and thorax in an adult and an infant. The *dashed line* represents the characteristic of lungs and thorax together. Transpulmonary pressure at the resting portion (functional residual capacity) is less in the infant, and thoracic compliance is greater in the infant.

The volumes and capacities of the lungs are determined by many factors, including muscle strength, static-elastic characteristics of the chest wall and lungs, airway status, and patient age and cooperation. TLC is reached when the force generated by maximal voluntary contraction of the inspiratory muscles equals the inward recoil of the lung and chest wall. FRC occurs when the respiratory muscles are relaxed and no external forces are applied; it is therefore the volume at which the inward recoil of the lung is exactly balanced by the outward recoil of the chest wall (see Fig. 4-9).

In healthy children and young adults, end-expiratory lung volume is equivalent to FRC. This is not the case in infants, who breathe at a lung volume higher than FRC. This higher volume seems to be a sensible solution to the infants' problem of having an airway closing volume that exceeds FRC. An infant maintains the expiratory lung volume higher than FRC by a combination of postinspiratory diaphragmatic activity and laryngeal adduction.

The factors determining RV vary with age. In adolescents and young adults, RV occurs when the expiratory muscles cannot compress the chest wall further. In young children and older adults, RV is a function of the patency of small airways and the duration of expiratory effort.

Measurement

Tidal volume and VC can be determined by measuring the expired volume. The measurement of FRC and RV requires another approach. Because both volumes include the air in the lungs that the patient does not normally exhale, they must be measured indirectly. One method uses the principle of dilution of the unknown volume with a known concentration of a gas that is foreign to the lung and only sparingly absorbed, such as helium. The patient breathes from a container with a known volume and concentration of helium in oxygen-enriched air. After sufficient time has elapsed for the gas in the lung to mix and equilibrate with the gas in the container, the concentration of helium in the container is remeasured. Because initial volume × initial concentration of helium = final volume × final concentration of helium, the final volume, which includes gas in the lungs, can be calculated.

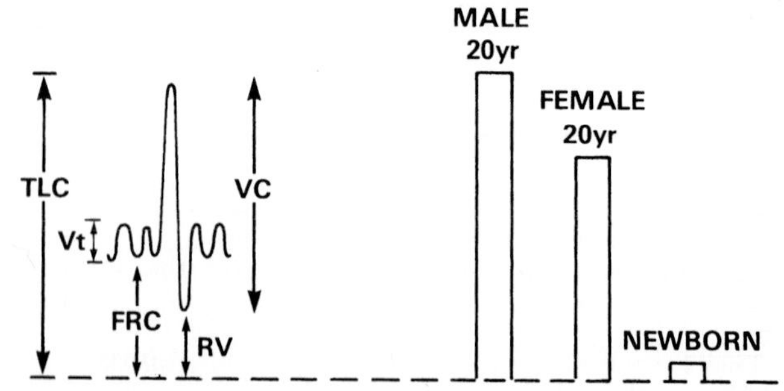

■ **FIGURE 4-11.** The lung volumes. The spirogram *(left)* demonstrates normal breathing followed by a maximal inspiratory effort and a maximal expiratory effort. FRC, functional residual capacity; RV, residual volume; TLC, total lung capacity (6.0 L in an average male, 4.2 L in an average female, and 160 mL in an average 3-kg infant; see histograms on *right*); VC, vital capacity; VT, tidal volume.

The helium dilution method will not measure gas behind closed airways ("trapped gas") or in regions of the lung that are poorly ventilated. There is, however, a method of measuring total gas volume within the thorax that depends on the change in volume that occurs with compression of the gas when breathing against an obstruction. Practically, this measurement requires the patient to be in a body plethysmograph and to pant against a closed shutter. The change in pressure can be measured in the mouthpiece; the change in volume can be recorded with a spirometer attached to the body plethysmograph: $V = P\Delta V/\Delta P$. This method has the advantage of being able to be repeated several times a minute. It has the disadvantage of including some abdominal gas in the measurement.

There have also been concerns about the validity of the plethysmographic technique in patients with obstructive lung disease. This issue has not yet been resolved because the technique has been reported to overestimate the lung volume in adults but underestimate the lung volume in infants with obstructive lung disease.

Interpretation

The major difficulty in detecting abnormalities in lung volumes is that the range of normal values is so large. For example, the mean TLC for a child 140 cm tall is 3.2 L; however, the statistical range of normal (mean ± 2 SD) is 1.9 to 4.3 L. This range of normal values, when expressed as percentage predicted, is even greater for younger children or smaller lung volumes (such as RV). Owing to this wide range of normality, care must be exercised in the interpretation of lung volumes. Measurement of lung volumes is of greatest benefit when repeated over several months to assess the progress of a chronic respiratory illness and the efficacy of treatment.

The VC is one of the most valuable measurements that can be made in a functional assessment, because it is highly reproducible and has a relatively narrow range of normal values. It can be decreased by a wide variety of disease processes, including muscle weakness, loss of lung tissue, obstruction of the airway, and decreased compliance of the chest wall. VC is therefore not a useful tool to discriminate between types of lesions. Its chief role is to assign a value to the degree of impairment and to document changes that occur with therapy or time. In order to decide whether obstructive or restrictive lung disease is present, it is useful to measure expiratory flow rates (see Chapters 9 and 10) and to observe the pattern of abnormalities in the other lung volumes. In obstructive lung disease (e.g., asthma), the smallest lung volumes are affected first: RV increases owing to abnormally high airway resistance at low lung volumes, and as the disease progresses, the FRC increases. Although the increase in FRC (hyperinflation) may rarely be due to loss of lung recoil, the overdistention is usually compensating for partial lower airway obstruction. When the lung volume is increased, intrathoracic airways enlarge, and widespread partial obstruction may be partially relieved by the assumption of a larger resting lung volume. Whereas the total lung capacity is only rarely affected in obstructive disease (such as asthma) in children (in contrast to emphysema in adults), TLC and VC are the first lung volumes to be affected in restrictive diseases of the chest wall (e.g., kyphoscoliosis) or lung (e.g., pulmonary fibrosis).

REGIONAL LUNG VOLUMES

During normal breathing, different areas of the lung have different regional lung volumes; the upper airspaces are inflated more than the lower airspaces. Because static-elastic properties are fairly constant throughout the lung, these different regional lung volumes result from the gradient of pleural pressure that exists from the top to the bottom of the lung. Although gravitational forces are thought to be largely responsible, the mechanisms responsible for this pleural pressure gradient are incompletely understood. In the erect adult lung, the pleural pressure is −8 cm H_2O at the apex and only −2 cm H_2O at the base. The significance of this phenomenon is that when a subject breathes in, the lowermost lung units will receive the majority of the inspired air (Fig. 4-12). This is advantageous because the majority of pulmonary blood flow also goes to the base of the lung, and thus blood flow and ventilation patterns are more closely matched.

DYNAMIC (FLOW-RESISTIVE) PROPERTIES OF THE LUNG

Gas Flow within Airways

The respiratory system must perform work to move gas into and out of the lungs. Because air moves into the lungs during inspiration and out of the lungs during expiration, and because the velocity of airflow increases from small airways to large airways, energy must be expended to accelerate the gas molecules. The respiratory system's resistance to acceleration (inertance) is minimal during quiet breathing and will not be considered further. In contrast, frictional resistance to airflow accounts for one third of the work performed during quiet breathing. The magnitude of pressure loss due to friction is determined by the pattern of flow. Flow may be laminar (streamlined) or turbulent, and which pattern exists depends on the properties of the gas (viscosity, density), the velocity of airflow, and the radius of the airway. In general, there is laminar flow in the small peripheral airways and turbulent flow in the large central airways.

The laws governing the frictional resistance to flow of gases in tubes apply to pulmonary resistance. The equation for

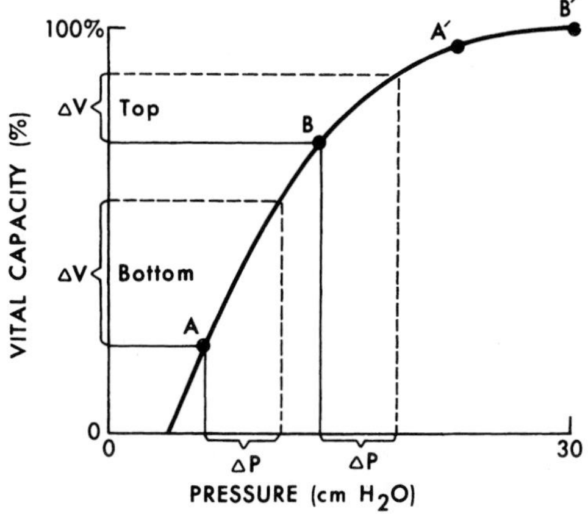

FIGURE 4-12. Pressure-volume curve of a normal lung *(heavy solid line)*. At functional residual capacity, distending pressure is less at the bottom than at the top; accordingly, alveoli at the bottom *(A)* are smaller (i.e., lower percentage regional vital capacity) than those at the top *(B)*. When a given amount of distending pressure (ΔP) is applied to the lung, alveoli at the bottom increase their volume (ΔV) more than alveoli at the top, owing to the varying steepness of the pressure-volume curve. When fully expanded to total lung capacity (100% VC), alveoli at the bottom *(A′)* are nearly the same size as alveoli at the top *(B′)*, because both points lie on the flat portion of the curve. (From Murray JF: The Normal Lung. Philadelphia: WB Saunders, 1976.)

calculating the pressure gradient required to maintain a laminar flow of air through a tube is given by Poiseuille's law:

$$P = \dot{V}\left(\frac{8l\eta}{\pi r^4}\right)$$

where P is pressure, $\dot{V}$ is flow, l is length, r is radius of the tube, and η is the viscosity of the gas. The viscosity of air is 0.000181 poise at 20°C, or only 1% that of water. Because resistance = pressure/flow, it is clear that the most important determinant of resistance in small airways will be the radius of the tube, which is raised to the fourth power in the denominator of the equation.

The pressure required to maintain turbulent flow is influenced by airway diameter and gas density and is proportional to the square of the gas velocity. The effect of gas density on turbulent flow has both therapeutic implications. Children with viral laryngotracheobronchitis have marked narrowing of the subglottic area, which greatly increases the resistance to airflow. The pressure required to overcome this increased resistance in the large airways, and hence the work of breathing, can be decreased by administering a low-density gas mixture (70% helium, 30% oxygen).

Measurement of Resistance

Resistance (R) is calculated from the equation

$$R = \frac{\text{driving pressure}}{\text{airflow}}$$

The pressure is measured at the two ends of the system—in the case of the lung, at the mouth and at the alveoli—and the corresponding flow is recorded. Measurement of alveolar pressure presents the greatest problem. Several methods have been used to measure alveolar pressure. The most common method employs a body plethysmograph. The subject sits in the airtight box and breathes through a tube connected to a pneumotachometer, an apparatus that measures airflow. When a shutter occludes the tube and airflow ceases, the mouth pressure is assumed to be equal to the alveolar pressure. Airway resistance can then be calculated because airflow, alveolar pressure, and ambient pressure are known.

Total pulmonary resistance can be measured in infants and children by the forced oscillation technique. This measurement includes airway resistance plus the tissue viscous resistance of the lung and chest wall. Nasal resistance is also included in the measurement if the infant is breathing through the nose. Although there are theoretical objections to this technique, it has several advantages. It does not require a body plethysmograph, estimates of pleural pressure, or patient cooperation, and it can be done quickly enough to be used on ill patients. A sinusoidal pressure applied at the upper airway changes the airflow, and the ratio of pressure change to flow change is used to calculate resistance. When the forced oscillations are applied at the so-called resonant frequency of the lung (believed to be 3 to 5 Hz), it is assumed that the force required to overcome elastic resistance of the lung and the force required to overcome inertance are equal and opposite, so that all of the force is dissipated in overcoming flow resistance. This technique has demonstrated that infants with bronchiolitis have about a twofold increase in inspiratory pulmonary resistance and a threefold increase in expiratory resistance.

Several new techniques have been developed that are capable of measuring lung function in infants and young children. Each has its advantages, underlying assumptions, and limitations, and these techniques are discussed in detail in Chapter 9.

Sites of Airway Resistance

The contribution of the upper airway to total airway resistance is substantial. The average nasal resistance of infants by indirect measurements is 13 cm H_2O/L/sec, or nearly half of the total respiratory resistance, as is the case in adults. It is hardly surprising that any compromise of the dimensions of the nasal airways in an infant who is a preferential nose breather will result in retractions and labored breathing. Likewise, even mild edema of the trachea or larynx will impose a significant increase in airway resistance.

In the adult lung, about 80% of the resistance to airflow resides in airways greater than 2 mm in diameter. The vast number of small peripheral airways provides a large cross-sectional area for flow and therefore contributes less than 20% to the airway resistance. Thus, these airways may be the sites of disease that may severely impair ventilation of distal airspaces without appreciably altering the total airway resistance. In the infant lung, however, small peripheral airways may contribute as much as 50% of the total airway resistance, and this proportion does not decrease until about 5 years of age. Thus, the infant and young child are particularly severely affected by diseases that affect the small airways (e.g., bronchiolitis).

Factors Affecting Airway Resistance

Airway resistance is determined by the diameter of the airways, the velocity of airflow, and the physical properties of the gas breathed. The diameter is determined by the balance between the forces tending to narrow the airways and the forces tending to widen them. One of the forces tending to narrow the airways is exerted by the contraction of bronchial smooth muscle. The neural regulation of bronchial smooth muscle tone is mediated by efferent impulses through autonomic nerves. Sympathetic impulses relax the airways, and the parasympathetic impulses constrict them. Bronchi constrict reflexly from irritating inhalants such as sulfur dioxide and some dusts; by arterial hypoxemia and hypercapnia; by embolization of the vessels; by cold; and by some vasoactive mediators, such as acetylcholine, histamine, and bradykinin. They dilate in response to an increase in systemic blood pressure through baroreceptors in the carotid sinus and to sympathomimetic agents such as isoproterenol and epinephrine. The large airways are probably in tonic contraction in health, because in unanesthetized adults, atropine or isoproterenol will decrease airway resistance.

Airway resistance changes with lung volume, but not in a linear manner. Increasing the lung volume to above FRC only minimally decreases airway resistance. In contrast, as lung volume decreases from FRC, resistance rises dramatically and approaches infinity at RV. Although alterations in bronchomotor tone play a role, it is the decrease in lung elastic recoil as lung volume declines that is the predominant mechanism for the change in airway resistance. The recoil of the lung provides a tethering or "guy wire" effect on the airways that tends to increase their diameter. Children of different ages will have different airway resistances owing to the different sizes of their lungs. Therefore, the measurement of airway resistance or its reciprocal, airway conductance, is usually corrected by dividing the airway conductance by the simultaneously measured lung volume.

The resultant specific airway conductance is remarkably constant regardless of the subject's age or height.

Dynamic Airway Compression

During a forced expiration, both the pleural and the peribronchial pressures become positive and tend to narrow the airways; forces tending to keep airways open are the intraluminal pressure and the tethering action of the surrounding lung. During active expiration, however, the intraluminal pressure must decrease along the pathway of airflow from the alveoli to the mouth, where it becomes equal to atmospheric pressure. Therefore, at some point in the airway, intraluminal pressure must equal pleural pressure—the equal pressure point (EPP) (see Chapter 10 and Fig. 10-6). Downstream from the EPP, pleural pressure exceeds intraluminal pressure and thus is a force that tends to narrow the airways. Indeed, during periods of maximum expiratory flow, pleural pressure exceeds the critical closing pressure of the airways, which become narrowed to slits. Despite the cartilaginous support of the larger airways, the membranous portion of the wall of the trachea and large bronchi invaginates under pressure to occlude the airways. Maximum flow under this circumstance is therefore determined by the resistance of the airways located upstream from the EPP, and the driving pressure is the difference between the alveolar pressure and the pressure at the EPP. In disease states in which there is an increased airway resistance, the EPP moves toward the alveoli because of the greater intraluminal pressure drop. Thus, small airways are now compressed during forced expiration with severe flow limitation. With the measurement of pressure-flow and flow-volume curves during forced expiration, it is possible to calculate resistance upstream and downstream from the point of critical closure, or EPP. Increasing the lung volume increases the tethering action of the surrounding lung on the airways, and therefore close attention must be paid to the lung volume at which resistance measurements are made during these studies.

Work of Breathing

The work performed by the respiratory pump is defined by the volume changes of the lungs when the respiratory muscles generate a given pressure. The volume-pressure relationships of the respiratory system depend on properties of the lung and chest wall tissues or the ease with which the airways allow the passage of air. A substantial portion of the pressure generated by the respiratory muscles is applied to produce reversible rearrangements of the structure of the alveolar gas-liquid interface and the fibrous network of the lungs. Another large portion of the effort of the respiratory muscles is directed at producing rearrangements or interactions that are not reversible. The energy spent in such an effort is directly transformed into heat, which is then dissipated into the atmosphere or carried away by the circulating blood. The magnitudes of the work and the pressures derived from these processes generally bear a relationship to the rate of gas flow in and out of the lungs. In this regard, the respiratory system exhibits a resistive behavior for which the driving pressure determines the flow of air. Both the elastic and the resistive components of the work of breathing are usually increased in children with respiratory disease. Establishing a diagnosis and formulating a therapy in these patients is almost always simplified when the clinician distinguishes between conditions that affect primarily the elastic (restrictive respiratory disease) and resistive (obstructive respiratory disease) behaviors of the respiratory system.

DISTRIBUTION OF VENTILATION

The distribution of ventilation will be influenced by several factors of normal lungs. The pleural pressure gradient results in a greater amount of the tidal volume going to the dependent areas of the lung (see Fig. 4-12). In addition, the rate at which an area of the lung fills and empties is related to both airway resistance and compliance. A decrease in airway dimension increases the time required for air to reach the alveoli; a region of low compliance receives less ventilation per unit of time than an area with high compliance. The product of resistance × compliance (time constant) is approximately the same in health for all ventilatory pathways. The unit of this product is time. Note:

$$\text{Resistance} = \frac{\text{pressure}}{\text{flow}} = \frac{\text{cm H}_2\text{O}}{\text{L/sec}}$$

and

$$\text{Compliance} = \frac{\Delta\text{volume (L)}}{\Delta\text{pressure (cm H}_2\text{O)}}$$

The product, then, is a unit of time, analogous to the time constant in an electrical system, that represents the time taken to accomplish 63% of the volume change.

As mentioned previously, peripheral airways contribute little to overall airway resistance after the age of 5 years. However, in the presence of small airway disease, some areas of the lung have long time constants but those of others are normal. This is particularly evident as the frequency of respiration increases. With increasing frequency, air goes to those areas of the lung with short time constants. These areas then become relatively overdistended, and a greater transpulmonary pressure is required to inspire the same volume of air because alveoli in these relatively normal areas are reaching their elastic limit. Thus, a decreased dynamic compliance with increasing frequency of respiration has been used as a test of small airway disease and indeed may be the only mechanical abnormality detectable in the early stages of diseases such as emphysema and cystic fibrosis.

Airway closure occurs in dependent areas of the lung at low lung volumes. The lung volume above RV at which closure occurs is called the closing volume. In infants, very young children, and older adults, airway closure occurs at FRC and therefore is present during normal tidal breathing. This results in intermittent inadequate ventilation of the respective terminal lung units and leads to abnormal gas exchange, notably to a lower Pa_{O_2} seen in these age groups. It also explains why oxygenation usually can be improved by placing the patient so that the good lung is uppermost in the infant with unilateral lung disease (in young healthy adults the opposite is true).

PULMONARY CIRCULATION

PHYSIOLOGIC CLASSIFICATION OF PULMONARY VESSELS

The pulmonary circulation is the only vascular bed to receive the entire cardiac output. This unique characteristic enables the pulmonary vascular bed to perform a wide variety of homeostatic physiologic functions. It provides an enormously large (80 m^2) yet extremely thin film of blood for gas exchange, filters the circulating blood, controls the circulating concentrations of many vasoactive substances, and provides a large surface area for the absorption of lung liquid at birth. The nomenclature of the pulmonary vessels is at times confusing because the anatomic classification of the vessels often does not correspond to their physiologic role.

Pulmonary vessels have been classified physiologically as extra-alveolar and alveolar vessels, fluid-exchanging vessels, and gas-exchanging vessels. When the outside of a vessel is exposed to alveolar pressure, it is classified as an alveolar vessel (capillaries within the middle of the alveolar septum), whereas extra-alveolar vessels (arteries, veins, and capillaries at the corner of alveolar septa) are intrapulmonary vessels that are subjected to a more negative pressure resulting from and approximating pleural pressure. The diameter of the extra-alveolar vessels is therefore greatly affected by lung volume, expanding as inspiration occurs. Although extra-alveolar vessels and alveolar vessels are subjected to different mechanical pressures, they are both classified as fluid-exchanging vessels because both leak water and protein and both can contribute to the production of pulmonary edema. The anatomic location of gas-exchanging vessels is unclear but is likely limited to the capillaries and smallest arterioles and venules.

PULMONARY VASCULAR PRESSURES

The pressure within the pulmonary circulation is remarkably low, considering that it receives the entire cardiac output (5 L/min in the adult human). Beginning a few months after birth, pulmonary arterial pressures are constant throughout life, with the average mean pulmonary arterial pressure being 15 mm Hg and the systolic and diastolic pressures being 22 and 8 mm Hg, respectively. The pulmonary venous pressure is minimally higher than the left atrial pressure, which averages 5 mm Hg. The pressure within human lung capillaries is unknown, but work in isolated dog lungs suggests it is 8 to 10 mm Hg, approximately halfway between the mean arterial and venous pressures. These values refer to pressures at the level of the heart in the supine position; because of gravity, pulmonary arterial pressures will be near zero at the apex of the upright adult lung and close to 25 mm Hg at the base. Depending on their location, vessels have different pressures on their outside walls. As defined previously, the alveolar vessels are exposed to alveolar pressure, which fluctuates during the respiratory cycle but will average out close to zero. In contrast, the extra-alveolar vessels are exposed to a negative fluid pressure on their outer walls, estimated to be between −6 and −9 cm H_2O. The pressure on the outside of the pulmonary vessel is not a trivial matter, because the transmural pressure (inside pressure–outside pressure), rather than the intravascular pressure, is the pertinent hydrostatic pressure influencing vascular distention and the transvascular movement of water and protein.

PULMONARY VASCULAR RESISTANCE

The resistance to blood flow through the lungs can be calculated by dividing the pressure across the lungs by the pulmonary blood flow.

$$R = \frac{\text{mean PA pressure} - \text{mean LA pressure}}{\text{pulmonary blood flow}}$$

A decrease in resistance to blood flow can occur only through (1) an increase in the blood vessels' diameters or (2) an increase in the number of perfused vessels, that is, an increase in the cross-sectional diameter of the pulmonary vascular bed. The diameter of an already open pulmonary vessel can be increased by decreasing the muscular tone of the vessel wall (e.g., with a vasodilating agent) or by increasing the transmural pressure (e.g., through increased pulmonary arterial or left atrial pressure). Previously unperfused pulmonary vessels may be opened up ("recruited") when their transmural pressure exceeds their critical opening pressure. This occurs when intravascular pressures are raised or when a vasodilator has decreased the vessels' critical opening pressure. An increase in cardiac output decreases the calculated pulmonary vascular resistance (PVR). This is important to remember when assessing vasodilating drugs; studies have been performed in which drugs were found to increase cardiac output substantially and to increase pulmonary arterial pressures minimally so that the calculated PVR falls. This permissive fall in resistance does not ensure that a particular drug has any direct vasodilating action at all, because the entire fall in PVR may have resulted from its cardiac effects.

The interrelationship between lung volume and PVR is complex and is influenced by pulmonary blood volume, cardiac output, and initial lung volume. The principal reason for this complex relationship is that a change in lung volume has opposite effects on the resistances of the extra-alveolar and alveolar vessels. As the lung is inflated, the radial traction on the extra-alveolar vessels increases their diameter, whereas the same rise in lung volume increases the resistance to flow through the alveolar vessels (which constitutes 35% to 50% of the total PVR). It is reasonable to say, however, that PVR is at its minimum at FRC, and any change in lung volume (increase or decrease) will increase the PVR (Fig. 4-13).

Active changes in the PVR can be mediated by neurogenic stimuli, vasoactive compounds, or chemical mediators. The normal adult pulmonary circulation appears to be maximally dilated, since no stimulus has been found that can further dilate the pulmonary vessels. In contrast, the neonatal lung or the vasoconstricted adult lung vasodilates in response to a variety of

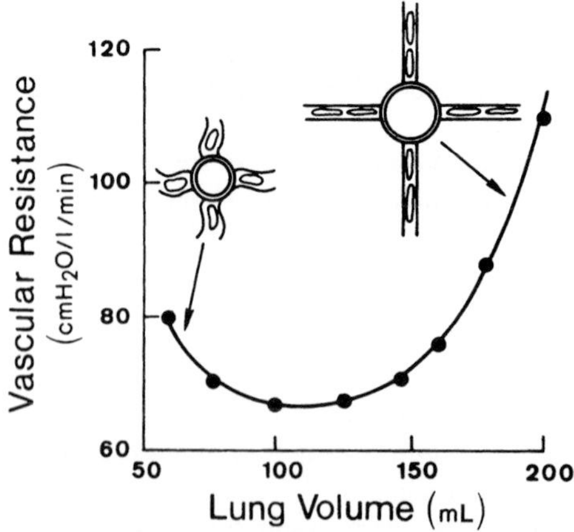

FIGURE 4-13. Effect of lung volume on pulmonary vascular resistance when the transmural pressure of the capillaries is held constant. At low lung volumes, resistance is high because the extra-alveolar vessels become narrow. At high volumes, the capillaries are stretched, and their caliber is reduced. (From West JB: Respiratory Physiology—the Essentials. Baltimore: Williams & Wilkins, 1974.)

agents, including nitric oxide, acetylcholine, β-agonist drugs, bradykinin, prostaglandin E, and prostacyclin.

The pulmonary circulation can undergo significant vasoconstriction, which is surprising in view of the paucity of muscle in the postnatal lung vessels. Hypoxia is the most common potent pulmonary vasoconstricting agent. Hypoxic vasoconstriction, which occurs when the alveolar PO_2 falls below 50 to 60 mm Hg, is a local response independent of neurohumoral stimuli. Although many suggestions have been made, the exact mechanism of hypoxia-induced vasoconstriction is unknown. Acidosis acts synergistically with hypoxia to constrict the pulmonary vessels; however, it is unlikely that CO_2 alone has any direct effect on the pulmonary circulation in humans. Stimulation of the pulmonary sympathetic nerves results in a weak vasoconstrictive response in the dog lung but little or no response in the normal human adult pulmonary circulation. Vasoactive substances such as histamine, fibrinopeptides, prostaglandins of the F series, and leukotrienes are capable of constricting the pulmonary vascular bed. It had been believed that vasoconstriction in the pulmonary circulation took place predominantly, if not exclusively, within the arterial section of the vascular bed. It has been demonstrated that other regions of the bed may narrow in response to stimuli. For example, hypoxia can constrict the pulmonary venules of newborn animals and might increase resistance within the capillary bed by inducing constriction of Kapanci cells that are located within the interstitium of the alveolar-capillary membrane. The fetal and neonatal pulmonary circulation contains a large amount of smooth muscle, which enhances the response to vasoconstrictive stimuli.

DISTRIBUTION OF BLOOD FLOW

Blood flow is uneven within the normal lung and is influenced by the vascular branching pattern and gravity which results in more blood flow being directed to the dorsal caudal regions and less to the cephalad regions. Gravitational forces are largely responsible for the increasing flow from apex to base because the intravascular pressure of a given blood vessel is determined by the pulmonary arterial pressure immediately above the pulmonary valve and the blood vessel's vertical distance from the pulmonary valve. Thus, with increasing height above the heart, the pulmonary arterial pressure decreases and less perfusion occurs. The opposite occurs for vessels located in the lung bases, and together these gravitational effects are responsible for a pressure difference of 23 mm Hg between apical and basal pulmonary arteries.

These regional differences in lung perfusion are best understood in terms of West's zones of perfusion (Fig. 4-14). West's zone I occurs when mean pulmonary arterial pressure is less than or equal to alveolar pressure, and as a result no blood flow occurs (except perhaps during systole). Zone I conditions are present in the apices of some upright adults and result in unperfused yet ventilated lung units (alveolar dead space). Moving down from the lung apices, pulmonary arterial pressure becomes greater than alveolar pressure, with the latter being greater than venous pressure. These are zone II conditions, and blood flow is determined by the difference between arterial and alveolar pressures and is not influenced by venous pressure; an appropriate analogy would be that of a vascular "waterfall," in which the flow rate is independent of the height of the falls. In zone III, left atrial pressure exceeds alveolar pressure, and flow is determined in the usual manner (i.e., by the arterial-venous pressure gradient).

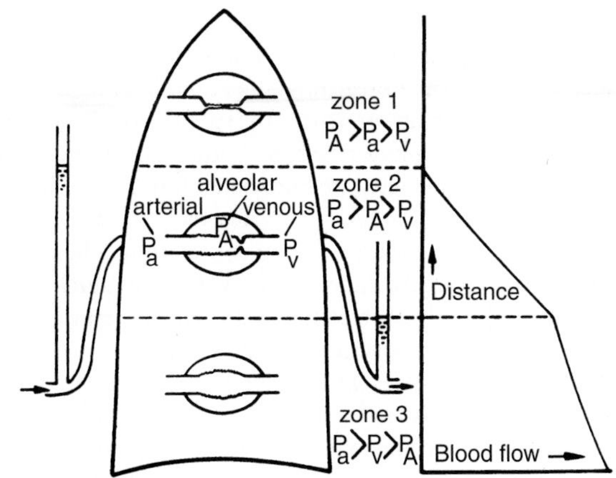

FIGURE 4-14. Model to explain the uneven distribution of blood flow in the lung based on the pressures affecting the capillaries. (From West JB, Dollery CT, Naimark A: Distribution of blood flow in isolated lung. Relation to vascular and alveolar pressures. J Appl Physiol 1964;19:713.)

METHODS OF EVALUATING THE PULMONARY CIRCULATION

The chest radiograph remains the most widely used tool for determining the possible presence of pulmonary vascular disease. Prominence of the pulmonary outflow tract and increased or decreased vascular markings may be noted radiographically. Regional pulmonary angiography further delineates localized disturbance in blood flow, although the procedure requires cardiac catheterization. Direct measurements of pulmonary artery and "wedge" pressures add further information. Occasionally, drugs can be infused into the pulmonary artery to evaluate the potential reversibility of pulmonary hypertension.

Noninvasive quantitative assessments of the pulmonary circulation are now available. Echocardiography is able not only to assess the structure and function of the right ventricle but also to provide a reasonable estimate of right ventricular pressure by assessing the small retrograde flow through the tricuspid valve that frequently occurs in significant pulmonary hypertension. Quantitative assessment of regional pulmonary blood flow can be made with intravenous injections of macroaggregates of albumin labeled with technetium 99m. The macroaggregates occlude a very small portion of the pulmonary vascular bed. The amount of regional blood flow can be determined by imaging the lungs with a large-field-of-view gamma camera and determining the count rate with a computer. The perfusion lung scintigram can be combined with a ventilation scintigram performed with either a radioactive gas (e.g., xenon 133 or krypton 81m) or a radiolabeled (^{99m}Tc–diethylenetriamine-pentacetic acid) aerosol that is distributed like a gas.

MUSCLES OF RESPIRATION

The importance of the muscles of respiration derives from the fact that these muscles, like the myocardium, can fail under abnormal circumstances and can induce or contribute to an impending or existing ventilatory failure. Although respiratory muscle fatigue has been suspected by clinicians at the bedside for a long time, it was only later demonstrated in human adults and newborn infants.

The principal muscle of respiration is the diaphragm, a thin musculotendinous sheet that separates the thoracic from the abdominal cavity. In adults its contraction causes descent of its dome and aids in elevation of the lower ribs. If the airway is occluded during normal breathing, the adult diaphragm is capable of generating airway pressures up to 150 to 200 cm H_2O during a maximal inspiratory effort. Some work indicates that the diaphragm has two separate but related functions. The costal part of the diaphragm (largely innervated by C5) acts to stabilize and elevate the lower rib cage during contraction. The vertebral (crural) portion (largely innervated by C3), a much thicker muscle, descends with contraction and is largely responsible for the volume change that occurs.

Other skeletal muscles located in the chest or abdominal wall, such as the intercostals, scalenes, and abdominal muscles, can play an important role in ventilation. During normal breathing, most of the accessory muscles are silent. However, during abnormal conditions or disease states, these muscles are recruited to stabilize the chest or abdominal wall so that the diaphragm may be more efficient. In addition, it has been demonstrated that the external intercostal muscles contract in acute asthmatic attacks not only during inspiration but also during expiration; this contraction maintains a higher lung volume and hence increases airway diameter. When airways are occluded during inspiration, abdominal muscles contract powerfully during expiration, pushing the abdominal contents and diaphragm toward the thoracic cavity. This action lengthens diaphragmatic fibers and enhances the capability of the diaphragm to generate force during the subsequent inspiration (length-tension curve).

The upper airways must be kept patent during inspiration, and therefore the pharyngeal wall muscles, genioglossus, and arytenoid muscles are properly considered muscles of respiration. There is an increase in neural output to these muscles immediately before diaphragmatic contraction during inspiration. The newborn also contracts these muscles during expiration to provide an expiratory outflow resistance and thus keeps end-expiratory volume greater than the FRC.

Respiratory muscles, whether the diaphragm, upper airway, intercostal, or abdominal muscles, are not homogeneous muscles in terms of their cellular structure, blood supply, metabolism, and recruitment patterns. Adult mature skeletal muscles have a mixture of fibers, and respiratory muscles are no different. The adult diaphragm, for instance, is made of fast- and slow-twitch fibers. Slow-twitch fibers are oxidative, and fast-twitch fibers are either glycolytic or moderately oxidative. Slow-twitch fibers are fatigue resistant—they are recruited first during a motor act; they generate low tensions; and they usually have a higher capillary/fiber ratio than fast fibers. Fast-twitch fibers can be either fatigue resistant (fast, moderately oxidative) or fast fatiguing (fast glycolytic); they are recruited during motor acts that require large force output. Thus, during normal quiet breathing, it is presumed that only the slow-twitch fibers in the diaphragm are active. In contrast, at the height of an acute attack of croup, asthma, or bronchiolitis during which muscle contractions are strong, both fiber types can be active, with the fast fibers generating the bulk of the force.

Muscle fiber composition, innervation, and metabolism are different in early life. The process of muscle fiber differentiation and interaction with the central nervous system is a continuous process, starting in utero and continuing postnatally. For example, slow oxidative fibers increase in utero and postnatally, whereas fast glycolytic fibers decrease postnatally. Polyneuronal innervation transforms into one motoneuron = one muscle fiber—the adult type of innervation—postnatally. Whether the young infant's ability to resist muscle fatigue is jeopardized by premature muscle fiber composition, innervation, and metabolism is not known and deserves further investigation.

Many factors predispose respiratory muscles to fatigue. Factors that increase fuel consumption (e.g., increased loads with disease); limit fuel reserves (e.g., malnutrition); alter acid-base homeostasis (e.g., acidosis); modify the oxidative capacity, glycolytic capacity, or both of the muscle (e.g., decreased activity of the muscle and possible atrophy after prolonged artificial ventilation); and decrease the oxygen availability to the muscle (e.g., anemia, low cardiac output states, hypoxemia) all predispose the diaphragm to failure. Reactive oxygen species (free radicals) produced by the contracting diaphragm are also thought to play a role in causing fatigue, particularly in conditions of ischemia/reperfusion and sepsis. In addition, changes in the external milieu of the muscle cell such as low phosphate levels or the presence of certain drugs (e.g., anesthetics) can limit the contractile ability and lead to premature muscle fatigue.

Diaphragmatic muscle function can be assessed clinically by observing the movements of the abdominal wall. During normal inspiration and with the contraction of the diaphragm, the abdominal contents are pushed away from the thorax. Because the abdominal wall is normally compliant during inspiration, the abdominal wall moves out to accommodate the increased pressure from the contracting diaphragm. With diaphragmatic fatigue, weakness, or paralysis, it is possible to observe an inward motion of the abdominal wall. Through the action of other respiratory muscles (intercostals), a drop in pressure occurs in the thorax during inspiration. Because of the "passive" behavior of the fatigued diaphragm, this pressure drop is transmitted to the abdomen, hence the movement of the abdominal contents toward the thoracic cavity.

The highly compliant chest wall in the newborn infant limits its expansion during inspiration. The chest wall becomes even more unstable during REM sleep, when intercostal muscle activity is inhibited and the rib cage is more prone to distortion. This creates an added load and the potential for diaphragmatic fatigue. In the laboratory, respiratory muscle function can be assessed using a number of techniques and tests, some more direct than others. Maximum airway pressure and fluoroscopic evaluation of the diaphragm are less invasive but may have less resolution than transdiaphragmatic pressure (Pdi, measured using balloon catheters across the diaphragm). Both the Pdi and electromyographic measurements can be useful in assessing change of muscle function over time, for example, when fatigue is suspected or after extubation and assisted ventilation.

To consider the main respiratory muscles—the diaphragm and the intercostal muscles—as the only respiratory muscles for breathing is insufficient, especially during stressful conditions or disease states. A number of muscles, such as the alae nasi, pharyngeal wall muscles, genioglossus, posterior cricoarytenoid, and thyroarytenoid, can play major roles in airway patency and hence in ventilatory output. Data indicate that upper airway muscles are strongly recruited during obstructive disease or during inspiratory occlusion, and that blood flow increases considerably to some of them (e.g., genioglossus). How prone these muscles are to fatigue under increased loads is unknown. How different these muscles are in terms of their structure, metabolism, and function in the neonate versus the adult is unclear and needs further research.

Because of the number of muscles involved, their location, and their function, the coordination of respiratory muscles becomes increasingly complex. The motor act of respiration should no longer be viewed as the result of one or two muscles contracting during inspiration and relaxing during expiration. At rest and even more so during disease states, the active coordination of various muscles becomes functionally very important. Defecation, sucking, and talking all involve the activation of several muscles that are shared by the respiratory apparatus for generating adequate ventilation. In some cases, obstructive apneas can actually be the result of muscle incoordination, with the diaphragm contracting when upper airway muscles that normally hold the airway open are relaxed.

GAS EXCHANGE

The vital process of gas exchange occurs in the terminal respiratory unit. The previous sections of this chapter deal with the problems of moving air and blood to and from these gas-exchanging units. This section focuses on the fate of gas once it is introduced into the lungs, how it is transferred from the alveolar space to the bloodstream, and how ventilation and perfusion are matched.

In Figure 4-15 the partial pressures of oxygen and carbon dioxide are depicted at various stages of the pathway from ambient air to the tissues. Because nitrogen is inert, changes in its partial pressure (PN_2) in the gas phase depend on changes in the partial pressures of oxygen and carbon dioxide, gases that are utilized and excreted, respectively. In contrast, PN_2 in blood and tissue is identical because nitrogen is inert. The rather complex influences of dead space, alveolar ventilation, ventilation-perfusion relationships, and tissue metabolism on the partial pressures of oxygen and carbon dioxide are discussed in some detail, and frequent reference to Figure 4-15 is useful in clarifying some of the concepts.

ALVEOLAR VENTILATION

The tidal volume (VT) consists of a portion that is in the conducting airways called the anatomic dead space, VD (consisting

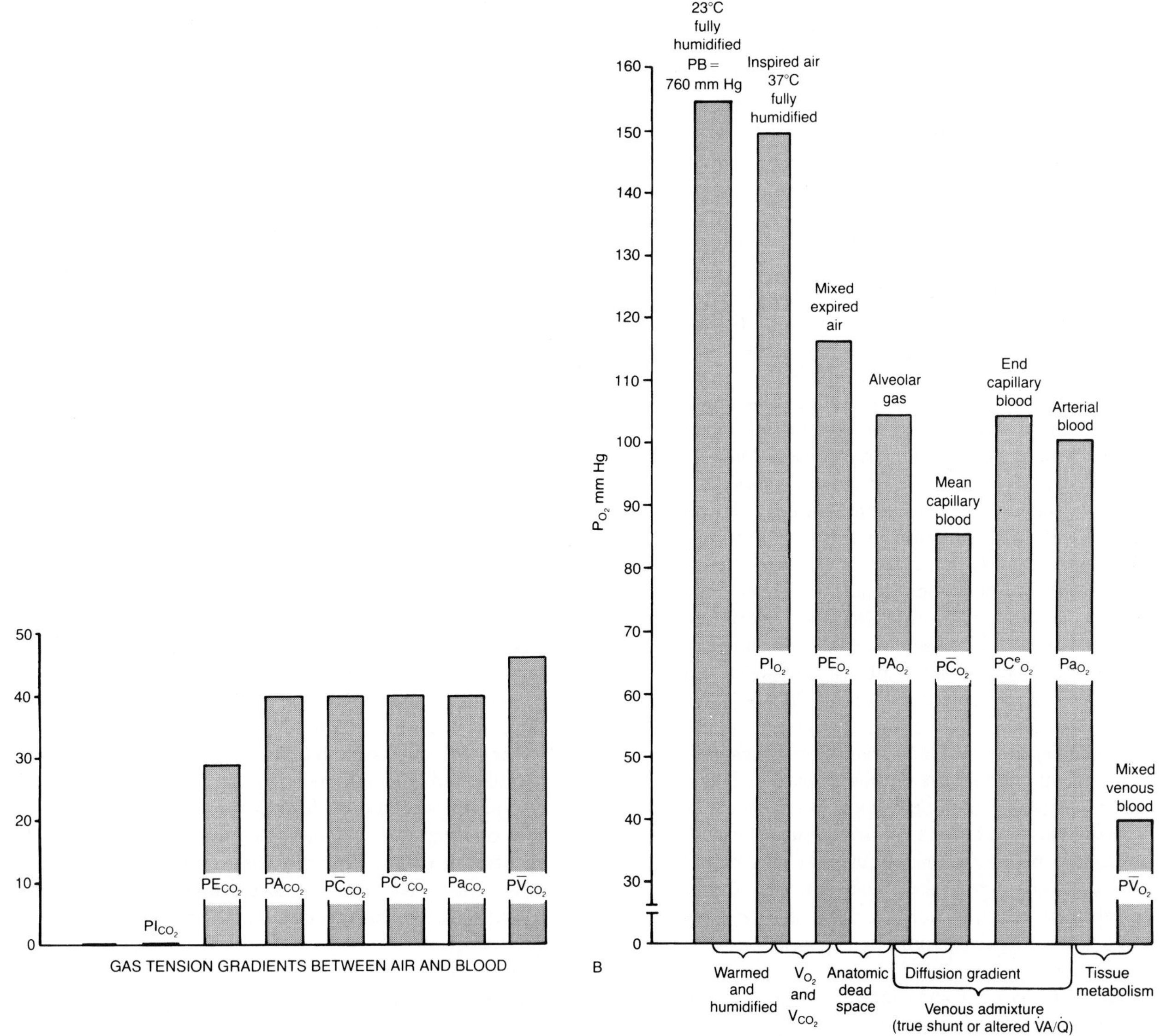

■ **FIGURE 4-15.** **A** and **B**, Partial pressures of oxygen and carbon dioxide in different portions of the airway and blood.

of the nose, mouth, pharynx, larynx, trachea, bronchi, and bronchioles), where no significant exchange of oxygen and carbon dioxide with blood takes place. A portion undergoes gas exchange in the alveoli (VA). Alveolar ventilation per minute is measured by the following equation:

$$V_A = V_T - V_D$$

In practice, VD is difficult to measure, so the alveolar ventilation equation is used. Since all expired CO_2 comes from the alveolar gas,

$$V_{CO_2} = V_A \times \%CO_2/100 \text{ or}$$

$$V_A = V_{CO_2} \times 100 \,/\, \%CO_2$$

The $\%CO_2/100$ is the fractional concentration of CO_2 in the alveolar gas (F_{ACO_2}), which can be measure by a rapid CO_2 analyzer. F_{ACO_2} can be converted to partial pressure of CO_2 by multiplying by, $P_B - 47$ mm Hg. Thus,

$$V_A = V_{CO_2} \,/\, P_{ACO_2}$$

In normal subjects the P_{CO_2} in alveolar gas (P_{ACO_2}) is the same as the arterial P_{CO_2} (P_{aCO_2}), which can be used to determine alveolar ventilation. Note the important relationship between alveolar ventilation and P_{aCO_2}. When VA is halved, then P_{aCO_2} must double at a constant V_{CO_2}; when VA is doubled, P_{aCO_2} is halved at a constant V_{CO_2}.

DEAD SPACE

The volume of the conducting airways is called the anatomic dead space (VDanat) and is filled by about 25% of each tidal volume (VT). Anatomic dead space in milliliters is roughly equal to the weight of the subject in pounds (for a 7-pound baby, 7 or 8 mL; for an adult, 150 mL) and is normally less than 30% of VT. In the normal premature infant, anatomic dead space is slightly higher than 30%. In practice, anatomic dead space is seldom measured but may be obtained by Fowler's method, which requires that a single breath of oxygen be inspired. On expiration, both the volume of expired gas and the percentage of nitrogen are measured. The first portion of the expired gas comes from the dead space and contains little or no nitrogen. As the breath is expired, the percentage of nitrogen increases until it "plateaus" at the alveolar concentration. By assuming that all the initial part of the breath comes from the anatomic dead space and all the latter portion from the alveoli, the anatomic dead space can be calculated. The same measurements can be made by monitoring the expired carbon dioxide concentration. In practice, anatomic dead space is difficult to define accurately, because it depends on lung volume (greater at large lung volumes when the airways are more distended) and on body position (smaller in supine position).

Physiologic dead space may be measured by making use of the argument originally developed by Bohr. Since all of the expired CO_2 (F_{ECO_2}) comes from the alveolar gas (F_{ACO_2}) and none from the dead space,

$$V_T \times F_{ECO_2} = V_A \times F_{ACO_2}$$

And since $V_A = V_T - V_D$, then

$$V_T \times F_{ECO_2} = (V_T - V_D) \times F_{ACO_2}$$

and

$$V_D/V_T = F_{ACO_2} - F_{ECO_2}/F_{ACO_2}$$

And since the partial pressure of a gas is proportional to its fractioned concentration (F),

$$V_D/V_T = P_{ACO_2} - P_{ECO_2}/P_{ACO_2} \text{ (Bohr equation)}$$

Or, since alveolar P_{CO_2} and arterial P_{CO_2} are identical in normal subjects,

$$V_D/V_T = P_{aCO_2} - P_{ECO_2}/P_{aCO_2}$$

It is now quite clear that VDphys must be defined according to the gas being measured. Because oxygen is more diffusible in the gas phase than is carbon dioxide, physiologic dead space using oxygen or various inert gases is different from the CO_2 dead space. However, VDphys measurements using CO_2 are helpful in assessing patients because they do reflect the portion of each breath that participates in gas exchange, particularly with respect to CO_2. An elevated VDphys indicates that areas of the lung are being underventilated in relationship to the amount of blood flowing through the region.

From the foregoing discussion, it is apparent that a VT must be chosen that will allow adequate alveolar ventilation. For example, an adult might breathe 60 times per minute with a VT of 100 mL for a minute ventilation of 6 L. Nevertheless, alveolar ventilation under these circumstances may be inadequate, because primarily the dead space is ventilated. In selecting suitable volumes and rates for patients on respirators, it is useful to approximate normal values and to consider adequate alveolar ventilation rather than total ventilation. A discussion of high-frequency ventilation is beyond the scope of this chapter.

Alveolar Ventilation and Alveolar Gases

The amount of alveolar ventilation per minute must be adequate to keep the alveolar P_{O_2} and P_{CO_2} at values that will promote the escape of carbon dioxide from venous blood and the uptake of oxygen by pulmonary capillary blood. In health at sea level, this means that P_{AO_2} is approximately 105 to 110 mm Hg and P_{ACO_2} is 40 mm Hg (Fig. 4-16).

Arterial P_{O_2} is markedly affected by the presence of right-to-left shunts, and therefore it is not a good measurement of the adequacy of pulmonary ventilation. P_{aCO_2} is minimally affected in the presence of shunts because $P_{\overline{v}CO_2}$ is 46 mm Hg and P_{aCO_2} is 40 mm Hg. If one third of the cardiac output is shunted, this raises P_{aCO_2} to only 42 mm Hg. Thus, the arterial P_{CO_2} is the optimum measurement of the adequacy of alveolar ventilation. When alveolar ventilation halves, P_{aCO_2} doubles; when alveolar ventilation doubles, P_{aCO_2} halves. Hyperventilation is defined as a P_{aCO_2} less than 35 mm Hg, and hypoventilation as a P_{aCO_2} greater than 45 mm Hg. Some of the causes of hypoventilation are listed in Box 4-1.

Inspired air has a fraction of inspired oxygen (F_{IO_2}) of 0.2093, and it is "diluted" in the alveoli by the FRC of air containing carbon dioxide and water vapor, so the partial pressure of oxygen in alveolar gas must be less than that of the inspired air (P_{IO_2}; see earlier discussion of Dalton's law). P_{AO_2} must be calculated from the alveolar air equation. When oxygen consumption equals carbon dioxide production, then,

$$P_{AO_2} = P_{IO_2} - P_{ACO_2}$$

$$P_{IO_2} = 0.2093 \times (P_B - 47 \text{ mm Hg}) = 150 \text{ mm Hg}$$

If P_{ACO_2} is 40 mm Hg, then P_{AO_2} is 110 mm Hg. Usually, the respiratory exchange ratio (R) is 0.8, or more oxygen is consumed than carbon dioxide eliminated, thereby decreasing

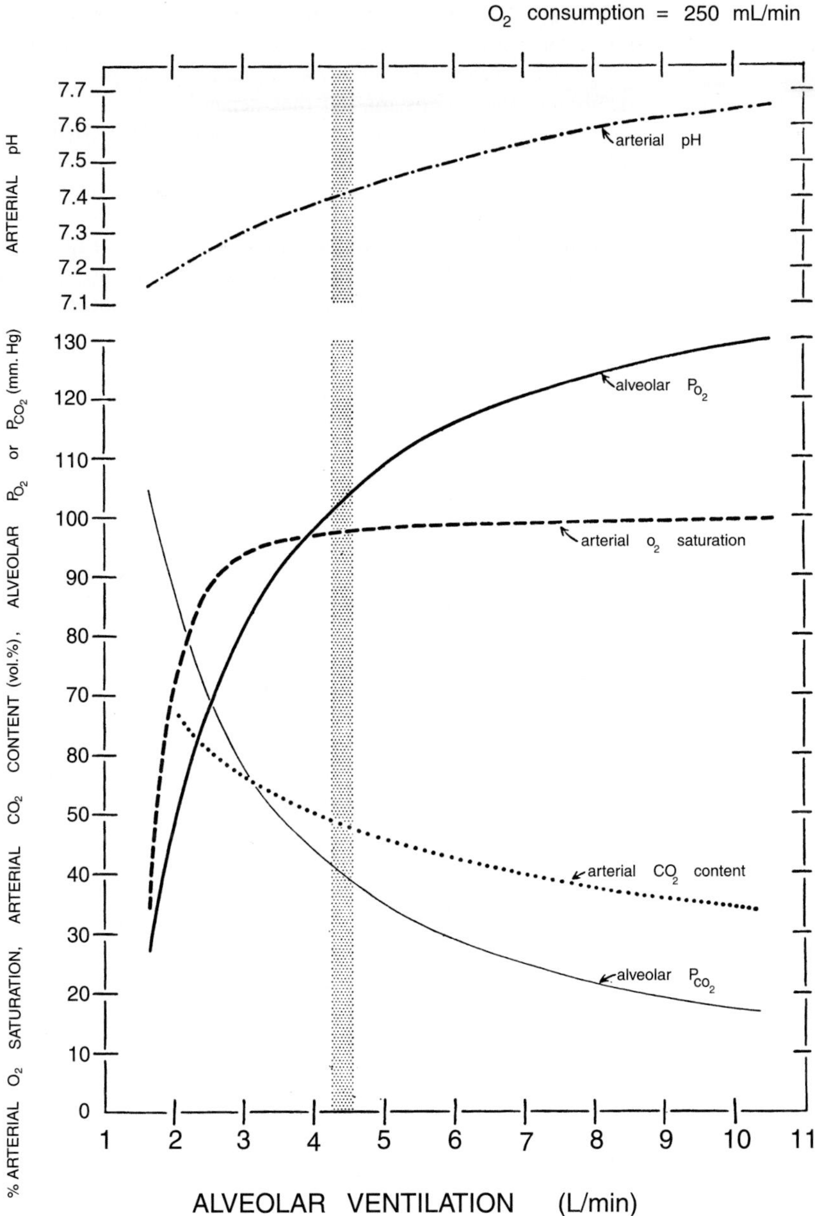

FIGURE 4-16. The effect of changing alveolar ventilation on alveolar gas and arterial blood oxygen, carbon dioxide, and pH. (From Comroe JH Jr, Forster RE II, Dubois AB, et al: The Lung, 2nd ed. Chicago: Year Book Medical, 1962.)

PAO_2 slightly more than would be expected from the dilution of $PACO_2$. To account for changes in R, a useful form of the alveolar air equation for clinical purposes is

$$PAO_2 = PIO_2 - \frac{PACO_2}{R}$$

When $PACO_2$ is 40 and R is 0.8, PAO_2 is 100 mm Hg. Note that breathing 40% oxygen raises PAO_2 to 235 mm Hg because FIO_2 is now 0.40. Note that this equation is less accurate during oxygen breathing when more arduous forms of the alveolar air equation may be used. However, this inaccuracy is seldom of importance in the clinical setting.

Because the partial pressures of alveolar gases must always equal the same total pressure, any increase in one must be associated with a decrease in the other. For example, If $PaCO_2$ is 80 mm Hg and the patient is breathing room air, assuming an R of 0.8, the highest that PAO_2 can be is 50 mm Hg.

DIFFUSION

Principles

According to Henry's law of diffusion, the diffusion rate for gases in a liquid phase is directly proportional to their solubility coefficients. For example, in water,

$$\frac{\text{solubility of } CO_2}{\text{solubility of } O_2} = \frac{0.592}{0.0244} = \frac{24.3}{1}$$

Therefore, carbon dioxide diffuses more than 24 times as fast as oxygen.

BOX 4-1 Illustrative Causes of Hypoventilation

Respiratory Center Depression

General anesthesia; excessive doses of drugs such as morphine, barbiturates, or codeine; severe or prolonged hypoxia, cerebral ischemia, high concentrations of CO_2; electrocution; cerebral trauma; increased intracranial pressure

Conditions Affecting the Airways and Lung

Upper or Lower Airway Obstruction

Foreign body, large tonsils and adenoids, vocal cord paralysis, croup, endobronchial tuberculosis, chronic bronchitis, emphysema, asthma, bronchiectasis, cystic fibrosis, bronchiolitis

Extensive Loss of Functioning Lung Tissue

Atelectasis, tumor, pneumonia, cystic fibrosis, surgical resection

Limitation of Movement of Lungs

Pleural effusion, pneumothorax, fibrothorax

Conditions Affecting the Thorax

Decreased Chest Wall Compliance

Arthritis, scleroderma, kyphoscoliosis, fractured ribs, thoracoplasty, thoracotomy, pickwickian syndrome, phrenic nerve paralysis

Diseases of Respiratory Muscles

For example, muscular dystrophy

Paralysis of Respiratory Muscles

Poliomyelitis, peripheral neuritis, spinal cord injury, myasthenia gravis; curare, succinylcholine botulinus, and nicotine poisonings

The diffusion rate of a gas in the gas phase is inversely proportional to the square root of molecular weight (Graham's law). Therefore, in the gas phase,

$$\frac{\text{rate for } CO_2}{\text{rate for } O_2} = 0.85$$

That is, carbon dioxide diffuses slower in the gas phase than does oxygen.

Combining Henry's and Graham's laws for a system with both a gas phase and a liquid phase (e.g., alveolus and blood): carbon dioxide diffuses 24.3 × 0.85 = 20.7 times as fast as oxygen.

The barriers through which a gas must travel when diffusing from an alveolus to the blood include the alveolar epithelial lining, basement membrane, capillary endothelial lining, plasma, and red blood cell. As observed on electron micrographs of lung tissue, the thinnest part of the barrier is 0.2 μm but may be as much as three times this thickness.

Fick's law of diffusion, modified for gases, states

$$Q/\text{min} = \frac{KS(P_1 - P_2)}{d}$$

The amount of gas (Q) diffusing through a membrane is directly proportional to the surface area available for diffusion (S), the pressure difference of the two gases on either side of the membrane, and a constant (K) that depends on the solubility coefficient of the gas and the characteristics of the particular membrane and liquid used, and is inversely proportional to the distance (d) through which the gas has to diffuse. In the lung of a given subject, exact values for K, S, and d are unknown. Therefore, for the lung, Bohr and Krogh suggested "diffusing capacity" (DL). DL is simply the inverse of the total resistance to diffusion and can be expressed as the sum of the individual component resistances:

$$\frac{1}{D_L} = \frac{1}{D_M} + \frac{1}{\theta V_c}$$

where $1/D_M$ is the resistance to diffusion of the gas across the alveolar-capillary membrane, plasma, and red blood cell membrane, θ is the reaction rate of the gas with hemoglobin, and Vc is the pulmonary capillary blood volume.

Measurement

Carbon monoxide and oxygen have been used to measure DL. Although the diffusing capacity of the lung for oxygen (D_{LO_2}) has been measured, the process is both complicated and fraught with technical problems because the average capillary oxygen tension must be determined. For this reason, and because a defect in D_{LO_2} is rarely the cause of hypoxemia, it is not used in the clinical setting. Carbon monoxide (CO), however, has been used extensively in children to test diffusing capacity. The advantage of using CO is its remarkable affinity for hemoglobin, some 210 times that of oxygen, and therefore the capillary PCO is negligible and offers no back-pressure for diffusion. To calculate the DLCO, one need know only the amount of CO taken up per unit time and the PACO.

Many techniques have been developed to measure the DLCO, but only two are discussed. The measurement of steady-state DLCO is performed by having the patient breathe a gas mixture containing 0.1% CO for several minutes. Although this measurement requires only a little patient cooperation, its disadvantage is that the value obtained is strongly influenced by maldistribution of the inspired air; if the inhaled gas mixture is not distributed properly to all parts of the lung, the measured DLCO will be decreased but not because of changes in DM, θ, or Vc.

The second technique, the measurement of single-breath DLCO, is less affected by airway disease. In this test, the subject takes a single large breath (from RV to TLC) of a CO-containing gas mixture. Following a 10-second breath-hold, the expired gases are collected so that PACO can be determined.

The difference between these two techniques is exemplified by the patient with acute asthma, in whom the steady-state DLCO value will be decreased, whereas the single-breath DLCO value will be normal or increased. Another advantage of the single-breath DLCO method results from the inclusion of helium in the inspired gas. This inert gas allows the DLCO to be corrected for the alveolar volume in which it was distributed, a measurement known as KCO:

$$K_{CO} = \frac{D_{LCO}\ \text{single} - \text{breath}}{\text{alveolar volume}}$$

The KCO is the most useful parameter for comparing the DL of children of different ages and hence different lung volumes. In addition, the KCO helps differentiate among simple loss of lung units (atelectasis), a decrease in pulmonary blood volume (emphysema), and the (albeit rarely seen) true diffusion defect.

The DLCO increases throughout childhood, is related to lung growth, and correlates best with subject height or body surface area. Clinically, a reduction in DLCO may occur for many reasons, including surgical lung resection, diffuse lung disease (pulmonary fibrosis, cystic fibrosis), and emphysematous destruction of the alveolar-capillary membrane. In addition, anemia may decrease the DLCO, and equations to correct the DLCO for anemia are available. Increases in DLCO rarely occur and usually result from pulmonary vascular engorgement (increased Vc) or pulmonary hemorrhage (e.g., Goodpasture's syndrome and idiopathic pulmonary hemosiderosis).

It is important to note that with a nonexercising patient, impaired diffusion of oxygen from the alveolar air to the pulmonary capillary is rarely the cause of a low PaO_2. Diffusion limitation may occur during exercise in patients with interstitial lung disease. Hypoxemia in pulmonary diseases usually results from alveolar hypoventilation or an imbalance between ventilation and perfusion of lung units. Thus, low DLCO values almost always reflect abnormalities in gas exchange rather than true diffusion defects.

SHUNT AND VENTILATION-PERFUSION RELATIONSHIPS

There are four pulmonary causes of arterial hypoxemia. Two of these, alveolar hypoventilation and diffusion defects, have already been discussed in this section. The remaining two, intrapulmonary shunt and ventilation-perfusion defects, result from abnormalities in the distribution of the ventilation and perfusion of the gas-exchanging units.

Shunt refers to blood that reaches the systemic circulation without coming in direct contact with a ventilated area of the lung. Because this blood is deoxygenated, it lowers the PaO_2. There are several causes of shunt. In normal lungs a small amount of shunt is present, because the thebesian veins and a portion of the bronchial vascular flow drain into the left side of the heart. Pathologic shunts result when abnormal vascular channels exist, as in cyanotic congenital heart disease or pulmonary arteriovenous fistula. Shunt, however, most commonly occurs in diseased lungs because alveoli are not ventilated but are still being perfused. This condition, known as intrapulmonary shunting, occurs in a variety of lung diseases, including pulmonary edema, atelectasis, and pneumonia.

A characteristic feature of shunt is that the resultant hypoxemia cannot be corrected by breathing pure oxygen, a reasonable consequence because, by definition, shunted blood does not pass ventilated lung units. This characteristic can be a useful clinical tool; if PaO_2 is less than 500 mm Hg while the subject is breathing 100% oxygen, a significant shunt is present. If mixed venous (pulmonary arterial) blood is available for measurement (or a mixed venous oxygen concentration is assumed), the amount of shunt can be calculated at any inspired oxygen concentration using the shunt equation:

the amount of oxygen in arterial blood = the amount of oxygen in blood that has passed through pulmonary capillaries ($\dot{Q}c$) + the amount of oxygen in shunted blood ($\dot{Q}s$),

and

the amount of oxygen = the content of oxygen per liter (CO_2) × the blood flow ($\dot{Q}$).

Therefore,

$$CaO_2\, \dot{c}\, \dot{Q}t = Cco_2\, \dot{Q}c + C\, \bar{v}o_2\, \dot{Q}s$$

(where t is total blood flow).

Since $Qc = \dot{Q}t - \dot{Q}s$,

$$CaO_2\, \dot{Q}t = Cco_2\, \dot{Q}t - Cco_2\, \dot{Q}s + C\bar{v}O_2\, \dot{Q}s$$

and

$$\frac{\dot{Q}s}{\dot{Q}t} = \frac{Cco_2 - CaO_2}{Cco_2 - C\bar{v}O_2}$$

where $\dot{Q}s/\dot{Q}t$ is the fraction of the total cardiac output that is shunted.

The average ratio between alveloar ventilation and blood flow (VA/Q) is 0.8, but even in the normal lung may range from near zero (not ventilated) to infinity (not perfused). Nevertheless, the most common cause of arterial hypoxemia is a result of mismatch of ventilation and perfusion within the lung, which increases the normal scatter of VA/Q values around the mean value. When a lung unit receives inadequate ventilation relative to its blood flow, $PACO_2$ rises (toward the mixed venous value of 46 mm Hg) and PAO_2 falls (toward the mixed venous value of about 40 mm Hg) and the oxygen content of the end-capillary blood falls. When this blood mixes with blood coming from normal VA/Q regions of the lung, the result is a lowering of oxygen concentration and arterial hypoxemia (so-called shunt-like effect). In contrast to what occurs in a true shunt, administration of an enriched oxygen mixture will correct the hypoxemia due to ventilation-perfusion mismatch, by raising PAO_2 (PN_2 must fall in order to keep the sum of the partial pressures of gases equal to PB). The increased PAO_2 results in an increased concentration of oxygen in the pulmonary capillary blood.

Whatever the absolute amount of regional ventilation and perfusion, the lung has intrinsic regularity mechanisms that are directed toward the preservation of normal $\dot{V}A/\dot{Q}$ ratios. When $\dot{V}A/\dot{Q}$ is high, the low carbon dioxide concentration results in local constriction of airways and tends to reduce the amount of ventilation to the area. When $\dot{V}A/\dot{Q}$ is low, the high alveolar carbon dioxide concentration results in local airway dilatation and tends to increase ventilation to the area. Furthermore, a low $\dot{V}A/\dot{Q}$ with an associated low alveolar oxygen concentration causes regional pulmonary vasoconstriction and produces a redistribution of blood flow to healthier lung units. These effects on airways and vessels from changing gas tensions tend to preserve a normal $\dot{V}A/\dot{Q}$, but they are limited mechanisms, and derangements are common with pulmonary disease.

SYSTEMIC GAS TRANSPORT

OXYGEN TRANSPORT

Once oxygen molecules have passed from the alveolus into the pulmonary capillary, they are transported in the blood in two ways. A small proportion of the oxygen exists as dissolved oxygen in the plasma and water of the red blood cell. For 100 mL of whole blood equilibrated with a PO_2 of 100 mm Hg, 0.3 mL of oxygen is present as dissolved oxygen. If this represented the total oxygen-carrying capacity of blood, cardiac output would have to be greater than 80 L/min to allow 250 mL of oxygen to be consumed per minute. During 100% oxygen breathing, PaO_2 is approximately 650 mm Hg, and 100 mL of blood contains 2.0 mL of dissolved oxygen; a cardiac output of about 12 L/min would be required if no hemoglobin were present and if the tissues could extract all of the oxygen.

Because 1 g of hemoglobin can combine with 1.39 mL of oxygen, between 40 and 70 times more oxygen is carried by hemoglobin than by the plasma, enabling the body to achieve a cardiac output at rest of 5.5 L/min with an oxygen uptake of 250 mL/min.

The potential usefulness of hyperbaric oxygen (i.e., oxygen under very high pressures) for a variety of clinical conditions is due to the fact that at a pressure of 3 atmospheres (absolute) (PAO_2 of about 1950 mm Hg), approximately 6.0 mL of oxygen is dissolved in 100 mL of whole blood, and this amount can meet the metabolic demands of the tissues under resting conditions even when no hemoglobin is present.

The remarkable oxygen-carrying properties of blood depend not on the solubility of oxygen in plasma but on the unusual properties of hemoglobin. Figure 4-17 illustrates the oxyhemoglobin dissociation curve, showing that hemoglobin is nearly 95% saturated at a PO_2 of 80 mm Hg. The steep portion of the curve, up to about 50 mm Hg, permits large amounts of oxygen to be released from hemoglobin with small changes in PO_2. Under normal circumstances, 100% oxygen breathing will raise the amount of oxygen carried by the blood by only a small amount, because at a PO_2 of 100 mm Hg, hemoglobin is already 97.5% saturated. Even with air breathing, one is on the flat portion of the curve. The presence of a right-to-left shunt markedly affects PO_2 but may reduce the percentage saturation only minimally. For example, a 50% shunt with venous blood containing 15 mL of oxygen/100 mL will reduce the oxygen content of 100 mL of blood only from 20 mL to 17.5 mL. The blood is still 88% saturated, but PaO_2 is now 60 mm Hg instead of 100 mm Hg. Thus, the change in oxygen content is linearly related to the amount of right-to-left shunt, but the change in PO_2 is not, because the oxyhemoglobin dissociation curve is S shaped. It is also apparent that at levels greater than 60 mm Hg, PaO_2 is a more sensitive measure of blood oxygenation because neither percentage saturation nor oxygen content changes as much as PO_2 in this range. However, at PO_2 below about 60 mm Hg, relatively small changes of PO_2 produce large changes in saturation and content, and in this range the measurement of content may be more reliable than the measurement of PO_2.

The oxyhemoglobin dissociation curve is affected by changes in pH, PCO_2, and temperature. A decrease in pH, an increase in PCO_2 (Bohr effect), or an increase in temperature shifts the curve to the right, particularly in the 20 to 50 mm Hg range. Thus, for a given PO_2, the saturation percentage is less under acidotic or hyperpyrexic conditions. In the tissues, carbon dioxide is added to the blood, and this facilitates the removal of oxygen from the red blood cells. In the pulmonary capillaries, carbon dioxide diffuses out of the blood, facilitating oxygen uptake by hemoglobin. An increase in temperature has an effect similar to that of an increase in PCO_2 and thus facilitates oxygen removal from the blood by the tissues. Note that a patient who is pyrexic with carbon dioxide retention could not have a normal oxygen saturation during air breathing because of the Bohr and temperature effects on the oxyhemoglobin dissociation curve.

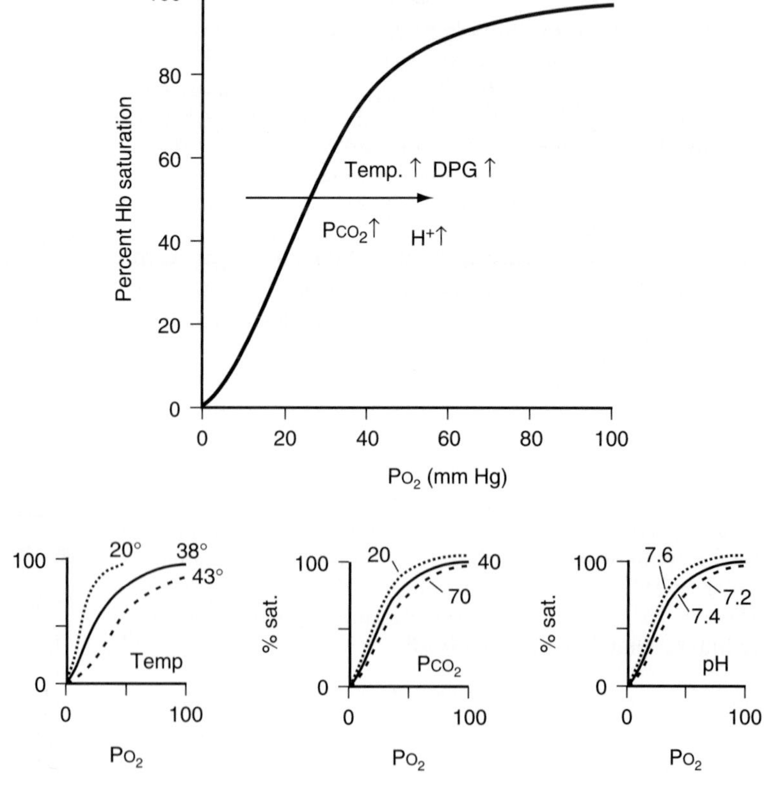

■ **FIGURE 4-17.** Oxyhemoglobin dissociation curves. The large graph shows a single dissociation curve, applicable when the pH of the blood is 7.40 and temperature is 38°C. The blood oxygen tension and saturation of patients with carbon dioxide retention, acidosis, alkalosis, fever, or hypothermia will not fit this curve because it shifts to the right or left when temperature, pH, or PCO_2 is changed. Effects on the oxyhemoglobin dissociation curve of change in temperature *(upper left)* and in PCO_2 and pH *(lower right)* are shown in the smaller graphs. A small change in blood pH occurs regularly in the body (i.e., when mixed venous blood passes through the pulmonary capillaries, PCO_2 decreases from 46 to 40 mm Hg, and pH rises from 7.37 to 7.40). During this time, blood changes from a pH of 7.37 dissociation curve to a pH of 7.40 dissociation curve. Note that increased 2,3-diphosphoglycerate also shifts the curve to the right. (From West JB: Respiratory Physiology—the Essentials, 5th ed. Baltimore: Lippincott Williams & Wilkins, 1995.)

The erythrocyte concentration of 2,3-diphosphoglycerate (DPG) plays a major role in shifting oxyhemoglobin dissociation curves. DPG and hemoglobin are present in about equimolar concentrations in adult human red blood cells. There is strong binding between DPG and the β chain of hemoglobin, and this complex is highly resistant to oxygenation. Shifts of the dissociation curve to the right associated with an increased DPG concentration (e.g., in anemia) facilitate the release of oxygen to the tissues. Because erythrocyte DPG concentration can change within a matter of hours, a regulatory role for DPG in maintaining optimal tissue oxygenation has been suggested.

The fetal oxyhemoglobin dissociation curve is to the left of the adult curve at a similar pH. Thus, at a given PO_2, fetal hemoglobin contains more oxygen than adult hemoglobin. This property ensures that an adequate amount of oxygen will reach fetal tissues, since the fetus in utero has a PaO_2 of about 20 to 25 mm Hg in the descending aorta. The different affinity of fetal hemoglobin for oxygen results from its interaction with DPG. Both fetal and adult red blood cells have similar intracellular concentrations of DPG, but fetal hemoglobin, which has a γ chain instead of a β chain, interacts less strongly with this molecule; therefore, the fetal oxyhemoglobin curve is to the left of the adult curve. Fetal hemoglobin disappears from the circulation shortly after birth, and by a few months of age less than 2% is present. Normal fetal development is not dependent on differences in maternal and fetal hemoglobins, because in some species they are identical.

Abnormal hemoglobins differ in their oxygen-carrying capacity. For example, hemoglobin M is oxidized by oxygen to methemoglobin, which does not release oxygen to the tissues; a large amount is incompatible with life. The formation of methemoglobin by agents such as nitrates, aniline, sulfonamides, acetanilid, phenylhydrazine, and primaquine may also be life threatening. Congenital deficiency of the enzyme hemoglobin reductase is also associated with large amounts of methemoglobin, and affected patients are cyanotic in room air. Similarly, sulfhemoglobin is unable to transport oxygen. Carbon monoxide has 210 times more affinity for hemoglobin than oxygen, so it is important to note that PO_2 may be normal in carbon monoxide poisoning but oxygen content will be reduced markedly.

Thus, a variety of factors may affect the position of the oxyhemoglobin dissociation curve. The position of the curve may be described by measuring the PO_2 at which there is 50% saturation, the so-called P_{50}. When the curve is shifted to the left, the P_{50} is low; when the curve is shifted to the right, the P_{50} is elevated. Although the P_{50} is the traditional method of describing the affinity of hemoglobin for oxygen (see Fig. 4-17), a more appropriate clinical measurement is the P_{90}. This is the PaO_2 at which the hemoglobin is 90% saturated and, as outlined below, corresponds to the goal of oxygen therapy (Table 4-3).

TABLE 4-3. Effect of temperature and acute respiratory acidosis and alkalosis on hemoglobin oxygen affinity

Temperature*		P_{50}	P_{90}
28°C		16.5	35
32°C		20.5	44
40°C		32.0	68
Respiratory Acidosis and Alkalosis†			
pH	**PCO_2**	**P_{50}**	**P_{90}**
7.56	20	22	48
7.48	30	24.5	52.5
7.40	40	27	58
7.32	50	29.5	63
7.26	60	31	67

* PCO_2 = 40 mm Hg, pH = 7.40.

† Temperature = 37°C.

P_{50} and P_{90}: PO_2 at which 50% or 90% of the hemoglobin is saturated.

Data from Rebuck AS, Chapman KR: The P_{90} as a clinically relevant landmark on the oxyhemoglobin dissociation curve. Am Rev Respir Dis 1988;137:962–963.

Oxygen Delivery to Tissues

The cardiopulmonary unit not only must oxygenate the blood but also must transport oxygen to the systemic tissues in adequate amounts. The total oxygen delivery to the systemic tissues is determined by the PaO_2, the amount of saturated hemoglobin, and the left ventricular output (see the equation that follows). For an average adult with a PaO_2 of 100 mm Hg, a hemoglobin (Hb) concentration of 15 g/100 mL (97.5% saturation), and a cardiac output (C.O.) of 5 L/min, approximately 1000 mL of oxygen is delivered to systemic tissues each minute. This large delivery of oxygen provides a significant margin of safety, because under normal circumstances the systemic tissues use only one fourth of the available oxygen; mixed venous PO_2 is 40 mm Hg and hemoglobin is 73% saturated. The systemic oxygen transport equation is useful to emphasize a therapeutic principle: the three practical ways to improve oxygenation of peripheral tissues are to increase hemoglobin saturation, to increase hemoglobin concentration, and to augment cardiac output.

$$\text{oxygen delivery} = \text{blood oxygen content} \times \text{cardiac output}$$
$$\text{where}$$
$$\text{blood oxygen content/100 mL} = \text{dissolved oxygen}$$
$$(0.003\ \text{mL/100 mL blood} \times PaO_2)$$
$$\text{plus}$$
$$\text{oxygen carried by hemoglobin} = 1.39\ \text{mL/g} \times \text{g Hb/100 mL}$$

Cyanosis is one clinical sign of inadequate oxygenation of systemic tissues. The degree of visible cyanosis depends on the amount of unsaturated hemoglobin present in the blood perfusing the superficial vessels. In polycythemia adequate amounts of oxygen may be present, but the patient appears cyanotic because not all the hemoglobin is saturated. Conversely, in anemia, the patient may be inadequately oxygenated without appearing cyanotic. The clinical assessment of oxygenation is hazardous in part because poor peripheral circulation may result in peripheral cyanosis when the arterial blood is well oxygenated. Thus, the most reliable estimate of the oxygen content of arterial blood requires direct measurement, because neither hypoxemia nor hyperoxemia can be assessed reliably by clinical observation.

OXYGEN THERAPY

Increased Inspired Mixtures

Increased inspired mixtures of oxygen are required when tissue oxygenation is inadequate. The response to increased inspired oxygen depends on which cause of hypoxia is present (Box 4-2). Most of the conditions characterized by hypoxemia respond well to added oxygen. Patients with venoarterial shunts will respond

BOX 4-2 Four Types of Hypoxia and Some Causes

Hypoxemia (Low Po_2 and Low Oxygen Content)

Deficiency of oxygen in the atmosphere
Hypoventilation (see Box 4-1)
Uneven distribution of alveolar gas and/or pulmonary blood flow
Diffusion impairment
Venous to arterial shunt

Deficient Hemoglobin (Normal Po_2 and Low Oxygen Content)

Anemia
Carbon monoxide poisoning

Ischemic Hypoxia (Normal Po_2 and Oxygen Content)

General or localized circulatory insufficiency
Tissue edema
Abnormal tissue demands

Histotoxic Anoxia (Normal Po_2 and Oxygen Content)

Poisoning of cellular enzymes so that they cannot use the available oxygen (e.g., cyanide poisoning)

less well, because the shunted blood does not perfuse alveoli. Even so, tissue oxygenation may be improved slightly by the addition of dissolved oxygen to the blood, which does undergo gas exchange in the lung. A direct attack on the underlying disorder in anemia, ischemia, and poisonings is clearly indicated; oxygen therapy may be a life-saving measure during the time required to treat the disease.

Oxygen therapy can be utilized to facilitate the removal of other gases loculated in body spaces, such as air in pneumothorax, pneumomediastinum, and ileus. High inspired oxygen mixtures effectively wash out body stores of nitrogen. With air breathing, the blood that perfuses the tissue spaces has an arterial oxygen tension of 100 mm Hg and a venous tension of 40 mm Hg. With oxygen breathing, although arterial tensions rise to 600 mm Hg, venous oxygen tensions do not rise above 50 to 60 mm Hg because of oxygen consumption and the shape of the dissociation curve. With air breathing, arterial and venous nitrogen tensions are the same, about 570 mm Hg. If the loculated gas were air at atmospheric pressure, the gradient for the movement of nitrogen to the blood would be very small. After nitrogen washout, with oxygen breathing, the lack of high elevation in venous oxygen tension permits movement of both nitrogen and oxygen into the blood. The increased pressure differences increase the rate of absorption of loculated air some 5- to 10-fold.

Administration of Oxygen

There are several methods of delivering enriched oxygen gas mixtures to nonintubated patients. Known concentrations of oxygen can be piped into chambers that surround the infant's head, such as an oxygen tent or a head box. Usually, these chambers allow significant leakage of gases, so it is imperative that the O_2 concentration be measured inside the chamber near the patient's face. Another method is to run pure oxygen through nasal prongs or cannulae at specified flow rates. Although this method can be efficacious in improving the PaO_2, it must be remembered that it does not provide a constant FIO_2 during the breath, nor can the FIO_2 be accurately calculated or measured. The reason is that patients will "beat the system," because their inspiratory flow rates exceed the rate at which the pure oxygen is being piped toward their faces. A simple calculation illustrates the point. If a 70-kg man breathes at 30 breaths/min with an inspiratory/expiratory time ratio of 1:1, his duration of inspiration will be 1 second. Given a tidal volume of 0.5 L, his average inspiratory flow rate will be 0.5 L/sec or 30 L/min. Given that nasal prongs are usually set at 2 to 6 L/min for the average 70-kg man, it is immediately obvious that his initial portion of inspiration will be 100% oxygen but that the percentage will fall quickly toward that of room air by the end of inspiration. This pattern is applicable not only to adults but also to infants.

Thus, although one can "guestimate" what flow rate of oxygen the patient will require to normalize the blood oxygen tension, the actual FIO_2 will vary within and between breaths, especially if the patient changes the depth or pattern of breathing. In practice today in hospitalized children, oxygen flow rate is titrated by measurement of pulse oxymetry.

Hazards of High Oxygen Mixtures

Hypoxemia in conditions associated with alveolar hypoventilation, such as chronic pulmonary disease and status asthmaticus, may be overcome by enriched oxygen mixtures without concomitant lessening of the hypercapnia. The patient may appear pink but become narcotized under the influence of carbon dioxide retention. In chronic respiratory acidosis, respiration may be maintained chiefly by the hypoxic drive. This is a condition that is rarely seen in pediatric patients but may occur in the terminally ill patient with cystic fibrosis.

With the institution of oxygen therapy, there is usually a small drop in minute ventilation as the hypoxic stress is relieved with a concomitant small increase in the PaO_2. Rarely, a patient with chronic respiratory failure may cease breathing if excessive oxygen is given. It is therefore essential to measure the pH and $PaCO_2$ in addition to the PaO_2 or saturation in these groups of patients. The goal of oxygen therapy is to give just enough oxygen to return the arterial oxygen saturation to 90%.

Excessive oxygenation of the blood can be dangerous. Human volunteers in pure oxygen at 1 atmosphere experience symptoms in about 24 hours, chiefly substernal pain and paresthesias. Laboratory animals exposed for longer periods die of pulmonary congestion and edema in 4 to 7 days. The toxicity of oxygen is directly proportional to its partial pressure. Symptoms occur within minutes under hyperbaric conditions and yet are not present after 1 month in pure oxygen at 1/3 atmosphere. Some of the acute effects of oxygen are a slight decrease of minute ventilation and cardiac output and constriction of retinal and cerebral vessels and the ductus arteriosus. Retinal vasoconstriction does not seem to be a significant problem in mature retinas that are fully vascularized. In premature infants, however, the vasoconstriction may lead to ischemia. After the cessation of oxygen therapy, or with maturation of the infant, neovascularization of the retina occurs. The disorderly growth and scarring may cause retinal detachments and fibroplasia, which appears behind the lens; hence the names *retrolental fibroplasia* and *retinopathy of prematurity*, as it is now known. Experimental data have shown that the retinal disease is worse in newborn kittens that are made mildly hypoxemic or normoxemic after exposure to high oxygen, relative to kittens that have been kept in a slightly enriched oxygen environment following hyperoxic exposure.

This suggests that an overaggressive approach to decreasing the level of oxygen therapy in premature infants may actually enhance rather than decrease the risk for severe retinal disease.

As the care of premature infants with acute lung disease has improved, the survival rate has increased impressively. Regrettably, chronic lung disease of prematurity or bronchopulmonary dysplasia has emerged (see Chapter 19). At the present time it is difficult to determine the relative contributions of prematurity, ventilator-induced barotrauma, oxygen toxicity, and the preceding acute lung injury in the evolution of this serious disorder. It does seem prudent, however, to minimize the FIO_2 in these patients, given the damage that occurs in totally normal lungs exposed to very high concentrations of oxygen.

CARBON DIOXIDE TRANSPORT AND ACID-BASE BALANCE

Buffering and Transport

Acids are normally produced in the body at the rates of 15 to 20 moles of carbonic acid and 80 mmol of fixed acids per day. For the cells to maintain their normal metabolic activity, the pH of the environment of the cells must be close to 7.40. The understanding of the regulation of hydrogen ion concentration requires knowledge of the buffering action of the chemical constituents of the blood and of the role of the lungs and kidneys in the excretion of acids from the body.

The most important constituents for acid-base regulation are the sodium bicarbonate and carbonic acid of the plasma, the potassium bicarbonate and carbonic acid of the cells, and hemoglobin.

The concentration of carbonic acid is determined by the partial pressure of carbon dioxide and the solubility coefficients of carbon dioxide in plasma and in red blood cell water. Carbonic acid in aqueous solution dissociates as follows:

$$CO_2 + H_2O \leftrightarrow H_2CO_3$$

$$H_2CO_3 \leftrightarrow H^+ + HCO_3^-$$

The law of mass action describes this reaction:

$$\frac{[H^+][HCO_3^-]}{[H_2CO_3]} = K$$

In plasma, K has the value of $10^{-6.1}$. An equivalent form of this equation is

$$pH = pK + \log\frac{[HCO_3^-]}{H_2CO_3}$$

By definition, pH = –log [H^+]; pK = –log K = 6.1 for plasma. Applied to plasma, in which dissolved carbon dioxide exists at a concentration 1000 times that of carbonic acid, the equation becomes

$$pH = 6.1 + \log\frac{[HCO_3^-]}{0.03\,PCO_2}$$

This form of the equation is known as the Henderson-Hasselbalch equation. A clinically useful form of this equation is

$$H^+ = (nmol/L) = 24 \times \frac{PCO_2}{HCO_3^-}$$

Thus, at a normal bicarbonate concentration of 24 mEq/L, when PaO_2 is 40 mm Hg, hydrogen ion concentration is 40 nM.

Just as oxygen has a highly specialized transport mechanism in the blood to ensure an adequate delivery to tissues under physiologic conditions, carbon dioxide produced by the tissues has a special transport system to carry it in the blood to the lung, where it is expired. The amount of carbon dioxide in blood is related to the PCO_2 in a manner shown in Figure 4-18. Unlike the relation of oxygen content to PO_2, the relation of carbon dioxide content to PCO_2 is nearly linear; therefore, doubling alveolar ventilation halves $PaCO_2$. Oxygenated hemoglobin shifts the carbon dioxide dissociation curve to the right (Haldane effect), so that at a given PCO_2 there is a lower carbon dioxide content. This effect aids in the removal of carbon dioxide from the blood in the lung when venous blood becomes oxygenated. The average arterial carbon dioxide tension ($PaCO_2$) in adults is 40 mm Hg and in infants is closer to 35 mm Hg; venous levels in both are normally 6 mm Hg higher. The small difference between arterial and venous PCO_2 is why the effect of venous admixture on arterial PCO_2 is very small.

Carbon dioxide is transported in the blood in three ways: dissolved in the blood, as bicarbonate, and as carbamino compound. At the tissue level the processes involved in the uptake of carbon dioxide into the blood are as follows (Fig. 4-19):

1. Carbon dioxide diffuses into the blood from the tissue. Some carbon dioxide is dissolved in the plasma water in physical solution.
2. Carbon dioxide hydrates slowly in the plasma to form a small amount of carbonic acid.
3. Most of the carbon dioxide enters the red blood cells. A small amount is dissolved in the intracellular water. A fraction combines with hemoglobin to form a carbamino compound.
4. A larger fraction in the red blood cell hydrates rapidly, because of the presence of carbonic anhydrase, to form carbonic acid, which dissociates into H^+ plus HCO_3^-.
5. Bicarbonate diffuses into plasma because of the concentration gradient, and Cl^- ions enter the cell to restore electrical neutrality.

Hemoglobin is important in the transport of carbon dioxide because of two properties of the molecule. First, it is a good buffer, permitting blood to take up carbon dioxide with only a small change in pH. Second, hemoglobin is a stronger acid when oxygenated than when reduced; thus, when oxyhemoglobin is reduced, more cations are available to neutralize HCO_3^-. Carbon dioxide exists in two forms in the red blood cell because of this property of hemoglobin: as bicarbonate ion and as hemoglobin carbamate ($HbNHCOO^-$).

$$KHbO_2 + H_2CO_3 \leftrightarrow HHb + O_2\uparrow + KHCO_3$$

$$KHbO_2NH_2 + CO_2 \leftrightarrow HHb\dot{c}\ NHCOOK + O_2\uparrow$$

An enzyme in the red cell, carbonic anhydrase, accelerates the reaction

$$CO_2 + H_2O \leftrightarrow H^+ + HCO_3^-$$

some 13,000 times. A concentration gradient between red cell and plasma causes the bicarbonate ion to leave the red cell.

CARBON DIOXIDE DISSOCIATION CURVES FOR WHOLE BLOOD

P_{CO_2}	CO_2 CONTENT OF WHOLE BLOOD when O_2 saturation is 0%	70%	97.5%
10	31.6	28.2	26.5
20	42.2	38.0	36.3
30	49.3	45.1	43.3
40	54.6	50.2	48.4
50	59.1	54.9	53.1
60	63.0	58.6	57.0
70		62.1	60.2
80		65.3	63.6

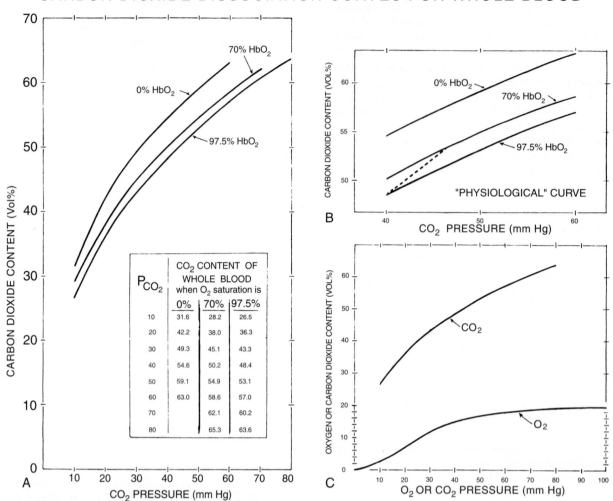

■ **FIGURE 4-18.** The carbon dioxide dissociation curve. The large graph (**A**) shows the relationship between P_{CO_2} and carbon dioxide content of whole blood; this relationship varies with changes in saturation of hemoglobin with oxygen. Thus, P_{CO_2} of the blood influences oxygen saturation (Bohr effect), and oxygen saturation of the blood influences carbon dioxide content (Haldane effect). The oxygen–carbon dioxide diagram gives the correct figure for both carbon dioxide and oxygen at every P_{O_2} and P_{CO_2}. **B,** Greatly magnified portion of the large graph to show the change that occurs as mixed venous blood (70% oxyhemoglobin, P_{CO_2} 40 mm Hg). *Dashed line* is a hypothetical transition between the two curves. **C,** Oxygen and carbon dioxide dissociation curves plotted on same scale to show the important point that the oxygen curve has a steep and a flat portion and that the carbon dioxide curve does not. (From Comroe JH Jr: The Lung, 2nd ed. Chicago: Year Book Medical, 1963.)

Because the red blood cell membrane is relatively impermeable to Na^+ and K^+, the chloride ion and water move into the red cell to restore electrical neutrality (chloride shift or Hamburger shift). Thus, although the larger portion of the buffering occurs within the red cell, the largest amount of carbon dioxide is in the plasma as HCO_3^- (Table 4-4). The shift of chloride and HCO_3^- was previously thought to be passive, that is, to occur by diffusion due to a concentration gradient. It is now known to be an active process dependent on a specific transport protein within the red blood cell membrane. This anion transport occurs rapidly, with a half-time of 50 msec.

In the lung a process the reverse of that just described takes place, because carbon dioxide diffuses out of the blood and into the alveoli. Diffusion of CO_2 is rapid, so the equilibrium between the P_{CO_2} of the pulmonary capillary and that of alveolar air is promptly achieved. About 30% of the CO_2 that is exchanged is given up from hemoglobin carbamate.

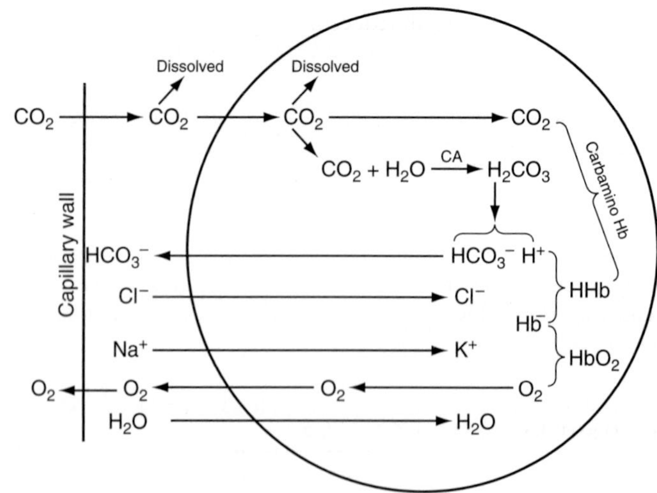

■ **FIGURE 4-19.** CO_2 transport in blood. See text for further explanation.

When hemoglobin is oxygenated in the pulmonary capillary, chloride and water shift out of the red cell, and bicarbonate diffuses in to combine with hydrogen ion to form H_2CO_3, which is in turn dehydrated to form carbon dioxide. Carbon dioxide then diffuses out of the cell into the plasma and alveolar gas.

Although red blood cells from newborn infants have less carbonic anhydrase activity than adult cells, no defect in carbon dioxide transport is apparent. However, when breathing 100% oxygen, there is less reduced hemoglobin present in venous blood, and therefore less buffering capacity for H^+ is present, leading to an increased PCO_2. This is an important consideration during hyperbaric oxygenation, when the venous blood may remain almost completely saturated with oxygen, H^+ is less well buffered, and tissue PCO_2 rises.

Acid-Base Balance

To understand acid-base balance within the body, it is important to differentiate between the processes that promote a change in acid-base state and the end result of all these primary and secondary processes. *Acidemia* and *alkalemia* refer to the final acid-base status within the blood (hence the suffix *-emia*). Two processes can promote the development of acidemia: metabolic acidosis (loss of HCO_3^- or gain of H^+) and respiratory acidosis (increase in PCO_2, which increases H^+ via carbonic acid). Two processes can promote the development of alkalemia: metabolic alkalosis (gain of HCO_3^- or loss of H^+) and respiratory alkalosis (decrease in PCO_2). Obviously, if there is a primary acidotic process, the body will try to maintain homeostasis by promoting a secondary alkalotic process and vice versa. Therefore, to understand the patient's acid-base balance, one must first measure the pH of the blood, and if it is abnormal, determine what primary and secondary (or compensatory) processes are involved. This is illustrated in Table 4-5; note, however, that the HCO_3^- shown in Table 4-5 is the standard HCO_3^- (i.e., corrected to a PCO_2 of 40 mm Hg; see later section on the Difference between Additions of CO_2 to Blood In Vitro and In Vivo).

Metabolic acidosis occurs in such conditions as diabetes (in which there is an accumulation of keto acids); renal failure, when the kidney is unable to excrete hydrogen ion; diarrhea from loss of base; and tissue hypoxia associated with lactic acid accumulation. When pH falls, respiration is stimulated so that PCO_2 will fall and tend to compensate for the reduction in pH. This compensation is usually incomplete, and pH remains below 7.35. The pH, carbon dioxide content (HCO_3^- PCO_2), HCO_3^-, and PCO_2 are all reduced.

TABLE 4-4. Carbon dioxide in the blood

	ARTERIAL BLOOD		VENOUS BLOOD	
	M M/L BL	%	M M/L BL	%
Total	21.9		24.1	
Plasma dissolved CO_2	0.66	3	0.76	3
HCO_3^-	14.00	64	15.00	63
Cells dissolved CO_2	0.44	2	0.54	2
HCO_3^-	5.7	26	6.1	25
$HbNHCOO^-$	1.2	5	1.8	7

Note: The table gives normal values of the various chemical forms of CO_2 in blood with an assumed hematocrit level of 46. Approximately twice as much CO_2 exists in the plasma as the red blood cells, chiefly as HCO_3^-

TABLE 4-5. Blood measurements in various acid-base disturbances

	pH	$PaCO_2$ (mm Hg)	Standard HCO_3^- (mEq/L)	CO_2 Content (mEq/L)
Metabolic acidosis	↓	↓	↓	↓
Acute respiratory acidosis	↓	↑	↔	Slight↑
Compensated respiratory acidosis	(↔ or slight ↓)	↑	↑	↑
Metabolic alkalosis	↑	Slight ↑	↑	↑
Acute respiratory alkalosis	↑	↓	↔	Slight ↓
Compensated respiratory alkalosis	(↔ or slight ↑)	↓	↓	↓
Normal values	7.35–7.45	35–45	24–26	25–28

Metabolic alkalosis occurs most commonly after excessive loss of HCl due to vomiting (as in pyloric stenosis) or after an excessive citrate or bicarbonate load. The carbon dioxide content is elevated, and the PCO_2 will be normal or elevated, depending on the chronicity of the alkalosis.

Acute respiratory acidosis is secondary to respiratory insufficiency and accumulation of carbon dioxide within the body. The associated acidosis may be compensated for by renal adjustments that promote retention of HCO_3^-. Compensation may require several days. Patients with chronic respiratory acidosis, in whom therapy may improve alveolar ventilation, often have a rapid fall of $PaCO_2$. The adjustment in bicarbonate may be much slower, with a resultant metabolic alkalosis of several days' duration. Such a sequence of events has been noted in emphysema and cystic fibrosis.

Similarly, acute respiratory alkalosis, for example, secondary to fever, psychogenic hyperventilation, or a pontine lesion with meningoencephalitis, is associated with high pH, low PCO_2, and normal bicarbonate level. Renal compensation in time leads to excretion of bicarbonate and return of pH toward normal.

It is important to point out that the lung excretes some 300 mEq/kg of acid per day in the form of carbon dioxide, and the kidney excretes 1 to 2 mEq/kg/day. Thus, the lung plays a large role in the acid-base balance of the body, in fact providing rapid adjustment when necessary. The Henderson-Hasselbalch equation may be thought of as

$$\text{pH} \alpha \frac{\text{kidney}}{\text{lung}}$$

Difference between Additions of CO_2 to Blood In Vitro and In Vivo

An appreciation of the difference between the so-called in vitro and in vivo CO_2 dissociation curves is necessary to clarify the confusion that has arisen regarding the interpretation of measurements of acid-base balance, particularly during acute respiratory acidosis (acute hypoventilation). When blood in vitro is equilibrated with increasing concentrations of CO_2, bicarbonate concentration also increases because of the hydration of carbon dioxide. If, for example, blood with a PCO_2 of 40 mm Hg and a bicarbonate concentration of 24 mEq/L were equilibrated with a PCO_2 of 100 mm Hg, the actual bicarbonate concentration would be measured as 34 mEq/L. In the commonly used Astrup nomogram, a correction for this increased bicarbonate due to CO_2 alone is made, and the standard bicarbonate (bicarbonate concentration at P_{CO_2} of 40 mm Hg) is considered to be 24 mEq/L, or a base excess of zero. With this correction, one can readily see that the metabolic (renal) component of acid-base balance is normal. However, confusion has arisen because the in vitro correction figures have been incorrectly applied to the situation in vivo. Unlike equilibration in the test tube, the additional bicarbonate generated during in vivo acute hypercapnia not only is distributed to water in red cells and plasma but also equilibrates with the interstitial fluid space; that is, bicarbonate ion equilibrates with extracellular water. If the interstitial fluid represents 70% of extracellular water, then 70% of the additional bicarbonate generated will be distributed to the interstitial fluid. Thus, an arterial sample taken from a patient with an acute elevation of P_{CO_2} to 100 mm Hg would have an actual bicarbonate concentration of 27 mEq/L. If 10 mEq/L were subtracted according to the in vitro correction, the standard bicarbonate would be reported as 17 mEq/L, or a base excess of −7, indicating the presence of metabolic as well as respiratory acidosis. This conclusion would be incorrect; actually, the bicarbonate concentration in vivo is appropriate for the P_{CO_2}. The situation is worse in the newborn infant because of the high hematocrit and large interstitial fluid space. Base excess values of as much as −10 mEq/L (standard bicarbonate 14 mEq/L) may be calculated despite the fact that the in vivo bicarbonate concentration is appropriate for the particular P_{CO_2} and there is no metabolic component to the acidosis. Thus, the appropriate therapy is to increase alveolar ventilation and not to administer bicarbonate.

TISSUE RESPIRATION

Aerobic Metabolism

The ultimate function of the lung is to provide oxygen to meet the demands of the tissues and to excrete carbon dioxide, a by-product of metabolic activity. Thus, respiratory physiologists have been concerned with the assessment of respiration at the tissue level and the ability of the cardiopulmonary system to meet the metabolic demands of the body.

One method is to measure the amount of oxygen consumed by the body per minute ($\dot{V}_{O_2}$). This is equal to the amount necessary to maintain the life of the cells at rest, plus the amount necessary for oxidative combustion required to maintain a normal body temperature, as well as the amount used for the metabolic demands of work above the resting level. The basal metabolic rate is a summation of many component energy rates of individual organs and tissues and is defined as the amount of energy necessary to maintain the life of the cells at rest, under conditions in which there is no additional energy expenditure for temperature regulation or additional work.

In practice, O_2 is measured after an overnight fast, the subject lying supine in a room at a comfortable temperature. This "basal" metabolic rate has a wide variability (±15% of predicted $\dot{V}_{O_2}$). Since absolutely basal conditions are difficult to ensure, the measurement of basal metabolic rate is not widely used at present.

The performance of the cardiopulmonary system can be more adequately assessed and compared with normal measurements under conditions of added work, such as exercise. During exercise, healthy subjects demonstrate an improvement in pulmonary gas exchange, cardiac output, and tissue oxygen extraction. Performance can be increased by physical fitness, and athletes are able to increase their cardiac output by six- or sevenfold. In children the relationship between work capacity, ventilation, and oxygen consumption is the same as that in the adult. The maximal $\dot{V}_{O_2}$ that can be achieved increases throughout childhood, reaches its peak of 50 to 60 mL/min/kg between 10 and 15 years of age, and thereafter declines slowly with age.

At the tissue level, the ability of a given cell to receive an adequate oxygen supply depends on the amount of local blood flow, the distance of the cell from the perfusing capillary, and the difference between the partial pressures of oxygen in the capillary and in the cell. The critical mean capillary P_{O_2} appears to be in the region of 30 mm Hg for children and adults. Exercising muscle has 10 to 20 times the number of open capillaries as resting muscle does.

The body's response to exercise therefore is complex and depends on the amount of work, the rate at which the workload is increased, and the subject's state of health and degree of physical fitness. A detailed description of the physiologic response to exercise and its use in diagnosing cardiorespiratory disease is beyond the scope of this chapter, but exercise testing is now an essential tool in clinical medicine (see Chapter 11).

Anaerobic Metabolism

The adequacy of oxygen supply to the tissues has been assessed by measuring blood lactate, a product of anaerobic metabolism (Embden-Meyerhof pathway). When there is an insufficient oxygen supply to the tissues due to either insufficient blood flow or a decrease in blood oxygen content, lactic acid concentration within the tissues and blood rises. In the blood this accumulation leads to a metabolic acidosis.

During moderate to heavy muscular exercise, cardiac output cannot meet the demands of the muscles, and an oxygen debt is incurred, which is repaid on cessation of exercise. During this period, lactic acid accumulates, and therefore rigorous exercise is often associated with metabolic acidosis. There is an excellent correlation between the serum lactate level and the oxygen debt. Oxygen debt is not measurable at rest and is difficult to measure during exercise, but the adequacy of tissue oxygenation appears to be accurately reflected in the serum lactate level. In adult humans, blood lactate is less than 1 mEq/L but may rise to 10 to 12 mEq/L during very heavy exercise.

Relationship between $\dot{V}_{O_2}$ and $\dot{V}_{CO_2}$

In the normal subject in a steady state, the amount of carbon dioxide excreted by the lung per minute depends on the basal metabolic activity of the cells and the type of substrate being oxidized. The volume of carbon dioxide exhaled divided by the amount of oxygen consumed is known as the respiratory exchange ratio (R). For the body as a whole, the ratio is 1 if primarily carbohydrate is being metabolized, 0.7 if fat, and 0.8 if protein. Normally, the ratio is 0.8 at rest, approximately 1.0 during exercise, and greater than 1 at exhaustion. The respiratory exchange ratio may vary considerably with changes in alveolar ventilation and metabolism and therefore must be measured in the steady state (i.e., with a steady alveolar ventilation and a steady metabolic rate). For an individual organ, the metabolic respiratory quotient (R.Q.) is nearly constant but may vary from 0.4 to 1.5, depending on the balance of anabolism and catabolism in that organ. Thus, the measurement of R represents the result of many component metabolizing organs and tissues. In the first few days after birth, R falls from nearly 1 to 0.7, indicating a loss of carbohydrate stores; when feeding has started, R approaches 0.8.

With breath-by-breath CO_2 and O_2 concentrations, R can now be calculated on a breath-by-breath basis. Using this technique it is possible to define more precisely the workload at which anaerobic metabolism begins (threshold for anaerobic metabolism). As lactic acid begins to accumulate in the blood, the carbon dioxide dissociation curve shifts to the right, and there is a sudden increase in expired CO_2. R therefore suddenly increases from about 1.0 to above 1.0. It has been shown that the threshold for anaerobic metabolism in both adults and children can be increased by training. This technique is particularly useful in children, because it does not require blood sampling and can be readily applied to cooperative subjects with a variety of pulmonary and cardiac problems.

■ REGULATION OF RESPIRATION

Over the past 20 years, the classic concepts regarding the respiratory control system have been challenged and broadened in many areas. It is appropriate for pediatricians to have an understanding of the normal respiratory control mechanisms, because alterations in respiratory frequency or alveolar ventilation are common to many diseases in infancy and childhood.

The study of the regulation of respiration centers around three main ideas: (1) the generation and maintenance of a respiratory rhythm, (2) the modulation of this rhythm by a number of sensory feedback loops and reflexes, and (3) the recruitment of respiratory muscles that can contract appropriately for gas exchange (Fig. 4-20). The central controller requires reflexes to make "online" adjustments of the pattern of breathing not only to minimize energy costs but also to adapt to a variety of conditions and situations. These conditions may be behavioral, nonhomeostatic (e.g., sucking, speech production), and homeostatic (metabolic rate, oxygenation).

■ CENTRAL PATTERN GENERATION

It is clear now that the central nervous system, particularly the brainstem, has the inherent ability to function as the respiratory "sinus node," or the central pattern generation (CPG).

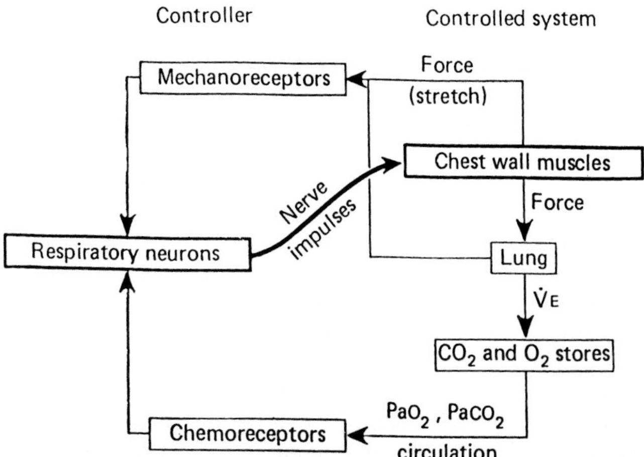

■ **FIGURE 4-20.** Schematic diagram of the respiratory control system. (From Fishman AP: Pulmonary Diseases and Disorders. New York: McGraw-Hill, 1980.)

Although not well defined, the CPG for breathing is most likely composed of several groups of cells in the brainstem that have the property of a pacemaker. By analogy with rhythmic oscillatory systems, such as locomotion in vertebrates or other rhythmic behavior in invertebrates, this property of pacemaking is thought to be brought about in one of two ways: (1) Endogenous burster cells in the brainstem may have an inherent pacemaker property. These cells fire rhythmically in the absence of input or drive by virtue of their membrane properties and ion currents. (2) Alternatively, none of the respiratory-related cells may have the capability of bursting without synaptic input, but it is by virtue of their interconnections and their network properties that the output of the respiratory system oscillates rhythmically.

Whether respiratory pacemaking is the result of endogenous burster neurons or of synaptically driven neurons, two other properties have to be added to the respiratory CPG to explain its function. First, because both peripheral input (e.g., stretch receptors from the lungs and oxygen receptors from the carotid bodies) and central input (e.g., hypothalamus, amygdala) converge on the brainstem and make synapses with respiratory neurons, the CPG has to be able to integrate input from phasic or tonic excitatory or inhibitory influences. Moreover, because phrenic output is absent between inspiratory efforts, an inspiratory off-switch mechanism must be incorporated in the system. This off-switch mechanism is excited by the generator and in turn inhibits the CPG for the duration of expiration.

Little is known about the interconnections of the various respiratory groups of cells or nuclei or about the respiratory CPG. We know, however, that the medullary respiratory-related neurons are concentrated in two columns of cells that are not totally separate, one dorsally and the other ventrally located. Most cells in these two columns are located rostral to the obex, the dorsal column being just lateral to the central canal or the floor of the fourth ventricle and the ventral being lateral and ventral to the dorsal column.

Pontine neurons located in the rostral pons (pneumotaxic nucleus) also play an important role in shaping respiratory output. Sectioning the pons below this group of neurons induces a slower and deeper respiration. Although inherent rhythmicity cannot be ruled out totally for other pontine cell groups, the pneumotaxis (rostral) pontine cells cannot spontaneously generate respiratory rhythmicity.

The respiratory control areas are also influenced by higher centers. Tachypnea, associated with fever or changes in behavioral states or emotion, is presumably mediated by the influence of the hypothalamus, cortex, or the limbic system on the brainstem centers. Furthermore, voluntary control of ventilation has been demonstrated in adult humans and is based on the influence of forebrain structures on brainstem or spinal cord nuclei.

■ SENSORY FEEDBACK SYSTEM

The respiratory system is endowed with a wealth of afferent pathways to maintain control over several functional variables and adjust them at appropriate times. These pathways inform the central pattern generator about instantaneous changes that take place in, for example, the lungs, the respiratory musculature, the blood (acid-base), and the environment. The terms *sensory* and *afferent* refer not only to peripheral but also to central systems converging on the brainstem respiratory neurons.

Studies performed on adult animals have strongly suggested that the afferent receptor system is important not only to signal changes but also to provide an excitatory driving influence on the CPG. This sensory system might be even more significant in early life than in more mature subjects. The best illustration is in the newborn infant, who begins to breathe spontaneously in association with various sensory stimuli of the birth process.

Upper Airways and Lung Receptors

Cutaneous or mucocutaneous stimulation of the area innervated by the trigeminal nerve (e.g., face, nasal mucosa) decreases respiratory frequency and may lead to generation of respiratory pauses. These respiratory effects become less important with age, their strengths are species specific, and they depend on the state of consciousness. Because cortical inhibition of the trigeminal afferent impulses is more pronounced during REM sleep, trigeminal stimulation has a greater effect on respiration during quiet (non-REM) sleep.

The laryngeal receptor reflex is probably the most inhibitory reflex on respiration known. Sensory receptors are present in the epithelium of the epiglottis and upper larynx. Introduction into the larynx of small amounts of water or solutions with low concentrations of chloride results in apnea. The duration and severity of the respiratory changes depend on the behavioral state and are exacerbated by the presence of anesthesia. They are also worse if the subject is anemic, hypoglycemic, or a premature infant. In the unanesthetized subject, the reflex effects are almost purely respiratory and are mediated by the superior laryngeal nerve, which joins the vagal trunk after the nodose ganglion.

Stretch, irritant, and J receptors (vagal) are present in the tracheobronchial tree and lung interstitial space and were described earlier in this chapter. These play an important role in informing the central nervous system about the status of lung volume, tension across airways, and lung interstitial pressure. The secondary neurons (where vagal afferents first synapse) are located in the nucleus tractus solitarius in the medulla. Stretch receptors, when stimulated by inflation of the lungs, prolong expiratory duration and delay the start of the next inspiration. However, the effect of lung inflation on the activity of inspiratory neurons in the medulla is not uniform. Some of the neurons are inhibited but others are excited, and it is on the basis of lung inflation that some have categorized brainstem neurons. Stimulation of vagal afferents at low current intensities (i.e., stretch receptor afferents) inhibits inspiration, hence the term *inspiration-inhibiting reflex*. Cooling the whole vagus nerve, thus eliminating stretch, irritant, and J receptors, induces an increase in the duration of both inspiration and expiration and in tidal volume. J receptors appear to be stimulated by lung edema. They produce tachypnea with interspersed short periods of respiratory pauses.

Vagal afferents carrying impulses from the lungs and airways have to be differentiated from vagal axons of vagal motoneurons, also located in the dorsal medulla (dorsomedial nucleus of the vagus) or in the ventral medulla (part of the nucleus ambiguus). Vagal motoneurons, which innervate upper airway musculature, are important in determining the tone of these muscles and thus the patency of the upper airways. The interconnections between these neurons and others in the medulla are not well defined, but later studies have indicated that vagal motoneurons are relatively small, have high input resistance, and are probably recruited with relatively small synaptic currents.

O_2 and CO_2

The respiratory control system also receives information about O_2 and CO_2 tensions from sensory receptors located in specialized neural structures in blood vessels, airways, and the central nervous system. These tensions seem to be sensed, compared with "programmed" values, and acted on by the controller to increase or decrease ventilation accordingly. Although these structures help maintain acid-base homeostasis in the blood and the cerebrospinal fluid (CSF), one could view the brainstem ventilatory control apparatus as a way the brain adjusts its own CSF acid-base medium for neuronal function at large.

The exact location of the central chemoreceptors is uncertain. Evidence suggests that chemoreceptive tissue is located superficially along the ventral lateral medulla. Direct stimulation of this area by an increase in P_{CO_2} or H^+ concentration produces an increase in ventilation, and conversely, a decrease in P_{CO_2} or H^+ concentration causes a depression of ventilation. It has been suggested that this area is influenced primarily by the acid-base composition of CSF and that the delay in ventilatory response to changes in arterial P_{CO_2} and bicarbonate is due to the time required to change the CSF H^+ concentration. Carbon dioxide, which diffuses into the CSF in a few minutes, has a rapid effect on the central chemoreceptors. Changes in blood bicarbonate are much less rapidly reflected in the CSF (24 to 48 hours). Thus, with acute metabolic acidosis, arterial P_{CO_2} falls along with CSF P_{CO_2}. Hyperventilation is produced by the H^+ stimulation of peripheral chemoreceptors, but this stimulus is inadequate to compensate fully for the metabolic acidosis because of inhibition from the decreased H^+ concentration in the CSF. After 24 hours, CSF bicarbonate falls and restores CSF pH to normal. There is a further fall in arterial P_{CO_2}, and arterial pH returns toward normal. From these observations it has been suggested that the control of alveolar ventilation is a function of the central chemoreceptors, which are under the influence of CSF or brain interstitial fluid H^+, acting in association with the peripheral chemoreceptors, which are directly under the influence of the arterial blood.

The peripheral chemoreceptors are found in the human along the structures associated with the branchial arches. Two sets of chemoreceptors appear to be of greatest physiologic importance: (1) the carotid bodies, located at the division of the common carotid artery into its internal and external branches, and (2) the aortic bodies, which lie between the ascending aorta and the pulmonary artery. Afferent nerves from the carotid body join the glossopharyngeal (IX) nerve; those from the aortic bodies join the vagosympathetic trunk along with the recurrent laryngeal nerves.

The carotid and aortic bodies are responsive primarily to changes in the partial pressure of oxygen. At rest they are tonically active, signifying that some ventilatory drive exists even at a Pa_{O_2} of 100 mm Hg. Inhalation of 33% oxygen reduces ventilation; inhalation of low oxygen mixtures is associated with a significant increase in ventilation when the Pa_{O_2} is less than 60 mm Hg. Potentiation of the hypoxic stimulus is achieved by an increase in Pa_{CO_2}. For example, at a Pa_{CO_2} of 50 mm Hg, ventilation is significantly increased when Pa_{O_2} is lowered to 80 mm Hg. Hypoxia and hypotension presumably act together to decrease the oxygen supply of the chemoreceptor tissue, resulting in a greater ventilatory response to hypoxia.

The response of the peripheral chemoreceptors to P_{CO_2} is rapid (within seconds), and ventilation increases monotonically with $Paco_2$. This increase in ventilation can be substantial (two- to threefold), with a 5- to 10-mm Hg increase in $Paco_2$. More important than the amplitude may be the rate of the change in $Paco_2$. Further evidence supports the hypothesis that the carotid bodies respond more to an oscillating $Paco_2$ than to a steady $Paco_2$ at the same mean level, because these chemoreceptors adapt to a constant stimulus in the same manner as to thermal or touch sensory receptors of the skin. Part of the hyperventilation of exercise may be accounted for on this basis, because oscillations of arterial Pco_2 of about 7 mm Hg accompany moderate exercise. Another important concept related to carotid body function is the "gated" nature of its responsiveness. Stimulation of the carotid sinus nerve has no effect during expiration, only during inspiration. The peripheral chemoreceptors play a minor role in the stimulation of respiration when there is central depression, and respiration is maintained for the most part by the hypoxic drive alone.

The peripheral chemoreceptors, also responsive to changes in arterial pH, increase ventilation in association with a fall of 0.1 pH unit and produce a two- to threefold increase with a fall of 0.4 pH unit. Some investigators believe that the peripheral chemoreceptor response is mediated through changes in intracellular hydrogen ion concentration.

Recently, a system of oxygen sensing neurons in the central nervous system has been described extending from the thalamus to the brainstem. They probably play a role in the adaptation to physiologic conditions (ascent to high altitude) and in clinical conditions associated with chronic hypoxemia.

Other Reflexes

A variety of peripheral reflexes are known to influence respiration. Hyperpnea may be produced by stimulation of pain and temperature receptors or mechanoreceptors in limbs. Visceral reflexes, such as those resulting from distention of gallbladder or traction on the gut, are usually associated with apnea. Afferent impulses from respiratory muscles (e.g., intercostals) may play a role in determining the optimum response of the muscles of ventilation to various respiratory stimuli. In newborn infants an inspiratory gasp may be elicited by distention of the upper airways. This reflex is mediated by the vagus nerve and is known as the Head reflex. It has been suggested that this inspiratory gasp reflex is important in the initial inflation of the lungs at birth.

The Newborn Infant

There is special interest in the control of breathing in the newborn period because it is the period of transition from the intrauterine state, when the lungs are not required for gas exchange, to extrauterine existence, which depends on the lung as the organ of gas exchange.

A number of studies have demonstrated that the responsiveness to stimuli in newborn infants is different from that of older or mature adult subjects. Although the exact mechanisms for these differences have generally been elusive, the rapid maturational changes that occur in key control systems could serve as the bases for the different responses seen in early life.

Infants, like adults, increase ventilation in response to inspired carbon dioxide. However, a comparison of ventilation per kg in infants (premature and full term) and adults shows that all infants breathe more at a given Pco_2 than do adults. Presumably, this is because infants have a higher CO_2 production per kilogram; yet the change in ventilation per mm Hg change in Pco_2 is the same in full-term infants and adults, suggesting that their neurochemical apparatus have the same sensitivity but that the ventilatory response is a function of body mass. This concept has been challenged; it has been pointed out that the ventilatory response to CO_2 may be impaired because of mechanical factors, such as stiffness of a lung, or because of a very compliant chest wall. However, measurements of respiratory center output by mouth pressure during brief airway occlusion (presumably eliminating mechanical factors) indicate that premature infants may not respond as well as the full-term infant or adult to inspired CO_2. Maturation of this response is a function of gestational as well as postnatal age.

Peripheral chemoreceptors are functional in newborn infants, as demonstrated by a slight decrease in $\dot{V}_E$ with 100% oxygen breathing. The effect of hypoxia as a stimulant may differ in the first 12 hours of life; 12% oxygen in the first 12 hours of life fails to stimulate ventilation. Presumably, the atypical response reflects the persistence of fetal shunts that affect the oxygen tensions of blood perfusing the carotid body. In addition, the newborn infant has been found to increase ventilation only transiently in response to a hypoxic stimulus; ventilation rapidly falls below baseline. In adults the increase in ventilation is maintained above basal levels, although lessening with time.

The mechanisms responsible for this different response to hypoxia in the newborn are not well understood. It has been suggested that the biphasic hypoxic response is multifactorial and may be due to one or more of the following: (1) reduction in dynamic lung compliance, (2) reduction in chemoreceptor activity during sustained (>1 to 2 min) hypoxia, (3) central neuronal depression due to either an actual drop in excitatory synaptic drive other than carotid input or changes in neuronal membrane properties reducing excitability, and (4) decrease in metabolic rate.

Whether this decrease in respiration during phase 2 is mediated by certain neurotransmitters is not clear. Adenosine, prostaglandins, and endorphins have been tested as potential mediators, but results have not been conclusive. It is known, however, that endorphins may play an important modulator role during severe hypoxia in animals or humans, in newborns or adults. Primary apnea, for example, is markedly shortened by administration of naloxone in asphyxiated newborn animals.

Of great importance is the fact that newborn animals rely on carotid body function for O_2 responsiveness and survival more than adults do. This may seem paradoxical to conventional teaching. However, a number of newborn animal species (lambs, rats, piglets) have died within days to weeks of carotid body denervation when performed during a certain time window in early life. This does not happen in the more mature animal.

Other key systems are also maturing in the newborn and may be important to the overall output of the respiratory system. For example, it is well known that the chest wall in the newborn infant is very compliant. During REM sleep, when intercostal muscles are inhibited and chest wall stability is jeopardized, a load is added on the respiratory muscles. Whether this leads to respiratory muscle fatigue or predisposes the infant to it depends on a number of variables, including oxygenation, cellular composition of the respiratory muscles, general nutritional status, hemoglobin content, cardiovascular function, electrolyte concentrations, phosphate and acid-base status, and the presence or absence of anesthetics or depressant drugs.

Although the maturation of the central nervous system and its activities have been thought to be at the basis of some responses observed in early life, few studies have been done to test this hypothesis. Studies have demonstrated that neurons in the medulla oblongata of newborn animals have different electrophysiologic properties than the neurons of adult animals. This finding may have profound implications on the capabilities of neurons for synaptic integration and repetitive firing in early life.

DERANGEMENTS OF RESPIRATORY REGULATION

Periodic Breathing

Periodic breathing is commonly seen in otherwise normal premature infants and rarely seen in full-term infants. It is characterized by a period of apnea lasting from 3 to 10 seconds followed by a period of ventilation for 10 to 15 seconds. The average respiratory rate is 30 to 40 per minute; the rate during the ventilatory interval is 50 to 60 per minute. It is rarely seen during the first 24 hours of life and disappears by 38 to 40 weeks' postconceptual age. Periodic breathing may appear intermittently, interspersed with long periods of regular breathing. During periodic breathing infants appear more wakeful, with tremors of the tongue and extremities and movements of the eyes. This resembles the REM stage of sleep in the adult, which can also be associated with periodic or Cheyne-Stokes respiration. Also, as in the adult with Cheyne-Stokes respiration, periodic breathing is associated with mild hyperventilation, resulting in slightly alkalotic arterial blood (mean pH 7.44) compared with regular breathing (mean pH 7.39). Average arterial P_{CO_2} is approximately 3 to 4 mm Hg lower during periodic breathing. During the apneic period P_{CO_2} increases by 6 to 7 mm Hg, and the increased cyclic change in Pa_{CO_2} may be responsible for the slight hyperventilation.

The cause of periodic breathing is unknown. Some believe that it is the result of an immature brainstem. It is interesting to note that Cheyne-Stokes breathing, which is a form of periodic breathing, is prevalent in the elderly, who are at the other end of the age spectrum.

Respiratory Pauses and Apneas

The term *apnea* has been variously defined by different investigators and clinicians. Pauses of more than 2 to 3 seconds, 6 seconds, 10 seconds, 15 seconds, or 20 seconds have all been considered apneas. Because long respiratory pauses are more likely to be associated with life-threatening alterations in cardiovascular, metabolic, and neurologic functions, it may be more appropriate to categorize or define respiratory pauses by the presence or absence of associated changes. In addition, because infants have higher O_2 consumption per unit of body weight and a relatively smaller lung volume and O_2 stores than adults, it is possible that relatively short pauses (up to several seconds) that are not clinically important in the adult can induce consequential clinical effects in the newborn infant. Evidence in young animals has shown that hemoglobin saturation starts to decrease within 5 to 10 seconds of a pause. By 20 to 30 seconds, electroencephalographic changes have started to occur, and by 60 seconds after the start of the pause, the electroencephalogram is almost isoelectric. Although the study of the sequence of events during prolonged apneas may not be feasible in infants for ethical reasons, it is important to investigate the pauses that are considered clinically "safe" and possibly redefine what constitutes a prolonged apnea that needs attention.

Although the pathogenesis of respiratory pauses is controversial, there is a consensus about some observations. For example, normal infants, children, and adult humans exhibit respiratory pauses and apneas, mostly during sleep. Pauses are more frequent during REM sleep, and the average pause is longer in quiet sleep. Paradoxical as it may seem, the presence of respiratory pauses and breathing irregularities is a healthy sign; the complete absence of such pauses may be indicative of respiratory control abnormalities.

Prolonged apneas, in comparison, can be life threatening. Some of these apneas, called apneic spells, are associated with overt clinical symptoms of distress, including cyanosis and marked bradycardia. These spells occur generally in premature infants, suggesting serious underlying disease and requiring treatment. The lack of air movement in the chest and apnea can be related to either an obstructive condition or a failure to generate breathing. Obstruction has been described in infants, and it occurs mostly during sleep. The site of obstruction can vary; most often it is at the level of the posterior pharyngeal wall. In infants and children this obstruction can be due to enlarged tonsils and adenoids, excess fat in the pharyngeal wall, reduced tone in a large genioglossus muscle, or short retracted jaws. Obstruction can also occur in the nose or in the larynx.

Failure to generate breathing, called central apnea, is probably due to either failure of the excitatory mechanisms or the drive to terminate a normally occurring respiratory pause, or active inhibition or obstruction of central mechanisms that initiate breathing. Examples of conditions that are associated with central apnea include activation of laryngeal receptors (e.g., during aspiration); hypoventilation syndromes; carotid body immaturity or degeneration (loss of excitatory input); presence of anesthetics or depressant drugs; and, in certain instances, seizures.

Upper Airway Obstruction

This condition occurs mostly in sleep and is being recognized with increased frequency in children, from infancy to adolescence. In contrast to the pathophysiology of upper airway obstruction (UAO) in adults, anatomic abnormalities often prove to be the cause of UAO in children. Such abnormalities include enlarged tonsils and adenoids, malformations (Crouzon's disease), micrognathia (Pierre Robin syndrome), and muscular hypotonia. The usual site of obstruction is the oropharynx, between the pharyngeal wall, the soft palate, and the tongue.

Snoring is commonly present with UAO in children. Pauses are usually terminated by a loud snore and arousal. In older children, disturbed sleep habits include restlessness and arousals during the night, enuresis, failure to thrive, developmental delays, and poor school performance. Long-standing UAO can first become evident with right ventricular failure and cor pulmonale. Treatment varies, depending on the underlying cause of obstruction.

Sudden Infant Death Syndrome

This syndrome is not uncommon, occurring between the ages of 1 month and 1 year, with a peak incidence at about 3 months of age. The terminal episode is presumed to occur during sleep. Thus, investigators have been led to suspect that sudden infant death syndrome (SIDS) results from a conglomeration of events, some related to abnormal or immature control systems and others to environmental factors. The pathophysiology of SIDS seems to involve the cardiorespiratory control system, and abnormalities in the autonomic nervous system and in arousal from sleep have been proposed (see Chapter 73).

Dysautonomia (Riley-Day Syndrome)

This rare disease, first recognized in 1949, is characterized by some degree of mental and physical retardation, deficient lacrimation, excessive sweating, transient hypertension, postural hypotension, attacks of cyclic vomiting, absence of the knee jerk reflex and of tongue papillae, and blotchy skin. It occurs predominantly in Jewish children and may or may not be associated with mental deficiency. Recurrent pulmonary infiltrations are thought to be the result of a defective swallowing mechanism with associated aspiration. Studies of the control of breathing in these patients show that they are less responsive than normal subjects to changes in Pa_{CO_2} and oxygen tensions, perhaps because of peripheral chemoreceptor dysfunction. Since they do not have a normal ventilatory drive prompted by changes in arterial P_{CO_2} and P_{O_2}, protection from high altitude and a warning against breath holding during swimming may be important considerations.

METABOLIC FUNCTIONS OF THE LUNG

The lungs have important nonrespiratory functions, including phagocytosis by alveolar macrophages, filtering of microemboli from blood, biosynthesis of surfactant phospholipids, and excretion of volatile substances. An equally important nonrespiratory function is the pharmacokinetic function of the pulmonary vascular bed: the release, degradation, and activation of vasoactive substances. The lung is ideally situated for regulating the circulating concentrations of vasoactive substances, since it receives the entire cardiac output and possesses an enormous vascular surface area. As Table 4-6 illustrates, the pulmonary vascular bed not only handles a wide variety of compounds (amines, peptides, lipids), but in addition is highly selective in its metabolic activity. For example, norepinephrine is metabolized by the lung, whereas epinephrine, which differs from it only by a methyl group, is unaffected by passage through the pulmonary circulation.

The physiologic consequences of the metabolic functions of the lung can be illustrated by angiotensin-converting enzyme (ACE). A peptidase located on the surface of the endothelial cell, ACE is responsible for the degradation of bradykinin, a potent vasodilator and edematogenic peptide, and for the conversion of angiotensin I to angiotensin II, a potent vasoconstrictor. Angiotensin II production influences systemic blood pressure at all ages but is especially important during the neonatal period, because sympathetic innervation is incompletely developed.

TABLE 4-6. Handling of biologically active compounds by the lung

Metabolized at the endothelial surface without uptake	Bradykinin Angiotensin I Adenine nucleotides
Metabolized after uptake by the endothelial cell	Serotonin Norepinephrine Prostaglandins E and F
Unaffected by passage through the lung	Epinephrine Dopamine Angiotensin II Vasopressin PGA
Released by the lung	Prostaglandins (e.g., prostacyclin) Histamine SRS-A ECF-A Kallikrein

SUGGESTED READING

Normal Lung Anatomy and Cell Function

Barnes PF: Neural control of airways in health and diseases. Am Rev Respir Dis 1986;134:1289.

Derenne JP, Macklem PT, Roussos C: The respiratory muscles. Mechanics, control and pathophysiology. Am Rev Respir Dis 1978;118(Part I):119 and 118(Part II):373.

Van Hayek H: The Human Lung. Trans. Krahl VE. New York: Hafner, 1960.

Weibel ER: Morphometry of the Human Lung. New York: Academic Press, 1963.

Weibel ER: Lung cell biology. In: Fishman AP, ed: The Respiratory System: Handbook of Physiology, Section 3, Vol. 1. (American Physiologic Society.) Baltimore: Williams & Wilkins, 1985.

Growth and Development of the Lung

American Thoracic Society: Mechanisms and Limits of Induced Postnatal Lung Growth. Workshop Report. Am J Respir Crit Care Med 2004;170:319–343.

Burri PH: Development and growth of the human lung. In: Fishman AP, ed: The Respiratory System: Handbook of Physiology, Section 3, Vol. 1. (American Physiologic Society.) Baltimore: Williams & Wilkins, 1985.

De Mello DE, Reid LM: Prenatal and postnatal development of the pulmonary circulation. In: Hadad G, Abman S, Chernick V, eds: Chernick-Mellins Basic Mechanisms of Pediatric Respiratory Disease, 2nd ed. London: BC Decker Hamilton, 2002.

Ochs M, Nyengaard JR, Jung A, et al: The number of alveoli in the human lung. Am J Respir Crit Care Med 2004;169:120–124.

Olver RE, Ramsden CA, Strang LB, Walters DV: The role of amiloride blockable sodium transport in adrenaline induced lung liquid reabsorption in the fetal lamb. J Physiol 1986;376:321.

Polger G, Weng TR: The functional development of the respiratory system. Am Rev Respir Dis 1979;120:625.

Reid LM: The pulmonary circulation. Remodelling in growth and disease. Am Rev Respir Dis 1979;119:531.

Schachtner S, Taichman D, Baldwin HS: Mechanisms of lung vascular development. In: Hadad G, Abman S, Chernick V, eds: Chernick-Mellins Basic Mechanisms of Pediatric Respiratory Disease, 2nd ed. London: BC Decker Hamilton, 2002.

Shannon J, Hyatt BA: Tissue interactions in lung organogenesis. In: Hadad G, Abman S, Chernick V, eds: Chernick-Mellins Basic Mechanisms of Pediatric Respiratory Disease, 2nd ed. London: BC Decker Hamilton, 2002.

Van Golde L, Batenburg JJ, Robertson P: The pulmonary surfactant system. Biochemical aspects and functional significance. Physiol Rev 1988;68:374.

Ventilation

Bates DV: Respiratory Function in Disease, 3rd ed. Philadelphia: WB Saunders, 1989.

Bryan AC, Wohl MD: Respiratory mechanics in children. In: Fishman AP, ed: The Respiratory System. Handbook of Physiology, Section 3, Vol. 3. (American Physiologic Society.) Baltimore: Williams & Wilkins, 1986.

Burrows B (chairman), Huang N, Hughes R, et al: Pulmonary terms and symbols. A report of the ACCP-ATS Joint Committee on Pulmonary Nomenclature. Chest 1975;67:583–593.

Murray JF: The Normal Lung, 2nd ed. Philadelphia: WB Saunders, 1986.

Nunn VF: Applied Respiratory Physiology. London: Butterworth, 1977.

Weibel ER, Bachofen H: How to stabilize the alveoli. Surfactant or fibers. News Physiol Sci 1987;2:72.

West JB: Ventilation/bloodflow and gas exchange. Oxford, UK: Blackwell Scientific, 1970.

Pulmonary Circulation

Barer GR: The physiology of the pulmonary circulation and methods of study. Pharmacol Ther 1976;2:247.

Culver BH, Butler J: Mechanical influences on the pulmonary circulation. Ann Rev Physiol 1980;42:187.

Hughes JMB: Pulmonary circulation and fluid balance. In: Widdicombe JG, ed: Respiratory Physiology, Vol II. (International Review of Physiology Series, Vol. 14.) Baltimore: University Park Press, 1977.

Moser KM: Pulmonary Vascular Diseases. (Lung Biology in Health and Disease Series, Vol. 14.) New York: Marcel Dekker, 1979.

Permutt S: Mechanical influences on water accumulation in the lung. In: Fishman AP, Renkin E, eds: Pulmonary Edema. (American Physiologic Society.) Baltimore: Williams & Wilkins, 1979.

Muscles of Respiration

Bazzy-Asaad A: Respiratory muscle function: Implications for ventilatory failure. In: Hadad G, Abman S, Chernick V, eds: Chernick-Mellins Basic Mechanisms of Pediatric Respiratory Disease, 2nd ed. London: BC Decker Hamilton, 2002.

Grassino A, Macklem PT: Respiratory muscle fatigue and ventilatory failure. Ann Rev Med 1984;35:625.

Haddad GG, Akabas SR: Adaptation of respiratory muscles to acute and chronic stress. Considerations on energy and fuels. Clin Chest Med 1986;7:70.

Gas Exchange

Single-breath carbon monoxide diffusing capacity (transfer factor). Recommendations for a standard technique. Am Rev Respir Dis 1987; 136:1299.

Gas Transport to the Systemic Vasculature

Astrup P, Jorgensen K, Anderson OS, Engel K: The acid-base metabolism. A new approach. Lancet 1960;1:1035.

Davenport H: The ABC of Acid Base Chemistry, 4th ed. Chicago: University of Chicago Press, 1958.

Jones NL: Blood gases and acid-base physiology. New York: Thieme-Stratton, 1980.

Winters RW: Terminology of acid-base disorders. Ann Intern Med 1965;63:873.

Regulation of Respiration

Berger AJ, Mitchell RA, Severinghaus JW: Regulation of respiration. N Engl J Med 1977;297:92.

Haddad GG, Mellins RB: The role of airway receptors in the control of respiration in infants. A review. J Pediatr 1977;91:281.

Harper RM, Gozal D: Sleep and respiratory control. In: Hadad G, Abman S, Chernick V, eds: Chernick-Mellins Basic Mechanisms of Pediatric Respiratory Disease, 2nd ed. London: BC Decker Hamilton, 2002.

Neubauer JA, Sunderram J: Oxygen-sensing neurons in the central nervous system. J Appl Physiol 2004;96:367–374.

Phillipson EA: Control of breathing during sleep. Am Rev Respir Dis 1978;118:909.

Nonrespiratory Aspects of the Lung

Bakhle YS, Vane JR, eds: Metabolic Functions of the Lung. New York: Marcel Dekker, 1977.

Brain JD, Proctor DV, Reid LM, eds: Respiratory Defense Mechanisms. New York: Marcel Dekker, 1978.

Parker JC, Guyton AC, Taylor AC: Pulmonary transcapillary exchange and pulmonary edema. In: Guyton AC, Young DB, eds: Cardiovascular Physiology, Vol. III. (International Review of Physiology Series, Vol. 18.) Baltimore: University Park Press, 1979.

Staub NC, ed: Lung Water and Solute Exchange. New York: Marcel Dekker, 1978.

5 Biology and Assessment of Airway Inflammation

Peter J. Barnes, DM

INTRODUCTION

Inflammation is classically characterized by four cardinal signs: calor and rubor (due to vasodilatation), tumor (due to plasma exudation and edema), and dolor (due to sensitization and activation of sensory nerves). It is now recognized that inflammation is also characterized by an infiltration with inflammatory cells and that these will differ depending on the type of inflammatory process. It is important to recognize that inflammation is an important defense response that defends the body against invasion from microorganisms and against the effects of external toxins. Allergic inflammation is characterized by the fact that it is driven by exposure to allergens through immunoglobulin E (IgE)–dependent mechanisms, resulting in a characteristic pattern of inflammation. The inflammatory response seen in allergic diseases is characterized by an infiltration with eosinophils and resembles the inflammatory process mounted in response to parasitic and worm infections. The inflammatory response not only provides an acute defense against injury, but is also involved in healing and restoration of normal function after tissue damage as a result of infection of toxins. In allergic disease, the inflammatory response is activated inappropriately and is harmful rather than beneficial. For some reason allergens, such as house dust mite and pollen proteins, activate an eosinophil inflammation. Normally, such an inflammatory response would kill the invading parasite (or vice versa) and would therefore be self-limiting, but in allergic disease the inciting stimulus persists and the normally acute inflammatory response becomes converted into a chronic inflammation which may have structural consequences in the airways and skin. Cystic fibrosis (CF) and bronchiectasis are characterized by a neutrophilic pattern of inflammation, driven in part by chronic bacterial infection. In this chapter most emphasis is placed on allergic inflammation because this underlies the most common diseases of the respiratory tract in children.

ACUTE INFLAMMATION

Acute inflammation in the respiratory tract is an immediate defense reaction to inhaled allergens, pathogens, or noxious agents. Inhalation of an allergen, such as house dust mite, activates surface mast cells by an IgE-dependent mechanism. This releases various bronchoconstrictor mediators, resulting in rapid contraction of airway smooth muscle and wheezing. These mediators also results in plasma exudation and swelling of the airways and attract inflammatory cells from the circulation, particularly eosinophils, neutrophils (transiently), and T lymphocytes, which are mainly of the T-helper 2 (Th2) type. This accounts for the so-called late response occurring 4 to 6 hours after allergen exposure and resolving within 24 hours, which should be regarded as an acute inflammatory reaction. The acute inflammatory response in the respiratory tract is usually accompanied by increased mucus secretion, which is a part of the defense system to protect the delicate mucosal surface of the airways.

CHRONIC INFLAMMATION

Many inflammatory conditions of the respiratory tract are chronic and may persist for many years. This inflammation may persist even in the absence of causal mechanisms. This is well illustrated in patients with occupational asthma who continue to have asthma despite complete avoidance of sensitizing agents, and in adult patients with chronic obstructive pulmonary disease who have continued inflammation, even after stopping smoking for many years. This molecular and cellular mechanism for the persistence of inflammation in the absence of its causal mechanisms is not yet understood, but presumably involves some type of long-lived immunologic memory that drives the inflammatory process.[1] Structural cells, such as airway epithelial cells, that make up the airway wall may also drive the chronic inflammatory process. This is an important area of research, because understanding these mechanisms might lead to potentially curative therapies in the future.

STRUCTURAL CHANGES AND REPAIR

The acute inflammatory response is usually followed by a repair process that restores the tissue back to normal. This may involve proliferation of damaged cells, such as airway epithelial cells and fibrosis to heal any breach in the mucosal surface. These repair processes may also become chronic in response to continued inflammation, resulting in structural changes in the airways that are referred to as remodeling. These structural changes in asthma and CF may result in irreversible narrowing of the airways, with a fixed reduction in airflow. In asthma there are several structural changes found in the airway wall, including fibrosis, increased amount of airway smooth muscle and increases numbers of blood vessels (angiogenesis).[2] There is much debate about the importance of airway remodeling in asthma because this is not seen in all patients. It may contribute to airway hyperresponsiveness (AHR) in asthma, but may also have some beneficial effects in limiting airway closure.[3]

INFLAMMATORY CELLS

Many different inflammatory cells are involved in airway inflammation, although the precise role of each cell type is not yet certain[4] (Fig. 5-1). In children with asthma, the same kind of inflammation is seen in bronchial biopsies, compared with adults, indicating that similar pathophysiologic mechanisms

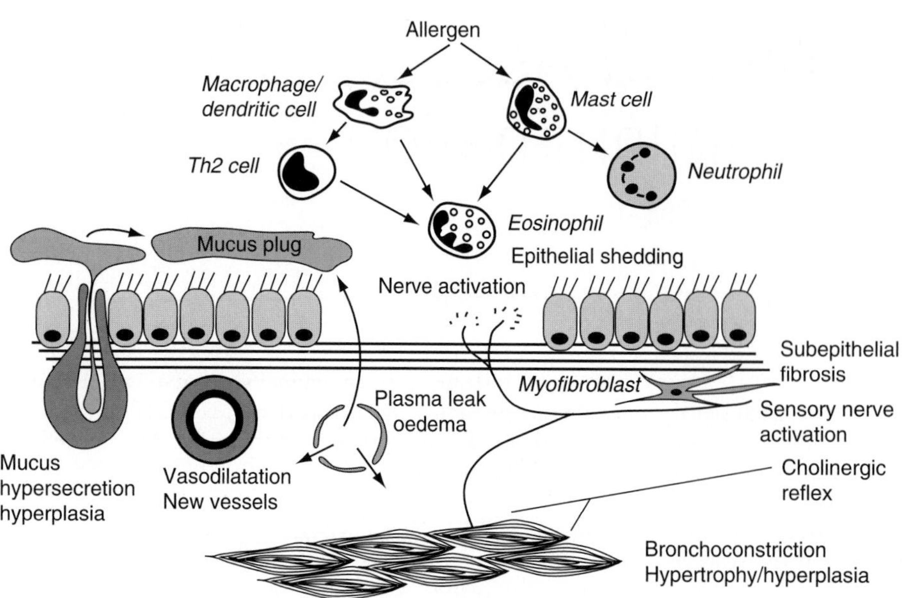

FIGURE 5-1. The pathophysiology of asthma is complex, with participation of several interacting inflammatory cells, which results in acute and chronic inflammatory effects on the airway. Th2, T-helper 2 cell.

are operative.[5] It is evident that no single inflammatory cell is able to account for the complex pathophysiology of asthma, but some cells predominate in allergic inflammation, whereas the pattern of inflammation in CF is different, resulting in different pathophysiologic consequences and different response to therapy.

MAST CELLS

Mast cells are important in initiating the acute bronchoconstrictor responses to allergen and probably to other indirect stimuli, such as exercise and hyperventilation (via osmolality or thermal changes) and fog. Treatment of asthmatic patients with prednisone results in a decrease in the number of tryptase-positive mast cells. Furthermore, mast cell tryptase appears to play a role in airway remodeling, because this mast cell product stimulates human lung fibroblast proliferation. Mast cells also secrete certain cytokines, such as interleukin-4 (IL-4) and eotaxin, which may be involved in maintaining the allergic inflammatory response, and tumor necrosis factor-α (TNF-α). Mast cells are found in increased numbers in airway smooth muscle of asthmatic patients and this appears to correlate with AHR, suggesting that mast cell mediators mediate AHR.[6] Interestingly, it appears to be the presence of mast cells in the smooth muscle layer that distinguishes between the pathology of asthma and eosinophilic bronchitis in adults.

However, there are questions about the role of mast cells in more chronic allergic inflammatory events, and it seems more probable that other cells, such as macrophages, eosinophils, and T lymphocytes, are more important in the chronic inflammatory process, including AHR. Classically, mast cells are activated by allergens through an IgE-dependent mechanism, mediated through the high-affinity IgE receptor. The importance of IgE in the pathophysiology of asthma has been highlighted by recent clinical studies with humanized anti-IgE antibodies, which inhibit IgE-mediated effects. Anti-IgE therapy is effective in patients, including children, with severe asthma who are not well controlled with high doses of corticosteroids and is particularly effective in reducing exacerbations.[7]

MACROPHAGES

Macrophages, which are derived from blood monocytes, traffic into the airways in inflammatory diseases under the direction of specific chemokines. In the airways these monocytes differentiate into macrophages, which have the capacity to secrete many inflammatory proteins, chemotactic factors, lipid mediators, and proteinases. In asthma they may be activated by allergen via low-affinity IgE receptors ($Fc_{\varepsilon}RII$). The enormous immunologic repertoire of macrophages allows these cells to produce at least 100 different products, including a large variety of cytokines that may orchestrate the inflammatory response. Macrophages have the capacity to initiate a particular type of inflammatory response via the release of a certain pattern of cytokines. Macrophages may both increase and decrease inflammation, depending on the stimulus. Alveolar macrophages normally have a suppressive effect on lymphocyte function, but this may be impaired in asthma after allergen exposure. One anti-inflammatory protein secreted by macrophages is IL-10, and its secretion is reduced in alveolar macrophages from patients with asthma. Macrophages may therefore play an important anti-inflammatory role, by preventing the development of allergic inflammation. There may be subtypes of macrophages that perform different inflammatory, anti-inflammatory, or phagocytic roles in airway disease, but at present it is difficult to differentiate these subtypes.

DENDRITIC CELLS

Dendritic cells are specialized macrophage-like cells that have a unique ability to induce a T lymphocyte–mediated immune response and therefore play a critical role in the development of asthma.[8] Dendritic cells in the respiratory tract form a network that is localized to the epithelium, and act as very effective antigen-presenting cells.[9] It is likely that dendritic cells play an important role in the initiation of allergen-induced responses in asthma. Dendritic cells take up allergens, process them to peptides, and migrate to local lymph nodes where they present the allergenic peptides to uncommitted T lymphocytes, and with the aid of costimulatory molecules, such as B7.1, B7.2, and CD40, they program the production of allergen-specific T cells. Animal studies have demonstrated that myeloid dendritic cells are critical to the development of Th2 cells and eosinophilia.

EOSINOPHILS

Eosinophil infiltration is a characteristic feature of allergic inflammation. Asthma might more accurately be called chronic eosinophilic bronchitis (a term first coined as early as 1916). It should be noted that mixed cellularity and neutrophilic forms of asthma have been described, and indeed there is some evidence that neutrophil dominated asthma may be part of the severe end of the spectrum. Allergen inhalation results in a marked increase in eosinophils in bronchoalveolar lavage fluid at the time of the late reaction, and there is a correlation between eosinophil counts in peripheral blood or bronchial lavage and AHR. Eosinophils are linked to the development of AHR through the release of basic proteins and oxygen-derived free radicals.[10] Several mechanisms are involved in recruitment of eosinophils into the airways. Eosinophils are derived from bone marrow precursors, and the signal for increased eosinophil production is presumably derived from the inflamed airway. Eosinophil recruitment initially involves adhesion of eosinophils to vascular endothelial cells in the airway circulation, their migration into the submucosa, and their subsequent activation. The role of individual adhesion molecules, cytokines, and mediators in orchestrating these responses has been extensively investigated. Adhesion of eosinophils involves the expression of specific glycoprotein molecules on the surface of eosinophils (integrins) and their expression of such molecules as intercellular adhesion molecule-1 (ICAM-1) on vascular endothelial cells. An antibody directed at ICAM-1 markedly inhibits eosinophil accumulation in the airways after allergen exposure and also blocks the accompanying hyperresponsiveness, although results in other species are less impressive. However, ICAM-1 is not selective for eosinophils and cannot account for the selective recruitment of eosinophils in allergic inflammation. The adhesion molecule very late antigen-4 (VLA-4) expressed on eosinophils, which interacts with VCAM-1, appears to be more selective for eosinophils, and IL-4 increases the expression of VCAM-1 on endothelial cells. Granulocyte-macrophage colony-stimulating factor (GM-CSF) and IL-5 may be important for the survival of eosinophils in the airways and for "priming" eosinophils to exhibit enhanced responsiveness.

There are several mediators involved in the migration of eosinophils from the circulation to the surface of the airway. The most potent and selective agents appear to be chemokines, such as RANTES (released on activation, normal T cell expressed and secreted), eotaxins 1 through 3, and macrophage chemotactic protein-4 (MCP-4), which are expressed in epithelial cells. There appears to be a cooperative interaction between IL-5 and chemokines, so that both cytokines are necessary for the eosinophilic response in airways. Once recruited to the airways, eosinophils require the presence of various growth factors, of which GM-CSF and IL-5 appear to be the most important. In the absence of these growth factors, eosinophils may undergo programmed cell death (apoptosis).

After a humanized monoclonal antibody to IL-5 is administered to asthmatic patients, there is a profound and prolonged reduction in circulating eosinophils and eosinophils recruited into the airway after allergen challenge. However, there is no effect on the response to inhaled allergen and no reduction in AHR. A clinical study with anti-IL-5-blocking antibody showed a similar profound reduction in circulating eosinophils, but no improvement in clinical parameters of asthma control. However, the eosinophils are not completely eradicated in the airway wall after this therapy, suggesting that they may still be exerting effects on the airways.

NEUTROPHILS

Neutrophils are the predominant inflammatory cells in patients with CF, but appear to be involved only in severe asthma, when increased numbers of neutrophils are found in the sputum and bronchial biopsies. It is not certain whether these neutrophils play a pathophysiologic role or whether they are a response to high does of corticosteroid therapy, which increases the survival of neutrophils. However, these neutrophils may generate oxidative stress, which may play an important role in the pathophysiology of severe asthma.

T LYMPHOCYTES

T lymphocytes play a very important role in coordinating the inflammatory response in asthma through the release of specific patterns of cytokines, resulting in the recruitment and survival of eosinophils and in the maintenance of mast cells in the airways.[11] T lymphocytes are coded to express a distinctive pattern of cytokines, which are similar to that described in the murine Th2 type of T lymphocytes, which characteristically express IL-4, IL-5, IL-9, and IL-13. This programming of T lymphocytes is presumably due to antigen-presenting cells, such as dendritic cells, which may migrate from the epithelium to regional lymph nodes or which interact with lymphocytes resident in the airway mucosa. The naïve immune system is skewed to express the Th2 phenotype; data now indicate that children with atopy are more likely to retain this skewed phenotype than normal children. There is some evidence that early infections or exposure to endotoxins might promote Th1-mediated responses to predominate and that a lack of infection or a clean environment in childhood may favor Th2 cell expression and thus atopic diseases.[12] Indeed, the balance between Th1 cells and Th2 cells is thought to be determined by locally released cytokines, such as IL-12, which tip the balance in favor of Th1 cells, or IL-4 or IL-13, which favor the emergence of Th2 cells (Fig. 5-2). Regulatory T (Tr) cells suppress the immune response through the secretion of inhibitory cytokines, such as IL-10 and transforming growth factor-β (TGF-β), and play an important role in immune regulation with suppression of Th1 responses,[13] and there is some evidence that regulatory T-cell function may be defective in asthmatic patients.[14]

B LYMPHOCYTES

In allergic diseases, B lymphocytes secrete IgE, and the factors regulating IgE secretion are now much better understood.[15] IL-4 is crucial in switching B cells to IgE production, and CD40 on T cells is an important accessory molecule that signals through interaction with CD40 ligand on B cells. There is increasing evidence for local production of IgE, even in patients with intrinsic asthma.

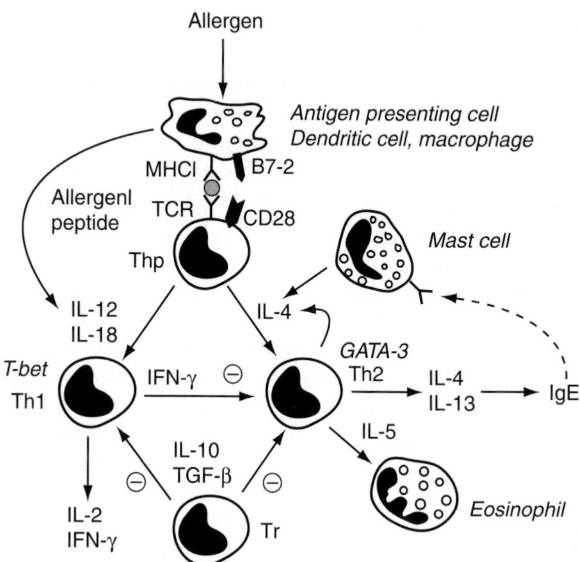

■ **FIGURE 5-2.** Asthmatic inflammation is characterized by a preponderance of T-helper 2 (Th2) lymphocytes over Th1 cells. The transcription factors T-bet and GATA-3 may regulate the balance between Th1 and Th2 cells. Regulatory T cells (Tr) have an inhibitory effect. IFN, interferon; IL, interleukin; TCR, T-cell receptor; TGF, transforming growth factor; Tp, T progenitor.

■ BASOPHILS

The role of basophils in asthma is uncertain, because these cells have previously been difficult to detect by immunocytochemistry. Using a basophil-specific marker, a small increase in basophils has been documented in the airways of asthmatic patients, with an increased number after allergen challenge. However, these cells are far outnumbered by eosinophils (approximately 10:1 ratio), and their functional role is unknown. There is also an increase in the numbers of basophils, as well as mast cells, in induced sputum after allergen challenge.

■ PLATELETS

There is some evidence for the involvement of platelets in the pathophysiology of allergic diseases, since platelet activation may be observed and there is evidence for platelets in bronchial biopsies of asthmatic patients. After allergen challenge there is a significant fall in circulating platelets, and circulating platelets from patients with asthma show evidence of increased activation and release the chemokine RANTES.

■ STRUCTURAL CELLS AS A SOURCE OF MEDIATORS

Structural cells of the airways, including epithelial cells, endothelial cells, fibroblasts, and even airway smooth muscle cells, may be an important source of inflammatory mediators, such as cytokines and lipid mediators in asthma and CF. Indeed, because structural cells far outnumber inflammatory cells in the airway, they may become the major source of mediators driving chronic airway inflammation. Epithelial cells may have a key role in translating inhaled environmental signals into an airway inflammatory response and are probably the major target cell for inhaled glucocorticoids in asthma (Fig. 5-3). Epithelial cells may also play an important role in CF in driving the neutrophilic inflammatory response. Airway epithelial cells, through the release of growth factors, may also be important in driving the structural changes that occur in chronic airway inflammation.[16]

■ INFLAMMATORY MEDIATORS

Many different mediators have been implicated in asthma, and they may have a variety of effects on the airways, which account for all of the pathologic features of asthma (Fig. 5-4). Although less is known about the mediators of CF, it is becoming clear that they differ from those implicated in asthma. Because each mediator has many effects, the role of individual mediators in the pathophysiology of airway inflammatory disease is not yet clear. The multiplicity and redundancy of effects of mediators makes it unlikely that preventing the synthesis or action of a single mediator will have a major impact in the therapy of these diseases. However, some mediators may play a more important role if they are upstream in the inflammatory process. The effects of single mediators can only be evaluated through the use of specific receptor antagonists or mediator synthesis inhibitors.

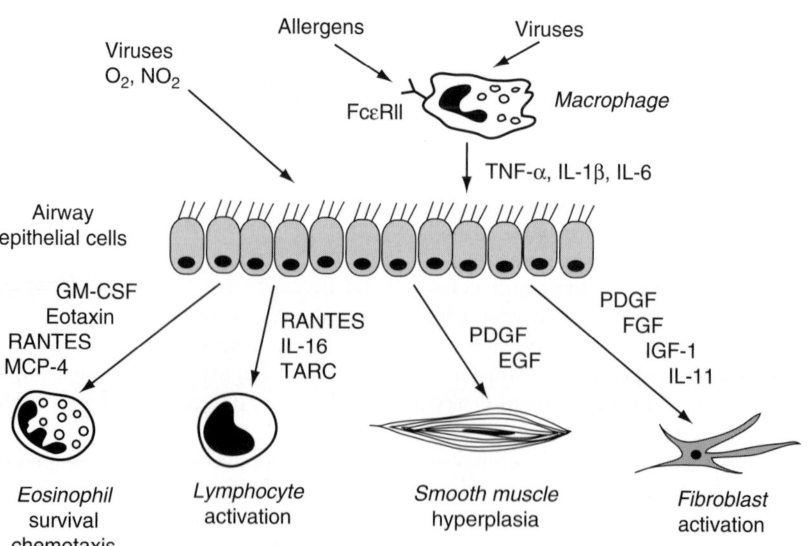

■ **FIGURE 5-3.** Airway epithelial cells may play an active role in asthmatic inflammation through the release of many inflammatory mediators, cytokines, chemokines, and growth factors.

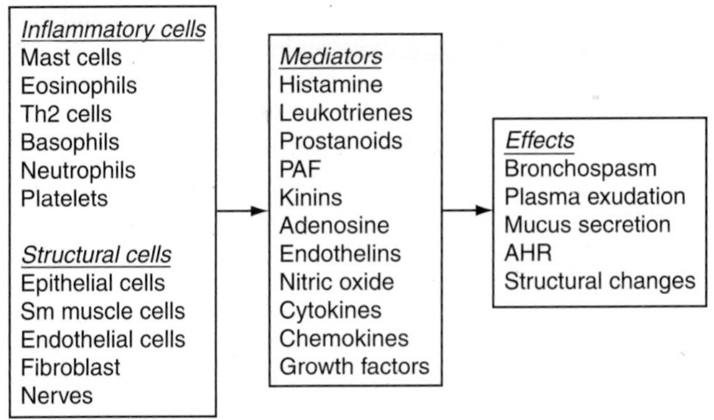

FIGURE 5-4. Many cells and mediators are involved in asthma and lead to several effects on the airways. AHR, airway hyperresponsiveness; PAF, platelet-activating factor.

LIPID MEDIATORS

The cysteinyl-leukotrienes (LTs) LTC_4, LTD_4, and LTE_4 are potent constrictors of human airways and may also increase AHR. The introduction of potent specific leukotriene antagonists has recently made it possible to evaluate the role of these mediators in asthma. Potent LTD_4 antagonists protect (by about 50%) against exercise- and allergen-induced bronchoconstriction, suggesting that leukotrienes contribute to bronchoconstrictor responses. Chronic treatment with anti-LTs improves lung function and symptoms in asthmatic patients, although the degree of lung function improvement is not as great as with inhaled corticosteroids, which have a much broader spectrum of effects.[17] In addition to their effects of airway smooth muscle and vessels, cys-LTs have weak anti-inflammatory effects. Platelet-activating factor (PAF) is a potent inflammatory mediator that mimics many of the features of asthma, including eosinophil recruitment and activation and induction of AHR, yet even potent PAF antagonists, such as modipafant, do not control asthma symptoms, at least in chronic asthma. Prostaglandins (PGs) have potent effects on airway function, and there is increased expression of the inducible form of cyclo-oxygenase 2 (COX-2) in asthmatic airways, but inhibition of their synthesis with COX inhibitors, such as aspirin or ibuprofen, does not have any effect in most patients with asthma. PGD_2 is a bronchoconstrictor prostaglandin produced predominantly by mast cells that activates a novel chemoattractant receptor termed chemoattractant receptor of Th2 cells (CRTH2), which is expressed on Th2 cells, eosinophils, and basophils and mediates chemotaxis of these cell types and may provide a link between mast cell activation and allergic inflammation.

CYTOKINES

Cytokines are cell-signaling molecules that are increasingly recognized to be important in chronic inflammation and to play a critical role in orchestrating this type of inflammatory response and are the target for the development of new asthma therapies[18] (Fig. 5-5). Many inflammatory cells (macrophages, mast cells, eosinophils, and lymphocytes) and airway structural cells are capable of synthesizing and releasing cytokines. While inflammatory mediators like histamine and leukotrienes may be important in the acute and subacute inflammatory responses and in exacerbations of asthma, it is likely that cytokines play a dominant role in maintaining chronic inflammation in airway diseases. Research in this area is hampered by a lack of specific antagonists, although important observations have been made using specific neutralizing antibodies that have been developed as novel therapies.[18]

The cytokines that appear to be of particular importance in asthma include the lymphokines secreted by T lymphocytes. There is increased gene expression of IL-5 in lymphocytes in bronchial biopsy samples from patients with symptomatic asthma and allergic rhinitis. However, as discussed above, a blocking antibody to IL-5, while profoundly reducing circulating eosinophils, has no effect on the allergic response or on asthma control. IL-4 and IL-13 both play a key role in the allergic inflammatory response since they determine the isotype switching in B cells that result in IgE formation. IL-4, but not IL-13, is also involved in differentiation of Th2 cells and therefore may be critical in the initial development of atopy, whereas IL-13 is much more abundant in established disease and may therefore be more important in maintaining the inflammatory process. Another Th2 cytokine, IL-9, may play a critical role in sensitizing the response to cytokines IL-4 and IL-5.

Other cytokines, such as IL-1β, IL-6, TNF-α, and GM-CSF, are released from a variety of cells, including macrophages and epithelial cells, and may be important in amplifying the inflammatory response. TNF-α may be an amplifying mediator in

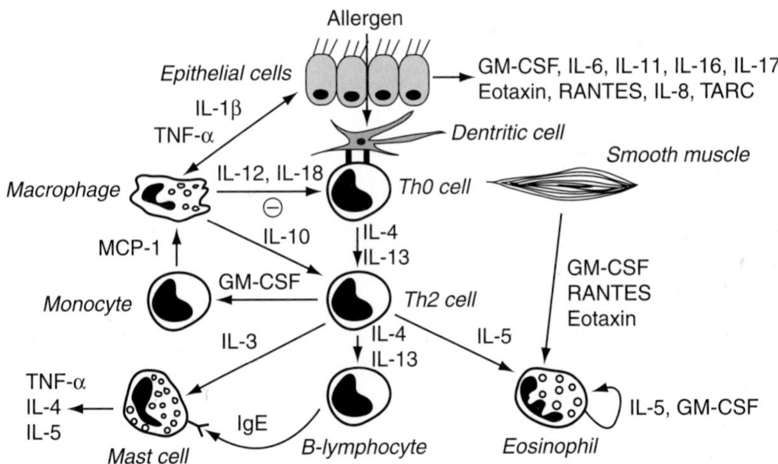

FIGURE 5-5. The cytokine network in asthma. Many inflammatory cytokines are released from inflammatory and structural cells in the airway and orchestrate and perpetuate the inflammatory response. GM-CSF, granulocyte-macrophage colony-stimulating factor; IL, interleukin; MCP, monocyte chemotactic protein; SCF, stem cell factor; TARC, thymus- and activation-regulated chemokine; TNF, tumor necrosis factor.

asthma and is produced in increased amounts in asthmatic airways. TNF-α and IL-1β both activate the proinflammatory transcription factors nuclear factor-κB (NF-κB) and activator protein-1 (AP-1), which then switch on many inflammatory genes in the asthmatic airway. Other cytokines, such as interferon-γ (IFN-γ), IL-10, IL-12, and IL-18, play a regulatory role and inhibit the allergic inflammatory process.

CHEMOKINES

Many chemokines are involved in the recruitment of inflammatory cells in the airways.[19] Chemokines are low molecular weight compounds (typically 8 to 10 kd) that regulate leukocyte trafficking across cellular barriers. There are four groups, defined by the number of amino acids separating the first two cysteine residues at the N-terminal end. There are four families: XCL; CXCL (ligand) and CXCR (receptor); CX3CL; and CCL. Over 50 different chemokines are now recognized, and they activate more than 20 different surface receptors. Chemokine receptors belong to the seven-transmembrane receptor superfamily of G protein–coupled receptors, and this makes it possible to find small molecule inhibitors, which has not been possible for classical cytokine receptors. Some chemokine receptors appear to be selective for single chemokines, whereas others are promiscuous and mediate the effects of several related chemokines. Chemokines appear to act in sequence in determining the final inflammatory response, and so inhibitors may be more or less effective depending on the kinetics of the response.

Several chemokines, including eotaxin, eotaxin-2, eotaxin-3, RANTES, and MCP-4, activate a common receptor on eosinophils termed CCR3. There is increased expression of eotaxin, eotaxin-2, MCP-3, MCP-4, and CCR3 in the airways of asthmatic patients, and this is correlated with increased AHR. Although it was thought that CCR3 receptors were restricted to eosinophils, there is now evidence for their expression on Th2 cells and mast cells, so that these inhibitors may have a more widespread effect than on eosinophils alone, making them potentially more valuable in asthma treatment. RANTES, which shows increased expression in asthmatic airways, also activates CCR3, but also has effects on CCR1 and CCR5, which may play a role in T-cell recruitment.

MCP-1 activates CCR2 on monocytes and T lymphocytes. Blocking MCP-1 with neutralizing antibodies reduces recruitment of both T cells and eosinophils in a murine model of ovalbumin-induced airway inflammation, with a marked reduction in AHR. MCP-1 also recruits and activates mast cells, an effect that is mediated via CCR2. MCP-1 instilled into the airways induces marked and prolonged AHR in mice, associated with mast cell degranulation. A neutralizing antibody to MCP-1 blocks the development of AHR in response to allergen. MCP-1 levels are increased in bronchoalveolar lavage fluid of patients with asthma. This has led to a search for small molecule inhibitors of CCR2.

CCR4 are selectively expressed on Th2 cells and are activated by the chemokines monocyte-derived chemokine (MDC) and thymus- and activation-regulated chemokine (TARC). Epithelial cells of patients with asthma express TARC, which may then recruit Th2 cells. Increased concentrations of TARC are also found in bronchoalveolar lavage fluid of asthmatic patients, whereas MDC is only weakly expressed in the airways. TARC may thus induce a sequence of responses resulting in coordinated eosinophilic inflammation. Inhibitors of CCR4 may therefore inhibit the recruitment of Th2 cells and thus persistent eosinophilic inflammation in the airways.

Different chemokines are involved in the recruitment of neutrophils. IL-8 and related CXC chemokines such as growth-related oncogene-α (GRO-α) play an important role and may be generated by macrophages and airway epithelial cells in CF patients.

OXIDATIVE STRESS

As in all inflammatory diseases, there is increased oxidative stress, as activated inflammatory cells, such as macrophages, neutrophils, and eosinophils, produce reactive oxygen species. Evidence for increased oxidative stress in asthma is provided by the increased concentrations of 8-isoprostane (a product of oxidized arachidonic acid) in exhaled breath condensates and increased ethane (a product of oxidative lipid peroxidation) in exhaled breath of asthmatic patients.[20] Increased oxidative stress is related to disease severity and may amplify the inflammatory response and reduce responsiveness to corticosteroids, particularly in severe disease and during exacerbations. One of the mechanisms whereby oxidative stress may be detrimental in asthma is through the reaction of superoxide anions with nitric oxide (NO) to form the reactive radical peroxynitrite, which may then modify several target proteins.

ENDOTHELINS

Endothelins are potent peptide mediators that are vasoconstrictors and bronchoconstrictors. Endothelin-1 levels are increased in the sputum of patients with asthma; these levels are modulated by allergen exposure and steroid treatment. Endothelins induce airway smooth muscle cell proliferation and promote a profibrotic phenotype and may therefore play a role in the chronic inflammation of asthma.

NITRIC OXIDE

NO is produced by several cells in the airway by NO synthases (NOS). The inducible from of NOS (iNOS) shows increased expression, particularly in airway epithelial cells and macrophages of asthmatic airways. Other constitutive NOS isoforms include neuronal (nNOS) and endothelial (eNOS). Although the cellular source of NO within the lung is not known, inferences based on mathematical models suggest that it is the large airways that are the source of NO. The combination of increased oxidative stress and NO may lead to the formation of the potent radical peroxynitrite that may result in nitration of proteins in the airways.

GROWTH FACTORS

Many growth factors are released in airway diseases from inflammatory cells and structural cells and these may play a critical role in the structural changes that occur in chronic inflammation, including fibrosis, airway smooth muscle thickening, angiogenesis, and mucous hyperplasia. While the role of individual mediators is not yet established, there is evidence for increased expression of TGF-β, a mediator associated with fibrosis; vascular-endothelial growth factor (VEGF), a mediator associated with angiogenesis; and epidermal growth factor, a mediator that induces mucous hyperplasia and expression of mucin genes (Fig. 5-6).

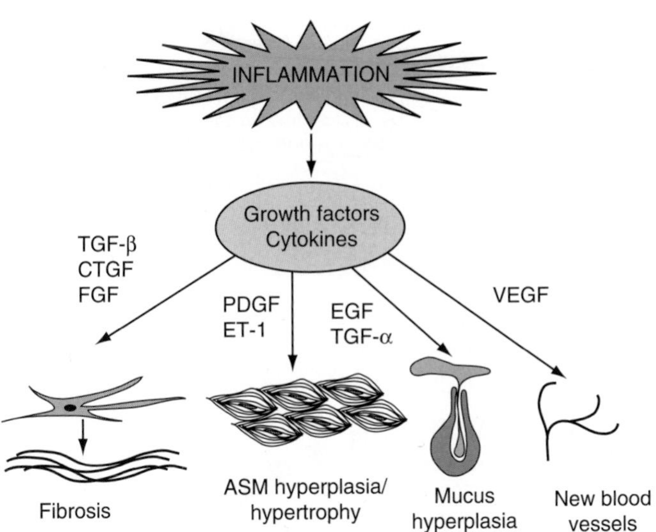

FIGURE 5-6. Growth factors and airway structural changes in asthma. CTGF, connective tissue growth factor; EGF, epidermal growth factor; ET, endothelin; FGF, fibroblast growth factor; PDGF, platelet-derived growth factor; TGF, transforming growth factor; VEGF, vascular-endothelial growth factor.

NEURAL MECHANISMS

Neural mechanisms may play an important role in the inflammatory response of airways. Neural reflexes may be activated by inflammatory signals, resulting in reflex bronchoconstriction, and airway nerves may release neurotransmitters, particularly neuropeptides, that have inflammatory effects.[21] There is a close interaction between nerves and inflammatory cells in allergic inflammation, because inflammatory mediators activate and modulate neurotransmission, whereas neurotransmitters may modulate the allergic inflammatory response. Inflammatory mediators may act on various prejunctional receptors on airway nerves to modulate the release of neurotransmitters. Inflammatory mediators may activate sensory nerves, resulting in reflex cholinergic bronchoconstriction or release of inflammatory neuropeptides (Fig. 5-7).

Inflammatory products may also sensitize sensory nerve endings in the airway epithelium, so that the nerves become hyperalgesic. Hyperalgesia and pain (dolor) are cardinal signs of inflammation, and in the asthmatic airway may mediate cough and chest tightness, which are characteristic symptoms of asthma. The precise mechanisms of hyperalgesia are not yet certain, but mediators such as prostaglandins, certain cytokines, and neurotrophins may be important. Neurotrophins, which may be released from various cell types in peripheral tissues, may cause proliferation and sensitization of airway sensory nerves.[22] Neurotrophins, such as nerve growth factor (NGF), may be released from inflammatory and structural cells in asthmatic airways and then stimulate the increased synthesis of neuropeptides, such as substance P, in airway sensory nerves, as well as sensitizing nerve endings in the airways. Thus, NGF is released from human airway epithelial cells after exposure to inflammatory stimuli. Neurotrophins may play an important role in mediating AHR in asthma.

Airway nerves may also release neurotransmitters that have inflammatory effects. Thus neuropeptides such as substance P, neurokinin A, and calcitonin gene-related peptide (CGRP) may be released from sensitized inflammatory nerves in the airways, which increases and extends the ongoing inflammatory response in asthma and other types of chronic inflammation.[23] There is increasing experimental evidence linking neurogenic inflammation with postrespiratory syncytial virus airway dysfunction, at least in rodents.

TRANSCRIPTION FACTORS

The chronic inflammation of asthma and CF is due to increased expression of multiple inflammatory proteins (cytokines, enzymes, receptors, adhesion molecules). In many cases, these inflammatory proteins are induced by transcription factors, DNA-binding factors that increase the transcription of selected target genes (Fig. 5-8). One transcription factor that may play a critical role in asthma is NF-κB, which can be activated by multiple stimuli, including protein kinase C activators, oxidants, and proinflammatory cytokines (such as IL-1β and TNF-α). There is evidence for increased activation of NF-κB in asthmatic airways, particularly in epithelial cells and macrophages. NF-κB regulates the expression of several key genes that are overexpressed in asthmatic and CF airways, including proinflammatory cytokines (IL-1β, TNF-α, GM-CSF), chemokines (IL-8, RANTES, macrophage inhibitory protein-1α [MIP-1α], eotaxin), adhesion molecules (ICAM-1, VCAM-1), and inflammatory enzymes (COX-2 and iNOS). The c-Fos component of AP-1 is also activated in asthmatic airways and often cooperates with NF-κB in switching on inflammatory genes. Many other

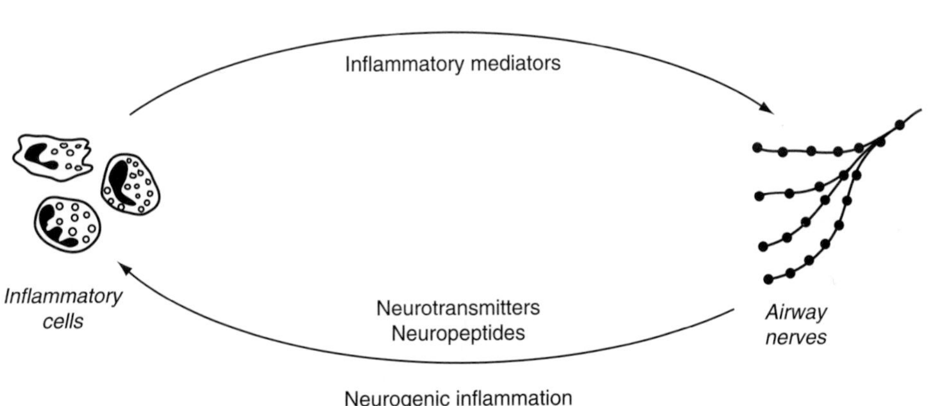

FIGURE 5-7. Two-way interaction between inflammation and neural control of the airways.

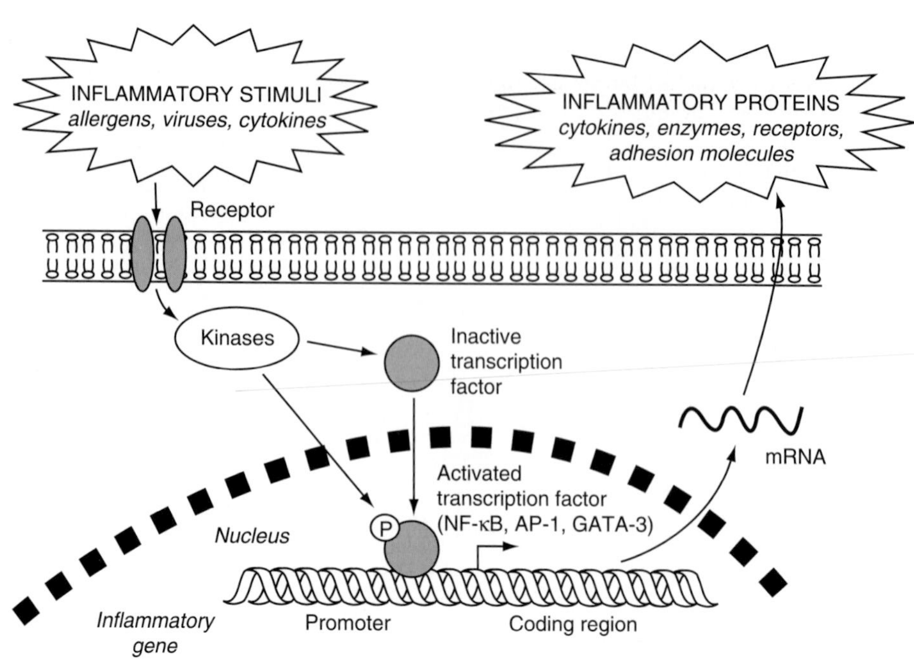

■ **FIGURE 5-8.** Transcription factors play a key role in amplifying and perpetuating the inflammatory response in asthma. Transcription factors, including nuclear factor-κB (NF-κB), activator protein-1 (AP-1), and GATA-3 are activated by inflammatory stimuli and increase the expression of multiple inflammatory genes.

transcription factors are involved in the abnormal expression of inflammatory genes in asthma, and there is growing evidence that there may be a common mechanism that involves activation of coactivator molecules at the start site of transcription of these genes that are activated by transcription factors to induce acetylation of core histones around which DNA is wound in the chromosome. This local unwinding of DNA opens up the chromatin structure and allows RNA polymerase and other transcription factors to bind, thus switching on gene transcription.[24]

Transcription factors play a critical role in determining the balance between Th1 and Th2 cells. The transcription factor GATA-3 determines the differentiation of Th2 cells and the expression of Th2 cytokines and shows increased expression in asthmatic patients.[25] The differentiation of Th1 cells is regulated by the transcription factor T-bet. Deletion of the T-bet gene is associated with an asthma-like phenotype in mice, suggesting that it may play an important role in regulating against the development of Th2 cells.

■ ANTI-INFLAMMATORY MECHANISMS

Although most emphasis has been placed on inflammatory mechanisms, there may be important anti-inflammatory mechanisms that may be defective in asthma, resulting in increased inflammatory responses in the airways.[26] Endogenous cortisol may be important as a regulator of the allergic inflammatory response, and nocturnal exacerbation of asthma may be related to the circadian fall in plasma cortisol. Blockade of endogenous cortisol secretion by metyrapone results in an increase in the late response to allergen in the skin. Cortisol is converted to the inactive cortisone by the enzyme 11β-hydroxysteroid dehydrogenase, which is expressed in airway tissues. It is possible that this enzyme functions abnormally in asthma or may determine the severity of asthma.

Various cytokines have anti-inflammatory actions. IL-1 receptor antagonist (IL-1ra) inhibits the binding of IL-1 to its receptors and therefore has a potential anti-inflammatory potential in asthma. It is reported to be effective in an animal model of asthma. IL-12 and IFN-γ enhance Th1 cells and inhibit Th2 cells. IL-12 promotes the differentiation and thus the suppression of Th2 cells, resulting in a reduction in eosinophilic inflammation, and its expression may be reduced in asthmatic airways.

IL-10, which was originally described as cytokine synthesis inhibitory factor, inhibits the expression of multiple inflammatory cytokines (TNF-α, IL-1β, GM-CSF) and chemokines, as well as inflammatory enzymes (iNOS, COX-2). There is evidence that IL-10 secretion and gene transcription are defective in macrophages and monocytes from asthmatic patients; this may lead to enhancement of inflammatory effects in asthma and may be a determinant of asthma severity.[27] IL-10 secretion is lower in monocytes from patients with severe compared with mild asthma, and there is an association between haplotypes associated with decreased production and severe asthma.

Other mediators may also have anti-inflammatory and immunosuppressive effects. PGE_2 has inhibitory effects on macrophages, epithelial cells, and eosinophils; exogenous PGE_2 inhibits allergen-induced airway responses, and its endogenous generation may account for the refractory period after exercise challenge. However, it is unlikely that endogenous PGE_2 is important in most asthmatics since nonselective cyclo-oxygenase inhibitors only worsen asthma in a minority of patients (aspirin-induced asthma), and aspirin-sensitive asthma is in any case rare in children.

■ NONINVASIVE ASSESSMENT OF AIRWAY INFLAMMATION

Inflammation plays a key role in the pathophysiology of airway diseases, and suppression of this inflammation is a major aim of therapy. This implies that the degree of inflammation needs to be assessed during clinical management. Physiologic measurements, such as spirometry, measure the outcome of inflammation, but only indirectly reflect inflammation. Furthermore, treatment with bronchodilators makes it difficult to interpret changes in spirometry. Direct measurement of inflammation by bronchial biopsy or bronchoalveolar lavage is used in research studies, but is clearly inappropriate for routine assessment and repeated measurements, especially in children. This means that less invasive procedures need to be devised for assessing airway inflammation.

INDUCED SPUTUM

Sputum may be induced by nebulized hypertonic saline for analysis of inflammatory cells and mediators in the supernatant. This technique has been applied successfully to children, but is difficult to use in clinical practice. Under age 6 years, very few children will produce a sputum sample, but in children over 12, 75% can produce a satisfactory sample.[28] Furthermore, induced sputum may induce wheezing in asthmatic patients, is uncomfortable, and may induce inflammation in the airways, making repeated measurements difficult. Although induced sputum has proved to be a useful research technique in investigating airway inflammation in children, it is unlikely to be of use in clinical practice due to the technical issues involved in obtaining samples.

EXHALED GASES

There has been considerable recent progress in the measurement of exhaled gases that may reflect the inflammatory process in the airways.[29] This technique is technically simple and is feasible even in young children. Repeated measurements are possible and it is also feasible in patients with severe disease.

EXHALED NITRIC OXIDE

Most progress has been made with NO, which may be detected in exhaled breath by chemiluminescence analyzers. The concentration of NO is increased in exhaled breath of children, including infants, with asthma and decreases with inhaled corticosteroid therapy. It is important to pay meticulous attention to the details of technique when making the measurements. On- or offline measurements can be made, including during a slow exhalation, tidal breathing, or even as part of the squeeze technique for measuring expiratory flow rates in infants. Exhaled NO is correlated with other markers of inflammation such as eosinophils in induced sputum and airway hyperresponsiveness in children. The relationship between NO and sputum eosinophils is closest in steroid-naïve children. There is increasing evidence that it may be useful in monitoring the control of inflammation in asthma and that it may predict exacerbations. Exhaled NO is paradoxically reduced in CF, and this may reflect the high degree of oxidative stress and generation of superoxide anions, which combine avidly with NO to form peroxynitrite, high concentrations of which are detectable in CF airways.

Much of the early work was done by measuring FeNO using a single expiratory flow rate. It is well known that FeNO levels are inversely proportional to flow rate. Recently, sophisticated mathematical modeling combined with measurements of FeNO at different expiratory flow rates has allowed the partition of NO production to an airway and alveolar components. This technique requires a considerable degree of cooperation, and is not suited to young children. At the moment it remains in the realm of research.

OTHER EXHALED GASES

There are other exhaled volatile markers of inflammation, but they are less well characterized than NO. Exhaled carbon monoxide reflects the activation of heme oxygenase-1 an enzyme induced by stress. Concentrations of CO are increased in asthmatic and CF children, but there is a large degree of overlap with values in normal children, and environmental factors interfere with the measurements, so it is less useful than exhaled NO. Ethane is formed by lipid peroxidation in response to oxidative stress, and levels are increased in asthma and CF, but this requires complex measurements by gas chromatography/mass spectrometry so that it is not practical in clinical studies. Indeed, exhaled breath contains multiple hydrocarbons, and there is emerging evidence that these may show different patterns in different diseases, reflecting the different components of inflammation, so that each disease may have a unique "breathogram."

EXHALED BREATH CONDENSATE

Another technique that is gaining popularity is exhaled breath condensate (EBC) which is formed through condensation of cooled exhaled breath for analysis of a variety of mediators, including hydrogen peroxide, lipid mediators, purines, and cytokines.[30] Differences in the patterns of mediators are found between asthma and CF, reflecting the different inflammatory mediators in the respiratory tract. Exhaled 8-isoprostane has been found to be a useful measurement of oxidative stress with increased concentrations in severe asthma and CF. The concentrations of mediators in EBC are low, so that sensitive assays are needed and great attention needs to be paid to the collection procedure and avoidance of salivary contamination. New approaches in the future include metabonomic analysis, where multiple metabolites are monitored, giving unique patterns for each disease.

CONCLUSIONS

Airway inflammation is a critical component of many chronic airway diseases in children. The inflammatory response involves many different inflammatory cells, which are recruited to and activated in the airways. Each of these cells releases multiple mediators, which then exert effects on the airway wall. In asthma the major effects are bronchoconstriction and plasma exudation, whereas in CF the predominant response is mucus hypersecretion. Among the multiple mediators of inflammation, cytokines play an important role in orchestrating the inflammatory response and amplifying and perpetuating inflammation, whereas chemokines play a key role in selective recruitment of inflammatory cells to the airway. The molecular basis of inflammation is now better understood, with increased expression of multiple inflammatory genes, switched on by transcription factors, such as NF-κB and AP-1. Endogenous anti-inflammatory mechanisms counteract these inflammatory mechanisms, and there is some evidence that they may be defective in asthma, allowing inflammation to become more severe or to persist longer. Neural mechanisms and neurotrophins may also be involved in amplifying the inflammatory response. This complex inflammatory process needs to be monitored in the management of the disease, and there are several new noninvasive approaches to monitory inflammation in the airway by breath analysis, including exhaled NO and exhaled breath condensate, which look promising in children.

REFERENCES

1. Cohn L, Elias JA, Chupp GL: Asthma: Mechanisms of disease persistence and progression. Annu Rev Immunol 2004;22:789–815.
2. Vignola AM, Mirabella F, Costanzo G, Di Giorgi R, Gjomarkaj M, Bellia V, Bonsignore G: Airway remodeling in asthma. Chest 2003;123(Suppl): 417–422.
3. McParland BE, Macklem PT, Pare PD: Airway wall remodeling. Friend or foe? J Appl Physiol 2003;95:426–434.
4. Barnes PJ: Pathophysiology of asthma. Eur Respir Mon 2003;8:84–113.
5. Payne DN, Rogers AV, Adelroth E, Bandi V, Guntupalli KK, Bush A, Jeffery PK: Early thickening of the reticular basement membrane in children with difficult asthma. Am J Respir Crit Care Med 2003;167:78–82.
6. Brightling CE, Bradding P, Pavord ID, Wardlaw AJ: New insights into the role of the mast cell in asthma. Clin Exp Allergy 2003;33:550–556.
7. Lanier BQ: Newer aspects in the treatment of pediatric and adult asthma. Monoclonal anti-IgE. Ann Allergy Asthma Immunol 2003;90:13–15.
8. Banchereau J, Briere F, Caux C, Davoust J, Lebecque S, Liu YJ, Pulendran B, Palucka K: Immunobiology of dendritic cells. Annu Rev Immunol 2000;18:767–811.
9. Holt PG, Stumbles PA: Regulation of immunologic homeostasis in peripheral tissues by dendritic cells. The respiratory tract as a paradigm. J Allergy Clin Immunol 2000;105:421–429.
10. Robinson DS, Kay AB, Wardlaw AJ: Eosinophils. Clin Allergy Immunol 2002;16:43–75.
11. Larche M, Robinson DS, Kay AB: The role of T lymphocytes in the pathogenesis of asthma. J Allergy Clin Immunol 2003;111:450–463.
12. Liu AH, Murphy JR: Hygiene hypothesis. Fact or fiction? J Allergy Clin Immunol 2003;111:471–478.
13. Umetsu DT, Akbari O, DeKruyff RH: Regulatory T cells control the development of allergic disease and asthma. J Allergy Clin Immunol 2003;112:480–487.
14. Ling EM, Smith T, Nguyen XD, Pridgeon C, Dallman M, Arbery J, Carr VA, Robinson DS: Relation of $CD4^{+}CD25^{+}$ regulatory T-cell suppression of allergen-driven T-cell activation to atopic status and expression of allergic disease. Lancet 2004;363:608–615.
15. Gould HJ, Beavil RL,Vercelli D: IgE isotype determination. Epsilon-germline gene transcription, DNA recombination and B-cell differentiation. Br Med Bull 2000;56:908–924.
16. Knight DA, Holgate ST: The airway epithelium. Structural and functional properties in health and disease. Respirology 2003;8:432–446.
17. Barnes PJ: Anti-leukotrienes. Here to stay? Curr Opin Pharmacol 2003;3:257–263.
18. Barnes PJ: Cytokine modulators as novel therapies for asthma. Ann Rev Pharmacol Toxicol 2002;42:81–98.
19. Panina-Bordignon P, D'Ambrosio D: Chemokines and their receptors in asthma and chronic obstructive pulmonary disease. Curr Opin Pulmon Med 2003;9:104–110.
20. Paredi P, Kharitonov SA, Barnes PJ: Analysis of expired air for oxidation products. Am J Respir Crit Care Med 2002;166(Suppl):31–37.
21. Joos GF, De Swert KO, Schelfhout V, Pauwels RA: The role of neural inflammation in asthma and chronic obstructive pulmonary disease. Ann NY Acad Sci 2003;992:218–230.
22. Freund V, Frossard N: Expression of nerve growth factor in the airways and its possible role in asthma. Prog Brain Res 2004;146:335–346.
23. Barnes PJ: Neurogenic inflammation in the airways. Respir Physiol 2001;125:145–154.
24. Barnes PJ, Adcock IM: How do corticosteroids work in asthma? Ann Intern Med 2003;139:359–370.
25. Zhou M, Ouyang W: The function role of GATA-3 in Th1 and Th2 differentiation. Immunol Res 2003;28:25–37.
26. Barnes PJ: Endogenous inhibitory mechanisms in asthma. Am J Respir Crit Care Med 2000;161(Suppl):176–181.
27. Barnes PJ: IL-10. A key regulator of allergic disease. Clin Exp Allergy 2001; 31:667–669.
28. Gibson PG, Henry RL, Thomas P: Noninvasive assessment of airway inflammation in children. Induced sputum, exhaled nitric oxide, and breath condensate. Eur Respir J 2000;16:1008–1015.
29. Kharitonov SA, Barnes PJ: Exhaled markers of pulmonary disease. Am J Respir Crit Care Med 2001;163:1693–1772.
30. Montuschi P, Barnes PJ: Analysis of exhaled breath condensate for monitoring airway inflammation. Trends Pharmacol Sci 2002;23:232–237.

6 The History and Physical Examination

Hans Pasterkamp, MD

At the beginning of the 21st century the diagnosis of disease still requires a detailed medical history and a thorough physical examination. For the majority of patients in many areas of the world, additional information from laboratory tests and other data are of rather limited availability. Modern science and technology have changed the situation considerably in the industrialized nations, but we are paying a high price. Cost containment in health care has become essential, and physicians have to be skillful in their history taking and physical examination techniques to collect a maximum of information before ordering expensive medical-technical investigations. The relevance of these skills in pediatric respiratory medicine is exemplified by clinical severity scores that are widely used in care maps for asthma, bronchiolitis, and croup in children, or in scores developed to manage patients suspected to have severe acute respiratory syndrome (SARS).

The diagnosis of disease in children even more than in older patients has to rely on the patient's history and on observations gathered during the physical examination. Young children cannot follow instructions and participate in formal physiologic testing, and physicians hesitate before subjecting their pediatric patients to invasive diagnostic procedures. Diseases of the respiratory tract are among the most common in children, and in the majority of cases they can be correctly identified from medical history data and physical findings alone. The following review of the medical history and physical examination in children with respiratory disease includes some observations that were made with the help of modern technology. These technologic aids do not lessen the value of subjective perceptions but rather emphasize how new methods may further our understanding, sharpen our senses, and thereby advance the art of medical diagnosis.

THE HISTORY

GENERAL PRINCIPLES

The medical history should be taken in an environment with comfortable seating for all, a place for clothing and belongings, and some toys for younger children. Formula should be on hand to help quiet infants and toddlers. Privacy has to be assured, without the usual interruptions by phone calls and other distractions. If possible, the physician should see one child at a time because the presence of young siblings or other children in the room tends to be distracting. Data that should be recorded at the beginning include the patient's name and address, the parents' or guardians' home and work phone numbers, the name of the referring physician, and information on the kindergarten or school if this is relevant. In many cases the history will be given by someone other than the patient, but the physician should still ask even young children directly about their complaints. When asking about the history of the present illness, the physician should encourage a clear and chronologic narrative account. Questions should be open ended, and at intervals the physician should give a verbal summary to confirm and clarify the information. Past medical data and system review are usually obtained by answers to direct questions.

STRUCTURE OF THE PEDIATRIC HISTORY

The source of and the reason for referral should be noted. On occasion, the referral may have been made by someone other than the patient or the parents, such as a school teacher, a relative, or a friend. The *chief complaint* and the person most concerned about it should be identified. The *illness at presentation* should be documented in detail regarding its onset and duration, the environment and circumstances under which it developed, its manifestations and their treatments, and its impact on the patient and the family. Symptoms should be defined by their qualitative and quantitative characteristics as well as by their timing, location, aggravating or alleviating factors, and associated manifestations. Relevant past medical and laboratory data should be included in the documentation of the present illness.

This general approach is also applicable when the emphasis is on a single organ system, such as the respiratory tract. The onset of disease may have been gradual (e.g., with some interstitial lung diseases) or sudden (e.g., with foreign body aspiration). The physician should ask about initial manifestations and who noticed them first. The age at first presentation is important because respiratory diseases that manifest soon after birth are more likely to have been inherited or to be related to congenital malformations. Depending on the duration of symptoms, the illness will be classified as acute, subacute, chronic, or recurrent. These definitions are arbitrary, but a disease of less than 3 weeks duration is generally called acute, between 3 weeks and 3 months subacute, and longer than 3 months chronic. If symptoms are clearly discontinuous, with documented intervals of well-being, the disease is recurrent. This distinction is important because many parents may perceive their child as being chronically ill, not realizing that young normal children may have six to eight respiratory infections per year, particularly during the first 2 years if the child is in a daycare setting or if they have older siblings.

Respiratory diseases are often affected by environmental factors. There should be a careful search for seasonal changes in symptoms to uncover possible allergic causes. Exposure to noxious inhaled agents, for example, from industrial pollution or more commonly from indoor pollution by cigarette smoke, can sustain or aggravate a patient's coughing and wheezing. Similarly, a wood-burning stove used for indoor heating may be a contributing factor. The physician should therefore obtain a detailed description of the patient's home environment. Are there household pets, such as dogs, cats, and hamsters, or birds, such as budgies, pigeons, or parrots? What are the plants in and around the house? Are there animal or vegetable fibers in the bedclothes or in the floor and window coverings (e.g., wool, feathers)? Are there systems in use for air conditioning and humidification?

There may be a relationship between respiratory symptoms and daily activities. Exercise is a common trigger factor for cough and wheezing in many patients with hyperreactive airways. A walk outside in cold air may have similar effects. Diurnal variation of symptoms may be apparent, and attention should be paid to changes that occur at night. These changes may also be related to airway cooling, or they may reflect conditions that are worse in the recumbent position, such as postnasal drip or gastroesophageal reflux. Food intake may bring on symptoms of respiratory distress when food is aspirated or when food allergies are present.

A large proportion of children presenting with respiratory symptoms will be suffering from infection, most often viral. It is important to know whether other family members or persons in regular contact with the patient are also affected. When unusual infections are suspected, questions should be asked about recent travel to areas where exotic infective organisms may have been acquired. Drug abuse by parents or by older patients and others with high-risk lifestyles may lead the physician to consider the possibility of the acquired immunodeficiency syndrome (AIDS).

Descriptions of respiratory disease manifestations may come from the parents or directly from an older child. Common symptoms are fever, cough and sputum production, wheezing or noisy breathing, dyspnea, and chest pain. Most of these are discussed in more detail at the end of this chapter.

The previous medical history will provide an impression of the general health status of the child. First, the birth history should be reviewed, including prenatal, natal, and neonatal events. The physician should inquire about the course of pregnancy, particularly whether the mother and fetus suffered from infections, metabolic disorders, or exposure to noxious agents, such as nicotine. The duration of pregnancy, possible multiple births, and circumstances leading to the onset of labor should be noted. Difficult labor and delivery may cause respiratory problems at birth (e.g., asphyxia and meconium aspiration), and the physician should ask about birth weight and Apgar scores. The neonatal course has to be reviewed carefully because many events during this period may have an impact on the patient's respiratory status in later years. Were there any signs of neonatal respiratory distress, such as tachypnea, retractions, and cyanosis? Treatment with oxygen or endotracheal intubation should be recorded. Some extrathoracic disorders provide valuable clues for diagnosis, such as the presence of eczema in atopic infants or neonatal conjunctivitis in a young patient with chlamydia pneumonia, particularly if there was a documented infection of the mother.

Much is learned from a detailed feeding history, which should include the amount, type, and schedule of food intake. The physician should ask whether the child was fed by breast or bottle. For the newborn and young infant, feeding is a substantial physical exercise and may, in the presence of respiratory disease, lead to distress, much as climbing stairs does in the older patient. The question of exercise tolerance in an infant is therefore asked by inquiring how long it takes the patient to finish a meal. The caloric intake of infants with respiratory disease is often reduced despite an increased caloric need, to support the work of breathing. This reduced caloric intake commonly results in a failure to thrive. Older patients with chronic respiratory disease and productive cough may suffer from a continuous exposure of their taste buds to mucopurulent secretions and may quite understandably lose their appetites, but medical treatment (e.g., with certain antibiotics) may have similar effects. Patients with food hypersensitivity may react with bronchospasm or even with interstitial lung disease on exposure to the allergen (e.g., to milk). Physical irritation and inflammation occur if food is aspirated into the respiratory tract. This happens frequently in patients with debilitating neurologic diseases and deficient protective reflexes of the upper airways but may also occur in neurologically intact children.

The physical development of children with chronic respiratory diseases may be retarded. Malnutrition in the presence of increased caloric requirements is common, but the effects of some long-term medical treatments (e.g., with steroids) should also be considered. Previous measurements of body growth should be obtained and plotted on standard nomograms. Psychosocial development may be affected if chronic lung diseases, such as asthma or cystic fibrosis, limit attendance and performance at school or if behavioral problems arise in children and adolescents subjected to chronic therapy. More severely affected patients may also be delayed in their sexual development.

Many diseases of the respiratory tract in children have a genetic component, either with a clear mendelian mode of inheritance (e.g., autosomal recessive in cystic fibrosis, homozygous deficiency of α_1-antitrypsin, sex-linked recessive in chronic granulomatous disease, and autosomal dominant in familial interstitial fibrosis) or with a genetic contribution to the cause. Examples of familial aggregation of respiratory disease are chronic bronchitis and bronchiectasis or familial emphysema in patients with heterozygous α_1-antitrypsin deficiency, in which the susceptibility of the lung to the action of irritants (e.g., cigarette smoke) is increased. A mixed influence of genetic and environmental factors exists in polygenic diseases, such as asthma or allergic rhinitis.

When inquiring about the family history, the physician should review at least two generations on either side. The parents should be asked whether they are related by blood, and information should be obtained about any childhood deaths in the family. The health of the patient's siblings and also of brothers and sisters of both parents should be documented. Particular attention should be paid to histories of asthma, allergies and hay fever, chronic bronchitis, emphysema, tuberculosis, cystic fibrosis, and sudden unexpected infant death.

A detailed report of prior tests and immunizations should be obtained. Quite often this requires communication with other health care providers. Results of screening examinations (e.g., tuberculin and other skin tests, chest radiographs, and sweat chloride measurements) should be noted. Similarly, childhood illnesses, immunizations, and possible adverse immunization reactions should be documented. If the history is positive for allergic reactions, these have to be confirmed and defined. Previous hospital admissions and their indications should be listed, and the patient's current medications and their efficacy should be documented. If possible, the drug containers and prescriptions should be reviewed. The physician may use the opportunity to discuss the pharmacologic information and the technique of drug administration, particularly with inhaled bronchodilator medications.

One of the most important goals in taking a history is to become more aware of the particular psychological and social situation of the patient. It is impossible to judge current complaints or responses to medical interventions without an individual frame of reference for each patient. The physician should encourage the child and the parents to describe a typical day at home, daycare, kindergarten, or school. This will provide valuable information about the impact of the illness on daily routines, the financial implications, the existing or absent social support structures, and the coping strategies of the family. Compliance with medical treatment is rarely better than 50%, and physicians are generally unable to predict how well their patients follow and adhere to therapeutic regimens. Compliance can improve if the patient and the parents gain a better understanding of the disease and its treatment. It is important to recognize prior experiences that the family may have had with the health care system and to understand individual religious and health beliefs. Particularly in children with chronic respiratory ailments whose symptoms are not being controlled or prevented, the effort and unpleasantness (e.g., of chest physiotherapy) may limit the use of such interventions. The physician should also consider the social stigma associated with visible therapy, especially among peers of the adolescent patient.

A review of organ systems is usually the last part of the history and may actually be completed during the physical examination. Although the emphasis is on the respiratory system, questions about the general status of the child will be about appetite, sleep, level of activity, and prevailing mood. Important findings in the region of the head and neck are nasal obstruction and discharge, ear or sinus infection, conjunctival irritation, sore throat, and swallowing difficulty. The respiratory manifestations of coughing, noisy breathing, wheezing, and cyanosis are discussed in detail at the end of this chapter. Cardiovascular findings may include palpitations and dysrhythmia in hypoxic patients; there may be edema formation and peripheral swelling with cor pulmonale. Effects of respiratory disease on the gastrointestinal tract may appear with cough-induced vomiting and abdominal pain. There may be a direct involvement with diarrhea, cramps, and fatty stools in patients with cystic fibrosis. The physician should ask about hematuria and about skin manifestations, such as eczema or rashes, and about swellings and pain of lymph nodes or joints. Finally, neurologic symptoms, such as headache, lightheadedness, or paresthesia, may be related to respiratory disease and cough paroxysms or hyperventilation.

THE PHYSICAL EXAMINATION

Traditionally, the physical examination is divided into inspection, palpation, auscultation, and percussion. The sequence of these steps may be varied depending on the circumstances, particularly in the assessment of the respiratory tract in children. The classic components of the physical examination and some modern aids and additions are discussed in the following sections.

INSPECTION

Much can be learned from simple observation, particularly during those precious moments of sleep in the young infant or toddler, who when awake can be a challenge even for the skilled examiner. First, the pattern of breathing should be observed. This includes the respiratory rate, rhythm, and effort. The respiratory rate decreases with age and shows its greatest variability in newborns and young infants (Fig. 6-1). The rate should be counted over at least 1 minute, ideally several times for the calculation of average values. Because respiratory rates differ among sleep states and become even more variable during wakefulness, a note should be made describing the behavioral state of the patient. Observing abdominal movements or listening to breath sounds with the stethoscope placed before the mouth and nose may help in counting respirations in patients with very shallow thoracic excursions.

Longitudinal documentation of the respiratory rate during rest or sleep is important for the follow-up of patients with chronic lung diseases, even more so for those too young for standard pulmonary function tests. Abnormally high breathing frequencies or tachypnea can be seen in patients with decreased compliance of the respiratory apparatus and in those with metabolic acidosis. Other causes of tachypnea are fever (approximately five to seven breaths per minute increase per degree above 37°C), anemia, exertion, intoxication (salicylates), and anxiety and psychogenic hyperventilation. The opposite, an abnormally slow respiratory rate or bradypnea, can occur in patients with metabolic alkalosis or central nervous system depression. The terms *hyperpnea* and *hypopnea* refer to abnormally deep or shallow respirations. At given respiratory rates, this determination is a subjective clinical judgment and is not easily quantified unless the pattern is obvious, such as the Kussmaul type of breathing in patients with diabetic ketoacidosis.

Significant changes in the rhythm of breathing occur during the first months of life. Respiratory pauses of less than 6 seconds are common in infants under 3 months of age. If these pauses occur in groups of three or more that are separated by less than 20 seconds of respiration, the pattern is referred to as periodic breathing. This pattern is very common in premature infants after the first days of life and may persist until 44 weeks postconceptional age. In full-term infants, periodic breathing is usually observed between 1 week and 2 months of age and

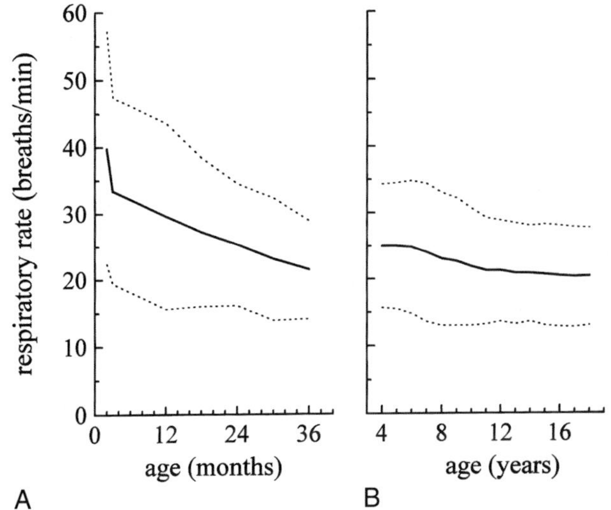

■ **FIGURE 6-1.** **A** and **B,** Mean values *(solid line)* ± 2 SD *(dotted lines)* of the normal respiratory rate at rest (during sleep in children under 3 years of age). There is no significant difference between the sexes, and the regression lines represent data from both boys and girls. The respiratory rate decreases with age and shows the greatest normal variation during the first 2 years of life. (**A,** Data from Rusconi F, Castagneto M, Gagliardi L, et al: Reference values for respiratory rate in the first 3 years of life. Pediatrics 1994;94:350. **B,** Data from Hooker EA, Danzl DF, Brueggmeyer M, Harper E: Respiratory rates in pediatric emergency patients. J Emerg Med 1992;10:407.)

is normally absent by 6 months. Apnea with cessation of air flow lasting more than 15 seconds is uncommon and may be accompanied by bradycardia and cyanosis. In preterm infants, a drop in oxygen saturation may be seen up to 7 seconds after a respiratory pause when in room air and up to 9 seconds later when on supplemental oxygen.

Other abnormal patterns include Cheyne-Stokes breathing, which occurs as cycles of increasing and decreasing tidal volumes separated by apnea (e.g., in children with congestive heart failure and increased intracranial pressure). Biot breathing consists of irregular cycles of respiration at variable tidal volumes interrupted by apnea and is an ominous finding in patients with severe brain damage.

After noting the rate and rhythm of breathing, the physician should look for signs of increased respiratory effort. The older child will be able to communicate the subjective experience of difficult breathing, or dyspnea. Objective signs that reflect distressed breathing are chest wall retractions; visible use of accessory muscles and the alae nasi; orthopnea; and paradoxical respiratory movements. The more negative intrapleural pressure during inspiration against a high airway resistance leads to retraction of the pliable portions of the chest wall, including the inter- and subcostal tissues and the supraclavicular and suprasternal fossae. Conversely, bulging of intercostal spaces may be seen when pleural pressure becomes greatly positive during a maximally forced expiration. Retractions are more easily visible in the newborn infant, in whom intercostal tissues are thinner and more compliant than in the older child.

Visible contraction of the sternocleidomastoid muscles and indrawing of supraclavicular fossae during inspiration are among the most reliable clinical signs of airway obstruction. In young infants, these muscular contractions may lead to head bobbing, which is best observed when the child rests with the head supported slightly at the suboccipital area. If no other signs of respiratory distress are present in an infant with head bobbing, however, central nervous system disorders, such as third ventricular cysts, should be considered. Older patients with chronic airway obstruction and extensive use of accessory muscles may appear to have a short neck because of hunched shoulders. Orthopnea exists when the patient is unable to tolerate a recumbent position.

Flaring of the alae nasi is a sensitive sign of respiratory distress and may be present when inspiration is abnormally short (e.g., under conditions of chest pain). Nasal flaring enlarges the anterior nasal passages and reduces upper and total airway resistance. It may also help to stabilize the upper airways by preventing large negative pharyngeal pressures during inspiration.

The normal movement of chest and abdominal walls is directed outward during inspiration. Inward motion of the chest wall during inspiration is called paradoxical breathing. This is seen when the thoracic cage loses its stability and becomes distorted by the action of the diaphragm. Classically, paradoxical breathing with a seesaw type of thoracoabdominal motion is seen in patients with paralysis of the intercostal muscles, but it is also commonly seen in premature and newborn infants who have a very compliant rib cage. Inspiratory indrawing of the lateral chest is known as Hoover's sign and can be observed in patients with obstructive airway disease. Paradoxical breathing also occurs during sleep in patients with upper airway obstruction. The development of paradoxical breathing in an awake, nonparalyzed patient beyond the newborn period usually indicates respiratory muscle fatigue and impending respiratory failure.

Following inspection of the breathing pattern, the examiner should pay attention to the symmetry of respiratory chest excursions. Unilateral diseases affecting lungs, pleura, chest wall, or diaphragm may all result in asymmetric breathing movements. Trauma to the rib cage may cause fractures and a "flail chest" that shows local paradoxical movement. Pain during respiration usually leads to "splinting" with flexion of the trunk toward and decreased respiratory movements of the affected side. The signs of hemidiaphragmatic paralysis may be subtle and are usually more noticeable in the lateral decubitus position with the paralyzed diaphragm placed up. This position tends to accentuate the paradoxical inward epigastric motion on the affected side.

Other methods to augment inspection of chest wall motion use optical markers. In practice, this technique is done by placing both hands on either side of the patient's lateral rib cage with the thumbs along the costal margins. Divergence of the thumbs during expansion of the thorax supposedly aids in the visual perception of the range and symmetry of respiratory movements. This technique is of little use in children. A more accurate method of documenting the vectors of movement at different sites (but one that is not yet practical for bedside evaluation) is to place a grid of optical markers on the chest surface and film their positional changes during respiration relative to a steady reference frame. A similar concept is used in optical studies of chest deformities. Projection of raster lines onto the anterior chest surface allows stereographic measurement of deformities, such as pectus excavatum, and augments the visual image of the surface shape (Fig. 6-2). In practice and without such tools,

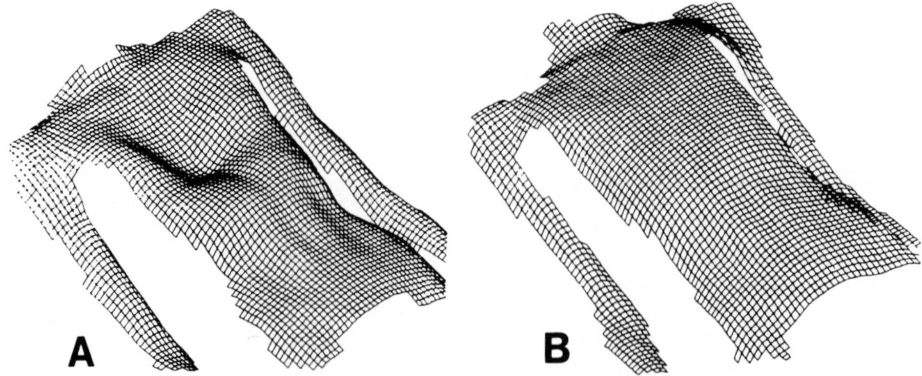

FIGURE 6-2. Optical markers augment the visual perception of chest wall deformities. In this example of rasterstereography, lines are projected onto the anterior thorax, and the surface image is computed as a regular network. The change of the funnel chest deformity before **(A)** and after surgery **(B)** is easily appreciated. In practice and at the bedside, the physician should inspect at different angles of illumination to enhance the visual perception of chest wall deformities. (From Hierholzer E, Schier F: Rasterstereography in the measurement and postoperative follow-up of anterior chest wall deformities. Z Kinderchir 1986;41:267–271.)

however, the physician should inspect the chest at different angles of illumination to enhance the visual perception of chest wall deformities. Their location, size, symmetry, and change with respiratory or cardiac movements should be noted.

The dimensions of the chest should be measured. Chest size and shape are influenced by ethnic and geographic factors that should be taken into account when measurements are compared with normative data. Andean children who live at high altitudes, for example, have larger chest dimensions relative to stature than children in North America. The chest circumference is usually taken at the mamillary level during midinspiration. In practice, mean readings during inspiration and expiration should be noted (Fig. 6-3*A*). Premature infants have a greater head circumference than chest circumference, while these measurements are very similar at term (see Fig. 6-3*B*). Malnutrition can delay the time at which chest circumference begins to exceed head circumference.

Further objective documentation of the chest configuration may include measurements of thoracic depth (anteroposterior [AP] diameter) and width (transverse diameter). The thoracic index, or the ratio of AP over transverse diameter, is close to unity in infants and decreases during childhood. Measurements should be taken with a caliper at the level of the nipples in upright subjects. Normative values for young children are available but

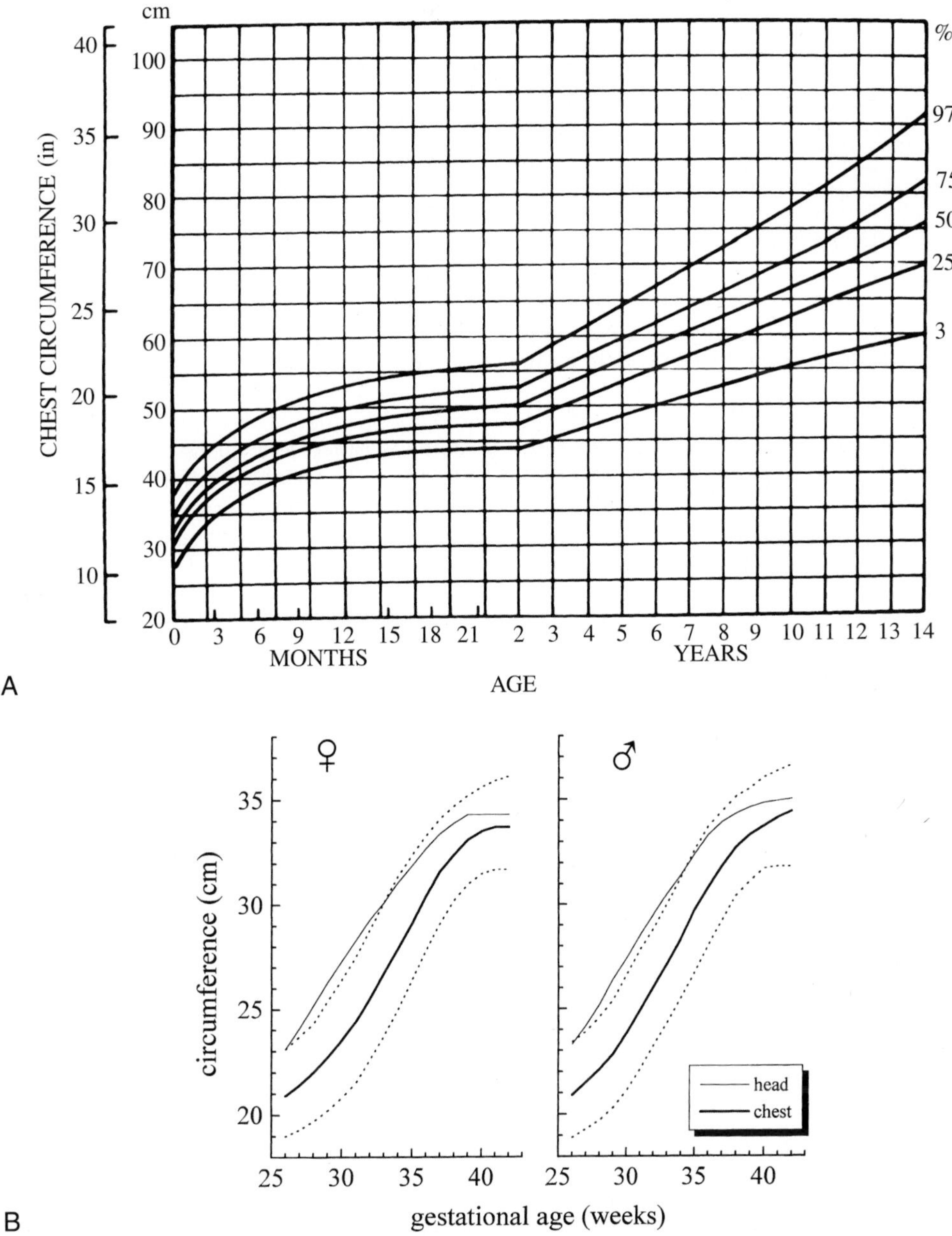

■ **FIGURE 6-3.** **A,** Normal distribution of chest circumference from birth to 14 years. Tape measurements are made at the mamillary level during midinspiration. Before plotting the values on the graph, one should add 1 cm for males and subtract 1 cm for females between 2 and 12 years of age. **B,** Normal distribution of chest circumference from 26 to 42 weeks of gestation. The dotted lines indicate the 10th and 90th percentiles, respectively. Note that chest circumference is close to head circumference at term. (**A,** From Feingold M, Bossert WH: Normal values for selected physical parameters. An aid to syndrome delineation. Birth Defects 1974;10(13):14. **B,** Data from Britton JR, Britton HL, Jennett R, et al: Weight, length, head and chest circumference at birth in Phoenix, Arizona. J Reprod Med 1993;38:215.)

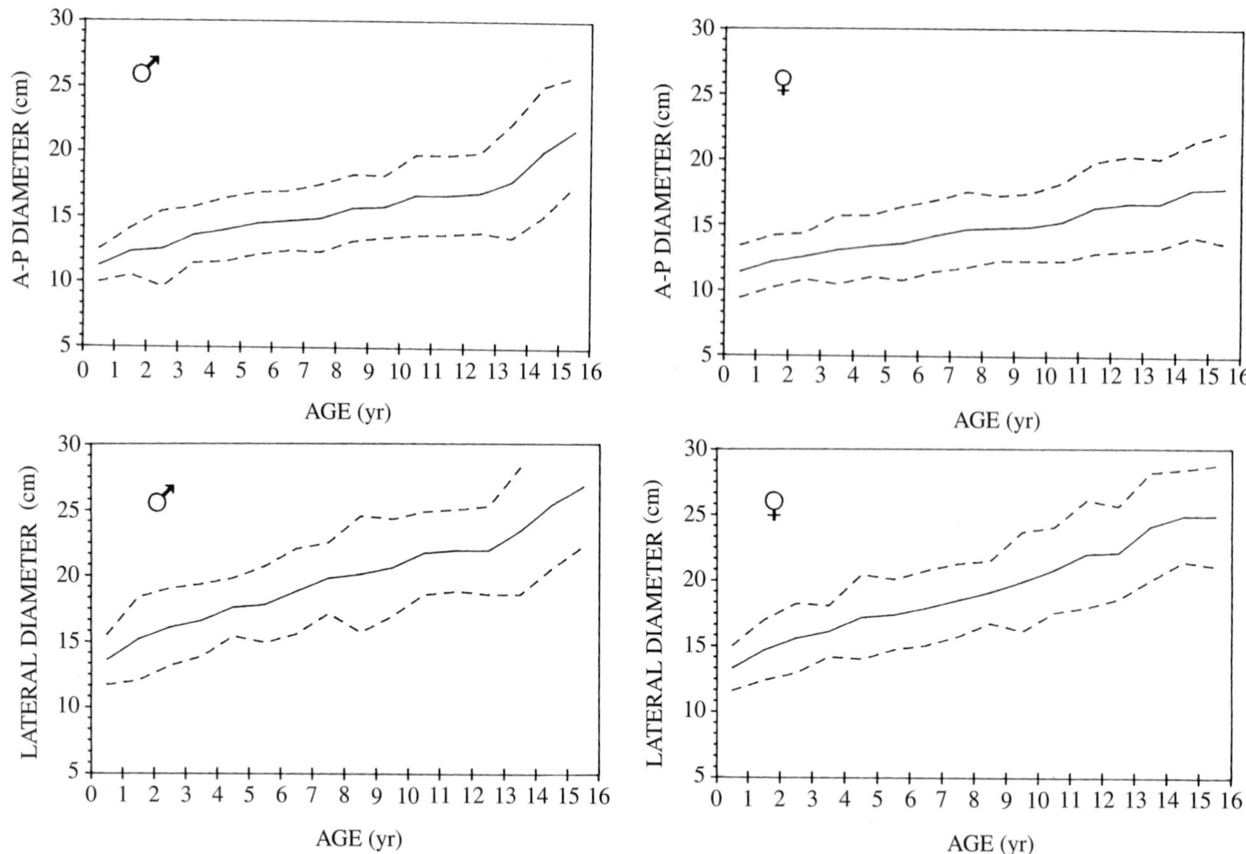

■ **FIGURE 6-4.** Mean values *(solid line)* ± SD *(dashed lines)* of the normal distribution of anteroposterior (AP) and lateral chest diameters in boys and girls. Caliper measurements are made at the mamillary level during midinspiration. (Data from Lucas WP, Pryor HB: Range and standard deviations of certain physical measurements in healthy children. J Pediatr 1935;6:533–545.)

dated (Fig. 6-4). Most of the configurational change of the chest occurs during the first 2 years and is probably influenced by gravitational forces after the upright position becomes common. Disease-related changes in thoracic dimensions occur either as potential causative factors (e.g., the elongated thorax with a stress distribution that favors spontaneous pneumothorax in lanky adolescents, particularly males who increase their thoracic height vs. width more than females) or as a secondary event (e.g., the barrel-shaped chest in patients with emphysema and chronic hyperinflation of the lung).

Inspection of the patient should also be directed to the extrathoracic regions. Many observations on the examination of the head and neck provide valuable clues to the physical diagnosis. Bluish coloration of the lower eyelid ("allergic shiners"); a bilateral fold of skin just below the lower eyelid (Dennie lines); and a transverse crease from "allergic salutes," running at the junction of the cartilaginous and bony portion of the nose, may all be found in atopic individuals. The nose should always be examined, and bilateral patency should be documented by occluding each side while feeling and listening for airflow through the other nostril. Even without a speculum one can assess the anterior half by raising the nose tip with one thumb and shining a light into the nasal passageways. Color and size of the mucosa should be noted. The frequency of asymptomatic nasal polyps seems to be high. Most polyps arise from the mucosa of the ostia, clefts, and recesses in the ostiomeatal complex. Easily visible nasal polyps are common in patients with cystic fibrosis. Nasal polyposis may also be familial or associated with allergy, asthma, and aspirin intolerance.

The oropharynx should be inspected for its size and signs of malformation, such as cleft palate, and for signs of obstruction by enlarged tonsils. Evidence of chronic ear infections should be documented, and the areas over frontal and maxillary paranasal sinuses should be tested for tenderness. Inspection of the skin is important and may reveal the eczema of atopy. The finding of a scar that typically develops at the site of a successful bacillus Calmette-Guérin (BCG) vaccination may be relevant. Common physical findings such as cyanosis, clubbing, and the cardiovascular signs of pulmonary disease are discussed in more detail at the end of this chapter.

■ PALPATION

Palpation follows chest inspection to confirm observed abnormalities, such as swellings and deformations; to identify areas of tenderness or lymph nodal enlargement; to document the position of the trachea; to assess respiratory excursions; and to detect changes in the transmission of voice sounds through the chest. Chest palpation may offer the first physical contact with the patient, and it is very important for the physician to perform this procedure with warm hands.

Palpation should be done in an orderly sequence. Commonly, one begins with an examination of the head and neck. Cervical lymphadenopathy and tenderness over paranasal sinuses should be noted. Palpation of the oropharynx may be indicated to find malformations such as submucosal clefts or to identify causes of upper airway obstruction. The position of the trachea must be documented in every patient. This is a very important part of the physical chest examination because tracheal deviation most often indicates significant intra- or extrathoracic abnormalities.

In the older child, the tracheal position is assessed by placing the index and the ring fingers on both sternal attachments of the sternocleidomastoid muscles. The trachea is then felt between these landmarks with the middle finger on the suprasternal notch. In small children, palpation is done with one index finger sliding gently inward over the suprasternal notch. Looking for asymmetry, the physician should always make sure that the patient is in a straight position, and deformities, such as scoliosis, should be taken into account.

A very slight deviation of the trachea toward the right is normal. Marked deviations may indicate a pulling force toward the side of displacement (e.g., atelectasis) or a pushing force on the contralateral side (e.g., pneumothorax). The physician should note whether the displacement is fixed or whether there is a pendular movement of the trachea during inspiration and expiration that may suggest obstruction of a large bronchus. Posterior displacement of the trachea may occur with anterior mediastinal tumors or barrel chest deformities, whereas an easily palpable anteriorly displaced trachea is sometimes seen with mediastinitis. In patients with airway obstruction and respiratory distress, retractions of the suprasternal fossa may be seen, and a "tracheal tug" may be felt by the examiner.

Placing the hands on both sides of the lateral rib cage, the physician should feel for symmetry of chest expansion during regular and deep breathing maneuvers. Slight compression of the chest in the transverse and anteroposterior directions may help to localize pain from lesions of the bony structures. Voice-generated vibrations are best felt with the palms of both hands just below the base of the fingers placed over corresponding sites on the right and left hemithorax. Asymmetric transmission usually indicates unilateral intrathoracic abnormalities. The patient is asked to produce low-frequency vibrations of sufficient amplitude by saying "ninety-nine" in a loud voice. In young infants, crying may produce the vibrations that are felt as tactile fremitus over the chest wall. This fremitus is decreased if an accumulation of air or fluid in the pleural space reduces transmission. Small consolidations of the underlying lung will not diminish the tactile fremitus as long as the airways remain open, whereas collapse of the airways and atelectasis will reduce the transmission of vibratory energy if larger portions of the lung are affected.

■ AUSCULTATION

Auscultation is arguably the most important part of the physical chest examination. The subjective perception of respiratory acoustic signs is influenced by the site and mode of sound production; by the modification of sound on its passage through the lung, chest wall, and stethoscope; and finally by the auditory system of the examiner. Knowledge about these factors is necessary to appreciate fully the wealth of information that is contained in the acoustic signs of the thorax.

Thoracic Acoustics

Observations on sound generation in airway models and electronic analyses of respiratory sounds suggest a predominant origin from complex turbulences within the central airways. The tracheal breath sound heard above the suprasternal notch is a relatively broad-spectrum noise, ranging in frequency from less than 100 Hz to greater than 2000 Hz. Resonances from the trachea and from supraglottic airways "color" the sound (Fig. 6-5). Lengthening of the trachea with growth during childhood causes lower tracheal resonance frequencies. A dominant source of tracheal breath sounds is turbulence from the jet flow at the glottic aperture. However, narrow segments of the supraglottic passages also contribute to sound generation. There is a very close relationship between airflow and tracheal sound intensity, particularly at high frequencies. In the presence of local narrowing (e.g., in children with subglottic stenosis), flow velocity at the stenotic site is increased, and so is the tracheal sound intensity. Relating tracheal sound levels to airflow measured at the mouth can provide information about changes during therapy. Auscultation over the trachea will provide some information under these circumstances, but objective acoustic measurements are required for accurate comparisons.

Basic "normal" lung sounds heard at the chest surface are lower in frequency than tracheal sounds because sound energy is lost during passage though the lungs, particularly at higher frequencies. However, lung sounds extend to frequencies higher than traditionally recognized. New observations on the effects of gas density indicate that lung sounds at frequencies above 400 Hz are mostly generated by flow turbulence. At lower frequencies, other mechanisms that are not directly related to air flow (e.g., muscle noise and thoracic cavity resonances) have

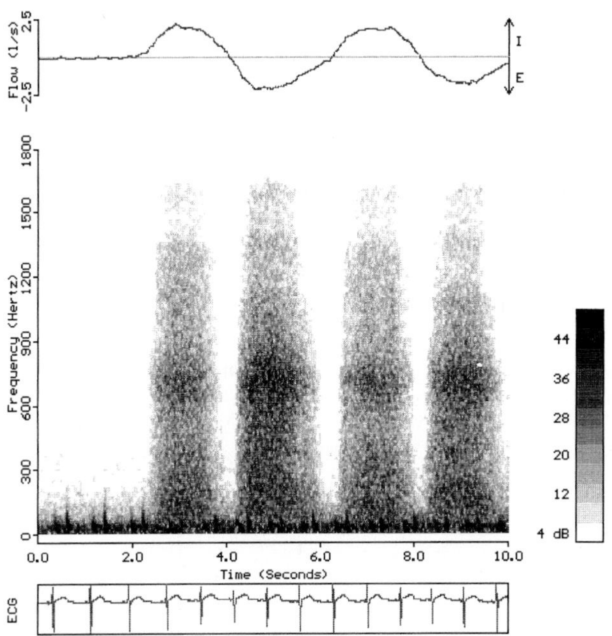

■ **FIGURE 6-5.** Digital respirosonogram of sounds recorded over the trachea of a healthy young man. Time is on the horizontal axis, frequency is on the vertical axis, and sound intensity is shown on a scale from black (loud) to white (low). Airflow is plotted at the top, with inspiration above and expiration below the zero line. The sonogram illustrates the broad range of tracheal sounds during both inspiration and expiration. There is a distinct pause between the respiratory phases. Expiration is louder than inspiration, and resonance is apparent around 700 Hz. In this example, the subject was holding his breath at the beginning. During this respiratory pause, heart sounds below 200 Hz are easily identified by their temporal relation to the simultaneously recorded electrocardiogram (ECG).

prominent effects on lung sounds and gas density effects are less obvious. Inspiratory lung sounds show little contribution of noise generated at the glottis. Their origin is likely more peripheral (i.e., in the main and segmental bronchi). Expiratory lung sounds appear to have a central origin and are probably affected by flow convergence at airway bifurcations (Fig. 6-6).

Sound at different frequencies takes different pathways on the passage through the lung. Low-frequency sound waves propagate from central airways through the lung parenchyma to the chest wall. At higher frequencies, the airway walls become effectively more rigid and sound travels further down into the airways before it propagates through lung tissue. This information cannot be gathered on subjective auscultation but requires objective acoustic measurements. A trained ear, however, will recognize many of the findings that are related to these mechanisms. For example, lung sounds in healthy children and adults are not necessarily equal at corresponding sites over both lungs. In fact, expiratory sounds are typically louder at the right upper lobe compared with the left side. Similar asymmetry has been recognized when sound is introduced at the mouth and measured at the chest surface. A likely explanation for this asymmetry is the effect on sound propagation by the cardiovascular and mediastinal structures to the left of the trachea. Asymmetry of lung sounds is also noticeable in most healthy subjects during inspiration when one listens over the posterior lower chest. The left side tends to be louder here, probably because of the size and spatial orientation of the larger airways due to the heart.

Objective acoustic measurements have also helped to clarify the difference between lung sounds in newborn infants and in older children. The most obvious divergence occurs in lung sounds at low frequencies where newborn infants have much less intensity. This may be explained by thoracic and airway resonances at higher frequencies in newborn infants and perhaps also by their lower muscle mass. Lung sounds at higher frequencies are similar between newborn infants and older children (Fig. 6-7).

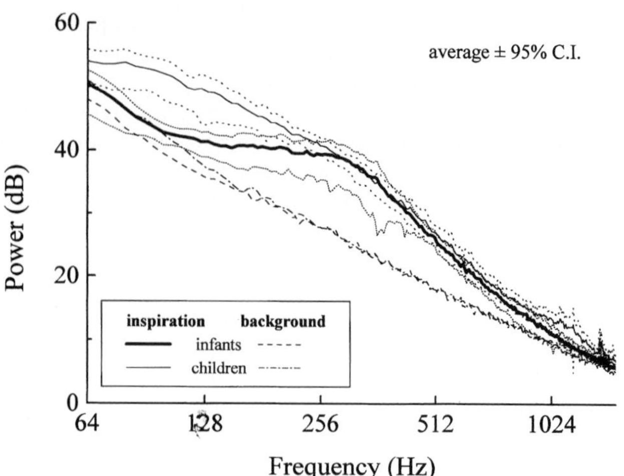

■ **FIGURE 6-7.** Average spectra of inspiratory lung sounds, recorded over the posterior basal segment of the right lung in healthy newborn infants (n = 10) and children (n = 9) at airflows of 15 mL/s/kg. The spectra of background noise at resting end expiration are plotted for comparison. Dotted lines mark the 95% confidence intervals (C.I.). Note the similarity of spectral slopes in newborn infants and older children at frequencies above 300 Hz and the significantly reduced sound power at lower frequencies in newborns. (Data from Pasterkamp H, Powell RE, Sanchez I: Lung sound spectra at standardized air flow in normal infants, children, and adults. Am J Respir Crit Care Med 1996;154:424–430.)

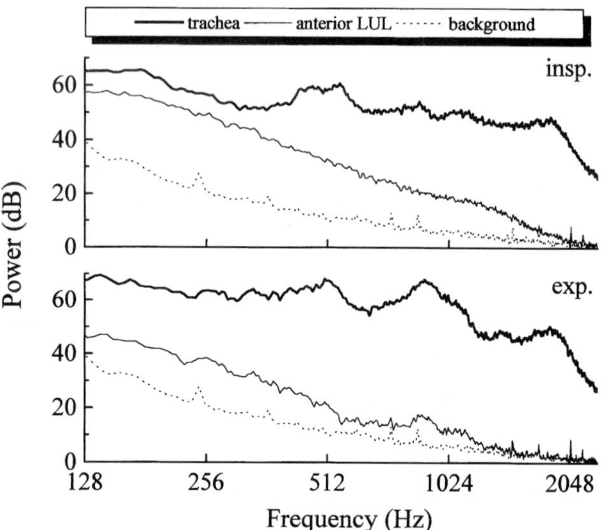

■ **FIGURE 6-6.** Average spectra of respiratory sounds at airflow of 1.5 ± 0.3 L/sec, recorded simultaneously at the suprasternal notch (trachea) and at the second intercostal space in the midclavicular line on the left (anterior left upper lobe [LUL]) of a healthy 12-year-old boy. The average sound spectrum during breath holding at resting end expiration (background) is plotted for comparison. Inspiratory lung sounds are louder than expiratory sounds, while the opposite is true for tracheal sounds. Lung sound intensity is clearly above background at frequencies as high as 1000 Hz. Expiratory lung sounds show some of the same spectral peaks that are present in tracheal sounds.

Adventitious respiratory sounds usually indicate respiratory disease. Wheezes are musical, continuous (typically longer than 100 msec) sounds that originate from oscillations in narrowed airways. The frequency of the oscillation depends on the mass and elasticity of the airway wall as well as on local airflow. Widespread narrowing of airways in asthma leads to various pitches, or polyphonic wheezing, whereas a fixed obstruction in a larger airway produces a single wheeze, or monophonic wheezing. Expiratory wheezing is related to flow limitation and can be produced by normal subjects during forced expiratory maneuvers. The situation is less clear for wheezing during inspiration, which is common in asthma but cannot be produced by healthy subjects unless it originates from the larynx (e.g., in vocal cord dysfunction). Very brief and localized inspiratory wheezes may be heard over areas of bronchiectasis.

Crackles are nonmusical, discontinuous (less than 20 msec duration) lung sounds. Crackle production requires the presence of air-fluid interfaces and occurs either by air movement through secretions or by sudden equalization of gas pressure. Another mechanism may be the release of tissue tension during sudden opening or closing of airways. Crackles are perceived as fine or coarse, depending on the duration and frequency of the brief and dampened vibrations created by these mechanisms. There may be a musical quality to the sound if a short oscillation occurs at the generation site. This has been called tinkling crackle or squawk and may appear during inspiration, typically in patients with interstitial lung diseases. Fine crackles during late inspiration are common in restrictive lung diseases and in the early stages of congestive heart failure, whereas coarse crackles during early inspiration and during expiration are frequently heard in chronic obstructive lung disease. Fine crackles are usually inaudible at the mouth, whereas the coarse crackles of widespread airway obstruction can be transmitted through the large airways and may be heard as clicks with the stethoscope held in front of the patient's open mouth. Some crackles over the anterior chest may occur in normal subjects who were breathing at low lung volumes, but they will disappear after a few deep breaths.

Several other abnormal respiratory sounds are not generated in intrathoracic airways. Pleural rubs originate from mechanical stretching of the pleura, which causes vibration of the chest wall and local pulmonary parenchyma. These sounds can occur during both inspiration and expiration. Their character is like that of creaking leather and is similar in some ways to pulmonary crackles. Stridor refers to a more or less musical sound that is produced by oscillations of critically narrowed extrathoracic airways. It is therefore most commonly heard during inspiration. Grunting is an expiratory sound, usually low pitched and with musical qualities. It is produced in the larynx when vocal cord adduction is used to generate positive end-expiratory pressures, such as in premature infants with immature lungs and surfactant deficiency. Snoring originates from the flutter of tissues in the pharynx and has less musical qualities. It may be present during both inspiration and expiration.

There may also be cardiorespiratory sounds. These are believed to occur when cardiac movements cause regional flows of air in the surrounding lung. Because of its synchronicity with the heart beat, this sound may be mistaken for a cardiac murmur. It can be identified by its vesicular sound quality and its exaggeration during inspiration and in different body positions.

At the boundary between different tissues, reflection of sound may occur and sound transmission may decrease, depending on the matching or mismatching of the tissue impedances. Many of the acoustic signs of the chest are explained on the basis of impedance matching alone. The stethoscope is basically an impedance transformer that reduces sound reflection at a mismatched interface, namely, body surface to air. Because it is the only part of the sound transmission pathway that can be kept constant, it is best to always use the same stethoscope. The choice of a bell- or a diaphragm-type stethoscope depends on individual preference. Diaphragm chest pieces can be placed more easily and with less pressure on small chests with narrow intercostal spaces. Compared with bell-type stethoscopes, they tend to deemphasize frequencies below 100 Hz. Both the bell-type and the diaphragm stethoscopes show some attenuation at frequencies above 400 Hz.

Technique of Auscultation

Ideally, auscultation of the chest should be performed in a quiet room; however, with pediatric patients the usual setting may be anything but quiet. Fortunately, the human auditory system allows selective evaluation of acoustic signals even when they are masked by much louder surrounding noises. This psychoacoustic phenomenon, known as the "cocktail party effect," at present cannot be reproduced by modern electronic techniques, which is but one of the reasons for the lasting popularity of the stethoscope.

This instrument, the most widely used in clinical medicine since its introduction almost 200 years ago, carries symbolic value for the health care profession, much like a modern staff of Aesculapius. Every child knows that doctors have stethoscopes. The physician should use this to advantage when assessing pediatric patients by encouraging children to listen themselves to their heartbeats and breathing sounds. Even infants may be fascinated as long as the stethoscope is shiny. Ice cold chest pieces, on the other hand, scare off most patients.

The patient should be in a straight position during auscultation because incurvature of the trunk may lead to artificial side differences of sound production and transmission. In newborns and young infants, a straight position may be best achieved when they are supine. Infants and toddlers will often be assessed while their parents hold them on their laps. Beginning auscultation on the back of these young patients will provoke less anxiety than a frontal approach. Older children can be examined in the sitting or standing position. The number of sites over the chest that are assessed during auscultation will be determined by the clinical situation. Ideally, all segments of the lung should be listened to, but this may not be possible, particularly in very young children.

Because the intensity of respiratory sounds is related to airflow, sufficiently deep respirations (with flow >0.5 L/sec) are needed for a good sound signal. An older patient will cooperate and breathe deeply through an open mouth. With infants and young children, however, one may have to rely on sounds made during sighs or deep inspirations in between crying. On the other hand, normal breath sounds can mask the presence of some adventitious sounds (e.g., fine crackles of low intensity). Asking the patient to take very slow, deep breaths with less airflow than is needed to generate normal breath sounds can help to unmask these adventitious sounds.

The physician should make note of the lung sound intensity over different areas of the chest in a qualitative way, keeping in mind that this intensity reflects both local sound generation and sound transmission characteristics of the thorax. It is therefore not correct to speak of local "air entry" when one actually refers to local breath sound intensity. Decreased breath sounds, for example, are common in asthma even when normal blood gases indicate that air entry has to be adequate. Obviously, a qualitative distinction between absence or presence of local breath sounds will be easier than attempts at quantification. Also, when the stethoscope is placed over any given location, it is not known how large an area of the underlying lung is actually being assessed. In adult subjects, moving the chest piece of the stethoscope by 10 cm will position it to receive sound from entirely different lung units, but similar data for children are not available.

Assessment of regional ventilation by thoracic acoustic signs becomes more meaningful when two sites are compared simultaneously. Differential auscultation with special stethoscopes that employ two chest pieces or a single divided chest piece has not become popular in clinical practice. Comparative auscultation is absolutely essential for airway management in the emergency room and intensive care unit for assessment of endotracheal tube position or for identification of the side of a pneumothorax. Listening simultaneously to two homologous sites over both lungs may also help to detect local abnormalities. Atelectatic areas will transmit sound more slowly than inflated lung tissue, but the resulting phase shift is too small to be detectable on subjective auscultation. With local airway narrowing, however, the maximum sound intensity over the affected side may become sufficiently delayed to be perceived as "phase heterophony." In some cases, breath sounds may still be audible over the affected side after inspiratory efforts have ceased. This "post-effort" breath sound is a sign of incomplete airway obstruction.

There are special circumstances in which only the presence or absence of breath sounds is of interest (e.g., during transportation of critically ill patients in noisy vehicles and during resuscitation in the emergency department). Under these conditions, and when a firm attachment of the chest piece is important, a self-adhering stethoscope, based on negative suction pressure within the bell of the chest piece, may be applied. New techniques of adaptive electronic filtering are soon to be employed in stethoscopes that are optimized for use in very noisy environments.

Respiratory sounds should be documented according to their location and character. Normal projections of lobar borders to the surface of the chest are shown in Figure 6-8. These may be distorted by local pulmonary disease, and mapping of respiratory sounds should therefore be done with reference to external anatomic landmarks (Fig. 6-9). The examiner should be familiar with the segmental structure of the underlying lung.

Respiratory sound characteristics include the intensity (amplitude), pitch (predominant frequency), and timing during the respiratory cycle. Also, sounds will have a particular timbre (character) caused by the presence of resonances and overtones. Unfortunately, the terminology in use for the description of respiratory sounds is still confusing and imprecise. During a symposium on lung sounds in Tokyo in 1985, an attempt was made to achieve a global and uniform nomenclature for breath sounds. The resulting recommendations for classification of adventitious lung sounds are presented in Figure 6-10, and Table 6-1 summarizes mechanisms and sites of generation, acoustic characteristics, and clinical relevance of the major categories of respiratory sounds.

A basic grouping into musical, continuous sounds of long duration and nonmusical, discontinuous sounds of short duration is made, with the former being referred to as wheezes and the latter as crackles. Furthermore, musical adventitious sounds or wheezes may be classified as high or low pitched. Some use the term *rhonchus* for low-pitched wheezes (<200 Hz), whereas others describe the poorly characterized "secretion sounds," which share musical and nonmusical qualities, as rhonchi. Crackles are subclassified as fine or coarse. Regular breath sounds include tracheal/bronchial, bronchovesicular, and vesicular/normal sounds. Finally, other respiratory sounds should be specified, such as pleural rubs, expiratory grunting, and inspiratory stridor. Historical terms such as *rales* and *crepitations* should

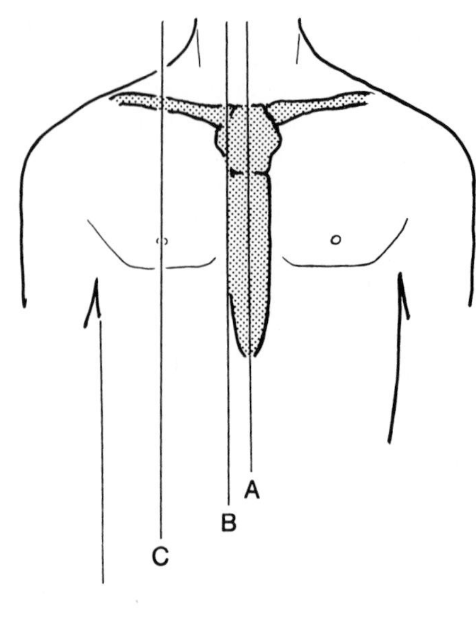

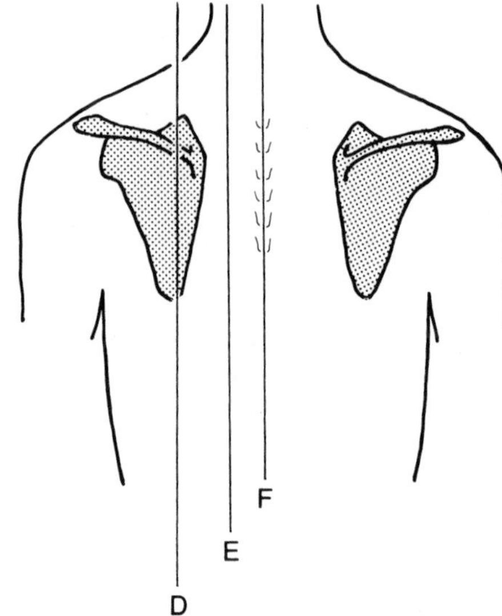

■ **FIGURE 6-9.** Vertical reference lines of the chest. The center line is indicated anteriorly by the suprasternal notch *(A)* and posteriorly by the spinous processes *(F)*. The sternal *(B)* and midclavicular *(C)* lines over the front and the scapular *(D)* and paravertebral *(E)* lines over the back provide longitudinal landmarks of the thorax. From a lateral view, the midaxillary line is used for orientation. Horizontal reference points are the supra- and infraclavicular fossae, Ludwig's angle (junction of the second rib at the sternum), the mammillae (normally at the fourth rib), and the epigastric angle. Posteriorly, the prominent spinous process of the seventh cervical vertebra and the supra- and infraspinous fossae of the scapulae provide markers for orientation.

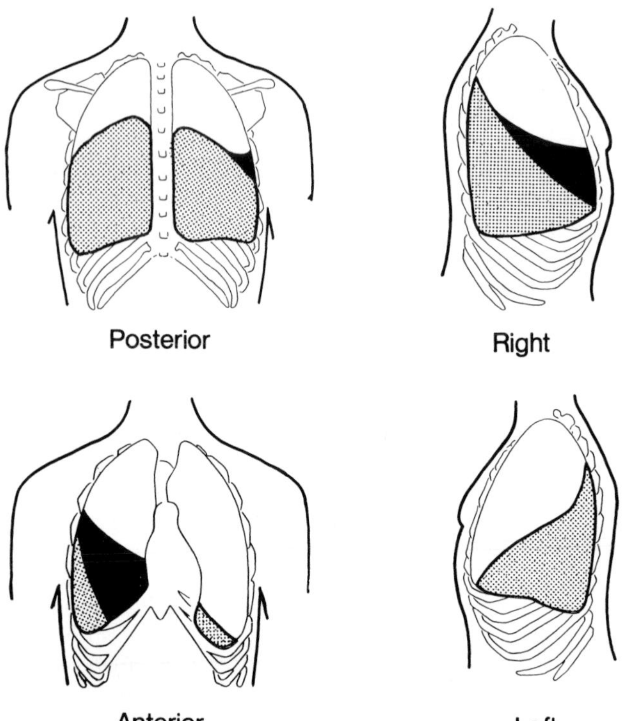

■ **FIGURE 6-8.** Projections of the pulmonary lobes on the chest surface. The upper lobes are white, the right-middle lobe is black, and the lower lobes are dotted.

LUNG SOUND NOMENCLATURE

	English	French	German	Japanese	Portuguese	Spanish
Discontinuous						
Fine (high pitched, low amplitude, short duration)	Fine crackles	Râles crepitants	Feines Rasseln	捻髪音	Estertores finos	Estertores finos
Coarse (low pitched, high amplitude, long duration	Coarse crackles	Râles bulleux ou Sous-crepitants	Grobes Rasseln	水泡音	Estertores grossos	Estertores gruesos
Continuous						
High pitched	Wheezes	Râles sibilants	Pfeifen	ふえ(笛)音	Sibilos	Sibilancias
Low pitched	Rhonchus	Râles ronflants	Brummen	いびき(鼾)音	Roncos	Roncus

■ **FIGURE 6-10.** Recommendation from the 1985 International Symposium on Lung Sounds in Tokyo for a unified nomenclature of adventitious sounds. (Reproduced with permission from Cugell DW: Lung sound nomenclature. Am Rev Respir Dis 1987;136:1016.)

be abandoned, and flowery descriptions such as "raspy" or "blowing" breath sounds should not be used because these adjectives are even less well defined than the suggested terms.

Several auscultatory signs are based on the transmission of voice sounds. Speech sounds have a fundamental note of about 130 Hz in men and 230 Hz in women, with overtones from 400 to 3500 Hz. Vowels are produced when particular pairs of overtones or formants are generated. On passage through the lung, the higher frequency formants are filtered, and speech heard over the chest becomes a meaningless mumble. With consolidation and transmission of higher frequency components, however, speech may become intelligible. This occurs with normal speech (bronchophony) and with whispered voice (pectoriloquy). There may be a change in vowels from e to a over areas of lung consolidation. The acoustic basis for these phenomena is the same as for bronchial breath sounds. The American Thoracic Society and the American College of Chest Physicians recommend the term *egophony* for all of these findings.

■ PERCUSSION

Percussion is used to set tissues into vibration with an impulsive force so that their mechanical and acoustic response can be studied. If the vibrations are undamped and continue for a significant amount of time, the perceived sound will be resonant or "tympanic," whereas rapid attenuation of the vibrations will lead to a flat or "dull" percussion note. The former occurs when there is a large acoustic mismatch (e.g., tissue overlying an air-filled cavity), whereas the latter occurs when the underlying tissue is similar to the surface tissue and vibratory energy propagates away quickly. Structures that absorb energy when struck by a sound at their natural frequency continue vibrating after the

■ **TABLE 6-1.** Respiratory sounds

	Mechanisms	Origin	Acoustics	Relevance
Basic Sounds				
Lung	Turbulent flow, vortices, other	Central (expiration), lobar to segmental airways (inspiration)	Low pass filtered noise (<100 to >1000 Hz)	Regional ventilation, airway caliber
Tracheal	Turbulent flow, flow impinging on airway walls	Pharynx, larynx, trachea, large airways	Noise with resonances (<100 to >3000 Hz)	Upper airway configuration
Adventitious Sounds				
Wheezes	Airway wall flutter, vortex shedding, other	Central and lower airways	Sinusoidal (<100 Hz to >1000 Hz, duration typically >80 msec)	Airway obstruction, flow limitation
Rhonchi	Rupture of fluid films, airway wall vibration	Larger airways	Series of rapidly dampened sinusoids (typically <300 Hz and duration <100 msec)	Secretions, abnormal airway collapsibility
Crackles	Airway wall stress-relaxation	Central and lower airways	Rapidly dampened wave deflections (duration typically <20 msec)	Airway closure, secretions

Modified from Pasterkamp H, Kraman SS, Wodicka GR: State of the art. Respiratory sounds—advances beyond the stethoscope. Am J Respir Crit Care Med 1997;156:974–987.

initial sound is gone and are called resonant. The fundamental resonance of the thorax depends on body size and is about 125 Hz for adult males, between 150 and 175 Hz for adult females, and between 300 and 400 Hz for small children.

Chest percussion in children is performed by light tapping with the index or middle finger (the plexor) on the terminal phalanx of the other hand's middle finger (the pleximeter). The pleximeter should be placed firmly but not hard, and care should be taken that other fingers do not touch the chest wall, which may cause artificial damping of the percussion note. Percussion should be gentle, with quick perpendicular movements of the plexor originating from the wrist (Fig. 6-11). The patient should be relaxed during the examination because tension of the chest wall muscles may alter the percussion note. More important, chest deformities and scoliosis in particular will have a significant effect on percussory findings.

Symmetric sites over the anterior, lateral, and posterior surface of the chest should be compared in an orderly fashion. As with chest auscultation, findings should be reported with reference to standard external landmarks (see Fig. 6-9). The ribs and vertebral spinous processes are used for horizontal mapping. The level at which the tympanic lung resonance changes to a dull percussion note should be defined over the posterior chest during maximal inspiration and expiration to delineate the lung borders and their respiratory excursions.

Subjective assessment of percussion note differences includes both acoustic and tactile perception. Tympanic, lower-pitched percussion notes mean less-damped vibrations of longer duration, which are felt by the pleximeter finger. Dull sounds with higher frequencies correspond to vibrations that die away quickly. Dullness replaces the normal chest percussion note when fluid accumulates in the pleural space or when consolidation close to the chest wall occurs in the underlying pulmonary parenchyma. Similar to the vibrations generated by percussion, the vibrations from the patient's voice ("say 'ninety-nine'") will also not be felt under these circumstances. However, the tactile fremitus is equally absent over areas of pneumothorax, whereas the percussion note may have a hyperresonant quality.

Conventional percussion cannot detect small pulmonary lesions located deeply within the thorax. Auscultatory percussion has been proposed to overcome this limitation. This technique combines light percussion of the sternum with simultaneous auscultation over the posterior chest. A decrease in sound intensity is believed to indicate lung disease. The method is of little value, however, because even large intrathoracic lesions can remain undetected since percussion sounds either may be totally absorbed within the lung or may travel as transverse waves along the thoracic bones. Propagation along the thoracic bones is believed to explain the "coin sound," a sign that is used to detect a pneumothorax. It is elicited by creating a high-pitched sound impulse that propagates into the body, using a coin placed flat on the chest, which is then struck with another coin edge on. On auscultation of the opposite side of the thorax, a distinct click is heard if air separates the ribs from the lung and sound travels along these bones. Under normal circumstances with ribs and parenchyma in contact, however, the sound will be absorbed and no click will be heard.

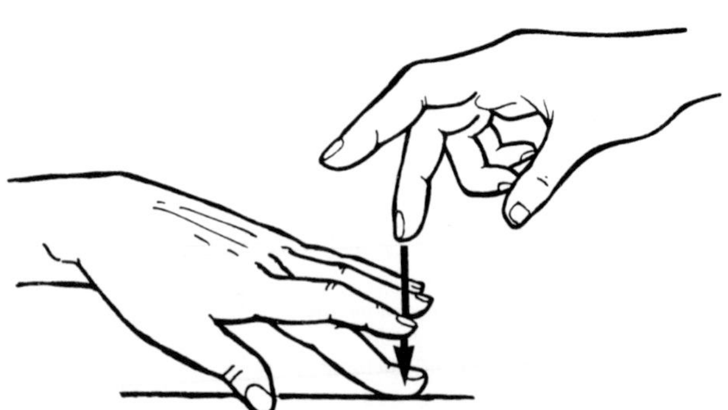

FIGURE 6-11. Percussion in children should be done with gentle perpendicular movements from the wrist and tapping of the plexor finger *(right)* on the terminal phalanx of the pleximeter finger *(left)*. The contact area of the pleximeter on the chest should be small, and other fingers should not touch the surface to avoid damping of the percussory vibrations.

TASTE AND SMELL

A complete physical examination extends beyond the perception of vision, hearing, and touch. Olfactory impressions should also be documented, even if they are subtle. Malodorous breath is easily noticed and may, particularly if chronic, indicate infection within the nasal or oral cavity (e.g., paranasal sinusitis), nasal foreign body, or dental abscess. Bad breath may also originate from intrathoracic infections, such as lung abscess or bronchiectasis, and it may also be noted in patients with gastroesophageal reflux. Nowadays physicians rarely use their tastebuds to make a medical diagnosis. One particular disease of the respiratory tract in children, however, lends itself to gustatory diagnosis. Most often the discovery is made by the mother of a patient with cystic fibrosis who notices that the skin of her child tastes abnormally salty.

COMMON SIGNS AND SYMPTOMS OF CHEST DISEASE IN CHILDREN

There are several common complaints and presentations of children with chest diseases that deserve a more detailed description. In particular, cough and sputum production, noisy breathing, wheezing, cyanosis, digital clubbing, cardiovascular signs, and chest pain need to be discussed.

COUGH AND SPUTUM PRODUCTION

Cough is not an illness by itself, but it is a cardinal manifestation in many chest diseases. Cough is probably the single most common complaint in children presenting to the physician. The act of coughing is a reflex aimed at removal of mucus and other material from the airways that follows the stimulation of cough or irritant receptors. These receptors are located anywhere between the pharynx and the terminal bronchioles. They send their afferent impulses via branches of the glossopharyngeal and vagus nerves to the cough center in the upper brainstem and pons. The efferent signals travel from the cough center via vagus, phrenic, and spinal motor nerves to the larynx and diaphragm as well as to the muscles of the chest wall, abdomen, and pelvic floor. Cortical influences allow the voluntary initiation or suppression of cough.

There are three phases of coughing: (1) deep inspiration; (2) closure of the glottis, relaxation of the diaphragm, and contraction of expiratory muscles; and (3) sudden opening of the glottis. During the second phase, intrathoracic pressures up to 300 mm Hg can be generated and may be transmitted to the vascular and cerebrospinal spaces. Airflow velocity during the third phase is highest in the central airways and may reach three fourths the speed of sound. This speed depends on the sudden opening of the glottis and influences the success of expectoration. Patients with glottic dysfunction and those with tracheostomies may therefore have a less effective cough.

Stimuli that cause coughing may originate centrally, such as in psychogenic cough, or they may be pulmonary, located either in the major airways or in the pulmonary parenchyma. Also, cough can be provoked by nonpulmonary causes, such as irritation of pleura, diaphragm, or pericardium and even through stimulation of Arnold's nerve (a branch of the vagus) by wax or foreign bodies in the external ear.

A detailed history should define the nature of the cough, whether it is dry, hacking, or brassy, and whether it is productive by sound and appearance. In young children, expectoration is unusual, but if observed, the quantity and quality of sputum should be noted. In particular, the physician should inquire about the color and odor of the expectorate and about the presence of blood in the sputum. The yellow-green color of purulent sputum results from the cellular breakdown of leukocytes and the liberation of myeloperoxidase from these cells. This finding indicates a retention of secretions and does not necessarily reflect an acute infection.

The timing of coughing is important, and its relationship to daily routines should be sought. Cough during or after feeding occurs with aspiration. Nighttime cough may be related to asthma or to postnasal drip, whereas productive cough early in the morning is typical for bronchiectasis. Cough following exercise or exposure to cold air points toward airway hyperreactivity. Seasonal worsening or coughing on exposure to potential allergens should be documented, as should the association of coughing and wheezing. The physician should ask about active and passive smoking, keeping in mind that, regrettably, there are quite a few children as young as 8 years of age who smoke regularly.

A detailed diary kept by the parents or the patient to note the frequency and timing of cough can be of value. Technology to record, quantify, and characterize cough is being developed. Some acoustic characteristics of cough are quite specific for certain diseases, such as the sound of a barking seal in viral croup or the whooping noise in pertussis. In patients with chronic cough, the physician should weigh the possible causes in view of their prevalence at different ages (Table 6-2). Also, complications of severe coughing paroxysms, such as pneumothorax, cough syncope, or nonsyncopal neurologic manifestations, should be considered. Regarding the last, the physician should inquire about lightheadedness, headache, visual disturbance, paresthesia, and tremor.

TABLE 6-2. Causes of chronic cough

Infant	Preschool	School Age/ Adolescence
Congenital anomalies	Foreign body	Reactive
Tracheoesophageal fistula	Infections	Asthma
Neurologic impairment	Viral	Postnasal drip
Infections	Mycoplasma	Infections
Viral (RSV, CMV)	Bacterial	Mycoplasma
Chlamydia	Reactive	Irritative
Bacterial (pertussis)	Asthma	Smoking
Cystic fibrosis	Cystic fibrosis	Air pollution
	Irritative	Psychogenic
	Passive smoking	

Data modified from Eigen H: The clinical evaluation of chronic cough. Pediatr Clin North Am 1982;29:67.

NOISY BREATHING

Quite frequently a child is brought to the physician's attention because of abnormal breathing noises. This noise may be a nonmusical hiss, much like the one produced in normal subjects at increased rates of ventilation, or it may have the musical qualities of stridor and snoring. Also, bubbling and crackling noises may be heard, and the tactile perception may contribute to the impression of a "rattly" chest in these patients.

Attention should be focused on the noise-generating structures of the extrathoracic airways that are located at points of anatomic narrowing (e.g., the nasal vestibule, the posterior nasal orifices, and the glottis). The most common cause of noisy breathing in toddlers and young children is nasopharyngeal obstruction; in young infants, laryngomalacia is a leading cause. It is uncertain to what degree sounds from large intrathoracic airways contribute to the noise of breathing. Placing the stethoscope within the airstream in front of the mouth, one hears predominantly those sounds that are produced locally in the mouth and larynx. Noisy breathing is a common finding in patients with asthma and bronchitis and does not necessarily reflect intrathoracic airway pathology because the upper airways are also frequently affected in these patients.

To clarify the causes of noisy breathing, the parents or patient should describe their own perceptions of the noise: does it occur during inspiration, expiration, or both? Is it just an exaggeration of the normal breath sound noise, or does it have musical qualities? Did an episode of choking precede the onset of noisy breathing? Is the abnormal sound more prominent during certain activities, such as exercise? At what times of day or night and in which body positions is it most noticeable? The physician should also inquire about associated cough, sputum production, and dyspnea.

Children may suffer from partial obstruction of the upper airways during sleep; complete obstruction, which is found in adult patients with sleep apnea, is less common. Invariably, these children are heavy snorers at night, whereas normal children's snoring is largely confined to times of upper respiratory tract infection. Usually enlarged adenoids and tonsils cause the breathing disturbance. The physician should inquire about the typical signs and symptoms found in patients with increased work of breathing and abnormal sleep patterns at night (Box 6-1).

In the older child and adolescent, the physician should first inspect the nasal passageways and proceed to an examination of the oropharynx before auscultation of the neck and thorax. The acoustic signs should be checked while the patient breathes first with the mouth open, then closed. In younger children, examination of the nose and mouth is unpopular and often results in agitation and crying. It is better to start with auscultation before inspection in these children. Noisy breathers should be examined when they are sitting or standing upright and when they are lying down because upper airway geometry is position dependent and may influence the respiratory sounds. The examiner should also note abnormal crying or speech in the patient, as this may point to laryngeal disease.

WHEEZING

Wheezing is a common respiratory symptom and refers to musical, adventitious lung sounds that are often heard by the patient

BOX 6-1 **Clinical Symptoms in Children with Heavy Nocturnal Snoring**

Nighttime Manifestations

Profuse nocturnal sweating
Restless sleep
Abnormal movements during sleep
Special sleeping position
Enuresis

Problems with Growth and Nutrition

Anorexia
Weight <3rd percentile
Nausea with or without vomiting

Behavioral and Learning Problems

Hyperactivity
Aggression
Social withdrawal

Minor Motor Problems

Lack of coordination
Clumsiness

Other Manifestations

Frequent upper airway infections
Frequent morning headaches
Excessive daytime somnolence

Data modified from Guilleminault C, Winkle R, Korobkin R, Simmons B: Children and nocturnal snoring. Evaluation of effects of sleep related respiratory resistive load and daytime functioning. Eur J Pediatr 1982;139:165.

as well as the physician. Stridor is even more noticeable. Essentially, it is a very loud inspiratory wheeze originating from extrathoracic airways. When asking the patient or the parents about wheezing and stridor, one should keep in mind that the use of lung sound terminology among nonprofessionals is no better standardized than it is among health care providers. Therefore, the physician should inquire about musical, whistling noises during respiration, and, if necessary, demonstrate stridor or the forced expiratory wheeze that can be produced even by healthy individuals.

Most typically, wheezing is associated with hyperreactive airway disease, but any critical narrowing of the airways can produce wheezing. Box 6-2 lists conditions other than asthma that may be associated with wheezing and stridor. The wheezing typical in asthma originates from oscillations of airways at many sites. On auscultation, one hears many different tones simultaneously, which is called polyphonic wheezing. Obstruction of a single airway can produce a single monophonic wheeze or, in the obstruction of extrathoracic airways, stridor. Both inspiratory and expiratory wheezes are present in the majority of asthmatic patients. The audible expiratory phase (expirium) is typically prolonged because of wheezing. Objectively measured expiratory time (expiration), however, is rarely prolonged except in very severe airway obstruction. Under these circumstances, airflow is minimal, and thus wheezing is absent. Respiration becomes ominously silent, and the patient may have carbon dioxide retention and cyanosis. In less severe cases, however, the proportion of inspiration and expiration occupied by wheezing correlates to some extent with the degree of airflow obstruction. Objective and reproducible wheeze quantification can be achieved by computer-assisted techniques, but in practice the quantification of wheezing severity is made by subjective assessment at the bedside.

Wheezes are often high pitched and will therefore attenuate during their passage through lung tissue, particularly if the lungs are hyperinflated. Auscultation over the neck may give a better impression of respiratory sounds and should be included as a part of the routine physical examination. Tracheal auscultation to determine if and when there is wheezing after methacholine inhalation challenge has been advocated instead of spirometry in young children who are thought to have bronchial hyperreactivity. However, wheezing may be absent even if airways become significantly obstructed during bronchial provocation (Fig. 6-12). In our experience, wheezing heard at the chest but not necessarily at the trachea is very suggestive of airway narrowing and hyperresponsiveness. Listening to respiratory sounds over the neck may help to identify patients who are thought to be asthmatic but

BOX 6-2 **Causes of Wheezing and Stridor Other than Asthma**

Malformation

Cardiovascular anomalies (e.g., vascular ring)
Airway anomalies (e.g., web, cyst, hemangioma, malacia, stenosis)
Esophageal anomalies (e.g., enteric cyst)

Inflammation

Tracheitis
Bronchitis
Bronchiolitis
Bronchiectasis
Cystic fibrosis

Compression

Extrinsic

Esophageal foreign body
Lymphadenopathy
Malignancy

Intrinsic

Endobronchial foreign body
Tumor (rare)

Extrathoracic Disease

Laryngitis
Epiglottitis
Vocal cord paralysis
Retropharyngeal abscess
Peritonsillar abscess
Laryngomalacia
Polyps, adenoids

Other

Metabolic disturbances (e.g., hypocalcemia, hypokalemia)
Psychosomatic illness (e.g., emotional laryngeal wheezing, factitious asthma)

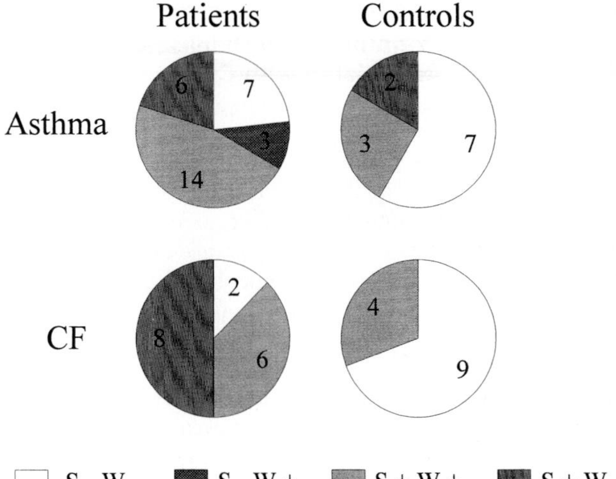

■ **FIGURE 6-12.** Summary of findings regarding wheeze as an indicator of significant flow obstruction during methacholine bronchial provocation in children. Negative responses, i.e., less than 20% decline in forced expiratory volume in 1 second (FEV) at a dose of 8 mg/mL (spirometry) and no wheeze (acoustic monitoring), are indicated by a minus sign, positive responses by a plus sign. Note the low sensitivity of wheeze as an indicator of airflow obstruction, particularly in children with cystic fibrosis. S, spirometry; W, wheezing. (Data from Sanchez I, Powell RE, Pasterkamp H: Wheezing and airflow obstruction during metacholine challenge in children with cystic fibrosis and in normal children. Am Rev Respir Dis 1993;147:705, and Sanchez I, Avital A, Wong I, et al: Acoustic vs. spirometric assessment of bronchial responsiveness to metacholine in children. Pediatr Pulmonol 1993;15:28.)

who generate the wheezing noises solely in the larynx. These are usually older children and adolescents who may have emotional problems and vocal cord dysfunction.

■ CYANOSIS

Cyanosis refers to a blue color of the skin and mucous membranes due to excessive concentrations of reduced hemoglobin in capillary blood. The oxygen content of capillary blood is assumed to be midway between that of arterial and that of venous blood. Areas with a high blood flow and a small arteriovenous oxygen difference (e.g., the tongue and mucous membranes) will not become cyanotic as readily as those with a low blood flow and a large arteriovenous oxygen difference (e.g., the skin of cold hands and feet). A distinction is therefore made between peripheral cyanosis (acrocyanosis), which is confined to the skin of the extremities, and central cyanosis, which includes the tongue and mucous membranes. Circumoral cyanosis is not an expression of central cyanosis and is rarely pathological. The absolute concentration of reduced hemoglobin in the capillaries necessary to produce cyanosis is between 4 and 6 g/100 mL of blood. This level is usually present when the concentration of reduced hemoglobin in arterial blood exceeds 3 g/100 mL. Clinical cyanosis will occur at different levels of arterial oxygen saturation, depending on the amount of total hemoglobin (Fig. 6-13).

Physiologically, there are five mechanisms that can cause arterial hemoglobin desaturation in the patient who breathes room air at normal altitude: (1) alveolar hypoventilation, (2) diffusion impairment, (3) right-to-left shunting, (4) mismatch of ventilation and perfusion, and (5) inadequate oxygen transport by hemoglobin. Clinically, diffusion impairment is of little importance as a single cause. Imbalance of ventilation and perfusion is by far the most common mechanism and is correctable by administration of 100% oxygen. The physician should therefore look for a change in cyanosis while the patient breathes oxygen.

Observer agreement regarding cyanosis was found to range from poor when assessing acrocyanosis to very good in the evaluation of young children with bronchiolitis. To minimize the variability of this finding, cyanosis is best observed under daylight and with the patient resting in a comfortably warm room. The distribution of cyanosis and the state of peripheral perfusion should be noted. Patients with decreased cardiac output and poor peripheral perfusion can be cyanotic despite normal arterial hemoglobin saturation. Some patients may become cyanotic only during exercise, a not uncommon response when restrictive lung disease reduces the pulmonary capillary bed and the transit time of erythrocytes becomes too short for full saturation during episodes of increased cardiac output. Congenital heart disease in infants may lead to differential cyanosis, which affects only the lower part of the body (e.g., in patients with preductal coarctation of the aorta). Less commonly, only the upper part of the body is cyanotic, for example, in patients with transposition of the great arteries, patent ductus arteriosus, or pulmonary hypertension.

The clinical impression of cyanosis is usually confirmed by an arterial blood gas analysis or more commonly by pulse oximetry. Pulse oximetry, however, will not take into account the presence of abnormal hemoglobin. For example, in methemoglobinemia the oxygen-carrying capacity of blood is reduced and patients may appear lavender blue, but pulse oximetry may overestimate oxygen saturation in arterial blood (SaO_2). The blood of newborn infants, conversely, can be well saturated and not cyanotic at lower arterial oxygen tensions because of the different oxygen-binding curve of fetal hemoglobin. In the patient with hypoxemia who does not present with cyanosis (e.g, the anemic patient), the physician has to pay particular attention to other clinical signs and symptoms of hypoxia. These include tachypnea and tachycardia, exertional dyspnea, hypertension,

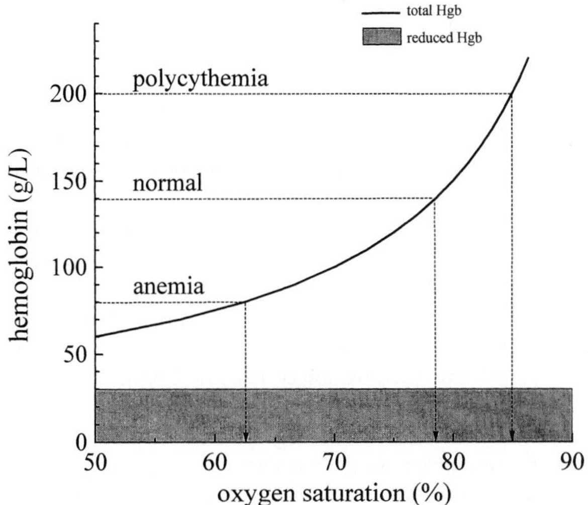

■ **FIGURE 6-13.** Cyanosis requires at least 30 g/L of reduced hemoglobin (Hgb) in arterial blood or 4 to 6 g/100 mL in capillary blood. The arterial oxygen saturation (SaO_2) at which cyanosis occurs is dependent on the amount of total Hgb. As illustrated, a child with 30 g/L of Hgb plus 110 g/L of oxyhemoglobin has an SaO_2 of 78%. In the anemic patient (i.e., total Hgb of 80 g/L with Hgb of 30 g/L), SaO_2 will drop much lower (to less than 65% in this example) before cyanosis occurs, whereas in the patient with polycythemia (i.e., total Hgb of 200 g/L), cyanosis appears at a higher SaO_2 (85%).

headache, and behavioral changes. With more severe hypoxia there may be visual disturbance, somnolence, hypotension, and ultimately coma. In addition, the patient may have an elevated level of carbon dioxide. Depending on how rapidly and to what extent the level of carbon dioxide has risen, the clinical signs of hypercarbia will largely reflect vascular dilatation. These signs include flushed, hot hands and feet; bounding pulses; confusion or drowsiness; muscular twitching; engorged retinal veins; and, in the most severe cases, papilledema and coma.

DIGITAL CLUBBING

Digital clubbing refers to a focal enlargement of the connective tissue in the terminal phalanges of fingers and toes, most noticeably on their dorsal surfaces. This sign was first described by Hippocrates, and the term *Hippocratic fingers* is used by some to denote simple digital clubbing. The pathogenesis of clubbing is still not entirely clear. Vascular endothelial growth factor from the continued impaction of shunted megakaryocytes and platelets in the digital vasculature, potentiated by hypoxia, is considered to drive the cellular and stromal changes in clubbing. Platelet-derived growth factor may contribute to the stromal changes, including the maturation of new microvessels.

Clubbing of the digits may be idiopathic, acquired, or hereditary. Cystic fibrosis, bronchiectasis, and empyema are the most common pulmonary causes of acquired digital clubbing in children. Clubbing is also seen infrequently in extrinsic allergic vasculitis, pulmonary arteriovenous malformations, bronchiolitis obliterans, sarcoidosis, and chronic asthma. Box 6-3 shows a list of nonpulmonary diseases associated with clubbing. A systemic disorder of bones, joints, and soft tissues known as hypertrophic osteoarthropathy (HOA) includes digital clubbing. In the majority of cases, HOA is associated with bronchogenic carcinoma and other intrathoracic neoplasms, but the pediatrician may see HOA in patients with severe cystic fibrosis or chronic empyema and lung abscess. In addition to clubbing, these patients may have periosteal thickening; symmetric arthritis of ankles, knees, wrists, and elbows; neurovascular changes of hands and feet; and increased thickness of subcutaneous soft tissues in the distal portions of arms and legs. The primary idiopathic or hereditary form of HOA—pachydermoperiostosis—appears with prominent furrowing of the forehead and scalp. Approximately half of the reported cases have a positive family history. Genetic studies suggest an autosomal-dominant inheritance with variable expression and a predilection for males.

Digital clubbing is not only an important indicator of pulmonary disease but also may reflect the progression or resolution of the causative process. Pulmonary abscess and empyema may lead to digital clubbing over the course of only a few weeks. In this case, clubbing will resolve if effective treatment is instituted before connective tissue changes become fixed. Interestingly, even long-standing finger clubbing seems to resolve in patients after successful heart and lung transplantation. In patients with cystic fibrosis, progression of finger clubbing suggests a suboptimal control of chest infections. It is therefore useful to quantify the degree of digital clubbing. Measurements have focused on the hyponychial (Lovibond) angle and on the phalangeal depth ratio (Fig. 6-14). Changes of the hyponychial angle are quantified on "shadowgrams"—projections of the finger's lateral profile onto a magnifying screen—whereas the phalangeal depth ratio is measured from plaster casts. Computerized analysis from digital photographs has provided information on the distribution of the hyponychial angle in healthy subjects and in patients with various diseases. Almost 80% of adult patients with cystic fibrosis have a hyponychial angle greater than 190 degrees, the upper limit of normal.

For routine clinical practice, the sign described by Schamroth, a cardiologist who himself developed finger clubbing during several attacks of infective endocarditis, is a most useful method of measuring finger clubbing (see Fig. 6-14). Another way is to place a plastic caliper with minimal pressure over the interphalangeal joint. If it is easy to slide the caliper from this joint across the nail fold, the distal phalangeal diameter to interphalangeal diameter ratio must be less than 1, and the patient has no clubbing.

BOX 6-3 Nonpulmonary Diseases Associated with Clubbing

Cardiac

Cyanotic congenital heart disease
Subacute bacterial endocarditis
Chronic congestive heart failure

Hematologic

Thalassemia
Congenital methemoglobinemia (rare)

Gastrointestinal

Crohn disease
Ulcerative colitis
Chronic dysentery, sprue
Polyposis coli
Severe gastrointestinal hemorrhage
Small bowel lymphoma
Liver cirrhosis (including α_1-antitrypsin deficiency)

Other

Thyroid deficiency (thyroid acropachy)
Chronic pyelonephritis (rare)
Toxic (e.g., arsenic, mercury, beryllium)
Lymphomatoid granulomatosis
Fabry's disease
Raynaud's disease, scleroderma

Unilateral Clubbing

Vascular disorders (e.g., subclavian arterial aneurysm, brachial arteriovenous fistula)
Subluxation of shoulder
Median nerve injury
Local trauma

CARDIOVASCULAR SIGNS

Pulmonary heart disease, or cor pulmonale, is a consequence of acute or chronic pulmonary hypertension and appears as right ventricular enlargement. The progression of chronic cor pulmonale to ultimate right ventricular failure is accompanied by certain physical signs. Initially, the right ventricular systolic pressure and muscle mass increase as pulmonary artery pressure rises. During this stage, cardiac auscultation may be normal or may reveal an increased pulmonary component of the second heart sound, caused by an increase in diastolic pulmonary

NORMAL

CLUBBING

Phalangeal Depth Ratio

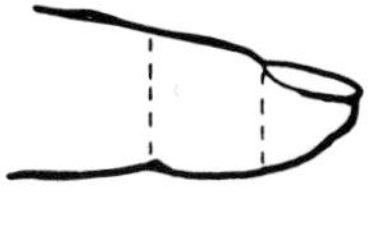

IPD>DPD

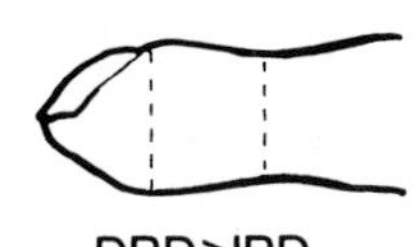

DPD>IPD

Hyponychial Angle

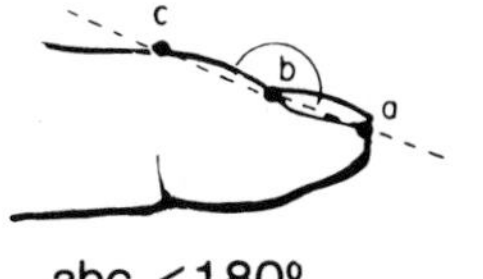

abc <180°

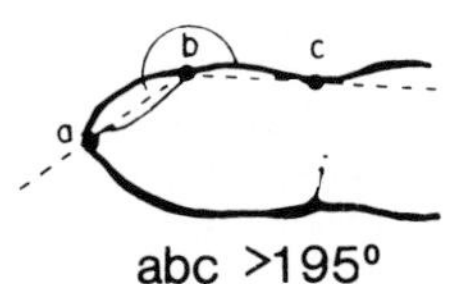

abc >195°

Schamroth's Sign

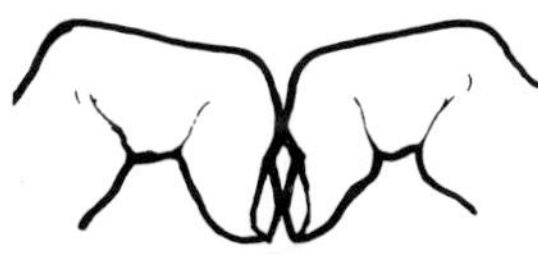

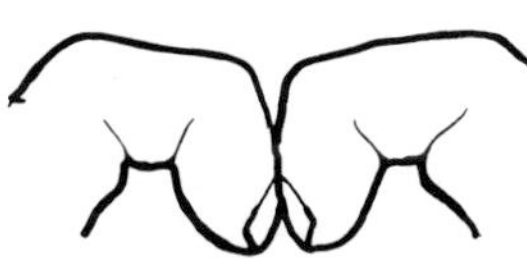

■ **FIGURE 6-14.** Finger clubbing can be measured in different ways. The ratio of the distal phalangeal diameter (DPD) over the interphalangeal diameter (IPD), or the phalangeal depth ratio, is less than 1 in normal subjects but increases to greater than 1 with finger clubbing. The DPD/IPD can be measured with calipers or more accurately with finger casts. The hyponychial angle can be measured from lateral projections of the finger contour on a magnifying screen and is usually less than 180 degrees in normal subjects but greater than 195 degrees in patients with finger clubbing. For bedside clinical assessment, Schamroth's sign is useful. The dorsal surfaces of the terminal phalanges of similar fingers are placed together. With clubbing, the normal diamond-shaped aperture or "window" at the bases of the nail beds disappears, and a prominent distal angle forms between the end of the nails. In normal subjects this angle is minimal or nonexistent.

arterial pressure. The physician should look for a parasternal right ventricular heave. As pulmonary hypertension progresses, there is an increase in right ventricular end-diastolic volume. Dilation of the main pulmonary artery and right ventricular outflow tract lead to systolic pulmonary ejection clicks and murmurs. Diastolic murmurs appear when pulmonary or tricuspid valves or both become insufficient. Third and fourth heart sounds at the left lower sternal border are signs of decreased right ventricular compliance. Most of these right-sided cardiovascular findings are accentuated during inspiration, which augments venous return. Finally, cardiac output falls while end-diastolic pressure and volume increase further in the failing right ventricle.

Clinical findings at this stage include hepatic engorgement, jugular venous distention, and peripheral edema. Occasionally, there may be cyanosis and intracardiac right-to-left shunting through a patent foramen ovale. The physician should exclude the possibility of congenital cardiac defects or acquired left-sided heart disease before making the diagnosis of cor pulmonale. Hyperinflation of the lungs should be taken into account as a cause of the attenuation of cardiovascular sounds and the lowering of the subcostal liver margin, which may be misinterpreted as hepatic enlargement.

Complete assessment of the cardiovascular system includes a careful auscultation and palpation of the pulse to detect cardiac arrhythmia. This problem is not uncommon in patients with chronic lung disease and may appear as sinus or paroxysmal supraventricular tachycardia, atrial premature contractions, or ventricular ectopic beats. Causes include hypoxemia, acid-base imbalance, and enlargement of the right heart, but effects of common drugs such as aminophylline, beta sympathomimetics, or diuretics should not be overlooked.

During quiet spontaneous respiration there is a phasic variation of arterial blood pressure. The widening of this normal respiratory variation is known as pulsus paradoxus. Increased respiratory resistance may exaggerate the normal inspiratory-expiratory difference in left ventricular stroke volume. This is mediated by effects of intrathoracic pressures on ventricular preload. Clinically, pulsus paradoxus is first assessed by palpation of the radial pulse and then is measured at the brachial artery with a sphygmomanometer as the difference in systolic pressure between inspiration and expiration. The pressure cuff is deflated from above systolic level, and the highest pressure during expiration at which systolic pulse sounds are heard is recorded. Similarly, the highest pressure at which every pulse is just audible throughout inspiration is also noted. In general, a drop of greater than 10 mm Hg during inspiration is taken as clinically significant but only a severe paradox of greater than 24 mm Hg is a reliable indicator of severe asthma. The poor correlation between pulsus paradoxus and objective measurements of airflow obstruction may be explained by other factors that affect pleural pressure swings (e.g., the degree of pulmonary hyperinflation and the airflow rate). Furthermore, the accurate measurement of pulsus paradoxus is a challenge in tachypneic, tachycardic, and uncooperative young children. A work group on behalf of the British Thoracic Society Standards of Care Committee found pulsus paradoxus to be absent in one third of patients with the severest obstruction. In contrast to North American practice guidelines, it was therefore recommended that pulsus paradoxus be abandoned as an indicator of severity of asthma attack. In children, wheeze seems to be the clinical parameter of respiratory severity scores that correlates best with pulsus paradoxus, most likely because wheeze requires critical intrathoracic pressures. Perhaps the application of new plethysmographic methods using pulse oximeters will improve the diagnostic value of this clinical sign.

■ CHEST PAIN

Chest pain is relatively common in older children and adolescents but may also present in younger children. The occurrence rate in an emergency department approaches 2.5 per 1000 patient visits, and chest pain accounts for an estimated 650,000 physician visits of patients between the ages of 10 and 21 years annually in the United States. Chest pain in children is most often benign and self-limited. Typical origins are musculoskeletal problems and idiopathic, dysfunctional, and psychogenic causes (Table 6-3). Younger children more frequently have underlying cardiorespiratory problems, whereas children over the age of 12 years are more likely to have psychogenic pain.

■ **TABLE 6-3.** Causes of chest pain in children

Thorax	**Cardiovascular System**
Costochondritis	Structural lesions (e.g., mitral valve prolapse, idiopathic hypertrophic subaortic stenosis [IHSS], coronary disease)
Tietze's syndrome	Acquired cardiac disease (e.g., carditis, arteritis, tumor involvement)
Muscular disease	Arrhythmia
Precordial catch	**Esophagus**
Trauma	Gastroesphageal reflux
Connective tissue disorders	Foreign body
Xiphoid-cartilage syndrome	Achalasia
Rib tip syndrome	**Vertebral Column**
Leukemia	Deformities (e.g., scoliosis)
Herpes zoster	Vertebral collapse
Breast development or disease (e.g., gynecomastia, mastitis)	**Psychogenic Causes**
Lungs, Pleura, and Diaphragm	Anxiety
Asthma	Hyperventilation
Cystic fibrosis	Unresolved grief
Infection (e.g., bronchitis, pneumonia, epidemic pleurodynia)	Identification with another person suffering chest pain
Inhalation of irritanta (e.g., chemical pneumonitis, smoking)	
Stitch (associated with exercise)	
Foreign body	
Pneumothorax	
Pleural disease (e.g., pleurisy, effusion)	
Diaphragmatic irritation (e.g., subphrenic abscess, gastric distention)	
Sickle cell anemia	

The history is most important in the assessment of these patients, who usually have few physical findings and rarely any laboratory data of diagnostic value. The physician should recognize a clinical profile suggestive of psychogenic pain but should also keep in mind that psychogenic and organic causes are not mutually exclusive. A substantial number of patients have a family history of chest pain. Parents of younger children should explain how they know that their child is in pain. It is important to determine whether sleep is affected, because organic pain is more likely than psychogenic pain to awaken the patient or to prevent the child from falling asleep. The duration of symptoms may be an indicator; acute, short-lasting pain is more likely to be organic than pain of many months duration. Localized, sharp, and superficial pains suggest an origin in the chest wall, whereas diffuse, deep, substernal, and epigastric pains are likely to be visceral, originating in the thorax if the pain affects dermatomes T1 to T4 and in the diaphragm or abdomen if it affects dermatomes T5 to T8. The physician should inquire about cough or asthma, recent exercise or trauma, heart disease in the patient and the family, cigarette smoking, and emotional problems.

A close inspection and careful palpation of the chest and abdomen are essential. Common abnormal findings include chest wall tenderness, fever, or both. The physician should use pressure on the stethoscope to elicit local tenderness while the patient is distracted by the auscultation. Cardiac murmurs with or without a midsystolic click may be found in patients with mitral valve prolapse but this condition is rarely associated with chest pain, at least in children. More commonly there are noncardiac causes of chest pain in children with mitral valve prolapse (e.g., orthopedic or gastroesophageal disorders). In general, the presence of systemic signs such as weight loss, anorexia, or syncopal attacks will direct the attention to organic causes of chest pain in children.

SUGGESTED READING

General Reading

Seidel HM: Mosby's Guide to Physical Examination, 4th ed. St. Louis, MO: CV Mosby, 1999.

Swartz MH: Textbook of Physical Diagnosis. History and Examination, 4th ed. Philadelphia: WB Saunders, 2001.

Inspection of the Respiratory System

Britton JR, Britton HL, Jennett R, et al: Weight, length, head and chest circumference at birth in Phoenix, Arizona. J Reprod Med 1993;38:215.

Carlo WA, Martin RJ, Bruce EN, et al: Alae nasi activation (nasal flaring) decreases nasal resistance in preterm infants. Pediatrics 1983;72:338.

Carse EA, Wilkinson AR, Whyte PL, et al: Oxygen and carbon dioxide tensions, breathing and heart rate in normal infants during the first six months of life. J Dev Physiol 1981;3:85.

Commey JO, Levison H: Physical signs in childhood asthma. Pediatrics 1976;58:537.

DeGroodt EG, van Pelt W, Borsboom GJ, et al: Growth of lung and thorax dimensions during the pubertal growth spurt. Eur Respir J 1988;1:102.

Edmonds ZV, Mower WR, Lovato LM, Lomeli R: The reliability of vital sign measurements. Ann Emerg Med 39:233,2002.

Feingold M, Bossert WH: Normal values for selected physical parameters. Birth Defects 1974;10:14.

Gadomski AM, Permutt T, Stanton B: Correcting respiratory rate for the presence of fever. J Clin Epidemiol 1994;47:1043.

Gagliardi L, Rusconi F: Respiratory rate and body mass in the first three years of life. The working party on respiratory rate. Arch Dis Child 1997;76:151.

Gilmartin JJ, Gibson GJ: Mechanisms of paradoxical rib cage motion in patients with chronic obstructive pulmonary disease. Am Rev Respir Dis 1986; 134:683.

Hierholzer E, Schier F: Rasterstereography in the measurement and postoperative follow-up of anterior chest wall deformities. Z Kinderchir 1986;41:267.

Larsen PL, Tos M: Origin of nasal polyps. An endoscopic autopsy study. Laryngoscope 2004;114:710.

Lees MH: Cyanosis of the newborn infant. J Pediatr 1970;77:484.

Peters RM, Peters BA, Benirschke SK, Friedman PJ: Chest dimensions in young adults with spontaneous pneumothorax. Ann Thorac Surg 1978;25:193.

Robotham JL: A physiological approach to hemidiaphragm paralysis. Crit Care Med 1979;7:563.

Staats BA, Bonekat HW, Harris CD, Offord KP: Chest wall motion in sleep apnoea. Am Rev Respir Dis 1984;130:59.

Stinson S: The physical growth of high altitude Bolivian Aymara children. Am J Phys Anthropol 1980;52:377.

Taylor JA, Del Beccaro M, Done S, Winters W: Establishing clinically relevant standards for tachypnea in febrile children younger than 2 years. Arch Pediatr Adolesc Med 1995;149:283.

Usen S, Webert M: Clinical signs of hypoxaemia in children with acute lower respiratory infection. Indicators of oxygen therapy. Int J Tuberc Lung Dis 2001;5:505.

Warwick WJ, Hansen L: Chest calipers for measurement of the thoracic index. Clin Pediatr 1976;15:735.

Watkin SL, Spencer SA, Pryce A, Southall DP: Temporal relationship between pauses in nasal airflow and desaturation in preterm infants. Pediatr Pulmonol 1996;21:171.

Respiratory Sounds

Ackerman NB, Bell RE, deLemos RA: Differential pulmonary auscultation in neonates. Clin Pediatr 1982;21:566.

Baughman RP, Loudon RG: Sound spectral analysis of voice transmitted sound. Am Rev Respir Dis 1986;134:167.

Cugell DW: Lung sound nomenclature. Am Rev Respir Dis 1987;136:1016.

Forgacs P: Lung Sounds. London: Baillière Tindall, 1978.

Gavriely N, Palti Y, Alroy G, Grotberg JB: Measurement and theory of wheezing breath sounds. J Appl Physiol 1984;57:481.

Guilleminault C, Winkle R, Korobkin R, Simmons B: Children and nocturnal snoring. Evaluation of the effects of sleep related respiratory resistive load and daytime functioning. Eur J Pediatr 1982;139:165.

Hopkins RL: Differential auscultation of the acutely ill patient. Ann Emerg Med 1985;14:589.

Kiyokawa H, Greenberg M, Shirota K, Pasterkamp H: Auditory detection of simulated crackles in breath sounds. Chest 2001;119:1886.

Morrison RB: Post-effort breath sound. Tex Med 1971;67:72.

Pasterkamp H, Kraman SS, Wodicka GR: Respiratory sounds. Advances beyond the stethoscope. Am J Respir Crit Care Med 1997;156:974.

Wodicka GR, Shannon DC: Airway sound transmission analysis. In: Roberts JT, ed: Clinical Management of the Airway. Philadelphia: WB Saunders, 1994, pp 87–97.

Yernault JC, Bohadana AB: Chest percussion. Eur Respir J 1995;8:1756.

Pulsus Paradoxus

Clark JA, Lieh-Lai M, Thomas R, et al: Comparison of traditional and plethysmographic methods for measuring pulsus paradoxus. Arch Pediatr Adolesc Med 2004;158:48.

Frey B, Freezer N: Diagnostic value and pathophysiologic basis of pulsus paradoxus in infants and children with respiratory disease. Pediatr Pulmonol 2001;31:138.

Pearson MG, Spence DP, Ryland I, Harrison BD: Value of pulsus paradoxus in assessing acute severe asthma. British Thoracic Society Standards of Care Committee. BMJ 1993;307:659.

Digital Clubbing

Atkinson S, Fox SB: Vascular endothelial growth factor (VEGF)-A and platelet-derived growth factor (PDGF) play a central role in the pathogenesis of digital clubbing. J Pathol 2004;203:721.

Augarten A, Goldman R, Laufer J, et al: Reversal of digital clubbing after lung transplantation in cystic fibrosis patients. A clue to the pathogenesis of clubbing. Pediatr Pulmonol 2002;34:378.

Bentley D, Moore A, Schwachman H: Finger clubbing. A quantitative survey by analysis of the shadowgraph. Lancet 1976;2:164.

Dickinson CJ: The aetiology of clubbing and hypertrophic osteoarthropathy. Eur J Clin Invest 1993;23:330.

Husarik D, Vavricka SR, Mark M, et al: Assessment of digital clubbing in medical inpatients by digital photography and computerized analysis. Swiss Med Wkly 2002;132:132.

Nakamura CT, Ng GY, Paton JY, et al: Correlation between digital clubbing and pulmonary function in cystic fibrosis. Pediatr Pulmonol 2002;33:332.

Schamroth L: Personal experience. S Afr Med J 1976;50:297.

Waring WW, Wilkinson RW, Wiebe RA, et al: Quantitation of digital clubbing in children. Measurements of casts of the index finger. Am Rev Respir Dis 1971;104:166.

Cough and Wheezing

Eigen H: The clinical evaluation of chronic cough. Pediatr Clin North Am 1982;29:67.

Lalloo UG, Barnes PJ, Chung KF: Pathophysiology and clinical presentations of cough. J Allergy Clin Immunol 1996;98(Suppl):91.

Mountain RD, Sahn SA: Clinical features and outcome in patients with acute asthma presenting with hypercapnia. Am Rev Respir Dis 1988;138:535.

Pasterkamp H: Acoustic markers of airway responses during inhalation challenge in children. Pediatr Pulmonol Suppl 2004;26:175.

Shim CS, Williams MH: Relationship of wheezing to the severity of asthma. Arch Intern Med 1983;143:890.

Stern RC, Horwitz SJ, Doershuk CF: Neurologic symptoms during coughing paroxysms in cystic fibrosis. J Pediatr 1988;112:909.

Chest Pain

Owen TR: Chest pain in the adolescent. Adolesc Med 2001;12:95.

Selbst SM, Ruddy R, Clark BJ: Chest pain in children. Follow-up of patients previously reported. Clin Pediatr (Philadelphia) 1990;29(7):374–377.

Woolf PK, Gewitz MH, Berezin S, et al: Noncardiac chest pain in adolescents and children with mitral valve prolapse. J Adolesc Health 1991;12:247.

Cyanosis

Salyer JW: Neonatal and pediatric pulse oximetry. Respir Care 2003;48:386.

Wang EE, Law BJ, Stephens D, et al: Study of interobserver reliability in clinical assessment of RSV lower respiratory illness. A Pediatric Investigators Collaborative Network for Infections in Canada (PICNIC) study. Pediatr Pulmonol 1996;22:23.

7 Bronchoscopy and Bronchoalveolar Lavage in Pediatric Patients

Robert E. Wood, MD • Cori Daines, MD

Visualization of the interior of the body is often the most effective and efficient way to evaluate a patient's problem. As an old Chinese proverb says, "A picture is worth a thousand words." Recent advances in endoscopic techniques and instrumentation have greatly enhanced the pulmonary specialist's ability to visualize the interior of the respiratory tract. This in turn has led to improvements in diagnosis and treatment.

Bronchoscopy—the visual examination of the airways—is usually performed for diagnostic purposes but is also useful for certain therapeutic maneuvers. Bronchoscopy can be performed with either rigid or flexible (fiberoptic) instruments, depending on the particular needs of the patient and the skills and instrumentation available to the bronchoscopist. In general, most procedures that can be done with a rigid bronchoscope can be carried out with a flexible instrument, and vice versa. However, there are some notable exceptions. For example, a rigid instrument cannot be passed through an endotracheal tube, and a flexible instrument is quite unsuited for removal of aspirated foreign bodies from the lungs of children. For the most effective care of pediatric patients, both rigid and flexible instruments must be available, and there must be practitioners trained in the use of each type of instrument (though not necessarily the same person). In many patients, the combined use of both instruments may yield the most optimal result.

In addition to visualization, bronchoscopes also provide an effective means to obtain specimens from the lungs and airways. Tissue samples can be obtained by biopsy forceps, secretions can be aspirated from the airways, and bronchoalveolar lavage (BAL) yields samples of the fluid resident on the surfaces of the alveoli and distal airways. Bronchoscopy is primarily a clinical tool, but it is increasingly being used for investigational purposes as well. Although pediatric patients present special challenges (technical as well as ethical) to the investigative use of bronchoscopy, age alone is no contraindication to the use of bronchoscopy for research.[1]

Bronchoscopy involves the examination of at least part of the upper airway as well as the trachea and bronchi; this is especially true with (and an advantage of) flexible instruments. Rigid bronchoscopes are generally passed through the patient's mouth, whereas flexible bronchoscopes are generally passed through the patient's nose. Bronchoscopes can also be used to examine just the upper airway, although the high incidence of concurrent upper and lower airway lesions[2,3] makes it wise to examine both upper and lower airways unless there is a good reason not to do so.

■ INSTRUMENTATION

The rigid ("open tube") bronchoscope, a metal tube of appropriate diameter and length, is passed into the trachea; through this tube the operator can look and the patient can breathe. The instrument is not a simple metal tube; it is equipped to deliver anesthetic gases and light to the distal tip.

The large open channel, through which instruments may be passed, is one of the major advantages of rigid bronchoscopes. However, visualization is challenging, especially when passing an instrument (such as a biopsy forceps). A major advance in bronchoscopic technique came with the development of the glass rod telescope.[4] This device yields exceptionally fine optical performance, and various instruments such as biopsy and foreign body forceps have been designed specifically to work with the telescopes. Rigid bronchoscopes have holes in the side along the distal tip to allow ventilation of the contralateral lung when the bronchoscope is advanced into one main stem bronchus.

The rigid bronchoscope must be an appropriate size for the patient. Therefore, a variety of instruments must be available to the pediatric bronchoscopist, ranging in diameters from 3 to 7 mm or larger, and in length from 20 to 50 cm. There must be a full range of telescope lengths for the different lengths of bronchoscopes. In addition, glass rod telescopes may be made with a prism on the distal end to facilitate observation of the upper lobes (typically, 30, 70, or even 120 degrees).

Likewise, the auxiliary instruments (e.g., biopsy or foreign body forceps) must match the telescopes and/or bronchoscopes. A large variety of forceps and other devices has been devised for specialized purposes. Perhaps the most valuable are the "optical forceps," which are matched with a glass rod telescope and allow the bronchoscopist to operate the forceps under close and direct visualization.

The nomenclature of bronchoscope sizes can be confusing. In general, rigid instruments are defined by the diameter of the largest instrument that will pass through the bronchoscope, while flexible bronchoscopes are defined by their outer diameter. For example, a 3.5-mm flexible bronchoscope will easily pass through a "3.5-mm" rigid bronchoscope.

The flexible bronchoscope is essentially a solid instrument composed of thousands of glass fibers that carry the light for illumination and the image. The tip of the instrument can be deflected to guide it into the desired path or location. Most flexible bronchoscopes have a small suction channel, through which secretions can be aspirated, fluids can be delivered to the airways, or small flexible instruments can be passed.

The typical pediatric flexible bronchoscopes are 3.5 or 2.8 mm in diameter, with a suction channel approximately 1.2 mm in diameter. Smaller instruments (2.2 mm) have no suction channel and thus have somewhat limited utility when there are secretions or blood in the airways; they also cannot be used to obtain diagnostic specimens. Larger instruments, ranging from

4.9 to 6.3 mm in diameter, are used in adults. These instruments have suction channels ranging from 2.0 mm to 3.2 mm.

In contrast to the rigid bronchoscope, through which the patient breathes (either spontaneously or by positive pressure), the flexible bronchoscope forces the patient to breathe around the instrument. Therefore, the instrument must be small enough not only to fit into the airway but to allow the patient to breathe. Most full-term newborn infants can breathe around the 3.5-mm instrument (the 2.8-mm instrument can allow spontaneous breathing in infants as small as 1.5 kg), but great care must be taken to ensure the adequacy of ventilation during procedures.

Flexible bronchoscopes are quite limited in their capacity for instruments to be passed through them. The most common instruments used with flexible bronchoscopes are flexible biopsy forceps and cytology or microbiology brushes. Small grasping forceps and folding retrieval baskets are also available but have limited usefulness, especially in pediatric patients. Suctioning is done directly with the bronchoscope, rather than by passing a device through the channel, as is the case with rigid bronchoscopes.

Flexible bronchoscopes are limited in their optical performance by the number of glass fibers that compose the image. Although larger, adult-size instruments now mostly utilize a video chip at the working tip (and thus generate an image with greater resolution), pediatric instruments, because of their small diameter, continue to rely on glass fibers to transmit the image. While the images obtained by flexible instruments are quite satisfactory for most clinical purposes, the glass rod telescope gives much greater resolution and image quality.

CARE AND MAINTENANCE OF BRONCHOSCOPES

Bronchoscopy is not a sterile procedure, since the instruments pass through a nonsterile area (the nose and/or mouth). However, bronchoscopes and associated instruments must be cleaned and sterilized before use in a patient.[5] Transmission of infectious agents from patient to patient due to inadequate cleaning or sterilization procedures has been well documented.[6,7] In general, bronchoscopic equipment should be cleaned as soon as possible after use, because dried blood and/or mucus is much more difficult to remove and will prevent adequate sterilization by any method.[8] At a minimum, the instruments should be flushed with water immediately after use and, if possible, soaked in an enzymatic detergent until formal cleaning can be done.

Rigid bronchoscopes are cleaned by vigorous brushing with detergent, followed by rinsing; they can be sterilized by steam autoclaving. Glass rod telescopes and other associated components must not be exposed to steam, however, and must be sterilized with ethylene oxide or with liquid agents such as glutaraldehyde or peracetic acid.[9]

Flexible bronchoscopes are cleaned by careful scrubbing of the exterior with a soft cloth and enzymatic detergent. The suction channel must be cleaned by multiple passes of an appropriate cleaning brush. Thorough rinsing is followed by high-level disinfection[8,9] (with glutaraldehyde or peracetic acid) or sterilization (with ethylene oxide).

The lenses of rigid telescopes and flexible bronchoscopes must be carefully scrubbed and polished with a soft cloth during cleaning. Otherwise, small amounts of protein left on the lens will accumulate over time, making the image progressively less satisfactory.

Flexible bronchoscopes and glass rod telescopes are made of glass and are fragile (not to mention expensive). They must never be dropped and must not be subjected to forces that will cause breakage. Flexible bronchoscopes should never be passed through a patient's mouth unless protected by a rigid bite block; an endotracheal tube will not protect the bronchoscope from severe damage by teeth.

The care with which instruments are cleaned and handled must match the care with which they are utilized in the patient's airway. Individuals responsible for cleaning and preparing the instruments must be well trained and supervised.

INDICATIONS FOR DIAGNOSTIC BRONCHOSCOPY

It is difficult to categorize the indications for diagnostic bronchoscopy without a great deal of overlap. In a given situation, there may be more than one indication for bronchoscopy. In general, however, one can utilize a bronchoscope to define airway anatomy and/or airway dynamics, and to obtain specimens for further diagnostic study. The diagnostic result of a particular procedure can include anatomic findings, definition of abnormal airway dynamics, or the results of microbiologic and/or microscopic evaluation of specimens obtained during the procedure. Bronchoscopy performed for diagnostic purposes may also have therapeutic benefit, such as the removal of a mucus plug causing atelectasis.

It should be noted that there is often great value in a normal bronchoscopic examination; the definitive exclusion of suspected problems (e.g., foreign body aspiration[2]) may be as important as a specific diagnostic finding. Bronchoscopy (rather than simple laryngoscopy) is often performed in patients in whom the suspected lesion is in the upper airway. Since effective laryngoscopy in children usually requires sedation and laryngeal anesthesia, it adds very little to the risk of the procedure to continue the examination into the lower airways. Unsuspected lesions in the lower airways are not uncommonly found.[2,3]

Airway obstruction is one of the most common general indications for diagnostic bronchoscopy and may involve the upper or lower airways or both. The extent of anatomic obstruction, especially fixed obstruction in the subglottic space, is often much greater than would be suspected from clinical examination. If a patient is stridulous during the examination, the vibrating structures causing the noise will always be visible, if one is looking in the right place.

Imaging techniques, such as computed tomography or magnetic resonance imaging scans, can yield considerable diagnostic information about the lungs and even the airways. In some cases, such techniques may make bronchoscopy unnecessary. However, imaging studies are quite limited and cannot provide specimens or (in most cases) define abnormal airway dynamics. In general, radiologic studies should be performed before bronchoscopy, because it may be important to direct the focus of the bronchoscopy (e.g., BAL site) to a specific region of the lungs.

In general, there is only one indication for diagnostic bronchoscopy—when there may be information in the lungs or airways that is necessary to the care of the patient and that is best obtained by bronchoscopy.

Care must be taken to ensure that airway dynamics are not altered by positive pressure ventilation, which will often prevent

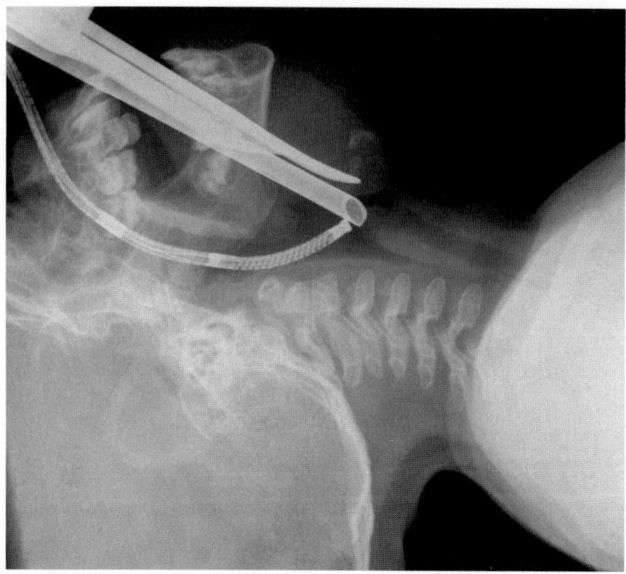

■ **FIGURE 7-1.** The rigid bronchoscope approaches the larynx directly, with mandibular lift. The flexible instrument approaches the larynx from behind, making it difficult to evaluate the subglottic space and posterior cervical trachea.

dynamic airway collapse. The depth of sedation may also influence the airway dynamics; if the patient is too deeply sedated, abnormal dynamics may not be visible.

The choice between rigid and flexible instruments should be made with some care, if there is a choice available. In many patients, the combined use of both rigid and flexible instruments can add immeasurably to the value of the procedures. Rigid instruments often distort the airway, while at the same time allowing better visualization of the anatomic details. This is especially true in the larynx and upper trachea. Rigid instruments lift the mandible and hyoid, but allow a much better view of the posterior aspects of the larynx and cervical trachea. Flexible instruments do not distort the anatomy (they follow the natural curvature of the airway) but approach the larynx from behind and are, therefore, less capable of viewing details of the posterior aspects of the larynx, subglottic space, and cervical trachea (Fig. 7-1).

■ BRONCHOALVEOLAR LAVAGE

In many cases, bronchoscopic visualization alone is not sufficiently informative. BAL[10,11] yields a specimen that can give representative data from the distal airways and alveolar surfaces, and has become one of the more important aspects of diagnostic bronchoscopy. BAL can be defined as the instillation into and recovery from the distal airways of a volume of saline sufficient to ensure that the fluid returned contains at least some fluid that was originally present on the alveolar surface. Both soluble and cellular constituents of the alveolar (and small airway) surface fluid are contained in the effluent. This epithelial surface fluid is diluted to an unknown but significant degree by the saline used in its collection. Therefore, the concentrations of substances measured in the BAL fluid do not give an accurate estimate of the concentration at the epithelial surface. Various methods have been used to derive a reasonable measure of the dilution,[12] although none are free of problems, since the epithelial fluid is not static. There is constant flux of fluid and soluble constituents across the epithelial surface, and the duration and volume of the fluid used for lavage may have substantial impact on the concentration of substances in the effluent.[13–15] Fortunately, for clinical purposes, and especially in pediatric patients, the information in most cases need not be quantitative. The primary value of BAL is to obtain a specimen from the distal airways that is relatively representative and that can yield information about infectious and/or inflammatory processes. However, the interpretation of BAL data is rarely totally free of ambiguities.

■ INDICATIONS FOR BRONCHOALVEOLAR LAVAGE

Bronchoalveolar lavage is performed primarily for diagnostic purposes, although it can also be performed for therapeutic reasons. The main indications are listed in Table 7-1. BAL may be indicated for the diagnosis of infectious processes when a sputum specimen cannot be obtained or the results from sputum analysis are equivocal. In immunocompetent individuals, this may include the infant or young child with cystic fibrosis[16,17] or pneumonia with pulmonary symptoms requiring therapy. These children may be unable to produce spontaneous sputum, and cultures from the upper airway may either yield no pathogens when the bronchi are infected or yield pathogens when the lungs are sterile. In immunocompromised individuals, the diagnosis of potential infections in the face of pulmonary infiltrates is valuable and often unable to be attained without BAL.[18–20] In either immunocompetent or immunocompromised individuals, BAL may help to distinguish infectious from noninfectious processes in the child with radiographic abnormalities. In general, however, if a satisfactory sputum specimen can be obtained, bronchoscopy solely to obtain cultures from the distal airways is not indicated as a primary approach. It may, however, be indicated when therapy geared toward suspected pathogens based on a sputum sample fails to provide therapeutic response. BAL should ideally be performed before antibacterial therapy is started but may still be informative if there is a lack of clinical response or clinical deterioration.

Bronchoalveolar lavage is often indicated to distinguish infectious from noninfectious processes, such as alveolar hemorrhage (which may occur without frank hemoptysis), pulmonary alveolar proteinosis,[21,22] or interstitial lung diseases.[23,24] BAL may lead to a diagnosis of pulmonary histiocytosis documented by the presence of more than 5% CD1a-positive cells.[25,26] BAL is also indicated in the evaluation of patients with suspected aspiration, both to obtain microbiologic specimens to guide antibiotic therapy and to obtain evidence for the aspiration. Although a specific exogenous marker is not available, the presence of significant numbers of macrophages heavily laden with lipid[27] is a strong correlate of aspiration. In patients who have undergone lung transplant, BAL is often used in conjunction with transbronchial biopsy to distinguish rejection from infection.[28] BAL alone, however, is not sufficient to establish a diagnosis of rejection in these patients (Box 7-1).

In addition to diagnostic indications, BAL is occasionally indicated for the therapeutic removal of materials from the airway. This may include the removal of mucus plugs or blood clots to aid ventilation, the removal of bronchial casts in plastic bronchitis, or whole-lung lavage as a therapy in pulmonary alveolar proteinosis.[29,30] Additionally, BAL may be therapeutic for the removal of foreign lipoid material from the lung to prevent damage to the alveolar structures.

TABLE 7-1. Indications for diagnostic bronchoscopy

Indication	Rigid Instruments	Flexible Instruments
Stridor	May alter airway dynamics	Preferred
Persistent wheeze (not responsive, or poorly responsive to bronchodilator therapy)		Preferred
Atelectasis (persistent, recurrent, or massive)	May be needed to remove airway obstruction	
Localized hyperinflation		Preferred
Pneumonia		Preferred (much better to obtain BAL specimens)
• Recurrent		
• Persistent		
• Patients unable to produce sputum		
• Atypical or in unusual circumstances (e.g., immunocompromised patients)		
Hemoptysis	May be best if there is brisk bleeding	Preferred to evaluate distal airways
Foreign body aspiration	Mandatory for removal of foreign bodies	May be useful to examine for the possibility of foreign body; rarely useful for removal
• Known		
• Suspected		
Cough (persistent)		Preferred
Suspected aspiration	Preferred to evaluate posterior larynx and cervical trachea	Preferred to obtain BAL
Evaluation of patients with tracheostomies	Preferred to evaluate posterior larynx and subglottic space	Preferred to evaluate tube position and airway dynamics
Suspected mass or tumor	Preferred for laryngeal or tracheal lesions	Preferred for lesions in distal airways
Suspected airway anomalies		
Complications of artificial airways		

BAL, bronchoalveolar lavage.

TECHNIQUES FOR BRONCHOALVEOLAR LAVAGE

Bronchoalveolar lavage is most conveniently performed during flexible bronchoscopy. Care must be taken to avoid contamination of the lower airway specimen with upper airway secretions during passage of the bronchoscope through the upper airway (or by aspiration following topical laryngeal anesthesia). For routine procedures, it is helpful to gently suction away excessive nasal and oral secretions before inserting the bronchoscope, and to flush oxygen through the suction channel (flow rate approximately 2 L/min) while passing the bronchoscope through the upper airway. Excessive volumes of topical anesthetic should be avoided. Suction should not be performed through the bronchoscope until the tip of the instrument is deep within the lungs.

BOX 7-1 Indications for Bronchoalveolar Lavage

Diagnosis of suspected infection
Pulmonary infiltrates
Dyspnea
Hypoxia
Tachypnea
Recurrent pulmonary infiltrates
Persistent pulmonary infiltrates
Interstitial infiltrates
Diffuse alveolar inflammation
Pulmonary hemorrhage
Alveolar proteinosis
Pulmonary histiocytosis
Aspiration
Lung transplant
Hypereosinophilic lung diseases
Therapeutic removal of materials

In immunocompromised patients or those in whom it is vital to minimize ambiguity in the results, it is useful to electively intubate the patient and pass the flexible bronchoscope through the endotracheal tube. The upper airway can then be examined after removing the endotracheal tube. In children who already have a tracheostomy tube in place, performing the BAL through the tracheostomy tube before examining the upper airway may lead to less contamination.

After the bronchoscope has been introduced into the lower airway, it should be gently wedged into the selected bronchus. Site selection is based on clinical, bronchoscopic, or radiographic findings. If there is diffuse disease, however, it is advantageous to wedge the bronchoscope into the lingula or right middle lobe bronchus. These bronchi are relatively long and horizontal; the tip of the bronchoscope is more likely to remain wedged into these bronchi during coughing than in a lower lobe bronchus. When the bronchoscope does not remain wedged, saline may spill into other bronchi, producing coughing and possibly respiratory distress.

With the bronchoscope wedged into the bronchus, normal sterile saline is instilled through the suction channel of the bronchoscope and immediately withdrawn. Enough air should be instilled after each aliquot to ensure clearance of the saline from the suction channel. The volume of the channel can be as high as 2 mL in bronchoscopes with larger suction channels. The fluid can be withdrawn by hand suction with a syringe or aspirated into a trap. Although sufficient suction must be applied to overcome the resistance of the channel in the bronchoscope, too much negative pressure will cause the bronchus to collapse, preventing efflux of fluid and possibly causing trauma to the airway mucosa. Fluid return may also be impaired if the patient is not breathing spontaneously. In some patients, almost any amount of negative pressure will result in collapse of the bronchus, and fluid return may be challenging. In such situations, it may be necessary to instill additional volumes of saline to recover a representative specimen. The suction port of a flexible bronchoscope is offset from the optical axis of the instrument, so that if the bronchus into which the instrument is wedged is centered in the image, the suction port may be partially occluded by the bronchial wall. Positioning the bronchoscope so that the image of the bronchus is off center may improve fluid return.

Some centers utilize saline that has been warmed to body temperature (37°C) to minimize bronchospasm and increase return, although with small-volume BAL there is little risk and room temperature saline may be safely used. There is no consensus about the number and volume of aliquots that should be used in BAL. In adult patients, it is common to utilize three aliquots of 100 mL or five aliquots of 50 mL.[11] In children, various protocols have been used. Some bronchoscopists use a standard volume of 10 to 20 mL in two to four aliquots regardless of body weight and age[31]; others adjust the volume to the patient's functional residual capacity based on weight[18] or adjust the volume based on weight using 3 mL/kg divided into three aliquots with a maximum of 20 mL per aliquot.[21,32] Given the great variability in alveolar surface area being sampled based on the child's size, the size of the bronchoscope and the location of the wedge, no technique is truly capable of standardization. For clinical purposes, the precise volume is probably of little relevance, since the primary application in children is the detection of infectious agents and examination of the cellular constituents. There should be uniformity in technique within a given institution. For clinical research, consistent protocols may be helpful, but no technique will ensure that the dilution of specimens is truly uniform.

Generally, 40% to 60% of the instilled fluid will be recovered; the remainder of the fluid will be absorbed over a few hours. The first aliquot returned is relatively enriched in fluid from the surface of the conducting airways and may have a higher percentage of inflammatory cells.[33] Some bronchoscopists separate out this first aliquot for culture rather than pooling it with subsequent aliquots, although the bronchial surface fluid will be washed into the alveolar spaces by each aliquot, therefore "contaminating" the subsequent aliquots with bronchial contents. For routine purposes, the small differences in content from one aliquot to the next do not warrant different handling.

Performing a BAL usually prolongs the bronchoscopic procedure by 1 to 3 minutes, minimally increasing the risks of hypoxia or hypercarbia, but is well tolerated by most patients, even those who are critically ill. If a patient is thrombocytopenic, BAL could theoretically increase the risk of bleeding, but it can be performed relatively safely in children with platelet counts of more than 20,000 platelets/mL.[34] Some children do develop transient fever after BAL, especially if their airways were significantly inflamed, but this is almost always transient and self-limited. A theoretical risk of spreading infection and causing iatrogenic pneumonia exists[6] but is rarely proven. The most problematic complication of BAL is not obtaining the correct information by not preparing for and adequately performing the procedure, or by failing to perform the appropriate analysis of the specimen.

PROCESSING OF BRONCHOALVEOLAR LAVAGE SPECIMENS

Fluid from BAL should be processed promptly. Some centers keep the sample at 4°C before processing to maintain cell viability,[35] although this is most important if the sample will not be promptly transported to or processed by the laboratory and is not generally necessary. The sample should routinely be processed for microbiology and cytologic studies. Some research protocols call for filtering of the BAL fluid before processing (to remove mucus plugs, etc.). However, this procedure may alter the diagnostic value of the specimen, because cells and microorganisms may adhere to the filter, and there may be important information hidden within mucus plugs. The bronchoscopist should organize a routine technique for processing with the institutional laboratory service; pediatric specimens may require different processing and interpretation than do specimens from adult patients.

Microbiologic studies are performed according to the clinical indications for the procedure. Because of the potential for contamination of BAL specimens by secretions from the oropharynx, semiquantitative culture techniques may help in the interpretation of results. In addition to cultures, other techniques such as special stains or polymerase chain reaction may help to identify pathogens; the bronchoscopist should consult with the laboratory to determine what analyses may be available and the specific requirements for specimen volume and handling.

The basic cytologic analysis of a BAL specimen involves a cellular differential, which can be performed with simple stains such as Wright's or a Giemsa. The specimen is centrifuged onto a slide[36]; most centers perform cytospins at 250 to 500 *g* for 5 to 10 minutes.[35] Special stains are performed according to the clinical indications (i.e., lipid or iron stains, methamine silver stains, etc.). Total cell counts may be performed, but because of the variable dilution of the specimen, these are of relatively limited value in interpretation. Flow cytometry can be done for special processing. Although all BAL samples should routinely be processed for microbiologic studies and cytology, there is wide variability in practice as to the specific tests that are considered routine. This variability stems from differences in patient population, in institutional capabilities and preferences, and in advancing technologies. Box 7-2 lists some potential tests for BAL fluid.

INTERPRETATION OF BRONCHOALVEOLAR LAVAGE FINDINGS

Interpretation of BAL findings must be undertaken with the knowledge that both technique and disease state play a large role in results. For instance, wedging more proximally increases both cell number and percentage of neutrophils. Small volumes sample mainly the airway. BAL samples the bronchial and alveolar surfaces and does not necessarily reflect parenchymal processes; it is best at identifying what does not belong. In general, cell numbers in normal children will range between 100,000 and 250,000 cells/mL. Normal BAL fluid contains less than 5% neutrophils (usually 1% to 2%).[32,37,38] Patients with an active bacterial infection may have up to 95% neutrophils, and rarely less than 25%. Patients with bacterial infection often have bacterial forms visible in the cytoplasm of neutrophils recovered in BAL[39]; this may be a useful measure to differentiate between infection and contamination of the specimen with oral secretions. Increased neutrophils can also be seen in chronic inflammatory states associated with aspiration or cystic fibrosis, in acute respiratory distress syndrome, in alveolitis, in scleroderma, and even in asthma. Normally, 80% to 90% of the nonepithelial cells in BAL are alveolar macrophages. Lymphocytes are the next most common cell type, comprising 5% to 10% of the BAL cells in normal children. Although increased percentages of

BOX 7-2 **Potential Bronchoalveolar Lavage Assays**

Microbiologic Studies

Gram Stain

Cultures
Bacterial (quantitative)
Viral
Fungal
Mycobacterial
Anaerobic

Stains

Grocott-Gomori methenamine–silver nitrate stain
Ziehl-Neelsen stain (acid-fast bacteria)

Immunoassays

Chlamydia
Mycoplasma
Legionella
Fungi
Viruses

Polymerase Chain Reaction

Viruses
Chlamydia
Mycoplasma
In situ viruses

Cytologic Studies

Total Cell Count

Stains for Differential Cytology

Giemsa, Wright's, hematoxylin & eosin

Flow Cytometry

Trypan Blue Exclusion for Cell Viability

Lymphocyte Subsets

Special Stains

Lipid Stains

Oil Red O
Sudan IV

Iron Stain

Prussian blue

Stains for Pulmonary Alveolar Proteinosis

Periodic acid–Schiff

Electron Microscopy

Noncellular Components

Surfactant Proteins

Cytokines

lymphocytes are not diagnostic of any specific disease, increased numbers are seen in sarcoidosis (20% to 50%), *Mycobacterium tuberculosis* infection, interstitial lung disease, *Pneumocystis carinii* infection, or nontuberculosis mycobacterial infection. Eosinophils are rare in normal subjects (0% to 1%); significant numbers suggest an allergic state, eosinophilic pneumonia, parasitic infection, interstitial lung disease, drug-induced lung disease, *P. carinii* infection, or a foreign body reaction. Large numbers are seen in eosinophilic pneumonia. Epithelial cells are common in BAL fluid but are not counted in the differential. Squamous cells from the upper airway, often covered in oral bacteria, and ciliated columnar cells from the lower airway can be seen.

Opinions vary with respect to what numbers of bacteria constitute adequate evidence of infection. In general, for common bacterial species such as *Staphylococcus aureus*, *Haemophilus influenzae*, and *Streptococcus pneumoniae*, concentrations of more than 100,000 organisms/mL of BAL fluid,[40] in association with significant numbers of neutrophils, are adequate evidence of infection. In the absence of neutrophils (except in neutropenic patients), bacteria are more likely to represent contamination than infection. Numbers of bacteria in excess of 500,000 organisms/mL are common in clear-cut bacterial infection, as is the finding of intracellular bacteria. However, the interpretation is not always straightforward, especially if significant numbers of "oral flora" are also recovered. In pediatric patients, it is possible to obtain BAL specimens that are sterile, but the majority will have at least some oral flora even if there are no pathogens. In immunocompromised patients, the finding of pathogens that are not normally in the lung may be diagnostic, regardless of numbers. *Pneumocystis carinii*, *M. tuberculosis*, *Legionella pneumophila*, *Nocardia*, *Histoplasma*, *Blastomyces*, *Mycoplasma*, influenza virus, and respiratory syncytial virus would therefore be true pathogens, whereas herpes simplex virus, cytomegalovirus, *Aspergillus*, atypical mycobacteria, bacteria, and *Candida* may not be pathogens but merely contaminants or colonizing agents.

Viruses can be grown from BAL fluid, but the process may require weeks, limiting the utility of this assay.[41] Using polymerase chain reaction to detect viruses can speed diagnosis and may be more sensitive. Another indication of viral infection is the finding of viral cytopathic effect on stains. This is caused by nuclear inclusion bodies that on stain result in a halo or "owl's eye" around the nucleus. This is not specific but can be helpful in suggesting that an isolated virus is truly a pathogen.

Fungi can be seen on stain as well as grown in culture. Distinguishing contamination or colonization from true infection can be difficult, however. Mycobacteria must be cultured on special medium and may take up to 8 weeks to grow. With significant infection, the acid-fast bacteria smear may be positive as well. Newer molecular methods such as nucleic acid probes[42] or DNA amplification[43] can speed detection.

A Grocott-Gomori (methenamine–silver nitrate) stain helps in the detection of fungi, especially *P. carinii*, for which it can be diagnostic. Periodic acid–Schiff (PAS) staining is used to characterize the diffuse proteinaceous material in pulmonary alveolar proteinosis. The lamellar bodies defining the material as surfactant can be seen on electron microscopy. Prussian blue stains detect iron in macrophages from pulmonary hemorrhages or hemosiderosis. Macrophages become positive for iron staining about 50 hours after bleeding occurs, not immediately. If no further bleeding occurs, iron will clear in 12 to 14 days from the airways and in 2 to 4 weeks from the parenchyma. It can be normal to have up to 3% of macrophages staining positive for iron.[44]

Lipid stains (Oil Red O or Sudan IV) are meant to detect lipid-laden macrophages in an attempt to diagnose aspiration of food (from swallowing or gastroesophageal reflux). Although this technique is plagued by a lack of sensitivity and specificity,[45] the use of a "lipid index"[27] may increase the utility of the test. A positive lipid stain does not reveal the source of the lipid (aspiration vs. endogenous sources). Also, lipid stains do not identify children who aspirate oral secretions but who are not being fed orally.

For illustrative examples of BAL cytology, see Figures 7-2 through 7-10.

SPECIAL TECHNIQUES

One extension of bronchoalveolar lavage is whole-lung ("bronchopulmonary") lavage, used therapeutically in individuals with pulmonary alveolar proteinosis. Alveolar proteinosis is less common in children than adults, and special techniques may be required for whole-lung lavage.[29] Whole-lung lavage can be performed with partial cardiopulmonary bypass or by sequential single-lung lavage.

Another special technique is nonbronchoscopic BAL. This involves blindly placing a catheter through an endotracheal or tracheostomy tube into a distal "wedged" position, instilling normal saline, and then withdrawing that saline into a trap or syringe.[46] The suction catheter should have only one hole at the end. This is truly a blind procedure and will likely only yield useful results in diffuse lung disease. Although some groups have advocated use of this technique routinely in neonates intubated with small endotracheal tubes,[35] the wide availability of a 2.8-mm flexible bronchoscope that can be used through endotracheal tubes as small as 3.5 mm has significantly decreased the need for nonbronchoscopic procedures.

RESEARCH APPLICATIONS

A widely untapped arena for BAL is its use in clinical, translational, and basic science research. In recent years, many new assays for detection of inflammatory markers, for the function of bronchoalveolar cells, and for the detection of a wide array of noncellular BAL components have been developed. Some of these are used sporadically in clinical assays, such as the determination of lymphocyte subpopulations and the identification of surfactant proteins, but most are used strictly for research purposes. One of the limitations of such assays is the lack of control data, because normal children do not ordinarily undergo flexible bronchoscopy with BAL. Development of collaborations and specimen banks may help define the normal population, allowing research to proceed more rapidly.

THERAPEUTIC INDICATIONS FOR BRONCHOSCOPY

Therapeutic indications for bronchoscopy in infants and children primarily involve the restoration of airway patency. While the majority of such applications will involve the use of a rigid bronchoscope, considerable therapeutic benefit can often be achieved with flexible instruments as well. Therapeutic bronchoscopy is indicated when it is the best way to achieve the desired therapeutic goals.

The removal of foreign bodies is one of the more common therapeutic applications of bronchoscopy in children. It is also one of the more difficult and potentially dangerous bronchoscopic procedures in children. Only under the most unusual circumstances should foreign body removal be attempted with a flexible bronchoscope. The devices that can be passed through a flexible instrument and used for foreign body retrieval are rudimentary at best, and airway management is difficult. Small, peripherally located foreign bodies[47] may best be reached with a flexible bronchoscope but may yet be difficult to remove.

Mass lesions in the airways can often be dealt with effectively with a bronchoscope. Granulation tissue is the most common such lesion and may result from foreign bodies, mycobacterial infection, or mechanical trauma associated with artificial airways. Less commonly, tumor masses may be found in children, usually a hemangioma or a bronchial carcinoid tumor.

Benign mass lesions can be resected, if appropriate, with either forceps or a laser. Malignant lesions, or lesions that extend through the bronchial wall, are usually best approached surgically rather than endoscopically, although endoscopic resection may be used for temporary relief of obstruction in selected cases. In general, the use of endobronchial forceps is easier with rigid bronchoscopes; there is better potential for control of bleeding, and the forceps are larger and more readily manipulated than the small, flexible instruments that can be used with flexible bronchoscopes. Laser applications may utilize either rigid or flexible instruments. In the subglottic space and upper trachea, carbon dioxide lasers are often used; these lasers require a direct line of sight between the laser and the lesion and are thus much more difficult to use in the distal airways. Lasers within the near-infrared or visible light spectrum (neodymium:yttrium aluminum-garnet [Nd:YAG], argon, potassium-titanyl-phosphate [KTP], etc.) can be operated through a flexible fiber (as small as a few hundred microns in diameter). Therefore, these lasers are more appropriate for use in distal airway lesions. Depending on the amount of laser energy delivered, tissue may be vaporized or merely desiccated. A potential risk of vaporization is that the heat produced may injure surrounding normal tissue; lasers should not be used exuberantly. Desiccation, rather than vaporization, of benign lesions may lead to less scarring afterward.

Tracheal or bronchial stenosis, or severe localized tracheomalacia or bronchomalacia can be treated endoscopically. Depending on the nature of the lesion, the airway may be dilated,[48] treated with a laser,[49,50] or subjected to stent placement. The effect of dilation or laser therapy may be temporary, however, and follow-up examinations (and repeated treatments) are almost always required. A variety of endobronchial stents are available that may be placed to ensure airway patency under certain conditions. However, none of these devices is truly appropriate for pediatric patients, and there is little experience with such devices in children, especially young infants. Great caution should be taken when considering stenting in pediatric patients. Stents are associated with numerous problems, such as mucus retention, formation of granulation tissue, and migration of the stent. In growing children, a stent will have to be replaced periodically; otherwise, the child will develop an iatrogenic stenosis. However, if the stent has become embedded in the airway mucosa, it may be nearly impossible to remove safely.[51] Nevertheless, in highly selected patients, stenting may be the only way to achieve and maintain airway patency.

Mucus plugs or blood clots in the airways causing atelectasis will usually yield to endoscopic treatment. Localized trauma from endotracheal suctioning is a common cause of mucus plugs. Children with small (usually organic) foreign bodies, cystic fibrosis, asthma, or allergic bronchopulmonary aspergillosis may also develop central mucus plugs. In some cases, mucus plugs must be removed with forceps, much as though they were a foreign body. Most mucus plugs, however, will yield to suctioning through a flexible bronchoscope. By touching the tip of the flexible bronchoscope to the proximal surface of the mucus plug and applying constant suction, plugs much larger than the diameter of the suction channel can often be removed, even if in pieces. Local lavage with saline or a mucolytic agent (1% *N*-acetylcysteine) can also be helpful to dislodge a mucus plug.

Alveolar filling disorders such as alveolar proteinosis or lipid aspiration are treated by bronchopulmonary lavage. Although this may be accomplished, after a fashion, directly through a bronchoscope, it is more effective to utilize large volumes of saline and to lavage relatively large areas of the lung at one time. In adults, a double-lumen endotracheal tube is used[52]; this is not feasible in smaller patients. A flexible bronchoscope can be used to position a single-lumen cuffed endobronchial catheter through which an entire lung can be lavaged with large volumes, while ventilation is maintained with a nasopharyngeal tube.[29]

Flexible bronchoscopes are valuable in the management of tracheostomy and endotracheal tubes. The difficult or complicated intubation can be readily accomplished by passing the endotracheal tube over a flexible bronchoscope.[53] Problems with tube positioning or tube patency can be resolved quickly with a flexible instrument.

Bronchoscopy can be used in the management of intractable air leaks.[54] A systematic search for the bronchus leading to the air leak can be made with a Fogarty catheter, which is inflated in a bronchus while observing the air leak from the chest tube. When the site of the leak is defined, fibrin glue or Gelfoam can be packed into the bronchus leading to the site of the air leak. More proximal leaks, as from the stump of a resected bronchus, can be treated directly by application of tissue adhesive.[55]

■ CONTRAINDICATIONS TO BRONCHOSCOPY

Bronchoscopy should not be performed in the absence of a suitable indication or appropriate equipment and personnel skilled in its use. Otherwise, there are no absolute contraindications to bronchoscopy. However, if the same diagnostic information can be obtained by a less expensive, less invasive, or potentially less dangerous technique, then bronchoscopy is not indicated.

Relative contraindications to bronchoscopy include any variable that will increase the risk. Specific risk factors should be treated and, if possible, alleviated before bronchoscopy. Cardiovascular instability, bleeding diatheses (thrombocytopenia or hypoprothrombinemia), severe bronchospasm, and hypoxemia are primary examples. Some conditions that increase the risk are themselves indications for bronchoscopy, such as severe airway obstruction. In these cases, the procedure is performed with both diagnostic and therapeutic intent, and can be lifesaving. Appropriate modifications must be made in the techniques chosen for anesthesia and monitoring when there are additional risk factors.

■ ANESTHESIA FOR BRONCHOSCOPY

Safe and effective bronchoscopy requires that the patient be comfortable and remain reasonably still during the procedure. Adequate oxygenation and ventilation must be maintained, and the patient must be carefully and continuously monitored. These criteria can be met with either general anesthesia or sedation (usually performed by the intravenous administration of a narcotic and/or a benzodiazepine[56] and administered by the bronchoscopist), depending on the individual child's situation and the procedure planned. Sedation and general anesthesia are merely points on a continuum between the fully awake state and surgical anesthesia; it matters little how the desired, safe state is achieved. Furthermore, "conscious sedation," in which reflexes are preserved and the patient may respond to verbal instructions, is not appropriate for most pediatric procedures. Deep sedation and light "general anesthesia" are virtually indistinguishable. An advantage of general anesthesia is that an anesthesiologist takes full responsibility for monitoring the patient. Current practice guidelines for sedation[57] mandate the presence of a trained individual whose sole responsibility is to monitor the patient, although this person does not have to be an anesthesiologist. Our current practice at Cincinnati Children's Hospital is to utilize an anesthesiologist, and the child is sedated with general anesthetic agents (inhaled or given intravenously) to a point that maintains spontaneous breathing but ensures safe comfort. Another significant advantage of using "general anesthetic" agents for sedation is rapid induction and relatively rapid emergence.

Sedation and/or anesthesia diminish or abolish protective reflexes. To reduce the risk for aspiration of gastric contents, patients should be given nothing by mouth for several hours before the procedure. Clear liquids may be given up to 2 hours before the procedure.[58,59] It is prudent to aspirate the stomach with a catheter before proceeding with the bronchoscopy. Young infants may become dehydrated or hypoglycemic if kept on nothing by mouth for too long, and intravenous fluid may be necessary before a procedure.

General anesthesia should be used in any situation in which intravenous sedation is not suitable. Children who have undergone numerous invasive procedures are often difficult to sedate, and there should be a low threshold for switching to general anesthesia. Likewise, those children who have a history of difficult sedation are poor candidates for repeated attempts at sedation. Unstable upper airway obstruction is a prime indication for general anesthesia, because sedation may result in significant hypoxemia or a sudden need for an artificial airway. In this case, the use of a very-short-acting agent such as propofol or an inhalational agent may reduce the risk, whereas the usual agents used for intravenous sedation prolong the risk. General anesthesia should be considered for complicated and/or prolonged procedures such as the extraction of extensive mucus plugs or laser procedures.

When general anesthesia is utilized for diagnostic bronchoscopy, careful attention must be given to airway dynamics. If the patient does not breathe spontaneously, then the usual airway dynamics are reversed; airway pressure during inspiration exceeds that during expiration. This may result in diagnostic confusion in patients with tracheomalacia and/or bronchomalacia. During therapeutic procedures, positive pressure ventilation is often utilized.

Flexible bronchoscopes are sufficiently small to allow the patient to usually breathe around them. Spontaneous breathing is the rule for most flexible procedures. However, in some circumstances it may be necessary to provide for positive pressure ventilation. This is simple if the patient is intubated with an endotracheal tube large enough to accommodate the flexible bronchoscope, but this approach may present problems in very small children. Ventilation may be assisted via a mask (through which the flexible bronchoscope is passed), a laryngeal mask airway, or a nasopharyngeal tube.[60] The introduction of 2.8-mm flexible bronchoscopes dramatically extended downward the size of endotracheal tubes through which a flexible bronchoscope can be passed while maintaining positive pressure ventilation (3.5 mm vs. 5.0 mm with the 3.5-mm instrument; Table 7-2).

Many techniques are suitable for effective general anesthesia during bronchoscopy. Traditional inhalational agents such as halothane are being replaced by newer, short-acting agents such as sevoflurane and propofol. The safety record of general anesthesia in recent years has removed many of the earlier objections to its use, and pediatric patients should not be deprived of its benefits when appropriate.

Sedation, like general anesthesia, can be produced by a variety of agents and techniques.[56] Important principles of sedation include careful preparation of the patient; the use of fractional doses of short-acting agents with titration of total dose to the needed effect; appropriate monitoring before, during, and after the procedure; and careful selection of agents.

The drugs chosen for sedation should be matched to the specific needs of the child and the procedure. For totally noninvasive procedures such as magnetic resonance imaging, purely sedative agents such as chloral hydrate[61] or a barbiturate can be used.[62] However, invasive procedures that involve any discomfort are best performed with an analgesic agent such as a narcotic, as well as an amnesic agent such as a benzodiazepine.

Sedative agents have a variety of physiologic effects in addition to reducing the level of consciousness. The most important of these is depression of respiratory drive, and this effect may last longer than the sedation. Children who have undergone sedation for procedures may be at greater risk after the procedure is completed than during the procedure itself due to the absence of the stimulation of the procedure and diminished staff awareness and alertness. Effective monitoring must be continued until all the effects of sedation have resolved.[57]

Pharmacologic agents to reverse the effect of narcotics and benzodiazepines are available, and some physicians utilize these agents routinely at the completion of procedures.[63] This is not necessarily a good idea, however, because their effect is considerably shorter than the respiratory depression induced by the sedative agents. Furthermore, patients awakened abruptly from sedation are often disturbed and may become combative. Monitoring must be continued whether or not a reversal agent has been given; indeed, it may be argued that monitoring must be continued longer after reversal than without it. On the other hand, such agents should always be readily available in the event of serious respiratory depression.

Sedation, no matter how administered, involves more than giving drugs. Children are often very responsive to suggestion—whether positive or negative, whether intentional or inadvertent. Simple distraction or more formal methods of focusing attention on something other than the procedure[64,65] may be surprisingly effective in children, especially in the 3- to 8-year age group. Even infants respond to tone of voice and the atmosphere around them. Careful preparation of the child and the parents, focusing on positive aspects and creating positive expectation, can be powerful adjuncts to chemical sedation. On the other hand, negative suggestions can make even the most powerful drugs less effective. A screaming, upset child will require much higher doses of virtually any agent to achieve effective sedation, and that child's recovery will be prolonged. For this reason, presedation with oral drugs such as chloral hydrate or midazolam and careful attention to atmosphere and language can often facilitate deeper sedation with minimal doses of other agents.

During the process of sedation or induction of anesthesia, many children experience a phase of disinhibition or excitement, during which their behavior may be difficult to control. This should be expected and not be interpreted as an adverse or allergic reaction to the drug used. In fractional dosing for sedation, a sufficient dose should be given initially to get beyond the disinhibition phase; if very small doses are given initially, disinhibition may be prolonged, and the total sedative dose required may be significantly increased.

TABLE 7-2. Artificial airways and flexible bronchoscopes used in pediatric patients

Instrument Diameter (mm)	Smallest Tube That Can Be Used* (mm)	Smallest Tube for Assisted Ventilation (mm)	Smallest Tube for Spontaneous Ventilation (mm)
2.2	2.5	3.0	3.5
2.8	3.0	3.5	4.0
3.5	4.5	5.0	5.5
4.7	5.5	6.0	6.5

*For intubation only.

TECHNIQUES FOR BRONCHOSCOPY

FACILITIES FOR BRONCHOSCOPY

It is important that bronchoscopy be performed in a suitable venue. Because of the need for general anesthesia, rigid bronchoscopy is almost always performed in an operating room. The relative ease with which flexible bronchoscopy can be done makes it tempting to use the instrument in nonconventional places such as at the bedside or in an emergency room. While there are clearly circumstances in which such practice is justified, bronchoscopy is a serious procedure with the potential for lethal complications and should be performed only by physicians who are well trained in the necessary cognitive and technical skills, and with full preparation for all contingencies. Therefore, a fully equipped and staffed endoscopy suite or operating room is the most appropriate venue. With suitable preparation, bronchoscopy (rigid or flexible) can be performed at the bedside in an intensive care unit, but this may still place the bronchoscopist at a disadvantage in terms of access to equipment and supplies in the event of difficulties. If bronchoscopy is performed in an intensive care unit, the bronchoscopist must take along everything that will possibly be needed and have it readily at hand.

RIGID BRONCHOSCOPY

The appropriate rigid bronchoscope (length and diameter) is chosen for the patient. Under a satisfactory level of general anesthesia, the patient is positioned supine with the shoulders supported and the head slightly extended. The larynx is exposed with a laryngoscope, and the tip of the bronchoscope is gently advanced through the glottis and into the trachea. With the proximal end of the bronchoscope closed with a lens cap or with a telescope in place, the side port is attached to the anesthesia circuit and the patient can be ventilated with positive pressure.

The bronchoscope is manipulated to visualize the tracheal and bronchial anatomy; the head and neck may be turned to help direct the bronchoscope into the main stem bronchi. Telescopes greatly facilitate inspection, and can be used in conjunction with a video camera. Angulated telescopes make it much easier to visualize the upper lobe segments. The telescope must be removed and cleaned if the lens becomes covered with secretions; suctioning is performed with a suction pipe or a suction catheter. During these times ventilation is momentarily interrupted. It is also possible to work for extended periods with an open proximal end, while maintaining ventilation with a Venturi jet injector.[66]

When instrumentation is required, such as the removal of a foreign body, the instruments may be passed through the open channel of the bronchoscope. Unfortunately, this significantly impairs the view of the operative site, because the instruments obstruct the line of vision. Optical forceps, which incorporate the glass rod telescope and allow direct visualization of the operative site, are in most cases the preferred instrument for biopsy and for foreign body extraction. Very small flexible forceps can also be passed through a side arm and alongside the telescope, but the tip of these instruments may be difficult to control.

At Cincinnati Children's Hospital, the vast majority of rigid bronchoscopic procedures (including foreign body removal) are performed using only the glass rod telescopes; the open tube sheath is used in special circumstances. This technique requires that the patient breathe spontaneously, so anesthetic technique is critical, but it is much easier to evaluate airway dynamics. Because the overall size of the instruments is smaller, mechanical complications are less frequent.

FLEXIBLE BRONCHOSCOPY

Most diagnostic procedures can be performed in most pediatric patients with the standard 2.8-mm or 3.5-mm pediatric flexible instrument. In older children, a 4.9-mm instrument can be used (especially if a larger suction channel is needed), whereas in very small infants it may be appropriate to use a 2.2-mm ultrathin bronchoscope. The patient is properly prepared for the procedure, and positioned supine with the head and neck in a neutral position. It is possible to perform flexible bronchoscopy in a sitting or some other position in special circumstances.

Flexible bronchoscopes are usually inserted transnasally. This avoids the potential for the patient to bite (and thus destroy) the instrument and also affords a view of the nasal and nasopharyngeal anatomy. Another advantage of this approach is that the bronchoscope does not contact the tongue; the tongue is a very powerful muscle and can readily move the bronchoscope in ways contrary to the intent of the bronchoscopist. A flexible bronchoscope can also be inserted orally if desired, always with a suitable bite block, even with the patient under general anesthesia, or through an artificial airway such as an endotracheal tube (with a bite block) or tracheostomy tube.

The tip of the flexible bronchoscope can be flexed or extended in a single plane; movement to one side or another is accomplished by rotation. The instrument is directed to the site of interest by advancing the shaft while controlling the angulation and rotation at the tip. This combination of three simultaneous movements requires good hand-eye coordination on the part of the bronchoscopist. In contrast to glass rod telescopes, the image rotates as the instrument is rotated; this may produce disorientation on the part of operators unaccustomed to using rigid instruments. As the instrument is advanced through the airway, secretions may be removed by suctioning, and topical anesthetic can be applied, also through the suction channel.

The patient must be able to breathe around the instrument; most infants 3 kg or larger can breathe satisfactorily around the standard 3.5-mm pediatric flexible bronchoscope (infants larger than about 1.5 kg can usually breathe around the 2.8-mm instrument). Smaller infants will not be able to do so, and their procedures must be performed with an ultrathin instrument or with apneic technique. If the patient is intubated, the bronchoscope must be small enough to pass readily through the tube (see Table 7-2).

Flexible bronchoscopes are much smaller than rigid instruments (although the glass rod telescopes, if used alone, are equally small) and can be advanced much farther into the distal airways. Depending on the instrument used and the size of the patient, airways as small as 2 mm and as far as 14 to 16 generations from the carina may be inspected.

The instruments that can be passed through a flexible bronchoscope are quite limited because of the small diameter of the suction channel (1.2 mm in pediatric instruments, 2.0–3.2 mm in "adult" instruments). Cup or "alligator" biopsy forceps, brushes, grasping forceps, expandable basket retrieval devices, balloon catheters (for dilation of stenoses), and laser fibers are the most common such instruments.

SPECIAL PROCEDURES

Transbronchial biopsies can be obtained through flexible or rigid bronchoscopes for the investigation of localized or diffuse lung disease.[67–69] The forceps are passed through the bronchoscope into the selected bronchus and advanced to the desired depth, opened, advanced, closed, and withdrawn. This is best done with fluoroscopic guidance, both to reduce the risk of complications such as penetration of the pleura and to maximize success in obtaining adequate specimens from the desired area. Such specimens are very small, even with the largest available instruments, but are useful in the diagnosis and management of selected lung diseases. Because of the small size of the specimens and the nature of pediatric lung disease, as well as for technical reasons, transbronchial biopsy is performed much less frequently in children than in adults. Complications of transbronchial biopsy include bleeding (which may be massive), pneumothorax, and perforation of other organs.

Biopsy of endobronchial lesions is more straightforward and can yield useful diagnostic information. Such lesions are less common in pediatric than in adult patients (where malignant lesions are much more frequent). Small biopsy specimens can be obtained with flexible forceps via a flexible bronchoscope, under direct vision. Because of the very small size of such specimens and the risk of bleeding, biopsy of endobronchial lesions may be best done with a rigid instrument, which allows use of larger forceps and perhaps better control of hemorrhage, should it occur. Endobronchial lesions in pediatric patients are most often granulation tissue, but tumors such as hemangiomas or carcinoid tumors may also be found. These bleed rather vigorously when biopsied.

Bronchial brushing is performed to obtain specimens of bronchial epithelial cells for a variety of studies—morphologic, physiologic, and molecular. Flexible cytology brushes are passed through the bronchoscope, and the bronchial surface is gently abraded to obtain the specimen. One potential problem with brushing is the loss of much of the specimen (or contamination of the specimen) when the brush is withdrawn through the bronchoscope. To minimize this problem, many cytology brushes are packaged with an outer sheath and have very short bristles. The sheath is passed through the bronchoscope, the brush is extended to collect the specimen, then withdrawn into the sheath. With conventional technique, up to several hundred thousand epithelial cells can be obtained in this fashion.

Brushes are also used to obtain specimens for microbiologic diagnosis. One potential advantage of bronchoscopy is that specimens can be obtained from the lower airways without contamination by mouth flora. Unfortunately, however, there is a significant risk of such contamination by passage of the bronchoscope through the nose and/or mouth on the way to the distal airways. Specimens obtained by simple aspiration through the bronchoscope often show evidence of oral flora. To surmount this problem, a protected microbiology specimen brush has been developed[70] that is protected by two concentric sheaths; the outer sheath is plugged with wax to prevent secretions in the bronchoscope channel from contaminating the brush. This specimen collection system functions very well to avoid contamination of the brush specimen by secretions present in the suction channel of the bronchoscope. Unfortunately, however, it does not guarantee freedom from contamination by upper airway flora. If during the preparation for the procedure and insertion of the bronchoscope any oral secretions are aspirated into the trachea and bronchi, then the site from which the specimen is collected will be contaminated, and it makes relatively little difference what technique is used to obtain the specimen. Topical laryngeal anesthesia almost always results in contamination of the trachea and at least central bronchi to some extent with oral flora.

Foreign body extraction should be performed with a rigid bronchoscope.[71,72] When the foreign body is a manufactured object, it is helpful to practice on a duplicate object to ensure that the forceps chosen will secure a firm grasp on the object. There is a great variety of forceps available for use with different types of foreign bodies. It may be helpful to pass a balloon catheter beyond the foreign body and then use the inflated balloon to pull the object proximally.[73] Foreign body extraction may be complicated by the presence of inspissated secretions or granulation tissue. Foreign bodies such as nuts, which may fragment, may be present in multiple sites, and a very thorough examination of all bronchi should be made after removing a foreign body. In rare circumstances, such as a straight pin lodged in the periphery of the lung,[47] a flexible bronchoscope may be useful in foreign body removal.

Laser applications in bronchoscopy[74] (other than for subglottic or high tracheal lesions) are relatively uncommon in pediatric patients. However, in selected circumstances[50] a laser can be used to ablate tissue in a very controlled, hemorrhage-free manner. A quartz laser fiber can be passed through a rigid or flexible bronchoscope to direct the laser energy very precisely. Lesions as small as 0.5 mm can be created, but care must be taken to ensure that the energy delivered does not create enough steam to injure surrounding normal tissue.

Balloon dilation of bronchial or tracheal stenoses is a useful technique that can eliminate the need for thoracotomy in some patients.[48,75] An angioplasty balloon catheter is used; these devices can be inflated at very high pressure (up to 15 atm). A catheter with a predetermined inflated diameter is positioned in the desired location under direct vision. The balloon is then inflated, and a pressure of several atmospheres is maintained for 30 to 60 seconds before deflating the balloon. In most cases, such catheters cannot easily be passed through the suction channel of a pediatric flexible bronchoscope, but a flexible instrument can be used to guide the positioning of a catheter that has been passed alongside the bronchoscope, through either an endotracheal tube or a rigid bronchoscope.

Bronchoscopic intubation is a technique that facilitates difficult or complicated intubations,[53,76,77] and should almost always be successful if the right instruments are available and the operator is skilled in their use. A flexible bronchoscope is passed through a suitable endotracheal tube. The bronchoscope is then passed into the trachea (usually through the nose, but an oral approach may be used instead). With the tip of the bronchoscope held just above the carina, the endotracheal tube is advanced over the flexible bronchoscope until its tip is seen through the bronchoscope. The bronchoscope must be held so that its shaft is straight while the endotracheal tube is advanced over it; otherwise, damage to the bronchoscope may result. The bronchoscope is withdrawn, the patient is ventilated, and then the bronchoscope again inserted to verify the position of the endotracheal tube and to ensure that the anatomy and patency of the distal airways are adequate.

COMPLICATIONS OF BRONCHOSCOPY

Every procedure has potential for complications, ranging from trivial to lethal. Bronchoscopy is no exception, although reported lethal complications of bronchoscopy in pediatric patients are rare. The risk of complications is a function of inherent risk factors in the patient (disease state, severity of disease, age, etc.), the procedure performed, the skill and experience of the bronchoscopist and the bronchoscopy team, and the patient's preparation for the procedure.

In general, the risk is greater with rigid bronchoscopy than with flexible bronchoscopy. This is because foreign body extraction is perhaps the most challenging, difficult, and risky bronchoscopic procedure commonly performed in pediatric patients, and is always done with a rigid instrument. In addition, the relatively large diameter and rigid nature of the rigid bronchoscope make it more likely to traumatize the mucosa of the subglottic space or airways. However, flexible bronchoscopy is not immune to serious complications, and at least one death has been reported in association with a flexible bronchoscopy in a pediatric patient.[78] Disaster lurks around the corner for the unwise or unwary.

Mechanical complications of bronchoscopy result from direct trauma to the airway. Pneumothorax or pneumomediastinum, subglottic edema, and hemorrhage are most common. Such complications are more likely when auxiliary instruments such as biopsy forceps are used. The greatest risk is incurred during the extraction of foreign bodies and in the performance of transbronchial biopsy. The risk of mechanical complications can be reduced by careful selection of instruments and procedures. Epistaxis is common in thrombocytopenic patients; consideration should be given to passing the flexible bronchoscope via an orotracheal tube instead of transnasally. Because most such patients are also immunosuppressed, this practice will also reduce the risk of contamination of the BAL specimen with oral secretions and flora. Patients with large adenoids often develop epistaxis when a nasopharyngeal tube is passed to facilitate ventilation during the procedure; nasopharyngeal tubes should only be placed after examination of the nasopharyngeal airway.

Physiologic complications of bronchoscopy include hypoxia, hypercapnia, hypotension, laryngospasm, bronchospasm, cardiac arrhythmias, and aspiration. There is a constant risk of hypoventilation during bronchoscopy, due to anesthesia or to airway obstruction. Smaller patients are at greater risk of airway obstruction. All bronchoscopes (rigid as well as flexible) produce some degree of airway obstruction. Vagal stimulation due to inadequate topical anesthesia or catecholamine release due to inadequate sedation/anesthesia may result in cardiac arrhythmia. Laryngospasm or bronchospasm are usually due to inadequate topical anesthesia. Seizures can result from lidocaine toxicity. The risk of physiologic complications can be reduced by careful attention to patient preparation as well as anesthetic and monitoring techniques.

Bacteriologic complications of bronchoscopy include the introduction of infectious agents into the lung from the patient's own upper airway or from another patient if the instruments are not adequately cleaned and sterilized. Infection in one part of a patient's lung can be spread to other areas. Although the risk appears to be low, it is possible that susceptible patients could develop bacterial endocarditis after bronchoscopy; appropriate antibiotic prophylaxis should be considered for the patient at risk. However, if a BAL specimen is to be obtained for culture, the prophylactic antibiotics should not be administered until after the BAL specimen is obtained. Bronchoscopy can also result in spread of infectious agents from the patient to the personnel performing the bronchoscopy; sensible precautions should be taken to protect personnel. Older patients known to have cavitary tuberculosis, for example, represent very high risk to the bronchoscopy team, and bronchoscopy should in most cases be delayed until appropriate therapy has been given for a sufficient time to greatly reduce this risk.

There are also cognitive risks of bronchoscopy: the failure to obtain useful information or making the wrong diagnosis. Even failure to perform bronchoscopy when it is the best or only way to obtain information necessary for the patient's care could be considered an error or complication. The bronchoscopist must be aware of the many pitfalls that await the unwary.[77] Video recording the procedure allows later review of the observations, and sometimes leads to a revision of the diagnosis. Serious consideration should be given to recording all procedures, to augment teaching, consultative reports, and even research data acquisition.

Cognitive risks are reduced by adequate training and experience on the part of the bronchoscopist and support staff. There is no simple guideline regarding the requirements for training of a bronchoscopist; obviously, inherent aptitude varies greatly from individual to individual. The bronchoscopist must develop both manual skills and an effective knowledge of anatomy, pathology, indications for bronchoscopy, and techniques for anesthesia/sedation so as to safely and effectively perform procedures. A formal, comprehensive training program should be a prerequisite, but there is no substitute for good judgment and experience. Most authorities suggest that a minimum of 50 to 100 procedures performed with a suitable mentor are required before an individual should be certified to do bronchoscopy independently.[79,80]

Complications of bronchoscopy may include more than adverse effects on the patient or personnel. Failure to utilize a bite block when a flexible bronchoscope is passed through a patient's mouth, for example, can result in destruction of the instrument. Flexible bronchoscopes currently cost in excess of $18,000 (USD). The smaller the bronchoscope, the more fragile the instrument. Flexible bronchoscopes are often damaged during passage through endotracheal tubes. Biopsy forceps can also perforate the suction channel, thus decommissioning the instrument.

■ ECONOMIC ASPECTS OF BRONCHOSCOPY

Bronchoscopy is not a simple, inexpensive procedure. Total cost will depend on institutional variables as well as the nature and extent of the procedure performed. Specific costs include support for equipment and procedure rooms, consumable supplies, laboratory charges for processing of diagnostic specimens, monitoring of the sedated patient before and after the procedure, record keeping, support of ancillary staff, and professional fees. When general anesthesia is used instead of sedation performed by the bronchoscopist, costs are generally higher, but this should not be significant in decision making if the services of an anesthesiologist significantly enhance the safety of the patient. In large part because of the need for general anesthesia, rigid bronchoscopy may be more expensive than flexible bronchoscopy,[81] but again, the decision about which technique to use should be made on the basis of the patient's medical needs.

Although definitive studies of cost effectiveness in pediatric practice have not been reported, bronchoscopy is often a cost-saving procedure. For example, the early identification of a specific infectious agent in the immunocompromised patient with pneumonia can mean that more expensive, multiple antimicrobial therapy can be avoided (thus also reducing potential risk of complications of such treatment). Young patients with cystic fibrosis admitted to hospital for intensive therapy are not infrequently discovered at bronchoscopy to have no evidence of bacterial infection; evidence may be found instead for other causes of the persisting symptoms (such as gastroesophageal reflux with microaspiration). The definitive identification of causes of pulmonary symptoms such as stridor can reduce "doctor shopping" and multiple expensive diagnostic evaluations. The cost associated with missed diagnoses (when bronchoscopy is not performed) can be enormous.

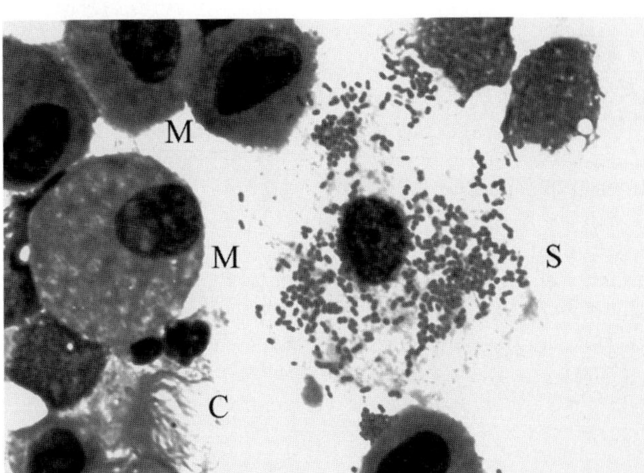

■ **FIGURE 7-2.** Alveolar macrophages (*M*). Squamous epithelial cell (*S*) with adherent bacteria. Such cells usually represent contamination of the specimen with oral secretions. Ciliated epithelial cell (*C*); these cells are often seen in normal BAL specimens and are of little diagnostic significance. (See Color Plate 1.)

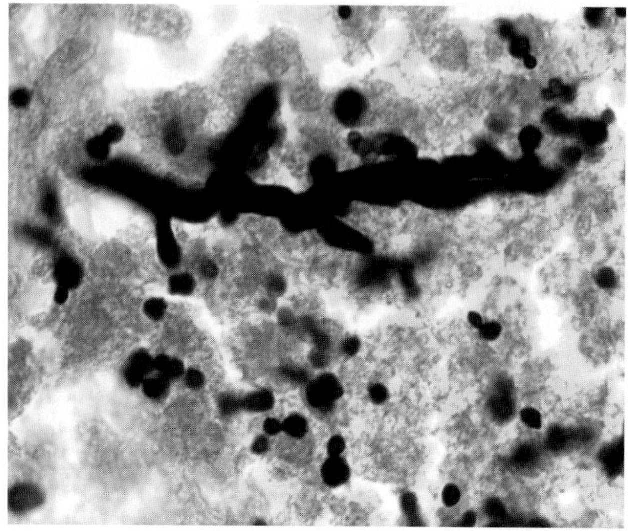

■ **FIGURE 7-3.** Budding yeast on methenamine silver stain. (See Color Plate 2.)

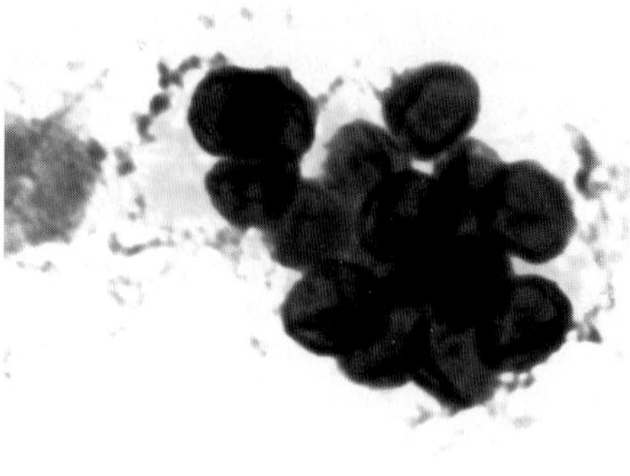

■ **FIGURE 7-4.** Pneumocysts (methenamine silver stain). (See Color Plate 3.)

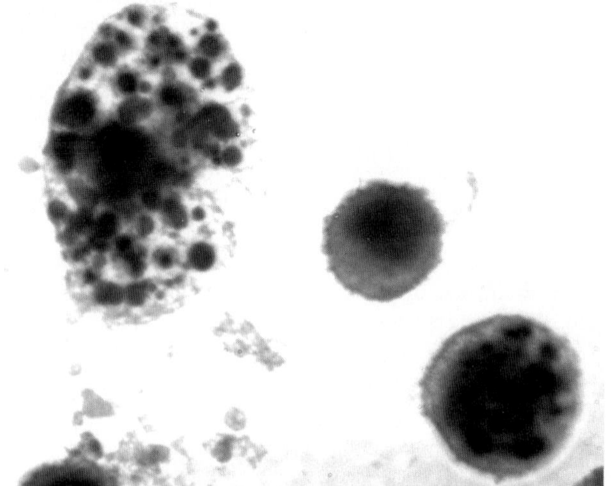

■ **FIGURE 7-5.** Lipid-laden macrophages (Oil Red O stain). (See Color Plate 4.)

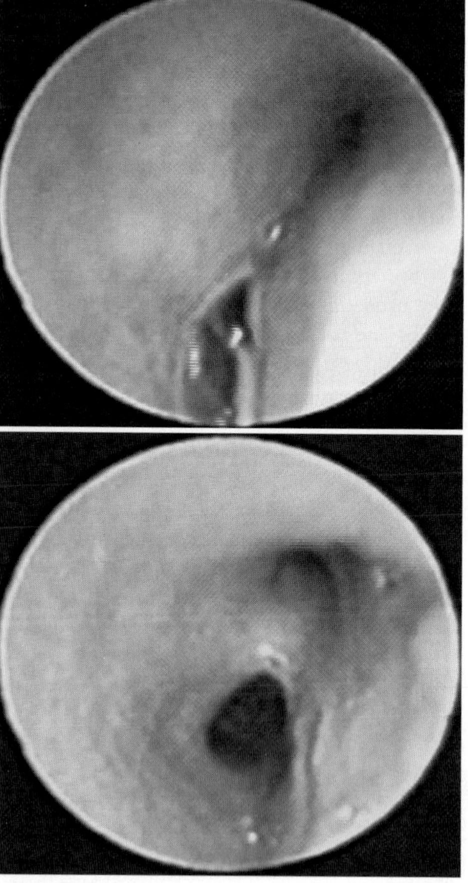

■ **FIGURE 7-6.** Bronchomalacia, right main bronchus. *Top:* During expiration. *Bottom:* During inspiration. (See Color Plate 5.)

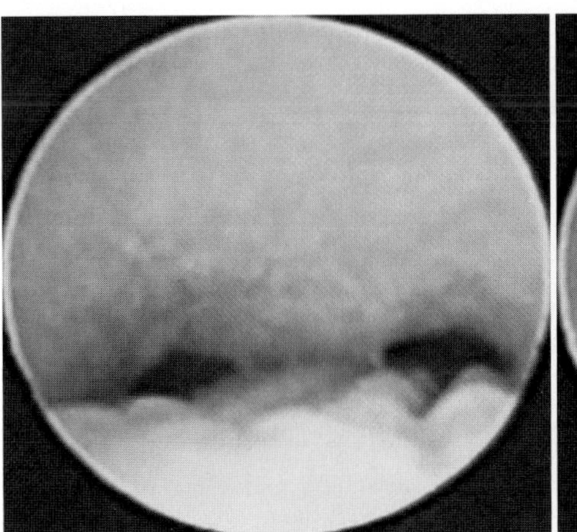

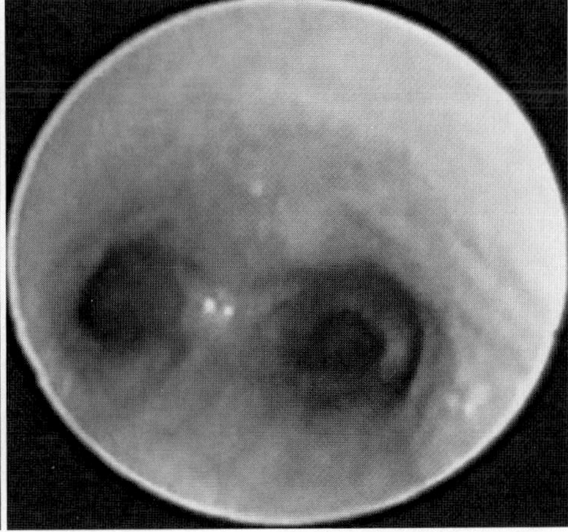

■ **FIGURE 7-7.** Tracheomalacia. *Left:* During expiration. *Right:* During inspiration. (See Color Plate 6.)

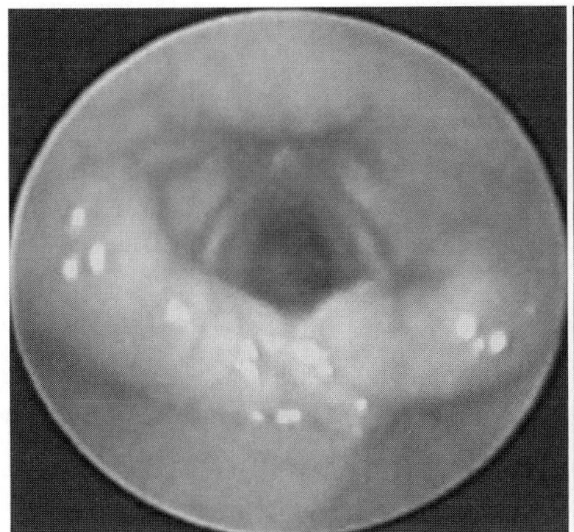

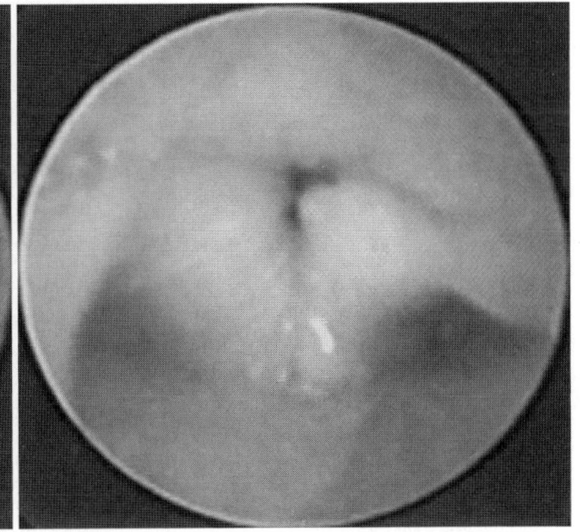

■ **FIGURE 7-8.** Laryngomalacia. *Left:* During expiration. *Right:* During inspiration, the arytenoids prolapse into the glottis. (See Color Plate 7.)

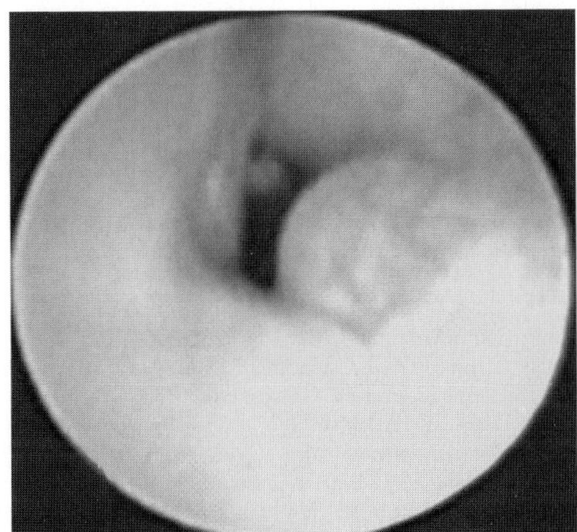

■ **FIGURE 7-9.** Infant with persistent stridor, beginning 3 months after intubation. Large subglottic cyst arises from the right side of the subglottic space. (See Color Plate 8.)

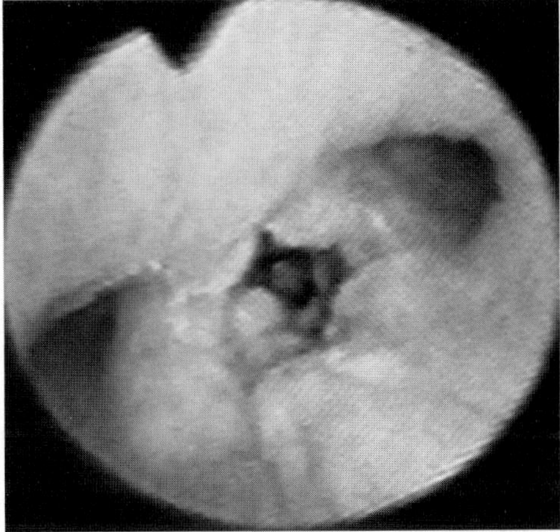

■ **FIGURE 7-10.** Endobronchial damage (granulation tissue) resulting from deep endotracheal suctioning. The right middle lobe *(on left)* and the superior segment of the right lower lobe *(on right)* are relatively unaffected; the orifice leading to the basal segments (the direct path of the catheter) is nearly occluded. Continued injury may lead to atelectasis or even complete bronchial stenosis. (See Color Plate 9.)

REFERENCES

1. Workshop summary and guidelines: Investigative use of bronchoscopy, lavage, and bronchial biopsies in asthma and other airway diseases. J Allergy Clin Immunol 1991;88:808–814.
2. Wood RE, Gauderer MW: Flexible fiberoptic bronchoscopy in the management of tracheobronchial foreign bodies in children. The value of a combined approach with open tube bronchoscopy. J Pediatr Surg 1984;19: 693–698.
3. Gonzalez C, Reilly JS, Bluestone CD: Synchronous airway lesions in infancy. Ann Otol Rhinol Laryngol 1987;96:77–80.
4. Gans SL, Berci G: Advances in endoscopy of infants and children. J Pediatr Surg 1971;6:199–223.
5. MacDonald E, Blair KC: Care and maintenance of endoscopic equipment. In: Holinger LD, Lusk RP, Green CG, eds: Pediatric Laryngology and Bronchoesophagology. Philadelphia: Lippincott-Raven, 1997.
6. Prakash UB: Does the bronchoscope propagate infection? Chest 1993;104: 552–559.
7. Spach DH, Silverstein FE, Stamm WE: Transmission of infection by gastrointestinal endoscopy and bronchoscopy. Ann Intern Med 1993; 118:117–128.
8. Rutala WA, Clontz EP, Weber DJ, Hoffmann KK: Disinfection practices for endoscopes and other semicritical items. Infect Control Hosp Epidemiol 1991;12:282–288.
9. Martin MA, Reichelderfer M: APIC guidelines for infection prevention and control in flexible endoscopy. Am J Infect Control 1994;22:19–38.
10. Reynolds HY: State of the art. Bronchoalveolar lavage. Am Rev Respir Dis 1987;135:250–263.
11. Baughman RP: Bronchoalveolar Lavage. St. Louis: Mosby–Year Book, 1992.
12. Rennard SI, Basset G, Lecossier D, et al: Estimation of volume of epithelial lining fluid recovered by lavage using urea as marker of dilution. J Appl Physiol 1986;60:532–538.
13. Kelly CA, Fenwick JD, Corris PA, et al: Fluid dynamics during bronchoalveolar lavage. Am Rev Respir Dis 1988;138:81–84.
14. Cheng PW, Boat TF, Shaikh S, et al: Differential effects of ozone on lung epithelial lining fluid volume and protein content. Exp Lung Res 1995;21: 351–365.
15. Von Wichert P, Joseph K, Muller B, Franck WM: Bronchoalveolar lavage. Quantitation of intraalveolar fluid? Am Rev Respir Dis 1993;147:148–152.
16. Wood RE: Treatment of CF lung disease in the first two years. Pediatr Pulmonol Suppl 1989;4:68–70.
17. Balough K, McCubbin M, Weinberger M, et al: The relationship between infection and inflammation in the early stages of lung disease from cystic fibrosis. Pediatr Pulmonol 1995;20:63–70.
18. deBlic J, McKelvie P, Le-Bourgeois M, et al: Value of bronchoalveolar lavage in the management of severe acute pneumonia and interstitial pneumonitis in the immunocompromised child. Thorax 1987;42:759–765.
19. Pattishall EN, Noyes BE, Orenstein DM: Use of bronchoalveolar lavage in immunocompromised children with pneumonia. Pediatr Pulmonol 1988;5:1–5.
20. Frankel LR, Smith DW, Lewiston NJ: Bronchoalveolar lavage for diagnosis of pneumonia in the immunocompromised child. Pediatrics 1988;81: 785–788.
21. Ratjen F, Bruch J: Adjustment of bronchoalveolar lavage volume to body weight in children. Pediatr Pulmonol 1996;21:184–188.
22. Wang B, Stern E, Schmidt RA, Pierson DJ: Diagnosing pulmonary alveolar proteinosis. Chest 1997;111:460–466.
23. deBlic J, Blanche S, Danel C, et al: Bronchoalveolar lavage in HIV infected patients with interstitial pneumonitis. Arch Dis Child 1989;64:1246–1250.
24. Fan LL, Langston C: Chronic interstitial lung disease in children. Pediatr Pulmonol 1993;16:184–196.
25. Stephan J: Histiocytoses. Eur J Pediatr 1995;154:600–609.
26. Refabert L, Rambaud C, Mamou-Mani T, et al: Cd 1a-positive cells in bronchoalveolar lavage samples from children with Langerhans cell histiocytosis. J Pediatr 1996;129:913–915.
27. Colombo JL, Hallberg TK: Recurrent aspiration in children. Lipid-laden alveolar macrophage quantitation. Pediatr Pulmonol 1987;3:86–89.
28. Guilinger RA, Paradis IL, Dauber JH, et al: The importance of bronchoscopy with transbronchial biopsy and bronchoalveolar lavage in the management of lung transplant recipients. Am J Respir Crit Care Med 1995;152:2037–2043.
29. McKenzie B, Wood RE, Bailey A: Airway management for unilateral lung lavage in children. Anesthesiology 1989;70:550–553.
30. deBlic J: Pulmonary alveolar proteinosis in children. Paediatr Respir Rev 2004;5:316–322.
31. Pingleton AK, Harrison GF, Stechschulte DJ, et al: Effect of location, pH and temperature of instillate in bronchoalveolar lavage in normal volunteers. Am Rev Respir Dis 1983;128:1035–1037.
32. Riedler J, Grigg J, Stone C, et al: Bronchoalveolar lavage cellularity in healthy children. Am J Respir Crit Care Med 1995;152:163–168.
33. Rennard SI, Ghafouri M, Thompson AB, et al: Fractional processing of sequential bronchoalveolar lavage to separate bronchial and alveolar samples. Am Rev Respir Dis 1990;141:208–217.
34. Weiss S, Hert R, Gianola F, et al: Complications of fiberoptic bronchoscopy in thrombocytopenic patients. Chest 1993;104:1025–1108.
35. de Blic J, Midulla F, Barbato A, et al: Bronchoalveolar lavage in children. ERS Task Force on bronchoalveolar lavage in children. European Respiratory Society. Eur Respir J 2000;15:217–231.
36. Mordelet-Dambrine M, Arnoux A, Stanislas-Leguern G, et al: Processing of lung lavage fluid causes variability in bronchoalveolar cell count. Am Rev Respir Dis 1984;130:305–306.
37. Ratjen F, Bredendiek M, Brendel M, et al: Differential cytology of bronchoalveolar lavage fluid in normal children. Eur Respir J 1994;7:1865–1870.
38. Midulla F, Villani A, Merolla R, et al: Bronchoalveolar lavage studies in children without parenchymal lung disease. Cellular constituents and protein levels. Pediatr Pulmonol 1995;20:112–118.
39. Sole-Violan J, Rodriguez de Castro F, Rey A, et al: Usefulness of microscopic examination of intracellular organisms in lavage fluid in ventilator-associated pneumonia. Chest 1994;106:889–894.
40. Thorpe JE, Baughman RP, Frame PT, et al: Bronchoalveolar lavage for diagnosing acute bacterial pneumonia. J Infect Dis 1987;155:855–861.
41. Naber SP: Molecular medicine. Molecular pathology—diagnosis of infectious disease. N Engl J Med 1994;331:1212–1215.
42. Roth A, Schaberg T, Mauch H: Molecular diagnosis of tuberculosis. Current clinical validity and future perspectives. Eur Respir J 1997;10: 1877–1891.
43. Delacourt C, Proveda JD, Chureau C, et al: Use of polymerase chain reaction for improved diagnosis of tuberculosis in children. J Pediatr 1995;126: 703–709.
44. Sherman JM, Winnie G, Thomassen MJ, et al: Time course of hemosiderin production and clearance by human pulmonary macrophages. Chest 1984; 86:409–411.
45. Moran JR, Block SM, Lyerly AD, et al: Lipid-laden alveolar macrophage and lactose assay as markers of aspiration in neonates with lung disease. J Pediatr 1988;112:643–645.
46. Koumbourlis AC, Kurland G: Nonbronchoscopic bronchoalveolar lavage in intubated, mechanically ventilated infants. Technique, efficacy, and applications. Pediatr Pulmonol 1993;15:257–263.
47. Castro M, Midthun DE, Edell ES, et al: Flexible bronchoscopic removal of foreign bodies from pediatric airways. J Bronchol 1994;1:92–98.
48. Bagwell CE, Talbert JL, Tepas JJ III: Balloon dilatation of long-segment tracheal stenosis. J Pediatr Surg 1991;26:153–159.
49. Rimell FL, Shapiro AM, Mitskavich MT, et al: Pediatric fiberoptic laser rigid bronchoscopy. Otolaryngol Head Neck Surg 1996;114:413–417.
50. Azizkhan RG, Lacey SR, Wood RE: Acquired symptomatic bronchial stenosis in infants. Successful management using an argon laser. J Pediatr Surg 1990;25:19–24.
51. Lim LH, Cotton RT, Azizkhan RG, et al: Complications of metallic stents in the pediatric airway. Otolaryngol Head Neck Surg 2004;131: 355–361.
52. Kariman K, Kylstra JA, Spock A: Pulmonary alveolar proteinosis. Prospective clinical experience in 23 patients over 15 years. Lung 1984;162: 223–231.
53. Rucker RW, Silva WJ, Worcester CC: Fiberoptic bronchoscopic nasotracheal intubation in children. Chest 1979;76:56–58.
54. McManigle JE, Fletcher GL, Tenholder MF: Bronchoscopy in the management of bronchopleural fistula. Chest 1990;97:1235–1238.
55. Wood RE, Lacey SR, Azizkhan RG: Endoscopic management of large, postresection bronchopleural fistulae with methacrylate adhesive (Super Glue). J Pediatr Surg 1992;27:201–202.
56. Cote CJ: Sedation for the pediatric patient. A review. Pediatr Clin North Am 1994;41:31–58.
57. American Academy of Pediatrics Committee on Drugs: Guidelines for monitoring and management of pediatric patients during and after sedation for diagnostic and therapeutic procedures. Pediatrics 1992;89:1110–1115.
58. Sandhar BK, Goresky GY, Malt by JR, Shaffer EA: Effect of oral liquids and ranitidine on gastric fluid volume and pH in children undergoing outpatient surgery. Anesthesiology 1989;71:327–330.
59. Schreiner MS, Triebwasser A, Keon TP: Ingestion of liquids compared with preoperative fasting in pediatric outpatients. Anesthesiology 1990;72: 593–597.

60. Bailey AG, Valley RD, Azizkhan RG, Wood RE: Anaesthetic management of infants requiring endobronchial argon laser surgery. Can J Anaesth 1992; 39:590–593.
61. American Academy of Pediatrics Committee on Drugs and Committee on Environmental Health. Use of chloral hydrate for sedation in children. Pediatrics 1993;92:471–473.
62. Pereira JK, Burrows PE, Richards HM, et al: Comparison of sedation regimens for pediatric outpatient CT. Pediatr Radiol 1993;23:341–344.
63. Baktai G, Szekely E, Marialigeti T, Kovacs L: Use of midazolan ('Dormicum') and flumazenil ('Anexate') in paediatric bronchology. Curr Med Res Opin 1992;12:552–559.
64. Olness K: Hypnosis in pediatric practice. Curr Prob Pediatr 1981;12:1–47.
65. Bullock EA, Shaddy RE: Relaxation and imagery techniques without sedation during right ventricular endomyocardial biopsy in pediatric heart transplant patients. J Heart Lung Transplant 1993;12:59–62.
66. Sloan IA, McLeod ME: Evaluation of the jet injector in paediatric fibreoptic bronchoscopes. Can Anaesth Soc J 1985;32:79–81.
67. Fitzpatrick SB, Stokes DC, Marsh B, Wang KP: Transbronchial lung biopsy in pediatric and adolescent patients. Am J Dis Child 1985;139:46–49.
68. Kurland G, Noyes BE, Jaffe R, et al: Bronchoalveolar lavage and transbronchial biopsy in children following heart-lung and lung transplantation. Chest 1993;104:1043–1048.
69. Shure D: Transbronchial biopsy and needle aspiration. Chest 1989;95: 1130–1138.
70. Wimberley N, Faling LJ, Bartlett JG: A fiberoptic bronchoscopy technique to obtain uncontaminated lower airway secretions for bacterial culture. Am Rev Respir Dis 1979;119:337–343.
71. Cohen SR, Herbert WI, Lewis GB, Geller KA: Foreign bodies in the airway. Five-year retrospective study with special reference to management. Ann Otol Rhinol Laryngol 1980;89:437–442.
72. Patterson EJ: History of bronchoscopy and esophagoscopy for foreign body. Laryngoscope 1926;36:157–175.
73. Kosloske AM: The Fogarty balloon technique for the removal of foreign bodies from the tracheobronchial tree. Surg Gynecol Obstet 1982;155: 72–73.
74. Personne C, Colchen A, Leroy M, et al: Indications and technique for endoscopic laser resections in bronchology. A critical analysis based upon 2,284 resections. J Thorac Cardiovasc Surg 1986;91:710–715.
75. Dab I, Malfroot A, Goossens A: Therapeutic bronchoscopy in ventilated neonates. Arch Dis Child 1993;69:533–537.
76. Ovassapian A: Fiberoptic Airway Endoscopy in Anesthesia and Critical Care. New York: Raven Press, 1990.
77. Wood RE: Pitfalls in the use of the flexible bronchoscope in pediatric patients. Chest 1990;97:199–203.
78. Wagener JS: Fatality following fiberoptic bronchoscopy in a two year-old child. Pediatr Pulmonol 1987;3:197–199.
79. Dull WL: Flexible fiberoptic bronchoscopy. An analysis of proficiency. Chest 1980;77:65–67.
80. Green CG, Eisenberg J, Leong A, et al: Flexible endoscopy of the pediatric airway. Am Rev Respir Dis 1992;145:233–235.
81. Squires RH, Morriss F, Schluterman S, et al: Efficacy, safety, and cost of intravenous sedation versus general anesthesia in children undergoing endoscopic procedures. Gastrointest Endosc 1995;41:99–104.

8 Diagnostic Imaging of the Respiratory Tract

Øystein E. Olsen, PhD •
Catherine M. Owens, BSc

Pediatric chest radiology is a complex subject, and a full understanding of all relevant pathologies with which it aids diagnosis are dealt with in the clinical sections of this book. This chapter gives a brief overview of the imaging modalities used to help achieve an accurate and timely diagnosis, thus enabling prompt treatment of the many varied pathologic entities encountered within the pediatric thorax. The dedicated reader may wish to consult more specialized and comprehensive texts.[1–3]

The utility of imaging modalities is often uncertain because of: (1) an increasing number of available techniques and (2) the presence of numerous rare disease entities in children. Nevertheless, modern clinical practice is highly dependent on radiology.

Areas of specific concern within the pediatric age group will be discussed, in particular: (1) radiation protection; (2) technical challenges, such as motion and breathing artifacts; (3) developing anatomy and pathophysiology; and (4) to a certain degree, different interpretation of images compared with images obtained in adults.

PLAIN RADIOGRAPHY

The plain chest radiograph remains the basis for the evaluation of the chest in childhood. In the neonate, satisfactory films can be obtained in incubators using modern mobile x-ray apparatus. The baby lies on the cassette and the film is exposed. Although automatic triggering of the exposure can be made, an experienced radiographer will usually be able to judge the end of inspiration. An adequate inspiration occurs with the right hemidiaphragm at the level of the eighth rib posteriorly. Films in expiration frequently show a sharp rightward kink in the trachea and varying degrees of opacification of the lung fields, with apparent enlargement of the heart. Films should be well collimated, with the baby positioned as straight as possible. Lordotic films should be avoided, especially if the size of the heart is of particular interest. As much monitoring equipment as possible should be removed.

Computed radiography is particularly useful in intensive care, and the facility of data manipulation (e.g., edge enhancement) improves visualization of supportive apparatus, such as tubes and lines.

Children older than 5 years of age can usually cooperate sufficiently to stand for a posteroanterior film in the same way as adults. In younger children, some form of chest stand is needed in which an assistant, preferably the caregiver, can hold the child in front of a cassette while standing behind a suspended protective lead apron. With proper collimation, the dose to the caregiver is small, and this position allows straighter positioning of the child than a position to the side. The difference between a posteroanterior projection and an anteroposterior projection in the small child is usually negligible. High-kilovoltage technique, with added filtration and the use of a grid, allows evaluation of the trachea and major bronchi, which is important in stridor.

SPECIFIC FEATURES OF THE CHEST RADIOGRAPH IN CHILDREN

The Thymus (Fig. 8-1)

The normal thymus is a frequent cause of widening of the anterior mediastinum during the first years of life. The lateral margin often shows an undulation, the thymic wave, which corresponds to the indentations of the ribs on the inner surface of the thoracic cage. Particularly on the right, the thymus may have a triangular, sail-like configuration. The thymus may involute in times of stress, and steroids can induce a decrease in size. At times, the differentiation of a physiologic thymus from pathology in the anterior mediastinum can be difficult. Ultrasound examination will usually differentiate cystic lesions from the homogeneous normal thymic tissue. Occasionally, the normal thymus can act as a significant space-occupying lesion in the superior mediastinum, and in such cases, differentiation may be helped by either ultrasound or magnetic resonance imaging (MRI), which shows homogeneous echogenicity/signal within a normal thymus. On MRI, a normal thymus has intermediate signal on T2-weighted images (similar to the spleen and lymph nodes) and shows minimal uniform enhancement on T1-weighted images after intravenous contrast medium injection (Fig. 8-2).

The Cardiothoracic Ratio

In toddlers, the cardiothoracic ratio can at times exceed 0.5, and care should be exercised in overdiagnosis of cardiomegaly, particularly if the film may be expiratory.

Kink of the Trachea to the Right

Kinking of the trachea to the right is a frequent feature of a chest film taken at less than full inspiration. This is a physiologic buckling and does not represent a mass lesion.

Soft Tissue

Soft tissue may be prominent in children, and the anterior axillary fold that crosses the chest wall can at times mimic pneumothorax. Similarly, skin folds can at times cast confusing shadows. Plaits of hair over the upper chest can mimic pulmonary infiltrations in the upper lobes.

Pleural Fluid

Whereas in adults an early sign of pleural effusion is blunting of the costophrenic angles, in childhood it is more common to see separation of the lung from the chest wall, with reasonable preservation of the clarity of the costophrenic angles and accentuation of the lung fissures. In the supine position, an apical rim

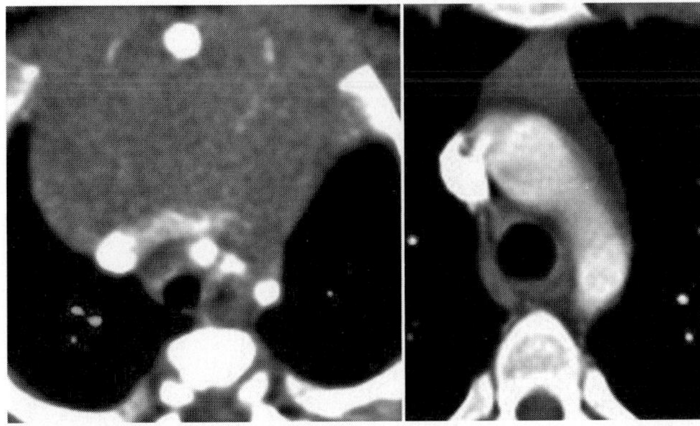

■ **FIGURE 8-1.** Axial contrast-enhanced computed tomography shows the considerable difference in thymic size in a 3-month-old child compared with a 10-year-old child.

of soft tissue density is seen, and if a moderate to large unilateral effusion is present, the affected hemithorax has a diffuse increase in density, with preservation of vascular markings simulating ground-glass parenchymal opacification. This is due to pleural fluid collecting in the dorsal (dependent) pleura.

SYSTEMATIC REVIEW OF THE CHEST RADIOGRAPH

Without a systematic analytical approach to the pediatric chest radiograph, the possibility of missing relevant radiologic information is high. To combat this, knowledge of the various pitfalls in interpretation, anatomic variants, and pathologic processes relevant to the specific age group are vital. This is particularly important when there is one very conspicuous abnormal imaging finding, which can result in cessation of more intense scrutiny of the remainder of the film. Image review should therefore follow a strict systematic order, including checking the putative identity of the radiograph, and include the following.

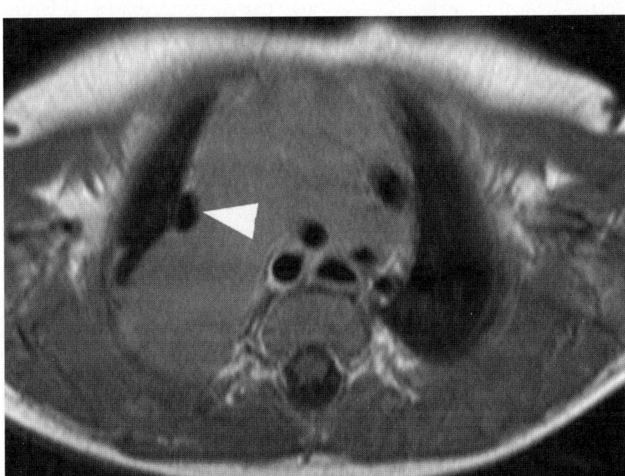

■ **FIGURE 8-2.** Chest radiograph (not shown) in a 3-month-old child showed an unusual upper mediastinal contour. Magnetic resonance imaging (T1-weighted spin echo after intravenous injection of gadolinium chelate) shows normal signal and no abnormal contrast enhancement from a normal, but large thymus, extending posterior to the right brachiocephalic vein *(arrowhead)*. There is no sign of vascular or airway compression.

General Degree of Lung Inflation

Flattening of the diaphragm or diaphragmatic domes below the level of the eighth posterior ribs, elongation of the mediastinum, and widening of the intercostal spaces are all signs of pulmonary overinflation. Intercostal bulging of the pleura or lung parenchyma may be a sign of high ventilator pressures in an intubated child.

Generalized pulmonary underinflation is usually due to radiographic exposure during expiration, but may be a real finding confirming small lung volumes, as in cases of idiopathic respiratory distress syndrome, in which the lung parenchyma is noncompliant, or in bilateral pulmonary hypoplasia or associated with lobar collapse.

Elevation of the diaphragm, with consequential lung compression due to bowel distention, pneumoperitoneum, or the presence of a large abdominal mass, should also be considered. Hence, the periphery of the radiograph (e.g., the area under the diaphragm) should always be carefully and routinely inspected as part of a systematic review.

Asymmetrical Lung Volume

Mediastinal shift toward a lung with uniformly increased density compared with the contralateral lung, in the absence of pneumothorax, is a sign of differential inflation of the two lungs. This may be caused by overinflation of the more lucent lung (e.g., due to a ball-valve mechanism in the central airways), in which case the ipsilateral hemidiaphragm would be flattened (Fig. 8-3).

Alternatively, it may be caused by volume loss in the denser lung, in which case the diaphragm of the denser hemithorax would be elevated. This may be a sign of unilateral pulmonary hypoplasia, aplasia, or agenesis (Figs. 8-4 to 8-6), in which case the mediastinum is shifted toward the hemithorax containing the small lung and ipsilateral elevation of the hemidiaphragm is seen.

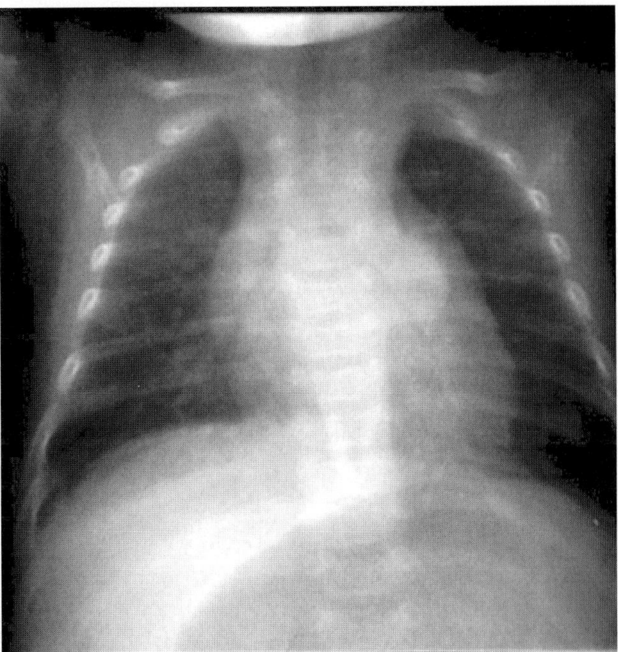

■ **FIGURE 8-3.** Chest radiograph in a young child shows a semicircular left convex distortion of the left mediastinal outline due to a bronchogenic cyst and secondary overinflation of the left lower lobe.

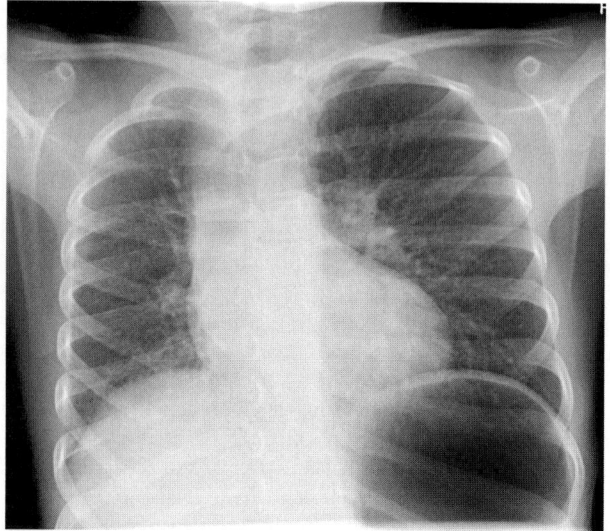

■ **FIGURE 8-4.** In a 10-year-old girl who presented with shortness of breath, chest radiograph shows a small right hemithorax (rib crowding, diaphragmatic elevation, compensatory large left lung), but no lung opacification. This was later diagnosed as an interrupted right pulmonary artery (see Figs. 8-34 and 8-54).

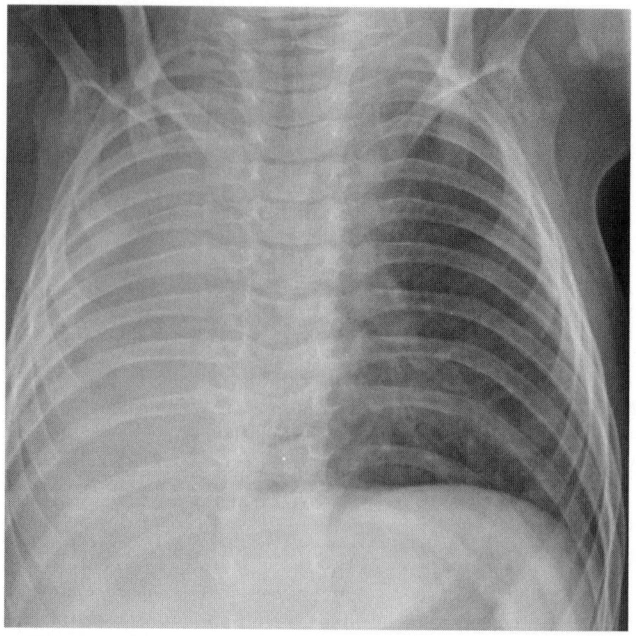

■ **FIGURE 8-6.** The right hemithorax is opacified by the mediastinal structures that are shifted to the right. However, there is no overexpansion of the left lung or pleura. On computed tomography, the right lung was aplastic (see Fig. 8-36).

Combined overinflation of one lung and volume loss of the other can sometimes be seen secondary to mass lesions that affect the central airways (Fig. 8-7).

Other causes of asymmetrical lung volumes include diaphragmatic pareses/paralysis and a large abdominal mass lesion that causes elevation of the ipsilateral hemidiaphragm. The diaphragm may also be apparently elevated secondary to a subpulmonic fluid collection. In congenital diaphragmatic hernia, the multicystic appearance of bowel content may or may not be obvious within the thorax (Fig. 8-8). If seen, it may sometimes be difficult to distinguish from congenital cystic adenomatoid malformation (Table 8-1).

Lobar Overinflation

Lobar inflation may have a similar appearance to whole-lung overinflation. However, there is usually evidence of lobar confinement because the lobar outline can be identified as it herniates across

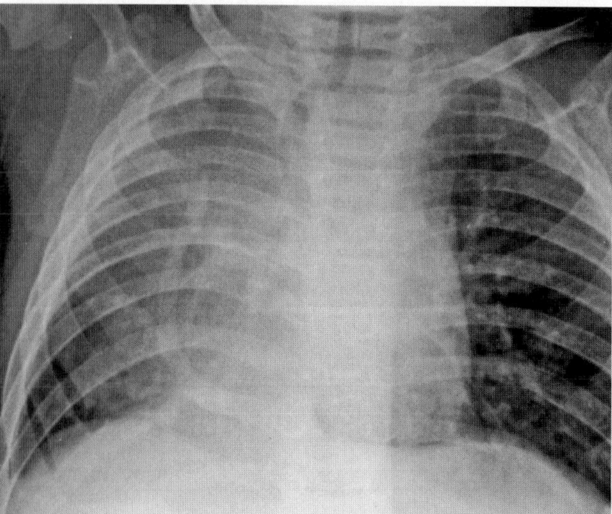

■ **FIGURE 8-5.** Chest radiograph shows a hypoplastic right lung with an abnormal vascular structure running toward the diaphragmatic level medially. This represents systemic venous drainage of the right lung. The shape of the abnormal vein resembles a Turkish scimitar (bowed sword), hence, the denotation *scimitar syndrome* (see Figs. 8-33 and 8-35).

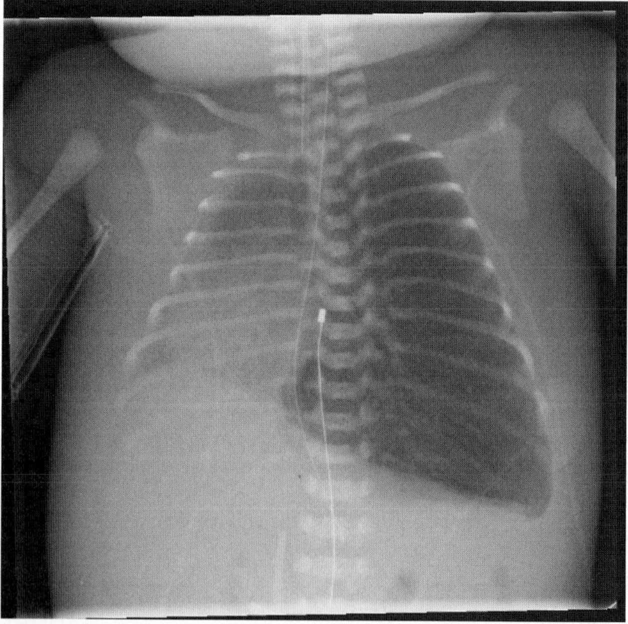

■ **FIGURE 8-7.** Chest radiograph of a neonate with respiratory distress shows an overexpanded left lung (inverted left hemidiaphragm, intercostal bulging of the left lung) as well as a small right hemithorax (elevated right hemidiaphragm, crowding of the right ribs). Both were secondary to a central bronchogenic cyst (see Fig. 8-32).

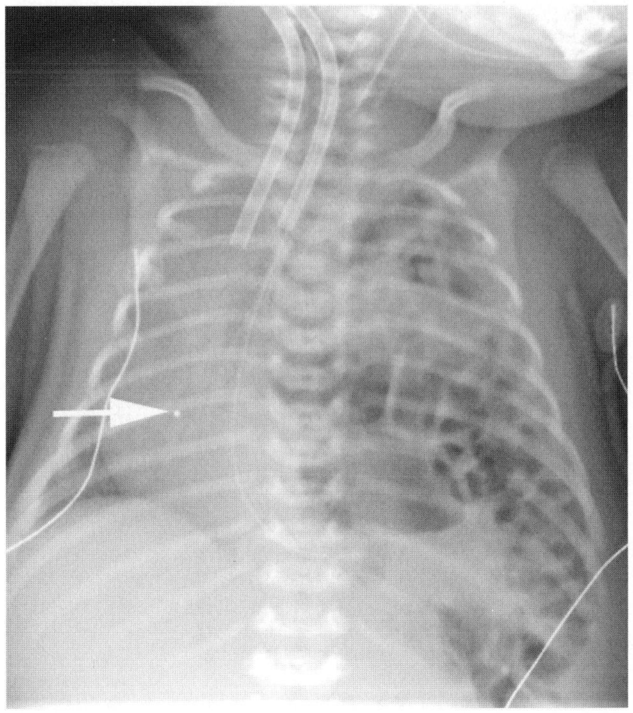

■ **FIGURE 8-8.** An infant with antenatally diagnosed left congenital diaphragmatic hernia. Chest radiograph shows disruption of the lateral left diaphragmatic outline, bowel in the left hemithorax, and mediastinal shift to the right. Note venous-arterial extracorporeal membrane oxygenation with a metal marker on the tip of the venous cannula *(arrow)*. The endotracheal tube is too high.

the midline, and the remaining ipsilateral pulmonary lobes show compressive atelectasis or collapse (Fig. 8-9). The left upper, right middle, or left lower lobe is usually affected as a consequence of congenital lobar overinflation. A lateral radiograph may be helpful in deciding which lobe is involved, although computed tomography (CT) of the chest is required in most cases to clarify the anatomy and identify a potential underlying causative abnormality, such as an extrinsic lesion causing partial bronchial compression (e.g., mediastinal bronchogenic cyst) or a mass within the bronchial lumen causing a ball-valve effect (e.g., endobronchial granuloma or adenoma).

■ **TABLE 8-1.** Differential diagnoses in asymmetrical lung volume

	Increased Ipsilateral Density	Decreased Ipsilateral Density	Normal Density
Small lung	Atelectasis Central airway obstruction Congenital venolobar syndrome Diaphragmatic elevation/paresis	Swyer-James syndrome (Macleod's syndrome)	Hypoplasia Interrupted pulmonary artery
Large lung		Primary/secondary congenital overinflation Central airway obstruction with ball-valve effect	

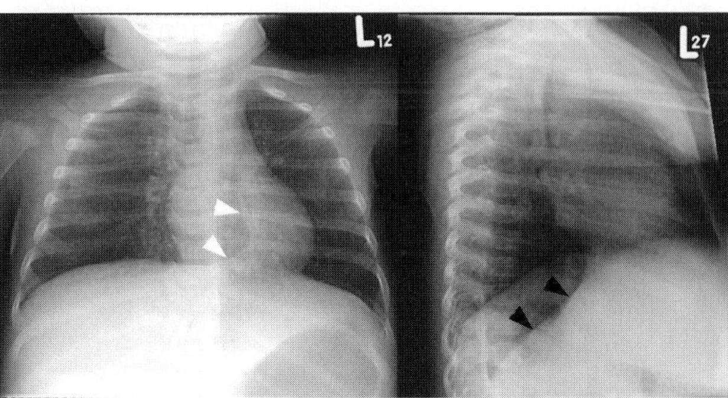

■ **FIGURE 8-9.** The lateral view is not part of a routine chest radiograph. In this case, the anteroposterior view shows probable lobar overexpansion of the right lung *(white arrowheads)*, but it is not clear which lobe is involved. The lateral view is helpful, showing depression of the posterior diaphragm *(black arrowheads)* and thereby clarifying right lower lobe involvement, which is uncommon in lobar overinflation (emphysema).

Mediastinal Distortion

Mediastinal distortion may occur secondary to a mediastinal mass. Therefore, the normal outline of the mediastinum should always be reviewed. This constitutes, on the left, thymus, aortic arch, pulmonary outflow tract, pulmonary hilum, and the left heart border; and on the right, thymus, azygos vein, hilum, and the right heart border. In young children, the outline of the superior structures may be obscured by a normal thymus (discussed earlier), which because the thymus lies in the anterior mediastinum, should never obscure the posterior paraspinal lines. Any distortion of the airways, such as narrowing, deviation, and splaying of the main bronchi, suggests extrinsic mass effect or functional/structural abnormalities of the airways (Fig. 8-10).

Mass lesions disrupting the paraspinal lines or involving the apices of the chest are most likely localized in the posterior

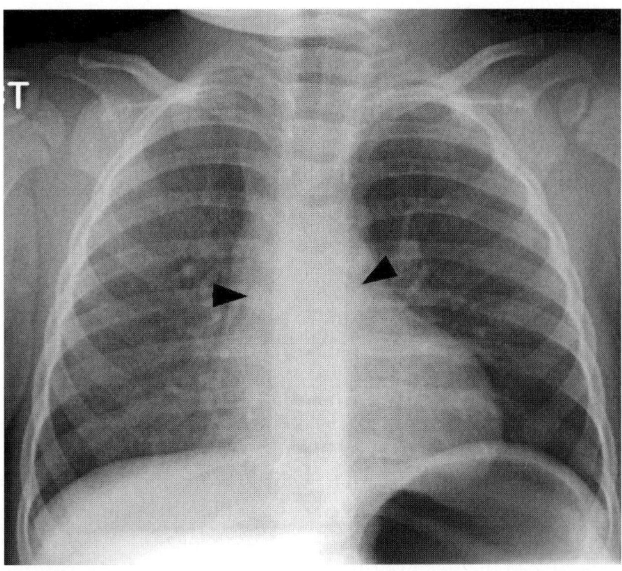

■ **FIGURE 8-10.** A 2-year-old boy presented with pyrexia. Chest radiograph shows displacement of the left main and lower lobe bronchi by a subcarinal mass *(between arrowheads)* and associated reduced radiopacity of the left lung due to air trapping. The mass was later proven to be lymphadenopathy caused by *Mycobacterium avium-intracellulare.*

mediastinum, and the list of differential diagnostic possibilities includes congenital abnormalities (lateral meningocele, neurenteric cyst, duplication cyst), neoplasm (neurogenic tumor), and infection (spondylodiscitis). Rib or vertebral body erosion suggests an aggressive lesion, such as infection or malignancy (e.g., neuroblastoma).

Any abnormal appearance of the thymus (discussed earlier), such as inappropriate size or shape or evidence of associated airway compression, suggests an anterior mediastinal mass lesion. Diagnostic differentials include rebound thymic hyperplasia, germ cell tumor, T-cell lymphoma, and thymoma.

Any other mass lesion in the mediastinum usually originates from the middle mediastinum. In the young child, the diagnosis is more likely to be a congenital abnormality (e.g., bronchogenic cyst), and in the older child, enlarged lymph nodes, which may be reactive or due to malignant disease (lymphoproliferative disease, which is rarely metastatic), sarcoidosis (rare, usually paratracheal), or idiopathic hyperplasia.

Lung atelectasis (discussed earlier) should be considered when there is loss of the upper mediastinal outline, even without apparent lung opacification.

Hilar Expansion

Unlike in adults, where bronchogenic carcinoma is a common cause of hilar adenopathy, in children, hilar enlargement almost always represents lymphadenopathy. However, prominent hili can also be seen due to enlargement of the pulmonary arteries, and in infants, due to a bronchogenic cyst (see Fig. 8-3). Distinguishing vascular from nodal enlargement can be difficult, but pulmonary arterial enlargement should result in a concave lateral hilar outline, whereas soft tissue masses are said to cause a convex lateral hilar margin, with a noticeable increase in soft tissue density at the enlarged hilum.

False impressions of hilar enlargement occur when the child is rotated on the film cassette: a hilum that is pointing away from the detector becomes more distinct from the heart shadow and consequently appears more prominent. A repeat exposure may be necessary in some difficult inconclusive cases, and cross-sectional imaging may be performed if there is doubt.

Peribronchial markings should not be prominent in children, unlike in adults. More distinct markings in the perihilar regions, particularly with coexisting general overinflation, often represent bronchial inflammation, such as asthma or viral infection. Other conditions included in the differential diagnosis are discussed in the section on high-resolution computed tomography (HRCT) [discussed later]. Patchy perihilar opacification, with air bronchograms, is usually due to radiographic summation of peribronchial thickening, but may be difficult to distinguish from airspace opacification (consolidation).

Lung Opacities

The plain radiograph usually allows distinction between atelectasis, which is defined as parenchymal opacification with loss of volume, and consolidation, which is opacification without volume loss and with the outline of gas-filled bronchi (air bronchograms) [Fig. 8-11]. Opacities in the lungs can be localized according to the neighboring structure that is obscured (silhouette sign). Loss of the upper mediastinal outline is consequent on upper lobe opacification, loss of the heart borders is caused by right middle lobe or lingular opacification, and loss of diaphragmatic definition is due to lower lobe pathology.

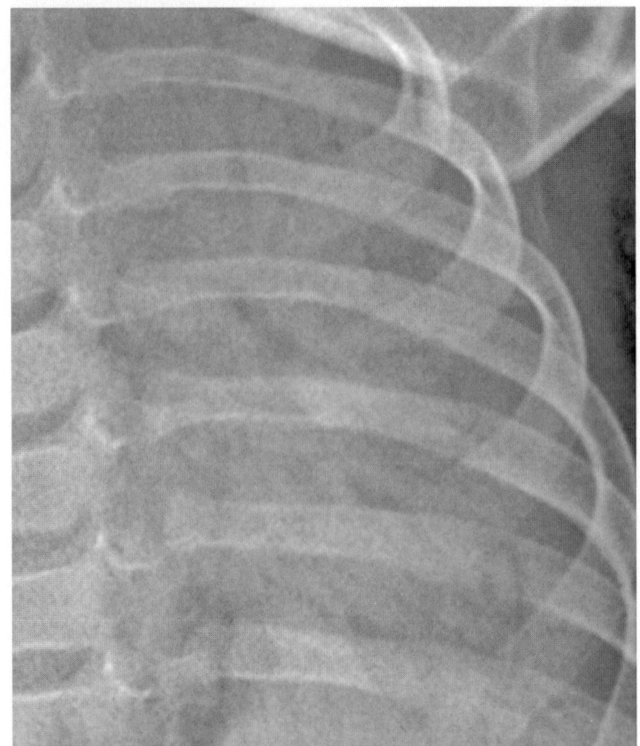

■ **FIGURE 8-11.** Consolidation. The lung parenchyma is opacified with air bronchograms, which are seen, but there are no vascular markings.

There are several important signs of volume loss. First, the entire hemithorax may appear shrunken, with ipsilateral mediastinal shift, diaphragmatic elevation, and crowding of the ribs. Second, adjacent noncollapsed lung may show compensatory overinflation and appear hypertranslucent due to dilution of vascular shadows. Third, the hilum may be displaced, either cranially or caudally, toward the atelectasis (Fig. 8-12).

It is important to recognize these signs, even with no apparent lung opacity, particularly in upper lobe atelectasis, where the affected segments, or the whole lobe, may be collapsed against the mediastinum and therefore difficult to identify.

The clinical and radiographic history of atelectasis may give important clues as to the causative pathology. Acute atelectasis may be due to a dislodged endotracheal tube, an aspirated foreign body, or mucous plugging (Fig. 8-13), and may therefore require further nonradiologic investigation and intervention. Chronic atelectasis is more likely caused by extrinsic airway obstruction (e.g., bronchogenic cyst, mediastinal lymphadenopathy, neoplasms) or chronic infection (e.g., tuberculosis), and may therefore require cross-sectional imaging. In a febrile infant with respiratory distress and multifocal segmental atelectases that change location over the course of hours, infection with respiratory syncytial virus causing bronchiolitis may be suspected.

Consolidation has many causes, as in adults, and is due to any process that replaces air in the terminal airspaces with fluid, mucus, or cellular material. The clinical history, the distribution of abnormality, and the presence of associated calcification, lymphadenopathy, or pleural effusion may assist in interpretation of the specific cause (Figs. 8-14 and 8-15). Typically, pulmonary edema causes bilateral patchy consolidation in a perihilar distribution as well as pleural fluid (discussed earlier), although there may be lateral predominance.

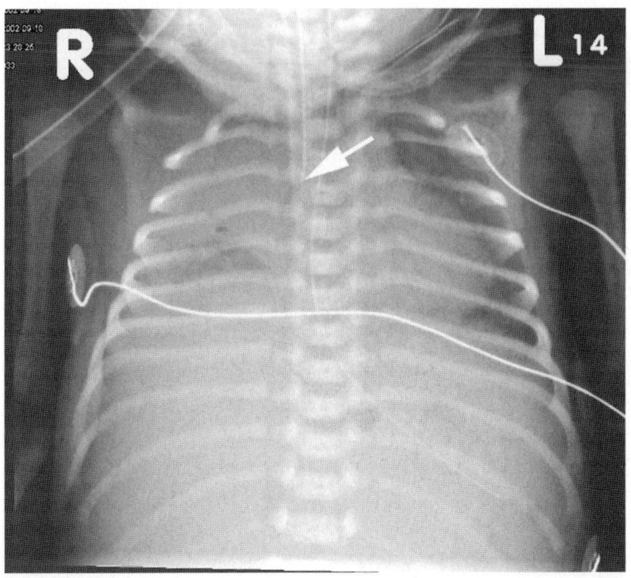

■ **FIGURE 8-12.** The tip of the endotracheal tube is in the proximal right main stem bronchus *(arrow)*. There is associated atelectasis of the right upper lobe (loss of definition of the right upper mediastinal border, opacification of the right upper hemithorax, elevation of the right hemidiaphragm, and crowding of the right ribs).

Ground-glass change, a description initially confined to HRCT, is now also used to describe radiographic lung opacification with partial preservation of vascular markings, with or without air bronchograms (Fig. 8-16). This sign is nonspecific and may be caused by interstitial or partial airspace opacification processes. In the neonatal setting, it is often used in the description of respiratory distress syndrome (Fig. 8-17), usually combined with generally decreased lung volumes. Pleural fluid may give a similar appearance (discussed earlier).

Focal and Multifocal Lung Densities

Focal and multifocal lung densities often require additional cross-sectional imaging for their definitive underlying cause to be elucidated, except in cases with clear clinical evidence of infective pneumonia. In children, pneumonic consolidation often has a more distinct, rounded appearance (round pneumonia),

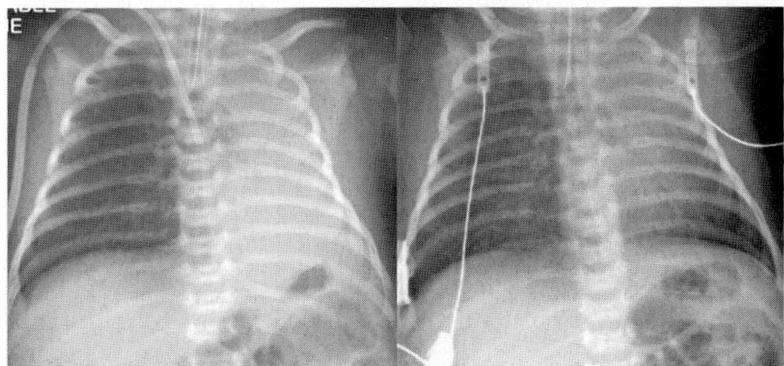

■ **FIGURE 8-13.** A neonate in the intensive care unit had increasing oxygenation problems. Chest radiograph *(left)* shows loss of the left cardiomediastinal and diaphragmatic outlines, opacification of the left hemithorax without air bronchograms, and mediastinal shift to the left. These findings strongly suggest left lung collapse, and at bronchoscopy, a mucous plug was removed from the left main stem bronchus. Immediately afterward *(right)*, there is considerably improved aeration of the left lower lobe (diaphragm now seen), but persistent collapse of the left upper lobe (persisting mediastinal blurring and shift).

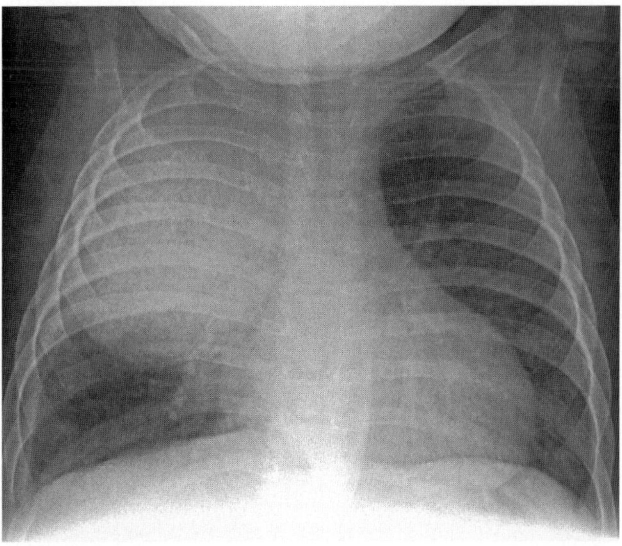

■ **FIGURE 8-14.** In a 1-year-old girl with cough, chest radiograph shows a calcified mass in the right upper and mid zones. Also seen is pleural fluid, which was caused by infection with *Mycobacterium tuberculosis* (see Fig. 8-51).

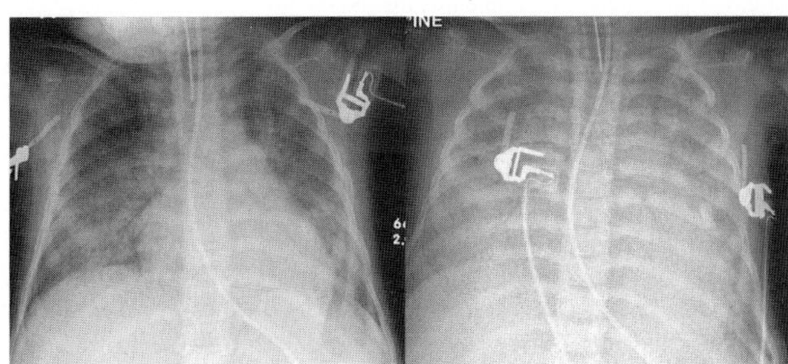

■ **FIGURE 8-15.** A 3-year-old boy who was treated in the intensive care unit after a traffic accident had increasing difficulty with oxygenation. Chest radiograph on admission *(left)* shows patchy areas of consolidation. Hemorrhagic fluids returned via the endotracheal tube. The second day *(right)*, there was almost complete whiteout of both lungs, with air bronchograms and loss of the cardiomediastinal and diaphragmatic outlines. The findings confirm extensive pulmonary hemorrhage.

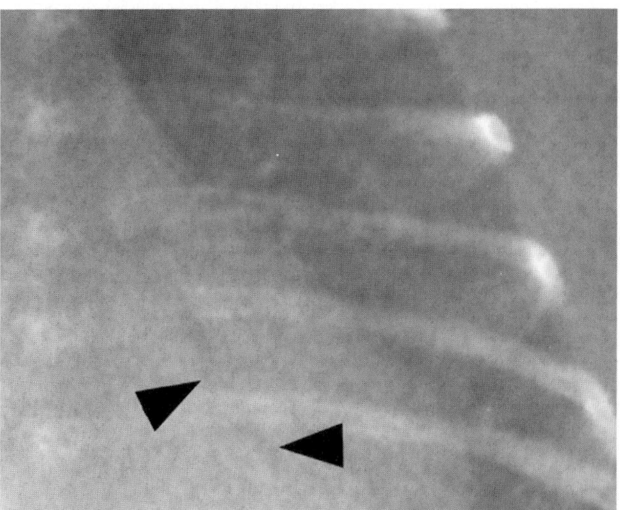

■ **FIGURE 8-16.** Ground-glass change. There is moderately increased opacity of the lung with air bronchograms *(arrowheads)*, but preservation of vascular markings.

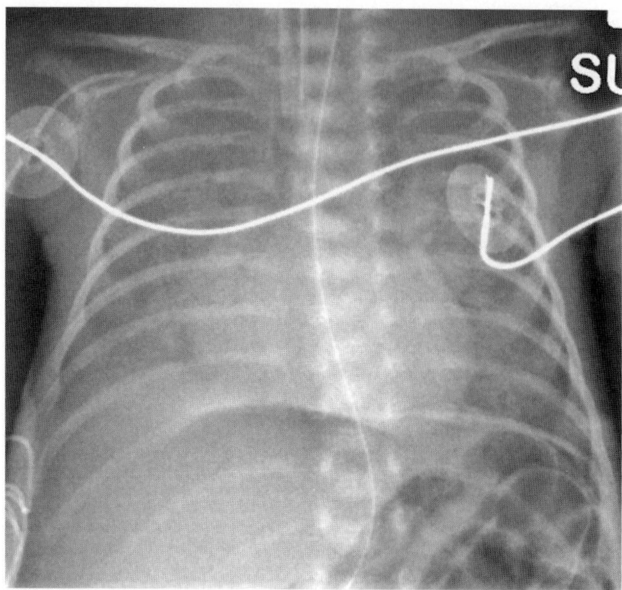

■ **FIGURE 8-17.** In a 3-week-old infant born at 32 weeks' gestation on ventilator support, there is bilateral diffuse ground-glass change (opacification, blurring of the cardiomediastinal and diaphragmatic outlines, preserved vascular markings), in keeping with respiratory distress syndrome. Note the lucency overlying the liver, outlining the right hemidiaphragm as well as bowel wall in the upper left quadrant. This is diagnostic of pneumoperitoneum. The child had bowel perforation secondary to necrotizing enterocolitis.

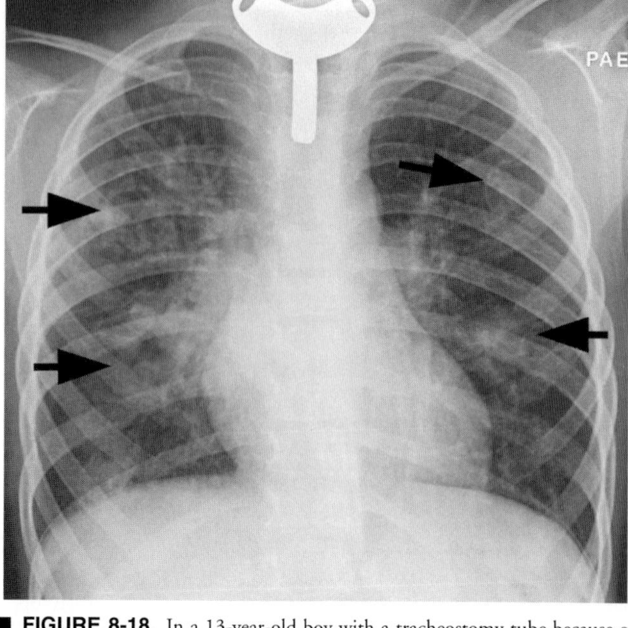

■ **FIGURE 8-18.** In a 13-year-old boy with a tracheostomy tube because of laryngeal papillomatosis, chest radiograph shows multiple nodular processes, some of which are cavitating, caused by parenchymal dissemination of the papillomatosis (*arrows;* see Fig. 8-37).

which should be recognized and followed with plain radiographs only. In equivocal cases, cross-sectional imaging is necessary for further characterization of the lesion. Differential diagnoses for a solitary parenchymal lesion may include congenital malformation, such as sequestration (usually in the posterobasal left lower lobe), microcystic congenital cystic adenomatoid malformation, and vascular malformation. A lung abscess may have no apparent gas-fluid level.

Multifocal lesions may represent infectious processes (e.g., fungus, tuberculosis, papillomatosis) [Fig. 8-18], granulomatous disease, Langerhans' cell histiocytosis, other inflammatory disease (Figs. 8-19 and 8-20), diffuse interstitial lung disease (Fig. 8-21), or metastases (e.g., nephroblastoma, hepatoblastoma, malignant germ cell tumor, sarcoma).

Some lung lesions tend to be predominantly cystic in radiographic terms (containing a gas-filled cavity). Pneumatoceles usually follow pneumonia, classically caused by infection with *Staphylococcus aureus.*

Multifocal multicystic parenchymal lesions may represent congenital cystic adenomatoid malformation, Langerhans' cell histiocytosis nodules at the cavitating stage, Wegener's granulomatosis, disseminated laryngeal papillomatosis (see Fig. 8-18), or necrotizing vasculitis (see Fig. 8-20).

Pulmonary Interstitial Emphysema

Pulmonary interstitial emphysema is a complication that occurs when high ventilatory pressures are used to ventilate stiff lungs. It appears as lace-like lucencies in a linear pattern radiating from the pulmonary hilum to the surface of the lung, and may be further complicated by pneumothorax or pneumomediastinum (Figs. 8-22 to 8-24). In some cases, this may be difficult to distinguish radiologically from ventilator-induced central bronchial dilation.

Lung Abscess

A lung abscess is a cavitated lesion that normally contains both fluid and gas. The consequent gas-fluid level is easily recognized, but may be missed unless the x-ray beam is tangential (i.e., horizontal) to the gas-fluid interface. With a diverging beam, the fluid level appears more blurred and meniscoid (Fig. 8-25).

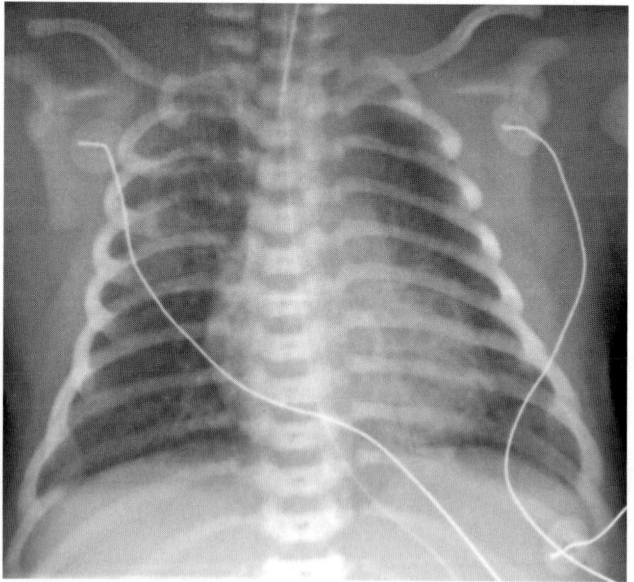

■ **FIGURE 8-19.** Radiograph of male neonate shows patchy consolidation in the right upper zone and behind the heart on the left, with overinflated lungs. This picture is commonly seen in meconium aspiration.

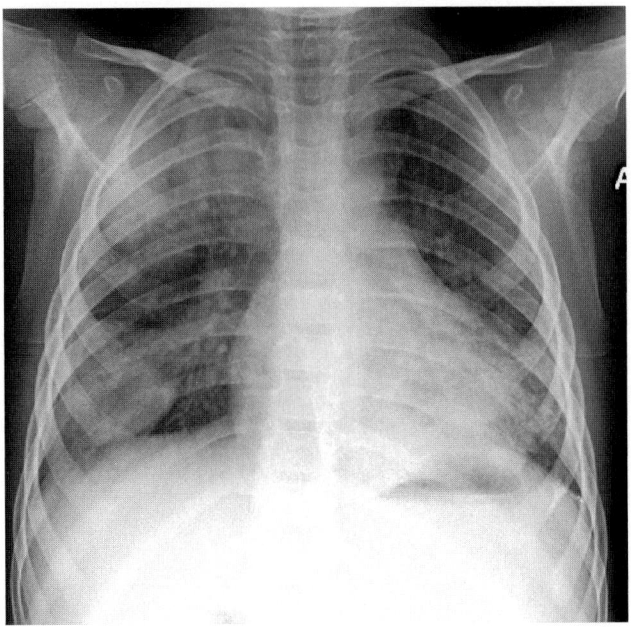

■ **FIGURE 8-20.** A 6-year-old boy presented with difficulty breathing. Inflammatory markers were increased. Chest radiograph shows areas of opacification in the right upper and mid zones and the left mid zone that represent vasculitic lesions (see Fig. 8-48). On plain film, this is indistinguishable from multifocal pneumonia.

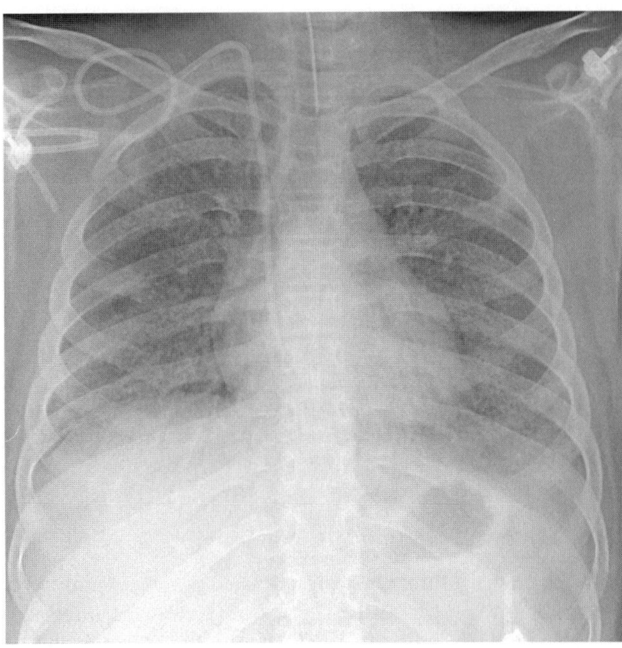

■ **FIGURE 8-21.** A 4-year-old boy undergoing chemotherapy had respiratory failure acutely. Chest radiograph shows globally increased density of both lungs in a granular pattern, with preservation of vascular markings. This was due to diffuse interstitial pneumonitis caused by bleomycin (see Fig. 8-40).

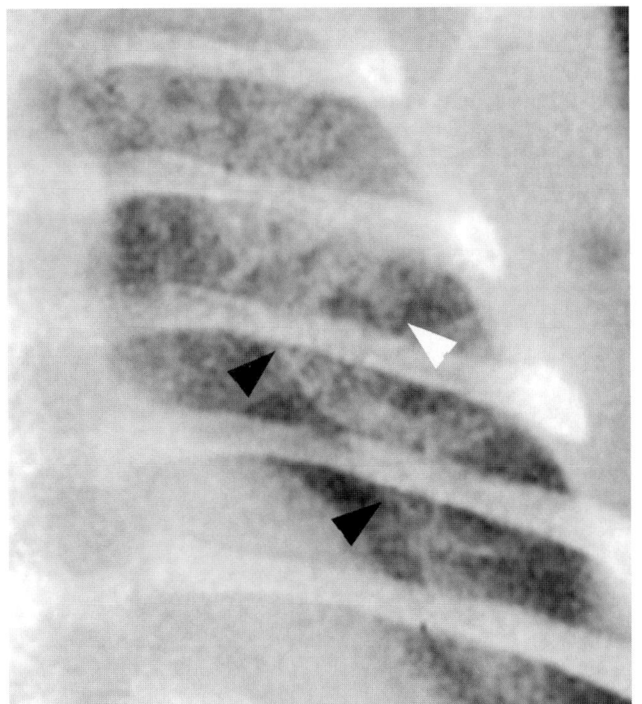

■ **FIGURE 8-22.** Detail from a chest radiograph in an infant after long-standing ventilatory support shows monotonous tubular lucencies *(white arrowhead)* suggestive of pulmonary interstitial emphysema. The mediastinal border is seen very crispl, with a medial lung edge *(black arrowheads)* due to anterior pneumothorax.

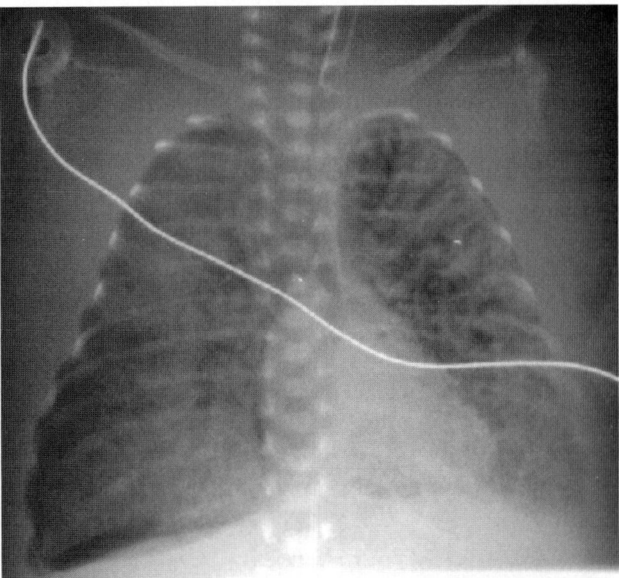

■ **FIGURE 8-23.** A 6-week-old girl born at 30 weeks' gestation was ventilated with great difficulty. Chest radiograph shows overexpanded lungs that are seen bulging out intercostally, with the diaphragm flattened. Concurrently, there is increased opacification of the lungs, which is presumed to be due to respiratory distress syndrome. Linearly arranged bubbly lucencies can be seen radiating from the hila, suggesting pulmonary interstitial emphysema secondary to high-pressure ventilation. There is also a pneumothorax seen at the base of the right lung.

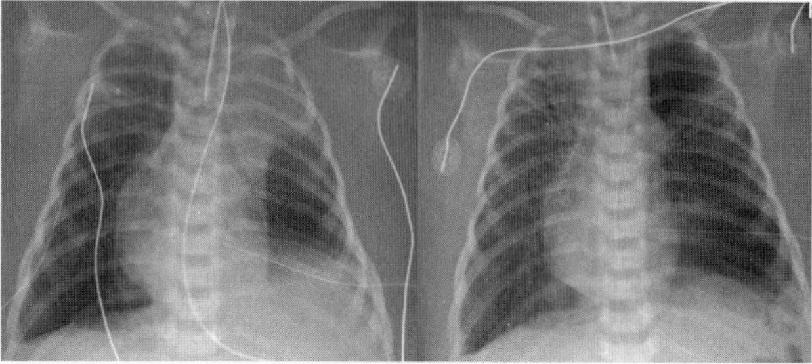

■ **FIGURE 8-24.** A 6-week-old girl was ventilated with high-pressure settings (chest radiographs show a flattened diaphragm and splayed ribs). After an acute exacerbation *(left)*, the radiograph showed collapse of the left upper lobe (opacification without air bronchograms, increased interlobar fissure, and elevated diaphragm). The next day *(right)*, the left upper lobe had reexpanded, but a left pneumothorax is seen. Linear bubbly lucencies can be seen from the hili to the lung edges, suggesting pulmonary interstitial emphysema.

Diffuse Interstitial Lung Disease

Diffuse interstitial lung disease is discussed in more detail in the section on HRCT (discussed later). More advanced interstitial processes may be appreciated radiographically as peribronchial thickening, ground-glass change, or interstitial nodules (Figs. 8-21 and 8-26).

Pneumothorax

In young children, the appearance of pneumothorax differs from the typical adult appearance. The variation is due to differences in lung parenchymal elasticity. In children, there is often no peripheral lucent zone on supine radiographs, which is the typical appearance in adults, because in the child, gas collects anteriorly in the anterior pleural reflection (Figs. 8-27 and 8-28). Increased clarity of the cardiac outline may be the only finding, and it should be assessed carefully. If there is clinical doubt, a lateral shoot-through or decubitus x-ray should be performed. These are more sensitive for detecting small-volume pneumothoraces.

Skeletal Abnormalities Associated with Respiratory Disorders

On conventional radiographs, undermineralization of the skeleton can be diagnosed confidently only in severe cases. Associated with prematurity, this metabolic bone condition is commonly seen in infants with idiopathic respiratory distress syndrome. Bone mineral loss is also a feature of a multitude of constitutional disorders, and may be seen secondary to systemic corticosteroid therapy.

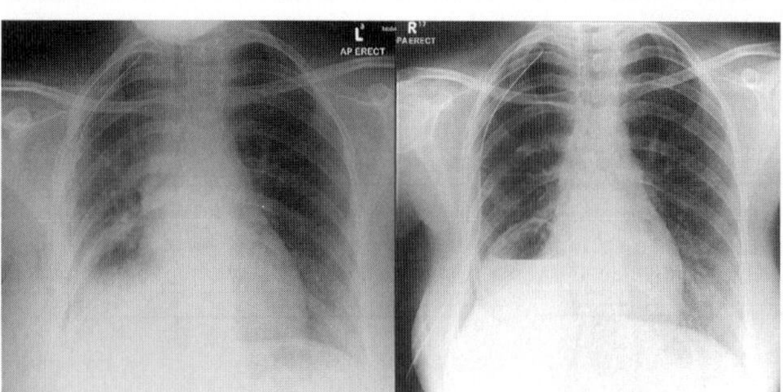

■ **FIGURE 8-25.** Two chest radiographs obtained in the same patient on the same day. The *right* is a true erect exposure showing the gas-fluid level of an abscess within the right lung, whereas the *left* is semierect and does not show the gas-fluid level of the abscess.

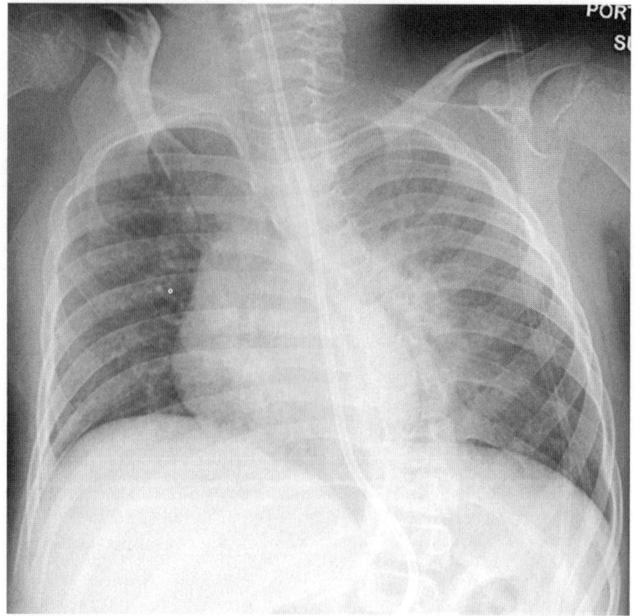

■ **FIGURE 8-26.** Chest radiograph of a 9-year-old girl with gastroesophageal reflux and chronic aspiration shows bilateral perihilar bronchial wall thickening, particularly in the upper zones (see Fig. 8-47). Apparent rotation is caused by scoliosis.

Scoliosis may be caused by vertebral abnormalities, which may be part of the VATER (*V*ertebral, *A*norectal, *T*racheo-*E*sophageal, *R*enal/*R*adial malformations) or VACTERL (like VATER, but including *C*ardiovascular malformations) sequences, or more commonly, may be caused by neuromuscular disorders. In addition, it may be secondary to chest conditions, such as hypoplastic lung, atelectasis, or empyema, in which case, the resultant spinal curvature is concave toward the side of the abnormality.

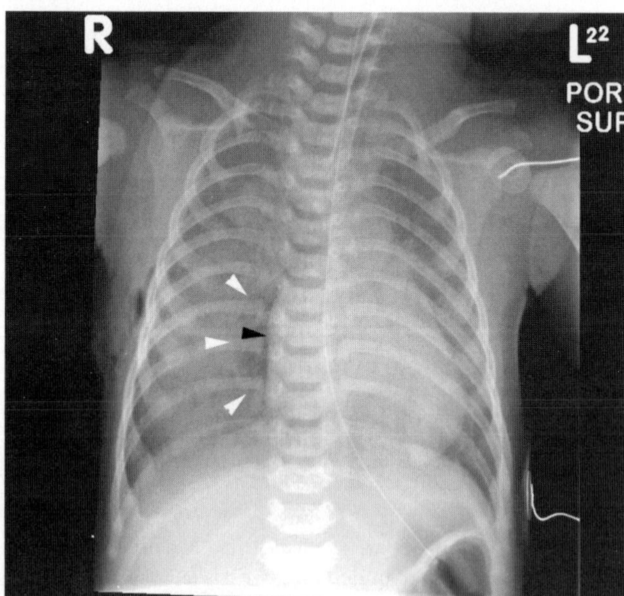

■ **FIGURE 8-27.** An anterior pneumothorax as seen typically in infants. The *white arrowheads* show the lateral boundary of the lucency. Gas adjacent to the right heart border causes a crisp outline *(black arrowhead)*.

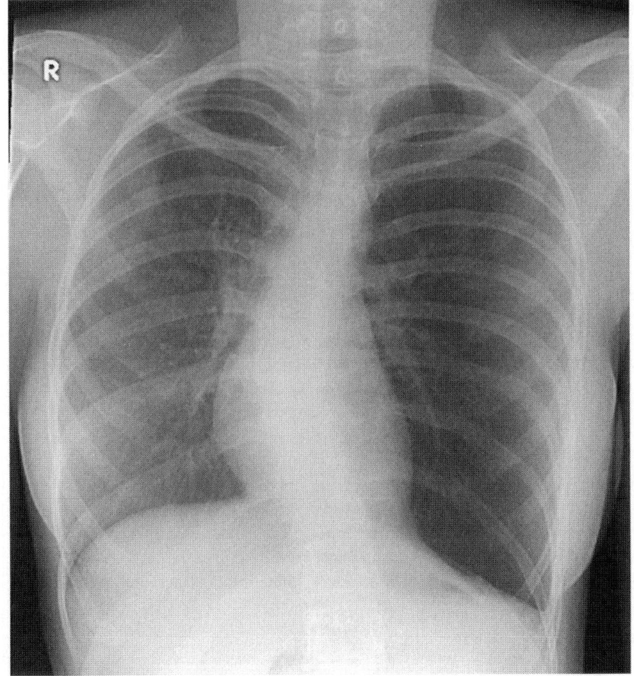

■ **FIGURE 8-28.** Chest radiograph in a 12-year-old girl shows a hyperlucent left hemothorax, inversion of the left hemidiaphragm, and a very crisp cardiodiaphragmatic outline. This is suggestive of anterior tension pneumothorax. Scoliosis is noted.

Both focal and multifocal osseous lesions may be associated findings in conditions that also involve the lungs. Well-defined lytic ("punched out") lesions in the ribs or scapulae and collapse of vertebral bodies are features of Langerhans' cell histiocytosis. More ill-defined lesions are seen in primary neoplasms (e.g., Askin's tumor), lymphoma, infection (e.g., tuberculosis), or infection associated with chronic granulomatous disease. Erosion of posterior rib elements, with splaying, is seen with thoracic paraspinal neuroblastoma.

■ FLUOROSCOPIC TECHNIQUES

Limitation of radiation exposure is vital in childhood, but a quick fluoroscopic screening examination (using pulsed rather than continuous fluoroscopy) of the chest can frequently prove extremely useful, in particular, in the evaluation of differing lung radiolucencies in suspected foreign body aspiration and generally in stridor.[4] With obstructive overinflation, the affected lung will show little volume change with respiration, and the mediastinum will swing contralaterally on expiration. Fluoroscopic lateral views may also be valuable for dynamic evaluation of tracheomalacia, where the trachea may be seen to collapse during expiration.

Barium swallow is still the primary study in patients with suspected vascular ring, which abnormally indents the contrast column in the esophagus. This test may also be valuable for assessing extrinsic masses. Laryngeal cleft and tracheoesophageal fistula can be excluded with a good-quality single-contrast study when a water-soluble contrast medium with a high iodine concentration is delivered under pressure via a nasal tube to the esophagus. The child is kept prone and screened with a horizontal beam to facilitate visualization of contrast leakage into the trachea or bronchi.

Thin-section CT has almost eliminated the need for bronchography in children; however, the technique is still used in functional studies for assessing the dynamics of intermittent airway obstruction (Fig. 8-29). With this technique, the mucosa of the trachea and the first to third generations of bronchi are coated with water-soluble contrast medium, which is instilled with a repeat small-bolus technique via a fine tube at the subglottic level in the intubated child.[5]

■ SPIRAL COMPUTED TOMOGRAPHY

Computed tomography is an invaluable technique in many pediatric chest diseases.[6] However, it is vital to assess the diagnostic benefit versus the radiation risk to the patient. CT is currently the most sensitive way of imaging the lungs due to its high spatial resolution. High-speed scanning allows for superb depiction of even small vessels after delivery of an intravenous bolus of iodinated contrast medium. In the younger child (younger than 5 years of age), sedation or general anesthesia may be required, although this need has reduced with the introduction of multi-detector-row, or multislice, CT (MDCT) scanners with faster acquisition times.

Unlike HRCT, spiral CT acquires volumetric data on the whole chest, usually after intravenous injection of contrast medium, which allows detailed anatomic depiction of the mediastinal and pulmonary vasculature and distinction between vascularized and cystic/necrotic mass lesions.

Spiral CT potentially shows the thoracic anatomy in a multiplanar manner and has increased sensitivity over a conventional chest radiograph. CT is ideal for visualizing chest/pleural lesions and can detect extension of mediastinal masses through the chest wall. The trachea and major bronchi are well visualized, and extrinsic and intrinsic airway masses are easily diagnosed. The increased sensitivity of chest CT versus chest x-ray for the detection of pulmonary nodules has been studied extensively.

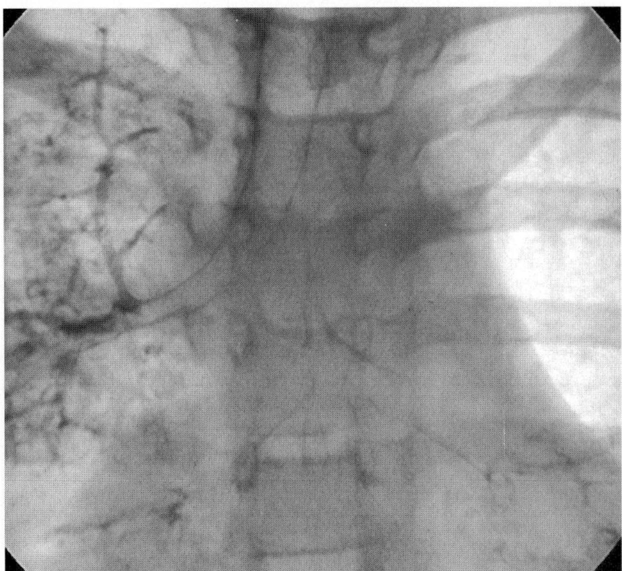

■ **FIGURE 8-29.** Bronchogram in a girl with stridor shows a long stenosis of the distal trachea, with an abnormal origin of the right upper lobe bronchus from the trachea (see Figs. 8-30 and 8-31). (Image courtesy of Dr. D. Roebuck, London.)

There are many advantages of conventional CT over plain chest x-ray; however, cardiac and respiratory motion artifacts may significantly degrade image quality. The paucity of mediastinal fat in children compared with adults may deter depiction of small mediastinal lesions. Spiral CT and ultrafast electron beam CT are particularly useful for investigating the major intrathoracic airways and cardiovascular and mediastinal abnormalities. The advantage of quick scan times in children is particularly useful, reducing the need for sedation and giving excellent vascular opacification with relatively lower contrast volumes.

ISOTROPIC COMPUTED TOMOGRAPHY

The main advantages of MDCT over conventional single-detector CT are the decreased acquisition time (increased temporal resolution) and the ability to acquire isotropic data (increased spatial resolution). The term *isotropic* implies that image resolution in all three dimensions is almost equal, so that post hoc image construction in all planes is possible without loss of structural detail. These benefits have dramatically expanded the application of CT in the evaluation of cardiovascular and airway diseases. MDCT is now commonly used in place of conventional angiography because the images are acquired more safely, without the need for arterial puncture, and often without the need for general anesthesia or sedation because acquisition times are very rapid (6–8 seconds). The additional benefit over angiography is that superb anatomic images of the mediastinum and lung parenchyma are acquired in the same data set, without additional radiation. The overall dose in MDCT is significantly lower than that in conventional angiography. Thus, MDCT can aid in the diagnosis of pulmonary embolus, arteriovenous malformation, aneurysm, and dissection. Images of the airway acquired simultaneously can ascertain the presence of airway stenosis and narrowing as well as show the cause of possible extrinsic compression.

REVIEW OF FINDINGS

The interpretation of findings requires systematic review of all anatomic structures and areas, including those shown in Table 8-2 (Figs. 8-30 to 8-38).

Depiction of parenchymal anatomy and abnormality with spiral CT is inferior to that done with HRCT. On the other hand, the spiral scan covers the whole volume of the lungs; therefore, it is more sensitive for demonstrating solitary lesions, such as metastasis or a fungal lesion.

Computed tomography performs poorly in differentiating between pleural effusion and empyema.[7] Pleural thickening and enhancement are often present in reactive effusions. Plain radiography, followed by ultrasound, is the investigation of choice, because ultrasound has the ability to visualize the fibrinous septations of an infectious process. However, CT is useful in distinguishing between empyema and lung abscess. Empyema shows a wide pleural base (see Fig. 8-38), whereas a lung abscess is usually seen partially separated from the pleura, with a wedge of lung on either side in the imaging plane.

PITFALLS

Technical factors may confound interpretation. Some artifacts may impede detection of significant lesions. In young children, there is invariably some degree of dependent lung opacification. When the distinction between atelectatic lung and nodular change is difficult, it may be helpful to repeat a few slices of the scan with the child in the prone position. Streak artifacts may be seen, and are caused by high-concentration contrast medium in the innominate vein at the side of delivery. This may degrade the imaging of structures in the upper mediastinum.

TABLE 8-2. Main review areas for spiral computed tomography of the chest

Structure/Area	Abnormalities
Airways	Extrinsic compression (see Figs. 8-30 and 8-31) Caliber change
Vessels	Vascular rings Aberrant vessels
Anterior mediastinum	Thymic enlargement, nodularity, heterogeneous enhancement
Middle mediastinum	Enlarged lymph nodes Bronchopulmonary foregut malformations (see Fig. 8-32) Cardiac abnormalities
Posterior mediastinum	Benign lesions: Duplication cyst, meningocele, ganglioneuroma, abscess, extramedullary hematopoiesis Malignant lesions: Neuroblastoma
Hila	Enlarged lymph nodes
Lung parenchyma	Lung/lobar aplasia, agenesis, hypoplasia, overinflation (see Figs. 8-33 to 8-36) Focal lesions: Nodules, consolidation, atelectasis (see Fig. 8-37)
Pleura	Transudate, exudates, pus, hemorrhage, lymph (see Fig. 8-38)
Chest wall and spine	Osseous or soft tissue lesions: Infection, benign and malignant tumors Abnormal configuration: Scoliosis, pectus deformities
Upper abdomen	Lesions of the liver, spleen, adrenal glands, and upper poles of kidneys Retroperitoneal, peritoneal, and abdominal wall lesions

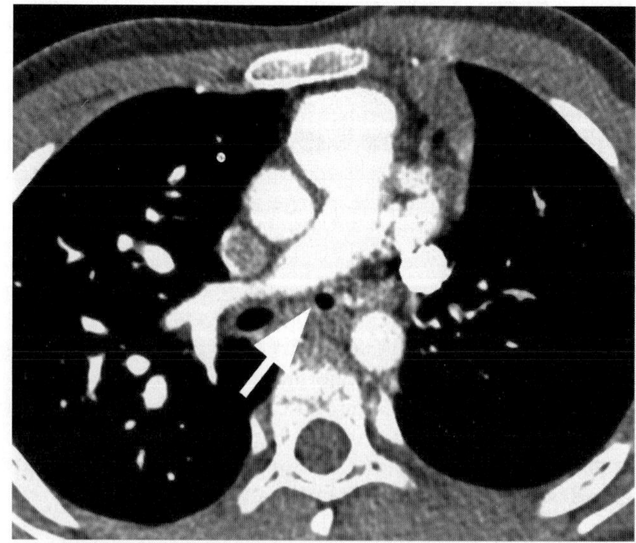

FIGURE 8-30. On arterial phase computed tomography of the same girl as in Figure 8-29 there is narrowing of the trachea *(arrow)* where it passes between the right pulmonary artery and the descending aorta.

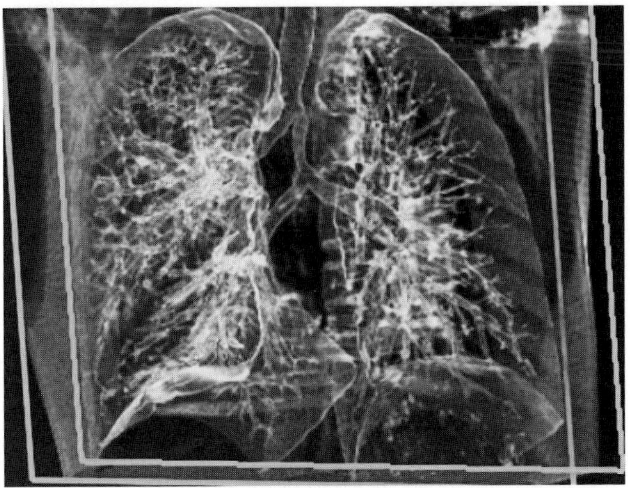

■ **FIGURE 8-31.** Volume rendering of the computed tomography volume data in the same child as in Figures 8-29 and 8-30 shows the anatomy of both the central and peripheral airways, with distal tracheal stenosis.

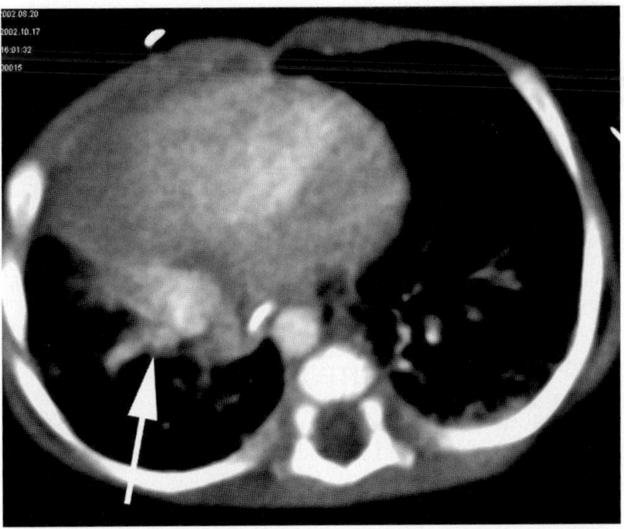

■ **FIGURE 8-33.** Contrast-enhanced spiral computed tomography shows systemic drainage of the hypoplastic right lung into the right atrium (*arrow;* see Figs. 8-5 and 8-35).

The peridiaphragmatic areas are also difficult to assess because lesions are difficult to depict separately from the diaphragm in the transaxial plane. Whenever possible, therefore, multiplanar reconstructions in the coronal and sagittal planes should be reviewed.

On the other hand, some artifacts mimic pathology. Tachypnea or motion will inevitably blur the final image, and this phenomenon is easily confused with ground-glass change. Apparent bronchiectases in the lingula and right middle lobe may sometimes be an artifact due to motion in which a single airway branch is represented twice in the image. Small parenchymal nodules (<5 mm) usually represent benign processes, even in children with known malignant disease. Therefore, such findings should not automatically be interpreted as lung metastases.[8]

■ DOSE

Dose considerations are particularly important in pediatric imaging. CT delivers the largest radiation burden of all imaging modalities. Therefore, its indications should be restricted and the dose kept as low as reasonably achievable.[9,10] Depending on the collimation (e.g., slice thickness of 0.75 or 1.5 mm with a 16-slice scanner), tube current, and length of the scan, the absorbed dose varies in equivalence to between 25 and 50 chest radiographs for a 2-month-old infant. In pediatric applications, the tube current should be substantially reduced, and image

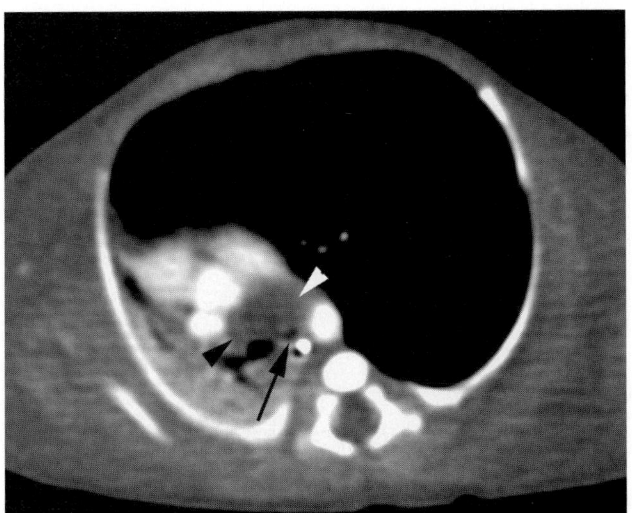

■ **FIGURE 8-32.** Contrast-enhanced spiral computed tomography shows a precarinal bronchogenic cyst *(arrowheads)*, with associated narrowing of the left main stem bronchus *(arrow)*, a hyperinflated left lung, and a collapsed right lung (see Fig. 8-7).

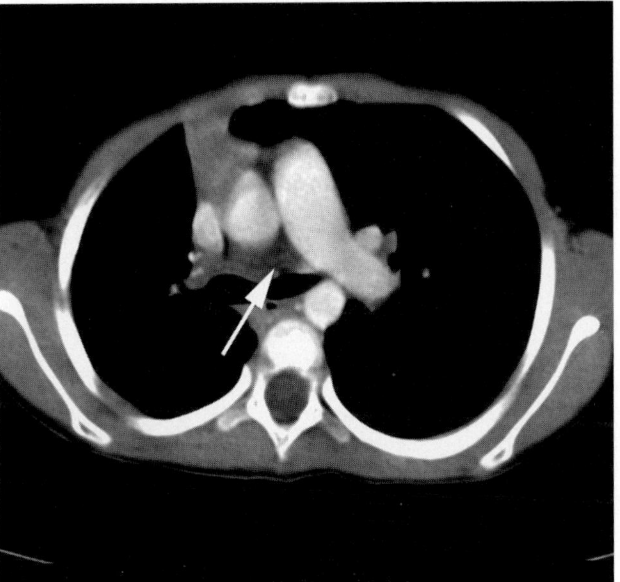

■ **FIGURE 8-34.** Contrast-enhanced computed tomography throughout the mediastinum shows a small right lung and no enhancement in the normal situs of the right pulmonary artery *(arrow)*. Due to the absent right pulmonary artery, the right lung receives systemic supply, but the collaterals cannot be seen (see Figs. 8-4 and 8-54).

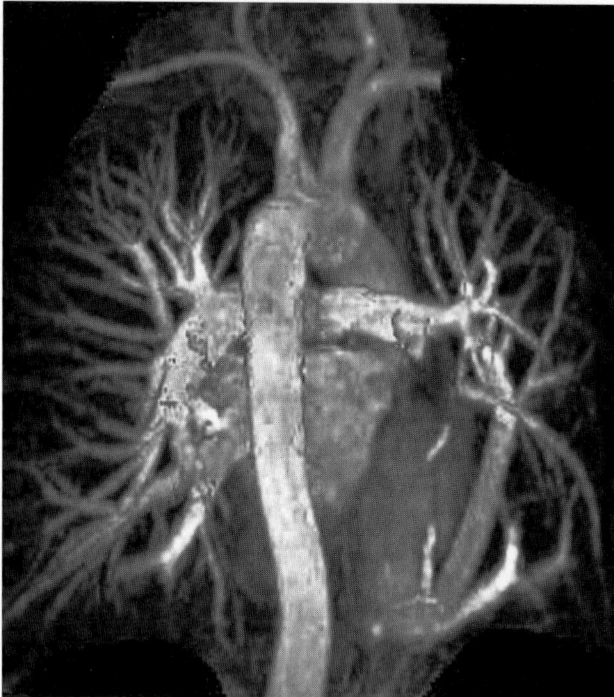

■ **FIGURE 8-35.** Three-dimensional magnetic resonance imaging scan shows the infra-atrial drainage of a scimitar vein (posterior view; see Fig. 8-5 and 8-33).

quality can usually be dropped (lower signal-to-noise ratio) without loss of relevant diagnostic information. Some suggested settings and dose calculations are given in Table 8-3.

■ HIGH-RESOLUTION COMPUTED TOMOGRAPHY

High-resolution computed tomography is the modality of choice in suspected interstitial lung disease. It allows a detailed structural assessment of secondary pulmonary lobules and intrapulmonary interstitium, thereby aiding diagnostic work-up. HRCT usually allows a confident radiologic diagnosis in cases of alveolar proteinosis, pulmonary lymphangiectasia, and idiopathic pulmonary hemosiderosis.[11] It also contributes guidance during lung biopsy and thoracoscopic procedures by targeting areas of active disease. HRCT allows early detection of diffuse pulmonary parenchymal disease to the level of the secondary pulmonary lobule, and is also useful in the characterization of opportunistic infection in the immunocompromised patient. Serial imaging may be useful in monitoring disease activity.

The recommended technique in children with diffuse pulmonary disease includes HRCT slices of approximately 1- to 2-mm thickness at 1- to 2-cm intervals from the lung apices to the lung bases (depending on the size of the thorax). A high-resolution image construction algorithm is mandatory. If possible, CT slices should be obtained at full inspiration to diminish

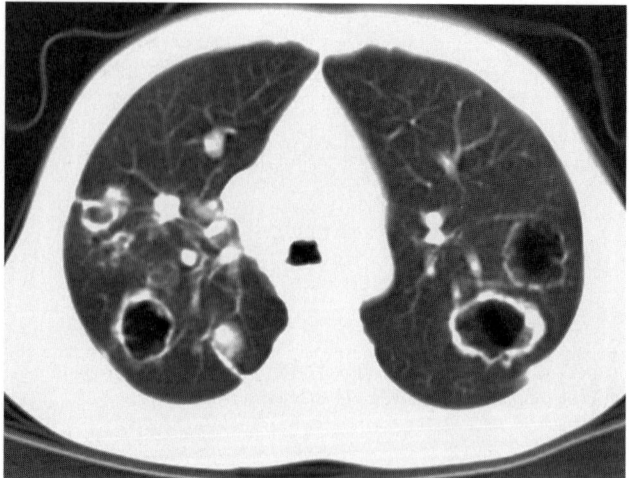

■ **FIGURE 8-37.** Chest computed tomography of an 8-year-old girl with laryngotracheal papillomatosis shows multiple peripheral nodules and cavities with posterior dominance, in keeping with pulmonary dissemination (see Fig. 8-18).

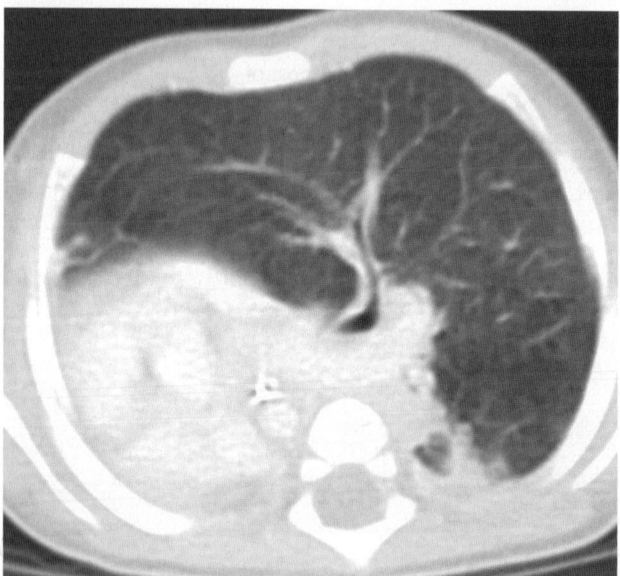

■ **FIGURE 8-36.** Contrast-enhanced computed tomography shows agenesis of the right lung and compensatory increased volume of the left lung, which appears structurally normal (see Fig. 8-6).

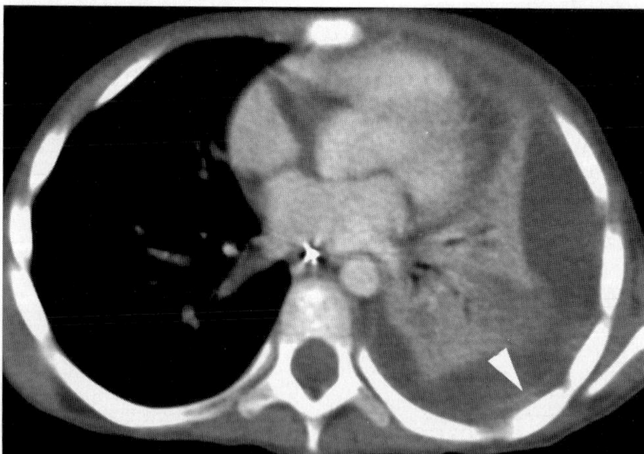

■ **FIGURE 8-38.** Contrast-enhanced computed tomography confirms the ultrasound finding of consolidated lung (note air bronchograms) and pleural fluid. There is mild pleural thickening and enhancement that is nonspecific *(arrowhead)*. Computed tomography did not show calcification. Acid-fast bacilli were cultured from the pleural fluid. This case shows the currently nonspecific role of computed tomography in imaging of pleural fluid (see Fig. 8-39).

TABLE 8-3. Suggested pediatric chest protocol for a Siemens 16-detector-row scanner with phantom measured computed tomography dose index (CTDI), and estimated effective dose (and equivalent number of chest radiographs), based on a tube collimation of 1.5 mm

Body Weight (kg)	Tube Voltage (kV)	Tube Current (mA-s)	CTDI (mGy)	Estimated Effective Dose (mSv)
<15	120	17	1.2	M: 0.6 (×24 CXR)* F: 0.8 (×32 CXR)*
15–24	120	20	1.4	
25–34	120	30	2.1	M: 0.9 (×36 CXR) F: 1.1 (×44 CXR)
35–44	120	50	3.5	
45–54	120	70	4.9	

*Conversion factor for an 8-week-old infant (scan range, 10 cm).
†Conversion factor for a 7-year-old child (scan range, 15 cm).

vascular crowding, particularly in the dependent areas of the lung, where atelectasis is more common in children than in adults.

Knowledge of the anatomic basis for HRCT is a prerequisite for understanding abnormal features. Supplying arterial and bronchiolar branches pass in the core of the secondary pulmonary lobule; draining veins and lymphatics pass in the connective tissue between lobules, the interlobular septa. The subpleural interstitium connects to the interlobular septa, constituting the peripheral fiber system. Extending from the hila, the bronchovascular interstitium extends centripetally.

DOSE

Adjustment of the radiation dose to the size of the child is crucial for radiation protection. The dose can be substantially reduced from a standard adult dose without loss of diagnostic information. Suggested settings and calculated doses are given in Table 8-4.

CONTROLLED VENTILATION TECHNIQUE

A method for noninvasive controlled ventilation in sedated children may be particularly useful in HRCT. Positive pressure is applied at a facemask, and the pressure applied is adjusted by changing the setting of a pressure pop-off valve. Respiratory pauses are induced by means of a step increase in ventilation, combined with rapid lung inflation at a pressure of 25 cm water, given synchronously with spontaneous tidal inspiration. Lung inflations are repeated approximately three to six times until a respiratory pause occurs. Inspiratory or expiratory scans can then be acquired with minimized motion artifact.[12]

INTERPRETATION

Interpretation of HRCT images is based on the presence and distribution of certain findings (e.g., septal thickening, ground-glass change, nodular change), which may represent a variety of histopathologic processes.

Regional or Generalized Increased Density

Consolidation (Fig. 8-39) and atelectasis may appear alike on plain radiographs, as discussed earlier. On HRCT, subsegmental atelectasis may be recognized by the traction it exerts on adjacent bronchi (traction bronchiectasis).

Ground-glass change is increased pulmonary attenuation, with preservation of vascular markings (Figs. 8-40 and 8-41). This may be due to partial airspace filling or may represent dense intralobular septal thickening that is too subtle to be resolved due to the inherent resolution of the HRCT scanner. Thus, the concept of partial volume effects comes into play when HRCT images show hazy opacification resembling airspace opacification when the abnormality lies in the interstitium.

Lung attenuation differs substantially between full inspiration and expiration. Diffuse, global ground-glass change may therefore be difficult to distinguish from a normal expiratory phase in the lungs. The posterior tracheal membrane is a helpful indicator because it is posteriorly convex on inspiration and horizontal or slightly anteriorly convex on expiration.

Regional or Generalized Decreased Density

Circulating blood accounts for most of the normal parenchymal radiopacity. Consequently, decreased radiodensity is most commonly caused by abnormally reduced perfusion due to reflex vasoconstriction in small airway disease. This can be regional (mosaic attenuation) or global (Fig. 8-42).

Differentiation between mosaic attenuation and regional ground-glass change is often difficult. In this case, acquisition of expiratory scans to document air trapping associated with small airway disease can be useful (Figs. 8-43 and 8-44). In uncooperative children, if breathing cannot be controlled voluntarily (normally younger than 5 years of age), a few slices can be

TABLE 8-4. Suggested pediatric high-resolution chest settings with calculated computed tomography dose index (CTDI) and estimated absorbed dose with dose equivalent number of chest radiographs, based on a tube collimation of 1.0 mm in the Siemens 16-detector-row scanner

Body Weight (kg)	Tube Voltage (kV)	Tube Current (mA-s)	CTDI (mGy)	Estimated Effective Dose (mSv)
<35	120	25	0.5	M/F: 0.2 (×8 CXR)
≥35	120	65	1.1	M/F: 0.4 (×16 CXR)

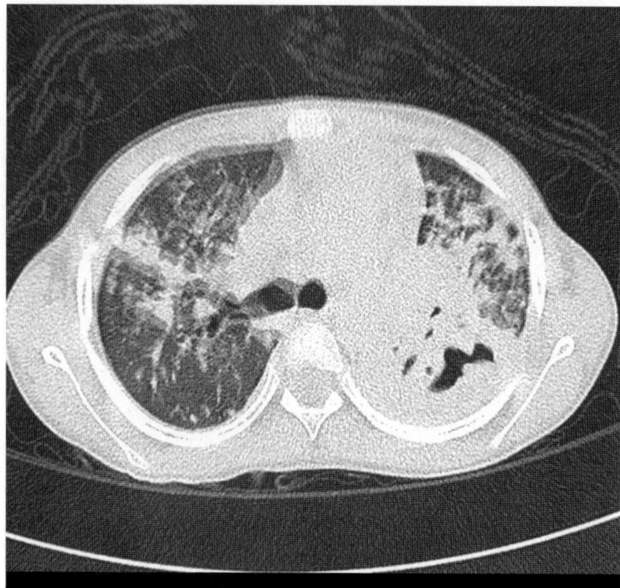

■ **FIGURE 8-39.** High-resolution computed tomography at a higher level in the same child as in Figure 8-38 additionally shows cavitation within the left upper lobe consolidation. This was later proven to be due to *Mycobacterium tuberculosis*. Abundant motion artifacts are noted.

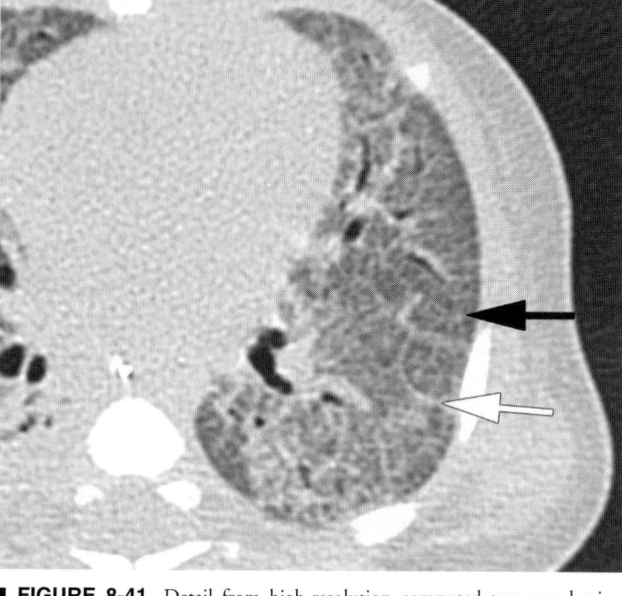

■ **FIGURE 8-41.** Detail from high-resolution computed tomography in a 3-month-old boy with chronic pneumonitis of infancy shows homogeneous ground-glass change, interlobular septal thickening *(white arrow)*, and discrete centrilobular nodules *(black arrow)*.

acquired in alternating decubitus positions. The dependent lung simulates expiration as the dependent hemithorax is splinted and its motion restricted, causing underaeration of the dependent lung and hyperaeration of the nondependent lung, effectively providing an expiration view of the dependent lung and an inspiration view of the nondependent lung.[13]

This is useful in practice for the detection of air trapping in the dependent lung. In small airway disease, the contrast between underperfused and more normal tissue increases on expiration due to air trapping, enforcing the mosaic appearance.

Septal Thickening

Intralobular interstitial thickening appears as fine web-like outlines, representing abnormal thickening of the lobular connective tissue or lobular bronchovascular interstitium due to inflammation or edema. If it is coarser, it resembles ground-glass change (discussed earlier).

Interlobular septal thickening is best appreciated in the subpleural lung, where it outlines the secondary lobules. It may be the result of interstitial edema, hemorrhage, fibrosis, cellular infiltration, or lymphangiectasia (Figs. 8-41 and 8-45). Diseases that affect the peripheral acini of two adjacent lobules may give the same appearance.

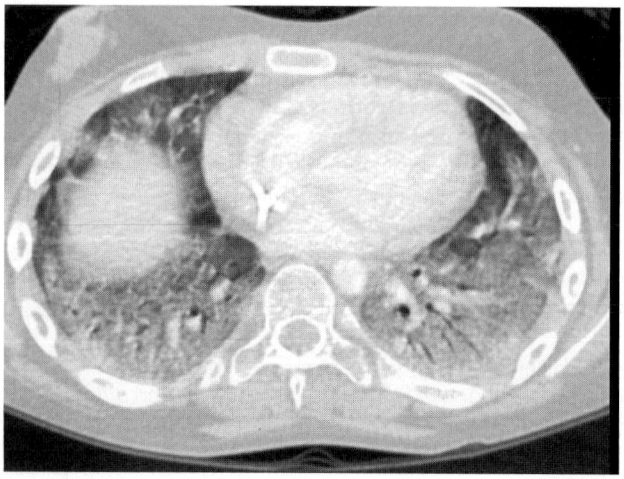

■ **FIGURE 8-40.** High-resolution computed tomography in a 4-year-old boy undergoing chemotherapy shows widespread ground-glass change whose cause cannot be determined. However, in this setting, it is suggestive of drug-induced pneumonitis, in this case, probably bleomycin (see Fig. 8-21).

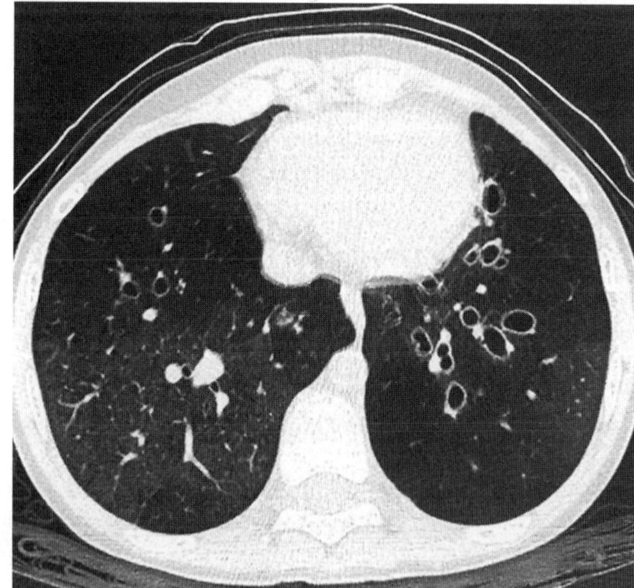

■ **FIGURE 8-42.** High-resolution computed tomography slice shows bronchial dilation with mild bronchial wall thickening (large airway disease), as well as almost globally hypoattenuating lung parenchyma and associated hypovascularity (small airway disease) in a 9-year-old boy with constrictive bronchiolitis.

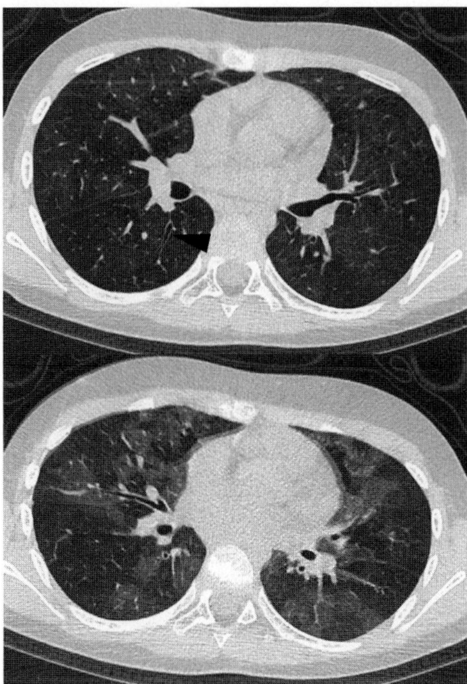

■ **FIGURE 8-43.** In an 11-year-old girl who received a bone marrow transplant, on inspiration *(top)*, there are global attenuation differences seen in a mosaic pattern, as well as bronchial dilation *(arrowhead)*. The mosaic pattern is accentuated on expiration *(bottom)*, suggesting air trapping within low-attenuating segments.

Peribronchovascular thickening is prominence of the bronchial walls or pulmonary arteries, usually with conspicuous centrilobular arteries. In the more extreme forms, this is caused by cellular infiltration (tends to appear nodular) or edema (smooth).

Interlobular septal thickening superimposed on ground-glass change is termed the *crazy paving* pattern, which is typically seen in childhood-type pulmonary alveolar proteinosis.

Nodules

Centrilobular nodules are nodular densities that are located centrally in the secondary pulmonary lobule. They represent small infiltrates associated with bronchioles and alveolar ducts (e.g., infection, hypersensitivity pneumonitis).

Centrilobular nodules (Figs. 8-41 and 8-46) may coexist with peribronchial inflammation and impaction of fluid, cells, or mucus in the centrilobular bronchioles (see Fig. 8-44). The nodular branching patterns cause the characteristic tree-in-bud finding. This is a sign in infectious bronchitis/bronchiolitis, bronchiectasis, and tuberculosis.

Perilymphatic nodules are small infiltrates associated with the visceral pleura, interlobular septa, and bronchovascular bundles (e.g., sarcoidosis).

Random nodules are small infiltrates with no predominant anatomic association, typically seen in hematogenously spread disease (e.g., metastatic disease, miliary tuberculosis).

Bronchial Change

Bronchiectasis is dilation of the bronchus. The commonly used cutoff point for normal/abnormal equals the diameter of the

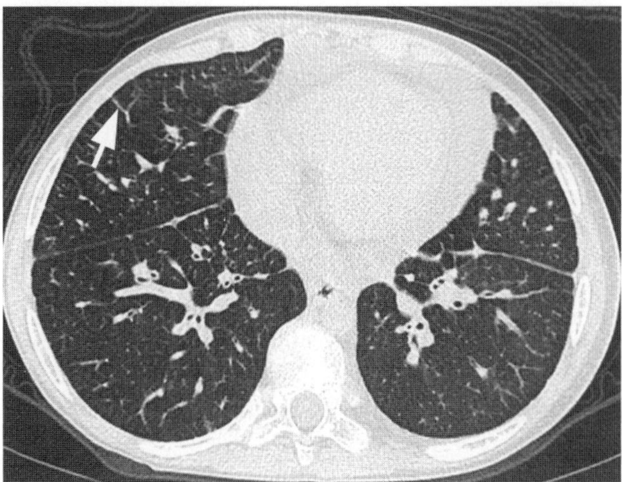

■ **FIGURE 8-45.** In a 13-year-old boy with known enteric lymphangiectasia, high-resolution computed tomography shows thickening of the oblique fissures, interlobular septal thickening *(arrow)*, and peribronchovascular thickening. This suggests mild pulmonary involvement.

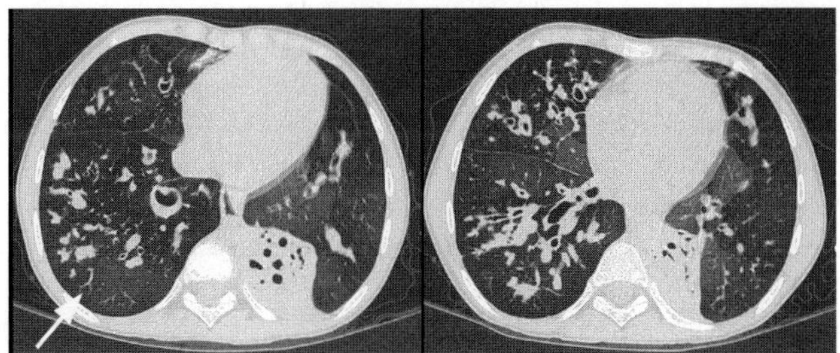

■ **FIGURE 8-44.** High-resolution computed tomography in an adolescent girl with end-stage cystic fibrosis shows mosaic attenuation, dilation, and wall thickening of the bronchi; mucus within the bronchi; and terminal branches with tree-in-bud sign *(arrow)*. On expiration *(right)*, there is accentuation of the mosaic pattern, confirming small airway obstruction.

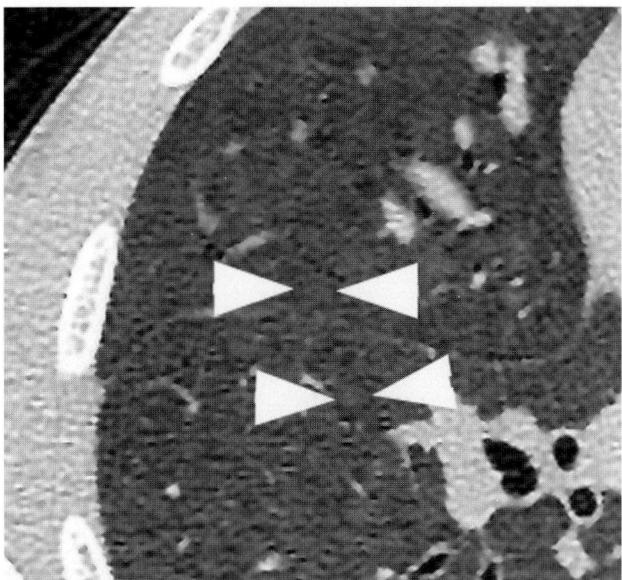

■ **FIGURE 8-46.** In an 8-year-old girl with intermittent hemoptysis, high-resolution computed tomography shows centrilobular ground-glass nodules *(arrowheads)* and mild fissural thickening. This is suggestive of idiopathic pulmonary hemosiderosis, which was confirmed histologically.

adjacent artery. In early phases of cystic fibrosis, small airway disease represented by mosaic attenuation may be the only finding evident on HRCT. With advancing disease, the typical pattern is seen: bronchial dilation accompanied by bronchial wall thickening, mucus impaction, and architectural distortion (see Fig. 8-44). Bronchial dilation with minimal bronchial wall change and coexisting severe small airway disease usually points toward constrictive bronchiolitis (see Fig. 8-42). Bronchial wall thickening without dilation, often with patchy consolidation, is often seen in chronic aspiration (Fig. 8-47). It is sometimes difficult to distinguish between bronchial distention secondary to high ventilator pressure and genuine bronchial dilation.

Architectural Distortion

Fibrosis and altered elasticity of the tissues permanently alters the structure of the lung parenchyma. This is seen as reduced parenchymal attenuation, cysts, deviation of vessels, bronchi and interlobular septa, and traction bronchiectasis (see Fig. 8-44).

Cyst formation may also be caused by cystic resolution of pneumonia, forming a pneumatocele, or necrotic change of a preexisting parenchymal nodule (e.g., degeneration of granulomatous change in Langerhans' cell histiocytosis, vasculitis, or Wegener's granulomatosis) [Fig. 8-48].

Seen in end-stage disease, honeycombing is the result of clusters of thick-walled air cysts, representing structurally distorted, dilated respiratory bronchioles lined by fibrotic tissues, collapsed alveoli, and vessels.

■ ANGIOGRAPHY

In noncardiac chest pathology, angiography is used relatively infrequently. Magnetic resonance angiography is a useful noninvasive technique with no radiation burden.

Interventional techniques, such as embolization of bronchial arteries, are performed in cases of severe hemorrhage/hemoptysis in cystic fibrosis. Therapeutic embolization of feeding vessels to intralobar or extralobar sequestrations or to pulmonary arteriovenous malformations can be obtained using metallic coils. Thoracotomy can thereby be avoided.

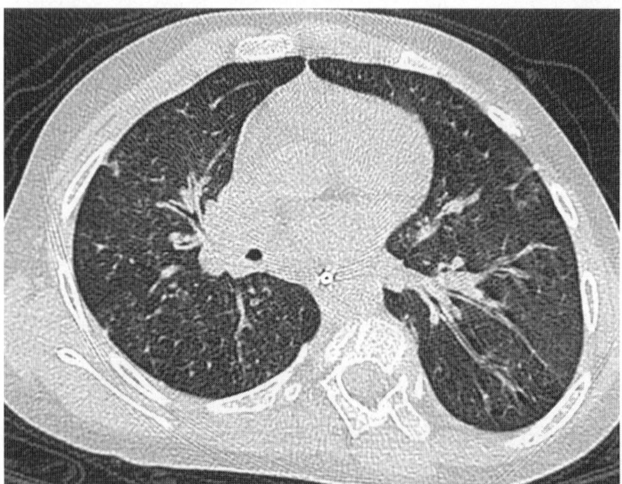

■ **FIGURE 8-47.** High-resolution computed tomography confirms bronchial wall thickening and shows small foci of subpleural interlobular septal thickening in a 9-year-old girl with gastroesophageal reflux and chronic aspiration (see Fig. 8-26).

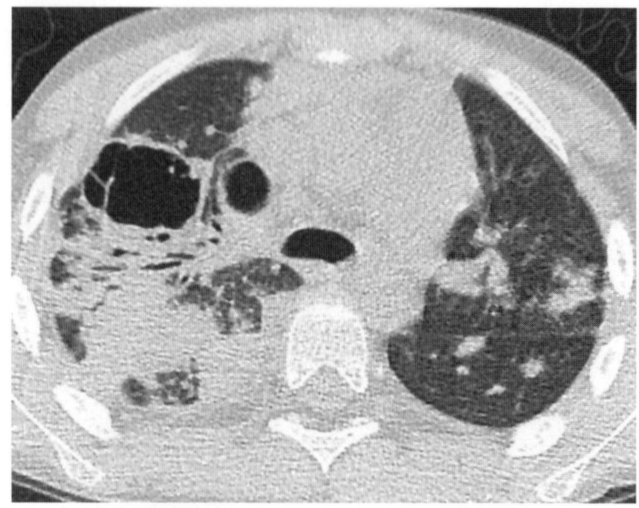

■ **FIGURE 8-48.** High-resolution computed tomography shows architectural distortion with large nodular change, air cyst, traction bronchiectasis, and pleural thickening in the right lung, and nodular change in the left. Histopathology verified nonspecific necrotizing vasculitis (see Fig. 8-20).

■ MAGNETIC RESONANCE IMAGING

The importance of nonionizing radiation techniques in pediatrics cannot be overemphasized, and MRI is a highly desirable diagnostic tool for use in children, although drawbacks include the increased use of sedation or general anesthesia due to prolonged scan times and usually closed imaging systems.

The multiplanar imaging capabilities of electrocardiogram gated MRI and magnetic resonance angiography make these important methods for evaluating cardiac lesions, anomalies of the mediastinal vessels, and masses, such as bronchopulmonary foregut malformations, chest wall masses, bone marrow infiltrations, tracheobronchial abnormalities, and neurogenic masses. The multiplanar capability of MRI, combined with its superb soft tissue contrast resolution, allows more specific diagnosis of some mediastinal masses. Ongoing refinements, with improved gating techniques and shorter scan times, are under continuous development and continue to enhance the role of MRI in evaluating the pulmonary hili, lung parenchyma, heart, and diaphragm.

Although it is well established in cardiac imaging, experience with lung MRI is still limited. The main technical problems are: (1) low proton density in the lungs and hence a very weak signal return (echo) from the lung parenchyma and (2) pulse and motion artifacts from the heart, from the great vessels, and from breathing, causing significant degradation of the images. Breathing hyperpolarized helium allows detection of signal from within the airspaces. Unfortunately, the gas has a short half-life and is not readily available in most imaging centers.

Magnetic resonance imaging achieves tissue contrast first by adjusting the train of excitation, refocusing radiofrequency pulses, and switching magnetic field gradients. A T1-weighted MRI sequence takes advantage of the relatively fast realignment with the main magnetic field of fat molecules, so that fat appears bright on the acquired images. Such images are generally useful for studying anatomy. T2-weighted MRI sequences play on the relatively slow realignment of water molecules with the main magnetic field. Because water appears bright on these images, they are particularly helpful in detection of fluid collections and edema.

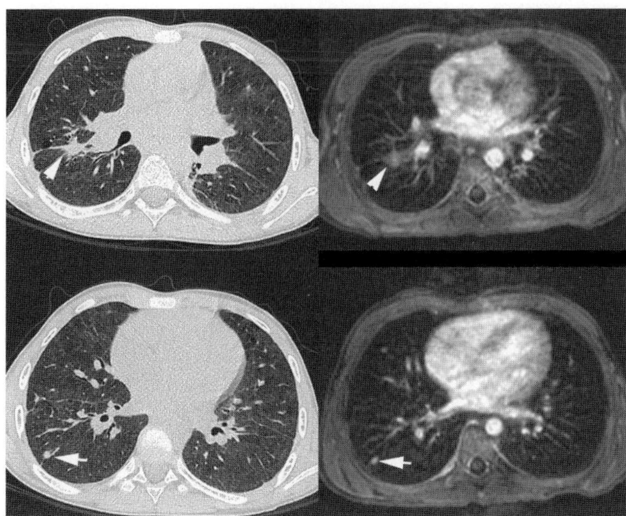

■ **FIGURE 8-49.** In a 12-year-old boy with chronic granulomatous disease, high-resolution computed tomography *(left)* and contrast-enhanced three-dimensional gradient echo magnetic resonance imaging *(right)* acquired on the same day show corresponding findings of spiculated, enhancing lesions near the right hilum *(arrowheads)* and subpleurally in the right lower lobe *(arrows)*.

A second facility for creating image contrast or enhancing inherent tissue imaging contrast is the administration of intravenous MRI contrast medium, which is usually gadolinium chelate. This is typically combined with a T1-weighted pulse sequence and gives superb images of vascular structures, even potentially including the most peripheral vessels. Additionally, contrast media are useful for detecting contrast enhancement in inflammatory or neoplastic lesions (Figs. 8-49 to 8-51). Ultrafast pulse sequences, with three-dimensional acquisition of volumetric MRI data, are diagnostically promising and can be implemented on most modern scanners. Although the diagnostic accuracy is still unknown, MRI potentially may be used for imaging parenchymal lung lesions.[14]

■ ULTRASONOGRAPHY

Ultrasound is particularly important in pediatric practice because it obviates the need for ionizing radiation. The real-time

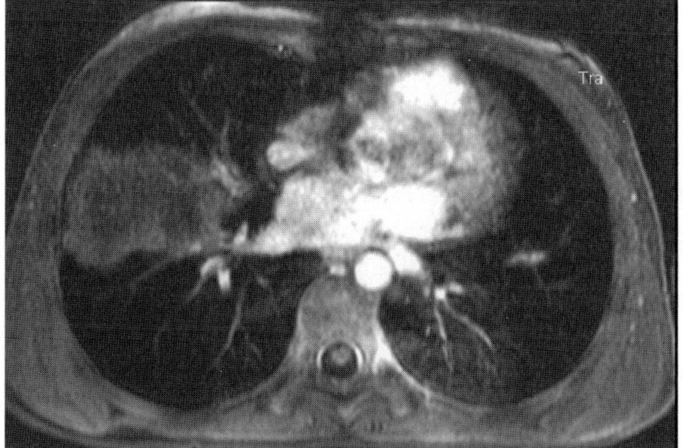

■ **FIGURE 8-50.** A 12-year-old boy who received a heart-lung transplant had a right-sided density on chest radiographs. Magnetic resonance imaging (T1-weighted gradient echo, breath-hold, gadolinium-enhanced) shows an enhancing mass lesion in close relation to the right oblique fissure. Histopathologically, this was diagnosed as (post-transplant) lymphoproliferative disease.

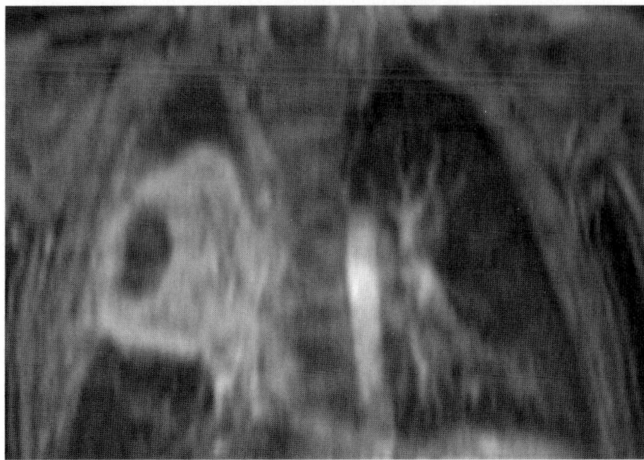

■ **FIGURE 8-51.** Contrast-enhanced magnetic resonance imaging scan (gradient echo) in a 1-year-old boy with cough and pyrexia shows enhancement in the right upper lobe, except in a presumed necrotic focus, and mediastinal enhancement. *Mycobacterium tuberculosis* was later confirmed microbiologically (see Fig. 8-14).

and portable application of ultrasound makes it even more useful, especially in intensive care units. Because air is highly reflective, the applications of chest ultrasound are limited; however, ultrasound is useful in patients with complete radiographic opacification of a hemithorax because it can distinguish between pleural fluid, consolidation, atelectasis, and parenchymal masses (Fig. 8-52). It also allows characterization of pleural fluid collections as simple, complicated, or fibroadhesive, which is important information for planning thoracocentesis or thoracotomy. It also can be used to study a prominent thymus and thereby obviate unnecessary CT scanning.[15]

Doppler ultrasound with color flow and power Doppler aid in the evaluation of vascular status and patency and abnormal vascular anatomy. Ultrasound is useful in the diagnosis of bronchopulmonary foregut malformations, particularly intralobar and extralobar sequestrations in which the systemic arterial supply to the lesion can be traced with color Doppler in real time, thus both verifying the diagnosis and acting as a road map for the surgeon (Fig. 8-53).

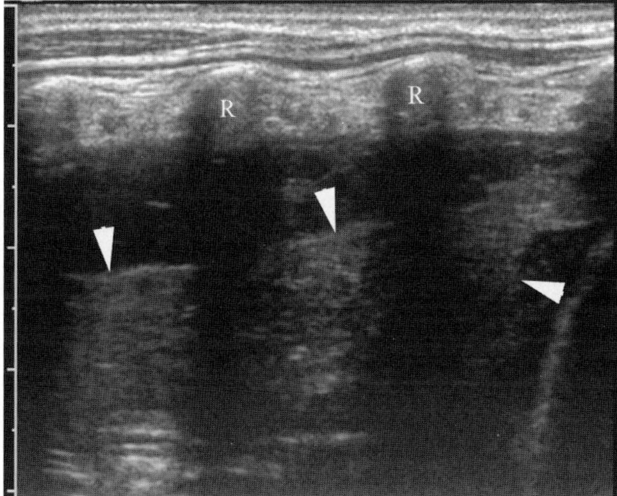

■ **FIGURE 8-52.** Coronal ultrasound image of the left hemithorax shows consolidated lung *(arrowheads)* surrounded by fluid, which is mainly anechoic, but with some echogenic strands. Note the acoustic shadows from the ribs (R). Acid-fast bacilli were cultured from the pleural fluid.

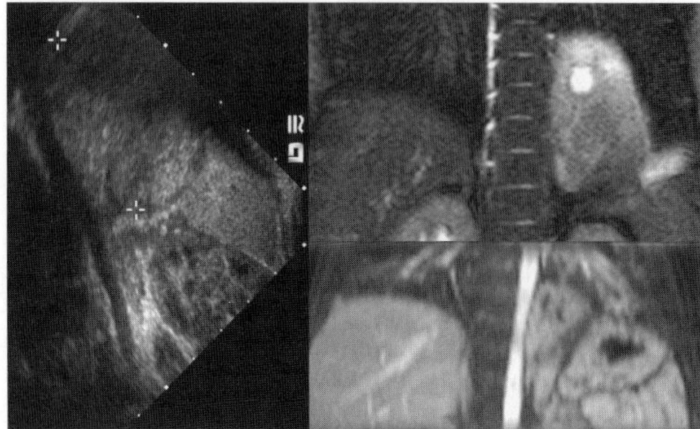

■ **FIGURE 8-53.** A neonate with an antenatally diagnosed chest mass was scanned with ultrasound *(left)*, which showed a nonaerated, noncalcified mass lesion *(between calipers)* paraspinally, immediately above the left hemidiaphragm. The magnetic resonance images also show a cyst (*upper right,* inversion recovery), seen as high signal, and confirm the close relation to the aorta and the intrathoracic position of the mass (*lower right,* contrast-enhanced gradient echo), where the diaphragm *(dark line)* is seen separating the lesion from the stomach (intermediate signal ellipsoid). There was no change in size over time, and the systemic supply from the aorta to this sequestration was later verified. The differential diagnosis for a paraspinal mass in this age group would include neuroblastoma.

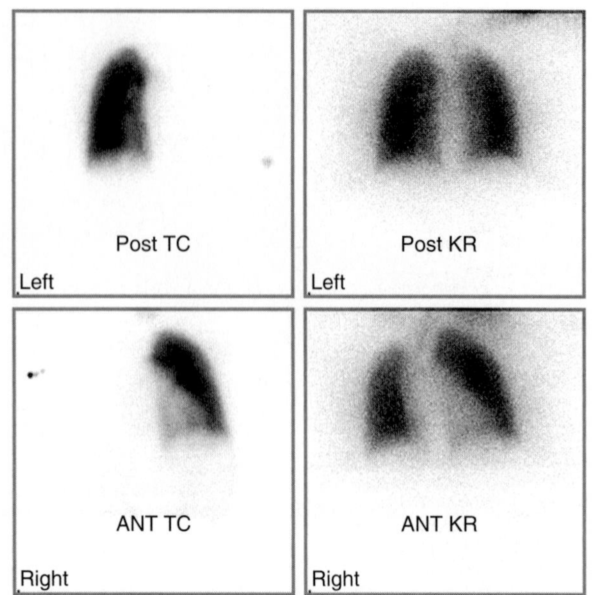

■ **FIGURE 8-54.** A ventilation/perfusion isotope study in a patient with absent right pulmonary artery on computed tomography confirms interrupted pulmonary arterial supply to the right lung *(left)*. The hypoplastic right lung has preserved ventilation (*right;* see Figs. 8-4 and 8-34).

Ultrasound has a role in assessing spontaneous diaphragmatic movement, and can easily be performed at the bedside. The skilled operator will be able to assess paresis and paradoxical movement and also evaluate the differential diagnoses of upper abdominal mass and subpulmonary collection, although the accuracy of assessing diaphragmatic function per se compared with phrenic nerve stimulation is unknown.

■ RADIONUCLIDE IMAGING

Nuclear medicine techniques are used to help delineate cardiac function, right-to-left shunts, pulmonary embolism, inflammatory lung disease, and lung ventilation/perfusion (Fig. 8-54). However, although in the past, nuclear medicine was the sole means of functional assessment of the heart and lung, the technique is gradually being replaced by CT for assessment of pulmonary embolism and small airway disease and by MRI for combined assessment of cardiac morphology and function.

Positron emission tomography (PET) is a promising modality. It uses biologically interesting radionuclides (e.g., carbon 11, oxygen 15, nitrogen 13) to mark biochemical substrates (e.g., glucose). PET is therefore a modality for metabolic rather than structural studies, and in patients with malignant disease, PET uses the relatively high glucose metabolism in malignant cells for imaging. Combined with CT, anatomic and functional data can be fused into one image. The clinical efficacy of the technique is being explored.

■ CONCLUSION

Radiologic evaluation of the child cannot be extrapolated from adult imaging. Particular awareness of the issues of radiation protection, developmental anatomy and physiology, and the range of pediatric disorders is crucial.

REFERENCES

1. Lucaya J, Strife JL: Pediatric chest imaging. Chest imaging in infants and children. Berlin: Springer-Verlag, 2002.
2. Siegel MJ: Pediatric Body CT. Philadelphia: Lippincott Williams & Wilkins, 1999.
3. Owens CM, Thomas KE: The paediatric chest. In: Sutton D, ed: Textbook of Radiology and Imaging, 7th ed. New York: Churchill Livingstone, 2003, pp 247–263.
4. Rudman DT, Elmaraghy CA, Shiels WE, Wiet GJ: The role of airway fluoroscopy in the evaluation of stridor in children. Arch Otolaryngol Head Neck Surg 2003;129:305–309.
5. Burden RJ, Shann F, Butt W, Ditchfield M: Tracheobronchial malacia and stenosis in children in intensive care. Bronchograms help to predict outcome. Thorax 1999;54:511–517.
6. Thomas KE, Owens CM, Britto J, Nadel S, Habibi P, Nicholson R: Efficacy of chest CT in a pediatric ICU. A prospective study. Chest 2000;117: 1697–1705.
7. Donnelly LF, Klosterman LA: CT appearance of parapneumonic effusions in children. Findings are not specific for empyema. AJR Am J Roentgenol 1997;169:179–182.
8. Grampp S, Bankier AA, Zoubek A, Wiesbauer P, Schroth B, Henk CB, et al: Spiral CT of the lung in children with malignant extra-thoracic tumors. Distribution of benign vs malignant pulmonary nodules. Eur Radiol 2000;10:1318–1322.
9. Frush DP, Donnelly LF, Rosen NS: Computed tomography and radiation risks. What pediatric health care providers should know. Pediatrics 2003; 112:951–957.
10. Donnelly LF, Frush DP: Pediatric multidetector body CT. Radiol Clin North Am 2003;41:637–655.
11. Koh DM, Hansell DM: Computed tomography of diffuse interstitial lung disease in children. Clin Radiol 2000;55:659–667.
12. Long FR, Castile RG: Technique and clinical applications of full-inflation and end-exhalation controlled-ventilation chest CT in infants and young children. Pediatr Radiol 2001;31:413–422.
13. Choi SJ, Choi BK, Kim HJ, Lee SH, Choi SH, Park SJ, et al: Lateral decubitus HRCT. A simple technique to replace expiratory CT in children with air trapping. Pediatr Radiol 2002;32:179–182.
14. Karabulut N, Martin DR, Yang M, Tallaksen RJ: MR imaging of the chest using a contrast-enhanced breath-hold modified three-dimensional gradient-echo technique. Comparison with two-dimensional gradient-echo technique and multidetector CT. AJR Am J Roentgenol 2002;179:1225–1233.
15. Kim OH, Kim WS, Kim MJ, Jung JY, Suh JH: US in the diagnosis of pediatric chest diseases. Radiographics 2000;20:653–671.

9 Pulmonary Function Tests in Infants and Preschool Children

Janet Stocks, PhD

Measurement of lung function is an integral component of respiratory physiology and clinical assessment of lung diseases in school-aged children and adults. Despite the heightened vulnerability to respiratory diseases in infants and young children, until recently, assessments of pulmonary function in this group have been restricted to specialized research establishments. This was largely attributable to the lack of suitable equipment and difficulties in undertaking such measurements in small, potentially uncooperative subjects. The realization that insults to the developing lung may have lifelong effects and that much of the burden of respiratory disease in childhood and later life has its origins in infancy and early childhood emphasized the need to develop more sensitive methods of assessing respiratory function in infants and preschool children that could be used as objective outcome measures to identify early determinants of lung and airway function, distinguish changes due to disease from those related to growth and development, and evaluate the effects of new diagnostic and therapeutic advances. Indeed, it is now realized that assessment of respiratory function in the very young has major implications for our understanding of respiratory health and disease, not only during childhood, but also throughout life.

■ HISTORICAL BACKGROUND

The first recorded attempts to measure lung function in infants were made more than 100 years ago, but relatively little progress was made thereafter until the 1960s, when many of the tests originally developed for assessing adults, including plethysmography and esophageal manometry, were adapted for use in infants. During the 1980s, many new tests were developed specifically for use in infants, including occlusion techniques for assessing passive respiratory mechanics and the squeeze, or rapid thoracoabdominal compression (RTC), technique for measuring partial forced expiratory maneuvers in infants. It was during this period that the first commercially available equipment designed for use in infants became available. With the release of more automated and computerized systems, infant pulmonary function tests (PFTs) were no longer restricted to specialized physiology laboratories, but began to be used in a wider range of settings, including neonatal intensive care units. This was accompanied by an exponential increase in publications in this area. As the diversity of users and applications increased, so did the need for international standardization of equipment and techniques, a challenge that eventually led to the formation of the European Respiratory Society–American Thoracic Society (ERS-ATS) Task Force on infant lung function. This task force has been responsible for a large number of publications and postgraduate courses over the last 10 years, including recommendations for both users and manufacturers of infant lung function equipment.[1,2]

In contrast to the rapid developments in the field of infant lung function testing during the last decade, the preschool years (approximately 3–6 years), when the child is too old to sedate, yet too young to cooperate with conventional PFTs, continued to be regarded as the dark ages of pediatric pulmonology. Accurate evaluation of respiratory function in this age group is crucial in many contexts. Children commonly present with asthma-like symptoms during this period. Although many of these children will stop having symptoms as they grow, others will continue to have asthma that persists into adult life. The treatment implications of these two clinical patterns are different, yet we are currently hampered by a lack of objective assessments to help distinguish between them. This is a particular problem when treatment with inhaled steroids is contemplated, without any objective means of measuring benefit or side effects. Such assessments would be equally valuable in children recovering from chronic neonatal lung disease and those with diseases such as cystic fibrosis (CF), who are prone to recurrent or persistent respiratory symptoms and (in the case of CF) a progressive decline of lung function during later childhood. Continuous, longitudinal assessments of pulmonary function from birth throughout early childhood in both healthy children and those with respiratory disease, whereby changes in lung volume and mechanics due to disease could be distinguished from those due to the rapid growth and development of the respiratory system during this period, would greatly facilitate understanding of the evolution and natural history of respiratory diseases and could contribute to better monitoring of current treatments and the development of more effective therapeutic interventions for use in young children.

During the last 5 years, attention has been increasingly focused on trying to adapt equipment, methods, and measurement conditions to improve the feasibility of assessing lung function in preschool children. These efforts have been met with remarkable success in that, with specially trained operators and a suitable environment, many PFTs now appear to be feasible in at least 50% of 3-year-olds and in the majority of children older than 4 years of age. Techniques that have been recently adapted for the preschool age group include spirometry, the forced oscillation technique (FOT), the interrupter technique, plethysmographic assessments of specific airway resistance (sR_{aw}), and measures of functional residual capacity (FRC) and gas-mixing efficiency using gas dilution and washout techniques. A joint ATS-ERS Task Force is working to produce recommendations for the use of these tests in preschool children that will highlight the current state of knowledge and indicate where further data are needed before definitive guidelines can be developed.[3]

"Pulmonary Function Tests in Infants and Preschool Children," by Janet Stocks: The contributor retains the copyright to her original artwork. There are no other exceptions to the copyright.

OVERVIEW

This chapter provides an overview of the following:

- Differences in assessing lung function in infants and young children compared with older, cooperative subjects
- Which tests are now feasible in infants and young children
- The limitations of applying these tests, an understanding of which is essential when reviewing the ever-increasing literature in the field or deciding whether to refer an infant or young child for lung function tests
- What has been learned from clinical and epidemiologic studies that have included infant or preschool PFTs as outcome measures
- The problems associated with interpreting results in this age group, including those related to the lack of reliable reference or repeatability data with which to separate the effects of disease from those of growth and development
- Key areas for future clinical and research applications

This chapter focuses on the most widely used PFTs for this age group, with only brief mention of applications that are limited to a few specialized research departments. Similarly, due to the complexity of the subject, only brief mention is made of applications in the intensive care unit. For simplicity, the term *infant PFTs* is used to refer to all measurements obtained in sleeping infants and young children (generally younger than 2 years of age), whereas *preschool PFTs* is used to refer to those tests used in awake young children (generally 3–6 years of age). Although some limited success has been obtained in 2- to 3-year-olds, such children are generally too old to sedate, and yet are insufficiently coordinated or cooperative to participate in most of the tests designed for awake subjects. This results in a substantially higher failure rate, with most operators preferring to defer testing until after the third birthday.

Detailed descriptions of individual techniques with respect to theory, equipment, data collection, analysis, and quality control, all of which have been described in detail previously, will not be provided. Instead, the emphasis is on the application and interpretation of these tests and their role in pediatric pulmonology. References are generally limited to those published during the last few years, with the reader directed toward representative examples, the bibliographies of which will provide a wider literature, if required.

DIFFERENCES IN ASSESSING LUNG FUNCTION IN INFANTS AND PRESCHOOL CHILDREN

INFANTS AND TODDLERS YOUNGER THAN 2 YEARS OF AGE

In addition to the marked developmental changes in respiratory physiology that occur during the first years of life and affect both the measurement and the interpretation of results, the major differences in undertaking PFTs in children younger than 2 years of age relate to sleep state, sedation, ethical issues, posture, and the need to miniaturize and adapt equipment for measurements in small subjects who cannot be asked to undertake any special breathing maneuvers and who tend to be preferential nose breathers.[4,5]

DEVELOPMENTAL CHANGES

Certain developmental changes affect the assessment of lung function in infants.

Influence of the Upper Airways

Infants are preferential nose breathers, with nasal resistance representing approximately 50% of total airway resistance. Consequently, changes in lower airway resistance as a result of disease or therapeutic interventions may be masked, especially if there has been a recent upper respiratory infection. For this reason, it is usually necessary to postpone lung function testing for at least 3 weeks after the onset of any respiratory infection. This can be disruptive to scheduling of infant lung function tests. Because the nose also acts as a very efficient filter, less aerosolized material (whether delivered as a challenge or a therapeutic intervention) may reach the lung than in a mouth-breathing adult.[5] As discussed later, the upper airways also play an important role in modulating expiratory flow and lung volume. A facemask rather than a mouthpiece is generally used in infant (and some preschool) testing. This must be taken into account when calculating apparatus dead space as well as when interpreting longitudinal changes in lung function.

Compliance of the Chest Wall and Dynamic Elevation of End-Expiratory Level

During infancy, the highly compliant chest wall results in minimal outward elastic recoil, such that during passive expiration, the lungs recoil to a much lower volume in relation to total lung capacity (TLC) than in older subjects. The potential difficulties imposed by the compliant chest wall, which include instability of FRC and the tendency for small airway closure during tidal breathing, are at least partially compensated for by the dynamic elevation of end-expiratory level, whereby infants breathe in before they reach their passively determined resting lung volume. This occurs whenever the duration of expiration is less than three expiratory time constants, in other words, in the presence of either a short expiratory time (rapid respiratory rate) or a long time constant (usually associated with elevated expiratory resistance). Because the expiratory time constant is the product of compliance and resistance, typical values in a healthy 4-kg neonate with total respiratory compliance of 40 mL•cm H_2O^{-1} and total resistance of 40 cm H_2O•L^{-1}•sec would be 0.16 seconds. In the presence of airway disease with a resistance of 80 cm H_2O•L^{-1}•sec, this time constant would double, requiring duration of expiration to be at least 0.96 seconds (i.e., a respiratory rate of less than 30/min in the presence of an inspiratory/expiratory ratio of 1:1) for complete lung emptying. By contrast, in an infant with respiratory distress syndrome in whom compliance is very low (e.g., <10 mL•cm H_2O^{-1}), the high elastic recoil and short time constant will result in rapid lung emptying and potential atelectasis. During the first months of life, infants modulate both expiratory time and flow to maintain an adequate FRC. This is mediated through tonic and phasic vagal stretch receptors that are exquisitely sensitive to changes in resting lung volume. In contrast to adults, the Hering-Breuer inflation reflex is physiologically active over the tidal range during the first year of life. The instantaneous change in breathing rate and pattern in response to small changes in resting lung volume can be seen during the application of continuous negative or positive pressure, as well as after an apneic pause. In addition to changes in respiratory rate, infants often use postinspiratory diaphragmatic and laryngeal activity to slow (or brake) expiratory flow. The latter is particularly noticeable in those with respiratory distress syndrome, who may exhibit audible grunting. Intubation removes this defense mechanism and can lead to rapid deterioration unless compensated for by an appropriate level of positive end-expiratory pressure.

Although this ability to modulate expiratory flow and timing, and hence resting lung volume, may be physiologically beneficial to the infant, it can complicate attempts to assess respiratory function. Whereas the active Hering-Breuer inflation reflex facilitates assessment of passive respiratory mechanics in infants (discussed later), the variability of end-expiratory level may impede assessment and interpretation, not only of lung volumes, but also of respiratory mechanics and forced expiratory flow (FEF), which are highly volume-dependent. As discussed later, changes in respiratory rate, expiratory time, and the emptying time of the lung with growth may all have significant effects on the interpretation of longitudinal changes in various indices, such as timed forced expired volumes.[6,7]

SLEEP STATE, SEDATION, AND DURATION OF THE TESTING PROCEDURE

Although there have been a few attempts to assess lung function in awake infants, measurements are normally limited to periods of sleep so that the infant will tolerate maneuvers such as positioning of a facemask for measurements of airflow, brief airway occlusions (for assessment of passive respiratory mechanics and plethysmographic lung volume), and application of thoracoabdominal pressure via an inflatable jacket (for forced expiratory maneuvers). If reproducible measures of resting lung volume or respiratory mechanics are to be obtained, it is essential that a representative and stable end-expiratory level be established first. To achieve this, it is usually necessary for the child to be in quiet, rather than rapid eye movement, sleep. Because the duration of these periods is inversely proportional to postconceptional age[8] and may last 10 minutes or less in a preterm infant, this can present a real challenge when undertaking measurements in very young or immature infants. Testing during the first 48 hours after delivery, although tempting due to the increased availability of the mother and infant before hospital discharge, is similarly difficult due to the instability of breathing patterns and lung mechanics during this period, as the infant adapts to extrauterine respiration.

Studies in Unsedated Infants

Unless clinically indicated, sedation is generally contraindicated for PFTs in newborn infants, but successful measurements using a full range of tests can usually be achieved during natural sleep after a feed in all infants up to at least 44 weeks postconceptional age. Tests that are primarily based on tidal breathing recordings (including the FOT and assessments of FRC and ventilation inhomogeneity by multiple-breath washout [MBW]) may also be applicable in the unsedated infant up to approximately 4 to 6 months postnatal life, whereas tests such as forced expiratory maneuvers and plethysmography generally require sedation, certainly beyond 3 months of age. Studies that can be performed without sedation are more readily acceptable to both parents and some ethics committees (discussed later). The drawback of such studies is that the range of investigations is more limited, the duration of testing is longer, and the success rate of achieving useful data is lower than in sedated infants. The rate of success will be influenced by the age of the infant and the invasiveness of the procedure, but is typically approximately 60% in both home-based and hospital studies, compared with approximately 90% for most sedated studies.

Studies in Sedated Infants

Sedation is usually achieved using oral chloral hydrate in a dose of 50 to 100 mg/kg. The hospital-specific protocol for sedation should always be followed. With the exception of a small proportion of "high-risk" children (e.g., those with known or suspected upper airway obstruction, in whom sedation is generally contraindicated due to the risk of exacerbating symptoms[8]), chloral hydrate has been shown to have an excellent safety record and has been administered to thousands of infants worldwide, without adverse side effects. Nevertheless, its action can be unpredictable, with the time taken to fall asleep after administration ranging from 15 minutes to more than 2 hours. The duration of subsequent induced sleep can be equally variable, such that the operators rarely have longer than 45 minutes in which to collect all of the required measurements. Furthermore, the bitter taste of this agent is not appreciated by the recipients, who may object loudly, making this the most stressful aspect of infant lung function testing for infants and their parents and the major reason why parental consent to participate in research studies requiring repeated measurements is withheld. Caution with respect to repeated sedation also limits the frequency with which serial measurements can be undertaken, potentially limiting their clinical usefulness in individual infants, as discussed later.

The need to administer sedation may limit the extent to which healthy infants can be recruited for the establishment of reference data or as control subjects. Some research ethics committees will not give approval for healthy children to be recruited for studies that require sedation, but others consider it unethical to apply these tests to infants with respiratory disease unless results can be properly interpreted, after all other factors that determine lung function, such as age, sex, and body size, are taken into account. Such committees consider the study of healthy infants perfectly acceptable, provided all necessary safety measures are observed. Further discussions of ethical issues relating to lung function testing in infancy have been reported previously.[8,9]

Total Duration of the Testing Procedure

Given the time required to obtain informed parental consent and for the infant to fall asleep, the testing procedure may last up to 4 hours and is commonly at least 2 hours after the child has arrived in the department, which may limit the parents' ability or willingness to attend if repeat measurements are scheduled at intervals of less than every 4 to 6 months. The relatively short time that an infant spends asleep, with or without sedation, means that important decisions have to be made regarding which respiratory function test or tests should be used on any particular occasion. In the past, regrettably, such decisions have often been based primarily on what equipment happened to be available within any given center, without due consideration of the underlying pathophysiology, clinical question, or hypothesis that was being investigated. This, in turn, has led to many inconclusive or contradictory reports in the literature.

POSTURE

During infancy, most PFTs are obtained in the supine position, which will influence not only the position of the diaphragm and efficiency of the respiratory musculature, but also the FRC, lung mechanics, and distribution of ventilation. Such changes must be taken into account when interpreting results, particularly when reporting longitudinal changes in lung function within individuals. The high compliance of the upper airways in infants and the ease with which upper airway obstruction can occur must continually be borne in mind. Hence, throughout the testing procedure, the neck or shoulders should be supported in the midline in slight extension, with the position stabilized by a neck roll or head ring, and no depression of the jaw or upper airway obstruction during placement of the facemask. The latter is particularly important during assessments of plethysmographic airway resistance, when the weight of recording equipment must be adequately supported, and during tests such as the raised volume technique, when firm pressure on the facemask may be required to eliminate air leaks under conditions of elevated airway pressure (discussed later).

SAFETY ISSUES

For all studies involving infants, strict safety precautions must be followed. Resuscitation equipment, including suction, must be available, and two skilled operators, fully trained in basic life support, one of whom has prime responsibility for monitoring the well-being of the infant, must be present. Pulse oximetry is usually used for continuous monitoring throughout the testing session.

EQUIPMENT REQUIREMENTS

One of the greatest difficulties in assessing respiratory function in infancy and early childhood has been that of obtaining suitable equipment. Until recently, a lack of commercially available, well-validated systems meant that most research establishments used their own custom-built equipment and software. While facilitating high standards within such centers, this impeded not only training, but also attempts to establish multicenter trials or any meaningful comparison of results between different centers. As a result of close collaboration between scientists and manufacturers, led by the ERS-ATS Task Force, together with technologic advances in terms of improved frequency response, miniaturization of equipment, and increasingly sophisticated software, facilities for performing infant PFTs are no longer limited to specialized research establishments. The series of manuscripts published by the ERS-ATS Task Force[1,10–14] provides some guidance and recommendations to both users and manufacturers regarding suitable specifications for infant lung function equipment, although these will need constant review and update. Users and potential purchasers of such equipment should ensure not only that it meets the basic requirements specified by the ERS-ATS Task Force with respect to characteristics such as dead space, resistance, frequency response, and ease with which it can be dismantled for cleaning between every subject studied, but also that its use is limited to the range of body size and measurement conditions specified by the manufacturer, as previously validated. Of particular note is that much of the commercially available equipment has not yet been validated for use either in preterm infants or in those receiving assisted ventilation. Frequent calibration checks, regular maintenance of equipment, including validation of calibration tools, and a good supply of spare parts are even more essential when assessing infants than when testing older subjects, given the time-consuming nature of these investigations and the impossibility of repeating the measurements in the event of equipment failure or error in this age group.

LEAKS AND DEAD SPACE

The fact that infants must be studied using an oronasal mask rather than a mouthpiece may introduce both physiologic problems, in that the relatively large apparatus dead space may cause changes in the end-expiratory level, and technical problems, in that it may be difficult to estimate the true effective dead space of the mask (i.e., that which is not occupied by the child's face during use and must therefore be subtracted from the total measured volume to calculate FRC). In the past, such errors may have contributed to the variability of FRC results reported from different laboratories or with different techniques.[15] Of even greater importance is the potential influence of leaks around the facemask, which can be difficult to identify and are the most common source of error when undertaking infant PFTs. Although these are most likely to occur during tests that require airway occlusion or administration of positive airway pressure (e.g., plethysmography, occlusion techniques, and the raised volume technique), they also invalidate all other assessments, including FRC by gas dilution and tidal breathing parameters. Many centers use therapeutic putty to create an airtight seal between face and mask (Fig. 9-1), whereas others depend on an air-filled, cushioned mask, particularly in very young and unsedated infants. Whatever the approach, operators must be vigilant at all times if serious errors caused by leakage are to be avoided. Warning signs of such leakages include low tidal volume (V_T; with volumes <6 mL/kg being very rare when an infant is breathing through a mask and a pneumotachometer [PNT], unless the child is very tachypneic), a drift of the V_T signal wherein expiratory volume is less than that inspired through the flowmeter, or failure of the end-expiratory level to return to baseline after a brief airway occlusion (Fig. 9-2).

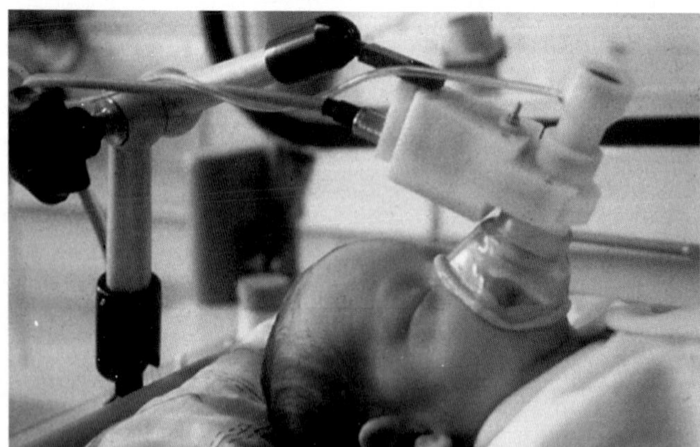

FIGURE 9-1. Infant lung function tests using a facemask and a pneumotachometer. Note the use of a ring of silicone putty to create an airtight seal during the recordings. (Copyright © VIASYS Healthcare Gmb H.)

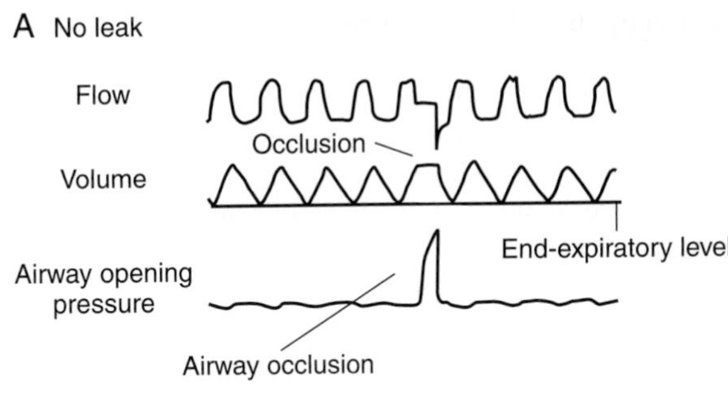

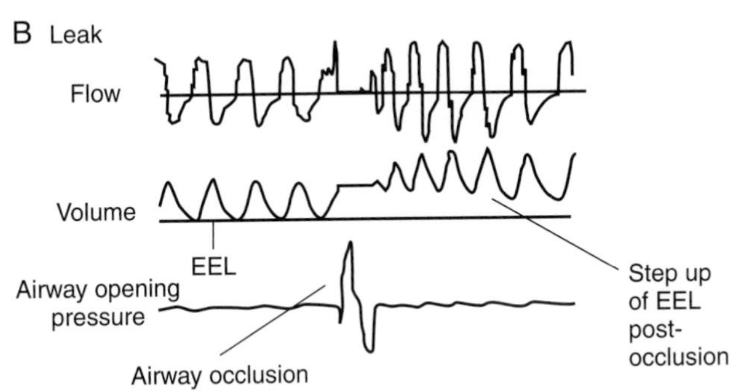

FIGURE 9-2. Occlusion test to check for leaks around the facemask. Time-based recording of flow, volume, and pressure at the airway opening during spontaneous tidal breathing. **A,** When there is no leak through or around the facemask, there will be a period a zero flow during a brief airway occlusion, and a stable end-expiratory level, as seen from a tidal volume trace, will be maintained after release of the occlusion. **B,** By contrast, if air escapes around the side of the mask during such an occlusion, there will be a step-up of the end-expiratory level (EEL), as shown here. (Copyright © Janet Stocks.)

PRESCHOOL CHILDREN

Assessment of preschool children presents a number of special challenges. Such children are generally too old to sedate for lung function testing, and they may not have the necessary coordination or concentration to perform many of the physiologic maneuvers required for lung function tests used in older subjects. They also have a short attention span and are easily distracted and thus need to be engaged and encouraged by the operator to participate in the test. Although measurement conditions for testing preschool children are broadly similar to those required for older subjects, every effort should be made to make the environment as child-friendly (and safe!) as possible. This includes provision of suitable furniture, games, and wall coverings as well as adaptation of the normal lung function terminology, with terms such as *blowing games* and *puffing playrooms* replacing the more familiar *spirometry* and *lung function lab.*

To this end, the most important acquisition for any preschool setup is personnel with suitable temperaments (i.e., a love of children, infinite patience and stamina, and a good sense of humor). Adaptability, meticulous attention to detail, and a thorough background in respiratory physiology are also essential requirements because appropriate criteria for acceptable tests in the preschool child may differ markedly from those established for older subjects.[16] The criterion for a successful preschool session should be not so much that valid respiratory function results have been obtained, but that the child (and the parents) want to return for subsequent visits. Because young children tire easily, visits should be timed carefully (i.e., preferably in the morning or early afternoon, but not coinciding with the time of a regular nap) to maximize success. The emotional and developmental stage of the child will be an important determinant of the child's success with PFTs, with this influence being greatest in tests that require more active cooperation from the child, such as spirometry. The child's medical history may also be highly relevant. Those delivered extremely prematurely or with extended hospital stays during the neonatal period may display considerable antipathy toward hospital environments in general as well as to electronic equipment or facial attachments. Such children will need particular understanding, and it may be helpful to send the parents home with equipment such as a mask, tubing, or mouthpieces with which to familiarize the child before subsequent appointments are arranged. The need to gain the child's confidence, provide coaching in the various techniques and maneuvers, and allow time for rest or games between the different PFTs when necessary means that plenty of time should be set aside for preschool PFTs, particularly when testing those younger than 4 years of age or those who are attending for the first time. The use of computer games and appropriate incentives to help the child understand what is required during special maneuvers, such as forced expirations, can be extremely helpful,[16] whereas encouragement to sit quietly during more prolonged periods of data collection (such as when using the MBW technique to assess gas-mixing efficiency) can be provided by the opportunity to watch a favorite video. The choice of such videos, however, must be considered carefully. Those that lead to overt laughter, breath-holding, or vocal participation are not conducive to high-quality PFTs!

In contrast to the situation when lung function tests were first adapted for infants, commercial equipment is available for most preschool tests, albeit not specifically designed for this age group. The potential effects of using equipment developed for older and larger individuals, particularly with respect to dead space and resistance, needs to be considered. Adaptations of both hardware and software will be necessary in the near future if the use of such equipment is to be optimized in very young children, and a joint ATS-ERS Task Force is currently working to produce preliminary recommendations in this field.[3]

ANTHROPOMETRY AND BACKGROUND DETAILS

Given the rapid rate of somatic growth during infancy and early childhood, accurate measurements of height and weight using a calibrated stadiometer and scales are essential. Two trained operators are required to obtain valid measurements in infants, and these procedures can be equally challenging in lively preschoolers. For accurate interpretation of lung function tests, it is also essential to record data on environmental, genetic, and socioeconomic factors that are likely to affect lung growth, including sex; ethnic group; family history of asthma and atopy; cigarette smoke exposure, both prenatal and postnatal; allergen exposure, including pets; relevant current and past medical history; and medication use.

METHODS OF ASSESSING PULMONARY FUNCTION IN INFANTS AND YOUNG CHILDREN

The emphasis placed on the assessment of airway function during early life, using techniques to assess airway or respiratory resistance and forced expired maneuvers, reflects the fact that wheezing disorders of either a transient or persistent nature dominate most of the respiratory problems encountered in infants and young children beyond the neonatal period. Nevertheless, there is increasing awareness that these measurements are determined not only by the caliber of the airways, but also by the compliance of the airway wall and the elastic recoil of the surrounding parenchyma, leading to the search for suitable parameters that will reflect these characteristics and hence improve the interpretation of results.

An ideal lung function test for infants and young children would be one that meets the following criteria:

- It is acceptable both to the child and the parents
- It is applicable to any age and arousal state
- It is independent of subject cooperation
- It is simple and involving no risk
- It is reproducible
- It is sensitive enough to distinguish between health and disease
- It is able to reflect the clinical situation or provide accurate and specific information about the structure and function of the lungs

No such test currently exists, and even if it did, no single test is ever likely to provide all of the necessary information for a clinical or research study. Nevertheless, there are a wide variety of techniques now available for measuring lung volume, respiratory mechanics, ventilation inhomogeneity, and the control of breathing. Details of most of the commonly used infant PFTs have been summarized previously,[1,4,10–14,17] whereas those relating to preschool tests have been emerging at an increasing rate during the last few years.[3] As summarized in Table 9-1, some of these tests can be applied to both age groups, whereas others are applicable only in a sleeping infant or a relatively cooperative preschool child.

When designing a protocol for assessing lung function in either clinical or research studies, it is vital to consider not only which combination of tests is most appropriate to address the underlying question, but also the order in which these should be performed. Given the potential effect of lung inflations or deep inspirations on underlying respiratory mechanics, it is generally advisable to undertake tests based on tidal breathing recordings (including those used to measure resting lung volume, gas trapping, ventilation inhomogeneity, and respiratory mechanics) before any forced expiratory maneuvers. This can present difficulties when the primary outcome measures are derived from forced expiratory maneuvers, which therefore must take precedence in any protocol. It is particularly important to consider what is feasible in the time available. Although this is largely dictated by the duration of the sleep period in infants and that of concentration and cooperation in preschoolers, it is also dependent on the age and clinical status of the subject and, very importantly, the expertise of the operators. Hence, when setting up new facilities for either infant or preschool testing, it is wise to commence with a relatively simple baseline protocol that can be successfully completed in the majority of subjects, and then to gradually introduce new techniques or interventions as expertise and confidence develop.

ASSESSMENT OF LUNG VOLUME AND VENTILATION

Many of the techniques for measuring lung volume in older children and adults have been successfully adapted for use in infants and young children. Because infants cannot be

TABLE 9-1. Feasibility of various pulmonary function tests in children of different ages

Measurement Conditions	Infant and Toddlers* (0–2 yr)	Preschool Children (3–6 yr)	Children (6–18 yr)
	Sleeping, with or without sedation	Awake, with some active cooperation possible	Awake, with full cooperation
Technique			
Tidal breathing parameters	✓	✓	✓
Plethysmographic FRC	✓	×	✓
Plethysmographic TLC, RV, etc.	Specialized laboratory only	×	✓
FRC by gas dilution or multiple-breath washout (MBW)	✓	✓	✓
Gas-mixing efficiency by MBW	✓	✓	✓
Plethysmographic R_{aw}	If a heated rebreathing system is available	×	✓
Plethysmographic sR_{aw}	(✓)	✓	✓
Occlusion technique: respiratory mechanics (R_{rs}, C_{rs}, time constant)	✓	×	×
Interrupter technique (R_{int})	(✓) not yet validated	✓	✓ (but rarely used)
Forced oscillation (Z_{rs})	✓	✓	✓
Forced expiratory maneuvers using tidal or RVRTC	✓	×	×
Voluntary forced expiratory maneuvers (i.e., spirometry)	×	✓	✓

*The suggested age range provides a rough indication only, and feasibility will depend on the developmental as well as the chronologic age of the child. Some tests, such as specific airway resistance or interrupter resistance, may be feasible in children between 2 and 3 years of age, but the success rate is generally much lower than in those older than 3 years of age.

C_{rs}, compliance of the total respiratory system; FRC, functional residual capacity; R_{aw}, airway resistance; R_{int}, interrupter resistance; R_{rs}, respiratory resistance; RV, residual volume; RVRTC, raised volume rapid thoracoabdominal compression; sR_{aw}, specific airway resistance; TLC, total lung capacity; Z_{rs}, impedance of the respiratory system.

instructed to undertake special breathing maneuvers, lung volume measurements in this age group have primarily been those that can be undertaken during tidal breathing (i.e., FRC using either plethysmographic or gas dilution/washout techniques). In recent years, it has also become possible to obtain measurements over the full range of lung volume in specialized centers, using what has become known as the *raised volume technique*.[18]

Introduction

As in older subjects, measurement of lung volume may be essential for accurate interpretation of volume-dependent pulmonary mechanics, such as lung compliance, resistance, or FEF, as well as for defining normal lung growth. It must, however, be remembered that current methods of assessing lung volume provide only a global measure of total volume and provide no information on the number and size of alveoli or the surface area available for gas exchange, which may be critical when investigating the effects of preterm delivery or prenatal and postnatal interventions on subsequent lung growth. Furthermore, potential evidence of congenital lung hypoplasia from lung volume measurements may be masked by the ability of the lung to expand rapidly to fill the available space, as, for example, after surgical repair of congenital diaphragmatic hernia. Whereas a low TLC is the primary criterion for diagnosis in older children, lung volume assessments in preschool children and infants are usually limited to FRC, which may limit their diagnostic value. Reduced lung volume due to restrictive lung disease may be found in children with rare lung conditions, such as fibrosing alveolitis or hypoplasia, but this pattern is more common in children with disorders affecting the chest wall, such as scoliosis, pectus excavatum, or myopathy, or in those with surfactant deficiency or atelectasis due to conditions such as respiratory distress syndrome or chronic lung disease of infancy. The most common abnormality of lung volume during infancy is that associated with airway obstruction, wherein both hyperinflation (due to dynamic elevation of lung volume in the presence of elevated airway resistance and a long expiratory time constant) and gas trapping (due to peripheral airway closure) result in elevated FRC values in wheezy infants and those with diseases such as CF. The ability to detect such hyperinflation will depend on both the underlying pathophysiology and the measurement technique selected. One of the greatest potential uses for lung volume measurements is with respect to optimizing ventilator and continuous positive airway pressure settings in infants and children requiring ventilatory support. Although there is growing interest and research activity in this field, considerable technologic difficulties must be overcome before such measures are likely to influence the clinical management of individual children (discussed later).

Tidal Breathing Parameters

Measurement of tidal breathing is fundamental to many of the PFTs that can be applied during infancy and early childhood. Requirements for noninvasive methods of assessing lung function during natural sleep or prolonged periods of monitoring have resulted in persistent efforts to analyze tidal breathing parameters, whether derived from changes in flow and volume at the airway opening or from body surface measurements. Although superficially appearing to be one of the simplest investigations to undertake, such measurements and their interpretation are in fact highly complex,[10] and it is therefore important to have a basic appreciation of the numerous factors that may influence these recordings. Tidal breathing parameters have been used in both clinical and research settings:

- To determine VT and breathing frequency
- To determine minute ventilation
- To investigate the control of breathing
- To establish regularity of breathing patterns before assessments of lung volume and mechanics
- As an integral part of sleep staging
- In combination with clinical information
- In combination with monitoring of CO_2, O_2, exhaled nitric oxide, and SaO_2
- As an indirect measure of airway mechanics
- To trigger equipment

Patterns of tidal flow-volume loops can yield potentially important information about the likely site of obstruction (Fig. 9-3). Peripheral airway narrowing generally produces a concave pattern of the expiratory flow-volume loop, with peak tidal flow occurring early in expiration. This pattern probably reflects a reduction in postinspiratory diaphragmatic or laryngeal braking (which, in health, normally slows lung emptying) in the presence of a prolonged expiratory time constant due to elevated airway resistance. Flattening of the expiratory limb is suggestive of a fixed extrathoracic airway obstruction, whereas marked convexity of the volume axis may reflect physiologic braking of expiratory flow. A pattern of inspiratory fluttering may be associated with laryngomalacia, whereas stiff lungs (low

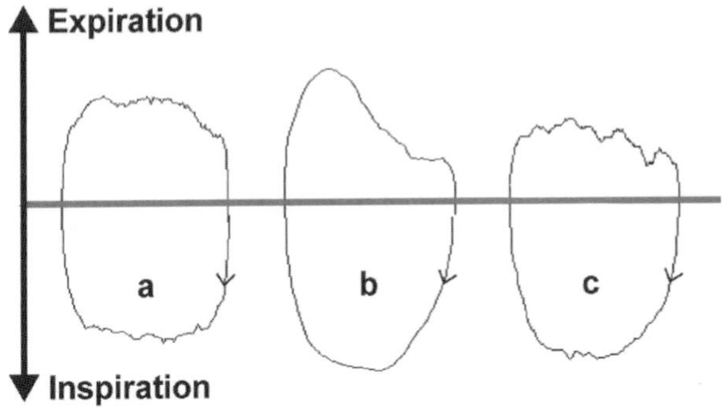

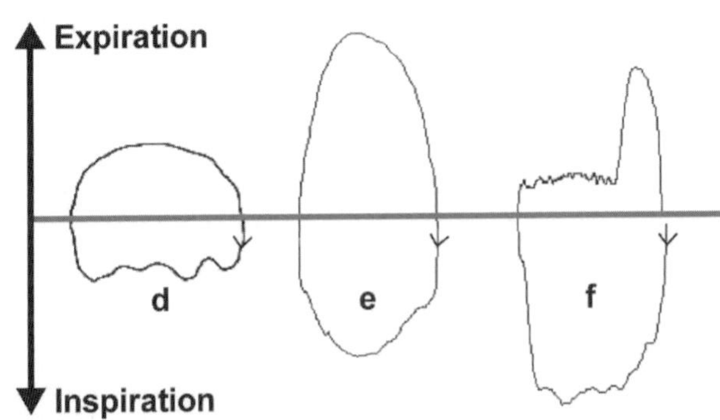

FIGURE 9-3. Patterns of tidal flow-volume loops. Normal *(a)*; flow limitation or airway obstruction *(b)*; laryngeal braking or fixed intrathoracic obstruction *(c)*; fixed extrathoracic obstruction *(d)*; reduced compliance (i.e., rapid lung emptying due to stiff lungs or increased elastic recoil) *(e)*. Marked expiratory grunting may occur in the presence of decreased functional residual capacity or stiff lungs to increase the expiratory time constant *(f)*. (Copyright © Janet Stocks.)

compliance and high elastic recoil) may be reflected by a relatively small VT, with high peak flow and rapid lung emptying. Considerable caution is required when interpreting such loops due to natural physiologic variability, particularly during early infancy. Attempts to quantify such patterns have resulted in numeric descriptors of the tidal flow pattern, such as the time to peak tidal expiratory flow as a ratio of total expiratory time (t_{PTEF}:t_E) [Fig. 9-4]. This index, which is sometimes referred to as the *tidal breathing ratio,* may be reduced in the presence of airway obstruction and has been shown to be a valuable outcome measure in various epidemiologic studies investigating early determinants of airway function.[19–23] However, this measurement is only distantly related to airway function and, as with most tidal breathing parameters, it conveys mixed information on the interaction between control of breathing and airway mechanics, thereby requiring cautious interpretation, especially within individual infants and children.[24]

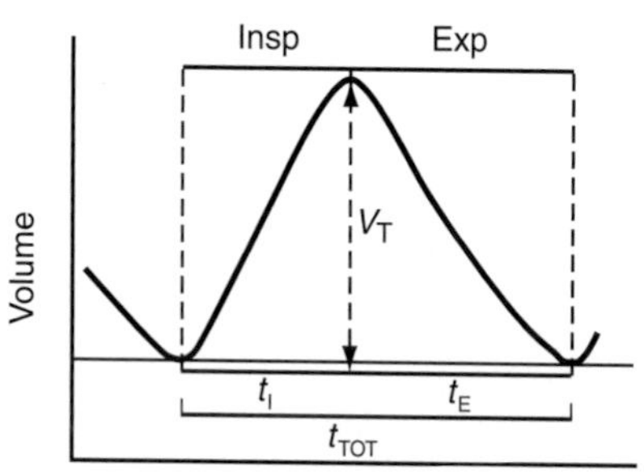

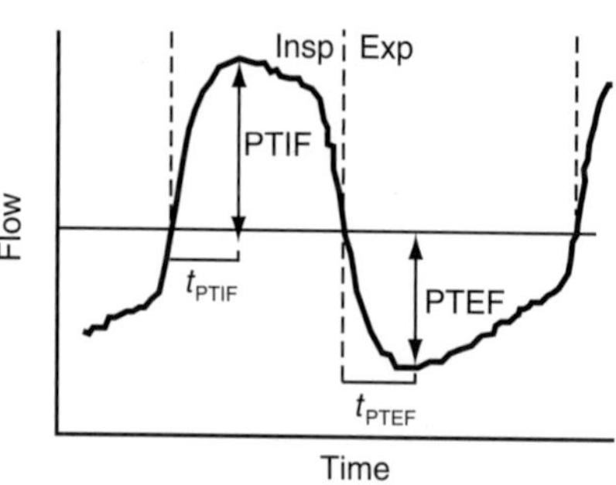

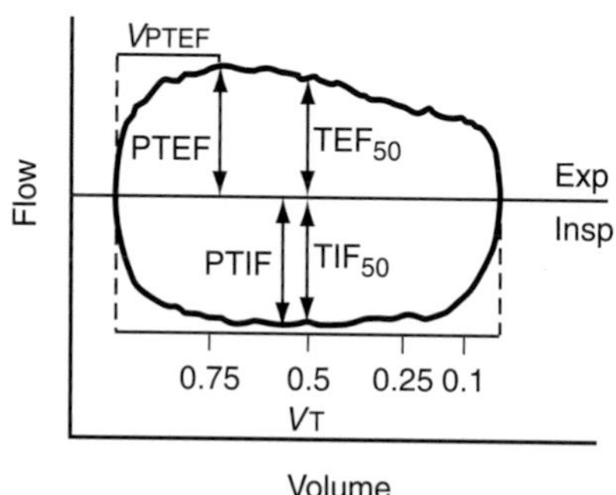

■ **FIGURE 9-4.** **A–C,** Tidal breathing parameters. In addition to tidal volume (VT) and respiratory rate, the following parameters are often calculated from recordings of tidal breathing: tidal expiratory (Exp) and inspiratory (Insp) flow when 50% VT remains in the lung (TEF_{50} and TIF_{50}, respectively); inspiratory time (t_I); expiratory time (t_E); total breath time (t_{TOT}); peak tidal inspiratory flow (PTIF); peak tidal expiratory flow (PTEF); time to peak expiratory flow (t_{PTEF}); time to peak inspiratory flow (t_{PTIF}); volume expired before PTEF is attained (V_{PTEF}); and tidal breathing ratio (t_{PTEF}:t_E). (Copyright © Janet Stocks.)

Equipment and Procedure

Various types of flowmeters (including pneumotachometers and, more recently, ultrasonic flowmeters) have been used to measure tidal flow in infants and preschool children. Each has its specific measurement principles, particularly with respect to the physical properties of the apparatus, and a specific measurement range. Physical properties of the flowmeter, together with apparatus resistance and dead space (including that of the facemask), can have a marked influence on tidal breathing parameters. Standardized measurement conditions are crucial in the assessment of tidal breathing parameters in infants. The pattern of tidal breathing will vary according to body and neck position and sleep state, as well as facial attachments, such as the mask. Similarly, technical factors (such as recording conditions; length of the data set; sampling rate and resolution; drifts; compensation to body temperature, pressure, saturated [BTPS] conditions; and signal-to-noise ratio) will all influence the accuracy of the tidal breathing parameters. When such measurements are taken, a recording period of at least 30 to 60 seconds (minimum of 20 breaths) is recommended, together with a robust algorithm for accurate breath detection.

Commercially available systems that have been developed and released for use in infants during the last 5 years generally adhere to recommended standards, and many have automated signal quality control measures, but this is not necessarily the case for older systems.[25] For those undertaking such measurements in preschool children, the potential influence of apparatus dead space and the relatively small signal-to-noise ratio when using equipment originally designed for much larger subjects must be taken into account. The most common factors that distort tidal breathing measurements are air leaks around the mask or mouthpiece, upper airway artifacts (head position) that lead to snoring or extrathoracic airway obstruction, secretions, and laryngeal braking. Sighs can significantly influence control of breathing and tidal waveform analysis, particularly in preterm and newborn infants.

Calculation and Reporting of Results

Tidal flow and volume waveforms can be described using time-based VT or tidal flow signals and the flow-volume loop. Apart from VT and respiratory rate, the most commonly reported parameters are illustrated in Figure 9-4.

Advantages and Limitations

The greatest advantage of undertaking tidal breath analysis during early life is undoubtedly the noninvasive nature of these recordings. Balanced against this is the fact that it is extremely difficult to record baseline values of tidal breathing when using any system that requires facial attachments, whereas attempts to use body surface measurements have met with limited success, except in large epidemiologic studies. In health, the pattern of tidal breathing is highly variable, and although assessments have been performed in awake, newborn infants, repeatable measures normally require that infants be in quiet sleep, by which time they are also likely to tolerate more direct measures of pulmonary function. In awake, preschool children, such problems may be even more marked. However, as discussed later, once the child is quiet and a reasonably regular pattern of breathing has been established, several other tests, including plethysmographic specific airway resistance and assessments of lung volume and ventilation inhomogeneity using MBW, can be performed almost as easily as simple tidal breathing recordings and are almost certainly more informative.

After initial reports in the 1980s regarding the potential value of t_{PTEF}:t_E in predicting subsequent wheezing in previously healthy infants,[22] a plethora of studies in both infants and preschool children used this simple index as an outcome variable. A review of the resultant literature reveals that, when used in large epidemiologic studies, significant group changes in t_{PTEF}:t_E can be observed, for example, in newborn infants after exposure to maternal smoking and in those most likely to have subsequent wheezing disorders, but that the clinical usefulness of this approach within individuals is limited by the marked within- and between-subject variability of breathing patterns, which is also strongly age-dependent. Even within epidemiologic studies, the discriminative ability of indices such as t_{PTEF}:t_E appears to diminish with increasing age.[4,23,24,26,27] Among infants and young children with CF, respiratory rate has been found to be elevated, but there were no differences in t_{PTEF}:t_E compared with healthy control subjects.[28] This illustrates the important, and often forgotten, principle that techniques that are eminently suited to studying large groups to derive information of potential mechanistic importance may be too variable to monitor individual children reliably. Nevertheless, careful recording of representative tidal breathing patterns may play a vital role in the interpretation of all other lung function tests.

Future Directions

Despite the problems discussed earlier, the potential for noninvasive methods, such as those that can be measured during tidal breathing in unsedated infants, has inspired several groups to continue the search for improved methods of analyzing and reporting such data. Fast Fourier transform of the recorded signals from the time to frequency domain has been used to quantify the harmonic content of the entire tidal flow waveform rather than depending on indices derived from a limited number of points.[29] This potentially exciting approach has recently been applied to flow-volume measurements derived from respiratory inductance plethysmography in spontaneously breathing preterm infants.[30] Given the nonintrusive nature of body surface measurements, this is an important area for future investigations. The potential limitations of deriving either qualitative or quantitative assessments of flow and volume from body surface recordings, particularly in the presence of marked asynchrony between chest wall and abdominal movements must, however, be borne in mind when attempting such measurements.

Electrical impedance tomography (EIT) is a rapidly developing technology that permits visualization of the spatial distribution of ventilation and hence any functional regional inhomogeneity. The basic principles of EIT have been described recently.[31] Briefly, EIT takes advantage of differences in conductance of electricity by different biologic tissues. The resistivity of lung tissue is approximately five times greater than that of most other soft tissues in the thorax, and it increases considerably when air moves into the alveoli during inspiration and the electrical current must flow around them. High-frequency, low-amplitude currents are passed between pairs of electrodes on the body, and the potentials between all of the other pairs of electrodes are simultaneously measured. The ratio of the potentials to the applied current are transfer impedances, with the EIT images being reconstructed from a set of transfer impedance measurements. Serial measurements using EIT in ventilated infants have been able to identify the redistribution of lung ventilation and changes in the magnitude of regional ventilation in response to alterations in ventilator settings, surfactant instillation, and changes in posture.[32,33] Several EIT systems have been described for thoracic imaging, although none is yet available commercially and analytic methods are still being developed. Provided further adaptations of hardware and software can be implemented to improve practical handling and facilitate stable and undisturbed measurements in the intensive care unit, this noninvasive method could become a useful bedside monitoring tool of regional lung ventilation in critically ill infants, with important implications for optimizing lung volume and minimizing lung injury.

The need to assess gas exchange and control of breathing when evaluating infants with respiratory disease, particularly those delivered prematurely or requiring ventilatory support, has been recognized in several recent publications.[34–37] Similarly, despite recognized difficulties in accurately interpreting measures of exhaled nitric oxide as a noninvasive marker of airway inflammation in infants due to the influence of nasal breathing and the marked flow dependency of such measures, there have been some interesting reports describing their potential utility in both clinical and epidemiologic studies that warrant further investigation.[38,39] Although further refinement and standardization of the technique is required, bedside equipment for evaluation of such markers is now available for use in infants and preschool children. As with such measurements in older children and adults, their clinical role has yet to be defined.

PLETHYSMOGRAPHIC ASSESSMENTS OF FUNCTIONAL RESIDUAL CAPACITY

Infants

The principles of plethysmography are identical for infants and older subjects (Fig. 9-5). Plethysmographic measurements of lung volume, which assess total thoracic gas volume at FRC, including any gas trapped behind closed airways, are well established in infants[14,18] and have been used in both clinical[40,41] and epidemiologic research.[27] Although several centers still employ their own custom-built equipment, gradual refinement of both the technique and the equipment has led to the release of commercially available equipment that is suitable for both clinical and research studies and that allows rapid access to the child, remote control of the shutter for airway occlusion, and an adequate frequency response and signal-to-noise ratio (at least for infants weighing more than 3–4 kg). It is now generally recommended that airway occlusion for FRC in infants be performed at end inspiration, with subsequent subtraction of the inspired VT. This has been found to be less disturbing to the infant, to cause less glottic closure, and to facilitate improved equilibration of pressures throughout the respiratory system compared with occlusion performed at end expiration. Critical quality control issues during data collection and analysis have been reported[15] and include the need to ensure adequate thermal equilibration of the box before the start of data recording, a stable end-expiratory level before and after the occlusion, absence of any

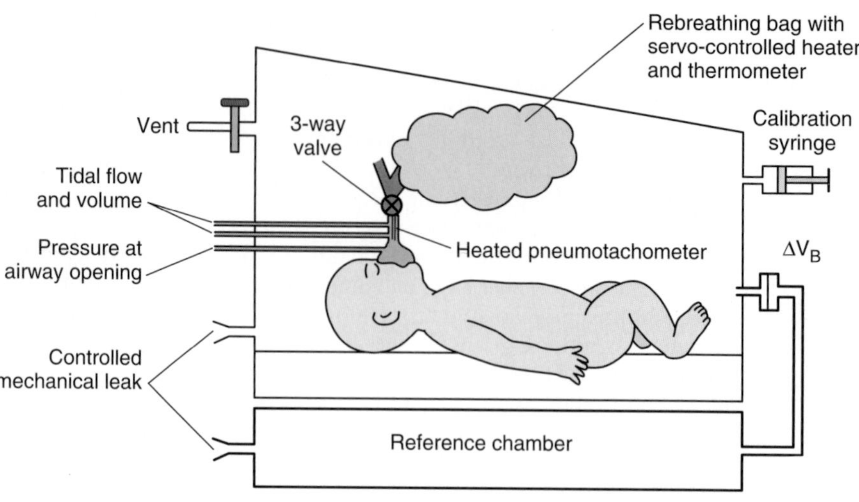

■ **FIGURE 9-5.** Infant plethysmography. Measurements of plethysmographic functional residual capacity are made while the infant sleeps within the plethysmograph and makes respiratory efforts against a closed shutter. Provision of a heated rebreathing bag or other means of compensating for changes in the temperature and humidity of respired gas allows simultaneous assessment of airway resistance. ΔV_B, changes in box volume. (Adapted from Stocks J, Sly PD, Tepper RS, Morgan WJ: Infant Respiratory Function Testing. New York: John Wiley & Sons, 1996, pp 1–577.)

air leak, and no phase lag (i.e., no looping on the X-Y plot) between the box and mouth pressure signals during the occlusion (Fig. 9-6). The shutter is usually closed for 6 to 10 seconds, or until at least two complete respiratory efforts have been made. The maneuver should be repeated until three to five technically satisfactory occlusions have been performed, with the mean and standard deviation (SD) FRC reported as the child's result. Such data can usually be obtained within 5 minutes. The coefficient of variation (100 × SD/mean) from three to five runs is, on average, less than 4% (range, 1%–10%).

Advantages and Limitations

The major disadvantages of infant plethysmographic measurements are the following:

- The equipment is expensive, relatively bulky, and not suitable for bedside assessments.
- Current commercially available plethysmographs have not been validated for use in infants weighing less than 3 kg.
- As in adults, overestimation of FRC may occur in the presence of severe airway obstruction.
- Published reference data may not be applicable for recently released commercially available equipment.[15]

The main advantages of infant plethysmography are the following:

- The rapidity and reproducibility with which measurements can be attained.
- That all gas within the lungs, including that in nonventilating or slowly ventilating areas, is measured. Paired measurements of FRC using both gas dilution and plethysmographic techniques may be useful in detecting the presence of nonventilating or poorly ventilating areas.

Preschool Children

Although there has been considerable success in obtaining plethysmographic measurements of specific airway resistance in preschool children (discussed later), such children are not generally amenable to panting against a closed shutter. FRC measurements in 3- to 5-year-olds are thus generally limited to those that can be obtained using one of the gas dilution or washout techniques, as described later.

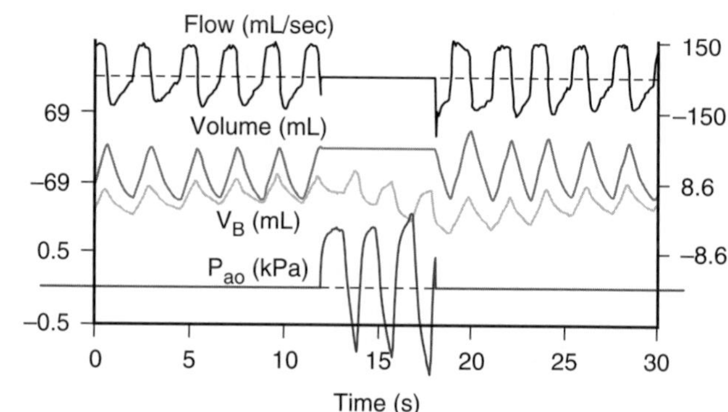

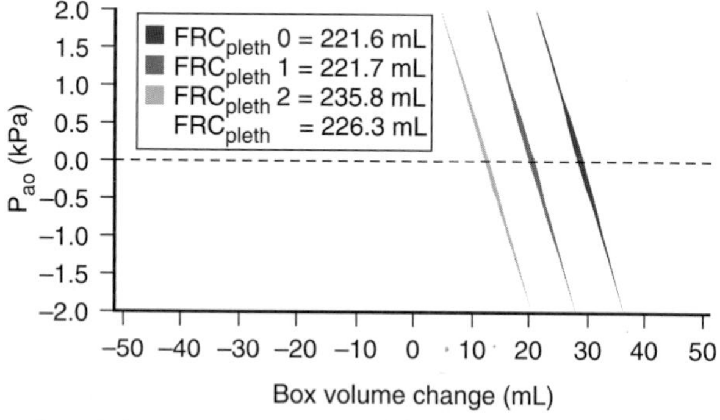

■ **FIGURE 9-6.** Criteria for technically acceptable measurements of plethysmographic functional residual capacity (FRC_{pleth}). **A,** Time-based trace of flow, tidal volume, box volume, and pressure at the airway opening before, during, and after shutter closure for measurement. As can be seen from the tidal volume trace, the shutter was closed at end inspiration. The infant made three respiratory efforts against the occlusion before shutter release. Note zero flow during the occlusion and stability of the tidal volume trace postocclusion, indicating absence of any leak. **B,** X-Y plot of pressure changes at the airway opening (P_{ao}) versus changes in box volume, which are used to calculate FRC. The slopes represent the three respiratory efforts against the shutter during a single occlusion, with FRC for that occlusion being reported as the mean of these efforts. Note the good phase relationship (no looping) between changes in box volume and P_{ao}. kPa, kilopascals; V_B, box volume signal. (Copyright © Janet Stocks.)

FUNCTIONAL RESIDUAL CAPACITY USING GAS DILUTION OR WASHOUT TECHNIQUES

Gas dilution techniques determine FRC by measuring areas of the lung that readily communicate with the central airways during tidal breathing. Apart from the differing measurement conditions discussed earlier and the need to miniaturize the equipment, methods of assessing FRC by gas dilution or washout are much the same in infants and preschool children as in older subjects. Full details of equipment specifications and techniques for performing these measurements in infants have been published previously.[13] Although closed circuit helium dilution has been widely used in the past, there are difficulties in reducing the circuit size sufficiently for use in infants, as well as challenges posed when an attempt is made to maintain a constant volume in the face of varying oxygen consumption and CO_2 production. Consequently, there has been increasing emphasis on the use of washout techniques in infants and young children, using either the bias flow nitrogen washout technique, which is based on a mixing chamber technique or, more recently, MBW (Fig. 9-7). The latter measures breath-to-breath changes in the concentration of an inert gas during the washout process and provides information on both lung volume and ventilation distribution.[42,43] Currently, there is no commercially available equipment to measure FRC in infants using either helium dilution or the mixing chamber technique. Among preschool children, equipment designed for older subjects can often be adapted, provided care is taken to minimize dead space of the circuitry.

Multiple-Breath Inert Gas Washout

The MBW test was introduced in the 1950s for measuring lung volume (FRC) and assessing overall ventilation inhomogeneity. It is generally performed during tidal breathing. The original test was the N_2 MBW test, using 100% O_2 for the washout. Although this is a valuable and simple technique for use in preschool and older children, the use of 100% O_2 may alter tidal breathing patterns in young infants and is therefore less suitable in this age group, particularly if measures of ventilation inhomogeneity are required. A wide range of alternative nonresident inert gases, including helium, argon, and sulfur-hexafluoride (SF_6), may be used as the tracer gas, with a range of appropriate devices, such as the catharometer, emission spectrometer, ultrasonic flowmeter (Fig. 9-8), or respiratory mass spectrometer (Fig. 9-9), being used to measure instantaneous gas concentrations.

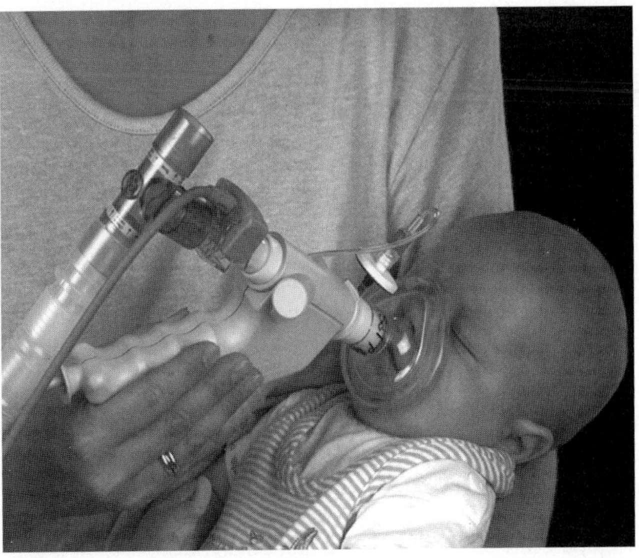

FIGURE 9-8. Multiple-breath inert gas washout in an infant using an ultrasonic flowmeter. (From Hammer J, Eber E: Paediatric Pulmonary Function Testing. Progress in Respiratory Research, Vol. 33. Basel: S. Karger AG, 2005. Permission granted by S. Karger AG, Basel.)

Methodologic Considerations

The MBW technique simply requires the child to breathe tidally through a facemask or mouthpiece attached to a flowmeter and gas analyzer and is therefore eminently suitable for both infants and preschool children. When an inert tracer gas is used, the subject initially rebreathes a gas mixture containing, for example, 4% SF_6 via a bias flow set to exceed the peak inspiratory flow. Wash-in continues until gas concentrations have equilibrated throughout the lung, as indicated by identical concentrations of the tracer gas throughout inspiration and expiration.

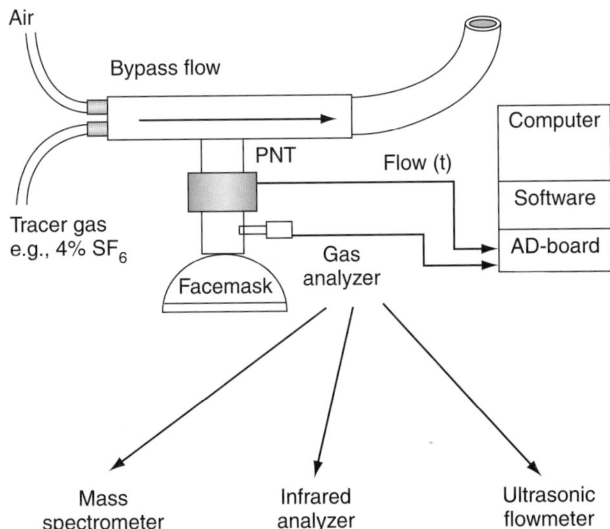

FIGURE 9-7. Multiple-breath inert gas washout. Schematic diagram of equipment used for measuring functional residual capacity and ventilation inhomogeneity using this technique. AD-board, analog to digital; PNT, pneumotachometer; SF_6, sulfur-hexafluoride. (Copyright © Janet Stocks.)

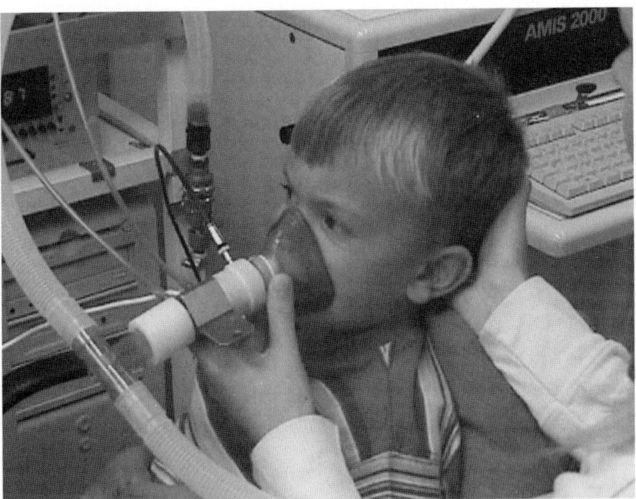

FIGURE 9-9. Multiple-breath inert gas washout in a preschool child using a mass spectrometer. Similar measurements can be made in sleeping infants. (Copyright © Janet Stocks.)

The gas supply is then disconnected during expiration so that the washout can commence, with the subject breathing room air until the end-tidal SF_6 concentration is less than 0.1% (i.e., 1/40th of the starting concentration) [Fig. 9-10]. Flow and gas concentration are measured continuously during inspiration and expiration, and the exhaled tracer gas volume is determined by integrating the product of flow and the tracer gas concentration over time.[42,43] FRC is calculated by dividing the BTPS-corrected volume of exhaled tracer gas by its concentration in the lungs just before washout. As in older subjects, values are corrected for apparatus dead space and volume inspired above the representative end-expiratory level at the time of switching. FRC should be calculated from at least two (ideally, three) technically acceptable measurements that are within 10% of each other.

Irrespective of technique, a mask is usually used for data collection in both infants and preschool children (see Figs. 9-8 and 9-9). Measurements in infants should be undertaken during periods of quiet sleep, whereas those in preschoolers are performed while the child is seated and awake. Cooperation is generally ensured by the ability to watch a favorite video during the recordings.[44] Care is required to maintain a leak-free seal at all times and to ensure that the child does not dribble into the equipment. Given suitable measurement conditions, technically satisfactory measurements of both FRC and indices of ventilation inhomogeneity using MBW can be obtained in at least 80% of children between 3 and 5 years of age (increasing from approximately 65% at 3 years to more than 90% by 5 years).[44]

With their rapid respiratory rate and higher ratio of VT/FRC, wash-in and washouts are generally much faster in infants and preschool children than in older subjects. Both phases of the technique are generally completed within 1 to 2 minutes in healthy infants and within 5 minutes in those with airway disease. Consequently, it is usually possible to complete three technically successful runs within 20 minutes. With the exception of measurements in unsedated neonates, in whom both measurement error and physiologic variability are likely to be slightly greater, the coefficient of variation for repeat within-occasion measures is approximately 5% (range, 2%–15%). The ultrasonic flowmeter, which simultaneously measures tidal flow and tracer gas concentration (see Fig. 9-8), provides a promising alternative to respiratory mass spectrometry during MBW and is currently undergoing evaluation for use in both infants and preschool children.[42,45]

The accuracy of recordings is dependent on the following:

- Accurate calibration
- Stability of the breathing pattern before switching into the tracer gas is performed
- Absence of leaks
- Ensuring that wash-in and washout continue for a long enough period

A potential cause of increased variability of results is the occurrence of sighs. These may mobilize gas in slowly ventilating or closed areas of the lungs, especially in subjects with marked ventilation inhomogeneity. The occurrence of such sighs should always be noted, and additional runs performed, if necessary.

Advantages and Disadvantages

Disadvantages of the MBW and gas dilution techniques include the following:

- They measure only the readily ventilated gas volume and not any gas trapped behind closed airways.
- They may require prolonged washout in those with severe disease.
- There is a paucity of commercially available equipment.

Advantages of the MBW technique include the following:

- It is suitable for bedside measurements.
- It can be undertaken at all ages, including unsedated newborn or preterm infants.
- It provides simultaneous assessments of gas-mixing indices as a measure of ventilation inhomogeneity.

GAS-MIXING EFFICIENCY

Although initially described many years ago, the use of MBW to assess gas-mixing efficiency or ventilation inhomogeneity has been used intermittently in infants and young children,[46] possibly reflecting the complexity of data analysis and the lack of

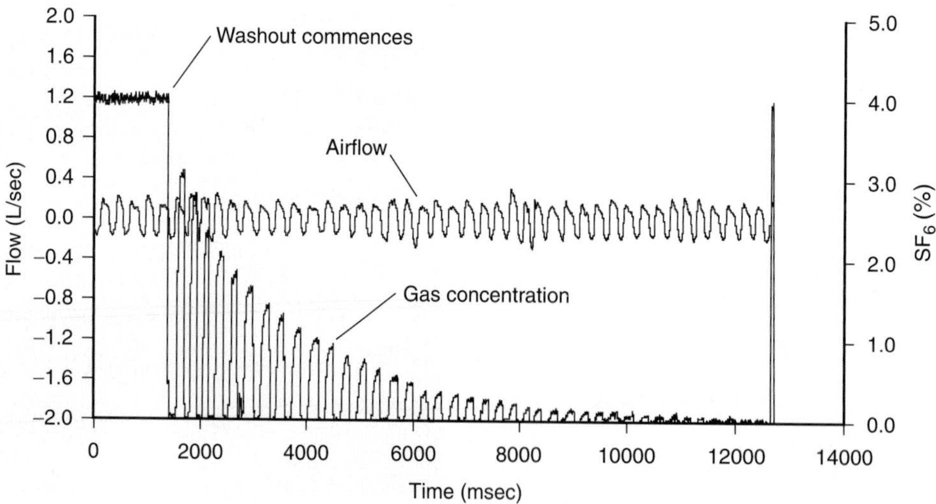

FIGURE 9-10. Time-based trace of airflow and inert gas concentration during multiple-breath washout of an inert gas. Washout commences once the concentration of inert gas in the lungs has equilibrated with that inspired during the wash-in phase, and continues until the tracer gas is cleared from the lungs, which in this example took approximately 110 seconds. SF_6, sulfur-hexafluoride. (Copyright © Janet Stocks.)

commercially available equipment and software. During recent years, technologic advances, combined with an increasing awareness that conventional measures of airway function may not detect early changes in peripheral airway function until lung disease is well established, have led to a resurgence of interest in this field. MBW is applicable to subjects of all ages, including unsedated infants, because measurements are performed during spontaneous tidal breathing.

Theoretical Background

The human lung is constructed for optimal mixing of fresh inspired air with the resident gas in the lungs. How well this works will determine the gas-mixing efficiency. Poor gas mixing is a consequence of increased ventilation inhomogeneity and is reflected both by the time or relative ventilation required to clear a tracer gas from the lungs, and by the magnitude of the phase III slope (alveolar plateau) of inert gas concentration during expiration.

A large number of parameters that reflect overall ventilation inhomogeneity have been defined. They are all calculated from the MBW in different ways, and generally, higher values signify increased ventilation inhomogeneity.

- The mixing ratio is calculated from the ratio between the actual and the estimated ideal number of breaths needed to lower the end-tidal tracer gas concentration to 1/40th of the starting value. The ideal number of breaths is proportional to the ratio between FRC and alveolar VT (i.e., VT minus equipment and airway dead space).
- The lung clearance index (LCI) is the number of turnovers of FRC (where turnover represents the expired volume equivalent to the subject's FRC) required to complete the washout (i.e., cumulative expired volume/FRC).
- Inhomogeneity of ventilation distribution may also be expressed by moment analysis of the washout curve. The zeroth moment is the area under the washout curve (end-tidal gas concentration plotted against lung volume turnover). The first and second moments give more weight to the latter part of the washout curve by multiplying the end-tidal gas concentration by the turnover (first moment) or the turnover squared (second moment). The ratios between the first and zeroth moments and between the second and zeroth moments are usually calculated over the first eight turnovers, with higher ratios indicating that a greater portion of the lungs is slowly ventilated (Fig. 9-11). Some of the other available indices have specific advantages, but indices such as the LCI and the mixing ratio are robust and relatively intuitive for patients and parents as well as medical personnel to understand. There is no consensus regarding which parameters should be reported, whether data should be reported as mean or median, or the ideal number of breaths on which to base reports, although an ATS-ERS Task Force is currently considering these issues.

An increased LCI results from differences in specific ventilation between parallel lung units. This can result from asymmetrical narrowing of the airway lumen at branch points throughout the airway tree, which in turn may be caused by inflammation, scarring, or obstruction by mucus, or may be secondary to changes in airway tone. Additionally, inhomogeneity may result from parenchymal changes in the subtended lung units, resulting in changes in compliance and differing time constants for filling and emptying.

Gas mixing in the lungs takes place through two mechanisms. Convective gas transport (bulk flow) predominates in the conducting airways (i.e., the central airways down to, and including, approximately the terminal bronchioles), whereas diffusion (molecular diffusion, or Brownian movement) predominates in the intra-acinar airways. The *quasi-stationary diffusion-convection front* is a transition zone where diffusive gas transport and convective gas transport are of similar magnitude. This occurs in the region of the entrance to the acinus and in its proximal portion. Poor gas mixing that occurs in the vicinity of this area as a result of interaction between convective and diffusive gas mixing is termed either *acinar-* or *diffusion-convection-dependent* inhomogeneity (S_{acin} or DCDI). Proximal to this front, inhomogeneity results from convective flow inhomogeneity, secondary to differences in specific ventilation between parallel lung units that fill and empty sequentially. This inhomogeneity of more proximal origin is termed either *conductive-* or *convection-dependent inhomogeneity* (S_{cond} or CDI).

Equipment and Procedure

Equipment and procedures for data collection when using the MBW technique are identical to those described earlier for measurements of lung volume using this technique. There are no guidelines for standardized measurements of ventilation inhomogeneity in infants, but the use of the technique in preschool and school-aged children has been described in some detail recently.[43,44,47] Attempts were made to use the MBW in preschool children more than 20 years ago, but met with only limited (<50%) success, possibly due to poor tolerance during relatively prolonged periods of data collection when using a mouthpiece and nose clip. More recent studies that have used a mask have reported technically successful results in more than 80% of 3- to 5-year-old children.

Advantages and Limitations

As with many lung function tests, errors will occur when using the MBW if there is too large an external dead space in relation to VT, if there are any leaks from the circuit, if there are faulty calibrations, or if there is a highly irregular breathing pattern. In addition, when using this technique, particular care must be taken to ensure the following:

- Correct alignment of signals from the gas analyzer and flowmeter during data collection
- Appropriate correction of the PNT signal for variations in the dynamic viscosity of the gas sample
- Switching into and out of the tracer gas mixture at the appropriate phase of the respiratory cycle

Some of these problems could easily be overcome with increasing automation and quality control feedback. There is an urgent need to establish recommendations with respect to data collection and analysis and to develop and validate commercially available equipment to facilitate widespread use of this technique. Due to the potential effect of sighs or deep inhalations, MBW should always be performed toward the beginning of any test protocol and certainly before any technique that requires lung inflation or forced expiratory maneuvers. Within-subject repeatability on the same occasion is good, but within-subject, between-occasion repeatability, as well as the ability of parameters such as LCI to detect changes in response to acute interventions, still need to be established.

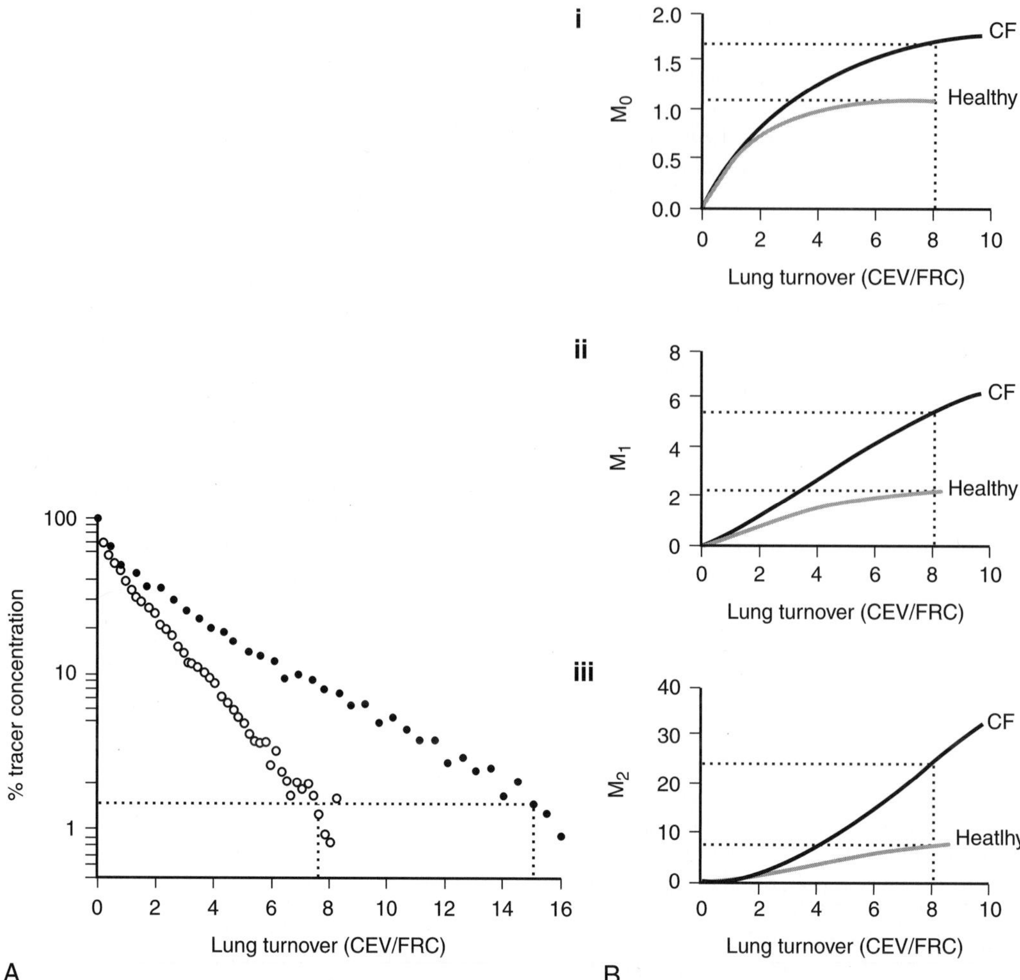

■ **FIGURE 9-11.** Calculation of indices of ventilation. **A,** Calculation of lung clearance index [LCI]. Representative traces from multiple-breath sulfur-hexafluoride washout (MBW_{SF6}) in a healthy infant *(open circles)* and one with cystic fibrosis (CF) *[solid circles]*, demonstrating the prolonged tail. *Dotted lines* show the number of turnovers required to reduce the tracer gas to 2% of the initial tracer concentration (equivalent to the LCI), which in this example was 7.7 for the healthy child and 15 for the child with CF. **B,** The concept of moments. The graph shows moments derived from MBW_{SF6} in a healthy infant and one with CF. The *horizontal dotted lines* indicate values for moments at eight lung turnovers. *i,* The zeroth moment (M_0) obtained from the area under the tracer concentration versus turnover; *ii,* the first moment (M_1) derived from the area under the curve described by panel *i; iii,* the second moment (M_2) derived from the area under the curve described by panel *ii.* As the moment number increases, there is increased weighting toward the end of the washout trace. CEV, cumulative expired volume; FRC, functional residual capacity. (Copyright © Janet Stocks.)

Clinical Applications

In health, gas-mixing efficiency appears to remain remarkably stable throughout the first 18 years of life (Fig. 9-12), thereby enabling the effects of disease to be distinguished from those of growth and development with greater confidence than when dealing with most parameters of lung function, which are highly dependent on age and body size. Indices of ventilation inhomogeneity are increased in children and adults with CF, asthma, chronic obstructive pulmonary disease, and post-transplant bronchiolitis obliterans, and in infants and preschool children with bronchopulmonary dysplasia and CF (Fig. 9-13). In older subjects, an increased LCI is usually reflected by a longer washout time. This is not necessarily true in infants and young children with lung disease, who may simply increase their minute ventilation (increased respiratory rate and VT) to compensate for less efficient gas mixing.[47] The MBW technique appears to be a more sensitive method of detecting early changes in lung function in infants and children with CF than conventional spirometry (Fig. 9-14).[43,44,47,48] Further work is needed, however, to establish the clinical role of these tests, particularly in subjects with more advanced lung disease, in whom this approach may be too sensitive to be of practical value.

MEASUREMENT OF OTHER STATIC LUNG VOLUMES

Until recently, it was possible to measure lung volume at FRC only in spontaneously breathing infants due to infants' inability to cooperate in special breathing maneuvers. Introduction of the raised volume technique in the mid-1990s, whereby a bias flow or pump is used to inflate the sleeping infant's lungs toward TLC before a small jacket is inflated and wrapped around the chest and abdomen to force expiration, means that it is now potentially possible to calculate quasi-values of TLC, expiratory reserve volume (ERV), and residual volume (RV).[18] Because accurate results are dependent on technical factors, such as the

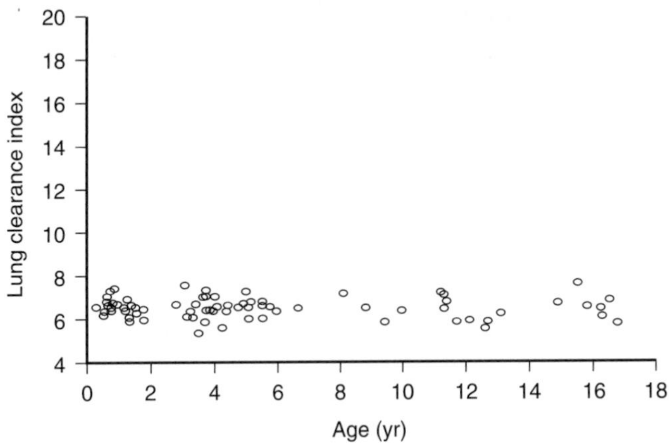

■ **FIGURE 9-12.** Lung clearance index (LCI) in healthy children from birth to 18 years of age. Note the stability of the LCI throughout childhood, making it one of the few parameters of lung function that is not dependent on age or body size. (Unpublished data, Institute of Child Health, London, 2004.)

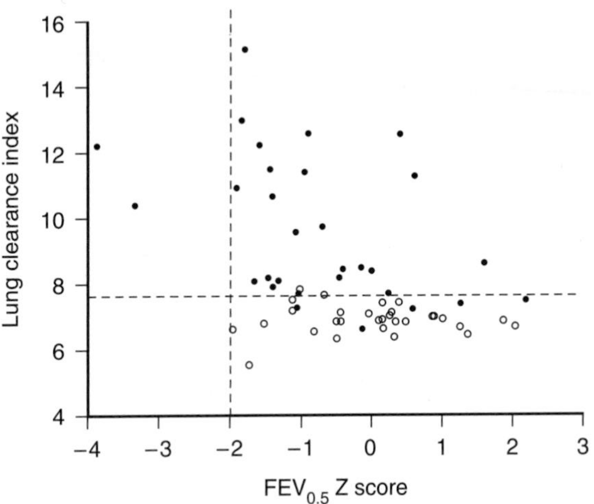

■ **FIGURE 9-14.** Lung clearance index (LCI) versus forced expired volume in 0.5 second ($FEV_{0.5}$) in healthy preschool children and those with cystic fibrosis (CF). LCI is plotted against $FEV_{0.5}$ and expressed as Z scores in 30 healthy preschool children (*open circles;* mean [SD] age, 4.1 [0.9] years) and 30 children of similar age with CF *(closed circles).* Results from all of the healthy children fell within normal limits (*dotted lines;* i.e., <7.8 for LCI and Z score greater than −1.96 for $FEV_{0.5}$). An abnormally low $FEV_{0.5}$ was observed in only two of the children with CF, whereas 22 of 30 children with CF had an abnormal LCI.[44] (Copyright © Janet Stocks.)

precise inflation pressure used, whether the infant makes an inspiratory effort before RV is attained, and the lack of significant volume drift throughout all of the recordings, this approach is currently limited to specialized testing centers. In addition, the lung volume achieved by inflating the lungs to 30 cm H_2O does not necessarily equate to the true TLC (infants have been observed to take a sigh, with considerable further volume increase, at the end of such inflations). Caution should therefore be exercised before an attempt is made to relate lung volumes obtained over an extended volume range using this approach to those recorded during spontaneous efforts later in childhood. Nevertheless, this approach has been shown to be discriminative when comparing lung function in infants with CF with that in healthy control subjects.[18]

As discussed earlier, preschool children are generally not capable of panting against an occlusion during plethysmographic assessments of lung volume. In addition, they may display a relatively uneven end-expiratory level during tidal breathing such that attempts to derive values for static lung volumes over an extended volume range by combining measures of FRC by gas dilution with spirometric assessments of forced expiration are likely to be highly unreliable. Similarly, the coordination required to perform a single-breath washout, which could potentially provide such information, generally precludes the use of this approach in those younger than 6 years of age.

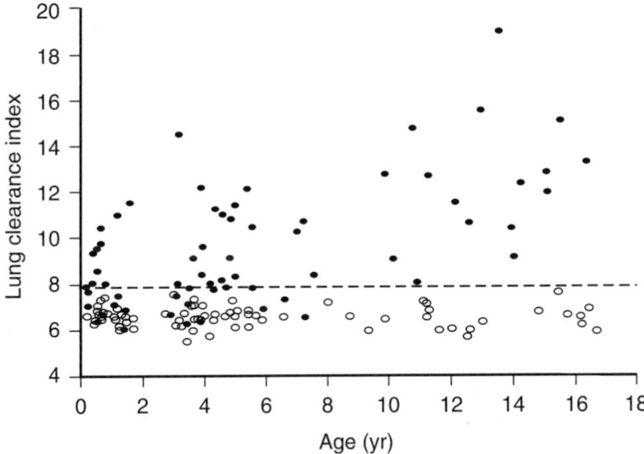

■ **FIGURE 9-13.** Comparison of lung clearance index (LCI) in healthy children and those with cystic fibrosis (CF). Collated data from studies performed at the Institute of Child Health, London, 2002–2004. The *dashed horizontal line* shows the 95% upper limit of normal (i.e., LCI, 7.8) derived from healthy children *(open circles).* Elevated LCI values were observed in many infants and preschool children with CF *(closed circles)* and in virtually all of those older than 7 years of age. (Copyright © Janet Stocks.)

■ RESPIRATORY MECHANICS: RESISTANCE AND COMPLIANCE

Assessments of respiratory resistance and, particularly, compliance are performed relatively more frequently in infants and young children than in older subjects. This probably reflects the relative ease with which such measurements can be performed in early life as well as the fact that, in contrast to older subjects, changes in the elastic properties of the lung often dominate the underlying pathophysiology of lung disease in newborn infants. A wide range of techniques is available, although those suitable for use in sleeping infants are rarely applicable to preschool children, as discussed later. The advantages of many of these techniques is that, in contrast to forced expiratory maneuvers, they are performed during tidal breathing and require little cooperation from the child, other than breathing through a facemask or mouthpiece. The term *airway resistance* should be reserved for techniques such as plethysmography, which relate changes in alveolar pressure to airflow. It should not be used to describe pulmonary (lung tissue plus airway) resistance, as calculated from changes in transpulmonary (esophageal) pressure, or respiratory (airway plus tissue plus chest wall) resistance, as measured from changes in pressure at the airway opening. Because infants are preferential nose breathers, measurements of resistance, which are performed while the infant breathes through a facemask, generally include nasal resistance (discussed earlier). It is therefore essential that these measurements be deferred for at least 3 weeks after the onset of a cold.

Esophageal manometry was once commonplace during assessments of lung function in infants,[49] but has generally been replaced by assessment of passive respiratory mechanics using one of the occlusion techniques. The exception to this is in ventilated or preterm infants, who may already have a nasogastric tube in situ for feeding purposes. Catheter tip transducers may be used instead of esophageal balloons or water-filled catheters to record changes in transpulmonary pressure in situations where esophageal manometry is still required.

PLETHYSMOGRAPHIC ASSESSMENTS OF AIRWAY RESISTANCE

Whole-body plethysmography is a well-established method for measuring lung volume and airway resistance (R_{aw}) in adults and older children, and it has been successfully adapted for measurements in both sleeping infants[4,14] and awake preschool children.[50] Measurements of airway resistance have been used to study normal airway growth and development in relation to lung volume during the first year of life and have demonstrated tracking of airway function during this period.[21,27] They have also been used to discriminate between healthy infants and those with respiratory disease or a history of wheezing.[27,40] Plethysmographic measurements of specific airway resistance (sR_{aw}, i.e., $R_{aw} \times$ FRC) are becoming an increasingly popular method of assessing both baseline airway function and bronchial responsiveness in preschool children with and without respiratory disease. Because resistance decreases as lung volume increases with growth, values of sR_{aw} remain relatively independent of changes in body size. This should facilitate attempts to distinguish changes in airway function due to disease from those resulting from growth and development, especially during early life, when somatic growth is so rapid. The sR_{aw} value has been used as an outcome measure in cross-sectional and longitudinal studies of healthy young children[51] and those with CF,[44,52,53] as well as being used to assess bronchial responsiveness to methacholine or cold, dry air and to document the effect of antiasthmatic therapies in preschool children.[54]

Methodologic and Theoretical Considerations

The principles of plethysmographic assessments of airway resistance measurements are identical in infants and preschool children and in older subjects.[4,14] The subject sits, or in the case of an infant, lies, inside a relatively airtight chamber, the whole-body plethysmograph, while changes in airflow are recorded at the airway opening using a mouthpiece or mask. By relating changes in plethysmographic pressure, which are inversely proportional to changes in alveolar pressure, to changes in flow throughout the breathing cycle, airway resistance can be calculated (Fig. 9-15). Changes in plethysmographic pressure during spontaneous breathing are calibrated in terms of alveolar pressure changes by using the relationship between the change in plethysmographic (box) signal and pressure at the airway opening during an airway occlusion. The latter is assumed to represent changes in alveolar pressure during periods of no airflow, such as occur during respiratory efforts against a closed shutter during plethysmographic assessments of FRC (discussed earlier). Although most sleeping infants will continue to make respiratory efforts against the shutter during a 6- to 10-second airway occlusion, this procedure is too demanding for most young children, thereby precluding direct measurement of R_{aw} in preschool children. Measurements of sR_{aw} can, however, be obtained by using a single-step procedure without the need to breathe against a closed shutter, making this an ideal test for young children. In recent years, this technique has been adapted in several ways to make it even more applicable to very young children, including the use of a specially adapted facemask and the option of having an adult accompany the child into the plethysmograph, if required.[50]

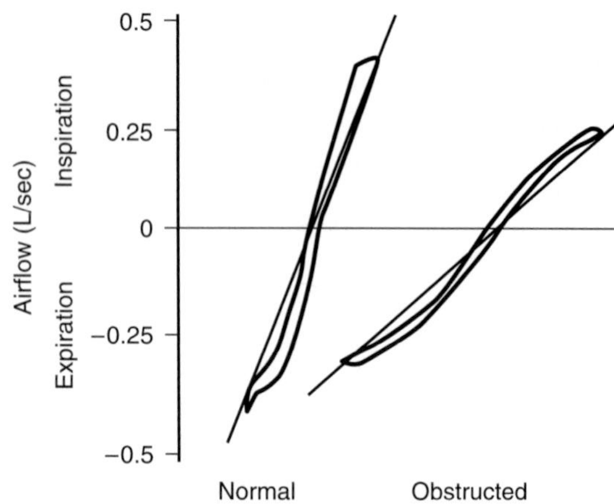

■ **FIGURE 9-15.** Specific airway resistance loops from a healthy child and one with airway obstruction. Changes in box volume are proportional to changes in alveolar pressure, reflecting the greater effort required to effect airflow *(flatter slope)* in the presence of airway obstruction. (Copyright © Janet Stocks.)

For reliable assessments of airway resistance, changes in box pressure must reflect only the changes in alveolar pressure required to drive flow, not those due to any changes in the temperature and humidity of the respired gas, which will distort the phase relationship between airflow at the mouth and box pressure. In the past, older children and adults either breathed heated, humidified air at BTPS conditions or were encouraged to pant during assessments of R_{aw} to minimize changes in gas temperature and humidity. Current commercially available adult plethysmographs, which are also being used for measurements in awake children as young as 2 years of age, have generally abandoned the use of rebreathing systems or the need for panting maneuvers. Instead, attempts are made to compensate electronically for phase lags between the box pressure signal and airflow that arise from changes in the temperature and humidity of the respired gas. Despite the recognized potential limitations and the finding of systematic differences between values of sR_{aw} obtained under true conditions and those derived after electronic compensation, this method has been successfully adapted to measure sR_{aw} in preschool children, but has yet to be validated in infants.

The majority of published studies that have undertaken plethysmographic assessments of R_{aw} in infants have used a heated rebreathing system to provide respired gas at BTPS conditions (see Fig. 9-5). This has proved to be an effective method, but is technically difficult to achieve, thereby limiting the use of infant plethysmography to specialized physiologic laboratories. In addition, recent concerns about both the potential infection risk, especially when studying infants with CF, and the fact that the buildup of CO_2 during rebreathing could cause physiologic changes in the very parameters being measured prompted a search for alternative solutions. Initial attempts to apply electronic thermal compensation to infant data similar to that used in preschool children have proved disappointing, suggesting that more sophisticated algorithms may be required to cope with the added complexities of undertaking these measurements during nose breathing. Efforts to resolve this problem are continuing in the hopes of making plethysmographic assessments of R_{aw} more generally applicable during infancy.

Equipment and Procedure

Infants

The equipment and technique used for undertaking plethysmographic assessments of R_{aw} have been described in detail previously.[1,4,14] Commercially available equipment that meets most of the ERS-ATS recommendations for plethysmographic measurements of lung volume in infants is now available, but none currently has a rebreathing bag to provide respired gas under BTPS conditions, and no system has a validated method of electronically compensating for thermal artifacts during airway resistance measurements. Hence, such measurements are currently limited to departments with their own custom-built equipment.

As with older subjects, it is important for thermal equilibrium to be established after the box is closed and before any recordings are started. Once the infant is breathing quietly and regularly, the infant is switched from breathing air from the box to a rebreathing system containing warmed, humidified air under BTPS conditions. Simultaneous changes in airflow and box pressure are then recorded. Technically acceptable loops are those in which there is minimal phase lag between these two signals at moments of zero flow (i.e., end inspiration and end expiration). Depending on the size of the bag and the child, each period of data collection should be limited to 20 to 30 seconds, with the bag being washed out between runs, to minimize CO_2 accumulation. The aim is to collect a minimum of 5 and preferably at least 20 breaths from which R_{aw} can be calculated. Despite these precautions, some hyperventilation or dynamic hyperinflation may occur when using a heated rebreathing bag. It is therefore recommended that baseline assessments of FRC_{pleth} be performed before R_{aw} recordings are obtained.

Specific airway resistance is calculated from the relationship of $\Delta V_{pleth}/\Delta Flow$ (usually displayed as an X-Y plot during spontaneous tidal breathing; see Fig. 9-15) multiplied by ambient pressure:

$$sR_{aw} = (\Delta V_{pleth}/\Delta Flow) \times (P_{amb} - PH_2O)$$

If technically acceptable measurements of FRC_{pleth} have been obtained, values of R_{aw} can subsequently be derived whereby:

$$R_{aw} = sR_{aw}/FRC$$

Full details of the derivation of these equations, together with the necessary correction factors (e.g., for apparatus resistance), have been published previously.[4]

Preschool Children

One of the advantages of plethysmographic assessments of sR_{aw} is that the same plethysmograph can be used in preschool children as in older subjects. Measurements can be carried out using either a mouthpiece and nose clips, as in older subjects, or a specially adapted facemask fitted with a flexible, noncompressible mouthpiece that prevents nose breathing and provides a stable opening of the airway.[50] Before the child is asked to enter the plethysmograph, all procedures must be demonstrated and explained. If the child is hesitant to enter the plethysmograph or to stay inside once the door is closed, measurements can be performed with the child sitting on an adult's lap. During measurements, the child should sit with the neck slightly extended. Children who do not spontaneously breathe at a respiratory rate of between 30 and 45 breaths·min^{-1} should be coached to do so. Lower rates will usually result in phase lags due to the inability of electronic compensation to correct adequately for thermal artifacts in the presence of slow, deep breathing, whereas higher rates may result in elevated values of sR_{aw} due to the flow and volume dependency of these measurements. Once the child is confident and comfortable, the plethysmograph door can be closed. Measurements should not be initiated for at least 1 minute after closure to allow thermal equilibrium of box pressure to be achieved. Once there is minimal drift of the box signal and the child is breathing regularly with a stable breathing pattern, measurements can begin. If measurements are made with an accompanying adult, the adult should breathe normally until the child's respiration has stabilized (as seen from the spirometric time-based recording) and then perform a deep inspiration followed by a slow expiration so that a constant low expiratory flow is generated during a 15- to 20-second period of data collection. Technical acceptability is based primarily on the respiratory rate, regularity of the breathing pattern, and absence of distortions due to leak, movement, or talking (Fig. 9-16).

As discussed earlier, sR_{aw} can be obtained simply by measuring changes in airflow relative to changes in plethysmographic volume without simultaneous measurement of FRC (see Fig. 9-15).

Reporting of Results

One of the potential limitations of plethysmographic measurement of airway resistance in infants and preschool children (in keeping with most other techniques available for use in this age group) is that there is no consensus regarding which parameters should be reported, whether data should be reported as mean or median, or the ideal number of breaths on which to base reports. Resistance changes throughout the breathing cycle due to a combination of factors, including the flow and volume dependency of airway resistance. Hence, there is no single value that represents resistance. Most commercially available systems have several ways of calculating R_{aw} and sR_{aw}, including the following:

- R_{aw} calculated from the slope of the line connecting the point of maximum ΔV_{pleth} swings during inspiration and expiration, often referred to as *total resistance* (R_{tot})
- R_{aw} calculated from the slope of $\Delta V_{pleth}/\Delta Flow$ between points of maximum flow, sometimes referred to as *resistance at peak flow* (R_{peak}) or *between points of maximum flow* ($R_{V'max}$)
- Mean R_{aw} calculated by the regression of $\Delta V_{pleth}/\Delta Flow$ throughout the entire breath, referred to as *effective resistance* (R_{eff})
- R_{aw} calculated at a fixed flow, usually 0.5 L•sec^{-1} during initial inspiration and expiration (R_I and R_E, respectively)

The latter approach is not recommended for use in young children due to the strong negative age dependency of this parameter, reflecting the fact that, in a 3-year-old child, 0.5 L•sec^{-1} will be similar to, or may even exceed, peak inspired or expired flow, whereas it will fall within the linear midflow range in an older subject. The relative advantages and limitations of these different approaches, especially in terms of within- and between-subject

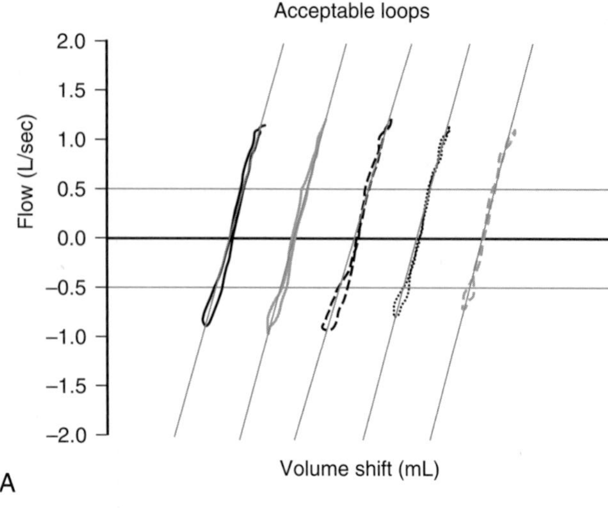

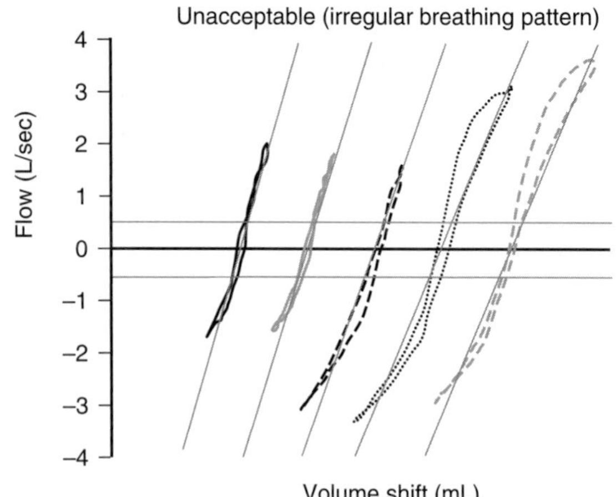

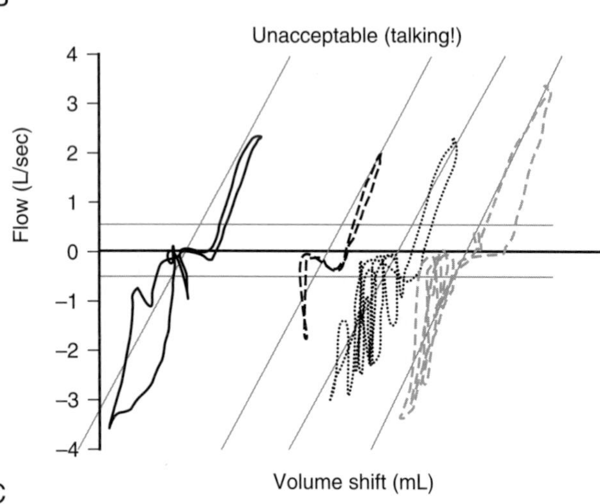

■ **FIGURE 9-16.** Specific resistance measurements and quality control criteria. **A,** A regular reproducible breathing pattern with a good phase relationship *(closed loops)*. **B,** By contrast, a variable respiratory rate and pattern resulted in highly variable values for specific airway resistance. **C,** The subject started to talk to the operator, thereby invalidating the recordings. (Copyright © Janet Stocks.)

variability and the ability to discriminate between children with and without lung disease, has yet to be ascertained. The user should be aware that reference values will vary according to which parameter is selected, with values of sR_{tot} generally exceeding those of sR_{eff}. It is also important to note that the default pediatric prediction equations used in many commercially available plethysmographs were derived from normative data collected under BTPS conditions or during panting. Such equations are totally inappropriate if data have been collected using electronic thermal compensation because they will result in gross overestimation of abnormalities. Preliminary reference values for sR_{aw} based on data collection with electronic compensation are currently being collated, with mean (95% limit of agreement) values for sR_{tot} approximating 1.3 (range, 1.0–1.6) and those for sR_{eff} approximating 1.15 (range, 0.85–1.45). Further studies will be required to confirm these findings.

Advantages and Limitations

The major advantages of plethysmographic assessments of airway resistance are that they represent a direct reflection of airway caliber that can be obtained during tidal breathing and that measurements using the same method can potentially be obtained at all ages. Although infant plethysmography provides valuable data in specialized centers, it remains limited by the lack of any validated method of obtaining reliable results without reliance on a heated rebreathing bag and the potential dominance of the upper airway in these nose-breathing subjects. Preschool plethysmography has the advantage that the necessary equipment is available in most secondary hospitals, thereby simplifying wide dissemination of this method, although its size precludes its use in field studies and most primary care facilities. Improvements in commercially available software, including computer animation and data storage, are required to facilitate both data collection and quality control in this age group. There remains an urgent need to develop a standard protocol for data collection, criteria for quality assurance, and methods for reporting results, as well as improved algorithms for calculating specific resistance to facilitate the comparison and collation of results collected in different centers. This in turn would facilitate the development of more reliable and appropriate reference data from healthy children.

■ PASSIVE RESPIRATORY MECHANICS

Measurements of passive respiratory mechanics (compliance, resistance, and expiratory time constant) are potentially possible if a state of relaxation can be induced in the respiratory system. This is feasible only in highly trained adults during spontaneous breathing and hence is not applicable to preschool children. However, in contrast to older subjects, the vagally mediated Hering-Breuer inflation reflex is active within the VT range throughout the first year of life. The occlusion technique for measuring passive respiratory mechanics is based on the ability to invoke this reflex by performing brief intermittent airway occlusions during spontaneous tidal breathing. Activation of vagally mediated pulmonary stretch receptors when the airway is occluded above FRC leads to inhibition of inspiration and prolongation of expiratory time (Fig. 9-17). Provided there is no respiratory muscle activity and rapid equilibration of pressures across the respiratory system during occlusion (as shown by the presence of a pressure plateau), alveolar pressure and hence elastic recoil of the respiratory system can be measured at the

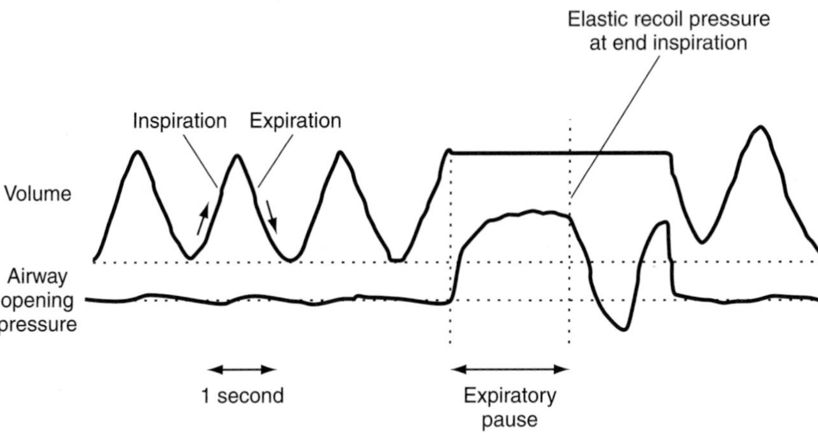

■ **FIGURE 9-17.** Passive respiratory mechanics. End-inspiratory occlusion was used to evoke the Hering-Breuer inflation reflex. Airway occlusion at end-tidal inspiration induces a respiratory pause (lengthening of expiratory time), during which the recoil pressure of the respiratory system can be measured at the airway opening if there is complete relaxation and sufficient time for pressures to equilibrate through the respiratory system. (Copyright © Janet Stocks.)

airway opening. By relating this recoil pressure to the volume above the passively determined end-expiratory volume at which the airway occlusion was performed or to the airflow occurring on release of the occlusion, the compliance and resistance of the respiratory system can be measured. The major limitation of this technique, as with all methods that use intermittent airway occlusions, is that pressures may not equilibrate rapidly enough in the presence of substantial airway obstruction to allow accurate measurements at the airway opening. Full details of data collection and analysis and quality control criteria have been reported previously, together with discussions of the relative advantages and limitations of this technique.[12]

Methodologic and Theoretical Considerations

Various adaptations of the occlusion technique have been developed since it was first described in the late 1970s. The most commonly used approach, and the one for which commercially available equipment is available, is the single-breath, or single-occlusion, technique (Fig. 9-18). When using this technique, resistance, compliance, and the passive expiratory time constant (τ_{rs}) of the respiratory system can potentially be calculated from a single airway occlusion (Fig. 9-19). Provided expiration is passive and there is no braking (slowing) of expiratory flow after release of the airway occlusion, a plot of the flow-volume relationship can be used to calculate τ (because time constant = volume/flow). Compliance of the total respiratory system (C_{rs}) is calculated by relating the volume above the passively determined lung volume at the moment of airway occlusion to the elastic recoil pressure measured during occlusion. Because infants frequently dynamically elevate FRC and may breathe in slightly earlier than usual after occlusion, it is necessary to extrapolate the linear portion of the flow-volume plot to zero flow to estimate the appropriate volume change when calculating C_{rs}. Because the respiratory time constant represents the product of resistance and compliance, respiratory resistance (R_{rs}) can simply be derived as C_{rs}/τ.

The optimal duration of airway occlusion is a compromise between ensuring sufficient time for pressure equilibration to occur, while making the occlusion brief enough to allow passive expiration after its release. A minimum occlusion time of 400 msec and a maximum of 1.5 seconds in which to attain a pressure plateau lasting at least 100 msec has been recommended.[12] Results are usually expressed as the mean of three to five valid measurements.

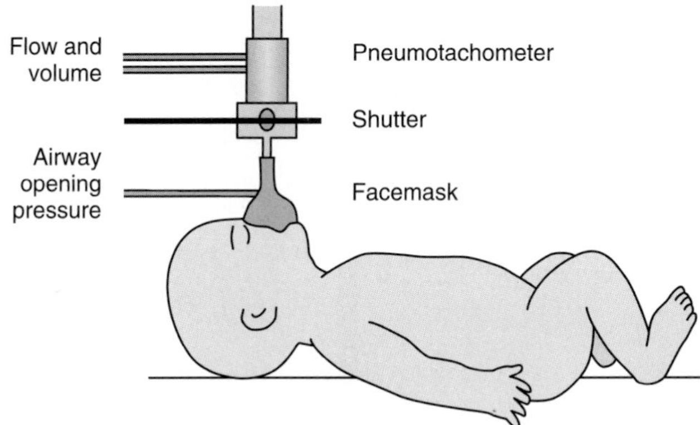

■ **FIGURE 9-18.** Occlusion technique. Schematic diagram of equipment used for passive mechanics using the occlusion technique in infants. (Copyright © Janet Stocks.)

Advantages and Limitations

The advantages of the single-occlusion technique are that the equipment is relatively simple and inexpensive, consisting of a flowmeter (usually a PNT) and shutter with which to effect the airway occlusion, attached to a facemask, and that measurements can easily be made at the bedside. As with all infant PFTs, attainment of a stable respiratory pattern and a leak-free seal around the mask are essential for successful data collection. Valid measurements also depend on three fundamental assumptions:

- There is complete relaxation of the respiratory system not only during the occlusion, but also during the subsequent expiration.
- Pressure measured at the facemask equilibrates rapidly and hence represents alveolar pressure.
- The lung can be treated as a single compartment that can be described by a single value of τ.

With persistence, these conditions can be achieved in the majority of healthy infants during quiet sleep, but they are much more difficult to satisfy in infants with severe airway disease, in whom pressure equilibration may not occur rapidly enough and in whom the respiratory system can rarely be described by a single time constant. It should also be remembered that results from the single-occlusion technique reflect the combined mechanics of the entire respiratory system (chest wall, lungs, and airway), which may reduce the ability to detect subtle changes in

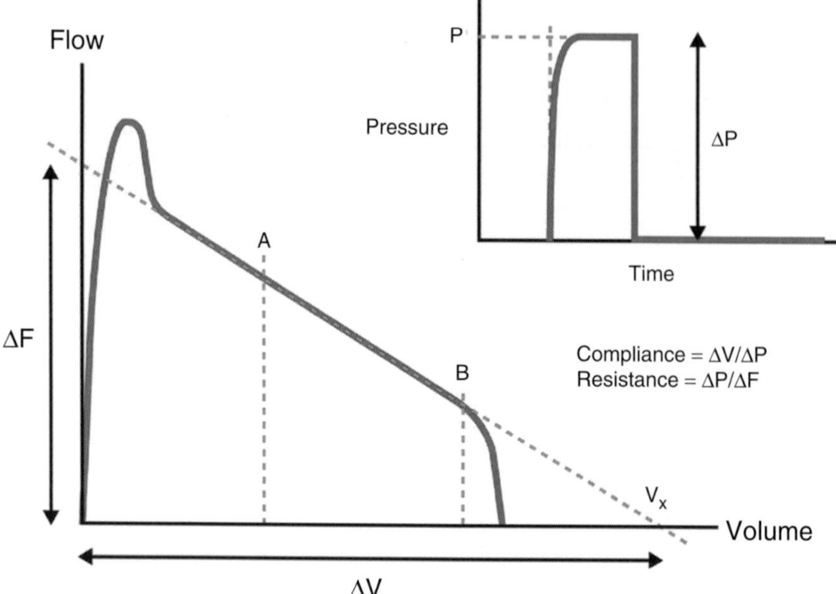

■ **FIGURE 9-19.** Assessment of passive respiratory mechanics using the single-breath occlusion technique. The volume of air in the lung above the passively determined end-expiratory level (i.e., ΔV) is calculated by extrapolating the linear portion of the descending flow-volume curve to zero flow [i.e., V_x]. During periods of no airflow (i.e., airway occlusion) and in the presence of complete respiratory muscle relaxation, as seen by the attainment of a pressure plateau, pressures equilibrate and the elastic recoil pressure of the respiratory system can be measured at the airway opening (ΔP). Respiratory system compliance can then be calculated as ΔV/ΔP. Similarly, by relating ΔP to ΔF, respiratory resistance is calculated. (Copyright © Janet Stocks.)

lung function in those with respiratory disease. Although significant changes in R_{rs} have been reported among groups of infants with airway disease, the major role of these measurements is probably with respect to assessing compliance in conditions in which there is likely to be restrictive pulmonary changes, such as respiratory distress syndrome, chronic lung disease of infancy, pulmonary hypoplasia, interstitial lung disease, and cardiac disease with pulmonary overperfusion.

■ INTERRUPTER TECHNIQUE

The occlusion techniques for assessing passive respiratory mechanics are not applicable in awake preschool children, because they will not relax the respiratory muscles either during or after release of the airway occlusion, thereby precluding reliable assessment of either elastic recoil pressure or the passive respiratory time constant. Nonetheless, resistance of the respiratory system can be assessed in this age group by using the interrupter technique, which relies on much shorter interruptions to airflow than those used during the occlusion techniques. Equipment for the interrupter technique is similar to that used for the occlusion techniques in infants, except that a shutter with much faster closure and opening times is required (Fig. 9-20). The interrupter technique was first reported in 1927 by von Neergaard and Wirz, who applied a sudden, brief (100-msec) occlusion to the airways during a normal respiratory cycle while recording flow and mouth pressure (P_m). Based on the assumption that pressures equilibrate rapidly throughout the respiratory system during periods of no airflow, such that P_m will reflect alveolar pressure during occlusion, interrupter resistance (R_{int}) was calculated by dividing the change in P_m after occlusion by the flow immediately before occlusion.

Despite initial setbacks due to the complexities of interpreting the postinterrupter pressure profile, technologic and engineering advances, together with an enhanced understanding of its physiologic basis, revived interest in the interrupter technique during the 1970s and 1980s. This has been further heightened during the last decade, as the potential use of the interrupter technique as a clinical tool for measuring lung function in young, "noncollaborating" children has been realized.[55]

Theoretical and Methodologic Considerations

Theoretically, when airflow at the mouth is suddenly interrupted, there will be a rapid initial change in P_m (P_{init}), followed by a slower change (P_{dif}) up to a plateau (P_{el}) [Fig. 9-21]. P_{init} is virtually instantaneous and reflects the pressure difference due to airway resistance at the time of interruption. During tidal breathing in preschool children, P_{init} and thus R_{int} will include a component of lung tissue and chest wall resistance, not just airway resistance. P_{dif} is due to the viscoelastic properties of the

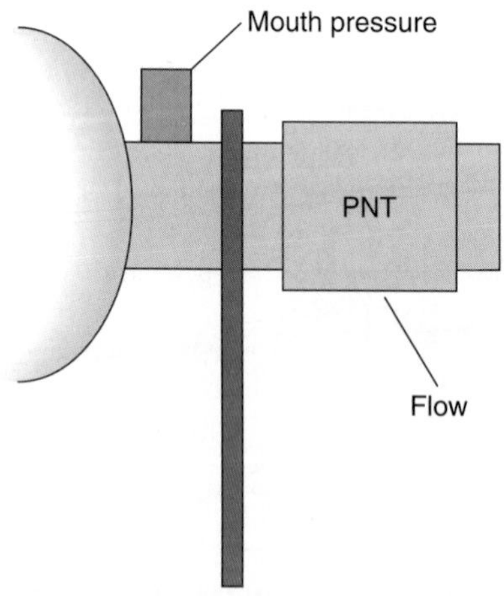

■ **FIGURE 9-20.** Schematic diagram of equipment used for the interrupter technique. PNT, pneumotachometer. (Copyright © Janet Stocks.)

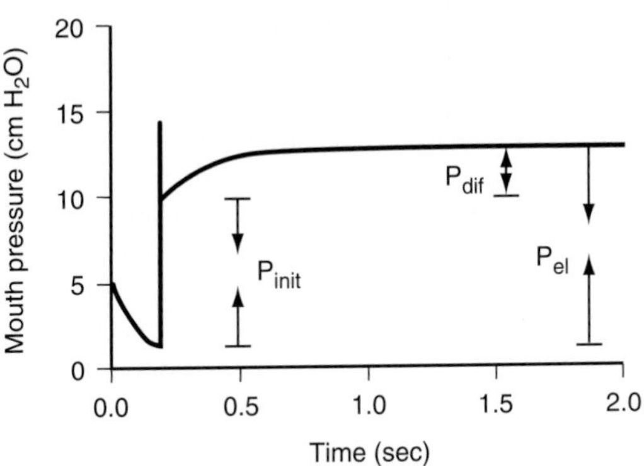

■ **FIGURE 9-21.** Schematic changes in mouth or mask pressure during the interrupter technique. Schematic description of the pressure-time curve showing mouth pressure changes after a sudden interruption of airflow at mid expiration. P_{init}, rapid initial change in mouth pressure (P_m); P_{dif}, secondary slower change in P_m; P_{el}, final plateau representing the pressure due to the elastic recoil of the respiratory system. (Copyright © Janet Stocks.)

respiratory tissues and reflects stress adaptation (relaxation or recovery) within the tissues of the lung and chest wall, plus gas redistribution (pendelluft) between pulmonary units with different pressures at the time of interruption. The final plateau represents the pressure due to elastic recoil of the respiratory system and may take several seconds to be reached, especially in the presence of airway obstruction. The total time of interruption should be less than 100 msec, to ensure that its duration is too short to be recognized, thereby preventing initiation of voluntary breathing against the occlusion. Consequently, a final pressure plateau is rarely observed with the interrupter technique, in contrast to occlusion techniques in infants.

When these measurements are performed, there is a series of rapid oscillations in pressure between the rapid and the slow change in P_m after airflow interruption (Fig. 9-22). This is due to the inertia and compressibility of the air column in the airways. These oscillations may be more or less damped depending on the time constant of the total system (including the chest wall, lungs, upper airways, and equipment), but their presence often makes it difficult to determine P_{init} accurately. Several methods have been proposed to extrapolate P_{init}. The greater the component of P_{dif} that is incorporated into the R_{int} measurement, the higher R_{int} will be with respect to pure airway resistance and the more it will approach the resistance of the total respiratory system. Even when P_m is linearly back-extrapolated to the beginning of the interruption, it is still partially dependent on the final part of the pressure-time curve. Therefore, it does not represent pure airway resistance.

The following preliminary recommendations have been developed by the ATS-ERS Task Force for data collection in preschool children:

- Measurements should be made with the child sitting upright, breathing through a mouthpiece and filter, wearing a nose clip, and with the cheeks supported.
- Airway occlusions should be made with a valve closing in approximately 10 msec and lasting for 100 msec.
- Occlusions should be triggered by a flow that is set to coincide with the child's peak expiratory flow and should be performed during expiration.
- Approximately 10 occlusions should be performed, with the aim of retaining a minimum of five technically acceptable maneuvers.
- The median and mean of all technically acceptable occlusions should be reported.
- All technical details, including the interruption trigger, the method for calculating P_m, the phase of respiration, and the means of determining technically acceptable occlusions should be reported.
- Linear back-extrapolation of P_m for R_{int} calculation should be used.

Advantages and Limitations

The major advantages of the interrupter technique are its portability and the simplicity of data collection, making it potentially ideal for use in fieldwork. The major limitation is that it is dependent on rapid equilibration between P_m and alveolar pressure after interruption. Ventilation inhomogeneities or severe bronchial obstruction, as well as compliance of the upper airways (mainly the cheeks), may delay this equilibration, such that alveolar pressure and hence R_{int} will be underestimated. Supporting the child's cheeks during R_{int} measurements is an effective method to reduce the influence of upper airway compliance when bronchial obstruction is mild to moderate, but will be insufficient to prevent underestimation of resistance in the presence of severe bronchial obstruction. This has led to some concerns about using R_{int} as an outcome measure in challenge tests. Furthermore, there is still some controversy about the best way to calculate and report results, particularly with respect to how to calculate pressure at the moment of interruption.

Several studies reporting reference values for the classic interrupter technique in preschool children have been published

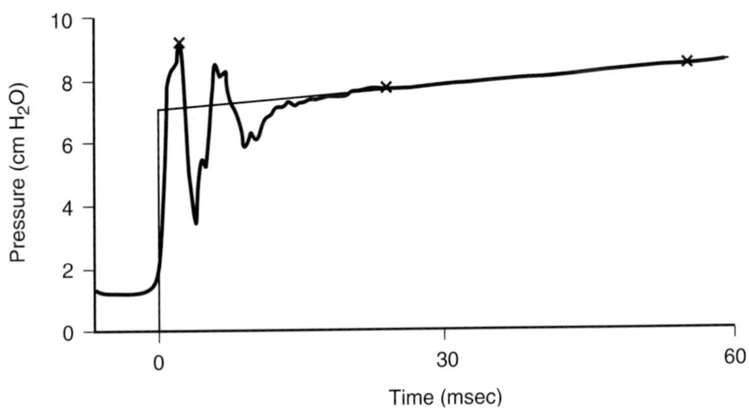

■ **FIGURE 9-22.** Technically acceptable interruption for assessing interrupter resistance. Actual pressure-time trace showing mouth pressure (P_m) during a 100-msec interruption. The *straight line* represents the linear back-extrapolation of P_m to the beginning of the interruption (T_0 = when P_m reaches 25% of the difference between the first peak and the baseline value) using pressures measured 30 msec and 70 msec later. (Copyright © Janet Stocks.)

recently, although comparison of these values is complicated by the variation in methods and equipment used in different laboratories. It is important to note that the intersubject variability of R_{int} in the general population is quite wide and that further large-scale longitudinal studies will be required to produce internationally applicable reference values for use in this age range. Further studies are required to determine the best algorithm to calculate P_m during the interruption and to establish the cutoff value for a decrease in R_{int} beyond which bronchodilator response should be considered clinically significant within an individual.[56,57] The role of R_{int} as the primary outcome in challenge tests and the usefulness of the interrupter technique in comparison with other techniques for lung function testing in preschool children remain to be determined. In contrast to its widespread use in preschool children, the application of R_{int} in infants is still in the early stages, and information on repeatability and guidelines for its use are still evolving.

FORCED OSCILLATION TECHNIQUE

With FOT, impedance of the respiratory system (Z_{rs}) is measured by superimposing small-amplitude pressure oscillations on the respiratory system and measuring the resultant oscillatory flow. This is another technique that has been adapted for use in infants and preschool children. Respiratory impedance describes the spectral (frequency domain) relationship between pressure and airflow throughout the respiratory cycle, providing a global measure of resistive, elastic (viscous), and inertial forces and the opportunity to investigate the frequency dependence of respiratory mechanics.

A detailed description of data collection and analysis, together with guidelines for the application and interpretation of FOT as a routine lung function test in the clinical setting, for both adult and pediatric populations, has been provided by a recent ERS Task Force Report.[58] As with the interrupter technique, FOT can be applied during spontaneous tidal breathing and requires no special maneuvers. It can also be used to define lung impedance in infants and older subjects, but because this requires an esophageal catheter to measure transpulmonary pressure, measurements in preschool children are generally limited to Z_{rs}, with transrespiratory pressure changes being measured at the mouth (P_m).

Methodologic and Theoretical Considerations

In most clinical setups, pressure and flow are measured at the mouth, with pressure oscillations that are generated by a loudspeaker being applied, either at the airway opening (the standard and most commonly used technique) or around the head (the head generator technique) [Fig. 9-23]. All complex time domain signals can be represented by a number of different sine waves that have different frequencies, amplitudes, and phases. After application of the sinusoidal oscillations, this is achieved by feeding the resultant pressure and flow signals into a Fourier analyzer for fast Fourier transform from the time domain to the frequency domain (Fig. 9-24). Data are then averaged over the measurement period (usually 8–16 seconds), and the component of P_m and flow caused by the applied oscillations is distinguished from changes due to tidal breathing, to calculate Z_{rs}. Impedance can be divided into the components of the P_m

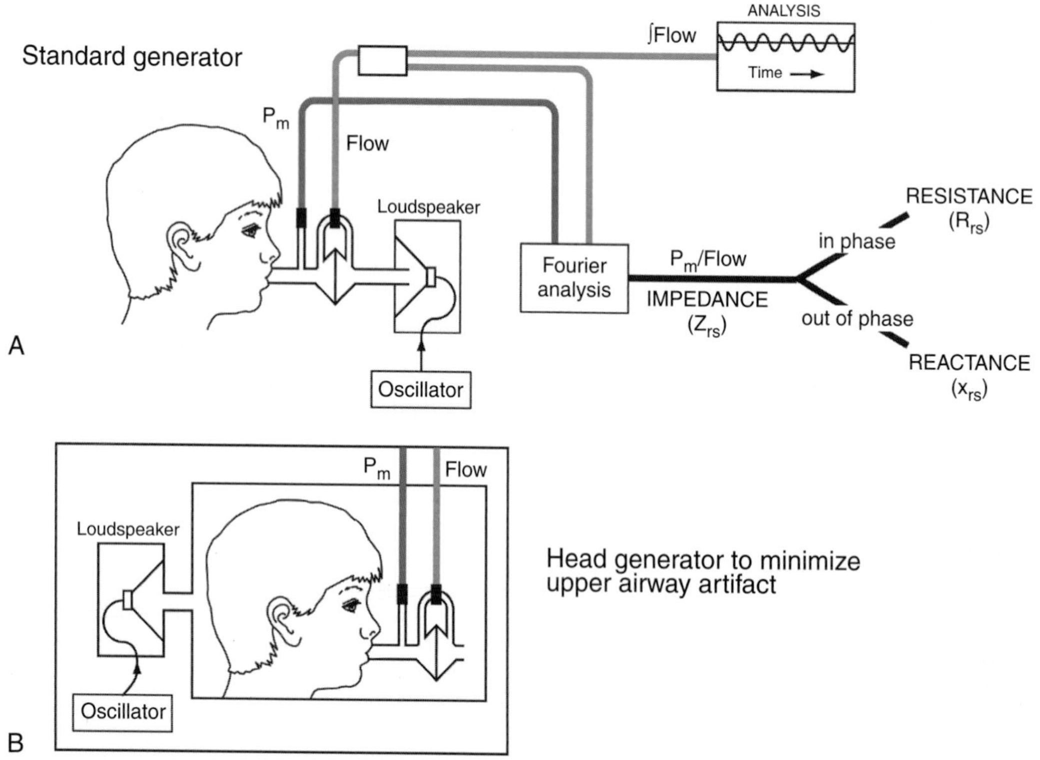

FIGURE 9-23. A, Schematic diagram of circuitry for the forced oscillation technique. The impedance of the respiratory system (Z_{rs}) can be measured by superimposing small-amplitude pressure oscillations on the respiratory system and measuring the resultant oscillatory flow. **B,** Pressure oscillations are applied either at the airway opening using a standard generator or around the entire head (head generator). The latter method is more cumbersome, but may reduce artifacts due to the compliance of the upper airway, which may be particularly important in young children. P_m, mouth pressure; R_{rs}, respiratory resistance; X_{rs}, respiratory reactance (i.e., elastance and inertance). (Copyright © Janet Stocks.)

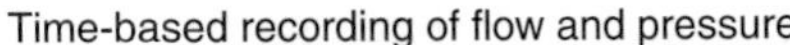

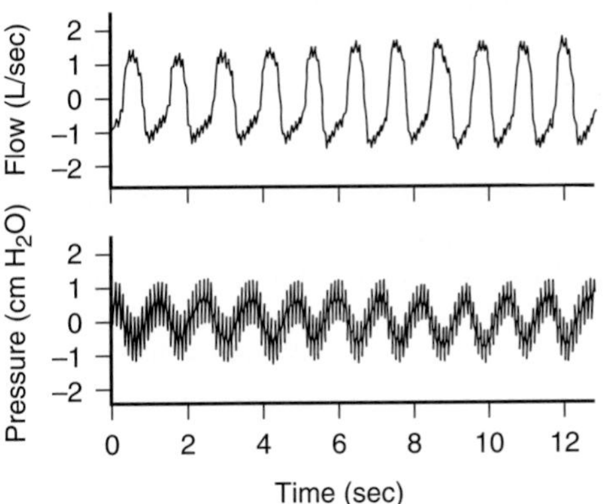

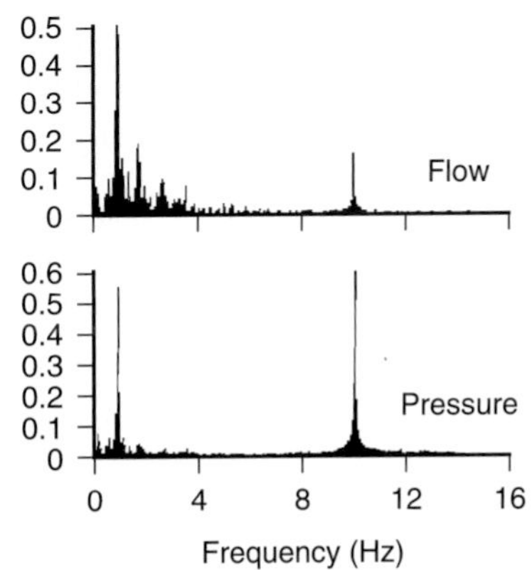

FIGURE 9-24. Time-based and fast Fourier transform (FFT) recordings during FFT. During application of sinusoidal oscillations, the resultant pressure and flow signals are fed into a Fourier analyzer, averaged over the measurement period (usually 8–16 seconds), and the component of mouth pressure (P_m) and flow caused by the applied oscillations distinguished from changes due to tidal breathing. Respiratory impedance is then calculated over a range of frequencies. Impedance is further divided into the components of the P_m signal that are in phase with flow, which represent the resistance of the respiratory system (also known as the *real* part), and the out-of-phase signal, or reactance, which is also sometimes referred to as the *imaginary* part. (From Stocks J, Sly PD, Tepper RS, Morgan WJ: Infant Respiratory Function Testing. New York: John Wiley & Sons, 1996, pp 1–577.)

signal that are in phase with flow and represent resistance of the respiratory system (also known as the *real* part) and the out-of-phase signal, reactance (elastance and inertance), sometimes referred to as the *imaginary* part.

The excitation signal may be either a single sine wave as shown in Figure 9-24 or, more commonly, a multifrequency signal, the classic approach being the use of a pseudorandom noise (i.e., mixing of a number of frequencies, usually harmonics of 2 Hz in the range 2–50 Hz). Although the use of a single sine wave may be ideal to track variations in Z_{rs} within a breath, with time or with changing breathing patterns, application of pseudorandom noise allows the frequency response of the respiratory system to be described and is therefore preferable in many situations. Most measuring systems have dynamic characteristics that allow measurements between 2 and 50 Hz. In clinical practice, however, the optimal frequency spectrum depends on the mechanical characteristics of the respiratory system within each subject, which will be determined by factors such as age, body size, and clinical status.

When using standard FOT, most of the clinically relevant information has been described with measurements at relatively low frequency (5–8 Hz). The lower frequency depends on the subject's breathing rate, and it may be difficult to obtain reliable data at less than 6 Hz in small children with breathing rates between 0.5 and 1 Hz. The higher limit of frequencies depends on the upper airway artifact. Cheek and pharyngeal wall compliance determine upper airway wall vibration during measurement of respiratory impedance at high frequencies, which can be a major technical issue with FOT. The effect is particularly important in small children because they have relatively low upper airway wall impedance relative to Z_{rs}, so the latter may be underestimated. The head generator technique has been designed to minimize upper airway wall motion by minimizing the pressure drop across it, but it requires more cumbersome equipment than the standard technique.[59,60] Impedance measurements should be used only if measured signals are of high quality because large errors and misinterpretation of data can occur with poor-quality signals.

Advantages and Limitations

Although some reference data have been reported for both infants and preschool children,[58] the wide degree of variability between healthy children of similar age or body size limits the extent to which this technique can be used to assess either the presence or the severity of airway disease within individuals. It may, however, be a valuable tool for detecting changes within individuals on the same occasion, particularly when assessing bronchial responsiveness.[53,61,62] In studies of young asthmatic children, parameters derived from FOT may provide a more reliable evaluation of bronchial obstruction and its reversibility than R_{int}, especially in those with high baseline values.[63] In addition, FOT facilitates noninvasive assessments of the bronchomotor response to deep inhalation, which may in turn be an important reflection of the degree and nature of airway obstruction.[62,64] These characteristics, together with the minimal requirement for the subject's cooperation, make FOT a suitable lung function test for epidemiologic and field studies. Preliminary data regarding within-subject variability have been published.[58]

Future Directions

During recent years, there have been two interesting modifications to FOT that, although currently remaining strictly in the specialist research arena, are of potential future clinical significance. As mentioned earlier, depending on the frequency of the applied pressure wave, the resultant impedance will contain different mechanical information. The response to very slow pressure oscillations (<2 Hz), during what has been referred to as *low-frequency FOT*, allows noninvasive partitioning of lung function into airway and tissue parameters.[65] This approach may be of particular interest for studies in preterm infants, where parenchymal disease is a major component of acute respiratory illness. By contrast, at very high frequencies, as are used in the high-frequency interrupter technique, the information derived is primarily related to airway wall mechanics, a particularly important consideration in wheezing disorders.[66]

CHEST WALL MECHANICS

A relatively neglected area of investigation, but one that has received more attention recently, is that relating to chest wall mechanics and the respiratory muscles.[67] Dysfunction of the respiratory muscles may not only result in disease, but also render an infant or child unable to compensate for the effects of such disease, with subsequent respiratory failure. Information regarding the strength of the respiratory muscles may be potentially useful in a number of clinical situations, including whether to wean an infant from the ventilator and the assessment of recovery from acute infections.[67] Methods of assessing respiratory muscle strength include determination of maximal inspired and expired pressure during respiratory efforts against brief airway occlusion.[68] Simple assessment of respiratory muscle strength does not, however, reflect either endurance or susceptibility to fatigue, and the marked within- and between-subject variability of this measure may limit its clinical usefulness. Consequently, work is being undertaken to evaluate the discriminative ability of alternative indices, such as the tension-time index of the respiratory muscles.[67] Although still to be evaluated in infants and young children, the latter has several advantages in that it is noninvasive, does not require placement of gastric or esophageal pressure transducers, and assesses muscle fatigue in all of the respiratory muscles, not simply the diaphragm.

Diaphragmatic function can also be assessed using nonvolitional tests, such as phrenic nerve stimulation. Original application of this technique using direct electrical stimulation was not only a highly skilled procedure, but also one that was relatively uncomfortable for the patient, thereby limiting its clinical applicability. Recent modifications of the technique, using magnetic rather than electrical stimulation, have overcome many of these problems. Although equipment remains expensive and is not yet widely available, this technique has been adapted for use in infants. By placing suitable catheters in the lower third of the esophagus and stomach, esophageal pressure (P_{es}) and gastric pressure (P_{gas}) can be measured using differential pressure transducers. This allows transdiaphragmatic pressure changes ($P_{di} = P_{es} - P_{gas}$) to be measured after magnetic stimulation of the left and right phrenic nerves.[69] It has been suggested that gestational age at birth and postconceptional age at the time of measurements must be taken into account when interpreting the results of such tests in infants.[70]

FORCED EXPIRATORY MANEUVERS

Beyond the neonatal period, most respiratory disorders are characterized by airway obstruction and narrowing, related to changes in airway caliber, airway wall thickness, secretions, inflammation, elastic recoil, or bronchial smooth muscle tone. Spirometry, whereby the subject inspires to TLC and exhales forcefully to RV, is the most frequently used method for measuring airway function in older children and adults. Among older subjects, spirometry has been used extensively to assess the nature and severity of airway disease, including degree of bronchial responsiveness and response to therapeutic interventions, and to monitor disease progression or resolution (see Chapter 10). The reliability of this technique is dependent on standardized methods, particularly with regard to achievement of flow limitation, rapidity with which flow increases at the beginning of expiration, sustained effort throughout the expiration, duration of the expiratory maneuver, and repeatability. Detailed criteria for data collection and interpretation have been published by the ATS and ERS, but even school-aged children may have difficulty meeting some of these quality control criteria. Despite earlier convictions that spirometric measurements were not routinely applicable to children younger than 6 years of age, recent reports have confirmed that the majority of preschool children are able to attempt these maneuvers, provided suitable modifications to data collection and analysis are introduced.[16] Similarly, by substituting voluntary effort with externally applied pressure to the chest and abdomen to force expiration, it has been possible to adapt these measurements and obtain both partial and full forced expiratory maneuvers in sleeping infants. Measurements of maximal expiratory flow at FRC (V'_{maxFRC}) have been used to help characterize the normal growth and development of the lungs during infancy and the pulmonary abnormalities associated with acute and chronic lung disorders during early childhood, whereas data derived from measuring forced flow and volume over an extended volume range have been found to discriminate clearly between those with and without respiratory disease, even in the absence of symptoms (discussed later).

ASSESSMENTS IN INFANTS

Partial Forced Expiratory Maneuvers

Infants cannot be instructed to perform forced expiratory maneuvers, but partial expiratory flow volume (PEFV) curves can be produced by wrapping a jacket around the chest and abdomen, which is inflated at the end of a tidal inspiration to force expiration. The resultant changes in airflow (and hence volume) are recorded through a flowmeter attached to a facemask, through which the child breathes (Fig. 9-25). This technique is usually referred to as the *squeeze*, or *tidal RTC*, technique.

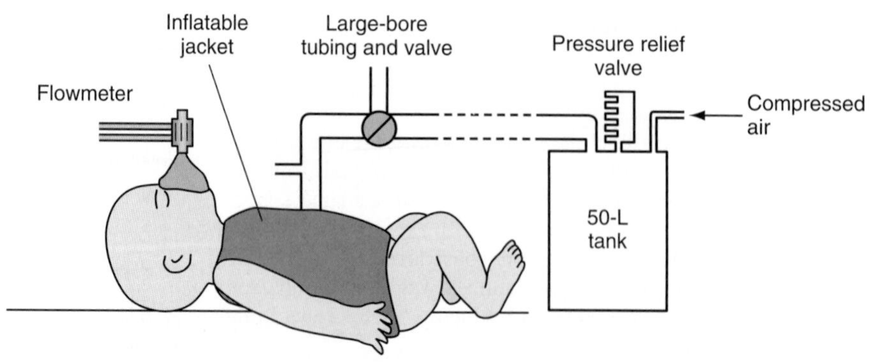

FIGURE 9-25. Tidal rapid thoracoabdominal compression (squeeze) technique for measuring partial forced expiratory maneuvers in infants. Airflow and volume are recorded while the infant breathes through a facemask and a flowmeter. At end-tidal inspiration, the jacket is inflated rapidly to force expiration. (Copyright © Janet Stocks.)

V'_{maxFRC}, which measures FEF at low lung volumes (i.e., similar to FEF_{75} or FEF_{85} in older children), is the most commonly reported parameter derived from this technique (Fig. 9-26). Guidelines regarding data collection and analysis for tidal RTC have been published by the ERS-ATS Task Force,[11] as have sex-specific collated reference data.[71] The validity of such reference equations for interpreting data collected with the new generation of commercially available infant lung function equipment has yet to be established.

Methodologic Considerations

To ensure that accurate and reproducible V'_{maxFRC} data are obtained, it is essential to do the following:

- Eliminate all leaks around the facemask.
- Establish a stable and representative end-expiratory level before forcing expiration.
- Ensure that flow limitation is achieved.

An initial jacket pressure of 20 to 30 cm H_2O is usually applied at the end of tidal inspiration, with the aim of transmitting approximately 10 cm H_2O to the pleural space. Jacket pressure is subsequently increased in increments of 10 to 20 cm H_2O until further increases do not elicit a further increase in flow at FRC. This is sometimes referred to as the *optimal pressure,* and it will vary considerably from child to child (i.e., 20–120 cm H_2O), depending not only on jacket efficiency, but also on the underlying respiratory mechanics, with infants with airway disease requiring far lower pressures to achieve flow limitation than healthy subjects. Measurements are repeated until at least three to five technically acceptable and reproducible maneuvers at optimal jacket pressure have been obtained. Because minor fluctuations in end-expiratory level can have marked effects on V'_{maxFRC}, it is generally recommended that V'_{maxFRC} be reported as the mean of the three highest technically acceptable results.

Advantages and Limitations

Measures of forced flow and volume reflect an integrated output of lung and airway mechanics and, as such, cannot be used to locate airway obstruction at any particular airway generation or anatomic location. Nevertheless, since V'_{maxFRC} is measured at low lung volumes, it is believed to reflect primarily airway caliber upstream of (i.e., distal to) the airway segment subjected to flow limitation. This makes it a useful measure of intrathoracic airway function in infants, in whom nasal resistance comprises such a large proportion of total resistance. However, because the caliber of the intrathoracic airways is determined not only by their anatomic dimensions, but also by the distending pressures surrounding them, full interpretation of results may require simultaneous measurement of lung volume and elastic recoil of the respiratory system. Whether flow limitation can be reached in healthy infants using this technique remains controversial. Nevertheless, this technique provides a useful forcing function that can provide a valuable measure of airway function in infants. As in older subjects, the shape of the loop and the numeric values derived contribute to the interpretation of results (Fig. 9-27). The tidal RTC technique has been used widely in clinical and epidemiologic research studies and remains one of the most practical techniques available for assessing response to bronchodilators or bronchial challenge in infants. Interpretation of results may, however, be confounded by numerous factors, as discussed later.

Forced Expiratory Maneuvers from Raised Lung Volume

Despite the popularity of tidal RTC, its value when assessing either baseline airway function or bronchial responsiveness may be limited by the dependence of reported values of V'_{maxFRC} on resting lung volume, which may not be stable in infants, particularly in the presence of disease or during intervention studies. During the 1990s, the tidal RTC technique was modified so that FEF and volume could be measured over an extended volume range in what rapidly became known as the *raised volume RTC* (RVRTC) technique (Fig. 9-28). Similar to spirometric assessments in older subjects, RVRTC allows the infant's lungs to be inflated toward TLC before rapid inflation of the jacket initiates forced expiration from this elevated lung volume, with the maneuver ending when the infant reaches residual volume (RV) (Fig. 9-29). During initial attempts to apply this technique, infants frequently inspired before reaching RV. Application of three to five augmented breaths to induce a respiratory pause before forced expiration subsequently overcame this problem.

Methodologic Considerations

The airway pressure used to augment inspiration is most commonly 30 cm H_2O, although some centers have used 20 cm H_2O. Jacket inflation must be maintained until lung emptying is complete, and care is required to ensure that air is not forced into the

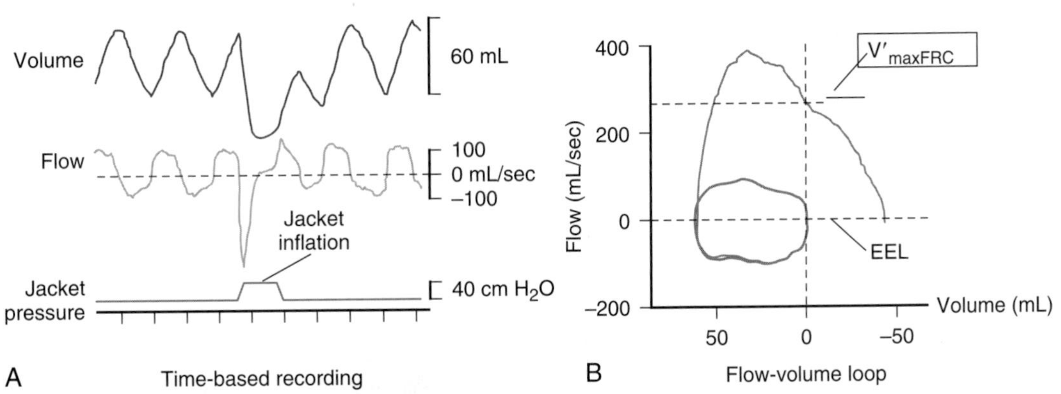

FIGURE 9-26. **A** and **B,** Partial expiratory flow volume maneuvers derived from the tidal rapid thoracoabdominal compression technique. Jacket pressure commences at approximately 30 cm H_2O and is increased in increments of 5 to 10 cm H_2O until further increases elicit no further increase in forced expiratory flow at functional residual capacity (i.e., when maximum flow at FRC [V'_{maxFRC}] is attained). EEL, end-expiratory level. (Copyright © Janet Stocks.)

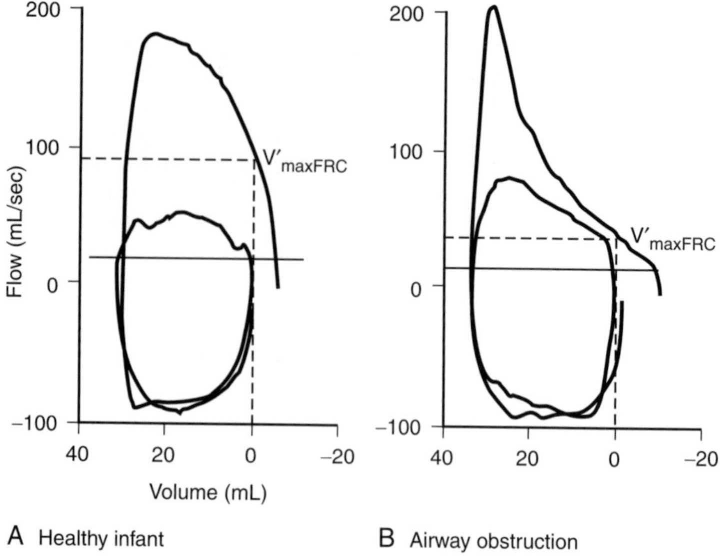

■ **FIGURE 9-27.** Comparison of partial flow-volume loops in health and disease. **A,** In a healthy newborn infant, maximal flow at FRC (V'_{maxFRC}) is 92 mL/sec. **B,** In an infant of similar age and weight, but with evidence of airway obstruction, much lower flows are recorded and the descending portion of the expiratory flow-volume loop has a characteristically scooped-out shape (concave to the volume axis). (Copyright © Janet Stocks.)

stomach during inflation. The procedure is repeated until at least two technically satisfactory and repeatable maneuvers have been recorded,[17] with values generally being reported from the best curve (i.e., that with the highest product of forced vital capacity (FVC) and either forced expiratory volume in 0.5 second ($FEV_{0.5}$) or forced expiratory flow at 75% of expired FVC ($FEF_{75\%}$) (discussed later). Figure 9-30 shows the relationship between a partial forced expiratory maneuver initiated from end-tidal inspiration and that recorded from the same infant after lung volume was raised with an inflation pressure of 30 cm H_2O.

Despite the increasing use of RVRTC in recent years, a wide range of methods that differ in terms of data collection, analysis, and presentation of results is still being used. Although there is insufficient evidence to produce firm guidelines, the ATS-ERS Task Force on infant lung function testing has recently produced a consensus statement that provides preliminary recommendations pertaining to equipment, study procedures, and reporting of data for the RVRTC, based on what is perceived to be current best practice.[17]

Analysis and Reporting of Results

The values that are most commonly reported from RVRTC include the following:

- FVC — Forced vital capacity from the applied inflation pressure (e.g., FVC_{30})
- $FEV_{0.4/0.5}$ — Forced expired volume at 0.4 or 0.5 seconds (or occasionally after 0.75 seconds)
- $FEF_{50\%/75\%/85\%}$ — Forced expiratory flow at 50%, 75%, or 85% of expired FVC (equivalent to maximal expired flow (MEF) 50%, 25%, and 15%, respectively, when using the European notation and relating MEF to the proportion of FVC remaining in the lungs
- $FEF_{25\%-75\%}$ — Forced expiratory flow between 25% and 75% of expired FVC

It should be noted that despite common use of the term FVC for the total volume expired during RVRTC, this does not necessarily equate to measures in older subjects, because infants

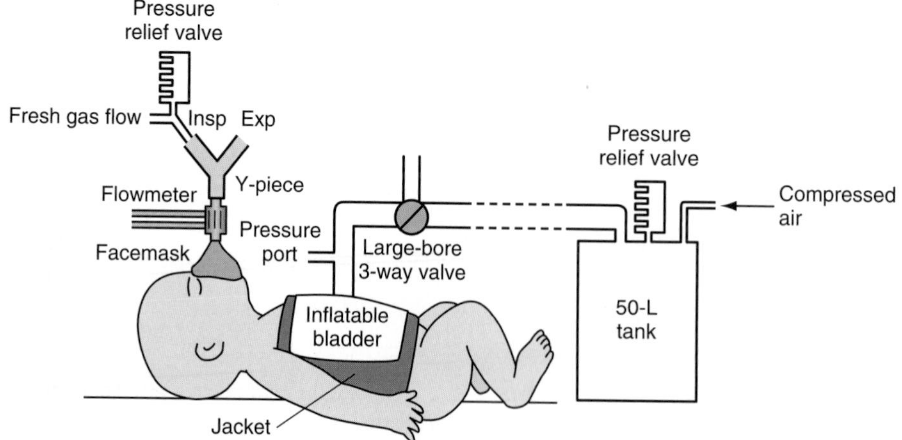

■ **FIGURE 9-28.** Forced expiratory maneuvers from increased lung volume. Using a system of valves or bias flow, the infant's lungs are inflated toward total lung capacity, using a preset standardized inflation pressure (usually 30 cm H_2O), before an external forcing function is applied. The latter is achieved by rapid inflation of a jacket wrapped around the thorax and abdomen. This allows forced measurement of expiratory flow and volume over a wide volume range, as in older subjects. Jacket pressure is increased incrementally until further increases elicit no further increase in forced expiratory flow and volume. Exp, expiration; Insp, inspiration. (Copyright © Janet Stocks.)

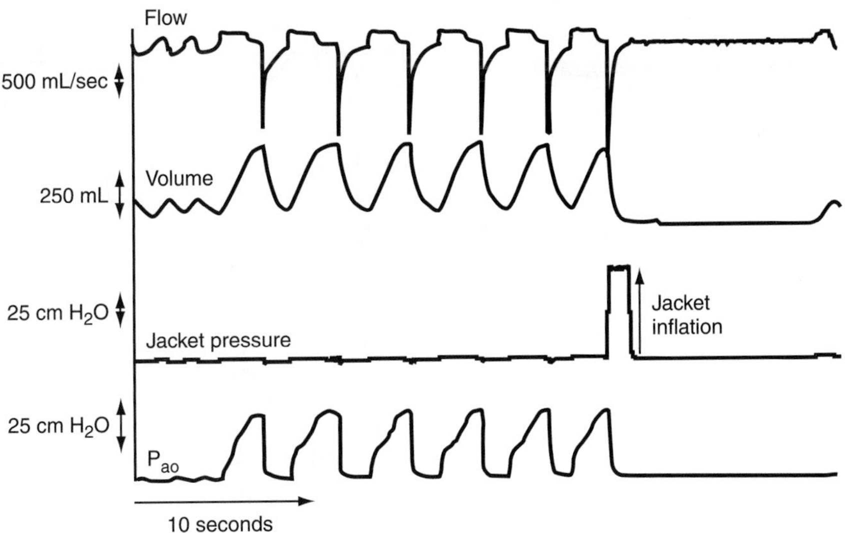

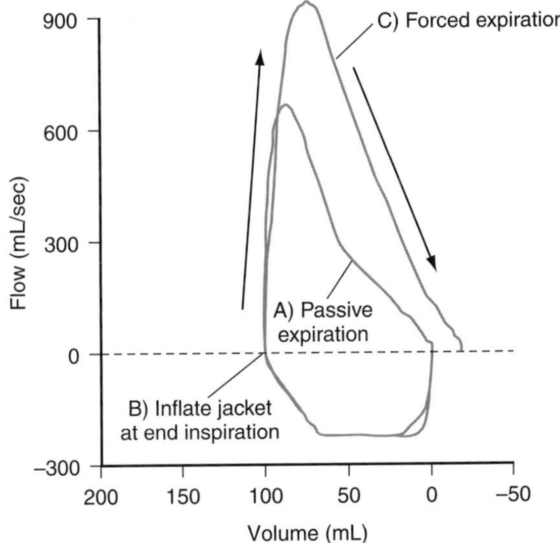

■ **FIGURE 9-29.** Forced expiratory maneuvers using the raised volume technique. **A,** Time-based trace. After an initial period of tidal breathing, a preset, standardized intermittent positive pressure of 30 cm H_2O is applied at the airway opening to inflate the lungs toward total lung capacity. The jacket is inflated at the end of the sixth augmented breath to force expiration from increased lung volume. **B,** Flow-volume curve obtained during passive and forced expiration from increased lung volume. (Copyright © Janet Stocks.)

have been observed to take a sigh at the end of an inflation to 30 cm H_2O, demonstrating that TLC has not actually been attained. Calculations of FEV_1, and to a lesser extent, $FEV_{0.75}$ are rarely feasible in young infants, except in the presence of marked airway obstruction, due to the very rapid lung emptying and short forced expiratory time (FET) that occurs during early life.[6,72] There is a marked age dependency of FEV/FVC ratios during infancy and early childhood, and in contrast to data from older subjects, such ratios discriminate poorly between infants with respiratory disease or impaired lung development compared with control subjects.[73,74] Although measures of timed forced expired volumes (FEV_t) are more reproducible than forced flows and have been found to be discriminative in both clinical and epidemiologic studies,[73–75] the latter may be equally sensitive when studying wheezy infants during both baseline measurements and assessments of bronchial responsiveness.[41,76,77]

Preliminary collation of data from healthy infants (3–149 weeks) studied in the United States ($n = 155$),[78] London ($n = 253$), and Brazil ($n = 25$), all of whom were measured using similar equipment and techniques, show an encouraging degree of overlap, with no marked intercenter differences (Fig. 9-31). More data, however, must be collected and formal statistical analyses undertaken before collated prediction equations can be developed for RVRTC.

Advantages and Limitations

As in older children and adults, assessment of $FEF_{\%}$ can be reported only when valid measurements of FVC have been obtained. Underestimation of FVC (with concomitant overestimation of $FEF_{\%}$) will occur if the child breathes in before RV has been reached. By contrast, underestimation of FVC because of failure to deliver the specified inflation pressure or because of

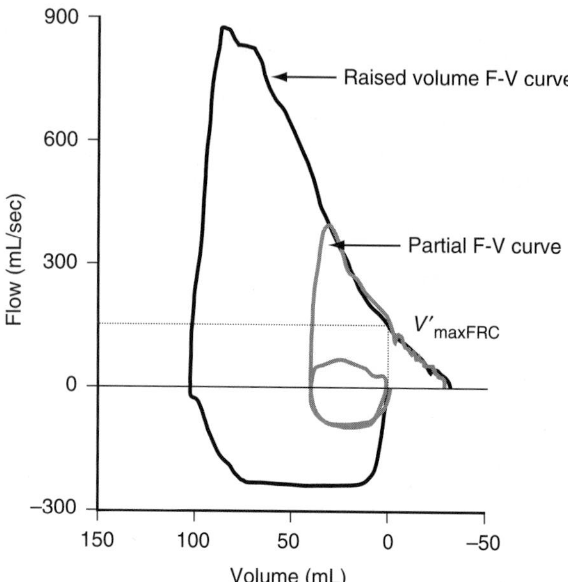

■ **FIGURE 9-30.** Overlay of tidal and increased volume forced expiratory flow volume (FEFV) curves from the same infant, illustrating the relative size of tidal and augmented breaths before forced expiration. F-V, flow-volume curve; V'_{maxFRC}, maximal flow at FRC. (Copyright © Janet Stocks.)

accumulation of gas in the stomach, with upward displacement of the diaphragm, will result in underestimation of both FEV_t and $FEF_{\%}$. Failure to reach flow limitation by using too low a jacket pressure may have minimal effect on FVC, provided the appropriate inflation pressure has been applied, but will underestimate both FEV_t and particularly flow. However, the choice of optimal jacket pressure remains debatable because the use of a high enough pressure to achieve flow limitation at high lung volumes may result in negative flow dependency at low lung volumes, particularly in infants prone to airway narrowing and closure.

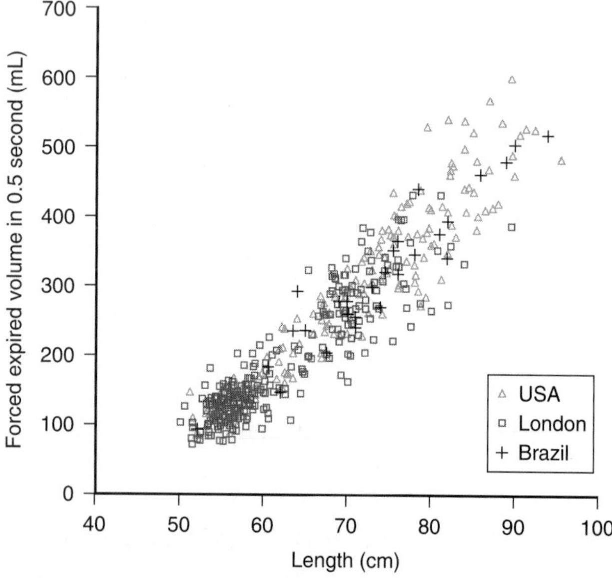

■ **FIGURE 9-31.** Collated data for forced expired volume in 0.5 second ($FEV_{0.5}$) during infancy. Scatter plot of $FEV_{0.5}$ versus length. Data collected using similar techniques from four centers. Note the increase in $FEV_{0.5}$ from approximately 100 mL in the first month of life to approximately 600 mL between 2 and 3 years of age. (Copyright © Janet Stocks.)

Flow-volume maneuvers from increased lung volume are more difficult to perform than partial flow-volume maneuvers. Extensive training and dedicated personnel who can ensure precision with respect to, for example, timing and inflation pressures are essential to assure accurate results. Leaks around the facemask will occur more easily because of the positive pressure within it. Some children, particularly those with severe airway disease, will not relax sufficiently or will consistently inspire before RV is reached, thereby invalidating calculations of both FVC and $FEF_{\%}$. Repeated inflations may result in accumulation of gas in the stomach, which not only is uncomfortable for the child, but also will invalidate the results. RVRTC may also affect subsequent measures of lung function, such that important decisions need to be made regarding the order of tests within a protocol.[79,80] Finally, considerable caution is required in infants who are oxygen-dependent, in whom repeated lung inflations might lead to prolonged apnea.

Potential advantages of RVRTC include the following:

- Forced flow and volume are measured from a more reproducible lung volume than when tidal maneuvers are performed.
- Flow can be assessed over an extended volume range from near TLC to RV.
- Flow limitation should be easier to achieve.
- Longitudinal assessment of similar values may be possible from infancy to adulthood (interpretation of such results is discussed later).

As with most infant lung function tests, the clinical utility of RVRTC in the individual infant has yet to be established. However, this technique has been used to improve the understanding of lung and airway growth in the healthy infant,[73,75,78] and several studies have indicated that RVRTC may be more discriminative than tidal RTC for distinguishing the effects of respiratory disease on airway function.[18,81] In clinical research studies, RVRTC has the potential to quantify the degree of airway obstruction,[18,41,76] monitor changes in airway mechanics over time,[73,74] and evaluate bronchial responsiveness (Fig. 9-32).[41,77,82]

Forced Expiratory Maneuvers in Preschool Children

Data Collection

With appropriate training and encouragement (Fig. 9-33), 60% to 80% of children between 3 and 6 years of age can achieve acceptable spirometry results, although a greater number of maneuvers than the maximum of eight recommended by the ATS may be necessary to achieve this due to the initial training required.[16] These measurements should generally be performed at the end of a test protocol, due to the potential and unpredictable effects of deep inhalation and forced expiration on other measures of respiratory function. Young children need to be taught what is meant by *taking a big breath in* or *blowing out as hard and fast as possible.* A variety of blowing games involving straws, bubbles, party whistles, and so forth can facilitate this process, as can demonstrations from the operator and the use of carefully selected computer incentives.[16,83] If such incentives are used, computerized games such as blowing out the candles must be used only to teach the child how to achieve peak

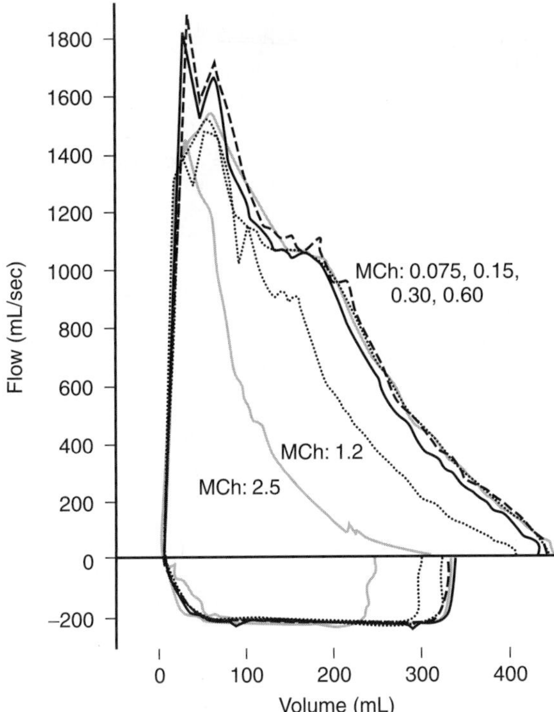

FIGURE 9-32. Use of the raised volume rapid thoracoabdominal compression technique to assess bronchial responsiveness in an infant. After baseline values for forced expired flow and volume were established using this technique, the maneuver was repeated after incremental doses of methacholine (MCh). Highly repeatable measurements were obtained with the first four doses, followed by a significant bronchoconstrictor response at higher doses. Note changes in the shape of the forced expiratory flow volume (FEFV) curve as well as reduction in flows. (Courtesy of R. Tepper, Indianapolis.)

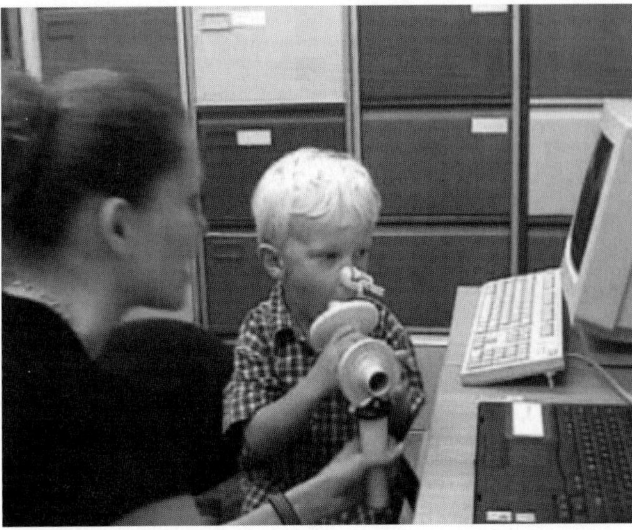

FIGURE 9-33. Preschool spirometry. Most preschool children older than 3 years of age will tolerate nose clips, although this is not imperative for acceptable results. As with all preschool tests, establishment of a good relationship between the technician and the child is vital. Judicious use of computerized incentives may improve both individual performance and success rates. (Copyright © Janet Stocks.)

expired flow because they provide no incentive for the child to continue blowing out to RV, and as a result, they may result in serious underestimation of FVC (Fig. 9-34). Considerable input is required from the investigator with respect to the targets that are set. If they are too low, the child will not make a maximum effort, and if they are too high, the child will become discouraged and may stop trying.[16]

Preschool spirometry can be performed with the subject either seated or standing, but the posture should be reported. Most preschool children tolerate nose clips quite happily, although their use does not appear to be mandatory for acceptable recordings.[84] As with older subjects, acceptable curves are those with a rapid rise to peak flow, smooth expiration, and no evidence of early inspiration (Fig. 9-35). It can be difficult to judge the quality of the results during data collection, and all loops should therefore be saved for review once the test has ended. Most young children appear to enjoy spirometry and will happily make repeated efforts to achieve their target. Although many of the curves may need to be rejected (Fig. 9-36), three technically satisfactory curves (discussed later) can usually be obtained with persistence.

Reporting of Results

Values that should be recorded when undertaking preschool spirometry include the following:

- FVC, FEV_1, $FEV_{0.75}$ (provided FET exceeds 1 and 0.75 seconds, respectively), $FEV_{0.5}$, $FEF_{25\%}$, $FEF_{50\%}$, $FEF_{75\%}$, and $FEF_{25\%-75\%}$
- Duration of forced expiration (FET)
- Back-extrapolated volume at the start of expiration (both as an absolute volume and as percent FVC)
- Timed expired volumes as fractions of FVC (e.g., $FEV_{0.5}$/FVC, $FEV_{0.75}$/FVC, and FEV_1/FVC)
- Absolute and percent differences between key parameters from the two "best" maneuvers, (e.g., ΔFVC, $\Delta FEV_{0.5}$, ΔFEV_1, $\Delta FEV_{0.75}$, $\Delta FEF_{25\%-75\%}$)

Quality Control

Preliminary recommendations regarding quality control for preschool children, including criteria for the start and end of testing, have been published recently.[16] Some examples of acceptable and unacceptable curves are shown in Figures 9-35

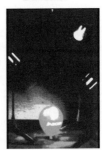

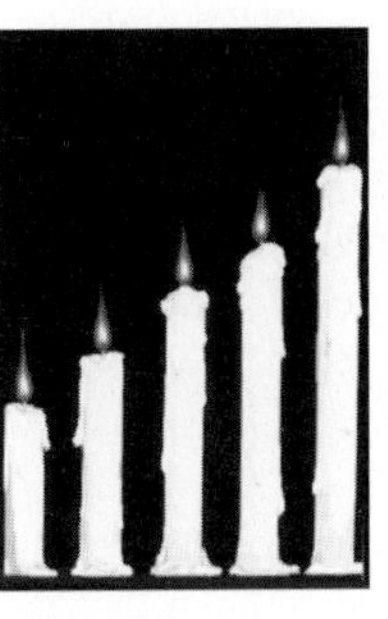

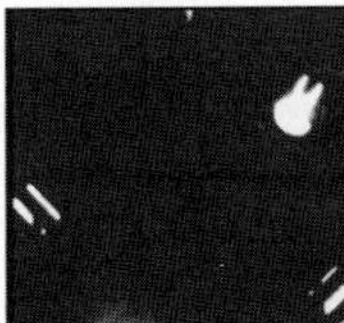

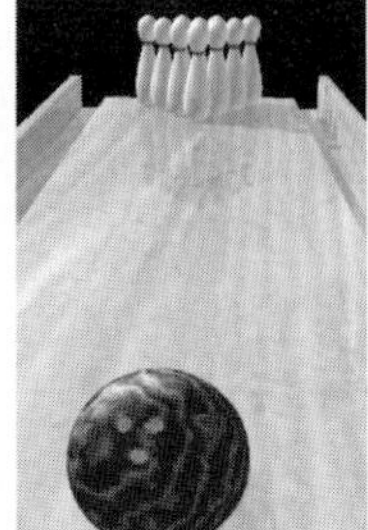

FIGURE 9-34. Choice of computerized incentive for preschool spirometry. Effective use of computerized incentive spirometry is dependent on selecting the appropriate game. Several of the choices, including the birthday cake candles, provide no incentive for the child to continue blowing once peak expired flow (PEF) has been achieved, whereas others may be too complex for the child (or, on occasion, the operator) to understand! Whichever game is selected, it is essential that appropriate targets be set and a sufficient number of trials be allowed to ensure that the child reaches true potential. (See Color Plate 10.) (Copyright © Janet Stocks.)

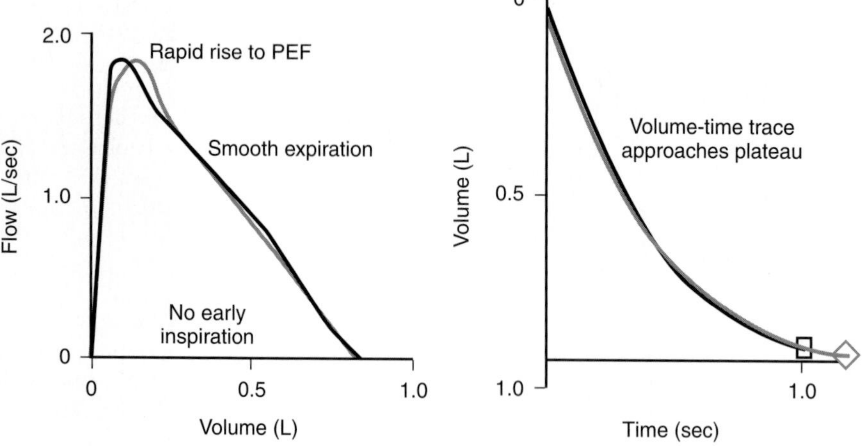

■ **FIGURE 9-35.** Technically acceptable spirometry data from a 3-year-old child. As with older subjects, acceptable curves are those with rapid rise to peak flow (PEF), smooth expiration, and no evidence of early inspiration on the flow-volume curve, as shown on the *left,* and with the volume-time trace *(right)* approaching a plateau. (Copyright © Janet Stocks.)

and 9-36. The main differences with respect to criteria used for adults are the following:

- Visual inspection is usually adequate to detect a slow start to the forced expiration, with the majority of children younger than 6 years of age being able to achieve a volume of back-extrapolation to the start of testing of less than 80 mL or less than 10% (Fig. 9-37).
- Technically acceptable data should not be judged by the duration of the effort because young children's lungs may empty extremely quickly (i.e., in <1 second).
- The ability to produce FEV_1 is age-dependent in both health and disease. Consequently, $FEV_{0.5}$ and $FEV_{0.75}$ should be calculated and reported in addition to FEV_1 for all children younger than 6 years of age. For many 2- to 4-year-old children, only the shorter timed volumes will be reportable.
- Even when FEV_1 is attainable, the clinical value of this measurement is questionable in this age group because the FEV_1/FVC ratio is more than 90% in the majority of preschool children.
- Further investigation of the discriminative ability of different spirometric parameters is an important area for future research.
- Evaluation of the end of the test by visual inspection is more difficult in preschool children, in whom there may be a relatively abrupt cessation of expiration. Modification of commercially available software to allow more objective evaluation of the change in the rate of lung emptying toward the end of expiration is required.
- Where incomplete expiration due to early inspiration is identified, timed expired volume and peak flow may still be reportable, even though FVC and FEF cannot be reported from such maneuvers.
- Repeatability can be assessed as for adults, but criteria of 100 mL or 10% of best effort for ΔFVC and ΔFEV_t between the two highest technically acceptable maneuvers may be more appropriate in this age group.

Interpretation of Results

It remains to be proven whether spirometric measures obtained during the preschool years are sensitive enough to influence clinical or research practice (discussed later). Several recent publications have reported normative data on spirometry from healthy preschool children.[85–87] These should be used with caution until they are further validated, because there are significant differences in predicted values according to which equations are selected, which could bias the interpretation of results from children with respiratory disease.[16] The rapidity with which FEV increases during early childhood is illustrated in Figure 9-38, which shows preliminary collated data for $FEV_{0.5}$ obtained with the RVRTC technique during infancy and with spirometry in young children between 3 and 9 years of age. With increasing consensus regarding the methods of data collection and analysis, it may soon be possible to collate such data on an international scale so that reliable reference data can be developed for this age group. In the meantime, it is recommended that any center undertaking preschool spirometry assess its own age-matched healthy control group before interpreting the results from those with lung disease. Although lack of appropriate control data can

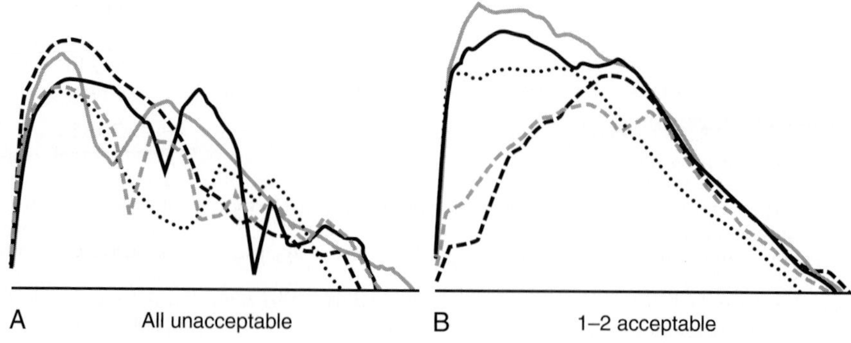

■ **FIGURE 9-36.** **A** and **B,** Technically unacceptable spirometry data. During initial attempts, this child was unable to produce any acceptable data, whereas during the second set of five maneuvers, one acceptable curve with a second of borderline quality was achieved, with reproducible overlay during the second half of forced expiration. (Copyright © Janet Stocks.)

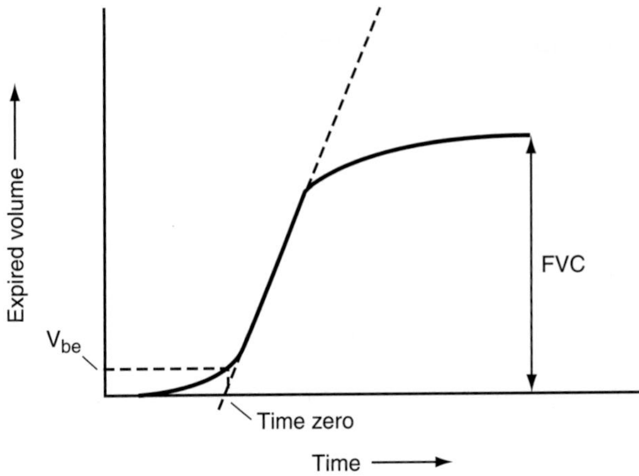

■ **FIGURE 9-37.** Start-of-test quality control criteria for preschool spirometry. Start-of-test quality control criteria for adults and older children specify a back-extrapolated volume (VBE) at the beginning of expiration that is less than 5% of forced vital capacity (FVC). This is not attainable by the majority of preschool children, whereas most can achieve a volume of back-extrapolation at the start of the test of less than 80 mL or less than 10%.[16] (Copyright © Janet Stocks.)

to some extent be circumvented if the child is used as his/her own control, for example, when assessing bronchial responsiveness, knowledge of the likely magnitude of response to such interventions in healthy children of similar age remains vital for meaningful interpretation of results.[56]

Similarly, despite the exciting potential for longitudinal assessments of parameters, such as $FEV_{0.5}$ from birth, caution will need to be exercised when interpreting results. As discussed earlier, during infancy, such measurements will be subject to differences in the precise methodologic details associated with the

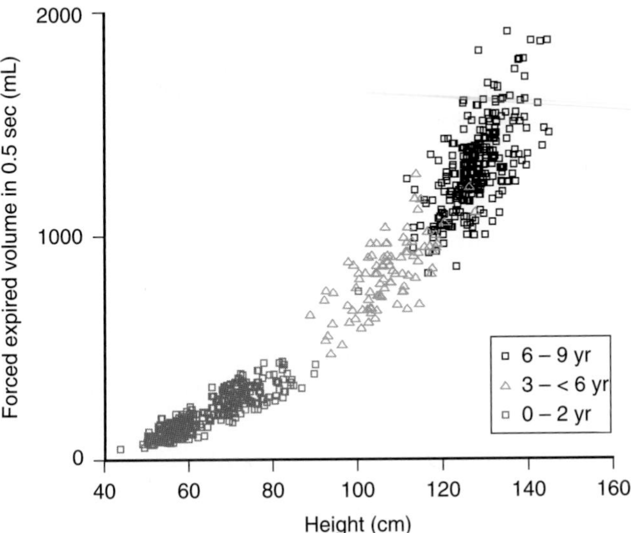

■ **FIGURE 9-38.** Collated measurements of forced expired volume in 0.5 second ($FEV_{0.5}$) from birth to 9 years of age. Measures of $FEV_{0.5}$ were collected in 413 healthy children (219 boys, 194 girls; 86% white) on 595 test occasions, using the raised volume rapid thoracoabdominal compression technique in supine, sedated infants and young children up to the age of 2 years and using spirometry in awake, seated children from 3 years of age onward. The main determinant of $FEV_{0.5}$ was height at the time of testing, which showed a strong curvilinear relationship (r^2 = 0.97). (Presented at the European Respiratory Society Conference 2004. Lum S, Castle R, Saunders C, Kozlowska WJ, Hoo AF, Aurora P, Stocks J: Forced expiratory volumes in healthy children from birth to school age. Eur Respir J 2004;24[Suppl 48]:158S.)

use of RVRTC. In addition, $FEV_{0.5}$ during the preschool years may reflect more central airway function than the same measure when recorded during infancy, due to the reduced rate of lung emptying with growth.[6,7] Although FEV_1 is routinely measured in older subjects, the underlying physiology of this parameter is complex. FEV_1 depends on the factors that determine maximum expiratory flow at a particular lung volume, the change in maximum expiratory flow with lung volume, and the change in intrapulmonary resistance with changes in lung volume. Although FEV_1 is considered to reflect primarily large and central airway function in older subjects, there is limited evidence to support this. Although it is likely that $FEV_{0.5}$ values in infants and preschool children reflect similar mechanical properties of the airways and alveoli, there is unlikely to be anatomic concordance with FEV_1 in older subjects. Similarly, longitudinal measurements of $FEV_{0.5}$ in the same infant are unlikely to provide physiologic information from the same airway generations on each occasion.

There are currently few data on within-subject, between-occasion repeatability of spirometry data in preschool children, which limits the interpretation of results from any intervention study.

ASSESSMENT OF BRONCHIAL RESPONSIVENESS

Assessing whether airway function improves after the use of bronchodilator drugs is probably one of the most important clinical investigations performed in older children and adults. The response to bronchoconstrictors is less frequently examined, and such measurements do not play such a central role in clinical management. The lack of evidence of bronchial hyperresponsiveness may, nonetheless, be useful in excluding a diagnosis of asthma. The role of such assessments during the first 5 years of life is less clearly defined, due to the difficulty in both performing and interpreting these tests during infancy and, until recently, the lack of available tests for use in preschool children. The effectiveness of bronchodilators in wheezy infants remains controversial, reflecting the fact that, in many infants who wheeze, the reduction in baseline airway function is not due to reversible bronchoconstriction, but is the result of transient conditions associated with diminished airway patency. There is, however, convincing evidence that the airways are fully innervated and capable of responding to a range of challenges during fetal and early postnatal life.[5,82] Bronchial hyper-responsiveness in early life has been found to be a risk factor for subsequent symptoms of asthma in some, but not all, reported studies,[88] and several studies have emphasized that bronchial responsiveness is likely to be more discriminative than baseline respiratory function in the assessment of preschool children and young school-aged children with persistent wheeze.[57,89–91] Important issues to address in the assessment of airway responsiveness include the technique used to assess the change in airway function, the agent used, the dosage and delivery efficacy of aerosol, quantification of the airway response, and the potential clinical utility of the information obtained.[92]

Methodologic Issues

Choice of Tests

The most commonly used test to assess airway response in older subjects is spirometry, although plethysmography is also a popular choice. In infants, the vast majority of studies have used partial, or more recently, raised volume flow-volume curves. By contrast, although spirometry has also been used in preschool children, this is a demanding test, and its use in intervention studies is usually reserved for slightly older children.[26,89] The most commonly used tests for assessing bronchial responsiveness in preschool children have been the interrupter technique, FOT, and plethysmographic assessments of specific resistance, although some investigators have used more indirect methods (particularly during bronchial challenge), including transcutaneous oxygen tension,[63] auscultation (wheeze),[93] or tidal breathing parameters[23,26] to assess responsiveness. The most important distinction is between techniques that require deep inflation to total lung capacity and those that are obtained during tidal breathing or at volumes close to FRC. Deep inflation can modify airway responses considerably,[64] and the difference in response before and after such maneuvers is sometimes used to localize the site of response in older subjects.

Technical problems related to the choice of method can influence the interpretation of airway responsiveness in early life. Thus, although the tidal RTC technique has been frequently used in infants during both bronchodilator and challenge tests, changes in FRC that may be induced by the intervention, but are not routinely measured during the procedure, may result in paradoxical changes in V'_{maxFRC} and an underestimation of airway responsiveness. Although the use of RVRTC should minimize problems associated with referencing flows to FRC, measured FVC can be underestimated secondary to accumulation of gas in the stomach from repeated maneuvers as well as by inspiration before RV is reached during forced expiration. Furthermore, the effect of repeated lung inflations on baseline respiratory mechanics and responsiveness has yet to be established in infants. Similarly, even though resistance is a more direct measure of airway caliber than maximal expiratory flow, a decrease in resistance may reflect changes in extrathoracic resistance, such as changes in the vocal cords or the pharyngeal airway. When tests such as the single-occlusion or interrupter techniques are used, bronchoconstriction after administration of a challenge may increase ventilation inhomogeneity or increase the time needed to reach pressure equilibration, resulting in a potentially dangerous underestimation of the change in resistance. When such tests are used, it is therefore recommended that transcutaneous oxygen tension be monitored, in addition to oxygen saturation. Given that marked reductions in airway function may occur during any challenge test, safety is of paramount importance. When such tests are performed in infants and preschool children, two fully trained operators, at least one of whom must be a nurse or physician, should always be present.

Choice of Provocative Stimulus

As in older subjects, many pharmacologic and physical stimuli have been used in challenge tests for infants and young children. Histamine and methacholine are the most commonly used agents that act directly on smooth muscle. Methacholine has been favored in most epidemiologic studies. Adenosine monophosphate and hypertonic saline cause bronchoconstriction via the release of mediators and have been used to provide a more indirect, and possibly more physiologic, stimulus. Exercise testing is obviously not appropriate for infants and does not appear to have been adapted for use in preschool children. The use of cold or dry air challenges is gaining popularity in this age range.[94] As in older subjects, inhalation of a β_2-adrenergic agonist drug, such as salbutamol (albuterol) or terbutaline, is routinely used both to reverse the effects of challenge tests and to assess bronchodilator response.

Administration of an Inhaled Agent

The method chosen to administer the inhaled pharmacologic agent will be influenced by the need for portability, the age and clinical status of the child, and the purpose of the assessment (clinical or research). The aerosol dose delivered to the airways will depend on the device used to generate the aerosol, the method of delivering the aerosol, and the location of aerosol deposition. Aerosol output varies according to the type and operating conditions of each nebulizer and the physical properties of the liquid to be aerosolized. The quantity of aerosol inhaled will depend on the size of the inhaled volume, whether inhalation is via the nasal or oral route, and whether the child is asleep, quietly awake, or crying, because different inspiratory flow patterns will accompany each of these states (see Chapter 16).[5] Whichever delivery system is used, an appropriate bronchodilator should be prepared before the first dose of challenge agent is administered.

Aerosols are generally delivered to infants during tidal breathing, whereas older, cooperative subjects often take deep inspirations to maximize aerosol delivery throughout the lung. Deep inspirations can also be used to deliver aerosols to sleeping infants, using techniques similar to those employed in ventilated subjects, or during RVRTC. The potential effect of deep inhalations on the lung function parameters being measured must be considered when choosing the mode of delivery. The effectiveness of the response to the generated aerosol will depend on the site of aerosol deposition. Only a small fraction of the pharmaceutical agent aerosolized by the nebulizer or metered-dose inhaler actually deposits within the airways.

There is currently no standardized dosage or method for delivery for the evaluation of bronchodilator responsiveness in infants and young children. Selection of dosage has varied among that used clinically; that demonstrated to reverse the acute effects of a bronchoconstricting agent; such as methacholine or histamine; and that required within an individual to effect an increase in heart rate.

Evaluation of Response

There is currently no consensus on how to evaluate whether an infant or young child has demonstrated an improvement in airway function after the administration of a bronchodilator. Different approaches include: (1) comparison of the best pretest and post-test values, (2) comparison of the premean and postmean values from several replicates, and (3) definition of a specific pre-to-post change for the individual, based on the variability of the measurement in the population. The importance of assessing within-subject variability between occasions, in the absence of any intervention, if such tests are to be interpreted in a meaningful fashion, has been stressed recently.[57,95]

As in older subjects, constructing a dose-response curve that quantifies the dose of agonist required to produce a specified reduction from baseline airway function has been used to summarize the degree of airway reactivity in infants and young children. When FEF is used to assess airway responsiveness in infants, the provocative concentration of the agonist needed to produce a 30% reduction from baseline (PC_{30}) in V'_{maxFRC}, or $FEF_{25\%}$, is often used. The magnitude of this decrease has been found to exceed the intrasubject within-test variability of the measurement, and it is frequently associated with a change in the shape of the flow-volume curve from convex to concave (see Fig. 9-32).[82] An alternative approach, based on the magnitude of response to a fixed intervention in relation to within-subject variability, is required when single-step tests, such as cold or dry air challenges, are used.

Age-Related Changes in Hyper-responsiveness

In infants, heightened responsiveness may result not only from anatomically small airways or increased smooth muscle tone, but also from relatively thicker airway walls, decreased chest wall recoil, or increased airway wall compliance. Together with the difficulties in estimating the dose of agonist that will actually be delivered to the lung in infants and young children, such factors make it virtually impossible to interpret apparent changes in bronchial reactivity during the first few years of life.[96] Any comparisons between results obtained in infancy and in later life, especially those derived from longitudinal studies, must consider not only all of the factors discussed earlier, but also the posture in which measurements are obtained.[82]

As discussed earlier, failure of infants and young children to respond to inhaled bronchodilators may be partially attributed to difficulties in delivering adequate amounts of aerosolized drugs in this age group, but may also reflect differences in the underlying pathology, with wheezing in younger children being due to factors such as congenitally small airways, airway wall edema, or secretions rather than to bronchial smooth muscle shortening. Whereas increased airway responsiveness is evident in most asthmatic adults and older wheezy children, this is not routinely the case in wheezy infants or preschool children. The degree of bronchodilator response appears to be age-related, and it is often (although not always) minimal or absent before 18 months of age, but well established by 6 to 8 years of age.

Future Directions

With increasing awareness of the importance of assessing the reversibility of a reduction in baseline airway function to improve the discriminative ability of currently available tests for preschool children, it is essential for international guidelines and standardized protocols for undertaking such tests to be developed as rapidly as possible, together with an assessment of which tests are most appropriate under specified conditions and for specific populations of young children.

The usefulness of assessing airway responsiveness must be approached in relation to how the information obtained will be used. Several research studies have been able to demonstrate bronchodilator and bronchoconstrictor responsiveness in healthy infants and young children, as well as those with various respiratory diseases. However, what is a clinically significant bronchodilator response for an individual child has not been defined. In addition, the clinical usefulness of assessing airway reactivity in individual patients who are not participating in a clinical research project has not been demonstrated.

APPLICATIONS OF PULMONARY FUNCTION TESTS IN INFANTS AND PRESCHOOL CHILDREN

EPIDEMIOLOGIC RESEARCH INTO EARLY DETERMINANTS OF RESPIRATORY FUNCTION

In recent years, there has been increasing use of lung function tests to provide objective outcome measures in population-based studies of respiratory health and disease during early life. Numerous studies have shown that the sex of an infant has a marked effect on airway function, as reflected by the lower maximal expiratory flow observed in boys compared with girls at any given height, both during infancy and in later childhood. This may contribute to the increased prevalence of wheezing in boys at all ages to puberty. Sex-specific reference data should therefore be used when predicting normal ranges of airway function.[71] Although less is known about the effect of ethnic group on lung function during early life, both nasal and airway resistance have been shown to be lower in Afro-Caribbean than in white infants. Preliminary data suggest that ethnic differences in spirometric values, long recognized among older children and adults, may also be detectable in preschool children.[16]

There is powerful evidence of the adverse effects of maternal smoking on infant lung function. This effect is apparent at least 7 weeks before the expected date of delivery and is independent of postnatal exposure, as demonstrated by studies that have assessed lung function in healthy infants before discharge from the neonatal unit. A recent review of the literature found conclusive evidence that smoking during pregnancy is associated with a reduction in FEF (by, on average, approximately 20%), as well as increases in both airway and total resistance.[97] There is also substantial evidence regarding the adverse effect of maternal smoking during pregnancy on postnatal control of breathing, particularly with respect to a blunted response to hypoxia, hypercapnia, and arousal stimuli.[35,98] In infants born to atopic mothers, exhaled nitric oxide levels are increased shortly after birth in those exposed to maternal smoking, whereas the reverse appears to be true among those delivered to nonatopic mothers.[39] It has recently been suggested that glutathione S-transferase may play a role in asthma and wheezing among those exposed to intrauterine tobacco smoke, because it functions in pathways that are possibly involved in asthma pathogenesis, such as xenobiotic metabolism and antioxidant defenses. A recent study of school-aged children indicated that the long-term effects of in utero exposure to maternal smoking on lung function and on asthma and wheezing were largely restricted to children with glutathione S-transferase null genotype.[99] Such studies underline the complex relationship between genetic and environmental factors on the development of airway disease and the importance of taking gene-environment interactions into account in future epidemiologic studies.

Although maternal smoking during pregnancy remains the most significant source of exposure to tobacco products in early life and is likely to be largely responsible for diminished airway function in the first few years of life, continuing postnatal exposure to tobacco smoke from either parent will increase the risk of respiratory infection, wheezing illnesses, and diminished lung function throughout childhood. The effect of parental smoking has an equally adverse effect on infants with lung disease,[100] thereby necessitating careful recording of such exposures if the results of either clinical or research studies are to be interpreted correctly.

A family history of atopy, particularly maternal asthma, has been shown to be associated with diminished airway function and increased airway responsiveness during both infancy and the preschool years.[21,51,88,101] Similarly, after adjustment for all known confounders, including age, sex, and current body size, timed FEV from increased lung volume was found to be significantly lower in infants born small for gestational age than in appropriately grown control subjects, with a similar tendency noted for FEF.[75]

These changes persisted throughout the first year of life.[73] Many of these epidemiologic studies have highlighted the complex interactions among birth weight, socioeconomic status, family history of atopy, parental smoking, and airway function in infants, and have emphasized the need for large numbers of infants to be recruited to studies such as these if meaningful conclusions are to be reached.

INFANT LUNG FUNCTION AS A PREDICTOR OF SUBSEQUENT RESPIRATORY MORBIDITY

The Tucson Children's Respiratory Study was the first longitudinal assessment of the natural history of asthma that included infant lung function tests. More than 1200 children were enrolled at birth. Eight hundred of these were still participating at 13 years of age,[22] although only 10% of these subjects had had lung function measured in the first few months of life. This study was the first to provide evidence that diminished airway function precedes wheezing illness, in that t_{PTEF}:t_E was significantly lower in boys (although not in girls) who subsequently wheezed with a lower respiratory illness in the first year of life. Although there was no significant difference in V'_{maxFRC} between those who did and did not wheeze when follow-up was limited to the first year of life, subsequent follow-up revealed a diminution of V'_{maxFRC} shortly after birth in those who wheezed during the first year and who had had at least one additional wheezing lower respiratory infection by 3 years of age.[22] Similar findings were reported from the East Boston study (which also used V'_{maxFRC} as an outcome measure) and in the East London study, which found elevated premorbid values of airway resistance in those who subsequently wheezed in the first year.[27] By contrast, the Perth longitudinal study suggested that reduced airway function in early life was associated with persistent wheeze at 11 years, but not with transient wheeze.[88] Discrepancies between results may reflect differences in techniques, methods of statistical analysis, population, and environment as well as the fact that, although a large number of children may be recruited to longitudinal studies during infancy, the number in whom repeated lung function measures can be made on all test occasions throughout childhood may be relatively small due to the inherent difficulties in conducting such studies. Nevertheless, despite the wide range of techniques used, all of these studies have provided evidence of diminished premorbid lung function shortly after birth among those with subsequent wheezing illness.

Although one of the major aims of these epidemiologic studies, namely, to predict which infants who wheeze are likely to progress to asthma in later life, has not yet been realized, considerable knowledge has been gleaned regarding the range of different wheezing phenotypes. It is now generally acknowledged that those with very early onset of wheeze (in the first year of life), whose mothers smoke, and in whom there is no family history of asthma or atopy have a relatively low risk of persistent asthma. By contrast, those in whom the onset of wheeze occurs later or in the absence of significant exposure to prenatal or postnatal tobacco smoke, where there is a maternal history of asthma, persistent personal atopy (eczema and allergy, initially to food, especially egg, and later to inhalants), and increased bronchial responsiveness (with or without diminished flow) in infancy, have a much higher risk of subsequent asthma. Interesting data are also beginning to emerge from large epidemiologic studies of "high-risk" preschool children (i.e., those with a family history of atopy or a history of persistent wheezing), many of which are designed to follow up large cohorts of young children into school age, which may shed further light on these associations.[51,52,63,102]

Although the extent to which tracking of lung function (i.e., the extent to which those with low initial levels of airway function for their age or body size subsequently retain this position) occurs in school-aged children is debatable, serial measurements of lung function have revealed considerable tracking during early life. This has been demonstrated in healthy term[73] and preterm[103] infants, in infants and young children with CF,[74,104] and between infancy and school age in those with bronchopulmonary dysplasia.[105]

APPLICATIONS DURING CLINICAL RESEARCH STUDIES

Difficulties in Assessing Lung Function in Infants and Young Children with Respiratory Disease

Despite numerous attempts to monitor changes in lung function as a means of identifying early onset of pulmonary disease during the first year of life, the natural course of pulmonary involvement in infants with respiratory disorders remains relatively poorly understood. As discussed earlier, problems encountered include the following:

- The need for sedation
- Difficulties in repeating measurements frequently enough
- Lack of appropriate reference data and information regarding within- and between-subject variability, especially in the presence of disease
- Confounding of measurements by developmental changes in respiratory physiology
- The fact that the assumptions underlying many of the tests (e.g., the presence of a single time constant or the need for rapid pressure equilibration during periods of no flow) are not valid in the presence of respiratory disease

Such problems are compounded if attempts are made to undertake measurements in the intensive care unit.[106–108] Additional factors include the following:

- The relative invasiveness of some of these techniques in clinically unstable infants
- Insensitivity of the test to changes in respiratory mechanics within individuals, due, for example, to the relative magnitude of resistance of the endotracheal tube
- Use of inappropriate tests to investigate the underlying pathophysiology
- Inaccuracies in displayed values of V_T[109]
- Confounding of results due to interactions between the ventilator and spontaneous breathing activity
- Leaks around the endotracheal tube
- The heterogeneous nature of the population with respect to maturity, body size, and clinical severity
- The multitude of possible treatment modalities to which ventilated infants and young children may be exposed
- Inappropriate adjustment of lung function results for body size

Despite these problems, many studies describe the application of infant lung function tests in clinical research, with the tidal RTC technique for measuring V'_{maxFRC} being the most commonly used method for assessing airway function in this age group. Due to the paucity of suitable tests for preschool children in the past, far fewer publications have reported the use of lung function tests as outcome measures in this age group, although this situation is changing rapidly and many such studies are in progress.

Clinical Research Studies

As discussed earlier, baseline airway function has been shown to be reduced in both infants and preschool children with recurrent wheeze, although in some studies, significant differences between such populations are evident only when bronchial responsiveness is compared.[89] Longitudinal studies in which preschool lung function is related to wheezing phenotypes are under way to assess the sensitivity and specificity of these tests in predicting subsequent outcome and discriminating those with airway disease from healthy control subjects. Serial measurements of lung function from infancy into the preschool or school-age years in recurrently wheezy children are also beginning to emerge.[23,24,105] The application and interpretation of PFTs in infants with CF have been summarized recently,[110,111] with most studies reporting diminished lung and airway function in symptomatic infants. It has recently been shown that airway function is reduced at an early stage in infants with CF, even in the absence of symptoms or clinically recognized previous lower respiratory illness,[100] and that this does not catch up during infancy and early childhood.[74] These findings have important potential implications for early interventions in CF.

Although several reports have suggested that RVRTC may be a more sensitive means of discriminating changes in lung function in infants with respiratory disease than either tidal breathing parameters[28] or V'_{maxFRC},[76,81] it should be remembered that this technique is more complex to apply and that guidelines to standardize data collection and analysis are only beginning to emerge.[17] A variety of techniques, including spirometry[16,44,104] plethysmography,[53] FOT and interrupter resistance,[112] and MBW,[43,44] have been used to assess pulmonary function in preschool children with CF, with some of these studies being longitudinal and beginning in infancy or early childhood. All have shown significant group differences between children with CF and healthy control subjects, although most show considerable overlap between the groups, with results from many young children with CF falling within the normal range. The exception is with respect to results obtained with MBW, wherein abnormal results were found in the majority of children with CF, despite normal results for other measures of lung function (see Fig. 9-13).

Relatively few studies have been designed wherein results from infant or preschool lung function tests have been used to assess response to therapeutic interventions, such as antibiotics or corticosteroids. As discussed earlier, interpretation of such studies is often limited by lack of knowledge regarding the natural disease process and within-subject repeatability of the measurements, as well as by the relatively small sample size and the heterogeneous nature of both disease severity and individual response to therapy. Further, preferably multicenter, randomized controlled trials using standardized equipment and protocols are necessary to determine the true role of lung function tests during early life in evaluating such interventions.

Applications during and after Intensive Care

Numerous studies have attempted to use parameters derived from infant lung function tests to assess the effects of preterm delivery, neonatal lung disease, and ventilatory support.[106] The most commonly used approaches in recent years have been assessments of passive respiratory mechanics and lung volume. The only volume that is routinely measured in infants during mechanical ventilation has been that at end expiration, with or without positive end-expiratory pressure, although determination of lung volume over an extended volume range, using the negative deflation technique, has also been described in a few specialized centers.[80]

Although some studies have suggested that measurements of respiratory mechanics may be predictive of subsequent bronchopulmonary dysplasia, this has not been confirmed in any randomized controlled studies, probably due to the enormous numbers of subjects that would be required to achieve sufficient power of study. Preterm delivery, even in the absence of any initial respiratory disease has been shown to have an adverse effect on subsequent lung growth and development, which persists, and may even worsen, throughout the first year of life.[46,103,113]

Most studies in infants with bronchopulmonary dysplasia or chronic lung disease of infancy have suggested that lung volumes are low early in infancy, but subsequently become normal or elevated. This has been attributed to the fact that, over time, pulmonary fibrosis may become less important relative to airway disease and lung volume may increase disproportionately with growth. Studies of infants with bronchopulmonary dysplasia/chronic lung disease of infancy have also reported reduced compliance, increased resistance, and decreased flow during the first year of life.[41] Follow-up to school age has shown that these changes may persist throughout early childhood.[105] Lung function tests have also been used as objective outcome measures to assess the effect of different types of ventilatory support, including extracorporeal membrane oxygenation and high-frequency oscillation during the neonatal period on subsequent lung growth and development [40,113–115]

Interpretation of Lung Function Results in Infants and Young Children and Their Role in Clinical Management

Within an individual infant or child, the clinical usefulness of any lung function test will always be enhanced if serial measures rather than a single assessment can be undertaken and if the choice of test is based on the question to be answered, clinical reasoning, and a knowledge of the suspected underlying pathophysiology, rather than simply on the equipment that happens to be available in any given center. Given the marked influence of factors such as preterm delivery, intrauterine growth retardation, sex, ethnic group, and maternal smoking during pregnancy, it is important to take a careful history from the parents when performing such tests in infants and young children with respiratory problems.

Reference Equations

Reference equations are essential to express pulmonary function in relation to expected values for healthy children of similar age, sex, body size, and ethnic group; to characterize and monitor disease severity; to expand knowledge regarding growth and development; and to study mechanisms of normal and abnormal function and the natural history of disease. Trends in predicted values can occur due to alterations in equipment and protocol[15] or to secular changes in population characteristics. The choice of reference equations directly influences the interpretation of pediatric lung function data, and this can have a significant effect on patient care and research.[116] The production or use of prediction equations based on percent predicted, without an accompanying prediction interval, is of minimal use in clinical practice and should be strongly discouraged because it gives no indication of the severity of change or of how unusual the finding is. The use of percentiles is preferable to that of percent predicted, but is of little value in describing the severity of change once the individual falls below the fifth percentile, and the expression of results as Z scores, as described later, is therefore recommended.

Most lung function data are normally distributed or can be transformed to a normal distribution, such that 90% of "normal" values are found within the range −1.65 to +1.65 SD (with 95% between −1.96 and +1.96 SD). In pediatrics, lung function variables of healthy subjects and those with respiratory symptoms or disease often overlap to such an extent that a normal lung function parameter does not exclude disease. Similarly, abnormal lung function parameters often, but not by definition, are associated with symptoms and disease. Z scores, or SD scores, are defined as:

$$Z = (\text{observed value} - \text{predicted value})/\text{RSD}$$

where RSD is the residual standard deviation of the reference population.

Z scores are by definition normally distributed with a mean of 0 and RSD of 1. Hence, the Z score indicates how many SDs an individual or group is below or above the predicted value for any given parameter. Z scores indicate how likely a result is to occur within a normal population and how far removed the result is from that predicted, having taken the natural variability of that parameter into account. Z scores are useful for tracking changes in lung function with growth or treatment, and they allow comparison of lung function results obtained with different techniques. Several recent publications have reported Z scores that can be used in infants and young children.[71,78,85,117]

When selecting reference data with which to interpret pediatric lung function results, it is essential to check how appropriate these data are, including the following:

- Whether the same equipment, technique, and methods of analysis were used
- Whether a comparable and sufficiently large population was studied, with even distribution of age and body size
- Whether raw data are available for inspection
- Whether appropriate statistical techniques were used

It is of practical importance to agree on the choice of reference equations on a national level and to aim for regular updated reference values for that specific population, because evaluation of medical treatment and study results heavily depend on that choice.

The need for sedation and the duration of studies limit the number of healthy infants who can be studied at any one center. Recent international collaborative efforts have led to the publication of sex-specific reference data for V'_{maxFRC} during infancy.[71] The development of more standardized equipment and techniques for both infant and preschool lung function testing should facilitate similar initiatives in the future. In the meantime, it is important to avoid back-extrapolation of spirometric reference data collected in older children and adults because these values will generally underestimate predicted values in those younger than 6 years old, resulting in loss of sensitivity with which to detect changes due to disease.

Use of Lung Function Tests in the Clinical Management of Individual Infants and Preschool Children

Although there is little doubt about the potential value of infant lung function tests as a means of providing objective outcome measures in clinical or epidemiologic research studies, their potential usefulness with respect to influencing clinical management within an individual infant remains debatable.[118–120] The clinical usefulness of any technique depends not only on its ability to measure parameters that are relevant to the underlying pathophysiology and to discriminate between health and disease, but also on within-subject repeatability both within and between test occasions. As discussed earlier, although highly reproducible measurements of lung function can be made in infants during the same test occasion, little is known about within-subject, between-test repeatability. Similar problems exist for preschool children, and considerable effort is required to collect data in this field if the goal is to identify what constitutes a clinically significant change within an individual as a result of disease progression or response to treatment.

Future Directions

If appropriate equipment were to be miniaturized or incorporated into the ventilatory circuit so that continuous online monitoring of relevant parameters could be undertaken, one major area in which infant lung function tests could influence clinical management in the future probably lies in the neonatal and pediatric intensive care unit. Given the current rate of technologic development, this is certainly feasible, but will demand a major commitment by all concerned, plus the recognition that many of the tests used previously are either too complex or insensitive to provide reliable and relevant information to guide treatment. Techniques that should be targeted include those that measure both absolute values and changes in lung volume, tissue mechanics, and distribution of ventilation, with results being carefully integrated with other relevant outputs. Meaningful interpretation and use of such data will also require an improved knowledge of respiratory physiology among pediatricians and intensive care physicians. Another area in which there may be a real role for lung function tests during early life is with respect to longitudinal measurements from birth and throughout the preschool years in high-risk groups, such as those with persistent wheezing, CF, and chronic lung disease of infancy. Rapid development in the understanding of the relevance of genetics and gene-environment interactions as determinants of airway function makes it likely that increasing attention will be paid to specific aspects of the individual's genotype in the future.

SUMMARY AND CONCLUSIONS

There has been remarkable progress in the field of infant and preschool lung function testing during the last decade. Commercially available equipment and international recommendations are now available for the most commonly used tests of infant lung function. Forced expiratory maneuvers can be performed over the full lung volume range throughout infancy and the preschool years, whereas noninvasive assessments of gas-mixing efficiency that are applicable from birth to old age offer the possibility of detecting (and hence potentially treating) early changes in airway function in children with respiratory disease. This field has also moved from an era when it was considered that the "dark ages" of pediatric pulmonary function extended from 2 to 5 years of age, to a situation where testing of preschool children from at least 3 years of age is seen to be increasingly feasible, using a wide variety of tests under both laboratory and field conditions.

Lung function testing in infants and young children will, nevertheless, always present a challenge, and it is therefore essential that the purpose of any test is clearly defined at the outset and that dedicated operators with the necessary expertise and patience are available to undertake and interpret such measurements. Despite its vital role in clinical and epidemiologic research, given the need for sedation, the specialized equipment, and the difficulty in repeating measurements at frequent enough intervals, it is unlikely that lung function testing will ever gain a routine place in the clinical assessment of infants with respiratory disease. By contrast, provided standardized protocols can be developed that incorporate appropriate quality control criteria for young children, together with reliable reference data and information regarding the relative sensitivity and specificity of the various tests in differentiating healthy children from those with respiratory disease, lung function tests in preschool children could soon assume a role similar to that of tests used in their school-aged counterparts. To achieve this goal, continuing international collaboration will be required, together with input from manufacturers to ensure that the available equipment and software is optimized for this very important age group.

REFERENCES

1. Frey U, Stocks J, Coates A, Sly P, Bates J: Standards for infant respiratory function testing. Specifications for equipment used for infant pulmonary function testing. Eur Respir J 2000;16:731–740.
2. Stocks J, Sly P, Morris MG, Frey U: Standards for infant respiratory function testing. What(ever) next? Eur Respir J 2000;16:581–584.
3. Sly P, Beydon N, Davies S, Gaultier C, Lombardi E, Morris MG, Stocks J: ATS-ERS consensus statement. Lung function testing in preschool children. The next frontier. Am J Respir Crit Care Med (in press).
4. Stocks J, Sly PD, Tepper RS, Morgan WJ: Infant Respiratory Function Testing. New York: John Wiley & Sons, 1996, pp 1–577.
5. Stocks J, Hislop AA: Structure and function of the respiratory system. Developmental aspects and their relevance to aerosol therapy. In Bisgaard H, O'Callaghan C, Smaldone GC, eds: Drug Delivery to the Lung. New York: Marcel Dekker, 2002, pp 47–104.
6. Ranganathan S, Hoo AF, Lum S, Goetz I, Castle R, Stocks J: Exploring the relationship between V'_{maxFRC} and parameters of forced expiration from raised lung volume in healthy infants. Pediatr Pulmonol 2002;33:419–428.
7. Tepper RS, Jones M, Davis S, Kisling J, Castile R: Rate constant for forced expiration decreases with lung growth during infancy. Am J Respir Crit Care Med 1999;160:835–838.
8. Gaultier C, Fletcher M, Beardsmore C, Motoyama E, Stocks J: Measurement conditions. In: Stocks J, Sly PD, Tepper RS, Morgan WJ, eds: Infant Respiratory Function Testing. New York: John Wiley & Sons, 1996, pp 29–44.
9. Beardsmore CS: Ethical issues in lung function testing in children. Paediatr Respir Rev 2000;1:342–346.
10. Bates J, Schmalisch G, Filbrun D, Stocks J: Tidal breath analysis for infant pulmonary function testing. Eur Respir J 2000;16:1180–1192.
11. Sly P, Tepper R, Henschen M, Gappa M, Stocks J: Standards for infant respiratory function testing. Tidal forced expirations. Eur Respir J 2000;16: 741–748.
12. Gappa M, Colin AA, Goetz I, Stocks J: Passive respiratory mechanics. The occlusion techniques. Eur Respir J 2001;17:141–148.
13. Morris MG, Gustafsson P, Tepper R, Gappa M, Stocks J: Standards for infant respiratory function testing. The bias flow nitrogen washout technique for measuring the functional residual capacity. Eur Respir J 2001;17: 529–536.
14. Stocks J, Godfrey S, Beardsmore C, Bar-Yishay E, Castile R: Standards for infant respiratory function testing. Plethysmographic measurements of lung volume and airway resistance. Eur Respir J 2001;17:302–312.
15. Hulskamp G, Hoo AF, Ljungberg H, Lum S, Pillow JJ, Stocks J: Progressive decline in plethysmographic lung volumes in infants. Physiology or technology? Am J Respir Crit Care Med 2003;168:1003–1009.
16. Aurora P, Stocks J, Oliver C, Saunders C, Castle R, Chaziparasidis G, Bush A, on behalf of the London Collaborative Cystic Fibrosis Study: Quality control for spirometry in preschool children with and without lung disease. Am J Respir Crit Care Med 2004;169:1152–1159.
17. Lum S, Stocks J, Castile R, Davies S, Henschen M, Jones M, Morris MG, Ranganathan S: ATS-ERS consensus statement: Raised volume forced expirations in infants. Guidelines for current practice. Am J Respir Crit Care Med (in press).
18. Castile R, Filbrun D, Flucke R, Franklin W, McCoy K: Adult-type pulmonary function tests in infants with respiratory disease. Pediatr Pulmonol 2000;30:215–227.
19. Stick SM, Burton PR, Gurrin L, Sly PD: Effects of maternal smoking during pregnancy and a family history of asthma on respiratory function in newborn infants. Lancet 1996;348:1060–1064.
20. Hoo A-F, Henschen M, Dezateux CA, Costeloe KC, Stocks J: Respiratory function among preterm infants whose mothers smoked during pregnancy. Am J Respir Crit Care Med 1998;158:700–705.
21. Dezateux C, Stocks J, Dundas I, Fletcher ME: Impaired airway function and wheezing in infancy. The influence of maternal smoking and a genetic predisposition to asthma. Am J Respir Crit Care Med 1999;159:403–410.
22. Taussig LM, Wright AL, Holberg CJ, Halonen M, Morgan WJ, Martinez FD: Tucson Children's Respiratory Study. 1980 to present. J Allergy Clin Immunol 2003;111:661–675.
23. Devulapalli CS, Haaland G, Pettersen M, Carlsen KH, Lodrup Carlsen KC: Effect of inhaled steroids on lung function in young children. A cohort study. Eur Respir J 2004;23:869–875.
24. Silverman M: Inhaled corticosteroids and the growth of lung function in children. Eur Respir J 2004;23:795–796.
25. Schmalisch G, Foitzik B, Wauer RR, Stocks J: In vitro assessment of equipment and software used to assess tidal breathing parameters in infants. Eur Respir J 2001;17:100–107.
26. Black J, Baxter-Jones AD, Gordon J, Findlay AL, Helms PJ: Assessment of airway function in young children with asthma. Comparison of spirometry, interrupter technique, and tidal flow by inductance plethsmography. Pediatr Pulmonol 2004;37:548–553.
27. Dezateux C, Stocks J, Wade AM, Dundas I, Fletcher ME: Airway function at one year. Association with premorbid airway function, wheezing and maternal smoking. Thorax 2001;56:680–686.
28. Ranganathan SC, Goetz I, Hoo AF, Lum S, Castle R, Stocks J: Assessment of tidal breathing parameters in infants with cystic fibrosis. Eur Respir J 2003;22:761–766.
29. Frey U, Silverman M, Suki B: Analysis of the harmonic content of the tidal flow waveforms in infants. J Appl Physiol 2001;91:1687–1693.
30. Habib RH, Pyon KH, Courtney SE, Aghai ZH: Spectral characteristics of airway opening and chest wall tidal flows in spontaneously breathing preterm infants. J Appl Physiol 2003;94:1933–1940.
31. Frerichs I, Dargaville A, Dudykevych T, Rimensberger PC: Electrical impedance tomography. A method for monitoring regional lung aeration and tidal volume distribution? Intensive Care Med 2003;29:2312–2316.
32. Brown BH: Electrical impedance tomography (EIT). A review. J Med Eng Technol 2003;27:97–108.
33. Frerichs I, Schiffmann H, Oehler R, Dudykevych T, Hahn G, Hinz J, Hellige G: Distribution of lung ventilation in spontaneously breathing neonates lying in different body positions. Intensive Care Med 2003;29:787–794.
34. Katz-Salamon M: Delayed chemoreceptor responses in infants with apnoea. Arch Dis Child 2004;89:261–266.
35. Sawnani H, Jackson T, Murphy T, Beckerman R, Simakajornboon N: The effect of maternal smoking on respiratory and arousal patterns in preterm infants during sleep. Am J Respir Crit Care Med 2004;169:733–738.
36. Bhat RY, Leipala JA, Singh NR, Rafferty GF, Hannam S, Greenough A: Effect of posture on oxygenation, lung volume, and respiratory mechanics in premature infants studied before discharge. Pediatrics 2003;112:29–32.
37. Galland BC, Taylor BJ, Bolton DP, Sayers RM: Respiratory responses to hypoxia/hypercapnia in small for gestational age infants influenced by maternal smoking. Arch Dis Child Fetal Neonatal Ed 2003;88: F217–F222.
38. Franklin PJ, Turner SW, Mutch RC, Stick SM: Measuring exhaled nitric oxide in infants during tidal breathing. Methodological issues. Pediatr Pulmonol 2004;37:24–30.

39. Frey U, Kuehni C, Roiha H, Cernelc M, Reinmann B, Wildhaber JH, Hall GL: Maternal atopic disease modifies effects of prenatal risk factors on exhaled nitric oxide in infants. Am J Respir Crit Care Med 2004;170: 260–264.
40. Beardsmore C, Dundas I, Poole K, Enock K, Stocks J: Respiratory function in survivors of the United Kingdom Extracorporeal Membrane Oxygenation Trial. Am J Respir Crit Care Med 2000;161:1129–1135.
41. Robin B, Kim YJ, Huth J, Klocksieben J, Torres M, Tepper RS, Castile RG, Solway J, Hershenson MB, Goldstein-Filbrun A: Pulmonary function in bronchopulmonary dysplasia. Pediatr Pulmonol 2004;37:236–242.
42. Pillow JJ, Ljungberg H, Hulskamp G, Stocks J: Functional residual capacity measurements in healthy infants. Ultrasonic flow meter versus a mass spectrometer. Eur Respir J 2004;23:763–768.
43. Gustafsson PM, Aurora P, Lindblad A: Evaluation of ventilation maldistribution as an early indicator of lung disease in children with cystic fibrosis. Eur Respir J 2004;22:972–979.
44. Aurora P, Bush A, Gustafsson P, Oliver C, Wallis CE, Price J, Stroobant J, Carr SB, Stocks J: London Collaborative Cystic Fibrosis Group. Multiple-breath washout as a marker of lung disease in preschool children with cystic fibrosis. Am J Respir Crit Care Med 2005;171:249–256.
45. Schibler A, Hall GL, Businger F, Reinmann B, Wildhaber JH, Cernelc M, Frey U: Measurement of lung volume and ventilation distribution with an ultrasonic flow meter in healthy infants. Eur Respir J 2002;20:912–918.
46. Hjalmarson O, Sandberg K: Abnormal lung function in healthy preterm infants. Am J Respir Crit Care Med 2002;165:83–87.
47. Aurora P, Oliver C, Lindblad A, Bush A, Wallis CE, Gustafsson P, Stocks J: Multiple-breath inert gas washout as a measure of ventilation distribution in children with cystic fibrosis. Thorax 2004;59:1068–1073.
48. Ljungberg H, Hulskamp G, Hoo AF, Lum S, Pillow JJ, Aurora P, Gustafsson P, Stocks J: Abnormal lung clearance index (LCI) is more common than reduced $FEV_{0.5}$ in infants with CF. Am J Respir Crit Care Med 2003;167:A41.
49. Coates AL, Stocks J, Gerhardt T: Esophageal manometry. In: Stocks J, Sly PD, Tepper RS, Morgan WJ, eds: Infant Respiratory Function Testing. New York: John Wiley & Sons, 1996, pp 241–258.
50. Klug B, Bisgaard H: Specific airway resistance, interrupter resistance, and respiratory impedance in healthy children aged 2–7 years. Pediatr Pulmonol 1998;25:322–331.
51. Lowe L, Murray CS, Custovic A, Simpson BM, Kissen PM, Woodcock A: Specific airway resistance in 3-year-old children. A prospective cohort study. Lancet 2002;359:1904–1908.
52. Woodcock A, Lowe LA, Murray CS, Simpson BM, Pipis SD, Kissen P, Simpson A, Custovic A: Early life environmental control. Effect on symptoms, sensitization, and lung function at age 3 years. Am J Respir Crit Care Med 2004;170:433–439.
53. Nielsen KG, Pressler T, Klug B, Koch C, Bisgaard H: Serial lung function and responsiveness in cystic fibrosis during early childhood. Am J Respir Crit Care Med 2004;169:1209–1216.
54. Nielsen KG, Bisgaard H: Discriminative capacity of bronchodilator response measured with three different lung function techniques in asthmatic and healthy children aged 2 to 5 years. Am J Respir Crit Care Med 2001;164: 554–559.
55. ATS-ERS Consensus statement: The interrupter technique in preschool children. Am J Respir Crit Care Med (in press).
56. Beydon N, Amsallem F, Bellet M, Boule M, Chaussain M, Denjean A, Matran R, Wuyam B, Alberti C, Gaultier C: Pre/postbronchodilator interrupter resistance values in healthy young children. Am J Respir Crit Care Med 2002;165:1388–1394.
57. Chan EY, Bridge PD, Dundas I, Pao CS, Healy MJ, McKenzie SA: Repeatability of airway resistance measurements made using the interrupter technique. Thorax 2003;58:344–347.
58. Oostveen E, MacLeod D, Lorino H, Farre R, Hantos Z, Desager K, Marchal F: The forced oscillation technique in clinical practice. Methodology, recommendations and future developments. Eur Respir J 2003;22:1026–1041.
59. Marchal F, Loos N: Lung function testing in preschool children. Pediatr Pulmonol 1999;18:21–23.
60. Mazurek H, Willim G, Marchal F, Haluszka J, Tomalak W: Input respiratory impedance measured by head generator in preschool children. Pediatr Pulmonol 2000;30:47–55.
61. Marchal F, Loos N, Monin P, Peslin R: Methacholine-induced volume dependence of respiratory resistance in preschool children. Eur Respir J 1999;14:1167–1174.
62. Schweitzer C, Moreau-Colson C, Marchal F: Respiratory impedance response to a deep inhalation in asthmatic children with spontaneous airway obstruction. Eur Respir J 2002;19:1020–1025.
63. Delacourt C, Benoist MR, Waernessyckle S, Rufin P, Brouard JJ, De Blic J, Scheinmann P: Relationship between bronchial responsiveness and clinical evolution in infants who wheeze. A four-year prospective study. Am J Respir Crit Care Med 2001;164:1382–1386.
64. Marchal F, Schweitzer C, Khallouf S: Respiratory conductance response to a deep inhalation in children with exercise-induced bronchoconstriction. Respir Med 2003;97:921–927.
65. Pillow JJ, Sly PD, Hantos Z: Monitoring of lung volume recruitment and derecruitment using oscillatory mechanics during high-frequency oscillatory ventilation in the preterm lamb. Pediatr Crit Care Med 2004;5:172–180.
66. Frey U, Makkonen K, Wellman T, Beardsmore C, Silverman M: Alterations in airway wall properties in infants with a history of wheezing disorders. Am J Respir Crit Care Med 2000;161:1825–1829.
67. Traeger N, Panitch HB: Tests of respiratory muscle strength in neonates. Neonatal Rev 2004;5:208–214.
68. Dimitriou G, Greenough A, Rafferty GF, Moxham J: Effect of maturity on maximal transdiaphragmatic pressure in infants during crying. Am J Respir Crit Care Med 2001;164:433–436.
69. Dimitriou G, Greenough A, Kavvadia V, Davenport M, Nicolaides KH, Moxham J, Rafferty GF: Diaphragmatic function in infants with surgically corrected anomalies. Pediatr Res 2003;54:502–508.
70. Dimitriou G, Greenough A, Moxham J, Rafferty GF: Influence of maturation on infant diaphragm function assessed by magnetic stimulation of phrenic nerves. Pediatr Pulmonol 2003;35:17–22.
71. Hoo AF, Dezateux C, Hanrahan J, Cole TJ, Tepper R, Stocks J: Sex-specific prediction equations for V'_{maxFRC} in infancy. A multi-center collaborative study. Am J Respir Crit Care Med 2002;165:1084–1092.
72. Lambert RK, Castile RG, Tepper RS: Model of forced expiratory flows and airway geometry in infants. J Appl Physiol 2004;96:688–692.
73. Hoo AF, Stocks J, Lum S, Wade AM, Castle RA, Costeloe KL, Dezateux C: Development of lung function in early life. Influence of birth weight in infants of nonsmokers. Am J Respir Crit Care Med 2004;170:527–533.
74. Ranganathan SC, Stocks J, Dezateux C, Bush A, Wade A, Carr S, Castle R, Dinwiddie R, Hoo AF, Lum S, Price J, Stroobant J, Wallis C: The evolution of airway function in early childhood following clinical diagnosis of cystic fibrosis. Am J Respir Crit Care Med 2004;169:928–933.
75. Dezateux C, Lum S, Hoo AF, Hawdon J, Costeloe K, Stocks J: Low birth weight for gestation and airway function in infancy. Exploring the fetal origins hypothesis. Thorax 2004;59:60–66.
76. Jones MH, Howard J, Davis S, Kisling J, Tepper RS: Sensitivity of spirometric measurements to detect airway obstruction in infants. Am J Respir Crit Care Med 2003;167:1283–1286.
77. Goldstein AB, Castile RG, Davis SD, Filbrun DA, Flucke RL, McCoy KS, Tepper RS: Bronchodilator responsiveness in normal infants and young children. Am J Respir Crit Care Med 2001;164:447–454.
78. Jones M, Castile R, Davis S, Kisling J, Filbrun D, Flucke R, Goldstein A, Emsley C, Ambrosius W, Tepper RS: Forced expiratory flows and volumes in infants. Am J Respir Crit Care Med 2000;161:353–359.
79. Lum S, Hulskamp G, Hoo AF, Ljungberg H, Stocks J: Effect of the raised lung volume technique on subsequent measures of V'_{maxFRC} in infants. Pediatr Pulmonol 2004;38:146–154.
80. Hammer J, Patel N, Newth CJ: Effect of forced deflation maneuvers upon measurements of respiratory mechanics in ventilated infants. Intensive Care Med 2003;29:2004–2008.
81. Ranganathan SC, Bush A, Dezateux C, Carr SB, Hoo AF, Lum S, Madge S, Price J, Stroobant J, Wade A, Wallis C, Wyatt H, Stocks J: Relative ability of full and partial forced expiratory maneuvers to identify diminished airway function in infants with cystic fibrosis. Am J Respir Crit Care Med 2002;166:1350–1357.
82. Weist A, Williams T, Kisling J, Clem C, Tepper RS: Volume history and effect on airway reactivity in infants and adults. J Appl Physiol 2002;93: 1069–1074.
83. Vilozni D, Barker M, Jellouschek H, Heimann G, Blau H: An interactive computer-animated system (SpiroGame) facilitates spirometry in preschool children. Am J Respir Crit Care Med 2001;164:2200–2205.
84. Chavasse R, Johnson P, Francis J, Balfour-Lynn I, Rosenthal M, Bush A: To clip or not to clip? Noseclips for spirometry. Eur Respir J 2003;21: 876–878.
85. Eigen H, Bieler H, Grant D, Christoph K, Terrill D, Heilman DK, Ambrosius WT, Tepper RS: Spirometric pulmonary function in healthy preschool children. Am J Respir Crit Care Med 2001;163:619–623.
86. Nystad W, Samuelsen SO, Nafstad P, Edvardsen E, Stensrud T, Jaakkola JJ: Feasibility of measuring lung function in preschool children. Thorax 2002;57:1021–1027.
87. Zapletal A, Chalupova J: Forced expiratory parameters in healthy preschool children (3–6 years of age). Pediatr Pulmonol 2003;35:200–207.

88. Turner SW, Palmer LJ, Rye P, Gibson NA, Judge PK, Cox M, Young S, Goldblatt J, Landau LI, Le Souef PN: The relationship between infant airway function, childhood airway responsiveness, and asthma. Am J Respir Crit Care Med 2004;169:921–927.
89. Joseph-Bowen J, de Klerk NH, Firth MJ, Kendall GE, Holt PG, Sly PD: Lung function, bronchial responsiveness, and asthma in a community cohort of 6-year-old children. Am J Respir Crit Care Med 2004;169: 850–854.
90. Merkus PJ: Effects of childhood respiratory diseases on the anatomical and functional development of the respiratory system. Paediatr Respir Rev 2003;4:28–39.
91. Silverman M: Interrupter resistance and wheezing at 4 years. Am J Respir Crit Care Med 2004;169:1335–1336.
92. Wilson NM, Lamprill JR, Mak JC, Clarke JR, Bush A, Silverman M: Symptoms, lung function, and beta2-adrenoceptor polymorphisms in a birth cohort followed for 10 years. Pediatr Pulmonol 2004;38:75–81.
93. Godfrey S, Uwyyed K, Springer C, Avital A: Is clinical wheezing reliable as the endpoint for bronchial challenges in preschool children? Pediatr Pulmonol 2004;37:193–200.
94. Nielsen KG, Bisgaard H: The effect of inhaled budesonide on symptoms, lung function, and cold air and methacholine responsiveness in 2- to 5-year-old asthmatic children. Am J Respir Crit Care Med 2000;162: 1500–1506.
95. Lagerstrand L, Ingemansson M, Bergstrom SE, Lidberg K, Hedlin G: Tidal volume forced expiration in asthmatic infants. Reproducibility and reversibility tests. Respiration 2002;69:389–396.
96. Le Souëf PN, Sears M, Sherrill D: The effect of size and age of subject on airway responsiveness in children. Am J Respir Crit Care Med 1995; 152:576–579.
97. Stocks J, Dezateux C: The effect of parental smoking on lung function and development during infancy. Respirology 2003;8:266–285.
98. Chang AB, Wilson SJ, Masters IB, Yuill M, Williams J, Williams G, Hubbard M: Altered arousal response in infants exposed to cigarette smoke. Arch Dis Child 2003;88:30–33.
99. Gilliland FD, Gauderman WJ, Vora H, Rappaport E, Dubeau L: Effects of glutathione-S-transferase M1, T1, and P1 on childhood lung function growth. Am J Respir Crit Care Med 2002;166:710–716.
100. Ranganathan S, Dezateux CA, Bush A, Carr SB, Castle R, Madge SL, Price JF, Stroobant J, Wade AM, Wallis CE, Stocks J: Airway function in infants newly diagnosed with cystic fibrosis. Lancet 2001;358:1964–1965.
101. Murray CS, Pipis SD, McArdle EC, Lowe LA, Custovic A, Woodcock A: Lung function at one month of age as a risk factor for infant respiratory symptoms in a high risk population. Thorax 2002;57:388–392.
102. Brussee JE, Smit HA, Koopman LP, Wijga AH, Kerkhof M, Corver K, Vos AP, Gerritsen J, Grobbee DE, Brunekreef B, Merkus PJ, de Jongste JC: Interrupter resistance and wheezing phenotypes at 4 years of age. Am J Respir Crit Care Med 2004;169:209–213.
103. Hoo AF, Dezateux C, Henschen M, Costeloe K, Stocks J: Development of airway function in infancy after preterm delivery. J Pediatr 2002;141: 652–658.
104. Marostica PJ, Weist AD, Eigen H, Angelicchio C, Christoph K, Savage J, Grant D, Tepper RS: Spirometry in 3- to 6-year-old children with cystic fibrosis. Am J Respir Crit Care Med 2002;166:67–71.
105. Filippone M, Sartor M, Zacchello F, Baraldi E: Flow limitation in infants with bronchopulmonary dysplasia and respiratory function at school age. Lancet 2003;361:753–754.
106. Schibler A, Frey U: Role of lung function testing in the management of mechanically ventilated infants. Arch Dis Child Fetal Neonatal Ed 2002; 87:F7–F10.
107. Sly PD, Lanteri C, Nicolai T: Measurement of respiratory function in the intensive care unit. In: Stocks J, Sly PD, Tepper RS, Morgan WJ, eds: Infant Respiratory Function Testing. New York: John Wiley & Sons, 1996, pp 445–484.
108. Stocks J: Infant respiratory function testing. Is it worth all the effort? Paediatr Anaesth 2004;14:537–540.
109. Castle R, Dunne C, Mok Q, Wade A, Stocks J: The accuracy of displayed values of tidal volume in the pediatric intensive care unit. Crit Care Med 2002;30:2566–2574.
110. Gappa M, Ranganathan S, Stocks J: Lung function testing in infants with cystic fibrosis. Lessons from the past and future directions. Pediatr Pulmonol 2001;32:228–245.
111. Gappa M: The infant with cystic fibrosis. Lung function. Paediatr Respir Rev (5 Suppl) 2004;1:S361–S364.
112. Beydon N, Amsallem F, Bellet M, Boule M, Chaussain M, Denjean A, Matran R, Pin I, Alberti C, Gaultier C: Pulmonary function tests in preschool children with cystic fibrosis. Am J Respir Crit Care Med 2002; 166:1099–1104.
113. Hofhuis W, Huysman MW, van der Wiel EC, Holland WP, Hop WC, Brinkhorst G, de Jongste JC, Merkus PJ: Worsening of V'_{maxFRC} in infants with chronic lung disease in the first year of life. A more favorable outcome after high-frequency oscillation ventilation. Am J Respir Crit Care Med 2002;166:1539–1543.
114. Habib RH, Pyon KH, Courtney SE: Optimal high-frequency oscillatory ventilation settings by nonlinear lung mechanics analysis. Am J Respir Crit Care Med 2002;166:950–953.
115. Thomas MR, Rafferty GF, Limb ES, Peacock JL, Calvert SA, Marlow N, Milner AD, Greenough A: Pulmonary function at follow-up of very preterm infants from the United Kingdom oscillation study. Am J Respir Crit Care Med 2004;169:868–872.
116. Stocks J, Quanjer PH: Reference values for residual volume, functional residual capacity and total lung capacity. Eur Respir J 1995;8:492–506.
117. Merkus PJ, Mijnsbergen JY, Hop WC, de Jongste JC: Interrupter resistance in preschool children. Measurement characteristics and reference values. Am J Respir Crit Care Med 2001;163:1350–1355.
118. Davis SD: Neonatal and pediatric respiratory diagnostics. Respir Care 2003;48:367–384.
119. Frey U: Clinical applications of infant lung function testing. Does it contribute to clinical decision making? Paediatr Resp Rev 2001;2: 126–130.
120. Godfrey S, Bar-Yishay E, Avital A, Springer C: What is the role of tests of lung function in the management of infants with lung disease? Pediatr Pulmonol 2003;36:1–9.

10 Pulmonary Function Testing in Children

Robert G. Castile, MD

INDICATIONS FOR TESTING

By far, the single most frequently performed test of pulmonary function in both children and adults is forced expiratory spirometry. To perform this maneuver, the subject takes the deepest possible breath and then expires as forcefully as possible into a spirometer via a mouthpiece to completely empty all of the exchangeable gas volume from the lungs as quickly as possible. The volume of gas expired and the rate at which it is expired are measured. These measurements can be done with a spirometer or by measuring expired flow with a pneumotachometer and then integrating the flow signal to obtain the expired volume. The maneuver is simple to perform and rapidly provides quantitative information about both lung volume and airway size. Because spirometry permits the assessment of only those volumes of air that can be voluntarily exchanged, additional techniques have been devised that allow the measurement of all of the gas contained in the lungs. Measurements of lung volume and forced expiratory flow form the foundations of pulmonary function testing in children and will be the primary focus of this chapter. The chapter also includes a description of two other tests that are performed routinely in the pulmonary function testing laboratory, measurement of maximal respiratory pressures and measurement of the diffusing capacity of the lung. These tests are useful in specific clinical situations.

Tests of pulmonary function in children enable clinicians to: (1) detect mechanical dysfunction of the respiratory system, (2) quantify the degree of dysfunction detected, and (3) define the nature of the dysfunction as obstructive, restrictive, or mixed obstructive and restrictive. Pulmonary function tests are also useful for objectively following the course of respiratory disease processes in children and documenting the effect of acute and long-term therapeutic interventions. These and other indications for performing pulmonary function tests in children are summarized in Box 10-1.

LUNG VOLUMES

SPIROMETRY

The earliest spirometric measurements of lung volume and its expirable subdivisions were made by Hutchinson in 1846.[1] Figure 10-1 shows a volume-time plot of a vital capacity maneuver. This diagram shows all of the major subdivisions of lung volume. The maneuver begins with normal tidal breathing. The subject then inhales to maximally fill the lungs. This is followed by a maximal expiratory effort and then a return to normal tidal breathing. Tidal volume (V_T) is the volume of air either inspired or expired with each normal tidal breath. The amount of air inspired from the resting expiratory level to full inflation is termed *inspiratory capacity* (IC). Inspiratory reserve volume (IRV) includes all of the extra volume that can be inspired above the tidal range (IC − V_T). Expiratory reserve volume (ERV) is the volume below the tidal end-expiratory level that can be forcefully expired from the lungs. Vital capacity (VC) is the maximal amount of air that can be expelled from the lungs after maximal inspiratory effort. VC represents the total voluntarily exchangeable lung volume. Even when the maximal amount of air has been expired from the lungs, some volume remains. The volume of air remaining in the lungs after maximal expiratory effort is referred to as *residual volume* (RV). The maximal amount of air that can be contained in the lungs at the end of maximal inspiration, total lung capacity (TLC), is the sum of RV and VC. Functional residual capacity (FRC) is the amount of air in the lungs at the end of normal tidal expiration. It represents the sum of ERV, which is expirable, and RV, which is not expirable. These various components of TLC are referred to as *fractional lung volumes.* All of these volumes, except RV, TLC, and FRC, can be measured with a spirometer.

MEASUREMENT OF RESIDUAL VOLUME, TOTAL LUNG CAPACITY, AND FUNCTIONAL RESIDUAL CAPACITY

Residual volume can be determined by measuring FRC and subtracting ERV. FRC can be measured by gas dilution techniques or by using a whole-body plethysmograph. Gas dilution techniques measure the communicating gas volume in the thorax. The plethysmographic method measures all gas contained in the thorax.

GAS DILUTION TECHNIQUES

Helium Dilution

Although it was recognized in the early 19th century that the nonexpirable volume of the lungs could be measured by gas dilution techniques,[2] it was not until the 1930s that these methods were applied clinically.[3] In the helium dilution method, the patient adds his or her lung volume to a closed-circuit spirometer system containing air and a known concentration of the inert gas helium (≈10%). The concentration of helium in the original closed system is diluted in direct proportion to the helium-free volume added to the circuit by the air from the patient's lungs. Specifically, the patient breathes into a closed circuit that contains a water-sealed spirometer, a helium analyzer, a blower fan for circulating gas throughout the system, a carbon dioxide absorber, and a regulated oxygen source to compensate for oxygen consumed during the measurements (Fig. 10-2). The patient's end-expiratory tidal breathing level is monitored using the spirometer, and oxygen is added to the system to maintain a constant volume. The patient continues to breathe while connected to the system until there is complete equilibration

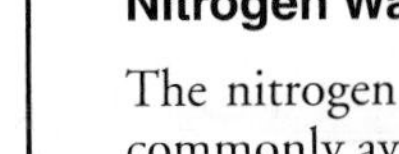

BOX 10-1 Uses of Pulmonary Function Studies in Children

- To establish pulmonary mechanical abnormality in children with respiratory symptoms
- To quantify the degree of pulmonary dysfunction
- To define the nature of pulmonary dysfunction (obstructive, restrictive, or mixed obstructive and restrictive)
- To aid in defining the site of airway obstruction as central or peripheral
- To differentiate fixed from variable and intrathoracic from extrathoracic central airway obstruction
- To follow the course of pulmonary disease processes
- To assess the effect of therapeutic interventions and guide changes in therapy
- To detect increased airway reactivity
- To evaluate the risk of diagnostic and therapeutic procedures
- To monitor for pulmonary side effects of chemotherapy or radiation therapy
- To aid in prediction of the prognosis and quantitate pulmonary disability
- To investigate the effect of acute and chronic disease processes on lung growth

between the gas in the spirometer system and the air in the patient's lungs. Equilibration is considered to have occurred when the helium concentration has fallen to a new steady-state level. FRC is determined based on the premise that the product of the initial helium concentration (C_i) and the volume of the system (V_{sys}) must equal the product of the final helium concentration (C_f) and the volume of the system after the child's lung volume (FRC) has been added.

$$C_i \times V_{sys} = C_f (V_{sys} + FRC)$$

Then FRC can be calculated from the known volume of the spirometer circuit and the initial and final helium concentrations in the circuit using the following formula:

$$FRC = V_{sys} (C_i - C_f)/C_f$$

Nitrogen Washout

The nitrogen washout technique for measuring FRC is now a commonly available component of many automated pulmonary function testing systems. Nitrogen is present in the lung in a known concentration (≈80%). With this method, nitrogen is washed from the child's lungs using a one-way flow of 100% oxygen by mouth. The total amount of nitrogen washed from the lungs provides a measure of the patient's resting FRC. Although the specific methods used in clinical practice vary in their details, volume is again measured in terms of gas dilution. FRC represents the unknown volume. The nitrogen concentration of the air in the lungs is either assumed or measured during expiration. The total volume of gas expired during washout and the concentration of nitrogen in the washout volume can be measured. As with the helium dilution method, the product of FRC and the nitrogen concentration in the lungs must equal the product of the total washout volume and the nitrogen concentration of the washout gas. FRC then equals the product of the washout volume and the nitrogen concentration of the washout volume divided by the nitrogen concentration of the air in the lungs.

In the open-circuit method (Fig. 10-3), 100% oxygen is inspired through a bias flow or one-way nonrebreathing system, and a mixture of nitrogen and oxygen is expired. The patient continues to breathe 100% oxygen until all of the nitrogen has been washed from the lungs. The amount of nitrogen exhaled is quantified by collecting the total volume of gas expired (V_{wo}) and measuring its nitrogen concentration (C_{wo}). FRC can then be calculated by dividing the volume of nitrogen exhaled ($C_{wo} \times V_{wo}$) by the concentration of nitrogen in the lungs (C_L). Alternatively, the nitrogen concentration in the expiratory limb of the circuit can be continuously integrated to obtain an index of the total amount of nitrogen expired. This integrated nitrogen system is calibrated using known volumes of air. FRC is calculated by dividing the integrated nitrogen value obtained from the patient washout by the nitrogen value obtained for the known calibration volume. This method assumes the mean nitrogen concentration in the lung to be equal to that of air. In practice, nitrogen continues to wash out from the blood and body tissues at a slow, nearly constant rate after all of the nitrogen has been washed from the lungs. At this point, the test is ended. Although the overwhelming majority of nitrogen

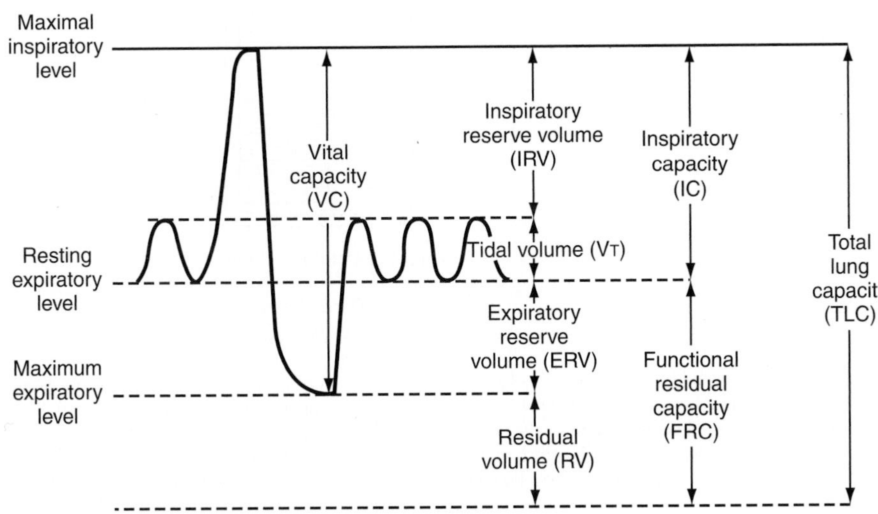

■ **FIGURE 10-1.** Tidal breathing followed by a vital capacity maneuver demonstrating the subdivisions of lung volume. (Modified from Murray JF, Nadel JA: Textbook of Respiratory Medicine, 2nd ed. Philadelphia: WB Saunders, 1994, p 801.)

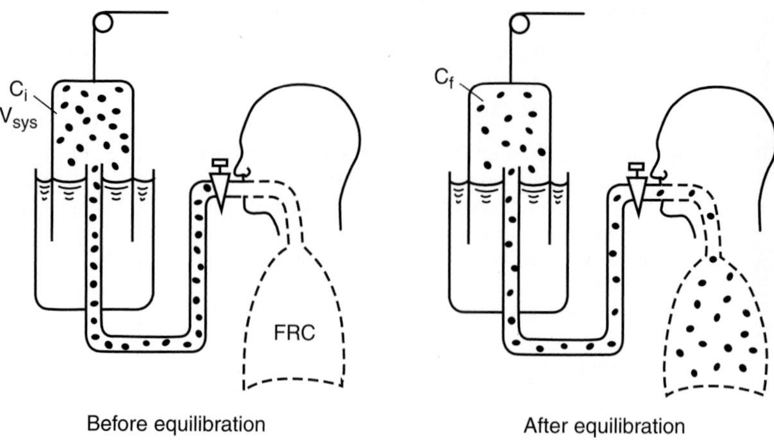

■ **FIGURE 10-2.** Helium dilution method for measuring functional residual capacity (FRC). C_f = final helium concentration; C_i = initial helium concentration; V_{sys} = system volume. *Dots* represent helium molecules, which, after equilibration, decrease in concentration in proportion to the patient's FRC. (Modified from West JB: Respiratory Physiology. The Essentials. Baltimore: Williams & Wilkins, 1974, p 15.)

washed out during testing comes from the air in the lungs, a small amount comes from blood and tissues. The rate of nitrogen washout from blood and tissues, measured at the end of lung washout, can be used to correct the washout FRC for nitrogen coming from the body. In practice, this small difference is often neglected. The results obtained with the open-circuit nitrogen washout method are comparable to those obtained with the closed-circuit helium dilution method.[4]

■ PLETHYSMOGRAPHY

The plethysmographic technique for measuring thoracic gas volume (TGV) was introduced by Dubois and colleagues in 1956[5] and depends on the principle of Boyle's law (pressure × volume = constant). Air is compliant: it can be compressed or expanded. The compliance of a volume of gas, such as the volume of air in the thorax, increases or decreases in proportion to the volume of that gas. The more air contained in the thorax, the more compressible, or compliant, it is. The smaller the volume of air, the stiffer it is. Thus, the quantity of air in the thorax can be measured by determining how stiff or compressible it is. The compliance of a gas is measured in terms of the volume change occurring in relation to a given pressure change.

To measure the pressure-volume relationship of the air contained in the thorax, the patient is placed in a closed box called a *whole-body plethysmograph* (Fig. 10-4). The patient breathes through a mouthpiece, and a shutter is closed at end-expiration. The patient is then asked to pant (make positive and negative

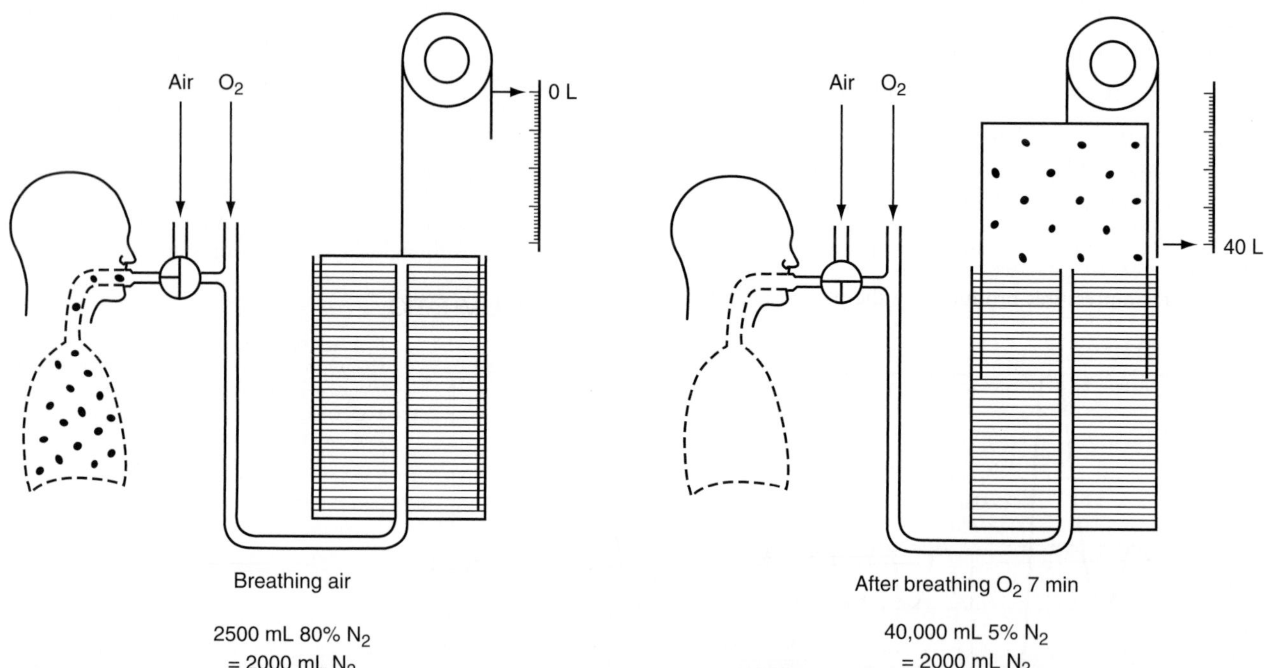

■ **FIGURE 10-3.** Nitrogen washout method for determining functional residual capacity (FRC). *Dots* represent molecules of nitrogen. Initially, all molecules are in the lungs as 80% nitrogen *(left)*. During 100% oxygen breathing, the nitrogen molecules are washed out of the lung and collected in the spirometer *(right)*. FRC is calculated from the total washout volume in the spirometer and the nitrogen concentration of the expired gas. In the example given, the expired volume is 40 L and the nitrogen concentration is 5%. Thus, the total amount of nitrogen expired is 2000 mL, which represents 80% of the patient's FRC. The patient's full FRC is, thus, 2500 mL. (Modified from Comroe JH, Forster RE, DuBois AB, et al: The Lung. Clinical Physiology and Pulmonary Function Tests, 2nd ed. Chicago: Year Book, 1974, p 14.)

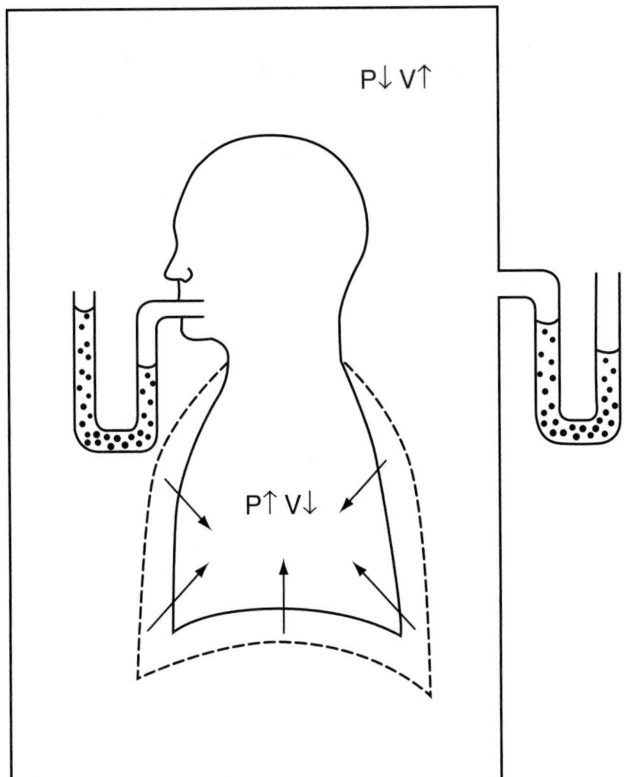

■ **FIGURE 10-4.** Plethysmographic method for measuring functional residual capacity. When the subject makes an expiratory effort against a closed airway, intrathoracic pressure (P) increases and lung volume (V) decreases. The increase in box volume results in a decrease in box pressure that allows the change in lung volume to be quantified. Lung volume is obtained from the ratio of the change in lung volume to the change in mouth pressure from Boyle's law. (Modified with permission from West JB: Respiratory Physiology. The Essentials. Baltimore: Williams & Wilkins, 1974, p 16.)

pressures against the closed shutter). These pressure changes are measured at the mouth, and it is assumed that they are transferred uniformly throughout the thoracic cavity. These pressure changes expand and compress the gas contained in the thorax.

The plethysmograph, or body box, allows measurement of the changes in TGV occurring in relation to the changes in intrathoracic pressure produced by the subject. When the positive intrathoracic pressures produced by the patient's expiratory efforts against the closed shutter compress and thereby cause a decrease in TGV, pressure in the closed plethysmograph becomes more negative. When the patient makes an inspiratory effort, TGV increases and box pressure increases. These changes in box pressure occur in direct proportion to the volume changes occurring in the thorax. The box itself can be calibrated (also using Boyle's law) such that the relationship of change in pressure to change in volume in the box surrounding the child is known. If, for example, 100 mL of air is injected into the box using a syringe and the box pressure increases by 1.0 cm H_2O, then for every 0.1-cm H_2O change in box pressure, box volume (whether occurring via injection of air into the box or as a result of volume change within the subject's thorax) has changed by 10 mL. In this manner, changes in TGV (as reflected by changes in box pressure) can be related to changes in mouth pressure, and the compliance of the air contained in the thorax can be determined. The magnitude of the ratio of the change in box pressure (ΔP_{box}) to the change in mouth pressure (ΔP_m) provides a measure of the volume of air contained in the thorax by the following formula:

$$TGV = (\Delta V/\Delta P_m) \times (P_{baro} - 47) \times (1.36\ \text{cm H}_2\text{O/mm Hg})$$

where P_{baro} = barometric pressure in millimeters of mercury, ΔV is measured as P_{box} calibrated in terms of volume in milliliters, ΔP_m is measured in centimeters of water, and the factor 1.36 converts barometric pressure from millimeters of mercury to centimeters of water.

Plethysmography measures the volume of air contained in the lungs when breathing is occluded. TGV is the gas volume in the lungs at the time of occlusion. If the shutter is closed at end-tidal expiration, then TGV equals FRC. Measurements of FRC can also be made with plethysmographs that measure volume change directly using a spirometer or obtain volume as the integral of flow from a pneumotachometer placed in the wall of the box. By convention, FRC measured plethysmographically is abbreviated as FRC_{pleth}, and the previously described measures of FRC by gas dilution are abbreviated as FRC_{helium} and $FRC_{nitrogen}$.

■ FORCED EXPIRATORY SPIROMETRY

■ HISTORICAL BACKGROUND

It was not until approximately 100 years after Hutchinson[1] first published spirometric measurements of lung volumes in 1846 that forced expiratory spirometry was recognized as a valuable tool for assessing lung function in patients with respiratory disease.[6] In the early 1950s, measurements of timed forced expiratory volumes, such as forced expiratory volume expired in 1 second (FEV_1), were recognized as useful measures of lung function.[7] By the mid-1950s, measurements of midexpiratory forced flow were noted to be highly reproducible (within a given individual), sensitive measures of early airway dysfunction.[8] In the late 1950s, Fry, Hyatt, and colleagues introduced the concept of the maximal expiratory flow-volume curve and demonstrated, with the use of isovolume pressure-flow plots, that forced expiratory flows were limited.[9–11] As a direct result of these physiologic insights, forced expiratory spirometry rapidly became the most widely used test of pulmonary function in both adults and children.

■ FLOW LIMITATION

In 1958, Hyatt and colleagues[11] demonstrated that expiratory flows were limited throughout most of the forced expiratory maneuver. They measured intrathoracic pressures with an esophageal catheter and plotted them against expiratory flows measured at the mouth at specific (iso) lung volumes. These isovolume pressure-flow curves (Fig. 10-5) demonstrated clearly that expiratory flow becomes limited or effort-independent at relatively modest positive intrathoracic pressure. Figure 10-5 demonstrates that flows over most of the descending portion of the maximal flow-volume curve are limited. The transpulmonary pressures required to achieve flow limitation increase somewhat at higher lung volumes. Pedersen and associates, in 1985,[12] demonstrated that even peak flow can be flow-limited with sufficient effort.

In 1967, Mead and colleagues[13] introduced the concept of an airway equal pressure point (EPP) [Fig. 10-6]. They pointed out that, during forced expiration, the driving pressure forcing flow

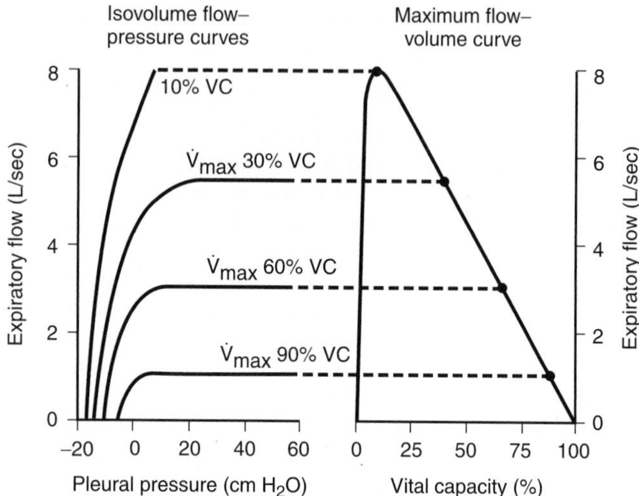

■ **FIGURE 10-5.** From a series of isovolume flow-pressure curves at varying percentages of expired vital capacity (VC) *[left]*, it is possible to construct a maximal expiratory flow-volume cure *(right)*. A similar flow-volume curve can be obtained by simply plotting expired flow against volume using an X-Y recorder during a single forced expiratory vital capacity maneuver. $\dot{V}_{max}$, maximal expiratory flow. (Modified with permission from Murray JF: The Normal Lung. Philadelphia: WB Saunders, 1976, p 102.)

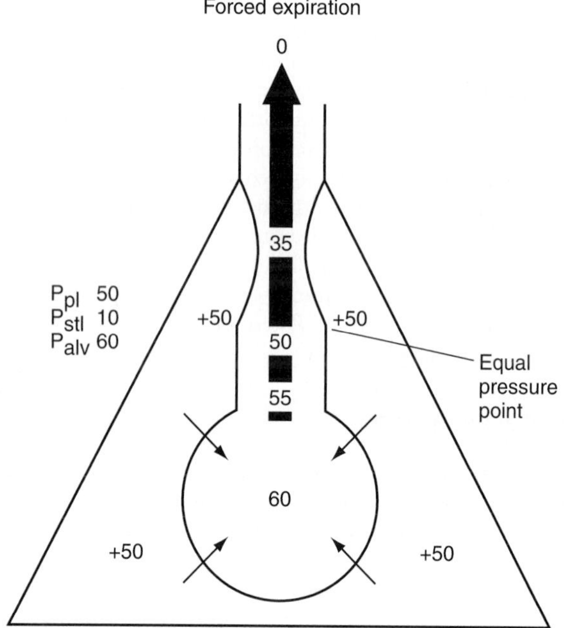

■ **FIGURE 10-6.** Schematic representation of the equal pressure point concept. Pleural pressure (P_{pl}), static elastic recoil pressure of the lung (P_{stl}), and alveolar pressure (P_{alv}) are expressed in centimeters of water. Pleural, alveolar, and airway pressures for a typical forced expiratory maneuver are shown. During forced expiration, muscular effort results in an increase in pleural pressure. The alveolar pressure driving flow is the sum of applied pleural pressure and lung elastic recoil pressure. As pressure is dissipated along the airways during airflow (60-55-50- . . . 0), there must be a point at which the pressures inside and outside the airway wall are equal (equal pressure point). Downstream from this point, the airways are compressed because lateral pressure in the lumen of the airway is lower than the pressure surrounding the airway wall. (Modified with permission from Murray JF: The Normal Lung. Philadelphia: WB Saunders, 1976, p 103.)

from the lungs was the sum of the pressure actively applied to the pleural space and lung recoil pressure. As the actively applied increase in pleural pressure is applied to both the alveoli and the airway walls, it is only the lung recoil pressure at any lung volume that allows pressure inside the airways to be higher than pressure outside the airways. During forced expiration, flow-related frictional and convective accelerative intrabronchial pressure losses occur. At some point along the airways from the alveoli to the mouth, flow-related pressure losses will equal the elastic recoil pressure and the difference between intrabronchial and extrabronchial pressures will be zero. This point along the path of flow is referred to as the *EPP*. Mouthward from this point, further intrabronchial airway pressure losses result in lower pressures within the airways than around them and, thus, dynamic compression of downstream airways. This model provided insight into the mechanical factors controlling airway dynamics during forced expiration, but did not explain the mechanism of flow limitation.

In 1977, Dawson and Elliott[14] pointed out that elastic tubes cannot carry a fluid or gas at a mean velocity greater than the speed at which pressures will propagate along the tube; that is, the mean rate at which gas molecules can flow through a flexible tube cannot exceed the speed at which the pressure driving the flow is propagated along the tube. This velocity of pressure propagation along the tube is referred to as the *tube wave speed*. The pertinent wave speed of pressure propagation in elastic tubes equals the inverse square root of the quotient of the tube wall specific compliance and gas density. The equation is

$$P_{ws} = (\rho dA/dPA)^{-1/2}$$

where P_{ws} is pressure wave speed, A is airway area, dA/dP is airway compliance, and ρ is gas density. During flow limitation, this wave speed, by definition, equals the speed of gas molecules flowing in the tube. Thus, bulk flow, limited by this mechanism, is the product of the tube wave speed and the cross-sectional area of the tube at the point of limitation. This point of limitation is referred to as the *choke point*. The bulk flow at wave speed is then the product of the speed limit of the gas molecules flowing in the tube (i.e., P_{ws}) and the cross-sectional area of the tube (A). Thus, the equation for the flow at wave speed is

$$V'_{ws} = (\rho dA/dPA)^{-1/2} \times A$$

where V'_{ws} is flow at wave speed limitation. Minimal algebraic rearrangement reveals that maximal flows at choke points are determined by gas density, airway-specific compliance, and airway area.

$$V'_{ws} = (\rho)^{-1/2} \times (dA/dPA)^{-1/2} \times A$$

Forced expiratory flows limited by this mechanism vary in inverse proportion to the square root of gas density and airway-specific compliance and will be directly proportional to the airway cross-sectional area at the site or sites of flow limitation. Increased airway wall compliance, such as occurs in bronchiectasis, will lower wave speed limits and forced expiratory flows. Reductions in the airway cross-sectional area, such as those occurring secondary to bronchospasm, will also decrease forced expiratory flows. Breathing a gas with lower density, such as helium-oxygen, permits higher maximal flows.

Figure 10-7 illustrates pressure wave speed (P_{ws}) flow limitation in a rigid tube (see Fig. 10-7*A*) and a compliant tube (see Fig. 10-7*B*). The gray circles represent air molecules, each with a cloud of negatively charged electrons surrounding a proton

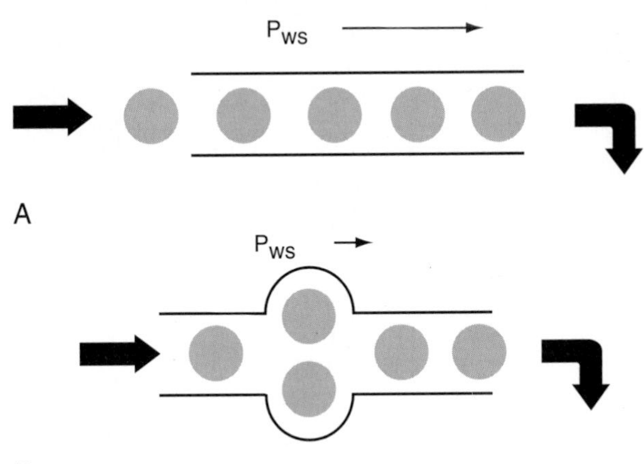

■ **FIGURE 10-7.** Pressure wave speed (P_{ws}) flow limitation in (**A**) a rigid tube and (**B**) a compliant tube. *Gray circles* represent air molecules. Flows are limited by the speed at which pressure is propagated along the tube (i.e., P_{ws}). In tube A, the speed of pressure propagation depends only on the compliance of the air in the tube. Thus, an increase in pressure driving flow proceeds from one end of the tube to the other at the speed of sound. In tube B, the speed of pressure propagation depends not only on the compliance of the air in the tube, but also on that of the walls of the tube. Because the walls of the tube are far more compliant than the air in the tube, P_{ws} and thus maximal possible flow velocities are much slower in tube B (see text).

and neutron core. In Figure 10-7*A*, pushing another air molecule instantaneously into the tube will result in expulsion of the last molecule in the line from the end of the tube. This does not, however, happen instantaneously. When the electron cloud of the first molecule moves forward, it "pushes" on the second negatively charged field. The second molecule then "springs" forward to influence the third, and so on down the line, until the last molecule moves out of the tube. This process of pushing together and springing forward is a pressure wave, and in air, pressure waves move at a finite speed, the speed of sound. The last air molecule in the line will not move out of the tube instantaneously, but rather in the time that it takes the pressure wave to move down the tube. The compressibility (i.e., compliance) of the gas in the tube controls the rate at which pressure is propagated. Thus, P_{ws} sets the limit on how quickly the molecules can flow through the tube. In Figure 10-7*B*, both the air in the tube and the walls of the tube are compliant and the compliance of the tube wall far exceeds that of the gas. When the first molecule is forced into the tube, the rate at which the pressure wave moves down the tube is slower because the walls of the tube stretch to absorb pressure and then rebound to return pressure to the tube. This markedly slows the rate at which the pressure wave moves down the tube. Again, P_{ws} sets the limit on how fast the last molecule in the line can be expelled, making the maximal velocities at which the air molecules can flow in the compliant tube much lower than for the rigid tube. In the lung, compliance of the airway wall plays a central role in determining the maximal velocities at which air molecules can flow. With the speed limits set by the wave speed, the airway cross-sectional area determines how many molecules can pass at that maximum velocity.

The elastic properties of the airway and its cross-sectional area thus interact to determine wave speed limits. Flow limitation occurs along airways where the product of airway elastance (i.e., stiffness, the inverse of compliance) and airway cross-sectional area is minimal. The site at which flow limitation occurs is thus dependent on the geometry of the bronchial tree and the manner in which changes in lung volume and flow-related pressure distributions affect that geometry. Flow limitation at wave speed limits is most likely to occur downstream of EPPs, where airways are dynamically narrowed and flow velocities are increased. At points where the velocities of the gas molecules flowing through these airway narrowings reach velocities equaling the speed of pressure propagation, flow limitation (choking) occurs.

At high lung volumes, the level of the bronchial tree with the smallest total cross-sectional area is in the trachea. In smaller airways, the airway cross-sectional area depends heavily on the elastic properties of the lung parenchyma. The total small airway cross-sectional area is large at high lung volumes and decreases steadily as forced expiration proceeds to lower lung volumes. Peripheral airway resistance thus increases steadily with decreasing lung volume. Both increases in resistive losses and declining lung elastic recoil pressures diminish intra-airway pressures as expiration proceeds. As a result, the EPP and the place (or places) where airways are dynamically compressed move toward the alveoli as lung volume decreases. Thus, the site of flow limitation, or choking, during a forced expiratory maneuver occurs initially in the trachea or central airways in normal subjects and moves progressively upstream toward the alveoli as forced expiration proceeds.

As the site of flow limitation moves from central to more upstream airways, the number of sites of choking must necessarily increase in an exponential manner. Only when all airways at a given level of the bronchial tree are choked will flow be limited at that level. Mead, in 1980,[15] pointed out that the manner in which global sites of flow limitation move from central to more peripheral airways must necessarily be complex. Figure 10-8 shows initial flow limitation in the trachea at high lung volumes. As lung volumes decrease and the wave speed limits of the airways upstream diminish, choking is likely to occur in some upstream segments. Mead[15] speculated, based on the complex nature of the bronchial tree, that it would be unlikely for all segments at a given level in the bronchial tree to reach their wave speed limits simultaneously. Thus, he postulated a sequential choking of airways upstream of the initial site of flow limitation. Upstream movement of the global site of flow limitation, he reasoned, would occur only when all upstream pathways were choked. Movement of the choke point according to this model in central and medium-sized airways was confirmed physiologically by McNamara and colleagues in 1987.[16] These sudden jumps of the global site of flow limitation that occur when the last remaining upstream airway chokes result in sudden decreases in flow, or "bumps" in the configuration of the flow-volume curve. This process probably repeats multiple times as forced expiration proceeds and the global site of flow limitation moves upstream from central to peripheral airways, with the number of sites of flow limitation increasing as lung volume decreases. Thus, in a general way, the flows measured during forced expiration reflect the functional anatomy of more central airways at high lung volumes and that of more peripheral airways at lower lung volumes.

As forced expiration proceeds, choke points multiply and cascade irregularly from central to peripheral airways. Flows measured at the mouth, however, reflect only the stepwise movement of global sites of flow limitation as these sites move from one level in the bronchial tree, where flow has become limited in all contributing pathways, to the next. In subsequent

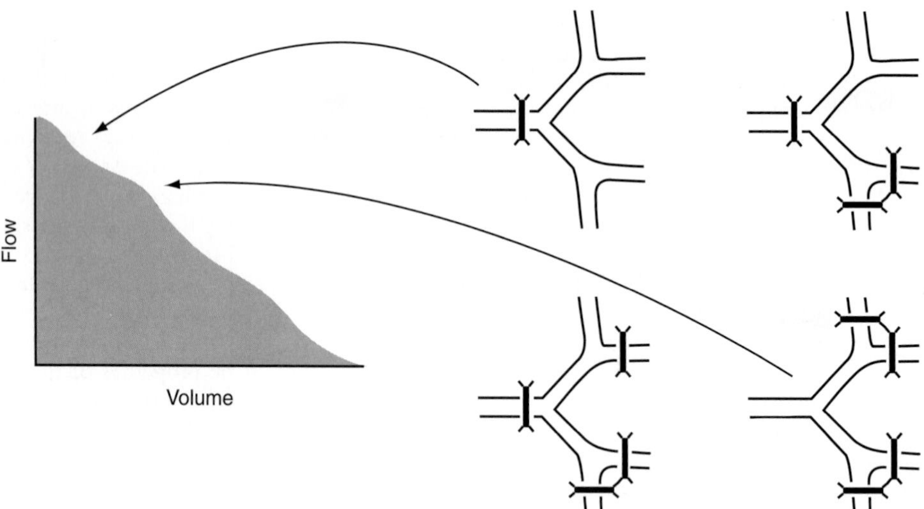

■ **FIGURE 10-8.** Movement of the global site of low limitation from the trachea to more peripheral airways. Flow limitation is shown occurring initially in the trachea at high lung volumes *(upper left)*. As lung volume decreases, segmental airways upstream from the controlling tracheal site of flow limitation become "choked" *(upper right)*. Eventually, only a single upstream pathway remains "unchoked" *(lower left)*. When the final pathway "chokes" *(lower right)*, the global site of flow limitation moves upstream, and this is accompanied by a sudden fall in maximal flow or a "bump" in the configuration of the maximal expiratory flow-volume curve. (Modified from Mead J: Expiratory flow limitation. A physiologist's point of view. Fed Proc 1980;39:2771–2775.)

work published in 1994, McNamara and colleagues[17] pointed out that this interdependent pattern of airway emptying inherently tends to hide airway nonhomogeneities. Because the global site of flow limitation does not move upstream until the upstream segment with the highest flow or wave speed has become flow-limited, the behavior of more slowly emptying segments is hidden. This may explain in part why even extensive nonhomogeneous small airway disease does not produce marked changes in forced expiratory flows measured at the mouth.

At low lung volumes, flow may not be limited by the wave speed mechanism, but rather by viscous flow limitation. In very small airways, viscosity-related pressure losses may result in decreases in the cross-sectional area and an effective limitation of flow at lower limits than those imposed by wave speed.[18] This possible change in the mechanism of flow limitation at low lung volume has no apparent clinical significance.

■ EQUIPMENT

Forced expiratory maneuvers in children are quantified using either a spirometer (dry rolling seal or water seal) or a pneumotachometer to measure flow and then integrating the flow signal to obtain volume. Most current devices provide immediate feedback on performance by plotting the maximal expiratory flow-volume curve. Devices that provide a continuous real-time plot of flow versus volume are the most useful in monitoring the efforts of children.

Equipment used for testing children should be capable of accurately measuring small volumes and low flows. Volume measurements should be accurate to within 30 mL or ± 3%. Flow measurements should be accurate to 0.1 L/sec or ± 5%.[19] Lemen and associates in 1982[20] assessed the frequency content of forced expiratory maneuvers in children. They recommended that equipment have a flat dynamic response through 12 Hz for flow and 6 Hz for volume to record flow and volume accurately during maximal expiratory maneuvers. Equipment should be calibrated frequently to ensure the accuracy of measurements. Equipment for testing children should permit adjustment of the size of the mouthpiece.

Equipment and test performance standards for spirometry were first published by the American Thoracic Society (ATS) in 1979.[21] These standards were updated twice in subsequent ATS statements published in 1987[22] and 1995.[23] Guidelines for testing children were published by Taussig and colleagues.[19]

■ TESTING PROCEDURE

The environment for pulmonary function testing in children should be quiet and free of distractions. Testing should be done in a room that is not used for other procedures that may cause distress in children. Parents may be present during testing to support the child emotionally, but the child's attention must be focused on the pulmonary function technician. The technician should engage the child in a friendly manner before beginning testing. The technician should be experienced in both pulmonary function testing and working with children.

Most children are able to perform a rudimentary forced expiratory maneuver by the age of 3 years.[24] Whether a child should be sent to the pulmonary function laboratory can be judged during a clinical examination. Children who are able to take deep breaths, cough, and blow out forcefully in response to the examiner's verbal instructions are likely to do better than expected forced expiratory maneuvers when sent to the laboratory. If they are able to perform respiratory maneuvers based on the examiner's verbal commands, they are likely to be able to perform even better with the additional visual feedback provided by real-time monitoring of the flow-volume curve. Most children, with practice, can perform adequate maneuvers by the time they are between 4 and 5 years of age.[25]

With a very young child, the initial goal of a visit to the pulmonary function laboratory is to provide a positive experience. The child should be praised and rewarded for any effort that he or she makes. Performance at subsequent visits to the laboratory will improve in relation to both experience and maturation. Children with chronic respiratory diseases, such as cystic fibrosis or asthma, who begin their laboratory experience at approximately 3 years of age are generally able to perform adequate forced expiratory maneuvers after two to four laboratory visits over 6 to 12 months. In children 5 years and older, it is important to spend significant time explaining and demonstrating the test to be performed and answering questions, because this can significantly improve initial performance.[26] Measurements made in children in this age range should be compared with measurements made in healthy children of similar ages.[27,28] Even if a child is unable to perform a full forced expiratory maneuver, a partial expiratory flow-volume maneuver can provide some measure of reserve airway function. Tidal flow-volume loops are monitored until FRC can be established, and then the child is asked to blow out forcefully to a level below FRC. The highest measure of flow at FRC (V'_{maxFRC}) is taken as the best estimate of reserve airway function at this volume level. These flow measurements can be compared with published standards.[29–31]

To perform a full maximal expiratory flow volume maneuver, young children must be able to do three things: (1) blow out forcefully, (2) take a deep breath to full inflation, and (3) continue to blow out forcefully until no more air can be expired. These three elements are most easily learned in that order. Most young children who blow using a mouthpiece quickly learn how to increase their effort in relation to the positive feedback of producing larger and larger partial flow-volume curves. Going to full inflation is also learned relatively easily, because taking deeper breaths also produces higher and wider monitored flow-volume curves. The third element is the most difficult to learn, because it provides little inherent sensory feedback and thus requires the child to follow the technician's instructions attentively. Only after the first two steps are mastered should a concerted effort be made to get the child to "continue blowing until the technician tells you to stop."

The forced expiratory maneuver may be done in either the sitting or the standing posture, with the head in a neutral erect position. Nose clips should be worn, but are not essential, because the velum closes voluntarily during forced expiratory maneuvers, thus preventing losses through the nose.[32] Thus, in younger children, nose clips may be omitted if they represent a source of distraction or a cause for concern.

Adequacy of performance is best judged by monitoring the expiratory flow-volume relationship. The level of effort is usually adequate to produce flow limitation if there is an initial rapid rise to a sharp peak in flow and the effort is smoothly sustained over the entire VC. An effort should be made to obtain three maximal expiratory flow-volume curves that appear similar in configuration and match within 5% of VC. Curves usually have small details, or "bumps," in configuration. These details of configuration should be similar on all curves if they are uniformly flow-limited.

The efforts of young children are frequently not rapid enough in onset to produce sharp initial peaks in flow, and thus it is more difficult to tell whether they have reached maximal flow limits. These limits may be outlined by asking the child to take a deep breath and then cough repeatedly until the lungs are empty. This maneuver produces repeated cough transients, followed by short, flow-limited segments (Fig. 10-9). This technique is useful in children of all ages for determining maximal flow limits. Some children, in a genuine effort to imitate the maneuver demonstrated by the technician, will voluntarily adduct the vocal cords to make a raspy respiratory sound during forced expiration. This "glottic" maneuver results in forced flows that are lower than the child's real flow-limited maximums. Such glottic flow-volume curves can appear to be fairly reproducible in configuration and may have a plausible "scooped" configuration. When glottic interference is suspected, the cough maneuver described earlier can be very helpful in defining the child's actual flow limits. Children who adopt this glottic pattern must be retrained to "blow quietly" until they can reproducibly produce curves that reach the limits defined by repeated coughing.

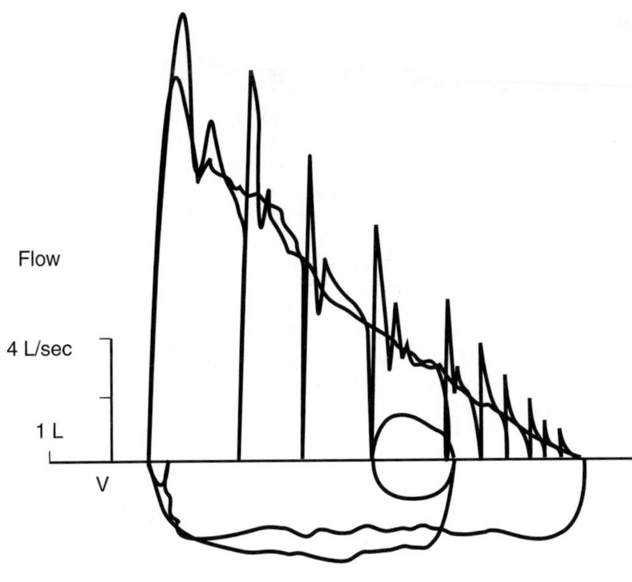

FIGURE 10-9. Repetitive coughing maneuver demonstrating maximal expiratory flow limits. From tidal end-expiration, the subject took a deep inspiration to total lung capacity (TLC) and then coughed repeatedly to residual volume (RV). From RV, the subject again took a deep breath to TLC and performed a maximal forced expiratory maneuver.

CALCULATION OF RESULTS

Forced expiratory maneuvers may be expressed as either volume-time spirograms or maximal expiratory flow-volume curves. Figure 10-10 shows volume-time spirograms from a normal child (see Fig. 10-10*A*) and from a child with moderate obstruction (see Fig. 10-10*B*). FEV_1, forced vital capacity (FVC), and forced expiratory flow between 25% and 75% of expired vital capacity (FEF_{25-75}) can be readily determined from spirograms. FEV_1 (see Fig. 10-10*A*) represents the volume of air expired in the first second of the forced expiratory maneuver. Ideally, departure of the volume-time spirogram from full inflation (zero expired volume) should occur abruptly, without delay. In many children, however, the onset of forced expiration is gradual, making the exact point in time when expiration had its onset, and thus FEV_1, difficult to determine. For this reason, the back-extrapolation method is used.[21] To designate a time of onset of the maneuver, a line drawn through the steepest portion of the spirogram is back-extrapolated through the time axis (see Fig. 10-10*A*). FVC (see Fig. 10-10*A*) is the entire volume of gas expired during the maneuver. FEF_{25-75} (see Fig. 10-10*B*) is obtained by connecting the points between 25% and 75% of expired FVC with a straight line. The slope of this line represents a coarse estimate of the rate of change of volume in relation to time (i.e., flow) during the midportion of the forced expiratory maneuver.

Instantaneous maximal flows at specific lung volumes are more easily measured from the maximal expiratory flow-volume plot. Figure 10-11 shows both maximal inspiratory and maximal expiratory flow-volume efforts from a normal child. This combination of maximal inspiratory and expiratory efforts is referred to as the maximal flow-volume loop. Instantaneous expiratory flows (FEFs) at 25%, 50%, and 75% of expired FVC are shown. These are standardly referred to as FEF_{25}, FEF_{50}, and FEF_{75}, respectively. The highest flow recorded is the peak flow, or FEF_{max}.

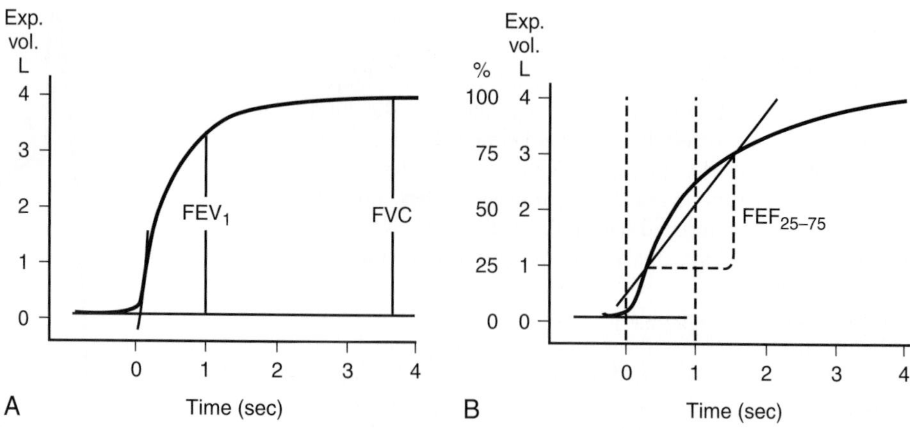

■ **FIGURE 10-10.** Volume-time spirograms from a normal child (**A**) and a child with obstructive airway disease (**B**). On the normal spirogram, zero time is determined by extrapolating the steepest part of the curve through the time axis. Forced expiratory volume in 1 second (FEV_1) and forced vital capacity (FVC) are measured directly from the tracings. Forced expiratory flow between 25% and 75% of expired vital capacity (FEF_{25-75}) is calculated by determining the slope of the line drawn connecting points on the spirogram at 25% to 75% of expiratory vital capacity. (Modified from Chernick V, Kendig EL: Kendig's Disorders of the Respiratory Tract in Children, 5th ed. Philadelphia, WB Saunders, 1990, p 150.)

Expired flows and volumes are standardly corrected to conditions of body temperature saturated with water. The final results are calculated from a minimum of three acceptable forced expiratory efforts that match within 5% for both FVC and FEV_1. The highest FVC and FEV_1 values from any of the three efforts are accepted as the final results. FEF_{25-75} and instantaneous flow values, such as FEF_{50} and FEF_{75}, are calculated from the single curve with the highest sum of FEV_1 and FVC. This is necessary because early termination of forced expiratory maneuvers can result in significantly higher measurements of FEF_{25-75} and instantaneous flows. The FEV_1/FVC ratio should be calculated from FEV_1 and FVC values obtained from a single effort.

Peak flow, or FEF_{max}, is often measured independently with a peak flow meter and reported separately from the results of forced spirometry. Peak flow is measured by instructing the patient to take the deepest possible breath and then blow out as quickly and as forcefully as possible. There is no need to sustain the effort through the complete FVC. Usually, the best effort of five attempts is recorded. Simple devices that allow the measurement of peak flow in the home setting are available and are widely used for monitoring variations in airway reactivity in patients with asthma. Measuring peak flow independently is important in establishing a baseline and helps to reinforce good measurement technique in the home setting.

Maximal inspiratory flows are not limited and are effort-dependent. This measurement is useful in distinguishing the nature of central airway obstructive lesions and should be performed whenever a central airway problem is suspected. To ensure maximal effort, this measurement should not be done immediately before or after a maximal expiratory effort. The patient should first be asked to push all of the air out of the lungs and then to inspire as rapidly as possible to full capacity. This should be done several times, until a consistent inspiratory flow-volume pattern is established. The curve shape shown in Figure 10-11 is typical of a normal maximal inspiratory effort. Only the forced inspiratory flow at 50% of vital capacity (FIF_{50}) is typically measured from these inspiratory curves. In normal individuals, FIF_{50} is approximately equal to FEF_{50}.

ASSESSING AIRWAY REACTIVITY

Airway reactivity is most frequently assessed by administration of an aerosolized bronchodilator (albuterol, metaproterenol, isoetharine, isoproterenol, or ipratropium bromide). The sixth edition of this text included a protocol for rapidly assessing bronchodilator responsiveness using isoetharine. With the decreasing availability of rapidly acting bronchodilators, albuterol has become the primary drug used to assess bronchial responsiveness in the pulmonary function laboratory. Ideally, the patient should not have taken β agonist or anticholinergic bronchodilators for 8 hours and sustained-release β agonists or methylxanthines for 12 hours before testing. Inhaled corticosteroids need not be discontinued. Resting heart rate should be recorded. After baseline spirometric measurements are obtained, albuterol is administered using either a nebulizer or a metered-dose inhaler with a spacer. The nebulized dose of albuterol is usually 2.5 or 5.0 mg in 3 mL normal saline. A nose clip should be worn during albuterol nebulization, but is not necessary when using a metered-dose system.[33] Albuterol can be delivered more rapidly using a metered-dose inhaler and a spacer. An inexpensive, disposable spacer can be made from a 6-inch length of ventilator tubing (Fig. 10-12). Good technique is essential when using the metered-dose inhaler and spacer. The patient first

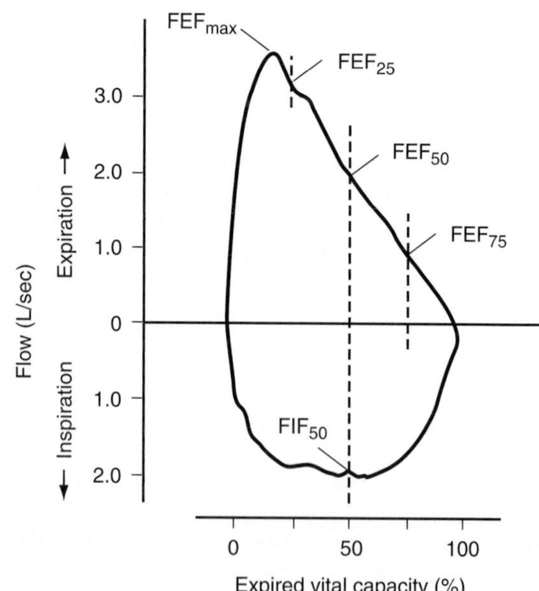

■ **FIGURE 10-11.** Maximal expiratory flow-volume loop in a normal child demonstrating instantaneous expiratory and inspiratory forced expiratory flow measurements. (Modified from Chernick V, Kendig EL: Kendig's Disorders of the Respiratory Tract in Children, 5th ed. Philadelphia: WB Saunders, 1990, p 151.)

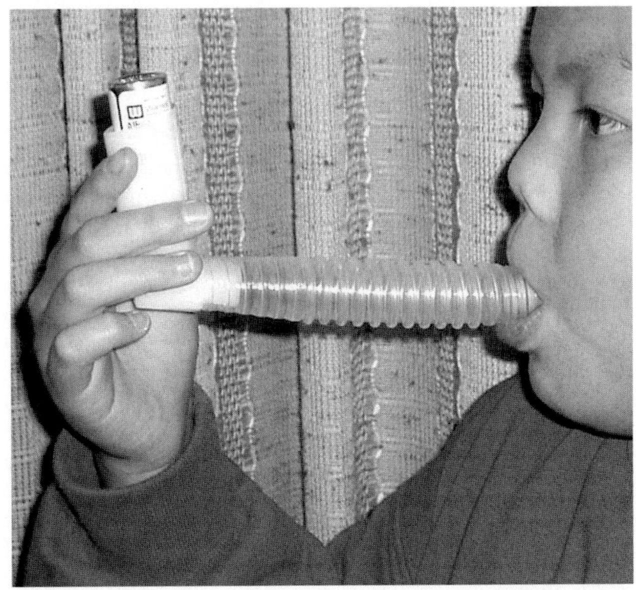

FIGURE 10-12. Child receiving metered-dose inhaled albuterol using a disposable spacer. The spacer is a 6-inch length of commercially available, corrugated ventilator tubing with a smooth internal surface (Smooth-Flo Corr-A-Tube II, Hudson Respiratory Care Inc., Temecula, CA).

exhales, then places the tubing in the mouth, inhales to TLC, and holds his or her breath for 5 to 10 seconds. The metered-dose inhaler is triggered just as inspiration begins. Doses of 2 to 10 puffs (180–1800 μg) have been used for testing. In practice, a dose of two to four puffs, properly inhaled, usually produces a brisk, sustained increase in heart rate. A 10% increase in heart rate that is sustained for 2 minutes is helpful in confirming effective drug delivery in children. Inhalation can be repeated if no increase in heart rate is seen. Spirometry is usually repeated beginning 15 to 20 minutes after the initiation of drug delivery. Although the onset of action of albuterol occurs in 5 to 15 minutes, this drug, when used for bronchodilator testing, has the disadvantage of having a peak response that occurs 30 to 60 minutes after drug delivery. After the administration of albuterol, forced expiratory maneuvers should be repeated every 1 to 2 minutes. Frequently, flows increase with subsequent maneuvers. Spirometry should be repeated until a plateau in FEV_1 is observed. For purposes of interpretation, it is helpful to record the time after albuterol administration when the best measurement was obtained. When postbronchodilator testing is terminated in less than 30 minutes, changes in function may be underestimated. The dose and route of administration of albuterol, change in heart rate, and pretest bronchodilator history should also be recorded and considered when interpreting the measured response.

Airway responsiveness can also be assessed by measuring changes in pulmonary function that occur after airway challenges that produce bronchoconstriction. These challenges include inhalation of methacholine, histamine, various specific antigens, ultrasonic nebulized distilled water, and hypertonic saline. Additional challenges include exercise and hyperventilation of subfreezing dry, cold air. Methacholine inhalation is the most common clinical method used for bronchoconstrictor challenge testing. Increasing concentrations of methacholine, from 0.025 to 25 mg/mL, are given by nebulization in a stepwise progression. Pulmonary function is measured at baseline and after each increasing dose of methacholine, until FEV_1 decreases by 20% or the maximum dose (25 mg/mL) is reached. Results are expressed in terms of the dose or concentration of methacholine that produces a 20% decline in FEV_1 (provocative dose or concentration, PD_{20} or PC_{20}). Lower provocative doses are indicative of greater degrees of airway reactivity. This method is reviewed in detail in the 1999 ATS guidelines on methacholine and exercise challenge testing.[34] Effective abbreviated methacholine challenge protocols have also been reported.[34–36]

Bronchial provocation tests should be done with caution, and all bronchoconstriction that is induced should be reversed at the end of the test with aerosolized bronchodilators. All patients who are considered for clinical assessment of airway reactivity with bronchoconstrictor stimuli should be assessed using bronchodilators before being scheduled for bronchoconstrictor challenge testing. Patients in whom increased airway reactivity has been clearly demonstrated using bronchodilators or in whom the diagnosis of asthma has been clearly established do not need to undergo clinical bronchoconstrictor challenge testing. This strategy should limit bronchoconstrictor challenge testing to patients with respiratory symptoms for which a specific etiology has not been found and also should minimize the risk of episodes of severe bronchoconstriction occurring in response to testing. Evaluations of airway responsiveness should be performed in laboratories with experience in airway challenge testing and should be conducted by highly trained personnel who are capable of assessing and managing patient responses.

INTERPRETATION OF RESULTS

Before an attempt is made to interpret pulmonary function test results in physiologic terms, the quality of the measurements made should be assessed. Tests should be evaluated in terms of patient effort, reproducibility, and freedom from artifacts. Less than optimal measurements should be interpreted with caution. After the measurements are evaluated for quality, the interpreter's job is to discern whether the results are normal or abnormal. If abnormality exists, the type and degree of abnormality must be established. Discerning abnormality from normality involves the comparison of test results with reference standards.

REFERENCE STANDARDS

Reference values serve two main purposes. First, they provide a large number of pulmonary function measurements made on children without respiratory disease with which individual patient measurements can be compared. Second, they provide the interpreter with an expectation of how lung function should change over time with normal growth.

Growth-related changes in pulmonary function test results correlate best with height. The patterns of change in pulmonary function with growth are significantly affected by sex and race. Most reference values provide independent prediction equations for boys and girls. The largest series of spirometric measurements in normal children was published by Wang and associates in 1993.[37] This longitudinal study, involving six representative cities in the United States, reported more than 80,000 measurements made in approximately 12,000 children 6 though 18 years of age. Figure 10-13 shows smoothed percentile plots for the growth of FEV_1 for white boys based on the longitudinal data of Wang and colleagues.[37] Similar plots and reference equations for boys and girls and for African American and white children for

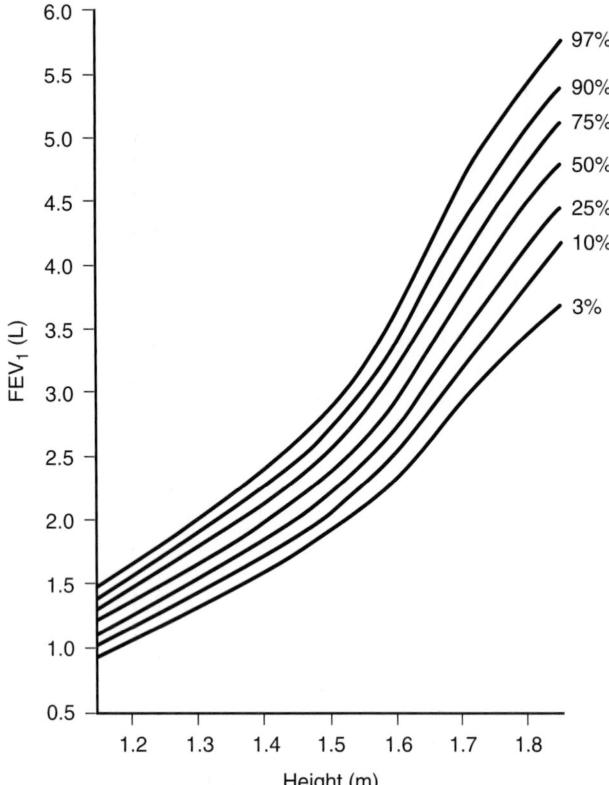

■ **FIGURE 10-13.** Smoothed percentiles of forced expiratory volume expired in 1 second (FEV_1) by height for white boys without respiratory disease from six cities in the United States. (From Wang X, Dockery DW, Wypig D, et al: Pulmonary function between 6 and 18 years of age. Pediatr Pulmonol 1993;15:75–88.)

FVC, FEV_1, FEF_{25-75}, and FEV_1/FVC are available in that publication. Both flow and volume measurements made in normal children grow along percentile curves. Children with large FEV_1 measurements relative to the mean, for example, continue to maintain those levels into adult life. Flow and volume measurements in given individuals track throughout childhood and adolescence along given percentiles. In children, the change in pulmonary function over time provides the most sensitive measure of respiratory disease. Children demonstrating decreasing levels of lung function in terms of percent predicted or percentile values can be presumed to have respiratory disease, even if all of their measured lung function values fall within two standard deviations of the mean for the reference population. Comparing serial measurements of lung function with percentile plots based on longitudinally collected reference values probably is the most sensitive way in which pulmonary function tests can be used to detect respiratory dysfunction in children.

Percentile plots, such as the one shown (Fig. 10-13), permit the interpreter to judge patient results in terms of the frequency of occurrence of similar results in the reference population. For the purpose of distinguishing abnormal from normal findings, test results are most commonly examined as percent of the predicted mean value. The 1991 ATS Statement[38] on interpretation of lung function tests recommends setting the lower limit of the normal range at the fifth percentile. Establishing approximate lower limits for spirometric measurements in terms of percentile of predicted values across the full range of heights is probably valid in children because the variability of spirometric measurements increases proportionally with the mean values of the measurements as height increases.[38] The results of Wang and colleagues[37] support this notion and provide percent of predicted values corresponding to the fifth percentile. Their results suggest that, as a general rule of thumb, FVC and FEV_1 values of less than 80% and FEF_{25-75} values of less than 67% of the predicted mean are below the normal range. Expressing pulmonary function results in terms of Z scores (predicted minus measured divided by standard deviation of predicted) has intrinsic value in that it identifies the patient's position in the predicted normal distribution, without reference to or the need to recall the lower limit for each different measure. Normality or abnormality of a given result cannot be determined completely by an arbitrary cutoff level. Because the normal range of most measures of lung function is wide, not knowing a child's initial or predisease level of lung function can also present problems. For example, children who have had disease-related decreases in lung function from one standard deviation above to one standard deviation below the mean value will be judged "normal" if their predisease level of function is not known. All results must be interpreted in light of the patient's clinical history.

Measurements of FVC and FEV_1 in relation to standing height are lower in African American children than in white children. This difference is substantially diminished by assessing lung function in terms of sitting height rather than standing height. This racial difference exists because leg lengths are proportionately longer in African American children. Thus, it is common practice to reduce predicted values for African American children by 12% to 15% to correct for these race-related differences in pulmonary function. This simple approach is, however, less than optimal, because race-related differences vary with age and height.[39,40] Currently, the use of race-specific prediction equations is the best way to account for racial differences in FVC and FEV_1 in children.[37–40] Reference measurements comparing differences in TLC between African American children and white children are inadequate. In relation to height, TLC measurements in African American adults are 12% lower than those in white adults.[38] Until more data become available, it would seem reasonable to predict TLC in African American children by reducing the predicted values derived from white reference populations by 12%.[41] When controlled for height, measurements of FVC and FEV_1 in normal Mexican American children and white children do not differ.[40] Other racial differences in pulmonary function have been reported,[42–45] but they are smaller than those between African American and white children, and must be more fully substantiated.

Reference values should be chosen that match the characteristics of the population being tested. Reference values should not be extrapolated beyond the age and height limits of the population studied.[46] Most reference standards, if extrapolated to predict normal values for children younger than 7 years of age, for example, significantly underestimate or overestimate the capabilities of these children. In children less than approximately 120 cm (≈47 inches) tall, predicted values should be derived from published normal measurements made on children 3 to 6 years of age.[27,28,47] Variation in the timing of the pubertal growth spurt may cause considerable deviation in percentile and percent of predicted pulmonary function values. This may be particularly problematic in children with chronic diseases, such as cystic fibrosis, in which the onset of puberty is often delayed.[48] Variations in the rates of change in measures of pulmonary function between reference equations may also influence a patient's apparent rate of change over time and thus affect clinical decisions.[48] Abrupt changes in predicted normal values are often seen at the transition from late adolescence to adulthood. Jumps in percent predicted values of lung function at this time are most often related to a change from pediatric to adult reference standards at a specific age. In patients with neuromuscular weakness and spinal deformities, arm span is often used to estimate height and calculate predicted values of pulmonary function.[49] For children whose arm span is difficult to determine accurately, FEV_1 and FVC can be predicted based on measurements of ulna length.[50]

TYPE OF PULMONARY DYSFUNCTION

Abnormalities of pulmonary function can be restrictive, obstructive, or a mixture of both categories. Restrictive disorders are characterized by a decrease in lung volume. This decrease may be caused by one of many mechanisms. Lung volume excursion may be decreased by chest wall deformity or increased chest wall stiffness, as in scoliosis. Respiratory muscle weakness may also reduce lung volume excursion. Increased elastic recoil of the lungs caused by an interstitial inflammatory process or fibrosis may also reduce lung volumes. Alveolar filling processes, such as lobar pneumonia, also reduce lung volume and, in that light, represent restrictive processes. Other space-occupying processes in the thoracic cavity, such as large bullae or congenital cysts, or processes that fill the pleural space, such as effusions, are restrictive. Any pulmonary process that reduces the amount of air filling the alveoli is restrictive.

Obstructive processes are characterized by reductions in airflow through the airways. These obstructions to airflow may occur at any level of the bronchial tree and may occur in relation to intrinsic narrowing or extrinsic compression. Reductions in airflow may also occur in relation to decreases in the integrity of the structure of airway walls, as in bronchiectasis, or in relation to global decreases in lung elastic recoil, as in emphysema. When small airways are narrowed, they frequently close at low lung volumes and thus result not only in reduced flow, but also in reduced FVC. Any process that causes a reduction in airway cross-sectional area at any level in the bronchial tree is obstructive.

Classically, restrictive and obstructive disorders have been distinguished by examining the ratio of airflow to lung volume. Airflow in restrictive disorders is usually reduced in proportion to reductions in lung volume. Thus, the ratio of FEV_1 to FVC, which is approximately 85% in normal individuals, remains unchanged (>80%) in restrictive disorders. In obstructive disorders, airflow is reduced proportionally more than lung volume. Thus, FEV_1/FVC decreases in obstructive processes.

Restrictive and obstructive processes can also be distinguished visually by examining the configuration of maximal expiratory flow-volume curves (Fig. 10-14). Patients with restrictive disorders have maximal expiratory flow-volume curves that are similar in shape to those of normal individuals, but smaller in terms of both flow and volume. The equal reduction of airflow and lung volume results in a flow-volume configuration that approximates a miniature of a normal curve configuration. In patients with increased elastic recoil, flow may actually increase slightly in proportion to lung volume. This relative increase in flow in relation to lung volume may produce a somewhat "bulging" appearance of the curve and an elevated FEV_1/FVC ratio. Obstructive processes produce a "scooped," or "sagging," appearance to the flow-volume curve. This scooped configuration occurs in relation to nonhomogenous airway emptying. With mild obstructive disease, this scooped appearance begins at low lung volumes. As obstructive diseases progress, the scooped configuration involves more and more of the descending portion of the curve.

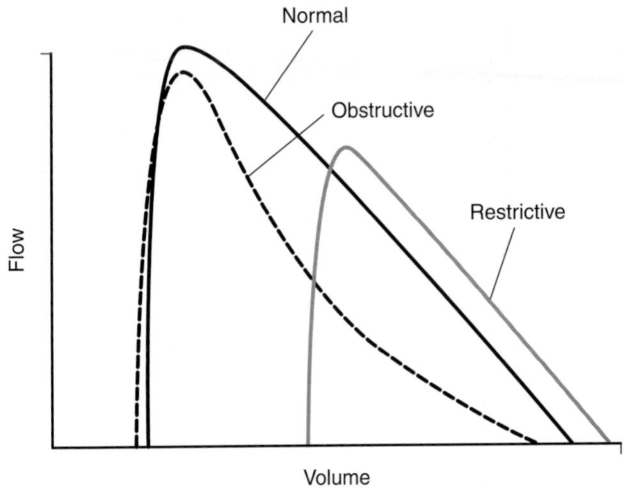

FIGURE 10-14. Changes in the maximal expiratory flow-volume curve configuration occurring with mild to moderate restrictive or obstructive respiratory dysfunction. (Data from Baum GL, Wolinsky E: Textbook of Pulmonary Diseases, 5th ed. Boston: Little, Brown, 1994, pp 115–116.)

Reductions in FVC in patients with obstruction occur at low lung volumes as affected airways close and trap gas. Dramatic reductions in FVC are not seen until the level of airway obstruction becomes fairly severe. Declines in FVC secondary to airway closure and gas trapping are accompanied by increases in the RV/TLC ratio. Reductions in lung volume in restrictive processes may occur at either high or low lung volumes. Patients with muscle weakness, for example, may not be strong enough to fully inflate the lungs. Similarly, chest wall deformities may prevent patients from either filling the lungs or completely emptying the air from the lungs at end expiration. Classically, RV/TLC ratios remain unchanged in restrictive disorders, but they may be either increased or decreased, depending on the etiology of the restriction.

Mixed restrictive and obstructive processes are difficult to distinguish using forced expiratory spirometry alone. When reductions in the magnitude of forced expiratory flow appear disproportionately large in relation to reductions in the FEV_1/FVC ratio or in relation to the degree of scooping seen on the maximal expiratory flow-volume curve, mixed obstructive and restrictive dysfunction should be suspected. The presence of a restrictive component can be confirmed by measurement of TLC, which will always be reduced in restrictive processes. Both plethysmographic and gas dilution measurements probably provide adequate measures of TLC in patients with pure restrictive disease. In patients with obstructive disease and air trapping, gas dilution methods underestimate FRC and TLC because they do not measure gas in noncommunicating, closed portions of the lungs. Plethysmography, however, is not without problems. Plethysmographic measurements may artificially overestimate lung volume in patients with airway obstruction.[51]

Central airway obstruction involving the larynx and trachea can be recognized because it produces distinctive changes in the configuration of maximal expiratory flow-volume loops (Fig. 10-15). Fixed central airway obstruction results in reductions in forced expiratory and forced inspiratory flow at high and mid lung volumes. If a lesion, such as a solid mass, produces an orifice-like reduction in central airway size, the flow produced through this orifice will remain approximately constant in relation to effort, producing a maximal flow-volume loop that is flattened on both inspiration and expiration (see Fig. 10-15*A*). Central airway obstructive lesions may also be variable. Variable extrathoracic lesions produce significantly greater reductions in inspiratory than in expiratory forced flows (see Fig. 10-15*B*). Variable intrathoracic lesions result in reductions in forced flows that are substantially greater during expiration than during inspiration (see Fig. 10-15*C*). Because the flows produced are at least partly effort-dependent, it is important to encourage the patient to make reproducible and maximal efforts, particularly while performing the maximal inspiratory maneuver. Normal values for maximal inspiratory flow at 50% of VC have been reported for children.[52]

DEGREE OF PULMONARY DYSFUNCTION

The degree of pulmonary dysfunction must necessarily be interpreted in relation to clinical experience. As noted in the earlier discussion of reference standards, values greater than 80% of predicted for FEV_1 are commonly considered to be within the normal range. Using FEV_1 in percent of mean predicted value, a rough and arbitrary guide to the degree of obstructive dysfunction is as follows: normal, 80% of predicted and above; mild dysfunction, 60% to 79% of predicted; moderate dysfunction, 40% to 59% of predicted; and severe, below 40% of predicted. For pulmonary processes characterized as restrictive, the same limits are useful approximations of the degree of deficit using the percent predicted value of FVC rather than FEV_1 to assess the degree of dysfunction. When available, the percent predicted value for TLC provides the best estimate of the degree of volume restriction.

This simplistic approach to estimating the degree of pulmonary dysfunction provides only a rough guide. Pulmonary function measures made on each patient must be interpreted individually and should guide patient management only in relation to the overall assessment of clinical status. A patient whose percent predicted FEV_1 is 80% of predicted may have mild or even moderate dysfunction if the predisease FEV_1 was 100% or 120% of predicted. Another individual whose FEV_1 is 80% may simply have relatively small lungs and be entirely normal. If this latter individual experiences a decrease in FEV_1 to 59% of predicted, he or she may have only mild airway obstruction.

Patients with progressive obstructive airway disease demonstrate progressive changes in the configuration of the flow-volume curve that correlate roughly with the degree of dysfunction (Fig. 10-16). With the exception of the purely central airway abnormalities discussed earlier, reductions in forced expiratory flows in patients with obstructive processes are first seen at low lung volumes. These reductions in flow occur first at low lung volumes because the portions of the lungs controlled by the affected airways empty more slowly and, thus, are still emptying at a low rate when most of the other, unaffected airways have completed the emptying process. As more airways or larger airways subtending greater portions of the lung volume become involved in the obstructive process, the reduction in flows and the scooping configuration of the maximal expiratory flow-volume curve begins at higher and higher lung volumes. A maximal expiratory flow-volume curve with a peak flow that is near normal, but with a scooping configuration over its entire descending portion, is typical of moderate dysfunction, with the obstructive process affecting approximately half of the air flowing from the lungs.

However, the scooped configuration of the flow-volume curve does not indicate the site of obstruction. Either severe obstruction of a single main stem bronchus or narrowing of approximately 50% of the small or medium airways could produce similarly scooped maximal expiratory flow-volume curves, typical of moderate obstruction. Nonhomogeneous emptying occurring at any level of the bronchial tree will produce scooping of the flow-volume curve. The site of nonhomogeneous obstruction may, however, be suspected clinically. Low flows at low lung volumes (scooping of the lower part of the maximal expiratory flow-volume curve) are often considered indicative of early small airway obstructive disease. Although this is most often the case clinically, a similar flow-volume curve configuration could also be observed in a patient with, for example, postpneumonic bronchiectasis involving a single segmental bronchus. This single involved segment of the lung will empty slowly and nonhomogeneously in relation to the remainder of the lung, and will result in low flows at the end of forced expiration. Diffuse obstruction involving the small airways subtending an equivalent portion of the lung volume would produce a maximal expiratory flow-volume curve with a virtually identical configuration. Thus, interpretations involving the site of airway obstruction, with the exception of the typical central

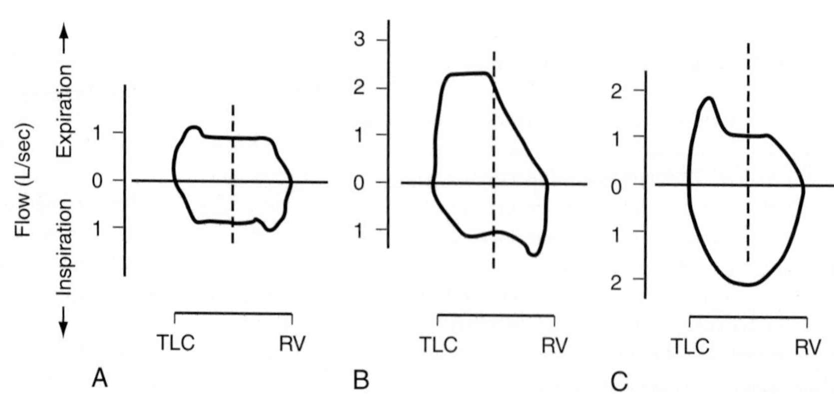

FIGURE 10-15. Maximal flow-volume curve loop configurations in central airway obstruction. **A,** Fixed central airway obstruction; **B,** variable extrathoracic central airway obstruction; **C,** variable intrathoracic central airway obstruction. RV, residual volume; TLC, total lung capacity. (Modified from Chernick V, Kendig EL: Kendig's Disorders of the Respiratory Tract in Children, 5th ed. Philadelphia: WB Saunders, 1990, p 151.)

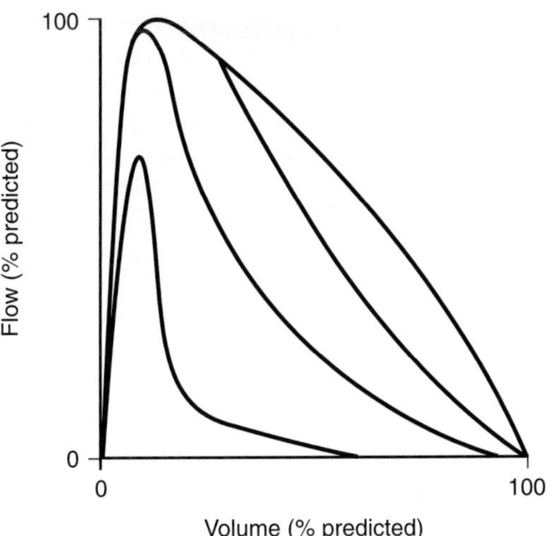

■ **FIGURE 10-16.** Typical changes in the maximal expiratory flow-volume curve configuration related to progressive obstructive pulmonary dysfunction. Curves are plotted superimposed at total lung capacity. The outer curve is representative of a normal configuration. Curves with progressively lower flows have configurations typical of mild, moderate, and severe dysfunction, respectively. (Modified from Rudolph AM, Kamei RK: Rudolph's Fundamentals of Pediatrics. Norwalk, Conn: Appleton & Lange, 1994, p 543.)

airway changes discussed earlier, should be made with appropriate caution.

As obstructive airway disease progresses, FVC, FEV_1, and FEF_{25-75} decline at different rates (Fig. 10-17). FEF_{25-75} and other measures of instantaneous flow (FEF_{50} and FEF_{75}) decline early in the course of progressive obstructive disease and are generally considered early indicators of airway dysfunction. FVC tends not to be affected until later in the course of obstructive airway disease, at which time it declines rapidly. FVC declines initially in relation to air trapping due to closure of the airways at end expiration. Reductions in FVC accelerate later in the course of disease as more airways close and diffuse fibrotic changes begin to add a restrictive component to the obstructive process. FEV_1 declines almost linearly in relation to disease progression and, thus, tends to be the best long-term measure of the degree of obstruction. In restrictive disorders, measures of airway function decline in concert with reductions in lung volume, making volume measurements, such as FVC or, if available, TLC, the best long-term measures of the degree of dysfunction.

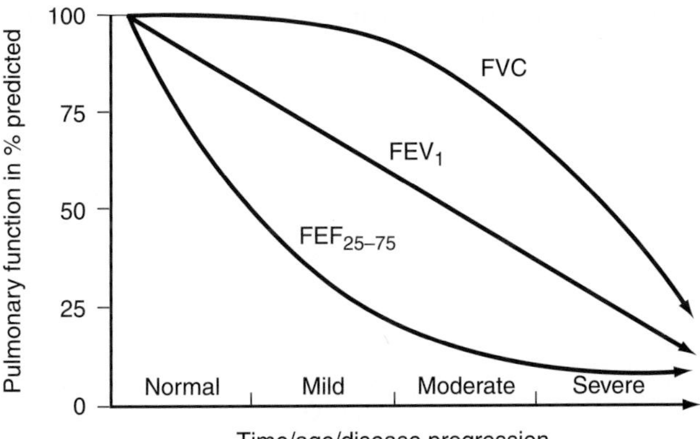

■ **FIGURE 10-17.** Course of pulmonary function test results in chronic obstructive pulmonary disease. Forced expiratory flow between 25% and 75% of expired vital capacity (FEF_{25-75}) declines early in the course of progressive obstructive lung disease. Forced vital capacity (FVC) remains nearly normal and then declines rapidly late in the course of the disease. Forced expiratory volume expired in 1 second (FEV_1) declines almost linearly as disease progresses.

ASSESSING CHANGES IN DEGREE OF PULMONARY DYSFUNCTION

Levels of change in measurements of pulmonary function that are indicative of clear changes in clinical condition are difficult to state in absolute terms. There is some general agreement regarding levels of change in function that are indicative of increased airway reactivity. As a rule of thumb, an increase in FEV_1 or FVC of 12% or 200 mL after the administration of a bronchodilator is considered a positive response.[38] Other studies done in various settings in adults and children have suggested that levels of change in FEV_1 of as low as 8% and as high as 25% indicate a positive response to bronchodilators.[38,53] Changes in FEF_{25-75} and instantaneous flows should be considered only secondarily when evaluating bronchodilator response. For these measures, increases of 35% to 50% are generally considered indicative of a positive response. There is also general agreement about the level of change in pulmonary function that constitutes a positive response to a bronchoconstrictor challenge. A 20% decline in FEV_1 after a bronchoconstrictor challenge is considered indicative of increased airway reactivity.

There is less agreement regarding the degree of change in pulmonary function that constitutes a significant improvement or decline over time in relation to therapeutic interventions or disease progression. Interpretation of disease-related changes is complicated by the fact that intrasubject variability related to the performance of pulmonary function tests varies significantly from one individual to the next. Changes in lung function of one standard deviation or more than 10% have been suggested as constituting a significant intrasubject change in lung function.[54] In 1990, Pattishall[55] reported that, in most pediatric laboratories, a 10% or 15% change in FVC or FEV_1 was considered significant. Interpretation of disease-related changes is complicated by the fact that intrasubject variability related to the performance of pulmonary function tests varies significantly from one individual to the next. Lemen, in the fifth edition of this book,[56] described a method for assessing significant changes in pulmonary function on an individual basis. He suggested estimating intrasubject variability of individual patients based on the variability that they demonstrated while performing the four to five maneuvers done as part of clinical testing. Subsequent measures that were more than two individual patient standard deviations from the baseline mean value were considered to be significantly changed.

Intrasubject variability (and, thus, the degree of change in function required to establish significance) also varies, depending on the pulmonary function parameter being measured, the interval between tests, and the type of patient being tested. In healthy subjects, changes in FEV_1 and FVC within a day of 5%, from week to week of 11% to 12%, and from year to year of 15% were generally considered significant by participants in the 1991 ATS Workshop on Lung Function Testing.[38] These critical limits approximately double in patients with chronic respiratory disease or when more variable measures of function, such as FEF_{25-75} or instantaneous flow, are being used. Intrasubject variability in adults and children with chronic respiratory disease is significantly higher than that in normal individuals.[57,58]

It is thus difficult to make general statements regarding the degree of change in lung function that constitutes a significant change in clinical status. In the final analysis, serial changes in pulmonary function must be interpreted in light of the individual patient's overall clinical situation.

OTHER TESTS OF FUNCTION

MAXIMAL RESPIRATORY PRESSURE

Respiratory muscle strength can be assessed by measuring maximal inspiratory and maximal expiratory pressures. These measurements are useful for assessing and following patients with respiratory muscle weakness due to neuromuscular problems, such as spinal cord injury, Guillain-Barré syndrome, diaphragmatic paralysis, muscular dystrophy, myasthenia gravis, and steroid myopathy. Measurements of respiratory pressure in humans were first recorded by Hutchinson in 1846.[1] Formal measurements of average maximal inspiratory and expiratory pressures in normal children and adults were reported in 1964 by Cook and associates.[59] In 1969, Black and Hyatt[60] described a simple hand-held device for assessing maximal respiratory pressures in the clinical setting and provided normal reference values for men and women.

Maximal respiratory pressure measurements are made by having the child make forceful inspiratory (Valsalva maneuver) and expiratory (Müeller maneuver) efforts into a closed system. The maximal pressures generated during brief 1- to 2-second efforts are recorded. The device used to measure these pressures is a short, cylindrical, metal or acrylic (Plexiglas) tube (diameter, ≈3 cm; length, ≈12 cm), with a firm, rubber mouthpiece that can be hand-held and pressed tightly against the lips (Fig. 10-18). The tube should have a 1- to 2-mm hole to permit a small air leak. This ensures that the pressures generated by the subject have not been made with the cheeks alone. A subject with a closed glottis can generate substantial negative pressure by sucking with the buccal muscles alone. The volume flowing in through the small hole fills the oral cavity rapidly. This makes it impossible to maintain high negative pressure for 2 seconds, and indicates that the glottis is closed. With the glottis open, the volume change occurring over 2 seconds due to the air leak is small relative to that of the lungs and upper airways, and has minimal effect on the measured pressures. The small air leak serves a similar function during expiratory maneuvers. Pressures are measured with the mouthpiece pressed firmly to the face, with the lips inside, as if blowing a bugle. This is most important for the measurement of expiratory pressures, which can exceed 200 cm H_2O. If pressures are measured with a scuba-type mouthpiece (lips around the mouthpiece), the maximal pressures generated are limited by the ability of the buccal muscles to tighten around the mouthpiece and prevent leaks. Individuals with normal muscle strength cannot prevent leaks at pressures above 120 to 150 cm H_2O. In patients with generalized muscle weakness, leaks may occur at even lower positive pressures. In patients with muscle weakness and limited buccal strength, measurements made with a facemask can provide an estimate of respiratory muscle strength.[61]

In the past, pressures have been assessed by observing maximal needle excursions on mechanical aneroid pressure gauges. More recently, pressure changes within the tube have been measured, using analog transducers, and recorded digitally. Pressures are measured with the child seated. Nose clips are generally placed, but are not absolutely necessary. The force generated by muscles varies in relation to muscle fiber length (i.e., length-tension characteristic). Figure 10-19 shows that the maximal inspiratory and expiratory pressures that can be generated are a function of VC.[62] For the respiratory system, the optimal length for force generation by the expiratory muscles (muscles of the chest wall and abdomen) occurs near TLC and by the inspiratory

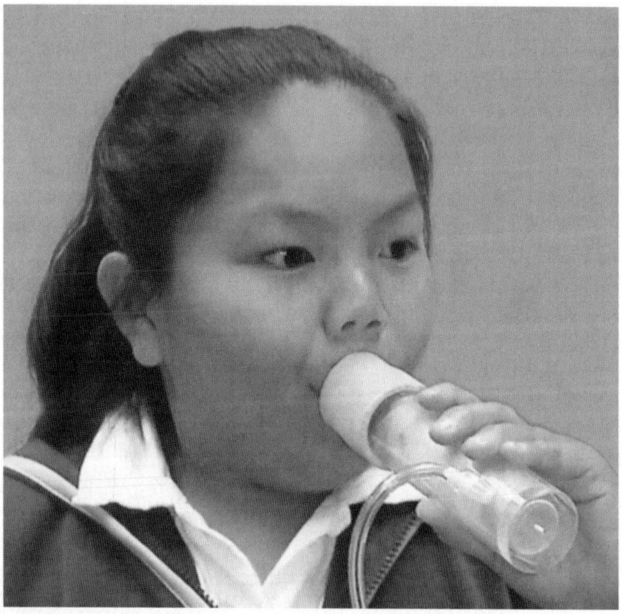

FIGURE 10-18. Child performing a maximal inspiratory pressure maneuver. The hand-held device consists of an acrylic (Plexiglas) cylinder with a 1.5-mm hole (air leak) at the distal end and a pressure port connected by clear tubing to a pressure transducer. The rubber mouthpiece is pressed firmly to the face, with the lips inside the device. Visual feedback is provided by a pressure-time plot on a computer monitor (not pictured).

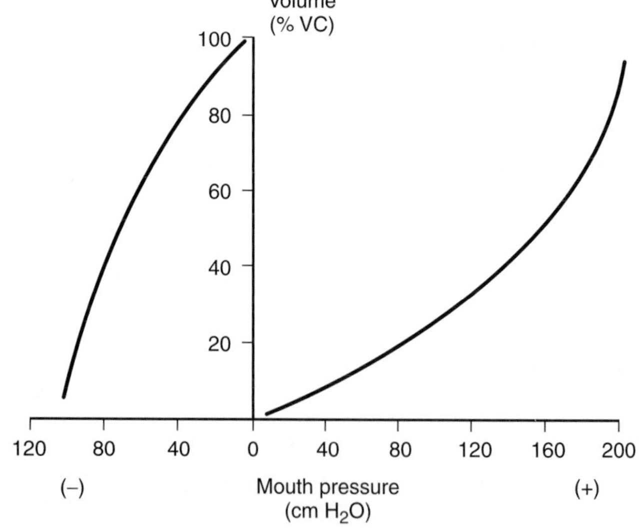

FIGURE 10-19. Plot of mouth pressure versus vital capacity (VC), showing how maximal inspiratory *(left)* and maximal expiratory *(right)* pressures change with lung volume. Inspiratory pressures are maximally negative near residual volume. Expiratory pressures are maximally positive near total lung capacity. (From Hyatt R, Scanlon P, Nakamura M: Interpretation of Pulmonary Function Tests. A Practical Guide. Philadelphia: Lippincott, 1997. By permission of Mayo Foundation for Medical Education and Research.)

muscles (primarily the diaphragm) near RV. For this reason, patients are asked to take a deep breath to near TLC before pressing the mouthpiece to the lips and making a forced expiratory effort, and then to breathe out maximally before making a forced inspiratory effort. Maximal pressures measured at mid lung volumes are generally lower and more variable. Inspiratory and expiratory maneuvers should be repeated at least five times because recorded pressures usually increase and plateau with repeated efforts. The highest pressure obtained in two to three serial measurements matching within 20% is recorded as maximal respiratory pressure.

Using this method, normal men can produce maximal expiratory pressures of 233 ± 84 cm H_2O and maximal inspiratory pressures of −124 ± 44 cm H_2O.[62] Normal women can produce maximal expiratory and inspiratory pressures of 152 ± 54 cm H_2O and −87 ± 32 cm H_2O, respectively.[62] Maximal pressures measured with the lips surrounding the mouthpiece are approximately 30% to 40% lower than those measured with the lips inside the mouthpiece, and may not reflect true respiratory muscle strength. Maximal inspiratory and expiratory pressures are similar in boys and girls. Maximal pressures in girls are similar to those measured in women. Pressures in boys are 80 to 100 cm H_2O lower than those in men, but increase to adult levels in adolescence.[63]

Although maximal respiratory pressures are variable between patients, they are very useful for assessing changes in respiratory muscle strength in individual patients, once they have become familiar with the measurement. Normal values for measurements of maximal pressures made at FRC have been published, making comparative assessments of respiratory strength possible in children who have difficultly performing maneuvers near TLC and RV.[64] The reference standards used to compare results should correspond to the method used to measure pressures. Tables summarizing normal reference standards for adults and children for all methods are available in the recent ATS-ERS statement on respiratory muscle testing.[65] Enthusiastic coaching by the technician is essential to ensure optimal results in children. In practice, a child who can generate a maximal expiratory pressure of 100 cm H_2O or more and a maximal inspiratory pressure of −80 cm H_2O or less is unlikely to demonstrate clinically significant respiratory muscle weakness. Children who are unable, with maximal effort, to produce maximal expiratory pressures greater than 40 cm H_2O are likely to have impaired ability to cough.

DIFFUSING CAPACITY FOR CARBON MONOXIDE

The diffusing capacity for carbon monoxide (DLCO) provides information about the rate at which oxygen is transferred from the lung to the pulmonary circulation. Oxygen travels from the alveoli to the red blood cells in the pulmonary capillaries by passive diffusion. The transfer of oxygen depends on the difference in oxygen tension between the alveolus and pulmonary capillary blood and on the area and thickness of the alveolar-capillary interface. Carbon monoxide follows the same pathway from the alveolus to the red blood cell, where it binds with hemoglobin. The transfer of carbon monoxide across the alveolar-capillary membrane is diffusion-limited. This means that the transfer of carbon monoxide is limited, not by pulmonary blood flow, but rather by the rate of diffusion across the alveolar-capillary membrane (and, to some extent, the red cell membranes). Carbon monoxide transfer is limited only by the rate of diffusion because the concentration of carbon monoxide in the lung during testing is low and the number of hemoglobin-binding sites is so high that they do not become saturated. DLCO is, thus, a measure of the impedance to gas flow across the alveolar-capillary interface. Although this measurement is widely available on commercial pulmonary function testing systems, it cannot be considered a routine test of function in children. Generally, DLCO is not useful as a screening test, but it can be helpful diagnostically, in combination with other tests of function. It is also useful for following some disease processes over time.

The simplest and most widely used technique for measuring DLCO is the single-breath method. This method was first described by Krogh in 1915,[66] and was subsequently developed as a clinical test of lung function by Forster and colleagues in 1954.[67] To perform this test, the child first breathes out to RV and then takes a deep breath (>90%–95% of VC) from a spirometer containing a mixture of 0.3% carbon monoxide, a tracer gas (e.g., 10% helium, 0.3% neon, or 0.3% methane), 21% oxygen, and the balance nitrogen. The breath is held at near full inspiration for 10 seconds, and the child then exhales completely. Concentrations of carbon monoxide and the tracer gas are measured in the alveolar fraction of the expired gas. The concentration of carbon monoxide reaching the alveoli at the beginning of the breath hold is lower than the inspired concentration (0.3%), because it is diluted by the volume in the lungs at the beginning of the maneuver (i.e., RV). The change in the concentration of the tracer gas is used to calculate mean alveolar carbon monoxide concentration at the start of the breath hold. It also provides a measure of alveolar volume by gas dilution. The volume of carbon monoxide taken up in 10 seconds is the product of the alveolar volume and the difference between the estimated starting concentration and the measured expired concentration of alveolar carbon monoxide. Diffusing capacity is the volume of carbon monoxide transferred from alveolar gas to blood in milliliters per minute divided by the difference between mean alveolar-capillary carbon monoxide pressure and mean pulmonary capillary carbon monoxide pressure. Mean capillary carbon monoxide pressure is assumed to be zero because carbon monoxide binds tightly to hemoglobin in the red blood cell. In North America, DLCO is expressed in milliliters per minute per milliliters of mercury. In Europe, the same measurement is referred to as the *transfer factor,* and it is expressed in millimoles per minute per kilopascal. Further details can be found in the 1995 ATS document on this technique.[68]

The DLCO value varies directly with lung size. Normal reference equations for adults predict DLCO based on height, sex, and age.[68] Published equations differ substantially in their predictions. In adults, the average normal single-breath DLCO is approximately 20 to 30 mL/min/mm Hg, is somewhat higher in men than in women, and declines with advancing age.[62] Normal reference values for children are limited.[69,70] Values in elementary school children range from 10 to 15 mL/min/mm Hg and increase with height, until they reach adult levels in late adolescence. The reference values selected should be appropriate to the methods used and the population undergoing testing. DLCO measurements differ substantially between laboratories. If predicted results consistently do not match the clinical situation, the reference equations and the details of testing should be reevaluated. In young children with VC of less than 1.5 to 2.0 L, methodologic modifications may be necessary to ensure the accuracy of measurement. This may also be true for older children who have restrictive disease and similarly small volumes.

The DLCO is increased in left-to-right shunts, pulmonary arteriovenous malformations, and hepatorenal syndrome. Most conditions for which DLCO is clinically useful, however, impair carbon monoxide transfer. DLCO is valuable in adults for assessing the degree and progression of emphysema, and may be helpful in distinguishing emphysema (low DLCO) from chronic obstructive pulmonary disease due predominantly to bronchiectasis (normal DLCO). There is, however, considerable overlap. DLCO is also low in intersitial lung disorders, including sarcoidosis, collagen vascular diseases (lupus erythematosus, scleroderma), hypersensitivity pneumonitis, histiocytosis X, and drug-induced lung disease (amiodarone, bleomycin, methotrexate). DLCO may be reduced in congestive heart failure, alveolar proteinosis, bronchial obstruction, bronchiolitis obliterans, pulmonary vascular obstruction (obliterative pulmonary vasculitis, pulmonary embolus), and pneumonectomy. DLCO monitoring in patients who undergo lung transplantation may aid in the early detection of bronchiolitis obliterans. DLCO is often most helpful when it detects abnormality in the face of otherwise normal spirometry findings and fractional lung volumes. DLCO may be reduced before the development of hypoxemia at rest or with exertion in patients with pulmonary vascular disorders, such as primary pulmonary hypertension, recurrent pulmonary emboli, or obliterative vasculopathy. DLCO should be measured in patients with unexplained dyspnea.

Although intended to be a measure of the size and thickness of the alveolar-capillary membrane, DLCO is affected by many factors that can complicate the interpretation of results. Increases in pulmonary capillary blood volume secondary to left-to-right intracardiac shunts increase DLCO. DLCO increases by approximately twofold during exercise because of recruitment of pulmonary capillaries and the related increase in the alveolar-capillary membrane surface area. DLCO may be elevated in patients with asthma or obesity, again probably because of increased pulmonary blood volume, but these increases are not of any clinical significance. DLCO is decreased in patients with anemia and increased in polycythemia. Hemoglobin levels should always be considered when interpreting results. When possible, hemoglobin levels should be measured and DLCO adjusted in accordance with ATS recommendations.[68] For children younger than 15 years of age (and all women), adjusted DLCO = measured DLCO × (9.38 + hemoglobin)/(1.7 × hemoglobin). For men and boys 15 years of age and older, adjusted DLCO = measured DLCO × (10.22 + hemoglobin)/(1.7 × hemoglobin). Severe anemia or anemia that develops in the course of chemotherapy should not be interpreted as lung disease. Intra-alveolar hemorrhage may result in substantial increases in DLCO related to the binding of carbon monoxide to hemoglobin in the airspaces. DLCO has been used to monitor the extent of intra-alveolar hemorrhage in Goodpasture's syndrome. Smoking in adults and adolescents can produce carboxyhemoglobin levels of as high as 10% to 12%. Each 1% increase in the level of carboxyhemoglobin results in approximately a 1% decrease in DLCO because of the reduction in the alveolar-to-capillary pressure gradient for carbon monoxide. The Valsalva maneuver reduces pulmonary blood volume and reduces carbon monoxide uptake. The Müeller maneuver, supine posture, and altitude produce increases in DLCO. Alveolar hypoxia and alveolar hypercarbia in patients with compensated respiratory failure reduce the alveolar-to-capillary gradient for oxygen, enhance the gradient for carbon monoxide, and increase DLCO. These later influences are modest or are not relevant in the normal clinical setting and, thus, usually do not affect the interpretation of results.

The interpretation of results is also confounded by disease-related factors that affect the distribution of ventilation and pulmonary blood flow. DLCO is measured only in areas of the lung into which gas and blood flow. Uneven distribution of ventilation and perfusion reduces the effective area for alveolar-capillary gas exchange. Results in patients with airway obstruction must be interpreted with caution. Global DLCO decreases if carbon monoxide does not reach an area of the lung or reaches an area in lower concentration. As with other dilutional methods, alveolar volume may be underestimated in patients with airway obstruction. Nonhomogeneous lung emptying can obscure the normal sharp demarcation between anatomic dead space and alveolar gas, resulting in a sample that does not reflect mean alveolar carbon monoxide concentration. If the pulmonary capillaries are obstructed, DLCO is generally decreased. DLCO is reduced in pulmonary capillary vasculopathy, but this may not be the case in pulmonary hypertension of precapillary origin. Large pulmonary emboli reduce perfusion to regions of the lung, but global changes in pulmonary vascular pressures may increase perfusion to other regions, blunting expected reductions in DLCO. Intuition would suggest that pneumonectomy should reduce DLCO by half. This is usually not the case, however, because when all of the cardiac output flows through a single lung, recruitment of pulmonary capillaries increases the surface area for gas exchange and results in a less than 50% reduction in DLCO. Interpretation of results requires careful consideration of multiple factors, including other measures of lung function, possible test-related and disease-related confounders, and the patient's clinical situation. DLCO should not be ordered routinely, but rather used only for specific clinical indications.

REFERENCES

1. Hutchinson J: On the capacity of the lungs, and on the respiratory movements, with the view of establishing a precise and easy method of detecting disease by the spirometer. Lancet 1846;1:630–632.
2. Davy H: Researches, chemical and philosophical, chiefly concerning nitrous oxide or dephlogisticated air and its respiration, 2nd ed. London: Briggs and Cottle, 1800.
3. Christie R: Lung volume and its subdivisions. J Clin Invest 1932;11: 1099–1118.
4. Tepper R, Asdell S: Comparison of helium dilution and nitrogen washout measurements of functional residual capacity in infants and very young children. Pediatr Pulmonol 1992;13:250–254.
5. Dubois A, Botelho S, Bedell G, et al: A rapid plethysmographic method for measuring thoracic gas volume. J Clin Invest 1956;35:322–326.
6. Tiffeneau R, Pinelli A: Air circulant et air captif dans l'exploration de la fonction ventilatrice pulmonaire. Paris Med 1947;133:624–628.
7. Gaensler E: Analysis of the ventilatory defect by timed capacity measurements. Am Rev Tuberc 1951;64:256–278.
8. Leuallen E, Fowler W: Maximal midexpiratory flow. Am Rev Tuberc Pulm Dis 1955;72:783–800.
9. Fry D, Hyatt R: Pulmonary mechanics. A unified analysis of the relationship between pressure, volume, and gas flow in the lungs of normal and diseased human subjects. Am J Med 1960;29:672–689.
10. Fry DL, Ebert RV, Stead WW, Brown CC: The mechanics of pulmonary ventilation in normal subjects and patients with emphysema. Am J Med 1954;16:89–97.
11. Hyatt R, Schilder D, Fry D: Relationship between maximum expiratory flow and degree of lung inflation. J Appl Physiol 1958;13:331–336.
12. Pedersen O, Lyager S, Ingram R Jr: Airway dynamics in transition between peak and maximal expiratory flow. J Appl Physiol 1985;59:1733–1746.

13. Mead J, Turner JM, Maclem PT, Little JB: Significance of the relationship between lung recoil and maximum expiratory flow. J Appl Physiol 1967;22:95–108.
14. Dawson S, Elliott E: Wave-speed limitation on expiratory flow. A unifying concept. J Appl Physiol Respir Environ Exercise Physiol 1977;43:498–515.
15. Mead J: Expiratory flow limitations. A physiologist's point of view. Fed Proc 1980;39:2771–2775.
16. McNamara JJ, Castile RG, Glass GM, Fredberg JJ: Heterogeneous lung emptying during forced expiration. J Appl Physiol 1987;63:1648–1657.
17. McNamara J, Castile R, Ludwig M, et al: Interdependent regional emptying during forced expiration before and after histamine inhalation of canines. J Appl Physiol 1994;76:356–360.
18. Wilson T, Hyatt R, Rodarte J: The mechanisms that limit expiratory flow. Lung 1980;158:193–200.
19. Taussig L, Chernick V, Wood R, et al: Standardization of lung function testing in children. J Pediatr 1980;97:668–676.
20. Leman R, Gerdes C, Wegmann M, et al: Frequency spectra of flow and volume events for forced vital capacity. J Appl Physiol 1982;53:977–984.
21. American Thoracic Society: ATS Statement. Snowbird Workshop on standardization of spirometry. Am Rev Respir Dis 1979;119:831–838.
22. American Thoracic Society: Standardization of Spirometry. 1987 Update. Am Rev Respir Dis 1987;136:1285–1293.
23. American Thoracic Society: Standardization of Spirometry. 1994 Update. Am J Respir Crit Care Med 1995;152:1107–1136.
24. Kanengiser S, Dozor A: Forced expiratory maneuvers in children aged 3 to 5 years. Pediatr Pulmonol 1994;18:144–149.
25. LeSouef P, Lafortune B, Landau L: Spirometric assessment of asthmatic children aged 2 to 6 years. Aust N Z Med J 1986;16:625.
26. Brough F, Schmidt C, Dickman M, Jackson B: Effect of two instructional procedures in the performance of the spirometry test in children 5 through 7 years of age. Am Rev Respir Dis 1972;106:604–605.
27. Eigen H, Bieler H, Grant D, et al: Spirometric pulmonary function in healthy preschool children. Am J Respir Crit Care Med 2001;163:619–623.
28. Zapletal A, Chalupova J: Forced expiratory parameters in healthy preschool children (3–6 years of age). Pediatr Pulmonol 2003;35:200–207.
29. Taussig L: Maximal expiratory flows at functional residual capacity. A test of lung function for young children. Am Rev Respir Dis 1977;116: 1031–1038.
30. Buist AS, Adams BE, Sexton GJ, Azzam AH: Reference values for functional residual capacity and maximal expiratory flow in young children. Am Rev Respir Dis 1980;122:15–18.
31. Wall M, Misley M, Dickerson D: Partial expiratory flow-volume curves in young children. Am Rev Respir Dis 1984;129:557–562.
32. Chavasse R, Johnson P, Francis J, et al: To clip or not to clip? Noseclips for spirometry. Eur Respir J 2003;21:876–878.
33. Gruber C, Moenkhoff M, Hamacher J, et al: The influence of a nose-clip on inhalation therapy in asthmatic children. Pediatr Asthma Allerg Immunol 2003;16:129–135.
34. American Thoracic Society: Guidelines for methacholine and exercise challenge testing. 1999. Am J Respir Crit Care Med 2000;161:309–329.
35. Chatham M, Bleecker E, Norman P, et al: A screening test for airways reactivity. An abbreviated methacholine inhalation challenge. Chest 1982;82:15–18.
36. Parker C, Bilbo R, Reed C: Methacholine aerosol as test for bronchial asthma. Arch Intern Med 1965;115:452–458.
37. Wang X, Dockery D, Wypij D, et al: Pulmonary function between 6 and 18 years of age. Pediatr Pulmonol 1993;15:75–88.
38. American Thoracic Society: Lung function testing. Selection of reference values and interpretation strategies. Am Rev Respir Dis 1991;144: 1202–1218.
39. Schwartz J, Katz SA, Fegley RW, Tockman MS: Sex and race differences in the development of lung function. Am Rev Respir Dis 1988;138: 1415–1421.
40. Hutchinson J: On the capacity of the lungs, and on the respiratory movements, with the view of establishing a precise and easy method of detecting disease by the spirometer. Lancet 1846;1:630–632.
41. Stocks J, Quanjer P: Workshop Report. Reference values for residual volume, functional residual capacity, and total lung capacity. Eur Respir J 1995;8:492–506.
42. Wall M, Olson D, Bonn B, et al: Lung function in North American Indian children. Reference standards for spirometry, maximal expiratory flow volume curves, and peak expiratory flow. Am Rev Respir Dis 1982;125: 158–162.
43. Neukirch F, Chasin R, Liard R, et al: Spirometry and maximal expiratory flow-volume curve reference standards for Polynesian, European, and Chinese teenagers. Chest 1988;94:792–798.
44. Berman S, Arnall D, Cornwall M: Pulmonary function test outcomes in healthy Navajo Native American adolescents. Am J Respir Crit Care Med 1994;150:1150–1153.
45. Ip M, Karlberg E, Karlberg J, et al: Lung function reference values in Chinese children and adolescents in Hong Kong. I. Spirometric values and comparison with other populations. Am J Respir Crit Care Med 2000;162:424–429.
46. Subbarao P, Lebecque P, Corey M, Coates AL: Comparison of spirometric reference values. Pediatr Pulmonol 2004;37:515–522.
47. Joseph-Bowen J, de Klerk, N, Firth M, et al: Lung function, bronchial responsiveness, and asthma in a community cohort of 6-year-old children. Am J Respir Crit Care Med 2004;169:850–854.
48. Rosenfeld M, Pepe M, Longton G, et al: Effect of choice of reference equation on analysis of pulmonary function in cystic fibrosis patients. Pediatr Pulmonol 2001;31:227–237.
49. Parker JM, Dillard TA, Phillips YY: Arm span-height relationships in patients referred for spirometry. Am J Respir Crit Care Med 1996;154: 533–536.
50. Gauld LM, Kapper J, Carlin JB, Robertson CF: Prediction of childhood pulmonary function using ulna length. Am J Respir Crit Care Med 2003;168:804–809.
51. Rodenstein D, Stanescu D, Francis C: Demonstration of failure of body plethysmography in airway obstruction. J Appl Physiol 1982;52:949–954.
52. Tomalak W, Radlinski J, Pogorzelski A, Doniec Z: Reference values for forced inspiratory flows in children aged 7–15 years. Pediatr Pulmonol 2004;38:246–249.
53. Dales R, Spitzer W, Tousignant P, et al: Clinical interpretation of airway response to a bronchodilator. Am Rev Respir Dis 1988;138:317–320.
54. Hilman B, Allen J: Clinical applications of pulmonary function testing in children and adolescents. In: Hilman B, ed: Pediatric Respiratory Disease. Diagnosis and Treatment, Philadelphia: WB Saunders, 1993.
55. Pattishall E: Pulmonary function testing reference values and interpretations in pediatric training programs. Pediatrics 1990;85:768–773.
56. Lemen R: Pulmonary function testing in the office and clinic. In: Kendig E, Chernick V, eds: Disorders of the Respiratory Tract in Children, 5th ed. Philadelphia: WB Saunders, 1990. pp 147–154.
57. Nickerson B, Lemen R, Gerdes C, et al: Within-subject variability and percent change or significance of spirometry in normal subjects and in patients with cystic fibrosis. Am Rev Respir Dis 1980;122:859–866.
58. Lebowitz M, Quackenboss J, Camilli A, et al: The epidemiological importance of intraindividual changes in objective pulmonary response. Eur J Epidemiol 1987;3:390–398.
59. Cook C, Mead J, Orzalesi M: Static volume-pressure characteristics of the respiratory system during maximal efforts. J Appl Physiol 1964;19: 1017–1022.
60. Black L, Hyatt R: Maximal respiratory pressure. Normal values and relationship to age and sex. Am Rev Respir Dis 1969;99:696–702.
61. Wohlgemuth M, van der Kooi EL, Padberg GW, Folgering HT: Face mask spirometry and respiratory pressures in normal subjects. Eur Respir J 2003; 22:1001–1006.
62. Hyatt R, Scanlon P, Nakamura M: Interpretation of pulmonary function tests. A practical guide. Philadelphia: Lippincott-Raven, 1997.
63. Szeinberg A, Marcotte JE, Roizin H, et al: Normal values of maximal inspiratory and expiratory pressures with a portable apparatus in children, adolescents, and young adults. Pediatr Pulmonol 1987;3:255–258.
64. Gaultier C, Zinman R: Maximal static pressures in healthy children. Respir Physiol 1983;51:45–61.
65. American Thoracic Society: Guidelines for methacholine and exercise challenge testing. 1999. Am J Respir Crit Care Med 2000;161:309–329.
66. Krogh M: The diffusion of gases through the lungs of man. J Physiol 1915;49:271–296.
67. Forster RE, Fowler WS, Bates DV, Van Lingen B: The absorption of carbon monoxide by the lungs during breathholding. J Clin Invest 1954;33: 1135–1145.
68. American Thoracic Society: Single-breath carbon monoxide diffusing capacity (transfer factor). Am J Respir Crit Care Med 1995;152:2185–2198.
69. Nasr S, Amato P, Wilmott R: Predicted values for lung diffusing capacity in healthy children. Pediatr Pulmonol 1991;10:267–272.
70. Stam H, van den Beek A, Grunberg K, et al: Pulmonary diffusing capacity at reduced alveolar volumes in children. Pediatr Pulmonol 1996;21:84–89.

11 Pulmonary Function Assessment in the Laboratory during Exercise

Dan M. Cooper, MD • Chaim Springer, MD

BIOLOGIC RELEVANCE OF EXERCISE IN THE GROWING CHILD

For both healthy children and those with chronic diseases, the ability to engage in play, exercise, and other physical activities is an essential component of daily life. For the pediatrician, precise assessment of the cardiorespiratory and metabolic responses to exercise can be a valuable tool in the diagnosis of disease, in the assessment of its impact, and for the recommendation of specific programs of physical activity. As has been noted in previous chapters, analysis of static pulmonary function can yield important information about the capability of the respiratory system in children. But testing the mechanical properties of the lung at rest does not reveal the consequences of disease on metabolic function when the organism is stressed. To accomplish this, respiration, in its fullest sense, must be assessed. By measuring gas exchange at the mouth ($\dot{V}O_2$, oxygen uptake; $\dot{V}CO_2$, carbon dioxide output; and $\dot{V}_E$, ventilation) and the heart rate (HR) responses to exercise-induced increases in metabolism, the relationship between respiration at the cells and respiration of the whole organism can be evaluated.

Since the last edition of this book, a striking new paradigm has emerged in which the health and possibly disease effects of exercise and physical activity can be viewed as a balance between pro- and antiinflammatory, catabolic and anabolic activity (Fig. 11-1). We now know that exercise can lead to a substantial perturbation of cellular homeostasis including a profound metabolic acidosis, markedly altered O_2 and substrate flux in tissue and mitochondria, and, on occasion, frank tissue injury. Exercise, even in healthy adults and children, results in what appears to be a "danger"-type activation of innate immune responses[1–4] that involves increased levels of circulating cytokines (e.g., interleukin-6 [IL-6]), leukocytosis, and leukocyte adhesion molecules that have been associated with such lung diseases as asthma and cystic fibrosis (CF).[5,6]

In contrast, the salient features of the healthy adaptation to repeated exercise are both anti-inflammatory and anabolic, consisting of increased muscle mass, angiogenesis and arteriogenesis, increased bone strength, and the formation of new mitochondria. In the years to come, an exercise test in a child may be used not only to gauge cardiorespiratory capacity, but also to gain insight into the broader stress, immunologic, and inflammatory state of that individual and its implication for physical performance.

PHYSICAL ACTIVITY AND GROWTH IN CHILDREN

The widely held but largely intuitive notion that vigorous physical activity occurs more frequently in children and adolescents than in adults is increasingly supported by scientific investigation.[7–9] Exercise in children is not merely play but rather contributes to long-term processes of growth, development, and risk factors for adult disease. Indeed, as demonstrated by Borer and colleagues[10] in some species, sedentary behavior is associated with reduced growth and growth hormone (GH) pulsatility (e.g., Fig. 11-2); whether or not physical activity alters somatic growth in humans is not yet known. As succinctly summarized recently by Rosenfeld, "Growth in any species is an extraordinarily complex process, but growth in humans is characterized by a number of unique features . . . [some of which] are characteristic only of *Homo sapiens* and are not replicated even in other primates."[11]

There is now a growing body of data supporting the idea that there exist "critical periods" of development during which a variety of stimuli can alter the overall programming of developmental processes.[12–14] The neonatal growth interval and puberty are critical periods of development, and there are increasing data showing long-term effects of physical activity (or inactivity) during these stages. Passive exercise in neonates can augment weight gain,[15] and bone mineralization is optimally enhanced by physical activity somewhere between the pre- and late pubertal period.[16] Type 2 diabetes and other insulin resistance syndromes become most manifest in physically inactive children during puberty as well.[17]

Closely tied to the concept of a critical period of growth and development is the theme of pediatric origins of adult disease. It is increasingly recognized that physical activity in children is not merely play but an essential component of healthy growth and development. Levels of physical activity markedly affect body composition, and sedentary lifestyles in children are a major cause of the current epidemic of childhood obesity and its accompanying morbidities.[18] In a recent American Heart Association Scientific Statement focused on the guidelines for the primary preventions of atherosclerotic cardiovascular disease beginning in childhood,[19] the data are summarized, and the authors conclude: "The existing evidence indicates that primary prevention of atherosclerotic disease should begin in childhood." As levels of physical activity progressively decline in children,[20] it is reasonable to speculate that sarcopenia, the debilitating loss of muscle mass observed in the elderly,[21] will ultimately be found to have roots in inadequate muscle development during childhood, a sad echo of our current understanding of osteoporosis.

A BIOLOGIC APPROACH TOWARD EXERCISE TESTING IN CHILDREN

The progressive exercise protocol in which power on a cycle ergometer or treadmill is increased until the subject reaches his

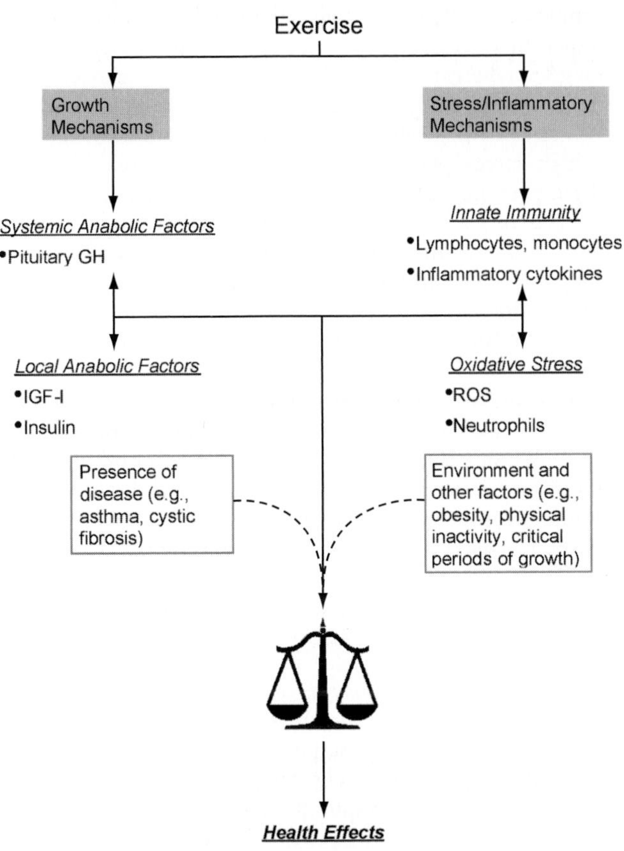

■ **FIGURE 11-1.** A schematic diagram relating exercise to health and growth in children. GH, growth hormone; IGF-1, insulin-like growth factor 1; ROS, reactive oxygen species.

or her maximal level of tolerance (e.g., Bruce protocol, Godfrey protocol, ramp protocol) remains the cornerstone of most exercise tests in children and adults.[22–25] Despite much discussion and debate about protocols and the advantages and disadvantages of treadmills and ergometers, there has yet to emerge a common, standardized approach for testing fitness and exercise capacity in children.[26,27] Most pediatric exercise tests last between 10 and 15 minutes, and usually about the last half of the test is performed at work rates (WRs) that are above the subject's lactate or anaerobic threshold (LAT). Our understanding of the maturation and development of the cardiorespiratory system in children has been greatly enhanced by investigations into maximal and supramaximal physiologic responses to exercise in children and adolescents.

It is becoming increasingly apparent, however, that peak or maximal exercise tests are not representative of patterns of physical activity actually encountered in the lives of children. While sustained heavy exercise rarely occurs in children, traditional exercise testing focuses largely on the peak or maximal O_2 uptake ($\dot{V}O_{2\,max}$), which can only be measured from sustained exercise precisely in the high-intensity range. $\dot{V}O_{2\,max}$ probably occurs only in the confines of the exercise laboratory, and a "true" $\dot{V}O_{2\,max}$ (i.e., a plateau or decrease in $\dot{V}O_2$ while the WR continues to increase) is observed in only about 28% of children and adolescents.[28] Because of this, cardiopulmonary exercise testing in children includes a growing variety of less effort-dependent protocols such as the physical work capacity at a specified HR. In the physical work capacity testing paradigm,[29–31] the subject performs a progressive exercise test in which the main variable is the WR achieved at a specified, submaximal HR (usually around 150–170 beats per minute).

Normal results of maximal exercise tests are obtained from studies done in large samples of healthy children. These values are profoundly effort dependent, and healthy subjects are routinely cajoled and prodded to continue exercising in the high-intensity range so as to achieve data of optimal quality. In contrast, patients with known or even suspected abnormalities are not encouraged as vigorously as are healthy subjects. Lactic acidosis and respiratory or cardiac insufficiency can accompany high WRs, and this causes reasonable concern regarding the safety of

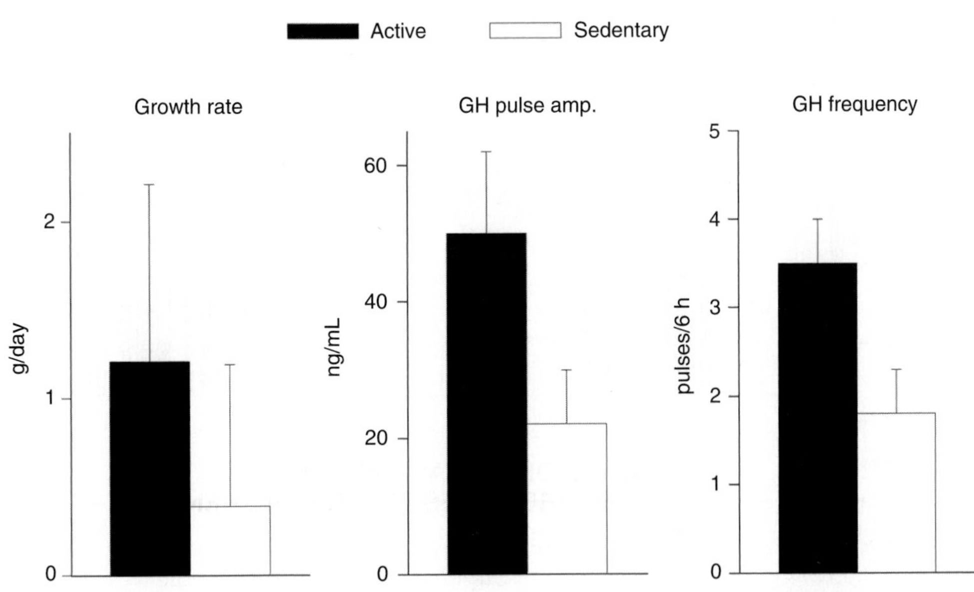

■ **FIGURE 11-2.** Comparison of three parameters in physically active versus sedentary growing hamsters. Active hamsters had significantly increased growth rate, growth hormone (GH) pulse amplitude, and GH pulse frequency compared with sedentary animals. The effect of physical activity on somatic growth in human children has yet to be determined; however, physically active children tend to have less fat and more lean tissue than their sedentary counterparts. (Data from Borer KT, Nicoski DR, Owens V: Alteration of pulsatile growth hormone secretion by growth-inducing exercise. Involvement of endogenous opiates and somatostatin. Endocrinology 1986;118:844–850.)

high-intensity exercise testing in individuals with heart or lung disease. As a consequence of such de facto differences in testing strategies, published "normal" maximal values may not be reliable for children with suspected impairments.

REAL PATTERNS OF PHYSICAL ACTIVITY IN CHILDREN

To better understand how formal exercise testing in children relates to actual patterns of physical activity observed in children under natural conditions, a direct observation system that quantifies the duration, intensity, frequency, and interval duration of children's physical activities was developed.[9,32] We used this system to assess the level and tempo of energy expenditure under free-ranging, natural conditions experienced by 15 children aged 6 to 10 years in southern California. Observations were recorded every 3 seconds during 4-hour time blocks from 8 AM to 8 PM. Using indirect calorimetry, calibration studies in the laboratory determined $\dot{V}O_2$ (mL/min/kg) during each coded activity, and activities were categorized by intensity (low, medium, or high). Subjects were found to engage in activities of low intensity 77.1% of the time and activities of high intensity 3.1% of the time (Fig. 11-3). The median duration of low- and medium-intensity activities was 6 seconds, of high-intensity activities only 3 seconds, with 95% lasting less than 15 seconds; however, different types of high-intensity activities were often strung together. Thus, it appears that under natural conditions of daily living, children engage in short bursts of intense physical activity interspersed with varying intervals of low and moderate intensity.

THE CARDIORESPIRATORY RESPONSE TO EXERCISE

Consider, for example, the important acts of fleeing from a predator or, in more modern terms, running to avoid an oncoming car. When sudden and large increases in metabolic demand are imposed by physical activity, the whole organism can successfully function only by means of an integrated response among several organ systems. At the very onset of exercise, before there has been sufficient time for an inincrease in environmental O_2 uptake, the healthy human must have sufficient stores of O_2, high-energy phosphates, nonaerobic metabolic capability, and supplies of substrate to perform significant amounts of physical activity. As exercise proceeds, cardiac output increases and blood flow is diverted to the working muscles without compromising the critical flow of O_2 and glucose to the brain.

Ventilation and pulmonary blood flow must increase to precisely match the energy demand of the working muscles, so that homeostasis for $PaCO_2$ and pH are maintained. There must be sufficient increase in substrate availability (glucose, fat, protein) but without depleting the peripheral blood glucose stores. Finally, the heat produced during exercise must be dissipated so that homeostasis for body temperature is maintained. In summary, as diagrammed in the late 1960s by Wasserman,[33] events at the cell are closely linked to events at the heart and lungs (Fig. 11-4).

MATURATION OF CARDIORESPIRATORY RESPONSES TO EXERCISE

The acute physiologic adjustments to physical activity in children are not simply scaled-down versions of those observed in adults. Maturation of cardiorespiratory, neurologic, and peripheral metabolic processes occur throughout childhood. These changes influence cardiorespiratory responses to physical activity rather profoundly and must be understood to properly interpret exercise tests.

CARBON DIOXIDE OUTPUT AND VENTILATORY RESPONSES

Breathing increases during exercise. The stimulus for the exercise hyperpnea is, to a large extent, the increased production of CO_2

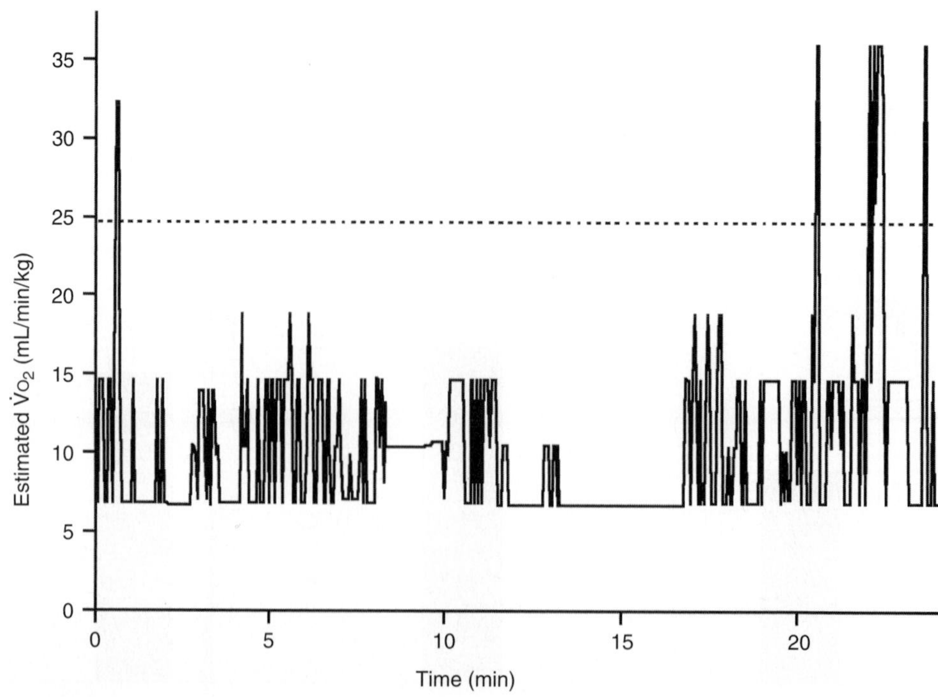

FIGURE 11-3. Representative example of activity patterns derived from direct observation in a 7-year-old boy during a 24-minute period. Bouts of physical activity are randomly spaced. Most bouts were in the low-intensity range (below the lactate threshold [LT], the dashed line, estimated for children this age); however, a substantial portion of the energy expenditure due to physical activity results from the less frequent, high-intensity bouts. (From Berman N, Bailey RC, Barstow TJ, Cooper DM: Spectral and bout detection analysis of physical activity patterns in healthy, prepubertal boys and girls. Am J Hum Biol 1998;10:289–297.)

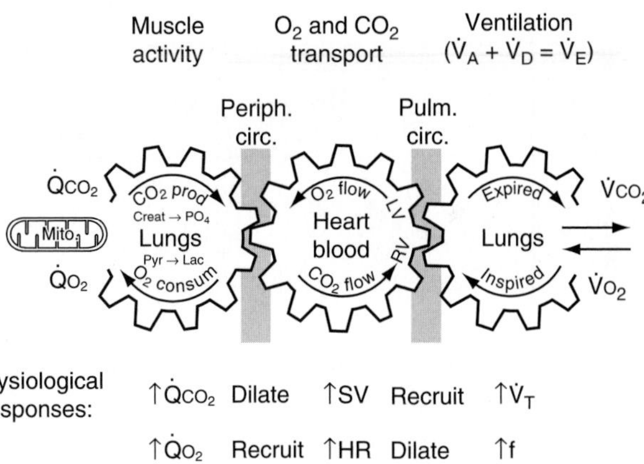

FIGURE 11-4. The renowned interlocking-gears figure showing the interconnection between mitochondrial and systemic respiration. This scheme was developed by Karl Wasserman in the late 1960s. Creat, creatinine; f, frequency; HR, heart rate; Lac, lactate; LV, left ventricle; Pyr, pyruvate; $\dot{Q}CO_2$, carbon dioxide production; $\dot{Q}O_2$, oxygen uptake; RV, right ventricle; $\dot{V}_A$, alveolar ventilation; $\dot{V}CO_2$, carbon dioxide output; $\dot{V}_D$ dead space; $\dot{V}_E$, ventilation; $\dot{V}O_2$, oxygen uptake; $\dot{V}_T$, tidal ventilation.

at the cells.[34,35] Thus, the relationship between $\dot{V}_E$ and $\dot{V}CO_2$ is significantly closer than is the relationship between $\dot{V}_E$ and $\dot{V}O_2$ during progressive exercise in adults.[33] The concentration of CO_2 in the arterial blood (measured as the $PaCO_2$) is held constant throughout most of progressive exercise despite large increases in metabolically produced CO_2. The control of breathing during exercise in adults has been reviewed elsewhere[36,37] and includes central and peripheral chemoreceptors. In addition, mechanoreceptors in the exercising muscles may also play a role, as suggested by Gozal and colleagues[38] from studies done in patients with congenital central hypoventilation syndrome. There is evidence that respiratory control does mature during childhood,[39] but much work needs to be done to fully understand the interaction between nervous system maturation and the control of breathing during exercise.

The robust nature of $PaCO_2$ homeostasis is reflected in healthy subjects at higher work intensities when additional CO_2 is liberated from the chemical combination of lactic acid (produced from anaerobic metabolism) and the ubiquitous buffer, bicarbonate. During this phase of isocapnic buffering,[40] $PaCO_2$ and pH remain constant as $\dot{V}_E$ increases in proportion to $\dot{V}CO_2$. Only at very high work intensities, when the pH begins to fall and the peripheral chemoreceptors are additionally stimulated, does hyperventilation occur and $PaCO_2$ fall ("respiratory compensation point").[41]

The ability to rapidly increase the metabolic rate is sustainable only if substantial cellular accumulation of metabolically produced CO_2 is prevented; otherwise, pH falls rapidly and adenosine triphosphate (ATP)–based energy metabolism pathways cannot operate. Redistribution of CO_2 from cells is facilitated by several mechanisms including: dissolution in body fluids and tissues, binding with hemoglobin, and, most importantly, rapid conversion to HCO_3^- with hemoglobin serving as a buffer for increased hydrogen ion concentration ($[H^+]$). There is evidence suggesting that the linkage between $\dot{V}CO_2$ and $\dot{V}_E$ undergoes a process of maturation during growth; in other words, there is a difference between children and adults in the ventilatory response to changes in metabolic rate. These differences can be readily seen from a variety of exercise protocols.

Progressive exercise provides a relatively simple way to gauge the coupling of $\dot{V}_E$ with $\dot{V}CO_2$ (Fig. 11-5). The alveolar gas equation suggests that the relationship is determined by the CO_2 "set point" (i.e., the level at which $PaCO_2$ is regulated) and the ratio of dead space to tidal volume (V_D/V_T):

$$\dot{V}_E = (863 \times PaCO_2^{-1} \times (1 - V_D/V_T)^{-1} \times \dot{V}CO_2$$

As shown in Figure 11-5, there is a linear relationship between $\dot{V}_E$ and $\dot{V}CO_2$ for most of the progressive test.[42] Variables such as elevated $PaCO_2$ will tend to lower the magnitude of the slope, while a high V_D/V_T will render the slope steeper.

We and others have found it helpful to quantify the relationship between $\dot{V}_E$ and $\dot{V}CO_2$ by calculating the slope of the best-fit line through the linear portion of the relationship (Figs. 11-5 and 11-6). Normal values have now been established for this parameter.[43,44] The slope of the relationship ($\Delta\dot{V}_E/\Delta\dot{V}CO_2$) decreases with increasing size among children and teenagers. Younger children need to breathe more than adults for a given increase in metabolic rate (i.e., $\Delta\dot{V}CO_2$). Whether this results from lower CO_2 stores in children associated with apparently lower $PaCO_2$ and lower hematocrit (i.e., less hemoglobin buffering capacity and consequently, less CO_2 "stored" in the blood) has not yet been determined.[45–47]

Additional data demonstrate substantial differences between children and adults in the $\dot{V}_E$ and $\dot{V}CO_2$ responses to, and recovery from, 1 minute of high-intensity exercise. We used these short exercise protocols because they more closely mimic patterns of activity actually observed in real life in children. Adults took longer than did children to recover from exercise, and $\tau\dot{V}CO_2$ (τ is the recovery time constant—the time required to reach about 63% of the end-exercise to pre-exercise steady-state values) and $\tau\dot{V}_E$ increased with work intensity in adults but not in children. These results are consistent with the hypothesis of a reduced anaerobic capability in children (see later). If high-intensity exercise in children results in a smaller increase in lactic acid concentrations, then, pari pasu, less CO_2 will be produced from bicarbonate buffering of H^+.

$PaCO_2$ seems to be controlled at lower levels in children than it is in adults.[39,48,49] These observations were corroborated

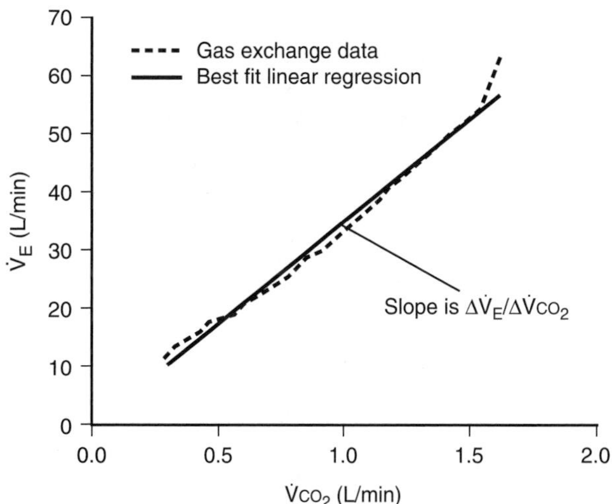

FIGURE 11-5. The relationship between $\dot{V}_E - \dot{V}CO_2$ during a progressive exercise test in a 9-year-old girl with CF. Since $\dot{V}_E$ is driven by $\dot{V}CO_2$, these data tend to have a high signal-to-noise ratio. The slope of the $\dot{V}_E - \dot{V}CO_2$ relationship is easily calculated using standard linear regression techniques.

indirectly by the measurements of end-tidal P_{CO_2} ($P_{ET}CO_2$) made in our 1-minute exercise studies showing that pre-exercise and peak-exercise values were significantly lower in children compared with adults, and more directly in a study of arterial Pa_{CO_2} in children by Ohuchi and colleagues.[47] A lower CO_2 set point may also explain, in part, the greater slopes of the $\dot{V}_E - \dot{V}CO_2$ relationship that we and others[50] observed in progressive exercise tests: If alveolar P_{CO_2} is lower, then greater $\dot{V}_E$ is needed to excrete a given amount of CO_2. Both the magnitude of the $\dot{V}_E - \dot{V}CO_2$ slopes and the growth-related decrease in them were quite similar to findings we obtained in a previous study of ventilatory responses in children and young adults.[42]

The coupling of $\dot{V}CO_2$ and $\dot{V}_E$ is closer in children than in adults. The rise in $P_{ET}CO_2$ with exercise seen in both children and adults indicates that $\dot{V}CO_2$ increased more rapidly than $\dot{V}_E$, but the exercise-induced jump in $P_{ET}CO_2$ was much smaller in children (from 37.8 ± 0.4 to 40.1 ± 0.3 mm Hg) compared with adults (from 40.5 ± 0.2 to 49.9 ± 0.4), suggesting that $\dot{V}_E$ kept pace with $\dot{V}CO_2$ better in children than in adults during exercise and early in recovery. Recently, Ratel and co-workers explored the implications of this closer coupling on acid-base balance during exercise in children.[51] Qualitatively similar observations have been made during recovery from exercise. While recovery $\tau\dot{V}_E$ was significantly longer than $\tau\dot{V}CO_2$ in adults following 1 minute of high-intensity exercise, the recovery times for $\dot{V}_E$ and $\dot{V}CO_2$ were indistinguishable in the children. Although $P_{ET}CO_2$ is only an indirect estimate of alveolar or arterial P_{CO_2}, the patterns in $P_{ET}CO_2$ appropriately reflected the disparity in the time constants of $\dot{V}_E$ and $\dot{V}CO_2$ in high-intensity exercise: In children, end-recovery $P_{ET}CO_2$ was virtually the same as pre-exercise, while in adults, a persistent hyperventilation manifested itself as significantly lower $P_{ET}CO_2$. Increasingly, investigators are using exercise tests to gauge how disease states (e.g., CF, bronchopulmonary dysplasia, or status post Fontan correction for single-ventricle congenital heart anomalies[52–56]) alter the relationship between CO_2 production and ventilatory control (Fig. 11-7).

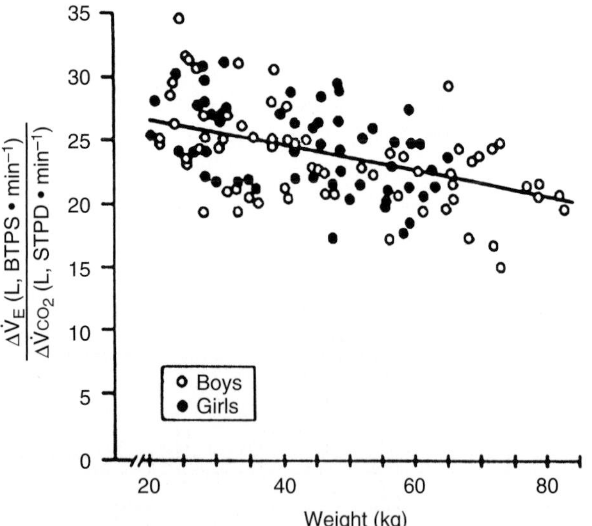

■ **FIGURE 11-6.** Slope of the $\dot{V}_E - \dot{V}CO_2$ relationship as a function of body weight in 128 healthy subjects ranging in age from 6 to 18 years old. The slopes significantly decreased with increasing weight. BTPS, body temperature, ambient pressure, and saturated with water vapor; STPD, standard temperature (0°C), barometric pressure at sea level (101.3 kPa), and dry gas.

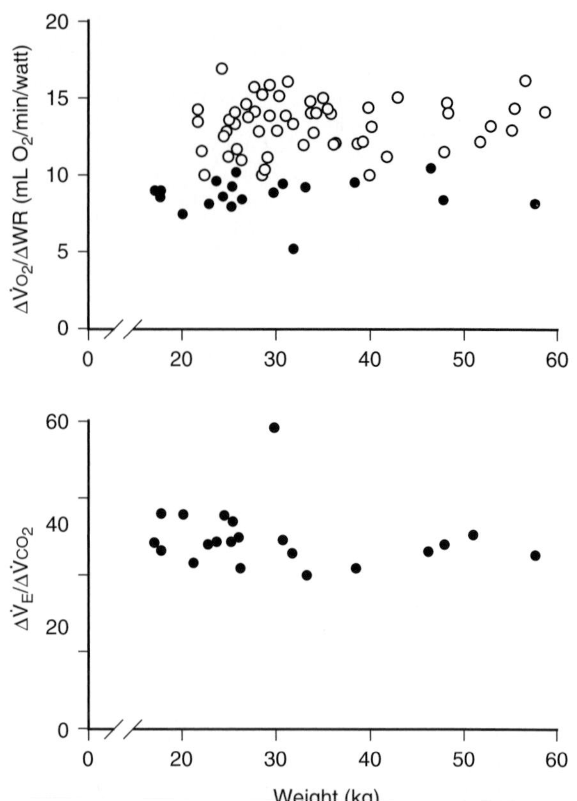

■ **FIGURE 11-7.** Dynamic variables of progressive exercise tests in CF children *(closed circles)* and controls *(open circles)* as a function of body weight. $\Delta\dot{V}O_2/\Delta WR$ data are shown in the upper panel, and $\Delta\dot{V}_E/\Delta\dot{V}CO_2$ in the lower panel. Both variables were significantly abnormal in CF subjects.

OXYGEN UPTAKE—AEROBIC AND ANAEROBIC CAPACITY

Bar-Or and co-workers were among the first to note maturational differences in exercise capacity (reviews are listed in the references),[57,58] even when appropriately scaled to body size. These investigators devised a protocol specifically for testing supramaximal, predominantly anaerobic, exercise (the Wingate test). Even differences between 8- and 11-year-old boys were observed, with the younger boys able to produce only 70% of the (size-adjusted) power generated by the older subjects. Much research still needs to be done to better explain the early-onset flow O_2 utilization in tests such as the Wingate, since technologies including near-infrared spectroscopy have demonstrated substantial O_2 utilization even in tests originally believed to be primarily anaerobic.[59]

As yet unexplained maturational differences in O_2 uptake responses to exercise have also been observed. Several lines of evidence suggest that the lower anaerobic capacity of children is associated with increased oxygen utilization during submaximal work. For example, we found significantly greater cumulative O_2 cost of exercise in children at virtually all WRs from a series of 1-minute exercise bouts (Fig. 11-8*A* and *B*).[60] In addition, the $\dot{V}O_2$ recovery time was prolonged in adults at the highest WR. (These observations have been expanded upon and updated by Hebestreit and colleagues,[61] who studied children at even higher WRs than those used in our studies, and by Fawkner and Armstrong.[62–64]) Finally, greater O_2 dependence of exercise in children is also seen in progressive exercise tests[24] in which both

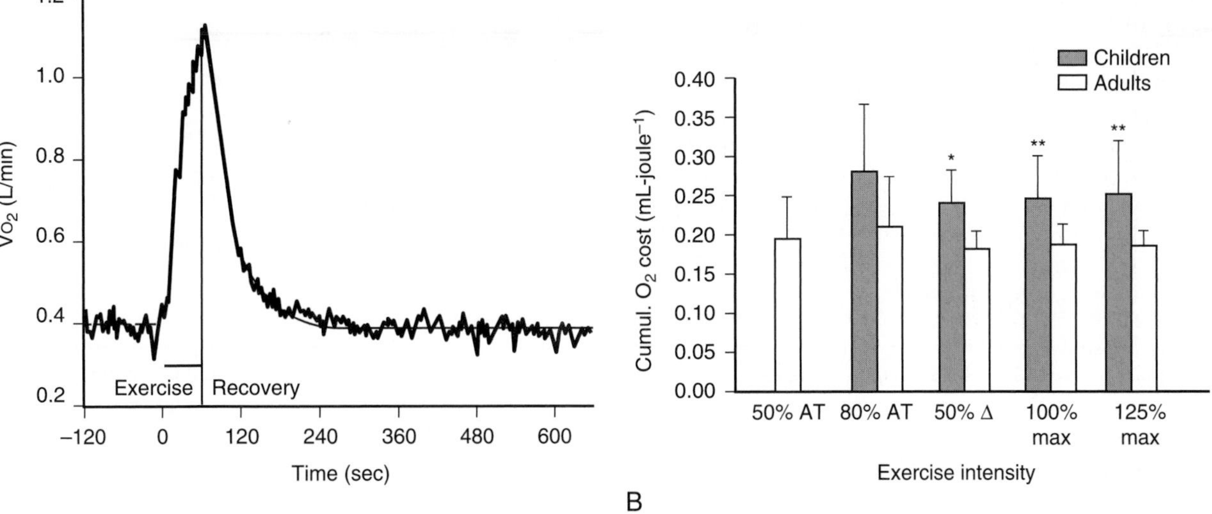

■ **FIGURE 11-8.** **A,** O_2 uptake response to 1 minute of high-intensity exercise (125% of the maximal WR) in an 8-year-old girl. Shown also is best-fit single exponential. *Vertical line* indicates end of 60-second exercise. Area under $\dot{V}O_2$ curve from time 0 to end of l-minute recovery period (mean baseline values *[dashed line]* were subtracted) is used to calculate cumulative O_2 cost of exercise. Area to the right of the vertical line to the end of recovery (again, mean baseline values were subtracted) represents O_2 cost for recovery period. **B,** Cumulative O_2 cost per joule at different work intensities in adults and children. Values are means ± SD. Cumulative O_2 cost was not affected by increasing work intensity in children and adults. However, cost was significantly higher in children than in adults at all WRs above the subject's lactate threshold: 50%Δ (*$P < .001$), 100% max, and 125% max (**$P < .01$).

the $\Delta\dot{V}O_2/\Delta WR$ and the ratio of $\dot{V}O_2$ to maximal WR[60] were higher in younger than in older subjects. While the mechanisms of these differences between children and adults remain unclear, recent work from Kaczor and colleagues[65] points toward lower levels of the key enzyme lactate dehydrogenase in the muscles of children. This might explain the generally lower lactate production in response to exercise in children as compared with adults.

We hypothesized that the growth-related changes in whole-body O_2 uptake and O_2 cost of exercise observed during high-intensity exercise reflect a maturation of the kinetics of high-energy phosphate metabolites in muscle tissue. This hypothesis was tested noninvasively in children and adults using ^{31}P magnetic resonance spectroscopy (MRS) to measure high-energy phosphate dynamics during exercise.

The current understanding of muscle energetics rests on the concept that the concentration of ATP is held constant in the muscle cell.[66] Chemical bond energy is converted to mechanical energy through the reaction:

$$ATP \rightarrow ADP + P_i + \text{energy}$$

where ADP is adenosine diphosphate and P_i is inorganic phosphate. Then, ADP is rephosphorylated by the reaction:

$$ADP + PCr \rightarrow ATP$$

where PCr is phosphocreatinine. Concentrations of ATP are constant throughout most of exercise except at the heaviest WRs, but the changes in PCr and P_i can now be examined in vivo. An example of high-energy phosphate dynamics during single-leg calf ergometer exercise in an 8-year-old child is given in Figure 11-9.[67]

In healthy adult subjects, the relationship between P_i/PCr and WR is characterized by an initial, almost linear portion. The slope of P_i/PCr to WR is a function of mitochondrial density and reflects the sensitivity of respiratory control at the cellular level[68] (Fig. 11-10). This is followed by a second, steeper slope that is associated with acceleration of glycolysis and increased lactic acid production suggestive of anaerobic metabolism.[69] Production of lactic acid, which is dissociated at physiologic pH, results in increasing [H^+]. Therefore, ^{31}P MRS can indirectly monitor glycolytic activity by measuring intracellular pH.

We found that during progressive exercise, muscle P_i/PCr ratio increases to a smaller extent in children compared with adults, even when the data are related to WR normalized to body weight. In addition, children showed a smaller drop in intramuscular pH. A slow and fast phase of P_i/PCr increase and pH decrease was noted in 75% of the adults and 50% of the children. The initial linear slope was the same in children and adults, suggesting a similar rate of mitochondrial oxidative metabolism during low-intensity exercise. But the different responses of the P_i/PCr

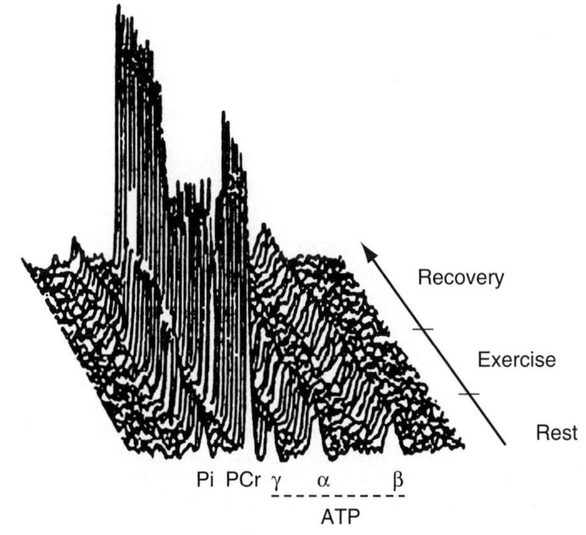

■ **FIGURE 11-9.** ^{31}P MRS spectra from right calf of 8-year-old boy at rest, during incremental exercise, and recovery.

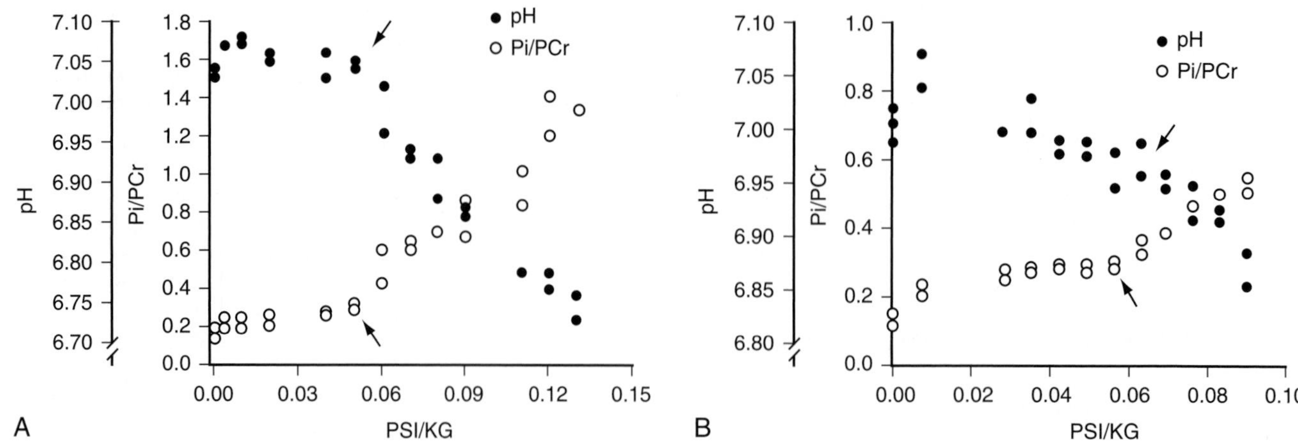

■ **FIGURE 11-10.** **A,** P_i/PCr and pH at rest and during incremental exercise in a 9-year-old girl. *Arrows,* transition points between slow and fast phases of P_i/PCr and pH changes. **B,** P_i/PCr and pH at rest and during incremental exercise in a 33-year-old man. *Arrows,* transition points between slow and fast phases of P_i/PCr increase and pH reduction.

ratio and pH during high-intensity exercise in children compared with adults indicate growth-related differences in energy metabolism (limited primarily to the high-intensity exercise range). In 1999, Petersen and co-workers[70] also suggested that muscle size itself may influence MRS assessment of muscle energy metabolism during exercise. Clearly, much research needs to be done to further understand high-energy phosphate metabolism and exercise during growth and maturation.

Our data might suggest that children may either deliver O_2 more effectively to the mitochondria than adults, be less able to facilitate anaerobic pathways, or have tissue O_2 requirements during exercise that are not found in adults. More effective O_2 utilization could result from variables that influence mitochondrial oxidative ATP resynthesis such as delivery of O_2 from the capillary blood, delivery of substrates, or greater density of mitochondria. Each of these variables might be responsible for a greater O_2-dependent ATP generation, lower P_i/PCr ratio, and higher pH during exercise in children. The mechanism of these intriguing O_2 cost differences between children and adults has yet to be fully elucidated (see the review by Boisseau and Delamarche[71]). Finally, little is known about the effect of childhood lung or heart disease, be it chronic or acute, on developmental aspects of high-energy phosphate dynamics in the exercising muscle.

Maturation of Heart Rate Responses

The dynamics of the HR response to exercise are proving to be increasingly useful in identifying abnormalities in a variety of disease states and as a simple, relatively noise-free data signal. The recovery time for HR was found to be greater for high-intensity compared with low-intensity exercise in both children and adults in our studies of 1-minute exercise[72] (Fig. 11-11), but the magnitude of the difference in children (e.g., τHR at 125% max was 27 ± 9 seconds compared with 16 ± 7 seconds at 80%

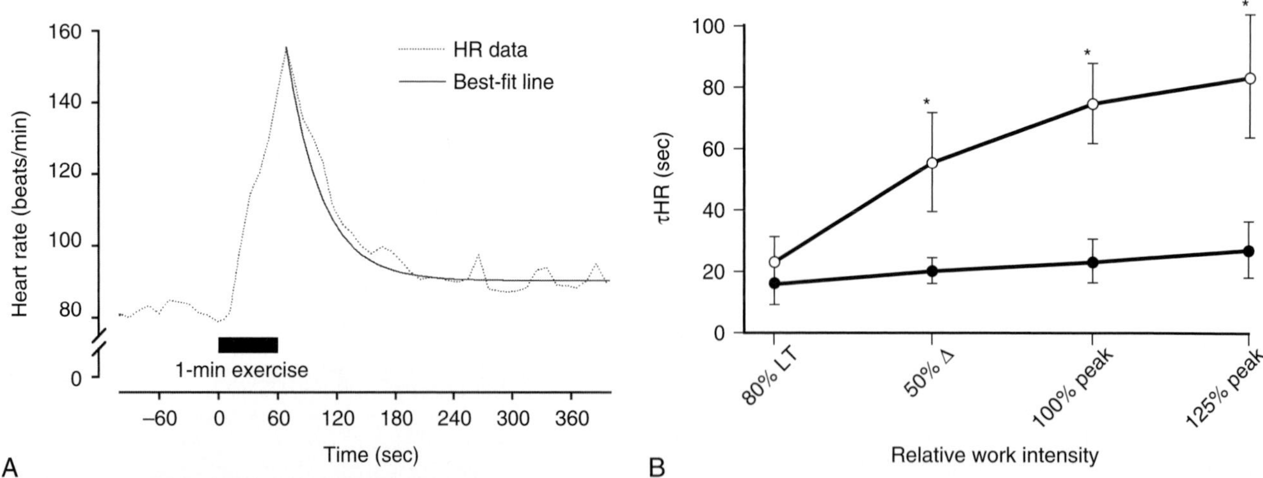

■ **FIGURE 11-11.** **A,** HR response before, during, and in the recovery from 1 minute of exercise in a 14-year-old Fontan subject. The recovery kinetics were quantified using a single exponential as shown. **B,** Recovery HR kinetics in children and adults. Each subject first performed a maximal WR test using a cycle ergometer. Following this, subjects exercised for 1 minute at constant WRs corresponding to: 80% LT (below-lactate threshold work); 50%Δ (the WR above the LT and halfway between the LT and peak WR); and at 100% and 125% of the peak WR. Iterative curve fitting was used to calculate the time constant (τ) from a best-fit single exponential function. Data are presented as mean ± SD. τHR tended to increase with work intensity in both adults and children. The recovery time constants were significantly (*$P < .001$) shorter in children compared with adults for all the LT work intensities just listed. (**A,** Data reprinted with permission from Troutman WB, Barstow TJ, Galindo AJ, Cooper DM: Abnormal dynamic cardiorespiratory responses to exercise in pediatric patients after Fontan procedure. J Am Coll Cardiol 1998;31:668–673.)

LAT) was substantially less than in adults (e.g., τHR at 125% max was 83 ± 20 seconds compared with 23 ± 8 seconds at 80% LAT). Moreover, HR recovered significantly faster in children compared with adults for each of the high-intensity exercise protocols. The maturation of the HR response reveals regulatory mechanisms associated with both metabolic rate per se and neuroendocrine modulation of physiologic function.

Indeed, previous work (done in adults) demonstrated that HR during dynamic exercise is regulated by a combination of neural, hormonal, and intrinsic mechanisms.[73–75] Immediately after exercise, accelerating influences from higher brain centers and peripheral nerve reflexes diminish, and HR is thought to be primarily regulated by restoration of vagal inhibitory tone and by prevailing levels of circulating catecholamines.[74] The role of neural control of HR response was also demonstrated in exercise studies of patients who had undergone heart transplants,[76,77] an in vivo model of a virtually denervated heart. In these individuals, treadmill exercise revealed a drastically slowed HR increase at the onset of exercise (HR increased only after the first 60–90 seconds) as well as a slowed decrease at the end of exercise (HR did not begin to slow for 1–2 minutes after exercise stopped). Moreover, there was a strong correlation between the HR response in these patients and plasma catecholamines. These observations indicate that sympathetic-parasympathetic factors are responsible for the rapid HR responses, while circulating catecholamines modulate HR responses more slowly. Interestingly, some degree of renervation in cardiac transplant patients with an improvement in HR responsiveness to exercise has been demonstrated recently.[78]

Thus, the growth-related differences in the HR response could be attributable either to maturation of sympathetic-parasympathetic neural regulation or to differences in the levels or effects of circulating modulators. Indirect evidence for the latter mechanism is provided by our data, and this may explain the prolongation of HR recovery with increasing exercise intensity in adults and children, as well as the large differences between the groups. As noted, low-intensity exercise revealed minimal differences in the HR recovery between adults and children. There is very little change in levels of circulating catecholamines during low-intensity exercise.[79] This, therefore, suggests that the purely neural control (i.e., sympathetic versus parasympathetic) of the HR response to exercise is similar between the children and adults tested.

By contrast, the largest differences in recovery τHR occurred following high-intensity exercise, and it is in the range above the anaerobic threshold where increases in $[H^+]$, lactate, and catecholamines are known to be smaller in children compared with adults.[67,80–83] Thus, we hypothesize that the growth-related changes in HR response to work intensity are a reflection of substantially different hormonal and metabolic responses to high-intensity exercise in adults compared with children. The mechanisms of the different lactate, catecholamine, and $[H^+]$ responses to high-intensity exercise have not been fully elucidated but are probably related to differences in the clearance of lactate, $[H^+]$, and catecholamines following exercise in children compared with adults.

USEFUL VARIABLES OF EXERCISE TESTING IN CHILDREN

In Table 11-1, the gas exchange and HR variables of exercise testing in children are briefly outlined. The gas exchange response to progressive, cycle ergometer exercise in a healthy 7-year-old boy tested in our laboratory is shown in Figure 11-12. Following a period of unloaded pedaling (0 watt), the WR increases in a linear manner. This protocol is known as a ramp WR input[84] and is one of several types of progressive exercise tests that can be used in children. Gas exchange is collected breath by breath and displayed online. Note that the increase in O_2 uptake does not immediately follow the onset of exercise. The response time of O_2 uptake is determined by the cellular, circulatory, and respiratory adaptations to the increase in energy demand in the muscle tissue. Following this, $\dot{V}O_2$ typically increases in a linear manner with increasing WR. However, the O_2 response may either "bend up" or "bend down" depending on the magnitude of change of the WR input.[85] In the data shown in Figure 11-12,

TABLE 11-1. Cardiorespiratory and metabolic variables obtained from exercise testing

Exercise Variable	Physiologic Importance
Maximal oxygen uptake ($\dot{V}O_{2\,max}$, peak $\dot{V}O_2$)	A plateau or decrease in $\dot{V}O_2$ despite a continuing increase in work rate. Care must be taken to distinguish the peak $\dot{V}O_2$ (the largest $\dot{V}O_2$ achieved by the subject) from the true $\dot{V}O_{2\,max}$.
Anaerobic, lactate, or ventilatory threshold (AT, LT, VAT)	The point during progressive exercise when lactate concentration begins to increase in the blood. The usual gas exchange manifestations of the AT are hyperventilation with respect to $\dot{V}O_2$ (increase in $\dot{V}_E/\dot{V}O_2$ and end-tidal PO_2), which occurs when $\dot{V}_E/\dot{V}CO_2$ and end-tidal PCO_2 are constant.
Work efficiency, or the O_2 cost of exercise (roughly, the inverse of efficiency; O_2 cost)	These variables are determined from the relationship of $\dot{V}O_2$ to the work rate.
Response time of gas exchange adaptations to exercise (mean response time, time constant—RT, MRT, τ)	The mathematically derived descriptor of the time required for $\dot{V}O_2$, $\dot{V}_E$, and $\dot{V}CO_2$ to achieve a steady state in response to or in recovery from a work rate input.
Ventilatory response to exercise ($\Delta\dot{V}_E/\Delta\dot{V}CO_2$)	Slope of the linear portion of the relationship between $\dot{V}_E/\dot{V}CO_2$ during progressive exercise. (Note that the ventilatory equivalent of CO_2 is the ratio $\dot{V}_E/\dot{V}CO_2$ and is not the same as the slope.)
Respiratory compensation point (RCP)	The point during heavy exercise when hyperventilation for $\dot{V}CO_2$ occurs. Presumably, at these heavy work loads, bicarbonate is no longer able to adequately buffer the lactic acid produced during high-intensity exercise, and pH changes. This stimulates the peripheral chemoreceptors.
O_2 pulse	The ratio $\dot{V}O_2$/HR. This ratio represents the amount of O_2 extracted per heart beat, which is not the same as the slope of the $\dot{V}O_2$-HR relationship during progressive exercise.
$\dot{V}O_2$-HR slope ($\Delta\dot{V}O_2/\Delta$HR)	This ratio represents the slope of the linear portion of the relationship between $\dot{V}O_2$ and HR during progressive exercise.

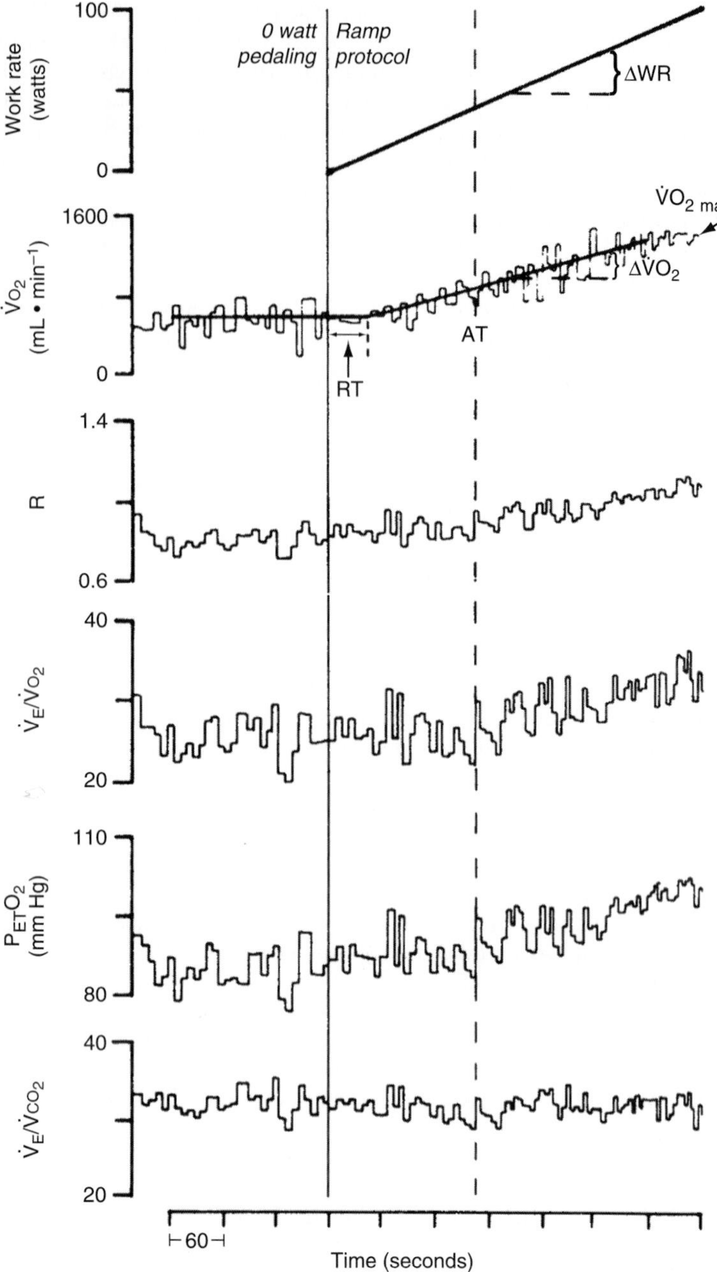

■ **FIGURE 11-12.** Breath-by-breath response of gas exchange to ramp exercise protocol in a 7-year-old boy. After a period of 0-watt pedaling, WR increases (ΔWR) in a linear manner. Note lag in response of O_2 uptake after WR has started (RT-$\dot{V}O_2$), linear increase of $\dot{V}O_2$ as WR increases, and plateau of $\dot{V}O_2$ despite an increasing WR ($\dot{V}O_{2\,max}$). Anaerobic threshold (AT) is determined by identifying $\dot{V}O_2$ where respiratory exchange ratio (R), ventilatory equivalent for O_2 ($\dot{V}_E/\dot{V}O_2$), and end-tidal O_2 ($P_{ET}O_2$) abruptly increase while ventilatory equivalent for CO_2 ($\dot{V}_E/\dot{V}CO_2$) and end-tidal CO_2 ($P_{ET}CO_2$) (not shown) remain unchanged or decrease. Work efficiency is determined from the ratio $\Delta WR/\Delta\dot{V}O_2$.

note that there was a plateau in $\dot{V}O_2$ at the end of exercise despite a continuing increase in the WR. The appearance of a plateau classically defines the $\dot{V}O_{2\,max}$. It is important to distinguish the $\dot{V}O_{2\,max}$ (i.e., where a plateau or reduction in $\dot{V}O_2$ occurs despite an increasing WR) from the peak $\dot{V}O_2$ (i.e., the highest $\dot{V}O_2$ achieved by a particular subject).

From cross-sectional population studies, the $\dot{V}O_{2\,max}$ changes in roughly direct proportion with body weight.[24,86] This is at odds with the empirically observed "three-fourths power law"—demonstrated most commonly in Kleiber's "mouse-to-elephant" curve[87]—and with the "surface area law." The surface area law stemmed from the belief that for mammals, all metabolic rates were determined by the rate of heat loss and heat production. Since heat loss was determined largely by the ratio of surface area to body mass and since for spheres and cylinders (geometrically close to the shape of animals) the ratio of surface area to body mass scaled to the two-thirds power of body mass, it was concluded that metabolic rate must be proportional to body mass to the two-thirds power; thus in mammals metabolic rates (note that the $\dot{V}O_{2\,max}$ can be considered a metabolic rate) must scale to the two-thirds power of body mass.[88]

The finding of a direct relationship between $\dot{V}O_{2\,max}$ and body weight in children (i.e., a scaling factor of one) suggests that the mechanism that links structure and function during the growth process within a species is different from the processes that determine the relationship between metabolic rates and body size in mature animals of different species. More recently, this idea was supported by a series of investigations of the relationship between $\dot{V}O_{2\,max}$ and muscle size in which the latter was measured using magnetic resonance imaging of muscle cross-sectional area in children and adults.[89]

Although $\dot{V}CO_2$ increases with progressive exercise, its pattern is not identical to that of $\dot{V}O_2$. Note in Figure 11-12 that the respiratory exchange ratio measured at the mouth (R, the ratio

$\dot{V}CO_2/\dot{V}O_2$) is constant at the beginning of exercise but begins to increase well before maximal exercise, indicating that $\dot{V}CO_2$ is increasing at a faster rate than $\dot{V}O_2$. The mechanism for the increase in R is the increased production of lactic acid, most likely consequent to anaerobic metabolism occurring at the muscle cells.[90] The buffering of the H^+ releases additional CO_2. Since ventilation is stimulated by the flow of CO_2 to the respiratory centers, $\dot{V}_E$ increases as well. Thus, as shown in Figure 11-12, the ratio of $\dot{V}_E$ to $\dot{V}O_2$ increases. The hyperventilation for $\dot{V}O_2$ results in an increase in the end-tidal PO_2 ($P_{ET}O_2$). However, since $\dot{V}_E$ and $\dot{V}CO_2$ increase proportionately, the ratio of these two variables remains constant. This constellation of findings—an increase in R, $\dot{V}_E/\dot{V}O_2$, and $P_{ET}O_2$ while the $\dot{V}_E/\dot{V}CO_2$ and $P_{ET}CO_2$ remain constant—constitutes the noninvasive measurement of the LAT.

Studies of the LAT have been made in large numbers of children using both treadmill and cycle ergometer exercise.[24,91] While the LAT in adults occurs at a metabolic rate (expressed as the $\dot{V}O_2$) equivalent to 40% to 60% of the subject's $\dot{V}O_{2\,max}$, this ratio is higher in children. Since the ratio of the LAT to $\dot{V}O_{2\,max}$ can be increased consequent to training programs,[92] one possible explanation is that children are generally "fitter" than adults. This, however, has not yet been substantiated.

Several theories have been proposed to explain the phenomenon of increasing blood lactate concentrations during progressive exercise.[93,94] Most prominent are: (1) oxygen lack at the muscle tissue level resulting in anaerobic metabolism and an increase in lactate production relative to uptake, (2) a reduction in lactate uptake independent of O_2 availability, and (3) an O_2-independent increase in lactate production due to increased "shuttling" of lactate associated with exercise.[95] Although the mechanisms of the LAT have not been entirely determined, its role as a physiologic marker distinguishing between low-intensity and high-intensity exercise is gaining use.[96,97]

The speed with which the WR increases during progressive exercise testing can influence the gas exchange response. In choosing the appropriate increment time and magnitude (or slope in the case of a ramp-type input), several variables must be considered. The first is the response time and delays that are known to occur in the gas exchange response. Because these times are different for $\dot{V}O_2$ and $\dot{V}CO_2$, care must be taken to ensure that observed changes in variables such as R do not result from these dynamic delays. If, for example, the slope is too steep for the capabilities of the subject being tested, then an increase in R may be observed that is not related to the production of lactic acid but instead results from differences in the dynamics of the gas exchange responses. In general, about 10 to 15 minutes of duration for a progressive exercise test in healthy children and adults is optimal.

For children 6 to 8 years old, a ramp slope of 5 watts/minute is used. For older children, 10 to 30 watts/minute ramp slopes are used. The selection of the magnitude of the WR input often involves an "educated guess" on the part of the investigator and requires some experience in assessing the capability of a particular child. A variety of maximal-type exercise protocols suitable for studies in children have been reviewed by Washington and colleagues.[98]

Much information can be gained from calculating the relationship of $\dot{V}O_2$ and HR. Fick's equation holds that:

$$\dot{V}O_2 = SV \cdot HR \cdot (a - \bar{v})O_2$$

where SV is the stroke volume and $(a - \bar{v})O_2$ is the arteriovenous O_2 difference. The relationship between $\dot{V}O_2$ and HR can therefore yield indirect information on changes occurring in stroke volume and the widening of the arteriovenous difference. During progressive exercise, the $\dot{V}O_2$-HR relationship can be viewed in two ways. First, the O_2 pulse represents the instantaneous ratio $\dot{V}O_2$/HR and when plotted against time is typically hyperbolic in shape.[99] However, because of the curvilinear nature, the O_2-pulse response is difficult to quantify. Another approach is to consider the slope of the linear portion of the $\dot{V}O_2$-HR relationship.[99] The slope of this response changes systematically with age, and normal values are available. In adult patients with congestive heart disease, a given increase in $\dot{V}O_2$ is accompanied by a more rapid HR response, most likely indicating a reduction in stroke volume.[100]

The vast majority of investigations focused on exercise in children utilize the $\dot{V}O_{2\,max}$ as the primary parameter of the overall exercise response. Another "maximal response" occasionally used in children is the maximal voluntary ventilation (MVV); this represents the greatest ventilation that a subject can perform while in the resting state. The maximal $\dot{V}_E$ during exercise is about 65% to 75% of the MVV. Some authors have suggested that this indicates a "ventilatory reserve," but the lung during maximal exercise has an increased blood volume and, therefore, the mechanics of breathing during these resting states and high-intensity exercise may not be completely comparable. Stein and co-workers recently presented data demonstrating the relationship between forced expiratory volume in 1 second (FEV_1) and MVV in children with CF.[101]

■ ALTERNATIVES TO MAXIMAL TESTING

Although the clinical utility of maximal values can be questioned, much useful information is available from progressive exercise protocols. Gas exchange and HR responses continuously change during progressive tests, and often the relationships between these changing variables (referred to as dynamic relationships) can be quantified using straightforward analytic techniques. As noted, the LAT in children and young adults can be determined noninvasively from the dynamic responses of gas exchange during progressive exercise. Simple linear regression analysis of HR and $\dot{V}O_2$ can provide noninvasive indicators of cardiac function.[24] The slope of the regression changes systematically with maturation and with diseases (e.g., heart failure). Similarly, linear regression analysis of $\dot{V}_E$ and $\dot{V}CO_2$ can be used to assess respiratory efficiency and control during exercise, and are abnormal in patients with diseases ranging from CF[55] to heart failure.[102] The real clinical value of progressive exercise testing for children may prove to be in the rich cardiorespiratory data obtained during the submaximal phases rather than from the final, single data point at peak or maximal power. As noted earlier, there are a variety of approaches to exercise testing that rely on submaximal values. In a recent and intriguing study, for example, Isasi and colleagues[103] found that fitness measured by the physical work capacity at 170 beats per minute was inversely correlated with resting levels of serum C-reactive protein, a known circulating indicator of inflammation. This supports the relationship between fitness and stress-inflammatory variables alluded to earlier.

The time course of the onset and recovery of gas exchange and HR in response to exercise may also prove in the years to come to be clinically useful in exercise testing in children. Investigations into the underlying mechanisms of these responses (e.g., the concepts of O_2 deficit and debt[104]) compose an important chapter of modern exercise physiology. In the 1970s, computing and other technologic advances permitted breath-to-breath measurement of gas exchange and facilitated much more precise kinetic analysis and modeling of the gas exchange responses than had been possible before.[90,105] One of the first attempts to gauge children's kinetic responses to exercise in a clinical setting was made in 1974, even before breath-by-breath measurements were widely available. Drakonakis and Halloran[106] measured O_2 uptake recovery from exercise in children with a variety of congenital heart lesions by (laboriously) collecting consecutive 1-minute samples of expired gas in balloons. The investigators found that children with cyanotic lesions showed markedly slowed recovery times following an exercise input.

Analysis of gas exchange and HR kinetic responses to exercise can be used to gain insight into cardiac, respiratory, and metabolic function[107–109] (see, for example, the use of this approach in children who have undergone Fontan surgical correction of congenital heart lesions[109]; Fig. 11-13). Since the pioneering work of Maćek and co-workers,[110] research into kinetic exercise responses in children has steadily advanced and will increasingly become part of standard exercise testing in children.[62,111]

■ THE PROBLEM OF SIZE

The evaluation and diagnosis of disease using exercise testing requires knowledge of adaptive mechanisms at both the cellular and organ systems levels. In children, interpretation of these adaptations is confounded by the rapid change in body size and development that characterizes the growth process. For example, how can one appropriately compare the $\dot{V}O_{2\,max}$ achieved by a 6-year-old child to that achieved by an 18-year-old? Should an obese 6-year-old who weighs as much as a normal 12-year-old be expected to have the same $\dot{V}O_{2\,max}$ as the older child?

The consequences of a particular strategy to normalize data among different-sized subjects is not inconsequential. For example, when body weight was used to compare exercise responses in lean and obese children, the obese children demonstrated low anaerobic thresholds per kilogram of body weight.[112] This type of observation has led to the suggestion that obese children are unfit and less physically active than leaner children. The problem here is that the LAT (like $\dot{V}O_{2\,max}$) is determined in large part by the active muscle mass. Body weight is only partially determined by muscle mass, and in the case of the obese child, the proportion of muscle mass to body weight is decreased.

Thus, normalization to body weight in the case of obese children might lead the clinician to conclude that these subjects were less fit than nonobese children. However, by contrast, if the normalization is made to body height, lean body mass, or by strategies that minimize the size dependence of the particular exercise parameter, then the degree of abnormality in the obese child is significantly reduced.[113] This determination is important; if the obese child is deemed "inactive," then the therapeutic approach ought to include programs of exercise. Such programs are expensive, require behavioral changes, and involve extensive supervision. For the obese child who is as physically active as leaner children, additional increases in physical activity may prove to be an impossible task.

In many areas of pediatrics, body surface area has been used to calculate drug dosages, energy expenditure, and other values. The use of body surface area stems from the surface area law, which, as noted earlier, was a popular concept in comparative physiology in the 19th century.[88] Much controversy surrounds the idea that metabolic rates in homeothermic animals are determined by the rate of heat loss, in turn dependent on the ratio of surface area to body mass. Moreover, the body surface area is a derived value that is based on the actually measured height and weight and then calculated using a set of assumptions that have not been rigorously tested.

As in the case of obesity, simple ratios of metabolic rates to body weight may lead to incorrect clinical conclusions unless the investigator clearly examines the underlying assumptions (e.g., to what extent body mass actually reflects muscle mass). On the other hand, height and weight are simple to obtain and are highly accurate assessments of body size. Moreover, in children, the correlation between height and weight is much higher than in adults,[24] probably because obesity in children is less prevalent than in adults, although obesity is increasing at an alarming rate in American children[114]; moreover, direct measurements of body size probably introduce less uncertainty than calculated values such as body surface area.

Many investigators have attempted to measure lean body mass as an estimate of muscle mass, and several techniques have been developed including: (cumbersome) underwater weighing, skinfold thickness calipers, computed tomography, magnetic resonance imaging, and dual x-ray absorptiometry.[115–119] Each of these techniques has advantages and disadvantages, and the choice of methodology ultimately depends not only on scientific factors (e.g., which component of lean body mass must be measured) but also on issues of expense, exposure to ionizing radiation, time required to complete the particular test, and the availability of facilities and personnel capable of performing the measurement accurately. Given the wide array of choices and the lack of a single "gold standard" for normalization, it behooves each investigator and clinician to precisely define how normalization was accomplished and the rationale for using any

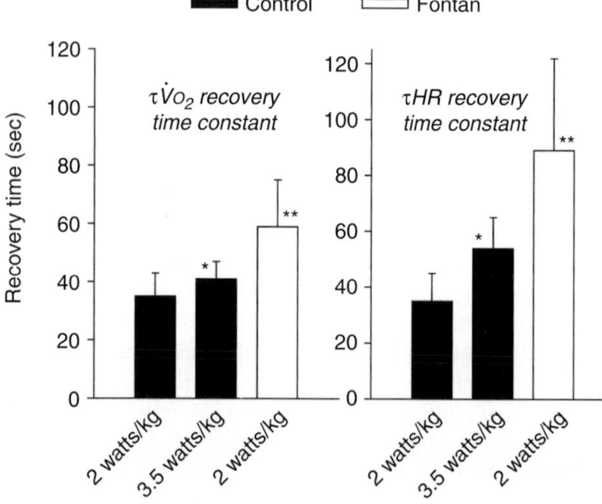

■ **FIGURE 11-13.** HR and $\dot{V}O_2$ recovery times for control and Fontan subjects. In controls, recovery times were longer following the higher WR protocols (*$P < .05$). In Fontan subjects, recovery times were prolonged compared with both the same absolute (2 watts/kg) and relative (3.5 watts/kg) protocols in control subjects (**$P < .001$).

particular approach. The interested reader may gain more in-depth understanding of the problem of size and scaling by consulting sources in the reference list.[120–125]

■ THE CONCEPT OF FITNESS

Another frequently used concept that lacks a universally accepted working definition is "fitness." Fitness refers to a task-specific capability of the cardiorespiratory system but is often used as a global indicator of the exercise response. In adults and children, the ability to perform a particular muscular activity is, to some extent, dependent on the individual's history of participation in that activity. The sedentary individual can improve his running distances or times by training programs. Thus, the terms *fit* and *trained* are often interchanged. The lack of precision in terminology can be confusing. For example, are differences in the LAT and $\dot{V}O_{2\,max}$ often observed between boys and girls indicative of differences in fitness, or do they represent gender-related biologic differences in mechanisms of O_2 transport? Is the normally active 6-year-old less fit than the child whose parents are grooming him to run a marathon? As with strategies for normalization, the investigator and clinician must attempt to be as specific as possible in applying the concept of fitness to a particular child.

■ METHODS OF ASSESSING EXERCISE RESPONSES IN CHILDREN

Sophisticated exercise systems that allow breath-to-breath measurement of gas exchange are commercially available, but these packages are invariably designed for adults. As a consequence, "off-the-shelf" exercise system components—ranging from the dimensions of the cycle ergometer to the dead space of breathing valves—are often inappropriate for children and increase the noise-to-signal ratio of the data obtained. Greater demand for exercise testing in children will eventually encourage manufacturers to market systems designed specifically for children.

Existing and new technologies must be applied imaginatively to develop strategies for testing exercise in individuals with physical disabilities and for young children between the ages of 1 and 6 years old. These populations are often ignored in research, because they are difficult to study. This is unfortunate, because exercise testing in these children could provide important clinical as well as basic biologic information about the fundamental interaction of respiration and growth and development in both health and disease. (Examples can be found in the reference list.[126,127])

There are a variety of methodologies that can be used successfully to measure cardiorespiratory or metabolic responses in children. The two most common testing devices are the cycle ergometer and the treadmill. With cycle ergometry, the WR input is determined by the load on the cycle's flywheel, and the subject pedals at a constant rate. In treadmill exercise, external WR is increased by various combinations of increasing treadmill speed and incline. Consequently, the fundamental difference between these two input devices is that with the cycle ergometer, the WR (power) input is known precisely, while with treadmill exercise the external WR can only be estimated. Hence, when one is attempting to relate gas exchange responses to specific WRs, the cycle ergometer is easier to use. Moreover, in studies of the transition between one level of exercise and another, the transition in WR on the cycle ergometer is brought about simply by changing the load on the flywheel, while on the treadmill, changing WR involves adjustments of the incline or treadmill speed. These changes often evoke an anxiety response and may change the muscle groups involved in the exercise.

There are certain disadvantages to cycle ergometer exercise. The child is asked to maintain a constant pedaling rate; this is difficult for younger children as yet unfamiliar with bicycles, particularly at low WRs. Variability in pedaling rate with a constant external load will result in variability in WR. This can be compensated for by specially designed ergometers in which the external load is adjusted to the pedaling rate to maintain a constant WR. In addition, not every child is adept at bicycle riding, and the investigator must always be aware that cardiorespiratory responses are "task specific." In other words, a trained swimmer may be quite fit yet perform poorly on a cycle ergometer.

Special skills are required on the part of the clinician to achieve successful exercise testing in children. Younger subjects easily succumb to the barrage of sensory input in the laboratory and have difficulty focusing on the exercise task at hand. They will come off the mouthpiece, vary pedaling rate, or change running speed on the treadmill. In addition, siblings often accompany the subject to be tested, and this can provide additional distraction. In our laboratory, we have attempted to deal with these problems in a systematic manner. First, there are always at least two trained individuals conducting the test; the role of one is to stay with the subject at all times. Usually, gentle, continuous verbal encouragement will help the child focus on the task at hand. We have also found that videocassettes and computer games are very helpful in occupying a sibling or the subject during breaks in the testing period.

Gas exchange analysis systems are of two general types: continuous measurement (breath by breath) and discrete measurement (requiring mixing chambers of the exhaled gas). Both systems can yield useful and accurate information on cardiorespiratory responses to exercise. For investigations of the dynamic or kinetic responses of gas exchange to various WR inputs, breath-to-breath systems offer the advantage of providing a sufficiently high density of data to permit subsequent mathematical analysis (e.g., curve fitting) that would be otherwise unavailable. Commercial systems are available that can be adapted to the needs of children (reduced system dead space, smaller crank radius for pedaling, adjustable seats). Moreover, while the mass spectrometer is still advantageous as a gas analyzer (rapid response, small sampling volume), advances in discrete gas analyzer technology have made these devices quite suitable for most systems designed for breath-by-breath analysis.

■ SAFETY OF EXERCISE TESTING IN CHILDREN

There has been little recent work on the importance question of the safety of exercise testing in children, particularly in those with chronic diseases of the cardiorespiratory system. Several investigators have examined the safety of maximal exercise testing in children. Alpert and co-workers[128] reviewed 1730 studies performed in their laboratory over a 9-year period in which children performed cycle ergometry testing to the point of fatigue. Included in their sample were a large number of children with congenital heart disease. There were no deaths, and the total complication rate was 1.79%. Complications included chest pain, dizziness or syncope, and decreased blood pressure. Hazardous arrhythmias occurred in only 0.46% of subjects. In the authors' laboratory, more than 400 healthy children have undergone progressive exercise testing with a similar low incidence of only mild complications. In addition, dozens of children with anemia, heart disease, diabetes, and lung disease have been tested, and no major complications have been observed. Nonetheless, appropriate monitoring devices (pulse oximetry, electrocardiograph, blood pressure manometers) must be close at hand, updated "crash carts" ought to be included in those laboratories where children with disease states are to be tested, and personnel should be experienced in the fundamentals of cardiopulmonary resuscitation in children.

Criteria for terminating exercise tests in the pediatric age group include symptoms of severe chest pain and signs of hypovolemia. Moreover, exercise should be terminated if ventricular or supraventricular tachycardia is noted or if ST-segmental depression exceeds 3 mm. Of course, either hypotension or hypertension are reasons to stop exercise. Contraindications for exercise testing in children with a variety of diseases are reviewed by the American Heart Association[129] and in the recent pediatric exercise treatise by Bar-Or and Rowland.[130] This list includes entities such as uncontrolled congestive heart failure, drug overdose, or a child with asthma and severe bronchoconstriction at the time of testing.

NORMAL VALUES

In all aspects of pulmonary function testing and exercise assessment, the clinician is faced with the problem of choosing normal values. As noted earlier, there are several large-series investigations of normal values for both pulmonary function testing and exercise results in children. But variations in methodology and in the racial and socioeconomic composition of population groups necessitate validation of normal values for any particular laboratory. For example, we compared the $\dot{V}O_{2\,max}$ obtained in our laboratory in 1984 with values obtained by Åstrand in Sweden in the 1950s. While the results for boys in our study ranging in age from 6 to 18 years were indistinguishable from the Swedish boys, the girls in our community demonstrated significantly lower values than did their Swedish counterparts.[24,86] A relentless reduction in physical activity has become apparent worldwide over the past two to three decades,[20] and, as noted earlier, represents a worrisome trend for the health of our nation in the years to come. Ideally, each laboratory should develop its own set of normal values. At the very least, a sample of local, healthy children can be tested to help choose an appropriate set of normal values.

THE CONCEPT OF FUNCTIONAL DISABILITY IN CHILDREN

In an adult, the concept of disability has both medical and economic significance. It can be assessed using the exercise laboratory by determining the extent to which cardiorespiratory impairment limits the performance of work-related tasks. The economic consequences of functional physical disability in children have not been addressed, yet they certainly exist. It is becoming increasingly clear that physical activity plays a role in subsequent growth and development. For example, there is growing awareness that patterns of activity established during childhood may profoundly affect health later in life.[4] The effects of cardiorespiratory, metabolic, and bone disease (e.g., osteoporosis) may be mitigated in the adult who was a physically active child or adolescent.

The concept of functional disability can be applied in pediatrics as well by recognizing that the major tasks of children are running, jumping, and activities associated with play. We believe that disability in children can be determined, in part, by measuring the cardiorespiratory response to exercise in the manners described earlier. In addition, an assessment of the level of physical activity in the life of the child would clearly be useful, but precisely what constitutes a healthy or normal amount of physical activity is not yet known. Part of the problem is that energy expenditure due to physical activity has proved to be difficult to quantify under field conditions (i.e., in the environment of the child, not the investigator).

It is becoming increasingly clear that physiologic indexes of fitness like $\dot{V}O_{2\,max}$ are influenced by both genetic and environmental factors, the latter most likely related to levels of habitual physical activity. Klissouras, using monoygotic and dizygotic twins, estimated that about 70% of the variance in maximal aerobic power is genetically determined.[131,132] Bouchard and co-workers proposed the genetic variance of aerobic fitness to be between 40% and 60%.[133–135] Consequently, it is not surprising that in most studies, the correlation between habitual physical activity and aerobic indexes of fitness such as $\dot{V}O_{2\,max}$ are weak.[136] Thus, the measurement of habitual physical activity level must be considered independently from physical fitness. Existing methodologies include a variety of questionnaires, interview techniques, HR monitoring, and sensors of limb acceleration and body trunk motion.[137–139] The data from these instruments must then be converted into units of metabolic energy metabolism (e.g., calories). In addition, more direct assessments of energy expenditure can be obtained from direct observation (as noted earlier) and/or from stable isotope methodologies such as the doubly labeled water technique.[140–142] Direct observation is noninvasive, but it is intrusive, arduous, and time consuming for the observer. Furthermore, while the doubly labeled water technique is now the generally accepted standard for accurately assessing energy expenditure over a period lasting about a week, its high cost prohibits its use as a routine tool. Interpreting the results of exercise tests will not be optimal until readily accessible and reasonably priced methods for assessing overall energy expenditure in children become available.

EXERCISE-INDUCED ASTHMA AND OTHER TESTS FOR BRONCHIAL REACTIVITY IN ASTHMATIC CHILDREN

The incidence of asthma, already the most common chronic disease of children, is rising.[143] Exercise-induced asthma (EIA) occurs in 60% to 80% of children[144,145] and leads to overall reductions in physical activity during childhood[146] during a critical period of growth and development. Because it is so common a finding in children with asthma, EIA has been used as one of the diagnostic tests to establish the disease. Figure 11-14 illustrates the pattern of the response of an asthmatic child to a 6-minute run.[147] During exercise, lung function changes little or may even improve. Toward the end of exercise or a few minutes afterward, lung function begins to fail. The maximum decrease in lung function occurs 5 to 10 minutes after the end of exercise, after which recovery in lung function will take

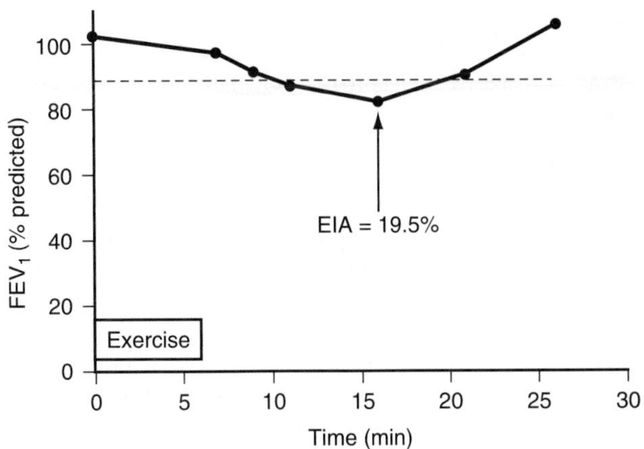

■ **FIGURE 11-14.** Changes in lung function expressed as a percentage of the predicted normal forced expiratory volume in 1 second (FEV_1) in response to 6 minutes of running on a treadmill by a 13-year-old boy with asthma. The *horizontal dashed line* indicates the lowest reduction seen in normal children. Note 13% fall in FEV_1. EIA, exercise-induced asthma.

place in about 30 to 45 minutes. In a small proportion of asthmatics, a late-phase reaction may develop.[148–150] Despite the importance of the phenomenon, the mechanism of EIA remains controversial.[151]

■ FACTORS AFFECTING THE SEVERITY OF EXERCISE-INDUCED ASTHMA

The upper limit of postexercise decrease in FEV_1 (mean ± 2 SD) was found to be 6% to 8% in normal children.[152] In asthmatic children the severity of EIA may be influenced by the severity of asthma[153] and by pre-exposure to allergens.[154] Moreover, the severity, duration, and type of exercise may influence the severity of EIA. Running, as compared with swimming under the same inspired-air conditions and work intensity, will result in much more EIA.[155] It is also important to note that the recovery from EIA differs in younger compared with older children. For example, Hofstra and co-workers[156] demonstrated that 7- to 10-year-olds with EIA improved FEV_1 by a mean of 1.60% per minute following the challenge, but improvement in 11- to 12-year-olds was significantly prolonged (0.54% per minute).

■ PATHOPHYSIOLOGY OF EXERCISE-INDUCED ASTHMA

The mechanism of EIA remains enigmatic. As noted, exercise has been demonstrated to be a vigorous stimulant of the stress-inflammatory immune system (Fig. 11-15),[157] involving increased levels of circulating IL-6 and intracellular adhesion molecules, many of which are involved in the pathophysiology of bronchoconstriction.[158,159] Moreover, hypoxia, such as can occur in the peripheral and pulmonary circulation during exercise, further stimulates IL-6 and pronounced systemic leukocytosis.[160] Hypoxia also stimulates endothelium to produce a variety of neutrophil attractants leading to neutrophil sequestration and activation.[161] Indeed, given the robust stress-inflammatory response in healthy children, one might wonder why all children do not wheeze when they exercise.

The effect of climate on EIA has been extensively studied. Breathing warm and humid air during exercise almost completely abolishes EIA, whereas breathing dry and cold air increases its severity.[162–164] Respiratory heat loss from the airway mucosa during exercise was suggested by Deal and his colleagues[165] as the trigger for bronchoconstriction, and they showed that exercise and hyperventilation with similar respiratory heat loss will result in similar bronchoconstriction. However, respiratory heat loss cannot entirely account for the triggering stimulus for EIA, since some asthmatic patients will develop EIA while breathing warm humid air at body temperature and humidity, which will not result in respiratory heat loss.[166–168] Also, Noviski and his colleagues[169] exercised a group of asthmatic children at two levels of exercise while the respiratory heat and water loss were kept constant by altering the inspired-air conditions. They found that the harder exercise with a mean $\dot{V}O_2$ of approximately 1.6 times greater than $\dot{V}O_2$ of the less strenuous exercise resulted in EIA that was greater by almost 1.7 times.

Anderson[170] has suggested that changes in osmolarity of the fluid lining the airways during exercise are the triggering stimulus for EIA. It has also been suggested that EIA and hyperventilation-induced asthma (HIA) are the result of cooling and rewarming of the airway mucosa, causing hyperemia and bronchial obstruction.[171,172]

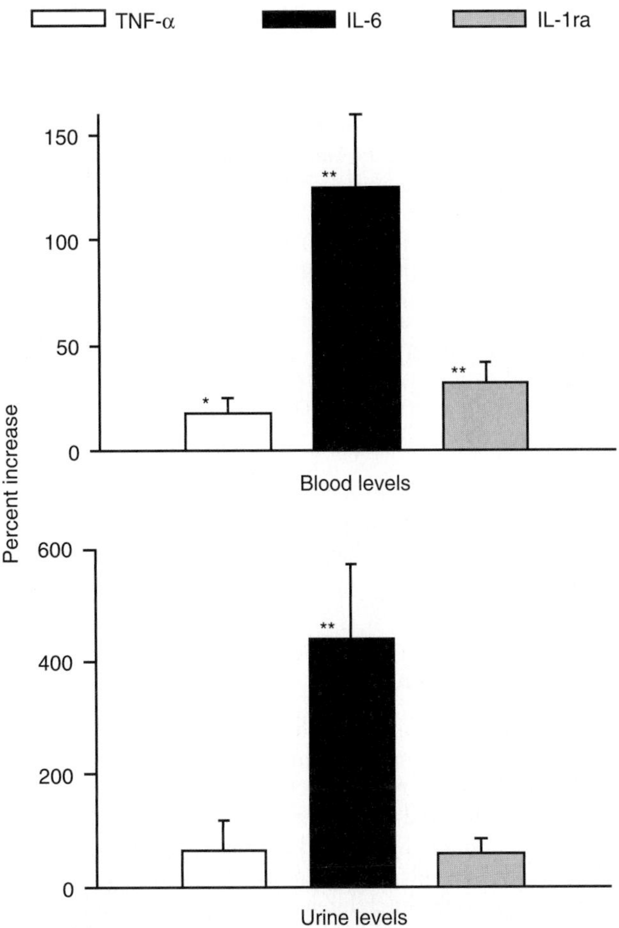

■ **FIGURE 11-15.** Effect of a soccer-practice type exercise protocol on serum (n = 9) and urine (n = 17) tumor necrosis factor α (TNF-α), interleukin 6 (IL-6), and IL-1ra. Data are expressed as the mean ± SE percentage change of each variable. In serum, there were significant elevations in all three of these cytokines with exercise, the most robust response observed for the inflammatory cytokine IL-6. In the urine, a statistically significant and quite substantial response was found for IL-6 alone (*$P < .05$; **$P < .001$).

Mediator release from circulating leukocytes and/or the airway mast cells was suggested as the intermediary pathway involved in EIA, HIA, and osmotic-induced asthma (OIA). Neutrophil chemotactic factor and histamine have been found to rise in blood after exercise,[173–175] as have intracellular adhesion molecules[176] and other inflammatory cytokines known to play a role in asthma even in healthy children.[158,177,178] Pre-exercise treatment with sodium cromoglycate (which has been shown to prevent mediator release from mast cells in vitro) prevented EIA.[179] Terfenadine, a H_1 histamine antagonist, has been shown to reduce the severity of EIA, HIA, and OIA.[180,181] It has been shown that the leukotriene LTD_4 may be one of the mediators released during exercise,[182] but leukotriene-blocking agents have only mixed success in blocking EIA.[183] As noted recently by McConnell and colleagues,[184] "Incidence of new diagnoses of asthma is associated with heavy exercise in communities with high concentrations of ozone, thus, air pollution and outdoor exercise could contribute to the development of asthma in children." Given recent research in the ways in which exposure to air pollutants can influence asthma and lung inflammation,[185,186] the association among ozone, exercise, and asthma further supports the idea that immune-inflammatory dysregulation may play a role in EIA.

The refractory period observed after EIA and sometimes after HIA and OIA was originally thought to be due to mediator depletion from mast cells.[187] However, neutrophil chemotactic factor was not found to be reduced after a second exercise when the subject was refractory.[188] It has recently been suggested that refractoriness to EIA and OIA but not to HIA may be due to the release of inhibitory prostaglandins whose effect persists for 30 to 60 minutes after the initial challenge.[179,189,190]

A MODEL OF THE PATHOPHYSIOLOGY OF EXERCISE-INDUCED ASTHMA

Ventilation is increased during exercise, causing cooling and drying of airway mucosa. The combination of osmotic changes and exercise itself is the trigger for EIA, causing mediator release that results in bronchoconstriction. The degree of bronchoconstriction is influenced by airway reactivity, which may be increased by viral infections or allergic stimulation. During exercise the stimuli for bronchoconstriction are opposed by increased sympathomimetic activity and by the release of prostaglandins that causes refractoriness to a subsequent exercise.

EXERCISE AND OTHER TESTS FOR BRONCHIAL REACTIVITY

Bronchial hyperreactivity to methacholine (MCH) or histamine is a characteristic feature of asthma[191–193] but is also present in patients with other types of chronic obstructive lung diseases.[194–199] Avital and co-workers[152] have compared bronchial reactivity to exercise, MCH, and adenosine 5′-monophosphate (AMP, which probably acts by increasing the release of mediators from mast cells) in children with asthma, in children with pediatric chronic obstructive pulmonary disease (PCOPD, including CF, bronchiolitis obliterans, primary ciliary dyskinesia, and bronchiectasis), and in healthy controls. While the asthmatics responded to all three challenges, the PCOPD patients responded only to MCH and the controls did not respond to any of the three challenges. MCH could distinguish both asthma and PCOPD from controls but could not distinguish asthma from PCOPD. Exercise and AMP not only distinguished asthma from controls but could also distinguish asthma from PCOPD. In a recent study involving 135 children and young adults with mild to moderate asthma, Avital and colleagues[200] compared the response to MCH, AMP, and exercise challenges and evaluated the relation between asthma severity and the response to these challenges. These investigators found that the sensitivity of MCH challenge in detecting bronchial reactivity was 98%, that of AMP challenge was 95.5%, and that of exercise was 65%. Logistic regression analysis and receiver operating characteristic curves of the three challenges showed that MCH was the best discriminator between severity groups. Therefore, it seems that exercise and AMP are specific stimuli for asthma and that AMP is more sensitive than exercise in the detection of bronchial hyperreactivity in asthmatic patients. In known asthmatics, MCH is the best challenge to predict the severity of the disease.

The diagnosis of asthma in preschool children may be difficult, since these children cannot usually perform reliable spirometric measurement of lung function. During recent years we have developed a new method to evaluate bronchial reactivity of preschool children to MCH and AMP. By this method, the response to inhaled MCH or AMP is assessed by the detection of wheeze—by auscultation to the chest or an increase in respiratory rate or desaturation.[201] We have shown that the efficacy of this method, using MCH, in diagnosing asthma is 95.5%. In the proper hands, challenge testing is virtually free of complications.[202]

PRACTICAL GUIDELINES FOR THE PERFORMANCE OF EXERCISE TESTING IN ASTHMATIC CHILDREN

Children should avoid physical activity for at least 3 hours before exercise testing, because they may show an attenuated response due to refractoriness. Medications that can influence the pulmonary response to exercise should be stopped before the test—6 and 12 hours for short- and long-acting β-adrenergic drugs, respectively, 8 hours for anticholinergic drugs, and 24 hours for cromolyn sodium. Caffeine-containing drinks or food should also be avoided before the test. Corticosteroids can be continued without any change, since their immediate effect on EIA is probably not significant. Baseline pulmonary function (FEV_1) should be at least 65% of the predicted value.[203] The exercise test can be performed by using either a bicycle ergometer or a treadmill. Our standard test for demonstrating EIA is a 6-minute run on a treadmill at a speed of 3 to 5 miles per hour with a slope of 10%. This will result in an O_2 consumption of about 60% to 80% of $\dot{V}O_{2\ max}$ and a HR of 170 to 180 beats per minute.[204] Lung function is measured before exercise and repeated until satisfactory reproducibility is demonstrated. Measurements are performed in duplicate after exercise (recording the best value) at 1, 3, 5, 10, and 15 minutes after exercise. Lung function is assessed by FEV_1 using a spirometer, but peak-flow measurements can also be used, especially in young children, since they are easier to perform. The asthmatic response is expressed by the percentage reduction in lung function from baseline. A 10% or greater reduction in FEV_1 or peak expiratory flow (PEF) is considered a positive response. Salbutamol nebulized solution should be prepared before the exercise test, since some children may respond with a severe asthmatic attack.

CLINICAL INDICATION FOR EXERCISE AND OTHER TESTS FOR BRONCHIAL REACTIVITY

Exercise testing may be useful in the assessment of the severity of bronchial obstruction that follows physical activity and to evaluate the efficacy of a specific therapy to prevent EIA. Because exercise and adenosine challenges are highly specific for asthma, they can help in the differentiation of asthma from other chronic obstructive lung diseases during childhood.

SUMMARY

The pediatrician, in attempting to assess the health status of his or her patients, frequently asks the question, "How is the child doing?" With exercise testing, a precise answer to this question can often be obtained. We have attempted to demonstrate that the cardiorespiratory response to exercise is a measurement of metabolism and growth and development as well as an index of the functional capabilities of the heart and lungs. Hopefully, child health care professionals will avail themselves of this resource. Finally, much more research has yet do be done before we fully understand the optimal role of physical activity in the life of healthy children or in those suffering from chronic diseases.

REFERENCES

1. Matzinger P: An innate sense of danger. Ann NY Acad Sci 2002;961:341–342.
2. Shephard RJ: Cytokine responses to physical activity, with particular reference to IL-6. Sources, actions, and clinical implications. Crit Rev Immunol 2002;22:165–182.
3. Pedersen BK, Hoffman-Goetz L: Exercise and the immune system. Regulation, integration, and adaptation. Physiol Rev 2000;80:1055–1081.
4. Cooper DM, Nemet D, Galassetti P: Exercise, stress, and inflammation in the growing child. From the bench to the playground. Curr Opin Pediatr 2004;16:286–292.
5. Simon D: Puberty in chronically diseased patients. Horm Res 2002;57 (Suppl 2):53–56.
6. De Benedetti F, Meazza C, Martini A: Role of interleukin-6 in growth failure. An animal model. Horm Res 2002;58(Suppl 1):24–27.
7. Cohen LA, Boylan E, Epstein M, Zang E: Voluntary exercise and experimental mammary cancer. In: Jacobs MM, ed: Exercise, Calories, Fat, and Cancer. New York: Plenum Press, 1992, pp 41–59.
8. Livingstone MB, Coward WA, Prentice AM, Davies PS, Strain JJ, McKenna PG, Mahoney CA, White JA, Stewart CM, Kerr MJ: Daily energy expenditure in free-living children. Comparison of heart-rate monitoring with the doubly labeled water ($2H_2{}^{(18)}O$) method. Am J Clin Nutr 1992;56:343–352.
9. Bailey RC, Olson J, Pepper SL, Barstow TJ, Porszasz J, Cooper DM: The level and tempo of children's physical activities. An observational study. Med Sci Sports Exerc 1995;27:1033–1041.
10. Borer KT, Nicoski DR, Owens V: Alteration of pulsatile growth hormone secretion by growth-inducing exercise. Involvement of endogenous opiates and somatostatin. Endocrinology 1986;118:844–850.
11. Rosenfeld R: Insulin-like growth factors and the basis of growth. N Engl J Med 2003;349:2184–2186.
12. Cameron N, Demerath EW: Critical periods in human growth and their relationship to diseases of aging. Am J Phys Anthropol (Suppl) 2002; 35:159–184.
13. Clark PM: Programming of the hypothalamo-pituitary-adrenal axis and the fetal origins of adult disease hypothesis. Eur J Pediatr 1998;157(Suppl 1):S7–S10.
14. Phillips D: Endocrine programming and fetal origins of adult disease. Trends Endocrinol Metab 2002;13:363–367.
15. Eliakim A, Dolfin T, Weiss E, Shainkin-Kestenbaum R, Lis M, Nemet D: The effects of exercise on body weight and circulating leptin in premature infants. J Perinatol 2002;22:550–554.
16. MacKelvie KJ, Khan KM, McKay HA: Is there a critical period for bone response to weight-bearing exercise in children and adolescents? A systematic review. Br J Sports Med 2002;36:250–257.
17. Goran MI, Ball GD, Cruz ML: Obesity and risk of type 2 diabetes and cardiovascular disease in children and adolescents. J Clin Endocrinol Metab 2003;88:1417–1427.
18. Nemet D, Cooper DM: Exercise, diet, and childhood obesity. The GH-IGF-I connection. J Pediatr Endocrinol Metab 2002;15(Suppl 2):751–757.
19. Kavey RE, Daniels SR, Lauer RM, Atkins DL, Hayman LL, Taubert K: American Heart Association guidelines for primary prevention of atherosclerotic cardiovascular disease beginning in childhood. J Pediatr 2003;142:368–372.
20. Tomkinson GR, Leger LA, Olds TS, Cazorla G: Secular trends in the performance of children and adolescents 1980—2000. An analysis of 55 studies of the 20m shuttle run test in 11 countries. Rev Environ Health 2003;33:285–300.
21. Roubenoff R: Sarcopenia. Effects on body composition and function. J Gerontol A Biol Sci Med Sci 2003;58:1012–1017.
22. Takken T, Spermon N, Helders PJ, Prakken AB, Van Der NJ: Aerobic exercise capacity in patients with juvenile dermatomyositis. J Rheumatol 2003; 30:1075–1080.
23. Jones S, Elliott PM, Sharma S, McKenna WJ, Whipp BJ: Cardiopulmonary responses to exercise in patients with hypertrophic cardiomyopathy. Heart 1998;80:60–67.
24. Cooper DM, Weiler-Ravell D, Whipp BJ, Wasserman K: Aerobic parameters of exercise as a function of body size during growth in children. J Appl Physiol 1984;56:628–634.
25. Godfrey S, Davies CT, Wozniak E, Barnes CA: Cardio-respiratory response to exercise in normal children. Clin Sci 1971;40:419–431.
26. Hebestreit H: Exercise testing in children—what works, what doesn't, and where to go? Paediatr Respir Rev 2004;5(Suppl A):S11–S14.
27. Williams CA, Armstrong N, Powell J: Aerobic responses of prepubertal boys to two modes of training. Br J Sports Med 2000;34:168–173.
28. Cooper DM, Weiler-Ravell D, Whipp BJ, Wasserman K: Growth-related changes in oxygen uptake and heart rate during progressive exercise in children. Pediatr Res 1984;18:845–851.
29. Trudeau F, Laurencelle L, Shephard RJ: Tracking of physical activity from childhood to adulthood. Med Sci Sports Exerc 2004;36:1937–1943.
30. Eisenmann JC, Katzmarzyk PT, Theriault G, Song TM, Malina RM, Bouchard C: Cardiac dimensions, physical activity, and submaximal working capacity in youth of the Quebec Family Study. Eur J Appl Physiol 2000;81:40–46.
31. Durant RH, Dover EV, Alpert BS: An evaluation of five indices of physical working capacity in children. Med Sci Sports Exerc 1983;15:83–87.
32. Berman N, Bailey RC, Barstow TJ, Cooper DM: Spectral and bout detection analysis of physical activity patterns in healthy, prepubertal boys and girls. Am J Hum Biol 1998;10:289–297.
33. Wasserman K, Van Kessel A, Burton GG: Interaction of physiological mechanism during exercise. J Appl Physiol 1967;22:71–85.
34. Phillipson EA, Bowes G, Townsend ER, Duffin J, Cooper JD: Role of metabolic CO_2 production in ventilatory response to steady-state exercise. J Clin Invest 1981;68:768–774.
35. Whipp BJ: Ventilatory control during exercise in humans. Ann Rev Physiol 1996;45:393–405.
36. Ward SA: Control of the exercise hyperpnoea in humans. A modeling perspective. Respir Physiol 2000;122:149–166.
37. Wasserman K: Breathing during exercise. N Engl J Med 1978;298:780–785.
38. Gozal D, Marcus CL, Davidson Ward SL, Keens TG: Ventilatory responses to passive leg motion in children with congenital central hypoventilation syndrome. Am J Resp Crit Care Med 1996;153:761–768.
39. Springer C, Cooper DM, Wasserman K: Evidence that maturation of the peripheral chemoreceptors is not complete in childhood. Respir Physiol 1988;74:55–64.
40. Whipp BJ, Davis JA, Wasserman K: Ventilatory control of the 'isocapnic buffering' region in rapidly-incremental exercise. Respir Physiol 1989;76:357–367.
41. Whipp BJ, Ward SA, Lamarra N, Davis JA, Wasserman K: Parameters of ventilatory and gas exchange dynamics during exercise. J Appl Physiol 1982;52:1506–1513.
42. Cooper DM, Kaplan MR, Baumgarten L, Weiler-Ravell D, Whipp BJ, Wasserman K: Coupling of ventilation and CO_2 production during exercise in children. Pediatr Res 1987;21:568–572.
43. Marinov B, Kostianev S, Turnovska T: Ventilatory efficiency and rate of perceived exertion in obese and non-obese children performing standardized exercise. Clin Physiol Funct Imaging 2002;22:254–260.
44. Marinov B, Kostianev S, Turnovska T: Ventilatory response to exercise and rating of perceived exertion in two pediatric age groups. Acta Physiol Pharmacol Bulg 2000;25:93–98.

45. Barstow TJ, Cooper DM, Sobel E, Landaw E, Epstein S: Influence of increased metabolic rate on ^{13}C-bicarbonate washout kinetics. Am J Physiol 1990;259:R163–R171.
46. Armon Y, Zanconato S, Barstow TJ, Cooper DM: Ventilatory response to bursts of exercise in children and adults. Pediatr Res 1989;25:363A.
47. Ohuchi H, Kato Y, Tasato H, Arakaki Y, Kamiya T: Ventilatory response and arterial blood gases during exercise in children. Pediatr Res 1999;45: 389–396.
48. Brady JP, Cotton EC, Tooley WH: Chemoreflexes in the newborn infant. Effect of 100% oxygen on heart rate and ventilation. J Physiol 1964;172: 332–334.
49. Brady JP, Ceruti E: Chemoreceptor reflexes in the newborn infant. Effect of varying degrees of hypoxia on heart rate and ventilation in a warm environment. J Physiol 1966;184:631–645.
50. Nagano Y, Baba R, Kuraishi K, Yasuda T, Ikoma M, Nishibata K, Yokota M, Nagashima M: Ventilatory control during exercise in normal children. Pediatr Res 1998;43:704–707.
51. Ratel S, Duche P, Hennegrave A, Van PE, Bedu M: Acid-base balance during repeated cycling sprints in boys and men. J Appl Physiol 2002;92:479–485.
52. Driscoll DJ, Staats BA, Heise CT, Rice MJ, Puga FJ, Danielson GK, Ritter DG: Functional single ventricle. Cardiorespiratory response to exercise. J Am Coll Cardiol 1984;4:337–342.
53. Santuz P, Baraldi E, Zaramella P, Filippone M, Zacchello F: Factors limiting exercise performance in long-term survivors of bronchopulmonary dysplasia. Am J Respir Crit Care Med 1995;152:1284–1289.
54. Reybrouck T, Boshoff D, Vanhees L, Defoor J, Gewillig M: Ventilatory response to exercise in patients after correction of cyanotic congenital heart disease. Relation with clinical outcome after surgery. Heart 2004;90: 215–216.
55. Moser C, Tirakitsoontorn P, Nussbaum E, Newcomb R, Cooper DM: Muscle size and cardiorespiratory response to exercise in cystic fibrosis. Am J Respir Crit Care Med 2000;162:1823–1827.
56. Pianosi PT, Fisk M: Cardiopulmonary exercise performance in prematurely born children. Pediatr Res 2000;47:653–658.
57. Inbar O, Bar-Or O: Anaerobic characteristics in male children and adolescents. Med Sci Sports Exerc 1986;18:264–269.
58. Bar-Or O: The wingate anaerobic test. An update on methodology, reliability, and validity. Sports Med 1987;4:381–394.
59. Nioka S, Moser D, Lech G, Evengelisti M, Verde T, Chance B, Kuno S: Muscle deoxygenation in aerobic and anaerobic exercise. Adv Exp Med Biol 1998;454:63–70.
60. Zanconato S, Cooper DM, Armon Y: Oxygen cost and oxygen uptake dynamics and recovery with one minute of exercise in children and adults. J Appl Physiol 1991;71:993–998.
61. Hebestreit H, Mimura K, Bar-Or O: Recovery of muscle power after high-intensity short-term exercise: comparing boys and men. J Appl Physiol 1993;74:2875–2880.
62. Fawkner S, Armstrong N: Oxygen uptake kinetic response to exercise in children. Sports Med 2003;33:651–669.
63. Fawkner SG, Armstrong N: Sex differences in the oxygen uptake kinetic response to heavy-intensity exercise in prepubertal children. Eur J Appl Physiol 2004;93:210–216.
64. Fawkner SG, Armstrong N: Longitudinal changes in the kinetic response to heavy-intensity exercise in children. J Appl Physiol 2004;97:460–466.
65. Kaczor JJ, Ziolkowski W, Popinigis J, Tarnopolsky MA: Anaerobic and aerobic enzyme activities in human skeletal muscle from children and adults. Pediatr Res 2005;57:331–335.
66. Sapega AA, Sokolow DP, Graham TJ, Chance B: Phosphorus nuclear magnetic resonance. A non-invasive technique for the study of muscle bioenergetics during exercise. Med Sci Sports Exerc 1993;25:656–666.
67. Zanconato S, Buchthal S, Barstow TJ, Cooper DM: ^{31}P-magnetic resonance spectroscopy of leg muscle metabolism during exercise in children and adults. J Appl Physiol 1993;74:2214–2218.
68. Dudley GA, Tullson PC, Terjung RL: Influence of mitochondrial content on the sensitivity of respiratory control. J Biol Chem 1994;262:9109–9114.
69. Chance B, Leigh JS, Kent J, McCully K: Metabolic control principles and ^{31}P NMR. Fed Proc 1986;45:2915–2920.
70. Petersen SR, Gaul CA, Stanton MM, Hanstock CC: Skeletal muscle metabolism during short-term, high-intensity exercise in prepubertal and pubertal girls. J Appl Physiol 1999;87:2151–2156.
71. Boisseau N, Delamarche P: Metabolic and hormonal responses to exercise in children and adolescents. Sports Med 2000;30:405–422.
72. Baraldi E, Cooper DM, Zanconato S, Armon Y: Heart rate recovery from 1 minute of exercise in children and adults. Pediatr Res 1991;29:575–579.
73. Carter JB, Banister EW, Blaber AP: Effect of endurance exercise on autonomic control of heart rate. Sports Med 2003;33:33–46.
74. Savin W, Davidson D, Haskell WL: Autonomic contribution to heart rate recovery from exercise in humans. J Appl Physiol 1982;53:1572–1575.
75. Darr K, Basset D, Morgan B, Thomas DP: Effects of age and training status of heart rate recovery after peak exercise. Am J Physiol 1988;254: H340–H343.
76. Cerretelli P, Grassi B, Colombini A, Caru B, Marconi C: Gas exchange and metabolic transients in heart transplant recipients. Respir Physiol 1988;74:355–371.
77. Degre SG, Niset GL, De Smet JM, Ibrahim T, Stoupel E, Le Clerc JL, Primo G: Cardiorespiratory response to early exercise testing after orthotopic cardiac transplantation. Am J Cardiol 1987;60:926–928.
78. Ferretti G, Marconi C, Achilli G, Caspani E, Fiocchi R, Mamprin F, Gamba A, Ferrazzi P, Cerretelli P: The heart rate response to exercise and circulating catecholamines in heart transplant recipients. Pflugers Arch 2002;443:370–376.
79. Cooper DM, Barstow TJ, Bergner A, Lee W-NP: Blood glucose turnover during high- and low-intensity exercise. Am J Physiol 1989;257:405–412.
80. Berthoin S, Allender H, Baquet G, Dupont G, Matran R, Pelayo P, Robin H: Plasma lactate and plasma volume recovery in adults and children following high-intensity exercises. Acta Paediatr 2003;92:283–290.
81. Dotan R, Ohana S, Bediz C, Falk B: Blood lactate disappearance dynamics in boys and men following exercise of similar and dissimilar peak-lactate concentrations. J Pediatr Endocrinol Metab 2003;16:419–429.
82. Matejkova J, Kropicova Z, Plachenta Z: Changes in acid-base balance after maximal exercise. In: Plachenta Z, ed: Youth and Physical Activity. Purkyne, Czechoslovakia: J.E. University, 1980, pp 191–199.
83. Lehmann M, Keul J, Korsten-Reck U: The influence of graduated treadmill exercise on plasma catecholamines, aerobic and anaerobic capacity in boys and adults. Eur J Appl Physiol 1981;47:301–311.
84. Whipp BJ, Davis JA, Torres F, Wasserman K: A test to determine parameters of aerobic function during exercise. J Appl Physiol 1981;50:217–221.
85. Hansen JE, Casaburi R, Cooper DM, Wasserman K: Oxygen uptake as related to work rate increment during cycle ergometer exercise. Eur J Appl Physiol 1988;57:140–145.
86. Astrand P-O: Experimental Studies of Physical Working Capacity in Relation to Sex and Age. Copenhagen: Ejnar Musckgaard, 1952.
87. Kleiber M: The Fire of Life. New York: Krieger, 1975.
88. Gray BF: On the surface law and basal metabolic rate. J Theor Biol 1981;93:757–762.
89. Zanconato S, Reidy G, Cooper DM: Calf muscle cross sectional area and maximal oxygen uptake in children and adults. Am J Physiol 1994;267: R720–R725.
90. Wasserman K, Whipp BJ, Koyal SN, Beaver WL: Anaerobic threshold and respiratory gas exchange during exercise. J Appl Physiol 1973;35:236–243.
91. Reybrouck T, Weymans M, Stijns H, Knops J, van der Hauwaert L: Ventilatory anaerobic threshold in healthy children. Age and sex differences. Eur J Appl Physiol Occup Physiol 1985;54:278–284.
92. Davis JA: Anaerobic threshold alterations caused by endurance training in middle aged men. J Appl Physiol 1979;46:1039–1046.
93. Katz A, Sahlin K: Regulation of lactic acid production during exercise. J Appl Physiol 1988;65:509–518.
94. Walsh ML, Bannister EW: Possible mechanisms of the anaerobic threshold. A review. Rev Environ Health 1988;5:269–273.
95. Brooks GA: Lactate shuttles in nature. Biochem Soc Trans 2002;30:258–264.
96. Coggan AR, Kohrt WM, Spina RJ, Kirwan JP, Bier DM, Holloszy JO: Plasma glucose kinetics during exercise in subjects with high and low lactate thresholds. J Appl Physiol 1992;73:1873–1880.
97. Svedahl K, MacIntosh BR: Anaerobic threshold. The concept and methods of measurement. Can J Appl Physiol 2003;28:299–323.
98. Washington RL, Bricker JT, Alpert BS, Daniels SR, Deckelbaum RJ, Fisher EA, Gidding SS, Isabel-Jones J, Kavey RE, Marx GR, et al: Guidelines for exercise testing in the pediatric age group. From the Committee on Atherosclerosis and Hypertension in Children, Council on Cardiovascular Disease in the Young, the American Heart Association. Circulation 1994;90:2166–2179.
99. Cooper DM, Weiler-Ravell D, Whipp BJ, Wasserman K: Oxygen uptake and heart rate during exercise as a function of growth in children. Pediatr Res 1984;18:845–851.
100. Samejima H, Omiya K, Uno M, Inoue K, Tamura M, Itoh K, Suzuki K, Akashi Y, Seki A, Suzuki N, Osada N, Tanabe K, Miyake F, Itoh H: Relationship between impaired chronotropic response, cardiac output during exercise, and exercise tolerance in patients with chronic heart failure. Jpn Heart J 2003;44:515–525.
101. Stein R, Selvadurai H, Coates A, Wilkes DL, Schneiderman-Walker J, Corey M: Determination of maximal voluntary ventilation in children with cystic fibrosis. Pediatr Pulmonol 2003;35:467–471.

102. Arena R, Myers J, Aslam SS, Varughese EB, Peberdy MA: Peak Vo_2 and VE/Vco_2 slope in patients with heart failure. A prognostic comparison. Am Heart J 2004;147:354–360.
103. Isasi CR, Deckelbaum RJ, Tracy RP, Starc TJ, Berglund L, Shea S: Physical fitness and C-reactive protein level in children and young adults. The Columbia University BioMarkers Study. Pediatrics 2003;111: 332–338.
104. Margaria R, Edwards HT, Dill DB: The possible mechanism of contracting and paying the oxygen debt and the role of lactic acid in muscular contraction. Am J Physiol 1933;106:689–695.
105. Beaver WL, Lamarra N, Wasserman K: Breath-by-breath measurement of true alveolar gas exchange. J Appl Physiol 1981;51:1662–1675.
106. Drakonakis AC, Halloran KH: Oxygen consumption during recovery from exercise in children with congenital heart disease. Am J Dis Child 1974;128:651–656.
107. Sietsema KE, Cooper DM, Perloff JK, Child JS, Rosove MH, Wasserman K, Whipp BJ: Control of ventilation during exercise in patients with central venous-to-systemic arterial shunts. J Appl Physiol 1988;64:234–242.
108. Giardini A, Donti A, Specchia S, Coutsoumbas G, Formigari R, Prandstraller D, Bronzetti G, Bonvicini M, Picchio FM: Recovery kinetics of oxygen uptake is prolonged in adults with an atrial septal defect and improves after transcatheter closure. Am Heart J 2004;147:910–914.
109. Troutman WB, Barstow TJ, Galindo AJ, Cooper DM: Abnormal dynamic cardiorespiratory responses to exercise in pediatric patients after Fontan procedure. J Am Coll Cardiol 1998;31:668–673.
110. Mac̆ek M, Vavra J, Mrzena B: Intermittent exercise of supermaximal intensity in children. Acta Paediat Scand 1971;217(Suppl):29–31.
111. McManus A, Leung M: Maximising the clinical use of exercise gaseous exchange testing in children with repaired cyanotic congenital heart defects. The development of an appropriate test strategy. Sports Med 2000;29:229–244.
112. Reybrouck T, Weymans M, Vinckx J, Stijns H, Vanderschueren Lodeweyckx M: Cardiorespiratory function during exercise in obese children. Acta Paediatr Scand 1987;76:342–348.
113. Cooper DM, Poage J, Barstow TJ, Springer C: Are obese children truly unfit? Minimizing the confounding effect of body size on the exercise response. J Pediatr 1990;116:223–230.
114. Slyper AH: The pediatric obesity epidemic. Causes and controversies. J Clin Endocrinol Metab 2004;89:2540–2547.
115. Sopher AB, Thornton JC, Wang J, Pierson RN Jr, Heymsfield SB, Horlick M: Measurement of percentage of body fat in 411 children and adolescents. A comparison of dual-energy X-ray absorptiometry with a four-compartment model. Pediatrics 2004;113:1285–1290.
116. Lohman TG: Advances in Body Composition Measurement. Champaign, Ill: Human Kinetics, 1992.
117. Seidell JC, Bakker CJ, van der Kooy K: Imaging techniques for measuring adipose-tissue distribution—a comparison between computed tomography and 1.5-T magnetic resonance. Am J Clin Nutr 1990;51:953–957.
118. Pietrobelli A, Peroni DG, Faith MS: Pediatric body composition in clinical studies. Which methods in which situations? Acta Diabetol 2003;40 (Suppl 1):S270–S273.
119. Goran MI: Measurement issues related to studies of childhood obesity. Assessment of body composition, body fat distribution, physical activity, and food intake. Pediatrics 1998;101:505–518.
120. Cooper DM, Berman N: Ratios and regressions in body size and function. A commentary. J Appl Physiol 1994;77:2014–2017.
121. Tanner JM: Fallacy of per-weight and per-surface area standards and their relation to spurious correlation. J Appl Physiol 1949;2:1–15.
122. Toth MJ, Goran MI, Ades PA, Howard DB, Poehlman ET: Examination of data normalization procedures for expressing peak Vo_2 data. J Appl Physiol 1993;75:2288–2292.
123. McMahon TA: Size and shape in biology. Science 1973;179:1201–1204.
124. Heusner AA: Energy metabolism and body size. II. Dimensional analysis and energetic non-similarity. Respir Physiol 1982;48:13–20.
125. Ekelund U, Yngve A, Brage S, Westerterp K, Sjostrom M: Body movement and physical activity energy expenditure in children and adolescents. How to adjust for differences in body size and age. Am J Clin Nutr 2004;79:851–856.
126. Tirosh E, Bar-Or O, Rosenbaum P: New muscle power test in neuromuscular disease. Feasibility and reliability. Am J Dis Child 1990;144: 1083–1087.
127. Takahashi CD, Nemet D, Rose-Gottron CM, Larson JK, Cooper DM, Reinkensmeyer DJ: Neuromotor noise limits motor performance, but not motor adaptation, in children. J Neurophysiol 2003;90:703–711.
128. Alpert BS, Verrill DE, Flood NL, Boineau JP, Strong WB: Complications of ergometer testing in children. Pediatr Cardiol 1983;4:91–96.
129. Gibbons RJ, Balady GJ, Beasley JW, Bricker JT, Duvemoy WF, Froelicher VF, Mark DB, Marwick TH, McCallister BD, Thompson PD Jr, Winters WL, Yanowitz FG, Ritchie JL, Gibbons RJ, Cheitlin MD, Eagle KA, Gardner TJ, Garson A Jr, Lewis RP, O'Rourke RA, Ryan TJ: ACC/AHA Guidelines for Exercise Testing. A report of the American College of Cardiology/American Heart Association Task Force on Practice Guidelines. J Am Coll Cardiol 1997;30:260–311.
130. Bar-Or O, Rowland TW: Pediatric exercise medicine. From physiologic principles to health care application. Champaign, Ill: Human Kinetics, 2004.
131. Klissouras V: Heritability of adaptive variation. J Appl Physiol 1971;31: 338–344.
132. Danis A, Kyriazis Y, Klissouras V: The effect of training in male prepubertal and pubertal monozygotic twins. Eur J Appl Physiol 2003;89: 309–318.
133. Bouchard C, Dionne FT, Simoneau JA, Boulay MR: Genetics of aerobic and anaerobic performances. Exerc Sport Sci Rev 1992;20:27–58.
134. Bouchard C, Rankinen T: Individual differences in response to regular physical activity. Med Sci Sports Exerc 2001;33:S446–S451.
135. Lakka TA, Bouchard C: Genetics, physical activity, fitness and health. What does the future hold? J R Soc Health 2004;124:14–15.
136. McMurray RG, Ainsworth BE, Harrell JS, Griggs TR, Williams OD: Is physical activity or aerobic power more influential on reducing cardiovascular disease risk factors? Med Sci Sports Exerc 1998;30:1521–1529.
137. Welk GJ, Corbin CB, Dale D: Measurement issues in the assessment of physical activity in children. Res Q Exerc Sport 2000;71(2 Suppl):S59–S73.
138. Sallis JF, Saelens BE: Assessment of physical activity by self-report. Status, limitations, and future directions. Res Q Exerc Sport 2000;71:S1–S14.
139. Treuth MS, Schmitz K, Catellier DJ, McMurray RG, Murray DM, Almeida MJ, Going S, Norman JE, Pate R: Defining accelerometer thresholds for activity intensities in adolescent girls. Med Sci Sports Exerc 2004;36:1259–1266.
140. Eliakim A, Barstow TJ, Brasel JA, Ajie H, Lee W-NP, Renslo R, Berman N, Cooper DM: The effect of exercise training on energy expenditure, muscle volume, and maximal oxygen uptake in adolescent females. J Pediatr 1996;129:537–543.
141. Abbott RA, Davies PS: Habitual physical activity and physical activity intensity. Their relation to body composition in 5.0–10.5-y-old children. Eur J Clin Nutr 2004;58:285–291.
142. Hoos MB, Gerver WJ, Kester AD, Westerterp KR: Physical activity levels in children and adolescents. Int J Obes Relat Metab Disord 2003;27: 605–609.
143. Redd SC: Asthma in the United States: Burden and current theories. Environ Health Perspect 2002;110(Suppl 4):557–560.
144. Cummiskey J: Exercise-induced asthma. An overview. Am J Med Sci 2001;322:200–203.
145. Godfrey S, Springer C, Noviski N, Maayan C, Avital A: Exercise but not methacholine differentiates asthma from chronic lung disease in children. Thorax 1991;46:488–492.
146. Lang DM, Butz AM, Duggan AK, Serwint JR: Physical activity in urban school-aged children with asthma. Pediatrics 2004;113:e341–e346.
147. Godfrey S: Series: Assessment of inflammation. Bronchial hyper-responsiveness in children. Paediatr Respir Rev 2000;1:148–155.
148. Speelberg B, van den Berg NJ, Oosthoek CH, Verhoeff NP, van den Brink WT: Immediate and late asthmatic responses induced by exercise in patients with reversible airflow limitation. Eur Respir J 1989;2:402–408.
149. Bahous J, Cartier A, Ouimet G, Pineau L, Malo JL: Nonallergic bronchial hyperexcitability in chronic bronchitis. Am Rev Respir Dis 1984;129: 216–220.
150. Crimi E, Balbo A, Milanese M, Miadonna A, Rossi GA, Brusasco V: Airway inflammation and occurrence of delayed bronchoconstriction in exercise-induced asthma. Am Rev Respir Dis 1992;146:507–512.
151. Anderson SD, Daviskas E: The mechanism of exercise-induced asthma is . . . J Allergy Clin Immunol 2000;106:453–459.
152. Avital A, Springer C, Bar-Yishay E, Godfrey S: Adenosine, methacholine, and exercise challenges in children with asthma or paediatric chronic obstructive pulmonary disease. Thorax 1995;50:511–516.
153. Fourie PR, Joubert JR: Determination of airway hyper-reactivity in asthmatic children. A comparison among exercise, nebulized water, and histamine challenge. Pediatr Pulmonol 1988;4:2–7.
154. Mussaffi H, Springer C, Godfrey S: Increased bronchial responsiveness to exercise and histamine after allergen challenge in asthmatic children. J Allergy Clin Immunol 1986;77:48–52.
155. Bar-Yishay E, Gur I, Inbar O, Neuman I, Dlin RA, Godfrey S: Differences between swimming and running as stimuli for exercise-induced asthma. Eur J Appl Physiol Occup Physiol 1982;48:387–397.

156. Hofstra WB, Sterk PJ, Neijens HJ, Kouwenberg JM, Duiverman EJ: Prolonged recovery from exercise-induced asthma with increasing age in childhood. Pediatr Pulmonol 1995;20:177–183.
157. Scheett TP, Mills PJ, Ziegler MG, Stoppani J, Cooper DM: Effect of exercise on cytokines and growth mediators in prepubertal children. Pediatr Res 1999;46:429–434.
158. Nemet D, Rose-Gottron CM, Mills PJ, Cooper DM: Effect of water polo practice on cytokines, growth mediators, and leukocytes in girls. Med Sci Sports Exerc 2003;35:356–363.
159. Peake JM: Exercise-induced alterations in neutrophil degranulation and respiratory burst activity. Possible mechanisms of action. Exerc Immunol Rev 2002;8:49–100.
160. Pedersen BK, Steensberg A: Exercise and hypoxia. Effects on leukocytes and interleukin-6-shared mechanisms? Med Sci Sports Exerc 2002;34:2004–2013.
161. Michiels C, Bouaziz N, Remacle J: Role of the endothelium and blood stasis in the development of varicose veins. Int Angiol 2002;21:18–25.
162. Bar-Or O, Neuman I, Dotan R: Effects of dry and humid climates on exercise-induced asthma in children and preadolescents. J Allergy Clin Immunol 1977;60:163–168.
163. Weinstein RE, Anderson JA, Sweet LC: Effects of humidification on exercise-induced asthma (EIA). J Allergy Clin Immunol 1976;57:250–251.
164. Ingram RH, Bishop JB: Ventilatory response to carbon dioxide after removal of chronic upper airway obstruction. Am Rev Respir Dis 1970;102:645–647.
165. Deal EC, McFadden ER, Ingram RH, Jaeger JJ: Hyperpnea and heat flux: Initial reaction sequence in exercise-induced asthma. J Appl Physiol 1979;46:476–483.
166. Ben-Dov I, Bar-Yishay E, Godfrey S: Exercise-induced asthma without respiratory heat loss. Thorax 1982;37:630–631.
167. Anderson SD, Schoeffel RE: Respiratory heat and water loss during exercise in patients with asthma. Effect of repeated exercise challenge. Eur J Respir Dis 1982;63:472–480.
168. Anderson SD, Schoeffel RE, Follet R, Perry CP, Daviskas E, Kendall M.: Sensitivity to heat and water loss at rest and during exercise in asthmatic patients. Eur J Respir Dis 1982;63:459–471.
169. Noviski N, Bar-Yishay E, Gur I, Godfrey S: Exercise intensity determines and climatic conditions modify the severity of exercise-induced asthma. Am Rev Respir Dis 1987;136:592–594.
170. Anderson SD: Is there a unifying hypothesis for exercise-induced asthma? J Allergy Clin Immunol 1984;73:660–665.
171. Gilbert IA, Fouke JM, McFadden ER Jr: Heat and water flux in the intrathoracic airways and exercise-induced asthma. J Appl Physiol 1987; 63:1681–1691.
172. Baile EM, Dahlby RW, Wiggs BR, Pare PD: Role of tracheal and bronchial circulation in respiratory heat exchange. J Appl Physiol 1985; 58:217–222.
173. Lee TH, Kay AB: Bronchial asthma and the neutrophil chemotactic factor. [Review]. Clin Allergy 1982;12(Suppl):39–45.
174. Lee TH, Brown MJ, Nagy L, Causon R, Walport MJ, Kay AB: Exercise-induced release of histamine and neutrophil chemotactic factor in atopic asthmatics. J Allergy Clin Immunol 1982;70:73–81.
175. Lee TH, O'Hickey SP: Exercise-induced asthma and late phase reactions. [Review]. Eur Resp J 1989;2:195–197.
176. Ando M, Shima M, Adachi M, Tsunetoshi Y: The role of intercellular adhesion molecule-1 (ICAM-1), vascular cell adhesion molecule-1 (VCAM-1), and regulated on activation, normal T-cell expressed and secreted (RANTES) in the relationship between air pollution and asthma among children. Arch Environ Health 2001;56:227–233.
177. Nemet D, Oh Y, Kim HS, Hill MA, Cooper DM: The effect of intense exercise on inflammatory cyotkines and growth mediators in adolescent boys. Pediatrics 2002;110:681–689.
178. Cengizlier R, Demirpolat E, Tulek N, Cakmak F: Circulating ICAM-1 levels in bronchial asthma and the effect of inhaled corticosteroids. Ann Allergy Asthma Immunol 2000;84:539–541.
179. O'Byrne PM, Jones GM: The effect of indomethacin on exercise-induced bronchoconstriction and refractoriness after exercise. Am Rev Respir Dis 1986;134:69–72.
180. Wiebicke W, Poynter A, Montgomery M, Chernick V, Pasterkamp H: Effect of terfenadine on the response to exercise and cold air in asthma. Pediatr Pulmonol 1988;4:225–229.
181. Finney MJ, Anderson SD, Black JL: Terfenadine modifies airway narrowing induced by the inhalation of nonisotonic aerosols in subjects with asthma. Am Rev Respir Dis 1990;141:1151–1157.
182. Manning PJ, Watson R, O'Byrne PM: The effects of H_2-receptor antagonists on exercise refractoriness in asthma. J Allergy Clin Immunol 1992; 90:125–126.
183. Berkman N, Avital A, Bardach E, Springer C, Breuer R, Godfrey S: The effect of montelukast on bronchial provocation tests and exhaled nitric oxide levels in asthmatic patients. Isr Med Assoc J 2003;5:778–781.
184. McConnell R, Berhane K, Gilliland F, London SJ, Islam T, Gauderman WJ, Avol E, Margolis HG, Peters JM: Asthma in exercising children exposed to ozone. A cohort study. Lancet 2002;359:386–391.
185. Delfino RJ, Zeiger RS, Seltzer JM, Street DH, McLaren CE: Association of asthma symptoms with peak particulate air pollution and effect modification by anti-inflammatory medication use. Environ Health Perspect 2002;110:A607–A617.
186. Adamkiewicz G, Ebelt S, Syring M, Slater J, Speizer FE, Schwartz J, Suh H, Gold DR: Association between air pollution exposure and exhaled nitric oxide in an elderly population. Thorax 2004;59:204–209.
187. Edmunds AT, Tooley M, Godfrey S: The refractory period after exercise-induced asthma. Its duration and relation to the severity of exercise. Am Rev Respir Dis 1978;117:247–254.
188. Belcher NG, Murdoch R, Dalton N, Clark TJ, Rees PJ, Lee TH: Circulating concentrations of histamine, neutrophil chemotactic activity, and catecholamines during the refractory period in exercise-induced asthma. J Allergy Clin Immunol 1988;81:100–110.
189. Mattoli S, Foresi A, Corbo GM, Valente S, Ciappi G: Effects of two doses of cromolyn on allergen-induced late asthmatic response and increased responsiveness. J Allergy Clin Immunol 1987;79:747–754.
190. Margolskee DJ, Bigby BG, Boushey HA: Indomethacin blocks airway tolerance to repetitive exercise but not to eucapnic hyperpnea in asthmatic subjects. Am Rev Respir Dis 1988;137:842–846.
191. Cockcroft DW, Killian DN, Mellon JJ, Hargreave FE: Bronchial reactivity to inhaled histamine. A method and clinical survey. Clin Allergy 1977;7:235–243.
192. Juniper EF, Frith PA, Dunnett C, Cockcroft DW, Hargreave FE: Reproducibility and comparison of responses to inhaled histamine and methacholine. Thorax 1978;33:705–710.
193. Townley RG, Bewtra AK, Nair NM, Brodkey FD, Watt GD, Burke KM: Methacholine inhalation challenge studies. J Allergy Clin Immunol 1979;64:569–574.
194. Avital A, Sanchez I, Chernick V: Efficacy of salbutamol and ipratropium bromide in decreasing bronchial hyperreactivity in children with cystic fibrosis. Pediatr Pulmonol 1992;13:34–37.
195. Price JF, Weller PH, Harper SA, Matthew DJ: Response to bronchial provocation and exercise in children with cystic fibrosis. Clin Allergy 1979;9:563–570.
196. Skorecki K, Levison H, Crozier DN: Bronchial lability in cystic fibrosis. Acta Paediat Scand 1976;65:39–44.
197. Ramsdale EH, Morris MM, Roberts RS, Hargreave FE: Bronchial responsiveness to methacholine in chronic bronchitis. Relationship to airflow obstruction and cold air responsiveness. Thorax 1984;39:912–918.
198. Ramsdell JW, Nachtwey FJ, Moser KM: Bronchial hyperreactivity in chronic obstructive bronchitis. Am Rev Respir Dis 1982;126:829–832.
199. Bahous J, Cartier A, Pineau L, Bernard C, Ghezzo H, Martin RR, Malo JL: Pulmonary function tests and airway responsiveness to methacholine in chronic bronchiectasis of the adult. Bull Eur Physiopathol Respir 1984;20: 375–380.
200. Avital A, Godfrey S, Springer C: Exercise, methacholine, and adenosine 5'-monophosphate challenges in children with asthma. Relation to severity of the disease. Pediatr Pulmonol 2000;30:207–214.
201. Avital A, Picard E, Uwyyed K, Springer C: Comparison of adenosine 5'-monophosphate and methacholine for the differentiation of asthma from chronic airway diseases with the use of the auscultative method in very young children. J Pediatr 1995;127:438–440.
202. Springer C, Godfrey S, Picard E, Uwyyed K, Rotschild M, Hananya S, Noviski N, Avital A: Efficacy and safety of methacholine bronchial challenge performed by auscultation in young asthmatic children. Am J Respir Crit Care Med 2000;162:857–860.
203. Silverman M, Anderson SD: Standardization of exercise tests in asthmatic children. Arch Dis Child 1972;47:882–889.
204. Eggleston PA, Rosenthal RR, Anderson SA, Anderton R, Bierman CW, Bleecker ER, Chai H, Cropp GJ, Johnson JD, Konig P, Morse J, Smith LJ, Summers RJ, Trautlein JJ: Guidelines for the methodology of exercise challenge testing of asthmatics. Study Group on Exercise Challenge, Bronchoprovocation Committee, American Academy of Allergy. J Allergy Clin Immunol 1979;64:642–645.

12 Lung Defenses: Intrinsic, Innate, and Adaptive

James M. Stark, MD • Giuseppe N. Colasurdo, MD

The practice of pediatric pulmonology often includes the child with "too many" respiratory infections. Considering the volume of air (and potential airborne pathogens) transiting the respiratory system daily, the question should actually be "why don't we get more infections?" The conducting airways branch 20 to 25 times between the trachea and the alveoli. The large surface area of the conducting airways and alveolar surfaces (>70 m^2 in the adult) poses a great challenge for the lung defenses. Because many of the particles that settle in the airways are potentially infectious, the airways have evolved several levels of defense to remove or kill these infectious agents. The anatomy of the lung, lung products, cell receptors, and subsequent signaling mechanisms activated, and host cellular responses all contribute to the normal lung defense and disease prevention. A defect in any of these defenses can result in an increased susceptibility to infection in the absence of classic immunodeficiencies. In this chapter we will review several aspects of the lung defenses. First, we will consider the contribution of the airway anatomy, physiology, and secretory products in limiting access of pathogens to the respiratory tract (intrinsic defenses). We will then consider the roles of the various "pattern recognition" proteins and receptors that provide the first line of antimicrobial and inflammatory defenses against invading pathogens (innate defenses) and orchestrate subsequent cellular immunity and antibody development (adaptive defenses). It must be emphasized that while there is a degree of redundancy in the function of the intrinsic, innate, and adaptive responses in the lung, defects in these defenses can "tip the scale" and place the host at increased risk for infection.

INTRINSIC LUNG DEFENSES

AERODYNAMIC FILTERING

The anatomy of the airways and the dichotomous branching of the lower airways make important contributions to the defense of the lungs against infection. The initial barrier is the nose, which acts as an effective filter because of its unusual structure and surface area. Very large particles are filtered by the nasal hairs, and particles larger than 10 μm collect on the surfaces of the turbinates and septum. Accumulation of these large particles is facilitated by their inertia, since they have a high linear velocity and do not easily change direction in the usual airflow. The tonsils and adenoids are strategically located to deal with larger soluble particles by specific local defenses. If the tonsils and adenoids are markedly enlarged, nasal resistance may be increased, resulting in mouth breathing, which bypasses the nasal anatomic defenses. Edema of the turbinates from viral infections or allergies may produce similar effects. Hydrophilic particles are enlarged by humidification of the inspired air, and this facilitates their accumulation in the upper airways.

Particles in the size range of 2 to 10 μm are removed from the airflow by accumulation on the walls of the branching airways beyond the nose and by sedimentation. Sedimentation occurs because the increasing cross-sectional area of the conducting airways leads to a decrease in the linear airflow velocity such that gravitational forces can act on the particles. Particles as small as 0.2 μm may not sediment at all and are exhaled. Particles in the size range of 2 to 0.2 μm generally penetrate the airways and can be deposited on the surface of the alveoli. Particles that are highly soluble are cleared from the lung in the lymphatic circulation. Particles in this size range include many bacteria, fungal spores, and larger (filamentous) viruses. Other physical factors may also be important in particle penetration. For example, an antigen such as *Alternaria* spp., which is 30 μm long and 10 μm wide, may penetrate deep into the lung because of its kitelike shape and efficient aerodynamic qualities. The electrostatic charges of particles may also affect lung penetration. Unipolar charged aerosols in high concentration may be deposited on the airway walls by electrostatic repulsion between the particles. Aerosolized drugs (generated by nebulizers or metered-dose inhalers) use particle size to direct deposition of the medication to different levels of the airway.

AIRWAY REFLEXES

Sneezing, bronchoconstriction, and coughing are airway reflexes that act as nonspecific host defenses. Sneezing is a forceful expulsion of air triggered by receptors in the nose and nasal pharynx that is effective in clearing the upper pharynx and nose. The mechanisms are similar to coughing (described later). Bronchoconstriction may also prevent entry of particles into the distal airways by decreasing airway caliber and redirecting airflow away from the irritated airways. It leads to increased pulmonary resistance, decreasing air velocity in the peripheral airways, thereby increasing the likelihood of sedimentation.

Coughing is a forceful expulsion of air from the lungs that is under both voluntary and involuntary control. The anatomic type of sensory nerves involved in the human cough reflex is unknown, but it seems likely the unmyelinated C fibers and the myelinated irritant receptors containing substance P and calcitonin gene–related peptide are involved.[1] Cough receptors appear to be located within the epithelium of the pharynx, larynx, trachea, and bifurcations of the major bronchi. These receptors can be stimulated by inflammatory mediators, chemical irritants, osmotic stimuli, and mechanical stimulation.

The cough reflex is initiated by stimulation of afferent fibers in the vagus nerve that connect to the cough center in the medulla oblongata in the upper brain stem. Some centrally acting cough suppressants, such as opiates, have their effect at this site. Efferent fibers transmit stimuli along the vagus nerve and spinal cord to the larynx, diaphragm, and abdominal muscles to produce cough.

MECHANICS OF COUGH AND ABNORMALITIES OF THE COUGH REFLEX

There are four important phases to cough that create the high velocities in the upper airway. These flow rates are necessary to create shear rates required to clear mucus from the airway walls and to promote its expulsion through the larynx. The phases of coughing are summarized here:

1. The inspiratory phase is initiated by a deep breath, which is usually 1.5 to 2 times the tidal volume and maximally dilates the respiratory tree.
2. The compression phase begins with closure of the larynx and is followed by contraction of the intercostal muscles and abdominal musculature that rapidly leads to increased intrathoracic pressure. Esophageal pressures can reach levels of 100 to 200 cm H_2O or more in normal adults.
3. The expressive phase is initiated when the glottis opens and high airflows are achieved. Following the glottic opening, the airways may collapse by as much as 80% in tracheal cross-sectional area, and this in turn increases the linear velocity of exhaled gas. Estimated velocities approach 25,000 cm/second (three fourths the speed of sound).
4. The relaxation phase is characterized by a fall in intrathoracic pressure associated with relaxation of the intercostal and abdominal muscles, and temporary bronchodilation.

Abnormalities of this cough mechanism can result in an ineffective cough. Cough receptors are not present in the alveoli or lung parenchyma, so that coughing may be absent in children with extensive alveolar disease or pneumonic consolidation. It is possible that repeated stimulation of cough receptors will eventually lead to a decrease in their sensitivity. This mechanism may explain why cough is sometimes absent in children with gastroesophageal reflux and recurrent aspiration. A decrease in the sensitivity of the cough center occurs in obtunded patients and individuals under the influence of opiates. The efferent nerves can be affected by poliomyelitis or infantile botulism. Muscles of coughing can be affected by neuromuscular diseases such as spinal muscular atrophy or muscular dystrophy leading to inadequate cough clearance of mucus from the airways and increased tendency toward atelectasis. Laryngeal disorders, such as vocal cord paralysis, or the presence of a tracheostomy tube prevent effective laryngeal closure so that the cough can lose its explosive quality and thereby decrease airway clearance. In patients with neuromuscular disorders, the use of cough-assist devices may be useful in enhancing airway clearance caused by decreased muscular force.

MUCUS AND LUNG WATER

Respiratory mucus and mucociliary clearance are a major component of lower respiratory defense. The airways between the larynx and the respiratory bronchioles are lined by ciliated columnar epithelium and covered by an airway surface liquid (ASL) layer 5 to 100 μm thick. With the advent of the capacity to fix or measure ASL in vivo and the development of well-differentiated human airway epithelial cultures that exhibit mucus transport in vitro, it has become possible to investigate the microanatomy of mucus transport in humans.[2] ASL has been described to consist of two distinct layers: the sol or periciliary liquid (PCL) layer adjacent to the epithelial surface, and the gel or surface mucus layer that appears to float on top of the sol layer. The PCL layer is a mucus-free zone at the cell surface approximately the height of the cilia. This layer is crucial because it provides a low-viscosity solution in which the cilia can beat rapidly (8–15 Hz) and shields the epithelial surface from the overlying mucus layer. The mucus layer consists of high molecular weight, heavily glycosylated macromolecules that are the products of at least two distinct genes (*MUC5AC* and *MUC5B*) that form tangled networks of polymers. Mucus glycoproteins are polymeric macromolecules with a protein core and branching oligosaccharide side chains that account for most the viscoelastic properties of normal mucus. Although cysteine accounts for less than 1% of the amino acid protein core, sulfhydryl bonds contribute to the polymerization of the glycoprotein and to the resulting viscous qualities of the mucus. The properties of this mucin gel are the product of the mucin and water contents, concentrations of monovalent and divalent ions, and the pH of the ASL. ASL water content is controlled by regulating levels of ion transport: Na^+ reabsorption and Cl^- secretion by the respiratory epithelial cell, with passive movement of water across the epithelial layer in response to ion transport. Dysregulation of both Na^+ and Cl^- contribute to the mucus and mucociliary transport abnormalities seen in cystic fibrosis (CF). Finally, in inflammatory states, large macromolecules such as DNA and polymerized actin from white cells can be present in large amounts and alter the viscoelastic properties of the mucus.

Mucus provides several important airway defense functions, including (1) a covering sheet that entraps particulate matter and microorganisms, (2) a movable medium that can be propelled by cilia (the tips of cilia drive the gel layer over the sol layer toward the oropharynx), (3) a waterproofing layer that acts to reduce fluid loss through the airways, and (4) a medium that transports essential secreted substances such as enzymes, defensins, collectins, antiproteases, and immunoglobulins (see later). The diversity of the carbohydrate side chains of the mucin macromolecules results, in effect, in a library of carbohydrate sequences that can provide binding to an enormous repertoire of particles that land on the mucus layer.[3]

Ciliary beat frequency and the effectiveness of the ciliary beat are primary determinants of clearance rate. Movement of the ASL on airway surfaces involves two steps: First, the ciliary power stroke acts to move the mucus layer unidirectionally on the airway surface; second, the frictional interaction of the mucus layer with the PCL allows this underlying layer to travel along with the overlying mucus. Ciliary dysfunction can therefore greatly diminish mucus clearance. Moreover, the physical properties of the ASL not only affect mucociliary clearance, but, along with the viscosity of mucus, they also alter the efficiency of airway clearance by cough (see earlier). The lubricating function of the PCL facilitates mucus movement along airway surfaces in response to coughing. In addition, the deficiency or absence of PCL allows adhesive interactions between the mobile mucins and mucus, and the airway epithelial cell surface mucins, effectively "tethering" the mucus and reducing the efficiency of cough in mucus clearance.

The mechanisms regulating the basal secretion of mucus and mucociliary clearance rates are unclear, as are the mechanisms regulating mucus clearance rates in response to airway stress. There is no efferent cholinergic innervation of the superficial airway epithelium. Moreover, tachykinin-mediated neural systems are present predominantly in the upper airways in humans, making it unlikely that these neural mechanisms regulate lung mucus production or transport. Systemic hormonal responses, such as response to epinephrine, have response times too long for it to accomplish this function. There is evidence supporting autocrine/paracrine airway epithelial signaling via 5′ nucleotides in the regulation of epithelial ion transport, ciliary beat frequency, and mucus secretion.[4] These data suggest that nucleotide release, in response to both ambient conditions and cough-induced shear stress, regulates mucus clearance rates.

DISORDERS OF THE MUCOCILIARY SYSTEM

Primary ciliary dyskinesia is a genetic disease associated with a defective ciliary structure and function, with resultant chronic otosinopulmonary disease, male infertility, and (in about half of patients) situs inversus. Two disease-causing mutations have been identified in the *DNAH1* (the human intermediate chain dynein) and *DNAH5* (human heavy chain dynein) genes.[5] Measurements of mucociliary clearance in patients with primary ciliary dyskinesia have revealed no basal, cilia-dependent mucus clearance, although cough-dependent clearance is nearly normal.[2] These patients maintain a nearly normal mucus clearance rate by increasing the dependence on cough. As a result, these patients exhibit milder airway disease than seen in CF (see later) and typically live into middle age.

Cystic fibrosis results from mutations in the respiratory epithelial inducible chloride channel (CFTR).[6] In patients with CF, mucus transport appears to be significantly altered by depletion of an isotonic ASL as the result of mutations in *CFTR*. Under basal conditions, Na^+ absorption by the normal respiratory epithelium regulates ASL volume; when ASL volumes are depleted, the airway epithelia can slow Na^+ absorption and increase Cl^- secretion. In CF, the airway epithelium has an accelerated basal rate of Na^+ and volume absorption that results from the absence of tonic inhibitory effects of CFTR on the epithelial Na^+ channel. In addition, the CF epithelium lacks active Cl^- transport through CFTR functioning as a Cl^- channel. These defects in Na^+ and Cl^- transport result in volume depletion on the airway surfaces, which, in turn, depletes the PCL, disrupts normal ciliary motion, and inhibits mucociliary clearance. Moreover, depletion of the PCL allows mucins in the mucus layer (MUC5AC and MUC5B) to contact mucins on the surface of the respiratory epithelium (MUC1 and MUC4), allowing molecular interactions that effectively "glue" the mucins together and further disrupt mucus clearance. This dual effect of PCL depletion and mucin tethering may partially explain differences in severity of lung disease between patients with primary ciliary dyskinesia and CF.[2]

INNATE LUNG DEFENSES

Innate immunity is an ancient system that provides multicellular organisms with the capability of immediate defense against a wide variety of pathogens (bacteria, fungi, viruses) without previous exposure. Hallmarks of this system are many capabilities: (1) recognition of structures present on a wide variety of pathogens that are distinct from self; (2) provision of early activation of host defenses and effector mechanisms that can destroy the pathogen within hours; (3) stimulation of the production of inflammatory cytokines and chemokines that recruit and activate other immune cells; (4) orchestration of the development of adaptive immune responses. The rapid inflammatory responses that follow exposure to infectious agents can be reproduced in the absence of traditional adaptive immune responses. Alexander Flemming first described the presence of antimicrobial substances in human secretions almost 80 years ago. Activation of cytokine expression within the lung can initiate a cascade of events resulting in cellular sequestration, recruitment, and activation at the site of infection. Several of these receptors function not only as adhesion proteins but also as receptors for various complement components. A new family of proteins has been described more recently: the Toll-like receptors (TLRs). The TLRs exhibit the ability both to recognize conserved patterns of molecular structures on pathogens (pathogen-associated molecular patterns [PAMPs]) and to activate a cascade of intracellular proinflammatory signals. A number of secreted proteins contribute to innate lung defenses. These include lectin-like proteins (collectin family) and antibiotic proteins secreted by a number of cell types within the lung. Together, these defenses protect the lung during the early phases of microbial invasion, before adaptive responses can contribute to the host defense.

COMPLEMENT

Several serum proteins reach the lung through transudation in response to inflammation, including the complement family and immunoglobulins (IgG, IgM, etc.; discussed later). The complement protein cascade is activated by two independent pathways: the classic pathway that is activated by antigen-antibody complexes (involving IgG or IgM) and the alternative pathway that is activated by foreign carbohydrates, such as bacterial and fungal components. The complement system functions to coat foreign particles with opsonin via the alternative pathway, thus making the particles more likely to be phagocytosed, to activate phagocytic cells by the local release of chemotactic agents such as C5a, and to lyse cells through the activation of the late complement components C5 through C9 (the membrane attack complex). Other important aspects of the complement pathway are the generation of anaphylatoxins, such as C3a and C5a, that cause the release of vasoactive mediators from mast cells, and the generation of C3b and C4 on the cell surface, where they interact with specific receptors on phagocytic cells.[7]

Complement deficiency is associated with recurrent infections, glomerulonephritis, or collagen vascular diseases such as systemic lupus erythematosus. Early complement deficiencies are associated with lupus, glomerulonephritis, or other rheumatologic diseases. Pneumonia has been described in association with C1 deficiency, although bacterial meningitis is a more common manifestation. Pneumonia complicated by empyema, pneumatoceles, and liver abscesses has been described as a consequence of C1r deficiency. Autoimmune disorders are associated with both C2 and C4 deficiency, although bacterial infections also occur in children with C2 deficiency (the most common complement deficiency). C3 deficiency (clinically the most severe and least common of the complement deficiencies) is associated with both autoimmune disorders and recurrent infections. C3 acts as an opsonizing agent and plays roles in both the classical and alternative pathways. C3 deficiency results in otitis media, pneumonia, sepsis, meningitis, and osteomyelitis, most commonly caused by *Streptococcus pneumoniae*, *Neisseria meningitidis*, *Klebsiella* spp., *Escherichia coli*, and *Streptococcus pyogenes*. C5 deficiency produces a complex defect due to the loss of chemotactic and anaphylatoxin activities; it leads to decreased lung clearance of *S. pneumoniae* but not *Staphylococcus aureus* in C5-deficient mice. The late complement deficiencies (C5–C9) impair serum bactericidal and cytolytic activities. This increases susceptibility to systemic infection with encapsulated organisms such as *N. meningitidis* and *S. pneumoniae*; however, pulmonary infections are relatively uncommon.

Defects of the alternative pathway of complement activity are very uncommon. Properdin factor deficiency usually is associated with infection with *N. meningitidis* but is also associated with pneumonia. Deficiency of factor H or I, regulatory proteins of both pathways, leads to autoimmune disorders and recurrent infections with *S. pneumoniae* and *Haemophilus influenzae*.

Most defects of complement synthesis are inherited as autosomal-recessive disorders with the exception of properdin deficiency, which is an X-linked condition. Symptoms do not usually occur unless the child is homozygous for the deficiency except in C2 and C4 deficiencies, in which the heterozygote may be symptomatic.

ADHESION PROTEINS

Adhesion and migration of circulating inflammatory cells (or their progenitors) are integral to cell recruitment and activation response to injury. Three major families of adhesion molecules participate in these processes in the lung: the immunoglobulin superfamily, the integrins, and the selectins (Table 12-1).

The immunoglobulin superfamily is a group of polypeptide genes characterized by the presence of one or more regions homologous to the basic structural unit of the immunoglobulin gene. Immunoglobulins and the T-cell receptors (TCRs) are the only members of this family that undergo somatic diversification for antigen recognition. These receptors can function as single peptide chains (e.g., intercellular adhesion molecule-1, CD4, leukocyte function-associated antigen 3) or may need to be associated as polypeptides for activity (TCRs, immunoglobulins, major histocompatibility complex [MHC] class I and II receptors, CD8). Several members of the immunoglobulin superfamily are involved in cell-cell adhesion and antigen presentation to T cells by several cell types discussed later. These adhesive interactions can be simple pairwise interactions or complex interactions involving several families of receptors as occurs in antigen presentation (the "immune synapse").

The integrins are a family of diverse molecules with a common structure that are involved in cell-substrate or cell-cell interactions. Members of this family are composed of two noncovalently associated polypeptide chains (α and β). Subgroups of this family are defined by common, shared β chains. β_1-integrins function primarily by interacting with matrix components (collagen, laminin, fibronectin). β_2-integrins (heterodimers of CD11a and CD18) are expressed almost exclusively on leukocytes and mediate cell-cell adhesion[8] (see Table 12-1). Leukocyte function-associated antigen 1 (LFA-1) is expressed by virtually all immune cells, with the exception of some tissue macrophages. Mac-1 and p150,95 are found on macrophages, monocytes, granulocytes, and some lymphocytes. The central role of the β_2-integrins in inflammation is demonstrated in patients with leukocyte adhesion deficiency, an inherited syndrome characterized by recurrent or progressive bacterial infections of skin and soft tissue, diminished pus formation, impaired wound healing, and delayed umbilical cord loss.[9] Despite systemic granulocytosis, granulocytes (pus) are absent in areas of infection, suggesting defective migration from vascular to extravascular sites. The disease phenotype and functional abnormalities affecting neutrophils and lymphocytes result from deficiency in CD18 production.

The selectin family of adhesion molecules mediates adhesion between leukocytes and vascular endothelium.[10] Three structurally related molecules have been identified: E-selectin, P-selectin, and L-selectin. E-selectin is expressed on endothelial cells following stimulation by cytokines such as interleukin-1 (IL-1) or tumor necrosis factor (TNF-α), and supports neutrophil adhesion. L-selectin is expressed on all leukocytes and is shed by

TABLE 12-1. Families of adhesion molecules in the lung

Immunoglobulin Superfamily	Integrins	Selectins
Members share the immunoglobulin domain structure.	Members consist of noncovalently associated heterodimers of two chains (α and β).	Consist of an extracellular signal sequence, a lectin-like domain, an epidermal growth factor–like domain, several short consensus repeats, and a membrane anchor.
Only immunoglobulins and the TCR undergo specific somatic diversification.	Responsible for interactions between cells, and between cells and matrix proteins (fibronectin, collagen).	Require Ca^{2+} for adhesion.
Peptides can be paired or unpaired.	Require divalent cations (Mg^{2+}, Mn^{2+}, Ca^{2+}).	Recognize and adhere to carbohydrate moieties like lectins.
Examples	**Examples**	**Examples**
Immunoglobulins	β_2-integrins:	ELAM-1
TCR (CD3)	LFA-1 (CD11a/CD18)	LECAM-1
MHC class I	Mac-1 (CD11b/CD18)	GMP-140
MHC class II	p150,95 (CD11c/CD18)	
ICAM-1 (CD54)	β_1-integrins:	
ICAM-2	VLA-4 ($\alpha 4\beta 1$, CD49d/CD29)	
VCAM-1	VLA-5 (fibronectin receptor, CD49c/CD29)	

ELAM-1, E-selection; GMP-140, P-selectin; ICAM-1, intercellular cell adhesion molecule 1; ICAM-2, intercellular cell adhesion molecule 2; LECAM-1, L-selectin; LFA-1, leukocyte function-associated antigen 1; MHC, major histocompatibility complex; TCR, T-cell receptor; VCAM-1, vascular cell adhesion molecule 1.

neutrophils following adhesion to endothelial cells. P-selectin mediates cellular adhesion of neutrophils and monocytes to activated platelets and endothelial cells. The N-terminal ends of these molecules are homologous and related to a number of calcium-dependent carbohydrate lectin molecules. The selectins also have similar lectin-binding ligands, which contain sialyl Lewis x and sialyl Lewis a antigens.

In addition to their role in orchestrating binding to cellular surfaces, adhesion proteins can function as pattern recognition binding receptors, working together with other cellular proteins to bind and internalize ligands. Moreover, the β_2-integrins function as complement receptors. Therefore, these proteins are capable of mediating migration of inflammatory cells into the airway and activation of these cells once they arrive.

TOLL-LIKE RECEPTORS

The Toll-like receptors are an ancient family of receptor proteins that have been evolutionally conserved and expressed in insects *(Drosophila)* and higher animals (humans). The TLRs play a central role in the initiation of cellular innate immune responses. A total of 10 human TLRs have been described. The TLR proteins have two functional regions. The extracellular domain (consisting of leucine-rich repeats and one or two cysteine-rich regions) recognizes an array of microbial components: sugars, proteins, lipids, DNA motifs, and double-stranded RNA. The intracellular region contains a Toll/IL-1 receptor domain, similar to the intracellular domain of the IL-1 receptor. The Toll/IL-1 receptor domain provides an intracellular scaffold that interacts with a number of "adapter" proteins to initiate and integrate well-defined signaling cascades resulting in cellular activation, and the production of a number of cytokines and chemokines.[11] Various TLRs are expressed on cell types involved in the first-line, innate immune defenses such as macrophages, neutrophils, and airway epithelial cells (Table 12-2). In addition, TLRs are expressed on macrophages, dendritic cells (DCs), and B and T lymphocytes, contributing to the adaptive immune responses that develop.

The individual TLR proteins have been found to associate as homodimers of identical protein chains and as heterodimers of different TLR proteins. These heterodimers exhibit different binding properties from those of parent chains, thereby extending the target repertoire of this relatively small family of proteins.[12] Table 12-2 demonstrates the types of ligands bound by the TLRs. These proteins utilize a variety of co-receptor molecules to further extend the versatility of the receptors. For example, TLR2 and TLR4 interact with MD-2 (soluble extracellular protein) and CD14 in binding with lipopolysaccharide (LPS).[13] Several additional immune recognition receptors are thought to cooperate with TLRs in response to products of pathogens. Dectin-1 (a lectin) is a major phagocytic receptor recognizing β-1,3-D-glucans thought to interact with TLR2 in binding and inflammatory response by macrophages or DCs to zymosan. Nucleotide oligomerization domain-2 (NOD2) is a cytosolic protein that recognizes muramyl dipeptide, a repeating structure in bacterial peptidoglycans. NOD2 is thought to amplify TLR-mediated signaling following LPS exposure. B-cell receptor binding to DNA-antigen complexes amplifies signaling in B cells following TLR9-DNA interactions. DC-SIGN is a lectin receptor that has been implicated in down-regulating the induction of IL-12 by TLRs. TLR interactions with Fcγ receptors has also been suggested.

In addition to inducing the production of inflammatory mediators such as TNF-α and IL-12, activation of TLRs has been implicated in the up-regulation of microbial killing mechanisms, including production of nitric oxide. In addition, differential TLR expression and signaling in different DC populations drive T-cell differentiation into a T-helper type 1 (Th1) or type 2 (Th2) phenotype. Thus, TLR-TLR and TLR–adapter protein interactions determine the specificity and activation properties of the interactions of the TLRs with their ligands.[11]

Toll-like receptor–mediated intracellular signaling has been shown to involve several intracellular pathways that result in the activation of nuclear transcription factors NF-κB, AP-1, and IRF-3, which, in turn, activate the transcription of messenger RNAs coding for several cytokines and chemokines.

TABLE 12-2. Toll-like receptors and their ligands

TLR	Cells Expressing	Ligand	Source
TLR1/TLR2	A, B, D, E, MC, MP, N, NK, PD, T	Triacylated lipoproteins	Bacteria
TLR2	A, D, MC, MP, N, T	Peptidoglycan, lipoteichoic acid	Gram-positive bacteria
		Glycolipids	Spirochetes
		Zymosan	Yeast
		HSP60, HSP70, HSPGp96	Host
TLR3	A, D, NK, PD	dsRNA	Viruses
TLR4	A, D, E, MC, MP, N, NK, PD	LPS, LTA	Gram-negative bacteria
		F protein	RSV
		HSP69, HSP70, HSPGp96, fibronectin	Host
TLR5	A, D, MP, N, T	Flagellin	Bacteria with flagella
TLR6/TLR2	A, B, D, E, MC, N	Diacylated lipoprotein	*Mycoplasma*
TLR7	B, E, MP, N, PD	Imidazoquinolines	Chemicals
TLR8	E, MP, N	?	
TLR9	D, E, N, PD, T	Unmethylated CpG DNA	Bacteria, viruses, insects
		Chromatin-IgG complexes	Host
TLR10	B, E, N, PD, T	?	

A, epithelial cells; B, B cells; D, dendritic cells; E, eosinophil; HSP, heat shock protein; LPS, lipopolysaccharide; LTA, lipoteichoic acid; MC, mast cells; MP, macrophages; N, neutrophils; NK, natural killer T cell; PD, plasmacytoid dendritic cells; RSV, respiratory syncytial virus; T, T-cells.

The expression of these proteins initiates the biologic and physiologic responses of the cell toward the invading pathogen. The best studied of these cascades is the interaction of the Toll/IL-1 receptor domain of the TLR with the adapter molecule MyD88, which links TLRs and other members of the IL-1 receptor family to the IL receptor–associated kinase family (described in Chapter 5). Activation of this family ultimately results in the phosphorylation of IκB, which then allows NF-κB nuclear translocation and the transcription of a number of proinflammatory genes (including those encoding TNF-α, IL-1, and IL-6).[14] TLR activation can also result in a MyD88-independent activation of the interferon regulatory factor IRF-3, followed by translocation to the nucleus and the transcriptional up-regulation of interferon-β (IFN-β) production. Other signaling adapters have been identified (TIRAP, TRIF) that contribute to the MyD88-dependent and MyD88-independent pathways.[13] Therefore, differential cytokine expression and cell activation depends on the presence of the receptor and its adapter proteins, the signaling cascade involved, and the presence of the various adapter proteins, which can vary with cell type and stage of differentiation.

Although the specific mechanisms involved in the regulation of TLR expression are not well understood, cytokines and growth factors appear to play important roles. Factors reported to affect TLR expression include IFN-γ, IL-1β, TNF-α, IL-2, IL-4, IL-15, granulocyte-macrophage colony-stimulating factor (GM-CSF), macrophage colony-stimulating factor, and macrophage migration inhibitory factor. Table 12-2 demonstrates differences in the cellular expression of the TLRs in various lung inflammatory cells. Note that there are different arrays of TLRs expressed by the different cell types. In addition, TLR expression levels are different in the various cell types listed. There are other differences in the levels of individual TLR expression that can vary with the stage of differentiation of an individual cell type. Finally, the cytokine and inflammatory milieu alters a cell's response to TLR activation. All of these features—the array of cells, the levels of TLR expression, the stage of development, and the cytokine environment—alter the quantity and responsiveness of these receptors, and the overall effects of innate TLR activation on the development of both innate and adaptive immune responses.

COLLECTINS

The collectins are members of a superfamily of collagenous, calcium-dependent (C-type) lectins. The family included mannose-binding lectin (also known as mannose-binding protein), and surfactant-associated proteins A and D (SP-A and SP-D, respectively). As part of the innate immune system, the collectins have a key role as first line of defense against invading microorganisms. We will briefly discuss the role of SP-A and SP-D in innate lung defenses in this chapter. More in-depth discussion of these pulmonary collectins can be found in Chapter 2 of this text.

Lung collectins are synthesized by alveolar type II cells and subsets of bronchiolar epithelial cells. Both SP-A and SP-D are secreted into the airspaces by alveolar type II cells. However, nonciliated bronchiolar cells contain secretory granules containing SP-A and SP-D, suggesting these cells also secrete collectins into the airway. The basic functional unit of collectins is a trimer of proteins. In the monomeric subunit there are four functional domains: the N-terminal cysteine-rich domain, a collagen domain, a coiled-coil neck domain, and a C-terminal C-type lectin domain (also known as a carbohydrate recognition domain). Selective binding of collectins to specific complex carbohydrates is mediated by the carbohydrate recognition domain and requires calcium. Human SP-A is assembled as heterotrimers or homotrimers of two genetically different chain types, whereas SP-D is assembled as homotrimers. Multimerization of the trimers influences the binding affinity and ligand selectivity of SP-A and SP-D. SP-A preferentially forms hexamers of trimeric units ($6 \times 3 = 18$ chains), whereas SP-D forms tetramers ($4 \times 3 = 12$ chains).[15] This N-terminal association and cross-linking of the trimeric subunits permits bridging between spatially separated ligands via the C-terminal lectin domains, increasing binding affinity and specificity.

SP-A and SP-D bind to a variety of polysaccharides, phospholipids, and glycolipid ligands. SP-A binds to polysaccharides containing *N*-acetylmannosamine or mannose preferentially to glucose, and the surfactant lipid dipalmatoylphosphatidylcholine. SP-D shows preferential binding to polysaccharides containing inositol, maltose, and glucose preferentially to mannose, and the surfactant lipid phosphatidylinositol.[15] The three-dimensional trimeric and oligomeric structures give SP-A and SP-D additional orders of specificity for particulate antigens and invading pathogens. Several carbohydrate recognition domains in the collectin oligomer can simultaneously bind to different ligands on a single polysaccharide chain, increasing the binding avidity of the complex to greater levels than could be attained by binding to single ligands. SP-A and SP-D interact with a variety of gram-negative and gram-positive organisms, fungi (*Aspergillus fumigatus*, *Cryptococcus neoformans*, and *Candida albicans*), *Pneumocystis carinii*, several respiratory viruses including respiratory syncytial virus, influenza A virus, and cytomegalovirus, and *Mycobacterium tuberculosis*. SP-A and SP-D interact with the glycoconjugate and/or lipid moieties present on invading pathogens and with receptors on host cells and, through these interactions, provide a number of host defense functions. First, they can agglutinate microorganisms by formation of bridges between various carbohydrate ligands on the cell surface. Mannose-binding lectin can lead to activation of the complement cascade, whereas SP-A can bind C1q, preventing the formation of active complement complex. Lung collectins can lead to opsonization through activation of complement and deposition of C3 (mannose-binding lectin) or directly opsonized microorganisms (SP-A and SP-D). Opsonization mediated by SP-A can lead to stimulation of phagocytosis and killing of pathogens. However, some organisms can increase their efficiency of infection by using SP-A as a Trojan horse to gain entry into cells. SP-A and SP-D can alter viral infectivity, presumably by blocking binding of virus to their surface receptors or by enhancing cellular uptake and killing. Finally, SP-A and SP-D can alter the permeability of bacterial and fungal cell membranes, resulting in enhanced cell killing.[16]

Several cell surface receptors have been described for SP-A and SP-D, but few have been characterized to the point of understanding how collectin-receptor interactions lead to cellular responses. SPR-210 (surfactant protein receptor, 210 kd) is the best-characterized SP-A receptor. It is found on type II cells and alveolar macrophages. C1q receptors bind mannose-binding lectin and SP-A, although their presence and function in the lung are unclear. SP-A has been found to interact with CD14 and TLR4, suggesting a role of SP-A in LPS-mediated cell responses. In addition, the SP-A–TLR4 interactions may be important in the uptake of respiratory syncytial virus–F protein in the lung. Gp340 is an SP-D binding protein belonging to the family of scavenger receptors (see later) that may also bind SP-A. SP-D has also been shown to interact with CD14 and function in the modulation of LPS-elicited cytokine release. The mode of signaling through these receptors and the role of SP-A and SP-D in this signaling is currently under investigation.[16]

In addition to their roles in binding to microorganisms or their products, collectins have several other activities. They are anti-inflammatory, functioning in the regulation of responses to LPS and other microbial products, uptake of apoptotic cells, and modulation of oxidant metabolism and metalloproteinase expression. Collectins are immunomodulatory, decreasing proliferative responses of T cells and altering signaling via TLRs. Collectins are proinflammatory, enhancing migration or airspace retention of phagocytes. Finally, SP-A and SP-D play roles in surfactant homeostasis, helping to regulate cellular uptake and metabolism of surfactant lipid and altering the spatial organization of surfactant lipid. Therefore, SP-A and SP-D play key roles in both the innate and adaptive immune responses in the lung.[15]

ANTIMICROBIAL PEPTIDES

Recent studies have confirmed Alexander Flemming's observations made almost 80 years ago that human airway secretions possess intrinsic microbicidal and microbistatic properties. These activities lie in several cationic polypeptide constituents: lysozyme, lactoferrin, secretory leukoprotease inhibitor, and neutrophil and epithelial defensins. These antimicrobial proteins and peptides differ in their molecular specificity and mechanisms of action: acting as hydrolyzing enzymes, creating pores in the bacterial wall, or chelating iron. They would therefore be expected to act cooperatively and possibly synergistically against a broad spectrum of organisms, making it unlikely that these organisms would develop resistance to the group.

Lysozyme is one of the most abundant antimicrobial proteins (14 kd) in the airways, with concentrations estimated at 0.1 to 1 mg/mL, levels sufficient to kill important pulmonary pathogens such as *S. aureus* and *Pseudomonas aeruginosa*. Lysozyme damages the walls of bacteria and fungi by hydrolyzing the β1-4 glycosidic bond between *N*-acetylmuramic acid and *N*-acetylglucosamine, which are structural components of bacterial peptidoglycan and fungal chitin.[17] In humans, lysozyme is secreted predominantly by the serous cells of submucosal glands in the conducting airways, and, to a lesser extent, by airway epithelial cells and alveolar macrophages. It is also a component of both phagocytic and secretory granules of neutrophils. Its role in defending the human lungs from infection is still unclear, but recent studies in rodents suggest it is an important component of the respiratory defenses.[17]

Lactoferrin is an iron-binding protein present in secretions such as tears, saliva, and bronchial secretions. It is present in ASL at concentrations similar to those of lysozyme (0.1–1 mg/mL). It is produced by the submucosal glands and neutrophils, and has activity against both gram-positive and gram-negative bacteria, as well as *Candida* spp. It binds iron and sequesters it from microorganisms. Lactoferrin is an iron-binding glycoprotein found in exocrine secretions of mammals and released from neutrophil granules during inflammation. Lactoferrin's antimicrobial actions result from chelation of iron, which is required by many bacteria for optimal growth, or by destabilization of bacterial membranes.[18] Some of the antimicrobial activities of lactoferrin are related to its ability to bind LPS with high affinity. Indeed, recent in vitro studies indicate that lactoferrin is able to compete with the LPS-binding protein for LPS binding and prevent the transfer of LPS to CD14 present at the surface of monocytes.[19]

Secretory leukoprotease inhibitor is a 12-kd protein about 10-fold less abundant than lysozyme and lactoferrin in ASL. The N-terminal domain has modest activity against both gram-positive and gram-negative organisms. The C-terminal domain is an effective inhibitor of neutrophil elastase.

Human defensins are present in bronchoalveolar lavage (BAL) fluid from uninflamed lungs at a concentration of about 100 ng/mL. However, in the inflamed airways these concentrations are increased to about 1 μg/mL. Expression of defensins (peptides 3–5 kd in size) is modulated locally by inflammation. Although 20 potentially expressed genes have been identified by the Human Genome Project, relatively few proteins have been isolated and characterized. Four human neutrophil peptides (HNP-1 through HNP-4) are located in neutrophil azurophilic granules (HNP-4 is less abundant than the other three). Two other defensins (HD-5 and HD-6) are located in gastrointestinal epithelial cells. Three recently characterized defensins (HBD-1, HBD-2, and HBD-3) are β-defensins, differing from the neutrophil defensins in the organization of their cysteines. All three of these defensins are detectable in the respiratory epithelium and are inducible by LPS and cytokines. The defensins are microbicidal under low-salt conditions.

Calthecidins are members of a family of peptides with a conserved N-terminal region of 100 amino acid residues and a heterogeneous C-terminal region (10–40 amino acid residues). The human peptide LL-37 displays LPS-binding activity and broad-spectrum microbicidal activity.

CELLULAR DEFENSES: AT THE CROSSROADS OF INNATE AND ADAPTIVE IMMUNITY

INFLAMMATORY CELLS IN THE LUNG

Our knowledge of the cellular constituents in the lung, their activation state, and their function have been considerably augmented in the last 20 years by the ability to safely perform flexible fiberoptic bronchoscopy and biopsy in both control subjects and clinical patients. Using BAL, the "normal" cellular constituents of the alveolar space have been determined in a number of studies in both adults and children. Macrophages are the major cellular component of BAL fluid, constituting 81% to 95% of the cells obtained. The remainder of the cells is made up of lymphocytes, neutrophils, and eosinophils, whose total cell numbers and percentage composition vary greatly with disease state. Data obtained from BAL and biopsy studies provide direct evidence of the role of inflammatory cells, adhesion molecules, and cellular mediators in humans, and confirm cell culture and animal studies. This technique is discussed in further detail in Chapter 7.

THE RESPIRATORY EPITHELIUM

The airway epithelium is more than a passive barrier to airway water loss or a passive fortification against bacterial and viral infection. Published data support the active participation of the airway epithelium in the regulation of airway smooth muscle tone, the physical removal of inhaled substances through ciliary clearance, and secreting or transporting broad-spectrum antimicrobial substances. Finally, the respiratory epithelium is a functional interface between the pathogen and innate or adaptive immune response. This makes the airway epithelium a pivotal structure in respiratory physiology and pathology.

The respiratory epithelium participates in "passive" lung immunity in many different ways. The epithelium presents a physical barrier to viral and bacterial invasion, lining the respiratory tract from the nose to the alveoli with a wide range of cell phenotypes.[20,21] Ciliated epithelial cells are important in moving mucus up the airway, thereby removing particulate material, and injury to these by agents such as oxidants can alter ability to remove mucus from the airway. Tracheobronchial glands and goblet cells are important sources of airway mucus, which serves to nonspecifically trap particulates (see earlier). The respiratory epithelium also serves functions in the regulation of water and ion movement into the airway mucus.[2] The respiratory epithelium serves as its own reservoir for injury repair, presumably using the basal cell layers for progenitor cells.[21] Finally, the respiratory epithelium serves to regulate airway smooth muscle tone through several mechanisms, thereby restricting ventilation to injured areas. Through the mechanisms listed earlier, the respiratory epithelium helps nonspecifically to protect the lung from inhaled toxins or microorganisms.

Additionally, the respiratory epithelium performs more specific interactions with the innate and adaptive immune systems. Alveolar type II cells manufacture SP-A and SP-D (described in more detail later).[15,22] The respiratory epithelium can also be induced to produce a number of bioactive cytokines, including IL-1, IL-6, IL-8, GM-CSF, and RANTES (for "regulated upon activation, normal T-cell expressed and secreted"[23]; discussed in greater detail in Chapter 5 of this text). The respiratory epithelium also can up-regulate expression of several adhesion molecules (see later) that support interactions between the epithelial cell and inflammatory cells recruited to the lung, including neutrophils, eosinophils, and lymphocytes. Epithelial cells metabolize arachidonic acid and produce a number of bioactive eicosanoids either directly or through transcellular metabolism with airway inflammatory cells. Moreover, the respiratory epithelium is able to respond to a number of inflammatory mediators with production of cytokines and adhesion molecules. Bacterial or viral binding to TLRs on the epithelial surface can result in activation of NF-κB or other transcription factors, as well as signal cytokine production and expression of new cellular receptors on the epithelial surface, facilitating interaction with inflammatory cells with protective, or potentially injurious, consequences. The inflammation resulting from airway injury is thought to be responsible for the airway hyperresponsiveness and obstruction that accompanies a number of diseases, such as asthma.

RESIDENT CELL DEFENSES: AT THE INTERFACE OF INNATE AND ADAPTIVE IMMUNITY

Three major groups of inflammatory cells reside primarily within the lung parenchyma itself: mast cells, DCs, and macrophages. Although these cells are recruited and expand from bone marrow–derived precursors, and (particularly in the case of macrophages) are capable of some degree of migration, they reside primarily within the lung itself. Other inflammatory cells are recruited from the circulation in their mature form (neutrophils, eosinophils, and lymphocytes) and, once activated, are capable of their mature functions.

Mast Cells

Mast cells and basophils have long been recognized as the major effector cells of allergic reactions, by virtue of their expression of the high-affinity Fc receptors for immunoglobulin E (IgE) ($Fc_{\varepsilon}RI$) and the vast array of mediators they produce. They share a number of properties: (1) similar staining of cytoplasmic granules; (2) synthesis of chemical mediators; (3) expression of $Fc_{\varepsilon}RI$; (4) activation of the cells resulting in degranulation or exocytosis, with release of both preformed and newly generated chemical mediators. Despite these similarities, mast cells and basophils are clearly different: Basophils differentiate and mature in the bone marrow and are found primarily in the circulation. In contrast, mast cells are distributed throughout normal tissues throughout the body in close proximity to blood vessels and do not circulate in the blood. Both cell types are found in both atopic and nonatopic subjects, and can synthesize and release cytokines in response to both IgE-mediated and non-IgE-mediated stimuli. It has been postulated that they play a role in host defense against parasites, in wound healing, in immunoregulation, and in tumor angiogenesis. Therefore, though small in number, mast cells and basophils play an important role in health and disease.

Human mast cells have been demonstrated to originate in the bone marrow from $CD34^+$ c-Kit^+CD13^+ progenitor cells. Early mast cell differentiation can occur in bone marrow–derived cells grown in the presence of recombinant human IL-3 (although IL-3 alone cannot lead to complete mature mast cell maturation). However, $CD34^+$ precursor cells cultured with fibroblasts (stromal cells) mature to IgE receptor-positive, tryptase-positive mast cells with granular morphologic patterns found in mature human tissue mast cells. Subsequently, these fibroblasts (stromal cells) have been demonstrated to produce mast cell growth factor/stem cell factor, which reacts with the receptor c-Kit located on the surface of the $CD34^+$ progenitor cells.[24] Acquisition of IgE receptors appears to occur early in mast cell development.

Mast cells originate from bone marrow stem cells and reside in connective tissues and at mucosal surfaces, but they cannot be morphologically identified in the peripheral circulation. The means by which mast cells home into tissues is unclear. Presumably, the first point of interaction with the target tissue or organ occurs between the mast cell and the vascular endothelium, and subsequently between mast cells and interstitial components such as collagen, laminin, and fibronectin. Although there are limited data on mast cell adhesion molecules involved in the specific endothelium or lymphocyte interactions, several known adhesion molecules have been described on the mast cell surface. These include β_2-integrins such as leukocyte function-associated antigen 1 (CD11a/CD18), Mac-1 (CD11b/CD18), and p150,95 (CD11c/CD18), β_1-integrins (CD49d/CD29), the laminin receptor (CD49f/CD29), and others.[24] In fact, mast cell adherence to laminin appears to be the major mechanism of cell retention in the subendothelial interstitium. Once recruited from the circulation, mast cells acquire their mature phenotype in the tissue microenvironment. Several cytokines produced by fibroblasts (primarily IL-3 and stem cell factor) determine the final mast cell phenotype (tissue vs. mucosal mast cells). Once in the interstitial spaces, several other cytokines influence the production of a number of serine proteases, which differ between mast cell phenotypes (mucosal vs. serosal).

IgE Receptor

Immunoglobulin E is the principal antibody responsible for type I allergic responses in humans. Two major receptors for the Fc receptors of IgE exist: $Fc_εRI$ (receptor for Fc portion of IgE I) and $Fc_εRII$ (receptor for Fc portion of IgE II). $Fc_εRII$ receptors are absent on basophils and mast cells and will not be discussed here. There are many $Fc_εRI$ receptors on mature mast cells, and these receptors have an extremely high affinity for IgE. Cross-linking of $Fc_εRI$ results in mast cell triggering. The major biologic effect of $Fc_εRI$ aggregation is release of allergic mediators. In addition, $Fc_εRI$ activation results in production of several proinflammatory cytokines, including IL-4, IL-5, IL-6, IL-3, IFN-γ, and TNF- α. The intracellular signaling pathways leading to mast cell activation following $Fc_εRI$ aggregation are presently under investigation.

Mast cell granules are the major distinguishing morphologic feature of this cell type. These granules contain a large number of preformed mediators (Table 12-3), which are released within minutes of cell activation. In addition, mast cells secrete several lipid mediators produced via both the cyclo-oxygenase (prostaglandin D_2 [PGD_2]), and lipoxygenase (leukotriene C_4 [LTC_4] and leukotriene B_4 [LTB_4]) pathways of arachidonic acid metabolism; production of these products persists for as long as 30 minutes following mast cell activation. That mast cells in airways lie adjacent to nerves, blood vessels, and lymphatics highlights their pivotal importance in regulating allergic inflammatory processes. Mast cell proteases stimulate tissue remodeling, neuropeptide inactivation, and enhanced mucus secretion. Histamine stimulates smooth muscle cell contraction, vasodilatation and increased venular permeability, and further mucus secretion. Histamine induces IL-16 production by $CD8^+$ cells and airway epithelial cells. Leukotrienes C4 and B4, and prostaglandin D_2 affect venular permeability and can regulate the activation of immune cells. Finally, mast cells produce a diverse array of cytokines both constitutively (GM-CSF, TNF-α, and IL-6) and following mast cell activation (IL-1, IL-2, IL-3, IL-4, IL-5, IL-10, IL-13, IL-14, IL-16, and IFN-γ).[24] The best-characterized mast cell cytokine in asthmatic inflammation is TNF-α, which induces adhesion molecules on endothelial cells and subsequent transmigration of inflammatory leukocytes. IL-13 is critical to the development of allergic asthma. This process requires the synthesis of new messenger RNA and occurs hours after the initial stimulus.

It had been argued that mast cells present a host system that evolved primarily to fight parasites. However, current research suggests that mast cells are more central to both innate and adaptive responses in the lung. Mast cells can phagocytose particles, present antigens, produce cytokines, and release vasoactive substances.[24] In addition, mast cells exhibit a wide array of adhesion and other receptors that enable them to react to both nonspecific and specific stimuli. Finally, the antigen-specific responses via IgE-dependent responses make mast cells part of the adaptive immune responses within the lung.

TABLE 12-3. Mediators released by activated human mast cells

Mediator	Circumstances of Release
Granular Mediators	
Histamine	Major biogenic amine of mast cells and basophils Potent vasoactive and smooth muscle spasmogenic activities Rapidly metabolized
Heparin	Proteoglycans
Chondroitin sulfate E and A	Bind histamine, neutral proteases, and acid hydrolases May stabilize granular products
Tryptase	Located in secretory granules Uniquely stabilized with heparin Rapidly cleaves and inactivates fibrinogen Hydrolyzes several neuropeptides (VIP, CGRP, and PHM)
Chymase	Serine class neutral proteases Converts angiotensin I to II Attacks lamina lucida of basement membrane (possibly) Contributes to blister formation seen in mastocytosis
Carboxypeptidase	Zinc metalloprotease
Cathepsin-G-like protease	
Arachidonic Acid–Derived Mediators	
PGD_2	
LTC_4	
LTB_4	
PAF	
Cytokines	
TNF-α, GM-CSF, SCF, IL-3, IL-4, IL-5, IL-6, IL-10, IL-13, IL-14, IL-16, IFN-γ	Produced constitutively or following activation.
Chemokines	
MIP-1α. T-cell activation gene 3, lymphotactin, JE/mcp-1, IFN-γ	

CGRP, calcitonin gene–related peptide; GM-CSF, granulocyte-macrophage colony-stimulating factor; IFN-γ interferon-γ; IL-3, IL-4, etc., interleukin-3, interleukin-4, etc.; LTB_4, leukotriene B_4; LTC_4, leukotriene C_4; MCP-1, monocyte chemotactic protein 1; MIP-1α, macrophage inflammatory protein 1α; PAF, platelet-activating factor; PGD_2, prostaglandin D_2; PHM, peptide histidine-methionine; SCF, stem cell factor; TNF-α, tumor necrosis factor-α; VIP, vasoctive intestinal peptide.

Dendritic Cells

Dendritic cells are the primary resident antigen-presenting cell population in the lung and airway wall.[25] However, activation of DCs in response to innate stimuli is essential to initiate the adaptive response to lung-acquired antigens. In these processes, the phenotype and function of DCs play an important role in initiating tolerance, memory, and polarized Th1 and Th2 differentiation. Antigen presentation to T cells is actively and tightly regulated in vivo by soluble factors produced by mature tissue macrophages. In addition to suppressing DC antigen presentation functions, tissue macrophages elaborate cytokines that suppress T-cell proliferation. Therefore, the phenotype of the DCs, responses to innate stimuli and cytokines produced by macrophages, and the lung microenvironment play important roles in determining the host adaptive response to antigen.[25]

Although DC precursors are detectable in fetal airways,[26] MHC class II Ia^+ DCs are not present in the mucosa of the conducting airways or alveolar septae at birth. This suggests that, like the mast cell, DCs initially migrate into the airway in an immature form. MHC class II Ia^+ cells develop in the airway throughout the birth-to-weanling period. Exogenous stimuli appear to play a central role in the postnatal development of DCs: This is inferred from "direction" of MHC class II Ia$^+$ DC development—initially in the nasal turbinate and then progressively down to the level of the alveolus. Inflammation plays a role in this development: cytokines such as IFN-γ promote the maturation of MHC class II Ia$^+$ DCs, whereas steroids prevent maturation.

Dendritic Cell Phenotypes and Recruitment to the Lung

In humans, three distinct subtypes of DCs have been described. Langerhans DCs and interstitial DC both are derived from CD34$^+$ myeloid precursors (CD11c$^+$ CD13$^+$ CD33$^+$ CD14$^{+/-}$). In the presence of GM-CSF and either IL-4 or TNF-α, the precursor matures into interstitial DCs. Langerhans DCs arise from CD11c$^+$ D14$^+$ or CD11c$^+$ D14$^-$ precursors and require transforming growth factor-β for maturation. Plasmacytoid DCs (ultrastructurally resembling plasma cells) are found in the T-cell zones of lymphoid organs and in the thymus. These cells have a unique phenotype (CD11c$^-$ D4$^+$ D123$^+$ D45RA$^+$ HLADR$^+$) and are able to secrete large amounts of IFN-α upon viral stimulation (see the 2002 review by Lipscomb and colleagues).[25] DCs are migratory cells that move between various environments in the lung and lymphoid organs and perform specific functions at each site. Bone marrow precursors enter blood and enter tissues, including the lung, where they become resident DCs. Interstitial and Langerhans DCs are found at the interface with the external environment (mucosal surfaces, skin). In these tissues they have the ability to migrate to inflammatory foci, where they can take up antigen, process the antigen, then emigrate through the lymphatics to the draining lymph nodes, where they associate with areas rich in T cells and initiate the immune response. This migration is accompanied by alterations in the repertoire of adhesion proteins and chemokine receptors on the DC surface: As the DCs mature, they lose responsiveness to inflammatory chemokines and gain responsiveness to lymphoid chemokines. This loss of inflammatory chemokine receptors is at least partially regulated by ligand-induced down-regulation by autocrine secretion of macrophage inflammatory protein-1α, macrophage inflammatory protein-1β, and RANTES by maturing DCs.[25]

Dendritic Cells, Innate Recognition, and Adaptive Responses

As the initiator of T-cell responses, DCs recognize and respond to danger signals, mature (alter their function), and initiate the adaptive immune response. DC receptors sample the environment, and the "danger signals" (as described in this "danger model," proposed by Matzinger in 1992)[27,28] result in activation of the DC to migrate and mature, process antigen for expression, and release cytokines to further modulate the immune response. These danger signals can arise from cell necrosis and tissue destruction (such as necrotic cells, intracellular ATP and UTP, matrix degradation products, endogenous heat shock proteins) or from foreign substances. Microorganisms (bacteria, fungi) display motifs referred to as PAMPs—LPS (gram-negative organisms), peptidoglycans and lipoteichoic acids (gram-positive organisms), microbial DNA (rich in CpG motifs), microbial heat shock proteins, and double-stranded viral RNA—that stimulate the DCs to undergo maturation.[25,28] The TLRs (described earlier) are the most important receptors on DCs that recognize these microbial products and signal the message to initiate the adaptive responses. TLR1 through TLR5 are expressed on DCs and are down-regulated during maturation. After binding to their ligands, TLR-2 (peptidoglycans, lipoteichoic, acids, and lipopeptides), TLR-4 (LPS), and TLR-9 (CpG) signal through a number of molecules resulting in the translocation of the transcription factor, NF-κB, and subsequent transcriptional activation of the expression of a number of proinflammatory/regulatory molecules.[25] In addition, a family of intracellular proteins, called NOD receptors also respond to injury- and pathogen-related signals.[28] These innate signals cause the maturation and activation of DCs that result in the adaptive T- and B-cell responses discussed later.

Macrophages

An extensive literature has developed over the last decade supporting the concept that macrophages are important regulators of airway inflammation. Alveolar macrophages have four important attributes that contribute to their functional capacity: mobility, phagocytosis, receptor expression for signal recognition, and production and release of a number of bioactive mediators.[29] They are capable of several activities: scavenging particulates, removing macromolecules, killing microorganisms, acting as accessory and regulatory cells for a number of immune functions, recruiting and activating other inflammatory cells, maintaining and repairing injured lung tissues, removing apoptotic cells, and modulating normal lung physiology. Many of these functions are "turned off" in the resting state but are up-regulated with macrophage activation. The regulation of macrophage activation and turnover is undoubtedly important in determining pulmonary health or disease, because the activated functions of this cell not only can help to kill invading organisms, or recruit other inflammatory cells, but they also can result in pulmonary inflammation or fibrosis. Moreover, macrophages can cooperate with other cell types (DCs and lymphocytes) by means of cell-cell interactions and cytokine signals to orchestrate development of cell-mediated immunity consisting of delayed-type hypersensitivity and cytotoxic T cells, and humoral immunity.[29]

Macrophages are present in the interstitium and at epithelial surfaces in the lung.[29] They are far more abundant in the distal respiratory tract, particularly the alveolus, than in the tracheobronchial tree. Various macrophage subpopulations may exist, based on differences in morphology, density, surface markers, and function.

Origin, Kinetics, and Development

The macrophage population is usually constant in size, but this is the result of a dynamic steady state of cellular recruitment, cell division, and cell turnover. The turnover time for alveolar macrophages has been calculated to be 21 to 28 days in animal models. At the end of this period there is an efflux of cells from the lungs up the mucociliary escalator, although the mechanisms for this efflux are still unknown. Speculation also exists that a subpopulation of alveolar macrophages may cross the alveolar epithelium to return to the interstitium, or to migrate to regional lymph nodes. During acute inflammation, it is clear that monocyte influx is the major contributor to the expansion of the macrophage population, although local proliferation of resident macrophages contributes to a lesser degree. Following this acute inflammatory response, the number of alveolar macrophages returns to normal resting levels by removal through mucociliary transport mechanisms and by migration to peribronchial or perivascular connective tissue or regional lymph nodes.

Macrophage Characteristics and Functions

Ultrastructural analysis predicts that macrophages are metabolically active cells. They have a well-developed vacuolar apparatus and many mitochondria. The prominent cytoplasmic organelles in the alveolar macrophage are the secondary lysosome and the Golgi apparatus. The alveolar macrophage is exposed to an aerobic environment with a partial pressure of O_2 of approximately 100 torr, unlike the peritoneal macrophage that functions in an environment of 5 torr. Alveolar macrophages have a resting rate of metabolism 3 times that of monocytes and almost 10 times that of polymorphonuclear leukocytes, which increases by nearly twofold following phagocytosis. Alveolar macrophages produce several oxygen metabolites, including O_2^- (superoxide anion), H_2O_2 (hydrogen peroxide), and OH (hydroxyl radical). They can be activated to produce these reactive oxygen intermediates by several substances, including zymosan, IgG, immune complexes, and several cytokines (IFN-γ, GM-CSF, TNF, and platelet-derived growth factor). These reactive oxygen intermediates play an important role in host antimicrobial defense: Defects in the ability to generate these oxygen products lead to a high susceptibility to infections, as in chronic granulomatous disease. Moreover, uncontrolled production of these reactive oxygen intermediates may play a role in lung injury.

Traditionally, the alveolar macrophage has been viewed chiefly as a phagocytic cell. In the lung, macrophages ingest inorganic and organic particles such as viruses, bacteria, and fungi. It has been speculated that the predominant mechanism by which insoluble particles are removed from the lung is ingestion by alveolar macrophages followed by clearance up the mucociliary ladder. However, in order for macrophages to ingest microorganisms, receptor-mediated uptake is necessary. Three groups of receptors play important roles in opsonization: Fc (immunoglobulin) receptors, complement receptors, and the pattern recognition receptors (Table 12-4).

Three receptors for the Fc portion of IgG have been described on alveolar macrophages: FcγRI (high-affinity Fc receptor for monomeric IgG), FcγRII (a low-affinity receptor for IgG and aggregated IgG), and FcγRIII (a low-affinity receptor for aggregated IgG). On human alveolar macrophages, FcγR for IgG subclasses IgG1 and IgG3 are present in greater numbers than receptors for IgG2 and IgG4. In addition, Fc receptors for IgE (Fc_εRII) and IgA have been described. The macrophage has access to any molecules recognized by these immunoglobulins through their Fc receptors. In addition, alveolar macrophages have membrane-bound, cytophilic IgG and IgA, which play a role in nonopsonic phagocytosis.

Three complement receptors have been described on alveolar macrophages. The most important is CR1 (CD35), which mediates high-affinity binding to C3b and low-affinity binding to iC3b and C4b. CR3 (Mac-1) is the CD11b/CD18 (member of the β_2-integrin family, described earlier) that binds iC3b with high affinity and C3dg and C3d with low affinity. CR4 (CD11c/CD18, also a member of the β_2-integrin family) binds iC3b. SP-A is thought to bind to the macrophage complement receptors, thereby nonspecifically opsonizing microorganisms.

New classes of receptors have been recently been delineated on macrophages. These receptors have been named pattern recognition receptors, because they share in common the ability to recognize certain patterns of molecules produced by microbes, not by hosts (see Table 12-4).[13,30] These molecules, called PAMPs, are invariant molecular constituents of infectious agents that are evolutionarily conserved—that is, shared by large groups of pathogens. These PAMPs include LPS (a component of gram-negative organisms), lipoteichoic acid, a component of gram-positive organisms, mannans (component of yeast), and glycolipids (component of mycobacteria). The pattern recognition receptors are limited in number and are encoded in the germline (innate). Several of these receptors signal the cell that binding has occurred and activate the macrophage, or contribute to phagocytosis.[13] In contrast, the phosphatidylserine receptor allows the macrophage to recognize and phagocytose apoptotic cells but does not result in inflammation.[31] The TLRs have been discussed earlier. The remaining receptors (see Table 12-4), including the TLRs, share the ability to discriminate between self and infectious agents by recognition of the molecular epitopes (PAMPs). In some cases and circumstances, these molecules facilitate uptake of the pathogen or cell; in other situations they function in cell signaling and activation.

TABLE 12-4. Macrophage receptors involved in clearance of lung pathogens

"Classic" Macrophage Opsonic Receptors	Pattern Recognition Receptors	
Ig Receptors	*Receptor*	*Ligand*
Fc_γ Receptors	CD36	Apoptotic cells
Fc_γRI	CD14	LBP/LPS
Fc_γRII	Mannose receptor	Carbohydrates
Fc_γRIII		
Fc_εRII	Sialadhesin	Sialic acid
Fc_α	Integrins	Glucans, RGD
	PS Receptor	Apoptotic cells
Complement Receptors	**TLRs**	
CR1 (CD35)	*Receptor*	*Ligand*
CR3 (Mac-1; CD11b/CD18)	TLR2	pg, LTA, LPS
CR4 (CD11c/CD/18)	TLR4	SP-A
	TLR9	CpG
	SRs	
	Receptor	*Ligand*
	SR-AI, SR-AII	LPS, LTA, CpG
	MARCO	
	LOX-1	Polyanion
	SR-PSOX	Phosphatidylserine

CpG, bacterial DNA-containing unmethylated CpG; Ig, immunoglobulin; LBP, lipopolysaccharide-binding protein; LPS, lipopolysaccharide(s); LTA, lipoteichoic acid; pg, peptidoglycan; RGD, a three-residue peptide composed of arginine-glycine-aspartic acid; SP-A, surfactant-associated protein A; SRs, scavenger receptors; TLRs, Toll-like receptors.

Macrophage Products

In addition to the reactive oxygen intermediates discussed earlier, macrophages produce many intracellular and secreted products that are responsible for several of their bactericidal and cell-activating activities (Table 12-5). Human alveolar macrophages have been shown to produce metabolites of arachidonic acid by both the cyclo-oxygenase and lipoxygenase pathways, and mediators from both pathways play a role in the modulation of inflammatory reactions. Cyclo-oxygenase products secreted by

TABLE 12-5. Secretory products of alveolar macrophages that mediate inflammatory and immune responses

Enzymes	Arachidonic Acid Metabolites	Cytokines	Other Bioactive Peptides
Acid Hydrolases	Prostaglandin E_2	IL-1α	Endothelin 1
Proteases	Prostaglandin $F_{2\alpha}$	IL-1β	Endothelin 3
Lipases	Thromboxane A_2	TNF-α	Defensins
Deoxyribonucleases	Leukotriene B_4	TGF-β	Plasmin Inhibitors
Glycosidase	Leukotriene C_4	PGDF	α_2-macroglobulin
Sulfatases	5-HETE	IL-6	Fibronectin
Phosphatases	**Bioactive Lipids**	IL-8	
Neutral Hydrolases	Platelet-activating factor	MIP-1α	
Plasminogen activator	**Reactive Oxygen Metabolites**	MIP-1β	
Collagenase	Superoxide anion	MIP-2	
Elastase	Hydrogen peroxide	MCP-1	
Lysozyme	Hydroxyl radical	IFN-α	
	Reactive Nitrogen Metabolites	IFN-β	
	Nitric oxide, peroxynitrite		

5-HETE, 5-hydroxyeicosatetraenoic acid; IFN-α, interferon-α; IFN-β, interferon-β; IL-1α, IL-1β, etc., interleukin-1α, interleukin-1β, etc.; MCP-1, monocyte chemotactic protein 1; MIP-1α, MIP-1β, etc., macrophage inflammatory protein 1α, macrophage inflammatory protein 1β, etc.; PGDF, platelet-derived growth factor; TGF-β, transforming growth factor-β; TNF-α, tumor necrosis factor-α.

alveolar macrophages include thromboxane A_2, prostaglandin E_2, prostaglandin D_2, and prostaglandin $F_{2\alpha}$. Thromboxane A_2 is produced in the greatest amount. Lipoxygenase products include LTB_4 and 5-hydroxyeicosatetraenoic acid. The precise activities of these products are diverse and complex, and the precise mechanisms of macrophage activation that lead to the production of arachidonic acid metabolites are presently unclear.

Alveolar macrophages produce a large, diverse array of enzymes that can be divided into three major groups: acid hydrolases, neutral hydrolases, and lysozyme (see Table 12-5). Acid hydrolases function primarily as intracellular digestive enzymes but can be secreted into the extracellular environment, where they have several functions such as microbial killing, degradation of connective tissue, activation of complement components, and lysis of fibrin. Lysozyme is a major secretory product of macrophages, and it is bactericidal for a many microorganisms.

Several cytokines and chemotactic factors are produced by alveolar macrophages (see Table 12-5). The proinflammatory cytokine IL-1 is one of the most important regulatory products of the macrophage. Transforming growth factor-β also has many biologic functions, including chemoattraction for fibroblasts and effects on the composition of the extracellular matrix. Through the generation of cytokines, the macrophage plays a central role in phagocyte recruitment and activation, wound healing, fibrosis, and modulation of actions of other innate and adaptive immune responses in the lung.[23] Therefore, the regulation of cytokine production must be precisely balanced in the normal lung to prevent the ongoing activity of these cytokines.

Defensins are major components of neutrophil and macrophage granules. Production of these proteins is regulated in a tissue- and age-specific manner. They have been demonstrated to have a wide range of activity against bacteria, fungi, and some viruses, but can also damage host tissues.[32]

Antimicrobial Activity of Alveolar Macrophages

The alveolar macrophage plays an essential role in the killing of invading microorganisms in the lung. Under normal conditions there are no bacterial infections in the lung despite ongoing environmental exposures, demonstrating the high efficiency of this protective system. The efficiency of microbial killing by alveolar macrophages depends on the specific organism involved and the size of the initial inoculum. Small quantities of organisms (10^5) can be eliminated by alveolar macrophages alone. Slightly larger quantities of organisms (10^6–10^7) require additional assistance (influx) of polymorphonuclear granulocytes, but large inocula (10^8 organisms) overcome this phagocytic barrier. Different species of invading organism are cleared and killed with different efficiencies by alveolar macrophages. Immunocompromised hosts are particularly susceptible to infections by intracellular organisms (i.e., *Mycobacterium*, *Listeria*, and *Legionella*) that can be phagocytosed normally but cannot be killed without T-lymphocyte-derived macrophage-activating cytokines. Similar observations have been made with fungi and viruses. These studies indicate the necessity of interactions between the various components of the immune system in fighting microbial invasion in the lung. Despite the wide armamentarium of enzymes, reactive oxygen products, and other products, the alveolar macrophage must interact with other components of the immune system to phagocytose and kill foreign invaders.

RECRUITED CELLULAR DEFENSES

All pulmonary inflammatory cells are initially derived from bone marrow precursors, recruited from the circulation. The cells discussed so far migrate to the lung in an "immature form" and mature or differentiate within the lung in response to local cytokines or through activation by pathogens. The cells discussed in this section are recruited from the pulmonary circulation in their mature, active forms. In the process of recruitment, these cells transform from a "quiescent" resting state into a state where they are fully "activated" or "primed" for further cellular activities. The major cell types discussed in this section include neutrophils, eosinophils, and lymphocytes.

Neutrophils

Neutrophils are characterized by their multilobed nucleus and distinctive cytoplasmic granules containing an arsenal of enzymes and proteins that contribute to neutrophil function. Neutrophils constitute about half the circulating white cell population, and their primary function is phagocytosis and killing of invading pathogens. To accomplish this, the neutrophil must respond to signals in the area of injury, adhere and transmigrate through the vascular endothelium, migrate to the area of infection, then recognize, phagocytose, and kill the pathogen. Interruption of any of these steps will leave the host susceptible to infections. Patients with leukocyte adhesion deficiency are unable to recruit neutrophils into sites of inflammation, and, as a result, they sustain recurrent, life-threatening infections.[9] These leukocyte adhesion deficiency patients lack the normal β_2-integrins to allow neutrophil recruitment from the circulation. In chronic granulomatous disease the neutrophils lack components of the NADPH oxidase system, and, therefore, neutrophils that have engulfed organisms cannot efficiently kill them. The processes of neutrophil recruitment and activation, followed by neutrophil removal (cell death, or apoptosis) after the resolution of the infectious process or injury, must be closely regulated at several levels. Disruption of these regulatory processes leads to acute or ongoing lung injury.

Origin, Kinetics, and Development

Neutrophils are short-lived cells; their life span from stem cell to removal in the tissues is 12 to 14 days. A normal adult weighing 70 kg produces about 1×10^{11} neutrophils each day, derived from $CD34^+$ myeloid progenitor cells. Neutrophil development from these progenitors is regulated by three major hematopoietic growth factors: Granulocyte colony-stimulating factor (G-CSF), GM-CSF, and IL-3. G-CSF can be produced by a wide number of cell types, and appears to be involved in maintenance of normal neutrophil numbers and stressed granulopoiesis. GM-CSF operates locally and functions as a multilineage growth factor, stimulating the proliferation and maturation of neutrophils, eosinophils, and monocytes. IL-3 has similar activities but appears to function in earlier stages of hematopoiesis than either G-CSF or GM-CSF.

Granulocyte progenitor cells in the bone marrow produce myeloblasts, which then differentiate through several recognizable morphologic stages into mature, nondividing polymorphonuclear neutrophils. It normally takes about 14 days for the neutrophil precursor to mature and be released into the blood.[33] Once in the circulation, neutrophil half-life is quite short (approximately 6–7 hours). The pulmonary capillary bed is unique in its ability to "concentrate" neutrophils. The term *margination* has been proposed to describe this increased concentration of neutrophils in noninflamed lungs. Margination is proposed to result from discordance between the diameter of neutrophils (6–8 μm) and that of the capillary segments (2–15 μm). Morphometric and videomicroscopic studies have suggested that the neutrophil must change shape within 40% to 60% of these capillary segments to traverse the pulmonary circulation. The increased concentration of neutrophils present within the pulmonary capillary bed results from the structural characteristics of the capillary bed and the mechanical properties of the neutrophils that cause them to deform more slowly than red blood cells, increasing the pulmonary capillary transit time. This prolonged transit time is proposed to allow neutrophils time to sense and respond to the presence of inflammatory processes.[33]

In response to inflammatory stimuli, neutrophils further accumulate in preparation for migration ("sequestration"). In much of the systemic circulation, neutrophil sequestration occurs in postcapillary venules in the form of rolling, and is mediated by selectins. In the lungs, the known adhesion molecules do not appear to mediate the initial events of sequestration. Rather, in the pulmonary capillary, inflammatory mediators alter the mechanical properties of the neutrophils, resulting in changes in deformability thought to be induced by polymerization of actin beneath the plasma membrane. This "stiffening" reduces the neutrophil deformability, lengthening the capillary transit times or stopping the movement of the neutrophil altogether in the sites of inflammation.[33] Once sequestration has occurred, the neutrophils can adhere via selectin or CD11/CD18–intercellular adhesion molecule-1 mechanisms used elsewhere in the circulation and migrate across the vascular endothelium into the lung.

Neutrophil Function

Once the neutrophil has migrated into the tissue, its primary purpose is to recognize, ingest, and destroy pathogens. Phagocytosis consists of two steps: recognition and internalization of the foreign material into the phagosome. Killing or neutralization then involves a secretory response. Materials may bind directly to the neutrophil, resulting in ingestion. However, as in the case with macrophages (described earlier), opsonization by serum proteins usually occurs. Neutrophils exhibit both specific Fc-mediated binding and nonspecific binding using complement receptors CR1, CR3, as used by macrophages.[34] Intracellular killing is generally associated with the initiation of the respiratory burst. The importance of this process is demonstrated by patients with chronic granulomatous disease, whose neutrophils cannot undergo the oxidative burst.[35] In addition, alternative mechanisms of killing exist, including secretion of granular proteins into the phagosome (Table 12-6).

Secretion of granule contents from the neutrophil into its local environment is usually referred to as degranulation. In addition, the cell actively releases a number of other materials to the outside, including lipid mediators of inflammation (platelet-activating factor [PAF], LTB_4). The signals initiating neutrophil degranulation and secretion are still unclear. During inflammatory reactions, the earliest responses involve neutrophil emigration, with subsequent degranulation and secretion of granule contents. Degranulation involves the fusion of the granule membrane with either the developing or the formed phagosome. Neutrophils contain different classes of granules: primary (or azurophilic) and secondary (or secretory, or specific) granules[36] (see Table 12-6). Degranulation and secretion of the two major classes of granules are regulated separately. Exposure of the neutrophil to a wide variety of stimuli produces little overt activity, as measured by secretion or oxidative burst. Rather, this stimulation raises the cell to a higher level of responsiveness to a second set of activating agents. The physiologic consequence of this process is that neutrophils can be recruited

TABLE 12-6. Secretory products of neutrophils that mediate inflammatory and immune responses

Neutrophil Granular Proteins	*Specific (Secondary) Granules*	**Reactive Oxygen Intermediates**
Azurophil (Primary) Granules	β_2 microglobulin	Superoxide anion (O_2^-)
Granulophysin (CD63)	Lysozyme	Hydrogen peroxide
Acid β-glycerophosphatase	Lactoferrin	Hypochlorous acid
Acid mucopolysaccharide	Vitamin B_{12}-binding protein	Nitric oxide
Azurocidin	Cytochrome b_{558}	**Lipid Mediators/Arachidonic Acid Metabolites**
α_1-antitrypsin	Collagenase	PAF
BPI	Gelatinase	LTB_4
Myeloperoxidase	hCAP-18	
Lysozyme	Histaminase	
Cathepsins (A, D, E, F, G)	NGAL	
N-acetyl-β-glucosaminidase	uPA	
β-glucuronidase	Sialidase	
β-glycerophosphatase	Transcobalamin-I	
α-mannosidase	*Gelatinase Granules (Tertiary Granules)*	
Defensins	Gelatinase	
Sialidase	β_2 microglobulin	
Ubiquitin-protein	CRISP-3	
Serprosidins	Lysozyme	
Proteinase-3		
Elastase		
Cathepsin G		

BPI, bactericidal/permeability-inducing peptide; hCAP-18, human cathelicidin-18; LTB_4, leukotriene B_4; NGAL, neutrophil gelatinase-associated lipocalin; PAF, platelet-activating factor; uPA, urokinase-type plasminogen activator.

through the vasculature into the interstitium or tissues without damage to normal tissues along the way. However, the cell is "primed" for a second set of signals at the site of infection or inflammation.

Eosinophils

Eosinophils are the second largest group of granulocytic cells in the circulation. They can be morphologically distinguished from neutrophils by their ability to be stained by negatively charged dyes, such as eosin. They are 8 μm in diameter and typically have two nuclear lobes. Their biologic function was unclear for most of the 20th century, but in the late 1960s and early 1970s the possibility was raised that eosinophils might be involved in immunity to parasites. This received experimental support in the middle 1970s, in a report of eosinophil-dependent killing of schistosomula of *Schistosoma mansoni*. Since that time, a great deal has been discovered about the biologic functions and mediators of this important cell. Current research has focused on the role of the eosinophil in pulmonary inflammation associated with asthma. Eosinophil-derived products (see later) have the functional ability to produce the pathologic and physiologic features of asthma. Eosinophils and/or eosinophil products are present in the blood, sputum, and autopsy samples from patients with active asthma (or dying from acute asthma), and there is a correlation between the presence of eosinophils and asthma severity. Finally, eosinophils and/or their products are characteristic features of airway mucosa and BAL specimens following antigen challenge in humans and animals. These lines of evidence indicate that eosinophilic infiltration in asthma may play a major role in the pathogenesis of the disease, and that prevention of eosinophil influx or release of eosinophil products may be major targets for asthma therapy. However, the failure of anti-eosinophil therapies to eradicate asthma has resulted in a reevaluation of the role of eosinophils.[37]

Origin, Kinetics, and Development

Eosinophils arise from bone marrow precursor cells. The nature of the cytokine interactions in eosinophil maturation in vivo is unclear. In vitro studies demonstrate that IL-3, GM-CSF, and IL-5 are important in eosinophil maturation, and there is increasing evidence that IL-5 has the major role. The migration of eosinophils from the bone marrow takes about 3.5 days after DNA synthesis has been completed. In the blood, the half-time of eosinophils is 18 hours. Like neutrophils, there appears to be a marginated pool of eosinophils, which are in dynamic equilibrium with the circulating pool. Eosinophils marginate and emigrate into the tissues through postcapillary venules, probably through interactions with a number of adhesion molecules, unlike the margination of neutrophils in the pulmonary circulation discussed earlier. However, eosinophils, but not neutrophils, adhere to the ligand vascular cell adhesion molecule-1 on the endothelial surface and, once adherent, can be attracted by a specific array of chemotactic agents into the lung. The nature of eosinophil interactions with respiratory epithelium is still not completely defined but involves interaction between epithelial intercellular adhesion molecule-1 and the eosinophil β_2-integrins. The life span of eosinophils in the lung is unknown, although it is assumed that they survive for several days. In vitro studies demonstrate that eosinophils can survive for over a week in the presence of IL-3, GM-CSF, and IL-5. Eosinophils are removed from the tissues by macrophages following apoptosis.

Eosinophil Function

As described earlier, protection against parasitic infections has been speculated to be the "biologic mission" of the eosinophil. Over the last decade, there has been a growing body of evidence that implicates the eosinophil as an important element in the pathogenesis of asthma and allergies, although recently the role of the eosinophil in asthma is being reevaluated.[37] Many of our concepts of the biologic roles of eosinophils have been derived from studies of their mediators and biologic functions (Table 12-7).

Eosinophil granules contain several unique proteins with extensive biologic activities that contribute to the role of the eosinophil in lung inflammation, including major basic protein, eosinophil peroxidase, eosinophil cationic protein, and eosinophil-derived neurotoxin. Major basic protein accounts for over 50% of the eosinophil granule protein. Major basic protein is a potent toxin for mammalian cells and parasites in vitro and has been localized in tissues in hypersensitivity diseases, such as bronchial asthma. Eosinophil peroxidase is an abundant protein in the matrix of the human eosinophil granule and differs from neutrophil myeloperoxidase structurally. Like myeloperoxidase, eosinophil peroxidase catalyzes the oxidation of halides by H_2O_2 to form highly reactive intermediates, which have antibacterial and antihelmintic activities. Eosinophil cationic protein and eosinophil-derived neurotoxin are closely related proteins that are located in the granule matrix and that demonstrate neurotoxic properties. The cytotoxic action of eosinophil cationic protein involves the formation of channels in cell membranes, like complement-membrane interactions. Eosinophil cationic protein is part of the growing family of pore-forming proteins that includes lymphocyte perforin. Collectively, these eosinophil proteins have potent activity that implicates the role of the eosinophil in the control of parasitic diseases. However, these proteins also have activities that are associated with the pathogenesis of obstructive lung disorders. Other peptide products of eosinophils are elastase, histaminase, phospholipase, and arylsulfatase (see Table 12-7). In conclusion, eosinophils and eosinophil mediators play a role in the airway obstruction found in many common pediatric pulmonary diseases. It is likely that understanding the roles of eosinophils and eosinophil granular proteins in airway obstruction will be important in designing new therapies for common diseases such as asthma.

Eosinophils produce two principal lipid mediators with biologic effects implicating them in asthma and allergic disease: PAF and LTC_4 (see Table 12-7). PAF is capable of eliciting many of the characteristic features of the asthmatic airway. In a guinea pig model, PAF is one of the most potent inducers of airway microvascular leakage. It is also a potent bronchoconstrictor that can lead to airway hyperresponsiveness. Eosinophils also elaborate many products of arachidonic acid metabolism. Thromboxane B_2 and prostaglandin E_2 are the major cyclo-oxygenase pathway products, and LTC_4 is the major 5-lipoxygenase product of eosinophils. A great deal of attention has been paid to the roles of LTC_4 and the other sulfidopeptide leukotrienes in the airway. They increase vascular permeability and enhance mucus production in animal and human models. Moreover, the sulfidopeptide leukotrienes have a major effect on airway smooth muscle contraction: administration of LTD_4 augmented response to methacholine in normal subjects that persisted 2 to 3 weeks. Moreover, sulfidopeptide leukotrienes increase histamine responsiveness in asthmatic subjects. It seems clear that these eosinophil-derived lipid products (particularly PAF and LTC_4) have the potential to contribute to the pathophysiologic features found in asthma and bronchiolitis.

Activated eosinophils undergo a "respiratory burst" like that exhibited by neutrophils, and produce a similar repertoire of reactive oxygen intermediates following activation (see Table 12-7).

TABLE 12-7. Secretory products of eosinophils that mediate inflammatory and immune responses

Eosinophil Granular Proteins	**Eicosanoids**	**Cytokines**
MBP	*Cyclo-oxygenase products*	GM-CSF
EPO	TXB_2	IFN-γ
ECP	PGE_2	IL-1α
EDN	6-keto-$PGF_{1\alpha}$	IL-2
Other Granular Proteins	5-lipoxygenase products	IL-3
	LTC4	IL-4
Collagenase	15-lipoxygenase products	IL-5
Elastase	15-HETE	IL-6
Histimanase	**Peptide Mediators**	IL-9
Phospholipase		IL-10
Arylsulfatase B	Substance P	IL-11
	VIP	IL-12
Lipid Mediators/Arachidonic Acid Metabolites		IL-16
	Reactive Oxygen Intermediates	TGF-α
PAF		TGF-β
	Superoxide anion	**Chemokines**
	Hydrogen peroxide	
	Hypochlorous acid	Eotaxin
	Hypobromous acid	IL-8
	Hydroxyl radical	MIP-1α
		MCP-1, 3, 4
		RANTES

ECP, eosinophil cationic protein; EDN, eosinophil-derived neurotoxin; 15-HETE, 15-hydroxyeicosatetraenoic acid; GM-CSF, granulocyte-macrophage colony-stimulating factor; IFN-γ, interferon-γ; IL-1α, IL-1β, etc., interleukin-1α, interleukin-1β, etc.; LTC_4, leukotriene C_4; MBP, major basic protein; MCP-1, monocyte chemotactic protein; MIP-1α, macrophage inflammatory protein 1α; PAF, platelet-activating factor; PGE_2, prostaglandin E_2; $PGF_{1\alpha}$, prostaglandin $F_{1\alpha}$; RANTES, regulated upon activation, normal T-cell expressed and secreted; TGF-α, transforming growth factor-α; TGF-β, transforming growth factor-β; TxB_2, thromboxane B_2; VIP, vasoactive intestinal peptide.

Mechanisms of damage by eosinophil-produced oxidants are not well established, but peroxidation of lipids in the plasma membrane by O_2^- may be important. In the lung, oxygen radicals may cause increased vascular permeability and edema formation through effects on vascular endothelium, and they may cause increased smooth muscle contractility by effects on the airway epithelium.

Eosinophils have recently been demonstrated to produce a number of bioactive cytokines (see Table 12-7). The biologic relevance and roles of these cytokines in eosinophil-effector cell interactions remains to be elucidated in vivo.[38]

In summary, eosinophils synthesize a number of biologically active peptides that contribute to their ability to destroy parasites in vivo. However, these products, and other eosinophil products such as PAF, LTC_4, and reactive oxygen intermediates have the potential to disrupt the airways, and they have physiologic activities that implicate the eosinophil as a primary effector cell in asthma, although the extent of eosinophil involvement has recently come under greater scrutiny.[37] Additional research will be necessary to further define the role of the eosinophil and to develop pharmacologic interventions that block production or prevent the activity of these bioactive products in human subjects.

Innate Lymphocyte Responses in the Lung: Natural Killer, Natural Killer T cells, and γδ T Cells

Although lymphocyte populations are generally regarded as part of adaptive immunity, several subsets function in innate responses including recognition and elimination of tumor cells and certain pathogens. They accomplish this through the use of limited sets of conserved recognition receptors. Three major lymphocyte populations will be considered in this context. Natural killer (NK) cells are bone marrow–derived lymphocytes that are distinct from either B or T cells. Natural killer T (NK-T) cells are T cells that express the NK cell marker, NK1, a highly restricted/limited repertoire of the CD3/T-cell receptor (TCR) complex with specificity for antigens presented in association with CD1. These cells most closely resemble CD4 T cells in terms of cytokine production. Finally, γδ T cells have a limited diversity of TCRs that recognize self and bacterial/protozoan antigens. These innate lymphocytes are considered to be a first-line of defense against tumors and infection, and in modulating inflammation in the lung.

NK cells are capable of lysing certain tumor cells without prior sensitization (thus the name natural killer). They were originally thought to primarily provide protection against tumor cells. Subsequently, they have been demonstrated to provide defense against viral infections (e.g., humans deficient in NK cells have difficulty in controlling herpesviruses).[39] NK cells express several distinctive surface receptors that influence cell function: CD56; the killer cell immunoglobulin-like receptors, which are inhibitory receptors that recognize specific MHC class I receptors; NK receptors NKR-P1, CD161, NKG2A-NKG2E, and CD94, which are inhibitory receptors; CD16 (FcγRIII [Fc receptor for target-bound IgG]), which mediates antibody-dependent cell-mediated cytotoxicity; CD2; and the β_2-integrins (discussed earlier).

Natural killer cells develop in the bone marrow and require stem cell factor (c-Kit ligand), IL-7, flt-3 ligand, IL-15, ILF-12, IL-18, and IFN-γ for maturation. NK cells constitute only a small population of cells (2.5% of splenic leukocytes). This population, however, can respond and expand quickly in response to infection, contributing significantly to innate defenses. One mechanism of early innate response is the presence of multiple activation receptors on the surface of individual NK cells. In addition, NK cells have constitutive expression of many cytokine receptors that allow these cells to be stimulated by proinflammatory cytokines early in the course of response to injury or infection. Stimulation of NK cells can lead to production of cytokines (IFN-γ, TNF-α, GM-CSF). Moreover, activated or infected macrophages and DCs produce a number of cytokines that can stimulate NK cells to produce cytokines and chemokines. IFN-α/β enhances NK cell cytotoxicity, through mechanisms discussed later for T lymphocytes. In addition, NK cells appear to play an important role in attenuation or resolution of immune responses through action on CD8 T cells or indirect control of DCs.

The NK-T cells are CD4 T cells that express a unique set of cellular receptors. These receptors include the NK receptors (including CD16) and a unique invariant TCR α chain and a limited Vβ repertoire. This unique TCR allows the NK-T cell to recognize molecules associated with CD1. Ligands for this complex include glycosyl phosphatidylinositol, hydrophobic peptides, and α-galactosylceramide. NK-T cells appear to function primarily in regulating autoimmunity and malignancy. In addition, they appear to be important in processing of lipids from mycobacteria.[40]

γδ T lymphocytes are innate T-lymphocyte populations that express the γδ TCR with limited diversity. In humans the Vγ2Vδ2 TCR is utilized by the majority of γδ T cells. These cells recognize small organic phosphate antigens from microbes. This population expands significantly in protozoal infections such as malaria, toxoplasmosis, and mycobacterial infections.[40] Differential expression of IFN-γ and IL-4 influences the development of Th1 and Th2 responses, respectively.

■ ADAPTIVE LUNG DEFENSES

Most pathogens gain entry to the lung across mucosal surfaces. An important aspect of inflammatory and immune responses to the entry of respiratory pathogens is the ability to mount an appropriate, regulated immune response that can clear the infection rapidly and efficiently, yet not expose the surrounding tissues or the entire host to chronic inflammation. Innate immunity provides the first level of protection. Adaptive or specific immunity provides specific responses to antigens during the acute infection and provides specific immune memory that protects against subsequent exposure. A number of cell types contribute to airway mucosal defense, as discussed earlier. As part of the mucosal surface from the nasal airway to the conducting airways, the bronchial-associated lymphoid tissue functions in the development of adaptive lung defense. The bronchial-associated lymphoid tissue is made up of intraepithelial lymphocytes, macrophages, DCs, NK cells, and NK-T cells that recognize foreign substances, invading organisms or their exoproducts, and products of cell injury using the receptor systems discussed earlier. The DCs or macrophages interact with them and interact with lymphocytes to create the cellular immune responses or to signal antibody production. These cells migrate to local lymph nodes, tonsils, or adenoids, process antigens, generate cytokines, and generate the adaptive immune responses. While extensive reviews of humoral (B-cell mediated) and cellular (T-cell mediated) immunity, antigen presentation, and cellular activation are well beyond the scope of this chapter, we will briefly discus the roles of humoral and cellular immunity with respect to lung defense.

T LYMPHOCYTES (T CELLS) AND LUNG DEFENSE

Several types of T lymphocytes contribute to lung immunity and tissue pathology. Two major types of antigen receptors are used by T lymphocytes: the δγ TCR (discussed earlier) and the αβ receptor (making up the CD4 and CD8 T-cell populations). The αβ T-cell mounts cytolytic responses to infected cells, makes cytokines, and stimulates B-cell responses (later). αβ T cells expressing the receptor protein CD4 are termed Th cells. CD4 T cells recognize antigens presented via the MHC class II antigen and provide effector function primarily by the release of cytokines. Th cells can be further differentiated phenotypically into Th1 and Th2 populations according to their profiles of cytokine production. Th1 cells differentiate in the presence of IL-12 and IL-18 and produce IFN-γ, IL-2, and TNF-α in response to antigen. These cells have been regarded as responsible for the delayed hypersensitivity response to viral or bacterial infection, stimulating local macrophage activation and neutrophil recruitment, and altering specific T-cell responses. Th2 cells are driven to differentiate by the presence of IL-4, and, in the presence of antigen they respond by making Il-4, ILF-5, IL-10, and IL-13. These cytokines are responsible for driving B lymphocytes to make antibodies, and they lead to the recruitment and activation of basophils and eosinophils. The Th2 phenotype has been associated with an allergic/asthmatic phenotype in mouse models and human studies.[41]

αβ T cells expressing CD8 are cytotoxic cells. In response to peptides presented by the MHC class I molecules, CD8 T cells function in target cell toxicity. CD8 T-cell toxicity is mediated by the release of cellular granules containing perforin (perturbs the cell membrane) and granzymes (disrupt target cells by altering intracellular targets). In addition, CD8 T cells can initiate apoptosis in target cells by Fas-FasL interactions. CD8 cells reinforce viral defenses by rendering adjacent cells resistant to infection, presumably by release of interferons.

T-cell responses are tightly regulated. Whereas responses are necessary to eliminate pathogens, uncontrolled responses can cause autoimmune inflammatory diseases.[41]

B LYMPHOCYTES (B CELLS)

Humoral immunity is mediated by antibodies produced by B lymphocytes. Antibodies are proteins that function to eliminate or neutralize the antigens that specifically induce their production. The interaction of antigens with B lymphocytes triggers the production of antibodies specific to that antigen and establishes the potential for a rapid release of large amounts of antibody upon future stimulation (immune memory).

As B cells differentiate, one of the first changes is the rearrangement of information coded in the variable (V), diversity (D), and joining (J) regions of the gene. Through genetic rearrangement, DNA for one discrete V region is opposed to that of specific D J regions. This rearrangement is responsible for the specific affinity (idiotype) of the antibodies produced by B cells. The commitment of B cells to make antibodies of certain antigens is established before exposure to those antigens.

Initially, B cells express IgM and IgD isotypes on the cell surface. Upon interaction of an antigen with the membrane-bound IgM, the clone of B cells with the genetic information coding for the antigen-specific antibodies undergoes two changes: proliferation resulting in clonal expansion, and differentiation resulting in production of antibodies of different isotypes. In addition, the B cells begin to express MHC class II molecules on their cell surface, which allows them to interact with Th cells. This hypermutation and class switching of immunoglobulin genes, and the generation of memory B cells and plasma cell precursors occurs in the germinal centers of secondary lymphoid follicles, in the presence of DCs, Th cells, and macrophages. The organization of these structures provides an immune microenvironment that maximizes generation of antibody responses by bringing all the relevant cell types into close contact for cell-cell signaling, recently named the immune synapse. Depending on the type of antigen, the B-cell response may be classified as T-cell dependent or independent. The T-cell-independent pathogens can stimulate B cells without assistance from T cells. Examples of T-cell-independent antigens include polysaccharides and polymerized flagellin, which provide numerous repeating epitopes. T-cell-independent antigens do not induce the formation of germinal centers and thus cannot induce the generation of memory B cells or somatic hypermutation that results in the production of high-affinity antibodies. The extent of class switching from IgM to other classes of antibodies is also severely limited in the absence of Th cell–generated cytokines. In general, protein antigens are T-cell dependent, and these peptide-MHC complexes on CD4 T cells provide the cytokine signals that initiate somatic hypermutation and immunoglobulin class switching.[42]

HUMORAL IMMUNITY

Immunoglobulin Isotypes

Depending on the stage of development of the B lymphocyte, different immunoglobulin isotypes are produced. Before antigenic stimulation, the "naive" B lymphocyte expresses IgM (and IgD) on its surface. Early in the antigenic response, IgM, IgG3, and IgG1 are produced by B lymphocytes. In the chronic response, the predominant isotypes produced are IgG2 and IgG4. In addition, IgA is important in the mucosal immune response. The relative concentrations of immunoglobulin isotypes present in the BAL fluid of healthy individuals are listed in Table 12-8.

Immunoglobulin A

Secretory IgA is the predominant immunoglobulin isotype present in airway secretions.[43] Secretory IgA is composed of two IgA molecules (dimeric IgA), a joining protein (J chain), and secretory component. The dimeric IgA-J chain complex is produced by B lymphocytes in the submucosal space. Secretory

TABLE 12-8. Relative concentration of immunoglobulin subclass protein in serum and bronchoalveolar lavage*

	IgG1	IgG2	IgG3	IgG4	IgA	IgE
Serum	4.5	2.1	0.03	0.1	2	200
BAL	50	22	1.4	4	183	9

* The values for serum are given in mg/mL; those for BAl are in mg/mL, except for IgE, for which all values are given in mg/mL.

BAL, bronchoalveolar lavage.

component is produced by mucosal epithelial cells and acts as a receptor for dimeric IgA. After IgA binds to secretory component, the entire complex undergoes endocytosis and is transported to the apical surface of the cell, where the secretory IgA complex is released into the mucosal environment. Secretory component serves to protect the secretory IgA complex from proteases present in the mucosal environment.

Secretory IgA serves several functions including neutralization of viruses and exotoxin, enhancement of lactoferrin and lactoperoxidase activities, and inhibition of microbial growth. Because dimeric IgA is able to bind two antigens simultaneously, it is capable of forming large antigen-antibody complexes. In this manner, IgA neutralizes microbes and facilitates their removal by mucociliary clearance, inhibits microbial binding to epithelial cells, and inhibits uptake of potential allergens.

Selective IgA deficiency, defined by a serum IgA concentration of less than 0.05 mg/mL, is often detected in healthy individuals during routine blood donor screening. Symptomatic individuals present with varied manifestations including recurrent sinusitis, otitis media, pharyngitis, bronchitis, pneumonia, chronic diarrhea, and autoimmune syndromes. Individuals with associated IgE deficiency tend to have less serious pulmonary disease in contrast to individuals with normal or high IgE, who in addition to the disorders already mentioned suffer from allergic respiratory problems and pulmonary hemosiderosis.

As mentioned earlier, one of the roles of secretory IgA is to inhibit uptake of allergenic antigens. If these antigens are not removed in individuals who have enhanced IgE responses, then increased allergic problems would be expected. Patients with IgA deficiency tend to have a high incidence of antibodies to milk. Exposure to cow's milk can result in cow's milk allergy and, in severe cases, secondary pulmonary hemosiderosis. There is an increased incidence of selective IgA deficiency in individuals with asthma and CF.

In general, patients with selective IgA deficiency are treated symptomatically for respiratory, gastrointestinal, and allergic problems. Since most preparations of γ-globulin contain IgA; the use of γ-globulin increases the risk of anaphylaxis if the recipient has antibodies to IgA. Transfusion of blood products presents a similar problem for these individuals. In patients with a combined IgA and IgG deficiency who need immunoglobulin therapy or the transfusion of blood products, it is essential to ensure that the recipient does not have IgA antibodies or use a preparation that does not contain IgA.

Immunoglobulin G

Although concentrations of IgG in the airway are less than those of IgA, all IgG subclasses are detectable in respiratory secretions. As opposed to IgA, which is actively transported into the airway, IgG reaches the airway largely by transudation through the mucosa. IgG functions by opsonizing microbes for phagocytosis and killing, activating the complement cascade, and neutralizing many bacterial endotoxins and viruses.

IgG deficiency, as in X-linked agammaglobulinemia or common variable hypogammaglobulinemia, is associated with recurrent otitis media, sinusitis, bronchitis, and pneumonia. Recurrence of airway infections may result in chronic airway injury with bronchiectasis. The combination of altered opsonic activity and bronchiectasis results in chronic colonization with respiratory pathogens such as *P. aeruginosa*.

In patients suspected of IgG deficiency, IgG subclasses should be quantified and the antibody response to polysaccharide vaccines (*S. pneumoniae, H. influenzae*) should be measured. IgG-deficient patients with recurrent respiratory tract infections often benefit from prophylactic antibiotics, intravenous γ-globulin therapy, and the use of airway clearance techniques.

The identification of a selective IgG subclass deficiency, or combined subclass deficiency, is not predictive of the capacity to produce antibody to pneumococcal polysaccharide or tetanus toxoid antigen. However, failure to demonstrate an antibody response to pneumococcal polysaccharide or tetanus toxoid is an indication of a potentially serious problem. Children with deficiency of all isotypes (e.g., Bruton's agammaglobulinemia) uniformly develop chronic airways infection and lung dysfunction unless treated aggressively.

Immunoglobulin E

Immunoglobulin E appears to participate in immunity to parasites. It binds to the parasites, and eosinophils then bind to the opsonized organisms via the IgE Fc receptors. Eosinophils are stimulated to release granular contents, resulting in lysis of the parasite. Isolated IgE deficiency has not been reported. IgE deficiency in combination with IgG4 deficiency has been described in a patient who suffered from recurrent otitis media and sinusitis.

Job's syndrome (or hyper-IgE syndrome) is characterized by recurrent skin and lower respiratory tract infections, eczema, elevated IgE levels, and eosinophilia. Associated facial and bone abnormalities are common. Symptoms occur within the first month of life with severe eczema, mucocutaneous infections, sinusitis, and lower respiratory tract infections with *S. aureus* or *H. influenzae*. Development of empyema, lung abscesses, and pneumatoceles is common.

Immunoglobulin M

Most IgM remains in the vascular space because of its high molecular weight. However, IgM does gain access to the airway by exudation or by active secretion via secretory component. IgM is capable of agglutinating bacteria and activating the complement cascade. Therefore, even though low levels of IgM are detected in airway secretions, it plays a role in mucosal defense.

Isolated IgM deficiency is not associated with recurrent respiratory infections. Individuals with IgM deficiency appear to have a specific defect in B-lymphocyte maturation, but the B lymphocytes are capable of secreting other antibody isotypes.

■ SUMMARY

The lung is continuously exposed to potential pathogens. The multilayered defenses provided by the intrinsic, innate, and adaptive systems protect the lung from invasion yet are able to limit inflammatory responses and resolve lung inflammation after the pathogen has been eliminated. Although there is considerable overlap in the activities of these various defenses, defects can result in either recurrent infection or persistent inflammation.

REFERENCES

1. Chung KF: Cough. In: Crystal RG, West JB, Barnes PJ, Weibel ER, eds: The Lung. Scientific Foundations. Philadelphia: Lippincott-Raven, 1997, pp 2309–2323.
2. Knowles MR, Boucher RC: Mucus clearance as a primary innate defense mechanism for mammalian airways. J Clin Invest 2002;109:571–577.

3. Lamblin G, Degroote S, Perini JM, Delmotte P, Scharfman A, Davril M, Lo-Guidice JM, Houdret N, Dumur V, Klein A, Rousse P: Human airway mucin glycosylation. A combinatory of carbohydrate determinants which vary in cystic fibrosis. Glycoconj J 2001;18:661–684.
4. Morse DM, Smullen JL, Davis CW: Differential effects of UTP, ATP, and adenosine on ciliary activity of human nasal epithelial cells. Am J Physiol Cell Physiol 2001;280:C1485–C1497.
5. Noone PG, Leigh MW, Sannuti A, Minnix SL, Carson JL, Hazucha M, Zariwala MA, Knowles MR: Primary ciliary dyskinesia. Diagnostic and phenotypic features. Am J Respir Crit Care Med 2004;169:459–467.
6. Davis PB, Drumm M, Konstan MW: Cystic fibrosis. Am J Respir Crit Care Med 1996;154:1229–1256.
7. Watford WT, Ghio AJ, Wright JR: Complement-mediated host defense in the lung. Am J Physiol Lung Cell Mol Physiol 2000;279:L790–L798.
8. Sheppard D: Functions of pulmonary epithelial integrins. From development to disease. Physiol Rev 2003;83:673–686.
9. Anderson DC, Schmalsteig FC, Finegold MJ, Hughes BJ, Rothlein R, Miller LJ, Kohl S, Tosi MF, Jacobs RL, Waldrop TC, Goldman AS, Shearer WT, Springer TA: The severe and moderate phenotypes of heritable Mac-1, LFA-1 deficiency. Their quantitative definition and relation to leukocyte dysfunction and clinical features. J Infect Dis 1985;152:668–689.
10. Ley K: The role of selectins in inflammation and disease. Trends Mol Med 2003;9:263–268.
11. Underhill DM: Toll-like receptors. Networking for success. Eur J Immunol 2003;33:1767–1775.
12. Vasselon T, Detmers PA: Toll receptors. A central element in innate immune responses. Infect Immun 2002;70:1033–1041.
13. Akira S, Sato S: Toll-like receptors and their signaling mechanisms. Scand J Infect Dis 2003;35:555–562.
14. Cook DN, Hollingsworth JW II, Schwartz DA: Toll-like receptors and the genetics of innate immunity. Curr Opin Allergy Clin Immunol 2003; 3:523–529.
15. Crouch E, Wright JR: Surfactant proteins A and D and pulmonary host defense. Annu Rev Physiol 2001;63:521–554.
16. Van De Wetering JK, van Golde LM, Batenburg JJ: Collectins. Eur J Biochem 2004;271:1229–1249.
17. Skerrett SJ: Lysozyme in pulmonary host defense. New tricks for an old dog. Am J Respir Crit Care Med 2004;169:435–436.
18. Baveye S, Elass E, Mazurier J, Spik G, Legrand D: Lactoferrin. A multifunctional glycoprotein involved in the modulation of the inflammatory process. Clin Chem Lab Med 1999;37:281–286.
19. Elass-Rochard E, Legrand D, Salmon V, Roseanu A, Trif M, Tobias PS, Mazurier J, Spik G: Lactoferrin inhibits the endotoxin interaction with CD14 by competition with the lipopolysaccharide-binding protein. Infect Immun 1998;66:486–491.
20. Breeze RG, Wheeldon EB: The cells of the pulmonary airways. Am Rev Respir Dis 1977;116:705–777.
21. Evans MJ, Van Winkle LS, Fanucchi MV, Plopper CG: Cellular and molecular characteristics of basal cells in airway epithelium. Exp Lung Res 2001;27:401–415.
22. Shepherd VL: Distinct roles for lung collectins in pulmonary host defense. Am J Respir Cell Mol Biol 2002;26:257–260.
23. Strieter RM, Belperio JA, Keane MP: Cytokines in innate host defense in the lung. J Clin Invest 2002;109:699–705.
24. Mekori YA, Metcalfe DD: Mast cells in innate immunity. Immunol Rev 2000;173:131–140.
25. Lipscomb MF, Masten BJ: Dendritic cells. Immune regulators in health and disease. Physiol Rev 2002;82:97–130.
26. Nelson DJ, McMenamin C, McWilliam AS, Brenan M, Holt PG: Development of the airway intraepithelial dendritic cell network in the rat from class II major histocompatibility (Ia)-negative precursors. Differential regulation of Ia expression at different levels of the respiratory tract. J Exp Med 1994;179:203–212.
27. Matzinger P: Tolerance, danger, and the extended family. Annu Rev Immunol 1994;12:991–1045.
28. Matzinger P: The danger model. A renewed sense of self. Science 2002;296: 301–305.
29. Gordon SB, Read RC: Macrophage defences against respiratory tract infections. Br Med Bull 2002;61:45–61.
30. Peiser L, Mukhopadhyay S, Gordon S: Scavenger receptors in innate immunity. Curr Opin Immunol 2002;14:123–128.
31. Savill J, Gregory C, Haslett C: Cell biology. Eat me or die. Science 2003; 302:1516–1517.
32. Ganz T: Antimicrobial polypeptides in the host defense of the respiratory tract. J Clin Invest 2002;109:693–697.
33. Doerschuk CM: Mechanisms of leukocyte sequestration in inflamed lungs. Microcirculation 2001;8:71–88.
34. Lee WL, Harrison RE, Grinstein S: Phagocytosis by neutrophils. Microbes Infect 2003;5:1299–1306.
35. Kobayashi SD, Voyich JM, DeLeo FR: Regulation of the neutrophil-mediated inflammatory response to infection. Microbes Infect 2003;5: 1337–1344.
36. Faurschou M, Borregaard N: Neutrophil granules and secretory vesicles in inflammation. Microbes Infect 2003;5:1317–1327.
37. Alam R, Busse WW: The eosinophil—quo vadis? J Allergy Clin Immunol 2004;113:38–42.
38. Lacy P, Moqbel R: Immune effector functions of eosinophils in allergic airway inflammation. Curr Opin Allergy Clin Immunol 2001;1:79–84.
39. Yokoyama WM, Kim S, French AR: The dynamic life of natural killer cells. Annu Rev Immunol 2004;22:405–429.
40. Jameson J, Witherden D, Havran WL: T-cell effector mechanisms. Gammadelta and CD1d-restricted subsets. Curr Opin Immunol 2003;15: 349–353.
41. Boyton RJ, Openshaw PJ: Pulmonary defences to acute respiratory infection. Br Med Bull 2002;61:1–12.
42. Delves PJ, Roitt IM: The immune system. First of two parts. N Engl J Med 2000;343:37–49.
43. Pilette C, Ouadrhiri Y, Godding V, Vaerman JP, Sibille Y. Lung mucosal immunity. Immunoglobulin-A revisited. Eur Respir J 2001;18:571–588.

13 Acute Respiratory Failure

Emily L. Dobyns, MD • Todd C. Carpenter, MD • Anthony G. Durmowicz, MD • Kurt R. Stenmark, MD

Acute respiratory failure (ARF) is a term used to describe any disruption of the respiratory system (including malfunctions in the central nervous system respiratory control center; the nerves, muscles, or pleura; or the lungs themselves) that impairs its primary functions of delivering oxygen to and removing carbon dioxide from the pulmonary capillary bed. Factors other than respiratory system dysfunction can also affect oxygen and carbon dioxide tension in a given patient and need to be taken into consideration. These include environmental factors, such as the ambient barometric pressure (altitude) as well as patient age, the temperature, and the fraction of inspired oxygen (FIO_2). Earlier arterial blood gas determinations of oxygen and carbon dioxide tension, especially in patients with underlying chronic lung disease or significant metabolic derangements, may also determine whether ARF is present. Ultimately, however, most clinicians agree that, in the absence of an intracardiac shunt, ARF is present if partial pressure of oxygen in arterial blood (PaO_2) is less than 50 mm Hg or if partial pressure of carbon dioxide in arterial blood ($PaCO_2$) is greater than 50 mm Hg.

Acute respiratory failure requiring mechanical ventilation is a common problem in the pediatric age group. A recent study, and the largest performed to date in children, demonstrated that 17% (1096 of 6403) of children admitted to the pediatric intensive care unit (ICU) required mechanical ventilator support for a minimum of 24 hours.[1] Other studies suggest that acute hypoxemic respiratory failure accounts for approximately 16% of all ICU patient days. The morbidity and mortality rates in these patients has not been as well defined as in adult studies, where current mortality rates, at least for acute respiratory distress syndrome (ARDS), are approximately 30% to 40%. Reports in the 1990s, based on small sample sizes, placed the mortality rate at anywhere from 30% to 70% for children with ARDS.[1,2] However, in the recent large series mentioned earlier, the overall mortality rate was far lower than that reported in adult patients.[1]

There are developmental physiologic differences between the respiratory systems of children and adults that help to explain why respiratory failure is a common problem in the pediatric patient. An infant's thoracic cage is soft and therefore less able to withstand the large increases in negative intrathoracic pressure that must be generated to inflate the noncompliant lung. The intercostal muscles of the infant and young child are also poorly developed, and because the young child's ribs are aligned more in the horizontal plane across the chest wall, there is a lack of "bucket-handle" motion in the rib cage to augment chest expansion during inspiration. The child's diaphragm is shorter than that of the adult, making it less effective in generating force, and it has decreased numbers of type I muscle fibers, making it more prone to fatigue. In addition, a child's airway is much smaller than that of the adult, and in accordance with Poiseuille's law, the same degree of airway narrowing causes a much greater increase in airflow resistance. Finally, growing children have fewer air-exchanging units (respiratory bronchioles and alveoli) than adults, and the alveoli that are present are smaller. This, combined with the decreased amount of collateral ventilation in a child's lung compared with that of the adult, contributes to the decreased stability of the air-exchanging units, with an increased likelihood of collapse.

■ CLINICAL CLASSIFICATION OF ACUTE RESPIRATORY FAILURE

By convention, respiratory failure has previously been categorized as either type I or type II failure, although many pediatric patients with severe respiratory failure have a component of both types of failure. Type I failure, also termed *nonventilatory,* or *normocapnic, respiratory failure*, is characterized by abnormally low PaO_2 with normal to low $PaCO_2$. Type II failure, also known as *ventilatory,* or *hypercapnic, failure,* is distinguished by elevated $PaCO_2$ as well as a variable degree of hypoxemia. Some of the causes of types I and II respiratory failure are listed in Table 13-1.

The most common cause of hypoxemia in type I respiratory failure is the mismatch of alveolar ventilation relative to perfusion. When an unventilated area of the lung is perfused, blood is not oxygenated. This is referred to as an *intrapulmonary shunt,* and the total amount of pulmonary blood flow that perfuses nonventilated or underventilated areas is known as the *shunt fraction.* Another term for shunt fraction is *venous admixture.* It is the calculated amount of mixed venous blood that would need to mix with arterial blood to account for an observed difference between alveolar and arterial partial pressure of oxygen (PO_2). The shunt fraction can be calculated using the following equation:

$$\dot{Q}s/\dot{Q}t = (Cc'O_2 - CaO_2)/(Cc'O_2 - CvO_2)$$

where $Cc'O_2$ is the oxygen content of pulmonary capillary blood, CaO_2 is the oxygen content of arterial blood, and CvO_2 is the oxygen content of mixed venous blood. The oxygen content of pulmonary capillary blood is approximated by the alveolar oxygen content. Although it does not define the anatomic pathway of the shunt, the calculation of shunt fraction, or venous admixture, is a convenient index with which to follow changes in ventilation and perfusion matching and, thus, the overall efficiency of pulmonary gas exchange. If $PaCO_2$, hemoglobin, and the difference between arterial oxygen content and mixed venous oxygen content are held constant, then arterial PaO_2 is determined mainly by the inspired oxygen concentration and the amount of venous admixture. A small amount of venous admixture is normally present and is the result of drainage of the bronchial and thebesian veins into the pulmonary veins and left ventricle, respectively. Pathologic admixture can be caused by atelectasis, edema, pneumonia, or congenital heart disease characterized by intracardiac right-to-left shunting. In the normal lung, shunt fraction is less than 5%. Shunt fraction of greater than 15% results in significant impairment of oxygenation.

TABLE 13-1. Causes of acute respiratory failure

Type I Failure	Type II Failure
Acute respiratory distress syndrome Aspiration Atelectasis Bronchiolitis Cardiogenic pulmonary edema Cystic fibrosis Embolism (air, blood, fat) Interstitial lung disease Postobstruction pulmonary edema Radiation Sepsis Severe pneumonia (bacterial, viral, fungal, parasitic) Toxin or toxic gas inhalation Transfusion-related acute lung injury Trauma (pulmonary contusion)	Respiratory center Drugs (opiates, barbiturates, anesthetic agents) Central alveolar hypoventilation syndrome (Ondine's curse) Upper motor neuron Cervical spinal cord trauma Syringomyelia Demyelinating diseases Tumors Anterior horn cell Poliomyelitis Werdnig-Hoffmann syndrome Lower motor neuron Post-thoracotomy phrenic nerve damage Guillain-Barré syndrome Neuromuscular junction Botulism, multiple sclerosis, myasthenia gravis Neuromuscular blocking antibiotics (kanamycin, streptomycin, polymyxin) Organophosphate poisoning Tetanus Chest wall and pleura Contracted chest burn scars, flail chest, kyphoscoliosis Massive pleural effusion, morbid obesity Muscular dystrophy, pneumothorax Increased airway resistance Laryngeal obstruction (croup, diphtheria, epiglottitis, foreign body aspiration, postextubation edema, vocal cord paralysis) Lower airway obstruction (asthma, emphysema)

The hypoxemia caused by a true shunt does not respond to oxygen administration because the supplemental oxygen never reaches the blood that perfuses the nonventilated areas.

In contrast to shunt, or venous admixture, areas of the lung that are ventilated but not perfused are referred to as *dead space.* The portion of a tidal volume breath (VT) that is dead space (VD) is presented as the ratio VD/VT and is calculated in clinical situations using the following equation:

$$V_D/V_T = (PaCO_2 - PetCO_2)/PaCO_2$$

where $PaCO_2$ is arterial partial pressure of carbon dioxide (PCO_2) and $PetCO_2$ is end-tidal PCO_2. This is essentially the wasted part of the breath, and in the normal lung, it consists almost entirely of the volume of each breath that fills the conducting airways (i.e., anatomic dead space). The VD/VT ratio in the normal lung is approximately 0.30. VD/VT has a tendency to increase slightly with age and also increases slightly when going from the supine to the upright position (0.30–0.34). *Alveolar dead space,* defined as that part of the inspired gas that passes through the anatomic dead space to mix with gas at the alveolar level but which does not take part in gas exchange, is negligible in the normal lung; however, under pathologic conditions, such as pulmonary embolus, acute lung injury/acute respiratory distress syndrome (ALI/ARDS), and emphysema, it may increase dramatically. In severe ARDS, for example, VD/VT may increase to 0.75 due to the increase in alveolar dead space. The hypoxemia caused by an increase in dead space can usually be corrected by a corresponding increase in minute ventilation. If, for example, minute ventilation is 5 L/min and VD/VT is 0.30, then true alveolar ventilation is 3.5 L/min. If VD/VT were to increase to 0.50, minute ventilation would need to be increased to 7.0 L/min to maintain the same alveolar ventilation of 3.5 L/min.

Another potential cause of arterial hypoxemia in type I failure is impairment of oxygen diffusion across the alveolar-capillary membrane. In this situation, equilibrium between alveolar gas and pulmonary capillary blood is not achieved during the normal transit time of blood through the pulmonary capillary bed and, thus, oxygenation is incomplete. Disease processes such as severe lung fibrosis or pulmonary edema can potentially create a barrier to diffusion across the alveolar-capillary membrane. In resting normal subjects, a diffusion equilibrium is achieved for oxygen early (0.25–0.30 sec) in the course of the normal pulmonary capillary transit time of an erythrocyte (≈0.75 sec) and, as such, oxygen uptake by pulmonary capillary blood is limited, not by diffusing capacity, but by the amount of pulmonary blood flow. It is only under conditions of exercise at high altitude (hypoxia plus decreased transit time) that oxygen uptake is limited by diffusion in the normal subject. Even though an increase in the barrier to oxygen diffusion at times appears an attractive rationale for arterial hypoxemia, many believe that, even in disease states, such as pulmonary edema or lung fibrosis, the primary cause of hypoxemia remains maldistribution of ventilation relative to perfusion (shunt) as a result of the pathologic process and not diffusion limitation per se.

Regardless of the cause of hypoxemia in the setting of ARF, calculation of the alveolar-arterial oxygen tension difference (A-a difference) is a sensitive and clinically relevant measure of impairment of oxygen exchange from lung to blood. Alveolar oxygen tension (PAO_2) is estimated by the alveolar gas equation:

$$PAO_2 = [(PB - PH_2O)FIO_2] - [PaCO_2/RQ]$$

where PB is barometric pressure, PH_2O is partial pressure of water vapor (47 mm Hg), and RQ is the respiratory quotient (usually assumed to be 0.8). The A-a difference, then, is equal to $PAO_2 - PaO_2$. Although measurable at any given FIO_2, the A-a difference is commonly determined with the patient breathing an FIO_2 of 1.00 for 20 minutes. When the patient is breathing 100% oxygen, PAO_2 is the same in all ventilated alveoli. Under these circumstances, the A-a difference is a reflection of physiologic shunting of blood in the lung (in the absence of cyanotic congenital heart disease). The normal A-a difference is less than 50 mm Hg at an FIO_2 of 1.00 (<30 mm Hg when breathing room air). An A-a difference of greater than 450 mm Hg is indicative of severe respiratory failure. Another way of defining the severity of lung injury is by dividing PaO_2 by FIO_2. As defined by the American-European Consensus Conference on Acute Respiratory Distress Syndrome, ALI exists when PaO_2/FIO_2 is less than 300 mm Hg. ARDS exists when PaO_2/FIO_2 is less than 200 mm Hg, signifying a more severe impairment of oxygenation.[3] Importantly, the pulmonary disease process must be of acute onset, must affect both lungs (bilateral densities on radiographic films of the chest), and must not be due to cardiac failure.

Type II, or hypercapnic, respiratory failure is characterized by increased alveolar and arterial carbon dioxide. This type of respiratory failure is associated with a malfunction of the structures that ventilate the lung, including major airways, bronchi, respiratory muscles, and thoracic cage. Thus, the final common pathway for type II respiratory failure is alveolar hypoventilation. The usually mild degree of hypoxemia that can be associated with pure type II failure (i.e., in the absence of significant lung parenchymal disease) is explained by the same alveolar gas equation used to determine P_{AO_2} that was described earlier. Essentially, as the carbon dioxide concentration increases in alveolar gas as a result of hypoventilation, there is less space available for oxygen and nitrogen. When the patient breathes room air, as Pa_{CO_2} rises, P_{AO_2} gradually diminishes, resulting in a relatively mild degree of hypoxemia. The hypoxemia can easily be overcome with the administration of small amounts of oxygen. For example, breathing an inspired oxygen concentration of 30% will restore alveolar P_{O_2} to normal in a hypoventilating patient with an alveolar P_{CO_2} of approximately 100 mm Hg. It is important to remember that in pure type II failure, the use of supplemental oxygen can prevent hypoxia, even in a patient with severe hypoventilation. This carries the risk of causing iatrogenic hypercarbia by removing the hypoxic stimulus to respiration. The child who is already in some degree of parenchymal lung failure (type I) is also at increased risk for type II failure. Hypoxemia secondary to parenchymal lung damage may decrease the available energy supply to the respiratory muscles, leading to suboptimal function. The resulting alveolar hypoventilation is a result of the diminished capacity of the respiratory muscles to keep up with the demands placed on them. In addition, the principal causes of lung parenchymal failure ($\dot{V}/\dot{Q}$ mismatch, intrapulmonary shunt, and diffusion defects) also diminish the efficiency of carbon dioxide exchange across the alveolar capillary membrane. Although large amounts of carbon dioxide can easily be eliminated by the normal respiratory system, the failing lung parenchyma may find it difficult to eliminate carbon dioxide effectively, especially in the face of increased metabolic demands, such as during fever, when there is a 14% increase in carbon dioxide production per degree Celsius increase in temperature.

Respiratory failure may also be classified as acute or chronic, depending on the rapidity of its onset and the ability of the body to compensate for it. Chronic respiratory failure presupposes an underlying chronic respiratory disease that is associated with either type I or type II failure. The patient may be able to lead a relatively normal life, depending on his or her ability to adjust to the work of breathing and on the adequacy of the body's ability to compensate for retained carbon dioxide. However, the patient with chronic respiratory insufficiency may quickly progress to ARF as the result of a minor respiratory illness, such as a viral infection. Assessment of the patient's acid-base balance helps in the evaluation of carbon dioxide retention over time and helps to determine whether the process is acute or chronic (i.e., after adequate renal compensation has occurred). Although it is not perfect, a clinically useful method of ascertaining acid-base balance is by the calculation of base excess (BE), which compares the buffering capacity of a patient's blood with normal capacity. It is calculated as follows:

$$BE = -1.2(24 - \text{measured bicarbonate})$$

where −1.2 is a correction factor for nonbicarbonate blood buffering capacity (e.g., hemoglobin, plasma proteins) and 24 is the normal bicarbonate level. Metabolic alkalosis is associated with a positive value, whereas metabolic acidosis is associated with a negative value, often reported as a base deficit. The distinction between respiratory and nonrespiratory causes of acid-base disturbances is crucial because the approaches to treatment differ. For example, a patient with severe respiratory acidosis will likely require mechanical ventilation, whereas nonrespiratory acidosis is more likely due to decreased cardiac output and perfusion and would respond more effectively to medical management aimed at increasing cardiac output.

It should be noted that there is an ever-changing demographic of patients in the ICU and, thus, of patients with respiratory failure. At least 43% of children recently enrolled in the study of respiratory failure by Randolph and colleagues[1] had one or more chronic underlying conditions, including pulmonary, cardiac, oncologic, hematologic, and neurologic conditions. The nature and severity of the underlying condition have significant effects on the severity and type of respiratory failure, the management approaches taken, and ultimately, the outcome. For instance, although the overall mortality rate for ALI/ARDS was recently reported as very low (<5%), the mortality rate in patients who undergo bone marrow transplantation ranges from 70% to 100%. ALI/ARDS is the most serious and also the most well-studied form of respiratory failure encountered; thus, the remainder of the chapter will focus on this particular condition.

PATHOPHYSIOLOGY AND PATHOGENESIS OF ACUTE LUNG INJURY/ACUTE RESPIRATORY DISTRESS SYNDROME

GENERAL DESCRIPTION AND PATHOLOGY OF ACUTE LUNG INJURY/ACUTE RESPIRATORY DISTRESS SYNDROME

Acute lung injury is the term used to describe the pulmonary response to a broad range of injuries occurring either directly to the lung or as a consequence of injury or inflammation at other sites in the body. As suggested earlier, ARDS represents the more severe end of this condition, in which there are widespread inflammatory changes throughout the lung. In some cases, these changes can be accompanied by an aggressive fibrotic response.

Trauma, sepsis, aspiration, pneumonia, ischemia or reperfusion, and other clinical catastrophes (Table 13-2)[4] are well known to contribute to the development of acute lung injury (ALI or ARDS). ARDS is associated with severe gas exchange and mechanical abnormalities of the lung, typically necessitating mechanical ventilation with positive end-expiratory airway pressure. Depending on the age group studied and the inciting cause, it has a significant mortality rate. Conversely, ALI/ARDS may itself contribute to morbidity and mortality in the critically ill patient in the ICU. The basic underlying abnormality, when attributed to either exogenous (indirect, e.g., sepsis) or

TABLE 13-2. Conditions associated with the development of acute lung injury or acute respiratory distress syndrome

Direct Insult Pulmonary Etiology	Indirect Insult Extrapulmonary Etiology
Pneumonia	Sepsis
Aspiration	Severe trauma with multiple fractures
Inhalation injury	Shock
Pulmonary contusion	Acute pancreatitis
Fat emboli	Cardiopulmonary bypass
Near-drowning	Disseminated intravascular coagulation
Reperfusion injury	Burn
	Head injury
	Transfusion

endogenous (direct, e.g., pneumonia, aspiration) causes, is an increase in alveolar-capillary permeability, resulting in pulmonary edema, which is more severe in ARDS than in ALI. It is also well recognized that some of the lung injury observed in the patient with ALI/ARDS is created and exacerbated by mechanical ventilation, which was necessitated by the pulmonary insult. As discussed later, however, mortality from ARDS has improved significantly in recent years. Some, but not all, of this improvement in mortality is believed to be due to improvements in the ventilatory support mechanisms used to support these patients.

Currently, ALI/ARDS is defined clinically by gas exchange and chest radiographic abnormalities that occur shortly after a known predisposing injury and in the absence of heart failure. The pathophysiology of ARDS is driven by an aggressive inflammatory reaction. Indirect injury can occur in an ongoing fashion as part of a systemic inflammatory response syndrome, which can be due to either infective or noninfective causes. ARDS can thus occur in conjunction with failure of other organs, a condition that has been termed *multiorgan dysfunction syndrome*. It should also be noted that a number of endogenous anti-inflammatory mechanisms are initiated to counterbalance the effects of this aggressive inflammatory response. This has been termed a *compensatory anti-inflammatory response syndrome*. Some have suggested that these responses can be excessive and contribute to a state of immunoparesis that predisposes the patient to secondary infections that cause further lung injury.[5]

From a pathologic point of view, lung injury is believed to be an evolving condition and has been described as passing through three overlapping phases: (1) an inflammatory, or exudative, phase; (2) a proliferative phase; and (3) a fibrotic phase (Table 13-3). These phases may be complicated by other variables, for example, episodes of nosocomial pneumonia as well as the previously mentioned deleterious effects of ventilator-induced lung injury. Moreover, it is important to note that recent studies have suggested that the initiating insults themselves may influence the pathophysiologic picture. Radiographic differences have been identified between patients with ARDS arising from direct pulmonary injuries and those with ARDS caused by indirect injuries.[6] Emerging studies have suggested greater areas of alveolar collapse and edema in patients who die of ARDS caused by direct rather than indirect injuries. Interestingly, it is possible that these differences may not only translate into differences in outcome, but also may ultimately dictate differences in treatment approaches (discussed later).

The exudative phase in acute lung injury is believed to persist for the first week after the onset of symptoms. The histologic changes have been termed *diffuse alveolar damage*. This phase is characterized by significant proteinaceous and often hemorrhagic interstitial and alveolar edema, with accompanying hyaline membrane formation. The hyaline membranes may be eosinophilic, and they contain fibrin, immunoglobulin, and complement. The microvascular and alveolar barriers have focal areas of damage, and the alveolar wall is edematous, with areas of necrosis observed in the epithelial lining. Neutrophils are found increasingly during the initial phases in capillaries and interstitial tissue and progressively within the airspace.

The proliferative phase has typically been described as beginning 7 days after the onset of respiratory failure and lasting 1 to 2 weeks. However, recent evidence suggests that this phase may actually begin within the first 48 hours and therefore accompany the inflammatory phase (discussed later). The proliferative phase is characterized by organization of the exudates and by fibrosis. The lung is very heavy and fluid-filled, appearing almost solid. Microscopically, the lung architecture becomes steadily more deranged. The capillary network is often severely damaged, and there is a progressive decline in the number of intact capillaries. In the later stages of this phase, there may even be intimal proliferation in the small vessels, which can lead to a further reduction in the vascular luminal area and, thus, to potential increases in blood flow resistance and persistence of increased pulmonary artery pressure. The interstitial space becomes grossly dilated, with necrosis of type I pneumocytes often observed. Apoptosis or necrosis of type I pneumocytes exposes areas of the epithelial basement membrane that can initiate and perpetuate fibroproliferative responses. The alveolar lumen may fill with leukocytes, red cells, fibrin, and other cellular debris. During this period, alveolar type II cells proliferate, presumably in an attempt to cover the denuded epithelial surfaces, and ultimately differentiate into type I cells. This proliferation may not be well controlled and may not use the typical mechanisms that control type II cell proliferation and differentiation during normal lung development. In addition, fibroblasts and myofibroblasts accumulate in the interstitial space and, later, even in the alveolar lumen. This excessive and sometimes uncontrolled proliferation of fibroblasts can result in extreme

TABLE 13-3. Summary of histopathologic changes in acute respiratory distress syndrome

Appearance of the Lungs	Exudative Phase	Proliferative Phase	Fibrotic Phase
Macroscopic	Heavy, rigid, dark	Heavy, gray	Cobblestone
Microscopic	Hyaline membranes Edema Neutrophils Epithelial damage greater than endothelial damage	Barrier disruption Edema Proliferation of alveolar type II cells Myofibroblast infiltration Neutrophils Alveolar collapse Alveoli filled with cells and an organizing matrix Epithelial apoptosis Fibroproliferation	Fibrosis Macrophages Lymphocytes Matrix organization Deranged acinar architecture Patchy emphysematous change
Vasculature	Local thrombus	Loss of capillaries Pulmonary hypertension	Myointimal thickening Tortuous vessels

narrowing or even obliteration of the airspaces. Ultimately, fibrin and cell debris are replaced by collagen fibrils in the intra-alveolar space and lung interstitium.

The fibrotic stage is the final stage of lung injury. It has been described as beginning approximately 10 days after the initiating injury, although current evidence suggests that it may begin much earlier, perhaps even accompanying the early proliferative phase. At this time, there may be a decline in the number of neutrophils and a relative accumulation of lymphocytes and macrophages. The most dramatic (although often unpredictable) changes are those in the accumulation of collagen in the lung. Total lung collagen in some cases has been reported to double within the first 2 weeks. During this period, the vasculature appears grossly abnormal, with vessels often narrowed due to mural fibrosis and even myointimal thickening. Many studies suggest that the degree of fibrosis is the key predictor of outcome. High levels of procollagen peptides detected early in ARDS have been shown to predict a poor outcome. Further, fibrosis, once established, can lead to a persistent reduction in lung compliance, thereby increasing the work of breathing and decreasing VT, thus resulting in increased carbon dioxide retention. Gas exchange is reduced because alveolar obliteration and interstitial thickening contribute to continued hypoxia and ventilator dependence. The patients therefore may have long stays in the ICU and become ventilator-dependent. These patients are at high risk for nosocomial infections, especially pneumonia, which can ultimately contribute to increased mortality.

As mentioned earlier, there may be a much greater overlap between the exudative and fibroproliferative phases than previously believed. Many mediators are common to both processes. For instance, early increases in procollagen III peptide levels (a marker for collagen turnover, which is an indication of the proliferative phase) have been observed in bronchoalveolar lavage (BAL) fluid within 24 hours of ventilation for ARDS and consistently have been shown to be associated with poor outcome. Myofibroblasts have also been shown to appear in increased numbers in the alveolar wall early in the process. Interestingly, BAL fluid obtained from patients with ARDS within 48 hours of diagnosis is intensely mitogenic for fibroblasts. These observations suggest that the fibrotic characteristic of ARDS may not be a late event, but rather one initiated early in the disease process. This is important because inflammatory and fibroproliferative processes, although closely overlapping, may be regulated through independently regulated signaling pathways. This observation offers the possibility of early treatment directed against fibrosis, independent of treatment directed against inflammation.

PULMONARY HYPERTENSION IN ACUTE LUNG INJURY/ACUTE RESPIRATORY DISTRESS SYNDROME

Pulmonary hypertension due to vasoconstriction and occlusion of the pulmonary microvasculature is widely recognized as a characteristic feature of ARDS. Mild to moderate elevations in pulmonary artery pressure (mean, 30–40 mm Hg) have been consistently reported in adult patients with ARDS. Pulmonary hypertension is probably a ubiquitous complication of the syndrome. Some investigators have suggested that ARDS is unlikely in patients with pulmonary artery pressure of less than 20 mm Hg. Although the degree of pulmonary arterial hypertension may be mild to moderate in most patients with ARDS, in this setting of diffuse alveolar damage, it can promote the accumulation of extravascular water in the lung and cause right ventricular dysfunction, thus reducing ejection fraction and cardiac output. In fact, the presence and degree of pulmonary hypertension have been shown to be adverse prognostic indicators in patients with ARDS.[7]

In the exudative, or acute, phase of ARDS, a number of factors may contribute to the increase in pulmonary artery pressure that is observed. Increased circulating levels of vasoactive mediators, such as serotonin, endothelin-1, thromboxane, leukotrienes, and platelet-activating factor (PAF), may contribute to the increase in pulmonary vascular tone. There may also be important contributions from increased activity of the sympathetic nervous system. The role of hypoxic pulmonary vasoconstriction in contributing to the elevations in pulmonary artery pressure observed in ARDS is controversial. Although hypoxic pulmonary vasoconstriction might play some role in increasing pulmonary vascular resistance locally, generally, the pulmonary vascular response to hypoxia has been described as being reduced in patients with ARDS. Administration of 100% oxygen to patients with ALI/ARDS does not significantly alter pulmonary hemodynamics. In later (fibroproliferative) phases of ARDS, structural changes in the small pulmonary arteries (vascular remodeling) develop, as described earlier. The intimal changes have been described as correlating with the duration and severity of lung injury. Initially, there is evidence of endothelial injury, and thromboemboli are described almost universally. These initial changes precede (and lead to) later fibrocellular intimal obliteration of arteries, veins, and sometimes even lymphatic vessels. Such changes are observed in patients who live for more than 10 days. The fibroproliferative changes cause continued elevations in pulmonary artery pressure, which may or may not be amenable to vasodilator therapy (discussed later).

Because pulmonary hypertension is such a frequent complication of ARDS, many interventions to decrease pulmonary artery pressure have been attempted to ameliorate the syndrome. Currently, pharmacologic manipulation of pulmonary vascular tone is feasible in patients with ARDS, but unfortunately, none of these treatments has a proven mortality benefit. Research aimed at further elucidating the mechanisms underlying pulmonary hypertension in ARDS may lead to improvements in the outcome of pharmacologic interventions.

ROLE OF INFLAMMATORY CELLS IN THE GENERATION AND AMPLIFICATION OF LUNG INJURY

Acute inflammation may be initiated by a specific stimulus (transient or persistent) derived from either the injurious event itself or the lungs' resident cell population. For example, aspiration of acid or exposure to high concentrations of oxygen may directly cause lung cell necrosis and resultant inflammation secondary to the release of cytokines from the dying lung cells. In other instances, inhaled bacteria, drugs, or even other particulates may be phagocytized by alveolar macrophages. The alveolar macrophages may then release proinflammatory cytokines, such as tumor necrosis factor (TNF), and chemotaxins, such as macrophage-derived neutrophil chemotactic factor, hydroxyeicosatetraenoic acids, leukotriene B (LTB_4), and complement components (C5a and C5a[HETE]-des-Arg), initiating the lung inflammatory process. Polymorphonuclear neutrophils (PMNs) may be recruited into the lung interstitium and alveoli within hours of injury and are capable of releasing many injurious agents that perpetuate the cycle of injury.

Polymorphonuclear neutrophils are the cells most often implicated as playing an important pathogenetic role in many different forms of lung injury. Many forms of acute lung injury (especially ARDS) are characterized by marked accumulation of PMNs in the lung. Further, in many animal models, the degree of lung injury is reduced if neutrophil influx is ablated. Of note, ARDS can develop in neutropenic patients, leading to the idea that neutrophils are an important, but not essential, component of the injury response.

Typically, the inciting injury or stimulus activates PMNs or endothelial cells, resulting in marked changes in their interaction in the vascular space. Activated PMNs aggregate and adhere to the luminal surface of endothelial cells. PMN adhesion occurs, at least partially, through specific interactions of proteins on the plasma membranes of both PMNs and endothelial cells. PMN membranes have integrin receptors that are members of either the immunoglobulin gene superfamily or the "selectin" family of lectin–endothelial cell adhesion molecules (LECAMs). Three relevant integrins on PMNs that are known to be important in PMN-endothelial interaction are LFA-1, MAC-1 (also known as Mol, or CR3), and P150,95. On the endothelial surface, intracellular adhesion molecules types 1 and 2 (ICAM1 and ICAM2), vascular cell adhesion molecule type 1 (VCAM), and endothelial leukocyte adhesion molecule type 1 are some of the ligands to which the PMN-integrins bind. The quantities of cell surface integrins on PMNs, as well as intracellular adhesion molecules and vascular cell adhesion molecule type 1 on endothelial cells, are increased by several different mediators, including TNF, interleukin-1 (IL-1), endotoxin, and thrombin. After activation and adhesion, PMNs generate oxidants and proteases that cause direct injury to resident lung cell populations, including the endothelium and epithelium. Furthermore, it appears that activated PMN-endothelial interaction leads to marked increases in vascular capillary permeability. This, in turn, leads to leakage of plasma proteins into the lung interstitium and sometimes into the alveolar space.

Subsequent to PMN influx, blood monocytes appear to be recruited into the lung. In a period of 1 to 2 days, newly recruited monocytes mature into activated macrophages. Studies have demonstrated that the recruitment of monocytes seems to require the presence of PMNs, although this is certainly not an absolute requirement. Macrophages produce a variety of cytokines, procoagulants, and growth factors capable of causing further lung injury. Macrophages are a heterogeneous cell population, and specialized subpopulations of macrophages with different functional capabilities likely exist. For example, some macrophages may be more specialized for lysosomal enzyme synthesis, whereas others may be especially cytocidal for tumor cells. A complex interaction between activated macrophages and lymphocytes that promotes inflammation can develop. Activated macrophages release IL-1β and IL-8. IL-1β is chemotactic for lymphocytes and stimulates the production of lymphokines and monokines (interferon-γ and macrophage inhibitory factor [MIF]) by helper T lymphocytes. The cytokine IL-2 stimulates the replication of T-lymphocyte clones, promotes B-lymphocyte differentiation and immunoglobulin production, and activates killer T cells. The IL-8 chemokines are potent PMN chemotaxins and activators. Thus, it is likely that macrophages can both initiate and amplify lung injury. Furthermore, it is clear that numerous inflammatory cells interact and participate in the ongoing inflammatory response seen in acute lung injury.

SPECIFIC MEDIATORS OF LUNG INJURY

Accumulation of inflammatory cells can clearly result in tissue injury (Fig. 13-1). This presumably occurs as a result of the combined effects of increased production of cytokines, oxidants, proteases, and cationic proteins. PMNs can secrete proteases and produce oxidants in regulated fashion without causing their own death. Activated oxygen metabolites (hypochlorite [OCl^-], superoxide anion [O_2^-], hydroxyl radical [OH], hydrogen peroxide [H_2O_2], and chloramines) are produced and released outside the PMN. It is not known exactly how these highly reactive compounds reach the extracellular space, except for hydrogen

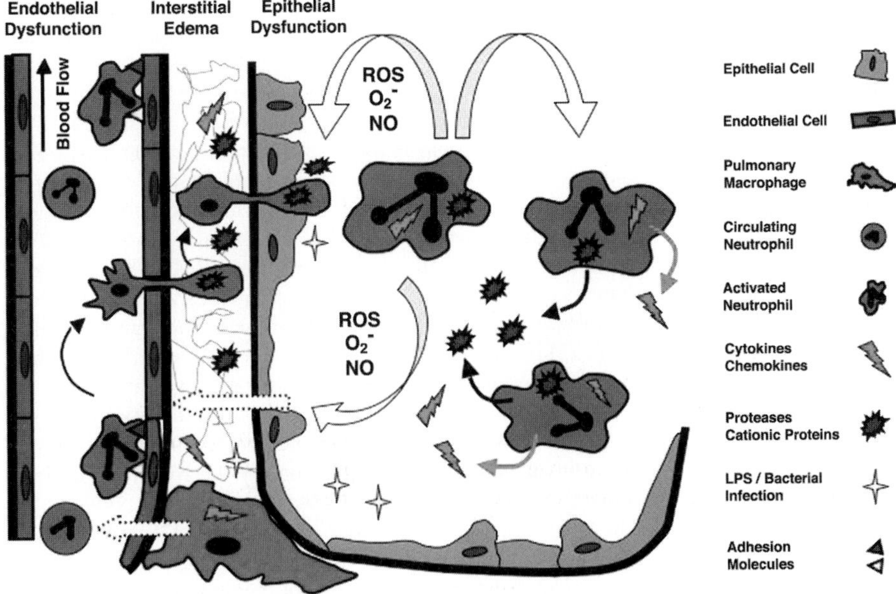

FIGURE 13-1. Mechanisms of lung injury. Step 1: In response to an inciting event or injury, the pulmonary macrophages and endothelium become activated and up-regulate surface expression of adhesion molecules. Step 2: This leads to neutrophil adhesion and subsequent transmigration from the intravascular space into the alveolus. Step 3: The activated neutrophil produces a plethora of inflammatory mediators that include reactive oxygen species (ROS) such as OH^- and O_2^- and nitric oxide (NO), cytokines, chemokines, proteases, and cationic proteins. In addition to the activated neutrophil, the other cells that make up the alveolar unit, including the pulmonary monocytes and macrophages and the pulmonary endothelial and epithelial cells, also contribute significantly to the production of inflammatory mediators. The neutrophil, however, is the major cause of ROS production in the context of acute lung injury and acute respiratory distress syndrome. LPS, lipopolysaccahride.

peroxide, which readily crosses cell membranes. It is important to note that the relatively high alveolar oxygen concentrations used to treat the hypoxemia observed in acute lung injury may act to "feed the fire" and promote increased production of further reactive oxygen metabolites.

Cytokines

The inflammatory process is driven in part by cytokines, including TNF-α and IL-1β, IL-6, and IL-8. All have been found in the BAL fluid and plasma of patients with ARDS. These cytokines are produced by inflammatory cells, and they can promote neutrophil-endothelial adhesion, induce increases in permeability, and amplify other anti-inflammatory responses. However, despite their well-known presence and role in bacterial or toxin-mediated sepsis, the importance of these cytokines in the actual pathogenesis of ARDS remains unclear. Levels of TNF-α are not uniformly increased in patients with lung injury, and therapeutic trials using anti-TNF-α and IL-1 have been disappointing and inconclusive. Many believe that the huge redundancy in the proinflammatory mediator system is responsible for failure of single-anticytokine therapeutic agents and suggest that the search for a "common pathway" that is susceptible to single-drug inhibition is overly simplistic. Other proinflammatory mediators, including vascular endothelial growth factor, high-mobility group 1 protein, and thrombin, have also been implicated, either directly or indirectly, in the increased vascular permeability that contributes to edema and lung injury. The etiologic role of these mediators in ARDS is even less well established than that of the cytokines. The balance of anti-inflammatory "cytokines" and mediators must also be considered in the context of ALI/ARDS. There is good evidence that mediators, such as soluble TNF receptors (sTNF-r), IL-4, and IL-10, and even other molecules, such as carbon monoxide, at very low concentrations, are powerful down-regulators of the inflammatory response and are commonly observed in the setting of acute lung injury.

The factors responsible for the intense neutrophilic infiltrate that is often observed in ALI/ARDS remain unclear. Although early studies implicated complement, more recently, the focus has been on chemokines, specifically IL-8. IL-8 levels are raised in the BAL fluid of at-risk patients who ultimately go on to have ARDS. It is a powerful neutrophil chemoattractant derived from alveolar macrophages and other cells, and it may be regulated by hypoxia or hyperoxia. Future studies are needed to determine the exact chemokines responsible for initiating and then amplifying the neutrophilic response.

Reactive Oxygen Species

Free radicals damage a variety of cell components, including deoxyribonucleic acid, membrane lipids, and proteins (see Fig. 13-1). At the most extreme end of the spectrum, oxygen radicals, at least in vitro, have even been shown to lyse endothelial cells and fibroblasts. The more subtle damaging effects of oxidants are complex and incompletely defined. When exposed to hydroxyl radicals or superoxide anions, membrane lipids undergo peroxidation of polyunsaturated fatty acids in a self-perpetuating chain reaction, resulting in markedly decreased cell membrane fluidity. Nucleic acids are rapidly nicked by hydroxyl radicals, resulting in abnormal cross-linkages and mutations. Glyceraldehyde-3-phosphate dehydrogenase, a requisite enzyme for glycolysis, is inhibited both directly by oxidants and by the resulting increase in intracellular redox potential (ratio of nicotinamide adenine dinucleotide$^+$ to nicotinamide adenine dinucleotide [reduced form]). The resulting depletion of adenosine triphosphate prevents other essential cellular functions, such as ion transport, from being carried out. Increases in free intracellular calcium are observed. This can activate phospholipases, endonucleases, and calcium-dependent proteases, resulting in cell lysis. Many enzymes, including membrane transport proteins, are also inactivated because their sulfhydryl groups are subject to oxidation. Oxidants may also directly oxidize the cellular cytoskeleton and interfere with exocytosis. For example, H_2O_2 alters β-adrenergic and purinergic receptor-mediated signal transduction in alveolar type II cells. In addition, oxidation of proteins may also make them more susceptible to proteolytic degradation.

There are a number of lines of evidence supporting a significant role for activated oxygen species in contributing to lung injury in the setting of ARDS. First, the large numbers of PMNs present provide the capability for generating many oxidants within the alveolar space. Second, expired gas contains increased H_2O_2. Third, BAL fluid in patients with ARDS contains nonfunctional α_1-antitrypsin because of oxidation of the active-site methionine to a sulfoxide, cleavage of the active site, or both. Fourth, myeloperoxidase is often present in BAL fluid obtained from patients with ARDS, consistent with the ability to form hypochlorous acid. Fifth, alveolar glutathione levels are markedly depleted. Fortunately, BAL fluid from patients with ARDS has also been shown to contain increased functional antioxidant activity, due predominantly to increases in transferrin and ceruloplasmin. The influx of serum antioxidant proteins that occurs with increased permeability pulmonary edema may help to protect the lung from additional oxidant damage.

Proteolytic Enzymes

Proteolytic enzymes are another major class of compounds capable of causing damage to the lung. Most of the important proteases involved in lung injury are endoproteases (Table 13-4) that are released both by circulating inflammatory cells (especially PMNs) and by resident lung cells and that function extracellularly at neutral pH. Proteases can injure cells directly, degrade components of the extracellular matrix, and break down extracellular and cell surface macromolecules. However, proteases have also been demonstrated to be important in normal growth and development of the lung as well as in lung host defense.

The majority of proteases that cause lung injury are generated by PMNs. Macrophages, T lymphocytes, eosinophils, mast cells, fibroblasts, type II alveolar epithelial cells, and basophils also release proteases, but usually in much smaller quantities. Proteases are classified based on whether they contain metal ions (metalloenzymes) and on the essential amino acid at the active site (serine- and cysteine-proteases). PMNs contain more than six proteases that are stored within at least three types of cytoplasmic granules—azurophilic, specific, and tertiary. Neutrophil elastase is recognized as the most injurious of these proteases because of its activity against a broad range of extracellular matrix molecules and its ability to injure many types of lung cells directly. It is made and stored during neutrophil maturation and is not subsequently actively synthesized. A primary action of neutrophil elastase is lysis of the elastic fiber. The resulting elastin peptides are chemotactic, calling more neutrophils to the region, thus propagating the injury. The name *elastase* is somewhat of a misnomer because, in addition to

■ **TABLE 13-4.** Proteases relevant to the lung

Protease	Category	Cell Source	ECM Substrates
Neutrophil elastase	Serine-proteinase	PMN (Az) Mast cells Basophils	Elastin, FN, LM, tI–IV collagen, PG
Cathepsin G	Serine-proteinase	PMN (Az) Eosinophils	FN, PG, elastin, tIV collagen
Collagenase	Metalloproteinase	PMN (Sp) Fibroblasts Macrophages Eosinophils	tI, III–V, and VII collagens; gelatin; FN; PG
Gelatinase	Metalloproteinase	PMN (Sp and 3) Fibroblasts Macrophages Eosinophils	LM; elastin; FN; gelatin; tIV, V, VII, and X collagen
Proteinase-3	Serine-proteinase	PMN (Az)	tI and III collagen
Plasminogen activator	Serine-proteinase	PMN (surface) Macrophages Type II cells	Elastin, plasminogen
Cathepsin D	Aspartic-proteinase	Monocytes PMN (Az) Fibroblasts Macrophages	PG, tIV collagen, FN
Cathepsin L	Cysteine-proteinase	Macrophages	tIV collagen, FN
Cathepsin B	Cysteine-proteinase	Macrophages PMN (Az)	Elastin
Stromelysins	Metalloproteinase	Macrophages Fibroblasts	PG, LM
Punctuated metalloproteinases	Metalloproteinase	Monocytes	Elastin, PG
Granzymes	Serine-proteinase	T cells	Cellular matrix
Chymase	Serine-proteinase	Mast cells Basophils	FN, PG, collagen

Az, azurophilic granules; ECM, extracellular matrix; FN, fibronectin; LM, laminin; PG, proteoglycans; PMN, polymorphonuclear neutrophil; Sp, specific granules; t, type; 3, tertiary.

Adapted from Hubbard RC, Brantly ML, et al: Proteases. In: Crystal RG, West JB, eds: The Lung. Scientific Foundations. New York: Raven Press, 1991.

cleaving elastin, it cleaves collagen types I through IV, fibronectin, laminin, proteoglycan core proteins, plasminogen, immunoglobulin G, immunoglobulin M, C3, C5, and many coagulation factors. Consistent with these effects, neutrophil elastase has been shown to compromise the integrity of the endothelial barrier and promote microvascular injury, with resultant increased permeability and interstitial edema. Many of the peptide fragments generated by lysis of these proteins are also chemotactic for PMNs. Neutrophil elastase can also potentiate the inflammatory response indirectly by increasing the expression and release of IL-8, a potent neutrophil chemoattractant and activating agent. Based on these properties, neutrophil elastase is believed to be an important pathogenetic factor in many lung diseases causing respiratory failure, including ARDS, idiopathic pulmonary fibrosis, emphysema, cystic fibrosis, chronic bronchitis, and immune complex injury.

Under normal physiologic conditions, antiprotease defenses in the lung limit the action of protease to the desired physical location for a short, specified period. Lung antiprotease defenses include α_1-antitrypsin, α_2-macroglobulin, secretory leukoprotease inhibitor, tissue inhibitor of metalloproteases, and α_1-antichymotrypsin. Because the levels of antiproteases in the bloodstream are usually high, most lung tissue injury is likely secondary to proteases generated locally in the lung rather than coming from the bloodstream.

Evidence for the role of proteases in acute lung injury is circumstantial, but strong. In ARDS, large numbers of PMNs are usually present in BAL fluid. Elastase activity has been reported to be increased in the lavage fluid of many, but not all, patients. Neutrophil collagenase and myeloperoxidase are also frequently present. Macrophages from patients with ARDS have been shown to release a peptide, probably IL-8, that promotes neutrophil protease secretion. Importantly, antiprotease inhibitors, specifically α_1-antiprotease inhibitor, have been shown to be inactivated in the setting of acute lung injury through oxidation of active-site methionine to a sulfoxide. In many patients with ARDS, much of the α_1-antiprotease inhibitor that is antigenically present in the alveolar space has been shown to be no longer functionally active. In experimental models, protease instillation or localized activation produces a lung injury characterized by edema, inflammation, and hypoxemia. Pharmacologic inhibition of proteases using a variety of inhibitors in a number of animals has consistently reduced lung injury.

Proteases and oxidants may act synergistically in causing injury to lung tissue. Oxidants can inactivate antiprotease defenses and allow proteases to act in an "unchecked" fashion. Oxidation of proteins may also alter their secondary or tertiary structure and allow them to be more easily degraded by proteases. This mechanism is probably operative in the destruction of the extracellular matrix that is observed in lung injury. Furthermore, damage or degradation of lung extracellular matrix proteins by proteases or oxidants results in the generation of more neutrophil chemotactic factors. The resulting influx of more neutrophils increases the local generation of both proteases and oxidants. Thus, a vicious cycle of lung inflammation, release of oxidants and proteases, and destruction of antiprotease defenses can be initiated, which, under the right conditions, perpetuates a cycle of ongoing lung injury.

Other Mediators

A plethora of other mediators also appear to be important causes of tissue damage in different types of lung injury. These include bacterial lipopolysaccharide (endotoxin), activated coagulation proteins, arachidonic acid–derived lipids, and cations. Studies implicating these mediators in acute lung injury again are somewhat circumstantial. One approach has been to assess or document increased levels of particular compounds in blood or lavage fluid from animals with experimental lung injury or humans with lung disease. Another approach has been to use pharmacologic inhibitors to demonstrate the importance of a particular mediator or pathway in lung injury due to specific stimuli. However, most inhibitors are not completely specific. Furthermore, given the multiple interactions of mediators, oxidants, and proteases, and the redundancies in biologic systems, particularly in response to injury in the lung, it is likely that whatever the initiating abnormality, changes in many mediators will follow rapidly. Thus, it would seem simplistic to expect to identify a single mediator that is of primary importance in acute lung injury states. Furthermore, once injury has been initiated, it is unlikely that inhibiting one mediator system will prevent further lung damage.

Complement activation, either within the lung or within the circulation, is associated with lung injury. C5 fragments (C5a and C5a-des-Arg) are especially potent PMN chemotaxins and activators. Experimental models have used an infusion of C5a and demonstrated rapid activation of PMNs, with aggregation and trapping in the pulmonary microvasculature. In some cases, a morphologic picture similar to that of diffuse alveolar damage or ALI develops. Other investigators have found that a second or additional stimulus, such as hypoxemia, is needed to cause lung injury. For instance, in combination with complement activation, short periods of hypoxia were sufficient to increase lung permeability to albumin. If complement activation is extensive, with large amounts of C5a and C5a-des-Arg generated, endothelial and type II epithelial damage can occur, and may be accompanied by edema, hemorrhage, and fibrin deposition.

Several lipid mediators have also been evaluated and discussed as potential mediators in acute lung injury. Phosphatidylcholine, the principal component of the cell membrane, is metabolized to arachidonic acid by either phospholipase A_2 or phospholipase C. In turn, arachidonic acid is metabolized by either the lipoxygenase or the cyclo-oxygenase pathway to generate a series of biologically active compounds, the leukotrienes and the prostaglandins, respectively. Leukotriene B_4, leukotriene C_4, and leukotriene D_4 concentrations are increased in the BAL fluid of patients at risk for ARDS as well as in those in whom the syndrome exists. Urinary excretion of leukotriene E_4 is increased for at least the first 5 days of ARDS, which suggests persistent leukotriene generation. The leukotrienes, especially leukotriene B_4, probably recruit and activate PMNs, but clearly, they are not sufficient to account for the entire syndrome of diffuse alveolar damage or ARDS. Changes in the balance of vasodilating and vasoconstricting prostaglandins have been reported in experimental models of ALI and human ARDS. Thromboxane appears to be particularly important in the early increase in pulmonary artery pressure that is often observed in at least the early phase of acute lung injury.

Platelet-activating factor is a phospholipid with a broad range of biologic activities. Many different resident and nonresident lung cell types have been reported to make PAF, including PMNs, alveolar macrophages, mast cells, platelets, fibroblasts, endothelial cells, and epithelial cells. PAF has a broad range of effects on many different lung cell types at very low concentrations. It can prime PMNs to respond more readily and more aggressively to other stimuli. PAF induces smooth muscle constriction, and both bronchoconstriction and vasoconstriction can occur in the lung. In addition, PAF promotes edema formation, possibly through induction of the secondary release of other mediators, such as leukotrienes.

Recently, a variety of highly charged compounds have also been recognized as potential contributions to ALI. For example, polycations (e.g., poly-L-lysine) cause pulmonary edema and respiratory failure in animals. Inflammatory cells contain a variety of cationic proteins that increase vascular permeability. These highly positively charged molecules appear to bind to endothelial cells, which normally exhibit a highly negative charge, and alter capillary permeability.

MANAGEMENT OF ACUTE RESPIRATORY FAILURE

RECOGNITION AND EARLY INTERVENTIONS

Acute respiratory failure is often preceded by a compensated state in which the patient, through increased effort, is able to maintain adequate gas exchange at the expense of increased work of breathing. Normal values of frequently determined respiratory parameters (Table 13-5) and clinical signs of respiratory failure are listed (Table 13-6). Tachypnea is often the first manifestation of respiratory distress in infants. Increased work of breathing is manifest by chest wall retractions and flaring of the alae nasi. Inspiratory stridor is a sign of obstruction in the upper airway, occurring anywhere from the supraglottic space to the lower trachea. Common causes of stridor in the pediatric

TABLE 13-5. Approximate normal values

Parameter	Newborn	Older Infant and Child
Respiratory frequency (breaths/min)	40–60	20–30 (≤6 yr)
		15–20 (>6 yr)
Tidal volume (mL/kg)	5–6	7–8
Arterial blood		
pH	7.30–7.40	7.30–7.40 (≤2 yr)
		7.35–7.45 (>2 yr)
P_{CO_2} (mm Hg)	30–35	30–35 (≤2 yr)
		35–45 (>2 yr)
Standard HCO_3^- (mEq/L)	20–22	20–22 (≤2 yr)
		22–24 (>2 yr)
P_{O_2} (mm Hg)	60–90	80–100
Heart rate (beats/min)	100–200	100–180 (≤3 yr)
		70–150 (>3 yr)
Blood pressure (mm Hg)		
Systolic	60–90	75–130 (≤3 yr)
		90–140 (>3 yr)
Diastolic	30–60	45–90 (≤3 yr)
		50–80 (>3 yr)

TABLE 13-6. Signs of respiratory failure

Clinical Signs
Respiratory
Tachypnea Altered depth and pattern of respiration (deep, shallow, irregular, apnea) Retractions of the chest wall Flaring of the alae nasi Cyanosis Decrease or absence of breath sounds Expiratory grunting Wheezing or prolonged expiration
General
Fatigue Excessive sweating
Cardiac
Tachycardia Hypertension Bradycardia Hypotension Cardiac arrest
Cerebral
Restlessness Irritability Headache Mental confusion Papilledema Seizures Coma
Laboratory Findings
Hypoxemia (acute or chronic) Hypercapnia (acute or chronic) Acidosis (metabolic or respiratory)

population are laryngomalacia, laryngotracheobronchitis (croup), epiglottitis, aspiration of a foreign body, and congenital airway abnormalities, such as vocal cord cysts. Prolonged expiration with wheezing is a sign of lower airway obstruction, most likely at the bronchial or bronchiolar level. Viral bronchiolitis and asthma are two conditions commonly associated with lower airway obstruction. Expiratory grunting is another clinical sign of respiratory failure in infants and children; it is caused by premature epiglottic closure accompanying active chest wall contraction during early expiration. Infants grunt to increase airway pressure, thus trying to preserve or increase functional residual capacity. Cyanosis is a fairly late sign of respiratory failure. It should be noted that since the presence of cyanosis depends on the quantity of desaturated hemoglobin in blood, respiratory failure can exist in the presence of anemia without any sign of cyanosis. Therefore, arterial blood oxygen saturation or tension should be measured whenever a question of serious respiratory impairment exists, even in the absence of cyanosis. It should also be noted that the manifestations of respiratory failure are not always clinically evident and that some of the signs and symptoms discussed earlier, when present, may have a nonrespiratory etiology. For instance, tachypnea without respiratory distress commonly results from an attempt to compensate for metabolic acidosis (e.g., the patient with diabetic ketoacidosis). Thus, clinical assessment of arterial hypoxemia and hypercapnia is not always reliable. The clinician should therefore have a low threshold for measuring arterial blood gases or performing a pulse oximetry study.

The goals in the management of respiratory failure are to anticipate and recognize respiratory problems and to support those functions that are compromised or lost. Although measurement of arterial blood gases and pH is necessary for obtaining precise information about gas exchange in the lung, in an emergency situation, clinical judgment is paramount and the clinician must be able to assess the patient for respiratory compromise and initiate therapeutic measures appropriately. Table 13-7 outlines the American Heart Association's rapid cardiopulmonary assessment, which should be applied to any child with suspected respiratory or circulatory insufficiency. Restoration of airway patency and institution of ventilation are the first steps in resuscitation of the patient with suspected respiratory failure. Initially, the airway should be cleared of secretions or mechanical obstructions, such as foreign materials. A child who shows signs of adequate gas exchange should be allowed to maintain a neutral "sniffing" position. Hyperextension of the neck should be avoided because it may increase upper airway obstruction. Artificial airways may be useful in maintaining upper airway patency in the pediatric patient. An oropharyngeal airway is useful in an unconscious infant or child, but may stimulate retching and vomiting in the conscious child. Nasopharyngeal airways, available commercially in a variety of sizes, are better tolerated by a conscious patient. In the absence of a commercial nasopharyngeal airway, an appropriately sized endotracheal tube (ETT) may be used. A complication of small-diameter nasopharyngeal airways is that they may become obstructed by mucus, vomitus, or the soft tissue of the pharynx.

Once airway patency has been achieved, assisted ventilation may be necessary if adequate air entry and breath sounds are not observed. Assisted ventilation should not be delayed until placement of an ETT is accomplished, because the vast majority of infants and children with respiratory failure can be successfully ventilated and oxygenated with a bag-valve-mask (BVM) device, even in the setting of airway obstruction as a result of conditions such as epiglottitis. Assisted ventilation with a BVM device must

TABLE 13-7. Rapid cardiopulmonary assessment

Respiratory Assessment	Cardiovascular Assessment
A. Airway Patency	**C. Circulation**
B. Breathing Rate Air entry Rising chest Breath sounds Stridor Wheezing Mechanics Retractions Grunting Accessory muscle use Nasal flaring Color	Heart rate Blood pressure Peripheral pulses Present/absent Volume Skin perfusion Capillary refill time Temperature Color Mottling Central nervous system perfusion Recognition of parents Reaction to pain Muscle tone Pupil size

From Chameides L, Hazinski MF, eds: Textbook of Pediatric Advanced Life Support. Dallas: American Heart Association, 1994.

be done with caution while chest and abdominal motion is observed carefully because excessive pressure may produce pneumothorax, pneumomediastinum, or gastric distention, with subsequent vomiting. Facemasks are available in a variety of sizes; a proper facemask should provide an airtight seal on the face, enveloping the nose and mouth, but avoiding depression of the eyes. Gastric distention, with a subsequent increase in respiratory embarrassment, can be minimized during assisted ventilation by application of gentle cricoid pressure by an assistant. During assisted BVM ventilation, monitoring of inflation pressure with a manometer is also important to reduce traumatic complications, such as pneumothorax.

A laryngeal mask airway (LMA) may be used when a facemask is difficult to fit or tracheal intubation is difficult. An LMA is made of a silicone rubber tube connected to a miniature mask with an inflatable cuff. The LMA is placed in the larynx and used to lift the epiglottis away, leaving the airway lumen open. Rescue ventilation can be provided to the child with the LMA in place, or the trachea can be intubated through the LMA using a stylet or bronchoscope.

The patient with suspected respiratory failure should be administered high levels of oxygen. Methods of oxygen administration and maximal achievable FIO_2 are listed in Table 13-8. The use of a nasal cannula as an oxygen delivery device is unsuitable in emergency situations for children with suspected respiratory failure, because the inspired oxygen concentration cannot be controlled adequately. Many children do not tolerate oxygen facemasks, although some may accept soft pediatric masks. Many times, a child may tolerate a face shield better than a mask. Oxygen concentration up to 40% can be delivered with high flow through the shield. When BVM ventilation is performed in an emergency situation, 100% oxygen should be used to flow through the bag. In addition to oxygen administration, rapid assessment of both respiratory drive and the ability to maintain an open airway is necessary in the child with suspected respiratory failure. As mentioned earlier, if the child is hypoventilating, administering high concentrations of oxygen to correct hypoxemia will mask the development of hypercarbia if the practitioner does not correctly assess inadequate alveolar ventilation or measure arterial PCO_2 concentrations.

Endotracheal intubation is indicated in the patient with ARF who has continued severe hypoxemia despite supplemental oxygen administration, who has worsening hypercapnia with acidosis, or who requires airway protection (Table 13-9). By linking the respiratory system directly to a ventilator, therapies such as the use of high oxygen concentrations, hyperventilation, and the delivery of positive end-expiratory pressure (PEEP) can be administered. The equipment required for ETT intubation includes an appropriately sized ETT (and one size larger and one size smaller), a stylet, a laryngoscope with an appropriately sized blade and a functioning light, a resuscitation bag and mask connected to a high-flow oxygen source, and suction. Optimally, the patient should be monitored by pulse oximetry and a cardiorespiratory monitor, and the appropriate staff and equipment should be available in case cardiopulmonary resuscitation is needed. ETT size can be estimated with the use of a Broselow tape or the following formula:

$$\text{ETT size (in millimeters)} = (16 + \text{age in years})/4$$

Generally, a newborn infant would require an ETT with an internal diameter of 3.0 to 3.5 mm, and a 1-year-old child would need a 4.0-mm ETT. Children younger than 8 years old should, under most circumstances, be intubated with an uncuffed ETT, because their narrow subglottic space usually forms a good seal around an appropriately sized ETT. For placement of the ETT, in the absence of possible traumatic spine injury, the child's head and neck should be placed in a "sniffing" position to allow better visualization of the glottis. Preoxygenation with 100% oxygen should be performed next. At this time, premedications, such as atropine, may be given, and a sedative/amnestic, such as a benzodiazepine, should be given. If desired, and when appropriate, a muscle relaxant, such as succinylcholine (depolarizing muscle relaxant) or pancuronium, vecuronium, or rocuronium (nondepolarizing muscle relaxants), should be administered. After administration of a muscle relaxant, it is necessary to provide complete support of the patient's ventilation by BVM with 100% oxygen. Gentle cricoid pressure should be maintained during this time to prevent gastric distention. After suctioning, the glottis should be visualized and the ETT passed through the vocal cords. Intubation attempts should be limited to 15 to 30 seconds, depending on the patient's level of oxygenation and hemodynamic condition. If unsuccessful, the patient should again be preoxygenated with BVM

TABLE 13-8. Methods of oxygen administration

Method	Maximum Achievable FIO_2 (at 6–10 L/min O_2)
Nasopharyngeal catheter	50%
Nasal prongs	50%
Masks	
Without a reservoir bag	50%
With a reservoir bag (partial rebreathing)	70%
With a reservoir bag (nonrebreathing)	95%
Venturi	24%, 28%, 35%, and 40%
Incubator	40%
Canopy tent	50%
Head box	95%

FIO_2, fractional concentration of inspired oxygen.

TABLE 13-9. Criteria for intubation and mechanical ventilation

Parameter*	Findings
Clinical†	
Respiratory	Apnea, decreased breath sounds despite rigorous chest wall movement, weakening ventilatory effort
Cardiac	Asystole, peripheral collapse, severe bradycardia or tachycardia
Cerebral	Coma, lack of response to physical stimuli, uncontrolled restlessness
General	Limpness, loss of ability to cry
Laboratory‡	
$PaCO_2$	Newborn: >60–65 mm Hg Older infant or child: >55–60 mm Hg Rapidly rising (>5 mm Hg/hr)
PaO_2 (FIO_2 = 100%)	Newborn: <40–50 mm Hg Older infant or child: <50–60 mm Hg

*Clinical or laboratory findings may dictate the need for mechanical ventilation.
†More than one episode of apnea with bradycardia or an episode of cardiac arrest is adequate indication for initiating mechanical ventilation, even in the absence of blood gas data.
‡Laboratory values less extreme than those indicated must be supplemented by clinical evidence of severity to warrant initiating mechanical ventilation.

ventilation before another attempt is made. After successful placement of the ETT, its proper position in the trachea should be assessed by use of a colormetric filter (attached to the ETT at the time of intubation) that shows a change in color from purple to yellow, by listening for equal breath sounds, by obtaining a chest x-ray, or by direct bronchoscopic visualization, if available.

OBJECTIVES OF MECHANICAL VENTILATION

Mechanical ventilation is a method of supporting the failing respiratory system until its function can return; it is not, of itself, curative or therapeutic. Therefore, the primary objective should be to avoid iatrogenic lung injury, which undoubtedly adds to the cascade of injurious inflammatory processes that contribute to ALI, as described earlier. Because there have been few randomized studies of most aspects of respiratory care, there is no universal agreement on an optimal mode of mechanical ventilation for any specific pulmonary disease state. Thus, to apply mechanical ventilation in a rational manner, the clinician must have an understanding of the pathophysiology underlying the cause of respiratory failure in each patient. Table 13-10 lists basic physiologic goals that mechanical ventilation can help to achieve. From a clinical viewpoint, these goals translate to: (1) relieving potentially life-threatening hypoxia, (2) reversing life-threatening respiratory acidosis, (3) preventing or reversing atelectasis, (4) reversing ventilatory muscle fatigue, (5) decreasing systemic or myocardial oxygen consumption, and (6) stabilizing the chest wall. In the process of achieving these objectives, it is important to remember that the underlying pathophysiology of a disease state varies with time and, thus, the methods and intensity of mechanical ventilation should be reassessed frequently. Mechanical ventilation is associated with a number of adverse consequences, including hemodynamic and ventilator-induced lung injury (Table 13-11), and measures to minimize such complications should be implemented whenever possible. In addition, to minimize potential side effects, the physiologic endpoints of mechanical ventilation do not have to be in the normal range (e.g., permissive hypercapnia; discussed later).

Basic Modes of Mechanical Ventilation

As alluded to earlier, specific recommendations regarding the particular mode of ventilation in ARF are lacking. Therefore, it is important to choose a method that has been shown to be capable of supporting patients with ARF and with which the clinician is familiar. The two basic modes of positive-pressure mechanical ventilation are: (1) volume-limited, time-cycled ventilation and (2) pressure-limited, time-cycled ventilation. In the past, it was recommended that young children weighing less than 10 kg be ventilated in the pressure-limited mode. However, now, with improved technology and the decreased working volumes of ventilators, even premature infants may be successfully supported using an appropriate volume-limited mode. In the support of patients with ARF, there are specific advantages and disadvantages to both the volume-limited and pressure-limited modes of ventilation (Table 13-12). In the volume-limited mode, VT, or minute ventilation (VT × rate [breaths/min]), gas flow rate, and inspiratory time are the variables set by the clinician. The resultant end-inspiratory pressure observed in the patient is therefore dependent on the compliance and airflow resistance of the ventilated lung. By maintaining constant minute ventilation, this mode of ventilation tends to allow better control of $PaCO_2$, and changes in lung compliance are easily detected by monitoring end-inspiratory pressure. A disadvantage, however, is that, as lung compliance decreases, higher end-inspiratory pressures result, thereby putting the already injured lung at risk for further injury. In the pressure-limited mode, end-inspiratory pressure limit, gas flow, and inspiratory time are the variables controlled. Therefore, VT becomes the dependent variable that will increase or decrease with changes in lung compliance or airflow resistance. The obvious advantage of this mode is the ability to keep end-inspiratory pressures low,

TABLE 13-10. Physiologic goals of mechanical ventilation

Support pulmonary gas exchange
Alveolar ventilation ($PaCO_2$ and pH)
Arterial oxygenation (PaO_2 and SaO_2)
Increase lung volume
End-inspiratory lung inflation
Functional residual capacity
Reduce work of breathing
Unload respiratory muscles

TABLE 13-11. Complications associated with mechanical ventilation

Respiratory
Tracheal lesions (erosion, edema, stenosis, granuloma, obstruction, perforation)
Accidental displacement of the endotracheal tube (into the main stem bronchus, esophagus, or hypopharynx) or actual extubation
Infection (tracheitis, pneumonitis)
Air leaks (pneumothorax, pneumomediastinum, interstitial emphysema)
Trapping of gas (hyperinflation)
Excessive secretions (atelectasis)
O_2 hazards (depression of ventilation, bronchopulmonary dysplasia)
Pulmonary hemorrhage
Perpetuation of inflammation
Direct injury to the alveolar-capillary unit
Circulatory
Impairment of venous return (decreased cardiac output, systemic hypotension)
O_2 hazard (retrolental fibroplasia, cerebral vasoconstriction)
Septicemia
Intracranial hemorrhage (intraventricular, subarachnoid)
Hyperventilation (decreased cerebral blood flow)
Metabolic
Increased work of breathing ("fighting" the ventilator)
Alkalosis (potassium depletion, excessive bicarbonate therapy)
Renal and Fluid Balance
Antidiuresis
Excess water in inspired gas
Equipment Malfunction (Mechanical)
Failure of the power source
Malfunction of the ventilator (leak, value dysfunction)
Improper humidification (overheating of inspired gas, condensation in the inspiratory line)
Improper tubing connections (kinked line, disconnection)

■ **TABLE 13-12.** Comparison of volume-controlled and pressure-controlled ventilation

Volume-Controlled Ventilation	Pressure-Controlled Ventilation
Advantages	Advantages
Guaranteed tidal volume and minute ventilation	Precise control of peak volume (end-inspiratory/alveolar volume)
Precise control of the flow pattern	Decelerating flow pattern reported to:
Changes in respiratory impedance easily detected	Improve distribution of ventilation
Clinician familiarity	Decrease dead space ventilation
	Decrease peak airway pressure
	Have higher initial flows that more readily match the patient's demands
Disadvantages	Disadvantages
Variable peak airway and alveolar pressures and volumes	Tidal volume varies with changes in impedance
Constant flow may not meet patient's initial flow demands (flow dyssynchrony)	Changes of respiratory impedance not easily detected
	Minute ventilation is a complex function of pressure, impedance, and frequency

From Martin LD: New approaches to ventilation in infants and children. Curr Opin Pediatr 1995;7:250.

thereby decreasing the risk of ventilator-induced lung injury. Disadvantages include more difficulty in detecting changes in lung compliance and the risk of constantly changing V_T and, subsequently, less control over carbon dioxide elimination.

Many of the strategies currently applied to the treatment of pediatric ARDS have come directly from the adult literature, with little experience in pediatric patients. This approach of applying new ideas and therapies learned from adults to pediatric patients must be tempered by the realization that a child with ARF may be very different from an adult with ARF. In a recent descriptive study of pediatric patients with respiratory failure, Randolph and associates found that only 17.1% of all patients admitted to the pediatric ICU required mechanical ventilation for 24 hours or longer, much less frequently than in the adult population.[1] They also found that there were differences between diagnoses and chronic conditions in children older than and younger than 1 year of age, again emphasizing the heterogeneity of the population across the broad age range seen in pediatrics. They also noted that, despite meeting American-European Consensus Conference criteria for ALI/ARDS, mortality was rare (1.6%), again much lower than the mortality rate in most adult studies. Therefore, although the same treatment is used in pediatric patients, the response and outcomes may be very different from those in adult trials.

General Concepts of Acute Lung Injury Relevant to Mechanical Support

Two main concepts have changed the perception and approach to ARDS over the last decade. The lung injury in ARDS had been viewed as being very homogenous, most likely related to diffuse pulmonary edema that caused the lungs to be stiff and poorly compliant. The approach to mechanical ventilation was to use high pressures to inflate the stiff, noncompliant lungs. Gattinoni and colleagues were among the first to demonstrate that the lung injury in ARDS is actually very heterogeneous, with areas of dependent collapse and edema, areas of regional hyperinflation, and normal-appearing areas.[9] Gattinoni further proposed that ventilation with high pressures to inflate the entire lung not only may be unsuccessful in inflating the densely collapsed areas, but also might injure the normal areas by overstretching them. These findings led to the "baby lung" concept of ARDS, in which the injured lung is viewed as being small rather than stiff. The concept of the lung as small rather than stiff began the trend of altering how these injured lungs should be ventilated.

The second major concept that has contributed to the change in the approach to ventilator use has been the emergence of the concept of ventilator-induced lung injury (VILI).[10] There is a growing body of literature based on animal studies and now human trials that demonstrates that mechanical ventilation can exert physical forces on the normal lung that result in a picture of acute lung injury. This ARDS-like injury is characterized by pulmonary edema, altered surfactant production, and production of proinflammatory cytokines, all of which may contribute to extrapulmonary organ failure and ongoing lung injury.[11]

Two primary factors appear to damage the lung in VILI. The first is "volutrauma," which is seen when the lung is overdistended at high inspiratory lung volumes. This injury is probably not the result of high airway pressure, but rather the result of mechanical stretching of the tissue and perhaps elevations in vascular pressure. The second factor is the generation of shear forces as a result of repeated opening and closing of edematous, surfactant-deficient alveoli throughout the respiratory cycle.

Combining the concept of a small, rather than stiff, lung with the realization that mechanical ventilation alone can directly injure the lung radically altered the approach to mechanical ventilation of the patient with ALI/ARDS.[12] The goals of oxygenation and ventilation are no longer to normalize gas exchange at any cost. Rather, the approach taken is to provide adequate oxygenation and ventilation while protecting the lung from further injury. The "open-lung," or "lung-protective," strategy of ventilation is directed at recruiting and then maintaining open, collapsed, and dependent portions of the lung, reducing overdistention in nondependent areas, and decreasing the frequency of repetitive opening and closing of the alveolar airspaces, thus reducing shear-induced injury. Higher arterial P_{CO_2} values (permissive hypercapnia) and lower arterial P_{O_2} values (permissive hypoxemia) are tolerated to achieve a less damaging pattern of ventilation. Although the precise manner by which these goals can be achieved remains somewhat controversial, the general principles and goals of open-lung ventilation are widely accepted and constitute the basis for most currently accepted approaches to this problem.

Low-Tidal-Volume Ventilation

The combination of the use of elevated levels of applied PEEP to recruit and maintain patency of the lung and airways with limitation of inspiratory pressures or volumes forms the foundation of lung-protective strategies of ventilation. In experimental settings, end-inspiratory plateau or pause pressures greater than 25 to 30 cm H_2O have been found to be most closely associated with alveolar overdistention and lung injury. Limitation of V_T to a level that generates plateau pressures of less than 30 cm H_2O has been proposed to assist in lung-protective ventilation.

The U.S. National Institutes of Health ARDSNET trial is the largest study to date comparing the open-lung approach to ventilation in the patient with ARDS with traditional modes of ventilatory support.[13] The effect on mortality was compared in a cohort of adult patients with ARDS ($n = 861$) randomized to receive VT limited to 6 mL/kg or standard treatment with 12 mL/kg VT. Although not targeted, the plateau pressures in the group with limited VT were lower (24 vs. 32 cm H_2O). PEEP and FIO_2 were titrated to arterial oxygenation in both treatment groups. There was a 25% reduction in the mortality rate in the group with limited VT (6 mL/kg). The investigators also found significant reductions in days of mechanical ventilation, circulating cytokine levels, and incidence of extrapulmonary organ failure in the limited VT group. This study and several others provide evidence to suggest that low VT can reduce VILI and systemic inflammatory response in adults with ARDS.[14]

Although the use of low VT is being extrapolated to pediatrics, there are no published trials comparing low with standard VT ventilation in pediatric ARDS. Indeed, some recent data suggest that young animals may be less susceptible than adults to ventilation with high VT. It remains uncertain whether VT between 6 and 12 mL/kg provides intermediate degrees of protection. The conclusion that can be drawn is that ventilation of the injured mature lung with high VT (≥12 mL/kg) may cause further damage and should be avoided.

Using Pressure-Volume Curves to Guide Mechanical Ventilation

Despite the simplicity of application and the existing clinical evidence supporting the use of low VT, another approach used to adjust ventilator settings is based on assessment of an individual patient's respiratory mechanics, which can take into account the often marked differences in respiratory mechanics observed between patients with ALI/ARDS. Pressure-volume curves generated during the respiratory cycle can be used to target ventilator settings. The static pressure-volume curve generated by the injured lung differs from that observed in the normal patient (Fig. 13-2). It is characterized by a lower inflection point, a linear range, an upper inflection point, and significant hysteresis. The lower inflection point is believed to represent a point of widespread alveolar recruitment, whereas the upper inflection point is believed to represent widespread alveolar overdistention. The initial level of PEEP is set to equal the pressure just above the lower inflection point to prevent alveolar collapse at end expiration. VT is set to limit peak inspiratory pressures below the upper inflection point to prevent alveolar overdistention.

Setting PEEP just above the lower inflection point has been demonstrated to improve oxygenation in patients with acute lung injury, and may reduce VILI. In a cohort ($n = 53$) of adults with ARDS, the mortality rate and the incidence of barotrauma were reduced in the group whose ventilator parameters were set using this strategy.[15] Additionally, patients treated with a protective ventilation strategy based on pressure-volume curve analysis showed a reduction in both airway and cytokine levels. These findings suggest that a lung-protective strategy of ventilation based on pressure-volume curve analysis may reduce VILI and improve patient outcome.

Recruiting Maneuvers in the Open-Lung Strategy of Mechanical Ventilation

Prolonged or high-pressure inflation (a recruiting maneuver) may improve lung recruitment and oxygenation by reopening fluid-filled or collapsed alveoli. Intermittent application of prolonged or high-pressure inflations may be less damaging to the lung than constant ventilation with high VT or inspiratory pressures. These maneuvers are often used as part of an open-lung strategy of ventilation.[16,17] Recruiting maneuvers may also reverse the atelectasis that may occur with the lower VT used in a lung-protective strategy of ventilation. Recruiting maneuvers may be administered as a sustained high level of continuous positive airway pressure (30–40 cm H_2O for 30–40 sec) as often as needed to maintain oxygenation, or they may be added into the ventilator cycle as high-pressure (40–60 cm H_2O) sigh breaths.

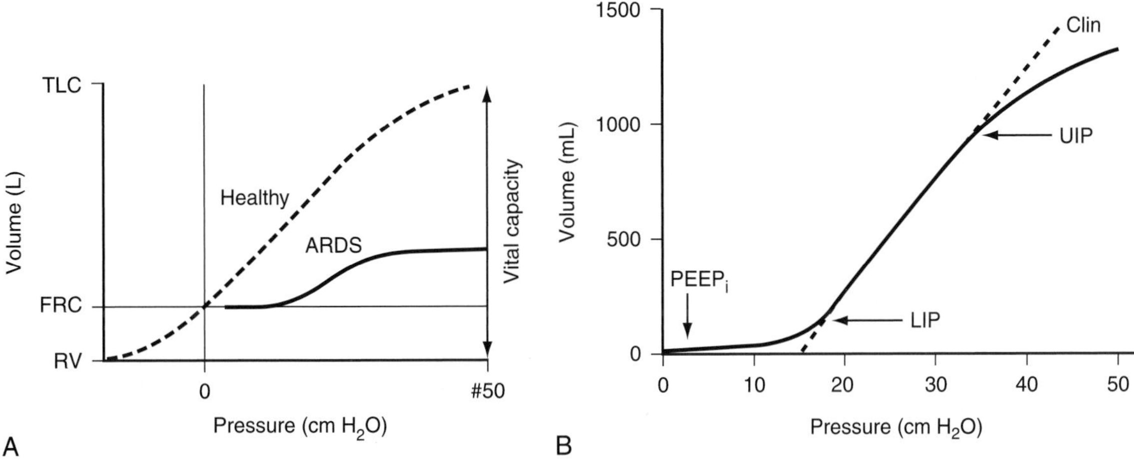

■ **FIGURE 13-2.** Lung pressure-volume curves help to direct mechanical ventilation. **A,** Pressure-volume curve of the respiratory system in a healthy subject and in a patient with acute respiratory distress syndrome. Example of the pressure-volume relation of the respiratory system in a patient with acute respiratory distress syndrome (ARDS) *(solid line)* compared with the pressure-volume curve of the respiratory system and the respiratory volumes in a healthy subject *(dashed line)*. FRC, functional residual capacity; RV, residual volume; TLC, total lung capacity. **B,** Typical inspiratory pressure-volume curve of the respiratory system in a patient with acute respiratory distress syndrome. Volumes are expressed relative to the end-expiratory lung volume at zero end-expiratory pressure. The curve consists of three segments identified by a lower inflection point (LIP) and an upper inflection point (UIP). The intermediate linear segment has the steeper slope *(dashed line)*, or the greater compliance (chord compliance, or Clin). Note the presence of intrinsic positive end-expiratory pressure ($PEEP_i$), causing a rightward shift of the curve. (From Maggiore SM, Brochard L: Pressure-volume curve in the critically ill. Curr Opin Crit Care 2000;6:1–10, figs. 1 and 2.)

Transient hypoxemia and reversible hemodynamic changes have been reported as adverse events with recruiting maneuvers.

There are no published trials evaluating the use of recruiting maneuvers in pediatric patients. Reports from adults show highly variable oxygenation responses in patients treated with recruiting maneuvers. There may be some benefit in combining recruiting maneuvers with different lung recruitment strategies. Combining prone positioning and recruiting maneuvers in adults with ARDS produced significantly greater improvement in oxygenation and end-expiratory lung volume than either strategy alone.[12,18]

Prone Positioning in the Patient with Acute Respiratory Failure

The use of prone positioning as a maneuver to enhance oxygenation through lung recruitment was first reported in 1974. Changes in lung recruitment are frequently cited as the cause of improved oxygenation. Gattinoni and associates have demonstrated that patients in the prone position have more recruitment of the dorsal lung regions on computed tomography scan, but additional factors must contribute to the improvement in oxygenation because oxygenation can improve without an increase in lung volume.[19] These other factors could include redistribution of pulmonary blood flow to provide better ventilation-perfusion matching and improved aeration of the larger dorsal lung areas, decreases in abdominal compression, and mobilization of secretions. Concerns about patient safety during turning have proven to be manageable, and early successful case reports have led to the use of prone positioning in many ICUs.

Few pediatric studies have been published evaluating the effects of prone positioning in ARDS. The technique was reported to improve oxygenation and to be well tolerated in an early case series of seven pediatric patients. Curley and colleagues evaluated 25 children with ARDS who were placed in the prone position for 20 hours a day and found that 84% demonstrated improvement in oxygenation.[20] However, 24% had pressure ulcers, and the mortality rate of 24% was not significantly improved. An observational study of 23 consecutive children with ARDS also showed an improvement in oxygenation with prone positioning; however, the mortality rate remained high, suggesting no significant effect on overall outcome. In a retrospective series of pediatric patients with ARDS, the improvement in oxygenation increased when they were left prone for 20 hours rather than just 6 hours, suggesting a time dependence of the effect.

Prone positioning is a simple, noninvasive procedure that may improve oxygenation in patients with ARDS, in conjunction with conventional mechanical ventilation. Prone positioning appears to be safe and effective in pediatric patients with ARDS. It also appears that longer periods in the prone position are more effective than shorter periods in improving oxygenation.

NONCONVENTIONAL METHODS OF VENTILATORY SUPPORT

INVERSE-RATIO VENTILATION

Another approach that has been used to improve oxygenation in the patient with hypoxemic respiratory failure, especially in the setting of ARDS, is inverse-ratio ventilation. In this approach, the inspiratory time of the ventilator is adjusted to exceed the expiratory time, thus "inverting" the inspiratory-to-expiratory ratio. Although the mechanism by which this approach improves oxygenation is uncertain, most evidence indicates that it leads to the generation of air trapping and intrinsic PEEP, effectively increasing total PEEP levels as well as mean airway pressure. The reported advantage of inverse-ratio ventilation is improved oxygenation at lower plateau airway pressures, thereby potentially reducing VILI. Additionally, the use of a longer inspiratory time allows for better recruitment of collapsed and atelectatic lung units. Successful use of this technique in a child with ARDS was reported in the early 1980s, but few data in children have since been reported.[21] Factors that limit the use of inverse-ratio ventilation include the need for heavy sedation and hemodynamic compromise. Studies in animals and humans have suggested that inverse-ratio ventilation reduces cardiac output, does not improve lung recruitment, and does not improve gas exchange compared with volume-controlled, normal-ratio ventilation, when total PEEP levels are matched.

HIGH-FREQUENCY VENTILATION

High-frequency ventilation is defined by the use of supraphysiologic ventilatory rates with VT values that are lower than the anatomic dead space. Three types of high-frequency ventilation devices have been used clinically: high-frequency positive pressure ventilation, high-frequency jet ventilation, and high-frequency oscillatory ventilation (HFOV). HFOV provides an active exhalation phase, whereas the others rely on lung recoil or passive exhalation. Because HFOV has been used more commonly in pediatric clinical trials, the following discussion is limited to HFOV.

An HFOV device has three components. The bias flow provides a source for the continuous flow of fresh gas. A piston or diaphragm generates high-frequency oscillations of the column of gas in the circuit and airways. An exhalation port exerts a "low-pass filter effect" that is critically important in maintaining mean airway pressure throughout the respiratory cycle.

The low-pass filter effect occurs as the initial peak pressure wave amplitude that is generated during inspiration is progressively decreased or dampened as the pressure wave moves down the airways into the alveoli. As a result, the alveoli are exposed to lower-amplitude pressure waveforms. The degree of dampening depends on the resistive forces generated by the HFOV circuit, the diameter of the ETT, the respiratory frequency, the percentage of inspiratory time, airway resistance, lung compliance, and the region of the lung that is affected. In a computer model of respiratory distress in preterm animals, respiratory mechanics have been shown to significantly alter intrapulmonary pressure amplitudes and, thus, mean airway pressure. Furthermore, this experimental model demonstrated that distal transmission of the driving pressure amplitude may be increased in conditions of low lung compliance (e.g., in ARDS).[22] This is important because mean airway pressure is the main determinant of oxygenation during HFOV. Increases in mean airway pressure lead to increased lung recruitment and, ultimately, improved oxygenation. However, if mean airway pressure is increased to the point where the lung becomes hyperinflated, PaO_2 and SpO_2 (oxygen saturation measured by pulse) will fall as the alveolar capillaries are compressed.

The to-and-fro displacement of the piston produces pressure amplitude changes above and below the set mean airway pressure, or ΔP. The frequency (Hertz) of oscillation determines the time for piston displacement. These two variables determine the

VT delivered and facilitate carbon dioxide exchange. Gas exchange is determined by facilitated diffusion (direct alveolar ventilation, pendelluft, convective streaming, augmented dispersion, cardiogenic mixing, and molecular diffusion) rather than the bulk flow of gas seen in conventional ventilation.

Early experience with HFOV was mainly in neonatal respiratory distress syndrome. One of the early trials that compared HFOV (used in a strategy to minimize total pressure) with conventional mechanical ventilation showed no difference in outcome. Additionally, concern was raised regarding adverse events in the HFOV group. A subsequent trial using a recruitment strategy of HFOV in the treatment of neonatal respiratory distress syndrome showed improved gas exchange and outcome compared with conventional mechanical ventilation, and there were no adverse events noted in the HFOV group. As a result, HFOV is most commonly applied in a lung recruitment strategy.

A trial of HFOV may be considered in a patient with relatively homogeneous disease on chest x-ray whose oxygenation index ([mean airway pressure × FIO_2 × 100]/PaO_2) is 13 to 15 on maximal conventional ventilator settings. The initial mean airway pressure is set 3 to 5 cm H_2O higher than the mean airway pressure set on the conventional ventilator. Mean airway pressure is increased in increments of 2 to 3 cm H_2O until SpO_2 shows significant improvement (≥90%) and there is no deterioration in systemic blood pressure. The amplitude of piston displacement (ΔP) is adjusted to achieve adequate chest movement. The frequency is set at 8 or 10 Hz (use of a lower frequency increases the VT that is delivered and may result in stacking of breaths, which may result in an injurious pattern of ventilation). Once SpO_2 is stable at greater than 90%, FIO_2 is decreased preferentially to 0.60 or less before mean airway pressure is decreased. The degree of lung inflation is assessed with frequent chest x-rays. Hyperinflation is defined as nine-rib or greater expansion on an anteroposterior chest x-ray. If hyperinflation is present, mean airway pressure should be decreased by 1 or 2 cm H_2O and reassessed by chest x-ray.

In a randomized prospective trial comparing HFOV and conventional mechanical ventilation in pediatric respiratory failure, the HFOV-treated group showed improved oxygenation and lower oxygen requirements at 21 days.[23] Additionally, the 30-day survival rate without lung disease was significantly higher in the group receiving HFOV only compared with the group treated with conventional mechanical ventilation.

HFOV should be considered in patients with severe ARDS requiring high mean airway pressures and FIO_2. The results of HFOV will be improved in the future, when actual measurements of lung volume, compliance, and delivered VT can be made.

BILEVEL POSITIVE AIRWAY PRESSURE

Bilevel positive airway pressure (BiPAP) ventilation is a noninvasive technique used to provide ventilatory support to a spontaneously, but insufficiently, breathing patient using a facemask or nasal mask. With this mode of ventilation, BiPAP cycles between two levels of continuous positive airway pressure. BiPAP has been used successfully in adults with respiratory failure of diverse etiologies, such as pneumonia, chronic obstructive pulmonary disease, and pulmonary edema. This mode of ventilation in adults has resulted in shorter duration of ventilation, less need for sedation, and fewer complications than intubation and positive pressure ventilation.[24]

The data in pediatric patients are less clear. In a retrospective chart review of pediatric patients with mild to moderate hypoxemic respiratory insufficiency, BiPAP was found to improve gas exchange and decrease respiratory rate. Three of 28 children treated with BiPAP required intubation. Nine of the patients had severe underlying neurologic disease or immunocompromise, leading the authors to conclude that it may be a particularly useful adjunct in "patients whose underlying condition warrants avoidance of intubation."[25] A randomized trial of pediatric patients with ARF compared BiPAP with synchronized intermittent mechanical ventilation and found no differences in the duration or complications of ventilation or the need for sedation.

As a noninvasive mode of ventilation, BiPAP may be useful in patients with mild to moderate respiratory failure, especially if they have underlying conditions in which avoiding intubation is preferable. There appear to be few complications associated with BiPAP. However, one potential complication deserves mention: tachypnea may be relieved by BiPAP, but gas exchange may not be significantly improved. This can result in unexpected respiratory failure and arrest, if blood gases are not monitored closely.

NONVENTILATORY METHODS OF RESPIRATORY SUPPORT

A large number of pharmacologic therapies have been employed to aid in the treatment of ALI/ARDS. These include agents with vasoactive, anti-inflammatory, and anticoagulant effects as well as drugs directed at promoting alveolar fluid resorption (Table 13-13). The agents that have received the most attention will be discussed briefly.

Nitric Oxide

Nitric oxide (NO) is an endogenous vasodilator. In the vascular endothelial cell, the enzyme NO synthase acts on L-arginine to release NO. NO diffuses rapidly into the adjacent underlying vascular smooth muscle cells and activates soluble guanylate cyclase, which stimulates the conversion of guanosine triphosphate to cyclic guanosine monophosphate (cGMP) and ultimately results in cGMP-mediated smooth muscle relaxation and, thus, vasodilation. Endothelial NO synthase can be activated by circulating and locally produced factors, such as acetylcholine and bradykinin, and also by physical forces, such as shear stress. Due to its rapid binding to hemoglobin, its half-life is extremely short.

The delivery of inhaled NO (iNO) to ventilated lung regions results in vasodilation of adjacent pulmonary arteries. Thus, NO dilates vessels only where there is gas exchange. This can lead to an improvement in ventilation-perfusion ratios, thus decreasing shunt and improving oxygenation. Importantly, iNO has no effect on systemic blood vessels and, thus, systemic blood pressure because of the rapid inactivation of NO on contact with hemoglobin. Other potential benefits of iNO include regulation of immune and inflammatory function, reduction of pulmonary capillary pressure, decreased pulmonary edema formation, and reduction of neutrophil sequestration in the lung. One potential downside of iNO therapy, especially in the patient receiving high FIO_2, is that NO may interact with superoxide (generated under high FIO_2 conditions) to form the free radical peroxynitrite, which may damage the lung or inactivate surfactant.

Inhaled NO has been shown to acutely lower pulmonary artery pressure and improve gas exchange in neonates, children,

TABLE 13-13. Nonventilatory therapies for acute lung injury or acute respiratory distress syndrome

Systemic	Inhalation
Vasoactive Drugs	
Prostacyclin Almitrine Dobutamine Cyclic guanosine 3′,5′-monophosphate phosphodiesterase inhibitors (sildenafil) Endothelin antagonists	Nitric oxide Prostacyclin
Anti-inflammatory Agents	
Corticosteroids *N*-acetylcysteine Lisofylline Ketoconazole Superoxide dismutase Catalase Antiadhesion molecules Matrix metalloproteinase and elastase inhibitors	
Anticoagulant Agents	
Activated protein C Tissue factor pathway inhibitors Antithrombin Heparin	Heparin
Alveolar Fluid Resorption	
β-adrenergic agents Dopamine Glucocorticoids	β-adrenergic agents
Supportive Measures	
Fluid restrictin Starches Extracorporeal membrane oxygenation	Surfactant

and adults with acute hypoxemic respiratory failure.[26,27] Inhalation of NO by neonates with respiratory failure and persistent pulmonary hypertension of the newborn resulted in a decreased need for extracorporeal membrane oxygenation (ECMO). However, the improvement in oxygenation in patients with persistent pulmonary hypertension of the newborn who were treated with iNO is often directly related to a decrease in extrapulmonary shunting of blood across the ductus arteriosis or foramen ovale, due to the decrease in pulmonary vascular resistance. Although pulmonary artery pressure is elevated in ARDS, hypoxemia is the result of intrapulmonary shunting of blood due to lung parenchymal disease (inflammation, edema), which may or may not be improved with iNO.

However, early studies did suggest that intrapulmonary shunting could be decreased and oxygenation improved in patients with ARDS who were treated with inhaled NO.[26] Two subsequent randomized trials of inhaled NO in the treatment of adults with ARDS have shown acute improvement in oxygenation and a decrease in the intensity of mechanical ventilatory support.[28,29] Neither, however, showed any difference in mortality rate.

The first study reported in children showed that iNO improved oxygenation, decreased pulmonary artery pressure, and reduced intrapulmonary shunt in patients with acute hypoxemic respiratory failure.[27] A randomized trial of iNO in the treatment of pediatric patients with ARDS showed acute improvement in oxygenation in the group treated with iNO and also showed that two subgroups (patients with OI > 25 at entry and immunocompromised patients) had a more sustained improvement in oxygenation with iNO.[30]

Responsiveness to iNO may be enhanced by therapies that promote lung recruitment (especially HFOV). Biochemical inactivation of NO (by increased phosphodiesterase-5 activity or increased O_2^- production) may occur in the setting of lung injury and may be amenable to complementary pharmacologic strategies, such as phosphodiesterase-5 inhibition with agents such as sildenafil. In some patients, the underlying disease may not be amenable to NO therapy (e.g., anatomic cardiac disease, left ventricular dysfunction, structural vascular disease). Therefore, further studies are needed to better identify the role of iNO in specific patient groups with hypoxemic respiratory failure.

Prostacyclin

Endothelial cells produce prostaglandins using the cyclo-oxygenase pathway. These prostaglandins have vasodilatory, anti-inflammatory, and antiplatelet activities. Prostacyclin has been used as a pulmonary vasodilator in ARDS.[31] When given intravenously, prostacyclin has reduced pulmonary pressures, but worsened ventilation-perfusion mismatch, resulting in a deterioration of gas exchange. Aerosolized prostacyclin has been used to treat ARDS and has resulted in reductions in pulmonary artery pressure and increases in oxygenation similar to those achieved with iNO. The selectivity of vasodilation with prostacyclin is dependent on the dose applied, which is dependent on the nebulizer used. Additionally, there is no way to precisely measure the concentration of prostacyclin that is absorbed. Currently, there are few controlled data evaluating the use of inhaled prostacyclin in ARDS.

Inhibition of Phosphodiesterases

As stated earlier, NO activates soluble guanylate cyclase, generating cGMP and resulting in smooth muscle relaxation and vasodilation. Phosphodiesterases degrade cGMP. The balance between production of cGMP and degradation by phosphodiesterases affects vascular tone. The phosphodiesterase-5 isoform specifically hydrolyzes cGMP and may augment NO-induced pulmonary vasodilation. Sildenafil is a selective phosphodiesterase-5 inhibitor that is easily absorbed orally. In animal models and now human case reports, sildenafil has been shown to augment the pulmonary vasodilating effects of low-dose iNO, with few systemic effects.[32] Whether it will have an effect on the long-term outcome of patients with ARDS remains to be determined.

Surfactant Administration

Endogenous surfactant is produced by type II alveolar epithelial cells. Surfactant is composed of phospholipids and four phospholipid-associated proteins, surfactant proteins A, B, C, and D. The phospholipid components of surfactant reduce alveolar surface tension, thereby stabilizing the alveoli and preventing collapse. Injury to the alveolar-capillary membrane, as is seen in ARDS, results in pulmonary edema and alteration in surfactant homeostasis and function. This causes alveolar instability and collapse, ventilation-perfusion mismatch, hypoxemia, and decreased lung compliance, all of which characterize ALI/ARDS.

Although the existence of surfactant proteins has been recognized for more than 20 years, their functions have been determined only recently.[33] These proteins enhance spreading of surfactant, define the organization of surfactant into lamellar bodies and tubular myelin, regulate surfactant homeostasis, and play an important role in host defense. Exogenous surfactants differ in their surfactant protein content and their surface-tension-lowering capabilities.

Exogenous surfactant administration has been associated with a significant decrease in the mortality rate in the treatment of neonatal respiratory distress. Success in neonates prompted the use of exogenous surfactant in the treatment of ARDS. Respiratory distress syndrome in neonates is due to a deficiency of surfactant, but unlike respiratory distress syndrome in neonates, ARDS in children is associated with disturbance in surfactant composition and function. Adult patients who have ARDS or are at risk for ARDS have reduced concentrations of surfactant proteins A and B in lavage fluid, and recovery of the surfactant protein A level appears to correlate with the severity of lung injury.

The goal of surfactant administration in ARDS is to reverse functional impairment of the surfactant system by instilling an excess of surface-active material.[34] Several factors affect the efficacy of surfactant administration. The composition of the exogenous surfactant is important, and protein-containing surfactants appear to be superior to protein-free surfactants. In a large randomized trial comparing two types of surfactant for the treatment of neonatal respiratory distress, the natural surfactant containing surfactant proteins B and C was associated with a lower mortality rate. The mode of administration of surfactant and the ventilation strategy used during instillation also play roles in surfactant efficacy. Aerosolized surfactant tends to deposit preferentially in the more compliant portions of the lung, not the stiff, atelectatic areas. The use of an open-lung strategy of ventilation appears to allow for better distribution of surfactant within the lung. Finally, surfactant is inactivated rapidly by plasma proteins; therefore, large doses may be needed before a response is seen.

Exogenous surfactant administration for the treatment of ARDS has been studied in adults and pediatric patients, with less favorable results than those seen in the treatment of neonatal respiratory distress.[35] In a large trial, 725 adults with ARDS were randomized to receive aerosolized saline (placebo) or surfactant for up to 5 days. There were no differences in 30-day mortality rates or in oxygenation between the two groups. Shortcomings of this study were the lack of detail on the method of mechanical ventilation used and the fact that previous studies have shown that only a very small amount of aerosolized surfactant actually reaches the alveolus.

In a multicenter trial of pediatric patients with acute hypoxemic respiratory failure who were randomized to receive intratracheally instilled surfactant or conventional treatment (no placebo), there was a rapid improvement in oxygenation in the surfactant-treated group.[36] Additionally, the surfactant group spent less time on mechanical ventilation and had shorter ICU stays. This was a fairly heterogeneous population of patients with ARDS and non-ARDS respiratory failure. There was no difference in the mortality rate between groups. Two other smaller randomized studies have also demonstrated an immediate improvement in oxygenation in pediatric patients with ARDS who were randomized to receive surfactant therapy.[37]

In summary, although the advantages of surfactant administration in the neonate with respiratory distress syndrome are well known, its benefits in the older child and adult with ARDS have not yet been proven. Thus, it remains an experimental form of rescue therapy.

Extracorporeal Membrane Oxygenation

Extracorporeal membrane oxygenation uses partial cardiopulmonary bypass to support gas exchange. Two types of ECMO are used: (1) venoarterial, in which the outflow of blood from the venous system is returned to the arterial circulation, and (2) venovenous, in which the outflow of blood from the venous system is returned to the venous circulation. Venoarterial ECMO provides cardiac as well as pulmonary support. It requires cannulation of a central artery (usually the carotid) and therefore is associated with an increased risk of complications.

Extracorporeal membrane oxygenation does not "treat" ARDS; it provides lung "rest," allowing time for the lungs to heal. Therefore, before a patient is placed on ECMO, two criteria must be met. The lung disease must be reversible, and the prognosis with conventional therapy must be extremely poor. Assessment of whether the patient meets these criteria is one of the most difficult aspects of ECMO. Reversibility of disease in the setting of lung failure has never been directly addressed. Therefore, selection of patients for ECMO is based primarily on the patient's failure to respond to maximal therapy. Unfortunately, maximal therapy differs from institution to institution and with access to other therapies. No pre-ECMO predictors of death have been identified. Recovery of lung function by day 7 of ECMO was shown in a retrospective study by Morton[38] to correlate with good outcome; however, in this instance, the patients are already receiving ECMO. The complications of ECMO can be devastating (e.g., central nervous system bleed). The challenges facing the clinician are to define the patient population most likely to benefit from ECMO and to better assess the true effect of ECMO on patient survival.

Glucocorticoids

Although corticosteroids have been shown to be effective in ameliorating disease in a variety of animal models of acute lung injury, most human studies evaluating the effect of early steroid administration in patients with ARDS have not shown a beneficial effect. However, a single trial by Meduri and colleagues suggests a potential beneficial effect of prolonged glucocorticoid administration, when started later (>7 days) in the course of ARDS.[39] In these patients, high-dose methylprednisolone was given for 2 weeks, followed by tapering of the dosage for another 2 weeks. The dose, time of administration, length of treatment, and evaluation of success in pediatric patients have not been systematically studied. The ARDS clinical trials network of the National Institutes of Health, National Heart, Blood, and Lung Institute is currently conducting a trial of methylprednisolone for adults with nonresolving (7–28 days) ARDS to help resolve this question.

Activated Protein C

Fibrin deposition occurs in the alveoli and interstitium of the lung early in ARDS. Fibrin is a potent inhibitor of surfactant function and may be an important contributor to supporting the fibroproliferative phase of ARDS.[40] Thus, due to the excessive coagulation and reduced fibrinolysis reported in ARDS, anticoagulation strategies have been considered in the treatment of ARDS.[41] In a recent multicenter randomized trial of activated protein C in the treatment of patients with severe sepsis, there was an increase in ventilator-free days in those treated with activated protein C. This has led to further interest in the use of activated protein C to treat ARDS. There is currently a large multicenter randomized pediatric trial examining the role of activated protein C in sepsis, with a secondary outcome being the effect of activated protein C in pediatric patients with ARDS. Until the results of this study are completed, the role of activated protein C in the treatment of patients with ARDS remains undetermined.

Alveolar Fluid Resorption–Promoting Drugs

Resorption of alveolar fluid is mediated through active sodium and chloride transport by alveolar pneumocytes.[42] This is accomplished through epithelial sodium channels on the apical surface of the pneumocyte and adenosine triphosphate–regulated sodium pumps on the basal surface. Under normal conditions, this system operates to keep the alveolar space free of excess water. In the setting of ARDS, this system is often damaged, either directly, by the loss of alveolar pneumocytes (discussed earlier), or indirectly, impaired by hypoxia and the products of viral or bacterial infection. Current studies are directed at stimulating fluid transport by increasing the activity of sodium channels in the remaining pneumocytes. Both β_2-adrenergic agents (e.g., terbutaline) and dopamine have been shown to stimulate sodium channel activity. In animal studies, these agents have been shown to promote lung epithelial liquid clearance. Ongoing trials in humans will determine whether these agents will be beneficial in the setting of ALI/ARDS.

REFERENCES

1. Randolph AG, Meert KL, et al: The feasibility of conducting clinical trials in infants and children with acute respiratory failure. Am J Respir Crit Care Med 2003;167:1334–1340.
2. Wang JD, Wang TM, et al: Clinical spectrum of acute respiratory distress syndrome in a tertiary pediatric intensive care unit. Acta Paediatr Taiwan 2003;44:202–207.
3. Artigas A, Bernard GR, et al: The American-European Consensus Conference on ARDS, part 2. Ventilatory, pharmacologic, supportive therapy, study design strategies, and issues related to recovery and remodeling. Acute respiratory distress syndrome. Am J Respir Crit Care Med 1998;157:1332–1347.
4. Frutos-Vivar F, Nin N: Epidemiology of acute lung injury and acute respiratory distress syndrome. Curr Opin Crit Care 2004;10:1–6.
5. Bellingan GJ: The pulmonary physician in critical care * 6. The pathogenesis of ALI/ARDS. Thorax 2002;57:540–546.
6. Gattinoni L, Vagginelli F, et al: Physiologic rationale for ventilator settings in acute lung injury/acute respiratory distress syndrome patients. Crit Care Med 2003;31(4 Suppl):S300–S304.
7. Dreyfuss D, Saumon G: From ventilator-induced lung injury to multiple organ dysfunction? Intensive Care Med 1998;24:102–104.
8. Groeneveld AB: Vascular pharmacology of acute lung injury and acute respiratory distress syndrome. Vascul Pharmacol 2002;39:247–256.
9. Gattinoni L, D'Andrea L, et al: Regional effects and mechanism of positive end-expiratory pressure in early adult respiratory distress syndrome. JAMA 1993;269:2122–2127.
10. Dreyfuss D, Saumon G: Ventilator-induced lung injury. Lessons from experimental studies. Am J Respir Crit Care Med 1998;157:294–323.
11. Brower RG, Rubenfeld GD: Lung-protective ventilation strategies in acute lung injury. Crit Care Med 2003;31(4 Suppl):S312–S316.
12. Grasso S, Mascia L, et al: Effects of recruiting maneuvers in patients with acute respiratory distress syndrome ventilated with protective ventilatory strategy. Anesthesiology 2002;96:795–802.
13. Acute Respiratory Distress Syndrome Network: Ventilation with lower tidal volumes as compared with traditional tidal volumes for acute lung injury and the acute respiratory distress syndrome. The Acute Respiratory Distress Syndrome Network. N Engl J Med 2000;342:1301–1308.
14. Ranieri VM, Suter PM, et al: Effect of mechanical ventilation on inflammatory mediators in patients with acute respiratory distress syndrome. A randomized controlled trial. JAMA 1999;282:54–61.
15. Amato MB, Barbas CS, et al: Effect of a protective-ventilation strategy on mortality in the acute respiratory distress syndrome. N Engl J Med 1998; 338:347–354.
16. Brower RG, Morris A, et al: Effects of recruitment maneuvers in patients with acute lung injury and acute respiratory distress syndrome ventilated with high positive end-expiratory pressure. Crit Care Med 2003;31: 2592–2597.
17. Barbas CS, de Matos GF, et al: Lung recruitment maneuvers in acute respiratory distress syndrome. Respir Care Clin North Am 2003;9:401–418, vii.
18. Pelosi P, Bottino N, et al: Sigh in supine and prone position during acute respiratory distress syndrome. Am J Respir Crit Care Med 2003;167:521–527.
19. Gattinoni L, Tognoni G, et al: Effect of prone positioning on the survival of patients with acute respiratory failure. N Engl J Med 2001;345:568–573.
20. Curley MA, Thompson JE, et al: The effects of early and repeated prone positioning in pediatric patients with acute lung injury. Chest 2000;118: 156–163.
21. Goldstein B, Papadakos PJ: Pressure-controlled inverse-ratio ventilation in children with acute respiratory failure. Am J Crit Care 1994;3:11–15.
22. Pillow JJ, Sly PD, et al: Dependence of intrapulmonary pressure amplitudes on respiratory mechanics during high-frequency oscillatory ventilation in preterm lambs. Pediatr Res 2002;52:538–544.
23. Arnold JH: High-frequency ventilation in the pediatric intensive care unit. Pediatr Crit Care Med 2000;1:93–99.
24. Antonelli M, Conti G, et al: A comparison of noninvasive positive-pressure ventilation and conventional mechanical ventilation in patients with acute respiratory failure. N Engl J Med 1998;339:429–435.
25. Fortenberry JD, Del Toro J, et al: Management of pediatric acute hypoxemic respiratory insufficiency with bilevel positive pressure (BiPAP) nasal mask ventilation. Chest 1995;108:1059–1064.
26. Rossaint R, Gerlach H, et al: Efficacy of inhaled nitric oxide in patients with severe ARDS. Chest 1995;107:1107–1115.
27. Abman SH, Kinsella JP: Inhaled nitric oxide therapy for pulmonary disease in pediatrics. Curr Opin Pediatr 1998;10:236–242.
28. Dellinger RP, Zimmerman JL, et al: Effects of inhaled nitric oxide in patients with acute respiratory distress syndrome. Results of a randomized phase II trial. Inhaled Nitric Oxide in the ARDS Study Group. Crit Care Med 1998;26:15–23.
29. Lundin, S, Mang H, et al: Inhalation of nitric oxide in acute lung injury. Results of a European multicentre study. The European Study Group of Inhaled Nitric Oxide. Intensive Care Med 1999;25:911–919.
30. Dobyns EL, Cornfield DN, et al: Multicenter randomized controlled trial of the effects of inhaled nitric oxide therapy on gas exchange in children with acute hypoxemic respiratory failure. J Pediatr 1999;134:406–412.
31. Pappert D, Busch T, et al: Aerosolized prostacyclin versus inhaled nitric oxide in children with severe acute respiratory distress syndrome. Anesthesiology 1995;82(6):1507–1511.
32. Toward TJ, Smith N, et al: Effect of phosphodiesterase-5 inhibitor, sildenafil (Viagra), in animal models of airways disease. Am J Respir Crit Care Med 2004;169:227–234.
33. Whitsett, JA, Weaver TE: Hydrophobic surfactant proteins in lung function and disease. N Engl J Med 2002;347:2141–2148.
34. Lewis JF, Brackenbury A: Role of exogenous surfactant in acute lung injury. Crit Care Med 2003;31(4 Suppl):S324–S328.
35. Haitsma JJ, Papadokos PJ, et al: Surfactant therapy for acute lung injury/acute respiratory distress syndrome. Curr Opin Crit Care 2004;10:18–22.
36. Willson DF, Zaritsky A, et al: Instillation of calf lung surfactant extract (calfactant) is beneficial in pediatric acute hypoxemic respiratory failure. Members of the Mid-Atlantic Pediatric Critical Care Network. Crit Care Med 1999;27:188–195.
37. Moller JC, Schaible T, et al: Treatment with bovine surfactant in severe acute respiratory distress syndrome in children. A randomized multicenter study. Intensive Care Med 2003;29:437–446.
38. Morton A, Dalton H, et al: Extracorporeal membrane oxygenation for pediatric respiratory failure. Five-year experience at the University of Pittsburgh. Crit Care Med 1994;22:1659–1667.
39. Meduri GU, Chinn AJ, et al: Corticosteroid rescue treatment of progressive fibroproliferation in late ARDS. Patterns of response and predictors of outcome. Chest 1994;105:1516–1527.
40. Idell S: Coagulation, fibrinolysis, and fibrin deposition in acute lung injury. Crit Care Med 2003;31(4 Suppl):S213–S220.
41. Laterre PF, Wittebole X, et al: Anticoagulant therapy in acute lung injury. Crit Care Med 2003;31(4 Suppl):S329–S336.
42. Hastings RH, Folkesson HG, et al: Mechanisms of alveolar protein clearance in the intact lung. Am J Physiol Lung Cell Mol Physiol 2004; 286:L679–L689.

14 Chronic Respiratory Failure

Raouf S. Amin, MD

CHRONIC RESPIRATORY FAILURE

OVERVIEW

Respiratory failure is defined as the condition in which arterial oxygen tension (PaO_2) is less than 60 torr or arterial carbon dioxide tension ($PaCO_2$) is higher than 45 torr. This condition occurs when the respiratory system does not receive sufficient alveolar ventilation to meet the metabolic demands of cellular respiration.[1] When respiratory failure persists for longer than 1 month, necessitating ventilatory support or oxygen supplementation to provide adequate gas exchange for the support of vital functions, it is considered chronic.

The respiratory system comprises two anatomic components: the lungs, which are the gas exchange organs, and the pump, which ventilates the lungs. The respiratory pump consists of the chest wall, including the respiratory muscles, the respiratory controllers in the central nervous system, and the pathways connecting these controllers with the respiratory muscles (spinal cord, peripheral nerves).

Respiratory failure is commonly classified as hypoxic, hypercapnic, or a combination of the two. Hypoxic respiratory failure is characterized by improper gas exchange, whereas hypercapnic failure is characterized by ventilatory pump dysfunction. Respiratory failure secondary to lung disease manifests predominantly with hypoxemia, whereas dysfunction of the ventilatory pump manifests primarily with hypercapnia. In nonprogressive conditions, such as some forms of muscular dystrophy or chronic parenchymal lung disease, hypercapnic and hypoxic chronic respiratory failure remain distinct entities. In many cases, however, multiple factors contribute to the development of chronic respiratory failure (Fig. 14-1), and hypoxic and hypercapnic respiratory failure may coexist.

This chapter discusses the various types of chronic respiratory failure, their course of progression, and their clinical management.

PATHOPHYSIOLOGY

Oxygen-Carbon Dioxide Diagram

The basic distinctions between various types of respiratory failure are depicted in the oxygen-carbon dioxide diagram (Fig. 14-2). Proposed by Fenn and colleagues,[2] this diagram shows the relationship between the alveolar partial pressure of oxygen (P_AO_2) [abscissa] and that of carbon dioxide (P_ACO_2) [ordinate]. Under steady-state conditions, the ratio of carbon dioxide elimination to oxygen uptake, measured at the mouth, is considered the metabolic respiratory quotient. The slope of the line connecting the two axes represents the respiratory exchange ratio. This graphic approach is useful in conceptualizing the interaction between partial pressure of oxygen (PO_2) and that of carbon dioxide (PCO_2) in the presence of a large alveolar arterial gradient, such as that in hypoxic respiratory failure, and in the absence of an alveolar arterial gradient, such as that in hypercapnic respiratory failure. Figure 14-2 shows several examples of respiratory failure. When failure is predominantly hypercapnic, the relationship between PO_2 and PCO_2 follows the slope of the respiratory exchange ratio. The three levels of hypercapnic respiratory failure associated with normal lung function are designated as A1 to A3. Mild (A1) to moderate (A2) degrees of hypercapnia are usually associated with no hypoxemia or mild hypoxemia. In severe hypoventilation that increases $PaCO_2$ to 100 torr, alveolar PO_2 decreases to close to 60 torr (A3). Central hypoventilation syndrome exemplifies conditions of hypoventilation with normal lung structure and function. In these conditions, alveolar hypoventilation is usually the sole cause of hypercapnia. Based on the oxygen-carbon dioxide diagram, hypercapnia secondary to central hypoventilation is usually associated with moderate to severe hypoxemia only at high levels of PCO_2. Thus, despite the presence of alveolar hypoventilation that results in significant hypercapnia, hypoxemia is not a predominant feature when lung function is normal. In hypoxic respiratory failure, the compensatory increase in minute ventilation secondary to low PO_2 maintains PCO_2 in the eucapnic level (see Fig. 14-2*B*). Chronic interstitial lung diseases are typical examples of hypoxic respiratory failure occurring when the diffusion defect fails to maintain normal oxygen conditions, but well-preserved function of the ventilatory pump maintains normal PCO_2. In chronic progressive lung disease or neuromuscular disorders associated with significant impairment of lung function, both components of the respiratory system fail to maintain adequate oxygenation and ventilation. This dual failure leads to significant hypoxemia and a variable degree of hypercapnia (see Fig. 14-2*C*). In children, severe obstructive lung disease secondary to cystic fibrosis and bronchopulmonary dysplasia are common examples of respiratory failure secondary to both lung and ventilatory pump failure.

Hypercapnic Respiratory Failure

The hallmark of ventilatory pump failure is carbon dioxide retention. At steady state, the volume of carbon dioxide eliminated per minute is equal to the volume produced by the body ($\dot{V}CO_2$). This is dependent on both P_ACO_2 and alveolar ventilation (V_A). The relationship between V_A and carbon dioxide production and elimination is expressed in the following equations:

$$VCO_2 = V_A \times P_ACO_2$$

$$P_ACO_2 = VCO_2/V_A$$

$$PCO_2 = K(VCO_2)/V_A$$

where K is a constant of proportionality.

Because V_A is equal to minute ventilation (V_E) minus dead space ventilation (V_D), and V_E is the product of tidal volume (V_T) and breathing frequency (f), the last equation may be presented as

$$PCO_2 = K(VCO_2)/V_T \times f\,(1 - V_D/V_T)$$

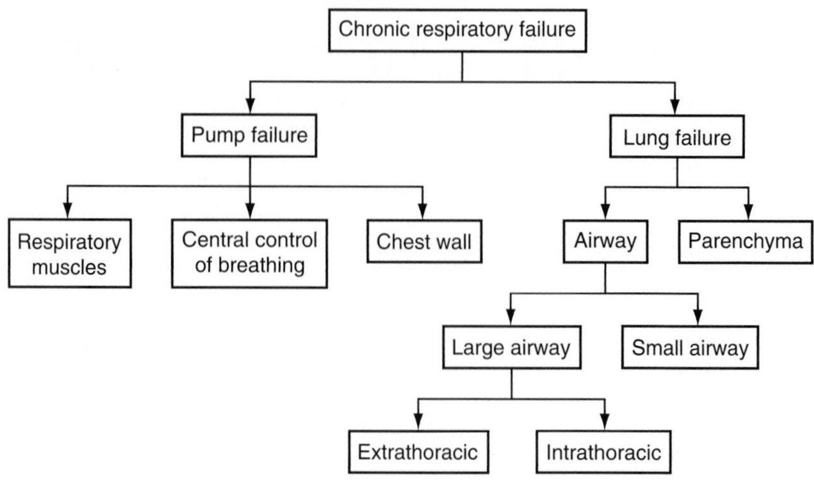

FIGURE 14-1. Different compartments of the respiratory system that may contribute to chronic respiratory failure.

The respiratory equation offers insight into the pathophysiology of hypercapnic respiratory failure. Accordingly, the following factors contribute to hypercapnia in patients with pump failure: (1) a decrease in minute ventilation by virtue of a decrease in breathing frequency or tidal volume, which leads to perfusion of units with low ventilation or right-to-left shunting; (2) increased dead space ventilation by virtue of an increase in the VD/VT ratio; and (3) increased carbon dioxide production.

At constant carbon dioxide production and a fixed dead space volume, alveolar ventilation changes when tidal volume or breathing frequency is altered. Under normal conditions, a decrease in the frequency of breathing is associated with an increase in tidal volume to maintain constant minute ventilation. This will decrease the VD/VT ratio, thereby increasing alveolar ventilation. On the other hand, when breathing frequency increases, tidal volume decreases to maintain constant minute ventilation. This increases the VD/VT ratio as well as dead space ventilation, thereby decreasing alveolar ventilation.

Two distinct breathing patterns can contribute to hypercapnic respiratory failure. The first is failure to increase tidal volume when breathing frequency decreases, which leads to a reduction of minute ventilation. The second is persistently fast breathing frequency, coupled with small tidal volumes, which leads to an increase in dead space ventilation. A third factor in the respiratory equation that can contribute to hypercapnia is the rate of carbon dioxide production. Although this rate is not usually measured in clinical settings, it is essential to recognize its role in the development of hypercapnia. Carbon dioxide production increases with hyperthermia, during muscular activity, and during inspiratory resistive breathing. Under normal conditions, an increase in carbon dioxide production is compensated for by increasing minute ventilation. Hypercapnia secondary to increased carbon dioxide production will develop in patients with impaired ventilatory capacity. A change in the level of nutritional support can alter carbon dioxide production and greatly stress the ventilatory system. Patients may adapt to chronic malnutrition through a decrease in the metabolic rate, and the resultant decrease in carbon dioxide production lowers ventilatory requirements. When nutritional support is reestablished, there is an abrupt increase in carbon dioxide production, especially if carbohydrates account for a high proportion of total calories, because carbohydrates have a high respiratory quotient. If such patients can handle only low carbon dioxide production in a malnourished state, hypercapnic respiratory failure will result from the increase in metabolic rate.

Hypoxic Respiratory Failure

Hypoxemia is the primary manifestation of hypoxic respiratory failure. Carbon dioxide exchange is also affected, but usually can be compensated for by increasing alveolar ventilation. Thus, in the absence of superimposed ventilatory pump failure, hypercapnia is not a feature of gas exchange failure. In many cases of gas exchange failure, respiratory alkalosis occurs secondary to dyspnea-associated increases in ventilatory drive and minute ventilation. In chronic respiratory failure, hypoxemia can be caused by one or more of the following basic mechanisms:

- Ventilation-perfusion mismatch
- Incomplete diffusion equilibrium
- Global alveolar hypoventilation

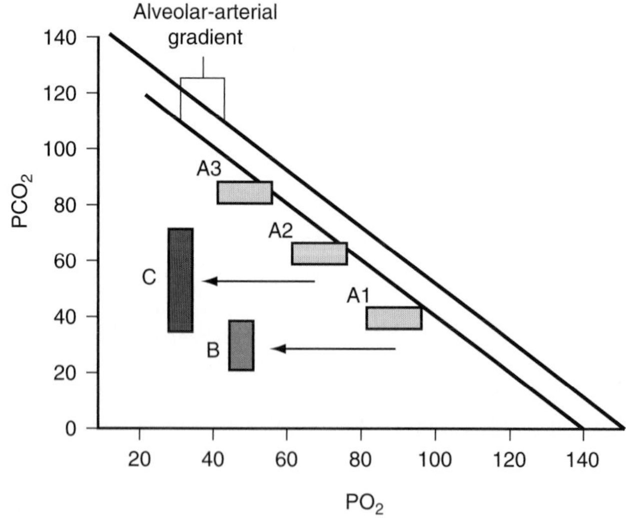

FIGURE 14-2. Oxygen-carbon dioxide depicts the relationship between the alveolar partial pressure of oxygen (abscissa) and that of carbon dioxide (ordinate). A1, A2, and A3 represent three levels of hypercapnic respiratory failure associated with normal lung function. B represents hypoxic respiratory failure associated with normal partial pressure of carbon dioxide. C is an example of hypoxic and hypercapnic respiratory failure.

Ventilation-Perfusion Mismatch

Ventilation-perfusion mismatch is mismatched distribution of ventilation and perfusion, with some lung units receiving disproportionately high ventilation and others receiving disproportionately high perfusion. In units with a low ratio of ventilation to perfusion, alveolar oxygen is taken up by the perfusing blood at a high rate and is refreshed by ventilation at a slow rate. The result is shunt-like mixing of poorly oxygenated blood from units with low perfusion with well-oxygenated blood from high-perfusion units. The well-oxygenated blood from lung units with a high ventilation-perfusion ratio cannot fully compensate for the poorly oxygenated blood from units with a low ventilation-perfusion ratio for the same reasons that oxygen supplementation does not alter the degree of hypoxemia in the presence of right-to-left shunt. Consequently, supplemental oxygen is expected to increase oxygen delivery to units with a low ventilation-perfusion ratio, with minimal effect on units with a high ventilation-perfusion ratio.

Incomplete Diffusion Equilibrium

When red blood cells in alveolar capillaries do not achieve full PaO_2 equilibrium with alveolar gas, incomplete diffusion equilibrium occurs. Incomplete equilibrium can develop under four conditions: (1) when there is a thickened alveolar-capillary membrane that blocks diffusion or slows the rate of diffusion of oxygen from alveolus to capillary; (2) when there is abnormally low oxygenation of mixed venous blood, as in anemia; (3) when there is significant destruction of parenchymal lung tissue, leading to a reduction in alveolar capillary volume, which in turn reduces the red cell transit time through alveolar capillaries; and (4) when there is increased cardiac output that also reduces alveolar-capillary transit time. Destruction of parenchymal lung tissue, with the resulting loss of capillary surface area, is the major factor leading to incomplete diffusion equilibrium.

Hypoxic respiratory failure in children can develop secondary to obstructive, restrictive, or interstitial lung disease. The effect of each group of disorders on gas exchange and respiratory control will be discussed separately.

CLINICAL PRESENTATION OF HYPERCAPNIC RESPIRATORY FAILURE

Ventilatory pump dysfunction can result from inadequate central neural ventilatory drive, inadequate performance of the respiratory muscles, or excessive respiratory load.

INADEQUATE CENTRAL DRIVE

The most common causes of inadequate central drive leading to chronic respiratory failure in children are related to congenital or acquired central hypoventilation syndromes. Congenital syndromes may present as isolated hypoventilation or may be associated with various genetic and metabolic abnormalities. Acquired hypoventilation occurs secondary to central nervous system infection, tumor, or trauma.

Congenital Central Hypoventilation Syndrome

Congenital central hypoventilation syndrome (CCHS) is failure of automatic control of breathing; its etiology is unknown.[3] This condition involves an integration abnormality of chemoreceptor input to the central controllers of respiration. Because breathing during non–rapid eye movement sleep is almost entirely controlled by the automatic system, ventilation is most compromised during non–rapid eye movement sleep.[4,5] The clinical presentation of CCHS varies depending on the severity of the disorder. Infants with severe CCHS do not breathe spontaneously and require ventilatory assistance.[6–8] Those with milder forms of the disorder often remain undiagnosed until they present with pulmonary hypertension and heart failure.[9] Because more severely affected children hypoventilate during both wakefulness and sleep, they are diagnosed at an earlier age. During sleep, children with CCHS have absent or negligible ventilatory sensitivity to both hypercarbia and hypoxemia.[10,11] This abnormal chemoreceptor response is also observed in patients with adequate daytime ventilation.

Patients with CCHS often have other abnormalities of autonomic nervous system functioning. Several reports have described the presence of decreased heart rate variability,[9] decreased nocturnal blood pressure dipping,[12] and diminished pupillary light response.[13,14] There are also reports of esophageal achalasia[15] and Hirschsprung's disease.[16–18] Recent studies[19–25] describing the genetics of isolated CCHS found that 40% to 96% of children with this syndrome had mutations of the *PHOX2b* gene, with the large majority occurring as de novo mutations.

A wide spectrum of genetic syndromes can be associated with central hypoventilation. These include myelomeningocele with Arnold-Chiari deformity,[26–29] skeletal dysplasia,[30] Möbius' syndrome,[31–33] Joubert[34–36] and Prader-Willi syndromes,[37,38] and inborn errors of metabolism, such as pyruvate dehydrogenase complex deficiency,[39] Leigh disease,[40] and carnitine deficiency.[41–43]

Acquired Central Hypoventilation Syndrome

Abnormal central control of breathing can develop secondary to chronic respiratory failure caused by chronic lung disease.[44] Persistent hypercapnia can blunt the ventilatory response to carbon dioxide in the presence of chronic lung disease. A similar effect can also develop from metabolic alkalosis and hypochloremia associated with diuretic therapy.[45–47]

INADEQUATE PERFORMANCE OF THE RESPIRATORY MUSCLES

Respiratory neuromuscular diseases are conditions in which there is a dysfunction of the pathway connecting the respiratory centers and the respiratory muscles, leading to respiratory muscle weakness. Muscle disorders can be broadly subdivided into myopathies, neuropathies, and neurogenic atrophies. In myopathies, pathology is confined to the muscle itself, with no associated structural abnormalities in the peripheral nerves. In neuropathies and neurogenic atrophies, muscle weakness is secondary to an abnormality in the peripheral nerve, between the anterior home cell and the neuromuscular junction. Further categorization is based on the characteristic features of particular disorders. Thus, the term *muscular dystrophy* is used to describe progressive, degenerative, genetic myopathies; these are subdivided on the basis of clinical distribution, severity of weakness, and mode of inheritance. Spinal muscular atrophies and neuropathies are neurogenic disorders in which the lesion is in the anterior horn cell or the peripheral nerve. These disorders are further characterized on the basis of their clinical features, modes of inheritance, and structural changes. Metabolic myopathies comprise syndromes in which a specific metabolic abnormality has been identified. These disorders include glycogenoses, mitochondrial myopathies, disorders of lipid metabolism, and iron-channel defects. Less common forms of respiratory neuromuscular disease include acquired injuries to the spinal cord as a result of traumatic injury or encephalomyelitis.

Chronic Respiratory Failure in Neuromuscular Disorders

Neuromuscular disorders associated with slow progression of muscle weakness allow examination of the long-term effect of respiratory muscle dysfunction on lung volume and pulmonary and chest wall mechanics. In patients with these disorders, there is evidence that respiratory failure is due not only to the direct effect of weakness, but also to a variety of additional pathogenic mechanisms. These mechanisms include: (1) the effect of respiratory muscle weakness on lung volume, (2) changes in the mechanical properties of the lungs, (3) changes in the mechanical properties of the chest wall, (4) changes in ventilatory drive, and (5) impaired coughing mechanism (Table 14-1). To understand the pathophysiology of respiratory failure, it is essential that clinicians adequately assess the role of each of these mechanisms.

Effect of Respiratory Muscle Weakness on Lung Volumes

Several studies[48–50] in patients with neuromuscular disorders have demonstrated that respiratory muscle weakness results in decreased vital capacity. As the underlying disorder progresses, this decline increases. This relationship is illustrated in a study[51] of 25 boys with Duchenne's muscular dystrophy (DMD). An inverse relationship was found between age and forced vital capacity and forced expiratory volume in 1 second (FEV_1). The absolute values of forced vital capacity and FEV_1 increase until the mean age of 14 years and decrease thereafter. Forced vital capacity and FEV_1 decreased annually by 5.6% and 4.2% of predicted values, respectively. Studies of functional residual capacity and residual volume show that patients with neuromuscular disorders have decreased functional residual capacity, but normal residual volume.[48,52] Therefore, the ratio of residual volume to total lung capacity is elevated.

Based on the sigmoid shape of the pressure-volume curve of normal respiratory systems, substantial changes in pressure produce slight changes in volume at the extremes of vital capacity. It would thus be expected that a significant decline in vital capacity would occur only when muscle weakness becomes severe. However, observations made in adolescents and adults with neuromuscular disorders indicate that the reduction in vital capacity is greater than would be anticipated for the degree of respiratory muscle weakness. The disproportionate reduction in lung volume relative to the degree of muscle weakness is the result of the change in the mechanical properties of the lung and chest wall.[49,52,53]

Changes in the Mechanical Properties of the Lungs

De Troyer and Deisser[54] examined the static expiratory pressure-volume curves obtained from patients with chronic respiratory muscle weakness. These studies showed that static lung recoil pressure is increased at all absolute lung volumes, indicating a decrease in pulmonary compliance. Other studies[48,54] have shown that values of compliance obtained during inspiration are also markedly reduced. The specific cause of decreased lung elasticity in patients with long-standing respiratory muscle weakness has not yet been determined. Several mechanisms have, however, been proposed to explain abnormal lung compliance in the normal lungs of patients with long-term respiratory muscle weakness. One such mechanism is a decrease in alveolar surface tension caused by breathing at low lung volume. This mechanism has been demonstrated in animals in which breathing at low constant tidal volume led to a decrease in lung compliance.[55] Changes in lung compliance were, nevertheless, rapidly reversed after a few deep breaths.[56] In contrast, it has also been shown that decreased lung compliance in patients with chronic respiratory muscle weakness is not reversed by short periods of positive pressure mechanical hyperinflation of the lungs.[54,57] This lack of reversibility suggests that alteration in surface tension is not the primary determinant of decreased lung compliance in humans. The second postulated mechanism of decreased lung compliance is a change in lung tissue elasticity resulting from chronic respiratory muscle weakness. Although this mechanism has not been proven, it remains the most plausible because patients with neuromuscular disorders have normal gas exchange and exhibit no structural lung abnormalities when evaluated by computed tomography of the chest.[49]

Changes in the Mechanical Properties of the Chest Wall

To explain the greater reduction of vital capacity relative to the degree of respiratory muscle weakness, several studies have examined chest wall compliance.[53] Because the methods used to measure chest wall mechanics require full patient cooperation, they have been limited to adults. Despite differences in methods,

TABLE 14-1. Factors contributing to chronic respiratory failure in neuromuscular disorders

Performance of the Ventilatory Pump	Functional Changes	Outcome
Inadequate performance of the respiratory muscles		
Weakness of the inspiratory muscles	Decreased inspiratory flow Decreased inspiratory capacity Increased dead space ventilation	Restrictive ventilation Decreased airway clearance
Weakness of the expiratory muscles	Decreased expiratory flow Increased residual volume/total lung capacity	Decreased airway clearance
Abnormal elastic properties of the lung	Decreased lung compliance	Decreased inspiratory flow Restrictive ventilation
Abnormal chest wall mechanics	Decreased compliance Increased compliance Loss of the sense of dyspnea	Restrictive ventilation Increased chest wall distortion Rapid respiratory decompensation
Central control of breathing	Decreased respiratory drive in selective disorders	Sleep-disordered breathing

results show that long-term neuromuscular disorders lead to a reduction in chest wall compliance.[53,58] These functional changes have been attributed to ankylosis in the costosternal and costovertebral joints. A reduction in chest wall compliance was observed independent of the presence of scoliosis. These observations have not, however, been reproduced in children with neuromuscular disorders. In a study by Papastamelos and colleagues,[59] 18 children with neuromuscular disorders who ranged in age from 3 months to 3.8 years were found to have a significantly greater increase in chest wall compliance than control subjects. This study concluded that an increase in chest wall compliance might also contribute to respiratory dysfunction resulting from an increased propensity for rib cage deformation and reduced end-expiratory lung volume.

Changes in Ventilatory Drive

Breathing Patterns

Patients with neuromuscular disorders tend to breathe at a faster frequency and with a smaller tidal volume. This breathing pattern manifests before the development of abnormal blood gas values, suggesting that it is not necessarily mediated via the chemoreceptors. The elevated breathing frequency in such patients could be related to signals received from the respiratory muscles themselves. This observation is supported by the finding that partial curarization in healthy subjects is associated with shallow, rapid respiration.[60]

Ventilatory Control

Although breathing patterns in patients with various neuromuscular disorders are similar, central ventilatory control differs. In patients with muscular dystrophy, a number of studies[61,62] have shown significant reduction in both hypercapnic and isocapnic hypoxic ventilatory responses. Studies have used mouth occlusion pressure as an index of central respiratory output that is independent of respiratory muscle function.[61,62] These studies demonstrate a well-preserved mouth occlusion pressure response. Additional data from the dystrophic diaphragm have also been obtained from electromyography signals.[63] These studies have found an increase, rather than a decrease, in central respiratory output. In contrast, patients with high spinal cord transection have gross carbon dioxide insensitivity during wakefulness; this insensitivity is further increased during sleep.[64] These findings are similar to those in patients with CCHS. Patients with myotonic dystrophy differ in several important aspects from those with other neuromuscular disorders. Studies in these patients have shown that both hypercapnic and hypoxic responses are reduced.[65,66] Mouth occlusion pressure is also abnormally low.

Impaired Coughing Mechanism

Contraction of the normal expiratory muscles elicited by coughing produces increased positive pleural pressure that results in dynamic compression of the central intrathoracic airways. The compression induces high flow velocity, mobilizing the secretions adhering to the airway walls. The physiologic correlate of this dynamic airway compression is a brief spike in airflow that adds to the sustained flow coming from the lungs. This brief spike is referred to as the *peak flow transient.* In the presence of expiratory muscle weakness, the pleural pressure generated during coughing is decreased. Dynamic airway compression is thereby reduced in magnitude, eventually leading to disappearance of the peak flow transient. The cough is also defective because of a decrease in both maximum expiratory flow and maximum inspiratory flow. In patients with neuromuscular disorders, the impaired clearance of secretions associated with a defective coughing mechanism contributes to the high prevalence of pulmonary infection. Such infection can become an important factor in the development of chronic respiratory failure.

STAGES OF RESPIRATORY FAILURE

Early evidence of respiratory muscle dysfunction is noted when muscles fail to perform their function under conditions of stress, such as respiratory infection, recovery from general anesthesia, exercise, and sleep. In many instances, the onset of early respiratory insufficiency occurs after the patient has lost ambulation. Detecting respiratory muscle dysfunction during exercise, thus, is not feasible. In these patients, evaluation of breathing during sleep might allow identification of the early stages of respiratory muscle dysfunction. Figure 14-3 outlines the stages of hypercapnic respiratory failure in patients with progressive neuromuscular disorders. The gradual transition from stage 1 to stage 3 respiratory failure is characteristic of DMD, in which there is a gradual progression of respiratory muscle weakness over two decades. In some disorders, such as congenital muscular dystrophy, if respiratory insufficiency is present, it might not progress beyond stage 1 or 2. In other disorders, respiratory muscle weakness is extremely severe, with patients presenting in stage 3 respiratory failure.

EFFECT OF SLEEP ON THE RESPIRATORY SYSTEM

Several changes in ventilatory control and respiratory muscle function occur with sleep onset, and familiarity with these changes provides a framework for understanding the pathophysiology of the early stages of chronic respiratory failure manifesting during sleep. These changes are discussed later.

Reduction in Muscle Tone

There is a sleep-stage-related decrease in postural muscle tone that reaches its nadir during rapid eye movement sleep. Muscle hypotonia is attributed to supraspinal suppression of the gamma motor neuron drive and presynaptic inhibition of skeletal muscle spindle afferents.[67–69] This muscle hypotonia clearly involves the

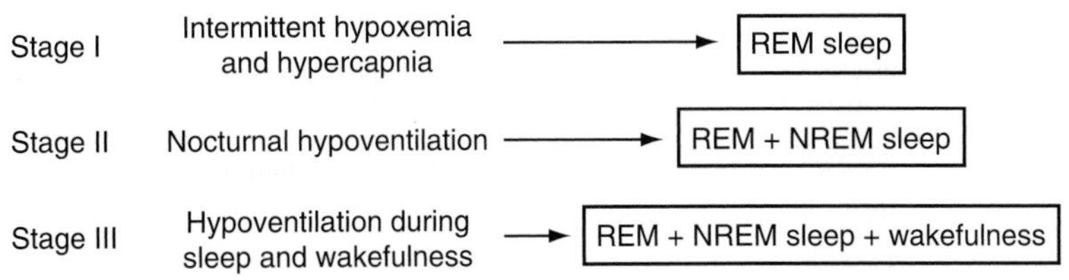

Stage I	Intermittent hypoxemia and hypercapnia →	REM sleep
Stage II	Nocturnal hypoventilation →	REM + NREM sleep
Stage III	Hypoventilation during sleep and wakefulness →	REM + NREM sleep + wakefulness

FIGURE 14-3. Stages of hypercapnic respiratory failure in patients with progressive neuromuscular disorders. NREM, non–rapid eye movement; REM, rapid eye movement.

intercostal and dilator muscles of the upper airway. In contrast, the diaphragm muscle, with its scant muscle spindles, is less subject to central inhibition and is therefore crucial in maintaining respiration during rapid eye movement sleep.[70–72] As such, the degree of alveolar hypoventilation during sleep and the accompanying hypoxemia and hypercapnia are dependent on diaphragmatic function.

Restrictive Ventilatory Defect

During normal sleep, there is a decrease in functional residual capacity and a consequent reduction in oxygen storage.[73] In patients with neuromuscular disorders, these changes are often exaggerated during sleep.[74,75]

Upper Airway Resistance

Muscular hypotonia during sleep involves the dilator muscles of the upper airway and leads to loss of tonic activity in the musculature of the tongue, pharynx, and larynx.[76–78] A fall in functional residual capacity further reduces the cross-sectional area of the upper airway and contributes to further increases in upper airway resistance.[79] Some patients with neuromuscular disorders experience rapid weight gain as a result of the loss of ambulation. This weight gain leads to a significant degree of airway obstruction and possibly to obstructive sleep apnea or obstructive hypoventilation during sleep. With the increase in upper airway resistance that occurs during sleep, patients with significant diaphragmatic weakness are sometimes unable to generate sufficient force to overcome the physiologic changes in the caliber of the upper airway. As a result, they are unable to generate inspiratory flow.

Central Respiratory Drive

In normal sleep, hypercapnic and hypoxic responses are diminished because of an increase in upper airway resistance and a decrease in the sensitivity of the chemoreceptors. This decline in chemosensitivity can contribute to sleep apnea in patients with neuromuscular diseases.[80–84] Arousal from sleep during obstructive sleep apnea is partly due to an increase in respiratory effort that stimulates mechanoreceptors in the chest. Prolonged obstructive sleep apnea is frequently caused by the inability of weak respiratory muscles to trigger an arousal response from the mechanoreceptor and by the blunted central respiratory response to chemoreceptor input.

NEUROMUSCULAR DISORDERS

Although several neuromuscular disorders show a wide spectrum of severity of weakness or respiratory insufficiency, many disorders exhibit specific characteristics of symptom onset, age at loss of ambulation, and age at death. This discussion will be limited to the most common neuromuscular disorders that present with respiratory insufficiency during childhood, including muscular dystrophies, spinal muscle atrophy, and quadriplegia.

THE MUSCULAR DYSTROPHIES

The muscular dystrophies are a group of degenerative disorders of the skeletal muscles that develop secondary to abnormalities of dystrophin or dystrophin-associated proteins. Most muscular dystrophies follow a progressive clinical course, culminating in respiratory insufficiency. Some milder forms may, however, follow a static course or may even show functional improvement; these types do not lead to significant respiratory compromise.

Duchenne's Muscular Dystrophy

Duchenne's muscular dystrophy is the most common neuromuscular disorder in childhood.[85] Because it is associated with severe respiratory complications, historically, it has received extensive attention in the literature. As early as 1879, Gowers stated: "the disease is one of the most interesting, and at the same time most sad. Manifesting itself at the transition from infancy to childhood, it develops with the child's development, grows with his growth so that every increase in stature means increase in weakness, and each year takes a step further on the road to helpless infirmity and, in most cases, to an early and inevitable death."[86] One of the most common causes of early death in DMD is respiratory insufficiency, which usually progresses gradually during the second or third decade of life.

Duchenne's muscular dystrophy is an X-linked disorder that is characterized by progressive weakness of the skeletal muscles, with associated pathologic changes in muscles due to protein dystrophin deficiency. The estimated incidence of DMD is approximately 1 in 3500 male births, with one third of cases due to new mutations. The onset of the disorder is usually insidious. Muscle weakness is commonly unrecognized before the child begins to walk. However, according to one series,[87] approximately two thirds of cases are diagnosed before age 4 years. The most frequent presenting symptoms are abnormal gait, frequent falls, and difficulty climbing steps. Infants often have generalized hypotonia and poor head control. Pain in the muscles, especially in the calves, is a common complaint; this is usually exacerbated with exercise. Enlargement of the muscles, particularly the calves, is also a common feature. Typically, there is a steady progression of muscle weakness; however, the rate of progression is variable. Immobilization for any reason may lead to a marked decline in muscle strength. Loss of ambulation generally occurs between the ages of 9 and 11 years. Before this loss, children with DMD have minimal skeletal deformity secondary to contractures of the Achilles tendon and the knee flexors. Although these skeletal deformities can contribute to the early onset of scoliosis, most patients have progressive scoliosis soon after the loss of ambulation. In the early stages of DMD, muscle biopsy shows increased variation in fiber size, splitting of muscle fibers, and proliferation of connective and adipose tissue. In the terminal stage of the disease, muscle is largely replaced by adipose tissue, with residual islets of muscle fibers. Myocardial involvement has also been demonstrated through abnormal electrocardiographic findings in 80% of affected boys. Although autopsy studies are limited, there is evidence of extensive myocardial fibrosis.[88]

SPINAL MUSCLE ATROPHY

Spinal muscle atrophy consists of a group of hereditary proximal symmetrical muscular atrophies associated with degeneration of the anterior horn cells of the spinal cord.[89] In 1971, Fried and Emery[90] proposed a classification of spinal muscle atrophies, dividing the disorder into three clinically and genetically distinct forms, as discussed in the following sections.

Type I (Werdnig-Hoffman Disease)

Type I spinal muscle atrophy manifests in utero or within the first few months of life. The onset might appear more acutely, with sudden loss of motor function in the extremities. However, there is commonly a period of complete normal motor function before the onset of disease. Infants typically show generalized hypotonia and rapidly progressive paralysis of the extremities. The lower extremities are usually more affected than the upper extremities, and the disorder involves more proximal than distal muscles. There is also significant weakness of the trunk muscles, leading to poor head control, and these children can never sit without support. The intercostal muscles are severely affected so that breathing is dependent almost exclusively on diaphragmatic function. As a result of the severe degree of muscle weakness, infants with type I muscle atrophy have a weak cry and an ineffective cough. They are susceptible to recurrent atelectasis, with volume loss involving the upper and lower lobes, as well as to recurrent pulmonary infection. Death often occurs before 2 years of age.

Because the function of the intercostal muscles is to stabilize the chest wall during diaphragmatic contraction, infants with spinal muscle atrophy have a characteristic paradoxical respiration pattern with loss of intercostal muscle function. During inspiration, the upper chest retracts inward and the lower chest expands outward. During expiration, the upper chest expands outward and the lower chest retracts inward. This distinctive breathing pattern gives the chest a typical bell-shaped appearance.

Type II (Intermediate)

Type II spinal muscle atrophy manifests between 3 and 15 months of age. Infants with this disorder usually have normal motor function for the first 6 months of life and are usually able to sit without support. However, they are never able to stand independently or walk. As with type I spinal muscle atrophy, the lower extremities and more proximal muscles are affected more severely than the upper extremities and distal muscles. The intercostal muscles are also affected, but usually not as severely as in type I. The diaphragm tends to be spared, and breathing depends primarily on diaphragmatic function. The most important factor in determining the long-term prognosis is respiratory function. Patients often survive beyond 4 years of age.

Type III (Kugelberg-Welander Disease)

Type III spinal muscle atrophy generally manifests after 24 months of age and follows a more benign clinical course. Children with this disorder usually achieve normal milestones in the first year of life and are able to walk at a normal age or at a slightly delayed age. They usually present in a similar fashion to children with muscular dystrophy, with a wide, waddling gait and difficulty climbing steps. Weakness is usually confined to the muscles of the pelvic girdle, but the arms may be involved as well. Patients with type III spinal muscle atrophy usually maintain ambulation over many years. In some cases, subjects show improvement in function as a result of compensatory reinnervation of the affected muscles. Loss of ambulation may, however, be precipitated by an incidental injury or fracture. As in all patients confined to wheelchairs, these children are susceptible to contractures and postural deformities.

RESPIRATORY MUSCLE WEAKNESS IN QUADRIPLEGIA

The rib cage and abdomen normally expand in phase during inspiration, with the increase in rib cage dimension predominating over the increase in abdominal dimension in both the seated and supine postures. Expansion of the rib cage provides the largest contribution to tidal volume. The diaphragm causes expansion of the lower portion of the rib cage. This action is the result of two mechanisms. The first mechanism, the appositional component of diaphragmatic action, is related to the fact that there is a zone where the diaphragm is directly apposed to the rib cage. As a result, the increase in abdominal pressure that takes place during diaphragmatic contraction is transmitted through the apposed diaphragm, thus expanding the lower rib cage. The magnitude of that appositional force depends on the size of the zone of apposition and the increase in abdominal pressure. The second mechanism by which the diaphragm expands the lower rib cage is related to the insertion of the diaphragmatic muscle fibers to the upper margin of the lower six ribs. From these insertions, the fibers of the costal diaphragm run cranially. When they contract, they exert a force that elevates the lower ribs and rotates them outward. The magnitude of diaphragmatic contraction is related to the resistance provided by the abdominal contents against diaphragmatic descent. When abdominal compliance is low, the resistance against diaphragmatic descent is high and the dome shape of the diaphragm is preserved. The diaphragm can then lift the lower ribs more effectively. In contrast, when the abdomen is more compliant, the dome of the diaphragm descends more easily during inspiration, the zone of apposition decreases markedly in size, and the increase in abdominal pressure is small. To the extent that the transaction of the cervical cord makes the abdomen more compliant, the diaphragm is less effective in expanding the lower rib cage.

Transections of the spinal cord denervate the muscles that are innervated by segments situated below the lesion. After transection of the upper cervical cord (C1–C3), the intercostal, abdominal, scalene, and diaphragmatic muscles are paralyzed. Very few muscles, such as the sternocleidomastoid, are spared and can be used during breathing. Patients with high spinal cord injury always require ventilatory assistance. Transection of the lower cervical cord (C5–C8) causes paralysis of the intercostal and abdominal muscles, but spares the diaphragm. Preservation of diaphragmatic function allows spontaneous respiration. Patients with spinal transection have a distinct pattern of breathing, depending on the level of injury. In quadriplegic patients, paralysis of the inspiratory muscles of the rib cage, especially the scalenes and intercostals of the parasternal area, is associated with delayed and reduced rib cage expansion relative to abdominal expansion.

Quadriplegia causes a reduction in lung volume secondary to paralysis of the inspiratory muscles. As in patients with other neuromuscular disorders, the reduction in lung volume measured in those with long-standing quadriplegia is greater than would be expected for the degree of muscle weakness. These changes are believed to be secondary to a decrease in lung and chest wall compliance. Traumatic transection of the lower cervical cord causes paralysis of all primary muscles of expiration, including those of the lateral wall of the abdomen, the expiratory intercostals, and the triangularis sterni muscles. Nevertheless, quadriplegic patients have small end-expiratory reserve volume, indicating that they are still able to activate some muscles that have expiratory action. Studies[91,92] demonstrate that the clavicular portion of the pectoralis major muscle, which is innervated by nerve fibers originating in the fifth through seventh cervical segments, becomes active during expiration. This muscle also becomes active during expiration and coughing.

In summary, traumatic transection of the lower cervical cord produces paralysis of all of the inspiratory intercostal muscles, leaving the diaphragm as the major inspiratory muscle. In quadriplegic patients, the inability to fully expand the lungs is associated with recurrent pulmonary collapse and infection. Additionally, the loss of expiratory muscle function is associated with a defective cough that hampers the clearance of bronchial secretions and predisposes patients to an increased risk of pulmonary infection.

CHRONIC RESPIRATORY FAILURE IN OBSTRUCTIVE PULMONARY DISEASE (BOX 14-1)

Obstructive pulmonary disease is associated with increased airway secretions and altered viscoelastic properties of the lung, leading to an increase in airway resistance during both inspiration and expiration. The altered rheologic properties of airway fluid compromise ciliary removal of inhaled particles and further diminish flow rates. Associated destruction of the lung interstitium increases pulmonary compliance. Hence, the lungs are more easily inflated and functional residual capacity is increased. The loss of lung elasticity allows the airways to be more compressible, thus slowing airflow during expiration and leading to air trapping. Inspiration may begin when there is alveolar positive end-expiratory pressure.[93] Thus, at the start of inspiration, contraction of the inspiratory muscles is necessary to reduce the positive pressure before air can enter the lungs. This increases the work of breathing.[94–96] The associated hyperinflation of the lung shortens the inspiratory muscles, thereby diminishing the maximum generated force. In addition, the diaphragm is flattened so that its contraction is wasted in retracting the lateral rib cage rather than expanding the lungs. An increase in respiratory drive requires the intercostal muscles and the ancillary muscles of the neck to assist the diaphragm. These respiratory muscles use energy less efficiently than the diaphragm, which increases oxygen consumption.

Several changes in the function of respiratory muscles and in ventilatory control take place in patients with obstructive pulmonary disease, allowing them to compensate for the adverse effects of airway obstruction on the respiratory system. Respiratory muscles generate a stronger force when stretched by loads. Hyperinflation elongates the expiratory muscles, leading to more forcible contraction. Similarly, the increase in airway resistance slows respiratory muscle shortening and subsequently increases the contractile forces. The spindles present in the intercostal muscles ensure that the muscles shorten adequately. The gamma motor fibers, which signal central respiratory demands from muscle fibers, stretch the spindles. These spindles then reflexively produce greater activity in the alpha motor fibers that supply the contracting muscles. The diaphragm has no spindles; however, reflexes originating in the intercostal muscles can augment phrenic motor discharge to the diaphragm.[70,72] PaO_2 and $PaCO_2$ in the arterial blood and brain are monitored by the peripheral and central chemoreceptors that act on the respiratory centers, leading to an increased drive to the respiratory muscles. In most patients with obstructive pulmonary disease, measures of respiratory drive indicate that the hypoxic and hypercapnic responses are within normal limits.[97] However, some patients with obstructive pulmonary disease have a reduced hypercapnic response.[98] In these patients, failure of the compensatory mechanism leads to progression from hypoxic respiratory failure to hypercapnic or hypoxic failure. Two factors lead to progressive respiratory failure. The first is a persistent increase in the work of breathing, leading to excessive metabolic consumption and reducing the strength and endurance of the respiratory muscles. The second is decreased chemosensitivity secondary to the use of medication, metabolic alkalosis, and sleep-disordered breathing. In addition, destruction of the capillary bed, aggravated by pulmonary vasoconstriction secondary to hypoxia, produces right ventricular failure that contributes to respiratory insufficiency.

BOX 14-1 Factors Contributing to Respiratory Insufficiency in Patients with Obstructive Pulmonary Disease

- Increased airway resistance
- Shortening of the length of inspiratory muscles secondary to hyperinflation
- Air-trapping with alveolar positive end-expiratory pressure
- Increased oxygen consumption
- Ventilation-perfusion mismatch
- Reduced diffusion capacity
- Increased dead space ventilation

CHRONIC RESPIRATORY FAILURE IN RESTRICTIVE PULMONARY DISEASE

Interstitial lung diseases encompass a heterogeneous group of disorders involving the alveolar interstitium and epithelium, the airways, and the pulmonary vasculature. In disorders in which the predominant structural abnormality is derangement of the alveolar interstitium, lung volumes, which comprise total lung capacity, functional residual capacity, residual volume, and vital capacity, are reduced. The elastic work of breathing is increased as a result of reduced static lung compliance. Additionally, gas exchange is impaired, as evidenced by a reduction in diffusion capacity. The changes in pulmonary mechanics result in a breathing pattern characterized by rapid breathing frequency and normal to small tidal volume. The magnitude of changes in the breathing pattern mirrors the changes in lung elastance.[99,100] The increase in breathing frequency is accomplished by a reduction in inspiratory time (T_i) and expiratory time (T_e). Smaller tidal volume, coupled with a shorter T_i, allows ventilation to be achieved with less work and lower oxygen consumption. Despite the decrease in tidal volume, ventilation is increased at rest and during exertion in patients with interstitial lung disease.[99] An increase in ventilation is necessary to overcome the increased respiratory dead space and abnormal distribution of ventilation. The relationship between minute ventilation (V_E), tidal volume (V_T), and duration of the respiratory cycle (T_{TOT}), as shown in the following equation, helps to conceptualize the factors that govern the control of breathing: $V_E = (V_T/T_i)\,(T_i/T_{TOT})$

The V_T/T_i ratio represents inspiratory flow, and T_i/T_{TOT} represents the ratio of inspiratory time to the total duration of the respiratory cycle. In patients with interstitial lung disease, V_E increases because of an increase in inspiratory flow, because the T_i/T_{TOT} ratio remains the same as that in normal subjects.[100,101]

When patients with interstitial lung disease are unable to maintain a higher than normal inspiratory flow, chronic respiratory failure will develop.

Respiratory failure in children with chronic lung disease is rarely the result of isolated obstructive or interstitial lung disease. In obstructive lung disease, there is usually associated involvement of the alveolar interstitium, whereas in interstitial lung disease, there is usually an associated airway obstruction. The pathophysiology of chronic respiratory failure in children with chronic lung disease is complex, and includes failure of the adaptive breathing patterns that are seen in both disorders.

CHRONIC RESPIRATORY FAILURE SECONDARY TO CHEST WALL DYSFUNCTION

Hypoventilation has been described in infants with congenital disorders affecting the development of the chest wall, such as asphyxiating thoracic dystrophy,[102] short-limb dwarfism,[103] and giant omphalocele.[104] Idiopathic scoliosis can lead to significant restrictive lung disease when the spinal angle exceeds 70 degrees, when a large number of vertebrae are involved, with cephalad location of the curve, and with loss of the normal thoracic kyphosis.[105–108]

METHODS OF EVALUATION OF CHRONIC RESPIRATORY FAILURE

EVALUATION OF THE CHEMICAL CONTROL OF BREATHING

The primary function of breathing is to supply oxygen and remove carbon dioxide from the body in response to changes in arterial blood gas values. The negative feedback chemical control system is considered the fundamental mechanism of respiratory regulation. Chemical control of breathing is evaluated by ventilatory responses to hypercapnia and hypoxia. The changes in PaO_2 are sensed by the peripheral chemoreceptors. The carotid body plays a predominant role in regulating PaO_2. Changes in PCO_2 are sensed by the central chemoreceptors and the carotid body. The stimulus to the central chemoreceptor is most closely approximated by the concentration of hydrogen ions in the cerebrospinal fluid rather than in arterial blood. Input from the chemoreceptors is integrated by the respiratory centers in the brain stem.

HYPERCAPNIC VENTILATORY RESPONSE

A linear relationship exists between $PaCO_2$ and alveolar ventilation. A hypercapnic ventilatory response is measured by the slope of the relationship between $PaCO_2$ and minute ventilation. Two standardized tests for hypercapnic response have been described.[109,110] The first test, which is no longer used, involves a steady-state method in which subjects breathe several different concentrations of mixed carbon dioxide, each for 5 to 15 minutes, until ventilation becomes stable. In the commonly used rebreathing method, the subject rebreathes from a bag that contains a gas mixture consisting of 7% carbon dioxide and 93% oxygen. Equilibration is achieved between mixed venous, arterial, and alveolar carbon dioxide levels and that inside the bag soon after rebreathing. After this initial period of equilibration, the changes in end-tidal carbon dioxide reflect the changes in PCO_2 at the chemoreceptor level. The hypercapnic ventilatory response is obtained by measuring minute ventilation simultaneously with end-tidal carbon dioxide. The test is usually completed in 4 to 5 minutes, when the end-tidal carbon dioxide reaches 74. The relationship between end-tidal carbon dioxide and minute ventilation is linear, and the hypercapnic ventilatory response curve is a straight line in the physiologic range. The slope S of the regression line and its intercept B on the end-tidal carbon dioxide axis are obtained from the following equation: $V_E = S$ (end-tidal carbon dioxide − B). S is expressed as the change in minute ventilation per change in end-tidal carbon dioxide. This equation provides an index of respiratory chemosensitivity to hypercapnia. Normal values for the hypercapnic ventilatory response have been reported in children.[111]

HYPOXIC VENTILATORY RESPONSE

In contrast to the ventilatory response to PCO_2, minute ventilation does not change until PaO_2 decreases to 50 to 60 torr. The difference in the shapes of the hypoxic and hypercapnic ventilatory response curves explains why alveolar ventilation and arterial blood gas levels are determined by hypercapnic rather than hypoxic chemosensitivity. Two methods have been described for the measurement of ventilatory response to isocapnic hypoxia. The first relies on end-tidal oxygen as the stimulus parameter.[112] The second relies on oxygen saturation as the stimulus parameter. Linear regression can be applied to express the hypoxic chemosensitivity. Normal values for the hypoxic ventilatory response have also been reported.[113]

Many factors can affect the values of the ventilatory response. The following precautions should be taken to minimize confounding effects on the results:

- The use of stimulants, such as caffeine-containing beverages, or medications known to have a stimulant effect on the respiratory system should be avoided.
- Subjects should rest for at least 20 minutes before the examination.
- Subjects should fast and should have an empty bladder. (The urge to urinate could stimulate breathing.)
- The examination room should be quiet.
- The body temperature should be measured. Fever can affect ventilatory response.
- Preferably, the test is repeated during the same session, with at least a 10-minute interval between tests.

TESTS OF RESPIRATORY MUSCLE STRENGTH

The force generated by the respiratory muscles leads to displacement of the structures of the chest wall and, ultimately, to an increase or decrease in lung volume. This force is estimated as changes in pressure, and the shortening of muscle fibers is estimated as changes in lung volume. To test respiratory muscle strength, pressure can be measured either during a voluntary maneuver or during involuntary contractions, particularly in response to phrenic nerve stimulation.

Volitional tests of respiratory muscle strength include the following:

- Maximum static inspiratory and expiratory pressures
- Maximum static transdiaphragmatic pressure

- Maximum sniff pressure
- Maximum cough pressure

Nonvolitional tests of respiratory muscle strength include the following:

- Electrical phrenic nerve stimulation
- Magnetic phrenic nerve stimulation
- Twitch transdiaphragmatic pressure
- Abdominal muscle stimulation

The following section primarily discusses volitional tests of respiratory muscle strength, since nonvolitional tests have little clinical application in children.

Volitional Tests of Respiratory Muscle Strength

Maximum Static Inspiratory and Expiratory Pressures

Measurement of static inspiratory and expiratory pressures at the mouth reflects the muscle strength of the inspiratory and expiratory muscles. The pressure measured at the mouth reflects the pressure developed by the respiratory muscle and the passive elastic recoil pressure of the respiratory system, including the lung and chest wall. At functional residual capacity, the passive elastic recoil pressure of the respiratory system is negligible. However, at residual volume, where maximum inspiratory pressure is usually measured, the passive elastic recoil pressure can significantly contribute to maximum inspiratory pressure. In a similar fashion, peak expiratory pressure, when measured at total lung capacity, can also be affected by the positive elastic recoil pressure of the chest wall. It is essential to recognize that the relationship between the force generated by the respiratory muscle and the pressure produced in the thorax or mouth is complex, and that multiple factors, independent of respiratory muscle strength, can affect maximum inspiratory and expiratory pressures. Because of the force-length relationship and the varying contribution of the elastic recoil pressure of the respiratory system, maximum static inspiratory and expiratory pressures depend on lung volume. Inspiratory effort is maximized at low lung volume, and expiratory effort is maximized at total lung capacity. Therefore, maximum inspiratory pressure is usually measured at, or close to, residual volume, whereas peak expiratory pressure is measured at, or close to, total lung capacity. Patients with an abnormally high lung volume, as in obstructive pulmonary disease, may have a low maximum inspiratory pressure. This is partially due to the shortening of inspiratory muscle fiber length that is associated with increased lung volume rather than to reduced inspiratory muscle strength. Maximum inspiratory and expiratory maneuvers are often simple for patients to perform. Normal values are available for children as well as adults. However, because these tests require full cooperation from the patient, it is sometimes difficult to ascertain whether the maximum effort has been made.[114] This can lead to difficulty in the interpretation of test results.

Maximum Static Transdiaphragmatic Pressure

Transdiaphragmatic pressure is defined as the difference between pleural and abdominal pressures. Given that the diaphragm is the only muscle in which contraction simultaneously reduces pleural pressure and increases abdominal pressure, an increase in transdiaphragmatic pressure is, in principle, the result of diaphragmatic contraction. Because changes in esophageal pressure reflect changes in pleural pressure, the difference between esophageal and abdominal pressures equals transdiaphragmatic pressure.

Esophageal and abdominal pressures are typically measured by passing a pair of balloon catheters through the nose, after administration of local anesthesia of the nasal mucosa and pharynx. The position of the catheters is usually assessed by asking the subject to perform sharp sniffing maneuvers while the signal is monitored on an oscilloscope or a computer screen. Placing the probes becomes more difficult when the subject cannot inspire voluntarily, as in anesthetized patients and those with diaphragmatic paralysis, cognitive impairment, or muscle incoordination.

The lack of normal values in the pediatric age range prohibits the use of this method in evaluating children with respiratory muscle weakness.

Maximum Sniff Pressure

A sniff is a short, sharp, voluntary inspiratory maneuver performed through one or both unconcluded nostrils. The sniff test reflects the force generated by contraction of the diaphragm and other inspiratory muscles. Patients are required to make maximum effort during a sniff maneuver. Pressure is measured by wedging a catheter in one nostril, which can be done by various techniques, including the use of foam and dental impression molding. The pressure in the obstructed nostril reflects the pressure in the nasopharynx, which is a reasonable indication of alveolar pressure. The sniff test is easily performed by most patients, requires little practice, and is relatively reproducible. As with other volitional tests, the pressure measured during the sniff is dependent on maximum effort. This pressure is, however, difficult to obtain if there is upper airway distortion or nasal obstruction. Normal values for sniff pressure in children have been reported.[115]

Maximum Cough Pressure

Measurement of pressure during cough is a reflection of the muscles in the abdomen, which function as the main expiratory muscles. The use of cough pressure in the assessment of respiratory muscle strength is limited, because normal pediatric values are not available.

MANAGEMENT OF CHRONIC RESPIRATORY FAILURE

LONG-TERM MECHANICAL VENTILATION

The goal of long-term mechanical ventilation is to correct chronic respiratory failure, allowing patients to reach their maximum developmental potential. This option is presented when it is believed that long-term ventilation will enhance the patients' ability to develop cognitively or physically. The decision to use long-term mechanical ventilation and the choice of method of ventilatory support are personal decisions that are made by patients and their families.

Methods of long-term mechanical ventilation of pediatric patients fall into two classifications—invasive and noninvasive.

Invasive Methods of Mechanical Ventilation

Invasive mechanical ventilation can be achieved via a permanent tracheostomy or electrophrenic pacing device. As a general principle, patients with chronic respiratory failure who require constant mechanical ventilation are most often treated with a permanent tracheotomy and positive pressure ventilation.

Positive Pressure Ventilation via Tracheotomy

A number of positive pressure ventilators have been designed specifically for use in the home. Most such ventilators are microprocessor-controlled volume ventilators. They are not driven by air compressors and therefore offer portability. Although older prototypes had limits on the lowest tidal volume delivered to patients, most modern units can deliver appropriate tidal volumes to small infants. Some ventilators also offer a pressure limit function. This function is similar to the assisted control mode, except that the inspiratory phase is terminated when a set pressure is reached, thus putting a limit on the tidal volume delivered to the patient. However, a major disadvantage of microprocessor-controlled volume ventilators is the absence of constant flow. When used in a synchronized intermittent mandatory ventilation mode or in an assisted control mode, a significant load is imposed on the respiratory muscles because of the difficulty in triggering an assisted breath. External sources of flow have been used to circumvent this difficulty, decreasing the work of breathing in triggering the ventilator.[116]

Constant-flow nonportable ventilators have also been used for infants and children who require long-term home mechanical ventilation.[117] These ventilators have an optional compressor, an external air-oxygen blender, and a gas outlet port that can power a nebulizer during inspiration. The work of breathing needed to trigger a spontaneous ventilator-assisted breath is lower than that needed with microprocessor-controlled volume ventilators (Box 14-2).

Noninvasive Methods of Mechanical Ventilation

Positive Pressure Ventilation via a Nasal Mask

Noninvasive positive pressure ventilation can be provided by a nasal or full-face mask; however, a full-face mask carries the risk of pulmonary aspiration or gastric perforation. This mode of ventilation has several advantages, including avoidance of the need for a tracheotomy, portability, and relative simplicity of the equipment and setup. The ventilators that are most commonly used via a nasal mask are bilevel pressure ventilators. These ventilators are electrically powered, driven by a compressor or blower, and controlled by a microprocessor that modulates the delivered flow. They are usually triggered when there is a change in flow for a specific duration. Bilevel pressure ventilators are capable of compensating for leaks. This is accomplished by the flow control valve, which adjusts the level of leak present by measuring flow at the end of exhalation, and then readjusts the trigger sensitivity to the new baseline flow.

A drawback of noninvasive positive pressure ventilation using a bilevel ventilator is patient-ventilator asynchrony. Asynchrony can develop from a gross air leak, from the inability of the ventilator to meet the patient's inspiratory flow demands at the onset of inspiration, or from the lack of patient-ventilator coordination during termination of inspiration. The last two causes can be resolved by adjusting the rate of increase to peak pressure (rise time) and the end-inspiratory flow pressure that terminates each breath. Unfortunately, however, these adjustment options are not available on all types of bilevel ventilators. Another important drawback of this type of ventilator is its pressure-dependent exhalation system, which has the potential risk of carbon dioxide rebreathing and secondary hypercapnia.

Negative Pressure Ventilators

Negative pressure ventilators are designed to apply external subatmospheric pressure to expand the rib cage. Several methods for negative pressure ventilation are available.

Chest Cuirass. The chest cuirass is designed to be placed over the patient's thorax and abdomen and secured with wide straps. The negative pressure generator is attached at the opening on the top of the shell. The major problem with the commercial shell is its fit, especially in children.

Raincoats. The raincoat is a modified poncho that is worn over a shell-like grid. The grid is an accessory to prevent the negative pressure attachment from being applied directly to the thorax. The primary problem with this chamber is leakage. Additionally, many patients complain of being cold when using the raincoat, because room air is drawn into it when negative pressure is generated.

Modes of Ventilation

Patients with different diagnoses may benefit from different modes of positive pressure ventilation. Synchronized intermittent mandatory ventilation, with or without pressure support, is a mode of ventilation that is frequently used during the hospital stay. Hospital ventilators require compressed air or other gas sources that can generate high continuous gas flow rates. Home ventilators do not have continuous gas flow; therefore, a synchronized intermittent mandatory ventilation dial on a home unit does not provide the same support as that provided by a hospital ventilator. An external source of continuous flow, such as in units typically used for continuous positive airway pressure, can be attached to the circuit, providing the same flow rate and volume as that provided by a hospital ventilator.[108] A one-way valve placed proximal to a pass-over humidifier is needed to minimize the work of breathing. In addition, the exhalation valve must be placed as close to the tracheostomy as feasible to minimize dead space during spontaneous respiration. Positive end-expiratory pressure can be applied to all positive pressure ventilators by attaching a disposable positive end-expiratory pressure valve to the exhalation valve. Whenever positive end-expiratory pressure is applied to a volume preset home care ventilator, the effort required to draw gas spontaneously from outside the circuit is increased. Careful adjustment of the sensitivity of the unit is therefore necessary.

BOX 14-2 Equipment Required during Invasive Positive Pressure Ventilation

Primary ventilator
Oxygen source
Remote alarm
Backup ventilator
System humidifier
Ventilator circuits
Suction apparatus
Suction supplies
Spare tracheostomy tube
Battery charger

Ventilator Settings

One of the main goals of long-term mechanical ventilation in children is to meet their ventilatory demands, so as to leave sufficient energy available for other activities. In the absence of parenchymal lung disease, ventilators are adjusted to maintain oxygen saturation greater than 95% and $PaCO_2$ tension of 35 to 40 torr during wakefulness and sleep. In the presence of parenchymal lung disease, oxygen supplementation may be needed to maintain normal oxygen saturation. Normal $PaCO_2$ tension in the presence of parenchymal lung disease might not be achievable with safe ventilator settings that could be used at home. Positive pressure ventilation via a tracheotomy is complicated by the fact that, during sleep, because of the generalized muscle atonia that develops, children can have a greater degree of leakage from around the tracheostomy tube than during wakefulness.[118] Qualitative assessment of ventilation and the degree of leakage from around the tracheostomy tube can be performed by examining the changes in inspiratory and expiratory flows obtained from a pneumotachograph. End-tidal carbon dioxide can be measured by a capnograph, and changes in tidal volume can be measured by respiratory inductive plethysmography. Accurate measurements of leakage can be obtained by measuring inhaled and exhaled volumes during different stages of sleep.

Correction of the leakage from around the tracheostomy tube can be made by making further adjustments to the ventilator settings or by using a cuffed tracheostomy tube and inflating the cuff with different volumes during wakefulness and sleep.

Choosing between Noninvasive and Invasive Ventilation

Noninvasive positive pressure ventilation is usually the first choice for patients who require long-term ventilation. However, as outlined in Box 14-3, there are conditions in which this approach is neither safe nor practical.

Outcomes of Long-Term Mechanical Ventilation in Children

Several studies have examined both the short- and long-term effects on the survival and quality of life of children who require long-term mechanical ventilation.[106,119–128] Similarly, research examining the effect of providing long-term care for ventilator-dependent children on the quality of life of home caregivers has been limited.

Safety

All studies show that infants and children who are rigorously selected to receive long-term mechanical ventilation can be safely managed at home. These studies have demonstrated that failure of ventilator equipment rarely occurs. A survey of 150 ventilator-assisted patients conducted over a 1-year period found that there was one mechanical failure of the equipment for every 1.25 years of continuous use.[129]

Quality of Life and Developmental Potential

The main goals of home mechanical ventilation in children are to optimize quality of life, rehabilitation, and growth and development. The primary outcome measure of quality of life of technology-dependent children is reintegration into the school system. Multiple studies have demonstrated that ventilator-dependent children have been successfully attending school for years.[122,130–132] However, further studies are needed to reevaluate children's perceptions of their quality of life and to evaluate the quality of life of their caregivers.

Survival

The long-term survival of children treated with mechanical ventilation is primarily dependent on the clinical course of the underlying disease. In general, a better outcome is observed when the underlying disease is reversible (e.g., bronchopulmonary dysplasia) than in progressive disorders. The management of patients with severe bronchopulmonary dysplasia with long-term mechanical ventilation is substantiated by several studies showing a short-term survival rate of greater than 90%, eventual weaning from ventilatory support, and decannulation in the majority of cases.[112,126] The mean 5-year survival rate in pediatric patients with central hypoventilation syndromes was found to approach 90%, whereas that of children with progressive neuromuscular disorders was found to be 75%.[119,130,131,133–135]

BOX 14-3 Indications for and Contraindications to Different Modes of Ventilation

Indications for Invasive Ventilation

- Failure to ventilate adequately with noninvasive ventilation
- Failure to tolerate noninvasive ventilation
- High level of dependence on assisted ventilation (16–20 hr/day)

Contraindications to Noninvasive Ventilation

- Swallowing disorders
- History of pulmonary aspiration secondary to gastroesophageal reflux or vocal cord paralysis
- Inability to tolerate noninvasive ventilation

Tracheotomy in Children

Indications

Over the last three decades, tracheotomy in children has become an increasingly common procedure and one that is performed in all major pediatric hospitals. Over the last decade, the number of children requiring tracheotomy due to neurologic disorders has increased, whereas the number who required it due to prematurity has decreased.[136]

Recent reviews show that the primary reasons for tracheotomy[124,125,137–139] include upper airway obstruction secondary to anatomic abnormalities (38%–75%), the anticipated need for prolonged ventilation (24%–53%), and the need for effective pulmonary toilet.

The majority of children who require tracheotomy are younger than 1 year of age, with a higher incidence in boys. Congenital conditions associated with upper airway obstruction contribute to this observation. Because the incidence of laryngeal trauma secondary to intubation and subsequent upper airway obstruction has decreased from 20% to 8%, tracheotomy in infants requiring prolonged ventilation can now be performed at several months of age. In older children, it is still recommended that tracheotomy be performed if intubation is expected to last longer than 2 to 3 weeks.[124,137–139]

Complications

Although tracheotomy is performed to alleviate airway compromise or provide safe access for ventilation or pulmonary toilet, it also runs the risk of significant complications, especially in the pediatric population. Reports of urgent tracheotomy procedures list more complications than those performed electively.[136,137,140] Reported complication rates range from 19% to 85%.[138,139,141–143] Most authors categorize these as either early complications (intraoperative complications and those occurring up to the first tracheostomy tube change) or late complications (occurring after the first tube change). Recent studies have shown that cannula obstruction is the most common early complication. Less common early complications include local infection, accidental decannulation, false passage formation, pneumomediastinum, pneumothorax, acute hemorrhage, and death.[139,142]

Late complications include recurrent tracheitis, accidental decannulation, cannula obstruction, subglottic stenosis, suprastomal obstruction, tracheal ulceration or granuloma, persistent tracheocutaneous fistula, tracheomalacia, delayed tracheoesophageal fistula, tracheal innominate fistula, and hemorrhage.[137,140] Although many of these complications can be prevented or minimized, some (e.g., suprastomal granulation, collapse, and stenosis; persistent tracheocutaneous fistula; and tracheomalacia) correlate with the duration over which tracheotomy is required. In children requiring long-term tracheotomy and ventilatory support, the weight and torque of the ventilator tubing can contribute to accidental decannulation, irritation of the site of the stoma, and ulceration and hemorrhage in the lower trachea. Increased dry airflow and increased secretions can cause obstruction of the cannula. Granulation can form at the inferior end of the tracheotomy tube secondary to copious secretions and recurrent tracheitis. Long-term tracheotomies often lead to epithelialization of the stoma and a persistent tracheocutaneous fistula when the child is ready for decannulation.

Types of Tracheotomy Tubes

It is common to use the smallest possible plastic tracheotomy tube. This ensures adequate ventilation and allows sufficient laryngeal airflow to maintain audible speech, while minimizing potential damage to the cartilaginous framework at the tracheostoma. Neonatal tracheostomy tubes are usually used for infants weighing up to 7 kg. A standard pediatric tube is adequate for most infants and children. However, customized longer tubes can be used when standard tubes do not maintain the patency of the airway adequately.

Pediatric tracheotomy tubes can be metal or plastic, although the latter are preferred due to their flexibility and conformity to the airway. A disadvantage of plastic tubes is that they have a single cannula. When an inner cannula is needed, such as after reconstructive surgery of the airway, or when copious, tenacious secretions cause mucous plugging, a metal tracheotomy tube with an inner cannula is preferred.[137]

There are several types of pediatric cuffed tracheostomy tubes. Some are sized in neonatal, pediatric, and pediatric long lengths. Most tubes have high-volume, low-pressure cuffs that minimize tracheal mucosal irritation when inflated. Some tubes have low-volume, high-pressure cuffs that are generally used in ventilator-dependent children who have significant leaks during sleep. Different degrees of cuff inflation may be needed during wakefulness and sleep. To prevent irritation of the tracheal mucosa, caution should be taken to ensure that cuff pressure does not exceed 20 cm H_2O. There is limited experience with tracheostomy tubes with foam cuffs, because they are technically difficult to use.

Fit of the tracheostomy tube is best assessed with rigid or flexible endoscopy, because positioning of the child during radiographic assessment often puts undue pressure and distortion on the tube.[137,140]

REFERENCES

1. Kurzner SI, Garg M, Bautista DB, Sargent CW, Bowman CM, Keens TG: Growth failure in bronchopulmonary dysplasia. Elevated metabolic rates and pulmonary mechanics. J Pediatr 1988;112:73–80.
2. Fenn WO, Rahn H, Otis AB: A theoretical study of the composition of the alveolar air at altitude. Am J Physiol 1946;146:637–653.
3. Mellins RB, Balfour HH Jr, Turino GM, Winters RW: Failure of automatic control of ventilation (Ondine's curse). Report of an infant born with this syndrome and review of the literature. Medicine (Baltimore) 1970;49: 487–504.
4. Fleming PJ, Cade D, Bryan MH, Bryan AC: Congenital central hypoventilation and sleep state. Pediatrics 1980;66:425–428.
5. Shannon DC, Marsland DW, Gould JB, Callahan B, Todres ID, Dennis J: Central hypoventilation during quiet sleep in two infants. Pediatrics 1976;57:342–346.
6. Deonna T, Arczynska W, Torrado A: Congenital failure of automatic ventilation (Ondine's curse). A case report. J Pediatr 1974;84:710–714.
7. Guilleminault C, McQuitty J, Ariagno RL, Challamel MJ, Korobkin R, McClead RE Jr: Congenital central alveolar hypoventilation syndrome in six infants. Pediatrics 1982;70:684–694.
8. Haddad GG, Mazza NM, Defendini R, Blanc WA, Driscoll JM, Epstein MA, Epstein RA, Mellins RB: Congenital failure of automatic control of ventilation, gastrointestinal motility and heart rate. Medicine (Baltimore) 1978;57:517–526.
9. Hunt CE, Brouillette RT: Abnormalities of breathing control and airway maintenance in infants and children as a cause of cor pulmonale. Pediatr Cardiol 1982;3:249–256.
10. Paton JY, Swaminathan S, Sargent CW, Keens TG: Hypoxic and hypercapnic ventilatory responses in awake children with congenital central hypoventilation syndrome. Am Rev Respir Dis 1989;140:368–372.
11. Weese-Mayer DE, Silvestri JM, Menzies LJ, Morrow-Kenny AS, Hunt CE, Hauptman SA: Congenital central hypoventilation syndrome. Diagnosis, management, and long-term outcome in thirty-two children. J Pediatr 1992;120:381–387.
12. Trang H, Boureghda S, Denjoy I, Alia M, Kabaker M: 24-hour BP in children with congenital central hypoventilation syndrome. Chest 2003;124: 1393–1399.
13. Goldberg DS, Ludwig IH: Congenital central hypoventilation syndrome. Ocular findings in 37 children. J Pediatr Ophthalmol Strabismus 1996;33: 175–180.
14. Lambert SR, Yang LL, Stone C: Tonic pupil associated with congenital neuroblastoma, Hirschsprung disease, and central hypoventilation syndrome. Am J Ophthalmol 2000;130:238–240.
15. Faure C, Viarme F, Cargill G, Navarro J, Gaultier C, Trang H: Abnormal esophageal motility in children with congenital central hypoventilation syndrome. Gastroenterology 2002;122:1258–1263.
16. Nakahara S, Yokomori K, Tamura K, Oku K, Tsuchida Y: Hirschsprung's disease associated with Ondine's curse. A special subgroup? J Pediatr Surg 1995;30:1481–1484.
17. Croaker GD, Shi E, Simpson E, Cartmill T, Cass DT: Congenital central hypoventilation syndrome and Hirschsprung's disease. Arch Dis Child 1998;78:316–322.
18. Sakai T, Wakizaka A, Nirasawa Y: Congenital central hypoventilation syndrome associated with Hirschsprung's disease. Mutation analysis of the RET and endothelin-signaling pathways. Eur J Pediatr Surg 2001;11: 335–337.
19. Van Limpt V, Schramm A, Van Lakeman A, Sluis P, Chan A, Van Noesel M, Baas F, Caron H, Eggert A, Versteeg R: The Phox2B homeobox gene is mutated in sporadic neuroblastomas. Oncogene 2004;23(57):9280–9288.
20. Trang H, Laudier B, Trochet D, Munnich A, Lyonnet S, Gaultier C, Amiel J: PHOX2B gene mutation in a patient with late-onset central hypoventilation. Pediatr Pulmonol 2004;38:349–351.
21. Kijima K, Sasaki A, Niki T, Umetsu K, Osawa M, Matoba R, Hayasaka K: Sudden infant death syndrome is not associated with the mutation of PHOX2B gene, a major causative gene of congenital central hypoventilation syndrome. Tohoku J Exp Med 2004;203:65–68.

22. Matera I, Bachetti T, Puppo F, Di Duca M, Morandi F, Casiraghi GM, Cilio MR, Hennekam R, Hofstra R, Schober JG, Ravazzolo R, Ottonello G, Ceccherini I: PHOX2B mutations and polyalanine expansions correlate with the severity of the respiratory phenotype and associated symptoms in both congenital and late onset central hypoventilation syndrome. J Med Genet 2004;41:373–380.
23. Trochet D, Bourdeaut F, Janoueix-Lerosey I, Deville A, de Pontual L, Schleiermacher G, Coze C, Philip N, Frebourg T, Munnich A, Lyonnet S, Delattre O, Amiel J: Germline mutations of the paired-like homeobox 2B (PHOX2B) gene in neuroblastoma. Am J Hum Genet 2004;74:761–764.
24. Gaultier C, Amiel J, Dauger S, Trang H, Lyonnet S, Gallego J, Simonneau M: Genetics and early disturbances of breathing control. Pediatr Res 2004;55: 729–733.
25. Dauger S, Pattyn A, Lofaso F, Gaultier C, Goridis C, Gallego J, Brunet JF: Phox2b controls the development of peripheral chemoreceptors and afferent visceral pathways. Development 2003;130:6635–6642.
26. Weese-Mayer DE, Brouillette RT, Naidich TP, McLone DG, Hunt CE: Magnetic resonance imaging and computerized tomography in central hypoventilation. Am Rev Respir Dis 1988;137:393–398.
27. Kirk VG, Morielli A, Gozal D, Marcus CL, Waters KA, D'Andrea LA, Rosen CL, Deray MJ, Brouillette RT: Treatment of sleep-disordered breathing in children with myelomeningocele. Pediatr Pulmonol 2000;30: 445–452.
28. Montserrat JM, Picado C, Agusti-Vidal A: Arnold-Chiari malformation and paralysis of the diaphragm. Respiration 1988;53:128–131.
29. Rabec C, Laurent G, Baudouin N, Merati M, Massin F, Foucher P, Brondel L, Reybet-Degat O: Central sleep apnoea in Arnold-Chiari malformation. Evidence of pathophysiological heterogeneity. Eur Respir J 1998;12:1482–1485.
30. Harding CO, Green CG, Perloff WH, Pauli RM: Respiratory complications in children with spondyloepiphyseal dysplasia congenita. Pediatr Pulmonol 1990;9:49–54.
31. Holve S, Friedman B, Hoyme HE, Tarby TJ, Johnstone SJ, Erickson RP, Clericuzio CL, Cunniff C: Athabascan brainstem dysgenesis syndrome. Am J Med Genet 2003;120A:169–173.
32. Sarnat HB: Watershed infarcts in the fetal and neonatal brainstem. An aetiology of central hypoventilation, dysphagia, Moibius syndrome and micrognathia. Eur J Paediatr Neurol 2004;8:71–87.
33. Fujita I, Koyanagi T, Kukita J, Yamashita H, Minami T, Nakano H, Ueda K: Moebius syndrome with central hypoventilation and brainstem calcification. A case report. Eur J Pediatr 1991;150:582–583.
34. Saito Y, Ito M, Ozawa Y, Obonai T, Kobayashi Y, Washizawa K, Ohsone Y, Takami T, Oku K, Takashima S: Changes of neurotransmitters in the brainstem of patients with respiratory-pattern disorders during childhood. Neuropediatrics 1999;30:133–140.
35. Maria BL, Boltshauser E, Palmer SC, Tran TX: Clinical features and revised diagnostic criteria in Joubert syndrome. J Child Neurol 1999;14:583–590, discussion 590–591.
36. Mercado A, Pedraza L, Mayol PM, Rodriguez Santana R, Tejeda C: Joubert syndrome. Respiratory failure requiring home mechanical ventilation. Bol Asoc Med P R 1991;83:451–455.
37. MacDonald JT, Camp D: Prolonged but reversible respiratory failure in a newborn with Prader-Willi syndrome. J Child Neurol 2001;16:153–154.
38. Manni R, Politini L, Nobili L, Ferrillo F, Livieri C, Veneselli E, Biancheri R, Martinetti M, Tartara A: Hypersomnia in the Prader Willi syndrome. Clinical-electrophysiological features and underlying factors. Clin Neurophysiol 2001;112:800–805.
39. Johnston K, Newth CJ, Sheu KF, Patel MS, Heldt GP, Schmidt KA, Packman S: Central hypoventilation syndrome in pyruvate dehydrogenase complex deficiency. Pediatrics 1984;74:1034–1040.
40. Arii J, Tanabe Y: Leigh syndrome. Serial MR imaging and clinical follow-up. AJNR Am J Neuroradiol 2000;21:1502–1509.
41. Vergani L, Angelini C: Infantile lipid storage myopathy with nocturnal hypoventilation shows abnormal low-affinity muscle carnitine uptake in vitro. Neuromuscul Disord 1999;9:320–322.
42. Del Carmen Sanchez M, Lopez-Herce J, Carrillo A, Moral R, Arias B, Rodriguez A, Sancho L: Late onset central hypoventilation syndrome. Pediatr Pulmonol 1996;21:189–191.
43. Katz ES, McGrath S, Marcus CL: Late-onset central hypoventilation with hypothalamic dysfunction. A distinct clinical syndrome. Pediatr Pulmonol 2000;29:62–68.
44. Katz-Salamon M, Jonsson B, Lagercrantz H: Blunted peripheral chemoreceptor response to hyperoxia in a group of infants with bronchopulmonary dysplasia. Pediatr Pulmonol 1995;20:101–106.
45. De Broe ME, De Backer WA: Pathophysiology of hemodialysis-associated hypoxemia. Adv Nephrol Necker Hosp 1989;18:297–315.
46. Javaheri S, Shore NS, Rose B, Kazemi H: Compensatory hypoventilation in metabolic alkalosis. Chest 1982;81:296–301.
47. Hazinski TA: Furosemide decreases ventilation in young rabbits. J Pediatr 1985;106:81–85.
48. De Troyer A, Borenstein S, Cordier R: Analysis of lung volume restriction in patients with respiratory muscle weakness. Thorax 1980;35:603–610.
49. Estenne M, Gevenois PA, Kinnear W, Soudon P, Heilporn A, De Troyer A: Lung volume restriction in patients with chronic respiratory muscle weakness. The role of microatelectasis. Thorax 1993;48:698–701.
50. De Bruin PF, Ueki J, Bush A, Manzur Y, Watson A, Pride NB: Inspiratory flow reserve in boys with Duchenne muscular dystrophy. Pediatr Pulmonol 2001;31:451–457.
51. Tangsrud S, Petersen IL, Lodrup Carlsen KC, Carlsen KH: Lung function in children with Duchenne's muscular dystrophy. Respir Med 2001;95: 898–903.
52. Gibson GJ, Pride NB, Davis JN, Loh LC: Pulmonary mechanics in patients with respiratory muscle weakness. Am Rev Respir Dis 1977;115:389–395.
53. Estenne M, Heilporn A, Delhez L, Yernault JC, De Troyer A: Chest wall stiffness in patients with chronic respiratory muscle weakness. Am Rev Respir Dis 1983;128:1002–1007.
54. De Troyer A, Deisser P: The effects of intermittent positive pressure breathing on patients with respiratory muscle weakness. Am Rev Respir Dis 1981;124:132–137.
55. Williams JV, Tierney DF, Parker HR: Surface forces in the lung, atelectasis, and transpulmonary pressure. J Appl Physiol 1966;21:819–827.
56. Ferris BG Jr, Pollard DS: Effect of deep and quiet breathing on pulmonary compliance in man. J Clin Invest 1960;39:143–149.
57. McCool FD, Mayewski RF, Shayne DS, Gibson CJ, Griggs RC, Hyde RW: Intermittent positive pressure breathing in patients with respiratory muscle weakness. Alterations in total respiratory system compliance. Chest 1986;90:546–552.
58. Estenne M, De Troyer A: The effects of tetraplegia on chest wall statics. Am Rev Respir Dis 1986;134:121–124.
59. Papastamelos C, Panitch HB, Allen JL: Chest wall compliance in infants and children with neuromuscular disease. Am J Respir Crit Care Med 1996;154:1045–1048.
60. Fucharoen S, Ketvichit P, Pootrakul P, Siritanaratkul N, Piankijagum A, Wasi P: Clinical manifestation of beta-thalassemia/hemoglobin E disease. J Pediatr Hematol Oncol 2000;22:552–557.
61. Begin R, Bureau MA, Lupien L, Lemieux B: Control of breathing in Duchenne's muscular dystrophy. Am J Med 1980;69:227–234.
62. Gigliotti F, Pizzi A, Duranti R, Gorini M, Iandelli I, Scano G: Control of breathing in patients with limb girdle dystrophy. A controlled study. Thorax 1995;50:962–968.
63. Scano G, Gigliotti F, Duranti R, Gorini M, Fanelli A, Marconi G: Control of breathing in patients with neuromuscular diseases. Monaldi Arch Chest Dis 1993;48:87–91.
64. Burns SP, Kapur V, Yin KS, Buhrer R: Factors associated with sleep apnea in men with spinal cord injury. A population-based case-control study. Spinal Cord 2001;39:15–22.
65. Begin P, Mathieu J, Almirall J, Grassino A: Relationship between chronic hypercapnia and inspiratory-muscle weakness in myotonic dystrophy. Am J Respir Crit Care Med 1997;156:133–139.
66. Zifko UA, Hahn AF, Remtulla H, George CF, Wihlidal W, Bolton CF: Central and peripheral respiratory electrophysiological studies in myotonic dystrophy. Brain 1996;119(Pt 6):1911–1922.
67. Holstege JC, Bongers CM: A glycinergic projection from the ventromedial lower brainstem to spinal motoneurons. An ultrastructural double labeling study in rat. Brain Res 1991;566:308–315.
68. Takakusaki K, Kohyama J, Matsuyama K, Mori S: Medullary reticulospinal tract mediating the generalized motor inhibition in cats. Parallel inhibitory mechanisms acting on motoneurons and on interneuronal transmission in reflex pathways. Neuroscience 2001;103:511–527.
69. Kodama T, Lai YY, Siegel JM: Changes in inhibitory amino acid release linked to pontine-induced atonia. An in vivo microdialysis study. J Neurosci 2003;23:1548–1554.
70. Duron B, Jung-Caillol MC, Marlot D: Myelinated nerve fiber supply and muscle spindles in the respiratory muscles of cat. Quantitative study. Anat Embryol (Berl) 1978;152:17–92.
71. De Troyer A, Brunko E, Leduc D, Jammes Y: Reflex inhibition of canine inspiratory intercostals by diaphragmatic tension receptors. J Physiol 1999; 514(Pt 1):255–263.
72. Jammes Y, Arbogast S, De Troyer A: Response of the rabbit diaphragm to tendon vibration. Neurosci Lett 2000;290:85–88.
73. Hudgel DW, Devadatta P: Decrease in functional residual capacity during sleep in normal humans. J Appl Physiol 1984;57:1319–1322.

74. Matsumoto H, Osanai S, Onodera S, Akiba Y, Nakano H, Oomatsu H, Matsuura T, Yahara O, Tobise K, Sakai E: [Respiratory pathophysiology during sleep in patients with myotonic dystrophy]. Nihon Kyobu Shikkan Gakkai Zasshi 1990;28:961–970.
75. Ragette R, Mellies U, Schwake C, Voit T, Teschler H: Patterns and predictors of sleep disordered breathing in primary myopathies. Thorax 2002;57:724–728.
76. Rowley JA, Zahn BR, Babcock MA, Badr MS: The effect of rapid eye movement (REM) sleep on upper airway mechanics in normal human subjects. J Physiol 1998;510(Pt 3):963–976.
77. White DP, Edwards JK, Shea SA: Local reflex mechanisms. Influence on basal genioglossal muscle activation in normal subjects. Sleep 1998;21: 719–728.
78. Rowley JA, Sanders CS, Zahn BR, Badr MS: Effect of REM sleep on retroglossal cross-sectional area and compliance in normal subjects. J Appl Physiol 2001;91:239–248.
79. Stanchina ML, Malhotra A, Fogel RB, Trinder J, Edwards JK, Schory K, White DP: The influence of lung volume on pharyngeal mechanics, collapsibility, and genioglossus muscle activation during sleep. Sleep 2003;26:851–856.
80. Wiegand L, Zwillich CW, White DP: Sleep and the ventilatory response to resistive loading in normal men. J Appl Physiol 1988;64:1186–1195.
81. Douglas NJ, White DP, Weil JV, Pickett CK, Martin RJ, Hudgel DW, Zwillich CW: Hypoxic ventilatory response decreases during sleep in normal men. Am Rev Respir Dis 1982;125:286–289.
82. White DP: Occlusion pressure and ventilation during sleep in normal humans. J Appl Physiol 1986;61:1279–1287.
83. Nakayama H, Smith CA, Rodman JR, Skatrud JB, Dempsey JA: Effect of ventilatory drive on carbon dioxide sensitivity below eupnea during sleep. Am J Respir Crit Care Med 2002;165:1251–1260.
84. Dempsey JA, Smith CA, Przybylowski T, Chenuel B, Xie A, Nakayama H, Skatrud JB: The ventilatory responsiveness to CO(2) below eupnoea as a determinant of ventilatory stability in sleep. J Physiol 2004;560:1–11.
85. Davies SW, Emery TM, Watling MI, Wannamethee G, Lipkin DP: A critical threshold of exercise capacity in the ventilatory response to exercise in heart failure. Br Heart J 1991;65:179–183.
86. Gowers W: Clinical lecture on pseudohypertrophic muscular paralysis. Lancet 1879;1:113.
87. Dubowitz V: Progressive muscular dystrophy of the Duchenne type in females and its mode of inheritance. Brain 1960;83:432–439.
88. Moriuchi T, Kagawa N, Mukoyama M, Hizawa K: Autopsy analyses of the muscular dystrophies. Tokushima J Exp Med 1993;40:83–93.
89. Emery AE, Hausmanowa-Petrusewicz I, Davie AM, Holloway S, Skinner R, Borkowska J: International collaborative study of the spinal muscular atrophies. Part 1. Analysis of clinical and laboratory data. J Neurol Sci 1976;29: 83–94.
90. Fried K, Emery AE: Spinal muscular atrophy type II. A separate genetic and clinical entity from type I (Werdnig-Hoffmann disease) and type 3 (Kugelberg-Welander disease). Clin Genet 1971;2:203–209.
91. Estenne M, Van Muylem A, Gorini M, Kinnear W, Heilporn A, De Troyer A: Evidence of dynamic airway compression during cough in tetraplegic patients. Am J Respir Crit Care Med 1994;150:1081–1085.
92. Fujiwara T, Hara Y, Chino N: Expiratory function in complete tetraplegics. Study of spirometry, maximal expiratory pressure, and muscle activity of pectoralis major and latissimus dorsi muscles. Am J Phys Med Rehabil 1999;78:464–469.
93. Ranieri VM, Grasso S, Fiore T, Giuliani R: Auto-positive end-expiratory pressure and dynamic hyperinflation. Clin Chest Med 1996;17:379–394.
94. Rochester DF: The respiratory muscles in COPD. State of the art. Chest 1984;85:47S–50S.
95. Yan S, Kaminski D, Sliwinski P: Inspiratory muscle mechanics of patients with chronic obstructive pulmonary disease during incremental exercise. Am J Respir Crit Care Med 1997;156:807–813.
96. Sexton WL, Poole DC: Effects of emphysema on diaphragm blood flow during exercise. J Appl Physiol 1998;84:971–979.
97. Montes de Oca M, Celli BR: Mouth occlusion pressure, CO_2 response and hypercapnia in severe chronic obstructive pulmonary disease. Eur Respir J 1998;12:666–671.
98. Van de Ven MJ, Colier WN, Van der Sluijs MC, Kersten BT, Oeseburg B, Folgering H: Ventilatory and cerebrovascular responses in normocapnic and hypercapnic COPD patients. Eur Respir J 2001;18:61–68.
99. Gaultier C, Perret L, Boule M, Tournier G, Girard F: Control of breathing in children with interstitial lung disease. Pediatr Res 1982;16:779–783.
100. Renzi G, Milic-Emili J, Grassino AE: The pattern of breathing in diffuse lung fibrosis. Bull Eur Physiopathol Respir 1982;18:461–472.
101. DiMarco AF, Kelsen SG, Cherniack NS, Gothe B: Occlusion pressure and breathing pattern in patients with interstitial lung disease. Am Rev Respir Dis 1983;127:425–430.
102. Reiterer F, Muller WD, Wendler H: [Variance in the clinical picture and course of asphyxiating thoracic dysplasia (Jeune syndrome)]. Klin Padiatr 1986;198:340–343.
103. Hunter AG, Bankier A, Rogers JG, Sillence D, Scott CI Jr: Medical complications of achondroplasia. A multicentre patient review. J Med Genet 1998;35:705–712.
104. Tsakayannis DE, Zurakowski D, Lillehei CW: Respiratory insufficiency at birth. A predictor of mortality for infants with omphalocele. J Pediatr Surg 1996;31:1088–1090, discussion 1090–1091.
105. Shneerson JM, Simonds AK: Noninvasive ventilation for chest wall and neuromuscular disorders. Eur Respir J 2002;20:480–487.
106. Splaingard ML, Frates RC Jr, Jefferson LS, Rosen CL, Harrison GM: Home negative pressure ventilation. Report of 20 years of experience in patients with neuromuscular disease. Arch Phys Med Rehabil 1985;66:239–242.
107. Gonzalez Lorenzo F, Diaz Lobato S, Perez Grueso F, Villamor Leon J: Noninvasive mechanical ventilation and corrective surgery for treatment of a child with severe kyphoscoliosis. Pediatr Pulmonol 2001;32:403–405.
108. Paditz E, Reitemeier G, Leupold W, Paul KD, Heinicke D, Reuner U, Dinger J, Schwarze R: [Noninvasive nocturnal nasal mask ventilation (NIPPV) in childhood and adolescence. Dresden experiences with 11 patients]. Med Klin (Munich) 1996;91(Suppl 2):31–33.
109. Stefanutti D, Fitting JW: Sniff nasal inspiratory pressure. Reference values in Caucasian children. Am J Respir Crit Care Med 1999;159:107–111.
110. van Limpt V, Schramm A, van Lakeman A, Sluis P, Chan A, van Noesel M, Baas F, Caron H, Eggert A, Versteeg R: The Phox2B homeobox gene is mutated in sporadic neuroblastomas. Oncogene 2004;23:9280–9288.
111. Dahan A, Berkenbosch A, DeGoede J, Olievier IC, Bovill JG: On a pseudorebreathing technique to assess the ventilatory sensitivity to carbon dioxide in man. J Physiol 1990;423:615–629.
112. Read DJ: A clinical method for assessing the ventilatory response to carbon dioxide. Australas Ann Med 1967;16:20–32.
113. Pianosi P, Wolstein R: Carbon dioxide chemosensitivity and exercise ventilation in healthy children and in children with cystic fibrosis. Pediatr Res 1996;40:508–513.
114. Weil JV, Zwillich CW: Assessment of ventilatory response to hypoxia. Methods and interpretation. Chest 1976;70(1 Suppl):124–128.
115. Bernardi L, Hilz M, Stemper B, Passino C, Welsch G, Axelrod FB: Respiratory and cerebrovascular responses to hypoxia and hypercapnia in familial dysautonomia. Am J Respir Crit Care Med 2003;167:141–149.
116. Zinman R, Ness V: How to modify a volume-cycled home ventilator to satisfy a child's need for pressure-limiting and continuous positive airway pressure during spontaneous breathing. Respiration 1996;63:363–367.
117. Wheeler WB, Maguire EL, Kurachek SC, Lobas JG, Fugate JH, McNamara JJ: Chronic respiratory failure of infancy and childhood. Clinical outcomes based on underlying etiology. Pediatr Pulmonol 1994;17:1–5.
118. Gilgoff IS, Peng RC, Keens TG: Hypoventilation and apnea in children during mechanically assisted ventilation. Chest 1992;101:1500–1506.
119. Schreiner MS, Downes JJ, Kettrick RG, Ise C, Voit R: Chronic respiratory failure in infants with prolonged ventilator dependency. JAMA 1987;258: 3398–3404.
120. Schreiner MS, Donar ME, Kettrick RG: Pediatric home mechanical ventilation. Pediatr Clin North Am 1987;34:47–60.
121. Oren J, Kelly DH, Shannon DC: Long-term follow-up of children with congenital central hypoventilation syndrome. Pediatrics 1987;80:375–380.
122. Gilgoff IS, Kahlstrom E, MacLaughlin E, Keens TG: Long-term ventilatory support in spinal muscular atrophy. J Pediatr 1989;115:904–909.
123. Stjernqvist K, Svenningsen NW: Extremely low-birth-weight infants less than 901 g. Development and behaviour after 4 years of life. Acta Paediatr 1995;84:500–506.
124. Burr BH, Guyer B, Todres ID, Abrahams B, Chiodo T: Home care for children on respirators. N Engl J Med 1983;309:1319–1323.
125. Frates RC Jr, Harrison GM, Splaingard ML: Home care for children on respirators. N Engl J Med 1984;310:1126–1127.
126. Adams AB, Whitman J, Marcy T: Surveys of long-term ventilatory support in Minnesota. 1986 and 1992. Chest 1993;103:1463–1469.
127. Weese-Mayer DE, Silvestri JM, Kenny AS, Ilbawi MN, Hauptman SA, Lipton JW, Talonen PP, Garcia HG, Watt JW, Exner G, Baer GA, Elefteriades JA, Peruzzi WT, Alex CG, Harlid R, Vincken W, Davis GM, Decramer M, Kuenzle C, Saeterhaug A, Schober JG: Diaphragm pacing with a quadripolar phrenic nerve electrode. An international study. Pacing Clin Electrophysiol 1996;19:1311–1319.

128. Trenchard D, Meanock C: Obstructive apnea and paradoxical rib cage movements induced by diaphragm pacing. A probable mechanism and suggestions for treatment. Am Rev Respir Dis 1982;125:784–785.
129. Srinivasan S, Doty SM, White TR, Segura VH, Jansen MT, Davidson Ward SL, Keens TG: Frequency, causes, and outcome of home ventilator failure. Chest 1998;114:1363–1367.
130. Canlas-Yamsuan M, Sanchez I, Kesselman M, Chernick V: Morbidity and mortality patterns of ventilator-dependent children in a home care program. Clin Pediatr (Phila) 1993;32:706–713.
131. Khan Y, Heckmatt JZ, Dubowitz V: Sleep studies and supportive ventilatory treatment in patients with congenital muscle disorders. Arch Dis Child 1996;74:195–200.
132. Appierto L, Cori M, Bianchi R, Onofri A, Catena S, Ferrari M, Villani A: Home care for chronic respiratory failure in children. 15 years experience. Paediatr Anaesth 2002;12:34–50.
133. Frates RC Jr, Splaingard ML, Smith EO, Harrison GM: Outcome of home mechanical ventilation in children. J Pediatr 1985;106:850–856.
134. Rutherford MA, Heckmatt JZ, Dubowitz V: Congenital myotonic dystrophy. Respiratory function at birth determines survival. Arch Dis Child 1989;64:191–195.
135. Heckmatt JZ, Loh L, Dubowitz V: Night-time nasal ventilation in neuromuscular disease. Lancet 1990;335:579–582.
136. Ward RF: Current trends in pediatric tracheotomy. Pediatr Pulmonol Suppl 1997;16:290–291.
137. Sherman JM, Davis S, Albamonte-Petrick S, Chatburn RL, Fitton C, Green C, Johnston J, Lyrene RK, Myer C 3rd, Othersen HB, Wood R, Zach M, Zander J, Zinman R: Care of the child with a chronic tracheostomy. This official statement of the American Thoracic Society was adopted by the ATS Board of Directors, July 1999. Am J Respir Crit Care Med 2000;161:297–308.
138. Goldenberg D, Golz A, Netzer A, Joachims HZ: Tracheotomy. Changing indications and a review of 1,130 cases. J Otolaryngol 2002; 31:211–215.
139. Carr MM, Poje CP, Kingston L, Kielma D, Heard C: Complications in pediatric tracheostomies. Laryngoscope 2001;111:1925–1928.
140. McMurray JSaP, Christopher AJ: Tracheotomy in the pediatric patient. In: Practical Pediatric Otolaryngology. Philadelphia: Lippincott-Raven, 1999.
141. Carron JD, Derkay CS, Strope GL, Nosonchuk JE, Darrow DH: Pediatric tracheotomies. Changing indications and outcomes. Laryngoscope 2000;110:1099–1104.
142. Wetmore RF, Marsh RR, Thompson ME, Tom LW: Pediatric tracheostomy. A changing procedure? Ann Otol Rhinol Laryngol 1999;108:695–699.
143. Donnelly MJ, Lacey PD, Maguire AJ: A twenty year (1971–1990) review of tracheotomies in a major paediatric hospital. Int J Pediatr Otorhinolaryngol 1996;35:1–9.

15 Pediatric Lung Transplantation

Blakeslee E. Noyes, MD

With reports of successful heart-lung and lung transplantation in adults in the early 1980s,[1,2] the application of lung transplantation to the pediatric population became an appealing prospect. Early reports of success in children undergoing lung transplantation[3–5] led to a marked increase in such procedures beginning in the early 1990s. Since 1986 and through June 2003, nearly 800 lung and 500 heart-lung transplantations, in patients younger than 17 years, have been reported to the Registry for the International Society for Heart and Lung Transplantation.[6] In these children, the number of lung transplant procedures performed annually over the past decade has varied between 60 and 80, although recent data show closer to 60 performed per year. The number of heart-lung transplants performed has dropped below 20 per year worldwide with the recognition that lung transplantation or isolated heart transplantation can be used in many conditions once thought to be amenable only to heart-lung transplantation. Heart-lung transplant procedures are rarely performed in the United States and now are concentrated in a few centers in England and France. From a high of 30 to 35 centers performing lung transplant procedures in the mid-1990s, the number has dropped to 25 in recent years, yielding a statistical average of two to three transplantations per center annually. In reality, a few centers perform the majority of these procedures, while most centers perform very few. The number of lung transplantations performed yearly is less than one tenth the number of other solid-organ transplantations, such as heart, liver, and kidney transplantation. Explanations for this relative paucity include the lower harvest rate of donor lungs and the small number of pediatric lung transplant centers in the United States and worldwide.[7] Notwithstanding changes in the allocation of lung allografts, a mortality rate approaching 50% in candidates awaiting lung transplantation underscores the need to expand the potential donor pool and perhaps the number of centers performing this procedure.[8]

■ INDICATIONS AND TIMING

Indications for lung transplantation in children have undergone considerable change in the past two decades as experience with this procedure has grown. Lung transplantation has been performed successfully even in young infants with distinctly uncommon problems such as surfactant protein B deficiency or alveolar capillary dysplasia. The most common diagnoses for which children undergo transplantation are listed in Table 15-1 according to the age in years at time of transplantation. In children younger than 1 year, the most common indications are congenital heart disease, primary pulmonary hypertension, and pulmonary vascular disease; about two thirds of children have one of these diagnoses. In this age group, rare indications include pulmonary alveolar proteinosis (including surfactant protein B deficiency), interstitial lung disease, and bronchopulmonary dysplasia.[4] In patients 1 to 10 years of age, cystic fibrosis (CF) becomes the most common indication, and in the 11- to 17-year-old group, fully 68% of pediatric lung transplantations are performed in CF patients. In the 1- to 10-year-old group, disorders leading to pulmonary hypertension remain a common indication, accounting for 31% of patients. Although primary pulmonary hypertension has been a common indication in children in the past, recent statistics show that the number is quite small, largely because of the successful use of chronic intravenous (IV) infusion with epoprostenol (Flolan, GlaxoSmithKline, Triangle Park, North Carolina) and the availability of alternative therapies such as sildenafil (Viagra, Pfizer, New York).[6]

Timing of referral for lung transplantation has been predicated on predictions of mortality in a 2-year time span and the typical waiting time of 2 years for donor lungs. For example, studies in CF led to recommendations for referral for lung transplantation once the forced expired volume in one second (FEV_1) declined below 30% predicted.[9] More recent studies have suggested using the rate of decline in pulmonary function, rather than any given value, but the idea remains that predicted 2-year survival is an important criterion. In other diseases leading to lung transplantation, criteria are less clear, and serial assessments of lung and heart function and the quality of life are necessary as the child receives maximal medical therapy.

New guidelines for all children older than 12 years have recently been promulgated (Spring 2005) by the United Network of Organ Sharing and the Organ Procurement and Transplantation Network, based on each candidate's medical urgency.[10] This new system will attempt to replace waiting time as the sole criterion for allocating donor lungs and replace it with a "lung allocation score" based on diagnosis and other factors, including age, height/weight, need for supplemental oxygen, pulmonary arterial pressures, 6-minute walk distance, and lung function. Using the lung allocation score, the higher the score, the more likely a lung allograft will be offered. Transplant centers will be required to update each candidate's information semi-annually. At the time of this writing, it is difficult to predict the outcome and pitfalls of this new allocation system. It is of note that children younger than 12 years will continue to have donor lungs allocated according to recipient size, blood type, and length of time on the waiting list.

■ CONTRAINDICATIONS

As experience with pediatric lung transplantation has grown, the number of absolute contraindications has declined to just a few, with most considered relative contraindications based on each transplant center's experience and expertise (Box 15-1).

■ **TABLE 15-1.** Indications for pediatric lung transplantation (%)

	AGE (YEARS)		
Underlying Disease	**<1**	**1–10**	**11–17**
Cystic fibrosis	0	36	68
PPH	14	14	10
CHD	47	11	2
Pulmonary vascular disease	12	3	0
IPF	0	7	4
Graft failure	6	10	6
BO (not for retransplantation)	0	4	4
Other	20	15	6

Note: Because of rounding, columns do not add to 100%.

BO, bronchiolitis obliterans; CHD, congenital heart disease; IPF, idiopathic pulmonary fibrosis; PPH, primary pulmonary hypertension.

Data from January 1991 to June 2003, modified from Boucek MM, Edwards LB, Keck BM, Trulock EP, Taylor DO, Hertz MI: Registry for the International Society for Heart and Lung Transplantation. Seventh official pediatric report–2004. J Heart Lung Transplant 2004;23(8): 933–947.

Absolute contraindications to pediatric lung transplantation include systemic disease affecting other organ systems such as malignancy; human immunodeficiency virus (HIV) infection; hepatitis B or C; tuberculosis; or liver, renal, or left ventricular failure. In some transplant centers, however, multiorgan transplantation (e.g., liver-lung transplantation) may be an option in selected patients with failure of an organ other than the lung. It is not uncommon for lung transplant candidates to present unique and complex challenges to the transplant center, including malnutrition, diabetes, osteoporosis or osteopenia, vertebral compression fractures, and the use of systemic corticosteroids. These are considered relative, and not absolute, contraindications. Infection or colonization with *Aspergillus,* atypical mycobacteria, or multiresistant organisms are relative contraindications in patients with CF. Some transplant centers consider *Burkholderia cepacia* complex infection in CF an absolute contraindication because of its inherent resistance to most available antimicrobial agents, while other centers will accept candidates with *B. cepacia* provided they are not infected with genomovar III (also known as *B. cenocepacia*), a particularly virulent organism that is associated with poor outcomes in the immediate posttransplantation period.[11] Prior pleurodesis (either chemical or surgical), although not a contraindication to transplantation, prolongs surgical time because of excessive bleeding from the parietal pleura, particularly when cardiopulmonary bypass and attendant heparinization is employed. Psychosocial problems and their potential impact on long-term graft survival are generally addressed by both the referring and transplant center. In families where nonadherence to a recommended treatment regimen is recognized by the referring physician, some centers recommend formulation of a contract between the referring physician and family that outlines the need for strict adherence to a treatment program over a 3- to 6-month period prior to referral for lung transplantation. A significant psychiatric or mental health disorder in either the primary caregiver or the patient is considered a contraindication to transplantation. Financial concerns may pose a significant burden for many families since travel to the transplant center before transplantation and a long stay near the transplant center are often necessary.

BOX 15-1 Contraindications to Pediatric Lung Transplantation

Absolute

1. Active infection with HIV, tuberculosis, hepatitis B or C
2. Malignancy
3. Renal, liver, or left ventricular failure
4. Irreversible or progressive CNS or neuromuscular disease

Relative

1. Severe malnutrition
2. Diabetes
3. Osteoporosis or osteopenia
4. Vertebral compression fracture
5. Systemic corticosteroids
6. *B. cepacia* infection* or multiply resistant organisms
7. Severe psychological disorder—patient or caregiver, psychosocial issues

*For some transplant centers, an absolute contraindication, particularly with genomovar III *(B. cenocepacia).*

■ SURGICAL TECHNIQUE

Potential donor lungs are evaluated using arterial blood gases, chest radiography, airway cultures, and airway examination by bronchoscopy. In addition, the donor is routinely screened for hepatitis A, B, and C; HIV; varicella-zoster virus; cytomegalovirus (CMV); Epstein-Barr virus (EBV); and herpesvirus.

In virtually all pediatric transplant procedures, cardiopulmonary bypass with heparinization is used for the implantation procedure. The surgical approach is via a bilateral anterolateral transsternal incision (the "clamshell" incision), which optimizes visualization and access to both pleural spaces. The great majority of children undergo bilateral sequential lung transplantation with telescoped bronchial-to-bronchial anastomoses. Peribronchial lymphatic tissue from the donor and recipient is used to cover the anastomosis. This may reduce the exposure of adjacent vascular structures to infection, in the event of airway infection and subsequent dehiscence. In patients with CF, careful attention to maintaining sterility of the donor allograft requires vigorous washing of the recipient trachea and bronchial stumps with an antibiotic solution prior to implantation.

Heart-lung transplantation is rarely used in children in the United States at this time. Even in the presence of marked right ventricular hypertrophy associated with pulmonary hypertension, successful bilateral lung transplantation is generally associated with resolution of right ventricular dysfunction.[12,13] In patients with pulmonary hypertension caused by a congenital heart defect, intracardiac repair of the anatomic defect typically takes place at the time of bilateral lung transplantation, obviating the need for heart-lung transplantation. Single lung transplantation is used infrequently among children, and much less than in adults.[6]

Success with living donor lobar lung transplantation was first reported by Starnes in 1994.[14] In this procedure, a right lower lobe from one healthy donor and a left lower lobe from another (generally family members) are implanted in the recipient. Typically, this technique has been used in both adults and children in the setting of rapidly progressive respiratory failure where cadaveric lung allografts were judged unlikely to be available or where further deterioration in clinical status would make the patient ineligible for cadaveric transplantation. In a procedure where three individuals are at risk and the potential donors may be under pressure from family members, obvious ethical concerns arise, and careful evaluation by an independent, established team of generalists, pulmonologists, psychologists, social workers, ethicists, and clergy is essential. This approach remains controversial, but shortage of potential donors may make living donor allografts an option in selected circumstances.

■ POSTTRANSPLANTATION MANAGEMENT

■ IMMUNUOSUPPRESSIVE REGIMEN

In the immediate preoperative period, triple-drug immunosuppression and directed antimicrobial therapy is begun. In virtually all circumstances, immunosuppression consists of a calcineurin inhibitor (either tacrolimus or cyclosporine), azathioprine or mycophenolate mofetil, and corticosteroids. Because lung transplant recipients have a higher risk for rejection episodes than other solid-organ transplant recipients, more intense immunosuppression regimens have been developed.[15] For example, the targets for trough levels for tacrolimus and cyclosporine are typically maintained in a range of 10 to 20 mg/mL and 300 to 500 mg/mL, respectively. Initial dosing for prednisone is typically 0.5 to 1.0 mg/kg/day, with the goal of 0.25 to 0.5 mg/kg/day by 3 to 4 months after transplantation, depending on the clinical course. Nearly all patients remain on prednisone at 1 and 5 years posttransplantation.[6] In addition, the use of induction immunotherapy at the time of transplantation has become more widely used in pediatric lung transplantation; recent data indicate that over 50% of patients receive either a polyclonal agent (antilymphocyte or antithymocyte globulin) or, more commonly, an interleukin-2 receptor antagonist (daclizumab or basiliximab).[6]

■ ANTIMICROBIAL REGIMEN

Most patients receive IV antibiotics before and after lung transplantation based on the most likely potential infecting organisms. Cultures from the donor may allow precise choices of antibiotics. In patients *without* CF, a first-generation cephalosporin is often used for 7 to 10 days posttransplantation. In recipients with CF, their pretransplantation sputum flora cultures help guide therapy; in most cases, antimicrobial therapy directed against *Pseudomonas aeruginosa* is selected, although some patients will need treatment for other pathogens. In CF patients in whom *Aspergillus fumigatus* has been isolated, many transplant centers use IV amphotericin or voriconazole postoperatively and, in some circumstances, aerosolized amphotericin, oral itraconazole, or oral voriconazole.[7] Prophylaxis against *Pneumocystis carinii* is begun shortly after transplantation with trimethoprim-sulfamethoxazole (TMP-SMZ) and is administered three times weekly. In patients unable to tolerate TMP-SMZ, nebulized pentamidine or oral dapsone are alternatives. Oral nystatin is begun in the early posttransplantation period to reduce the likelihood of candidal disease.

The approach to CMV prophylaxis in the pediatric transplant recipient is controversial, varying considerably among transplant centers.[16] Typically, ganciclovir or valganciclovir are administered for 4 to 12 weeks posttransplantation if either the donor or recipient is seropositive for CMV. Depending on the center preference, this may include a combination of IV ganciclovir followed by oral valganciclovir. In most instances, CMV prophylaxis is not administered when both recipient and donor are CMV seronegative.[16] In addition, some pediatric centers administer CMV hyperimmune globulin (Cytogam, MedImmune, Gaithersburg, Maryland) in conjunction with ganciclovir, based on reports of improved outcomes with CMV disease in adult patients.[17]

■ COMPLICATIONS

Complications following lung transplantation occur in predictable time lines: the first month after transplantation accounts for many complications related to the surgical procedure; an early phase, 1 to 6 months after transplantation, when infectious complications become more prevalent; and a late phase, greater than 6 months after transplantation, when bronchiolitis obliterans (BO) and malignancies are observed more frequently (Fig. 15-1).

■ IMMEDIATE POSTTRANSPLANTATION PHASE

Since virtually all pediatric lung transplant procedures are performed with cardiopulmonary bypass, postoperative bleeding, particularly in the pleural space or at the site of the vascular anastomoses, is common.[4] Other complications of the surgical procedure include injury of the phrenic or recurrent laryngeal nerve, causing diaphragmatic or vocal cord dysfunction. Dehiscence at either the vascular or bronchial anastomoses may require prompt surgical attention and an early return to the operating room. Fortunately, dehiscence of the airway anastomosis has become much less common with the use of a telescoping bronchial anastomosis. This type of anastomosis does not prevent other airway complications, however, such as fibrotic strictures, excessive granulation tissue, or airway collapse at the site of the anastomosis.[18] Most transplant centers perform flexible bronchoscopy within 24 to 48 hours of transplantation to obtain cultures from the lower airways and to assess the integrity of the airway anastomosis. In the event of the development of stenosis of the airway lumen, balloon dilation or stent placement by bronchoscopy may be necessary.

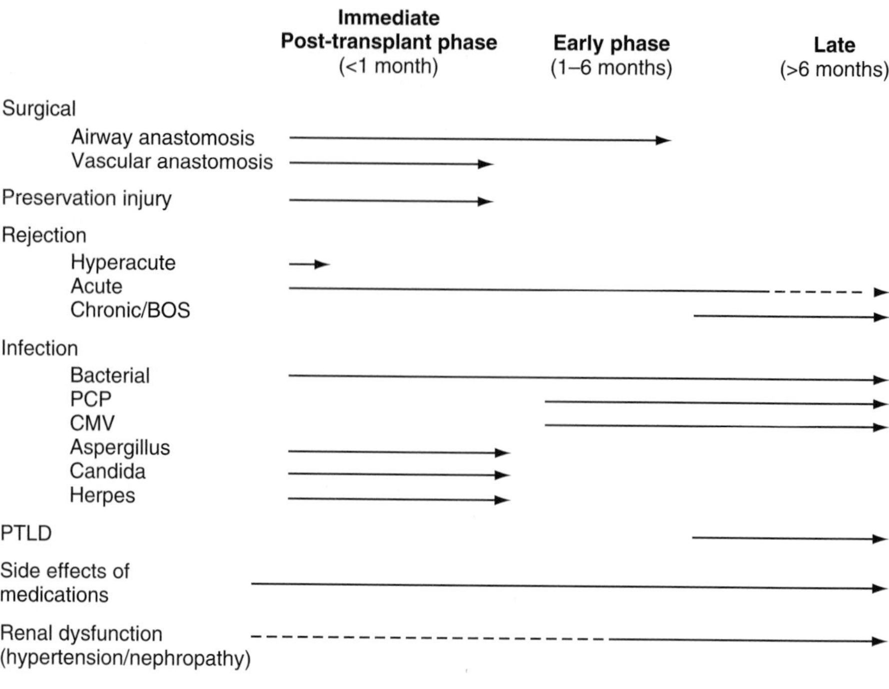

■ **FIGURE 15-1.** Timing of complications after lung transplantation.

Mechanisms invoked to explain the development of anastomotic narrowing include donor airway ischemia, impaired airway healing, and barotrauma if prolonged ventilation is needed after transplantation.[18]

Lung allograft rejection remains problematic, representing an important obstacle to long-term success of transplantation, particularly in comparison with other solid-organ transplant procedures. A variety of mechanisms have been proposed to explain this discrepancy, including the richness of immune effector cells resident in the pulmonary vasculature and lymphatic system, the ongoing daily exposure of the vast epithelial surface of the lung allograft to potential environmental pathogens, and the fact that the lungs are exposed to the entire cardiac output.[19]

Hyperacute rejection within hours of transplantation is a rare complication in the immediate posttransplantation period. It is associated with circulating recipient antibodies that bind to donor tissue antigens, and the severity of the immune response can lead to early graft loss.[4]

Acute rejection is much more common than hyperacute rejection and can occur as early as 1 week after transplantation or as long as 2 to 3 years later. Most commonly, episodes of acute rejection occur 2 to 12 weeks after transplantation.[19] Nonspecific signs and symptoms of acute rejection include cough, fever, dyspnea, hypoxemia, and radiographic changes. Lung function studies, if available, tend to show an obstructive pattern. Chest examination may show tachypnea and crackles. Since these symptoms are not specific for rejection and are difficult to differentiate from infection, evaluation by bronchoscopy with bronchoalveolar lavage and transbronchial biopsy is warranted. Histologically, biopsy specimens in acute rejection show perivascular lymphocytic infiltrates with or without airway inflammation. They are classified according to a standardized scoring system.[20] Since patients with acute rejection may also be asymptomatic, many transplant centers advocate surveillance bronchoscopy with transbronchial biopsy on a scheduled basis (e.g., at 2 weeks; 1, 2, and 3 months after transplantation; at quarterly intervals for the first year; and semiannually thereafter).[21] A smaller number of transplant centers perform bronchoscopy and biopsies only when symptoms of lower respiratory tract disease become manifest, arguing that long-term outcomes are unaffected with this approach.[22]

Treatment of acute rejection consists of 10 mg/kg of IV methylprednisolone daily for 3 days. For persistent or recurrent acute rejection, lympholytic therapy with, for example, antithymocyte globulin may be administered or the daily immunosuppressive regimen may be altered or enhanced. Although episodes of acute rejection are common after lung transplantation (and even expected), there are data which suggest that younger transplant recipients (<3 years) may have fewer episodes of acute rejection than older children or adults.[23]

In addition to rejection and early anastomotic complications, another problem that occurs in the first week is early graft dysfunction related to reimplantation lung injury. It is associated with the harvesting procedure and duration of ischemia prior to implantation; the generation of hydroxyl radicals and proinflammatory cytokines during ischemia may be causative factors.[24] Complications related to graft dysfunction vary from mild, noncardiogenic pulmonary edema to a picture of acute respiratory distress syndrome histologically characterized as diffuse alveolar damage. Patients generally have marked hypoxemia and diffuse infiltrates. Treatment is supportive with careful fluid management and ventilatory support; early retransplantation may be necessary and provides the only hope for survival in a small number of patients.

Sources of increased risk for infection in the immediate posttransplantation period (and beyond) are multifactorial and include the intensity of immunosuppression, loss of a normal cough reflex owing to both postoperative pain and the disruption of afferent and efferent nerves responsible for coordinating the cough response, impairment of mucociliary transport, and alteration in trafficking of immune effector cells to regional lymph nodes.[25] Despite the use of prophylactic antibiotics in the perioperative period (discussed earlier), recipient factors (particularly in patients with CF) and donor factors (e.g., active viral infection) may lead to significant infectious complications early in the postoperative period. In CF transplant recipients, the chronically infected lungs may cause seeding of the blood or mediastinum with recipient airway flora during explantation. Furthermore, chronic sinus disease typical of CF is a potential source of infection to the allograft and has led some transplant centers to advocate pretransplantation sinus surgery coupled with antibiotic washing of the sinuses.[26,27]

EARLY PHASE (1–6 MONTHS)

Infection

Infectious complications in this period include those due to opportunistic *(Pneumocystis, Candida)* and viral (CMV) pathogens as well as organisms carried with the donor organs during implantation. Bacterial pathogens are the leading cause of infection, and CMV disease is the next most common infection. Patients who are seropositive for CMV or who are seronegative and receive lungs from a CMV-positive donor are at particular risk for CMV disease during this early phase since most prophylactic regimens against CMV have been completed by this time. The incidence of CMV disease in these transplanted lungs reaches 75% or higher in the first 6 months after transplantation.[28] The long-term impact of CMV disease in the lung transplant population has been controversial, although there are reported associations of CMV with the subsequent development of BO.[29] Other investigators have cast doubt on this association.[30] In addition, CMV has detrimental effects on airway mucosal immunity, which increases the risk for superinfection with bacteria and fungi.[25]

Clinical manifestations of CMV infection vary from a febrile, viral syndrome associated with leukopenia to invasive disease with viremia affecting, most commonly, the lung but also other organs, particularly the gastrointestinal (GI) tract. In CMV pneumonitis, patients may develop a constellation of symptoms including cough, fever, chills, respiratory distress, crackles, and diffuse interstitial infiltrates. Isolation of CMV by bronchoalveolar lavage (BAL) or transbronchial biopsy in the setting of a typical clinical picture is strongly suggestive of CMV pneumonia, although it is worth noting that asymptomatic shedding of CMV occurs. Treatment for CMV includes IV ganciclovir for 2 to 4 weeks and, in some hands, adjunctive therapy with CMV hyperimmune globulin. Oral valganciclovir may be administered for 2 to 3 months after completion of the IV ganciclovir course.

Pneumocystis carinii was a common problem in lung transplant recipients in the early phase after transplantation before routine administration of TMP-SMZ began in the late 1980s. As with other solid-organ recipients, TMP-SMZ prophylaxis has resulted in a marked decline in disease attributable to this fungus in lung transplant recipients. Patients ill with *Pneumocystis* present with acute onset of fever, respiratory distress, hypoxemia, and interstitial infiltrates. Silver or fluorescent staining of BAL specimens will demonstrate organisms with a typical morphology and is diagnostic of disease. IV TMP-SMX is the treatment of choice.

Medication Side Effects

Triple-drug immunosuppressive therapy has offered a therapeutic approach that allows long-term success in solid-organ transplantation. However, the side effects of these medications can be troublesome enough in some patients to ultimately affect functional outcome and quality of life. The degree of immunosuppression is a delicate balance between too much, with risks for the development of opportunistic infections, and too little, with its attendant risks of allograft rejection.

Cyclosporine and tacrolimus are both associated with hypertension and nephropathy, although these may be less severe with tacrolimus.[31] The risks for renal dysfunction with cyclosporine or tacrolimus is compounded by the frequent use of other nephrotoxic drugs such as aminoglycosides, ganciclovir, or amphotericin. One year after lung transplantation, 38% of patients have hypertension and 7% renal dysfunction (serum creatinine >2.5 mg/dL); this rises to 72% and 22%, respectively, 5 years after transplantation.[6] Hirsutism and gingival hyperplasia appear to occur more frequently in cyclosporine-based immunosuppression.[31] Calcineurin inhibitors also cause neurologic toxicity, and seizures, headache, and sleep disturbance are common problems in the first months after transplantation.[32] In patients with CF, inconsistent and erratic metabolism and absorption of cyclosporine can occur and underscores the need for close monitoring of blood levels. Routine blood counts are necessary for patients receiving azathioprine because of its effect on white blood cell counts. Systemic and oral corticosteroids have the potential to cause a host of well-known side effects. For example, daily use of oral corticosteroids may lead to glucose intolerance and diabetes, particularly in patients with CF, with prevalence rates of nearly 25% in long-term survivors of lung transplantation.[6]

LATE PHASE (>6 MONTHS)

Ongoing complications in the late phase include those related to infection, drug toxicity, acute rejection, and the airway anastomosis. Posttransplantation lymphoproliferative disease (PTLD) and BO, two very serious complications, also become apparent.

Posttransplantation Lymphoproliferative Disease

The incidence of malignancy after lung transplantation in children is 5.7% 1 year after transplantation and rises to 8.7% at 5 years; PTLD is by far the most common malignancy.[6] PTLD is understood to be an EBV-driven lymphoma in an immunosuppressed patient.[33,34] PTLD appears to occur more commonly in lung transplant recipients than other solid-organ transplant recipients, in patients with CF, and in children as compared with adults.[35] These findings are probably explained by the intensity of immunosuppression in lung transplant recipients and the fact that many pediatric patients are EBV seronegative at the time of transplantation.

Manifestations of PTLD are protean, often vague, and often confusing. A high index of suspicion is required since early diagnosis and treatment improves the likelihood of resolution of disease. The most common site of PTLD involvement in lung transplant patients is the allograft, so symptoms of cough, fever, and dyspnea are not surprising. The most common radiographic finding is single or multiple pulmonary nodules that are round or ovoid.[36] Other sites of involvement in PTLD include the lymph nodes, GI tract, skin, and other organs. Histologic diagnosis can be made by transbronchial biopsy or direct sampling of a lymph node. A monomorphous histologic pattern has a worse prognosis.

If PTLD is identified early, the mainstay of treatment is reduction in immunosuppression alone. This is successful in greater than 80% of patients. Unfortunately, this approach appears to put patients at increased risk for developing bronchiolitis obliterans syndrome (BOS). In those patients with PTLD who fail to respond to reduced immunosuppression, most transplant centers administer the chemotherapeutic agents used in non-Hodgkin's lymphoma. Rituximab, an anti-CD20 monoclonal antibody shown to be effective in non-Hodgkin's lymphoma, has been promising in a small number of patients with PTLD. Since rituximab appears to induce a rapid remission in PTLD lesions, the time that immunosuppression needs to be reduced is shortened, hopefully decreasing the likelihood of developing BOS.[37]

Bronchiolitis Obliterans and Bronchiolitis Obliterans Syndrome

BO is the greatest obstacle to long-term success of adult and pediatric lung transplantation. By 6 years after lung transplantation in children, only 40% of survivors are free of BO, a worrisome figure since BO is the leading cause of death after the first year posttransplantation.[6] Histologic analyses of lesions of BO show progressive and irreversible stenosis of the bronchiolar lumen, eventually resulting in fibrosis and near occlusion of the airway lumen with collagen.[30]

It is generally accepted that BO is the end stage of a process of chronic rejection for which the immunologic basis is poorly understood. Tissue obtained by transbronchial biopsy may not be diagnostic of BO because of the patchy and uneven distribution of the disease. As a result, the term *bronchiolitis obliterans syndrome* (BOS) has evolved as the physiologic surrogate for BO.[38] Among the criteria used to establish a diagnosis of BOS is an otherwise unexplained fall in FEV_1 of greater than 20% from the best previous baseline studies.

A variety of risk factors have been identified for the development of BOS, including acute rejection, CMV disease and other respiratory viruses (respiratory syncytial virus, influenza, adenovirus), anastomotic complications, and noncompliance with the immunosuppressive regimen.[39] BO is felt to result from an inflammatory reaction induced by one or more of these risk factors, which leads to epithelial airway damage and eventually severe airway obstruction.[40] Of the risk factors identified, the frequency and severity of episodes of acute rejection seem to correlate best with the development of BO, supporting an immunologically mediated inflammatory response as a causative factor. This finding would suggest both the importance of routine surveillance bronchoscopy to detect subclinical acute rejection, and the need for aggressive treatment of acute rejection. Further support for this approach is recent information from Hopkins and colleagues, who found that very mild episodes of acute rejection (grade A1) were a risk factor for early-onset BO.[41] Although the usual approach to the finding of minimal or grade A1 rejection in asymptomatic patients is observation, Hopkins and colleagues suggest careful clinical assessment of the patient and possibly altering or enhancing immunosuppression, in an effort to reduce the risk for early development of BO. Other factors thought to enhance the risk for developing BO include CMV and stenosis or ischemia of the airway. Noncompliance with the posttransplantation medication regimen is clearly a contributory factor to the onset of BOS in lung transplant recipients, including children and adolescents. There are center-specific data showing that younger children[42] and patients receiving living related lobar transplants[43] are at lower risk for developing BOS.

Treatment of BO is problematic at best, with augmented immunosuppression the general recommendation. Some transplant centers endorse changing the immunosuppressive regimen from cyclosporine to tacrolimus, with anecdotal reports of success.[44] Antilymphocyte agents such as antithymocyte globulin or OKT3 may be effective adjunctive therapy in some patients.[19] As with PTLD, early identification and treatment is most likely to be effective. In many patients, however, progression of disease is inexorable and often complicated by infection with bacterial or viral pathogens. The goal of therapy is to ameliorate the chronic rejection, reduce the risk for infectious complications, and prevent further deterioration in lung function.

OUTCOMES

SURVIVAL

Survival after pediatric lung transplantation is depicted in Figure 15-2 for patients who underwent transplantation between January 1990 and June 2002. There is no statistical difference in survival rates among the different age groups shown, with a 50% survival rate of 3.7 years collectively. This does not compare favorably with pediatric patients undergoing heart transplantation, where the half-life is closer to 12 to 13 years.[6] However, most deaths after pediatric lung transplantation occur shortly after transplantation, so that if survival data are analyzed for survivors at 1 year posttransplantation, the 50% survival rate increases to 6.7 years.[6] As a group, survival at 1 year for pediatric recipients is 75% and at 5 years, nearly 50% (see Fig. 15-2). Analysis by procedure type for patients who underwent transplantation for primary pulmonary hypertension shows a marked and statistically significant difference in survival favoring double-lung over single-lung transplantation.[6] In patients with primary pulmonary hypertension, survival for those patients receiving double-lung transplantation at 5 years after transplantation was nearly 65% versus 25% for those patients receiving single-lung transplantation.

FUNCTIONAL OUTCOME AND QUALITY OF LIFE

Over 80% of lung transplant survivors report no activity limitations at 1, 3, and 5 years posttransplantation. About half of patients require hospitalization at 2 or more years after transplantation, with infection being the most common reason.[6] Several assessment tools are available to provide more objective measurements of quality of life following lung transplantation in adults and children. Perhaps not surprisingly, the quality of life and survival in adult lung transplant recipients were better than those of candidates who remained on the waiting list.[45] There are few well-controlled studies regarding quality of life in children undergoing lung transplantation. Nixon found a 24% improvement in quality of

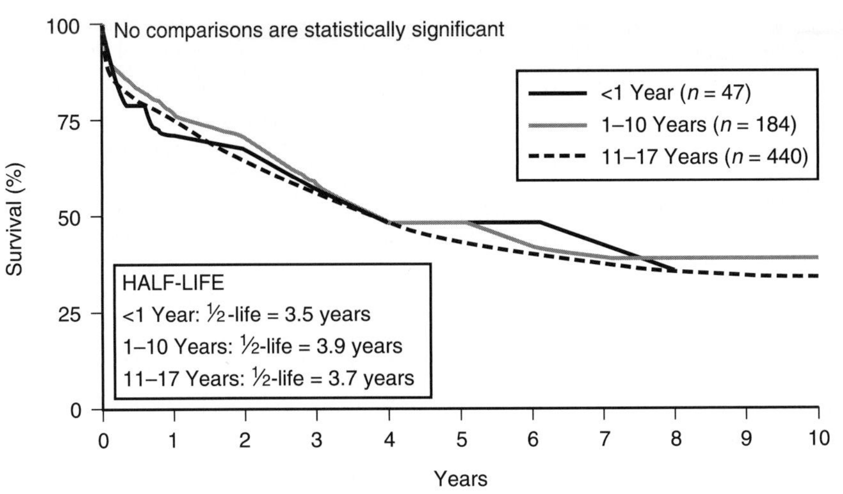

■ **FIGURE 15-2.** Survival after pediatric lung transplantation is depicted for patients undergoing transplantation between January 1990 and June 2002. (From Boucek MM, Edwards LB, Keck BM, Trulock EP, Taylor DO, Hertz MI: Registry for the International Society for Heart and Lung Transplantation. Seventh official pediatric report—2004. J Heart Lung Transplant 2004; 23(8):933–947.)

well-being in a small number of recipients after transplantation.[46] More recently, a group of 47 thoracic organ recipients (of whom 6 were lung transplant recipients) scored lower on a health status questionnaire administered to the parent or caregiver compared with a normal population but were similar to children with asthma, juvenile rheumatoid arthritis, or intractable epilepsy.[47] It is worth emphasizing that assessments of quality of life are difficult and affected by the child's baseline capabilities prior to transplantation and their expectations after transplantation.[46]

■ GROWTH

Somatic growth after lung transplantation is an ongoing problem for most patients, partly because of substandard pretransplantation nutritional status and the continued use of systemic corticosteroids after the transplant procedure. Improving nutritional status and maximizing growth is an important goal after transplantation.

Since early reports of successful lung transplantation in young children, concerns have been raised concerning the potential for lung allograft growth.[3] Animal data indicate that allogeneic lung transplantation is associated with an increase in lung volumes and airway size with age.[48] Work in young children by Cohen and colleagues has provided reassuring data with regard to lung allograft growth. These authors performed infant lung function studies in 23 lung transplant recipients who were younger than 3 years at the time of transplantation.[21] They demonstrated that in infants without airway obstruction, the functional residual capacity, as a surrogate for lung growth, increased in parallel with height acquisition, and the increase was comparable with that of normal children, suggesting normal growth of the allograft. Further support comes from Ro and co-workers, who used serial computed tomography scan measures to document airway growth of intrathoracic airways over time.[49]

■ CAUSES OF DEATH

Causes of death after pediatric lung transplantation are depicted in Table 15-2. Graft failure and infection are important causes of death in the first year after transplantation. In the first 30 days after transplantation, surgical complications are an important cause of death. After the first 30 days and before 1 year posttransplantation, infection from any cause accounts for nearly 50% of deaths. By 1 to 3 years after transplantation, BO becomes the leading cause of death, accounting for 37% to 46% of mortality. Infection remains an important cause of death throughout the follow-up period. Although these represent the most recent data available from the International

■ **TABLE 15-2.** Causes of death after pediatric lung transplantation (%)

	TIME AFTER TRANSPLANTATION			
Cause of Death	**0–30 days**	**31 days to 1 year**	**>1–3 years**	**>3 years**
Graft failure	44.4	18.7	19.8	10.9
Technical	13.3	1.3	0	0
Cardiovascular	13.3	2.7	2.5	0
Acute rejection	0	4.0	0	1.9
Bronchiolitis	0	6.7	37.0	45.6
Lymphoma	0	4.0	4.9	6.5
CMV	0	6.7	0	0
Infection, not CMV	13.3	41.3	21.0	19.6
Other	15.6	14.7	14.8	15.2

Note: Because of rounding, some columns do not add to 100%.

CMV, cytomegalovirus.

Data from January 1991 to June 2003, modified from Boucek MM, Edwards LB, Keck BM, Trulock EP, Taylor DO, Hertz MI: Registry for the International Society for Heart and Lung Transplantation. Seventh official pediatric report—2004. J Heart Lung Transplant 2004;23(8):933–947.

Society of Heart and Lung Transplantation, there has been little shift in the distribution of causes of death over previous registry data.[6]

FUTURE DIRECTIONS

Lung transplantation has offered hope to a number of children with a variety of diseases in whom early death was otherwise inevitable. The shortage of organ donors and of lung transplant centers will likely cause this procedure to be limited to fewer than 100 children annually. It is unclear whether living related lobar transplantation will be adopted by more transplant centers and increase the number of potential recipients or will remain a procedure offered at just a few centers. At the time of this writing, xenotransplantation is still a theoretical method of expanding the potential donor pool. National efforts to increase awareness about organ donation will likely remain the cornerstone in efforts to increase the number of transplantations performed in the United States and worldwide. BO will remain a major stumbling block to long-term success of lung transplantation in the absence of better methods to detect early infection and rejection and in the absence of improved treatment strategies. Elucidating the immunologic mechanisms in the development of BO will provide an important opportunity to improve the success of pediatric lung transplantation. Bacterial and viral infections are important causes of death after lung transplantation, and efforts to tailor antimicrobial therapy to specific situations will continue to be important. In spite of these obstacles, over 1300 children in the past two decades have been given a chance for long-term survival because of the success of lung transplantation.

REFERENCES

1. Reitz BA, Wallwork JL, Hunt SA, Pennock JL, Billingham ME, Oyer PE, Stinson EB, Shumway NE: Heart-lung transplantation. Successful therapy for patients with pulmonary vascular disease. N Engl J Med 1982;306(10):557–564.
2. Grossman RF, Frost A, Zamel N, Patterson GA, Cooper JD, Myron PR, Dear CL, Maurer J: Results of single-lung transplantation for bilateral pulmonary fibrosis. The Toronto Lung Transplant Group. N Engl J Med 1990;323(8):551–552.
3. Noyes BE, Kurland G, Orenstein D, Fricker FJ, Armitage JM: Experience with pediatric lung transplantation. J Pediatrics 1994;124(2):261–268.
4. Sweet SC: Pediatric lung transplantation. Update 2003. Pediatr Clin North Am 2003;50;1393–1417.
5. Métras D, Shennib H, Kreitmann B, Camboulives J, Viard L, Carcassonne M, Giudicelli R, Noirclerc M, and the Joint Marseille-Montréal Lung Transplant Program: Double-lung transplantation in children. A report of 20 cases. Ann Thorac Surg 1993;55:352–357.
6. Boucek MM, Edwards LB, Keck BM, Trulock EP, Taylor DO, Hertz MI: Registry for the International Society for Heart and Lung Transplantation. Seventh official pediatric report—2004. J Heart Lung Transplant 2004;23(8):933–947.
7. Mallory GB, Spray TL: Paediatric lung transplantation. Eur Respir J 2004; 24:839–845.
8. Whitehead BF, De Leval MR: Paediatric lung transplantation. The agony and the ecstasy. Thorax 1994;49(5):437–439.
9. Kerem E, Reisman J, Corey M, Canny GJ, Levison H: Prediction of mortality in patients with cystic fibrosis. N Engl J Med 1992; 326(18):1187–1191.
10. United Network for Organ Sharing: Information for Transplant Professionals about the Lung Association Score System. Accessed April 18, 2005 at www.unos.org.
11. Chaparro C, Maurer J, Gutierrez C, Krajden M, Chan C, Winton T, Keshavjee S, Scavuzzo M, Tullis E, Hutcheon M, Kesten S: Infection with *Burkholderia cepacia* in cystic fibrosis. Am J Respir Crit Care Med 2001;163(1):43–48.
12. Carere R, Patterson GA, Liu P, Williams T, Maurer J, Grossman R: Right and left ventricular performance after single and double lung transplantation. J Thorac Cardiovasc Surg 1991;102:115–122.
13. Katz WE, Gasior TA, Quinlan JJ, Lazar JM, Firestone L, Griffith BP, Gorcsan J: Immediate effects of lung transplantation on right ventricular morphology and function in patients with variable degrees of pulmonary hypertension. J Am Coll Cardiol 1996;27:384–391.
14. Starnes VA, Barr ML, Cohen RG: Lobar transplantation. Indications, technique, and outcome. J Thorac Cardiovasc Surg 1994;108(3):403–411.
15. Mendeloff EN: Pediatric lung transplantation. Chest Surg Clin North Am 2003;13:485–504.
16. Danziger-Isakov LA, Faro A, Sweet S, Michaels MG, Aurora P, Mogayzel PJ Jr, Mallory GB Jr, Boyer DM, Rice TB, DelaMorena M, DeBaun MR, IPLTC Group: Variability in standard care for cytomegalovirus prevention and detection in pediatric lung transplantation. Survey of eight pediatric lung transplant programs. Pediatr Transplant 2003;7:469–473.
17. Valantine HA, Luikart H, Doyle R, Theodore J, Hunt S, Oyer P, Robbins R, Berry G, Reitz B: Impact of cytomegalovirus hyperimmune globulin on outcome after cardiothoracic transplantation. A comparative study of combined prophylaxis with CMV hyperimmune globulin plus ganciclovir versus ganciclovir alone. Transplantation 2001;72(10): 1647–1652.
18. Kaditis AG, Gondor M, Nixon PA, Webber S, Keenan RJ, Kaye R, Kurland G: Airway complications following pediatric lung and heart-lung transplantation. Am J Respir Crit Care Med 2000;162:301–309.
19. Trulock EP: Management of lung transplant rejection. Chest 1993;103(5): 1566–1576.
20. Yousem SA, Berry GJ, Cagle PT, Chamberlain D, Husain AN, Hruban RH, Marchevsky A, Ohori NP, Ritter J, Stewart S, Tazelaar HD: Revision of the 1990 working formulation for the classification of pulmonary allograft rejection. Lung Rejection Study Group. J Heart Lung Transplant 1996;15(1 part 1):1–15.
21. Cohen, AH, Mallory GB Jr, Ross K, White DK, Mendeloff E, Huddleston CB, Kemp JS: Growth of lungs after transplantation in infants and in children younger than 3 years of age. Am J Respir Crit Care Med 1999;159:1747–1751.
22. Valentine VG, Taylor DE, Dhillon GS, Knower MT, McFadden PM, Fuchs DM, Kantrow SP: Success of lung transplantation without surveillance bronchoscopy. J Heart Lung Transplant 2002;21(3):319–326.
23. Sweet SC, Spray TL, Huddleston CB, Mendeloff E, Canter CE, Balzer DT, Bridges ND, Cohen AH, Mallory GB Jr: Pediatric lung transplantation at St. Louis Children's Hospital, 1990–1995. Am J Resp Crit Care Med 1997;155(3):1027–1035.
24. Kurland G, Orenstein DM: Complications of pediatric lung and heart-lung transplantation. Curr Opin Pediatr 1994;6:262–271.
25. Alexander BD, Tapson VF: Infectious complications of lung transplantation. Transplant Infect Dis 2001;3:128–137.
26. Lewiston N, King V, Umetsu D, Starnes V, Marshall S, Kramer M, Theodore J: CF patients who have undergone heart-lung transplantation benefit from maxillary sinus antrostomy and repeated sinus lavage. Transplant Proc 1991;23:1207–1208.
27. Holzmann D, Speich R, Kaufmann T, Laube I, Russi E, Simmen D, Weder W, Boehler A: Effects of sinus surgery in patients with cystic fibrosis after lung transplantation. A 10-year experience. Transplantation 2004;77(1):134–136.
28. Smyth RL, Scott JP, Borysiewicz LK, Sharples LD, Stewart S, Wreghitt TG, Gray JJ, Higenbottam TW, Wallwork J: Cytomegalovirus infection in heart-lung transplant recipients. Risk factors, clinical associations, and response to treatment. J Infect Dis 1991;164:1045–1050.
29. Sharples LD, McNeil K, Stewart S, Wallwork J. Risk factors for bronchiolitis obliterans. A systemic review of recent publications. J Heart Lung Transplant 2002;21(2):271–281.
30. Tamm M, Aboyoun CL, Chhajed PN, Rainer S, Malouf MA, Glanville AR: Treated cytomegalovirus pneumonia is not associated with bronchiolitis obliterans syndrome. Am J Respir Crit Care Med 2004;170:1120–1123.
31. Armitage JM, Fricker FJ, del Nido P, Starzl TE, Hardesty RL, Griffith BP: A decade (1982 to 1992) of pediatric cardiac transplantation and the impact of FK 506 immunosuppression. J Thorac Cardiovasc Surg 1993; 105(3):464–473.
32. Wong M, Mallory GB, Goldstein J, Goyal M, Yamada KA: Neurologic complications of pediatric lung transplantation. Neurology 1999;53: 1542–1549.
33. Purtilo DT, Strobach RS, Okano M, Davis JR: Epstein-Barr virus–associated lymphoproliferative disorders. Lab Invest 1992;67(1):5–23.
34. Boyle GJ, Michael MG, Webber SA, Knisly AS, Kurland G, Cipriani LA, Griffith BP, Fricker FJ: Posttransplantation lymphoproliferative disorders in pediatric thoracic organ recipients. J Pediatr 1997;131(2):309–313.

35. Cohen AH, Sweet SC, Mendeloff E, Mallory GB, Huddleston CB, Kraus M, Kelly M, Hayashi R, DeBaun MR: High incidence of posttransplant lymphoproliferative disease in pediatric patients with cystic fibrosis. Am J Respir Crit Care Med 2000;161:1252–1255.
36. Lim GY, Newman B, Kurland G, Webber SA: Posttransplantation lymphoproliferative disorder. Manifestations in pediatric thoracic organ recipients. Radiology 2002;222:699–708.
37. Verschuuren EA, Stevens SJ, van Imhoff GW, Middeldorp JM, de Boer C, Koeter G, The TH, van der Bij W: Treatment of posttransplant lymphoproliferative disease with rituximab: The remission, the relapse, and the complication. Transplantation 2002;73(1):100–104.
38. Estenne M, Maurer JR, Boehler A, Egan JJ, Frost A, Hertz M, Mallory GM, Snell GI, Yousem S: Bronchiolitis obliterans syndrome 2001. An update of the diagnostic criteria. J Heart Lung Transplant 2002; 21(3):297–310.
39. Boehler A, Kesten S, Weder W, Speich R: Bronchiolitis obliterans after lung transplantation. A review. Chest 1998;114(5):1411–1426.
40. Vilchez RA, Dauber J, Kusne S: Infectious etiology of bronchiolitis obliterans: The respiratory viruses connection—myth or reality? Am J Transplant 2003;3:245–249.
41. Hopkins PM, Aboyoun CL, Chhajed PN, Malouf MA, Plit ML, Rainer SP, Glanville AR: Association of minimal rejection in lung transplant recipients with obliterative bronchiolitis. Am J Respir Crit Care Med 2004;170:1022–1026.
42. Ibrahim JE, Sweet SC, Flippin M, Dent C, Mendeloff E, Huddleston CB, Trinkhaus K, Canter CE: Rejection is reduced in thoracic organ recipients when transplanted in the first year of life. J Heart Lung Transplant 2002; 21(3):311–318.
43. Woo MS, MacLaughlin EF, Horn MV, Szmuszkovicz JR, Barr ML, Starnes VA: Bronchiolitis obliterans is not the primary cause of death in pediatric living donor lobar lung transplant recipients. J Heart Lung Transplant 2001;20(5):491–496.
44. Roman A, Bravo C, Monforte V, Reyes L, Canela M, Morell F: Preliminary results of rescue therapy with tacrolimus and mycophenolate mofetil in lung transplant patients with bronchiolitis obliterans. Transplant Proc 2002;34(1):146–147.
45. Yacoub MH, Gyi K, Khaghani A, Dyke C, Hodson M, Radley-Smith R, Banner NR: Analysis of 10-year experience with heart-lung transplantation for cystic fibrosis. Transplant Proc 1997;29(1–2):632.
46. Nixon PA, Morris KA: Quality of life in pediatric heart, heart-lung, and lung transplant recipients. Int J Sports Med 2000;21(Suppl 2): 109–112.
47. Hirshfeld AB, Kahle AL, Clark BJ, Bridges ND: Parent reported health status after pediatric thoracic organ transplant. J Heart Lung Transplant 2004;23:1111–1118.
48. Hislop AA, Rinaldi M, Lee R, McGregor CGA, Haworth SG: Growth of immature lung transplanted into an adult recipient. Am J Physiol 1993; 264:L60–L65.
49. Ro PS, Bush DM, Kramer SS, Mahboubi S, Spray TL, Bridges ND: Airway growth after pediatric lung transplantation. J Heart Lung Transplant 2001; 20(6):619–624.

16 Drug Administration by Aerosol in Children

Allan L. Coates, MDCM • Christopher O'Callaghan, FRCP

The administration of drugs directly into the respiratory tract for the treatment of lung disease seems a logical choice, since, in theory, the drug will have its maximal effect on the diseased lung and side effects on other organs should be minimized. However, fundamental to the evolution of the species from single-celled organisms has been the selective ability to exclude all but a tiny part of the external environment from the body. In the context of delivering medication, this becomes a significant challenge. The lungs are generally considered to be a sterile environment, with the alveoli protected by a series of barriers to penetration for all but gas. It is within this context that drug delivery by aerosol must be achieved. By definition, successful delivery means noninvasively overcoming the protective mechanisms of the airway for distal lung deposition. These barriers include the nose, the posterior pharynx, and the dividing points of the airways. For drugs that are not rapidly absorbed, this also includes mucociliary clearance and alveolar macrophages. Hence, the design of an appropriate therapeutic aerosol requires not only the delivery of an adequate amount of drug but also the ability to avoid the various defense mechanisms of the respiratory system.

The purpose of this chapter is fourfold. The first purpose is to help caregivers develop a greater understanding of the underlying principles and practical concerns of drug administration by aerosol. The second is to provide some information on which informed decisions can be based regarding the appropriate choice of devices. The third goal is to raise the clinicians' consciousness of the need for the development of standards for aerosol therapy. Surprisingly, the amount of the prescribed (nominal) dose of drug available for a child to inhale may vary by a factor of five or more depending on the type of drug delivery device chosen and, in the case of valved holding chambers (VHCs), how they are maintained. This is particularly worrying for nebulizers and VHCs that may be bought over the counter with the prescriber and parent unaware that their choice may so markedly affect the dose of drug the child receives. Finally, there are a number of newer and very innovative concepts being developed for future use that will be discussed briefly. Drugs may be administered directly to the respiratory system as liquids or solids so as to treat pulmonary diseases or for systemic treatment of administration for nonpulmonary diseases. The benefits of aerosol therapy are briefly outlined in Box 16-1.

■ ANATOMY AND INHALED MEDICATION

The body's defense against "foreign" material entering the respiratory system begins with the filtering process of the upper airway. The nasal passages with hairs and turbinates force inspired airborne particles to flow though a series of convoluted turns, and some come into contact with the mucosa, which is lined with ciliated columnar epithelial cells and a blanket of mucus, becoming entrapped. This arrangement can be highly effective and may extract particulate matter as small as 1 μm.[1] While delivery of the aerosol via the mouth typically results in significantly greater lung deposition, larger aerosol particles (>5 μm) are often unable to negotiate the curves in the posterior pharynx and the vocal cords, and become deposited there following impact. This is normally referred to as "inertial impaction," which could loosely be defined as the inability of a particle to remain suspended in a moving column of air as it flows around relatively sharp corners. Implicit in this definition of inertial impaction is the effect of inspiratory flow and particle density.[2] Once particles successfully reach the lung, carried in the inspired gas flow, they settle by sedimentation, wherein gravity causes them to fall to the surface. For particles much smaller than 1 μm, transportation by diffusion rather than bulk flow and deposition by electrostatic forces becomes important. On account of their large surface areas relative to their mass, small particles settle very slowly and may be exhaled before they contact the respiratory epithelium. The ideal particle size for entry and deposition in the lungs in adults breathing through their mouths is in the range of 1 to 5 μm. Avoiding aerosol loss in the upper airway requires a combination of aerosol design (primarily a size factor) and appropriate administration techniques. The obvious corollary is that administration of aerosols by mouthpiece is much more efficient[3] than administration by a mask to a patient breathing through the nose. Use of a facemask may result in unwanted side effects from drugs that may be readily absorbed from the nasal mucosa while also diminishing the therapeutic effects because of decreased pulmonary deposition.[3,4]

For aerosolized soluble pharmaceuticals, the volume of the droplet and hence the amount of drug carried is proportional to the third power of the radius. Small particles, such as those smaller than 1 μm, may be numerous but carry little drug. Larger particles, such as those larger than 5 μm, while carrying much more drug, may be too large to penetrate below the vocal cords in adults.[5,6] The fraction of the drug carried in particles sufficiently small as to enter the lungs when inhaled is known as the respirable fraction (RF). The data supporting an RF as the fraction of the mass particles of 5 μm and less for adults or fully grown children are[6] derived from deposition studies that looked at this factor specifically. There are supportive data from recalculating a deposition study of Wildhaber and colleagues[7] for a choice of 4 μm for children who are 4 years of age. There is little direct in vivo evidence in small children and infants, but there are signs that the choice of a 5-μm cutoff appropriate in adults would be too large,[7] especially for infants inhaling through a facemask.[3] This is supported by data from an ingenious

> **BOX 16-1 Benefits of Using Aerosol Drug Delivery**
>
> - Has a rapid onset of action.
> - Increased therapeutic index: Side effects are reduced since aerosolized dose given directly to lungs is lower than systemic doses required for a similar effect.
> - Aerosolized drugs may overcome barriers such as first-pass metabolism of drug by the liver and poor gastrointestinal availability.
> - May be used as a portal of entry to the systemic circulation. Allows rapid systemic delivery of a variety of proteins and peptides (e.g., insulin).
> - There is a potential reduction in the use of injections (e.g., aerosolized measles vaccine).

in vitro model[8] of the upper airway of a 9-month-old infant that would suggest that the RF would be 3 μm or less and inversely dependent on inspiratory flow.

When dealing with solid particles that may be of irregular shape, defining diameter is more problematic than with a spheric droplet of water. By convention, particle size is defined as the aerodynamic behavior equivalent of a sphere of unit density. This takes both size and shape into consideration. As an example of conditions affecting inertial impaction, one can think of driving at night through a light snowfall. The snowflakes, while much larger than small raindrops, are very light and are carried over the car in the slipstream of the air without hitting the windshield. In contrast, tiny rain droplets will hit the windshield. In this case, the rain droplets, while very much smaller than the snowflakes, have a larger aerodynamic diameter.

Taking advantage of the fact that some large particles may be very light and more likely to follow the airstream into the lung and thus avoid impaction, drug designers have produced large porous particles. Their low density allows them to behave similarly to much smaller aqueous droplets.[2] It has been suggested that systemic protein delivery could be facilitated by these large particles, because they resist phagocytosis by alveolar macrophages, thereby allowing slow release of peptides such as insulin.[2]

PARTICLE SIZE DISTRIBUTION MEASUREMENTS

Given that size is one of the major determinants of both the likelihood of particles entering the lung and the amount of drug carried by each particle, it is essential to know the particle size distribution of a medical aerosol to make any prediction of the amount of drug that is likely to be deposited in the lungs. While an extensive review of the technology is beyond the scope of this chapter, a recent detailed review covers virtually all aspects in detail.[9] Unfortunately, particle size may be measured in a variety of ways that may give very different results; this makes it difficult for the clinician to interpret promotional material.

Most medical nebulizers and many other aerosol devices produce droplets with a variable size range, exhibiting a Poisson distribution that contains a large quantity of small particles and a progressively smaller quantity of larger particles (Fig. 16-1). For both wet and dry aerosols, the amount of drug depends on the volume of the particle. Since particle volume as opposed to particle number is the important variable, a more useful characterization can be obtained by plotting the logarithm of the diameter against the probability distribution of volume (or mass). For most aerosols produced by medical nebulizers, this distribution results in an approximation of a bell-shaped curve, which is referred to as log normal (Fig. 16-2).[1] The diameter of particles or droplets wherein 50% of the mass of the aerosol is contained in smaller (or larger) particles is referred to as the mass median diameter (MMD). The MMD is usually derived by laser measurement and cannot be used to size aerosolized drug suspensions, since not all of the droplets will contain a particle of drug. Measurement of the mass median aerodynamic diameter helps to define the behavior of inhaled particles of different density and has the advantage of permitting the measurement of the particle size of nebulized suspensions. The degree to which the aerosol is polydisperse is given by the geometric standard deviation (σ_g), which is the ratio of the diameter at 84.3% of the mass of the aerosol to that at 50% of the distribution.[10] The larger the σ_g, the more the aerosol is polydisperse. If the cumulative amount of aerosol is plotted against the logarithm of diameter, the slope of the line at the midpoint of the mass distribution is related to the σ_g (see Fig. 16-2). A vertical line would indicate a monodisperse aerosol with a σ_g of unity.

There are two principal methods of determining the size distribution of an aerosol. One is based on the aerodynamic behavior of the particle, and the second is the physical measurement of size. The latter technique, using laser diffraction technology, is frequently based on the ability of small particles to diffract light at their edges. As an example of the former, the aerosol is drawn into a device wherein it is forced to undergo a series of turns in the airstream. At each turn there is a collection system; a plate as used in a cascade impactor[11] or a pool of liquid as used in a liquid impinger or Next Generation Pharmaceutical Impactor.[12] Failure of the particle to remain in suspension in the airstream results in the impaction of the particle on the plate

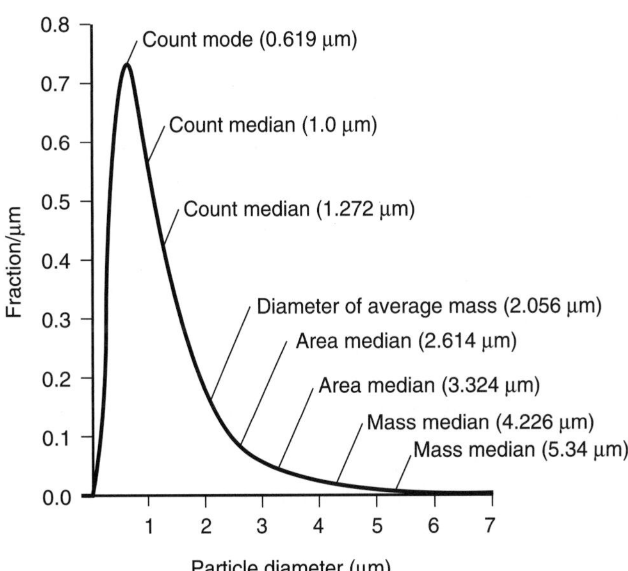

FIGURE 16-1. Probability distribution for most aerosols, which is a Poisson curve that contains a large number of small droplets and progressively smaller numbers of larger droplets. (From Morrow PE: Aerosol characterization and deposition. Am Rev Respir Dis 1974;110[Suppl]:88–99.)

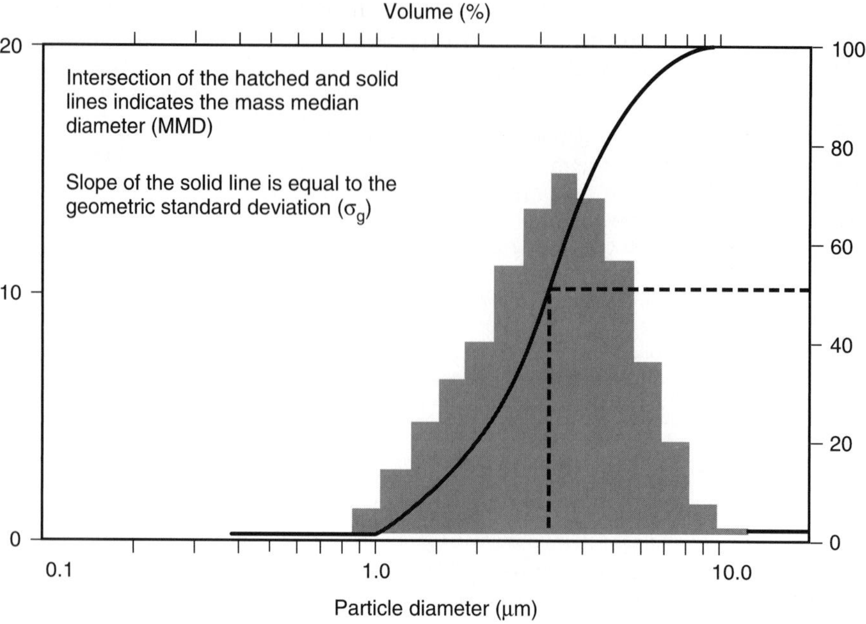

■ **FIGURE 16-2.** Particle size distribution of a medical aerosol generator as measured by laser diffraction. Each bar in the histogram represents a size band of particles, and the height of the bar in the histogram represents the percentage of that sample that is within that band. The scale at the left is used to read the histogram. The scale at the right is used to read the cumulative plot represented by the solid line going through the histogram. The particle size that corresponds to 50% on the cumulative curve is the MMD, in this case 3.3 μm. The slope of the line at the 50% point corresponds to the geometric standard deviation (σ_g).

or into the liquid. By eluting the drug from each plate and assaying the amount, or by directly measuring the concentration at each liquid stage in the impinger or the Next Generation Pharmaceutical Impactor, it is possible to calculate the particle size distribution, since each plate or stage removes a specific size range of particles from the flow of aerosol. A major advantage of these systems is that they allow a separate measurement of the drug of interest and ignore the particle size of any excipient added to enhance dispersion.

The second method is the one of choice for measuring the particle size distribution of droplets produced by nebulization. For this purpose, a laser beam is passed through the cloud of aerosol droplets and the degree of light diffraction measured. As long as there are no changes to the aerosol between the time of generation and the moment of measurement introduced by either the measuring techniques—specifically, drying of the droplets or allowing heat transfer to the droplets—inertial impaction techniques agree well with the laser light diffraction techniques.[13,14] Particle size measurements by laser diffraction measure droplet volume only. For drugs such as albuterol that are dissolved in the aqueous solution, droplet volume reflects drug distribution particle size. However, for suspensions of budesonide, many of the drug particles are on the order of 2 μm in size, so that some droplets may be too small to carry any drug and laser diffraction particle sizing is erroneously small.[15] In such cases, accurate particle sizing depends on using inertial impaction methods to separate droplets of various sizes and chemical quantification of the drug contained in each size range.

Another area of confusion is that some nebulizer manufacturers report the performance of their devices in terms of particle size distribution measured by inertial impaction techniques, whereas others use light diffraction techniques. Unless care is taken to prevent heat transfer between the cool aerosol and the warmer temperature of the impactor or Next Generation Pharmaceutical Impactor, the former results in an artificially smaller distribution.[14] Such information is frequently not made available by the marketing personnel, making appropriate choices for the clinician difficult.

Proper interpretation of particle size data is often also an area of difficulty. Most often, the manufacturer will specify an MMD with a σ_g measured at a particular flow driving the nebulizer. The interpretation of these data hinges on the assumption that the particle size distribution is log normal. While this is not usually totally correct, it is a reasonable approximation. If the RF is defined as the mass of aerosol contained in particles whose diameters are 5 μm or less, then an MMD of 5 μm would imply that 50% of the mass (not number of particles), if inhaled, would pass through the upper airway and be deposited below the vocal cords in the airways (or alveoli if <2 μm). In general, medical nebulizers will generate aerosols with a MMD that is less than 5 μm, but the σ_g will frequently be greater than 2. Knowing the MMD and the σ_g, it is possible to calculate the mass of aerosol contained in any particle size range of interest, using the Hatch-Choate equation,[10,16] and hence derive the RF.[16] Figure 16-2 is an example of an aerosol distribution with an MMD of 3.3 μm and a σ_g of 1.7.

To reproduce the specified MMD and σ_g, a nebulizer must be driven by the flow that is specific for that device. A higher nebulizing flow results in a smaller MMD,[17] with the converse also being true. For instance, if the MMD is reported when using a flow of 8 L/minute, but the compressor used to drive the nebulizer is only capable of delivering 5 L/minute, the MMD of the aerosol particles that the patient receives at home will be larger than the reported MMD and the RF smaller. In the hospital setting, where the utilization of a dry gas source is usual, gas flow exiting the nebulizer may be as much as 2 L/minute less than actually indicated by the rotameter as a result of inadequate "back pressure" compensation of the flow meter.[18] In both these situations, producing a larger MMD will lead to a smaller RF and decreased pulmonary deposition.

■ PATIENT BREATHING PATTERNS

The major issue with breathing pattern is the difference between nose breathing and mouth breathing. The nose is very good at both removing inhaled particulate matter before it reaches the lungs[3] and absorbing soluble drugs through the nasal mucosa. In a recent article comparing delivery systems in the emergency department setting, increased nasal deposition of albuterol with systemic absorption from a "mask/nebulizer" delivery system resulted in increased tachycardia compared with administration through a mouthpiece with similar degrees of bronchodilation.[4] Rapid inspiratory flows will increase inertial impaction of drugs on the posterior pharynx (and the nasal turbinates if nose breathing) but for conventional dry powder inhalers (DPIs) used in the treatment of asthma, high flows are necessary to disperse the drug being inhaled. Holding one's breath after a single inhalation from a DPI or metered-dose inhaler (MDI) increases the time available for pulmonary deposition by sedimentation, thereby reducing drug loss due to exhalation of smaller particles. In a similar fashion, slow deep inspirations both increase deposition through enhanced sedimentation and lead to more peripheral drug deposition. On the other hand, for nebulizers that have a constant output, prolonged breath holding after each inspiration would be very wasteful of drug, since nebulization continues whether the patient is breathing in or not. Thus, it is of concern that some devices work at cross-purposes. There are devices being marketed that will allow a combination of positive end-expiratory pressure chest physiotherapy coupled with nebulization of drugs to treat cystic fibrosis (CF). In this situation, the short inspiration but prolonged expiration necessary for successful positive end-expiratory pressure therapy is not what is ideal for inhaled drug therapy. Hence, because many devices work with different principles, teaching of proper technique depends on both the capabilities of the child and the requirements of the device.

One of the biggest challenges is that in obstructive lung disease, no matter what the breathing pattern is, it leads to increased deposition in the central airways and reduced deposition in the peripheral airways, a challenge when trying to deliver antibiotics or other agents to the areas most affected in diseases such as CF.

Finally, all instructions to the patients are to no avail if there is little or no adherence to recommended therapy. Adherence to asthma medications is poor.[19] Underuse of prescribed medications occurs approximately 50% of the time. There is no evidence that adherence is improved by changing to a different inhaler device, be it small or unobtrusive, even though such devices are often marketed on the basis that they are more acceptable to a patient and they will, therefore, be used more. With improvement in technology, there is increasing likelihood of drug delivery devices being available that can both monitor and prompt patient use.

■ METERED-DOSE INHALERS

The MDI has a pressurized chamber that holds a propellant and the drug, usually in suspension. Previously, the propellant was a chlorofluorocarbon (CFC), which was a liquid under pressure, but as soon as it was released to atmospheric pressure, it "flashed" and became a gas. More recently, in keeping with the Montreal Protocol to reduce the harmful affects of fluorocarbons on the ozone layer, the propellant has been changed to hydrofluoroalkane. It cannot be assumed that CFC inhalers and the replacement, hydrofluoroalkane inhalers, are equivalent in every situation. For example, the 3M CFC-free beclomethasone dipropionate MDI emits drugs in much smaller particles, around 1 μm, which is likely to result in an increased lung dose and more peripheral deposition of the medication. It is still unclear what effect this will have on the dose equivalence or side effect profiles of this hydrofluoroalkane formulation, particularly in children under the age of 5 years. The emitted aerosol from some hydrofluoroalkane formulations is warmer and less dense than that from the CFC-containing MDIs, and patients may experience a different feel and taste when using their inhalers. They should be warned about this and reassured that it does not mean that the inhaler is not working properly.[20] A further advantage of the non-CFC MDI may be its enhanced dose reproducibility.[21] In addition, the dose released is unaffected by storage orientation or ambient temperature, unlike CFC inhalers.[22]

Before use, the device must be shaken to disperse the propellant and suspended drugs evenly so as to have consistent amounts of drug emitted with activation. Additions of surface-active material and manipulations of polarity further facilitate the dispersion of the suspension. Some MDIs use soluble agents such as beclomethasone-hydrofluoroalkane preparations, which reduce the risk of inconsistency with drug delivery due to settling.

As well as a reservoir, there is a metering chamber of a fixed volume. The actual amount of drug contained in this chamber depends on the volume of the chamber and the concentration of drug within the propellant. While rigorously controlled at the time of manufacture, multiple activations without shaking can result in higher concentrations of drug if the device is held in the operating position and the drug settles, or lower concentrations if the propellant is concentrated around the opening to the metering chamber at the time of refilling after activation.

The flashing process that occurs when the aerosol propellant mixture leaves the inhaler is never instantaneous, and until it has occurred completely, the drug particles contained in droplets have a greater particle size distribution than the particles alone. The velocity of the plume leaving the orifice is in the order of 25 to 30 m/second but is rapidly slowed by the resistance of the air. If the device is activated when held between the lips during a vigorous inspiration, whether or not the particles in the plume will have become small enough through loss of propellant and slow enough not to strike the posterior pharynx depends on the device plume velocity as well as the particle size and the distance traveled (which depends on the size of the patient). An MDI alone, especially for inhaled steroids, should never be used in childhood, since coordination between inhalation and actuation of the MDI is rarely perfect and upper airway deposition may result in thrush or in a hoarse voice. For inhaled steroids absorbed via the gastrointestinal tract, upper airway deposition may result in an added systemic steroid burden with no therapeutic gain. Clearly, alternative delivery systems are needed for both children and for many if not most adults, especially the elderly.

Unlike early dry powder preparations wherein high levels of relative humidity became a problem, in an MDI, the drug is completely protected from the environment. However, flashing requires energy, specifically heat; perhaps more important, the pressure inside the reservoir is very dependent on the ambient temperature. Hence, in cold climates, the MDI may be too cold to empty the metering chamber completely and the droplets may not flash but may "rain out" in the mouth or VHC.

Since the development of the MDI in the 1960s, perhaps the most important change in thinking has been the appreciation of the need to use VHCs, often incorrectly referred to as "spacers." The word "spacers" refers to devices that increase the volume between the MDI and the patient. This reduces the "ballistic" component by both allowing complete flashing of the propellant and letting friction of the air slow down the particles, but it has no valves and requires active coordination of the patient. VHCs are regarded as the best drug delivery device for the delivery of antiasthma drugs to children under the age of 5 years and in older children for the delivery of inhaled corticosteroids. They present the child with a relatively static cloud of aerosolized drug, reducing the need to coordinate actuation of the MDI with inhalation. The lack of a ballistic component markedly reduces the oropharyngeal deposition of drug, reducing the likelihood of local side effects such as thrush and hoarseness. In the case of steroids with significant gastrointestinal absorption, such as beclomethasone dipropionate, use of a VHC significantly reduces systemic absorption of drug from the gastrointestinal tract where it has no therapeutic benefit. A recent study revealed no advantage of using a nebulizer to deliver bronchodilator medications in an emergency room setting over the delivery of an appropriate bronchodilator drug given by VHC.[4] On account of the variability in VHCs, particularly their size and antistatic properties, drug delivery may vary considerably. Indeed, as with nebulizers the prescribed (nominal dose) may bear little resemblance to the amount of drug inhaled if different spacers are used to deliver the same drug. The addition of a facemask to VHCs has revolutionized the treatment of young children with asthma. However, drug will only be delivered if the facemask fits the child's face, forming a complete seal without leaks. It has recently been shown that a facemask recommended for many years for use with an inhaled steroid may have delivered little if any drug to young children because of problems in obtaining a seal between the child's face and the mask.[23] Delivery by a mouthpiece is more efficient, and patients should use this in preference to a facemask where possible.

In an attempt to slow the aerosol emitted from MDIs, or to reduce the need for coordination between inhalation and actuation, researchers have developed several modifications of the MDI. The Spacehaler (Evans Medical Ltd, Lower Head, UK) is a pressurized MDI with a novel actuator design that reduces the velocity of the aerosol cloud that emerges from the inhaler. This has the effect of reducing impaction of the aerosol in the oropharynx and the amount of nonrespirable drug delivered to the patient. Although the device appears to be as effective in the delivery of albuterol to adults as an MDI and large-volume holding chamber, there are no published studies on the use of this device by children or for the delivery of corticosteroids.[24] The Synchroner (Fisons plc, Loughborough, UK) is an open spacer that was designed as a training aid. The spacer has an open section on its upper surface and folds up like a clasped knife when not in use. When open, the Synchroner places the MDI 10 cm from the subject's mouth, and if inhalation is not coordinated with MDI actuation, an aerosol cloud can be seen to plume up from the top of the spacer. This gives visual feedback to the patient of poor technique. Although the spacer increases lung deposition and reduces oropharyngeal deposition of sodium cromoglycate compared with an MDI, it does not function as a VHC and good coordination is still required to use it.[25]

Both MDIs and VHCs have advantages and disadvantages. Pressurized MDIs are cheap, convenient to carry, and quick to use. However, they are very difficult to use correctly. For optimum drug delivery, the MDI requires a high degree of coordination and psychomotor skill, with inhalation, actuation, and breath holding all occurring in a precise sequence. In practice, few adults and even fewer children can use a pressurized MDI correctly, and less than 15% of the emitted drug enters the typical patient's lungs. The variability of drug delivery to the lower respiratory tract between patients is extremely high. It is also surprisingly high within the same subject. Apart from counting the number of actuations from an MDI, there is no reliable way a patient can detect when the device is running out. MDIs should not be used alone in the treatment of children under the age of 5. Because of coordination problems, they are not considered the first-choice delivery device for children of any age.

One attempt to address problems with coordination in MDIs has been the development of breath-actuated MDIs. Devices such as the Autohaler (3M Reicher) and the Easi-Breathe (Baker Norton, UK) incorporate a mechanism that is activated during inhalation, which triggers the MDI. In theory this reduces the need for the patient or caregiver to coordinate MDI actuation with inhalation.[26] However, patients may stop breathing when the MDI is actuated because of the cold propellant effect.[27] Use of these devices for delivery of albuterol should be restricted to older children and adults. Evaluation of their efficacy in children under the age of 5 years is limited in one study[28] to eight children. We are unaware of any trials that have been performed on the use of inhaled steroids from such devices in children or adults. Oropharyngeal deposition of steroids using the devices is still very high and is minimized by the use of the conventional MDI and VHC instead. One of the devices, the Easi-Breathe, may also be used with a short open tube spacer. Although this addition may be expected to reduce extrathoracic drug deposition, there are no published evaluations of its use.

While MDIs are easy to carry and conceal for the self-conscious adolescent, VHCs are not. Side effects from systemic absorption of albuterol that deposited outside the lung are rare. In contrast, it is sensible to reduce the deposition of steroids in the upper airway. One issue that is often neglected is that the plastic used in some VHCs, when taken straight out of the box, carries a high static electrical charge that will remove most of the medication. However, rinsing in mild detergent followed by a water rinse and air drying will remove much of the static electricity.[29] Failure to do this will mean that many days of multiple doses may be administered until the plastic has completely discharged. This often results in the diagnosis of refractory asthma that has resolved by the time the patient reaches the pediatric respiratory physician. In reality, what has really happened is that, while the patient was waiting for the appointment, the static charge was reduced by repeated dosing, so the medication was delivered effectively and the asthma treated. Newer VHCs that are made of material that eliminates static electricity can be used very effectively "right out of the package."[30] Pulmonary deposition correctly results in a pulmonary delivery in the order of 2% in infants using an MDI with a VHC,[31] and even the best of devices in adults achieve delivery of less than 50% of the released dose with much variation in between. However, as Tal and colleagues have argued,[31] on a milligram per kilogram of body weight basis, 20% deposition from an MDI and VHC in a 70-kg adult is very similar to 2% in a 7-kg infant. In children, there are large variations, even when technique is good.[7] As mentioned earlier, nose breathing will remove more of the aerosol particles than mouth breathing, so as soon as a child is old enough to use a mouthpiece rather than a facemask, he or she should be switched.

■ DRY POWDER INHALERS

Dry powder inhalers are widely used to deliver both bronchodilator and anti-inflammatory drugs. The common characteristic of both the MDIs and the DPIs is that a single activation results in the release of a known ("metered") dose of drug from the device. Unfortunately, there is a common misconception that precision in the amount of drug released translates into a similar level of precision in the amount of drug delivered. This is far from the case. DPIs require the patient to generate the necessary energy both to disperse and to deliver the drug. For children with less than adequate inspiratory efforts, delivery can be quite variable, although numerous clever features have been incorporated into many devices so that there is consistency after a certain minimal inspiratory flow has been achieved. As with any other aerosol, the size of the particle is fundamental to the eventual site of delivery. While there are several ways to produce particles of less than 5 μm, including milling and spray drying, these particles tend to be bound together by electrostatic, van der Waals, and capillary forces. Hence, fine particles have poor flow characteristics and tend to be quite difficult to disperse. One way around this is to bind the small particles loosely to a larger excipient particle such as lactose. These particles, in the range of 30 to 60 μm, have much better flow characteristics. The preparation is then packaged in some form of metering device. Common are blister packs, gelatin capsules, or small cavities containing a fixed volume. The device is prepared for use by piercing the blister pack or capsule, or loading the outflow track; the patient then inhales. The inspiratory air is forced to go through some system that generates high turbulence so as to separate the drug and the excipient. The drug then deposits below the vocal cords, while the excipient strikes the posterior pharynx. Flows required are generally in the range of 30 L/minute or higher. Most devices are designed so that flows in excess of the minimum do not give rise to variable deposition. However, flows less than the minimum can result in failure to separate the excipient from the drug and poor pulmonary deposition. Studies suggesting that younger children, under the age of 5 years, can reliably inhale with sufficient inspiratory flow and volume to use DPIs have tended to use children selected by their ability to perform other complicated respiratory maneuvers. Their use in this age group should be avoided. Advantages of DPIs over MDIs and VHCs include compactness and ease of transport as well as ambient temperature insensitivity. The latter feature is a particular advantage when treating exercise-induced asthma in children doing sports in a cold environment. DPIs used to deliver steroids still have the disadvantage of significant upper airway deposition of drug.

A guide to device choice in relationship to the child's age is given in Table 16-1.

■ **TABLE 16-1.** Inhaler devices for children under 5 years of age

Device	AGE: 1–3 Years	3–5 Years
MDI plus VHC and facemask	First choice	Second choice
MDI plus VHC	Second choice	First choice
Nebulizer	Third choice	Third choice
Breath-activated MDI	Avoid	Avoid
DPIs		
β_2 agonists	Avoid	Not recommended
Corticosteroids	Avoid	Not recommended

DPIs, dry powder inhalers; MDI, metered-dose inhaler; VHC, valved holding chamber.

■ NEBULIZERS

Metered-dose inhalers and DPIs tend to be somewhat complex and very dependent on the physical properties of the agents being aerosolized. The development of this type of drug device is both expensive and lengthy, and as a result, is largely restricted to agents that are in widespread use (e.g, agents used in the treatment of asthma). For diseases with less prevalence, such as CF, few pharmaceutical companies are willing to invest the resources necessary to develop specific agents using complex aerosol delivery systems. Consequently, many physicians treating patients with CF have resorted to using commercially available nebulizers to aerosolize drugs that may not have been originally intended for aerosol delivery. This practice results in the generation of a cloud of droplets for inhalation whose characteristics are dependent on a combination of the physical attributes of the drug and the performance of the nebulizer. Since the decision to institute this type of aerosol therapy is usually made by the individual prescribing physician, this "off-label" method of drug administration may circumvent the quality control mechanisms of the governmental drug-regulating bodies (e.g., the U.S. Food and Drug Administration). The failure to match the delivery device to the agent being nebulized[18] and the use of the aerosol route of administration for agents not intended for this purpose[32] can, and sometimes do, lead to problems. Hence, the need to administer medication by aerosol, despite the lack of an appropriate delivery system, can result in a variety of clinical situations in which drug efficacy is less than optimal.

Basically, nebulization can be accomplished by ultrasound, by jet nebulization, by vibrating membrane technology, by using a piston to force droplets through tiny holes, and by electrostatic devices. These last systems are discussed later in the section on Future Directions. The ultrasonic method uses a piezoelectric crystal that rapidly vibrates the nebulizing solution placed in a compartment directly above. The liquid vibrates to the extent that droplets become separated from the surface (Fig. 16-3). The cloud of droplets can be carried to the patient for inhalation by directing a flow of air across the surface of the solution. Depending on the type of ultrasonic nebulizer, the particle size distribution may be quite appropriate for inhalation, and many of these nebulizers are capable of producing large amounts of aerosol per unit time. In general, ultrasonic nebulizers tend to have larger particle size distributions than jet nebulizers, but there is considerable overlap that is very device dependent. However, there are some disadvantages of ultrasonic nebulization. Some devices have a relatively large residual volume (V_r) at the end of effective nebulization, which results in a large quantity of wasted drug. A second theoretic disadvantage is the heat generated by the ultrasonic process, which can denature the proteins in the agents being nebulized.[33] Another limitation of this method is that some drugs (e.g., budesonide) are available only as suspensions rather than solutions. Since the vibrations of the ultrasonic nebulizer are at the surface of the liquid, suspended particles below the surface can settle, thus reducing the concentration of drug in the output. Viscosity of the agent being nebulized can affect output. These devices are not disposable and may require a complicated sterilization process for use with more than one patient.

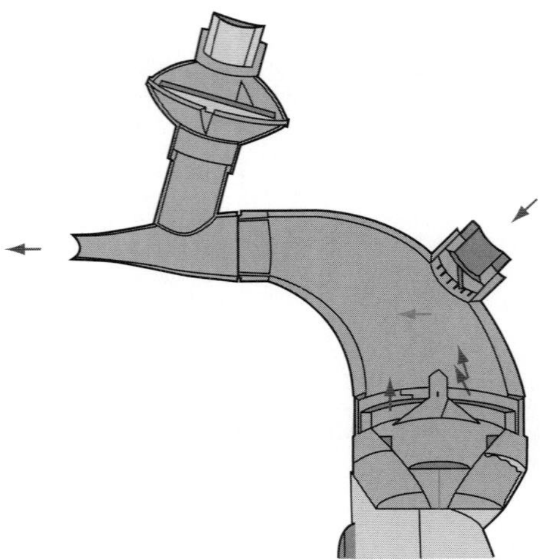

■ **FIGURE 16-3.** Schematic drawing of an ultrasonic nebulizer, which relies on the vibration of a piezoelectric crystal to produce an aerosol. When the patient inhales, air is entrained through this device, capturing the aerosol that is generated for inhalation. When the patient breathes out, he or she does so through the filter at the top, which prevents drug-laden air from contaminating the surroundings.

Somewhat analogous to ultrasonic nebulizers, but clearly an advance, are vibrating-membrane devices. Several of these devices are available, each with similarities and differences. All have an electronic circuit that senses both the membrane and the drug being nebulized and adjusts the frequency of the membrane to the resonant frequency. This results in high energy efficiency for aerosol production, since each droplet is nebulized only once (see later for the contrast with jet nebulizers), allowing battery-operated portable systems to be used efficiently. The aerosols generated tend to be more monodisperse than those produced by jet nebulizers, and the MMD is determined by a combination of the hole sizes in the membrane and the physical properties, largely viscosity, of the agent being nebulized. Because of the absence of a baffling system and other areas to trap droplets, these devices have very low residual volumes and can be highly efficient.[34] Because of efficiency, they can often shorten treatment time compared with other devices. For diseases such as CF, wherein lack of adherence to medically recommended therapies is common—often because of the time requirements of the therapy—devices could reduce total treatment time, hopefully promoting better adherence to all aspects of CF treatment. However, there are some drawbacks. One is the initial cost, which clearly makes these devices reusable rather than disposable. If they are going to be shared among different patients, complicated cleaning and sterilization procedures may be necessary. As long as the drug being nebulized is a solution with relatively low viscosity, good output rates are easily achieved so nebulization times can be minimized. However, increasing viscosity may compromise efficiency, so that performance of these devices, even more than jet nebulizers, is linked to the drug being nebulized. Finally, if the drug of choice is a suspension, the particles may be too large to pass through the membrane, resulting in clogging, low output, or both.

A widely accepted alternative is jet nebulization. Jet nebulizers range widely in cost and performance, but the less expensive ones are disposable so complicated cleaning procedures are unnecessary. Jet nebulization is a comminution process wherein a high-velocity gas jet fragments a film of liquid into droplets of varying sizes (Fig. 16-4). Passing compressed air through an extremely small orifice generates the high-velocity jet. At the exit of this orifice are one or two capillary "feed" tubes that lead to the well of the reservoir containing the nebulizing solution. Forcing a jet of gas to travel at high velocity will result in a reduction of air pressure at the sides of this jet stream. As a result of this Bernoulli effect, liquid from the reservoir will be drawn up the capillary tube, spread out to the exit of the jet orifice, and be fragmented by the stream jet. Another method of shearing the liquid film into aerosol is employed by the Ventstream and Sidestream nebulizers (both by Medic-Aid Ltd., Pagham, UK). Rather than shearing the liquid film at a 90-degree angle, the shearing takes place over the surface of the liquid film, resulting in a less violent process. In both these methods, the range of particle sizes is considerable, ranging from 0.1 to 30 μm. Forcing this air containing aerosol droplets through a series of baffles causes the larger particles to be removed by inertial impaction and to run back to the reservoir to be renebulized—the fate of 99% of the droplets generated.[35] With increasing nebulizing flow, a larger number of small particles are generated by the jet and fewer large particles survive the baffling process, giving rise to a smaller particle size distribution. The goal is to have the majority of the remaining particles within the respirable fraction ($\leq$5 μm diameter). Particles that are small enough to escape inertial impaction may leave the nebulizer and deposit in the airway during inspiration, or are lost to the atmosphere during the expiratory phase. Particles can also rain out in the nebulizer. Since the internal volume of the nebulizer and gas flow through it determine the suspension time of a particle within the nebulizer, higher nebulizing flow will increase output and reduce rainout. In general, higher nebulizing flows such as those that can be achieved by the use of tanks of compressed gas or hospital medical gases result in increased rates of output and smaller particle size distributions than home-based compressor units. These differences, depending on their magnitude, may have to be considered with regard to the choice of dose so as to achieve a desired pulmonary deposition.

The process of jet nebulization is very violent and may destroy complex molecules, such as lipid-DNA complexes or proteoliposomes.[36] This places considerable physical demands

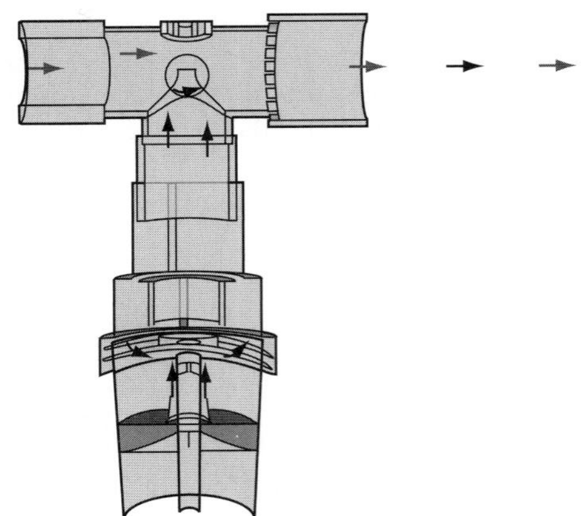

■ **FIGURE 16-4.** Schematic drawing showing the inside of the Cirrus jet nebulizer. Air under high pressure passes through a small hole as it expands, and the negative pressure generated sucks the drug solution or suspension up the feeding tube, where it is atomized. The atomized drug either strikes the baffle and returns for renebulization, or leaves the nebulizer.

on the equipment. Repetitive use of disposable devices in the laboratory can lead to degradation of the particle size distribution when the device is driven hard from a 50-psi source of compressed air, although, with the use of a compressor in the home environment, the clinical significance of this is questionable.[37] However, the plastic in disposable devices may not stand up to proper cleaning, and failure to clean the device adequately leads to significant bacterial contamination.[37] On the other hand, reusable devices are built with material that will withstand the high flows and pressures over a prolonged period of time as well as repetitive cleaning.

In the standard unvented nebulizer (see Fig. 16-4), the only inlet to the nebulizer (once charged) is the driving flow, and the only outlet is the exit of this flow carrying the suspended droplets. This outlet is usually connected to a combination of a T-piece and a mouthpiece (or a facemask for children too small to use a mouthpiece). The aerosol output of this type of device is independent of any respiratory activity of the patient. The output will remain constant during inspiration, when drug is inhaled into the patient's airway, and also during expiration when the aerosolized drug is lost to the atmosphere. The Sidestream nebulizer incorporates an adaptation to increase the rate of output by allowing air to be drawn into the device by the Venturi action of the flow from the compressor (Fig. 16-5). This greatly increases the rate of aerosol leaving the device but does nothing to reduce the waste of aerosol during expiration.

One way to minimize drug loss during expiration is to entrain the inspiratory flow of the patient through the nebulizer (Fig. 16-6). This causes particles that would normally rain out when using a standard unvented nebulizer to be swept into the airway because of the enhanced flow through the nebulizer during inspiration. During expiration, increased rainout occurs, and the drug returns to the reservoir for renebulization. Such vented nebulizers increase aerosol output during inspiration and become "quiescent" during expiration, hence minimizing drug waste. Figure 16-7 shows the comparison of a standard unvented to a vented, or "breath-enhanced" nebulizer, both widely used in the treatment of CF. The difference can be seen in the rate of output within the RF for both types of nebulizers. For an adult with CF, it is estimated that the breath-enhanced Pari LC Jet Plus nebulizer would double the deposition of inhaled tobramycin compared with the unvented device.[38] Similar results have been shown in vivo by direct comparison of the unvented Hudson 1730 and the breath-enhanced Ventstream nebulizer.[39] There are other methods that minimize drug loss by producing aerosol only during inspiration. However, these devices either require

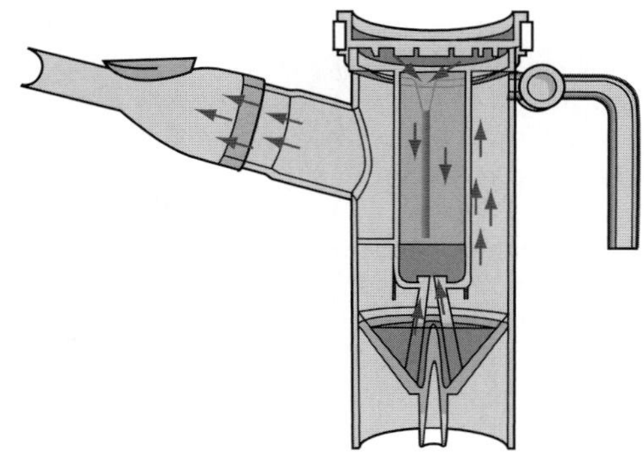

■ **FIGURE 16-6.** Schematic drawing showing the inside of the Pari LC Plus nebulizer. This differs from a conventional nebulizer, in that when the patient breathes in, a vent at the top of the nebulizer opens, allowing extra air to be entrained through the device. This extra air carries with it more aerosol that would normally have been deposited within the device and renebulized. Drug delivery is increased, since proportionately more drug is inhaled during inspiration than is lost during the expiratory phase when the valve at the top of the nebulizer closes.

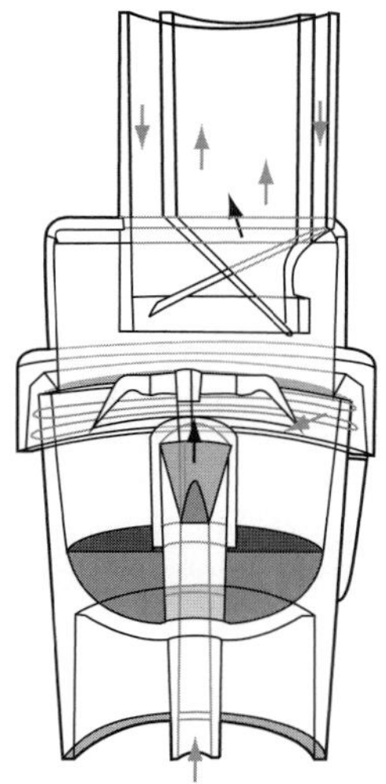

■ **FIGURE 16-5.** Cutaway drawing of a Sidestream nebulizer. This nebulizer is similar to a conventional jet nebulizer except that there is a vent in the top of the device. As air under high pressure from the compressor passes through the small hole known as the Venturi within the device, it expands rapidly, creating a negative pressure. The open vent allows extra air to be drawn through the nebulizer as a result of this negative pressure. The extra air entrained through the nebulizer captures more drug aerosol from the device that would normally have impacted within the device and would in time be renebulized. This device does not necessarily deliver more drug aerosol, but it significantly shortens nebulization times.

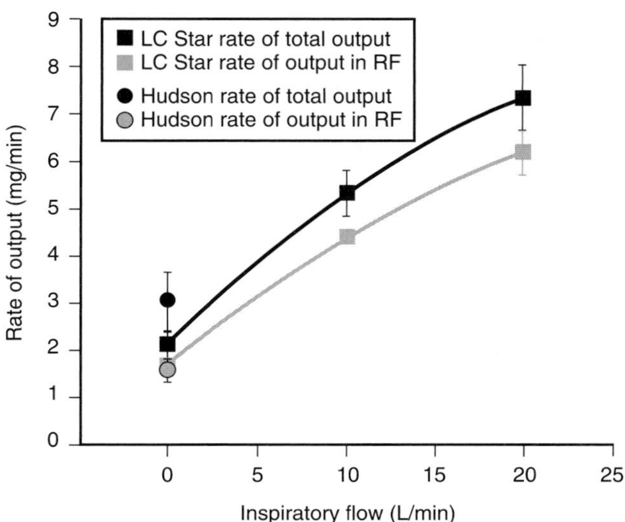

■ **FIGURE 16-7.** Rate of output of colistin from an unvented (Hudson Updraft II) and a breath-enhanced nebulizer (Pari LC Star) in relation to entrained flow. The breath-enhanced nebulizer dramatically increases the rate of output (both total and that in the RF), whereas inspiratory flow (entrained flow plus nebulizer driving flow) has no effect on the unvented nebulizer. (Modified from Katz SL, Ho SL, Coates AL: Nebulizer choice for treatment of cystic fibrosis patients with inhaled colistin. Chest 2001;119:250–255.)

complicated sensing devices (Halolite Medic-Aid Ltd., Pagham, UK), or manual triggering devices (Pari LL, Pari Respiratory Equipment Inc., Midlothian, Va., USA) requiring considerable patient coordination. One advantage of the Halolite is that it can deliver a precise dose of medication to the airway, an advantage for a drug with a narrow therapeutic safety profile.[40] Recently new, simple, disposable breath-actuated nebulizers requiring only normal breathing from the mouthpiece have become available. This type of device[40] produces no aerosol during expiration, virtually eliminating environmental contamination, a significant issue with aerosolized antibiotics, especially in a hospital setting. The only drug wastage that occurs with the breath-actuated devices is from that remaining in the device at the end of nebulization.

The total aerosol output of a jet nebulizer is the difference between the initial dose of drug placed in the nebulizer and that remaining after nebulization has ceased. Ideally, the particle size of the aerosol and the amount of the specific drug in each particle size range under conditions of use should be determined. The amount of drug likely to be inhaled may be determined by collecting drug on a filter at the exit of the mouthpiece or mask with a breathing simulator, or better still a patient, breathing as he or she normally would do through the device. This allows an estimation of the total drug available for inhalation and that contained in particles likely to reach the lower respiratory tract. Estimating the drug output based on residual volume tells only half the story, and the use of weight loss to determine drug output is often totally misleading, since evaporation during nebulization is not taken into account.

Several other variables influence drug output from a jet nebulizer. Various geometric configurations of different nebulizers will result in different V_r values.[18] Furthermore, solutions with lower surface tension will have less tendency to remain on the nebulizer walls, causing further V_r reduction.[18] The relative humidity of the driving-gas flow is another variable. For example, most home compressors are considered a "wet" gas source, since ambient water vapor is compressed to the saturation point. In contrast, tanks of compressed air and oxygen, or hospital gases from a wall outlet are dry gas sources. When utilizing a wet source, there is less evaporative loss and less concentration of the drug in the V_r, thus nebulized drug output is increased.[41] Unfortunately, not all investigators report output taking into consideration evaporative losses,[42] despite the recognition that failure to do so can lead to significant errors.[43]

There are several types of nebulizers with highly variable levels of efficiency. Drug dosing that does not consider the nebulizer/compressor efficiency can result in marked underdosing or very significant overdosing.[40,44] Hence, most drugs that are commonly administered by nebulization have a very wide therapeutic safety margin.

One of the principal advantages of using jet nebulizers is that little cooperation from the patient is required, especially when the nebulizer is directed to a facemask, which is then strapped to the face of a small child. However, Everard and colleagues[45] have shown that moving the mask just 2 cm from the face may reduce the delivery of the nebulized drug by up to 85%. A mouthpiece should be used whenever possible. Another general recommendation involves the use of the appropriate fill volume. All devices have a V_r, which may be somewhat reduced by tapping the nebulizer walls during nebulization. The variables already mentioned ultimately determine the V_r of a particular nebulizer.

BOX 16-2 Therapeutic Indications for Nebulized Therapy in Children

Asthma

β_2 agonists
Anticholinergics
Corticosteroids

Croup

Nebulized budesonide
Nebulized epinephrine

Cystic Fibrosis

Nebulized antibiotics
Nebulized antifungals
Nebulized recombinant human DNase
Nebulized hypertonic saline

Bronchiectasis

Nebulized antibiotics

Pulmonary Hypertension

Nebulized prostacyclin

Immunization

Nebulized measles vaccine

The amount of drug that is nebulized is inversely proportional to the concentration of the drug in the V_r. Hence, aerosolized output can be increased for a given dose of drug by minimizing the concentrating effects of nebulization through increasing the charge volume, although the cost will be a longer nebulization time. For most devices, a charge volume of 4 mL is ideal,[46] since drug output for volumes of 3 mL or less are lower and device dependent.[46]

Finally, in this age of increasing concern about health care expenses, cost-effective considerations must be taken into account. In the hospital, the actual cost of treatment is a combination of the cost of the nebulizer, the cost of the medication being nebulized, and the labor costs of administration. At home, costs include those of the compressor. While labor may be less of an issue, inefficient nebulizers that require longer nebulization times may reduce adherence to recommended treatment, with its own associated costs. For any agent other than the least expensive drugs, the cost of the drug and the efficiency of the nebulizer, rather than the cost of the device, is the determinant for the cost effectiveness of drug delivery.

The benefits of nebulizer therapy are outlined in Box 16-2.

NEBULIZER USE FOR VENTILATED PATIENTS

Many patients receive inhaled therapy during mechanical ventilation. They range from tiny infants receiving inhaled surfactants to older children receiving medication for treatment of acute severe asthma. Unfortunately, the use of aerosolized medications for ventilated patients is largely supported by anecdotal evidence. One of the biggest issues is optimizing the amount of drug delivered to the lung. Variables affecting drug deposition can be classified into those related to the ventilator, those related to the ventilator circuit, those affected by the choice of nebulizer or drug delivered, and finally those variables determined by the patient and his or her disease.[47–50]

Optimized deposition occurs during synchronized ventilation but is reduced if the patient inappropriately triggers ventilation or is fighting the ventilator. Increasing the patient's tidal volume will increase drug deposition from a nebulizer. Increase in the respiratory rate, while keeping the minute volume constant, decreases the lung delivery of aerosol, since a greater proportion of the inspired air is used to move aerosol in the functional dead spaces of the circuit and the respiratory tract. Nebulized aerosol is delivered to the patient only during inspiration. Therefore, if the patient has a short inspiratory phase or a prolonged expiratory phase, aerosol delivery will be reduced. This may be a result of either inappropriate settings of the ventilator or the patient's illness; for example, a patient with airways obstruction such as asthma will have prolonged expiration. The inspiratory waveform will differ according to the mode of ventilation chosen.

Other influences on the deposition of aerosol include the endotracheal tube (ETT), heating and humidification of inspired gases, and gas density. The ETT provides a significant obstruction to aerosol delivery if it is coated with secretions, since these promote turbulent airflow. Ventilated gases are normally heated and humidified to reduce the risk of airway damage, but high humidity may cause a rapid increase in particle size. A small number of studies demonstrate that using nonhumidifying gases while delivering nebulized drugs can double aerosol delivery to the lung. However, this is not generally recommended. Low-density gases are less likely to demonstrate turbulent flow, and several studies have shown that using low-density gases such as heliox can improve lung deposition of drug up to 50%. The ventilator must be designed for use with heliox. If heliox is used to power the nebulizer, the effect on drug output must be determined.

Many different nebulizers are available for use with ventilated patients. Aerosols may be generated continuously throughout ventilation or timed to coincide with inspiration. Aerosol delivery may be given continuously or intermittently. Some nebulizers run off the ventilated driving-gas flow and are synchronized so that the driving gas flows only during inspiration. However, the timing of the gas flow may be such that there is a delay between the start of the inspiration and aerosol production. The most efficient position of a nebulizer in a ventilatory circuit is in the inspiratory limb at least 30 cm from the ETT. In this position, the inspiratory tube appears to act as a reservoir for nebulized drug. Several patient-related variables may also affect drug deposition. These include the severity of the disease (e.g., more central deposition of inhaled drugs with airways obstruction), as well as the presence of hyperinflation and ventilatory retractions. Drug delivery is enhanced if the patient and ventilator are working in synchrony and is reduced if the patient is "fighting" the ventilator.

In addition to conventional jet and ultrasonic nebulizers, two other devices have been proposed for use with ventilated patients. The first is a mesh-based system wherein liquid is forced through a rapidly vibrating mesh and aerosol droplets are formed as the liquid extrudes through the pores in the mesh. No gas flow is needed, and these devices are small and highly efficient. A different approach is to force liquid through a fine catheter that has been passed through the ETT, thus bypassing the upper airway. Production of aerosol occurs at the end of the catheter. High delivery rates have been found with the system during in vitro experiments.

Pressurized MDIs may also be used with adapters that attach directly to the ETT or elsewhere in the inspiratory ventilator circuit. Impaction on surrounding structures after actuation means that much drug is lost on the walls of the tubing and ETT. Incorporating a spacer device into the circuit increases the drug delivery from the MDI considerably and, like the nebulizer, the spacer may best be placed in the inspiratory limb approximately 30 cm from the ETT.[51–54]

It is important that any devices used to deliver inhaled medicines are thoroughly tested and their efficacy understood, both in the clinical setting for which they are intended and with the drugs that will be used. Unfortunately, research into the delivery of aerosolized medications to children on ventilators has been limited.

FUTURE DIRECTIONS

Several issues must be addressed in the future of aerosol delivery systems. These include developing systems that are far more energy efficient, and hence compact, and developing methods of using the lung for the delivery of systemic drugs such as insulin, growth hormone, and analgesics. One of the problems with jet nebulizers is the energy requirements, since most particles are nebulized an estimated 100 times before entering a droplet with a particle size small enough to avoid either impaction on the baffles or raining out in the device.[35] While breath-enhanced devices are more energy efficient, it is the vibrating membranes that are the most efficient devices, with the advantage that they can be powered by either disposable or rechargeable batteries. One of the more interesting concepts is using electrical fields to draw an aqueous solution through pores into a column that is so microscopically thin that droplets of uniform size break off because of surface tension. Both vibrating membranes and electrostatic devices also have a major advantage of energy efficiency. In both cases, the other advantage is a fairly uniform particle size distribution that can be manipulated by pore size, physical properties of the solution, and the electric field.

Another area that is rapidly developing is systemic delivery of drugs. As mentioned earlier, one of the difficulties with DPIs is the dispersal of tiny particles of powder. One approach has been to place the particles of drug on large porous particles with very low density that, because of their low density, will behave in a way that is aerodynamically similar to a very much smaller droplet of unit density. However, because of their relatively large size, these large porous particles have excellent dispersal characteristics, making them ideal for DPIs. New complex formulations have avoided many of the traditional pitfalls of dry powders, allowing much more uniform dose delivery—clearly an asset if a drug such as insulin is being delivered. In another device, a piston drives the drug through microscopic pores in blister packs while sensors monitor breathing. This creates a small cloud of aerosol during inspiration, so that virtually all of the drug is deposited below the vocal cords, satisfying the requirement for precision in dosing. Needless to say, the more complex the system, the greater the cost. Hence, high-technology formulation systems are more likely to find application in the delivery of drugs wherein dose precision is essential. Asthma treatment needs are met by the combination of MDIs and VHCs for small children, with a switch to DPIs, if preferred, when the child is capable of the inspiratory maneuvers required.

TABLE 16-2. Comparison of advantages and disadvantages of one device over others

Device	Advantages	Disadvantages
Nebulizer	Use of quiet tidal breathing May be used by patients of any age May be used to deliver large doses Wide range of medications (e.g., rhDNase, nebulized antibiotics)	Unless the patient concentrates, he or she may inadvertently breathe through the nose as opposed to the mouth (inappropriate nasal inhalation), resulting in little or no drug deposition in the lung. Expensive and often very noisy Time consuming Usually require power supply Require regular servicing Drugs often require preservatives. Osmolality and pH may vary. Large variability in drug output depending on the device chosen (e.g., dose of inhaled steroid may vary by a factor of four depending on nebulizer bought by parent).
Ultrasonic devices	May be hand-held and quieter in operation Portable and may be run by rechargeable batteries	Very poor delivery of steroid suspensions by conventional ultrasonic devices
Pressurized MDI	Convenience	Requires good coordination Results in high oropharyngeal deposition of drugs such as steroids Cannot be recommended for children of any age when used alone
Breath-actuated MDI	Convenience Tends to overcome coordination difficulties Popular with children over the age of 5 requiring bronchodilator therapy	Cold propellant effect may still halt inspiration in some patients. Relatively high deposition of drugs (e.g., inhaled corticosteroids in the oropharynx) Cannot be recommended for children under 5 years of age
pMDI plus spacer	Convenience Use with spacer holding chambers allows drugs to be given to patients of any age. Use with facemask, providing seal is obtained, allows delivery to the youngest of children. Markedly reduces oropharyngeal deposition of drug Use of antistatic spacers reduces variability of drug delivery. May be used to administer bronchodilators in emergency situations	Many devices are affected by the static on the spacer walls resulting in variable deposition of drug. Holding chambers are recommended. Spacer devices without a valve tend to require coordination, which is difficult for young children.
DPIs	Convenience Useful in the delivery of bronchodilators in children over the age of 5	Effort-dependent efficiency Cannot be recommended for children under the age of 5 years Significant oropharyngeal deposition of inhaled corticosteroids

DPIs, dry powder inhalers; MDI, metered-dose inhaler; pMDI, pediatric MDI; rhDNase, recombinant human deoxyribonuclease.

CONCLUSIONS

Aerosol therapy in the treatment of respiratory diseases in children has had a long and increasingly successful history, especially in CF and asthma. Relative advantages a disadvantage of devices are summarized briefly in Table 16-2. However, safe and effective treatment depends on understanding the advantages and limitations of both the medication and the delivery device. The use of the respiratory tract to deliver systemic pharmaceuticals such as insulin, growth hormone, or morphine is becoming a reality as delivery systems with high degrees of efficiency and reproducibility are becoming available.

REFERENCES

1. Brain JD, Blanchard JD: Mechanisms of particle deposition and clearance. In: Moren F, Dolovich MB, Newhouse MT, Newman SP, eds: Aerosols in Medicine. Principles of Diagnosis and Therapy, 2nd ed. Amsterdam, London, New York, Tokyo: Elsevier, 1993, pp 117–156.
2. Edwards DA, Ben-Jebria A, Langer R: Recent advances in pulmonary drug delivery using large, porous inhaled particles. J Appl Physiol 1998;85:379–385.
3. Chua HL, Collis GG, Newbury AM, Chan K, Bower GD, Sly PD, LeSouëf PN: The influence of age on aerosol deposition in children with cystic fibrosis. Eur Respir J 1994;7:2185–2191.
4. Schuh S, Johnson DW, Stephen D, Callahan S, Winders P, Canny GJ: Comparison of albuterol delivered by a metered dose inhaler with spacer versus a nebulizer in children with mild asthma. J Pediatr 1999;135: 22–27.
5. Clay MM, Pavia D, Newman SP, Clarke SW: Factors influencing the size distribution of aerosols from jet nebulisers. Thorax 1983;38:755–759.
6. Coates AL, MacNeish CF, Dinh L, Rollin T, Gagnon S, Ho SL, Lands LC: Accounting for radioactivity before and after nebulization of tobramycin to insure accuracy of quantification of lung deposition. J Aerosol Med 2000;13:169–178.
7. Wildhaber JH, Dore ND, Wilson JM, Devadason SG, LeSouëf PN: Inhalation therapy in asthma. Nebulizer or pressurized metered-dose inhaler with holding chamber? In vivo comparison of lung deposition in children. J Pediatr 1999;135:28–33.
8. Janssens HM, Jongste JC, Fokkens WJ, Robben SGF, Wouters K, Tiddens HAM: The Sophia anatomical infant nose-throat (Saint) model. A valuable tool to study aerosol deposition in infants. J Aerosol Med 2001;14:433–441.
9. Mitchell JP, Nagel MW: Particle size analysis of aerosols from medicinal inhalers. Kona-Powder and Particle 2004;No. 22:32–65.
10. Hinds WC: Particle Size Statistics. Aerosol Technology. Properties, Behaviour, and Measurements of Airborne Particles. New York, Chichester, Brisbane, Toronto, Singapore: Wiley, 1982, pp 69–103.
11. Marple VA, Olson BA, Miller NC: The role of inertial particle collectors in evaluating pharmaceutical aerosol delivery systems. J Aerosol Med 1998;11: S139–S153.
12. Marple VA, Roberts DL, Romay FJ, Miller NC, Truman KG, Holroyd MJ, Mitchell JP, Hochrainer D: Next generation pharmaceutical impactor (a new impactor for pharmaceutical inhaler testing). Part 1. Design. J Aerosol Med 2003;16:283–299.
13. Clark AR: The use of laser diffraction for the evaluation of the aerosol clouds generated by medical nebulizers. Int J Pharm 1995;115:69–78.

14. Kwong WTJ, Ho SL, Coates AL: Comparison of nebulized particle size distribution with Malvern laser diffraction analyzer versus Andersen cascade impactor and low-flow Marple personal cascade impactor. J Aerosol Med 2000;13:303–314.
15. Keller M, Lintz F-C, Walther E, Knoch M: Effect of novel pharmaceutical formulation on nebulisation efficiency of an air jet and new electronic nebuliser [Abstract]. J Aerosol Med 2003;14:390.
16. Morrow PE: Aerosol characterization and deposition. Am Rev Respir Dis 1974;110(Suppl):88–99.
17. Nikander K: Some technical, physiochemical and physiological aspects of nebulizer therapy. Eur Respir Rev 1997;7:168–172.
18. MacNeish CF, Meisner D, Thibert R, Kelemen S, Vadas EB, Coates AL: A comparison of pulmonary availability between Ventolin (albuterol) nebules and Ventolin (albuterol) Respirator Solution. Chest 1997;111:204–208.
19. Coutts JA, Gibson NA, Paton JY: Measuring compliance with inhaled medication in asthma. Arch Dis Child 1992;67:332–333.
20. Partridge M, Woodcock A: Metered dose inhalers free of chlorofluorocarbons. BMJ 1995;310:684–685.
21. June D, Carlson S, Ross D: The effect of temperature on drug delivery characteristics of chlorofluorocarbon (CFC) and hydrofluoroalkane (HFA) metered dose inhalers. Respir Drug Delivery 1996;5:133–144.
22. Everard ML, Devadason SG, Summer QA, LeSouëf PN: Factors affecting total and respirable dose delivered by a Salbutamol metered dose inhaler. Thorax 1995;50:746–749.
23. Haden M, Barry PW, O'Callaghan C: Randomised control study of facemask efficiency. Thorax 2004;89:72–73.
24. Gunawardena KA, Sohal T, Jones JI, Upchurch FC, Crompton GK: Spacehaler for delivery of Salbutamol. A comparison with a standard metered dose inhaler plus volumatic spacer device. Respir Med 1997;91:313–316.
25. Newman SP, Clark AR, Talaee N, Clark SW: Pressurized aerosol deposition in the human lung with and without an "open" spacer device. Thorax 1989;44:706–710.
26. Newman SP, Weisz AW, Galaee N, Clarke SW: Improvement of drug delivery with a breath actuated pressurised aerosol for patients with poor inhaler technique. Thorax 1991;46:712–716.
27. Pedersen S, Frost L, Arnfred T: Errors in inhalation technique and efficiency in inhaler use in asthmatic children. Allergy 1986;41:118–124.
28. Ruggins NR, Milner AD, Swarbrick A: An assessment of a new breath actuated inhaler device in acutely wheezy children. Arch Dis Child 1993; 68:477–480.
29. Wildhaber JH, Devadason SG, Hayden MJ, Everard ML, Summer QA, LeSouëf PN: Effect of electrostatic charge, flow, delay and multiple actuations on the delivery of salbutamol from different small volume spacers for infants. Thorax 1996;51:985–988.
30. Louca E, Leung K, Coates AL, Mitchell JP, Nagel MW: Comparison of Three Valved Holding Chambers for the Delivery of Fluticasone Propionate to an Infant Face Model. J Aerosol Med (in press).
31. Tal A, Golan H, Grauer N, Aviram M, Albin D, Quastel MR: Deposition pattern of radiolabeled salbutamol inhaled from a meter-dose inhaler by means of a spacer with mask in young children with airway obstruction. J Pediatr 1996;128:479–484.
32. Dodd M, Abbott J, Maddison J, Moorcroft AJ, Webb AK: Effect of tonicity of nebulized colistin on chest tightness and pulmonary function in adults with cystic fibrosis. Thorax 1997;52:656–658.
33. Cipolla DC, Clark AR, Chan H-K, Gonda I, Shire SJ: Assessment of aerosol delivery systems for recombinant human deoxyribonuclease. S T P Pharma Sciences 1994;4:50–62.
34. Geller DE, Rosenfeld M, Waltz DA, Wilmott RW, and AeroDose TOBI Study Group: Efficiency of pulmonary administration of tobramycin solution for inhalation in cystic fibrosis using an improved drug delivery device. Chest 2003;123:28–36.
35. Dennis JH, Hendrick DJ: Design characteristics for drug nebulizers. J Med Eng Technol 1992;16:63–68.
36. Schwarz LA, Johnson JL, Black M, Cheng SH, Hogan ME, Waldrep JC: Delivery of DNA-cationic liposome complexes by small-particle aerosol. Hum Gene Ther 1996;7:731–741.
37. Rosenfeld M, Emerson J, Astley S, Joy P, Williams-Warren J, Standaert TA, Yim DL, Crist D, Thykkuttatihil M-J, Torrence M, FitzSimmons SC, Ramsey BW: Home nebulizer use among patients with cystic fibrosis. J Pediatr 1998;132:125–131.
38. Coates AL, MacNeish CF, Lands LC, Meisner D, Kelemen S, Vadas EB: A comparison of the availability of tobramycin for inhalation from vented versus unvented nebulizers. Chest 1998;113:951–956.
39. Newnham DM, Lipworth BJ: Nebuliser performance, pharmacokinetics, airways and systemic effects of salbutamol given via a novel nebuliser delivery system ("Ventstream"). Thorax 1994;49:762–770.
40. Leung K, Louca E, Coates AL: Comparison of breath enhanced to breath actuated nebulizers for rate, consistency and efficiency. Chest 2004;26: 1619–1627.
41. Coates AL, MacNeish CF, Lands LC, Smountas A, Meisner D, Kelemen S, Vadas EB: Factors influencing the rate of drug output during the course of wet nebulization. J Aerosol Med 1998;11:101–111.
42. Weber A, Morlin G, Cohen M, Williams-Warren J, Ramsey BW, Smith AL: Effect of nebulizer type and antibiotic concentration on device performance. Pediatr Pulmonol 1997;23:249–260.
43. O'Callaghan C, Clarke AR, Milner AD: Inaccurate calculation of drug output from nebulisers. Eur J Pediatr 1989;148:473–474.
44. Coates AL, Allen PD, MacNeish CF, Ho SL, Lands LC: Effect of size and disease on expected deposition of drugs given by jet nebulization to children with cystic fibrosis. Chest 2001;119:1123–1130.
45. Everard ML, Clark AR, Milner AD: Drug delivery from jet nebulizers. Arch Dis Child 1992;67:586–591.
46. Coates AL, MacNeish CF, Meisner D, Kelemen S, Thibert R, MacDonald J, Vadas EB: The choice of jet nebulizer, nebulizing flow and the addition of Ventolin Respiratory Solution affects tobramycin aerosols used in cystic fibrosis. Chest 1997;111:1206–1212.
47. Fok TF, Al-Essa M, Monkman S, Dolovich MB, Girard L, Coates G, Kirpalani H: Pulmonary deposition of Salbutamol aerosol delivered by metered dose inhaler, jet nebuliser and ultrasonic nebuliser in mechanically ventilated rabbits. Pediatr Res 1997;42:721–727.
48. Coleman DM, Kelly HW, McWilliams BC: Determinants of aerosolised albuterol delivery to mechanically ventilated infants. Chest 1996;109: 1607–1613.
49. Coleman DM, Kelly DH, McWilliams BC: Therapeutic aerosol delivery during mechanical ventilation. Ann Pharmacother 1996;30:644–655.
50. Dhand R, Tobin MJ: Bronchodilator delivery with metered dose inhalers in mechanically ventilated patients. Eur Respir J 1996;9:585–595.
51. Dhand R, Tobin MJ: Inhaled bronchodilator therapy in mechanically ventilated patients. Am J Respir Crit Care Med 1997;156:3–10.
52. Denjean A, Guimaraes H, Migdal M, Mirammand JL, Dehan M, Gaultier C: Dose-related bronchodilator response to aerosolised Salbutamol (albuterol) in ventilator-dependent premature infants. J Pediatr 1992;120:974–979.
53. O'Callaghan C, Hardy JG, Stammers J, Stephenson TJ, Hull D: Evaluation of techniques for delivery of steroids to lungs of neonates using a rabbit model. Arch Dis Child 1992;67:20–24.
54. Lee H, Arnon S, Silverman M: Bronchodilator aerosol administered by metered dose inhaler and spacer in subacute neonatal respiratory distress syndrome. Arch Dis Child 1994;70:F218–F222.

Respiratory Disorders in the Newborn

17 Congenital Lung Disease

Robin Michael Abel, FRCS • Andrew Bush, MD • Lyn S. Chitty, PhD • Jonny Harcourt, FRCS • Andrew G. Nicholson, DM

The increased skill and widespread application of antenatal ultrasound has allowed precise early diagnosis of many congenital malformations but has brought new problems with it. Recent UK national guidelines recommend that all women be offered a detailed fetal anomaly scan at around 20 weeks' gestation to confirm the gestational age and examine the fetal anatomy in detail. Many parents are now faced with having to decide what to do for a baby affected by an abnormality, some of which would have previously escaped detection. The natural history for many of these malformations is unknown, and so health professionals can have difficulty offering accurate information to parents faced with the unexpected diagnosis of an abnormality in their baby. The diagnosis of fetal lung lesions is one good example. Early reports published in the 1980s described a poor outcome for fetuses with lung masses detected in the second trimester. However, these studies were biased by a high incidence of intervention, including termination of pregnancy. With increasing use of antenatal ultrasound and the detection of many less obvious lesions it has become clear that, if conservative management is followed, many may disappear or regress considerably by term. Indeed, as we will demonstrate in this chapter, the outcome for such fetuses is in general very good, and the dilemma now is one that faces the pediatricians—namely, whether to pursue conservative or surgical management. Further confusion arises as to how these malformations should be described. The nomenclature of congenital lung disease was never very clear, with terms such as *sequestrated segment, cystic adenomatoid malformation, hypoplastic lung,* and *malinosculation* being used to describe abnormalities that often overlap. Now, however, they are used inconsistently before and after birth. For example, congenital cystic adenomatoid malformation (CCAM) is used by perinatologists to describe a lesion that may well disappear before birth but is used postnatally to describe an abnormality that may require lobectomy. CCAM may have a pulmonary arterial supply or be supplied like a sequestration from systemic arteries, and histologic features of these lesions may overlap. New imaging modalities such as magnetic resonance imaging (MRI) now allow delineation of blood supply with increasing precision. New treatment options, such as fetal surgery and postnatal embolization of feeding vessels, have become available; however, the availability of a procedure is not necessarily the best indication for its performance. A complete reappraisal of the diagnosis, investigation, and management of congenital lung disease is thus timely.

■ CLINICAL APPROACH

To clarify dialogue among various professionals (obstetricians, perinatologists, pediatric surgeons, pathologists, pediatricians), it is suggested that these principles be followed[1]:

1. What is actually seen should be described without indulgence in embryologic speculation, which may later be proved wrong. Clinical descriptions should not include assumptions of pathology, since the same clinical appearance (e.g., a multicystic mass) may have different pathologic etiologies.
2. The description should be in common language, discarding Latin.
3. The lung and associated organs should be approached in a systematic manner, because abnormalities are often multiple and associated lesions will be missed unless carefully sought.
4. Pathologic descriptions should describe what is actually seen (epithelial and mesenchymal elements), which may then be related to a diagnostic category (CCAM).

■ DESCRIBE WHAT IS ACTUALLY SEEN

The recommendation to describe what is actually seen should be followed both before and after birth. In principle, antenatal ultrasound abnormalities should be described using such terms as *increased echogenicity* with large, small, or multiple cysts rather than as CCAM. The presence or absence of abnormal feeding vessels may be defined using color or power Doppler. Other features such as mediastinal shift should also be described. In the postnatal period, a radiographic abnormality should be described as solid or cystic. If cystic, the cysts are either single or multiple, and the uniformity and thickness of the walls should be described. They may be filled with air, or partially or completely with fluid; moreover, their size should be recorded. Postnatally, an air-fluid level suggests that the abnormality is ventilated, albeit with a long time constant. If the lesion has been excised, the pathologist should describe the tissues found (epithelial, mesenchymal) and the contents of any cysts that may be present, thus giving a simple description of what is seen under the microscope. Only then is it relevant to make a pathologic diagnosis such as one of the various histologic types of CCAM (see subsequent sections). Any classification system that is to be robust cannot be based on embryologic speculation.

USE COMMON LANGUAGE

Many terms are ambiguous and are best avoided. For example, *hypoplastic lung* could be taken as meaning a lung that is small but otherwise normal, or small because the underlying structure is abnormal; the term *congenital small lung* (CSL) avoids such ambiguity. The use of the term *emphysema* in congenital lobar emphysema is another source of confusion, since it implies lung destruction, whereas in at least some variants (e.g., polyalveolar lobe) there may be too many, not too few alveoli. What is actually seen is a *congenital large hyperlucent lobe* (CLHL), which term should be used in clinical practice. Throughout this chapter, unwarranted established terms will be given in parentheses after the proposed new term; for the convenience of the reader, the new terms will be spelled out in full, with the abbreviated form being given in parentheses. A summary comparison of old and new nomenclature is provided in Table 17-1.

USE A SYSTEMATIC APPROACH

The lung can be considered to be formed from six "trees": bronchial, arterial (systemic and pulmonary), venous (systemic and pulmonary), and lymphatic. There are no known abnormalities of bronchial venous drainage, so in practice, only five trees have to be considered. There are three other areas wherein malformations may affect the respiratory system and that should thus also be assessed. These are (1) the heart and great vessels; (2) the chest wall, including the respiratory neuromuscular apparatus; and (3) the abdomen. Finally, the possibility of multisystem disease (e.g., tuberous sclerosis) should be considered. Each patient suspected of having a congenital lung malformation should be systematically evaluated along these lines, if important coexistent abnormalities are not to be missed. The importance of a systematic approach to treatment, with an appropriate evaluation of all trees and associated systems before embarking on treatment, cannot be overstated.

TABLE 17-1. Comparison of new and old terms used to describe the clinical, but not pathologic, appearances of congenital lung malformations

New Nomenclature	Old Terms Superseded
Congenital large hyperlucent lobe	Congenital lobar emphysema Polyalveolar lobe
Congenital thoracic malformation (CTM)	Cystic adenomatoid malformation (types 0–4 pathologically) Sequestration (intra- and extrapulmonary) Bronchogenic cyst Reduplication cyst Foregut cyst
Congenital small lung (CSL)	Pulmonary hypoplasia
Absent lung, absent trachea	Agenesis of lung, tracheal aplasia
Absent bronchus	Bronchial atresia

KEEP CLINICAL AND PATHOLOGIC DESCRIPTIONS SEPARATE

This is an extension of the principle of describing what is seen. Black-and-white images on a scan are unlikely to be pathognomonic of a single histologic entity. It is more logical to describe the clinical appearances and construct a pathologic differential diagnosis. Only after excision of the lesion can the pathologist construct an appropriate classification from examination of the excised specimen.

AGE-RELATED PRESENTATIONS OF CONGENITAL LUNG DISEASE

A complete review of congenital lung disease might also include a few disorders that are acquired in utero, such as congenital pneumonias (discussed in Chapter 18), but this chapter is limited to the stricter definition of developmental disorders. We first describe the age-related clinical presentations of congenital lung disease (summarized in Table 17-2) and then consider, tree by tree, the important abnormalities encountered.

TABLE 17-2. Presentation of congenital lung disease by age

Age	Presenting Feature
Antenatal	Intrathoracic mass Pleural effusion Fetal hydrops Oligohydramnios or polyhydramnios Other associated abnormalities discovered
Newborn period	Respiratory distress Stridor Bubbly secretions in mouth, not able to swallow Failure to pass nasogastric tube Unable to establish an airway Cardiac failure Chance finding Cyanosis in a well infant Poor respiratory effort
Later childhood/ adulthood	Recurrent infection (including tuberculosis, *Aspergillus*) Hemoptysis, hemothorax Bronchiectasis, bronchopleural fistula Steroid-resistant airway obstruction Cardiac failure Malignant transformation Cyanosis Coughing on drinking Chance finding of mass or hyperlucent area on chest radiograph

ANTENATAL PRESENTATION

Antenatal presentation is usually associated with an abnormality detected at the time of a routine fetal anomaly scan as described in detail later. However, abnormalities of amniotic fluid volume may also indicate underlying pulmonary pathology. This may be secondary, as in bilateral CSL (pulmonary hypoplasia) associated with both early-onset oligohydramnios for whatever reason (bilateral renal dysplasia/agenesis, first- or early second-trimester rupture of the membranes, etc.), or polyhydramnios associated with conditions such as the Pena-Shokeir phenotype or antenatal onset of severe spinal muscular atrophy, wherein severe neuromuscular disease prevents normal respiratory movements and lung development; another possibility is compression of the fetal esophagus by a mass, preventing normal swallowing of amniotic fluid. In other situations there is a primary pulmonary anomaly (e.g., tracheoesophageal fistula or laryngeal/tracheal agenesis) that causes the polyhydramnios. Other presentations include short limbs in those skeletal dysplasias associated with bilateral CSL secondary to small chests and short ribs (e.g., Jeune's asphyxiating thoracic dystrophy), or talipes and polyhydramnios in congenital myotonic dystrophy.

PRESENTATION IN THE NEWBORN PERIOD

Not all lesions are detected prenatally, although with increasing use and improvements in technology and sonographic skills, postnatal presentation is becoming less common. Late detection may particularly be an issue in diaphragmatic hernias, some of which do not present with sonographic findings until after the time of the routine anomaly scan or indeed well after birth. Large airway obstruction as the primary problem is suggested by stridor, failure to pass an endotracheal tube (ETT), or successful passage of the ETT but inability to establish ventilation. This last may be due to a tracheoesophageal fistula, as well as to large airway stenosis or complete obstruction. Respiratory distress in the absence of major airway disease may be due to disorders of the lung parenchyma. These include a large cystic or solid congenital thoracic malformation (CTM), the presence of unilateral or bilateral small lungs, and congenital pleural effusion or lymphatic disorder. Vascular abnormalities may present at this time. One such group are aortopulmonary collaterals supplying either a CSL or a CTM. These act hemodynamically as systemic arteriovenous malformations and cause high-output heart failure. Abnormalities of venous drainage, such as "scimitar" syndrome (hemianomalous pulmonary venous drainage to the inferior caval vein), may also present as heart failure or enter the differential diagnosis of pulmonary hypertension in the newborn period. Other vascular problems that may present at this time include alveolar-capillary dysplasia (discussed in Chapter 18). and pulmonary arteriovenous malformation (PAVM), which may present as cyanosis in a well infant (not with heart failure, unless there is an associated systemic, usually cerebral, arteriovenous malformation). Chest wall disease such as diaphragmatic hernia and asphyxiating dystrophy presents as respiratory distress with difficulty in establishing ventilation. By contrast, neuromuscular disease, such as severe spinal muscular atrophy or myotonic dystrophy with maternal inheritance, is characterized by inadequate or absent respiratory effort but with ease of establishing ventilation, unless there are associated unilateral or bilateral CSLs. This last group of conditions is covered in Chapter 18.

LATER PRESENTATION OF CONGENITAL LUNG DISEASE

Congenital lung disease may present later in childhood, or even in adult life. Respiratory distress as the sole presenting feature of congenital lung disease is rare after infancy. Many CTMs can present as an asymptomatic radiologic abnormality, including a focal solid or cystic mass, or hyperlucency. Unilateral CSL may also be a chance finding. A cystic CTM enters the differential diagnosis of recurrent pneumonia in the same location, with failure of radiologic clearing between bouts or atelectasis due to large airway compression. More rarely, a cystic CTM may present as a lung abscess, focal bronchiectasis, pneumothorax, hemoptysis, or hemothorax, or even with malignant transformation, although it must be stressed that this last is very rare. The occurrence of any of this formidable but rare list of complications is extremely unusual in the first 2 years of life. Other conditions presenting with hemoptysis are any abnormalities characterized by abnormal systemic arterial supply and PAVM. The latter may also present with progressive cyanosis in a well person, which may lead to polycythemia, or with systemic abscess or embolism, including cerebral, due to bypass of the pulmonary vascular filter.

Another important presentation of congenital lung disease is as "steroid-resistant asthma." Large airway narrowing such as tracheomalacia, vascular ring, or pulmonary artery sling, or complete cartilage rings enter the differential diagnosis; important physiologic clues come from the inspiratory and/or expiratory amputation of the flow volume curve, and the presence of a normal residual volume in the face of a greatly reduced FEV_1/FVC ratio (ratio of forced expiratory volume in 1 second to forced vital capacity).

Tracheoesophageal fistula and diaphragmatic hernia are considered the archetypal conditions presenting in the newborn period. However, both can present late. Tracheoesophageal fistula may present with recurrent bouts of coughing after drinking, or hemoptysis. Symptoms may have been present for more than 15 years.[2] Diaphragmatic hernia usually presents with gastrointestinal symptoms later on, although abrupt presentation with respiratory distress has been described. Whether some of these late-presenting hernias are truly congenital has been disputed.

It can be seen from the foregoing that congenital lung disease is not necessarily rare and esoteric and important only up to the stage of early infancy, but that in many clinical scenarios it is worth asking, "Could there be a congenital thoracic disease present?" when considering the differential diagnosis.

ANTENATAL DIAGNOSIS

WHAT CAN WE DIAGNOSE AND WHEN?

Fetal lung abnormalities are increasingly detected prenatally as a result of advances in ultrasound imaging improving diagnosis and also because fetal anomaly scanning is now routinely offered to many women in the developed world. A fetal lung lesion is suspected either when a mass (cystic or solid) is identified in the thorax or because of mediastinal shift (Table 17-3). The opportunity to identify an intrathoracic anomaly in the antenatal period permits further investigations and occasionally offers the potential for intrauterine therapy. It also identifies fetuses that may benefit from delivery in a center offering tertiary-level

TABLE 17-3. The differential diagnosis of fetal intrathoracic lesions

Solid Lesions	Cystic Lesions
Microcystic adenomatoid malformation	Macrocystic adenomatoid malformation
Pulmonary sequestration	Congenital diaphragmatic hernia
Right-sided diaphragmatic hernia	Bronchogenic cyst
Tracheal/laryngeal atresia	Mediastinal encephalocele
Rhabdomyoma	Pleural and pericardial effusions
Mediastinal teratoma	

neonatal support and the option of early postnatal surgical intervention. Many of these lesions can be detected around 20 weeks' gestation, but for some, in particular diaphragmatic hernias and pleural effusions, late presentation is well recognized. Such lesions may not be detected until an incidental scan in the third trimester is undertaken, or indeed until after birth when the neonate or infant presents clinically. It must also be recognized that a sonographic diagnosis can only describe the macroscopic nature of the lesion, and a definitive diagnosis for many anomalies must await definitive radiologic or histologic diagnosis after birth. Many reported studies are seriously limited, because they base conclusions solely on prenatal ultrasound or postnatal imaging. While advances in technology have improved antenatal diagnosis of lesions that may benefit from early postnatal intervention, many of the abnormalities detected appear to resolve spontaneously or are clinically silent. The pediatrician is frequently faced with a new dilemma—how to manage the well infant with a lesion that would not have been brought to medical attention were it not for antenatal imaging. What is the natural history of some of these lesions; do they require intervention, or are they benign variants? This section will present an overview of the antenatal diagnosis and management of the more common types of congenital intrathoracic abnormalities. Postnatal management of the abnormalities is discussed in subsequent sections.

CONGENITAL DIAPHRAGMATIC HERNIA

The prenatal incidence of congenital diaphragmatic hernia (CDH) is around 1 in 2000. There are a wide variety of abnormalities associated with CDH, including aneuploidy, in particular trisomies 18 and 13, genetic syndromes, and structural abnormalities. Many of these will result in a stillbirth or the pregnancy being terminated, so isolated CDH is much more common in neonates. Anomalies associated with this condition include neural tube defects (e.g., myelomeningocele), cardiac defects, and midline anomalies such as cleft lip and palate. Genetic syndromes such as Fryn's syndrome can account for up to 10% of cases in some series.

The herniation of abdominal contents into the chest inhibits normal lung development, resulting in pulmonary hypoplasia,[3] which, in isolated lesions, is the main cause of death.

The diagnosis of a left-sided CDH is usually first suspected when mediastinal shift is observed and abdominal viscera are seen within the fetal thorax (Fig. 17-1*A* and *B*). The most useful clue is usually the identification of a cystic structure (the stomach) in the chest together with absence of an intra-abdominal stomach. The observation of peristalsis in the chest can also be a useful clue, since loops of bowel may be difficult to distinguish from other cystic lesions. Paradoxical movements of the viscera in the chest with fetal breathing movements are also occasionally seen. Once alert to the possible diagnosis, the clinician doing a careful examination of the fetus in the coronal and parasagittal planes will fail to identify the diaphragm. Right-sided CDHs are more difficult to recognize, because in these cases it is usually only the liver that is herniated, and this is of similar echogenicity to lung tissue. Often the only clue is mediastinal shift, and this can be overlooked at the time of a routine anomaly scan unless the degree of shift is great. The diagnosis is sometimes made in the third trimester when a scan is performed because of polyhydramnios caused by increased intrathoracic pressure due to the presence of herniated abdominal contents in the chest. This prevents normal swallowing movements and results in late onset of increased amniotic fluid.

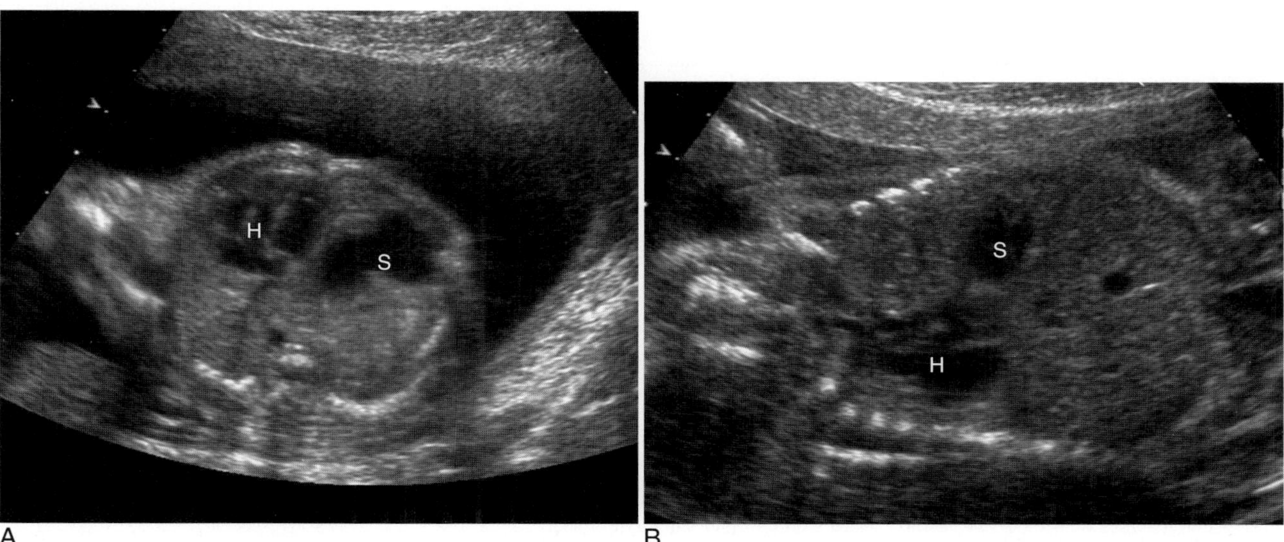

FIGURE 17-1. **A,** Transverse view through the thorax at 20 weeks' gestation in a fetus with a diaphragmatic hernia. The stomach (*S*) is seen displacing the heart (*H*) to the right. **B,** In the longitudinal plane no diaphragm can be seen, and the stomach is in the chest.

The overall prognosis for fetuses with CDH is poor, with the major causes of death being pulmonary hypoplasia and/or the associated abnormalities. The time of diagnosis is related to outcome, with those diagnosed early faring the worst. Other poor prognostic indicators include evidence of liver within the chest and cardiac disproportion before 24 weeks' gestation. Isolated left-sided hernias, an intra-abdominal stomach, and diagnosis after 24 weeks are favorable prognostic factors. Survival in these cases is now reported to be in excess of 60% (Table 17-4).[18]

Following the prenatal diagnosis of CDH, management should include a detailed search for other anomalies and fetal karyotyping. Expert fetal echocardiography is indicated, since examination of the heart is complicated by distortion of intrathoracic contents. Consultation with a pediatric surgeon should be offered and, given the variable prognosis in terms of perinatal mortality as well as morbidity, termination of pregnancy is an option that should be discussed. Delivery of ongoing pregnancies should be planned in a center with neonatal intensive care and pediatric surgical facilities. In the event of fetal or perinatal death, a postmortem examination is to be recommended. This should include a genetic opinion to facilitate an accurate diagnosis of any possible underlying syndrome, which may confer an increased risk of recurrence in future pregnancies. Intrauterine surgery has been performed for CDH. In principle, the airway is occluded and the continued secretion of lung liquid beyond the obstruction leads to expansion of the lung. The procedure is demanding and carries significant maternal risks as well as the possibility of precipitating preterm labor. A recent randomized controlled trial failed to show any benefit for this approach.[19]

CONGENITAL THORACIC MALFORMATION, SUBSEQUENTLY DIAGNOSED PATHOLOGICALLY AS CONGENITAL CYSTIC ADENOMATOID MALFORMATION

Congenital cystic adenomatoid malformation is traditionally classified according to histologic and clinical findings; however, sonographic classification is best achieved by considering these malformations as either macrocystic (Fig. 17-2*A* and *B*) or microcystic (Fig. 17-3*A* and *B*).[20] The main differential diagnosis to consider with a macrocystic CCAM is diaphragmatic hernia. Differentiating features have been described earlier. However, in a series of 87 fetuses seen in the Fetal Medicine Unit at University College London Hospitals with a prenatal diagnosis of CCAM, 3 in fact had a diaphragmatic hernia and 1 an eventration of the diaphragm (Table 17-5). In two of those with a diaphragmatic hernia, the correct diagnosis was made prenatally after serial scanning. In the other case of diaphragmatic hernia and that of the eventration, the correct diagnosis was made only on postnatal imaging.

Most CCAMs occur in isolation, although other abnormalities including bronchopulmonary sequestration and CDH have been reported to occur in association with CCAM, as have a broad range of extrapulmonary malformations including renal and cardiac anomalies.[21,22] Aneuploidy is not a recognized association.

In general, the prognosis for a fetus with a CCAM is good, with only a small number going on to develop hydrops, which is a poor prognostic sign, particularly if evident at the initial presentation in the second trimester. Traditionally, both polyhydramnios and mediastinal shift were considered poor prognostic indicators, but more recent data suggest that these signs are less reliable than once thought. Accurate prediction of outcome for prenatally diagnosed lesions can be difficult following a single scan, because spontaneous in utero improvement is often observed. Serial scans should be undertaken to detect those lesions that progress in size or display adverse prognostic features that may warrant consideration of intervention. The King's College Hospital group have reported on 67 fetuses with an antenatally diagnosed congenital lung malformation.[23] Of the 64 who were born alive, 42 underwent postnatal surgery. Surgery was performed in 45% of lesions showing late-gestation "resolution." Although there was some correlation between the antenatal appearances and the need for surgery, this was not usefully predictive for an individual, and the need for operation was judged on postnatal features rather than clinical need. At University College London Hospitals, we have seen 87 fetuses with cystic lung lesions in the last 12 years, of whom 71 are alive, 20 having

TABLE 17-4. Prognosis for antenatally diagnosed congenital diaphragmatic hernia*

Authors	Number	Chromosome Abnormality *n* (%)	% Survival Overall	% Survival at <24 Weeks	% Survival at >24 Weeks	% Survival in Isolated Cases
Thorpe-Beeston and colleagues[4]	36	11 (31)	25			60
Adzick and colleagues[5]	38	6 (16)	24	0	38	38
Sharland and colleagues[6]	55	2 (4)	27	26	40	28
Manni and colleagues[7]	28	3 (11)	14	0	100	30
Bollman and colleagues[8]	33	6 (18)	18			44
Dommergues and colleagues[9]	135	14 (10)	19			30
Howe and colleagues[10]	48	13 (34)	27	24	30	50
Geary and colleagues[11]	34	5 (15)	18	31	33	38
Bahlmann and colleagues[12]	19	1 (7)				
Betremieux and colleagues[13]	31	4 (13)	38			60
Garne and colleagues[14]	187	20 (11)	71			
Laudy and colleagues[15]	26†	0 (0)	50			
Dott and colleagues[16]	249	18 (7)	19/54§			
Hendrick and colleagues[17]	22‡	0 (0)	70			
Total	941	103 (13)	32/35	16	48	42

*Where there is no figure for the survival, data were not given in the publication.
†Only isolated left-sided congenital diaphragmatic hernia (CDH) cases were included in study.
‡Only right-sided CDHs were included in study.
§Overall survival has increased during the time period of the study from 19% (1968–1971) to 54% (1996–1999).

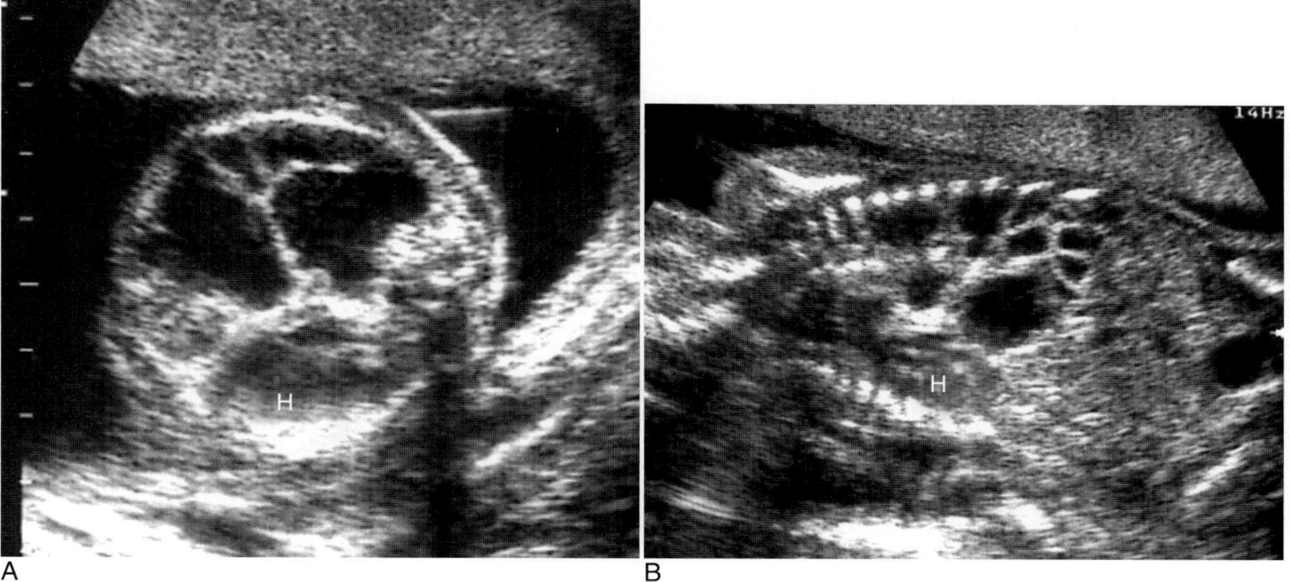

■ **FIGURE 17-2.** Axial (**A**) and longitudinal (**B**) views through the thorax in a fetus referred at 21 weeks' gestation with skin edema and increased liquor. The heart (*H*) can be seen displaced to the left, and the whole chest appears to be full of abnormal lung tissue. In the longitudinal view (**B**), the diaphragm is displaced downward by the abnormally expanded lung tissue. The large cysts were aspirated and pleuroamniotic shunts inserted, after which the skin edema resolved. The pregnancy continued to term; respiratory support was required at birth, with surgery in the neonatal period. The child is now alive and well at the age of 3 years.

had surgery. This is a much lower proportion than in the King's series and demonstrates the varying approach to management. Table 17-5 shows the type of cystic lung lesion, other sonographic findings, diagnosis, and outcome for the University College London Hospitals cohort. In all cases, early consultation with neonatal and pediatric surgical staff is helpful for parents. Where there are single or multiple large cysts (see Fig. 17-2*A* and *B*) with associated hydrops or polyhydramnios, improvement has been reported with in utero decompression by thoracocentesis or the insertion of a shunt.[24] Intrauterine surgery to remove these lesions has also been reported.[24] Where a lesion has persisted or increased in size and mediastinal shift persists in the third trimester, delivery in a center with neonatal intensive care and surgical facilities should be considered. In all cases careful postnatal follow-up should be undertaken, with computed tomography (CT) being offered to all. Lesions that have apparently involuted completely in utero are well documented to still be present when examined by CT after birth.

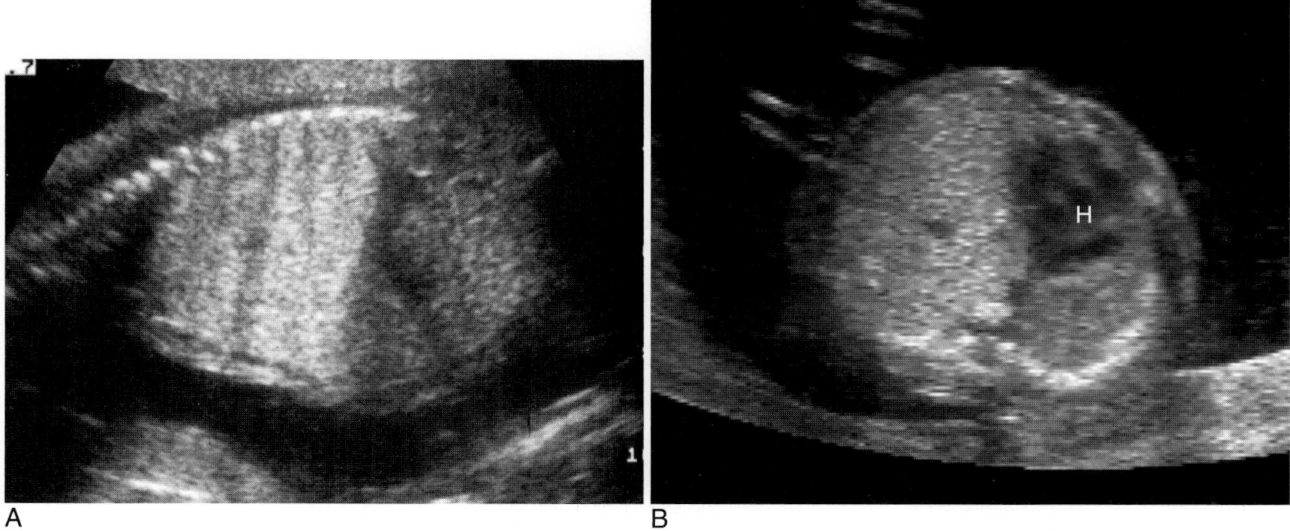

■ **FIGURE 17-3.** **A,** Parasagittal view through the chest at 21 weeks' gestation showing the echogenic wedge-shaped left lower lung behind the chest in a fetus with a microcystic lesion. **B,** In the axial view of the fetal chest, the abnormal lung can be seen causing marked mediastinal shift, with the heart (*H*) lying in the right chest. The mediastinal shift resolved as pregnancy progressed, and the infant was well at birth. Postnatal imaging confirmed the presence of the lesion, and a conservative management policy was followed.

TABLE 17-5. Summary of cohort of patients with cystic lung lesions seen at University College London Hospitals in 12 years*

			POSTNATAL MANAGEMENT					POSTNATAL DIAGNOSIS‖					
Ultrasound Findings	Total†	LB	Surgical (Emergency)	Surgical (Elective)	Conservative	ToP‡	Perinatal Death§	CCAML	No evidence of pathology	PS	Other	No diagnosis	LTFO/ WFI
Macrocystic	40	35	7	5	22	2	0	28	2	0	6	4	1/2
Microcystic	47	39	5	3	23	4	3	22	6	5	11	3	1/0
Mediastinal shift	55	44	11	11	23	6	2	33	5	3	13	5	1/2
Hydrops	14	7	4	0	3	5	2	6	0	1	7	0	0
Intrauterine therapy	9	9	4	0	5	0	0	6	0	0	3	0	0
Apparent resolution in utero	19	19	1	4	12	0	0	15	2	0	1	1	0
Total cases seen	87	74	12	8	46	6	3	50	8	5	17	7	2/2

*Others included: Congenital diaphragmatic hernia (3); pulmonary lymphangiectasis (2); Fraser syndrome (3); eventration of the left diaphragm, teratoma, congenital intradiaphragm cystic lung abnormality, Sturge-Weber syndrome, intra-abdominal calcification, echogenic mass below abdomen, unclassified abnormal lung, neuroblastoma, Peters anomaly with pulmonary hypoplasia.

†Total cases in cohort.

‡Pregnancies were terminated for the following reasons: 45,XO with pulmonary lymphangiectasis, severe hydrops, congenital pulmonary lymphangiectasis, Fraser syndrome (2 cases), Fraser syndrome and extralobar sequestration.

§Perinatal deaths were secondary to Fraser syndrome, severe hydrops, and pulmonary sequestration with hydrops.

‖Some cases with conservative management do not have a definitive diagnosis.

CCAML, cystic adenomatoid malformation of the lung; LB, live birth; LTFO, lost to follow-up; PS, pulmonary sequestration; ToP, termination of pregnancy; WFI, waiting for information (in some cases details of outcome are awaited or the pregnancy is ongoing).

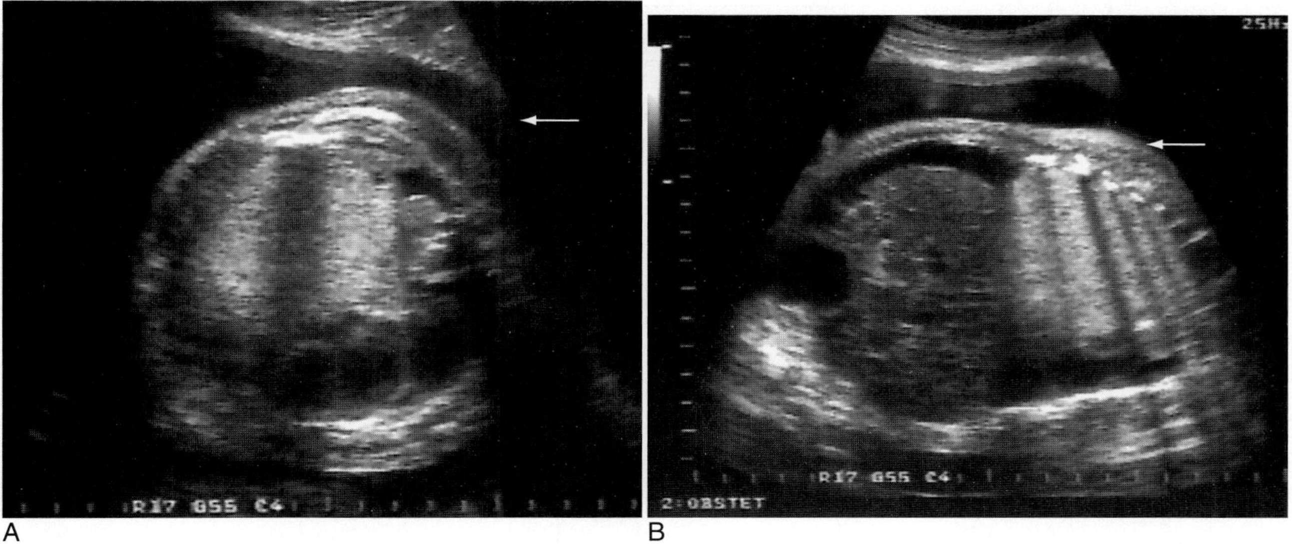

■ **FIGURE 17-4.** Axial (**A**) and longitudinal (**B**) view through the thorax of a fetus that presented at 34 weeks' gestation with hydrops and polyhydramnios. The large echogenic mass can be seen occupying most of the chest. There is a significant rim of ascitic fluid visible in the abdomen, as well as pleural effusions in the chest. Preterm labor ensued after amniodrainage. Resuscitation failed, and a postmortem examination demonstrated a sequestrated lobe with associated pulmonary hypoplasia.

CONGENITAL THORACIC MALFORMATION, SUBSEQUENTLY DIAGNOSED PATHOLOGICALLY AS BRONCHOPULMONARY SEQUESTRATION

In the fetus a sequestrated lobe of lung is most often identified as a mass of uncertain origin in the chest or subdiaphragmatic area. Prenatally it is not possible to make a definitive diagnosis unless an independent blood supply is demonstrated using Doppler ultrasound, although it should be noted that a CCAM might also have an aortic blood supply. The use of the generic term *CTM* may thus be appropriate in this context. The sequestrated lobe usually appears as an echogenic mass in the chest (Fig. 17-4*A* and *B*) or abdomen (Fig. 17-5*A* and *B*). It can be associated with hydrops, mediastinal shift, and polyhydramnios (see Fig. 17-4). The prenatal management of fetuses with lesions suspected to be a sequestration is much as for those with a suspected CCAM; serial scanning should be undertaken, and the

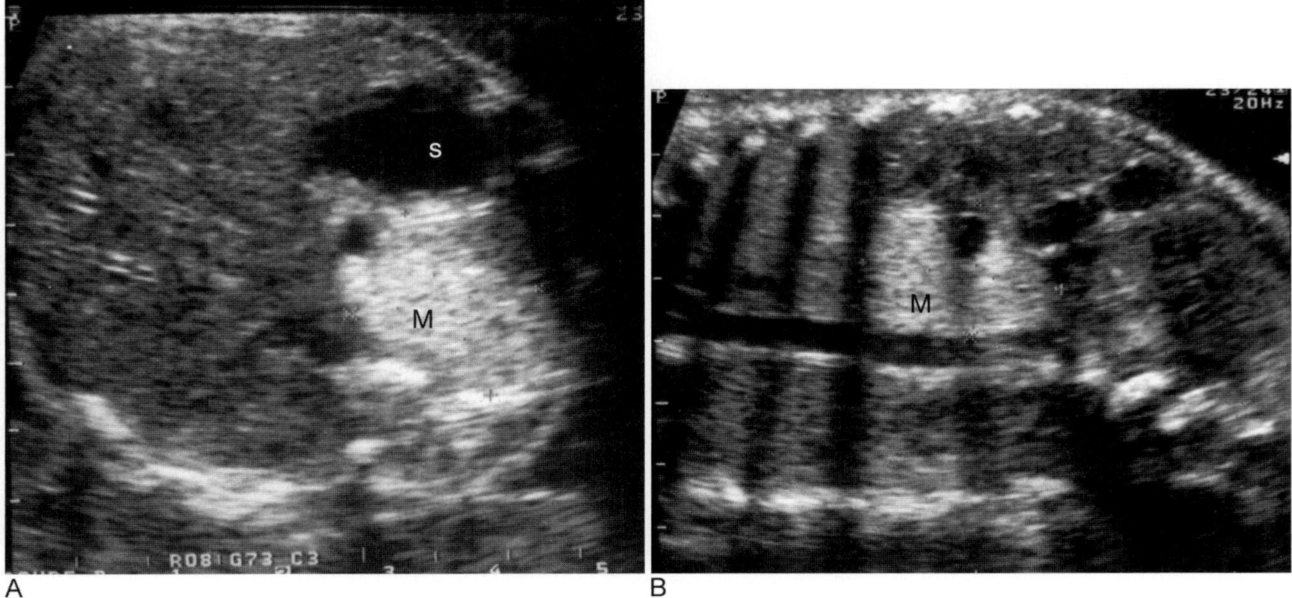

■ **FIGURE 17-5.** Axial (**A**) and longitudinal (**B**) views through the abdomen of a fetus at 22 weeks' gestation. Note the echogenic mass (*M*) related to the diaphragm lying behind the stomach (*s*). An ultrasound-guided needle biopsy after birth confirmed this to be a pulmonary sequestration. This subsequently resolved spontaneously in early childhood.

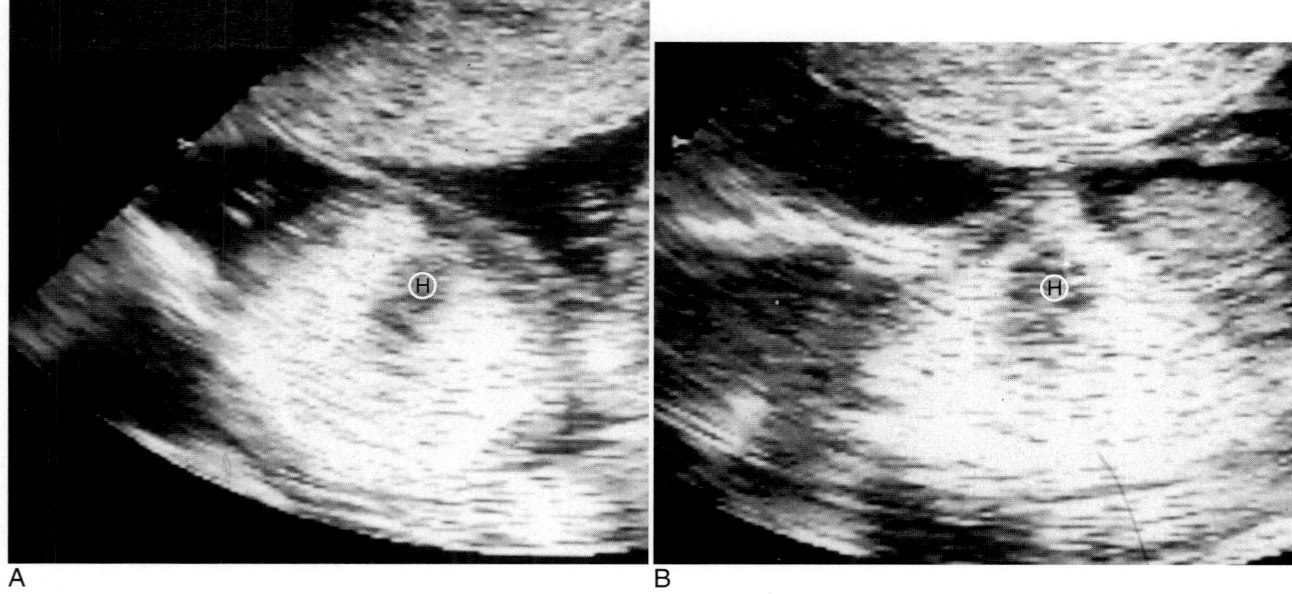

■ **FIGURE 17-6.** Axial (**A**) and longitudinal (**B**) views of the thorax of a fetus at 19 weeks' gestation with tracheal agenesis. The lungs are completely bright and can be seen compressing the heart (*H*) in **A**. In the longitudinal plane (**B**) the diaphragm is displaced downward by the expanded lung issue.

fetus should be delivered in a tertiary unit if there is significant mediastinal shift in the third trimester. Spontaneous improvement in utero has also been reported.

■ UPPER RESPIRATORY TRACT ATRESIA

Laryngeal or tracheal atresia are rare malformations that may be isolated or found in association with other abnormalities or genetic syndromes, the most common of which is Fraser syndrome. The diagnosis of laryngeal or tracheal obstruction should be suspected when enlarged, uniformly hyperechogenic lungs are seen on ultrasound (Fig. 17-6). Other sonographic features include cardiac and mediastinal compression, flattening or convexity of the diaphragms, hydrops, and polyhydramnios. A dilated, fluid-filled upper trachea can also be seen in tracheal atresia (Fig. 17-7). The differential diagnosis of laryngeal or tracheal atresia includes subglottic stenosis and bilateral microcystic CCAM. When associated with Fraser syndrome there may be renal anomalies, syndactyly of fingers and toes, and cryptophthalmos. The prognosis is invariably poor, and the option of termination of pregnancy should be discussed. Parents should also have the opportunity to discuss the prognosis with a pediatric surgeon, and, if the pregnancy is continued, delivery should be planned in a unit with neonatal intensive care and pediatric surgical facilities. Ex utero intrapartum treatment (EXIT procedure) has been reported (see later).

■ POSTNATAL FEATURES OF CONGENITAL LUNG DISEASE: AIRWAY AND LUNG PARENCHYMA

■ CONGENITAL ABNORMALITIES OF THE UPPER AIRWAY

This section will detail the variety of different congenital abnormalities that involve the upper airway. It will deal with clinical problems involving the larynx and trachea. Although we will not cover the complete spectrum of congenital disorders that can cause respiratory disorder in neonates, the pediatric otolaryngologist will be experienced in dealing with airway problems due to congenital abnormalities involving the whole airway from the anterior nares to the bronchi. The abnormalities may be intrinsic or extrinsic to the airway and be single or multiple. The spectrum of disorders is detailed in Tables 17-6 and 17-7.

These abnormalities may present with immediate respiratory distress at delivery but may also be subtle in their clinical symptoms and signs. Airway abnormalities should be considered in the presence of an abnormal cry; a breathy, weak, or husky voice;

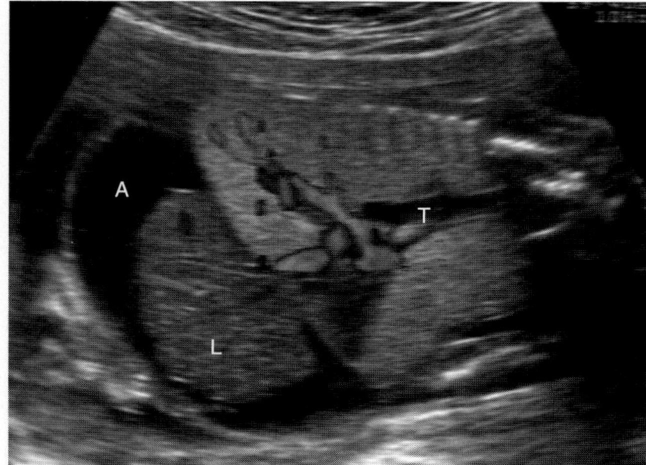

■ **FIGURE 17-7.** Longitudinal view of a fetus with tracheal agenesis. The abnormally dilated trachea (*T*) is seen as a fluid-filled structure in the mediastinum. The lungs bulge downward into the ascites (*A*) in the abdominal cavity, in which the liver (*L*) can be seen. (See Color Plate 11.)

■ **TABLE 17-6.** Congenital conditions above the larynx and trachea causing neonatal airway obstruction

Intrinsic	
Nose	Atresia (absence), e.g., arhinia Choanal atresia (complete obstruction) Piriform aperture stenosis (narrowing) Severe craniofacial abnormalities, e.g., hemifacial microsomia (Goldenhar's syndrome) and the midfacial syndromes (e.g., Apert's syndrome or Crouzon's syndrome) Tumors (e.g., teratoma, dermoid, or glioma)
Oral cavity and oropharynx	Macroglossia (e.g., Pierre Robin sequence) Retrognathia (e.g., Treacher Collins syndrome)
Extrinsic	
Viscerocranial and neck masses	Lymphatic malformations (e.g., cystic hygroma) Vascular malformations (e.g., arteriovenous malformation) Vascular tumors (e.g., capillary hemangiomas) Encephaloceles

or recurrent crouplike episodes. Difficulties with feeding may also be a feature of airway abnormalities such as laryngomalacia or laryngeal cleft. In these situations there may be recurrent episodes of aspiration with feeding (laryngeal cleft) or respiratory distress and gastroesophageal reflux (laryngomalacia).

■ MANAGEMENT OF NEONATAL RESPIRATORY DISTRESS

Severe Distress at Birth

Immediate examination in the delivery room may provide an obvious diagnosis by the pediatric staff, such as a major craniofacial abnormality. Severe airway problems such as congenital tracheal stenosis may, however, have no external physical signs.

It is not unusual for children to be intubated for safety before a more definitive diagnosis is made. If the obstruction seems to be nasal (such as in choanal atresia), it may be confirmed by the inability to pass a nasal catheter on either side of the nose. The airway can be stabilized by using an oral airway to allow oral respiration while definitive diagnosis and surgical treatment is planned. Conversely, with oral or oropharyngeal obstruction, such as in Pierre Robin sequence, the airway may be improved by simply nursing the child prone. A nasopharyngeal airway might be necessary, however, if the obstruction is not easily relieved. This is a very reliable method and may avoid the necessity of a tracheostomy. As the child grows the nasopharyngeal airway may only be necessary when the child is asleep.

If intubation is extremely difficult it may be necessary to consider immediate tracheostomy to avoid the risk of the ETT becoming dislodged and subsequent failure to reintubate. This might be considered with a large cystic hygroma (Fig. 17-8). If the anatomy of the neck is very abnormal, it may be useful to pass a rigid bronchoscope that allows ventilation and acts as a marker for the trachea within the distorted anatomy of the neck, while tracheostomy is performed.

Assessment of the Nonintubated Neonate

A child who has chronic or episodic stridor may be examined with a flexible endoscope to assess the upper airway. This is a safe procedure provided that the following are available:

1. Small-diameter endoscope (ideally 1.8 mm)
2. Access to pediatric resuscitation equipment and personnel
3. Stable neonate—at most, minimal oxygen supplementation or pressure support

This is an excellent method for making a preliminary assessment of the airway. It will provide excellent views of the posterior choanae, naso-, oro-, and hypopharynx, as well as the laryngeal inlet and vocal cords. It will not, however, easily visualize the subglottis or upper trachea, and a variety of laryngeal abnormalities such as a laryngeal cleft may not be apparent. It does avoid the need for more formal endoscopic examination of the upper airway in many cases and has shown itself to be a safe and reliable method in experienced hands.

In cases wherein the symptoms are significant and flexible endoscopy or imaging has not made a diagnosis, a microlaryngoscopy and bronchoscopy are indicated. The preparation for the procedure includes a close discussion of the case with the pediatric anesthetist. It is ideal to have the child spontaneously breathing throughout and to avoid intubation, particularly if a subglottic stenosis is suspected, since this intervention may cause swelling within a compromised airway and lead to a sudden and severe obstruction. The larynx should be sprayed with

■ **TABLE 17-7.** Congenital abnormalities of the larynx and trachea

Organ	Abnormality
Larynx	Laryngeal atresia and webs Laryngeal cleft Laryngomalacia Vocal cord paralysis Saccular cysts and laryngoceles Subglottic hemangiomas Congenital subglottic stenosis
Trachea	Tracheomalacia Congenital tracheal stenosis (complete tracheal rings)

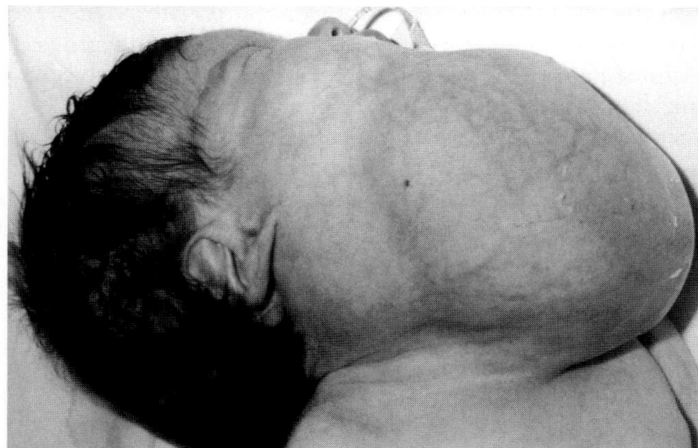

■ **FIGURE 17-8.** Severe neonatal upper airway obstruction due to cystic hygroma. (See Color Plate 12.) (Picture reproduced courtesy of Mr. C.M. Bailey.)

a metered dose of local anesthetic and a nasopharyngeal airway introduced to support the breathing with both adequate oxygenation and positive pressure if the mouth is closed or the laryngoscope occluded. The procedure should be done in a standardized fashion as listed here:

1. A global view of larynx within the pharynx should be established to visualize supraglottic lesions such as cysts or laryngomalacia.
2. Microlaryngoscopy should be performed. Using the microscope allows two-handed maneuvers. The larynx is probed to check for a laryngeal cleft and cricoarytenoid joint mobility. Glottic and subglottic lesions are usually self-evident.
3. Rigid bronchoscopy, including tracheoscopy and bronchoscopy, should be performed. Ventilation is supported through the sidearm of the bronchoscope.
4. Dynamic movements of the supraglottis and vocal cords should be studied with a 30-degree telescope while the child is waking up.

Assessment of the Intubated Neonate

Neonates whose respiratory distress is so severe that they need to be intubated represent a significant challenge for diagnosis. A child should be initially optimally managed for a trial of decannulation, including the following:

1. Systemic corticosteroid treatment if not contraindicated
2. Regular tracheobronchial toilet before trial of extubation
3. Treatment of gastroesophageal reflux, if present
4. Extubation onto a nasopharyngeal prong with continuous positive airway pressure
5. Early epinephrine nebulizer treatment if failing extubation

If the extubation fails the infant may merit a microlaryngoscopy and bronchoscopy. This is a potentially dangerous procedure in a child with a severely compromised airway and should be considered in conjunction with all the pediatric medical staff involved in the care as well as the family of the baby. The baby's medical condition may have to be optimized in readiness for surgery. An early discussion with the pediatric anesthetic staff is important to plan details of the procedure. Consent for an emergency tracheostomy will need to be obtained from the infant's family.

If the initial intubation was judged to be difficult, then the ETT should be left in situ for as long as possible. The infant should be self-ventilating and not paralyzed. With the infant in a supine position, the oral cavity, nose (if necessary), and pharynx should be examined with rigid endoscopes (and possibly a microscope). It may be possible to pass a fine rigid endoscope around the ETT and into the trachea to allow visualization of the lower airway without removing the tube. Alternatively, a rigid bronchoscope may be used once the tube has been removed. An alternative is to pass a flexible endoscope through the ETT, which has been gently withdrawn into the larynx or pharynx.

A microlaryngoscopy and bronchoscopy can be combined with any procedure that will improve the chances of extubation, such as aryepiglottoplasty in the presence of severe laryngomalacia. The child should be sent back to the intensive care unit with the ET tube in situ and a further trial of extubation attempted after a short period of recovery depending on the surgical insult of the procedure.

CONGENITAL ABNORMALITIES OF THE LARYNX

LARYNGEAL WEBS AND ATRESIA (ABSENT LARYNX)

The larynx develops in the embryo from the endodermal lining of the cranial end of the laryngotracheal tube and from the surrounding mesenchyme derived from the fourth and sixth pairs of branchial arches. The epithelium proliferates rapidly, and this leads to an occlusion of the laryngeal lumen, which recanalizes by the 10th week of gestation. Failure to reestablish a complete lumen leads to either a laryngeal web or, in extreme cases, to complete atresia.

Laryngeal Atresia

Although laryngeal atresia was once thought to be incompatible with life, with the advent of prenatal diagnosis there has been the possibility of planned immediate airway treatment. This type of anomaly (and similar gross abnormalities such as laryngeal cysts) have been given the label of congenital high-airway obstruction syndrome.[25] The early prenatal diagnosis provides two possible choices for airway intervention:

1. It has proved technically possible to introduce a tracheostomy while the fetus is still in utero, although in the one reported procedure the operation led to fetal distress and delivery of the child.[26]
2. With the EXIT procedure, the infant's oxygenation is allowed to be maintained on the uteroplacental circulation for as long as possible. This interval can be lengthened by anesthetic treatment to produce uterine relaxation and thus prolong the maternal-fetal circulation for as long as possible. Under optimal circumstances it is possible to maintain fetal oxygenation for as long as 30 minutes and so allow adequate time for bronchoscopy or simply tracheostomy to stabilize the airway.[27]

The EXIT survivors have shown a reasonably benign natural history with gradual recovery of diaphragmatic and pulmonary function. There are as yet no large series reports of long-term surgical reconstruction in these patients.

Laryngeal Webs

The majority of laryngeal web anomalies involve the anterior glottis (Fig. 17-9). There is a strong association with the velocardiofacial syndrome (chromosome 22q11.2 deletion), and the genetic abnormality is found in the majority of patients with anterior glottic webs, even those with no overt clinical features of the complete syndrome.[28] They present with either aphonia or an abnormal cry or airway obstruction. The web may be a thin band between the vocal cords of variable extent but may often involve an abnormal cricoid ring with an associated anterior subglottic stenosis. If the web is thin, then division is simple with either a laser or surgical instruments, but there is a high rate of restenosis. This can be prevented by temporarily placing a keel (a flat plastic stent) between the divided vocal cords, holding it in place with a looped suture through the soft tissues of the anterior neck. This is subsequently removed when epithelial healing is complete and the risk of restenosis is low.

If there is an associated anterior subglottic stenosis, conventional techniques of laryngotracheal reconstruction are appropriate. Posterior glottic webs are usually acquired from prolonged

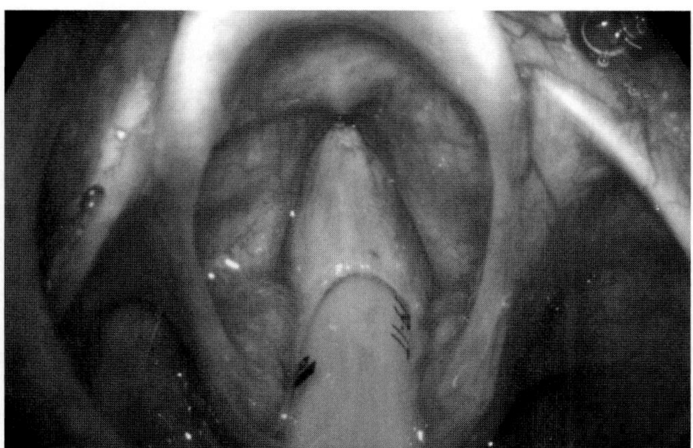

■ **FIGURE 17-9.** Congenital laryngeal web associated with anterior subglottic stenosis. (See Color Plate 13.) (Picture reproduced courtesy of Mr. C.M. Bailey.)

intubation but may rarely be congenital in origin. They are manifested as an interarytenoid web and usually present with airway obstruction. Tracheostomy is usually necessary for 3 to 5 years, since definitive corrective management has not been established.

LARYNGEAL CLEFT

The lower respiratory tract forms from the laryngotracheal diverticulum, which extends from the primitive pharynx. It becomes separated from the foregut by longitudinal ridges called tracheoesophageal folds, which fuse to form a partition known as the tracheoesophageal septum, which divides the laryngotracheal tube and the esophagus. It is a failure of the septum that leads to the formation of a laryngeal cleft.

Laryngeal clefts are associated with tracheoesophageal fistulas and may be a missed diagnosis as an explanation for recurrent aspiration following surgical repair of a tracheoesophageal fistula. They may also be a part of the G syndrome, the spectrum of which may also include cleft lip and palate, hypertelorism, and hypospadias.

Laryngeal clefts are variable in length and can be classified as follows:

Type 1. Interarytenoid
Type 2. Cricoid cleft (partial)
Type 3. Complete cricoid cleft (extending into the cervical trachea)
Type 4. Laryngotracheal cleft (extending into the thoracic trachea)

Patients with laryngeal clefts usually present with recurrent aspiration and cyanotic episodes with feeding, although neonates with more extensive clefts may demonstrate respiratory distress. The diagnosis may be made from videofluoroscopy, but endoscopic examination is the gold standard, and, indeed, during all routine rigid endoscopic examinations of the airway, a probe should be introduced between the arytenoid cartilages to screen for this defect.

Infants with laryngeal clefts should be assessed and aggressively treated for gastroesophageal reflux (including medical as well as surgical treatment such as Nissen fundoplication), since this significantly improves the outcome of surgical intervention.

Management of Type 1 Clefts

Conservative management of interarytenoid clefts should be the initial choice, with swallowing therapy, particularly aimed at thickening feeds to prevent aspiration. If this fails, endoscopic repair is advocated. Through a laryngoscope the mucosa is cut from the inner margins of the cleft, which are then sutured together (Fig. 17-10).[29]

Management of Types 2 and 3 Clefts

An anterior approach is most commonly used, since this avoids damage to the recurrent laryngeal nerves. A vertical laryngofissure is performed and the cleft closed with either direct suturing or interposition of a fascial graft. A tracheostomy may be necessary, but with shorter clefts 7 to 10 days of postoperative intubation may suffice to stent the surgical segment.

Management of Type 4 Clefts

To repair the thoracic segment, these patients require a thoracotomy, possibly via a posterolateral approach, and this may require the child to be maintained on extracorporeal membrane oxygenation (ECMO). This is combined with an anterior cervical approach to repair the upper cleft. If the tracheoesophageal folds are very basic, it may be necessary to close off the esophageal sphincters and to use the whole of the undivided foregut as the airway. With such severe abnormalities, there is a high mortality rate.

LARYNGOMALACIA (FLOPPY LARYNX)

Laryngomalacia is the most common congenital abnormality of the upper airway. Despite its relative frequency, the underlying pathologic mechanisms are poorly understood. The term *laryngomalacia* is a misnomer. There is no histologic evidence of an abnormality of the tissue of the supraglottis, and, in particular, the cartilage of the epiglottis is unremarkable. It is not an immature state of the supraglottis, since it is no more frequent among severely premature neonates than among full-term babies.

The larynges of children with this condition show a variable spectrum of characteristic macroscopic abnormalities, which

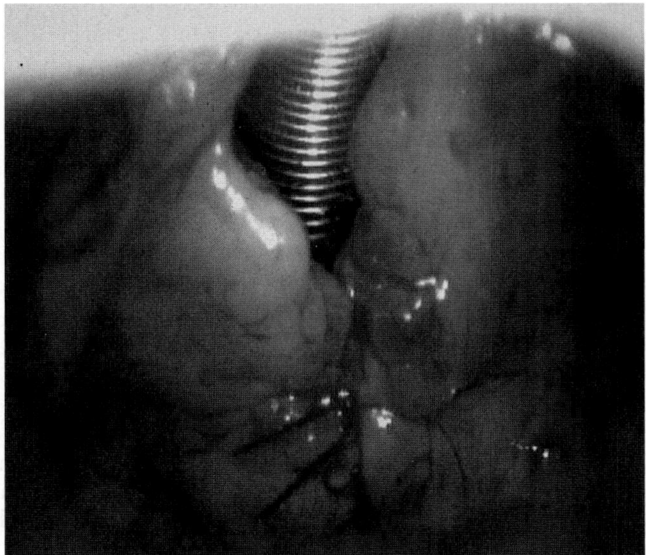

■ **FIGURE 17-10.** Endoscopic repair of laryngeal cleft type 1. (See Color Plate 14.)

cause or are caused by a dynamic anomaly of the supraglottis. These abnormalities include the following:

1. The aryepiglottic folds are short and very vertical, curling the epiglottis into an Ω shape.
2. Prominent cuneiform and corniculate cartilages lie over the arytenoid cartilage and prolapse into the airway.
3. Loose, redundant mucosal covering of the aryepiglottic fold prolapses into the airway.

It has been suggested that these facets of laryngomalacia are produced by an incoordination of the laryngeal muscles due to neuromuscular immaturity. This leads to a mistiming of laryngeal movements and tends to cause indrawing and lengthening of the supraglottic structures. It may be just a structural variation, however.

The principal symptom of laryngomalacia is inspiratory stridor with noisy respiration. The onset of the stridor is usually within the first week of life but characteristically is not with the first breath. The reason for the delayed onset of symptoms is unclear. There may be associated feeding problems, with the child becoming distressed and regurgitating from the efforts of inspiration. Feedings are often short, and if laryngomalacia is severe the child may fail to thrive. The vast majority of affected infants progress very well despite the stridor, and the management will be expectant with reassurance for the parents; typical cases may not require any further investigation, but the diagnosis can be confirmed with flexible endoscopy. It should be noted that one group has suggested that the application of topical anesthesia to the larynx may exaggerate the appearances of laryngomalacia.[30] Flexible endoscopy should involve inspection of the whole airway and allows the identification of multiple causes of stridor, which is reported in 10% to 15% of cases. The symptoms tend to resolve in the second year of life, although the stridor may become louder as the child becomes more active, particularly at the stage of crawling. The laryngeal abnormality may persist into adulthood, and occasionally the condition will present as inspiratory stridor in teenagers undertaking extremes of exercise.

Laryngomalacia—Active Treatment

In the minority of cases (≤10%), the child will fail to adequately gain weight, and in this situation the traditional treatment had been tracheostomy. A surgical alternative has been popularized in the last 10 years. Aryepiglottoplasty ("supraglottoplasty") involves surgical relief of the tight aryepiglottic folds and/or removal of the cuneiform/corniculate and/or redundant mucosal covering.[31] This can be performed with microscissors or a laser. With the latter there is virtually no bleeding, but the infant may suffer more postoperative pain and be more reluctant to feed postoperatively; this can be a major problem in neonates with other established feeding problems. There are serious potential complications of excessive removal of the supraglottic tissues, including supraglottic stenosis and aspiration. To avoid these, the surgery should be as limited as possible and if necessary unilateral, with the option to repeat if there is inadequate symptom improvement.

VOCAL CORD PARALYSIS

Congenital vocal cord paralysis (VCP) may be unilateral or bilateral. When only one side is affected, it is usually the peripheral nerve that is nonfunctioning. Moreover, it is far more commonly found on the left than on the right because of the longer course of the left recurrent laryngeal nerve. It may be associated with cardiac or great vessel abnormalities or be due to birth trauma. Bilateral VCP is more likely to be associated with a lesion of the central nervous system such as hydrocephalus or the Arnold-Chiari abnormality.

Diagnosis of VCP may be made using a flexible endoscope, but an assessment of vocal cord movement should be part of a standardized endoscopic evaluation of the pediatric airway. At completion of the laryngoscopy and tracheoscopy/bronchoscopy, the vocal cords should be visualized with a 30-degree telescope, while the child's level of anesthesia is progressively lightened. It is only in the first stages of anesthesia that active abduction of the vocal cords is seen. Movements of the vocal cords in deeper stages of anesthesia are usually passive. During inspiration the high velocity of air movement reduces lateral pressure at the glottis (as a result of Bernoulli's principle), and the elastic vocal cords passively adduct. During expiration the opposite movement is seen. Activity of the vocal fold is typified as abduction during inspiration (to reduce the upper airways' resistance), and the anesthetist should call out when the child is inspiring so that the active movements can be identified.

Unilateral VCP may be a delayed diagnosis, since there will often be no associated airway obstruction. The voice will be breathy and hoarse, but there may be remarkably good compensation, with good apposition by the mobile vocal cord to the paralyzed side, allowing reasonable phonation. It is mandatory to image the whole length of the left recurrent laryngeal nerve to screen for anomalies in the skull base, neck, and thorax. If compensation is inadequate, improved apposition with the contralateral vocal cord may be achieved by vocal cord bulking with collagen, fat, or other materials injected into the vocal cord, or by medialization of the whole cord by laryngeal framework surgery.

Bilateral VCP will produce immediate stridor at birth, which may be biphasic but is usually predominantly inspiratory. If the infant is intubated, ventilation should be very straightforward; this in fact gives the clue to the diagnosis. Treatment with a tracheostomy while awaiting spontaneous resolution of the VCP is the traditional treatment for this condition. It is not, however, inevitable that all children with bilateral VCP will need airway intervention. Treatment of the primary neurologic abnormality will obviously be of potential benefit. If the child is closely monitored and provided with adequate home support, it may be possible to avoid a tracheostomy in nearly 50% of cases.[32]

The upper airways resistance associated with bilateral VCP can be reduced by excising part of the vocal cord and/or arytenoid cartilage on one side. The cord can also be lateralized with open surgery. This will obviously affect the potential for vocal quality but may allow decannulation for those who have a tracheostomy. There is not universal agreement about the age at which one should abandon hope of spontaneous recovery of vocal cord movement and consider further surgery. There are reports of this occurring as late as 11 years of age, although many suggest that if there has been no evidence of activity by the age of 2 years, then it can be assumed that this is a permanent condition and that cord surgery should be considered in an attempt to reverse the tracheostomy. There is a minor risk of aspiration after vocal cord resection, and so this intervention should only be considered with caution in the presence of significant feeding problems.

SACCULAR CYSTS AND LARYNGOCELES

The saccule is a blind ending structure that opens into the laryngeal ventricle, the lateral space between the true and false vocal cord. It runs in an anterosuperior direction and is usually of modest size in the normal larynx. It is lined by pseudostratified columnar epithelium and contains serous and mucous glands. A laryngocele is an abnormally enlarged laryngeal saccule and is filled with air. The condition is a rare congenital abnormality but may produce significant airway obstruction. It may be entirely within the confines of the larynx or extend into the neck via the thyrohyoid membrane. If the lesion is small in size, it can be excised by an endoscopic approach. Alternatively, an open operation may be necessary for larger lesions, with the possible need for a covering tracheostomy.

Saccular cysts are filled with mucus and are found in the false vocal cord or aryepiglottic fold (Fig. 17-11). They are presumed to arise from a part of the saccule that has become sealed off from its outlet into the ventricle. They may be massive and cause immediate and severe airway obstruction. Standard endoscopic procedure is aspiration and marsupialization with scissors or laser. There is quite a high rate of recurrence, and open resection may eventually become necessary.[33]

SUBGLOTTIC HEMANGIOMA

Subglottic (and tracheal) hemangiomas (Fig. 17-12) are benign vascular tumors that may be multiple in site in the head and neck and may be enormous in size. Their natural history is of a rapid growth phase for 12 to 18 months followed by a period of involution and final resolution. They are more common on the left side than the right. They are usually asymptomatic at birth but cause increasing airway obstruction from about 3 months of age. They are usually diagnosed during endoscopic examination of the upper airway, precipitated by the onset of stridor or other airway symptoms. Diagnosis does not require formal biopsy, since the presence of an asymmetric compressible bluish mass in the subglottis is highly characteristic and biopsy will precipitate brisk bleeding, although this should be easily manageable with compression from an ETT.

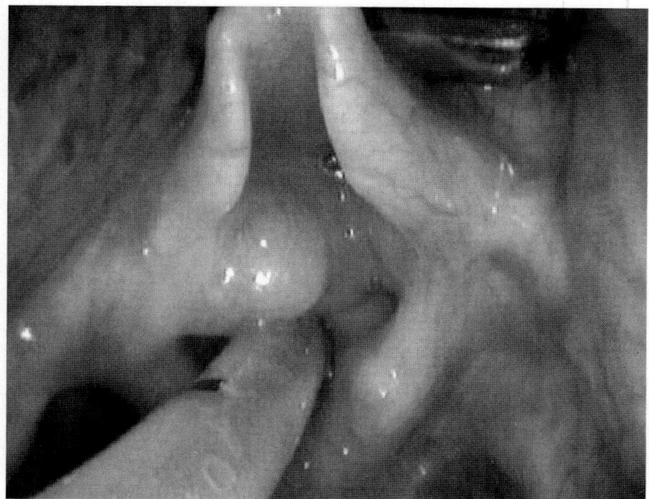

FIGURE 17-11. Congenital saccular cyst of aryepiglottic fold. (See Color Plate 15.)

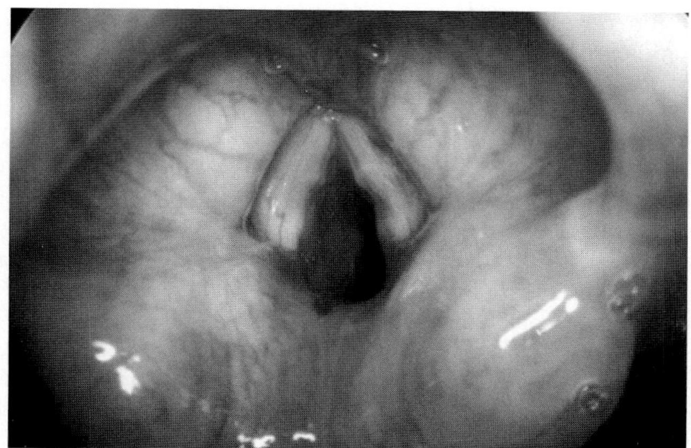

FIGURE 17-12. Subglottic hemangioma. (See Color Plate 16.) (Picture reproduced courtesy of Mr. C.M. Bailey.)

Management of this condition remains very controversial. Traditional treatment relies on tracheostomy with the aim of relieving the obstruction but at the cost of the risk of tubal blockage or dislodgement and severe or even fatal airway obstruction as well as the inevitable risk of secondary subglottic stenosis, feeding problems, and speech delay. The alternatives are varied:

1. Systemic or intralesional corticosteroids. The tumor is sensitive to steroids, although the effect is not rapid. With systemic treatment there is the risk of growth retardation and immunosuppression, and so intralesional injection is an alternative. This can be combined with intubation with an oversized ETT for a few days to compress the lesion. Note that subglottic hemangioma can present late as croup, with apparent response to dexamethasone, the standard treatment for this condition (see Chapter 23).[34] This apparent response has resulted in delayed diagnosis of the hemangioma.
2. Laser excision. This is a very effective method of reducing the size of the hemangioma, since it allows vaporization with minimal bleeding. There is a risk of scarring within the subglottis; this can lead to long-term obstruction, even after involution of the tumor.
3. Open excision via a vertical laryngofissure. There is no need for a covering tracheostomy, since the child can undergo postoperative intubation for 7 days or more (although the child will not need to have any ventilatory support during this period and should be fully awake). In experienced hands this can be curative with minimal morbidity. It may be considered in patients who have failed corticosteroid treatment.
4. Adjuvant treatment with α-interferon. This may be considered in patients with massive head and neck hemangiomas but not as a routine in isolated subglottic lesions.
5. Radiotherapy—external beam or brachytherapy. Though effective, this treatment with x-rays or radioactive gold implants has been largely abandoned because of the concern about irradiation in such young patients.

SUBGLOTTIC STENOSIS (NARROWING)

Differentiating between congenital and acquired subglottic stenosis may be difficult, particularly because any severe obstruction can lead to intubation, which is the single most common factor in acquired stenosis. Congenital stenosis is undoubtedly a separate entity and will often present in the first year of life with recurrent episodes of croup. The condition is typified by an abnormality of the cricoid cartilage, with prominent lateral shelves producing an elliptic subglottic space.

Diagnosis will be by endoscopic examination, and this should be combined with a careful inspection of the mobility of the vocal cords and cricoarytenoid joints. If the subglottic space only allows an ETT two sizes smaller than that expected for a child of its age, then surgical treatment should be considered. Performance of a tracheostomy should be avoided. A single-stage laryngotracheal reconstruction is appropriate. Rib cartilage is used to hold open a vertical slit in the cricoid and upper trachea, either in the anterior wall alone or as separate anterior and posterior grafts. The child is intubated for 7 to 10 days before a trial of extubation.

CONGENITAL ABNORMALITIES OF THE TRACHEA

TRACHEOMALACIA (FLOPPY TRACHEA)

Tracheomalacia is an abnormal collapse of the trachea due to localized or generalized weakness of the tracheal wall leading to respiratory obstruction (Fig. 17-13). This softening of the airways is commonly acquired as a complication of intubation of premature infants but may also be part of generalized chondrodystrophies. Microscopically, specimens show an increase in the ratio of muscle to cartilage. The condition occurs in primary or secondary forms, although either form can be congenital. In primary tracheomalacia there is an intrinsic abnormality of the tracheal wall, whereas in secondary cases there is extrinsic compression. In congenital cases, this is usually associated with cardiovascular abnormalities, which include the following:

1. Double aortic arch, which surrounds the trachea producing a concentric compression.
2. Anomalous innominate artery, which compresses the right anterior trachea.
3. Pulmonary artery sling, which compresses the right main bronchus.

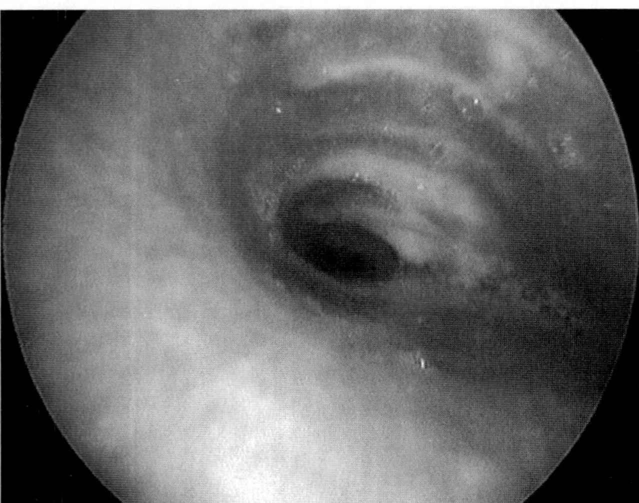

FIGURE 17-13. Tracheomalacia, acquired secondary to cardiac surgery. (See Color Plate 17.)

The differential diagnosis also includes mediastinal tumor, tracheal web, foreign body, and obstructive lesions of the upper airway. Congenital tracheomalacia may be associated with bronchomalacia, particularly in more generalized cases. It may also be found with other tracheal abnormalities such as tracheoesophageal fistula or laryngeal cleft. Although they may coexist, there is no connection with laryngomalacia.

The clinical manifestations of the condition are extremely variable, and it is often a diagnosis that can only be reliably made by endoscopy. There is likely to be stridor, which is usually expiratory because the obstruction is predominantly intrathoracic. There are usually recurrent acute episodes of stridor and dyspnea, during which the child may become cyanosed and moribund ("dying spells"). Such spells may be precipitated by severe crying, coughing, or even feeding. The symptoms are usually apparent in the immediate neonatal period but may deteriorate in the first and second year of life, in an almost stepwise manner.

Diagnosis is essentially by endoscopy. For the pediatric otolaryngologist this is most often with rigid bronchoscopy. The pediatric airway is very elastic and may collapse during effortful inspiration and certainly during coughing fits. The trachealis muscle also tends to bulge forward, giving the impression of a narrow airway. During endoscopy it is important that the child be adequately anesthetized to avoid coughing while there is still spontaneous respiration. There is no generally accepted definition of the degree of collapse that can be taken as abnormal, but it seems reasonable to suggest that more than 25% reduction of the lumen is a significant finding and that greater than 50% is likely to be symptomatic. As well as overdiagnosis, it is possible to miss the condition if the trachea is splinted by the bronchoscope or if there is excessive positive end-expiratory pressure applied by the anesthetist through the sidearm of the instrument. The procedure should involve a detailed laryngoscopy to screen for a laryngeal cleft, and active vocal cord movements should be confirmed, particularly if there has been tracheal surgery for a tracheoesophageal fistula or cardiovascular surgery for a vascular anomaly. An alternative diagnostic investigation is low contrast volume bronchography (see later). This technique has the advantage of allowing measurement of airway caliber during quiet breathing without the application of positive end-expiratory pressure.

Although the condition may progress in the first couple of years of life, it is generally self-limiting and if mild requires no active treatment. The patient's family should, however, be taught cardiopulmonary resuscitation, particularly if the acute episodes are severe; they can be provided with a facemask and ventilation bag. In general, "near-death" episodes are precipitated by a rise in intrapleural pressure leading to airway compression during, for example, crying. As the child becomes unconscious, pleural pressure falls to normal, airway compression is relieved, and the episodes are thus self-limiting, albeit frightening. In more severe cases active treatment might be considered, although many of the choices have severe potential complications and should only be utilized in the face of extreme circumstances:

1. Surgery for abnormal vasculature. If there is a vascular ring causing significant airway compression, then surgery is always indicated. However, this may relieve the compression, but once the tracheal wall has become weakened from external pulsatile pressure, it may not

immediately recover following removal of the anomalous vessel.

2. Aortopexy. A suture through the adventitial lining of the aortic arch and the periostium of the sternum is used to pull the arch forward, and because the anterior tracheal wall is intimately connected to the aortic arch with fascial tissue, it is also towed forward, widening the tracheal lumen. There may be a failure of the suture, and there is a risk of damage to the aortic arch itself.
3. Tracheostomy. This is very effective for short-segment tracheomalacia but is unsatisfactory when the distal trachea is involved. The tube tip must pass through the segment to stent it, and customized tubes can be manufactured to optimize the length. However, with a distal segment the tube tip may pass into the right main bronchus on neck flexion, and it may not adequately stent the tracheomalacic segment on neck extension.
4. Nasal or tracheostomy continuous positive airway pressure. A pneumatic splint of the segment can be achieved with continuous positive airway pressure via a tight-fitting facemask, or a tracheostomy if the former is not tolerated, particularly with collapse at the carina (and in association with bronchomalacia).
5. Segmental resection. This is suitable for short-segment collapse if the obstruction is severe. An end-to-end anastamosis is used to reconstitute the trachea.
6. Internal stents. These are typically made from siliconized plastic or are designed as expandable metal tubes. Stents may be highly effective at maintaining the lumen of the trachea but can be difficult to introduce down a bronchoscope and may be complicated by displacement, granulation, and infection.
7. Cartilage grafting. Rib cartilage grafts can be used to stiffen the tracheal wall, but if near to half of the tracheal wall is replaced, there can be slow or incomplete reepithelialization.

TRACHEAL AGENESIS (ABSENT TRACHEA) AND HYPOPLASIA (SMALL TRACHEA)

Atresia of the trachea is a rare anomaly that is probably due to a malformation in the development of the laryngotracheal groove and comprises either partial or complete absence below the larynx or cricoid cartilage, together with main stem bronchi that join in the midline and a bronchoesophageal or tracheoesophageal fistula in 80% of cases. Historically, cases have been incompatible with life, but isolated atresia may be amenable to surgical reconstruction. The lungs may show lobulation abnormalities or intrapulmonary hemorrhage. A minor degree of tracheal hypoplasia may be seen in Down syndrome, as well as many other airway abnormalities.

CONGENITAL TRACHEAL STENOSIS (COMPLETE TRACHEAL RINGS)

Congenital stenosis of the trachea can be either intrinsic or extrinsic in nature. Congenital extrinsic compression occurs with a variety of anomalies involving the great vessels. Intrinsic stenosis usually occurs as a fibrous stricture in the form of webs located in the subglottic area or just above the carina, although diffuse involvement has also been recorded. Intrinsic stenosis may lead to tracheal hypoplasia. An abnormally long and funnel-shaped trachea may also occur when the cartilage rings are complete with an absence of the posterior membranous portion. This very rare condition is often found in combination with other regional abnormalities, particularly cardiac. If the lumen of the trachea is small, this may not be compatible with life. Alternatively, the child may suffer immediate respiratory distress in the delivery room that is not relieved by intubation or even tracheostomy. Extracorporeal oxygenation may be necessary to allow time to consider a surgical remedy.

If the child's condition is relatively stable, it may not be necessary to consider any form of tracheal surgery, and there is potential for airway growth with the child. Surgery may, however, become necessary as the child grows if exercise tolerance is severely limited.

Surgical options include the following:

1. Resection of the stenotic segment. The innate elasticity of the pediatric trachea means that quite a long segment can be excised and the trachea reconstituted. It has been suggested that this is possible when up to eight rings are involved.
2. Reconstruction of the stenotic segment. There are many described procedures aimed at reconstructing the anterior wall of the stenotic segment after it has been opened in a vertical plane. These include: (a) pericardial patch tracheoplasty; (b) slide tracheoplasty; (c) homograft tracheal transplantation; (d) free tracheal autograft (partially excised segment used to patch the remainder); (e) costal cartilage autograft.
3. Tracheal transplant. This option is used in a few centers as treatment for complex tracheal disease. The transplanted scaffold is the cartilaginous structure of the donor trachea, denuded of all cells and thus not immunogenic. The scaffold is epithelialized by ingrowing recipient cells. However, although rejection is not a problem, airway obstruction needing bronchoscopic relief is common and repeated. Thus, the technique is very demanding, although it can be extremely successful.

The multiplicity of surgical techniques reflects the relatively poor outcome in the severely symptomatic patients,[35] and careful discussion with the family is imperative to come to a balanced view of the potential outcome of surgery.[36]

BRONCHIAL ABNORMALITIES

CONGENITAL BRONCHIAL STENOSIS AND ATRESIA

Congenital stricture of the bronchus occurs predominantly in a main stem or middle lobe bronchus and can produce acute and/or chronic pulmonary infection. Inflammatory scarring of the congenitally stenosed bronchus provides an ideal environment for distal suppuration, atelectasis, and bronchiectasis. Atresia is usually asymptomatic and detected incidentally on radiography. The airway may be blocked by a simple membrane, or there may be a discontinuity. It often results in cystic degeneration of the lobe distal to the obstruction before birth, since fetal lung liquid continues to be secreted and cannot drain into the amniotic cavity. The distal airspace is often cystic and filled with mucus, and is typically in continuity with an area of distal hyperinflation caused by collateral ventilation. Infection and scarring may ensue, with symptomatic presentation. Failure to identify the congenital nature of the problem may lead to a misdiagnosis of mucus plugging. Unlike the situation with absent bronchus, there is no focal opacity in congenital large hyperlucent lobe (congenital lobar emphysema). The continuity of the cyst with the distal airways and the hyperinflation of the distal lung distinguish absent bronchus from bronchogenic cyst (the nomenclature of which is discussed later), but the two conditions are occasionally associated.

ABNORMAL BRONCHIAL ORIGIN AND BRONCHIAL BRANCHING

Bronchi can arise from the gastrointestinal tract. Bronchial diverticula also possibly represent abnormal bronchial branching. The right upper lobe bronchus can arise from the trachea, particularly in association with the tetralogy of Fallot. An accessory cardiac lobe bronchus may arise from the intermediate bronchus. A tracheal origin of one or more of the right upper lobe bronchi is usually of no clinical significance but may be a cause of recurrent right upper lobe collapse in an intubated patient if the ETT is low. The right lower lobe bronchus may also arise from the left bronchial tree, a "bridging bronchus." Lung segments may also cross over, with bronchial and arterial connections from the opposite side, usually from right to left. The crossover may simply be of vessels and bronchi, or include a tongue of parenchymal tissue, the "horseshoe" lung, where there is fusion of the lungs behind the heart.[37]

DISORDERS OF BRONCHIAL LATERALITY

Abnormal arrangements require consideration of what makes, for example, a right lung a right lung. It is not because it is in the right hemithorax. In clinical practice, the two most useful determinants of right lung morphology are the presence of three lobes, not two, and a very short main bronchus before the take-off of the upper lobe bronchus. A third criterion is the presence of an eparterial bronchus. Mirror-image arrangement must be distinguished from the superficially similar congenitally small (hypoplastic) right lung with right-sided heart (dextroposition) by determining bronchial morphology. This is important, because each has a different implication and requires different investigation. Mirror-image arrangement may be a feature of primary ciliary dyskinesia (discussed in Chapter 63), whereas a CSL must have its vascular supply delineated (see later).

The term *isomerism* is so entrenched that it is probably not feasible to replace it with, for example, bilateral right lung, which would be more logical. Nearly 80% of children with right isomerism (bilateral right lung) lack a spleen, leading to a risk of overwhelming pneumococcal sepsis. A similar proportion with left isomerism (bilateral left lung) have multiple small spleens. Ivemark's syndrome consists of right isomerism (bilateral right lung), asplenia, a midline liver, malrotation of the gut, and a variety of cardiac abnormalities including a common ventricle, totally anomalous pulmonary venous drainage, and bilateral superior caval veins and right atria. Left isomerism (bilateral left lung) is associated with multiple small spleens (polysplenia), a midline liver, malrotation of the gut, partially anomalous pulmonary venous drainage, and cardiac septal defects. Although nonfamilial, Ivemark's syndrome is confined to males, whereas the other isomerism syndromes can affect either sex. Recently, a syndrome of left bronchial isomerism, normal atrial arrangement, and severe tracheobronchomalacia has been described,[38] extending the spectrum of left isomerism (bilateral left lung). Occasionally, a CSL may be so abnormal that its morphology can only be described as indeterminate. The contralateral lung morphology is, however, usually obvious. Quite commonly, minor deviations from the normal bronchial branching pattern may be seen, which one study suggested may be associated with spontaneous pneumothorax.[39]

OTHER DISORDERS OF THE BRONCHIAL WALLS

Abnormalities in bronchial wall caliber may result in all or part of the bronchial tree being too large or too small. These may present with recurrent infections, steroid-unresponsive wheeze, or stridor. Congenital tracheobronchomegaly (Mounier-Kuhn's syndrome) is characterized by tracheomalacia and bronchiectasis, with greatly dilated major airways. There are saccular bulges between the cartilages. Bronchial clearance is impaired, resulting in recurrent respiratory infection. This syndrome, which may be autosomally recessive, generally presents between the ages of 30 and 50 years, and is more common in males. It is occasionally associated with Ehlers-Danlos syndrome, cutis laxa, or Kenny-Caffey syndrome. True congenital bronchiectasis is much rarer than previously thought.

The lumen may be narrowed by complete cartilage rings (Fig. 17-14). There may be an associated pulmonary artery sling. A short segment, situated relatively distally in the airway, may require no treatment. If ventilation is critically compromised, surgical excision or a Z-plasty may be indicated. Bronchoscopic balloon dilatation should probably best be considered experimental. It is wise to ensure that the distal lung is normal before embarking on treatment; if the small airway is part of a generally maldeveloped segment, then enhancing ventilation may in fact only increase dead space ventilation.

Congenital bronchomalacia may be isolated, often with a good prognosis, at least in the short term, or associated with other congenital abnormalities including connective tissue disorders, and Larsen's and Fryn's syndrome. Williams and Campbell described a syndrome of diffuse bronchomalacia affecting the second to the seventh generations of bronchi.[40] Its occurrence in siblings and the very early onset of symptoms suggests a congenital etiology.

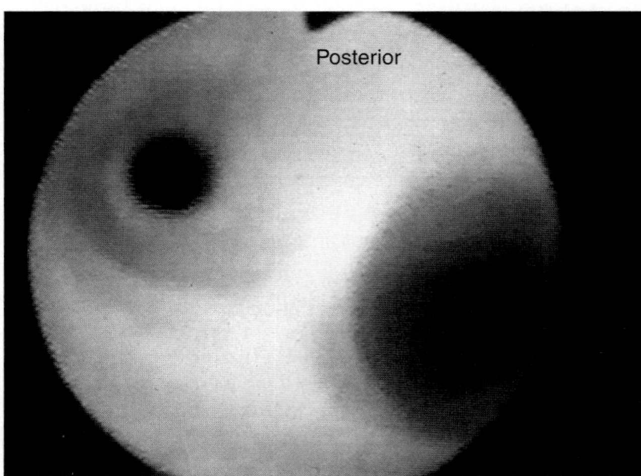

FIGURE 17-14. Bronchoscopic view of a single complete cartilage ring at the origin of the right main bronchus. (See Color Plate 18.)

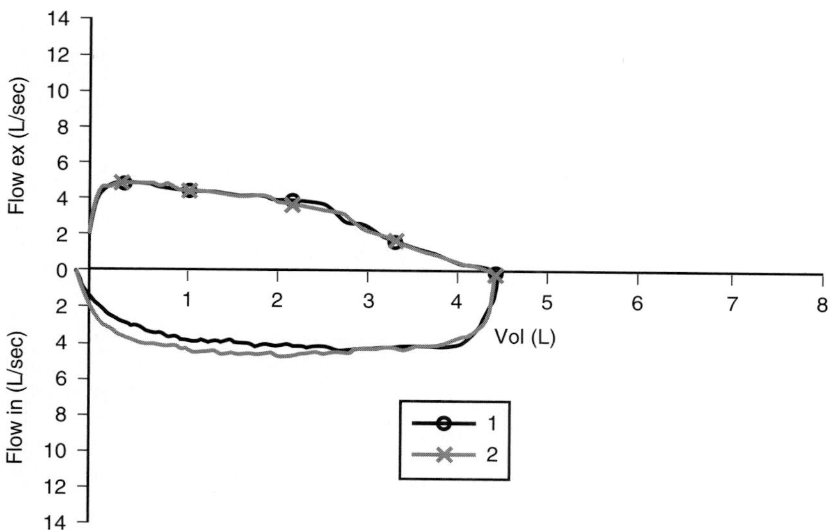

■ **FIGURE 17-15.** Typical appearance of the flow volume curve in fixed upper airway obstruction. There is marked abrupt attenuation of inspiratory and expiratory flow, persisting until late near-complete emptying, and then near-complete filling of the lungs.

Bronchomalacia may also be secondary to other congenital abnormalities, such as vascular rings. A rare cause of congenital tracheobronchomalacia is the presence of esophageal remnants in the wall of the trachea, generally associated with esophageal atresia and tracheoesophageal fistula. Fixed bronchial narrowing may be due to defects in the wall (e.g., complete cartilage rings) or extrinsic compression by an abnormal vessel or cyst. In older children, this may be suspected from the appearances of the spirometric flow volume loop (Fig. 17-15).

PULMONARY AGENESIS, APLASIA (ABSENT LUNG), AND HYPOPLASIA (SMALL LUNG)

Bilateral pulmonary agenesis is a rare malformation that may occur in anencephaly. Unilateral pulmonary agenesis is slightly more common, with absence of the carina and the trachea running directly into a single bronchus. Pathologically, the sole lung is larger than normal in pulmonary agenesis, and this enlargement is true hypertrophy and not emphysema. The mortality of right-sided agenesis is twice that of left-sided agenesis; this is probably a result of more severe mediastinal and cardiac displacement. Pulmonary aplasia, the most common variant, consists of a carina and main stem bronchial stump with absence of the distal lung. In this situation, secretions can pool in the stump, become infected, and possibly spill over to infect the sole lung. Lobar agenesis and aplasia are rarer than complete absence of one lung and usually affect the right upper and middle lobes together. Pulmonary hypoplasia (CSLs) consists of incompletely developed lung parenchyma connected to bronchi that may also be underdeveloped depending on when the presumed causal insult took effect in embryogenesis. There are a large number of causes of CSLs (Tables 17-8 and 17-9). The alveoli are reduced in number or size (numbers are assessed by counting alveolar wall intercepts on a line from the terminal bronchiole to the interlobular septum). However, hypoplasia is perhaps best considered to be present in term babies when the lung-to-body weight ratio is less than 0.012. There is a high incidence (>50%) of associated diaphragmatic, cardiac, gastrointestinal, genitourinary, and skeletal malformations, as well as frequent variations in the bronchopulmonary vasculature. Correction of any underlying abnormality, if feasible, either postnatally or antenatally, may permit growth of alveoli. However, airway branching is complete by 16 weeks, and so airways will not branch after a causal abnormality has been corrected, and since the airway pattern is abnormal, alveolar numbers are never likely to be normal.

ECTOPIA

Ectopia is growth of normal tissue in the incorrect anatomic position and, in relation to the lung, comprises either nonpulmonary tissues being present in the lung or lung tissue outside the thoracic cavity.[41,42] In relation to extrapulmonary tissues, ectopic

■ **TABLE 17-8.** Causes of bilateral congenital small lungs

System Fault	Examples
Lack of space	Abnormal thoracic, abdominal, or amniotic cavity contents (see Table 17-9)
Abnormal vascular supply	Pulmonary valve or artery stenosis Tetralogy of Fallot
Neuromuscular disease	CNS, anterior horn cell, peripheral nerve, or muscle disease (particularly severe spinal muscular atrophy and myotonic dystrophy inherited from mother) reducing fetal breathing movements

CNS, central nervous system.

■ **TABLE 17-9.** Congenital small lungs due to extrapulmonary mechanical factors

Extrapulmonary Mechanical Factor	Examples
Abnormal thoracic contents	Diaphragmatic hernia Pleural effusion Large CTM
Thoracic compression from below	Abdominal tumors Ascites
Thoracic compression from the sides	Amniotic bands Oligohydramnios (any cause) Asphyxiating dystrophy/scoliosis or other chest wall deformity

CTM, congenital thoracic malformation.

glial tissue is well recognized within the lung, with nodules of glial tissue being implanted in anencephalics or due to embolization in relation to intrauterine trauma. Adrenocortical tissue, thyroid, liver, and skeletal muscle have also been described in the lung, and pancreatic tissue has been found in intralobar sequestrations. Ectopic lung tissue may be found in the neck, chest wall, and even in the abdomen, although some ectopias represent extralobar sequestrations. Alternative terms for this occurrence include *congenital pneumatocele* and *congenital pulmonary hernia*, although they are best regarded as true ectopias. Entire kidneys may also be intrathoracic in location.

■ CONGENITAL CYSTIC LESIONS

Numerous pathologic conditions present with cystic changes in the lung, with acquired lesions outnumbering those that are developmental in origin. This section discusses the pathology of developmental lesions. It usually only after surgical excision that sensible pathologic diagnoses can be made.

FOREGUT (BRONCHOGENIC) CYSTS (CLINICALLY, CYSTIC CONGENITAL THORACIC MALFORMATIONS)

Foregut cysts can be defined as closed epithelium-lined sacs developing abnormally in the thorax from the primitive developing upper gut and respiratory tract. When these structures differentiate toward airway and contain cartilage in the wall, they are termed bronchogenic cysts, while those developing toward the gut are termed enterogenous cysts, although they are most likely of common origin from abnormal division of the embryonic foregut.[43] Bronchogenic cysts are the most common cysts in infancy, although many do not present until adulthood. About 50% are situated in the mediastinum close to the carina, and less frequently adjacent to the esophagus and alongside the tracheobronchial tree. More rarely, they are found within the lung parenchyma and exceptionally in sites such as below the diaphragm, pericardium, presternal tissues, and skin. Foregut cysts are usually single, unilocular, and more common on the right. They may have a systemic blood supply. Symptoms often relate to compression of the airways or complications such as hemorrhage or infection, which may be reflected in the macroscopic appearance when the wall is thickened by fibrous scarring and shows brown discoloration due to chronic bleeding (Fig. 17-16). Microscopic examination shows a cyst lined by respiratory-type epithelium, although there may be squamous metaplasia and even ulceration with a foreign body–type granulomatous reaction depending on secondary phenomena. The wall is often fibrous and inflamed, and it may contain seromucous glands and cartilage plates (Fig. 17-17). In the absence of cartilage, such a cyst should be termed a simple foregut cyst.

Enterogenous cysts are subdivided into esophageal and gastroenteric (duplication) cysts, the former being more common. Esophageal cysts are intramural and do not involve the mucosa. They are lined by either squamous or respiratory-type epithelium. Gastroenteric cysts, in contrast, are typically unconnected to the esophagus but may be in close association with the vertebrae, often in the region of the sixth to the eighth. Symptoms are typically due to pressure, infection, or hemorrhage, and there may also be symptoms in association with the vertebral anomalies. In infants, they are a common cause of a posterior mediastinal mass and are typically paravertebral in location.

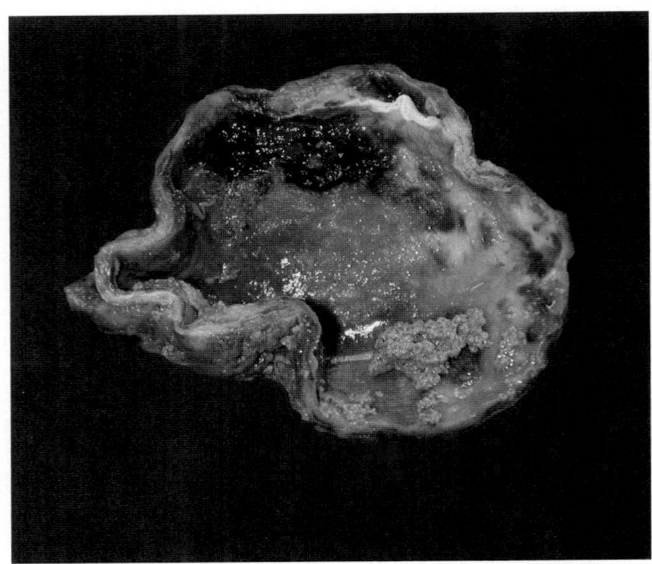

■ **FIGURE 17-16.** Mediastinal bronchogenic cyst. The inner surface of this unilocular cyst is partly hemorrhagic and partly covered by purulent debris, indicative of recurrent infection. (See Color Plate 19.)

They may extend across the diaphragm. The cysts are often saccular and are lined by gastric or intestinal mucosa with a muscle layer akin to the muscularis propria. Gastric mucosa may cause symptoms due to ulceration. Malignant transformation is exceptionally rare but is reported in gastroenteric cysts.

CONGENITAL CYSTIC ADENOMATOID MALFORMATION (CLINICALLY, CYSTIC CONGENITAL THORACIC MALFORMATION)

This term encompasses a spectrum of variably sized cysts with differing histology. The reported incidence is between 1 in 25,000 and 1 in 35,000, although as with many conditions, the advent of antenatal ultrasound is causing us to revise upward our

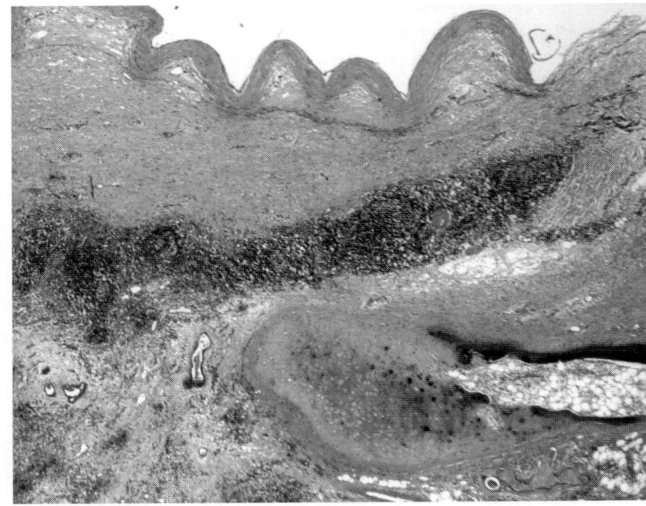

■ **FIGURE 17-17.** Mediastinal bronchogenic cyst. The lining of the cyst is mainly denuded, while the wall is chronically inflamed. Note the cartilage plate that indicates bronchogenic origin. (See Color Plate 20.)

estimations of prevalence. The relationship between different types and with other malformations is contentious and their etiology is obscure, although some view them as defects relating to insults to the pulmonary airways during maturation—hence the proposed alternative term *congenital pulmonary airway malformation*, or here, the more generic *CTM*. Pathologically, there are five types (types 0–4), the speculation being that they represented malformations of five successive groups of airways. Thus, type 0 (a condition formerly described as acinar dysplasia) is described as bronchial, type 1 as bronchial/bronchiolar, type 2 as bronchiolar, type 3 as bronchiolar/alveolar duct, and type 4 as peripheral.[44] Although lesions are not obviously distributed along the bronchial pathway, there is a high incidence of associated abnormalities of the bronchial tree on detailed analysis, and furthermore, vascularity and cellular composition in CCAMs corresponds to that seen in airways during gestation. This histologic classification is useful, because it permits identification of certain histologic patterns that rarely undergo malignant transformation in association with certain subtypes. However, it is still not ideal (see later) and will probably undergo revision with greater insight into pathogenesis.[45]

Type 0 CCAMs (also termed acinar dysplasia) are rare, incompatible with life, and typically associated with other abnormalities. The lungs are small and firm, and histology shows bronchial-type airways with cartilage, smooth muscle, and glands that are separated only by abundant mesenchymal tissue. This condition is discussed in more detail in Chapter 18.

Type 1 is the most common type of CCAM and has the best prognosis, because these malformations are usually localized and affect only part of one lobe. Most present in the perinatal period or in utero, but rare cases can present later. Cysts are usually multiloculated and range considerably in size, although type 1 CCAMs are larger than 2 cm in diameter by definition (Fig. 17-18). There is no relationship between age and cyst size. Microscopically, there is a sharp boundary between the lesion and the adjacent normal lung but no capsule. The cystic spaces are lined by pseudostratified ciliated columnar epithelium, and mucous cell hyperplasia is seen in 35% to 50% of cases (Fig. 17-19). Arbitrarily, hyperplasia is defined as mucous cell proliferation confined to the cyst, while extensions of this process into the alveolar parenchyma with lepidic growth pattern is classified as bronchioloalveolar carcinoma.[46] This latter complication is considerably rarer, and it has been argued that such proliferations are not neoplastic. However, occasional cases have metastasized, and recent comparative genomic hybridization studies have shown chromosomal aberrations in the mucous cells similar to those seen in adenocarcinomas of nonsmokers. Therefore, such proliferations should be regarded as bronchioloalveolar carcinomas with a very good prognosis following complete resection.

Type 2 CCAMs are the second most frequent type. They generally cause respiratory distress in the first month of life and may be associated with renal agenesis, cardiovascular defects, diaphragmatic hernia, and syringomyelia, which often have an

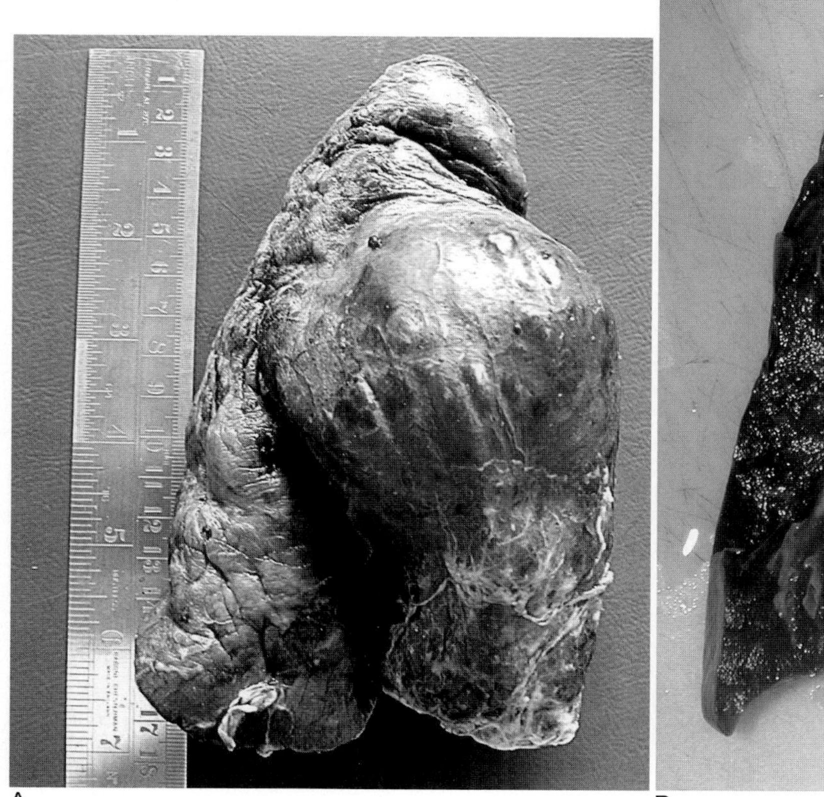

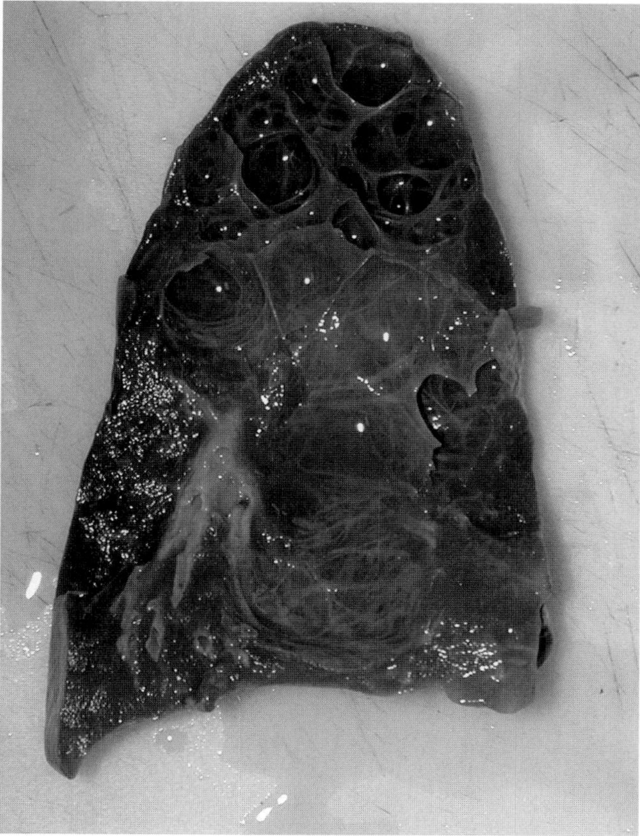

A B

■ **FIGURE 17-18.** Type 1 CCAM. **A,** A cystic lesion bulges to fill most of the lower lobe. **B,** The cut surface shows a multiloculated cyst replacing most of the parenchyma. (See Color Plate 21.)

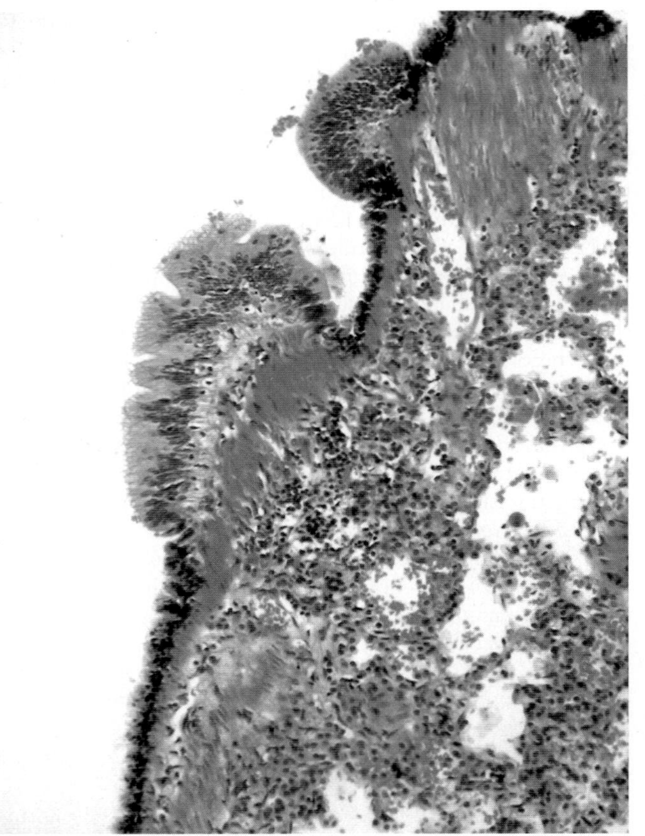

■ **FIGURE 17-19.** Type 1 CCAM. The cyst lining is mainly of respiratory type, although mucous cell hyperplasia is not infrequently seen. (See Color Plate 22.)

additional adverse effect on the prognosis. Occasional cases present later in childhood with infection. Macroscopically, the lesions are spongelike, comprising multiple small cysts. Microscopically, the cystic airspaces relate to a relative overgrowth of dilated bronchiolar structures that are separated by alveolar tissue, which appears comparatively underdeveloped. Occasional examples contain striated muscle, although this has no clinical significance.

Type 3 CCAMs are uncommon and occur almost exclusively in male infants. They typically involve and expand a whole lobe, the others being compressed. It may cause hypoplasia in the remaining pulmonary tissue. Macroscopically, lesions appear solid and not cystic. Microscopically, there is an excess of bronchiolar structures separated by airspaces that resemble late fetal lung. There is also a virtual absence of small, medium, and large pulmonary arteries within the lesion. Some regard this lesion as identical to pulmonary hyperplasia.[45]

Type 4 CCAMs are also very rare and comprise peripheral thin-walled cysts that are often multiloculated. The cystic spaces are typically lined by alveolar type I or type II cells, with the intervening stroma being thin and comprising loose mesenchymal tissue (Fig. 17-20). Their etiology is obscure, but there may be a spectrum of disease between these lesions and type 1 pleuropulmonary blastomas. Indeed, if the stroma of a suspected type 4 CCAM is even focally hypercellular, classification and management as type 1 pleuropulmonary blastoma is recommended by some groups.[45,46]

TREATMENT DECISIONS IN CONGENITAL CYSTIC LUNG DISEASE

Definitive treatment is surgical excision. If the cystic lesion is causing significant symptoms, then the decision is easy. Once a previously asymptomatic cystic lesion has become infected, it is safe to assume that recurrent infections are inevitable, and the

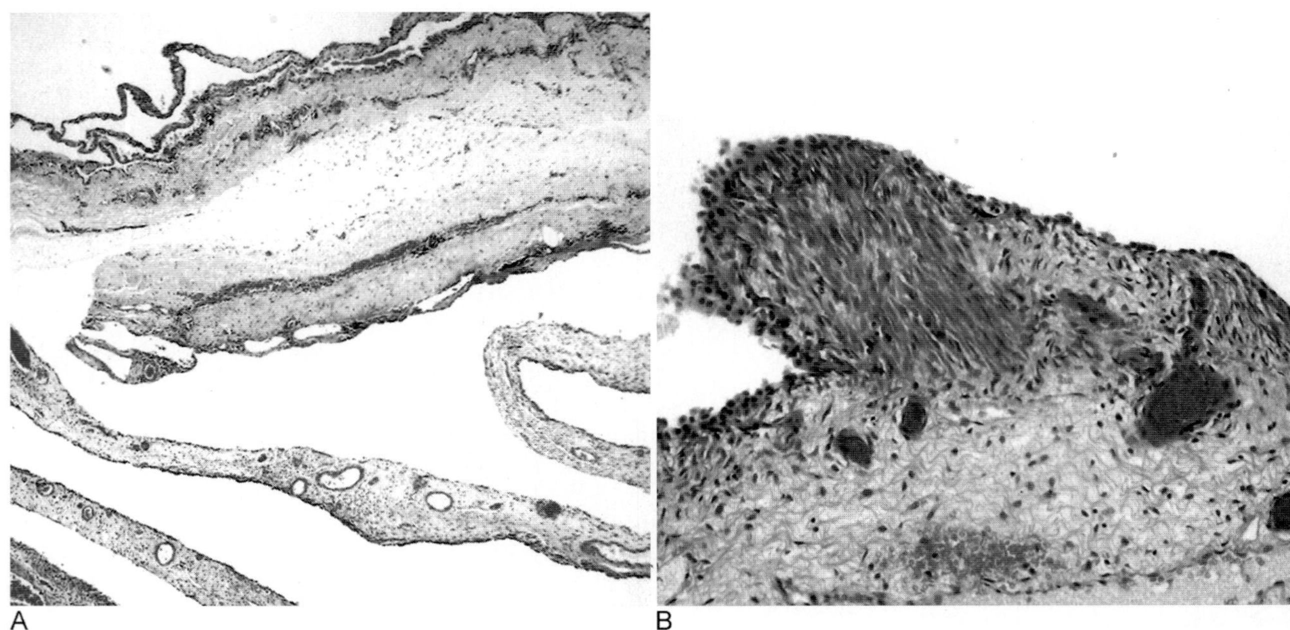

■ **FIGURE 17-20.** Type 4 CCAM. **A,** These cysts are lined typically by pneumocytes with loose and myxoid fibrous stroma comprising the walls of variably sized thin-walled cysts. **B,** Care must be taken to ensure that no blastematous elements are present, which would then indicate a diagnosis of pleuropulmonary blastoma. (See Color Plate 23.)

lesion should be excised (Fig. 17-21). If the lesion is discovered as a chance finding on a chest radiograph, it is likely to be excised to establish the diagnosis and exclude a malignancy. It is in the area of the small, asymptomatic CTM discovered on antenatal ultrasound that most difficulty is encountered. If it is cystic, then it is likely (but unproven) that infection will occur sooner or later, and prophylactic excision is recommended by many.[47] It is said that all lesions should be excised to prevent malignant transformation, but there is little evidence in favor of this view (see later).

PULMONARY SEQUESTRATION

The classical definition of sequestration is pulmonary tissue that is isolated from normal functioning lung and is nourished by systemic arteries, although the separation may be purely vascular. The intrapulmonary variant is contained within otherwise normal lung parenchyma. The less common extralobar sequestration is divorced from and accessory to the lung. Sequestrations may also connect to the esophagus or stomach, as well as contain pancreatic tissue; they also may show histologic features of adenomatoid malformations. These complicated lesions are perhaps best classified pathologically as complex "bronchopulmonary-foregut malformation," if the simpler term *CTM* is not to be used.

Their etiology is far from understood, with various proposed theories. Some workers have suggested that intralobar sequestration is acquired when a focus of infection or scarring acquires its blood supply from a systemic collateral, basing this on the relative sparsity of other malformations associated with this type of sequestration and its rarity in perinatal autopsies. Those who believe sequestration to be congenital generally propose that accessory lung buds are fundamental to both forms of pulmonary sequestration and liken them to intestinal duplications, with subsequent acquisition of a blood supply from the nearest and most convenient source, which happens to be systemic.

Intralobar sequestrations are usually found in the posterior basal segment of the left lower lobe and extralobar sequestrations beneath the left lower lobe. About 15% of extralobar sequestrations are abdominal. The intralobar sequestration is encircled by visceral pleura and has no pleural separation from the rest of the lobe. The remainder of the affected lobe and lung is normal, unless secondary changes such as infection have supervened. More than half the cases of intralobar sequestration are diagnosed after adolescence, and symptoms in neonates and infants are uncommon. Extralobar sequestration is generally detected in infancy because of associated malformations and affects males four times more frequently than females. Though much rarer, intralobar sequestrations may also be associated with other malformations.

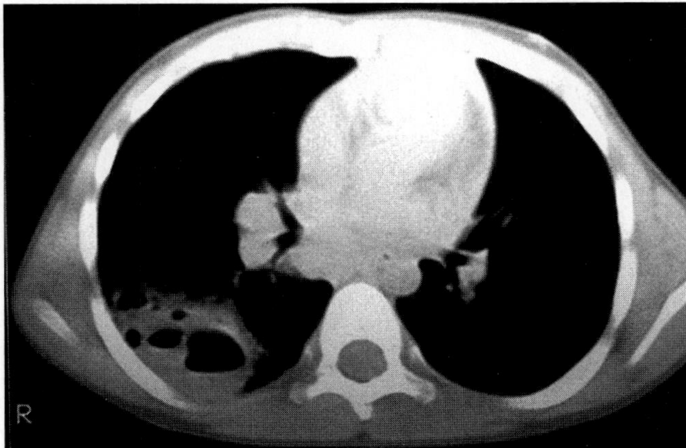

FIGURE 17-21. CT scan of a right-sided, thin-walled, multicystic CTM with air-fluid levels. The CTM is the seat of recurrent infection.

Both types of sequestration have certain similar pathologic characteristics as well as clear-cut differences. In both types, the pulmonary tissue is largely cystic and contains disorganized, airless alveoli, bronchi, cartilage, respiratory epithelium, and a systemic artery. It is often secondarily infected, bronchiectatic, or atelectatic, and may show histology of a CCAM, particularly type 2 CCAM in extralobar variants.[48] The aberrant arteries may arise from the thoracic or abdominal aorta and, in the latter instance, may pierce the diaphragm and run through the pulmonary ligament before reaching the sequestration. The elastic vessel walls may become atherosclerotic, and the lumen varies considerably in size. In intralobar sequestrations, the systemic arteries are likely to be large, and the veins drain into the pulmonary system, while in extralobar variants, the systemic arteries are small and the venous drainage is likewise systemic through the azygos system.

Treatment of sequestration is surgical excision. As with CTMs, the vascular supply should be carefully delineated by preoperative investigations (see later) and embolization of aortopulmonary collaterals considered.

CONGENITAL LARGE HYPERLUCENT LOBE (CONGENITAL LOBAR EMPHYSEMA)

A rare condition, congenital large hyperlucent lobe presents in 50% of cases in the neonatal period, otherwise in early infancy. Some cases are caused by easily identifiable partial obstruction such as mucosal flaps or twisting of the lobe on its pedicle. However, in many cases, a deficiency of bronchial cartilage is thought to be the cause, leading to inappropriate collapse of the airway and the trapping of air. Histologically, the majority of cases show normal radial alveolar counts but with no apparent maturation with age when compared to age-matched controls, suggesting a postpartum arrest of acinar development within affected lung tissue. A minority of cases, however, show true alveolar hyperplasia with increased radial alveolar counts, this sometimes being referred to as a polyalveolar lobe.[49] The condition affects the left upper (42%), right middle (35%), right upper (21%), and lower lobes (2%). The affected lobe cannot deflate, but overdistends and displaces adjacent lobes, and subsequently the mediastinal structures. The emphysematous lobe may herniate into the contralateral hemithorax, usually through the anterior mediastinum. The condition may be diagnosed antenatally (see earlier), present as respiratory distress (often with consequent failure to thrive in infancy), or be a chance finding on a chest radiograph taken later in life.

Presentation in Infancy

Clinical features of infantile lobar emphysema are those suggestive of a tension pneumothorax: hyperresonance of the affected hemithorax associated with diminished breath sounds and deviation of mediastinal structures to the contralateral side. Usually, a chest radiograph will demonstrate a hyperlucent lobe with features of compression and collapse

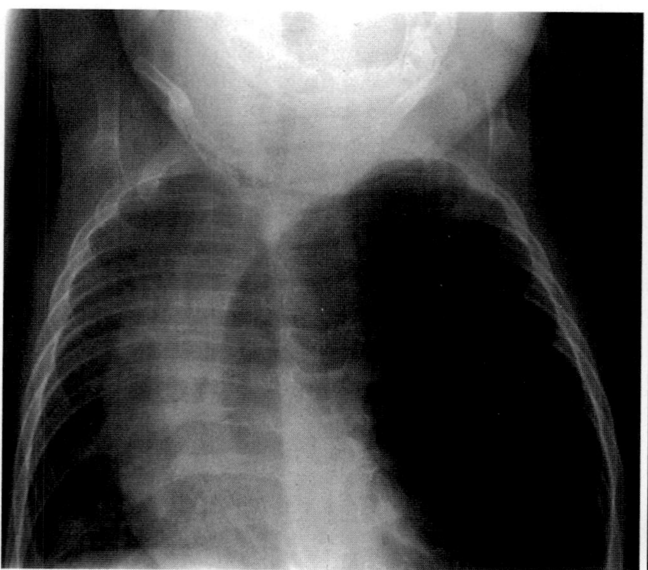

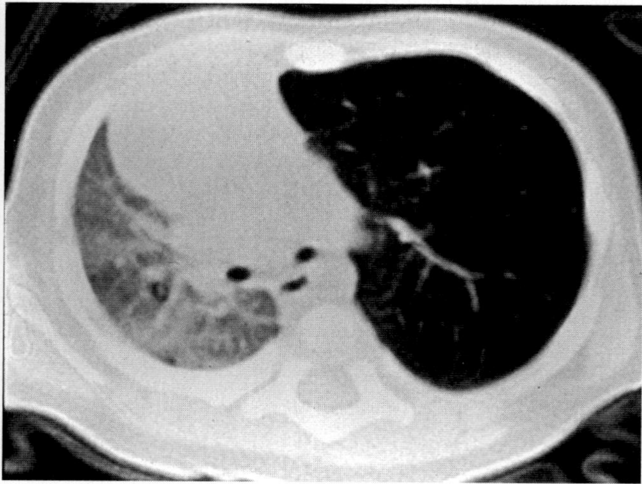

■ **FIGURE 17-22.** Chest radiograph and CT scan of a congenital large hyperlucent lobe (congenital lobar emphysema).

of adjacent lung and depression of the ipsilateral diaphragm (Fig. 17-22). The mediastinum is deviated, and the contralateral lung may be collapsed. Occasionally, initial chest radiographs may demonstrate an opaque lung field. This then clears and the affected lung becomes overinflated and hyperlucent on the radiograph. Ventilation-perfusion (V/Q) scanning may demonstrate delayed uptake and clearance of isotope and reduced blood flow in the affected lobe. This investigation is particularly useful if it is unclear whether the problem is a pathologically distended lobe on one side or a congenitally small contralateral lung, with secondary physiologic overexpansion. Bronchoscopy may reveal causes of intrinsic obstruction and permit the removal of a foreign body or inspissated secretions. An echocardiogram is valuable in evaluating the heart and great vessels, while a contrast CT scan is useful in evaluating the anatomy of the emphysematous lobe—its size and relations, and whether it has herniated into the contralateral hemithorax. It is useful in demonstrating the nature of adjacent lobes of the lung. This investigation is also useful in excluding contralateral pulmonary hypoplasia.

Differential Diagnosis

There are two broad groups of differential diagnoses. The first is any intrinsic or extrinsic cause of failure of airspace emptying. Intrinsic partial obstruction may result from inspissated mucus or aspirated material. Endobronchial granulomas due to endotracheal suction may result in obstruction of the airway as well.[50] Intrinsic obstruction due to bronchial atresia of the affected lobe is well recognized (Fig. 17-23). The affected parenchyma is ventilated collaterally, through the pores of Kohn, from adjacent normal lung. Extrinsic compression of bronchi due to congenital heart disease or anomalies of the great vessels usually presents as emphysematous changes of more gradual onset, often after the neonatal period. Less common causes of extrinsic compression include bronchogenic cysts. The second big group is any cause of loss of lung volume on the contralateral side. Other causes include absent lung, and lobar or lung collapse due to bronchial obstruction. Mediastinal shift with an opaque large lung, an occasional early finding in congenital large hyperlucent lobe, should be distinguished from other causes of unilateral opacification and contralateral mediastinal shift in the neonate, such as chylothorax, CDH, or airless congenital CTM.

Treatment

Those children who do not suffer respiratory compromise can be managed conservatively. Their outcome is comparable to that of those children managed by resection of an emphysematous lobe (Fig. 17-24); the distended emphysematous lobe does not compromise the growth and development of adjacent lung.[51] Lobectomy is indicated in the event of respiratory distress. The actual surgical technique is as for any other lobectomy.

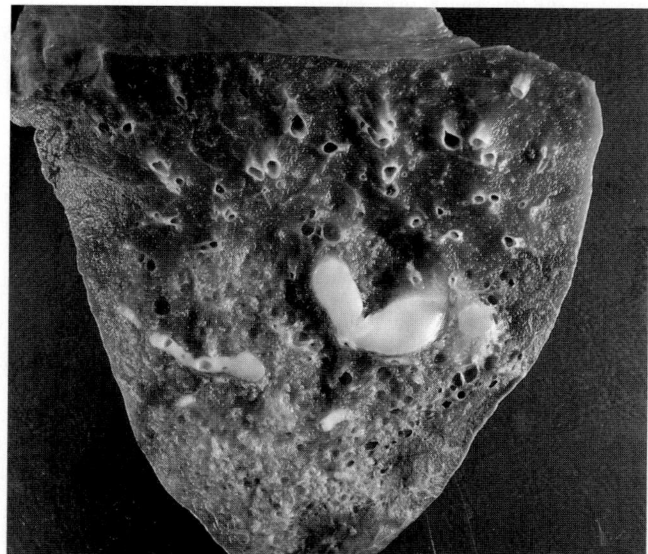

■ **FIGURE 17-23.** Bronchial atresia. The cut surface of the lung shows dilated airways plugged with mucus with surrounding microcystic changes. Dissection showed atresia at the origin of the apical segmental bronchus. (See Color Plate 24.)

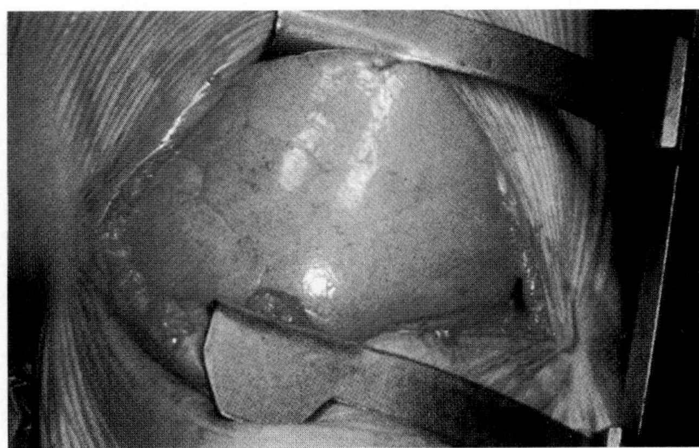

■ **FIGURE 17-24.** Surgery for congenital large hyperlucent lobe (congenital lobar emphysema). The hyperexpanded lobe protrudes out of the thoracotomy incision. (See Color Plate 25.)

Ventilation in this circumstance may be difficult. Low-pressure high-frequency oscillation has been advocated to prevent barotrauma to the affected lobe and further respiratory compromise to the adjacent lung.

■ ABNORMAL CONNECTIONS BETWEEN THE BRONCHIAL TREE AND OTHER STRUCTURES

■ TRACHEOESOPHAGEAL FISTULA AND ESOPHAGEAL ATRESIA

Pathology

If there is incomplete mesodermal separation of the primitive foregut, then a fistula may develop between the esophagus and the trachea (Fig. 17-25). Most commonly, they are associated with esophageal atresia, with about 85% of such cases being associated with a fistula. Typically, the proximal part of the esophagus ends in a blind sac and the distal part takes origin from the lower part of the trachea. The upper blind pouch is large and substantial, and usually ends about 8 cm from the superior alveolar ridge in the region of the azygos vein. Conversely, the lower esophageal segment is small and originates from the region of the distal posterior membranous trachea, carina, or right main stem bronchus.

Instances of communication between the trachea and the esophagus with an otherwise normal esophagus occur in about 3% of tracheoesophageal fistulas. Although symptoms from this congenital abnormality are fairly gross, the diagnosis is often delayed, with considerable respiratory morbidity due to aspiration and infection. The tracheoesophageal connection is almost always small, and the majority are found in the neck, from below the larynx to the thoracic inlet. Occasionally, a bronchus may communicate with the esophagus.

Associations

Tracheoesophageal fistula is more common in first and twin pregnancies of mothers of increasing age. About two thirds have an associated abnormality of some sort.[52] Of the live births, 20% have birth weight below the fifth centile. More than 50% of infants with esophageal atresia have associated anomalies. These are most common in pure esophageal atresia without fistula and least common in H-type fistula. The acronym VATER initially described vertebral, anal, tracheoesophageal, radial, and renal anomalies. This was then modified to VACTERL to include cardiac and limb problems. Infants with this association have a high mortality rate. Almost 80% have cardiac anomalies, these being the principal cause of death. Esophageal disease is also part of the CHARGE syndrome (coloboma, heart disease, choanal atresia, retarded growth, genital hypoplasia, and ear [deafness] abnormalities), which carries a high mortality. Chromosomal abnormalities are reported in 6% of cases, in trisomy 13, 18, and 21 in particular.[53] Other associations include Potter's syndrome (bilateral renal agenesis), Pierre Robin, polysplenia, and DiGeorge sequences. The incidence of cardiac anomalies has been reported to be between 30% and 50% in various series. There is also a significant incidence (47%) of tracheobronchial anomalies[54] ranging from tracheomalacia, abnormal nonciliated epithelium, lung agenesis, and hypoplasia or ectopic bronchi, to glossoptosis and airway obstruction. Pharyngeal function and aspiration on deglutition is common. The incidence of vertebral and skeletal anomalies, ranging from sacral agenesis, hemivertebrae, and rib and radial anomalies is 20% to 50% overall. Cases with associated cleft lip[55] and duodenal atresia are higher risk.

Presentation

The incidence of esophageal atresia is 1 in 2500. Maternal polyhydramnios has been reported in 85% of cases with pure esophageal atresia and 32% of those associated with tracheoesopheal fistula. Diagnosis by antenatal ultrasound is unreliable, with up to 50% false positives.[52] At birth the baby is commonly frothing, choking, and suffering cyanotic episodes despite oral suction. If the condition is suspected, the initial examination

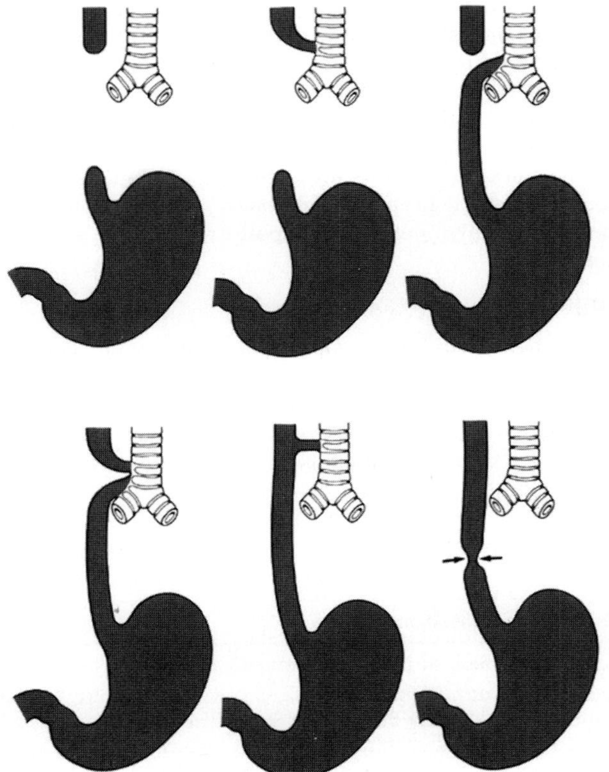

■ **FIGURE 17-25.** Types of tracheoesophageal fistulas.

TABLE 17-10. Waterson classification of esophageal atresia, with survival figures

Group	Classification	Survival
A	Birth weight >2500 g, otherwise well	100%
B	Birth weight 2000–2500 g, otherwise well Birth weight >2500 g, moderate anomalies Noncardiac anomalies including patent ductus arteriosus Ventricular septal defect and atrial septal defect	85%
C	Birth weight <2000 g, severe cardiac anomalies	65%

should be carefully performed to identify any associated anomalies. The effect of birth weight and associated anomalies on survival is given in Tables 17-10 and 17-11. An attempt should be made to pass an orogastric tube. Acid fluid may be aspirated from the tube if gastric contents reflux into the upper pouch across the fistula. A plain radiograph will demonstrate the tube coiled in the upper pouch and may identify pulmonary abnormalities such as consolidation of the right upper lobe due to aspiration, plethoric lung fields due to cardiac anomalies, and vertebral and rib anomalies. The radiograph will reveal the presence or absence of gas in the stomach, indicating the presence or absence of a tracheoesophageal fistula. The intestinal gas pattern should be carefully examined on the abdominal radiograph to try to exclude distal intestinal atresia. An echocardiogram is useful to identify intracardiac structural anomalies and the possibility of a right-sided aortic arch.

Preoperative Care

The preoperative care for this condition should start from the moment it is suspected. Continuous suction of the oropharynx is important to reduce the risk of aspiration and thus protect the airway. A sump sucker such as a replogle tube is useful, since it permits continuous suction and protects the esophageal mucosa from direct suction-related trauma.[56] Cyanotic episodes have been reported with the use of this form of suction of the upper pouch. This is thought to be due to the generation of excessive negative pressure causing ineffective inspiration. The infant should be nursed prone. If pulmonary consolidation is identified, then physiotherapy and postural drainage should be employed.

Surgery

A right thoractomy[57] by extrapleural approach with end-to-end single-layer anastomosis and division of fistula remains the most common technique for the majority of children presenting with esophageal atresia and tracheoesophageal fistula. Routinely, the infant is fed by a transanastomotic tube. The use of intercostal drains and postoperative contrast studies varies between institutions and cases.[58] A variety of approaches have been proposed for those cases of esophageal atresia with a large distal fistula presenting with respiratory compromise due to gastric distention: endotracheal intubation beyond the fistula orifice, Fogarty balloon occlusion of the fistula, and formation of gastrostomy. More recently, urgent thoracotomy and fistula ligation with primary or subsequent repair of the atresia has gained wider acceptance. Several pre- and perioperative techniques have been proposed for cases wherein the distance between the proximal and distal segments is wide. The absolute length of the gap is not so relevant as its relation to the size and strength of the wall of the esophageal segments. Per pouch bougienage either pre- or perioperatively to shorten the gap has been widely described and more recently modified.[59] Perioperative techniques to facilitate primary anastomosis include the use of circular, transverse, or spiral myotomies of the upper pouch. More recently, alternative techniques have been proposed to repair long-gap esophageal atresia.[59] An alternative approach, described by Scharli,[60] is to mobilize the gastric cardia into the chest by thoracoabdominal approach, permitting division of the left gastric artery. Favorable long-term results of this approach have been reported.[61] The primary thoracoscopic repair of esophageal atresia and tracheoesophageal fistula is well described. The possible advantages of this approach are being assessed.[62] Failing these techniques, then the only option may be esophageal replacement by colonic, ileocolic, or gastric interposition. Each technique is associated with vagotomy and requires a gastric drainage procedure. Proponents of each approach have described good results. More recently, gastric transposition has become a well-established substitute for esophageal replacement.[63]

TABLE 17-11. Spitz classification of esophageal atresia, with survival figures

Group	Classification	Survival
I	Birth weight >1500 g without congenital heart disease	97%
II	Birth weight <1500 g or major congenital heart disease	59%
III	Birth weight <1500 g and major congenital heart disease	22%

Postoperative Course

Even after completely successful surgery, tracheomalacia is common, and the well-known brassy "tracheoesophageal fistula cough" (TOF-cough) a feature. Recurrent aspiration leading to bronchitis and bronchopneumonia is frequent. A missed diagnosis of laryngeal cleft should always be considered (see earlier). Occasionally, tracheomalacia may be so severe as to be life threatening, but generally the cough sounds more impressive than the consequences. Up to 17% of patients may require fundoplication for postoperative gastroesophageal reflux, and 25% have dysphagia at 2 years.[52] The early mortality associated with this condition is often related to the associated malformations. The long-term outcome is good.[64]

OTHER ABNORMAL CONNECTIONS

Rare cases of direct communication between the bronchial tree and congenital cysts have been described. Congenital bronchobiliary fistula as part of upper gastrointestinal tract duplication is a source of bile in respiratory secretions. Rarely, a CTM may connect with the stomach and be associated with abdominal visceral malrotation.

CONGENITAL DISEASE OF THE PULMONARY ARTERIAL TREE

When surgery is contemplated for any CTM, it is important that any abnormal vasculature is identified in advance. Inadvertent severing of anomalous systemic arteries has led to fatal hemorrhage, whereas ligation of anomalous veins from adjacent nonsequestered lung has led to infarction of normal tissue. The pulmonary and systemic arterial trees must be considered separately. Systemic arterial abnormalities of the great vessels of the mediastinum can be separated into those of the bronchial circulation (normally 1% to 2% of the left ventricular output) and other pathologic collaterals. The pulmonary capillary bed may be bypassed, leading to direct arteriovenous communication, or absent, resulting in minimal pulmonary arteriovenous connections.

DISORDERS OF PULMONARY ARTERY ARRANGEMENT

Pulmonary arterial and venous arrangement generally mirrors bronchial arrangement. Exceptions to this rule include congenital origin of the left pulmonary artery from the right (pulmonary artery sling) (Fig. 17-26). Presentation is as with any vascular ring (see earlier). In this condition, the left pulmonary artery has to traverse the mediastinum from left to right, compressing the trachea as it does so. There may also be a crossover arterial segment, with the right upper lobe supplied by a branch from the left pulmonary artery, so preoperative pulmonary angiography is essential. Surgical repair of a sling with a crossover may result in infarction of the right upper lobe if the abnormal vessel has not been discovered. Another association is complete cartilage rings, and the infant should be evaluated for this anomaly, probably before undergoing surgery. Isolated crossover pulmonary artery branches in the absence of bronchial crossover are occasionally seen. They cross the mediastinum to supply lung segments, which often are abnormal in other ways.

ABSENT OR SMALL PULMONARY ARTERY

Either lung may be affected by unilateral absence of a pulmonary artery, and the defect may be isolated or associated with other cardiovascular anomalies, typically tetralogy of Fallot with an absent left pulmonary artery and patent ductus arteriosus with an absent right pulmonary artery. There is an association with absent pulmonary valve syndrome. Symptoms may not arise until adult life, when they are generally due to pulmonary infection or hemorrhage. When there is only a short section absent, patients may be amenable to surgical correction, but usually the pulmonary vasculature is absent in much of the lung; histologic examination reveals hypertrophied bronchial arteries and often areas of dense fibrous scarring (Fig. 17-27). Normal pulmonary blood flow in utero and in the early postnatal period is needed for normal lung development. Before birth, less than 5% of the cardiac output reaches distal to the arterial duct, so it may seem surprising that interference with this small flow leads to underdevelopment of the alveolar bed and its vasculature, but there is considerable experimental evidence and clinical observation to confirm that this is so. Congenitally small unilateral pulmonary artery is usually seen in association with an ipsilateral small lung. However, it is unclear whether the primary abnormality is related to blood flow or whether both the small lung and the abnormal blood supply are due to an unknown primary event.

Pulmonary stenosis may affect lobar and segmental vessels as well as the main pulmonary arteries, and the narrowings may be multiple. Unilateral absence of a pulmonary artery leads to the lung on that side receiving only systemic blood, either through anomalous systemic arteries or enlarged bronchial arteries. People with isolated unilateral absence may lead a normal life, or

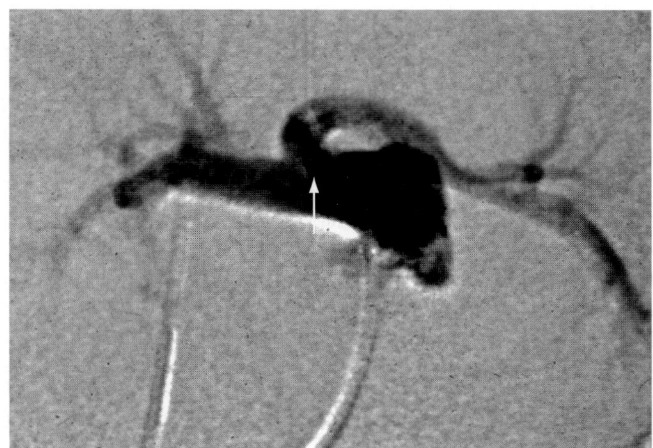

FIGURE 17-26. Digital subtraction angiogram of a pulmonary artery sling. The left pulmonary artery takes origin from the right pulmonary artery *(arrow)*.

symptoms may not arise until adult life; one third remain completely asymptomatic. Symptoms include pulmonary infection or bleeding from bronchopulmonary anastomoses. Ipsilateral lung tumor and pulmonary hypertension have been reported.[65] Clinically, the condition may be difficult to distinguish from embolic occlusion and obliterative bronchiolitis. The presence of other congenital defects would militate against these, and the absence of mosaic attenuation on CT scan would point away from obliterative bronchiolitis.

It is worth noting an iatrogenic complication related to an abnormal pulmonary blood supply in children with pulmonary valve atresia and supply of the lungs solely by systemic arterial blood. In the surgical procedure of unifocalization, the

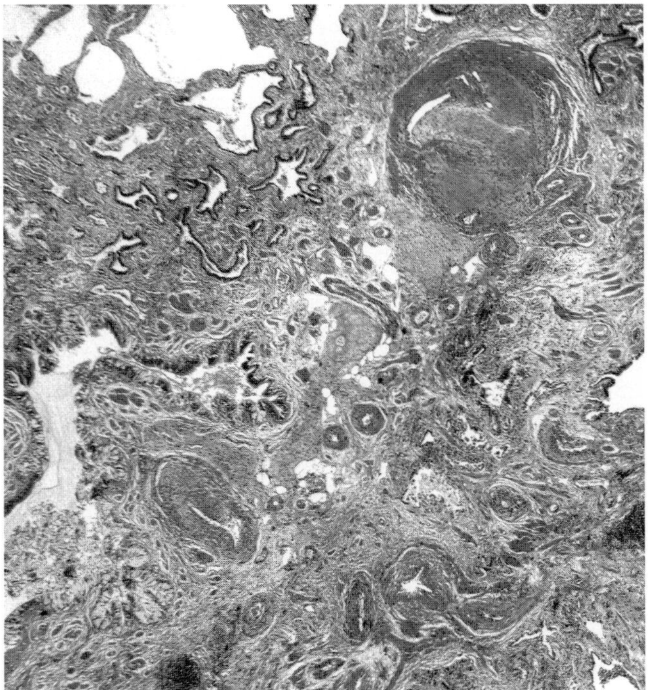

FIGURE 17-27. Absence of the pulmonary artery. The parenchyma lacks pulmonary arteries but instead shows very prominent bronchial arteries. (See Color Plate 26.)

collateral circulation is used to create an artificial trunk supplying the whole of the lung, which can then be anastomosed to the right ventricle via a conduit. We have reported on children with severe postoperative bronchial ischemia and even total infarction, as a result of excessively vigorous stripping of the bronchial circulation from the airways (Fig. 17-28).[66]

Anomalous systemic arteries supplying the lung may be associated with any CTM or even be an isolated finding.[67] They are also found if the pulmonary artery is absent and may also be part of complex arteriovenous malformations. They may also be an isolated finding. One or both pulmonary arteries may take origin from the aorta.[68] Bilateral origin from the aorta is part of the spectrum of common arterial trunk and usually will present to the pediatric or fetal cardiologist. Unilateral origin of a pulmonary artery from the aorta may be an isolated abnormality, sometimes presenting with persistent tachypnea.

CONGENITAL DISEASE OF THE SYSTEMIC ARTERIAL TREE

Two groups of abnormalities are relevant to the lung. The first includes those producing a vascular ring. Although numerous variations from the normal aortic arch development have been reported, only a few distinct patterns can produce extrinsic tracheal obstruction, and even these may be incidental findings without clinical correlation. The most likely types that compromise the trachea and esophagus, singly or together, are (1) right aortic arch with left ligamentum arteriosum or patent ductus arteriosus, (2) double aortic arch, (3) anomalous innominate or left carotid artery, (4) aberrant right subclavian artery, usually in association with a diverticulum of Kommerell (Fig. 17-29), and (5) pulmonary artery sling (see Fig. 17-26) (origin of left pulmonary artery from right pulmonary artery, sometimes with a crossover segment from the left artery supplying the right upper lobe). Right aortic arch and double aortic arch account for the largest number. The common denominator in these arch anomalies is compression and narrowing of the tracheoesophageal complex. Presentation is with stridor, or steroid-resistant asthma, and surgical treatment is recommended. If there is doubt about the extent of any compression, for example, in the case of right aortic arch and aberrant right subclavian artery, which may be a normal variant, then a preoperative bronchoscopy should be performed. The second group of systemic arterial abnormalities includes collateral vessels arising from the aorta and supplying all or part of one or both lungs, or a CTM. These vessels may be hypertrophied bronchial arteries or abnormal nonbronchial arteries; there may be multiple collaterals.[69] This last group may be seen in association with direct pulmonary arteriovenous connections ("PAVMs"). Aneurysm of aortopulmonary collateral vessels has been described.

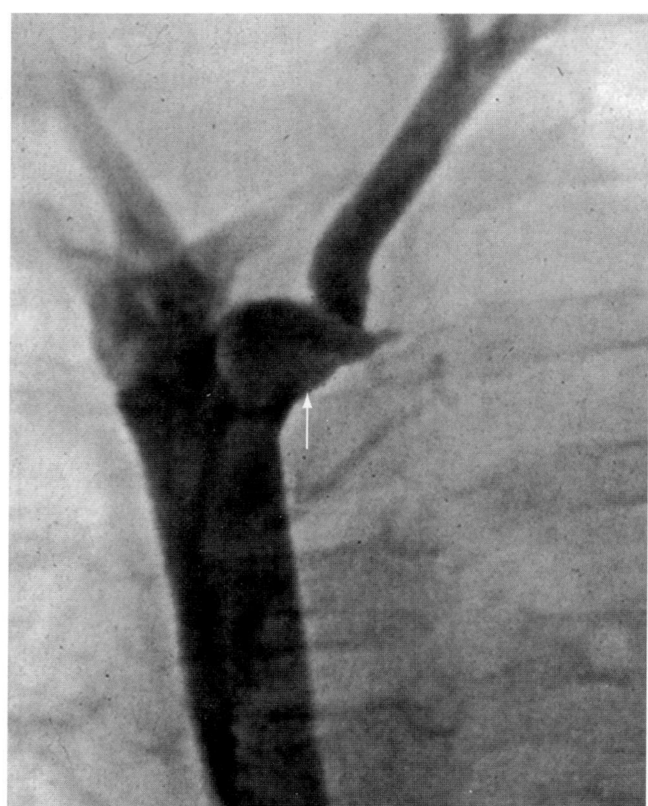

FIGURE 17-29. Digital subtraction angiogram showing a right-sided aortic arch, with aberrant origin of left subclavian artery from a diverticulum of Kommerell *(arrow)*. A left-sided ligamentum arteriosum completed the vascular ring.

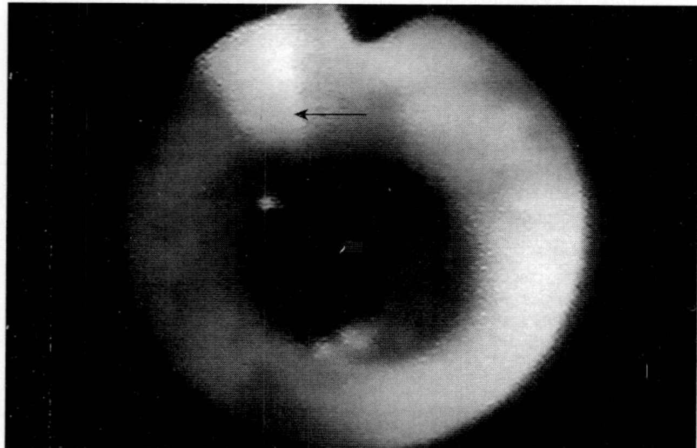

FIGURE 17-28. Iatrogenic complete infarction of the trachea, which is black and necrotic. The child had undergone a unifocalization procedure, in which the bronchial arteries had been stripped from the airways and anastomosed to create a pulmonary trunk. The child is intubated, and the line *(arrowed)* marks the endotracheal tube. (See Color Plate 27.)

Dieulafoy's disease is most commonly found in the gastrointestinal tract, but a few cases have been reported in the lung. Patients generally present with massive hemoptysis and are found to have an isolated bronchial artery that is often dilated and tortuous, running within the subepithelial stroma.

CONGENITAL DISEASE OF THE PULMONARY VENOUS TREE

ABNORMAL PULMONARY VENOUS DRAINAGE

Anomalous pulmonary veins result in blood from the lungs returning to the right side of the heart rather than entering the left atrium. The anomalous veins may join the inferior caval vein or hepatic, portal, or splenic veins below the diaphragm, or above the diaphragm they may drain into the superior caval vein or its tributaries, the coronary sinus, or the right atrium. Anomalous pulmonary venous drainage may be obstructed

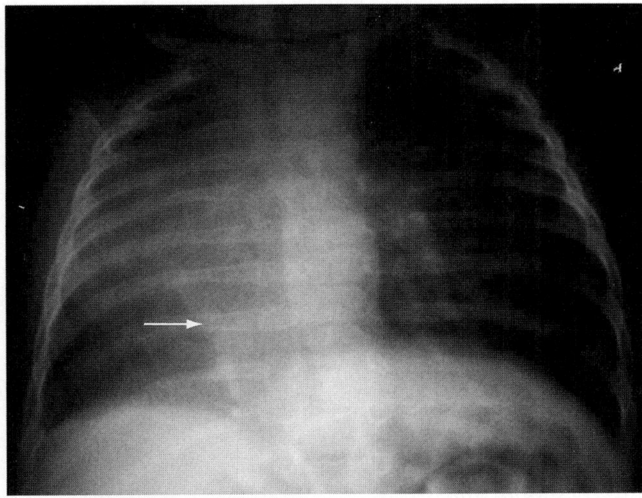

■ **FIGURE 17-30.** Scimitar syndrome (congenital small right lung, venous drainage to the inferior caval vein). The abnormal right-sided venous drainage is *arrowed.*

or unobstructed. The anomaly may be total or partial, unilateral or bilateral, and isolated or associated with other cardiopulmonary developmental defects. These include bronchial isomerism, mirror-image arrangement, asplenia, pulmonary stenosis, patent arterial duct, and a small interatrial communication. The type of isomerism gives a good indication as to whether the anomaly is total or partial, right-sided isomerism suggesting totally anomalous veins and left-sided isomerism suggesting a partial anomaly. Occasionally, the anomalous vein runs much of its course buried within the lung substance. Anomalous pulmonary venous connections are often narrow, and this may cause relatively mild pulmonary hypertension. Unilateral anomalous venous drainage may be part of complex lung malformations; it may also be seen in association with what appears to be a simple lung cyst. This underscores the need for accurate delineation of all abnormalities even in straightforward-appearing cases. Minor abnormalities of venous connection, such as a segment draining directly into the azygos system, are not uncommon and usually not of practical significance.

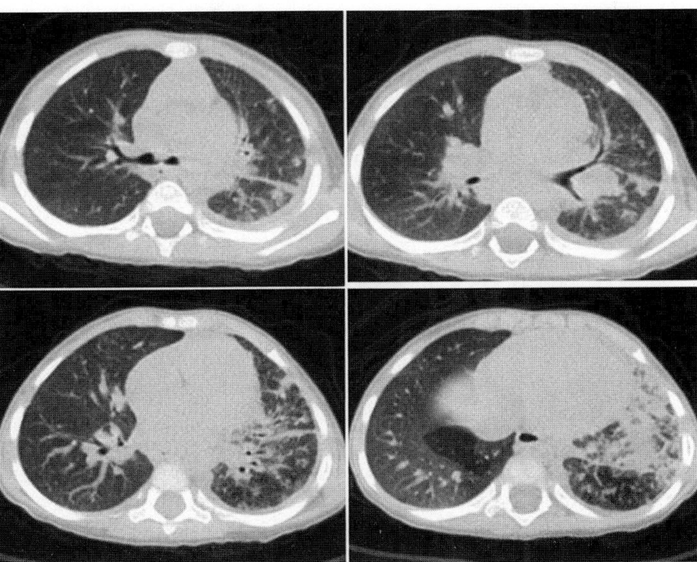

■ **FIGURE 17-31.** CT scan showing changes associated with absent left pulmonary veins. The left lung is engorged, with dilated lymphatic vessels and a left-sided pleural effusion.

The scimitar syndrome is a particular clinical problem characterized by a small right lung, resulting in the heart moving to the right (cardiac dextroposition), and an abnormal band shadow representing the abnormal venous drainage to the systemic veins (Fig. 17-30), fancifully compared to a scimitar (a sign that is in fact often absent). Infants with this condition presenting in heart failure have a worse prognosis, often because of associated abnormalities, among which may be malformations in the left side of the heart. Aortopulmonary collaterals should be sought and occluded. More invasive treatment options include reimplantation of the vein or pneumonectomy. Severe pulmonary hypertension is an adverse prognostic feature. An association with horseshoe lung has been described; this usually causes early death, but occasional long-term survival has been reported.[70,71]

CONGENITAL ABSENCE OF THE PULMONARY VEINS

Absence of the pulmonary veins or narrowing of their ostia into the left atrium results in pulmonary venous obstruction. It may also be associated with partial anomalous pulmonary venous drainage. The atresia may be unilateral (Fig. 17-31) or bilateral, but in either case severe hypertensive changes develop in both lungs. Congenital pulmonary vein atresia carries a very poor prognosis; few children with the condition survive longer than a year. Stenting open the ostia via cardiac catheterization has been reported.

ABNORMALITIES OF THE CONNECTIONS BETWEEN THE PULMONARY ARTERIAL AND VENOUS TREES

Congenital alveolar capillary dysplasia (misalignment of lung vessels) represents a failure of capillaries to grow in appropriate number and location within the alveolar tissue of the lung, often associated with abnormally sited pulmonary veins within bronchovascular bundles, and is an unusual cause of congenital pulmonary hypertension, persistent fetal circulation, and respiratory distress in the newborn. It is discussed in detail in Chapter 18.

PAVMs constitute an important group of abnormalities that potentially involves systemic and pulmonary arterial and venous trees (Fig. 17-32). They represent a direct intrapulmonary connection between pulmonary artery and vein without an intervening capillary bed. This cavernous arteriovenous aneurysm is an uncommon cause of symptoms in the pediatric age group and is often diagnosed in adults. Presentation is with cyanosis, hemoptysis, or neurologic complications (see later). The chest radiograph may be normal, but more usually well-defined single or multiple opacities are seen, with vessels connecting them to the hila, which are strongly suggestive of the diagnosis.

Fistulas occur in the lower lobes in about 60% of cases; they are single in 60% and unilateral in 75%. Many cases of pulmonary arteriovenous fistulas are associated with hereditary hemorrhagic telangiectasia (HHT; Osler-Weber-Rendu disease). HHT is a genetic vascular disorder characterized by epistaxis, telangiectases, and visceral manifestations including PAVMs. The two known disease types, HHT1 and HHT2, are caused by mutations in the endoglin *(ENG)* and *ACVRL1 (ALK-1)* genes, respectively.[72,73] Macroscopically, lesions can be peripheral or central and may simulate a saccular, cavernous hemangioma because of its aneurysmal swelling. The fistula is fed by at least one afferent artery, usually pulmonary and less often bronchial, and may be drained by several veins, almost always pulmonary. In 80%, there is a single feeding pulmonary artery and a single draining pulmonary vein. There are numerous communications between artery and vein in this tortuous, dilated, wormlike vessel mass. On microscopic examination, the arteriovenous fistula is lined with vascular endothelium. Diagnosis is suspected on imaging (see earlier) and confirmed by documenting an abnormal right-to-left shunt at the pulmonary vascular level, either by contrast echocardiography (the contrast being a peripheral injection of microbubbles) or a technetium Tc 99m macroaggregate lung perfusion scan, with shunt quantification by counting over the kidneys and brain. Contrast echocardiography should be used to screen patients with HHT for PAVMs.

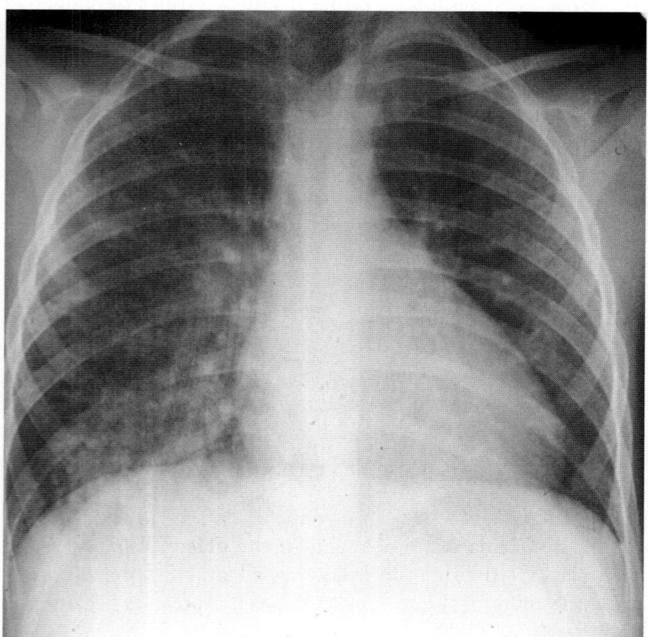

FIGURE 17-32. Chest radiograph showing several pulmonary arteriovenous fistulas, in particular in the right lower lobe.

The large connections may have both a systemic and a pulmonary arterial supply (see earlier). It is important to know if there is a systemic component, since this may cause high-output cardiac failure. Furthermore, whereas embolization of an abnormal pulmonary arteriovenous connection via the feeding pulmonary artery may be curative, more extensive procedures may be needed to deal with systemic arterial components.

Complications of PAVMs are related to the bypassing of the filtration function of the pulmonary circulation, and hyperviscosity due to the polycythemia secondary to systemic arterial hypoxemia. Pulmonary hypertension does not develop, because there is no alveolar hypoxemia. The patient may develop systemic, in particular cerebral, abscess or thrombosis.

Embolization of PAVMs is the preferred treatment option, even if they are extensive. If the child is treated before puberty, further embolizations may be needed after the pubertal growth spurt. Although lung transplantation has been reported for this condition, the results are clearly inferior. Multiple procedures may be necessary. In one series, one third of patients obtained normal oxygen saturation and 15% an improved exercise tolerance, and generally embolization, even of major, multiple PAVMs is preferable to transplantation.[74] Diffuse microscopic disease is more difficult to treat, but there is some evidence that embolization may reduce the prevalence of neurologic complications.

CONGENITAL DISEASE OF THE LYMPHATIC TREE

This tree is the hardest to delineate, and in most malformations it will not be relevant. Lymphatic tree disorders usually require histologic confirmation. Lymphatic hypoplasia of varied distribution underlies the yellow nail syndrome in which lymphedema is accompanied by discoloration of the nails and pleural effusions. Though inherited, it may not be manifest until adult life. The Klippel-Trenaunay syndrome, usually characterized by varicosities of systemic veins, cutaneous hemangiomas, and soft tissue hypertrophy, is another congenital disorder in which pleuropulmonary abnormalities are described, including pulmonary lymphatic hyperplasia, pleural effusions, pulmonary thromboembolism, and pulmonary vein varicosities. Congenital chylothorax is described in Chapter 18.

Congenital pulmonary lymphangiectasia may be either secondary to obstruction to pulmonary lymphatic or venous drainage, or primary, the latter either limited to the lung or part of generalized lymphangiectasia. There is a high association of primary pulmonary lymphangiectasia with other congenital abnormalities, particularly asplenia and cardiac anomalies. It causes severe respiratory distress and has been generally thought to be fatal in the neonatal period, but milder cases with prolonged survival have been described, and indeed presentation may be delayed until adult life.[75,76] The lungs are heavy, with widened interlobular septa, and on the visceral pleural surface there is a pronounced reticular pattern of small cysts that accentuates the lobular architecture of the lungs. The cysts measure up to 5 mm in diameter and are situated in the interlobular septa and about the bronchovascular bundles. Near the hila of the lungs, the cysts are elongated. Microscopy confirms that the cysts are located in connective tissue under the pleura, in the interlobular septa, and about the bronchioles and arteries. Serial sections show that they are part of an intricate network of intercommunicating channels that vary greatly in width and are devoid of valves. The cysts are lined by an attenuated simple endothelium. The absence of multinucleate foreign body giant cell reaction distinguishes this condition from interstitial emphysema. The clinical history is also usually quite different; interstitial emphysema is usually a complication of positive pressure ventilation in a very preterm infant.

OTHER RELEVANT ISSUES

CONGENITAL DISORDERS OF THE CHEST WALL

Disorders of the bony ribcage and scoliosis are described in Chapter 51. Here we concentrate on diaphragmatic disorders. Disorders of fetal breathing movements are beyond the scope of this chapter, but these are essential for normal lung development. The abdomen is part of the chest wall, and any disorder that increases abdominal contents before birth, such as fetal ascites or a large tumor, will impede lung development and cause bilateral CSL.

Congenital Diaphragmatic Hernia

Pathologic Anatomy

Eighty percent of CDHs are left-sided, through the left pleuroperitoneal canal. Bilateral CDHs are rare. The defect is within the diaphragm itself; there is usually no associated membranous sac. The diaphragm itself may be well developed or significantly deficient, especially at its origin from the 12th rib. Intestine, stomach, liver, and spleen may all herniate into the chest. A nonmuscular membranous sac is present in 10% to 15% of cases, signifying the early occurrence of this lesion before closure of the pleuroperitoneal canal. Associations of this condition are discussed under antenatal presentation (see earlier).

Postnatal Presentation

The diagnosis of CDH is usually made antenatally. From birth infants may present with a variety of symptoms and signs. Typically, the abdomen is scaphoid (Fig. 17-33), the chest funnel-shaped, the trachea and mediastinum deviated to the contralateral side. The infant may be entirely well or suffer from several problems ranging from choking episodes to apneas to acute respiratory failure. Rare late presentation may be associated with

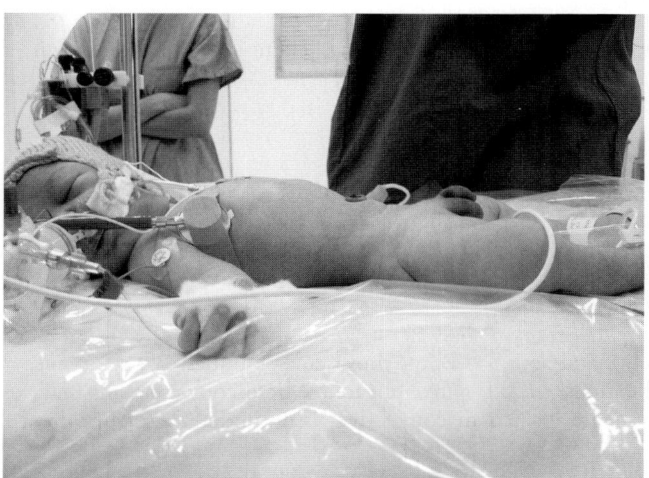

FIGURE 17-33. Scaphoid abdomen in CDH.

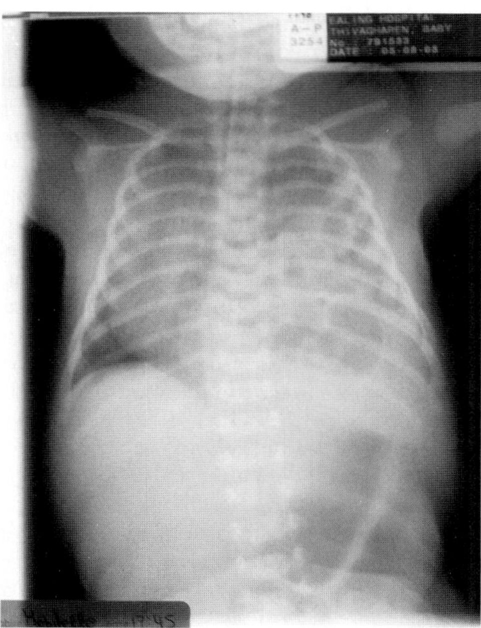

FIGURE 17-34. Plain radiograph demonstrating left-sided CDH. There are obvious gas-filled loops of bowel in the chest.

chronic gastrointestinal symptoms.[77] The diagnosis of CDH is confirmed by a plain radiograph of the chest and abdomen (Fig. 17-34), after the passage of a nasogastric tube. The plain film is a poor indication of the degree of pulmonary hypoplasia.[78] If doubt persists, then an ultrasound scan of the chest demonstrating intrathoracic intestinal peristalsis is helpful. An echocardiogram should be performed to exclude intracardiac anomalies; fetal echocardiography should, however, have been part of the antenatal diagnostic work-up. The postnatal differential diagnosis of CDH is similar to the prenatal one and includes extensive congenital cystic disease of the lung, Morgagni anterior diaphragmatic hernia, paraesophageal hiatus hernia, and eventration of the diaphragm.

Surgery

The management of CDH is no longer regarded as a surgical emergency. The initial management is to stabilize the baby and optimize respiratory function. Delayed surgical repair has become generally more accepted, with lower mortality rates than have been seen with immediate repair. The exact timing of surgery remains controversial. Many studies have reported varying periods of delay before surgery. One of the principal advantages of this strategy has been related to pulmonary artery pressures falling toward more normal values.[79] The operative repair may be by thoracotomy, or by subcostal or transverse abdominal approaches. The advantage of an abdominal approach is that it permits identification and correction of an associated intestinal malrotation. The laparoscopic repair of CDH has been described.[80] The principle of repair is as with any other hernia: reduction of herniated viscera, identification and excision of any hernia sac, and repair of the defect. Usually, repair may be achieved primarily following adequate mobilization of the defect's margins. Occasionally, this is not possible because the size of the defect prevents primary suture repair. In these circumstances, a prosthetic patch may be required. An autologous muscle flap is preferred by many surgeons.[81] Should anticoagulation therapy be required, if ECMO therapy is anticipated, then some surgeons would prefer to minimize any dissection to reduce the risk of postoperative bleeding secondary to anticoagulation for ECMO. In these circumstances, the mobilization of the defect margins is less and the use of prosthetic patches is greater. For the same reason, malrotation will not be corrected. An intercostal chest drain is placed in the ipsilateral hemithorax by some surgeons to drain any subsequent pneumothorax or chylothorax. The negative pressure associated with such a device has been reported to increase barotrauma to the hypoplastic lung.[82] Some surgeons will leave the drain in situ, only to have negative pressure applied in the event of an accumulation that requires drainage. Chylothorax complicating repair of CDH is well recognized. It may be a persistent complication associated with significant morbidity. Recently, octreotide has been advocated in the management of this complication.[83]

Outcome

Survival of neonates reportedly varies between 39% and 95% after repair of CDH.[41] The large variation in mortality reflects the varying severity of the pulmonary hypoplasia and abnormal pulmonary vascularity, as well as variations in the period and technique of preoperative stabilization, peri- and postoperative mechanical ventilation, and the use of ECMO. If ECMO has to be used, the outlook is not good. Only about one third of patients thus treated survive to a year of life, and substantial comorbidity (respiratory, gastrointestinal, neurodevelopmental) is common.[84] Stege and colleagues have demonstrated that the survival of this condition within one well-circumscribed geographic locus has remained unchanged over 11 years despite the advent of new therapies. The mortality increased with the presence of other malformations.[85] A variety of neurologic abnormalities, including motor and cognitive anomalies as well as gastroesophageal reflux and foregut dysmotility and skeletal anomalies, have been reported in infants surviving management of this condition.[86] Significant respiratory and nutritional problems associated with gastroesophageal reflux can occur but often tend to improve with time. Respiratory findings reported in survivors include a range of abnormalities on imaging, from a complete normal examination to ipsilateral lucency on the chest radiograph. Lung function may be normal, or there may be obstructive or restrictive disease. V/Q scans are almost invariably abnormal. Bronchial hyperreactivity is also described, but the pattern of challenge testing suggests distal airway dysfunction rather than airway inflammation. It is suggested that most of these functional abnormalities relate to the intensity of ventilation in the perioperative period, rather than the degree of pulmonary hypoplasia at birth. However, pulmonary hypoplasia is obviously a critical determinant of survival. The incidence of gastroesophageal reflux has been reported as higher in those diaphragmatic hernias that were repaired directly.[87] Postoperative failure to thrive due to gastroesophageal reflux and oral dysfunction is common. The overall outcome of the condition is known to be worse when it is found to occur within certain syndromes such as Fryn's.[41]

Anterior Diaphragmatic Hernia

Anterior diaphragmatic hernias occur through the foramen of Morgagni (Fig. 17-35)—a potential space that transmits the internal mammary artery, lying between the sternal and costal attachments of the diaphragm. They are much rarer than Bochdalek's hernia and tend not to present in the neonatal period. If unilateral, they occur more often on the right than the left and are almost always associated with a hernial sac. Often, these hernias are bilateral, and the hernial sacs may communicate with each other or with the pericardium.[88] Anterior diaphragmatic hernias may occur as an isolated morphologic malformation but are often associated with cardiac anomalies and are the diaphragmatic defect associated with the pentalogy of Cantrell. The principles of repair are similar to those for Bochdalek's hernia. Since the diaphragmatic defect is smaller and more easily repaired, prosthetic patches or autologous grafts are far less frequently required than with Bochdalek's hernia. Abdominal and thoracic approaches have been described for open repair.[89] Laparoscopic repair is now well established.[90] The long-term outcome following repair is excellent, principally determined by the nature of any associated anomalies. There may be mild airflow obstruction and bronchial hyperreactivity to methacholine, possibly related

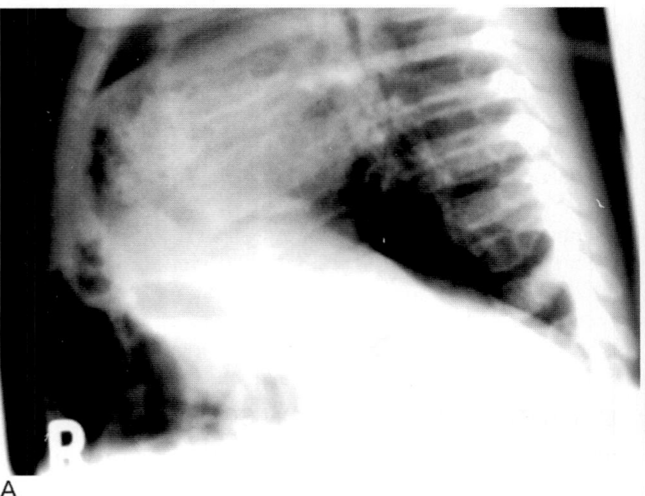

A

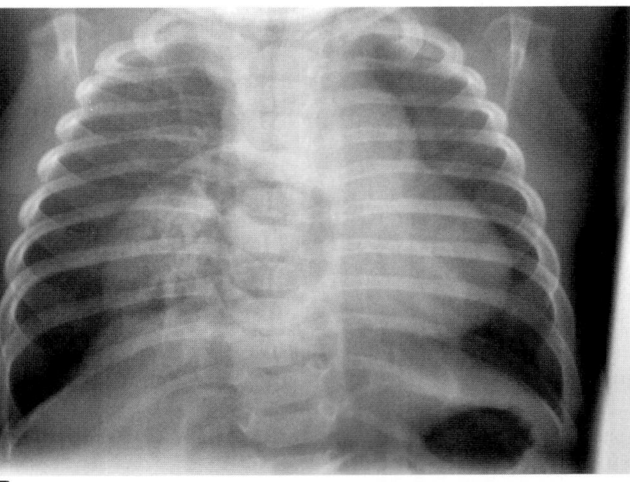

B

FIGURE 17-35. Lateral (**A**) and posteroanterior (**B**) chest radiographs showing a Morgagni hernia.

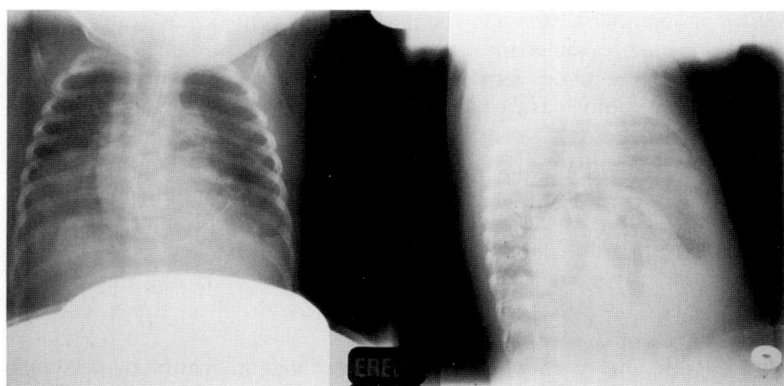

FIGURE 17-36. Bilateral eventrations of the diaphragm.

to distal airway dysfunction. Chest asymmetry and scoliosis are also not uncommon.

Diaphragmatic Eventration

Eventration of the diaphragm may be congenital or acquired (Fig. 17-36). The congenital lesion is far rarer than the acquired one, which is most often either an injury to the phrenic nerve acquired during difficult instrumental delivery, insertion of chest drain for pneumothorax, or cardiac surgery. Should the lesion result from difficult, often breech delivery, then it may be associated with Erb's palsy. The congenital lesion results from an incomplete development of the muscular portion of the diaphragm or its innervation. This has been described in neonatal cases of fetal rubella and cytomegalovirus infection. The defect is more common on the left than the right side and usually presents as a moderate to complete thinning of the diaphragmatic muscle fibers. In extreme cases, it may be very difficult pathologically to differentiate the lesion from a CDH. Bilateral lesions are rare. Several associated anomalies have been described with the congenital form of diaphragmatic eventration: rib and cardiac anomalies, renal ectopia, and exomphalos. Presentation is usually as a chance finding on a chest radiograph taken for other purposes. The diagnosis is confirmed by ultrasound examination demonstrating paradoxical movement of the diaphragm. Usually, no treatment is needed, and the radiologic appearance improves with time. Bilateral large eventrations may need repair, and the best approach is through the chest, followed by radial incision and plication of the diaphragm using a nonabsorbable suture.

CONGENITAL CARDIAC DISORDERS

Cardiac malformations may be coincidental to or a fundamental part of a pulmonary malformation. They are sufficiently common that echocardiography should be a routine part of the work-up of most suspected congenital lung abnormalities. Coincidental malformations are seen with, for example, congenital large hyperlucent lobe. Around 10% have an atrial or ventricular septal defect. Lung abnormalities in which heart disease is fundamental include those with the pulmonary atresia spectrum (see earlier). By definition, lung blood supply is abnormal. However, these cases usually present to the pediatric cardiologists and are beyond the scope of this chapter. It should be noted that vascular compression of the airways in the setting of congenital heart disease is not uncommon and may be referred to the pediatric pulmonologist.

MULTISYSTEM CONGENITAL DISORDERS THAT AFFECT THE LUNG

Most congenital lung abnormalities are isolated, but a few are part of a more generalized disorder. Tuberous sclerosis may affect the lung as well as kidneys, heart, and brain. Complex abnormalities of lung development may be associated with chromosomal abnormalities. Micronodular type II pneumocyte hyperplasia is largely though not exclusively confined to patients with tuberous sclerosis, of which it is a particularly rare manifestation. It is a multifocal microscopic lesion that usually has no clinical significance, but in rare cases the lesions are of an appreciable size and so numerous that pulmonary function is compromised and the patient complains of breathlessness. The hyperplastic cells show no atypia and appear to be devoid of any malignant potential. Micronodular type II pneumocyte hyperplasia may be seen in otherwise normal lungs or in association with pulmonary lymphangioleiomyomatosis. Unlike lymphangioleiomyomatosis, it affects tuberous sclerosis patients of either sex, and the hyperplastic type II cells fail to stain for HMB-45.

Rare metabolic diseases may affect the lung. These include Niemann-Pick, and lysinuric protein intolerance. They also enter the differential diagnosis of pediatric interstitial lung disease (see Chapter 47).

ROLE OF SPECIFIC INVESTIGATIONS

CHEST RADIOGRAPHY

All infants in whom any suggestion of a lung malformation has been made antenatally will require a chest radiograph before discharge. In many it will be normal, but subsequent, more detailed imaging may reveal tiny malformations. Specific points in the chest radiograph in the context of congenital lung disease include the determination of bronchial arrangement and the side of the aortic arch (Fig. 17-37); a right-sided arch may be a normal variant of no concern but may give a clue to the presence of a vascular ring.[91] A normal chest radiograph does not exclude a significant CTM.

VENTILATION-PERFUSION SCANNING

This technique gives useful functional information. Unilateral absent perfusion and ventilation is seen in complete absence of one lung. Unilateral absence of perfusion, which may be

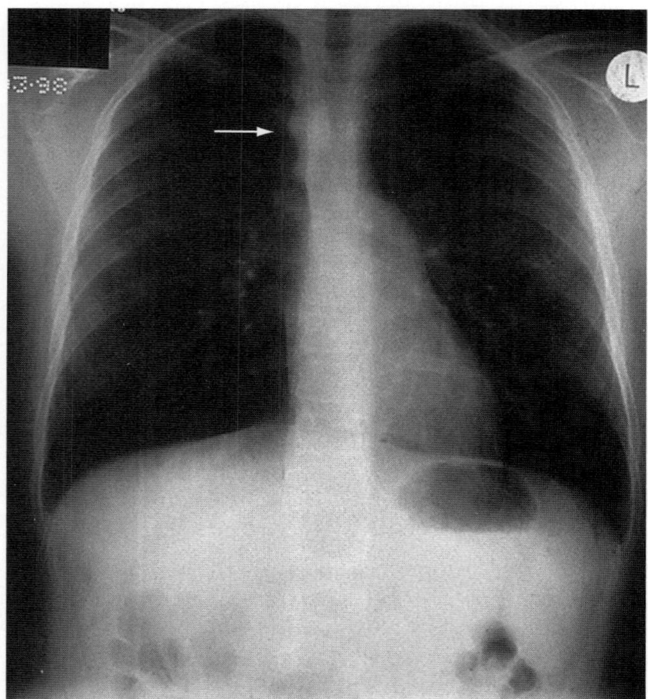

■ **FIGURE 17-37.** Right-sided aortic arch *(arrowed)*. Note the tracheal compression by the associated vascular ring.

combined with secondary abnormalities in ventilation, is seen in unilateral absence of the pulmonary artery, unilateral origin of pulmonary artery from aorta, and unilateral absence of pulmonary veins. Bilateral absent or greatly reduced perfusion is seen in common arterial trunk ("truncus arteriosus"); the pattern of ventilation is normal. Focal defects are seen with large CTMs. Increased uptake of radiolabeled microspheres given by peripheral vein injection is seen in the brain and kidneys as a feature of PAVMs (as well as in congenital heart disease with right-to-left shunt) and has been used to quantitate shunt. Split lung function may be useful in determining whether operation on a unilateral bronchial or pulmonary artery stenosis is advisable. In cases of doubt, V/Q scanning can differentiate congenital large hyperlucent lobe from hyperinflation of a normal lobe secondary to contralateral CSL or lobar atelectasis; in this case, the lucent area is functional, whereas congenital lobar emphysema causes a filling defect.

ULTRASOUND SCANNING (INCLUDING ECHOCARDIOGRAPHY)

Cardiac abnormality is so important when considering congenital lung malformations that it is wise to include an echocardiogram as part of the investigation of many if not most infants with suspected congenital lung disease. Indeed, antenatal ultrasound will have already detected many cardiac abnormalities. Echocardiography detects relevant abnormalities of the systemic arteries in the mediastinum, such as double aortic arch and aberrant origin of subclavian artery. The pulmonary arteries and veins should be imaged and unilateral abnormal (hemianomalous) venous drainage excluded. Injection of saline into a peripheral vein allows detection of a right-to-left shunt; in such cases, bubbles appear in the left atrium. Pulmonary artery pressure may be estimated from the Bernoulli equation if there is physiologic tricuspid or pulmonary regurgitation. It may be possible to image abnormal collateral arteries arising from the abdominal aorta. Parenchymal ultrasound imaging is generally less helpful. Defects in the diaphragm may be identified and pleural disease confirmed. Ultrasound is useful in differentiating thymic abnormalities from mediastinal cysts.

COMPUTED TOMOGRAPHY

Computed tomography gives the best images of parenchymal abnormalities and is currently probably the first investigation of choice in an adult with suspected CTM. A cystic CTM large enough to have the potential to be infected may be invisible on chest radiographs, so CT is recommended for all infants in whom an antenatal diagnosis of a lung malformation has been made, even if the chest radiograph after birth appears normal. Scanning after contrast injection, especially using modern reconstruction techniques, may delineate abnormal aortopulmonary collaterals, obviating the need for angiography.

MAGNETIC RESONANCE IMAGING

At present, MRI requires general anesthesia in small children, but the lack of radiation exposure and ability to reconstruct vascular anatomy make this an attractive technique. MRI is the best way of detecting extension of a neurogenic tumor into the spinal canal. It can also be used to image any airway compression and its cause.

BARIUM SWALLOW

A barium swallow investigation is used in this context to diagnose a vascular ring (Fig. 17-38). If the appearances are those of an anomalous subclavian artery, which may be a variant of no consequence, airway compression may be confirmed with a bronchoscopy. A barium swallow cannot rule out an H-type tracheoesophageal fistula.

ESOPHAGEAL TUBE INJECTION

Abnormal connections between the esophagus and the trachea or a CTM are best delineated by a tube esophagram. The pressure injection of barium will reveal a connection that a simple barium swallow will miss. This investigation is only needed in selected cases, in which either the malformation is close to the bronchial tree, or severe infection (particularly anaerobic) is a feature.

ANGIOGRAPHY

In complex cases, angiography may be necessary before surgery. However, the increasing use of CT and MRI to delineate vascular anatomy means that invasive investigation is now needed much less often. The operator must completely delineate the anatomy of the pulmonary and systemic trees, including establishing whether there are any arterial collaterals (see earlier). It should be remembered that a CTM may be supplied from the coronary, internal mammary, intercostals, or subclavian arteries. At the same time, any embolization that might be indicated can be performed, including occlusion of PAVMs and systemic

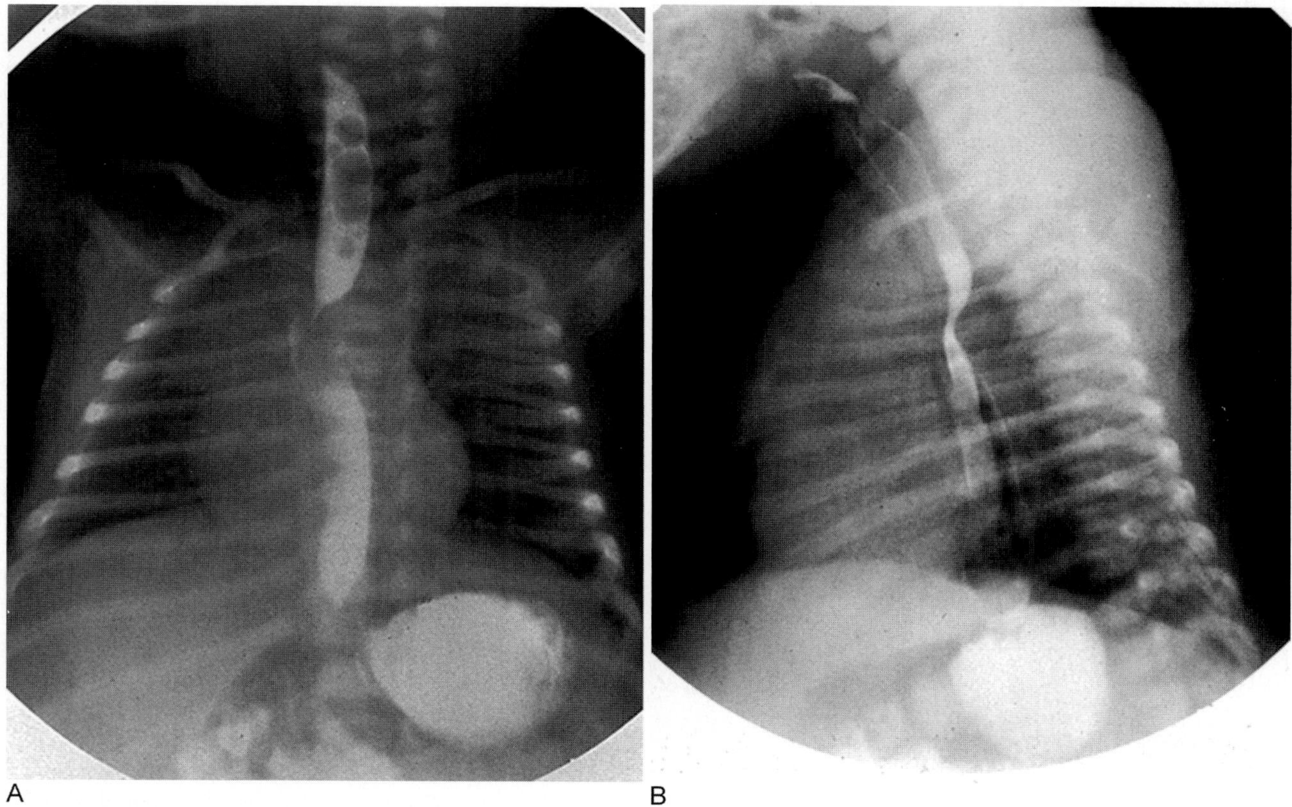

■ **FIGURE 17-38.** Barium swallow showing the indentation of a vascular ring (double aortic arch). **A,** Posteroanterior view. **B,** Lateral view.

arterial collaterals (Fig. 17-39). This may be the only treatment required, or the occlusion of large aortopulmonary collaterals to a CTM may make subsequent surgery safer. It should be stated that the role of embolization in congenital disorders of the lung, other than pulmonary arteriovenous fistula, is controversial.

■ BRONCHOSCOPY

The most clear-cut use of bronchoscopy is in the investigation of stridor (see earlier). In all but typical cases of laryngomalacia, this investigation should be performed at an early stage. Multiple causes of stridor are not uncommon, and all of the accessible respiratory tract should be examined. Bronchoscopy should not be delayed by performing a series of nondiagnostic imaging studies. In other contexts, bronchoscopy is probably best combined with other procedures requiring a general anesthetic, such as angiography (see earlier). Other than for the investigation of stridor, an anesthetic can rarely be justified solely for bronchoscopy in the context of congenital lung disease. Ideally, the procedure should be performed under general anesthesia via a facemask, so that the whole of the airway can be inspected, including the larynx, under conditions of quiet respiration. First, bronchial arrangement can be verified. Second, abnormalities of the bronchial wall such as complete cartilage rings or compression by a vascular ring can be ascertained. Finally, the presence of blind-ending bronchial stumps can be determined; these may act as a sump for infection. Another role for bronchoscopy is the assessment of airway narrowing in the case of aberrant origin of the left subclavian artery. This may be a harmless normal variant or may cause significant airway narrowing, if a left arterial ligament completes a vascular ring. In doubtful cases, bronchoscopic inspection of the airway is indicated.

■ LOW CONTRAST VOLUME BRONCHOGRAPHY

Airway malacia can be visualized directly and further documented by performing a limited bronchogram with a soluble contrast medium.[92] Unlike the bronchograms carried out before the advent of CT scanning, the purpose is to delineate the major airways, not to achieve alveolar filling, and only very small volumes of water-soluble contrast are required.

■ SPECIFIC TREATMENT ISSUES

Details of the treatment of specific conditions can be found in the foregoing sections. For many abnormalities, surgery is the best and definitive treatment. For all but the smallest, sickest infants, lobectomy is a safe and well-tolerated procedure, with few if any significant sequelae. However, pneumonectomy carries a significant mortality in infancy. There is also considerable long-term morbidity, in particular scoliosis, which may worsen dramatically during the pubertal growth spurt. In general, asymptomatic congenital cystic disease merits surgery, because it is likely that there will be a complicating infection of the cyst eventually, which may make the operation more difficult.[47]

It should be remembered that children with complex malformations (e.g., unilateral CSL with abnormal vasculature) may be asymptomatic for long periods despite a formidable list of abnormalities. A conservative approach, perhaps occluding any aortopulmonary collaterals, may be adequate.

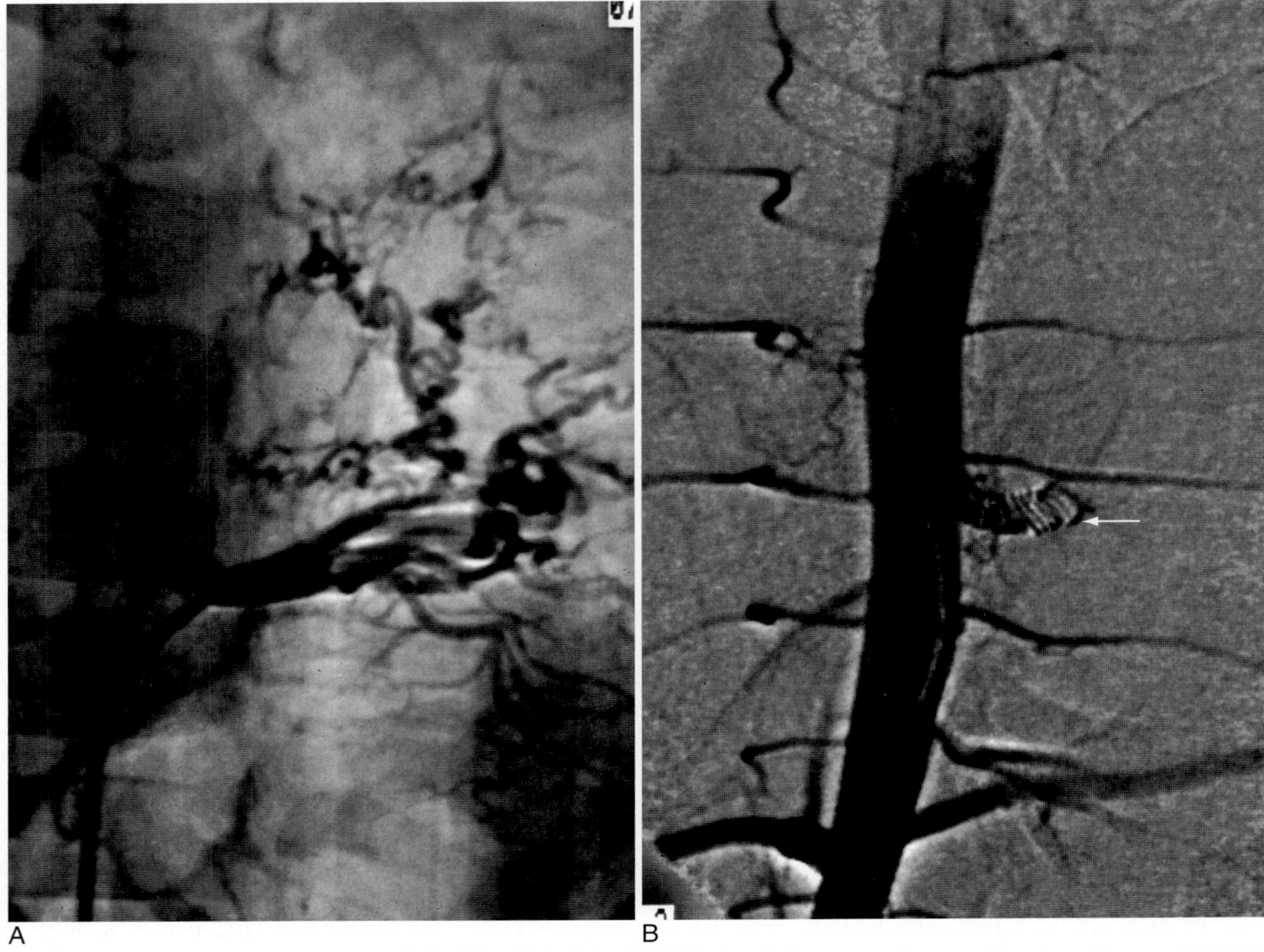

FIGURE 17-39. Digital subtraction angiogram before (**A**) and after (**B**) coil embolization of a large aortopulmonary collateral supplying a cystic CTM in the left lower lobe. The *arrow* (**B**) points to the site of the coil occlusion.

LONG-TERM FOLLOW-UP

There are several issues to be considered, including the effects of previous treatment (usually lung resection) and the needs of the child with a malformation that is being managed conservatively.

In general, lobectomy is well tolerated. The effects of lung resection have been reviewed[64]; issues include the total amount of resection and the age at operation (and thus the possibility of new lung tissue formation). Human and animal data are difficult to interpret, but in general it is extent, not age of resection that is important. A related issue is whether a large malformation, such as a congenital large hyperlucent lobe (congenital lobar emphysema), can so compress normal lung as to interfere with its growth. The evidence would seem to be that this is not the case and that even very large lobes can be left intact unless the infant is symptomatic. Sacrifice of lung tissue is not inevitable during surgery for malformations; simple cysts may be resected in their entirety without the need for a pulmonary resection.

In some cases, a malformation may be so small that conservative management is offered. This strategy is not without risk, although the exact risk is impossible to quantitate at the present time. There are isolated case reports of malignant tumors in children with a CTM, typically bronchioloalveolar carcinoma in type 1 CCAMs, but the risk attributable to the malformation is not known. Furthermore, malignant disease may develop in sites distant from the original malformation,[93] implying that the malformation is merely a marker of increased malignant potential throughout the lungs, in which case removing the malformation would not address the underlying problem. Some advocate removal of even the tiniest malformations, while others are more conservative. Further information on the relationship between CCAM and pleuropulmonary blastoma can be found at http://www.ppbregistry.org. It is suggested that a higher incidence of suspicion is justified in those with bilateral disease, a family history of pleuropulmonary blastoma, pulmonary cysts or renal anomalies, or a close relative with a childhood malignancy, especially Wilms' tumor or medulloblastoma. Fortunately, malignant transformation appears to be very rare; but there is insufficient evidence on which to base definitive recommendations.

SUMMARY AND CONCLUSIONS

Congenital lung disease can present at any time from 20 weeks of gestation to old age and should at least be considered as part of the differential diagnosis in many clinical situations. The lesions may regress to virtually nothing, or require relatively straightforward surgery, or be among the most complex therapeutic challenges encountered. The chief need is for information about the long-term consequences of many of the lesions diagnosed antenatally, so that more precise counseling can be provided. Children with congenital lung disease should be enrolled in registries and followed up in a systematic manner. Another need is for refinement of MRI scanning so that it can be performed without need of general anesthesia and also give more precise information about parenchymal abnormalities, to obviate the need for radiation exposure.

REFERENCES

1. Bush A: Congenital lung disease. A plea for clear thinking and clear nomenclature. Pediatr Pulmonol 2001;32:328–337.
2. Azoulay D, Regnard JF, Magdeleinat P, Diamond T, Rojas-Miranda A, Levasseur P: Congenital respiratory-esophageal fistula in an adult. Report of 9 cases and review of the literature. J Thoracic Cardiovasc Surg 1992; 104:381–384.
3. Falconer AR, Brown RA, Helms P, Gordon I, Baron JA: Pulmonary sequelae in survivors of congenital diaphragmatic hernia. Thorax 1990;45:126–129.
4. Thorpe-Beeston JG, Gosden CM, Nicolaides KH: Prenatal diagnosis of congenital diaphragmatic hernia. Associated malformations and chromosomal defects. Fetal Ther 1989;4:21–28.
5. Adzick NS, Vacanti JP, Lillehei CW, O'Rourke PP, Crone RK, Wilson JM: Fetal diaphragmatic hernia. Ultrasound diagnosis and clinical outcome in 38 cases. J Pediatr Surg 1989;24:654–657.
6. Sharland GK, Lockhart SM, Heward AJ, Allan LD: Prognosis in fetal diaphragmatic hernia. Am J Obstet Gynecol 1992;166:9–13.
7. Manni M, Heydanus R, Den Hollander NS, Stewart PA, De Vogelaere C, Wladimiroff JW: Prenatal diagnosis of congenital diaphragmatic hernia. A retrospective analysis of 28 cases. Prenat Diagn 1994;14:187–190.
8. Bollmann R, Kalache K, Mau H, Chaoui R, Tennstedt C: Associated malformations and chromosomal defects in congenital diaphragmatic hernia. Fetal Diagn Ther 1995;10:52–59.
9. Dommergues M, Louis-Sylvestre C, Mandelbrot L, Oury JF, Herlicoviez M, Body G, Gamerre M, Dumez Y: Congenital diaphragmatic hernia. Can prenatal ultrasonography predict outcome? Am J Obstet Gynecol 1996; 174:1377–1381.
10. Howe DT, Kilby MD, Sirry H, Barker GM, Roberts E, Davison EV, McHugo J, Whittle MJ: Structural chromosome anomalies in congenital diaphragmatic hernia. Prenat Diagn 1996;16:1003–1009.
11. Geary MP, Chitty LS, Morrison JJ, Wright V, Pierro A, Rodeck CH: Perinatal outcome and prognostic factors in prenatally diagnosed congenital diaphragmatic hernia. Ultrasound Obstet Gynecol 1998;12:107–111.
12. Bahlmann F, Merz E, Hallermann C, Stopfkuchen H, Kramer W, Hofmann M: Congenital diaphragmatic hernia. Ultrasonic measurement of fetal lungs to predict pulmonary hypoplasia. Ultrasound Obstet Gynecol 1999;14:162–168.
13. Betremieux P, Lionnais S, Beuchee A, Pladys P, Le Bouar G, Pasquier L, Loeuillet-Olivo L, Azzis O, Milon J, Wodey E, Fremond B, Odent S, Poulain P: Perinatal management and outcome of prenatally diagnosed congenital diaphragmatic hernia. A 1995–2000 series in Rennes University Hospital. Prenat Diagn 2002;22:988–994.
14. Garne E, Haeusler M, Barisic I, Gjergja R, Stoll C, Clementi M, Euroscan Study Group: Congenital diaphragmatic hernia. Evaluation of prenatal diagnosis in 20 European regions. Ultrasound Obstet Gynecol 2002;19:329–333.
15. Laudy JA, Van Gucht M, Van Dooren MF, Wladimiroff JW, Tibboel D: Congenital diaphragmatic hernia. An evaluation of the prognostic value of the lung-to-head ratio and other prenatal parameters. Prenat Diagn 2003;23:634–639.
16. Dott MM, Wong LY, Rasmussen SA: Population-based study of congenital diaphragmatic hernia. Risk factors and survival in Metropolitan Atlanta, 1968–1999. Birth Defects Res Clin Mol Teratol 2003;67:261–267.
17. Hedrick HL, Crombleholme TM, Flake AW, Nance ML, von Allmen D, Howell LJ, Johnson MP, Wilson RD, Adzick NS: Right congenital diaphragmatic hernia. Prenatal assessment and outcome. J Pediatr Surg 2004;39:319–323.
18. Geary MP, Chitty LS, Morrison JJ, Wright V, Pierro A, Rodeck CH: Perinatal outcome and prognostic factors in prenatally diagnosed congenital diaphragmatic hernia. Ultrasound Obstet Gynecol 1998;12:107–111.
19. Harrison MR, Keller RL, Hawgood SB, Kitterman JA, Sandberg PL, Farmer DL, Lee H, Filly RA, Farrell JA, Albanese CT: A randomised trial of fetal endoscopic tracheal occlusion for severe fetal congenital diaphragmatic hernia. N Engl J Med 2003;349:1916–1924.
20. Stocker JT, Madewell JE, Drake RM: Congenital cystic malformation of the lung. Classification and morphologic spectrum. Hum Pathol 1977;8:155–171.
21. Samuel M, Burge DM: Management of antenatally diagnosed pulmonary sequestration associated with congenital cystic adenomatoid malformation. Thorax 1999;54:701–706.
22. Thorpe-Beeston JG, Nicolaides KH: Cystic adenomatoid malformation of the lung. Prenatal diagnosis and outcome. Prenat Diagn 1994;14:677–688.
23. Davenport M, Warne SA, Cacciaguerra S, Patel S, Greenough A, Nicolaides K: Current outcome of antenatally diagnosed cystic lung disease. J Pediatr Surg 2004;39:549–556.
24. Adzick NS, Harrison MR, Crombleholme TM, Flake AW, Howell LJ: Fetal lung lesions. Management and outcome. Am J Obstet Gynecol 1998;179: 884–889.
25. Lim FY, Crombleholme TM, Hedrick HL, Flake AW, Johnson MP, Howell LJ, Adzick NS: Congenital high airway obstruction. Natural history and management. J Pediatric Surg 2003;38:940–945.
26. Paek BW, Callen PW, Kitterman J, Feldstein VA, Farrell J, Harrison MR, Albanese CT: Successful fetal intervention for congenital high airway obstruction syndrome. Fetal Diagn Ther 2002;17:272–276.
27. Collins DW, Downs CS, Katz SG, Gatt SP, Marsland C, Abrahams N, Turner RJ: Airway management on placental support (AMPS)—the anaesthetic perspective. Anaesth Intensive Care 2002;30:647–659.
28. Miyamoto RC, Cotton RT, Rope AF, Hopkin RJ, Cohen AP, Shott SR, Rutter MJ: Association of anterior glottic webs with velocardiofacial syndrome (chromosome 22q11.2 deletion). Otolaryngol Head Neck Surg 2004;130:415–417.
29. Watters K, Russel J: Diagnosis and management of type 1 laryngeal cleft. Int J Pediatr Otorhinolaryngol 2003;67:591–596.
30. Nielson DW, Ku PL, Egger M: Topical lidocaine exaggerates laryngomalacia during flexible bronchoscopy. Am J Respir Crit Care Med 2000;161: 147–151.
31. Toynton SC, Saunders MW, Bailey CM: Aryepiglottoplasty for laryngomalacia. J Laryngol Otol 2001;115:35–38.
32. Daya H, Hosni A, Bejar-Solar I, Evans JN, Bailey CM: Pediatric vocal fold paralysis. A long-term retrospective study. Arch Otolaryngol Head Neck Surg 2000;126:21–25.
33. Civantos FJ, Holinger LD: Laryngocoeles and saccular cysts in infants and children. Arch Otolaryngol Head Neck Surg 1992;118:296–300.
34. Kiff KM, Mok Q, Dunne J, Tasker RC: Steroids for intubated croup masking airway haemangioma. Arch Dis Child 1996;74:66–67.
35. Backer CL, Mavroudis C, Holinger LD: Repair of congenital tracheal stenosis. Semin Thorac Cardiovasc Surg Pediatr Card Surg Annu 2002;5:173–186.
36. Rutter MJ, Willging JP, Cotton RT: Nonoperative management of complete tracheal rings. Arch Otolaryngol Head Neck Surg 2004;130:450–452.
37. Frank JL, Poole CA, Rosas G: Horseshoe lung. Clinical, pathologic, and radiologic features and a new plain film finding. AJR Am J Roentgenol 1986;146:217–226.
38. Bush A: Left bronchial isomerism, normal atrial arrangement and bronchomalacia mimicking asthma. A new syndrome? Eur Respir J 1999;14: 475–477.
39. Bense L, Eklund G, Wiman LG: Bilateral bronchial anomaly. A pathogenetic factor in spontaneous pneumothorax. Am Rev Respir Dis 1992;146:513–516.
40. Williams H, Campbell P: Generalized bronchiectasis associated with deficiency of cartilage in the bronchial tree. Arch Dis Child 1960;35:182–190.
41. Marchevsky AM: Lung tumors derived from ectopic tissues. Semin Diagn Pathol 1995;12:172–184.
42. Kershisnik MM, Kaplan C, Craven CM, Carey JC, Townsend JJ, Knisely AS: Intrapulmonary neuroglial heterotopia. Arch Pathol Lab Med 1992;116: 1043–1046.
43. Nobuhara KK, Gorski YC, La Quaglia MP, Shamberger RC: Bronchogenic cysts and esophageal duplications. Common origins and treatment. J Pediatr Surg 1997;32:1408–1413.
44. Stocker JT: Congenital pulmonary airway malformation—a new name and an expanded classification of congenital cystic adenomatoid malformations of the lung. Histopathology 2002;41:424S–431S.
45. Langston C: New concepts in the pathology of congenital lung malformations. Semin Pediatr Surg 2003;12:17–37.
46. MacSweeney F, Papagiannopoulos K, Goldstraw P, Sheppard MN, Corrin B, Nicholson AG: An assessment of the expanded classification of congenital cystic adenomatoid malformations, and their relationship to malignant transformation. Am J Surg Pathol 2003;27:1139–1146.

47. Papagiannopoulos K, Hughes S, Nicholson AG, Goldstraw P: Cystic lung lesions in the pediatric and adult population. Surgical experience at the Brompton Hospital. Ann Thorac Surg 2002;73:1594–1598.
48. Conran RM, Stocker JT: Extralobar sequestration with frequently associated congenital cystic adenomatoid malformation, type 2. Report of 50 cases. Pediatr Dev Pathol 1999;2:454–463.
49. Mani H, Suarez E, Stocker JT: The morphologic spectrum of infantile lobar emphysema. A study of 33 cases. Paediatr Respir Rev 2004;5(Suppl 1): S313–S320.
50. McShane D, Nicholson AG, Goldstraw P, Ladas G, Travis WD, Ramanan R, Balfour-Lynn IM, Rosenthal M, Bush A: Inflammatory endobronchial polyps in childhood. Clinical spectrum and possible link to mechanical ventilation. Pediatr Pulmonol 2002;34:79–84.
51. Stigers KB: The clinical and imaging spectrum of findings in patients with congenital lobar emphysema. Pediatr Pulmonol 1992;14:160–170.
52. Sparey C, Jawaheer G, Barrett AM, Robson SC: Esophageal atresia in the Northern Region Congenital Anomaly Survey 1985–1997. Prenatal diagnosis and outcome. Am J Obstet Gynecol 2000;182:427–431.
53. Bianca S, Bianca M, Ettore G: Oesophageal atresia and Down syndrome. Downs Syndr Res Pract 2002;8:29–30.
54. Usui N: Anomalies of the tracheobronchial tree in patients with esophageal atresia. J Pediatr Surg 1996;31:258–262.
55. Spitz L, Yang X, Pierro A, Kiely EM, Drake D: Adverse association of oesophageal atresia and cleft lip and palate [Comment]. Br J Surg 2003; 90:716–717.
56. Barlev DM, Nagourney BA, Saintonge R: Traumatic retropharyngeal emphysema as a cause for severe respiratory distress in a newborn. Pediatr Radiol 2003;33:429–432.
57. Singh SJ, Kapila L: Denis Browne's thoracotomy revised. Pediatr Surg Int 2002;18:90–92.
58. Patel SB, Ade-Ajayi N, Kiely EM: Oesophageal atresia. A simplified approach to early management. Pediatr Surg Int 2002;18:87–89.
59. Gauderer MW: Delayed blind-pouch apposition, guide wire placement, and nonoperative establishment of luminal continuity in a child with long gap esophageal atresia. J Pediatr Surg 2003;38:906–909.
60. Scharli AF: Esophageal reconstruction in very long atresias by elongation of the lesser curvature. Pediatr Surg Int 1992;7:101.
61. McCollum MO, Rangel SJ, Blair GK, Moss RL, Smith BM, Skarsgard ED: Primary reversed gastric tube reconstruction in long gap esophageal atresia. J Pediatr Surg 2003;38:957–962.
62. Lorincz A, Langenburg S, Klein MD: Robotics and the pediatric surgeon [Review]. Curr Opin Pediatr 2003;15:262–266.
63. Ludman L, Spitz L: Quality of life after gastric transposition for oesophageal atresia. J Pediatr Surg 2003;38:53–57.
64. Zach MS, Eber E: Adult outcome of congenital lower respiratory tract malformations. Thorax 2001;56:65–72.
65. Wang TZ, Lin YM, Hwang JJ: Unilateral pulmonary artery agenesis in adulthood—not always a benign disease. Chest 1997;111:832–833.
66. Schulze-Neick I, Ho Y, Bush A, Rosenthal M, Franklin RC, Redington A, Penny DJ: Severe airflow limitation after the unifocalization procedure. Clinical and morphological correlates. Circulation 2000;102(Suppl 111): III-142–III-147.
67. Yamanaka A, Hirai T, Fujimoto T, Hase M, Noguchi M, Konishi F: Anomalous systemic supply to normal basal segments of the left lower lobe. Ann Thorac Surg 1999;68:332–338.
68. Nashef SAM, Jamieson MPG, Pollock JCS, Houston AB: Aortic origin of right pulmonary artery. Successful surgical correction in three consecutive patients. Ann Thorac Surg 1987;44:536–538.
69. Nakamura H, Makihara K, Taniguchi Y, Ishigo K, Ohgi S: Thoracoscopic surgery for intralobar pulmonary sequestration. Ann Thorac Cardiovasc Surg 1999;5:405–407.
70. Najm HK, Williams WG, Coles JG, Rebeyka IM, Freedom RM: Scimitar syndrome. 20 years' experience and results of repair. J Thorac Cardiovasc Surg 1996;112:1161–1168.
71. Huddleston CB, Mendelhoff EN: Scimitar syndrome. Adv Cardiac Surg 1999;11:161–178.
72. Abdalla SA, Geisthoff UW, Bonneau D, Plauchu H, McDonald J, Kennedy S, Faughnan ME, Letarte M: Visceral manifestations in hereditary haemorrhagic telangiectasia type 2. J Med Genet 2003;40:494–502.
73. Berg J, Porteous M, Reinhardt D, Gallione C, Holloway S, Umasunthar T, Lux A, McKinnon W, Marshuk D, Guttmacher A: Hereditary haemorrhagic telangiectasia. A questionnaire based study to delineate the different phenotypes caused by endoglin and ALK1 mutations. J Med Genet 2003;40:585–590.
74. Begbie ME, Wallace GM, Shovlin CL: Hereditary haemorrhagic telangiectasia (Osler-Weber-Rendu syndrome). A view from the 21st century. Postgrad Med J 2003;79:18–24.
75. Barker PM, Esther CR Jr, Fordham LA, Maygarden SJ, Funkhouser WK: Primary pulmonary lymphangiectasia in infancy and childhood. Eur Respir J 2004;24:413–419.
76. Wagenaar SS, Swierenga J, Wagenvoort CA: Late presentation of primary pulmonary lymphangiectasis. Thorax 1978;33:791–795.
77. Mei-Zahav M, Solomon M, Trachsel D, Langer JC: Bochdalek diaphragmatic hernia. Not only a neonatal disease. Arch Dis Child 2003;88: 532–535.
78. Cloutier R, Allard V, Fournier L, Major D, Pichette S, St-Onge O: Estimation of lungs' hypoplasia on postoperative chest x rays in congenital diaphragmatic hernia. J Pediatr Surg 1993;28:1086–1089.
79. Haugen SE: Congenital diaphragmatic hernia. Determination of the optimal time for operation by echocardiographic monitoring of the pulmonary artery pressure. J Pediatr Surg 1991;26:560–562.
80. Karamanoukian HL, Glick PL: Congenital diaphragmatic hernia. Ann Thorac Surg 2003;75:1059–1060.
81. Sydorak RM, Hoffman W, Lee H, Yingling CD, Longaker M, Chang J, Smith B, Harrison MR, Albanese CT: Reversed latissimus dorsi muscle flap for repair of recurrent congenital diaphragmatic hernia. J Pediatr Surg 2003;38:296–300.
82. Wung JT, Sahni R, Moffitt ST, Lipsitz E, Stolar CJ: Congenital diaphragmatic hernia. Survival treated with very delayed surgery, spontaneous respiration, and no chest tube. J Pediatr Surg 1995;30:406–409.
83. Goyal A, Smith NP, Jesudason EC, Kerr S, Losty PD: Octreotide for treatment of chylothorax after repair of congenital diaphragmatic hernia. J Pediatr Surg 2003;38:E19–E20.
84. Davis PJ, Firmin RK, Manktelow B, Goldman AP, Davis CF, Smith JH, Cassidy JV, Shekerdemian LS: Long-term outcome following extracorporeal membrane oxygenation for congenital diaphragmatic hernia. The UK experience. J Pediatr 2004;144:309–315.
85. Stege G, Fenton A, Jaffray B: Nihilism in the 1990s. The true mortality of congenital diaphragmatic hernia. Pediatrics 2003;112:532–535.
86. D'Agostino JA: Outcome for infants with congenital diaphragmatic hernia requiring extracorporeal membrane oxygenation. The first year. J Pediatr Surg 1995;30:10–15.
87. Kamiyama M, Kawahara H, Okuyama H, Oue T, Kuroda S, Kubota A, Okada A: Gastroesophageal reflux after repair of congenital diaphragmatic hernia. J Pediatr Surg 2002;37:1681–1684.
88. Ikeda K, Hokuto I, Tokieda K, Nishimura O, Ishimoto H, Morikawa Y: A congenital anterior diaphragmatic hernia with massive pericardial effusion requiring neither emergency pericardiocentesis nor operation. A case report and review of the literature. J Perinat Med 2002;30:336–340.
89. Mouroux J, Venissac N, Alifano M, Padovani B: Morgagni hernia and thoracic deformities. Thorac Cardiovasc Surg 2003;51:44–45.
90. de Vogelaere K, de Backer A, Delvaux G: Laparoscopic repair of diaphragmatic Morgagni hernia. J Laparoendosc Adv Surg Tech A 2002;12: 457–460.
91. Payne DNR, Lincoln C, Bush A: Lesson of the week. Right sided aortic arch in children with persistent respiratory symptoms. Br Med J 2000;321: 687–688.
92. Inwald DP, Roebuck D, Elliott MJ, Mok Q: Current management and outcome of tracheobronchial malacia and stenosis presenting to the paediatric intensive care unit. Intensive Care Med 2001;27:722–729.
93. Papagiannopoulos KA, Sheppard M, Bush A, Goldstraw P: Pleuropulmonary blastoma. Is prophylactic resection of congenital lung cysts effective? Ann Thorac Surg 2001;72:604–605.

18 Respiratory Disorders in the Newborn

Anne Greenough, MD

Respiratory disorders are the most common cause of neonatal unit admission and a major cause of neonatal mortality and morbidity. In this chapter, the etiology, presentation, management, and outcome of neonatal respiratory disorders are described, as is the initiation of respiration at birth and resuscitation; relevant congenital anomalies are described in Chapter 17.

RESPIRATORY DEPRESSION AT BIRTH

INITIATION OF RESPIRATION AT BIRTH

Fetal breathing activity is essential for normal lung growth. It can be detected as early as 14 weeks of gestation in the human, and the amount of time the fetus spends breathing increases with advancing gestational age. Fetal breathing activity ceases during labor. At birth, one of the most important stimuli to initiate breathing is cooling. In addition, audiovisual, proprioceptive, and touch stimuli recruit central neurons and increase central arousal. The central chemoreceptor areas are activated at birth, as indicated by the expression of genes, such as *c-fos*; skin cooling may be involved in this activation. In addition, there is a switching on of genes encoding neurotransmitters involved in respiratory control. Hypoxia mediated by central chemoreceptors is important to the onset of respiration, but peripheral chemoreceptor activity is not critical. Birth is also associated with the removal of respiratory inhibitory mechanisms, including prostaglandins and adenosine. Prostaglandin E_2 inhibits fetal breathing movements (FBMs), and prostaglandin inhibitors, such as indomethacin, stimulate FBMs. Plasma concentrations of prostaglandin E_2 decrease at birth, and it has been suggested this may be important for the onset of respiration. In the neonate, prostaglandin E_1 and E_2 depress ventilation. The median time for the onset of respiratory activity is 10 seconds. A high negative inspiratory pressure, greater than 20 cm H_2O, is required to overcome the high flow resistance and inertia of liquid in the airways, as well as the surface tension at the air-liquid interface. Expiration is also active for the first few breaths to aid the distribution of ventilation and further fluid clearance from the lungs. A functional residual capacity (FRC) is formed following the first breath in over 95% of infants. Following a vaginal delivery, the FRC is usually fully formed by 2 hours, but compliance increases more slowly over the first 24 hours as lung liquid is gradually absorbed.

RESPIRATORY DEPRESSION AT BIRTH

Failure of adequate initiation of respiration at birth can occur because of birth depression (asphyxia), drugs depressing respiration, trauma to the central nervous system, anemia, sepsis, and congenital malformations. It is more common in prematurely born infants, and the requirement for active resuscitation is inversely related to gestational age at birth. In newborn animals, after acute postnatal asphyxia there is an early period of apnea, which is called primary apnea. Primary apnea can last up to 10 minutes, but usually after 1 or 2 minutes gasps occur with increasing frequency until the last gasp. The period of apnea that follows is called secondary or terminal apnea; during this time the heart rate falls rapidly, but may continue for at least 10 minutes after the last gasp. The blood pressure falls, paralleling the changes in heart rate, and a severe mixed acidemia and hyperkalemia develop. If the infant is in primary apnea, he or she can be provoked to breathe by peripheral stimuli such as being rubbed with a warm towel, whereas in secondary apnea active resuscitation by positive pressure ventilation is required. The newborn can survive at least 20 minutes of complete oxygen deprivation because the neonatal brain can metabolize lactate and ketones. In addition, infants have large glycogen stores in their brain, liver, and myocardium, which can be metabolized anaerobically to produce energy; growth-retarded infants, who have low glycogen stores, are less able to withstand oxygen deprivation. Birth depression can result in hypoxic ischemic encephalopathy, convulsions, and abnormal neurodevelopmental outcome. Affected infants may also suffer myocardial ischemia and heart failure, pulmonary hemorrhage, and acute tubular necrosis. Respiratory distress is worsened by asphyxia because pulmonary blood flow declines during asphyxia, but after the asphyxia has ceased, there is a reactive hyperemia. This is associated with fluid transudation and edema, the protein-rich edema fluid inhibits surfactant function, and any persisting acidemia inhibits surfactant synthesis. At 1 and 5 minutes following birth, the infant's color, respiratory activity, heart rate, tone, and response to a stimuli are assessed and the Apgar scores calculated. A low Apgar score at 5 minutes is associated with the development of long-term neurologic problems.

DELIVERY ROOM RESUSCITATION

Approximately 10% of infants require some form of resuscitation, and 2% require intubation and positive pressure ventilation. The International Liaison Committee on Resuscitation (ILCOR) and American Heart Association/American Academy of Pediatrics (AHA/AAP) have produced a consensus statement on the procedures that should be followed if a newborn fails to breathe adequately; the following remarks reflect their recommendations.[1] Infants who have failed to establish regular respiration by 1 minute, but who have a heart rate in excess of 80 beats/min, should be provided with facial oxygen. Routine oropharyngeal suction should not be undertaken, as it will inhibit the onset of respiratory effort if too vigorously applied. If the infant fails to show an immediate response, but still has a heart rate in excess of 80 beats/min, facemask resuscitation should be commenced. Intubation and ventilation should be undertaken in infants in whom facemask ventilation fails to produce an improvement in oxygen saturation or respiratory efforts within 15 to 30 seconds or who have a heart rate which is either below 60 beats/min at birth or falls, despite basic resuscitation. Inflation pressures of 25 to 30 cm H_2O, rates of approximately 30 beats/min, and an inspiratory to expiratory ratio of 1:1 should be used for the resuscitation of full-term infants. Results from two randomized trials have highlighted that the onset of spontaneous breathing and crying were significantly delayed in infants being resuscitated with 100% oxygen rather than air. As a consequence, the current consensus is that resuscitation with air is probably as good as 100% oxygen for most asphyxiated full-term infants, but some infants may require supplementary oxygen. External cardiac massage should be commenced in all infants whose heart rate is below 60 beats/min and fail to improve within 30 seconds of the onset of adequate ventilatory support. Cardiac massage is best achieved by placing both hands round the chest so that the thumbs are over the lower part of the sternum and the fingertips close to the spine. The sternum is then depressed by one third of the diameter of the chest, approximately 2 cm. A ratio of three compressions to one inflation, with a rate of 120 "events" (that is 90 compressions and 30 inflations) per minute is recommended. Chest compressions can be discontinued once the heart rate exceeds 80 beats/min. If the heart rate fails to improve on commencing external cardiac massage, 0.1 to 0.3 mL/kg of 1:10,000 adrenaline (epinephrine) should be injected down the endotracheal tube. If endotracheal adrenaline fails to produce a response, a further dose of adrenaline (0.1 to 0.3 mL/kg of 1:10,000 strength) should be given via an umbilical vein catheter or the intraosseous route. Administration of sodium bicarbonate (a dose of 1 to 2 mEq/kg of a 0.5 mEq/mL solution given over at least 2 minutes[2]) should be restricted to those with prolonged arrest, since giving bicarbonate may reduce cerebral blood flow and may lead to intracranial hemorrhages in preterm infants, because of the large osmotic load. Naloxone (0.1 mg/kg intravenously or via the endotracheal tube[2]) should only be given to infants who are receiving adequate ventilatory support and if the infant's respiratory depression has resulted from maternal opiate administration. The intramuscular route leads to a slower response. Naloxone should not be given to the newborns of opiate-addicted mothers, because this will precipitate acute withdrawal symptoms. Group O Rhesus negative blood (10 mL/kg body weight) should be given over 5 to 10 minutes if the infant is hypotensive due to blood loss. If there is no response to 30 minutes of full resuscitation, then consideration should be given to stopping resuscitative measures, because the infant's prognosis is very poor. It is important, however, to consider underlying conditions, such as congenital diaphragmatic hernia (CDH), pneumothorax, or hypoplastic lungs, which may make the infant difficult to resuscitate.

CONTROL OF BREATHING

A loose complex of respiratory neurons ("center"), which lie within the ventrolateral region of the brainstem, generate the respiratory cycle. The phasic transition from inspiration to expiration is modulated by input from the slowly adapting pulmonary stretch receptors and pontine neurons; suppression of either input prolongs inspiration (apneusis). The rhythm is transmitted to spinal motor neurons and cranial premotor neurons; the latter control the activity of airway muscles. Afferents from the forebrain, hypothalamus, central and peripheral chemoreceptors, muscles, joints, and pain receptors are integrated into the "center." The number of intersynaptic connections reaches a peak toward the end of fetal life. The excitatory neurotransmitter glutamate excites receptors involved in generating and transmitting respiratory rhythms to spinal and cranial respiratory neurons. Opioids (endorphins and exogenous drugs) decrease respiration by peripheral and central actions, the latter are due to suppression of recurrent excitation by glutaminergic inputs within the primary respiratory network. Both γ-aminobutyric acid (GABA) and glycine are essential for generating respiratory rhythm; they are released by late and postinspiratory neurons and turn off inspiratory neurons, so facilitating the transition from inspiration to expiration. Deficiency of glycinergic inhibition in knockout mice results in a slower frequency of breathing.

Central and peripheral chemoreceptors modify respiratory activity in response to changes in blood gases. The central chemoreceptors are situated near the ventral surface of the medulla and respond to changes in carbon dioxide/pH and oxygen. The peripheral chemoreceptors are situated at the bifurcation of the common carotid arteries (carotid bodies) and above and below the aortic arch (aortic bodies). In the fetus, the arterial chemoreceptors are active, but have reduced sensitivity. The peripheral chemoreceptors are not essential for the initiation of respiration and are virtually silenced when the arterial oxygen level rises at birth. Resetting of the carotid chemoreceptors to hypoxia occurs within 24 to 48 hours of birth; this may result from changes in dopamine levels. The fetus responds to hypoxia with a suppression of ventilation, which is most marked in growth-retarded fetuses; the hypoxic suppression of ventilation is mediated by the lateral part of the lower pons. In response to hypoxia, there is redistribution of the circulation to favor the heart, brain, and adrenals; this minimizes oxygen consumption and conserves oxygen supplies for vital organs. Hyperoxia stimulates continuous fetal breathing. In the perinatal period, the newborn has a biphasic response to hypoxia, a transient increase in minute ventilation followed by a decrease to or below baseline levels. The initial increase in ventilation is probably due to activation of peripheral chemoreceptors, and the subsequent reduction in ventilation may result from a fall in carbon dioxide tensions following the initial hyperventilation or the suppressant effect of hypoxia, which occurs in the fetal state, persisting into the neonatal period. The decrease in ventilation is the predominating response to hypoxia if the infant is in non–rapid eye movement (non-REM) sleep or nursed in a cold environment. Very immature infants respond to hypoxia in a similar fashion to fetuses, that is, with apnea. The biphasic response to hypoxia disappears at 12 to 14 days and the adult pattern is then seen, that is, stimulation of breathing without depression. Exposure to a hyperoxic gas causes a temporary suppression of breathing due to withdrawal of peripheral chemoreceptor drive. After a few minutes of hyperoxia, ventilation increases to above control levels probably because of hyperoxic cerebral vasoconstriction, resulting in increased brain tissue carbon dioxide. Immaturity and prolonged exposure to supplementary oxygen reduce the response to hyperoxia.

The fetus and newborn respond to increased carbon dioxide levels with an increase in breathing activity. If the newborn inhales a low percentage (<2%) of carbon dioxide, the main response is an increase in tidal volume, whereas a higher percentage provokes an increase in both frequency and tidal volume. The slope of ventilatory response to carbon dioxide is less in full-term infants during active than quiet sleep and in preterm infants, but increases with postnatal growth.

Respiratory activity is also affected by stimulation of respiratory reflexes. Hering and Breuer described three respiratory reflexes: an inflation, an expiratory, and a deflation reflex. The Hering-Breuer inflation reflex is stimulated by lung inflation and results in cessation of respiratory activity. In the newborn, the reflex produces a pattern of rapid, shallow tidal breathing and operates within the tidal volume range. In older subjects, the reflex prevents excessive tidal volumes and can only be stimulated if the inflating volume is increased above a critical threshold. The Hering-Breuer expiratory reflex is stimulated if inflation is prolonged; the active expiration seen in infants ventilated at slow rates and long inflation times, and which may result in pneumothoraces, may be a manifestation of this reflex. In animal models, the Hering-Breuer deflation reflex is evidenced by a prolonged inspiration generated in response to deflating the lung rapidly or following an unusually vigorous expiratory effort which takes the lung below its end-expiratory level. In the newborn this reflex may have a role in maintaining the FRC. Head's paradoxical reflex, also called the inspiratory augmenting reflex or provoked augmented inspiration, is the underlying mechanism of the first breath and sighing. A rapid inflation stimulates a stronger diaphragmatic contraction. The reflex improves compliance and reopens partially collapsed airways; it has an important role in promoting lung expansion during resuscitation. Rapid chest wall distortion, via the intercostal phrenic inhibitory reflex, results in a shortening of inspiratory efforts. This reflex response is inhibited by an increase in FRC or applying continuous positive airway pressure (CPAP), the mechanism may be improved chest wall stability. Inhalation of toxic gases such as nitrogen dioxide and sulfur dioxide causes a change in the frequency and depth of respiration via stimulation of subepithelial chemoreceptors in the trachea, bronchi, and bronchioles. The response is less in REM sleep and in the premature infant. The presence of upper airway reflexes results in cold exposure stimulating breathing via trigeminal afferents in the facial skin, whereas irritant stimuli to the nasal mucosa cause inhibition of breathing. The laryngeal chemoreceptors defend the lower airway from inhalation.

PERIODIC BREATHING

Periodic breathing is characterized by regular cycles of breathing of 10 to 18 seconds' duration, interrupted by pauses of at least 3 seconds in duration; this pattern recurs for at least 2 minutes. Periodic breathing is a benign condition and not a precursor of significant apnea. The frequency of periodic breathing decreases with increasing postmenstrual age and administration of methylxanthines.

APNEA

Apnea is defined as cessation of breathing for at least 10 seconds; a duration of at least 20 seconds is frequently used to diagnose significant apneas, because normal infants do not have apneas of greater than 20 seconds. Apneas are classified as central, obstructive, or mixed. Central apnea is characterized by total cessation of inspiratory efforts without upper airway obstruction, whereas in obstructive apnea, the upper airway is obstructed so there is no airflow despite chest wall movements. Mixed apnea, a combination of central and obstructive apneas, accounts for 50% of all apneas; 40% are central and 10% are obstructive. Bradycardia may occur within a few seconds of the onset of apnea with accompanying changes in blood pressure and cerebral blood flow velocity. In infants without adequate cerebrovascular autoregulation, cerebral perfusion may decrease to very low levels during prolonged apnea and potentially exacerbate hypoxic-ischemic brain injury. The incidence of apnea of prematurity is inversely related to gestational age and usually resolves by about 37 to 40 weeks' postmenstrual age. Other causes of apnea include infection, intracranial abnormality or hemorrhage, anemia, metabolic disorders (especially hypoglycemia and temperature instability), and gastroesophageal reflux (GER). Certain pharmacologic agents can cause apnea, including barbiturates and sedatives.

Minor episodes of apnea respond to stimulation. Additional treatment is required if the apneas are frequent or severe or associated with prolonged desaturation. Methylxanthines, theophylline, and caffeine all may reduce apnea in preterm infants. Caffeine is the preferred agent, since once a day dosing is possible because of its longer half-life and it has a higher therapeutic index than theophylline. Side effects of theophylline include hyperactivity, tachycardia, cardiac dysrhythmias, feeding intolerance, and seizures. Doxapram, a respiratory stimulant, has been used to treat apnea and appears helpful if given in addition to a methylxanthine in refractory cases. In two randomized controlled trials[3,4] (both involving small numbers of infants), doxapram appeared to be as effective as methylxanthines in reducing apnea in preterm infants, but it has many side effects. Infants who have troublesome apnea despite treatment with methylxanthines may benefit from CPAP, which decreases the frequency of apnea by increasing the functional residual capacity, stabilizing oxygenation, and/or splinting the upper airway. CPAP is effective in infants whose episodes are precipitated or prolonged by pharyngeal obstruction. CPAP distends both the pharynx and laryngeal aperture and so prevents mixed and obstructive apneas, but has no effect on central apnea. Infants with severe and refractory apnea may need to be intubated and supported by mechanical ventilation; minimal ventilator settings should be used to reduce the risk for volutrauma.

GASTROESOPHAGEAL REFLUX

GER should be suspected in neonates with recurrent respiratory problems, especially if there is troublesome apnea unresponsive to treatment with a methylxanthine or right upper lobe collapse or consolidation on the chest radiograph. The diagnosis can be confirmed by the demonstration of fat-laden macrophages in the tracheobronchial secretions, or more usually by radiologic or pH probe demonstration of reflux. Apnea preceded by a fall in pH to less than 4, recorded by a probe placed in the esophagus, is diagnostic of reflux-stimulated apnea. Although pH monitoring is often considered the standard diagnostic test, its use is limited in preterm infants, because their gastric pH is greater than 4 for 90% of the time. As a consequence, before undertaking a Nissan fundoplication, a contrast study is usually undertaken to confirm reflux. In the future, impedence testing may provide a more accurate tool. The widespread practice of treating GER in preterm infants is not justified, because often, continuous pH monitoring demonstrates a poor temporal relationship between the GER and apnea, indicating that their occurrence in the same patient is coincidental and treatment for the GER will not influence the apneas. If, however, episodes of troublesome apnea with complications such as recurrent aspiration are attributed to reflux, the volume of feed given at any one time should be reduced and the infant given small frequent feeds or given very low volumes continuously. If the signs persist, the feeds should be thickened or given nasojejunally. Nursing the infant prone can reduce the amount of reflux. Antacids should be given if there is evidence of esophagitis. Prokinetic agents are used in infants with GER if they remain symptomatic despite use of thickened feeds. Erythromycin binds to neural motilin receptors and stimulates gastric antral contractions and induces antral migrating motor complexes, which are important for gastric emptying. Two randomized trials have reported a more rapid establishment of full oral feeds in infants treated with erythromycin,[5] but this treatment has potential side effects, including cardiac arrhythmias. It is also possible that erythromycin may be less effective in inducing migrating motor complexes in infants younger than 32 weeks of gestational age. Infants who have troublesome GER resistant to all the above treatments may require a fundoplication; however, in our experience such a need is extremely unusual in prematurely born infants.

RESPIRATORY DISTRESS SYNDROME

Approximately 1% of infants develop respiratory distress syndrome (RDS). The risk for RDS is inversely proportional to gestational age, with 50% of babies younger than 30 weeks of gestational age developing RDS, but only 2% of those with a gestational age between 35 and 36 weeks developing RDS. Babies with RDS have noncompliant lungs that contain less surfactant than normal. Hyaline membranes line the terminal airways, hence the alternative name of hyaline membrane disease.

PATHOPHYSIOLOGY

RDS is due to immaturity of the lung resulting in surfactant deficiency. The infant's problems are compounded by poor clearing of lung fluid, inadequate respiratory efforts due to a poorly developed respiratory center, and an underdeveloped chest wall and respiratory muscles. Surfactant is produced in alveolar type II cells, cuboidal cells covering about 2% of the alveolar surface, and account for 15% of the cell numbers. They differentiate from the columnar epithelium during the canalicular phase of development, but are not prominent until about 24 weeks of gestation. Surfactant is a complex mixture of substances, including phospholipids, neutral lipids, and proteins. Lipids are the major constituent of surfactant; the most important are phosphatidylcholine and phosphatidylglycerol, representing 70% to 80% and 5% to 10% of the lipids, respectively. Approximately 60% of the phosphatidylcholine is saturated, and the primary saturated fatty acid is palmitic acid; hence it is called disaturated palmityl phosphatidylcholine (DPPC). It has been suggested that only 50% of the DPPC is synthesized directly from saturated diacylglycerols as precursors, and the rest is produced by two remodeling mechanisms. Both remodeling mechanisms involve deacylation of de novo synthesized 1-saturated-2-unsaturated phosphatidylcholine and acyl-2-lysophosphatidylcholine. Acyl-2-lysophosphatidylcholine is then either reacylated by reaction with a saturated acyl coenzyme A or transacylated; only the reacylation mechanism is quantitatively important. These processes are activated during fetal lung development and after corticosteroid administration. Several other hormones, including thyroid hormones and insulin and epidermal growth factor (EGF), influence this sequence of events. For example, in nonhuman primates, in utero treatment with EGF has been shown to result in higher surfactant protein A (SP-A) levels and lecithin:sphingomyelin (L:S) ratios. Phosphatidylinositol, phosphatidylserine, and phosphatidylethanolamine make up a further 10% of the lipids in surfactant. About 10% of the total lipids in surfactant are neutral lipids; cholesterol, triacylglycerols, and free fatty acid. Cholesterol alters the fluidity and organization of lipid rich membranes. Sphingomyelin represents less than 2% of surfactant lipid. Surfactant is synthesized in the endoplasmic reticulum; the phospholipid then moves via intracellular pathways to the lamellar bodies, which unravel to highly surface-active tubular myelin. There is direct transition from the tubular myelin to the surface film, with absorption of a mixture of saturated and unsaturated phospholipids. The surface film is then refined by selectively squeezing out unsaturated phopholipids, generating small vesicular forms of surfactant, which have poor surfactant activity. They are mainly taken up by type II cells, although some are degraded by macrophages or lost from the airways. The loss of surfactant into the airways is proportional to the rate and depth of respiration and can be reduced by addition of CPAP. Surfactant lost in this way is swallowed or, in fetal life, moves into the amniotic fluid. Surfactant may be degraded locally in the alveoli and small airways, the breakdown products being absorbed and recycled by the alveolar cells. The surface of the type II cell facing the alveolus is covered with microvilli and lectin receptors, and aerosolized DPPC can rapidly enter type II cells. More than 90% of the phosphatidylcholine on the alveolar surface is reprocessed, the turnover time being approximately 10 hours. There is negative feedback regulation of surfactant production mediated by surfactant protein A binding to type II cells. Surfactant secretion is controlled by stretch receptors and stimulated by alveolar distention. Beta-adrenergic receptors on alveolar type II cells, which increase in number toward the end of gestation, also control secretion. The palmitic acid residues of DPPC are nonpolar and hydrophobic and orient toward the air, whereas the head group of phosphatidylcholine is polar and hydrophilic and associates with the liquid phase. DPPC is a symmetrical molecule, and the two straight hydrophobic fatty acid chains allow close packing of the monolayer. Compression of such a monolayer results in it being changed from a liquid to a condensed gel or solid state. As the radius decreases, the presence of an insoluble surface film means that the surface tension is reduced and the "solid" monolayer formed in expiration promotes stability of the alveoli and prevents atelectasis. The reduction in surface tension decreases the work of breathing and prevents transudation of fluid as, in conditions of high surface tension, fluid is sucked into the alveolar spaces from the capillaries. DPPC is relatively rigid at body temperature and cannot move rapidly enough to maintain a surface monolayer during the respiratory cycle, and hence a "spreading" agent such as phosphatidylglycerol is required. Initially, phosphatidylinositol (PI) is the primary acidic phospholipid, but with increasing lung maturation, PI is replaced by phosphatidylglycerol. In RDS, phosphatidylglycerol is absent and there are also low levels of phosphatidylcholine, which is relatively unsaturated. As a consequence, the resulting monolayer formed in expiration is unstable and does not reduce surface tension effectively; once the monlayer has been refined, there is so little DPPC available the alveoli are of small size. Thus, infants with RDS have a low FRC and noncompliant lungs and their work of breathing is increased. The alveolar hypoventilation results in ventilation perfusion imbalance and hypoxia. The increased alveolar surface tension secondary to the lack of surfactant promotes the flow of protein-rich fluid from the intravascular space to the interstitium and the alveolar spaces. This leak is increased as hypoxia damages the integrity of the alveolar capillary membrane. These plasma proteins inhibit surfactant function by adsorbing onto the alveolar surface, and the infant's lungs become stiffer and more atelectatic and a vicious cycle occurs.

The four surfactant-associated proteins—SP-A, SP-B, SP-C, and SP-D—comprise 5% to 10% of surfactant by weight. SP-A is composed of 248 amino acids and belongs to the calcium-dependent collectin family of proteins. The human gene is located on chromosome 10; gene expression occurs exclusively in type II pneumocytes. Synthesis of SP-A increases after 28 weeks of gestation. The roles of SP-A include determining the structure of tubular myelin, the stability and rapidity of spreading, and recycling of phospholipids. SP-A and SP-D form part of the innate host defense against infection. As collectins, they target carbohydrate structures on invading microorganisms, particularly bacteria, resulting in agglutination and enhanced clearance. SP-A binds endotoxin and a wide range of gram-positive and -negative organisms, promoting phagocytosis and killing of microorganisms by alveolar macrophages. It acts also as an opsonin for the phagocytosis of viruses, such as herpes simplex, influenza A, and respiratory syncytial virus (RSV). SP-A increases nitric oxide production by macrophages to promote pathogen killing. SP-A polymorphisms have been associated with severe RSV infection and an increased risk for bronchopulmonary dysplasia (BPD). The SP-B gene is located on chromosome 2. The messenger RNA (mRNA) for SP-B is detectable in the epithelial cells of bronchi and bronchioles at 12 to 14 weeks of gestation and after 25 weeks in the type II cells. SP-B is required for the formation of tubular myelin and increases the spreading of surfactant phospholipids onto an air-water interface. SP-B is important for surface activity; SP-C and -B together are more effective. SP-B can also protect the pulmonary surfactant film from inactivation by serum proteins. The absence of SP-B is associated with markedly decreased phosphatidylglycerol and an additional aberrant SP-C peptide. DPPC synthesis is preserved in SP-B deficiency, but SP-C cannot be processed to its active peptide and no secretion of normal surfactant occurs. In SP-B knockout mice, lamellar bodies are absent and tubular myelin structures are absent. SP-B deficiency is an autosomal recessively inherited disorder and causes lethal hypoxemic respiratory failure. Partial deficiencies of SP-B with less severe clinical courses have now been reported. These conditions are reviewed in more detail in Chapter 20. SP-B polymorphisms may explain differences in the risk for RDS between black and white subjects and between males and females. The SP-C gene is located on chromosome 8. The mRNA for SP-C is present early in lung development at the distal tips of the branching airways, but subsequently occurs only in the type II cells. SP-C enhances surface adsorption and spreading of phospholipids and may play a role in enhancing the reuptake of phospholipids. SP-C deficiency has been associated with an interstitial lung disease. SP-D production begins in the bronchiolar and terminal epithelium from about 21 weeks of gestation. SP-D expression is widely distributed in epithelial cells in the body; in the lung, SP-D expression occurs in the type II cells, Clara cells, and other airway cells and glands. Glucocorticoids increase SP-D expression. SP-D is involved in the immune function of the lung, binding to a variety of complex carbohydrates and glycolipids and may have a role in host defense functions in the lung by interacting with the surfaces of bacteria and other microorganisms. An SP-D polymorphism has been associated with severe RSV infection.

There are many factors that influence lung maturation and surfactant production and hence whether an infant develops RDS. Both cortisol and thyroxine increase lung maturation. Beta-adrenergic drugs increase the amount of intracellular cyclic adenosine monophosphate, hence increasing the production and secretion of surfactant. EGF may also be important, because EGF infusion into lambs prevents RDS. Prolactin levels are lower in infants who do rather than do not develop RDS, but its role in surfactant production regulation remains speculative. Insulin delays the maturation of alveolar type II cells, decreasing the proportion of saturated phosphatidylcholine and inhibiting SP-A and SP-B mRNA accumulation and SP-A and SP-B gene expression in vitro. In addition, infants of diabetic mothers have delayed appearance of phosphatidylglycerol. Pulmonary maturity may also be delayed in infants with severe hemolytic disease of the newborn; this may be because of increased levels of insulin due to beta-islet cell hypertrophy. Boys are much more likely to develop RDS than girls, with a male-to-female ratio of 1.7:1; boys are also more likely to die from the disease. Boys' lungs are approximately 1 week more immature than girls', they have delayed maturation of the L:S ratio, and they have late appearance of phosphatidylglycerol due to inhibition of synthesis by fetal androgens. Black compared with white babies have a lower incidence of RDS, 60% to 70% of that of white babies of the same gestational age; in one series, only 40% of African infants younger than 32 weeks of gestational age developed RDS compared with 75% of the white infants.[6] Allelic variation in the surfactant protein A gene has been reported between white Americans and Nigerians. Asphyxia, hypoxia, hypotension, and hypothermia can impair surfactant synthesis and/or increase alveolar capillary leakiness. Exposure to cold results in impaired surfactant function; below 34°C, DPPC cannot spread to form an adequately functioning monolayer. Cesarean section carried out before labor increases the risk for both RDS and transient tachypnea of the newborn (TTN). There appears to be a genetic predisposition, because families in which several relatively mature babies have developed RDS have been reported. Specific alleles of the SP-A and SP-B genes associate interactively to increased susceptibility to RDS.[7]

CLINICAL PRESENTATION

Infants with RDS present within 4 hours of birth, they are tachypneic (respiratory rate >60 breaths/min) and have intercostal and subcostal indrawing, sternal retraction, nasal flaring, and an expiratory grunt. During expiration, the infant continues to contract the diaphragm in an attempt to delay any reduction in thoracic volume and simultaneously contracts the constrictor muscles of the larynx to close the upper airway. Contraction of the abdominal muscles then results in an explosive exhalation of air, the grunt. The lungs are noncompliant and of small volume; in severe disease, the FRC may be as low as 3 mL/kg, whereas the FRC is 25 to 30 mL/kg in recovering babies. Over the first 24 to 36 hours after birth, the dyspnea worsens due to the disappearance of the small quantities of surfactant present in an infant with RDS and the inhibitory effect of plasma proteins on surfactant, which leak onto the alveolar surface in the early edematous stage of lung damage. The pulmonary artery pressure (PAP) remains high throughout the first week; at least during systole, the PAP can be higher than systemic pressure and there is then right to left ductal shunting. At approximately 36 to 48 hours of age, endogenous surfactant synthesis commences and the infant's respiratory status improves; this is associated with a spontaneous diuresis. A full recovery from RDS can be expected by 1 week of age, although respiratory support may still be required because of the development of complications. Nowadays, this classical presentation is unusual, because exogenous surfactant is given; relatively mature infants so treated are frequently in room air by 48 hours of age.

DIAGNOSIS AND DIFFERENTIAL DIAGNOSIS

The diagnosis is made on the clinical history, including premature birth and the chest radiograph appearance; there is diffuse atelectasis resulting in fine granular opacification in both lung fields and an air bronchogram where the air-filled bronchi stand out against the atelectatic lungs (Fig. 18-1). If the disease is severe, the lungs may be so opaque that it is impossible to distinguish between the lung field and the cardiac silhouette, a "whiteout." If the radiograph is taken in the first 4 hours, interpretation may be difficult because of retention of fetal lung fluid; as the fluid clears, the chest radiograph appearance may show marked improvement. Antenatally, fetal lung maturity can be assessed by sampling amniotic fluid, because as the fluid secreted by the fetal lung moves out into the amniotic fluid it carries with it surfactant. As the lung matures, the amount of DPPC (lecithin) in the amniotic fluid increases, but the amount of sphingomyelin remains unchanged throughout gestation; thus, lung maturity can be assessed from the ratio of lecithin to sphingomyelin (L:S ratio). The lower the L:S ratio, the more likely the infant is to develop RDS: 21% of infants with an L:S ratio of 1.5 to 2.0 being affected, compared with 80% with an L:S ratio below 1.5, but an L:S ratio less than 2.0 predicts RDS with an accuracy of only 54%. An L:S ratio greater than 2.0 is usually associated with lung maturity and in 95% of cases will predict the absence of RDS. A mature L:S ratio, however, can be associated with RDS in the infants of diabetic mothers or those with rhesus disease; in those cases, the abnormality is deficiency of phosphatidylglycerol. Further problems in interpreting the L:S ratio can occur when the specimen is contaminated with blood, meconium, or vaginal secretions. The L:S ratio can also be assessed in fluid from the pharynx or stomach. Pulmonary maturity can be estimated by measuring the level of serum SP-A in cord blood using an enzyme-linked immunosorbent assay system, but the tests are expensive and time consuming. Tests of surfactant maturity are now rarely used, and because of the proven efficacy of prophylactic surfactant administration, many clinicians give exogenous surfactant very soon after birth to all infants born below a certain gestational age; the exact cut off depends on local resource issues, but usually infants younger than 29 weeks of gestational age receive prophylactic surfactant. Rapid assessments of lung maturity may, however, be useful in situations where supplies of surfactant are limited.

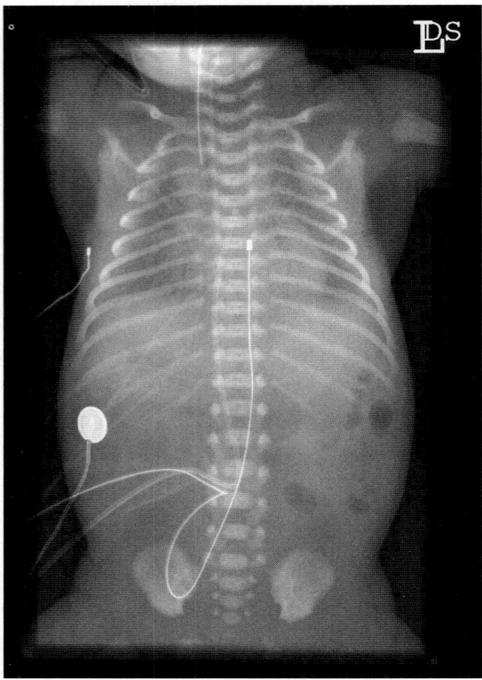

FIGURE 18-1. Chest radiograph of an infant with severe respiratory distress syndrome—diffuse reticulogranular appearance with an air bronchogram.

It is impossible to differentiate severe early-onset septicemia from RDS, and both conditions may coexist. All dyspneic newborn babies, therefore, should have appropriate bacterial cultures taken and antibiotics administered from the earliest signs of respiratory illness, because without treatment early-onset septicemia can be fatal within hours. Penicillin and gentamicin act synergistically against group B streptococcus (GBS) and are also effective against many of the organisms causing early-onset septicemia and pneumonia. In babies with RDS who are stable or are improving, antibiotics should be stopped when negative culture results are notified at 48 to 72 hours. Infants with RDS may have coexistent pulmonary hypertension, their oxygen requirement will be out of proportion to their chest radiograph appearance, and they frequently have a poor response to surfactant therapy. Respiratory distress presenting after 4 to 6 hours of age is usually due to pneumonia, and the differential diagnosis includes air leak, heart failure secondary to congenital heart disease, or aspiration.

MANAGEMENT

The management of an infant who is at high risk for RDS begins in the labor suite. Practice differs regarding whether preterm babies are placed immediately on nasal CPAP or are intubated to be given surfactant; if the latter option is chosen, then some clinicians would then immediately extubate the infant onto nasal CPAP, whereas others prefer the infant to remain intubated until further assessment can take place on the neonatal intensive care unit (NICU). On arrival in the NICU, the infant must be put into an incubator prewarmed to 35° to 36°C or placed under a radiant heater. The infant should be carefully examined, including measurement of the head circumference and weight. Appropriate monitoring should be put in place to measure blood pressure and an umbilical arterial catheter (UAC) or a peripheral arterial cannula inserted to facilitate measurements of partial pressure of oxygen in arterial blood (PaO_2), $PaCO_2$, and pH. A blood sample should be obtained to estimate the hemoglobin level, white blood cell count, and coagulation status and for culture. A chest radiograph should be taken, preferably after inserting the UAC. Vitamin K and antibiotics should be given and surfactant administered, if it has not been given in the labor ward. It is then important to handle the infant as little as possible, which can result in hypoxia and irregular respiration. As a consequence, chest physiotherapy and routine endotracheal suctioning are contraindicated in the first 24 to 48 hours, particularly because secretions are not a problem unless infection develops. If the blood pressure monitoring reveals the infant to be hypotensive and this is due to anemia, the first transfusion (15 mL/kg) usually should be given by infusion over 10 to 15 minutes; thereafter, transfusions should be given more slowly at a rate guided by the condition of the neonate. Blood loss after birth is usually iatrogenic, but a sudden drop in the hemoglobin level in an infant with RDS suggests the development of an intracerebral hemorrhage. Ventilated preterm neonates tolerate hemoglobin levels of less than 13 g/dL poorly and should be transfused with blood from a CMV-negative donor, which is routine NICU practice; the blood should be irradiated to avoid the risk for graft-versus-host disease. Only if the infant has a clinically important patent ductus should he or she receive furosemide (1.0 mg/kg) during the transfusion. If the hypotensive neonate's hemoglobin is not low, saline should be given rather than albumin; the response to albumin is no better than that to saline, and albumin has more adverse effects. If the neonate is severely hypoxic or acidemic, their cardiac function may be impaired, this would usually be confirmed by echocardiography examination. In such circumstances, volume expansion will be poorly tolerated, in which case inotropes are the preferred treatment for hypotension. Renal function is often impaired in RDS, and urine production may be less than 1.0 mL/kg/hr; peripheral edema, however, is usually due to leaky capillaries. Infants with RDS should start on 40 to 60 mL/kg/24 hours[1] of a 10% dextrose solution and fluid intake subsequently guided by the electrolye levels and the change in the infant's weight. Ill neonates lose about 1% to 3% of their body weight per day, and a greater loss may indicate dehydration, whereas static or increased weight suggests too much fluid has been given. Sodium and potassium do not usually need to be added to the fluid intake for the first 36 to 48 hours, but calcium should usually be given. Characteristically, a diuresis occurs around the time the infant's lung function improves; then the fluid input should be increased to prevent dehydration. Since the protein and caloric reserves of the very low birth weight neonate are small, it is essential that some form of nutrition be given as soon as possible after birth. Neonates with severe respiratory illness may have an ileus and delayed gastric emptying; consequently, enteral feeding is initially not feasible. Parenteral nutrition should be given until an adequate enteral intake has been achieved. However, it is important to introduce enteral feeds as soon as possible because the prolonged absence of enteral feeding compromises gut growth and development. Thus, once bowel sounds are present in a ventilated neonate, who is appropriately grown and has passed meconium, enteral feeding should be started.

Surfactant given as "rescue" therapy (i.e., to infants with established RDS) improves the outcome of babies with established RDS, resulting in reductions in pneumothorax, mortality, and the combined outcome of mortality and BPD. There are a number of commercially available surfactant preparations, and they can be divided into two groups: natural surfactants (derived from animals' lungs) and synthetic surfactants. Natural surfactants more closely mimic the physiologic mixture of lipids and proteins (SP-B and SP-C) and have a more rapid effect on oxygenation than the older synthetic surfactants. Meta-analysis of the results of randomized trials highlighted that administration of natural rather than synthetic surfactant was associated with significant reductions in mortality (odds ratio [OR] 0.66, 95% confidence intervals [CI] 0.76–0.96) and pneumothorax (OR 0.63, CI 0.53–0.78).[8] More recently, a synthetic surfactant containing a polypeptide KL4 composed of lysine and leucine, which mimics the effects of SP-B, has been produced and appears to be as resistant to the inhibitory effects of proteins on the alveolar surface as natural surfactants. Although beneficial effects are seen after a single dose of surfactant, better results are obtained with more than one dose. Multiple doses compared with a single dose were associated with an approximately 50% reduction in the pneumothorax rate. The Osiris (1992) trial,[9] however, showed no benefit of three or four doses of a synthetic surfactant (colfosceril palmitate [DPPC], hexadecanal and tyloxapol, Exosurf Neonatal, Burroughs Wellcome) compared with two doses. Many clinicians usually now give two doses of a natural surfactant. Not all babies, including those with a PDA, cardiogenic shock, pulmonary hypertension, or an air leak respond to surfactant; failure to respond marks out a group of babies with a poorer prognosis. During the administration of the surfactant, there may be transient hypoxemia and bradycardia, but if care is taken with the surfactant instillation, there is only a transient perturbation in cerebral hemodynamics and either no effect or a slight reduction in the incidence of cerebral hemorrhage. No increased risk for infection has been found, although instilling surfactant could theoretically swamp the alveolar macrophages. Massive pulmonary hemorrhage, however, has been noted following surfactant administration, and the occurrence noted to be doubled by the use of a synthetic surfactant. Follow-up studies have demonstrated that surfactant treatment is not associated with additional neurologic deficits or an increase in severe retinopathy of prematurity, but better long-term lung function.

Some infants have relatively mild RDS and require only warm humidified supplementary oxygen. If their disease is more severe, continuous distending pressure is required to prevent atelectasis and improve oxygenation. CPAP can be delivered via an endotracheal tube, a facemask, a tube into one nostril, a pair of tubes into both nostrils, or a binasal tube. The devices can be connected via a T-piece circuit to a standard neonatal ventilator or a dedicated device. The method of administration of the CPAP influences its efficacy and side effects. Nowadays, a binasal system is most frequently employed. Increasing the level of CPAP increases lung volume and hence improves oxygenation, but it is possible to cause overdistention and carbon dioxide retention; infants may also suffer an air leak. In many centers, use of nasal CPAP (nCPAP) was restricted to relatively mature infants with moderate RDS; immature infants or those with a supplementary oxygen requirement in excess of 60% are intubated and mechanically ventilated. There are now reports of use of nCPAP in the labor suite and to provide ongoing respiratory support, in preference to intubation and ventilation. Such a policy has been described as a gentler form of ventilation, because it has been reported to be associated with a lower incidence of BPD, but this has not been confirmed in the randomized trials performed to date. In other centers, immature infants are intubated in the labor suite to receive prophylactic surfactant, and then ongoing respiratory support is provided by mechanical ventilation; more mature infants (older than 28 weeks of gestational age) are intubated and ventilated because of worsening respiratory distress and/or a major or recurrent troublesome apnea. Conventional mechanical ventilators deliver intermittent positive pressure inflations and positive end-expiratory pressure (PEEP). The ventilator inflations are delivered at a preset rate, which may be out of synchrony to the infant's respiratory efforts, leading to the development of an air leak. As a consequence, ventilators that are patient triggered have been developed for neonatal use. Although the results of physiologic studies demonstrated that that form of ventilation was associated with improvements in gas exchange, a lower work of breathing, and less asynchrony, meta-analysis of the results of randomized trials failed to demonstrate that patient-triggered ventilation reduced BPD or intracerebral hemorrhage or improved survival.[10] Volutrauma/barotrauma has been incriminated in the causation of BPD; consequently, forms of ventilatory support that deliver smaller tidal volumes than during conventional ventilation have been investigated.[11] To maintain minute volume using such techniques, fast frequencies are used. During high-frequency jet ventilation (HFJV), high velocity "bullets" of gas are fired at rates of 200 to 600 per minute and this entrains gas down the endotracheal tube. High-frequency oscillatory ventilation (HFOV) is usually delivered at frequencies between 10 and 15 Hz. Randomized trials have yielded conflicting results regarding whether use of HFJV reduces BPD; HFJV, however, may be helpful in infants who have already suffered the consequences of barotrauma, and its use has been associated with more rapid resolution of pulmonary interstitial emphysema (PIE). Randomized trials comparing HFOV to conventional ventilation have also yielded conflicting results regarding the impact on BPD and intracerebral hemorrhage. Meta-analysis of the results of those trials, however, demonstrated no advantage or disadvantage of prophylactic HFOV, that is, ventilation commencing within the first 12 hours after birth.[12] In infants with severe RDS, transfer to HFOV can improve oxygenation if a high-volume strategy is used (i.e., if the mean airway pressure is increased to optimize lung volume). There has been only one randomized trial comparing HFOV to conventional ventilation in prematurely born infants with severe respiratory failure; HFOV use was associated with a significant reduction in new pulmonary air leaks, but an increase in intracerebral hemorrhage. Pulmonary hypertension should be suspected in infants with RDS, whose hypoxia is more severe than would be anticipated from their chest radiograph appearance. The management of affected infants is described in the later section on Pulmonary Hypertension of the Newborn.

PREVENTIVE STRATEGIES

Administration of antenatal steroids matures the fetal lung, inducing the enzymes for surfactant synthesis and the genes for the surfactant proteins. As a consequence, antenatal administration of dexamethasone or betamethasone to pregnant women significantly reduces the incidences of RDS (OR 0.63, CI 0.44–0.82), neonatal death (OR 0.60, CI 0.48–0.75), cerebral hemorrhage (OR 0.48, CI 0.32–0.72), and necrotizing enterocolitis (OR 0.58, CI 0.32–1.09).[13] Benefit is maximal in infants delivered within 24 to 168 hours of maternal therapy being started; a smaller benefit is seen in infants whose mothers have received less than 24 hours of treatment. Antenatal steroids do not increase the risk for infection in pregnancies complicated by premature rupture of the membranes; indeed, they have a beneficial effect. Glucocorticoids should also be given in diabetic pregnancies, and the insulin regimen altered as necessary during the brief period of hyperglycemia resulting from the steroid treatment. There are, however, doubts about the safety of multiple courses of corticosteroids; although data from animal models have highlighted that repeated doses have beneficial effects on lung function, they may have adverse effects on brain function and fetal growth. The safety and efficacy of multiple versus single courses are currently being investigated in randomized trials.[14] Guidelines for antenatal steroid usage have been produced by the Royal College of Obstetricians and Gynaecologists and the National Institutes of Health in the United States. Their recommendations include that antenatal treatment with corticosteroids should be considered for all women at risk for preterm labor between 24 and 36 weeks. Betamethasone (two doses 24 hours apart) rather than dexamethasone (four doses 12 hours apart) is preferred, since in an observational study betamethasone was associated with a lower occurrence of cystic periventricular leukomalacia.[15] Corticosteroids should be given unless immediate delivery is anticipated. In the absence of chorioamnionitis, antenatal corticosteroids are recommended in pregnancies complicated by preterm and prolonged rupture of the membranes and in other complicated pregnancies, unless there is evidence that corticosteroids will have an adverse effect on the mother. Thyroid hormones induce surfactant synthesis, but meta-analysis of the results of 11 trials demonstrated that antenatal administration of thyrotrophin-releasing hormone (TRH), which unlike T_4, T_3, or thyroid-stimulating hormone does cross the placenta, did not reduce the risk of neonatal respiratory distress or BPD. Indeed, there were adverse effects: an increase in requirement for ventilation and a greater likelihood of the treated infants having a low Apgar score at 5 minutes.[16] Antenatally administered TRH can also produce transient suppression of the pituitary thyroid axis and complications in the mother, including nausea, vomiting, and increased blood pressure. Other drugs, including aminophylline and ambroxol, have been used in animal experiments to mature the surfactant synthetic pathways. The effect of antenatal betamimetics on the human neonate appears to be small, although in a randomized controlled trial, infants whose mothers had received an infusion of terbutaline prior to elective delivery had significantly better lung function. Benefit from ambroxol has been reported, but this is not a consistent finding.

A large number of studies have been carried out to assess the impact of surfactant given prophylactically, that is, within the first few minutes after birth. Meta-analyses of the results of trials comparing administration of surfactant prophylactically or selectively, or early versus late, have demonstrated that prophylactic/early administration is more effective. Prophylactic versus selective surfactant administration has been associated with significant reductions in neonatal mortality (OR 0.61, CI 0.28–0.77), BPD and death (OR 0.85, CI 0.76–0.95), pneumothorax (OR 0.54, CI 0.42–0.84), and early versus late reductions in neonatal mortality (OR 0.87, CI 0.77–0.99) and pneumothorax (OR 0.70, CI 0.58–0.82).[17] Positive effects of both synthetic and natural surfactants have been reported. Prophylactic use of natural surfactant results in significant reductions in pneumothorax (OR 0.35, CI 0.26–0.49), mortality (OR 0.60, CI 0.44–0.83), and the combined outcome of mortality and BPD (OR 0.84, CI 0.75–0.93), but not BPD alone.

MORTALITY AND MORBIDITY

Overall, the mortality from RDS is between 10% and 15%; the mortality rate is inversely proportional to gestational age. The acute complications of RDS include air leaks, patent ductus arteriosus (PDA), and pulmonary hemorrhage, and these are discussed in the relevant sections below. Bronchopulmonary dysplasia, defined as oxygen dependency beyond 36 weeks' postmenstrual age, develops in more than 50% of infants born prior to 29 weeks of gestation. This condition is described in detail in Chapter 19. In addition, infants with RDS may suffer an intracerebral hemorrhage or periventricular leukomalacia, both conditions increasing the risk for adverse neurodevelopmental outcome. The latter is particularly common in infants born prior to 26 weeks of gestational age.[18]

ACUTE RESPIRATORY DISTRESS SYNDROME

Acute respiratory distress syndrome (ARDS) can occur following asphyxia, shock, sepsis, or meconium aspiration syndrome. Asphyxia results in damage to the myocardium, and the associated severe metabolic acidemia in depressed myocardial contractility. This leads to heart failure and pulmonary edema. Asphyxia also damages the pulmonary blood vessels and, if the leak of protein-rich fluid onto the alveoli is large, ARDS develops. ARDS is a disease of full-term babies who, within the first hour or two, usually present with tachypnea (respiratory rate of at least 100 breaths/min) rather than with retraction or grunting. Respiration is stimulated by metabolic acidemia, damage to the central nervous system, and/or pulmonary edema. Infants with ARDS are severely hypoxemic. The chest radiograph demonstrates diffuse pulmonary infiltrates and in severe cases there will be a "whiteout." Surfactant administration can improve oxygenation in ARDS and is most effective if given early and in larger doses than used in RDS. In adults and children with ARDS, prone positioning has been shown to improve oxygenation. A high level of PEEP should be used in an attempt to restore the FRC to normal values, and this will also increase the mean airway pressure (MAP) level and hence oxygenation. High-volume strategy HFOV can also improve oxygenation, particularly in those patients who had a positive response to PEEP elevation. Fluid intake should initially be restricted to 40 mL/kg/24 hours, and if heart failure is present, furosemide should be administered. If the infant is anemic and there is coexisting myocardial asphyxial injury, a blood transfusion should be given slowly with a diuretic, but if the anemia is severe, then a single-volume exchange transfusion using packed red blood cells should be undertaken. Broad-spectrum antibiotics, usually penicillin plus an aminoglycoside, should be administered, but aminoglycoside levels must be carefully monitored because these infants are at risk for renal dysfunction. The mortality of ARDS is high, particularly in infants who develop secondary infection or do not respond to elevation of their PEEP level. Air leaks and infection are commonly seen in infants with ARDS.

TRANSIENT TACHYPNEA OF THE NEWBORN

TTN occurs in 4 to 6 per 1000 full-term infants. TTN may be more common in prematurely born infants (an incidence of 10 per 1000 has been reported), but in prematurely born infants, coexisting problems such as RDS may mask the presentation. TTN is due to delayed fetal lung fluid clearance and hence has also been called retained fetal lung fluid or wet lungs. In fetal life, the lung is filled with liquid, increasing from 4 to 6 mL/kg body weight at midgestation to about 20 mL/kg near term. Fetal lung fluid is produced initially at a rate of 2 mL/kg/hr, increasing to 5 mL/kg/hr at full term. It contributes one third to one half of the daily turnover of amniotic fluid. Compared with either amniotic fluid or plasma, lung liquid has a high chloride but low bicarbonate and protein concentration. The secondary active transport of chloride ions from the interstitial space into the lung is the main force for lung liquid secretion, sodium ions, and water following passively down electrical and osmotic gradients. The presence of lung liquid is essential for normal lung development; chronic drainage results in pulmonary hypoplasia. The volume of fetal lung liquid is regulated by the resistance to lung liquid efflux through the upper airway; a pressure in the lumen of the lung is generated that is approximately 1 cm of water greater than that in the amniotic cavity; the pressure is essential for lung growth. During labor and delivery, the concentration of epinephrine increases, the chloride pump responsible for lung liquid secretion is inhibited, and lung liquid secretion ceases. In addition, lung liquid resorption commences as the raised epinephrine levels stimulate sodium channels on the apical surface of the pulmonary epithelium, via which fetal lung liquid absorption occurs. Thyroid hormone and cortisol are necessary for maturation of the normal response of the fetal lung to epinephrine. Exposure to postnatal oxygen tensions increases sodium transport across the pulmonary epithelium. Although some liquid is squeezed out under the high vaginal pressure during the second stage of labor, the majority is absorbed into the pulmonary lymphatics and capillaries. Air entry into the lung displaces liquid from the terminal respiratory units into the perivascular space; the hydraulic pressure in the pulmonary circulation is reduced and blood flow is increased. As a consequence, the effective vascular surface area for fluid exchange is increased, facilitating water absorption into the pulmonary vascular bed. The replacement of lung liquid by air is largely accomplished within a few minutes of birth.

TTN is more common in infants who are born by cesarean section without labor,[19] because lung fluid clearance will not have occurred. Respiratory distress is more likely to occur if a cesarean section without labor is performed at 37 rather than 38 weeks of gestation.[19] Surfactant deficiency may be important in the pathogenesis of TTN. Other risk factors for TTN include male sex and a family history of asthma. Infants of asthmatic mothers may have a genetic predisposition to β-adrenergic hyporesponsiveness.

Infants with TTN are tachypneic, with respiratory rates up to 120 breaths/min, but they rarely grunt, because their lungs are not atelectatic. The chest may be barrel shaped as a result of hyperinflation, and the liver and spleen palpable because of downward displacement of the diaphragm. Peripheral edema is often present, and affected babies lose weight more slowly than controls. There is usually only a mild hypoxia; if there is a marked respiratory or metabolic acidosis, the diagnosis should be reviewed. The chest radiograph shows hyperinflation, prominent perihilar vascular markings due to engorgement of the periarterial lymphatics (Fig. 18-2), edema of the interlobar septae, and fluid in the fissures. Cerebral irritation from subarachnoid blood or perinatal hypoxic ischemia should be considered in the differential diagnosis of a tachypneic infant, but affected infants have a respiratory alkalemia. The chest radiograph appearance of TTN may mimic that of heart failure.

Management includes supplementary oxygen; very unusually, infants with TTN have been reported to require very high concentrations of oxygen or even mechanical ventilation. Intravenous antibiotics should be administered until infection has been excluded and nasogastric tube feeds withheld until the respiratory rate settles. Diuretics are of no proven benefit.[20] In a randomized trial, infants given furosemide lost more weight than the placebo group, but there were no significant differences between groups with regard to duration of tachypnea or hospitalization. By definition, TTN is self-limiting, and affected infants have usually made a complete recovery within a few days of birth. Complications are rare, although air leaks may occur, particularly if the infant has required CPAP or intermittent positive pressure ventilation (IPPV). There is debate as to whether infants who had TTN are more likely to wheeze at follow-up. Finally, it should be noted that respiratory distress for no good reason in a full-term infant, especially if associated with rhinorrhea, should prompt consideration of the diagnosis of primary ciliary dyskinesia (see Chapter 63) irrespective of whether mirror-image organ arrangement is present. This is rare (1 in 15,000 live births), but is probably one of only a few causes of coughing on the neonatal unit. Some of these babies develop only mild neonatal respiratory distress or rhinorrhea, insufficient to merit admission to the NICU.

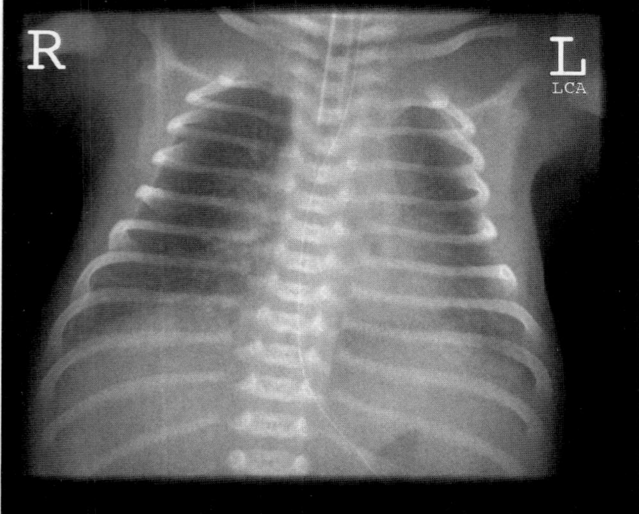

FIGURE 18-2. Transient tachypnea of the newborn. Severe changes with widespread consolidation indistinguishable radiologically from infection, the rapid clearance of the abnormalities within 24 hours confirmed the diagnosis.

PNEUMONIA

EARLY-ONSET PNEUMONIA

Early-onset pneumonia is acquired transplacentally or during labor or delivery; ascending infection is particularly likely if there is prolonged rupture of the membranes. Transplacentally acquired organisms that can cause pneumonia include *Listeria monocytogenes, Mycobacterium tuberculosis, Treponema pallidum,* rubella virus, cytomegalovirus (CMV), herpes simplex virus (HSV), adenovirus, and influenza A virus. Sixty percent to 70% of cases of pneumonia caused by ascending infection are due to *Streptococcus agalactiae* (GBS). There are seven identifiable subtypes of GBS based on capsular polysaccharide antigens, and most neonatal infections are caused by types I, II, and III. The incidence of early-onset GBS sepsis is 1.8 per 1000 live births in the United States and 0.3 to 1 per 1000 in the United Kingdom. *Escherichia coli* is the second most common cause of early neonatal sepsis. Approximately 40% of *E. coli* strains causing early-onset sepsis possess the capsule type K1, which confers antiphagocytic properties and resistance to complement-mediated killing. Pregnancy is associated with an increased carriage of K1 strains, which are then vertically transmitted. Other organisms that cause ascending infection include *Haemophilus influenzae, Streptococcus pneumoniae, Listeria monocytogenes, Klebsiella pneumoniae, Candida albicans,* adenovirus, CMV, HSV, and echovirus.

Risk factors for early-onset pneumonia include prolonged rupture of the membranes, premature labor, and organisms present in the vagina. Other risk factors for GBS infection include chorioamnionitis, prolonged labor, and frequent pelvic examinations in labor. Vaginal and rectal carriage rates of GBS are reported to be between 7% and 23%. Infants at highest risk for GBS infection are those whose mothers, although having GBS in their vagina, have little or no circulating anti-GBS immunoglobulin. Approximately 1% of infants born vaginally to mothers who carry GBS at the time of birth become infected. The most important reservoir for transmission of *Listeria monocytogenes* to humans is food, especially dairy products, contaminated by infected farm animals. Women infected with HIV are considerably more susceptible to *L. monocytogenes* than the general population.

CLINICAL PRESENTATION AND DIAGNOSIS

Infants with transplacentally acquired infection present at birth, and those infected with organisms acquired from the birth canal present within the first 48 hours after birth. The infant typically suffers progressive respiratory distress and has signs of systemic sepsis, which develop within a few hours of birth. Infants who are frankly septicemic with poor peripheral perfusion, cyanosis, and inadequate respiration have a poor prognosis. Most cases of GBS pneumonia present within the first 4 to 6 hours; if the infant does not receive prompt treatment, their condition rapidly deteriorates such that they require intubation and ventilation for apnea and develop pulmonary hypertension. Infants with congenitally acquired listerial infection are often extremely ill at birth with severe pneumonia and hepatomegaly. Diarrhea and an erythematous skin rash may occur. Characteristically, affected infants have small pink-gray cutaneous granulomas; these granulomas are widespread in the lung, liver, and nervous system. More typically infants with early-onset pneumonia have respiratory distress with nonspecific signs, such as poor feeding and irritability; they may be febrile or hypothermic.

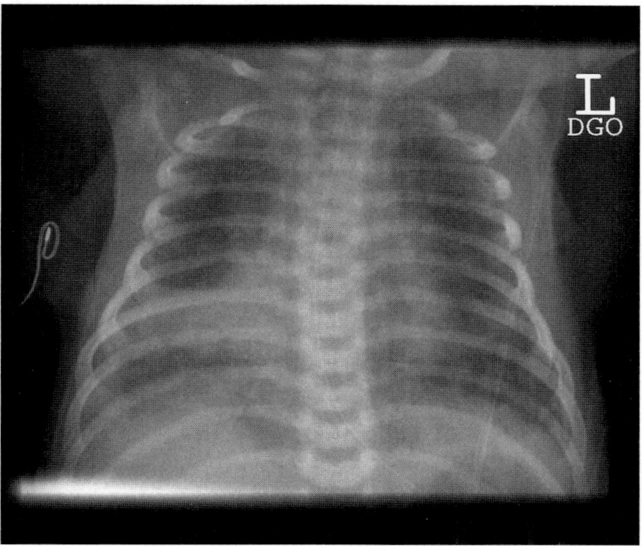

■ **FIGURE 18-3.** Right-sided lobar pneumonia.

The chest radiograph appearance is varied; there can be lobar (Fig. 18-3) or segmental consolidation, atelectasis, or diffuse haziness or opacification (Fig. 18-4). In addition, pleural effusions may occur, particularly if the pneumonia is the result of bacterial or fungal infection. Rarely, there is abscess or pneumatocele formation, and these complications are most likely to occur with staphylococcal or coliform pneumonia. GBS is easy to culture and will usually grow from surface swabs and the gastric aspirate. Listeria can be isolated from the first meconium passed. In addition to the appropriate cultures from the infant, histologic evaluation and culture of the placenta should be undertaken, and serologic testing of the mother and infant for syphilis or viral agents should be considered. If infection due to herpes is likely, viral cultures from the maternal lesions and the infant should be obtained.

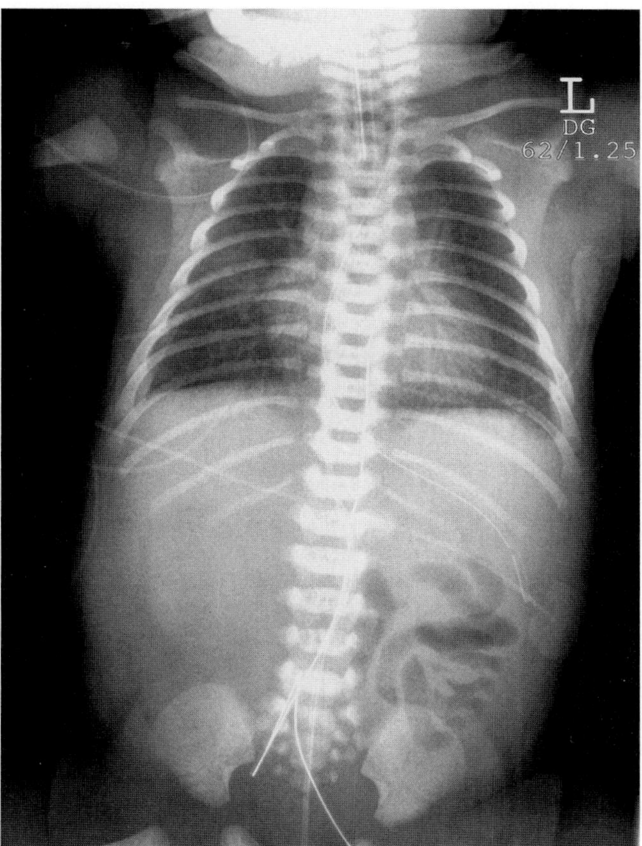

■ **FIGURE 18-4.** Group B *Streptococcus* (GBS) pneumonia mimicking respiratory distress syndrome. The focal consolidation in the posterior segment of the right upper lobe is more suggestive of GBS pneumonia.

■ TREATMENT

All infants with respiratory distress should receive antibiotic treatment. Initial treatment for early-onset pneumonia should be a combination of ampicillin or benzylpenicillin and an aminoglycoside. Modification to that regimen may be necessary once the culture results are known or there is good reason to suspect a particular organism; for example, *H. influenzae* with ampicillin resistance are emerging and cefotaxime should be added if *H. influenzae* sepsis is suspected. Cefotaxime and ceftriaxone are used for *E. coli* sepsis, but for infection with *Listeria*, the most effective antibiotic therapy is ampicillin plus gentamicin, since *Listeria* organisms are resistant to all third-generation cephalosporins. Antibiotic therapy should continue for at least 10 days, but for 3 weeks if the pneumonia is due to *Staphylococcus aureus*. Long-term intravenous therapy should be given if there is abscess formation. Empyemas should be drained and intravenous antibiotics administered for at least 2 weeks. It is important to prevent vertical transmission of GBS by giving intrapartum antibiotic prophylaxis (penicillin or ampicillin) to women identified by screening in pregnancy to carry GBS and/or have risk factors. Risk factors include a previous infant with GBS disease, GBS in the maternal urine during pregnancy, preterm labor, ruptured membranes for more than 18 hours prior to delivery, and intrapartum fever. The mortality rate for early-onset disease is 15%, but higher for low birth weight infants.

■ LATE-ONSET PNEUMONIA

The majority of cases of late-onset pneumonia on a neonatal intensive care unit occur in ventilated, prematurely born infants. The most common responsible bacteria are coagulase-negative staphylococci, *S. aureus,* and gram-negative bacilli, including *Klebsiella, E. coli,* and *Pseudomonas*. Viruses can also cause late-onset pneumonia, and these include RSV, influenza virus, parainfluenza virus, adenovirus, and rhinovirus; viral pneumonia usually occurs when there are high levels of infection in the community, resulting in nosocomial infection. Fungal infections are a significant problem if infants have had prolonged exposure to antibiotics, particularly third-generation cephalosporins; pneumonia occurs as a result of blood-borne spread.

The development of pneumonia in a ventilated infant will present as an increasing requirement for ventilatory support. Initial treatment should be a third-generation cephalosporin and vancomycin, because the most likely infecting organism will be a coagulase-negative staphylococci. Clearly, this choice should be modified according to local knowledge and, if necessary, according to culture results. If the infant is already on antibiotics, the regimen should usually be changed and the spectrum of cover broadened. Ventilator-associated pneumonia

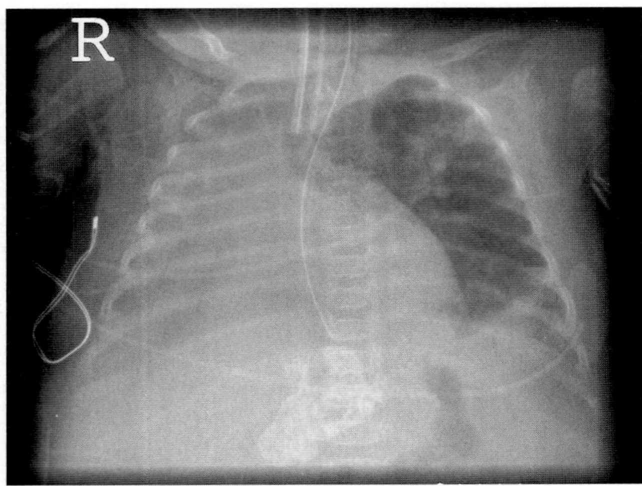

■ **FIGURE 18-5.** Aspiration with right lung collapse and herniation of the left lung across the mediastinum.

increases morbidity (prolonged length of NICU stay) and mortality, particularly in infants born prior to 28 weeks of gestation.[21]

■ ASPIRATION PNEUMONIA

This occurs in infants with GER or sucking or swallowing incoordination. Aspiration can result in physical obstruction because inhaled curd is particulate. The resultant airway obstruction can lead to lung collapse (Fig. 18-5) and/or consolidation and predispose to infection. Chemical irritation occurs with the aspiration of acidic gastric contents. The infant may initially be asymptomatic if the aspiration is due to GER, but if there is massive regurgitation, the infant may be found cyanosed and apneic or gasping. On auscultation crepitations, rhonchi may be heard. A new area of consolidation, particularly in the right upper lobe, on the chest radiograph is suggestive of aspiration (Fig. 18-6).

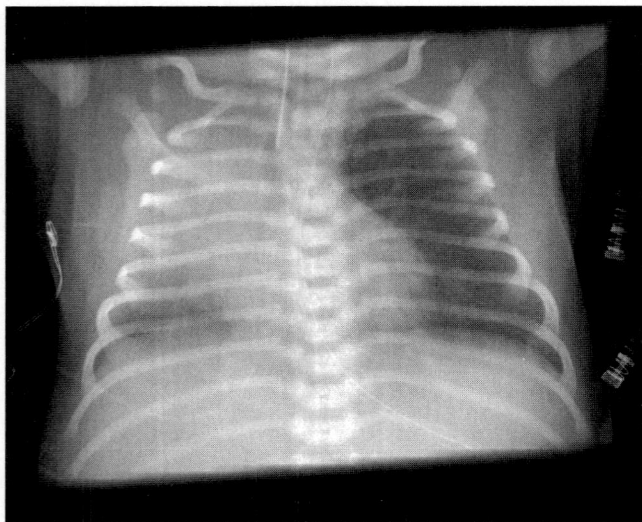

■ **FIGURE 18-6.** Aspiration with predominantly right upper lobe changes in an infant with sucking and swallowing incoordination following severe birth depression.

Following the episode of aspiration, the airway should be cleared and the infant may require supplementary oxygen or even ventilatory support. Broad-spectrum antibiotic cover should be given, usually flucloxacillin and an aminoglycoside, for at least 5 days. If the infant has an area of consolidation, regular physiotherapy should be undertaken, and the infant positioned to optimize drainage from the affected lobe.

■ INTERSTITIAL LUNG DISEASE

Interstitial lung disease is an uncommon cause of respiratory distress in neonates and is covered in detail in Chapter 47. Familial interstital lung disease has been reported in association with mutations of the surfactant protein B and C genes. Chronic pneumonitis of infancy, characterized by type II cell hyperplasia and alveolar filling by proteinaceous material, occurs only in the pediatric age range. In addition, it has been suggested that interstital lung disease may occur as a developmental disorder, particularly due to an abnormality in differentiation of pulmonary mesenchyme.[22] In seven neonates with atypical neonatal lung disease, lung biopsies revealed expansion of the interstitium by spindle-shaped cells containing periodic acid-Schiff-positive diastase-labile material consistent with glycogen. Electron microscopy demonstrated primitive interstitial mesenchyme cells with few cell organelles and abundant monoparticulate glycogen. Abundant glycogen is not normally found in pulmonary interstital cells; therefore, the infants were suggested to be suffering from a developmental disorder, which was named pulmonary interstitial glycogenosis.[22] There was no evidence of a generalized abnormality of glycogen metabolism or storage.

Infants with interstital lung disease can present in the first weeks after birth with tachypnea. Their chest radiographs demonstrate bilateral interstitial infiltrates. All the infants diagnosed as having pulmonary interstital glycogenosis (PIG) presented with tachypnea and hypoxemia; their chest radiographs demonstrated a diffuse fine interstital reticular pattern with overinflated lungs, resembling early diffuse infectious pneumonia.[22] High-resolution computed tomography (CT) scans showed nonspecific patchy ground glass opacification. Infants with PIG[22] were treated with pulse corticosteroids and, in one case, hydroxychloroquine was also given, but no clinical benefit was seen from adding that therapy. Clinical resolution and radiographic improvement was noted in most of the infants, which would indicate that PIG has a more favorable prognosis than other idiopathic interstitial lung diseases.[22]

■ MECONIUM ASPIRATION SYNDROME

Meconium staining of the amniotic fluid occurs in 8% to 20% of pregnancies, and 5% of babies born through meconium-stained amniotic fluid develop meconium aspiration syndrome (MAS). Prolonged severe fetal hypoxia can stimulate fetal breathing with inhalation of amniotic fluid containing meconium, or the inhalation may occur perinatally if the airway contains meconium-stained amniotic fluid. Meconium aspiration is a disease of full-term or post-term babies, as the prevalence of meconium-stained liquor is 10% or more after 38 weeks of gestation but 22% in babies with a gestational age of 42 weeks. Meconium staining of the liquor occurs in less than 5% of preterm pregnancies and suggests infection in these cases. Passage of meconium relates to motilin levels. Motilin is produced mainly by the jejunum and stimulates peristalsis. Levels are very low in preterm infants and nonasphyxiated full-term infants, but elevated in asphyxiated full-term babies who pass meconium intrapartum.

Meconium is sticky and composed of inspissated fetal intestinal secretions. When it is inhaled, it creates a ball valve mechanism in the airways: air can be sucked in, but cannot be exhaled. The result is gas trapping and lung overdistention, predisposing to air leaks. Meconium is also an irritant, and inflammatory cells and mediators are released in response to the presence of meconium in the airways. An inflammatory pneumonitis with alveolar collapse develops. The pulmonary artery pressure is increased, because the inflammatory response results in release of vasoactive substances, which cause vasoconstriction. Although meconium is initially sterile, because of its organic nature, its presence in the airway predisposes to pulmonary infection, particularly with *Escherichia coli*. In addition, because meconium may inhibit phagocytosis and the neutrophil oxidative burst, bacteria can grow in meconium-stained amniotic fluid. Meconium (particularly the chloroform soluble phase, composed of free fatty acids, triglycerides, and cholesterol) inhibits surfactant function and production in a concentration-dependent manner.

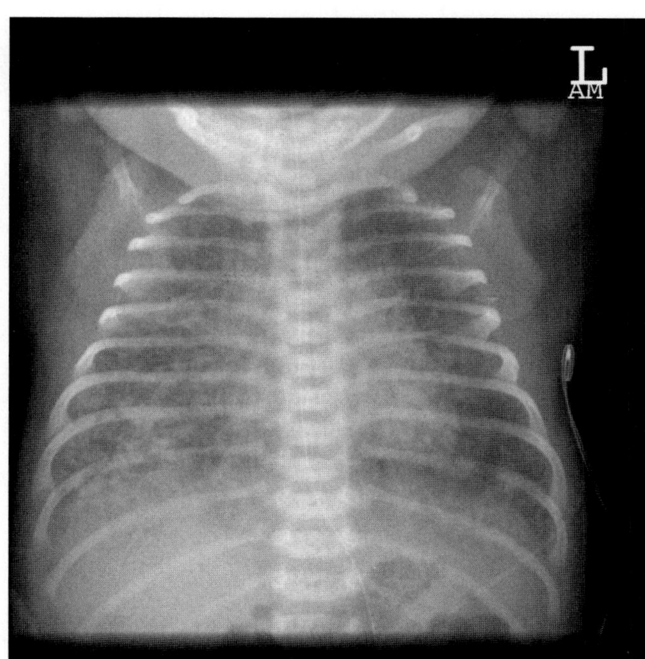

FIGURE 18-7. Meconium aspiration syndrome with diffuse patchy infiltration bilaterally.

CLINICAL PRESENTATION

Infants with MAS are tachypneic, their respiratory rate may exceed 120 breaths/min, and they have intercostal and subcostal recession and use their accessory respiratory muscles. They are frequently hypoxic due to ventilation-perfusion mismatch and pulmonary hypertension, but unless the disease is severe, carbon dioxide levels are not usually elevated. Meconium in the airways causes widespread crackles, and affected infants have an overdistended chest due to air trapping. In mild cases, recovery may occur within 24 hours, but those who require ventilation are frequently still symptomatic at 2 weeks of age and may remain oxygen dependent beyond the neonatal period. Early chest radiographs demonstrate widespread patchy infiltration (Fig. 18-7) and overexpansion; small pleural effusions occur in approximately 20% of patients. In severe cases, by 72 hours of age the appearance is often changed to that of diffuse and homogeneous opacification of both lung fields because of pneumonitis and interstitial edema. The changes gradually resolve over the next week, but in severe cases the chest radiograph appearance may merge into the pattern seen in BPD. Air leaks, particularly pneumothorax and pneumomediastinum, are common, occurring in approximately 20% of infants. If there has been severe intrapartum asphyxia, there may be echocardiogram changes, suggesting subendocardial ischemia, and the echocardiogram will show reduced cardiac contractility. In those with pulmonary hypertension, echocardiography will demonstrate right to left shunting at ductal and atrial levels.

MANAGEMENT

In the initial stages of the illness, sufficient supplementary oxygen should be given to maintain the oxygen saturation levels at 95% or the arterial oxygen level greater than 10 kPa. Warmed, humidified oxygen should be delivered into a headbox, even if the infant requires an oxygen concentration of up to 80%, providing there is no respiratory acidosis. Intubation and ventilation are indicated if the $PaCO_2$ rises above 8 kPa (60 mm Hg), particularly if the infant is hypoxic. If, however, the infant has hypoxic ischemic encephalopathy (HIE), more rigid control of the blood gases is required. CPAP may improve oxygenation, but will increase the risk for pneumothorax and thus is not recommended in MAS. Babies with MAS can be very difficult to ventilate; theoretically, a long expiratory time and a low level of PEEP should be used, but elevation of PEEP may be necessary to improve oxygenation, although that maneuver will increase the risk for a pneumothorax. A neuromuscular blocking agent should be administered, because infants with MAS often “fight the ventilator,” hence increasing their risk for an air leak. In infants with severe disease and pulmonary hypertension, HFOV, particularly if used with nitric oxide (NO), and NO used in conjunction with conventional ventilation can improve oxygenation and reduce the need for extracorporeal membrane oxygenation (ECMO). When the oxygenation index was greater than 40, results of a randomized trial demonstrated that ECMO improved survival by 50% (UK Collaborative ECMO Trial Group 1996).[23] Overall, more than 90% of babies with MAS managed with ECMO survive. Meta-analysis of the results of the two randomized trials demonstrated that surfactant administration also reduces the risk for requiring ECMO (RR 0.64, CI 0.46–0.91).[24] Administering the surfactant by dilute surfactant lavage may be particularly effective in improving gas exchange.[25] The efficacy of corticosteroids in MAS, however, is controversial. Broad-spectrum antibiotics, such as penicillin and gentamicin, should be given.

PREVENTIVE STRATEGIES

Avoidance of postterm delivery is the most important factor in reducing MAS. In uncontrolled studies, meticulous clearing of the airway at delivery has been reported to reduce the incidence of MAS. No significant benefit of routine endotracheal intubation and suctioning at birth over routine resuscitation, including oropharyngeal suction of vigorous full-term meconium stained babies, however, was demonstrated by the meta-analysis of the results of four randomized trials[26]; but the rates of MAS, HIE, and mortality in that systematic review were low, thus making reliable estimates of the treatment effect impossible. On the evidence to date, intubation and suctioning should be restricted to newborns who are depressed, that is, those who have a heart rate less than 100 beats/min, poor respiratory effort, and poor tone. It is important that an experienced pediatrician attend such deliveries. As soon as possible after delivery, the pediatrician should gently insert a laryngoscope and clear the upper airway of any meconium-stained material present. Direct endotracheal suctioning is only indicated if meconium is seen below the cords. Compression of the neonatal thorax is not recommended, because it is unlikely to prevent gasping, and compression of the thorax can stimulate respiratory efforts. Whether instillation of water or saline into the lower respiratory tract is useful is controversial; an increase in wet lung has been noted following this procedure. If the infant requires mechanical ventilation, then tracheal suction with saline lavage can result in an improvement in airway resistance. Aspiration of the stomach is frequently undertaken to prevent subsequent inhalation following vomiting or reflux of previously swallowed meconium. Routine gastric lavage prior to feeding in one study, however, did not decrease the incidence of MAS in babies born through meconium-stained liquor. There is an inverse relationship between amniotic fluid volume and fetal heart rate decelerations, possibly due to either cord or head compression. Amnioinfusion to maintain amniotic fluid volume during labor is undertaken to try and stop such compression and hence reduce the likelihood of MAS. Results of a meta-analysis suggested that amnioinfusion, particularly in settings of limited perinatal surveillance, improved perinatal outcome with significant reductions in MAS, HIE, and neonatal intensive care unit admission.[27] There are, however, adverse outcomes of amnioinfusion, including increased incidences of cord prolapse, infection, and requirement for instrumental delivery. Suppression of fetal breathing movements by maternal narcotic administration, although successful in a baboon model, did not reduce the incidence of MAS in two clinical series.

MORTALITY AND MORBIDITY

Mortality rates are between 4% and 12%; the majority of deaths are from respiratory failure, pulmonary hypertension, or air leaks. Fifty percent of babies who require mechanical ventilation because of MAS suffer an air leak. Bronchopulmonary dysplasia is a rare complication of MAS. Neurologic sequelae occur in infants with coexisting HIE. MAS is associated with long-term respiratory morbidity; lung function abnormalities, including increased bronchial hyperreactivity, have been reported, and up to 40% of those who have had severe MAS go on to develop asthma at school age.

PULMONARY HYPERTENSION OF THE NEWBORN

Infants with persistent pulmonary hypertension of the newborn (PPHN) have pulmonary hypertension, producing right to left shunts at the level of the ductus arteriosus and the foramen ovale. PPHN has been called persistent fetal circulation, but this is inaccurate because the high-flow, low-resistance circuit through the placenta present in the fetal circulation is missing.

CHANGES IN THE CIRCULATION AT BIRTH

In the fetus, the pulmonary vascular resistance (PVR) is high, but within the systemic circulation there is a low-resistance component, the placenta. As a consequence, there is shunting across the PDA and only approximately 10% of the right ventricular output enters the pulmonary circulation. At birth, removal of the placenta from the circulation reduces venous return through the inferior vena cava to the right atrium. This results in lowering of the right atrial pressure at a time when the left atrial pressure is increased because of the increased pulmonary venous return; hence, the foramen ovale closes. The flow through the ductus venosus is diminished, and passive closure of the ductus venosus occurs within 3 to 7 days after birth. PVR falls rapidly in the first minutes after birth, then more gradually over the next days. The fall in PVR is associated with a structural reorganization and thinning of the vessel walls. It is a consequence of lung aeration, which results in opening up the pulmonary capillary bed, an acute lowering of PVR, and an increase in pulmonary blood flow. This is due both to a mechanical effect and oxygenated blood passing through the pulmonary circulation. Inflation of the lungs stimulates pulmonary stretch receptors, which leads to reflex vasodilation of the pulmonary vascular bed. Mechanical expansion creates surface forces at the gas-liquid interface within the alveoli, which physically expand small blood vessels and decrease perivascular pressure. The majority of the changes in cardiopulmonary hemodynamics occur by 8 hours, although some degree of right to left ductal shunting may be found up to 12 hours after birth. In most infants, the ductus arteriosus closes by 24 hours of age, but there is a significant delay in ductal closure in infants with pulmonary hypertension. PVR is high in the fetus because of the low oxygen tension and low prostaglandin (PGI_2) and NO levels and the presence of vasoconstrictor substances, such as endothelin-1 (ET-1). PGI_2 production and release is increased by pulmonary tissue stretch. PGI_2 participates in the reduction of PVR accompanying ventilation, but it is not essential for maintaining low PVR once it is established. The vasodilator effects of exogenous PGI_2 are blocked by NO synthase inhibitors, which suggests that NO modulates PGI_2 activity. NO is produced by the vascular endothelial cells; NO synthase acts on L-arginine to form citrulline and NO. NO then diffuses into the smooth muscle cells, stimulating guanylate cyclase and increasing guanosine-monophosphate production; this results in smooth muscle relaxation. Increased fetal oxygen tensions augment endogenous NO release, and pharmacologic NO blockade attenuates the rise in pulmonary blood flow after birth. Decreased production of endogenous vasoconstrictors, such as thromboxane and ET-1, may also participate in the decrease in PVR at birth. In neonates with hypoxia and severe pulmonary hypertension, ET-1 levels are elevated. In the pulmonary hypertension which accompanies sepsis due to GBS or other organisms, thromboxane A_2 may cause initial severe arterial spasm followed by increased vascular permeability and an increased lung fluid content. The increased capillary permeability in sepsis-induced pulmonary hypertension appears to also be due to the action of bacterial endotoxins sequestering white cells in the lungs, where they release vasoactive agents such as tumor necrosis factor. Elevated levels of other vasoconstrictors, such as the leukotrienes LTC4 and LTD4, have been found in some neonates with pulmonary hypertension; the levels fell with successful therapy.

PATHOPHYSIOLOGY

Pulmonary hypertension in the neonate may be primary or secondary to a number of conditions, including severe intrapartum asphyxia, infection, pulmonary hypoplasia, drug therapy (e.g., the use of nonsteroidal anti-inflammatory drugs before delivery), alveolar capillary dysplasia, congenital heart disease, or overventilation. The neonatal pulmonary vasculature is extremely sensitive to changes in pH, $Pa{O_2}$, and $Pa{CO_2}$; perinatal or postnatal hypoxemia and metabolic or respiratory acidemia can cause marked pulmonary arterial spasm and pulmonary hypertension. A rise in the hematocrit can cause pulmonary hypertension, but polycythemia is not a consistent feature of neonates with pulmonary hypertension. Pulmonary hypertension in the neonate is often characterized by varying degrees of vascular remodeling and decreased arteriolar number. The pulmonary hypertension, which occurs in infants with CDH or in other conditions associated with pulmonary hypoplasia, is due to a reduction in the number of intralobar arteries and increased muscularity of the arteries. Following chronic hypoxia in utero, excessive muscularization of the pulmonary arterioles is found and muscle extends into the normally muscle-free intra-acinar arteries; such changes are seen in extremely small for gestational age infants. In other infants, there is a normal arteriolar number and muscularization, but the normal decrease in PVR after birth fails to occur. Persistent pulmonary hypertension may also be due to alveolar capillary dysplasia with congenital misalignment of the pulmonary veins. This condition is usually sporadic, but rarely family occurrence has been reported. Alveolar capillary dysplasia is an uncommon condition; in a 3-year retrospective study, the diagnosis was made in 5 of 173 infants treated with ECMO in the United Kingdom.

CLINICAL PRESENTATION

Infants with PPHN usually present within 12 hours of birth; affected infants are cyanosed but have only mild respiratory distress, and grunting is rare. The second heart sound is loud because of the rise in pulmonary artery pressure. There may be a soft systolic murmur due to tricuspid or occasionally mitral incompetence. In neonates who are critically ill, because of GBS infection, severe asphyxia, and CDH, pulmonary hypertension appears within 6 hours of birth; the infants additionally have the clinical features of their underlying condition.

DIAGNOSIS AND DIFFERENTIAL DIAGNOSIS

Pulmonary hypertension is diagnosed in an infant with severe hypoxemia. When the hypoxemia is disproportionately severe for the radiologic abnormalities, there is evidence of a right-to-left ductal shunt with a lower level of oxygenation in the distal aortic blood (obtained from an umbilical artery catheter) compared with the preductal blood (obtained from the right radial artery), and the echocardiograph demonstrates a structurally normal heart. Echocardiography is important not only to establish the diagnosis, but also to exclude cyanotic congenital heart disease. In primary pulmonary hypertension, the chest radiograph changes are often minimal and, although in secondary pulmonary hypertension the chest radiograph appearance will be that of the underlying lung disease, the appearance will be less severe than anticipated for the severity of the hypoxemia. The most important differential diagnosis is cyanotic congenital heart disease, but when this presents in the first 12 hours, it is usually with heart failure, distinctive murmurs, and obvious changes on the chest radiograph and electrocardiogram. The response to ventilation with 100% oxygen can help to distinguish the two conditions; in some infants with pulmonary hypertension, the arterial oxygen level will increase to above 13 kPa (100 mm Hg), whereas in cyanotic congenital heart disease it will not rise above 5 to 6 kPa (37.5–45 mm Hg). However, not all neonates with pulmonary hypertension, especially those with sepsis or a CDH, have a large improvement in oxygenation in response to 100% oxygen. Alveolar capillary dysplasia should be suspected in infants with pulmonary hypertension unresponsive to maximal cardiorespiratory support, who cannot be weaned from ECMO; in such cases a lung biopsy can establish the diagnosis.

TREATMENT

Minimal handling is important, because it is easy to precipitate severe hypoxemia in infants with pulmonary hypertension. As a consequence, endotracheal tube suctioning should only be performed when essential to maintain endotracheal tube patency, and chest physiotherapy is contraindicated. Monitoring must be continuous. The size of the right-left shunt is in part dependent on the systemic blood pressure; thus, aggressive therapy should be used to achieve an appropriate systemic blood pressure. The hemoglobin level should be kept greater than 13 g/dL (PCV 40%) in order to maximize oxygen transport to the tissues, but if polycythemia (central packed cell volume greater than 70%) is present, a dilutional exchange transfusion should be undertaken. Broad-spectrum antibiotic cover should be given. Infants should be ventilated if their $Pa{O_2}$ is less than 5 to 6 kPa (37 to 45 mm Hg) in 70% oxygen. If mechanical ventilation is needed, the level of inspired oxygen should be sufficient to achieve a $Pa{O_2}$ of at least 8 to 9 kPa (56 to 63 mm Hg), the pH should be kept above 7.25, and the $Pa{CO_2}$ in the range of 4.8 to 5.5 kPa (35 to 40 mm Hg). Hyperventilation to reduce the $Pa{CO_2}$ to 2.5 to 3.5 kPa is no longer recommended, because it may result in a 50% reduction in cerebral blood flow. Although no long-term adverse sequelae have been described in babies born at full term, hypocapnia in preterm babies has been linked to the development of periventricular leukomalacia. Hyperventilation can also cause barotrauma, resulting in air leaks and BPD. High inflating pressures and PEEP levels can result in lung overdistention and worsen PVR. Alkalosis can promote pulmonary vasodilation; hence, some clinicians give infants with pulmonary hypertension infusions of sodium bicarbonate or tromethamine (THAM). Such a strategy, however, should not be maintained for a prolonged period, because persisting alkalemia increases the hypoxic reactivity of the pulmonary vasculature, thus tending to perpetuate the pathophysiology of pulmonary hypertension. Neuromuscular blocking agents should be administered to full-term babies to prevent them from fighting the ventilator. Anecdotally, high-frequency oscillatory and jet ventilation have been used with improvements in oxygenation. ECMO is an effective rescue therapy for infants with pulmonary hypertension.

A variety of vasodilator drugs have been used to treat infants with pulmonary hypertension. Between 25% and 50% of affected babies respond to tolazoline hydrochloride, but this is not a specific vasodilator, and hypotension is a common side effect. Other side effects include renal failure and gastrointestinal hemorrhage. Prostacyclin (PGI_2) is an effective pulmonary vasodilator, but also is nonselective and has side effects. Tolazoline and PGI_2 have been given via inhalation to avoid the side effects associated with systemic administration, but as yet there is no long-term experience with this mode of delivery. Magnesium sulfate administration improves oxygenation, but is less effective than NO and has more side effects. Magnesium levels must be carefully monitored, because hypermagnesia can cause sedation, muscle relaxation, hyporeflexia, hypotension, and calcium and potassium disturbances. NO is a vasodilator substance that relaxes vascular smooth muscle. When NO is inhaled, it diffuses across the capillary membrane and activates guanylate cyclase in the pulmonary arteriolar smooth muscle. The resulting increase in cyclic guanosine monophosphate causes smooth muscle relaxation. NO then binds rapidly to hemoglobin and once bound is inactivated and therefore produces no systemic effects. Levels of up to 80 ppm have been used, but in full-term infants 5 ppm appears as effective as higher doses. Administration of NO to infants with pulmonary hypertension improves oxygenation, but not all babies respond. A poor response, which occurs in infants with severe parenchymal disease, systemic hypotension, myocardial dysfunction, or structural pulmonary abnormalities such as pulmonary hypoplasia or dysplasia, is predictive of a poor outcome. In full-term babies, meta-analysis of the results of randomized trials demonstrated that use of inhaled NO was associated with an improvement in oxygenation and a reduction in the combined outcome of death or need for ECMO; the effect was due to a reduction in the need for ECMO. The combined intervention of inhaled NO and HFOV may be more successful than use of inhaled NO or HFOV alone in rescuing infants at or near full term with severe respiratory failure, reflecting that the efficacy of inhaled NO is improved if combined with a strategy to improve lung volume. No significant long-term benefits of inhaled NO have been demonstrated in babies with CDH. Only one randomized trial has demonstrated that inhaled NO has any significant long-term benefit for preterm babies.[28] There is currently insufficient evidence to recommend routine use of NO in prematurely born babies or in full-term babies with CDH. It is important to wean infants from inhaled NO as soon as oxygenation has improved and they have stabilized; otherwise, tolerance may occur. Unfortunately, NO has side effects; it reacts rapidly with oxygen to form nitrogen dioxide, which is toxic to the lung. The nitrosylhemoglobin produced by NO binding to hemoglobin is rapidly converted to methemoglobin, which is then reduced by methemoglobin reductase in erythrocytes. Immature infants and those of certain ethnic groups (including those of Turkish and American Indian origin) have low levels of methemoglobin reductase. These problems are more likely if high concentrations of NO are used for prolonged periods in high inspired oxygen concentrations. NO administration has been associated with an increased bleeding time. Other potential side effects include surfactant dysfunction and mutagenicity.

MORTALITY AND MORBIDITY

The mortality rate varies according to the underlying condition. The mortality rates are 10% to 20% in infants who require ECMO because of primary pulmonary hypertension or pulmonary hypertension complicating RDS or MAS. In babies with GBS sepsis, the mortality rate ranges from 10% to 50%, with most babies dying from irreversible hypoxia or myocardial failure. Alveolar capillary dysplasia is a uniformly fatal condition. BPD occurs in infants who have required a high level of respiratory support, and neurologic damage may be sustained in infants who have suffered severe hypoxia.

SECONDARY PULMONARY HYPOPLASIA

Secondary pulmonary hypoplasia can result in utero from reductions in intrathoracic space, FBMs, or amniotic fluid volume. Reduction in intrathoracic space occurs with small chest syndromes (particularly asphyxiating thoracic dystrophy or Jeune's syndrome), cystic adenomatoid malformation or sequestration of the lung, CDH, and pleural effusions. Infants with anterior abdominal wall defects (AWDs) can have abnormal lung growth because in utero they have a reduction in viscera in the upper part of the abdominal cavity and hence an inadequate framework for chest wall development. Intrathoracic compression by pleural effusions may explain the association of hydropic fetuses due to rhesus isoimmunization and pulmonary hypoplasia, but an immune mechanism may also be a factor. Cessation or reduction of FBMs is responsible for the abnormal lung growth in certain neurologic or neuromuscular diseases presenting in utero, for example, Werdig-Hoffman disease and myotonic dystrophy inherited from the mother. There is, however, considerable debate regarding the relevance of absent FBMs in other conditions associated with abnormal lung growth, for example, oligohydramnios resulting from premature rupture of the membranes (PROM). Experimental production of oligohydramnios, by chronic drainage of amniotic fluid or urinary tract obstruction, is associated with the development of pulmonary hypoplasia. Reduction in the production of amniotic fluid can occur with fetal renal abnormalities, for example, Potter's syndrome or uteroplacental insufficiency. Loss of amniotic fluid following PROM or amniocentesis has also been associated with pulmonary hypoplasia or at least lung function abnormalities suggestive of abnormal lung growth. The timing of onset of the oligohydramnios in pregnancies complicated by PROM is critical; pulmonary hypoplasia only occurs if the onset of membrane rupture is prior to 26 weeks of gestation. Abnormal lung development, however, is not an invariable consequence of early-onset oligohydramnios; in one cohort, 23% of patients who had membrane rupture prior to 20 weeks of gestation had no clinical signs suggestive of pulmonary hypoplasia. Pulmonary hypoplasia has also been described in infants with trisomy 18 or 21.

The clinical signs are similar to those seen with primary pulmonary hypoplasia. Some with mild pulmonary hypoplasia are apparently asymptomatic but on inspection are tachypneic. Others suffer severe respiratory distress from birth and require ventilatory support. Infants with pulmonary hypoplasia have small-volume, noncompliant lungs, and their chest wall is disproportionately small with respect to the abdomen. In addition, infants with secondary pulmonary hypoplasia may have associated congenital anomalies, for example, diaphragmatic hernia/eventration, an anterior abdominal wall defect, a dislocated hip, and/or talipes. They may also have the features of neuromuscular diseases such as Werdig-Hoffman disease or congenital dystrophia myotonica inherited from the mother. The "dry lung syndrome" has been described following oligohydramnios due to premature rupture of the membranes and is likely to be due to functional compression. Affected infants are difficult to resuscitate, requiring high peak inflating pressures; the requirement for high pressures may continue for 48 hours, but then the infants make a spontaneous recovery, indicating they have no structural abnormality.

On antenatal ultrasound examination, oligohydramnios and abnormalities (e.g., pleural effusion and CDH) commonly associated with pulmonary hypoplasia can be identified. A variety of techniques to diagnose pulmonary hypoplasia have been investigated, including the development of reference ranges of fetal chest growth related to gestational age, relating the thoracic to the abdominal circumference, and calculating the thoracic to heart ratio or the thoracic to head ratio. In addition, fetal lung volume can be assessed by echoplanar magnetic resonance imaging (MRI) or three-dimensional ultrasonography. The usefulness of the absence of FBMs as a marker of pulmonary hypoplasia is controversial. On the chest radiograph, the ribs may appear crowded with a low thoracic to abdominal ratio (Fig. 18-8) and a classically bell-shaped chest (Fig. 18-9), but the lung fields are clear unless there is coexisting RDS. Pneumothorax or other forms of air leak are frequently present. The chest radiograph may also demonstrate features of the infant's underlying condition (Figs. 18-10 and 18-11). Pathologically, pulmonary hypoplasia is diagnosed if the lung weight to body weight ratio is less than 0.015 in infants born before 28 weeks of gestation and less than 0.012 in infants born after 28 weeks of gestation; in addition, there is a radial alveolar count of less than 4.

Antenatally diagnosed pleural effusions can be chronically drained by thoracoamniotic shunts, which will facilitate ease of resuscitation. In utero surgery has been undertaken for infants with CDH, but this has been problematic. As a consequence, the efficacy of reversible tracheal "obstruction" is being investigated in cases predicted to be at high risk for fatal pulmonary hypoplasia. The rationale for that approach follows from the observation that obstruction of the upper respiratory tract, as occurs in laryngeal atresia, results in larger than normal lungs. If an infant with pulmonary hypoplasia requires ventilatory support, the minimum pressures compatible with acceptable gases should be used because these infants are at high risk for air leaks. Low pressure, fast rate ventilation or HFOV can be helpful in some infants, but ECMO would usually be contraindicated because the infants do not have a reversible condition. Pulmonary vasodilators can be useful if there is coexisting pulmonary hypertension. Home oxygen therapy allows early

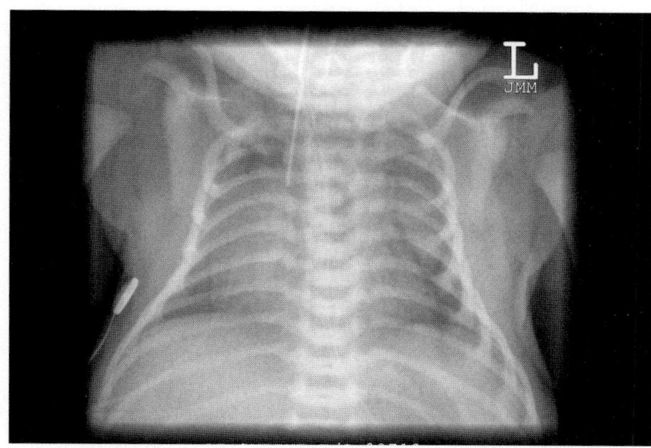

■ **FIGURE 18-9.** Bell-shaped chest characteristic of pulmonary hypoplasia. The infant had bilateral renal agenesis. The trachea appears deviated to the right because of some secondary right-sided collapse.

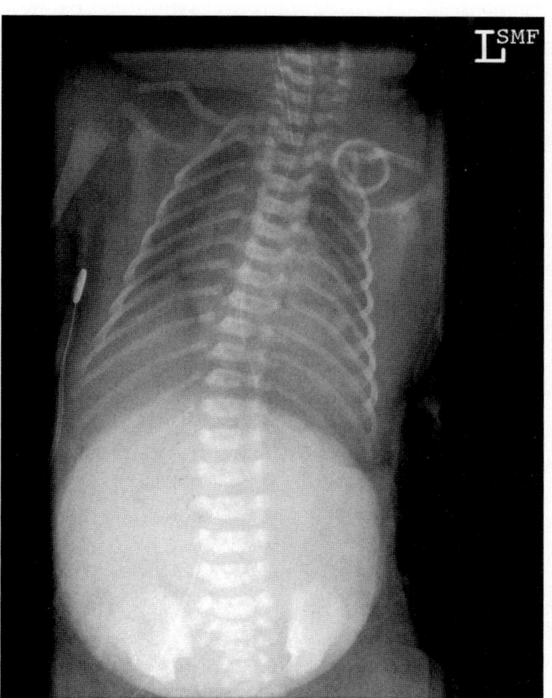

■ **FIGURE 18-8.** Pulmonary hypoplasia in association with an abdominal wall defect. The radiopaque area is the silo containing the gastroschisis.

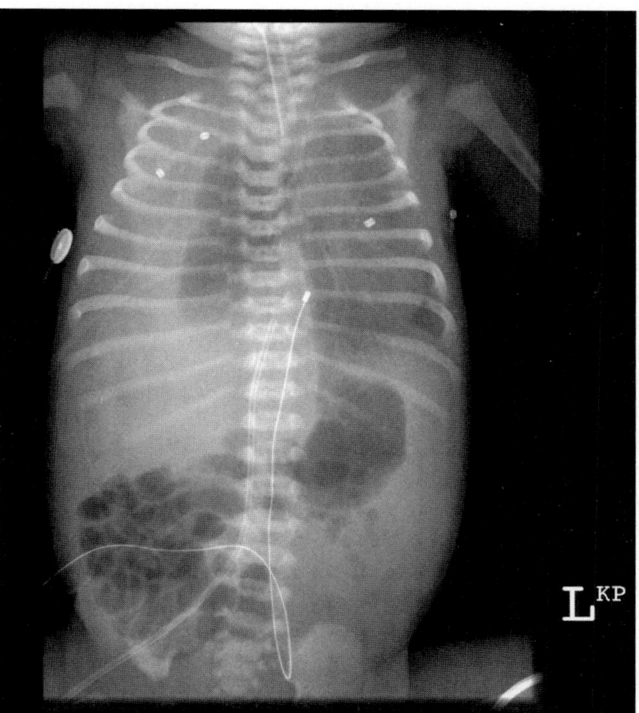

■ **FIGURE 18-10.** Chest radiograph of an infant with a right-sided pleural effusion. The two radiopaque dots on each side of the chest represent the ends of the thoracoamniotic shunts; the shunt on the right side is lying entirely within the chest, resulting in a large effusion accumulating and pushing the mediastinum across to the left. Umbilical arterial and umbilical venous catheters are in place.

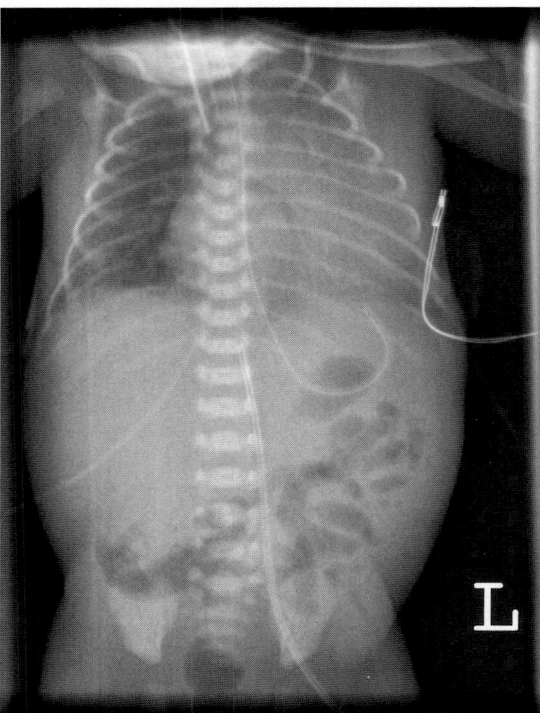

FIGURE 18-11. Pulmonary hypoplasia in an infant with trisomy. The infant has the characteristic gracile ribs and has a large heart due to critical pulmonary stenosis.

discharge, but parents need to be counseled that supplementary oxygen may be required for many months. Every attempt should be made to reduce further compromise to the lungs; full immunization is essential, and RSV prophylaxis should be considered.

Infants with Potter's syndrome (large low-set ears, prominent epicanthic folds, and a flattened nose) and postural limb defects die in the neonatal period. There is also a 100% mortality rate in infants with the oligohydramnios syndrome (pulmonary hypoplasia, abnormal facies, and limb abnormalities) due to PROM. In less severely affected infants, the perinatal mortality rate is approximately 50% if membrane rupture occurs between 15 and 28 weeks.[29] Infants with pulmonary hypoplasia who remain on high-pressure ventilation and high inspired oxygen concentrations at the end of the first week are in an extremely bad prognostic group. It is our experience that such infants rarely go home, and if they do, only with home oxygen therapy, and they die within the first 2 years following infection. Infants born following oligohydramnios can suffer limb abnormalities due to the compression, and the reported incidence varies from 27% to 80%; they also suffer from long-term respiratory problems, including BPD and recurrent episodes of wheezing and coughing. In addition, neurologic or developmental deficits are more common, being reported in 28% of infants born after preterm rupture of the membranes prior to 26 weeks of gestation.

AIR LEAKS

PNEUMOTHORAX

Spontaneous pneumothoraces occur immediately after birth due to the high transpulmonary pressure swings generated by the first spontaneous breaths. Chest radiographs obtained on consecutive newborns demonstrated that 1% of newborns had an air leak, but only 10% of the affected infants were symptomatic. Pneumothoraces more usually occur as a complication of respiratory disease or a congenital malformation, particularly if there is uneven ventilation, alveolar overdistention, and air trapping, and the infant is receiving ventilatory support. Approximately 5% to 10% of ventilated babies develop an air leak; they are particularly likely to occur in babies who fight the ventilator and actively exhale during ventilator inflation (active expiration). Rarely, pneumothoraces occur as a result of a direct injury to the lung, for example, via perforation by suction catheters or introducers passed through the endotracheal tube or via central venous catheter placement.

Small pneumothoraces may be asymptomatic and diagnosed on a chest radiograph taken for other reasons. If an infant suffers a large pneumothorax, he or she frequently deteriorates dramatically with marked respiratory distress, pallor, shock, and deterioration in the oxygenation. A tension pneumothorax results in a shift of the mediastinum and abdominal distention due to displacement of the diaphragm. Pneumothorax causes and aggravates hemorrhage into the germinal layer and cerebral ventricles of preterm infants. A chest radiograph should be obtained if a pneumothorax is suspected, unless the infant's clinical condition makes emergency drainage mandatory. A large pneumothorax is associated with absent lung markings and a collapsed lung on the ipsilateral side. If the pneumothorax is under tension, there will also be eversion of the diaphragm, bulging intercostal spaces, and mediastinal shift (Fig. 18-12). A small pneumothorax, however, may only be recognized by a difference in radiolucency between the two lung fields (Fig. 18-13).

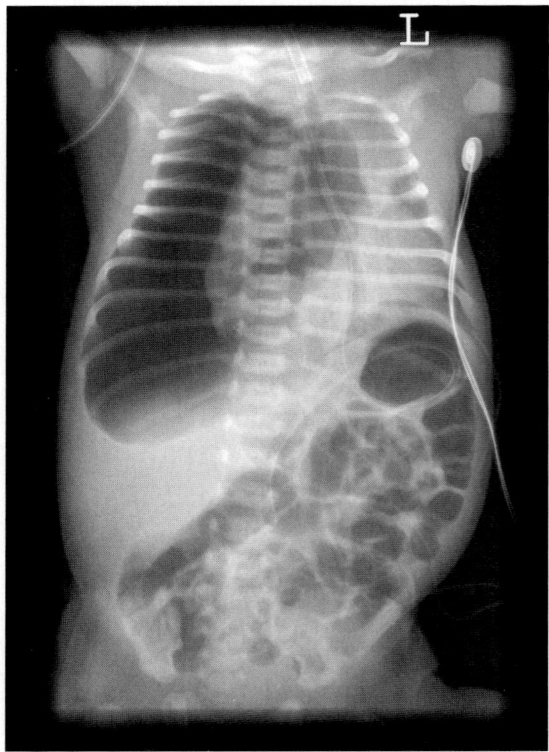

FIGURE 18-12. Tension right pneumothorax with eversion of the diaphragm.

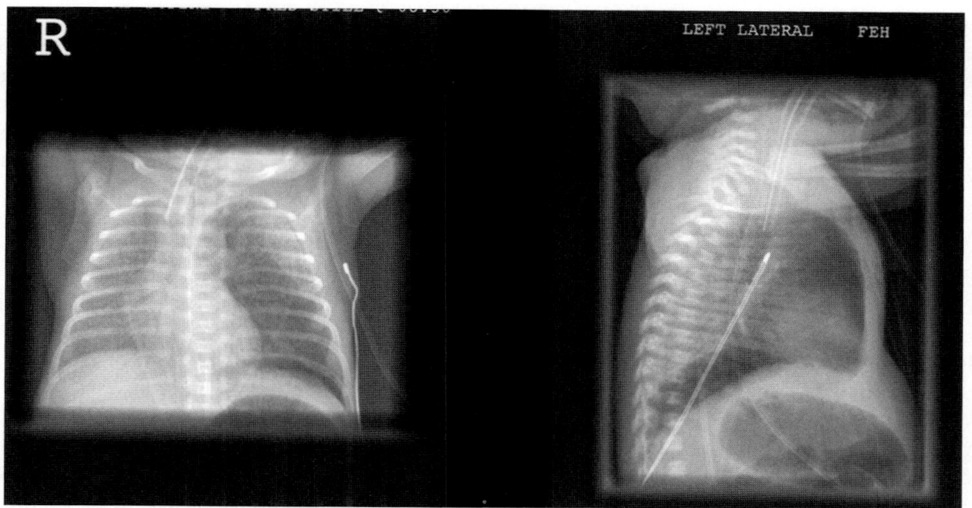

■ **FIGURE 18-13.** Left-sided pneumothorax, demonstrated by the discrepancy in the translucency of the two lung fields and small rim of basal free air. The lateral chest radiograph demonstrates the free air.

Unusually the appearance of either lobar emphysema or cystic adenomatoid malformation of the lung may resemble a pneumothorax. In a preterm infant with a thin chest wall, transillumination with an intense beam from a fiberoptic light will demonstrate an abnormal air collection by an increased transmission of light, but PIE can give a similar appearance.

Asymptomatic pneumothoraces do not require treatment, but the infant should be carefully observed. Nursing an infant with a pneumothorax in an inspired oxygen concentration of 100% favors resorption of the extra-alveolar gas, but this strategy should not be used in infants at risk for retinopathy of prematurity. If the infant is symptomatic or has a tension pneumothorax, the pneumothorax must be drained. If the infant is in extremis and there is no time for insertion of a chest drain, emergency aspiration should be undertaken with a butterfly needle (18-gauge), which is attached to a three-way tap held under water in a small sterile container. The needle is inserted through the skin in the second intercostal space anteriorly, and then the skin and needle moved sideways before advancing the needle through the underlying muscle; this reduces the likelihood of leaving an open needle track for entry of air once the needle has been removed. Following emergency drainage, a chest tube (French gauge 10–14) should be inserted under local anesthesia through either the second intercostal space just lateral to the midclavicular line or the sixth space in the midaxillary line. The tip of the chest tube should lie retrosternally to achieve the most effective drainage; whether the drain has been positioned correctly should be checked on a lateral chest radiograph (Fig. 18-14). Complications of malpositioned tubes include traumatization of the thoracic duct resulting in a chylothorax, cardiac tamponade due to a hemorrhagic pericardial effusion, and phrenic nerve injury. Once inserted, the tube should be connected to an underwater seal drain with suction of 5 to 10 cm H_2O. Heimlich valves are useful during transport, but they should not be used for long-term drainage because they can become blocked. The chest drain can be removed 24 hours after there is no further bubbling of air into the water seal.

To prevent air leaks from occurring, it is important to stop infants from breathing out of phase with the ventilator (active expiration or asynchrony). This can be achieved by administration of a neuromuscular blocking agent, but because this has side effects, including fluid retention, many clinicians prefer to administer analgesics and/or sedatives to try to suppress respiratory activity. Administration of analgesics and/or sedatives such as fentanyl, morphine, diamorphine, midazolam, or chloral hydrate, however, although having benefits, has not been demonstrated in randomized trials to reduce the pneumothorax rate, and they too have side effects. An alternative strategy to prevent pneumothoraces is to use a form of ventilatory support, which encourages the infant to breathe synchronously with the ventilator (i.e., inspiration and inflation coinciding). Use of a faster (60 breaths/min) rather than a slower (30–40 breaths/min) rate during conventional ventilation has been associated with a reduced risk for pneumothorax development (relative risk

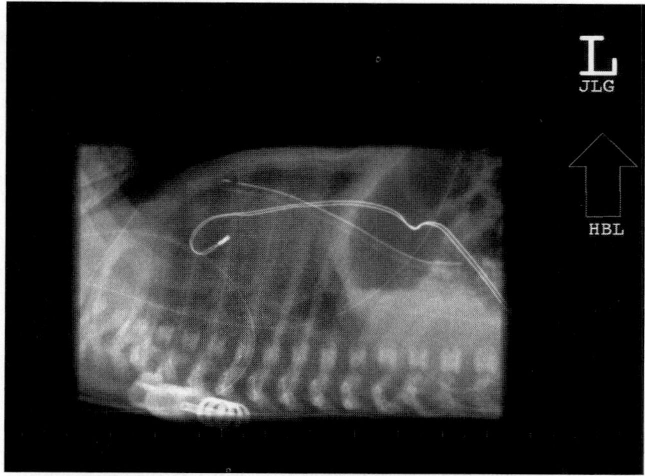

■ **FIGURE 18-14.** Lateral chest x-ray demonstrating appropriate retrosternal placement of the chest drainage tube.

0.69, CI 0.51–0.93),[5] but randomized trials have failed to demonstrate that either patient-triggered ventilation or high-frequency oscillation is efficacious in that respect. Surfactant administration is associated with a lower risk for pneumothorax development.

PULMONARY INTERSTITIAL EMPHYSEMA

The incidence of PIE is inversely related to birth weight. It has rarely been described in spontaneously breathing infants and occurs mainly in neonates with RDS, supported by positive-pressure ventilation and exposed to high peak inspiratory pressures and/or malpositioned endotracheal tubes. PIE commonly involves both lungs, but may be lobar in distribution. It frequently occurs with either a pneumothorax or pneumomediastinum. In surfactant deficient infants, rupture of the small airways can occur distal to the termination of the fascial sheath. Gas then dissects into the interstitium and becomes trapped within the perivascular sheaths of the lung, resulting in PIE. The trapped gas reduces pulmonary perfusion by compressing the vessels and interfering with ventilation; as a result, affected infants are profoundly hypoxemic and hypercarbic. PIE is usually diagnosed when a chest radiograph is obtained on a severely ill neonate. The chest radiograph demonstrates hyperinflation and a characteristic cystic appearance, which may be diffuse, multiple, or small, nonconfluent cystic radiolucencies (Fig. 18-15). At a later stage, large bullae may appear. The appearance may be confused with lobar emphysema or with cystic adenomatoid malformation of the lung, especially if localized.

If the PIE is localized, the infant should be nursed in the lateral decubitus position with the affected lung dependent and hence underventilated, this promotes partial or complete atelectasis. Selective bronchial intubation to bypass the affected lung for 24 to 48 hours may also be associated with resolution of the PIE; selective intubation of the left main bronchus can be difficult, and adequate blood gases cannot be maintained in some infants if only one lung is ventilated. Despite such maneuvers, if the PIE persists and compresses adjacent normal lung parenchyma, resection of the affected area may be necessary to alleviate respiratory distress. If the infant has widespread PIE, the PEEP and peak inflating pressure should be reduced to the minimum compatible with acceptable gases and the infant paralyzed to try to avoid extension of the air leak. Transfer to high-frequency jet, flow interruption, or oscillatory ventilation, or to continuous negative pressure with intermittent mandatory ventilation have all been anecdotally described as improving gas exchange in infants with PIE and respiratory failure poorly responsive to conventional ventilation. If such strategies fail and the infant is in extremis, linear pleurotomies, scarifying the lung through the chest wall to create an artificial pneumothorax, may help to decompress the PIE. The mortality rate from diffuse PIE has been reported to be high, but the studies generally predated the routine use of antenatal steroids and postnatal surfactant. The incidence of BPD is increased following diffuse PIE.

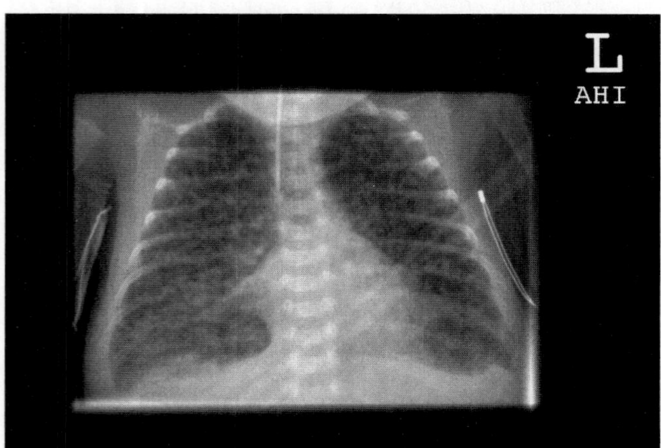

FIGURE 18-15. Severe bilateral pulmonary interstitial emphysema.

PNEUMOMEDIASTINUM

Pneumomediastinum occurs in approximately 2.5 per 1000 live births. An isolated pneumomediastinum rarely causes severe symptoms. Pneumomediastinum, however, usually coexist with multiple air leaks in severely ill ventilated babies. On the chest radiograph, a pneumomediastinum appears as a halo of air adjacent to the borders of the heart, and on the lateral view there is marked retrosternal hyperlucency. The mediastinal gas may elevate the thymus away from the pericardium, resulting in a crescentic configuration resembling a spinnaker sail (Fig. 18-16). An isolated pneumomediastinum usually requires no treatment. In full-term infants, use of a high inspired oxygen concentration is associated with resorption of extra-alveolar air. Drainage of a pneumomediastinum is difficult because the gas is collected in multiple independent lobules and multiple needling and tube drainage may be required.

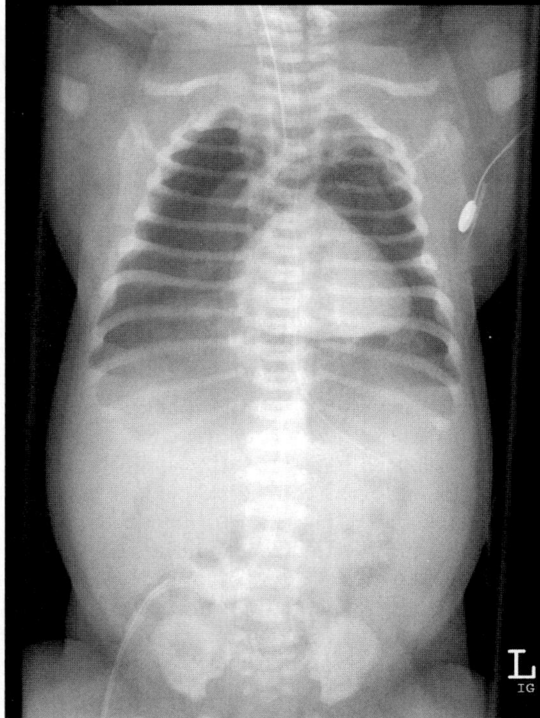

FIGURE 18-16. Bilateral pneumothoraces with elevation of the thymic shadow indicating air in the mediastinum and air inferior to the diaphragmatic surface of the heart.

PNEUMOPERICARDIUM

A pneumopericardium is usually accompanied by other air leaks such as a pneumomediastinum, widespread PIE, or a tension pneumothorax, which suggests that the gas enters the pericardium through a defect in the pericardial sac, probably at the pericardial reflection near the ostia of the pulmonary veins. The majority of cases occur in ventilated, prematurely born babies. A pneumopericardium causes cardiac tamponade with sudden hypotension, bradycardia, and cyanosis. The chest radiograph demonstrates gas completely surrounding the heart, outlining the base of the great vessels and contained within the pericardium. Gas can be seen inferior to the diaphragmatic surface of the heart, differentiating this abnormality from a pneumomediastinum, in which the mediastinal gas is limited inferiorly by the attachment of the mediastinal pleura to the central tendon of the diaphragm (see Fig. 18-16). All symptomatic pneumopericardia should be drained immediately by direct pericardial tap via the subxyphoid route. The blood pressure should be monitored continuously, and the tap repeated if bradycardia or hypotension recur. Catheter drainage may be necessary if the pericardial air reaccumulates. The mortality of symptomatic pneumopericardia is between 80% and 90%, and many survivors have neurologic sequelae.

PNEUMOPERITONEUM

A pneumoperitoneum may result from perforation of the gut or by gas dissecting from the chest through the diaphragmatic foramina into the peritoneum; the latter scenario is particularly likely in ventilated babies who have a pneumothorax and a pneumomediastinum. If the pneumoperitoneum is large, the diagnosis can be made from the anteroposterior radiograph (Fig. 18-17), but a horizontal-beam lateral or right lateral radiograph may be required to demonstrate smaller leaks (Fig. 18-18). Treatment is only necessary if the abdomen is under sufficient tension to cause respiratory embarrassment, then the pneumoperitoneum should be drained either by needle aspiration or by inserting a drainage tube.

SYSTEMIC AIR EMBOLISM

The majority of infants who suffer a systemic air embolism have other air leaks. Affected infants deteriorate suddenly, with pallor, cyanosis, hypotension, and bizarre irregularities on their echocardiogram. On the chest radiograph, gas can be seen in the systemic and pulmonary arteries and veins. Early withdrawal of air from the umbilical artery catheter may be of benefit, particularly if the leak is small or has been introduced through an intravascular line, but the condition is usually fatal.

PATENT DUCTUS ARTERIOSUS

In fetal life, blood is shunted from the right heart via the pulmonary artery through the ductus arteriosus to the aorta, and the lungs are "bypassed." At birth, the ductus arteriosus begins to constrict with the onset of breathing. In the majority of infants, the ductus arteriosus has closed by 24 hours of age, and in 90% will have closed by 60 hours of age. Ductal closure is delayed in infants with pulmonary hypertension and respiratory failure as a consequence of acidosis or persistence of low oxygen tensions; in such circumstances, PGE_2 levels remain high. The incidence of PDA is inversely related to gestational age, reflecting the association between maturity at birth and respiratory distress syndrome.

CLINICAL PRESENTATION AND DIAGNOSIS

A hemodynamically significant PDA presents as failure of improvement in an infant with RDS or an acute deterioration necessitating an increase in respiratory support. Some infants will present when they are extubated from the ventilator. The increased pulmonary blood flow is associated with a decrease in pulmonary compliance, and without PEEP the infant is unable to maintain small airway patency and hence collapses on extubation. Infants with a hemodynamically significant PDA have tachycardia, bounding pulses, an active precordium, and sometimes a murmur, although the latter might be absent. The typical ductal murmur is systolic (in about 75% of cases), but can be continuous and is best heard at the upper left sternal edge, under the clavicle. As the PVR falls, the left to right shunt through the ductus increases and the peripheral pulses become bounding; this reflects the widened pulse pressure due to the "steal" of blood being shunted from the high-pressure systemic circulation into the lower-pressure pulmonary circulation. The left to right shunt means higher blood flow in the lungs, and the infant is tachypneic and crackles can be heard at the lung bases. The chest radiograph demonstrates cardiomegaly, pulmonary plethora, and a wide angle between the left and right main bronchi due to left atrial dilatation. The diagnosis can be confirmed by echocardiography;

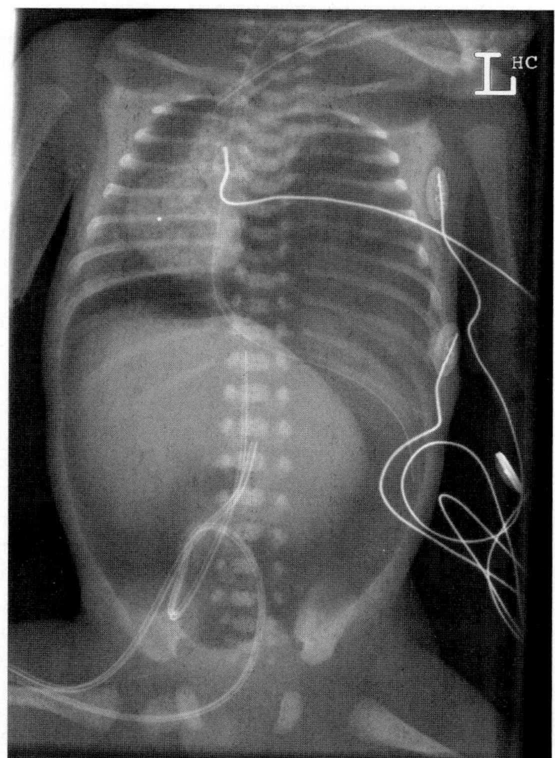

FIGURE 18-17. Large pneumoperitoneum. The mediastinum is pushed to the right by free air in the left chest. Umbilical arterial and umbilical venous catheters are in place.

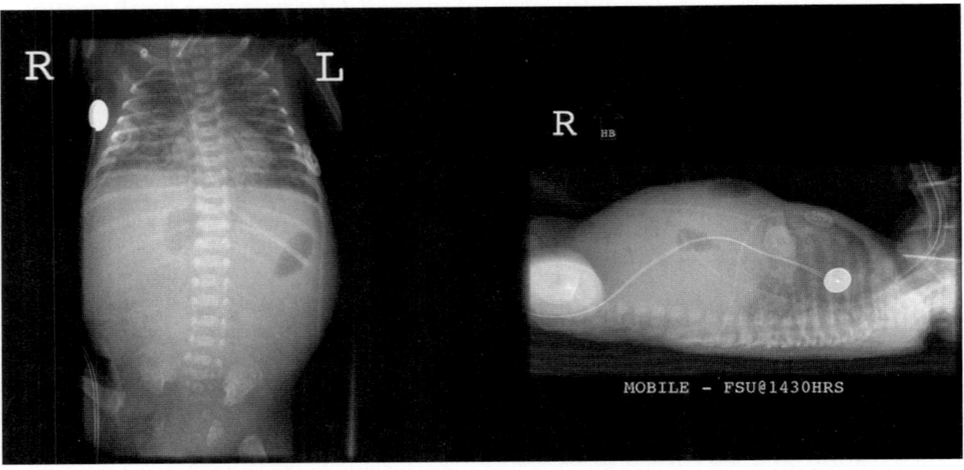

FIGURE 18-18. Anterior posterior abdominal radiograph shows a small pocket of nonanatomic air. The horizontal beam demonstrates a free collection, confirming the diagnosis of a pneumoperitoneum.

echocardiographic signs of a ductal shunt precede the development of overt clinical signs by 3 days on average. Typical echocardiographic findings of a moderate to large left to right ductal shunt are bowing of the interatrial septum to the right with enlargement of the left atrium and ventricle and left atrium enlargement with a left atrial:aortic root (LA:Ao) ratio greater than 1.4:1. In addition, color Doppler examination reveals a continuous flare-up in the main pulmonary artery from the arterial duct. The size of the shunt can be determined from the ductal size on color Doppler examination, the LA:Ao ratio, and whether the diastolic flow in the descending aorta is reversed during diastole. If the shunt is large, flow reversal will be throughout diastole. Echocardiographic examination is also important to exclude other congenital heart abnormalities.

MANAGEMENT

Initial management of an infant with a PDA usually includes fluid restriction, although there have been no randomized trials demonstrating that fluid restriction in infants with a hemodynamically significant PDA promotes ductal closure. Diuretics are frequently given, but theoretically furosemide might promote ductal patency via its effect on renal prostaglandin synthesis. Early randomized trials demonstrated that fluid restriction reduced the likelihood of a PDA; those results, however, have not been confirmed by recent studies, which have included infants routinely exposed to antenatal corticosteroids and postnatal surfactant.[30] If there is no improvement following fluid restriction for 24 hours, providing there are no contraindications, such as poor renal function or a low platelet count, indomethacin is given. Indomethacin, a cyclooxygenase inhibitor, inhibits the synthesis of prostaglandin E. Ductal closure is achieved with indomethacin treatment in 48 hours in approximately 70% of infants. Indomethacin can be given in three doses 12 hours apart or for 6 or 7 days at 24 hourly intervals; results from randomized trials have highlighted that there is more sustained closure with the longer course.[31] Indomethacin treatment has a number of side effects, including gastric or bowel perforation and reduction in renal function. Recently, there has been increasing use of ibuprofen rather than indomethacin, because ibuprofen appears to have fewer side effects than indomethacin, particularly less impact on urine output. Chronic lung disease, however, has been reported to be more common in ibuprofen- than indomethacin-treated infants.[32] There have now been a number of randomized trials assessing the efficacy of indomethacin given prophylactically, presymptomatically, or to treat a symptomatic PDA. Meta-analysis[33] of the results of those trials has demonstrated that prophylactic treatment with indomethacin, started in the first 24 hours, is associated with significant reductions in severe intracerebral hemorrhage. All trials, including those in which treatment was given presymptomatically on ultrasound evidence or when the PDA was hemodynamically significant, have shown such treatment results in a decreased need to treat a subsequent PDA. In addition, use of indomethacin for asymptomatic ducts has been associated with a small but statistically significant reduction in the duration of supplementary oxygen.[34] Overall, however, there has been no significant reduction in mortality regardless of the timing of the indomethacin administration. Surgical closure has been reserved for infants in whom there is a contraindication to indomethacin administration or the treatment has been ineffective. Surgery is now often performed safely on the neonatal intensive care unit, and this has the advantage of avoiding the risks inherent in patient transfer.[35]

MORTALITY AND MORBIDITY

BPD is significantly increased in infants who had a PDA, particularly if they have also suffered from nosocomial infection. If there is a large PDA, there is a diastolic steal, and retrograde diastolic flow develops in the cerebral circulation and the descending aorta, renal, and mesenteric blood vessels; hence, the incidence of necrotizing enterocolitis is increased in infants who have had a PDA, the mechanism being compromised gut (diastolic) blood flow.

PULMONARY EDEMA

Pulmonary edema occurs when there is leakage of fluid from pulmonary capillaries into the interstitium and alveoli. This can occur when the pulmonary capillary pressure is greater

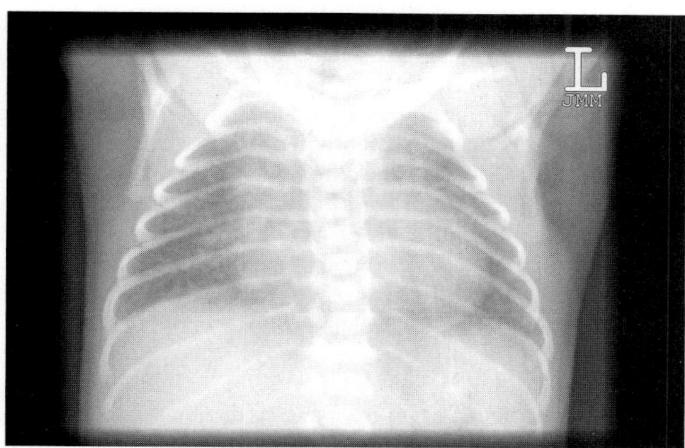

■ **FIGURE 18-19.** Pulmonary edema due to a large ventricular septal defect. Note also the gracile ribs of an infant with trisomy 13.

than the plasma oncotic pressure or there is disruption of the barriers between the vascular space and the lung interstitium. Increased lung microvascular pressure occurs most commonly if there is a large left to right shunt from a PDA, but can occur in infants with cardiac disease (e.g., severe forms of total anomalous pulmonary venous drainage). In addition, cardiac arrhythmias, particularly tachyarrhythmias, can result in an acute onset of heart failure and pulmonary edema. Myocardial dysfunction or an over-rapid infusion will exacerbate these problems. Altered capillary permeability occurs in ARDS or following any hypoxic insult. Fluid accumulates if the lymphatic system is overloaded, and thus pulmonary edema also occurs if there are abnormalities of the pulmonary lymphatic drainage. Initially, any excess fluid builds up in the interstitium, but as the fluid accumulates, this disrupts the alveolar membrane, and fluid fills the alveoli.

The infant with pulmonary edema is tachycardic, pale, and sweaty and has poor volume peripheral pulses with reduced cardiac output. The chest radiograph demonstrates perihilar shadowing obscuring the vascular structures (Fig. 18-19) and linear septal shadows (Kerley B lines) in the lower part of the lungs; in the most severe cases, there may be fluid visible in the horizontal and oblique fissures, cardiomegaly, and pericardial effusions. Cardiac causes of pulmonary edema can be diagnosed from the echocardiogram or electrocardiogram.

Fluid input should be restricted and fluid overload avoided. Diuretic treatment is given to reduce the circulating volume and the clinical manifestations of pulmonary edema, but may critically lower the cardiac output. Positive pressure ventilation may be needed to acutely stabilize the patient and, in infants already ventilated, oxygenation can be improved by increasing the PEEP. Treatment of any underlying structural or functional cause is essential.

■ PULMONARY HEMORRHAGE

Pulmonary hemorrhage occurs most commonly in very low birth weight babies who have heart failure secondary to a large pulmonary blood flow due to a PDA. Surfactant administration may increase the risk for pulmonary hemorrhage, particularly if a synthetic rather than a natural surfactant is used and the surfactant is given prophylactically rather than as rescue therapy. Pulmonary hemorrhage also occurs following severe birth depression and in infants with hydrops due to rhesus hemolytic disease, left heart failure, congenital heart disease, sepsis, fluid overload, and clotting abnormalities. Infants who are growth retarded are more likely to suffer a pulmonary hemorrhage. Pulmonary hemorrhage is a severe form of lung edema with leakage of red cells and is better named hemorrhagic pulmonary edema. In most cases, however, the amount of blood lost is small, and the hematocrit of the lung effluent is less than 10%.

Infants who suffer a massive pulmonary hemorrhage deteriorate suddenly with copious bloody secretions appearing from the airway. The infant is hypotensive, because of blood and fluid loss and heart failure, and usually limp and unresponsive. If the hemorrhage is secondary to heart failure, the infant may be tachycardic, and have the murmur of a PDA, hepatosplenomegaly, and a triple rhythm. Affected infants are dyspneic and cyanotic with widespread crackles and reduced air entry into their lungs. The chest radiograph usually demonstrates a "whiteout," with just an air bronchogram visible (Fig. 18-20). Rarely, a lobar pattern of consolidation is found, suggesting that the hemorrhage has occurred only in part of the lung.

All infants with a massive pulmonary hemorrhage should be intubated and ventilated; frequently, peak inflating pressures above 30 cm H_2O are necessary to achieve acceptable blood gases. A high PEEP should be used to help redistribute fluid back into the interstitial space and to improve oxygenation. Neuromuscular blockade and sedation should be used until the hemorrhage is controlled. Although surfactant administration has been incriminated in increasing the risk for a pulmonary hemorrhage, once a hemorrhage has occurred, a single dose of surfactant has been shown to improve oxygenation. Frequent suctioning is initially required to prevent the copious bloody secretions blocking the endotracheal tube. Physiotherapy, however, is not of proven value. Infection may cause a pulmonary hemorrhage; thus, broad-spectrum antibiotics should be administered, ensuring coverage against infection by

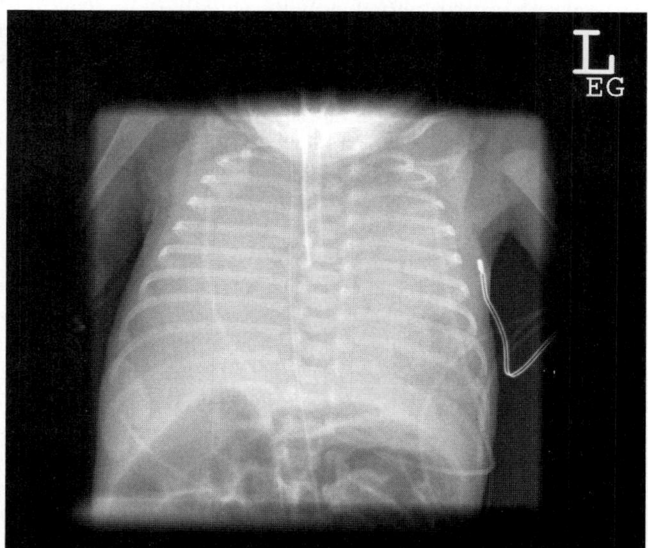

■ **FIGURE 18-20.** Chest radiograph of an infant with a patent ductus arteriosus who suffered a massive pulmonary hemorrhage. The endotracheal tube tip is too low, as it abuts the carina.

Staphylococcus and *Pseudomonas*. Blood transfusions may be required, and it is important to support the blood pressure. Fluid input should be restricted, particularly if there is a coexisting patent ductus, and diuretics given if there is evidence of fluid overload.

The mortality rate of pulmonary hemorrhage has been reported to be as high as 40%, but many of the studies predate the modern era of neonatal intensive care. Affected babies frequently require high-pressure ventilation; thus, air leaks and BPD are common sequelae. The occurrence of cerebral bleeds is doubled in babies who suffer pulmonary hemorrhage, and seizures are also more common.

UPPER AIRWAY OBSTRUCTION

The presentation of upper airway obstruction depends on the site and the magnitude of the obstruction. Tachypnea may be the only manifestation of a partial obstruction, whereas those with a complete obstruction will present with severe respiratory failure, which will be fatal if not promptly relieved. This subject is discussed in more detail in Chapter 17.

NASAL

Infants are obligate nasal breathers, and thus, any anatomic or functional obstruction will result in respiratory distress. Choanal atresia is the most common cause of true nasal obstruction, but occurs in only 1 in 10,000 live births. It can be unilateral or bilateral, isolated or associated with other congenital abnormalities, such as in CHARGE syndrome (coloboma of the iris and retina, heart disease, atresia choanae, retarded growth, genital hypoplasia, and ear defects). Infants with unilateral choanal atresia may be asymptomatic until the nonaffected nares becomes blocked (e.g., with secretions). Infants with bilateral choanal atresia classically appear normal when crying and mouth breathing, but respiratory difficulty appears as soon as they try to breathe through their nose. Less common causes of nasal obstruction include midnasal stenosis and choanal stenosis. Choanal atresia or stenosis can be diagnosed on a CT scan, but MRI should also be employed to determine whether there are intracranial connections in suspected encephalocele, meningocele, and nasal glioma. Nasal causes of obstruction are relieved by an oral airway. Surgical intervention for choanal atresia includes opening the bony membrane that is blocking the airway and inserting tubes to maintain the airway; these are sutured in place for at least 4 weeks.

PHARYNGEAL

Pharyngeal obstruction can occur if there is macroglossia or micrognathia. Craniofacial syndromes associated with oropharyngeal obstruction include Pierre Robin syndrome, hemifacial microsomia, and Crouzon's syndrome. If the tongue is too large or there is inadequate space for the tongue, it is displaced posteriorly into the hypopharynx, causing obstruction, particularly if the infant is nursed supine. As a consequence, affected infants should be nursed prone.

LARYNGEAL

Laryngeal obstruction can result from laryngeal polyps or cysts and dynamic causes, such as vocal cord palsy and severe laryngomalacia. Birth injury is responsible for 20% of vocal cord palsy; traction on the infant's neck during delivery can result in damage to the recurrent laryngeal nerve; it can also occur following cardiac surgery such as duct ligation. Stridor occurring immediately after delivery should always raise the suspicion of a vocal cord palsy, but may also be due to a laryngeal web, cyst, or stenosis. Bilateral vocal cord palsy can occur in infants with severe neurologic abnormalities; affected infants have pharyngeal incoordination, and aspiration is common. Laryngomalacia presents during the first few days after birth. Laryngomalacia is most commonly due to prolapse of the aryepiglottic folds, which collapse on inspiration due to the negative airway pressure; the stridor, therefore, is worse on crying and feeding, but tends to be better when the infant is at rest. Management is usually supportive, since the condition resolves over 12 to 24 months. Subglottic stenosis can be congenital, resulting from a malformation of the cricoid cartilage, but is more commonly acquired secondary to intubation. Infants with acquired subglottic stenosis present with respiratory distress due to upper airway obstruction after extubation, and this condition should be suspected if there are intubation difficulties, particularly difficulty in siting an appropriately sized endotracheal tube. Hoarseness suggests a laryngeal lesion, such as a laryngeal web or vocal cord palsy. Laryngeal obstruction is relieved by intubation, but not by an oral airway.

Lesions within the laryngotracheobronchial tree, such as stenosis, are sometimes visible on a chest radiograph or a penetrated filtered (Cincinnati) view. MRI is the investigation of choice for extrinsic lesions, particularly if vascular compression is suspected. Laryngoscopy can be used to diagnose dynamic conditions, but rigid laryngotracheobronchoscopy is the investigation of choice for all complex airway lesions.

Vocal cord palsy resulting from a birth injury or following an operative procedure is usually due to edema and inflammation and usually resolves with time. Spontaneous resolution is not the case if bilateral cord palsy is associated with a neurologic condition; consequently, affected infants may require a tracheostomy to protect their airway and the siting of a gastrostomy feeding tube, because they have pharyngeal incoordination. The occurrence of acquired subglottic stenosis can be minimized by using appropriately sized endotracheal tubes (i.e., there should be a leak around the tube). If there is no leak, airway edema should be suspected and pre-extubation corticosteroids and adrenaline nebulizers should be given. Nevertheless, some neonates require reintubation because of stridor and airway compromise, and such infants should then remain intubated for a period of "laryngeal rest." If after such a period extubation still fails, an endoscopic examination should be performed to determine the diagnosis. Surgical intervention for subglottic stenosis consists of a cricoid split or immediate laryngeal reconstruction using rib cartilage; rarely a tracheostomy is required.

REFERENCES

1. Kattwinkel J, Niermeyer S, Nadkarni V, Tibballs J, Phillips B, Zideman D, et al: Resuscitation of the newly born infant. An advisory statement from the Paediatric Working Group of the International Liaison Committee on Resuscitation. Resuscitation 1999;40(2):71–88.
2. Niermeyer S, Kattwinkel J, van Reempts P, Nadkarni V, Phillips B, Zideman D, et al: International guidelines for neonatal resuscitation. An excerpt from the Guidelines 2000 for Cardiopulmonary Resuscitation and emergency cardiovascular care. International consensus on science. Pediatrics 2000;106:e29.

3. Eyal F, Alpan G, Sagi E, Glick B, Arad I: Aminophylline versus doxapram in idiopathic apnea of prematurity. A double-blind controlled study. Pediatrics 1985;75:709–713.
4. Peliowski A, Finer N: A blinded, randomized placebo-controlled trial to compare theophylline and doxapram for the treatment of apnea of prematurity. J Pediatrics 1990;116:648–653.
5. Ng E, Shah V: Erythromycin for feeding intolerance in preterm infants (Cochrane Review). In: The Cochrane Library, Issue 3, 2004. Chichester, UK: John Wiley & Sons.
6. Kavvadia A, Greenough A: Influence of ethnic origin on respiratory distress in very premature infants. Arch Dis Child 1998;78:F25–F28.
7. Hallman M, Haataja R: Genetic influences and neonatal lung disease. Semin Neonatol 2003;8(1):19–27.
8. Soll RF, Blanco F: Natural surfactant extract versus synthetic surfactant for neonatal respiratory distress syndrome (Cochrane Review). In: The Cochrane Library, Issue 3, 2004.
9. OSIRIS Collaborative Group: Early versus delayed neonatal administration of a synthetic surfactant—the judgement of OSIRIS. Lancet 1992;340: 1363–1369.
10. Greenough A, Milner AD, Dimitriou G: Synchronised mechanical ventilation for respiratory support in newborn infants (Cochrane Review). In: The Cochrane Library, Issue 3, 2004.
11. Greenough A: Update on modalities of mechanical ventilators. Arch Dis Child Fetal Neonatal Ed 2002;87:F3–F6.
12. Henderson Smart DJ, Bhuta J, Cools F, Offringa M: Elective high frequency oscillatory ventilation versus conventional ventilation for acute pulmonary dysfunction in preterm infants (Cochrane Review). In: The Cochrane Library, Issue 3, 2004.
13. Crowley P: Prophylactic corticosteroids for preterm birth (Cochrane Review). In: The Cochrane Library, Issue 3, 2004.
14. Aghajafari F, Murphy K, Matthews S, Ohlsson A, Anankwan K, Hannah M: Repeated doses of antenatal corticosteroids in animals. A systemic review. Am J Obstet Gynecol 2002;186(4):843–849.
15. Baud O, Foix-L'Helias L, Kaminski M, Audibert F, Jarreau PH, Papiernik E, et al: Antenatal glucocorticosteroid treatment and cystic periventricular leukomalacia in very premature infants. N Engl J Med 1999;341: 1190–1196.
16. Crowther CA, Alfirevic Z, Haslann RR: Thyrotropin-releasing hormone added to corticosteroids for women at risk of preterm birth for preventing neonatal respiratory disease (Cochrane Review). In: The Cochrane Library, Issue 3, 2004.
17. Soll RF, Morley CJ: Prophylactic versus selective use of surfactant for preventing morbidity and mortality in preterm infants (Cochrane Review). In: The Cochrane Library, Issue 3, 2004.
18. Costeloe K, Hennessy E, Gibson AT, Marlow N, Wilkinson AR, for the EPICure Study Group: The EPICure study. Outcomes to discharge from hospital for infants born at the threshold of viability. Pediatrics 2000; 106:659–671.
19. Morrison JJ, Rennie JM, Milton PJ: Neonatal respiratory morbidity and mode of delivery at term. Influence of timing of elective caesarian section. Br J Obstet Gynaecol 1995;102(2):101–106.
20. Lewis V, Whitelaw A: Furosemide for transient tachypnoea of the newborn (Cochrane Review). In: The Cochrane Library, Issue 3, 2004.
21. Katzenstein AL, Gordon LP, Oliphant M, Swender PT: Chronic pneumonitis of infancy. A unique form of interstitial lung disease occurring in early childhood. Am J Surg Pathol 1995;101;1065–1069.
22. Schroeder SA, Shannon DC, Mark EJ: Cellular interstitial pneumonitis in infants. A histopathological study. Chest 1992;101:1065–1069.
23. UK Collaborative ECMO Trial Group: UK Collaborative randomized trial of neonatal extracorporeal membrane oxygenation. Lancet 1996;348:75–82.
24. Soll RF, Dargaville P: Surfactant for meconium aspiration syndrome in full term infants (Cochrane Review). In: The Cochrane Library, Issue 3, 2004.
25. Wiswell T, Knight GR, Finer NN, Donn SM, Desai H, Walsh WF, et al: A multicentre randomized controlled trial comparing Surfaxin (Lucinactant) lavage with standard care for treatment of meconium aspiration syndrome. Pediatrics 2002;109:1081–1087.
26. Halliday HL: Endotracheal intubation at birth for preventing morbidity and mortality in vigorous, meconium-stained infants born at term (Cochrane Review). In: The Cochrane Library, Issue 3, 2004.
27. Hofmeyer GJ: Amnioinfusion for meconium stained liquor in labour (Cochrane Review). In: The Cochrane Library, Issue 3, 2004.
28. Schreiber MD, Gin-Mestan K, Marks JD, Huo D, Lee G, Srisuparp P: Inhaled nitric oxide in premature infants with respiratory distress syndrome. N Engl J Med 2003;349:2099–2107.
29. Winn HN, Chen M, Amom E: Neonatal pulmonary hypoplasia and perinatal mortality in mid-trimester rupture of the membranes—a critical analysis. Am J Obstet Gynecol 2000;182:1638–1644.
30. Kavvadia V, Greenough A, Dimitriou G, Hooper R: Randomised trial of fluid restriction in ventilated very low birthweight infants. Arch Dis Child 2000;83:F91–F96.
31. Herrera C, Holberton J, Davis P: Prolonged versus short course of indomethacin for the treatment of patent ductus arteriosus in preterm infants (Cochrane Review). In: The Cochrane Library, Issue 3, 2004.
32. Ohlsson A, Walia R, Shah S: Ibuprofen for the treatment of a patent ductus arteriosus in preterm and/or low birthweight infants (Cochrane Review). In: The Cochrane Library, Issue 3, 2004.
33. Fowlie PW, Davis PG: Prophylactic intravenous indomethacin for preventing mortality and morbidity in preterm infants. Cochrane Database Systemic Review 2002;(3):CD000174.
34. Cooke L, Steer P, Woodgate D: Indomethacin for asymptomatic patent ductus arteriosus in preterm infants (Cochrane Review). In: The Cochrane Library, Issue 3, 2004.
35. Gould DS, Montenegro LM, William Gaynor J, Lacey SP, Ittenbach R, Stephens P, et al: A comparison of on-site and off-site patent ductus arteriosus ligation in premature infants. Pediatrics 2003;112:1298–1301.

19 Bronchopulmonary Dysplasia

Steven H. Abman, MD • Jonathan M. Davis, MD

Bronchopulmonary dysplasia (BPD) is the chronic lung disease of infancy that follows mechanical ventilation and oxygen therapy for acute respiratory distress after birth in premature newborns.[1–5] As first characterized by Northway and colleagues in 1967, BPD has traditionally been defined by the presence of persistent respiratory signs and symptoms, the need for supplemental oxygen to treat hypoxemia, and an abnormal chest radiograph at 36 weeks corrected age[1] (Fig. 19-1). With the introduction of surfactant therapy, maternal steroid use, new ventilator strategies, aggressive management of the patent ductus arteriosus (PDA), improved nutrition, and other treatments, the clinical course and outcomes of premature newborns with RDS have dramatically changed over the past 30 years. During the presurfactant era, BPD was directly related to the severity of acute RDS and was often described in larger (mean birth weight 2200 g) and more mature (mean gestational age 34 weeks) premature infants. In striking contrast, BPD is now more commonly found in smaller and less mature newborns who initially have very mild or no clinical signs of RDS,[6,7] and is currently characterized by disruption of normal lung development, rather than the marked fibroproliferative changes in the lung (Fig. 19-2). Thus, the so-called "new BPD" represents the inhibition of lung development with altered growth, structure, and function of the distal airspaces and vasculature.

Despite these changes in perinatal care, chronic lung disease after premature birth remains a major clinical problem. With increasing survival of extremely premature newborns, BPD is one of the most significant sequelae of neonatal intensive care, with an estimated 7000 to 10,000 affected infants in the United States each year. The medical and socioeconomic impact of BPD is substantial, with many infants requiring frequent hospitalizations due to recurrent respiratory infections, reactive airways disease, upper airway obstruction, cor pulmonale, neurologic-related issues, and related problems. In addition, some infants with BPD have persistent respiratory problems, as manifested by recurrent wheezing and exercise intolerance, and in some cases, signs and symptoms continue into adolescence and adulthood (Fig. 19-3). This chapter will briefly review changes in the epidemiology of BPD, current concepts in its pathogenesis and pathophysiology, and therapeutic strategies for the treatment or prevention of BPD in at-risk infants.

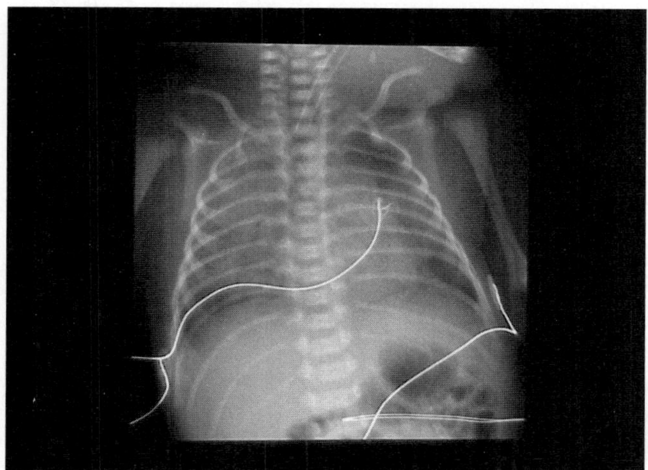

■ **FIGURE 19-1.** Chest x-ray demonstrating typical features of severe bronchopulmonary dysplasia in a young infant.

■ DEFINITION

Despite extensive clinical studies of premature babies with chronic lung disease, the definition of BPD remains problematic. BPD is generally defined by the presence of chronic respiratory signs, a persistent oxygen requirement, and an abnormal chest radiograph at 1 month of age or at 36 weeks' corrected age. Unfortunately, this definition lacks specificity and fails to account for important clinical distinctions related to extremes of prematurity and wide variability in criteria for the use of prolonged oxygen therapy. For example, Shennan and colleagues suggested that the need for oxygen supplementation at 36 weeks' postconceptual age may be a better predictor of late pulmonary disease during infancy than the need for oxygen at 28 days of life.[8] Oxygen use at 1 month of age may not adequately account for differences between the effects of delayed lung maturation versus lung injury, since the need for supplemental oxygen at 28 days of life in premature infants born at 24 or 25 weeks' gestation may represent lung immaturity and not the results of "lung injury." However, many of these infants may not ultimately develop chronic respiratory disease or have an abnormal chest radiograph. Additionally, chest x-ray findings can be subtle and are generally not sensitive or specific for BPD. Recently, a consensus conference of the National Institutes of Health suggested a new definition of BPD that incorporates many elements of previous definitions and attempts to categorize the severity of BPD[3] (Table 19-1). Finally, wide variability exists in defining the need for supplemental oxygen, which has a marked impact on the incidence of BPD.[9] For example, a recent report showed for a given study population, the incidence of BPD decreased from 37% to 24% if the need for supplemental oxygen was defined by accepting oxygen saturations above 92% or 88% while breathing room air, respectively.[10] Further work is needed to better identify early physiologic, structural, and genetic or biochemical markers of BPD, in order to better associate early features of BPD with critical long-term endpoints, such as the presence of late respiratory disease

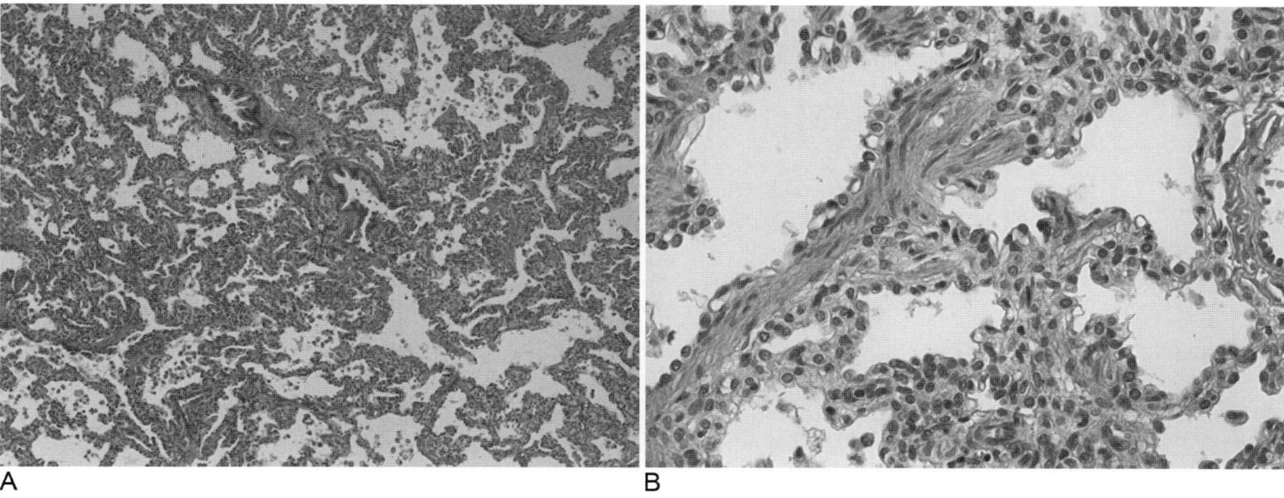

■ **FIGURE 19-2.** Lung histology from an infant who died with severe bronchopulmonary dysplasia (BPD) following prolonged mechanical ventilation. **A,** Classic features of thickened interstitium, increased cellularity, and fibroproliferative changes. **B,** A higher-powered view that illustrates distal fibroproliferative changes in severe BPD. (See Color Plate 28.)

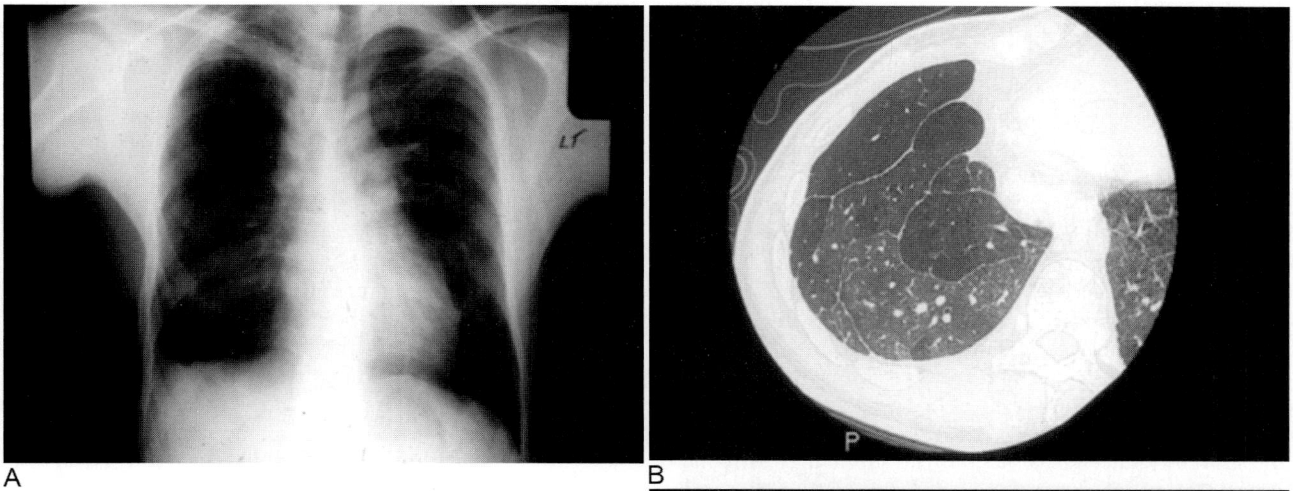

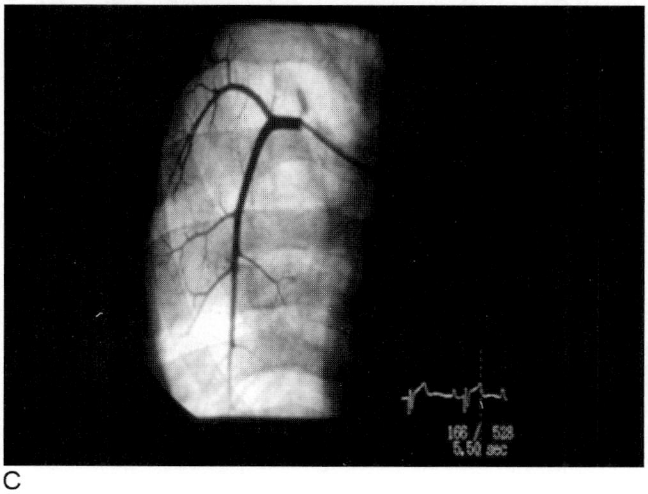

A

B

C

■ **FIGURE 19-3.** **A–C,** Chest x-ray, chest computed tomography and right pulmonary artery angiogram from a 26-year-old adult patient who was born at 26 weeks' gestation, and required mechanical ventilation for 6 months during his first year of life.

TABLE 19-1. NIH Consensus Conference: Diagnostic criteria for establishing bronchopulmonary dysplasia (BPD)

	GESTATIONAL AGE	
	<32 Weeks	**>32 Weeks**
Time point of assessment	36 weeks PMA or discharge to home, whichever comes first	>28 days but <56 days postnatal age or discharge to home, whichever comes first
	Treatment with oxygen >21% for at least 28 days	
Mild BPD	Breathing room air at 36 wk PMA or discharge, whichever comes first	Breathing room air by 56 days postnatal age, or discharge, whichever comes first
Moderate BPD	Need for <30% O_2 at 36 wk PMA or discharge, whichever comes first	Need for <30% O_2 to 56 days postnatal or discharge, whichever comes first
Severe BPD	Need for >30% O_2 ± PPV or CPAP at 36 wk PMA or discharge, whichever comes first	Need for >30% O_2 ± PPV or CPAP at 56 days postnatal age or discharge, whichever comes first

CPAP, continuous positive airway pressure; PMA, postmenstrual age; PPV, positive pressure ventilation.

From Jobe AH, Bancalari E: Bronchopulmonary dysplasia. Am J Respir Crit Care Med 2001;163:1723–1729.

(e.g., recurrent hospitalizations, reactive airways disease, the need for prolonged oxygen or respiratory medications, exercise intolerance, and others) during infancy and early childhood.

EPIDEMIOLOGY AND INCIDENCE

The epidemiology and incidence of BPD have changed dramatically over the past 40 years. In the early 1960s, oxygen and mechanical ventilation was first selectively used for premature infants with acute respiratory failure due to apnea and "hyaline membrane disease." At that time, infants who survived for 72 hours generally went home without apparent chronic lung disease. However, as these therapies were applied more widely, there was a growing recognition of premature infants who developed chronic pulmonary symptoms, hypoxemia, and chest radiographic abnormalities. Shepard and colleagues reported that 50% of premature neonates who received oxygen and mechanical ventilation developed chronic lung disease beyond 6 months of age.[11] In 1967, Northway and co-workers provided a comprehensive characterization of the clinical, radiologic, and pathologic features of chronic lung disease in 32 infants who had received high concentrations of oxygen and mechanical ventilation from birth.[1] On average, these premature infants were born at 34 weeks' gestation and weighed 2200 g, yet the mortality rate was 67%, and the surviving infants had persistent respiratory distress and abnormal chest radiographs beyond the first 4 weeks of life. This study first applied the term *bronchopulmonary dysplasia*, emphasizing abnormalities of the airways, parenchyma, and vasculature in the pathology of chronic lung disease. This seminal report identified the interactive role of three key factors: (1) lung immaturity; (2) acute lung injury caused by oxygen, mechanical ventilation, and other factors; and (3) inadequate repair of the initial lung injury, which still serves as an important paradigm for our current understanding of BPD. Although much has been learned about BPD since its initial description, the disease continues to change with time due to improved treatment strategies and survival. Mortality has dramatically decreased over the past few decades, with survival increasing from less than 10% in the past to over 50% in the most extremely preterm newborn (24–26 weeks' gestation). In 1967, the average gestational age and birth weight of surviving BPD infants was 34 weeks and 2234 grams, but now BPD is rare in infants older than 32 weeks of gestation. Currently, most infants developing BPD are much smaller and less mature at birth, averaging less than 1000 g in 75% of cases.[4,7,9] The risk of BPD rises with decreasing birth weight; the incidence has been reported as high as 85% of neonates between 500 and 699 g but decreases to 5% in infants with birth weights over 1500 g. In these immature infants, even minimal exposure to oxygen and mechanical ventilation may be sufficient to contribute to BPD. A recent report demonstrated that about two thirds of infants who develop BPD have only mild respiratory distress at birth.[7] Although the overall incidence of BPD is reported at about 20% of ventilated newborns, wide variability exists between centers.[12] This variability likely reflects regional differences in the clinical definitions of BPD, the number of inborn versus outborn populations, the proportion of newborns with extreme prematurity, and specific patient management.

There is now growing recognition that infants with persistent lung disease after premature birth have a different clinical course and pathology than had been traditionally observed in infants dying with BPD during the presurfactant era[13–15] (Fig. 19-4). The classic progressive stages that first characterized BPD are often absent due to changes in clinical management. The disease has clearly changed from being predominantly defined by the severity of acute lung injury to its current characterization, which can be predominantly defined by a disruption of distal lung growth. In contrast with "classic BPD," the "new BPD" develops in preterm newborns who often require minimal ventilatory support with low fractions of inspired oxygen (FIO_2) during the early postnatal days.[3,6,7] As a result, the term *chronic lung disease of infancy* has often been used interchangeably with *BPD* to describe the chronic respiratory disease that can develop after premature birth. In addition to its changing epidemiology, the nature of BPD has evolved as well, such that pathologic signs of severe lung injury with striking fibroproliferative changes have become more rare. More typically, infants with BPD now have less severe acute respiratory disease early in their course. At autopsy, lung histology displays more uniform and milder regions of injury, and signs of impaired alveolar and vascular growth are more prominent. The implications for how these changes in BPD will alter long-term pulmonary outcomes is unknown.

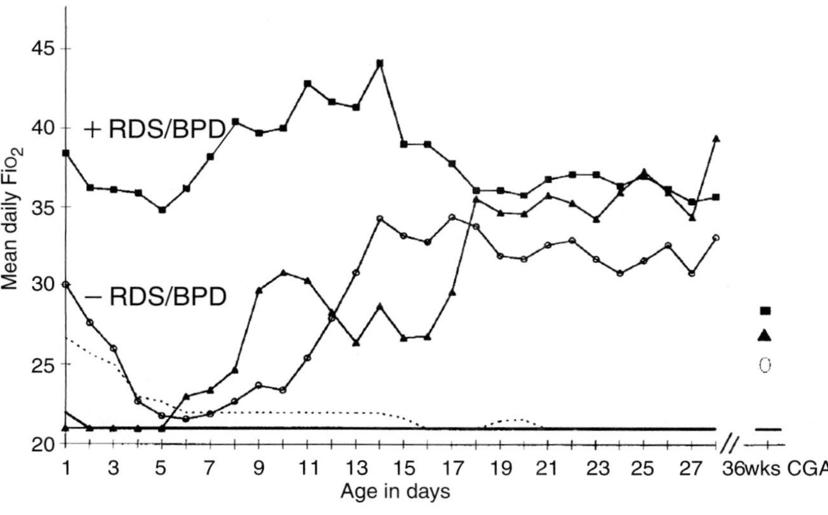

■ **FIGURE 19-4.** Variable clinical courses in infants with bronchopulmonary dysplasia (BPD). This figure is adapted from the work of Charafeddine and colleagues[6] and illustrates serial changes in oxygenation in patients with BPD who present with and without acute respiratory distress syndrome (RDS). As shown, lung disease can progressively increase and can later appear indistinguishable from the clinical features of "typical" BPD that follows RDS.

■ RADIOLOGIC AND PATHOLOGIC FEATURES

Radiographic abnormalities characteristic of BPD were first described by Northway and associates in 1967, documenting the progression of the disease process through four distinct stages. The radiographic progression of BPD is now seldom categorized by these four stages. Although persistent chest x-ray abnormalities remain a major part of the diagnostic criteria for BPD and were once considered useful for staging disease progression, the chest x-ray has proven to be less useful than in the recent past. Overall, radiographic changes are widely variable, scoring systems are somewhat subjective, and clinical disease severity appears to correlate poorly with x-ray findings, which are relatively insensitive for predicting late complications. Growing use of other imaging approaches, such as computerized axial tomography (CT) or magnetic resonance imaging (MRI), in addition to direct measurements of infant lung function, will play a more critical role in assessing disease severity and course. These findings can be important in determining ultimate pulmonary morbidity. CT scans often show regional heterogeneity, with regions of hyperinflation and sparse arterial density alternating with relatively normal appearing regions. MRI of ventilated premature newborns demonstrate striking regional variations in lung disease, with marked gravity-dependent atelectasis and edema. More studies of the role of CT and MRI in BPD are needed to quantify and correlate structural and functional changes.

The changing pathologic features of BPD continues to provide important insights into the pathobiology and epidemiology of BPD over time[15] (Table 19-2). Original studies of BPD described a continuous process through distinct stages of disease, progressing from acute lung injury, or an "exudative phase" with diffuse pulmonary edema, proteinaceous debris, and inflammation, to a "proliferative phase" with structural features of chronic lung disease. Older reports described the gross "cobblestone" appearance of the lungs, representing alternating areas of atelectasis, marked scarring, and regional hyperinflation (or "emphysema"). Typical histologic features of BPD include marked airway changes, such as squamous metaplasia of large and small airways, increased peribronchial smooth muscle and fibrosis, chronic inflammation and airway edema, and hyperplasia of submucosal glands. Parenchymal disease is characterized by volume loss from atelectasis and alveolar septal fibrosis alternating with overdistention or "emphysematous" regions. Mesenchymal thickening with increased cellularity and destruction of alveolar septae with alveolar hypoplasia is present, suggesting a marked reduction in surface area available for gas exchange. Growth of capillary beds is reduced, and small pulmonary arteries have hypertensive structural remodeling, which includes smooth muscle hyperplasia and distal extension of smooth muscle growth into vessels that are normally nonmuscular. In addition, the vessels are often described as "dysmorphic" due to their centralized location in the thickened mesenchyme, which may further impair gas exchange. Although reductions in alveolar number was described in older infants dying with BPD, this pattern of "alveolar simplification" has become the most striking pathologic feature of the "new BPD"[11] (Fig. 19-5). In contrast with past reports, recent studies of infants dying with BPD describe fewer signs of airway injury

■ **TABLE 19-2.** Pathologic features of bronchopulmonary dysplasia (BPD)

Presurfactant ("Old BPD")	Postsurfactant ("New BPD")
Alternating atelectasis with hyperinflation	Less regional heterogeneity of lung disease
Severe airway epithelial lesions (e.g., hyperplasia, squamous metaplasia)	Rare airway epithelial lesions
Marked airway smooth muscle hyperplasia	Mild airway smooth muscle thickening
Extensive, diffuse fibroproliferation	Rare fibroproliferative changes
Hypertensive remodeling of pulmonary arteries	Fewer arteries but "dysmorphic"
Decreased alveolarization and surface area	Fewer, larger and simplified alveoli

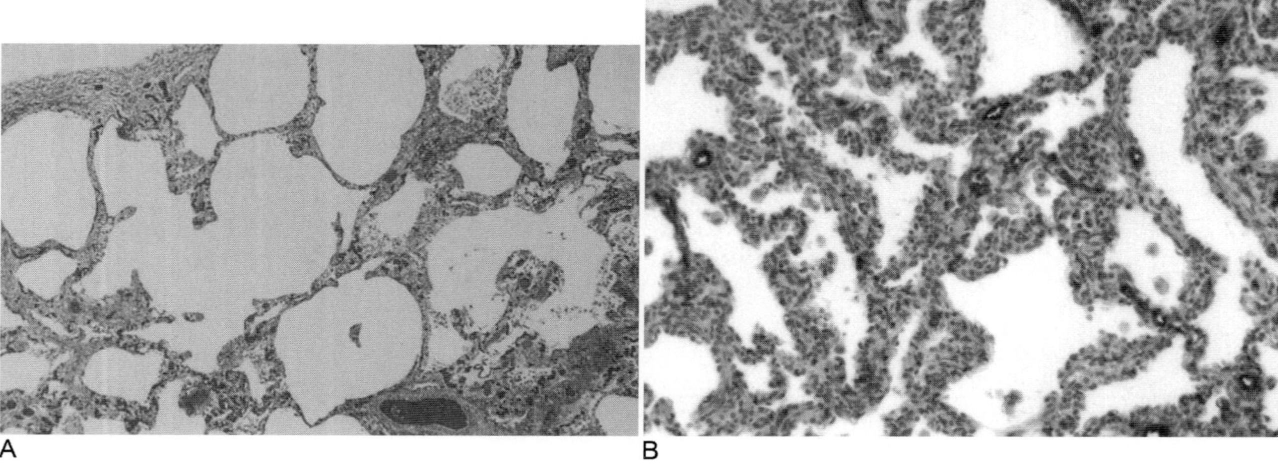

■ **FIGURE 19-5.** Lung histology illustrating decreased alveolarization in an older child who died with severe bronchopulmonary dysplasia (BPD) in the postsurfactant period. As shown in **A,** there is a dramatic reduction of septation and alveolarization, with distension of distal airspaces. **B** shows factor VIII immunostaining for vascular endothelium, illustrating "dysmorphic" lung vascular growth in BPD.

and interstitial fibrosis, but emphasize persistent reductions of distal airspace and vascular growth. Decreased alveolarization and impaired growth of small pulmonary arteries results in decreased lung surface area for gas exchange, which has important functional implications regarding late cardiopulmonary sequelae.

In addition to changes in the distal lung, the pathology of BPD is further characterized by abnormal airway structure. Upper airways (i.e., trachea and main bronchi) of infants with BPD often reveal significant lesions, depending on the frequency and duration of endotracheal intubation. Grossly, mucosal edema or necrosis can be focal or diffuse. The earliest histologic changes include patchy loss of cilia from columnar epithelial cells, which can then become dysplastic or necrotic, resulting in breakdown of the epithelial lining. Ulcerated areas may involve the mucosa or extend into the submucosa. Infiltration of inflammatory cells (neutrophils and lymphocytes) into these areas may be prominent. Goblet cells appear hyperplastic, suggesting greater capacity for increased mucous production that can mix with cellular debris. Granulation tissue often develops in the subglottis due to damage from endotracheal intubation or more distally throughout the airway due to trauma from repeated suctioning. Significant narrowing of the trachea and main bronchi secondary to injury can lead to subglottic stenosis, tracheal cysts and polyps, and related acquired lesions. Tracheomalacia, often complicating the course of severe BPD, can appear as marked redundancy of the posterior wall of the trachea, due to chronic ventilation of the compliant premature airway.

Changes in the smaller airways and distal airspace constitute the most striking pathologic changes in severe BPD. Early RDS is characterized by proteinaceous debris in the distal airspaces (hyaline membranes), while the epithelium appears as a thin, dysplastic lining, made up primarily of type II alveolar cells. These membranes become incorporated into the underlying airway. Edema, inflammation, exudate, and necrosis of epithelial cells are often found, along with a necrotizing bronchiolitis. Later in the clinical course, cellular debris, inflammatory cells, and proteinaceous exudate can accumulate and obstruct many of the terminal airways and the distal lung. It has been suggested that this process, with associated atelectasis, may actually protect the distal airspaces from further damage due to high oxygen levels and stretch-induced injury during mechanical ventilation. Fibroblast proliferation and activation leads to peribronchial fibrosis, smooth muscle thickening, and, in advanced cases, obliterative bronchiolitis. In more recent cases, these changes in airway morphology have been less striking.

In the chronic phase of BPD (usually in infants older than 2 months of age), the cobblestone appearance of the lung's surface is much more pronounced, as hyperexpanded units are present alongside atretic and fibrotic units to impart a "pseudofissuring" to the surface of the lung. With time and growth of relatively normal areas of the lung, the cobblestone effect disappears, but large pseudofissures remain, and normal lobes are impossible to identify. Tracheomegaly, tracheomalacia, and ciliary dysfunction may be present as either focal or diffuse abnormalities.[16–18] Granulomatous nodules, concentric fibrosis, and polyps may also be present and may cause tracheal or bronchial obstruction. On microscopic examination, the hallmark of this phase of BPD is alveolar septal fibrosis such that the width of the alveolar septa is 10 times greater than normal. The focal nature of BPD is still present with fibrotic, hyperexpanded, and normal lung units adjacent to one another. There is mucous gland hypertrophy in the bronchial mucosa, and squamous metaplasia is more pronounced. In addition, muscular hyperplasia around pulmonary arteries and especially around bronchioles can now be identified in more than 80% of infants who die during this phase of the disease; however, even these abnormalities may be focal, and normal bronchovascular anatomy may be seen in many lung regions. Cardiac involvement has also been demonstrated in infants with BPD, including evidence of myocardial ischemia or fibrosis, right ventricular hypertrophy, and left ventricular or biventricular hypertrophy.

■ PATHOGENESIS

BPD represents the response of the lung to acute injury during a critical period of lung growth, that is, during the canalicular period, in which airspace septation and vascular development increases dramatically. Lung injury after premature birth and the

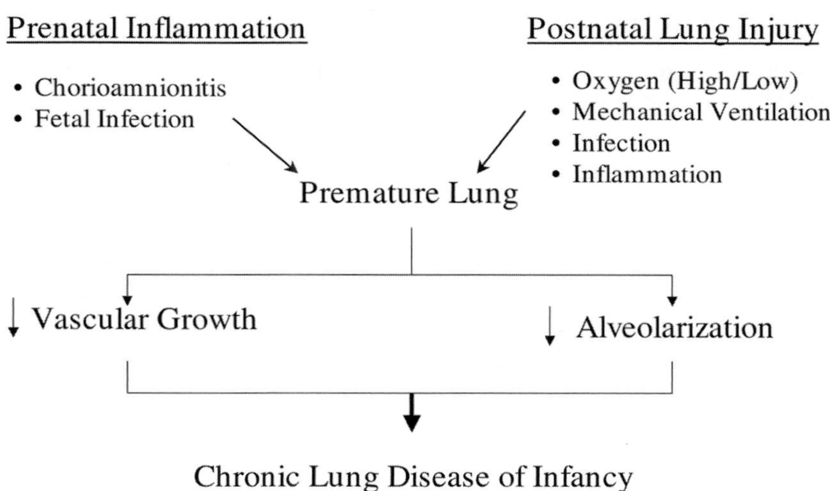

■ **FIGURE 19-6.** Pathogenesis of bronchopulmonary dysplasia.

subsequent inhibition of lung growth results from complex interactions between several adverse stimuli, including inflammation, hyperoxia, mechanical ventilation, and infection, on the poorly defended developing lung (Fig. 19-6). This contributes to the long-term abnormalities of lung structure and function that characterize BPD. Several characteristics of the immature lung initially increase the susceptibility of the premature newborn to the development of BPD. One of the most critical factors relates to deficiency and dysfunction of lung surfactant. Surfactant dysfunction causes atelectasis, impairs ventilation and gas exchange, aggravates lung injury, and promotes inflammation. Maturational related decreases in host antioxidant defenses and impaired epithelial function also contribute to lung injury, abnormal ion and water transport, and increased lung edema. In addition, lung structural immaturity due to decreased connective tissue may increase susceptibility for barotrauma and air leaks, and centralization of capillaries in mesenchyme or septae decreases the efficiency of gas exchange. Severe prematurity is associated with a markedly increased compliance of the chest wall, which hinders spontaneous breathing and increases susceptibility for overdistention of the lung during mechanical ventilation. Thus, multiple intrinsic factors that are associated with prematurity increase the susceptibility for BPD. Major pathogenetic mechanisms that cause BPD are discussed below.

■ PRENATAL EVENTS

Subclinical intrauterine infection and the ensuing inflammatory response have been clearly implicated in the etiology of preterm labor and premature rupture of membranes.[19–23] Growing evidence also supports the concept that prenatal infection and inflammation are major risk factors for BPD. While several investigators have found a lower incidence of acute RDS in preterm infants born to mothers with chorioamnionitis and funisitis (possibly due to an adaptive response to in utero stress), a significantly higher incidence of BPD was also observed in these same infants.[21] This suggests that although intrauterine infection may accelerate lung maturation, inflammation may also "prime the lung," causing lung injury, progressive inflammation, and subsequent inhibition of lung growth. Antenatal exposure of the lung to proinflammatory cytokines has been found to be a major risk factor for the development of BPD. Clinically, amniotic fluid interleukin-8 (IL-8) and tumor necrosis factor-α (TNF-α) levels in mothers whose fetuses developed BPD are higher in comparison with levels from mothers whose newborns did not develop BPD.[19–22] Injection of endotoxin into the amniotic fluid of pregnant sheep 6 days before delivery markedly increases lung compliance (59%), gas volume (twofold), and concentrations of surfactant lipids and proteins,[24] which were greater effects than those achieved with steroid treatment. White blood cell counts and several inflammatory cytokines are increased in fetal membranes and lungs after endotoxin exposure that hastens maturation, suggesting that endotoxin-induced inflammation may induce lung maturation through increased inflammation. Despite these acute physiologic effects, however, early endotoxin and cytokine exposure may also impair later lung growth. Similar patterns of cytokine expression have been observed in newborns who subsequently develop cerebral palsy, suggesting that prenatal exposure to cytokines may represent a common pathway for the initiation of preterm labor, injury to the lung, and damage to the developing central nervous system of the fetus.

The use of antenatal corticosteroids has been shown to enhance fetal lung maturation and lower the risk for developing acute RDS, while the effects on the incidence of BPD are more controversial. Antenatal treatment with betamethasone has multiple, direct beneficial effects on the fetal lung, including improved lung compliance, lung volumes, surfactant production and antioxidant enzyme activity.[25,26] Betamethasone may also prevent lung damage in the fetus indirectly by reducing maternal cytokine production and exposure in the fetus or by altering gene expression of critical growth factors and their receptors. Repetitive courses of prenatal corticosteroids have also been used routinely and are associated with further improvements in lung mechanics and reduced oxidative stress in the lung. However, multiple courses of antenatal steroids do appear to significantly reduce both somatic and lung growth in the fetus, which may be detrimental to long-term pulmonary function.[27] Recent clinical data have failed to confirm a previous report that antenatal glucocorticoid treatment reduces the risk for chronic lung disease in premature newborns and may worsen long-term neurodevelopmental outcomes.

HYPEROXIA AND OXIDANT STRESS

Postnatal exposure to adverse stimuli, such as hyperoxia or ischemia-reperfusion injury after asphyxia, contributes to the development of BPD. Under normal conditions, a delicate balance exists between the production of reactive oxygen species (ROS) and protective antioxidant defense systems. Damage caused by ROS ranges from cell membrane destruction to mitochondrial injury, protein nitration, inactivation of growth factors, and modification of nucleic acids. The premature infant appears to be especially susceptible to ROS-induced damage due to the lack of adequate antioxidants after premature birth. Antioxidant enzymes (e.g., superoxide dismutase [SOD], catalase, and glutathione peroxidase) markedly increase in the rabbit lung during late gestation.[28] Increase in antioxidant enzymes during the latter part of gestation parallels the maturation pattern of pulmonary surfactant, and increases in both systems are critical for the normal transition to postnatal life. In addition, the ability to increase synthesis of antioxidant enzymes in response to hyperoxia is decreased in preterm animals, suggesting that premature birth may precede the normal up-regulation of antioxidants, which persists during early postnatal life. Premature birth precedes the normal up-regulation of these antioxidant systems and other ROS scavengers (e.g., vitamin E, ascorbic acid, glutathione, and ceruloplasmin) and may result in an imbalance between oxidants and antioxidants and an increased risk for the development of BPD. Experimental models have shown that hyperoxia, in the absence of ventilation, can induce lung injury that mimics RDS and late sequelae that are similar to BPD. Endothelial and alveolar type II cells are both extremely susceptible to hyperoxia and ROS-induced injury leading to increased permeability edema, cellular dysfunction, and impaired survival and growth. Hyperoxia also impairs mucociliary function, promotes inflammation, and inactivates antiprotease, further complicating clinical outcome. Clinical studies suggest that ROS are involved in the pathogenesis of BPD. Expired pentane and ethane have been measured as indirect evidence of free radical–induced lipid peroxidation in the first week of life and found to be significantly elevated in neonates subsequently developing BPD.[29]

Further evidence for the role of ROS in lung injury comes from several studies which have shown that antioxidant supplementation with SOD and catalase reduces cell damage, increases survival, and prevents lung injury from prolonged hyperoxia and mechanical ventilation.[30] In addition, genetically engineered mice overexpressing either CuZnSOD, MnSOD, or extracellular SOD survive longer, whereas mice with disrupted CuZnSOD or ecSOD genes have higher mortality and worse lung growth in hyperoxia than normal controls.[31–33] These studies confirm the critical role of the intricate balance between the production of ROS and antioxidant defenses in the development of lung injury.

VOLUTRAUMA

The treatment of premature newborns with RDS with positive pressure mechanical ventilation contributes to lung injury, provoking a complex inflammatory cascade that leads to BPD. Pneumothorax and pulmonary interstitial edema are strongly associated with BPD, suggesting that ventilator-induced lung injury can cause chronic lung disease.[34,35] However, even in the absence of overt signs of air leak, treatment of premature neonates with mechanical ventilation can initiate or promote lung injury with inflammation and permeability edema, and contribute to high risk for developing BPD.

Nilsson and colleagues have shown that even brief periods of positive pressure ventilation cause bronchiolar epithelial damage in the lung, with the severity of the injury correlating with the amount of peak pressure used.[36] Positive pressure ventilation exposes the lung to cyclical stretch stress, due to changes in both airway pressure and volume, which damage small airways and distal airspaces. Surfactant deficiency further contributes to persistent atelectasis, causing more injury due to cyclic reinflation and overdistention of inflated lung regions. Even with normal tidal volumes, ventilation of the immature or injured newborn lung results in nonuniform inflation and relative overdistention of ventilated segments, especially in the presence of low functional residual capacity (FRC). Stretching of capillary endothelium and distal lung epithelium increases permeability to serum proteins that may further inhibit surfactant function, creating a vicious cycle that promotes lung injury. Mechanical ventilation with high tidal volumes, especially with poorly recruited lung due to low positive end-expiratory pressures (PEEP), stimulates lung cytokine production.[37]

The adverse effects of tidal volume breaths in lungs with low FRC can be decreased with better lung recruitment after the application of higher levels of PEEP. Experimental studies have clearly shown that overdistention of these lung regions, and not pressure, is responsible for lung injury in the surfactant-deficient lung.[34] For example, strapping the chest wall to restrict overexpansion increased lung pressure but limited lung stretch, and inhibited lung injury in rats and neonatal lambs.[38] Tremblay and associates have observed that mechanical ventilation with high tidal volumes and low PEEP markedly increases lung edema and cytokine expression production.[37] In this same model, lung injury increases cytokine release from the lungs into the systemic circulation, suggesting a potential mechanism linking multiorgan dysfunction and sepsis syndrome with lung injury. An National Institutes of Health (NIH)–sponsored trial showed improved survival of adults with acute respiratory distress syndrome by using a ventilator strategy that used low tidal volumes with high PEEP levels in order to recruit atelectatic lung regions and to maintain FRC.[39] This suggests that the damaging effects of oxygen and mechanical ventilation in the lung occur via similar pathways primarily involving activation of the inflammatory cascade that ultimately leads to the development of acute lung injury and BPD. Lung protective strategies, including the use of high-frequency ventilation, permissive hypercapnia, prone position, and inhaled nitric oxide, are currently under investigation.

Strategies to prevent lung injury have included changes in methods of ventilation. Even brief exposure to large volume breaths during resuscitation shortly after birth can initiate early lung injury, which decreases the subsequent response to surfactant therapy.[40] With the increased use of nasal continuous positive airway pressure (nCPAP), many preterm infants can be managed without the need for endotracheal intubation and mechanical ventilation, which may lessen the risk for lung injury. Although well substantiated in laboratory and single center reports, ongoing multicenter trials are under way to determine whether nCPAP can decrease the incidence of BPD.

Whether more rapid removal of endotracheal tubes and switching to mechanical ventilation with nasal prongs will reduce the incidence of BPD is unknown. Synchronized intermittent mechanical ventilation (SIMV) and high-frequency devices have been extensively studied. Bernstein and associates reported that infants (<1000 g) who were treated with SIMV developed less BPD than those receiving conventional ventilation.[41] Several multicenter trials have demonstrated that high-frequency oscillatory ventilation (HFOV) or high-frequency jet ventilation (HFJV) using high-volume, alveolar recruitment strategies in conjunction with surfactant replacement therapy reduced complications of mechanical ventilation (pulmonary interstitial emphysema, pneumothorax) and lowered the incidence of BPD compared with conventional ventilation.[42,43] However, these findings have not been consistently found in other trials.

Regardless of the type of ventilation strategy used, it is imperative to avoid even brief periods of overdistention, since high tidal volumes and hypocarbia are associated with a greater risk for developing both lung and neurologic injury in critically ill neonates. A retrospective study of 1105 newborns who were born with weights below 2000 g between 1984 and 1987 demonstrated a strong relationship between prolonged cumulative exposure to hypocapnia (partial pressure of carbon dioxide in arterial blood [$PaCO_2$] <35 torr) with "disabling" cerebral palsy.[44] This study also noted that hypocapnia, hyperoxia, and duration of mechanical ventilation were independently associated with a two- to threefold increase in risk for cerebral palsy.

The use of surfactant replacement therapy has reduced some complications of mechanical ventilation. Surfactant permits more equal distribution of pressures and ventilation to all alveoli, prevents overdistention of distal airspaces and bronchioles, and stabilizes lung volume. A major benefit of surfactant therapy has been the ability to reduce airway pressures without causing atelectasis, to maintain greater uniformity of lung recruitment, and to reduce air leak. However, BPD continues to be an important problem despite the widespread use of exogenous surfactant and strategies to minimize lung injury using mechanical ventilation (i.e., permissive hypercapnia).[45] A recent study compared the outcomes of premature infants weighing 500 to 1500 g at birth who were treated in either Boston or New York, and reported that the incidence of BPD was significantly higher in Boston (22%) compared with New York (4%), even after adjusting for baseline risk factors, such as severity of prematurity.[46] Using multivariate analyses to examine differences in specific respiratory care practices during the first week of life, most of the increased risk for BPD was associated with the early initiation of mechanical ventilation and may be decreased with early nCPAP therapy. This suggests that attempts to minimize the use of mechanical ventilation using nCPAP (with or without exogenous surfactant) may lower the incidence and severity of BPD in high-risk infants.

INFLAMMATION

Although hyperoxia and volutrauma directly injure the neonatal lung, these effects are partly mediated and potentiated by the recruitment and activation of inflammatory cells and the release of potent inflammatory products.[47–50] A sustained increase in the neutrophil number in tracheal fluid samples distinguishes infants who develop BPD from those with mild RDS. In addition, the presence of activated macrophages, high concentrations of lipid products, oxidant-inactivated α_1-antitrypsin activity, and other markers of active inflammation are strongly linked with the development of BPD. More recently, increased proinflammatory cytokines, including IL-6 and IL-8, and decreased IL-10 levels, have been recovered in the tracheal fluid of infants who subsequently developed BPD.[51] Release of early-response cytokines, such as TNF-α, IL-1β, IL-8, and transforming growth factor-β (TGF-β) by macrophages and the presence of soluble adhesion molecules (i.e., selectins) may impact other cells to release chemoattractants and recruit neutrophils that further amplify the inflammatory response.[49–53] Elevated concentrations of proinflammatory cytokines in conjunction with reduced anti-inflammatory products (i.e., IL-10) usually appear in tracheal aspirates within a few hours of life in infants subsequently developing BPD. Proinflammatory cytokines and the activated leukocytes that accompany them cause significant pulmonary damage, including breakdown of capillary endothelial integrity and leakage of larger molecules (e.g., albumin) into alveolar spaces. Albumin leakage and associated pulmonary edema are known to inhibit surfactant function and have been postulated to be important factors in the development of BPD.[54]

The release of elastase and collagenase from activated neutrophils may directly destroy the elastin and collagen framework of the lung. Markers of collagen and elastin degradation have been recovered in the urine of infants with BPD.[55] The major defense against the action of elastase activity is α_1-proteinase inhibitor, which may be inactivated by ROS.[56] Increased elastase activity accompanied by compromised antiproteinase function may result in an imbalance that has been demonstrated in tracheal aspirates and sera of infants developing BPD. Therapy with exogenous antiproteases could potentially restore this delicate balance and prevent the development of BPD. This hypothesis has been tested in a pilot study in which treatment of premature neonates with intravenous doses of α_1-proteinase inhibitor over the first 2 weeks of life had a trend toward reductions in the incidence of BPD and the duration of ventilator support.[57] These mechanisms may play a major role in the disruption of alveolar septae or saccules, contributing to regional emphysema.

Marked inflammation in the lung and inhibition of alveolarization appear to begin a cascade of destruction and abnormal repair that develops into BPD. The initial trigger that activates lung inflammation may be ROS, mechanical ventilation, infectious agents, or other adverse stimuli that attract and activate inflammatory cells, including leukocytes, macrophages, and fibroblasts. Neutrophils and macrophages cause additional release of ROS and diverse mediators, thereby amplifying injury.[47–50] Recent evidence suggests that eosinophils may also play a role in the development of BPD. Fibroblast activation can lead to striking fibroproliferation and remodeling of the immature lung after injury, including altered matrix production in the airway, vasculature, and interstitium. As the acute cycle of injury continues with further production and accumulation of inflammatory mediators, significant injury to the lung can occur during a particularly critical period of rapid growth (i.e., six divisions from 24 to 40 weeks' gestation). Watterberg and associates have demonstrated that extremely premature infants have evidence of adrenal insufficiency at birth, with the lowest serum cortisol concentrations during the first week of life correlating with increased lung inflammation and adverse respiratory outcome.[58] Pilot studies examining early treatment with low-dose hydrocortisone in extremely low birth weight infants increased the likelihood of survival without BPD, a benefit that was particularly apparent in infants born to mothers with chorioamnionitis.[59] The mechanisms underlying this observation are uncertain, but may include suppression of lung inflammation with less inhibition of lung growth than observed with higher doses of steroids, avoidance of the harmful effects of steroid insufficiency, or enhancing the beneficial effects of low-dose hydrocortisone on lung development, or others. A recent multicenter trial was halted, however, due to an increased risk for gastrointestinal perforation.

INFECTION

Colonization with *Ureaplasma urealyticum* is associated with an increased risk for subsequent development of BPD. *U. urealyticum* has been recovered from cervical cultures of pregnant women and implicated as a possible cause of chorioamnionitis, prematurity, and BPD.[60] Several investigators have cultured the upper genital tract of mothers prior to delivery and tracheal aspirates from preterm infants after delivery and found that BPD developed significantly more often in infants colonized with ureaplasma compared to those with negative cultures. In addition, premature infants born to mothers with premature rupture of the membranes who had received prenatal erythromycin (which is often effective against ureaplasma) had a lower incidence of BPD compared with untreated controls. In contrast, other studies have found that while *Ureaplasma* was frequently detected (by culture or polymerase chain reaction) in many low birth weight infants, its presence was not associated with the development of BPD. Other investigators have suggested that both prenatal and postnatal infections act as a potent stimulus for the inflammatory response, with recruitment of leukocytes, release of ROS, and activation of the arachidonic cascade ultimately leading to BPD. Since preterm infants are relatively immunodeficient at birth (both cellular and humoral arms), they are much more susceptible to colonization and subsequent infection with a variety of infectious agents (e.g., virus, bacteria, fungi) that may affect the severity of BPD. Bacteremia with low virulence organisms, in addition to the persistence of a patent ductus arteriosus, and the degree of prematurity, are strongly associated with development of BPD in the postsurfactant era.[7]

NUTRITION

Premature infants have increased nutritional requirements due to increased metabolic needs and rapid growth requirements. Severe lung disease may further increase energy expenditures (i.e., increased work of breathing) in infants with limited nutritional reserves. If these increased energy needs are not met by exogenous sources, the infant will develop a catabolic state, which is probably a major contributing factor to the pathogenesis of BPD. Inadequate nutrition, which could interfere with normal growth and maturation of the lung, may potentiate the deleterious effects of oxygen. Newborn rats with inadequate caloric intake have decreased lung weights, protein levels, and DNA content.[61] These abnormalities were even greater in pups that were nutritionally deprived at birth and then exposed to hyperoxia.

Antioxidant enzymes play a vital role in the protection of the lung, and many of these enzymes have trace elements (e.g., copper, zinc, selenium) that are an integral part of their structure. Deficiencies in these elements may predispose the lung to further injury, while supplementation may provide protection to the lung and prevent hyperoxic lung damage. The repair of elastin and collagen is limited in animals that are undernourished, and copper and zinc may be necessary for this repair. Vitamin E and A deficiency have also been postulated to be important in the development of BPD. Current nursery feeding and hyperalimentation regimens appear to provide adequate amounts of vitamin E for preterm infants. However, concentrations of vitamin A may be deficient in premature neonates, and this vitamin appears to be important in maintaining cell integrity and in tissue repair. Several investigators have found lower serum retinol levels in cord blood and in the first month of life in infants who subsequently developed BPD.[62] Despite adequate supplementation, some infants remain vitamin A deficient, presumably from increased absorption of parenteral vitamin A into the tubing of the intravenous administration set or due to higher nutritional requirements. A multicenter trial of vitamin A supplementation in premature infants at risk for developing BPD recently demonstrated that large doses of intramuscular vitamin A given three times per week was associated with a small (7%), but significant, reduction in the incidence of BPD, suggesting that vitamin A deficiency is one contributor to lung injury.[63]

Large volumes of intravenous fluids are often administered to premature infants to provide adequate fluid requirements (due to increased insensible water losses) and sufficient calories. Excessive fluid administration can be associated with the development of a patent ductus arteriosus and pulmonary edema leading to increased oxygen and ventilator requirements and the development of BPD. Early closure of the ductus using indomethacin or surgical ligation has been associated with improvements in pulmonary function, but these approaches have not affected the incidence of BPD.

GENETIC FACTORS

Past studies have implied that preterm neonates were more likely to develop BPD if there was a strong family history of atopy and asthma. Nickerson and Taussig found a positive family history of asthma in 77% of infants with RDS who subsequently developed BPD, compared with only 33% who did not.[64] Bertrand evaluated the relationship between prematurity, RDS, and the need for mechanical ventilation to a family history of airway hyperactivity.[65] The severity of lung disease was directly related to the degree of prematurity and the duration of oxygen exposure. However, siblings and mothers of infants with the most significant lung disease had evidence of airway reactivity, suggesting that all three factors are involved in determining long-term outcome. When histocompatibility loci (HLA) were examined, Clark and associates found that only infants with HLA-A2 developed BPD, again suggesting that other underlying factors that are poorly understood may be important in the pathogenesis of BPD.[66] More recently, Hagan reported that a family history of asthma is associated with an increase in the overall severity of BPD in premature infants, but does not appear to be a causative factor.[67] With recent technologic advances in genomics, proteomics, and bioinformatics, more information on the contribution of genetic factors to the risk of developing BPD are under vigorous study.[68]

ABNORMAL GROWTH FACTOR SIGNALING

Multiple growth factors, including vascular endothelial growth factor (VEGF), have been shown to play critical roles in normal lung growth and cellular differentiation throughout development[69]; VEGF is a potent endothelial cell mitogen and survival factor, which is essential for angiogenesis and vascular growth and remodeling. Bhatt and co-workers first demonstrated decreased lung expression VEGF in the lungs from premature infants who died with BPD.[70] Experimentally, hyperoxia down-regulates VEGF expression, and pharmacologic inhibition of VEGF signaling in newborn rats impairs lung vascular growth and inhibits alveolarization.[71] Lung VEGF expression down-regulation has also been observed in primate and ovine models of BPD induced by mechanical ventilation after premature birth, further supporting the hypothesis that impaired VEGF signaling contributes to lung hypoplasia and the pathogenesis of BPD.[72] Ongoing studies of the regulation and activities of diverse growth factors are likely to lead to greater understanding of the pathobiology and treatment of BPD.

PATHOPHYSIOLOGY

AIRWAY DISEASE AND LUNG MECHANICS

Chronic respiratory signs in children with BPD include tachypnea with shallow breathing, retractions, and paradoxical breathing pattern, with coarse rhonchi, crackles, and wheezes typically heard on auscultation. Persistent abnormalities in lung mechanics and impaired gas exchange often require treatment with oxygen and ventilator support. Increased airway resistance and bronchial hyperreactivity can be demonstrated even during the first week of life in preterm neonates at risk for BPD.[73] These abnormalities are common in older infants with BPD and can cause dynamic airway collapse and expiratory flow limitation. Other abnormalities of lung function include increased dead space ventilation, decreased lung compliance, maldistribution of ventilation, and abnormal ventilation-perfusion matching. FRC is often reduced early in the course due to atelectasis, but increases during the later stages of BPD due to gas trapping with hyperinflation. Increased respiratory rate with shallow breathing increases dead space ventilation that results from marked regional variability of time constants and decreased lung surface area. Nonuniform damage to the airways and distal lungs results in variable time constants for different areas of the lungs, altering the distribution of inspired gas to relatively poorly perfused lung and worsening ventilation-perfusion matching.

Two methods used to measure lung compliance include dynamic measurements and passive expiratory techniques after airway occlusion.[74] Both methods show a reduction of lung compliance in infants with BPD. The decrease in lung compliance appears to correlate well with morphologic and radiographic changes in the lung. Compliance can be reduced because of increased resistance, with frequency dependence of compliance when infants are breathing rapidly. The use of pulmonary function testing to follow the progression of BPD and the response of the lung to various therapeutic interventions has become widespread. However, care must be exercised in the interpretation of results because of inherent variability in the measurements and possible error from excessive chest wall distortion.

Infants with BPD at 28 days of age have an increased total respiratory resistance, expiratory resistance, and severe flow limitation, especially at low lung volumes.[74,75] The presence of tracheomalacia may also result in airflow limitation, which may actually be worsened by bronchodilator therapy.[17] Indeed, in some studies, an elevated pulmonary resistance in infants younger than a week old accurately predicts those infants who will go on to develop chronic BPD.[73] Dynamic lung compliance is also markedly reduced in infants with BPD,[74] even in those who no longer require oxygen therapy. The reduction in compliance is due not only to small airway narrowing but also to interstitial fibrosis, edema, and atelectasis. FRC is usually decreased but may be increased or normal. These dynamic abnormalities lead to an increase in the work of breathing and to ventilation-perfusion mismatching. Highly unusual ventilation-perfusion patterns have been observed during ventilation-perfusion scanning studies.[76] Nitrogen washout is prolonged, particularly in hyperexpanded regions.

A few studies have assessed the changes in pulmonary function of BPD infants beyond the first few months of life.[77] Most infants with BPD show improvement of pulmonary function with time, so that lung function is usually in the low-normal range by 2 to 3 years of age. Whether this improvement represents repair of damaged lung or growth of new lung (or both) has not been determined. Infants with severe BPD may have evidence of chronic obstructive pulmonary disease, and about one half of these infants will have reversible airway obstruction. Infants whose lung function remains unchanged or worsens are usually those whose somatic growth is markedly delayed, but the relationship between abnormal lung repair and delayed somatic growth is unclear. Some neonatologists have used this latter observation to justify aggressive nutritional supplementation for infants with BPD, with unproven success. Indeed, it may be equally likely that the delay in somatic growth in these severely affected infants is the result of chronic hypoxemia or an adaptive response to delayed lung repair.

Studies of pulmonary function in older children who were born prematurely have indicated that although subtle defects of small airway function may be present in childhood, these abnormalities are not more frequent in infants with BPD than in premature infants without BPD.[65,77] These studies suggest that prematurity per se may have a small but measurable impact on lung growth, which may predispose an individual to the development of lung disease later in life.

PULMONARY CIRCULATION IN BRONCHOPULMONARY DYSPLASIA

In addition to adverse effects on the airway and distal airspace, acute lung injury also impairs growth, structure, and function of the developing pulmonary circulation after premature birth.[78,79] Endothelial cells have been shown to be particularly susceptible to oxidant injury due to hyperoxia or inflammation. The media of small pulmonary arteries may also undergo striking changes, including smooth muscle cell proliferation, precocious maturation of immature pericytes into mature smooth muscle cells, and incorporation of fibroblasts into the vessel wall.[80] Structural changes in the lung vasculature contribute to high pulmonary vascular resistance (PVR) due to narrowing of the vessel diameter and decreased vascular compliance. In addition to these structural changes, the pulmonary circulation is further characterized by abnormal vasoreactivity, which also increases PVR.[81,82] Finally, decreased angiogenesis may limit vascular surface area, causing further elevations of PVR, especially in response to high cardiac output with exercise or stress.

Overall, early injury to the lung circulation leads to the rapid development of pulmonary hypertension, which contributes significantly to the morbidity and mortality of severe BPD. Even from the earliest reports of BPD, pulmonary hypertension and cor pulmonale were recognized as being associated with high mortality.[83,84] Walther and colleagues showed that elevated pulmonary artery pressure in premature newborns with acute RDS (determined from serial echocardiograms) was associated with severe disease and high mortality.[83] Past studies have also shown that persistent echocardiographic evidence of pulmonary hypertension beyond the first few months of life is associated with up to 40% mortality in infants with BPD.[84] High rates of mortality have also been reported in infants with BPD and pulmonary hypertension who require prolonged ventilator support.[85] Although pulmonary hypertension is a marker of more advanced BPD, elevated PVR also causes poor right ventricular function, impaired cardiac output, limited oxygen delivery, increased pulmonary edema, and perhaps a higher risk for sudden death.

Physiologic abnormalities of the pulmonary circulation in BPD include elevated PVR and abnormal vasoreactivity, as evidenced by the marked vasoconstrictor response to acute hypoxia.[81,82,86] Cardiac catheterization studies have shown that even mild hypoxia causes marked elevations in pulmonary artery pressure, even in infants with modest basal levels of pulmonary hypertension. Treatment levels of oxygen saturations above 92% to 94% effectively lower pulmonary artery pressure.[82] Strategies to lower pulmonary artery pressure or limit lung injury to the pulmonary vasculature may limit the subsequent development of pulmonary hypertension in BPD.

In addition to pulmonary hypertension, clinical studies have also shown that metabolic function of the pulmonary circulation is impaired, as reflected by the impaired clearance of circulating norepinephrine (NE) across the lung. Normally, 20% to 40% of circulating NE is cleared during a single passage through the lung, but infants with severe BPD have a net production of NE across the pulmonary circulation. It is unknown whether impaired metabolic function of the lung contributes to the pathophysiology of BPD by increasing circulating catecholamine levels, or if it is simply a marker of severe pulmonary vascular disease. It has been speculated that high catecholamine levels may lead to left ventricular hypertrophy or systemic hypertension, which are known complications of BPD.

CARDIOVASCULAR ABNORMALITIES IN BRONCHOPULMONARY DYSPLASIA

In addition to pulmonary vascular disease and right ventricular hypertrophy, other cardiovascular abnormalities that are associated with BPD include left ventricular hypertrophy (LVH), systemic hypertension, and the development of prominent systemic-to-pulmonary collateral vessels. An early report described infants with severe BPD and LVH in the absence of right ventricular hypertrophy, and suggested that left ventricular dysfunction may contribute to recurrent edema in BPD.[87] Steroid therapy can cause LVH, which tends to be transient and resolves with cessation of steroid therapy.

A high incidence of systemic hypertension can occur in BPD,[88] but its etiology remains obscure. Systemic hypertension may be mild, transient, or striking and usually responds to pharmacologic therapy. On occasion, further evaluation of such infants may reveal significant renal vascular or urinary tract disease. Whether the high incidence of systemic hypertension in BPD reflects altered neurohumoral regulation or increased catecholamine, angiotensin, or antidiuretic hormone levels is still unknown.

Prominent bronchial or other systemic-to-pulmonary collateral vessels were noted in early morphometric studies of infants with BPD, and can be readily identified in many infants during cardiac catheterization. Although these collateral vessels are generally small, large collaterals may contribute to significant shunting of blood flow to the lung, causing edema and need for higher FIO_2. Collateral vessels have been associated with high mortality in some patients with severe BPD who also had severe pulmonary hypertension. Some infants have improved after embolization of large collateral vessels, as reflected by a reduced need for supplemental oxygen, ventilator support, or diuretics. However, the actual contribution of collateral vessels to the pathophysiology of BPD is poorly understood.

TREATMENT

In addition to chronic respiratory disease, infants with BPD have significant growth, nutritional, neurodevelopmental, and cardiovascular problems. The severity of respiratory disease varies widely among infants with BPD. In its most severe presentation, children with BPD require home ventilation or prolonged home oxygen therapy. Most infants, even those who have weaned off supplemental oxygen therapy, have recurrent hospitalizations caused by lower respiratory exacerbations due to viral infections, with respiratory syncytial virus (RSV) or influenza, reactive airways disease, or pulmonary hypertension accompanied by congestive heart failure. In addition, persistent or recurrent respiratory exacerbations may also be due to structural lesions (i.e., tracheomalacia, subglottic stenosis, bronchomalacia), chronic aspiration (gastroesophageal reflux or swallowing dysfunction), or others. In addition to supplemental oxygen therapy, chronic treatment with bronchodilators, diuretics, inhaled or systemic steroids, and nutritional supplements are commonly used as supportive therapy. Although some studies have suggested that the early use of postnatal steroids may reduce the incidence and severity of BPD, significant concerns exist regarding adverse effects, including bowel perforation and worsened neurodevelopmental outcomes.[89,90] Therapeutic approaches to infants with BPD are described below.

OXYGEN THERAPY

Supplemental oxygen to avoid intermittent or prolonged periods of hypoxemia remains the mainstay of BPD therapy. Adverse effects of hypoxemia include pulmonary hypertension with cor pulmonale, poor growth, impaired lung growth, bronchoconstriction, and a greater frequency of apnea or cyanotic episodes.[91–94] During long-term therapy, frequent assessments of oxygenation are needed to ensure adequate levels of supplemental O_2 therapy. In general, supplemental oxygen is administered to target O_2 saturations at greater than 92% while awake, during feedings, and with sleep. Higher O_2 saturation levels (>94%–96%) are generally recommended for patients with right ventricular hypertrophy, pulmonary hypertension, poor growth, apneic episodes, and other problems.[93] A recent study (the STOP-ROP trial) examined the role of oxygen therapy in retinopathy of prematurity, and suggested that infants who were treated with hyperoxia to maintain high oxygen saturations had a higher risk for chronic lung disease than infants treated with supplemental oxygen that targeted lower saturations.[95] However, interpretation of these data in the setting of preventing or treating infants with pulmonary hypertension are limited, since the targeted ranges for the low and high oxygen saturation groups fell between typical recommendations for oxygen therapy. That is, the current recommendation for treatment of patients with BPD and pulmonary hypertension is to maintain oxygen saturations at 92% to 96%. Whether higher oxygen saturations induce more lung injury remains unproven, but the adverse effects of hypoxemia are clear, and common practice is to target O_2 saturations to avoid hypoxemia.

Past studies have suggested that most infants with BPD show steady improvement in the level of supplemental O_2 therapy, and are off supplemental oxygen by 6 to 12 months. Patients who fail to wean off supplemental oxygen, especially those with recurrent hospitalizations, poor growth, RVH, and other signs, should be evaluated for unsuspected cardiac or pulmonary problems that are slowing their recovery. Such evaluations should include prolonged pulse oximetry (especially during sleep); assessment of compliance with O_2 therapy in outpatients; sleep studies; laryngoscopy and bronchoscopy; swallowing studies; pH probes; echocardiograms; sweat test; serum immunoglobulins; and others.

MECHANICAL VENTILATION

With established disease, patients with BPD who require prolonged ventilatory assistance generally require larger tidal volume breaths and a slower rate to enhance the distribution of gas due to heterogeneity of lung units. Ventilation of infants with severe BPD with fast rates and smaller tidal volumes increases dead space ventilation and may worsen gas exchange and increase gas trapping. Slow weaning of ventilatory support should allow for better assessments of respiratory muscle strength and lung function over time. Flexible bronchoscopy is useful to determine whether structural airway disease is complicating the clinical course. Criteria for tracheostomy and chronic mechanical ventilation are controversial, but are indicated in patients with BPD and severe respiratory failure, as reflected by chronic hypoventilation and hypercarbia. Additional findings of severe retractions, problems handling secretions due to neurologic disease, vocal cord paralysis, severe tracheomalacia, persistent signs of pulmonary hypertension, and other signs provide clinical markers for assessing the need for chronic support.

PHARMACOLOGIC THERAPY

Many pharmacologic agents have been used in the treatment of infants with BPD, including diuretics, bronchodilators, and corticosteroids, reflecting the complex nature of the disease.[96] Despite extensive investigations of drug therapy of BPD, controversy persists regarding the role of these agents in the overall management of BPD. This is partly due to the problem that most of the data from drug studies often only examine acute, transient responses in lung function, which may be statistically significant but may not lead to sustained improvement despite chronic therapy. The balance between benefits and potential toxicities with prolonged therapy are critical. In addition, the treatment of premature infants with pharmacologic agents generally targets three different time periods in the evolution of BPD. These include (1) prophylaxis and the prevention of BPD; (2) treatment of evolving BPD; and (3) treatment of established BPD. In each case, the goals of therapy must be carefully considered, along with assessment of potential adverse effects from long-term use. In general, medications should be added one at a time for careful assessments of efficacy and discontinued if an adequate clinical response is not observed after a few days of observation.

DIURETICS

Diuretic therapy, including furosemide, hydrochlorothiazide, and spironolactone, are commonly used in infants with BPD. The overall rationale for therapy is to treat recurrent pulmonary edema that can worsen lung compliance and gas exchange. Increased fluid and salt retention, due to hyperaldosteronism and elevated antidiuretic hormone release, can contribute to the development of pulmonary edema. Past studies have shown that diuretic therapy can acutely improve lung mechanics in infants with BPD, but the effects of some drugs may be independent of the diuretic response. However, such adverse effects as nephrocalcinosis, osteopenia, ototoxicity, hyponatremia, hypokalemia, hypochloremia, alkalosis, and impaired growth commonly complicate the course of treated infants. Metabolic alkalosis may impair respiratory drive and contribute to CO_2 retention. Using furosemide therapy on alternate days, rather than as daily treatment, may optimize lung mechanics and gas exchange in infants with BPD while decreasing the frequency or severity of side effects.[97] The use of spironolactone in combination with furosemide or a thiazide diuretic may sustain the diuretic response and minimize potassium and calcium depletion. However, initial reports that low doses of thiazides can prevent furosemide-induced hypercalciuria have not been confirmed. Potassium chloride and arginine hydrochloride supplements may be needed to replace K^+ and Cl^- losses. The use of sodium chloride supplements to treat electrolyte imbalance induced by diuretics should be discouraged. During the acute phase of BPD in hospitalized infants, diuretic therapy is used intermittently when symptoms of acute fluid intolerance occur, such as rapid weight gain, systemic edema, and increased respiratory symptoms or oxygen requirements that cannot be explained by infection. Doses of furosemide (1 mg/kg) are given intramuscularly or intravenously every 12 hours (or 2 mg/kg/dose every 12 hours by mouth) for 2 to 3 days, then discontinued, and the patient is reassessed. Long-term furosemide therapy with close monitoring of serum electrolyte, pH, and clinical response should be considered for hospitalized, ventilator-dependent infants with severe BPD and persistent need for high FIO_2, and perhaps unventilated infants on high supplemental oxygen. The role for continuous diuretic therapy in infants with mild to moderate BPD is unclear, especially in view of the risks of diuretic therapy and the lack of long-term studies.

BRONCHODILATORS

Bronchodilator therapy, using β agonists, can reverse acute bronchospasm and improve airway resistance and respiratory system compliance in infants with BPD.[94,98] These physiologic abnormalities may be present as early as the first week of life in preterm neonates during mechanical ventilation.[73] However, the role of β agonists for chronic therapy is unproven, since most of the effects on lung mechanics are transient. Similarly, anticholinergic and theophylline therapies can improve lung mechanics in BPD infants, but whether prolonged therapy causes sustained improvement is uncertain. Older patients with BPD often have asthma, characterized by intermittent and reversible airways obstruction during acute respiratory exacerbations, and seem to be highly responsive to bronchodilator therapy. Short-term β-agonist therapy is effective when acute bronchospasm is present. Any infant with BPD and acute wheezing or hypercarbia deserves a therapeutic trial of these agents. However, the physician should be mindful of their short duration of action, their cardiac side effects, and the possibility of rebound bronchospasm. The clinician must consider that when BPD is accompanied by tracheomalacia, bronchodilator therapy may worsen lung function, probably by increasing large airway instability.[17]

CORTICOSTEROIDS

Corticosteroid therapy is perhaps the most controversial area of BPD care. Corticosteroids, especially dexamethasone, have long been used to reduce lung inflammation during the treatment of infants with severe BPD. Clinical studies have consistently shown that steroids acutely improve lung mechanics and gas exchange, and reduce inflammatory cells and their products in tracheal samples of patients with BPD.[99,100] Despite these studies, there have been multiple experimental and clinical studies that have raised concerns that high-dose and prolonged use of corticosteroids can impair head growth, neurodevelopmental outcomes, and lung structure. Additionally, a recent multicenter study was halted prior to completion due to a high incidence of gastrointestinal perforation.[89] Other side effects include systemic hypertension, hyperglycemia, cardiac hypertrophy, poor somatic growth, sepsis, intestinal bleeding, and myocardial hypertrophy. Currently, the routine use of steroids in premature newborns is strongly discouraged, as reflected in strong editorial statements from the American Academy of Pediatrics.[101] However, these findings are generally based on data from studies that have used extremely high doses of dexamethasone for prolonged periods of time, and many questions persist regarding the risk-benefit relationship with the use of other steroids for shorter study periods. In addition, there is a need to better define the potential role of steroids in the prevention of BPD, treatment of evolving BPD or treatment of severe, established BPD. As a result, some centers recommend the selective use of steroids at lower doses and shorter durations (5–7 days) in ventilator-dependent infants with severe, persistent lung disease beyond 3 to 4 weeks of age. Inhaled steroids have been studied, but the major effect of inhaled steroid therapy in a multicenter randomized trial was to simply decrease the perceived need for the use of systemic steroids.[102]

OUTCOME

Most follow-up data were obtained from patients from the presurfactant era, with only limited studies describing the clinical course of patients who have reached adolescence and young adulthood. Late respiratory morbidity is common in infants and young children born prematurely, especially in those with BPD. Approximately 50% of infants with BPD will require readmission to the hospital during early childhood for respiratory distress, often with lower respiratory tract infections. This high rate of hospitalization generally declines during the second and third year of life, but lung function studies often show limited reserve even in patients with minimal overt respiratory signs.[103–105] This observation likely explains the severity of presentation in some infants with BPD after acquiring RSV or other infections. During infancy, lung growth and remodeling can result in progressive improvement of pulmonary function and weaning from oxygen therapy. However, other respiratory problems (e.g., reactive airway disease and recurrent pulmonary infections) and abnormal neurologic development are additional abnormalities that may occur and require careful follow-up.

Infants with BPD demonstrate improvements in clinical status and lung mechanics during the first year, yet persistent airflow abnormalities may remain. In some infants, lung volumes during tidal breathing approaches expiratory flow limitations, suggesting limited reserve. Infants with BPD have reduced measurements of absolute and size corrected flow rates in comparison with age- and size-matched control patients, suggesting poor airway growth with age.[105] A 2-year follow-up study that compared BPD and premature newborns without BPD showed late airway obstruction in most infants (80%) with BPD versus 40% in the non-BPD group.[105] Overall, lung volume progressively increases with age, but airflow obstruction persists during early childhood.

Chest radiograph findings during follow-up are generally nonspecific, demonstrating typical findings as hyperinflation with peribronchial cuffing and scattered or focal interstitial infiltrates consistent with fibrosis or atelectasis. These findings tend to clear with age, but are very insensitive markers of changes in lung function. CT scans can also demonstrate regional variations in lung disease, often displaying hyperinflated or emphysematous areas with diminished arterial density. The utility for serial CT scans during follow-up is uncertain, but may help to identify localized area of disease, such as large cysts, that may require surgical resection.

Although pulmonary function in most survivors with BPD improves over time with continued lung growth and permits normal activity, abnormalities detected by pulmonary function testing may remain through adolescence. Follow-up studies of children with BPD have shown an increased incidence of wheezing and other clinical respiratory symptoms that may continue into later years.[106] In addition, pulmonary function studies have demonstrated increased airway resistance and reactivity, decreased lung compliance, ventilation-perfusion mismatch, abnormal exercise tolerance, and blood gas abnormalities (e.g., increased $PaCO_2$) in older children with a history of BPD.[107] The most significant abnormalities were found in children who had clinical respiratory symptoms such as wheezing and repeated pulmonary infections, especially early in their childhood (<2 years of age).[108] Baraldi and colleagues demonstrated progressive improvements in pulmonary function tests over the first 2 years of life in infants with BPD, although evidence of airway dysfunction continued to persist.[105] It appears that abnormal pulmonary function and distress are greatest in the first 2 years of life in infants with BPD. Improvement in lung function can occur between years 7 and 10, but over

25% of adolescents with a history of BPD have abnormal lung function. More recently, Filipone and colleagues showed a strong correlation between maximal flows at FRC ($\dot{V}_{max}$ FRC) at 2 years of age with forced expiratory volume in 1 second (FEV_1) at school age, suggesting persistent airflow limitation in selected patients with BPD.[109] Comprehensive longitudinal studies following patients into adulthood are currently lacking.

Despite increases in lung volumes of infants with BPD during childhood, morphometric studies have shown that older patients who die with BPD fail to demonstrate compensatory alveolar growth. These observations suggest that distal airspaces remain relatively hypoplastic, with marked reductions in alveolar number, and impaired gas exchange is likely to persist due to reduced alveolar numbers and microvascular growth. Functionally, the loss of surface area impairs gas exchange and contributes to prolonged oxygen requirements, frequent respiratory exacerbations, and late physiologic abnormalities, including exercise intolerance.[110]

Finally, there are few data on pulmonary function of adult patients with a previous history of premature birth and severe BPD. Northway and colleagues reported persistent evidence of gas trapping and airway reactivity in young adults and adolescents with BPD who were treated nearly three decades ago.[110] Clinical experience suggests that increasing numbers of older survivors with severe BPD are only beginning to reappear as young adult patients. More studies are needed to determine the long-term respiratory course of premature neonates, with or without severe BPD, and their relative contribution to the growing adult population with chronic obstructive pulmonary disease.

PREVENTION STRATEGIES

A multidisciplinary approach to the prevention of BPD in infants is needed. The use of antenatal steroids in mothers at high risk for delivering a premature infant may reduce the severity and incidence of BPD.[25] The early use of nasal or mask CPAP (with or without prior surfactant treatment) may eliminate the need for mechanical ventilation in some premature infants or facilitate successful extubation in others.[111] Aggressive treatment of symptomatic patent ductus arteriosus with fluid restriction, diuretics, indomethacin, or surgical closure may reduce the severity of BPD. Tidal volumes and inspired oxygen concentrations should be reduced as low as necessary in order to reduce hypocarbia, volutrauma, and oxygen toxicity, while using more aggressive lung recruitment strategies, such as more liberal PEEP, HFOV, or perhaps prone positioning. The early use of synchronized mechanical ventilation or high-frequency ventilation (HFV) in newborn infants with significant RDS may reduce the severity and incidence of BPD.[42,43] The combined use of HFV and surfactant replacement may prevent significant lung damage in premature and full-term infants with significant lung disease unresponsive to surfactant replacement and conventional mechanical ventilation.[112] Further conclusive evidence of the beneficial effects of both synchronized ventilation and HFV in premature infants is needed.

Aggressive nutritional support is critical in helping to promote normal lung growth, maturation, and repair. It also protects the lung from the damaging effects of hyperoxia, infection, and barotrauma. Systemic supplementation with vitamin A in sufficient quantities to establish normal serum retinol concentrations has been reported to reduce the incidence of BPD, although the need to administer repeated doses through the intramuscular route has limited the widespread use of this therapy.

Recent studies have suggested that the early use of low doses of hydrocortisone may reduce the incidence of BPD, presumably by treating cortisol deficiency and minimizing inflammation. However, early dexamethasone should not be used to prevent BPD because of significant concerns regarding increased mortality, side effects (i.e., ileal perforation), and long-term sequelae (cerebral palsy).[89,113,114] The most promising method for preventing the development of BPD appears to be prophylactic supplementation of human recombinant antioxidant enzymes. This seems to be a logical strategy in preventing BPD, because ROS appear to play a major role in the pathogenesis of lung injury and premature infants are known to be relatively deficient in these enzymes at birth. Several animal studies have shown that prolonged exposure to high oxygen concentrations can cause severe lung damage and death, and administration of antioxidants can prevent many of these complications. Recombinant human CuZnSOD (rhSOD) has been administered prophylactically to the lungs of premature infants at high risk for developing BPD. In preliminary studies in premature infants, the prophylactic use of both single and multiple intratracheal doses of rhSOD appeared to mitigate inflammatory changes and severe lung injury from oxygen and mechanical ventilation with no apparent associated toxicity. In animal studies, the rhSOD appeared to localize both in intracellular and extracellular compartments following intratracheal instillation with significant quantities of active protein present 48 hours after the dose is given. Multicenter collaborative trials using prophylactic, intratracheal rhSOD in premature infants at high-risk for developing BPD have recently been completed. Premature infants (birth weight 600–1200 g) receiving intratracheal instillation of rhSOD at birth had significantly (44%) fewer episodes of respiratory illness (wheezing, asthma, pulmonary infections) severe enough to require treatment with bronchodilators or corticosteroids at 1 year corrected age compared with placebo controls.[115] This suggests that rhSOD did prevent long-term pulmonary injury from ROS in high-risk premature infants. Further therapeutic intervention trials are needed in order to ultimately develop a therapy that can prevent or significantly ameliorate this important chronic lung disease.

In addition, protecting the pulmonary vasculature from injury may not only lower PVR and improve gas exchange, but it may also enhance distal lung growth and improve long-term outcome. Extensive laboratory and clinical studies suggest that inhaled nitric oxide (iNO) lowers PVR and improves oxygenation in patients with pulmonary hypertension in different settings, including premature infants with severe RDS and BPD.[116,117] However, there are persistent concerns about potential toxicity and adverse effects of iNO therapy in the premature infant. Experimental data have suggested that iNO therapy may be "lung protective" in several animal models, including premature lambs with RDS and increases alveolar growth in injured neonatal rats.[118,119] Whether iNO therapy has a potential role in the prevention of pulmonary vascular injury in premature newborns at risk for BPD is unknown. A multicenter clinical trial of low-dose iNO therapy (5 ppm) was recently performed in severely ill premature newborns with RDS who had marked hypoxemia despite surfactant therapy (i.e., a/A O_2 ratio <0.10), with an estimated mortality rate of 53%.[116] In this study, iNO acutely improved PaO_2, but did not improve survival.

Notably, there was no increase in the frequency or severity of intracranial hemorrhage or BPD, and the duration of mechanical ventilation was reduced.[120] Based on findings, a multicenter trial is now under way to determine whether early treatment with low-dose iNO therapy will prevent the early inflammatory changes that contribute to BPD, and protect the pulmonary circulation from injury during this critical time period.

■ CONCLUSIONS

Thirty years after its original description, BPD remains a significant complication of premature birth and a persistent challenge for the future. BPD has evolved from the classical stages described in the past to a disease characterized largely by inhibition of lung development. Future strategies that improve long-term outcomes will be dependent on the successful integration of basic research on fundamental mechanisms of lung development and the response to injury, as well as studies that test novel interventions to lower the frequency and severity of the cardiopulmonary sequelae of BPD.

REFERENCES

1. Northway WH Jr, Rosan RC, Porter DY: Pulmonary disease following respirator therapy of hyaline-membrane disease. N Engl J Med 1967; 276:357–368.
2. Bland RD, Coalson JJ: Chronic lung disease in early infancy. New York: Marcel Dekker, 2000.
3. Jobe AH, Bancalari E: Bronchopulmonary dysplasia. Am J Respir Crit Care Med 2001;163:1723–1729.
4. Bancalari E, Abdenour GE, Feller R, Gannon J: Bronchopulmonary dysplasia. Clinical presentation. J Pediatr 1979;95:819–823.
5. Jobe AH: The new BPD: An arrest of lung development. Pediatr Res 1999; 46:641–643.
6. Charafeddine L, D'Angio CT, Phelps DL: Atypical chronic lung disease patterns in neonates. Pediatrics 1999;103:759–760.
7. Rojas MA, Gonzalez A, Bancalari E, et al: Changing trends in the epidemiology and pathogenesis of chronic lung disease. J Pediatr 1995;126:605–610.
8. Shennan AT, Dunn MS, Ohlsson A, et al: Abnormal pulmonary outcomes in premature infants. Prediction from oxygen requirement in the neonatal period. Pediatrics 1988;82:527–532.
9. Ellsbury DL, Acarregui MJ, McGuinness GA, et al: Controversy surrounding the use of home oxygen for premature infants with BPD. J Perinatol 2004;24:36–40.
10. Walsh MC, Wilson-Costello D, Zadell A, et al: Safety, reliability and validity of a physiologic definition of BPD. J Perinatol 2003;23: 451–456.
11. Shepard F, Gray J, Stahlman MT: Occurrence of pulmonary fibrosis in children who had idiopathic RDS. J Pediatr 1964;65:1078.
12. Avery ME, Tooley WH, Keller JB, et al: Is chronic lung disease in low birth weight infants preventable? A survey of eight centers. Pediatrics 1987; 79:26–30.
13. Hussain AN, Siddiqui NH, Stocker JT: Pathology of arrested acinar development in postsurfactant BPD. Hum Pathol 1998;29:710–717.
14. Bancalari E, Gonzalez A: Clinical course and lung function abnormalities during development of chronic lung disease. In: Bland RD, Coalson JJ, eds: Chronic Lung Disease in Early Infancy. New York: Marcel Dekker, 2000.
15. Coalson JJ: Pathology of chronic lung disease of early infancy. In: Bland RD, Coalson JJ, eds: Chronic Lung Disease in Early Infancy. New York: Marcel Dekker, 2000, pp 85–124.
16. Panitch HB, Allen JL, Alpert BF, Schidlow DV: Effects of CPAP on lung mechanics in infants with acquired tracheomalacia. Am J Respir Crit Care Med 1994;150:1341–1346.
17. Panitch HB, Keklikian EN, Motely RA, Schidlow DV: Effects of altering smooth muscle tone on expiratory flows in patients with tracheomalacia. Pediatr Pulmonol 1990;9:170–176.
18. O'Brodovich H, Forrest JB, Newhouse MT: Ciliary defects associated with the development of BPD. Am Rev Respir Dis 1984;129:190–193.
19. Yoon BH, Romero R, Jun JK, et al: Amniotic fluid cytokines (interleukin-6, tumor necrosis factor-alpha, interleukin-1 beta, and interleukin-8) and the risk for the development of bronchopulmonary dysplasia. Am J Obstet Gynecol 1997;177:825–830.
20. Hitti J, Krohn MA, Patton DL, et al: Amniotic fluid tumor necrosis factor-alpha and the risk of respiratory distress syndrome among preterm infants. Am J Obstet Gynecol 1997;177:50–56.
21. Watterberg KL, Demers LM, Scott SM, Murphy S: Chorioamnionitis and early lung inflammation in infants in whom bronchopulmonary dysplasia develops. Pediatrics 1996;97:210–215.
22. Ghezzi F, Gomez R, Romero R, et al: Elevated interleukin-8 concentrations in amniotic fluid of mothers whose neonates subsequently develop bronchopulmonary dysplasia. Eur J Obstet Gynecol Reprod Biol 1998;78:5–10.
23. Jobe AH: Antenatal factors in the development of BPD. Semin Neonatol 2003;8:9–17.
24. Jobe AH, Newnham JP, Willet KE, et al: Effects of antenatal endotoxin and glucocorticoids on the lungs of preterm lambs. Am J Obstet Gynecol 2000;18:401–408.
25. Crowley PA: Antenatal corticosteroid therapy: A meta-analysis of the randomized trials, 1972 to 1994. Am J Obstet Gynecol 1995;173:322–335.
26. Polk DH, Ikegami M, Jobe AH, et al: Preterm lung function after retreatment with antenatal betamethasone in preterm lambs. Am J Obstet Gynecol 1997;176:308–315.
27. Banks BA, Cnaan A, Morgan MA, et al: Multiple courses of antenatal corticosteroids and outcome of premature neonates. North American Thyrotropin-Releasing Hormone Study Group. Am J Obstet Gynecol 1999;181:709–717.
28. Frank L, Groseclose EE: Preparation for birth into an O_2-rich environment. The antioxidant enzymes in the developing rabbit lung. Pediatr Res 1984;18:240–244.
29. Ogihara T, Okamoto R, Kim HS, et al: New evidence for the involvement of oxygen radicals in triggering neonatal chronic lung disease. Pediatr Res 1996;39:117–119.
30. Davis JM, Rosenfeld WN, Sanders RJ, Gonenne A: Prophylactic effects of recombinant human superoxide dismutase in neonatal lung injury. J Appl Physiol 1993;74:2234–2241.
31. White CW, Avraham KB, Shanley PF, Groner Y: Transgenic mice with expression of elevated levels of copper-zinc superoxide dismutase in the lungs are resistant to pulmonary oxygen toxicity. J Clin Invest 1991; 87:2162–2168.
32. Wispe JR, Warner BB, Clark JC, et al: Human Mn-superoxide dismutase in pulmonary epithelial cells of transgenic mice confers protection from oxygen injury. J Biol Chem 1992;267:23937–23941.
33. Ahmed MN, Suliman HR, Folz RJ, et al: Extracellular superoxide dismutase protects lung development in hyperoxia-exposed newborn mice. Am J Respir Crit Care Med 2003;167:400–405.
34. Dreyfuss DD, Saumon G: Ventilator induced lung injury. Lessons from experimental studies. Am J Respir Crit Care Med 1998;157:294–323.
35. Hodson WA: Ventilation strategies and BPD. In: Bland RD, Coalson JJ, eds: Chronic Lung Disease in Early Infancy. New York: Marcel Dekker, 2000, pp 173–208.
36. Nilsson R, Grossman G, Robertson B: Lung surfactant and the pathogenesis of neonatal bronchiolar lesions induced by artificial ventilation. Pediatr Res 1978;12:249–255.
37. Tremblay L, Valenza F, Ribeiro SP, et al: Injurious ventilatory strategies increase cytokines and c-fos m-RNA expression in an isolated rat lung model. J Clin Invest 1997;99:944–952.
38. Carlton DP, Cummings JJ, Scheerer RG, et al: Lung overexpansion increases pulmonary microvascular protein permeability in young lambs. J Appl Physiol 1990;69:577–583.
39. Acute Respiratory Distress Syndrome Network. Ventilation with lower tidal volumes as compared with traditional tidal volumes for acute lung injury and the ARDS. N Engl J Med 2000;342:1301–1308.
40. Bjorklund LJ, Ingimarsson J, Curstedt T, et al: Manual ventilation with a few large breaths at birth compromises the therapeutic effect of subsequent surfactant replacement in immature lungs. Pediatr Res 1997;42:348–355.
41. Bernstein G, Mannino FL, Heldt GP, et al: Randomized multicenter trial comparing synchronized and conventional intermittent mandatory ventilation in neonates. J Pediatr 1996;128:453–463.
42. Clark RH, Gerstmann DR, Null DM, deLemos RA: Prospective, randomized comparison of high-frequency oscillatory and conventional ventilation in respiratory distress syndrome. Pediatrics 1992;89:5–12.
43. Keszler M, Modanlou HD, Brudno DS, et al: Multicenter controlled clinical trial of high-frequency jet ventilation in preterm infants with uncomplicated respiratory distress syndrome. Pediatrics 1997;100: 593–599.
44. Collins MP, Lorenz JM, Jetton JR, Paneth N: Hypocapnia and other ventilation-related risk factors for cerebral palsy in low birth weight infants. Pediatr Res 2001;50:712–719.

45. Mariani G, Cifuentes J, Carlo WA: Randomized trial of permissive hypercapnia in preterm infants. Pediatrics 1999;104:1082–1088.
46. Van Marter LJ, Allred EN, Pagano M, et al: Do clinical markers of barotrauma and oxygen toxicity explain interhospital variation in rates of chronic lung disease? The Neonatology Committee for the Developmental Network. Pediatrics 2000;105:1194–1201.
47. Groneck P, Gotz-Speer B, Opperman M, et al: Association of pulmonary inflammation and increased microvascular permeability during the development of bronchopulmonary dysplasia. A sequential analysis of inflammatory mediators in respiratory fluids of high-risk neonates. Pediatrics 1994;93:712–718.
48. Pierce MR, Bancalari E: The role of inflammation in the pathogenesis of bronchopulmonary dysplasia. Pediatr Pulmonol 1995;19:371–378.
49. Groneck P, Speer CP: Inflammatory mediators and bronchopulmonary dysplasia. Arch Dis Child Fetal Neonatal Ed 1995;73:F1–F3.
50. Ozdemir A, Brown MA, Morgan WJ: Markers and mediators of inflammation in neonatal lung disease. Pediatr Pulmonol 1997;23:292–306.
51. Jones CA, Cayabyab RG, Kwong KY, et al: Undetectable interleukin (IL)-10 and persistent IL-8 expression early in hyaline membrane disease. A possible developmental basis for the predisposition to chronic lung inflammation in preterm newborns. Pediatr Res 1996;39:966–975.
52. Ramsay PL, O'Brian SE, Hegemier S, Welty SE: Early clinical markers for the development of bronchopulmonary dysplasia. Soluble E-Selectin and ICAM-1. Pediatrics 1998;102:927–932.
53. Munshi UK, Niu JO, Siddiq MM, Parton LA: Elevation of interleukin-8 and interleukin-6 precedes the influx of neutrophils in tracheal aspirates from preterm infants who develop bronchopulmonary dysplasia. Pediatr Pulmonol 1997;24:331–336.
54. Bland RD, Albertine KH, Carlton DP, et al: Chronic lung injury in preterm lambs. Abnormalities of the pulmonary circulation and lung fluid balance. Pediatr Res 2000;48:64–74.
55. Alnahhas MH, Karathanasis P, Kriss VM, et al: Elevated laminin concentrations in lung secretions of preterm infants supported by mechanical ventilation are correlated with radiographic abnormalities. J Pediatr 1997;131:555–560.
56. Merritt TA, Cochrane CG, Holcomb K, et al: Elastase and α_1-proteinase inhibitor activity in tracheal aspirates during respiratory distress syndrome. Role of inflammation in the pathogenesis of bronchopulmonary dysplasia. J Clin Invest 1983;72:656–666.
57. Stiskal JA, Dunn MS, Shennan AT, et al: Alpha-1-proteinase inhibitor therapy for the prevention of chronic lung disease of prematurity. A randomized, controlled trial. Pediatrics 1998;101:89–94.
58. Watterberg KL, Scott SM, Backstrom C, et al: Links between early adrenal function and respiratory outcome in preterm infants. Airway inflammation and patent ductus arteriosus. Pediatrics 2000;105:320–324.
59. Watterberg KL, Gerdes JS, Gifford KL, Lin HM: Prophylaxis against early adrenal insufficiency to prevent chronic lung disease in premature infants. Pediatrics 1999;104:1258–1263.
60. Wang EE, Ohlsson A, Kellner JD: Association of Ureaplasma urealyticum colonization with chronic lung disease of prematurity. Results of a meta-analysis. J Pediatr 1995;127:640–644.
61. Frank L, Groseclose E: Oxygen toxicity in newborn rats. The adverse effects of undernutrition. J Appl Physiol 1982;53:1248–1255.
62. Shenai JP: Vitamin A supplementation in very low birth weight neonates. Rationale and evidence. Pediatrics 1999;104:1369–1374.
63. Tyson JE, Wright LL, Oh W, et al: Vitamin A supplementation for extremely-low-birth-weight infants. National Institute of Child Health and Human Development Neonatal Research Network. N Engl J Med 1999;340:1962–1968.
64. Nickerson BG, Taussig LM: Family history of asthma in infants with bronchopulmonary dysplasia. Pediatrics 1980;65:1140–1144.
65. Bertrand JM, Riley SP, Popkin J, Coates AL: The long-term pulmonary sequelae of prematurity. Rhe role of familial airway hyperreactivity and the respiratory distress syndrome. N Engl J Med 1985;312:742–745.
66. Clark DA, Pincus LG, Oliphant M, et al: HLA-A2 and chronic lung disease in neonates. JAMA 1982;248:1868–1869.
67. Hagan R, Minutillo C, French N, et al: Neonatal chronic lung disease, oxygen dependency and a family history of asthma. Pediatr Pulmonol 1995;20:277–283.
68. Hallman M, Haatja R: Genetic influences and neonatal lung disease. Semin Neonatol 2003;8:19–27.
69. Kumar VH, Ryan RM: Growth factors in the fetal and neonatal lung. Front Biosci 2004;9:464–480.
70. Bhatt AJ, Pryhuber GS, Huyck H, et al: Disrupted pulmonary vasculature and decreased VEGF, flt-1, and Tie 2 in human infants dying with BPD. Am J Respir Crit Care Med 2000;164:1971–1980.
71. Jakkula M, Le Cras TD, Gebb S, et al: Inhibition of angiogenesis decreases alveolarization in the developing rat lung. Am J Physiol Lung Cell Mol Physiol 2000;279:L600–L607.
72. Abman SH: BPD. A vascular hypothesis. Am J Respir Crit Care Med 2001;164:1755–1756.
73. Goldman SL, Gerhardt T, Sonni R, et al: Early prediction of chronic lung disease by pulmonary function testing. J Pediatr 1983;102:613–617.
74. Tepper RS, Morgan WJ, Cota K, Taussig LM: Expiratory flow limitation in infants with bronchopulmonary dysplasia. J Pediatr 1986;109:1040–1046.
75. Wolfson MR, Bhutani BK, Shaffer TH, Bowen FW: Mechanics and energetics of breathing helium in infants with bronchopulmonary dysplasia. J Pediatr 1984;104:752.
76. Slavin JD, Mathews J, Spencer RP: Pulmonary ventilation/perfusion and reverse mismatches in an infant. Acta Radiol Diagn 1986;27:708–709.
77. Hakulinen AL, Järvenpaa AL, Turpeinan M, Sorijavi A: Diffusing capacity of the lung in school-age children born very preterm with and without BPD. Pediatr Pulmonol 1996;21:353–360.
78. Abman SH: Pulmonary hypertension in chronic lung disease of infancy. Pathogenesis, pathophysiology and treatment. In: Bland RD, Coalson JJ, eds: Chronic Lung Disease in Infancy. New York: Marcel Dekker, 2000, pp 619–668.
79. Parker TA, Abman SH: The pulmonary circulation in BPD. Semin Neonatol 2003;8:51–62.
80. Tomashefski JF, Opperman HC, Vawter GF: BPD: A morphometric study with emphasis on the pulmonary vasculature. Pediatr Pathol 1984;2:469–487.
81. Halliday HL, Dumpit FM, Brady JP: Effects of inspired oxygen on echocardiographic assessment of pulmonary vascular resistance and myocardial contractility in BPD. Pediatrics 1980;65:536–540.
82. Abman SH, Wolfe RR, Accurso FJ, et al: Pulmonary vascular response to oxygen in infants with severe BPD. Pediatrics 1985;75:80–84.
83. Walther FJ, Bender FJ, Leighton JO: Persistent pulmonary hypertension in premature neonates with severe RDS. Pediatrics 1992;90:899–904.
84. Fouron JC, LeGuennec JC, Villemont D, et al: Value of echocardiography in assessing the outcome of BPD. Pediatrics 1980;65:529–535.
85. Goodman G, Perkin R, Anas N: Pulmonary hypertension in infants with BPD. J Pediatr 1988;112:67–72.
86. Mourani PM, Ivy DD, Gao D, Abman SH: Pulmonary vascular effects of inhaled NO and oxygen tension in BPD. Am J Respir Crit Care Med 2004;170:1006–1013.
87. Apkon M, Nehgme RA, Lister G: Cardiovascular abnormalities in BPD. In: Bland RD, Coalson JJ, eds: Chronic Lung Disease in Infancy. New York: Marcel Dekker, 2000, pp 321–356.
88. Abman SH, Warady BA, Lum GM, Koops BL: Systemic hypertension in infants with BPD. J Pediatr 1984;104:928–931.
89. Stark AR, Carlo WA, Tyson JE, et al: Adverse effects of early dexamethasone treatment in extremely low birth weight infants. N Engl J Med 2001; 344:95–101.
90. Murphy BP, Inder TE, Huppi PS, et al: Impaired cerebral cortical gray matter after treatment with dexamethasone for neonatal chronic lung disease. Pediatrics 2001;107:217–221.
91. Abman SH, Accurso FJ, Koops BL: Experience with home oxygen in the management of infants with BPD. Clin Pediatr 1984;23:471–476.
92. Groothius JR, Rosenberg AA: Home oxygen promotes weight gain in infants with BPD. Am J Dis Childhood 1987;141:992–995.
93. Abman SH: Monitoring cardiovascular function in infants with chronic lung disease of prematurity. Arch Dis Child 2002;87:F15–F18.
94. Subcommittee of the Assembly of Pediatrics, American Thoracic Society: Statement on the care of the child with chronic lung disease of infancy and childhood. Am J Respir Crit Care Med 2003;168:356–396.
95. Supplemental Therapeutic Oxygen for Prethreshold Retinopathy of Prematurity (STOP-ROP), a randomized controlled trial. Pediatrics 2000;105:295–310.
96. Hazinski TA: Drug therapy for established BPD. In: Bland RD, Coalson JJ, eds: Chronic Lung Disease in Infancy. New York: Marcel Dekker, 2000, pp 257–284.
97. Rush MG, Englehardt B, Parker RA, et al: Double blind, placebo controlled trial of alternate day furosemide therapy in infants with chronic BPD. J Pediatr 1990;117:112–118.
98. De Boeck K, Smith J, Van Lierde S, Devlieger H: Response to bronchodilators in clinically stable 1 year old patients with BPD. J Pediatr 1998;157:75–79.
99. Yoder MC, Chua R, Tepper R: Effect of dexamethasone on pulmonary inflammation and pulmonary function of ventilator-dependent infants with BPD. Am Rev Respir Dis 1991;143:1044–1048.
100. Halliday HL: Clinical trials of postnatal corticosteroids. Inhaled and systemic. Biol Neonate 1999;76(Suppl 1):29–40.

101. Committee on Fetus and Newborn: Postnatal corticosteroids to treat or prevent chronic lung disease in premature infants. Pediatrics 2002; 109:330–338.
102. Cole CH, Colton T, Shah BL, et al: Early inhaled glucocorticoid therapy to prevent BPD. N Engl J Med 1999;340:1005–1010.
103. Tepper RS, Morgan WJ, Cota K, Taussig LM: Expiratory flow limitation in infants with BPD. J Pediatr 1986;109:1040–1046.
104. Gerhardt T, Hehre D, Feller R, et al: Serial determinations of pulmonary function in infants with CLD. J Pediatr 1987;110:448–456.
105. Baraldi E, Filippone M, Trevisanuto D, et al: Pulmonary function until two years of life in infants with bronchopulmonary dysplasia. Am J Respir Crit Care Med 1997;155:149–155.
106. Jacob SV, Coates AL, Lands LC, et al: Long-term pulmonary sequelae of severe bronchopulmonary dysplasia. J Pediatr 1998;133:193–200.
107. Gross SJ, Iannuzzi DM, Kveselis DA, Anbar RD: Effect of preterm birth on pulmonary function at school age. A prospective controlled study. J Pediatr 1998;133:188–192.
108. Mitchell SH, Teague G: Reduced gas transfer at rest and during exercise in school age survivors of BPD. Am J Respir Crit Care Med 1998; 157:1406–1412.
109. Filipone M, Sartor M, Zacchello F, Baraldi E: Flow limitation in infants with BPD and respiratory function at school age. Lancet 2003; 361:753–754.
110. Northway WH, Moss RB, Carlisle KB, et al: Late pulmonary sequelae of BPD. N Engl J Med 1990;323:1793–1799.
111. Higgins RD, Richter SE, Davis JM: Nasal continuous positive airway pressure facilitates extubation of very low birth weight neonates. Pediatrics 1991;88:999–1003.
112. Davis JM, Richter SE, Kendig JW, Notter RH: High frequency jet ventilation and surfactant treatment of newborns with severe respiratory failure. Pediatr Pulmonol 1992;13:108–112.
113. Yeh TF, Lin YJ, Lin H, et al: Outcomes at school age after postnatal dexamethasone therapy for lung disease of prematurity. N Engl J Med 2004;350:1304–1313.
114. Jobe AH: Postnatal corticosteroids for preterm infants—do what we say, not what we do. N Engl J Med 2004;350:1349–1351.
115. Davis JM, Parad RB, Michele T, et al: Pulmonary outcome at 1 year corrected age in premature infants treated at birth with recombinant CuZn superoxide dismutase. Pediatrics 2003;111:469–476.
116. Kinsella JP, Walsh WF, Bose C, et al: Randomized controlled trial of inhaled nitric oxide in premature neonates with severe hypoxemic respiratory failure. Lancet 1999; 354:1061–1065.
117. Banks BA, Seri I, Ischiropoulos H, et al: Changes in oxygenation with inhaled nitric oxide in severe bronchopulmonary dysplasia. Pediatrics 1999;103:610–618.
118. Kinsella JP, Parker TA, Galan H, et al: Effects of inhaled NO on pulmonary edema and lung neutrophil accumulation in severe experimental HMD. Pediatr Res 1997; 41:457–463.
119. Tang JR, Markham NE, Lin YJ, et al: Inhaled NO attenuates pulmonary hypertension and improves lung growth in infant rats after neonatal treatment with a VEGF receptor inhibitor. Am J Physiol Lung Cell Mol Physiol 2004; 287:L344–L351.
120. Schreiber MD, Gin-Mestan K, Marks JD, et al: Inhaled NO in premature infants with respiratory distress syndrome. N Engl J Med 2003;349: 2099–2107.

20 Genetic Causes of Surfactant Deficiency

Lawrence M. Nogee, MD

Pulmonary surfactant is the mixture of lipids and proteins that reduces alveolar surface tension at the air-liquid interface and prevents end-expiratory atelectasis. Surfactant deficiency due primarily to impaired production associated with pulmonary immaturity is the principal cause of the respiratory distress syndrome (RDS) observed in premature infants. Surfactant replacement therapy is now routine in the treatment of infants with RDS and has resulted in improvements in RDS-related morbidity and mortality. While the causal relationship of surfactant deficiency to RDS was first made over 45 years ago, in the past decade it has been recognized that surfactant deficiency may also result from single gene disorders that disrupt normal surfactant production and metabolism. In contrast to premature infants with RDS, infants with these disorders are usually full term, and have a much more severe and often fatal course. With modern neonatal intensive care, infants affected with these disorders may survive for many months, often requiring prolonged mechanical ventilation, sustaining considerable morbidity and consuming significant medical resources. Moreover, milder forms of these disorders may be the molecular basis for some forms of interstitial lung disease in older children and adults. While these genetic illnesses are rare, and therapeutic options for affected children limited at the current time, it is important for physicians to recognize affected infants and arrive at an accurate diagnosis in order to properly counsel parents regarding prognosis and recurrence risk. From a scientific standpoint, an understanding of the pathophysiology of these disorders potentially provides both insights into normal surfactant metabolism, and how genetic mechanisms may contribute to the development of surfactant deficiency in more common diseases such as neonatal RDS. This chapter will summarize current knowledge concerning the clinical and laboratory findings associated with the three currently recognized genetic disorders involving surfactant metabolism that result in acute and chronic lung disease. It is highly likely, given recent scientific advances in the understanding of lung development and surfactant metabolism in combination with data available from the human genome project, that additional genetic mechanisms for neonatal and pediatric lung disease will continue to be identified.

■ OVERVIEW OF SURFACTANT COMPOSITION AND METABOLISM

Pulmonary surfactant is a complex mixture of phospholipids, neutral lipids, and specific proteins that is produced by the alveolar type II cell, stored intracellularly in organelles known as lamellar bodies, and secreted by exocytosis. The major lipid is phosphatidylcholine (PC), a large fraction of which contains two palmitic acid side chains that are fully saturated, termed either dipalmitoyl phosphatidylcholine (DPPC) or disaturated phosphatidylcholine (DSPC), and is critical for surface tension reduction. The effective lowering of surface tension also requires the presence of one or both of two extremely hydrophobic surfactant proteins, SP-B and SP-C. Addition of either SP-B or SP-C to surfactant lipids results in a surfactant preparation that effectively lowers surface tension in vitro and can effectively treat surfactant deficiency in animal models. Both SP-B and SP-C are present in varying amounts in the mammalian-derived exogenous surfactant preparations used to treat infants with RDS. Pulmonary surfactant also contains two larger glycoproteins, SP-A and SP-D, which are members of the collectin family, having both a collagenous domain and a carbohydrate-binding domain. The principal roles for SP-A and SP-D appear to be in local host defense, since both molecules can bind to a wide variety of microorganisms and facilitate their uptake and killing by alveolar macrophages.[1] SP-A also interacts with surfactant phospholipids, calcium, and SP-B in order to form tubular myelin. Mice genetically engineered to be unable to produce SP-A lack tubular myelin in their lungs, but do not develop RDS or spontaneous lung disease with age, and have increased susceptibility to infection with a number of different microorganism.[2] Genetically engineered mice unable to produce SP-D are also more susceptible to infection with certain organisms, and develop an accumulation of surfactant lipids in their lungs and emphysema as they age.[3–5] However, genetic abnormalities of SP-A or SP-D production resulting in human lung disease have not yet been recognized.

■ SURFACTANT PROTEIN B AND HEREDITARY SURFACTANT PROTEIN B DEFICIENCY

SP-B is a 79–amino acid hydrophobic protein that facilitates adsorption to the air-liquid interface and enhances the surface tension–lowering properties of surfactant phospholipids.[6] SP-B is encoded on a single gene spanning approximately 10,000 base pairs (bp) on human chromosome 2 and which contains 11 exons, the last of which is untranslated. The gene is transcribed into a 2-kb messenger RNA (mRNA), which is translated into a 381–amino acid preproprotein. The first 23 amino acids comprise a signal peptide that is removed cotranslationally. The remaining proprotein (pro-SP-B) undergoes several proteolytic processing steps to yield the mature peptide found in the airspaces, with the mature peptide domain corresponding to exons 6 and 7 of the gene[7] (Fig. 20-1). SP-B is primarily produced by alveolar type II epithelial cells, routed to lamellar bodies, the intracellular storage organelle for surfactant, and secreted along with surfactant phospholipids into the airspaces. The gene is also expressed within the lung in nonciliated bronchiolar epithelial cells, although only type II cells fully process pro-SP-B to mature SP-B.

Hereditary SP-B deficiency was the first recognized genetic cause of surfactant deficiency.[8] The proband was a full-term infant who presented with clinical and radiographic signs of RDS,

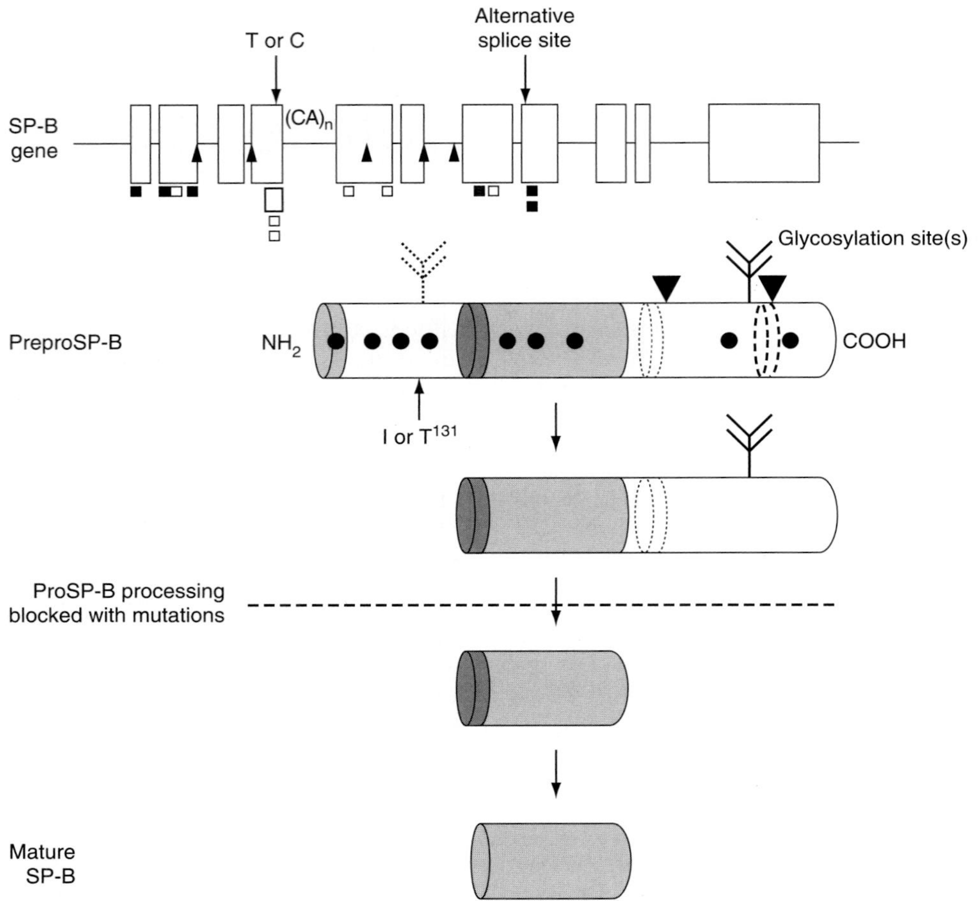

■ **FIGURE 20-1.** Mutations resulting in SP-B deficiency. The SP-B gene is diagramed at top, with the exons indicated by rectangles and the introns by lines. The locations of known nonsense *(solid squares)* and frameshift mutations *(open squares)*, which completely preclude pro-SP-B production, are indicated below the corresponding exon, and the locations of mutations affecting mRNA splicing are indicated by *triangles*. An *arrow* indicates the position of an alternative splice site at the beginning of exon 8. The locations of a nonsynonymous single nucleotide polymorphism (T or C) in exon 4 that encodes either isoleucine (I) or threonine (T) in the proprotein and affecting a potential glycosylation site are shown. The SP-B preproprotein is diagrammed in the middle, with the locations of missense mutations *(closed circles)* or small in-frame deletions *(dashed line in proprotein)* or insertions *(triangles)* indicated, which would allow for pro-SP-B production, but which would not be efficiently processed to mature SP-B in the steps outlined at the bottom.

but who did not improve despite maximal medical support, including extracorporeal membrane oxygenation (ECMO).[8] The family history was notable for a previous child, also born at full term, who had died in the neonatal period from lung disease. An open lung biopsy revealed an accumulation of granular, eosinophilic material that filled distal airspaces. This pathology, which is similar to that seen in alveolar proteinosis in adults, had been observed in other full-term neonates with refractory respiratory failure, some of whom also had a family history of neonatal respiratory disease inherited in an autosomal-recessive fashion.[9,10] The proteinosis material represented an abnormal accumulation of pulmonary surfactant, and suggested that a disruption of normal surfactant metabolism was responsible for the disease. SP-B was undetectable in lung tissue from the affected infants, which contained abundant amounts of SP-A and the SP-C precursor protein (pro-SP-C).[8] A frameshift mutation in the SP-B gene that accounted for the lack of SP-B was subsequently identified in affected infants, establishing an inherited deficiency of SP-B as the basis for their lung disease.[11]

SP-B deficiency has subsequently been recognized as the cause of lung disease in over 75 infants and 50 families worldwide[11–22] (and L.M. Nogee, unpublished observations). Affected infants are typically full term and generally present with symptoms and signs of surfactant deficiency, with chest radiographs resembling those of premature infants with RDS. The initial lung disease in SP-B-deficient infants may be quite severe, with hypoxic respiratory failure and associated pulmonary hypertension, often requiring treatment with high-frequency ventilation, inhaled nitric oxide, and even ECMO. However, some infants may have an initial milder course and not require mechanical ventilation for several days to weeks. However, their respiratory disease is progressive, and death usually results from hypoxic respiratory failure within 3 to 6 months, even with maximal medical management. Transient improvement may be seen in response to treatment with systemic steroids or exogenous surfactant; however, the only effective treatment is lung transplantation.[23]

SP-B deficiency is inherited in an autosomal-recessive fashion with affected infants having loss-of-function mutations on both alleles. The most common mutation involves a net 2 base insertion in codon 121 (termed 121ins2), which results in a frameshift and premature termination codon. The 121ins2 mutation has accounted for approximately two thirds of the mutant alleles identified to date, and has been found principally in individuals of Northern European descent. A common ancestral origin likely accounts for the finding of a common mutation. Over two dozen other SP-B mutations have been identified[12,13,20,21] (see Fig. 20-1). Most of these mutations are unique to a given family, thus limiting the sensitivity of genetic testing, although several mutations have been identified in more than one unrelated family in certain ethnic groups. These include the 122delT (Lebanese ancestry), c.479G>T mutation (French-Canadian), R295X (Hispanic), and 1043ins3 (Asian) mutations.[12]

While complete deficiency of SP-B is invariably lethal, partial deficiency, due to mutations in which pro-SP-B is unable to be efficiently processed to mature SP-B, resulting in a reduction but not absence of SP-B, can be associated with more prolonged survival.[14,17] This finding suggests that there is a critical level of SP-B needed for normal lung function. This is supported by experiments with genetically engineered mice in which SP-B production was able to be turned off, with the development of lung disease when SP-B levels fell below 20% to 25% of control values.[24] Having a loss of function SP-B mutation on only one allele (haploinsufficiency) could thus be a risk factor for the development of lung disease if other factors further reduce SP-B expression. This hypothesis is supported by the observation that genetically engineered mice with one null SP-B allele were more susceptible to pulmonary oxygen toxicity than their wild-type littermates.[25] However, adult carriers for one SP-B null allele had normal pulmonary function in one study,[26] and whether carriers for one SP-B mutation have an increased risk for lung disease will require further study.

Pathology findings in lung tissue from SP-B-deficient infants include nonspecific findings of interstitial fibrosis and alveolar type II epithelial cell hyperplasia. While findings of alveolar proteinosis were prominent in the lungs of some of the first infants identified with this disorder, this finding has not been universal in the lungs of SP-B-deficient infants. The histopathology of alveolar proteinosis may result from mechanisms other than SP-B deficiency, including SP-C gene abnormalities and ABCA3 deficiency, and a recent study found that SP-B gene mutations actually accounted for a minority of children with the histopathologic findings of alveolar proteinosis.[20] While the histologic finding of alveolar proteinosis may be suggestive of an inherited surfactant abnormality, the term *congenital alveolar proteinosis* should not be used synonymously with SP-B deficiency (Fig. 20-2).

Inactivation of the SP-B gene in genetically engineered mice also resulted in a neonatal lethal respiratory phenotype, further indicating an essential role for SP-B in normal lung function.[27] Interestingly, both SP-B-deficient infants and animals have secondary changes in the metabolism of other surfactant components, indicating a role for SP-B beyond lowering surface tension in the airspaces. These secondary changes include markedly abnormal lamellar bodies and accumulation of aberrantly processed SP-C peptides.[28,29] Mature SP-C is also derived by proteolytic processing of a precursor protein (pro-SP-C). The abnormal SP-C-related peptides observed in SP-B-deficient infants result from incomplete processing of pro-SP-C to mature SP-C.[30] This block in SP-C processing may result in SP-B-deficient infants also being deficient in mature SP-C, and the partially processed pro-SP-C peptides are not very surface active, further contributing to surfactant dysfunction in SP-B-deficient infants.[31] The lamellar bodies in SP-B-deficient mice and infants are poorly organized, with loosely packed lamellae and vacuolar inclusions, having the appearance more of multivesicular or composite bodies (Fig. 20-3).

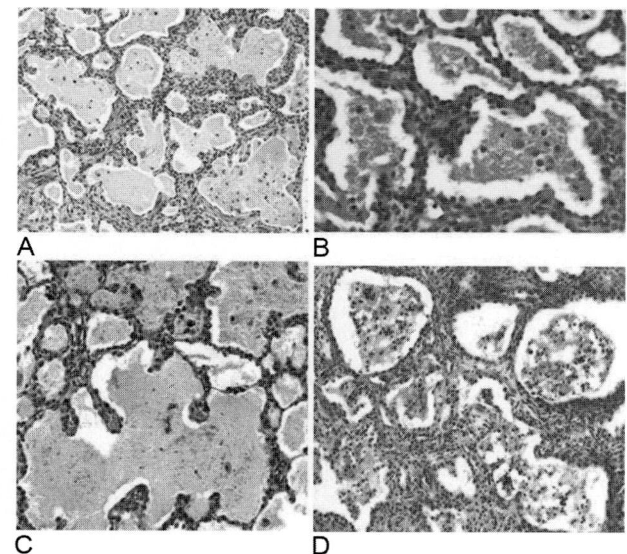

■ **FIGURE 20-2.** Variable and overlapping histology associated with mutations in genes important in surfactant metabolism. **A,** Results from an SP-B-deficient infant, demonstrating marked accumulation of granular proteinaceous material with entrapped macrophages filling distal airspaces. **B,** Similar pathology from a patient with ABCA3 deficiency **(B)** and from a patient with an SP-C mutation **(C),** although with better preservation of the alveolar architecture in **C. D,** Results from a patient with a different SP-C mutation, demonstrating interstitial thickening and accumulations of foamy macrophages in the airspaces, but with scant amounts of proteinaceous material. (See Color Plate 29.)

This appearance is consistent with a role for SP-B in membrane fusion of smaller vesicles in order to pack and organize lipid bilayers into lamellar bodies.[32] The final processing steps for mature SP-C occurs in lamellar bodes, and the failure to properly form this intracellular organelle is thus likely related to the SP-C processing abnormality.

The incidence of SP-B deficiency is unknown, although it is likely that the disease is rare. The carrier frequency of the 121ins2 mutation has been estimated to be approximately 1 in 1000 individuals in the United States, which when combined with the relative frequency of this mutation would be expected to result in a disease incidence of 1 in 1.5 million live births.[33] However, the relative incidence in other countries and subpopulations may be very different. In two recent studies, SP-B deficiency was the basis for lung disease in 12% to 18% of selected full-term infants with severe lung disease of unclear etiology.[20,34]

The diagnosis of SP-B deficiency should be considered in a full-term infant who presents with clinical or radiographic features of surfactant deficiency that fails to improve after the first 7 to 10 days of life, or when there is a family history of severe neonatal lung disease. Confirmation of the diagnosis requires finding a mutation on both alleles of the SP-B gene; such clinical genetic testing is currently available in several laboratories. Findings of alveolar proteinosis and accumulations of macrophages in airspaces in combination with interstitial thickening and fibrosis are consistent with the diagnosis, but not diagnostic. Examination of lung tissue by electron microscopy may be useful in establishing the diagnosis, but such studies are not routinely performed, and the sensitivity of such analyses has not been evaluated (see Fig. 20-3).

Because a critical level of SP-B expression is essential for normal lung function, SP-B is a reasonable candidate gene for

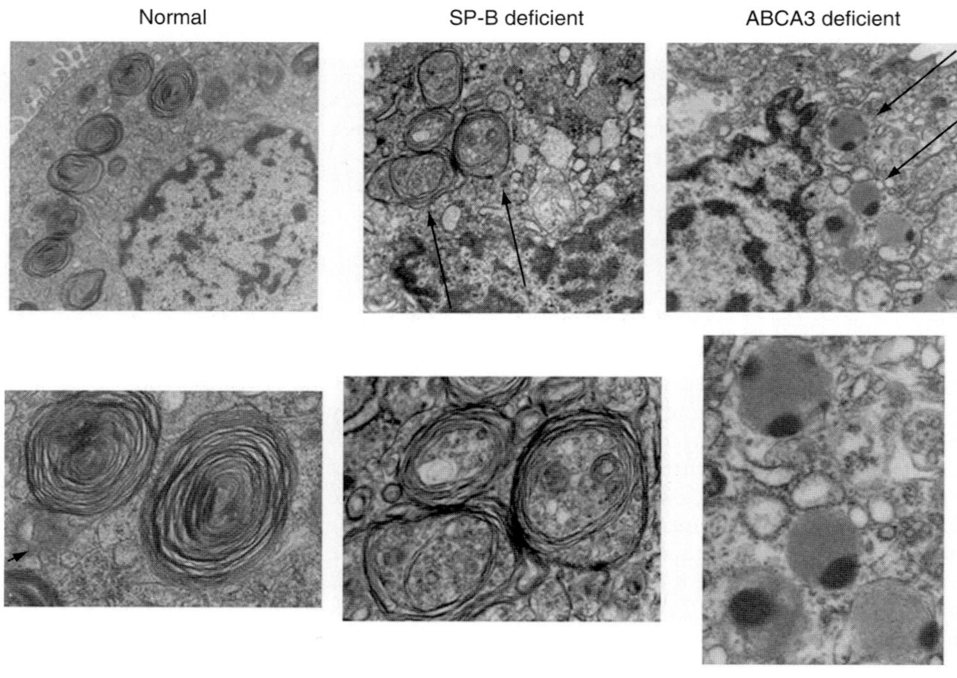

■ **FIGURE 20-3.** Ultrastructural findings associated with SP-B and ABCA3 deficiency. *Top left,* A portion of a type II cell with normal lamellar bodies. *Top middle,* A type II cell from an SP-B-deficient patient contains abnormally formed lamellar bodies with large whorls and vacuolar inclusions *(arrows)*. *Top right,* The lamellar bodies in the type II cells of a patient with ABCA3 deficiency are small and dense, with eccentrically placed inclusions *(arrows)*. Higher-power views of normal *(bottom left)*, SP-B-deficient *(bottom middle)*, and ABCA3-deficient *(bottom right)* lamellar bodies.

contributing to more common lung diseases such as RDS and acute respiratory distress syndrome (ARDS). Identified genetic variants, including a variable tandem nucleotide repeat region in intron IV and multiple single nucleotide polymorphisms (SNPs) have been characterized in the SP-B gene. Several studies have linked alleles with different lengths of the intron IV tandem repeat region with an increased risk for RDS, but because this sequence does not affect the SP-B coding sequence and it is not known to regulate SP-B expression, the mechanism for this association and the significance of these associations remain unclear.[35,36] A relatively common SNP results in either isoleucine or threonine being encoded in codon 131, and the allele encoding threonine at this position (131T) has an additional potential site for N-linked glycosylation.[37] An increased risk for either RDS or ARDS in association with the 131T allele has been observed, but the effect is relatively modest and often in combination with other SP-B variants.[38–40] The relationship between different SP-B genetic variants and different lung diseases requires further study.

■ SURFACTANT PROTEIN C GENETIC ABNORMALITIES AND LUNG DISEASE

SP-C is an extremely hydrophobic 35–amino acid peptide that is encoded by a single gene (referred to as *SFTPC*) spanning approximately 3500 bp on human chromosome 8, containing six exons, of which the sixth is untranslated. The gene is transcribed into a 900-bp mRNA, which is alternatively spliced at the beginning of exon 5, thus yielding after translation either a 191– or 197–amino acid proprotein (Fig. 20-4). Posttranslational modifications include palmitoylation of cysteine residues in the mature peptide such that SP-C is a proteolipid.[41–43] SP-C, like SP-B, enhances the surface tension–lowering properties of surfactant lipids and is present in mammalian-derived exogenous surfactant preparations used to treat infants with RDS.[6,7] Whereas SP-B deficiency generally results in neonatal-onset lung disease that is rapidly fatal, the phenotype associated with abnormalities of SP-C expression is much more variable.

SP-C gene abnormalities were first recognized in an infant whose family history was notable for a three-generation history of interstitial lung disease (ILD) characterized as desquamative interstitial pneumonitis that was inherited in an autosomal-dominant fashion.[44] The child was free of respiratory symptoms at birth, but because of the family history was closely monitored and underwent lung biopsy at 3 months of age after developing cyanosis in room air and increased interstitial markings on chest radiographs. The lung histology was consistent with nonspecific interstitial pneumonitis or chronic pneumonitis of infancy (CPI).[45] Mature SP-C was undetectable in her lung tissue, and DNA sequence analysis of her SP-C gene revealed a single base substitution in the first base of intron IV of the SP-C gene that resulted in the skipping of exon 4 and a shortened proprotein. The same mutation was identified in the child's mother, who along with the child also had reduced levels of pro-SP-C expression as evaluated by immunohistochemical staining. A mutation was identified on only one allele of the SP-C gene. While this was consistent with the autosomal-dominant inheritance pattern, it did not readily explain the lack of mature SP-C in the child's lung tissue. However, SP-C has been demonstrated to self-associate in the secretory pathway.[46] A dominant-negative effect on SP-C production from the abnormal pro-SP-C that resulted from the mutation could then account for the lack of mature SP-C. Recent studies in which pro-SP-C containing this mutation was expressed in different cell lines in vitro provide support for this mechanism, because the abnormal pro-SP-C was not processed to mature SP-C, not routed appropriately in the cells, and was rapidly degraded.[47,48]

Subsequent studies have confirmed and extended these observations linking SP-C genetic abnormalities to lung disease. Thomas and colleagues reported a large five-generation kindred affected by familial pulmonary fibrosis associated with an SP-C missense mutation (L188Q).[49] There was considerable

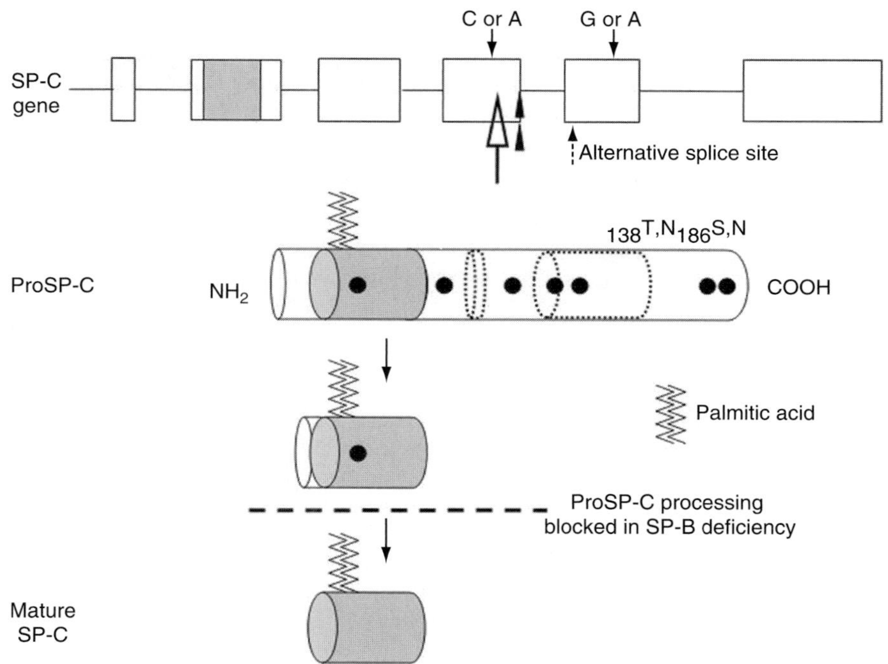

■ **FIGURE 20-4.** SP-C mutations associated with interstitial lung disease. The SP-C gene is diagramed at *top*, with the exons indicated by rectangles and the introns by lines. A *large arrow* indicates the location of a frameshift mutation, and *triangles* indicate the location of splicing mutations, which result in the skipping of exon 4. The SP-C proprotein is diagrammed *below*, with *closed circles* indicating the locations of missense mutations and *dashed lines* in the proprotein indicating locations of an in-frame deletion and the results of the skipping of exon 4 due to splice site mutations. The locations of two nonsynonymous single nucleotide polymorphisms in exons 4 and 5 that result in variations in codons 138 (threonine [T] or asparagine [N]) and 186 (serine [S] or asparagine [N]) in the proprotein are shown.

heterogeneity in both the lung pathology, with features of both nonspecific interstitial pneumonitis and usual interstitial pneumonitis in older patients associated with the mutation, and clinical severity of disease, with the age of onset ranging from early infancy to the sixth decade, as well as asymptomatic adults with the mutation, consistent with incomplete penetrance. Both genetic linkage and the observation of cellular toxicity due to expression of the mutation in cell lines in vitro supported that the identified mutation was causally related to disease. Hamvas and colleagues reported an infant who had no family history of lung disease and who underwent lung transplantation for progressive interstitial lung disease most consistent with chronic pneumonitis of infancy, who had an apparent de novo SP-C mutation resulting in a 3–amino acid deletion in pro-SP-C.[50] Sporadic disease due to an SP-C missense mutation (I73T) has also been reported in a child whose lung pathology also included features of alveolar proteinosis.[51] The I73T mutation has also been found in multiple other unrelated individuals with both familial and sporadic interstitial lung disease, and on SP-C alleles of apparently diverse genetic backgrounds, suggesting that this region in the SP-C gene may be a "hot spot" for mutation.[52] The lung disease due to SP-C mutations can thus be familial with a pattern of autosomal-dominant inheritance with variable penetrance, or occur in the absence of a family history due to de novo mutations, and associated with variable onset of symptoms and lung pathology. The incidence and prevalence of lung disease associated with SP-C gene mutations are unknown.

The pathophysiology of lung disease due to SP-C mutations is complex and incompletely understood. The lack of mature SP-C due to a putative dominant-negative effect on SP-C production likely contributes to the lung disease. Mice that are unable to produce SP-C due to targeted inactivation of their SP-C gene can develop progressive airspace enlargement and interstitial inflammation as they age.[53] Because the surfactant isolated from such SP-C-deficient mice is unstable at low lung volumes, SP-C deficiency could thus result in recurrent atelectasis, with subsequent development of chronic lung disease.[54] However, the phenotype of SP-C null mice is strain dependent, suggesting that genetic modifiers may be important in the development of SP-C-related lung disease. Human lung disease resulting from null mutations on both alleles of the SP-C gene has not yet been reported. However, familial ILD associated with markedly reduced SP-C expression in lung tissue and undetectable SP-C in bronchoalveolar lavage, but without any mutations in the SP-C gene of affected individuals identified to account for these findings, has been observed.[55] These observations both support a role for SP-C deficiency in the pathogenesis of ILD, and indicate that genes other than *SFTPC* may result in SP-C deficiency (i.e., locus or genetic heterogeneity).

Alternatively, SP-C mutations may cause lung disease due to toxicity from an abnormally formed pro-SP-C, a "toxic gain-of-function" mechanism. All of the SP-C mutations associated with human lung disease that have been identified to date would be predicted to result in the production of an abnormal proprotein, which is likely misfolded.[56] The exposure of hydrophobic epitopes in the misfolded proprotein may be directly toxic to alveolar epithelial cells, especially if produced in sufficient amounts to be unable to be efficiently degraded. This possible mechanism is supported by in vitro and animal experiments as well as data from patients with SP-C mutations. When pro-SP-C lacking the residues encoded by exon 4 (corresponding to the effect of the mutation identified in the index family) was expressed in a pulmonary epithelial cell line, it accumulated in perinuclear aggregates, whereas pro-SP-C corresponding to the wild-type sequence was routed to cytoplasmic granules.[47] In a different set of experiments, transgenic mice expressing pro-SP-C lacking exon 4 sequences had markedly disrupted lung development that correlated with the level of abnormal transgene expression, supporting the potential toxic effects of SP-C mutations. The severe disruption in lung development in these animals also suggested a mechanism whereby SP-C mutations could cause severe, early-onset lung disease, which has been observed in some infants with SP-C mutations.[48] Abnormal perinuclear accumulation of pro-SP-C observed by immunofluorescence, along with intense immunohistochemical staining for pro-SP-C, were observed in the explanted lung tissue of an infant with a different SP-C mutation, supporting a mechanism of toxicity of abnormal pro-SP-C.[50] The amount of SP-B in bronchoalveolar lavage fluid obtained at the time of lung transplantation from this child was markedly reduced compared with control samples, suggesting a more global degree of disruption of surfactant metabolism. These observations indicate that the pathophysiology of lung disease associated with SP-C mutations is complex, and different features may occur with different types of mutations and account for some of the clinical heterogeneity (Fig. 20-5).

Clinical features in children and adults with SP-C mutations have included chronic respiratory symptoms (tachypnea, cough, cyanosis in room air) and failure to thrive, although a systematic analysis of the clinical and laboratory features associated with SP-C-related lung disease is not currently available. The age of onset is variable, with some infants developing respiratory distress immediately after birth, and other individuals remaining apparently asymptomatic well until adulthood.[56] The lung disease in some children appears to have been triggered or exacerbated by viral infections.[49] The diagnosis should be considered in an infant with progressive forms of interstitial lung disease, particularly with biopsy findings interpreted as desquamative interstitial pneumonitis, chronic pneumonitis of infancy, or nonspecific interstitial pneumonitis.

There is currently no specific therapy for patients with SP-C mutations. Treatment has included corticosteroids and hydroxychloroquine, but the efficacy of these agents in lung disease due to SP-C mutations is unknown and complicated by the variability in the natural history of the disease. Because mutations likely result in misfolded protein that is either rapidly degraded or accumulates early in the secretory pathway, therapies designed to improve protein folding and routing may eventually prove to be beneficial to patients with SP-C mutations.[47,57,58] However, if an agent increases the production of pro-SP-C that is not efficiently routed and accumulates intracellularly, this could prove more toxic than therapeutic. The generation of an animal model of the disease will be critical in order to test different evolving therapies. Misfolded pro-SP-C due to genetic or other mechanisms could contribute to other lung diseases when pro-SP-C expression is increased in association with alveolar type II cell hypertrophy following lung injury, thus hindering recovery. Finally, misfolding of proteins other than SP-C in the secretory pathway of the alveolar type II cell could be a general mechanism causing cellular injury and resulting in interstitial or other lung diseases.

Two SNPs in the SP-C gene that alter the SP-C coding sequence have been identified, one of which results in either threonine or asparagine being encoded in codon 138, and the other encoding either serine or asparagine in codon 186. A recent study found an increased risk for RDS in patients with the variants encoding asparagines, particularly at position 186, an effect

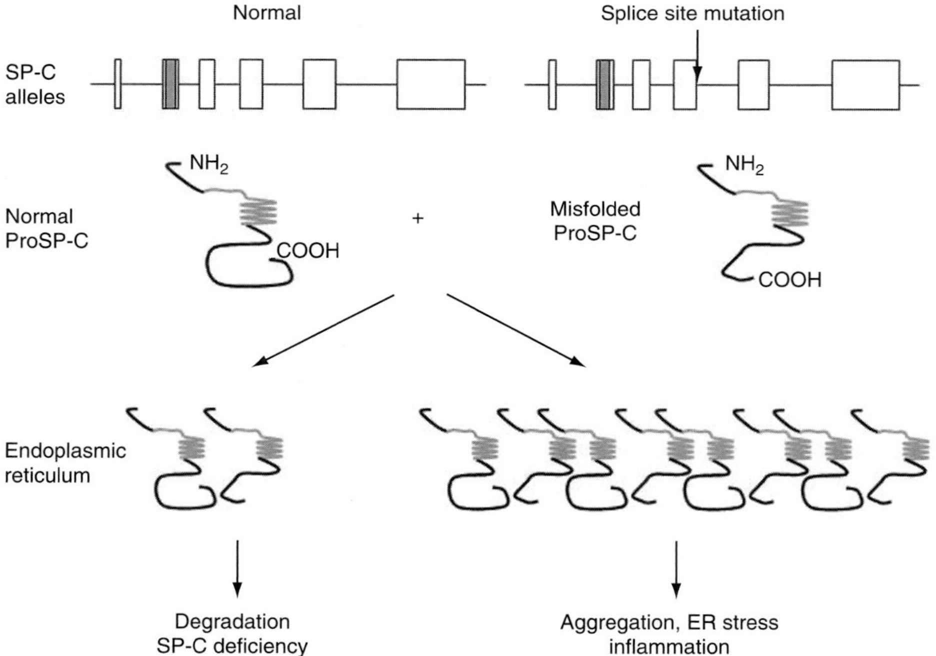

■ **FIGURE 20-5.** Proposed pathophysiology of SP-C mutations. *Top,* The two SP-C gene alleles, one encoding normal SP-C, and the other with a mutation resulting in production of abnormal pro-SP-C (in this example resulting in the skipping of exon 4 in the mRNA and deletion of corresponding sequence in the proprotein). *Middle,* The pro-SP-C molecules arising from each allele interact in the ER. The abnormal pro-SP-C is unstable and targeted for degradation, which also results in degradation of normal SP-C, which, depending on the balance between SP-C production and degradation, can lead to SP-C deficiency *(bottom left)* or to accumulations of abnormally folded pro-SP-C complexes in the endoplasmic reticulum, leading to a stress response and secondary cell injury and inflammation *(bottom right).*

that was more pronounced in premature infants and also influenced by gender.[59] Because mice completely deficient in SP-C do not develop neonatal lung disease, the mechanism by which these SNPs would affect the risk for RDS is unclear.

■ ABCA3 DEFICIENCY

ABCA3 is a member of the ATP-binding cassette family, a large group of transmembrane proteins that transport substances across biologic membranes. The gene for ABCA3 is located on human chromosome 16 and contains 33 exons, of which the first three are untranslated. The gene encodes a 1704–amino acid protein, which is primarily expressed within lung, although it is also expressed in a number of other tissues, including kidney, intestine, thyroid, and brain.[34] ABCA3 expression is developmentally regulated, with expression increasing in later gestation in rats, and its expression is also increased by glucocorticoids.[60,61] Within the lung, ABCA3 is primarily expressed in alveolar type II cells and localized to the limiting membrane of lamellar bodies by immunogold studies.[61,62] The function of ABCA3 is unknown, but because other ABCA subclass proteins are involved in lipid transport, its expression in the lung and localization within the type II cell suggest that it has a role in surfactant metabolism. It is a reasonable hypothesis that ABCA3 either transports lipids essential for surfactant function into lamellar bodies or transports lipids deleterious to surfactant function out of these organelles. Mutations in different genes encoding other ABC proteins have been linked to a number of diverse human genetic diseases.[63] Given its potential role in surfactant metabolism, ABCA3 was thus an attractive candidate gene for contributing to neonatal lung disease due to surfactant deficiency.

ABCA3 deficiency has now been recognized as a cause of lung disease with the identification of disease-causing mutations in 16 of 21 infants with clinical and or radiographic signs of severe neonatal surfactant deficiency.[34] The group of infants studied was highly selected, with the majority of infants having had either a family history of severe neonatal lung disease or a history of consanguinity, or both, thus making a genetic mechanism for their lung disease likely. The lung histology from nine infants in whom tissue was available was similar to what had been observed in patients with SP-B or SP-C mutations, with accumulations of proteinaceous material filling distal airspaces (alveolar proteinosis), and collection of foamy macrophages in distal airspaces with variable amounts on interstitial thickening (DIP, CPI). SP-B and SP-C gene abnormalities were excluded by a combination of protein expression and genetic studies.

The clinical phenotype of ABCA3-deficient infants was similar to that of those with SP-B deficiency, with 15 of 16 dying within the first 3 months of life. The identified mutations were scattered throughout the gene, and included nonsense and frameshift mutations, as well as missense mutations in codons that had been highly conserved during evolution. The disease was inherited in an autosomal-recessive manner. No common mutations were identified, although infants from consanguineous unions were homozygous for the mutation identified in their family. The one infant with prolonged survival (7 years at the time of the report) had a missense mutation on one allele and an unidentified mutation on the other allele, suggesting that some alleles may be associated with milder disease. Since the initial group of infants selected for analysis was one that largely had fatal disease, whether ABCA3 deficiency frequently results in chronic lung disease will require further study.

ABCA3 is localized to lamellar bodies, and abnormal lamellar body formation was observed in those infants from whom appropriate material was available for analysis, including a pair of siblings previously identified as having abnormal lamellar bodies due to an unknown mechanism.[64] The lamellar bodies were often much smaller and dense appearing, although on higher magnification, densely packed membranes were observed. Eccentrically placed dense inclusions were often observed within the abnormal lamellar bodies, sometimes giving a "fried-egg" appearance. The ultrastructural appearance was distinct from that of SP-B deficiency, in which the abnormal lamellar bodies are larger and loosely packed with vesicular inclusions, often with the appearance of composite or multivesicular bodies[28,29] (see Fig. 20-3). These findings indicate that ultrastructural examination of lung tissue obtained at biopsy or autopsy may be helpful in establishing the diagnosis of ABCA3 deficiency and distinguishing it from other inborn errors of surfactant metabolism.

The incidence and prevalence of ABCA3 deficiency are unknown. Because the ABCA3 gene is much larger (containing 30 coding exons spanning almost 60,000 bases) than those encoding SP-B and SP-C, it would not be surprising if it was a more frequent cause of lung disease than SP-B deficiency or SP-C-related disease. The large percentage of infants with lung disease of unknown etiology in this first study who had ABCA3 mutations suggests that ABCA3 deficiency may account for a significant fraction of children with apparent genetic neonatal lung disease for whom the underlying cause is unknown. In two studies that examined the roles of first SP-B and then SP-C gene mutations in 40 infants with severe unexplained respiratory disease, only 5 patients had such mutations identified, and the characteristics of many of the patients without identified mutations were consistent with ABCA3 deficiency.[20,65] Additional studies will be needed to determine the contribution of ABCA3 mutations to neonatal and childhood lung disease, and to clarify the role of ABCA3 in surfactant metabolism, as well as the potential roles of other ABC transporters in alveolar type II cell and surfactant metabolism.

■ SUMMARY

Three single gene disorders resulting in disruptions in surfactant metabolism and surfactant deficiency have been identified to date, and the features of these illnesses are summarized in Table 20-1. The phenotype of SP-B and ABCA3 deficiencies is usually that of severe surfactant deficiency in the neonatal period, while SP-C gene abnormalities have a much more variable course. There is considerable overlap in the histopathology associated with each of these disorders. Because surfactant is composed principally of lipids, accumulations of foamy macrophages that have ingested the abnormal surfactant are common in these disorders. While such lipid-laden macrophages may be observed in association with aspiration, in a very young infant whose disease dates to the neonatal period they may represent an abnormality in endogenous lung lipid metabolism. Ultrastructural examination of lung tissue may provide invaluable information as to the cause of the disorder, and should be included with the studies obtained when performing a lung biopsy in a young infant with unexplained respiratory failure or interstitial lung disease. Finally, given the complexity of the surfactant system, it is highly likely that other genetic disorders disrupting surfactant metabolism

TABLE 20-1. Genetic abnormalities of surfactant

	Hereditary SP-B Deficiency	ABCA3 Deficiency	SP-C Mutations
Age of Onset	Newborn	Newborn	Newborn to adult
Mode of Inheritance	Autosomal recessive	Autosomal recessive	Autosomal dominant or sporadic
Mechanism	Loss-of-function mutations in *SFTPB* (chromosome 2)	Loss-of-function mutations in *ABCA3* (chromosome 16)	Toxic gain-of-function mechanism in *SFTPC* (chromosome 8)
Pathology	PAP Alveolar type II cell hyperplasia Pulmonary fibrosis	DIP CPI PAP	CPI DIP NSIP Pulmonary fibrosis
Electron Microscopy	Absent lamellar bodies Poorly formed multivesicular bodies	Absent lamellar bodies with small dense bodies with dense, eccentric inclusions	Normal lamellar bodies
Outcome	Fatal in newborn period	Often fatal in neonatal period	Variable

CPI, chronic pneumonitis of infancy; DIP, desquamative interstitial pneumonitis; NSIP, nonspecific interstitial pneumonitis; PAP, pulmonary alveolar proteinosis.

will be identified, providing new insights into normal surfactant metabolism, and suggesting new candidate genes for both pediatric interstitial lung disease, as well as contributing to more common lung diseases such as neonatal RDS.

Acknowledgments

The author gratefully acknowledges the collaboration and contributions of Jeffrey Whitsett, Susan Wert, and Timothy Weaver, Cincinnati Children's Hospital and University of Cincinnati College of Medicine, Cincinnati, Ohio; Aaron Hamvas and F. Sessions Cole, St. Louis Children's Hospital and Washington University, St. Louis, Missouri; and Michael Dean, NCI, Frederick, Maryland. This work was supported by grants from the National Institutes of Health, HL-54703, HL-56387, HL-65174, and the Eudowood Foundation.

REFERENCES

1. Crouch E, Wright J: Surfactant proteins a and d and pulmonary host defense. Annu Rev Physiol 2001;63:521–554.
2. Korfhagen TR, LeVine AM, Whitsett JA: Surfactant protein A (SP-A) gene targeted mice. Biochim Biophys Acta 1998;1408:296–302.
3. Korfhagen TR, Sheftelyevich V, Burhans MS, et al: Surfactant protein-D regulates surfactant phospholipid homeostasis in vivo. J Biol Chem 1998;273: 28438–28443.
4. Botas C, Poulain F, Akiyama J, et al: Altered surfactant homeostasis and alveolar type II cell morphology in mice lacking surfactant protein D. Proc Natl Acad Sci U S A 1998;95:11869–11874.
5. Wert SE, Yoshida M, LeVine AM, et al: Increased metalloproteinase activity, oxidant production, and emphysema in surfactant protein D gene-inactivated mice. Proc Natl Acad Sci U S A 2000;97:5972–5977.
6. Weaver TE, Conkright JJ: Function of surfactant proteins B and C. Annu Rev Physiol 2001;63:555–578.
7. Weaver TE: Synthesis, processing and secretion of surfactant proteins B and C. Biochim Biophys Acta 1998;1408:173–179.
8. Nogee LM, de Mello DE, Dehner LP, Colten HR: Brief report. Deficiency of pulmonary surfactant protein B in congenital alveolar proteinosis. N Engl J Med 1993;328:406–410.
9. Schumacher RE, Marrogi AJ, Heidelberger KP: Pulmonary alveolar proteinosis in a newborn. Pediatr Pulmonol 1989;7:178–182.
10. Moulton SL, Krous HF, Merritt TA, et al: Congenital pulmonary alveolar proteinosis. Failure of treatment with extracorporeal life support [see comments]. J Pediatr 1992;120:297–302.
11. Nogee LM, Garnier G, Dietz HC, et al: A mutation in the surfactant protein B gene responsible for fatal neonatal respiratory disease in multiple kindreds. J Clin Invest 1994;93:1860–1863.
12. Nogee LM: Alterations in SP-B and SP-C expression in neonatal lung disease. Annu Rev Physiol 2004;66:601–623.
13. Nogee LM, Wert SE, Proffit SA, et al: Allelic heterogeneity in hereditary surfactant protein B (SP-B) deficiency. Am J Respir Crit Care Med 2000; 161:973–981.
14. Ballard PL, Nogee LM, Beers MF, et al: Partial deficiency of surfactant protein B in an infant with chronic lung disease. Pediatrics 1995;96: 1046–1052.
15. Andersen C, Ramsay JA, Nogee LM, et al: Recurrent familial neonatal deaths. Hereditary surfactant protein B deficiency. Am J Perinatol 2000;17: 219–224.
16. Ball R, Chetcuti PA, Beverley D: Fatal familial surfactant protein B deficiency [Letter]. Arch Dis Child Fetal Neonatal Ed 1995;73:F53.
17. Dunbar AE III, Wert SE, Ikegami M, et al: Prolonged survival in hereditary surfactant protein B (SP-B) deficiency associated with a novel splicing mutation. Pediatr Res 2000;48:275–282.
18. Somaschini M, Wert S, Mangili G, et al: Hereditary surfactant protein B deficiency resulting from a novel mutation. Intensive Care Med 2000;26: 97–100.
19. Williams GD, Christodoulou J, Stack J, et al: Surfactant protein B deficiency. Clinical, histological and molecular evaluation. J Paediatr Child Health 1999;35:214–220.
20. Tredano M, Griese M, de Blic J, et al: Analysis of 40 sporadic or familial neonatal and pediatric cases with severe unexplained respiratory distress. Relationship to SFTPB. Am J Med Genet 2003;119A:324–339.
21. Tredano M, van Elburg RM, Kaspers AG, et al: Compound SFTPB 1549C<ra>GAA (121ins2) and 457delC heterozygosity in severe congenital lung disease and surfactant protein B (SP-B) deficiency. Hum Mutat 1999;14:502–509.
22. Lin Z, deMello DE, Wallot M, Floros J: An SP-B gene mutation responsible for SP-B deficiency in fatal congenital alveolar proteinosis. Evidence for a mutation hotspot in exon 4. Mol Genet Metab 1998;64:25–35.
23. Hamvas A, Nogee LM, Mallory GB Jr, et al: Lung transplantation for treatment of infants with surfactant protein B deficiency. J Pediatr 1997;130:231–239.
24. Melton KR, Nesslein LL, Ikegami M, et al: SP-B deficiency causes respiratory failure in adult mice. Am J Physiol Lung Cell Mol Physiol 2003;285: L543–L549.
25. Tokieda K, Iwamoto HS, Bachurski C, et al: Surfactant protein-B-deficient mice are susceptible to hyperoxic lung injury [see comments]. Am J Respir Cell Mol Biol 1999;21:463–472.
26. Yusen RD, Cohen AH, Hamvas A: Normal lung function in subjects heterozygous for surfactant protein-B deficiency. Am J Respir Crit Care Med 1999;159:411–414.
27. Clark JC, Wert SE, Bachurski CJ, et al: Targeted disruption of the surfactant protein B gene disrupts surfactant homeostasis, causing respiratory failure in newborn mice. Proc Natl Acad Sci U S A 1995;92:7794–7798.
28. deMello DE, Heyman S, Phelps DS, et al: Ultrastructure of lung in surfactant protein B deficiency. Am J Respir Cell Mol Biol 1994;11:230–239.
29. Stahlman MT, Gray MP, Falconieri MW, et al: Lamellar body formation in normal and surfactant protein B–deficient fetal mice. Lab Invest 2000; 80:395–403.
30. Vorbroker DK, Profitt SA, Nogee LM, Whitsett JA: Aberrant processing of surfactant protein C in hereditary SP-B deficiency. Am J Physiol 1995;268: L647–L656.
31. Li J, Ikegami M, Na CL, et al: N-terminally extended surfactant protein (SP) C isolated from SP-B-deficient children has reduced surface activity and inhibited lipopolysaccharide binding. Biochemistry 2004;43:3891–3898.

32. Weaver T, Na C, Stahlman M: Biogenesis of lamellar bodies, lysosome-related organelles involved in storage and secretion of pulmonary surfactant. Semin Cell Dev Biol 2002;13:263.
33. Hamvas A, Trusgnich M, Brice H, et al: Population-based screening for rare mutations. High-throughput DNA extraction and molecular amplification from Guthrie cards. Pediatr Res 2001;50:666–668.
34. Shulenin S, Nogee LM, Annilo T, et al: ABCA3 gene mutations in newborns with fatal surfactant deficiency. N Engl J Med 2004;350:1296–1303.
35. Floros J, Veletza SV, Kotikalapudi P, et al: Dinucleotide repeats in the human surfactant protein-B gene and respiratory-distress syndrome. Biochem J 1995;305:583–590.
36. Floros J, Fan R: Surfactant protein A and B genetic variants and respiratory distress syndrome. Allele interactions. Biol Neonate 2001;80(Suppl 1):22–25.
37. Wang G, Christensen ND, Wigdahl B, et al: Differences in N-linked glycosylation between human surfactant protein-B variants of the C or T allele at the single-nucleotide polymorphism at position 1580. Implications for disease. Biochem J 2003;369:179–184.
38. Haataja R, Ramet M, Marttila R, Hallman M: Surfactant proteins A and B as interactive genetic determinants of neonatal respiratory distress syndrome. Hum Mol Genet 2000;9:2751–2760.
39. Marttila R, Haataja R, Ramet M, et al: Surfactant protein B polymorphism and respiratory distress syndrome in premature twins. Hum Genet 2003; 112:18–23.
40. Lin Z, Pearson C, Chinchilli V, et al: Polymorphisms of human SP-A, SP-B, and SP-D genes. Association of SP-B Thr131Ile with ARDS. Clin Genet 2000;58:181–191.
41. Curstedt T, Johansson J, Persson P, et al: Hydrophobic surfactant-associated polypeptides. SP-C is a lipopeptide with two palmitoylated cysteine residues, whereas SP-B lacks covalently linked fatty acyl groups. Proc Natl Acad Sci U S A 1990;87:2985–2989.
42. ten Brinke A, Posthuma G, Batenburg JJ, et al: The transmembrane domain of surfactant protein C precursor determines the morphology of the induced membrane compartment in CHO cells. Eur J Cell Biol 2003;82: 285–294.
43. Vorbroker DK, Dey C, Weaver TE, Whitsett JA: Surfactant protein C precursor is palmitoylated and associates with subcellular membranes. Biochim Biophys Acta 1992;1105:161–169.
44. Nogee LM, Dunbar AE, Wert SE, et al: A mutation in the surfactant protein C gene associated with familial interstitial lung disease. N Engl J Med 2001;344:573–579.
45. Katzenstein AL, Gordon LP, Oliphant M, Swender PT: Chronic pneumonitis of infancy. A unique form of interstitial lung disease occurring in early childhood. Am J Surg Pathol 1995;19:439–447.
46. Conkright JJ, Bridges JP, Na CL, et al: Secretion of surfactant protein C, an integral membrane protein, requires the N-terminal propeptide. J Biol Chem 2001;276:14658–14664.
47. Wang WJ, Mulugeta S, Russo SJ, Beers MF: Deletion of exon 4 from human surfactant protein C results in aggresome formation and generation of a dominant negative. J Cell Sci 2003;116:683–692.
48. Bridges JP, Wert SE, Nogee LM, Weaver TE: Expression of a human surfactant protein C mutation associated with interstitial lung disease disrupts lung development in transgenic mice. J Biol Chem 2003;278: 52739–52746.
49. Thomas AQ, Lane K, Phillips J III, et al: Heterozygosity for a surfactant protein C gene mutation associated with usual interstitial pneumonitis and cellular nonspecific interstitial pneumonitis in one kindred. Am J Respir Crit Care Med 2002;165:1322–1328.
50. Hamvas A, Nogee LM, White FV, et al: Progressive lung disease and surfactant dysfunction with a deletion in surfactant protein C gene. Am J Respir Cell Mol Biol 2004;30:771–776.
51. Brasch F, Griese M, Tredano M, et al: Interstitial lung disease in a baby with a de novo mutation in the SFTPC gene. Eur Respir J 2004;24:30–39.
52. Cameron HS, Somaschini M, Carrera P, et al: A common mutation in the surfactant protein C gene associated with lung disease. J Pediatr 2005;146:370–375.
53. Glasser SW, Detmer EA, Ikegami M, et al: Pneumonitis and emphysema in sp-C gene targeted mice. J Biol Chem 2003;278:14291–14298.
54. Glasser SW, Burhans MS, Korfhagen TR, et al: Altered stability of pulmonary surfactant in SP-C-deficient mice. Proc Natl Acad Sci U S A 2001;98: 6366–6371.
55. Amin RS, Wert SE, Baughman RP, et al: Surfactant protein deficiency in familial interstitial lung disease. J Pediatr 2001;139:85–92.
56. Nogee LM, Dunbar AE III, Wert S, et al: Mutations in the surfactant protein C gene associated with interstitial lung disease. Chest 2002; 121(Suppl):20–21.
57. Rubenstein RC, Zeitlin PL: A pilot clinical trial of oral sodium 4-phenylbutyrate (Buphenyl) in deltaF508-homozygous cystic fibrosis patients. Partial restoration of nasal epithelial CFTR function. Am J Respir Crit Care Med 1998;157:484–490.
58. Burrows JA, Willis LK, Perlmutter DH: Chemical chaperones mediate increased secretion of mutant alpha 1-antitrypsin (alpha 1-AT) Z. A potential pharmacological strategy for prevention of liver injury and emphysema in alpha 1-AT deficiency. Proc Natl Acad Sci U S A 2000;97:1796–1801.
59. Lahti M, Marttila R, Hallman M: Surfactant protein C gene variation in the Finnish population—association with perinatal respiratory disease. Eur J Hum Genet 2004;12:312–320.
60. Yoshida I, Ban N, Inagaki N: Expression of ABCA3, a causative gene for fatal surfactant deficiency, is up-regulated by glucocorticoids in lung alveolar type II cells. Biochem Biophys Res Commun 2004;323:547–555.
61. Mulugeta S, Gray JM, Notarfrancesco KL, et al: Identification of LBM180, a lamellar body limiting membrane protein of alveolar type II cells, as the ABC transporter protein ABCA3. J Biol Chem 2002;277:22147–22155.
62. Yamano G, Funahashi H, Kawanami O, et al: ABCA3 is a lamellar body membrane protein in human lung alveolar type II cells. FEBS Lett 2001;508:221–225.
63. Dean M, Rzhetsky A, Allikmets R: The human ATP-binding cassette (ABC) transporter superfamily. Genome Res 2001;11:1156–1166.
64. Tryka AF, Wert SE, Mazursky JE, et al: Absence of lamellar bodies with accumulation of dense bodies characterizes a novel form of congenital surfactant defect. Pediatr Dev Pathol 2000;3:335–345.
65. Tredano M, Griese M, Brasch F, et al: Mutation of SFTPC in infantile pulmonary alveolar proteinosis with or without fibrosing lung disease. Am J Med Genet 2004;126A:18–26.

Disorders of the Pleura

21 Air and Liquid in the Pleural Space

Mark Montgomery, MD • David Sigalet, MD

The pleura plays an integral role in respiration. The pleural space couples the lung with the chest wall and provides an integrated respiratory system. Consequently, disorders of the pleura constitute an important cause of morbidity and mortality in infants and children. Prompt recognition and appropriate management can avert a more serious cardiorespiratory catastrophe. This chapter discusses the anatomic features of the pleural membranes and fluid, the physiology of liquid transport in the potential space, and the various disorders of liquid and air accumulation and their management.

■ ANATOMY OF THE PLEURAL SPACE

■ ANATOMIC FEATURES

The pleural space is a potential space, 10 to 24 μm wide, defined by the parietal and visceral pleurae.[1,2] The parietal pleura covers the inner aspect of the chest wall and diaphragm. The visceral pleura is tightly adherent to the surface of the lungs and to interlobar fissures. A thin film of liquid separates the two surfaces. An understanding of pleural function requires an appreciation of the structure of these membranes.

Parietal Pleura

The parietal pleura consists of a single layer of flat, cuboidal, mesothelial cells, 1 to 4 μm thick, supported by loose connective tissue.[3] Blood vessels, nerves, and lymphatic vessels invest the connective tissue. The arterial supply is derived from the intercostal and internal mammary arteries. Venous blood drains to the systemic circulation. The parietal pleura possesses nervous innervation from the sensory branches of the intercostal and phrenic nerves. The parietal pleura has direct connection to the lymphatic vessels. The surface of the parietal pleura contains stomas, 2 to 12 μm in diameter, that exhibit preferential caudal distribution.[4] The stomas may exhibit a 10-fold increase in size with inspiratory maneuvers. Stomas are instrumental in clearing fluid and particle accumulations via the lymphatics. Lymphatic vessels are located in the submesothelial layer of the parietal pleura. The anterior parietal pleura drains to the internal intercostal lymph nodes, and the posterior parietal pleura drains to the lymph nodes located along the internal thoracic artery. The presence of sensory innervation and stomas distinguishes the parietal pleura from the visceral pleura.[5]

Visceral Pleura

The visceral pleura is a complex and delicate membranous structure. There is a single mesothelial layer of cuboidal cells overlying the basement membrane, and there are multiple subepithelial layers of connective tissue. Microvilli, 0.1 μm wide and 3 to 6 μm long, are evident on the apical surfaces of the visceral mesothelial cells. The microvilli participate in the homeostasis of the pleural fluid and contribute to transmembrane solute and fluid movement. Further, vesicles contained within the microvilli trap particles and glycoproteins, thereby reducing friction between the visceral and parietal pleurae.[6] Blood supply to the visceral pleura is via the bronchial arteries, with a minor contribution from the pulmonary circulation. The connective tissue underlying the mesothelial layer is richly endowed with type 1 collagen and provides much of the tensile strength of the pleura. The lymphatics drain to the mediastinal nodes, following the course set by the pulmonary veins or arteries. The visceral pleura has no sensory innervation, but it is supplied by branches of the vagus and sympathetic trunks.

■ PHYSIOLOGY OF THE PLEURAL SPACE

■ FORMATION AND ABSORPTION OF PLEURAL FLUID

The pleural membranes are permeable to liquid. Normally, the influx and outflow of pleural fluid is balanced to result in a small, but measurable, amount (0.1–0.2 mL/kg) of sterile, colorless liquid.[7] The pleural liquid is thickest over dependent areas of the thorax. The fluid provides union and prevents friction between the visceral and parietal pleurae. Normal pleural fluid contains

1.5 g/dL protein. Normally, pleural liquid is alkaline (pH 7.60). There are approximately 1700 cells/mm^3, consisting of 75% macrophages, 23% lymphocytes, and 2% mesothelial cells.[8] Pleural fluid homeostasis is a balance among production of pleural fluid, competence of the pleural membrane, and absorption of pleural fluid via microvilli, capillary membranes, and lymphatic stomas.

A rational understanding of the accumulation of excess pleural liquid requires knowledge of normal liquid transport into and out of the pleural cavity. Fluid influx and outflow are described by Starling forces and also determined by clearance via lymphatic stomas.[9] Nearly 90% of the original amount of pleural liquid filtered out of the arterial end of the capillaries is reabsorbed at the venous end. The remainder of the filtrate (10%) is returned via the lymphatics. The balance between filtration and reabsorption forces determines the direction of liquid movement. Starling described a classic approach to convective (bulk) liquid movement between vascular and extravascular compartments, which can be expressed as:

$$Q_v = K_f[(P_c - P_{is}) - (\pi_{pl} - \pi_{is})]$$

where Q_v = rate of net liquid movement per unit surface area of a capillary; K_f = capillary filtration coefficient; P_c = capillary hydrostatic pressure; P_{is} = hydrostatic pressure in the interstitial space (equivalent to intrapleural pressure); π_{pl} = plasma oncotic pressure; and π_{is} = oncotic pressure in the interstitial space (equivalent to oncotic pressure of the pleural liquid).[10] The movement of liquid across the pleural capillaries obeys this law of transcapillary liquid exchange. The filtration coefficient (K_f) is an index of capillary wall permeability that depends on the structural integrity of the intercellular junctions of the endothelial lining. Oncotic pressure (π) is a function of the molal concentration of protein, mainly albumin. Normal plasma with a protein concentration of 7.0 g/dL has an oncotic pressure of 32 to 35 cm H_2O, whereas pleural liquid with a protein concentration of 1.5 to 1.77 g/dL has an estimated oncotic pressure of approximately 6 cm H_2O. Mean hydrostatic pressures (P_c) in the parietal and visceral pleural capillaries are 30 and 11 cm H_2O, respectively. Intrapleural pressure (equivalent to hydrostatic pressure in the interstitial space) at resting lung volume is approximately 5 cm H_2O subatmospheric, so there is a net pressure of 9 cm H_2O (filtration pressure) at the parietal pleural capillary level, tending to drive liquid into the pleural space. In contrast, a net driving pressure of $^-$10 cm H_2O (absorption pressure) is acting on the visceral pleural capillaries, driving liquid from the pleural space into the capillaries (Table 21-1). Net liquid absorption from the pleural space occurs because absorption pressure is slightly greater than filtration pressure. Increased negative pressure develops in the liquid between the contact points of the visceral and parietal pleurae because of increased stretching and deformation at these sites. Ultimately, the negative pleural liquid pressure equilibrates with the absorption pressure. Thus, the pleural space is kept virtually liquid-free, a state that represents an equilibrium between filtration and absorption.

Pleural absorption of liquid is augmented by intercostal and diaphragmatic activity (e.g., deep breathing exercises), which results in increased vascular and lymphatic uptake owing to dilation of the lymphatic stomas and the dehiscences formed between mesothelial cells of the visceral pleura. Predictably, hypoventilation decreases absorption of particulate matter from the pleural space. Moreover, markedly negative intrapleural pressures throughout the respiratory cycle, such as those occurring with atelectasis or with continuous suction on closed thoracostomy tubes, will contribute to the generation of pleural fluid.

The parietal pleura plays a vital role in the clearance of excess pleural fluid. The capacity of the lymphatic system to drain the pleural space is tremendous via stomas in the parietal pleura. The rate of fluid transport from the pleural space through the lymphatics increases in a linear fashion to exceed the usual rate of fluid production by almost 30-fold. The ability of the parietal pleura to markedly enhance fluid absorption is crucial to preventing fluid accumulation.

MAINTENANCE OF AN AIR-FREE PLEURAL SPACE

The pleural membranes are permeable to gas, yet the pleural space is free of air. The difference between total gas pressure in the venous system and that in the pleural space accounts for this fact. Partial pressures of gases in the venous blood at sea level are: partial pressure of oxygen (PO_2) = 40 torr, partial pressure of carbon dioxide (PCO_2) = 46 mm Hg, partial pressure of nitrogen (PN_2) = 573 mm Hg, and PH_2O = 47 mm Hg. The sum of these is 706 mm Hg, which is 54 mm Hg (73 cm H_2O) less than atmospheric pressure (at sea level). Because total gas pressure in venous blood is approximately 73 cm H_2O subatmospheric and intrapleural pressure at resting lung volume is approximately 5 cm H_2O subatmospheric, there is a pressure gradient of approximately 68 cm H_2O, favoring continuing absorption of gas from the pleural space into the circulation. Thus, provided there is no continuing air leak to the pleural space from the atmosphere, gas volume within the pleural space diffuses out until all of the gas disappears, at a rate of 100 mL/wk, so normally, the pleural space is kept totally gas-free. The clinical practice of using supplemental oxygen therapy to speed resorption of a small pneumothorax is based on this principle.

TABLE 21-1. Starling relationship in the parietal and visceral pleura

	Parietal Pleura	Visceral Pleura
Force Moving Liquid into the Pleural Space (cm H_2O)		
Capillary hydrostatic pressure	30	11
Interstitial hydrostatic pressure (pleural pressure)	−5	−5
Oncotic pressure of the pleural liquid	−6	−6
Total (cm H_2O)	41	22
Force Moving Liquid into the Pleural Capillaries (cm H_2O)		
Plasma oncotic pressure	32	32
Net Force (cm H_2O)	−9 (out)	10 (in)

■ ACCUMULATION OF EXCESS PLEURAL LIQUID

■ PATHOGENESIS

The normal state of a nearly liquid-free pleural cavity represents equilibrium between pleural liquid formation (filtration) and removal (absorption). Fundamentally, excess liquid accumulates in the pleural cavity (effusion) whenever filtration exceeds removal as a result of: (1) increased filtration associated with normal or impaired absorption, (2) normal filtration associated with inadequate removal, or (3) addition of exogenous fluid (peritoneal cavity or intravenous fluid extravasation).[10,11] Thus, disequilibrium may be due to disturbances in the Starling forces that govern filtration and absorption, alterations in lymphatic drainage, or both.

Various clinical disorders can alter vascular filtration and absorption in the pleural capillaries as well as lymphatic flow (Table 21-2).[6] Inflammation (e.g., pleural infection, rheumatoid arthritis, systemic lupus erythematosus, pulmonary infarction) or direct toxic damage to the endothelium may increase the filtration coefficient. The increase in the filtration coefficient allows protein loss from the capillaries and accumulation in the pleural cavity, thereby increasing oncotic pressure in the interstitial space. Local blood flow may increase in response to inflammation, resulting in an increase in capillary hydrostatic pressure. The net consequence of these changes is increased liquid and protein transudation into the pleural cavity that exceeds the normal capacity of lymphatic drainage. In all conditions that result in pleural effusion due to abnormality in the pleural membrane, there will be an excess of protein or other large molecules in the pleural fluid.

Pleural fluid formation is enhanced in the face of increased capillary hydrostatic pressure or more negative hydrostatic pressure in the interstitial space.[11] Hydrostatic pressure increases with systemic venous hypertension (e.g., pericarditis, right-sided heart failure caused by overinfusion of blood or fluid, superior vena cava syndrome) or because of pulmonary venous hypertension (e.g., congestive heart failure). The resulting increased accumulation of pleural liquid (hydrothorax) is due to increased driving pressure in the systemic capillaries. The creation of a markedly subatmospheric pleural pressure (e.g., persistent high negative pressures occasionally used during tube thoracostomy drainage), even in the presence of normal hydrostatic pressure in the pleural capillaries, may also result in increased fluid filtration from the pleural capillaries. This mechanism also explains effusions that occur after pneumonectomy, recurrence of effusion after repeated thoracenteses, and the increasing effusion that occurs in tuberculosis, with visceral pleural thickening, fibrosis, and permanently atelectatic lungs. Oncotic pressure (π) determines how effectively fluid is reabsorbed. Net absorption by the visceral pleura is reduced to zero by an increase in the pleural liquid protein concentration of more than 4 g/dL (40 g/L, an exudate) in the presence of a normal plasma protein concentration. When plasma oncotic pressure is significantly reduced (e.g., hypoalbuminemia due to nephrosis), parietal pleural filtration is increased and visceral pleural absorption is reduced. In all of these conditions, excess pleural fluid remains an ultrafiltrate, with normal concentrations of pleural fluid protein.

Proper functioning of the lymphatic stomas and system are essential in clearing the pleural space of excess fluid. If lymphatic channels are unable to provide adequate drainage, pleural effusion ensues. Lymphatic drainage may be impeded as a result of: (1) systemic venous hypertension; (2) mediastinal lymphadenopathy (e.g., lymphoma or fibrosis); (3) fibrosis of the parietal pleura (e.g., tuberculosis); (4) obstruction of the thoracic duct (e.g., chylothorax); and (5) developmental hypoplasia of the lymphatic channels (e.g., hereditary lymphedema). On occasion, the lymphatic system is overloaded by absorption of peritoneal fluid (e.g., liver cirrhosis with ascites, peritoneal dialysis) via the diaphragmatic lymphatics.[12] The result is escape of excess lymphatic fluid under increased pressure into the pleural cavity, where pressure is normally subatmospheric, and development of a hydrothorax. The contribution of an abnormality in the lymphatic system must be considered in the evaluation of ongoing development of a pleural effusion.

This discussion shows that a single clinical disorder may cause pleural effusion through one or several mechanisms. Moreover, clinical disorders may coexist. These facts explain the varying characteristics of pleural effusion seen clinically.

■ TABLE 21-2. Pathophysiology of pleural liquid accumulation

Primary Mechanism	Clinical Disorders	Pleural Effusion
Altered Starling Forces		
Increased capillary permeability (K_f)	Pleuropulmonary infection; circulating toxins; systemic lupus erythematosus; rheumatoid arthritis; sarcoidosis; tumor; pulmonary infarction; viral hepatitis	Exudate
Increased capillary hydrostatic pressure (P_c)	Overhydration; congestive heart failure; venous hypertension; pericarditis	Transudate
Decreased hydrostatic pressure of the interstitial space (P_{is})	Trapped lung with chronic pleural space; post-thoracentesis	Transudate
Decreased plasma oncotic pressure (π_{pl})	Hypoalbuminemia; nephrosis; hepatic cirrhosis	Transudate
Increased oncotic pressure in the interstitial space (π_{is})	Pulmonary infarction	Exudate
Inappropriate Lymphatic Flow		
Inadequate outflow	Hypoalbuminemia; nephrosis	Transudate
Excessive inflow	Hepatic cirrhosis with ascites; peritoneal dialysis	Transudate
Impared flow (mediastinal lymphadenopathy and fibrosis; thickening of the parietal pleura; obstruction of the thoracic duct; developmental hydroplasia or defect)	Mediastinal radiation, superior vena caval syndrome, pericarditis; tuberculosis; lymphoma, mediastinal hygroma; hereditary lymphedema, congenital chylothorax	Exudate, transudate, or chyle
Disruption of the diaphragmatic lymphatics	Pancreatitis; subphrenic abscess	Exudate
Vascular Leak	Trauma; spontaneous rupture; vascular erosion by a neoplasm; hemorrhagic disease	Blood

FUNCTIONAL PATHOLOGY

The degree of dysfunction is determined by the rapidity of development of pleural effusion and the quantity of pleural fluid, as well as by the nature of the underlying disorder and the status of cardiopulmonary reserve. The usual result of pleural effusion is limited lung inflation, with a resultant decrease in vital capacity. Pleural inflammation is associated with pain that worsens with deep breathing, limiting full lung expansion. Pleuritic pain may resolve as pleural fluid increases, because contact between the irritated pleural membranes is reduced. In all cases of pleural fluid accumulation, the underlying lung and corresponding chest wall are uncoupled and function may not be coordinated. Further, elastic resistance to lung distention increases, thereby limiting lung expansion. Compressive atelectasis may contribute to decreased lung expansion, ventilation-perfusion mismatch, and hypoxemia. Pleural fluid may also distort the chest wall. The chest wall may bulge outward, with downward displacement of the ipsilateral hemidiaphragm. Inspiratory muscles are placed at a mechanical disadvantage, compromising inspiratory efforts. Rarely, a large pleural effusion will produce mediastinal shift, decreasing venous return and compromising cardiac output. Therapy may also contribute to ongoing pulmonary compromise. Pain caused by thoracentesis or indwelling chest tubes may limit full inspiration. Ongoing suctioning for chest tube drainage may promote continued development and removal of pleural fluid. Chronic loss of protein or lipids as a result of chest tube drainage may result in malnutrition.

HISTORY AND PHYSICAL EXAMINATION

Pleural effusion is usually secondary to an underlying disorder. The underlying disease determines the predominant systemic symptoms. Until accumulation of pleural liquid increases enough to cause cardiorespiratory difficulties (e.g., dyspnea, orthopnea), pleural effusion may be asymptomatic.[13] Symptoms of direct pleural involvement include chest pain, chest tightness, and dyspnea. Older children may have sharp pleuritic pain on inspiration or with cough that is due to stretching of the parietal pleura. The locus of pleurisy determines the site of pain, which may be felt in the chest overlying the site of inflammation or may be referred to the shoulder, if the central diaphragm is involved, or to the abdomen, if the peripheral diaphragm is involved. Severe chest pain inhibits respiratory movement and causes dyspnea. As effusion increases and separates the pleural membranes, pleuritic pain becomes a dull ache and may disappear.

Attention to chest findings on physical examination is important, particularly if only a small amount of pleural fluid is present. Pleural rub due to roughened pleural surfaces may be the only finding early in the course of disease, and may be heard during inspiration and expiration. As pleural effusion increases, pleural rub is lost. Thus, pleural rub indicates the absence of significant pleural effusion. Diminished thoracic wall excursion, fullness of the intercostal spaces, dull or flat percussion, decreased tactile and vocal fremitus, diminished whispering pectoriloquy, and decreased breath sounds are easily demonstrated over the involved site in an older child with moderate effusion. However, breath sounds in a neonate with moderate pleural effusion may be deceptively loud and clear throughout both lung fields because of the small chest volume. Additional signs of pleural effusion include displacement of the trachea and cardiac apex toward the contralateral side and splinting of the involved hemithorax, resulting in scoliosis concave to the affected side.

Frequent reassessment must continue after the detection of pleural fluid. The underlying condition resulting in pleural disease must be determined. Knowledge of the mechanisms that resulted in pleural effusion and the expected natural history or response to therapeutic interventions are essential to monitor the progress of the child with pleural effusion.

CHEST IMAGING

A standard posteroanterior chest radiograph is relatively insensitive in detecting pleural effusion. In general, a minimum of approximately 400 mL pleural liquid is required for roentgenographic visualization in upright views of the chest.[14] An expiratory view may accentuate pleural fluid, which is seen as a straight, radiodense line.[15] Obliteration of the costophrenic sinus (Fig. 21-1) is the earliest radiologic sign of pleural liquid accumulation. When effusion is moderate, chest radiographs demonstrate uniform water density and widened interspaces on the affected side, with displacement of the mediastinum to the contralateral hemithorax. In acutely ill children, when only a supine view is available, detection of pleural fluid is problematic. Generalized haziness of the affected hemithorax or accentuated pleural reflection may be the only clue to this disorder (Fig. 21-2). Standard posteroanterior chest radiographs may be inadequate to evaluate pleural fluid fully.

Lateral decubitus films provide valuable information about the quantity and quality of effusions, allow evaluation of the underlying parenchyma, and assist in planning investigations and therapy. Thin, mobile (nonloculated) pleural fluid will layer out on the dependent side (Figs. 21-3 and 21-4). Lateral decubitus views with the unaffected side inferior may enhance visualization of the underlying parenchyma on the affected hemithorax.

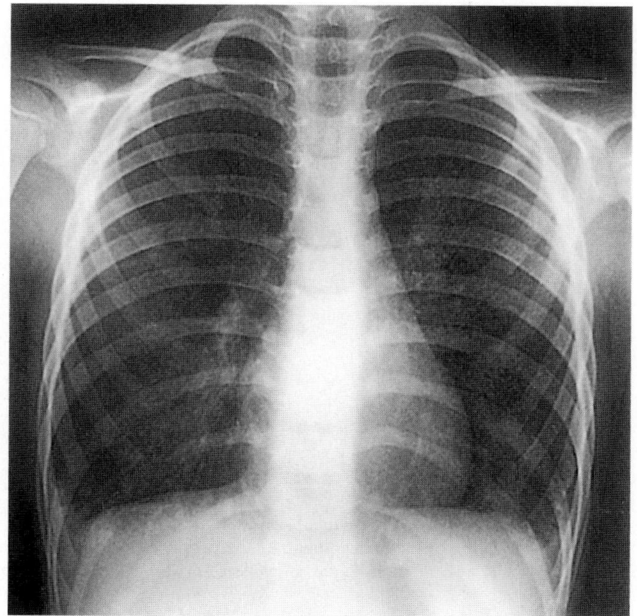

FIGURE 21-1. Posteroanterior chest radiograph demonstrating lung hyperinflation and perihilar interstitial infiltrates, consistent with *Mycoplasma* pneumonia. Blunted costophrenic angles indicate small bilateral pleural effusions.

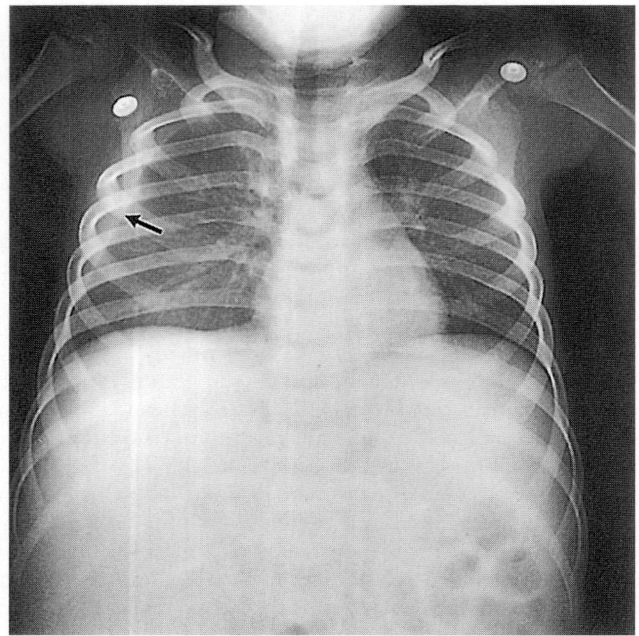

■ **FIGURE 21-2.** Anteroposterior supine chest radiograph, with pleural fluid evident between the chest wall and the lung *(arrow)*. Note the generalized increased haziness of the right hemithorax due to the accumulation of pleural fluid.

Placing the unaffected side superior enhances the evaluation of pleural effusion. As little as 50 mL pleural liquid can be detected with properly exposed lateral decubitus views; this liquid is seen as a layering of liquid density in the dependent portion of the thoracic cavity. Moreover, a decubitus film demonstrating more than 10 mm pleural fluid between the inside of the chest wall and the lung indicates an effusion of sufficient volume for thoracentesis. Decubitus films may also demonstrate infrapulmonary pleural effusion (Figs. 21-5 and 21-6). Failure of the liquid to shift from the upright to the decubitus view indicates loculation, as commonly seen in staphylococcal empyema (Figs. 21-7 and 21-8). Evaluation of the parenchyma and differentiation of loculated effusion caused by pleural fibrosis or infiltration may require adjunctive imaging modalities.

Ultrasonography can differentiate pleural thickening from effusion, preventing fruitless attempts at diagnostic thoracentesis, and identify the best site for thoracentesis, or insertion of a thoracostomy tube. Moreover, ultrasound will detect loculations and identify the quality of effusion. Anechoic pleural fluid (Fig. 21-9*A*) may be either a transudate or an exudate. Demonstrable multiple echogenic foci indicate an exudate or an empyema (see Fig. 21-9*B*). There may be accentuation of the visceral pleura with an empyema, due to thickening of the visceral pleura, compressive atelectasis, or consolidation of the adjacent parenchyma. Thus, the border between the pleural fluid and the parenchyma may be accentuated. Differentiation of a solid mass from echogenic pleural fluid is apparent by variations in the latter with breaths. A wealth of information is available from sonographic evaluation of a pleural disorder.

Computed tomography (CT) scans are extremely helpful in evaluating the pleura and the underlying parenchyma in large loculated effusions.[16] Pleural thickening or a mass is readily apparent (Fig. 21-10). The parietal pleura readily enhances in the presence of an empyema (Fig. 21-11). A loculated parapneumonic effusion is differentiated from a lung abscess by the angle made between the fluid-filled mass and the chest wall. An empyema usually creates an obtuse angle where it meets the chest wall, in contrast to the acute angle produced by an abscess. CT scan may be extremely helpful in making a differential diagnosis. Magnetic resonance imaging has not demonstrated an advantage over CT scans in the evaluation of pleural disorders.

Further thoracic imaging techniques are required to demonstrate bronchopleural fistulas. One approach is by sinography. Radiopaque contrast material is injected into the affected pleura

■ **FIGURE 21-3.** Posteroanterior erect chest radiograph demonstrating bilateral pleural effusions, with that on the left greater than that on the right. Also evident are atelectasis in the right upper lobe and consolidation in the left lower lobe.

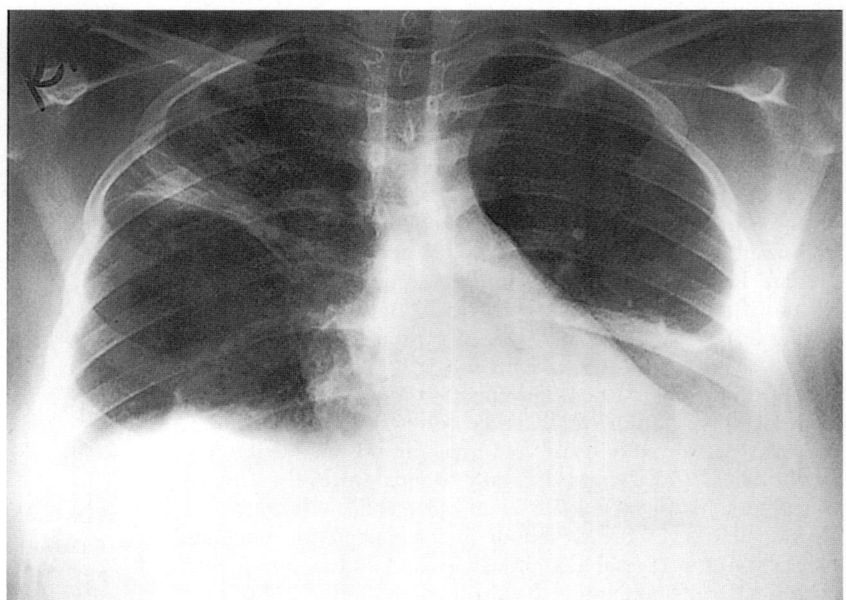

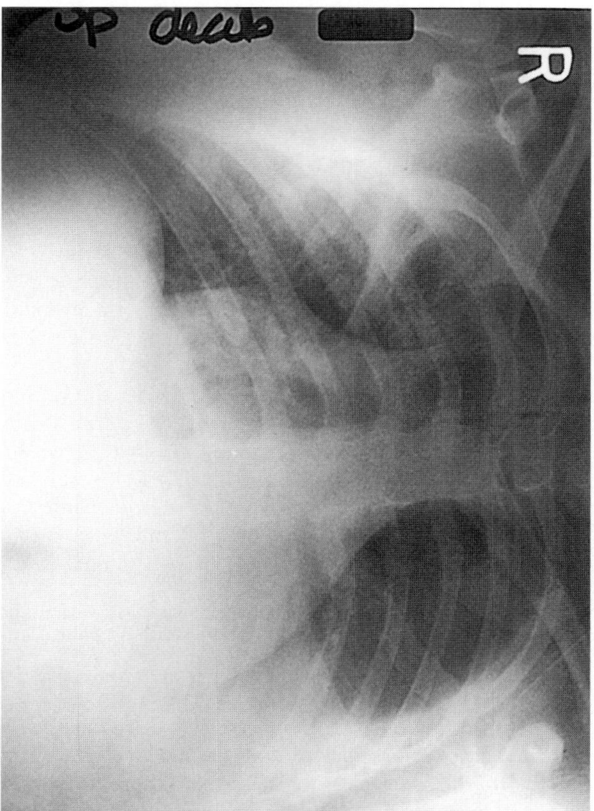

■ **FIGURE 21-4.** Left lateral decubitus image of the chest showing the layering of a nonloculated left pleural effusion.

through a needle or an existing chest tube (Fig. 21-12). As the patient coughs, the contrast material opacifies the fistula and spreads throughout the bronchial tree. This is the procedure of choice for peripherally situated small fistulas. Selective bronchography is used to delineate multiple, centrally located fistulas.

EXAMINATION OF PLEURAL FLUID

Evacuation of liquid by thoracentesis confirms the clinical and radiologic diagnosis of effusion. The specimen may provide the only evidence on which to make the diagnosis of certain disease states or to exclude others.[17]

There are multiple techniques used for obtaining pleural fluid by thoracentesis. Regardless of the procedure used, similar principles apply. The clinician must be knowledgeable about the procedure and the anatomy of the pleural space. The child and parents should be aware of the need for thoracentesis and knowledgeable about the procedure. Consideration should be given to the use of short-duration sedation, if needed. The child should have vascular access, and supplemental oxygen should be available. The site of thoracentesis may be determined clinically or by ultrasound. The site should be 1 to 2 cm below the site of onset of dullness to percussion in the midaxillary line or posteriorly. The site should be selected carefully. In cases of pleural irritation, there may be diaphragmatic splinting, elevating the hemidiaphragm, and dullness to percussion may be due to fluid or subdiaphragmatic organs. If ultrasound is used to locate the pleural fluid to be tapped, then thoracentesis should be performed at the time of ultrasound. Localization of the fluid may be lost if the site is only marked at the time of ultrasound, because the same body position may not be duplicated later. After the site of thoracentesis is determined, adequate analgesia is provided. With strict aseptic technique, a thoracentesis needle or large-bore intravascular catheter is introduced just above the rib. This placement avoids the intercostal nerve and vascular bundle. Attention must be paid to ensure that the needle is not introduced beyond the fluid, into the lung. A chest radiograph should be obtained after thoracentesis to ensure that a pneumothorax has not been created and to evaluate the underlying lung parenchyma.

The gross appearance of the liquid may be a clue to the cause of effusion.[18] Pale, clear, yellow liquid suggests a transudate. Aspiration of chylous liquid (Box 21-1) suggests injury to the lymphatic channels (e.g., neoplasm, tuberculosis, surgery) or spontaneous anatomic leakage of chyle (e.g., congenital chylothorax).

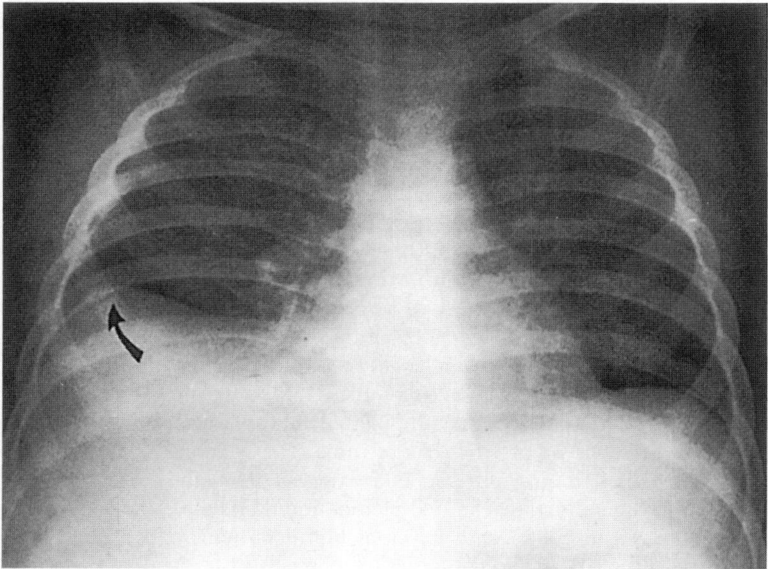

■ **FIGURE 21-5.** Upright chest radiograph of a child with nephrotic syndrome, demonstrating right infrapulmonary pleural effusion. The right hemidiaphragm shows peak elevation laterally *(arrow)* and relative lucency of the costophrenic sinus, signs that indicate an intrapulmonary location of the liquid.

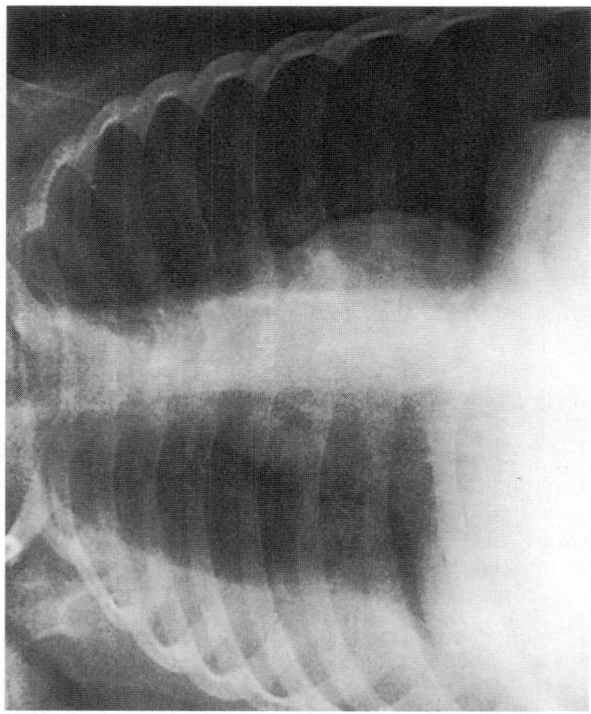

■ **FIGURE 21-6.** Decubitus chest radiograph with the right side dependent, obtained in the same patient as in Figure 21-5, confirming the presence of a free-flowing right pleural effusion.

In congenital chylothorax, a characteristic milky appearance of the liquid and the presence of chylomicrons are seen only after oral feedings have been started. Pleural liquid may assume the appearance of chyle, which is milky white and opalescent. If further analysis does not show fat globules, chylomicrons, or a turbid supernatant, the effusion is called *chyliform*. The milky appearance represents fatty degeneration of pus and endothelial cells.

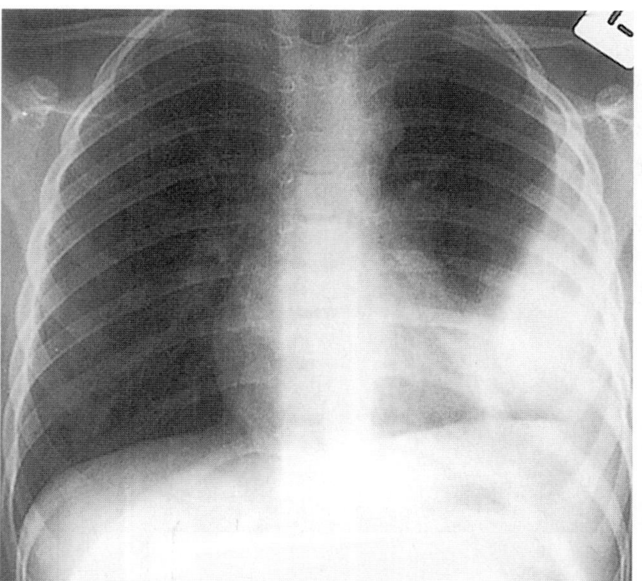

■ **FIGURE 21-7.** Posteroanterior erect chest radiograph demonstrating a large left empyema. Concomitant passive atelectasis of the adjacent lung is noted.

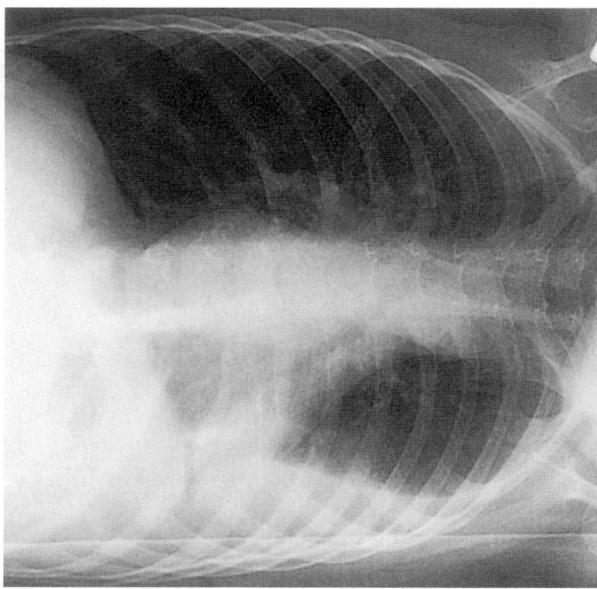

■ **FIGURE 21-8.** Left lateral decubitus chest radiograph showing no change in the configuration of the left empyema, indicating that it is loculated.

It may be seen in long-standing cases of purulent effusion. Bloody fluid implies vascular erosion from a malignant tumor or trauma to the intercostal or chest wall vessels. Brisk and massive bleeding is seen when the systemic circulation is involved, because systemic pressure is sixfold higher than pulmonary pressure. A purulent specimen indicates bacterial infection of the pleura. Fluid with a chocolate brown or anchovy paste appearance suggests amebiasis, usually on the right side. Anaerobic pleural infections have a characteristic putrid odor.

Laboratory evaluation of pleural fluid will allow evaluation of the integrity of the pleural membrane. The first point in clinical decision making regarding pleural effusion is to establish whether the effusion is a transudate or an exudate. If the pleural membrane is intact, then a transudate results. There is aberration in the Starling forces (altered hydrostatic or oncotic pressure) or fluid movement from the peritoneal cavity across the diaphragmatic pores. In clinical scenarios in which the pleural membranes are intact, the fluid is an ultrafiltrate, whereby the concentration of protein and large molecules is not increased. In contrast, exudative pleural effusion results when the integrity of the pleural membrane is impaired. There is leakage of protein or other large molecules across the membrane. Inflammation of the pleural membrane, pleural or mediastinal malignancy, and infection in the pleural space are the most likely causes of exudative effusion. The criteria used to characterize pleural effusion as an exudate (Light's criteria) include: (1) the ratio of pleural fluid to serum protein level is greater than 0.5; (2) the ratio of pleural fluid to serum lactate dehydrogenase (LDH) level is greater than 0.6; and (3) the ratio of pleural fluid to LDH level is greater than two thirds of the upper limit of normal for serum levels (Table 21-3).[19–21] Absence of all three criteria indicates that the pleural fluid is a transudate, and the presence of any one of the three criteria indicates an exudate. Other minor criteria that suggest that an effusion is an exudate include elevated pleural liquid cholesterol (>45 mg/dL, 1.16 mmol/L) and a pleural liquid protein level greater than 3.0 g/dL. In clinical scenarios in which a transudate is expected,

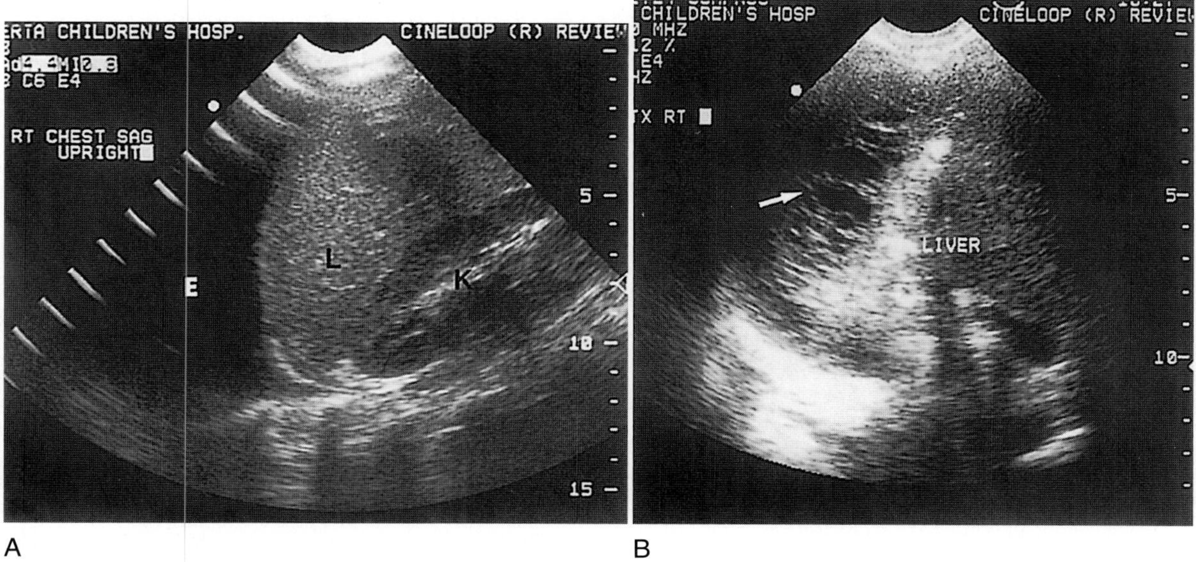

■ **FIGURE 21-9.** **A,** Sagittal sonogram of the lower right hemithorax and upper quadrant. A large anechoic right pleural effusion (E), the liver (L), and the kidney (K) are identified. This is the appearance of a nonloculated uncomplicated pleural effusion. **B,** Transverse sonogram of the right upper quadrant 6 days later demonstrates a lesion of mixed echogenicity *(arrow)* posterolateral to the liver, consistent with an empyema.

yet the pleural effusion is characterized as an exudate by Light's criteria, further biochemical analysis can be helpful. Serum and pleural fluid albumin levels will be substantially different in an exudate. In a transudate, the serum albumin level is greater than the pleural level by at least 1.2 mg/dL (12 g/L). At a minimum, pleural fluid levels of total protein, LDH, and glucose should be determined on all samples. Further, bacterial culture, cell count, and differential are required on all samples. The need for cytology and further biochemical analysis is dictated by the clinical scenario.

A red blood cell count of 5000 to 10,000/μL imparts a bloody appearance to the pleural fluid. Automated determination of the red blood cell count in pleural fluid is often inaccurate, possibly due to the confusing assortment of debris in the fluid. Blood in the pleural fluid due to thoracentesis tends to vary in intensity during the procedure. Further, platelets are present in pleural fluid obtained during a traumatic tap. Hemothorax is present if the hematocrit of the pleural fluid is more than 50% of the hematocrit of peripheral blood. In the absence of trauma, the usual causes of bloody pleural effusion include malignancy, lung infarction, and postpericardiotomy syndrome.

Obtaining the number and type of white blood cells in the pleural fluid assists in determining the etiology of effusion.[22,23] Eighty percent of transudates have white blood cell counts of up

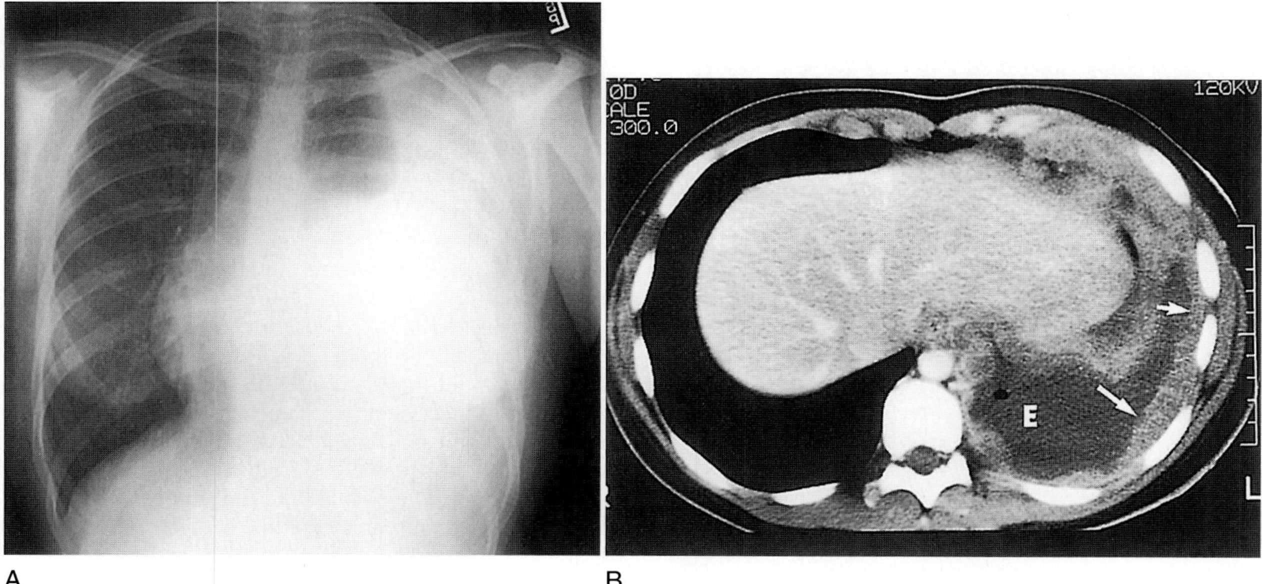

■ **FIGURE 21-10.** **A,** Posteroanterior erect chest radiograph illustrating a large left pleural effusion. The pleural fluid obscures evaluation of the underlying left lung. Mass effect, with shift of the mediastinum to the right, is noted. **B,** Axial enhanced computed tomography scan of the lower chest demonstrates a lobulated mass along the left pleural surface *(arrows)*, surrounding the left hydrothorax (E).

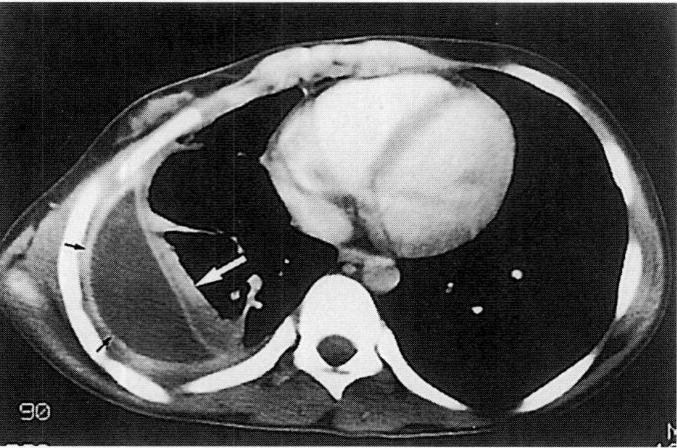

■ **FIGURE 21-11.** Axial enhanced computed tomography image of the chest. A loculated empyema with a peripheral enhancing rim *(small black arrows)* is identified within the lower right hemithorax. The rim is smooth in contour and of minimal thickness. Concomitant atelectasis of the adjacent lung is noted *(large white arrow)*.

to 1000/μL. Monocytes, lymphocytes, and macrophages are the predominant white blood cells in a transudate. Lymphoma and tuberculosis characteristically produce pleural effusions with white blood cell counts of less than 10,000/μL, of which approximately 85% are lymphocytes. Lymphocytes are also commonly seen in the pleural fluid of patients with sarcoidosis, chronic rheumatoid arthritis, chylothorax, and yellow nail syndrome. White blood cell counts in patients with parapneumonic effusion, empyema, acute pancreatitis, and lupus pleuritis are usually greater than 10,000/μL. Frank pus is due to the combination of leukocytes, fibrin, and cellular debris. Consequently, the white blood cell count of a grossly purulent effusion may be lower than expected. Eosinophilia, greater than 10% eosinophils, usually results from pleural injury and signifies recent hemothorax or pneumothorax. Pulmonary infarction, parasitic or fungal infection, and drug hypersensitivity reactions are other causes of eosinophilic pleural effusions. Basophils usually represent leukemic involvement of the pleura. Cytology of the pleural fluid is essential for an undiagnosed lymphocytic effusion, a basophilic effusion, or an exudate in the presence of malignancy at another site.

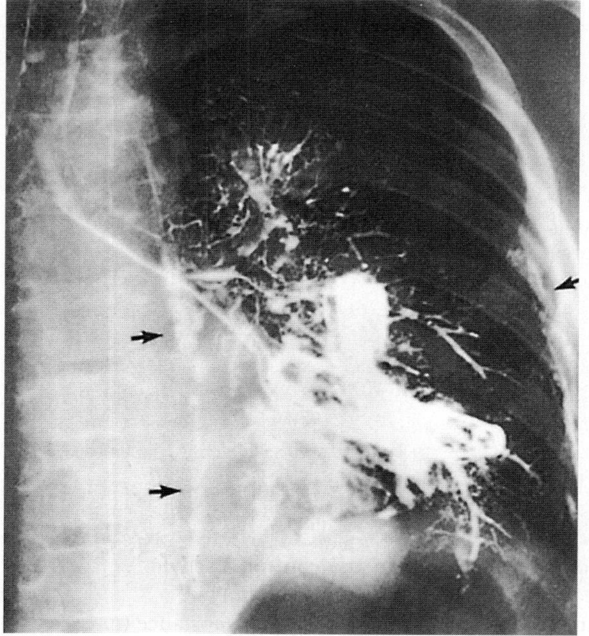

■ **FIGURE 21-12.** Pleurogram of a child with a bronchopleural fistula, demonstrating the contrast material in the pleural cavity *(arrows)* and airways. Lipiodol was injected through a chest tube.

BOX 21-1 Physical and Chemical Characteristics of Chyle

Sterile
Ingested lipophilic dyes stain the effusion
Cells are predominantly lymphocytes
Sudan stain shows fat globules
Total fat content exceeds that of plasma (e.g., ≤660 mg/dL)
Protein content is half of or the same as that of plasma (usually ≥3.0 g/dL)
Electrolyte count is the same as that of plasma
Blood urea nitrogen level is the same as that of plasma
Glucose level is the same as that of plasma

Biochemical analysis of a pleural effusion provides further information regarding its nature and etiology.[21,24] Moreover, pleural fluid pH that is greater than 7.45 or greater than blood pH is consistent with a transudate. Samples sent for pleural fluid pH should be handled, transported, and analyzed in the same way as arterial blood samples. Pleural fluid pH less than 7.30 occurs in the presence of increased carbon dioxide production (e.g., infection), acid leak into the pleural space (e.g., esophageal rupture), or a decrease in normal hydrogen ion transport from the pleural space (e.g., pleuritis, pleural fibrosis). The pH of the pleural fluid supplies prognostic information. It differentiates between causes of high pleural fluid amylase: pH less than 7.3 indicates esophageal rupture, and pH greater than 7.3 indicates pancreatitis. A nontuberculous parapneumonic effusion with a pH of less than 7.20 indicates a high probability of loculation. Pleural effusions with pH of less than 7.10, an LDH level of greater than 1000 IU/L, and a glucose level of less than 50% of blood glucose should be considered parapneumonic effusions. LDH levels provide additional information beyond the characterization of transudates or exudates. A high LDH level in the face of normal or near-normal levels of pleural fluid protein suggests malignancy or pleural infection. Pleural fluid glucose is less than 50% of blood values in cases of decreased transport to the pleural space or increased uptake. Empyema, tuberculosis, rheumatoid arthritis, lupus pleuritis, pancreatitis, malignancy, and esophageal rupture reduce pleural fluid glucose levels. All pleural fluid samples should be cultured appropriately, including tuberculosis and fungal cultures, in the proper clinical setting.

A chylous effusion is characterized by a normal pleural fluid/serum glucose concentration ratio (<0.5), the presence of chylomicrons, the presence of triglycerides, and an abundance of T lymphocytes. The pleural fluid pH is normal.[25]

Extravasated infusates or effusions secondary to peritoneal dialysis produce a characteristic biochemical picture. The milky appearance or color may be similar to that of the infusate. The pleural liquid glucose level is greater than the blood glucose level. Nevertheless, the pleural glucose level is less than that of the infusate due to active transport. Pleural liquid LDH levels

TABLE 21-3. Chemical separation of transudates and exudates*

	PLEURAL LIQUID CONCENTRATION		PLEURAL/SERUM CONCENTRATION RATIO	
Type of Effusion	**Protein**	**LDH**	**Protein**	**LDH**
Transudate	<3 g/dL	<2/3*	<0.5	<0.6
Exudate	≥3 g/dL	>2/3	≥0.5	≥0.6

*Pleural lactate dehydrogenase levels should be less than two thirds of the upper level of serum lactate dehydrogenase.

LDH, lactate dehydrogenase.

are low. The fluid may have a neutrophilic predominance or may be hemorrhagic, as shown by cell counts.

Pleuritis due to collagen vascular disease can be further evaluated by assays of the pleural fluid. Pleural fluid rheumatoid factor levels exceeding blood levels and pleural fluid titers greater than 1:320 are positive for rheumatoid arthritis. Similarly, pleural fluid antinuclear antibody titers of greater than 1:160, or greater than serum levels, are positive for lupus pleuritis.

PLEURAL BIOPSY

Parietal pleural biopsy is indicated in patients with unexplained inflammatory pleural effusion. This typically occurs in the context of malignancy; either as a primary cause or as a precursor for infection during periods of immunosuppression.[26] The procedure may be performed either percutaneously at the bedside with a specially designed needle, during thoracoscopy, or by open thoracotomy under general anesthesia. Although a variety of special cutting needles have been developed for bedside use, the majority of these procedures are now done in the operating room with thoracoscopy.

The specific needles used for percutaneous sampling, namely, the Cope, Abrams Ballestero, Vim-Silverman, and Harefield needles, vary slightly, but in general, obtain a sample of pleural tissue via a side-biting mechanism. The Harefield needle allows aspiration of liquid at the time of pleural biopsy. The tissue specimen includes portions of intercostal muscle and the adjoining parietal pleura. It is approximately 4 mm in diameter and is sent for histologic and culture studies. The liquid in the pleural space prevents the needle from puncturing the lung. Thus, biopsy is most easily accomplished at the time of initial thoracentesis, when there is the least chance of lacerating the underlying lung. The greatest value of percutaneous parietal biopsy is in clinical disorders that cause lymphocytic pleural effusions and widespread involvement of the pleural surface (e.g., tuberculosis, tumors).

MANAGEMENT OF NONINFLAMMATORY PLEURAL EFFUSIONS

Treatment of transudates and hemorrhagic and chylous pleural effusions is directed at supportive therapy of the functional disturbances and at specific management of the underlying disorder. Evacuation of a transudate after the initial diagnostic thoracentesis is indicated only for relief of dyspnea and other cardiorespiratory disturbances caused by mediastinal displacement. Intercostal tube drainage may be provided in lieu of repeated thoracenteses, depending on the child's tolerance of the procedures and the progression of the underlying disorder. Diuretics administered to some patients may slow reaccumulation of the transudate and may decrease or eliminate the need for frequent thoracentesis. Specific treatment of the underlying disorder emphasizes the need for thorough history taking and meticulous physical examination to arrive promptly at an accurate clinical diagnosis. Cardiovascular and renal causes (e.g., congestive heart failure, nephrosis) and lymphatic disorders that cause inappropriate lymphatic flow are managed accordingly. Pleural transudates due to fluid overload (e.g., from intravenous infusion) or overload of lymphatic drainage (e.g., ascites, peritoneal dialysis) may require only diuresis or may resolve spontaneously.

The treatment of hemothorax associated with shock requires immediate expansion of the vascular volume and direct surgical repair of bleeding vessels. In general, a requirement for blood transfusion of more than 20 mL/kg or ongoing blood loss of greater than 3 mL/kg/hr is an indication for immediate thoracotomy. Smaller bleeds should be evacuated, because healing may be associated with pleural adhesions. Fibrinolytic enzymes instilled into the pleural cavity may help if clots have formed. Chest pain is relieved by analgesics.

Chylothorax poses unique problems in management.[27,28] Immediate thoracentesis is required for life-threatening cardiorespiratory embarrassment. In the absence of a life-threatening situation, the initial treatment of neonatal and most cases of postsurgical or traumatic chylothorax includes: (1) single thoracentesis, with complete drainage of chyle; (2) nutritional support; and (3) close surveillance of the patient's nutritional status and immune competency. Flow through the thoracic duct must be reduced enough to allow the defect to heal. The use of a medium-chain triglyceride diet, with avoidance of fatty meals containing long-chain fatty acids, significantly reduces lymph flow (up to tenfold) because medium-chain triglycerides are absorbed directly into the portal venous blood and contribute little to chylomicron formation. Cessation of chylous effusion should occur by the end of the second week of treatment. However, even with the use of medium-chain triglycerides and avoidance of long-chain fatty acids, there may still be substantial flow through the thoracic duct and continued development of the chylothorax. Discontinuation of oral feeding and the use of total parenteral nutrition are often required. Vitamin supplements are added to avoid deficiency states. No surgical treatment is permitted for 4 to 5 weeks to allow sufficient time for closure of lymphatic channel fistulas. With the foregoing therapeutic program, most patients respond favorably, with progressive weight gain and cessation of the chylothorax.[29] The use of intravenous somatostatin or octreotide has shown some promise in assisting in the control of chylothorax. In the few treatment-resistant cases, thoracotomy is required. Giving the patient a small amount of a high-fat substance (e.g., cream) preoperatively assists in the detection of the thoracic duct defect at thoracotomy. Rarely, chylothorax is due to lymphangiomatosis involving the ribs. In these cases, abnormalities are detected on chest radiograph, and there is little response to the dietary manipulations discussed earlier.

MANAGEMENT OF EXUDATES AND EMPYEMA

Inflammation of the pleural membranes (e.g., pleurisy, pleuritis) is usually a consequence of diseases elsewhere in the body and, rarely, of disturbances residing primarily in the pleura. The inciting process may be infection, neoplasm, trauma, pulmonary vascular obstruction, systemic granulomatous disease, or a generalized inflammatory disorder affecting the serous membranes. Table 21-4 classifies clinical disorders that may cause pleurisy and empyema according to the original site and nature of the inciting process. Infection from adjacent pulmonary and subdiaphragmatic foci reaches the pleura by contiguous spread. Bacteria occasionally reach the pleural cavity via a bronchopleural fistula, through a traumatic breach of the chest wall, or by way of the circulation from distant sites of suppuration. Trauma after certain diagnostic and therapeutic cardiothoracic procedures irritates the pleura, which may become secondarily infected. Pulmonary embolism (thrombus, fat, or gas) results in focal parenchymal necrosis that spreads to involve the pleural surface, causing pleurisy, with or without effusion. Connective tissue disorders, such as systemic lupus erythematosus and rheumatoid arthritis, may involve the pleura as part of the more widespread inflammatory process.

Primary neoplasms of the pleura, including benign and malignant mesothelioma, are rare causes of exudative pleural effusions in children. Metastatic involvement of the pleura may arise directly from pulmonary parenchymal lesions or through contiguous spread of a metastatic lung lesion. Neoplastic masses may obstruct the lymphatic channels, decreasing the removal of proteins from the pleural space. Pleural irritation may occur after certain diagnostic procedures (e.g., needle aspiration of the lung, percutaneous pleural biopsy) or therapeutic interventions (e.g., radiation therapy for mediastinal malignancy, cardiothoracic surgery). Fortunately, the risk of occurrence of secondary purulent pleurisy due to medical intervention is low.

Thoracoabdominal infections are the major origin of pleurisy with effusion.[29,30] Up to 20% of children with viral and *Mycoplasma* pneumonia have effusions. These are usually transient and of minor importance.[31,32] On occasion, however, the effusions may be massive and cause respiratory distress, necessitating prompt drainage, or they may be recalcitrant and cause prolonged morbidity in infants with concurrent malnutrition. Nonetheless, the effusions do not become loculated.

Pulmonary tuberculosis usually causes fibrinous, or "dry," pleurisy until the caseous materials containing the tuberculous antigen leak into the pleura via the pleural circulation.[33] Considerable effusion then occurs as a result of the specific allergic reaction of the pleural membranes. The onset of effusion is within 6 months of the primary infection, coincident with the development of cell-mediated immunity.[34] The cellular character of the exudate is lymphocytic. Effusion is usually on the side of the primary parenchymal focus. Bilateral effusions indicate hematogenous dissemination from a remote focus. Frank tuberculous empyema is rare, occurring in only approximately 2% of cases of tuberculous pleurisy, particularly those complicated by bronchopleural fistula.

Nontuberculous bacterial pneumonias are the most frequent origin of inflammatory pleural effusions, or parapneumonic effusions.[35–37] Such an effusion may loculate owing to pleural adhesions, or may be purulent. Box 21-2 lists, in order of descending prevalence, the predominant aerobic and anaerobic isolates of empyema. The opportunity to establish a specific etiologic agent depends on the patient's age, the nature of the underlying disease, the laboratory culture methods used, and the timing of the initiation of antimicrobial therapy. *Staphylococcus aureus* is the single most common pathogen causing empyema in infants younger than 2 years of age. Superficial skin lesions, osteomyelitis, and cystic fibrosis are other conditions associated with staphylococcal empyema. *Haemophilus influenzae* type b is now an infrequent causative agent for empyema, due to the widespread use of immunization. *Streptococcus pneumococcus* is commonly responsible for empyema. Group A streptococcus has reemerged as a significant agent that causes empyema in later childhood and adolescence. Antimicrobial therapy for community-acquired loculated parapneumonic effusion must provide coverage for these agents.[38] Additional coverage for gram-negative infections should be considered in children with nosocomial pneumonia, particularly that caused by *Pseudomonas aeruginosa*.

TABLE 21-4. Etiologic spectrum of pleurisy and empyema

Origin and Nature of Inflammation	Clinical Examples
Primary in the Pleura	
Neoplasm	Primary pleural mesothelioma
Trauma	After cardiothoracic surgery, lung aspiration and percutaneous pleural biopsy, thoracic irradiation therapy
Contiguous Structures	
Lung infection	Pneumonia (aerobic and anaerobic bacterial, tuberculous, fungal, viral, mycoplasmal, echinococcal), bronchopleural fistula
Chest wall and subdiaphragmatic infection	Chest wall contusion and abscess, intra-abdominal abscess (subphrenic and hepatic), acute hemorrhagic pancreatitis, pancreaticopleural fistula
Mediastinal infection and neoplasm	Acute mediastinitis (secondary to esophageal rupture), mediastinal tumors
Systemic Diseases	
Septicemia	Distant sites of suppuration
Malignancy	Lymphoma, leukemia, neuroblastoma, hepatoma, multiple myeloma
Vascular obstruction	Pulmonary infarction
Connective tissue or collagen disorder	Systemic lupus erythematosus, polyarteritis, Wegener's granulomatosis, rheumatoid arthritis, scleroderma, rheumatic fever
Granulomatous disease	Sarcoidosis

BOX 21-2 Bacteriology of Nontuberculous Empyema

Aerobic Bacteria

Streptococcus pneumoniae
Staphylococcus aureus
Streptococcus pyogenes
Haemophilus influenzae type b
Escherichia coli
Klebsiella species
Pseudomonas aeruginosa

Anaerobic Bacteria

Microaerophilic streptococci
Fusobacterium nucleatum
Bacteroides melaninogenicus
Bacteroides fragilis
Peptococcus
Peptostreptococcus
Catalase-negative, non-spore-forming, gram-positive bacilli

Anaerobic pleuropulmonary infections, which are uncommon in children, have distinctive clinical characteristics. More than 90% of patients have periodontal infections, altered consciousness, and dysphagia.[39] Aspiration of a large volume of oropharyngeal secretions occurs in the presence of disturbed clearing mechanisms. It is therefore not surprising that the three predominant pleural anaerobic isolates—microaerophilic streptococci, *Fusobacterium nucleatum*, and *Bacteroides melaninogenicus*—compose the normal flora of the upper respiratory tract and that the primary pulmonary disease (e.g., lung abscess, necrotizing pneumonia) is usually located in gravity-dependent lung segments. The clinical course is generally insidious and indolent. Mediastinal and subdiaphragmatic foci of infection are also common sites of origin for anaerobic empyema.

Except for septicemia from contiguous or distant sites of suppuration, the systemic origins of pleurisy generally produce nonpurulent effusion. Effusion secondary to pulmonary embolism of venous thrombi, fat, or gas is rare in childhood, although it may be a serious consequence of malignancy. Pleurisy may be associated with connective tissue disorders, such as lupus erythematosus and rheumatoid arthritis, and in this case, it is part of a more widespread inflammatory process.

In summary, various clinical disorders resulting from a myriad of inflammatory origins can induce pleurisy and empyema. Certain clinical settings are distinctive for specific bacterial isolates. Treatment of inflammatory pleural disorders is aimed at specific management of the underlying cause as well as relief of functional disturbances caused by the inciting clinical disorder, associated pleural involvement, and concurrent complications. Therapy is both medical and surgical. A prompt, specific etiologic diagnosis is optimal for management.

General supportive measures include bed rest for the acutely ill child and appropriate analgesia. Fluid management must be sufficient to replace increased losses due to fever and tachypnea. Supplemental oxygen should be administered to the child with hypoxia or increased work of breathing. It is imperative to recognize that irritability may be due to pain, high fever, distressing cough, or hypoxia. Lying on the affected side may provide temporary relief by splinting the involved thorax.

The development of effusion after "dry" pleurisy usually provides relief from pain. However, accumulation of an excessive amount of pleural liquid necessitates thoracentesis to relieve dyspnea. Repeated thoracentesis and, eventually, continuous chest tube drainage are indicated if rapid reaccumulation of effusion induces dyspnea and dominates the clinical picture, as commonly occurs in neoplasm. Although most effusions due to a noninfectious inflammatory process require only drainage to relieve dyspnea, additional specific measures may be indicated in the presence of certain underlying systemic diseases. Systemic and intrapleural instillation of chemotherapeutic agents and mediastinal irradiation of the involved nodes or primary tumor sites are used to control pleural effusion in lymphoma. Prednisone ameliorates dyspnea as well as cough, anorexia, and weight loss in sarcoidosis. Corticosteroids increase the rate at which tuberculous effusion resolves and fever returns to normal, but definitive proof of their value on eventual ventilatory function has not been shown. If steroids are to be used to help alleviate dyspnea, concomitant antituberculous chemotherapy is essential. Tuberculous effusions usually clear within 6 months of treatment with isoniazid, rifampin, and pyrazinamide. Asymptomatic noninfectious pleural exudates require only management of the underlying disorder. Improvement in the underlying systemic disease is paralleled by resolution of the accompanying pleural exudate.

Pleural effusions due to infection require specific antimicrobial treatment and certain surgical considerations. Significant early morbidity and mortality rates are associated with uncontrolled infection of the pleural space. The management of loculated parapneumonic effusions is variable and evolving with the development of new surgical modalities.[40–44] The principal underlying treatment is to control and evacuate infection and balance the benefits of treatment with the risks and complications. Hence, treatment approaches must be individualized based on the child's current condition and preexisting health status and the characteristics of the pleural fluid. Parenteral antimicrobial therapy is required. The initial choice of antimicrobial agents is based on the clinical data, the bacterial epidemiology in the community, and the known pharmacologic properties of the drugs. Dosage must be adequate, and initial administration should be by the intravenous route. Infection may be polymicrobial, so more than one antimicrobial drug must be given initially. Subsequent changes in antimicrobial coverage are guided by the results of culture and sensitivity tests. A guide to antimicrobial therapy for nontuberculous bacterial pleurisy and empyema is presented in Table 21-5. Physicians must always be aware of the potential side effects of the drugs on various target organs and must be prepared to use alternative drugs, if necessary. Unlike adults, children with empyema usually do not have the long-term sequelae of fibrothorax or trapped lung.[45–48] Children, regardless of the interventions used or avoided, do not have long-term sequelae. Management decisions revolve around strategies to promote prompt control of infection and resolution of respiratory compromise.

Removal of infected pleural fluids should be considered in all cases. Thoracentesis is performed to relieve dyspnea during the acute stage, and is repeated as required; it may be all that is necessary for free-moving effusions with pH greater than 7.20. When the fluid is still mobile and is not loculated, diagnostic

TABLE 21-5. A guide to antimicrobial therapy for bacterial pleurisy and empyema

Infecting Agent	Drug and Dosage (per Kilogram per Day) Route and Duration*
A. Aerobic bacteria	
1. Staphylococci	a. Cloxacillin, 100–200 mg, divided in 3–6 doses, IV initially, for 3–4 weeks
	b. Clindamycin, 24–40 mg/kg, divided in 3–4 doses
2. *Haemophilus influenzae*	a. Cefotaxime, 200 mg/kg, maximum of 8 g/day divided in 4 doses
	or
	b. Ceftriaxone, 80–100 mg/kg, divided in 1–2 doses
	or
	c. Chloramphenicol, 50–100 mg/kg, divided in 4 doses
3. Pneumococcus and streptococci	Penicillin G, 250,000–400,000 units/kg, divided in 4–6 doses
4. *Escherichia coli* and *Klebsiella*	Cefotaxime, same as A.2.a.
5. *Pseudomonas aeruginosa*	a. Ticarcillin, 200–300 mg/kg, divided in 4–6 doses
	or
	b. Ceftazidime, 30–50 mg/kg, maximum of 6 g/day divided in 3 doses with
	c. Tobramycin, 5–7 mg/kg, divided in 3 doses
B. Anaerobic bacteria†	
1. *Bacteroides fragilis*	Clindamycin, 24–40 mg/kg, divided in 3–4 doses
2. All except *B. fragilis*	a. Same as B.1
	or
	Penicillin G, same as A.3.

*The lower dose in the dosage range and less frequent intervals of administration are recommended for neonates.
†The duration of therapy for anaerobic pneumonitis requires an adjustment if the lung lesions go on to cavitate. Often 6 to 12 weeks of therapy is required before the lung lesions clear or only a small, stable residual lesion is left.

IV, intravenously; kg, kilogram body weight.

thoracentesis can also be therapeutic. An attempt should be made to remove as much fluid as possible. The technique for thoracentesis is as previously described, with important modifications. The initial thoracentesis should be performed with a large-bore intravenous catheter. A large-bore needle is required for drainage of thick secretions. However, a large-bore needle increases the risk of trauma to the chest wall and lung. The provision of appropriate sedation and analgesia is paramount to successful initial drainage of infected fluid. Consultation with anesthesia colleagues is important to ensure that appropriate analgesia, sedation, and patient monitoring are provided for the procedure. Immediate closed-tube thoracostomy is indicated when examination shows frank pus in the pleural fluid, a positive Gram stain, pH less than 7.20 or more than 0.05 units below arterial pH, or massive effusion associated with overwhelming sepsis. Application of negative pressure to the tube enhances obliteration of the empyema space and reexpansion of the lung. A thoracostomy tube has a larger bore than an intravenous catheter and, theoretically, improves drainage from the pleural space. The vast majority of pleural drainage occurs in the first 12 to 24 hours. An empyema or a parapneumonic effusion can loculate within 24 to 48 hours of the initiation of appropriate antibiotics. Once the pleural fluid is loculated, further attempts at thoracentesis or chest tube drainage are fruitless, and the benefits of instrumenting the pleural space must be weighed carefully with the risks. If the child is responding to antibiotic therapy, with improved appetite, increased energy level, and defervescence, then surgical intervention is not required. The child with ongoing respiratory compromise and constitutional symptoms should be considered for video-assisted thoracoscopic surgery. In some centers, the safety and tolerability of video-assisted thoracoscopic surgery has lead to earlier introduction of surgery to evacuate the pleural space. Another option is the use of streptokinase or urokinase to lyse pleural adhesions and promote tube thoracostomy drainage. The usual method with urokinase is age dependent. For children under the age of 1 year, 10,000 units in 10 mL normal saline is instilled through the chest tube, and for children over 1 year of age, 40,000 units in 40 mL normal saline is used. The drug is administered twice daily with 4 hour dwell time for 3 days.[49] With specific parenteral antimicrobial therapy and timely provision of appropriate pleural drainage, patients should recover completely from an episode of bacterial pleurisy and empyema. Invasive procedures, such as thoracotomy and decortication, are rarely required. Symptoms usually resolve in stages, with improved energy and appetite preceding the resolution of fever. Once chest drainage is less than 30 mL/day and the patient's constitutional symptoms have improved, the chest tube may be removed. Intravenous antibiotics should be used until the constitutional symptoms have resolved for several days. The total duration of antibiotic administration, intravenous and oral, is at least 3 to 4 weeks. Findings on chest radiograph will resolve slowly, lagging behind clinical improvement. The clinician must take care to follow radiographic improvement in a child who is asymptomatic. Obtaining occasional chest radiographs to follow the resolution of empyema is appropriate. Residual pleural thickening will be present on chest radiographs taken 6 months after the acute event. As long as the child is asymptomatic, infrequent imaging to follow resolution of empyema is appropriate.

PROGNOSIS

The outlook in inflammatory pleural disorders depends on the nature of the underlying clinical problem, the nature and extent of pleural disease, the age of the patient, the timing of the initiation of therapy, and the occurrence of complications. Noninfectious pleurisy and effusions resolve with resolution of the underlying systemic problem. Malignant pleurisy carries an extremely grave prognosis, whereas viral and *Mycoplasma* pleural diseases generally resolve spontaneously with time. Patients with empyema have a more prolonged and complicated hospital course and may require longer follow-up after returning home than do patients with nonempyemic, free-moving pleural liquid. Parapneumonic effusions and empyema still produce significant morbidity and mortality. Only 30 years ago, the mortality rate associated with empyema approximated 100%. Most recent series report case fatality rates of 6% to 12%, with the highest rates among infants younger than 1 year of age. Prompt and adequate therapy during the acute phase should result in complete recovery. Complications, such as bronchopleural fistula and tension pneumatocele, are rare, but may delay full recovery. Fibrothorax is extremely rare. In contrast to adults, infants and children have a remarkable ability to resolve pleural thickening, with no effect on subsequent lung growth and function.

AIR IN THE PLEURAL SPACE

ETIOLOGY AND PATHOGENESIS

Intrapleural accumulation of air (pneumothorax) ensues whenever the pleural space has a free communication with the atmosphere, either from a chest wall defect through the parietal pleura or from alveolar rupture. Rarely, pneumothorax results from infection with gas-producing microorganisms. A chest wall defect can result from surgical procedures or from a penetrating injury from a missile or projectile.[50] Thoracic trauma, including compressive blunt injury caused by vehicular accidents, falls, and external cardiac massage, can rupture the lung. Infants and children are prone to internal injury from blunt trauma because of the greater compressibility of the chest wall. Thus, laceration or transection of major airways may accompany chest trauma, even without fractured rib fragments or obvious external injury.

Fundamentally, three factors determine the extent of alveolar distention: (1) the degree of transpulmonary pressure exerted, (2) the duration of pressure applied, and (3) the ratio of inexpansible to expansible portions of the lung.[51] Alterations of these factors, with concomitant lung rupture, can occur during the patient's own respiratory efforts. More commonly, lung rupture occurs during resuscitation and artificial ventilation and in the presence of incomplete obstruction of the airways and parenchymal consolidation, seen in a variety of diseases of the lower respiratory tract. Positive intra-alveolar inflation pressure increases air volume, but decreases blood volume in the adjacent vessels. Given this disproportionate change in blood volume and air volume, the tissue that tethers the perivascular sheath to the alveolar wall tends to attenuate. Because the mechanical forces in the alveolar wall and the tethering elements are angular to each other, rupture of the base of the alveoli occurs when critical shear or traction force is exceeded, allowing gas to escape into the perivascular space. The escaping air dissects along perivascular planes centrifugally, to the hilum, where it ruptures into the mediastinum (pneumomediastinum) and then through the visceral pleura, into the pleural space (Fig. 21-13). Alternatively, when under tension in the interstitial space, air may rupture directly through the visceral pleura, into the pleural space. When the air leak is confined to the interstitium, the condition is known as *pulmonary interstitial emphysema* (Fig. 21-14). When under sufficient pressure, air may dissect out of the thorax, along subcutaneous tissue planes (subcutaneous emphysema), or into the peritoneal cavity (pneumoperitoneum) [Fig. 21-15].[52] Air may become loculated in lobar fissures to produce pulmonary pseudocysts. Less commonly, air that ruptures into the mediastinum may dissect into the pericardial space (pneumopericardium). Box 21-3 lists the clinical entities that result from air leak due to lung rupture.

In the neonatal period, lung rupture can result from prolongation of the high transpulmonary pressure required during the first few breaths to inflate an airless lung, which opens sequentially. Prolonged application of high transpulmonary pressure across the normally aerated portions of the lung occurs because some of the airways may be occluded by aspirated blood, mucus, meconium, or squamous epithelium. The incidence of symptomatic spontaneous pneumothorax in the newborn period is approximately 0.5%, whereas a radiographic survey of neonates detected an incidence of approximately 3%. The newborn is particularly susceptible to uneven alveolar distention because the pores of Kohn, which normally allow interalveolar air distribution, are underdeveloped.

Hyaline membrane disease, with multiple areas of atelectasis, can also lead to rupture of alveoli. The incidence of air leak in hyaline membrane disease varies, depending on the severity of lung disease, peak and end-expiratory pressures, and the use of exogenous surfactant therapy.

The pathogenesis of pneumothorax in the older child can be disease-specific.[53] Parenchymal necrosis adjacent to the visceral pleura produces a small tear in the pleural membrane. In cavitary or progressive tuberculosis, subpleural caseous infiltrates undergo liquefaction, resulting in pleural necrosis and rupture. Although an inflammatory response is elicited that attempts to seal off the rupture, bronchopleural fistula often persists. Pneumothorax that is sometimes seen in miliary pulmonary tuberculosis is unexplained. Pulmonary metastases of a sarcoma have been postulated to grow very rapidly, outgrow their blood supply, and become necrotic, rupturing the bronchus and pleural space and creating a bronchopleural fistula. Alternatively, tumor emboli cause lung infarction, necrosis, and, eventually, air leak.

Alternatively, disruption of the visceral pleura may occur in the presence of parenchymal overdistention. Primary or metastatic pulmonary tumor may cause lung rupture by ball-valve obstruction of an airway. In cystic fibrosis, pneumothorax results from rupture of subpleural blebs and large bullae as a result of chronic air trapping in patients with long-standing, more advanced obstructive lung disease. Rupture of blebs and bullae usually occurs during exacerbation of pulmonary infection. In asthma, it is postulated that the visceral pleura is thinner and thus has increased susceptibility to rupture at transpulmonary pressures that would not allow rupture under normal circumstances. Moreover, mucoid impaction may be associated with expiratory obstruction, leading to overdistention and rupture of alveoli. Normally, alveoli in the upper lobes are more distended than those in dependent lung regions. This distention is accentuated in tall individuals, and may appear on CT scan as an area of cystic dilation of the apical airspaces. Spontaneous pneumothorax, with or without these physical "blebs," is most common in tall, lean individuals (e.g., Marfan's syndrome) [Fig. 21-16].

FUNCTIONAL PATHOLOGY

Regardless of the age of the patient and the underlying cause of pneumothorax, massive or continued air leak elevates the intrapleural pressure to above atmospheric pressure, a condition known as *tension pneumothorax*. The ipsilateral lung collapses

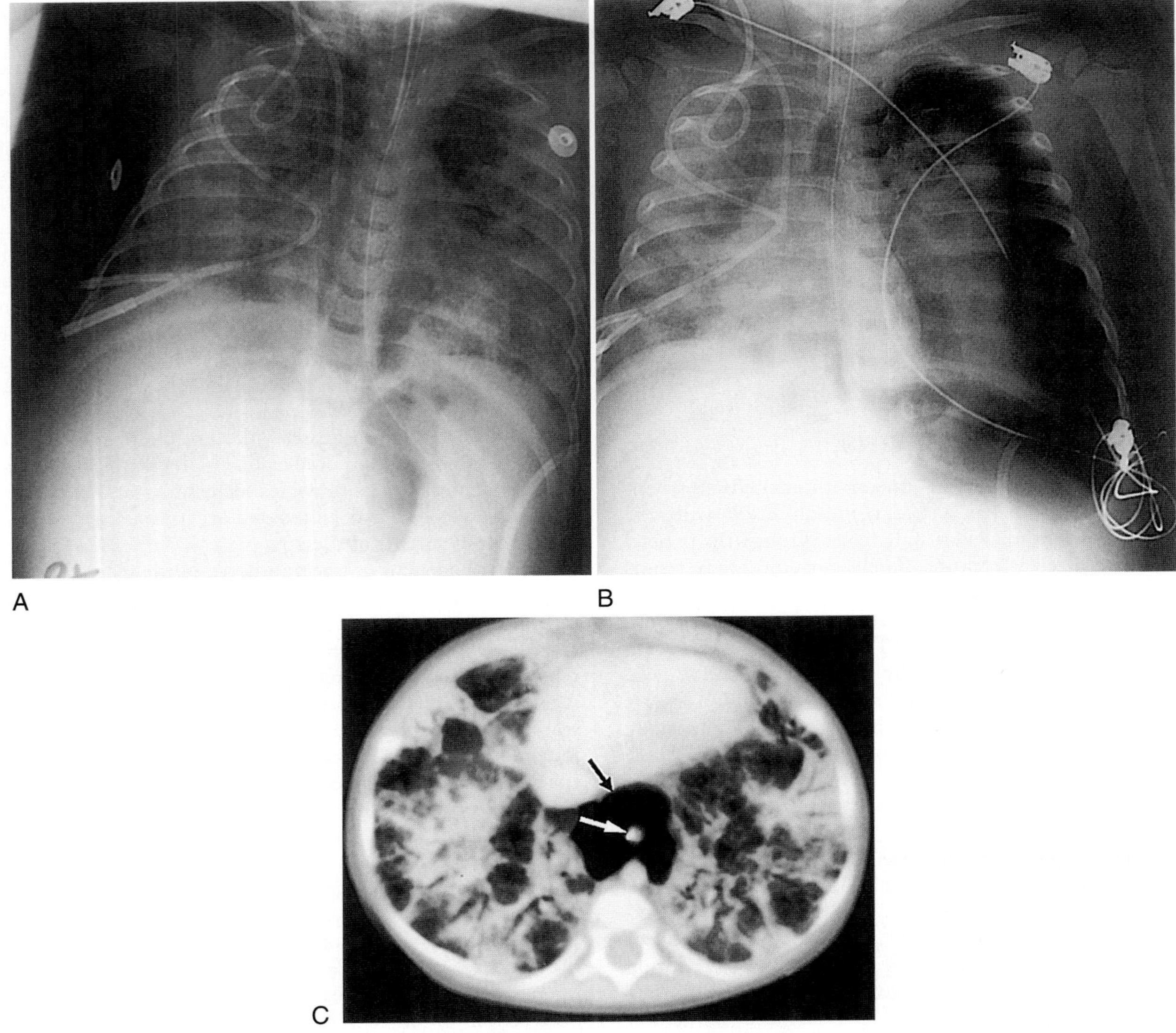

■ **FIGURE 21-13. A,** Anteroposterior chest radiograph in a patient with acute myelocytic leukemia and acute respiratory distress syndrome (ARDS). A large pneumomediastinum is evident from the hyperlucency overlying the thoracic vertebrae. **B,** Chest radiograph 1 day later demonstrates a large left tension pneumothorax and increasing pneumomediastinum, highlighting the left border of the heart. **C,** Enhanced axial chest computed tomography using lung windows demonstrates diffuse alveolar opacities throughout both lungs, consistent with ARDS, and a large pneumomediastinum, as depicted by the air *(black arrow)* encircling the esophagus *(white arrow).*

because its elastic recoil can no longer be counteracted by the outward pull of a previously subatmospheric pleural pressure. The contralateral lung is overexpanded during inspiration, and as a result, greater retractive force develops, pulling the mediastinum toward it during expiration and impeding venous return to the heart. Because ventilation is impaired, greater inspiratory efforts develop in an attempt to generate sufficient negative pleural pressure to ventilate the normal lung, aggravating the tension pneumothorax, shifting the mediastinum further, and severely impeding systemic venous return to the heart. Hypoxemia and hypercapnia result. Compensatory tachycardia occurs and further decreases diastolic filling and ventricular output, with cardiac standstill imminent unless pulmonary tamponade is decompressed. Lung collapse per se does not contribute in a major way to poor gas exchange because there is redistribution of pulmonary blood flow to the normal lung, which will have lower vascular resistance.

In addition to the intrapleural pressure that develops and the inherent elastic recoil of the lung, the degree of lung collapse also varies with the cause of pneumothorax and the presence of visceroparietal adhesions. Chronic lung disease that decreases lung elastic recoil and concomitant pleural adhesions prevents total collapse.

HISTORY AND PHYSICAL EXAMINATION

Symptoms of pneumothorax vary according to the extent of lung collapse, the degree of intrapleural pressure, the rapidity of onset, and the age and respiratory reserve of the patient. A patient may have sudden cardiorespiratory collapse without

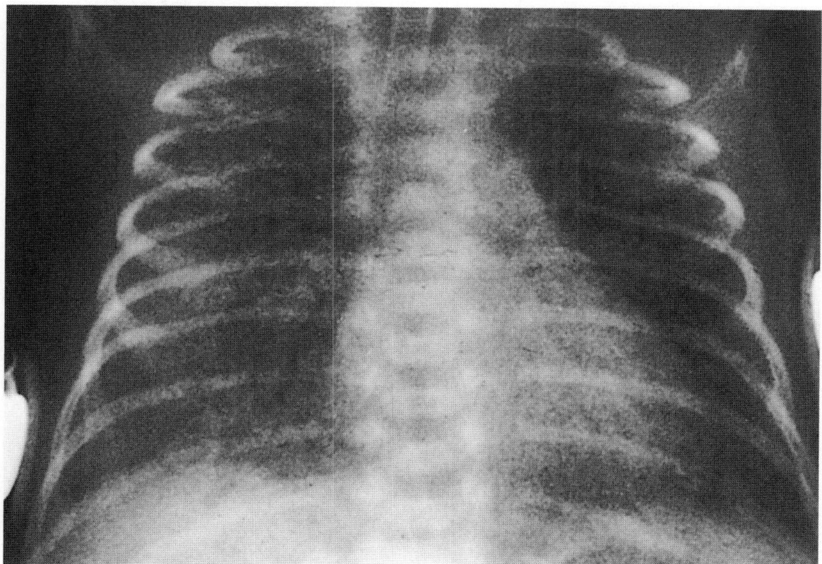

■ **FIGURE 21-14.** **A,** Chest radiograph of a neonate with hyaline membrane disease, demonstrating interstitial emphysema of the right lung.

clinical warning or antecedent roentgenographic changes, or may be asymptomatic, with the diagnosis made initially on the basis of chest roentgenogram. Early recognition of lung rupture requires keen awareness of its possibility, particularly in patients with conditions known to be associated with this complication (Box 21-4). Pneumothorax may also be a spontaneous event, unrelated to any known cause, particularly in the newborn infant.

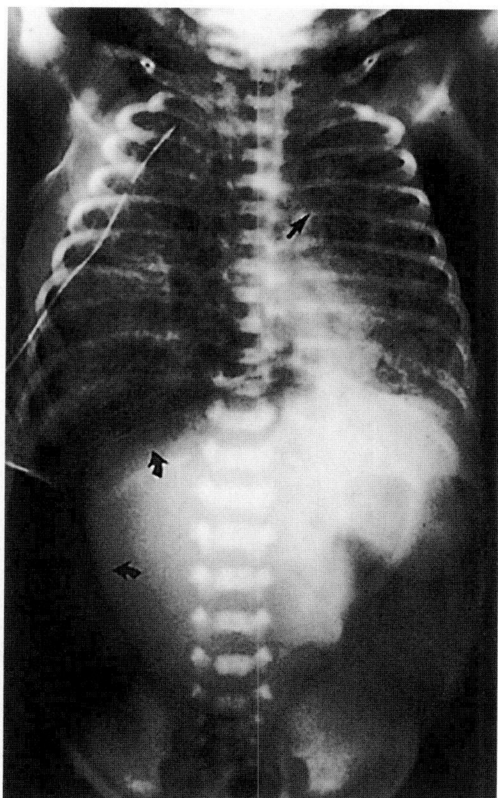

■ **FIGURE 21-15.** Chest radiograph of a neonate with hyaline membrane disease, demonstrating pneumomediastinum *(straight arrow)*, massive subcutaneous emphysema, and pneumoperitoneum that is pushing the liver down *(curved arrows)*.

In an otherwise normal neonate, symptoms of spontaneous pneumothorax are often subtle, and physical findings are misleading because no abnormalities may be immediately discernible. Certain clinical features, however, have been seen on close observation: (1) the infant is unusually irritable; (2) tachypnea with a respiratory rate greater than 60 breaths/min is invariably seen; and (3) chest bulging is usually noticeable, especially with unilateral pneumothorax. A shift of the cardiac impulse away from the site of pneumothorax is a useful sign, but often, it cannot be detected confidently. It is also difficult to identify diminished air entry on the ipsilateral side because of the small size of the newborn chest. Grunting, retraction, and cyanosis are noted late in the progression of the complication.

In a newborn with underlying lung disease requiring mechanical respiratory assistance, certain observations are useful to note. Sudden deterioration, accompanied by decreased compliance of the respiratory system and the need for increased inspiratory pressure, suggests a diagnosis of tension pneumothorax, which necessitates prompt needle decompression. Changes in vital signs include decreases in heart rate, blood pressure, and respiratory rate, and narrowing of pulse pressure. An ominous clinical presentation is cardiorespiratory arrest. Even when deterioration is gradual, auscultation is often unreliable, because breath sounds from the remaining expansible areas of the lungs are clearly transmitted across the small newborn chest during mechanical ventilation. Serial chest roentgenograms taken at least daily are essential during the early phase of ventilatory treatment of the newborn, even in the absence of clinical signs of pneumothorax, because these signs can occur without warning. Moreover, in the presence of interstitial emphysema, pneumomediastinum, or hyperlucency of any lung zone, particularly when the infant is receiving continuous distending pressure, the clinician must be alert to the increased threat of impending serious air leak and pneumothorax.

Although certain limitations of physical examination of the chest have been alluded to, periodic physical reappraisal remains important, and must be done whenever a patient shows clinical

BOX 21-3 Clinical Spectrum of Air Leak Phenomena Secondary to Rupture of Alveoli

Interstitial emphysema
Pneumomediastinum
Pneumothorax
Subcutaneous emphysema
Pneumoperitoneum
Pneumopericardium
Pulmonary pseudocyst
Pulmonary venous gas embolism

worsening, deterioration in arterial gas tensions, or both. Additional nonroentgenographic tools for monitoring infants for pneumothorax in high-risk situations (e.g., in hyaline membrane disease or meconium aspiration, during mechanical ventilation) should be used; they include continuous electrocardiographic display on the oscilloscope[54] and intermittent electrocardiographic recordings. A sudden decrease (≥40%) or variability in the QRS voltage in the left precordial lead and standard leads I, II, and III suggests pneumothorax. Care must be taken to avoid misdiagnosis as a result of electronic artifacts, such as a change in standardization. Chest transillumination with a powerful fiberoptic light probe has been effectively applied to the diagnosis of pneumothorax at the bedside, and has a distinct advantage. These techniques allow for more focused use of the chest radiograph in following these patients.

Roentgenographic confirmation is essential when the physical findings are minimal and cardiorespiratory function is only modestly altered. An anteroposterior chest film supplemented by a horizontal beam cross-table lateral view, with the patient supine or in the decubitus position, can detect even relatively small amounts of intrapleural or mediastinal air. Pneumothorax must be differentiated from lung cyst and lobar emphysema. In both of these conditions, the lower border of the radiolucency is crescentic; in addition, attenuated lung markings may appear lateral to this line. A congenital diaphragmatic hernia is readily identified in the following way: a nasogastric tube with a radiopaque tip is used for decompression and left in place while a radiograph is taken; if the radiograph shows the tip in the thoracic cavity, then a diaphragmatic hernia is present.

In an older child, certain conditions, including bronchiolitis, asthma, cystic fibrosis, pertussis syndrome, hydatid cyst, progressive primary pulmonary tuberculosis, metastatic sarcoma, staphylococcal pneumonia, and blunt thoracic injury, alert the clinician to the risk of pneumothorax. The diagnosis is suspected when a patient has sudden, severe cardiorespiratory collapse, or less seriously, shallow breathing and sudden pain in the chest or referred to the shoulder. Contributory factors include frequent paroxysms of cough, severe underlying lung disease, and the use of a respirator. Pneumothorax is not as difficult to detect in older children as it is in the newborn because abnormal physical findings are easier to detect in the older child. Nonetheless, in children with diffuse, obstructive lung disorders, the physical signs of the underlying disease may be similar to those of pneumothorax, and may be unchanged by the development

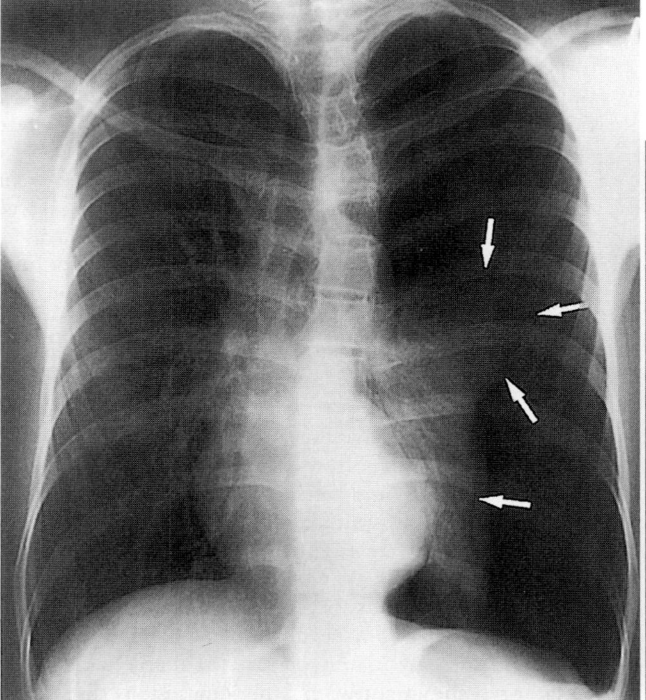
A

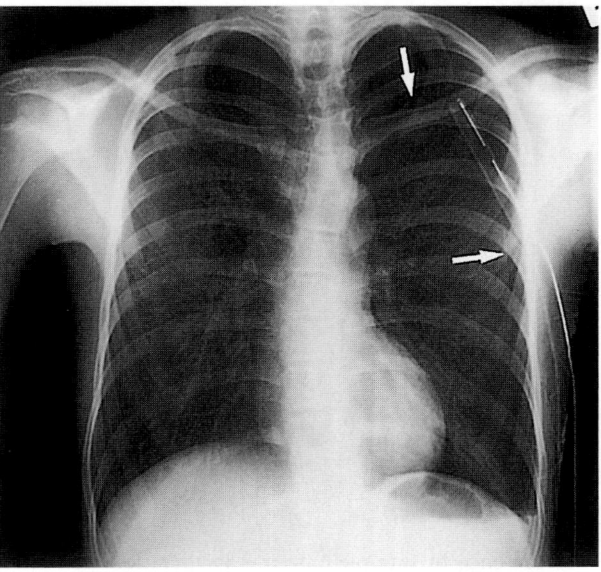
B

■ **FIGURE 21-16.** **A,** Posteroanterior chest radiograph demonstrating a spontaneous left tension pneumothorax, with shift of the cardiac silhouette and the mediastinum to the right. The left hemidiaphragm is flattened. The left lung is completely collapsed. **B,** Posteroanterior chest radiograph after insertion of a chest tube on the left shows a residual moderately sized pneumothorax. A small bleb is identified along the superior aspect of the left upper lobe. This patient has Marfan's syndrome. *Arrows* on each film indicate lung margins.

BOX 21-4 Conditions Associated with Alveolar Rupture

First breath
Diagnostic and therapeutic maneuvers
Thoracentesis
Aspiration lung biopsy
Percutaneous pleural biopsy
Cardiothoracic surgery
Resuscitation
Ventilator therapy, especially with positive end-expiratory pressure
Lower respiratory tract diseases
Hyaline membrane disease
Aspiration syndrome
Asthma
Cystic fibrosis
Tuberculosis (cavitary, miliary)
Pneumonia and bronchiolitis
Malignancy (primary or metastatic)
Blunt thoracic trauma

of this complication, except for the shift of the trachea and the apical beat. Even the latter may be difficult to locate in light of overinflation. The scratch sign, which is a loud, harsh sound heard over the midsternum when the affected side is stroked with a dull instrument or a finger, may be elicited.

Radiologic confirmation during full expiration is helpful. Bullae, a massive lung cyst, or partial obstruction with secondary overinflation may be mistaken for chronic pneumothorax. Careful attention to the patient's history and assessment of the edge of the lung on chest film usually clarify the diagnosis. Another consideration is traumatic diaphragmatic hernia, which usually occurs on the left side because of the shielding effect of the liver on the right side and possible inherent weakness of the left leaf of the diaphragm. Attention should be directed to the convex shadow cast by the upper border of the stomach and to the linear opacities representing the bowel wall. The size of the pneumothorax can be estimated from the following formula[33]:

$$\text{Size of pneumothorax (\%)} = (1 - [L^3/H^3]) \times 100$$ [55]

where L is the diameter of the lung and H is the diameter of the hemithorax on upright inspiratory chest radiograph. Collapse of the lung halfway to the lung border can also approximate a "medium" pneumothorax.

Definitive diagnosis is made with a chest roentgenogram taken after barium swallow. Errors in diagnosis may lead to trauma to the stomach, spleen, or other abdominal organs located in the chest cavity or to the development of tension pneumothorax during attempts to insert a needle into an intrapulmonary airspace.

Arterial gas tensions and pH may be normal initially, with P_{CO_2} even below normal at times. In the presence of unrelieved tension, however, acidosis, hypoxemia, and hypercapnia are invariably present.

In the presence of intrapleural air, consideration should be given to other air leak phenomena. Pneumomediastinum rarely results in cardiopulmonary compromise, but may precede pneumothorax. Air may also dissect to the pericardium, producing tamponade, or to the peritoneum, where differentiation from a ruptured abdominal viscus is essential. With subcutaneous emphysema, palpable crepitations over the neck and torso may be present.

MANAGEMENT

In room air, the pleural space is cleared of 1.25% of the volume of the hemithorax every 24 hours.[56] When pneumothorax is present, intrapleural gas absorption can be hastened considerably (approximately sevenfold, to almost 10%/day), if the gas is loculated (there is no continuous air leak), by breathing 100% oxygen. Breathing 100% oxygen washes out nitrogen from the body without significantly increasing venous P_{O_2}. Under ordinary circumstances, arterial blood is almost completely saturated with oxygen during air breathing; therefore, oxygen breathing changes the arterial oxygen content by increasing only the amount of oxygen dissolved in plasma. The increase in dissolved oxygen that occurs with a change from air to oxygen breathing is approximately 1.5 volumes percent. Because the difference in arteriovenous oxygen content remains, on average, 5 volumes percent, and the steep part of the oxyhemoglobin dissociation curve is in effect, breathing 100% oxygen increases venous P_{O_2} from 40 to, say, 50 torr. This increase in venous P_{O_2} is accomplished while P_{N_2} goes to nearly zero, and therefore total venous gas pressure is approximately 143 mm Hg, or 617 mm Hg (800 cm H_2O) less than atmospheric pressure. Thus, breathing 100% oxygen will hasten the absorption of loculated gas.[56]

The functional consequences of tension pneumothorax or even a small pneumothorax in patients with respiratory insufficiency pose an immediate threat to life unless the intrapleural air is immediately evacuated. Effective management requires early clinical recognition and prompt radiologic investigation. Frequent use of electrocardiographic monitoring and chest transillumination hastens confirmation of the diagnosis and increases the chance of successful treatment.

A rational approach to the therapeutic management of air leak complications should take into account the clinical severity, presence, and nature of the underlying lung disease; the patient's gestational and postnatal age; the precipitating event; and the history of recurrence. Attention must be directed equally to the treatment of the underlying disease process. With a small, nonprogressive, asymptomatic, or mildly symptomatic pneumothorax that is not associated with underlying disease, expectant care is frequently satisfactory, because the gas eventually will be absorbed. In neonates, conservative measures include frequent, small feedings; mild sedation to minimize crying; and administration of oxygen-enriched air. Spontaneous resolution is usually achieved in 1 to 3 days. Absorption of the loculated pneumothorax is hastened sevenfold by oxygen inhalation, which increases the pressure gradient of gases between the pleura and venous blood. Administration of high concentrations of oxygen to premature infants must be closely monitored because of the dangers of retrolental fibroplasia. In the absence of a definitive roentgenographic picture that excludes the usual differential diagnoses, it is best to defer needle aspiration unless clinical worsening requires a different approach. Needle perforation of a tension pulmonary cyst, congenital lobar emphysema, or traumatic tear of the lung can cause or worsen tension pneumothorax, resulting in a more precarious clinical situation.

In the presence of underlying disease, direct mechanical evacuation of intrapleural air should be performed unless the pneumothorax is very small, the underlying disorder is mild, and the patient's clinical status is stable. Close clinical and blood gas monitoring is an integral part of management. Appropriate measures must be taken as soon as clinical or biochemical deterioration is detected.

Specific clinical settings mandate decompression and evacuation of intrapleural air.[57] Evacuation of intrapleural air is essential in all patients before air transport. The reduction in barometric pressure with ascent increases the volume of intrapleural air, possibly converting a small pneumothorax to tension pneumothorax in transit. Tube thoracostomy provides an escape for intrapleural air should the volume increase. Similarly, any child with a moderately sized or larger pneumothorax, or one associated with cardiorespiratory compromise, requires aspiration or drainage (see Fig. 21-16). Proper site selection will facilitate evacuation of the air. Generally, unless loculated, air will reside in the superior and anterior aspect of the hemithorax. However, placement of the chest tube in an interlobar fissure does not necessarily render the tube ineffective. The operator should be familiar with chest wall and pleural anatomy. Direct needle aspiration using the second or third intercostal space, along the midclavicular line, is warranted for prompt decompression of severe tension pneumothorax. The fourth or fifth intercostal space, in the midaxillary line, is often selected for placement of a chest tube. There are a variety of catheters available for use in drainage of intrapleural air. Pigtail catheters inserted using a modified Seldinger approach have been used, even in neonates. This technique offers theoretical advantages in reducing trauma to the chest wall and lungs. The catheter should be connected to an underwater seal, and suction applied at −5 to −15 cm H_2O. Shortly after the procedure, a chest film should be taken to assess lung expansion. The drainage tube is left in place for an average period of 3 days, until there has been no air leak for 24 hours. Suction is then discontinued. Cessation of air leak is recognized by cessation of bubbling in the drainage collection system during the respiratory cycle. Observing the swing of the water meniscus, which normally oscillates during respiration, ensures patency of the tube. After cessation of air leak is established and complete lung expansion is confirmed by roentgenography, the tube is withdrawn. The tube may be clamped for 2 to 4 hours, and then unclamped, with absence of air leak confirmed again. The tube should not remain in place, clamped, for an extended period before withdrawal. Narcotic analgesics are indicated to reduce pleuritic pain associated with tube removal. If possible, based on the child's age, understanding, and cooperation, the tube should be removed during an expiratory breath-hold. This maneuver maintains positive pleural pressure, reducing the incidence of recurrence of pneumothorax with chest tube removal.

Management of pneumothorax in patients with cystic fibrosis involves several considerations. With the first occurrence of a small, asymptomatic, unilateral pneumothorax, resolution is typical after expectant care in the hospital and treatment of the acute pulmonary infection. If spontaneous resolution does not occur or if the initial episode is a large pneumothorax, chest tube drainage is required. After most of the intrapleural air has been evacuated, CT scan is recommended in patients with persistent or recurrent pneumothorax. If an apical bleb is found, then thoracoscopic resection is indicated. If no bleb is found, then either thoracoscopic or sclerosing pleurodesis is indicated. Due to the advent of lung transplantation in cystic fibrosis, discussion should be held with the transplant center before any procedure that obliterates the pleural space is performed. Moreover, new forms of chest physiotherapy that involve positive expiratory therapy should be withheld for 2 to 3 months to ensure that the ruptured bleb has healed. The long-term prognosis in cystic fibrosis after pneumothorax is poor, with a median survival time of 30 months.

PROGNOSIS

Recurrence of spontaneous pneumothorax is common, ranging in incidence from 40% to 87%. The risk of recurrence is increased if the initial episode is slow to resolve (>7 days). Moreover, each recurrence increases the incidence of further recurrence. To decrease the risk of recurrence, children should avoid scuba diving. On a temporary basis, 4 weeks after resolution of pneumothorax, all air travel, contact sports, and playing brass or woodwind musical instruments is to be avoided. Both CT scans and thoracoscopy have proven useful in detecting inciting blebs in cases of recurrent or slow-to-resolve air leak. Consideration should be given to these further investigations and to pleurodesis if the initial pneumothorax occurs in individuals whose habitus or underlying lung disease places them at increased risk for recurrence.

REFERENCES

1. Light RW: Anatomy of the pleura. In: Light RW, ed: Pleural Diseases, 3rd ed. Baltimore: Williams & Wilkins, 1995.
2. Davila RM, Crouch EC: Anatomic organization and function of the human pleura. Semin Respir Crit Care Med 1995;16(4):261–268.
3. Sahn SA: The pleura. Am Rev Respir Dis 1988;138:184–234.
4. Wang N: The preformed stomas connecting the pleural cavity and the lymphatics in the parietal pleura. Am Rev Respir Dis 1975;111:12.
5. Wang NS: Anatomy and physiology of the pleural space. Clin Chest Med 1985;6:3–16.
6. Müller K-M: Principles of anatomy and pathology of the pleura. Eur Respir Mon 2002;22:1–27.
7. Zocchi L: Physiology and pathophysiology of pleural fluid turnover. Eur Respir Mon 2002;22:28–49.
8. Rossi GA: Cells of the pleural space. In: Crystal RG, West JB, eds: The Lung. Scientific Foundations. New York: Raven Press, 1991.
9. Agostini E, Zocchi L: Starling forces and lymphatic drainage in pleural liquid and protein exchanges. Respir Physiol 1991;86:271–281.
10. Kinasewitz GT, Groome LJ, Marshall RP, Diana JN: Role of pulmonary lymphatics and interstitium in visceral pleural fluid exchange. J Appl Physiol 1984;56:355–363.
11. Wiener-Kronish JP, Broaddus VC: Interrelationship of pleural and pulmonary interstitial liquid. Annu Rev Physiol 1993;55:209–226.
12. Broaddus VC: Transudative pleural effusions. Eur Respir Mon 2002;22:157–176.
13. Yernault JC: History, symptoms and clinical examination in pleural diseases. Eur Respir Mon 2002;22:60–75.
14. Conces DW Jr, Tarver RD: Pleural imaging. Semin Respir Crit Care Med 1995;16:279–287.
15. Moskowitz H, Platt RT, Schachar R, Mellins H: Roentgen visualization of minute pleural effusion. Radiology 1973;190:33.
16. Bittner RC, Teichgraeber UK: Imaging techniques in the diagnosis of pleural diseases. Eur Respir Mon 2002;22:76–109.
17. Collins TR, Sahn SA: Thoracentesis. Complications, patient experience and diagnostic value. Chest 1987;91:817–822.
18. Sahn SA: The diagnostic value of pleural fluid analysis. Semin Respir Crit Care Med 1995;16:269–278.
19. Light RW, Macgregor MI, Luchsinger PC, Ball WC: Pleural effusions. Diagnostic separation of transudates and exudates. Ann Intern Med 1972; 77:507.
20. Romero S, Candela A, Martin C, et al: Evaluation of different criteria for the separation of pleural transudates from exudates. Chest 1993; 104:399–404.
21. Schoenfeld N: Critical issues in pleural fluid examinations. Laboratory parameters, tumour markers and cytological methods. Eur Respir Mon 2002;22:110–119.

22. Light RW, Erozan YS, Ball WC: Cells in pleural fluid. Their value in differential diagnosis. Arch Intern Med 1973;132:854–860.
23. Dines D, Pierre RV, Franzen S: The value of cells in the pleural fluid in the differential diagnosis. Mayo Clin Proc 1975;50:571.
24. Light RW: Diagnostic approach in a patient with pleural effusion. Eur Respir Mon 2002;22:131–145.
25. Prakash UBS: Chylothorax and pseudochylothorax. Eur Respir Mon 2002;22:249–265.
26. Van Hoff DD, LiVolsi V: Diagnostic reliability of needle biopsy of the parietal pleura. Am J Clin Pathol 1975;64:200–203.
27. Chernick V, Reed MH: Pneumothorax and chylothorax in the neonatal period. J Pediatr 1970;76:624.
28. Kosloke AM, Martin LW, Schubert WK: Management of chylothorax in children by thoracentesis and medium-chain triglyceride feedings. J Pediatr Surg 1974;9:365.
29. Goto M, Kawamata K, Kitano M, et al: Treatment of chylothorax in a premature infant using somatostatin. J Perinatol 2003;23:563–564.
30. Bechamps GJ, Lynn HG, Wenzl JE: Empyema in children. Review of Mayo Clinic experience. Mayo Clin Proc 1970;45:43.
31. Fine NL, Smith LR, Sheedy PF: Frequency of pleural effusions in mycoplasma and viral pneumonias. N Engl J Med 1970;288:790.
32. Griz A, Giammona ST: Pneumonitis with pleural effusion in children due to *Mycoplasma pneumoniae*. Am Rev Respir Dis 1974;109:665.
33. American Thoracic Society: Treatment of tuberculosis and tuberculosis infection in adults and children. Am J Respir Crit Care Med 1994; 149:1359–1374.
34. Berger HW, Mejia E: Tuberculous pleurisy. Chest 1973;63:88.
35. McLaughlin FJ, Goldmann DA, Rosenbaum DM, et al: Empyema in children. Clinical course and long-term follow-up. Pediatrics 1984;73:587–593.
36. Freij BJ, Kusmiesz H, Nelson JD, McCracken GH: Parapneumonic effusions and empyema in hospitalized children. A retrospective review of 227 cases. Pediatr Infect Dis 1984;3:578.
37. Stiles QR, Lindesmith GG, Tucker BL, et al: Pleural empyema in children. Ann Thorac Surg 1970;10:37.
38. Eichenwald HF: Antimicrobial therapy in children. Curr Probl Pediatr 1974;4:3.
39. Bartlett JG, Finegold SM: Anaerobic infections of the lung and pleural space. Am Rev Respir Dis 1974;100:56.
40. Chen LE, Langer JC, Dillon PA, et al: Management of late-stage parapneumonic empyema. J Pediatr Surg 2002;37:371.
41. Hoff SJ, Neblett WW, Edwards KM, et al: Parapneumonic empyema in children. Decortication hastens recovery in patients with severe pleural infections. Pediatr Infect Dis J 1991;10:194–199.
42. Henke CA, Leatherman JW: Intrapleurally administered streptokinase in the treatment of acute loculated nonpurulent parapneumonic effusions. Am Rev Respir Dis 1992;145:680–684.
43. Gocmen A, Kiper N, Toppare M, et al: Conservative treatment of empyema in children. Respiration 1993;60:182–185.
44. Sahn SA, Antony VB, Good JTJ: Decortication is rarely necessary following empyema. Clin Res 1981;29:88A.
45. Neff CC, van Sonnenbert E, Lawson DW, Patton AS: CT follow-up of empyemas. Pleural peels resolve after percutaneous catheter drainage. Radiology 1990;176:195–197.
46. Redding GJ, Walund L, Walund D, et al: Lung function in children following empyema. Am J Dis Child 1990;144:1337–1342.
47. Smith LP, Gerald B: Empyema in childhood followed roentgenographically. Decortication seldom needed. Radiology 1969;106:114–117.
48. Light RW: Management of parapneumonic effusions. Chest 1991;100: 892–893.
49. Balfour-Lynn IM, Abrahamson E, Cohen G, et al: BTS guidelines for the management of pleural infection in children. Thorax 2005;60(Suppl 1): i1–i21.
50. Noppen M, Schramel F: Pneumothorax. Eur Respir Mon 2002;22: 279–296.
51. Chernick V, Reed NH: Pneumothorax and chylothorax in the neonatal period. J Pediatr 1970;76:624–632.
52. Lichter I, Gwynne JF: Spontaneous pneumothorax in young subjects. Thorax 1971;26:409–417.
53. Summers RS: The electrocardiogram as a diagnostic aid in pneumothorax. Chest 1973;63:127.
54. Light RW: Physiology of the pleural space. In: Light RW, ed: Pleural Diseases. Baltimore: Williams & Wilkins, 1995, p 13.
55. Light RW: Management of spontaneous pneumothorax. Am Rev Respir Dis 1993;148:245–248.
56. Northfield TC: Oxygen therapy for spontaneous pneumothorax. BMJ 1971;4:86–88.
57. Baumann MH, Strange C, Heffner JE, et al: Management of spontaneous pneumothorax. An American College of Chest Physicians Delphi consensus statement. Chest 2001;119:590–602.

Infections of the Respiratory Tract

22 Diagnosis of Viral Respiratory Illness: Practical Applications

Stelios Psarras, PhD •
Nikolaos G. Papadopoulos, MD •
Sebastian L. Johnston, MD

Laboratory methods for the detection of respiratory viruses allow for not only the identification, but also the exclusion of a specific etiology underlying a given pathogenic state of the respiratory system. They complement and support the clinical diagnosis and provide a basis for clinical decision making and further treatment. They are also useful for epidemiologic studies.

Like all viruses, respiratory viruses can be detected by one or a combination of the three major viral detection methods:

- Direct detection of the virus or its genetic material or proteins
- Culture of the virus in a suitable host or cell line and assessment of its presence and effects on the host or cell line
- Serologic evidence of infection in the organism

Direct detection methods include detection of whole viruses with electron microscopy and detection of inclusion bodies by light microscopy. In addition, a virus can be detected by means of specific antibodies against its antigens, either in body fluids or after its culture in host cells. Polymerase chain reaction (PCR) seems to be the most powerful of the molecular biologic techniques used to detect viral genetic material directly. A recent development of this technique, real-time PCR, also allows calculation of the number of copies of the virus present in a given biologic sample.

Culture of a respiratory virus in a host allows both its direct detection, as described earlier, and its indirect detection, based on the biologic effects it may trigger in the host. Thus, respiratory viruses can be detected and titrated from the cytopathic effect (CPE) that they trigger in cultured cells; for example, orthomyxoviruses and paramyxoviruses, such as influenza and parainfluenza, can be detected by their ability to trigger erythrocytes to aggregate (hemagglutination).

Serologic studies can be used in many ways for virus detection. In one approach, the presence of specific antibodies in the organism can lead to inhibition of a biologic effect that a stock viral solution elicits in target cells (e.g., inhibition of hemagglutination). In addition, the ability to assess immunoglobulin M (IgM)–specific antibodies in the patient's blood during the acute phase or changes in immunoglobulin G (IgG) antibody titers between the acute phase and convalescence is a valuable tool that can identify ongoing viral infection and, in some cases, discriminate between recurrent and latent infection.

■ BRIEF OVERVIEW OF VIRUSES INVOLVED IN RESPIRATORY ILLNESS

Viral agents with a tropism for the respiratory system infect or produce symptoms in both the upper and lower airways. Although it is frequently mentioned that hundreds of different viruses can produce respiratory symptoms, this is due to the large number of picornavirus (>150) and adenovirus (>50) serotypes. Because there are small differences in clinical presentation between these serotypes, seven to eight types of agents can be described separately. The majority of them are ribonucleic acid (RNA) viruses (influenza A and B; respiratory syncytial virus [RSV] types A and B; parainfluenza 1, 2, 3, and 4 viruses; human rhinoviruses [RVs]; human coronaviruses [HCVs] OC43 and 229E), including the newly identified NL63 and severe acute respiratory syndrome (SARS) coronaviruses and the also recently identified human metapneumovirus (MPV).

The most prevalent pathogenic microorganisms are probably human RVs. These "common cold" viruses belong to the picornavirus (small RNA) family, which also includes the enteroviruses, such as poliovirus, echovirus, and Coxsackie virus, and cardiovirus and aphthovirus. More than 100 RV serotypes have been identified and numbered. These are divided into major (90% of serotypes) and minor groups; the former use intercellular adhesion molecule-1 as their cellular receptor, whereas the latter use the low-density lipoprotein receptor. The epidemiology of RV-induced colds is closely related to social contact, and peaks are usually seen when children return to school after a vacation period. One of the most prominent roles of RV is in triggering asthma exacerbations.[1] Comparative titrations of nasal, pharyngeal, and oral secretions have shown that replication is more active in the nose. However, studies comparing nasal and throat swabs with sputum samples obtained during asthma exacerbations showed that the viral isolation rate was higher in sputum, suggesting that RVs may also replicate in the lower airway. This was later clearly demonstrated with the use of molecular biology-based detection techniques.[2] Although the severity of upper respiratory tract symptoms after RV infection does not differ between patients with asthma and normal subjects, both the duration and the severity of lower respiratory tract symptoms are more pronounced in patients with asthma.[3] The lower respiratory tract epithelial cells infected by RVs are rich sources of inflammatory mediators that may trigger or propagate airway inflammation and obstruction.

Respiratory syncytial virus belongs to the Pneumovirinae subfamily and is a medium-sized (100–300 nm) RNA virus. Variations in the attachment glycoprotein of the viral envelope give rise to the two antigenically distinct strains of RSV, A and B. Although there have been conflicting data, the majority of studies report that A strains are more common and produce more severe disease. A wide range of species can be experimentally infected with human RSV, but natural infection is species-specific. RSV enters the body through the eye or nose and, to a lesser extent, through the mouth. The virus subsequently spreads along the airway mucosa, mostly by cell-to-cell transfer along intracytoplasmic bridges, and also through aspiration from the upper to the lower airway. RSV follows a well-characterized epidemiologic pattern, with yearly outbreaks occurring between October and May in temperate climates. At least half of the infant population becomes infected during their first RSV epidemic, and almost all children have been infected by 2 years of age. Although infection usually leads to mild respiratory illness, some infants have more severe disease. Bronchiolitis is the characteristic clinical manifestation of such a complication. There is evidence that hospitalizations for bronchiolitis have considerably increased during recent decades and that hospitalized children have increased probability of wheezing later in life,[4] with the immune status of the host probably playing an important role in the process.[5] The relationship between RSV infection, atopy, subsequent symptoms, and the development of asthma is discussed in detail in Chapter 55.

Three types of influenza viruses, designated A, B, and C, and belonging to the orthomyxoviruses, have been identified. They are negative-stranded segmented RNA viruses. The two influenza envelope glycoproteins hemagglutinin and neuraminidase determine both viral entry into target cells, by binding to sialic acids and fusing with cellular membrane elements, and the release of the virus. Infection with influenza virus occurs by inspiration of contaminated droplets from infected persons. Infected cells become round and swollen with pyknotic nuclei. Edema and polymorphonuclear infiltration are seen in the surrounding tissues. The progressive changes in epithelial cells suggest that infection starts in the trachea and then ascends or descends. The epidemiology of influenza viruses is characterized by yearly epidemics lasting for 6 to 8 weeks during late winter; each year, there is usually only one dominant type or subtype. Illnesses initially appear in children, whereas later in the epidemic, more adults are affected. Viruses are present in the community before and after the epidemic, causing illness at a low frequency. Antigenic variation readily occurs in H and N primary structures, giving rise to new subtypes (antigenic shift) and to intrasubtype changes (antigenic drift). Only type A influenza viruses have been associated with pandemics that have been occurring every 10 to 40 years. The last potentially pandemic strains to emerge were recorded in 1997 and 2003, and were of avian origin.[6] The currently circulating type A human isolates are H1N1 and H3N2 subtypes. The avian isolates were of H5N1 and H7N7 subtypes and were able to be transmitted to and infect humans[7] by entering the cells through different cellular receptors.[8]

Human parainfluenza viruses (PIVs) include four members, numbered 1 to 4, and belong to the Paramyxoviridae subfamily, together with mumps and measles. Each PIV has distinct epidemiologic and clinical characteristics, as well as different age distribution patterns. PIV 1 and PIV 2, members of the *Respirovirus* genus, are generally associated with laryngotracheobronchitis (croup), upper respiratory tract illness, and pharyngitis, whereas PIV 3, a member of the *Rubulavirus* genus, is also a major cause of infant bronchiolitis and is associated with the development of pneumonia in susceptible subjects. PIV 4 is rare and less well studied. PIV 1 occurs in biennial epidemics during autumn, coinciding with croup outbreaks; its peak incidence occurs in children 2 to 3 years of age. PIV 2 epidemics are less predictable; however, they more or less follow the biennial pattern of PIV 1, affecting mostly children younger than 5 years of age. PIV 3 is unique among PIVs in its propensity to infect infants younger than 6 months of age in spring epidemics. PIV 3 infections are more frequent and occur yearly, with peaks seen during spring and summer. Infection is initiated by attachment of the virus to the host cell through interaction of the viral H and N glycoproteins with cellular sialic acid receptors, followed by uncoating of the virus, its translocation into the cytoplasm, and transcription, leading to replication. For transmission, aerosol spread is considered important, although deposition on surfaces and subsequent self-inoculation may also be relevant. Virus replication can occur throughout the tracheobronchial tree, causing local inflammation; however, only mild and rapidly repaired focal tissue destruction is observed in vivo. However, in immunocompromised hosts, fatal giant cell pneumonia may develop. Central to the pathogenesis of PIV infection is the ability of these viruses to escape interferon-mediated immune responses.[9]

In contrast to the rest of the respiratory viruses, adenoviruses are deoxyribonucleic acid (DNA) viruses. This large family of viruses includes six subgenera and more than 50 serotypes. Their overall size is 70 to 90 nm; the virion is naked and contains 36 to 38 kb double-stranded DNA, encoding more than 50 polypeptides from both strands. Some of these proteins allow efficient endosomal lysis and escape, leading to genome entrance into the host cell nucleus. The propensity of adenoviruses to shut off the expression of host messenger RNA and induce excess synthesis of adenoviral proteins leads to an accumulation of such proteins as intranuclear bodies, which are incompatible with normal cell function. In upper airway epithelial cells, ciliary and microtubular abnormalities lead to defective mucociliary clearance. An important feature of adenovirus is its ability to persist in the host for a long time, through low-grade replication, or for even longer periods, with production of adenoviral proteins without replication of a complete virus.

Human coronaviruses were isolated during the mid-1960s. The majority of HCVs studied to date are related to one of two reference strains, designated OC43 and 229E, which differ extensively. Recently, coronavirus NL63 was isolated from an infant with bronchiolitis and conjunctivitis.[10] It shares 65% sequence identity with 229E, but several prominent differences indicate that NL63 is a new group I coronavirus. Human aminopeptidase N, which is present on lung, intestinal, and kidney epithelial cells, has been identified as a receptor for HCV-229E. OC43 binds to major histocompatibility complex class I molecules. Viral replication has been demonstrated in the nasal mucosa, inducing inflammation, ciliary damage, and epithelial cell shedding. Its in vivo CPE is not pronounced, as in the case of RV infections. HCV replication in the lower airway has not been confirmed. Volunteers can be successfully infected by intranasal inoculation. HCV causes approximately 15% of common colds. The disease is generally mild, and there is evidence that HCV-induced colds may cause milder lower respiratory tract symptoms than other viruses. However, there have been reports of more severe lower respiratory tract involvement in young children and the elderly.

The recent Eastern Asia-based SARS epidemic has been attributed to a new coronavirus that shares limited homology with the other known coronaviruses.[11] The virus causes diffuse alveolar damage, with interstitial infiltrates. After 3 to 7 days of fever, a nonproductive cough may progress to breathlessness and hypoxemia in 15% of patients. This serious infection is characterized by a 3% to 6% mortality rate (or even as high as 43%–55% when patients older than 60 years of age are considered).[12] In children, the illness is much more mild (see Chapter 33). Although SARS-CoV is a coronavirus, it differs phylogenetically from all other known HCVs, and there is evidence that it is not derived from any other characterized coronavirus. In addition, sequence of the Tor2 isolate showed a number of distinctive features of its genome (e.g., several small, open reading frames between its genes) that are of potential biologic significance.[13]

Finally, a new respiratory virus, MPV, was recently isolated from nasopharyngeal aspirates of young children in the Netherlands,[14] and was later shown to be present worldwide. MPV is the first human respiratory pathogen classified as a member of the *Metapneumovirus* genus. The new virus proved to have paramyxovirus-like pleomorphic particles on electron microscopy. Phylogenetic analyses showed some sequence variation between isolates and the existence of two potential genetic clusters of MPV. The clinical symptoms of the children from whom the virus was isolated in the Netherlands ranged from upper respiratory airway disease to severe bronchiolitis and pneumonia.[14] Subsequent studies, conducted in different locations and using mixed patient populations with various respiratory symptoms, established the association of this virus with acute respiratory illness in both the upper and lower tracts, and in all age groups.[15,16]

DIAGNOSTIC TECHNIQUES

VIRUS CULTURES

Treatment of Clinical Samples

A major prerequisite for the successful application of a detection method is the appropriate collection, transport, and maintenance of the clinical sample. In general, samples collected during the first days of symptoms lead to higher recovery rates of viruses. Upper respiratory samples include nasopharyngeal and oropharyngeal swabs, with the former providing a lower rate of contamination by lower respiratory components. The swabs can then be placed in viral transport medium for further culture or can be used to prepare slides for immunofluorescent detection, either by rolling the swab directly on the slide or after recovery of cells by centrifugation. Nasopharyngeal aspirates (NPAs) are considered better sources for viral isolation than swabs. Although induced sputum is often contaminated by oropharyngeal components and microbial agents that hinder viral recovery, it is an easily obtainable sample, at least in older children, in whom the success rate is greater than 70%. Therefore, it is often used after either filtering through 200-nm membrane filters or dilution, usually in the presence of a reducing agent, such as 0.1% dithiothreitol, to reduce its viscosity. Transtracheal aspirates, bronchial biopsy specimens, and bronchial wash samples are all considered better sources than sputum for both culture and direct immunodetection of viruses in pelleted cells. Similarly, after centrifugation under mild conditions (10 min/500 × *g*), both the supernatant and the pellet of bronchoalveolar lavage provide good sources for isolation and immunofluorescent detection of respiratory viruses. However, the invasiveness of these procedures precludes their routine use in children. A detailed description of this issue is beyond the scope of this chapter, and a variety of comprehensive articles are available within this textbook and elsewhere.

Cell Culture

For each respiratory virus, there are a number of cell lines and strains that allow its replication in vitro (Table 22-1). Susceptible cell cultures may undergo degenerative processes on exposure to respiratory viruses. The most common CPE patterns include syncytia formation (fusion of many cells in multinucleated structures), vacuolation (generation of large, bubble-like regions in the cytoplasm), and granular degeneration. Rounding and detachment are also common features (Fig. 22-1). The dose that causes the CPE in 50% of inoculated wells ($TCID_{50}$) is used to express the content of a given viral preparation (titer).

When the cell monolayer is permitted to grow covered by a solid (agar) medium, the foci of virus-infected cells form plaques that may be able to be stained by specific dyes (e.g., neutral red) in a manner different from uninfected cells; thus, they can be readily identified and counted. Viruses can also be plaque-purified with this technique.

Viruses that possess hemagglutinins (e.g., influenza and parainfluenza viruses) may be able to adhere to erythrocytes of the host cells in which they replicate. When a suspension of erythrocytes derived from a suitable species is added to the infected cell culture, these adhere in clumps after a certain period, revealing virus.

Rotation enhances both the yield and the effectiveness of the CPE of a cultivated virus. Liposomal and other agents added in the media, as well as centrifugation protocols, may increase the detection rate. In addition, a virus can be isolated by culturing cells derived from a biopsy sample, although coculture with helper cells often leads to higher recovery rates, because this technique overcomes the viral inhibitory activity of certain tissue homogenates.

Cell culture can be used in two additional ways for the identification of respiratory viruses. First, sera from patients

TABLE 22-1. Cell lines commonly used for identification of respiratory viruses

Cell Line	Origin	Type	Virus
A549	Human alveolar adenocarcinoma	Continuous	AdV, RSV
HeLa	Human cervical carcinoma	Continuous	AdV, RSV, RV
Hep-2	HeLa contaminant	Continuous	AdV, RSV
HEK	Human embryonic kidney	Primary	AdV
LLC-MK_2	Monkey kidney	Continuous	IFV, PIV, HCV-NL63
MDCK	Canine kidney	Continuous	IFV
MRC-5	Human fibroblasts	Cell strain	AdV, HCV
MRC-c/C16	Human fetal lung fibroblasts	Continuous	HCV
Mv1Lu	Mink lung	Continuous	IFV
PMK	Monkey kidney	Primary	IFV, PIV
tMK	Monkey kidney	Continuous	MPV
Vero E6	Monkey kidney	Continuous	SARS-CoV
WI-38	Human lung fibroblasts	Cell strain	RV, HCV

can be assessed for the ability to inhibit the CPE, plaque formation, or hemadsorption activity normally triggered by a stock viral solution of known infectivity. Conversely, virus strains isolated from patients can be exposed to specific immune sera known to prevent such activities, and the final result assessed on the cell culture.

Although cell culture remains, in many cases, the gold standard, achieving the highest sensitivity scores in the detection of several viruses, it has the major disadvantage of being a rather time-consuming process, demanding several days or even weeks before some results can be obtained. This is obviously unacceptable in clinical practice, in particular, whenever decisions about, or alterations in, antiviral treatment must be made. Recently, more rapid protocols, using a combination of cell culture with another detection method, such as immunofluorescence, electron microscopy, or PCR-based methods, have been developed. With these techniques, rather than monitoring the appearance of CPE, the sample is inoculated onto the culture and the presence of replicating virus is verified after 24 to 48 hours by the second method.

Mixtures of cell lines have also been used to improve detection rates. In an interesting recent advance, influenza-susceptible, mink-lung-derived Mv1Lu cells and the human adenocarcinoma A549 cell line were used in combination to detect respiratory viruses. Coculture of these two cell lines in shell vials has been shown to detect respiratory viruses synergistically, with greater sensitivity than single cultures. The R-mix monolayers that can be used directly from cryopreserved vials are inoculated on coverslips with the clinical sample, and the vial is centrifuged at $700 \times g$ for 60 minutes. Serum-free medium is added, and 24 hours later, the coverslip is removed and stained with a mixture of antisera against many respiratory viruses. If a positive signal is present, cells from a parallel coverslip can be dispersed onto a suitable chamber containing multiple coverslips that can be examined separately for the presence of individual respiratory viruses using monoclonal antibodies. Using this method, definitive results (positive and negative) can be obtained within 2 days,[17] whereas in conventional, single-cell-culture CPE observation, the final result takes approximately 10 days; moreover, positive results can be obtained up to 4 days earlier with this method. Although of similar sensitivity to conventional cell culture and direct immunofluorescence with respect to most respiratory viruses (influenza, parainfluenza, and RSV), this method is less sensitive in detecting adenovirus; RV has not been tested so far.[18]

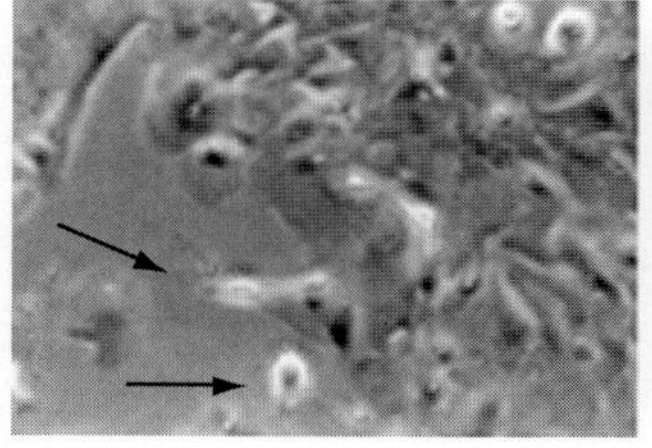

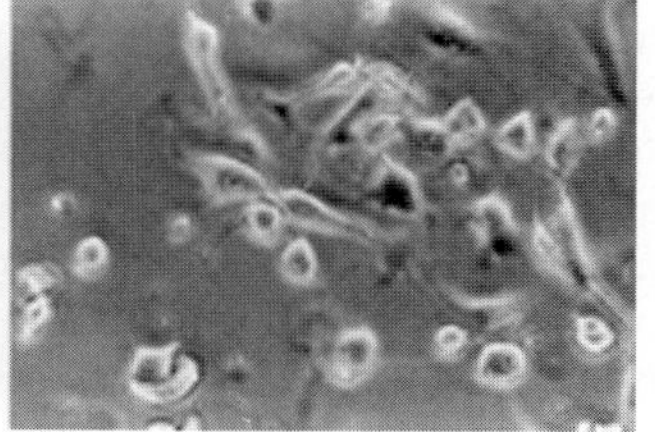

FIGURE 22-1. Cytopathic effect caused by human rhinoviruses in vitro. **A,** Primary cultures of human bronchial epithelial cells were infected by RV7 at a multiplicity of infection of 10, and 24 to 48 hours later, characteristic shrinkage and rounding can be seen in some cells *(arrows),* whereas the rest of the monolayer remains intact. **B,** At later time points, fully developed cytopathic effect gradually leads to cellular detachment, cell debris, and detachment of the cell layer.

Eggs

Fertile eggs are used for the culture of respiratory viruses, such as influenza. Inoculation into the amniotic cavity is used mainly for the isolation of such viruses from clinical samples. Harvesting is usually conducted 48 to 72 hours after inoculation. The eggs should have been previously chilled to prevent the release of red blood cells, which would lead to loss of virus due to absorption to the cells.

Animals

Inoculation of a susceptible animal is a common practice for the detection of many viruses. In the recent SARS epidemics, for instance, one of the first crucial tests to identify the virus was intracranial and intraperitoneal injection of clinical samples into suckling mice, with observation of the mice for 14 days for pathologic findings.[11] Other examples include AdV serotype 5, which, when given intravenously to adult mice, kills them within 3 to 4 days, whereas other adenoviruses, when administered subcutaneously to newborn hamsters, cause their death within 4 to 12 days.

DETECTION OF WHOLE VIRUSES BY ELECTRON MICROSCOPY

Nasopharyngeal aspirates and lavages, as well as lung biopsy specimens, are suitable material for the detection of respiratory viruses by electron microscopy.

Fluid Samples

In a typical protocol, a 300- or 400-mesh grid is placed on a drop of sample for 5 to 15 minutes. After it is drained with filter paper, the grid can be stained. Fluid samples should be placed on support films on the grid. Films made from 0.3% to 0.5% polyvinyl formal in ethylene dichloride (Formvar solution) are mechanically stronger than collodion films (2% solution in isoamyl acetate). The films are cast on a glass slide by experienced personnel, and grids are made by pressing the grid onto the film slide appropriately in the presence of water. A silver-gray rather than charcoal-gray or gold color coincides with optimal film thickness, and additional carbon coating under vacuum facilitates spreading of the sample, improving the results. Glow discharging under the vacuum or treatment of the grids with a suitable agent (e.g., poly-L-lysine, Alcian blue, cytochrome C, or bovine serum albumin) is commonly used to overcome spreading problems.

No viral transport medium should be added to NPA or bronchoalveolar lavage specimens before electron microscopy because it includes salts and proteins that may obscure the electron microscopy field; in addition, it dilutes the particles. In contrast, concentration of particles contained in lavage and NPA samples is recommended. This can be achieved with ultracentrifugation, ultrafiltration, or agar diffusion. With agar diffusion, a drop of suspension is placed on top of 2% agar and allowed to diffuse freely. At the end of this procedure, liquid and salts are diffused into the agar, leaving a film-coated grid containing the virus that can be drained on filter paper and stained for electron microscopy. The pseudoreplica technique is a variation of the agar diffusion method, whereby the drop is allowed to diffuse into the agar, irradiated, and covered by Formvar film. Then the Formvar membrane is carefully removed and allowed to float onto a water surface. Grids are then applied on the replica membrane and picked up with the aid of filter paper.

Antibodies are also used for the concentration of viruses in suspension (clumping), as well as their attachment onto grids. For aggregation, the samples can be incubated with the antiserum, centrifuged, and placed onto grids with the pseudoreplica technique; alternatively, antiserum is mixed with agar, and a grid is placed onto the gel. Then virus suspension is added and allowed to absorb, followed by removal and staining of the grid. In solid-phase immunoelectron microscopy, the film is coated with antibodies before incubation with virus suspension.

Immunoprecipitation techniques are particularly helpful when picornaviruses are to be detected. These viruses are so small that they sometimes appear similar to lipid droplets. In addition, these techniques allow the specific identification of virus in a biologic fluid, provided that the viral etiology of the pathogenic state under investigation is suspected or known; however, some viruses tend to clump in the absence of antiserum, reducing the specificity of this procedure. Viruses in suspension or on grids can be incubated with primary antiserum, allowed to aggregate, and after the antibody has been washed out, the preparation can be treated with a colloidal gold-labeled secondary antibody. Gold labeling has been used specifically to detect immune complexes in serum, as well as subviral particles. In a somewhat different approach, viruses are exposed to excess antibodies, resulting in extensive coating rather than aggregation of the viruses. This method allows specific identification and serotyping of viruses and can serve to assess the reactivity of convalescent serum against known viruses.

Finally, short-term culture of virus in vitro, if possible, with harvesting before the appearance of the CPE, is a good alternative for the enrichment of a sample that contains unacceptably low numbers of viral particles for electron microscopy. Adenoviruses and paramyxoviruses belong to the group of viruses that can be detected in supernatants before a massive CPE occurs. On the other hand, adenovirus is membrane-associated and may be lost on removal of the debris with centrifugation.

An additional problem with NPA specimens is the presence of mucus, which inhibits spreading of the samples. These specimens can be treated with an equal volume of a buffer containing an appropriate dithiothreitol concentration to break down the mucus.

Biopsy Specimens

Specimens should be placed in 2% to 5% glutaraldehyde in cacodylate or phosphate buffer and stored in a refrigerator at –20° C, rather than frozen, to maintain the tissue architecture and specifically localize the virus. Osmium fixation (1%–2% OsO_4 in a 4-[2-hydroxyethyl]-1-piperazineethanesulfonic acid [HEPES]- or a piperazine diethanesulfonic acid [PIPES]-based buffer) is also used. En bloc staining can then be conducted with uranyl acetate in veronal buffer. Otherwise, dehydration and embedding in resins should follow the fixation step. Although it is not optimal, formalin-fixed material and paraffin-embedded sections can also be used for electron microscopy, under some circumstances, after suitable treatment. Because the sample area used for electron microscopy is limited, it is wise first to stain sections with suitable stains, such as toluidine blue; to select areas of particular interest (e.g., those with a CPE); and to trim the sections further for thin sectioning. Viruses can also be seen by extracting solid tissue with a suitable buffer, after homogenization or repeated freezing and thawing and further treatment as a liquid sample. Thin sectioning is also the method of choice for identification of virus in cell culture. If the virus has triggered cell lysis, it can be detected in cell supernatant or medium, after ultracentrifugation is performed to remove the debris, followed by negative staining of the pellet. Cells can also be embedded in agar and further treated as tissue blocks.

Electron Microscopic Appearance of Respiratory Viruses

Electron microscopy of liquid samples containing respiratory viruses aims to identify particles based on their morphologic characteristics (Table 22-2). Picornaviruses and adenoviruses are the two types of respiratory viruses with naked virions of icosahedral symmetry; they have a round appearance on electron microscopy. In contrast to adenoviruses, which have the higher size ranges among naked virions, picornaviruses are very small, and can be often confused with some tail-less bacteriophage species. If available, immunoprecipitation techniques can be used in such cases, and clumping, coating, or concentration of spherical structures is a prerequisite for a given sample to be characterized as positive. In addition, adenoviruses can degenerate, and individual capsomers may appear separately, forming hexagonal lattices. Adenoviruses also resemble herpesviruses in appearance, and differentiation may be based on the larger size of the latter. Enveloped respiratory viruses, such as influenza viruses, parainfluenza viruses, and coronaviruses, have a soft membrane that can become deformed during drying for negative staining. Thus, the particles may appear pleomorphic, and may vary in size. The enveloped respiratory viruses are spiked, rather than smooth. Coronaviruses have long (20-nm) spikes on the surface, whereas paramyxoviruses and orthomyxoviruses contain

TABLE 22-2. Main morphologic characteristics of respiratory viruses

Virus	Envelope	Capsid Symmetry	Genome	Virion Size (nm)	Projections (nm)	Nucleocapsid Size (nm)
AdV	No	I	ds DNA	70–90		
RV	No	I	+ sRNA	24–30		
HCV	Yes	C	+ sRNA	80–150	20	10–20
SARS-CoV	Yes	C	+ sRNA	80–140	20–40	
IFV	Yes	H	– sRNA	80–120		9–15
PIV	Yes	H	– sRNA	150–250		12–18
MPV	Yes	H	– sRNA	150–600	13–17	
RSV	Yes	H	– sRNA	100–300	12	6–7

C, complex; H, helical; I, icosahedral; –/+ sRNA, negative or positive sense single-stranded RNA.

projections that appear as a fringe on the outer side. However, even these forms can sometimes be confused with mitochondria or inverted bacterial membrane debris. Finally, a major problem with the orthomyxovirus and paramyxovirus families is that they have a similar electron microscopic appearance, and additional information is usually required to discriminate between them.

Another feature that may facilitate the identification of a particular respiratory virus is the appearance of the nucleocapsid. This structure is present in enveloped viruses and contains the nucleic acids and some viral proteins. It can be spherical, helical, or complex. Parainfluenza viruses, for instance, have helical filamentous nucleocapsids.

Information obtained from electron microscopic study of thin sections of solid tissues is not limited to the appearance of viral particles. The cellular location also provides important evidence of their properties. For instance, viruses replicating in the nucleus are DNA viruses, whereas RNA viruses replicate in the cytoplasm. Naked viruses, such as adenoviruses, cause cell lysis and can be seen as round shells with a core of different density surrounded by dead cells. If the cytopathology is advanced, adenoviruses may be seen in both the nucleus and the cytoplasm. Picornaviruses cause swelling of the endoplasmic reticulum, and the ribosomes may appear as large beads on a string. Enveloped viruses acquire their membranes by budding through the nuclear envelope, through the plasma membrane, or into vesicles within the cells. There are some difficulties in discriminating virions from normal cell organelles, such as lysosomes and Golgi complexes; however, viruses with spikes appear to have a thicker membrane than the cellular compartments. The size and shape of the nucleocapsid are also of importance. In thin sections, spherical nucleocapsids have a round appearance and resemble small, naked virions, whereas those acquiring a filamentous (helical) shape are thin, elongated structures that are seen going into and out of the plane of section. Adenoviruses can be discriminated from the otherwise similar herpesviruses by the smaller size of their nucleocapsid.

Transmission electron microscopy is a method of reference for the identification and measurement of many viruses (e.g., used as an immediate indicator in the outbreak of the recent SARS epidemic). However, it needs specialized and expensive instrumentation and skilled technicians, a fact that does not facilitate its use in smaller laboratories. Moreover, it is unable to discriminate among viruses of the same family or among particular subtypes, and in many cases, an additional method, such as fluorescence, is necessary to overcome this obstacle. In addition, it cannot distinguish between infectious and noninfectious particles, in contrast to culture-based methods. However, even one virus particle can be identified in a sample, whereas other methods (e.g., antigen detection) require a greater number of viral elements.

Other Whole-Virus Detection Methods

Fluorescent dyes can be used to stain a purified virus preparation and allow enumeration of virus in a solution. OliGreen, for instance, a dye that specifically binds to nucleotides, has been successfully used for the enumeration of adenovirus 5, RSV, and influenza A. This method can be performed within 1 hour.[19] To that end, density-gradient-purified virus preparations are incubated with the dye and subjected to analysis in a modified flow cytometer. Although it has not yet been tested in clinical samples, this method provides information about the genome size of the virus. Its measurements have been consistent with data obtained with transmission electron microscopy enumeration of the same viral stocks.

ANTIGEN DETECTION

Antigen-based detection methods for respiratory viruses presuppose the knowledge or suspicion that a particular virus is present in the sample and preclude the discovery of unknown viruses. However, these methods are rapid and accurate. These features are of major importance for the surveillance and control of epidemic diseases (e.g., influenza, RSV). Viral antigens can be revealed based on the ability of the antigen to interact with an antibody or to elicit a specific immune response. In addition, specific functional assays, such as hemagglutination tests, assessing the presence of particular proteins that are found in the envelope of orthomyxoviruses and paramyxoviruses, can be conducted to reveal the respective virus. These are described in the section on serologic methods. Sputum and nasal aspirates are considered better than throat swabs for the detection of viruses, such as RSV and influenza, with these methods.

Immunoassays

Immunofluorescence

Immunofluorescence is based on the chemical conjugation of a fluorochrome with an antibody, without compromising either the ability of the fluorochrome to fluoresce or the specificity of the antibody. Fluorescein isothiocyanate and tetramethyl rhodamine isothiocyanate are the most widely used fluorochromes; the former fluoresces yellowish-green, whereas the latter appears reddish-orange. Fluorescein isothiocyanate seems to be more suitable for clinical samples because the background is more often red than green. In addition, red-fluorescing dyes, such as Congo red, can be used to stain all cellular components red and provide a contrast to the green fluorescence of fluorescein isothiocyanate. A fluorescence microscope is required for the detection of light emitted by excited fluorochrome. In modern fluorescence microscopes with epi-illumination systems, light of selected wavelengths is deflected through the objective to the top surface of the sample. The resulting emitted light is directed through the objective, a dichroic mirror, a barrier filter, and the oculars, to the observer. Each fluorochrome has specific fluorescence characteristics. For instance, fluorescein isothiocyanate absorption is at 495 nm and emission is at 525 nm. With the available interference filters in fluorescence microscopes, 85% of transmitted light is between 400 and 500 nm (i.e., the visible part of the spectrum).

Practically, first, the sample should be fixed onto a slide. Thereafter, it is incubated, either with a specific antibody conjugated with a fluorochrome (direct detection) or with a primary specific antibody and thereafter with a secondary antibody raised against the primary one that has been conjugated with the fluorochrome (indirect detection). The first method is less sensitive, but it avoids nonspecific staining of negative samples, as is often seen with the indirect method. However, the generation of primary conjugates for many viruses is laborious and costly, whereas secondary conjugates may be common for several antigens. Incubation times are short for both procedures (30–45 minutes at 37°C), making immunofluorescence an advantageous method for rapid virus detection.

Viral samples can also be detected by immunofluorescence with spin cultures, whereby suitable cell monolayers are grown on coverslips within flat-bottom vials. The sample is then applied on top of the coverslip, and the vial is centrifuged (650–900 × *g* for 30–60 minutes). This technique facilitates virus entry into the target cells, and 18 to 24 hours later, or longer (depending on the virus), the coverslip is removed, fixed, and stained for immunofluorescence.

Direct and indirect immunofluorescence has been used for the development of a number of rapid tests for the detection of respiratory viruses. These can be accomplished within a few minutes, and they have become very popular due to their rapidity and ease of performance. Usually, a spot or slide containing the sample is prepared for every virus being tested, cytospun, and incubated with the monoclonal antibody. In a recent advance, a single spot can be used for the simultaneous detection of seven respiratory viruses (RSV, influenza A and B, adenovirus, and parainfluenza 1–3 viruses). A rhodamine label is used with the RSV antibody system, whereas fluorescein is used in all other cases. Thus, the development of a reddish-gold color in the spot suggests the presence of RSV particles in the sample, whereas a green color (fluorescein) is followed by a second reaction in another spot to determine which of the other viruses is present. The sensitivity of this method was greatly enhanced by centrifugation and was superior to that of enzyme immunoassay (EIA)–based protocols, but inferior to that of cell culture in that study.[20] Another indirect fluorescence method proved more efficient than cell culture in detecting respiratory viruses in nasopharyngeal swabs.[21]

Radioimmunoassay

There are two types of radioimmunoassays (RIAs). In competitive RIA methods, a known quantity of radioactivity-labeled antigen competes with unlabeled antigen that is added (test sample). The inhibition of binding of labeled antigen depends on the concentration of unlabeled antigen in the clinical sample. The labeled antigen that is finally bound to antibody is measured and referred to as *bound antigen,* whereas the unconjugated labeled antigen is referred to as *free antigen.* To circumvent problems arising from the separation of bound from free antigen in solid-phase RIA, the immunoreactant that is used first (antibody or antigen) is immobilized on a solid support. After each step, unwanted reactants can be removed readily by washing. In contrast to the laborious and expensive generation of labeled viral antigens, many of which are labile, noncompetitive RIA methods use labeled antibodies instead of viral antigens. The former are more stable, with more predictable structures and biochemical properties. Noncompetitive RIAs are, therefore, more popular in diagnostic virology. In a technique known as *sandwich RIA,* unlabeled viral antibodies adsorbed to a solid-phase support are allowed to capture viral antigens present in the clinical sample. Then a radiolabeled antibody (indicator antibody) is allowed to bind to the captured viral antigens. This procedure can be either direct or indirect. In the latter case, a primary unlabeled indicator antibody is used initially, followed by incubation with a secondary radiolabeled antibody. In all of these procedures, free antibody is removed after the final incubation and bound iodine-125-labeled antibody is measured.

Nasal aspirates are a suitable source for assessing the presence of respiratory viruses, such as RSV, with RIA. For the direct detection of viruses in tissue or cell culture, ^{125}I-labeled viral antibody is incubated with the cell monolayers or tissue sections and unbound labeled antibody is removed. The bound radioactivity is then measured. The radioactivity bound to the infected tissue or culture is then compared with the radioactivity bound to uninfected control samples. Ratios exceeding 2:1 are considered positive. In the indirect version of this technique, the sample is first incubated with unlabeled antibody, followed by ^{125}I-labeled secondary antibody.

Enzyme Immunoassays

As indicated by their name, EIAs are based on the conjugation of suitable enzymes (e.g., horseradish peroxidase, alkaline phosphatase) to antibodies and their subsequent use for the qualitative and quantitative detection of antigens. Enzyme-labeled antibodies are coupled to substrates that give insoluble color products and used to detect viral antigens, directly or indirectly, in tissues or cell cultures in cytoimmunoenzymatic staining. Colored substrates can be observed with the naked eye, with light microscopy, and even with electron microscopy, in the case of electron-dense products. As in the immunofluorescence methods described earlier, infected and control cell monolayers and tissue sections on slides are fixed and incubated directly with enzyme-coupled antibody (or with an uncoupled primary and an enzyme-coupled secondary antibody, in the indirect approach). Unbound enzyme conjugate is removed by washing, and the slides are incubated with enzyme substrates. After development of the colored product, the slides are rinsed, counterstained, and mounted in mounting medium to be observed under a light microscope.

A modification of the indirect approach includes an additional step whereby an antibody raised against the enzyme is incubated with the sample. Because this antibody is also conjugated with enzyme, its sensitivity is greatly enhanced. Both peroxidase-antiperoxidase and alkaline phosphatase–antialkaline phosphatase are being used, and the final reaction products can be either soluble color complexes or insoluble substrates that can be observed with the naked eye, observed with a light microscope, or measured in a spectrophotometer. In a typical peroxidase-antiperoxidase protocol, the sample and control are incubated with rabbit antiviral antibody and subsequently with a secondary antibody raised in a different species (e.g., sheep, goat). Subsequently, the sample is incubated with peroxidase-antiperoxidase raised in rabbit and, finally, with the substrate, followed by a stopping reaction.

Avidin-biotin is another system that is widely used to increase sensitivity in such approaches. The binding reaction between these two molecules is strong, and it occurs independently of the immune reactions in the assay. In a typical avidin-biotin complex protocol, biotin-conjugated primary antibodies are incubated with the samples, and after the unbound antibodies have been washed out, enzyme-conjugated avidin or streptavidin is added. The complex formed is monitored, with the final addition of substrate and mounting of the slide. In the indirect approach, an unlabeled primary antibody is first incubated with the sample, followed by secondary incubation with biotinylated antibody and the biotin-avidin enzyme complex incubation.

To assess the presence of viral antigens quantitatively, heterogenous EIA assays are used in which enzymatic activity is independent of the interaction of the antigen with the enzyme-conjugated antibody (or vice versa, if enzyme-conjugated antigen is used). To that end, the unbound enzyme-labeled antibody should be removed and the incubation should be relatively long. Like viral RIA assays, quantitative EIAs use unlabeled antiviral antibody bound to a solid phase (e.g., microtiter plates, cuvettes). Unbound antibody is removed after adsorption, and nonspecific binding sites are blocked by blocking agents, such as bovine serum albumin. After samples are added, unbound material is removed and enzyme-conjugated antibody is added. This antibody binds to antigen captured by solid-phase bound antibody. After removal of unbound material, enzyme substrate is added and the formation of the reaction product is measured. This measurement reflects the amount of enzyme bound to antigen that is retained in the solid phase. Control samples are always included to define the background levels of each modification. Influenza, adenovirus, and RSV can be measured by these methods.

The cassette EIA method is based on the fact that large amounts of antibody can be bound to nitrocellulose, nylon, and other membranes. Such a membrane is attached to a plastic well, and the entire system is attached to a cassette containing a material that can absorb all waste fluid generated during the assay. The antibody and the controls can be dotted or slotted onto the membrane in separate wells. The method offers the advantages of increased sensitivity and reduced time required for its completion. Based on the same principle, numerous variations are used, with different sensitivity scores. The solid phase, for instance, can be substituted by beads coated with antibody. After incubation with the sample, the beads can be transferred to the membranes and the assay can go on as a standard EIA. Alternatively, a classic dot-blot apparatus can be used to place an antibody in dots on the membrane. The additional binding sites on the membrane are then blocked. Samples and controls can then be added as serial dilutions for quantitation, and waste fluids are collected from the associated vacuum system. However, such systems, although able to discriminate between serotypes of the same species (e.g., influenza A vs. B), may not be as sensitive as cell culture or direct immunofluorescence in detecting virus.

Fluoroimmunoassay

In time-resolved fluoroimmunoassay, the unusually long fluorescence decay time of the lanthanide element europium (Eu^{+3}) is used to discriminate the fluorescence decay characteristics of europium-conjugated antibodies from the background fluorescence decay of clinical samples. Europium is first chelated with ethylenediaminetetraacetic acid and then conjugated to antibody. In a representative protocol, a microtiter plate or strip is coated with antibody and the remaining binding sites of the plates blocked. The clinical sample is then added simultaneously with the europium-conjugated antibody, and after incubation, the unbound material is washed out. Adenovirus, RSV, influenza virus, and parainfluenza virus have been detected with time-resolved fluoroimmunoassay. There are, however, reports of limited sensitivity of this method in detecting respiratory viruses in clinical samples.[22]

Optical Immunoassay

A recent advance in the field of antigen detection is optical immunoassay technology. This allows direct visual detection of a macromolecule that is bound onto a molecular thin film. This binding will result in an increase in the thickness of the optical surface (silicon wafer film) that will alter the reflected light path and will be perceived as a color change that is observable with the naked eye. Practically, viral-specific antibodies are immobilized on the surface and allowed to capture extracted viral antigens that are placed directly onto the surface and incubated at room temperature for a short period. After addition of a suitable substrate, a positive result appears as a color spot, whereas in the absence of antigens in the sample, the background color remains unchanged. Commercially available tests for influenza virus and RSV can take as little as 15 minutes to be completed and do not require sophisticated laboratory equipment, providing obvious advantages. An influenza-specific optical immunoassay test has been reported to be as good as cell culture in detecting influenza A or B from clinical samples[23]; however, others found low sensitivity scores with this method compared with those obtained by direct fluorescence or cell culture.[24]

Agglutination Assays

In the latex agglutination assay, antibody-coated nanoparticles from polystyrene, polyacrylamide and other latexes, agarose beads, or colloidal gold agglutinate in the presence of viral antigens. In a typical protocol for respiratory viruses, a clarified and diluted NPA sample is mixed with antibody-coated latex particles on a microscope slide. An agglutination reaction can be readily observed, usually after 10 to 15 minutes. Although these methods are simple and rapid, they are usually characterized by low sensitivity, and many control clinical samples show nonspecific agglutination.

SEROLOGIC METHODS

As indicated by the name, serologic methods attempt to detect viruses in the host by assessing the presence of specific antibodies in blood samples. In most cases, during the course of an illness, blood samples should be collected at least twice: in the acute phase and during convalescence. Comparison of the antibody pattern in these two states allows safe demonstration of diagnostically significant active virus. Acute-phase blood should be collected as soon as possible after the onset of disease (no later than

1 week), whereas the convalescent sample should be collected at least 2 weeks after onset. These requirements make serologic testing more relevant for epidemiologic studies than for clinical use, because the long delay before a definite diagnosis is made limits its use in urgent decision making in clinical practice. However, in many cases in which rapid methods of antigen detection are inefficient (e.g., RSV detection in adults), serologic testing is considered a reference method; moreover, it remains the method of choice for archival material; for example, it is as sensitive as PCR in detecting influenza infections.[25]

Among the five classes of human immunoglobulins (IgG, IgM, IgA, IgE, and IgD), the four IgG subclasses (IgG1–4) have a longer half-life (22 days) than the others and are associated with long-term protection. In addition, IgG antibodies exert their protective role against infection by triggering complement fixation and improve the specificity of the immune response by binding to the surface of cytotoxic effector cells. Most viruses induce mainly IgG1 and IgG3 responses. IgM antibodies represent approximately one tenth of serum immunoglobulins and are the first to be produced after exposure to a foreign antigen. Secretory IgA constitutes the first line of defense against mucosal viral infections.

On first encounter with the foreign antigen, the IgM class of antibodies is primarily produced, whereas IgG may be produced subsequently and may dominate the later phase of the response. On repeat encounter, memory B cells produce high levels of high-affinity IgG antibodies. When the antigen is localized in the mucosa, the immune response, driven by B cells of the interstitial lymphoid follicles (e.g., tonsils, Peyer's patches) also produces high quantities of IgA.

There are many potential antigens in each virus that may be presented at different time points in the course of infection. The primary antibody response to a virus is typically characterized by early onset of IgM production (peaking at 2 weeks) that declines later, followed by IgG production (reaching a plateau 2 weeks later) that may persist for years. Reinfection may result in overproduction of IgG, together with low or undetectable production of IgM.

Another major issue in antibody measurement is the type of antibodies targeted by the test. Thus, antibodies detected by EIAs may be different from those that confer neutralization activity. Neutralizing antibodies persist after viral infection; their measurement aims to determine vaccine efficacy and is used in epidemiologic studies rather than for the diagnosis of primary infection. Neutralizing antibodies are raised against particular epitopes, usually found on the surface of the virus, and on binding to the virus, render it noninfectious by blocking its attachment to receptors or preventing uncoating of the virus. In tests assessing neutralizing antibody, the serum sample is usually incubated with a viral preparation of known titer, and its ability to inhibit $TCID_{50}$ during CPE development in cell culture is assessed. Alternatively, the reduction in the ability of the viral preparation to form plaques can be measured.

There are three main ways to detect respiratory virus in the host serologically. Immunoassays, conducted in a manner similar to that described earlier for the detection of viral antigens, directly measure antibody-virus interaction through the use of labeled reagents. Complement fixation and passive agglutination assays are based on the ability of virus-antibody interactions to interfere with the functions discussed earlier, but do not allow differentiation between antibody classes. Finally, assays, such as hemagglutination inhibition, allow the measurement of particular antibodies that specifically interact with viral surface proteins.

Immunoassays

As in the antigen detection immunoassays described earlier, reporter molecules conjugated with antibodies (or antigens) allow the assessment of virus-antibody interactions. The reporter molecules may fluoresce (immunofluorescence), may have enzymatic activity for color-developing substrates (EIA), or may have radioactivity (RIA).

Immunofluorescence

In immunofluorescence assays, purified hyperimmune animal sera or monoclonal antibodies are labeled with a fluorescent dye (e.g., fluorescein isothiocyanate). In a typical protocol, a serum sample is incubated with virus-infected cells that are fixed on a slide. After unbound material is washed out, the slide can be dried, mounted, and observed under a fluorescence microscope. Streptavidin-biotin and similar systems that are currently used provide greater flexibility and sensitivity in antibody detection. Background fluorescence is a common obstacle in immunofluorescence procedures. In solid-phase fluoroimmunoassay, the viral antigen is immobilized on an opaque solid-phase surface rather than a slide, and fluorescence is measured in a fluorometer, allowing quantitation and automation of the method. However, fluoroimmunoassay instrumentation cannot discriminate between background and positive fluorescence.

Enzyme Immunoassays

Enzyme immunoassays are used to detect and quantitate antibody raised against viral antigens. Antigens are obtained from various sources, such as lysates from virus-infected cells. To that end, cells are washed, resuspended in serum-free medium, and subjected to repeated freeze-thaw cycles. Virus is then clarified with ultracentrifugation, providing a rich source of antigens. Synthetic peptides also may be used for antigen preparation.

For indirect EIA, the antigen is bound to a solid-phase surface, and after incubation with the serum sample, bound antibodies are detected with an anti-human antibody enzyme conjugate. The more abundant IgG antibodies compete for antigens with the other classes and, thus, should have been removed before IgM measurement. Nonspecific binding is common in this method, and impurities present in the antigen preparation may cause false-positive results. Preincubating the sera with uninfected cells may reduce this problem.

To increase the specificity of this method, inhibition, or competitive, EIAs have been used. In this case, serum antibodies are detected by their ability to block the binding of a known antibody conjugate to the antigen. The detector antibody can be added simultaneously, with or after the antigen and the serum sample. False-negative results can be caused, in this case, by serum antibodies that do not compete with the conjugated antibody, but inhibit the ability of the antibody that is being tested to do so.

In the capture EIA method, anti-human immunoglobulin class-specific antibodies are first bound on a solid-phase (capture-phase) surface. After incubation with the serum sample, viral antibodies are bound on the capture phase, together with viral-unrelated antibodies. Viral antigens are added last and subsequently detected with an antigen-specific antibody conjugate. Due to the selective class-specific adsorption in the first step, this method avoids the problems caused by competition between antibody classes, particularly improving IgM detection. On the other hand, low-level IgG detection may be less sensitive due to the presence of large quantities of total IgG antibodies in serum.

Other Immunoassays

When it is necessary to detect low levels of virus-specific antibodies in serum, standard immunoblot techniques (Western blot) can be used. Briefly, the protein content of semipurified virus propagated in cell culture is applied onto a nondenaturing polyacrylamide gel, and after electrophoretic separation, protein bands are transferred to a nitrocellulose or nylon membrane that can be cut into narrow strips and stored in the freezer. Serum samples can be diluted in buffer containing a protein that blocks free binding sites to reduce nonspecific binding, and then incubated with the membrane. After a washing step, bound antibodies are measured with the use of a radioactive or enzyme-labeled conjugate bound to a suitable secondary antibody. In dot immunobinding assays, viral antigens are bound in a dotted membrane. The membrane is then treated so that the potential protein-binding sites remaining in the membrane are blocked. The dots are then covered with small (e.g., 3-mm) strips saturated with the test serum. After a washing step, anti-human IgG conjugated with the appropriate enzyme is added, followed by incubation with the appropriate chromogen substrate. The intensity of the color spots is compared with that produced by the control sera to reveal specific antiviral antibodies. Dot immunobinding assays serve as qualitative rather than quantitative assays and are also subject to problems with nonspecific binding.

In radioimmunoprecipitation assays, antigen-antibody complexes formed after incubation of the serum being tested with viral antigens are cross-linked and immunoprecipitated with protein A or anti-human IgG antibody. The quantity of radioactivity bound in the precipitate can be measured, and is proportional to the concentration of specific antibodies in the serum.

Avidity assays measure the relative degree of dissociation between specific antiviral antibodies and their respective antigens. During maturation of the immune response, the avidity (strength of the combined interaction of an antiserum with a pattern of antigens) of IgG antibodies remains high, whereas their concentration declines. Thus, sera from recent infection are characterized by high-avidity antibodies and sera from reinfection have low-avidity antibodies. Practically, serum is incubated first with antigen bound to a solid-phase surface. The complex is then allowed to dissociate in the presence or absence of urea, and the relative degree of antibody dissociation (ratio of absorbance in the presence of urea to absorbance in the absence of urea) is measured by standard EIA methods.

Finally, three types of methods have been used to specifically measure IgM antibodies that typically are transiently expressed during primary infection and may facilitate its identification. First, in IgG absorption methods, an IgG absorbent (e.g., staphylococcal protein A, streptococcal protein G) is incubated with the serum, and after a centrifugation step, so that IgM antibodies can be measured in the supernatant. These absorbents are believed to be superior to anti-human IgG antibodies for this method, because the latter may also remove some types of IgM. However, staphylococcal protein cannot bind IgG3, and this could interfere with the accuracy of the method because viral antibodies may be significantly represented in this subclass. Streptococcal protein G, on the other hand, binds all IgG subclasses, but not IgM; accordingly, combinations of streptococci and protein A have been used to remove all IgG and IgA from serum samples before IgM measurement. IgA can interfere with IgM measurement, resulting in false-negative findings by competing with IgM for antigenic sites. Second, in one of the early IgM separation methods, rate zonal centrifugation allowed purification of the IgM subclass based on its higher sedimentation coefficient compared with that of the other antibody classes. Gel filtration takes advantage of the higher molecular weight of IgM compared with the other classes (900 vs. 150–400 kd). However, serum lipoproteins and nonspecific cell agglutinins may be fractionated, together with IgM, and could interfere with the assay. Ion-exchange chromatography, based on the differential binding of IgM and IgG classes to anion-exchange resins, has been used, but the IgM yield is relatively low, whereas IgG and IgA may still be present in the IgM fraction after elution from the column. Third, in the popular IgM immunoassays, anti-human IgM-specific antibodies are employed. Indirect immunofluorescence and EIA are the methods typically used for IgM detection. Capture IgM assays show reduced nonspecific binding; in this method, solid-phase, fixed anti-human IgM antibodies separate IgM after incubation with the serum sample. The potential presence of antiviral elements is further detected using labeled viral antigen or unlabeled antigen, followed by a labeled antigen-specific antibody. Detection of antiparainfluenza IgM has been also reported with the use of hemadsorption.

Complement Fixation

Complement fixation systems take advantage of the fact that complement proteins bind, or "fix," to antigen-antibody complexes during the host immune response to a foreign antigen. If this antigen is cell localized, then the deposition of complement elements will cause cell lysis. Complement fixation to IgM is stronger (>1000 times/antibody molecule) than that to IgG. Complement fixation antibodies can be raised against some or all viral proteins. Their titers increase slowly during primary infection, reaching lower levels than antibody titers detected by the other methods. In addition, they decline gradually, making this method less sensitive than others for the detection of viral infection. An additional problem is the interference of some serum elements (heparin, IgG aggregates) with complement formation. In a typical complement fixation assay, the serum sample is incubated with a particular antigen in the presence of a known amount of guinea pig complement. If a specific antibody is present in the serum, the complement will be bound and depleted from the solution. Subsequently, sheep erythrocytes coated with hemolysin (anti-sheep erythrocyte antibody) are added, and their lysis is proportional to the availability of complement proteins that did not react with the specific antibody during the first step. However, complement fixation assays are considered less sensitive than virus isolation and antigen detection methods in revealing the presence of a respiratory virus in patients.

In immune adherence agglutination assay, a rapid and more sensitive variation, aggregation, rather than lysis, of erythrocytes occurs and is measured. In this detection method, complement that is bound to antigen-antibody complexes is allowed to bind to C′3b receptors in human primate erythrocytes. Thus, agglutination of the erythrocytes reveals specific antibodies in the sample.

A simple technique used earlier for the detection of hemagglutinating activity–containing viruses, such as influenza and parainfluenza, is the hemolysis-in-gel test. Erythrocytes from sheep or chicken were first sensitized by coupling to a viral antigen in a chromium chloride solution. After a washing step, the erythrocytes were suspended in an agarose gel containing guinea pig complement. The serum sample was then loaded onto a well in the gel and allowed to diffuse. The presence of antibodies against the virus would lead to the formation of a zone of hemolysis around the well.

Anticomplement antifluorescence is a modified immunofluorescence assay for the detection of complement fixation antibodies. In this assay, complement is added during or after exposure of virus-infected cells to the serum being tested. Any complement that is bound can then be detected with anti-C′3 antibody. Because nonspecifically bound IgG cannot trigger complement fixation, anticomplement antifluorescence assays do not have the common background problems associated with conventional immunofluorescence.

Agglutination Assays

Hemagglutinin or hemagglutinin-neuraminidase proteins expressed in the envelopes of viruses, such as influenza and parainfluenza, are able to bind to specific erythrocyte surface receptors and cause their agglutination. Practically, erythrocyte cross-linking leads to observable cell clumping. Hemagglutination inhibition tests measure the presence of specific antibodies in the sera that inhibit virus-mediated agglutination of erythrocytes. This is a sensitive assay that is affected, however, by both nonspecific hemagglutinins and agglutinin inhibitors present in the serum. Nevertheless, it is a particularly reliable method in influenza surveillance protocols.[26]

Fusion proteins present in the envelope of viruses, such as parainfluenza and RSV, allow their entry into cells by triggering fusion of the viral surface with the cell surface membrane. In the case of erythrocytes, fusion may lead to hemolysis. Hemolysis inhibition assays take advantage of these properties to measure the presence of antibodies in a serum sample that bind and block viral antigens and inhibit hemolysis. In this way, the hemolysis inhibition assay detects both antihemagglutinin and antifusion antibodies in the serum. In a typical protocol, serum dilutions are mixed and incubated with purified virus. A 10% suspension of suitable erythrocytes is then added. After some hours of incubation, the erythrocytes are removed by centrifugation and the optical density of the "cleared" supernatant is read with a spectrophotometer. A classic endpoint titer can then be calculated by defining the highest serum dilution that causes 50% inhibition of hemolysis.

In passive agglutination assays, sera are incubated with viral antigens attached to erythrocytes or to materials such as latex or bentonite. The particles or cells agglutinate in the presence of a specific antibody, forming precipitates in the bottom of the tubes. In the passive hemagglutination method, aggregates of erythrocytes develop due to "antibody bridges" formed between antigen-coated erythrocytes. These can be visible, even with the naked eye, and may detect low levels of antibodies.

DETECTION OF VIRAL NUCLEIC ACIDS

A constellation of methods that gained increasing attention during recent years due to their increased sensitivity, ease of use, and accuracy are genetic material-based methods, with PCR in the leading position. The common element in these methods is the isolation and partial purification of viral RNA or DNA and its subsequent detection and analysis in suitable molecular biology systems.

Hybridization

Hybridization-based protocols require the presence of single-stranded RNA or DNA. Because the majority of respiratory viruses are single-stranded RNA, these viruses are believed to be suitable for detection with hybridization techniques. In this approach, a suitable oligonucleotide probe sharing a certain degree of homology that allows base pair matching with the single-stranded viral nucleic acid is allowed to anneal under stringent reaction conditions (hybridization). Whereas single-stranded RNA viruses provide ready-made, yet labile, genetic material, the double-stranded DNA content of adenovirus must first be denatured or dissociated by chemical (e.g., sodium hydroxide) or physical (heat) means. The resulting single-stranded DNA would return to its double-stranded configuration on removal of the dissociation agent. The probe can be labeled directly with enzymes or other reporter molecules; alternatively, linker moieties, such as biotin or digoxigenin, can be attached to probes and serve as bridges for the attachment of reporter molecules. Digoxigenin-labeled probes are believed to be more sensitive for in situ hybridization than those using the biotin-streptavidin system. In a typical protocol, the viral nucleic acid is isolated, purified, denatured, and bound to a nitrocellulose or nylon membrane. The probe, denatured and labeled, is incubated with the viral nucleic acid, under carefully defined conditions, and unbound material is thoroughly washed out. A reporter molecule is then added (e.g., alkaline phosphatase-labeled streptavidin), and after a second incubation period, the unbound reporter is washed out and the final chromogen or other suitable substrate is added to give rise to a measurable signal.

Several hybridization-based techniques are used for viral nucleic acid detection, such as the molecular biology dot-blot and Southern blot protocols and liquid and in situ hybridization. As suggested by its name, liquid hybridization allows the detection of nucleic acid that is free in solution rather than attached to a solid-phase surface. Microtiter plates and strips can be used in this method, increasing the ease of handling. In situ hybridization allows the detection of virus in a variety of sources, including cells and tissues grown or fixed on slides, respectively. RNA hybridization proved to be a sensitive method for detecting influenza replication in culture, being clearly superior to hemagglutination assays.[27] It shows high sensitivity in detecting RNA viruses (detection limits, 30–100 copies of viral genome/cell). For example, in situ hybridization-based detection of RV is shown in biopsy specimens from human bronchi (Fig. 22-2). In some cases, hybridization can be superior even to PCR in detecting a respiratory virus in the airway.[28]

Hybridization techniques are also used in combination with PCR-based methods to increase the overall sensitivity of respiratory virus detection protocols.

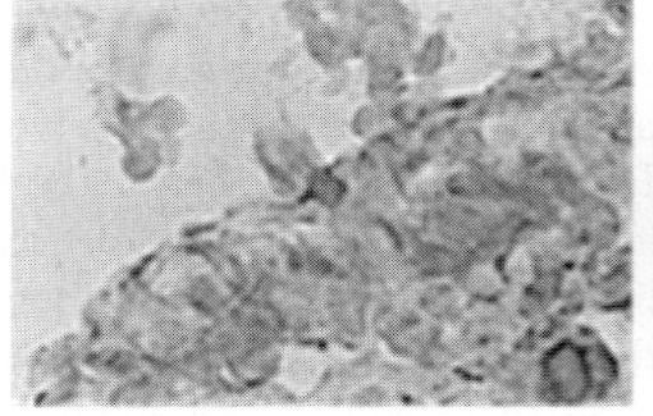
A

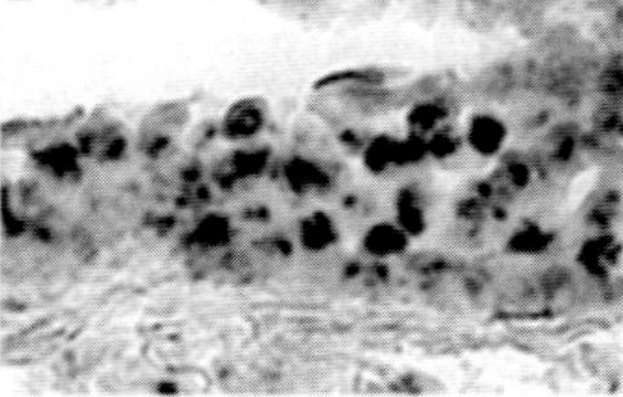
B

FIGURE 22-2. Detection of rhinovirus ribonucleic acid with in situ hybridization, in a bronchial biopsy specimen obtained from a volunteer, **(A)** at baseline and **(B)** after experimental inoculation with rhinovirus. No signal could be observed in the baseline biopsy specimen, whereas an intense signal (*black spots*), located at the bronchial epithelium, is present 3 days after nasal inoculation with the virus.

Polymerase Chain Reaction

Polymerase chain reaction methods allow specific amplification of defined DNA sequences and their subsequent detection and assessment. They have become a common practice in detection protocols during the last few years. This section discusses recent innovations in the field, but does not describe PCR basics in detail. Many existing handbooks describe this method. The majority of respiratory viruses are RNA viruses; therefore, reverse transcription PCR is required for their detection in clinical samples. First, total RNA is extracted from NPA samples or throat swabs by standard molecular biologic techniques. The samples should be kept at −70°C to avoid deterioration of the genetic material. A good practice is to store samples at −70°C in an appropriate virus transport medium (e.g., Hank's balanced salt solution enriched with 0.5% bovine serum albumin). If throat swabs are the source, they can be placed directly into a denaturing solution to inactivate ribonuclease enzyme activity, and then stored or transported at room temperature. Extracted RNA is then reverse transcribed into complementary DNA (cDNA; e.g., with reverse transcriptase isolated from a retrovirus, such as murine MoMuLV) and further amplified by PCR using virus-specific oligonucleotides (primers) that have been designed with the aid of computer software. These primers are usually planned to amplify sequences that are 100 to 1000 base pairs long (amplicons), and can be designed so that they discriminate between different serotypes of the same virus. Nucleotide diversity that is frequently observed among different strains of a given virus species should also be taken into account, and areas of high homology should be selected for serotype-specific primer pairs design. The amplicons can then be electrophoresed in a 1% to 2.5% agarose gel and visualized as DNA bands under an ultraviolet transilluminator after they are stained with ethidium bromide or another DNA dye. This is readily accomplished within 1 working day, a fact that is of particular importance for the clinical diagnostic laboratory.

To further improve the specificity and sensitivity of the test, the amplicons can be hybridized with labeled synthesized DNA probes directed against regions of the amplicon. For instance, Southern blot has been successfully used for the identification of picornaviruses. Alternatively, reverse transcriptase PCR can be combined with EIA techniques, consisting of hybridization of the amplicon with biotinylated RNA probes directed against the internal sequences of the amplicon. Time-resolved fluorometry has also been combined with PCR for the detection of picornaviruses.[29] PCR amplicons can also be used as a source for a second round of PCR in the "nested" PCR that usually shows increased sensitivity. In this approach, a second set of primers is designed against sequences that were localized internally in the sequences that were amplified in the first round. The method can be so sensitive as to detect a few particles of respiratory virus.[30] Nested-type PCR not only may increase sensitivity, but also may discriminate between serotypes within viral species that are of similar size and thus are difficult to separate with gel from the first round of PCR. Discrimination within or between species can be also accomplished by digesting the amplicons with restriction endonucleases. Human RVs, for instance, can be discriminated from enteroviruses based on the specific pattern produced after digestion of the PCR product with BglI restriction endonuclease.[31] Enteroviruses lack a BglI recognition site in their respective amplified sequence. Thus, their product remains undigested, retaining its original size (Fig. 22-3).

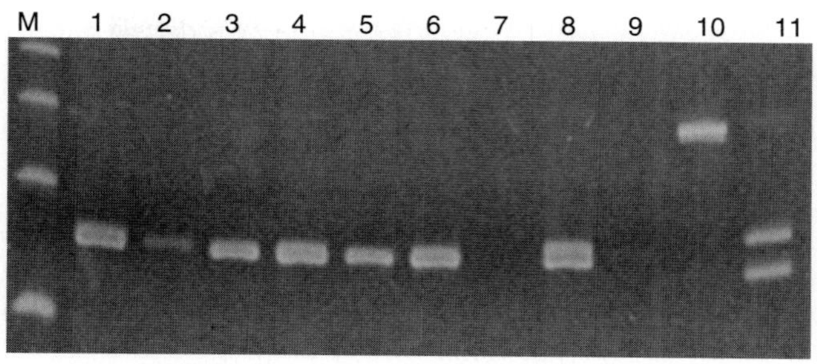

■ **FIGURE 22-3.** Detection of rhinovirus genetic material by reverse transcriptase polymerase chain reaction and its differentiation from enteroviruses. Picornavirus amplicons generated by the OL26-OL27 primer pair were digested with BglI. Rhinovirus (lanes 1–6) is detected as a single band with approximately 190 base pairs (bp) [consisting of two almost identical bands]. This easily allows differentiation from a poliovirus isolate (lane 10), whose amplicon remains undigested (~380 bp), and from a coxsackie virus (lane 11), which produces a duplet (~175 and 200 bp, respectively). M, DNA size marker.

In multiplex PCR, a mix of primer pairs is used, allowing simultaneous amplification and detection of several serotypes or viruses. There are many such examples in the literature; the formulation of Hexaplex (Prodesse, Waukesha, Wisconsin), for instance, allows the detection of H1N1, H3N2, influenza A, influenza B, both RSV subtypes, and three of the four human parainfluenzas.[32] This multiplex PCR has been tested in clinical samples and seems to achieve high rates of sensitivity and specificity. In addition, this highly sensitive and rapid type of test not only allows simultaneous detection of many viruses, providing obvious advantages for clinical practice, but also may reveal the presence of virus in samples with few viral copies or the presence of viral RNA without live virus, both of which may be missed with conventional cell culture techniques. The detection limits of multiplex reverse transcriptase PCR protocols allow the identification of as few as 100 to 140 copies of virus/mL, or one $TCID_{50}$. This method can be at least as sensitive as combined tissue culture and immunofluorescence methods. Combination with hybridization may further improve detection scores. In a combination of multiplex reverse transcriptase PCR and enzyme hybridization assay, the amplicons of seven respiratory viruses (RSV A and B, influenza A and B, parainfluenza 1–3 viruses) were purified and hybridized with peroxidase-labeled probes into avidin-coated, 96-well microplates. The signal emitted after incubation of the complex with the substrate allowed the detection of almost twice as many positive clinical samples compared with conventional culture and indirect immunofluorescence methods.[33] The performance of multiplex PCR assays may vary, depending on the virus tested. For instance, a multiplex PCR enzyme-linked immunosorbent assay that can detect seven respiratory viruses, in addition to the common respiratory pathogens *Mycoplasma pneumoniae* and *Chlamydia pneumoniae,* although it proved to be more sensitive than cell culture in detecting parainfluenza 3 virus, adenovirus, and influenza virus, was less efficient (by at least a factor of 10) in revealing RSV and parainfluenza 1 virus. Recent developments in this method include primers specific for additional viral and bacterial species (e.g., *Reovirus, Bordetella pertussis*), allowing for the detection of as many as 19 different microorganisms in a clinical sample.[34] Finally, multiplex PCR assays have been designed to discriminate between multiple subtypes within one species, as is the case with adenoviruses and picornaviruses.[35,36] In another approach, degenerate primers have been used to discriminate between adenovirus serotypes.[37]

Amplicons can also be subjected to sequence analysis to identify potential point mutations or deletions or specific serotypes. Cloning of PCR fragments that are generated with a series of partially overlapping or degenerate primers into bacterial plasmids allows sequencing of the entire viral genome, a laborious activity that is not necessary for usual clinical practice, but is indispensable when a previously unknown viral species is characterized (e.g., MPV) or when a high-risk epidemic from an initially unknown viral strain or mutation must be confronted efficiently and quickly (e.g., SARS). Heteroduplex formation between the amplicons may result in differential mobility of the product when run in a gel, and can be used for subtyping viral genomes. By combining, for instance, reverse transcriptase PCR and heteroduplex formation, variant strains of influenza can be differentiated.[38]

In situ PCR allows detection of viral genetic material and, furthermore, its localization at the cellular and tissue levels, providing information that is of particular importance for clinical pathology. Thus, paraffin-embedded, fixed cells or tissue sections are xylene-treated and then digested with protease and deoxyribonuclease solutions. The PCR mixture containing Taq polymerase is placed on top of it, and the entire slide is placed on an aluminium foil boat, transferred onto a conventional or modified PCR apparatus, and subjected to PCR amplification. If the one of the four deoxynucleoside 5′-triphosphates (dNTPs) that is present in the PCR mixture and is providing the nucleotide source is reduced and replaced by a modified nucleotide (e.g., biotinylated or digoxigenin-coupled deoxyuridine 5-triphosphate), then the emerging amplicons can be detected by incubation with an enzyme-labeled probe (e.g., alkaline phosphatase, antidigoxigenin). Alternatively, in the absence of modified nucleotides, the amplified DNA can be detected by conventional in situ hybridization, conducted as described earlier. Alternatively, the PCR mixture can be transferred to a test tube and run in an agarose gel or subjected to Southern analysis to identify the viral genomic fragments.

Real-Time Polymerase Chain Reaction

Recent advances in PCR technology allowed the development of real-time PCR. Real-time PCR can be more sensitive and time-efficient than conventional PCR, cell culture, and immunofluorescence in detecting respiratory viruses in clinical samples[39,40]; further, it is quantitative, allowing for assessment of the exact number of viral copies in a clinical sample. This is of particular importance because, in some cases, the actual viral load may determine the course of a disease. The final detection step employs either a dye able to bind to double-stranded DNA (e.g., SYBR Green I) or a more specific hybridization probe (e.g., TaqMan, Molecular Beacons, Light Cycler probes) to monitor the presence and quantity of amplicons. For quantitative analysis as well as determination of the detection limits, serial dilutions of plasmid DNA containing a known amount of viral genome (virus genome equivalent) per microliter can be used as a standard reference solution.

In fluorescent dye SYBR Green protocols, the dye is incorporated into the amplicons in each cycle and assessment of fluorescing DNA is collected during each extension phase. However, such dyes bind to DNA, independent of the specific sequence, and thus can also detect undesired, nonspecifically amplified DNA. Thus, the specificity of the method is tested by the melting curves at which the final amplicon is briefly heated to denature (e.g., 95°C), allowed to reassociate at a lower temperature (e.g., 65°C for 15 seconds), and finally re-denatured to 95°C by gradually increasing the temperature at a defined rate (e.g., 0.1°C/sec). The continuously measured fluorescence data recorded during this last stage are plotted against the temperature and allow calculation of the melting peak that characterizes a given amplicon under the conditions used. When the melting peak of a particular product coincides with the standard, it is considered specific. Highly sensitive one- and two-step, real-time PCR assays for the qualitative and quantitative detection of most respiratory viruses, including SARS-CoV, have been reported.[41–43]

In hybridization-based protocols, a specific probe sharing consensus homology with the sequenced strains of a viral species is labeled with a reporter fluorogenic dye (e.g., 6-carboxyfluoroscein) at the 5′ end and a quencher dye (e.g., carboxytetramethylrhodamine) at the 3′ end. The probe is present in the conventional PCR master mix (containing buffer, magnesium^{+2} salts, dNTPs, water, and the primers) during PCR, and the real-time apparatus records the fluorescence emerging during time. The reporter dye fluorescence (e.g., 6-carboxyfluoroscein) is considered positive and compared with the fluorescence emitted by a reference dye present in the PCR master mix to normalize for non-PCR-related fluorescence fluctuations among samples. A threshold is usually set, above which a signal is considered positive.

Recent approaches to the detection of respiratory viruses include the development of multiplex real-time PCR protocols. A SYBR Green–based reaction, for instance, allowed simultaneous detection of influenza A and B, together with RSV, with specificity comparable to that achieved with commercially available rapid antigenic tests and considerably higher sensitivity scores.[44] Discrimination between the particular species was based on the specific melting temperature curves elicited by the amplicons. This method, however, was not designed to discriminate between A and B subtypes of RSV. Limitations in the number of viruses and viral serotypes are inherent in the real-time approach, especially in the protocols using a labeled probe, because most platforms do not allow the simultaneous use of more than two fluorochromes. Using a more advanced apparatus that can detect up to four fluorochromes, Templeton and colleagues[45] succeeded in detecting both influenza serotypes, RSV, and all four parainfluenza subtypes in a two-tube reaction. In their approach, the specific probes were labeled with different fluorochromes (i.e., 6-carboxyfluoroscein, Texas red, hexachlorofluoroscein, and cyanin 5); the overall reaction could be accomplished within 6 hours and proved to be more sensitive than cell culture in detecting these seven respiratory viruses in clinical samples. The detection limits ranged from 0.1 to 0.0001 $TCID_{50}$ of viral stocks of known titer, depending on the virus.

Other Methods

Advances in molecular biology continuously offer additional PCR- and hybridization-based methods. In a recent study, as few as 100 RNA copies of parainfluenza virus (or one TCID50) could be detected by probe hybridization and electrochemiluminescence or by using molecular beacons.[46] The first step in this approach, nucleic acid sequence–based amplification, was used. This technique employs avian myeloblastosis virus reverse transcriptase, together with ribonuclease H and T7 RNA polymerase, under isothermal conditions, and is able to directly amplify RNA. The use of nucleic acid sequences to amplify RNA with primers directed against the 5′ noncoding region of RV serotypes allows discrimination between RV subgroups.[47]

Complementary DNA-amplified restriction fragment length polymorphism allows the identification of previously unknown viral sequences. In this method, double-stranded cDNA is synthesized from viral RNA and digested with frequently cutting restriction endonucleases. Double-stranded adaptors are then ligated to the ends of the emerging restriction fragments and provide primer sites during PCR amplification. A second selective fragment amplification step is conducted by adding one or more bases to the PCR primers. If the complementary bases are present in the viral sequence, then successful amplification will occur. A modification of this method was successfully employed in the recent discovery of the new coronavirus NL63.[10]

Recently, Wang and colleagues used the powerful microarray technology to detect approximately 140 distinct viral genomes simultaneously, including most respiratory viruses.[48] To that end, 1600 oligonucleotides with a relatively greater length than those commonly used in array technology (70 vs. 20–25 bases) were selected after a genome-wide BLAST (Basic Local Alignment Search Tool, a method for rapid searching of nucleotide and protein databases) analysis and ranked according to shared homology to regions of the viral genomes. Using an ink-jet oligonucleotide synthesizer, these oligonucleotides are synthesized in situ and placed onto directed locations of a glass wafer.[49] The glass surfaces can then be hybridized, under strict conditions, with cDNA, PCR amplicons, RNA, or another form of genetic material derived from viral stocks, virally infected cells in cultures, or clinical samples. Human and cellular transcripts are also included to normalize against nonspecific hybridization. This material is labeled with cyanin 5 or cyanin 3, which provides red or green coloring, respectively, to allow color visualization of microarray data that are obtained after the arrays are scanned with confocal laser scanners and analyzed with suitable instrumentation and software. This method allows the detection of paramyxoviruses, orthomyxoviruses, adenoviruses, and picornaviruses from clinical samples. It can also detect and discriminate among all 102 RV serotypes, based on the hybridization pattern obtained from each serotype. After human volunteers were experimentally infected with RV, the array could detect as few as 100 infectious RV particles in NPA samples.[48] Analysis of a small number of samples from naturally acquired colds showed different RV serotypes and parainfluenza 1 virus, which has also been confirmed by conventional reverse transcriptase PCR. Although it is extremely promising, this technique needs further evaluation, including cost-effectiveness, before being applied in clinical practice.

Practical Considerations in the Use of Nucleic Acid–Based Techniques

Nucleic acid–based virus detection is both rapid and accurate. The identification of a particular virus can be further, and without doubt, confirmed by restriction analysis or sequencing of the product and further comparison with published genome databases. In addition, the PCR-based methods have proved to be very sensitive, usually exceeding the sensitivity scores of cell culture techniques. However, false-positive or false-negative findings can be a problem with these methods, if certain practical measures in the handling of viral genetic material are not meticulously followed. First, preservation of the sample is of particular importance for the integrity of the viral genomic material. RNA, the genomic material of most respiratory viruses, is particularly vulnerable to degradation by ribonucleases that are present in all biologic samples and fluids. Ribonuclease-free vials, solutions, and buffers should be used in designated areas of the laboratory, and all material should be used by specialized personnel. In addition, if it takes too long for an NPA sample to be transported from the clinic to the laboratory, or if the sample remains on ice for too many hours instead of being placed in the freezer immediately, the sensitivity of the method, even that of a PCR-based protocol, can be unexpectedly low. Further, biologic fluids often contain substances that can inhibit PCR amplification (e.g., mucus). In this case, dilution of the sample or treatment with a suitable agent (e.g., dimethyl sulfoxide) may facilitate detection of the virus. The use of clinical samples spiked with stock virus or the inclusion of synthetic heterologous competitor RNA in the reaction may facilitate normalization of PCR outcomes.

On the other hand, PCR-based techniques are also subject to problems with contamination, especially if large numbers of samples are handled simultaneously. In the case of a nested PCR protocol, the first and second rounds of PCR should be conducted in separate areas, with separate sets of pipettes, and of course, with different plasticware. Nested PCR protocols include several negative controls to monitor for the presence of contamination. If it occurs, replacement of the pipettes is required, as well as a review of laboratory and handling practices.

TECHNIQUES TO DIAGNOSE RESPIRATORY VIRUSES IN CLINICAL PRACTICE

Respiratory infections cause a major health problem, with huge associated costs and mortality rates worldwide. In addition, threatening influenza pandemics and mortal epidemics of previously unknown respiratory viruses, such as SARS-CoV, require the use of rapid and reliable detection methods in clinical practice. Moreover, large epidemiologic studies are required to better define the involvement of these viruses in noninfectious diseases, such as asthma, in the short and long term. This analysis will help in drug development and the implementation of intervention strategies, even during an outbreak. Because many respiratory symptoms are common among these viruses, clinical examination does not determine the etiology of particular cases. On the other hand, drugs are being developed that specifically block infection by individual viruses (i.e., anti-influenza neuraminidase inhibitors), but they are useless if the patient has been infected by another virus. Thus, all of these methods are of major and increasing importance and use in clinical practice. It is not possible to determine which is the optimal method for virus detection because many parameters vary, depending on the particular conditions and the scope of the analysis (cost-effectiveness, time required, sensitivity, availability of skilled personnel and laboratory equipment). It is a combination of methods, rather than a single one, that is practically used in particular cases because most protocols are not ideal. Even electron microscopy is still recognized as an indispensable method in some cases.[50] Although cell culture remains the gold standard, it is time consuming and tends to be replaced by antigen-detecting methods and molecular biologic techniques. Their commercial availability, ease of performance, and rapidity have made the newly developed antigen-based methods increasingly popular. Actually, these tests tend to be preferred in routine analysis, especially in small units lacking advanced facilities. They can be accomplished within 15 minutes to a few hours. However, they can be inferior to cell culture in terms of sensitivity,[51] and are of limited value for the detection of some respiratory viruses, such as RSV, in older population groups.[52]

On the other hand, PCR has been widely used as a research tool during the last decade, and its clinical use is steadily increasing. PCR cannot, however, replace the use of cell culture in worldwide influenza surveillance, an aspect of classic virology that is vital for informing vaccine constituents.[53]

■ FUTURE DIRECTIONS

Rapidity, high sensitivity and specificity, ease of use, and cost-effectiveness are the major requirements imposed on the respiratory viral detection assay field. In particular, the need for rapid diagnostics is likely to increase as more specific antiviral therapies enter the market. Many of the whole-virus, antigen, serologic, and molecular methods have been extensively tested and used in clinical practice. Although PCR-based analysis was the major breakthrough in recent years, none of the existing methods can be considered ideal, and usually, a combination of techniques is used for more accurate results, increasing the costs, time, and skills required for analysis. Rapid antigen detection tests are, for the moment, the easiest to apply and are expected to be further improved in the future. Electronic microscopy is still useful in many cases, as, for example, in the crucial first screening and characterization of the previously unknown SARS-CoV.

Simultaneous and reliable detection of as many viruses as possible, in the shortest time possible, and ideally, in a single test, is the goal of any novel and future technique. Although it is specific, sensitive, and reliable, multiplex real-time PCR can detect only limited numbers of viruses simultaneously. This may, however, improve in the future. Nevertheless, detection of up to 19 microorganisms seems to be achievable with conventional multiplex PCR methods, retaining PCR approaches in a leading position. On the other hand, the rapidly developing gene array field is promising, but without clinical relevance. This technique can also be combined with assays revealing expression patterns of target genes in the host, thus providing an overall picture not only of viral presence, but also of host response. This pattern could provide additional information regarding the immediate effects of a specific treatment that would obviously be of tremendous importance in clinical practice.

REFERENCES

1. Johnston SL, Pattemore PK, Sanderson G, Smith S, Lampe F, Josephs L, et al: Community study of role of viral infections in exacerbations of asthma in 9–11 year old children. BMJ 1995;310:1225–1228.
2. Papadopoulos NG, Bates PJ, Bardin PG, Papi A, Leir SH, Fraenkel DJ, et al: Rhinoviruses infect the lower airways. J Infect Dis 2000;181:1875–1884.
3. Corne JM, Marshall C, Smith S, Schreiber J, Sanderson G, Holgate ST, et al: Frequency, severity, and duration of rhinovirus infections in asthmatic and non-asthmatic individuals. A longitudinal cohort study. Lancet 2002;359: 831–834.
4. Shay DK, Holman RC, Newman RD, Liu LL, Stout JW, Anderson LJ: Bronchiolitis-associated hospitalizations among US children, 1980–1996. JAMA 1999;282:1440–1446.
5. Psarras S, Papadopoulos NG, Johnston SL: Pathogenesis of respiratory syncytial virus bronchiolitis-related wheezing. Paediatr Respir Rev 2004; 5(Suppl A):S179–S184.
6. Peiris JS, Yu WC, Leung CW, Cheung CY, Ng WF, Nicholls JM, et al: Re-emergence of fatal human influenza A subtype H5N1 disease. Lancet 2004;363:617–619.
7. Fouchier RA, Schneeberger PM, Rozendaal FW, Broekman JM, Kemink SA, Munster V, et al: Avian influenza A virus (H7N7) associated with human conjunctivitis and a fatal case of acute respiratory distress syndrome. Proc Natl Acad Sci U S A 2004;101:1356–1361.
8. Matrosovich MN, Matrosovich TY, Gray T, Roberts NA, Klenk HD: Human and avian influenza viruses target different cell types in cultures of human airway epithelium. Proc Natl Acad Sci U S A 2004;101:4620–4624.
9. Psarras S, Papadopoulos NG, Johnston SL: Parainfluenza viruses. In: Zuckermann AJ, Banantvala JE, Pattison JR, Griffiths PD, Scoub BD, eds: Principles and Practice of Clinical Virology, 5th ed. Chichester, UK: John Wiley & Sons, 2004, pp 299–321.
10. van der Hoek L, Pyrc K, Jebbink MF, Vermeulen-Oost W, Berkhout RJ, Wolthers KC, et al: Identification of a new human coronavirus. Nat Med 2004;10:368–373.
11. Ksiazek TG, Erdman D, Goldsmith CS, Zaki SR, Peret T, Emery S, et al: A novel coronavirus associated with severe acute respiratory syndrome. N Engl J Med 2003;348:1953–1966.
12. Poutanen SM, Low DE, Henry B, Finkelstein S, Rose D, Green K, et al: Identification of severe acute respiratory syndrome in Canada. N Engl J Med 2003;348:1995–2005.
13. Rota PA, Oberste MS, Monroe SS, Nix WA, Campagnoli R, Icenogle JP, et al: Characterization of a novel coronavirus associated with severe acute respiratory syndrome. Science 2003;300:1394–1399.
14. van den Hoogen BG, de Jong JC, Groen J, Kuiken T, de Groot R, Fouchier RA, et al: A newly discovered human pneumovirus isolated from young children with respiratory tract disease. Nat Med 2001;7:719–724.
15. Osterhaus A, Fouchier R: Human metapneumovirus in the community. Lancet 2003;361:890–891.
16. Xepapadaki P, Psarras S, Bossios A, Tsolia M, Gourgiotis D, Liapi-Adamidou G, et al: Human metapneumovirus as a causative agent of acute bronchiolitis in infants. J Clin Virol 2004;30:267–270.
17. Barenfanger J, Drake C, Mueller T, Troutt T, O'Brien J, Guttman K: R-Mix cells are faster, at least as sensitive and marginally more costly than conventional cell lines for the detection of respiratory viruses. J Clin Virol 2001;22:101–110.
18. Dunn JJ, Woolstenhulme RD, Langer J, Carroll KC: Sensitivity of respiratory virus culture when screening with R-mix fresh cells. J Clin Microbiol 2004;42:79–82.
19. Ferris MM, McCabe MO, Doan LG, Rowlen KL: Rapid enumeration of respiratory viruses. Anal Chem 2002;74:1849–1856.
20. Landry ML, Ferguson D: Suboptimal detection of influenza virus in adults by the Directigen Flu A+B enzyme immunoassay and correlation of results with the number of antigen-positive cells detected by cytospin immunofluorescence. J Clin Microbiol 2003;41:3407–3409.
21. Hopkins PM, Plit ML, Carter IW, Chhajed PN, Malouf MA, Glanville AR: Indirect fluorescent antibody testing of nasopharyngeal swabs for influenza diagnosis in lung transplant recipients. J Heart Lung Transplant 2003;22: 161–168.
22. Raty R, Kleemola M, Melen K, Stenvik M, Julkunen I: Efficacy of PCR and other diagnostic methods for the detection of respiratory adenoviral infections. J Med Virol 1999;59:66–72.
23. Covalciuc KA, Webb KH, Carlson CA: Comparison of four clinical specimen types for detection of influenza A and B viruses by optical immunoassay (FLU OIA test) and cell culture methods. J Clin Microbiol 1999;37:3971–3974.
24. Schultze D, Thomas Y, Wunderli W: Evaluation of an optical immunoassay for the rapid detection of influenza A and B viral antigens. Eur J Clin Microbiol Infect Dis 2001;20:280–283.
25. Frisbie B, Tang YW, Griffin M, Poehling K, Wright PF, Holland K, et al: Surveillance of childhood influenza virus infection. What is the best diagnostic method to use for archival samples? J Clin Microbiol 2004;42: 1181–1184.
26. Zambon M, Hays J, Webster A, Newman R, Keene O: Diagnosis of influenza in the community. Relationship of clinical diagnosis to confirmed virological, serologic, or molecular detection of influenza. Arch Intern Med 2001;161: 2116–2122.
27. Rimmelzwaan GF, Baars M, Claas EC, Osterhaus AD: Comparison of RNA hybridization, hemagglutination assay, titration of infectious virus and immunofluorescence as methods for monitoring influenza virus replication in vitro. J Virol Methods 1998;74:57–66.
28. Pitkaranta A, Puhakka T, Makela MJ, Ruuskanen O, Carpen O, Vaheri A: Detection of rhinovirus RNA in middle turbinate of patients with common colds by in situ hybridization. J Med Virol 2003;70:319–323.
29. Lonnrot M, Sjoroos M, Salminen K, Maaronen M, Hyypia T, Hyoty H: Diagnosis of enterovirus and rhinovirus infections by RT-PCR and time-resolved fluorometry with lanthanide chelate labeled probes. J Med Virol 1999;59:378–384.
30. Myatt TA, Johnston SL, Rudnick S, Milton DK: Airborne rhinovirus detection and effect of ultraviolet irradiation on detection by a semi-nested RT-PCR assay. BMC Public Health 2003;3:5.

31. Papadopoulos NG, Hunter J, Sanderson G, Meyer J, Johnston SL: Rhinovirus identification by BglI digestion of picornavirus RT-PCR amplicons. J Virol Methods 1999;80:179–185.
32. Kehl SC, Henrickson KJ, Hua W, Fan J: Evaluation of the Hexaplex assay for detection of respiratory viruses in children. J Clin Microbiol 2001;39:1696–1701.
33. Liolios L, Jenney A, Spelman D, Kotsimbos T, Catton M, Wesselingh S: Comparison of a multiplex reverse transcription-PCR-enzyme hybridization assay with conventional viral culture and immunofluorescence techniques for the detection of seven viral respiratory pathogens. J Clin Microbiol 2001;39:2779–2783.
34. Weigl JA: Pediatric Infectious Diseases Network on Acute Respiratory Tract Infection. Available at http://pid-ari.net/#.
35. Adhikary AK, Inada T, Banik U, Numaga J, Okabe N: Identification of subgenus C adenoviruses by fiber-based multiplex PCR. J Clin Microbiol 2004;42:670–673.
36. Billaud G, Peny S, Legay V, Lina B, Valette M: Detection of rhinovirus and enterovirus in upper respiratory tract samples using a multiplex nested PCR. J Virol Methods 2003;108:223–228.
37. Mitchell S, O'Neill HJ, Ong GM, Christie S, Duprex P, Wyatt DE, et al: Clinical assessment of a generic DNA amplification assay for the identification of respiratory adenovirus infections. J Clin Virol 2003;26:331–338.
38. Ellis JS, Zambon MC: Combined PCR-heteroduplex mobility assay for detection and differentiation of influenza A viruses from different animal species. J Clin Microbiol 2001;39:4097–4102.
39. Dagher H, Donninger H, Hutchinson P, Ghildyal R, Bardin P: Rhinovirus detection. Comparison of real-time and conventional PCR. J Virol Methods 2004;117:113–121.
40. Nijhuis M, van Maarseveen N, Schuurman R, Verkuijlen S, de Vos M, Hendriksen K, et al: Rapid and sensitive routine detection of all members of the genus enterovirus in different clinical specimens by real-time PCR. J Clin Microbiol 2002;40:3666–3670.
41. Ng LF, Wong M, Koh S, Ooi EE, Tang KF, Leong HN, et al: Detection of severe acute respiratory syndrome coronavirus in blood of infected patients. J Clin Microbiol 2004;42:347–350.
42. Maertzdorf J, Wang CK, Brown JB, Quinto JD, Chu M, de Graaf M, et al: Real-time reverse transcriptase PCR assay for detection of human metapneumoviruses from all known genetic lineages. J Clin Microbiol 2004;42:981–986.
43. Hu A, Colella M, Tam JS, Rappaport R, Cheng SM: Simultaneous detection, subgrouping, and quantitation of respiratory syncytial virus A and B by real-time PCR. J Clin Microbiol 2003;41:149–154.
44. Boivin G, Cote S, Dery P, De Serres G, Bergeron MG: Multiplex real-time PCR assay for detection of influenza and human respiratory syncytial viruses. J Clin Microbiol 2004;42:45–51.
45. Templeton KE, Scheltinga SA, Beersma MF, Kroes AC, Claas EC: Rapid and sensitive method using multiplex real-time PCR for diagnosis of infections by influenza A and influenza B viruses, respiratory syncytial virus, and parainfluenza viruses 1, 2, 3, and 4. J Clin Microbiol 2004;42:1564–1569.
46. Hibbitts S, Rahman A, John R, Westmoreland D, Fox JD: Development and evaluation of NucliSens basic kit NASBA for diagnosis of parainfluenza virus infection with 'end-point' and 'real-time' detection. J Virol Methods 2003;108:145–155.
47. Loens K, Ieven M, Ursi D, De Laat C, Sillekens P, Oudshoorn P, et al: Improved detection of rhinoviruses by nucleic acid sequence-based amplification after nucleotide sequence determination of the 5' noncoding regions of additional rhinovirus strains. J Clin Microbiol 2003;41:1971–1976.
48. Wang D, Coscoy L, Zylberberg M, Avila PC, Boushey HA, Ganem D, et al: Microarray-based detection and genotyping of viral pathogens. Proc Natl Acad Sci U S A 2002;99:15687–15692.
49. Hughes TR, Mao M, Jones AR, Burchard J, Marton MJ, Shannon KW, et al: Expression profiling using microarrays fabricated by an ink-jet oligonucleotide synthesizer. Nat Biotechnol 2001;19:342–347.
50. Biel SS, Madeley D: Diagnostic virology. The need for electron microscopy. A discussion paper. J Clin Virol 2001;22:1–9.
51. Weinberg A, Zamora MR, Li S, Torres F, Hodges TN: The value of polymerase chain reaction for the diagnosis of viral respiratory tract infections in lung transplant recipients. J Clin Virol 2002;25:171–175.
52. Casiano-Colon AE, Hulbert BB, Mayer TK, Walsh EE, Falsey AR: Lack of sensitivity of rapid antigen tests for the diagnosis of respiratory syncytial virus infection in adults. J Clin Virol 2003;28:169–174.
53. Ellis JS, Zambon MC: Molecular diagnosis of influenza. Rev Med Virol 2002;12:375–389.

23 Acute Infections Producing Upper Airway Obstruction

Ian M. Balfour-Lynn, MD •
Jane C. Davies, MD

Upper airway obstruction due to acute infection is not uncommon in children, and many parents have experienced an anxious night with a "croupy" child. Although infants and young children are most commonly affected, due to their relatively narrow upper airways, older children and adults can also have significant symptoms. Fortunately, these are mostly due to self-limiting viral laryngotracheobronchitis (LTB), but there is also a group of bacterial infections (epiglottitis, bacterial tracheitis, diphtheria, retropharyngeal abscess) that can occasionally cause significant obstruction. It is the job of the emergency physician, pediatrician, pediatric pulmonologist, or otorhinolaryngologist to diagnose more serious infections promptly so that treatment can be instituted early and disastrous obstruction avoided. It is also important to recognize when a simple viral LTB is causing significant problems so that appropriate treatment can be given immediately. This chapter is clinically orientated and outlines the principal infective causes of upper airway obstruction, with an emphasis on diagnosis and treatment. Confusion exists regarding the nomenclature for these disorders, with some using the term *croup* to refer to any inflammatory disorder of the upper airway, whereas others restrict its use to subglottic disease (i.e., LTB, which is usually of viral origin). The term *croup* will be largely avoided in this chapter, for the sake of clarity.

The consequence of these upper airway infections is usually stridor, which is a clinical sign and should not be considered a definitive diagnosis. This chapter briefly outlines the principles behind what causes stridor, which should clarify why this condition mostly affects infants and young children. The appendix in Holinger, Lusk, and Green's book *Pediatric Laryngology & Bronchoesophagology* discusses the physics of airflow and fluid dynamics.[1] The laws of fluid dynamics are based on flow through fixed tubes and may not always apply to dynamic airways in vivo. Normally, airflow through the upper airways is laminar, and the moving column of air produces slight negative pressure on the airway walls.[2] Inflammation resulting from infection causes a degree of airway narrowing, which increases the flow rate through the narrowed segment (Venturi effect). This, in turn, causes a reduction in the pressure exerted on the airway wall (Bernoulli principle); in other words, negative intraluminal pressure increases. This enhances the tendency of the airway to collapse inward, further narrowing the airway and causing turbulent airflow. The respiratory phase (inspiration or expiration) has a differential effect on airflow, depending on whether the obstruction is intrathoracic or extrathoracic (Fig. 23-1). Stridor is the sound made by rapid, turbulent flow of air through a narrowed segment of a large airway. It is most often loud, with medium or low pitch, and inspiratory. It usually originates from the larynx, upper trachea, or hypopharynx.[3] Progression of the disease process may make stridor softer, higher-pitched, and biphasic (inspiratory and expiratory). With the onset of complete obstruction, stridor may become barely audible as minimal air moves across the critically narrowed airway.[4]

The laryngeal anatomy of children makes them particularly susceptible to narrowing of the upper airways. The larynx of a neonate is situated high in the neck, and the epiglottis is narrow, omega-shaped (ω), and vertically positioned. The narrowest segment of the pediatric airway is the subglottic region (in adults, it is at the glottic level), which is encircled by the rigid cricoid cartilage ring. There is nonfibrous, loosely attached mucosa in this region that is easily obstructed in the presence of subglottic edema. Additionally, the cartilaginous support of the infant airway is soft and compliant, easily allowing dynamic collapse of the airways during inspiration. Further, young children have proportionally large heads and relatively lax neck support; this combination increases the likelihood of airway obstruction when supine.[5] Their tongues are also relatively large for the size of the oropharynx. Simple mathematics shows why a small amount of edema has such a profound effect on the cross-sectional area and, hence, airflow. The diameter of the subglottis in a normal newborn is approximately 5 mm, and 0.5 mm edema in that region reduces the cross-sectional area to 64% of normal (area $= \pi \times \text{radius}^2$). Airflow is directly proportional to the airway radius to the fourth power (Poiseuille's law), so a small reduction in caliber has a major effect on flow rate. The same 5-mm airway with 0.5 mm edema will have a flow rate of only 41% of baseline, assuming that pressure remains unchanged, a situation that is not necessarily the case if the Bernoulli principle (discussed earlier) is in play. Because the caliber of the airway is almost inevitably reduced further, in accord with the Bernoulli principle, and Poiseuille flow is not established, the flow rate is much further reduced and the work of breathing is greatly increased to maintain ventilation.

■ VIRAL LARYNGOTRACHEOBRONCHITIS

ETIOLOGY

The most common etiologic agents are the parainfluenza viruses (PIVs), of which PIV 1 is found most frequently and leads to epidemics. PIV 2 may account for many sporadic cases, and PIV 3 is a less common cause of viral LTB, usually targeting the epithelium of the smaller airways, leading to bronchiolitic illness. The PIVs belong to the Paramyxoviridae family, along with respiratory syncytial virus, measles, mumps, and the recently identified human metapneumovirus.[6] Together, the PIVs account for more than 75% of cases of viral LTB, although

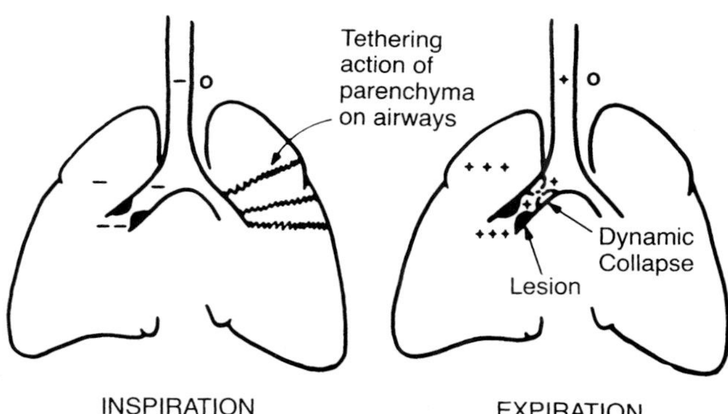

■ **FIGURE 23-1.** The effect of the respiratory phase on extrathoracic and intrathoracic obstruction. During inspiration, the negative intratracheal pressure (relative to atmospheric pressure) leads to dynamic collapse of the extrathoracic airway, thus worsening the effects of an extrathoracic obstructive lesion. In contrast, intrathoracic obstruction improves during inspiration because of the tethering effect of the lung parenchyma opening the intrathoracic airways. During expiration, intratracheal pressure is positive relative to atmospheric pressure, opening the extrathoracic trachea and lessening the obstructive effect of lesions. In contrast, intrathoracic obstruction worsens because of lower pressure in the airways relative to the surrounding parenchyma, collapsing the airways. (From Loughlin GM, Taussig LM: Upper airway obstruction. Semin Respir Med 1979;1:131–146. Thieme Medical Publishers, Inc.)

other respiratory viruses, such as respiratory syncytial virus, influenza virus, and adenovirus, can produce a similar clinical syndrome. Herpesviruses tend to cause a more severe and protracted form of the disease. LTB can also occur with some systemic infections, such as measles, and less commonly, *Mycoplasma.* In general, however, it is not usually possible to identify the cause of infection from the child's symptoms, because severity does not consistently correlate with any particular etiologic agent.

■ EPIDEMIOLOGY

Viral LTB is the most common cause of infective upper airway obstruction in the pediatric age group. Affected children are usually of preschool age, with a peak incidence between the ages of 18 and 24 months.[7] Reported incidence rates vary from 1.5% to 6%, but only approximately 2% of these require hospital admission, and fewer than 2% of those admitted require endotracheal intubation and intensive care.[8] This proportion has fallen dramatically since the use of corticosteroids has become routine. There is a male preponderance in children younger than 6 years of age (1.4:1), although at an older age, both sexes appear to be affected equally. Cases may occur in epidemics, with those due to PIV 1 particularly presenting in autumn and winter and infection with other organisms, including PIV 2, occurring more commonly as isolated infections. Infection is via droplet spread or direct inoculation from the hands. Viruses can survive for long periods on dry surfaces, such as clothes and toys, emphasizing the importance of infection control practices.

■ PATHOPHYSIOLOGY

Infection affects the larynx, trachea, and bronchi, although swelling and inflammation in the subglottic area leads to the characteristic clinical features of viral LTB. In addition to relative differences in airway size (discussed earlier), it is suggested that poor cell-mediated immunity in younger age groups also accounts for differences observed between adults and children.[9] The epithelium of the subglottis possesses abundant mucous glands, secretions from which can further narrow the airway lumen in response to infection. The PIVs are trophic for the respiratory epithelium, binding in particular to ciliated cells via an interaction between the viral hemagglutinin-neuraminidase protein and its receptor, sialic acid. Other viral proteins, in particular, the F protein, are important in membrane fusion and the passage of viral particles between cells. Many strains of PIV are cytopathic, with infection leading to the formation of giant cells and cell death. As with many infective processes, the ensuing inflammatory response is heavily involved in the evolution of symptoms. Both polymorphonuclear and monocytic leukocytes infiltrate the subepithelium, which leads to vascular congestion and airway wall edema. In addition, the symptoms of viral LTB are believed to be caused by the release of spasmogenic mediators, leading to decreased airway diameter. This may result from a type I hypersensitivity response to PIV, and some authors have postulated a role for anti-PIV-specific immunoglobulin E (IgE) in the development of airway narrowing.[10] These factors may play a relatively greater role in patients with recurrent (spasmodic) croup, and these patients may have hyperreactivity of the extrathoracic and intrathoracic airways.[11] The etiology of recurrent, spasmodic croup remains unclear, with authors expressing differing views on whether it is a separate disease entity.

■ CLINICAL PRESENTATION AND DIAGNOSIS

Mild

Most children are affected mildly by viruses that cause LTB.[7] The exact incidence remains unknown because many of them do not receive medical attention, but are managed by parents at home. Children have a barking cough and a hoarse cry or voice; these symptoms are worse in the evening and at night. They may also have inspiratory stridor on exertion, but stridor at rest is usually absent, as are other signs of respiratory distress. There is most commonly a coryzal prodrome, accompanied

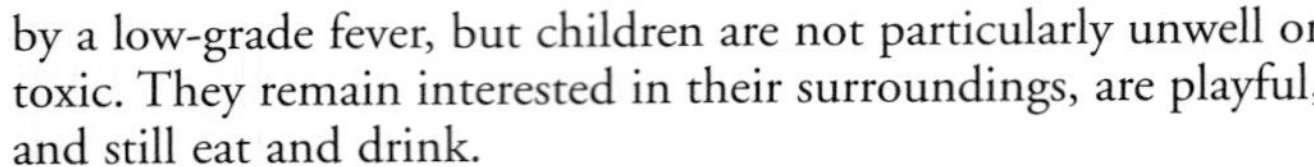

by a low-grade fever, but children are not particularly unwell or toxic. They remain interested in their surroundings, are playful, and still eat and drink.

Moderate

Features of moderate viral LTB include those discussed earlier, but with inspiratory stridor present at rest, as well as a degree of respiratory distress manifest by chest wall recession, tachypnea, and the use of accessory muscles of respiration. There is usually accompanying tachycardia, but children remain interactive and are able to take at least liquids orally.

Severe

Progression from moderate to severe infection can occur rapidly, and may be precipitated by the distress caused by clinical examination. Worrisome signs include those of increasing respiratory distress, with the child appearing anxious or preoccupied and tired. Drooling may occur, and the child will often refuse liquids or be unable to coordinate swallowing and breathing. However, the child with viral LTB will not appear toxic, with high fever and flushed face, as do those with the classic signs of bacterial epiglottitis (Table 23-1). Another difference is in the nature of the cough; a harsh, barking cough is not commonly associated with epiglottitis (in which there is often a muffled cough and cry). Restlessness and agitation are late signs of airway obstruction of any cause, as is cyanosis, pallor, or decreased level of consciousness. Pulse oximetry should be performed, but limitations must be recognized. Oxygen saturation may be well preserved until the late stages of severe viral LTB, and may lead to significant underestimation of respiratory compromise in a patient who is receiving supplementary oxygen. Conversely, desaturation may be seen in children with relatively mild airway obstruction (presumably reflecting lower airway involvement and ventilation-perfusion mismatch).[12] Pulsus paradoxus is present in this group with severe disease, but in clinical practice, it is difficult to assess, and attempts to do so could worsen symptoms by causing distress.

Recurrent or Spasmodic Croup

Symptoms are similar to those of the more typical forms of confirmed viral LTB, but children are often older, do not have the same coryzal prodrome, and may be afebrile during the episode. There may be links with atopy. Attacks often occur suddenly, at night, and may resolve equally quickly. Treatment must be guided by the degree of severity, and is similar to that for viral LTB. Some practitioners prescribe inhaled corticosteroids (via a spacer device) to be kept at home and administered by the parents in case of an episode, although there is a paucity of evidence for or against this practice.

Noninfective Causes of Acute Airway Obstruction

There are a number of noninfective causes of upper airway obstruction, and these must be considered in the differential diagnosis of infective causes (Box 23-1). Foreign body inhalation

TABLE 23-1. Differentiation of principal infective causes of upper airway obstruction

	Viral Laryngotracheobronchitis	Epiglottitis	Bacterial Tracheitis	Diphtheria	Retropharyngeal Abscess
Principal Organisms	Parainfluenza 1–3 Influenza Adenovirus Respiratory syncytial virus	*Haemophilus influenzae* *Streptococcus*	*Staphylococcus aureus* *Moraxella catarrhalis* *H. influenzae*	*Corynebacterium diphtheria*	Mixed flora, including *S. aureus*, *Streptococcus*, *H. influenzae*, anaerobes
Age Range	6 mo–4 yr (peak, 1–2 yr)	2–7 yr	6 mo–8 yr	All ages	<6 yr
Incidence	Common	Rare	Rare	Rare if vaccinated	Uncommon
Onset	Insidious Usually follows upper respiratory tract infection	Rapid	Slow, with sudden deterioration	Insidious	Gradual
Site	Below the vocal cords	Supraglottis	Trachea	Tonsils, pharynx, larynx, nose, skin	Retropharyngeal space
Clinical Manifestations	Low-grade fever Nontoxic Barking (seal-like) cough Stridor Hoarseness Restlessness	High fever Severe sore throat Minimal nonbarking cough Toxic Stridor Drooling Dysphagia Muffled voice Sits in the tripod position	High fever Toxic Brassy cough Stridor Hoarse voice Neck pain Choking	Fever Toxic Stridor Sore throat Fetor oris Cervical lymphadenopathy Bull neck	Fever Sore throat Neck pain and stiffness (especially on extension) Dysphagia Stridor (less common) Drooling Retropharyngeal bulge
Endoscopic Findings	Deep red mucosa Subglottic edema	Cherry-red or pale and edematous epiglottis Edematous aryepiglottic folds	Deep red mucosa Ulcerations Copious, thick tracheal secretions Subglottic edema, with normal epiglottis and arytenoids	Gray, adherent membrane on the pharynx	N/A
Intubation	Occasional	Usual	Usual	Occasional	Unusual
Therapy	Corticosteroids Nebulized epinephrine	Intubation (1–3 days) IV antibiotics	Intubation (3–7 days) IV antibiotics Tracheal suction	Diphtheria antitoxin IV antibiotics Immunization during convalescence	IV antibiotics ± surgery

IV, intravenous.

BOX 23-1 Infectious and Noninfectious Causes of Acute Upper Airway Obstruction

Infectious

Viral laryngotracheobronchitis
Epiglottitis
Bacterial tracheitis
Diphtheria
Retropharyngeal abscess
Peritonsillar abscess

Noninfectious

Foreign body
Trauma
Caustic burns
Spasmodic croup
Angioneurotic edema

is the most common noninfective cause in children. Symptoms, which may partly mimic those of viral LTB, depend on the location of the foreign body, the degree of resultant airway obstruction, and to a lesser extent, the nature of the foreign body. Onset of symptoms may be either acute or insidious; a large foreign body may cause severe obstruction, whereas a smaller one may simply lead to laryngeal and tracheal irritation and airway edema. In cases of severe airway obstruction, the voice may be lost and breath sounds quiet. This condition is an emergency, requiring immediate visualization of the larynx and trachea and removal of the foreign body by a physician or surgeon experienced in this procedure. Occasionally, an unrecognized inhaled foreign body leads to chronic stridor. Acute upper airway obstruction may also result from the ingestion of caustic substances, with resulting pharyngeal burns, edema, and inflammation of the epiglottis, aryepiglottic folds, larynx, and trachea. This diagnosis is usually clear from the history. Rarely, angioneurotic edema may cause acute laryngeal swelling and airway obstruction. Patients appear nontoxic and may exhibit other signs of allergic disease, such as urticaria and abdominal pain. In hereditary angioneurotic edema due to C1 esterase deficiency, the family history may be positive, although first presentation is more common in adults than in children.

There are numerous causes of chronic airway obstruction that are discussed elsewhere in this book. Confusion may arise when an upper respiratory tract infection unmasks a previously asymptomatic congenital abnormality. For example, mild subglottic stenosis may cause symptoms only with the additional burden of airway edema due to a simple viral upper respiratory illness. It is important to ensure that there is no history of intubation, which may have been brief, as in resuscitation of a newborn in the maternity unit, or of any coexisting signs, such as a cutaneous hemangioma, which may increase the index of suspicion for a congenital airway abnormality.

WHO SHOULD BE EVALUATED?

Most children with viral LTB were previously well; have short, self-limiting symptoms; and make a full recovery. The lack of complete immunity and the variety of agents that can cause viral LTB mean that more than one episode is not uncommon, particularly in separate seasons. However, some children have symptoms that should lead to further clinical evaluation. These include multiple episodes, particularly if they are severe or frequent, symptoms that are particularly slow to resolve, and symptoms that occur between or in the absence of obvious infections. Evaluation of patients in this group is aimed at identifying an underlying airway abnormality that would predispose the child to more severe airway narrowing in response to viral infection or that could cause problems independently of such infection. Investigation is usually centered on airway endoscopy. This must be performed in a unit and by an operator experienced in the technique, because there is a risk in many of these conditions of exacerbating the airway obstruction. Spontaneous breathing is necessary to identify vocal cord problems or airway malacia, and anesthetic techniques must be carefully considered. If an inhaled foreign body is considered likely, rigid bronchoscopy is the study of choice. Additional studies that might be considered once the acute episode has resolved include plain lateral neck and chest radiographs, computed tomography or magnetic resonance imaging scan, contrast assessment of the upper airway (e.g., videofluoroscopy, barium swallow), and pH study. Polysomnography may help to determine the severity of chronic symptoms. Rarer causes of recurrent stridor, such as hypocalcaemia or angioneurotic edema, are diagnosed on blood testing.

MANAGEMENT OF VIRAL LARYNGOTRACHEOBRONCHITIS

Management must be based on clinical assessment of severity. Such assessment should be based on the clinical features described earlier; there is no role for radiography in the assessment of acute airway obstruction. In skilled hands, plain lateral neck radiographs may demonstrate sites of obstruction, but this rarely influences management; it also wastes time and can be dangerous. The neck extension that is required could precipitate sudden worsening of airway obstruction, which can be fatal in severe cases. Several scoring systems have been devised,[13] and the most commonly applied, the 17-point Westley scale (which assesses degree of stridor, chest retractions, air entry, cyanosis, and level of consciousness), has been well validated. However, these are mainly used in the context of clinical trials, and are not a substitute for experienced clinical assessment.

Supportive Care

Children with mild croup can be managed at home. They should be treated with plenty of fluids and antipyretics as required. Because the vast majority of cases are of viral etiology, there is no role for the routine use of antibiotics in the absence of other features suggestive of bacterial infection. Parents should be told that symptoms are often worse at night.

Humidification

Both at home and in the hospital setting, humidified air (either steam or cool mist) has been used for more than a century to produce symptomatic relief from croup. Despite this, there is very little supportive published evidence, with most studies suggesting no benefit. The first randomized controlled study, published in 1984, compared humidified air with no treatment.[14] The authors reported no difference in croup score, heart and respiratory rates, and transcutaneous gas values at various time points, up to 12 hours. This study was probably underpowered to detect differences, given its small size (n = 16) and the relatively mild symptoms at baseline. An even smaller study of seven children showed no benefit of nebulized water.[15] A third, larger, double-blind randomized study (n = 71), showed no immediate (2-hour) benefit from humidified air, in combination with systemic steroid treatment.[16] Thus, although anecdotally, humidified air is still used by parents at home, it may be the calming effect of the warm, steamy bathroom that is helping, without a measurable effect on symptoms. Case reports have described severe burns caused by spilling of boiling water and facial scalds from the use of steam, so this type of treatment is not without the potential for harm.[17]

Corticosteroids

The use of corticosteroids has received much attention over the last few years, and their therapeutic role is no longer in doubt. Their mechanism of action, however, remains unclear, although is believed to relate to rapid-onset anti-inflammatory or vasoconstrictive properties. The cumulative evidence strongly supports their use in children with moderate to severe symptoms, although there are still outstanding questions, including the optimal route of administration, the most appropriate dosing regimen, and the best oral agent.

The role of corticosteroids in the management of croup in children has been the subject of several Cochrane systematic reviews, with the most recent update in November 2003.[18] In this review, the authors identified 31 studies that fulfilled their criteria for inclusion, namely, randomized controlled trials in children measuring the effectiveness of corticosteroids (any route of administration) against either placebo or another treatment. A total of 3736 children were included, the majority from placebo-controlled trials. Outcome measures included the croup score (most commonly using the Westley scale), the requirement for admission or return visit, the length of stay, and the requirement for additional therapeutic interventions. Overall, treatment led to an improvement in the croup score at 6 and 12 hours, but the improvement was no longer apparent at 24 hours. The length of time spent in either the emergency department or the hospital was also significantly decreased, as was the requirement for nebulized epinephrine. Importantly, and in contrast to the previous version of the Cochrane review, the authors concluded with funnel plots and other statistical methods that these results were not influenced by publication bias.[18] Recently, a large randomized controlled trial (n = 720) studied mild croup (Westley score ≤ 2), and showed benefit of a single dose of dexamethasone, 0.6 mg/kg, in terms of return to medical care, resolution of symptoms, decreased loss of sleep by the child, and reduced parental stress.[19]

OUTSTANDING QUESTIONS

What Route of Administration and Dosing Regimen Is Best?

The studies included in the systematic review discussed earlier used the intramuscular, oral, or nebulized route to administer different corticosteroid preparations. A minority of studies sought to address the issue of which route of administration was optimal. Klassen and associates compared nebulized budesonide (2 mg) with oral dexamethasone (0.6 mg/kg); a third group received both treatments.[20] The croup score decreased significantly in each of the three groups, with no between-group differences, leading the authors to recommend the oral route because of cost and ease of administration. Two studies have compared dexamethasone administered by the oral or intramuscular route (0.6 mg/kg by either route).[21,22] Neither study reported significant differences, although they were probably underpowered to detect these. The authors of the Cochrane review calculated that, to answer this question, a further 513 patients would need to be studied; this is more than twice as many as were already reported. Johnson and associates compared nebulized budesonide with intramuscular dexamethasone.[23] The children (n = 144) had moderate croup and also received nebulized adrenaline. Both interventions produced significant improvements, although these were more marked in the dexamethasone group. Therefore, the question of which route of administration is optimal has yet to be answered. In clinical practice, on the basis of ease, time saving, and cost, the oral route appears to be widely favored (assuming that the child is not vomiting). With regard to the dosing regimen, most clinical studies have reported effects of a single dose of corticosteroid by any route. The question arises in practice whether children with a poor response or worsening of symptoms should receive further doses. According to the literature on intensive care management of children with croup, multiple doses are often routinely administered[24]; these also protect against postextubation airway edema. Outside the pediatric intensive care unit, there is no good-quality evidence to guide this decision. A child at home who shows continued deterioration after a single dose of corticosteroid should be evaluated again, preferably in a hospital setting, because treatment with nebulized epinephrine may be considered. In patients already admitted to the hospital, the decision will likely be between further doses of corticosteroids and nebulized epinephrine, with the latter approach supported by more trial data.

Which Oral Corticosteroid Preparation Should Be Used and at What Dose?

The majority of studies have used dexamethasone as the oral agent. However, many general practitioners visiting homes do not routinely carry this preparation, but do carry oral prednisolone. There have been no published studies comparing the two drugs, although some authors have advocated the use of oral prednisolone, 1 to 2 mg/kg.[25] In the case of dexamethasone, 0.6 mg/kg has been the dose most widely assessed. However, studies are beginning to suggest that this dose may be higher than required. Geelhoed and associates have reported that dexamethasone, 0.15 mg/kg, is just as effective as either 0.6 or 0.3 mg/kg.[26,27] This group, from Perth, Australia, adjusted their clinical guidelines to reflect this finding in the mid-1990s. Reassuringly, they have since published data confirming that this change has not negatively affected rates of admission to the pediatric intensive care unit or the need for intubation.[8] A practical approach might be to use dexamethasone, if available, at a dose of 0.15 mg/kg. If, for example, this preparation is not available at a home visit, prednisolone (at an equivalent dose of 1 mg/kg) can provide a useful substitute.

NEBULIZED EPINEPHRINE (ADRENALINE)

Most of the clinical trials have used the racemic form of this drug,[28] although there is now evidence that the L-isomer used alone (which is the only available formulation in some units) may be equally effective.[29] The mechanisms of action are believed to be a combination of rapid reduction in airway wall edema and bronchodilation. It has a rapid onset of action, within 30 minutes, and the effect lasts for 2 to 3 hours. The recommended dose is 0.4 to 0.5 mL/kg (to a maximum of 5 mL) of the 1:1000 preparation that is put undiluted into the nebulizer pot. According to these studies, nebulized epinephrine has been shown to improve the croup score and reduce the likelihood of hospital admission, but it is less clear whether, when given with corticosteroids, it reduces the need for intubation. It should be used in any child who has severe signs and symptoms, and should be considered for those with moderate signs and symptoms, depending on the signs of respiratory distress and, possibly, the response to corticosteroid administration. It can be administered in the home setting while awaiting an ambulance, but clearly, any child requiring this treatment at home must be transferred promptly to the hospital for monitoring. Multiple doses may be administered, although the requirement for this must lead to consideration of the need for intensive care management. Although rebound worsening of symptoms after administration of nebulized epinephrine is often alluded to, in practice, this phenomenon does not appear to be a real risk. Traditionally, children treated with epinephrine have been admitted to the hospital, but recent studies have confirmed that discharge home is safe after 3 to 4 hours of observation, if the child has made a significant improvement.[30]

OTHER TREATMENTS FOR SEVERE CASES

Oxygen should be administered to any child with severe airway obstruction, even in the absence of severe hypoxia, because it will aid respiratory muscle function. As mentioned earlier, a child with severe respiratory distress and obstruction may have relatively normal pulse oximetry readings when breathing oxygen, which can be dangerous if misinterpreted by staff unaware of this limitation. Heliox (70%–80% helium with 20%–30% oxygen) has been used in both upper airway obstruction[31] and severe asthma, although its role in viral croup is not yet well defined. Helium, having a low viscosity, improves laminar airflow through the respiratory tract. Recently, a small randomized controlled study has compared heliox with nebulized epinephrine in children with croup, and reported equal benefit from both approaches.[32] More studies are required to determine the indications for use in this disease.

Some children with severe croup either do not respond to the usual therapies or are too severely compromised at presentation to permit their use. These children require urgent endotracheal intubation and mechanical ventilation to avoid potentially catastrophic complete airway obstruction and the serious sequelae of hypoxia and hypercapnia, such as hypoxic ischemic encephalopathy. Intubation should be performed by the most experienced person available, and should normally be attempted with an uncuffed endotracheal tube one size smaller than the usual size for the child.[24] Facilities for immediate tracheostomy must be available at the time of intubation. Children may have coexisting lower airway and parenchymal involvement that impairs gas exchange and may lead to slower than expected clinical improvement after intubation. Rarely, pulmonary edema may develop after relief of airway obstruction, particularly if the disease course has been prolonged. Most children without severe parenchymal involvement require respiratory support for 3 to 5 days.[24] As discussed earlier, corticosteroids are usually administered during this period, until after successful extubation, the timing of which depends on the development of an air leak, indicating resolution of airway narrowing.[24] Reintubation rates of approximately 10% have been reported.[33]

EPIGLOTTITIS

ETIOLOGY

Historically, *Haemophilus influenzae* type B (HiB) was responsible for almost all (approximately 99%) cases of epiglottitis in otherwise healthy patients. Since the introduction of HiB immunization, other organisms have been implicated, including groups A, B, C, and G β-hemolytic streptococcus. Other responsible organisms include *Haemophilus parainfluenzae, Staphylococcus aureus, Moraxella catarrhalis, Pneumococcus, Klebsiella, Pseudomonas,* candida, and viruses (herpes simplex, varicella, PIV, influenza).[2,34]

EPIDEMIOLOGY

H. influenzae type B vaccines were first licensed in the United States in 1988, with widespread immunization programs in place in the early 1990s. Since then, reported cases of invasive HiB disease (including epiglottitis) in children younger than 5 years of age have declined by 99%.[35] The same pattern has been repeated in Europe, with significant reductions in the United Kingdom.[36,37] Immunization was introduced in the United Kingdom in 1992, and with immunization coverage exceeding 90%, the decline in incidence was more than 95%.[37] In 1998, the incidence in those younger than 5 years of age was 0.6 per 100,000 compared with 31 to 36 per 100,000 in England and Wales before the introduction of the vaccine.[37] Ethnicity plays a part. Data from 1996–1997 in the United States show that the average annual incidence of HiB invasive disease per 100,000 children younger than 5 years of age was 0.5 among non-Hispanic whites, 0.6 among Asians and Pacific Islanders, 0.7 among non-Hispanic blacks, 0.7 among Hispanic Americans, and 12.4 among American Indians and Alaskan natives.[35] Nevertheless, cases of epiglottitis due to HiB continue to be reported,[38] as do cases due to other organisms.[34]

Cases of invasive HiB occur principally in nonimmunized children, but also rarely in some true vaccine failures. Clinical risk factors for vaccine failure include prematurity, Down syndrome, malignancy, developmental delay, and immunodeficiency, principally subnormal immunoglobulin concentrations (IgG2 subclass, IgA, IgM) and neutropenia.[39] However, these factors explain fewer than half of cases of vaccine failure.[39] An HiB IgG antibody titer of 0.15 μg/mL or greater has been considered to confer protection from disease, but given the natural waning in antibody levels, it is estimated that a titer of 1.0 μg/mL or greater should provide long-term protection.[38] However, there may also be qualitative functional problems with the antibody response that are not yet fully elucidated.

Epiglottitis tends to occur in children 2 to 7 years of age, but cases have been reported in those younger than 1 year.[2] Since the introduction of HiB vaccine, the peak age distribution has increased slightly.[40] Most cases occur in the fall and winter.

PATHOPHYSIOLOGY

Although HiB has a low point prevalence of nasopharyngeal carriage (1%–5%), most young children become colonized with

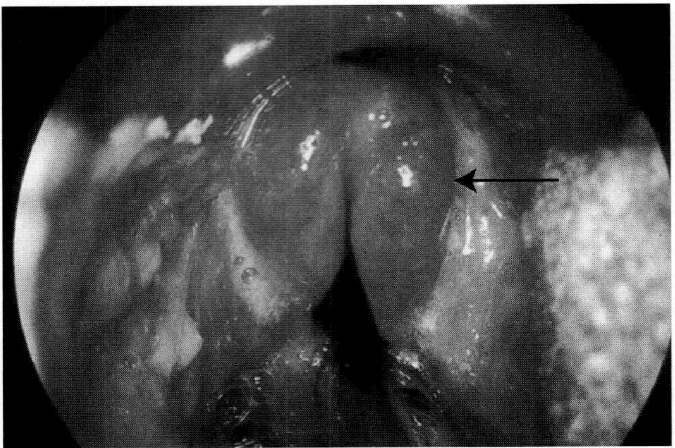

FIGURE 23-2. Swollen epiglottis *(arrow)* due to acute epiglottitis in an intubated child. (See Color Plate 30.) (From Benjamin B, Bingham B, Hawke M, Stammberger H: A Colour Atlas of Otorhinolaryngology. London: Taylor & Francis, 1995, p 292, with permission.)

HiB in the first 2 to 5 years.[41] The relationship between asymptomatic carriage, immunity, and the development of invasive disease is not clearly understood. Viral coinfection may have a role in the transition from colonization to invasion.[42] Colonies of HiB organisms reside in the nasal mucosal epithelium and submucosa. Invasive disease occurs when organisms disseminate from the mucosa of the upper respiratory tract via the bloodstream; bacteremia increases over a period of hours, and metastatic seeding can occur.[41] Thus, although situated in close proximity to the nose, the supraglottic area is likely to be affected via the bloodstream, although direct spread along mucosal surfaces may also play a part. This may account for the relatively high yield of positive blood cultures in epiglottitis and the relatively low incidence of epiglottitis among carriers of HiB.

Epiglottitis is more correctly called *supraglottitis.* It is a bacterial cellulitis of the supraglottic structures, particularly the lingual surface of the epiglottis and the aryepiglottic folds.[2] Destruction of the infected epithelial tissue results in mucosal ulcerations, which may appear on the epiglottis, larynx, and trachea. The submucosal glands are involved as well, with the formation of abscesses. Infection of the epiglottis itself causes a local inflammatory response resulting in a cherry-red edematous epiglottis when due to HiB (Fig. 23-2), although it tends to be pale and edematous and accompanied by edematous aryepiglottic folds when due to *Streptococcus.*[34,35] As supraglottic edema worsens, the epiglottis is displaced posteriorly, and may obstruct the airway.

CLINICAL PRESENTATION AND DIAGNOSIS

Classic epiglottitis due to HiB is a fulminant disease in an otherwise healthy child, who can be near death in a few hours. It is a medical emergency that can be alarming for the medical staff and devastating for the family. With the reduction in incidence, however, comes a lack of experience in recognition and management of this condition. Up to 20% of infants with epiglottitis are misdiagnosed initially, usually with viral LTB.[4] Typically, there is a short history of fever, severe throat pain, stridor, and respiratory distress, but the symptoms progress rapidly. Children become toxic and tend to sit anxiously in the classic tripod position (sitting upright, with the chin up, mouth open, bracing themselves on their hands) as air hunger develops (Fig. 23-3). They often drool because they cannot swallow their secretions, and the voice is muffled due to pain and soft tissue swelling. Stridor may progress, and when marked, signals almost complete obstruction of the airways. Complete, fatal airway obstruction may occur suddenly and without warning. The most serious complication of this disease process (and any infective upper airway obstruction) is hypoxic ischemic encephalopathy resulting from respiratory arrest due to severe airway obstruction. This tragic complication is almost always preventable with clinical suspicion, prompt diagnosis, and correct management. However, a recent 13-year case series demonstrated that cardiac arrest still occurred in 3 of 40 cases (7.5%), although there were no long-term sequelae.[38] Secondary sites of HiB infection may be present in approximately half of cases, and include meningitis, otitis media, pneumonia, and cellulitis; therefore, repeated physical examination during the admission is critical.[2] The pneumonia may contribute to poor gas exchange.

Generally, distinction from standard viral LTB is based on the older age of the child, the lack of a history of upper respiratory tract infection, the speed of progression, the degree of toxicity, the extent of drooling, the use of the tripod position, and minimal cough (see Table 23-1). However, it is important to remember that most of these symptoms can be present in acute severe upper airway obstruction from other causes.

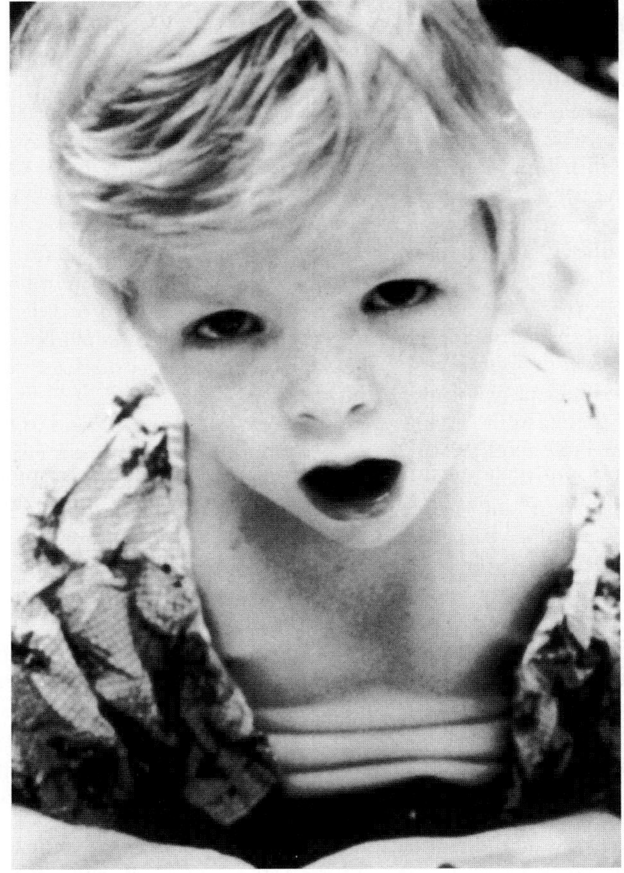

FIGURE 23-3. Characteristic posture in a patient with epiglottitis. The child is leaning forward and drooling, with a hyperextended neck. (Courtesy of Dr. Robert Berg.)

The presentation and clinical course of epiglottitis due to the various types of β-hemolytic streptococcal pathogens are similar to each other, but differ from those associated with HiB.[34] The onset of disease is more gradual, but the resolution of tissue damage and the time to recovery are longer, with a mean intubation time of 6 days.[34,43]

MANAGEMENT

The first priority and key response to the diagnosis must be to secure the airway in a controlled environment. Physical examination (especially of the throat) and cannulation or venipuncture should be deferred, because emotional upset and crying may precipitate complete airway obstruction. When epiglottitis is suspected clinically, the child (and parents) should be approached in a calm and reassuring manner. Oxygen should be given, even if the mask is held at a distance from the child's face. The child should be taken to the operating room, anesthetic room, or pediatric intensive care unit, and held by a parent. The child should be accompanied by a senior medical team skilled in airway management, carrying a laryngoscope, an endotracheal tube, and a percutaneous tracheostomy tray. If complete airway obstruction develops suddenly, performance of a Heimlich maneuver may relieve the obstruction temporarily; alternatively, forward traction may be applied to the mandible to relieve the obstruction.

Inhalational induction of anesthesia is preferred. Laryngoscopy should then be performed and the diagnosis confirmed, based on the appearance of the epiglottic region, as described earlier (erythema and edema of the supraglottis). Endotracheal intubation is then achieved using an orotracheal tube, which is later changed to a nasotracheal tube, because this is less likely to be displaced. Although tracheostomy is rarely necessary, a surgical team should be prepared to perform this immediately if intubation is unsuccessful. Once the airway is secured, the emergency is over, and the rest of the studies can be carried out. Intravenous cannulation and blood sampling can be done. The white cell count is increased, and blood culture findings are often positive (70% in one series[38]). Airway secretions and swabs from the epiglottic region should be sent for bacterial culture and viral detection. Urinary antigen testing may be useful for those already receiving antibiotics.[42]

Some authors have advocated the use of a lateral neck radiograph if the child is stable before intubation, claiming it to be the "single most useful study."[2,5] We strongly disagree, and this is not our recommendation, because it can precipitate respiratory arrest as a result of complete obstruction. We take the same view as Goodman and McHugh, who state, "plain radiographs have no role to play in the assessment of the critically ill child with acute stridor."[44]

Intravenous antibiotics are started and must cover HiB and *Streptococcus;* the response is usually rapid.[2] A third-generation cephalosporin, such as ceftriaxone or cefotaxime, is usually given, and may be changed once antibiotic sensitivities are available. Antibiotics have traditionally been given for 7 to 10 days; however, a randomized trial showed that a two-dose course of ceftriaxone was as efficacious as 5 days of chloramphenicol.[42] Contacts of patients with HiB should be given appropriate prophylaxis, usually rifampicin. There is some empiric evidence that corticosteroids may improve the course of epiglottitis; racemic epinephrine has not been shown to be of benefit, although it has been recommended. The duration of intubation for epiglottitis due to HiB averages 1 to 3 days,[5,38] but is longer when due to *Streptococcus,*[34] although as always, there is great individual variation. A decision to extubate may be made when an air leak develops around the endotracheal tube, but repeat endoscopy may be useful to aid this decision. Again, facilities for emergency tracheostomy must be available. Some give dexamethasone before extubation to reduce postextubation stridor.[4]

BACTERIAL TRACHEITIS

Bacterial tracheitis has also been known as *bacterial,* or *membranous LTB; nondiphtheritic laryngitis with marked exudate;* and *pseudomembranous croup.*

ETIOLOGY

The most common pathogen is *S. aureus*, although other organisms implicated include HiB, α-hemolytic streptococcus, pneumococcus, and *M. catarrhalis.*[5] Occasionally, gram-negative enteric organisms and *Pseudomonas aeruginosa* are isolated. In a recent case series, *M. catarrhalis* (27%) was more common than *S. aureus* (22%), although this represents data from a single center over the course of 14 months.[45] In addition, PIV and influenza viruses are commonly isolated from tracheal secretions; measles and enteroviruses have also been detected. Although it may be a primary bacterial infection, bacterial tracheitis is considered secondary to primary viral LTB, or perhaps a coinfection. Presumably, viral injury to the tracheal mucosa and impairment of local immunity predisposes to the bacterial superinfection.

EPIDEMIOLOGY

Bacterial tracheitis is a rare disease, with the largest recent case series describing only 46 cases.[45] The peak incidence is during the fall and winter, and it predominantly affects children 6 months to 8 years of age (mean, 5 years). Most affected children were previously well, but it has been reported as a complication of elective tonsillectomy and adenoidectomy.[46]

PATHOPHYSIOLOGY

Bacterial tracheitis is characterized by marked subglottic edema, with ulceration, erythema, pseudomembranous formation on the tracheal surface, and thick, mucopurulent tracheal secretions. The thick exudate and sloughed mucosa frequently obstruct the lumen of the trachea and the main stem bronchi.[2] The epiglottis and arytenoids are usually normal in appearance, although epiglottitis and bacterial tracheitis may coexist.

CLINICAL PRESENTATION AND DIAGNOSIS

The clinical picture is initially similar to that of viral LTB, with mild fever, cough, and stridor for several days. However, the patient's condition deteriorates rapidly, with a high fever and often a toxic appearance, with respiratory distress and airway obstruction. Other symptoms include choking episodes, orthopnea, dysphagia, and neck pain.[45] The clinical picture differs from that of epiglottitis in that its onset tends to be more insidious. Patients have a substantial brassy cough, are more able to lie flat, and tend not to drool (see Table 23-1).[5]

The children are more ill than with simple viral LTB, and do not respond to expected therapies, such as corticosteroids or nebulized epinephrine. There may be other coinfections, particularly pneumonia. Other reported complications include cardiopulmonary arrest, with subsequent hypoxic encephalopathy and seizures; pneumothorax; subglottic stenosis; septicemia; toxic shock syndrome; pulmonary edema; and adult respiratory distress syndrome.[47]

The white cell count shows polymorphonuclear leukocytosis, often with a left shift. A lateral neck radiograph may show a hazy tracheal air column, with multiple luminal soft tissue irregularities due to pseudomembrane detachment from the soft tissue, but radiographs should be taken only after the patient is stabilized and safe. There are, however, no clinical or radiographic features capable of confirming the diagnosis.[2] This must be confirmed by upper airway endoscopy and a positive bacterial culture.

MANAGEMENT

Diagnostic endoscopy, which should be done under general anesthesia, is also therapeutic because it enables removal of secretions and sloughed tissue from the airway lumen. Rigid endoscopy may be necessary, and sometimes the procedure must be repeated. Many patients require endotracheal intubation and mechanical ventilation to overcome airway obstruction, usually for 3 to 7 days. Frequent tracheal suction is necessary. In a recent series, 57% of patients required intubation, which is lower than the rate previously reported.[45] The decision to extubate is based on clinical improvement, with reduction of fever, decreased airway secretions, and the development of an air leak around the endotracheal tube. Corticosteroids may be given before extubation. Tracheostomy is required less often than in the past. Initially, intravenous broad-spectrum antibiotics are given, and these can be refined once cultures and antibiotic sensitivities are known, usually for 10 to 14 days. Mortality is now uncommon.

DIPHTHERIA

ETIOLOGY

Diphtheria is caused by toxigenic strains of the bacterium *Corynebacterium diphtheriae* and, less frequently, *Corynebacterium ulcerans*. The organism may be isolated on bacterial culture of nasal and pharyngeal swabs, and serologic studies may detect antibodies to diphtheria toxin. Polymerase chain reaction can confirm *Corynebacterium diphtheriae tox* genes.[48]

EPIDEMIOLOGY

Diphtheritic laryngitis was once the most common infectious cause of acute upper airway obstruction in children. Although it became uncommon due to widespread immunization programs started in the 1940s, it remains a serious disease in parts of the world. Large outbreaks occurred in the 1990s throughout Russia and the independent countries of the former Soviet Union. Most life-threatening cases occurred in unvaccinated or inadequately immunized persons, and it is important for children traveling to these countries, particularly for extended periods, to be vaccinated. A list of endemic countries is available on the Centers for Disease Control Web site (http://www.cdc.gov/travel/diseases/dtp.htm). Adults are particularly at risk because protective levels of diphtheria antibodies decrease progressively with time from immunization, so reimmunization is recommended before travel. The Third National Health and Nutrition Examination Survey of U.S. residents (1988–1994) indicated that fully protective levels (≥0.1 IU/mL) were found in 91% of children 6 to 11 years of age, but only in 30% of adults 60 to 69 years of age.[49]

PATHOPHYSIOLOGY

Diphtheria is an acute disease, primarily involving the tonsils, pharynx, larynx, nose, skin, and, occasionally, other mucous membranes. In the milder, catarrhal form, there is no membrane formation, but in the more severe, membranous form, there is a characteristic lesion of one or more patches of an adherent grayish-white membrane, surrounded by inflammation. The toxin causes local tissue destruction at the site of membrane formation, which promotes multiplication and transmission of the bacteria.[50]

CLINICAL PRESENTATION AND DIAGNOSIS

The incubation period is 1 to 6 days. Classic respiratory diphtheria is characterized by an insidious onset, and patients typically present with a 3- to 4-day history of upper respiratory infection. They have a fever, membranous pharyngitis with a sore throat, characteristic fetor oris, cervical lymphadenopathy, and sometimes edema of the surrounding soft tissues (bull-neck appearance). They may have a serosanguineous nasal discharge. Although not always present, the membrane is typically gray, thick, fibrinous, and firmly adherent, so it may bleed on attempted removal (Fig. 23-4). Laryngeal

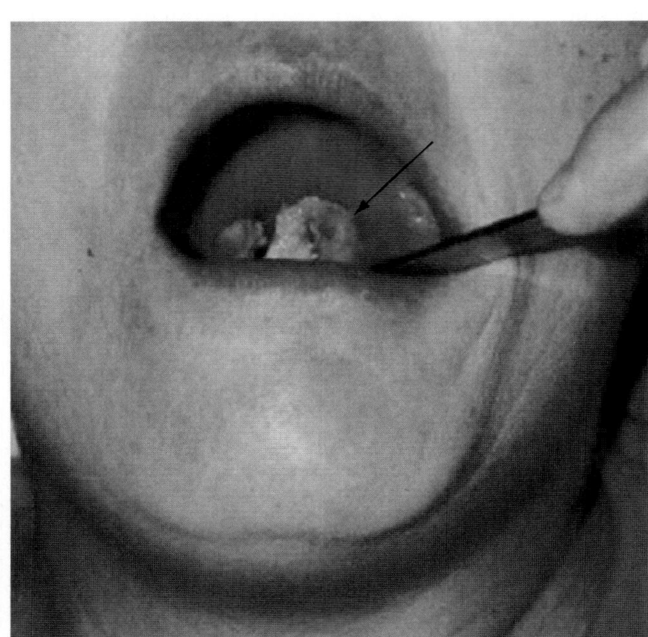

FIGURE 23-4. Diphtheritic membrane *(arrow)* extending from the uvula to the pharyngeal wall in an adult. (See Color Plate 31.) (From Kadirova R, Kartoglu HÜ, Strebel PM: Clinical characteristics and management of 676 hospitalized diphtheria cases. Kyrgyz Republic 1995. J Infect Dis 2000;181 [Suppl 1]:S110–S115. Photograph by P. Strebel.)

diphtheria most commonly occurs as an extension of pharyngeal involvement in children, leading to increasing hoarseness and stridor. The patient appears toxic, with symptoms of LTB, and signs of severe airway obstruction may develop quickly if the pharyngeal membrane dislodges and obstructs the airway. Complications include secondary pneumonia, toxin-mediated myocarditis, and less commonly, neuritis. Case fatality rates vary, and can reach 20%, but in a series of 676 patients (30% younger than 15 years of age) reported from the 1995 Kyrgyz Republic outbreak, the mortality rate was only 3%.[51] Deaths are usually due to airway obstruction or myocarditis.

MANAGEMENT

Because this condition is now rare, a high index of suspicion is important to make the diagnosis and institute prompt treatment. Patients should be strictly isolated. Diphtheria antitoxin, which is a hyperimmune equine antiserum (available from the Centers for Disease Control and Prevention), should be administered without waiting for laboratory confirmation, because it neutralizes circulating toxin, but not toxin bound to tissues. Antibiotics are not a substitute for antitoxin, but are given to eradicate the organism, stop toxin production, and reduce the likelihood of transmission.[50] Intravenous penicillin or erythromycin is used, and once the child can swallow comfortably, treatment can be given orally, for a total of 14 days.[50] Mechanical ventilation and tracheostomy may be required. Intravenous dexamethasone has been given to children with laryngeal diphtheria and airway obstruction, and a small case series suggested that it was beneficial.[52] Because the disease may not confer immunity, patients should be given a diphtheria toxoid-containing vaccine during convalescence. Antibiotic prophylaxis (penicillin or erythromycin) is recommended for close contacts after nasal and pharyngeal specimens are taken, and immunization should be given to those who have not been vaccinated in the preceding 5 years.[50]

RETROPHARYNGEAL ABSCESS

ETIOLOGY

Abscesses generally result from lymphatic spread of infection, although direct spread from adjacent areas, penetrating pharyngeal trauma (e.g., a fall with a pencil in the mouth), or foreign bodies can also play a role.[5] It has also been reported as a complication of adenoidectomy.[53] Infection is usually due to mixed flora, including *S. aureus*, various streptococcal species, HiB, and anaerobes.[54]

EPIDEMIOLOGY

The majority of cases occur in children younger than 6 years of age, probably due to the fact that retropharyngeal lymph nodes are so abundant at this age (they tend to atrophy later in life). A recent large series reported a median age of 3 years, with 75% of those affected younger than 5 years of age and 16% younger than 1 year.[54] Boys are more likely to be affected than girls.

PATHOPHYSIOLOGY

The retropharyngeal space (between the posterior pharyngeal wall and the prevertebral layer of deep cervical fascia) contains loose connective tissue and lymph nodes that drain the nasopharynx, paranasal sinuses, middle ear, teeth, and adjacent bones. The space extends from the base of the skull down to vertebra C7 or T1. Acute bacterial infection in this region may start as retropharyngeal cellulitis with localized thickening of the tissues, which can progress to purulent inflammation of the cellular tissue and retropharyngeal adenitis. However, when it is caused by lymphatic spread, it starts as adenitis. If liquefaction of one of the nodes occurs, an abscess can form and is usually contained within the inflammatory rind of the infected node.

CLINICAL PRESENTATION AND DIAGNOSIS

Presentation is often nonspecific, and there may be overlap with the presentation of croup, epiglottitis, tracheitis, and peritonsillar abscess (see Table 23-1).[5] Children with acute epiglottitis tend to appear more toxic and progress to respiratory distress more rapidly.[55] Excluding causes secondary to foreign bodies or trauma, patients usually have a history of viral upper respiratory infection that lasts several days and then worsens. Children then have high fever, sore throat, dysphagia, poor feeding, neck pain, and stiffness. Limitation of neck extension and torticollis are more common than limited neck flexion.[54] Although the occurrence of neck signs with fever may suggest meningitis, children tend not to be as toxic as those with meningitis. Further deterioration may lead to extrathoracic airway compromise, with drooling, stridor, and respiratory distress. The classically described picture of stridor and airway obstruction seems to be less common now, and in a recent series, only 3% of 64 children in Salt Lake City had stridor or wheezing.[54] Older series, however, have reported a higher incidence of stridor. Reported rates include 71% in patients younger than 1 year of age, 43% in patients older than 1 year of age, and no stridor in those older than 3 years of age in a series of 31 children from Sydney, Australia[56]; a rate of 56% in 17 patients in Denver[57]; and a rate of 23% in 65 children in Los Angeles.[58] It is possible that the spectrum of disease is changing, but it is more likely that the diagnosis is being made earlier, before the airways are compromised.[54] Sometimes a retropharyngeal mass is visible in the mouth, seen as an asymmetrical bulge of the posterior pharyngeal wall (Fig. 23-5), or a neck mass (marked lymphadenopathy or parapharyngeal abscess) is visible and palpable. Complications include rupture of the abscess with aspiration, asphyxiation or pneumonia, extension to a mediastinal abscess, and vascular complications, such as thrombophlebitis of the internal jugular vein and erosion through the carotid artery sheath.[53,55]

Once the child is stable and safe, a lateral neck radiograph with the neck in full extension may confirm the diagnosis. Widened prevertebral soft tissue and air or fluid levels in the retropharyngeal space are all indicators.[5] The radiograph must be taken in the correct position (true lateral orientation, with the neck in extension, and if possible, during full inspiration) to ensure that the retropharyngeal space is not falsely thickened.[54] A contrast-enhanced computed tomography scan is useful because it differentiates a fully developed abscess from cellulitis and delineates the full extent of the abscess. Blood culture findings are usually negative, but the white cell count will be increased.

MANAGEMENT

Traditionally, management involves surgical drainage of the abscess (plus antibiotics). However, currently, more cases are

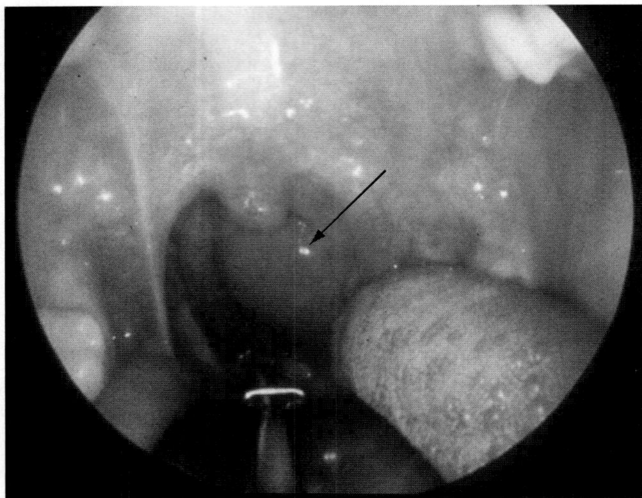

■ **FIGURE 23-5.** Retropharyngeal abscess behind and to the left of the uvula *(arrow)*. The tongue is pressed down and to the left with a tongue depressor. (See Color Plate 32.) (Photograph courtesy of the Otolaryngology Teaching Set, Department of Ear, Nose & Throat, Great Ormond Street Hospital for Children NHS Trust, London.)

being managed by intravenous antibiotics alone, although surgery must be considered early if there is a compromised airway. In one older series, 25% of patients required no surgery,[57] but in the Salt Lake City series that covered 1993–1998, 58% of 64 patients had antibiotics alone, with no treatment failures.[54] Many children start treatment with antibiotics before the diagnosis is made, and certainly, retropharyngeal cellulitis can be treated with antibiotics alone. When necessary, surgical drainage is performed through the intraoral route. Care must be taken to avoid aspiration of the infected material. Occasionally, if there is extension lateral to the great vessels, external drainage through the neck is necessary. Mortality is rare now, with no deaths in recent reports.

■ PERITONSILLAR ABSCESS (QUINSY)

■ ETIOLOGY

A peritonsillar abscess is usually a complication of acute tonsillitis, but may follow pharyngitis or a previous peritonsillar abscess. The infection usually involves mixed bacterial flora, with *Streptococcus pyogenes* the predominant organism. In a small series of children younger than 5 years of age, *Streptococcus viridans* was the most common organism detected.[59] Anaerobes may be present.

■ EPIDEMIOLOGY

Peritonsillar abscess is the most common deep-space head and neck infection in both adults and children. It is more common in young adults than in children, however. It tends to affect older children, and in one large, 10-year series, the mean age was 12 years, with two thirds of those affected older than 10 years of age.[60] In this series, 62% of cases occurred on the left side versus 38% on the right (with no obvious explanation).[60] There is no seasonal predilection.

■ PATHOPHYSIOLOGY

The infection is believed to arise from the spread of infection from the tonsil or the mucous glands of Weber, located in the superior tonsillar pole.[60] There is a spectrum of peritonsillar cellulitis that may then result in a collection of pus located between the tonsillar capsule (pharyngobasilar fascia), the superior constrictor, and the palatopharyngeus muscle.[60] There is a risk of spread through the muscle into the parapharyngeal space or other deep neck spaces. The abscess pushes the adjacent tonsil downward and medially, and the uvula may be so edematous as to resemble a white grape.

■ CLINICAL PRESENTATION AND DIAGNOSIS

The child, already affected by acute tonsillitis, becomes more ill, with a high fever, and has a severe sore throat or neck pain as well as marked dysphagia with referred earache. Absent or decreased oral intake can lead to dehydration, particularly in younger children.

Cervical lymphadenopathy is almost always present, the uvula is edematous and deviated to one side, there is fetor oris, and a striking feature may be trismus, with limited mouth opening. Examination may be difficult in a young, uncooperative child who refuses to open the mouth. The white cell count will be elevated

The relevance of this condition to pediatric pulmonologists is that acute enlargement of the tonsils can cause airway compromise, and a ruptured abscess can lead to aspiration of infected material and subsequent pneumonia.

■ MANAGEMENT

Children may need intravenous fluids. Antibiotics are necessary, and intravenous penicillin is as effective as broad-spectrum antibiotics, although additional anaerobic coverage should be considered.[61] Analgesia is important. Treatment often involves incision and drainage or needle aspiration, but an initial period of medical treatment in the absence of airway compromise and systemic toxicity is appropriate, especially in younger children.[62] There is some debate among otolaryngologists about the role and timing of tonsillectomy, and peritonsillar abscess is no longer considered an absolute indication for tonsillectomy.[62]

REFERENCES

1. Lusk RP, Khosla S: Principles of fluid dynamics. In: Holinger LD, Lusk RP, Green CG, eds: Pediatric Laryngology & Bronchoesophagology. Philadelphia: Lipincott-Raven, 1997, pp 381–391.
2. Stroud RH, Friedman NR: An update on inflammatory disorders of the pediatric airway. Epiglottitis, croup and tracheitis. Am J Otolaryngol 2001;22:268–275.
3. Holinger LD: Evaluation of stridor and wheezing. In: Holinger LD, Lusk RP, Green CG, eds: Pediatric Laryngology & Bronchoesophagology. Philadelphia: Lipincott-Raven, 1997, pp 41–48.
4. Schroeder LL, Knapp JF: Recognition and emergency management of infectious causes of upper airway obstruction in children. Semin Respir Infect 1995;10:21–30.
5. Rotta AT, Wiryawan B: Respiratory emergencies in children. Respir Care 2003;48:248–260.
6. Mackie PL: The classification of viruses infecting the respiratory tract. Paediatr Respir Rev 2003;4:84–90.
7. Klassen TP: Croup. A current perspective. Pediatr Clin North Am 1999;46:1167–1178.
8. Geelhoed GC: Sixteen years of croup in a Western Australian teaching hospital. Effects of routine steroid treatment. Ann Emerg Med 1996; 28:621–626.
9. Smith FS, Portner A, Leggiadro RJ, Turner EV, Hurwitz JL: Age-related development of human memory T-helper and B-cell responses toward parainfluenza virus type-1. Virology 1994;205:453–461.
10. Welliver RC, Wong DT, Middleton E Jr, Sun M, McCarthy N, Ogra PL: Role of parainfluenza virus-specific IgE in pathogenesis of croup and wheezing subsequent to infection. J Pediatr 1982;101:889–896.

11. Zach MS, Schnall RP, Landau LI: Upper and lower airway reactivity in recurrent croup. Am Rev Respir Dis 1980;121:979–983.
12. Stoney PJ, Chakrabarti MK: Experience of pulse oximetry in children with croup. J Laryngol Otol 1991;105:295–298.
13. Brown JC: The management of croup. Br Med Bull 2002;61:189–202.
14. Bourchier D, Dawson KP, Fergusson DM: Humidification in viral croup. A controlled trial. Aust Paediatr J 1984;20:289–291.
15. Lenney W, Milner AD: Treatment of acute viral croup. Arch Dis Child 1978;53:704–706.
16. Neto GM, Kentab O, Klassen TP, Osmond MH: A randomized controlled trial of mist in the acute treatment of moderate croup. Acad Emerg Med 2002;9:873–879.
17. Murphy SM, Murray D, Smith S, Orr D: Burns caused by steam inhalation for respiratory tract infections in children. BMJ 2004;328:757.
18. Russell K, Wiebe N, Saenz A, Ausejo SM, Johnson D, Hartling L, Klassen T: Glucocorticoids for croup. Cochrane Database Syst Rev 2004;(1):CD 001955. DOI: 10.1002/14651858.CD001955.pub2.
19. Bjornson CL, Klassen TP, Williamson J, Brant R, Mitton C, Plint A, Bulloch B, Evered L, Johnson DW, Pediatric Emergency Research Canada Network: A randomized trial of a single dose of oral dexamethasone for mild croup. N Engl J Med 2004;351:1306–1313.
20. Klassen TP, Craig WR, Moher D, Osmond MH, Pasterkamp H, Sutcliffe T, Watters LK, Rowe PC: Nebulized budesonide and oral dexamethasone for treatment of croup. A randomized controlled trial. JAMA 1998;279: 1629–1632.
21. Rittichier KK, Ledwith CA: Outpatient treatment of moderate croup with dexamethasone. Intramuscular versus oral dosing. Pediatrics 2000;106: 1344–1348.
22. Donaldson D, Poleski D, Knipple E, Filips K, Reetz L, Pascual RG, Jackson RE: Intramuscular versus oral dexamethasone for the treatment of moderate-to-severe croup. A randomized, double-blind trial. Acad Emerg Med 2003;10:16–21.
23. Johnson DW, Jacobson S, Edney PC, Hadfield P, Mundy ME, Schuh S: A comparison of nebulized budesonide, intramuscular dexamethasone, and placebo for moderately severe croup. N Engl J Med 1998;339:498–503.
24. Roe M, O'Donnell DR, Tasker RC: Respiratory viruses in the intensive care unit. Paediatr Respir Rev 2003;4:166–171.
25. Fitzgerald DA, Kilham HA: Croup. Assessment and evidence-based management. Med J Aust 2003;179:372–377.
26. Geelhoed GC, Macdonald WB: Oral dexamethasone in the treatment of croup. 0.15 mg/kg versus 0.3 mg/kg versus 0.6 mg/kg. Pediatr Pulmonol 1995;20:362–368.
27. Geelhoed GC, Turner J, Macdonald WB: Efficacy of a small single dose of oral dexamethasone for outpatient croup. A double blind placebo controlled clinical trial. BMJ 1996;313:140–142.
28. Kristjansson S, Berg-Kelly K, Winso E: Inhalation of racemic adrenaline in the treatment of mild and moderately severe croup. Clinical symptom score and oxygen saturation measurements for evaluation of treatment effects. Acta Paediatr 1994;83:1156–1160.
29. Waisman Y, Klein BL, Boenning DA, Young GM, Chamberlain JM, O'Donnell R, Ochsenschlager DW: Prospective randomized double-blind study comparing L-epinephrine and racemic epinephrine aerosols in the treatment of laryngotracheitis (croup). Pediatrics 1992;89:302–306.
30. Prendergast M, Jones JS, Hartman D: Racemic epinephrine in the treatment of laryngotracheitis. Can we identify children for outpatient therapy? Am J Emerg Med 1994;12:613–616.
31. Duncan PG: Efficacy of helium. Oxygen mixtures in the management of severe viral and post-intubation croup. Can Anaesth Soc J 1979;26:206–212.
32. Weber JE, Chudnofsky CR, Younger JG, Larkin GL, Boczar M, Wilkerson MD, Zuriekat GY, Nolan B, Eicke DM: A randomized comparison of helium-oxygen mixture (Heliox) and racemic epinephrine for the treatment of moderate to severe croup. Pediatrics 2001;107:E96.
33. Durward AD, Nicoll SJ, Oliver J, Tibby SM, Murdoch IA: The outcome of patients with upper airway obstruction transported to a regional paediatric intensive care unit. Eur J Pediatr 1998;157:907–911.
34. Isaacson G, Isaacson DM: Pediatric epiglottitis caused by group G beta-hemolytic *Streptococcus*. Pediatr Infect Dis J 2003;22:846–847.
35. CDC: Progress toward eliminating *Haemophilus influenzae* type b disease among infants and children. United States, 1987–1997. MMWR 1998;47(No.46):993–998.
36. Midwinter KI, Hodgson D, Yardley M: Paediatric epiglottitis. The influence of the *Haemophilus influenzae* b vaccine. A ten-year review in the Sheffield region. Clin Otolaryngol 1999;24:447–448.
37. Heath PT, Booy R, Azzopardi HJ, Slack MPE, Bowen-Morris J, Griffiths H, Ramsay ME, Deeks JJ, Moxon RE: Antibody concentration and clinical protection after HiB conjugate vaccination in the United Kingdom. JAMA 2000;284:2334–2340.
38. McEwan J, Giridharan W, Clarke RW, Shears P: Paediatric acute epiglottitis: Not a disappearing entity. Int J Ped Otolaryngol 2003;67:317–321.
39. Heath PT, Booy R, Griffiths H, Clutterbuck E, Azzopardi HJ, Slack MPE, Fogarty J, Moloney AC, Moxon RE: Clinical and immunological risk factors associated with *Haemophilus influenzae* type b conjugate vaccine failure in childhood. Clin Infect Dis 2000;31:973–980.
40. Gorelick MH, Baker MD: Epiglottitis in children, 1979 through 1992. Effects of *Haemophilus influenzae* type b immunization. Arch Pediatr Adolesc Med 1994;148:47–50.
41. Ward JI, Zangwill KM: *Haemophilus influenzae*. In: Feigin RD, Cherry J, eds: Textbook of Pediatric Infectious Diseases, 4th ed. Philadelphia: WB Saunders, 1998, pp 1464–1482.
42. Sawyer SM, Johnson PDR, Hogg GG, Robertson CF, Oppedisano F, MacIness SJ, Gilbert GL: Successful treatment of epiglottitis with two doses of ceftriaxone. Arch Dis Child 1994;70:129–132.
43. Lee TW, Sandoe JA: Epiglottitis caused by group C *Streptococcus*. Acta Paediatr 2001;90:1085.
44. Goodman TR, McHugh K: The role of radiology in the evaluation of stridor. Arch Dis Child 1999;81:456–459.
45. Bernstein T, Brilli R, Jacobs B: Is bacterial tracheitis changing? A 14-month experience in a pediatric intensive care unit. Clin Infect Dis 1998; 27:458–462.
46. Eid NS, Jones VF: Bacterial tracheitis as a complication of tonsillectomy and adenoidectomy. J Pediatr 1994;125:401–402.
47. Britto J, Habibi P, Walters S, Levin M, Nadel S: Systemic complications associated with bacterial tracheitis. Arch Dis Child 1996;74:249–250.
48. CDC: Fatal respiratory diphtheria in a U.S. traveller to Haiti. Pennsylvania, 2003. MMWR 2004;52(No. 53):1285–1286.
49. McQuillan GM, Kruszon-Moran D, Deforest A, Chu S, Wharton M: Serologic immunity to diphtheria and tetanus in the United States. Ann Intern Med 2002;136:660–666.
50. Farizo KM, Strebel PM, Chen RT, Kimbler A, Cleary TJ, Cochi SL: Fatal respiratory disease due to *Corynebacterium diphtheriae*. Case report and review of guidelines for management, investigation, and control. Clin Infect Dis 1993;16:59–68.
51. Kadirova R, Kartoglu HÜ, Strebel PM: Clinical characteristics and management of 676 hospitalized diphtheria cases. Kyrgyz Republic 1995. J Infect Dis 2000;181(Suppl 1):S110–S115.
52. Havaldar PV: Dexamethasone in laryngeal diphtheritic croup. Ann Trop Paediatr 1997;17:21–23.
53. Tuerlinckx D, Bodart E, Lawson G, De Wisplaere J-F, de Bilderling G: Retropharyngeal and mediastinal abscess following adenoidectomy. Pediatr Pulmonol 2003;36:257–258.
54. Craig FW, Schunk JE: Retropharyngeal abscess in children. Clinical presentation, utility of imaging, and current management. Pediatr 2003;111: 1394–1398.
55. Lee SS, Schwartz RH, Bahadori RS: Retropharyngeal abscess. Epiglottitis of the new millenium. J Pediatr 2001;138:435–437.
56. Coulthard M, Isaacs D: Retropharyngeal abscess. Arch Dis Child 1991;66:1227–1230.
57. Morrison JE Jr, Pashley NR: Retropharyngeal abscesses in children. A 10-year review. Pediatr Emerg Care 1988;4:9–11.
58. Thompson JW, Cohen SR, Reddix P: Retropharyngeal abscess in children. A retrospective and historical analysis. Laryngoscope 1988;98:589–592.
59. Friedman NR, Mitchell RB, Pereira KD, Younis RT, Lazar RH: Peritonsillar abscess in early childhood. Presentation and management. Arch Otolaryngol Head Neck Surg 1997;123:630–632.
60. Schraff S, McGinn JD, Derkay CS: Peritonsillar abscess in children. A 10-year review of diagnosis and management. Int J Ped Otorhinolaryngol 2001;57:213–218.
61. Prior A, Montgomery P, Mitchelmore I, Tabaqchali S: The microbiology and antibiotic treatment of peritonsillar abscesses. Clin Otolaryngol 1995; 20:219–223.
62. Blotter JW, Yin L, Glynn M, Wiet GJ: Otolaryngology consultation for peritonsillar abscess in the pediatric population. Laryngoscope 2000;110:1698–1701.

24 Bronchitis

Gerald M. Loughlin, MD

Bronchitis, a condition manifested primarily and at times exclusively by cough, is an inflammatory disease affecting the major airways. Even though the diagnosis is often based solely on the presence of cough, a symptom that is seen in many other respiratory diseases, both parents and primary care physicians seem comfortable in frequently making the diagnosis of bronchitis. A differential diagnosis based on the clinical presentations of bronchitis is presented in Box 24-1, and a diagnostic approach to the child with acute and chronic bronchitis is presented in Box 24-2.

ACUTE BRONCHITIS

Acute bronchitis is a transient inflammation of the trachea and major bronchi that is manifested primarily, and at times exclusively, by cough. It is seen most commonly by primary care physicians, is usually caused by viral infection, and typically resolves without therapy within 28 days.[1] Since viruses most often cause acute bronchitis, it is certainly possible for a child to experience several episodes of bronchitis during the fall and winter months.[2] However, there should be an asymptomatic period between infections, and no one episode should last longer than 28 days. Persistent symptoms and/or recurrent acute episodes that occur without obvious triggers and last more than 2 weeks are also considered abnormal. In addition, acute bronchitis occurring during the summer months is also a cause for concern about an underlying condition.[3]

Bronchitis is more common in younger children and in males, especially in children younger than 6 years of age. During an 8-year period, acute bronchitis accounted for approximately 40% of the total number of acute respiratory illnesses seen in a private practice setting.[4] Results from an Australia Morbidity and Treatment Survey indicate a relative frequency of acute bronchitis of 2.4%, making it the fifth most common clinical condition encountered by primary care physicians.[5] Again, the diagnosis is often based exclusively on the symptom of cough in a child with an upper respiratory tract infection.

Respiratory syncytial virus, influenza A and B, parainfluenza virus (especially type 3), adenovirus, rhinovirus, and the paramyxoviruses (including the recently identified metapneumovirus) have been linked to acute bronchitis.[2] Episodes can occur at any time, but they are most common in the winter months. However, adenovirus and rhinovirus infections may not follow a seasonal pattern. Rubeola is almost universally associated with acute bronchitis, the respiratory symptoms often preceding the more classic manifestations of this infection.

Most episodes of acute tracheobronchitis caused by bacteria occur as secondary infections during a period of vulnerability of the mucosal surface caused by a prior viral infection or other airway insult. Work by Ramphal and co-workers[5] in mice and ferrets provides experimental data that suggest a mechanism for secondary bacterial infections following either an acute viral infection or other injury to the respiratory epithelium. Influenza infection induces a widespread desquamation of the ciliated epithelium of the trachea. As a result, *Pseudomonas aeruginosa* organisms, which were previously swept out by motion of cilia, adhere to the injured cells and exposed basement membrane. Penetration of the mucosal barrier by bacteria causes a secondary bacterial bronchitis. Recovery of the ciliated epithelium occurs over 5 to 7 days in uncomplicated bronchitis.

Though far less common than viruses, *Streptococcus pneumoniae, Staphylococcus aureus, Haemophilus influenzae,* and *Mycoplasma pneumoniae* have been implicated as causative agents.[2] There are no characteristic clinical findings of bronchitis caused by *Mycoplasma.* It should be considered in an older child (>4 years) or adolescent. Recent work has also suggested that *Moraxella catarrhalis*[6] and *Chlamydia pneumoniae* (strain TWAR) are capable of producing acute bronchitis often associated with wheezing in adults.[7] There are limited data on the role of this latter organism in the pediatric or adolescent population. *Chlamydia* infections can also produce an acute tracheobronchitis and pneumonitis in young infants beginning at several weeks of age. Respiratory symptoms include a characteristic staccato cough, which may be preceded by blepharitis or conjunctivitis. Infection is acquired at birth. The diagnosis can be confirmed by culture and serology.[8] Treatment is largely supportive but also includes a trial of erythromycin.

Bordetella pertussis and *Corynebacterium diphtheriae* produce a characteristic illness marked by tracheobronchitis in nonimmunized children. Diphtheria is discussed in Chapter 23 and Pertussis in Chapter 36. Infection with *Mycobacterium tuberculosis* should also be considered as possible causes of acute and chronic bronchitis, especially in children from endemic areas. Tuberculosis is discussed in Chapter 34.

Cough associated with other constitutional symptoms can be seen in children with fungal respiratory tract infections. The cough is generally nonproductive and may be related to airway compression from lymph node enlargement. Fungal serology, delayed hypersensitivity skin testing, and cultures when available help establish a diagnosis. An important clue to the diagnosis is a history of a significant exposure to the fungus, residence in an endemic area, or a compromised immune status. These infections are discussed in more detail in Chapter 35.

CLINICAL MANIFESTATIONS

The cough associated with acute viral bronchitis usually appears 3 to 4 days after the onset of typical upper respiratory infection. Coughing indicates extension of the infection and inflammation to the trachea and bronchi. The cough is initially nonproductive, but several days into the illness may progress into a loose, congested cough with sputum production. Vomiting associated with coughing paroxysms may occur. The vomitus frequently contains mucus, confirming the productive nature of the cough in young children, who typically do not expectorate. In general, there are few constitutional symptoms, unless the bronchitis is secondary to a more severe systemic illness such as rubeola or a secondary bacterial infection. In the majority of children, symptoms usually resolve within 14 days and in most patients by 28 days. If the cough persists beyond this period, then one should suspect a previously unrecognized chronic condition.[9]

Auscultation of the chest is frequently unremarkable in the early stages. Coarse rhonchi may be heard as the illness progresses. Crackles are infrequent. Wheezing is not uncommon, and its presence has been thought to indicate bronchospasm and asthma (asthmatic or wheezy bronchitis), although it may simply reflect partial airway obstruction from airway inflammation.

Material for pathologic investigation of acute bronchitis is scanty, because the disease is usually mild and self-limited. As with other inflammatory processes affecting the airways, congestion of the mucosa develops early. Secretions are initially sparse, but mucous gland activity increases as the inflammatory process continues, resulting in mucus production. Migration of polymorphonuclear leukocytes into the airway wall and lumen contributes to the purulent appearance of the secretions. Desquamation of the ciliated epithelium occurs as well.[10]

"Plastic bronchitis" is an uncommon form of acute bronchitis characterized by acute severe obstruction of large airways with tenacious bronchial casts. Casts may be classified according to their composition. A type I cast is inflammatory, formed mostly of fibrin with cellular infiltrates. A type II cast consists mainly of mucus with few cells and often occurs after surgery for congenital heart disease. This condition is manifested by cough, wheezing, a toxic appearance, and respiratory distress. Symptoms are the consequence of large airway obstruction by thick tenacious mucus. Respiratory failure, a rare complication of most types of bronchitis, may be seen, especially in younger patients. It has

BOX 24-1 Differential Diagnosis of Bronchitis in Children

Acute

- Infection
  - Viral: Respiratory syncytial virus; parainfluenza 1, 2, 3; influenza A and B; adenovirus, rhinovirus, metapneumovirus
  - Chemical exposures: Aspiration of gastric contents, smoke inhalation, pollution (ozone, respirable particles)

Chronic/Recurrent

- Cystic fibrosis
- Asthma
- Dyskinetic cilia syndrome
- Tuberculosis
- Retained foreign body
- Aspiration: Anatomic abnormalities (tracheoesophageal fistula, laryngeal cleft); dysfunctional swallowing with and without gastroesophageal reflux
- Immunodeficiency: IgG, IgA, IgG subclasses, common variable immune deficiency, inability to respond to polysaccharide antigen
- Inhalation injury
  - Smoking—active
  - Indoor pollution: Cigarette smoke, woodstoves, cooking oils, chemicals (formaldehyde, nitrogen dioxide)
  - Outdoor pollution: soot, sulfur dioxide, ozone, nitrogen dioxide
- Chronic airway damage: Following infection or traumatic airway injury with delayed or incomplete healing
- Nonrespiratory causes: Psychogenic/functional or Gilles de la Tourette's syndrome

BOX 24-2 Approach to the Patient with Chronic/Recurrent Bronchitis

History

- Age at onset of symptoms
- Relationship of symptoms to feeding
- Associated symptoms (wheezing, fever)
- Characteristics of the cough: timing, productivity, influences that relieve or exacerbate cough
- Past history: respiratory illness, coughing, choking episodes, steatorrhea, failure to thrive
- Family history: asthma, bronchitis, cystic fibrosis, sinusitis
- Environmental exposures: smoking, use of wood-burning stoves, gas or oil cooking noxious chemicals, ozone

Physical Examination

- Growth and development
- Respiratory signs
  - Rales, rhonchi, wheezes
  - Sinus tenderness or swelling
  - Posterior pharyngeal secretions
  - Allergic shiners, rhinitis
  - Nasal polyps
  - Clinical response of respiratory symptoms to bronchodilators
  - Digital clubbing

Laboratory Evaluation

- Initial—should be obtained in all patients
  - Chest radiograph
  - Sputum culture: Gram and Wright stain (if available)
  - Purified protein derivative
  - Sweat chloride
- As indicated on basis of history, physical, and aforementioned laboratory data
  - Immunoglobulins
    - IgG, IgA, IgM, IgE
    - IgG subclasses
    - Functional antibody titers (diphtheria, tetanus)
    - Response to polysaccharide antigen challenge (Pneumovax)
  - Esophagram
  - Formal swallowing evaluation
  - pH probe
  - Technetium scan
  - Esophagoscopy
  - Sinus radiographs and/or computed tomography
  - Bronchoscopy
  - Cilia biopsy and function studies
  - Pulmonary function tests—before and after bronchodilators
  - Bronchial challenge—methacholine, exercise, cold air
  - Fungal serology/skin testing

also been reported in patients with asthma and acute chest syndrome seen in sickle cell anemia.[11]

DIAGNOSIS

The diagnosis of acute bronchitis is usually based on a clinical finding (cough), and laboratory tests are of limited value. A chest roentgenogram is not needed as a part of the initial evaluation of an isolated episode of acute bronchitis, unless a condition such as pneumonia, atelectasis, or a retained foreign body is suspected; if obtained, peribronchial thickening may be present. Hyperinflation suggests extension of the inflammation to involve the bronchioles. Viral cultures are infrequently obtained and are useful primarily for epidemiologic purposes. A sputum culture, as well as Gram and Wright staining of the sputum may be useful in cases in which a secondary bacterial infection or unusual etiology is suspected. Positive cold hemagglutination titers supported by a rise in specific *Mycoplasma* titers or polymerase chain reaction can be used to confirm this diagnosis.[12]

MANAGEMENT

Treatment of acute viral bronchitis is largely supportive. Adequate hydration, rest, and proper humidification of the ambient air are usually sufficient. Exposure to noxious agents such as cigarette smoke should be avoided. The usual mild case does not require antibiotics or other pharmacologic agents. Antibiotics should be reserved for conditions in which a bacterial infection is highly suspected on the basis of the clinical course or preferably proven by culture. Typically, treatment of a suspected bacterial infection is generally empiric, depending largely on the age of the patient, the organisms commonly encountered, and the sensitivity patterns of these organisms in the community.[2]

Since mucus production is common as the illness progresses, the use of a cough suppressant should be discouraged and in fact is contraindicated. In otherwise healthy children with an effective cough, chest physical therapy is not needed. If wheezing is detected on physical exam, then a trial of a β agonist should be considered. It is important that the response to an inhaled bronchodilator be assessed to identify wheezing due to bronchospasm and thus avoid overuse or inappropriate use of bronchodilators.[13] In the absence of wheezing, β_2 agonists in the acute phase of the illness are not routinely indicated.[14] Indications for steroids, either inhaled or systemic, are poorly defined, but they may be useful in those with severe symptoms (such as dyspnea and/or severe airflow obstruction) if there is a documented positive response to bronchodilators.

CHRONIC AND RECURRENT BRONCHITIS

The definition of chronic bronchitis in children is less clear, and the definition is not as well established as it is in adults.[15,16] Since symptoms of a typical episode of acute bronchitis infrequently last for more than 4 weeks, chronic bronchitis in children can be defined as persistence of symptoms (cough) for longer than 4 weeks following an acute insult. Similarly, there is cause for concern when a child has more than two episodes a year that occur without an obvious trigger and last longer than 2 weeks. Chronic/recurrent symptoms suggest that the stimulus of airway inflammation is still present; a complication of acute bronchitis may have developed, or a systemic disease such as cystic fibrosis, immune deficiency, or immotile cilia syndrome may be present. One concern with this definition is that an otherwise perfectly normal child could experience an isolated bad episode that has no lasting clinical significance. Despite these limitations, the yield in terms of early detection of chronic disease justifies an aggressive approach to the child with even a single episode of a cough that lasts for more than 28 days following a viral infection, and/or a recurrent cough, without an obvious cause. The reader is referred to specific chapters on conditions listed in Box 24-1 for detailed discussions of bronchitis associated with these conditions.

Notable exceptions to the rule that a chronic cough indicates underlying airway disease is the child who has a cough that is psychogenic or functional[17,18] or is a manifestation of Gilles de la Tourette's syndrome.[19] Psychogenic cough typically occurs in a healthy child without evidence of underlying lung disease. It is generally a loud, honking cough that usually attracts considerable attention. Characteristically, the cough stops during sleep or when the child believes he or she is unobserved. The child frequently appears quite unconcerned, whereas the parents are usually very anxious about the persistence of the cough. When a functional cough is suspected, initial efforts should focus on defining a treatable condition. However, once a reasonably comprehensive evaluation has been completed, attention should be turned to identifying the secondary gain accruing to the child by persistence of the cough. Similarly, cough without evidence of underlying airway pathology may be a manifestation of the involuntary vocalizations (cough, snorting, throat clearing) associated with Gilles de la Tourette's syndrome.[19]

PATHOLOGIC FINDINGS IN NONSPECIFIC CHRONIC BRONCHITIS

In children, data on the pathology of chronic/recurrent bronchitis is clouded by problems with definition and overlap with other diseases. Table 24-1 summarizes the findings of a study comparing biopsy material from children with asthma to material from children with nonspecific bronchial inflammation.[20] Work in a group of nonatopic children with recurrent bronchitis defined as one episode of clinically significant bronchitis per month confirms and extends these observations. This group demonstrated significant epithelial damage, with 87% of the biopsy samples showing a loss of 50% of the surface epithelium. Lymphocyte infiltration was noted and correlated with the degree of inflammation observed during bronchoscopy. These changes are also associated with decreased mucus transport.[21] The severity and acute nature of these findings was most likely influenced by the frequency of the episodes in the study population.

TABLE 24-1. Pathologic characteristics of chronic bronchitis and asthma in children

	PERCENTAGE OF CASES	
Characteristic	**Chronic Bronchitis**	**Asthma**
Round cell infiltration	100	100
Eosinophils	14	49
Hypertrophied submucosal glands	39	20
Increased mucus	20	12
Metaplasia of epithelium	0	6
Intact epithelium	86	86

Data from Székely E, Farkas E: Pediatric Bronchology. Baltimore: University Park Press, 1978.

Smith and colleagues, in a group of children whose chronic bronchitis was diagnosed by bronchoscopy, demonstrated increased numbers of neutrophils in bronchial secretions in almost all children evaluated.[22] Mucosal gland hypertrophy, a characteristic feature of chronic bronchitis in adults, was present in only 39% of the children studied. None of these studies has demonstrated in children a significant amount of metaplasia of the epithelium, another common pathologic feature of chronic bronchitis in adults. Additional studies are needed to determine the natural history of these pathologic findings. Fitch and colleagues performed a limited bronchial lavage on a group of children (mean age 6.7 years) with chronic unexplained cough and compared the results to normal controls and a group of atopic asthmatic children.[23] There was a small increase in percentage of eosinophils in those with cough compared with controls, but less than that seen in the children with asthma. There were no statistically significant differences in neutrophil counts among the three groups.

CHRONIC/RECURRENT BRONCHITIS AND ASTHMA

As noted earlier, wheezing is a nonspecific symptom reflecting airway narrowing without regard to mechanism. In bronchitis, airway narrowing may result from excessive mucus production, mucosal edema, and/or smooth muscle constriction. This overlap of the clinical presentations of asthma and bronchitis has made it difficult to distinguish between these conditions clinically, especially in young children. In an attempt to cope with this "gray zone" and to avoid labeling all children who cough and wheeze with viral infections as having asthma, the terms *asthmatic* and *wheezy bronchitis* have been applied to patients with predominant cough and mild and/or variable wheezing.[24] As with asthma episodes in children, coughing and wheezing illnesses in children are frequently triggered by viral infections or exposure to cigarette smoke. An increased incidence of airway hyperreactivity has also been observed in patients with wheezy bronchitis and their first-degree relatives. In young children, these episodes are most appropriately labeled as wheeze-associated respiratory illness as described by Martinez and colleagues.[25] Episodes that continue past the age of 6 years or are triggered by other influences such as exercise, cold air, or environmental exposures strongly suggest that the child with wheezy bronchitis actually has asthma.

In an unknown, but probably small number of patients, chronic/recurrent cough without wheezing may be a manifestation of an asthma exacerbation, "cough variant asthma."[26] Typically, this cough is nonproductive and may be exacerbated by exercise, cold air, or cigarette smoke. This relationship has recently been called into question, because in a number of studies, patients with presumed cough variant asthma lacked several key markers of the asthmatic state (bronchial hyperreactivity, family history, airway eosinophilia, and reversible airflow obstruction).[27–29] In addition, it is possible that wheezing has simply been missed on physical examination and may require more severe airway obstruction before it becomes detectable by physical examination.[30] Identifying the child who actually has cough variant asthma has proven to be a major challenge for clinicians. Yet, the common occurrence of chronic cough without an obvious cause has resulted in overdiagnosis and excessive treatment with asthma medications.[31] Nonetheless, application of the diagnosis of cough variant asthma has increased during the past decade.[32]

In most instances, the persistence of cough following an acute viral infection indicates delayed healing from certain infections such as influenza; however, the possibility that some children have unrecognized asthma as the etiology of the persistent cough after the acute phase of the upper respiratory infection has resolved should at least be considered. Several studies have suggested that children with cough variant asthma may be at increased risk for developing wheezing and when it develops may be seen only at higher levels of airflow obstruction.[30] Although a minority of children with chronic cough may have increased airway eosinophils, airway hyperreactivity, and a history of atopy, it is not clear who are candidates for asthma therapy (bronchodilators and steroids). A study by Chang and co-workers in children with a chronic cough without wheezing demonstrated that neither bronchodilators nor steroids were effective, even in those with associated airway hyperreactivity.[31] It may be that these are two distinct clinical entities. Children with chronic cough without wheezing have been shown to have a pattern of lung function that is different from children with asthma, and they also lack airway eosinophilia. Specifically, in response to methacholine challenge, some demonstrate a pattern of extrathoracic airway hyperreactivity as opposed to bronchial hyperreactivity.[33] In addition, evidence of airflow obstruction either clinically or on lung function testing, which is common in children who wheeze, may not be seen in some patients, whose cough is found to respond to asthma therapy.[26] In addition, theophylline, which is no longer a mainstay of asthma therapy, has been shown to be effective in treating cough variant asthma, possibly reflecting proposed anti-inflammatory properties of this medication. This medication needs more study in controlled clinical trials to establish efficacy and indications. As in children with asthma, caution should be advised in using this medication because of the potential for adverse side effects, drug interactions, and limited therapeutic range. In light of these data, it is still worth considering a trial of asthma therapy in a child with chronic/recurrent cough. However, if there is no improvement after a week of therapy, then it should be stopped. Furthermore, a positive response to treatment does not de facto indicate a diagnosis of asthma.

IMMUNE DEFICIENCY AND CHRONIC/RECURRENT BRONCHITIS

Children with selective deficiencies in immune system function have increased susceptibility to respiratory infections and to delayed resolution of symptoms.[34] Chronic recurrent bronchitis has been reported in selective immunoglobulin A (IgA) deficiency, in IgA deficiency associated with IgG subclass deficiency (especially IgG2), and in combined deficiency of IgG2 and IgG4 in the presence of normal total IgG and IgA. Common variable IgG deficiency, a disorder of B-lymphocyte function associated with inadequate production of immunoglobulins, has also been associated with chronic/recurrent pulmonary disease including tracheobronchitis. Children who are unable to respond to the capsular polysaccharide have been shown to have an increased frequency of respiratory tract infections (pneumonia, sinusitis, and otitis). Similarly, children who cannot respond to the polysaccharide antigen contained in the wall of certain bacteria have also been reported to develop recurrent episodes of bronchitis. The measurement of the specific response to the *H. influenzae* type b capsular polysaccharide vaccine or to the subtypes of the pneumococcal vaccine can be used to identify these children. Bronchitis obliterans has been reported as a complication of immune deficiency in children.[35]

Recognition of these immune deficiencies can have important therapeutic implications. More aggressive antibiotic therapy coupled with antibody replacement therapy is indicated to control symptoms.

FOCAL AIRWAY INJURY OR COMPRESSION

In children who present with chronic/recurrent productive cough, at times associated with fever and a focal infiltrate (atelectasis or pneumonia), fiberoptic bronchoscopy may reveal underlying airway pathology. This includes localized inflammation involving a segmental or subsegmental bronchus, bronchomalacia, and retained foreign body.[27,36] Exacerbations of chronic symptoms are usually triggered by viral infections that are often followed by secondary bacterial infection due to compromise of airway clearance function. Secretions are increased and frequently contain many neutrophils. Culture of these secretions may reveal a variety of bacterial pathogens such as *H. influenzae* and *M. catarrhalis*. Extended antibiotic coverage is frequently required for effective therapy. The prevalence and natural history of this disorder are not known. Most patients improve with therapy, but an occasional patient suffers permanent injury and requires resection of the damaged segment to control symptoms and prevent recurrences.

AIRWAY IRRITANTS AND CHRONIC/RECURRENT BRONCHITIS

Aspiration

Aspiration in children occurs secondary to anatomic defects of the trachea and esophagus, swallowing dysfunction, gastroesophageal reflux, and accidents. The presence of a retained foreign body must always be considered in evaluating children with chronic cough, even with lack of a history of foreign body aspiration (Chapter 41).

The respiratory manifestations of tracheoesophageal fistula and esophageal atresia are discussed in Chapter 17. Gastroesophageal reflux has been linked to pulmonary disease such as bronchitis, asthma, and pneumonia. This topic is discussed in detail in Chapter 40.

In children without significant gastroesophageal reflux, accidental aspiration of large amounts of gastric contents is usually an isolated event generally occurring in association with another condition such as endotracheal intubation or a seizure. The resulting bronchitis is usually an acute self-limited process that may be followed by a secondary bacterial infection.

Chronic bronchitis (cough) can also result from swallowing dysfunction.[37] This problem is encountered most often in children with central nervous system injury, but it is also seen in neurologically and developmentally normal children, especially former premature infants. Clinical experience suggests that this diagnosis is frequently delayed in this population. Fluoroscopic evaluation of swallowing using a modified barium meal of varying consistencies is useful in detecting both an abnormal swallowing pattern and associated aspiration. Even if aspiration is not noted, the finding of a dysfunctional swallow is highly suggestive that respiratory symptoms are related to aspiration during swallowing. Clinical observation of feeding is essential in establishing a diagnosis, because these patients frequently have more difficulty with thinner liquids, and thicker barium may minimize symptoms during the study. Treatment of this disorder generally involves thickening feedings in otherwise normal children, but in some children even thickened feedings may not relieve the symptoms. Although nasogastric or nasoduodenal feedings can be used on a temporary or trial basis to see if symptoms resolve and tube feedings are tolerated, placement of a gastrostomy offers a more permanent and perhaps safer solution.

Aspiration of a foreign substance produces an inflammatory response in the airways similar to that in viral tracheobronchitis. The intensity of this response is related to the composition of the aspirated substance. For example, aspiration of material with a low pH is more likely to produce a vigorous inflammatory reaction. Inert materials usually produce less inflammation. Aspiration of gastric contents produces a loss of ciliated epithelium, a situation that reduces the defenses of the respiratory epithelium and may predispose to infection. If the insult is recurrent, as it can be in several of these situations, then there may not be sufficient time for healing to occur, and the patient may become predisposed to chronic disease.

Air Pollution

There is increasing evidence that exposure to air pollution both indoors and outdoors should be considered in evaluating a child with chronic cough. Breathing polluted air may either produce chemical bronchitis or predispose to recurrences of infectious bronchitis. In the past, variability in the types of pollutants, inadequate measures of lengths of exposure, and an inability to separate the effects of pollution alone from interactions between pollution and other provocative influences, have contributed to some confusion in the literature regarding the relationship between pollution and bronchitis. However, recent data have provided convincing evidence of the link between air pollution and the occurrence of bronchitis and other respiratory symptoms in children.[38,39] Substances of concern include respirable particles, sulfur dioxide, nitrogen dioxide, ozone, and organic carbon products.

Long-term exposure to high levels of atmospheric pollution composed of reducing substances increases the incidence of chronic and recurrent lower respiratory tract disease, including bronchitis. Both upper and lower respiratory tract illnesses occurred more frequently in children who lived in highly polluted areas. A recent study from Germany demonstrated dramatic reductions in reporting of bronchitis associated with reductions in industrial air pollution.[40] At high concentrations, oxidizing agents can cause airway injury and clinical disease in animals and humans. Available clinical data on exposure to concentrations of these pollutants encountered routinely suggest that ozone exposure does not increase the incidence of bronchitis or the predisposition to lower respiratory tract illness in children.

An extensive review of the current status of the health effects of indoor air pollution is provided by Samet and co-workers.[41] Table 24-2, adapted from this review, summarizes data on potential sources of indoor air pollution commonly encountered by children. An increased occurrence of bronchitis and asthma has been reported in children living in homes heated by wood-burning stoves and in those using gas cooking. Use of these stoves, especially in modern energy-efficient homes, increases a child's exposure to the byproducts of combustion. Children are at increased risk because they are often "trapped" indoors during the winter months, when the stoves are in routine operation. In general, families should be discouraged from using these stoves,

■ TABLE 24-2. Common sources of air pollution in the home

Source	Pollutants
Cigarette smoke	Respirable particles, carbon monoxide, volatile organic substances
Gas stoves	Nitrous oxide, carbon monoxide
Wood-burning stoves, fireplaces	Respirable particles, carbon monoxide, polycyclic aromatic hydrocarbons
Kerosene heaters	Nitrous oxide, carbon monoxide, sulfur dioxide
Building materials	Formaldehyde
Dust	Inhaled allergens (mites, cockroach, etc.)

Adapted from Samet JM, Marbury MC, Spengler JD: Health effects of indoor air pollution. Part I. Am Rev Respir Dis 1987;136:1486, with permission.

especially if their children have asthma or chronic bronchitis. However, if economic pressures dictate their use, every effort should be made to minimize the volume of combustion products released into the indoor environment.

Cigarette smoke is perhaps the most common pollutant predisposing children to bronchitis.[42] Exposure to cigarette smoke occurs in either an active or a passive manner. The latter occurs when children inhale air polluted by smokers, usually parents and/or relatives. The case for active smoking as an influence in producing tracheobronchitis is quite clear. Cigarette smoking among children and adolescents increases chronic cough as well as the frequency of bronchitis produced by respiratory viruses. The effects of involuntary (passive) smoking on the lungs are perhaps more subtle but just as real. Work by several investigators has documented an association between bronchitis and pneumonia on the one hand, and parental, especially maternal, smoking on the other. This effect appears to be age dependent and is more apparent in the first year of life. Cessation of parental smoking may produce dramatic relief of symptoms in certain children. The smoking habits of all the adults in the household, as well as the child, should be assessed as a component of the evaluation of chronic/recurrent bronchitis in children. A smoking history obtained from an older child or adolescent with parents present is frequently unreliable.

■ LONG-TERM CONSEQUENCES OF CHILDHOOD BRONCHITIS

Studies of children with wheezy bronchitis have demonstrated evidence of increased airway resistance and airway hyperreactivity; airflow obstruction was reversible in the older children but not in the infants. Long-term follow-up reveals attainment of normal lung function as young adults but a more rapid decline with aging than in a control population.[43]

Follow-up data from a study of preschool children referred for recurrent cough without wheezing, in the absence of infection, demonstrated that most children are asymptomatic, a third continue with cough, and only a small percentage subsequently develop wheezing.[44] This is in contrast to a study of new-onset asthma in children between 10 and 20 years of age, in which 31 of 36 subjects studied had a past history of respiratory symptoms or a diagnosis of rhinitis or chronic bronchitis,[45] and another study that demonstrated a link between cough and decreased lung function in a group of 7- and 8-year-old children.[46] More data, including appropriate controls and a consistent definition of chronic cough, are needed to determine the natural history of chronic/recurrent cough in children.

REFERENCES

1. Hay AD, Wilson A, Fahey T, Peters TJ: The duration of acute cough in preschool children presenting to primary care. A prospective cohort study. Fam Pract 2003;20:696–705.
2. Cherry JD: Acute bronchitis. In: Feigin RD, Cherry JD, Demmler GJ, Kaplan SL, eds: Textbook of Pediatric Infectious Diseases, Vol. 1. Philadelphia: WB Saunders, 2004, pp 262–269.
3. Chapman RS, Henderson FW, Clyde WA Jr, Collier AM, Denny FW: The epidemiology of tracheobronchitis in pediatric practice. Am J Epidemiol 1981;114:786–797.
4. Meza RA, Bridges-Webb C, Sayer GP: The management of acute bronchitis in general practice. Results from the Australia Morbidity and Treatment Survey, 1990–1991. Aust Fam Physician 1994;23:1550–1553.
5. Ramphal R, Small PM, Shands JW Jr, Fishlschweiger W, Small PA Jr: Adherence of *Pseudomonas aeruginosa* to tracheal cells injured by influenza infection or by endotracheal intubation. Infect Immun 1980;27:614–619.
6. Christensen JJ, Gadeberg O, Bruun B: *Branhamella catarrhalis*: Significance in pulmonary infections and bacteriological features. Acta Pathol Microbiol Immunol Scand [B] 1986;94:89–95.
7. Falck G, Heyman L, Gnarpe J, Gnarpe H: *Chlamydia pneumoniae* (TWAR). A common agent in acute bronchitis. Scand J Infect Dis 1994;26:179–187.
8. Beem MO, Saxon EM: Respiratory tract colonization and a distinctive pneumonia syndrome in infants infected with *Chlamydia trachomatis*. N Engl J Med 1977;296:306–310.
9. de Jongste JC, Shields MD: Cough-2. Chronic cough in children. Thorax 2003;58:998–1003.
10. Spencer H: Pathology of the Lung, Vol 1. Oxford: Pergamon Press, 1977.
11. Brogan TV, Finn LS, Pyskaty DJ, Redding GJ, Ricker D, Inglis A, Gibson RL: Plastic bronchitis in children. A case series and review of the medical literature. Pediatr Pulmonol 2002;34:482–487.
12. Kuroki H, Morozumi M, Chiba N, Ubukata K: Characterization of children with *Mycoplasma pneumoniae* infection detected by rapid polymerase chain reaction technique. J Infect Chemother 2004;10:65–76.
13. Thomson F, Masters IB, Chang AB: Persistent cough in children and the overuse of medications. J Paediatr Child Health 2002;38:578–581.
14. Smucny J, Flynn C, Becker L, Glazier R: Beta$_2$-agonists for acute bronchitis. Cochrane Database Syst Rev 2004;(1)CD001726.
15. Morgan WJ, Taussig LM: The chronic bronchitis complex in children. Pediatr Clin North Am 1984;31:851–864.
16. Taussig LM, Smith SM, Blumenfeld R: Chronic bronchitis in childhood. What is it? Pediatrics 1981;67:1–5.
17. Lokshin B, Lindgren S, Weinberger M, Koviach J: Outcome of habit cough in children treated with a brief session of suggestion therapy. Ann Allergy 1991;67:579–582.
18. Lavigne JV, Davis AT, Fauber R: Behavioral management of psychogenic cough. Alternative to the "bedsheet" and other aversive techniques. Pediatrics 1991;87:532–537.
19. Duncan KL, Faust RA: Tourette Syndrome manifest as chronic cough. Int J Pediatr Otolaryngol 2002;65:65–68.
20. Székely E, Farkas E: Pediatric Bronchology. Baltimore: University Park Press, 1978.
21. Gaillard D, Jouet JB, Egreteau L, Plotkowski L, Zahm JM, Benali R, Pierrot D, Puchelle E: Airway epithelial damage and inflammation in children with recurrent bronchitis. Am J Respir Crit Care Med 1994;150:810–817.
22. Smith TF, Ireland TA, Zaatari GS, Gay BB, Zwiren GT, Andrews HG: Characteristics of children with endoscopically proven chronic bronchitis. Am J Dis Child 1985;139:1039–1044.
23. Fitch PS, Brown V, Schock BC, Taylor R, Ennis M, Shields MD: Chronic cough in children. Bronchoalveolar lavage findings. Eur Respir J 2000;16: 1109–1114.
24. Horn ME, Brain EA, Gregg I, Inglis JM, Yealland SJ, Taylor P: Respiratory viral infection and wheezy bronchitis in childhood. Thorax 1979;34:23–28.
25. Martinez FD, Wright AL, Taussig L, Halonen WJ, Morgan WJ, and the Group Health Medical Associates: Asthma and wheezing in the first six years of life. N Engl J Med 1995;332:133–138.
26. Cloutier MM, Loughlin GM: Chronic cough in children. A manifestation of airway hyper-reactivity. Pediatrics 1981;67:6–12.
27. Wright AL, Holberg CJ, Morgan WJ, Taussig LM, Halonen M, Martinez FD: Recurrent cough in childhood and its relation to asthma. Am J Respir Crit Care Med 1996;153:1259–1265.
28. Faniran AO, Peat JK, Woolcock AJ: Persistent cough. Is it asthma? Arch Dis Child 1998;79:411–414.
29. Chang AB: Isolated cough; probably not asthma. Arch Dis Child 1999;80: 211–213.

30. Koh YY, Park Y, Jeong JH, Kim CK, Kim JT: Relationship of wheezing to airflow obstruction in asthmatic children and a history of cough-variant asthma. J Asthma 2002;39:307–314.
31. Chang AB, Phelan PD, Carlin JB, Sawyer SM, Robertson CF: A randomized, placebo controlled trial of inhaled salbutamol and beclomethasone for recurrent cough. Arch Dis Child 1998;79:6–11.
32. Kelly YJ, Brabin BJ, Milligan PJM, Reid JA, Heaf D, Pearson MG: Clinical significance of cough and wheeze in the diagnosis of asthma. Arch Dis Child 1996;75:489–493.
33. Turktas I, Dalgic N, Bostanci I, Cengizilier R: Extrathoracic airway responsiveness in children with asthma-like symptoms, including chronic persistent cough. Pediatr Pulmonol 2002;34:172–180.
34. Kattan M: AIDS and other immune deficiency states. In: Loughlin GM, Eigen H, eds: Respiratory Disease in Children. Diagnosis and Management. Baltimore: Williams & Wilkins, 1994, pp 657–669.
35. Perlman EJ, Lederman HM, Taylor GA, Fasano MB, Loughlin GM, Zeitlin PL: "Bronchitis" obliterans and prolonged transient hypogammaglobulinemia in a child. Pediatr Pulmonol 1993;16:375–379.
36. Wood RE: Localized tracheomalacia or bronchomalacia in children with intractable cough. J Pediatr 1990;116:404–406.
37. Arvedson JC, Lefton-Greif MA: Pediatric dysphagia. Complex medical, health and developmental issues. Semin Speech Lang 1996;117:257–330.
38. McConnell R, Berhane K, Gilliland F, Molitor J, Thomas D, Lurmann F, Avol E, Gauderman WJ, Peters JM: Prospective study of air pollution and bronchitis symptoms in children with asthma. Am J Respir Crit Care Med 2003;168:790–797.
39. Schwartz J: Air pollution and children's health. Pediatrics 2004;113: 1037–1043.
40. Heinrich J, Hoelscher B, Wichmann HE: Decline of ambient air pollution and respiratory symptoms in children. Am J Respir Crit Care Med 2000;161: 1930–1936.
41. Samet JM, Marbury MC, Spengler JD: Health effects of indoor air pollution. Part I. Am Rev Respir Dis 1987;136:1486–1508; Part II, 1988;137:221–242.
42. Manning P, Goodman P, Kinsella T, Lawlor M, Kirby B, Clancy L: Bronchitis symptoms in young teenagers who actively or passively smoke cigarettes. Irish Med J 1995;95:202–204.
43. Edwards CA, Osman LM, Godden DJ, Douglas JG: Wheezy bronchitis in childhood, a distinct clinical entity with lifelong significance? Chest 2003;124: 18–24.
44. Brooke AM, Lambert PC, Burton PR, Clarke C, Luyt DK, Simpson H: Recurrent cough. Natural history and significance in infancy and early childhood. Pediatr Pulmonol 1998;26:256–261.
45. Dodge R, Burrows B, Lebowitz MD, Cline MG: Antecedent features of children in whom asthma develops during the second decade of life. J Allergy Clin Immunol 1993;92:744–749.
46. Droste JHJ, Wieringa MH, Weyler JJ, Nelen VJ, Van Bever HP, Vermeire PA: Lung function measures and their relationship to respiratory symptoms in 7- and 8- year old children. Pediatr Pulmonol 1999;27:260–266.

25 Bronchiolitis

Mary Ellen B. Wohl, MD

Bronchiolitis means inflammation of the bronchioles. In a child younger than 2 years of age, the term is usually applied to a clinical syndrome characterized by rapid respiration, chest retractions, and wheezing.

■ CLINICAL PRESENTATION

Bronchiolitis is one of the major causes for hospital admissions of infants younger than 1 year of age; most commonly, it affects infants between the ages of 2 and 6 months.[1] The infant characteristically presents with a viral infection with mild rhinorrhea, cough, and, on occasion, a low-grade fever. Within 1 or 2 days, these symptoms are followed by the onset of rapid respiration, chest retractions, and wheezing. The infant may show irritability, poor feeding, and vomiting.

On physical examination, the respiratory rate is increased to rates often above 50 or 60 breaths per minute. The pulse rate is increased, and body temperature may be normal or elevated as high as 41°C. Mild conjunctivitis and/or otitis media is observed in many patients and pharyngitis in about 50% of patients.[2,3] Chest retractions are present. Expirations are frequently prolonged, but breath sounds may be normal. Wheezes and crackles may be heard throughout the lungs. Respiratory distress often prevents adequate oral fluid intake and causes dehydration. Although severe abnormalities in gas exchange can develop, cyanosis is detectable in only a minority of infants because of high cardiac outputs and rapid transit times through the capillary bed. Increased respiratory rate is an indicator of impaired gas exchange, and rates of 60 breaths per minute or higher are associated with reduced arterial saturations and elevation of carbon dioxide tensions. The ease of measuring oxygen saturation combined with rapid respiratory rates[4] may have contributed to the threefold increase in hospitalizations observed during the past 18 years.[5] Deaths from bronchiolitis have remained constant, in contrast to the overall decline in death rate for other respiratory diseases.[6,7]

The radiographic manifestations of bronchiolitis are nonspecific and include diffuse hyperinflation of the lungs, flattening of the diaphragm, prominence of the retrosternal space, and bulging of the intercostal spaces[8,9] (Fig. 25-1). Patchy or peribronchial infiltrates suggestive of interstitial pneumonia occur in the majority of infants. Atelectasis is observed in most infants, but consolidation is observed in only 24% of patients. Pleural fluid is rarely observed and, when present, is minimal. Some (13%) infants with illness severe enough to require hospitalization have normal chest roentgenograms.

■ ETIOLOGY

In 1957, Chanock and Finberg isolated respiratory syncytial virus (RSV) from two infants with lower respiratory tract disease.[10] Beem and co-workers in 1960 identified this virus, originally isolated from the chimpanzee and termed *chimpanzee coryza agent*, in 31 of 95 infants younger than 2 years of age with acute lower respiratory tract disease.[11] Subsequently, RSV has been found to be the etiologic agent in the majority of infants with bronchiolitis both in the past and currently.[1,12–18] Human metapneumovirus now accounts for about 8% of infants with bronchiolitis, previously RSV negative.[19] Infections with other viruses, primarily rhinovirus,[20,21] adenovirus, parainfluenza viruses of all types,[22–24] enterovirus, and influenza virus, have been summarized by Hall and Hall.[25]

In the Northern Hemisphere, epidemics of RSV disease occur yearly with some seasonal variation. Adults[26] as well as children are infected, and epidemics have been reported in newborn nurseries. In very young or premature infants, however, the presentation of disease is atypical and has features of severe pneumonia.[27] In general, only infants older than 1 month develop the clinical syndrome of bronchiolitis.[16] In large urban populations, the peak age incidence of RSV bronchiolitis is at 2 months[16]; in more rural settings it often appears later. The incidence of RSV infections is greater in males than females, and severe bronchiolitis is more likely to occur in male infants. Epidemiologic studies of RSV indicate that during an epidemic all ages have high rates of incidence. The lowest rate, 17%, is in adults.[28] High attack rates affect infants in daycare settings. Virtually all children in densely populated urban settings acquire infection by 2 years of age.[13–17] Once the virus is introduced into the family, most often by a school-aged child, 45% of family members acquire infection.[28] Groups at particular risk for infection are infants hospitalized for reasons other than RSV during an RSV epidemic, and hospital staff caring for infants.[29] Among infants hospitalized for 1 week, 45% become infected, and infection is related to the duration of hospitalization. Almost 40% of hospital staff acquire the infection, and these staff appear to be the source of spread. The major modes of transmission appear to be by large airborne particles or by self-inoculation after touching contaminated surfaces.[30] Severe and/or fatal disease may occur in hospitalized infants who acquire RSV infection.

Risk factors for the development of bronchiolitis include low levels of antibodies in cord blood, gender, birth month, absence of or minimal breastfeeding, crowded living conditions, being a twin or triplet, and low socioeconomic status.[31–33]

Two types of RSV exist: group A and group B. In a comparison of 134 infants hospitalized with group A infection and 131 infants hospitalized with group B infection, multivariant analysis indicated that prematurity, underlying medical conditions, group A RSV strains, and age younger than 3 months were independently associated with severe disease, with odds ratios for severe disease being 1.84, 2.84, 3.26, and 4.39, respectively, confirming that group A RSV infection results in greater severity than group B infection among hospitalized infants.[34] Furthermore, among 123 group A RSV isolates there were 5 genotypes and 22 subtypes, while among 81 group B isolates there were 4 genotypes and 6 subtypes. However, one or

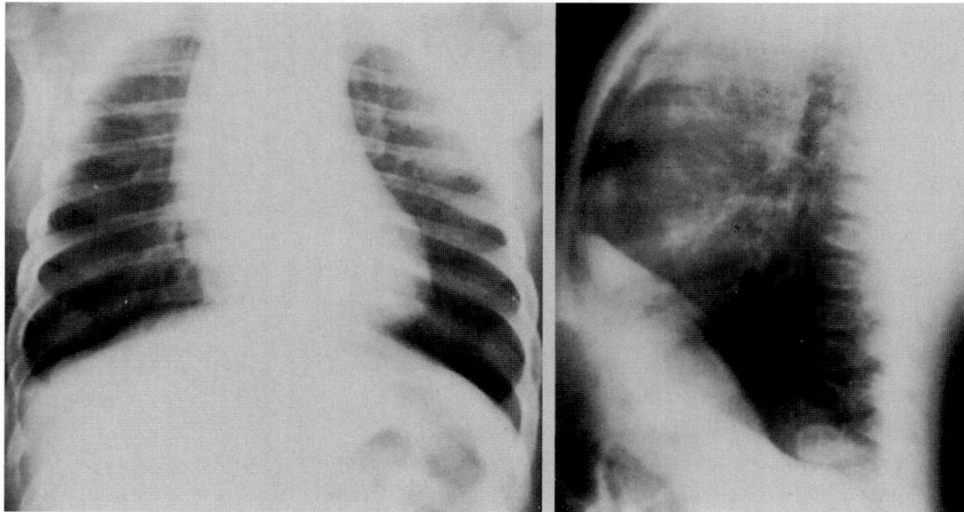

■ **FIGURE 25-1.** Chest radiographs of an infant with the clinical syndrome of acute bronchiolitis.

two genotypes or subtypes accounted for more than 50% of the isolates for a given year, and in no 2 years were these the same genotype or subtype isolated. It appears to be of benefit to the virus to modify its genotype or subtype yearly, suggesting that both group and genotype will be needed to characterize efficacy studies of candidate vaccines and to understand protective immunity after natural infection.[35]

Respiratory syncytial virus continues to be shed from the respiratory tract for an average of 9 days in children younger than 1 year of age. High titers of virus may remain in nasal washings despite clinical improvement.[36] Some infants, particularly those with immunodeficiency syndromes, shed virus for months after infection.[37] Among infants infected with human immunodeficiency virus, RSV is shed for a median of 30 days (range, 1–199 days).[38]

Circulating antibodies of the IgG class develop several days after infection. These are directed against the glycoprotein and fusion component of the viral surface and are protective in nature. Cell-mediated immunity develops and enhances clearing of the virus,[39] and cell-bound and cell-free antibody in nasal secretions help clear viral infection.[40] Experiments with formalin-killed RSV vaccine and subsequent infection with wild-type virus produced a severe disease in vaccinated infants.[41] Subsequent evidence suggests that the enhanced histopathology observed in those infants who died was related to the formalin inactivation of the virus leading to the production of nonfunctional titers of fusion and glycoprotein antibody that did not neutralize the virus.[42] The suggestion that high levels of antibody are associated with worse disease has largely been abandoned following the demonstration that maternal immunoglobulin is protective, that very young (but not premature) infants experience milder disease, and that subsequent infections with RSV tend to be milder than the initial one, all of which support the role of protection from neutralizing antibody.[31]

The innate immune response increases Toll-like receptor 4 expression[43]; macrophage inflammatory protein 1α and monocyte chemotactic protein 1, which are associated with worse disease, are also increased.[44] However, interferon-γ is decreased in nasopharyngeal secretions of infants with RSV infection.[45] Cell-bound immunoglobulin E (IgE) is present in the exfoliated nasopharyngeal epithelial cells of infants, and the persistence of IgE in the respiratory tract may contribute to ongoing wheezing. Virus-specific IgE and immunoglobulin G4 have been detected in infants.[46] Eosinophilic cationic protein has been observed in the serum of patients with RSV bronchiolitis, and levels greater than 8 μg/L are predictive of wheezing at age 5 years.[47]

The size of the infant's airway may contribute to the severity of bronchiolitis. In normal adults, the resistance of peripheral airways has little influence on the distribution of ventilation. This probably is not true for infants. One may speculate that a given amount of cellular debris and edema produces a greater degree of obstruction in an infant's small peripheral airways than in an older child's larger peripheral airways. The absence of effective collateral ventilation in infants contributes to the development of patchy atelectasis and abnormal gas exchange. Smooth muscle exists in the periphery of an infant's lung as it does in the lung of the older child, so the infant's airways may respond to mediator substances if these are released.

■ PATHOLOGY

The initial abnormalities of the lower respiratory tract in RSV bronchiolitis are necrosis of the respiratory epithelium and destruction of ciliated epithelial cells, followed by peribronchiolar infiltration with lymphocytes and neutrophils. The submucosa becomes edematous, but there is no destruction of collagen, muscle, or elastic tissue (Fig. 25-2). Cellular debris and fibrin form plugs within the bronchioles. The alveoli usually are normal, except those immediately adjacent to the inflamed bronchioles. Occasionally, there is more extensive alveolar involvement, and the increased cellularity of the subepithelial tissue of the bronchi and bronchioles extends to distant intra-alveolar walls. In such cases, edema fluid may accumulate within alveoli.[48,49]

In addition to these changes, RSV may cause severe pneumonia with extensive destruction of respiratory epithelium, necrosis of lung parenchyma, and formation of hyaline membranes, similar to the pneumonia that occurs in adenovirus infections.[49]

Recovery from acute bronchiolitis begins with regeneration of the bronchiolar epithelium after 3 or 4 days, but cilia do not

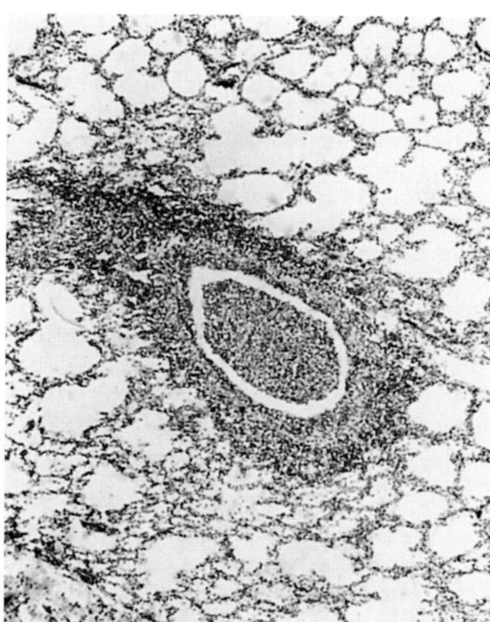

■ **FIGURE 25-2.** Histologic section of a bronchiole from an infant who later died of acute bronchiolitis. The RSV was grown from necropsy specimens. Peribronchiolar lymphoid infiltration and plugging of the lumen with exudate and cell debris can be seen. The surrounding alveoli are little affected. (Courtesy of Dr. W. Aherne.)

appear until much later, probably about 15 days. Mucous plugs are removed by macrophages.[49]

■ PATHOPHYSIOLOGY

As a result of the edema of the airway wall and the accumulation of mucus and cellular debris, many peripheral airways are narrowed, and some are partially and others totally occluded. The patchy distribution and variable degree of obstruction produce atelectasis in some areas of the lung and overdistention in others.

The mechanics of respiration are abnormal. The infant breathes at a high lung volume, and resting end-expiratory lung volume (functional residual capacity) is elevated. Dynamic compliance is decreased, in part because the infant is breathing at higher lung volumes and hence on a stiffer portion of the volume-pressure curve of the lung, and in part because of the uneven distribution of resistances within the lung. The decrease in compliance and increase in resistance result in increased work of breathing.

Serious alterations in gas exchange occur as a result of the airway obstruction and patchy distribution of atelectasis. Arterial hypoxemia develops as the result of mismatching of pulmonary ventilation and perfusion, with continued perfusion of underventilated units and overventilation of underperfused units. Modest increases in inspired oxygen (<40%) usually correct the ventilation-perfusion mismatch. The partial pressure of carbon dioxide in arterial blood is variable. In young infants in particular, some degree of carbon dioxide retention is noted sometime in the course of the disease. The probable mechanisms are severe ventilation-perfusion mismatch and hypoventilation secondary to the markedly increased work of breathing. Blood pH is variable. Some infants show a mild respiratory alkalosis. More commonly, metabolic acidosis is observed. Poor caloric and fluid intake contribute to the ketoacidosis in such infants. Finally, carbon dioxide retention produces acute respiratory acidosis.

■ DIAGNOSIS

New techniques such as real-time polymerase chain reaction and nested polymerase reaction have improved the diagnosis of RSV immeasurably. These techniques have been found to be superior to enzyme immunoabsorbent assays.[50–53] However, the U.S. Food and Drug Administration has as yet approved only enzyme immunoabsorbent assay techniques. As a result of these superior techniques, the diagnosis of multiple viruses contributing to the diagnosis of bronchiolitis has increased. In addition the sensitivities of respiratory virus cultures using culture with R-mix fresh cells is improved, particularly for influenza virus.[54]

The diagnosis of acute viral bronchiolitis is suggested by the clinical presentation, the age of the child, and the presence of an epidemic of RSV in the community. Routine laboratory tests are not specific. Chest roentgenograms, as noted earlier, may be normal or may show peribronchial thickening, patchy atelectasis, segmental collapse, or hyperinflation. The white blood cell count ranges from 5000 to 24,000 cells/mm^3. In patients with elevated white blood cell counts, there is a preponderance of polymorphonuclear leukocytes and band forms. A determination of hemoglobin concentration is not useful diagnostically but is helpful in assessing the effects of decreased oxygen saturation on cardiac output and tissue oxygenation.

Other causes of chest retraction and airway obstruction must be ruled out by careful physical and radiographic examination. These include obstruction of the nasopharynx by hypertrophied adenoids or a retropharyngeal abscess; laryngeal obstruction caused by abnormalities of the larynx, croup, a foreign body, and lobar emphysema. Occasionally, the hyperpnea of metabolic disorders such as salicylate poisoning mimics bronchiolitis. If salicylates have been given, measurements of pH, oxygen saturation, salicylate levels, and serum electrolytes aid in making the proper diagnosis. Congestive heart failure secondary to a congenital malformation or viral myocarditis may manifest clinical findings very similar to those of bronchiolitis, and the palpable liver and spleen found frequently in infants with bronchiolitis may contribute to the confusion. A history of normal growth and development and the absence of a cardiac murmur assist in the diagnosis. Infants with cardiac disease often develop congestive heart failure during viral infections, and the two conditions may coexist. The lung disease of cystic fibrosis may present as acute bronchiolitis.

■ TREATMENT

Mild bronchiolitis is often treated at home. For infants with mild respiratory distress, careful observation and adequate fluid administration are appropriate. Infants with moderate or severe respiratory distress should usually be hospitalized. The aims of hospital treatment are: (1) to support the infant, (2) to detect and treat possible complications, (3) to prevent the spread of infection to other patients and to staff, and (4) to treat with specific antiviral agents if indicated. Controversies in the treatment of bronchiolitis concern: (1) the use of bronchodilators, (2) the use of corticosteroids, (3) the use of antiviral agents, and (4) unfortunately, the use of antibiotics.

Supportive care for hospitalized infants with bronchiolitis includes the administration of oxygen and the appropriate fluids; careful monitoring to detect hypoxemia, apnea, and respiratory failure; and attention to temperature regulation.

The major consequence of the airway obstruction and the concomitant poor distribution of ventilation and perfusion is hypoxemia. Humidified oxygen should be administered to infants with all but the mildest illnesses. Any technique familiar to nursing personnel may be used, provided the oxygen is humidified and the flow rate of gas through the device is sufficient to prevent accumulation of carbon dioxide. The inspired oxygen concentration should be monitored frequently. Concentrations of 35% to 40% have been found to correct the arterial hypoxemia in most infants. In infants with no history of chronic obstructive pulmonary disease, oxygen can be safely administered without fear of significantly depressing respiration by blunting the hypoxic drive. However, a growing number of infants of very low birth weight are surviving respiratory distress syndrome of the newborn to be left with bronchopulmonary dysplasia of variable severity and higher mortality rates. Acute viral bronchiolitis presents special problems to those infants with chronic compensated carbon dioxide retention. Further impairment of gas exchange may make them severely hypoxemic. The administration of increased concentrations of inspired oxygen may be associated with additional carbon dioxide retention, because hypoxemia can be their major respiratory stimulus. Frequent measurement of oxygen saturation by pulse oximeter is required in these patients, and the minimum inspired concentrations consistent with an arterial saturation of 92% to 94% should be delivered. Care should be taken to measure saturations while the infant is quiet, because decreases in oxygen saturations can occur when an infant cries, for example. Unnecessarily high levels of inspired oxygen will be delivered if the goal is to prevent any episode of desaturation, however brief. Carbon dioxide retention should be monitored by periodic assessment of arterial blood gas tensions and serum bicarbonate. It should be noted that in patients with chronic carbon dioxide and bicarbonate retention, a decrease in the hypoxic drive associated with administration of oxygen usually produces additional carbon dioxide retention. This retention is to be expected and need not reflect worsening of the underlying disease.

With fever, chilling, or shivering, oxygen consumption is increased. Small infants should be nursed in incubators or under radiant warmers; care should be taken that temperature is controlled in oxygen tents or other devices used for the administration of oxygen.

The complications of RSV infection include apnea,[55] which appears to be the result of RSV G glycoprotein-CX3CR1 interacting with substance P depressing respiratory rates,[56] inappropriate antidiuretic secretion,[57,58] electrolyte abnormalities (which can present as seizures),[59] encephalopathy occurring in 1.8% of patients and usually presenting as seizures,[60] atrial tachycardias,[61] and respiratory failure requiring intubation and ventilation.

Because RSV causes extensive morbidity in infants with cardiac disease,[62] in children with compromised immunofunction,[63] and in neonates,[64] the spread of RSV infection must be minimized. RSV is shed in high titers for days after the onset of illness,[36] and hospital-acquired infections are common.[65–67] Therefore, careful attention must be directed to the prevention of transmission of infection both to other patients and to staff. Limitation of child-to-child contact, cohorting of patients, and careful hand washing are useful methods to limit nosocomial spread of RSV, but the most practical measure may be glove-and-gown precautions applied to all infants with suspected viral bronchiolitis.[68]

On admission to the hospital, some infants are not only dehydrated because of poor fluid intake but also have mild metabolic acidosis. Intravenous fluids should be given with care. It may be speculated that the presence of the large negative intrapleural pressures required to overcome the airway obstruction adds demands on the left ventricle. Furthermore, the negative intrathoracic pressures are probably transmitted to the interstitium surrounding the fluid-exchanging vessels, enhancing fluid accumulation in the lung. The uneven distribution of the airway obstruction amplifies these negative pressures, further enhancing fluid accumulation. The details of these mechanisms are discussed in Chapter 43.

The role of bronchodilators is controversial. The relative importance of mechanical obstruction secondary to edema, accumulated secretions, and cellular debris and potentially reversible smooth muscle contraction are unknown. Revival of interest in measurements of mechanics of respiration in infants has led to several studies evaluating the use of nebulized and inhaled sympathomimetic agents such as albuterol. Results for albuterol are either negative[69] or inconclusive,[70] and continuing the inpatient and outpatient therapy after documentation of no response serves only to increase the utilization of hospital resources and to increase costs.[71] Some well-designed controlled studies that have evaluated oxygen saturation following racemic epinephrine[72–75] demonstrate that racemic epinephrine produced greater improvement in oxygen saturation, clinical score, and/or pulmonary resistance than either saline or albuterol. However, other studies demonstrated no significant reduction in admission rates or changes in oxygen saturation,[76] and a recently reported randomized clinical trial of epinephrine versus placebo demonstrated no change in length of hospital stay or time to discharge.[77] However, these outcome measures may not be the most relevant to the baby's comfort.

Initial studies of the treatment of bronchiolitis with corticosteroids suggested that these drugs might favorably influence mortality and morbidity. However, large controlled studies have failed to demonstrate any significant clinical effect.[78–82] In particular, the response to corticosteroids in infants with a family history of allergy differed not at all from the response in infants without such a history. A relatively current meta-analysis does demonstrate a mean length of stay and duration of symptoms reduced by 0.43 days and a 1.60 clinical score reduction.[83] The use of oral dexamethasone at a single dose of 1 mg/kg demonstrated a reduction in respiratory assessment score and a reduction in hospitalizations.[84] A study using inhaled nebulized budesonide for 6 weeks failed to reduce the symptoms of acute bronchiolitis and failed to prevent postbronchiolitic wheezing.[85] A controlled trial of dexamethasone did not reduce the tracheal load of virus but did reduce the levels of interleukin-8 in the tracheal secretions without having any influence on white cell count.[86]

Ribavirin, a synthetic nucleoside analog resembling guanosine, has been shown to have a broad antiviral effect, probably by inhibiting viral protein synthesis. Delivered as a small-particle aerosol for 18 to 20 hours per day, it led to improvement in oxygenation and clinical state.[87–89] The American Academy of Pediatrics has revised its recommendations for treatment from "should be used" to "may be considered" in infants at high risk for severe disease such as those with complicated heart disease, including pulmonary hypertension; those with bronchopulmonary dysplasia or chronic pulmonary infection such as cystic fibrosis; those with underlying immunosuppressive diseases or therapy (those with acquired immunodeficiency syndrome, severe combined immunodeficiency disease, and organ transplantation); those infants who are severely ill with or without mechanical ventilation, or who are hypoxemic with increasing levels of carbon dioxide retention and poorly responsive to other therapies; and those hospitalized patients who are at increased risk of progressing from a mild to a more complicated course because they are younger than 6 weeks of age or have an underlying condition such as multiple congenital anomalies or certain neurologic or metabolic diseases.[90]

The routine administration of antibiotics has not been shown to influence the course of bronchiolitis,[91,92] and there is little rationale for their use. Lack of rapid diagnostic techniques to identify RSV or other viruses, the uncertainty about the cause of the disease in small, acutely ill infants, and the concern that viral infection may predispose to secondary bacterial invasion are arguments used to justify the administration of antibiotics. In children in whom a viral cause is established, who present with clinical features consistent with viral infection, including otitis media and segmental atelectasis, both common features of RSV infection, treatment with antibiotics is not recommended. A study of children younger than 2 years of age who were hospitalized with RSV lower respiratory infection reports that those children given parenteral antibiotics for 5 days or longer had a 9% incidence of secondary bacterial infection, in contrast to the overall incidence of 0.6% in those given no antibiotics at all.[92] The diversity of bacterial organisms reported in association with viral lower respiratory tract disease[92] makes it important that those infants who develop fever, elevated or shifted peripheral white blood cell counts, or clinical features suggesting sepsis should have bacterial cultures of blood, urine, and cerebrospinal fluid.

Other therapies have been reported as beneficial. All components of the surfactant system are involved during severe RSV infection, and therapy with surfactant has thus been suggested in infants who are severely ill.[93–95] Since helium increases the viscosity in distal airways, there is little evidence to support the administration of helium-oxygen mixtures, nor do such mixtures improve gas exchange in mechanically ventilated infants with bronchiolitis.[96]

■ PREVENTION

The prevention of RSV infection has been accelerated in recent years by the trials of RSV immune globulin administered intravenously monthly in doses of 750 mg to high-risk infants and of intramuscular palivizumab, a humanized respiratory monoclonal antibody that has demonstrated considerable efficacy in preventing the hospitalization of high-risk infants.[97] It is known commercially as Synagis, is administered IM at a dose of 15 mg/kg, and is distributed in 100-mg lyophilized vials.

Considerable work has been done to develop a viral vaccine. Estimated levels of protective antibody have been assessed,[98] but no effective vaccine for RSV has been developed.[99]

■ COURSE AND COMPLICATIONS

Although they may appear extremely ill on admission to the hospital, most infants with bronchiolitis, given adequate supportive care, are clinically improved within 3 or 4 days. By 2 weeks after the height of the illness, the respiratory rate is normal, and oxygen saturation and carbon dioxide tensions are within the normal range in most infants.

The major indications for intubation and mechanical ventilation are clinical deterioration (worsening respiratory distress, heart rates over 200 beats per minute, listlessness, and poor peripheral perfusion), apnea and/or bradycardia, and hypercarbia. Infants do not usually require intubation for oxygenation alone. The median duration of mechanical ventilation is relatively short, about 5 days more or less, but protracted courses of ventilation may be required.

■ RELATIONSHIP TO ASTHMA

Respiratory syncytial virus infection and its relationship to asthma appears to be well established, but the relationship is not clear. RSV lower respiratory tract illness is associated with an increased risk of frequent wheeze at age 6 years, but the risk decreases markedly with increasing age and is not significant at age 13 years.[100] There is no association with markers of atopy.[100] Lung function in the children who wheezed at age 6 was reduced at age 13 but reversed to normal when treated with salbutamol.[100] Lung function measured as maximum flow at functional residual capacity is depressed and symptoms of cough and wheeze are increased in infants who subsequently develop bronchiolitis, but there is no increase in airway responsiveness.[101] Martinez and co-workers[102,103] have explored initial lung function and its relationship to asthma. They found that 51% of children never wheezed, 20% had had at least one lower respiratory tract infection with wheezing during the first 3 years, 15% had wheezing at age 6 years, and 14% had wheezing at both ages 3 and 6. Twenty percent had lower levels of maximum expiratory flow at functional residual capacity both before 1 year and at age 6 and were more likely to have mothers who smoked. The 15% who had wheezing at age 6 and the 14% who wheezed at both 3 and 6—29% overall—had mothers who were more likely to have asthma and to have elevated serum IgE levels.[103]

■ LONG-TERM SEQUELAE

In some infants, lung function studies remain abnormal for months after the occurrence of bronchiolitis. However, until recently it was believed that no residual effects of the disease persist into late childhood except for a greater than expected incidence of asthma. Two studies now document that infants hospitalized with bronchiolitis and/or RSV infection continue to demonstrate abnormalities in lung function.[104,105] As a group, these children, when seen at 8 to 11 years and compared with control children, have experienced more frequent episodes of wheezing, demonstrate increased bronchial hyperreactivity, and have small but significant alterations in measurements of lung function. Lung function abnormalities are present even in those children who had no further episodes of wheezing. These abnormalities are not accompanied by skin test evidence of atopy. These studies have not been able to determine whether the bronchiolitis or RSV infection was responsible for the subsequent abnormalities. It may be that both hospitalizations for bronchiolitis and the subsequent abnormalities in lung function are manifestations of individual differences in airway reactivity, function, or size.[102] An excellent review of the relationship between RSV bronchiolitis and future obstructive airway diseases has recently been published.[106]

■ BRONCHIOLITIS OBLITERANS

Bronchiolitis obliterans, a chronic form of bronchiolitis first described in 1901 by Lange,[107] has been reported following inhalation of hydrochloric or nitric acids, and of sulfur dioxide, as well as in association with lupus erythematosus, rheumatoid arthritis, lung transplantation, heart-lung transplantation, bone marrow transplant (graft-versus-host disease), and severe infection, which is the subject of this section.

Severe bronchiolitis in particular is often observed following type 3 adenoviral infections,[108,109] type 7 adenoviral infections,[110,111] and type 21 adenoviral infections,[111,112] and the sequelae of these infections are often termed *bronchiolitis obliterans.* These adenovirus infections have been observed in native (Native American, Eskimo, Métis) children in Canada and in native (Maori) children in New Zealand and the South Pacific Islands. Bronchiolitis obliterans following Stevens-Johnson syndrome has been reported in two children and a young adult.[113,114] Sixty-five percent of the patients with pneumonia related to type 7 adenovirus and only 10% of the controls (patients with adenovirus type 7 upper respiratory tract infections) developed evidence of airways obstruction. Young age at the time of pneumonia and a "measles-like" illness is sometimes reported in adenovirus type 7 pneumonia and is associated with longer hospitalizations and more severe obstructive disease demonstrated both by reductions in forced expiratory volume in 1 second and maximum mid-expiratory flow rate.[110] In additional to adenovirus infections, influenza[115] and *Mycoplasma pneumoniae*[116] organisms cause bronchiolitis obliterans.

The presentation of infants and children with bronchiolitis obliterans does not differ from that of acute bronchiolitis caused by RSV, except that rhinorrhea is not a prominent feature and evidence for bronchopneumonia is more common. The infant becomes ill with cough and fever and subsequently develops dyspnea and wheezing. On physical examination, wheezes and crackles are heard. The radiographic features consist of peribronchial thickening and increased interstitial markings with areas of patchy bronchopneumonia. Collapse and consolidation of segments or lobes are common. The clinical and radiographic features of bronchiolitis obliterans wax and wane for several weeks or months. There are recurrent episodes of atelectasis, pneumonia, and wheezing. Recovery is not complete, and more than 60% of children with adenoviral pneumonia eventually develop chronic lung disease. Persistent atelectasis (of the right upper lobe in young children and of the left lower lobe in older children), bronchiectasis, recurrent pneumonias, generalized hyperinflation, increased pulmonary markings on chest radiographs, and development of the unilateral hyperlucent lung syndrome are among the reported long-term complications of adenovirus infection, particularly types 7 and 21.

Little is known about host factors that predispose to this unusual form of bronchiolitis. Maternal antibody may be protective, because the disease characteristically occurs in infants older than 6 months. In Canada it is seen more frequently in the Native American population, and in New Zealand in Polynesian children, suggesting that racial or socioeconomic variables may be important. No infectious agent has been clearly implicated in the bronchiolitis obliterans associated with bone marrow transplantation (graft-versus-host disease), heart-lung transplantation, and lung transplantation.

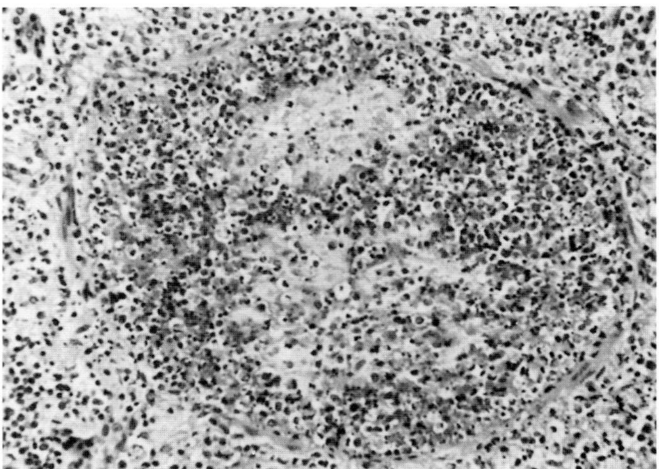

■ **FIGURE 25-3.** Necrotizing adenovirus bronchiolitis. The epithelial lining has been completely destroyed, and the lumen is filled with cellular debris. The smooth muscle is still largely intact. Adenovirus type 3 was recovered in tissue culture. (Original magnification ×240; courtesy of Dr. J. Hoogstraten.) (From Wohl ME, Chernick V: Bronchiolitis. Am Rev Respir Dis 1978;118:759.)

In lungs examined histologically, the abnormalities of large- and medium-sized bronchi may simply be hypertrophy and piling up of the bronchial epithelium. However, cellular infiltration of the wall extending to the peribronchial space, destruction and disorganization of the muscle and elastic tissue of the wall, and fibrosis of the wall and surrounding areas occur in the more severely affected. The most striking changes occur in the small bronchi and bronchioles; it is here that the mucosa is destroyed and the lumen is filled with fibrous tissue (Figs. 25-3 and 25-4). Typically, the terminal bronchioles are occluded and the distal respiratory bronchioles are dilated. The vessels are narrowed, and areas of overdistention,

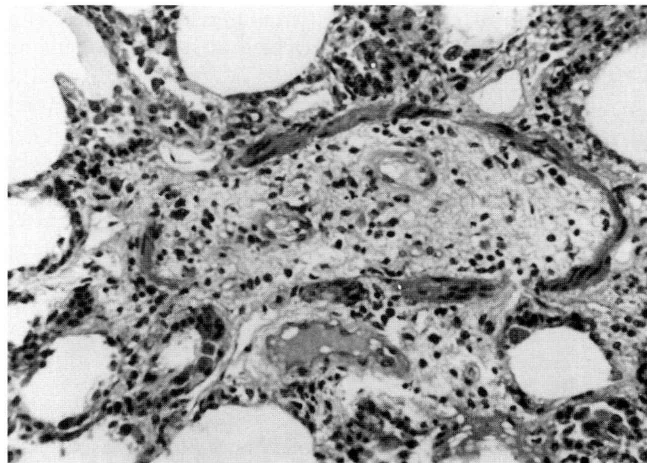

■ **FIGURE 25-4.** Obliterative bronchiolitis in a 1.5-year-old child who had had severe adenovirus bronchiolitis and pneumonia 1 year previously. The obliterated lumen of the bronchiole is filled with vascularized connective tissue. (Original magnification ×240; courtesy of Dr. J Hoogstraten.) (From Wohl ME, Chernick V: Bronchiolitis. Am Rev Respir Dis 1978;118:759.)

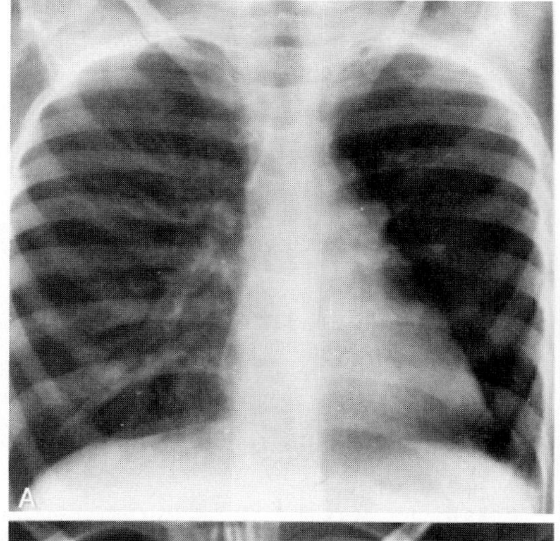

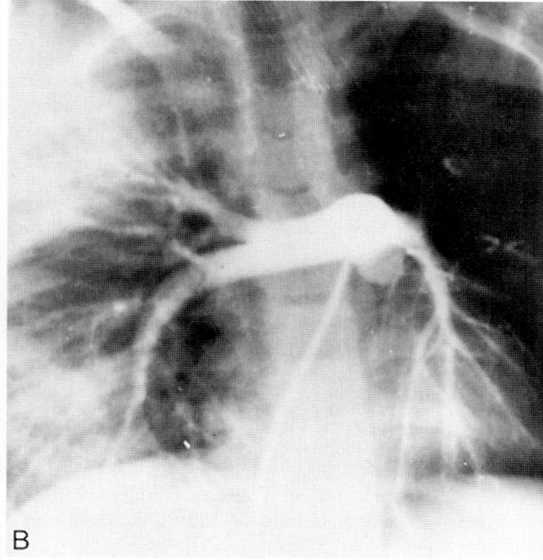

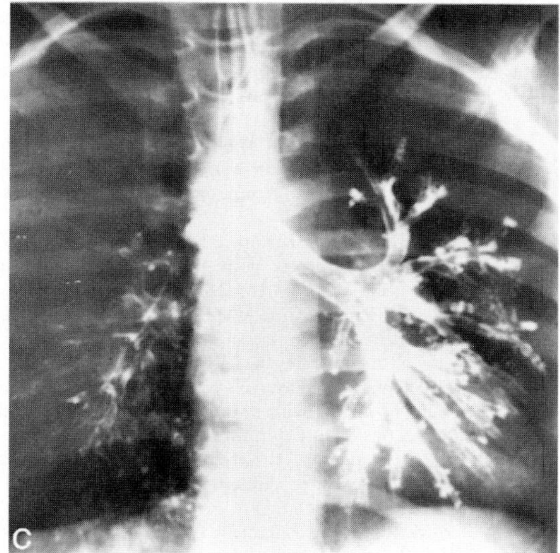

■ **FIGURE 25-5.** Left unilateral hyperlucent lung in a 4-year-old child secondary to adenovirus infection in early infancy. **A,** Plain chest film shows increased radiolucency of the left lung due to decreased bronchovascular markings. **B,** Decreased blood flow to the left lung is evident on the pulmonary angiogram. **C,** Bronchogram demonstrates a typical "pruned-tree" appearance. (From Wohl ME, Chernick V: Bronchiolitis. Am Rev Respir Dis 1978;118:759.)

atelectasis, and fibrosis occur within the alveolar region of the lung.

Bronchograms reveal marked pruning of the bronchial tree, and pulmonary angiograms reveal decreased vasculature in the involved lung (Fig. 25-5). These findings may be localized, as in those children who develop unilateral hyperlucent lung syndrome, or may be more diffuse. Similar sequelae, either diffuse or localized as described by Swyer and James,[117] have also been observed after other infections, including those involving influenza[115] and *Mycoplasma*.[116] These sequelae should be considered in the diagnostic evaluation of children who develop recurrent infections and fixed airway obstruction after what may be presumed to be severe viral bronchiolitis and pneumonia. However, there are few data to support the association of bronchiolitis obliterans with RSV infections, and bronchiolitis obliterans should not be considered a complication of RSV bronchiolitis.

The incidence of bronchiolitis obliterans in the pediatric population is not known. Patients who have persistent wheezing and cough following viral or *Mycoplasma* pneumonia, who have persistent localized physical findings after a respiratory insult, or who develop or are found to have unilateral or patchy regions of hyperlucency on chest radiographs should be considered for further investigation including ventilation-perfusion scans, bronchoscopy, computer tomographic scans of the chest, and lung biopsy. As this process is better understood and the clinical features better defined, therapeutic interventions may develop.

REFERENCES

1. Henderson FW, Clyde WA, Collier AM et al: The etiologic and epidemiologic spectrum of bronchiolitis in pediatric practice. J Pediatr 1979;95:183–190.
2. Reilly CM, Stokes J, McClelland L, et al: Studies of acute respiratory illnesses caused by respiratory syncytial virus. 3. Clinical and laboratory findings. N Engl J Med 1961;264:1176–1182.
3. Gardner PS: Respiratory syncytial virus infections. Postgrad Med J 1973; 49:788–791.
4. Mallory MD, Shay DK, Garret J, Bordley WC: Bronchiolitis management preferences and the influence of pulse oximetry and respiratory rate on the decision to admit. Pediatrics 2003;111:e45–e51.
5. Shay DK, Holman RC, Newman RD, et al: Bronchiolitis-associated hospitalizations among US children, 1980–1996. JAMA 1999;282:1440–1446.
6. Shay DK, Holman RC, Roosevelt GE, et al: Bronchiolitis-associated mortality and estimates of respiratory syncytial virus–associated deaths among US children, 1979–1997. J Infect Dis 2001;183:16–22.

7. Holman RC, Shay DK, Curns AT, et al: Risk factors for bronchiolitis-associated deaths among infants in the United States. Pediatr Infect Dis J 2002;22:483–490.
8. Simpson W, Hacking PM, Court SDM, Gardner PS: The radiological findings in respiratory syncytial virus infection in children. I. Definitions and interobserver variation in the assessment of abnormalities on the chest x-ray. Pediatr Radiol 1974;2:97–100.
9. Simpson W, Hacking PM, Court SDM, Gardner PS: The radiological findings in respiratory syncytial virus infection in children. II. The correlation of radiological categories with clinical and virological findings. Pediatr Radiol 1974;2:155–160.
10. Chanock R, Finberg L: Recovery from infants with respiratory illness of a virus related to chimpanzee coryza agent (CCA). II. Epidemiologic aspects of infection in infants and young children. Am J Hyg 1957;66:291–300.
11. Beem W, Wright FH, Hamre D, et al: Association of the chimpanzee coryza agent with acute respiratory disease in children. N Engl J Med 1960;263: 523–530.
12. Gardner PS, McQuillin J: Application of immunofluorescent antibody technique in rapid diagnosis of respiratory syncytial virus infection. BMJ 1968;3:340–343.
13. McClelland L, Hilleman MR, Hamparian VV, et al: Studies of acute respiratory illnesses caused by respiratory syncytial virus. 2. Epidemiology and assessment of importance. N Engl J Med 1961;264:1169–1176.
14. Brandt CD, Kim HW, Arrobio JO, et al: Epidemiology of respiratory syncytial virus infection in Washington, D.C. III. Composite analysis of eleven consecutive yearly epidemics. Am J Epidemiol 1973;98:355–364.
15. Kim HW, Arrobio JO, Brandt CD, et al: Epidemiology of respiratory syncytial virus infection in Washington, D.C. I. Importance of the virus in different respiratory tract disease syndromes and temporal distribution of infection. Am J Epidemiol 1973;98:216–225.
16. Parrott RH, Kim HW, Arrobio JO, et al: Epidemiology of respiratory syncytial virus infection in Washington, D.C. II. Infection and disease with respect to age, immunologic status, race and sex. Am J Epidemiol 1973; 98:289–300.
17. Glezen WP, Denny FW: Epidemiology of acute lower respiratory disease in children. N Engl J Med 1973;288:498–505.
18. McIntosh K: Pathogenesis of severe acute respiratory infection in the developing world. Respiratory syncytial virus and parainfluenza viruses. Rev Infect Dis 1991;13:S492–S500.
19. Williams JV, Harris PA, Tollefson SJ, et al: Human metapneumovirus and lower respiratory tract disease in otherwise healthy infants and children. N Engl J Med 2004;350:443–450.
20. Valenti WM, Clarke TA, Hall CB, et al: Concurrent outbreaks of rhinovirus and respiratory syncytial virus in an intensive care nursery. Epidemiologic and associated risk factors. J Pediatr 1982;100:722–725.
21. Papadopoulos NG, Moustake M, Tsolia M, et al: Association of rhinovirus infection with increased disease severity in acute bronchiolitis. Am J Respir Crit Care Med 2002;165:1285–1289.
22. Welliver RC, Wong DT, Sun M, McCarthy N: Parainfluenza virus bronchiolitis epidemiology and pathogenesis. Am J Dis Child 1986; 140:34–40.
23. Rubin EE, Quennec P, McDonald JC: Infections due to parainfluenza virus type 4 in children. Clin Infect Dis 1993;17:998–1002.
24. Knott AM, Long CE, Hall CB: Parainfluenza viral infections in pediatric outpatients. Seasonal patterns and clinical characteristics. Pediatr Infect Dis 1994;175:814–820.
25. Hall CB, Hall WJ: Bronchiolitis. In: Mandell GL, Bennett JE, Dolin R, eds: Principles and Practice of Infectious Diseases, 4th ed. New York: Churchill Livingstone, 1995, pp 612–619.
26. Hashem M, Hall CB: Respiratory syncytial virus in healthy adults. The cost of a cold. J Clin Virol 2003;27:14–21.
27. Hall CB, Kopelman AE, Douglas RG Jr, et al: Neonatal respiratory syncytial virus infection. N Engl J Med 1979;300:393–396,
28. Hall CB, Geiman JM, Biggar R, et al: Respiratory syncytial virus infections within families. N Engl J Med 1976;294:414–419.
29. Hall CB, Douglas RG, Geiman JM, Messner MK: Nosocomial respiratory syncytial virus infections. N Engl J Med 1975;293:1343–1346.
30. Hall CB, Douglas RG Jr, Schnabel KC, Geiman JM: Infectivity of respiratory syncytial virus by various routes of inoculation. Infect Immun 1981;33:779–783.
31. Glezen WP, Paredes A, Allison JE, et al: Risk of respiratory syncytial virus infections for infants from low-income families in relationship to age, sex, ethnic group and maternal antibody level. J Pediatr 1981;98: 708–715.
32. Spencer N, Logan S, Scholey S, Gentle S: Deprivation and bronchiolitis. Arch Dis Child 1996;74:50–52.
33. Jansson L, Nilsson, P, Olsson M: Socioeconomic environmental factors and hospitalization for acute bronchiolitis during infancy. Acta Paediatr 2002;91:335–338.
34. Walsh EE, McConnochie KM, Long CE, Hall CB: Severity of respiratory syncytial virus infection is related to virus strain. J Infect Dis 1997;175: 814–820.
35. Peret TC, Hall CB, Schnabel KC, et al: Circulation patterns of genetically distinct group A and B strains of human respiratory syncytial virus in a community. J Gen Virol 1998;79:2221–2229.
36. Hall CB, Douglas RG Jr, Geiman JM: Respiratory syncytial virus infections in infants. Quantitation and duration of shedding. J Pediatr 1979; 89:11–15.
37. Fishaut M, Tubergen D, McIntosh K: Cellular response to respiratory viruses with particular reference to children with disorders of cell-mediated immunity. J Pediatr 1980;96:179–186.
38. King JC Jr, Burke AR, Clemens JD, et al: Respiratory syncytial virus illnesses in human immunodeficiency virus-and noninfected children. Pediatr Infect Dis 1993;12:733–739.
39. McIntosh K, Masters HB, Orr I: The immunologic response to infection with respiratory syncytial virus in infants. J Infect Dis 1978; 138:24–32.
40. McIntosh K, McQuillin J, Gardner PS: Cell-free and cell-bound antibodies in nasal secretions from infants with respiratory virus infections. Infect Immun 1979;151:276–281.
41. Chanock RM, Parrott RH, Kapikian AZ, et al: Possible role of immunologic factors in pathogenesis of RS virus lower respiratory tract disease. Perspect Virol 1968;6:125–139.
42. Murphy BR, Prince GA, Walsh EE, et al: Dissociation between serum neutralizing and glycoprotein antibody responses of infants and children who received inactivated respiratory syncytial virus vaccine. J Clin Microbiol 1986;24:197–202.
43. Gagro A, Tominac M, Krsulovic-Hresic V, et al: Increased Toll-like receptor 4 expression in infants with respiratory syncytial virus bronchiolitis. Clin Exp Immunol 2004;135:267–272.
44. Garofalo RP, Patti J, Hintz KA, et al: Macrophage inflammatory protein-1· (not T helper type 2 cytokines) is associated with severe forms of respiratory syncytial virus bronchiolitis. J Infect Dis 2001;184:393–399.
45. Joshi P, Shaw A, Kakakios A, Isaacs D: Interferon-γ levels in nasopharyngeal secretions of infants with respiratory syncytial virus and other respiratory viral infections. Clin Exp Immunol 2003;131:143–147.
46. Bui RHD, Molinaro GA, Kettering JD, et al: Virus-specific IgE and IgG4 antibodies in serum of children with respiratory syncytial virus. J Pediatr 1987;110:87–90.
47. Pifferi M, Ragazzo V, Caramella D, Baldini G: Eosinophil cationic protein in infants with respiratory syncytial virus bronchiolitis. Predictive value for subsequent wheezing. Pediatr Pulmonol 2001;31:419–424.
48. Aherne W, Bird T, Court SDM, et al: Pathological changes in virus infections of the lower respiratory tract in children. J Clin Pathol 1970; 23:7–18.
49. McLean KH: The pathology of acute bronchiolitis—a study of its evolution. I. The exudative phase. Australas Ann Med 1956;5:254–267.
50. Ong GM, Wyatt DE, O'Neill HJ, et al: A comparison of nested polymerase chain reaction and immunofluorescence for the diagnosis of respiratory in children with bronchiolitis. J Hosp Infect 2001;49:122–128.
51. Boivin G, Cote S, Dery P, et al: Multiplex real-time PCR assay for detection of influenza and human respiratory syncytial viruses. J Clin Microbiol 2004;42:45–51.
52. Whiley DM, Syrmis MW, Mackay IM, Sloots TP: Detection of human respiratory syncytial virus in respiratory samples by LightCycler reverse transcriptase PCR. J Clin Microbiol 2002;40:4418–4422.
53. Gueudin M, Vabret A, Petitjean J, et al: Quantitation of respiratory syncytial virus RNA in nasal aspirates of children by real-time RT-PCR assay. J Virol Methods 2003;109:39–45.
54. Dunn JJ, Woolstenhulme RD, Langer J, Carroll KC: Sensitivity of virus culture when screening with R-mix fresh cells. J Clin Microbiol 2004; 42:79–82.
55. Bruhn FW, Mokrohisky ST, McIntosh K: Apnea associated with respiratory syncytial virus infection in young infants. Pediatrics 1977;90:382–386.
56. Tripp RA, Dakhama A, Jones LP, et al: The G glycoprotein of respiratory syncytial virus depresses respiratory rates through the CX3C motif and substance P. J Virol 2003;77:6580–6584.
57. Gozal D, Colin AA, Jaffe M, et al: Water, electrolyte and endocrine homeostasis in infants with bronchiolitis. Pediatr Res 1990;27:204–209.
58. van Steensel-Moll HA, Hazelzet JA, van der Voort E et al: Excessive secretion of antidiuretic hormone in infections with respiratory syncytial virus. Arch Dis Child 1990;65:1237–1239.

59. Hanna S, Tibby SM, Durward A, Murdoch IA: Incidence of hyponatremia and hyponatraemic seizures in severe respiratory syncytial virus bronchiolitis. Acta Paediatr 2003;92:430–434.
60. Ng YT, Cox C, Atkins J, Butler IJ: Encephalopathy associated with respiratory syncytial virus bronchiolitis. J Child Neurol 2001;16:105–108.
61. Donnerstein RL, Berg RA, Shehab Z, et al: Complex atrial tachycardias and respiratory syncytial virus infections in infants. J Pediatr 1994;125:23–28.
62. MacDonald NE, Hall CB, Suffin SC, et al: Respiratory syncytial virus infections in infants with congenital heart disease. N Engl J Med 1982;307:397–400.
63. Hall CB, Powell KR, MacDonald NE, et al: Respiratory syncytial viral infection in children with compromised immune function. N Engl J Med 1986;315:77–81.
64. Hall CB, Kopelman AE, Douglas RG Jr, et al: Neonatal respiratory syncytial virus infection. N Engl J Med 1979;300:393–396.
65. Hall CB, Douglas RG, Jr, Geiman JM, Messner MK: Nosocomial respiratory syncytial virus infection. N Engl J Med 1975;1343–1346.
66. Hall CB, Geiman JM, Douglas RG Jr, Meager MP: Control of nosocomial respiratory syncytial viral infections. Pediatrics 1978;62:728–732.
67. Isaacs D, Dickson H, O'Callaghan C, et al: Handwashing and cohorting in prevention of hospital acquired infection with respiratory syncytial virus. Arch Dis Child 1991;66:227–231.
68. Leclair JM, Freeman J, Sullivan BF, et al: Prevention of nosocomial respiratory syncytial viral infections through compliance with glove and gown isolation precautions. N Engl J Med 1987;317:329–334.
69. Dobson JV, Stephens-Groff SM, McMahon SR, et al: The use of albuterol in hospitalized infants with bronchiolitis. Pediatrics 1998;101:361–368.
70. Flores G, Horwitz RI: Efficacy of beta 2 agonists in bronchiolitis. A reappraisal and meta-analysis. Pediatrics 1997;100:233–239.
71. Lugo RA, Sallyer JW, Dean JM: Albuterol in acute broncholitis—continued therapy despite poor response? Pharmacotherapy 1998;18:198–202.
72. Krisjasansson S, Carlsen KCL, Wennergren G, et al: Nebulised racemic adrenaline in the treatment of acute bronchiolitis in infants and toddlers. Arch Dis Child 1993;69:650–654.
73. Sanchez I, De Koster J, Powell RE, et al: Effect of racemic epinephrine and salbutamol on clinical score and pulmonary mechanics in infants with bronchiolitis. J Pediatr 1993;122:145–151.
74. Reijonen T, Korppi M, Pitkakangas S, et al: The clinical efficacy of nebulized racemic epinephrine and albuterol in acute bronchiolitis. Arch Pediatr Adoles Med 1995;149:686–692.
75. Menon K, Sutcliffe T, Klassen TP: A randomized trial comparing the efficacy of epinephrine with salbutamol in the treatment of acute bronchiolitis. J Pediatr 1995;126:1004–1007.
76. Hariprakash S, Alexander J, Carroll W, et al: Randomized controlled trial of nebulized adrenaline in acute bronchiolitis. Pediatr Allergy Immunol 2003;14:134–139.
77. Wainwright C, Altamirano L, Cheney M, et al: A multicenter, randomized, double-blind controlled trial of nebulized epinephrine in infants with acute bronchilitis. N Engl J Med 2003;349:27–35.
78. Leer JA, Green JL, Heimlich EM, et al: Corticosteroid treatment of bronchiolitis. A controlled collaborative study in 297 infants and children. Am J Dis Child 1969;117:495–503.
79. Connolly JH, Field MB, Glasgow JF, et al: A double-blind trial of prednisone in epidemic bronchiolitis due to respiratory syncytial virus. Acta Pediatr Scand 1969;58:116–120.
80. Springer C, Bar-Yishay E, Uwayyed K, et al: Corticosteroids do not affect the clinical or physiological status of infants with bronchiolitis. Pediatr Pulmonol 1990;9:181–185.
81. Roosevelt G, Sheehan K, Grupp-Phelan J, et al: Dexamethasone in bronchiolitis. A randomized, controlled trial. Lancet 1996;348:292–295.
82. Klassen T, Sutcliffe T, Watters L, et al: Dexamethasone in albuterol-treated inpatients with acute bronchiolitis. A randomized, controlled trial. J Pediatr 1997;130:191–197.
83. Garrison MM, Christakis DA, Harvey E, et al: Systemic corticosteroids in infant bronchiolitis. A meta-analysis. Pediatrics 2000;105:1–6.
84. Schuh S, Coates AL, Binnie R, et al: Efficacy of oral dexamethasone in outpatients with acute bronchiolitis. J Pediatr 2002;140:27–32.
85. Richter H, Seddon P: Early budesonide in the treatment of bronchiolitis and the prevention of postbronchiolitic wheezing. J Pediatr 1998;132:849–853.
86. van Woensel JB, Lutter R, Biezeveld MH, et al: Effect of dexamethasone on tracheal viral load and interleukin-8 tracheal concentrations in children with respiratory syncytial infections. Pediatr Infect Dis J 2003;22:721–726.
87. Hall CB, McBride JT, Walsh EE, et al: Aerosolized ribavirin treatment of infants with respiratory syncytial viral infection. N Engl J Med 1983;308:1443–1447.
88. Smith DW, Frankel LR, Mathers LH, et al: A controlled trial of aerosolized ribavirin in infants receiving mechanical ventilation. N Engl J Med 1991;325:24–29.
89. Hall CB, McBride JT, Gala CL, et al: Ribavirin treatment of respiratory syncytial infection in infants with underlying cardiopulmonary disease. JAMA 1985;254:3047–3051.
90. Committee on Infectious Diseases: Reassessment of the indication for ribavirin therapy in respiratory syncytial virus infections. Pediatrics 1996;97:137–140.
91. Friis B, Anderson P, Brenoe E, et al: Antibiotic treatment of pneumonia and bronchiolitis. A prospective randomized study. Arch Dis Child 1984;59:1038–1045.
92. Hall CB, Powell KR, Schnabel KC, et al: Risk of secondary bacterial infection in infants hospitalized with respiratory syncytial viral infection. J Pediatr 1988;113:261–271.
93. Luchetti M, Casoraghi G, Valsecche R, et al: Porcine derived surfactant treatment of severe bronchiolitis. Arch Anaesthesiol Scand 1998;43:805–810.
94. Tibby SM, Hatherill M, Wright SM, et al: Exogenous surfactant supplementation in respiratory syncytial bronchiolitis. Am J Respir Crit Care Med 2000;162:1251–1256.
95. Haroon M: Can surfactant cure babies with severe bronchiolitis? Arch Dis Child 2003;88:834–835.
96. Gross MF, Spear RM, Peterson BM: Helium-oxygen mixture does not improve gas exchange in mechanically ventilated children with bronchiolitis. Crit Care 2000;4:188–192.
97. The Impact-RSV Study Group: Palivizumab, a humanized respiratory syncytial virus monoclonal antibody, reduces hospitalization from respiratory syncytial virus infections in high-risk infants. Pediatrics 1998;102:531–537.
98. Piedra PA, Jewell AM, Cron SG, et al: Correlates of immunity to respiratory syncytial virus (RSV)–associated hospitalization. Establishment of minimum protective threshold levels of serum neutralizing antibodies. Vaccine 2003;21:3479–3482.
99. Piedra PA: Clinical experience with respiratory syncytial virus vaccines. Pediatr Infect Dis J 2003;22:S94–S99.
100. Stein RT, Sherrill D, Morgan WJ, et al: Respiratory syncytial virus in early life and risk of wheeze and allergy at age 13 years. Lancet 1999;354:541–545.
101. Young S, O'Keeffe PT, Arnott J, Landau LI: Lung function, airway responsiveness and respiratory symptoms before and after bronchiolitis. Arch Dis Child 1995;72:16–24.
102. Martinez FD, Morgan WJ, Wright AL, et al: Initial airway function is a risk factor for recurrent wheezing respiratory illnesses during the first three years of life. Am Rev Resir Dis 1991;143:312–316.
103. Martinez FD, Wright AL, Taussig LM, et al: Asthma and wheezing in the first six years of life. N Engl J Med 1995;332:133–138.
104. Kattan M, Keens TC, Lapierre J-G, et al: Pulmonary function abnormalities in symptom-free children after bronchiolitis. Pediatrics 1977;59:683–688.
105. Sims DG, Downham MAPS, Gardner PS, et al: Study of 8-year-old children with a history of respiratory syncytial virus bronchiolitis in infancy. BMJ 1978;1:11–14.
106. Wennergren G, Krisjansson S: Relationship between respiratory syncytial bronchiolitis and future obstructive airway diseases. Eur Respir J 2001;18:1044–1058.
107. Lange W: Ùber eine eigentumliche Erkrankung der kleinen Bronchien und Bronchiolen (bronchitis et bronchiolitis obliterans). Deutsch Arch Klin Med 1901;70:342–364.
108. Herbert FA, Wilkinson D, Burchak E, Morgante O: Adenovirus type 3 pneumonia causing lung damage in childhood. Can Med Assoc J 1977;116:274–276.
109. Simila L, Lunna O, Lannig P, et al: Chronic lung damage caused by adenovirus type 7. A ten year follow-up study. Chest 1981;80:127–131.
110. Sly PD, Soto-Qiros ME, Landau LI, et al: Factors predisposing to abnormal pulmonary function after adenovirus type 7 pneumonia. Arch Dis Child 1984;59:935–939.
111. Becroft DMO: Bronchiolitis obliterans, bronchiectasis and other sequelae of adenvirus type 21 infection in young children. J Clin Pathol 1971;24:72–84.

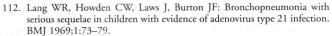

112. Lang WR, Howden CW, Laws J, Burton JF: Bronchopneumonia with serious sequelae in children with evidence of adenovirus type 21 infection. BMJ 1969;1:73–79.
113. Kim MJ, Lee KY: Bronchiolitis obliterans in children with Stevens-Johnson syndrome—follow up with high-resolurion CT. Pediatr Radiol 1996;26:22–25.
114. Yatsunami J, Natanishi Y, Matsuki H, et al: Chronic bronchiolitis obliterans associated with Stevens-Johnson syndrome. Intern Med 1995;34:772–775.
115. Laraya-Cuasay LR, DeForest A, Huff D, et al: Chronic pulmonary complications of early influenza virus infections in children. Am Rev Respir Dis 1977;16:617–625.
116. Ilses AF, Masel J, O'Duffy J: Obliterative bronchiolitis due to *Mycoplasma pneumoniae* in a child. Pediatr Radiol 1987;17:109–111.
117. Swyer PR, James GCW: A case of unilateral pulmonary emphysema. Thorax 1953;8:133–136.

26 Viral Pneumonia

James E. Crowe, Jr., MD

Viral pneumonia is one of the most common maladies affecting infants and children throughout the world. The World Health Organization and UNICEF report that acute respiratory infection continues to be a leading cause of mortality in young children; in 2000 it killed approximately 2 million children under the age of 5 in developing countries.[1] About 40% of these cases are due to viral infections. Pneumonia, a respiratory disease characterized by inflammation of the lung parenchyma, is usually caused by viruses, bacteria, or irritants. The term *pneumonia* refers to infection of the lung parenchyma and excludes the tissues of the airway such as the bronchi. However, acute viral lower respiratory tract infections in children are thought to affect all of the epithelial cells lining the airway, from the nasopharynx to the alveolar bed. Therefore, viral pneumonia is often a component of a more generalized respiratory tract infection syndrome.

INCIDENCE

It is well established that children younger than 5 years, especially infants, have a high burden of disease and hospitalization from respiratory syncytial virus (RSV), influenza virus, and parainfluenza virus (PIV). However, studies conducted during the last several decades have struggled to define precise quantitative models for the incidence of these diseases. Most large studies have been conducted in hospitals and thus lacked a known denominator of patients at risk. These studies also vary by differences in geographic location of the study, type of hospital, age of the patients, season, criteria for admission, severity of disease, and number and type of diagnostic tests performed. The relatively new use of molecular diagnostic tests has increased our ability to diagnose virus infection, but comparison of data from these studies with data from cell culture–based studies is problematic.

Prospective, active population-based surveillance is needed to define incidence. The U.S. Centers for Disease Control and Prevention sponsored studies in young children who were hospitalized for acute respiratory illness from October 1, 2000, to September 30, 2001, in Monroe County, New York (Rochester area), and Davidson County, Tennessee (Nashville area).[2] Eligible children younger than 5 years were those who resided in surveillance counties and were hospitalized for febrile or acute respiratory illness. Viral culture and polymerase chain reaction identification of viruses from nasal and throat samples were obtained from all surveillance children, providing population-based rates of hospitalization for RSV, influenza virus, and PIV, as well as demographic, clinical, and risk factor assessment for each virus. Of the 592 enrolled children, RSV was identified in 20%, influenza in 3%, PIV in 7%, other respiratory viruses in 36%, and no detectable virus in 39%. Population-based rates of acute respiratory illness hospitalizations in children younger than 5 years were 18 per 1000. Virus-positive hospitalization rates per 1000 children were 3.5 for RSV, 1.2 for PIV, and 0.6 for influenza virus. Younger age (particularly <1 year), black and Hispanic race/ethnicity, male gender, and presence of chronic underlying illness were associated with higher hospitalization rates.

ETIOLOGIC AGENTS

The etiologic agents that cause viral pneumonia are well defined. The cause of viral pneumonia varies depending on the age of the child, the setting in which the virus was acquired, the season, and the presence of medical or environmental risk factors. Although a very long list of viruses has been reported to cause pneumonia, the astute clinician can narrow the cause to a short list of potential agents using a careful medical history and physical examination. Common causes of viral pneumonia are shown in Box 26-1.

NEONATAL PNEUMONIA

PERINATAL/TRANSPLACENTAL ACQUISITION

Bacteria, viruses, and noninfectious conditions such as hyaline membrane disease can cause pneumonitis at the time of birth. Viruses are infrequently the cause of this presentation, and pneumonia often is only part of a more generalized presentation of a systemic disease. Rubella and cytomegalovirus (CMV) infection associated with systemic disease in the mother can be associated with severe congenital or neonatal disease that probably is acquired by the transplacental route, presumably through the hematogenous spread of virus. Pneumonia manifests with signs of respiratory distress such as retractions, grunting, tachypnea, and cyanosis, sometimes requiring immediate resuscitation and mechanical ventilation because of depressed respiration. Neonatal viral pneumonia can present with more nonspecific systemic signs of illness, such as apnea, bradycardia, poor peripheral perfusion, or temperature instability. These signs are also frequently found in bacterial pneumonia in the neonatal period. Usually, infants with congenital CMV or rubella pneumonia have additional signs of congenital infection, such as petechiae, hepatosplenomegaly, and low birth weight. CMV infection can be detected by testing of the urine of the infant in shell vial or traditional cell culture.

TRANSMISSION FROM THE BIRTH CANAL

Herpes simplex virus (HSV) type I or II infection of the mother's cervix can lead to exposure of the infant during labor or birth with infection by the mucosal route, including aspiration. HSV is capable of infecting the infant via an ascending route from the vaginal canal, because the risk of transmission from an infected mother is increased after a prolonged rupture of membranes during labor. The infection may be acquired without prolonged rupture of membranes during the passage through the birth canal. Transmission is more efficient if the mother is suffering a primary infection, as opposed to a reactivation. The presence of visible herpetic lesions is not needed for

BOX 26-1 Etiologic Agents of Acute Acquired Viral Pneumonia in Children, by Age

Perinatal

CMV
HSV types I and II
Enteroviruses
Rubella

3 Weeks to 3 Months

RSV, subgroups A and B
hMPV, subgroup A and B
PIV type 3

4 Months to 4 Years

RSV, subgroups A and B
hMPV, subgroups A and B
PIV types 1, 2, 3
Influenza A or B virus
Rhinoviruses
Adenoviruses

Older Children and Adults

Influenza A or B virus
Military recruits: adenovirus types 4 and 7

Viruses That Are Less Common or That Cause Pneumonia in Certain Settings

Adenovirus types 1, 2, 3, 5
Enterovirus spp.: echovirus, coxsackievirus
Coronaviruses, SARS-Coronavirus
Epstein-Barr virus, CMV, human herpesvirus 6 (in the immunocompromised)
Varicella-zoster virus
Developing world: measles virus, mumps viruses
Endemic areas: *Hantavirus*

transmission to the infant. Herpes simplex infection commonly presents in the second week of life. The medical history from the families of infants with pneumonia at this age should consider risk factors, and the physical examination should seek other manifestations of herpetic infection. The cytopathic effects of HSV have been observed in the lungs of infants with pneumonia caused by herpes infection. Systemic HSV infection should be treated with a prolonged course of intravenous acyclovir. Enteroviruses commonly cause symptomatic or asymptomatic infections of the gastrointestinal tract during the summer and fall. Infected mothers can transmit an enterovirus infection to the infant during birth, and these infections can cause severe systemic disease including pneumonia. When viral infection is acquired from contaminated amniotic fluid or in the birth canal, the infant may not be affected clinically in the first hours after birth.

TRANSMISSION IN THE NURSERY

Nosocomial transmission of viruses in the early postpartum period occurs, with surprising efficiency in some cases. The most common cause of nosocomial pneumonia is RSV, which occasionally causes nursery outbreaks.[3] Such outbreaks can be especially devastating in a neonatal intensive care unit if premature infants that require mechanical ventilation become infected. In this setting, infection is usually transmitted by fomites or directly from infected personnel via nasopharyngeal secretions.

INFECTION IN THE FIRST WEEKS OF LIFE

The most common causes of pneumonia in the developed world in the first weeks of life are RNA respiratory viruses, especially RSV. RSV causes yearly winter epidemics in the community that result in the hospitalization of between 0.5% and 3% of infants, depending on the population. During the winter, RSV is often the major cause of hospitalization of infants, and entire infant wards have been dedicated in many children's hospitals for cohorting of infants during the annual epidemics. Nosocomial spread of virus during the epidemics is common but can be minimized by strict attention to contact isolation and hand washing.

VIRAL PNEUMONIA DURING EARLY CHILDHOOD

A large panel of respiratory viruses is capable of causing pneumonia during childhood. RSV; human metapneumovirus (hMPV); PIV types 1, 2, and 3; influenza virus types A and B; and adenoviruses make up the majority of cases. RSV is still the most frequent cause of severe respiratory infections in infants after the first weeks of life and in young children, and it is responsible for 75,000 to 125,000 hospitalizations each year in the United States.[4,5] The role of rhinoviruses in causing lower respiratory tract illness such as pneumonia is under much discussion. Rhinovirus infection in children is so common that evidence for rhinovirus infection can be found frequently in children without symptoms of disease. Therefore, attributing causality to rhinovirus in cases of pneumonia is more difficult than with other viruses. Nevertheless, rhinovirus is present significantly more often in cases of childhood pneumonia, and some experts believe rhinovirus is the most common etiology of all types of lower respiratory tract illness in children. PIVs, commonly associated with laryngotracheitis, also cause pneumonia but in less discrete epidemics than those caused by RSV. PIV infections can occur at any time of the year. Influenza A or B viruses cause sharp winter epidemics. In the developing world, measles virus is still a major cause of pneumonia, especially in the setting of malnutrition or vitamin A deficiency, and mumps virus can cause lower respiratory tract illness. Influenza virus type C and PIV type 4 cause upper respiratory tract disease, but their ability to cause lower respiratory tract illness is less clear. Severe acute respiratory syndrome (SARS) is caused by the newly identified respiratory virus SARS-Coronavirus that was first recognized in Hong Kong during a 2003 epidemic, and this disease affected children.[6] Morbidity was high following SARS, with approximately one fourth of patients requiring intensive care and/or mechanical ventilation support. SARS morbidity and mortality are milder in children than they are in adults, and pneumonia is only one of the disease manifestations of what appears to be a systemic illness. It has been postulated that the other more conventional human coronaviruses, such as the OC43 and 229E strains, or the recently identified coronavirus NL strains, may also cause some cases of pneumonia.[7] Varicella-zoster virus can cause pneumonia during primary infection, especially in older subjects. Other viruses cause pneumonia less commonly, for example Epstein-Barr virus, CMV, and human herpesvirus 6.

CHAPTER 26

The immunocompromised are a special population at elevated risk for these infections, especially for CMV.

The major features of the epidemiology of respiratory virus pneumonia caused by common agents was determined in the United States in detail mostly during the 1960s through the 1980s in a series of seminal longitudinal studies, such as the D.C. Children's Hospital studies,[8–11] Chapel Hill Pediatrics surveillance study,[12] the Vanderbilt Vaccine clinic surveillance studies,[13,14] the Tecumseh study of respiratory illness (Tecumseh, Michigan), and the Tucson Children's Respiratory Study. The principal viruses identified in association with pneumonia in otherwise healthy infants and children were RSV, PIV, and influenza viruses. These studies used cell culture–based or serologic detection for the most part, and it is fair to say that most of these studies did not have optimal culture systems for rhinoviruses or coronaviruses. More recently, very large studies using database methods, such as the U.S. National Hospital Discharge Survey data system[15,16] or the Tennessee Medicaid Database[17] (~1% of U.S. children) have confirmed the earlier findings with larger numbers and added detail about the risk factors for severe disease. In the last several years, new data have emerged on the role of a newly identified paramyxovirus, hMPV,[18] which was shown to be one of the most common causes associated with lower respiratory tract infection in children.[19] Before 2001, studies could not address the epidemiology of this virus because it had not been discovered.

■ RISK FACTORS FOR PNEUMONIA

Most children are infected with the common respiratory viruses during the first years of life, but a minority suffers from lower respiratory tract disease or pneumonia to such an extent that it brings them to medical care. Studies have identified a number of risk factors for severe disease, especially young age, prematurity, preexisting lung disease (especially bronchopulmonary dysplasia), congenital heart disease, environmental exposure (smoking or wood fire heating), daycare, large number of siblings, low socioeconomic status, or birth near the start of the RSV season.[17] Exposures to infected children in the home or nosocomial exposure are pertinent historical risk factors.

■ PATHOGENESIS

Viral pneumonia is an infection of the cells surrounding the alveolar space. Alveolar walls thicken, and the alveolar space becomes occluded with exudates, sloughed cells, and activated macrophages. The clinical disease is distinguished by poor air exchange, first noted by poor oxygen intake (as detected by pulse oximetry or blood gas measurement) followed by CO_2 retention. The physiology of the disease reflects an inflammatory process resulting in an alveolar-capillary block that interferes with gas exchange, resulting in elevation of the alveolar-arterial PO_2 difference. Many cases of viral pneumonia in young children are also accompanied by inflammation of the bronchioles, and air trapping contributes to the poor level of gas exchange. Children compensate for respiratory compromise better than do adults, generally by increasing the respiratory rate. Children show a remarkable resilience when faced with respiratory compromise, even though their airways exhibit a much higher intrinsic level of resistance. Unrelieved tachypnea, however, can lead to exhaustion and respiratory failure. The histopathologic mechanisms underlying acute viral pulmonary disease in otherwise healthy children are not completely understood, because lung tissue is rarely obtained for histology before mechanical ventilation or other medical interventions in previously healthy patients.

■ LIFE CYCLE OF THE VIRUSES IN VIVO

Despite significant advances in our understanding of the basic virology and molecular biology of these viruses based on in vitro studies, relatively little is known about the life cycle and spread of these respiratory viruses to the lung parenchyma in vivo. It is thought that the initial infection occurs in the nasopharynx after inoculation with contaminated respiratory secretions (fomite transmission) or exposure to large-particle aerosols containing virus. The viruses that cause pneumonia all have surface fusion proteins that mediate both virus-cell fusion and cell-cell fusion in monolayer cell culture. The viruses cause cytopathic effects following infection by inducing necrosis or apoptosis of infected cells. The viral fusion peptides of these viruses cause multinucleated cell (syncytium) formation in cell monolayer cultures. It is presumed that they cause syncytium formation in vivo, but the direct evidence for this is scarce. In fact, viruses that cause syncytium in nonpolarized cultured cells (i.e., cells that do not form tight junctions and segregate apical and basolateral plasma membrane regions) often do not cause syncytia in polarized cell lines or primary cells in culture. Most of these viruses appear to infect both ciliated and nonciliated cells in culture. Impaired mucociliary clearance caused by infection of ciliated cells probably contributes to progression to pneumonia. Whether these viruses infect type I or II pneumocytes more efficiently is not known. Some of the respiratory viruses cause an abortive round of infection in cultured macrophages. Infection of alveolar macrophages may contribute to inflammatory disease of the lung.

The mechanism for spread of infection to the lower respiratory tract within days of inoculation is unknown. Virus probably spreads by microaspiration of infected secretions or by cell-to-cell spread of the virus. The rapid time course of spread in vivo suggests that aspiration of infected secretions results in direct inoculation of the lower respiratory tract. Autopsy cases of fatal RSV cases have demonstrated the presence of relatively little virus antigen, and pathologic changes in fatal cases can be patchy in distribution. Bronchoalveolar lavage and tissue specimens from bone marrow transplant patients or autopsies evaluated by direct immunofluorescence or immunoperoxidase stains revealed epithelial cells and macrophages that stain positive for RSV proteins, and electron microscopy revealed occasional epithelial cells with cytoplasmic inclusions composed of filamentous virions. There are limited autopsy data from PIV-infected or influenza-infected humans. In summary, the population(s) of cells that are the primary target of respiratory virus infections in humans are probably epithelial in origin but have not been fully defined in normal hosts.

■ VIRUS RECEPTORS ON HOST CELLS

The hemagglutinin protein of influenza virus mediates virus attachment to a glycoconjugate terminating in sialic acid and causes fusion with an intracellular membrane at low pH. The PIV hemagglutinin-neuraminidase glycoprotein mediates attachment to sialic acid–containing host cell receptors. The RSV surface protein that mediates attachment is the RSV G (glycosylated) glycoprotein. Its cellular receptor is not fully understood, but this glycosylated protein binds to heparan sulfates and to the CX3CR1 protein (the specific receptor for the CX3C chemokine fractalkine) through a CX3C motif in the viral protein.[20] The viability of mutant RSV strains lacking the glycosylated protein indicates that the attachment protein is not strictly required for replication in cell culture or in rodents. The RSV F protein binds to Toll-like receptor 4 (see the 2001 study by Haynes and colleagues)[21] and to heparan sulfates, and interacts with the cellular protein RhoA,[22] but whether any of these serves as a principal protein receptor is not clear at this time. An association between common Toll-like receptor 4 mutations and severity of RSV disease has been reported.

■ INFLAMMATION

The magnitude and character of the inflammatory response in the airway appear to be highly regulated by epithelial cell-derived cytokines and chemokines that attract and activate specific subsets of leukocytes associated with airway inflammation. Cytokine secretion appears to be highly regulated by nuclear factor κB (NF-κB) transcription factors, dimers of structurally related proteins that are retained in the cytoplasm by association with the inhibitory κB proteins. Upon various cellular stimulations usually related to stress or pathogens, the inhibitors are degraded and the nuclear factors κB translocate to the nucleus where they bind to κB DNA elements to induce transcription of a large number of genes, especially those associated with immune responses. Nuclear factor–interleukin 6 (NF-IL-6) regulates expression of cytokine and adhesion molecule genes without increased transcription. RSV infection induces increased expression of several cytokines, including IL-6 and IL-8, which are transcriptionally regulated by NF-κB and NF-IL-6. These cytokine-regulated pathways appear to contribute to airway inflammation during pneumonia.

Immune cells also probably play a major role in the pathogenesis of disease. The epithelial cells appear to initiate a cascade of events that represent components of the innate immune response. When epithelial cells secrete IL-6 and IL-8 and other soluble factors, they recruit and initiate activation of immune effectors. The chemokine RANTES (regulated upon activation, normal T-cell expressed and secreted) is a chemoattractant for eosinophils, monocytes, T cells, and basophils that is secreted in response to viruses such as RSV. Eventually, adaptive immune effectors such as $CD8^+$ T cells attack the virus-infected cells to eliminate the infection. This immune cytolysis is important to disease resolution but comes at the price of inducing some level of immunopathology. The cell surface factors that facilitate homing of lymphocytes to lung tissue are under investigation.

■ CLINICAL DISEASE

The clinical presentation of viral pneumonia is related principally to disease in the respiratory tract, including increased respiratory rate and supracostal, intercostal, or subcostal retractions. Infants show nasal flaring, grunting, and marked retractions during severe disease. Vital signs reveal fever in about half of cases at presentation; fever higher than 103°F is much less common than in bacterial pneumonia but can occur. Systemic toxicity is less common than with bacterial infection, because respiratory viruses (other than measles virus) rarely cause viremia. Of the conventional respiratory viruses, influenza virus is the one that most frequently causes high fever and toxic appearance. Respiratory failure, heralded by a change in alertness due to hypoxia and CO_2 retention or decreased respiratory effort due to exhaustion, requires immediate action. Physical examination reveals crackles on auscultation, generally more prominent on inspiration. RSV disease in infants is commonly a mixed presentation of bronchiolitis and pneumonia, in which case expiratory wheezing is present in addition to inspiratory crackles. The viruses that cause pneumonia also cause upper respiratory tract infection. Therefore, concomitant coryza is common, complicated in about a third of cases with otitis media. Nasal obstruction caused by purulent nasal secretions contributes to the respiratory distress, especially in infants. Mild to moderate dehydration is common as a result of increased respiratory and insensible losses, and poor oral fluid intake.

■ CLINICAL DIAGNOSIS OF PNEUMONIA

The terms *pneumonia* and *lower respiratory tract illness* have clinical, anatomic, and histologic definitions. *Lower respiratory illness* can be defined clinically as the presence of crackles, rhonchi, or wheezes on physical examination or as infiltrates on a chest radiograph, and anatomically is usually considered disease below the vocal cords. *Pneumonia* is an inflammation due to infection of the lung parenchyma, comprising alveoli and interstitial tissue with possible extension to the bronchioles. Viral pneumonia during childhood is often one component of a lower respiratory illness that also affects the small and large conducting airways. For example, the most common presentation of severe RSV infection of infants is bronchiolitis and pneumonia.

■ RADIOGRAPHIC FINDINGS

Chest radiographs using the posteroanterior view are the principal diagnostic radiologic test for pneumonias. Children who have an effusion or an empyema identified on chest radiograph may need a computed tomography scan to further define the scope of the problem, but these complications are rare in viral pneumonia. The radiologic findings on chest radiographs of viral pneumonia are similar to those of bronchiolitis and reactive airways disease. The usual findings on chest radiographs are hyperaeration, prominent lung markings due to bronchial wall thickening, and focal areas of atelectasis (Fig. 26-1). The hili may be somewhat prominent, but major hilar adenopathy is uncommon. The findings are commonly thought to differ from the typical case of bacterial pneumonia, which usually has been thought to present as lobar consolidation. It is true that most children with focal alveolar pneumonia have laboratory evidence of a bacterial infection, especially those with lobar infiltrates. However, half of the children with solely interstitial infiltrates on the chest radiograph had evidence of bacterial infection in some studies.[23] Therefore, radiologic presentation of interstitial infiltrates alone does not distinguish between bacterial and viral pneumonia. One also cannot differentiate viral pneumonia from bronchiolitis or reactive airways disease on the basis of radiologic findings alone. Differentiation is based on nonradiologic factors such as the age of the patient and the clinical history. The chest radiograph in newborns with viral pneumonia usually shows bilateral diffuse densities or may have a granular appearance, similar to that found in hyaline membrane disease. When infection is congenital, radiographic changes may be present at birth, whereas the radiographs of infants infected

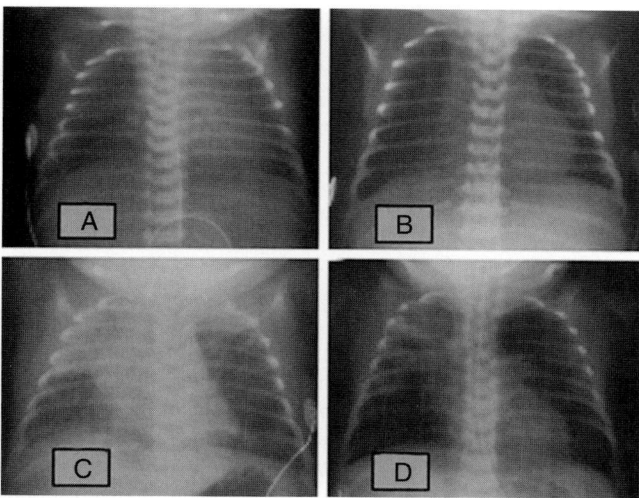

■ **FIGURE 26-1.** Chest radiographs from premature infant who suffered RSV pneumonia early in life. **A,** Infant presented with neonatal respiratory distress syndrome (RDS) requiring mechanical ventilation; radiograph shows ground-glass appearance and lung volume loss of RDS on day of birth. **B,** By 1 week of life, mechanical ventilation is discontinued, and the lung fields normalize. **C,** At 6 weeks of life, the child presented with RSV-positive test and respiratory distress requiring mechanical ventilation; radiograph shows diffuse interstitial infiltrates and atelectasis or pneumonia of the right upper lobe. **D,** By 7 weeks of life, the child remained on a mechanical ventilator, but infiltrates and atelectasis were improving. (Radiographs courtesy of James Crowe, MD, University of Texas Health Science Center at Houston.)

during birth may be normal initially but can rapidly progress during the first day of life.

■ DIFFERENTIAL DIAGNOSIS

The differential diagnosis for nonviral causes varies by age. In newborns, group B streptococcus infection and hyaline membrane disease are the most common considerations. In infants, atypical organisms such as *Chlamydia trachomatis* and *Ureaplasma urealyticum* must be considered, as well as *Pneumocystis carinii* in children with immunodeficiencies or in utero exposure to human immunodeficiency virus. Common bacterial causes of pneumonia are *Bordetella pertussis, Streptococcus pneumoniae, Haemophilus influenzae* (mostly nontypable species in the era of universal immunization against type B), and mycobacterial infections including tuberculosis. In young children, *Mycoplasma pneumoniae, S. pneumoniae,* and mycobacterial infections are important. In older children and adolescents, the atypical organisms *M. pneumoniae, C. trachomatis,* and *Chlamydia pneumoniae* remain important, and the bacteria *S. pneumoniae, B. pertussis,* and mycobacterial species are considerations. *Histoplasma capsulatum* infection is relatively common in certain areas of the United States and causes an atypical pneumonia. *Cryptococcus neoformans* infection is also a consideration in immunocompromised patients.

Many published studies have addressed the differentiation of bacterial from viral pneumonia using clinical, radiologic, and routine hematologic tests, but these methods have not been found to be sufficiently reliable in differential diagnosis.[23–33]

Chest radiographic findings, total white blood cell count, erythrocyte sedimentation rate, and serum C-reactive protein have been used widely in children with community-acquired pneumonia of varying etiology to discriminate between bacterial causes, but the specificities of these are not sufficient to determine the diagnosis in clinical practice. Lymphocytic predominance is usually present in the peripheral blood white blood cells during viral pneumonias, although this feature is also usually present in pertussis and atypical bacterial infections. Bacterial pneumonia requiring hospitalization on average causes higher fevers than viral pneumonia, and is more often associated with a fever higher than 103°F than is viral pneumonia. A lobar, segmental, or rounded well-defined pneumonia affecting a single lobe is more likely to be bacterial in etiology, as are cases associated with large pleural effusions, abscess, bullae, or pneumatoceles. A bedside cold agglutinins test may be positive in the case of viral pneumonia or mycoplasmal infection, and thus this test is not particularly helpful in distinguishing etiology.

■ LABORATORY DIAGNOSIS OF VIRAL ETIOLOGY

The specific cause of viral pneumonia can be identified by several methods with varying levels of stringency. Culture of virus in cell monolayer cultures is considered the gold standard. Viruses are identified by characteristic cytopathic effect and confirmed by immunodetection using virus-specific antibodies and fluorescence detection. Culture techniques require a high level of expertise and generally are best performed on fresh specimens, such as secretions obtained by nasopharyngeal aspiration or nasopharyngeal swab. Rapid diagnostic tests for RSV and influenza A and B based on the immunodetection of viral proteins in nasopharyngeal secretions are widely used, but their positive predictive value is most appropriate for use during epidemics when the prevalence of positive tests is expected to be high. Antigen detection tests are not sensitive enough to determine that a hospitalized patient is no longer shedding infectious virus; therefore, negative tests should not be used to justify termination of contact precautions in a patient with viral pneumonia. Increasingly, clinical detection of viruses is being performed by molecular genetic techniques, such as reverse transcriptase–polymerase chain reaction followed by hybridization or sequence analysis. This technique identifies the presence of viral nucleic acid. Polymerase chain reaction tests tend to be more sensitive than cell culture during the period of viral clearance (1–3 weeks after infection). It is not clear how long viral RNAs are present following active infections, but evidence to date shows that they may persist for weeks or months even when virus can no longer be cultured. Therefore, a positive polymerase chain reaction–based test must be used with caution, because in some cases it is possible that a positive test obtained during an acute pneumonia is actually related to a recent infection. Serology is helpful to diagnose or confirm infection, particularly in the clinical research setting. A fourfold rise in serum antibodies against a virus between the preinfection period and after infection, particularly when a serology testing functional antibodies is used, suggests a specific diagnosis. In practice, the use of serologic tests to diagnose the cause of pneumonia is difficult because the rise in antibodies in young children may not achieve a significant level until 6 to 8 weeks or more have passed.

■ COINFECTIONS

Single agents cause most cases of viral pneumonia, but coinfection does occur. Most careful studies in children have found evidence for the presence of two viruses in about 5% to 10% of cases of viral lower respiratory tract infection. There is little direct evidence in immunocompetent individuals that coinfection is characterized by a more severe clinical course than infection with a single agent. Bacterial superinfection does occur, but overt bacterial lung disease during viral pneumonia is unusual. Bacterial complication of viral pneumonia is suggested by an abrupt change in symptoms over several hours with appearance of generalized toxicity, and possibly with new radiographic findings of parenchymal consolidation or pleural effusions. Marked and changed leukocytosis (e.g., >20,000 cells/mm^3 white blood cells in the peripheral blood) is suggestive of a bacterial process, but not particularly sensitive or specific. *Streptococcus pneumoniae*, *H. influenzae*, and *Staphylococcus aureus* are the most common bacteria involved in complication of viral pneumonia, and influenza virus pneumonia is the most common viral pneumonia to be complicated by bacterial infection. Recent vaccine studies with a pneumococcal vaccine in a large population of children showed that a nine-valent bacterial polysaccharide vaccine prevented about a third of cases of viral pneumonia, suggesting frequent interactions of bacteria and viruses that are not apparent by current methods of clinical evaluation.[34]

■ THERAPY

Most infants and children with mild viral pneumonia can be treated symptomatically as outpatients. Oxygen is required if there is grunting, flaring, severe tachypnea, and retractions, or if pulse oximetry indicates oxygen saturation below 90% to 92%, or arterial blood gas measurement indicates depressed PO_2 (<60–70 mm Hg). Retention of CO_2 is particularly concerning, especially in the face of tachypnea. Severe respiratory distress, hypoxia, and dehydration are among the indications for hospitalization. Care in the hospital is principally supportive, such as the delivery of supplemental oxygen and intravenous fluids, and the use of mechanical ventilation in the case of respiratory failure. The youngest infants with RSV pneumonia may require monitoring for the risk of apnea, although apnea usually presents near the beginning of the illness. Chest physiotherapy and mucolytics may be of value, but their efficacy is uncertain in viral pneumonia. If a specific viral diagnosis is made early in the course of illness, there are some antiviral medications available. Licensed drugs for influenza infection include the M2 ion-channel inhibitors amantidine and rimantidine, and the neuraminidase inhibitors oseltamivir and zanamivir. These antiviral compounds work best when therapy is initiated in the first days of infection and are particularly relevant for those with immunosuppression or preexisting cardiopulmonary disease. Ribavirin delivered as an aerosol is licensed for treatment of severe RSV infection, but recent studies have questioned its value. Most centers do not routinely treat otherwise healthy infants with RSV pneumonia with ribavirin. RSV intravenous immune globulin and palivizumab, an intramuscular injectable humanized monoclonal antibody directed against the RSV fusion protein, are available for prophylaxis against RSV disease and are indicated for children with chronic cardiopulmonary disease and other serious risk factors. Clinical trials of therapy of acute disease using these antibody preparations, however, have not shown this treatment to be effective during hospitalization. Antibiotic therapy does not improve the outcome in viral pneumonia and has not been shown to alter the risk of bacterial complication of viral pneumonia as a superinfection. Indiscriminate use of antibiotics in the setting of viral infection causes the selection of antibiotic-resistant bacteria. If secondary infection does occur, usually in hospitalized patients in intensive care units, the selected infecting bacterium may not be susceptible to conventional antibiotics. Therefore, specific diagnosis of the etiology of severe pneumonia suspected to be of viral etiology is warranted even when an antiviral therapeutic option is not anticipated, so as to minimize inappropriate antibiotic exposure.

■ COMPLICATIONS

Many of the common sequelae of bacterial pneumonia, such as persistent effusions, empyemas, abscess formation, and pneumatoceles, are distinctly uncommon following viral pneumonia. Therefore, the prognosis for most forms of viral pneumonia caused by conventional respiratory viruses is excellent. Most otherwise healthy children with uncomplicated pneumonia recover without sequelae. Complications during influenza pneumonia in children range from acute otitis media, sinusitis, and bacterial tracheitis to rare episodes of encephalitis, myositis, myocarditis, febrile seizures, encephalopathy, or Reyes syndrome. RSV disease is commonly complicated by otitis media. Immunocompromised children, those with underlying cardiopulmonary disease, and neonates are at the highest risk for severe sequelae. Pulmonary hypertension can complicate the course of neonatal pneumonia, and concomitant pulmonary hemorrhage due to vascular damage may follow. Pulmonary interstitial emphysema and other types of gas leaks can occur, especially during mechanical ventilation. Mortality is high in neonatal viral pneumonia, especially in premature infants in whom the disease may resemble severe hyaline membrane disease. Infants with severe viral pneumonia early in life who require mechanical ventilation or treatment with high concentrations of supplemental oxygen are at increased risk of chronic lung disease. Some cases of viral pneumonia, especially those due to rapid-onset severe adenovirus infection, can lead to bronchiolitis obliterans and hyperlucent lung syndrome. The prognosis for pneumonia due to more uncommon causes of viral pneumonia such as varicella-zoster virus, SARS-*Coronavirus*, and measles virus can be guarded.

■ PROTECTIVE IMMUNITY

Serum neutralizing antibodies appear to be most protective of the lower respiratory tract against severe disease caused by viruses. Probably this is a result of the close association of the intravascular space with the alveolus. The gradient of antibody transfer to the nasopharynx is quite steep in that there are about 300-fold higher levels of immunoglobulin G (IgG) antibodies in the serum than in the nasopharynx, but levels of IgG in the alveolus and serum can be quite similar.

High levels of IgG in the alveolus are probably due to transudation. Higher in the airway, IgG antibodies are transported by the neonatal Fc receptor. Secretory IgA is uniquely suited for antiviral activity at the respiratory mucosal surface. Mucosal antibody secretion occurs locally, and polymeric IgA is taken up specifically by the polyimmunoglobulin receptor at the base of polarized epithelial cells, transcytosed in the apical direction, and secreted onto the mucosa. Antibodies may contribute to the resolution of acute primary infection of the lung. IgA and IgG RSV antibodies are present in the nasal secretions of infants early in infection, and the decrease in virus shedding in infants infected with RSV has been temporally associated with the detection of RSV-specific IgA in nasal washes. Laboratory studies and clinical trials provide strong evidence for the dominant role of antibodies in protection against reinfection. Maternal antibodies do not cross the placenta efficiently before 32 weeks' gestation; therefore, premature infants are lacking the serum antibody protection against viral pneumonia that is conferred to term infants.

Cell-mediated immunity probably plays a primary role in the clearance of established respiratory virus pneumonia in humans. The best evidence to support this concept is that patients with defects in cellular immunity such as recipients of bone marrow transplantation or patients with cancer undergoing immunosuppressive chemotherapy suffer more prolonged virus shedding or more frequent and more severe illnesses with RSV, influenza virus, or PIV type 3. The role in humans of cell-mediated immune effectors in protection against disease on reinfection or during virus challenge following immunization is less clear, however. Macrophages are abundant in the alveolar spaces of the lung. In vitro and in vivo data suggest that the resident pulmonary alveolar macrophage population actively suppresses the antigen-presenting function of lung dendritic cells (DCs) in situ. Low numbers of DCs and high numbers of macrophages have been noted in the human alveolar compartment, suggesting that the alveolar compartment may be less efficient for mounting an immune response. Human alveolar macrophages recovered during RSV infection can yield small amounts of RSV, but replication of RSV in alveolar macrophages is restricted. Inoculation of human alveolar macrophages with live or inactivated RSV induces increased secretion of cytokines, such as tumor necrosis factor, IL-6, IL-8, and IL-10.

Dendritic cells are widely distributed in the lung, where they are distinguished by their morphology and class II major histocompatibility complex antigen expression. DCs serve as potent pulmonary antigen-presenting cells. However, relatively little is currently known about how these cells respond to specific respiratory viruses at the mucosa. Recruitment of a wave of DCs into the respiratory tract mucosa appears to be a feature of the acute cellular response to local challenge with viral protein antigens or virus infection. Differentiation of DCs in the lung, homing of particular types of DCs to the lung, and crosstalk between adaptive immune cells and DCs in the lung are all areas of intense research.

■ PREVENTION

The viruses that commonly cause viral pneumonia are ubiquitous, and every child becomes infected in the first years of life with most of the common respiratory viruses. It is not feasible to avoid or prevent exposure or infection; therefore, the practical goal is to avoid infection at a time of high risk and to prevent severe disease or complications during infection. Thorough hand washing, the use of contact isolation, and patient or provider cohorting are critical to the prevention of the nosocomial spread of infection to high-risk individuals in the hospital. Vaccination of at-risk individuals with licensed vaccines for influenza virus (using trivalent H1N1/H3N2/B subunit or trivalent live attenuated virus vaccines) is wise. Amantidine or rimantidine can be used effectively as a prophylactic treatment in some for the prevention of symptomatic influenza disease during an epidemic or immediately following exposure. Polyclonal (RSV intravenous immune globulin) or monoclonal (palivizumab, IM) antibody prophylactic treatments can be used in infants at high risk of RSV disease, and these treatments prevent half or more of RSV hospitalizations during treatment. The combination of risk factors that best predicts susceptibility to hospitalization due to RSV is not entirely clear, but includes extreme prematurity, bronchopulmonary disease, and oxygen dependence. More subtle influences are important but they affect risk incrementally. The use of the live attenuated measles-mumps-rubella vaccine is effective against measles and mumps disease, and varicella vaccine prevents severe disease due to that virus. An adenovirus vaccine has been used effectively but only in the military to prevent epidemic disease in adults who live in close quarters.

■ EXPERIMENTAL VACCINES

Candidate vaccines have been developed and tested for prevention of viral pneumonia caused by RSV; PIV types 1, 2, and 3; and hMPV. Both subunit and live attenuated RSV vaccines have been tested in phase I or II trials, and the live attenuated vaccines appear promising. The challenge for investigators is to identify or generate attenuated viruses that are sufficiently immunogenic to induce a protective response in newborns without causing any signs or symptoms of respiratory disease. Cold-passaged or bovine strain PIV type 3 vaccines have been tested extensively in humans and appear promising. HMPV vaccine candidates have been generated but have not been tested in clinical trials to date.

REFERENCES

1. UNICEF Global Database on Prevalence and Treatment of Acute Respiratory Infection. Available at http://www.childinfo.org/areas/ari/countrydata.php/ UNICEF statistics. Accessed September 12, 2005.
2. Iwane MK, Edwards KM, Szilagyi PG, Walker FJ, Griffin MR, Weinberg GA, et al: Population-based surveillance for hospitalizations associated with respiratory syncytial virus, influenza virus, and parainfluenza viruses among young children. Pediatrics 2004;113:1758–1764.
3. Valenti WM, Clarke TA, Hall CB, Menegus MA, Shapiro DL: Concurrent outbreaks of rhinovirus and respiratory syncytial virus in an intensive care nursery. Epidemiology and associated risk factors. J Pediatr 1982;100:722–726.
4. Institute of Medicine: Prospects for immunizing against respiratory syncytial virus. In: New Vaccine Development. Establishing Priorities, Vol 1. Washington, DC: National Academy Press, 1985, pp 397–409.
5. Shay DK, Holman RC, Newman RD, Liu LL, Stout JW, Anderson LJ: Bronchiolitis-associated hospitalizations among US children, 1980–1996. JAMA 1999;282:1440–1446.
6. Leung CW, Kwan YW, Ko PW, Chiu SS, Loung PY, Fong NC, et al: Severe acute respiratory syndrome among children. Pediatrics 2004;113: e535–543.
7. Fouchier RA, Hartwig NG, Bestebroer TM, Niemeyer B, de Jong JC, et al: A previously undescribed coronavirus associated with respiratory disease in humans. Proc Natl Acad Sci U S A 2004;101:6212–6216.
8. Kim HW, Brandt CD, Arrobio JO, Murphy B, Chanock RM, Parrott RH: Influenza A and B virus infection in infants and young children during the years 1957–1976. Am J Epidemiol 1979;109:464–479.
9. Kim HW, Arrobio JO, Brandt CD, Jeffries BC, Pyles G, Reid JL, et al: Epidemiology of respiratory syncytial virus infection in Washington, D.C. I. Importance of the virus in different respiratory tract disease syndromes and temporal distribution of infection. Am J Epidemiol 1973;98:216–225.
10. Parrott RH, Kim HW, Arrobio JO, Hodes DS, Murphy BR, Brandt CD, et al: Epidemiology of respiratory syncytial virus infection in Washington, D.C. II. Infection and disease with respect to age, immunologic status, race and sex. Am J Epidemiol 1973;98:289–300.
11. Brandt CD, Kim HW, Arrobio JO, Jeffries BC, Wood SC, Chanock RM, et al: Epidemiology of respiratory syncytial virus infection in Washington, D.C. 3. Composite analysis of eleven consecutive yearly epidemics. Am J Epidemiol 1973;98:355–364.

12. Murphy TF, Henderson FW, Clyde WA Jr, Collier AM, Denny FW: Pneumonia. An eleven-year study in a pediatric practice. Am J Epidemiol 1981;113:12–21.
13. Reed G, Jewett PH, Thompson J, Tollefson S, Wright PF: Epidemiology and clinical impact of parainfluenza virus infections in otherwise healthy infants and young children <5 years old. J Infect Dis 1997;175:807–813.
14. Fisher RG, Gruber WC, Edwards KM, Reed GW, Tollefson SJ, Thompson JM, et al: Twenty years of outpatient respiratory syncytial virus infection. A framework for vaccine efficacy trials. Pediatrics 1997;99:E7.
15. Thompson WW, Shay DK, Weintraub E, Brammer L, Cox N, Anderson LJ, et al: Mortality associated with influenza and respiratory syncytial virus in the United States. JAMA 2003;289:179–186.
16. Shay DK, Holman RC, Roosevelt GE, Clarke MJ, Anderson LJ: Bronchiolitis-associated mortality and estimates of respiratory syncytial virus–associated deaths among US children, 1979–1997. J Infect Dis 2001;183:16–22.
17. Boyce TG, Mellen BG, Mitchel EF Jr, Wright PF, Griffin MR: Rates of hospitalization for respiratory syncytial virus infection among children in Medicaid. J Pediatr 2000;137:865–870.
18. van den Hoogen BG, de Jong JC, Groen J, Kuiken T, de Groot R, Fouchier RA, et al: A newly discovered human pneumovirus isolated from young children with respiratory tract disease. Nat Med 2001;7:719–724.
19. Williams JV, Harris PA, Tollefson SJ, Halburnt-Rush LL, Pingsterhaus JM, Edwards KM, et al: Human metapneumovirus and lower respiratory tract disease in otherwise healthy infants and children. N Engl J Med 2004;350: 443–450.
20. Tripp RA, Jones LP, Haynes LM, Zheng H, Murphy PM, Anderson LJ: CX3C chemokine mimicry by respiratory syncytial virus G glycoprotein. Nat Immunol 2001;2:732–738.
21. Haynes LM, Moore DD, Kurt-Jones EA, Finberg RW, Anderson LJ, Tripp RA: Involvement of Toll-like receptor 4 in innate immunity to respiratory syncytial virus. J Virol 2001;75:10730–10737.
22. Pastey MK, Crowe JE Jr, Graham BS: RhoA interacts with the fusion glycoprotein of respiratory syncytial virus and facilitates virus-induced syncytium formation. J Virol 1999;73:7262–7270.
23. Virkki R, Juven T, Rikalainen H, Svedstrom E, Mertsola J, Ruuskanen O: Differentiation of bacterial and viral pneumonia in children. Thorax 2002;57:438–441.
24. Turner RB, Lande AE, Chase P, Hilton N, Weinberg D: Pneumonia in pediatric outpatients. Cause and clinical manifestations. Pediatrics 1987; 111:194–200.
25. Bettenay FAL, de Campo JF, McCrossin DB: Differentiating bacterial from viral pneumonias in children. Pediatr Radiol 1988;18:453–454.
26. Isaacs D: Problems in determining the etiology of community-acquired childhood pneumonia. Pediatr Infect Dis J 1989;8:143–148.
27. Courtoy I, Lande AE, Turner RB: Accuracy of radiographic differentiation of bacterial from nonbacterial pneumonia. Clin Pediatr 1989;28: 261–264.
28. Tew J, Calenoff L, Berlin BS: Bacterial or nonbacterial pneumonia. Accuracy of radiographic diagnosis. Radiology 1977;124:607–612.
29. McCarthy PL, Spiesel SZ, Stashwick CA, Ablow RC, Masters SJ, Dolan TF Jr: Radiographic findings and etiologic diagnosis in ambulatory childhood pneumonias. Clin Pediatr 1981;20:686–691.
30. Swischuk LE, Hayden CK Jr: Viral vs. bacterial pulmonary infections in children (is roentgenographic differentiation possible?). Pediatr Radiol 1986;16:278–284.
31. Korppi M, Kiekara O, Heiskanen-Kosma T, Soimakallio S: Comparison of radiological findings and microbial aetiology of childhood pneumonia. Acta Paediatr 1993;82:360–363.
32. Shuttleworth DB, Charney E: Leukocyte count in childhood pneumonia. Am J Dis Child 1971;122:393–396.
33. Nohynek H, Valkeila E, Leinonen M, Eskola J: Erythrocyte sedimentation rate, white blood cell count and serum C-reactive protein in assessing etiologic diagnosis of acute lower respiratory infections in children. Pediatr Infect Dis J 1995;14:484–490.
34. Madhi SA, Klugman KP, The Vaccine Trialist Group: A role for *Streptococcus pneumoniae* in virus-associated pneumonia. Nat Med 2004; 10:811–813.

27 Community-Acquired Bacterial Pneumonia

Renato T. Stein, MD •
Paulo J.C. Marostica, MD

Community-acquired pneumonia (CAP) is one of the most important health problems affecting children all over the world. There are 4 to 5 million annual deaths reported in children younger than 5 years of age, especially in developing countries where it ranks among the most frequent causes of both mortality and morbidity.

Pneumonia can be broadly defined as inflammation of lung tissue due to an infectious agent that stimulates a response resulting in damage to lung tissue. Resolution of damage may be complete or only partial. Different definitions for pneumonia are found in the medical literature, varying from the finding of pulmonary pathogens in lung specimens, to the presence of pulmonary infiltrates on chest radiographs, or solely the clinical findings of tachypnea or retractions. The latter is the World Health Organization operational definition, which has to be applied to the vast majority of children worldwide, who do not have access to chest radiography. For practical reasons, most experts define pneumonia as an association of clinical findings and radiographic evidence of infiltrates.[1] In less affluent countries, the preferred term is sometimes *acute lower respiratory tract infection* (LRTI), possibly because of the difficulties in obtaining a chest radiograph. Not surprisingly, other common pediatric respiratory diseases may overlap this definition, especially viral bronchiolitis.

This chapter discusses bacterial pneumonias acquired in the community environment in children after the neonatal period. Pneumonias caused by viruses and other microorganisms are considered in Chapters 26, 31, 32, and 37. Although in many real-life situations viruses may coexist with typical and atypical bacteria in the same child as causal agents for CAP, these nonbacterial agents are mentioned in this chapter only for comparison with bacterial disease in the diagnosis and treatment of CAP. Complications of pneumonia such as pleural effusions and empyema are also discussed in Chapters 21 and 30. The upper airways are commensally colonized by a variety of pathogens, differently from the lower respiratory tract, which is considered to be sterile. Bacterial infections are frequently preceded by viral (especially respiratory syncytial virus, or rhinovirus) or *Mycoplasma pneumoniae* infections. Impairment of the cough reflex, interruption of mucociliary clearance because of virus-induced changes in ciliary structure and function, and virus-induced enhancement of bacterial adherence are some of the mechanisms believed to be contributory in this chain of events that may eventually lead to CAP.

EPIDEMIOLOGY

In North America, the annual incidence of pneumonia varies from 6 to 12 per 1000 children older than 9 years, to 30 to 45 per 1000 children younger than 5 years old. In Europe, approximately 2.5 million cases of childhood pneumonia occur yearly. The incidence of pneumonia is 10 times higher in developing than in developed countries, with as many as 5 million deaths occurring yearly in children younger than 5 years. Such variables as nutritional status, age, and the presence of an underlying condition (in particular measles in the developing world) influence morbidity and mortality rates due to CAP.[2–5]

Children attending daycare centers are also at increased risk of acquiring pneumococcal infections. Recent studies on the prevalence of capsulated *Haemophilus influenzae* serotype b infections show a significant decline after appropriate immunization, thus suggesting that this pathogen, which would have been responsible formerly for almost 20% of all CAPs, is less likely to cause CAP in vaccinated children.[6]

Respiratory syncytial virus and influenza infections usually occur in late fall and winter, and these pathogens may predispose infants and young children to bacterial CAP, especially if there are other risk factors present.

INFLUENCE OF AGE IN ETIOLOGY

There are significant age-related differences in the etiology of CAP during childhood (Table 27-1). From birth to 20 days of life, most pneumonias are caused by group B streptococci or gram-negative enteric bacteria. Viruses are the most frequent pathogens of CAP, especially in young children. *Chlamydia pneumoniae* and *M. pneumoniae* infections occur more often in school-aged children and during adolescence, although there are many reports of these agents causing CAP in younger children as well.[7–9] Infants in the first 3 months of life may present with a characteristic syndrome of low-grade or no fever, cough, and respiratory distress. This clinical picture may be caused by *Chlamydia trachomatis*, a variety of respiratory viruses, *Bordetella pertussis*, or possibly *Ureaplasma urealyticum* (the role of this last organism is less clear). *Staphylococcus aureus* was once a much more common pneumonia pathogen in the first year of life, but its prevalence has decreased. In young children, viruses are much more common causes of pneumonia than bacteria (see Chapter 26). In a study of 196 children from 2 to 5 years of age in Italy, Esposito detected a 24.5% prevalence of pneumococcal infections, 23.5% of atypical agents (*M. pneumoniae* and *C. pneumoniae*), and 8.2% of mixed infections.[10] Viral pathogens were not surveyed in this study. Other studies show similar distributions of agents in this age range.

Prevalence rates for *Streptococcus pneumoniae,* the most prevalent bacteria causing CAP, are less affected by age. *Streptococcus pneumoniae* is a common pathogen throughout both infancy and childhood, with the possible exception of the neonatal period. *Streptococcus pneumoniae* infections were less influenced by immunization, since many different serotypes, not all covered by vaccines, can cause disease. In any case, immunization against

■ **TABLE 27-1.** Most common agents causing community-acquired pneumonia, according to age group

	AGE			
Newborns	**1–3 Months**	**1–12 Months**	**1–5 Years**	**Older Than 5 Years**
Group B *Streptococcus* Enteric gram-negative	*Chlamydia trachomatis* *Ureaplasma urealyticum* Viruses *Bordetella pertussis*	Viruses *Streptococcus pneumoniae* *Haemophilus influenzae* *Staphylococcus aureus* *Moraxella catarrhalis*	Viruses *S. pneumoniae* *Mycoplasma pneumoniae* *C. trachomatis*	*S. pneumoniae* *M. pneumoniae* *C. pneumoniae*

this organism is not part of current routine infant schedules in most parts of the world.

Nontypable *H. influenzae* is less frequently associated with pneumonia than is *S. pneumoniae* in immunocompetent children, being occasionally found in case series from developing countries.[3–6,11,12] *Haemophilus influenzae* type b was once common in infants and young children before widespread use of the specific vaccine.[4]

■ CLINICAL FEATURES

Children with pneumonia are not necessarily acutely ill, and some of them may have no respiratory signs or symptoms.[13] Children with pneumonia may present with the clinical findings of fever, chills, abdominal and chest pain, and productive cough, all of which suggest typical bacterial pneumonia. A more gradual clinical onset associated with headache, malaise, nonproductive cough, and low-grade fever, on the other hand, is more commonly associated with infection by such atypical pathogens as *M. pneumoniae.*[12]

Wheezing is most frequently associated with viral, *Mycoplasma*, or *Chlamydia* infections, and true wheezing makes a bacterial cause unlikely in this setting. In the case series of pneumonias from Wubbel and colleagues, pneumococcal infection was the most frequent diagnosis among patients with a past history of wheezing when this was not a current clinical finding. On the other hand, viruses were the most frequent pathogens among those patients who wheezed.[5]

Tachypnea is a useful sign for the diagnosis of childhood pneumonia and is more specific and more reproducible than auscultatory signs. Usually, the cutoff points are a respiratory rate of 60 breaths per minute in infants younger than 2 months, 50 breaths per minute for infants from 2 to 12 months, and 40 breaths per minute for children 1 to 5 years old. Tachypnea is usually more sensitive and specific than crackles on auscultation. The positive predictive value of this finding is much greater in developing countries, where bacterial pneumonias are more prevalent. By contrast, in developed countries most children who present acutely with an increased respiratory rate have either bronchiolitis or asthma associated with a viral infection.[13–15]

In a recent Canadian series, of 570 pediatric patients with signs and symptoms suggestive of LRTI, fever was the most sensitive sign, while grunting and retractions were the most specific signs associated with alveolar infiltrates found on the chest radiograph.[16]

■ DIAGNOSIS

The diagnosis of pneumonia should be suspected in every child with fever, cough, tachypnea, respiratory distress, and crackles on chest auscultation. The presence of tachypnea, as defined earlier, is used by the World Health Organization in the diagnosis of pneumonia and is considered to have good sensitivity. To eliminate the effects of moment-to-moment variability, the best way to assess respiratory rate is over a 60-second period with the child alert and calm. Other respiratory signs such as retractions also indicate pneumonia, but no sign by itself can be used to diagnose or to rule out pneumonia. There is better interobserver agreement over signs that can be observed than for the ones that require auscultation of the chest, especially when examining infants; a high index of suspicion is paramount for this age group.[3]

Differential diagnosis includes viral bronchiolitis, asthma, cardiogenic causes of tachypnea, interstitial lung diseases, and chemical pneumonitis, especially secondary to aspiration syndromes. Infants and small children presenting with fever and respiratory signs are frequently sent for a chest radiograph and often receive antibiotic treatment for a presumptive diagnosis of bacterial pneumonia. Neither white blood cell counts nor radiology can differentiate reliably between viral and bacterial etiologies, which may indeed coexist. Radiologic signs of bilateral interstitial lung infiltrates or atelectasis, signs of bronchitis (true wheeze on auscultation), and generalized hyperinflation, though not definitive markers, are very likely to identify viral pneumonias correctly (Fig. 27-1*A* and *B*).

Tuberculosis should always be considered as a possible diagnosis, especially in endemic areas. The differential diagnosis of round pneumonias is important, and care should be taken, since secondarily infected congenital malformations or thoracic masses may have similar radiologic presentation (Fig. 27-2). Nonresolving pneumonia with persistence or recurrence of radiologic findings should alert the physician to noninfectious primary causes or infection with bacterial agents such as *Mycobacterium tuberculosis.*

■ LABORATORY TESTS

Esposito and co-workers demonstrated higher white blood cell counts and higher concentrations of C-reactive protein in children with bacterial pneumonias, but the results showed great overlap, meaning that these findings are of little help clinically in the individual child.[10] Korppi and colleagues found good specificity for cutoff levels of 60 mg/L for C-reactive protein and 35 mm/hr for erythrocyte sedimentation rate in pneumococcal pneumonias (83% and 73%, respectively), but the figures for sensitivity were much lower.[17] Other studies reported similar results.[5,13] Toikka and co-workers were able to show that higher levels of procalcitonin (≥2.0 ng/mL) and C-reactive protein (≥150 mg/mL) were associated with bacterial infection.[18]

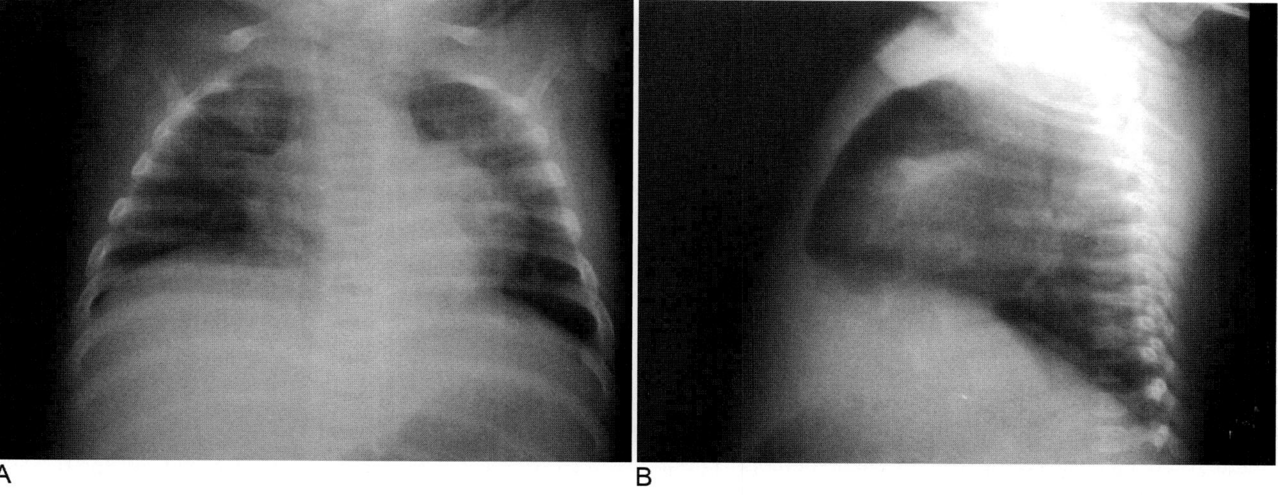

■ **FIGURE 27-1.** Viral pneumonia in a 6-month-old infant with respiratory syncytial virus–positive nasopharyngeal aspirate. **A,** Anteroposterior film with bilateral interstitial infiltrates, patchy atelectasis. **B,** Lateral film with hyperinflated lungs; increased anteroposterior volume, flattening of the diaphragm, mediastinal air cushion.

Unfortunately, in a clinical setting current laboratory tests have little value in differentiating bacterial from pneumonia caused by other agents.

ETIOLOGIC DIAGNOSIS

Different infectious agents present with similar clinical findings in CAP. Taking into account clinical and laboratory findings, in many cases a probable or possible agent can be inferred. On the other hand, only a small proportion of CAPs will have a definite pathogen identified. Various approaches have been used to try to resolve this issue.

Diagnostic methods for etiologic identification can be divided in microbiologic, immunologic, and DNA detection. The gold standard for etiologic diagnosis in CAP is either obtaining a lung puncture specimen or performing a bronchoalveolar lavage, but these are invasive methods and unacceptable for clinical purposes, with the possible exception of nosocomial or life-threatening infections.

Microbiology

Vuori-Holopainen and co-workers recently published a study in which transthoracic needle aspiration was used to obtain lung samples for viral and bacterial identification in Finnish children hospitalized for pneumonia.[19] These authors justified the procedure by citing the current increase in bacterial resistance, the change in the profile of organisms causing bacterial pneumonia secondary to the widespread use of vaccines, and the low yield of most other available techniques. The authors were able to identify a causative agent in 59% of 34 cases of CAP. Although 18% of patients developed a pneumothorax, recovery was complete in all cases. All samples were obtained from patients with unequivocal pulmonary consolidation on chest radiograph. This criterion may explain the lower yield of viruses and possibly *Mycoplasma*, as compared with other studies. Eighteen patients harbored *S. pneumoniae*, one patient had *M. pneumoniae*, and one patient had positive viral cultures (respiratory syncytial virus and parainfluenza). As in other studies after the introduction of *H. influenzae* type b vaccine, this agent was not detected in this study.

According to a Canadian consensus of experts, blood cultures should be performed in patients with suspected bacterial pneumonia or in those admitted to hospital. Although the test yield is between 1% and 30%, it may be the only chance to identify a causative pathogen.[3,13] However, worldwide, the majority of children with CAP are appropriately managed without recourse to this or any other investigation.

Sputum examination is a possible alternative for respiratory secretion sampling. It is practical for adolescent and school-aged children, but it should be interpreted with caution, since upper airway commensals, which can be pathogenic to lower airways, may contaminate the specimen. Furthermore, a child with lobar consolidation is unlikely to produce sputum in the acute phase of presentation. Zar and colleagues were able to recover pathogenic agents (*M. tuberculosis* and *Pneumocystis carinii*) from induced sputum samples (after 5% saline inhalation) in infants and young children with pneumonia from an area of high human immunodeficiency virus prevalence, suggesting a

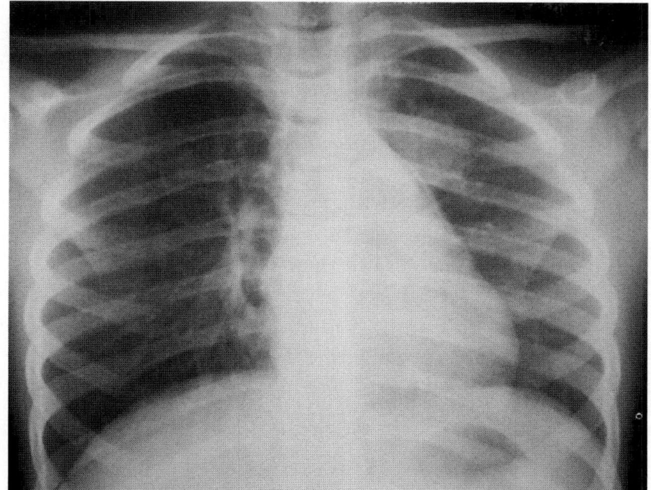

■ **FIGURE 27-2.** Round pneumonia. Opacity in the left upper segment, partially concealed by the mediastinal shadow.

causative relation between these agents and pulmonary manifestations.[20] These authors were also able to recover the more usual CAP bacteria (*S. pneumoniae, S. aureus, H. influenzae,* and *Moraxella catarrhalis*) but could not establish with certainty that the lower respiratory tract was the source in these cases, since these bacteria are also found in the upper respiratory tract. Bacterial cultures of throat or nasopharynx do not correlate well with lung parenchyma cultures and are more likely to confound than to help, with the known exception found in cystic fibrosis patients.[3,11,21] Interestingly, Zhao and co-workers, in China, were able to recover *S. pneumoniae* from tracheal aspirates in 11% of 1013 children under the age of 3 years with pneumonia or respiratory distress. These rates were much higher than 1% in control patients, suggesting a pathogenic relationship.[22] Tracheal aspirates are not without complications and should only be performed as an exception in the child with CAP.

Pleural fluid cultures may grow potential pathogens, but the usual practice of empiric antibiotic use in pneumonia decreases the sensitivity of this method. However, pleural fluid should be aspirated for culture whenever technically feasible, unless the effusion is small or the child is clinically recovering rapidly.

Serologic Tests

Detection of antigens in urine or plasma has been used, but the results are conflicting, and sensitivity and specificity are both low. In August 1999, the U.S. Food and Drug Administration approved a rapid immunochromatographic test for pneumococcal antigen detection. The sensitivity and specificity are, respectively, 86% and 94% in urine for adult patients.[11] In children, a positive test may be associated with clinical infection but may also be secondary to carriage or subclinical infection. One possible advantage of antigen detection methods is that they do not depend on bacterial viability. Serology is useful for some agents such as *M. pneumoniae, C. pneumoniae,* and *S. pneumoniae,* but paired acute and convalescent titers are needed, resulting in the diagnosis being retrospective in most cases. In children younger than 6 months of age there is only a weak immunologic response to capsular bacterial antigens, making this test less useful.[5,17] Antibodies to several different pneumococcal antigens can be measured. In a Finnish study, *S. pneumoniae* was considered to be the cause of CAP when increases in titers of these antibodies were detected (capsular polysaccharides, pneumolysin, or immune complexes specific to these antigens). The prevalence of these findings was significantly higher in children with the diagnosis of CAP than in healthy controls. Although all patients had radiologic or clinical findings suggestive of pneumonia, probably validating *S. pneumoniae* as causing the disease, the titers could have been secondary to infections at other sites as well or to nonspecific amnestic response to viral infection.[7,17,21]

An additional study showed that measuring circulating immune complexes to the pneumococcus was more sensitive than measuring either antigens or antibodies, with the exception of CAP in infants.[22]

Polymerase Chain Reaction

Polymerase chain reaction (PCR) has been used more recently as a diagnostic tool in respiratory infections. It may be applied to specimens from respiratory secretions, lung aspirate samples, or blood. Viruses, *M. pneumoniae, C. pneumoniae,* and other bacteria can be diagnosed through this method. It is a rapid diagnostic tool, but it does not differentiate carrier state from disease, except when lung aspirate samples are studied. Principi and co-workers were able to identify 194 patients with serologic evidence of acute infection with *M. pneumoniae* and 52 with *C. pneumoniae* in a cohort of 614 Italian children with LRTI.[9] Interestingly, 16 and 35 additional patients had positive PCR tests on nasopharyngeal aspirates for *M. pneumoniae* and *C. pneumoniae,* respectively. These findings suggest there may be asymptomatic carriers of these agents.[9,10] Similarly, in the series of Wubbel and colleagues of 168 pneumonia cases in children, two patients who were PCR positive for *Mycoplasma* from nasopharyngeal swab specimens had negative serology. On the other hand, none of their healthy controls had positive PCR results.[5] It is possible that quantitative PCR may solve these problems if cutoff levels can be adequately defined. More details of these and other tests for viral detection can be found in Chapter 22.

ETIOLOGY STUDIES USING DIFFERENT DIAGNOSTIC METHODS

In a prospective study, Clements and co-workers were able to diagnose the etiologic agent in 54% of CAPs.[1] They used a myriad of methods to obtain these results: blood cultures; acute serologic titers for respiratory viruses, *M. pneumoniae, Legionella,* and *Chlamydia* species; nasopharyngeal aspirates or swabs for direct immunofluorescence for the same pathogens; bacterial and viral culture and PCR on blood for *Mycoplasma* and *Chlamydia*; and nasopharyngeal aspirate for *Mycoplasma, Chlamydia,* and pertussis. Viruses, *M. pneumoniae,* and *S. pneumoniae* were the most common agents, with only 3 of 89 children showing evidence of dual infection.[1]

Juvén and colleagues studied, in a prospective fashion, 254 hospitalized Finnish children and adolescents with CAP at a mean age of 3.8 years.[23] They performed serologic tests for pneumococcus, *M. catarrhalis,* and nontypable *H. influenzae* antibodies. *Mycoplasma pneumoniae* immunoglobulin M and *Chlamydia pneumoniae* immunoglobulins M and G were measured at both acute and convalescent phases. Viral cultures and antigens were measured in nasopharyngeal secretions, and the same source was used for rhinovirus PCR testing. Blood samples for culture were obtained only when the patient appeared ill enough to warrant it. The authors were able to identify a possible causative agent in 85% of the patients. Bacteria were implicated as causal in 50% of the cases, while 30% had mixed viral-bacterial etiology, and viruses alone were responsible for 62% of the pneumonias. *Mycoplasma pneumoniae* was found in only 7% of the cases. There were significantly more viral infections (80%) in children younger than 2 years of age as compared with those who were older. Interestingly, the prevalence of individual pathogens varied from one year to the next, suggesting the occurrence of outbreaks. This was especially true for viruses and *M. pneumoniae.*

In a cohort of 613 children 2 to 14 years old, Principi and co-workers were able to identify *M. pneumoniae* and *C. pneumoniae* as the causative agents of 33.9% and 7.1%, respectively, of cases of CAP.[9] Even among younger patients, these were common ethiologic agents (20.4% and 5.2%, respectively).

Pathogens are not identified in nearly 85% of all cases of CAP, despite the use of modern diagnostic methods. This is actually the setting most physicians face in their daily practice.[11,21] In general, it is not necessary to order microbiologic investigations for children treated in ambulatory settings. Indeed, most hospitalized children should not need to undergo extensive investigations. Severe cases of presumed bacterial pneumonia should have blood and pleural fluid cultures, especially when pleural fluid is present. Acute serum samples should be saved in case a retrospective diagnosis becomes necessary.[3,14]

RADIOLOGIC FINDINGS

In general, chest radiographs are standard practice with hospitalized children for whom a diagnosis of pneumonia is being considered. The sensitivity of the test to diagnose pneumonia is approximately 75%. In early bacterial pneumonia, the finding of normal chest x-ray films is not uncommon. There is also significant variation in interpretation of these films in children. Specificity ranges from 42% to 100% in different studies because of varying definitions of pneumonia.[13]

A large proportion of children under the age of 5 with fever and leukocytosis, and without a definite source of infection have radiographic abnormalities consistent with pneumonia. In a study by Bachur and co-workers, 26% of the patients younger than 5 years who presented to the emergency department with fever, leukocytosis greater than 20,000 cells/mm^3, and no clinical findings suggestive of pneumonia actually had this diagnosis made after radiographs were done.[24] Therefore, a plain chest radiograph is part of the investigation of nonspecific clinical signs of infection in this age group.

Since chest radiographs do not change the outcome of LRTIs, recent British Thoracic Society guidelines on CAP do not recommend this examination for children older than 2 months of age cared for in an outpatient setting, whenever a clinical diagnosis of pneumonia is considered.[14,16,25] Conversely, recommendations published by Canadian experts state that chest radiographs are necessary for the diagnosis of pneumonia.[3] Certainly the degree of respiratory compromise and the child's general appearance should be included in the decision-making process. There is no evidence that performance of a chest radiograph improves outcome in children with a diagnosis of mild to moderate CAP.

Even though alveolar pneumonia is usually more frequently observed in infections by typical bacteria, compared with interstitial pneumonia, which occurs more frequently in viral pneumonias and after *Mycoplasma* and *Chlamydia* infections, it is usually impossible to make an etiologic diagnosis solely on the basis of chest radiographs.[3,12,13,17]

In the series by Clements and colleagues, no one radiologic finding was specific for any agent.[1] Similar findings were reported by Esposito and co-workers.[10] These researchers could not differentiate pneumococcal from atypical cases, although lobar and segmental consolidations were slightly more common in pneumococcal pneumonias whereas reticulonodular infiltrates were found in atypical cases. No differences were statistically significant.[10]

Kogan and co-workers observed 110 children between the ages of 1 month and 14 years with a diagnosis of CAP.[26] The first group consisted of 49 patients with clinical and radiologic findings of classic bacterial pneumonia (i.e., segmental, lobar, or alveolar consolidation). Of these patients, 9 had laboratory evidence of agents usually associated with atypical pneumonias (by positive cultures, serology, or PCR), and 10 patients had positive tests associated with typical bacterial pneumonias. In the second group, 30 out of 59 patients with a mixed alveolar-interstitial radiologic pattern had an atypical agent identified, and only two cases were caused by typical bacteria. These findings emphasize the protean radiologic findings of pneumonia agents, a situation that is particularly relevant for *M. pneumoniae*.[11,26] Similarly, Wubbel and co-workers were not able to differentiate viral, typical, or atypical on radiologic grounds alone.[5] Virkki and colleagues demonstrated in a series of 254 Finnish children that most children with an alveolar pneumonia had laboratory evidence of bacterial infection, but that interstitial infiltrates were seen on x-ray films of both viral and bacterial cases.[27]

In summary, even though alveolar infiltrates are more commonly found associated with typical bacteria, and interstitial pulmonary infiltrates with both viral infections and atypical agents, there is so much overlap of the findings that no identifiable pattern can be considered diagnostic of a specific agent.

Another important issue is that no follow-up radiographs are needed to evaluate a CAP with good clinical course. The recent British Thoracic Society guidelines suggest obtaining control radiographs only in cases of round pneumonias, lobar collapse, or clinical deterioration.[14]

STREPTOCOCCUS PNEUMONIAE

Streptococcus pneumoniae is the bacterial pathogen that most frequently causes pneumonia in children. It is responsible for more than half of the cases requiring hospital admissions.[13] In developing countries, it is estimated that 1 million children under the age of 5 years die yearly from bacterial pneumonias, most of those preventable with the use of simple and inexpensive antibiotics.

Various pneumococcus serotypes have been implicated, with distinct prevalence rates in different parts of the world.[13,22] The prevalence of penicillin resistance also varies widely throughout different countries and continents. It can be very low or higher than 40%, as found in countries such as Spain. Currently, there are websites at which anyone caring for children with CAP can check regional levels of pneumococcus resistance.[28–31]

In a Finnish series of 85 patients aged 0.4 months to 15.8 years with a diagnosis of pneumonia based on both positive blood cultures and radiographic findings, Toikka and co-workers observed that most children with a diagnosis of pneumonia had a typical illness with ill appearance, fever of 39°C or higher, leukocytosis, and lobar or segmental consolidation (Fig. 27-3).[8] However, 30% of the patients had an atypical illness, not showing all of the signs just mentioned.[8] It is interesting to note that one fourth of the patients did not have respiratory findings, presenting instead with mostly gastrointestinal symptoms. Likewise, Esposito found individuals with many different radiologic presentations for pneumococcal pneumonia, besides the typical alveolar infiltration.[10]

COMPLICATED PNEUMOCOCCAL COMMUNITY-ACQUIRED PNEUMONIAS

The most common complications associated with pneumococcal pneumonia are necrotizing pneumonia, pleural effusion, pleural empyema, and lung abscess. These complications are discussed in detail in Chapters 21 and 30. A study by Tan and colleagues compared clinical and laboratory data between patients with either complicated or uncomplicated pneumococcal pneumonia.[32] In this multicenter study in the United States,

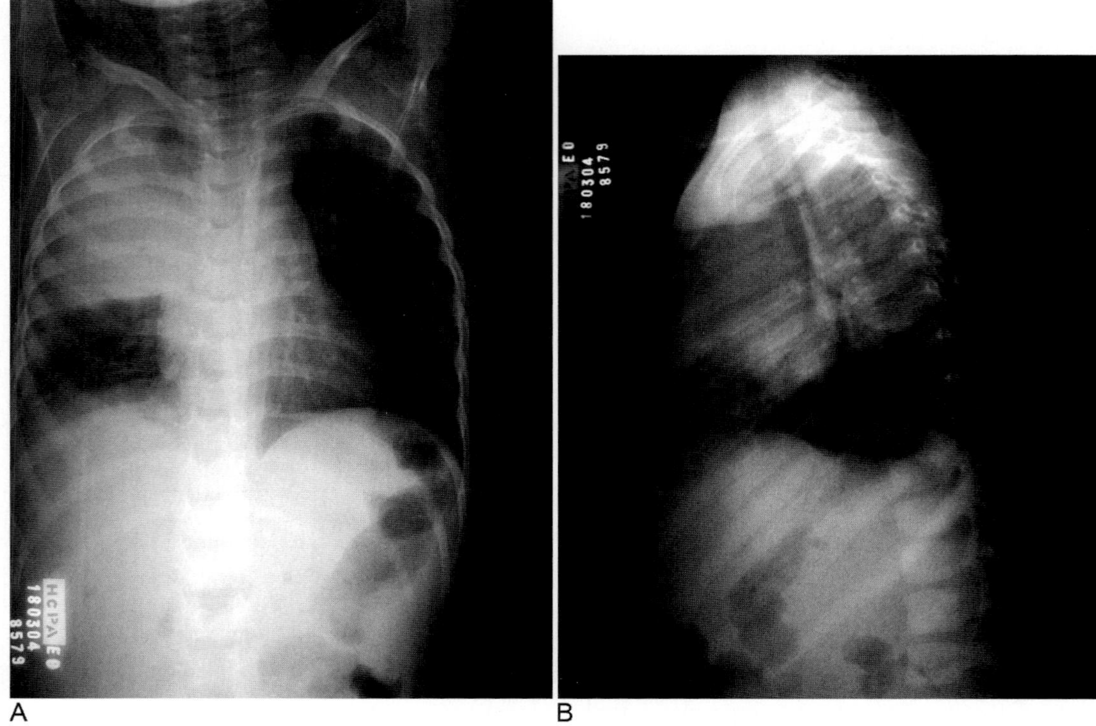

■ **FIGURE 27-3.** Pneumococcal pneumonia. Positive blood cultures for *Streptococcus pneumoniae.* Dense consolidation of upper and middle right lobes with air bronchogram. **A,** Anteroposterior view. **B,** Lateral view.

there was an increase in the proportion of complicated cases among hospitalized children. Patients with complicated disease were older (median age 45 months vs. 27 months) and were more likely to be white and have chest pain on presentation, but their disease was not more likely to be associated with antibiotic-resistant isolates. The antibiotic resistance profile is dependent on regional peculiarities, and every center should be encouraged to report local results.[17,32]

PNEUMOCOCCAL RESISTANT STRAINS

The National Committee for Clinical Laboratory Standards in the United States defines strains as resistant when the minimum inhibitory concentration (MIC) to penicillin is greater than or equal to 2 μg/mL, intermediate when the MIC is between 0.1 and 1 μg/mL, and sensitive when it is below 0.06 μg/mL. A recent report of the Drug-Resistant *Streptococcus pneumoniae* Therapeutic Working Group has suggested an upward shift on these levels, to 4, 2, and 1 μg/mL, respectively.[33] It should be emphasized, though, that the degree of penicillin resistance does not appear to cause adverse outcomes for pneumococcal CAP, since parenteral penicillin serum concentrations of as much as 15 to 18 μg/mL are achieved—much higher than the usual levels of resistance for these bacteria. Thus, it would be appropriate to modify MIC breakpoints, so that more pneumonia isolates would be classified as susceptible to penicillin.

Antibiotic resistance is usually associated with changes in the penicillin-binding sites of the transpeptidases of the bacteria. It may be associated with cross-resistance to other beta-lactams and carbapenems. In 1997, in the United States alone, 92% of resistant pneumococcus strains were serogroups 23, 6, 9, 19, and 14, which are covered by the recently available conjugated vaccines. A reduction of about 70% to 80% in the incidence of pneumococcal pneumonia after the introduction of these vaccines emphasizes the importance of this agent in these settings.[12,21,22,33]

In a study conducted in South America, penicillin resistance was associated with penicillin or amoxicillin use in the previous 3 months.[33]

Resistance to macrolides, which has increased lately, is associated with the alteration of the 50S ribosomal binding site, preventing the drug from inhibiting protein synthesis. Macrolide resistance is more likely to occur with the widespread use of this class of antibiotics in the community. An alternative mechanism explaining resistance to this group of antibiotics is the presence of efflux pumps to macrolides. The former mechanism is usually associated with high-level resistance and the latter with low-level resistance.[21,22,33]

In the Zhao series of hospitalized children, 51% of pneumococcus strains were penicillin intermediate and 8% were penicillin resistant. In addition, 86% were resistant to erythromycin, 67% to clindamycin, and 7% to ceftriaxone.[22]

OTHER BACTERIAL PATHOGENS

Haemophilus Influenzae Type B

This bacterium was once a more frequent cause of CAP, before the widespread use of appropriate *H. influenzae* type b immunization as part of the routine schedule of infant immunization. It is still an important cause of CAP in countries where these vaccines are not universally available. It affects mostly children younger than 5 years of age.

It is a fastidious gram-negative coccobacillus that requires factors V and X for growth. The most common mode of transmission is direct contact with respiratory secretions.

The radiologic findings vary from linear infiltrates and hyperinflation to bronchopneumonia. Pleural effusion is a common feature.

Group A Streptococcus and *Streptococcus Pyogenes*

This is an infrequent cause of CAP nowadays. Pneumonia is not the only presentation of group A streptococcal infections, with bacteremia and scarlet fever common, most significantly among small children. Varicella infections cause a transient immune paresis and predispose the patient to this type of pneumonia as well as skin and soft tissue infections, again mostly among young children. Measles and influenza are also associated with group A streptococcus, and a transient lessening in host defenses is believed to be the gateway to infection with previously commensal bacteria.

The radiologic presentation is protean, with unilateral or bilateral lobar, segmental, or interstitial involvement. Empyema may be observed in as many as one fourth of the cases. In some cases, serosanguineous pleural effusion may be a clinical finding. The initial manifestations are usually fever, chills, dyspnea, chest pain, and cough that are of abrupt onset. It can present with a severe clinical picture that can progress to death in almost three fourths of invasive infections.

Staphylococcus Aureus

Staphylococcus infection is currently a rare cause of pneumonia in immunocompetent children. It is almost exclusively a disease of infants. *Staphylococcus aureus* is a gram-positive coccus that looks like cluster of grapes under the microscope. The organism produces coagulase, which helps to differentiate it from other species of the same genus. Most pathogenic strains are capsulated. Most cases of pneumonia are secondary to inhalation of the infecting agent. In rare cases, it can be the result of bacteremic spread, usually in situations in which a predisposing factor is present (e.g., a catheter or intravenous drug use).

Staphylococcus aureus pneumonia tends to present as an acute and severe illness, especially because many antibiotics used to treat CAP do not provide appropriate coverage for this agent. Radiologic findings include bronchopneumonia with alveolar infiltrates, which is more commonly unilateral. The infiltrates may coalesce and may evolve to large areas of consolidation and cavitation. Destruction of bronchial walls may lead to air trapping and pneumatocele formation in about half of the cases. Pleural effusion and empyema are found in as many as 90% of the cases. Pneumothorax and pyopneumothorax are common complications. In the case of hematogenic spread of *S. aureus,* the radiologic picture is one of multiple bilateral pulmonary infiltrates that may cavitate. An increase in white blood cell count is usual but is not sufficiently sensitive or specific to suggest the etiologic diagnosis. Although the appearance of staphylococcal pneumatoceles may be dramatic, usually once the infection has been overcome, the pneumatoceles resolve completely over a few months.

Infrequent Agents

Moraxella catarrhalis, nontypable *H. influenzae, Legionella* sp., and *Klebsiella pneumoniae* are uncommon bacterial causes of CAP in immunocompetent patients, as are such other agents as fungi, rickettsia, and parasites.[4,5,7,11,12,17]

GENERAL MANAGEMENT

Infants and children with mild and moderate LRTIs can be safely cared for at home. In this situation, the child usually should be reexamined within 48 hours of the beginning of treatment.

According to the British Thoracic Society guidelines, an SaO_2 of 92% or less, cyanosis, respiratory rate greater than 70 breaths per minute, difficulty in breathing, intermittent apnea, grunting, inability to feed, and a family incapable of providing appropriate observation or supervision are indicators for hospital admission among infants.[14] In the case of older children, these indicators are an SaO_2 of 92% or less, cyanosis, respiratory rate greater than 50 breaths per minute, difficulty in breathing, grunting, signs of dehydration, or a family incapable of providing either appropriate observation or supervision. A Canadian board of experts includes also age younger than 6 months as lowering the threshold for admission.[3]

The World Health Organization has long been applying similar criteria in their worldwide programs aiming to prevent the mortality of CAP in children younger than 5 years of age. Studies carried out in Papua New Guinea[34] and in Gambia[35] suggested that pneumonia could be detected through simple signs and symptoms and yet present high sensitivity and specificity (i.e., using a cutoff respiratory rate of 50 breaths per minute and/or the presence of subcostal chest indrawing).

General management for hospital inpatients includes oxygen to keep saturation above 92%, antipyretics, and IV fluids if hydration is compromised by breathlessness or fatigue. Fluid intake should be carefully monitored, because pneumonia can be complicated by hyponatremia secondary to the syndrome of inappropriate antidiuretic hormone secretion. The benefit of nasogastric tube feeding should be weighed against its potential for respiratory compromise due to obstruction of a nostril, or by worsening gastroesophageal reflux by interfering with lower esophageal sphincter function.

There is no role for chest physiotherapy in the management of CAP, and it should thus not be performed. Some studies have even shown increase in fever duration with the use of this practice.[14,36]

TREATMENT WITH ANTIBIOTICS

Since viruses are the sole cause of many cases of pneumonia in childhood, it is appropriate not to treat every child with antibiotics. However, therapeutic decisions can be difficult, because most tests do not adequately differentiate viral from bacterial infection in the individual child. An additional issue is the knowledge that some patients harbor mixed viral and bacterial agents.[5,11]

The problem of bacterial resistance to antibiotics has increased steadily in the last few years, and it is certainly related to their overuse in situations in which viral involvement is quite probable or the illness is trivial and self-limiting, such as an upper respiratory infection. Hence, it is preferable to restrict antibiotics as much as possible and to use narrow-spectrum agents whenever appropriate. It is believed that less antibiotic pressure limits the emergence of bacterial resistance.[11,21] Prior antibiotic therapy, daycare attendance, travel, exposure to infections, and coexisting morbidities are risk factors for resistance.[21] It is also important to keep in mind that, in an era of vaccines against *H. influenzae* type b and *S. pneumoniae*, previously effective antibiotic regimens should be reevaluated.

Although no recent studies have addressed the issue of comparing use of antibiotics versus their nonuse, it is common sense to use them whenever a bacterial pneumonia is the most probable diagnosis. This diagnosis is especially probable when CAP develops after several days of nonspecific respiratory illness.[11]

Since a definitive etiologic diagnosis is more the exception than the rule, usually antibiotics are started on an empiric basis. Regional prevalences of CAP-causing agents should surely be taken into account. Macrolides, which are effective against *Mycoplasma* and *Chlamydia* spp., are especially attractive treatment options because they cover most common community-prevalent bacteria as well. A 3-day course of azithromycin was compared to a 5-day course in the treatment of CAP, without significant differences in outcomes.[37]

Randomized Controlled and Epidemiologic-Based Studies

Few studies compare, in a well-designed fashion, different classes of antibiotics for the treatment of childhood pneumonia. Since most children in the developed world do well with whatever treatment is given, randomized controlled studies would have to involve large numbers of patients to be able to detect significant differences between treatments. Most of the existing recommendations are based on expert opinion.

Vuori-Holopainen and colleagues randomly assigned 178 hospitalized Finnish children with evidence of either pneumonia or other acute nonmeningeal infections to receive either procaine penicillin or cefuroxime.[38] Of the 154 children completing the study, 59 had evidence of pneumococcal infection. The outcomes were similar between groups with full recovery in the great majority of the patients, and the authors concluded that penicillin remains a valid treatment for pneumonia. However, the adequacy of the sample size must be questioned.

Antibiotics for children with CAP can be given orally, since well-absorbed drugs can achieve the serum concentrations required for a good clinical outcome. Possible exceptions for this recommendation are gastric intolerance, severe signs and symptoms, or age younger than 2 months. In the study of Tsarouhas and co-workers, 170 children seen in outpatient clinics with presumed bacterial pneumonia were assigned to randomly receive either oral amoxicillin or IM procaine penicillin, and both groups had similar clinical outcomes.[39] In some situations an acceptable strategy could be an initial parenteral dose followed by an oral regimen. In yet another study, Chumpa and colleagues showed that for 110 patients with pneumonia and a positive blood culture for pneumococcus, one initial parenteral dose followed by oral antibiotics at discharge was associated with better outcomes in terms of fever improvement and a lower probability of hospital admission at follow-up, when compared with patients receiving oral antibiotics alone.[40] In a Latin America–based study, pneumococcal pneumonia in 274 children younger than 5 years responded well to either penicillin or ampicillin, independent of the resistant status of the bacterium. Seventy-eight percent of children with penicillin-resistant pneumococci pneumonia (MIC $\geq$ 2 μg/mL) were kept on either penicillin or ampicillin and had favorable outcomes. The authors do not mention the reason for changing antibiotics in the remaining 22% of children.[31]

Kogan and co-workers randomized 106 patients with pneumonia who could be treated as outpatients to receive either azithromycin or erythromycin as first choice of antibiotics whenever radiologic and clinical signs suggested an atypical causative agent, or amoxicillin (75 mg/kg/day) if the situation suggested a typical bacterial pathogen. Most clinical and radiologic outcomes were similar between the two treatment arms, with an earlier radiologic recovery in the azithromycin group.[26] Esposito and colleagues compared clinical response of pneumococcal and atypical pneumonias to macrolides and beta-lactams used either alone or in combination.[10] In that study, 196 patients were given antibiotic treatment without knowledge of etiology, since most cases were diagnosed retrospectively and followed the attending physician's choice of treatment. Pneumococcal infections had better clinical responses with beta-lactams used alone or in association with a macrolide (96.4% and 100%, respectively) than with the use of macrolides used alone (85.7%). Resistance of this microbial agent to macrolides is a possible explanation. On the other hand, atypical agents responded better to macrolides alone or combined with a beta-lactam (92.9% and 100%) than to a beta-lactam alone (52.4%). These authors suggest that this association should be considered when etiology is unknown.[10] Wubbel and co-workers randomized 168 pediatric patients to receive either azithromycin or amoxicillin-clavulanate if the patient was younger than 5 years, or erythromycin for older children. Using resolution of clinical signs and symptoms as their main outcome, antibiotic response was not significantly different among the three regimens, irrespective of CAP etiology.[5] Therapeutic failures with first-line oral beta-lactams are frequently due to *M. pneumoniae* infection, for which this class of antibiotics do not offer coverage. It is appropriate to treat even young children as outpatients. Shah and colleagues demonstrated that 580 children aged 2 to 24 months with pneumonia treated at home were at low risk for bacteremia if they did not have other signs of serious disease.[41]

Other studies reviewed the issue of treatment duration. A multicenter study from Pakistan, which enrolled 2188 children between the ages of 2 and 59 months, showed equivalence of a 3-day or 5-day course of amoxicillin in the treatment of nonsevere pneumonia, according to the World Health Organization's criteria. Of note were a low prevalence of positive radiographic findings (14%) and a relatively high rate of treatment failure (20%).[42]

Since most of the recommendations on antibiotic choice are a result of expert opinion, either alone or in consensus, the following recommendations are also based on the authors' view, based as much as possible on existing evidence.

Choice of Antibiotics

The choice of antibiotics is usually based on clinical features and most specifically on prevalence data for different organisms in different age groups. Though not a common feature, pneumococcus resistance rates of a specific locale also figure importantly in the decision-making process.

When a causative agent is known, narrow-spectrum antibiotics are preferred. Table 27-2 shows appropriate antibiotic choices, based on bacteriologic tests and MICs. As discussed earlier, penicillins can be used for most pneumococcal pneumonias, unless highly resistant strains are identified. In real-life situations, causative agents are rarely identified. In these cases, a model associating age and clinical presentation is probably the best guide.

Hospitalized patients with CAP caused by intermediate susceptible strains (0.1–1.0 μg/mL) respond well to adequate doses of beta-lactam antibiotics (e.g., 100,000–300,000 U/kg/day of penicillin). A possible exception, warranting precaution, would

TABLE 27-2. Choice of antibiotic treatment for community-acquired pneumonia when typical bacteria are identified

Pathogen	First Choice	Other
Streptococcus pneumoniae, penicillin susceptible or intermediate	Penicillin, ampicillin, or high-dose amoxicillin	Cefuroxime, ceftriaxone, azithromycin
S. pneumoniae, penicillin resistant (MIC > 2 μg/mL)	Second- or third-generation cephalosporins for sensitive strains; vancomycin	
Staphylococcus aureus	Methicillin/oxacillin	Vancomycin or teicoplanin (for MRSA)
Haemophilus influenzae	Amoxicillin	Amoxicillin/clavulanate, cefuroxime, ceftriaxone, other second- and third-generation cephalosporins
Moraxella catarrhalis	Amoxicillin/clavulanate	Cefuroxime

MIC, minimum inhibitory concentration; MRSA, methicillin-resistant *S. aureus*.

be the cases with very high resistance levels (MIC ≥ 2 μg/mL). Additional studies are required to determine at what level of penicillin resistance there should be a change in therapeutic strategy. Also, different sites of infection would warrant a different approach. This may be the case for middle ear or central nervous system infections. One of the reasons for the better response in pneumonia may be the increased blood perfusion in alveoli as compared with those organs.[33,37] A position paper by the U.S. Centers for Disease Control and Prevention was recently published supporting the findings that intermediate susceptible strains of pneumococcus respond well to high doses of beta-lactams.[33]

High doses of penicillin, ampicillin, and amoxicillin have been recommended whenever intermediate susceptible pneumococcus strains are considered. Some experts suggest an option with third-generation cephalosporins such as ceftriaxone or cefotaxime, since these beta-lactams have greater affinity to pneumococcus. Clinical outcomes data supporting these choices are lacking.

Children between 4 months and 5 years of age with CAP are most likely infected by pneumococcus, and amoxicillin, penicillin, or ampicillin are the drugs of choice (see Tables 27-1 and 27-2). Some experts suggest macrolides, such as azithromycin, clarithromycin, or roxithromycin as optional choices, because they are able to cover both typical and atypical bacteria. Lately, pneumococci have become increasingly macrolide resistant, so it is our suggestion to leave macrolides as a second-line treatment in situations where atypical infections are either probable or detected by laboratory tests.

In regions of the world where *H. influenzae* type b immunization is not available, clinicians should consider amoxicillin/clavulanate, cefprozil, cefdinir, cefpodoxime proxetil, cefuroxime, or ceftriaxone. The addition of a beta-lactamase inhibitor does not confer additional coverage for pneumococcus, since this is not the resistance-associated mechanism.

In recent years, *S. aureus* has become less frequently associated as an agent with CAP (especially among developed societies). In cases of positive cultures or a suggestive clinical picture, antibiotic coverage against this pathogen should be added (e.g., methicillin, oxacillin, clindamycin, or vancomycin in case of methicillin-resistant *S. aureus* [MRSA] strains). Thankfully, MRSA is generally not common in the community; however, expert advice should be sought in cases of CAP caused by suspected MRSA.

Neonates with CAP should have a combination of intravenous (IV) ampicillin and gentamicin. Methicillin/oxacillin may be needed if the clinical picture is suggestive of *S. aureus* infection. For children between 3 weeks and 3 months old with interstitial infiltrates visible on chest x-ray film, a macrolide should be used to cover for agents such as *C. trachomatis*, *B. pertussis*, and *U. urealyticum*.

Infants and young children with CAP can receive ampicillin, amoxicillin, penicillin, or even a third-generation cephalosporin orally, unless this is prevented by vomiting, or when the patient is so sick that hospitalization and parenteral antibiotics are needed. In cases of necrotizing pneumonia, coverage for *S. aureus* and gram-negative rods should include ceftriaxone or cefuroxime, plus oxacillin, nafcillin, cefazolin, or clindamycin, or even vancomycin in cases of MRSA. Atypical bacteria are not common agents in this age range and should be considered only for unresponsive cases. Vancomycin or teicoplanin should be reserved for severely ill patients, when coverage for high-resistant pneumococcus is desired, since overuse may lead to increased resistance in other pathogens. If the clinical and radiologic findings suggest the possibility of an atypical agent, then a macrolide is the first choice, and a beta-lactam will be added in cases of poor response.

Table 27-3 and Box 27-1 summarize the aforementioned recommendations, including suggested drug regimens.

SLOWLY RESOLVING PNEUMONIAS

This term refers to persistence of either clinical or radiologic findings of pneumonia beyond the normal time course during which one would expect the infection to resolve. One such

TABLE 27-3. Choice of antibiotic treatment for community-acquired pneumonia according to age and clinical picture

Age/Clinical Picture	Inpatient	Outpatient
Newborn	Ampicillin + gentamicin	—
3 weeks to 3 months, interstitial infiltrate, not toxic	Macrolides	Macrolides
4 months to 4 years	Penicillin or ampicillin; add macrolide if not responding	Amoxicillin
5 years or older: Alveolar infiltrate, pleural effusion, toxic appearance	Penicillin or ampicillin; add macrolide if not responding	Macrolide; amoxicillin
5 years or older: Interstitial infiltrate	Macrolides; consider adding a beta-lactam if not responding	Macrolide

BOX 27-1 **Suggested Antibiotic Dosages for the Treatment of Community-Acquired Pneumonia**

Penicillin

100,000 U/kg/day, q4h or q6h (if resistant strains are to be covered, up to 400,000 U/kg/day, for 7–10 days)

Ampicillin

50 mg/kg/day, q6h, for 7–10 days

Amoxicillin

50 mg/kg/day, q8h or q12h, for 7–10 days (if resistant strains are to be covered, dose can be increased up to 100 mg/kg/day)

Amoxicillin/clavulanate

40 mg/kg/day of amoxicillin for 7–10 days

Oxacillin/nafcillin

150 mg/kg/day, q6h, maximum 12 g/day, for 14–21 days

Cefuroxime

Oral

30 mg/kg/day, q12h, for 5–7 days

IV

150 mg/kg/day, q8h, for 7–10 days

Ceftriaxone

50–75 mg/kg/day, qd, for 7–10 days

Cefotaxime

200 mg/kg/day, q8h, for 7–10 days

Cefprozil

15–30 mg/kg/day, q12h, maximum 1 g/day, for 7–10 days

Cefdinir

14 mg/kg/day, q12h, for 7–10 days

Cefpodoxime proxetil

10 mg/kg/day, q12h, maximum 400 mg/day, for 7–10 days

Azithromycin

Oral

10 mg/kg/day, qd, for 3–5 days

Clarithromycin

15 mg/kg/day, q12h, maximum 1 g/day, for 5–7 days

Erythromycin

40 mg/kg/day, q6h, for 5–7 days

Vancomycin

40–60 mg/kg/day, q6h, for 7–10 days (14–21 days for *Staphylococcus aureus*)

Gentamicin

7.5 mg/kg/day, q8h, for 7–10 days

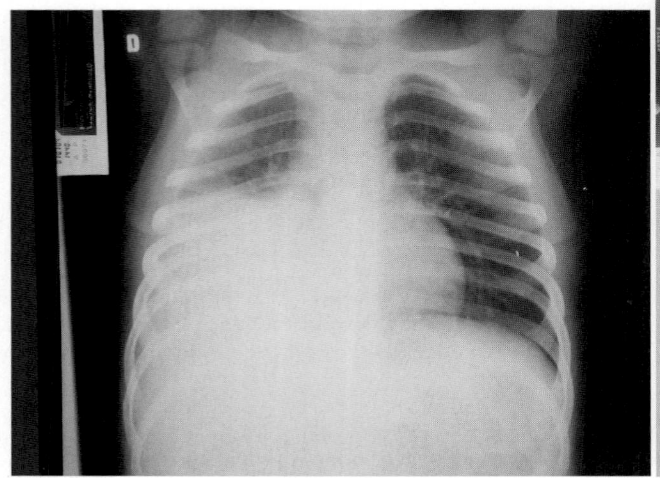

A

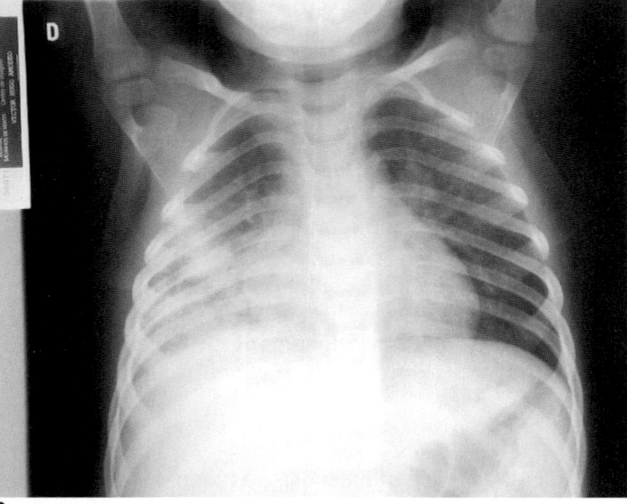

B

■ **FIGURE 27-4.** Slowly resolving pneumonia. **A,** A 3-year-old child with presumptive diagnosis of pneumococcal pneumonia. Lower and middle lobe consolidation, treatment started with IV benzyl penicillin. This evolved into a pleural effusion, which later necessitated a thoracotomy. **B,** The same child, radiographed 3 weeks after first diagnosis; good clinical condition on discharge. Aeration of previously consolidated areas.

situation is whenever patients fail to respond to conventional treatment, and another is when clinical symptoms or radiologic signs persist even in the presence of clinical improvement. It is generally accepted that between 48 and 96 hours after empiric "adequate" antibiotic treatment, patients with CAP should show significant clinical improvement. During this period, it is not recommended that antibiotics be changed unless there is clear evidence that other microorganisms not covered by the initial empiric choice of therapy are involved (e.g., *S. aureus* with developing pleural effusion or the presence of pneumatoceles, when initial therapy was with amoxicillin). Empyema or underlying lung abscess should be considered whenever there is persistence of fever with or without pleuritic pain (basal segment pneumonias may mimic acute abdominal pain). These situations often require additional management, rather than a change in antibiotic regimen (Fig. 27-4*A* and *B*). They are discussed in more detail in Chapters 21 and 30.

Such influences as inappropriate choice of drugs, unexpectedly resistant microorganisms, inadequate dosage, or poor compliance if oral therapy has been chosen can result in slowly resolving CAP and should always be considered.

Pneumonias that are either slow to resolve or unresponsive may be secondary to antibiotic failure. This may be the case with highly resistant strains of pneumococcus. In other instances, inappropriate choice of antibiotics may be an issue, as when there is inadequate coverage for atypical organisms. In endemic areas tuberculosis should always be considered, since its radiologic appearance may mimic usual bacterial pneumonia.

Inadequate host defenses or other coexisting diseases such as ciliary dyskinesia, cystic fibrosis, and noninfectious causes may also be associated with slowly responding or nonresponsive pneumonias. A number of differential diagnosis tests for such possible comorbidity should be considered, including bronchoscopy with bronchoalveolar lavage, chest computed tomography scan, and lung biopsies. Blood, pleural, and sputum cultures, as well as PCR should be considered for the diagnosis of possible atypical microorganisms.

When there is good clinical improvement but persistent radiographic findings, it should be remembered that in many cases complete radiographic resolution may take several months. Radiographic clearing after resolution of pneumococcal pneumonias may take as long as 3 months. Resolution time may be even longer for *S. aureus* pneumonia. Even viral pneumonias may lead to radiographic changes many months after the acute event.

Other conditions such as persistent alveolar collapse and/or atelectasis may be secondary to obstruction of the bronchial lumen, from either foreign body aspiration or lymph node enlargement. Congenital malformations such as pulmonary sequestration, bronchogenic cysts, or other mediastinal masses may also be causes for delayed radiologic improvement, especially if the appearance resembles round pneumonias. It is important to ensure adequate follow-up of all children with CAP who do not run a typical course with full resolution of their symptoms and signs.

REFERENCES

1. Clements H, Stephenson T, Gabriel V, Harrison T, Millar M, Smyth A, Tong W, Linton CJ: Rationalised prescribing for community-acquired pneumonia. A closed loop audit. Arch Dis Child 2000;83:320–324.
2. McCracken GH Jr: Etiology and treatment of pneumonia. Pediatr Infect Dis J 2000;19:373–377.
3. Jadavji T, Law B, Lebel MH, Kennedy WA, Gold R, Wang EEL: A practical guide for the diagnosis and treatment of pediatric pneumonia. Can Med Assoc J 1997;156:S703–S711.
4. Mulholland K: Magnitude of the problem of childhood pneumonia. Lancet 1999;354:590–592.
5. Wubbel L, Muniz L, Ahmed A, Trujillo M, Carubelli C, McCoig C, Abramo T, Leinonen M, McCracken GH Jr: Etiology and treatment of community-acquired pneumonia in ambulatory children. Pediatr Infect Dis J 1999;18:98–104.
6. Mulholland EK, Adegbola RA: The Gambian *Haemophilus influenzae* type b vaccine trial. What does it tell us about the burden of *Haemophilus influenzae* type B disease? Pediatr Infect Dis J 1998;17:S123–S125.
7. Heiskanen-Kosma T, Korppi M, Jokinen C, Kurki S, Heiskanen L, Juvonen H, Kallinen S, Stén M, Tarkiainen A, Rönnberg PR, Kleemola M, Mäkelä PH, Leinonen M: Etiology of childhood pneumonia. Serologic results of a prospective, population-based study. Pediatr Infect Dis J 1998; 17:986–991.
8. Toikka P, Juvén T, Virkki R, Leinonen M, Mertsola J, Ruuskanen O: *Streptococcus pneumoniae* and *Mycoplasma pneumoniae* coinfection in community-acquired pneumonia. Arch Dis Child 2000;83:413–414.
9. Principi N, Esposito S, Blasi F, Allegra L, and the Mowgli Study Group: Role of *Mycoplasma pneumoniae* and *Chlamydia pneumoniae* in children with community-acquired lower respiratory tract infections. Clin Infect Dis 2001;32:1281–1289.
10. Esposito S, Bosis S, Cavagna R, Faelli N, Begliatti E, Marchisio P, Blasi F, Bianchi C, Principi N: Characteristics of *Streptococcus pneumoniae* and atypical bacterial infections in children 2–5 years of age with community-acquired pneumonia. Clin Infect Dis 2002;35:1345–1352.
11. Nelson JD: Community-acquired pneumonia in children. Guidelines for treatment. Pediatr Infect Dis J 2000;19:251–253.
12. McIntosh K: Community-acquired pneumonia in children. N Engl J Med 2002;346:429–437.
13. Ruuskanen O, Mertsola J: Childhood community-acquired pneumonia. Semin Respir Infect 1999;14:163–172.
14. Coote NMA, Craig J, Heath PT, McKenzie AS, Saul P, Smyth R, Thomson AH for Pneumonia in Childhood Guideline Development Group of BTS Standards of Care. BTS guidelines for the management of community-acquired pneumonia in childhood. Thorax 2002;57(Suppl 1):i1–i24.
15. Russell G: Community-acquired pneumonia. Arch Dis Child 2001;85: 445–446.
16. Lynch T, Platt R, Gouin S, Larson C, Patenaude Y: Can we predict which children with clinically suspected pneumonia will have the presence of focal infiltrates on chest radiographs? Pediatrics 2004;113:e186–e189.
17. Korppi M, Heiskanen-Kosma T, Leinonen M: White blood cells, C-reactive protein and erythrocyte sedimentation rate in pneumococcal pneumonia in children. Eur Respir J 1997;10:1125–1129.
18. Toikka P, Irjala K, Juven T, Virkki R, Mertsola J, Leinonen M, Ruuskanen O: Serum procalcitonin, C-reactive protein and interleukin-6 for distinguishing bacterial and viral pneumonia in children. Pediatr Infect Dis J 2000;19: 598–602.
19. Vuori-Holopainen E, Salo E, Saxén H, Hedman K, Hyypiä T, Lahdenperä R, Leinonen M, Tarkka E, Vaara M, Peltola H: Etiological diagnosis of childhood pneumonia by use of transthoracic needle aspiration and modern microbiological methods. Clin Infect Dis 2002;34:583–590.
20. Zar HJ, Tannenbaum E, Hansio D, Hussey G: Sputum induction as a diagnostic tool for community-acquired pneumonia in infants and young children from a high HIV prevalence area. Pediatr Pulmonol 2003;36:58–62.
21. Bradley JS: Management of community-acquired pediatric pneumonia in an era of increasing antibiotic resistance and conjugate vaccines. Pediatr Infect Dis J 2002;21:592–598.
22. Zhao GM, Black S, Shinefield H, Wang CQ, Zhang YH, Lin YZ, Lu JL, Guo YF, Jiang QW: Serotype distribution and antimicrobial resistance patterns in *Streptococcus pneumoniae* isolates from hospitalized pediatric patients with respiratory infections in Shangai, China. Pediatr Infect Dis J 2003;22:739–742.
23. Juvén T, Mertsola J, Waris M, Leinonen M, Meurman O, Roivainen M, Eskola J, Saikku P, Ruuskanen O: Etiology of community-acquired pneumonia in 254 hospitalized children. Pediatr Infect Dis J 2000;19:293–298.
24. Bachur R, Perry H, Harper MB: Occult pneumonias. Empiric chest radiographs in febrile children with leukocytosis. Ann Emerg Med 1999;33: 166–173.
25. Swingler GH, Hussey GD, Zwarenstein M: Randomised controlled trial of clinical outcome after chest radiograph in ambulatory acute lower-respiratory infection in children. Lancet 1998;351:404–408.
26. Kogan R, Martiínez MA, Rubilar L, Payá E, Quevedo I, Puppo H, Girardi G, Castro-Rodriguez JA: Comparative randomized trial of azithromycin versus

erythromycin and amoxicillin for treatment of community-acquired pneumonia in children. Pediatr Pulmonol 2003;35:91–98.
27. Virkki R, Juven T, Rikalainen H, Svedström E, Mertsola J, Ruuskanen O: Differentiation of bacterial and viral pneumonia in children. Thorax 2002;57:438–441.
28. Eijkman-Winkler Centre for Medical Microbiology, Infectious Diseases and Inflammation. Available at http://www.ewi.med.uu.nl/ewi_en/.
29. Australian Government, Department of Health and Ageing. Available at http://www.health.gov.au/internet/wcms/Publishing.nsf/Content/Communicable+Diseases+Australia-1.
30. European Antimicrobial Resistance Surveillance System. Available at www.earss.rivm.nl.
31. Deeks SL, Palacio R, Ruvinsky R, Kertesz DA, Hortal M, Rossi A, Spika JS, Fabio JLD, The *Streptococcus pneumoniae* Working Group: Risk factors and course of illness among children with invasive penicillin-resistant *Streptococcus pneumoniae*. Pediatrics 1999;103:409–413.
32. Tan TQ, Mason EO Jr, Wald ER, Barson WJ, Schutze GE, Bradley, JS, Givner LB, Yogev R, Kim KS, Kaplan SL: Clinical characteristics of children with complicated pneumonia caused by *Streptococcus pneumoniae*. Pediatrics 2002;110:1–6.
33. Heffelfinger JD, Dowell SF, Jorgensen JH, Klugman KP, Mabry LR, Musher DM, Plouffe JF, Räkowsky A, Schuchat A, Whitney CG, and the Drug-Resistant *Streptococcus pneumoniae* Therapeutic Working Group: Management of community-acquired pneumonia in the era of pneumococcal resistance. Arch Intern Med 2000;160:1399–1408.
34. Shann F, Harta K, Thomas D: Acute lower respiratory tract infections in children. Possible criteria for selection of patients for antibiotic therapy and hospital admission. Bull WHO 1984;62:749–753.
35. Campbell H, Byass P, Forgie JM, O'Neill KP, Lloyd EN, Greenwood BM: Trial of cotrimoxazole versus procaine penicillin with ampicillin in treatment of community-acquired pneumonia in young Gambian children. Lancet 1988;2:1182–1184.
36. Wallis C, Prasad A: Who needs chest physiotherapy? Moving from anecdote to evidence. Arch Dis Child 1999;80:393–397.
37. Ficnar B, Huzjak N, Oreskovic K, Matrapazovski M, Klinar I: Azithromycin: 3-day versus 5-day course in the treatment of respiratory tract infections in children. Croatian Azithromycin Study Group. J Chemother 1997;9:38–43.
38. Vuori-Holopainen E, Peltola H, Kallio MJT for the SE-TU Study Group: Narrow versus broad-spectrum parenteral antimicrobials against common infections of childhood. A prospective and randomized comparison between penicillin and cefuroxime. Eur J Pediatr 2000;159:878–884.
39. Tsarouhas N, Shaw KN, Hodinka RL, Bell LM: Effectiveness of intramuscular penicillin versus oral amoxicillin in the early treatment of outpatient pediatric pneumonia. Pediatr Emerg Care 1998;14:338–341.
40. Chumpa A, Bachur RG, Harper MB: Bacteremia-associated pneumococcal pneumonia and benefit of initial parenteral antimicrobial therapy. Pediatr Infect Dis J 1999;18:1081–1085.
41. Shah SS, Alpern ER, Zwerling L, McGowan KL, Bell LM: Risk of bacteremia in young children with pneumonia treated as outpatient. Arch Pediatr Adolesc Med 2003;157:389–392.
42. Pakistan Multicentre Amoxicillin Short Course Therapy (MASCOT) Pneumonia Study Group: Clinical efficacy of 3 days versus 5 days of oral amoxicillin for treatment of childhood pneumonia. A multicentre double-blind trial. Lancet 2002;360:35–41.

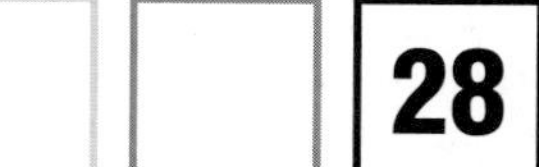

28 Pulmonary Infections in the Immunocompromised Pediatric Host

Dennis C. Stokes, MD

The diagnosis of pulmonary infections in immunocompromised pediatric patients remains a difficult challenge. Immunocompromised pediatric patients include the rare patients with congenital defects of host defense and defects in cell-mediated or humoral immunity, but the major expansion of this population has occurred with increased bone marrow and solid-organ transplantation, successful treatment of childhood malignancy, and the acquired immunodeficiency syndrome (AIDS) epidemic. These developments have significantly increased the population of children at risk for opportunistic infections, and the list of organisms that lead to pulmonary infections in these groups is extensive and growing. This chapter will review some of these common pulmonary infections and describe a rational diagnostic approach based on knowledge of the common pulmonary pathogens seen in various immunodeficiency disorders. The many diagnostic tools that are available, including bronchoscopy and open-lung biopsy (OLB), can generally be used to arrive at a specific diagnosis, although the specific yield of these procedures in pediatric patients continues to evolve as risk groups change and new pathogens arise.

The terms *opportunistic pathogens*, *immunodeficiency*, and *compromised host* have a relatively short history and were first used in the 1960s and 1970s, for patients with primary immunodeficiencies and when improved therapeutic programs for childhood malignancies (principally acute lymphocytic leukemia) resulted in longer survival and increased numbers of children at risk for opportunistic infections.[1] *Pneumocystis jirovecii* (previously *carinii*), previously identified as a pathogen primarily in outbreaks in malnourished infants, emerged as a major cause of pneumonia in the 1960s but then declined in importance in this population with the development of effective prophylaxis.[2] Varicella-zoster pneumonia also declined in frequency with effective preventive measures and antiviral therapy. Bacterial pneumonias were generally treatable with antimicrobial therapy, but fungal pneumonias such as those caused by *Aspergillus* and *Mucor* spp. became the major problem in children with prolonged neutropenia such as those receiving intensive chemotherapy for nonlymphocytic leukemias and bone marrow transplantation (BMT). The availability of trimethoprim-sulfamethoxazole (co-trimoxazole, TMP-SMZ) treatment for *Pneumocystis* pneumonia and broad-spectrum antibiotics for other pathogens provided a strong rationale for use of empiric treatment of pneumonia in immunocompromised patients, particularly when there was no effective antiviral therapy for cytomegalovirus (CMV) and other viral pathogens. This empiric treatment approach generated considerable debate on the role and timing of OLB that continues today. Pediatric flexible bronchoscopy has provided a specific diagnosis for many opportunistic infections, and newer minimally invasive techniques have reduced the low morbidity associated with OLB. The epidemic of human immunodeficiency virus infection in the 1980s resulted in a major new group of immunocompromised children, and *Pneumocystis* reemerged as the major pulmonary pathogen in this group, both as presenting infection and as cause of death. The introduction of highly active antiretroviral therapy for human immunodeficiency virus has changed the epidemiology of *Pneumocystis* pneumonia (PCP) and other pulmonary infections in AIDS with a dramatic reduction in risk.[3] Bone marrow and other tissue transplantation has continued to expand, and major noninfectious pulmonary complications have been described in these populations, including bronchiolitis obliterans in bone marrow and lung transplant patients and lymphoid interstitial pneumonia in pediatric AIDS. Ganciclovir/immunoglobulin has proved useful in the prevention and treatment of CMV pneumonitis in high-risk populations, increasing the importance of early diagnosis of CMV.[4] Fungal pathogens continue to be important, along with rarer saprophytic organisms resistant to antifungal therapy.[5]

CLINICAL PRESENTATION

Clinical presentations of pneumonia in the immunocompromised patient are often nonspecific and generally provide little help to the clinician seeking a specific diagnosis. Patients with an abnormal ability to deal with infection often have an atypical course when infected with a "usual" childhood respiratory pathogen. For example, the common respiratory viruses, respiratory syncytial virus and parainfluenza virus, commonly lead to more serious disease in immunocompromised patients.[6] Varicella-zoster, influenza, and measles are all potentially devastating pulmonary infections when they occur in immunocompromised hosts. Although adenovirus is capable of causing severe pneumonia in any child, it is particularly devastating in immunocompromised hosts and may exceed varicella-zoster virus (VZV) and *Pneumocystis* as a cause of fatal diffuse pneumonias in high-risk populations such as those undergoing BMT.[7]

The "opportunistic" pathogens are those typically not seen except in the patient with altered host defense, and when a patient is known or suspected to have an underlying immunodeficiency, these pathogens have to be considered. *Pneumocystis jirovecii* (previously *carinii*) pneumonia (or PCP) is probably the best example of infection due to an opportunistic pathogen and occurs in a variety of immunocompromised patients, including those with AIDS, T-cell disorders, agammaglobulinemia, cancer, as well as patients on high-dose corticosteroids.[2] The clinical course of opportunistic infections may be quite variable in these patients and is altered by the degree of residual host immunity.

For example, corticosteroid therapy accelerates the resolution of PCP in AIDS patients, suggesting that residual host inflammatory response to this organism is important in the pathogenesis of respiratory dysfunction with PCP even in profoundly immunosuppressed patients. Fungal pulmonary infections in patients with chemotherapy-induced neutropenia often result in mild clinical symptoms and radiographic findings until return of neutrophil counts results in significant inflammation, lung destruction, cavitation, and frequently clinical deterioration.

Another useful way to consider the types of pulmonary infections that occur in immunocompromised hosts is by the underlying host disorder. Childhood cancer therapy, bone marrow and organ transplantation, primary immunodeficiencies, and AIDS are each associated with specific pulmonary pathogens; Table 28-1 includes only a partial listing of the potential pathogens.

CHILDHOOD CANCER

Patients with childhood cancer are at high risk for respiratory infections for many reasons in addition to the immunosuppressive effects of chemotherapy and radiation, including mucosal disruption (gut, respiratory tract), neutropenia, malnutrition, radiation, and presence of chronic indwelling catheters. Among childhood cancer groups there are differing risks for various pathogens. For example, the major risk factor for pneumonia in patients with leukemia is chemotherapy-induced neutropenia. Because patients with nonlymphocytic leukemia undergo the most intensive chemotherapy and longest periods of neutropenia, they are at greatest risk for developing pneumonia. Bacterial pneumonias are most common, but respiratory syncytial virus, adenovirus, and enteroviruses are also significant causes of pneumonia in patients with leukemia. Fungal pneumonias typically occur in patients with prolonged neutropenia, hospitalization, and broad-spectrum antibiotic therapy. *Aspergillus* and Zygomycetes (*Mucor, Rhizopus, Cunninghamella*) are the two most common fungal pulmonary pathogens. *Candida* spp. frequently cause disseminated fungal infections, but their role in pulmonary disease is difficult to determine because they frequently contaminate sputum and bronchial washings of patients without *Candida* pneumonia. Primary isolated *Candida* pneumonia is relatively uncommon. *Pneumocystis* and VZV were major causes of pneumonia in leukemia patients in the 1970s, but use of prophylaxis and effective therapies have reduced their impact as causes of pneumonitis in oncology patients, although both still occur in this population. Patients with lymphoma are at risk for pneumonia because of neutropenia during therapy and from a variety of nonspecific immunologic defects, including anergy, and Hodgkin's disease patients are often infected with fungi such as *Cryptococcus neoformans* and parasitic infection with *Toxoplasma gondii.*

TISSUE TRANSPLANTATION: BONE MARROW AND SOLID ORGAN

Hematopoietic Stem Cell Transplantation (Bone Marrow Transplantation)

The types of pulmonary complications seen in allogeneic (nonidentical siblings or unrelated donors) BMT vary with the length of time following transplantation[8,9] (Table 28-2). Immediately following the BMT, patients are neutropenic from the conditioning regimen and at risk for bacterial pneumonias with *Pseudomonas aeruginosa* and *Staphylococcus aureus*. As the transplant becomes established and neutrophils return, acute graft-versus-host pulmonary disease becomes a serious concern. Immunosuppressive therapy for graft-versus-host disease with corticosteroids, cyclosporin A, or newer antirejection therapies adds to the risk of pneumonia with viral pathogens (CMV, herpes simplex virus [HSV], adenovirus) as well as *Pneumocystis* and fungi. If engraftment fails and prolonged neutropenia occurs, the risk of fungal pneumonia increases significantly. Idiopathic interstitial pneumonias also occur during this later time period,

TABLE 28-1. Typical pulmonary pathogens associated with immune disorders

Immune Disorder	TYPICAL PULMONARY PATHOGENS: Bacterial	Fungal	Viral	Protozoa/Other
Neutropenias				
Chronic Neutrophil function disorders	*H. flu., Streptococcus pneumoniae, Staphylococcus aureus, Klebsiella*			
Acute	Gram-negative organisms, including *Pseudomonas*	*Candida* sp.		
Prolonged, hospitalized patients		*Aspergillus* sp. *Mucor, Fusarium*		
Agammaglobulinemia, hypogammaglobulinemia	*S. pneumoniae, H. flu., Pseudomonas*	*Aspergillus,* PCP		
Congenital T-cell disorders	*Legionella, Nocardia, Listeria, Mycobacterium tuberculosis, Salmonella*	*Candida* sp. *Cryptococcus,* PCP	CMV, VZV, HSV, EBV, adenovirus	Toxoplasmosis
AIDS	*M. tuberculosis, Mycobacterium avium-intracellulare*	*Cryptococcus,* PCP	CMV	Toxoplasmosis
Complement deficiencies	Virulent encapsulated (e.g., *S.pneumoniae, H. flu.*)			
Immunosuppressive therapy (e.g., renal, liver, and lung transplant)	*S. aureus, Listeria, M. tuberculosis*	*Aspergillus, Mucor,* histoplasmosis, *Cryptococcus,* PCP	CMV, VZV, HSV	Toxoplasmosis
BMT				
Early	*Pseudomonas,* gram-negatives	*Candida* sp.	HSV	
Late	*S. aureus, S. pneumoniae*	*Aspergillus,* PCP	CMV, EBV, VZV	Toxoplasmosis

AIDS, acquired immunodeficiency syndrome; BMT, bone marrow transplant; CMV, cytomegalovirus; EBV, Epstein-Barr virus; *H.flu., Haemophilus influenzae;* HSV, herpes simplex virus; PCP, *Pneumocystis jirovecii* pneumonia; VZV, varicella-zoster virus.

Adapted from Stokes DC, Bozeman PM: Sinopulmonary infections in immunocompromised infants and children. In: Patrick CC, ed: Infections in Immunocompromised Infants and Children. New York: Churchill Livingstone, 1992, p 364.

TABLE 28-2. Pulmonary complications after bone marrow transplantation

Time after Transplant	Associations	COMPLICATIONS	
		Infections	**Noninfectious**
Early (<30 days)	Neutropenia, mucositis, antibiotics, radiation	Bacterial, HSV, RSV, *Candida*	Pulmonary edema, ARDS
Delayed (30–120 days)	Acute GvHD, failed engraftment	CMV, adenovirus, PC, *Aspergillus, Mucor,* herpesvirus 6, EBV	Interstitial pneumonias, lymphoproliferative syndrome
Late (>120 days)	Chronic GvHD, poor response to antigens	VZV, encapsulated bacteria, *PCP*	Bronchiolitis obliterans, BOOP

ARDS, acute respiratory distress syndrome; Boop, bronchiolitis with organizing pneumonia; CMV, cytomegalovirus; EBV, Epstein-Barr virus; GvHD, graft-versus-host disease; HSV, herpes simplex virus; *PCP, Pneumocystis jirovecii* pneumonia; RSV, respiratory syncytial virus; VZV, varicella-zoster virus.

possibly related to radiation or chemotherapy used in the preparative regimens before transplant. Organisms causing pneumonia late (>4–6 months following transplant) include *Haemophilus influenzae* and *Streptococcus pneumoniae* and are associated with persistent immune deficits to these encapsulated organisms. A frequent cause of morbidity in the late transplant period is bronchiolitis obliterans, thought to be an immunologic disorder related to chronic graft-versus-host disease, with infection potentially playing a role in provoking or exacerbating this devastating complication. CMV pneumonia is a major cause of morbidity and mortality in pediatric BMT and occurs more frequently in allogeneic than in autologous BMT patients and in patients who are seropositive before transplant or who receive marrow from seropositive donors. Risk of CMV pneumonitis is low in seronegative recipients who receive grafts from seronegative donors and screened blood products. T-cell depletion to prevent graft-versus-host disease in a CMV-seropositive recipient grafted from a nonimmune donor is associated with a higher risk of developing CMV interstitial pneumonia. Interstitial pneumonia in BMT patients may involve the complex interaction between CMV and graft-versus-host disease.

Solid-Organ Transplantation

The development of pulmonary infections following renal transplant is primarily attributable to chronic immunosuppression with cyclosporin A and corticosteroids.[8,10] CMV is the most significant pulmonary infection in all transplant patients, including those having heart and lung transplant. PCP and toxoplasmosis are also quite common, although prophylaxis has reduced the incidence of both infections. In pediatric renal transplant patients followed for as long as 72 months after transplant, CMV infection occurred in 40%, and CMV disease occurred in 15%. The highest risk for CMV infection occurs in the first 12 weeks after transplant, and donor CMV seropositivity, regardless of recipient CMV serum status, is significantly associated with CMV infection. Gram-negative and fungal infections are the most common pulmonary complications in liver transplant patients and occur primarily in the first month after transplant.

PRIMARY IMMUNODEFICIENCY

In patients with common variable immunodeficiency and X-linked agammaglobulinemia, repeated bacterial pneumonias are most common, with PCP occasionally seen in patients with severe hypogammaglobulinemia. Congenital T-cell disorders including severe combined immunodeficiency put patients at risk for most of the same opportunistic pathogens as AIDS patients, including PCP (see Table 28-1).[11] Fungi, primarily *Aspergillus* sp., and bacterial infections with *S. aureus* are the most common lung infections in children with chronic granulomatous disease. Extensive lung destruction and hilar adenopathy are also common in these patents. Although persistent and recurrent *Candida albicans* infection of the mucous membranes and skin is associated with the chronic mucocutaneous candidiasis, 50% of patients have recurrent bacterial pneumonias and are at risk for other opportunistic pathogens, including *P. jirovecii*, *Nocardia*, and VZV pneumonias. Pulmonary complications including bronchiectasis, empyema, and lung abscess frequently occur.

ACQUIRED IMMUNODEFICIENCY SYNDROME

The extensive list of pulmonary infections associated with AIDS includes *P. jirovecii*, CMV, bacterial pneumonias, and atypical mycobacteria (see Table 28-1).[12]

DIFFERENTIAL DIAGNOSIS OF PULMONARY INFILTRATES

NONINFECTIOUS PULMONARY DISEASE

Immunocompromised patients are at risk for a variety of noninfectious complications that simulate infection and complicate the diagnostic work-up (Table 28-3). These include pulmonary

TABLE 28-3. Noninfectious processes complicating or simulating pneumonia in the immunocompromised host

Process	Associations
Chemical pneumonitis	Aspiration syndromes
Atelectasis	Reactive airways disease, endobronchial or extrinsic obstruction
Hemorrhage	Thrombocytopenia, renal failure, coagulopathy, *Aspergillus*
Pulmonary edema	
Cardiogenic	Anthracycline cardiotoxicity, sepsis, myocarditis
Noncardiogenic	ARDS, pancreatitis, fluid overload
Drug-induced lung injury	Chemotherapy, azathioprine
Radiation pneumonitis	Radiation, 6–8 weeks previously
Leukostasis	Hyperleukocytosis, amphotericin B, WBC transfusions
Leukemia, lymphoma	Active disease
LIP	HIV infection in children
"Idiopathic pneumonitis" including pulmonary cytolytic thrombi	Allogeneic bone marrow transplantation, GVHD

ARDS, acute respiratory distress syndrome; GvHD, graft-versus-host disease; HIV, human immunodeficiency syndrome; LIP, lymphocytic interstitial pneumonitis; WBC, white blood cell.

hemorrhage (thrombocytopenia, infection, or idiopathic), radiation pneumonitis, atelectasis (endobronchial or external bronchial obstruction by nodes or tumor), drug-induced lung injury (chemotherapy), pulmonary edema (cardiac dysfunction due to anthracyclines or sepsis), acute respiratory distress syndrome, and active malignancy (leukostasis with hyperleukocystosis in leukemia, metastatic disease, lymphoma). Many of these processes produce nonspecific lung injury patterns that require a pathologic specimen and careful clinical correlation to make a correct diagnosis, although some (e.g., pulmonary hemorrhage or pulmonary involvement with leukemia) can be diagnosed by bronchoscopy alone. Idiopathic pneumonia syndrome is a diffuse lung injury syndrome occurring after BMT for which an infectious cause is not identified. Lung biopsy reveals diffuse alveolar damage and interstitial pneumonitis, and it is associated with a high mortality.[13]

COMMON INFECTIOUS PNEUMONIAS IN THE IMMUNOCOMPROMISED HOST

Viral

Cytomegalovirus

Cytomegalovirus is a herpesvirus that is a common infection of both neonates and older immunocompromised children.[4,14,15] Whether the virus results in disease depends on both the age and the immune status of the infected individual. The organism can be transmitted through an infected birth canal, as well as by breast milk, saliva, and blood (via infected white cells). Both humoral and cellular immune mechanisms are important in establishing protection against CMV. Individuals who are CMV-negative before acquired immunosuppression due to organ or marrow transplantation, and those who acquire the virus by transfusion are particularly at risk for disease. CMV-positive individuals who are then immunosuppressed also run a significant risk for "reactivation" pneumonia. CMV-infected cells typically contain nuclear inclusions that are deeply basophilic and surrounded by a clear halo, giving the "owl eye" appearance. Inclusions are typically seen in alveolar cells. The pathology varies from small hemorrhagic nodules scattered throughout the lung surrounded by relatively normal lung to diffuse alveolar damage or chronic interstitial pneumonitis. The radiographic pattern of the pneumonia is usually a diffuse reticulonodular pattern that is less alveolar in pattern than PCP. By high-resolution computed tomography (CT), patchy or diffuse ground-glass attenuation is most commonly seen with CMV. Approximately 50% of patients with aplastic anemia or hematologic malignancy treated by allogeneic BMT develop CMV infection, and CMV pneumonia caused a 90% mortality in this population before antiviral therapy. CMV frequently is also found as a co-pathogen with other opportunistic organisms, including *P. jirovecii* and *Aspergillus* sp., particularly in AIDS patients. The diagnosis of CMV pneumonia is usually made by demonstration of typical inclusions in lung tissue. Isolation of CMV from urine is not sufficient evidence that CMV is the cause of the pneumonia. Rapid diagnostic methods have become available using immunofluorescence, DNA hybridization, or shell vial culture combined with rapid detection methods, which provide rapid diagnosis of CMV from bronchoalveolar lavage (BAL). Such techniques, though highly sensitive, must be interpreted cautiously, since CMV can also be detected in asymptomatic individuals. The use of CMV-negative blood products has reduced the incidence of CMV pneumonia in seronegative (but not seropositive) transplant patients. Polymerase chain reaction for CMV has been used in BMT recipients to attempt to predict the development of CMV disease. Polymerase chain reaction detection precedes culture isolation of CMV and lasts longer than culture. Lack of polymerase chain reaction resolution or positive culture predicts development of CMV disease in BMT patients with a positive predictive value of 60%. IV immunoglobulin enriched for anti-CMV activity has been used for prophylaxis in high-risk populations without clear benefit. However, when CMV-IV immunoglobulin was combined with the antiviral drug ganciclovir, mortality in CMV pneumonitis in BMT patients was reduced.

Varicella-Zoster Virus and Herpes Simplex Virus

Varicella-zoster virus and HSV are DNA viruses that typically cause benign infections of the skin and mucous membranes. However, in certain high-risk groups, including neonates; patients with cancer and BMT, AIDS, and congenital defects of cell-mediated immunity; as well as transplant patients, VZV and HSV can lead to visceral dissemination and pneumonia.[15,16] In cancer patients with VZV, pneumonitis occurs in 85% of cases of visceral dissemination and is the principal cause of death. Before the availability of specific antiviral therapy, VZV pneumonitis mortality was 85%. Pneumonitis is much less common with reactivation of herpes zoster and HSV, but it is a potentially serious infection in BMT and oncology patients. The clinical presentation is nonspecific and includes fever, cough, dyspnea, and chest pain. Patients with VZV who have an increasing number of skin lesions, abdominal or back pain, or persistent fevers are at high risk for dissemination and pneumonia. HSV pneumonitis may be more subtle in its presentation, and pneumonitis can occur in the absence of mucocutaneous lesions in newborns and BMT patients. Chest radiographs of herpesvirus pneumonias typically show ill-defined nodular densities scattered through both lung fields, often beginning at the periphery. These nodules progress and coalesce into extensive infiltrates. Secondary infections such as staphylococcal pneumonia were more commonly seen in the preantibiotic era. Microscopically, the infection involves alveolar walls, blood vessels, and small bronchioles. Electron microscopy shows intranuclear inclusions of herpesvirus. Hemorrhage, necrosis, and extensive alveolar edema are seen in severe areas of involvement. The trachea and large bronchi are often involved. Varicella-zoster immune globulin can modify or prevent VZV infection in high-risk hosts exposed to the virus if given within 48 to 72 hours of exposure. VZV immune globulin, antiviral therapy with acyclovir and related drugs, and routine varicella vaccination have been the major influences accounting for the reduced incidence of serious VZV pneumonias in immunocompromised hosts.

Herpesvirus Type 6

Human herpesvirus 6 is a DNA virus that is the etiologic agent for roseola. It persists in normal hosts and can be isolated from lymphocytes and other sites. In the abnormal host, reactivation can lead to fever, hepatitis, bone marrow suppression, and interstitial pneumonia. Human herpesvirus 6 is commonly detected after solid-organ transplant and can cause fever, hepatitis, and encephalitis. Human herpesvirus 6 may also increase the risk of CMV and other infections. Antiviral compounds with activity against CMV such as ganciclovir, foscarnet, and cidofovir are active against human herpesvirus 6 as well.[17]

Adenovirus

Adenovirus is a DNA virus that is a common cause of community-acquired lower respiratory tract disease. Serotypes 3 and 7 are associated with epidemics of bronchiolitis and pneumonia in the general population, and in immunocompromised patients adenovirus is a major viral cause of serious morbidity and mortality.[17] Adenovirus typically causes fever, pharyngitis, cough, and conjunctivitis. Pneumonia is usually mild in normal hosts, but rapid progression can occur in immunocompromised patients with a necrotizing bronchitis and bronchiolitis. The radiographic picture is nonspecific and resembles other causes of diffuse pneumonia. The diagnosis is usually made by lung biopsy or brushings demonstrating typical adenoviral inclusions, or by culture, but the diagnosis may be delayed by institution of empiric antibiotic and antifungal therapy and delay in invasive procedures. Viral titers may provide a delayed diagnosis. Failure of pneumonia to respond despite therapy, particularly when there have been epidemics of typical acute respiratory disease in the community or hospital staff, should raise suspicion of adenovirus involvement. Unfortunately, there is no specific antiviral therapy for adenovirus. Supportive therapy includes oxygen, treatment of bacterial superinfections, intravenous (IV) immunoglobulin, and assisted ventilation.

Fungal

Pneumocystis Jirovecii (Formerly *Carinii*)

Pneumocystis jirovecii has been an organism of uncertain taxonomy and was regarded as a parasite because of its resemblance to cystic spore-forming protozoa. More recent studies using DNA hybridization methods place *P. jirovecii* with the fungi.[18] There are several animal models for infection with *Pneumocystis*, with no evidence of cross infection across species. The nomenclature *P. carinii* is now reserved for the organism infecting rats, while *P. jirovecii* is the organism isolated in humans.[19]

The organism exists in three forms in tissues: the trophozoite, the sporozoite, and the cyst. The trophozoites measure 2 to 5 μm and stain best with Giemsa stains but are not visible with Grocot-Gomori methenamine–silver nitrate or toluidine blue O stains, which stain the 5- to 8-μm cyst forms. The cysts are spheric or cup-shaped and often appear to contain up to eight 1- to 2-μm sporozoites within the cyst wall. The organism cannot be cultured from routine clinical specimens and must be identified in tissue, sputum, or alveolar lavage. The trophozoites appear to attach to type I cells through surface glycoproteins related to lectins and there undergo encystation. This interaction directly or through soluble factors leads to cell injury. The alveoli of lungs infected with *P. jirovecii* are filled with trophozoites and protein-rich debris, and the altered permeability produced by the organism contributes to the development of pulmonary edema and surfactant abnormalities, which lead to stiff lungs. Latent infection with *P. jirovecii* was thought to be common, since serologic studies indicated that 40% of children had antibodies to the organism, and more recent studies using sensitive polymerase chain reaction assays have found evidence of *P. jirovecii* in the nasopharynx and lungs of normal infants. Colonization appears to be common in immunocompromised patients but less common in normal hosts, and there is some evidence of patient-to-patient transmission.

In patients with congenital immunodeficiency or malignancy, the clinical features of PCP are nonspecific and include dyspnea, tachypnea, fever, and cough. Cyanosis occurs later, but early hypoxemia with a mild respiratory alkalosis is common. The most common chest radiographic finding is diffuse bilateral infiltrates. Since 1980, the most common underlying host defect in patients with *P. jirovecii* is AIDS, and the clinical features of PCP in this population differ from the pneumonias seen in non-AIDS populations. Patients with AIDS typically have a longer duration of symptoms and a more insidious presentation. Hypoxemia may be less intense. Organisms appear to be abundant in AIDS patients and can usually be identified in sputum, BAL, or even gastric lavage samples. Other superinfections (such as CMV) and pulmonary complications such as lymphoid interstitial pneumonia are often present in AIDS patients, however, and it is often difficult to know what role these complications play in the AIDS patient's symptoms. AIDS patients are also more likely to have spread of *P. jirovecii* to nodes, spleen, bone marrow, and other sites. They frequently have atypical chest radiographic findings, including lobar pneumonias, unilateral disease, and solitary nodules, although atypical radiographic presentations can also occur in other immunosuppressed patients.

Pneumocystis jirovecii pneumonia can be treated by several drugs. The earliest drug available for PCP was the dihydrofolate reductase inhibitor pentamidine, which was associated with a high rate of immediate reactions, such as hypotension, tachycardia, and nausea as well as hypoglycemia and nephrotoxicity. Pentamidine is also given by the aerosol route for treatment of mild to moderate pulmonary disease in AIDS patients, but its effectiveness is highly dependent on the delivery system used, and the aerosol route may predispose AIDS patients to extrapulmonary disease. Co-trimoxazole (TMP-SMZ) is the preferred treatment of PCP in children, but AIDS patients have a high incidence of reactions to TMP-SMZ. Of non-AIDS patients in whom TMP-SMZ treatment fails, 60% will respond to treatment with pentamidine. In addition to pentamidine and TMP-SMZ, several other drugs have been identified that are effective in PCP, including dapsone and trimetrexate. Corticosteroid administration during therapy improves outcome in PCP in AIDS patients. Typically, patients require 4 to 6 days before showing improvement with either pentamidine or TMP-SMZ, and failure to improve warrants consideration of other infections or a change to another anti-*Pneumocystis* drug. Patients at known risk for *P. jirovecii* generally receive prophylaxis. For pediatric oncology and immunocompromised patients, oral TMP-SMZ given on a schedule of 3 days per week is effective. However, if patients or parents are noncompliant there is a risk of breakthrough pneumonias on this schedule. For most patients TMP-SMZ remains the drug of choice, but other prophylactic regimens have been used, particularly in AIDS patients, including aerosolized and IV pentamidine and dapsone. IV pentamidine may be associated with a higher risk of failure. The success of highly active antiretroviral therapy for human immunodeficiency virus has allowed some patients to discontinue PCP prophylaxis.

Aspergillus Species

Aspergillus is a group of ubiquitous fungal organisms found in soil and other settings, including the hospital environment. *Aspergillus fumigatus* is the most common cause of pneumonia in immunocompromised hosts, but other pathogenic species include *A. niger* and *A. flavus.*[20] In tissue the organisms form septate hyphae with regular 45-degree dichotomous branching, best seen with methenamine silver staining. *Aspergillus* causes both acute invasive pulmonary aspergillosis and a more chronic necrotizing form. The former occurs most commonly in patients undergoing cancer therapy as well as other immunocompromised patients such as those with aplastic anemia. Aspergillosis of the lung is often preceded by or accompanied by invasion of the nose and paranasal sinuses in susceptible hosts. Confirmed risk factors for aspergillosis include prolonged neutropenia, concurrent chemotherapy and steroid therapy, and broad-spectrum antibiotic therapy. Cutaneous aspergillosis is often observed in patients with disseminated disease. In the lungs, *Aspergillus* can cause tracheobronchitis, pneumonia, abscesses and cavity formation, and diffuse interstitial pneumonia. The organisms often extend along blood vessels, and nodular lesions of necrosis surrounded by air often develop within an area of pneumonia, leading to the typical air crescent sign. CT of the chest is often very helpful in patients with disseminated fungal disease due to *Aspergillus* and other fungal pathogens. Two basic types of involvement are seen with CT—multiple nodules or fluffy masses—and cavitations occur commonly. CT is much more sensitive than plain radiographs and can reveal early evidence of cavitation. Diagnosis of *Aspergillus* pneumonia is generally made by tissue examination. *Aspergillus* can be isolated from BAL in approximately 50% of cases, and needle aspiration biopsy of peripheral lung lesions can also demonstrate typical fungal lesions.[21] Isolation of *Aspergillus* from a nasal culture in a patient with typical clinical risk features (prolonged neutropenia, progressive nodular infiltrates, cavitary lesion) may be helpful, but negative cultures do not exclude *Aspergillus*.

The treatment of *Aspergillus* pneumonia is amphotericin B, given at a dose of 1 to 1.5 mg/kg. Flucytosine or rifampin is sometimes added. The utility of surgical excision of *Aspergillus* lesions is somewhat controversial. Invasive pulmonaryaspergillosis during treatment of hematologic malignancy is generally considered a contraindication to subsequent BMT, but adult patients treated with amphotericin B and surgery have survived free of disease and without reactivation of *Aspergillus* following BMT. The outcome of *Aspergillus* pneumonia depends primarily on such host factors as degree of immunosuppression and recovery of neutrophil counts as well as early diagnosis and treatment.[22]

Mucor and *Rhizopus*

Mucormycosis includes fungal disease caused by organisms in the order Mucorales, including a variety of species in the genera *Rhizopus*, *Mucor*, and *Cunninghamella*.[23] In tissues they are differentiated from *Aspergillus* by their broad, nonseptate hyphae that branch at angles up to 90 degrees and have an appearance of "twisted ribbons." *Rhizopus* organisms cause disease only in patients with underlying disease. In adults, it is associated with chronic acidosis states, such as diabetes mellitus with ketoacidosis. Most pediatric cases of pneumonia occur in the oncology population, where the organism is found in the same risk groups as *Aspergillus*. Pneumonia due to *Rhizopus* is usually an insidious segmental pneumonia that is slowly progressive despite antifungal therapy. Persistent fever, chest pain, hemoptysis, and weight loss are typical. Cavitation may occur, and dissemination to brain and other sites occurs as a result of the propensity of the organism to invade blood vessels. Death may occur suddenly with massive pulmonary hemorrhage, mediastinitis, or airway obstruction. Specific diagnosis usually depends on demonstration of the organism in open, transbronchial, or needle aspiration lung biopsy specimens. As with *Aspergillus*, treatment with amphotericin B and possibly surgical resection as early as possible is critical to achieving a cure. Correction of chronic acidosis if present also appears to be important in some forms of *Rhizopus* disease.

Candida Species

Though important as a cause of fungal sepsis and secondary hematogenous pulmonary involvement, primary *Candida* pneumonia is unusual. *Candida albicans* and *Candida tropicalis* are the most important causes of fungal sepsis and secondary pulmonary involvement. Neutropenic children colonized with *C. tropicalis* are at 10-fold higher risk for dissemination than are children colonized with *C. albicans*. Patients with human immunodeficiency virus infection, primary immunodeficiencies, or prolonged neutropenia are at greatest risk, but other predisposing conditions include diabetes, corticosteroid administration, broad-spectrum antibiotic treatment, intravenous hyperalimentation, and presence of venous access devices. In tissue, silver stains show oval budding yeasts 2 to 6 μm in diameter with pseudohyphae. The prominent histologic features of primary *Candida* pneumonia include bronchopneumonia, intra-alveolar exudates, and hemorrhage. Amphotericin B is usually the treatment of choice for invasive *Candida* infections, along with flucytosine if synergism is desired. The imidazole antifungal agents, including ketoconazole, fluconazole, and itraconazole, have activity against *C. albicans* and have been used successfully. Use of the imidazole antifungal agents for prophylaxis has helped select out more resistant fungal organisms in high-risk populations, since *Candida* species other than *C. albicans* are frequently resistant to these agents.[24]

Histoplasmosis and Blastomycosis

Histoplasma capsulatum and *Blastomyces dermatitidis* are ubiquitous soil fungi endemic to the eastern and southeastern United States. Histoplasmosis is a common infection in immunocompetent children and may be asymptomatic or lead to an acute pneumonia with fever, hilar adenopathy, and pulmonary infiltrates. Blastomycosis is a less common, more serious infection. Both can cause chronic granulomatous pulmonary disease as well as disseminated disease. In the immunocompromised patient, including AIDS sufferers, the major risk for both organisms is dissemination with pulmonary infiltrates, hepatosplenomegaly, fevers, and adenopathy.[25] Histoplasmosis is much more common in the immunocompromised host than blastomycosis. Amphotericin B is indicated for both histoplasmosis and blastomycosis in immunocompromised hosts. Itraconazole is also effective for histoplasmosis and moderate blastomycosis without central nervous system involvement.

Cryptococcus Neoformans

Cryptococcus neoformans is a yeast that causes protean clinical manifestations in immunocompromised patients, particularly those with AIDS.[26] The meninges, endocardium, skin, and lymph nodes are often involved. The lungs are the portal of entry for *C. neoformans*, and pulmonary involvement may be minimal if dissemination occurs quickly. Pneumonia is typically accompanied by chest pain, fever, and cough. Pulmonary disease with *Cryptococcus* is rarer in pediatric AIDS patients than in adults. Treatment is IV amphotericin B and oral flucytosine, but fluconazole has also proven effective, particularly with central nervous system disease.

Rarer Fungal Pneumonias

Several recent trends have been noted in fungal infections, among them increased identification of rarer fungal pathogens including saprophytic fungi such as *Trichosporon beigelii* and *Fusarium* sp. These fungi cause skin and soft tissue infections and occasionally invade the lungs and sinuses. For example, *Scedosporium apiospermum* (formerly *Pseudallescheria boydii*) causes invasive disease in solid-organ transplant patients, with lung involvement in 50%.[27] These fungi are often difficult to diagnose, and their response to therapy with amphotericin B may be very poor.

Bacterial

The bacterial pathogens associated with pneumonia in immunocompromised hosts include those pathogens typically associated with pneumonia in children, such as *S. aureus* (particularly methicillin-resistant strains), *H. influenzae*, and *S. pneumoniae*. *Pseudomonas aeruginosa* is an important cause of pneumonia and sepsis in immunocompromised children, particularly hospitalized patients. Significant risk factors include neutropenia and perineal skin lesions. More unusual bacterial causes of pneumonia include *Listeria monocytogenes*, a gram-positive rod that causes primarily septicemia in immunocompromised patients, with subsequent pulmonary involvement. Corynebacteria (commonly called diphtheroids) are gram-positive bacilli or coccobacilli that exist as saprophytes on mucous membranes and skin. *Corynebacterium jeikeium* is a strain from this group that causes sepsis and pneumonia in oncology and BMT patients. *Listeria* infection can be treated by ampicillin plus an aminoglycoside, but newer cephalosporins are not active against *Listeria*, and *C. jeikeium* is resistant to most antibiotics except vancomycin. Other rare gram-negative organisms that cause pneumonia in the immunocompromised host include *Legionella pneumophila* and *Capnocytophaga* sp.

Mycobacteria

With the onset of the AIDS epidemic, disease due to both *Mycobacterium tuberculosis* and atypical strains such as *Mycobacterium avium-intracellulare* have been increasingly recognized in both AIDS and non-AIDS immunodeficient populations. Detailed discussion of mycobacterial infections in AIDS patients is beyond the scope of this chapter but is covered in recent reviews.[12]

Parasitic and Other Causes

Toxoplasma Gondii and *Cryptosporidium Parvum*

Toxoplasma gondii and *C. parvum* are both parasitic infections.[28] *Toxoplasma gondii* infects cats and other animals and secondarily infects humans, causing congenital toxoplasmosis during intrauterine infection; primary infection later in life usually causes only lymphadenopathy and mild systemic symptoms. *Cryptosporidium parvum* infects a variety of hosts and often occurs in waterborne outbreaks. In AIDS patients *Toxoplasma* primarily causes central nervous system disease, but disseminated disease with secondary pulmonary involvement can occur, presenting with shortness of breath, cough, fever, and bilateral interstitial infiltrates.[8] *Cryptosporidium parvum* causes severe diarrhea, but disseminated disease with pulmonary involvement can occur. Treatment of *T. gondii* is with pyrimethamine-sulfadiazine, while treatment of *C. parvum* is with azithromycin.

■ DIAGNOSTIC STUDIES

■ RADIOGRAPHY

Pneumonias in the immunocompromised host can be classified by their general radiologic appearance, including (1) diffuse alveolar and/or interstitial pneumonias; (2) localized alveolar lobar or lobular pneumonias, which may involve more than one lobe; and (3) nodular infiltrates, which may be cavitary or progress to frank lung abscess. The common causes of these general radiographic patterns are shown in Table 28-4, but it must be emphasized that radiographic appearances by plain chest radiograph are often deceptive in immunocompromised hosts and are usually not helpful in making a specific etiologic diagnosis. CT is much more sensitive than plain chest radiographs in revealing the extent of pulmonary disease and can demonstrate other findings such as early cavitation or visceral fungal lesions. CT can also help in planning approaches to bronchoscopy or biopsy.

Diffuse Interstitial and Alveolar Pneumonias

Although *P. jirovecii* is the prototypical organism associated with this radiographic pattern, "typical" *P. jirovecii* infection has declined significantly in patient populations receiving prophylaxis. Atypical radiographic appearances of *P. jirovecii* are more common, as, for example, when aerosolized pentamidine for prophylaxis of PCP in AIDS alters the radiographic presentation toward more upper lobe involvement. CMV is also associated with diffuse pneumonia in immunocompromised patients and is frequently seen with other infectious agents. In transplant patients, CT findings with CMV may be more heterogeneous, with nodules, consolidation, and ground-glass attenuation. Viral infections, including adenovirus, and influenza are also important causes of diffuse pneumonia.

■ **TABLE 28-4.** Radiographic patterns of pulmonary infections in immunocompromised hosts

Diffuse Interstitial/Alveolar	Lobar or Lobular (Bronchopneumonia)	Nodules, Cavity, or Lung Abscess
PCP	Bacteria, including *Streptococcus pneumoniae*, *Haemophilus influenzae*, *Staphylococcus aureus*, gram-negatives	Bacteria (including *S. aureus*, anaerobes, gram-negatives)
CMV	*Nocardia*	*C. neoformans*
Cryptococcus neoformans	*C. neoformans*	*Nocardia*
Aspergillus sp. (unusual)	*Aspergillus* sp.	*Aspergillus* sp.
Candida albicans and *other Candida* sp. (unusual)	*Mucor*	*L. pneumophila*
RSV	*Mycobacterium tuberculosis*	PCP (AIDS)
Varicella-zoster virus	*Legionella pneumophila*	*M. tuberculosis*
Adenovirus	Adenovirus	
Histoplasma capsulatum		

AIDS, acquired immunodeficiency syndrome; CMV, cytomegalovirus; PCP, *Pneumocystis jirovecii* pneumonia; RSV, respiratory syncytial virus.

Localized Alveolar Lobar or Lobular ("Bronchopneumonia") Pneumonias

Bronchopneumonias and lobar consolidation can occur in immunocompromised patients caused by the usual pathogens, such as *S. pneumoniae*, *H. influenzae*, and *S. aureus*. However, since the radiographic appearance is a product of the host's response to the organism as well as the organism, patients with abnormal host defenses often show an altered initial radiographic pattern and the radiographic findings may reflect poorly the extent of pulmonary involvement, particularly with profound neutropenia or immunosuppression.

Nodular, Cavitary, and Lung Abscess Lesions

Solitary pulmonary nodules, either unilateral or bilateral, are a less common presentation of infection in most immunocompromised patients but do occur frequently in pediatric oncology patients. Although most often these represent fungal pneumonias, other organisms including *Nocardia* can also present as pulmonary nodules. The development of a lung abscess generally indicates some degree of host immunity sufficient to localize an infection. The most common causes of cavitary lesions in pediatric cancer patients are fungi, especially *Aspergillus* sp. PCP and mycobacterial infections can also be associated with cavitary disease in AIDS patients.

INDIRECT DIAGNOSTIC TESTS

Sputum Examination and Cultures

Sputum produced by cough induced with inhalation of hypertonic saline aerosols has been useful in older children with AIDS and PCP. Gastric aspirates can be used in the younger child and are particularly helpful when the pathogen being considered is not a usual colonizing organism of the upper airway (e.g., tuberculosis). If the child requires endotracheal intubation for respiratory distress, endotracheal aspirates are easy to obtain. Diagnostic yield in complex immunocompromised patients is improved by using wax-protected microbiologic brushes or nonbronchoscopic BAL in the intubated patient. Although blood culture should be obtained in all immunocompromised children suspected of having a bacterial or fungal pneumonia, positive cultures are unusual though usually highly specific.

Antigen and Antibody Detection Methods

The ability to detect capsular polysaccharide antigens of bacterial pathogens even after antibiotics have been administered is occasionally helpful in hospitalized patients. Most hospitals routinely test for group B Streptococcus, *Neisseria meningitidis*, *S. pneumoniae*, and *H. influenzae* using latex agglutination or counterimmunoelectrophoresis. Concentrated urine samples are superior to serum samples. A number of tests for direct detection of fungal antigens have been described, but none are in widespread clinical use. Direct immunofluorescence can be used to detect *Legionella* sp. with a sensitivity of 50% and a specificity of 94%. Rapid diagnosis of respiratory syncytial virus, influenza A virus, parainfluenza viruses, and *Chlamydia* infections by enzyme-linked immunosorbent assay and direct immunofluorescence is also available. Viral cultures are generally available, and the shell vial technique for rapid identification of CMV is very useful. Genetic probes for detecting *P. jirovecii*, *Legionella*, *Mycobacterium*, and *Mycoplasma pneumoniae* are now commercially available, and the ability of the polymerase chain reaction to amplify specific regions of genomic DNA or RNA should allow a broader application of these sensitive diagnostic approaches in the immunocompromised patient, particularly when combined with BAL to obtain specimens.

INVASIVE DIAGNOSTIC STUDIES

Unfortunately, radiography and noninvasive diagnostic studies rarely produce a specific diagnosis in the immunocompromised child with pneumonia. In that circumstance, one is faced with either continuing empiric antimicrobial therapy or performing a more invasive diagnostic study to make a specific diagnosis. Fortunately, the safety and availability of these studies have improved significantly over the past few years.

Flexible Bronchoscopy

Flexible bronchoscopy is safe in experienced hands and provides excellent diagnostic material in the immunocompromised child with pneumonia.[29,30] Indications for bronchoscopy in children with pneumonia generally include (1) failure of pneumonia or fever to clear with appropriate antibiotic therapy, (2) suspicion of endobronchial obstruction by infection or tumor, (3) recurrent pneumonia in a lobe or segment, and (4) suspicion of unusual organisms. Although the yield of gastric aspiration is probably superior to bronchoscopy for suspected tuberculosis, bronchoscopy has the added value of allowing evaluation for endobronchial disease or bronchial compression. Simple cytology brushing obtained through the pediatric bronchoscope can be used for cytologic examination and viral cultures, but the yield is usually low. The bronchoscope suction channel is contaminated by upper airway organisms, and simple washings obtained through the bronchoscope channel are generally less useful than quantitative cultures of BAL. BAL is the most useful technique in the immunocompromised host, and a variety of infectious and noninfectious diagnoses can be made by BAL, including hemorrhage and pulmonary involvement with leukemia. BAL is generally safe, even in patients with reduced platelet counts.

Although the usefulness of bronchoscopy is well documented in this population, it is important to recognize the limitations of bronchoscopy. In immunocompromised patients on empiric broad-spectrum antibiotic therapy, the yield of bacterial pathogens will probably be low. In oncology patients and other non-AIDS immunocompromised patients, the number of *P. jirovecii* organisms is usually low compared with AIDS patients, and BAL may be falsely negative. In populations receiving prophylaxis for this infection, the yield for PCP will also probably be low. CMV can also be diagnosed rapidly by bronchoscopy, but patients may have other complicating infections such as fungi in addition to CMV that are more easily missed by bronchoscopy. *Aspergillus* and other fungi are often difficult to diagnose by bronchoscopy, particularly early in the infection when therapy is most likely to be effective. In pediatric BMT patients, fungal infections were the most commonly diagnosed infection by BAL, but the yield was only 17% in the early conditioning period (where broad-spectrum antibiotic coverage was common) compared with 82% in the period following transplant. Transbronchial biopsies can also be taken through the bronchoscope. Though safe in older patients, transbronchial lung biopsies may yield an unacceptable number of false-negative results in immunosuppressed patients and are most useful when organisms such as *P. jirovecii* or granulomatous lesions are probable. Reported experience with transbronchial biopsies in pediatric patients is limited, but transbronchial biopsy has a significant role in monitoring rejection and infections in the pediatric lung transplant patient, and in skilled hands can be done with conscious sedation and a transnasal approach in the older child. Obliterative bronchiolitis after transplantation can easily be missed by transbronchial biopsy, however.

Transthoracic Needle Aspiration Biopsy

Needle aspiration of the lung has been used for the diagnosis of PCP in pediatric cancer patients and for the diagnosis of localized infections in other immunosuppressed patients. Pneumothorax complicated 37% of the needle aspirates done for PCP, and this risk must be considered even with more modern "thin"-needle techniques. Use of CT or fluoroscopic guidance greatly improves the yield and safety of transthoracic needle aspiration biopsy, and it is the procedure of choice for many older children with suspected fungal peripheral lesions that can safely be aspirated, avoiding an open biopsy.[31] These peripheral lesions often have a poor diagnostic yield with bronchoscopy alone.

Open-Lung Biopsy

Open-lung biopsy is the "gold standard" by which other diagnostic modalities are judged. Using current surgical techniques, OLB is generally a procedure with a low morbidity that can be done rapidly and allows the surgeon to select optimal tissue for culture and microscopic examination. "Mini-thoracotomy" and lingular biopsy may be all that is necessary in patients with diffuse pulmonary processes, significantly reducing the morbidity of the procedure. Biopsy using fiberoptic pleuroscopy (also called thoracoscopy) may be adequate for pleural-based lesions and significantly reduces the morbidity associated with open biopsy in selected patients. Ventilated patients on high-pressure ventilator support are generally best managed by standard lung biopsy rather than thoracoscopy, and thoracoscopic techniques are not applicable to smaller children and infants. In immunocompromised patients it is difficult to make generalizations about OLB, and much depends on local influences such as availability of flexible bronchoscopy, age of the child, and the underlying condition. Complications such as respiratory failure, thrombocytopenia, or coagulopathies, and prior antibiotic/antifungal therapy may increase the risk of OLB or reduce the diagnostic yield. Some studies of OLB have questioned how often OLB results will lead to a change in therapy, if one excludes patients with organisms covered by empiric therapy such as *P. jirovecii* and nonspecific histologic findings without specific therapies such as fibrosis or nonspecific lung injury. Published results on OLB in immunocompromised pediatric patients have indicated yields that range from 36% to 94% for a specific diagnosis and generally support the utility of open biopsy[32–45] (Table 28-5). Although OLB is the procedure of choice for obtaining definitive diagnostic information in immunosuppressed patients with pulmonary infiltrates, timing of the biopsy is often difficult. The clinician does not want to commit the patient too early, especially if empiric therapy appears to be working and the patient is in good condition. On the other hand, the surgeon does not want to wait so long in the face of marginally successful therapy that the patient deteriorates and the risk of biopsy significantly increases. We generally recommend early bronchoscopy because

TABLE 28-5. Summary of open lung biopsy series in immunocompromised pediatric patients, 1980–2002

Reference	Number of Patients	Primary Diagnoses	Definitive Diagnosis	Change in Therapy
Mason and colleagues[32]	40	37 with malignancy	32 (80%), 25 with PCP	80%; mainly Rx for PCP
Imoke and colleagues[33]	34	30 with malignancy	21 (62%), 11 with PCP	50%; mainly Rx for PCP
Prober and colleagues[34]	44	Malignancy (59%); transplant (16%); immunodeficiency (34%)	43 (94%), 15 with PCP	65%; including Rx for PCP, discontinuing antibiotics
Early and colleagues[35]	35	22 immunocompromised	"All"; 10 of 22 (45%) infections; immunocompromised patients	55% of immunocompromised; mainly Rx for PCP
Doolin and colleagues[36]	56	42 with malignancy	46 (82%), 19 with PCP	18% benefit plus survival
Shorter and colleagues[37]	21	All BMT patients	8 of 22 (36%), 3 with CMV, 4 with PCP including 2 with mixed infection	10%; both with PCP
Foglia and colleagues[38]	26	50% immunocompromised	7 with PCP, 9 with nonspecific pneumonitis, 6 with CMV	58%
Snyder and colleagues[39]	87	94 biopsies; all BMTs	60% yield	49% (46 of 94); improved 18%
Bozeman and Stokes[40]	34	All immunocompromised	23 (67%), 14 (41%) with infection, 3 with PCP	Not noted; 11 (32%) with nonspecific histology
Gururangan and colleagues[41]	18	13 immunocompromised	14 of 19 (74%); 2 with PCP, 4 with measles	14 of 18 (78%)
Stefanutti and colleagues[42]	32	All immunocompromised; 17 primary, 19 secondary	22 (61%) specific histology; 2 PCP	Benefit from OLB in 33%
Kornecki and Shemie[43]	31	19 (59%) immunocompromised; all in respiratory failure	13 (39%) specific diagnosis; 20 (61%) with nonspecific histology; 6 PCP, 3 CMV, 1 PCP/CMV	25 of 33 bx (76%)
Shaikh and colleagues[44]	12	All BMT patients		3 of 12 (25%)
Hayes-Jordan and colleagues[45]	19	All BMT patients	6 with infection (30%), 5 with BOOP (26%)	17 of 19 (90%) only 8 (47.5%) with improved outcome

BMT, bone marrow transplant; BOOP, bronchiolitis obliterans organizing pneumonia; CMV, cytomegalovirus; OLB, open-lung biopsy; PCP, *Pneumocystis jirovecii* pneumonia; Rx, therapy.

Adapted from Bozeman PM, Stokes DC: Diagnostic methods in pulmonary infections of immunocompromised children. Bronchoscopy, needle aspiration and open biopsy. In: Patrick CC, ed: Infections in Immunocompromised Infants and Children. New York: Churchill Livingstone, 1992.

of the safety of this procedure when done early in the course of the pneumonia and the possibility of significant findings that may make open biopsy unnecessary. Any patient not clearly responding to therapy chosen on the basis of other diagnostic techniques (including bronchoscopy) or therapy chosen empirically will usually benefit from a specific diagnosis by open biopsy. In most centers this is a relatively safe procedure when performed before the need for respiratory support, and the risks only increase when the biopsy is delayed until the patient has become critically ill. In specific patient groups such as BMT and AIDS, the utility and timing of open biopsy may be different. In AIDS patients, OLB is rarely necessary, since a specific diagnosis can usually be made by BAL or transbronchial lung biopsy. If the disease process is progressing despite apparently adequate therapy or bronchoscopy is nondiagnostic, then OLB should be considered to rule out other co-pathogens. In BMT patients the approach may be modified to allow therapy of common noninfectious complications such as pulmonary edema before embarking on invasive diagnostic studies.

REFERENCES

1. Armstrong D: History of opportunistic infection in the immunocompromised host. Clin Infect Dis 1993;17:S318.
2. Thomas CF, Limper AH: *Pneumocystis* pneumonia. N Engl J Med 2004;350:2487.
3. Morris A, Lundgren JD, Masur H, et al: Current epidemiology of *Pneumocystis* pneumonia. Emerg Infect Dis 2004;10:1713.
4. Tamm M, Traenkle P, Grilli G, et al: Pulmonary cytomegalovirus infection in immunocompromised patients. Chest 2001;119:838.
5. Bag R: Fungal pneumonias in transplant recipients. Curr Opin Pulm Med 2003;9:193.
6. Welliver RC: Review of epidemiology and clinical risk factors for severe respiratory syncytial virus (RSV) infection. J Pediatr 2003;143:S112.
7. Leen AM, Rooney CM: Adenovirus as an emerging pathogen in immunocompromised patients. Br J Haematol 2005;128:135.
8. Kotloff RM, Ahya VN, Crawford SW: Pulmonary complications of solid organ and hematopoietic stem cell transplantation. Am J Respir Crit Care Med 2004;170:22.
9. Feinstein MB, Mokhtari M, Ferreiro R, et al: Fiberoptic bronchoscopy in allogeneic bone marrow transplantation. Findings in the era of cytomegalovirus antigen surveillance. Chest 2001;120:1094.
10. Fishman JA, Rubin RH: Infection in organ-transplant recipients. N Eng J Med 1998;338:1741.
11. Buckley RH: Pulmonary complications of primary immunodeficiencies. Paediatr Resp Rev 2004;5:5225.
12. Beck JM, Rosen MJ, Peavy HH: Pulmonary complications of HIV infection. Am J Respir Crit Care Med 2001;164:2160.
13. Clark JG, Hansen JA, Hertz MI, et al: Idiopathic pneumonia syndrome after bone marrow transplantation. Am Rev Respir Dis 1993;147:1601.
14. Sia IG, Patel R: New strategies for prevention and therapy of cytomegalovirus infection and disease in solid-organ transplant recipients. Clin Microbiol Rev 2000;13:83.
15. Pillay D: Management of herpesvirus infections following transplantation. J Antimicrob Chemother 2000;45:729.
16. Pacini-Edelstein S, Mehra M, Ament ME, et al: Varicella in pediatric liver transplant patients. A retrospective analysis of treatment and outcome. J Pediatr Gastroenterol Nutr 2003;37:183.
17. Clark DA, Griffiths PD: Human herpesvirus 6. Relevance of infection in the immunocompromised host. Br J Hematol 2003;120:384.
18. Edman JC, Kovacs JA, Masur H, et al: Ribosomal RNA sequence shows *Pneumocystis carinii* to be a member of the fungi. Nature 1988;344:519.
19. Miller R, Huang L: *Pneumocystis jirovecii* infection. Thorax 2004;59:731.
20. Muller FM, Trusen A, Weig M: Clinical manifestations and diagnosis of invasive aspergillosis in immunocompromised children. Eur J Pediatr 2002;161:563.
21. Hoffer FA, Gow K, Flynn PM, Davidoff A: Accuracy of percutaneous lung biopsy for invasive pulmonary aspergillosis. Pediatr Radiol 2001;31:144.
22. Marr KA: New approaches to invasive fungal infections. Curr Opin Hematol 2003;10:445.
23. Gleissner B, Schilling A, Anagnostopolous I, et al: Improved outcome of zygomycosis patients with hematological diseases? Leuk Lymphoma 2004;45:1351.
24. Abbas J, Bodey GP, Hanna HA, et al: *Candida krusei* fungemia: An escalating serious infection in immunocompromised patients. Arch Intern Med 2000;160:2659.
25. Adderson EE: Histoplasmosis in a pediatric oncology center. J Pediatr 2004;144:100.
26. Katz AS, Niesenbaurm I, Mass B: Pleural effusion as the initial manifestation of disseminated cryptococcosis in the acquired immune deficiency syndrome. Diagnosis by pleural biopsy. Chest 1989;96:440.
27. Idigoras P, Perez-Traillero E, Pineiro L, et al: Disseminated infection and colonization by *Scedosporium prolificans*. A review of 18 cases, 1990–1999. Clin Infect Dis 2001;32:E158.
28. Montoya JG, Liesenfeld O: Toxoplasmosis. Lancet 2004;363:1965.
29. Stokes DC, Shenep JL, Parham D, et al: Role of flexible bronchoscopy in the diagnosis of pulmonary infiltrates in pediatric patients with cancer. J Pediatr 1989;115:561.
30. Jain P, Sandur D, Meli Y, et al: Role of flexible bronchoscopy in immunocompromised patients with lung infiltrates. Chest 2004;125:712.
31. Cahill AM, Baskin KM, Kaye RD, et al: CT-guided percutaneous lung biopsy in children. J Vasc Interv Radiol 2004;15:955.
32. Mason WH, Siegel S, Tucker BL: Diagnostic open lung biopsy for diffuse pulmonary disease in immunocompromised patients. Am J Pediatr Hematol Oncol 1982;4:355.
33. Imoke E, Dudgeon DL, Colombani P, et al: Open lung biopsy in the immunocompromised pediatric patient. J Pediatr Surg 1983;18:816.
34. Prober C, Whyle H, Smith C: Open lung biopsy in immunocompromised children with pulmonary infiltrates. Am J Dis Child 1984;138:60.
35. Early GL, Williams TE, Kilman JW: Open lung biopsy. Its effect on therapy in the pediatric patient. Chest 1985;87:467.
36. Doolin EJ, Luck SR, Sherman JO, Raffensperger JG: Emergency lung biopsy. Friend or foe of the immunosuppressed child. J Pediatr Surg 1986;21:485.
37. Shorter NA, Ross AJ III, August C, et al: The usefulness of open lung biopsy in the pediatric bone marrow transplant population. J Pediatr Surg 1988;23:533.
38. Foglia RP, Shilyansky J, Fonkalsrud EW: Emergency open lung biopsy in immunocompromised pediatric patients. Ann Surg 1989;210:90.
39. Snyder CL, Ramsay NK, McGrave PB, et al: Diagnostic open lung biopsy after bone marrow transplantation. J Pediatr Surg 1990;25:871.
40. Bozeman PM, Stokes DC: Diagnostic methods in pulmonary infections of immunocompromised children. Bronchoscopy, needle aspiration, and open biopsy. In: Patrick CC, ed: Infections in Immunocompromised Infants and Children. New York: Churchill Livingstone, 1992, p 305.
41. Gururangan S, Lawson RAM, Morris Jones PH, et al: Evaluation of the usefulness of open lung biopsies. Pediatr Hematol Oncol 1992;9:107.
42. Stefanutti D, Morais L, Fournet J-C, et al: Value of open lung biopsy in immunocompromised children. J Pediatr 2000;137:165.
43. Kornecki A, Shemie SD: Open lung biopsy in children with respiratory failure. Crit Care Med 2001;29:1247.
44. Shaikh ZH, Torres HA, Walsh GL, et al: Open lung biopsy in bone marrow transplant patients has a poor diagnostic yield for a specific diagnosis. Transpl Infect Dis 2002;4:80.
45. Hayes-Jordan A, Benaim E, Richardson S, et al: Open lung biopsy in pediatric bone marrow transplant patients. J Pediatr Surg 2002;37:446.

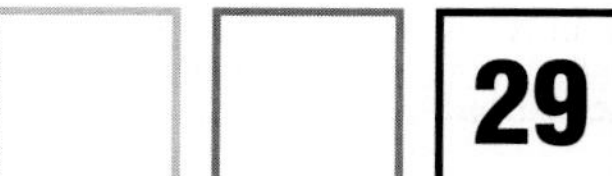

29 Bronchiectasis

Anne B. Chang, PhD •
Gregory J. Redding, MD

Bronchiectasis is a pathologic state of the conducting airways manifested by radiographic evidence of bronchial dilation and clinically by chronic productive cough. Although it develops transiently following pneumonia,[1] it is more often a persistent condition that can progress. Bronchiectasis can occur locally, producing recurrent cough and infectious exacerbations, or it can develop diffusely, resulting in additional generalized airway obstruction and destruction with eventual respiratory failure. The diagnostic criteria for bronchiectasis have changed, and the disease is now diagnosed on the basis of radiographic features of high-resolution computerized tomography (HRCT) rather than bronchography or chest radiographs.

Today the most important cause of clinically significant bronchiectasis in North America, Europe, and other affluent Western countries is cystic fibrosis (CF). Other causes of bronchiectasis, unrelated to CF, have been termed an *orphan disease* because of its low frequency, neglect in research, and treatment related to a lack of commercial interest.[2,3] Whether bronchiectasis is an orphan disease in other parts of the world remains unclear, but studies from Nigeria, New Guinea, India, and Turkey suggest it contributes substantially to respiratory morbidity in impoverished populations.[4–7] This chapter addresses bronchiectasis unrelated to CF and other underlying pulmonary host defense deficiencies such as ciliary dyskinesia syndromes and immunodeficiencies, which are covered elsewhere in this text.

EPIDEMIOLOGY AND PREVALENCE

PREVALENCE ACROSS TIME AND COUNTRIES

In most affluent countries, childhood bronchiectasis has almost disappeared.[8,9] Field reported on 160 children with bronchiectasis over a 20-year period from the 1940s to the 1960s, noting a decline in the incidence of bronchiectasis from 48 to 10 cases per 10,000 people.[10] By 1994, Nikolaizik and Warner had found that only 1% of 4000 children referred to a respiratory specialty service had bronchiectasis.[8] The reduced incidence over time has been ascribed to reduced crowding, improved immunization programs, better hygiene and nutrition, and early access to medical care.[8,9]

However, bronchiectasis remains common in less affluent countries[3,6,7] and among disadvantaged indigenous groups in affluent countries such as the Alaskan Yupik children in the United States,[11] aboriginal children in Australia,[12] and Maori and Pacific Islanders in New Zealand.[13] Among these populations, the incidence of childhood bronchiectasis is 147 to 200 per 10,000 children.[11,12] These estimates far exceed the prevalence of CF in mainstream communities in Australia and the United States (Australian CF prevalence is 3.5 per 10,000).[14] Nor has the prevalence of bronchiectasis decreased over time among Alaskan Native people despite dramatic reductions in tuberculosis and development of modern immunization programs. In this population, the prevalence of bronchiectasis among people born in the 1940s and among people born in the 1980s remained the same.[11] In most developing countries, obtaining prevalence estimates is difficult. Bronchiectasis is not mentioned in the World Health Organization (WHO) Bulletin on chronic respiratory disease,[15] despite recognition that a significant number (29% of 110) of adults with chronic obstructive pulmonary disease have underlying bronchiectasis[16] and that the majority of bronchiectasis in adulthood has its roots in childhood.[17,18]

ETIOLOGIC RISK FACTORS

Bronchiectasis is the end result of a variety of airway insults and predisposing conditions that ultimately injure the airways and lead to recurrent or persistent airway infection and destruction. Examples of these conditions are listed in Table 29-1. Bronchiectasis develops in some individuals when structural airway abnormalities, such as bronchomalacia, endobronchial tuberculosis, and retained aspirated foreign bodies, impair mucus and bacterial clearance. Similarly, persistent airway injury and narrowing associated with bronchiolitis obliterans (due to viral injury or following lung transplantation) can lead to bronchiectasis. Recurrent airway injury, such as occurs with aspiration syndromes, can also result in bronchiectasis. Pediatric cohorts published during the last decade that describe the frequencies of these associated conditions are summarized in Table 29-2.

Also predisposing to bronchiectasis is the presence of inhaled irritants, including indoor and outdoor pollutants, that stimulate mucus production in the presence of impaired airway clearance. Impaired upper airway defenses may also predispose to bronchiectasis based on the common association between rhinosinusitis and bronchitis/bronchiectasis. Indeed, the sinuses and eustachian tubes have been considered a "sanctuary site" by some for bacterial pathogens and cytokines that may predispose to recurrent lower airway infection. Finally, there are variations in host inflammatory responses (e.g., cytokine and matrix metalloproteinase [MMP] levels) and counterbalancing anti-inflammatory mechanisms (e.g., antioxidants and antiproteases), which may explain why some children develop bronchiectasis while others do not despite similar exposures and living conditions.

Previous Lower Respiratory Infections

It is well documented that respiratory infections in children can lead to later respiratory morbidity and lung function abnormalities.[19–22] Epidemiologic studies have linked acute lower respiratory infection in infancy with chronic bronchitis and productive cough later in childhood.[23–26] Children with the clinical findings of bronchiectasis whose chest HRCT scans do not meet the criteria for radiologic bronchiectasis are described as having chronic bronchitis or chronic suppurative lung disease (CSLD).[8,12] It is not known what fraction of

■ TABLE 29-1. Causes of bronchiectasis

Primary Pathophysiology	Diseases	Major Associations
Impaired immune function	Severe combined immunodeficiency	Gastrointestinal bacterial infections
	Common variable immunodeficiency	
	Natural killer cell deficiency	EBV infection
	Bare lymphocyte syndrome	
	X-linked lymphoproliferative disease	
	Ectodermal dysplasia	Teeth, hair, eccrine sweat glands
	Ataxia-telangiectasia	Cerebellar ataxia, telangiectases
	Bloom syndrome	Telangiectatic, altered pigmented skin
	DNA ligase I defect	Sun sensitivity
	T-cell deficiency	Thymus aplasia
	HIV	
Ciliary dyskinesia	Primary	Sinusitus
	Functional	
Abnormal mucus	CF	Pancreatic insufficiency
Clinical syndromes	Young's syndrome	Azoospermia
	Yellow nail lymphedema syndrome	Nail discoloration
	Marfan syndrome	Phenotypic appearance
	Usher's syndrome	Retinitis pigmentosa
Congenital tracheobronchomegaly	Mounier-Kuhn's syndrome	
	Williams-Campbell syndrome	
	Ehlers-Danlos syndrome	Phenotype appearance
Aspiration syndromes	Recurrent small-volume aspiration	Neurodevelopmental problems
	Primary aspiration	
	Tracheoesophageal fistula	
	Gastroesophageal reflux disease	
Obstructive bronchiectasis	Foreign body	
	Tumors (e.g., mucoepidermoid)	
	Lymph nodes, etc.	
Other pulmonary disease associations	Interstitial lung disease	
	Bronchiolitis obliterans	
	Allergic bronchopulmonary aspergillosis	
	Traction bronchiectasis	
	Bronchomalacia	
Others	α_1-Antitrypsin or protease inhibitor activity deficiency	Liver disease
	Post transplant	
	Autoimmune diseases	
	Post toxic fumes	
	Eosinophilic lung disease	

CF, cystic fibrosis; EBV, Epstein-Barr virus; HIV, human immunodeficiency virus.

■ TABLE 29-2. Etiologies of childhood bronchiectasis published in last 10 years

Study and Setting	Nikolaizik and Warner[8] *N* = 41 (%) London, England	Edwards and Co-workers[189] *N* = 60 (%) Auckland, New Zealand	Singleton and Co-workers[11] *N* = 46 (%) Remote, Indigenous Alaska	Karakoc and Colleagues[7] *N* = 23 (%) Adana, Turkey	Chang and Colleagues[12] *N* = 65 (%) Indigenous Australia
Postinfectious (severe pneumonia)	12 (29)	15 (15)	42 (92)	4 (17)	58 (90)
Tuberculosis	0	0	2 (4)	4 (17)	1 (1)
Inherited immune deficiency	8 (20)	7 (12)	0	4 (17)	2 (3)
Primary ciliary dyskinesia	7 (17)	0	0	3 (13)	0
Congenital malformations	6 (15)	1 (1)	0	0	1 (1)
Secondary immune defects	3 (7)	0	0	0	0
Aspiration of exogenous toxicants	2 (5)	1 (2)	1 (2)	0	0
GERD or aspiration	0	6 (10)	1 (2)	0	3 (5)
Unknown	2 (5)	30 (50)	0	0	0
CF-like or CF	1 (2)	0	0	4 (17)	0
"Asthma"	0	0	0	4 (18)	0

CF, cystic fibrosis; GERD, gastroesophageal reflux disease.

children with CSLD will eventually develop radiographic evidence of bronchiectasis nor how many will improve and become asymptomatic. The natural history of this population requires further study.

In non-CF cohort studies, the majority of children with bronchiectasis have had previous pneumonic events with lobar or diffuse alveolar infiltrates.[11,27] In a case-control study of childhood pneumonia and radiographically proven bronchiectasis, a strong association between hospitalized pneumonia and bronchiectasis was found.[27] Children who had been previously hospitalized for pneumonia were 15 times more likely to develop bronchiectasis. A dose effect was also shown; recurrent (more than one) hospitalization for pneumonia and more severe pneumonia (episodes with longer hospital stay or oxygen requirement) increased the risk of bronchiectasis later in childhood. Bronchiectasis was three times more likely in children with four or five episodes of pneumonia, and 21 times more likely if they had six or more pneumonia episodes. The overall number of pneumonia episodes rather than the site of pneumonia were associated with bronchiectasis. Specific infectious etiologies were not described in these studies.

Some authors have suggested that bronchiolitis is an important precursor of bronchiectasis.[28] However, in the Alaskan 5-year case-control follow-up of children hospitalized in infancy with severe respiratory syncytial virus infections, those with a previous respiratory syncytial virus hospitalization were not more likely to develop bronchiectasis.[29] In addition, hospitalizations for bronchiolitis among indigenous Australian infants were not risk factors for bronchiectasis.[12,27] Although measles, tuberculosis, pertussis, and severe viral pneumonia do not frequently cause bronchiectasis, they are so common in less affluent countries that these infections are still considered important antecedents to childhood bronchiectasis.[6,7]

Upper Airway Infection and Aspiration

Mechanisms by which upper respiratory tract infections predispose to lower airway inflammation and injury are reviewed elsewhere.[30] Bacterial pathogens colonizing the nose and mouth are shed into saliva and contaminate the lower airways. Proinflammatory cytokines from the oropharynx may also be aspirated and augment neutrophilic inflammatory responses in the lower airways. Hydrolytic enzymes in infected upper airway secretions impair protective secretory molecules such as mucins in the lower airways, and thereby predispose the lower airways to infection. In vitro studies have shown that some bacteria produce substances that cause ciliary slowing, dyskinesia, and stasis, setting the stage for chronic bacterial colonization of the lower airways.[31] Indigenous children in Central Australia have high and early rates of bacterial carriage in the nasopharynx, and simultaneous infection with two or more pathogens in acute lower respiratory tract infections is common.[32,33] Whether the concentration and/or persistence of these pathogens in upper airways constitute a significant risk factor for development or progression of bronchiectasis is unknown.

Bronchiectasis and other forms of suppurative lung disease have been described among individuals with neurologic and neuromuscular conditions that reduce the frequency and effectiveness of cough and also increase the risk of aspirating oropharyngeal contents. Brook reported on 10 children with such conditions who developed anaerobic pulmonary infections; 6 were notable for "poor oral hygiene."[34] Similar data have been reported in adults with chronic obstructive pulmonary disease, where periodontal disease was associated with more severe airway obstruction.[35]

Public Health Issues

In 1949, Field wrote, "Irreversible bronchiectasis is not commonly seen in the better social and economic classes. Good nutrition and home conditions probably give the child a better chance of more complete recovery from lung damaging disease."[36] Public health conditions, including malnutrition, crowding, and environmental pollution, increase the risk of acute respiratory infections (ARIs),[11,12,37,38] predispose children to persistent airway mucus production, and are likely to contribute to the prevalence of bronchiectasis in developing countries.

Macro- and selected micro-malnutrition increases infection risks, because it creates an immune deficiency state and leads to the malnutrition-infection-malnutrition cycle.[39] However, data on malnutrition specifically preceding bronchiectasis are limited and inconsistent. In Central Australia, children with bronchiectasis are three times more likely to have had malnutrition in early childhood before the diagnosis of bronchiectasis.[27] Seventeen percent of these children had weight Z scores below the 2 standard deviations of WHO-determined criteria.[12] In contrast, malnutrition is uncommon in Alaskan children.[11] One explanation for this difference may be the increased frequency of breastfeeding in Alaska, which approaches 80% among Alaskan Native mothers.[40] Breastfeeding is known to protect against development of bronchiectasis.[27] In addition, the role of micronutrient depletion such as zinc and vitamin A deficiency may increase the risk of ARIs, thus setting the stage for recurrent airway insults and subsequent long-term injury.[41,42]

Bronchiectasis may itself predispose to malnutrition as a result of chronic pulmonary infection, diminished appetite, and reduced caloric intake. This scenario is best described in patients with CF.[43] The caloric needs and daily oxygen consumption of children with bronchiectasis not associated with CF have not been reported.

Increased risk of ARI is associated with greater number of house occupants, housing with few rooms, and inadequate water supply.[37,38] No direct cause-and-effect relationship has been shown with bronchiectasis. In affluent countries, those communities with higher prevalences of bronchiectasis are also those where poverty and low standards of housing are common.[11,12] In a qualitative study, community members and health care providers believed that potential contributing variables to acute and chronic lung diseases were smoke, dust, feeding practices, socioeconomic conditions, and mold.[44]

The effects of environmental tobacco smoke (ETS) on children's respiratory systems are well known from both in utero and ex utero exposure and include reduced airway caliber, increased lower respiratory tract infections, and middle ear disease[45] Reviews on ETS and its effects on the developing lung and accelerated lung decline are available elsewhere.[46–49] ETS is a known contributor to the increased number of childhood respiratory illnesses. Exposure to indoor biomass combustion increases coughing illness associated with ARIs with a exposure-response effect.[50] Exposure to other ambient pollutants (nitrogen dioxide,[51,52] gas cooking[53]) is also associated with increased cough in children in both cross-sectional[51,52] and longitudinal studies.[54] There is no direct evidence of pollutants causing bronchiectasis, and the pathogenesis is probably indirect through an increased frequency of ARIs and increased airway mucus production.

■ GENETICS

The interplay between genotype and environment is increasingly recognized as the key in phenotypic expression of respiratory diseases.[55,56] An increased frequency of cystic fibrosis transmembrane regulator *(CFTR)* genotypes associated with cystic fibrosis, present in heterozygotes, has been described in several small series among patients with diffuse bronchiectasis.[57,58] Similarly, heterozygotes for α_1-antitrypsin have been described more frequently in those individuals with diffuse bronchiectasis.[59] Published guidelines suggest optional screening for α_1-antitrypsin deficiency for patients with idiopathic diffuse bronchiectasis.[60]

Aside from variations in specific gene frequencies, overexpression of innate pulmonary immune mechanisms, such as proinflammatory cytokine and adhesion molecule production and receptor expression, may contribute to the development of bronchiectasis in certain children. An increased or exaggerated neutrophilic response in Australian indigenous children as a group has been described.[61] Similarly, MMPs (e.g., MMP-2 and MMP-9) have been isolated from the sputum and bronchoalveolar lavage fluid of bronchiectatic subjects, suggesting a role in airway destruction by gelatinases and collagenases.[62,63] Among patients with allergic bronchopulmonary aspergillosis, increased concentrations of MMP-9 were associated with development of bronchiectasis as a specific feature of the infection.[64] Whether proinflammatory cytokine and collagenase overexpression are associated with early-onset disease or particularly progressive disease in childhood remains unknown.

■ PATHOLOGY AND PATHOPHYSIOLOGY

The histopathology of bronchiectasis was first described by Laënnec[65] in 1819. It includes alterations in subsegmental bronchial structure accompanied by neutrophilic inflammation, intraluminal secretion accumulation, and obliteration of distal airways. There are accompanying changes of peribronchial inflammation and fibrosis, distal lung collapse, bronchial and pulmonary vascular changes, and pleural adhesions. The macroscopic and microscopic features of bronchiectasis change as the disease progresses. Classical papers on bronchiectasis divided morphologic types of bronchiectasis into tubular or cylindrical, early fusiform, late fusiform, fusosaccular, and saccular types as different stages in the progression of disease.[17] The most commonly used classification is that of Reid's subtypes (cylindrical, varicose, and cystic[66]), which were based on bronchographic findings. The latter findings are illustrated in Figure 29-1. More recent HRCT scoring systems describe cylindrical and saccular changes as markers of disease severity.[67] Saccular and cystic changes tend to reflect clinically more advanced, severe, and irreversible disease, but there are no published data on whether these changes reflect ongoing disease activity and progression.[67]

Macroscopically, the airways are tortuous and dilated, at times extending to the pleural surface. Early histologic changes include bronchial wall thickening, edema, presence of inflammatory cells, development of lymphoid nodules and follicles, and mucous gland hyperplasia. Intraluminal secretions are purulent or mucopurulent. Microscopic changes include loss of ciliated epithelial cells and epithelial ulcerations. With time, chronic inflammation leads to squamous cell metaplasia and fibrotic obliteration of distal conducting airways and peribronchial tissue. As bronchiectasis becomes more severe, the airway walls are thin and saccular with destruction of the airway's muscular, elastic, and cartilaginous elements.[66,68] The saccular airway walls are composed of fibrous and granulation tissue with only remnants of normal tissue. In advanced disease, mucus-filled saccular airway changes can be severe enough to appear as cystic microabscesses.

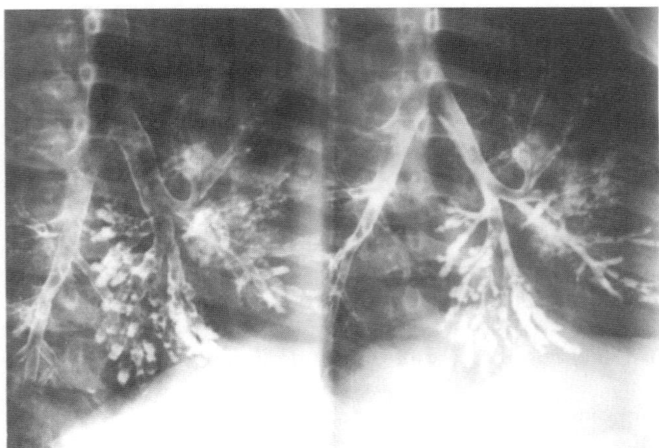

■ **FIGURE 29-1.** Varicose and cystic changes characteristic of severe bronchiectasis by bronchogram.

Vascular changes accompany bronchial structural changes in bronchiectasis. Large bronchopulmonary anastomosis can develop, and total bronchial arterial blood flow is increased. Extensive precapillary anastomoses between the two arterial systems can serve as a shunt between the pulmonary and systemic systems, increasing cardiac work.[68] Bronchopulmonary vascular anastomoses most often occur near distal subsegmental bronchi that have undergone saccular changes. Abnormal bronchopulmonary anastomoses and enlargement of aberrant bronchial arteries are thought to be associated with the metabolic demands of hypertrophied muscle, lymphoid tissue, and peribronchial granulation tissue during the course of the organizing pneumonitis that precedes the development of bronchiectasis.[69] Additional vascular remodeling of the pulmonary arteries and arterioles occurs in association with chronic airway obstruction and alveolar hypoxia, predisposing patients to pulmonary hypertension and cor pulmonale in severe cases.

The initial trigger for the bronchiectasis process is unknown. Animal models of bronchiectasis suggest that inadequate mucus clearance and persistent infection are necessary prerequisites.[70] Mucus clearance in bronchiectasis is reduced by a combination of factors including airflow limitation,[71,72] abnormal quantity and quality of mucus produced,[73] and substances produced by bacteria that cause ciliary slowing, dyskinesia, and mucus stasis.[31] Mucociliary clearance of the debris is enhanced by cough, exercise, and hyperventilation,[72,74,75] and is decreased in situations where airway caliber is diminished.[71,72] Decreased mucociliary clearance in turn leads to increased bacterial colonization and infection, setting up a vicious cycle. The role of bacteria in the pathogenesis of chronic lung infection has been reviewed by Stockley.[76]

Sputum markers of neutrophilic airway inflammation are found in adults with bronchiectasis, especially in those with chronic expectoration of mucopurulent sputum.[77,78] Angrill and colleagues found increased neutrophils, neutrophil elastase, myeloperoxidase, tumor necrosis factor-α (TNF-α), interleukin-8, and interleukin-6 in the sputum of adults with bronchiectasis.[77] The intensity of the inflammation was worse in colonized patients. However, even noncolonized subjects with bronchiectasis had a more intense bronchial inflammatory reaction than did control subjects. Although antibiotics have been shown to reduce airway inflammation in some studies over a period of weeks,[79] other studies using antibiotics showed no effect on the sputum markers of inflammation despite clinical improvement.[80,81] An upsurge in systemic inflammatory response has also been reported. However, there is a poor correlation between systemic and bronchial inflammatory mediators, suggesting that the inflammatory process is mostly compartmentalized to the airways.[80]

Exaggerated or persistent pulmonary inflammation present in bronchiectasis[78] leads to increased lung destruction by many mechanisms. The balance between proteases and antielastases are increasingly recognized in the protection of airways against hostile agents and destruction of lung tissue. Collagenase activity present in the bronchoalveolar lavage fluid of adults with moderately severe bronchiectasis originates from neutrophils as well as bacteria. These collagenolytic proteases are probable contributors to increasing tissue destruction.[82] Bronchoalveolar lavage specimens from adults with bronchiectasis contain MMPs (MMP-2, MMP-8, and MMP-9)[83] and collagenolytic proteinases of bacterial origin.[82] Endobronchial biopsies in adults with bronchiectasis demonstrate an overexpression of neutrophil MMPs.[83] Using sputum from adults with bronchiectasis, Shum and colleagues showed that serine proteases derived from neutrophils were responsible for degradation of proteoglycans in a model matrix and that the protease secretion was stimulated by TNF-α in the presence of cofactors isolated from bronchial secretions of bronchiectatic patients.[84]

There are additional pathogenic processes associated with bronchiectasis that contribute to persistence of airway inflammation and obstruction. For example, resolution of inflammation is normally associated with the orderly removal of apoptotic inflammatory cells, and impairment of this removal process has been described in adults with bronchiectasis.[85] Increased airway permeability has also been described with bronchiectasis when purulent sputum and significant colonization of the respiratory tract by bacterial pathogens are present.[86] Up-regulation of circulating adhesion molecules (E-selectin, intercellular adhesion molecule-1, and vascular adhesion molecule-1) have also been suggested to have a role in the pathogenesis of bronchiectasis.[83]

NATURAL HISTORY

Given the heterogeneity of etiologic factors and host responses, regional severity, and distribution of bronchiectasis, it is not surprising that the natural history is varied, ranging from mild respiratory morbidity to death from airway obstruction, pulmonary infection, and respiratory failure with hypercapnia. In some cases, bronchiectasis following pneumonia resolves radiographically.[1] More often, bronchiectasis persists on HRCT but becomes less severe clinically, with fewer infectious exacerbations and less evident cough later in childhood. In the series of 46 children with HRCT-documented bronchiectasis, one third improved, one third remained symptomatic but stable, and one third worsened while receiving medical therapy.[11] Both Field and Landau and co-workers reported reductions in exacerbations during the second and third decades of life despite persistence of bronchiectasis radiographically.[87,88]

Worsening bronchiectasis may become increasingly saccular in appearance within a local lung region, as illustrated in Figure 29-2. Alternatively, bronchiectasis can extend to additional airways as a result of either endobronchial spread of infection or evolution of disease at several airway sites. The frequency with which bronchiectasis extends to new lung regions varies from 2% to 35% with different series.[89,90] Local progression of disease rather than extension to new areas is probably more common.

The most severe cases of bronchiectasis have diffuse airway involvement and are accompanied by airflow limitation. Among those with obstructive changes on spirometry, 45% to 69% have some component of airway reversibility in response to inhaled β-adrenergic agents.[91,92] Unfavorable prognostic factors for patients with bronchiectasis include presence of asthma, bilateral lung involvement,[88,93] and saccular bronchiectasis.[93] The advent of better antibiotics, inhaled antibiotics, long-term oxygen therapy, and improved nutrition have improved prognosis. The use of long-term oxygen therapy has reduced the progression of pulmonary vascular disease among children with bronchiectasis due to CF. As a result, cor pulmonale and right heart failure associated with progressive airway obstruction are now uncommon complications of advanced bronchiectasis.[94] In one pediatric study in which echocardiography was performed in 50 children with bronchiectasis, only one child had pulmonary hypertension.[12] However, among indigenous groups, premature deaths in early adulthood (aged 30s and 40s) are unfortunately still common (unpublished Australian data). Current data indicate that the prognosis is worse among adults with bronchiectasis than among those with asthma, but it is better than adults with chronic obstructive pulmonary disease.[95]

CLINICAL FEATURES

PRESENTING CLINICAL FEATURES

The clinical case definition of bronchiectasis is imprecise, but the diagnosis should be considered when children have a chronic moist-sounding cough, exertional dyspnea, recurrent wheezing and chest infections, hemoptysis, growth failure, digital clubbing, and/or chest wall deformity (hyperinflation). The most common symptom is persistent or recurrent productive cough

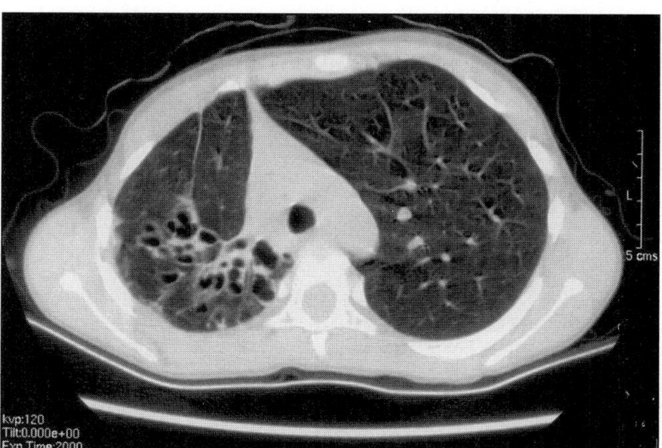

FIGURE 29-2. CT scan findings of saccular bronchiectasis in the right upper lobe of a 9-year-old boy.

of purulent or mucopurulent sputum. Sputum color has recently been shown to be a good reflection of neutrophilic airway inflammation.[96] The frequencies of hyperinflation and digital clubbing vary among case series (5% to 60%).[7,10,12,88] Digital clubbing can disappear after medical or surgical treatment in association with disappearance of purulent sputum.[10,88] Although hemoptysis is less common among children than in adults with bronchiectasis, a presenting finding of hemoptysis should raise the possibility of bronchiectasis as a cause. Chest auscultation may be entirely normal or reveal coarse inspiratory crackles over the affected regions. Hypoxemia by pulse oximetry and abnormal cardiac sounds associated with pulmonary hypertension are late signs in bronchiectasis. Like any other serious chronic respiratory illness, children with bronchiectasis may have growth failure.[12]

The median age of diagnosis of bronchiectasis unrelated to CF in affluent countries is 4 to 5 years.[11,12] A New Zealand cohort[13] was older at diagnosis (9–10 years old) but also experienced more advanced disease.[12] Idiopathic bronchiectasis is rare in infancy, but when present, it is likely to reflect congenital pulmonary malformations, such as cystic lung disease or tracheobronchomegaly,[97] or, alternatively, primary ciliary dyskinesia. Only half of those with ciliary dyskinesia have the Kartagener triad of situs inversus, bronchiectasis, and sinusitis.[98]

Risk factors of development of bronchiectasis are the presence on radiography of atelectasis[27,99] and of persistent lobar abnormalities.[29] In Alaska, children were more likely to develop bronchiectasis if chest radiographs obtained in children under 2 years of age showed lung parenchymal densities, persistent parenchymal densities greater than 6 months' duration, or parenchymal densities on several episodes.[29] Among aboriginal Australian children hospitalized with lobar changes on admission chest radiographs, children with alveolar abnormalities were more likely to have bronchiectasis on follow-up.[99] In a prospective radiographic study of alveolar changes (total of 179 lobes in 112 hospitalized children), the two most common involved lobes were the right upper lobe and left lower lobes.[99] Both lobes, however, had similar rates of radiologic clearance on follow-up (22% and 27%, respectively). Most studies, including those from the 1940s through the 1960s described the left lower lobe as the most commonly affected lobe in children with bronchiectasis.[11,12,88]

COMORBID CONDITIONS

Children with postinfectious bronchiolitis obliterans and CSLD share some common clinical features (airway limitation, chronic cough, recurrent ARIs) in addition to the same etiologic insult.[19,100] In a Brazilian study, clinical remission occurred in 23% of 31 children with postinfectious bronchiolitis obliterans, 10% died, and the remainder had persistent respiratory symptoms.[100] In another study, a third of 19 children with postinfectious bronchiolitis obliterans developed bronchiectasis.[19]

Several phenotypes of childhood wheeze have been recognized,[101] and airway hyperreactivity occurs in some individuals with bronchiectasis.[100] Inadequate treatment of asthma can lead to later significant morbidity and contribute to the prevalence and morbidity of adult chronic airway obstructive disease.[102] Indeed, the presence of features of asthma is an ominous prognostic factor in both children[10,88] and adults[95] with bronchiectasis. The frequency of reactive airway disease (RAD) varies from 26% to 74% in children with bronchiectasis.[11,12] As a corollary, clinicians must recognize that wheeze and cough may not be related to asthma but to increased airway secretions and airway collapse as features of bronchiectasis.

Gastroesophageal reflux disease (GERD) may coexist with any chronic respiratory illness and, when present, should be appropriately treated. There are published American and European pediatric guidelines on diagnosis and treatment of GERD.[103,104] However, data in adults indicate that GERD may resolve or significantly improve once the underlying respiratory disorder has been treated.[105] There is, however, no evidence-based approach to the management of GERD associated with bronchiectasis.

Hypertrophic osteoarthropathy (clubbing, periostosis of the tubular bones, and arthritis-like signs and symptoms) may occur in children with bronchiectasis.[106] Systemic amyloidosis has also been reported as a complication or comorbidity in bronchiectasis.[107] Cardiac dysfunction, though rare, has also been reported, and may or may not be accompanied by pulmonary hypertension. A study of 21 children with bronchiectasis showed that while ventricular systolic function was normal, some patients had changes in left ventricular diastolic function indices, characterized by abnormal E wave–to–A wave (E/A) ratios or isovolumic relaxation time values.[108] The authors also found that isovolumic relaxation time had a significant negative correlation with the clinical severity score. Other reported comorbid conditions associated with bronchiectasis are scoliosis, chronic suppurative ear disease, social problems, past urinary tract infections, and developmental delay.[11,12]

DIAGNOSTIC EVALUATIONS

The aims of evaluating children with suspected bronchiectasis are: (1) to confirm the diagnosis, (2) to define the distribution and severity of airway involvement, (3) to characterize extrapulmonary organ involvement associated with bronchiectasis (e.g., cor pulmonale), and (4) to identify familial and treatable underlying causes of bronchiectasis.

DIAGNOSTIC CRITERIA

Chest HRCT is the gold standard for diagnosis.[67,109] Plain chest radiographs are relatively insensitive in diagnosing bronchiectasis. In the study by Currie and colleagues, diagnosis of bronchiectasis by chest radiographs was present in only 49% of those with bronchographic evidence of bronchiectasis.[110] Radiologic features of bronchiectasis can also occur in the absence of CSLD as they are present in pulmonary fibrosis, congenital lesions such as Mounier-Kuhn's and Williams-Campbell syndrome,[67] and can occur as a result of traction in nonsuppurative lung disease.[111] Some children with CSLD may not yet have radiologically defined bronchiectasis, and airway dilatation presumably occurs at a later stage of the illness. Using ultrafast computed tomography (CT) scans, bronchiectasis was documented in only 43% of children with chronic productive cough.[112] Given that the gold standard to diagnose small-airway abnormalities including bronchiectasis is the HRCT scan,[67] the yield is likely to be higher if HRCT scans were used instead of standard CT scans.

The characteristic radiographic finding in bronchiectasis on HRCT is the presence of "signet ring," in which a dilated bronchus is greater than the diameter of the accompanying blood vessel in cross section.[67,109] This is illustrated in Figure 29-3.

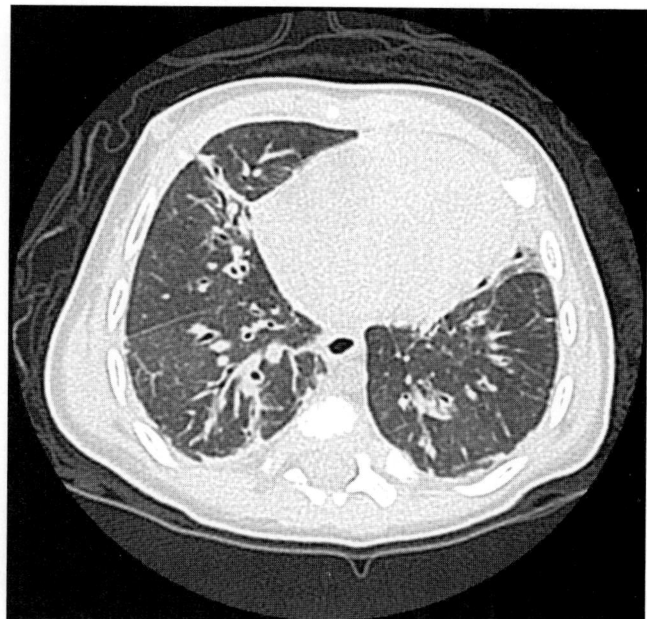

■ **FIGURE 29-3.** High-resolution finding of bronchiectasis illustrating the "signet ring" appearance of a dilated airway adjacent to smaller associated pulmonary vessels.

However, the absence of this characteristic finding does not exclude bronchiectasis. Box 29-1 lists other HRCT findings of bronchiectasis.[67,109] The presence of bronchial dilatation relative to the accompanying vessel does not always indicate the presence of bronchiectasis, because this finding can be present in the situations listed in Box 29-2. Abnormalities in the surrounding lung may be present (parenchyma loss, emphysema, scars, and nodular foci).[109] Chest HRCT signs of bronchiectasis include air-fluid levels in distended bronchi, a linear array or cluster of cysts, dilated bronchi in the periphery of the lung, and bronchial wall thickening due to peribronchial fibrosis.[113] Image quality and hence detection of bronchiectasis is dependent on the radiologic technique used (tube setting, radiation dose, collimation distance, and image intervals).[114] False-positive and false-negative situations that may occur are listed in Box 29-2. HRCT does not distinguish among the etiologies of bronchiectasis.[115] However, in adults bronchiectasis associated with CF, allergic bronchopulmonary aspergillosis, and atypical mycobacteria have some distinctive features.[67] Serial chest HRCT should also be performed to monitor changes in the distribution and severity of disease over time.

BOX 29-1 Features of Bronchiectasis on Chest HRCT Scans*

1. Signet ring sign: Internal diameter of bronchi is larger than accompanying vessel (diameters of both should be short axis).
2. Enlarged internal bronchial diameter.
3. Failure of airway to taper normally while progressing to lung periphery.
4. Presence of peripheral airways at CT periphery.
5. Presence of associated abnormalities:
   - Bronchial wall thickening
   - Mucoid plugging or impaction (seen as branching or rounded/nodular opacities in cross sections, tubular or Y-shaped structures or tree in bud appearance)
6. Mosaic perfusion.
7. Air trapping on expiration.

Compiled from references 67 and 190–192.

BOX 29-2 Pitfalls in Diagnosis of Bronchiectasis on Chest HRCT Scans

False Positives

1. Physiologic constriction of pulmonary artery (creates relative bronchial enlargement).
2. Artifacts from cardiac pulsation and respiratory motion (creates pseudocystic pattern).
3. Pseudobronchiectasis or transient bronchial atresia (related to acute pneumonia or atelectasis).
4. Increased bronchoarterial ratio in normals, asthmatics, or at high altitude.

False Negatives

1. Inappropriate HRCT protocol (incorrect electronic windows and/or collimation).
2. Poor image due to movement artifacts.
3. Nonuse of high-resolution techniques.

Compiled from references 67 and 190–192.

ETIOLOGIC EVALUATION

Pasteur and colleagues recently reported the etiologic causes of bronchiectasis in 150 newly diagnosed adults and identified one or more underlying cause in 47% of them.[18] They concluded that patients with bronchiectasis merit thorough investigation. Current best practices for investigating possible etiology for childhood CSLD are outlined in Table 29-3. Evaluation for primary ciliary dyskinesia syndrome, while ideal, is difficult to interpret in certain situations. Transient abnormal ciliary structure and orientation is commonly found in the presence of nasal space disease and infection.[116]

BRONCHOSCOPIC FINDINGS

Bronchoscopy is indicated to identify obstructive bronchiectasis, which can be intraluminal (tumors and foreign bodies[117]) or due to external airway compression. Bronchiectasis is a complication of inhaled foreign body and occurred in one study among 25% of patients whose diagnosis of foreign body aspiration was delayed by more than 30 days.[118] Airway mucosal changes typical of chronic bronchitis are usually present in bronchiectatic airways at bronchoscopy. Bronchoscopic findings include atrophic mucosa, increased secretions, and airway friability. Airway flaccidity, hypertrophy of elements in the wall, longitudinal corrugations, mucosal reddening, increased vascularity, dilated ducts, and displacement due to lobar collapse have also been described.[119] Five types of bronchoscopic findings of major airways related to bronchiectasis have been: type I, mucosal abnormality/inflammation only; type II, bronchomalacia

TABLE 29-3. Evaluation for underlying etiologies

Routine Investigation Type	Details	Subject of Evaluation
Baseline immune function	IgG, A, M, IgG subclasses, IgE, hemagglutinins, antibodies to vaccinations	Immune deficiency states
CBC	White cell count	Neutropenia
HIV status	HIV antibody, HIV PCR assay	HIV infection
Sweat test and consider genotype	Sweat chloride and CF genotype	CF
Radiology	Chest HRCT scan Chest radiograph	Diagnosis, congenital malformation, and disease severity
Aspergillosis serology	Aspergillosis specific IgE Skin test, total IgE	Allergic bronchopulmonary aspergillosis
Cilia biopsy	Electron microscopy and ciliary beat function	Ciliary dyskinesia
Sputum	Microscopy, sensitivity, and culture	Number of polymorphs, microbiology
Additional Tests, Depending on Clinical Characteristics		
Bronchoscopy	Airway abnormalities BAL	Obstructive bronchiectasis Congenital defect in bronchial walls
Investigations for GERD	Esophageal pH studies, manometry and/or upper endoscopy	GERD with or without aspiration syndromes
Barium meal		Tracheoesophageal fistula, esophageal abnormalities causing secondary aspiration such as achalasia
Mantoux	PPD tuberculin and atypical	Mycobacterium TB and atypical mycobacteria
Further immune tests	Neutrophil function, CH50, etc.	Immune function
Video fluoroscopy	Oropalatal function and assessment of laryngeal protection	Primary aspiration lung disease

BAL, bronchoalveolar lavage; CBC, complete blood count; CF, cystic fibrosis; GERD, gastroesophageal reflux disease; HIV, human immunodeficiency virus; HRCT, high-resolution computed tomography; PCR, polymerase chain reaction; TB, tuberculosis.

(Fig. 29-4*A*); type III, obliterative-like (see Fig. 29-4*B*); type IV malacia/obliterative-like combination; type V, no abnormality.[120] The frequencies of these findings among 28 children with non-CF bronchiectasis were 58%, 17%, 17%, 4%, and 2% for types I through V, respectively.[120] Structural airway lesions were present in 40% of the 33 children with postinfectious bronchiectasis and CSLD.[120] Bronchomalacia associated with bronchiectasis is related to chronic inflammation,[119] although it is unknown if bronchomalacia predates recurrent respiratory infections.

ASSESSMENT OF SEVERITY

Spirometry is insensitive in detecting early structural lung damage and even during disease progression.[121,122] Spirometric values may be normal, but when an abnormality is present, it is

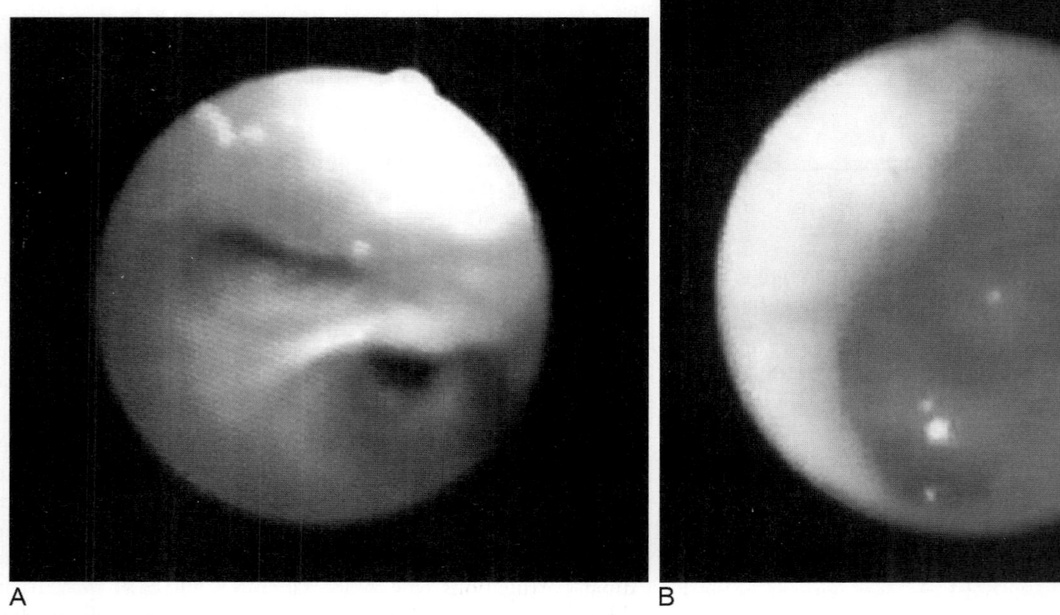

FIGURE 29-4. Major airway bronchoscopic findings where bronchiectasis is not present. **A,** Bronchomalacia (airway type II) of the right middle lobe. **B,** Obliterative-like lesion (airway type III) seen in the segmental bronchi (middle of picture) while the adjacent bronchi is widely patent and more inflamed. (See Color Plate 33.) (Reproduced from Chang AB, Boyce NC, Masters IB, Torzillo PJ, Masel JP: Bronchoscopic findings in children with non–cystic fibrosis chronic suppurative lung disease. Thorax 2002;57:935–938, with permission from the BMJ Publishing Group.)

classically obstructive in the earlier stages and later becomes a mixed obstructive and restrictive process. Although forced expiratory volume in 1 second (FEV_1) has been shown to correlate to chest HRCT abnormalities in some populations, it is not a sensitive measure, especially if bronchiectasis is localized. In contrast, when bronchiectasis is diffuse, spirometric abnormalities, though insensitive, better reflect disease severity.[123] Other pulmonary function test abnormalities described are a high residual lung volume, lower aerobic capacity, and lower maximal ventilation at maximal exercise.[124]

There are at least eight radiographic scoring systems to assess severity of bronchiectasis using plain films. However, given the insensitivity of chest radiographs in detecting bronchiectasis, these scoring systems have been superseded by chest HRCT scoring systems described by Webb and colleagues,[67] Bhalla and colleagues,[125] and Reiff and colleagues.[116] These chest HRCT scoring systems are based on composite scores of multiple radiologic findings. Some systems utilize expiratory scans,[126] others do not.[67] The Webb composite score[67] is a summation score of severity, extent, and additional features of emphysema and consolidation/atelectasis. The Bhalla score[125] comprises a sum of scores assigned to each of the nine categories: severity of bronchiectasis, peribronchial thickening, extent of bronchiectasis, extent of mucous plugging, sacculations, generations of bronchi involved, number of bullae, emphysema, and collapse/consolidation. One study compared these three scoring systems in a group of 59 children with non-CF bronchiectasis.[12] The correlation between the scores ranged from 0.61 to 0.8, but none related to FEV_1 values. This lack of correlation probably reflects the focal aspect of the disease and potential impairment of lung growth due to malnutrition and other variables.

Other evolving techniques to aid in diagnosis and assessment of severity of bronchiectasis include use of exhaled nitric oxide values,[127] breath condensate measurements,[128,129] and nuclear medicine scans. None of these as yet have defined roles in clinical practice.

ASSESSMENT OF DISEASE PROGRESSION

There is as yet little research on the most sensitive and appropriate method of assessing progression of bronchiectasis in children. Clinicians rely on frequency of acute pneumonias and on daily clinical symptoms, which may be perceived differently by children and their parents.[130] In bronchiectasis, a disease-specific pediatric quality-of-life assessment tool does not exist. The most sensitive objective assessment of disease progression is HRCT changes, because these precede pulmonary function changes.[12] Other assessments of disease progression include changes in chest radiographs, lung functions, markers of neutrophilic airway inflammation, and possibly assessments of airway proteases in stable outpatients. In pediatric bronchiectasis, there are no data relating these airway markers to imaging assessments of disease progression.

ASSESSMENT OF INFECTION

Sputum is the easiest method of obtaining an endobronchial microbiologic profile, and most older children with bronchiectasis readily produce sputum. In adults with bronchiectasis, sputum culture is generally reflective of lower airway organisms obtained by bronchoscopic protected brush brushings.[131] Common sputum pathogens in children with bronchiectasis are *Streptococcus pneumoniae* and *Haemophilus influenzae* non-type b. Other organisms include *Moraxella catarrhallis* and *Pseudomonas aeruginosa. Pseudomonas* is commonly found in adults with severe bronchiectasis, but it is uncommon in children. Its presence in sputum has been associated with more severe bronchiectasis and poorer quality of life.[132,133] Numerous patients with bronchiectasis are persistently colonized with potential pathogenic microorganisms, particularly those with early-onset disease, with varicose-cystic bronchiectasis, and FEV_1 less than 80% predicted.[131] Other methods of identifying airway pathogens from children with bronchiectasis are oropharyngeal swabs, bronchoalveaolar lavage, and induced sputum. Oropharyngeal cultures do not reliably predict the presence of bacterial pathogens in the lower airways of young CF patients.[134] No such correlative studies exists for children with non-CF bronchiectasis.

Symptomatic exacerbations, assumed to be infectious in nature, are characterized by increased sputum expectoration, cough severity, and change in sputum color—with or without reduction in exercise tolerance and energy. Like CF, fever and hemoptysis are uncommon in exacerbations of pediatric bronchiectasis. The endobronchial pathogens isolated during acute exacerbations have not been correlated with chronic endobronchial flora in children with bronchiectasis.

MANAGEMENT PRINCIPLES

As early as 1933, Roles and Todd emphasized the importance of early diagnosis and treatment in reducing mortality associated with bronchiectasis.[17] In bronchiectasis secondary to CF and primary ciliary dyskinesia, aggressive management of infections with antimicrobials, regular use of airway clearance methods, attention to nutrition, coupled with a vigilant monitoring of long-term clinical trends and proactive care, has led to improved survival and preservation of lung function.[135,136] CF produces a specific type of progressive bronchiectasis that differs from other forms of bronchiectasis with respect to mucus rheology, airway surface lining abnormalities, salt content, and extrapulmonary organ involvement. Nevertheless, management should be arguably as intensive in children with non-CF bronchiectasis to minimize acute exacerbations, daily symptoms, and functional limitations, if not to alter the natural history of the disease.[76,137,138] In addition, chronic lung infection and inflammation are independent risk factors of developing cardiovascular disease in adults.[139,140]

The aims of regular review include optimal postnatal lung growth, prevention of premature respiratory decline, maximal quality of life, and prevention of complications due to bronchiectasis. Ideally, a team approach with incorporation of allied health expertise (nursing, physiotherapy, nutritionist, social work) should be used, since this model has been shown to improve health outcomes for several chronic diseases.[135,141] Guidelines of management of bronchiectasis in certain minority groups have been published.[14] Issues that require regular monitoring are listed in Box 29-3.

ANTIMICROBIALS

There are few randomized controlled treatment trials on childhood bronchiectasis and only one trial that used antimicrobials for longer than 4 weeks.[142] Brief antimicrobial interventions significantly improve inflammatory profile in the airways[143,144] and

BOX 29-3 Management Issues for Regular Review

1. Accurate diagnoses of underlying etiology and conditions that aggravate bronchiectasis.
2. Philosophy of antibiotics use (maintenance, intermittent, regular hospitalizations).
3. Airway pathogens and drug sensitivity profiles.
4. Effectiveness of mucociliary clearance techniques.
5. Nutritional state and support.
6. Psychosocial support and adherence issues.
7. Pattern and frequency of acute respiratory exacerbations.
8. Presence of comorbid conditions.
9. Education and promotion of self-management.
10. Preventive measures (environment assessment, vaccines).
11. Indications for surgical resection of bronchiectatic regions.
12. Complications related to bronchiectasis (e.g., hemoptysis, lung abscess, pulmonary hypertension, sleep disorders, reactive airway disease).
13. Review of new therapies and therapeutic strategies as they emerge (e.g., macrolide use for anti-inflammatory antisecretagogue effects).

blood,[143,144] as well as improve quality-of-life measures.[132,144] In the study by Koh and colleagues, 25 children were randomized to receive 12 weeks of roxithromycin (4 mg/kg twice a day) or placebo.[142] A significant improvement in sputum features occurred after 6 weeks of treatment in the roxithromycin group, but improvements in FEV_1 were not observed in either group.[142] The roxithromycin group also had lesser degree of airway responsiveness than did the placebo group.[142] A 12-month trial in adults with non-CF *Pseudomonas*-colonized bronchiectasis showed that those on the continuous treatment had a reduced number of hospitalizations when compared with those in the symptomatic treatment arm.[145] Another 12-month trial using a randomized controlled design demonstrated that the symptoms of cough expectoration, hemoptysis, and general disability occurred significantly less in the those adults treated with tetracycline than in those treated with oral penicillin or placebo.[146] Long-term intervention trials have not been conducted in children with bronchiectasis.

The use of maintenance antimicrobials may be suitable in selected situations in which frequent exacerbations occur.[147] In adults, regular use of macrolides and trimethoprim has been shown to be beneficial in reducing pulmonary inflammation and infective exacerbations, and in improving lung function.[147,148] A review[81] on the prolonged use of antibiotics for purulent bronchiectasis in both children and adults also summarized elsewhere indicated a small benefit for its use.

ANTI-INFLAMMATORY AND ANTIOXIDANT AGENTS

In 18 children with CF and 15 children with idiopathic bronchiectasis, 6 months of β-carotene supplementation reduced plasma levels of TNF-α and malondialdehyde, a marker of lipid peroxidation.[149] However, clinical status did not improve, and its use is still speculative at this stage. In adults with bronchiectasis, nonsteroidal anti-inflammatory agents have a major effect on peripheral neutrophil function, significantly reducing neutrophil chemotaxis and fibronectin degradation by resting and stimulated neutrophils, but no effect on bacterial colonization of the airways or superoxide anion generation by neutrophils.[150]

ANTISECRETAGOGUES AND MUCOACTIVE AGENTS

Mucoactive agents are treatments that enhance mucus clearance from the respiratory tract in conditions of persistent mucus clearance impairment.[73] Mucolytics reduce mucus cross-linking and viscosity through disruption of polymer networks in the secretions by severing disulfide bonds, through depolymerizing mucopolysaccharides, and via liquefying proteins by degradation of DNA filaments and actin.[73] In adults, high doses of bromhexine used with antibiotics eased difficulty in expectoration and reduced sputum production.[151] The utility of DNase is less clear in non-CF bronchiectasis than among patients with CF. Several studies have shown no change in lung functions or quality of life in adults with bronchiectasis; another study reported more hospitalizations in the treatment group.[151–153]

Antisecretagogues reduce airway mucus production and secretion. These agents include anticholinergic agents, macrolide antibiotics, and bromhexine. Macrolides composed of 13-member rings are antibiotics with anti-inflammatory activities and reduce mucus hypersecretion in adults with bronchiectasis.[154] Although their benefit has also been shown in children with CF, there is currently insufficient evidence for recommending their use in all children with bronchiectasis.[155] Similarly, there is no evidence to indicate that anticholinergic therapy is either beneficial or harmful in the treatment of acute or stable bronchiectasis.[156] Some anticholinergic agents such as atropine and glycopyrrolate slow mucociliary transport and predispose to further mucus stasis. Others, such as ipratropium bromide, do not affect ciliary action in therapeutic doses.

AIRWAY CLEARANCE METHODS

Chest physiotherapy to improve mucociliary clearance is a standard treatment regimen in children with CF. Randomized controlled trials on the use of physiotherapy for idiopathic bronchiectasis are lacking. The rheologic properties of sputum differ in children with CF and those with idiopathic bronchiectasis.[157] Mucus from Alaskan Native children with bronchiectasis demonstrates decreased viscosity and elasticity as well as increased cough transportability compared with sputum from patients with CF. It is thus easier for them to expectorate. Cochrane and colleagues have shown that physiotherapy increases airway conductance among adults with airway obstruction and chronic sputum production.[158] There are many forms of physiotherapy, and these different methods have not been evaluated in children with bronchiectasis. Reviews on physiotherapy are available elsewhere.[159–161]

ASTHMA THERAPY

Asthma in children with bronchiectasis should be treated on its own merits. The use of inhaled corticosteroids for children with bronchiectasis who have demonstrated reversible airway obstruction following treatment with β-adrenergic agonists has not been evaluated. In adults, such studies are only of 4 to 6 weeks' duration and suggest a trend to improving lung function.[162,163] A Cochrane review on this subject concluded that there is insufficient evidence to provide guidelines to guide clinical practice.[162] Short- and long-acting β_2 agonists also have an indeterminate role in the management of bronchiectasis,[164,165] and their use must be individualized. Although the presence of asthma is associated with advanced bronchiectasis and a worse prognosis, treatment of asthma to alter long-term outcomes in children with bronchiectasis has not been studied. It may be that the asthmatic features associated with diffuse bronchiectasis reflect the disease itself rather than a concurrent condition. Increased cough in children with bronchiectasis should be initially treated as an exacerbation of bronchiectasis.

ENVIRONMENTAL MODIFICATION

In utero tobacco smoke exposure alters respiratory control,[166] pulmonary development, and physiology.[167,168] Whether it also influences the developmental aspects of local and systemic pulmonary immunity is unknown. Exposure to environmental smoke increases susceptibility to respiratory infections,[169,170] causes adverse respiratory health outcomes,[48] and increases coughing illnesses.[47,171] There are, however, no randomized controlled trials that have examined the impact of ETS reduction on children's cough or sputum production. A single report was found on cessation of parental smoking as a successful form of therapy for the children's cough.[172] Behavioral counseling for smoking mothers has been shown to reduce young children's ETS exposure in both reported and objective measures of ETS.[173]

PREVENTION THROUGH VACCINES

Vaccines are available to reduce the impact of *Pneumococcus* and influenza, particularly in high-risk groups. Currently, pneumococcal conjugate vaccine is recommended for all children younger than 24 months of age starting at 2 months and for high-risk children younger than 60 months old. Additional doses of 23-valent pneumococcal vaccine are recommended for high-risk children, including those with bronchiectasis.[174] These vaccines are expected to reduce the incidence of pneumonia by at least 30%.[175] There is controversy about whether the response of indigenous children to vaccination can be suboptimal,[176] and repeated immunization is necessary. This includes the response to the polysaccharide pneumococcal vaccine in targeted groups.[177] Yearly influenza vaccination is also recommended, although there are no published randomized controlled trials among children with CSLD, bronchiectasis, or CF. An excellent review evaluating vaccines for the prevention of pneumonia in children in developing countries has recently been published.[178]

SURGICAL CONSIDERATIONS

There are no controlled trials on the role of surgery in childhood bronchiectasis. Surgery is considered most often when bronchiectasis is focal and medical therapy has failed.[179] However, the role of surgery in the management of children with CSLD is controversial, with proponents for and against its use.[94,180] Perioperative mortality for lobectomy and pneumonectomy has dramatically fallen over the last 30 years.[181,182] In several reviews of surgical therapy for bronchiectasis, the compiled group of adult and pediatric patients experienced 1% mortality (6/597) and an operative complication rate of 8.5% (51/597).[62,181–183] Complications included empyema, bronchopulmonary fistulas, hypotension, and bleeding. Surgical treatment of bronchiectasis was more effective in patients with localized disease.[183] Appearance of new bronchiectasis following surgical management has previously been described among Australian aboriginal children.[12,184] Indications for surgical intervention are controversial, and data from the 1940s and 1950s cannot be applied given the major advances in antibiotics, physiotherapy techniques, and nutrition supplementation, as well as possible changes in socioeconomic standards among underserved populations. Our suggested indications for surgical intervention are outlined in Box 29-4. Although lung transplantation has been reported widely for patients with CF, this option has also been used for adults with end-stage suppurative disease unrelated to CF.[185,186] Outcomes following lung transplantation specifically for children with bilateral severe bronchiectasis without CF have not been reported.

BOX 29-4 Indications and Contraindications for Lobectomy

Indications

1. Poor control of symptoms (purulent sputum, frequent exacerbations) despite optimized medical therapy.
2. Poor growth despite optimized medical therapy.
3. Severe and recurrent hemoptysis uncontrolled by bronchial artery embolization.

Relative Indications

1. Localized disease with moderate persistent symptoms.

Contraindications

1. Widespread bronchiectasis.
2. Young child (<6 years).
3. Asymptomatic disease.

Finally, health cannot be isolated from social, economic, environmental, and educational issues. In developing nations, maternal education is closely linked to childhood health indices.[187,188] To effectively reduce the morbidity and mortality from CSLD and bronchiectasis in children, a multifaceted approach encompassing public health concerns requires consideration. Although it is beyond the scope of this chapter to address this important issue, future work must focus on the public health issues predisposing to childhood bronchiectasis if the disparity between developed and developing countries is to be reduced.

Acknowledgment

The authors are grateful to Dr. Rosalyn Singleton for her expert comments and critique.

REFERENCES

1. Gaillard EA, Carty H, Heaf D, Smyth RL: Reversible bronchial dilatation in children. Comparison of serial high-resolution computed tomography scans of the lungs. Eur J Radiol 2003;47:215–220.

2. Barker AF, Bardana EJ: Bronchiectasis. Update of an orphan disease. Am Rev Respir Dis 1988;137:969–978.
3. Callahan CW, Redding GJ: Bronchiectasis in children. Orphan disease or persistent problem? Pediatr Pulmonol 2002;33:492–496.
4. Adebonojo SA, Grillo IA, Osinowo O, Adebo O: Suppurative diseases of the lung and pleura. A continuing challenge in developing countries. Ann Thoracic Surg 982;33:40–47.
5. Anderson HR: Chronic lung disease in the Papua New Guinea Highlands. Thorax 1979;34:647–653.
6. Sethi GR, Batra V: Bronchiectasis. Causes and management. Indian J Pediatr 2000;67:133–139.
7. Karakoc GB, Yilmaz M, Altintas DU, Kendirli SG: Bronchiectasis. Still a problem. Pediatr Pulmonol 2001;32:175–178.
8. Nikolaizik WH, Warner JO: Aetiology of chronic suppurative lung disease. Arch Dis Child 1994;70:141–142.
9. Saynajakangas O, Keistinen T, Tuuponen T, Kivela SL: Bronchiectasis in Finland. Trends in hospital treatment. Respir Med 1997;91:395–398.
10. Field CE: Bronchiectasis. Third report on a follow-up study of medical and surgical cases from childhood. Arch Dis Child 1969;44:551–561.
11. Singleton R, Morris A, Redding G, Poll J, Holck P, Martinez P, et al: Bronchiectasis in Alaska Native children. Causes and clinical courses. Pediatr Pulmonol 2000;29:182–187.
12. Chang AB, Masel JP, Boyce NC, Wheaton G, Torzillo PJ: Non-CF bronchiectasis—clinical and HRCT evaluation. Pediatr Pulmonol 2003;35: 477–483.
13. Edwards EA, Metcalfe R, Milne DG, Thompson J, Byrnes CA: Retrospective review of children presenting with non cystic fibrosis bronchiectasis. HRCT features and clinical relationships. Pediatr Pulmonol 2003;36:87–93.
14. Chang AB, Grimwood K, Mulholland EK, Torzillo PJ: Bronchiectasis in indigenous children in remote Australian communities. Med J Aust 2002; 177:200–204.
15. Khaled NA, Enarson DA, Bousquet J: Chronic respiratory diseases in developing countries. The burden and strategies for prevention and management. Bull WHO 2001;79:971–979.
16. O'Brien C, Guest PJ, Hill SL, Stockley RA: Physiological and radiological characterisation of patients diagnosed with chronic obstructive pulmonary disease in primary care. Thorax 2000;55:635–642.
17. Roles FC, Todd GS: Bronchiectasis. Diagnosis and prognosis in relation to treatment. BMJ 1933;i:639–643.
18. Pasteur MC, Helliwell SM, Houghton SJ, Webb SC, Foweraker JE, Coulden RA, et al: An investigation into causative factors in patients with bronchiectasis. Am J Respir Crit Care Med 2000;162:1277–1284.
19. Chang AB, Masel JP, Masters B: Post-infectious bronchiolitis obliterans. Clinical, radiological and pulmonary function sequelae. Pediatr Radiol 1998;28:23–29.
20. Becroft DM: Bronchiolitis obliterans, bronchiectasis, and other sequelae of adenovirus type 21 infection in young children. J Clin Pathol 1971;24: 72–82.
21. Laraya-Cuasay LR, DeForest A, Huff D, Lischner H, Huang NN: Chronic pulmonary complications of early influenza virus infection in children. Am Rev Respir Dis 1977;116:617–625.
22. Penn CC, Liu C: Bronchiolitis following infection in adults and children. Clin Chest Med 1993;14:645–654.
23. Barker DJ, Osmond C: Childhood respiratory infection and adult chronic bronchitis in England and Wales. BMJ (Clin Res Ed) 1986;293: 1271–1275.
24. Cooreman J, Redon S, Levallois M, Liard R, Perdrizet S: Respiratory history during infancy and childhood, and respiratory conditions in adulthood. Int J Epidemiol 1990;19:621–627.
25. Singleton RJ, Redding GJ, Lewis TC, Martinez P, Bulkow L, Morray B, et al: Sequelae of severe respiratory syncytial virus infection in infancy and early childhood among Alaska Native children. Pediatrics 2003;112:285–290.
26. Cherniack NS, Dowling HF, Carton RW, McBryde VE: The role of acute lower respiratory infection in causing pulmonary insufficiency in bronchiectasis. Ann Intern Med 1967;66:489–497.
27. Valery PC, Torzillo PJ, Mulholland EK, Boyce NC, Purdie DM, Chang AB: A hospital-based case-control study of bronchiectasis in indigenous children in Central Australia. Pediatr Infect Dis J 2004;23:902–908.
28. Maxwell GM: Chronic chest disease in Australian aboriginal children. Arch Dis Child 1972;47:897–901.
29. Redding GJ, Singleton RJ, Lewis T, Martinez P, Butler JC, Bulkow L, et al: Early radiographic and clinical features associated with bronchiectasis in children. Pediatr Pulmonol 2004;37:297–304.
30. Scannapieco FA: Role of oral bacteria in respiratory infection. State of the art review. J Periodontol 1999;70:793–802.
31. Wilson R, Cole PJ: The effect of bacterial products on ciliary function. Am Rev Respir Dis 1988;138:S49–S53.
32. Torzillo P, Dixon J, Manning K, Hutton S, Gratten M, Hueston L, et al: Etiology of acute lower respiratory tract infection in Central Australian Aboriginal children. Pediatr Infect Dis J 1999;18:714–721.
33. Gratten M, Manning K, Dixon J, Morey F, Torzillo P, Hanna J, et al: Upper airway carriage by *Haemophilus influenzae* and *Streptococcus pneumoniae* in Australian aboriginal children hospitalised with acute lower respiratory infection. Southeast Asian J Trop Med Public Health 1994;25:123–131.
34. Brook I, Finegold SM: Bacteriology and therapy of lung abscess in children. J Pediatr 1979;94:10–12.
35. Scannapieco FA, Ho AW: Potential associates between chronic respiratory disease and periodontal disease. Analysis of National Health and Nutrition Examination Survey III. J Periodontol 2001;72:50–56.
36. Field CE: Bronchiectasis in childhood, III. Prophylaxis, treatment and progress with a follow-up study of 202 cases of established bronchiectasis. Pediatrics 1949;4:355–372.
37. Hoque BA, Chakraborty J, Chowdhury JT, Chowdhury UK, Ali M, el Arifeen S, et al: Effects of environmental factors on child survival in Bangladesh. A case control study. Public Health 1999;113:57–64.
38. Kolbe J, Wells AU: Bronchiectasis. A neglected cause of respiratory morbidity and mortality. Respirology 1996;1:221–225.
39. Gracey M: Nutrition and infections in Australian aboriginal children. Aust N Z J Med 1991;21:921–927.
40. Bulkow LR, Singleton RJ, Karron RA, Harrison LH: Risk factors for severe respiratory syncytial virus infection among Alaska native children. Pediatrics 2002;109:210–216.
41. Nacul LC, Arthur P, Kirkwood BR, Morris SS, Cameiro AC, Benjamin AF: The impact of vitamin A supplementation given during a pneumonia episode on the subsequent morbidity of children. Trop Med Int Health 1998;3:661–666.
42. Bhutta ZA, Black RE, Brown KH, Gardner JM, Gore S, Hidayat A, et al: Prevention of diarrhea and pneumonia by zinc supplementation in children in developing countries. Pooled analysis of randomized controlled trials. Zinc Investigators' Collaborative Group. J Pediatr 1999;135:689–697.
43. Peterson ML, Jacobs DR Jr, Milla CE: Longitudinal changes in growth parameters are correlated with changes in pulmonary function in children with cystic fibrosis. Pediatrics 2003;112:588–592.
44. Petersen KM, Singleton RJ, Leonard L: A qualitative study of the importance and etiology of chronic respiratory disease in Alaska native children. Alaska Med 2003;45:14–20.
45. International Consultation on Environmental Tobacco Smoke (ETS) and Child Health. Available athttp://tobacco who int/en/health/papers/ ets-report pdf 1999.
46. Ramsay MC, Reynolds CR: Does smoking by pregnant women influence IQ, birth weight, and developmental disabilities in their infants? A methodological review and multivariate analysis. Neuropsychol Rev 2000;10:1–40.
47. Couriel JM: Passive smoking and the health of children. Thorax 1994;49:731–734.
48. Li JS, Peat JK, Xuan W, Berry G: Meta-analysis on the association between environmental tobacco smoke (ETS) exposure and the prevalence of lower respiratory tract infection in early childhood. Pediatr Pulmonol 1999;27:5–13.
49. Haustein KO: Cigarette smoking, nicotine and pregnancy. Int J Clin Pharmacol Ther 1999;37:417–427.
50. Ezzati M, Kammen D: Indoor air pollution from biomass combustion and acute respiratory infections in Kenya. An exposure-response study. Lancet 2001;358:619–624.
51. Vedal S, Petkau J, White R, Blair J: Acute effects of ambient inhalable particles in asthmatic and nonasthmatic children. Am J Respir Crit Care Med 1998;157:1034–1043.
52. Hirsch T, Weiland SK, von Mutius E, Safeca AF, Grafe H, Csaplovics E, et al: Inner city air pollution and respiratory health and atopy in children. Eur Respir J 1999;14:669–677.
53. Holscher B, Heinrich J, Jacob B, Ritz B, Wichmann HE: Gas cooking, respiratory health and white blood cell counts in children. Int J Hyg Environ Health 2000;203:29–37.
54. Dodge R, Solomon P, Moyers J, Hayes C: A longitudinal study of children exposed to sulfur oxides. Am J Epidemiol 1985;121:720–736.
55. Kwiatkowski D: Science, medicine, and the future. Susceptibility to infection. BMJ 2000;321:1061–1065.
56. Kleeberger SR: Genetic aspects of susceptibility to air pollution. Eur Respir J Suppl 2003;40:52s–56s.
57. Pignatti PF, Bombieri C, Marigo C, Benetazzo M, Luisetti M: Increased incidence of cystic fibrosis gene mutations in adults with disseminated bronchiectasis. Hum Mol Genet 1995;4:635–639.

58. Tzetis M, Efthymiadou A, Strofalis S, Psychou P, Dimakou A, Pouliou E, et al: CFTR gene mutations—including three novel nucleotide substitutions—and haplotype background in patients with asthma, disseminated bronchiectasis and chronic obstructive pulmonary disease. Hum Genet 2001;108:216–221.
59. Varpela E, Koistinen J, Korhola O, Keskinen H: Deficiency of α1-antitrypsin and bronchiectasis. Ann Clin Res 1978;10:79–82.
60. ATS/ERS: Executive Summary. Standards for diagnosis and management of individuals with α1 antitrypsin deficiency. Am J Respir Crit Care Med 2003;168:820–822.
61. Gibson PG, Stuart JE, Wlodarczyk J, Olson LG, Hensley MJ: Nasal inflammation and chronic ear disease in Australian Aboriginal children. J Paediatr Child Health 1996;32:143–147.
62. Sepper R, Konttinen YT, Sorsa T, Koski H: Gelatinolytic and type IV collagenolytic activity in bronchiectasis. Chest 1994;106:1129–1133.
63. Maisi P, Prikk K, Sepper R, Pirila E, Salo T, Hietanen J, et al: Soluble membrane-type 1 matrix metalloproteinase (MT1-MMP) and gelatinase A (MMP-2) in induced sputum and bronchoalveolar lavage fluid of human bronchial asthma and bronchiectasis. APMIS 2002;110:771–782.
64. Gibson PG, Wark PA, Simpson JL, Meldrum C, Meldrum S, Saltos N, et al: Induced sputum IL-8 gene expression, neutrophil influx and MMP-9 in allergic bronchopulmonary aspergillosis. Eur Respir J 2003;21:582–588.
65. Laënnec RTH: De l'ausculatation médiate, un Traité du diagnostic des maladies des poumons et du coeur, fonde, principalement sur ce naveau moyen d'exploration. Paris, Brosson et Chande, 1819.
66. Reid LM: Reduction in bronchial subdivision in bronchiectasis. Thorax 1950;5:233–247.
67. Webb WR, Muller NL, Naidich DP: Airway Diseases. High-Resolution CT of the Lung. Philadelphia: Lippincott Williams & Wilkins, 2001, pp 467–546.
68. Spencer H: Diseases of the Bronchial Tree. Pathology of the Lung. Oxford: Pergamon Press Ltd, 1977, pp 116–149.
69. Chang AB, Ditchfield M, Robinson PJ, Robertson CF: Major hemoptysis in a child with cystic fibrosis from multiple aberrant bronchial arteries treated with tranexamic acid. Pediatr Pulmonol 1996;22:416–420.
70. Croxatto OC, Lanari A: Pathogenesis of bronchiectasis. Experimental study and anatomic findings. J Thorac Surg 1954;27:514–528.
71. Smaldone GC, Itoh H, Swift DL, Wagner HN: Effect of flow-limiting segments and cough on particle deposition and mucociliary clearance in the lung. Am Rev Respir Dis 1979;120:747–758.
72. Oldenburg FA, Dolovich MB, Montgomery JM, Newhouse MT: Effects of postural drainage, exercise and cough on mucus clearance in chronic bronchitis. Am Rev Respir Dis 1979;120:739–745.
73. King M, Rubin BK: Mucus-controlling agents. Past and present. Respir Care Clin N Am 1999;5:575–594.
74. Wolff RK, Dolovich MB, Obminski G, Newhouse MT: Effects of exercise and eucapnic hyperventilation on bronchial clearance. J Appl Physiol 1977; 43:46–50.
75. Bennett WD, Foster WM, Chapman WF: Cough-enhanced mucus clearance in the normal lung. J Appl Physiol 1990;69:1670–1675.
76. Stockley RA: Role of bacteria in the pathogenesis and progression of acute and chronic lung infection. Thorax 1998;53:58–62.
77. Angrill J, Agusti C, de Celis R, Filella X, Rano A, Elena M, et al: Bronchial inflammation and colonization in patients with clinically stable bronchiectasis. Am J Respir Crit Care Med 2001;164:1628–1632.
78. Hill SL, Burnett D, Hewetson KA, Stockley RA: The response of patients with purulent bronchiectasis to antibiotics for four months. Q J Med 1988; 66:163–173.
79. Stockley RA, Hill SL, Morrison HM: Effect of antibiotic treatment on sputum elastase in bronchiectatic outpatients in a stable clinical state. Thorax 1984;39:414–419.
80. Ip M, Shum D, Lauder I, Lam WK, So SY: Effect of antibiotics on sputum inflammatory contents in acute exacerbations of bronchiectasis. Respir Med 1993;87:449–454.
81. Evans DJ, Greenstone M: Long-term antibiotics in the management of non-CF bronchiectasis—do they improve outcome? Respir Med 2003;97: 851–858.
82. Sepper R, Konttinen YT, Ding Y, Takagi M, Sorsa T: Human neutrophil collagenase (MMP-8), identified in bronchiectasis BAL fluid, correlates with severity of disease. Chest 1995;107:1641–1647.
83. Zheng L, Lam WK, Tipoe GL, Shum IH, Yan C, Leung R, et al: Overexpression of matrix metalloproteinase-8 and -9 in bronchiectatic airways in vivo. Eur Respir J 2002;20:170–176.
84. Shum DK, Chan SC, Ip MS: Neutrophil-mediated degradation of lung proteoglycans. Stimulation by tumor necrosis factor-α in sputum of patients with bronchiectasis. Am J Respir Crit Care Med 2000;162: 1925–1931.
85. Vandivier RW, Fadok VA, Hoffmann PR, Bratton DL, Penvari C, Brown KK, et al: Elastase-mediated phosphatidylserine receptor cleavage impairs apoptotic cell clearance in cystic fibrosis and bronchiectasis. J Clin Invest 2002;109:661–670.
86. Chan TB, Arm JP, Anderson J, Eiser NM: Pulmonary epithelial permeability in bronchiectasis. Br J Dis Chest 1988;82:56–63.
87. Landau LI, Phelan PD, Williams HE: Ventilatory mechanics in patients with bronchiectasis starting in childhood. Thorax 1974;29:304–312.
88. Field CE: Bronchiectasis. A long term follow-up of medical and surgical cases from childhood. Arch Dis Child 1961;36:587–603.
89. Wilson JF, Decker AM: The surgical management of childhood bronchiectasis. Ann Surg 1982;195:354–363.
90. Clark NS: Bronchiectasis in childhood. BMJ 1963;1:80–88.
91. Bahous J, Cartier A, Pneau L, Bernard C, Ghezzo H, Martin RR, et al: Pulmonary function tests and airway responsiveness to methacholine in chronic bronchiectasis of the adult. Bull Eur Physiopathol Respir 1984;20: 375–380.
92. Ip M, Lam WK, So SY, Liong E, Chan CY, Tse KM: Analysis of factors associated with bronchial hyperactivity to methacholine in bronchiectasis. Lung 1991;169:43–51.
93. Perry KMA, King DS: Bronchiectasis. A study of prognosis based on follow-up of 400 patients. Am Rev Tuberculosis 1940;41:531.
94. Sanderson JM, Kennedy MC, Johnson MF, Manley DC: Bronchiectasis. Results of surgical and conservative management. A review of 393 cases. Thorax 1974;29:407–416.
95. Keistinen T, Saynajakangas O, Tuuponen T, Kivela SL: Bronchiectasis. An orphan disease with a poorly-understood prognosis. Eur Respir J 1997;10:2784–2787.
96. Stockley RA, Bayley D, Hill SL, Hill AT, Crooks S, Campbell EJ: Assessment of airway neutrophils by sputum colour. Correlation with airways inflammation. Thorax 2001;56:366–372.
97. Hubbard M, Masters IB, Chang AB: Rapidly progressing case of Mounier-Kuhn Syndrome in early childhood. Pediatr Pulmonol 2003;36:353–356.
98. Berdon WE, Willi U: Situs inversus, bronchiectasis, and sinusitis and its relation to immotile cilia. History of the diseases and their discoverers—Manes Kartagener and Bjorn Afzelius. Pediatr Radiol 2004;34:38–42.
99. Chang AB, Masel JP, Boyce NC, Torzillo PJ: Respiratory morbidity in central Australian Aboriginal children with alveolar lobar abnormalities. Med J Aust 2003;178:490–494.
100. Zhang L, Irion K, Kozakewich H, Reid L, Camargo JJ, da Silva PN, et al: Clinical course of postinfectious bronchiolitis obliterans. Pediatr Pulmonol 2000;29:341–350.
101. Silverman M, Wilson N: Wheezing phenotypes in childhood. Thorax 1997;52:936–937.
102. Ulrik CS, Backer V, Dirksen A: A 10 year follow up of 180 adults with bronchial asthma. Factors important for the decline in lung function. Thorax 1992;47:14–18.
103. Vandenplas Y, Ashkenazi A, Belli D, Boige N, Bouquet J, Cadranel S, et al: A proposition for the diagnosis and treatment of gastro-oesophageal reflux disease in children. A report from a working group on gastro-oesophageal reflux disease. Eur J Pediatr 1993;152:704–711.
104. Rudolph CD, Mazur LJ, Liptak GS, Baker RD, Boyle JT, Colletti RB, et al: Guidelines for evaluation and treatment of gastroesophageal reflux in infants and children: Recommendations of the North American Society for Pediatric Gastroenterology and Nutrition. J Pediatr Gastroenterol Nutr 2001;(32 Suppl)2:S1–S31.
105. Kerr P, Shoenut JP, Millar T, Buckle P, Kryger MH: Nasal CPAP reduces gastroesophageal reflux in obstructive sleep apnea syndrome. Chest 1992; 101:1539–1544.
106. Ozcay F, Ozbek N, Saatci U: Relapsing hypertrophic osteoarthropathy in a child with bronchiectasis. Indian Pediatr 2002;39:1152–1156.
107. Tuglular S, Yalcinkaya F, Paydas S, Oner A, Utas C, Bozfakioglu S, et al: A retrospective analysis for aetiology and clinical findings of 287 secondary amyloidosis cases in Turkey. Nephrol Dial Transplant 2002;17:2003–2005.
108. Akalln F, Koroglu TF, Bakac S, Dagli E: Effects of childhood bronchiectasis on cardiac functions. Pediatr Int 2003;45:169–174.
109. Westcott JL: Bronchiectasis. Radiol Clin North Am 1991;29:1031–1042.
110. Currie DC, Cooke JC, Morgan AD, Kerr IH, Delany D, Strickland B, et al: Interpretation of bronchograms and chest radiographs in patients with chronic sputum production. Thorax 1987;42:278–284.
111. Webb WR, Muller NL, Naidich DP: High-resolution computed tomography findings of lung disease. High-Resolution CT of the Lung. Philadelphia: Lippincott Williams & Wilkins, 2001, pp 71–193.

112. Coren ME, Ng V, Rubens M, Rosenthal M, Bush A: The value of ultrafast computed tomography in the investigation of pediatric chest disease. Pediatr Pulmonol 1998;26:389–395.
113. Naidich DP, McCauley DI, Khouri NF, Stitik FP, Siegelman SS: Computed tomography of bronchiectasis. J Comput Assist Tomogr 1982;6:437–444.
114. Yi CA, Lee KS, Kim TS, Han D, Sung YM, Kim S: Multidetector CT of bronchiectasis. Effect of radiation dose on image quality. AJR Am J Roentgenol 2003;181:501–505.
115. Reiff DB, Wells AU, Carr DH, Cole PJ, Hansell DM: CT findings in bronchiectasis. Limited value in distinguishing between idiopathic and specific types. AJR Am J Roentgenol 1995;165:261–267.
116. Meeks M, Bush A: Primary ciliary dyskinesia (PCD). Pediatr Pulmonol 2000;29:307–316.
117. Cataneo AJ, Reibscheid SM, Ruiz Junior RL, Ferrari GF: Foreign body in the tracheobronchial tree. Clin Pediatr (Phila) 1997;36:701–706.
118. Karakoc F, Karadag B, Akbenlioglu C, Ersu R, Yildizeli B, Yuksel M, et al: Foreign body aspiration. What is the outcome? Pediatr Pulmonol 2002;34:30–36.
119. Stradling P: Diagnostic Bronchoscopy. London: Longman Group, 1991, pp 1–185.
120. Chang AB, Boyce NC, Masters IB, Torzillo PJ, Masel JP: Bronchoscopic findings in children with non-cystic fibrosis chronic suppurative lung disease. Thorax 2002;57:935–938.
121. Tiddens HA: Detecting early structural lung damage in cystic fibrosis. Pediatr Pulmonol 2002;34:228–231.
122. de Jong PA, Nakano Y, Lequin MH, Mayo JR, Woods R, Pare PD, et al: Progressive damage on high resolution computed tomography despite stable lung function in cystic fibrosis. Eur Respir J 2004;23:93–97.
123. Marchant JM, Masel JP, Dickinson FL, Masters IB, Chang AB: Application of chest high-resolution computer tomography in young children with cystic fibrosis. Pediatr Pulmonol 2001;31:24–29.
124. Swaminathan S, Kuppurao KV, Somu N, Vijayan VK: Reduced exercise capacity in non-cystic fibrosis bronchiectasis. Indian J Pediatr 2003;70: 553–556.
125. Bhalla M, Turcios N, Aponte V, Jenkins M, Leitman BS, McCauley DI, et al: Cystic fibrosis. Scoring system with thin-section CT. Radiology 1991; 179:783–788.
126. Roberts HR, Wells AU, Milne DG, Rubens MB, Kolbe J, Cole PJ, et al: Airflow obstruction in bronchiectasis. Correlation between computed tomography features and pulmonary function tests. Thorax 2000;55: 198–204.
127. Narang I, Ersu R, Wilson NM, Bush A: Nitric oxide in chronic airway inflammation in children. Diagnostic use and pathophysiological significance. Thorax 2002;57:586–589.
128. Horvath I, Loukides S, Wodehouse T, Kharitonov SA, Cole PJ, Barnes PJ: Increased levels of exhaled carbon monoxide in bronchiectasis. A new marker of oxidative stress. Thorax 1998;53:867–870.
129. Loukides S, Horvath I, Wodehouse T, Cole PJ, Barnes PJ: Elevated levels of expired breath hydrogen peroxide in bronchiectasis. Am J Respir Crit Care Med 1998;158:991–994.
130. Juniper EF: How important is quality of life in pediatric asthma? Pediatr Pulmonol Suppl 1997;15:17–21.
131. Angrill J, Agusti C, de Celis R, Rano A, Gonzalez J, Sole T, et al: Bacterial colonisation in patients with bronchiectasis. Microbiological pattern and risk factors. Thorax 2002;57:15–19.
132. Wilson CB, Jones PW, O'Leary CJ, Hansell DM, Cole PJ, Wilson R: Effect of sputum bacteriology on the quality of life of patients with bronchiectasis. Eur Respir J 1997;10:1754–1760.
133. Evans SA, Turner SM, Bosch BJ, Hardy CC, Woodhead MA: Lung function in bronchiectasis. The influence of *Pseudomonas aeruginosa*. Eur Respir J 1996;9:1601–1604.
134. Armstrong DS, Grimwood K, Carlin JB, Carzino R, Olinsky A, Phelan PD: Bronchoalveolar lavage or oropharyngeal cultures to identify lower respiratory pathogens in infants with cystic fibrosis. Pediatr Pulmonol 1996;21:267–275.
135. Frederiksen B, Lanng S, Koch C, Hoiby N: Improved survival in the Danish center-treated cystic fibrosis patients. Results of aggressive treatment. Pediatr Pulmonol 1996;21:153–158.
136. Ellerman A, Bisgaard H: Longitudinal study of lung function in a cohort of primary ciliary dyskinesia. Eur Respir J 1997;10:2376–2379.
137. Tiddens H, Silverman M, Bush A: The role of inflammation in airway disease. Remodeling. Am J Respir Crit Care Med 2000;162:7S–10S.
138. Bush A, Tiddens H, Silverman M: Clinical implications of inflammation in young children. Am J Respir Crit Care Med 2000;162:S11–S14.
139. Jousilahti P, Vartiainen E, Tuomilehto J, Puska P: Symptoms of chronic bronchitis and the risk of coronary disease. Lancet 1996;348:567–572.
140. Kiechl S, Egger G, Mayr M, Wiedermann CJ, Bonora E, Oberhollenzer F, et al: Chronic infections and the risk of carotid atherosclerosis. Prospective results from a large population study. Circulation 2001;103:1064–1070.
141. De Boeck K: Improving standards of clinical care in cystic fibrosis. Eur Respir J 2001;16:585–587.
142. Koh YY, Lee MH, Sun YH, Sung KW, Chae JH: Effect of roxithromycin on airway responsiveness in children with bronchiectasis. A double-blind, placebo-controlled study. Eur Respir J 1997;10:994–999.
143. Hill SL, Morrison HM, Burnett D, Stockley RA: Short term response of patients with bronchiectasis to treatment with amoxicillin given in standard or high doses orally or by inhalation. Thorax 1986;41:559–565.
144. Lin HC, Cheng HF, Wang CH, Liu CY, Yu CT, Kuo HP: Inhaled gentamicin reduces airway neutrophil activity and mucus secretion in bronchiectasis. Am J Respir Crit Care Med 1997;155:2024–2029.
145. Orriols R, Roig J, Ferrer J, Sampol G, Rosell A, Ferrer A, et al: Inhaled antibiotic therapy in non-cystic fibrosis patients with bronchiectasis and chronic bronchial infection by *Pseudomonas aeruginosa*. Respir Med 1999;93:476–480.
146. Medical Council Research: Prolonged antibiotic treatment of severe bronchiectasis. BMJ 1957;255–259.
147. Honda T, Hayasaka M, Hachiya T, Kubo K, Katsuyama T, Nagata A: Two cases of severe bronchiectasis successfully treated with a prolonged course of trimethoprim/sulfamethoxazole. Intern Med 1996;35:979–983.
148. Tsang KW, Ho PI, Chan KN, Ip MS, Lam WK, Ho CS, et al: A pilot study of low-dose erythromycin in bronchiectasis. Eur Respir J 1999;13: 361–364.
149. Cobanoglu N, Ozcelik U, Gocmen A, Kiper N, Dogru D: Antioxidant effect of beta-carotene in cystic fibrosis and bronchiectasis. Clinical and laboratory parameters of a pilot study. Acta Paediatr 2002;91:793–798.
150. Llewellyn-Jones CG, Johnson MM, Mitchell JL, Pye A, Okafor VC, Hill SL, et al: In vivo study of indomethacin in bronchiectasis. Effect on neutrophil function and lung secretion. Eur Respir J 1995;8:1479–1487.
151. Crockett AJ, Cranston JM, Latimer KM, Alpers JH: Mucolytics for bronchiectasis (Cochrane Review). In: The Cochrane Library 2003; Issue 4. Chichester, UK: John Wiley & Sons, Ltd.
152. O'Donnell AE, Barker AF, Ilowite JS, Fick RB: Treatment of idiopathic bronchiectasis with aerosolized recombinant human DNase I. rhDNase Study Group. Chest 1998;113:1329–1334.
153. Wills PJ, Wodehouse T, Corkery K, Mallon K, Wilson R, Cole PJ: Short-term recombinant human DNase in bronchiectasis. Am J Respir Crit Care Med 1996;154:413–417.
154. Gorrini M, Lupi A, Viglio S, Pamparana F, Cetta G, Iadarola P, et al: Inhibition of human neutrophil elastase by erythromycin and flurythromycin, two macrolide antibiotics. Am J Respir Cell Mol Biol 2001;25: 492–499.
155. Jaffe A, Bush A: Anti-inflammatory effects of macrolides in lung disease. Pediatr Pulmonol 2001;31:464–473.
156. Lasserson T, Holt K, Evans D, Greenstone M: Anticholinergic therapy for bronchiectasis (Cochrane Review). In: The Cochrane Library 2003, Issue 4. Chichester, UK: John Wiley & Sons, Ltd.
157. Redding GJ, Ramirez O, Tomkiewicz RP, Kishioka C, Martinez P, Rubin BK: The properties of sputum from Alaska children with bronchiectasis. Am J Respir Crit Care Med 1997;155:A474.
158. Cochrane GM, Webber BA, Clarke SW: Effects of sputum on pulmonary function. BMJ 1977;2:1181–1183.
159. Oberwaldner B: Physiotherapy for airway clearance in paediatrics. Eur Respir J 2000;15:196–204.
160. Webber B, Hills SL: Mucus transport and physiotherapy. Eur Respir J 1999;13:949–950.
161. van der Schans CP, Postma DS, Koëter GH, Rubin BK: Physiotherapy and bronchial mucus transport. Eur Respir J 2000;13:1477–1486.
162. Kolbe J, Wells A, Ram FSF: Inhaled steroids for bronchiectasis (Cochrane Review). In: The Cochrane Library 2004, Issue 2. Chichester, UK: John Wiley & Sons, Ltd.
163. Tsang KW, Ho PL, Lam WK, Ip MS, Chan KN, Ho CS, et al: Inhaled fluticasone reduces sputum inflammatory indices in severe bronchiectasis. Am J Respir Crit Care Med 1998;158:723–727.
164. Sheikh A, Nolan D, Greenstone M: Long-acting beta-2-agonists for bronchiectasis (Cochrane Review). In: The Cochrane Library 2001, Issue 2. Chichester, UK: John Wiley & Sons, Ltd.
165. Franco F, Sheikh A, Greenstone M: Short acting beta-2 agonists for bronchiectasis (Cochrane Review). In: The Cochrane Library 2001, Issue 2. Chichester, UK: John Wiley & Sons, Ltd.

166. Lewis K, Bosque E: Deficient hypoxia awakening response in infants of smoking mothers: Possible relationship to sudden infant death syndrome. J Pediatr 1995;127:668–669.
167. Stick S: Pediatric origins of adult lung disease. 1. The contribution of airway development to paediatric and adult lung disease. Thorax 2000;55:587–594.
168. Le Souef PN: Tobacco related lung diseases begin in childhood. Thorax 2000;55:1063–1067.
169. Cohen S, Tyrrell DA, Russell MA, Jarvis MJ, Smith AP: Smoking, alcohol consumption, and susceptibility to the common cold. Am J Public Health 1993;83:1277–1283.
170. Wu-Williams AH, Samet JM: Environmental tobacco smoke. Exposure-response relationships in epidemiologic studies. Risk Anal 1990;10:39–48.
171. Lister SM, Jorm LR: Parental smoking and respiratory illnesses in Australian children aged 0–4 years. ABS 1989–90 National Health Survey results. Aust N Z J Public Health 1998;22:781–786.
172. Brand PL, Duiverman EJ: Coughing and wheezing children. Improvement after parents stop smoking. Ned Tijdschr Geneeskd 1998;142:825–827.
173. Hovell MF, Zakarian JM, Matt GE, Hofstetter CR, Bernert JT, Pirkle J: Effect of counselling mothers on their children's exposure to environmental tobacco smoke. Randomised controlled trial. BMJ 2000;321:337–342.
174. American Academy of Pediatrics: Pneumococcal Infections. In: Pickering LK, ed: Red Book: 2003 Report of the Committee on Infectious Diseases. Elk Grove Village, Ill: American Academy of Pediatrics, 2003, pp 490–500
175. Torzillo PJ, Gratten M: Conjugate pneumococcal vaccines for Aboriginal children in Australia. Med J Aust 2000;(173 Suppl):S51–S53.
176. Douglas RM, Hansman D, McDonald B, Paton J, Kirke K: Pneumococcal vaccine in aboriginal children—a randomized controlled trial involving 60 children. Community Health Stud 1986;10:189–196.
177. Moore RA, Wiffen PJ, Lipsky BA: Are the pneumococcal polysaccharide vaccines effective? Meta-analysis of the prospective trials. BMC Fam Pract 2000;1:1.
178. Mulholland K, Levine O, Nohynek H, Greenwood BM: Evaluation of vaccines for the prevention of pneumonia in children in developing countries. Epidemiol Rev 1999;21:43–55.
179. Lewinston NJ: Bronchiectasis in childhood. Pediatr Clin North Am 1984;31:865–878.
180. Williams H: Bronchiectasis. Its multiple clinical and pathological features. Arch Dis Child 1959;2:192–201.
181. Balkanli K, Genc O, Dakak M, Gurkok S, Gozubuyuk A, Caylak H, et al: Surgical management of bronchiectasis. Analysis and short-term results in 238 patients. Eur J Cardiothorac Surg 2003;24:699–702.
182. Agasthian T, Deschamps C, Trastek VF, Allen MS, Pairolero PC: Surgical management of bronchiectais. Ann Thorac Surg 1996;62:976–978.
183. Kutlay H, Cangir AK, Enon S, Sahin E, Akal M, Gungor A, et al: Surgical treatment in bronchiectasis. Analysis of 166 patients. Eur J Cardiothorac Surg 2002;21:634–637.
184. Hiller HG: The radiological follow-up of aboriginal children with bronchiectasis treated surgically or medically. Aust Paediatr J 1976;12:319–321.
185. Barlow CW, Robbins RC, Moon MR, Akindipe O, Theodore J, Reitz BA: Heart-lung versus double-lung transplantation for suppurative lung disease. J Thorac Cardiovasc Surg 2000;119:466–476.
186. Date H, Aoe M, Nagahiro I, Sano Y, Andou A, Matsubara H, et al: Living-donor lobar lung transplantation for various lung diseases. J Thorac Cardiovasc Surg 2003;126:476–481.
187. Cleland JG, Van Ginneken JK: Maternal education and child survival in developing countries. The search for pathways of influence. Soc Sci Med 1988;27:1357–1368.
188. Aaby P, Bukh J, Kronborg D, Lisse IM, da Silva MC: Delayed excess mortality after exposure to measles during the first six months of life. Am J Epidemiol 1990;132:211–219.
189. Edwards EA, Asher MI, Byrnes CA: Paediatric bronchiectasis in the twenty-first century. Experience of a tertiary children's hospital in New Zealand. J Paediatr Child Health 2003;39:111–117.
190. Hartman TE, Primack SL, Lee KS, Swensen SJ, Muller NL: CT of bronchial and bronchiolar diseases. Radiographics 1994;14:991–1003.
191. Kothari NA, Kramer SS: Bronchial diseases and lung aeration in children. J Thorac Imaging 2001;16:207–223.
192. McGuinness G, Naidich DP: Bronchiectasis. CT/clinical correlations. Semin Ultrasound CT MR 1995;16:395–419.

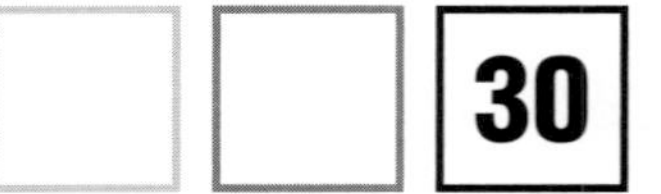

30 Lung Abscess and Pulmonary Infections Due to Anaerobic Bacteria

Itzhak Brook, MD

Pulmonary infections due to anaerobic bacteria include aspiration pneumonia, necrotizing pneumonia, lung abscess, and empyema that is associated with them, and pneumonia in mechanically ventilated and intubated patients. It usually occurs in children who are prone to aspiration of their oral secretions or refluxed gastric contents because of impaired cough reflex and other predisposing variables (Box 30-1).

The management of anaerobic pulmonary infections involves directing appropriate antimicrobial therapy against the potential bacterial pathogens. The increased recovery of anaerobic bacteria from pulmonary infections in children has led to greater appreciation of their role and to reevaluation of the proper treatment of this condition. This is not surprising, because anaerobes are part of the normal microflora of the oral mucous membranes and skin[1] and thus participate in many of the infections adjacent to those areas. Often, anaerobic organisms are present in combination with other facultative or aerobic organisms.

■ PATHOGENESIS

The microflora of the upper airways, including oral cavity, nasopharynx, and oropharynx, is complex and contains many types of obligate anaerobes. The distribution of bacteria within the mouth seems to be a function of their ability to adhere to the oral surfaces. The ratio of anaerobic bacteria to aerobic bacteria in saliva is approximately 10:1. The total count of anaerobic bacteria in the saliva reach 10^7 to 10^8 bacteria/mL.[1] The predominant anaerobic bacteria in the upper airways are *Fusobacterium* spp. (especially *F. nucleatum*), pigmented *Prevotella* and *Porphyromonas* spp., *Prevotella oralis*, and *Peptostreptococcus* spp. These organisms also predominate in oropharyngeal, otolaryngologic, and pulmonary infections.

Breakdown of normal host-protective mechanisms predisposes to anaerobic infection and is the common denominator in children who develop such infection. Aspiration of milk, food, oral secretions, regurgitated stomach contents, and vomitus is always associated with aspiration of aerobic and anaerobic oropharyngeal bacteria. If active or passive clearance of the aspirate is not achieved, there is a short latent period of several hours before the onset of pneumonia. The ensuing aspiration pneumonia can progress to necrotizing pneumonia, resulting in parenchymal damage and necrosis. This may lead to pneumatocele or abscess formation within 7 to 14 days. A lung abscess can also emerge from antecedent subacute or chronic airway infections. Secondary lung abscess can also arise from bacteremia, endocarditis, septic thrombophlebitis, or spread of infection from a subphrenic or hepatic infection. Infections below the diaphragm may extend to the lung or pleural space by way of the lymphatics, either directly through the diaphragm or via defects in it. An amebic lung abscess can be associated with a liver abscess as a result of perforation of the liver abscess into the lung.

Contributing to the development of these infections in children is the delay in their early recognition because of the patient's inability to complain.

Predisposing risk factors for aspiration and airways obstruction (see Box 30-1) include: (1) temporary or permanent depressed consciousness due to neurologic disease, debilitation, alcohol, anesthesia, or drugs; (2) neuromuscular disorders depressing the gag reflex or causing oropharyngeal incoordination; (3) congenital and acquired tracheoesophageal malformations; (4) obstruction due to aspirated foreign body; (5) lesions causing abnormal pulmonary drainage (e.g., congenital pulmonary sequestration, lobar emphysema, pneumatocele formation); (6) nasogastric tube feeding and gastroesophageal reflux; (7) prolonged tracheostomy; and (8) extended endotracheal intubation.

Intubation or tracheostomy predispose patients to infection, because they impair normal clearance of potential pathogens. Most infections of the lower respiratory tract are preceded by airway colonization with hospital-acquired enteric gram-negative bacteria and aerobic and anaerobic oral flora.[2,3] Colonization by these organisms occurs in all patients who undergo tracheostomy and intubation because of their inability to clear their secretions and their dependency on mechanical suctioning.

Poor oral hygiene, gingivitis, and periodontitis, as well as therapy with diphenylhydantoin contribute to the growth and increase the virulence of oral flora. This can lead to aspiration of larger amounts of "activated" oral flora.[4] Other conditions that increase the susceptibility to anaerobic lung infections include chronic airway disease, cystic fibrosis, congenital ciliary dysfunction, bronchiectasis, pulmonary instrumentation, and impairment of humoral or cellular immunity.

■ MICROBIOLOGY

Anaerobic bacteria are frequently recovered from aspiration pneumonia, necrotizing pneumonia, lung abscess, and empyema, which account for 30% to 70% of isolates.[5,6] The most common ones are pigmented *Prevotella* and *Porphyromonas*, *Bacteroides*, *Fusobacterium* (all gram-negative bacilli), *Peptostreptococcus* spp., microaerophylic streptococci, and *Veillonella* spp. (Box 30-2). More than half of the anaerobic gram-negative bacilli can produce the enzyme beta-lactamase. The predominant aerobic and facultative bacteria are *Streptococcus pneumoniae*, *Pseudomonas aeruginosa*, *Escherichia coli*, *Klebsiella pneumoniae*, *Haemophilus influenzae* type b,

BOX 30-1 Factors Predisposing Children to Develop Lower Respiratory Tract Infections Due to Their Endogenous Aerobic and Anaerobic Oral Bacterial Flora

Predisposing Risk Factors for Aspiration and Airways Obstruction

Temporary or permanent depressed consciousness that has depressed cough reflex due to neurologic disease, debilitation, alcohol, anesthesia, or drugs
Neuromuscular disorders depressing the gag reflex or causing oropharyngeal incoordination; congenital and acquired tracheoesophageal malformations
Obstruction due to aspirated foreign body
Lesions causing abnormal pulmonary drainage (e.g., congenital pulmonary sequestration, lobar emphysema, pneumatocele formation, bronchiectasis)
Nasogastric tube feeding and gastroesophageal reflux
Constant recumbent position
Prolonged tracheostomy
Extended endotracheal intubation
Pulmonary instrumentation

Change in Oropharyngeal Flora

Repeated administration of antibiotics
Poor oral hygiene, gingivitis, and periodontitis (also due to anticonvulsant therapy)
Poor oral hygiene
Long-term hospitalization and oral colonization with hospital flora

Impaired Immunologic and Other Defenses

Genetic disorders (i.e., Down syndrome, cystic fibrosis)
Congenital or acquired humoral or cellular immunity
Congenital ciliary dysfunction

Streptococcus pyogenes, alpha-hemolytic streptococci, and *Staphylococcus aureus*.[4,5,7] Cultures collected through percutaneous transtracheal aspirates (TTA) yielded an average of 4.9 organisms per patient (2.7 anaerobes and 2.2 aerobes).[4,5,8] Rare causes of lung abscess include *Mycoplasma pneumoniae.* In the neonatal period, group B streptococci, *K. pneumoniae*, and *E. coli* have been reported.

Pulmonary infections that develop in intubated infants and children reflect a mixed flora of oral anaerobes and nosocomial pathogens.[4] What often precedes the pneumonia in these patients is colonization with oral aerobic and anaerobic flora and nosocomial organisms. Some of these organisms can cause chronic tracheobronchitis and episodes of pneumonia.[2] Abscesses can also develop in the later stages of cystic fibrosis. In these cases *P. aeruginosa*, *S. aureus*, and oral anaerobes can be the cause.[9,10] Right-sided endocarditis, staphylococcal bacteremia, or Lemierre syndrome (necrotizing tonsillitis due to *Fusobacterium* spp.) can cause single or multiple lung abscesses.

The following organisms have been reported in lung abscess in adults but have yet to be described in children: *Campylobacter fetus, Corynebacterium equi, Legionella micdadei, Legionella pneumophila, Pasteurella multocida, Petriellidium boydii, Streptococcus milleri, Pseudomonas pseudomallei, Actinomyces,* and *Entamoeba histolytica.*

DIAGNOSIS

Anaerobic pneumonia is characterized by tachypnea, fever, and, rarely, apnea and hypotensive shock. A sudden onset of fever, chills, rapid respiration, cough, vomiting, diarrhea, abdominal distention, and elevated peripheral white blood cell count are the most common manifestations. The onset of the infection is sometimes more insidious than community-acquired pneumonia. Weeks to months of malaise, low-grade fever, and cough, with significant weight loss and anemia, may precede consolidation

BOX 30-2 Predominant Aerobic and Anaerobic Organisms Recovered in Aspiration Pneumonia, Lung Abscess, and Empyema in Children

Anaerobic Bacteria

Anaerobic Cocci

Peptostreptococcus spp.
Veillonella spp.
Microaerophilic streptococci

Gram-Positive Bacilli

Bifidobacterium spp.
Clostridium spp.

Gram-Negative Bacilli

Fusobacterium nucleatum
Fusobacterium spp.
Pigmented *Prevotella* and *Porphyromonas* spp.
Bacteroides ureolyticus
Prevotella oris-buccae
Prevotella oralis
Bacteroides spp.
Bacteroides fragilis group

Aerobic and Facultative Bacteria

Gram-Positive Cocci

Streptococcus pneumoniae
Alpha-hemolytic streptococci
Group A beta-hemolytic streptococci
Staphylococcus aureus
Staphylococcus epidermidis

Gram-Negative Bacilli

Proteus spp.
Pseudomonas aeruginosa
Klebsiella pneumoniae
Escherichia coli
Serratia marcescens
Citrobacter spp.
Enterobacter spp.
Haemophilus influenzae
Haemophilus parainfluenzae
Eikenella corrodens

and abscess formation. When an abscess develops, most children have fever, often as high as 40°C; malaise; and weight loss, and some have vomiting. Symptoms include cough, chest pain, dyspnea, sputum production, and hemoptysis. A putrid odor of the breath is occasionally noted. Signs localizing disease to the chest and within the chest are sometimes absent in lung abscess, particularly in very young children. Examination may reveal tachycardia, dyspnea with frequent expiratory grunts, dilated nostrils, flushed cheeks, cyanosis, rales, fine crackles, diminished breath sounds, dullness to percussion, retractions, decreased movement of the chest, bronchial breathing, and prolonged expiration. The presence of a pneumonic process in a posterior upper lobe or superior lower lobe suggests the presence of aspiration and lung abscess. Clubbing of the digits is rarely seen.

Children receiving steroids, and newborn infants, may have no fever or a subnormal temperature. Neonates may show less specific signs of illness, such as apnea, grunting, respiratory distress, diarrhea, and even hematemesis.

RADIOLOGIC MANIFESTATIONS

The chest radiograph in necrotizing pneumonia may show a radiolucent lesion, but computed tomography is more discerning; since decreased parenchymal contrast enhancement correlates with impending necrosis and cavitation.[11] Cavitation with an air-fluid level establishes the diagnosis of a lung abscess. The abscess usually appears as a solitary thick-walled cavity in the lung (Fig. 30-1). The most frequent sites of involvement are the posterior segments of the upper lobes and the superior segments of the lower lobes, especially on the right. This anatomic distribution in the segments that are the most dependent areas of the lung in the supine position supports the role of aspiration as a predisposing event. If aspiration occurs in the upright position, abscesses occur in the basilar segments of the upper lobes. A minority of patients have right middle lobe disease. Abscesses vary in size from 2 to 20 cm in diameter, and wall thickness can vary from 5 to 15 mm. An intrapulmonary abscess without communication with the bronchial tree is roentgenographically opaque. The abscess cavity becomes visible when air entering from a bronchus creates an air-fluid level over the pus. An air-fluid level is usually present but may be missed if only a supine film is taken. Abscess contents are usually uniloculated but may be multiloculated (Fig. 30-2). Compressive atelectasis is often seen around the abscess, especially if it is large. Most lung abscesses abut the pleural surface and are associated with overlying pleural thickening. A small amount of pleural fluid may be seen. Hilar and mediastinal adenopathy are sometimes present.

Ultrasound and computed tomography scanning may be used as diagnostic tools in lung abscess but are usually utilized to localize the lesion and guide drainage or transthoracic needle aspiration. This procedure is required only in complex cases or when the etiology cannot be ascertained reasonably from the clinical circumstances.[12] On ultrasound the abscess appears as a hyperechoic ring with irregular outer margins. The internal echo textures are inhomogeneous, and an air-fluid level is usually demonstrated. The diagnostic criteria for lung abscess on computed tomography scanning are: (1) the presence of a well-defined mass, (2) detection of a sharp angle between the lesion and the pleura, (3) density of the mass greater than that of water and normal pleural fluid, and (4) contrast enhancement showing an increase in density in tissue surrounding the lesion. Computed tomography scanning demonstrates the three-dimensional shape of the lesion and visualizes the pleuropulmonary interface, and is thus helpful for distinguishing lung abscess from empyema, pneumatocele, and fistula. Computed tomography can often define the extent of disease, underlying anomalies, and presence or absence of foreign body. Although magnetic resonance imaging appears to be effective in identifying lung abscess in children, its role in the diagnosis of this condition has yet to be defined.

LABORATORY FINDINGS

The white blood cell count is usually increased, with a predominance of polymorphonuclear leukocytes. In neonates, immature forms are observed more commonly. The erythrocyte sedimentation rate may be normal but usually is mildly increased, and values up to 150 mm in 1 hour have been reported. Mild anemia is sometimes present.

The determination of the organism responsible for lung abscesses is complicated because of the difficulty in obtaining uncontaminated specimens from the lower airways of patients. Therefore, the choice of antimicrobial therapy is often empiric.

Nasopharyngeal or sputum specimens are not reliable for identification of pulmonary pathogens, since these samples are contaminated by oropharyngeal aerobic and anaerobic bacteria.[2] Materials that are appropriate for culture should be obtained using a technique that bypasses the normal oropharyngeal flora in the upper airway. Invasive diagnostic techniques occasionally recommended to diagnose necrotizing pneumonia and lung abscesses include TTA, transthoracic aspiration, and fiberoptic bronchoscopy. Direct percutaneous aspiration of material in the infected lung or abscess is the most reliable mode of identification of the etiologic agent, but this technique is difficult unless the abscess is peripheral and in most situations appears unwarranted. TTA was a popular diagnostic test in the 1970s in both children[5] and adults[6]; however, the procedure is difficult to perform and requires an experienced operator. Obtaining specimens during fiberoptic bronchoscopy via a bronchial brush is much more widely used now than TTA. However, care must be taken not to contaminate the specimen with oral flora, the specimen obtained is usually very small, and bacterial growth can be inhibited by the local anesthetic agent. Relying on the microbiologic evaluation of pulmonary secretions is unreliable. The indications and comparative benefits of the aforementioned procedures are controversial and depend on the operator. Many pulmonologists believe that these diagnostic procedures should be reserved for patients with atypical presentations.

Bronchoscopy may be diagnostic and can be used to remove a foreign body or provide drainage of purulent fluid if this has not occurred spontaneously.

Quantitative culture of lower respiratory tract specimens obtained by bronchoalveolar lavage may improve the accuracy of identification of aerobic pathogens and has also been found to be useful in the diagnosis of anaerobic lung abscess.[4,12]

Empyema fluid, if available, provides a reliable specimen.[7] The role of quantitative culture in determining the causative agent has yet to be clarified. Blood cultures rarely detect the organism but occasionally may be positive in lung abscess associated with a septicemic illness.

Specimens should be cultured specifically for anaerobes and care taken to collect them in a satisfactory way. This is achieved

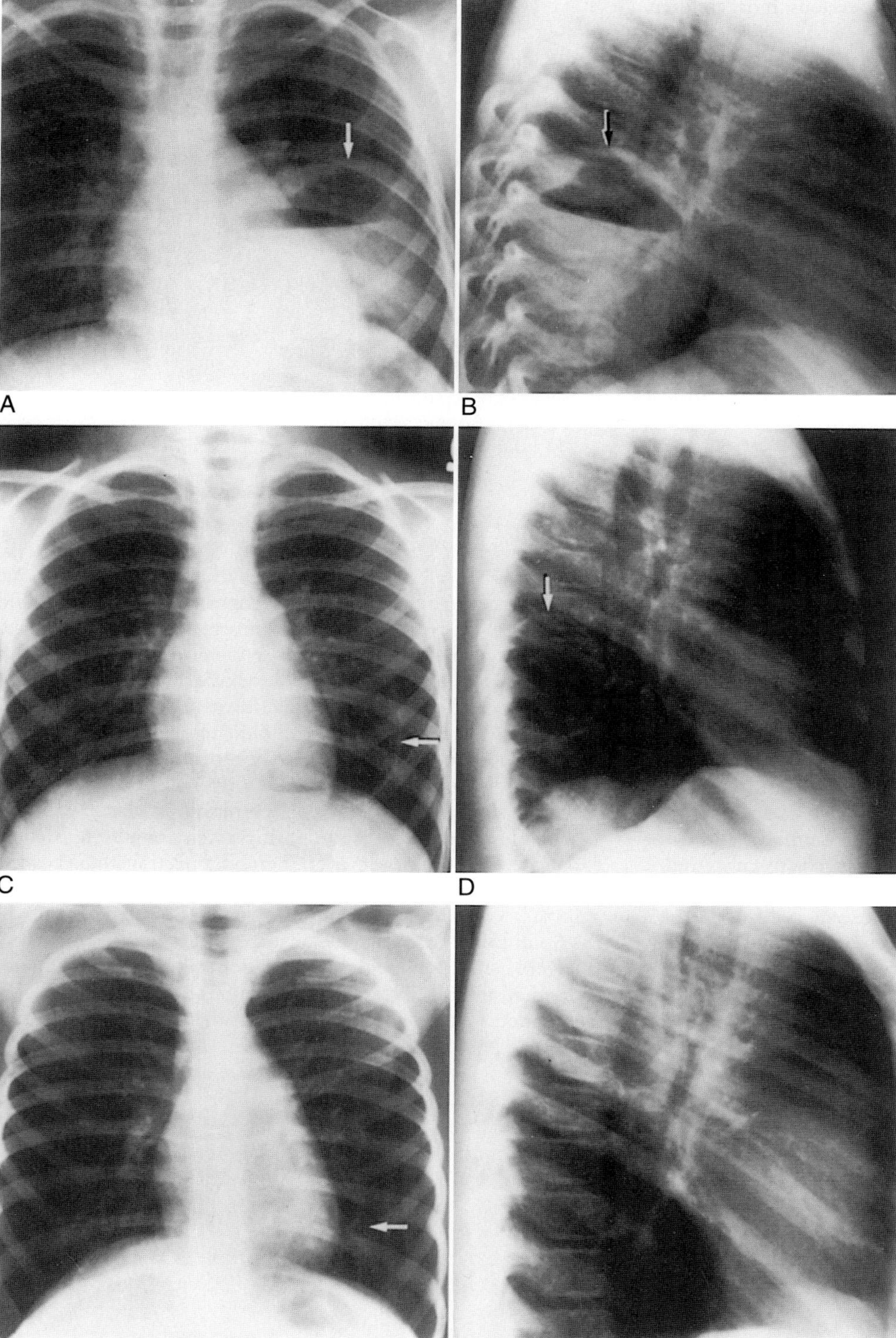

■ **FIGURE 30-1.** Primary lung abscess *(arrows)*. **A** and **B,** At presentation. **C** and **D,** One month after initiation of therapy. **E** and **F,** 1 year later.

Continued

by collecting the specimen in a sealed syringe or tube from which all air is expelled. If swabs are used, special transport swabs for anaerobic bacteria are required.[13] Prompt identification of the causative organisms can assist in the initiation of appropriate antimicrobial therapy.

■ DIFFERENTIAL DIAGNOSIS

The differential diagnosis of lung abscess includes congenital cysts or cystic adenomatoid malformation of the lung, traumatic pseudocyst, and noninfectious lesions such as pneumatoceles that may be associated with staphylococcal or viral pneumonia.

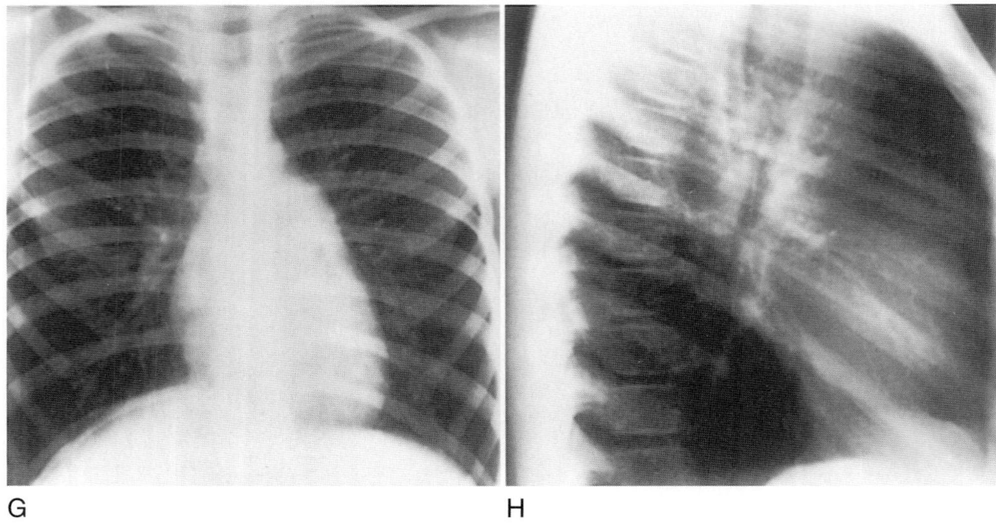

■ **FIGURE 30-1, cont'd.** **G** and **H,** 2 years later.

Infection of the lungs with *Echinococcus granulosus* causing a hydatid cyst may mimic a lung abscess. If the lesion on the chest roentgenograph fails to show a cavity and has a homogeneous density, the possibilities of simple pneumonia, primary or metastatic neoplasm, embolism, infarction, lymphoma, and loculated empyema must be entertained.

■ MANAGEMENT

Prolonged antibiotic therapy is the mainstay of treatment for aspiration pneumonia, necrotizing pneumonia, and lung abscess. The selection of antimicrobial agents is usually empiric and is based on age, history, physical examination, and radiographic findings, and by the organism recovered from reliable sources (i.e., blood, properly collected sputum, or pleural space). In severely ill patients, antimicrobial therapy may be guided by Gram stain of appropriate culture material, but treatment should not be withheld pending culture results.

There are no clear guidelines about the duration of antibiotic therapy required. The duration of treatment varies and depends on the type of pulmonary involvement. It would seem reasonable to use parenteral therapy until an effective program of oral therapy can be established, which should be continued until the child is asymptomatic. Initial response to therapy usually takes several days and complete resolution of the symptoms 1 to 3 weeks. Some authors recommend continuation of therapy until chest radiographs obtained at 2- to 4-week intervals show either complete resolution or a small, stable scar.[14] However, radiographic changes can lag up to 10 days behind clinical improvement. Anerobic infections may require therapy for prolonged periods (6–12 weeks or more) to prevent relapse.

Appropriate management of mixed pulmonary aerobic and anaerobic infections requires the administration of antimicrobials that are effective against both the aerobic and anaerobic components of the infection.[15] If such therapy is not given, the

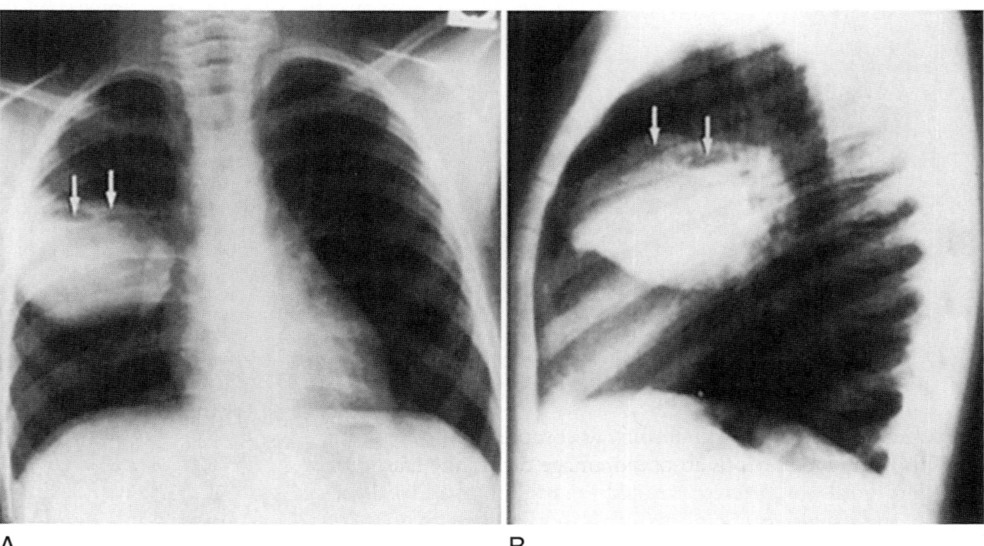

■ **FIGURE 30-2.** **A** and **B,** Multiloculated lung abscess *(arrows)*.

infection may persist and more serious complications may occur. However, even an appropriate antimicrobial selection may fail because of inability to penetrate the abscess, inactivation of a beta-lactam antibiotic by beta-lactamase-producing bacteria, low pH of the abscess, and binding of the agent(s) to protein.

When choosing antimicrobials for the therapy of mixed infections, an attempt should be made to cover most, or at least the most predominant, organisms (with the heaviest growth in culture) with a single agent or a combination of agents.

For children in whom aspiration is likely and thus anaerobes are the likely causative pathogens, clindamycin or high-dose penicillin G are recommended. Penicillin G may no longer be as effective in the treatment of pleuropulmonary infections, because more than half of the anaerobic gram-negative bacilli isolates recovered from these infections can produce the enzyme beta-lactamase.[16] This was demonstrated in two clinical trials in adults with lung abscess that have shown that clindamycin is more effective than penicillin, with fewer failures and relapses, shorter duration of fever, and shorter duration of putrid sputum following institution of treatment.[17,18] A recent retrospective study in 57 children illustrated the superiority of antimicrobials effective against penicillin-resistant anaerobic bacteria (ticarcillin-clavulanate or clindamycin) compared with an antibiotic lacking such coverage (ceftriaxone) in the therapy of aspiration or tracheostomy-associated pneumonia.[19]

Antimicrobials that are effective against penicillin-resistant anaerobic organisms are clindamycin, cefoxitin, chloramphenicol, metronidazole, a carbapenem (e.g., imipenem or meropenem), the combination of a penicillin with a beta-lactamase inhibitor, or metronidazole.[14,19–21] Since metronidazole is only effective against anaerobes and is ineffective against aerobic bacteria, it should be given in combination with penicillin to cover microaerophilic and anaerobic streptococci. Coverage against Enterobacteriaceae or *P. aeruginosa* may require the addition of an aminoglycoside, a quinolone (not yet approved for children in the United States) or a fourth-generation cephalosporin (e.g., cefepime). When antistaphylococcal coverage is needed, a penicillinase-resistant penicillin (e.g., oxacillin), vancomycin, or linezolid should be administered.[22]

In lung abscess associated with an immunocompromised state, a serious underlying illness or a nosocomial infection, aerobes and or facultatives are likely to be present, and specific antimicrobial therapy directed against the responsible organisms is indicated.

Children with lung abscess and necrotizing pneumonitis usually do well with antibiotic therapy alone, and it is unusual to require other therapy. Because these infections can drain spontaneously through the airway with postural drainage, surgical evacuation is not necessary if diagnosis is made early and appropriate therapy is instituted. Nonmedical treatments include drainage via bronchoscopy, percutaneous tube drainage, percutaneous needle aspiration, and wedge resection or lobectomy. Such interventions are indicated if there is clinical deterioration despite appropriate antibiotic therapy. Percutaneous drainage may be needed for a parapneumonic effusion.

Drainage may be necessary if an abscess is larger than 4 cm in diameter, causes mediastinal shift, or compresses the airway.[23] Even though percutaneous abscess drainage carries the hazard of bronchopleural fistula,[24,25] it should be considered for peripheral lesions that fail to respond to antimicrobial therapy or if bronchoscopy fails to drain a central lesion. Bronchoscopy may be helpful in relieving obstruction and is indicated if there is a history of foreign body aspiration.

■ COMPLICATIONS

In the preantibiotic era, complications of lung abscess were common, with 30% to 40% mortality and significant morbidity. Deaths still occur, particularly in developing countries, although they are usually attributable to the underlying disease process. Rare complications include overexpansion of the abscess with mediastinal shift, tension pneumothorax, spontaneous rupture of the abscess with seeding to other parts of the lung, empyema, bronchopleural fistula, septicemia, cerebral abscess, and inappropriate secretion of antidiuretic hormone.[26]

Complications also occur from aggressive investigations or therapies. Fiberoptic bronchoscopy has been complicated by massive intrabronchial aspiration of abscess contents. TTA has been complicated by hemoptysis and subcutaneous emphysema in children and by cardiac arrhythmias, bilateral pneumothorax, fatal hemorrhage, inadequate oxygenation, and intratracheal blood clots in adults. Complications of percutaneous tube drainage include the development of empyema and bronchopleural fistula. Percutaneous aspiration of the abscess can be complicated by a small pneumothorax, partial lobar collapse, or transient bacteremia. Lobectomy has been followed by empyema and pleural effusion.

■ COURSE AND PROGNOSIS

The outcome of lung abscess has dramatically improved since the introduction of antibiotics. Once adequate antibiotic therapy has been started, the fever resolves in about a week in most children, although it may last as long as 3 weeks. After complete clinical resolution of the illness, which averages 2 weeks, resolution of the cavity may take a variable amount of time. Progression of the infiltrates on chest radiograph during the first few days of therapy is not an indication of failure of medical therapy if the patient is otherwise responding well. Complete radiologic resolution may occur in 1 month but may take months or years (see Fig. 30-1). The rate of resolution of the cavity does not depend on its original size. During the resolution of the radiologic changes, children are well, do not seem prone to recurrent lower respiratory tract disease, and usually have normal pulmonary function.[22]

The outlook in lung abscess associated with immunocompromised children or in those with serious illness is more variable and depends on the underlying condition.

The availability of broad-spectrum, effective antibiotics has made the management of anaerobic lung infection more effective and much simpler. Drainage or excision of abscesses, with the attendant morbidity and mortality, seem no longer justified except in unusually complicated situations. Nevertheless, this condition still remains a challenge to pediatricians.

REFERENCES

1. Gibbons RJ: Aspects of the pathogenicity and ecology of the indigenous oral flora of man. In: Ballows RM, Dehaan V, Dowell R, Guze LB, eds: Anaerobic Bacteria. Role in Disease. Springfield, Ill: Charles C Thomas, 1974, pp 267–285.
2. Brook I: Bacterial colonization tracheobronchitis and pneumonia, following tracheostomy and long-term intubation in pediatric patients. Chest 1979;74:420–424.

3. Brook I: Pneumonia in mechanically ventilated children. Scand J Infect Dis 1995;27:619–622.
4. Brook I, Finegold SM: Bacteriology and therapy of lung abscess in children. J Pediatr 1979;94:10–12.
5. Brook I, Finegold SM: Bacteriology of aspiration pneumonia in children. Pediatrics 1980;65:1115–1120.
6. Bartlett JG, Finegold SM: Anaerobic pleuropulmonary infections. Medicine 1972;51:413–450.
7. Brook I: Microbiology of empyema in children and adolescents. Pediatrics 1990;85:722–726.
8. Brook I: Percutaneous transtracheal aspiration in the diagnosis and treatment of aspiration pneumonia in children. J Pediatr 1980;96:1000–1003.
9. Tan TQ, Seilheimer DK, Kaplan SL: Pediatric lung abscess. Clinical management and outcome. Pediatr Infect Dis J 1995;14:51–55.
10. Evans DA, Fiedler MA: Lung abscess in a patient with cystic fibrosis. Case report and review of the literature. Pediatr Pulmonol 1996;21:337–340.
11. Donnelly LF, Klosterman LA: CT appearance of parapneumonic effusions in children. Findings are not specific for empyema. AJR Am J Roentgenol 1997;169:179–182.
12. Henriquez AH, Mendoza J, Gonzalez PC: Quantitative culture of bronchoalveolar lavage from patients with anaerobic lung abscesses. J Infect Dis 1991;164:414–417.
13. Summanen P, Baron EJ, Ciron DM, et al: Wadsworth Anaerobic Bacteriology Manual, 6th ed. Belmont, Calif: Star Publishing, 2002.
14. Bartlett JG: Anaerobic bacterial infections of the lung and pleural space. Clin Infect Dis 1993;16(Suppl 4):S248–S255.
15. Finegold SM: Anaerobic bacteria in human disease. New York: Academic Press, 1977.
16. Brook I, Calhoun L, Yocum P: β-lactamase-producing isolates of *Bacteroides* species from children. Antimicrob Agents Chemother 1980;18:164–166.
17. Levison ME, Mangura CT, Lorber B, Abrutyn E, Pesanti EL, Levy RS, MacGregor RR: Clindamycin compared with penicillin for the treatment of anaerobic lung abscess. Ann Intern Med 1983;98:466–471.
18. Gudiol F, Manresa F, Pallares R, et al: Clindamycin vs. penicillin for anaerobic lung infections, high rate of penicillin failures associated with penicillin-resistant *Bacteroides melaninogenicus*. Arch Intern Med 1990; 150:2525–2529.
19. Brook I: Treatment of aspiration or tracheostomy-associated pneumonia in neurologically impaired children. Effect of antimicrobials effective against anaerobic bacteria. Int J Pediatr Otolaryngol 1996;35:171–177.
20. Brook I: Clindamycin in treatment of aspiration pneumonia in children. Antimicrob Agents Chemother 1979;15:342–345.
21. Brook I: Aspiration pneumonia in institutionalized children, a retrospective comparison of treatment with penicillin G, clindamycin, and carbenicillin. Clin Pediatr 1981;20:117–122.
22. Asher MI, Spier S, Beland M, et al: Primary lung abscess in childhood. The long-term outcome of conservative management. Am J Dis Child 1982; 136:491–494.
23. Rice TW, Ginsberg RJ, Todd TR: Tube drainage of lung abscesses. Ann Thorac Surg 1987;44:356–359.
24. Zuhdi MK, Spear RM, Worthen HM, Peterson BM: Percutaneous catheter drainage of tension pneumatocele, secondarily infected pneumatocele, and lung abscess in children. Crit Care Med 1996;24:330–333.
25. Hoffer FA, Bloom DA, Colin AA, Fishman SJ: Lung abscess versus necrotizing pneumonia. Implications for interventional therapy. Pediatr Radiol 1999;29:87–91.
26. Groskin SA, Panicek DM, Ewing DK, et al: Bacterial lung abscess. A review of the radiographic and clinical features of 50 cases. J Thorac Imaging 1991;6:62–67.

SUGGESTED READING

Baughman RP, Thorpe JE, Staneck J, et al: Use of the protected specimen brush in patient with endotracheal or tracheostomy tubes. Chest 1987;91:233–236.

Brook I: Aspiration pneumonia. Curr Treat Options Infect Dis 2001; 3:179–192.

Infections of the Respiratory Tract Due to Specific Organisms

31 Influenza

Margaret W. Leigh, MD

Influenza viruses have special features that distinguish them from other respiratory viruses. Most notably, influenza viruses alter their surface glycoproteins (hemagglutinin and neuraminidase) at irregular intervals. Previously formed antibodies often do not "recognize" the newly formed variants; consequently, repeated infections with influenza virus are common. Major antigenic shifts have been associated with widespread epidemics and pandemics characterized by overwhelming increases in the number of doctor visits, school and work absences, as well as hospitalizations and deaths attributable to respiratory illness. The typical illness from influenza virus infection, characterized by acute onset of high fever, headache, myalgia, anorexia, and malaise, is usually more debilitating than other respiratory viral infections. Superimposed bacterial infections (e.g., pneumonia, tracheitis, otitis media, and sinusitis) are much more common with influenza virus than with other respiratory viral infections. While most children without underlying disease recover uneventfully, children with chronic diseases are at risk for significant morbidity and mortality from influenza virus infection.

■ PROPERTIES OF INFLUENZA VIRUS

Influenza viruses, members of the family Orthomyxoviridae, contain negative, single-stranded RNA that is segmented into 8 pieces encoding 10 viral proteins. These include the structural proteins (hemagglutinin, neuraminidase, matrix protein, and nucleoprotein), as well as proteins needed for RNA synthesis. Virions are irregular spheric particles, 80 to 120 nm in diameter, that may be elongated or filamentous when first recovered from an infected host. The lipoprotein viral membrane is studded with numerous hemagglutinin and neuraminidase spikes. Hemagglutinin mediates viral attachment by binding to specific sialic acid residues on glycoproteins and glycolipids at the surface of host cells.

Influenza viruses are divided into three types, A, B, and C, based on their nucleoprotein and matrix protein content. Their hemagglutinin and neuraminidase antigens are variable and provide the basis for subtype classification used for the World Health Organization nomenclature. The influenza A subtypes associated with widespread human infection have distinct hemagglutinin proteins (H1, H2, or H3) and neuraminidase proteins (N1 or N2). Variation in antigenic composition occurs from time to time, primarily among A serotypes but also among the B serotypes. Major changes in hemagglutinin or neuraminidase are called antigenic shifts; minor changes within the same subtype are called antigenic drifts. The World Health Organization nomenclature for influenza A virus type and subtypes used to track antigenic drifts and shifts is shown in Table 31-1. While antigenic drifts occur almost annually, antigenic shifts occur at intervals of 10 years or more. Antigenic shifting is largely responsible for the ability of influenza to produce epidemics even in populations of persons who have previously been infected or immunized with influenza. The major antigenic shifts leading to pandemics in the last century occurred in 1918 (the Spanish flu pandemic, H1N1 strain), 1957 (Asian flu pandemic, H2N2 strain), and 1968 (Hong Kong flu pandemic, H3N2 strain). In the last quarter of a century, the prevalent strains in the United States have been H3N2 subtypes, which began to appear in 1968, and H1N1 subtypes, which were probably present from 1918 to 1956 and which reappeared in 1977.

For several decades, a worldwide surveillance program directed by the World Health Organization has been tracking the changes in influenza viruses. New strains are cultured and characterized in central laboratories. The spread of each new strain is tracked across continents. This information is used to determine which influenza virus strains to target in the next influenza vaccine. Influenza vaccines are modified each year to account for the antigenic alteration in the virus. Hosts for influenza viruses include birds, pigs, horses, and other mammals in addition to humans. Recent outbreaks of avian influenza, particularly the H5N1 subtype, have raised concerns that these new strains in birds may evolve into pandemic strains through reassortment with human strains.[1–3] In 1997, H5N1 influenza virus was transmitted to humans and killed 6 of the 18 known infected individuals. Since then, H5N1 has spread through domestic poultry in Asia, has been recovered from some wild migrating birds, has infected

TABLE 31-1. Severe influenza pandemics

Year	Virus Type (Subtype)	Common Name	Deaths Worldwide
1918	Influenza A (H1N1)	Spanish flu	40–100 million
1957	Influenza A (H2N2)	Asian flu	1 million
1968	Influenza A (H3N2)	Hong Kong flu	1 million

other humans with documented exposure to infected poultry, and has been transmitted to pigs and other mammals through reassortment with other strains. Particularly concerning are the high mortality rate in humans (~70%) and a 2004 report suggesting person-to-person transmission of H5N1 influenza in Thailand.[4] In addition to close surveillance, measures have been taken to control avian infection through monitoring of domestic and wild bird populations, vaccination of some domestic poultry, and disposal of infected poultry. The World Health Organization and other organizations are developing strategies to prevent spread of these strains as well as strategies to improve preparedness for a potential pandemic.

EPIDEMIOLOGY AND IMMUNITY

Influenza is spread readily from person to person through direct or indirect contact as well as inhalation of droplets of respiratory secretions dispersed by coughing and sneezing. The incubation period is short, usually 1 to 3 days. Groups maintained in confined areas, such as military barracks or airplane cabins, may be subjects of extensive and rapidly spread outbreaks. Influenza infection often occurs in epidemics that sweep through a community in a matter of 1 or 2 months. Morbidity is particularly severe in infants, persons over 65 years of age, and patients with immunosuppression or chronic diseases.[5,6]

Type-specific and subtype-specific immunity develops after natural infection, based on antibodies specific to HA and NA, but may not be adequate for prevention of reinfection; children may become infected several times within a matter of years by the same or related strains. Detectable strain-specific serum antibodies, however, do occur and persist. There is evidence that antibody developed against earlier strains may rise during a subsequent infection with a related strain of influenza virus. When an H1N1 influenza strain ("Russian" influenza) unexpectedly began to recirculate in 1977, illness was manifest primarily in persons who were too young to have been exposed to earlier H1N1 viruses.

The incidence of respiratory illnesses attributable to influenza virus infection is variable. Outbreaks of influenza in the United States usually peak in the winter months (January and February) but occasionally may be delayed until spring. Epidemiologic and surveillance studies have demonstrated that the highest attack rates for influenza virus occur in children; frequently outbreaks in school-aged children precede outbreaks in the adult population. Therefore, children are a major link in the spread of influenza infection throughout the community. The incidence of infection and illness in children of school age is 25% to 50% during interpandemic years and up to 70% during pandemic years.[7–10]

For a given year, the incidence of influenza virus may not exceed that for other respiratory viruses; however, during an outbreak, influenza virus is the most common etiologic agent recovered from patients with respiratory illnesses. For example, a 17-year study of hospitalized infants and young children from metropolitan Washington, D.C., demonstrated that 14% of 812 croup patients and 5% of 5313 hospitalized patients with respiratory infection showed evidence of influenza A or B virus infection; however, during the peak month of an influenza A virus outbreak, influenza A virus was demonstrated in 70% of croup patients and in 36% of all patients hospitalized for respiratory disease.[11]

LABORATORY DIAGNOSIS

The optimal time for demonstrating influenza virus in nasopharyngeal secretions by viral culture or antigen detection is during the first 72 hours of illness, because virus shedding drops abruptly with the activation of host defenses. For virus culture, nasopharyngeal secretions should be placed immediately in appropriate transport media and then inoculated into embryonated eggs or appropriate cell cultures (e.g., monkey kidney cell cultures). In 2 to 6 days, virus infection of these culture media can be detected by demonstration of hemagglutination or hemadsorption. Type-specific animal serums are used to identify the virus strain recovered. For rapid diagnosis, influenza antigen may be identified in either exfoliated cells on a slide with appropriate fluorescent-labeled antibody or in respiratory secretions by enzyme immunoassay. Several rapid diagnostic kits using these approaches are commercially available; however, the sensitivity and specificity of these rapid detection assays has been variable. Polymerase chain reaction assays to detect DNA produced by reverse transcription of unique influenza RNA has great potential as a sensitive and specific rapid diagnostic test. Several studies have used this approach to identify influenza virus in clinical specimens; but use in the clinical laboratory remains limited. Serology may be used to confirm the diagnosis retrospectively by demonstrating increased antibody titers in serum collected 3 weeks after the onset of illness compared with those in serum at the onset of illness. Antibodies to influenza virus may be determined by complement fixation, hemagglutination inhibition, enzyme immunoassay, or tissue culture neutralization methods.

PATHOGENESIS, PATHOLOGY

One of the predominant pathogenic characteristics of influenza viruses in susceptible hosts, such as chick embryos, ferrets, or humans, is a peculiar affinity for epithelial cells of the respiratory tract mucosa. Typically, influenza virus infects ciliated cells and causes widespread necrosis of these cells as early as 1 day after the onset of symptoms. Airway edema and infiltration of inflammatory cells into airway mucosa and epithelium are prominent pathologic features. Typically, repair and restoration of a ciliated, pseudostratified epithelium on the airway surface may take 2 to 4 weeks. Therefore, impaired mucociliary clearance and small airway obstruction may persist longer than the influenza illness. In some cases, infection may extend into the alveolar region, causing influenza virus pneumonia characterized by marked lymphocytic infiltration and distention of alveoli with a hyaline-like material. The immunologic responses to influenza infection include development of type- and subtype-specific serum and secretory antibody, an elevation in interferon levels in secretions and serum, a brief episode of lymphopenia, a depression in delayed hypersensitivity in general but an increase in influenza virus–specific cell-mediated responses, and some depression in the capacity of polymorphonuclear and mononuclear cells to respond to chemotaxis.

■ CLINICAL FEATURES

Influenza virus infection in children is characterized by a wide range of systemic, respiratory, and gastrointestinal symptoms[12] (Box 31-1). Infection in children may be subclinical but more typically is characterized by sudden onset of fever, chills, headache, malaise, and anorexia. Fever, ranging from 37.8°C to 40.5°C, typically lasts for 2 to 3 days but may last from 1 to 7 days. The most common respiratory tract symptoms in children include sneezing, sore throat with hoarseness, and a nonproductive cough. The influenza illness in young children differs from that in adolescents and adults; specifically, anorexia, abdominal pain, vomiting, and very high fever (>38.9°C) are more common in young children, whereas chills and myalgia are more common in adults. Usually, influenza virus infection is accompanied by a more sudden onset of these "toxic" signs than infections with parainfluenza virus, respiratory syncytial virus, or adenovirus. Infants with influenza virus infection often present with high fever and malaise suggesting sepsis. The respiratory illness may be limited to the upper respiratory tract or may present as tracheobronchitis, croup, bronchiolitis, or pneumonia. Subglottic croup is a common manifestation, especially in infants and typically is more severe than croup associated with parainfluenza virus. In uncomplicated cases, patients feel much better in 4 or 5 days; however, in patients with underlying cardiovascular disease or chronic lung disease, such as bronchopulmonary dysplasia, cystic fibrosis, or asthma, the respiratory illness may be more severe and prolonged.

Complications of influenza infection (Box 31-2) can be serious and life threatening. Bacterial superinfections (particularly pneumonia, tracheitis, otitis media, and sinusitis) are much more common with influenza virus than with other respiratory virus infections. Bacterial adherence in influenza-infected airways is enhanced. Multiple mechanisms have been proposed including stasis of mucus and entrapped bacteria because of influenza-mediated impairment of mucociliary clearance, desquamation of influenza-infected epithelial cells to expose basement membranes for bacterial attachment, exposure of bacterial receptors on the surfaces of influenza-infected cells, and presentation of new bacterial receptors during regeneration and remodeling of airways. Other conditions that may influence the likelihood of influenza-associated bacterial infections are impaired chemotaxis, phagocytosis, and bacterial killing by neutrophils and macrophages associated with influenza virus infection. Secondary bacterial pneumonia due to *Staphylococcus aureus, Streptococcus pneumoniae*, or *Haemophilus influenzae* is the most common life-threatening complication of influenza virus infection. In some cases, the bacterial pneumonia may become evident after partial recovery from the initial influenza virus illness, resulting in a biphasic disease pattern. In other cases, the bacterial illness may blend with the initial virus illness. Staphylococcal pneumonia associated with influenza virus may be especially severe and destructive. Other bacterial infections that have been reported in association with influenza virus infection are sepsis, bacterial tracheitis, and periorbital cellulitis.

Acute myositis has been associated with influenza infection, typically occurring during the early recovery phase from an otherwise uncomplicated influenza illness. The usual presentation is sudden onset of calf pain and refusal to walk. This condition is usually self-limited; however, rhabdomyolysis and associated renal failure from myoglobinuria have been reported. Other less common complications include neurologic disease (encephalitis, transverse myelitis, Guillain-Barré syndrome) and cardiac disease (myocarditis and pericarditis). Reye's syndrome, encephalopathy with fatty microvesiculation of the liver, was a frequent and life-threatening complication in children with influenza B virus infection treated with aspirin until this association was recognized and aspirin use was discontinued.

BOX 31-1 Clinical Features of Influenza Virus Infection in Children

Frequent (in >50% of patients)
Fever (>38.9°C)
Chills
Nonproductive cough
Headache
Anorexia
Malaise
Nasal stuffiness
Sore throat
Conjunctivitis
Common (in 25% to 50% of patients)
Sneezing
Prostration
Myalgia
Abdominal pain
Vomiting

BOX 31-2 Complications of Influenza Virus Infection

Common Complications

Otitis media
Sinusitis
Secondary bacterial pneumonia

Less Frequent Complications

Acute myositis
Rhabdomyolysis
Myocarditis
Pericarditis
Reye's syndrome
Encephalitis
Transverse myelitis
Guillain-Barré syndrome

■ PREVENTION

VACCINES

To be effective, influenza vaccines must contain antigens similar to those that will be encountered in nature within a few months following vaccine administration. Because influenza viruses show progressive antigenic variation, suitable vaccine strains are likely to be those recovered in the recent past. Typically, vaccines contain three virus strains, influenza A subtypes H1N1 and H3N2, and influenza B. In temperate climates, influenza vaccines should be administered in the fall months to allow time for antibody production before influenza outbreaks that typically occur in the winter months.

Because formulations and content of vaccines are likely to change yearly, the physician is advised to consult the most recent statements from the Public Health Service Advisory Committee on Immunization Practices or the American Academy of Pediatrics Committee on Infectious Diseases. Present target groups for vaccination include: (1) infants and children 6 months of age or older who would be at high risk if they contracted influenza, (2) medical care providers or household contacts of high-risk infants and children, (3) household contacts and out-of-home caregivers for children (aged 0–23 months) who are at increased risk for influenza-related hospitalization,[6,9,13,14] (4) children and adolescents receiving long-term aspirin therapy who are at increased risk for acquiring Reye's syndrome during influenza virus infection, and (5) other children whose families may wish to reduce their chances of acquiring influenza.[15,16] The high-risk category includes healthy children aged 6 to 23 months and children older than 6 months with chronic pulmonary disease (including moderate to severe asthma, bronchopulmonary dysplasia, and cystic fibrosis), cardiac disease that is hemodynamically significant, sickle cell disease or other hemoglobinopathies, chronic metabolic disease (including diabetes mellitus), renal dysfunction or immunosuppression (including immunosuppression caused by medications or by human immunodeficiency virus infection).[15,16]

If influenza vaccine supply is adequate, administration to all children may be appropriate. Surveillance studies demonstrate that outbreaks often begin in schools and then spread to the rest of the community. Administration of influenza vaccine to daycare children reduces influenza-related morbidity among household contacts.[17] Therefore, broad use of an effective vaccine in children, particularly those of preschool and school age, might well reduce the spread of virus and lessen the total impact of influenza in a community.

Two types of influenza vaccine are available: inactivated vaccine (administered by IM injection) and live, attenuated vaccine (administered by nasal spray). At present, the live, attenuated vaccine is approved only for healthy individuals aged 5 to 49 years, but the inactivated vaccine is approved for anyone older than 6 months of age including individuals with underlying conditions that increase their risk of complications from influenza infection.[12,15,16]

Inactivated Influenza Virus Vaccine

Inactivated influenza virus vaccines have been manufactured as whole-virus or split-virus preparations. For whole-virus vaccines, influenza virus is cultivated in eggs, harvested, inactivated, and purified by zonal centrifugation or chromatography to eliminate bacterial endotoxin or other reactive agents. Split-virus vaccines are prepared by treating the whole-virus preparation with organic solvents or detergents to disrupt the viral membrane and solubilize the viral proteins. Split-virus vaccines cause fewer side effects but may be less immunogenic than whole-virus vaccines. Since 2001, whole-virus vaccine preparations have not been available in the United States.

Dosage schedules for inactivated influenza vaccine incorporate strategies to minimize side effects and optimize antibody production.[12,15,16] Current recommendations include: (1) half the adult dosage for infants and children 6 to 35 months of age, (2) two doses 4 weeks apart for individuals under 9 years of age who have not had a prior influenza vaccine, and (3) single-dose vaccine for children who have had a prior influenza vaccine or who are older than 9 years of age. The only specific contraindication for the use of inactivated influenza vaccine is anaphylactic hypersensitivity to eggs. The most common symptoms associated with inactivated influenza vaccine administration are soreness at the injection site and fever (typically occurring 6 to 24 hours after injection and most prevalent in children younger than 2 years of age). Less common symptoms include nausea, lethargy, headache, muscle aches, and chills. In asthma patients, a brief impairment in airflow may follow administration of influenza vaccine; however, in large population studies, the frequency of asthma exacerbations is not increased following influenza vaccination.[18] Special consideration is needed for immunosuppressed and other immunocompromised children. Immune response may be limited and is best accomplished during periods of remission or when immunosuppressive drugs have been discontinued. In human immunodeficiency virus–infected individuals whose $CD4^+$ T-lymphocyte counts are greater than 100 cells/mm^3 and human immunodeficiency virus copies are fewer than 30,000 copies/mL, influenza vaccine is most effective[19]; it is ineffective in persons with advanced human immunodeficiency viral disease.[20]

Live, Attenuated Influenza Virus Vaccine

For decades, researchers have been developing and testing potential live, attenuated influenza vaccines that can be administered intranasally. The most effective approach for attenuation has been cold adaptation. This process involves cultivation of influenza virus in cell culture at successively lowered temperatures to select a strain that replicates efficiently at 25°C but not at human body temperature. In several human trials, these attenuated influenza viruses have maintained their antigenicity and phenotypic stability without reverting to wild-type infectious influenza strain and without significant side effects.[21–24] In 2004, a cold-adapted vaccine (FluMist manufactured by MedImmune, Inc.) was licensed for use in healthy individuals between the ages of 5 and 49 years. The target population is expected to expand as further experience with this vaccine is obtained. Because of the ease of administration, this vaccine could have widespread application. Side effects of the live, attenuated vaccine in healthy individuals include slight increase in nasal congestion, cough, headache, fever, vomiting, and myalgias compared with placebo recipients. Further study of potential side effects is needed in individuals with asthma and other chronic diseases. For live, attenuated vaccine, the efficacy in preventing laboratory-documented influenza illness in healthy individuals is comparable to the efficacy of inactivated vaccines (70% to 85%). Live, attenuated virus may be shed in low concentrations in the nasal secretions of individuals immediately after instillation; therefore, these vaccines should not be administered to close contacts of immunocompromised or immunosuppressed individuals. The live, attenuated vaccine is contraindicated in individuals with anaphylactic egg allergy.

The dosage schedule for live, attenuated vaccine is similar to inactivated vaccine.[12,15,16] Children younger than 9 years of age who have not had a prior influenza vaccine should receive two doses separated by 6 to 10 weeks; whereas children younger than 9 years with prior influenza vaccine and individuals older than 9 years require only one dose. The optimal time of administration is during the fall months. Because influenza antiviral agents reduce replication of influenza virus, these agents should not be administered within 48 hours before or within 2 weeks after administration of live, attenuated influenza vaccines.

ANTIVIRAL AGENTS FOR INFLUENZA

While immunization should be the primary method used to prevent influenza, several antiviral agents have been effective in preventing influenza illness. The agents should be considered when influenza infection is prevalent in a particular community and are recommended for (1) high-risk persons as an adjunct to late vaccination, (2) immunodeficient persons as a supplement to the protection afforded by vaccine, and (3) persons for whom influenza vaccine is contraindicated.[12,16] To prevent infection, these antiviral agents must be used before exposure and continued throughout the period of exposure (as long as 6–8 weeks).

Amantadine and Rimantadine (M2 Ion Channel Blockers)

The synthetic amine amantadine and its closely related analog, rimantadine, have been shown to be effective in preventing and possibly ameliorating influenza A but not influenza B infection. These agents are M2 ion channel blockers that inhibit influenza virus replication by blockade of hydrogen ion flow.[25] Amantadine and rimantadine appear to have similar prophylactic effectiveness against infection with influenza A virus, preventing illness in 70% to 90% of patients, but the incidence of adverse effects is lower with rimantadine. Side effects include insomnia, nervousness, impaired concentration, and gastrointestinal complaints such as nausea, vomiting, anorexia, and abdominal pain. Drugs that alter pharmacokinetics of amantadine and rimantadine include aspirin and acetaminophen, both of which may increase clearance of these agents. The recommended doses are the same for amantadine and rimantadine, as shown in Table 31-2. As of 2004, neither drug has been approved for use in infants younger than 1 year of age. Amantadine and rimantadine have not been effective in prevention or treatment of H5N1 influenza in animal models, and thus are unlikely to be effective if this virus strain evolves into a pandemic threat.

Zanamivir and Oseltamivir (Neuraminidase Inhibitors)

The neuraminidase inhibitors (zanamivir and oseltamivir) are effective for chemoprophylaxis of both influenza A and influenza B, preventing influenza illness in 80% to 85% of individuals. At this time oseltamivir has been approved for prophylaxis in children who are 13 years of age or older; zanamivir has not been approved by the U.S. Food and Drug Administration for prophylaxis. These agents inhibit release of influenza virions from infected cells, thereby inhibiting spread to other cells.[26,27] Adverse effects of orally administered oseltamivir include nausea, vomiting, and headache. Adverse effects of zanamivir, administered as an inhaled powder, include cough, nasal and throat irritation, and bronchospasm. These antiviral agents are effective for prophylaxis and treatment of avian influenza strains (H5N1, H7N7, and H9N2) in mouse models[28]; therefore, zanamivir and oseltamivir are options for prophylaxis and treatment of H5N1 influenza if this avian strain evolves into a human pathogen.

TABLE 31-2. Recommended dosages of agents for treatment and prophylaxis of influenza

Antiviral Agent	Prophylaxis Dosage	Treatment Dosage
Amantadine	*For children 1–9 years:* 5 mg/kg/day up to 150 mg in two divided doses *For children ≥10 years:* 100 mg twice daily	Same as prophylaxis
Rimantadine	*For children 1–9 years:* 5 mg/kg/day up to 150 mg in two divided doses *For children ≥10 years:* 100 mg bid	*For children ≥13 years* Same as prophylaxis
Zanamivir	Not FDA approved for prophylaxis	*For children ≥7 years:* 10 mg bid
Oseltamivir	*For children ≥13 years:* 75 mg bid	*For children ≥1 year:* ≤15 kg: 30 mg bid 16–23 kg: 45 mg bid 24–40 kg: 60 mg bid >40 kg: 75 mg bid

FDA, U.S. Food and Drug Administration.

TREATMENT

Symptomatic management of influenza virus illness includes bed rest, hydration, and control of fever and myalgias with anti-inflammatory agents not containing salicylates, such as acetaminophen or ibuprofen. Antibiotics should not be used in uncomplicated influenza but should be instituted for bacterial superinfections. Children with croup may benefit from humidified air and racemic epinephrine, but a substantial number of these patients require intubation and/or tracheostomy. Patients with significant lower respiratory disease may benefit from bronchodilators, especially patients with underlying lung disease; many may require supplemental oxygen, and some need continuous positive airway pressure or mechanical ventilation.

ANTIVIRAL AGENTS

Therapeutic use of antiviral agents may be considered for high-risk children and immunodeficient patients as well as for an infant or child with severe croup or pneumonia attributable to influenza virus infection.[12,16] Dosage recommendations for the specific agents are shown in Table 31-2. Amantadine and rimantadine may reduce symptoms and duration of illness if administered within 48 hours of onset of symptoms, based on studies in healthy adults. Currently, amantadine but not rimantadine is approved for therapeutic use in children who are 1 year of age or older. Drug-resistant strains of influenza virus develop rapidly in up to 30% of patients treated with amantadine or rimantadine and are easily transmitted to other individuals.[29,30] Therefore, use of these agents should be limited to high-risk individuals, and therapy should be stopped as soon as clinically warranted.

Zanamivir and oseltamivir can reduce the duration of uncomplicated influenza A and influenza B infection when administered within 48 hours of onset of symptoms. Zanamivir is approved for treatment of influenza virus–infected children who are 7 years of age or older. Oseltamivir is approved for treatment of children who are 1 year of age or older. Emergence of drug-resistant variants after treatment with NA inhibitors is relatively rare (in <1% of treated patients).[31]

REFERENCES

1. Lipatov AS, Govorkova EA, Webby RJ, et al: Influenza. Emergence and control. J Virol 2004;78:8951–8959.
2. Li KS, Guan Y, Wang J, et al: Genesis of a highly pathogenic and potentially pandemic H5N1 influenza virus in eastern Asia. Nature 2004;430:209–213.
3. Webby RJ, Webster RG: Are we ready for pandemic influenza? Science 2003;302:1519–1522.
4. Ungchusak K, Auewarakul P, Dowell SF, et al: Probable person-to-person transmission of avian influenza A (H5N1). N Engl J Med 2005;352: 333–340.
5. Glezen WP, Greenberg SB, Atmar RL, et al: Impact of respiratory virus infections on persons with chronic underlying conditions. JAMA 2000; 283:499–505.
6. Neuzil KM, Wright PF, Mitchel EF Jr, Griffin MR: The burden of influenza illness in children with asthma and other chronic medical conditions. J Pediatr 2000;137:856–864.
7. Glezen WP, Couch RB: Interpandemic influenza in the Houston area, 1974–76. N Engl J Med 1978;298:587–592.
8. Glezen WP, Keitel WA, Taber LH, et al: Age distribution of patients with medically-attended illnesses caused by sequential variants of influenza A/H1N1. Comparison to age-specific infection rates, 1978–1989. Am J Epidemiol 1991;133:296–304.
9. Neuzil KM, Zhu Y, Griffin MR, et al: Burden of interpandemic influenza in children younger than 5 years. A 25-year prospective study. J Infect Dis 2002;185:147–152.
10. Dunn FL, Carey DE, Cohen A, Martin JD: Epidemiologic studies of Asian influenza in a Louisiana parish. Am J Hyg 1959;70:351–371.
11. Kim HW, Brandt CD, Arrobio JO, et al: Influenza A and B virus infection in infants and young children during the years 1957–1976. Am J Epidemiol 1979;109:464–479.
12. 2003 Red Book: Report of the Committee on Infectious Diseases, 26th ed. Elk Grove Village, Ill.: American Academy of Pediatrics, 2003.
13. Izurieta HS, Thompson WW, Kramarz P, et al: Influenza and the rates of hospitalization for respiratory disease among infants and young children. N Engl J Med 2000;342:232–239.
14. Neuzil KM, Mellen BG, Wright PF, et al: The effect of influenza on hospitalizations, outpatient visits, and courses of antibiotics in children. N Engl J Med 2000;342:225–231.
15. American Academy of Pediatrics Policy Statement: Recommendations for Influenza Immunization of Children. Pediatrics 2004;113:1441–1447.
16. Harper SA, Fukuda K, Uyeki TM, et al: Centers for Disease Control and Prevention (CDC) Advisory Committee on Immunization Practices (ACIP): Prevention and control of influenza. Recommendations of the Advisory Committee on Immunization Practices (ACIP). MMWR Recomm Rep 2004;53(RR-6):1–40.
17. Hurwitz ES, Haber M, Chang A, et al: Effectiveness of influenza vaccination of day care children in reducing influenza-related morbidity among household contacts. JAMA 2000;284:1677–1682.
18. American Lung Association Asthma Clinical Research Centers: The safety of inactivated influenza vaccine in adults and children with asthma. N Engl J Med 2001;345:1529–1536.
19. Fine AD, Bridges CB, De Guzman AM, et al: Influenza A among patients with human immunodeficiency virus. An outbreak of infection at a residential facility in New York City. Clin Infect Dis 2001;32:1784–1791.
20. Kroon FP, van Dissel JT, de Jong JC, et al: Antibody response after influenza vaccination in HIV-infected individuals. A consecutive 3-year study. Vaccine 2000;18:3040–3049.
21. Belshe RB, Nichol KL, Black SB, et al: Safety, efficacy, and effectiveness of live, attenuated, cold-adapted influenza vaccine in an indicated population aged 5–49 years. Clin Infect Dis 2004;39:920–927.
22. Belshe RB, Mendelman PM, Treanor J, et al: The efficacy of live attenuated, cold-adapted, trivalent, intranasal influenzavirus vaccine in children. N Engl J Med 1998;338:1405–1412.
23. Clements ML, Makhene MK, Karron RA, et al: Effective immunization with live attenuated influenza A virus can be achieved in early infancy. J Infect Dis 1996;173:44–51.
24. Gruber WC, Darden PM, Still JG, et al: Evaluation of bivalent live attenuated influenza A vaccines in children 2 months to 3 years of age. Safety, immunogenicity and dose-response. Vaccine 1997;15:1379–1384.
25. Wang C, Takeuchi K, Pinto LH, Lamb RA: Ion channel activity of influenza A virus M2 protein. Characterization of the amantadine block. J Virol 1993;67:5585–5594.
26. Mendel DB, Tai CY, Escarpe PA, et al: Oral administration of a prodrug of the influenza virus neuraminidase inhibitor GS 4071 protects mice and ferrets against influenza infection. Antimicrob Agents Chemother 1998;42:640–646.
27. Sidwell RW, Huffman JH, Barnard DL, et al: Inhibition of influenza virus infections in mice by GS4104, an orally effective influenza virus neuraminidase inhibitor. Antivir Res 1998;37:107–120
28. Govorkova EA, Leneva IA, Goloubeva OG, et al: Comparison of the efficacies of RWJ-270201, zanamivir, and oseltamivir against H5N1, H9N2, and other avian influenza viruses. Antimicrob Agents Chemother 2001;45:2723–2732.
29. Iwahashi J, Tsuji K, Ishibashi T, et al: Isolation of amantadine-resistant influenza A viruses (H3N2) from patients following administration of amantadine in Japan. J Clin Microbiol 2001;39:1652–1653.
30. Shiraishi K, Mitamura K, Sakai-Tagawa Y, et al: High frequency of resistant viruses harboring different mutations in amantadine-treated children with influenza. J Infect Dis 2003;188:57–61.
31. McKimm-Breschkin JL: Resistance of influenza viruses to neuraminidase inhibitors—a review. Antivir Res 2000;47:1–17.

32 Atypical Pneumonias in Children

Misty Colvin, MD • L. Barry Seltz, MD • Leslie L. Barton, MD

In *Stedman's Medical Dictionary*, atypical is defined as "not typical; not corresponding to the normal form or type." The term *atypical pneumonia* was first used by Reimann in 1938 when he described several cases of "severe, diffuse, atypical pneumonia" clinically different from other commonly described pneumonias.[1] In 1944, Eaton isolated an agent that was believed to be the principal cause of atypical pneumonia; this agent was later placed in the genus *Mycoplasma* and given the name *Mycoplasma pneumoniae*.[2] Subsequently, other pathogens have been grouped under atypical pneumonias because of similar clinical presentations. This chapter reviews the atypical pneumonias.

HANTAVIRUS PULMONARY SYNDROME

Hantavirus pulmonary syndrome was first recognized in 1993 when a cluster of individuals living in the southwestern United States acquired an acute illness characterized by a febrile prodrome followed by rapid, diffuse pulmonary edema and cardiogenic shock, with an initial case fatality rate of 76%.[3]

VIROLOGY

Hantaviruses are RNA viruses from the family Bunyaviridae. Several hantaviruses pathogenic for humans have been identified in the United States. Sin Nombre virus is the primary causative agent of hantavirus pulmonary syndrome. Others include the Bayou, Black Creek Canal, Monongahela, and New York viruses. Several other hantaviruses are found in Europe, Asia, and South America.

EPIDEMIOLOGY

Rodents are the natural hosts of hantaviruses. In general, each virus has a single primary rodent host. The deer mouse (*Peromyscus maniculatus*) is the host for Sin Nombre virus; about 10% of deer mice tested show evidence of infection.[4] The rice rat is the host for Bayou virus; the cotton rat transmits Black Creek Canal virus, and the white-footed mouse is the host for the New York virus. Infection is associated with activities that bring individuals into contact with infected rodents, usually in rural settings, and most often follows inhalation of aerosolized saliva or excreta. It may also occur after an infected rodent bite or via contamination of broken skin. Person-to-person transmission has been documented only during an outbreak in Argentina.[4] The incubation period is 1 to 6 weeks after exposure. A total of 358 cases of hantavirus pulmonary syndrome had been reported in the United States through January 2004. The mean age of these cases is 37 years, with a range of 10 to 75 years.[5]

PATHOPHYSIOLOGY

After inhalation, the infectious particle is deposited in the terminal respiratory bronchiole or alveolus. Subsequent viremia results in widespread infection of pulmonary capillary endothelium and other cells.[6] Invasion results in induction of the immune response and the secretion of inflammatory mediators. Increased pulmonary capillary endothelial permeability results in pulmonary edema. These mediators are also thought to cause myocardial depression, resulting in cardiogenic shock.[6]

Histopathologic features are most consistent in the lungs and spleen. Pulmonary findings include an interstitial pneumonitis with mononuclear cell infiltration and intra-alveolar edema. Focal hyaline membranes, consisting of condensed fibrin apposed to alveolar walls, are also present. In the spleen, variable numbers of immunoblasts are seen in the red pulp and periarteriolar sheaths.[7]

CLINICAL MANIFESTATIONS

Hantavirus pulmonary syndrome typically begins with a 3- to 5-day prodrome characterized by fever, myalgias, malaise, and vomiting.[6] Respiratory symptoms begin after the prodrome with the onset of pulmonary edema. Patients develop a productive cough, and there is usually rapid decompensation. Mechanical ventilation may be necessary within 24 hours. Myocardial depression may lead to hypotension. The mortality rate is approximately 37%, despite intensive care; death generally occurs 24 to 48 hours after admission. Patients who survive recover quickly. Patients may show some degree of small airway obstruction as long as 1 year after recovery.[3] There are reports of infection in which patients had prodromal symptoms but never developed cardiopulmonary involvement. Renal disease and myositis are prominent features of infection with Bayou and Black Creek Canal viruses, similar to cases seen in South America. Hantaviruses in Europe and Asia also cause hemorrhagic fever with renal syndrome.

LABORATORY FINDINGS AND DIAGNOSIS

Diagnosis is confirmed by serology. The most widely used test is the enzyme immunoassay that detects IgM and IgG antibodies. Levels of both antibodies are present at the onset of clinical disease. Sin Nombre virus RNA can be detected by reverse transcriptase polymerase chain reaction (PCR) of peripheral blood cells during the first 10 days of illness.[6] Viral culture is enigmatically not useful for diagnosis. Characteristic laboratory findings include thrombocytopenia, elevated hematocrit, and circulating immunoblasts. Other laboratory findings may include elevated creatinine and lactate dehydrogenase, proteinuria, hematuria, normal to slightly prolonged partial thromboplastin time, and elevated prothrombin time.

Approximately one third of patients have airspace disease on initial radiographs; many are normal.[6] By 48 hours after hospital admission, virtually all patients have interstitial edema and two thirds develop worsening bibasilar or perihilar airspace disease. Pleural effusions are common.

TREATMENT

There is currently no specific therapy of hantavirus pulmonary syndrome. Supportive management of pulmonary edema, respiratory failure, and hypotension is critical. Extracorporeal membrane oxygenation appears to be beneficial, especially in critically ill patients. Anecdotal reports of corticosteroid use in South America suggest that they may be of value.[6] The utility of ribavirin is under investigation.[3]

PREVENTION

The best current approach for disease prevention is risk reduction through environmental modification and hygiene practices that deter rodents from colonizing home and work environments, together with safe cleanup of rodent waste. Measures include eliminating food sources and nesting sites, sealing holes, and using traps and rodenticides with careful disposal of dead rodents.

LEGIONNAIRE'S DISEASE

The original description of Legionnaire's disease followed an outbreak of atypical pneumonia at an American Legion convention in 1976. Legionnaire's disease continues to be an elusive diagnosis because of its indistinct clinical course and radiographic findings, the failure to suspect *Legionella* and obtain appropriate diagnostic studies, and the imperfections of available diagnostic tests.[8] Though rare in otherwise normal children, the incidence of Legionnaire's disease may be higher than previously estimated in those who are immunocompromised or who have underlying lung disease.

MICROBIOLOGY

Legionella species are obligate aerobic, mobile, gram-negative, intracellular bacilli that require special staining (Dieterle's stain) for visualization. Of the 14 known serotypes, only *Legionella pneumophila* types 1 (80% to 90% of clinical infection), 2, 4, and 6 are known to cause Legionnaire's disease. Infections with species other than *L. pneumophila* have also rarely been reported in both children and adults. The growth of *Legionella* requires 3 to 5 days' incubation on buffered charcoal yeast extract medium, enriched with both cysteine and ferric ions.

EPIDEMIOLOGY

Legionella are ubiquitous in the aqueous environment. Freshwater amoeba, such as *Acanthamoeba* and *Hartmannella*, are the natural hosts and probable reservoirs. Historically, epidemics have been linked to cooling towers, air conditioning, hot water tanks and plumbing, potable water devices, and air duct systems. Person-to-person transmission has not been documented. Legionnaire's disease is more common in adults than in children. Infection rates among men are twice those of women. Cigarette smoking, surgery, chronic lung disease, immunosuppression, and exposure to contaminated water sources are risk factors for Legionnaire's disease. Neonates are also susceptible. The incubation period for Legionnaire's disease is 2 to 14 days.

PATHOLOGY

Infection results from the inhalation of bacteria from an aerosolized contaminated water source or by microaspiration of a contaminated water source. Following phagocytosis by alveolar macrophages, *Legionella* multiply extensively, causing cell lysis. The ensuing inflammatory response attracts polymorphonuclear cells, fibrin, macrophages, and erythrocytes to the site. This exudate fills the alveoli and terminal bronchioles. Hemorrhage and microabscesses are observed. Lymph nodes are involved occasionally. Bacteria may also be recovered from extrapulmonary sites such as liver, spleen, and myocardium.

As with other intracellular organisms, the T cell—mediated response to infection confers immunity. Humoral immunity may aid in clearance of the organism by enhanced phagocytosis; otherwise its role is limited. The risk of reinfection is unknown.

CLINICAL MANIFESTATIONS

Infection with *L. pneumophila* results in two clinically distinct syndromes: Legionnaire's disease and Pontiac fever. Pontiac fever is an acute, self-limited, febrile illness without respiratory symptomatology. Legionnaire's disease is characterized by necrotizing multifocal pneumonia and a fulminant course.

Legionnaire's disease begins with a nonspecific prodrome of myalgias, fatigue, anorexia, malaise, headache, chills, vomiting, and watery diarrhea. The onset may be insidious or acute, but is usually followed by high fever. Relative bradycardia is well described in adults with Legionnaire's disease. Pleuritic chest pain and a dry cough ensue; the latter rarely becomes productive. Chest examination is consistent with a consolidating pneumonia: dullness to percussion, increased fremitus, bronchial breath sounds, and coarse crackles. A pleural friction rub may be heard, since nearly one third of patients with Legionnaire's disease will have pleural effusions. The extrapulmonary manifestations of *L. pneumophila* infection include neurologic (e.g., meningoencephalitis), cardiac (e.g., myocarditis), gastrointestinal (e.g., hepatitis), and renal (e.g., hypophosphatemia) abnormalities.[9] In more severe cases, patients become progressively ill, with confusion and delirium by the third to fourth day of illness. Shock, respiratory distress, or both develop by the fifth to sixth day of illness. The overall mortality is estimated to be 15%, although mortality rates may be as high as 60% for nosocomial infection and immunocompromised patients.[10]

LABORATORY FINDINGS AND DIAGNOSIS

Legionnaire's disease must be considered in any patient with severe progressive pneumonia of unclear etiology. Leukocytosis with a shift to the left, as well as lymphopenia, are common. Thrombocytosis and disseminated intravascular coagulation may also occur. Legionnaire's disease often results in elevated liver transaminases, creatine kinase, bilirubin, and alkaline phosphatase. Hyponatremia and hypophosphatemia are more frequent in Legionnaire's disease than in other bacterial pneumonias. Hypoxia is often more severe that would be predicted by the extent of the pneumonia.[9] Chest radiographs characteristically demonstrate early interstitial or patchy infiltrates (unilateral or bilateral) described as an acinar filling pattern, followed by nodular consolidation and cavitation.[10] The infiltrates often progress despite antibiotic therapy. Complete resolution of the lesions may take as long as 6 weeks.

Culture of sputum, and if available, lower respiratory secretions, pleural fluid, or lung biopsy specimens, is the definite diagnostic modality. *Legionella* antigen may also be detected in urine specimens, but this method is only established for serogroup 1. A combination of sputum culture and urine antigen detection may be the best diagnostic method.[8]

Indirect immunofluorescent antibody testing provides rapid results, requires specialized handling, and may yield false positives due to cross reactions with other bacteria (e.g., *Pseudomonas, Streptococcus, Candida, Bacteroides, Flavobacterium,* and *Stenotrophomonas*). Testing with monoclonal antibody improves the test's specificity. A positive immunofluorescent antibody test without other supporting evidence should not be considered diagnostic of legionellosis.[8] PCR testing is not commercially available.

Serologic testing does not yield results rapidly enough to be useful as a diagnostic tool. An antibody titer of 1:256 or higher suggests a recent infection but is not confirmatory. Seroconversion may take 9 to 12 weeks. When obtaining serologic studies, it is important to request testing for IgM as well as IgG, since some individuals will only demonstrate an IgM response. False-positive results may occur due to cross-reactivity with other bacterial causes of atypical pneumonia (e.g., *Francisella tularensis, Coxiella burnetti, Mycoplasma pneumoniae*).

TREATMENT

Azithromycin has replaced erythromycin as the antimicrobial of choice for the treatment of Legionnaire's disease. Tetracyclines and trimethoprim-sulfamethoxazole are therapeutic alternatives. Although fluoroquinolones have demonstrated efficacy in adults, their use in children is restricted. Rifampin is also recommended as adjunctive therapy in the presence of immunosuppression or severe illness.[9] Parenteral therapy should be administered until the patient responds clinically. The total duration of therapy is 5 to 10 days for azithromycin and longer when alternative therapies are utilized or in the presence of severe disease or immunosuppression.

PREVENTION

Prevention of legionellosis is best achieved by identification and eradication of the environmental source. Culture-positive water may be superheated (70°C to 80°C), hyperchlorinated, or ionized by copper-silver units. Unfortunately, no method is particularly successful.

PSITTACOSIS

The first human outbreak of psittacosis (ornithosis) was reported in 1879. All seven patients had contact with sick parrots and finches. All developed a febrile respiratory illness terminating in death in three.[11] The term *psittacosis* derives from the Greek word for parrot, *psittakos*.[12]

MICROBIOLOGY

Chlamydia psittaci is one of three *Chlamydia* species known to cause disease in humans. It is an obligate intracellular bacterium that contains both DNA and RNA within its cell wall.

EPIDEMIOLOGY

Psittacosis has a worldwide distribution and is generally sporadic. However, a serious epidemic occurred in the United States in 1929; 800 people were affected. It originated in a large shipment of infected parrots exported from Argentina.[12] From 1985 to 1995 there were 1132 cases of psittacosis reported to the Centers for Disease Control and Prevention.

Chlamydia psittaci has been isolated from approximately 100 bird species; it is most often found in psittacine birds, especially parrots, macaws, cockatiels, and parakeets. Pigeons, chickens, and turkeys have also been implicated as reservoirs. Transmission generally occurs as a result of inhalation of the organism, which has been aerosolized from feces or respiratory secretions of infected birds.[13] Humans have been infected after feeding and kissing infected sick or healthy-appearing birds, as well as after mouth-to-beak contact and handling of infected birds' plumage and tissues.[13] Infected mammals, including cattle, sheep, and goats, may also transmit organisms during parturition. Person-to-person transmission has not been proven. The incubation period is approximately 1 to 2 weeks.[12]

PATHOPHYSIOLOGY

After inhalation, the organism establishes infection in the epithelial cells of the respiratory tract. The organism spreads hematogenously to the liver and spleen, where replication occurs. Further hematogenous spread leads to invasion of the lungs and other organs. Noncaseating granulomas have been observed in the liver.[12]

CLINICAL MANIFESTATIONS

Clinical features range from an asymptomatic or mild influenza-like illness to systemic disease with severe pneumonia. Illness is generally of abrupt onset and is manifested by fever, headache, chills, myalgias, and a nonproductive cough. Relative bradycardia is a unique finding.[14] Splenomegaly may be seen in up to a third of patients.[12] A pink maculopapular rash, called Horder's spots, has been described.[14] Other organ involvement may manifest as endocarditis, myocarditis, hepatitis, arthritis, keratoconjunctivitis, and encephalitis. In the era before antibiotics became available, 15% to 20% of patients died.

The current mortality is less than 1% with appropriate treatment.

LABORATORY FINDINGS AND DIAGNOSIS

Diagnosis is usually serologic with documentation of a fourfold rise in complement fixation antibody titer between acute and convalescent specimens. In an appropriate setting, a single titer of 1:32 or greater is considered presumptive evidence of infection.[12] However, complement fixation tests do not distinguish between infections caused by the three *Chlamydia* species pathogenic in humans.[15] Microimmunofluorescence and PCR assays are more specific. The white blood cell count may be normal or mildly elevated. Mild anemia and elevated hepatic transaminases may be seen.

Chest radiographs are abnormal in about 75% of patients. Lower lobe consolidation is the most common finding.[14] Interstitial infiltrates and other patterns may be seen. The chest radiographic appearance is often worse than expected from the clinical examination.

TREATMENT

Tetracyclines are generally the treatment of choice. For children younger than 8 years of age, a macrolide (e.g., erythromycin, azithromycin) is recommended. Duration of therapy is 10 to 14 days following defervescence.[15] Remission of symptoms usually occurs within 48 to 72 hours.

PREVENTION

Individuals handling infected birds should wear protective clothing and respirator masks. Birds suspected of being infected should be examined and treated by a veterinarian. Deceased birds suspected of infection should be sealed in an impermeable container and transported to a veterinary laboratory for testing. Potentially contaminated cages should be disinfected. *Chlamydia psittaci* is susceptible to 70% alcohol, 1% Lysol, and a 1:100 dilution of household bleach.[13]

CHLAMYDIA PNEUMONIAE

In recent years, *C. pneumoniae* has been recognized as an increasingly common respiratory pathogen in both children and adults. Formerly known as the TWAR agent, *C. pneumoniae* was previously believed to be a strain of *C. psittaci*. As a result of improved diagnostic techniques and provider awareness, it has gained recognition as a distinct pathogen.

MICROBIOLOGY

Chlamydia pneumoniae is a genetically, morphologically, and antigenically distinct member of the genus *Chlamydia*. *Chlamydia pneumoniae* is an obligate intracellular pathogen with a cell wall similar to gram-negative bacteria. *Chlamydiae* spp. exhibit two forms: an intracellular dividing form (reticulate body) and an extracellular nondividing form (elementary body).[16]

EPIDEMIOLOGY

Chlamydia pneumoniae infection occurs worldwide. Initial infection peaks between the ages of 5 and 15 years of age in temperate developed regions, but earlier in tropical or less developed areas. There is no evidence of seasonality, although epidemics occur every 4 to 5 years. The infection is probably transmitted via respiratory secretions from person to person. No animal reservoir exists, although the organism has been isolated from several species. An estimated 2% to 5% of adults and children are asymptomatic nasopharyngeal carriers of *C. pneumoniae,* but it is unclear whether carriers are a reservoir of infection. Reinfection is common. Concurrent infection with *M. pneumoniae* or *Streptococcus pneumoniae* occurs frequently. The incubation period is 21 days.

PATHOLOGY

Following delivery to the respiratory mucosa, *C. pneumoniae* organisms are transported into the mucosal epithelial cells by endocytosis. *Chlamydiae* spp. prevent fusion of the phagosome with lysosomes, thus inhibiting their own death. Within the phagosome, the elementary bodies differentiate into reticulate bodies and undergo binary fission.[16] At 36 to 48 hours following inoculation, multiplication ceases and the reticulate bodies return to infectious elementary bodies. The contents of the phagosome are released by cytolysis, exocytosis, or extrusion of the entire inclusion.[16]

CLINICAL MANIFESTATIONS

Chlamydia pneumoniae infections often begin with a nonspecific prodrome of sore throat, malaise, headache, low-grade fever, and cough. The course is prolonged (2–6 weeks) and often biphasic. Patients may demonstrate upper respiratory tract infections such as pharyngitis, laryngitis, or sinusitis. A significant number will develop pneumonia or bronchitis. *Chlamydia pneumoniae* is a powerful inflammatory trigger and leads to an immunoglobulin E (IgE)–mediated bronchial reactivity.[17] Physical examination may reveal nonexudative pharyngitis, wheezes, and fine or coarse crackles.

The age of the patient often determines the severity of disease; adolescents more frequently develop lower respiratory tract infection.[18] Severe illness may affect previously healthy children and result in complications such as pneumatocele, pleural effusion, pneumothorax, interstitial fibrosis, or lung abscess. Other complications of *C. pneumoniae* infection include erythema nodosum, reactive arthritis, Guillain-Barrè syndrome, meningoencephalitis, myocarditis, and endocarditis. *Chlamydia pneumoniae* has also been isolated from middle ear fluid in children with acute otitis media, generally with other pathogens. Trials are currently under way to determine the relationship between *C. pneumoniae* infection and atherosclerotic heart disease.

Mortality is often associated with comorbid conditions or secondary infections.

LABORATORY FINDINGS AND DIAGNOSIS

Although quite ubiquitous, *C. pneumoniae* is diagnosed infrequently because of nonspecific radiographic and laboratory findings and a lack of reliable diagnostic tests. White blood cell counts are often normal or mildly elevated. Erythrocyte sedimentation rates are typically elevated. Chest radiography classically demonstrates a pattern of alveolar infiltrate or subsegmental pneumonitis without consolidation,[18,19] although it may also be normal. Pleural effusion is uncommon. Serologic testing is the primary diagnostic modality. Detection of antibody by microimmunofluorescence is the only currently acceptable test to diagnose an acute infection.[20] Newer Centers for Disease Control and Prevention criteria for serologic diagnosis require an IgM titer greater than 1:16 or a fourfold rise in the IgG titer.[16] Reliance on a single test for diagnosis is discouraged. *Chlamydia pneumoniae* may be cultured from the nasopharynx, sputum, or pleural fluid. Specimens must be placed in transport media, stored briefly at 4°C, and inoculated on cell-containing media. Identification of the bacteria by staining is difficult, since *C. pneumoniae*–specific reagent has limited availability.

PCR has not been standardized, nor has it been approved for commercial use.

TREATMENT

Few studies have investigated the response of *C. pneumoniae* infection to antimicrobial therapy. *Chlamydia pneumoniae* is susceptible to macrolides, tetracyclines, and quinolones; however, the latter two are not routinely recommended in children. For young children, a 14-day course of oral erythromycin is the treatment of choice. Acceptable alternatives include a 5-day course of oral azithromycin or a 10-day course of clarithromycin. Adolescent patients may be treated with a 5-day course of oral azithromycin, a 14- to 21-day course of oral doxycycline, or a 14- to 21-day course of oral tetracycline. Prolonged antimicrobial therapy (to 3 weeks) may be required. Parenteral therapy may be required for patients with severe disease.

PREVENTION

Chlamydia pneumoniae transmission may be decreased by avoidance of contact with persons with respiratory illness and their respiratory secretions. Antibiotics are not recommended either to eradicate carrier states or for postexposure prophylaxis. No vaccine exists for *C. pneumoniae* at this time.

MYCOPLASMA PNEUMONIAE

Mycoplasma were first identified in cattle over 100 years ago, and in 1937 they were identified in humans.[21] In 1944 Eaton recovered an organism from patients with atypical pneumonia.[2] Originally called the Eaton agent, it is now known as *M. pneumoniae.* Although 16 species of *Mycoplasma* are found in humans, only *M. pneumoniae, M. hominis*, and *Ureaplasma urealyticum* have been causally associated with disease in children.

MICROBIOLOGY

Mycoplasma pneumoniae are small, pleomorphic, cell wall–deficient organisms. They contain double-stranded DNA and grow in both anaerobic and aerobic environments. *Mycoplasma pneumoniae* grow relatively slowly; visible colony formation may take 3 weeks or longer.

EPIDEMIOLOGY

Infection occurs throughout the world and during all months of the year. Lower respiratory tract infection is more common beginning at school age (5 years). Although children younger than 1 year of age have demonstrable antibodies to *M. pneumoniae*, the rate of antibody positivity rises dramatically in children 5 to 15 years of age.[21] Under endemic conditions, the incidence of infection is about 4 per 1000 children per year.[22] In studies of children with community-acquired pneumonia, between 9% and 42% were due to *Mycoplasma*.[21] Reinfection may occur, although second episodes appear milder and reinfection is less common after pneumonia than after illness with milder symptoms; this has been attributed to rapidly falling antibody levels in patients who had mild disease.[22] *Mycoplasma pneumoniae* is transmitted by respiratory droplets during close contact.

The incubation period is 2 to 3 weeks.

PATHOPHYSIOLOGY

After respiratory secretions come in contact with the epithelial surface of the nasopharynx and perhaps the trachea and bronchi, the organisms attach to the host cell via neuraminic acid receptors. This attachment allows transport of a substance, perhaps hydrogen peroxide, involved in cell damage.[23] The manner in which infection extends throughout the respiratory tract is unknown. Additionally, it is unclear whether systemic symptoms are due to an immunologic response or direct spread of infection. Damage of the epithelial lining of the respiratory tract results in accumulation of debris and inflammatory exudates within the airway lumen.[23] Alveoli may also contain a similar exudate consisting of fibrin, mononuclear cells, and neutrophils.

CLINICAL MANIFESTATIONS

Approximately 20% of infections caused by *M. pneumoniae* are asymptomatic.[22] In symptomatic patients, the initial manifestation is usually pharyngitis followed by hoarseness. Cough subsequently develops that is generally constant and relatively nonproductive. Principi and colleagues studied children hospitalized for community-acquired lower respiratory tract infection due to mycoplasma.[24] Children were classified into three disease groups: acute bronchitis, wheezing, and pneumonia. In children with pneumonia, 60% had cough, 86% had fever, and 85% had crackles on chest examination.[24] Only 15% had evidence of rhinitis. Mean duration of illness in these children was 13 days, although cough has been reported to persist for 1 month or longer. More severe disease may be seen in normal children, as well as in certain high-risk groups (e.g., those with sickle cell anemia, immunodeficiency, and chronic cardiorespiratory disease). *Mycoplasma pneumoniae* has also been associated with several other disease processes including otitis media, sinusitis, mucocutaneous eruptions, myocarditis, pericarditis, hemolytic anemia, arthritis, glomerulonephritis, and nervous system disease (aseptic meningitis, encephalitis, cerebellar ataxia, transverse myelitis, peripheral neuropathy, psychosis, and Guillain-Barré syndrome).[21]

LABORATORY FINDINGS AND DIAGNOSIS

Diagnosis is generally confirmed by serology. IgM antibody appears 7 to 10 days after infection, and IgG appears about 3 weeks after infection.[22] The immunofluorescence antibody test and enzyme immunoassay detect *M. pneumoniae*–specific IgM and IgG antibodies. The presence of IgM antibodies confirms recent infection, although they may persist for several months. The complement fixation assay measures primarily IgM antibody; a fourfold or greater rise in titer between acute and convalescent specimens is considered positive.[22] False positives may occur as a result of cross-reactivity with other antigens, although these pathogens generally do not cause respiratory illness similar to that of *Mycoplasma*. Serum cold hemagglutinins may be present in about 50% of patients with pneumonia; however, other agents including adenovirus and Epstein-Barr virus may cause a positive test. PCR testing of nasopharyngeal or throat swab specimens has been utilized but is not universally available.

In a recent study of 68 children hospitalized with pneumonia due to mycoplasma, the most common radiographic finding was perihilar linear opacities seen in 60%; 40% had a reticulonodular infiltrate (Fig. 32-1), 28% had segmental or lobar consolidation, bilateral consolidation was found in 7%, and 6% had pleural effusions.[25] The authors concluded that the chest radiograph cannot be reliably used to predict mycoplasma infection. The white blood cell count, with an average of 13,000, was generally unremarkable.[25]

TREATMENT

The antimicrobials of choice for pneumonia caused by *M. pneumoniae* are the macrolides and the tetracyclines.[23] Because tetracycline has adverse effects on teeth, a macrolide (e.g., erythromycin, azithromycin) is the drug of choice in children. Therapy is administered for 10 days. Efficacy generally correlates with severity of illness and elapsed time before initiation of treatment. Treatment has not been adequately studied for the nonpulmonary manifestations of *M. pneumoniae* infection. Corticosteroids or intravenous immunoglobulin may be of benefit in patients with hemolytic anemia or encephalitis.[23]

PREVENTION

Vaccines have been developed with varying degrees of success. Jensen showed significant rises in antibody titers in 25 of 30 volunteers after vaccination.[26] However, more severe illness occurred in vaccinated subjects who did not have a significant immune response compared with the unvaccinated control group.[26] Since reinfection occurs commonly and sensitization may play a role in its pathogenesis, caution is indicated when promoting vaccines for *M. pneumoniae*. In certain circumstances (e.g., patients with sickle cell disease), prophylactic administration of antibiotics may be prudent.

INHALATIONAL ANTHRAX

Anthrax is a zoonotic disease that afflicts humans in causing three distinct disease patterns: dermatologic, gastrointestinal, and inhalational. The term *anthrax* is derived from the Greek word for coal (*anthrakos*) to depict the black eschar seen in cutaneous anthrax. Described in epidemics as woolsorter's disease, inhalational anthrax is extremely rare but often fatal. The potential of anthrax as a biological weapon was realized in 2001, when the distribution of the organism resulted in 22 human infections, of which 5 were fatal.[27]

MICROBIOLOGY

Bacillus anthracis is an aerobic, spore-forming, encapsulated, gram-positive, nonmotile bacillus. It grows optimally at 36°C, and colonies may appear 15 to 24 hours after the inoculation of sheep blood agar. Following incubation, the spores form chains of rods that resemble bamboo and then sporulate. *Bacillus anthracis* relies on three virulence factors: two exotoxins (lethal

FIGURE 32-1. Bilateral perihilar infiltrates, prominent on anteroposterior radiograph **(A)**, and reticulonodular infiltrates, prominent on lateral radiograph **(B)** of an adolescent with Mycoplasma pneumonia. (Courtesy of Rebecca Hulett, MD.)

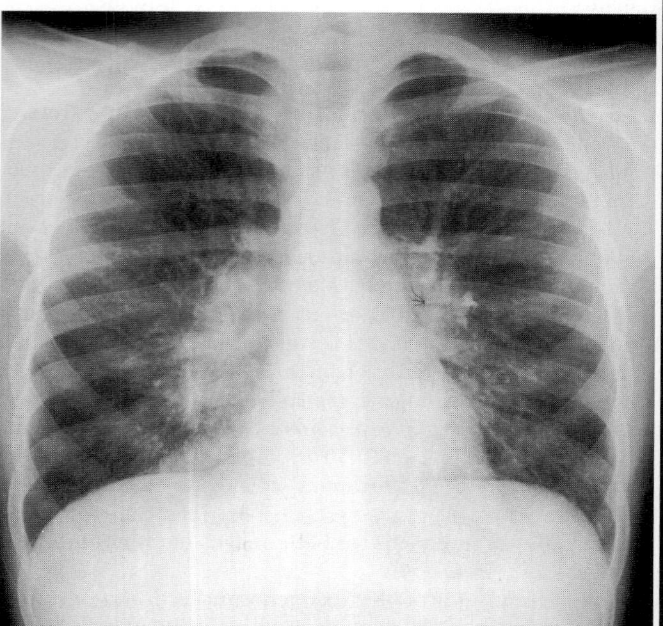

A

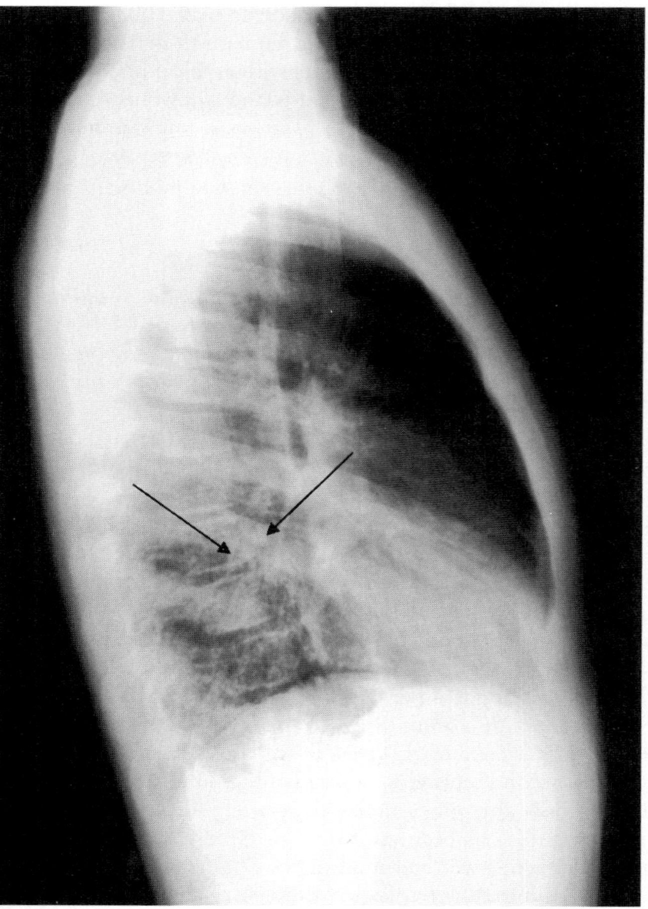

B

and edema toxins) and a specialized capsule. The capsule inhibits phagocytosis and the activation of neutrophils by lipopolysaccaride, to blunt the immune response. Lethal and edema toxins result in hemorrhage, edema, and necrosis.

EPIDEMIOLOGY

Bacillus anthracis and its extremely stable spores may be encountered worldwide. Anthrax is a zoonotic disease, infecting livestock subsequent to ingestion of spores. Humans are infected following contact with infected animals or contaminated animal products. Animal products that have been associated with infection apart from direct contact with the animal and/or carcass include hides, wool, hair, animal feeds, bone meal, and commercialized animal products. Rates of infection show neither seasonality nor gender preference. Cutaneous lesions are considered potentially infectious, but person-to-person transmission is rarely reported.

More than 95% of cases annually are primarily cutaneous in origin.[28] Gastrointestinal anthrax has occurred subsequent to the ingestion of raw or undercooked meat. Before 2001, inhalational anthrax was most recently reported in the United States following exposure to imported yarn.[28] In 2001, intentional contamination of the U.S. mail resulted in 11 cases of inhalational anthrax.[27]

The incubation period for anthrax is typically 1 to 7 days, but has been reported to be as long as several months for inhalational anthrax, because of spore dormancy and unpredictable clearance from the lungs.

PATHOLOGY

Following inhalation, spores are ingested by pulmonary macrophages and transported to hilar lymph nodes. Bacterial germination and toxin production occur in mediastinal lymph nodes. *Bacillus anthracis* infection results in lymphatic dilatation, interstitial edema, and necrosis that causes local hemorrhage. Hemorrhagic lymphadenitis, mediastinitis, and ultimately septicemia result.

Mechanisms of immunity are unclear. Humoral immunity against the toxin complex may play a role.

CLINICAL MANIFESTATIONS

The cutaneous form of *B. anthracis* infection is characterized by painless eschar formation and surrounding edema at the site of inoculation of abraded skin and a rarely fatal course. Gastrointestinal anthrax may affect the oropharynx or the intestinal tract. While gastrointestinal anthrax is associated with significant morbidity and mortality, inhalation anthrax is the most severe form of infection.

The disease begins with nonspecific symptomatology such as fever, myalgia, headache, cough, and abdominal and chest pain. Rhinorrhea is uncommon. The second phase of illness (second to fifth day) ensues rapidly with severe respiratory distress. The course is often marked by hemorrhagic mediastinitis, hemorrhagic pleural effusion, and bacteremia leading to dyspnea, hypoxemia, cyanosis, and shock. Inhalational anthrax is usually fatal within 24 hours.

The mortality of inhalational anthrax was previously estimated to be greater than 95%. In the most recent series, a 50% mortality rate was observed.[27]

Anthrax meningitis is a rarely reported complication of all forms of anthrax and follows dissemination of the organism via hematogenous or lymphatic routes. It is usually rapidly fatal.[29]

LABORATORY FINDINGS AND DIAGNOSIS

Chest radiography may reveal a widened mediastinum or prominent lymphadenopathy. Pulmonary hemorrhage and pleural effusions are frequently seen. Pulmonary infiltrates may be seen but should raise suspicion of superinfection. Computed tomography of the chest should be obtained in patients highly suspect for this infection to carefully evaluate the mediastinum and determine the presence of pleural fluid.

Identification of gram-positive bacilli on blood smear, in pleural fluid, in cerebrospinal fluid, or on skin biopsy suggests the diagnosis of anthrax. The infection may be confirmed by culture of the infected fluid or tissue and by serology. A single antibody titer measured by enzyme-linked immunosorbent assay greater than 1:32 or a fourfold rise in titer is diagnostic. PCR, immunofluorescence, and immunohistochemical assays are performed at the Centers for Disease Control and Prevention.

TREATMENT

Current regimens for treatment of inhalational anthrax are based on limited clinical experience; no controlled trial has been performed in humans. Though never routinely used in children, ciprofloxacin and doxycycline are considered the antimicrobials of choice as a component of a multidrug regimen for the treatment of inhalational anthrax in children. The risk-to-benefit ratio must be considered when treating with ciprofloxacin, since its use in children is restricted. One or two additional agents are also recommended for the treatment of inhalational anthrax; rifampin, ampicillin or penicillin, vancomycin, clindamycin, imipenem, chloramphenicol, and clarithromycin are reasonable additional agents.[30,31] Though active against *B. anthracis*, penicillin-resistant strains have been identified, and therefore penicillin should never be used as single-agent therapy. Clindamycin, an inhibitor of protein synthesis, is often utilized, because it disrupts both production and release of toxin by infected cells. Parenteral therapy for a recommended minimum of 14 days is given until the patient has improved; the recommended duration of therapy is 60 days. Corticosteroids have been suggested as adjunctive therapy for complications of inhalational anthrax such as severe edema, respiratory compromise, or meningitis. Cephalosporins and trimethoprim-sulfamethoxazole have no role in the treatment or prevention of anthrax.

PREVENTION

Ciprofloxacin and doxycycline are also recommended as initial postexposure antimicrobials of choice.[31] Once proven susceptible, amoxicillin can be used as a substitute for children. Antibiotic prophylaxis should begin as soon as possible and continue for 60 days, followed by careful observation. Some authorities recommend a 100-day course of prophylactic antimicrobials based on prolonged persistence of the organism in the experimental animal model.[32] Anthrax vaccine is available and is administered to military personnel. However, it is not approved for use in children. Livestock in enzootic areas may

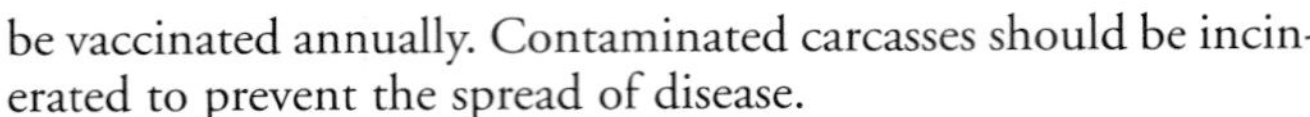

be vaccinated annually. Contaminated carcasses should be incinerated to prevent the spread of disease.

TULAREMIA

McCoy first identified tularemia in 1911 in Tulare County, California, as an illness that resembled bubonic plague in ground squirrels.[33] Originally, the causative agent was named *Bacterium tularense* for its site of discovery. Edward Francis, a public health surgeon, identified several infections with *B. tularense* in humans and confirmed the deer fly as a vector for the disease. Following his many contributions to the study of tularemia and a nomination for a Nobel Prize, Francis was honored when the genus name for the causative organism was changed to *Francisella*.[34]

MICROBIOLOGY

Francisella species are classified as aerobic, pleomorphic, gram-negative coccobacilli. *Francisella tularensis* is small, nonmotile, and does not produce any exotoxin; however, the bacterium has a nearly transparent cell wall and may contain endotoxin similar to other gram-negative bacilli. *Francisella tularensis* does not produce spores, yet it is resistant to freezing; the organism is readily killed by heat. Although it can be isolated on routine cultures, its growth is enhanced in a glucose-cysteine-enriched blood agar. There are two distinct groups of *F. tularensis*. Jellison type A (*F. tularensis* biovar *tularensis*) denotes those strains that are highly virulent for humans and account for 90% of *F. tularensis* isolated in the United States. Jellison type B (*F. tularensis* biovar *palaeantarctica*) is a group of less virulent strains found throughout Asia and Europe.[34]

EPIDEMIOLOGY

Francisella tularensis is ubiquitous in northern latitudes. It has been isolated from contaminated soil and water, infected ticks, and over 200 species of animals. Although tularemia occurs throughout the year, it peaks during the winter months (hunting season) in the northern and eastern United States and during the summer months (tick season) in the southern and more central states. From 1990 to 2000, a total of 1368 cases of tularemia were reported in the United States (only 59% were confirmed). Four states accounted for 56% of all reported tularemia cases: Arkansas (23%), Missouri (19%), South Dakota (7%), and Oklahoma (7%).[35] The incidence of tularemia was reported highest among males aged 5 to 9 years and older than 75 years.[35] It occurred more frequently in American Indians and Alaskan Natives (0.5 per 100,000) than in Caucasians (0.04 per 100,000) or African Americans and Asians/Pacific Islanders (0.01 or less).[35]

Contact with infected animals (or their carcasses) and bites by deer flies or ticks are the most common means of human infection. The organism infects various species of animals naturally, yet fewer than a dozen species have been known to transmit the infection. Rodents (e.g., squirrels) and classically, lagomorphs (rabbits and hares) transmit the infection, as well as sheep. Transmission of tularemia via cat bite has been reported, and it has been postulated that this may be an important source of infection in children. Ticks are the most common vectors, primarily *Dermacentor andersoni* (wood tick), *Dermacentor variabilis* (dog tick), and *Ambylomma americanum* (lone star tick). Deer flies more likely propagate disease among susceptible animals than among humans. Less commonly, humans are infected by the bite of an infected animal, via water, or by aerosolization. Person-to-person transmission has not been reported, since humans are considered the organism's terminal host.[34] The incubation period ranges from 1 to 21 days but is typically 3 to 5 days.

PATHOLOGY

Francisella tularensis may enter the body via the skin, mucous membranes, or respiratory or gastrointestinal tracts, but it typically infects the skin, lymph nodes, lungs, liver, and spleen. The bacterium spreads quickly to regional lymph nodes, causing a pattern of cellular changes characteristic of intracellular parasites. Organisms are rarely identified from lesions, which often demonstrate necrosis or granuloma formation. *Francisella tularensis* may also spread hematogenously, usually within the first week of infection. Reticuloendothelial hyperplasia is frequently observed. Although neutrophils are critical for the initial clearance of organisms, it is the T cell–mediated immune response, however, that is undoubtedly responsible for protective immunity. Reinfection is rare.

CLINICAL MANIFESTATIONS

Tularemia presents acutely with fever (typically higher than 103°F or 39.4°C), chills, myalgias, vomiting, and headache. Relative bradycardia is frequently described.[33] Physical findings often include lymphadenopathy, skin lesions or rashes, hepatosplenomegaly, and pharyngitis. Subcutaneous nodules may also be noted. Untreated tularemia may cause persistent fevers. The six clinical syndromes of tularemia are named to denote the site of organism entry: ulceroglandular, glandular, oculoglandular, oropharyngeal, typhoidal, and pneumonic.

Pneumonic tularemia is the most severe and lethal form of tularemia.[34] Although the disease is traditionally believed to be more common in adults, there have been an increasing number of reports in children. The primary form of the syndrome is acquired by inhalation. A secondary form of pneumonic tularemia may result from typhoidal tularemia. Signs and symptoms of pneumonic tularemia include sore throat, cough, dyspnea, chest pain, or pleuritic pain. Occasionally, a pleural effusion is present. These signs and symptoms of pneumonic tularemia are nonspecific and may be delayed. Thus, this disease is often confused with bronchiolitis, pneumonitis, or pharyngitis. Pneumonic tularemia is rare; a widespread outbreak should prompt concern for a bioterrorism event.[36]

LABORATORY FINDINGS AND DIAGNOSIS

The diagnosis of tularemia is confirmed by serologic testing. A single or initial titer of agglutinating antibody equal to or greater than 1:160 (by tube agglutination) or greater than 1:128 (by microagglutination) supports a presumptive diagnosis, and a fourfold increase in the titer 14 days later (minimum) confirms the diagnosis. An enzyme-linked immunosorbent assay exists that detects IgM, IgG, and IgA antibodies to *F. tularensis*.[34] Identification of the organisms in exudates and tissues may be accomplished by indirect fluorescent antibody or PCR assays. Immunoblotting and antigen detection assays are not commercially available. Routine cultures of sputum or exudates must be directed to the appropriate laboratory facility to ensure proper handling and safety of laboratory personnel.

The peripheral white blood cell count can range from 3000 to 15,000. Atypical lymphocytosis as well as sterile pyuria have also been reported. Nearly half of patients have elevated transaminase levels.

With pulmonic involvement, radiographic data may be difficult to interpret. Although a radiographic triad of findings (ovoid opacities, pleural effusion, and hilar adenopathy) associated with tularemic pneumonia has been well described, it is nonspecific. Radiographs of tularemia pneumonia in children may resemble community-acquired pneumonia, viral pneumonia, tuberculosis, fungal pneumonia, pneumonitis, and other atypical bacterial infections. In adults lymphoma and carcinoma may also be diagnostic considerations.

TREATMENT

Aminoglycosides are the preferred antimicrobials for treatment of tularemia. Although streptomycin was the classic therapeutic choice, it has been superseded by gentamicin. Resolution of signs and symptoms of infection is prompt and usually occurs within days. The duration of therapy is 7 to 10 days but may be extended in severe or complicated disease.

The tetracyclines and chloramphenicol (bacteriostatic agents) have also been used to treat tularemia. However, these antimicrobials are not as effective as streptomycin or gentamicin and are associated with a high relapse rate. Fluoroquinolones have demonstrated clinical efficacy, but their use in children is restricted. Beta-lactams are not effective.

Surgical intervention may be required for suppurative lesions.

PREVENTION

Tularemia may be avoided by eliminating exposure to infected animals and the vectors of disease. Deceased rodents and lagomorphs should be incinerated or buried. Children should be instructed not to handle sick or dead rodents and lagomorphs. Rubber gloves should be worn while preparing game animals, and the meat should be thoroughly cooked. Children and adults in endemic areas should wear protective clothing and consider the use of tick repellent (caution in young children because of possible toxicity). Following outdoor activities, inspection for ticks is mandatory, as is their careful removal.

A live vaccine, developed in 1960, remains unlicensed in the United States and for investigational use only. It has been successful in reducing the severity and incidence of tularemia in laboratory personnel, but its effect on naturally occurring disease is unknown. Doxycycline and fluoroquinolones have been utilized for postexposure prophylaxis.

Q FEVER

Q fever was first reported by E.H. Derrick in 1937 following investigation of a febrile illness in abattoir workers in Brisbane, Australia. He noted that the illness lasted 7 to 24 days and was characterized by fever, headache, malaise, anorexia, and myalgias. He named it Q (for query) fever, since the cause was then unknown.[37]

MICROBIOLOGY

The etiologic agent is *Coxiella burnetii*, a pleomorphic coccobacillus with a membrane similar to that of gram-negative bacteria. *C. burnetii* is an obligate intracellular microorganism.

EPIDEMIOLOGY

Q fever is a zoonosis with a worldwide distribution. In France, the annual incidence of acute Q fever has been estimated at 50 cases per 100,000 individuals. Limited seroepidemiologic data in children show that the highest prevalence rates are in The Netherlands, where 37% of boys and 70% of girls showed evidence of previous infection with *C. burnetii*.[38]

Cattle, sheep, and goats are the primary reservoirs, although pets including cats and dogs are also a source of infection. Tick vectors may be important in maintaining animal reservoirs but are not felt to be responsible for human disease. Humans are infected mainly via inhalation of contaminated aerosols as well as from contact with body fluids of infected livestock. Infection has been reported from consumption of raw milk, transplacental transmission, and blood transfusions.[38]

The incubation period is generally between 1 and 3 weeks. Humans are the only hosts known to develop disease from this infection.

PATHOPHYSIOLOGY

After inhalation, *C. burnetii* enters the host cell by phagocytosis. After fusion with the lysosome, the acidic pH activates organism enzymes allowing for replication within the phagolysosome. *Coxiella burnetii* undergoes sporogenesis, which allows it to survive for extended periods in the external environment.[33] It also undergoes a type of antigenic variation called phase variation, in which there is variable presentation of the lipopolysaccharide; anti–phase II antibodies are present primarily in early disease, and anti–phase I antibodies are present in chronic disease.

Liver biopsy in patients with hepatitis show characteristic doughnut-like granulomas due to the presence of a lipid-like vacuole that is surrounded by a fibrinoid ring.[33]

CLINICAL MANIFESTATIONS

Infected patients are asymptomatic in as many as half of cases, perhaps more in children. During an outbreak in Switzerland, 70 of 80 infected children were asymptomatic, as opposed to 121 of 335 adults.[38]

Q fever is clinically divided into two forms. Acute Q fever lasts less than 6 months; chronic Q fever lasts longer than 6 months. The most frequent presentation of acute Q fever in adults is a flulike illness. Pediatric illness is less well characterized. Most children appear to present with fever of unknown origin or pneumonia. Other manifestations in children include a flulike illness, myocarditis, central nervous system infection, pericarditis, and rhabdomyolysis.[38] In a series of 13 children hospitalized in Spain with Q fever, the predominant symptoms were fever lasting 5 to 10 days, headache, and abdominal pain with vomiting. A mild cough was present in about half of patients. All children completely recovered without specific therapy.[39]

Marrie recently reviewed *C. burnetii* pneumonia.[37] Between 82% and 100% of patients had fever. Headache is more common in patients with pneumonia from Q fever than from other etiologies. Cough, usually nonproductive, is found in 60% to 70% of patients. Other symptoms include anorexia, chills, myalgias, and arthralgias. Interestingly, only about one half of patients with Q fever pneumonia have clinical findings suggestive of pneumonia. Illness is generally mild and can last 10 days to 3 months.

Chronic Q fever occurs less commonly. In children, endocarditis and osteomyelitis are the primary clinical manifestations.

LABORATORY FINDINGS AND DIAGNOSIS

The diagnosis rests on serologic confirmation. The indirect immunofluorescence antibody test is most often used. Seroconversion usually is detected within 1 to 2 weeks after onset of disease. Antibody titers greater than 1:200 for anti–phase II IgG or greater than 1:50 for anti–phase II IgM suggest acute infection.[33] A fourfold rise in titers between acute and convalescent samples is diagnostic. Other serologic techniques include complement fixation and enzyme-linked immunoassay. Shell vial culture, immunohistochemistry, and PCR have also been utilized.

Laboratory findings are nonspecific. The white blood cell count is usually normal. Thrombocytopenia may be present initially in 10% of patients, with thrombocytosis occurring during the recovery phase.[37] Hepatic transaminases may be mildly elevated. Microscopic hematuria is present in about 50% of patients with Q fever pneumonia. A variety of autoantibodies have been described, including antibodies to mitochondria, to cardiolipin, and to smooth muscle.[33]

Chest radiographs are variable. Lower lobe involvement is the primary feature. One or several rounded opacities, segmental consolidation, and pleural effusions may be present.[37]

TREATMENT

The treatment of choice for Q fever pneumonia is doxycycline for 10 to 14 days; however, clinical studies, especially in children, are lacking.[37] A randomized study by Raoul found tetracyclines to be beneficial; however, adverse effects may limit their use in children.[33] Similar concerns arise with the use of fluoroquinolones. In a retrospective study of adult patients the mean time to defervescence was 2.9 days with doxycycline, 3.3 days with clarithromycin, 3.9 days with erythromycin, and 6.4 days with beta-lactams.[37] The authors conclude that macrolides may be adequate empiric therapy.

PREVENTION

In the United States, outbreaks have occurred mainly from occupational exposures. A vaccine has been developed and successfully protected at risk individuals in Australia; however, it is not currently available in the United States. Strict adherence to proper hygiene, especially when handling parturient farm animals, is recommended. Ensuring holding facilities for farm animals away from populated areas and proper disposal of birth products should decrease risk of infection.

REFERENCES

1. Reiman HA: An acute infection of the respiratory tract with atypical pneumonia. A disease entity probably caused by a filterable virus. JAMA 1938; 111:2377–2384.
2. Eaton MD, Meiklejohn G, Van Herick W: Studies on the etiology of primary atypical pneumonia. A filterable agent transmissible to cotton rats, hamsters, and chick embryos. J Exp Med 1944;79:649–668.
3. Graziano K, Tempest B: Hantavirus pulmonary syndrome. A zebra worth knowing. Am Fam Physician 2002;66:1015–1020.
4. Mills J, Corneli A, Young JC, et al: Hantavirus pulmonary syndrome—United States. Updated recommendations for risk reduction. MMWR Morbid Mortal Wkly Rep 2002;51(No. RR-9):1–10.
5. Case Information: Hantavirus Pulmonary Syndrome Case Count and Descriptive Statistics. Available at http://www.cdc.gov/ncidod/diseases/hanta/hps/noframes/caseinfo.htm.
6. Peters CJ, Khan A: Hantavirus pulmonary syndrome. The new American hemorrhagic fever. Clin Infect Dis 2002;34:1224–1231.
7. Zaki S, Greer PW, Coffield LM, et al: Hantavirus pulmonary syndrome. Pathogenesis of an emerging infectious disease. Am J Pathol 1995;146: 552–579.
8. Murdoch DR: Diagnosis of *Legionella* infection. Clin Infect Dis 2003; 36:64–69.
9. Stout JE, Yu VL: Legionellosis. N Engl J Med 1997;337:682–687.
10. Edelstein PH: Legionnaires' disease, Pontiac fever, and related illnesses. In: Feigen RD, Cherry JD, Demmler GJ, Kaplan SL, eds: Textbook of Pediatric Infectious Diseases. Philadelphia: WB Saunders, 2004, pp 1676–1687.
11. Harris R, Williams T: "Contribution to the question of *Pneumotyphus*." A discussion of the original article by J. Ritter in 1880. Rev Infect Dis 1985; 7:119–122.
12. Gregory D, Schaffner W: Psittacosis. Semin Respir Infect 1997;102:181–194.
13. Centers for Disease Control and Prevention: Compendium of measures to control *Chlamydia psittaci* infection among humans and pet birds. MMWR Morbid Mortal Wkly Rep 2000;49(RR-8):3–17.
14. Kirchner J: Psittacosis. Postgrad Med J 1997;102:181–194.
15. American Academy of Pediatrics: *Chlamydia (Chlamydophila) psittaci*. In: Pickering LK, ed: Red Book 2003 Report of the Committee on Infectious Diseases, 26th ed. Elk Grove Village, Ill: American Academy of Pediatrics, 2003, pp 237–238.
16. Hammerschlag MR: The intracellular life of *Chlamydia*. Semin Pediatr Infect 2002;13:239–248.
17. Hammerschlag MR: *Chlamydia* infections. In: Feigen RD, Cherry JD, Demmler GJ, Kaplan SL, eds: Textbook of Pediatric Infectious Diseases. Philadelphia: WB Saunders, 2004, pp 2482–2496.
18. Grayston JT: *Chlamydia pneumoniae* (TWAR) infections in children. Pediatr Infect Dis J 1994;13:675–685.
19. Kauppinen M, Saikku P: Pneumonia due to *Chlamydia pneumoniae*. Prevalence, clinical features, diagnosis, and treatment. Clin Infect Dis 1995; 21:S244–S252.
20. American Academy of Pediatrics: In: *Chlamydia (Chlamydophila) pneumoniae*. In: Pickering LK, ed: Red Book 2003 Report of the Committee on Infectious Diseases, 26th ed. Elk Grove Village, Ill: American Academy of Pediatrics, 2003, pp 235–237.
21. Nelson C: *Mycoplasma* and *Chlamydia* pneumonia in pediatrics. Semin Respir Infect 2002;17:10–14.
22. Ferwerda A, Moll H, de Groot R: Respiratory tract infections by *Mycoplasma pneumoniae* in children. A review of diagnostic and therapeutic measures. Eur J Pediatr 2001;160:483–491.
23. Cherry J, Ching N: *Mycoplasma* and *Ureaplasma* infections. In: Feigen RD, Cherry JD, Demmler GJ, Kaplan SL, eds: Textbook of Pediatric Infectious Diseases. Philadelphia: WB Saunders, 2004, pp 2516–2547.
24. Principi N, Esposito S, Blasi F, Allegra L: Role of *Mycoplasma pneumoniae* and *Chlamydia pneumoniae* in children with community acquired lower respiratory tract infections. Clin Infect Dis 2001;32:1281–1289.
25. Esposito J, Blasi F, Bellini F, Allegra L, Principi N: *Mycoplasma pneumoniae* and *Chlamydia pneumoniae* infections in children with pneumonia. Eur Respir J 2001;17:241–245.
26. Jensen KE, Senterfit LB, Chanock RM: An inactivated *Mycoplasma pneumoniae* vaccine. JAMA 1965;194:248–252.
27. Inglesby TV, Otoole T, Henderson DA, et al: Anthrax as a biological weapon, 2002-updated recommendations for management. JAMA 2002;287:2236–2252.
28. American Academy of Pediatrics: Anthrax. In: Pickering LK, ed: Red Book 2003 Report of the Committee on Infectious Diseases, 26th ed. Elk Grove Village, Ill: American Academy of Pediatrics, 2003, pp 196–199.
29. Dixon TC, Meselson M, Guillemin J, et al: Anthrax. N Engl J Med 1999;341:815–826.
30. Centers for Disease Control and Prevention: Update investigation of bioterrorism-related anthrax and interim guidelines for exposure management and antimicrobial therapy. MMWR Morbid Mortal Wkly Rep 2001;50:909–919.

31. Centers for Disease Control and Prevention: Interim recommendations for antimicrobial prophylaxis for children and breastfeeding mothers and treatment of children with anthrax. MMWR Morbid Mortal Wkly Rep 2001;50:1014–1016.
32. Bartlett JG, Inglesby TV, Borio L: Management of anthrax. Clin Infect Dis 2002;35:851–858.
33. Choi E: Tularemia and Q fever. Med Clin North Am 2002;86:393–417.
34. Feigin RD, Lau CC: Tularemia. In: Feigen RD, Cherry JD, Demmler GJ, Kaplan SL, eds: Textbook of Pediatric Infectious Diseases. Philadelphia: WB Saunders, 2004, pp 1628–1634.
35. Centers for Disease Control and Prevention: Update on emerging infections. Tularemia-United States, 1990–2000. MMWR Morbid Mortal Wkly Rep 2002;51:181–184.
36. Dennis D, Inglesby TV, Henderson DA, et al: Tularemia as a biological weapon. JAMA 2001;285:2763–2773.
37. Marrie TJ: *Coxiella burnetti* pneumonia. Eur Respir J 2003;21:713–719.
38. Maltezou H, Raoult D: Q Fever in children. Lancet Infect Dis 2002;2:686–691.
39. Ruiz-Contreras J, Montero R, Amador J, Corradi E, Vera A: Q Fever in children. Am J Dis Child 1993;147:300–302.

33 Pediatric Severe Acute Respiratory Syndrome

Albert Martin Li, MBBch • Ellis K.L. Hon, MBBS

Although severe acute respiratory syndrome (SARS) has wreaked havoc in Southeast Asia and other parts of the world, it appears to be a disease that predominantly affects adults. Less than 10% of the infected population were children. Among these infected children, only 5% required intensive care unit admission, and less than 1% required mechanical ventilation. In contrast to its adult counterpart, the clinical course of affected children is usually milder, the time to resolution is shorter, and the potential of children to infect others is low.

These very different features in children have led some to create the acronym "MARS" (mild acute respiratory syndrome). This chapter will discuss the clinical features, radiologic presentation, management, and outcome of children suffering from SARS based on our institutional experience.

■ EPIDEMIOLOGY

Severe acute respiratory syndrome was brought to Hong Kong on 21 February 2003 by an infected medical doctor from Guangdong, China, who stayed in a local hotel. It has been estimated that at least 12 guests and visitors to this hotel became infected through contact with this medical doctor directly or indirectly. The disease then spread from Hong Kong rapidly to Hanoi, Singapore, and Toronto when infected visitors and guests returned to their home countries. One of the infected visitors, the index case of Hong Kong's first outbreak, was admitted to the Prince of Wales Hospital in early March with pneumonia, and he subsequently infected 138 hospital staff, patients, and visitors.[1] The use of nebulized medications in the index case is believed to have caused this very extensive hospital outbreak, since nebulization could have generated a large amount of infective droplets. The first few pediatric cases were household contacts of the initial cohort of adult patients from the hospital outbreak. At that time, SARS had not yet been recognized as a highly infectious disease. The disease involving health care workers spread rapidly to the community by visitors to the hospital wards.

Most, if not all, children with SARS have either been in close contact with infected adults, as a household contact or in a health care setting. These are believed to be the important routes of transmission that put children at a particular risk. Surprisingly, in Hong Kong there has been no major spread of the disease among classmates in schools. This may partly be explained by the early strict hygiene precautions undertaken by schools following a large-scale educational program conducted by the local government.

■ VIROLOGY

Severe acute respiratory syndrome is now known to be caused by a novel coronavirus (SARS-CoV), and over 95% of well-characterized cohorts of SARS patients have evidence of recent SARS-CoV infection.[2–6] Coinfection with human metapneumovirus or other pathogens was also documented in a proportion of patients. Whether such coinfections contribute to enhancing the pathogenesis or transmission of the disease is still unclear.[7–9]

The genome of SARS-CoV indicates that it is a novel virus within the family of Coronaviridae, a group of enveloped positive-sense RNA viruses.[10] It is not related to any of the human or animal coronaviruses known to date. Viruses closely related to SARS-CoV have recently been isolated from animals such as civet cats.[11] It is postulated that SARS-CoV was an animal virus that had overcome the species barrier and adapted to human-to-human transmission. The presence of this animal reservoir may imply possible future animal-to-human transmission and the initiation of further disease outbreaks.

■ CLINICAL AND LABORATORY FEATURES

The incubation period of SARS is between 2 and 10 days, and the mean has been estimated to be 6.4 days (95% confidence interval, 5.2–7.7), with the mean time from onset of clinical symptoms to hospital admission between 3 and 5 days.[12] The frequency of common presenting symptoms from several pediatric series is summarized in Table 33-1.[13–15] The predominant and most consistent symptom is fever, which is present in most of the patients (>90%) so far diagnosed to have SARS. Other symptoms include coryza and cough. Chills, rigor, myalgia, and malaise, which are common in adult patients, may also be present in older children and adolescents, but are rare in young children. Some patients, adults and children alike, may present with diarrhea. Young children appear to have milder disease with shorter time period to resolution, while the course of disease in older children is more similar to that of the adults. It is unclear why children, especially those under the age of 12 years, would be less severely affected, but it might be because they have been exposed to many other respiratory viruses, which could make their immune systems more resilient. Others have proposed that young children are not able to mount a "heightened" mature immune response as seen in adult patients during the immune dysregulation phase of SARS and thus suffer less organ damage with its associated morbidity and mortality. Besides, children in general present with fewer comorbidities than adults. Physical examination is normal in most if not all young children, whereas inspiratory crackles over the lung bases are present in some adolescent and adult patients.

Laboratory features from the three published pediatric series of SARS are summarized in Table 33-2.[13–15] Lymphopenia is quite consistently present in children affected with SARS. There may also be thrombocytopenia, a moderately deranged clotting profile, as well as elevated concentrations of liver enzymes, lactate dehydrogenase, and creatinine kinase. These laboratory parameters, together with the presenting clinical features, may help in the clinical diagnosis of the disease. We have also studied

■ **TABLE 33-1.** Presenting clinical features (%) among pediatric series of severe acute respiratory syndrome

	Hon and Co-workers[13] (*N* = 10)	Chiu and Co-workers[15] (*N* = 21)	Bitnun and Co-workers[14] (*N* = 10)
Fever	100	91	100
Malaise	20	62	10
Chills or rigor	50	48	10
Myalgia	40	10	NR
Cough	80	43	60
Dyspnea	NR	14	10
Headache	40	14	10
Dizziness	10	38	NR
Sputum production	NR	14	NR
Sore throat	30	5	10
Coryza	60	33	40
Anorexia	NR	57	NR
Nausea and vomiting	20	NR	20
Diarrhea	NR	10	10
Chest pain	NR	NR	NR
Abdominal pain	10	NR	NR
Febrile convulsion	10	NR	NR
Rash	NR	5	NR

NR, not recorded.

■ **TABLE 33-2.** Abnormal laboratory findings (%) among pediatric series of severe acute respiratory syndrome

	Hon and Co-workers[13] (*N* = 10)	Chiu and Co-workers[15] (*N* = 21)	Bitnun and Co-workers[14] (*N* = 10)
Lymphopenia	100	91	40
Neutropenia	NR	NR	30
Thrombocytopenia	50	48	10
Leukopenia	70	24	20
High lactate dehydrogenase	NR	71	20
High creatinine kinase	10	43	10
High alanine transminases	50	24	20
High D-dimer	NR	14	NR
Prolonged activated partial thromboplastin time	NR	29	NR

NR, not recorded.

the inflammatory cytokine profile in SARS patients. They have markedly raised concentrations of circulating interleukin-1β, which may suggest the selective activation of the caspase-1-dependent pathway. Other key proinflammatory cytokines (interleukin-6 and tumor necrosis factor-α) were only mildly elevated; this is in sharp contrast to H5N1 influenza infection, in which these cytokines are significantly elevated.[16]

■ RADIOLOGIC FEATURES

The radiologic appearances of SARS are nonspecific, and differentiation from other commonly encountered childhood respiratory illnesses causing airspace disease is difficult. Similarly to adults, children with early SARS may have a normal chest radiograph but changes of typical airspace consolidation in their computed tomography (CT) thorax. However, routine CT thorax should not be carried out because of the significant radiation; more importantly, this might lead to overdiagnosis, since other viral infections could give rise to similar radiologic changes.

Based on our institutional experience, (1) the primary radiographic finding in pediatric patients with SARS is airspace opacification, which can be unilateral focal (two thirds of cases) or unilateral multiple/bilateral (one third of cases), (2) younger children and those with mild disease usually present with unilateral focal consolidation, while multifocal and bilateral involvement tend to occur in older patients and those with more severe disease, and (3) there is a higher prevalence of involvement of the lower lung zone.

In our patients with SARS, the airspace opacification is the worst on day 5 to day 7 after the onset of fever. Unlike adults whose radiographic findings usually progress to multiple areas of involvement, the majority of our children only showed an increase in extent of airspace opacification in the same lung zone (Figs. 33-1 and 33-2). The mean duration of time taken for complete radiographic resolution is 16 days (range, 8–30 days). No definite scarring, volume loss, bronchial thickening, or bronchiectasis has been identified in the follow-up radiographs of our pediatric patients who have recovered from the illness. Again, the initial report from adults that pulmonary complications in the form of pulmonary fibrosis and bronchiectasis may be as high as 20% stands in contrast to this.[5]

Similar to the findings on plain radiography, most patients presenting with a milder form of the disease show focal segmental airspace disease on high-resolution CT. Ground-glass opacification and consolidation are the two predominant features on high-resolution CT. It is common to find a combination of both findings. There is, however, no specific preference of distribution of the disease in children; approximately equal involvement of subpleural and peribronchial regions has been observed. In patients with multifocal disease, a mosaic pattern of lung attenuation with ground-glass and airspace infiltrates is observed, simulating the appearance of bronchiolitis obliterans organizing pneumonia. Again, the aforementioned radiologic appearances are nonspecific. Both ground-glass opacity and consolidation attenuation are common findings in children suffering from pneumonia of any etiology.[17] Pulmonary nodules, septal thickening, and lymphadenopathy are not features of SARS.

Babyn and colleagues[18] reviewed chest radiographs and thoracic CTs of 62 pediatric cases of SARS (25 suspect and 37 probable) and found that 35.5% of the patients had a normal chest radiograph. The most prominent radiologic findings observed were areas of consolidation (45.2%), often peripheral with multifocal lesions present in only 22.6% of the cases. Peribronchial thickening was noted on chest radiographs of 14.5% of patients. Pleural effusion was seen in one case, aged 17 years and 11.5 months. Interstitial disease was not observed in any patient.

■ DIAGNOSIS

Since the presentation is nonspecific and often indistinguishable from other childhood infections, the diagnosis is often difficult unless there is clear contact history with an infected patient. The U.S. Centers for Disease Control and World Health

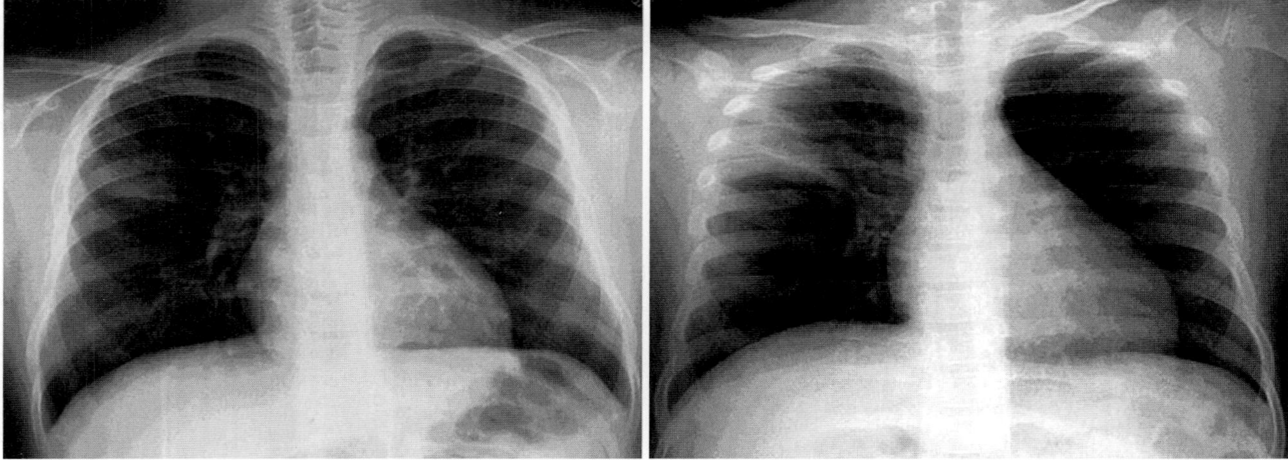

■ **FIGURE 33-1.** Radiologic progression over 3 days of focal consolidation affecting the right upper zone in a 13-year-old girl with SARS.

Organization have promulgated a case definition for SARS (Box 33-1). These definitions and criteria, while being applicable to both adults and children, are based mainly on adult experience.[19]

This case definition is useful in guiding clinicians in decision making regarding treatment. However, since the early symptoms of children affected with SARS are very much similar to those of other forms of upper or lower respiratory tract infections, the decision on admission, as to whether to isolate, and how to treat children presenting with fever but without a definite contact history remains difficult. Sometimes even the contact history might be misleading. In our hospital, we came across two children whose initial symptoms were suggestive of SARS and who had a definite history of contact with an affected individual, but who were later diagnosed to have bacterial septicemia.[20] The World Health Organization has subsequently revised the definition of a probable case to include a suspected case of SARS that is positive for SARS-CoV.

All suspected cases will be subjected to a battery of investigations: (1) Microbiologic studies to rule out common pathogens, including blood culture, nasopharyngeal aspirate for immunofluorescence and viral culture, and viral serology; (2) serial complete blood count and differential count; (3) serial liver and renal function tests, creatinine kinase and lactate dehydrogenase concentrations; (4) serial clotting profile including partial thromboplastin time, and D-dimer; and (5) serial chest radiograph. It is important to note that obtaining nasopharyngeal aspirate is an aerosol-generating procedure that may spread the virus. Staff performing the procedure should use adequate protection: mask, gloves, gown, and face shield.

The detection rates for SARS-CoV using reverse transcriptase–polymerase chain reaction are generally low in the first week of illness. The positivity rates on urine, nasopharyngeal aspirate, and stool samples have been reported to be 42%, 68%, and 97%, respectively, on day 14 of illness, and serology for confirmation may take up to 28 days for seroconversion.[5] Quantitative measurement of blood SARS-CoV RNA with real-time polymerase chain reaction technique has been developed with a detection rate of 87.5% to 100% within the first week

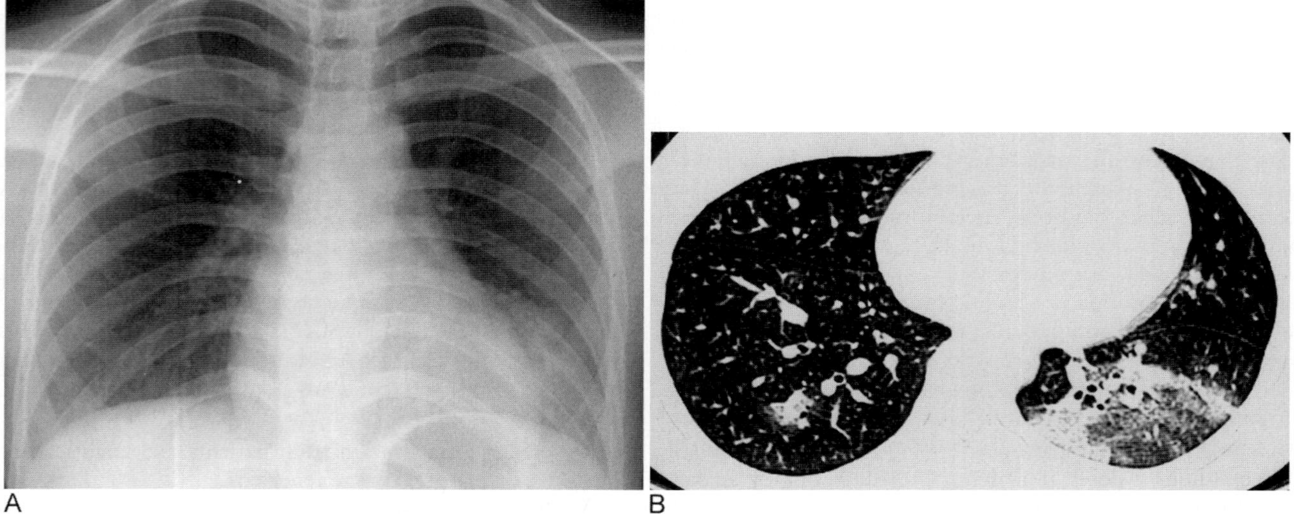

■ **FIGURE 33-2.** **A,** Chest radiograph of a 14-year-old girl presenting with fever and cough. There is ground-glass opacification in the left lower zone on admission. **B,** High-resolution CT of thorax on day 4 after onset of fever shows a combination of ground-glass opacification and consolidation in the left lower lobe.

BOX 33-1 Case Definition of Severe Acute Respiratory Syndrome

Suspect Case

1. A person presenting after 1 November 2002 with history of high fever (>38°C) and cough or breathing difficulty, and one or more of the following exposures during the 10 days before onset of symptoms:
   - Close contact with a person who is a suspect or probable case of SARS
   - History of travel to an area with recent local transmission of SARS
   - Residing in an area with recent local transmission of SARS
2. A person with an unexplained acute respiratory illness resulting in death after 1 November 2002, but on whom no autopsy has been performed, and one or more of the following exposures during the 10 days before onset of symptoms:
   - Close contact with a person who is a suspect or probable case of SARS
   - History of travel to an area with recent local transmission of SARS
   - Residing in an area with recent local transmission of SARS

Probable Case

1. A suspect case with radiographic evidence of infiltrates consistent with pneumonia or respiratory distress syndrome on chest radiograph
2. A suspect case of SARS that is positive for SARS coronavirus by one or more assays
3. A suspect case with autopsy findings consistent with the pathology of respiratory distress syndrome without an identifiable cause

after fever onset and then dropping to 62.5% at a mean of 14 days after fever onset.[21]

■ TREATMENT

The treatment of children with SARS is largely based on adult experience and has not been subject to controlled trials. The actual pathogenesis is poorly understood. SARS predominantly presents radiologically with ground-glass opacification and pathologically as revealed from autopsy results of fatal adult cases, diffuse alveolar damage, hyaline membrane formation, and scanty interstitial inflammatory-cell infiltrates.[22] Treatment during the outbreak therefore include agents against SARS-CoV as well as anti-inflammatory therapy to prevent viral replication-induced pneumonitis and subsequent pulmonary fibrosis.[23] Our initial practice is to treat children with suspect SARS with antibiotics covering organisms associated with both common bacterial and atypical pneumonia (e.g., *Streptococcus pneumoniae* and *Mycoplasma*). We would add oral ribavirin 40 to 60 mg/kg/day in three 8-hourly doses if a definite contact history makes SARS very likely. If the symptoms, especially fever and general well-being, do not respond to the treatment within 48 hours, corticosteroid will be commenced in the form of oral prednisolone 1 to 2 mg/kg/day in two divided doses or IV hydrocortisone 1 to 2 mg/kg/dose every 6 hours. If fever persists or when there is clinical deterioration or progressive chest radiograph change, pulse methylprednisolone 10 mg/kg/dose will be given every 24 hours for up to three doses, depending on clinical response. Oral ribavirin will at the same time be changed to 20 to 60 mg/kg/day intravenously given every 8 hours. Steroid will be continued for a total of 2 weeks in the form of prednisolone 1 to 2 mg/kg/day or hydrocortisone 1 to 2 mg/kg/dose every 6 hours after methylprednisolone. If the child's condition improves, the steroid will then be reduced to half the dose and gradually tapered off over a week. However, if the chest radiograph is still abnormal by day 21, low-dose steroid will be continued for a longer time and slowly tapered off according to clinical and radiologic assessment. In the younger children in whom the infection appears to run a milder course, an obvious question is whether treatment with either medication, either alone or in combination, is of any benefit. This question can only be answered by properly conducted randomized controlled trial.

The use of ribavirin has received considerable criticism from overseas and experts in Hong Kong; lack of in vitro antiviral efficacy[24] and common adverse reactions such as hemolysis[25] have been their major concerns. The efficacy of other possible agents against SARS-CoV such as Kaletra (ritonavir 400 mg and lopinavir 100 mg) has been assessed. The combination when used with concomitant ribavirin yielded significantly better clinical outcome in adult patients.[26] There are also strong advocates for not using corticosteroids at all, for fear of secondary sepsis and other complications (such as avascular necrosis). Not only is the efficacy of steroid therapy unproven in SARS, its timing and dosage regimens are also controversial. The general consensus is now to consider steroid therapy as second-line treatment to be reserved for those with severe or worsening disease.

Our policy requires that all patients with SARS, including children, be discharged home 21 days after the onset of symptoms provided their condition permits. Studies in adults suggest that over 50% of patients continue to excrete the virus in their stool and urine 3 weeks after onset of illness.[5] It is possible that the same might apply to children; therefore, instructions should be given to the parents on the proper disposal of excreta so as to prevent further transmission of the disease in the community.

■ PROGNOSIS, OUTCOME, AND SEQUELAE

The course of illness in adults has been described as triphasic.[27] Patients are relatively stable within the first week, which is the active viral replication phase. In the second week, about 80% of the patients will develop progressive pneumonic changes with increasing oxygen requirement ("immune response phase"). About 25% will develop acute respiratory distress syndrome, requiring intensive care unit admission. The mortality rate has been reported to be over 15% in adults, while the mortality rate may be as high as 50% for the elderly with comorbidities.[14] The clinical course in young children is markedly different. None of those younger than 12 years of age required intensive care unit admission, and most never required supplementary oxygen. In contrast, some adolescents may have a more progressive course, though less aggressive than that seen in adult patients. No fatalities among the pediatric age group were reported.

We have studied the radiologic and pulmonary function outcome of 47 serologically confirmed SARS pediatric patients at 6 months from diagnosis. Persistent radiologic abnormalities in the form of air trapping and ground-glass opacification were found in 34% of the study group. Need for oxygen supplementation and lymphopenia during the course of illness were found to be risk factors predisposing an individual to such abnormal radiology. Those with persistent radiologic abnormality had lung function similar to those with normal CT thorax. However, their oxygen consumption at peak exercise was significantly reduced compared with those with normal radiographs.

We will continue to see the effects of SARS on children long after the epidemic is over. Many children have experienced quarantine-imposed separation from their families and are not yet mature enough to understand the rationale. Some have lost many family members within a relatively short time period and have had their normal routines destroyed. In addition, they are bombarded daily with images of the disease in the form of the ubiquitous surgical masks, unprecedented media coverage, and community upheaval. The psychologic impact of this epidemic may become the major long-term sequelae as time goes by.

INFECTION CONTROL

Severe acute respiratory syndrome is a highly contagious disease, and the virus can remain stable and viable in urine and feces for as long as 4 days.[28] Transmission can occur via large droplets, by direct contact with infectious material, or by contact with fomites contaminated by infectious material.[27] In a few instances, potential airborne transmission was reported in association with endotracheal intubation, nebulized medications, and noninvasive positive pressure ventilation of SARS patients. Nosocomial transmission of the disease can effectively be stopped by enforcement of routine standard, contact, and droplet precautions in all clinical areas, and additional airborne precautions in all high-risk areas. During the SARS period, we adopted the policy of having a dedicated team of doctors and nurses providing care to all patients admitted to the designated SARS areas. We also have separate wards for patient triage, confirmed SARS cases, and step-down of patients in whom SARS has been ruled out. Designated changing rooms and areas for gowning and ungowning are also identified. We have summarized our experience in isolation procedures and the use of personal protection equipment in a recently published article.[29] An important lesson that we learned from this SARS epidemic relates to the need to enhance infection control programs in hospitals. A reliable alert mechanism, good communication among hospital staff members, efficient surveillance infrastructure, and continuing education to promote importance of appropriate patient care practices (especially hand washing) are vital ingredients for a successful infection control program. There are still many unanswered questions about the virus; its other possible modes of transmission, its infectivity during the incubation period and after clinical recovery, and whether it will become an endemic disease will have to be established.

REFERENCES

1. Lee N, Hui DS, Wu A, et al: A major outbreak of severe acute respiratory syndrome in Hong Kong. N Engl J Med 2003;348:1986–1994.
2. Peiris JS, Lai ST, Poon LL, et al: SARS Study Group. Coronavirus as a possible cause of severe acute respiratory syndrome. Lancet 2003;361:1319–1325.
3. Drosten C, Gunther S, Preiser W, et al: Identification of a novel coronavirus in patients with severe acute respiratory syndrome. N Engl J Med 2003;348: 1967–1976.
4. Ksiazek TG, Erdman D, Goldsmith CS, et al: SARS Working Group. A novel coronavirus associated with severe acute respiratory syndrome. N Engl J Med 2003;348:1953–1966.
5. Peiris JS, Chu CM, Cheng VC, et al: Clinical progression and viral load in a community outbreak of coronavirus associated–SARS pneumonia. A prospective study. Lancet 2003;361:1767–1772.
6. Chan KH, Poon LLM, Cheng VCC, et al: Detection of SARS coronavirus (SCoV) by RT-PCR, culture and serology in patients with severe acute respiratory syndrome (SARS). Emerg Infect Dis 2004;10(2):294–299.
7. Kuiken T, Fouchier RA, Schutten M, et al: Newly discovered coronavirus as the primary cause of severe acute respiratory syndrome. Lancet 2003;362: 263–270.
8. Fouchier RA, Kuiken T, Schutten M, et al: Aetiology: Koch's postulates fulfilled for SARS virus. Nature 2003;423:240.
9. Poutanen SM, Low DE, Henry B, et al: National Microbiology Laboratory Canada, Canadian Severe Acute Respiratory Syndrome Study Team. Identification of severe acute respiratory syndrome in Canada. N Engl J Med 2003;348:1995–2005.
10. Cavanagh D: Nidovirales. A new order comprising Coronaviridae and Arteriviridas. Arch Virol 1997;142:629–633.
11. Guan Y, Zheng BJ, He YQ, et al: Isolation and characterization of viruses related to the SARS coronavirus from animals in southern China. Science 2003;302:276–278.
12. Donnelly CA, Ghani AV, Leung GM, et al: Epidemiological determinants of spread of causal agent of severe acute respiratory syndrome in Hong Kong. Lancet 2003;361:1761–1766.
13. Hon K, Leung CW, Cheng W, et al: Clinical presentations and outcome of severe acute respiratory syndrome in children. Lancet 2003;361: 1701–1703.
14. Bitnun A, Allen U, Heurter H, et al: Children hospitalized with severe acute respiratory syndrome–related illness in Toronto. Pediatrics 2003;112: e261–e268.
15. Chiu WK, Cheung PC, Ng KL, et al: Severe acute respiratory syndrome in children. Experience in a regional hospital in Hong Kong. Pediatr Crit Care Med 2003;4:279–283.
16. Ng PC, Lam CWK, Li AM, et al: Inflammatory cytokine profile in children with severe acute respiratory syndrome. Pediatrics 2004;113:e7–e14.
17. Lucaya J, Le Pointe HD: High-resolution CT of the lung in children. In: Lucaya J, Strife JL, eds: Pediatric Chest Imaging. New York: Springer-Verlag, pp 55–91.
18. Babyn PS, Chu WC, Tsou IY, et al: Severe acute respiratory syndrome (SARS). Chest radiographic features in children. Pediatr Radiol 2004;34:47–58.
19. Centers for Disease Control and Prevention: Updated Interim U.S. Case Definition for Severe Acute Respiratory Syndrome (SARS). Available at http://www.cdc.gov/ncidod/sars/casedefinition.htm. Accessed June 19, 2005.
20. Li AM, Hon KLE, Cheng WT, et al: Severe acute respiratory syndrome. "SARS" or "not SARS." J Paediatr Child Health 2004;40:63–65.
21. Ng EK, Ng PC, Hon KL, et al: Serial analysis of the plasma concentration of SARS coronavirus RNA in pediatric patients with severe acute respiratory syndrome. Clin Chem 2003;49:2085–2088.
22. Nicholls JM, Poon LL, Lee KC, et al: Lung pathology of fatal severe acute respiratory syndrome. Lancet 2003;361:1773–1778.
23. Tsang KW, Lam WK: Management of severe acute respiratory syndrome. The Hong Kong University experience. Am J Respir Crit Care Med 2003;168:417–424.
24. Cyranoski D: Critics slam treatment for SARS as ineffective and perhaps dangerous. Nature 2003;423:4.
25. Booth CM, Matukas LM, Tomlinson GA, et al: Clinical features and short-term outcomes of 144 patients with SARS in the greater Toronto area. JAMA 2003;289:2801–2809.
26. Chu CM, Cheng VCC, Hung IFN, et al: Role of lopinavir/ritonavir in the treatment of SARS. Initial virological and clinical findings. Thorax 2004;59:252–256.
27. Wong GWK, Hui DSC: Severe acute respiratory syndrome (SARS). Epidemiology, diagnosis and treatment. Thorax 2003;58:558–560.
28. Seto WH, Tsang D, Yung RW, et al: Effectiveness of precautions against droplets and contact in prevention of nosocomial transmission of severe acute respiratory syndrome (SARS). Lancet 2003;361: 1519–1520.
29. Leung TF, Ng PC, Cheng FW, et al: Infection control for SARS in a tertiary paediatric centre in Hong Kong. J Hosp Infect 2004;56:215–222.

34 Tuberculosis and Nontuberculous Mycobacterial Disease

Anna M. Mandalakas, MD • Jeffrey R. Starke, MD

Despite the advances in diagnostic tests, availability of inexpensive curative treatment, and the nearly universal use of the bacillus Calmette-Guérin (BCG) vaccines, tuberculosis remains one of the three most important infectious diseases in the world in terms of mortality and morbidity. The World Health Organization (WHO) estimates that over 8 million people develop tuberculosis annually, and 1 to 3 million people die from the disease. As long as contagious tuberculosis persists in adults, children will be affected. However, many aspects of the epidemiology, pathophysiology, and natural history of childhood tuberculosis are fundamentally different from the features of the disease in adults. Thorough understanding of the disease is essential to treating individual children and designing effective interventions to control it.

While tuberculosis persists in many industrialized countries, disease caused by nontuberculous mycobacteria (NTM) represents an increasing proportion of all mycobacterial disease. The most common site for NTM disease in normal children is the superficial lymph nodes of the neck, but the most common site in adolescents and adults, and in children with cystic fibrosis (CF), is the lungs. The true incidence of NTM pulmonary disease likely has been vastly underestimated due to the low sensitivity of available diagnostic techniques and the fact that there is no mandatory public health reporting of NTM infections.

■ MYCOBACTERIOLOGY

The genus *Mycobacterium* consists of a diverse group of obligate aerobes that grow most successfully in tissues with high oxygen content, such as the lungs. These nonmotile, non-spore-forming, pleiomorphic rods range in length from 1 to 10 μm and in width from 0.2 to 0.6 μm. Their cell wall has a complex structure that includes a large variety of proteins, carbohydrates, and lipids. The mycolic acids are the most distinctive lipids. The lipid-rich cell wall makes them impermeable to many stains unless the dyes are combined with phenol. Once stained, the cells resist decolorization with acidified organic solvents, resulting in their hallmark trait of "acid-fastness." This property is demonstrated with basic fuchsin stain techniques, such as the Ziehl-Neelsen and Kinyoun methods, or the more sensitive fluorochrome method using auramine and rhodamine stains. It is not possible to distinguish one species of *Mycobacterium* from the others using only acid-fast staining.

Of the more than 60 species of *Mycobacterium* that have been described, about one half are pathogenic in humans.[1] The *M. tuberculosis* complex consists of five closely related species: *M. tuberculosis, M. bovis, M. microti, M. canetti,* and *Mycobacterium africanum.* The most commonly encountered NTM are classified together as the *Mycobacterium avium* complex (MAC) and include the species *M. avium, M. intracellulare, and M. scrofulaceum.* In 1959, Runyon proposed a classification system of NTM based on rate of growth and pigmentation. However, more sophisticated methods of species identification have become readily available. Mycolic acid and genetic analysis have more clearly delineated the species.[2]

Methods used for the isolation of *M. tuberculosis* from clinical samples also have proven useful for the isolation of NTM. Unfortunately, the NTM are very susceptible to killing by NaOH and other alkaline agents used for the liquification and decontamination of sputum and gastric aspirates, which may lead to negative cultures even when the acid-fast stain of the specimen is positive. Solid culture media for the isolation of *M. tuberculosis* and most NTM are either egg-potato-based (Lowenstein-Jensen) or agar-based (Middlebrook 7H10) media that contain antibacterial additives to prevent overgrowth. Unfortunately, these additives have some antimycobacterial effect, lowering culture yields from samples with few mycobacteria.

All mycobacteria are obligate aerobes that grow best in the presence of 5% to 10% CO_2. Most species of NTM grow best at neutral pH and a temperature of 35°C to 37°C, but *M. marinum* and *M. haemophilum* grow best at 28°C to 32°C. Isolation on solid media of slow-growing NTM takes 2 to 6 weeks; only the rapid growers (*M. fortuitum, M. chelonae, M. abscessus*) form visible colonies in less than 10 days. The radiometric Bactec system, which uses liquid Middlebrook medium, often leads to the isolation of all species of mycobacteria within 14 days. Sensitivity is increased and time for isolation is decreased by a larger specimen size. Addition of a simple chemical (NAT, paranitro-α-acetinamino-β-hydroxypropiophenone) to the culture bottle allows rapid distinction of *M. tuberculosis* from the NTM. The clinician caring for a child with a possible mycobacterial infection should be aware of the culture and isolation scheme being used and its limitations.

Traditional identification of NTM relied on statistical probabilities of a characteristic reaction pattern in a battery of biochemical tests. However, the slow speed of these tests has led to a search for more rapid methods of species identification. At present, many clinical laboratories use high-performance liquid chromatography analysis to speciate mycobacteria by determining the specific mycolic acid fingerprint of isolates grown in the laboratory.

Drug susceptibility testing for *M. tuberculosis* can be performed either on solid or liquid media that contain standard concentrations of antimicrobial agents.[2] However, drug susceptibility testing for NTM is far more complicated. In general, *M. kansasii, M. marinum, M. xenopi, M. ulcerans, M. gordonae,*

M. malmoense, M. szulgai, M. haemophilum, and some strains of MAC are susceptible to some or all standard antituberculosis drugs. For convenience, NTM organisms have been tested with the same methods, drugs, and critical concentration of drugs as are used for *M. tuberculosis*. However, the information generated is usually of little use in the management of NTM infections. For example, the drug concentrations used for testing susceptibility of *M. tuberculosis* are too low for use in testing MAC organisms. Drugs active against MAC and *M. kansasii* often have lower minimum inhibitory concentrations (MICs) in broth (Bactec) than on agar, so agreement between methods for these species has been poor. For the rapidly growing mycobacteria, routine susceptibility testing to antibiotics such as amikacin, cefoxitin, doxycycline, linezolide, sulfonamides, and the macrolides (erythromycin, clarithromycin, and azithromycin) should be performed on all clinically significant isolates. When and how MAC isolates should be subjected to susceptibility testing remains controversial.[3] Although determination of the MIC or synergy studies with various drugs may provide useful information, the meaning of these in vitro results and how to relate them to the testing of individual clinical isolates have yet to be determined in clinical trials. Because drug susceptibility testing of the NTM is not well standardized, interlaboratory variations in results are common and can be confusing for the clinician.

IMMUNOLOGY

The vast majority of studies on the human immune response to mycobacteria have centered on *M. tuberculosis*. Humans display a wide spectrum of immunologic responses to *M. tuberculosis*. The varied immunologic response is reflected in the diverse clinical manifestations ranging from asymptomatic infection with a positive tuberculin skin test to hematogenous dissemination with severe or fatal disease.[4–7]

Immunologically competent cells of the human host recognize *M. tuberculosis* by its antigens. An extraordinarily large number of these antigens have been described. In a few individuals, the innate immune system represented by macrophages, natural killer cells, and neutrophils control infection as part of the initial response to *M. tuberculosis*.[8] In the majority of infected persons, the acquired immune response is responsible for control of *M. tuberculosis* and the subsequent pathophysiologic events.

T cells, as antigen recognition units, have critical regulatory and effector roles in the immune response to *M. tuberculosis*. In the traditional model, macrophages present antigens from phagocytosed bacilli to T cells. Antigen-activated T cells secrete cytokines, which in turn stimulate macrophages, making them more effective at controlling mycobacterial growth. Recent advances in studies of the human immune response to mycobacteria have expanded on this simple model.[9] First, a large variety of circulating and tissue-bound T-lymphocyte subsets ($CD4^+$, $CD8^+$, and $\gamma\delta$T cells) have antigen receptors with high affinity for mycobacterial antigens.[5] Second, T cells also serve as cytotoxic effector cells against *M. tuberculosis*–infected macrophages. Third, after exposure to mycobacteria, macrophages produce a large number of cytokines (interleukin-1 [IL-1], IL-6, IL-10, IL-12, IL-15, IL-18, tumor necrosis factor-α, and transforming growth factor-β) that mediate further immune responses. The exact response is under genetic control, but is influenced by environmental factors such as nutrition and prior exposure to environmental NTM or a BCG vaccine. Of note, B lymphocyte–mediated humoral response to mycobacterial antigens occur in patients, but have no clearly demonstrated role in disease pathogenesis.

The course of infection is influenced largely by the host immune response to *M. tuberculosis*. Most children infected with *M. tuberculosis* develop a positive tuberculin skin test but no symptoms or radiographic abnormalities. These children have an effective macrophage- and lymphocyte-activated response with a rapid expansion of T cells and production of protective cytokines and mediators. In children who develop disease, the most common manifestation is pulmonary disease, including a Ghon focus, enlarged lymph nodes, or bronchial disease. However, the immune system in these children contains the disease which often resolves without chemotherapy.[10] A few children experience severe forms of disease, including progressive pulmonary tuberculosis, miliary tuberculosis, or tuberculous meningitis. These forms of disease result from an immune response that fails to contain the growth of the bacilli. The risk for disease development in childhood following primary infection is inversely related to age, suggesting an inadequate or immature immune response.[10,11]

Several lines of evidence suggest that the specific acquired host defenses against mycobacteria are genetically determined. Twin studies indicate that there is a higher concordance of tuberculosis among monozygotic compared with dizygotic twins.[12,13] Segregation analysis of tuberculosis in families indicates an oligogenic pattern of inheritance.[14] Homozygosity mapping of familial cases of NTM disease has identified mutations in the interferon-γ receptor 1 gene and IL-12 receptor that predispose to the serious and prolonged courses of disease.[15–17]

MYCOBACTERIUM TUBERCULOSIS

EPIDEMIOLOGY

Transmission

Transmission of *M. tuberculosis* is generally person-to-person and occurs via inhalation of mucous droplets that become airborne when an individual with pulmonary or laryngeal tuberculosis coughs, sneezes, speaks, laughs, or sings. After drying, the droplet nuclei can remain suspended in the air for hours. Only small droplets (<10 μm in diameter) can reach alveoli. Droplet nuclei also can be produced by aerosol treatments, sputum induction, aerosolization during bronchoscopy, and through manipulation of lesions or processing of tissue or secretions in the hospital or laboratory. Transmission occurs rarely by direct contact with infected body fluids or fomites.

There are many factors associated with the risk for acquiring *M. tuberculosis* infection.[18] The risk for acquiring infection has been associated with the extent of contact with the index case, the burden of organisms in the sputum, and the frequency of cough in the index case. Adults with pulmonary tuberculosis and bacilli present on acid-fast smear of sputum are more likely to transmit infection. In addition, the risk for transmission is directly correlated with the degree of contact with a contagious case. Most transmission to children occurs in the home. Markers of close contact such as urban living and overcrowding correlate with acquisition of infection. An increased risk for infection has been demonstrated in several institutional settings, including nursing homes, schools, correctional institutions, and homeless shelters. A growing problem concerns tuberculosis transmission in refugee and orphanage settings.[19,20] There is some evidence that the risk for acquiring infection increases with age from infancy to early adulthood, likely due to increasing contacts with infectious persons. In many populations, men are more likely to be infected than women. Although strains of *M. tuberculosis* show considerable variation in their virulence for guinea pigs, it is not clear that strain virulence is an important factor in human infection.

It has been noted for decades that children with tuberculosis rarely infect other children or adults.[21] The few documented cases of transmission from children have been in individuals with typical findings of adult-type tuberculosis, with lung cavities and sputum production, or infants with congenital tuberculosis, who have a large burden of organisms in the lungs. When transmission of *M. tuberculosis* has been documented in schools, orphanages, or children's hospitals, it almost invariably has come from an adult or adolescent with undiagnosed pulmonary tuberculosis. In fact, when a child is suspected clinically of having tuberculosis disease, the adults who accompany the child should undergo urgent testing (usually by chest radiograph) for tuberculosis to be sure they do not spread infection in the facility. In the typical case of childhood pulmonary tuberculosis, tubercle bacilli in endobronchial secretions are sparse. When young children with tuberculosis cough, they lack the tussive force of adults. Sputum production is rare in children, and collected specimens usually do not have acid-fast bacilli upon staining, indicating a low concentration of organisms. However, specimens from young infants with extensive tuberculosis infiltrates, children with cavitary lesions, or intubated children with tuberculosis should be handled as potentially infectious.

A few classic studies have investigated the factors that influence whether or not an infected person will develop tuberculosis. It is clear that the risk for disease is highest shortly after initial infection and declines thereafter. From infancy to age 10 years, age is inversely associated with the risk for developing disease. Most young children who develop tuberculosis disease do so within the first year after infection, with most cases occurring within 6 months of transmission of the organism. For unknown reasons, there is a second peak in the risk for developing disease during late adolescence and early adult life.

Incidence and Prevalence

It is instructive to examine the epidemiology of tuberculosis in the United States, where data collection and analysis are fairly complete. As a result of effective public health strategies in the United States, the incidence of tuberculosis steadily declined from the 1950s to 1985. However, rates of tuberculosis began to dramatically increase in the late 1980s and early 1990s, resulting in a peak incidence of 10.5 per 100,000 population in 1992.[22] Of note, case rates were consistently highest in racial and ethnic minorities. Asian and non-Hispanic blacks had the highest case rates of 46.6 and 31.7 cases per 100,000, respectively. In comparison, non-Hispanic whites had the lowest case rate of 4.0 per 100,000 persons. Multiple factors contributed to the resurgence of tuberculosis in the United States, including a large influx of foreign-born persons in the late 1970s, the human immunodeficiency virus (HIV) epidemic, homelessness, crowded living conditions, decreased access to medical care, cutbacks in funding of tuberculosis control programs, and increased incidence of multi-drug-resistant (MDR) tuberculosis.

During 1993 through 2002, the average year-to-year decrease in tuberculosis case rates was 6.8%, reaching 5.1 per 100,000 population in 2003 (Fig. 34-1). However, 2003 had a significantly smaller decrease of 1.9%, and the 2003 case rate remains higher than the national interim goal of 3.5 cases per 100,000 population that was set for 2000.[22] In 2003, 12 states (California, Texas, New York, Florida, Georgia, New Jersey, Arizona, Louisiana, Alabama, South Carolina, Hawaii, and Alaska) and the District of Columbia reported rates above the national average. Elevated rates continue to be reported in certain populations, including foreign-born persons and ethnic and racial minorities. Birth data were first collected by the tuberculosis surveillance system in 1986, when 21.8% of tuberculosis cases occurred among foreign-born persons. Since that time, the proportion has steadily increased, with the highest proportion being reported in 2003 (53.3%); this trend is enhanced by the steady decline in tuberculosis cases among U.S.-born persons (Fig. 34-2).

Childhood tuberculosis, defined as disease in children younger than 15 years, directly reflects the incidence of adult tuberculosis in a community. From 1992 through 2002, the trend in rates of tuberculosis varied by age group, with the largest decline occurring in children younger than 15 years (from 3.1 per 100,000 in 1992 to 1.5 in 2002) and in adults 25 to 44 years of age (from 12.7 to 6.2), 45 to 64 years of age (from 13.4 to 6.3), and 65 years and older (from 18.7 to 8.8), each group having decreased approximately 50%. In 2003, 6% of all reported cases in the United States occurred in children younger than 15 years as compared with 10% in 15- to 24-year-olds, 35% in 25- to 44-year-olds, 28% in 45- to 64-year-olds, and 21% in people 65 years and older. Over the past 30 years,

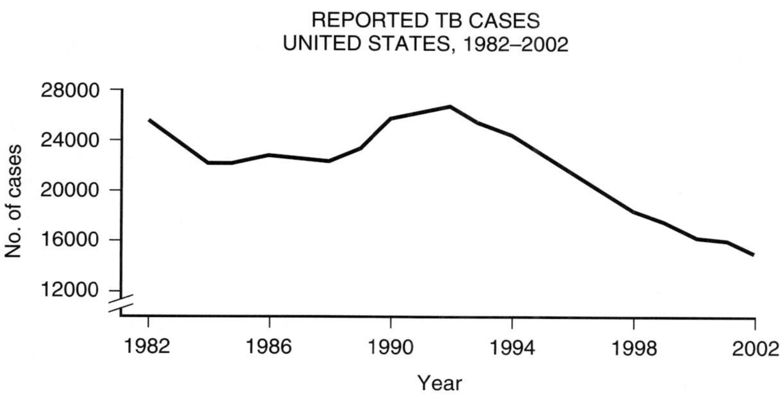

■ **FIGURE 34-1.** The number of reported tuberculosis cases in the United States from 1982 to 2002. (Data from the Centers for Disease Control and Prevention, Atlanta.)

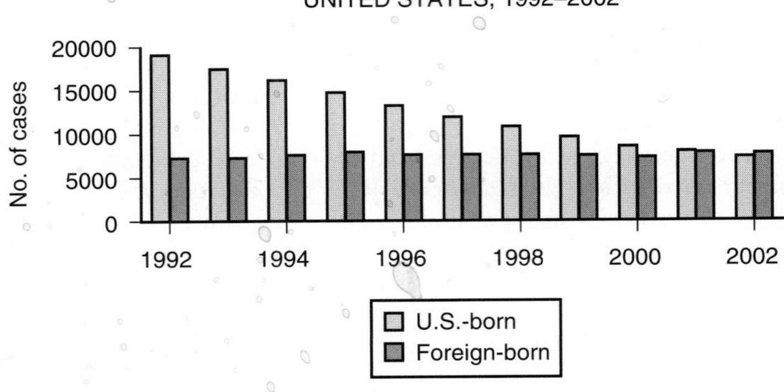

■ **FIGURE 34-2.** Number of tuberculosis cases in the United States—born vs. foreign-born persons, United States, 1992–2002. (Data from the Centers for Disease Control and Prevention, Atlanta.)

the proportion of tuberculosis cases reported in children has remained relatively stable at approximately 6%.

Analysis of all newly diagnosed, verified childhood tuberculosis cases reported to the National Tuberculosis Surveillance System between January 1993 and December 2001 offers important insight into the epidemiology of childhood tuberculosis in the United States.[23] A total of 11,480 cases of childhood tuberculosis were reported during this period. The highest annual case rates were consistently reported among those who were younger than 5 years, whose rates were 2.1 and 3.5 times higher than among children 5 to 9 and 10 to 14 years of age, respectively. Nearly 70% of all cases occurred in eight states (California, Texas, New York, Illinois, Georgia, Florida, New Jersey, and Pennsylvania). Urban areas reported over 70% of childhood tuberculosis cases, with one third of the total reported from New York City, Los Angeles, Chicago, San Diego, and Houston. Children who were racial or ethnic minorities comprised almost 90% of the cases. In 2001, the case rate for foreign-born children was 12.2 per 100,000 population compared with 1.1 per 100,000 population for U.S.-born children.[23] Between 1993 and 2001, nearly two thirds of all cases of pediatric tuberculosis in foreign-born children were reported in children from Mexico (40%), the Philippines (9%), Vietnam (6%), Somalia (4%), Russia and the newly independent states of the former Soviet Union (4%), and Haiti (3%). Sixty percent of all cases of tuberculosis reported in foreign-born children were diagnosed within 18 months of arrival in the United States. Children who immigrate legally into the United States are required to have neither a tuberculin skin test nor a chest radiograph. Although some of these children may have been infected with *M. tuberculosis* after immigration, most were already infected. Better screening of these children before immigration or access to medical care after immigration could have prevented many of these cases. HIV status was only reported in 24% of all cases, limiting the ability to measure the impact of HIV disease on childhood tuberculosis. Among adolescents 15 to 18 years of age, the annual number of reported cases remained stable (396 in 1993 and 386 in 2001) and case rates declined slightly. Other demographic features (geographic distribution, race and ethnicity, and birth country) mirrored tuberculosis in younger children.

Little is known about the epidemiology of childhood tuberculosis in the developing world. In the early 1990s, the WHO estimated there were 1.5 million cases and 450,000 deaths annually from childhood tuberculosis.[24] Unfortunately, in most resource-poor countries, the only means used to diagnose pulmonary tuberculosis is acid-fast strain of the sputum, which is positive in up to 70% of adults with pulmonary tuberculosis but less than 5% of children with pulmonary tuberculosis. As a result, most national tuberculosis programs grossly underestimate the rate of childhood tuberculosis. In regions where improved case finding has been examined, children often represent up to 40% of all cases, with a skew toward more serious and complicated cases. In most industrialized countries, children who are poor and who are immigrants or who have poor access to medical care carry the majority of the childhood tuberculosis burden.

■ CLINICAL MANIFESTATIONS

Pathophysiology

After inhaling *M. tuberculosis*, the majority of children do not develop disease, but rather develop latent tuberculosis infection (LTBI). These children have a positive tuberculin skin test result and no clinical or radiographic evidence of tuberculosis disease.[25] It is presumed that these children are infected with a low number of viable tubercle bacilli that are dormant and do not cause clinical disease or pathologic changes. Before an adequate immune response is mounted, bacilli located in the regional lymph nodes enter the systemic circulation directly or via the lymphatic duct. This occult hematogenous spread disseminates bacilli to a variety of organs where the bacilli may survive for decades.[26] If the dissemination is not controlled by the developing acquired immune response, disseminated tuberculosis results. The occult dissemination also provides the seed organisms for extrapulmonary tuberculosis, which accounts for 20% to 30% of childhood tuberculosis cases.

In a portion of children, infection results in pathologic changes and associated clinical disease. In these children, tubercle bacilli reach a terminal airway and induce a localized pneumonic inflammatory process referred to as the parenchymal (Ghon) focus. Bacilli originating from this focus drain via local lymphatics to the regional lymph nodes. The triad of the parenchyma focus, local tuberculous lymphangitis and enlarged regional lymph nodes, is referred to as the primary complex.

Evolution of Clinical Disease in Children

A review of information available from the prechemotherapy era provides a rich understanding of the natural evolution of clinical disease in children.[10,27] Following infection, all children progress through an asymptomatic incubation period generally lasting 3 to 8 weeks. The subsequent development of clinical disease is determined by the interaction of the host and the organism, and is highly age dependent (Table 34-1).[27]

Younger children (younger than 2 years) are at greatest risk for both the development of disease and severe manifestations of disease. After the age of 10 years, children are more likely to manifest adult-type disease. Recent data from the United States suggest that age-dependent disease presentation continues to persist despite available treatment for LTBI.[23] From 1993 to 2001, disseminated (1.4% of total cases) and meningeal (2.6%) tuberculosis were more frequently diagnosed in children younger than 5 years compared with children 5 to 9 years of age (miliary 0.4%, meningeal 1.4%) and children 10 to 14 years of age (miliary 1.4%, meningeal 1.4%). Children 5 to 9 years of age were more likely to have lymphatic tuberculosis (18.8%) compared with children younger than 5 years (14.1%) and children 10 to 14 years of age (15.6%). Among 190 children younger than 5 years in whom pulmonary and cavitary tuberculosis was reported, 54 (28%) were younger than 1 year and nearly all (90.5%) were U.S. born. Most adolescents (78%) had pulmonary disease and were more likely than adults and children to have pleural disease (5.2 % vs. 4.1% and 1.2%, respectively). More adolescents had cavitary disease on chest radiograph than adults or younger children.

The various manifestations of tuberculosis tend to occur in a predictable timetable.[26] Disseminated tuberculosis and tuberculous meningitis tend to be early manifestations, often occurring 2 to 6 months after initial infection has occurred. The primary complex and its complications occur most often 3 to 6 months after infection. It is not uncommon for untreated primary complex tuberculosis to result in calcification of the lung parenchyma and/or regional lymph nodes, a process that occurs at least 6 months after infection (Fig. 34-3). While pleural and lymph node tuberculosis often occur within 3 to 9 months after infection, other extrapulmonary forms of tuberculosis, especially skeletal and renal disease, may not occur for several years.

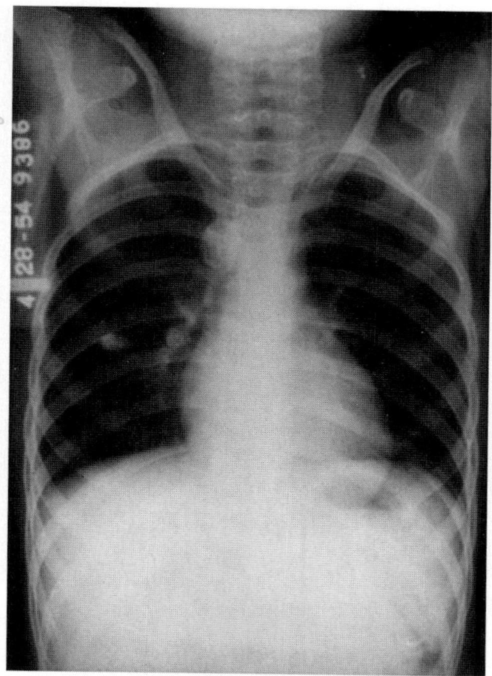

■ **FIGURE 34-3.** A calcified parenchymal lesion and lymph node in a child with tuberculosis infection. These lesions contain a small number of viable *M. tuberculosis.*

■ **TABLE 34-1.** Average age-specific risk for disease development following primary infection[10]

Age at Primary Infection	Immune-Competent Children (Dominant Disease Entity Indicated in Parentheses)	Risk of Disease following Primary Infection (%)
<1 year	No disease	50
	Pulmonary disease (Ghon focus, lymph node, or bronchial)	30–40
	TBM or disseminated disease	10–20
1–2 years	No disease	70–80
	Pulmonary disease (Ghon focus, lymph node, or bronchial)	10–20
	TBM or disseminated disease	2–5
2–5 years	No disease	95
	Pulmonary disease (lymph node or bronchial)	5
	TBM or disseminated	0.5
5–10 years	No disease	98
	Pulmonary disease (lymph node, bronchial, effusion, or adult-type)	2
	TBM or disseminated disease	<0.5
>10 years	No disease	80–90
	Pulmonary disease (effusion or adult-type)	10–20
	TBM or disseminated disease	<0.5

TBM, tuberculous meningitis.

Intrathoracic Tuberculosis

Intrathoracic tuberculosis consists of pulmonary infection and pulmonary disease. The primary complex that occurs after inhalation of *M. tuberculosis* includes the parenchymal Ghon focus with associated tuberculosis lymphangitis and affected regional lymph nodes. Approximately 70% of the primary foci are subpleural. Lobes are equally affected, and 25% of children have multiple parenchymal foci. When there are no clinical symptoms and the chest radiograph is normal, this is referred to as tuberculosis infection. Pulmonary tuberculosis occurs when tuberculosis infection is complicated by clinical symptoms and/or radiolographic abnormalities. Pulmonary disease may be associated with a diverse spectrum of pathology described in the following sections.

A Ghon focus with or without cavitation may accompany clinical disease, including weight loss, fatigue, fever, and chronic cough.[28] If the host is unable to contain the tubercle bacilli, progressive parenchymal caseation occurs in the lung parenchyma surrounding the Ghon focus. The area of caseation may discharge into a bronchus, resulting in the formation of a primary cavity with possible endotracheal spread (Fig. 34-4). The tubercle bacilli disseminate further to other parts of the lobe and can involve an entire lung. On rare occasions, an enlarging primary focus ruptures into the pleural cavity, creating a pneumothorax, bronchopleural fistula, or caseous pyopneumothorax. A severe progressive lesion is accompanied by profound fever, cough, and weight loss. Before the advent of chemotherapy, 25% to 65% of children with progressive primary disease died. However, with appropriate therapy, the prognosis is excellent.

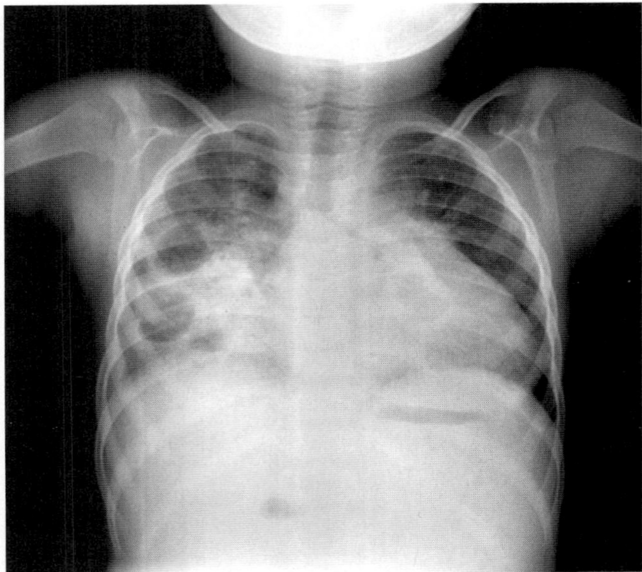

■ **FIGURE 34-4.** A young child with pulmonary tuberculosis has developed cavitation of the lung parenchyma.

The hallmark of pulmonary tuberculosis is enlargement of the regional hilar, mediastinal, or subcarinal lymph nodes (Fig. 34-5).[29,30] Isolated thoracic adenopathy usually causes few or no clinical signs or symptoms. In some children, particularly infants, the lymph nodes continue to enlarge, resulting in lymphobronchial involvement, where the affected bronchus may become partially or totally obstructed as a result of nodal compression, inflammatory edema, polyps, granulomatous tissue, or caseous material extruded from ulcerated lymph nodes (Fig. 34-6). While chest radiography rarely delineates the specific pathologic process causing the chest radiographic abnormalities, they are often apparent if bronchoscopy or a computed tomography scan of the chest is performed. The most frequently affected lobes are the right upper, the right middle, and the left upper lobe. Symptoms vary according to the degree of airway irritation and obstruction but frequently include a localized wheezing or persistent cough that may mimic pertussis. A common radiographic sequence is adenopathy followed by localized hyperinflation and then atelectasis of contiguous parenchyma, referred to as collapse-consolidation or segmental lesions (Fig. 34-7). The radiographic and clinical picture mimics foreign body obstruction and other obstructive disorders. Additional pathology that may accompany bronchial disease includes airway allergic consolidation, bronchopneumonia, and caseating consolidation. Children with allergic consolidation typically experience high fevers, acute respiratory symptoms, and signs of consolidation on chest radiograph. Children with caseating consolidation are very ill, with high undulating fevers, chronic cough, and occasional hemoptysis (Fig. 34-8).

In some children, an acute secondary bacterial infection that occurs distal to the obstructed bronchus plays a role in the clinical expression of disease. Children with secondary bacterial pneumonia often present with high fever, cough, and crackles. The clinical signs and symptoms often respond to antibiotics, but the chest radiographic findings do not clear because of the underlying tuberculosis.

Although segmental lesions and hyperaeration are the most common findings produced by enlarging thoracic lymph nodes, others occur. Enlarged paratracheal nodes may cause stridor and respiratory distress. Subcarinal nodes may impinge on the esophagus and cause difficulty swallowing, followed occasionally by the formation of an esophageal diverticulum; or the nodes may rupture directly into the esophagus and produce a bronchoesophageal fistula. Enlarged lymph nodes may compress the

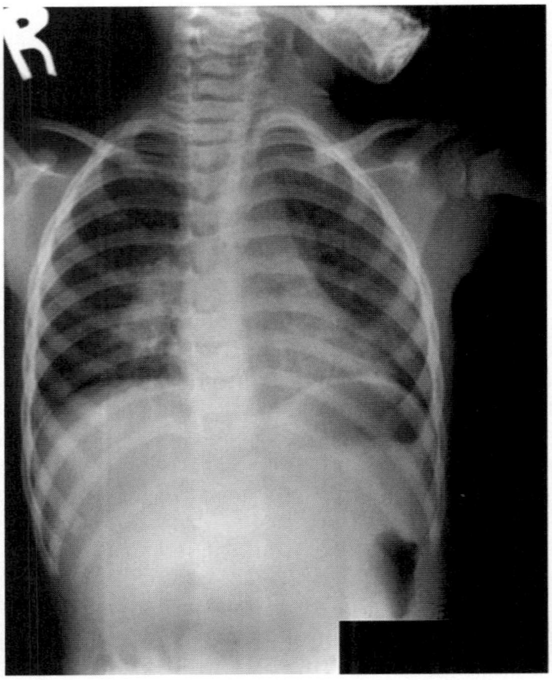

■ **FIGURE 34-5.** Hilar adenopathy in a child with early pulmonary tuberculosis. Most children with this radiographic appearance have few or no symptoms.

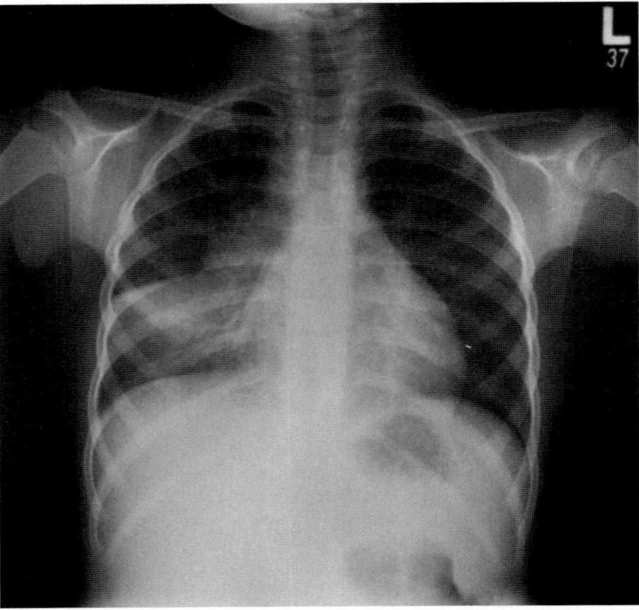

■ **FIGURE 34-6.** A classic collapse-consolidation lesion with hilar adenopathy in a child with pulmonary tuberculosis.

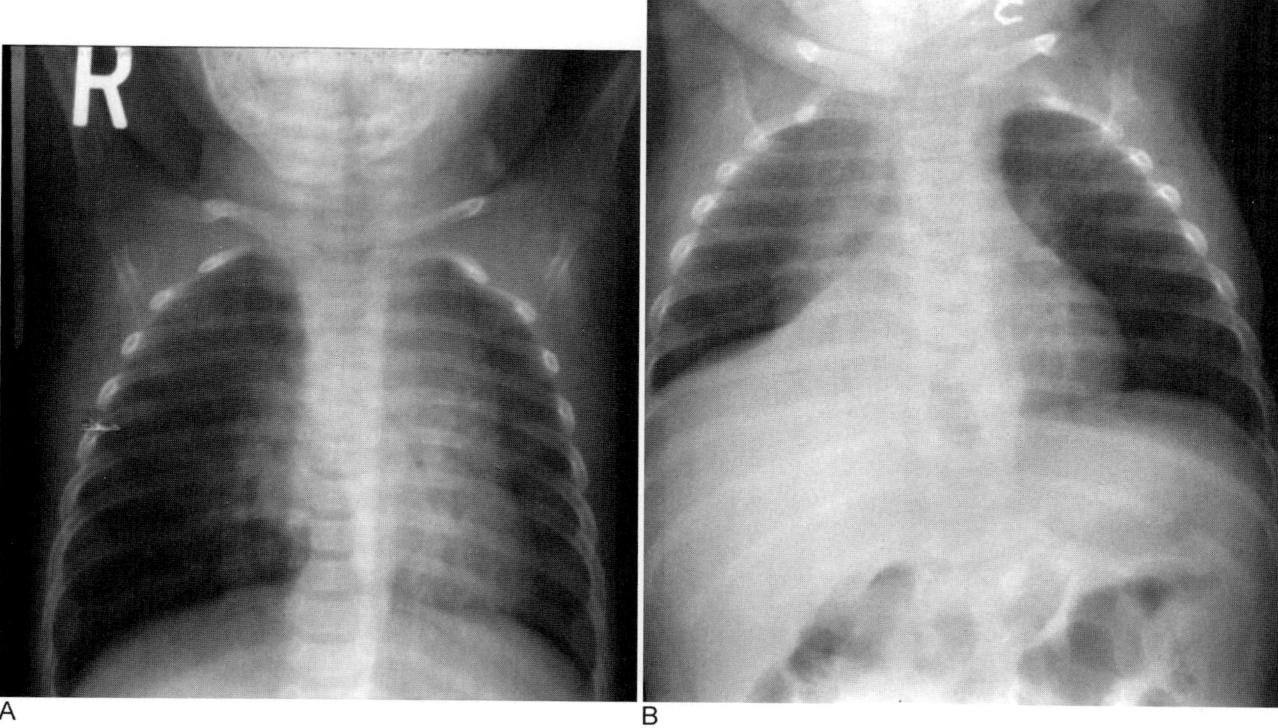

■ **FIGURE 34-7.** **A,** Hyperinflation of the right lower lobe in an infant with pulmonary tuberculosis and airway obstruction. At this point the child had respiratory distress. **B,** A chest radiograph from the same child several hours later shows complete collapse of the right lower lobe. At this point, the respiratory distress had ceased.

subclavian vein and produce edema of the hand and arm, or they may erode major blood vessels, including the aorta. They also may rupture into the mediastinum and point in the left, or more often the right, supraclavicular fossa. Compression of the left recurrent laryngeal nerve has been reported. Rupture into the pericardial sac causes tuberculous pericarditis. The late results of bronchial obstruction include the following possibilities: (1) complete reexpansion of the lung and resolution of the radiographic findings; (2) disappearance of the segmental lesion, with residual calcification of the primary focus or the regional lymph nodes; or (3) scarring and progressive contraction of the lobe or segment usually associated with bronchiectasis (Fig. 34-9). Permanent anatomic sequelae result from segmental lesions in approximately 60% of all cases, even though the abnormality usually is not apparent on plain radiographs. Cylindric (rarely saccular) bronchiectasis, sometimes stenoses, and elongation or shortening can be demonstrated on bronchography. Fortunately, most of these abnormalities are asymptomatic in the upper lobes.

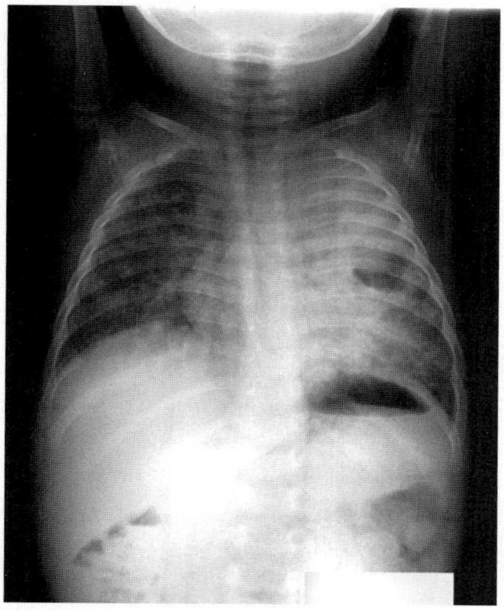

■ **FIGURE 34-8.** Pronounced caseating consolidation in a young child with pulmonary tuberculosis.

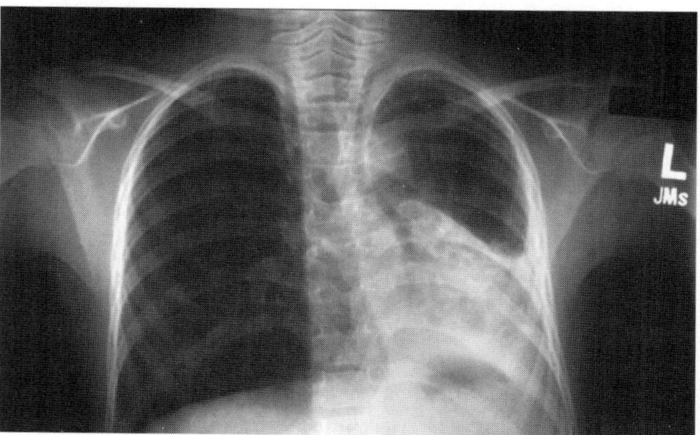

■ **FIGURE 34-9.** Bronchiectasis of the left lower lobe in a child with tuberculosis who was nonadherent to appropriate treatment.

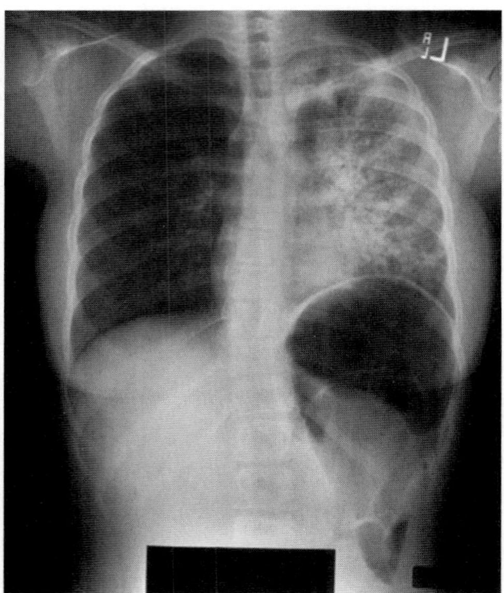

■ **FIGURE 34-10.** A chest radiograph of an adolescent girl with chronic pulmonary tuberculosis.

However, secondary infection may occur in the middle and lower lobes and cause the middle lobe syndrome.

Chronic pulmonary tuberculosis, often called adult type or reactivation tuberculosis, is the type of disease that occurs in pulmonary tissue that was sensitized to tuberculous antigens by an earlier tuberculous infection that became dormant or latent. Chronic pulmonary tuberculosis rarely develops in children who acquired infection with *M. tuberculosis* before 2 years of age, but is more common the closer infection occurs to the onset of puberty. It is rare in children younger than 10 years. The preponderance of evidence supports the concept that most cases of reactivation tuberculosis result from endogenous reinfection with the dormant bacilli. However, reinfection with a different strain of *M. tuberculosis*, leading to typical adult-type tuberculosis, has been documented.

Reactivation pulmonary tuberculosis arises from the small round foci of organisms in the apices of the lungs (often called Assman or Simon foci) that resulted from the lymphohematogenous spread at the time of the initial infection.[31] Fibronodular infiltrates in one or both upper lobe apices are most common, but more extensive pulmonary involvement leads to diffuse consolidation or cavitation (Fig. 34-10). Involvement of thoracic lymph nodes is usually absent. Cough, remitting fevers, night sweats, chest pain, sputum production, and hemoptysis are the most common clinical manifestations.

Pleural tuberculosis results from direct spread of caseous material from a subpleural parenchymal or lymph node focus, or from hematogenous spread.[32,33] Pleural tuberculosis is uncommon in children younger than 6 years and rare in those younger than 2 years. The presence of caseous material in the pleural space may trigger a hypersensitivity reaction, with the accumulation of serous straw-colored fluid containing few tubercle bacilli. This exudate has a high protein concentration and lymphocyte predominance; the amount of polymorphonuclear cells depends on the acuteness of onset. Although direct microscopy is usually negative, culture yields may be as high as 40% to 70%. Pleural biopsy often demonstrates caseating granulomas and increases the culture yield if ample tissue is collected. The clinical course associated with pleural involvement characteristically begins with acute chest pain, accompanied by high fever in the absence of acute illness, an ill-defined loss of vigor, and a dry cough. Active caseation in the pleural space may cause thick loculated pus, containing many tubercle bacilli (Fig. 34-11). The prognosis for children with tuberculous pleural effusion always has been good compared with other overt forms of tuberculosis, even before chemotherapy was available.

Tubercle bacilli from the lymphadenitis of the primary complex are disseminated during the incubation period in all cases of tuberculosis infection. The clinical picture produced by lymphohematogenous spread probably is determined by host susceptibility at the time of spread and by the quantity of tubercle bacilli released. Three clinical forms of dissemination can be recognized:

1. The lymphohematogenous spread may be occult, in which case it usually remains so, or it may be occult initially with metastatic, extrapulmonary lesions appearing months or years later (e.g., renal tuberculosis).
2. So-called protracted hematogenous tuberculosis, rarely seen today, is characterized by high, spiking fever, marked leukocytosis, hepatomegaly and splenomegaly, and general glandular enlargement, sometimes with repeated evidence of metastatic seeding in the choroid plexus, kidney, and skin. Calcifications may appear subsequently, often in large numbers, in the pulmonary apices (Simon foci) and in the spleen, thus attesting to the earlier dissemination of tubercle bacilli via blood. The tuberculin skin test usually is strongly positive. Bone marrow biopsy may confirm the clinical impression, but treatment often must be started on a presumptive basis. Although this type of tuberculosis in past years often ended tragically in tuberculous meningitis, today it is completely treatable if diagnosed in time.

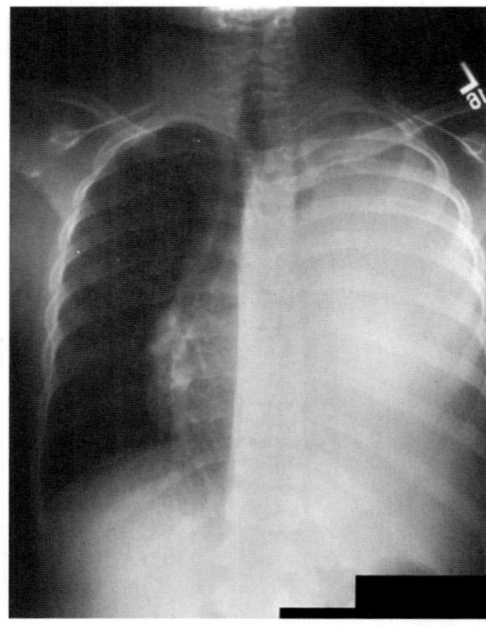

■ **FIGURE 34-11.** A large tuberculosis pleural effusion in an 11-year-old girl.

3. The third form of lymphohematogenous spread, analogous to sepsis with pyogenic bacteria, is miliary tuberculosis. It usually arises from discharge of a caseous focus, often a lymph node, into a blood vessel such as a pulmonary vein. It may be self-propagating, with repeated discharge arising at various sites. Most common during the first 2 to 6 months after infection in infancy, it can arise even in adults who have apparently well-healed, calcified lesions.

The clinical picture of miliary tuberculosis varies greatly, probably depending on the number of bacilli in the bloodstream.[34,35] Sometimes the patient is afebrile and appears to be well, and the condition is diagnosed by chance during contact investigation of another individual with infectious tuberculosis. The onset can be insidious, often occurring after the patient has had another precipitating infection. In rare cases, the onset is abrupt. Drowsiness, loss of weight and appetite, persistent fever, weakness, rapid breathing with a rustling sound on auscultation of the lungs, occasionally cyanosis, and almost always a palpable spleen are the clinical manifestations that lead the clinician to obtain a chest radiograph.

Usually within no more than 3 weeks after the onset of symptoms, tubercles, sometimes tiny and at times large, can be seen evenly distributed throughout both lung fields (Fig. 34-12). In the early stages, they often are detected best on a lateral view of the retrocardiac space. Recurrent pneumothorax, subcutaneous emphysema, pneumomediastinum, and pleural effusion are less serious but well-recognized complications of miliary tuberculosis. Cutaneous lesions, including painful nodules, papulonecrotic tuberculids, and purpuric lesions, may appear in crops.

The diagnosis usually is established by means of the clinical picture and a chest radiograph; sometimes by a liver or skin biopsy; by culturing *M. tuberculosis* from the gastric aspirate, urine, or bone marrow; or by fiberoptic bronchoscopy. Treatment usually is very successful.

Coinfection with HIV can change the clinical presentation of intrathoracic tuberculosis. In adults infected with both HIV and *M. tuberculosis*, the rate of progression from latent tuberculous infection to disease is increased greatly. Tuberculosis has typical clinical features when the patient's $CD4^+$ cell count is higher than 500/mm^3. As the $CD4^+$ cell count declines, the clinical picture changes; pulmonary cavities are rare, but lower lobe infiltrates or nodules often accompanied by thoracic adenopathy are common. Sputum is less often produced, and more invasive diagnostic techniques are often required to establish the diagnosis.

When pulmonary tuberculosis develops in an HIV-infected child, the clinical features tend to be typical of childhood tuberculosis in immunocompetent children, but the disease often progresses more rapidly and clinical manifestations are more severe.[36,37] There is also an increased tendency for the development of extrathoracic tuberculosis.

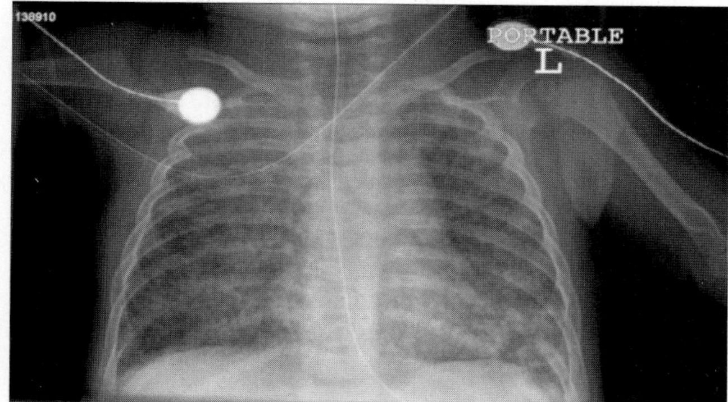

■ **FIGURE 34-12.** The appearance of miliary tuberculosis in the chest radiograph of an infant.

Extrathoracic Tuberculosis

A complete description of extrathoracic tuberculosis is beyond the scope of this book. However, pulmonologists may encounter this possibility when evaluating children with pulmonary involvement and other manifestations. The most common forms of extrathoracic disease in children include tuberculosis of the superficial lymph nodes (scrofula) and the central nervous system. Other rare forms of extrathoracic disease in children are osteoarticular, abdominal, gastrointestinal, genitourinary, cutaneous, and congenital disease.

Tuberculosis of the superficial lymph nodes (scrofula) is the most common form of extrathoracic tuberculosis.[38,39] Although this disease historically was associated with *M. bovis* obtained by drinking unpasteurized cow's milk, most current cases occur after primary pulmonary infection with *M. tuberculosis* and occur within 6 to 9 months of initial infection. Extension of primary lesions of the upper lung fields or abdomen leads to involvement of the supraclavicular, anterior cervical, tonsillar, and submandibular nodes. Rarely in children, tuberculosis of the skin or skeletal system can lead to involvement of the inguinal, epitrochlear, or axillary lymph nodes. Early during infection, lymph nodes are discrete, firm, and nontender. The lymph nodes become fixed to surrounding tissues and feel matted as the infection progresses. Low-grade fever may be the only systemic symptom. Although usually present, a primary pulmonary complex is visible radiologically only 30% to 70% of the time. Tuberculin skin test results are usually reactive. Although spontaneous resolution is possible, untreated lymphadenitis frequently progresses to caseating necrosis, capsular rupture, and spread to adjacent nodes and overlying skin. Rupture through the skin results in a draining sinus tract that may require surgical removal. Excisional biopsy and culture of lymph nodes are often required to differentiate between *M. tuberculosis* and NTM disease.

Central nervous system disease is the most serious complication of tuberculosis in children and complicates approximately 0.5% of untreated primary infections. It is most common in children 6 months to 4 years of age and generally occurs within 2 to 6 months of primary infection.[40] Central nervous system disease arises from the formation of a caseous lesion in the cerebral cortex or meninges that results from early occult lymphohematogenous spread.[41] Lesions enlarge and discharge bacilli into the subarachnoid space, leading to an exudate that infiltrates the cortical and meningeal blood vessels. This results in inflammation, obstruction, and subsequent infarction of the cerebral cortex. The clinical onset of tuberculous meningitis can be rapid or gradual. Infants and children are more likely to experience a rapid progression to hydrocephalus, seizure, and cerebral edema over several days (Fig. 34-13). In most children, signs and symptoms progress over several weeks, beginning nonspecifically with fever, headache, irritability, and drowsiness. Disease frequently advances abruptly with symptoms of lethargy, vomiting, nuchal rigidity, seizures, hypertonia, and

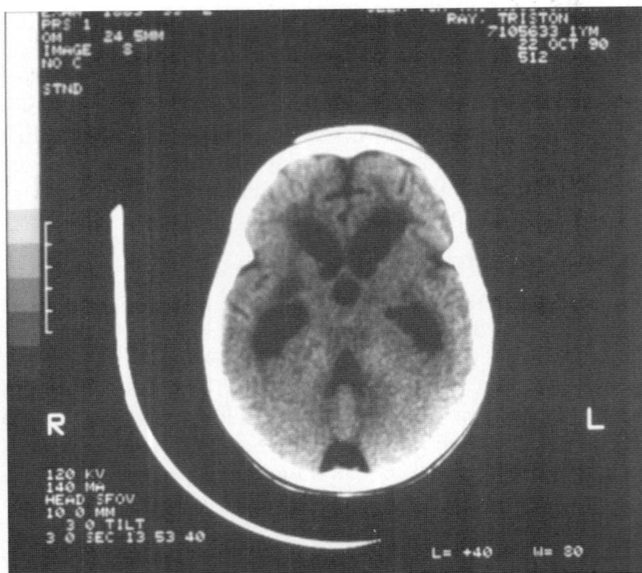

■ **FIGURE 34-13.** A computed tomography scan of the head demonstrating the communicating hydrocephalus that is typical of tuberculous meningitis.

focal neurologic signs. The final stage of disease is marked by coma, hypertension, decerebrate and decorticate posturing, and eventual death. Rapid confirmation of tuberculous meningitis can be extremely difficult with wide variability in cerebrospinal fluid characteristics and nonreactive tuberculin skin tests in 40% of cases. Although some older studies reported normal chest radiographs in 50% of cases, more recent reports have indicated that 80% of young children with tuberculous meningitis have significant abnormality on the chest radiograph. Since improved outcomes are associated with early treatment, empirical antituberculosis therapy should be instituted for any child with basilar meningitis and hydrocephalus or cranial nerve involvement that has no other apparent cause.

■ DIAGNOSIS

Tuberculin Skin Test

The tuberculin skin test is the most widely employed test for the diagnosis of tuberculosis and LTBI in children. Although currently available tuberculin skin test antigens are not 100% sensitive or specific, no better diagnostic test is widely available. The sensitivity and specificity of the tuberculin skin test are significantly affected by a number of factors that will be reviewed in this section.

Infection with *M. tuberculosis* produces a delayed-type hypersensitivity reaction to specific antigenic components of the bacilli that are contained in extracts of culture filtrates called "tuberculins." There are two types of tuberculin purified protein derivatives (PPDs) commercially available in the United States: Tubersol (Aventis Pasteur, Inc., Swiftwater, Pennsylvania) and Aplisol (Parke-Davis Pharmaceuticals, Morris Plains, New Jersey). A batch of PPD called PPD-S, produced by Siebert and Glenn in 1939, serves as the standard reference material worldwide. All PPD lots are bioassayed to demonstrate equal potency to PPD-S. The standard test dose of a commercially available preparation is defined as the dose of that product that is biologically equivalent to 5 tuberculin units (TU) of PPD-S. A small amount of Tween 80 is added to the diluent of PPD to reduce adsorption by glass and plastic. To minimize adsorption and subsequent loss of potency, tuberculin should never be transferred between containers and should be delivered as soon as possible after transfer to the syringe. Tuberculin should be stored refrigerated and in the dark.

The tuberculin reaction is the classic example of a delayed-type hypersensitivity reaction. In response to the antigen, previously sensitized T cells release lymphokines that induce local vasodilation, edema, fibrin deposition, and recruitment of other inflammatory cells.[42] The reaction to tuberculin typically begins 5 to 6 hours after injection and reaches maximal induration at 48 to 72 hours. In some individuals, the reaction may peak after 72 hours, and the largest reaction size should be considered the result. Vesiculation and necrosis rarely occur. In these cases, repeat tuberculin testing should be avoided.

Variability of the results of tuberculin skin test may be reduced by careful attention to details of administration and reading. A one-fourth to one-half inch, 27-gauge needle and tuberculin syringe are employed to inject 0.1 mL of 5-TU PPD intradermally (Mantoux method) into the volar or dorsal aspect of the forearm. If done correctly, a discrete, pale wheal 6 to 10 mm in diameter is produced. If the first test is administered improperly, another test dose may be employed at once in a site several centimeters from the original site.

The tuberculin skin test should be read 48 to 72 hours following injection. The diameter of induration should be measured transversely to the long axis of the forearm and recorded in millimeters. Use of the ball-point pen method developed by Sokal minimizes interobserver variability.[43] A dispassionate, trained health professional should interpret all skin tests.

A nonreactive tuberculin skin test does not exclude LTBI or tuberculosis. A number of factors can diminish tuberculin reactivity resulting in a false-negative reaction (Box 34-1) and decreased tuberculin test sensitivity. The administration of live-attenuated vaccines results in immune system suppression that appears more than 48 hours after vaccination. Tuberculin skin testing may be performed either on the same day as vaccination with live virus or 4 to 6 weeks later. Studies have demonstrated that up to 10% of immunocompetent children with reactive anergy tests and culture-confirmed tuberculosis have false-negative reactions to tuberculin testing.[44,45] In many of these children, tuberculin skin test conversion occurs after several months of treatment, suggesting that the infection was recently acquired or resulted in suppression of the immune response. Skin testing results were available in nearly all (95.4%) children reported to have newly diagnosed tuberculosis in the United States between 1993 and 2001. Eleven percent of these children had negative skin test results as defined by Centers for Disease Control and Prevention guidelines.[23] Of note, children who were diagnosed with disseminated or meningeal tuberculosis were less likely to have a positive tuberculin skin test result (57.6% and 54.6%, respectively) than those with pulmonary tuberculosis (90.6%).

A number of factors have been associated with false-positive tuberculin reactions and decreased tuberculin test specificity. Since some antigens in PPD are shared with other mycobacteria, false-positive reactions can occur in children who have been infected with other mycobacteria, including after receipt of BCG. Exposure to NTM varies geographically and generally results in smaller, transient indurations than those of *M. tuberculosis.* There is no reliable method of distinguishing BCG-induced

BOX 34-1 Factors Causing False-Negative Tuberculin Skin Tests

Factors Related to the Person Being Tested

- Infections
  - Viral (measles, mumps, chickenpox, HIV)
  - Bacterial (typhoid fever, brucellosis, typhus, leprosy, pertussis, overwhelming tuberculosis, tuberculosis pleurisy)
  - Fungal (blastomycosis)
- Live virus vaccinations (measles, mumps, polio, varicella)
- Metabolic derangements (chronic renal failure)
- Low protein states (severe protein depletion, afibrinogenemia)
- Diseases affecting lymphoid organs (Hodgkin's disease, lymphoma, chronic leukemia, sarcoidosis)
- Drugs (corticosteroids and other immunosuppressive agents)
- Age (newborns, elderly patients with "waned" sensitivity)
- Stress (surgery, burns, mental illness, graft-versus-host reactions)

Factors Related to the Tuberculin Used

- Improper storage (exposure to light and heat)
- Improper dilutions
- Chemical denaturation
- Contamination
- Adsorption (partially controlled by adding Tween 80)

Factors Related to the Method of Administration

- Injection of too little antigen
- Subcutaneous injection
- Delayed administration after drawing into syringe
- Injection too close to other skin tests

Factors Related to Reading the Test and Recording Results

- Inexperienced reader
- Conscious or unconscious bias
- Error in recording

cross-reactivity from reactivity secondary to mycobacterial infection. The degree of BCG cross-reactivity is dependent on a number of factors, including strain of BCG employed, age and nutritional status at vaccination, frequency of skin testing, and years since vaccination.[46–48] In most studies of children who received a BCG vaccine during the newborn period, only 50% react to tuberculin testing at 12 months and 80% to 90% lose reactivity within 2 to 3 years. Although BCG vaccination of older children or adults results in greater initial and more persistent cross-reactivity, most of these individuals lose cross-reactivity within 10 years of vaccination. In general, the tuberculin skin test should be interpreted the same for patients who have not received a BCG vaccination.

In any population, the likelihood that a positive tuberculin skin test represents true infection (positive predictive value) increases as the prevalence of infection with *M. tuberculosis* increases in that population.[49] The prevalence of LTBI is 5% to 10% in the general population of the United States and 0.1% to 1% for children entering school in many parts of the United States. Screening populations without a known or likely exposure to *M. tuberculosis* is likely to result in false-positive reactions. In contrast, the prevalence of LTBI in close contacts of individuals with infectious tuberculosis or immigrants from high-burden countries is much higher. The tuberculin skin test has high positive predictive value in these target populations.[49]

Interpretation of tuberculin skin test reactions is based on risk for infection (Box 34-2).[49] For children with the greatest risk for infection or developing tuberculosis after infection, or those with suspected tuberculosis disease, an induration greater than or equal to 5 mm is considered positive. For children with an increased risk for infection or progression to disseminated disease, an induration greater than or equal to 10 mm is considered positive. Children with low risk must have an induration greater than or equal to 15 mm to be considered positive. Varying interpretation of the tuberculin skin test based on a child's individual risk factors minimizes false-positive and false-negative readings.

In the United States, it is preferable to screen children for LTBI risk factors with a questionnaire and complete tuberculin

BOX 34-2 Definitions of a Positive Tuberculin Skin Test Results in Infants, Children, and Adolescents

Induration ≥5 mm

Children in close contact with known or suspected contagious case of tuberculosis disease

Children suspected to have tuberculosis disease:

- Findings on chest radiograph consistent with active or previously active tuberculosis
- Clinical evidence of tuberculosis disease

Children receiving immunosuppressive therapy or with immunosuppressive conditions, including HIV infection

Induration ≥10 mm

Children at increased risk for disseminated disease:

- Those younger than 4 years of age
- Those with other medical conditions, including Hodgkin's disease, lymphoma, diabetes mellitus, chronic renal failure, or malnutrition

Children with increased exposure to tuberculosis disease:

- Those born, or whose parents were born, in high-prevalence regions of the world
- Those frequently exposed to adults who are HIV infected, homeless, users of illicit drugs, residents of nursing homes, incarcerated or institutionalized, or migrant farm workers
- Those who travel to high-prevalence regions of the world

Induration ≥15 mm

Children 4 years of age or older without any risk factors

skin testing when risk factors are identified.[49] For this approach to be effective, clinicians performing tuberculin screening must be familiar with local tuberculosis case rates and community demographics. Local public health authorities should play an active role in determining interpretation of skin test reactions for individual communities.

Laboratory Diagnosis

Careful attention to the details of specimen collection and handling can optimize the isolation and identification of *M. tuberculosis.* A variety of specimens can be collected, including sputum, induced sputum, gastric aspirates, bronchial washings, bronchoalveolar lavage, transbronchial biopsy, urine, blood, cerebral spinal fluid, tissue, and other body fluids.[50,51] Since children cannot easily produce sputum, gastric aspirates are frequently obtained. Collection of gastric aspirates usually entails hospitalization to acquire about 50 mL of early morning gastric contents after the child has fasted for at least 8 to 10 hours, and preferably while he or she is still in bed.[52] Alternatively, trained public health nurses may perform this procedure in the home. *M. tuberculosis* may be recovered from gastric aspirates in roughly 40% of children with radiographic evidence of significant pulmonary disease.[53,54] The culture yields are as high as 70% in infants. Since many specimens will contain an abundance of bacteria other than mycobacteria, specimens should be collected in a sterile fashion and held under conditions that minimize growth of contaminating organisms.

Diagnostic tests for tuberculosis either detect the presence of *M. tuberculosis* in a clinical sample or demonstrate a host response to the organism. Methods for diagnosis of tuberculosis are summarized in Table 34-2.

Staining and Microscopic Examination

Acid-fast staining and microscopic examination are the easiest, quickest, and least expensive diagnostic procedures. However, these methods can only provide physicians with preliminary confirmation of the diagnosis due to the inability to differentiate between *M. tuberculosis* and NTM. Additionally, there must be 5000 to 10,000 bacilli present per millimeter of specimen to allow detection of the bacteria in stained smears, resulting in low sensitivity in children. Acid-fast stain of gastric aspirates are positive in fewer than 10% of children with pulmonary tuberculosis.

Culture

Culture is the most important laboratory test for the diagnosis and management of tuberculosis. A positive culture may result from as few as 10 organisms per milliliter of specimen. Growth of bacilli is necessary for precise speciation and drug susceptibility testing. Genotyping of the organism may be useful to identify epidemiologic links. Unfortunately, bacteriologic confirmation of tuberculosis in children is generally poor. For example, in the United States from 1985 to 1988, 90% of adult tuberculosis cases were bacteriologically confirmed, compared with 28% in children.[23] In three studies evaluating the role of bronchoscopy, only 13% to 62% of cultures in children with pulmonary tuberculosis were positive.[54–56] The yield from gastric aspirate was higher in these studies. Bronchoscopy can be useful to define anatomy or clarify the diagnosis, but it cannot be recommended solely to collect culture specimens in children.

Sputum smear or sputum culture were available for only 25% of children reported to have newly diagnosed tuberculosis in the United States between 1993 and 2001.[23] A small percentage of children were sputum smear or culture positive. Rates of positivity varied dramatically among age groups. Sputum smears were positive from 10.3% of 10- to 14-year-olds, 1.8% of 5- to 9-year-olds, and 1.6% of children under 5 years. Similarly, cultures were positive among 21.3% of 10- to 14-year-olds, 5% of 5- to 9-year-olds, and 4.2% of children under 5 years. Among all childhood tuberculosis cases, only 2.4% had positive gastric aspirate smears and 8.5% had gastric aspirate cultures positive for *M. tuberculosis.*[23] Since only positive gastric aspirate results were reported, it is impossible to know how many specimens were obtained or to determine the yield of this procedure.

It is clear that reliance on detection of *M. tuberculosis* using available methods will lead to misdiagnosis of the majority of cases of childhood pulmonary tuberculosis. Even in developed countries, the gold standard for diagnosis of childhood tuberculosis is a triad of (1) an abnormal chest radiograph and/or clinical findings consistent with tuberculosis; (2) a positive tuberculin skin test result; and (3) a history of recent (<1 year) contact with a person with contagious tuberculosis. The specificity of this triad is quite high. If the results of drug susceptibility testing on the organism isolated from the contact case are available, obtaining a culture from the child adds little sensitivity or specificity to the diagnosis if the triad is present.[50,51]

TABLE 34-2. Summary of laboratory methods for diagnosis of tuberculosis

Identification Method	Test System	Use
Culture		
Conventional media	Colony morphology (3–5 weeks)	Preliminary identification
	Biochemical tests	Species identification
Radiometric methods	Positive growth index (5–14 days)	Differentiates *Mycrobacterium tuberculosis* from nontuberculosis mycrobacteria species
Chromatography	HPLC mycolic acid profile	Speciates all common mycrobacteria
	Gas chromatography-fatty acid profile	Speciates all common mycrobacteria
DNA probes	Gen-Probe ACCUPROBES	Identifies *M. tuberculosis* complex, *M. avium, M. intracellulare-avium* complex, *M. kansasii, M. gordonae*
	Syngene SNAP probes	Identifies *M. tuberculosis* complex, *M. avium* complex
Rapid Direct Tests		
Direct smear	Acid-fast or fluorochrome stains	Easy, inexpensive, moderately sensitive
Antigen and Antibody	EIA agglutination tests	Simple, low-cost, modestly specific, but not highly sensitive
Nucleic acid detection	PCR amplification	Moderately sensitive, highly specific, technically complex

EIA, enzyme immunoassay; HPLC, high-performance liquid chromatography; PCR, polymerase chain reaction.

DNA Methodologies

DNA probe methods utilize nucleic acid hybridization with specifically labeled sequences to rapidly detect complementary sequences in the test sample. A variety of systems are commercially available. Although the *M. tuberculosis* complex probe tests have been 99% to 100% specific, the methods' dependence on large numbers of bacilli means they can be used in the laboratory only on cultured organisms.[57]

Direct detection of the DNA of *M. tuberculosis* directly in clinical samples has been performed using nucleic acid amplification, most often utilizing polymerase chain reaction (PCR). Most techniques have used the mycobacterial insertion element IS6110 as the DNA marker for *M. tuberculosis* complex organisms.[58] Evaluation of PCR for childhood tuberculosis has been limited. When compared with the clinical diagnosis of pulmonary tuberculosis in children, the sensitivity of PCR on sputum or gastric aspirates has varied from 25% to 83%, and the specificity has varied from 80% to 100%.[59–61] A negative PCR never eliminates tuberculosis as a diagnostic possibility, and a positive result does not completely confirm it. The major use for PCR in children may be when the diagnosis of tuberculosis is not readily established on clinical and epidemiologic grounds, and perhaps for children with HIV infection for whom a greater variety of causes of pulmonary disease must be considered.

Antibody and Antigen Detection

There has been some progress in the development of methods to detect *M. tuberculosis* antibodies and antigens. The use of enzyme immunoassay (EIA) has been reviewed extensively. Although a variety of serologic methods have been used to detect antibodies against *M. tuberculosis,* most of these tests lack sensitivity and specificity and are not available in the United States. Similarly, a large collection of techniques has been used to detect antigen, including competitive inhibition EIA, latex agglutination, reverse passive-hemagglutination, double-antibody sandwich EIA, and inhibition EIA. Three assays have been designed to detect specific protein antigen and offer the most promise with sensitivities and specificities ranging from 85% to 100% and 93% to 97%, respectively.[62–64]

THERAPY

Latent Tuberculosis Infection

The majority of children with *M. tuberculosis* infection have LTBI. These children have a reactive tuberculin skin test, normal chest radiograph, no clinical evidence of tuberculosis, and presumed infection with low numbers of viable tubercle bacilli. For the following reasons, children with LTBI should receive treatment: (1) infants and children less than 5 years of age have been infected recently, so risk for progression to disease is high; (2) risk for severe disease, including meningitis and disseminated disease, is inversely related to age; (3) children with LTBI have more years at risk for the development of disease later in life; and (4) children with LTBI become adults who may transmit organisms if they develop disease.[49]

Several large clinical trials have demonstrated the efficacy of isoniazid (INH) to reduce the risk for tuberculosis in children with LTBI. In 1958, the U.S. Public Health Service (USPHS) conducted a randomized trial to prevent tuberculosis disease in boarding schools in Alaska.[65] Two dosing regimens of INH were studied, 1.25 mg/kg/day versus 5 mg/kg/day given for 6 months to 1701 attendees 5 to 20 years of age either 5 days per week or daily. In 10 years of follow-up, participants who received the higher dose of INH had significantly less progression to tuberculosis (1.9%, 10 of 513) than participants receiving the lower dose (5.8%, 31 of 536). The study also demonstrated that an intermittent therapy course (5 days per week) was efficacious. Additional randomized controlled trials completed by the USPHS in the 1950s and 1960s found the protective efficacy of INH treatment of LTBI to be approximately 90% when analysis was restricted to compliant participants.[66] Secondary analysis of two USPHS household contact studies has suggested that the efficacy of INH treatment of LTBI plateaus at 9 to 10 months of therapy.[67] Similarly, in a study among the Inuit in Alaska, a second year of INH treatment did not result in additional benefit beyond that conferred by the first year of treatment.[68,69] Although the International Union against Tuberculosis and Lung Disease (IUATLD) has evaluated the efficacy of various durations of INH therapy in adults with LTBI, similar studies have not been conducted in children.[51] The current recommendation for treatment of LTBI in children is 9 months of INH given either daily (10–15 mg/kg, maximum 300 mg), or twice weekly (20–30 mg/kg, maximum 900 mg) under directly observed therapy (DOT).[49]

Rifampin has been used for the treatment of LTBI in children and adolescents when INH was not tolerated or the child was exposed to an INH-resistant, rifampin-susceptible source.[70] However, no controlled clinical trials have been completed. A 3- to 4-month regimen consisting of rifampin and INH has been used in England.[71] This observational study analyzing administrative data suggests that this regimen is effective, but no controlled trials have been reported.

LTBI treatment should be tailored according to host-immune factors, drug susceptibility, tolerance, and compliance (Table 34-3). If drug susceptibility is not available for either the child or source case, INH is recommended. No studies of the efficacy of LTBI treatment in HIV-infected children have been reported. Although some experts recommend extended treatment to 12 months, the American Academy of Pediatrics (AAP) currently recommends a 9-month INH regimen or at least a 6-month rifampin regimen. In most cases, treatment may be given daily without observation. If compliance is inadequate, intermittent DOT may be instituted. Treatment of MDR tuberculosis infection must be individualized and should be delivered via DOT.

Window Prophylaxis

After infection with *M. tuberculosis,* children may take up to 3 months to develop an immune response sufficient to produce a positive tuberculin skin test result.[72] Children younger than 5 years have a short incubation period and may develop severe disease prior to developing skin test reactivity.[73] Due to this risk, children with a negative tuberculin skin test and known or suspected exposure to an adult with contagious tuberculosis should receive treatment for LTBI. Tuberculin skin testing should be repeated 3 months after initial exposure. If the second tuberculin skin test result is negative, therapy may be discontinued. If skin test conversion occurs, therapy should be continued for the full 9 months.

Tuberculosis Disease

Principles of Treatment

Treatment of tuberculosis is designed to prevent the complications of disease in the host and the development of drug-resistance

TABLE 34-3. Preventive regimens for latent tuberculosis infection in children

Resistance Pattern of Source Case	Antimycobacterial Agent Dosage and Duration	Comments
INH susceptible or unknown	INH, 10 mg/kg as single daily dose × 9 mo (maximum 300 mg per dose) INH, 20–30 mg/kg twice weekly × 9 mo (maximum, 900 mg per dose)	Optimal duration for children is debated CDC and AAP recommend 9 mo Intermittent schedule should be given only by DOT
INH resistant or INH not tolerated	RIF, 10 mg/kg as single daily dose × 6 mo (maximum, 600 mg per dose)	
MDR-TB (resistant to INH and RIF)	Guided by susceptibility testing on a child or source case isolate	Should be provided in consultation with an expert DOT strongly recommended

AAP, American Academy of Pediatrics; ATS, American Thoracic Society; CDC, Centers for Disease Control and Prevention; DOT, directly observed therapy; IDSA, Infectious Disease Society of America; INH, isoniazid; MDR-TB, multidrug-resistant tuberculosis; RIF, rifampin.

in the organism. Antimycobacterial agents should be bactericidal and effective against intra- and extracellular organisms. Three or more drugs are used empirically for initial therapy and adjusted when susceptibility testing is available. Initial use of a single agent will select for emergence of a dominantly resistant population of bacilli. Therapy is provided for extended periods of time via DOT. Length of therapy is dependent on site of infection.

Pulmonary Tuberculosis

The first-line drugs used to treat tuberculosis in children are shown in Table 34-4.

Many therapeutic trials have been reported in children with pulmonary tuberculosis. A 6-month regimen consisting of INH and rifampin was effective in some patients with isolated hilar adenopathy.[74] Limited data are available to support a 6-month, INH-rifampin regimen for the treatment of pulmonary tuberculosis.[75] At least a dozen studies have examined the efficacy of 6-month regimens consisting of three or more drugs in children with pulmonary tuberculosis. The most common regimen studied consisted of INH and rifampin, supplemented with pyrazinamide during the first 2 months. Most trials used daily therapy for the first 2 months, followed by daily or twice weekly therapy to complete 6 months. In all of these trials, the overall success rate was greater than 95% for cure and 99% for significant improvement during a 2-year follow-up.

In children with suspected INH-susceptible pulmonary tuberculosis, the recommended treatment is a 6-month regimen consisting of INH and rifampin supplemented during the first 2 months with pyrazinamide. Daily administration of the drug during the first 2 weeks to 2 months may be followed by twice-weekly therapy to complete 6 months. All treatment for tuberculosis disease should be administered by DOT unless there is a compelling reason to avoid it.

In children or adolescents with adult-type pulmonary tuberculosis or epidemiologic circumstances suggesting an increased risk for infection with drug-resistant organisms, the American Thoracic Society (ATS) recommends an initial 2-month treatment

TABLE 34-4. Commonly used drugs for the treatment of tuberculosis in children

Drug	Dosage Forms	Daily Dose (mg/kg)	Twice Weekly Dose (mg/kg/day)	Maximum Dose
Ethambutol	Tablets: 100 mg 400 mg	15–20	50	Daily: 1 g Twice weekly: 2.5 g
Isoniazid*†	Scored tablets: 100 mg 300 mg Syrup: 10 mg/mL	10–15	20–30	Daily: 300 mg Twice weekly: 900 mg
Pyrazinamide	Scored tablets: 500 mg	15–30	50	2 g
Rifampin*	Capsules: 150 mg 300 mg Syrup: Formulated in syrup from capsules	10–20	10–20	Daily: 600 mg Twice weekly: 600 mg
Streptomycin (IM administration)	Vials: 1 g 4 g	20–40	20–40	Daily: 1 g

*Rifamate is a capsule containing 150 mg of isoniazid and 300 mg of rifampin. Two capsules provide the usual adult (>50 kg body weight) daily doses of each drug.

†Most experts advise against the use of isoniazid syrup due to instability and a high rate of gastrointestinal adverse reaction (diarrhea, cramps).

IM, intramuscular.

phase consisting of daily administration of four drugs, including INH, rifampin, pyrazinamide, and ethambutol, followed by 4 months of INH and rifampin twice-weekly therapy administered under DOT if the organism is susceptible to both drugs.[76] Although there have been concerns about the use of ethambutol in children, because it can cause optic neuritis that is difficult to detect in children, this adverse effect is extraordinarily rare in children and should not preclude the use of ethambutol with extensive or drug-resistant disease.

The optimal treatment of pulmonary tuberculosis in children and adolescents with HIV infection is unknown. The AAP and ATS recommend that initial therapy should consist of at least three drugs for the first 2 months and that total duration of therapy should be at least 9 months.[76]

Extrapulmonary Tuberculosis

Controlled trials have not been reported for children with extrapulmonary tuberculosis. In general, recommended treatment for extrapulmonary tuberculosis is the same as for pulmonary tuberculosis. Osteotuberculosis and tuberculous meningitis are exceptions. Recommended treatment of osteotuberculosis includes (1) 9 to 12 months of INH and rifampin or (2) 6 months of INH and rifampin supplemented by two other drugs during the first 2 months of therapy. There are inadequate data to support any 6-month treatment regimen for tuberculous meningitis. Recommended regimens consist of four-drug treatment during the initial 2 months followed by 7 to 10 months of therapy with INH and rifampin.

Drug-Resistant Tuberculosis

The incidence of drug-resistant tuberculosis is increasing in the United States and the world because of poor adherence by the patient, the availability of some antituberculosis drugs in noncontrolled over-the-counter formulations, and poor management by physicians. In the United States, approximately 10% of *M. tuberculosis* isolates are resistant to at least one drug. Certain epidemiologic factors—disease in an Asian, Eastern European or Hispanic immigrant to the United States, homelessness in some communities, and history of previous antituberculosis therapy—correlate with drug resistance in adult patients. Patterns of drug resistance in children tend to mirror those found in adult patients in the population.[77] Outbreaks of drug-resistant tuberculosis in children occurring at schools have been reported. Individual cases also have been recognized. The key to determining drug resistance in childhood tuberculosis usually comes from the drug susceptibility results of the infectious adult contact case's isolate.

Therapy for drug-resistant tuberculosis is successful only when at least two bactericidal drugs are given to which the infecting strain of *M. tuberculosis* is susceptible.[78] If only one effective drug is given, secondary resistance will develop. When INH resistance is considered a possibility on the basis of epidemiologic risk factors or the identification of an INH-resistant source case isolate, an additional drug—usually ethambutol—should be given initially to the child until the exact susceptibility pattern is determined and a more specific regimen can be designed. Exact treatment regimens must be tailored to the specific pattern of drug resistance. The duration of therapy usually is extended to at least 9 to 12 months if either INH or rifampin can be used and to at least 18 to 24 months if resistance to both drugs is present. Occasionally, surgical resection of a diseased lung or lobe is required. An expert in tuberculosis always should be involved in the management of children with drug-resistant tuberculosis infection or disease.

Adjunctive Therapy

Pyridoxine (25–50 mg/day) is recommended for infants, children, and adolescents treated with INH who have nutritional deficiencies, symptomatic HIV infection, and diets low in milk or meat products. Pyridoxine is also recommended for breastfeeding infants.

Corticosteroid administration is beneficial in the management of children when the host inflammatory reaction contributes significantly to tissue damage or impaired function. Administration of corticosteroids decreases mortality and morbidity in patients with tuberculous meningitis by reducing vasculitis, inflammation, and intracranial pressure. Corticosteroid administration may significantly reduce compression of the tracheobronchial tree caused by hilar lymphadenopathy, associated with miliary disease, and alveolar-capillary block, pleural effusion, and pericardial effusion.[76] Prednisone (1–2 mg/kg/day for 4 to 6 weeks) is most commonly employed.

Follow-up during Antituberculosis Therapy

The major goals of following children during treatment include promoting adherence, monitoring for toxicity and adverse effects of therapy, and assessing clinical response. Patients should be evaluated monthly and receive only enough medication for the interval between follow-up appointments. During the initial phase of treatment, clinicians should assess potential noncompliance. Children with missed appointments and poor compliance should be referred to the responsible public health agency that likely has programs incorporating incentives or behavioral modification.

Rates of adverse reactions caused by antituberculosis medications are low among children. INH and rifampin are associated with elevated serum alanine aminotransferase in less than 2% of children and rarely cause overt hepatitis. Elevated alanine aminotransferase levels are generally less than three times normal values, do not predict hepatotoxicity, and are not an indication for discontinuing treatment. Routine biochemical monitoring is not indicated if the child does not have liver disease and is not taking other hepatotoxic drugs. It is preferable to educate caregivers relative to potential adverse events and clinical symptoms (abdominal pain, vomiting, jaundice) necessitating medical evaluation and discontinuation of medication.

Frequent radiographic monitoring is not indicated. Since improvement of intrathoracic tuberculosis in children occurs slowly, chest radiographs are generally obtained at diagnosis, 1 or 2 months into therapy, and at completion of therapy. Radiographic resolution of hilar lymphadenopathy and associated pulmonary lesions may not occur for 2 to 3 years following treatment. A normal chest radiograph appearance is not necessary for completion of therapy. If resolution of radiographic abnormalities has not occurred by completion of therapy, radiographs may be obtained at 3- to 6-month intervals to assess continued improvement.

CONTROL AND PREVENTION

Bacillus Calmette-Guérin Vaccination

BCG vaccines have been administered to nearly 4 billion people and have been routinely administered to newborns in most countries except the United States and the Netherlands. Nevertheless, the immune response to BCG and its mechanism of action are not well understood. Large clinical trials have shown the efficacy of BCG vaccination to range from 0 to 80%. A number of factors contribute to the heterogeneity of results from these trials, including eligibility criteria, strain of vaccine employed, vaccine administration, diagnostic criteria, disease surveillance, and environmental factors.[79] Although BCG does not prevent primary pulmonary tuberculosis, studies have demonstrated that BCG vaccination decreases the risk for developing severe forms of disease, including meningitis and miliary tuberculosis.[80,81] The clinical presentation of tuberculosis disease in individuals who have received a BCG vaccination tends to be similar to that in nonimmunized persons.

Public Health Involvement

Childhood tuberculosis, defined as tuberculosis in children younger than 15 years, is a direct reflection of the incidence of adult tuberculosis within a community. Childhood tuberculosis usually represents recent transmission from an infectious adult or adolescent and is considered a sentinel event in public health. In response to a case of childhood tuberculosis, health departments should conduct an investigation to identify the source of infection and additional cases.

Health departments conduct several different types of investigations. Contact investigations evaluate all contacts of an infectious adult or adolescent for tuberculosis disease or LTBI. Contact investigations have the highest yield for finding infected persons and are considered the cornerstone of reducing the incidence of tuberculosis in developed nations. Source case investigations evaluate all contacts of a child with tuberculosis to identify an infectious adult or adolescent and other infected persons. Source case investigations are less successful because source cases frequently do not reside in the United States if the child is foreign born or has lived abroad. It is the health department's responsibility to ensure that all persons with suspected tuberculosis are identified and evaluated promptly and that appropriate treatment is prescribed and successfully completed. These responsibilities are accomplished through a number of activities, including epidemiologic surveillance and investigations, direct provision of diagnostic services and treatment, and monitoring of treatment decisions and outcomes. The health department should employ a tailored approach for each patient that accounts for individual needs to ensure completion of therapy. DOT is the preferred, core management strategy to assure adherence and involves providing the antituberculous drugs directly to the patients and watching that he or she swallows the medications.

PULMONARY DISEASE CAUSED BY NONTUBERCULOUS MYCOBACTERIA

EPIDEMIOLOGY

Several problems compound the epidemiologic description of NTM infections in humans.[82] The NTM rarely cause fatal infection, so mortality statistics are not helpful. There is no public health mandatory reporting of NTM infection. Smaller laboratories that isolate NTM often do not refer isolates to reference laboratories for identification and drug-susceptibility testing, so statistics from even these laboratories grossly underestimate the incidence of NTM disease. Finally, isolating an NTM from a clinical specimen often is not sufficient for the diagnosis of disease. Distinguishing among saprophytes, colonizers, and truly pathogenic organisms requires clinical correlation not available from laboratory reports.

Transmission of NTM to humans occurs from environmental sources, including soil, water, dust, and aerosols. There is some evidence that MAC strains more commonly isolated from persons with disease tend to be aerosolized preferentially from standing water, suggesting that aerosols from natural water are a primary source of NTM causing human infection. MAC species are found frequently in animals, particularly birds and swine, which may be an important natural reservoir for the organisms. There is little evidence to suggest that animal-to-human transmission is a major factor in human infection. There is no evidence supporting human-to-human transmission of NTM.

The number of reports of clusters of health care–associated disease caused by various species of NTM is growing. Most common are outbreaks by the rapid growers. Both clusters and sporadic NTM infections have been associated with a variety of surgical procedures, including sternal wound infections after open heart surgery, augmentation mammoplasty prostheses, corneal surgery, implantation of pressure equalizing tubes in the tympanic membranes, and insertion of central venous catheters. A number of outbreaks or pseudo-outbreaks of respiratory tract colonization caused by various NTM species have been associated with contaminated ice machines, showers, potable water supplies, infected laboratory supplies, contamination of topical anesthesia, or tap water in hospitals. Contamination of bronchoscopes or bronchoscopy supplies has been implicated in some of these outbreaks.[83] Isolation of the same NTM species from bronchoscopy samples in two or more patients in a short period of time should prompt an investigation to determine possible sources of contamination, especially if isolation of the NTM is a surprising finding.

The true incidence of disease caused by NTM is difficult to estimate. In the United States, there are marked geographic variations in rates and species. The best data come from a survey of state and major city health department laboratories conducted between 1981 and 1983.[82] Over 5000 patients diagnosed with NTM disease were investigated. The estimated annual prevalence of all NTM disease was 1.8 cases per 100,000 population, about 15% of the prevalence of tuberculosis. Rates were higher for MAC (1.3 per 100,000), *M. kansasii* (0.3 per 100,000), and the rapid growers (0.2 per 100,000).

The species of NTM causing infection and the anatomic site of disease vary by age. Among children, the majority of NTM infections are in the superficial cervical lymph nodes.[84] MAC is responsible for 95% of cases of NTM lymphadenitis in children. In contrast, the lung is the most common site of NTM disease in adults. MAC organisms account for about 60% of the respiratory isolates, and *M. kansasii* constitutes about 25% of isolates. Early reports of MAC pulmonary disease found that most patients were males who had some form of preexisting lung disease such as emphysema and frequent alcohol abuse. In contrast most recent reports have shown the majority of adults with MAC pulmonary disease to be women with no preexisting lung disease.[85] Up to 70% of adults with *M. kansasii* pulmonary infections have preexisting lung disease, while the majority of adults with pulmonary infection due to rapid grower NTM do not have chronic lung disease.[86] The majority of children with pulmonary infection by an NTM species have not had previous lung disease.[87,88]

An increasing number of cases of isolation of various NTM from the respiratory secretions of patients with CF has been reported recently.[89–98] It is difficult to compare these reports since the methods of ascertainment, culture methods, and definitions of colonization, infection, and disease differed widely. Since these patients have severe and progressive underlying pulmonary disease, it is difficult to assess the role of an NTM infection in an individual patient's clinical course. While the isolation of an NTM from a CF patient's sputum may be associated with a worsening clinical and radiographic course, in other patients the presence of an NTM may be an incidental finding. The CF patients from whom an NTM is isolated tend to be older and sicker patients. The incidence of isolation of an NTM has ranged from as high as 24% to a low of 3% in CF patients. MAC is isolated most frequently, but *M. kansasii, M. gordonae,* and the rapid growers also may be encountered. Repeated isolation of the same species of NTM from a CF patient with an otherwise unexplained decline in clinical scoring, who responds to appropriate antimycobacterial therapy, represents the strongest clinical definition of NTM lung disease in a CF patient.[90] However, a recent autopsy study showed that only two of six CF patients who had multiple respiratory cultures positive for an NTM had histologic evidence of disease (granuloma formation).[97]

Clinical disease due to NTM is common in adults and children with acquired immunodeficiency syndrome (AIDS). Occasionally, the NTM pulmonary infection mimics tuberculosis. Although isolated pulmonary infection with an NTM in patients with AIDS has been reported, pulmonary involvement usually is part of a widely disseminated infection. MAC accounts for 85% of cases, followed in incidence by *M. kansasii* and *M. gordonae*. Disseminated disease with pulmonary involvement caused by NTM has been described rarely in patients with other immunodeficiency states (leukemia, lymphoma, and other malignancies) and in otherwise normal children.[99,100] NTM disease also has been reported in adults and children after organ transplantation.

CLINICAL MANIFESTATIONS

The clinical manifestations of NTM infection depend on the species involved and the presence of underlying conditions in the patient. Although any organ system can be infected by NTM, certain organisms preferentially infect the lung (Table 34-5). This section will present the most common manifestations of pulmonary NTM infection in nonimmunocompromised hosts, then will present special considerations in patients with CF and immunocompromised hosts.

TABLE 34-5. Most common sites of infection for nontuberculous mycobacteria

Site	Most Common Organisms
Pulmonary	*M. kansasii, M. avium* complex, *M. xenopi, M. haemophilum, M. fortuitum, M. chelonae, M. gordonae* (rare), *M. szulgai* (rare), *M. malmoense* (rare)
Lymph node	*M. avium* complex, *M. kansasii, M. fortuitum, M. abscessus* (rare)
Disseminated	*M. avium* complex, *M. kansasii, M. fortuitum, M. chelonae, M. xenopi, M. haemophilum, M. gordonae* (rare)

Mycobacterium Kansasii

Mycobacterium kansasii is a mycobacterium that produces pigment when grown on solid media. This organism is antigenically and clinically most closely related to *M. tuberculosis*. Infection with *M. kansasii* usually occurs in adults with underlying pulmonary disease, especially smoking-related chronic obstructive pulmonary disease (COPD). Other predisposing lung conditions include bronchogenic carcinoma, bronchiectasis, silicosis, and prior tuberculosis. In contrast, most of the children and adolescents reported with *M. kansasii* pulmonary disease have not had underlying chronic conditions. In the United States, *M. kansasii* is most common in the Midwest and Southwest states, especially in Texas.[101] In the United States, the majority of cases of tuberculosis occur among racial and ethnic minorities, while the majority of cases of *M. kansasii* pulmonary disease occur among whites.

In adolescents and adults, the most common signs and symptoms associated with pulmonary disease due to *M. kansasii* are similar to those found with tuberculosis. Most patients experience significant cough and sputum production. About one third of patients have hemoptysis and about one fourth experience chest pain. Fever, chills, and night sweats occur in a minority of patients but over half of the patients experience significant weight loss. Younger children with pulmonary disease due to *M. kansasii* tend to have fewer systemic signs and symptoms and may present with only a cough and failure to gain weight.

The typical radiographic findings of *M. kansasii* pulmonary disease in adolescents and adults are similar to those found with tuberculosis (Fig. 34-14). About half of patients experience cavitation with or without fibrosis. Pleural scarring and nonspecific pulmonary infiltrates also are common. Adenopathy is rare, and pleural effusion is exceedingly rare. Most pulmonary findings occur in the apical regions, but abnormalities may be found throughout the lungs. Almost 40% of patients experience bilateral disease.

The chest radiographic findings of *M. kansasii* disease in children are similar to those found with primary tuberculosis. Adenopathy is common, and many children experience the type of collapse-consolidation lesion seen in primary tuberculosis. Calcification of enlarged hilar lymph nodes is common. It is likely that some cases of *M. kansasii* pulmonary disease in children are misdiagnosed as tuberculosis since *M. kansasii* often causes a positive tuberculin skin test result, and cultures from

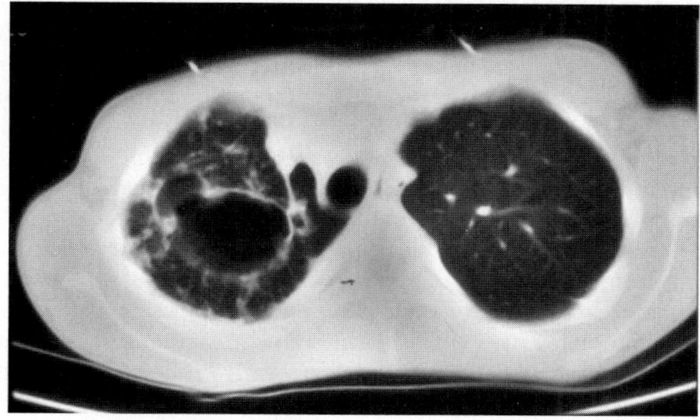

FIGURE 34-14. Computed tomography scan of an adolescent with pulmonary disease caused by *M. kansasii*.

children with either disease usually are negative. Fortunately, the treatment of pulmonary tuberculosis in children also is effective against most cases of *M. kansasii* disease.

Mycobacterium Avium Complex

Among immunocompetent hosts, pulmonary disease caused by MAC is much more common in adults than in adolescents or younger children. The average age of patients is about 60 years. About half the patients have preexisting pulmonary disease, including prior tuberculosis, COPD, silicosis, diabetes mellitus, or lung cancer. Patients without other pulmonary diseases tend to be younger and more frequently female.

Clinical features in adults tend to be similar in patients with or without predisposing conditions. Indolent productive cough with purulent sputum is the primary symptom in the majority of cases. It is common for patients to experience symptoms for up to 6 months or longer before the correct diagnosis is established. Hemoptysis is uncommon, and persistent fever is rare. Constitutional symptoms such as weight loss, night sweats, and malaise are uncommon.

The radiographic findings of MAC pulmonary disease in adults are similar to those with tuberculosis. About one third of patients have cavitation. However, a wide variety of radiographic findings can be seen, including lobar consolidation, interstitial disease, nodular or alveolar infiltrates, and involvement of multiple lobes. In one study among adults without preexisting lung disease, the most common presenting radiographic pattern was multiple discrete pulmonary nodules seen in 71% of patients.[85]

Because of the difficulty of proving the diagnosis by culture, the reported incidence of pulmonary MAC disease among children and adolescents is low. Almost all reported patients have been younger than 5 years, and the clinical and radiographic patterns of disease have been similar to that of primary tuberculosis in children.[87,88] Many of the reported cases have been treated initially as tuberculosis but were further investigated because of unusual clinical or radiographic findings or failure to respond to the usual antituberculosis chemotherapy. The majority of affected children have been immunocompetent with no underlying pulmonary disease. Most infected children have come to clinical attention due to fairly mild but persistent symptoms, including cough and low-grade fever; more severe systemic signs or symptoms are rare. Localized wheezing has been noted occasionally, and the diagnosis of an aspirated foreign body considered. Systemic symptoms such as fever, night sweats, and weight loss are uncommon.

The most common radiographic presentation of MAC pulmonary disease in children has been enlargement of the hilar or mediastinal lymph nodes, sometimes with accompanying atelectasis. Some children have experienced repeated episodes of fever and cough, interpreted as recurrent pneumonia or bronchitis. They have more extensive radiographic involvement, probably due to partial or complete obstruction of a bronchus caused by an enlarged lymph node. Several children have had the acute onset of pneumonia with extensive pulmonary infiltrates in one or several lobes, with a subsequent prolonged chronic course. Involvement of the pleura is exceedingly rare.

Several children with MAC pulmonary disease have undergone bronchoscopy, which generally demonstrates granulation tissue within one of the bronchi. Narrowing of the bronchus due to external compression from an enlarged lymph node can be seen occasionally. It is often the culture of this endobronchial material that leads to the isolation of MAC. Histologic examination of this tissue usually reveals caseating granulomas, which helps confirm the diagnosis of mycobacterial disease.

It becomes obvious that the diagnosis of pulmonary MAC disease in children is exceedingly difficult. MAC organisms can be isolated from the oral and gastric secretions of healthy children. Repeated isolation of the organism in association with an abnormal chest radiograph is suggestive but not diagnostic of significant infection. Definitive diagnosis usually requires invasive procedures such as bronchoscopy or pulmonary/endobronchial biopsy. It is likely that some cases of MAC pulmonary disease are misdiagnosed as tuberculosis on the basis of clinical and radiographic findings, a mild reaction to the tuberculin skin test, and spontaneous resolution over several months with or without appropriate chemotherapy. A key element in the differential diagnosis is the family investigation for tuberculosis. A case of "unusual" pulmonary tuberculosis in a child whose family has no risk factors for tuberculosis and whose other family members test negative for tuberculosis infection or disease should be investigated for the possibility of MAC pulmonary disease.[102]

Rapidly Growing Mycobacteria

Reports of pulmonary disease in children caused by the rapidly growing mycobacteria (*M. fortuitum, M. chelonae, M. abscessus*) are rare. The importance of these infections among adults was not well recognized until the 1970s. Adult patients with this infection are predominantly white, female nonsmokers who have prolonged periods from the onset of symptoms to the correct diagnosis of their disease. Cough is an almost universal presenting symptom, whereas constitutional symptoms become important only with progression of disease. In one study, the mean length of time from onset of symptoms to the first positive culture was 26 months.[103] The most common symptoms at diagnosis are cough, sputum production, and malaise. Fever eventually occurs in about one half of patients and hemoptysis occurs in about one third. About one third of patients have other pulmonary conditions, including preexisting tuberculosis, COPD, or bronchiectasis.

In contrast to other pulmonary mycobacterial infections, the most frequent patterns on chest radiograph of infections due to the rapidly growing mycobacteria are interstitial and alveolar densities. In many cases, the densities have a reticulonodular appearance. Cavitation is unusual, occurring in only 15% of patients. The upper lobes of the lung are involved in almost 90% of patients, but infiltrates may occur in any part of the lung.

Other Mycobacterial Species

Many other mycobacterial species have been associated with pulmonary disease. Pathogenic species of NTM that are rare causes of disease in the United States are *M. xenopi, M. malmoense,* and *M. szulgai.*[104] Most of the reported infections have been in adults; these infections appear to be exceedingly rare in children or not clinically detected. The pulmonary disease caused by these organisms tends to be similar to that caused by tuberculosis. The most common symptoms are productive cough, weight loss, and night sweats. The typical chest radiograph shows upper lobe densities, sometimes with cavitation. Pulmonary infections in children more often are similar to those caused by primary tuberculosis, including mild cough but a minimum of other signs and symptoms, and enlarged hilar or mediastinal lymph nodes, sometimes with associated pulmonary findings. The diagnosis of pulmonary disease in children caused by these other mycobacteria is exceedingly difficult. However, if any mycobacterium is isolated from a gastric or bronchoscopy specimen from a child, consideration must be given to the mycobacterium as a cause of pulmonary disease.

Mycobacterial Infection in Cystic Fibrosis

The incidence of finding various NTM organisms in the sputum of patients with CF appears to be increasing. It is not clear whether the apparent increase is due to changing conditions or treatments, or whether CF patients are living longer and having a greater opportunity of becoming colonized. Early retrospective reports of NTM in CF sputum indicated it to be an infrequent problem. However, the true incidence of NTM colonization or infection was not evaluated since not all patients were tested. More recent prospective studies suggested a much higher incidence of NTM in some CF centers.[88,89]

A fundamental problem in caring for CF patients with NTM in the sputum is determining the difference between colonization and disease. The ATS has published guidelines for the diagnosis of NTM disease in normal hosts. For individuals without cavitary lesions on chest radiography, the criteria include (1) two or more sputum smears being acid-fast positive and/or resulting in moderate to heavy growth on cultures; (2) failure of the sputum cultures to convert to negative with either bronchial hygiene or 2 weeks of antimicrobial drug therapy; and (3) other reasonable causes for pulmonary disease have been excluded. Unfortunately, these guidelines fail to differentiate among NTM species and are difficult to apply to CF patients with significant underlying pulmonary disease. The chronic suppurative lung disease present in patients with CF makes them likely hosts for NTM colonization. Malnutrition, diabetes mellitus, and frequent use of corticosteroids are additional risk factors for NTM infections in many CF patients. The signs and symptoms that may differentiate NTM colonization from disease in the healthy host include productive cough, dyspnea, hemoptysis, malaise, and fatigue. Older patients with advanced CF display these signs and symptoms much of the time, limiting the ability to use them as clinical indicators of NTM-related disease. Thus, in the CF patient, clinical indicators of tissue damage often cannot adequately differentiate between NTM colonization and disease. The differentiation can be made only at autopsy in some cases, and even patients with repeated positive sputum cultures for NTM may not have histologic evidence of mycobacterial disease.[97] The species of NTM found in the sputum of a CF patient may help in deciding whether colonization or disease is most likely present. Finding an unusual organism such as *M. kansasii* is more likely to reflect disease. While asymptomatic colonization with rapidly growing mycobacteria occurs, finding these organisms often is associated with a worsening course of pulmonary disease.[91] Of course, when a positive acid-fast stain of sputum from a CF patient is found, the possibility of disease caused by *M. tuberculosis* must be addressed immediately due to both personal and public health considerations. However, in general, patients with CF tend to have few risk factors for infection and disease caused by *M. tuberculosis*.

Because of the difficulty in distinguishing colonization from disease caused by NTM in CF patients, it is difficult to state specific clinical manifestations for NTM disease. Some patients experience an increase in cough and sputum production, weight loss, and other systemic symptoms such as night sweats or chronic low-grade fevers. Hemoptysis, which can occur in CF patients without NTM infection, appears to be no more frequent with NTM infection. Rarely, new cavitary lesions accompany the finding of an NTM in the sputum. Pleural involvement is exceedingly rare. There is some suggestion that NTM preferentially cause apical disease, but this is an inconsistent finding among various clinical reports. Some patients experience a decline in pulmonary function in association with the new acquisition of NTM in the sputum.

Unfortunately, a standard definition of NTM disease in CF patients, using clinical, radiographic, and pulmonary function testing results, is probably not possible. It is fairly clear that a single isolation of an NTM in the sputum of a CF patient who is not experiencing a decline in pulmonary function probably represents colonization, and treatment is not necessary. Repeated isolation of the same species of NTM from the sputum in association with declining pulmonary function is more suggestive, but not diagnostic, of invasive NTM infection of the lung.[89] In many cases, a fairly short (1–2 months) trial of antimycobacterial therapy, directed at the specific species of NTM isolated, may help to determine if significant infection is present.

DIAGNOSIS

Nonspecific laboratory tests such as blood counts, erythrocyte sedimentation rate, urinalysis, and serum chemistry tests usually are normal in children with NTM infections and have no diagnostic value. The key to diagnosis is a high level of suspicion based on epidemiologic factors and the clinical presentation. Acid-fast stains of appropriate specimens may give an early clue to the presence of NTM infection. However, the number of NTM in most fluids and tissues is small, and acid-fast smears are frequently negative when an infection is present. In pulmonary disease among adults and adolescents, a positive acid-fast smear of sputum is much more likely to indicate tuberculosis than an NTM infection. A negative acid-fast smear never should dissuade the clinician from considering the diagnosis of NTM disease in an appropriate setting. Similarly, histologic studies of involved tissues are helpful if classic granulomatous changes are demonstrated, but many NTM infections in immunocompetent hosts cause only nonspecific acute and/or chronic inflammation without granulomas, especially with infections due to the rapidly growing mycobacteria.

Skin testing with PPD from *M. tuberculosis* and other mycobacteria has been used to detect infection with NTM. Infections caused by MAC commonly are associated with reactions to a standard tuberculin skin test from 0 to 10 mm. Larger reactions are seen but rarely exceed 18 mm. Infections by *M. marinum, M. kansasii,* and *M. fortuitum* frequently are associated with tuberculin skin test reactions of 10 to 20 mm. Of course, similar reactions may be caused by infection with *M. tuberculosis.* Determining the source of the skin reaction to tuberculin can be difficult and is dependent largely on epidemiologic factors, especially the likelihood that the child has been exposed to an adult with pulmonary tuberculosis. Investigation of adults in the child's environment usually is necessary to help determine if a moderate (8–15 mm) reaction is due to infection with *M. tuberculosis* or a cross-reaction due to infection by NTM, and a negative skin test result never rules out NTM infection.

The most direct method for diagnosing NTM infection is appropriate mycobacterial culture of involved fluid or tissue specimens. Unfortunately, many NTM are plentiful in the environment and frequently are encountered as colonizers or agents that produce infection but not recognizable disease. The decision

BOX 34-3 Aids for Distinguishing Nontuberculous Mycobacterial Disease from Colonization

1. Quantity of growth—usually increased with disease
2. Repeated isolation of the same organism
3. Site of origin—from closed anatomic site more meaningful
4. Species of mycobacterium—is it a usual pathogen?
5. Host risk factors—immunocompromise, cystic fibrosis, smoking

whether or not NTM disease requiring treatment is present rests with the clinician's judgment of the extent of tissue invasion associated with isolation of the organism. Wolinsky[105] suggested considering five clinical facts (Box 34-3). Disease in the respiratory tract usually is associated with moderate to heavy growth of NTM, not with just a few colonies on the plate. However, light growth in normally sterile body fluids or tissues—such as a lung biopsy or bronchoscopy specimen—may indicate invasive disease. Repeated isolation of the same species of NTM, particularly if it is one known to be associated with pulmonary disease, is much more likely to indicate invasive infection. Finally, the risk factors of the host for significant NTM disease are a strong consideration in determining the clinical significance of a positive culture.

TREATMENT

Specific treatment of NTM disease depends on the location and extent of the infected tissue, the capability of the host's immune system, and the species of NTM involved. Surgery plays a more important role in the management of NTM disease than it does for tuberculosis because chemotherapy is relatively ineffective and most NTM infections are localized to one site. However, one important exception is the lung, where surgery is usually not employed, except in far advanced disease.

Many infections due to NTM are similar in clinical presentation to tuberculosis. An important initial consideration in managing all mycobacterial infections is to be certain that *M. tuberculosis* is not the actual pathogen. Usually, until an NTM is identified by culture, treatment is directed at tuberculosis for both therapeutic and infection control/public health reasons. This principle is especially important for young children with pulmonary disease, immunodeficiency, or AIDS, since dissemination of tuberculosis in these patients may have disastrous consequences. Fortunately, the clinical progression of most NTM infections is slow enough that a period of several weeks to several months of treatment directed at tuberculosis will not have a significant deleterious effect on the outcome of the NTM infection.

Determining the species of NTM causing infection is critical for directing chemotherapy. In general, *M. kansasii, M. marinum, M. xenopi, M. gordonae, M. malmoense, M. szulgai,* and *M. haemophilum* are susceptible to one or more of the standard antituberculosis drugs. Treatment of the rapidly growing mycobacterial and most strains of MAC require other antibiotics. The drugs used most commonly to treat NTM infections are listed in Table 34-6. Multiple-drug therapy is used for all infections because of the propensity of mycobacteria to develop resistance to single drugs. The treatment regimens that have been developed are based on either limited clinical trials in adults or anecdotal evidence from small series or case reports.

There have been no clinical trials published concerning the treatment of pulmonary NTM infections in children and adolescents. Treatment regimens are derived from clinical trials in adults or the best opinions of "experts." However, pulmonary

TABLE 34-6. Commonly used drugs for nontuberculous mycobacterial infections

Drug	How Supplied	Dosage (mg/kg/day) and Route of Administration*	Susceptible Pathogens
Amikacin	100-, 500-mg, 1-g vials	15–30 IM or IV in 3 doses; max: 1.5 g/day	*M. fortuitum, M. chelonae, M. ulcerans, M. avium* complex
Azithromycin			*M. avium* complex, *M. fortuitum, M. chelonae, M. abscessus*
Cefoxitin	1-, 2-, 10-g vials	100–200 IV in 4 doses; max:12 g/day	*M. fortiuitum, M. chelonae*
Ciprofloxacin	250-, 500-, 750-mg tabs	500–1500 total in 2 doses	*M. avium* complex
Clarithromycin	250-mg tabs, 25 mg/mL, 50 mg/mL suspension	10–30 PO in 2 doses	*M. avium* complex, *M. fortuitum, M. chelonae, M. abscessus, M. marinum*
Clofazamine	50-,100-mg caps	1–2 PO in 1 dose; max: 100 mg/day	*M. avium* complex
Doxycycline	100-mg tabs	2–4 PO in 2 doses; max: 200 mg/day	*M. marinum*
Erythromycin	250-, 500-mg tabs 250, 500 mg/mL suspensions	40 PO in 4 doses; max: 4 g/day	*M. fortuitum, M. chelonae*
Ethambutol	100-, 400-mg tabs	15–20 PO in 1 dose; max: 1 g/day	*M. kansasii, M. marinum, M. xenopi, M. ulcerans, M. gordonae, M. avium* complex
Isoniazid	100-, 300-mg caps	10–20 PO in 1 dose; max: 300 mg/day	*M. kansasii, M. xenopi, M. gordonae*
Rifampin	150-, 300-mg caps	10–20 PO in 1 dose; max: 600 mg/day	*M. kansasii, M. xenopi, M. marinum, M. ulcerans, M. gordonae, M. avium* complex
Streptomycin	1-, 4-g vials	20–40 IM in 1 dose; max: 1 g/day	*M. avium* complex
Trimethoprim-sulfamethoxazole	80-, 160-mg (TMP) tabs 40 mg/5 mL (TMP) suspension	8–20 mg of TMP PO in 2 doses; max: 2 g/day	*M. marinum, M. fortuitum, M. chelonae, M. ulcerans*

IM, intramuscular; IV, intravenous; PO, orally; TMP, trimethoprim.

disease tends to be more extensive in adults than in children, and the number of infecting organisms is probably much larger in adults. There is general agreement on which drug regimens should be used for initial treatment of NTM infections, but it is unclear what the optimal length of therapy is for children with NTM infection. There is no consensus about the proper treatment of NTM pulmonary infections in patients with CF. Most clinicians begin an initial regimen of appropriate therapy for several months to determine if a clinical response will occur.

Since *M. kansasii* is rarely a contaminant, all patients from whom *M. kansasii* is isolated in respiratory secretions should be considered to have disease and treated accordingly. There have been no randomized controlled trials of treatment for disease caused by *M. kansasii*. There have been, however, several retrospective and prospective studies of various treatment regimens.[9] A key drug for successful treatment has been rifampin. The current recommendation for treatment of pulmonary disease caused by *M. kansasii* is a regimen of INH, rifampin, and ethambutol given daily for 9 to 12 months. Clarithromycin also can be used in multidrug regimens. Although pyrazinamide is used commonly for the treatment of tuberculosis, all isolates of *M. kansasii* are resistant to it. The use of intermittent drug regimens or shorter courses have not been adequately studied to permit their recommendation. Untreated strains of *M. kansasii* are always susceptible to rifampin, INH, ethambutol, and streptomycin. Because the concentrations of drugs used in susceptibility testing were chosen for their usefulness with *M. tuberculosis* and not *M. kansasii*, some *M. kansasii* isolates may be reported to be resistant to streptomycin or INH. However, these isolates are susceptible to slightly higher drug concentrations, and laboratory reports showing resistance to the lower concentrations have no clinical or therapeutic significance as long as a rifampin-containing regimen is being used.

Recommended regimens for treatment of MAC pulmonary disease are based entirely on results of clinical trials in adults.[106] The traditional recommendation for initial therapy of patients with MAC pulmonary disease was a four-drug regimen consisting of INH, rifampin, ethambutol, and streptomycin. The usual recommendation for duration of therapy for the oral drugs was 18 to 24 months and for at least 12 months after sputum cultures became negative.

The recent advent of the new macrolides clarithromycin and azithromycin, and the successful use of these drugs for treatment of disseminated MAC infection in patients with AIDS, has led to their use in the treatment of pulmonary MAC disease in patients without AIDS. Preliminary results of several trials have shown that substituting clarithromycin for INH in an initial four-drug regimen leads to a more rapid conversion of sputum to negative, and higher cure and lower relapse rates. Resistance to clarithromycin emerges rapidly if the drug is used alone but does not occur frequently when combined with other drugs. Most experts now recommend inclusion of clarithromycin in the initial regimen for pulmonary disease due to MAC; the most commonly used other drugs are rifampin, ethambutol, and streptomycin. It is not yet known if the inclusion of clarithromycin in the initial regimen leads to a shorter necessary total length of therapy. Although there is only anecdotal information available for treatment of MAC pulmonary infections in children, the regimens used in adults seem to be effective in children.

Treatment of deep-seated infections due to the rapidly growing mycobacteria can be especially difficult. There have been no randomized clinical trials of various combination of antibiotics. Most treatment is based on susceptibility testing of the specific isolate because susceptibility patterns vary greatly even within a species. The most commonly used drugs include amikacin, cefoxitin, azithromycin, doxycycline, linezolide, sulfonamides, and clarithromycin. Successful treatment of disease due to *M. fortuitum* often can be accomplished with chemotherapy alone. The adult patients with *M. abscessus* infection who were cured usually received amikacin and cefoxitin or imipenem for 1 to 3 months followed by surgical excision.

Unlike tuberculosis, NTM infections of the lungs in adults often require resectional surgery for complete cure.[107] Even with optimal chemotherapy, eradication of the organism cannot be achieved in some patients. A combined approach with an initial period of chemotherapy to contain the infection followed by resectional surgery and a more prolonged course of chemotherapy leads to much higher cure rates. This is difficult surgery and it is important that the thoracic surgeon has some experience. There are no published guidelines about the need for resectional surgery in children with NTM pulmonary infection. In several case reports, excision of endobronchial lesions has been accomplished during bronchoscopy, but resection of lung parenchyma has seldom been performed and does not appear to be necessary in most cases.

PREVENTION

Little is known about the prevention of NTM infection in any group of individuals. Because these organisms are ubiquitous in nature, it is impossible to prevent exposure to them except under the most extreme circumstances. There has been no recommendation about the use of chemotherapy to prevent NTM infection in patients with CF. Until the risk factors for acquisition of NTM by CF patients are better delineated, chemoprophylaxis will not be a part of the management of these patients.

REFERENCES

1. Tortoli E: Impact of genotypic studies on mycobacterial taxonomy. The new mycobacteria of the 1990's. Clin Microbiol Rev 2003;16: 319–354.
2. Hale YM, Pfyfler GE, Salfinger M: Laboratory diagnosis of mycobacterial infections. New tools and lessons learned. Clin Infect Dis 2001;33: 834–845.
3. American Thoracic Society: Diagnosis and treatment of disease caused by nontuberculous mycobacteria. Am J Respir Crit Care Med 1997;156 (Suppl):1–25.
4. Schluger NW, Rom WN: The host immune response to tuberculosis. Am J Respir Crit Care Med 1998;157:679–691.
5. Smith S, Jacobs RF, Wilson CB: Immunobiology of childhood tuberculosis. A window on the ontology of cellular immunity. J Pediatr 1997;131:16–26.
6. Barnes PF, Grisso CL, Abrams JS, Band H, Rea TH, Modlin RL: Gamma delta T lymphocytes in human tuberculosis. J Infect Dis 1992;165:506–512.
7. Barnes P: Immunology of tuberculosis. Semin Pediatr Infect Dis 1993;4:232–245.
8. Vidal SM, Malo D, Vogan K, Skamene E, Gros P: Natural resistance to infection with intracellular parasites. Isolation of a candidate for Bcg. Cell 1993;73:469–485.
9. Daniel T, Boom W, Ellner J: Immunology of Tuberculosis. In: Reichman L, Hershfield E, eds: Tuberculosis. A Comprehensive International Approach. New York: Marcel Dekker, 2000, pp 187–214.
10. Marais BJ, Gie RP, Schaaf HS, Hesseling AC, Obihara CC, Starke JJ, Enarson DA, Donald PR, Beyers N: The natural history of childhood intrathoracic tuberculosis. A critical review of literature from the pre-chemotherapy era. Int J Tuberc Lung Dis 2004;8:392–402.
11. Horsburgh CR Jr: Priorities for the treatment of latent tuberculosis infection in the United States. N Engl J Med 2004;350:2060–2067.

12. Comstock GW: Tuberculosis in twins. A re-analysis of the Prophit survey. Am Rev Respir Dis 1978;117:621–624.
13. Kallman F, Reisner D: Twin studies on the significance of genetic factors in tuberculosis. Am Rev Respir Dis 1942;117:549–574.
14. Shaw MA, Collins A, Peacock CS, Miller EN, Black GF, Sibthorpe D, Lins-Lainson Z, Shaw JJ, Ramos F, Silveira F, Blackwell JM: Evidence that genetic susceptibility to Mycobacterium tuberculosis in a Brazilian population is under oligogenic control. Linkage study of the candidate genes NRAMP1 and TNFA. Tuberc Lung Dis 1997;78:35–45.
15. Newport MJ, Huxley CM, Huston S, Hawrylowicz CM, Oostra BA, Williamson R, Levin M: A mutation in the interferon-gamma-receptor gene and susceptibility to mycobacterial infection. N Engl J Med 1996;335: 1941–1949.
16. Jouanguy E, Altare F, Lamhamedi S, Revy P, Emile JF, Newport M, Levin M, Blanche S, Seboun E, Fischer A, Casanova JL: Interferon-gamma-receptor deficiency in an infant with fatal bacille Calmette-Guerin infection. N Engl J Med 1996;335:1956–1961.
17. Altare F, Durandy A, Lammas D, Emile JF, Lamhamedi S, Le Deist F, Drysdale P, Jouanguy E, Doffinger R, Bernaudin F, Jeppsson O, Gollob JA, Meinl E, Segal AW, Fischer A, Kumararatne D, Casanova JL: Impairment of mycobacterial immunity in human interleukin-12 receptor deficiency. Science 1998;280:1432–1435.
18. Comstock G: Epidemiology of tuberculosis. In: Reichman LB, Hershfield E, eds: Tuberculosis. A Comprehensive International Approach. New York: Marcel Dekker, 2000, pp 129–148.
19. Saiman L, Aronson J, Zhou J, Gomez-Duarte C, Gabriel PS, Alonso M, Maloney S, Schulte J: Prevalence of infectious diseases among internationally adopted children. Pediatrics 2001;108:608–612.
20. Sutter RW, Haefliger E: Tuberculosis morbidity and infection in Vietnamese in Southeast Asian refugee camps. Am Rev Respir Dis 1990;141:1483–1486.
21. Starke JR: Transmission of *Mycobacterium tuberculosis* to and from children and adolescents. Semin Pediatr Infect Dis 2001;12:115–123.
22. Centers for Disease Control and Prevention: Reported tuberculosis in the United States, 2003. Atlanta: U.S. Department of Health and Human Services, 2004.
23. Nelson LJ, Schneider E, Wells CD, Moore M: Epidemiology of childhood tuberculosis in the United States, 1993–2001. The need for continued vigilance. Pediatrics 2004;114:333–341.
24. Kochi A: The global tuberculosis situation and the new control strategy of the World Health Organization. Tubercle 1991;72:1–6.
25. American Thoracic Society, Centers for Disease Control and Prevention: Diagnostic Standards and Classification of Tuberculosis in Adults and Children. Am J Respir Crit Care Med 2000;161:1376–1395.
26. Wallgren A: Primary pulmonary tuberculosis in childhood. Am J Dis Child 1935;49:1105–1136.
27. Marais BJ, Grie RP, Schaaf HS, Starke JR, Hasseling AC, Donald PR, et al: A proposed radiologic classification of childhood intra-thoracic tuberculosis. Pediatr Radiol 2004;34:886–894.
28. Schaaf HS, Gie RP, Beyers N, Smuts N, Donald PR: Tuberculosis in infants less than 3 months of age. Arch Dis Child 1993;69:371–374.
29. Lincoln EM, Harris LC, Bovornkitti S, Carretero R: Endobronchial tuberculosis in children. Am Rev Tuberc Pulm Dis 1958;77:39–61.
30. Salazar GE, Schmitz TL, Cama R, Sheen P, Franchi LM, Centeno G, et al: Pulmonary tuberculosis in children in a developing country. Pediatrics 2001;108:448–453.
31. Lincoln EM, Gilbert L, Morales SM: Chronic pulmonary tuberculosis in individuals with known previous primary tuberculosis. Dis Chest 1960;38:473–482.
32. Lincoln EM, Davies PA, Bovornkitti S: Tuberculous pleurisy with effusion in children. Am Rev Tuberc 1958;77:271–289.
33. Levine H, Metzger W, Lacera D, Kay L: Diagnosis of tuberculous pleurisy by culture of pleural biopsy specimen. Arch Intern Med 1970;126:269–271.
34. Hussey G, Chisolm T, Kibel M: Miliary tuberculosis in children. A review of 94 cases. Pediatr Infect Dis J 1991;10:832–836.
35. Schuit KE: Miliary tuberculosis in children. Am J Dis Child 1979;133: 583–585.
36. Blusse van Oud-Alblas HJ, van Vliet ME, Kimpen JL, de Villiers GS, Schaaf HS, Donald PR: Human immunodeficiency virus infection in children hospitalized with tuberculosis. Ann Trop Paediatr 2002;22:115–123.
37. Chan SP, Birnbaum J, Rao M: Clinical manifestations and outcome of tuberculosis in children with acquired immunodeficiency syndrome. Pediatr Infect Dis J 1996;15:443–447.
38. Dandapat MC, Mishra BM, Dash SP, Kar PK: Peripheral lymph node tuberculosis. Review of 80 cases. Br J Surg 1990;77:911–912.
39. Schuit KE, Powell DA: Mycobacterial lymphadenitis in childhood. Am J Dis Child 1978;132:675–677.
40. Doerr CA, Starke JR, Ong LT: Clinical and public health aspects of tuberculous meningitis in children. J Pediatr 1995;127:27–33.
41. Rich A, McCodock H: The pathogenesis of tuberculosis meningitis. Bull Johns Hopkins Hosp 1933;52:5–9.
42. Tsicopoulos A, Hamid Q, Varney V, Ying S, Moqbel R, Durham SR, Kay AB: Preferential messenger RNA expression of Th1-type cells (IFN-gamma+, IL-2+) in classical delayed-type (tuberculin) hypersensitivity reactions in human skin. J Immunol 1992;148:2058–2061.
43. Sokol JE: Measurement of delayed skin test responses. N Engl J Med 1975;293:501–502.
44. Lincoln E, Gilbert L, Morales S: Chronic pulmonary tuberculosis in individuals with known previous primary tuberculosis. Chest 1960;38:473–478.
45. Steiner P, Rao M, Victoria MS, Jabbar H, Steiner M: Persistently negative tuberculin reactions. Their presence among children with culture positive for *Mycobacterium tuberculosis* (tuberculin-negative tuberculosis). Am J Dis Child 1980;134:747–750.
46. Karalliedde S, Katugaha LP, Uragoda CG: Tuberculin response of Sri Lankin children after BCG vaccination at birth. Tubercle 1987;68:33–38.
47. Menzies R, Vissandjee B, Amyot D: Factors associated with tuberculin reactivity among the foreign-born in Montreal. Am Rev Respir Dis 1992;146: 752–756.
48. Menzies R, Vissandjee B: Effect of bacille Calmette-Guerin vaccination on tuberculin reactivity. Am Rev Respir Dis 1992;145:621–625.
49. Pediatric Tuberculosis Collaborative Group: Targeted tuberculin skin testing and treatment of latent tuberculosis infection in children and adolescents. Pediatrics 2004;114:1175–1201.
50. Shingadia D, Novelli V: Diagnosis and treatment of tuberculosis in children. Lancet 2003;3:624–632.
51. Eamranond P, Jaramillo E: Tuberculosis in children. Reassessing the need for improved diagnosis in global control strategies. Int J Tuberc Lung Dis 2001;5:594–603.
52. Pomputius WF 3rd, Rost J, Dennehy PH, Carter EJ: Standardization of gastric aspirate technique improves yield in the diagnosis of tuberculosis in children. Pediatr Infect Dis J 1997;16:222–226.
53. Kendig J: Pulmonary and pleural tuberculosis. Semin Pediatr Infect Dis 1993;4:241–249.
54. Abadco DL, Steiner P: Gastric lavage is better than bronchoalveolar lavage for isolation of *Mycobacterium tuberculosis* in childhood pulmonary tuberculosis. Pediatr Infect Dis J 1992;11:735–738.
55. de Blic J, Azevedo I, Burren CP, Le Bourgeois M, Lallemand D, Scheinmann P: The value of flexible bronchoscopy in childhood pulmonary tuberculosis. Chest 1991;100:688–692.
56. Chan S, Abadco DL, Steiner P: Role of flexible fiberoptic bronchoscopy in the diagnosis of childhood endobronchial tuberculosis. Pediatr Infect Dis J 1994;13:506–509.
57. Musial CE, Tice LS, Stockman L, Roberts GD: Identification of mycobacteria from culture by using the Gen-Probe Rapid Diagnostic System for *Mycobacterium avium* complex and *Mycobacterium tuberculosis* complex. J Clin Microbiol 1988;26:2120–2123.
58. American Thoracic Society: Rapid diagnostic tests for tuberculosis. What is the appropriate use? Am J Respir Crit Care Med 1997;15:1804–1814.
59. Delacourt C, Poveda JD, Chureau C, Beydon N, Mahut B, de Blic J, et al: Use of polymerase chain reaction for improved diagnosis of tuberculosis in children. J Pediatr 1995;126:703–709.
60. Gomez-Postrana DG, Torronteras R, Caro P, Anguita ML, Lopez-Barrio AM, Andres A, et al: Comparison of Amplicor, in-house polymerase chain reaction and conventional culture for the diagnosis of tuberculosis in children. Clin Infect Dis 2001;332:17–22.
61. Smith KC, Starke JR, Eisenach K, Ong LT, Denby M: Detection of *Mycobacterium tuberculosis* in clinical specimens from children using a polymerase chain reaction. Pediatrics 1996;97:155–160.
62. Wadee AA, Boting L, Reddy SG: Antigen capture assay for detection of a 43-kilodalton *Mycobacterium tuberculosis* antigen. J Clin Microbiol 1990;28:2786–2791.
63. Sada E, Aguilar D, Torres M, Herrera T: Detection of lipoarabinomannan as a diagnostic test for tuberculosis. J Clin Microbiol 1992;30:2415–2418.
64. Sada E, Brennan PJ, Herrera T, Torres M: Evaluation of lipoarabinomannan for the serological diagnosis of tuberculosis. J Clin Microbiol 1990;28: 2587–2590.
65. Comstock GW, Hammes LM, Pio A: Isoniazid prophylaxis in Alaskan Boarding schools. A comparison of two doses. Am Rev Respir Dis 1969; 100:773–779.
66. Ferebee SH: Controlled chemoprophylaxis trials in tuberculosis. A general review. Bibl Tuberc 1970;26:28–106.
67. Comstock GW: How much isoniazid is needed for prevention of tuberculosis among immunocompetent adults? Int J Tuberc Lung Dis 1999;3:847–850.

68. Comstock GW, Ferebee SH: How much isoniazid is needed for prophylaxis? Am Rev Respir Dis 1970;101:780–782.
69. Comstock GW, Baum C, Snider DE Jr: Isoniazid prophylaxis among Alaskan Eskimos. A final report of the bethel isoniazid studies. Am Rev Respir Dis 1979;119:827–830.
70. Villarino ME, Ridzon R, Weismuller PC, Elcock M, Maxwell RM, Meador J, Smith PJ, Carson ML, Geiter LJ: Rifampin preventive therapy for tuberculosis infection. Experience with 157 adolescents. Am J Respir Crit Care Med 1997;155:1735–1738.
71. Ormerod LP: Rifampicin and isoniazid prophylactic chemotherapy for tuberculosis. Arch Dis Child 1998;78:169–171.
72. Jacobs RF, Starke JR: Tuberculosis in children. Med Clin North Am 1993;77:1335–1351.
73. Nolan RJ Jr: Childhood tuberculosis in North Carolina. A study of the opportunities for intervention in the transmission of tuberculosis to children. Am J Public Health 1986;76:26–30.
74. Jacobs RF, Abernathy RS: The treatment of tuberculosis in children. Pediatr Infect Dis 1985;4:513–517.
75. Reis FJ, Bedran MB, Moura JA, Assis I, Rodrigues ME: Six-month isoniazid-rifampin treatment for pulmonary tuberculosis in children. Am Rev Respir Dis 1990;142:996–999.
76. American Thoracic Society/Centers for Disease Control and Prevention/Infectious Diseases Society of America. Treatment of tuberculosis. Am J Respir Crit Care Med 2003;167:603–662.
77. Steiner P, Rao M, Mitchell M: Primary drug-resistant tuberculosis in children: Correlation of drug-susceptibility patterns of matched patient and source-case strains of Mycobacterium tuberculosis. Am J Dis Child 1985;139:780–782.
78. Swanson DS, Starke JR: Drug-resistant tuberculosis in pediatrics. Pediatr Clin North Am 1995;42:553–581.
79. Colditz G, Brewer T, Berkey C, Wilson ME, Burdick E, Fineberg HV, et al: Efficacy of BCG vaccine in the prevention of tuberculosis. Meta-analysis of the published literature. JAMA 1994;271:698–702.
80. Smith PG: Retrospective assessment of the effectiveness of BCG vaccination against tuberculosis using the case-control method. Tubercle 1982;63:23–35.
81. Wunsch Filho V, de Castilho EA, Rodrigues LC, Huttly SR: Effectiveness of BCG vaccination against tuberculous meningitis. A case-control study in Sao Paulo, Brazil. Bull WHO 1990;68:69–74.
82. O'Brien RJ, Geiter LJ, Snider DE Jr: The epidemiology of nontuberculous mycobacterial disease in the United States. Am Rev Respir Dis 1987;135:1007–1014.
83. Tobin-D'Angelo MJ, Blass MA, de Rio C, Halvosa JS, Blumberg HM, Horsburgh CR Jr: Hospital water as a source of *Mycobacterium avium* complex isolates in respiratory specimens. J Infect Dis 2004;189:98–104.
84. Wolinsky E: Mycobacterial lymphadenitis in children. A prospective study of 105 nontuberculous cases with long-term follow-up. Clin Infect Dis 1995;20:954–963.
85. Prince DS, Peterson DD, Steiner RM, Gottlieb JE, Scott R, Israel HL, et al: Infection with *Mycobacterium avium* complex in patients without predisposing conditions. N Engl J Med 1989;321:863–868.
86. Daley CL, Griffith DE: Pulmonary disease caused by rapidly growing mycobacteria. Clin Chest Med 2002;23:623–632.
87. Fergie JE, Milligon TW, Henderson BM, Stafford WW: Intrathoracic *Mycobacterium avium* complex infection in immunocompetent children. Case report and review. Clin Infect Dis 1997;24:250–253.
88. Nolt D, Michaels MG, Wald ER: Intrathoracic disease from nontuberculous mycobacteria in children. Two cases and a review of the literature. Pediatrics 2003;112:e434–e439.
89. Olivier KN, Weber DJ, Wallace RJ Jr, Faiz AR, Lee J-H, Zhang Y, et al: Nontuberculous mycobacteria. I. Multicenter prevalence study in cystic fibrosis. Am J Respir Crit Care Med 2003;167:828–834.
90. Olivier KN, Weber DJ, Lee J-H, Handler A, Tudor G, Molina PL, et al: Nontuberculous mycobacteria. II. Nested-cohort study of impact on cystic fibrosis lung disease. Am J Respir Crit Care Med 2003;167:835–840.
91. Sermet-Garudelus I, Le Bourgeois M, Pierre-Audigier C, Offredo C, Guillemot D, Halley S, et al: *Mycobacterium abscessus* and children with cystic fibrosis. Emerg Infect Dis 2003;9:1587–1591.
92. Oliver A, Maiz L, Canton R, Escobar H, Baquero F, Gomez-Mampaso E: Nontuberculous mycobacteria in patients with cystic fibrosis. Clin Infect Dis 2001;32:1298–1303.
93. Fauroux B, Delaisi B, Clement A, Saizou C, Maissonet D, Truffot-Pernot C, et al: Mycobacterial lung disease in cystic fibrosis. A prospective study. Pediatr Infect Dis J 1997;16:354–358.
94. Aitken ML, Burke W, McDonald G, Wallis C, Ramsey B, Nolan C: Nontuberculosis mycobacterial disease in adult cystic fibrosis patients. Chest 1993;103:1096–1099.
95. Hjelt K, Hojlyng N, Howitz P, Ilum N, Munk E, Valerius NH, et al: The role of mycobacteria other than tuberculosis (MOTT) in patients with cystic fibrosis. Scand J Infect Dis 1994;26:569–575.
96. Kilby JM, Gilligan PH, Yankaskas JR, Highsmith WE Jr, Edwards LJ, Knowles MR: Nontuberculous mycobacteria in adult patients with cystic fibrosis. Chest 1992;102:70–75.
97. Tomashefski JF Jr, Stern RC, Demko CA, Doershuk CF: Nontuberculous mycobacteria in cystic fibrosis. An autopsy study. Am J Respir Crit Care Med 1996;154:523–528.
98. Whittier S, Hopfer RL, Knowles MR, Gilligan PH: Improved recovery of mycobacteria from respiratory secretions of patients with cystic fibrosis. J Clin Microbiol 1993;31:861–864.
99. Doucette K, Fishman JA: Nontuberculous mycobacterial infection in hematopoietic stem cell and solid organ transplant recipients. Clin Infect Dis 2004;38:1428–1439.
100. Lincoln EM, Gilbert LA: Disease in children due to mycobacteria other than *Mycobacterium tuberculosis.* Am Rev Respir Dis 1972;105:638–714.
101. Lillo M, Orengo S, Cernoch P, Harris RL: Pulmonary and disseminated infection due to *Mycobacterium kansasii.* A decade of experience. Rev Infect Dis 1990;12:760–767.
102. Starke JR: Nontuberculous mycobacterial infections in children. Adv Pediatr Infect Dis 1992;7:123–159.
103. Griffith DE, Girard WM, Wallace RJ Jr: Clinical features of pulmonary disease caused by rapidly growing mycobacteria. An analysis of 154 patients. Am Rev Respir Dis 1993;147:1271–1278.
104. Woods GL, Washington JA: Mycobacteria other than *Mycobacterium tuberculosis.* Review of microbiologic and clinical aspects. Rev Infect Dis 1987;9:275–295.
105. Wolinsky E: When is an infection disease? Rev Infect Dis 1981;3:1025–1027.
106. Benson CA, Williams PL, Currier JS, Holland F, Mahon LF, MacGregor RR, et al: A prospective randomized trial examining the efficacy and safety of clarithromycin in combination with ethambutol, rifabutin or both for the treatment of disseminated *Mycobacterium avium* complex disease in persons with acquired immunodeficiency syndrome. Clin Infect Dis 2003;37:1234–1243.
107. Pomerantz M, Madsen L, Goble M, Iseman M: Surgical management of resistant *Mycobacterium tuberculosis* and other mycobacterial pulmonary infections. Ann Thorac Surg 1991;52:1108–1011.

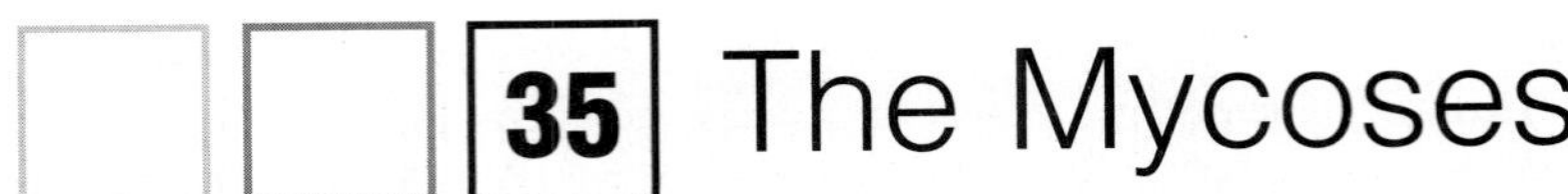

35 The Mycoses

Joseph J. Nania, MD • Peter F. Wright, MD

ENDEMIC MYCOSES

HISTOPLASMOSIS

Histoplasmosis is a fungus found in soil that is a significant cause of pulmonary and systemic disease in the geographic regions in which it occurs. In the United States, this area is broadly classified as the basins of the Mississippi and Ohio Rivers and their tributaries. The disease is acquired by airborne or dust transmission and is seen more frequently in people living in rural areas. In such areas the majority of adults, at least historically, have had evidence of exposure to the microbe.

In many ways the disease mimics tuberculosis in its pathogenesis and clinical manifestations.[1] It was originally described in military recruits from the south central United States who had x-ray films interpreted as consistent with tuberculosis but negative tuberculin tests.[2] The acquisition of histoplasmosis is most often asymptomatic. Symptomatic histoplasmosis involves four major clinical scenarios. In infants there can be a disseminated disease with hepatosplenomegaly, anemia, and a picture clinically most analogous to leukemia.[3] In the 1940s to 1960s there was rarely a time that such children were not hospitalized at Vanderbilt, an institution closely associated with the initial recognition of the disease. Clearly, the disease is less common now and, when found, may be associated with disorders in the innate immune system.[4] The second presentation, which can occur in all ages but most commonly in childhood, is of acute histoplasmosis with fever and pulmonary symptoms.[5] One classical pulmonary sign is unilateral wheezing with radiographic evidence of compression of a bronchus. A third presentation is with diffuse fibrosis of the mediastinum, occasionally with pericardial involvement.[6] This can be a life-threatening disease that is difficult to approach clinically. A fourth presentation is of recrudescent disease in children and adults in the face of malignancy, acquired or congenital immunodeficiency, or immunosuppression.

Histoplasmosis—the Microbe

Histoplasma capsulatum is a dimorphic fungus with a mycelial phase at ambient temperature and a yeast phase at body temperature. It is acquired by inhalation of spores from the soil. In the respiratory tract, the organism assumes an oval to pear-shaped yeast form in infected tissue that is distinctive (2- to 4-μm organisms often in clusters with a large vacuole and condensed protoplasm at one end of the cell), seen primarily in cells of the reticuloendothelial system (Fig. 35-1*E* and *F*). It can be recovered from sputum and gastric washings, but samples obtained at bronchoscopy or surgical biopsy offer the best diagnostic option. *Histoplasma* in the disseminated form of the disease can sometimes be seen in cells of the monocyte lineage on a peripheral blood smear. *H. capsulatum* is slowly growing and can be isolated on Sabouraud's dextrose agar or on an agar incorporating a beef heart infusion. It is identified as a white, fluffy mold that darkens in color with age. Microscopically, the mold has long slender hyphae with round smooth microconidia. With further incubation, the large 7- to 25-μm distinctive tuberculate macroconidia are usually seen. Polymerase chain reaction (PCR)–based diagnosis of culture extracts and from tissue has been introduced but is not widely available.[7,8]

Epidemiology

Acquisition is obviously governed by the geographic distribution of the fungus. Within a known area of histoplasmosis prevalence, specific scenarios can be elicited that point to the possibility of acquisition of histoplasmosis. The well-recognized association of the disease with exposure to blackbird and starling roosts relates to the bird droppings forming a fertile environment for growth of the fungus. Other scenarios include nearby soil disruption for farming or construction, cleaning of poultry houses, spelunking, and cutting of decayed wood. Globally, there are reports of histoplasmosis from a number of countries in the Caribbean and South and Central America (Costa Rica, Jamaica, and Brazil). Its impact as a tropical disease, particularly in the context of acquired immunodeficiency syndrome (AIDS), is not well defined.

Pathogenesis

As already indicated, the pathogenesis of the disease parallels that of tuberculosis. The initial focus is in the peripheral lung, where the spores are taken up by macrophages and begin to replicate in the nonimmune host. They probably disseminate before there is a systemic immune response, because recrudescent disease in adults can present far from the respiratory tract, for example, as tongue ulcers or epididymal thickening. As in tuberculosis, there is early transport to regional lymph nodes with formation of a primary complex. During this time there may be persistent fever, respiratory symptoms, and, as the regional lymph nodes enlarge, compression of the major airways or pulmonary vessels. This is largely a tissue reaction to the microbe that may rarely progress to a diffuse fibrosis. Occasionally, if the initial inoculum is very large, there is diffuse pneumonia and with resolution a lung with a radiographic appearance resembling buckshot with multiple calcifications.

Clinical Manifestations

Pulmonary Histoplasmosis

The presenting signs in patients with acute histoplasmosis include fever, cough, and chest pain. The duration of fever is impressive, with over one half of the patients in a series from Vanderbilt having fever of more than 2 weeks' duration.[5] On auscultation more than 50% had wheezing that was often unilateral. The radiologic picture of acute histoplasmosis is well defined (Fig. 35-2*A*).[9] The diagnostic dilemma when there is mediastinal adenopathy is to distinguish it from lymphoma or tuberculosis (see Fig. 35-2*B*).[10] Pericardial involvement is seen, though not commonly. The fluid in these cases is often serosanguinous.

Acute Disseminated Histoplasmosis

There is an impression that disseminated histoplasmosis is on the decline. There were only 2 occurrences after 1970 in a series of 19 cases reported from Memphis.[3] Between 1932 and 1978 there were 84 cases of disseminated histoplasmosis documented at Vanderbilt.[5] In the past 30 years there have been less than a handful of cases. In the recent cases, we have had a child who clearly had an immune defect and another instance in which both a father and his daughter were hospitalized as neonates with disseminated histoplasmosis strongly indicative of a genetic predisposition. There is a recent description that histoplasmosis along with other granulomatous diseases may be associated with the delivery of tumor necrosis factor antagonists, particularly infliximab (Remicade), a monoclonal antibody directed against tumor necrosis factor.[11] Inherited defects in innate immunity associated with granulomatous disease are also being described. Disseminated histoplasmosis has been described as the presenting symptom in pediatric human immunodeficiency virus (HIV) infection.[12]

Fibrosing Mediastinitis

Mediastinal disease in childhood differs from that in adults. In childhood, mediastinal involvement is an acute adenopathy. In the Vanderbilt experience, surgical intervention can be successful in relieving bronchial compression. In adults and occasionally older children, the diffuse fibrosis is a late complication of histoplasmosis and has no evidence of continued active replication of histoplasmosis.[6] Patients present with pulmonary ischemia and infarction with arterial involvement, pulmonary edema with venous involvement and hemoptysis, and hypoxemia with bronchial obstruction. There is little evidence of ongoing infection, and the surgical approach is extremely difficult because of loss of surgical planes and little hope of relieving the vascular or bronchial compression. Steroids and other anti-inflammatories have no role, and until recently there have been few options as vascular and airway compression set in. A recent promising development has been the insertion of stents in the pulmonary veins and/or arteries as described by Doyle and colleagues.[13] No effective way of relieving bronchial compression has yet been described. The description of a calcium-binding protein in histoplasmosis is proposed to contribute to the calcification of many older lesions.

Chronic Disseminated Histoplasmosis

The recrudescence of histoplasmosis is well recognized in adults with age, malignancy, or immunosuppression. Histoplasmosis is well recognized as confounding the diagnosis and care of pediatric patients with malignancy. St. Jude Children's Research Hospital has reported the largest series of histoplasmosis in the setting of malignancy.[14] These included cases of acute pulmonary disease,[10] disseminated disease,[14] and acute pulmonary disease mimicking malignancy.[15]

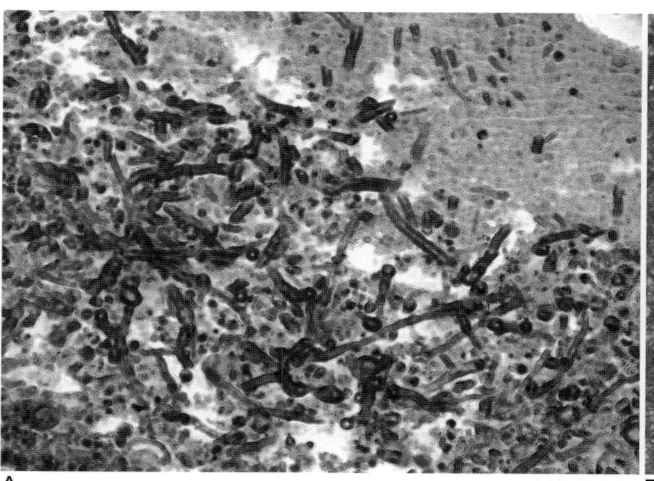
A

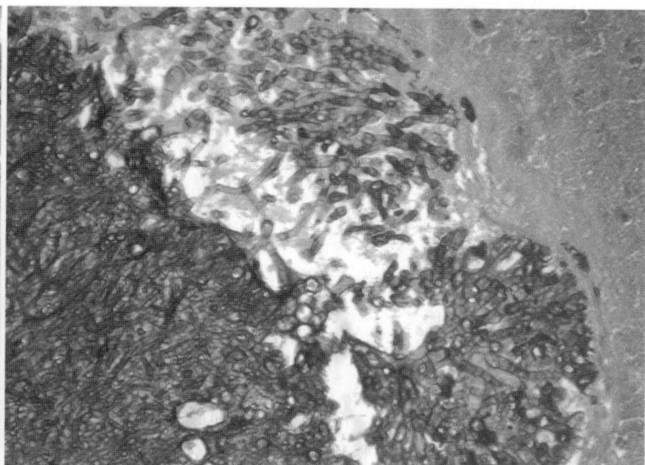
B

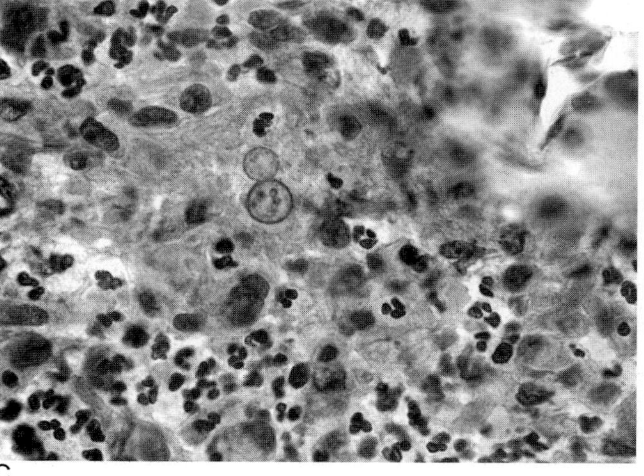
C

■ **FIGURE 35-1.** Panels showing the typical morphology of invasive aspergillosis (**A** and **B**), blastomycosis (**C** and **D**), and histoplasmosis (**E** and **F**). **A, C,** and **E,** Hematoxolyn and eosin. **B, D,** and **F,** Gomori's methenamine silver stain. (See Color Plate 34.)

Continued

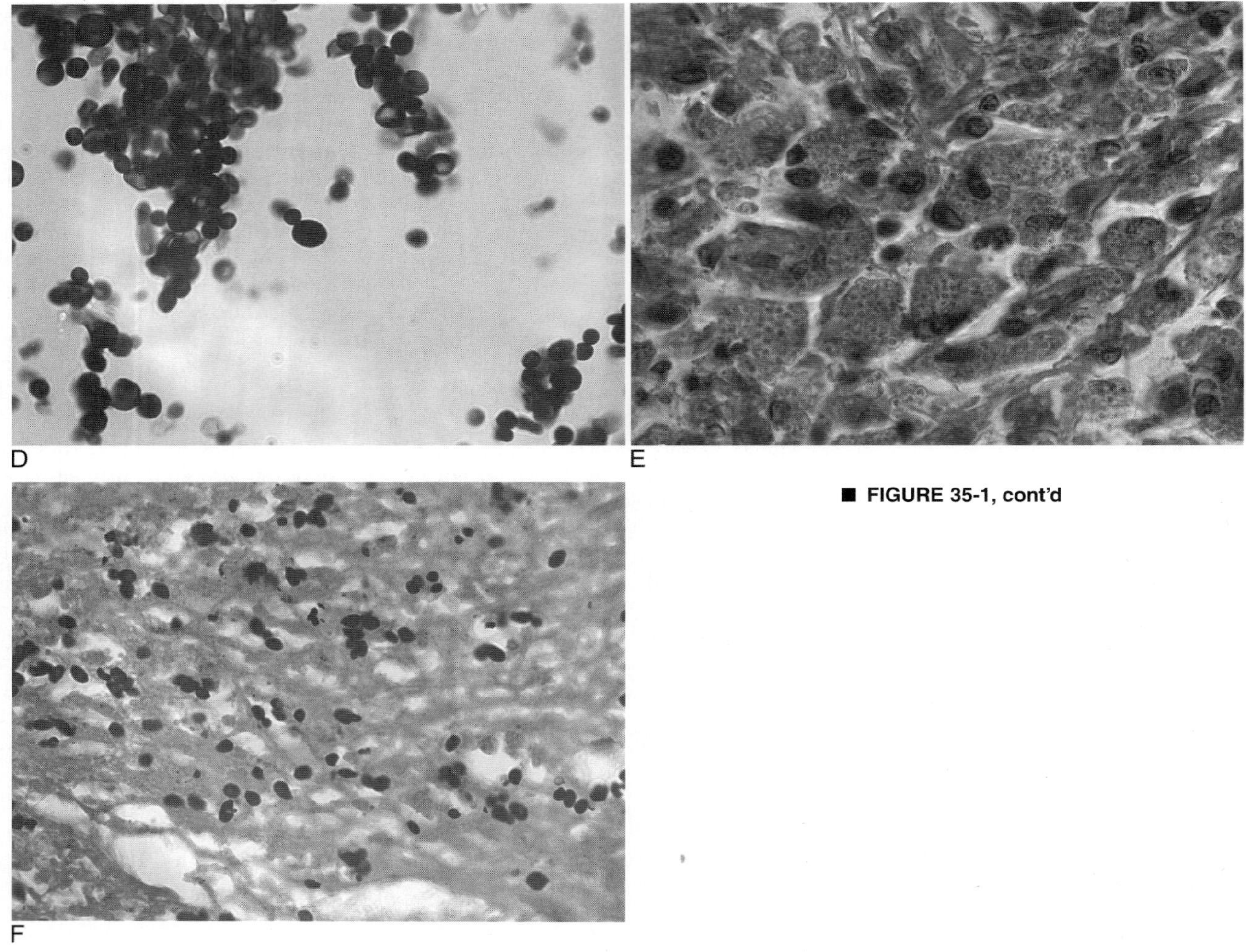

■ **FIGURE 35-1, cont'd**

Rarer Clinical Presentations

Involvement of a number of organ systems besides the lung has been described in histoplasmosis. Joint involvement is seen in approximately 10% of cases of histoplasmosis and may be accompanied by erythema nodosum. Pericarditis is recognized both during the acute disease and as a complication of the fibrotic progression of the disease. Adrenal calcification and insufficiency can be seen. In AIDS, central nervous system (CNS) disease is seen frequently. Ocular involvement is described but uncommon. Transplacental transmission has been reported.

Diagnosis

The diagnosis of histoplasmosis is problematic. An intradermal skin test was available and in the pediatric population seemed very useful. A positive test read in a manner analogous to a tuberculin test was indicative of exposure. In an urban population in Nashville a positive test was rarely (1 in 187 children tested) observed in children under 5 years of age. In contrast, it was positive in 22 of 23 children with documented histoplasmosis in an earlier pediatric series from Vanderbilt.[5] The skin test was taken off the market because of the high rate of positivity seen in adults from rural areas—for example, 80% positivity in naval recruits from middle Tennessee. This led to concerns that it was not indicative of current or recent infection and hence of little diagnostic value, although quite the opposite appears to be true in the pediatric age range. There are continued reports of the utility of the test from other countries.

The serologic diagnosis of histoplasmosis is fraught with dangers. A test does not become positive until 2 to 6 weeks after infection. A positive test may reflect disease at any point during life. There is cross reaction with other fungal diseases (blastomycosis, coccidiomycosis, and paracoccidiomycosis) and a background rate of positivity in unexposed people. Two different types of assays are available: an immunodiffusion test that measures H and M bands and a complement fixation test. In acute infection the complement fixation test is the most sensitive and in the immunodiffusion assay M bands are more common than H bands. The complement fixation test is usually interpreted as being positive when the result exceeds a cutoff of 1:32. The complement fixation test has been helpful in the differential diagnosis of a mediastinal mass between lymphoma and histoplasmosis.[10] It is concerning that in the Vanderbilt series there were a number of children with histologically proven histoplasmosis whose complement fixation serology was negative.[5]

A uniquely important test in disseminated disease is the *H. capsulatum* antigen assay. Antigen is most consistently detected in urine but may also be positive in serum or bronchial lavage fluid.[16] The antigen test is usually not positive in localized

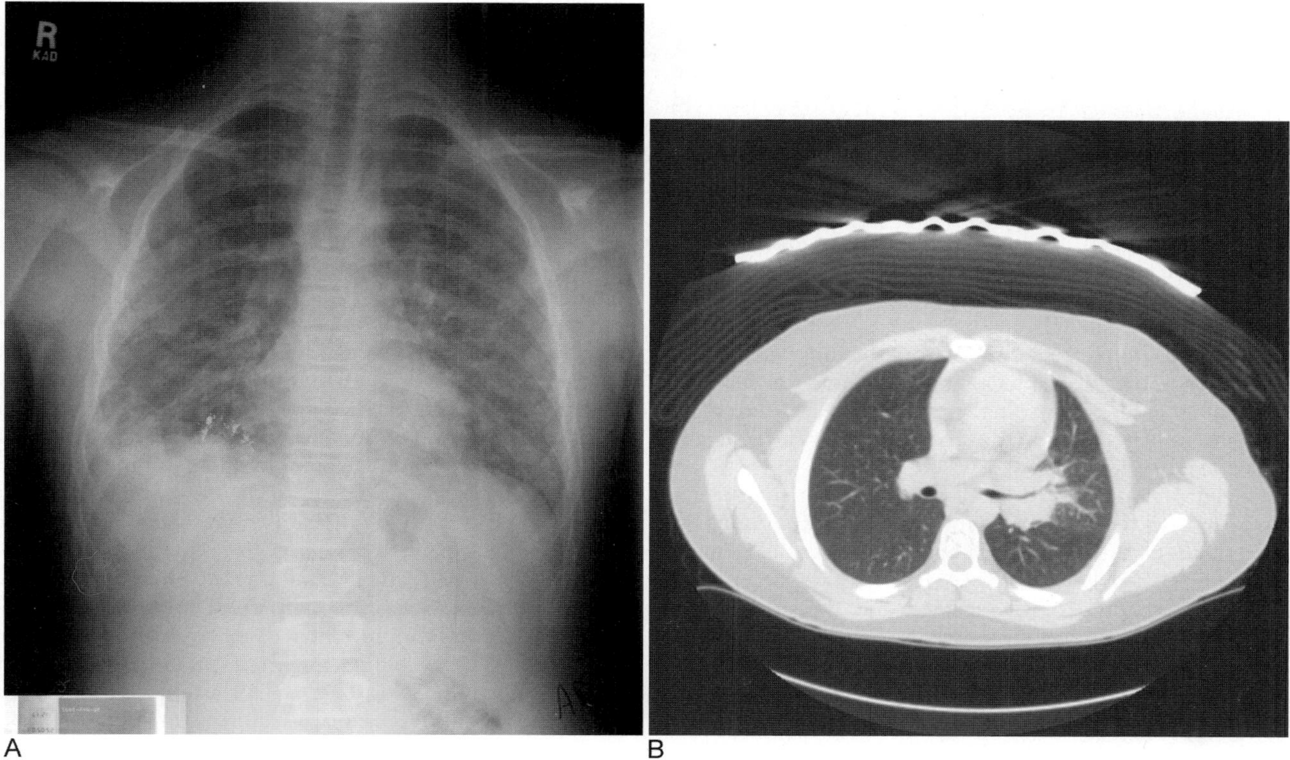

■ **FIGURE 35-2.** **A,** Chest x-ray in acute histoplasmosis showing a diffuse interstitial process. **B,** Cross-sectional CT with narrowing of the right main stem bronchus attributable to hilar adenopathy in histoplasmosis.

pulmonary disease, but in primary disseminated disease in childhood or in the face of immunosuppression it is both a strong indicator of disease and a useful parameter to follow as a measure of response to and duration of therapy once treatment is undertaken. The test is available through MiraVista Diagnostics, Indianapolis, Indiana.

The most reliable way of making a diagnosis of histoplasmosis is with tissue histology or culture of tissue. The sample is incubated for up to 6 weeks at 30°C in Sabouraud's dextrose agar or brain-heart infusion agar. The diagnosis in the mycelial phase can be confirmed by PCR probe. Tissue samples should also be stained using Grocot-Gomori methenamine–silver nitrate stain. The organism can occasionally be seen in the peripheral blood using a Wright-Giemsa stain in disseminated disease. In tissue, *H. capsulatum* has a narrow-necked budding yeast form in contrast to the broader-based blastomycosis (see Fig. 35-1*E* and *F*).

The radiographic manifestations of histoplasmosis are well described. They include evidence of peripheral airway disease and mediastinal adenopathy very analogous to tuberculosis (see Fig. 35-2*A*). Bronchial or vascular compression is best defined by computed tomography (CT) scan (see Fig. 35-2*B*). Pericarditis can be appreciated by an enlarged cardiac silhouette. On resolution of disease there is often residual calcification.

Treatment

Histoplasmosis in the normal host is usually a self-limited disease, and the indications for treatment are not clear. With prolonged fever, radiographic evidence of a large inoculum, or bronchial compression, we have instituted treatment with oral itraconazole in a dose of 5 to 10 mg/kg/day for 4 to 6 weeks. Ketoconazole is an alternative therapy. In disseminated disease the use of amphotericin B remains the gold standard with prolonged therapy to a total dose of 30 to 35 mg/kg over 2 to 3 months. Liposomal amphotericin has been shown to be comparable and less toxic though more expensive.[17] With AIDS, continued suppressive therapy with itraconazole is utilized, although recent evidence suggests it can ultimately be stopped.[15] As indicated, the urine histoplasma antigen if initially positive can be used to monitor the response to antifungal therapy, and treatment should be continued until the antigen is below the lower limit of detection.

■ COCCIDIOMYCOSIS

Coccidiomycosis[18] is a fungal disease caused by *Coccidioides immitis*. It is confined largely to parts of the southwestern United States. Geographically, infection is seen in regions of low rainfall, high summer heat, and alkaline soil. This defines its distribution in the central valleys of California, Arizona, New Mexico, and adjacent parts of Mexico. Apart from a differing geographic distribution, there are many similarities between coccidiomycosis and histoplasmosis. *C. immitus* is a dimorphic fungus that exists as either a mycelium or a unique spherule form in the human body. In culture, the infectious forms, referred to as arthrospores or arthroconidia, are seen, but there is not person-to-person spread. In many of the endemic regions, skin test positivity exceeds 50% and there is an estimated 3% risk of acquisition of infection per year. Infection is acquired via the respiratory tract through inhaled arthrospores. Outbreaks of coccidiomycosis are seen in connection with dust storms and thus, although the largest number of arthrospores is found in the soil at the time of rain, the greatest at risk of acquisition of disease is in the dry, dusty seasons of the year. The illness is characterized by an incubation period of 7 to 21 days, after which is the onset of cough and chest pain. About one third of sufferers will have clinically significant shortness of breath, and fever is present in three quarters of the patients. Extrapulmonary manifestations are relatively rare but can involve bones, joints, and skin. Rare, but clinically severe is meningeal disease, which is seen in less than 1% of patients. Late complications include a chronic fibrocavitary pneumonitis.

The diagnosis of the disease is based on a variety of serologic tests, including complement fixation tests or direct identification of the organism. It is quite a rapidly growing fungus, with visible colonies in 5 to 7 days, so that if culture material from an affected site can be obtained, the likelihood of recovering the organism is quite high.

Treatment is not indicated for all patients. If patients are not at particular risk (i.e., not pregnant or immunocompromised and without evidence of severe pulmonary disease), treatment can effectively be withheld. With severe disease, amphotericin B is considered the drug of first choice, but the organism is sensitive to azole antifungal agents, including fluconazole and itraconazole.

BLASTOMYCOSIS

Blastomycosis[19] is another disease caused by a dimorphic fungus that exists in nature in a mycelial form and converts to a yeast at body temperature. The disease has an endemic geographic localization rather similar to histoplasmosis. It is found in the Ohio River Valley, with disease reported along the borders of the Great Lakes and the St. Lawrence River. It appears to grow best in warm, moist soil with decaying organic matter but has been difficult to isolate from nature. Spelunking has been identified as a particular risk factor.

Blastomyces dermatitidis is almost always acquired as a pulmonary infection, but hematogenous spread is seen quite frequently with involvement of the skin, osseous structures, and genitourinary tract among the most common sites of extrapulmonary disease. Approximately 50% of presentations are with pulmonary disease and the rest with extrapulmonary manifestations. The presenting pulmonary lesion is most frequently as an alveolar infiltrate or mass lesion. The presenting picture may also be that of a persistent pneumonia with a productive cough similar to that seen in histoplasmosis. The skin manifestations can include verrucous lesions and ulcerated lesions with friable granulation tissue. The bony lesions appear as osteolytic lesions. Involvement of the genitourinary tract in the male is seen as a prostatitis or epididymitis. The disease is considered relatively rare in children but is certainly seen. The diagnosis is best based on visualization of the yeast in smears, in tissue specimens, or by culture (see Fig. 35-*1C* and *D*). Growth of the organism is achieved by culture of the mycelial form at 30°C, with a shift to 37°C being used to see the more distinctive yeast forms. There is no reliable serology. Positive tests have considerable cross reaction with histoplasmosis. Nor is there a reliable skin test.

Treatment of acute pulmonary blastomycosis is generally recommended, although spontaneous resolution is frequent. Once blastomycosis becomes a chronic or extrapulmonary infection, treatment is clearly indicated. No large controlled trials of therapy have been done, but amphotericin B is the drug of choice in life-threatening infections and itraconazole is considered the optimal azole drug for therapy of less severe illness. The duration of therapy is recommended to be at least 6 months.

OPPORTUNISTIC PULMONARY FUNGAL INFECTIONS

Despite recent promising advances in diagnosis and treatment, fungal infections continue to be a major cause of morbidity and mortality in immunocompromised hosts. Children with altered immunity constitute a growing proportion of pediatric patients. Great improvements in survival of patients with malignancies and other life-threatening conditions have been achieved through increased use and maximized intensity of therapies, such as transplantation and cytotoxic chemotherapy, which lead to altered host immunity. Such therapies lead to suppression of function and numbers of lymphocytes and phagocytes. Susceptibility to opportunistic fungi is also increased in these patients by frequent use of broad-spectrum antibacterial agents, disruption of normal mucosal barriers to infection, and frequent need for indwelling catheters and invasive procedures. Although rates of perinatally acquired HIV/AIDS have fallen in the United States with improved screening of pregnant women and the widespread availability of highly active antiretroviral therapy, HIV/AIDS continues to be a global health crisis and a major cause of immunosuppression in children worldwide.

The lungs are frequent sites of infection in immunocompromised patients. The respiratory tract is the portal of entry for most of the fungi that cause invasive disease including the opportunistic mycoses. Pulmonary fungal infections require a high index of suspicion. As is the case with most pulmonary infections in children, radiographic patterns lack etiologic specificity, and microbiologic diagnosis is seldom made without the use of invasive procedures to obtain a culture. Procedures such as bronchoscopy and lung biopsy have to be carefully timed, since they may become too risky because of rapid progression of underlying disease.

ASPERGILLOSIS—INVASIVE PULMONARY DISEASE

The inflammatory syndrome of allergic bronchopulmonary aspergillosis and the superinfection of preexisting lung lesions with *Aspergillus* spp., commonly referred to as an aspergilloma, occur in patients without impaired host defenses. The invasive forms of pulmonary aspergillosis, however, occur almost exclusively in immunocompromised hosts. Only the invasive form of infection will be discussed in this section.

Aspergillosis—the Microbe

Aspergillus is a ubiquitous environmental mold that lives primarily in the soil and decomposing plant matter. Exposures as varied as proximity to hospital construction/renovation and marijuana smoking have been implicated as sources of infection with *Aspergillus*.[20,21] The infective components of the organism are conidia, which are readily aerosolized from the end of hyphal stalks. Inhalation and subsequent germination of conidia leads to the formation of hyphae in the distal airways. Next, hyphal forms invade pulmonary blood vessels and parenchyma, with resulting pathology characterized by thrombosis and ischemic necrosis of the affected lung (see Fig. 35-1*A* and *B*). This sequence of events necessary to the pathogenesis of invasive *Aspergillus* infection may occur over a highly variable period of time, since the incubation period is estimated to be between 2 days and 3 months.[20] After invasion of pulmonary tissue, spread to contiguous thoracic structures or hematogenous dissemination may occur.

Of about 180 species in the *Aspergillus* genus, 5 account for the vast majority of invasive disease reported. *A. fumigatus* causes about 90% of invasive disease and is the species about which the most is known in terms of virulence factors and host immune response.[22] *A. flavus* is the principal species found in sinusitis and accounts for up to 10% of all invasive isolates. *A. niger*, *A. terreus*, and *A. nidulans* are less common causes of invasive disease. *A. terreus* is resistant to amphotericin B, and infection is associated with high rates of mortality.[20] *A. nidulans* is uncommon in patients with hematologic malignancies but is well described as a cause of invasive infections in patients with chronic granulomatous disease.[23] The varying pathogenicities of different species are thought to be related to variables such as the ability to grow at 37°C; conidial size; growth rate; and the production of enzymes, toxins, and other virulence factors.[22]

Immunity

Innate immunity is clearly an important part of the defense against *Aspergillus.* Anatomic barriers, including an intact mucosa, bronchial mucus, surfactant, and ciliated respiratory epithelium eliminate conidia and prevent their germination after inhalation. Alveolar macrophages are responsible for ingestion of conidia, although killing after ingestion appears to be slow and incomplete. Although neutrophils do have some activity against conidia as well, their primary role is in adherence to and damage of hyphae. Oxidants are certainly important in hyphal damage, but neutrophils also have nonoxidative factors that are thought to contribute to an effective response. It appears that complement and platelets also have a role in the response to *Aspergillus*, albeit not as well characterized as the role of phagocytes. Although studies in humans are lacking, there is evidence from animal models to suggest a role for both T-cell and humoral immunity. The clinical observation has been made that AIDS patients without neutropenia or predisposing therapies such as corticosteroids are at risk for invasive aspergillosis, but whether impaired T-cell immunity is the key in the pathogenesis of invasive aspergillosis in these patients remains unclear.[22]

Predisposing Factors

The risk for developing invasive aspergillosis (IA) is associated with several immunocompromising conditions and therapies. The most common predisposing situations are neutropenia, corticosteroid therapy, cytotoxic chemotherapy, broad-spectrum antibiotics, and acute leukemia. A large multicenter review of 595 patients with IA reported the proportion of cases with various underlying diagnoses. Bone marrow transplant (BMT) was the diagnosis in 32% of patients, leukemia or lymphoma in 29%, solid-organ transplant in 9%, AIDS in 8%, solid-organ tumor in 4%, chronic granulomatous disease in 2%, and unspecified pulmonary or other miscellaneous underlying conditions in 14%. Only 2% had no identifiable predisposing risk factors.[24] Among patients who have received BMT, IA occurs in roughly 5% to 10% of patients and is the leading cause of death. Recipients of allogeneic BMT were not neutropenic at the time of diagnosis of IA in 72% of cases in one large series.[25] Other risk factors for invasive disease in BMT included underlying diagnosis of hematologic malignancy, graft-versus-host disease, and corticosteroid therapy.

Whereas many patients with cancer undergo chemotherapy with cytotoxic agents, have periods of neutropenia, and receive broad-spectrum antibiotics, patients with leukemia carry a high risk of developing IA as a result of both the greater intensity of these factors in comparison with patients with other tumors and malignant transformation of immune cells. Patients with other tumors carry a lower risk of IA.

The risk of IA in recipients of solid-organ transplants varies depending on the type of transplant. Lung and heart transplant recipients have higher risks, with reported prevalence of 8.4% and 6.2%, respectively. Prevalence estimates in other organ transplants are lower: 1.7%, liver; 1.0%, pancreas; and 0.7%, kidney.[26] Precise rates specific to pediatric solid-organ transplant patients are not known. Although later cases do occur, the period of 1 to 6 months after solid-organ transplantation is the time of highest risk of IA. Other than type of transplant and timing, risk factors in these patients include cytomegalovirus infection, smoking, poor graft function, and renal failure requiring hemodialysis. Receipt of the monoclonal antilymphocyte agent OKT3 is also identified as a risk factor.[26]

As mentioned earlier, HIV-infected patients are known to be at risk for IA. Although most cases occur in the setting of advanced AIDS, the well-known risk factors for IA are not consistently present. In one retrospective review of mostly adult HIV-infected patients with pulmonary IA, only 24% of patients had documented absolute neutrophil counts under 500/mm^3. All patients with IA for whom clinical information was available, however, had other risk factors or comorbidities that have been proposed as predisposing to IA. Corticosteroids were being used in 15%, broad-spectrum antibiotics in 15%, and chemotherapy in 13%. Comorbid conditions included cytomegalovirus (63%), *Pneumocystis jiroveci* (previously *P. carinii*) (28%), bacterial and/or other fungal pneumonias (20%), lymphoma (13%), Kaposi sarcoma (10%), and atypical mycobacterial infection (10%).[27]

In a review of 473 HIV-infected children followed in the Pediatric Branch of the National Cancer Institute from 1987 to 1995, IA was diagnosed in 1.5% of patients.[28] Although five of the seven patients were neutropenic in the 4 weeks preceding diagnosis, two patients had no well-established risk factors. One of the two non-neutropenic patients had concurrent varicella and a history of lymphoid interstitial and recurrent bacterial pneumonia. The other had no comorbidities other than HIV infection.

Aspergillus infection is well described in premature neonates. In addition to commonly possessing risk factors such as therapy with broad-spectrum antibiotics and corticosteroids, low birth weight neonates have immature phagocyte and cellular immune function and often have compromised skin barrier function due to prematurity.[29,30] *Aspergillus* organisms more commonly gain entry in these patients via the skin and mucous membranes than in other patient populations. Associations with *Aspergillus* infection in neonates include skin maceration from adhesive tape or venous arm boards, percutaneous catheter insertion sites, and necrotizing enterocolitis, all reflecting mucocutaneous portals of entry.[29,30] Although primary cutaneous aspergillosis occurs in neonates, IA with cutaneous dissemination is described, as is primary invasive pulmonary disease. A high index of suspicion for aspergillosis is necessary in these patients, since diagnosis has commonly been made only after death.[29]

Of primary immunodeficiencies, chronic granulomatous disease has the best-characterized association with IA. There is a 33% lifetime risk of IA in chronic granulomatous disease.[31] Although *A. fumigatus* is the most common cause, *A. nidulans* occurs with unusually high frequency, was more likely to be fatal than *A. fumigatus*, and is rarely seen in patients without chronic granulomatous disease.[23] Severe combined immune deficiency is the other primary immunodeficiency for which the risk of IA is known to be significant. IA occurs in about 4% of severe combined immune deficiency patients and is usually fatal.[32]

Of immunosuppressive medications, corticosteroids are the agents whose administration is most clearly a risk factor for developing IA. Although the mechanisms are still incompletely understood, steroids have been shown to impair the anticonidial activity of macrophages and suppress neutrophils, both in recruitment and antifungal activity.[22] Steroids also are known to directly increase the growth rate of *A. fumigatus* and *A. flavus*. Less is known about the risk for IA conferred by immunosuppressant medications, such as cyclosporine A and tacrolimus, which act through the calcineurin pathway. Interestingly, these agents have been shown to enhance the effects of several antifungal medications in vitro, but the clinical implications of this observation remain to be seen.[33] Newer immunomodulating drugs with indications primarily for autoimmune diseases such as Crohn's and rheumatoid arthritis are known to predispose to a number of infections. Pulmonary aspergillosis has been reported in patients taking etanercept and infliximab, medications that interfere with the action of tumor necrosis factor-α.[34,35] Further experience with these and similar immunosuppressive drugs will be needed to define more precisely the risk of IA during therapy.

Clinical Presentation

Invasive aspergillosis can be classified into four clinical presentations: pulmonary aspergillosis, tracheobronchitis, rhinosinusitis, and disseminated disease.[21] Of these forms, pulmonary aspergillosis is the most common. In a study of aspergillosis in children with cancer, 70% of the 66 children with culture-proven disease had lung involvement.[36] In children with either chronic granulomatous disease or HIV/AIDS, pulmonary disease is also the most common manifestation.[27,31] Invasive pulmonary aspergillosis (IPA) has protean manifestations, presenting as hemorrhagic infarction, lobar pneumonia, lung abscess, solitary or multiple nodules, or pleural-based disease with effusion. The presenting symptoms are often nonspecific as well, with the most common complaints being fever, cough, and dyspnea. Findings that are more concerning for the diagnosis (albeit still not pathognomonic) are pleuritic chest pain and hemoptysis, both of which occur in the minority of patients with IPA.

Aspergillus tracheobronchitis associated with pseudomembrane formation and/or necrosis is a well-described entity in adults with HIV/AIDS, BMT, and lung transplant. This entity is thought to occur less commonly in children with the same underlying diagnoses.[28] The clinical presentation varies from hemoptysis, wheezing, and obstruction, or fever and cough to a lack of symptoms with findings on bronchoscopy.[37]

Diagnosis

Diagnosis of IA is proven only by biopsy and culture. Morphologic identification of the mold in culture of tissue from a sterile site is definitive evidence. Visualization of tissue-invasive hyphal forms typical of the mold in conjunction with positive culture from the same organ (e.g., lung tissue and culture of airway secretions) is also considered proof of aspergillosis (see Fig. 35-1*A* and *B*).[32] When lung biopsy is performed, tissue from both the peripheral and central areas of the affected lung should be sampled.[32] Thoracoscopic biopsy for diagnosis of IPA has not been systematically studied in children but has been reported. Given that biopsy is often not possible in patients at risk for aspergillosis as a result of thrombocytopenia and other conditions related to their underlying diseases, alternate methods of diagnosis are often relied on.

The radiographic appearance of IPA is variable. Plain chest radiographs yield nonspecific findings: segmental consolidation, multilobar consolidation, perihilar infiltrates, pleural effusions, and/or nodular lesions.[38] The latter is more highly suggestive of fungal disease. Since plain radiographs can be completely normal in up to 10% of patients with IPA, CT is the imaging of choice for early diagnosis. Classic CT findings of the "halo sign" (distinct nodular lesion with surrounding area of decreased attenuation) and the "air crescent sign" (a late finding of nodular cavitation, usually occurring after recovery of neutrophil counts) appear to be less common in children with IPA than adults.[38] However, the presence of these findings is highly suggestive of the diagnosis of aspergillosis or other invasive mold infection.

Despite the angioinvasive nature of *Aspergillus* spp., positive blood cultures for the mold are rarely reported in IA. However, detection of galactomannan, a polysaccharide cell wall antigen of *Aspergillus* spp., in blood has been used in Europe and Canada for years in the diagnosis of IA and was approved for use in the United States in 2003. The antigen is detected by a double-sandwich enzyme-linked immunosorbent assay that recognizes circulating galactomannan in patients with IA. In some series the sensitivity and specificity of the assay has been high, and detection of galactomannan has preceded the radiologic findings by 8 or 9 days in patients with IA. The sensitivity was 81% and the specificity was 89% in studies that led to Food and Drug Administration approval in the United States.[39] Although data are limited, high false-positive rates and sensitivity rates as low as 66.7% have been documented in children.[32] Variables such as cutoff values for positivity, specimen treatment, preceding antifungal treatment, pretest probability of IA based on risk factors, and false-positive results in patients receiving piperacillin/tazobactam are thought to contribute to variability of results.[40]

Detection of *Aspergillus* spp. in respiratory tract secretions has been used as a surrogate method of diagnosis in patients at risk for aspergillosis with clinical and radiographic findings consistent with the diagnosis. Both direct examination for hyphal elements (via staining with calcofluor and methenamine silver) and fungal culture should be performed on respiratory specimens. Although a negative culture of sputum or bronchoalveolar lavage fluid cannot rule out the diagnosis, a positive culture in a neutropenic or BMT patient with new pulmonary infiltrates is putative evidence of IPA.[29,41] In solid-organ transplant patients, non-neutropenic patients with chronic lung disease, and HIV-infected patients, however, the positive predictive value of respiratory tract cultures is much lower. Detection of *Aspergillus* spp. in bronchoalveolar lavage fluid by both galactomannan assay and PCR technology has been studied, but the precise role of these techniques in diagnosis remains to be seen. Though very sensitive, the low specificity of bronchoalveolar lavage fluid PCR is probably due to the ubiquitous nature of *Aspergillus* spp. conidia.[32]

Treatment and Prognosis

For over 40 years, amphotericin B was recommended as primary therapy for IA. The toxicities of amphotericin B are well known, with nephrotoxicity being the most common dose-limiting side effect. Additionally, amphotericin B has only had modest success historically in the treatment of IA. Overall response rates to amphotericin B have been estimated at 55% and less than 40% in severely immunosuppressed patients.[24,42] Mortality with amphotericin B as sole therapy for IA was 65% in one large retrospective review.[24] Although the newer lipid formulations of amphotericin B offer reduced toxicity, they provide no proven increase in efficacy relative to the parent compound, amphotericin B deoxycholate.

Approved in an oral formulation in 1992, itraconazole was the first triazole antifungal with a spectrum of activity that included *Aspergillus* spp. and other filamentous fungi. Retrospective review has shown response rates to itraconazole, both as primary therapy and after an initial course of amphotericin B, to be better than those of amphotericin B as the sole therapy.[24] However, the numbers of severely immunosuppressed patients in the amphotericin B–treated group was markedly higher than those treated with itraconazole, probably reflecting the unwillingness of clinicians to use a relatively unproven new therapy on their patients at highest risk. Although itraconazole is certainly less toxic than amphotericin B, the dependence of oral absorption of itraconazole capsules on a low gastric pH limits its use in some patients. The availability of an oral solution of itraconazole with higher bioavailability and an intravenous formulation of the medication has circumvented this problem; however, the development and approval of other new antifungal agents that are effective against *Aspergillus* spp. have relegated itraconazole to a minor position in the treatment of aspergillosis.

Caspofungin acetate was approved for use in 2001 for salvage therapy of IA. It is the first echinocandin antifungal approved for use in the United States, and the mechanism of action targets the synthesis of β-1,3-D-glucan, an essential part of the fungal cell wall. Caspofungin is available only for intravenous administration and has not been studied for (nor should it be used for) initial therapy of aspergillosis.

In 2002, voriconazole was approved for use in the United States. It possesses broad activity against most *Aspergillus* spp. (including species such as *A. terreus* and *A. nidulans*, against which amphotericin B has been ineffective) and is available in both intravenous and highly bioavailable oral formulations. Shortly after approval of voriconazole, a landmark randomized comparative study, in 277 patients 12 years or older (including 240 patients with IPA), was published that established the agent as the treatment of choice for IA.[42] Compared with amphotericin B deoxycholate as primary therapy of IA, voriconazole showed a significantly higher rate of successful outcomes (52.8% vs. 31.6%), higher rates of survival (70.8% vs. 57.9%), and lower toxicity. Although no randomized trials have been published in pediatric patients, review of experience at the National Cancer Institute using voriconazole on a compassionate release basis offers the largest published series of children in whom the drug has been used. In the treatment of pediatric patients refractory to or intolerant of standard antifungal therapy given for aspergillosis and other invasive fungal infections, voriconazole was well tolerated and produced relatively satisfactory outcomes.[43] Two other triazole antifungals, ravuconazole and posaconazole, are anticipated for approval and possess potent anti-*Aspergillus* activity, as well. They are expected to be effective for treatment of IA.

Combination therapy for IA with agents listed above and other antifungal agents such as 5-flucytosine has not been studied in clinical trials. In vitro and animal studies show promise for improved efficacy of a combination of an echinocandin and either a broad-spectrum triazole or amphotericin B in the treatment of IA. In a retrospective study of 47 patients with IA after cancer chemotherapy or BMT, patients receiving the combination of voriconazole and caspofungin for salvage therapy had a lower rate of mortality than historical controls who received voriconazole only.[44] Other than this single small, nonrandomized study, there is only anecdotal clinical evidence to support use of such combinations, and further investigations are needed before such combination therapy can be recommended.

Therapeutic surgical excision of IPA has been advocated by some for debulking of primary lesions and preventing disseminated infection or pulmonary hemorrhage. One retrospective review of 43 pediatric patients with IPA, most of whom were highly immunosuppressed, found a significantly higher survival rate in the 18 patients who underwent surgical intervention compared with those who received medical therapy only.[45] The retrospective nature of the study, high overall mortality rate in the series (91%), and limitations of medical therapy available at the time of the study (i.e., before approval of voriconazole) make it difficult to know if such findings can be generalized to current care.

Adjunctive therapies such as colony-stimulating factors, interferon-γ, and infusions of granulocytes harvested from donors pretreated with granulocyte colony-stimulating factor have promise in the treatment of aspergillosis. These modalities have not yet been well studied and are not yet recommended.[46]

Optimal length of medical therapy for any form of IA, including pulmonary disease, is not known. Recommendations stress the need to determine length of treatment based on clinical and radiographic resolution of the disease, combined with consideration of the underlying immunosuppressive condition and the likelihood of its improvement or resolution.[46]

CRYPTOCOCCOSIS

Cryptococcosis—the Microbe

Cryptococcus neoformans is an encapsulated yeast that has a worldwide distribution. Although the organism has been isolated from soil, trees, and fruit, there has long been recognition of a unique role of dried pigeon droppings as a naturally occurring culture medium for *Cryptococcus*.[47] Desiccated *C. neoformans* yeast and basidiospores from the organism's sexual state (*Filobasidiella neoformans*) are both about 2 μm. This size makes aerosolization and alveolar deposition the probable route of infection in humans. After inhalation, the organism initially grows in the alveoli without significant inflammatory response, probably because of the antiphagocytic effect of the polysaccharide capsule. Before development of cellular immunity, *C. neoformans* disseminates widely, most commonly manifesting as meningitis or parenchymal brain infection.[48] The reason for the tropism of *C. neoformans* for the CNS is not known.

Immunity

Cellular immunity is generally agreed to be the most important component of an effective immune response to *C. neoformans*. Pathologically, this is demonstrated by the formation of granulomatous inflammation in response to infection. T cells activate alveolar macrophages, via cytokines such as interferon-γ, and promote transformation of macrophages into giant cells that are able to ingest the encapsulated yeast.[47] Humoral immunity plays a role in opsonization, activation of natural killer cells, and clearing of capsular polysaccharide. Although natural killer cells, neutrophils, and eosinophils are all thought to contribute to the immune response, patients with isolated defects in any of these components of immunity are not thought to be predisposed to symptomatic cryptococcosis. In contrast, conditions associated with defective cellular immunity are associated with an increase in symptomatic cryptococcal infections.

AIDS is clearly the underlying condition with which cryptococcosis has been seen most often and remains an AIDS-defining illness in HIV-infected persons. $CD4^+$ lymphocyte counts are often fewer than 100 cells/μL. In adults with AIDS, *C. neoformans* disease occurs in about 5% of patients annually, but in children with AIDS a considerably lower rate, not quite 1%, has been reported.[49] Reasons for the lower incidence in children with AIDS are not known, but it is not thought to be due to differential exposure to the organism.[50] In the pre-AIDS era, symptomatic cryptococcosis was a rare condition, occurring in less than one per a million persons per year in the United States.[47] At that time, high-risk patients were those with defects in cellular immunity: patients with malignancies, particularly Hodgkin's disease and other hematologic cancers, and recipients of organ transplants. *Cryptococcus neoformans* infection is also reportedly associated with sarcoidosis, diabetes mellitus, hyper–immunoglobulin M (IgM) syndrome, and hyper-IgE syndrome.[51]

Clinical Manifestations

Although it is commonly thought of as an opportunistic infection that affects immunocompromised patients, particularly those with AIDS, *C. neoformans* infection may occur most commonly as subclinical or mild pulmonary disease in normal hosts. Evidence from a series of pediatric patients with pulmonary cryptococcosis[51] and a serologic survey of healthy urban children[50] support this notion. Cough, chest pain, and fever are common presenting complaints for symptomatic individuals. An isolated pulmonary nodule may be the only manifestation in immunocompetent individuals, at times associated with hilar adenopathy, but masslike and consolidative lesions with a particular predilection for the lower lobes are also well described.[48,51]

Even in immunocompromised hosts, the pulmonary component of cryptococcosis may be mild or asymptomatic on presentation. Although the respiratory tract is the portal of entry for infection, it is estimated that less than 10% of patients with disseminated cryptococcosis have pulmonary symptoms at the time of diagnosis.[48] When symptoms are present, the presentation varies considerably, from a subacute cough with fever, chest pain, and weight loss, to rapidly progressive pulmonary disease with adult respiratory distress syndrome.[47] Highlighting the tendency for *C. neoformans* to disseminate, it is estimated that only about one third of HIV-negative patients with cryptococcosis have isolated pulmonary involvement. Similarly, 90% of AIDS patients have concomitant meningitis or parenchymal brain lesions ("cryptococcomas") on presentation.[47] Virtually any organ can be infected in disseminated cryptococcosis, but in addition to the CNS, the skin, prostate, and eyes are particularly important sites of extrapulmonary infection. As with normal hosts, there is no typical radiographic pattern for pulmonary cryptococcal infection. Pulmonary nodules, mass lesions, lobar consolidations, and diffuse infiltrates with effusion have all been described in compromised patients.[51]

Diagnosis

Although cultures may take up to a week to become positive, *C. neoformans* grows on most clinical media, including standard radiometric blood culturing systems. However, in the diagnosis of pulmonary disease both the sensitivity and specificity of cultures of respiratory secretions are questionable.[51] The majority of cryptococcal isolates from sputum are thought to represent colonization.[48] Conversely, isolation of the organism from blood, cerebrospinal fluid (CSF), or other sterile body sites is reasonably sensitive and would be putative evidence of pulmonary cryptococcosis when clinical or radiographic signs are suggestive. It is important to note, however, that in immunocompromised hosts, other pulmonary (and nonpulmonary) opportunistic infections may be present simultaneously. *Mycobacterium tuberculosis*, nontuberculous mycobacteria, cytomegalovirus, *Nocardia*, and *P. jiroveci* (formerly *P. carinii*) have all been reported as co-pathogens, highlighting the need for appropriate studies to rule out such diagnoses in severely compromised patients.[47] Direct histopathologic identification of *C. neoformans* from biopsy specimens is both sensitive and specific for the diagnosis of pulmonary infection. Several different stains can be used to identify the yeast in tissue, including the nonspecific Grocot-Gomori methenamine–silver nitrate and others such as mucicarmine, which stains the polysaccharide capsule red.[47,48] Additionally, a monoclonal antibody against the main capsular polysaccharide antigen (GXM) has been used for specific identification of the yeast in tissue.[51] In examination of CSF, India ink has long been used to identify *C. neoformans*. The sensitivity is about 80% for AIDS patients and 50% for non-AIDS patients with cryptococcal meningitis, and it has been used on other clinical specimens as well.[47]

Detection of the capsular polysaccharide of *C. neoformans* in blood or CSF by latex agglutination or enzyme immunoassay is a reliable method of diagnosing disseminated infection. For the diagnosis of cryptococcal meningitis, CSF antigen detection assays are at least 90% sensitive and specific.[47] However, these techniques are thought to be less sensitive in the patient with isolated pulmonary cryptococcosis.[51]

Antibodies to *C. neoformans* can develop in response to either colonization or infection and are not useful in diagnosis.[47,50,51]

As described earlier, imaging of the chest by plain radiograph and CT is not diagnostic. Isolated or multiple nodules, pulmonary masses, lobar consolidation, cavitary lesions, pleural effusion, diffuse interstitial infiltrates, and adult respiratory distress–like appearance have all been described with pulmonary cryptococcosis.[47–49,51] If signs of increased intracranial pressure or other signs suggestive of CNS infection are present, magnetic resonance imaging or CT of the head to rule out hydrocephalus and cryptococcomas is indicated.

Given the limitations of noninvasive methods, invasive procedures are often necessary to confirm the diagnosis of cryptococcosis, especially when involvement is limited to the lungs. Either fine-needle aspiration or biopsy may be required to confirm the diagnosis. When pleural effusions are present, cultures of thoracentesis fluid are positive in about 40% of AIDS patients.[52] Some authors have questioned the need for examination of spinal fluid in nonimmunocompromised patients with pulmonary cryptococcosis, no overt signs of CNS infection, and a negative serum antigen.[53] However, given the frequency of concomitant meningitis, lumbar puncture with measurement of opening pressure, CSF India ink preparation, a cryptococcal antigen assay, and routine studies are generally recommended.[54]

Treatment

Since there is a paucity of data in children, recommendations for treatment of cryptococcosis are extrapolated from studies and recommendations in adult patients.[54] For asymptomatic patients with normal immunity and a positive culture for *C. neoformans* from the respiratory tract, observation without antifungal treatment or fluconazole for 3 to 6 months are both reasonable options. For normal hosts with mild-to-moderate symptoms, fluconazole (either intravenous or oral) is recommended for a period of 6 to 12 months. If fluconazole cannot be used, itraconazole and amphotericin B are effective alternatives. Patients with severe symptoms and all immunocompromised patients should be treated as CNS cryptococcal infection would be. Based on relatively large studies in both HIV-negative and HIV-positive patients, the preferred regimen is amphotericin B plus flucytosine for 2 weeks (or until CSF cultures are negative) followed by a minimum of 10 additional weeks of fluconazole. An alternative regimen in immunocompromised HIV-negative hosts is amphotericin (with or without flucytosine) for 6 to 10 weeks. Fluconazole for primary therapy is discouraged because of unsatisfactory outcomes in preliminary studies. For HIV-infected patients, more studies have been done to justify alternative regimens. Amphotericin (with or without flucytosine) for 6 to 10 weeks, fluconazole plus flucytosine for 6 weeks, fluconazole alone for 10 to 12 weeks, or itraconazole alone for 10 to 12 weeks are all satisfactory options. Additionally, lifelong maintenance therapy is recommended for all HIV-positive patients with cryptococcosis. Outcomes for patients with cryptococcosis have been studied for those with CNS involvement, and mortality is predicted by several CSF parameters, such as organism load, opening CSF pressure, low CSF glucose or leukocyte count, and high titer of cryptococcal antigen in CSF or blood. Additionally, those being treated with corticosteroids or with an underlying diagnosis of lymphoreticular malignancy also have higher mortality with cryptococcosis. Prognosis for patients with isolated pulmonary cryptococcosis has not been studied thoroughly, but in the absence of dissemination, outcomes appear to be more favorable.[51,53]

■ CANDIDIASIS

Candida species are yeast and common human commensals that most often colonize the gastrointestinal tract. Of about 150 known species of *Candida*, only about 10 cause human disease. *C. albicans* is by far the most common species and causes the majority of human infections. *Candida* species other than *C. albicans*, however, do account for almost half of isolates in some series. Infections occur primarily via tissue invasion from endogenously acquired strains rather than by person-to-person spread. The immune response to *Candida* is complex, but the most important components in preventing invasive disease appear to be normal number and function of neutrophils and intact complement pathways. T lymphocytes are clearly important in controlling mucosal and cutaneous candidiasis, but patients with defects of cellular immunity are not at increased risk for invasive infection.[55]

Although *Candida* spp. are the most common of fungal pathogens and a frequent cause of nosocomial infections, true pulmonary infection with *Candida* spp. is relatively rare. When pulmonary candidiasis does occur, it is usually in the setting of disseminated infection with hematogenous seeding or with aspiration of oropharyngeal secretions heavily colonized with *Candida*.[56] Neutropenic patients, low birth weight infants, or premature neonates whose mothers have *Candida* chorioamnionitis are the patients in whom pulmonary dissemination has occurred most often.[29]

The clinical manifestations and radiologic findings of pulmonary candidiasis are nonspecific. Fever, cough, and septic appearance are common. Patterns on chest radiographs have been described most often as multilobar consolidation, widespread bronchopneumonia, or nodular infiltrates. Rarely, cavitary lesions, adult respiratory distress syndrome, and pleural effusion have been encountered in histologically proven pulmonary candidiasis.[56]

It is clear that the diagnosis of pulmonary candidiasis cannot be made reliably in the absence of histopathologic confirmation.[29,55–57] Isolating *Candida* spp. from a culture of the airways has poor predictive value for the presence of true disease. In a large study of adult cancer patients, the positive predictive value of a culture of the sputum for pulmonary candidiasis was 42% and just 29% for bronchoalveolar lavage specimens, using histopathology from autopsy specimens as the gold standard.[56] Similarly, in a study of non-neutropenic patients, nearly 90% of bronchoalveolar lavage cultures positive for *Candida* spp. were judged to be probable or definite contaminants, despite the majority of the cultures having been done on protected brush specimens.[58]

It has even been reported that limiting identification of yeast in respiratory specimens by diagnostic microbiology laboratories has led to improved outcomes and reduced costs in patients.[59] The authors assert that fewer erroneous diagnoses of pulmonary candidiasis resulted in shorter length of stay and avoidance of unnecessary antifungal therapy.

When true pulmonary candidiasis occurs, high rates of mortality have been reported in neutropenic patients. Choice of antifungal agent and length of therapy for pulmonary disease specifically have not been well studied, but generally amphotericin has been used.[57] Consideration can be given to the use of flucytosine in combination with amphotericin or fluconazole as the primary agent, given a susceptible strain.[29] For *C. albicans*, 95% or more of strains are susceptible to fluconazole, but resistance is more common among strains of *C. krusei, C. glabrata*, and *C. tropicalis*. Standards for susceptibility to fluconazole have been set for *Candida* spp., and testing is available commercially. In disseminated candidiasis, other sites of infection may dictate the type and length of treatment (e.g., endocarditis or endophthalmitis).

■ ZYGOMYCOSIS

The causative agents of zygomycosis belong to the order Mucorales and class Zygomycetes. Human disease caused by these filamentous fungi is most often due to *Rhizopus* but can also be due to *Mucor*, *Absidia*, *Cunninghamella*, *Rhizomucor*, and a number of other species reported occasionally. These environmental molds are found primarily in soil and organic matter in a near worldwide distribution. Although percutaneous and ingestional acquisitions are known to occur, the main route of transmission is inhalation of spores from an environmental source. Outbreaks of disease have been linked to construction, excavation, and contaminated air-conditioning filters.[60] The Zygomycetes share hyphal morphology characterized by sparse or absent septation and variable size (but wider than *Aspergillus* spp. hyphae). As with *Aspergillus* spp., angioinvasion is a typical finding on histopathology.

People with intact innate immunity are not at significant risk for invasive zygomycosis. Early observations of patients with impaired immune systems gave insight into the mechanisms of protection against these fungi. Diabetic patients have long been known to be at risk for developing rhinocerebral zygomycosis, most often during ketoacidosis. Dysfunctions of macrophage phagocytosis, neutrophil chemotaxis, and oxidative killing by neutrophils have been demonstrated in diabetic ketoacidosis. Similar to the response to *Aspergillus*, macrophages are primarily responsible for aborting the germination of spores through phagocytosis. Once germination has occurred, neutrophils are responsible for damaging fungal hyphae through attachment and oxidative damage without phagocytosis.[60] Given the importance of the innate immune response, it is not surprising that neutropenia is the single most common risk factor for developing zygomycosis. Other important risk factors include use of corticosteroids and broad-spectrum antibiotics and organ transplantation. One other well-established group of patients at risk is those receiving iron chelation therapy.[60] It is thought that the Zygomycetes are able to use iron bound to chelators as a growth factor. Hemochromatosis itself may also be a minor risk factor for developing zygomycosis.

Zygomycosis can be classified into a few predominant forms: rhinocerebral, pulmonary, cutaneous, gastrointestinal, and disseminated disease. Pulmonary zygomycosis is clinically indistinguishable from pulmonary aspergillosis and associated with similarly high rates of mortality. Common factors predisposing to pulmonary zygomycosis include leukemia, lymphoma, BMT, and diabetes mellitus. The clinical presentation is commonly fever and pulmonary infiltrates that persist despite treatment for presumed bacterial pneumonia. In advanced disease, hemoptysis can occur due to angioinvasion and hemorrhagic infarction that characterize this group of infections.[61]

Radiographic findings, as in aspergillosis, are quite variable. Isolated nodules, lobar consolidation, cavitary lesions, and disseminated pulmonary involvement have all been described.[60] The sensitivity of cultures of respiratory tract specimens is low, and fungemia is not usually detected with clinical cultures. Serology is not useful clinically, and antigen detection and molecular diagnostic techniques have not been developed for clinical diagnostic purposes.[60] These factors make early diagnosis of invasive zygomycosis very difficult, and in fact, the diagnosis is often preterminal or made at autopsy.[60,61] This makes a high index of suspicion and aggressive, tissue-based approach essential, assuming the patient can tolerate the necessary procedure.

The treatment for zygomycosis is aggressive debridement and high-dose intravenous amphotericin B. In a retrospective review of 255 cases of pulmonary mucormycosis, mortality of patients treated surgically was significantly lower than those who received medical treatment alone.[62] These data must be interpreted keeping in mind the potential for selection bias that exists in a retrospective analysis, but it supports strong consideration of surgical intervention for therapeutic reasons.

In addition to attempting reversal of the predisposing condition leading to the infection, antifungal therapy with amphotericin B is indicated. Initial doses of amphotericin B deoxycholate should be 1.0 to 1.5 mg/kg/day and at least 5 mg/kg/day if using lipid formulations of amphotericin B.[61] Itraconazole has variable activity against this class of fungi. It is of note that newer triazole and echinocandin antifungals, including voriconazole and caspofungin, have no appreciable activity against the Zygomycetes.[63] In fact, an increase in zygomycosis in stem cell transplant patients receiving voriconazole as antifungal prophylaxis has been reported.[64] The investigational triazole agent posaconazole has in vitro activity against Zygomycetes, but clinical efficacy has not yet been demonstrated. Length of treatment with antifungals has not been studied for pulmonary zygomycosis, but a course of therapy lasting many months is indicated for survivors, based on clinical response and reversal of the underlying immunocompromised state.

OTHER UNCOMMON PULMONARY MYCOSES

Sporothrix schenckii is a dimorphic fungus with a worldwide distribution in soil and decaying organic material. Sporotrichosis is most commonly a cutaneous or lymphocutaneous infection that manifests as a chronic, ulcerated skin lesion, often with regional lymphadenopathy.[65] In addition to cutaneous disease, sporotrichosis can occasionally occur as osteoarticular, meningeal, and pulmonary infection. Pulmonary disease and other forms of disseminated sporotrichosis are rare in children. Pneumonia occurs most commonly in middle-aged men with alcoholism and chronic obstructive pulmonary disease.[65] The presentation is subacute or chronic in most cases, and nonspecific. Signs and symptoms include cough, fever, weight loss, and hemoptysis. Radiographs often reveal chronic cavitary fibronodular disease, but no specific pattern is typical.[52] The combination of surgical resection and amphotericin B is preferred for life-threatening or extensive pulmonary sporotrichosis. Itraconazole also has activity against *S. schenckii* and can be considered for less serious disease.[65]

Trichosporon spp. are yeasts related to *Cryptococcus* that cause an infection of the distal hair shaft called white piedra and a hypersensitivity pneumonia that occurs in summer months in Japan.[61] The yeasts of this genus also occasionally cause disseminated infections in immunocompromised hosts. *Trichosporon beigelii* (also referred to as *T. asahii)* has been reported as a cause of pneumonia in neutropenic patients, particularly in those with hematologic malignancies.[61,66] Although there are descriptions of isolated pulmonary infection (presumably from aspiration of the organism), most cases of pulmonary trichosporonosis have been reported as part of disseminated disease, including involvement of the bloodstream, kidneys, liver, skin, and retina.[66] Cough, dyspnea, and hemoptysis are typical. Radiographs often show diffuse alveolar infiltrates, but diffuse interstitial infiltrates, patchy reticulonodular infiltrates, lobar consolidation, bronchopneumonia, and cavitary lesions have also been described.[66] Diagnosis is based on isolation of the organism from the respiratory tract, but because *Trichosporon* spp. can colonize the oropharynx, sputum cultures are not by themselves diagnostic. It is also notable that, as a result of the relatedness of *Trichosporon* spp. to *Cryptococcus*, false-positive serum cryptococcal antigen tests have been reported in confirmed cases of trichosporonosis. Preferred treatment for invasive infection is fluconazole, because decreased susceptibility to amphotericin B has been demonstrated.[67] The addition of flucytosine may also be considered.[29] Newer triazole antifungal agents, such as voriconazole, also have activity against *Trichosporon* spp., but the echinocandins do not.[61]

Fusarium spp. have been recognized as an infrequent but important cause of disseminated infection in neutropenic patients. This filamentous fungus, which is primarily a plant pathogen, has long been known to cause infections of the nails, skin, and cornea of humans. In recent years, it has been appreciated that *Fusarium* spp. such as *F. solani*, *F. oxysporum*, and *F. moniliforme* are important causes of infections of the lungs and sinuses, and of disseminated infection in patients undergoing leukemia chemotherapy and hematopoietic stem cell transplant patients.[52] In addition to neutropenia, corticosteroid therapy seems to be an important predisposing factor in developing fusariosis. The clinical presentation is similar to other opportunistic mold infections in that sinusitis and pulmonary infiltrates are common; however, fusariosis differs in that metastatic skin lesions and isolation of the organism from blood culture are much more common. Diagnosis can be made with certainty only by isolation of the organism from culture of infected tissues or blood. Distinguishing *Fusarium* spp. from *Aspergillus* spp. or other septate hyaline molds by histopathology is unreliable.[52] Mortality from fusariosis has historically been greater than 50%, and amphotericin B treatment generally has been, at best, only modestly successful. Adjunctive treatment with colony-stimulating factors and/or granulocyte transfusions has been used as well.[52] Voriconazole has potent activity against *Fusarium* spp.; it is approved for treating fusariosis, and there exist anecdotal reports of its use in successful treatment in immunocompromised hosts.[68] Definitive data for the best therapeutic approach to fusariosis are lacking.

Phaeohyphomycosis is an invasive infection due to one of the dematiaceous molds, a group characterized by darkly pigmented cell walls.[52] As with many molds, the respiratory tract is the usual portal of entry for these fungi and extrapulmonary dissemination is common. Infections generally occur in neutropenic hosts, as with the other opportunistic mold infections, and localize to the CNS, sinuses, and lungs. *Pseudallescheria boydii* and the closely related *Scedosporium* spp. are important causes of pulmonary infection, since they are difficult to treat and associated with high rates of mortality.[52] *Scedosporium apiospermum* has been reported as a cause of pulmonary infection in children with chronic granulomatous disease.[69] Another dematiaceous mold, *Bipolaris*, can cause pulmonary infection as well, although its most frequent manifestation is sinusitis. As with fusariosis, the diagnosis of phaeohyphomycosis must be established by culture, because the activity of amphotericin B is not consistently fungicidal and in some cases depends on the specific species.[52] Newer triazole agents such as voriconazole have activity in vitro and have been used successfully in a small number of patients, including children intolerant or refractory to conventional therapy.[43] Surgical resection of fungal lesions and adjunctive colony-stimulating cytokine therapies can both be considered in difficult cases.[52]

Penicillium marneffei is a dimorphic fungus that has been identified as an important opportunistic infection in HIV-infected patients who live in or have traveled to eastern Asia. The lungs are the portal of entry, and it is thought that impaired cell–mediated and alveolar phagocytic function is the main predisposing factor in AIDS patients.[52] The clinical syndrome commonly includes fever, lymphadenopathy, hepatosplenomegaly, pulmonary infiltrate, weight loss, anemia, and generalized rash similar to that associated with molluscum contagiosum virus. Amphotericin B is favored for induction therapy, with itraconazole given long-term as maintenance/suppressive therapy.[52]

Acknowledgments

The authors wish to recognize the contributions of the following collaborators for their roles in obtaining radiographs and pathologic specimens used for the figures in this chapter: Richard M. Heller, Sharon M. Stein, and James D. Chappell.

REFERENCES

1. Goodwin RA, Des Prez RM: State of the art. Histoplasmosis. Am Rev Respir Dis 1978;117:929–956.
2. Schwarz J, Baum GL: The history of histoplasmosis, 1906 to 1956. N Engl J Med 1957;256:253–258.
3. Leggiadro RJ, Barrett FF, Hughes WT: Disseminated histoplasmosis of infancy. Pediatr Infect Dis J 1988;7:799–805.
4. Casanova JL, Laurent A: The human model. A genetic dissection of immunity to infection in natural conditions. Nat Rev Immunol 2004;4:55–66.
5. Butler JC, Heller R, Wright PF: Histoplasmosis during childhood. South Med J 1994;87:476–480.
6. Davis AM, Pierson RN, Loyd JE: Mediastinal fibrosis. Semin Respir Infect 2001;16:119–130.
7. Bracca A, Tosello ME, Girardini JE, et al: Molecular detection of *Histoplasma capsulatum* var. *capsulatum* in human clinical samples. J Clin Microbiol 2003;41:1753–1755.
8. Martagon-Villamil J, Shrestha N, Sholtis M, et al: Identification of *Histoplasma capsulatum* from culture extracts by real-time PCR. J Clin Microbiol 2003;41:1295–1298.
9. Kirchner SG, Hernanz-Schulman M, Stein SM, et al: Imaging of pediatric mediastinal histoplasmosis. Radiographics 1991;11:365–381.
10. Woods WG, Singher LJ, Krivit W, Nesbit ME Jr: Histoplasmosis simulating lymphoma in children. J Pediatr Surg 1979;14:423–425.
11. Wallis RS, Broder MS, Wong JY, et al: Granulomatous infectious diseases associated with tumor necrosis factor antagonists. Clin Infect Dis 2004; 38:1261–1265.
12. Beyers M, Feldman S, Edwards J: Disseminated histoplasmosis as the acquired immunodeficiency-syndrome defining illness in an infant. Pediatr Infect Dis J 1992;11:127–128.
13. Doyle TP, Loyd JE, Robbins IM: Percutaneous pulmonary artery and vein stenting. Am J Respir Crit Care Med 2001;164:657–660.
14. Adderson EE: Histoplasmosis in a pediatric oncology center. J Pediatr 2004;144:100–106.
15. Goldman M, Zackin R, Fichtenbaum CJ, et al: Safety of discontinuation of maintenance therapy for disseminated histoplasmosis after immunologic response to antiretroviral therapy. Clin Infect Dis 2004;38:1485–1489.
16. Wheat LJ, Kohler RB, Tewari RP: Diagnosis of disseminated histoplasmosis by detection of *Histoplasma capsulatum* antigen in serum and urine specimens. N Engl J Med 1986;314:83–88.
17. Johnson PC, Wheat LJ, Cloud GA, et al for the U.S. National Institute of Allergy and Infectious Diseases Mycoses Study Group: Safety and efficacy of liposomal amphotericin B compared with conventional amphotericin B for induction therapy of histoplasmosis in patients with AIDS. Ann Intern Med 2002;137:105–109.
18. Stevens DA: Coccidioidomycosis. N Engl J Med 1995;332:1077–1082.
19. Bradsher RW, Chapman SW, Pappas PG: Blastomycosis—review article. Infect Dis Clin North Am 2003;17:21–40.
20. Marr KA, Patterson T, Denning D: Aspergillosis pathogenesis, clinical manifestations and therapy. Infect Dis Clin North Am 2002;16:875–894.
21. Denning DW. *Aspergillus* species. In: Mandell GL, Bennett JE, Dolin R, eds: Mandell, Douglas and Bennett's Principles and Practice of Infectious Diseases. Philadelphia: Churchill Livingstone, 2000, pp 2674–2685.
22. Latge JP: *Aspergillus fumigatus* and aspergillosis. Clin Microbiol Rev 1999;12:310–350.
23. Segal BH, DeCarlo ES, Kwon-Chung KJ, et al: *Aspergillus nidulans* infection in chronic granulomatous disease. Medicine 1998;77:345–354.
24. Patterson TF, Kirkpatrick WR, White M, et al: Invasive aspergillosis. Disease spectrum, treatment practices, and outcomes. Medicine 2000;79:250–260.
25. Wald A, Leisenring W, van Burik J-A, Bowden RA: Epidemiology of *Aspergillusi* infections in a large cohort of patients undergoing bone marrow transplantation. J Infect Dis 1997;175:1459–1466.
26. Patterson JE: Epidemiology of fungal infections in solid organ transplant patients. Transpl Infect Dis 1999;1:229–236.
27. Mylonakis E, Barlam TF, Flanigan T, Rich JD: Pulmonary aspergillosis and invasive disease in AIDS. Chest 1998;114:251–262.
28. Shetty D, Giri N, Gonazalez CE, et al: Invasive aspergillosis in human immunodeficiency virus-infected children. Pediatr Infect Dis J 1997;16: 216–221.
29. Walsh TJ, Gonzalez C, Lyman CA, et al: Invasive fungal infections in children. Recent advances in diagnosis and treatment. Adv Pediatr Infect Dis 1996;11:187–290.
30. Herron MD, Vanderhooft SL, Byington C, King JD: Aspergillosis in a 24-week newborn. A case report. J Perinatol 2002;23:256–259.

31. Winkelstein JA, Marino MC, Johnston RB Jr, et al: Chronic granulomatous disease. Report on a national registry of 368 patients. Medicine 2000;79: 155–169.
32. Muller FC, Trusen A, Weig M: Clinical manifestations and diagnosis of invasive aspergillosis in immunocompromised children. Eur J Pediatr 2002;161:563–574.
33. Steinbach WJ, Schell WA, Blankenship JR, et al: In vitro interactions between antifungals and immunosuppressants against *Aspergillus fumigatus*. Antimicrob Agents Chemother 2004;48:1664–1669.
34. Lassoued S, Billey T, Sire S, et al: Pulmonary aspergillosis in a patient with rheumatoid arthritis treated by etanercept. Clin Exp Rheumatology 2004;22:267–268.
35. Warris A, Bjorneklett A, Gaustad P: Invasive pulmonary aspergillosis associated with infliximab therapy. N Engl J Med 2001;344:1099–1100.
36. Abbasi S, Shenep JL, Hughes WT, Flynn PM: Aspergillosis in children with cancer. A 34-year experience. Clin Infect Dis 1999;29:1210–1219.
37. Mehrad B, Paciocco G, Martinez FJ, et al: Spectrum of *Aspergillus* infection in lung transplant recipients. Chest 2001;119:169–175.
38. Thomas KE, Owens CM, Veys PA, et al: The radiological spectrum of invasive aspergillosis in children. A 10-year review. Pediatr Radiol 2003; 33:453–460.
39. Wheat LJ: Rapid diagnosis of invasive aspergillosis by antigen detection. Transpl Infect Dis 2003;5:158–166.
40. Marr KA, Balajee SA, McLaughlin L, et al: Detection of galactomannan antigenemia by enzyme immunoassay for the diagnosis of invasive aspergillosis. Variables that affect performance. J Infect Dis 2004;190: 641–649.
41. Horvath JA, Dummer S: The use of respiratory-tract cultures in the diagnosis of invasive pulmonary aspergillosis. Am J Med 1996;100:171–178.
42. Herbrecht R, Denning DW, Patterson TF, et al: Voriconazole versus amphotericin B for primary therapy of invasive aspergillosis. N Engl J Med 2002;347:408–415.
43. Walsh TJ, Lutsar I, Driscoll T, et al: Voriconazole in the treatment of aspergillosis, scedosporiosis and other invasive fungal infections in children. Pediatr Infect Dis J 2002;21:240–248.
44. Marr KA, Broeckh M, Carter RA, et al: Combination antifungal therapy for invasive aspergillosis. Clin Infect Dis 2004;39:797–802.
45. Gow KW, Hays-Jordan AA, Billups CA, et al: Benefit of surgical resection of invasive pulmonary aspergillosis in pediatric patients undergoing treatment for malignancies and immunodeficiency syndromes. J Pediatr Surg 2003;38:1354–1360.
46. Stevens DA, Kan VL, Judson MA, et al: Practice guidelines for diseases caused by *Aspergillus*. Clin Infect Dis 2000;30:696–709.
47. Perfect JR, Casadevall A: Cryptococcosis. Infect Dis Clin North Am 2002;16:837–874.
48. Sarosi GA: Cryptococcal pneumonia. Semin Respir Infect 1997;12:50–53.
49. Gonzalez CE, Daiva S, Lewis LL, et al: Cryptococcosis in human immunodeficiency virus-infected children. Pediatr Infect Dis J 1996;15:796–800.
50. Goldman DL, Khine H, Abadi J, et al: Serologic evidence for *Cryptococcus neoformans* infection in early childhood. Pediatrics 2001;107:1–6.
51. Sweeney DA, Caserta MT, Korones DN, et al: A ten-year-old boy with a pulmonary nodule secondary to *Cryptococcus neoformans*. Case report and review of the literature. Pediatr Infect Dis J 2003;22:1089–1093.
52. Wheat LJ, Sarosi G, Goldman M: State-of-the-art review of pulmonary fungal infections. Semin Respir Infect 2002;17:158–181.
53. Nadrous HF, Antonios VS, Terrell CL, Ryu JH: Pulmonary cryptococcosis in nonimmunocompromised patients. Chest 2003;124:2143–2147.
54. Saag MS, Graybill RJ, Larsen RA, et al: Practice guidelines for the management of cryptococcal disease. Clin Infect Dis 2000;30:710–718.
55. Hostetter MK: *Candida* species. In: Long SS, Pickering LK, Prober CG, eds: Principles and Practice of Pediatric Infectious Diseases. New York: Churchill Livingstone, 2003, pp 1203–1213.
56. Kontoyiannis DP, Reddy BT, Torres HA, et al: Pulmonary candidiasis in patients with cancer. An autopsy study. Clin Infect Dis 2002;34:400–403.
57. Pappas PG, Rex JH, Sobel JD, et al: Guidelines for treatment of candidiasis. Clin Infect Dis 2004;38:161–189.
58. Rello J, Esandi ME, Diaz E, et al: The role of *Candida* sp. isolated from bronchoscopic samples in nonneutropenic patients. Chest 1998;114:146–149.
59. Barenafanger J, Arakere P, Cruz RD, et al: Improved outcomes associated with limiting identification of *Candida* spp. in respiratory secretions. J Clin Microbiol 2003;41:5645–5649.
60. Ribes JA, Vanover-Sams CL, Baker DJ: Zygomycetes in human disease. Clin Microbiol Rev 2000;13:236–301.
61. Groll AH, Walsh TJ: Uncommon opportunistic fungi: new nosocomial threats. Clin Microbiol Infect 2001;7(Suppl 2):8–24.
62. Tedder M, Spratt JA, Anstadt MP, et al: Pulmonary mucormycosis. Results of medical and surgical therapy. Ann Thorac Surg 1994;57:1044–1050.
63. Dannaoui E, Meletiadis J, Mouton JW, et al: In vitro susceptibilities of zygomycetes to conventional and new antifungals. J Antimicrob Chemother 2003;51:45–52.
64. Imhof A, Balajee SA, Fredricks DN, et al: Breakthrough fungal infections in stem cell transplant recipients receiving voriconazole. Clin Infect Dis 2004;39:743–746.
65. Kauffman CA, Hajjeh R, Chapman SW: Practice guidelines for the management of patients with sporotrichosis. Clin Infect Dis 2000;30: 684–687.
66. Tashiro T, Nagai H, Nagaoka H, et al: *Trichosporon beigelii* pneumonia in patients with hematologic malignancies. Chest 1995;108:190–95.
67. Walsh TJ, Melcher GP, Rinaldi MG, et al: *Trichosporon beigelii*, an emerging pathogen resistant to amphotericin B. J Clin Microbiol 1990;28: 1616–1622.
68. Baden LR, Katz JT, Fishman JA, et al: Salvage therapy with voriconazole for invasive fungal infections in patients failing or intolerant to standard antifungal therapy. Transplantation 2003;76:1632–1637.
69. Jabado N, Casanova JL, Haddad E, et al: Invasive pulmonary infection due to *Scedosporium apiospermum* in two children with chronic granulomatous disease. Clin Infect Dis 1998;27:1437–1441.

36 Pertussis and Other *Bordetella* Infections of the Respiratory Tract

Ulrich Heininger, MD

Pertussis ("whooping cough") is an acute bacterial infection of the respiratory tract. The illness occurs worldwide and affects all age groups, but it is most serious in young, unprotected infants. It is caused by *Bordetella pertussis* (first described in 1906) and, though less frequently, by *B. parapertussis* (1937), *B. bronchiseptica* (1962), and *B. holmesii* (1998).[1–3] The term *pertussis* was coined in 1670 and means "violent cough." The clinical picture was described for the first time in 1640 by Guillaume de Baillou, based on a 1578 epidemic in Paris.[3]

■ MICROBIOLOGY, PATHOGENESIS, AND IMMUNITY

Bordetella organisms are small, aerobic, gram-negative coccobacilli. Today, the genus comprises eight different species, of which five have been shown to cause respiratory tract illness in humans: *B. pertussis* and *B. parapertussis*, the causative agents of whooping cough; *B. bronchiseptica* and *B. holmesii*, which can cause variable respiratory symptoms; *B. trematum*, which has been found in ear and wound infections.[1] However, the overwhelming majority of *Bordetella* infections are caused by *B. pertussis* and *B. parapertussis*, to which the following discussion pertains.

The organism is transmitted by aerosol droplets from infected to susceptible humans. After transmission, adhesion of the bacteria to ciliated cells of the upper and lower respiratory tract establishes colonization, followed by multiplication and spread on the epithelium, local mucosal damage, and finally, induction of respiratory symptoms. Invasiveness is extremely rare.[4] Asymptomatic, transient colonization frequently occurs during reinfection in immune individuals.[5] Animal studies suggest that a variety of virulence factors is involved in the various steps of infection of the respiratory tract (Table 36-1). Expression of these factors is regulated in response to environmental changes by BvgAS, a two-component signal transduction system.[6] The precise mechanisms during *B. pertussis* and *B. parapertussis* infection in the human host are unknown. Laboratory studies suggest that several factors working in concert allow adherence of the organisms to the epithelium and filamentous hemagglutinin (FHA) inhibits phagocytosis. Later on, effects caused by adenylate cyclase toxin and pertactin expression allow effective phagocytosis and killing of the bacteria by the host.[7] The popular belief that pertussis is a single-toxin illness caused by pertussis toxin (PT), exclusively produced by *B. pertussis*, is refutable by the observation that a similar illness results from infection with *B. parapertussis*, which does not express PT.[8] Further insight in the pathogenesis of *Bordetella* infection will be gained in the future now that several members of the genus have been sequenced.[9]

The pathology of pertussis has been characterized by studies of *B. pertussis* infection. It causes inflammation, congestion, and infiltration of the respiratory mucosa with lymphocytes and granulocytes and leads to accumulation of viscous secretions in the lumen of the bronchi, bronchiolar obstruction, and occasional atelectasis.[3] Later in infection, necrosis of the midzonal and basilar parts of the bronchial epithelium results in necrotizing bronchitis (Fig. 36-1). Subsequently, bronchopneumonia may develop and is either caused by *B. pertussis* itself or by secondary infections with other pathogenic bacteria.

Infection with *B. pertussis* of a previously naïve host results in production of serum and salivary antibodies against a number of antigens such as PT, FHA, pertactin, and adenylate cyclase toxin.[10–12] Enzyme-linked immunosorbent assay techniques allow discrimination of class-specific antibodies, with IgG being more reliably detectable than IgA, IgE, and IgM. In individuals who have been "primed" by *B. pertussis* infection or immunization, reinfection will elicit a secondary immune response with or without concomitant symptoms.[5] Of note, infection with *B. pertussis* does not provide lifelong immunity, and apparently no cross protection between different species of *Bordetella* exists.[13,14] After natural infection, sustained IgG and IgA serum antibody levels against FHA, pertactin, and—though less—PT have been observed for several years before they return close to baseline values after approximately 5 years.[15,16] Yet, the precise role of serum antibodies in immunity against pertussis is a matter of ongoing debate, and various studies show conflicting results.[17,18]

Cell-mediated immune responses to *B. pertussis* have been shown to play an important role in protection against pertussis. In mice, challenge with *B. pertussis* resulted in a predominant T-helper 1 cell–mediated immune response followed by complete bacterial clearance.[19] Specific protection could be conferred by adoptive transfer of immune spleen cells into immunosuppressed mice, further underlining the role of T-helper 1 cells. Interestingly, persistent vaccine efficacy has been documented in young children several years after immunization despite significant antibody decline, and it was also preferentially mediated by T-helper 1 cells.[20]

■ EPIDEMIOLOGY

Pertussis occurs worldwide, and humans are the only host of *B. pertussis.* Transmission occurs effectively by droplets, with secondary attack rates close to 100% in exposed susceptible individuals.[3] The incubation period is usually 7 to 10 days but may vary substantially. In a household contact study, secondary cases were noted to have their onset up to 6 weeks after the onset of illness in the primary case, especially when antibiotics were used.[21]

TABLE 36-1. Virulence factors of *Bordetella pertussis* and their specific characteristics

Factor (gene)	Bvg Regulation	Molecule	Major Role	Other Functions	Comments
Pertussis toxin *(ptx)*	Yes	"A" protomer and "B" subunits	Toxin and first-line adhesion factor	Causes leukocytosis by lymphocytosis	Precise role in disease unknown
Filamentous hemagglutinin *(fha)*	Yes	Large, filamentous protein (220 kd)	Major adhesin; predominantly in trachea	Not known	Need for inclusion in vaccine questionable
Fimbriae 2 and 3 *(fim2, fim3, fimX)*	Yes	Small, filamentous proteins (≈23 kd)	Adhesion factor; predominantly in trachea	Agglutinogens; sustain infection	Important stimulator of host's immune response
Pertactin *(prn1, prn2, prn3)*	Yes	69-kd outer membrane protein	Adhesion factor, induces type-specific antibody	Major protective antigen (mouse model)	Important vaccine antigen, used for genotyping
Adenylate cyclase *(cyaA)*	Yes	Protein toxin	Toxin; inhibits phagocytosis by ↑ cAMP	Inhibits chemotaxis and induces apoptosis of macrophages	Candidate for future vaccines!
Tracheal cytotoxin *(tct)*	No	Peptidoglycan derivative	Toxin; paralyzes mucociliary clearance system	Inhibits DNA synthesis and cell death	Nonimmunogenic → not suitable for vaccine
Dermonecrotic toxin *(dnt)*	Yes	Heat-labile toxin (140 kd)	Toxin; dermal necrosis and vasoconstriction	Effect only after injection in skin	Role in human disease unknown
Tracheal colonization factor *(tcfA)*	Yes	Proline-rich protein	Adhesion factor; predominantly in trachea	Not known	C-terminal homology to *prn, brkA,* and *vag-8*
Bordetella resistance to killing factor *(brkA)*	Yes	Outer membrane protein (32 kd)	Adhesion factor	Provides resistance to complement	C-terminal homology to *prn, tcfA,* and *vag-8*
Virulence-activated gene 8 *(vag-8)*	Yes	Outer membrane protein (95 kd)	Adhesion factor (?)	Not known	C-terminal homology to *prn, tcfA,* and *brkA*
Lipooligosaccharide *(wlb)*	Yes	Lipid A and trisaccharide	Presumably required for nasal colonization	Not known	Substantially species-specific structure within *Bordetella*
Bvg intermediate-phase protein A *(bipA)*	Yes	Outer membrane protein (137 kd)	Transmission (?) and adhesion factor	Not known	First of a new class of *Bordetella* antigens ("intermediate phase")
Type III secretion system *(bsc)*	Yes	Several, not yet specified proteins	Secretes effector proteins into host cells	Down-regulation of the host immune system	Appears to be functional only in *B. bronchiseptica* (and some *B. parapertussis* strains)

CAMP, cyclic adenosine monophosphate.

Modified and updated from Heininger U: Recent progress in clinical and basic pertussis research. Eur J Pediatr 2001;160:203–213.

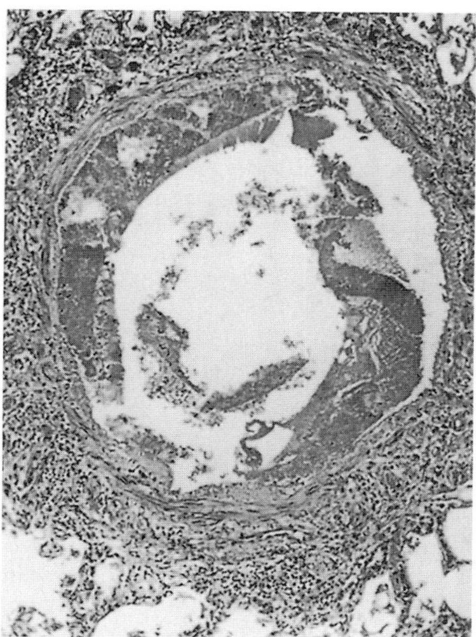

■ **FIGURE 36-1.** Necrotizing bronchitis (×100).

The epidemiology of pertussis caused by *B. pertussis* infection is greatly influenced by immunization, which not only provides individual protection but to some extent also confers group protection. In the absence of immunization, pertussis mainly affects infants and young children, whereas comparatively few cases occur in adolescents and adults. Yet, pertussis in adolescents and adults is an important source of infection in young, unprotected children, especially because disease in older age groups often is mild and may not be recognized as pertussis.[13] In contrast to *B. pertussis*, *B. parapertussis* infections appear to occur independent of immunization activities, and their relative frequency varies considerably by geography and time.[8,22]

In the 1930s and 1940s the annual incidence of pertussis was approximately 150 per 100,000 population, and the case fatality rate was 4% in the United States.[23] After the introduction of pertussis vaccines in the 1950s, significant changes in the epidemiology of pertussis occurred: overall, reported cases decreased by approximately 150-fold to a low of one case and less than 0.01 deaths per 100,000 by the mid-1970s. However, a resurgence of cases and a gradual shift toward an increase of pertussis in adolescents and adults has recently been noted in North America and elsewhere.[24] It is still a matter of debate whether this increase is caused by waning vaccine immunity and a decreased chance for natural boosters, a consequence of increased awareness and diagnostic tools, or both. It should be noted that pertussis in adolescents and adults frequently is atypical, and true numbers of cases are probably higher than reported.[25,26] Furthermore, in support of a true change in epidemiology, a rise in fatalities due to pertussis has been observed in infants in the United States during the last decade. Whereas 1.67 deaths per million infants per year were reported in the 1980s, the rate increased to an average of 2.40 in the 1990s. The increased incidence almost exclusively affected infants under 4 months of age.[27]

The crucial role that mass immunization plays in controlling pertussis has been clearly demonstrated in countries such as Japan, England, and Sweden, where infant pertussis vaccination was either discontinued or markedly curtailed as a result of unsubstantiated concerns about vaccine-related adverse events. In Japan, after two children died within 48 hours of the receipt of the same lot of pertussis vaccine, the percentage of infants immunized decreased rapidly from 78% in 1974 to 14% in 1976. During the 4-year period before 1975 there were 400 cases of pertussis annually, and a total of 10 deaths. In contrast, from 1976 to 1979, following the dramatic drop in vaccine use for infants, the number of pertussis cases increased to 13,000 per year and there were a total of 113 deaths. When pertussis immunization was reintroduced in 1981, the number of cases fell back to the pre-1975 rates.[3]

In the prevaccine era pertussis had been endemic, with occurrence of epidemics every 2 to 5 years. It has previously been noted that the epidemic cycle remained basically unchanged after introduction of routine immunization in childhood.[28] Thus, it appeared that immunization effectively controlled disease but had only a limited effect on the circulation of the organism in the population. Recently, data from the United Kingdom have challenged this proposal; there, the interepidemic cycle of pertussis increased from 2 years in the prevaccination era to 4 years after introduction of pertussis immunization—a situation that can best be explained by reduced circulation of *B. pertussis* in a highly immunized population.[29] Moreover, this observation is in accordance with the concept of waning immunity in adolescents and adults that has been recognized over the last few decades.

Several studies have shown that females and males are equally affected by pertussis in childhood, whereas a female preponderance (55% to 69%) is noted in adolescents and adults.[23,30,31] Most likely, this is due to more frequent contact of females with young children, from whom they acquire infection. The seasonal pattern of pertussis is variable between different geographic locations.[30,31]

■ CLINICAL CHARACTERISTICS

Typical pertussis is a three-stage illness, comprising catarrhal, paroxysmal, and convalescent phases.[3] The catarrhal stage lasts for about 1 to 2 weeks and is characterized by flulike symptoms such as coryza, sneezing, lacrimation, conjunctival injection, malaise, unspecific cough, and occasionally a low-grade fever. It is followed by the paroxysmal stage, which is marked by an increase of frequency and severity of cough with paroxysms as the most typical feature; characteristically, repetitive series of 5 to 10 or more hacking spells of cough occur during a single expiration. At the end of a paroxysm, a typical whoop is noted which is caused by the sudden inrush of inspired air through a narrowed glottis. Cyanosis, neck vein distention, bulging eyes, tongue protrusion, salivation, lacrimation, sweating, and also frequently post-tussive vomiting of food or viscous mucus occur. Fever is usually minimal or absent during this stage. Paroxysms may occur several times per hour, during both day and night, triggered by various stimuli such as eating and drinking, and physical or emotional stress. The paroxysmal stage may last from a few days to several weeks, until the convalescent stage with gradual improvement is reached; this phase is marked by a decrease in the frequency and severity of coughing spells. However, over a period of several months, similar coughing episodes may again occur, often associated with other respiratory tract infections. Notably, *B. pertussis* infections present with considerable variability that primarily depends on age, previous immunization, or infection. Other variables, including the presence of passively acquired antibody (in young infants), degree of exposure, specific bacterial inoculum, host genetic and acquired factors, and genotype of the organism, may contribute to attenuation of symptoms.

The variability of symptoms is exemplified by results from a study of 1860 culture-positive cases in unvaccinated children and adolescents in Germany. In that study, 38% of patients had a total cough illness duration of 4 weeks or less, 18% had nonparoxysmal cough, 21% did not whoop, and 47% did not have post-tussive vomiting.[31]

On rare occasions, *B. pertussis* infection has been found to cause otitis media and to be associated with unilateral hyperlucent lung (MacLeod's or Swyer-James syndrome) and the hemolytic uremic syndrome.[32–34]

There is a wide spectrum of complications of pertussis, most of which predominantly occur in young infants (Table 36-2). Respiratory complications include bronchopneumonia with or without atelectasis, pulmonary hypertension, and otitis media mainly secondary to other respiratory tract pathogens. Pertussis also has been associated with activation of latent tuberculosis. Additional complications that have been observed as a consequence to pertussis include ulcer of the frenulum of the tongue, epistaxis, melena, subconjunctival hemorrhages, meningoencephalitis, encephalopathy with cerebral seizures, tetanic seizures caused by severe alkalosis as a result of loss of gastric contents due to persistent vomiting, subdural hematomas, spinal epidural hematoma, rupture of the diaphragm, rib fracture, umbilical hernia, inguinal hernia, rectal prolapse, dehydration, syndrome of inappropriate antidiuretic hormone secretion, apnea, and nutritional disturbances.[3] Death secondary to pneumonia and/or pulmonary hypertension or sudden death, probably due to severe hypoxemia, occurs mainly in infants, for whom the rate is 0.6%.[30,35] There is no evidence for long-term sequelae such as allergic sensitization after pertussis.[36]

Overall symptoms with *B. parapertussis* infection are similar to those caused by *B. pertussis*, but illness usually is less severe and of shorter duration.[8] Dual infections of *B. pertussis* and *B. parapertussis* have been observed.[37] On rare occasions, *B. bronchiseptica* and *B. holmesii* have been isolated from children with pertussis-like illness.[38,39]

DIAGNOSIS AND DIFFERENTIAL DIAGNOSIS

In typical cases, a diagnosis of pertussis can be established on the basis of characteristic symptoms. However, several microorganisms other than *B. pertussis* or *B. parapertussis* can cause cough illnesses that can occasionally be confused with pertussis. In one study from Germany, which was conducted within a protective efficacy trial of an acellular pertussis vaccine, the frequency of serologic evidence for an infection with microorganisms other than *B. pertussis* was assessed in children with pertussis-like coughs.[40] Of 149 such children, a diagnosis of adenovirus ($n = 33$); parainfluenza viruses 1, 2, and 3 ($n = 18$); *Mycoplasma pneumoniae* infection ($n = 15$); and respiratory syncytial virus infection ($n = 14$) was made. In studies of concurrent outbreaks of *Mycoplasma* and *B. pertussis* infections it has been shown that clinical symptoms alone lacked adequate specificity to distinguish pertussis from mycoplasmal infection.[41] Moreover, in populations with high immunization rates, atypical presentations of *B. pertussis* may be more frequent than classical illness, and a high index of clinical suspicion is imperative in the diagnosis of pertussis.[30] These observations underscore the need for appropriate laboratory tests if there is any doubt about the diagnosis.[42]

Isolation of *B. pertussis* or *B. parapertussis* from a person with a cough illness provides certainty of its causative role. Nasopharyngeal secretions, obtained by aspiration or calcium alginate or Dacron swabs, and specific media (Regan-Lowe or Bordet-Gengou agar and modified Stainer-Scholte broth) are necessary to recover *Bordetella* spp. The organisms are distinguished from each other by specific latex agglutination tests or by specific fluorescent antibody staining of suspicious colonies. Alternatively, direct fluorescent antibody tests can be applied. Sensitivity of culture is optimal (≥95%) in unvaccinated, untreated individuals early in the course of the illness, when clinical suspicion is frequently low. During the paroxysmal phase, sensitivity of culture rapidly declines to 50% or lower. Over the last decade, polymerase chain reaction (PCR) technique has markedly improved the diagnosis of pertussis. It is particularly useful in oligosymptomatic cases, in patients who have been started on antibiotics, and in patients with progressed illness. It should be noted that calcium alginate swabs should not be used for collection of nasopharyngeal secretions for PCR

TABLE 36-2. Complications in 1640 unvaccinated patients with *Bordetella pertussis* infections by age group as reported in follow-up questionnaires

	AGE					
Complication	**<6 Months ($N = 63$) N (%)**	**6–12 Months ($N = 59$) N (%)**	**1–4 Years ($N = 610$) N (%)**	**4–9 Years ($N = 846$) N (%)**	**>9 Years ($N = 62$) N (%)**	**Total ($N = 1640$) N (%)**
Pneumonia	2 (3.2)	–	8 (1.3)	18 (2.1)	–	28 (1.7)
Apnea/cyanosis	10 (15.9)	1 (1.7)	–	1 (0.1)	–	12 (0.7)
Otitis media	–	–	6 (0.9)	4 (0.5)	–	10 (0.6)
Poor feeding/severe vomiting	2 (3.2)	–	2 (0.3)	2 (0.2)	1 (1.6)	7 (0.4)
Cardiopulmonary failure	1 (1.7)	–	–	–	–	1 (0.1)
Death	–	1 (1.6)	–	–	–	1 (0.1)
Others*	–	2 (3.4)	5 (0.8)	15 (1.8)	–	22 (1.3)
Unspecified	1 (1.6)	–	8 (1.3)	5 (0.6)	2 (3.2)	16 (1.0)
Any	15 (23.8)	3 (5.1)	29 (4.8)	45 (5.3)	3 (4.8)	95 (5.8)

* Includes cases of epistaxis, inguinal hernia, frequent paroxysms, and bronchitis.

From Heininger U, Klich K, Stehr K, Cherry JD: Clinical findings in *Bordetella pertussis* infections. Results of a prospective multicenter surveillance study. Pediatrics 1997;100:e10.

because of assay inhibition, whereas Dacron swabs are suitable. Advanced technology today allows discrimination between different species of the *Bordetella* genus, and recent developments such as real-time detection of the amplification products and Light Cycler PCR now provide results within a few hours.[43,44] Concerns about the specificity of PCR have led to the formulation of consensus recommendations proposing that "a PCR-positive result in someone with mild or no symptoms should be interpreted with caution and, if possible, other markers such as serology or epidemiology should be added."[45] Several studies have since been carried out, and rates of sensitivity varied between 21% and 65%. False-positive results were found to be rare.[1]

Serologic tests are the most sensitive technique for the diagnosis of *Bordetella* infections. Enzyme immunoassays have most widely been applied, and although whole-cell preparations of *B. pertussis* can be used as antigens, purified proteins such as PT, FHA, and pertactin are preferable for their better specificity. IgG antibody assays provide sufficient sensitivity, but addition of IgA assays is helpful.[46] Although paired acute and convalescent phase serum samples are optimal, analysis of a single serum specimen is more appropriate for routine purposes. Unfortunately, however, serology tests are not standardized and interpretation of results is difficult in the presence of vaccine-induced preexisting antibodies. Therefore, test results have to be interpreted cautiously, and cutoff values derived from age-matched control groups are required. IgA antibodies have traditionally been considered to be reliable indicators of recent or acute infection.[47] A recent study, however, has shown persistently high IgA antibodies against FHA, pertactin, and, though less pronounced, PT for as long as 30 months after infection.[16] This observation further complicates the serologic diagnosis of *B. pertussis* infection in single-serum analyses.

Most cases of pertussis caused by primary *B. pertussis* infection in unvaccinated individuals will demonstrate leukocytosis due to lymphocytosis. This is caused by the effects of PT, which appears to reduce L-selectin expression by the T cells and thus prevents their homing to the lymphoid tissues.[48] In contrast, secondary infections and breakthrough cases of pertussis in vaccinated patients (with preexisting IgG antibodies to PT) frequently lack leukocytosis, as do patients infected with *B. parapertussis* (which does not express PT).[8]

The role of radiographic imaging in pertussis is limited. The most frequent abnormalities are consolidation, atelectasis, and hilar lymphadenopathy. In a case series of 238 hospitalized patients with pertussis, radiographic abnormalities were detected in 63 patients (26%). Pulmonary consolidation was seen in 50 patients (21%), atelectasis in 9 (4%), and lymphadenopathy in 22 (9%). Most consolidations were peribronchial (72%). For unknown reasons, both atelectasis and consolidation were more common on the right and predominantly involved the lower and middle lobes of the lung. Radiographic abnormalities were more common beyond infancy. Follow-up radiographs after 1 month demonstrated no significant radiographic sequelae.[49] One can conclude that chest radiographs should be limited to severe cases and when pulmonary complications are suspected on the basis of clinical findings.

■ TREATMENT

Several antibiotics have proven in vitro activity against *B. pertussis* and *B. parapertussis*.[1] Sufficient minimal inhibitory concentrations have been demonstrated for macrolides and for fluoroquinolones. In contrast, minimal inhibitory concentrations of oral beta-lactam antibiotics, including cephalosporins, are unacceptable and render them unsuitable for treatment of pertussis. Oral erythromycin (succinate formulation at 50 mg/kg body weight/day given every 6–8 hours or estolate formulation at doses of 40 mg/kg/day in 12-hour intervals for 14 days) still is the preferred treatment. When given in the catarrhal or early paroxysmal stage of the illness, this will ameliorate the symptoms, eradicate the bacteria from the nasopharynx within a few days, and terminate contagiousness of the patient. Of the different formulations, erythromycin is favored by most experts. The following recent observations should be noted. First, some erythromycin-resistant strains of *B. pertussis* have been isolated in the United States during the 1990s.[50] However, because these observations have so far been limited to single cases, erythromycin remains the first-line drug, although ongoing surveillance of antibiotic susceptibility of isolated strains is necessary. The mechanism underlying resistance is currently unknown. Second, 7 days of erythromycin estolate was shown to be equally effective as 14 days in a large Canadian study.[51] It should be noted, though, that this investigation was carried out in a highly vaccinated community, and results may have been different in unvaccinated children. Third, when erythromycin is used in young infants the occurrence of a hypertrophic pyloric stenosis as an adverse event should be borne in mind, and parents need to be educated about the symptoms of this rare but significant risk.[52]

New macrolide antibiotics with improved gastrointestinal tolerability, such as clarithromycin or azithromycin, appear to be acceptable alternatives with effects comparable to those with erythromycin. Clinical efficacy studies, however, are still limited. In Canada, the microbiologic and clinical efficacy and the clinical safety of a 7-day course of clarithromycin (15 mg/kg/day in two doses for 7 days) was compared to a 14-day course of erythromycin (40 mg/kg/day in three doses for 14 days) in a prospective, randomized, single-blind (investigator) trial in children from 1 month to 16 years of age with culture-proven pertussis.[53] Nasopharyngeal cultures for *B. pertussis* were performed at enrollment and after the end of treatment. Microbiologic eradication and clinical cure rates were equal: 100% (31/31) for clarithromycin and 96% (22/23) for erythromycin. Patients on clarithromycin had significantly fewer adverse events (45%) than those on erythromycin (62%).

In an open, uncontrolled study in the United States, 34 subjects (most of them children) with culture or PCR-proven *B. pertussis* infection received a 5-day course of azithromycin (10 mg/kg in a single dose on the first day and 5 mg/kg/day as single doses on the following 4 days). *B. pertussis* was eradicated from the nasopharynx in 33 (97%) of 34 patients after 72 hours, and all were negative on follow-up after 2 to 3 weeks.[54]

The role of intravenous antipertussis immunoglobulin treatment remains controversial. In one recent study, a hyperimmunoglobulin was prepared as a 4% IgG solution from the pooled plasma from donors immunized with inactivated pertussis toxoid, resulting in IgG PT antibody concentrations more than sevenfold higher than those in conventional intravenous immunoglobulin products.[55] Twenty-six children with laboratory-confirmed pertussis received one of three doses (1500, 750, or 250 mg/kg). All three treatment groups demonstrated a decrease of lymphocytosis ($P < .05$) and clinical improvement (paroxysmal coughing) by the third day after antipertussis immunoglobulin treatment. No serious adverse events occurred, but one patient experienced transient hypotension that responded to a decreased infusion rate. Unfortunately, no information on concomitant antibiotic treatment was provided. Prospective, controlled trials must be conducted before any firm conclusions on the value of immunoglobulin treatment of pertussis can be drawn.

General supportive medical treatment is important for patients with pertussis. Young infants, who are threatened by hypoxemia associated with apneic spells, should be hospitalized and their blood oxygen saturation closely monitored. Careful removal of respiratory secretions and oxygen supplementation may be necessary. Pneumonia, frequent apneic spells, and significant respiratory distress may require assisted ventilation, especially in neonates and young infants.[3] Physicial and emotional stress, which may trigger paroxysms, should be avoided. Further, if post-tussive vomiting is present, careful attention should be paid to adequate fluid and food intake. Respiratory isolation precautions should be implemented until 5 days of effective antibiotic treatment have been received.

Uncontrolled observations indicate that corticosteroids and/or β-adrenergic drugs adjunctive to antibiotics may ameliorate symptoms of pertussis, but evidence of efficacy is lacking.[3]

PREVENTION

Prevention of pertussis is possible by avoidance of exposure, post-exposure antibiotic treatment, and immunization. Avoidance of exposure is usually impossible in clinical practice, given that contagiousness is highest during the early stage of illness in the primary case where a diagnosis of pertussis commonly has not yet been made. Prophylactic use of erythromycin (or clarithromycin or azithromycin) has been shown to protect from *B. pertussis* infection when given to close contacts and is most useful when administered before the occurrence of the first secondary case.[56] Recommended duration of treatment is 14 days and should be given to all close contacts regardless of age and immunization status according to recommendations by the American Academy of Pediatrics.[57] Moreover, children younger than 7 years of age who are unimmunized or incompletely immunized should receive a dose of pertussis vaccine.

Active immunization of infants, preschool children, and possibly adolescents is the most effective way to prevent pertussis. Over the last two decades, acellular pertussis vaccines (containing various numbers and quantities of *B. pertussis* antigens) have been developed and studied for safety, immunogenicity, and efficacy. They have substituted conventional whole-cell pertussis vaccines, mainly because they cause less unpleasant side effects.[1] Virtually all countries recommend a primary series of two or three vaccine doses in infancy and usually also a reinforcing dose in the second year of life. Timely initiation of the immunization series, usually at 2 months of age, is crucial, because the risk for severe pertussis in immunized infants decreases from dose to dose when compared with unimmunized infants.[58] The optimal timing and number of further booster immunizations is a matter of ongoing debate. Since vaccine-induced efficacy is sustained despite declining antibody values, observational studies are needed to answer these questions. Investigations conducted so far indicate ongoing efficacy after three or four doses of acellular pertussis vaccine for several years.[1] Today, most countries still recommend a fifth dose at preschool age, but postponing it to adolescence is an interesting concept that has already been adapted by some countries such as Canada, France, and Germany.

Overall, when compared to conventional whole-cell pertussis vaccines, acellular component vaccines have been shown to cause lower rates of local and systemic reactions such as fever.[3] Also, severe reactions such as febrile seizures and hypotonic-hyporesponsive episodes declined significantly (79% and 60%, respectively) with the broad dissemination of acellular pertussis vaccines.[59] Of some concern is that local reactions after pertussis immunization increase from dose to dose, and whole-limb swelling at the site of injection may occur. Yet, these side effects are only temporary, usually not interfering with the child's well-being, and without sequelae. Furthermore, they are considered to be less severe than those seen after five consecutive doses of whole-cell vaccine.[60]

Providing timely and complete immunizations against pertussis for all infants, young children, and possibly adolescents and adults will help to better control pertussis in the future.

REFERENCES

1. Heininger U: Recent progress in clinical and basic pertussis research. Eur J Pediatr 2001;160:203–213.
2. Woolfrey BF, Moody JA: Human infections associated with *Bordetella bronchiseptica*. Clin Microbiol Rev 1991;4:243–255.
3. Cherry JD, Heininger U: Pertussis and other *Bordetella* infections. In: Feigin RD, Cherry JD, eds: Textbook of Pediatric Infectious Diseases. Philadelphia: WB Saunders, 2004, pp 1588–1608.
4. Centers for Disease Control and Prevention: Fatal case of unsuspected pertussis diagnosed from a blood culture—Minnesota, 2003. MMWR Morb Mortal Wkly Rep 2004;53:131–132.
5. Long S, Lischner H, Deforest A, Clark J: Serologic evidence of subclinical pertussis in immunized children. Pediatr Infect Dis J 1990;9:700–705.
6. Weiss AA, Falkow S: Genetic analysis of phase change in *Bordetella pertussis*. Infect Immun 1984;43:263–269.
7. Heininger U: Pertussis. An old disease that is still with us. Curr Opin Infect Dis 2001;14:329–335.
8. Heininger U, Stehr K, Schmitt-Grohé S, Lorenz C, Rost R, Christenson P, et al: Clinical characteristics of illness caused by *Bordetella parapertussis* compared with illness caused by *Bordetella pertussis*. Pediatr Infect Dis J 1994;13:306–309.
9. Parkhill J, Sebaihia M, Preston A, Murphy LD, Thomson N, Harris DE, et al: Comparative analysis of the genome sequences of *Bordetella pertussis, Bordetella parapertussis* and *Bordetella bronchiseptica*. Nat Genet 2003;35: 32–40.
10. Thomas M, Redhead K, Lambert H: Human serum antibody responses to *Bordetella pertussis* infection and pertussis vaccination. J Infect Dis 1989; 159:211–218.
11. Zackrisson G, Lagergard T, Trollfors B, Krantz I: Immunoglobulin A antibodies to pertussis toxin and filamentous hemagglutinin in saliva from patients with pertussis. J Clin Microbiol 1990;28:1502–1505.
12. Cherry JD, Xing DX, Newland P, Patel K, Heininger U, Corbel MJ: Determination of serum antibody to *Bordetella pertussis* adenylate cyclase toxin in vaccinated and unvaccinated children and in children and adults with pertussis. Clin Infect Dis 2004;38:502–507.
13. Mortimer EA: Pertussis and its prevention. A family affair. J Infect Dis 1990;161:473–479.
14. Taranger J, Trollfors B, Lagergard T, Zackrisson G: Parapertussis infection followed by pertussis infection. Lancet 1994;2:1703.
15. Isacson J, Trollfors B, Hedvall G, Taranger J, Zackrisson G: Response and decline of serum IgG antibodies to pertussis toxin, filamentous hemagglutinin and pertactin in children with pertussis. Scand J Infect Dis 1995;27: 273–277.
16. Heininger U, Cherry JD, Stehr K: Serologic response and antibody-titer decay in adults with pertussis. Clin Infect Dis 2004;38:591–594.
17. Hewlett EL, Halperin SA: Serological correlates of immunity to *Bordetella pertussis*. Vaccine 1998;16:1899–1900.
18. Taranger J, Trollfors B, Lagergard T, Sundh V, Bryla DA, Schneerson R, et al: Correlation between pertussis toxin IgG antibodies in postvaccination sera and subsequent protection against pertussis. J Infect Dis 2000;181: 1010–1013.
19. Mills KH, Barnard A, Watkins J, Redhead K: Cell-mediated immunity to *Bordetella pertussis*. Role of Th1 cells in bacterial clearance in a murine respiratory infection model. Infect Immun 1993;61:399–410.

20. Ausiello CM, Lande R, Urbani F, Di Carlo B, Stefanelli P, Salmaso S, et al: Cell-mediated immunity and antibody responses to *Bordetella pertussis* antigens in children with a history of pertussis infection and in recipients of an acellular pertussis vaccine. J Infect Dis 1995;181:1989–1995.
21. Heininger U, Cherry JD, Stehr K, Schmitt-Grohé S, Überall MA, Laussucq S, et al: Comparative efficacy of the Lederle/Takeda acellular pertussis component DTP (DTaP) vaccine and Lederle whole-cell component DTP vaccine in German infants following household exposure. Pediatrics 1998;102: 546–553.
22. Liese JG, Renner C, Stojanov S, Belohradsky BH, Munich Vaccine Study Group: Clinical and epidemiological picture of *B pertussis* and *B parapertussis* infections after introduction of acellular pertussis vaccines. Arch Dis Child 2003;88:684–687.
23. Cherry JD: The epidemiology of pertussis and pertussis immunization in the United Kingdom and the United States. A comparative study. Curr Probl Pediat 1984;14:1–78.
24. Wirsing von König CH, Halperin S, Riffelmann M, Guiso N: Pertussis of adults and infants. Lancet Infect Dis 2002;2:744–750.
25. Cherry JD: Epidemiological, clinical, and laboratory aspects of pertussis in adults. Clin Infect Dis 1999;28(Suppl 2):S112–S117.
26. Schmitt-Grohé S, Cherry, JD, Heininger U, Überall MA, Pineda E, Stehr K: Pertussis in German adults. Clin Infect Dis 1995;21:860–866.
27. Vitek CR, Pascual FB, Baughman AL, Murphy TV: Increase in deaths from pertussis among young infants in the United States in the 1990s. Pediatr Infect Dis J 2003;22:628–634.
28. Fine PEM, Clarkson JA: Reflections on the efficacy of pertussis vaccines. Rev Infect Dis 1987;9:866–883.
29. Rohani P, Earn DJD, Grenfell BT: Impact of immunisation on pertussis transmission in England and Wales. Lancet 2000;355:285–286.
30. Farizo KM, Cochi SL, Zell ER, Brink EW, Wassilak SG, Patriarca PA: Epidemiological features of pertussis in the United States, 1980–1989. Clin Infect Dis 1992;14:708–719.
31. Heininger U, Klich K, Stehr K, Cherry JD: Clinical findings in *Bordetella pertussis* infections. Results of a prospective multicenter surveillance study. Pediatrics 1997;100:e10.
32. Decherd ME, Deskin RW, Rowen JL, Brindley MB: *Bordetella pertussis* causing otitis media. A case report. Laryngoscope 2003;113:226–227.
33. Trimis G, Theodoridou M, Mostrou G, Kakavakis K: Swyer-James (MacLeod's) syndrome following pertussis infection in an infant. Scand J Infect Dis 2003;35:197–199.
34. Berner R, Krause MF, Gordjani N, Zipfel PF, Boehm N, Krueger M, et al: Hemolytic uremic syndrome due to an altered factor H triggered by neonatal pertussis. Pediatr Nephrol 2002;17:190–192.
35. Heininger U, Stehr K, Cherry JD: Serious pertussis overlooked in infants. Eur J Pediatr 1992;151:342–343.
36. Henderson J, North K, Griffiths M, Harvey I, Golding J, Avon Longitudinal Study of Pregnancy and Childhood Team: Pertussis vaccination and wheezing illnesses in young children. Prospective cohort study. BMJ 1999;318: 1173–1176.
37. Lautrop H: Observations on parapertussis in Denmark 1950–1957. Acta Pathol Microbiol Scand 1958;43:255–266.
38. Stefanelli P, Mastrantonio P, Hausman SZ, Giuliano M, Burns DL: Molecular characterization of two *Bordetella bronchiseptica* strains isolated from children with coughs. J Clin Microbiol 1997;35:1550–1555.
39. Yih WK, Silva EA, Ida J, Harrington N, Lett SM, George H: *Bordetella holmesii*-like organisms isolated from Massachusetts patients with pertussis-like symptoms. Emerg Infect Dis 1999;5:441–443.
40. Wirsing von König CH, Rott H, Bogaerts H, Schmitt HJ: A serologic study of organisms possibly associated with pertussis-like coughing. Pediatr Infect Dis J 1998;17:645–649.
41. Davis SF, Sutter RW, Strebel PM, Orton C, Alexander V, Sanden GN, et al: Concurrent outbreaks of pertussis and *Mycoplasma pneumoniae* infection. Clinical and epidemiological characteristics of illnesses manifested by cough. Clin Infect Dis 1995;20:621–628.
42. Müller FM, Hoppe JE, Wirsing von Konig CH: Laboratory diagnosis of pertussis. State of the art in 1997. J Clin Microbiol 1997;35:2435–2443.
43. Templeton KE, Scheltinga SA, Van Der Zee A, Diederen BM, Kruijssen AM, Goossens H, et al: Evaluation of real-time PCR for detection of and discrimination between *Bordetella pertussis*, *Bordetella parapertussis*, and *Bordetella holmesii* for clinical diagnosis. J Clin Microbiol 2003;41: 4121–4126.
44. Kösters K, Reischl U, Schmetz J, Riffelmann M, Wirsing von Konig CH: Real-time LightCycler PCR for detection and discrimination of *Bordetella pertussis* and *Bordetella parapertussis*. J Clin Microbiol 2002;40:1719–1722.
45. Meade BD, Bollen A: Recommendations for use of the polymerase chain reaction in the diagnosis of *Bordetella pertussis* infections. J Med Microbiol 1994;41:51–55.
46. Hallander HO: Microbiological and serological diagnosis of pertussis. Clin Infect Dis 1999;28(Suppl 2):S99–S106.
47. Viljanen MK, Ruuskanen O, Granberg C, Salmi TT: Serological diagnosis of pertussis. IgM, IgA and IgG antibodies against *Bordetella pertussis* measured by enzyme-linked immunosorbent assay (ELISA). Scand J Infect Dis 1982;14:117–122.
48. Hudnall SD, Molina CP: Marked increase in L-selectin-negative T cells in neonatal pertussis. The lymphocytosis explained? Am J Clin Pathol 2000;114:35–40.
49. Bellamy EA, Johnston ID, Wilson AG: The chest radiograph in whooping cough. Clin Radiol 1987;38:39–43.
50. Korgenski EK, Daly JA: Surveillance and detection of erythromycin resistance in *Bordetella pertussis* isolates recovered from a pediatric population in the Intermountain West region of the United States. J Clin Microbiol 1997;35:2989–2991.
51. Halperin SA, Bortolussi R, Langley JM, Miller B, Eastwood BJ: Seven days of erythromycin estolate is as effective as fourteen days for the treatment of *Bordetella pertussis* infections. Pediatrics 1997;100:65–71.
52. Honein MA, Paulozzi LJ, Himelright IM, Lee B, Cragan JD, Patterson L, et al: Infantile hypertrophic pyloric stenosis after pertussis prophylaxis with erythromycin. A case review and cohort study. Lancet 1999;354: 2101–2105.
53. Lebel MH, Mehra F, Mehra S: Efficacy and safety of clarithromycin versus erythromycin for the treatment of pertussis. A prospective, randomized, single blind trial. Pediatr Infect Dis J 2001;20:1149–1154.
54. Pichichero ME, Hoeger WJ, Casey JR: Azithromycin for the treatment of pertussis. Pediatr Infect Dis J 2003;22:847–849.
55. Bruss JB, Malley R, Halperin S, Dobson S, Dhala M, McIver J, et al: Treatment of severe pertussis. A study of the safety and pharmacology of intravenous pertussis immunoglobulin. Pediatr Infect Dis J 1999;18: 505–511.
56. De Serres G, Boulianne N, Duval B: Field effectiveness of erythromycin prophylaxis to prevent pertussis within families. Pediatr Infect Dis J 1995; 14:969–975.
57. American Academy of Pediatrics: Active immunization. Pertussis. In: Pickering LK, ed: 2003 Red Book. Report of the Committee on Infectious Diseases. Elk Grove Village, Ill: American Academy of Pediatrics, 2003, pp 472–486.
58. Juretzko P, von Kries R, Hermann M, Wirsing von König CH, Weil J, Giani G: Effectiveness of acellular pertussis vaccine assessed by hospital-based active surveillance in Germany. Clin Infect Dis 2002;35: 162–167.
59. Le Saux N, Barrowman NJ, Moore DL, Whiting S, Scheifele D, Halperin S, et al: Decrease in hospital admissions for febrile seizures and reports of hypotonic-hyporesponsive episodes presenting to hospital emergency departments since switching to acellular pertussis vaccine in Canada. A report from IMPACT. Pediatrics 2003;112:e348.
60. Halperin SA, Scheifele D, Mills E, Guasparini R, Humphreys G, Barreto L, et al: Nature, evolution, and appraisal of adverse events and antibody response associated with the fifth consecutive dose of a five-component acellular pertussis–based combination vaccine. Vaccine 2003;21:2298–2306.

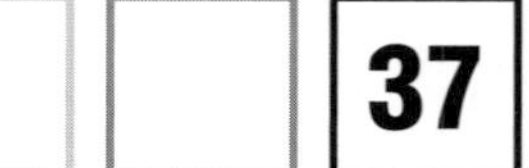

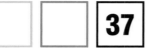

37 Pneumonia Secondary to Varicella and Measles

Joanne Embree, MD • Samira Mubareka, MD • Victor Chernick, MD

Measles and varicella viruses cause the two childhood exanthematous febrile illnesses that are the most commonly associated with severe pneumonia. They may both be responsible for primary pneumonias in the healthy child, as well as among those who are immunosuppressed. Vaccines are available to prevent illness due to both of these viruses; therefore, with universal vaccine coverage, pneumonia due to measles and varicella should ultimately become the subject of medical historical textbooks. These two viruses, their epidemiology, the diseases, and the primary pneumonia syndromes they cause are reviewed in this chapter. Secondary pneumonias due to superinfection with bacterial or other pathogens are covered elsewhere in this book (see Chapters 27, 28, and 30).

VARICELLA

VARICELLA VIRUS CHARACTERISTICS

While investigating an outbreak of chickenpox in prisoners in 1904, Tyzzer first described the now classic pathologic findings of multinucleated giant cells, differentiating varicella-zoster virus (VZV) infection from smallpox.[1] Also known as human herpes virus type 3, VZV is a member of the subgroup alphaherpes, which also includes herpes simplex types 1 and 2 (HSV-1 and -2). It is the etiologic agent for chickenpox and herpes zoster. VZV is a double-stranded DNA virus surrounded by a nucleocapsid. The nucleocapsid is derived from the host cell, and is embedded with viral glycoproteins.[2] The entire genome of VZV has been sequenced, and it shares similarities with the linear sequence of HSV-1. At least five glycoproteins are produced (gB, gC, gE, gH, and gL), and particularly gE may be seen on the surface of infected host cells. Functions of these glycoproteins include viral entry into the host cell (gB), antibody binding (gE), and fusion (gH). Thymidine kinase plays a central role in replication and is the target for acyclovir.[3] Infectious virions are fragile and must be enveloped. Disruption of the envelope by drying or detergent will affect the virion's viability.[4] There is limited variability in the sequence of the virus, but recent phylogenetic studies confirm the existence of three genotypes (A, B, and C), with predominance of genotype C in the United Kingdom, and genotype A in certain African countries, the Indian subcontinent, and the Far East.[5] Humans are the only reservoir for this virus.[6]

EPIDEMIOLOGY

In temperate climates, childhood illness secondary to VZV infection is common. Seasonality is observed, with more cases occurring in late winter and spring. Prior to vaccination, the incidence of varicella and the birth rate were very close. The transmission rate is high, with 80% to 90% transmission to susceptible household members.[7] The seroprevalence in Germany, for example, was noted to be 79.4% in the first 3 months of life, to fall with a nadir at 8.6% by 12 months, and then to subsequently rise to reach 94.2% in 10- to 11-year-olds. Ninety-six percent of women of childbearing age in this study were noted to be seropositive for VZV-specific immunoglobulin G (IgG), and by the age of 40 years, 99% of all individuals surveyed were seropositive.[8] In a recent study by Brisson, the incidence of primary VZV infection in the general population in the United Kingdom was estimated to be 1291 cases per 100,000 person-years, with 84% of cases occurring in children younger than 15 years, and the highest rate being in the 0- to 5-year-old age group. In addition, the younger than 15 years age group also accounted for 70% of hospitalizations. In another study, infants younger than 12 months accounted for 17% of pediatric admissions for varicella, and admission followed the expected seasonality for varicella, where over 90% of admissions were between the last week of December until late June.[9] Eighty-five percent of deaths attributable to primary VZV infection were in adults. Rates of hospitalization for zoster were similar as for primary infection; however, mortality rates were higher (0.566 vs. 0.05 deaths per 100,000 person-years for zoster and primary VZV infection, respectively).[10] Although congenital infection has been well described, a study of a prospective cohort of 362 pregnant women infected with VZV (347 with primary infection) revealed that only one case of confirmed congenital varicella syndrome was noted.[11] Severe neonatal varicella occurs predominantly in neonates born of mothers with chickenpox 5 days prior to or 2 days after birth. The mortality rate is 20% to 30% in these cases.[12]

The incidence of herpes zoster increases with age. In patients older than 65 years, the incidence was found to be 11.8 per 1000 person-years.[13] Patients infected with the human immunodeficiency virus (HIV) are also at risk for developing herpes zoster, with an incidence of 29.4 cases per 1000 person-years.[14]

CLINICAL PRESENTATIONS OF VARICELLA

The origin of the term *chickenpox* has been postulated to be derived from the French word for chickpea, *chiche-pois*, used to describe varicella skin lesions.[7] The cutaneous eruption of chickenpox is characterized by a pruritic vesicular rash with areas of confluence distributed over the whole body, and may involve mucous membranes. Vesicles initially appear on the head and neck, and subsequently spread to the trunk and extremities.[15] Lesions have been described as "dewdrop on a rose petal" in appearance. Typically, 100 to 300 lesions can be counted, with higher numbers noted in adults. A prodrome may be experienced 1 to 2 days prior to the onset of rash, and consists of headache, fever, and a feeling of general unwellness. Hepatic disease with elevated enzymes may occur but seldom progresses to hepatic failure in the absence of Reye's syndrome. Although complications of primary VZV infection occur in immunocompromised individuals, in one series of 182 patients hospitalized for varicella, the 14 immunocompromised patients did not differ significantly in length of stay or admission to a critical care unit, compared with immunocompetent patients.[16] Severe complications of varicella in children include bacterial superinfection, neurologic sequelae, and thrombocytopenia. In an American study, two thirds of patients hospitalized for complicated varicella experienced more than one complication.[17] In a German study of 119 otherwise healthy children with complicated varicella, 61.3% had neurologic complications. Overall, 1 to 3 per 10,000 cases may be complicated by neurologic problems. Ataxia most often accompanies the onset of rash; however, the onset may be up to 2 weeks after the cutaneous eruption. Cerebrospinal fluid analysis is frequently normal, and the condition is generally self-limited. Encephalitis tends to complicate varicella in infants and older adults, with one to two episodes per 10,000 cases of varicella. The mortality rate may be as high as 10%, and neurologic deficits persist in 20%.[18] Ten percent of patients hospitalized for varicella in an Israeli study experienced febrile seizures.[19] Cellulitis was the most common bacterial complication, and thrombocytopenia was noted in five patients. Fortunately, no patients had developed Reye's syndrome.[20] Varicella gangrenosa is a rare complication associated with autoimmune-mediated protein S deficiency.[7] Among HIV-infected children, recurrent varicella, either disseminated (32%) or zoster (61%), was noted in over half of one cohort studied.[21]

The mortality rate is high (30%) in infants who acquire varicella perinatally. Visceral involvement is not uncommon.[18]

Zoster

Zoster, also known as shingles, is the clinical manifestation of VZV reactivation in sensory ganglia. Reactivation may be associated with stress and age, reflecting changes in immune status. The incidence of zoster is higher in older individuals and children who contracted chickenpox as infants. Involvement is most likely to be at the site of severe skin disease during primary infection.[7] Frequently, a prodrome of pain in the affected dermatome is reported, followed by a vesicular eruption on an erythematous base. These crust in 7 to 10 days in immunocompetent patients. In the immunocompromised host, new lesions may continue to form for a longer period of time, and may continue for up to 2 weeks.[4] In addition, these patients may develop visceral involvement.[18] Dermatomes most commonly involved include T1 to L2 and V1.[13] Hutchinson's sign (lesion on the tip of the nose) should prompt an effort to rule out ocular involvement.[7] Persistence of pain 30 days after resolution of shingles defines postherpetic neuralgia. The incidence increases with age, with an overall prevalence of 8% at 30 days.[14] Delayed contralateral hemiparesis carries a high mortality rate (20%–25%) and can follow an episode of zoster ophthalmicus by weeks to months. Other complications of zoster include chronic encephalitis secondary to demyelination, and zoster sine herpete, where neuropathic pain is reported in the absence of a cutaneous eruption. In HIV-infected patients, acyclovir-resistant strains may cause a chronic skin eruption. Multidermatomal zoster is an acquired immunodeficiency virus (AIDS)–defining illness.[7] Lesions in this population may be atypical and present with large ulcers.[18] Patients with altered cell-mediated immunity have a 20-fold higher risk for developing herpes zoster.[7]

Disseminated Zoster

Disseminated zoster in the absence of cutaneous lesions has been described. In one Canadian case, an 8-year-old child with acute myeloid leukemia presented with back pain, hematuria, and elevated liver enzymes. She eventually developed tachypnea and hypoxia, with evidence of pneumonia on chest radiography. The diagnosis was confirmed by polymerase chain reaction (PCR) of the bone marrow, liver, and serum. Unfortunately, the outcome was fatal.[22] Disseminated varicella-zoster in an undiagnosed adolescent with HIV has been reported after vaccination after the patient presented with fever, respiratory distress, cough, and leg weakness. Of note in this case was a protracted (1-month) history of a papular rash.[23] In a series of bone marrow transplant recipients, disseminated visceral VZV infection presented with abdominal pain in all cases, and carried a high mortality rate of 50%.[24] A chronic varicella syndrome has been described in HIV-infected children. This syndrome is characterized by persistently culture-positive unresolving skin lesions. Acute retinal necrosis has been described in HIV-infected patients, and follows an episode of herpes zoster weeks to months afterward. Blindness is the result in 75% to 85% of cases and is due to retinal necrosis and detachment.[18]

VARICELLA PNEUMONIA

Pathophysiology

VZV is transmitted by direct contact or droplet spread, with a period of communicability of as long as 5 days prior to the onset of cutaneous lesions, until all lesions are crusted.[6] The virus is thought to enter the host through the respiratory tract[2] and to then be disseminated through the bloodstream. A secondary viremic stage exists following infection of the reticuloendothelial system, where replication takes place. Transportation to the periphery manifests in the form of chickenpox. VZV is able to circulate in B lymphocytes, T lymphocytes, and monocytes.[25] Latency is established in sensory dorsal root ganglia, and some investigators believe that this may represent a low level of persistent infection where VZV gene expression is down-regulated.[26] Peripheral blood mononuclear cell–associated viremia has been detected in half of patients with varicella, but only 16% of patients with herpes zoster.[27]

A cytopathic effect is exerted on tissue cultures infected with VZV, producing syncytial formation, followed by the formation of a "viral highway," where virions form rows when exiting an infected cell. This characteristic is unique for VZV.[28] The host cell is lysed subsequent to infection, and some cell lines (e.g., Vero cells) undergo apoptosis.[2] Pneumonitis is postulated to be secondary to alveolar epithelial infection by VZV, and electron microscopy has demonstrated the presence of herpesvirus. Desquamated alveolar cells subsequently contribute to poor gas exchange and hypoxemia.[3]

Epidemiology

Among patients hospitalized with VZV infection in Israel, 17% had pneumonia. For patients over 15 years of age, pneumonitis may be the most common complication.[19] Prior to vaccination, lower respiratory tract infection complicated 7.93 per 10,000 cases of varicella cases in hospitalized persons where viral pneumonitis was responsible in 5.59 per 10,000 cases of complicated varicella infection.[17] Mortality in one series of 22 adults admitted to a critical care unit was 13.6%.[29] A 10-year experience with varicella pneumonia has been examined in Stockholm County, Sweden.[30] Twelve percent of adults admitted with VZV infection had varicella pneumonia, with an overall mortality rate of 1%. The male:female ratio was 3:1, with a mean age of 31 years. In another series, 3.5% of community-acquired pneumonia requiring admission to an intensive care unit over a 10-year period in South Africa was secondary to varicella infection.[31] Among children requiring hospitalization for varicella infection, 19% had comorbidities.[9] In this study, 10 patients experienced respiratory infections, whereas 3 patients had documented bacterial pneumonia and the remainder did not have a microbiologic etiology identified. Varicella pneumonitis has been described in pediatric burn patients, where 2 of 15 cases of primary varicella infection were associated with pneumonia in one series.[32]

Approximately half of cases of VZV infection in pregnancy occur during the third trimester. Among pregnant women with varicella, independent predictors for the development of pneumonia include smoking and greater than 100 skin lesions.[33] It has been suggested that low-dose and short-course steroids, as well as nasal corticosteroids, may be associated with disseminated varicella.[34]

Clinical Presentation

Varicella pneumonia is likely to manifest early during the course of infection, with symptoms developing within 4 days after the onset of cutaneous lesions. Patients tend to be febrile (mean temperature 39°C) with elevated white blood cell counts.[19] Leukopenia has been described in an otherwise healthy adult with varicella pneumonia, and five of six patients in one small series were thrombocytopenic.[35] In addition to cough and dyspnea, chest pain and hemoptysis have also been described, along with abdominal and/or back pain in 50% to 75% of patients with varicella pneumonitis.[34] Cough and dyspnea were described in over 80% in a series of adult patients.[36] In the same study, physical examination of the chest was normal in 23%. Conversely, of all patients with abnormal chest radiographs, two thirds may be asymptomatic.[18] Tachypnea (respiratory rate of over 30 breaths/min) is a feature in approximately 25% of adult patients.[30] The diagnosis may be delayed in the absence of typical skin lesions.[31] In a study of 18 pregnant women, the diagnosis of varicella pneumonia was generally made within 6 days after the onset of rash. Dyspnea lasted an average of 5.5 days in this study.[33] In a study of 347 cases of primary varicella infection during pregnancy, 25.9% of women reported dyspnea, but only 5.2% had chest radiographs consistent with varicella pneumonia.[11]

Complications secondary to VZV pneumonia include prolonged mechanical ventilation and bacterial superinfection of the lower respiratory tract or skin. Up to 25% of patients will develop bacterial superinfection, and the etiologic organism depends on immune status. In patients with normal neutrophil function, gram-positive organisms predominate, and as neutrophils fall, gram-negative bacteria and yeast may be the causative agents.[34] One case of pulmonary hypertension has been described in a patient with a protracted and complicated course.[37] In addition, a case of biopsy-proven interstitial pneumonitis responsive to steroid therapy has been described as a complication of varicella pneumonia.[38] A case of biopsy-proven pulmonary granuloma formation with a miliary pattern on chest radiography has also been published. In this case, pathology revealed 1- to 2-mm granulomas with necrotic centers with calcification.[39] Of note, at least one case of recurrent varicella pneumonia in an adult patient with HIV has been documented.[40] Other rare pulmonary complications include thromboembolic phenomena, hemorrhage, and the syndrome of inappropriate antidiuretic hormone secretion. Few studies describe the effects of varicella pneumonitis on pulmonary function. Diffusion defects and restrictive patterns on pulmonary function tests have been described in immunocompromised children with varicella.[34] In a series of 10 patients with varicella pneumonia, vital capacity was normal and there were no studies consistent with airway obstruction. Diffusion abnormalities were described in all of these patients. With time, diffusing capacity at rest and with exercise improved, but abnormalities persisted for months to years and returned to normal in only three patients.[41]

Diagnosis

A history of exposure and a characteristic cutaneous eruption should be sought. The chest radiograph may reveal bilateral, diffuse acinar opacities acutely, with resolution anticipated after 7 to 14 days.[42] The apices may be spared.[43] The lung periphery and lateral view should be examined for nodules. Infiltrates form as nodules enlarge.[34] Approximately 2% of patients may develop small (<3 mm) calcified nodules in the mid and lower lung zones.[42] High-resolution CT scan may reveal bilateral nodules that may be 1 to 10 mm in diameter, and in some cases these may coalesce. A ground-glass appearance has also been described.[44] On gross examination, the lung may be plum colored, and lesions similar to those seen on the skin during chickenpox have been described.[34] Pathology may reveal hyaline membranes, eosinophilic intranuclear inclusions of desquamated septal cells, and focal necrosis of blood vessels and alveolar cells in severe cases.[2] Diffuse alveolar damage may be noted with type II cell hyperplasia.[44] Other features may include hyaline membranes, fibrosis, and necrotizing bronchiolitis and bronchitis. Postinfectious changes include the formation of encapsulated nodules, which may be calcified.[44] Viral particles consistent with herpesvirus may be evident on electron microscopy.[34] A novel shell vial tissue culture method utilizing CV-1 and MRC-5 cells has been used for the simultaneous detection of HSV and VZV from vesicular fluid obtained from skin lesions. This method was more sensitive than conventional tissue culture with MRC-5 or A-549 cell lines for the isolation of VZV. A cytopathic effect was noted by days 3 to 4 and positive staining with a VZV-specific monoclonal antibody by day 2 (prior to the appearance of a cytopathic effect).[45] The RETCIF method (rapid enhanced tissue culture immunofluorescence) has been applied to respiratory specimens (not exclusively), including bronchoalveolar lavage, nasopharyngeal aspirates, and nasal and throat swabs. This method used tissue culture combined with staining with monoclonal antibodies to obtain results prior to the development of a cytopathic effect.[46] It is important to recall that virions are fragile and susceptible to drying and temperature. Specimens intended for culture should be transported to the diagnostic laboratory in a timely manner and in the appropriate viral culture media.

Direct immunofluorescence assay is frequently used in clinical laboratories for the detection of VZV in vesicular fluid from skin lesions. Intact epithelial cells are necessary; therefore, vesicles should be unroofed and the base of the lesion scraped vigorously. Fluorescein-conjugated monoclonal antibodies specific for VZV are used to detect viral antigens in the clinical specimen. Assays capable of simultaneously detecting HSV-1 and -2, and VZV, have been developed. VZV monoclonal antibodies are specific for VZV glycoprotein gp1 and the immediate early antigen. Correlation with conventional methods was 87.1% in one study, with a turnaround time of 1.5 hours.[47] Although electron microscopy (EM) is not helpful in differentiating herpesviruses from each other, it is useful to rule out other infections presenting as vesiculopustular rashes, such as smallpox.[48] Unfortunately, the sensitivity of EM is limited and was only 16% when compared with PCR when applied to cutaneous lesions.[49]

Whereas tissue culture methods are time consuming and EM nonspecific, molecular methods may offer both timely and specific results. Unfortunately, they are not readily available in most clinical laboratories, but may be accessible through reference centers. PCR has been applied in a variety of clinical situations. Primers specific for HSV-1, HSV-2, and VZV run on the cerebrospinal fluid (CSF) of 2700 patients presenting with symptoms of encephalitis revealed a sensitivity of 94% and specificity of 100% for the detection of VZV in the CSF.[50] PCR on dermal swabs was found to be sensitive and specific compared with conventional shell vial culture techniques,[51] and when compared with tissue culture, proved to be substantially more sensitive.[52] VZV PCR has also been used on paraffin-embedded tissue.[53] Quantitative assays have been developed for herpesviruses, including VZV, in the CSF.[54] In addition, quantitative assays for whole blood as well as serum and plasma have been developed.[55] The rapid and definitive diagnosis of a case of disseminated varicella with pneumonitis using PCR was demonstrated by amplifying a region of the VZV gene 29 from a bronchoalveolar lavage sample.[56] The versatility of the PCR method has been demonstrated using parallel detection of several human herpesviruses simultaneously using real-time PCR[57] and consensus PCR methods.[58] Although studies have focused on central nervous system disease, these methods have been applied to respiratory specimens, including bronchoalveolar lavages, sputum, and throat swabs from patients with signs and symptoms of viral encephalitis.[59] The sensitivity of real-time PCR appears to be inferior to conventional nested PCR for VZV.[60] PCR has also been used successfully to diagnose visceral disseminated VZV in immunocompromised patients without typical skin lesions.[61] Other molecular methods, such as restriction fragment length polymorphism, have been used to distinguish wild-type VZV and varicella vaccine viral infection.[62] The use of serology in the diagnosis of acute VZV infection is limited, where less than half of patients with an acute infection will have elevated VZV IgM or IgA, although paired sera (acute and convalescent) will demonstrate a rise in approximately 85%.[52] Serology is helpful in determining susceptibility to VZV infection after exposure, and to assess response to vaccination.[63]

Treatment

An excellent review of the management of VZV infection has been published. Among immunocompetent children 2 to 12 years old and adolescents, the administration of acyclovir shortened the time to healing of cutaneous lesions and shortened the duration of fever. In addition, there was no alteration of antibody response to VZV infection. Selection of an appropriate dose is emphasized, because it differs from the dose used in HSV infection.[64] Acyclovir has been used to successfully treat varicella pneumonia.[65] Defervescence was noted within 1 to 2 days after therapy was initiated for one series of six otherwise healthy adults with varicella pneumonia.[35] Oral acyclovir has also been administered to immunocompromised children with chickenpox to prevent dissemination. In one study, acyclovir (800 mg orally five times daily) was initiated in 25 children with chickenpox.[66] Two children had to be changed to intravenous therapy (one patient developed pneumonia, and the other continued to develop new lesions). There was no evidence of dissemination in the remainder of the patients. Foscarnet is recommended in cases of acyclovir-resistant VZV.[67] Cidofovir has been used in rare case of foscarnet resistance.[7] Mutations in the thymidine kinase gene are felt to be responsible for acyclovir resistance.[68] Assays have been developed to identify strains of VZV resistant to acyclovir[69]; however, these methods are not generally available in most clinical microbiology laboratories. Valacyclovir is currently available in Canada but has not been licensed for use in children. Due to its greater bioavailability compared with acyclovir, however, it has been used in the United States to complete a course of treatment for VZV infection in pediatric heart transplant recipients.[70] In an uncontrolled study of 15 adults admitted to hospital with respiratory failure secondary to varicella pneumonia, patients who received corticosteroids (40%) reportedly recovered rapidly, with improved ventilation parameters and chest radiography.[71] The use of extracorporeal life support for VZV pneumonia in children who were ventilator dependent has been described.[37] The use of noninvasive positive pressure ventilation in the form of continuous positive airway pressure (CPAP) has been advocated.[31]

PREVENTION

Prevention of postnatally acquired neonatal varicella is the result of transplacentally delivered VZV-specific IgG with cord:maternal blood ratios of antibody titers between 1.2:1 and 1.8:1, with higher ratios noted after 38 weeks of gestation.[72] Two varicella vaccines composed of a live attenuated vaccine strain are currently available. The first was licensed in the United States in 1995, and since that time, data exist demonstrating the persistence of antibodies in 99.5% of vaccinees after 6 years, with an annual varicella infection breakthrough rate between 0.2% and 2.3%.[73] The Canadian Immunization Guide recommends the vaccination of the following susceptible individuals: 12- to 18-month-old infants; older children and adolescents; health care workers and other individuals at risk for occupational exposure; family members of susceptible immunocompromised individuals; women of childbearing age (contraindicated during pregnancy); and other susceptible individuals (e.g., immigrants from a tropical country who may not have had prior exposure).[74] Evidence exists to support the simultaneous administration of the varicella vaccine with the measles, mumps, and rubella (MMR) vaccine.[75] Modeling studies indicate that mass infant vaccination is anticipated to reduce inpatient hospital days by 50%, the benefit of reduced pediatric hospitalizations being offset by increased adult admissions for zoster.[76]

The approach to VZV exposure begins with history taking. Studies reveal that the positive predictive value of a history of chickenpox is 73.7%.[77] For VZV-susceptible children, the administration of immune globulins with high titers of VZV-specific antibodies (VZIG) is protective over a period of 3 to 4 weeks.[63] Indications for VZIG in susceptible exposed individuals include immunocompromised children; pregnant women; newborns where the mother developed chickenpox within 5 days prior to delivery or 48 hours after delivery; hospitalized premature infants older than 28 weeks' gestation where maternal susceptibility is noted; and hospitalized premature infants younger than 28 weeks' gestation (or <1000 g birth weight) regardless of maternal susceptibility.[67] Acyclovir prophylaxis is used in subpopulations of immunocompromised patients, notably bone marrow transplant recipients. In addition, isolation in laminar airflow rooms during periods of profound immunosuppression also contributes to the prevention of VZV infection in this population.[78]

MEASLES

MEASLES VIRUS CHARACTERISTICS

The measles virus is a single-stranded RNA member of the Paramyxoviridae family, subfamily Paramyxoviridae, genus *Morbillivirus*.[2] It is closely related to the bovine rinderpest and canine distemper viruses.[79,80] It is a relatively large spherical enveloped virus with a diameter of 100 to 250 nm. There are six structural proteins. Three (nucleoprotein or N protein, large or L protein, and phosphoprotein or P protein) are found in complex form with the viral RNA and form the nucleocapsid. The other three (fusion or F protein, H glycoprotein, and the matrix or M protein) make up the viral envelope. The virus is considered to be genetically stable, but there are detectable differences in nucleotide sequences among wild virus strains.[81] The measles virus is sensitive to heat and is inactivated after 30 minutes at 56°C and following a few days at room temperature. It is easily destroyed by solvents, acids, alkalis, and both ultraviolet and visible light. It survives freeze drying well and may survive in storage at −70°C with a protein stabilizer for several decades. Humans are thought to be the only naturally infected host, but monkeys can be infected experimentally.[82,83]

EPIDEMIOLOGY

In the past, measles was the most common contagious exanthematous disease in childhood and remains a frequent cause of childhood illness in many medically developing countries. Since the introduction of measles vaccine programs in the 1960s, the incidence and complications of measles has decreased. However, measles has yet to be eliminated and continues to cause intermittent epidemics in all areas of the world.[84] The World Health Organization estimated that there were greater than 40 million cases of measles worldwide in 2001 with more than a million deaths as a result of this infection.[85] With effective immunization programs, the age distribution of cases has changed to involve more children older than 5 years and adults in areas with high vaccination rates.[86,87] However, in regions of low vaccination coverage or under situations of crowding, the majority of children affected are younger than 1 year and the rate of pulmonary complications remains high.[88]

In many underdeveloped countries, measles remains a serious and life-threatening disease, frequently with pulmonary complications. Increased susceptibility to infection has been associated with unvaccinated status, crowded conditions, and time since vaccination among vaccinated individuals.[89] In both the prevaccination and postvaccination eras, severe illness and pneumonia has been associated with the following factors: young age, malnutrition, crowded conditions, unvaccinated status, congenital or acquired immunodeficiency, and coexistence of other severe infections.[90–98]

One of the reasons measles continues to be a significant problem in developing countries is primarily due to the continuing high incidence of infection prior to the time of scheduled vaccination at 9 months of age.[99] These infants also have the highest rates of pulmonary and other complications as well as the highest mortality rates. Infants become susceptible to measles once the passively transferred maternal antimeasles antibodies fall below protective levels, which occurs generally between 5 and 11 months of age.[100–102] Infants in developing countries generally lose maternal antimeasles antibodies at a higher rate than do infants in more developed countries.[103] The factors that determine the age of the infant at which this will occur are not known. Infant nutrition and associated diarrheal diseases likely play a role. Maternal factors such as the status of the mother's immune system are also important. Infants born to HIV-infected mothers have been noted to be more susceptible in infancy regardless of their own HIV infection status and to have lower antimeasles titers at birth compared with infants born to seronegative mothers.[104] Also, infants become susceptible to measles earlier if they are born to mothers who acquired their immunity through vaccination as opposed to natural infection.[105–107] The effect of the infant's relatively immature cell-mediated immune system to adequately respond to measles has not been completely investigated. Finally, infants are more likely to acquire measles within the home. Therefore, as secondary contacts, they are more likely to have more severe disease possibly due to the effect of a higher inoculum of virus.[108]

The adverse effect of dehydration and malnutrition on patients with measles has frequently been emphasized by reports of the disease in the tropics and is often described in patients who died due to measles infection. Malnutrition may contribute to the increased severity of measles due to its inhibitory effect on both humoral and cell-mediated immunity. Chandra[109] studied the effect of malnutrition on the antibody response to live, attenuated measles vaccine in 20 malnourished children and 20 matched healthy controls. In the malnourished group, the time of the first appearance of secretory IgA antibody was delayed and the maximum level reached was lower. Whittle and colleagues[110] showed depression of cell-mediated immunity during measles in South African malnourished children. Vitamin A deficiency is also associated with more severe measles disease, and studies are in progress to more clearly determine the role of supplementation with this vitamin in enhancing the immune response to measles and other viral infections.[111]

Patients with immunologic defects, whether genetic or related to disease, may have severe and often fatal measles. Patients with leukemia and lymphoma have increased susceptibility to infection by the measles virus because of lowered resistance, which is a function of their disease and of their therapy, whether they are receiving antimetabolites, chemotherapy, or irradiation.[112–118] Many deaths from measles pneumonia in leukemic patients have been reported. In addition, measles pneumonia is now looming as an important and severe complication in children with HIV infection.[119–122]

Measles is a highly infectious virus that attacks almost all susceptible individuals. It is spread rapidly through close contact with infectious large-droplet aerosols, and dispersion is increased with coughing and sneezing. Airborne transmission is less common but has been described in a doctor's office setting.[123] Infected individuals can transmit the virus from 4 days before to 4 days after the appearance of the rash.

CLINICAL PRESENTATION OF MEASLES

Clinically, measles can be diagnosed by the history of a prodromal illness involving a low to moderate fever, slight dry "hacking" cough, coryza, conjunctivitis, and photophobia. Koplik spots appear during the day that the rash first erupts and disappear quickly, and therefore are frequently not observed. There is usually a high fever (40°C–40.5°C) associated with the appearance of the rash. Typically, the rash begins on the head as faint macules along the hairline. During the first 24 hours it spreads rapidly over the face, neck, and upper chest and becomes maculopapular in appearance. During the next 24 hours, it spreads down the body to the arms, trunk, and upper legs. At 3 to 4 days, it reaches the feet while starting to fade on the face. As the rash fades, the skin feels like fine sandpaper and desquamates over a 7- to 10-day period. In instances where the rash is not typical or not present at all, the diagnosis can be difficult to make with certainty on clinical grounds alone, and serologic laboratory confirmation is necessary.[124]

Inflammation of the conjunctivae and mucous membranes of the nasopharynx may occur at the time of the infection associated with mild transient respiratory symptoms. However, usually the prodromal signs occur 10 to 12 days following the initial infection. As the rash develops, the fever increases and the inflammation of the tracheobronchial tree progresses. The cough increases in frequency and often develops a "barking" quality. Transient crackles and rhonchi may be heard in the lungs. Most patients recover within a few days of the onset of the rash, although a mild cough may linger for a few days longer. In some patients, a recrudescence of the disease or increasing severity of the initial symptoms is noted along with the development of high fevers. These patients need careful examination and monitoring for the development of complications such as encephalitis, otitis media, lymphadenitis, sinusitis, and pulmonary disease—either bronchitis, tracheobronchitis, bronchiolitis, or pneumonia. Excessive mucoid and mucopurulent secretions may be found in the posterior pharyngeal spaces. A hoarse voice or barking cough may call attention to increased involvement of the larynx. Physical findings suggesting obstruction of bronchi, either partial or complete, may be detected. Hyperresonance and decreased breath sounds suggest areas of hyperaeration and large bullae. These areas clear quickly if they are due to endobronchial obstruction by mucoid secretions and desquamated epithelial material, but they remain longer if they are also associated with bronchopneumonia and peribronchial inflammation. Similarly, complete obstruction with segmental collapse may clear rapidly or remain for a prolonged period, depending on the underlying disease.

Bacterial pneumonia during the course of measles should be suspected if there is an increase in the respiratory distress and areas of consolidation found on examination of the lungs, most often, but not always, in association with a toxic appearance, return of fever or prolonged fever, and changes in the peripheral blood counts.

A killed measles vaccine (KMV) was used from 1963 to 1967 and originally was given to patients to whom live viral vaccines were postulated to have a possible harmful effect.[125] Withdrawal of KMV followed a report by Rauh and Schmidt,[126] who described the findings in 125 children immunized 2½ years previously with KMV when they were subsequently exposed in a measles epidemic. Fifty-four of these children developed measles, predominantly in a modified form. A distinctive atypical presentation was reported in eight (6.4%) of those infected. Similar reports of small numbers of these atypical measles cases also were documented from the United States, Canada, and Sweden.[127–129] In these cases, more than half of the patients had pneumonia, a much higher incidence than in natural measles infection. Three patients who failed to develop a rash had atypical measles pneumonia as confirmed by an increase in antibody titer to measles. The onset of the illness was abrupt after exposure to measles virus. High fever, cough, headache, myalgia, and abdominal pain preceded the rash by 2 to 3 days. The other atypical features were an unusual rash (in appearance, location, and progression), severe pneumonia, and the absence of catarrhal symptoms and conjunctivitis. The rash appeared first on the palms and soles and in the creases of the body, and progressed from the extremities to the trunk, often sparing the face, rather than following the usual sequence of face to body and extremities. As such, the rash could be confused with Rocky Mountain spotted fever.[130] The exanthem was maculopapular, with petechial and purpuric lesions, sometimes also vesicular without progression to crusting; it was occasionally urticarial. Edema of the extremities was often observed. Pulmonary symptoms and signs soon developed, suggesting pneumonia, which if present can be confirmed by roentgenographic findings (Fig. 37-1). The roentgenographic findings of pneumonia were chiefly that of a lobular infiltration, but more diffuse and segmental lesions were occasionally seen. Hilar adenopathy was a common finding, as was pleural effusion.[131–134] Although the pneumonia was usually severe, all patients recovered, and the associated pleural effusion cleared within a short time. The acute illness usually subsided within 4 to 7 days. White blood cell counts were low, ranging from 2700 to 10,000 cells/mm^3. The differential count varied, sometimes showing a mild eosinophilia of 4% to 13% and returned to normal in 4 to 6 days. The platelet count was normal. In general, the pulmonary lesions cleared completely, but some patients had residual nodular lesions measuring 1.5 to 4 cm that remained for many months before they gradually disappeared.[132,135–138] Calcification in these nodules has been described and, when this occurs, poses a critical diagnostic problem of ruling out the possibility of tuberculosis. There is no specific treatment. Neither antibiotics nor antipyretics altered the disease course. Because KMV is no longer available, this type of measles should gradually disappear. However, because the syndrome can appear several years after vaccination, counseling vaccinees on the potential for this disease syndrome is suggested.[139]

This atypical reaction has been attributed, in part, to delayed hypersensitivity and to Arthus reactions.[140] Administration of KMV results in delayed hypersensitivity to measles virus antigen and to specific serum antibodies.[141–143] With the passage of time, vaccinated persons may lose more of their protective antibody compared with their hypersensitivity. Bellanti and colleagues,[144] in a comparative study of children receiving attenuated and inactivated measles vaccines, reported a difference in antibody responses. Recipients of inactivated measles virus showed a reduced amount of nasal secretory gamma A antibody but an adequate production of serum antibodies. The differences in the antibody response of the respiratory tract may account for the altered or atypical response of a child receiving inactivated vaccine to measles virus infection. When they were subsequently exposed to wild virus, an exaggerated Arthus-type reaction

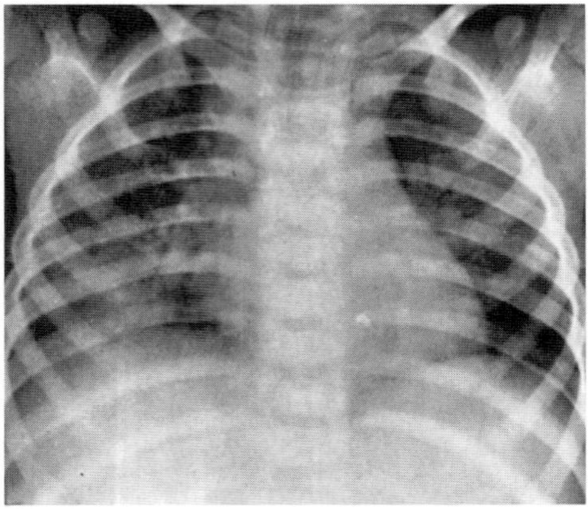
A

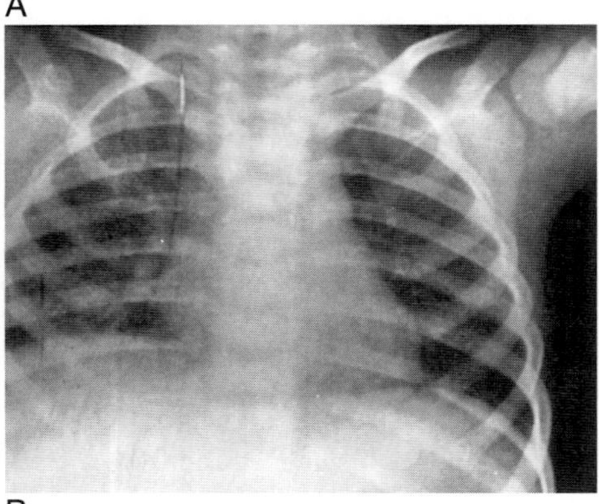
B

FIGURE 37-1. **A,** Four days after admission, pulmonary infiltration is seen in the right base above the diaphragm. There are also mottled soft lesions of irregular size in the right lung near the hilus and in the left upper lobe. **B,** There is complete clearing of the lungs 6 days later.

occurred in the pulmonary mucous membranes; this explains the severe and frequent atypical pneumonia. An Arthus-like phenomenon is also observed locally in skin reactions of persons vaccinated with KMV upon retesting with live measles virus. This may also account for the unusual skin manifestations. Another study by Annunziato and colleagues[134] involving histopathologic and serologic investigations of 17 adolescents with atypical measles syndrome with pneumonia 14 years after vaccination with KMV indicated an inadequate production of antibody to hemolysin (protein F). This antibody acts to prevent cell-to-cell spread of paramyxovirus. Absence of antibody to protein F resulted because KMV lacked the protein F antigen.[143] This phenomenon also is a significant factor in the development of atypical measles.

MEASLES PNEUMONIA

Pneumonia related to measles infection is still the most common complication and may be caused by direct invasion of the lungs by the measles virus (primary measles pneumonia), or may occur due to a secondary infection by other viral or bacterial pathogens. In some individuals, a virulent form of pneumonia, giant cell pneumonia, may develop. In addition, bronchitis, laryngotracheitis, or bronchiolitis may occur in severe measles illness. The following discussion includes the presentation and pathophysiology of pneumonia related to measles infection in both the immunocompetent and immunosuppressed host as well as giant cell pneumonia. The pneumonia described as part of the atypical measles syndrome associated with previous immunization by the killed measles vaccine is detailed above.

Pathophysiology

Even when uncomplicated by pneumonia, measles should be considered a respiratory disease as well as a systemic infection that begins with infection of the upper respiratory tract and conjunctivae. The infectious droplets from the nasopharyngeal secretions of a patient with an acute infection lodge on the respiratory epithelium of the new host. From this site, the virus then invades the bloodstream, producing a primary viremia. This primary viremia was demonstrated by Enders and colleagues,[145] who inoculated monkeys with measles virus from tissue culture and recovered the virus from blood within 5 to 7 days after inoculation; Sergiev and associates[82] recovered the virus as early as the third day using blood from patients with measles to inoculate monkeys. Following the primary viremia, the virus progresses to the reticuloendothelial system and generalized lymphadenopathy develops. There is a short period of decrease in virus titer in the blood after inoculation, followed by a rise (secondary viremia) that can be detected 6 to 11 days before the appearance of the rash and which persists for 1 to 2 days following the rash onset. The prodromal signs of measles occur during the period of secondary viremia. Measles virus may be cultured from the respiratory tract during the early prodromal period. Tracheobronchitis is usually found at this time, and pneumonia occasionally occurs. Roentgenograms taken during the first days of the rash show increased hilar markings that correlate with the peribronchial infiltration present in the first few days of the posteruptive stage of measles.

During the eruptive stage of measles, the inflamed epithelial lining of the respiratory tract with its disturbed physiology is ripe for secondary bacterial infection and the consequent development of bacterial complications. Accumulated bronchial secretions, desquamated giant cells, and epithelial cells often fill the lumen of the bronchi and produce obstruction of the bronchial tree, thus promoting areas of atelectasis, areas of hyperaeration, and the growth of bacterial pathogens in the pulmonary tissues, resulting in a superimposed bacterial pneumonia.

In measles, all epithelial cells of the respiratory tract from the nasal mucosa to the bronchioles are inflamed (Fig. 37-2). In affected areas, hyperplasia of the lymphoid tissue is seen. In primary pneumonia, there is an interstitial pneumonia with peribronchial infiltration by mononuclear cells (Fig. 37-3). Two types of giant cells are found: (1) large multinucleated syncytial cells containing inclusion bodies; and (2) Warthin-Finkeldey cells found in the lymph nodes and the reticuloendothelial system.[146] Warthin-Finkeldey cells are probably formed by the clumping and fusion of lymphoid cells and rarely contain inclusion bodies. Warthin-Finkeldey cells are pathognomonic for measles infection and were first described in the tonsils and appendix; they have subsequently been found in lymph nodes throughout the respiratory and gastrointestinal tracts and in the spleen, thymus, and bone marrow of infected patients.[147] The alveoli may become filled with the syncytial giant cells, and these together with desquamated degenerative cells may line the alveolar wall like a hyaline membrane (Fig. 37-4). In some instances, obstruction of the bronchioles may occur, which results in hyperaeration and bullae.

Epithelial multinucleated cells are seen in "giant cell" pneumonia and are diagnostic of this illness.

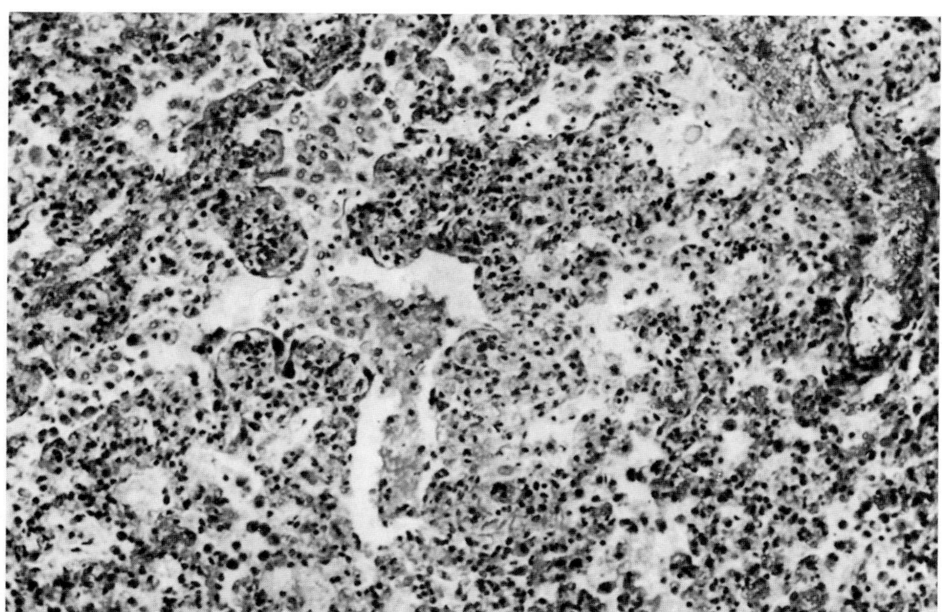

■ **FIGURE 37-2.** Measles pneumonia. Section of a lung showing extensive interstitial inflammation. Desquamated bronchial epithelium, giant cells, and mononuclear cells are present in the alveoli and ducts. (Hematoxylin and eosin, original magnification ×150.) (Courtesy of Dr. Renata Dische.)

Epidemiology

The frequency of pulmonary complications varies from epidemic to epidemic and from country to country and has been heavily influenced by the use of the measles virus vaccine. Prior to the use of measles vaccine, Miller[148] reviewed the experience in England and Wales in 1963 and reported that pneumonia, severe bronchitis, and/or croup occurred in 1 of every 26 cases reported, mostly among young infants and children. Little information is available concerning the actual risk for pulmonary complications in developed countries in the postvaccine era. One epidemic reported in Aberdeen, SD, between October 1970 and mid-January 1971 resulted in 292 cases (patients 1–14 years of age). From one group in this area, pneumonia was diagnosed in more than a third of the patients, three of whom died. Another epidemic, reported from the Naval Hospital in Great Lakes, IL, in the winter of 1974 listed 32 naval recruits 17 to 27 years of age admitted for acute measles, with 50% having pneumonia. A third measles outbreak in the winter of 1980 was of unusual interest because the source cases resulted from the importation of the virus into the United States (Westchester County, NY) by persons arriving from Portugal and Venezuela. There were 116 reported patients, mostly 10 years of age and over, one half of whom had previously been immunized. Only one person, an adult, developed pneumonia. By contrast, a fourth epidemic in southern Texas in 1981 largely affected infants younger than 15 months (42 of the 94 cases). Pneumonia was a frequent complication, occurring in 16%, all of whom were younger than 2 years. One patient with pneumonia died.[149]

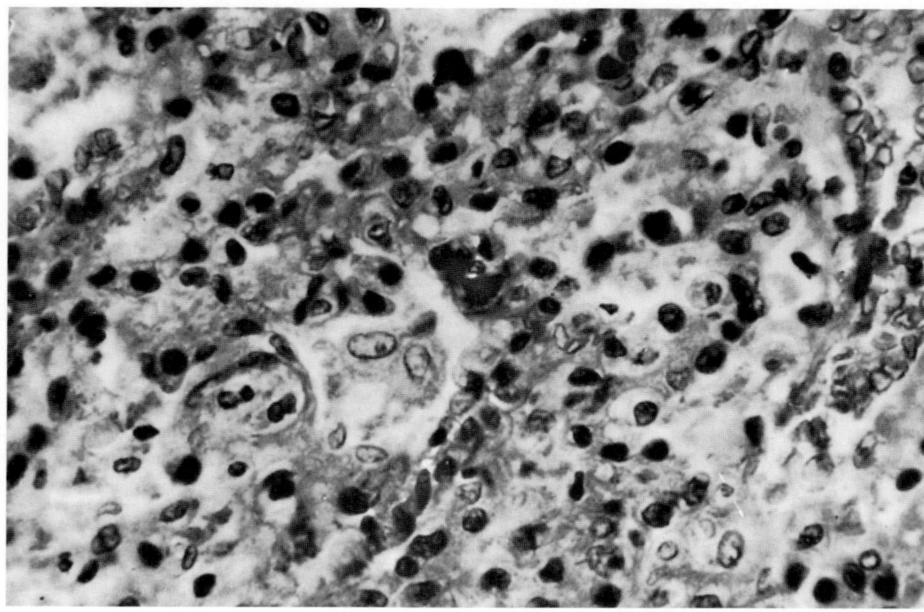

■ **FIGURE 37-3.** Measles pneumonia. Alveolar septa infiltrated by mononuclear cells. (Hematoxylin and eosin, original magnification ×500.) (Courtesy of Dr. Renata Dische.)

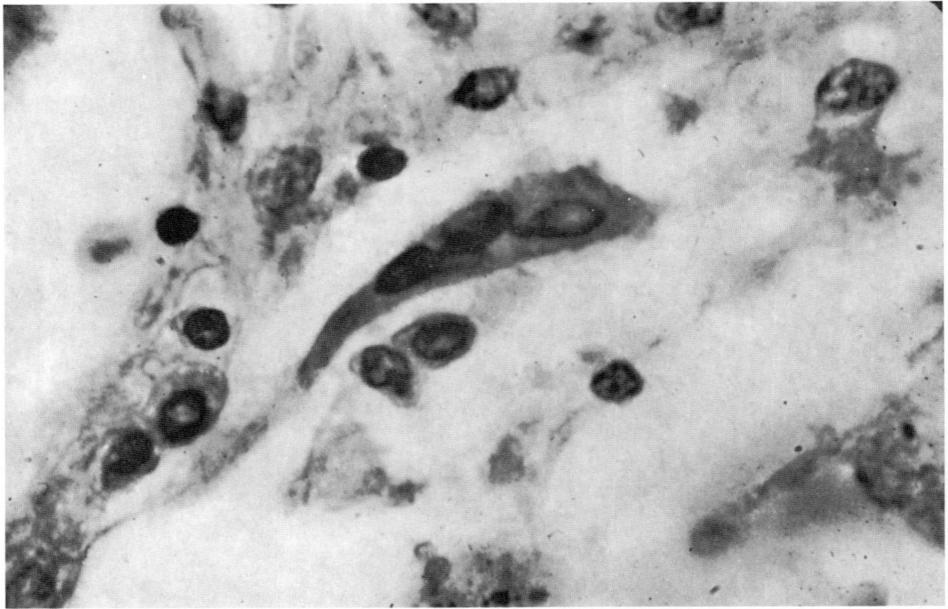

■ **FIGURE 37-4.** Measles pneumonia. Giant cell lining alveolus. (Hematoxylin and eosin, original magnification ×1500.) (Courtesy of Dr. Renata Dische.)

A measles outbreak was sustained in Los Angeles from 1987 through 1990 and, in a review of 440 patients seen at one children's hospital during this time, 36% of the children had radiographically proven pneumonia of which 12 were admitted to intensive care, 9 required intubation and assisted ventilation, and 3 died of pulmonary complications.[150] During the winter of 1990 to 1991, a large measles outbreak with 1424 reported cases occurred in Philadelphia. The outbreak involved 486 children who, for religious reasons, had not been vaccinated. Six of these children died of pneumonia, one with giant cell pneumonia.[151]

Clinical Presentation

Primary measles pneumonia occurs early in the course of the illness. The white blood cell count is not diagnostic. A chest roentgenogram is the most important laboratory examination. Because the tracheobronchial tree (Figs. 37-5 and 37-6) and the bronchopulmonary lymph nodes are always infected in measles, it is not unexpected that chest roentgenograms will show some evidence of this involvement. The majority of chest roentgenograms show a picture commonly seen in viral pneumonia, and there is no pathognomonic finding specific for

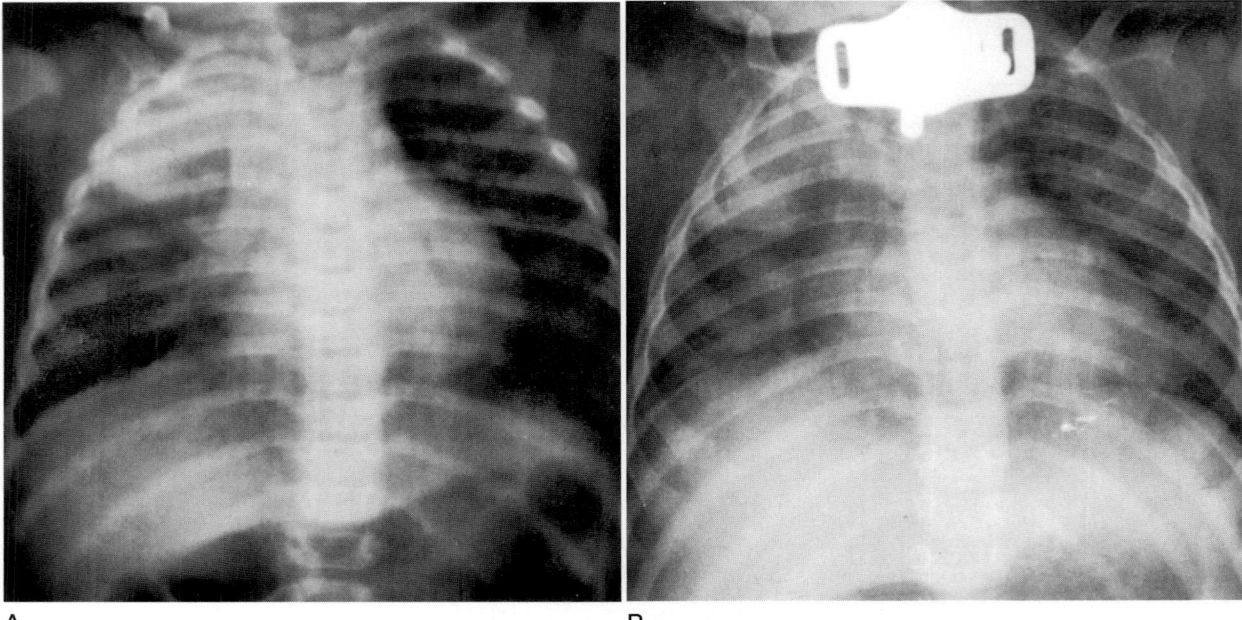

■ **FIGURE 37-5.** **A,** A chest radiograph taken on admission 3 days after an onset of measles rash, showing homogeneous density in the right upper lobe and some prominence of the right root. **B,** A chest radiograph taken 3 days after admission and 2 days after tracheostomy. Respiratory distress was relieved, although the right upper lobe pulmonary shadow remains.

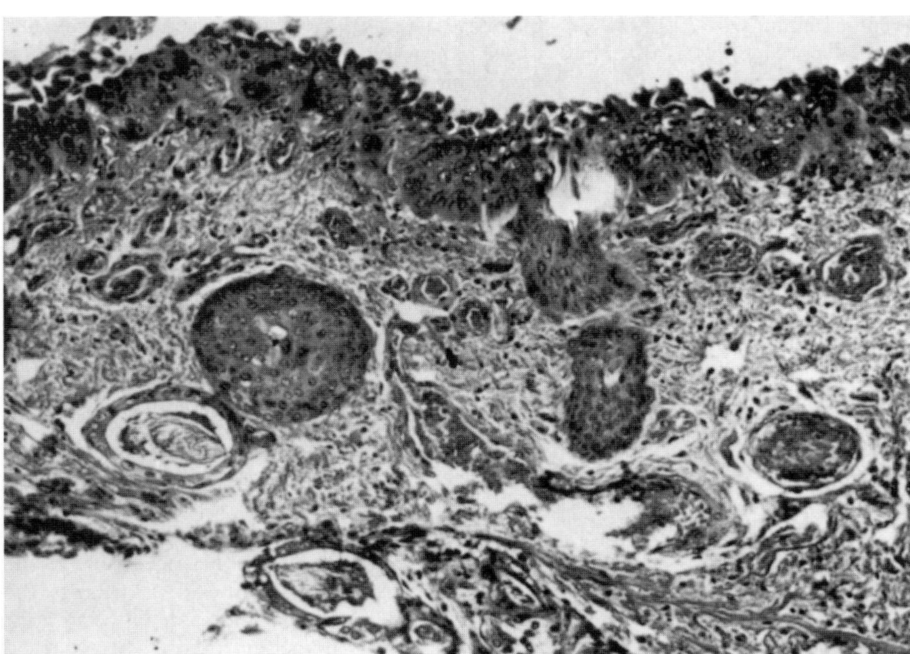

■ **FIGURE 37-6.** Measles tracheitis (original magnification ×150).

measles (Fig. 37-7).[152,153] There are increased bronchovascular markings radiating out from the hilar areas, especially into the lower lobes, and there is enlargement of the bronchopulmonary nodes in the hilar areas. These radiographic findings may persist several weeks after the patient has recovered clinically from measles. Rarely, pronounced enlargement of the superior mediastinum, similar to that in childhood tuberculosis, may be seen. When bronchopneumonia becomes established, the areas of increased density may coalesce. Patchy areas of unequal aeration with blebs and atelectasis may appear and disappear; emphysematous blebs may also be a complication. Segmental collapse occasionally occurs, but usually clears as the infection subsides.

Pneumonia due to bacterial secondary pulmonary infection occurs later in the course and often presents as a biphasic illness.[154] In general, the patients have a recurrence of fever and may take on a toxic appearance. The most common bacterial pathogens implicated include coagulase-positive staphylococci, hemolytic streptococci, pneumococci, and *Haemophilus influenzae*. Secondary bacterial pneumonia is often accompanied by a lobar infiltrate on the chest radiograph, but the appearance will vary depending on the bacterial pathogen involved. There is usually an increase in polymorphonuclear cells, including the appearance of a significant number of band forms in peripheral white blood counts.

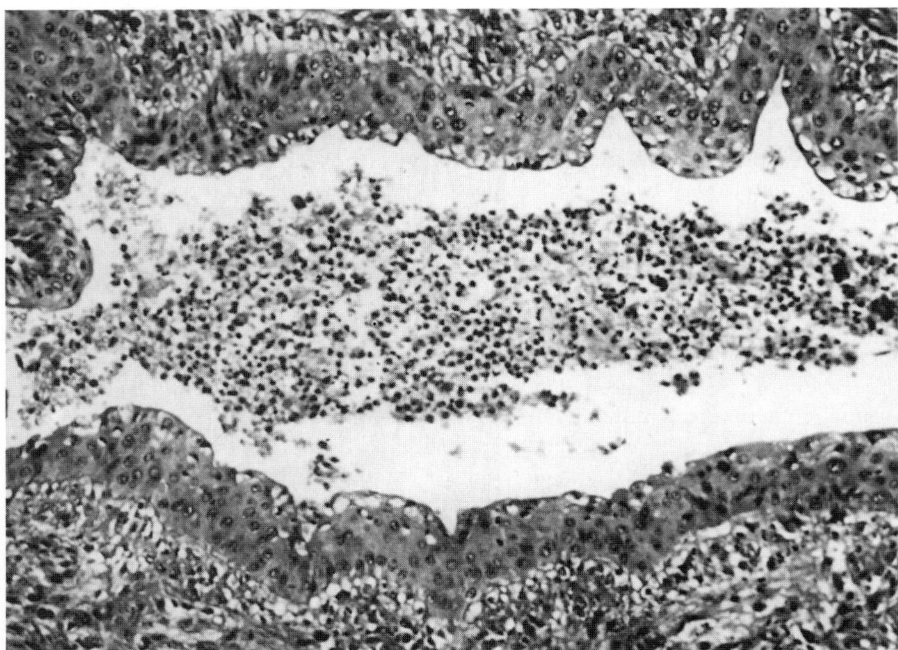

■ **FIGURE 37-7.** Extensive bronchitis and squamous cell metaplasia seen in autopsy material of a patient who died of measles pneumonia (original magnification ×150).

A persisting pulmonary shadow in the roentgenogram that does not coincide with the criteria for a bacterial pneumonia may be due to a collapsed segment or lobe of the lung secondary to the measles infection, due to tuberculous bronchopulmonary nodes, or it may represent a tuberculous pulmonary infiltrate. Tuberculosis cannot be excluded on the basis of a negative tuberculin skin test reaction. The skin reaction to tuberculin is greatly reduced during an active measles infection; therefore, if tuberculosis is suspected, other tests should be done and the tuberculin skin test should be repeated 3 to 6 weeks after resolution of the measles illness.[155]

Rarely, obstructive lesions in the diseased lower respiratory tract may lead to pneumomediastinum. Three of the 897 patients studied by Fawcitt and Parry[152] had pneumomediastinum, and the condition is periodically described in case reports. The mechanism for the development of air in the mediastinum was described by Macklin and Macklin.[156] Rupture of diseased alveoli with blebs and the coalescence of adjacent blebs into large bullae form the framework for pulmonary interstitial emphysema. The trapped air follows the path of least resistance and proceeds along the sheaths of blood vessels and adjacent bronchi, either the usual route along the structures upward to the mediastinum and around the heart or peripherally toward the pleura, producing a pneumothorax.

Atelectasis in single or multiple lobes of the lungs occurs in patients of all ages with measles, although less frequently than in patients with pertussis. Fawcitt and Parry[152] obtained roentgenographic evidence of atelectasis in 28.4% of patients in their series, most of whom were older than 1 year. If atelectasis persists for a time and secondary bacterial infection occurs, bronchiectasis may be the ultimate outcome. Any patient with long-standing atelectasis should be considered as a potential candidate for bronchiectasis and followed prospectively.

Except for staphylococcal infection, empyema is a rare complication of measles pneumonia. In a study of 100 patients in 1937 prior to the availability of antibiotics, Degen[157] described empyema in 13% and pleurisy in 27%. In this same series, four patients were described with exudative pericarditis.

Aaby and associates[158] have noted that infants exposed to measles during the first 6 months of life have a 5.7 times increased risk for mortality from another infectious disease in the next 60 months of life, implying a prolonged effect of measles infection on the developing immune system. The deleterious effect of measles on active tuberculosis infection is well known, with many reports of tuberculous meningitis, bronchogenic spread of tuberculosis, and miliary spread of tuberculosis following measles.[159] One recommendation that has been made is that untreated children with a positive tuberculin reaction should receive isoniazid (INH) during the high-risk period associated with the measles illness. Fortunately, at present, the spread of tuberculosis disease in association with measles epidemics is not seen. The second effect of measles and the administration of measles vaccine is the suppression of the tuberculin skin reaction.[155,160–165] Considerable variation in time occurs in the return of tuberculin sensitivity, ranging from 10 days to 5 weeks, with an average of 18 days after the onset of the rash.

Clinically, giant cell pneumonia cannot be distinguished from other viral-associated pneumonia, and the diagnosis depends solely on histologic examination of lung tissue.[166] Giant cell interstitial pneumonia was first described by Hecht in 1910 in a report of autopsy findings in 27 children. In 19 of these cases, there was a history of measles. When not associated with measles, this illness is referred to as Hecht's pneumonia.

This disease is most commonly associated with measles illness in the normal host. It may also be associated with typical and nontypical cases of measles in the immunocompromised host such as those with underlying disease of the reticuloendothelial or hematopoietic system, children treated with antimetabolites, and those with congenital or acquired immunodeficiency including HIV infection.[167–174] It has also been reported in association with paramyxovirus infections such as respiratory syncytial virus and influenza virus type 3 in immunocompromised children.[175]

The most valuable contribution in elucidating the cause of giant cell pneumonia was made by McCarthy and associates.[125,176] A virus indistinguishable from the measles virus was isolated from autopsy from each of three cases of giant cell pneumonia. There had been no clinical manifestations of measles in these patients. All had other serious illnesses, which were cystic fibrosis, leukemia, and Letterer-Siwe disease. This report suggests that in cases of giant cell pneumonia occurring in the course of other serious disease, but with no clinical measles, the host response to the measles infection is altered. The reason for this atypical host response is not clear, although it has been reported in patients already affected with chronic debilitating disease and with impaired immune response.

Diagnosis

When pneumonia occurs during the typical clinical picture of measles, there is usually no difficulty in making the diagnosis. The diagnosis of measles pneumonia is more difficult in the patient presenting with pneumonia but without the typical exanthem of measles. In these instances, performing serologic tests for measles, obtaining respiratory secretions for PCR testing, viral cultures, and testing for underlying immunodeficiencies are necessary.

Serologic testing for measles can be done by testing for IgM antibody or checking for a significant rise in IgG antibody titers in paired acute and convalescent serum specimens. Antibody formation in measles can be measured by the hemagglutination inhibition test; by measurement of complement fixation antibodies, which appear within 2 to 3 days of the rash; by the measurement of neutralizing antibodies, which appear as the rash begins to subside; or by enzyme-linked immunosorbent assay (ELISA) antibody techniques.[177–180] IgM antibodies may not be detectable in the first few days of the illness, and the test should be repeated if measles is strongly suspected on clinical or epidemiologic grounds. The usual antibody response may be suppressed in patients who are debilitated secondary to chronic disease or who have illnesses that directly affect the immune system. The measles outbreak in Greenland in 1951, which was a virgin area for measles infection, furnished a unique opportunity for the study of antibody responses to infection. Bech[181] showed that one third of 71 patients had complement-fixing antibodies on the first day following onset of the rash, and the titers generally reached levels from 1:32 to 1:512 within a few days. A more rapid rise in antibody level in immune individuals occurred on reexposure to measles.

Virus can be recovered from blood, urine, nasopharygeal samples, broncoscopy samples, or lung tissue. Van Binnendijk and colleagues[182] described the usefulness of detection of measles virus RNA through reverse-transcriptase PCR testing from clinical samples during a recent measles outbreak in the

Netherlands. Measles virus RNA was detectable in throat swab specimens from 93% of patients with clinical symptoms of measles. Eighty-eight percent of patients excreted the virus in urine. Measles virus RNA was detectable in specimens collected from 5 days before the onset of rash until 12 days afterward.

Laboratory diagnostic methods now available for the detection of measles virus may permit the clinical recognition of giant cell pneumonia. The importance of making the diagnosis is to appropriately choose therapy and prevent measles in contacts.

Treatment

Treatment of measles is primarily supportive. Cough medication should only be provided with caution, and codeine products should be avoided. Patients with signs of obstructive laryngotracheitis should be observed closely in hospital and may need intubation if increased respiratory distress and restlessness suggest impending serious airway obstruction.

There is no specific antiviral treatment for primary measles pneumonia. Oxygen therapy is used as is indicated by hypoxemia. Early administration of ribavirin potentially may have some benefit for certain patients, but reports of its use are anecdotal and it is not currently recommended.[183] Prophylactic antibiotic therapy for prevention of secondary bacterial pneumonia is not indicated.[184,185] Unnecessary use of antibiotics may result in selection of antibiotic-resistant organisms, which then necessitates more complicated antimicrobial therapy. Blood and tracheal cultures (if intubated) in severely ill patients should be taken early in the course of a suspected secondary bacterial illness and prior to antibiotic administration.

The survival of two immunocompromised patients who received large doses of γ-globulin at the time of exposure suggests that this therapy may modify the course of measles pneumonitis. Furthermore, high-titer measles antibody administration may mitigate established giant cell pneumonia. In populations where there is endemic malnutrition, the use of vitamin A supplements has been shown to reduce the mortality and complications associated with measles.[186]

PREVENTION

Prevention of measles primarily involves provision of immunization to susceptible adults and children prior to exposure to the virus. Secondary methods of prevention include the provision of specific immune globulin, infection prevention procedures in the health care settings designed to minimize droplet and airborne transmission, and, when necessary, quarantine. In many countries, measles is a reportable disease and public health officials will assist in the process of identification and notification of contacts. When possible, identified susceptible contacts should be immunized. Nonimmune individuals at high risk for serious disease who are known to have been exposed to measles within a period of 4 days and for whom vaccination would be problematic (infants and nonimmunized children with leukemia or with symptomatic HIV infection) should be given either high-dose measles immune globulin or, if that is not available, γ-globulin.[187,188] This will reduce their risk for developing serious infection. In addition, older children and adults traveling to endemic areas should consider being revaccinated prior to departure.[189]

The dramatic decline in measles in countries that have introduced universal immunization of young children has been dramatic and represents one of the successes of targeted public health programs. Extensive experience with the use of measles vaccine in a worldwide program has shown that measles immunization is safe, effective, and generally long lasting.[83,190–196] In theory, measles could be completely eliminated, because it is a virus that affects only humans. Many studies have shown a high level of immunity (95%–98%) obtained from live measles vaccination. Krugman,[197] in a 10-year follow-up of children immunized with live measles vaccine, observed clinical protection against measles and a rise in protective antibody titer when these children were exposed in measles epidemics 8½ years later.

Outbreaks of measles among highly immunized population in the 1980s and 1990s prompted a reevaluation of the immunization programs with the recommendation that children receive two doses of a measles-containing vaccine for optimal protection.[67,198,199] There were multiple reasons for the failure of the single-dose vaccination program to eliminate measles including earlier susceptibility to the disease of infants born to vaccinated mothers, either nonimmunization or poor response to the vaccine in a significant proportion of children, and the theoretical concern of waning immunity among vaccinated populations no longer repeatedly reexposed to the wild virus. The ultimate duration of protection from illness provided by vaccination alone is still unknown. In those outbreaks of measles in the United States, two thirds of the patients had been previously immunized with a single dose of vaccine. The relative contributions to epidemics among "immunized populations" of "cold chain" failure and degradation of the vaccine prior to administration, primary nonresponse to the single-dose vaccine, or decay in immunity with time are not known.[200–202] It remains to be seen how effective a two-dose vaccination program will be on a significant exposure of the population with measles in the future. There is conflicting evidence concerning whether individuals who do not respond to one dose will have an effective response to additional doses.[203] Unfortunately, although trials of high-dose vaccines showed improved response to the virus in young infants, the subsequent finding of increased mortality among vaccinees has halted the use of this vaccine strategy.[204] Earlier immunization of infants prior to the current age of recommended vaccination (15 months of age in the United States, 12 months in Canada, and 9 months in most developing countries) may be feasible in some areas.[205] It is hoped that the goal of worldwide measles elimination can be attained within the next two decades.

In 1998, an article written by Andrew Wakefield and colleagues[206] that detailed 12 children with chronic enterocolitis and regressive developmental disorder and which suggested a causal association of this condition with receipt of the MMR vaccine generated considerable controversy in both the lay and the medical press.[83] This association has since been successfully disputed, but the deleterious effect of the controversy on measles immunization programs has been felt worldwide.[207–214] It has, however, served to demonstrate the importance of systematic monitoring for measles and other vaccine-preventable diseases, ongoing evaluations of immunization programs for safety and efficacy, as well as the need for health care providers to be knowledgeable about vaccine-preventable diseases and immunization issues.

REFERENCES

1. Weller TH: Varicella. Historical perspective and clinical overview. J Infect Dis 1996;174(Suppl 3):306–309.

2. Fields BN, Knipe DM, Howley PM, Griffin DE: Fields Virology, 4th ed. Philadelphia: Lippincott Williams & Wilkins, 2001.
3. Arvin A: Varicella-zoster virus. Clin Microbiol Rev 1996;9(3):361.
4. Mandell GL, Douglas RG, Bennett JE, Dolin R: Mandell, Douglas, and Bennett's Principles and Practice of Infectious Diseases, 5th ed. Philadelphia: Churchill Livingstone, 2000.
5. Barrett-Muir W, Scott FT, Aaby P: Genetic variation of varicella-zoster virus. Evidence for geographical separation of strains. J Med Virol 2003;70(Suppl 1):42.
6. Chin J: Control of Communicable Diseases Manual. An Official Report of the American Public Health Association, 17th ed. Washington, DC: American Public Health Association, 2000.
7. Chen TM, George S, Woodruff CA, Hsu S: Clinical manifestations of varicella-zoster virus infection. Dermatol Clin 2002;20(2):267.
8. Wutzler P, Farber I, Wagenpfeil S, et al: Seroprevalence of varicella-zoster virus in the German population. Vaccine 2001;20(1–2):121.
9. Jackson MA, Burry VF, Olson LC: Complications of varicella requiring hospitalization in previously healthy children. Pediatr Infect Dis J 1992; 11(6):441.
10. Brisson M, Edmunds WJ: Epidemiology of varicella-zoster virus in England and Wales. J Med Virol 2003;70(Suppl 1):9.
11. Harger JH, Ernest JM, Thurnau GR, et al: Frequency of congenital varicella syndrome in a prospective cohort of 347 pregnant women. Obstet Gynecol 2002;100(2):260.
12. Unknown: National advisory committee on immunization (naci) update on varicella. Can Commun Dis Rep 2004;30:1–26.
13. Schmader K: Herpes zoster in older adults. Clin Infect Dis 2001;32(10): 1481.
14. Gnann JWJ, Whitley RJ: Clinical practice. herpes zoster. N Engl J Med 2002;347(5):340.
15. Cohen JI, Brunell PA, Straus SE, Krause PR: Recent advances in varicella-zoster virus infection. Ann Intern Med 1999;130(11):922.
16. Maharshak N, Somekh E: Hospitalization for varicella in central Israel. Acta Paediatr 1999;88(11):1279.
17. Galil K, Brown C, Lin F, Seward J: Hospitalizations for varicella in the United States, 1988 to 1999. Pediatr Infect Dis J 2002;21(10):931.
18. Gnann JWJ: Varicella-zoster virus. Atypical presentations and unusual complications. J Infect Dis 2002;186(Suppl 1):91.
19. Somekh E, Maharashak N, Shapira Y, et al: Hospitalization for primary varicella-zoster virus infection and its complications in patients from southern Israel. Infection 2000;28(4):200.
20. Ziebold C, von Kries R, Lang R, et al: Severe complications of varicella in previously healthy children in Germany. A 1-year survey. Pediatrics 2001;108(5):E79.
21. von Seidlein L, Gillette SG, Bryson Y, et al: Frequent recurrence and persistence of varicella-zoster virus infections in children infected with human immunodeficiency virus type 1. J Pediatr 1996;128(1):52.
22. Grant RM, Weitzman SS, Sherman CG, et al: Fulminant disseminated varicella zoster virus infection without skin involvement. J Clin Virol 2002;24(1–2):7.
23. Kramer JM, LaRussa P, Tsai WC, et al: Disseminated vaccine strain varicella as the acquired immunodeficiency syndrome–defining illness in a previously undiagnosed child. Pediatrics 2001;108(2):E39.
24. David DS, Tegtmeier BR, O'Donnell MR, et al: Visceral varicella-zoster after bone marrow transplantation. Report of a case series and review of the literature. Am J Gastroenterol 1998;93(5):810.
25. Koenig A, Wolff MH: Infectibility of separated peripheral blood mononuclear cell subpopulations by varicella-zoster virus VZV. J Med Virol 2003;70(Suppl 1):59.
26. Hay J, Ruyechan W: Varicella-zoster virus—a different kind of herpesvirus latency? Semin Virol 1994;5:241.
27. Mainka C, Fuss B, Geiger H, Wolff MH: Characterization of viremia at different stages of varicella-zoster virus infection. J Med Virol 1998;56(1):91.
28. Padilla JA, Nii S, Grose C: Imaging of the varicella zoster virion in the viral highways. Comparison with herpes simplex viruses 1 and 2, cytomegalovirus, pseudorabies virus, and human herpes viruses 6 and 7. J Med Virol 2003; 70(Suppl 1):103.
29. Gregorakos L, Myrianthefs P, Markou N, et al: Severity of illness and outcome in adult patients with primary varicella pneumonia. Respir Int Rev Thorac Dis 2002;69(4):330.
30. Nilsson A, Ortqvist A: Severe varicella pneumonia in adults in Stockholm county 1980–1989. Scand J Infect Dis 1996;28(2):121.
31. Potgieter PD, Hammond JM: Intensive care management of varicella pneumonia. Respir Med 1997;91(4):207.
32. Sheridan RL, Weber JM, Pasternak MM, et al: A 15-year experience with varicella infections in a pediatric burn unit. Burns 1999;25(4): 353.
33. Harger JH, Ernest JM, Thurnau GR, et al: Risk factors and outcome of varicella-zoster virus pneumonia in pregnant women. J Infect Dis 2002; 185(4):422.
34. Feldman S: Varicella-zoster virus pneumonitis. Chest 1994;106(1 Suppl):22.
35. Schlossberg D, Littman M: Varicella pneumonia. Arch Intern Med 1988;148(7):1630.
36. Jones AM, Thomas N, Wilkins EG: Outcome of varicella pneumonitis in immunocompetent adults requiring treatment in a high dependency unit. J Infect 2001;43(2):135.
37. Lee WA, Kolla S, Schreiner RJJ, et al: Prolonged extracorporeal life support ECLS for varicella pneumonia. Crit Care Med 1997;25(6):977.
38. Keane J, Gochuico B, Kasznica JM, Kornfeld H: Usual interstitial pneumonitis responsive to corticosteroids following varicella pneumonia. Chest 1998;113(1):249.
39. Meyer B, Stalder H, Wegmann W: Persistent pulmonary granulomas after recovery from varicella pneumonia. Chest 1986;89(3):457.
40. Fraisse P, Faller M, Rey D, et al: Recurrent varicella pneumonia complicating an endogenous reactivation of chickenpox in an HIV-infected adult patient. Eur Respir J 1998;11(3):776.
41. Bocles J, Ehrenkranz N, Marks A: Varicella pneumonia. Ann Intern Med 1964;60(2):183.
42. Grainger R: Grainger and Allison's Diagnostic Radiology. A Textbook of Medical Imaging, 4th ed. Orlando, FL: Churchill Livingstone, 2001.
43. Picken G, Booth AJ, Williams MV: Case report. The pulmonary lesions of chickenpox pneumonia—revisited. Br J Radiol 1994;67(799):659.
44. Kim JS, Ryu CW, Lee SI, et al: High-resolution CT findings of varicella-zoster pneumonia. AJR Am J Roentgenol 1999;172(1):113.
45. Huang Y, Hite S, Duane V, Yan H: CV-1 and MRC-5 mixed cells for simultaneous detection of herpes simplex viruses and varicella zoster virus in skin lesions. J Clin Virol 2002;24:37.
46. Alexander R, Lamb D, White D, et al: "RETCIF." A rapid, sensitive method for detection of viruses, applicable for large numbers of clinical samples. J Virol Methods 2001;97(1–2):77.
47. Chan E, Brandt K, Horsman G: Comparison of Chemicon SimulFluor direct fluorescent antibody staining with cell culture and shell vial direct immunoperoxidase staining for detection of herpes simplex virus and with cytospin direct immunofluorescence staining for detection of varicella-zoster virus. Clin Diagn Lab Immunol 2001;8(5):909.
48. Besser J, Crouch N, Sullivan M: Laboratory diagnosis to differentiate smallpox, vaccinia, and other vesicular/pustular illnesses. J Lab Clin Med 2003; 142(4):246.
49. Jain S, Wyatt D, McCaughey C, et al: Nested multiplex polymerase chain reaction for the diagnosis of cutaneous herpes simplex and herpes zoster infections and a comparison with electron microscopy. J Med Virol 2001;63(1):52.
50. Sauerbrei A, Wutzler P: Laboratory diagnosis of central nervous system infections caused by herpesviruses. J Clin Virol 2002;25(Suppl):45.
51. Espy M, Teo R, Ross T, et al: Diagnosis of varicella-zoster virus infections in the clinical laboratory by LightCycler PCR. J Clin Microbiol 2000; 38(9):3187.
52. Sauerbrei A, Eichorn U, Schacke M, Wutzler P: Laboratory diagnosis of herpes zoster. J Clin Virology 1999;14:31.
53. DeBiasi R, Kleinschmidt-DeMasters B, Weinberg A, Tyler K: Use of PCR for the diagnosis of herpesvirus infections of the central nervous system. J Clin Virol 2002;25(Suppl):5.
54. Aberle S, Puchhammer-Stockl E: Diagnosis of herpesvirus infection of the central nervous system. J Clin Virol 2002;25(Suppl):79.
55. de Jong MD, Weel JF, Schuurman T, et al: Quantitation of varicella-zoster virus DNA in whole blood, plasma, and serum by PCR and electrochemiluminescence. J Clin Microbiol 2000;38(7):2568.
56. Cowl C, Prakash U, Mitchell P, Migden M: Varicella-zoster virus detection by polymerase chain reaction using bronchoalveolar lavage specimens. Am J Respir Crit Care Med 2000;161:753.
57. Stocher M, Leb V, Bozic M, et al: Parallel detection of five human herpes virus DNAs by a set of real-time polymerase chain reactions in a single run. J Clin Virol 2003;26:85.
58. Minjolle S, Arvieux C, Gautier A, et al: Detection of herpesvirus genomes by polymerase chain reaction in cerebrospinal fluid and clinical findings. J Clin Virol 2002;25(Suppl):59.
59. Calvario A, Bozzi A, Scarasciulli M, et al: Herpes consensus PCR test. A useful diagnostic approach to the screening of viral diseases of the central nervous system. J Clin Virol 2002;25(Suppl):71.
60. Nicoll S, Brass A, Cubie H: Detection of herpes viruses in clinical samples using real-time PCR. J Virol Methods 2001;96:25.
61. de Jong MD, Weel JF, van Oers MH, et al: Molecular diagnosis of visceral herpes zoster. Lancet 2001;357(9274):2101.

62. Lässker U, Harder T, Hufnagel M, Suttorp M: Rapid molecular discrimination between infection with wild-type varicella-zoster virus and varicella vaccine virus. Infection 2002;30(5):320.
63. Rah DL: Assays for antibodies to varicella-zoster virus. Infect Dis Clin North Am 1996;10(3):507.
64. Balfour HHJ: Current management of varicella zoster virus infections. J Med Virol 1993;(Suppl 1):74.
65. Gogos CA, Bassaris HP, Vagenakis AG: Varicella pneumonia in adults. A review of pulmonary manifestations, risk factors and treatment. Respiration 1992;59(6):339; Comment in Respiration 1993;60(4):254.
66. Meszner Z, Nyerges G, Bell AR: Oral acyclovir to prevent dissemination of varicella in immunocompromised children. J Infect 1993;26(1):9.
67. American Academy of Pediatrics, Committee on Infectious Diseases: Red book. 2003 Report of the Committee on Infectious Diseases, 26th ed. Elk Grove Village, Ill: American Academy of Pediatrics, 2003.
68. Morfin F, Thouvenot D, De-Turenne-Tessier M, et al: Phenotypic and genetic characterization of thymidine kinase from clinical strains of varicella-zoster virus resistant to acyclovir. Antimicrob Agents Chemother 1999;43(10):2412.
69. Sahli R, Andrei G, Estrade C, et al: A rapid phenotypic assay for detection of acyclovir-resistant varicella-zoster virus with mutations in the thymidine kinase open reading frame. Antimicrob Agents Chemother 2000; 44(4): 873.
70. Dodd DA, Burger J, Edwards KM, Dummer JS: Varicella in a pediatric heart transplant population on nonsteroid maintenance immunosuppression. Pediatrics 2001;108(5):E80.
71. Mer M, Richards GA: Corticosteroids in life-threatening varicella pneumonia. Chest 1998;114(2):426.
72. Sauerbrei A, Wutzler P: Placental boost to varicella-zoster antibodies in the newborn. J Perinat Med 2002;30(4):345.
73. Vessey SJ, Chan CY, Kuter BJ, et al: Childhood vaccination against varicella. Persistence of antibody, duration of protection, and vaccine efficacy. J Pediatr 2001;139(2):297.
74. Canadian Immunization Guide, 6th ed. Ottawa, Ontario, Canada: Canadian Medical Association, 2002.
75. Shinefield HR, Black SB, Staehle BO, et al: Vaccination with measles, mumps and rubella vaccine and varicella vaccine. Safety, tolerability, immunogenicity, persistence of antibody and duration of protection against varicella in healthy children. Pediatr Infect Dis J 2002;21(6):555.
76. Brisson M, Edmunds W, Gay N: Varicella vaccination. Impact of vaccine efficacy on the epidemiology of VZV. J Med Virol 2003;70(Suppl):31.
77. Murray DL, Lynch MA: Determination of immune status to measles, rubella, and varicella-zoster viruses among medical students. Assessment of historical information. Am J Public Health 1988;78(7):836.
78. Masaoka T, Hiraoka A, Teshima H, Tominaga N: Varicella-zoster virus infection in immunocompromised patients. J Med Virol 1993;(Suppl 1):82.
79. Adams JM, Imagawa DT: The relationship of canine distemper to human respiratory disease. Pediatr Clin North Am 1957;4:193.
80. Carlstrom G: Neutralization of canine distemper virus by serum of patients convalescent from measles. Lancet 1957;273:344.
81. Rota PA, Bellini WJ: Update on the global distribution of genotypes of wild-type measles virus. J Infect Dis 2003;187(Suppl 1):270.
82. Sergiev PG, Ryazantseva NE, Shroit IG: The dynamics of pathological processes in experimental measles in monkeys. Acta Virol 1960;4:265.
83. Rall GF: Measles virus 1998–2002: Progress and controversy. Annu Rev Microbiol 2003;57:343.
84. Miller MA: Introducing a novel model to estimate national and global measles disease burden. Int J Infect Dis 1999;4:14.
85. World Health Organization: The World Health Report. Available at http://www.who.int/whr/2002/whr2002_annex3.pdf.
86. Khuri-Bulos NA: Measles in Jordan: A prototype of the problems with measles in developing countries. Pediatr Infect Dis J 1995;14:22.
87. Duclos P, Redd SC, Varughese P, Hersh BS: Measles in adults in Canada and the United States: Implications for measles elimination and eradication. Int J Epidemiol 1999;28:141.
88. Porter JDH, Gastellu-Etchegorry M, Navarre I, et al: Measles outbreaks in the Mozambican refugee camps in Malawi. The continued need for an effective vaccine. Int J Epidemiol 1990;19:1072.
89. Aaby P, Leeuwenburg J: Patterns of transmission and severity of measles infection. A reanalysis of data from the Machakos area, Kenya. J Infect Dis 1990;161:171.
90. Aaby P, Bukh J, Leerhoy J, et al: Vaccinated children get milder measles infection. A community study from Guinea-Bissau. J Infect Dis 1986; 154:858.
91. Baratta RO, Ginter MC, Price MA, et al: Measles (rubeola) in previously immunized children. Pediatrics 1970;46:397.
92. Barkin RM: Measles mortality. Analysis of the primary cause of death. Am J Dis Child 1975;129:307.
93. Bwibo NO: Measles in Uganda. An analysis of children with measles admitted to Mulago Hospital. Trop Geogr Med 1970;22:167.
94. DeBuse PJ, Lewis MG, Mugerwa JW: Pulmonary complications of measles in Uganda. J Trop Pediatr 1970;16:197.
95. Diaz T, Nunez JC, Rullan JV, et al: Risk factors associated with severe measles in Puerto Rico. Pediatr Infect Dis J 1992;11:836.
96. Josan K, Suciu O, Iepureau A, et al: On the gravity of the complications of measles after the epidemic that occurred in the winter of 1968–1969 in patients hospitalized in the infectious diseases clinic of Cluj. Pediatria (Bucur) 1970;19:41.
97. Markowitz LE, Nieburg P: The burden of acute respiratory infection due to measles in developing countries and the potential impact of measles vaccine. Rev Infect Dis 1991;13(Suppl 6):555.
98. Morley DC: Measles in Nigeria. Am J Dis Child 1962;103:230.
99. Taylor WR, Kalisa R, Madisu M, et al: Measles control efforts in urban Africa complicated by high incidence of measles in the first year of life. Am J Epidemiol 1988;127:788.
100. Dabis F, Waldman RJ, Mann GF, et al: Loss of maternal measles antibody during infancy in an African city. Int J Epidemiol 1989;18:264.
101. Halsey NA, Boulos R, Mode F, et al: Response to measles vaccine in Haitian infants 6 to 12 months old. Influence of maternal antibodies, malnutrition, and concurrent illnesses. N Engl J Med 1985;313:544.
102. Johnson CE, Nalin DR, Chui L, et al: Measles vaccine immunogenicity in 6- versus 15-month-old infants born to mothers in the measles vaccine era. Pediatrics 1994;93:939.
103. Hartter HK, Oyedele OI, Dietz K, et al: Placental transfer and decay of maternally acquired antimeasles antibodies in Nigerian children. Pediatr Infect Dis J 2000;19:635.
104. Embree JE, Datta P, Stackiw W, et al: Increased risk of early measles in infants of human immunodeficiency virus type 1-seropositive mothers. J Infect Dis 1992;165:262.
105. Lennon JL, Black FL: Maternally derived measles immunity in era of vaccine protected mothers. J Pediatr 1986;108:671.
106. Pabst HF, Spady DW, Marusyk RG, et al: Reduced measles immunity in infants in a well-vaccinated population. Pediatr Infect Dis J 1992;11:525.
107. Markowitz LE, Albrecht P, Rhodes P, et al: Changing levels of measles antibody titres in women and children in the United States. Impact on response to vaccination. Pediatrics 1996;97:53.
108. Pison G, Aaby P, and Knudsen K: Increased risk of death from measles in children with a sibling of opposite sex in Senegal. BMJ 1992;304:284.
109. Chandra RK: Reduced secretory antibody response to live attenuated measles and poliovirus vaccines in malnourished children. BMJ 1975; 2:583.
110. Whittle HC, Dossetor A, Oduloju A, et al: Cell-mediated immunity during natural measles infection. J Clin Invest 1977;62:678.
111. Cherian T, Varkki S, Raghupathy P, et al: Effect of vitamin A supplementation on the immune response to measles vaccination. Vaccine 2003; 21:2418.
112. Meadow SR, Weller RO, Archibald RWR: Fatal systemic measles in a child receiving cyclophosphamide for nephrotic syndrome. Lancet 1969;2:876.
113. Kemahan J, McQuillin J, Craft AW: Measles in children who have malignant disease. BMJ 1987;295:15.
114. Breitfeld V, Hashida Y, Sherman FE, et al: Fatal measles infection in children with leukaemia. Lab Invest 1973;28:279.
115. Siegel MM, Walter TC, Ablin AR: Measles pneumonia in childhood leukaemia. Pediatrics 1977;60:38.
116. Gray MM, Glass S, Eden OB, et al: Mortality and morbidity caused by measles in children with malignant disease attending four major treatment centers. A retrospective review. BMJ 1987;295:19.
117. Mawhinney H, Allen IV, Beare JM, et al: Dysgammaglobulinemia complicated by disseminated measles. BMJ 1971;2:380.
118. Weitzman S, Manson D, Wilson G, Allen U: Fever and respiratory distress in an 8-year-old boy receiving therapy for acute lymphoblastic leukemia. J Pediatr 2003;142:714.
119. Lauzon D, Delage G, Brochu P, et al: Pathogens in children with severe combined immunodeficiency disease or AIDS. Can Med Assoc J 1985; 135:33.
120. Markowitz LE, Chandler FW, Roldan EO, et al: Fatal measles pneumonia without rash in a child with AIDS. J Infect Dis 1988;158:480.
121. Krasinski K, Borokowsky W: Measles and measles immunity in children infected with human immunodeficiency virus. JAMA 1989;261:2512.
122. Palumbo P, Hoyt L, Demasio K, et al: Population-based study of measles and measles immunization in human immunodeficiency virus-infected children. Pediatr Infect Dis J 1992;11:1008.

123. Bloch AB, Orenstein WA, Ewing WM, et al: Measles outbreak in pediatric practice. Airborne transmission in an office setting. Pediatrics 1985; 75:676.
124. Makhene MK, Diaz PS: Clinical presentations and complications of suspected measles in hospitalized children. Pediatr Infect Dis J 1993;12:836.
125. Mitus A, Holloway A, Evans AE, et al: Attenuated measles vaccine in children with acute leukaemia. Am J Dis Child 1962;103:413.
126. Rauh LW, Schmidt R: Measles immunization with killed virus vaccine. Am J Dis Child 1965;109:232.
127. Brodsky AL: Atypical measles. Severe illness in recipients of killed measles virus vaccine upon exposure to natural infection. JAMA 1972;222:1415.
128. McLean DM, Kettyls GDM, Kingston J, et al: Atypical measles following immunization with killed measles vaccine. Can Med Assoc J 1970;103:743.
129. Nader PR, Horwitz MS, Rousseau J: Atypical exanthem following exposure to natural measles. Eleven cases in children previously inoculated with killed vaccine. J Pediatr 1968;72:22.
130. Nieburg PI, D'Angelo LJ, Herrmann KL: Measles in patients suspected of having Rocky Mountain spotted fever. JAMA 1980;244:808.
131. Fulginiti VA, Eller JJ, Downie AW, et al: Altered reactivity to measles virus. Atypical measles in children previously immunized with inactivated measles virus vaccines. JAMA 1967;202:1075.
132. Young LW, Smith DI, Glasgow LA: Pneumonia of atypical measles. Residual nodular lesions. AJR Am J Roentgenol 1970;110:439.
133. Young LW, Ross DW: Radiological case of the month. Giant cell pneumonia. Am J Dis Child 1980;134:511.
134. Annunziato D, Kaplan MH, Hall VW, et al: Atypical measles syndrome. Pathologic and serologic findings. Pediatrics 1982;70:203.
135. Laptook AWE, Nussbaum M, Shenker IR: Pulmonary lesions in atypical measles. Pediatrics 1978;62:42.
136. Margolin F, Gandy TK: Pneumonia of atypical measles. Pediatr Radiol 1979;131:653.
137. Sherkow L: Pulmonary residuum 14 months after skin rash and pneumonia. JAMA 1980;243:65.
138. Mitnick J, Becker MH, Rothberg M, et al: Nodular residua of atypical measles pneumonia. AJR Am J Roentgenol 1980;134:257.
139. Fulginiti VA, Helfer RE: Atypical measles in adolescent siblings 16 years after killed measles vaccine. JAMA 1980;244:804.
140. Buser F: Side reaction to measles vaccination suggesting the Arthus phenomenon. N Engl J Med 1967;277:250.
141. Norrby E, Lagercrantz R, Gard S: Measles vaccination. IV. Responses to two different types of preparations given as a fourth dose of vaccine. BMJ 1965;1:813.
142. Norrby E, Lagercrantz R, Gard S: Measles vaccination. VI. Serological and clinical follow-up analysis 18 months after a booster injection. Acta Paediatr Scand 1966;55:457.
143. Norrby E, Enders-Ruckle G, ter Meulen V: Difference in the appearance of antibodies to structural components of measles virus after immunization with inactivated and live virus. J Infect Dis 1975;132:262.
144. Bellanti JA, Sanga RL, Kluntinis B, et al: Antibody responses in serum and nasal secretions of children immunized with inactivated and attenuated measles-virus vaccines. N Engl J Med 1969;280:628.
145. Enders JF, McCarthy K, Mitus A, et al: Isolation of measles virus at autopsy in cases of giant-cell pneumonia without rash. N Engl J Med 1959;261:875.
146. Archibold WR, Weller RO, Meadow SR: Measles pneumonia and the nature of the inclusion-bearing giant cells. A light and electron microscope study. J Pathol 1971;103:27.
147. Corkett EU: The visceral lesions in measles. Am J Pathol 1945;21:905.
148. Miller DL: Frequency of complications of measles, 1963. BMJ 1964;2:75.
149. Centers for Disease Control: MMWR Morb Mortal Wkly Rep 1989;38:205, 456.
150. Mason WH, Ross LA, Lanson J, et al: Epidemic measles in the postvaccine era. Evaluation of epidemiology, clinical presentation and complications during an urban outbreak. Pediatr Infect Dis J 1993;12:42.
151. Rogers DV, Gindler JS, Atkinson WI, et al: High attack rates and case fatality during a measles outbreak in groups with religious exemption to vaccination. Pediatr Infect Dis J 1993;12:288.
152. Fawcitt J, Parry HE: Lung changes in pertussis and measles in childhood. A review of 1894 cases with a follow-up study of the pulmonary complications. Br J Radiol 1957;30:76.
153. DeCarlo J Jr, Startzman HH Jr: The roentgen study of the chest in measles. Radiology 1954;63:849.
154. Weinstein L, Franklin W: The pneumonia of measles. Am J Med Sci 1949; 217:314.
155. Helms S, Helms P: Tuberculin sensitivity during measles. Acta Tuberc Scand 1956;35:166.
156. Macklin MT, Macklin CC: Malignant interstitial emphysema of the lungs and mediastinum as an important occult complication in many respiratory diseases and other conditions. An interpretation of the clinical literature in the light of laboratory experience. Medicine 1944;23:281.
157. Degen JA: Visceral pathology in measles. A clinicopathologic study of 100 fatal cases. Am J Med Sci 1937;194:104.
158. Aaby P, Bukh J, Kronborg D, et al: Delayed excess mortality after exposure to measles during the first six months of life. Am J Epidemiol 1990;132:211.
159. Kohn JL, Koiransky H: Relation of measles and tuberculosis in young children. A clinical and roentgenographic study. Am J Dis Child 1932;44:1187.
160. Brody JA, McAlister R: Depression of tuberculin sensitivity following measles vaccination. Am Rev Respir Dis 1964;90:607.
161. Brody JA, Overfield T, Hammes LM: Depression of the tuberculin reaction by viral vaccines. N Engl J Med 1964;271:1294.
162. Lennon RG, Isacson P, Rosales T: Skin tests with measles and poliomyelitis vaccines in recipients of inactivated measles virus vaccine. Delayed dermal hypersensitivity. JAMA 1967;200:275.
163. Starr S, Berkovich S: Effects of measles, gamma-globulin-modified measles, and vaccine measles on tuberculin test. N Engl J Med 1964;270:386.
164. Tamashiro VG, Perez HH, Griffin DE: Prospective study of the magnitude and duration of changes in tuberculin reactivity during uncomplicated and complicated measles. Pediatr Infect Dis J 1987;6:451.
165. Zweiman B, Pappagianis D, Maibach H, et al: Effect of measles immunization on tuberculin hypersensitivity and in vitro reactivity. Int Arch Allergy 1971;40:834.
166. Janigan DT: Giant cell pneumonia and measles. An analytical review. Can Med Assoc J 1961;85:741.
167. McConnell EM: Giant-cell pneumonia in an adult. BMJ 1961;2:289.
168. Pinkerton H, Smiley WL, Anderson WAD: Giant-cell pneumonia with inclusions. Pediatrics 1952;10:681.
169. Rossipal E, Falk W, Zanger J: Atypical measles with giant cell pneumonia under treatment with chlorambucil [author's translation]. Verh Dtsch Ges Pathol 1972;56:388.
170. Shah KJ, Lewis MJ, Cameron AH, et al: Giant cell pneumonia complicating acute lymphocytic leukaemia in remission. Ann Radiol 1977;20:79.
171. Nadel S, McGann K, Hodinka RL, et al: Measles giant cell pneumonia in a child with human immunodeficiency virus infection. Pediatr Infect Dis J 1991;10:542.
172. Akhtar M, Young I: Measles giant cell pneumonia in an adult following long-term chemotherapy. Arch Pathol 1973;96:145.
173. Koffler D: Giant cell pneumonia. Arch Pathol 1964;78:267.
174. Clinicopathologic Exercises, Case 34-1988. N Engl J Med 1988;319:495.
175. Weintraub PS, Sullender WM, Lombard C, et al: Giant cell pneumonia caused by parainfluenza type 3 in a patient with acute myelomonocytic leukaemia. Arch Pathol Lab Med 1987;111:569.
176. McCarthy K, Mitus A, Cheatham W, et al: Isolation of virus of measles from three fatal cases of giant cell pneumonia. Am J Dis Child 1958; 96:500.
177. Bech V: Studies on the development of complement fixing antibodies in measles patients. J Immunol 1959;83:267.
178. Krugman S, Giles JP, Friedman H, et al: Studies on immunity to measles. J Pediatr 1965;66:471.
179. Norrby E: Hemagglutination by measles virus. A simple procedure for production of high potency antigen for hemagglutination-inhibition (HI) tests. Proc Soc Exp Biol Med 1962;111:814.
180. Health Canada: Measles Surveillance. Guidelines for Laboratory Support. Can Commun Dis Rep 1999;25:201.
181. Bech V: Measles epidemics in Greenland. Am J Dis Child 1962;103:252.
182. Van Binnendijk RS, van den Hof S, van den Kerkhof H, et al: Evaluation of serological and virological tests in the diagnosis of clinical and subclinical measles virus infections during an outbreak of measles in The Netherlands. J Infect Dis 2003;189:898.
183. Gururangan S, Stevens RF, Morris DJ: Ribavirin response in measles pneumonia. J Infect 1990;20:219.
184. Hussey G, Simpson J: Nosocomial bacteremias in measles. Pediatr Infect Dis J 1990;9:715.
185. Olson RW, Hodges GR: Measles pneumonia. Bacterial suprainfection as a complicating factor. JAMA 1975;232:363.
186. Hussey GD, Klein M: A randomized control trial of vitamin A in children with severe measles. N Engl J Med 1990;323:160.
187. Levine AS, Graw RG Jr, Young RC: Management of infections in patients with leukaemia and lymphoma. Current concepts and experimental approaches. Semin Hematol 1972;9:141.
188. Stokes J Jr, Maris EP, Gellis SS: Chemical, clinical, and immunological studies in the products of human plasma fractionation. XI. The use of concentrated normal human serum gamma globulin (human immune serum

globulin) in the prophylaxis and treatment of measles. J Clin Invest 1944;23:531.
189. Hill DR, Pearson RD: Measles prophylaxis for international travel. Ann Intern Med 1989;111:699.
190. Black FL, Woodall J, Pinheiro De P: Measles vaccine reactions in a virgin population. Am J Epidemiol 1969;89:168.
191. Hull HF, Williams PJ, Oldfield F: Measles mortality and vaccine efficacy in rural West Africa. Lancet 1983;1:972.
192. Kim SK, Son BK, Chung CY, et al: Efficacy of measles vaccine during the 1993 measles epidemic in Korea. Pediatr Infect Dis J 1995;14:346.
193. Koenig MA, Khan MA, Wojtyniak B, et al: Impact of measles vaccination on childhood mortality in rural Bangladesh. Bull WHO 1990;68:441.
194. McCormick JB, Halsey N, Rosenberg R: Measles vaccine efficacy determined from secondary attack rates during a severe epidemic. J Pediatr 1977;90:13.
195. Malfait P, Jataou IM, Jollet M-C, et al: Measles epidemic in the urban community of Niamey. Transmission patterns, vaccine efficacy and immunization strategies, Niger, 1990 to 1991. Pediatr Infect Dis J 1994; 13:38.
196. Markowitz LE, Preblud SR, Fine PEM, et al: Duration of live measles vaccine-induced immunity. Pediatr Infect Dis J 1990;9:101.
197. Krugman S: Present state of measles and rubella immunization in the United States. A medical progress report. J Pediatr 1977;90:1.
198. Gindler JS, Atkinson WL, Markowitz LE, et al: Epidemiology of measles in the United States in 1989 and 1990. Pediatr Infect Dis J 1992;11:841.
199. Markowitz LE, Preblud SR, Orenstein WA, et al: Patterns of transmission in measles outbreaks in the United States 1985–1986. N Engl J Med 1989;320:75.
200. Gustafson TL, Lievens AW, Brunell PA, et al: Measles outbreak in a fully immunized secondary-school population. N Engl J Med 1987; 316:771.
201. Hull HF, Montes JM, Hays PC, et al: Risk factors for measles vaccine failure among immunized students. Pediatrics 1985;76:518.
202. Matson DO, Byington C, Canfield M, et al: Investigation of a measles outbreak in a fully vaccinated school population including serum studies before and after revaccination. Pediatr Infect Dis J 1993;12:292.
203. Cohn M, Robinson ED, Faerber M, et al: Measles vaccine failures. Lack of sustained measles-specific immunoglobulin G responses in revaccinated adolescents and young adults. Pediatr Infect Dis J 1994;13:34.
204. Halsey NA: Increased mortality after high titre measles vaccines. Too much of a good thing. Pediatr Infect Dis J 1993;12:462.
205. Carson MM, Spady DW, Albrecht P, et al: Measles vaccination of infants in a well-vaccinated population. Pediatr Infect Dis J 1995;14:17.
206. Wakefield AJ, Murch SH, Anthony A, et al: Ileal-lymphoid-nodular hyperplasia, non-specific colitis, and pervasive developmental disorder in children. Lancet 1998;351:637.
207. Peltola H, Patja A, Leinikki P, et al: No evidence for measles, mumps, and rubella vaccine. No epidemiological evidence for a causal association. Lancet 1999;353:2026.
208. Kaye JA, del Mar Melero-Montes M, Jick H: Mumps, measles, and rubella vaccine and the incidence of autism recorded by general practitioners. A time trend analysis. BMJ 2001;322:460.
209. Dales L, Hammer SJ, Smith NJ: Time trends in autism and in MMR immunization coverage in California. JAMA 2001;285:1183.
210. Taylor B, Miller E, Lingham R, et al: Measles, mumps, and rubella vaccination and bowel problems or developmental regression in children with autism. Population study. BMJ 2002;324:393.
211. Fombonne E, Chakrabarti S: No evidence for a new variant of measles-mumps-rubella-induced autism. Pediatrics 2001;108:E58.
212. Halsey NA, Hyman SL, Conference Writing Panel: Measles-mumps-rubella vaccine and autistic spectrum disorder: Report from the New Challenges in Childhood Immunizations Conference convened in Oak Brook, Illinois, June 12–13, 2000. Pediatrics 2001;107:E84.
213. Horton R: The lessons of MMR. Lancet 2004;363:747.
214. Murch SH, Anthony A, Casson DH, et al: Retraction of an interpretation. Lancet 2004;363:749.

38 Toxocariasis, Hydatid Disease of the Lung, Strongyloidiasis, and Pulmonary Paragonimiasis

Mobeen H. Rathore, MD

TOXOCARIASIS (VISCERAL LARVA MIGRANS)

Toxocariasis is a soil-transmitted zoonotic infection that causes two main diseases in humans: visceral larva migrans (VLM) that can involve many major organs and characteristically cause eosinophilia, hepatomegaly, and pneumonitis, and ocular larva migrans (OLM). Humans are aberrant or incidental hosts and not necessary for the life cycle of the *Toxocara*. VLM results from the inflammatory response to the migration of immature, second-stage larvae through the viscera of a host that is not suitable for completion of the parasite's life cycle.

ETIOLOGY

Two species of *Toxocara* are primarily responsible for most cases of VLM: *Toxocara canis* and *Toxocara cati*, transmitted from dogs and cats, respectively. Other *Toxocara* species have been implicated in human infection, including *T. vulpis,* while the role of *T. lyncus* and *T. malaysiensis* in causing human infection is not clear. In addition, *Bayliascaris procyonis*, *Capillaria hepatica*, *Ascaris suum*, and rarely *Ascaris lumbricoides*, hookworm larvae, and *Strongyloides stercoralis* can also cause the VLM-like syndrome.

EPIDEMIOLOGY

Toxocara are found worldwide in domesticated and wild dogs and cats. *T. canis* is a common parasite of dogs found throughout the world. Prevalence of infected dogs varies from country to country, but levels above 40% are not uncommon. Infection with *Toxocara* is more prevalent than realized because many individuals do not express the complete VLM syndrome. In one study of children from different regions of the United States, the seroprevalence of *Toxocara* antibodies, as measured by enzyme-linked immunosorbent assay (ELISA), varied from 4.6% to 7.3%. One rural Pennsylvania community with poor sanitation had a 54% seropositive rate as measured by ELISA, versus 9% for a nearby community with better sanitation. The seroprevalence of *Toxocara* antibodies was 7% among young adults in Sweden. As in the United States, rural areas had a higher rate than urban areas. Puppies are especially dangerous because transplacental infection results in 77% to 100% of puppies becoming infected. By the time the animals are 3 weeks old, mature egg-laying worms can be present. In the United States, the infection rate decreases to under 20% in dogs older than 1 year. Adult female worms shed 200,000 ova per day and are passed unembryonated onto the soil in the feces of the infected animal. Under suitable soil conditions, the ova become embryonated and infectious after a minimum of 2 to 3 weeks. Because of the thick shell, the embryonated ova can survive in humid soil for months. Most infections arise in children with a history of pica, or in individuals who have accidentally ingested contaminated soil. Animals are not directly infectious because of the time lag before the ova become infectious.

PATHOGENESIS

In the natural host, infectious ova are ingested and hatch in the upper alimentary tract. The second-stage larvae then migrate through the intestinal walls into the bloodstream and then into the liver and lungs of the infected animal. From the lungs the larvae mature by migrating through the tracheobronchial tree and passing into the upper alimentary tract. There, the mature worm can begin laying eggs, which pass out in the feces to begin the cycle anew.

In aberrant hosts such as humans, the initial stages of infection are identical: infectious second-stage larvae hatch in the small intestine and then begin migrating through blood and lymphatics to the liver, lung, brain, and other organs such as the eye. However, before the larvae can complete their transtracheal passage and maturation to adult worms, host defenses block further migration of the larvae by encasing them within a granulomatous reaction, which is generally eosinophilic in nature. The pathogenesis of VLM is the direct result of the immunologic response of the body to the dead and dying larvae. Multiple eosinophilic abscesses may develop in the infected tissues. The larvae remain alive, infective, and antigenic for an indefinite period of time. The inflammation appears as an eosinophilic granuloma and an open biopsy of a granulomatous lesion will often show the *Toxocara* larva. Host antibodies are generated against excretory-secretory (ES) antigens of the larvae. These are glycoprotein antigens that contain protease, acetylcholinesterase, and eosinophil-stimulating activity.

CLINICAL MANIFESTATIONS

Toxocara is mainly an infection of young children, since they have a greater opportunity of ingesting the infectious ova while in playgrounds and sandboxes. Children are also less likely to follow good hygienic practices. The classic case occurs in a male child, younger than 6 years, with a history of pica and exposure to dogs. A child with fever of unknown etiology and eosinophilia should be assumed to have *Toxocara* infection until proven otherwise. The extent of signs and symptoms depends on the number and location of granulomatous lesions as well as the host's immune response. The initial symptoms include a prodrome of anorexia, fever, and lassitude. More recently, the so-called "covert toxocariasis" has been implicated as responsible for many subtle clinical manifestations. In a study of children in Ireland, the most frequent clinical manifestations were fever, headache, anorexia, abdominal pain, nausea, vomiting, lethargy, sleep and behavior disorders, pharyngitis, pneumonia, cough, wheeze, limb pain, cervical lymphadenitis, and hepatomegaly. In VLM the specific signs and symptoms depend on the organ affected. Liver invasion is an early event; hepatomegaly of varying degrees is almost always present. With more severe involvement, various combinations of abdominal pain, arthralgias, myalgias, weight loss, high intermittent fevers, pulmonary disease, and neurologic disturbance may be seen. It is the immediate hypersensitivity response to the larvae that manifests as symptoms of VLM. In addition to being an environmental risk factor for asthma, these include idiopathic seizure disorder, functional intestinal disorders, skin diseases (prurigo and chronic urticaria), eosinophilic and reactive arthritis, and angioedema.

Pulmonary involvement has been reported in anywhere from 20% to 80% of infected children. Cough, if present, is generally nonproductive. Wheezing is the most frequent finding on chest examination, although rhonchi and crackles have also been described. Because of the wheezing, some patients are diagnosed initially as suffering from asthma. There is no typical chest radiograph. Descriptions of imaging studies range from patchy airspace disease with pseudonodular infiltrates on computed tomography (CT), to diffuse interstitial pneumonitis, to an asymptomatic pulmonary mass. A pattern similar to miliary tuberculosis has been reported in severe cases. The varied patterns seen on film may reflect whether direct larval invasion of lung tissue or a hypersensitivity reaction to larval antigens is the primary pathologic process present in that particular patient. Although pulmonary symptoms are generally mild, acute respiratory failure has been reported from *Toxocara* infection.

The time course for VLM may be quite prolonged. The initial stage of the illness lasts several weeks, beginning with low-grade fevers and nonspecific symptoms, and progressing to eosinophilia and hepatomegaly. Episodes of bronchitis, asthma, or pneumonia may occur. Over the next month, intermittent high fevers occur along with the major manifestations of the disease. Recovery may take as long as 1 to 2 years, during which time the eosinophilia resolves along with the hepatomegaly. Resolution of pulmonary infiltrates occurs more rapidly.

COMPLICATIONS

Neurologic disturbances have been described in severe cases from invasion of the central nervous system by larvae. Seizures, encephalopathy, meningoencephalitis, and transverse myelitis have been reported. Ocular involvement occurs when a larva enters the anterior vitreous of the eye. This can be difficult to differentiate from retinoblastoma, especially when hepatomegaly and eosinophilia are absent. Renal, pancreatic, and cardiac invasion rarely occur. The few deaths described with VLM have resulted from myocardial, neurologic, or overwhelming systemic involvement.

DIAGNOSIS

Neutrophilia occurs during the first few days but rapidly gives way to the eosinophilia classically seen in the disease. Eosinophilia can range up to 50% to 90% of the total white blood cell count. Levels above 30% were considered essential for the diagnosis in early studies. Leukocytosis is generally present, with extreme values of over 100,000 cells/mm^3 occasionally reported.

Other laboratory findings may also be helpful in supporting a diagnosis of VLM. Serum immunoglobulin E (IgE) levels are above 900 IU/mm in 60% of patients tested. Hypergammaglobulinemia is frequently reported, characterized by elevations of any one or all of the immunoglobulin classes. Because of cross-reactivity between larval and blood group antigens, many patients will develop high anti-A and anti-B isohemagglutinin titers that persist for months after the initial infection. Bronchoalveolar lavage fluid may also exhibit a relative eosinophilia.

Once VLM is clinically suspected, an ELISA using the larval ES antigens to detect the host's antibodies is the most widely available and accepted test for confirmation. If a titer above 1:32 is considered, the diagnostic sensitivity is approximately 78%, with a specificity of over 92%. Because antibodies against *Toxocara* are present for years, an antigen-capture ELISA has been developed to separate acute from dormant infection, but it is not commercially available.

Examination of the stool for ova and parasites is not helpful because the larva rarely mature in humans. Before the ELISA against ES antibodies was developed, tissue biopsy to demonstrate the larva in eosinophilic granulomas was the definitive test for diagnosis. Skin tests, other serologic testing, and fluorescent antibody techniques were troubled by low sensitivities and unacceptably high cross-reactivity with other parasitic infections.

Differential diagnosis should include the visceral lesions that may be produced by other nematode worms, as well as immature stages of certain spiroid nematodes and filarial worms. Invasion of the liver by *Fasciola hepatica*, a nematode worm, or *Capillaria hepatica*, a trematode, might also be included. *Toxocara canis* may also produce the PIE syndrome (pulmonary infiltrates and eosinophilia). Also to be considered in the diagnosis are trichinosis, hepatitis, leukemia, the many causes of intense eosinophilia, tuberculosis, asthma, lead poisoning, and the leukemoid reaction occurring in severe bacterial pneumonia.

TREATMENT

Albendazole or mebendazole are the recommended treatments of choice for *Toxocara* infections. Albendazole is used at a dose of 10 mg/kg per day in two divided doses for 5 days was better than thiabendazole. Most patients recover without specific anthelmintic therapy. Corticosteroids have been useful in patients with severe pulmonary involvement, possibly by treating the hypersensitivity component of the disease. Otherwise, treatment is symptomatic.

PREVENTION

Measures that decrease the ingestion of contaminated soil reduce the incidence of the disease. Anticipatory guidance should focus on the risks of pica and elimination of the behavior. Regular deworming of puppies and lactating or pregnant bitches should be performed, and the risks of indiscriminate disposal of dog feces, especially in children's play areas, needs to be emphasized.

HYDATID DISEASE OF THE LUNG (PULMONARY HYDATIDOSIS)

The lung is involved in human hydatidosis caused by the cystic larval stage of the tapeworm *Echinococcus*: cystic hydatid disease, caused by *Echinococcus granulosus*, which is worldwide in distribution, and alveolar hydatid disease, associated with *Echinococcus multilocularis*, which is commonly seen in the Northern Hemisphere, and polycystic disease caused by *E. vogeli* seen in Central and South America.[1]

The life cycles of *E. granulosus*, *E. multilocularis*, and *E. vogeli* are similar.[1] The first developmental stage is the tapeworm, which reaches sexual maturity only in the intestinal tract of its definitive mammalian host, usually a carnivore. Infectious ova are released during defecation, contaminating fields, irrigated lands, and wells. *Echinococcus* eggs are extremely resistant to climatic conditions, and in northern regions will survive for at least 2 years. When eggs are swallowed by humans, the outer shell is digested and the embryos penetrate the intestine and are hematogenously disseminated to various parts of the body, mostly to the liver and lung. In the lung the embryos form hydatid cysts. Under ideal conditions, tapeworm heads, or protoscoleces, develop within the cysts.

CYSTIC HYDATID DISEASE

Classic, or pastoral, cystic hydatidosis is most commonly seen in the sheep- and cattle-raising areas of the Mediterranean, Middle East, South America, Russia, Eastern Europe, India, Australia, and Africa. In North America, it is seen among the California Basque sheep herders, and in Utah, New Mexico, and Arizona, particularly among the Native American populations.

Humans become infected from contaminated water and food or through close contact with infected dogs. Lung cysts develop when embryos pass through the liver, through lymphatic ducts bypassing the liver, by contiguous extension from the liver, or through the bronchi.

The hydatid slowly enlarges, and its rate of growth is dependent on the distensibility of the tissue and the age of the host. Pulmonary cysts grow fast, and they grow faster in children. At a size of 1 cm, three layers can be identified within the cyst: (1) an inner layer of germinal epithelium or endocyst that is responsible for formation of daughter cysts by endogenous vesiculation; (2) a middle noncellular, laminated layer or ectocyst; and (3) an adventitia or pericyst, an outer capsule of fibrous tissue, vasculature, giant cells, and eosinophils resulting from a weak host reaction. With time, blood capsules and daughter cysts may develop and disintegrate, liberating free scoleces or "hydatid sand."

Echinococcus granulosus is known to affect all age groups and any body cavity, organ, or site, and it most frequently affects the liver and the lungs, with the lung more commonly affected in children.[2] Infection occurs mostly during childhood, although years may elapse before manifestations are seen. There is no gender preference, and the slight differences in gender incidence are probably due to activity or occupation. Asymptomatic hydatidosis in family members is seen in 5% to 18% of cases.

In cystic hydatid disease, 17% to 75% of cases occur in children. After the age of 4 years, the distribution throughout childhood is even. In Tunis, of 643 children with pulmonary hydatid cysts, the mean age was 5 years (2 to 15 years).[2]

Involvement of the diaphragm and transdiaphragmatic extension into the lung has been described in patients with primary hydatid cysts of the liver. Other tissues that may be affected are the brain, eye, heart, mediastinum, blood vessels, pleura, diaphragm, pancreas, spleen, endocrine glands, bone, and genitourinary tract. The central nervous system is affected more often in children than in adults.

Clinical Features

Cyst size, location, and the potential for impairment of vital structures determine the clinical manifestations. The primary infection may remain asymptomatic for years. The slowly enlarging hydatid cyst is usually well tolerated. An awareness of symptoms is due to pressure from the enlarging cyst, secondary infection, and cyst rupture. The intact cyst is most commonly asymptomatic and may account for a third of all cases.

The more common manifestations of pulmonary cysts are cough, chest pain, hemoptysis, fever, and malaise. Retarded growth patterns have been observed in many children. Other manifestations are sputum production, chest discomfort, loss of appetite, dyspnea, vomiting of cyst elements, dysphagia, and hepatic pain. Bronchospasm has been reported with relief of bronchial asthma after removal of the cyst.[3]

Children with echinococcosis may present as emergency cases because of complications of the disease. These complications may be mechanical, with hydatid growth affecting the bronchial tree or pleura; they may also result from hematogenous spread, infection, or allergic reaction. Cyst rupture, pneumothorax, atelectasis, bronchopleural fistula, empyema, residual cavity, bronchiectasis, secondary cysts, and superimposed infection including saprophytic mycosis have been reported. A rare complication is rupture into the cardiovascular system with dissemination or sudden death.

Up to 30% of lung cysts may be complicated by rupture into the pleural space or bronchus, precipitated by coughing, sneezing, trauma, or increased abdominal pressure. Chills, fever, increased cough, mild hemoptysis, and change in appearance on radiographs suggest rupture. Coughing up of hydatid cyst elements, described as "coughing up grape skins," is diagnostic. Secondary hydatidosis in the pleura, acute asphyxia by bronchial obstruction, and allergic reactions, including anaphylaxis, may follow cyst rupture and leakage.

Bronchobiliary fistula occurs in 2% of cases and is commonly, but not always, preceded by suppuration. The right side and posterior basal segment are most frequently affected. Pyrexia and weight loss may mimic malignancy, but bile expectoration is pathognomonic.

Rarer complications caused by the cysts' unusual location have been reported: arterial emboli, portal hypertension, systemic venous obstruction, paraplegia, pleural effusion, phrenic nerve paralysis, transitory paralysis of cervical sympathetic chain, lower extremity thrombophlebitis, and stress ulcer.[4]

Diagnosis

Awareness of the disease is most important. Lung involvement is very likely if a cyst is present elsewhere in the body. Cystic hydatid disease is suspected based on a history of current or previous residence in an endemic area, clinical observations, and radiographic evidence. In 10% a diagnosis is suspected on routine radiographic study alone. A history of contact with possibly infected dogs may be obtained in only 29% to 48% of cases.

Physical examination is rarely definitive. Occasionally, a hydatid thrill (fluid wave) can be felt while percussing a large cyst. Demonstration of scoleces and hooklets of the parasite in vomitus, stool, urine, or sputum is pathognomonic but is rarely observed and may be seen only during surgery. Fine-needle aspiration under ultrasonographic or CT guidance may be successful with few complications in adults. However, observations in children are sparse, and the procedure carries a substantial risk, since leakage may induce anaphylactic shock.

Hepatic function may be abnormal in one half of patients with liver cysts. An increased specific serum IgE may be observed, but eosinophilia is more often absent than present and is completely unreliable in areas endemic for other parasites.

The basis for serologic tests is the formation of antibodies to the parasite that develop in the host tissue. False-negative results may be found in 10% to 30% of tests and are more common in children and with pulmonary cysts. The Casoni skin test involves injection of hydatid fluid in the dermis, which produces an erythematous papule in 50% to 80% of patients in less than 60 minutes. A Casoni test can be helpful if the results are strongly positive, but positive test results in known cases vary considerably, from 38% to 81%. False-negative results, sometimes due to infected cysts, and false-positive results occur in 30% of those tested. The Casoni test results remain positive for life.

Other serologic tests include latex agglutination, indirect hemagglutination, complement fixation, agar gel diffusion, enzyme immunoassay, and immunoblot. Cross-reactivity between echinococcosis and cysticercosis (*Taenia solium* infection) is a problem with any test that employs whole-cyst antigens. Serum antibody testing by indirect hemagglutination is 91% sensitive and 83% specific at a titer greater than or equal to 1:128. Immunoblot is 86% sensitive and 99% specific. After surgical removal of the cyst, there is generally a rapid decline in antibody within 3 months. Failure to observe the decline suggests incomplete cyst removal. Antibodies may persist for years after surgical removal of a hydatid cyst. Serum antibody tests can be referred to the Centers for Disease Control and Prevention (CDC), Atlanta, GA. However, up to 50% of patients with hydatid cysts in the lung or calcified cysts are seronegative. Laboratory tests may be more sensitive in complicated cysts, but at present, no single test is infallible, and there is still no serologic test that can effectively rule out the disease. Thus, disease awareness is most important.

The main diagnostic tool is the radiographic study, which is 98% to 100% accurate. However, with miniature screening radiographic studies, only 40% of cases are diagnosed. On occasion, inflammatory reactions and secondary infections may mask both closed and ruptured cysts, and the cysts are discovered after inflammation subsides.

On radiography, lung cysts are readily detected, and the possibility of a hydatid cyst in an endemic area should always be considered. An intact cyst is seen as a round or oval homogeneous lesion with a sharply defined smooth border surrounded by normal lung or a zone of atelectasis. It may be located in the periphery, center, or hilum; may be single or multiple, unilateral or bilateral; and may be of various size (Fig. 38-1). The final form depends on the location and neighboring structures. With an increase in size, bronchial dislocation occurs but no obstruction, as has been demonstrated by tomography or bronchography. On fluoroscopy, good elasticity of the cyst wall is demonstrable, and there is no interference with movement of the diaphragm.

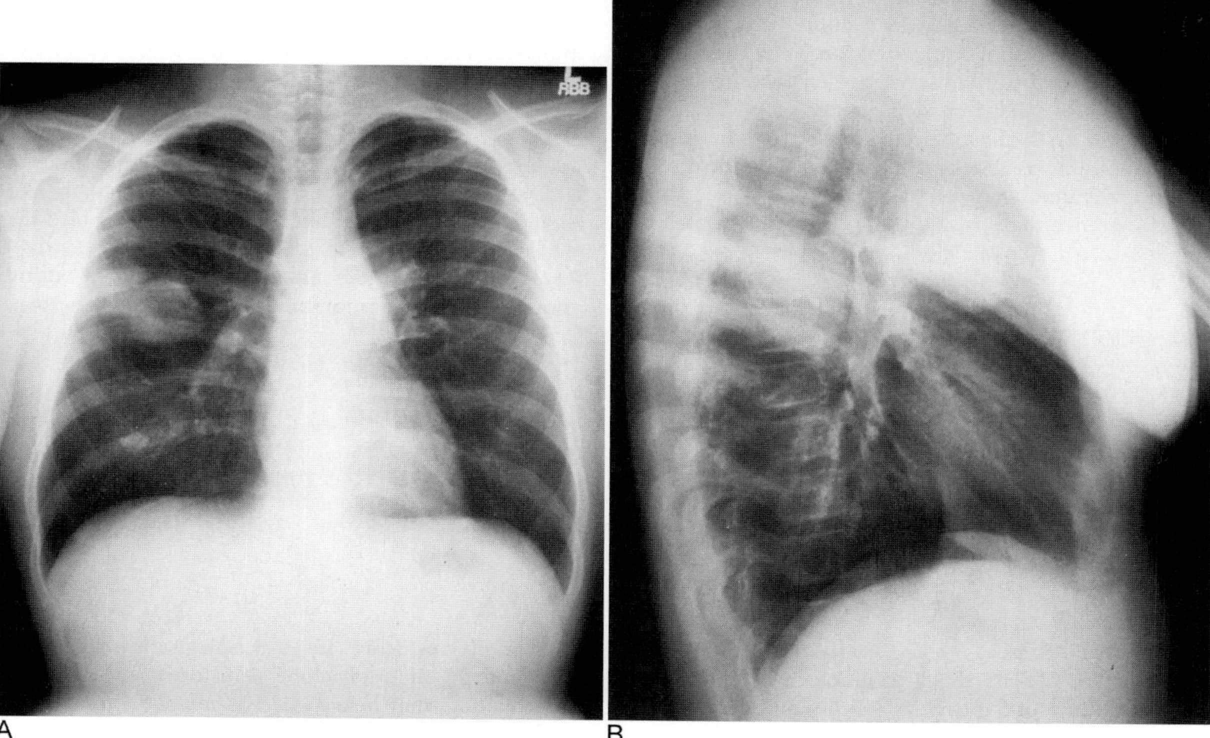

FIGURE 38-1. The posteroanterior (**A**) and lateral (**B**) chest radiographs from a 15-year-old boy with cough of several months' duration show bilateral circumscribed densities in the anterolateral right upper lobe and the superior left lower lobe. Histopathology after excision confirmed the diagnosis of hydatid cysts.

As the cyst grows, air passages and surrounding vessels are eroded, producing bronchial air leaks into the cyst adventitia. The bronchial air leak is actually nonfunctional before rupture because of pressure of the endocyst against bronchial passages and may be recognized only during surgery. With varying stages of air dissection into the cyst, different classic radiologic signs may be seen. A pericystic emphysema is seen in cysts before rupture. A "meniscus sign" or "crescent sign" is a crescentic radiolucency above the homogeneous cyst shadow on deep inspiration that is seen when air penetrates between adventitia and ectocyst. As air dissection continues, the parasite's membrane is torn, and some hydatid fluid flows out. An air-fluid level is seen within the cyst lumen as well as an air cup between ectocyst and adventitia, known as "double air-layer appearance" or the Cumbo sign. With free connection to a bronchus, the cyst wall is detached from adventitia, crumbles, collapses, and floats on remaining cyst fluid. This result is seen on the radiograph as air between the collapsed floating cyst wall and the adventitia, known as the "water lily sign" or Camellote sign. The adventitial wall does not collapse at once, so the obliteration of the cyst cavity is not an immediate outcome.

Cystic hydatidosis of the lung occurs most often as a single unilocular cyst. Only about 7% to 38% occur as multiple unilocular cysts. The inferior lobes are most commonly affected. In children, the ratio of intact to ruptured cysts is 3:1, which is the inverse of that in adults. Unlike in liver and spleen hydatid cysts, calcification of lung cysts is rare. A high right hemidiaphragm and right basal bronchiectasis suggest bronchobiliary fistula. A tract on sinugram or bronchogram is diagnostic.

CT should be performed preoperatively to better define and localize the cysts. CT may aid in diagnosing pulmonary hydatid cysts, although radiography can often make the diagnosis (Fig. 38-2). CT can demonstrate the water density in the intact cyst and can differentiate pleural from parenchymal lung or chest wall pathology. CT is especially helpful in complicated lung disease when more than one compartment of the chest is involved.[5] The ability of CT, however, to demonstrate characteristic hydatid anatomy, such as detached or collapsed membrane and daughter cysts, allows specific diagnosis to be made.[6]

Ultrasonography helps distinguish cystic lesions from solid tumors. Pathognomonic signs on ultrasonography are multiple daughter cysts within a cyst, separation of the laminated membrane from the wall of the cyst, and collapsed cysts.[7] A simple cyst with a thick wall in patients from an endemic area is suggestive. Abdominal ultrasonography is also recommended for liver cyst detection. Angiography can sometimes demonstrate a characteristic halo effect around the cyst and may help determine the number and location of cysts.

Differential diagnoses include abscess, hamartoma, pulmonary arteriovenous fistula, benign granuloma, malignant tumor, metastasis, and cysts of different origin. The presence of the Cumbo sign is confirmatory.

Histopathology

Histopathology depends on the size of cyst, the time after rupture, and the allergic reactivity of the host. With intact hydatid cysts, minimal atelectasis and compression are seen. A strong allergic eosinophilic reaction in surrounding lung tissue can be found with a recently ruptured cyst. Cysts ruptured for less than 10 days show reversible inflammatory infiltrates of lymphocytes or giant cell granulomata around parasite components. When the rupture is older than 10 days, severe fibrosis starts to develop, leading to dense scarring with subsequent tendency toward bronchiectasis and superinfection.

Treatment

Spontaneous cure is possible after coughing out the cyst and its contents, but more commonly infection and toxemia from the residual cyst may follow. Up to two thirds of symptomatic patients may die without intervention. When possible, surgery is the recommended treatment for all cases, although conservative management with benzimidazoles may be equally effective in asymptomatic patients. The success of surgery is dependent on the size and location of the cyst and on the skill of the surgeon. It is important to perform surgery immediately after diagnosis because the weak adventitial reaction and occurring bronchial communications may lead to rupture with intrapulmonary dissemination. Only in the benign Alaskan-Canadian variant is conservative treatment recommended.

The aims of surgery are total eradication of the parasite with evacuation of the cyst and removal of the endocyst, prevention of cyst rupture and consequent dissemination during the operation, and extirpation of the residual cavity. The lung parenchyma should be preserved and resection should be avoided in children

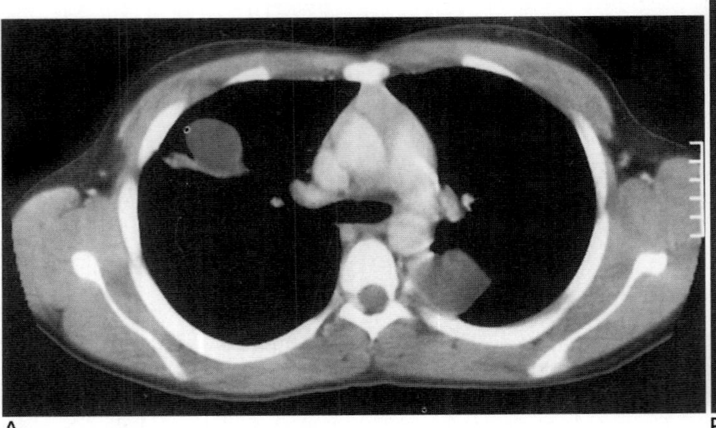

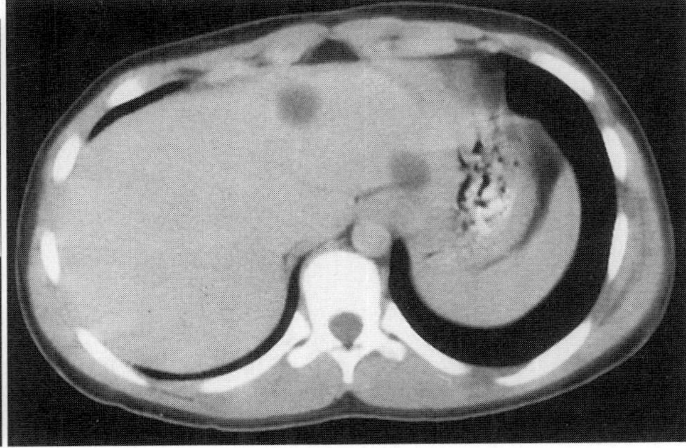

FIGURE 38-2. Computed tomography (CT) of the chest **(A)** confirms the location of fluid-filled cysts in the anterior right upper lobe and the superior left lower lobe (same patient as in Fig. 38-1), and liver involvement is seen on abdominal CT in this case **(B)**.

if possible because the damaged lung parenchyma has great capacity for recovery. Lung resection may be done in cases with bronchiectasis, severe inflammation, and large or multiple cysts that have destroyed lung parenchyma.

The posterolateral approach is favored. Surgical techniques to eradicate the parasite may include puncture and aspiration of cyst in situ, excision of the entire cyst by enucleation, wedge resection, segmentectomy, lobectomy, or pneumonectomy.

Such surgical procedures as enucleation with or without obliteration of the residual cavity by sutures (capitonnage) and cystectomy are mainly used for uncomplicated cysts. Lobectomy or segmental resection is reserved for lung destroyed by large cysts or bronchobiliary and biliary-pleural fistulas. One favored procedure is subtotal cystopericystectomy with total extirpation of the parasite or its rests in ruptured cysts, followed by closure of bronchial leaks and washing with a scolicidal solution. Subtotal extirpation of the pericyst or adventitia is then performed, leaving the hilar portion in place, because total resection of the adventitia in its hilar pole carries some considerable risk. In many cases of cystic hydatid disease of the lung, Keystone[8] has found it possible to eliminate the intact cyst by positive-pressure ventilation to force the cyst from the surgical opening in the lung.

Rupture and spillage may occur and may lead to dissemination and anaphylaxis, which may be fatal. This complication, although uncommon even with spillage during surgery, is greatly feared. The differences in surgical techniques therefore reflect the desire to prevent spillage of viable cyst contents. Commonly, the operative field is protected with saline-moistened gauzes, and the cysts are gently manipulated.

After extirpation of the parasite, bronchial fistulas are closed. To prevent recurrence, the residual cavity is injected with scolicidal agents, such as formalin, hypertonic saline, povidone-iodine, or absolute alcohol; silver nitrate has been used to freeze the cyst wall. Because of extremely grave complications with the use of formalin and hypertonic solutions, others have used hydrogen peroxide with good results. The residual cavity is then either obliterated by sutures or left open to communicate with the pleural space. Alternatively, the pericystic membrane is resected with repair of bronchial leakage. With a bronchobiliary fistula, the usually accompanying biliary hypertension is corrected, and the hepatic cavity is obliterated or drained. In cases with bronchobiliary fistula, the operative mortality rate is between 5% and 50%.

The more common surgical complications in children include atelectasis, hydropneumothorax, wound infection, pleural reaction, and hemothorax. Other reported complications from surgery are chest infection, abscess, empyema, septic shock, bronchial rupture, pneumothorax, bronchobiliary fistula, biliary-pleural fistula, hemorrhage, massive aspiration, prolonged drainage, bronchiectasis, and allergic reactions, including anaphylactic shock and death with rupture. The perioperative morbidity rate is 3% to 10%, and the mortality rate is 0 to 5%. The recurrence rate is 0 to 5%.

When surgery is impractical or impossible, treatment with benzimidazoles (i.e., mebendazole or albendazole) is recommended.[9] The dose for mebendazole is typically 50 to 60 mg/kg/day for several months, often up to a year. This medication interferes with uptake of glycogen by cestodes but is poorly absorbed and produces low blood concentrations of the drug. High-dose treatment with mebendazole 100 to 200 mg/kg/day for 3 months has been used in children successfully and without serious side effects. A peak in the therapeutic blood level of 80 ng/mL, measured by high-pressure liquid chromatography or radioimmunoassay, is recommended. Absorption is enhanced with meals, and mebendazole should therefore be taken with meals in three divided doses. Repeated courses may be necessary. Cure of hydatid disease has been achieved in 35% to 75% of patients and recurrence rates have been low.

Adverse reactions to mebendazole may occur within the first month. Febrile and allergic reactions, alopecia, glomerulonephritis, and reversible leukopenia have been reported. With hepatobiliary disease, increased blood levels and toxicity have been observed. Monitoring of clinical status, liver function, renal function, and complete blood count should be done weekly for the first month and biweekly thereafter.

In adult patients, albendazole has been as effective or even better than mebendazole. High blood and tissue levels of this benzimidazole derivative can be achieved. Further enhancement of drug concentration in target tissues may be possible with the concurrent use of cimetidine. Only a few observations in children have been reported. For those who are 10 years of age and older, 28-day courses of 10 to 14 mg/kg/day, separated by 14-day drug-free periods, have been recommended. Albendazole is usually well tolerated. Liver function may be abnormal in as much as 20% of patients during treatment with this anthelmintic, but side effects are rarely severe. In addition to treatment with benzimidazole derivatives, percutaneous drainage of hydatid cysts under sonographic guidance with irrigation of the cavity using hypertonic saline and with scolicidal instillation of absolute alcohol has been successful in adult patients who were ineligible for surgery.

Prevention and Follow-up

Hydatid lung disease is preventable. Preventive measures include the use of veterinary taeniacides for dogs; the proper disposal of carcasses and entrails of animals to prevent dogs from gaining access and proper hand, food, and drink care to prevent contamination from dog excrement.

Follow-up abdominal ultrasonography should be done annually for 5 years or more. Chest radiographs and CT scans should be repeated after 2 or 3 years and at 5 years. A cyst cavity may remain, and serologic findings may be positive for several years.

SYLVATIC ALASKAN-CANADIAN VARIANT

Among the sylvatic cycles, the Alaskan-Canadian variety is clinically and morphologically distinct and has been named *E. granulosus* var. *canadensis*. It is seen in the tundra and northern coniferous forests of North America to the Great Lakes, mainly among the native population, including the Eskimo, Aleut, and other Native American Indians, 75% of whom live in areas where *E. granulosus* occurs. The wolf is the definitive host, and sometimes the dog, which ingests the tapeworm by eating the viscera of infected deer. Intermediate hosts are large deer, elk, reindeer, moose, and caribou. Pig, sheep, and cattle have been shown in experiments to resist the infection. Humans are not very suitable hosts.

The Alaskan-Canadian sylvatic infection is more benign; the cysts are smaller, more delicate, do not grow as rapidly, and produce fewer symptoms than the classic or pastoral *E. granulosus*. The risk of anaphylaxis with rupture is less, and the prospect for spontaneous cure without significant complications seems excellent.

Most commonly affected organs are the liver and the lung, with lung involvement in 61% of the cases. Most cysts are simple, intact, and uninfected. The mean age for pulmonary cysts is younger than that for liver cysts. For pulmonary cysts, the mean age is 22 years (5 to 77 years), and for liver cysts, it is 65.3 years (24 to 96 years). In patients with lung cysts, 71% are younger than 20 years.

Only 6% to 8% of cases are symptomatic, mostly because of cyst rupture, which may occur in some 26% of patients. Cough, purulent expectoration, and hemoptysis are usual complaints. Serious complications are rare, and no cases of anaphylaxis or seeding have been seen in the Alaskan[10,11] or Canadian experience.[12,13]

Diagnosis is based on a history of residence in an endemic area, association with dogs, and routine radiographic study. Typically, a round or oval homogeneous water-like density with clear-cut borders and no surrounding reaction is seen. Such classic signs as water lily and crescent sign are rare. Laboratory tests are of little value. Eosinophilia is positive in only 29% of cases, hemagglutination in 10%, and the Casoni test in 56%. With cyst leak or rupture, test results are usually but not always positive.

The surgical risk is minimal. Extrusion of the intact vesicle is not appropriate, and an open wedge resection of adventitia with intact cyst is favored. Gentleness is very important. The bronchial stump should be closed, and the defect in the lung is obliterated. Alternatively, cystectomy may be performed.

Quite commonly, the cyst evacuates into the bronchi, and the symptoms disappear. Thus, surgery is not recommended for asymptomatic patients, who are managed by observation. No serious morbidity and mortality have been reported with this approach.

ALVEOLAR HYDATID DISEASE

Echinococcus multilocularis is a cestode that differs morphologically and biologically in its larval and adult stages from *E. granulosus*. The usual definitive host is the fox, with dogs and cats acting as sources of human infection in endemic areas. Intermediate hosts are rodents and humans. The larval stage develops normally in rodents, but humans are unusual and poor intermediate hosts. The disease is usually found across much of the Soviet Union, central Europe, northern Japan, Alaska, and northern Canada. Human disease is rare in the Western Hemisphere, but the cestode is endemic in the north-central United States and Canada.

The infection usually occurs during childhood. A case-control study has identified the following risk factors: having a lifetime pattern of dog ownership, tethering dogs near the house, and living in a house built directly on the tundra rather than on gravel or permanent foundations, thus allowing contact with contaminated dog feces.[14] Other implicated factors are the drinking of unboiled melted snow and the skinning of foxes. The disease manifests usually between the ages of 19 and 40 years but has been seen in those as young as 5 years. The mean age at diagnosis in Alaska is 53 years. The disease favors neither sex.

The larval cestode persists in its proliferative phase because of the inability of humans to provide the conditions necessary for normal development. Instead of developing a thick, laminated layer and growing into large, single cysts, the parasite has a thin, deficient ectocyst that grows and infiltrates into the surrounding tissues. The growing cyst may have several small, fluid-filled pockets containing protoscoleces. Because of its structure, this larval form is called an alveolar or multilocular hydatid. It provokes a severe host reaction and becomes surrounded by an inflammatory or granulomatous reaction, instead of the fibrous host response seen with *E. granulosus*. A central area of necrosis is always seen.

The cyst is slow growing, behaves like a malignancy, and has been mistaken for carcinoma, which it can mimic clinically and microscopically. Untreated it can be just as devastating, with mortality rates as high as 80%. The primary site of infection is the liver, where a dense honeycomb of small, multilocular cysts is formed. The cyst appears as a solid cancer-like growth that may cavitate and attain massive size. Through the inferior vena cava it may metastasize to distant organs. Alveolar hydatid disease of the lung is invariably a metastatic focus.

Diagnosis is based on history of exposure, elevated serologic titers, and characteristic changes on radiographic studies. Physical signs are confusing, and subjective symptoms may be mild, vague, and ill defined. Patients present usually with asymptomatic hepatomegaly. When symptoms are present, they are commonly related to the abdomen: mild epigastric and right upper-quadrant abdominal pain or distress, intermittent fever, and jaundice.

On radiologic examination, hepatomegaly and hepatic calcification are the most common findings. Typically, the diagnosis is made with abdominal radiographs that show scattered radiolucent areas surrounded with calcification, sometimes referred to as the "Swiss cheese" liver calcification pattern. This finding is pathognomonic, but at least 5 years of illness must elapse before calcification can be demonstrated. Without the characteristic radiographic study, the diagnosis is rarely made preoperatively.

CT and ultrasonography will demonstrate an indistinct mass with a necrotic center. Serologic tests used are the same as those for *E. granulosus* but tend to produce more positive findings with high titers. Indirect hemagglutination titers decline markedly during the first year after radical surgical resection but not after chemotherapy. The EM2 ELISA, using a semipurified homologous antigen fraction, is more sensitive and specific than tests using heterologous *E. granulosus* antigen fractions.[15] Results may still be positive, however, even when the parasite is no longer viable.[16] Needle biopsy confirms the diagnosis. There is no risk for anaphylaxis or spillage of protoscoleces because the tumor is essentially solid.

Treatment is by surgery. Early diagnosis is very important to permit resection before infiltration becomes too extensive. However, many cases are undiagnosed until they are well advanced and the hepatic lesions are unresectable.

At surgery, liver invasion is often more extensive than suggested by the degree of calcification on the radiograph. Complete excision is the only hope. Cure is possible when partial hepatectomy or hepatic lobectomy can remove all multilocular cysts and still preserve enough organ function. Still, radical hepatic resection is curative in only 20% of cases. Palliative measures are designed to ensure adequate bile drainage.

If surgery is unsuccessful or impractical, mebendazole is recommended at 40 mg/kg/day in divided doses for life, which may prevent progression of the primary lesion and metastasis and prolong life. Mebendazole's lethal effect on the larval cestode, however, has not been demonstrated conclusively. Albendazole has been shown to be effective in killing the larval cestode. Hepatic toxicity with the use of this drug can develop without warning, however, and does not seem to be dose related or likely due to hypersensitivity. Hepatic function should then be monitored the entire time the drug is administered. Monitoring should be done weekly during the first month and monthly thereafter.

Though not fulminating, the disease is ultimately fatal unless early surgical interference can remove the parasite cyst. Patients have survived at least 16 years after diagnosis. Death is due to liver failure; invasion of contiguous areas; and metastases to the lung, brain, and distant organs. The best means of preventing alveolar hydatid disease remains the control of the cestode in domestic animals, the primary source of human infection.

POLYCYSTIC HYDATID CYST

Polycystic hydatid cyst disease is caused by *E. vogeli* and *E. oligarthrus*. Only *E. vogeli* causes pulmonary disease and it is polycystic in nature. Polycystic echinococcosis occurs only in Central and South America and because of that is also called neotropical echinococcosis. Ninety-nine human cases of polycystic hydatic cyst have been diagnosed in 11 countries.

Bush dog is the definitive host, and pacas and agoutis are intermediate hosts. Domesticated dogs can also get infected naturally and experimentally.[1] It is speculated that domesticated dogs play a role in transmission of the infection to humans.[17]

After liver, lung is the second most common organ involved in polycystic hydatid disease.[18] After establishing infection in the liver, the infection spreads to other organ systems, including the lungs.[19]

Clinically polycystic hydatid disease is similar to alveolar hydatid disease caused by *E. multilocularis*. The severity of the disease is between cystic and alveolar infections.[18] The typical clinical scenario is an infection lasting a long time and manifesting as chronic disease. The reported range before diagnosis is 1 month to 22 years. Clinical manifestations primarily include abdominal pain and a palpable abdominal mass, usually hepatomegaly. Patient may have jaundice, fever, weight loss, and anemia. Patients with pulmonary involvement will have hemoptysis and may have other chest symptoms depending on the size and location of the cyst. Eosinophilia is often present.

Serologic tests cannot differentiate between infections caused by *E. vogeli* and other echinococci.[20] Antibodies against *Echinococcus* can be detected in 75% of the infected individuals using indirect hemagglutination assay.[21] An ELISA in one study could specifically diagnose *E. vogeli* infection.[22] Pulmonary involvement can be diagnosed by the polycystic structures on chest radiography, ultrasonography, or CT. Identification of protoscoleces or rostellar hooks by the shape and dimension is diagnostic.[23]

Medical treatment is preferred over surgical intervention because of high risks with surgery. Albendazole is the drug of choice. Although experience in the treatment of polycystic hydatid disease is limited, it has shown success in small series. In operable cases, prolonged or even lifelong therapy with albendazole or mebendazole may be needed.

STRONGYLOIDIASIS

Strongyloidiasis is caused by the nematode *Strongyloid stercoralis*. The helminth is 2 to 3 mm long and 30 to 50 μm wide.[24] The life cycle of *S. stercoralis* is not completely understood. The female worm is infectious and it lays its embryonated eggs in the intestine; the rhabditiform larvae hatch in the mucosa and then bore through the epithelium and migrate into the intestinal lumen and are excreted in stool. The rhabditiform larvae, in the soil and under suitable warm and moist conditions, develop into filariform larvae (direct developmental cycle). However, the rhabditiform larvae can also develop into free-living (nonparasitic) adult male and female helminthes who can mate and lay eggs in the soil (indirect developmental cycle), and these eggs hatch into rhabditiform larvae which can develop into infectious filariform larvae. Similar to the hookworm, these infectious larvae can penetrate human skin, enter the bloodstream, and reach the heart and lungs. In the lung they molt, climb up the bronchi and trachea, and are swallowed. Once in the intestinal mucosa and crypts they complete their life cycle.[25] Internal autoinfection can occur, when rhabditiform larvae in the lower bowel develop directly into filariform larvae which in turn penetrate the intestinal mucosa and gain access into lymphatic and hematogenous systems and reach the lung and bowel to complete their life cycle. Massive autoinfection can induce hyperinfection syndrome. Another phenomenon referred to as external autoinfection occurs when the filariform larvae penetrate the perianal skin.

Strongyloidiasis is widely present endemically in the tropical and subtropical parts of the world; the larvae are sensitive to dryness and extreme temperatures. It also occurs sporadically in the temperate areas. Humans are the primary hosts, but primates, cats, and dogs are also frequently infested. A prevalence of 0.4% to 4% has been estimated in the southern United States.[26,27] The infection occurs more frequently in rural areas and in lower socioeconomic groups.

The site of *S. stercoralis* skin penetration is inflamed, with lymphocytic and eosinophilic infiltration. The organism causes inflammation and ulceration of the intestinal tract. The penetration of the larvae in lungs causes an inflammatory reaction.

Clinical manifestations of strongyloidiasis can range from an asymptomatic infection (one third of the infected) to a fatal outcome. Because of the autoinfection phenomenon, many patients will have a chronic infection and symptoms may continue for years. Hyperinfection is the most serious and potentially fatal manifestation. Symptoms fall into three broad categories: cutaneous, intestinal, and pulmonary. These can be present during acute or chronic disease and during hyperinfection syndrome.[28,29]

The acute disease is often recognized by its cutaneous manifestations followed by pulmonary and intestinal symptomatology. The hallmark of cutaneous symptoms is pruritis at the site of larval entry, usually at the foot or ankle but sometimes also the perianal area. The site of entry has erythema and edema with a petechial or urticarial localized skin rash. Within a week or so the migration of larvae into the tracheobronchopulmonary tree causes itching of the throat, dry cough, and Loffler-like pneumonia with eosinophilia. This is followed by intestinal manifestations that include colicky abdominal pain (often epigastric), diarrhea, flatulence, and malaise.

Acute infection is followed by the stage when the symptoms may be recurrent or continuous as the patient enters the chronic stage of the disease. This stage of the disease, if not treated, can last decades. With chronic infection the cutaneous features include stationary urticaria and larva currens (similar to larva migrans). Gastrointestinal symptoms are similar to those in the acute disease and can range from mild to severe. Burning or colicky abdominal pain can accompany diarrhea that can contain blood and mucus and alternate with constipation. In addition, patients may complain of anorexia, nausea, vomiting, flatulence, and perianal pruritis. There may also be epigastric tenderness. The pulmonary manifestations include dry cough and wheezing. With worsening infection, patients may complain of fever, malaise, dyspnea, weakness, and weight loss.

The hyperinfection syndrome is disseminated strongyloidiasis from massive autoinfection, resulting in an overwhelming larval burden and increased dissemination of the larvae to the lungs and other organ systems.[30,31] This results in severe pulmonary and extrapulmonary systemic symptoms. Although this syndrome can occur without a predisposing cause, it is usually associated with depressed cellular immunity. Malnourished and debilitated individuals are at increased risk, especially if they are on immunosuppressive therapy (e.g., steroids). Human immunodeficiency virus (HIV)–infected patients do not seem to be at risk unless they are on steroids.[32] Pulmonary manifestations are increasing cough and dyspnea along with an odorless mucopurulent or blood-tinged sputum. Pulmonary changes include pneumonia, bronchitis, and pleural effusion. Rarely, miliary abscesses may form. Eosinophilia is absent in hyperinfection syndrome.

As for other helminthic infections, the diagnosis of strongyloidiasis is best made by visual identification. For *S. stercoralis,* identifying the characteristic rhabditiform larvae in stool, sputum, or duodenal fluid is diagnostic. Serologic tests (gel diffusion and ELISA) are not useful.

The chest radiograph is normal in most infected patients. During pulmonary larval migration, there may be irregular and transient patches of pneumonitis or fine nodularity. Hyperinfection is accompanied by chest radiographic changes that range from focal to diffuse pulmonary infiltrates, to cavitation and abscess formation.

The combination of cutaneous, intestinal, and pulmonary symptoms, with eosinophilia on peripheral smear, and potential exposure in an endemic area provide essential clues for making the diagnosis. Pulmonary symptoms should be differentiated from pneumonitis due to tuberculosis, mycoses, paragonimiasis, ascariasis, tropical pulmonary eosinophilia, and Loffler's syndrome due to other causes.

The treatment is medical, and the goal is elimination of all the worms; therefore, repeated treatment is sometimes needed. Even after completion of treatment, patients must be followed for years to assure complete eradication of all worms. Thiabendazole 25 mg/kg/dose twice a day for 2 or 3 days, or for 2 to 3 weeks for hyperinfection syndrome (if started early), is usually effective.[33] The duration of therapy should be determined by clinical response and worm burden. Ivermectin appears to be as effective as thiabendazole with fewer side effects.[34] Albendazole also appears to be as effective as thiabendazole.[35] Alternatives include mebendazole and pyrvinium pamoate. Pyrantel pamoate is not effective and should not be used for treatment.

PULMONARY PARAGONIMIASIS (LUNG FLUKE DISEASE)

Paragonimiasis, also known as lung fluke disease, endemic hemoptysis, oriental lung fluke, and pulmonary distomiasis, is caused by genus *Paragonimus.* Most human disease is caused by *Paragonimus westermani.* Other species of *Paragonimus,* such as *P. skrjabini, P. heterotremus,* and *P. miyazakii* can also cause human disease. Paragonimiasis is a zoonotic infection of carnivorous animals, including those in the canine and feline families (which also serve as reservoir hosts). The animals are more likely the cause of infection than fresh water, although certain culinary habits (eating fresh or pickled crustaceans) also cause many infections. In humans the organism primarily infects the lungs, although brain and liver infections have also been reported.[36,37]

Paragonimus westermani is reddish brown in color, 7 to 16 mm long, 4 to 8 mm wide, and 2 to 5 mm thick.[38] Lung cysts have two adult flukes in them, and eggs reach the bronchi either by penetrating the intact cyst wall or after rupture of the cyst wall. From the bronchi the eggs reach the mouth and are either spit out or swallowed and then excreted in stool. In the water these eggs embryonate and hatch in approximately 3 weeks. The hatched miracidium invades the first intermediate host (one of several families of snails)[39] and after a protracted asexual cycle they form sporocytes that turn into cercarie, which enter the second intermediate host (crustaceans), where they encyst and form the infectious metacercarie that reach the definitive host. Once eaten by the definitive host, the metacercarie encyst in the duodenum, penetrate the intestinal wall to reach the liver, and change into flukes. These flukes migrate through the diaphragm into the lung. Once in the lung, over a period of 5 to 6 weeks they mature into adult flukes and are encysted as a result of host immune response. Adult flukes begin to lay eggs 8 to 10 weeks after the infection.[40]

Paragonimiasis is seen in the Far East, Southeast Asia, the Indo-Pakistan subcontinent, some Pacific Islands, Africa, and parts of South and Latin America.[41]

As the life cycle of the fluke suggests, it can cause both pulmonary and extrapulmonary disease.

The pathogenesis of pulmonary disease is a result of parasite and host factors. The lesions are a result of direct mechanical damage by the flukes or their eggs or by the toxins released by the flukes. The host response also adds to the damage in the lungs when the host immune response takes the form of eosinophilic infiltration and the subsequent development of a cyst of host granulation tissue around the flukes. Besides the adult flukes, the cyst also contains eggs and Charcot-Leyden crystals. The cysts are in the parenchyma of the lungs close to the bronchioles. The release of cyst contents can cause bronchopneumonia, and the cyst wall may fibrose and become calcified. In extrapulmonary infections the flukes may form cysts, abscesses, or granulomata.

The symptoms depend on the site infected and the infectious burden. Some individuals may remain asymptomatic because of low inoculum burden. Pulmonary paragonimiasis has acute and chronic stages with different clinical manifestations. The main clinical manifestations of paragonimiasis are respiratory symptoms and eosinophilia. Once the flukes reach the lungs, the patient can have cough, dyspnea, or chest tightness (or even pain), and systemic symptoms of fever malaise and night sweats may be present. The patient may recall being sick days or weeks prior to their current illness with fever, diarrhea, and abdominal pain. Chills and urticarial rash may occur, leading to the diagnosis of a viral syndrome. A peripheral smear at this time shows eosinophilia. The diagnosis of paragonimiasis is frequently not made in the acute stage of the disease. The chronic stage usually follows 2 to 4 months later. Most patients look well, and the disease may resemble chronic bronchitis or bronchiectasis with a worsening cough that starts out dry and becomes productive and profuse. The sputum is gelatinous and blood streaked or rusty brown in color. Hemoptysis can be frequent and life threatening. Low-grade fever along with vague pleuritic chest pain may be present. Patients may also have weight loss and complain of muscular weakness. In uncomplicated pulmonary paragonimiasis, the chest examination may be remarkably normal. Children rarely have digital clubbing. Pulmonary paragonimiasis can be complicated by lung abscess, pneumothorax, pleural adhesions, empyema, and interstitial pneumonia. Pulmonary manifestations may be associated with abdominal (hepatic or peritoneal) and cerebral manifestations.[42]

Paragonimiasis is rare in children because they are less likely to indulge in consumption of exotic food, and because this helminth is not transmitted by fecal-oral transmission, by person-to-person contact, or from consumption of infested water. In the United States the most likely patient is a refugee, a recent immigrant, or someone who has traveled to an endemic region.

Like other protozoal infections, the definitive diagnosis can be made by identifying the protozoal eggs. The characteristic operculated eggs can be identified in sputum or stool specimens. Bronchoalveolar lavage has also been successful in identifying the eggs and making the diagnosis.[43] In complicated pulmonary paragonimiasis the eggs can be identified in pleural fluid or lung abscess material. Rarely, adult flukes can be identified in the sputum. Serologic tests using various techniques (Immunoblot, counterimmunoelectrophoresis, complement fixation, and ELISA) are sensitive and specific.[44] They are more useful in diagnosing extrapulmonary paragonimiasis. Skin testing cannot be used to make a diagnosis.

Chest radiography may be normal in acute pulmonary paragonimiasis or it may show peribronchitis and hilar lymphadenopathy. However, in chronic paragonimiasis chest radiography may show various abnormalities, including patchy nodular or linear infiltration, well-defined homogeneous densities, pleural thickening, effusion, and calcification. The pathognomonic radiographic picture shows a ring shadow with a crescent-shaped opacity along one side of the border.[45–48] CT scan may define the cavities much better.[43,48]

Pulmonary tuberculosis is the major differential diagnosis since the same endemic areas have a high prevalence of tuberculosis. Other conditions to consider include pulmonary neoplasm and other parasitic infections endemic for the region.

Prevention efforts should be aimed at educating against the use of untreated fresh water for drinking or cooking (since this water may contain the infected crustaceans which may infect the human host even though the water itself does not support the infectious metacercarie) and not to eat improperly prepared or raw crustaceans. Eradication of reservoirs is not practical.

Treatment is praziquantel 25 mg/kg/dose three times daily after meals for 3 days. Bithionol has also been used with some success but has more adverse effects.

REFERENCES

1. Eckert J, Deplazes P: Biological, epidemiological and clinical aspects of Echinococcus. A zoonosis of increasing concern. Clin Microbiol Rev 2004;17(1):107.
2. Chaouachi B, Nouri A, Ben Salah S, et al: Les kystes hydatiques du poumon chez l'enfant. A propos de 643 cas. Pediatrie 1988;43(9):769.
3. Bakir F: Serious complications of hydatid cyst of the lung. Am Rev Respir Dis 1967;96(3):483.
4. Ayuso LA, de Peralta GT, Lazarao RB, et al: Surgical treatment of pulmonary hydatidosis. J Thorac Cardiovasc Surg 1981;82(4):569.
5. Erdem CZ, Erdem LO: Radiological characteristics of pulmonary hydatid disease in children. Less common radiological appearances. Eur J Radiol 2003;45:123.
6. Saksouk FA, Fahl MH, Rizk GK: Computed tomography of pulmonary hydatid disease. J Comput Assist Tomogr 1986;10(2):226.
7. Pant CS, Gupta RK: Diagnostic value of ultrasonography in hydatid disease in abdomen and chest. Acta Radiol 1987;28(6):743.
8. Keystone JS: Larval tapeworm infections. In: Nelson JD, ed: Current Therapy in Pediatric Infectious Disease, 2nd ed. Toronto, Ontario, Canada: BC Decker, 1988.
9. Senyuz OF, Yesildag E, Celayir S: Albendazole in the treatment of hydatid liver disease. Surg Today 2001;31:487.
10. Wilson JF, Diddams AC, Rausch RL: Cystic hydatid disease in Alaska. A review of 101 autochthonous cases of *Echinococcus granulosus* infection. Am Rev Respir Dis 1968;98(1):1.
11. Pinch LW, Wilson JF: Non-surgical management of cystic hydatid disease in Alaska. A review of 30 cases of *Echinococcus granulosus* infection treated without operation. Ann Surg 1973;178(1):45.
12. Webster GA, Cameron TWM: Epidemiology and diagnosis of echinococcosis in Canada. Can Med Assoc J 1967;96:600.
13. Moore RD, Urschel JD, Fraser RE, et al: Cystic hydatid lung disease in northwest Canada. Can J Surg 1994;37(1):20.
14. Stehr-Green JK, Stehr-Green PA, Schantz PM, et al: Risk factors for infection with *Echinococcus multilocularis* in Alaska. Am J Trop Med Hyg 1988; 38(2):380.
15. Lanier AP, Trujillo DE, Schantz PM, et al: Comparison of serologic tests for the diagnosis and follow-up of alveolar hydatid disease. Am J Trop Med Hyg 1987;37(3):609.
16. Rausch RL, Wilson JF, McMahon BJ, O'Gorman MA: Consequences of continuous mebendazole therapy in alveolar hydatid disease—with a summary of a ten-year clinical trail. Ann Trop Med Parasitol 1986;80(4):403.
17. Basset D, Girou C, Nozais P, et al: Neotropical echinococcosis in Surinam. *Echinococcus oligarthrus* and *Echinococcus vogeli* in the abdomen. Am J Trop Med Hyg 1998;59:787.
18. D'Alessandro A: Polycystic echinococcus in tropical America. *Echinococcus vogeli* and *E. oligarthrus*. Acta Trop 1997;67:43.
19. Rausch RL, D'Alessandro A: Histogenesis in the metacestode of *Echinococcus vogeli* and mechanism of pathogenesis in polycystic hydatid disease. J Parasitol 1999;85:410.
20. Morar R, Feldman C: Pulmonary echinococcosis. Eur Respir J 2003;21: 1069.
21. Meneghelli UG, Martinelli ALC, Bellucci AD, et al: Polycystic hydatid disease (*Echinococcus vogeli*). Treatment with Albendazole. Ann Trop Med Parasitol 1992;86:151.
22. Gottstein B, D'Alessandro A, Rausch RL: Immunodiagnosis of polycystic hydatid disease/polycystic echinococcosis due to *Echinococcus vogeli*. Am J Trop Med Hyg 1995;53:558.
23. Rausch RL, D'Alessandro A, Rausch RV: Characteristic of the larval *Echinococcus vogeli* in the natural intermediate host, the paca, *Cuniculus paca* L (Rodentia: Dasyproctidae). Am J Trop Med Hyg 1981;30:1043.
24. Centers for Disease Control and Prevention: Parasite Image Library. Available at http://www.dpd.cdc.gov/dpdx/HTML/ImageLibrary/Strongyloidiasis_il.htm.
25. Centers for Disease Control and Prevention. Available at http://www.dpd.cdc.gov/dpdx/HTML Strongyloidiasis.htm.
26. Centers for Disease Control and Prevention: Publication of CDC Surveillance Summaries. MMWR Morb Mortal Weekly Rep 1992; 41(8):145.
27. Genta RM: Global prevalence of strongyloidiasis. Critical review with epidemiologic insights into the prevention of disseminated disease. Rev Infect Dis 1989;11:755.
28. Hiroshi T: Strongyloidiasis. In: Goldsmith R, Heyneman D, eds: Tropical Medicine and Parasitology. East Norwalk, Conn: Appleton & Lange, 1989, p 368.
29. Mahmoud AAF: Intestinal nematodes (roundworms), strongyloidiasis. In: Mandell GL, Douglas RG, Bennet JE, eds: Principles and Practice of Infectious Diseases, 3rd ed. New York: Churchill Livingstone, 2003, p 2135.
30. Scowden EB, Schaffer W, Stone WJ: Overwhelming strongyloidiasis. An unappreciated opportunistic infection. Medicine 1978;57:527.
31. Igra-Siegman Y, Kapila R, Sen P, et al: Syndrome of hyperinfection with *Strongyloides stercoralis*. Rev Infect Dis 1981;3:397.
32. Genta RM: Dysregulation of strongyloidiasis. A new hypothesis. Clin Microbiol Rev 1992;5:345.
33. Groves DI: Treatment of strongyloidiasis with thiabendazole. An analysis of toxicity and effectiveness. Trans R Soc Med Hyg 1982;76:114.
34. Salazar SA, Berk SH, Howe D, Berk SL: Ivermectin vs thiabendazole in the treatment of strongyloidiasis. Infect Med 1994;11:50.
35. Liu LX, Weller PF: Strongyloidiasis and other intestinal nematode infections. Infect Dis Clin North Am 1993;7:665.

36. Harinasuta KT, Bunnag D: Lung fluke disease. In: Goldsmith R, Heyneman D, eds: Tropical Medicine and Parasitology. East Norwalk, Conn: Appleton & Lange, 1989, p 472.
37. Blair D, Xu ZB, Agatsuma T: Paragonimiasis and the genus Paragonimus. Adv Parasitol 1999;42:113.
38. Centers for Disease Control and Prevention: Parasite image. Available at http://www.dpd.cdc.gov/dpdx/HTML/Image_Library.htmDavis.
39. GM, Chen CE, Kang ZB, Liu YY: Snail hosts of Paragonimus in Asia and the Americas. Biomed Environ Sci 1994;7:369.
40. Centers for Disease Control and Prevention: Life cycle. Available at http://www.dpd.cdc.gov/dpdx/HTML/Paragonimiasis.htm.
41. Goldsmith R, Bunnag D, Bunnag T: Lung fluke infections. Paragonimiasis. In: Strickland GT, ed: Hunter's Tropical Medicine, 7th ed. Philadelphia: WB Saunders, 1991, p 827.
42. Kagawa FT: Pulmonary paragonimiasis. Semin Respir Infect 1997;12:149.
43. Mukae H, Taniguchi H, Matsumoto N, et al: Clinicoradiologic features of pleuropulmonary *Paragonimus westermani* of Kyusyu Island Japan. Chest 2001;120:514.
44. Slemenda SB, Maddison SE, Jong EC, Moore DD: Diagnosis of paragonimiasis by immunoblot. Am J Trop Med Hyg 1988;39:469.
45. Fraser RG, Pare JAP, Pare PD: Parasitic infestation of the lung. In: Fraser RG, Pare JAP, Pare PD, et al, eds: Diagnosis of Diseases of the Chest, 3rd ed. Philadelphia: WB Saunders, 1995, p 1081.
46. Johnson RJ, Johnson JR: Paragonimiasis in Indochinese refugees. Roentgenographic findings with clinical correlations. Am Rev Respir Dis 1983;128:534.
47. Im JG, Whang HY, Kim WS, et al: Pleuropulmonary paragonimiasis. Radiologic findings in 71 patients. AJR Am J Roentgenol 1992;159:39.
48. Singcharoen T, Silprasert W: CT findings in pulmonary paragonimiasis. J Comput Assist Tomogr 1987;11:1101.

SUGGESTED READING

American Academy of Pediatrics: Red Book. 2003 Report of the Committee on Infectious Diseases. Elk Grove Village, Ill: American Academy of Pediatrics, 2003.

Bartelink AK, Kortbeek LM, Huidekoper HJ, et al: Acute respiratory failure due to toxocara infection. Lancet 1993;342:1234.

Bastid C, Azar C, Doyer M, et al: Percutaneous treatment of hydatid cysts under sonographic guidance. Dig Dis Sci 1994;39(7):1576.

Beaver PC: The nature of visceral larva migrans. J Parasitol 1969;55:3.

Beaver PC, Snyder CH, Carrera GM, et al: Chronic eosinophilia due to visceral larva migrans. Pediatrics 1952;9:7.

Beshear JR, Hendley JO: Severe pulmonary involvement in visceral larva migrans. Am J Dis Child 1973;125:599.

Bhatia V, Sarin SK: Hepatic visceral larva migrans. Evolution of the lesion, diagnosis, and role of high-dose albendazole therapy. Am J Gastroenterol 1994;89:624.

Borrie J, Shaw JHF: Hepatobronchial fistula caused by hydatid disease. The Dunedin experience 1952–79. Thorax 1981;36(1):25.

Bouzid A, Nekmouche L, Benallegue S: Les kystes hydatiques multifocaux de l'enfant. Chir Pediatr 1986;27(1):33.

Buijs J, Borsboom G, van Gemund JJ: Toxocara seroprevalence in 5-year old elementary school children. Relation with allergic asthma. Am J Epidemiol 1994;140:839.

Burke JA: Visceral larval migrans. J Ky Med Assoc 1977;75:62.

Cypress RH, Karol MH, Zidian JL, et al: Larva-specific antibodies in patients with visceral larva migrans. J Infect Dis 1977;135:633.

de Savigny DH: In vitro maintenance of *Toxocara canis* larvae and a simple method for the production of *Toxocara* ES antigen for use in serodiagnostic tests for visceral larva migrans. J Parasitol 1975;61:781.

Dogan R, Yuksel M, Cetin G, et al: Surgical treatment of hydatid cysts of the lung. Report on 1055 patients. Thorax 1989;44(3):192.

Door J, Houel J, Dor V, et al: Le kyste hydatique du poumon considerations anatomo-chirurgicales. A propos d'une observation recente chez un enfant et d'une statistique de plus de 500 cas operes. Ann Chir Thorac Cardiovasc 1967;6(2):369.

Elburjo M, Gani EA: Surgical management of pulmonary hydatid cysts in children. Thorax 1995;50(4):396.

Feldman GJ, Parker HW: Visceral larva migrans associated with the hypereosinophilic syndrome and the onset of severe asthma. Ann Intern Med 1992;116:838.

Gillespie SH, Bidwell D, Voller A, et al: Diagnosis of human toxocariasis by antigen capture enzyme linked immunosorbent assay. J Clin Pathol 1993; 46:551.

Glickman LT, Schantz PM, Dombroske RL, Cypress R: Evaluation of serodiagnostic tests for visceral larval migrans. Am J Trop Med Hyg 1978;27:492.

Gocmen A, Toppare MF, Kiper N: Treatment of hydatid disease in childhood with mebendazole. Eur Respir J 1993;6(2):253.

Grunebaum M: Radiological manifestations of lung echinococcus in children. Pediatr Radiol 1975;3(2):65.

Hartleb M, Januszewski K: Severe hepatic involvement in viscerallarva migrans. Eur J Gastroenterol Hepatol 2001;13:1245.

Horton RJ: Chemotherapy of *Echinococcus* infection in man with albendazole. Trans R Soc Trop Med Hyg 1989;83(1):97.

Hotez PJ: Visceral and ocular larva migrans. Semin Neurol 1993;13:175.

Jones WE, Schantz PM, Foreman K, et al: Human toxocariasis in a rural community. Am J Dis Child 1980;134:967.

Lampkin BC, Mauer AM: Clinical manifestations of visceral larva migrans variability as related to duration of ingestion. Clin Pediatr 1970;9:683.

Lamy AL, Cameron BH, Le Blanc JG, et al: Giant hydatid lung cysts in the Canadian northwest. Outcome of conservative treatment in three children. J Pediatr Surg 1993;28(9):1140.

Lightowlers MV: Immunology and molecular biology of *Echinococcus* infections. Int J Parasitol 1990;20(4):471.

Ljungström I, Van Knapen F: An epidemiological and serological study of toxocara infection in Sweden. Scand J Infect Dis 1989;21:87.

Magnaval JF, Galindo V, Glickman LT, Clanet M: Human Toxocara infection of the central nervous system and neurological disorders. A case control study. Parasitology 1997;115:537.

Masuda Y, Kishimoto T, Ito H, Tsuji M: Visceral larva migrans caused by *Trichuris vulpis* presenting as a pulmonary mass. Thorax 1987;42:990.

Mistrello G, Gentili M, Falagiani P, et al: Dot immunobinding assay as a new diagnostic test for human hydatid disease. Immunol Lett 1995;47(1–2):79.

Mok CH: Visceral larva migrans. A discussion based on review of the literature. Clin Pediatr 1968;7:565.

Mottaghian H, Mahmoudi S, Vaez-Zadeh K: A ten-year survey of hydatid disease (*Echinococcus granulosus*) in children. Prog Pediatr Surg 1982;15:113.

Mutaf O, Arikan A, Yazici M, et al: Pulmonary hydatidosis in children. Eur J Pediatr Surg 1994;4(2):70.

Nahmias J, Goldsmith R, Soibelman M, el-On J: Three- to 7-year follow-up after albendazole treatment of 68 patients with cystic echinococcosis (hydatid disease). Ann Trop Med Parasitol 1994;88(3):295.

Nelson S, Greene T, Ernhart CB: *Toxocara canis* infection in preschool age children. Risk factors and the cognitive development of preschool children. Neurotoxicol Teratol 1996;18(20):167.

Novick RJ, Tchervenkov CI, Wilson JA, et al: Surgery for thoracic hydatid disease. A North American experience. Ann Thorac Surg 1987;43(6):681.

Oteifa NM, Moustafa MA, Elgozamy BM: Toxocariasis as a possible cause of allergic diseases in children. J Egypt Soc Parasitol 1998;28:365.

Ozcelik C, Inci I, Toprak M, et al: Surgical treatment of pulmonary hydatidosis in children. Experience in 92 patients. J Pediatr Surg 1994;29(3):392.

Ozer Z, Cetin M, Kahraman C: Pleural involvement by hydatid cysts of the lung. Thorac Cardiovasc Surg 1985;33(2):103.

Patterson R, Huntley CC, Roberts M, Irons JS: Visceral larva migrans. Immunoglobulins, precipitating antibodies and detection of IgG and IgM antibodies against *Ascaris* antigen. Am J Trop Med Hyg 1975;24:465.

Perrin J, Boxerbaum B, Doershuk CF: Thiabendazole treatment of presumptive visceral larva migrans (VLM). Clin Pediatr 1975;14:147.

Rausch RL, Wilson JF, Schantz PM, McMahon BJ: Spontaneous death of *Echinococcus multilocularis*. Cases diagnosed serologically (by EM2 ELISA) and clinical significance. Am J Trop Med Hyg 1987;36(3):576.

Roig J, Romeu J, Riera C, et al: Acute eosinophilic pneumonia due to toxocariasis with bronchoalveolar lavage findings. Chest 1992;102:294.

Sadrieh M, Dutz W, Navabpoor S: Review of 150 cases of hydatid cyst of the lung. Dis Chest 1967;52(5):662.

Saenz-Santamaria J, Moreno-Casado J, Nunez C: Role of fine needle biopsy in the diagnosis of hydatid cyst. Diagn Cytopathol 1995;13(3):229.

Schantz PM: Toxocara larva migrans now. Am J Trop Med Hyg 1989;41 (Suppl):21.

Seah SKK, Hucal G, Law C: Dogs and intestinal parasites. A public health problem. Can Med Assoc J 1975;112:1191.

Snyder CH: Visceral larval migrans. Pediatrics 1961;28:85.

Struchler D, Schubarth P, Gualzata M: Thiabendazole vs albendazole in the treatment of toxocariasis. A clinical trial. Ann Trop Med Parasitol 1989; 83:473.

Taylor MR, Keane CT, O'Connor P: The expanded spectrum of toxocaral disease. Lancet 1988;1:692–694.

Teggl A, Lastilla MG, De Rosa F: Therapy of human hydatid disease with mebendazole and albendazole. Antimicrob Agents Chemother 1993;37(8):1679.

Thompson WM, Chisholm DP, Tank R: Plain film roentgenographic findings in alveolar hydatid disease—*Echinococcus multilocularis*. Am J Roentgenol Radium Ther Nucl Med 1972;116(2):345.

Thornieporth NG, Disko R: Alveolar hydatid disease (*Echinococcus multilocularis*)—review and update. Prog Clin Parasitol 1994;4:55.

Tuncel E: Pulmonary air meniscus sign. Respiration 1984;46(1):139.

Wen H, Zhang HW, Muhmut M, et al: Initial observation on albendazole in combination with cimetidine for the treatment of human cystic echinococcosis. Ann Trop Med Parasitol 1994;88(1):49.

Wilson JF, Rausch RL, McMahon BJ, et al: Albendazole therapy in alveolar hydatid disease. A report of favorable results in two patients after short-term therapy. Am J Trop Med Hyg 1987;37(1):162.

Wilson JF, Rausch RL, Wilson FR: Alveolar hydatid disease. Review of the surgical experience in 42 cases of active disease among Alaskan Eskimos. Ann Surg 1995;221(3):315.

Worley G, Green IA, Forthingham TE. *Toxocara canis* infection. Clinical and epidemiological associations with seropositivity in kindergarten children. J Infect Dis 1991;149:591.

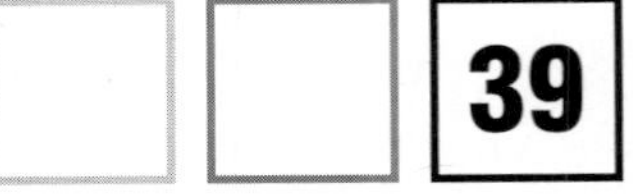

39 Respiratory Disorders in Pediatric HIV Infection

Meyer Kattan, MD

The first cases of acquired immunodeficiency syndrome (AIDS) in children were described in 1982.[1] Human immunodeficiency virus type 1 (HIV-1) was established as the cause of AIDS.[2,3] At the onset of the pandemic, respiratory complications were the most common presenting problem in children. Acute pulmonary infections were a major cause of morbidity and mortality throughout the world. Since then, significant strides have been made in understanding the virus and developing medications that slow the progression of disease. In developed countries where early identification of HIV-infected infants is possible and medications are readily available for both treatment of HIV-1 infection and prophylaxis of opportunistic infections, there has been a marked reduction in the rates of opportunistic infections and the rates of acute pulmonary disease.[4]

The emerging countries in Africa and Asia have the majority of HIV-1-infected patients worldwide. In these areas, early identification and treatment of HIV-1 infection and its complications is not the standard of care and the pulmonary manifestations of HIV-1 infection remain a significant problem. Malnutrition complicates the clinical outcomes of pulmonary disease. The spectrum of respiratory illnesses in these countries at the present time does not differ greatly from that reported earlier from developed countries except for a higher incidence of tuberculosis (TB).

■ DEFINITION

HIV-1 infection results in a disease spectrum ranging from asymptomatic infection to severely symptomatic cases meeting the Centers for Disease Control and Prevention (CDC) surveillance case definition for AIDS.[5] The definition of AIDS was established not for the practical care of patients but for surveillance purposes. Infected patients who are asymptomatic are classified as CDC category N. Asymptomatic patients may have abnormal immune function. Symptomatic patients are classified as CDC category A, B, or C depending on the severity of the signs and symptoms. The CDC surveillance definition for AIDS is an illness characterized by the presence of an indicator disease (e.g., encephalopathy, *Pneumocystis* pneumonia, lymphoid interstitial pneumonia) and documentation of HIV-1 infection. Any condition listed in the surveillance case definition for AIDS except for lymphoid interstitial pneumonitis or pulmonary lymphoid hyperplasia places the child in category C.

■ ETIOLOGY AND PATHOGENESIS

HIV-1 is a retrovirus, which is a heterogeneous group of lipid-enveloped RNA viruses. HIV-1 comprises several subtypes designated as A through J with different geographic distributions. In the United States, Europe, Japan, and the Caribbean, subtype B is the primary subtype found in infected individuals, while other subtypes predominate in Africa and parts of Asia. Recombinant subtypes (mosaics) have been described. Another retrovirus, HIV-2, is relatively rare and causes a less severe AIDS-like syndrome.

Through the action of its enzyme, reverse transcriptase, DNA is synthesized from RNA, which is then integrated into the host DNA genome. Most retroviruses contain only three gene regions. The group antigen gene (*gag*) encodes the core nucleocapsid proteins. The viral core contains four nucleocapsid proteins, p24, p17, p9, and p7. The envelope genes (*env*) encode the surface core proteins of the virus. HIV-1 has two major viral envelope proteins, the external glycoprotein 120 (gp120) and the transmembrane gp41 (Fig. 39-1). The polymerase gene (*pol*) gives rise to viral enzymes (e.g., reverse transcriptase, protease, and endonuclease). In addition to the *gag, pol,* and *env* genes, the 9-kilobase RNA genome of HIV-1 contains at least six additional genes (*vif, vpu, vpr, tat, rev,* and *nef*) that code for proteins involved in the regulation of gene expression.

The human CD4$^+$ T lymphocyte is the major cellular target for HIV-1. The HIV-1 gp120 envelope protein binds to the CD4 molecule on the host cell membrane with strikingly high affinity. This leads to entry of the virus into the T cell and integration of the viral genome into the host DNA. HIV-1 also infects monocytes and macrophages but has much less pronounced cytopathic effects in these cells. Therefore, infected monocytes serve as a reservoir for HIV-1, allowing further dissemination of the virus throughout the body.

Infection with HIV-1 results in profound changes in T-lymphocyte function. There is progressive depletion of the CD4$^+$ helper lymphocytes. CD4$^+$ depletion is an indicator of severity of HIV-1 infection since the incidence of opportunistic infections and other complications correlates with the number and percentage of CD4$^+$ lymphocytes. In the first 9 months of life, the rate of decline of CD4$^+$ cells in HIV-1-infected infants is double that of noninfected infants.[6] Possible mechanisms for depletion of CD4$^+$ lymphocytes include death of infected cells, increased susceptibility to apoptosis, and decreased generation of T lymphocytes.[7,8]

Two CD4$^+$ lymphocyte subsets, T-helper 1 (TH1) lymphocytes and TH2 lymphocytes have been identified by their ability to release different types of cytokines. TH1 lymphocytes produce cytokines that are responsible for delayed-type hypersensitivity, and TH2 lymphocytes produce cytokines that are responsible for antibody production. The ability to produce type 1 cytokines such as interleukin-2 and interferon-γ is progressively lost in HIV-1-infected children.[9] This may account for decreased lymphocyte proliferation responses against certain antigens. Production of interferon-γ is necessary for macrophage activation and effective cellular defense against intracellular organisms. The inability to elaborate this predicts progression of disease.[10] There is a delayed and weak cytotoxic T-lymphocyte

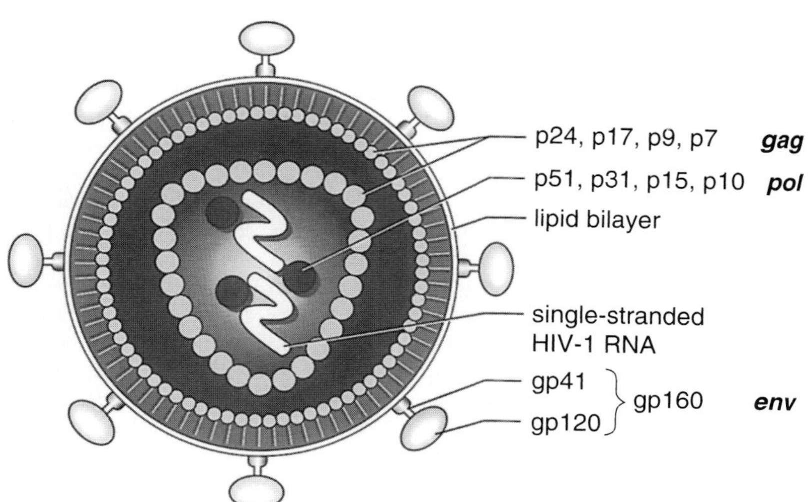

■ **FIGURE 39-1.** Schematic representation of the human immunodeficiency virus (HIV-1). Two single-stranded RNA chains are surrounded by a nucleocapsid polypeptide. A lipid envelope surrounding the viral core contains the viral envelope proteins gp 41 and gp 120. *Gag, env,* and *pol* are the gene regions coding for the respective proteins. (Adapted from Graham BS, Wright PF: Candidate AIDS vaccines. N Engl J Med 1995; 333:1332.)

response in HIV-1-infected children, which may explain the higher viral loads observed in children.[11] Natural killer cells are a subpopulation of T lymphocytes. Natural killer cell–mediated cytotoxicity is reduced in infected children.[12]

B-cell dysfunction with defective humoral immunity occurs in untreated infants.[13] If there is defective B-cell function early in life, before the development of specific memory cells, severe infection with otherwise common organisms may result. Studies indicate that HIV-1-infected children have an impaired ability to produce and maintain antibodies to pediatric vaccines, and this inability appears early in life.[14,15]

■ EPIDEMIOLOGY

An estimated 2.5 million children under 15 worldwide are living with HIV-1 infection in 2003, 90% of whom reside in developing countries. There were 700,000 children newly infected that year. HIV-1 infection and AIDS have disproportionately affected minority populations in the United States. The rates of AIDS cases per 100,000 population reported among adults and adolescents in 1999 were 84.2 for African Americans, 34.6 for Hispanics, 9.0 for whites, 11.3 for American Indians/Alaska Natives, and 4.3 for Asian/Pacific Islanders.

The identifiable risk factors associated with HIV-1 infection in children include a mother who was an intravenous drug user or who was a heterosexual partner of an intravenous drug user, bisexual fathers, and transfusion of blood or blood products to the mother or directly to the child. Perinatal transmission accounts for virtually all new cases of HIV-1 infection in children younger than 13 years since the initiation of screening of blood products. Of the reported cases of AIDS in children younger than 13 years in the United States, approximately 90% were born to mothers who were HIV-1 infected or who were at risk for HIV-1 infection and, in approximately 60% of those cases, the mother was either an intravenous drug abuser or the heterosexual partner of an intravenous drug abuser. Perinatal transmission can occur in utero, intrapartum, and through breastfeeding. Although most transmission of HIV-1 occurs during pregnancy and at birth, breastfeeding may account for 5% to 15% of infants becoming infected after delivery.[16] This is an important modality of transmission of HIV-1 infection in developing countries, particularly where mothers continue to breastfeed for prolonged periods. Sexual abuse is another mode of infection in young children.[17] Adolescents, like adults, acquire HIV-1 infection primarily through sexual transmission and intravenous drug abuse.[18]

Unlike women in other regions of the world, African women are more likely to be infected with HIV-1 than men. The prevalence rates vary in different parts of the continent. More than one in five pregnant women are HIV-1 infected in most countries in southern Africa. In sub-Saharan Africa, median HIV-1 prevalence in antenatal clinics exceeds 10% in only a few countries. The HIV-1 seroprevalence rate in childbearing women in the United States is estimated to range between 1.5 and 1.7 per 1000 women.[19] The highest seroprevalence rates are seen in urban areas, but high rates have also been observed in some rural areas.[20]

The transmission rate from mother to infant varied in different regions of the world from 13% to 39% in the absence of intervention.[21–25] The maternal viral load is the major risk factor for perinatal transmission. The use of zidovudine during pregnancy after the first trimester, during labor, and for the first 6 weeks of neonatal life reduced the transmission rate from 26% to 8%.[26] Subsequent cohort studies have reported lower transmission rates when zidovudine is combined with elective cesarean section or use of highly active antiretroviral regimens that reduce maternal viral load to very low levels. The risk for transmission is approximately 2% with perinatal antiretroviral regimens and maternal viral load levels below 1000 copies/mL by RNA-polymerase chain reaction (PCR).[27,28]

Despite success in reducing perinatal transmission in industrialized countries, there have been barriers to the implementation of perinatal HIV-1 regimens in resource-poor countries. Barriers include poor access to care, lack of prenatal testing programs, cost of antiretroviral therapy, and the necessity of breast feeding.

■ DIAGNOSIS

A screening enzyme-linked immunosorbent assay (ELISA) detects specific immunoglobulin G (IgG) antibody to the virus. This test has a specificity of 99%.[29] The test is confirmed using an immunoblot analysis (Western blot). In this assay, HIV-1 antigens are electrophoretically separated into bands. Antibodies to HIV-1 can be identified when bound to specific antigenic bands. Maternal HIV-1 antibodies usually become undetectable in infants by 10 months but may be present until 18 months of age. Therefore, standard HIV-1-IgG serologic assays cannot be used in detecting HIV-1 infection in the first 18 months of life. Diagnosis of HIV-1 infection in nearly all infants by 2 months of age is now possible by other viral detection assays.[30] DNA PCR can detect HIV-1 DNA in peripheral blood monocytes and lymphocytes and is the diagnostic method of choice for infants younger than 2 years. The sensitivity and specificity is 95% and 97%, respectively, for infants older than 1 month.[31] RNA PCR is used for quantitation of plasma virion RNA and is widely used to assess response to therapy and predict the clinical course. It may detect infection earlier than DNA PCR. Detection of p24 viral core protein by an ELISA is most likely to detect infection in early stages before antibody formation, and in the later stages of disease when viral load is highest. False-negative p24 antigen results can be reduced by using a modified assay that dissociates immune complexes formed with maternal antibodies. The limited sensitivity and specificity of this test in infants reduce its usefulness in infant diagnosis. Cell culture has an equivalent diagnostic profile compared with DNA PCR but is more costly.

NATURAL HISTORY OF HIV-1 INFECTION IN CHILDREN

Perinatally acquired HIV-1 infection differs from infection in adults in that it occurs in the setting of an immature and developing immune system. In adults, HIV-1 is carried to the regional lymph nodes and then disseminated throughout the lymphoid tissues where viral replication occurs. This results in a viremic stage with high HIV-1 RNA levels that decline rapidly over the subsequent few months and remain at a steady-state level for a variable period of time. Eventually, the cytopathic effect of the virus results in disruption of the cells and release of the virus into the blood. In perinatally infected children, there is a rapid rise in HIV-1 RNA levels to several hundred thousand copies per milliliter within a month of birth that then fall very slowly in the first 2 years of life. Higher HIV-1 RNA levels are associated with rapid progression of disease.[32]

Immunologic dysfunction occurs early in untreated infants, and symptoms and opportunistic infections are prevalent in the first year of life. HIV-1 disease progression is most rapid in the first year of life. Studies from Western countries in the era before aggressive antiviral therapy show that approximately 70% of infected children develop some HIV-1-related symptoms by 1 year of age and 25% to 28% die by age 5 years.[33–35] With earlier diagnosis and the more widespread use of potent antiretroviral therapy, the natural history of HIV-1 infection has changed, but the data are limited in children. More recent cohorts of infected children followed prospectively from birth show that the majority has slowly progressive disease. Over time, acute lung disease has become less problematic in resource-rich countries and the pulmonary manifestations have become part of a chronic multiorgan disease.

HIV-1 AND LUNG DEFENSE

The profound immunologic alterations caused by HIV-1 result in a spectrum of infectious and noninfectious lung diseases (Box 39-1). In the lung, as in peripheral blood, HIV-1 infects pulmonary lymphocytes and infection can be identified in lymphocytes obtained from bronchoalveolar lavage (BAL) fluid.[36] The virus decreases numbers of lung $CD4^+$ cells and also causes infiltration of $CD8^+$ cells in the interstitial and alveolar spaces. This is mediated by cytokines, including interleukin-15 from alveolar macrophages that induce T-cell proliferation and stimulate T-cell migration.[37] The number of natural killer cells are increased in BAL fluid of HIV-1-infected individuals, but they lose their functional capabilities with progression of disease.[38] Alveolar macrophages obtained by BAL can also be infected with HIV-1.[39] Although some components of macrophage defense are preserved during HIV-1 infection, lack of activation signals from T lymphocytes impairs effective defense by macrophages. The T lymphocytes from HIV-1-infected individuals do not produce interferon-γ normally in response to antigens, which is necessary for macrophage activation. The inability to elaborate this predicts progression of disease.[10]

PULMONARY DISORDERS

Infants who are infected by vertical transmission have no recognizable pulmonary disease at birth attributable to the infection.[40] The incidence of respiratory distress syndrome and

BOX 39-1 Pulmonary Complications of HIV Infection

Infections

Viruses

- Cytomegalovirus
- Respiratory syncytial virus
- Herpes simplex virus
- Parainfluenza virus
- Influenza virus
- Adenovirus

Bacteria

- Encapsulated organisms (e.g., *Streptococcus pneumoniae, Haemophilus influenzae, Staphylococcus aureus*)
- Gram-negative organisms (e.g., *Escherichia coli, Klebsiella, Pseudomonas aeruginosa*)
- *Mycobacterium tuberculosis*
- *Mycobacterium avium-intracellulare*

Fungi

- *Pneumocystis jiroveci*
- *Candida albicans*
- *Histoplasma capsulatum*
- *Cryptococcus neoformans*
- *Aspergillus species*
- *Coccidioides immitis*

Interstitial pneumonia

- Lymphoid interstitial pneumonia
- Pulmonary lymphoid hyperplasia
- Desquamative interstitial pneumonia

Malignancies

- Kaposi sarcoma
- Lymphoma

bronchopulmonary dysplasia is similar in infected and uninfected children born to HIV-1-infected mothers.[41] In untreated infants, the initial symptoms and signs of HIV-1 infection include hepatosplenomegaly, lymphadenopathy, pulmonary disease, and sepsis.[33,42] Pulmonary problems have been the predominant causes of morbidity and mortality in HIV-1-infected children under 13 years of age.[42,43] *Pneumocystis* pneumonia (PCP), lymphocytic interstitial pneumonia (LIP), and bacterial pneumonia were the pulmonary complications most frequently encountered. With earlier diagnosis, new medications, and longer survival during the past decade of the AIDS pandemic, the spectrum of disease, the course and character of the disease, and its complications have changed.

In a prospective cohort followed from birth in the United States, the rate of lower respiratory tract infections in HIV-1-infected children in the first year of life was approximately 2.8 times greater than the rate in uninfected children born to HIV-1-infected mothers.[44] In a prospective study from Rwanda, the risk for developing severe pneumonia among infected children was three times greater than among uninfected children.[45] The highest incidence of pneumonia occurs in the first 12 months of life. The incidence rate for pneumonia (excluding PCP) is between 20 and 25 per 100 child-years during the first 12 months.[44,46] In a prospective cohort enrolled at a mean age of 40 months, 25% of the children developed an acute pneumonia over 3 years, and multiple episodes occurred in 34% of children.[46]

A prior history of an AIDS-defining recurrent bacterial infection and a lower $CD4^+$ count are risk factors for the development of acute pneumonia.[46] In a subgroup of these patients, higher levels of baseline HIV-1 RNA titers (especially when RNA was >1 million copies/mL) were associated with a higher rate of acute pneumonia. In children younger than 12 months, a low $CD4^+$ cell count in the infant and low maternal $CD4^+$ cell count appear to be risk factors for pneumonia.[44] The rate of decline of $CD4^+$ cells during the first year of life is also associated with development of lower respiratory tract infections (Table 39-1).

The etiology of the pulmonary infections is varied. Bacterial pneumonias with both gram-negative and -positive organisms and viral pneumonias occur more frequently in HIV-1-infected children. Mixed infections with multiple bacterial isolates or bacterial and viral isolates are sometimes found. In many cases no organisms are isolated. This is partially a result of the difficulty in obtaining diagnostic specimens in children. The incidence of PCP has declined with highly active antiretroviral therapy (HAART), but the effect of antiretroviral therapy on the rates of bacterial and viral pneumonia is not known. The rates of PCP and TB remain high in regions with a poor medical infrastructure and limited availability of drugs.

With the successful prevention of mother-to-infant transmission with antiretroviral regimens, there is a growing population of uninfected infants born to HIV-1-infected mothers. Prospective studies indicate that the uninfected children born to HIV-1-infected mothers are not more susceptible to pulmonary disease than those born to uninfected mothers.[44] In areas where there is a high rate of pneumonia, the rates and types of pneumonia are similar in uninfected children born to infected and uninfected mothers.[45]

TABLE 39-1. Mean rate of decline of CD4 lymphocyte count in first year of life prior to developing lower respiratory tract infection (LRI) or *Pneumocystis* pneumonia (PCP)

	Cells/mm³/month
HIV-uninfected	55 ± 9
HIV-infected, no LRI	134 ± 20
HIV-infected, with LRI	266 ± 61
HIV-infected, with PCP	375 ± 112

HIV, human immunodeficiency virus.

From Kattan M, Platzker A, Mellins RB, Schluchter MD, Chen XC, Peavy H, et al: Respiratory diseases in the first year of life in children born to HIV-1-infected women. Pediatr Pulmonol 2001;31(4):267–276.

■ BACTERIAL PNEUMONIA

Bacterial pneumonia occurs more frequently in HIV-1-infected children because of defects of both cellular and humoral immunity. Recurrent pneumonia is one of the clinical conditions included in the Centers for Disease Control AIDS surveillance case definition. The symptoms are nonspecific and include fever, respiratory distress, and cough and accompanied by hypoxemia. Bacterial pneumonia can be focal or diffuse. The bacterial isolates reported in Western countries and Africa are remarkably similar.[47,48] *Streptococcus pneumoniae* and *Staphylococcus aureus* are the most commonly documented gram-positive organisms. Using postmortem percutaneous lung aspirates from children in Zimbabwe, Ikeogu found *Klebsiella* and *Pseudomonas* species to be the most common gram-negative organisms.[48] In hospitalized HIV-1-infected children in Thailand, bacterial coinfection was observed in 33% of children with PCP.[49] *Bordetella pertussis* has been recovered in children with respiratory distress and cough.[50]

Isolation of bacterial organism in cases of pneumonia is problematic in young children because invasive procedures are often required. Children do not often have a productive cough, and induced sputum for bacterial pneumonia is not reliable. A positive blood culture with a new radiographic infiltrate may establish the cause of pneumonia. An organism other than common oral flora accompanied by neutrophils obtained from bronchial lavage fluid strongly suggests a bacterial cause of pneumonia.

Intravenous immune globulin (IVIG) may be effective in reducing some bacterial infections in patients with symptomatic HIV-1 infection and peripheral $CD4^+$ cell counts of 200/mm³ or greater. Data from the National Institute of Child Health and Human Development IVIG Clinical Trial conducted in an era with no antiretroviral therapy and limited PCP prophylaxis indicated that IVIG was associated with a 48% reduction in the rate of acute laboratory-proven bacterial or clinically diagnosed pneumonia episodes per 100 patient-years in those with $CD4^+$ cell counts of 200/mm³ or higher.[51] The AIDS Clinical Trials Group reported that the beneficial effect of IVIG was limited to those children not receiving trimethoprim-sulfamethoxazole (TMP-SMZ) prophylaxis.[52] IVIG is currently recommended in HIV-1-infected children in combination with antiretroviral agents only for hypogammaglobinemia (IgG < 400 mg/dL), children with two or more serious bacterial infections in a 1-year period, those who fail to form antibodies to common antigens, or those with chronic parvovirus B19 infections.[53]

Pneumococcal vaccination is indicated for children 2 months and older with asymptomatic or symptomatic HIV-1 infection in view of the high incidence of invasive pneumococcal infection.[53] Reimmunization after 3 to 5 years is recommended. Adolescents with a $CD4^+$ count of greater than 200/μL should receive the 23-valent polysaccharide vaccine. HIV-1-infected children should be immunized with *Haemophilus influenzae* type b vaccine according to the routine childhood immunization schedule.

TUBERCULOSIS

TB remains a major public health problem throughout the world. An increase in the incidence of TB has paralleled the AIDS epidemic, and the two diseases are strongly related.[54] In one report from Zambia, the HIV-1 seroprevalence rate in children with TB disease was 55.8% compared with 9.6% in a control population at the same hospital.[55] Birth cohorts of perinatally HIV-1-infected infants and children followed prospectively in the United States have found only a small number of cases of TB, but there are reports of TB and HIV-1 infection in the United States.[56,57] Because of the association of TB and HIV-1 infection, children with TB disease should be tested for HIV-1 disease.

It is not clear if HIV-1 infection increases susceptibility to TB. Children with HIV-1 infection are more likely to be in contact with HIV-1-infected adults with TB and therefore are increasingly susceptible to tuberculous infection and disease. Control of TB in children with HIV-1 infection rests predominantly with adequate public health measures to control TB in the community by contact and source tracing and ensuring adherence to medication regimens.

Pulmonary TB is the predominant clinical presentation, although extrapulmonary disease can occur.[57] Fever, cough, lobar pneumonia, and lymphadenopathy may indicate *Mycobacterium tuberculosis* disease.

Annual screening of HIV-1-infected children for TB infection or disease is recommended with the Mantoux tuberculin skin test. A reaction greater than 5 mm is considered positive.[58] Many children with HIV-1 infection have negative skin test results to control antigens; therefore, a negative tuberculin skin test result may not rule out infection. If there is a high index of suspicion for pulmonary TB (e.g., contact with TB) in an HIV-1-infected child with a pulmonary infiltrate who is anergic, attempts to isolate the organism may be warranted to rule out *M. tuberculosis* infection.

Bacteriologic confirmation of pulmonary TB in infants and children remains difficult. Examination of expectorated sputum is the initial test performed to diagnose TB in the older child with a productive cough. In the younger child, gastric lavage is a common procedure to obtain specimens for staining and culture. The organism can be isolated from bronchial lavage fluid or from lung tissue obtained from biopsy. Some studies suggest that the yield for *M. tuberculosis* is higher with gastric lavage compared with bronchoalveolar lavage.[59,60] In a report from South Africa, sputum induction for isolation of the organism was successful in infants and children with HIV-1 infection.[61] In that study, induced sputum had a better yield for pulmonary TB than gastric lavage.

The recommended treatment regimen of pulmonary infections in children with a sensitive strain is isoniazid, rifampin, and pyrazinamide for 2 months followed by isoniazid and rifampin for a total of 12 months of therapy.[53] In areas where there is a high prevalence of multiple drug-resistant strains, infection should be treated with four drugs if the susceptibility pattern is unknown—isoniazid, rifampin, pyrazinamide, and ethambutol for 2 months followed by isoniazid and rifampin if the patient has responded well to the initial treatment. Streptomycin, cycloserine, or ethionamide may be substituted for ethambutol. If the isolate is known to be isoniazid and rifampin resistant, two or three drugs to which the organism is sensitive should be given for 18 to 24 months after culture conversion. Second-line drugs such as clarithromycin, azithromycin, and ciprofloxacin may be required. Daily or twice weekly regimens are acceptable. Directly observed therapy should be used where possible to ensure administration of the medication. Contact tracing is an essential part of the management.

Mortality with this disease is high either from the tuberculous infection itself or by acceleration of the natural history of HIV-1 disease. In a comparison of children with TB with and without HIV-1 infection, those with coinfection had a poorer clinical and radiologic response to treatment at 6 months. Mortality was higher in the HIV-1-infected group.[62]

There are limited data on the efficacy of prophylaxis in the context of HIV-1 infection. A study in HIV-1-infected adults has demonstrated the efficacy of a 1-year course of isoniazid prophylaxis in decreasing the frequency of active TB in symptom-free HIV-1-seropositive adults with a positive tuberculin skin test.[63]

Preventive therapy for HIV-1-infected children with a positive tuberculin skin test result but no evidence of active disease is 9 months of isoniazid. In patients where the source case is likely to have an isoniazid-resistant strain, rifampin should be added. If the child is anergic but has a history of exposure, isoniazid is recommended. If the contact is known to have a multidrug-resistant strain, the child should be treated with two drugs to which the strain is susceptible.[64]

The role of bacillus Calmette-Guérin (BCG) in preventing infection in HIV-1-seropositive children is unknown. In areas of low TB prevalence, the BCG vaccine is not recommended. However, in areas where the prevalence is high, the World Health Organization recommends that BCG be given at birth.

MYCOBACTERIUM AVIUM COMPLEX

Mycobacterium avium complex (MAC) is ubiquitous in the environment and is found in water, soil, and dairy products. Before the HIV-1 epidemic, MAC infrequently caused disease. MAC most commonly resulted in pulmonary infections in immunologically normal persons with chronic lung disease or cervical adenitis in children. In contrast, MAC is a frequent opportunistic infection in patients with HIV-1 infection and can occur in conjunction with other opportunistic infections. The organism can be found in the blood, lung, liver, and bone marrow. Localized disease caused by MAC includes cervical adenitis, pneumonitis, hepatic dysfunction, and abscesses. In HIV-1-infected patients, respiratory symptoms are not a prominent feature, and the clinical manifestations are usually due to extrapulmonary disease. The significance of the organism in the bronchial secretions is unclear, but most likely reflects disseminated disease rather than pulmonary infection. Symptoms are often nonspecific, with intermittent fever, weight loss, night sweats, cachexia, and diarrhea. Respiratory symptoms are not usually the prominent feature, but tachypnea and chronic infiltrates may be present. None of 22 children with MAC in one series of children with AIDS had respiratory symptoms.[65] Children with MAC were older and had lower CD4+ cell counts than non-MAC children. Patients with disseminated MAC have a poor prognosis.[66] In one report of children who died, 42% had disseminated MAC and in 24% it was the underlying cause of death.[67]

Recommendations for prophylaxis and therapy for disseminated MAC disease in patients with HIV-1 have been published.[64] With any regimen, a minimum of two agents is recommended to minimize the risk for proliferation of resistant strains. Every treatment regimen should include either azithromycin or clarithromycin. Ethambutol is recommended as a second drug. The addition of a third or fourth drug from one of the following is suggested: clofazimine, rifabutin, rifampin, ciprofloxacin, and amikacin. Prophylaxis with clarithromycin or azithromycin to prevent a first episode is recommended for children 6 years of age and older with a CD4+ count of less than 50/μL, 2 to 6 years of age with a CD4+ count of less than 75/μL, 1 to 2 years of age with a CD4+ count of less than 500/μL, and younger than 1 year with a CD4+ count of less than 750/μL.

■ VIRAL INFECTION

Pneumonia associated with common viral pathogens, such as respiratory syncytial virus (RSV), parainfluenza, herpes simplex, and adenovirus occurs in HIV-1-infected children.[42,68] Prolonged duration of RSV antigen shedding for up to 90 days has been observed in HIV-1-infected children.[69] Concomitant bacterial or opportunistic infection must be ruled out in those patients with persistent symptoms or clinical deterioration with RSV. Measles virus and varicella-zoster virus can cause severe pulmonary disease in this group of patients.[70] In a report from Côte d'Ivoire, Africa, measles giant cell pneumonia was more common in children older than 15 months who were HIV-1 positive than in children who were HIV-1 negative.[43] Acyclovir or valacyclovir are the agents of choice for varicella infection. Measles virus is susceptible in vitro to ribavirin, but there are no controlled clinical studies.

Cytomegalovirus (CMV) is a herpesvirus that can cause retinitis, encephalitis, colitis, and pneumonitis in HIV-1-infected patients. HIV-1-infected and -uninfected infants born to HIV-1-infected mothers have similar rates of in utero infection (4.5%), but HIV-1-infected infants have higher rates of CMV acquired during the first 4 years of life. More than 50% of HIV-1-infected infants have CMV infection by 12 months compared with 40% of uninfected infants born to HIV-1-positive mothers.[71] CMV infection is more likely to occur in children with low CD4+ counts. In cell culture, coinfection with CMV stimulates HIV-1 replication.[72] The occurrence of coinfection of HIV-1-infected children with CMV early in life is associated with more rapid disease progression to class C disease.

CMV pneumonia was found in 7% of HIV-1-seropositive infants from Zimbabwe on autopsy.[48] The virus has been isolated in bronchial lavage fluid in 35% to 78% of HIV-1-infected adults with respiratory illness and has also been found in bronchial lavage fluid in children, but its isolation does not necessarily indicate pneumonitis.[73–75] Proposed criteria for a tentative clinical diagnosis of CMV pneumonitis include (1) CMV recovered in culture, (2) CMV inclusions in BAL cells or from biopsy specimens, (3) no other pathogens, and (4) progressive pneumonitis.[54] CMV is often found with other pathogens in the lung. The presence or absence of CMV with PCP made no difference in the short-term outcome or long-term survival in adults and children.[76,77]

Histologically, alveolar macrophages, type II pneumocytes, bronchial and bronchiolar epithelial cells, and capillary endothelial cells may manifest cytomegaly and nuclear and cytoplasmic inclusions. The degree of interstitial pneumonitis varies because of the presence of concomitant infections. Ganciclovir appears to be the most effective drug in the treatment of CMV infection.

Prevention of viral infection when feasible may be useful. Yearly influenza vaccine should be considered for children 6 months or older. HIV-1-infected children mount antibody responses to influenza vaccinations, but the titers are lower than in HIV-1-negative controls.[78] Routine immunization with measles vaccine is recommended. Varicella vaccine should be considered for those having no or mild signs or symptoms of disease.

■ FUNGAL INFECTION

Opportunistic fungal infections can cause severe pulmonary disease in children with HIV-1 infection, but the number of reported cases is small. The most common infections are with *Candida* species, *Aspergillus* species, *Cryptococcus neoformans, Histoplasma capsulatum, Coccidioides immitis,* and *Penicillium marneffei.* Dissemination of infection is common and treatment is difficult. Constitutional symptoms such as weight loss and fever may reflect extrapulmonary involvement.

Cryptococcus usually presents as meningitis but can involve the lungs, causing an interstitial pneumonia.[79] *Histoplasma capsulatum* most commonly affects the lungs but is likely to become disseminated in HIV-1-infected patients.[80,81] Standard serologic test results can be positive for both coccidiomycosis and histoplasmosis, but false-negative tests occur in the most profoundly immunocompromised patients.[82] Skin testing is not useful because of problems with anergy and lack of standardization of most fungal skin test preparations. Cultures of bone marrow, cerebrospinal fluid, and lymph node or lung biopsy can make the diagnosis. *Candida* species are often found in the oropharynx and esophagus in HIV-1-infected children. Tracheobronchial candidiasis and pulmonary infection are less common. Isolation of *Candida* from BAL fluid most likely represents an oropharyngeal contaminant because pulmonary infection is rarely confirmed on lung biopsy. Tissue invasion should be demonstrated on bronchial or lung biopsy to confirm the diagnosis.

Aspergillus infection has been reported in patients with HIV-1 infection. It occurs late in the course of HIV-1 infection and usually follows corticosteroid use or neutropenia.[83] Aspergilloma and invasive cavitary aspergillosis have been described.[84,85] *Aspergillus* infection can cause necrosis of the tracheobronchial tree, with formation of a fungal pseudomembrane resulting in severe airway obstruction.[86] Transmural and peribronchial extension of the infection occurs (Fig. 39-2). The most prominent symptoms are cough and fever. In the obstructive form, dyspnea is noted.

Amphotericin B is the drug of choice for most life-threatening fungal infections. Alternative regimens include fluconazole and itraconazole. However, even with treatment, relapse and mortality rates are high. Some form of chronic suppressive therapy is often given following infection.

■ *PNEUMOCYSTIS JIROVECI* PNEUMONIA

Untreated children with HIV-1 infection have a high propensity to develop *Pneumocystis* pneumonia. *Pneumocystis jiroveci*

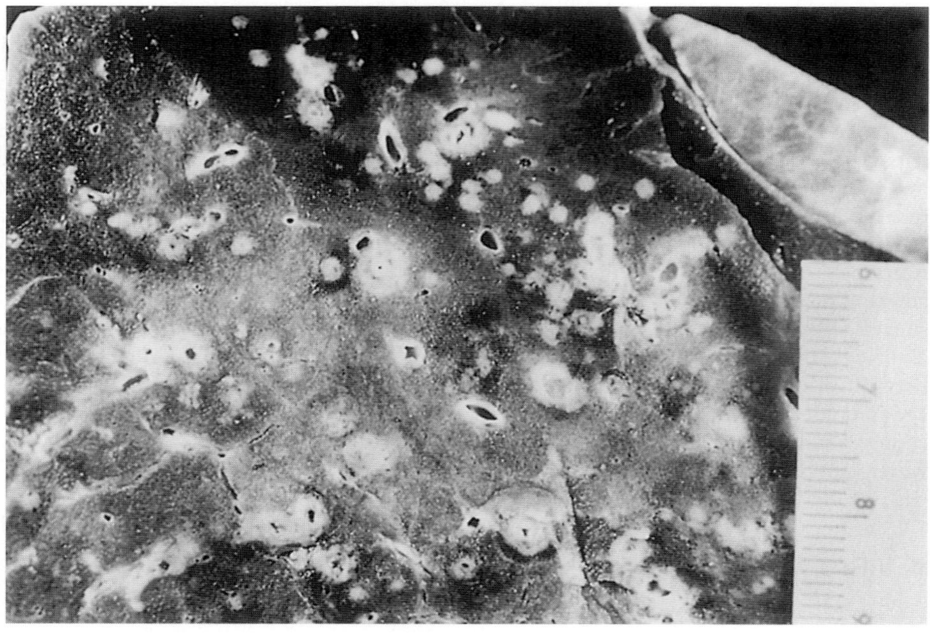

■ **FIGURE 39-2.** Cut section of lung from a 15-year-old with hemophilia and human immunodeficiency virus infection who developed airway obstruction from *Aspergillus* infection. Diffuse peribronchial and peribronchiolar cuffing is noted. (From Pervez NK, Kleinerman J, Kattan M, Freed JA, Harris MB, Rosen MJ, et al: Pseudomembranous necrotizing bronchial aspergillosis. A variant of invasive aspergillosis in a patient with hemophilia and acquired immune deficiency syndrome. Am Rev Respir Dis 1985; 131:962.)

(previously *Pneumocystis carinii*) was originally classified as a protozoan. Analysis of ribosomal RNA sequences suggest a homology between fungi and *P. jiroveci.*[87,88] The organism is now classified as a fungus. Two morphologic forms of the organism are found in infected lungs: thin-walled single-nucleated trophozoites adherent to type I pneumocytes and thick-walled cysts containing four to eight single-nucleated sporozoites. The organism attaches to the alveolar epithelium, resulting in desquamation of alveolar cells. As the infection progresses, a diffuse desquamative alveolitis ensues, and alveoli become filled with a foamy exudate consisting of alveolar macrophages and cysts containing sporozoites. Interstitial inflammation becomes evident.

The incidence of PCP among perinatally infected children during the first year of life has been estimated at 12% to 25%.[35,89,90] PCP can be the initial presentation of HIV-1 infection. The median age of presentation is 5 months.[91] Children with PCP most commonly have acute onset of cough, fever, tachypnea, and retractions. Decreased breath sounds or crackles may be present on auscultation. The children are commonly markedly hypoxemic. An important risk factor for the development of PCP in adults is a $CD4^+$ cell count of less than 1000 cells/mm^3. However, 18% to 26% of children younger than 12 months have $CD4^+$ counts greater than 1500 cells/mm^3 at the time of PCP diagnosis.[92,93] A rapid rate of decline in $CD4^+$ is associated with the development of PCP in children.[44]

There is a high rate of respiratory failure and need for mechanical ventilation among children with PCP. Early reported experience indicated a mortality rate exceeding 40% with the initial episode and the majority surviving less than a year subsequent to the episode.[94,95] In reports from Africa, where malnutrition is a complicating factor for the expression of pulmonary disease, the prevalence is high and the mortality rate is approximately 50%.[96] The survival rate in HIV-1-infected children following PCP is lower than with other disease manifestations.[91] A possible explanation for decreased survival after PCP is that the presence of *P. jiroveci* can increase HIV-1 replication. It has been demonstrated that HIV-1 production by alveolar lymphocytes obtained from BAL fluid is increased during PCP.[97] Alternatively, acquiring PCP may simply be a marker for a lower $CD4^+$ cell count and progression of disease.

The usual laboratory findings with PCP include a normal white blood cell count, an elevated lactic dehydrogenase (LDH), and normal IgG. LDH levels of greater than 1000 IU/L are frequently associated with PCP but not exclusively.[42] The chest radiograph typically shows a diffuse reticulonodular infiltrate most prominent in the perihilar region and extending peripherally (Fig. 39-3). Air bronchograms, focal infiltrates, and pneumotoceles can also be present on the radiograph. Radionuclide scans with intravenous gallium 67 or aerosolized technetium 99m diethylenetriamene pentacetate (^{99m}Tc-DTPA) have added little to the chest radiograph and arterial blood gas in predicting PCP in children.

Empirical treatment for PCP in children with typical clinical presentation may no longer be justifiable in areas where PCP has become less common in relation to other infections with use of prophylactic therapy. The diagnosis of PCP relies on the identification of the organism from bronchial washings or lung tissue. Bronchoalveolar lavage with fiberoptic bronchoscopy is a reliable method for establishing the diagnosis.[68] In intubated patients, instillation of 2 to 3 aliquots of 5 to 10 mL of saline into the endotracheal tube followed by suctioning also provides a high yield in isolating PCP. False-negative results rarely occur with lavage using the bronchoscope or via the endotracheal tube. Sputum induction has been used to diagnose PCP in children older than 2 years. The patient inhales a mist of 3% saline generated by an ultrasonic nebulizer for 10 to 30 minutes.[98] The diagnostic yield using this technique is variable and is dependent on the experience of those collecting and interpreting the specimen. Nasopharyngeal aspirates have been used to identify *P. jiroveci,* but the yield is lower than with induced sputum.[96,99,100]

Methenamine silver, toluidine blue O, and fluorescein-conjugated monoclonal antibody are stains that identify the

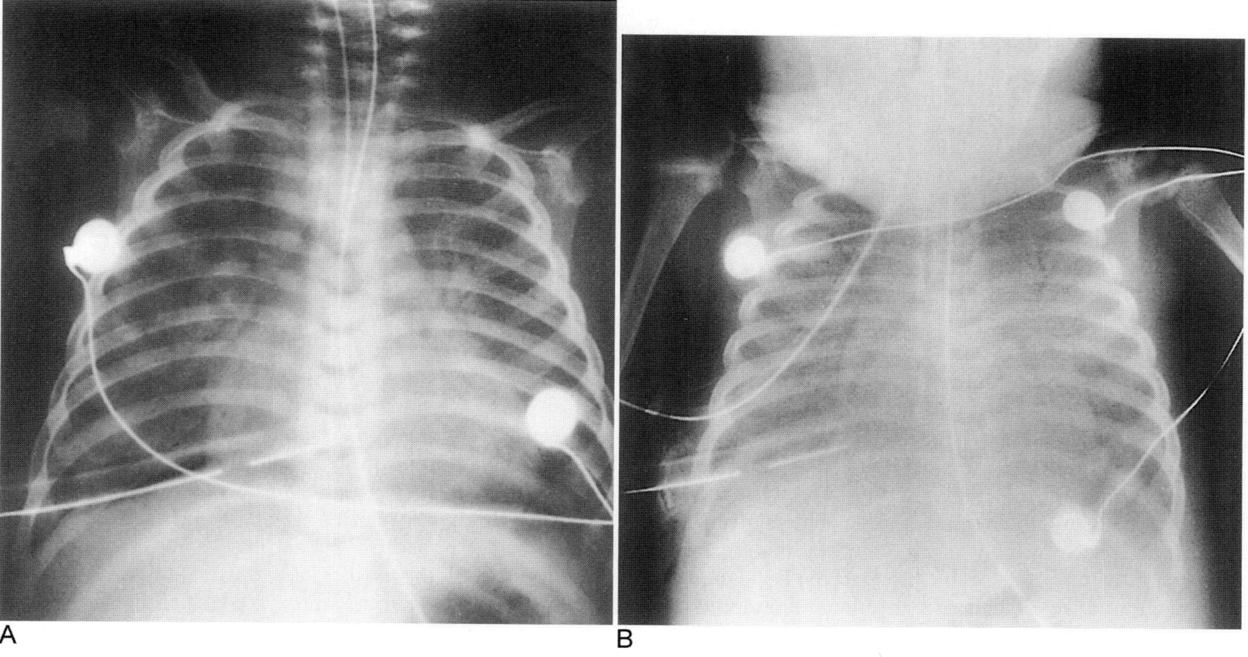

FIGURE 39-3. Chest radiograph of a 3-month-old infant presenting with *Pneumocystis carinii* pneumonia. **A,** The initial radiograph shows a bilateral infiltrate most prominent in the perihilar region. **B,** Chest radiograph taken 1 week later shows progression of disease with opacification of both lung fields.

thick-walled cysts of *P. jiroveci*. Trophozoite forms are identified with Giemsa stain, modified Wright-Giemsa stain, or fluorescein-conjugated monoclonal antibody. Use of PCR technology may be more sensitive in detecting low burdens of the organism.[101,102]

High-dose intravenous TMP-SMZ is the treatment of choice for PCP. The conventional dose is trimethoprim, 15 to 20 mg/kg/day, and sulfamethoxazole, 75 to 100 mg/kg/day for 21 days. A clinical response is usually observed by 5 to 7 days, although there can be a deterioration in the patient's condition in the first few days of therapy. Side effects of TMP-SMZ include rashes and thrombocytopenia. An alternative treatment for PCP is pentamidine administered intravenously or intramuscularly (4 mg/kg/dose once daily) if the TMP-SMZ is not well tolerated or there does not appear to be a response after 1 week of treatment with TMP-SMZ. The intramuscular route is painful and can cause sterile abscesses and should be avoided if possible. Side effects from pentamidine include pancreatitis, renal dysfunction, and both hyperglycemia and hypoglycemia.

A National Institutes of Health consensus panel has recommended that corticosteroids be used as an adjunct to therapy in adults with severe PCP based on studies showing improved survival and decreased incidence of respiratory failure.[103] Moderate to severe infection has been defined for this purpose as a partial pressure of oxygen in arterial blood (PaO_2) of less than 70 mm Hg or an alveolar-arterial oxygen gradient of more than 35 mm Hg. Controlled clinical trials using corticosteroids in children with PCP have not been conducted, but uncontrolled data suggest that corticosteroids are beneficial.[104] Extrapolation from adult studies to children is limited by the fact that the immune system is still developing. In addition, PCP is likely a primary infection in infants, whereas in adults some cases of PCP may represent reactivation.

Early treatment with HAART and PCP prophylaxis have had a dramatic effect on reducing the incidence of the disease.[44] Because of the high mortality and morbidity associated with PCP, prevention should be the primary objective. Prophylaxis is so effective that failure to adhere to the prophylactic regimen is considered to be the most likely cause of PCP in an HIV-1-infected child. In recent prospective studies of HIV-1-infected children who have access to antiretroviral therapy and prophylaxis, the incidence of PCP is less than 10%. Guidelines for prophylaxis against PCP for children infected with or prenatally exposed to HIV-1 are shown in Table 39-2.[64] Prophylaxis for PCP is recommended in all infants born to HIV-1-infected mothers beginning at 4 to 6 weeks of age. Once HIV-1 infection in the infant has been excluded, the prophylaxis can be stopped. For HIV-1-infected children, prophylaxis should be continued throughout the first year of life. Cessation of primary prophylaxis for PCP can be considered in adolescents if the $CD4^+$ lymphocyte count is greater than 200 cells/μL.[105] Children with a history of PCP should receive prophylaxis for life.

TABLE 39-2. CDC guidelines for PCP prophylaxis for HIV-exposed and HIV-infected children

Age	PCP Prophylaxis
Birth to 4–6 wk, HIV exposed	No
4–6 wk to 4 mo, HIV exposed	Yes
4–12 mo	
HIV infected or indeterminate	Yes
HIV exposed, not infected	No
1–5 yr, HIV infected	CD4 count <500 cells/μL or CD4% <15%
≥5 yr, HIV infected	CD4 count <200 cell/μL or CD4% <15%

CDC, Centers for Disease Control and Prevention; HIV, human immunodeficiency virus; PCP, *Pneumocystis* pneumonia.

TMP-SMZ substantially reduces the risk for PCP among HIV-1-infected children. The recommended regimen is TMP-SMZ 150/750 mg/m^2/day administered orally in two divided doses three times weekly on consecutive days. If TMP-SMZ is not tolerated, alternative prophylactic regimens include dapsone 2 mg/kg (not to exceed 100 mg) administered orally once daily or, in children 5 years of age and above, aerosolized pentamidine 300 mg administered via nebulizer monthly. If neither dapsone nor aerosolized pentamidine is tolerated, some clinicians use intravenous pentamidine (4 mg/kg) administered every 2 or 4 weeks.

CHRONIC LUNG DISEASE

The introduction of highly active combination antiretroviral therapy has resulted has resulted in a reduction of the viral load and a better prognosis. In children receiving antiretroviral treatment, the spectrum of lung disease has changed. There are fewer opportunistic pulmonary infections, and pulmonary manifestations of HIV-1 are more likely to be chronic. The identification of chronic lung disease usually relies on interpretation of the chest radiograph. In a prospective birth cohort of HIV-1-infected children, the cumulative incidence of chronic radiographic lung changes was 33% by 4 years of age.[106] Parenchymal consolidation persisting for 3 or more months was present in 8% of HIV-1-infected children, nodular changes persisting 3 or more months in 8%, and reticular changes or increased bronchovascular markings persisting for 6 or more months in 14%. These radiographic changes were associated with an increased frequency of clubbing, crackles, tachypnea, and decreased oxygen saturation. Resolution of these chronic changes occurred in 50% to 60% of the cases over the period of the study. This resolution was associated with a declining CD4$^+$ cell count but not with lower rates of clinical abnormalities or viral load, and thus may be an indication of progression of the HIV-1 infection. Mortality rates in HIV-1-infected children with chronic radiographic changes were not different from mortality rates in HIV-1-infected children without these changes.

The etiology of chronic lung disease in HIV-1-infected children is varied. LIP/PLH, nonspecific interstitial pneumonitis, bronchiectasis, and diffuse alveolar damage are reported causes. Pulmonary infections can also be a cause of chronic lung disease. In reports from Africa, TB is one of the most common causes of chronic lung disease.[107] Chronic PCP infection can result in chronic interstitial disease and cysts.[108,109]

LYMPHOCYTIC INTERSTITIAL PNEUMONIA/PULMONARY LYMPHOID HYPERPLASIA

The most commonly reported chronic lung disease is LIP/PLH complex. The presence of this condition in an HIV-1-infected child places a child in the moderately symptomatic category (category B) of the CDC classification. A report from a prospective birth cohort indicates that chronic nodular densities are observed in 8% of patients by 4 years of age.[106] In HIV-1-infected children 5 years of age or younger who died at home in Zimbabwe, 9% had LIP on autopsy.[48]

The pathology consists of a diffuse infiltration of lymphocytes in the interstitium and scattered nodules of mononuclear cells 0.5 mm in diameter. The mononuclear cells consist of lymphocytes, plasma cells, immunoblasts, and histiocytes. In LIP the infiltration is diffuse throughout the parenchyma. In PLH the infiltration is primarily adjacent to the bronchial and bronchiolar walls and consists of bronchial associated lymphoid tissue hyperplasia (Fig. 39-4). The etiology of the abnormal lymphoproliferative response is unclear. The principal hypotheses are that lymphoproliferation is a response to the HIV-1 alone or superinfection with another virus. Epstein-Barr viral DNA has been found in lung biopsies of children with LIP, and HIV-1 RNA has been identified in the lungs of infants with LIP.[110–112] However, a causal relationship between Epstein-Barr virus and LIP/PLH has not been confirmed.

The onset of LIP/PLH is insidious and the course slowly progressive. It usually becomes evident after the first year of life,

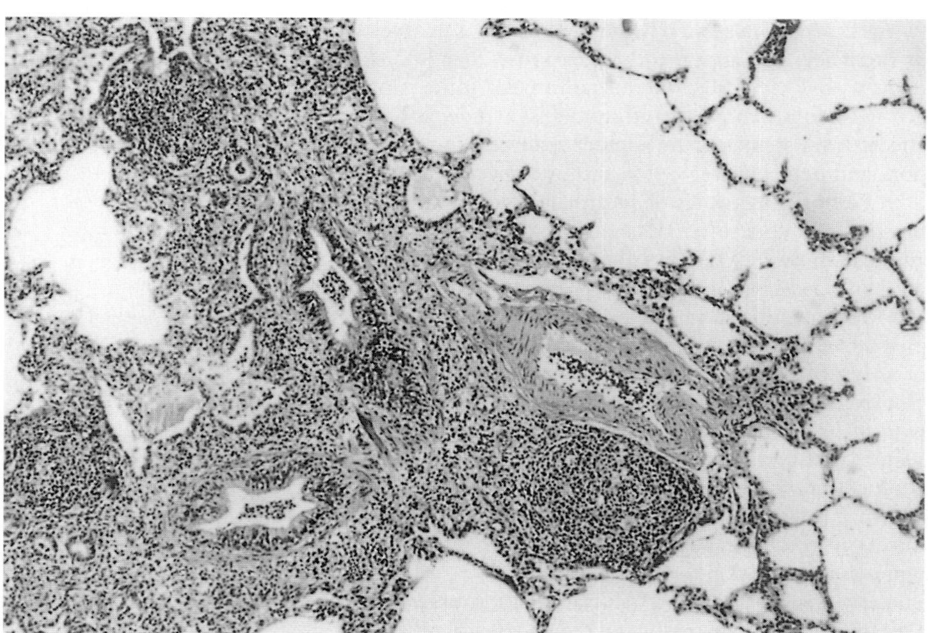

FIGURE 39-4. Lung biopsy from a child with pulmonary lymphoid hyperplasia. There is interstitial and peribronchiolar lymphoid infiltration.

with a median age of onset of 2.5 to 3.0 years.[91] However, reticulonodular changes on chest radiographs may be observed before 12 months of age.[106] Cough or tachypnea may be present. Auscultation of the chest may be normal or reveal crackles and wheezes. Generalized lymphadenopathy, hepatosplenomegaly, clubbing, and parotid gland enlargement are commonly associated physical findings. Admission rates for lower respiratory tract illness are higher for children with LIP/PLH compared with HIV-1-infected children without LIP/PLH.[113]

The chest radiograph typically shows a bilateral diffuse interstitial reticulonodular pattern with or without hilar adenopathy. Elevated serum immunoglobulin levels are associated with LIP/PLH.[42] Serum IgG levels of greater than 2500 mg/dL are strongly associated with LIP/PLH. Lung biopsy establishes the diagnosis. However, a presumptive diagnosis of LIP/PLH can be made based on the clinical findings and the typical reticulonodular radiographic pattern lasting more than 2 months without another documented cause. In a longitudinal study, resolution of the chronic nodular radiographic findings occurred in 61% of children.[106]

Treatment of LIP/PLH is nonspecific. Oxygen is administered for hypoxemia as required. Although treatment of LIP/PLH with corticosteroids has been reported to improve hypoxemia in a small number of patients, controlled clinical trials have not been carried out.[114]

Some cases of LIP/PLH progress to a lymphoproliferative disorder characterized by polyclonal, polymorphic B-cell content without evidence of cellular atypia, necrosis, or prominent mitotic activity but with extranodal systemic and prominent pulmonary involvement[115] (Fig. 39-5). Some cases have progressed to malignant lymphoma.

BRONCHIECTASIS

With increasing survival of HIV-1-infected children with lung disease, additional complications are becoming apparent. An important cause of chronic infiltrates and atelectasis on chest radiographs is bronchiectasis. This should be suspected when radiographs show persistent abnormalities in the same lobe for more than 6 months. The diagnosis can be confirmed with a computed tomography scan demonstrating dilated tubular structures (see Fig. 39-5). Bronchiectasis with HIV-1 infection has been associated with LIP.[116] It is possible that the lymphocytic infiltration into the mucosa and submucosa of the bronchiole leads to destruction, fibrosis, atelectasis, and, subsequently, bronchiectasis. Other mechanisms of development of bronchiectasis include acute or chronic infection, a direct effect of HIV-1 on the lung and persistent atelectasis. Some children who are symptomatic despite the standard medical regimen of cyclic antibiotics and aggressive pulmonary therapy might benefit from adjunctive IVIG therapy at 600 mg/kg per dose, given monthly.

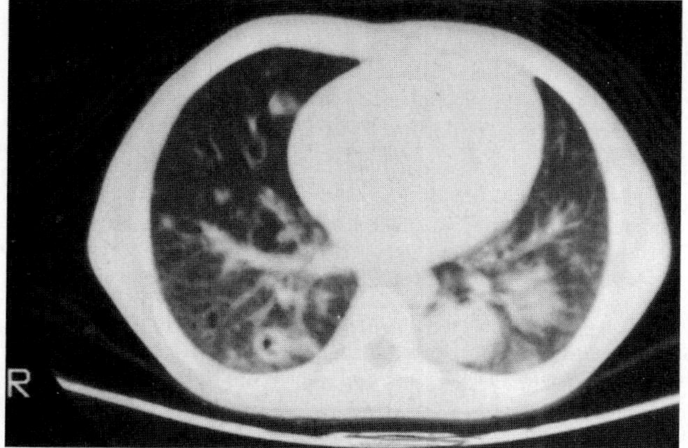

FIGURE 39-5. Computed tomography scan of a child with a polyclonal lymphoproliferative disorder. Nodular infiltrates are present bilaterally with large nodules evident in the left lower lobe.

DIFFUSE ALVEOLAR DAMAGE

Diffuse alveolar damage (DAD) describes a sequence of events following severe acute lung injury caused by any one of a variety of insults. Possible etiologies in HIV-1-infected patients include viral or opportunistic infections such as PCP, adult respiratory distress syndrome, and oxygen toxicity. This is characterized clinically by respiratory distress and diffuse pulmonary infiltrates. This entity should be suspected if there is persistent hypoxemia following acute respiratory failure from PCP or other opportunistic infections. Recurrent episodes of respiratory failure may represent viral infections superimposed on a lung with DAD.

The early exudative stage of DAD occurring over 2 or 3 days is characterized by alveolar and interstitial edema and hyaline membrane formation. This progresses to a proliferative stage after 1 week in which there is hyperplasia of type II pneumocytes and desquamation of alveolar lining cells and thickening of the interstitium with fibroblast proliferation.

PULMONARY TUMORS

Kaposi sarcoma has been associated with HIV-1 infection. It occurs predominantly in homosexual men and is uncommon in children. Although cases have been reported in infants, most cases of Kaposi sarcoma in the pediatric age group have occurred in adolescents.[117] The clinical presentation varies from indolent skin disease to disseminated visceral involvement. The most common manifestation is violaceous plaques of the skin. Pulmonary involvement causes dyspnea, cough, and fever. Examination of the lungs reveals multiple hemorrhagic nodules and/or violaceous endobronchial lesions. The chest radiograph can show an interstitial pattern that is usually homogeneous or nodular infiltrates. Pleural effusions are common. The diagnosis is made by biopsy.

Pulmonary tumors of smooth muscle origin in children have been reported. The airways, lungs, and pulmonary veins have been found to have nodular masses that on biopsy have been leiomyoma and leiomyosarcoma.[118] Pseudolymphomas and lymphomas have also been reported.

UPPER AIRWAY DISEASE

Lymphoid proliferation occurs with HIV-1 infection, and it is therefore not surprising that tonsillar and adenoidal hypertrophy and pharyngeal infiltration is observed. This has resulted in upper airway obstruction in children with HIV-1 infection. It has not been determined if upper airway obstruction occurs with greater frequency in HIV-1-infected children compared with those not infected.

Candida supraglottitis has been described with a slowly progressive course and lesions on the epiglottis, arytenoid cartilages, and aryepiglottic folds.[119] Noninfectious infiltration of the epiglottis has also been described with gradual onset of droolingand dysphagia. Biopsy shows acute and chronic inflammation, with granulation tissue and lymphoid follicles in the submucosa.[120]

PULMONARY DISEASE AND MORTALITY

Pulmonary disease is an important cause of HIV-1-related deaths. Development of PCP is associated with shorter survival and LIP with longer survival.[91,121] Infection is the most prevalent underlying cause (the single cause that initiated the events resulting in death) of death for children younger than 6 years. Two-thirds of these infections are pulmonary infections. Children with HIV who survive longer are less likely to die of pulmonary disease or infection and more likely to die of cardiac causes or with wasting syndrome. In the prospective Pediatric Pulmonary and Cardiovascular Complications of Vertically Transmitted HIV-1 Study, chronic lung disease (diagnosed by case by case mortality review) was present in 58% of children who died but was rarely an underlying cause of death.[67]

APPROACH TO THE HIV-1-INFECTED PATIENT WITH PULMONARY DISEASE

The child with HIV-1 infection is often seen with fever and tachypnea. The differential diagnosis is large, and a systematic approach based on current knowledge of HIV-1 infection is helpful. The majority of severe complications are infectious, and the likelihood increases with decreasing $CD4^+$ cell counts. Ventricular dysfunction and cardiomyopathy have been observed in pediatric HIV-1 infection.[122,123] The ventricular dysfunction is slowly progressive and is associated with immune dysfunction.[124] Therefore, it is important to rule out cardiac disease with congestive heart failure as a cause of the respiratory symptoms. If the patient has acute respiratory symptoms, a chest radiograph, arterial blood gas or oxygen saturation, complete blood count, and blood culture should be obtained. The majority of patients with a normal or unchanged chest radiograph and normoxia will have a self-limited viral illness. A nasopharyngeal specimen for identification of respiratory viruses including RSV may be indicated. Serum immunoglobulins and LDH may be helpful in distinguishing PCP from LIP/PLH. A positive blood culture and a lobar infiltrate support the diagnosis of a bacterial pneumonia. Persistent lobar infiltrates of more than 6 months' duration may be indicative of bronchiectasis. In such cases, a computed tomography scan of the chest is helpful in establishing the diagnosis. A diffuse nodular infiltrate with hilar adenopathy in the absence of hypoxemia suggests LIP/PLH. If hypoxemia is present with a diffuse interstitial infiltrate, PCP is the most likely possibility. If the patient is hypoxemic, a bronchial lavage should be performed. The predominance of neutrophils in the presence of a culture that is not the usual oral flora in the BAL is strong evidence for a bacterial pneumonia. If the BAL is negative, an open lung biopsy may be indicated to establish the diagnosis. Increased clearance of inhaled ^{99m}Tc-DTPA has been noted in the absence of radiographic abnormalities in HIV-1-infected children, but the role of this technique for detection of early lung disease remains to be determined.

SUMMARY

Respiratory diseases play a major role in morbidity and mortality in HIV-1-infected children, particularly in countries with a poor medical infrastructure. The spectrum of pulmonary diseases in industrialized and emerging countries is similar, but preventable complications such as PCP, TB, and measles pneumonia are more common in the latter. In the emerging countries, underlying malnutrition complicates the clinical outcome.

REFERENCES

1. Centers for Disease Control and Prevention: Unexplained Immunodeficiency and Opportunistic Infections in Infants. New York, New Jersey, California. MMWR Morb Mortal Wkly Rep 1982;31:665–667.
2. Barre-Sinoussi F, Chermann JC, Rey F, Nugeyre MT, Chamaret S, Gruest J, et al: Isolation of a T-lymphotropic retrovirus from a patient at risk for acquired immune deficiency syndrome (AIDS). Science 1983;220(4599):868–871.
3. Gallo RC, Salahuddin SZ, Popovic M, Shearer GM, Kaplan M, Haynes BF, et al: Frequent detection and isolation of cytopathic retroviruses (HTLV-III) from patients with AIDS and at risk for AIDS. Science 1984;224(4648):500–503.
4. Palella FJ Jr, Delaney KM, Moorman AC, Loveless MO, Fuhrer J, Satten GA, et al: Declining morbidity and mortality among patients with advanced human immunodeficiency virus infection. HIV Outpatient Study Investigators. N Engl J Med 1998;338(13):853–860.
5. Centers for Disease Control and Prevention. 1994 Revised classification system for human immunodeficiency virus infection in children less than 13 years of age. MMWR Morb Mortal Wkly Rep 1994;43(RR-12):1–10.
6. Shearer WT, Rosenblatt HM, Schluchter MD, Mofenson LM, Denny TN: Immunologic targets of HIV infection. T cells. NICHD IVIG Clinical Trial Group, and the NHLBI P2C2 Pediatric Pulmonary and Cardiac Complications of HIV Infection Study Group. Ann NY Acad Sci 1993;693:35–51.
7. Nielsen SD, Sorensen TU, Ersboll AK, Ngo N, Mathiesen L, Nielsen JO, et al: Decrease in immune activation in HIV-infected patients treated with highly active antiretroviral therapy correlates with the function of hematopoietic progenitor cells and the number of naive $CD4^+$ cells. Scand J Infect Dis 2000;32(6):597–603.
8. McCloskey TW, Oyaizu N, Bakshi S, Kowalski R, Kohn N, Pahwa S: CD95 expression and apoptosis during pediatric HIV infection. Early upregulation of CD95 expression. Clin Immunol Immunopathol 1998;87(1):33–41.
9. Hyjek E, Lischner HW, Hyslop T, Bartkowiak J, Kubin M, Trinchieri G, et al: Cytokine patterns during progression to AIDS in children with perinatal HIV infection. J Immunol 1995;155(8):4060–4071.
10. Murray HW, Hillman JK, Rubin BY, Kelly CD, Jacobs JL, Tyler LW, et al: Patients at risk for AIDS-related opportunistic infections. Clinical manifestations and impaired gamma interferon production. N Engl J Med 1985;313(24):1504–1510.
11. Luzuriaga K, Holmes D, Hereema A, Wong J, Panicali DL, Sullivan JL: HIV-1-specific cytotoxic T lymphocyte responses in the first year of life. J Immunol 1995;154(1):433–443.
12. Bonagura VR, Cunningham-Rundles SL, Schuval S: Dysfunction of natural killer cells in human immunodeficiency virus-infected children with or without Pneumocystis carinii pneumonia. J Pediatr 1992;121(2):195–201.
13. Bernstein LJ, Ochs HD, Wedgwood RJ, Rubinstein A: Defective humoral immunity in pediatric acquired immune deficiency syndrome. J Pediatr 1985;107(3):352–357.
14. Brena AE, Cooper ER, Cabral HJ, Pelton SI: Antibody response to measles and rubella vaccine by children with HIV infection. J Acquir Immune Defic Syndr Hum Retrovirol 1993;6(10):1125–1129.
15. Rutstein RM, Rudy BJ, Cnaan A: Response of human immunodeficiency virus-exposed and -infected infants to Haemophilus influenzae type b conjugate vaccine. Arch Pediatr Adolesc Med 1996;150(8):838–841.
16. Dunn DT, Newell ML, Ades AE, Peckham CS: Risk of human immunodeficiency virus type 1 transmission through breastfeeding. Lancet 1992;340(8819):585–588.
17. Siegel R, Christie C, Myers M, Duma E, Green L: Incest and Pneumocystis carinii pneumonia in a twelve-year-old girl. A case for early human immunodeficiency virus testing in sexually abused children. Pediatr Infect Dis J 1992;11(8):681–682.

18. Lindegren ML, Hanson C, Miller K, Byers RH Jr, Onorato I: Epidemiology of human immunodeficiency virus infection in adolescents, United States. Pediatr Infect Dis J 1994;13(6):525–535.
19. Davis SF, Rosen DH, Steinberg S, Wortley PM, Karon JM, Gwinn M: Trends in HIV prevalence among childbearing women in the United States, 1989–1994. J Acquir Immune Defic Syndr Hum Retrovirol 1998;19(2): 158–164.
20. Wasser SC, Gwinn M, Fleming P: Urban-nonurban distribution of HIV infection in childbearing women in the United States. J Acquir Immune Defic Syndr Hum Retrovirol 1993;6(9):1035–1042.
21. Blanche S, Rouzioux C, Moscato ML, Veber F, Mayaux MJ, Jacomet C, et al: A prospective study of infants born to women seropositive for human immunodeficiency virus type 1. HIV Infection in Newborns French Collaborative Study Group. N Engl J Med 1989;320(25):1643–1648.
22. Andiman WA, Simpson BJ, Olson B, Dember L, Silva TJ, Miller G: Rate of transmission of human immunodeficiency virus type 1 infection from mother to child and short-term outcome of neonatal infection. Results of a prospective cohort study. Am J Dis Child 1990;144(7):758–766.
23. Leroy V, Newell ML, Dabis F, Peckham C, Van de Perre P, Bulterys M, et al: International multicentre pooled analysis of late postnatal mother-to-child transmission of HIV-1 infection. Ghent International Working Group on Mother-to-Child Transmission of HIV. Lancet 1998;352(9128): 597–600.
24. European Collaborative Study: Mother-to-child transmission of HIV infection. The European Collaborative Study. Lancet 1988;2(8619):1039–1043.
25. European Collaborative Study: Children born to women with HIV-1 infection. Natural history and risk of transmission. European Collaborative Study. Lancet 1991;337(8736):253–260.
26. Connor EM, Sperling RS, Gelber R, Kiselev P, Scott G, O'Sullivan MJ, et al: Reduction of maternal-infant transmission of human immunodeficiency virus type 1 with zidovudine treatment. Pediatric AIDS Clinical Trials Group Protocol 076 Study Group. N Engl J Med 1994;331(18):1173–1180.
27. Garcia PM, Kalish LA, Pitt J, Minkoff H, Quinn TC, Burchett SK, et al: Maternal levels of plasma human immunodeficiency virus type 1 RNA and the risk of perinatal transmission. Women and Infants Transmission Study Group. N Engl J Med 1999;341(6):394–402.
28. Cooper ER, Charurat M, Mofenson L, Hanson IC, Pitt J, Diaz C, et al: Combination antiretroviral strategies for the treatment of pregnant HIV-1-infected women and prevention of perinatal HIV-1 transmission. J Acquir Immune Defic Syndr Hum Retrovirol 2002;29(5):484–494.
29. Weiss SH, Goedert JJ, Sarngadharan MG, Bodner AJ, Gallo RC, Blattner WA: Screening test for HTLV-III (AIDS agent) antibodies. Specificity, sensitivity, and applications. JAMA 1985;253(2):221–225.
30. Kalish LA, Pitt J, Lew J, Landesman S, Diaz C, Hershow R, et al: Defining the time of fetal or perinatal acquisition of human immunodeficiency virus type 1 infection on the basis of age at first positive culture. Women and Infants Transmission Study (WITS). J Infect Dis 1997;175(3):712–715.
31. Bremer JW, Lew JF, Cooper E, Hillyer GV, Pitt J, Handelsman E, et al: Diagnosis of infection with human immunodeficiency virus type 1 by a DNA polymerase chain reaction assay among infants enrolled in the Women and Infants' Transmission Study. J Pediatr 1996;129(2):198–207.
32. Shearer WT, Quinn TC, LaRussa P, Lew JF, Mofenson L, Almy S, et al: Viral load and disease progression in infants infected with human immunodeficiency virus type 1. Women and Infants Transmission Study Group. N Engl J Med 1997;336(19):1337–1342.
33. Galli L, de Martino M, Tovo PA, Gabiano C, Zappa M, Giaquinto C, et al: Onset of clinical signs in children with HIV-1 perinatal infection. Italian Register for HIV Infection in Children. AIDS 1995;9(5):455–461.
34. Barnhart HX, Caldwell MB, Thomas P, Mascola L, Ortiz I, Hsu HW, et al: Natural history of human immunodeficiency virus disease in perinatally infected children. An analysis from the Pediatric Spectrum of Disease Project. Pediatrics 1996;97(5):710–716.
35. European Collaborative Study: Natural history of vertically acquired human immunodeficiency virus-1 infection. Pediatrics 1994;94(6 Part 1): 815–819.
36. Landay AL, Schade SZ, Takefman DM, Kuhns MC, McNamara AL, Rosen RL, et al: Detection of HIV-1 provirus in bronchoalveolar lavage cells by polymerase chain reaction. J Acquir Immune Defic Syndr Hum Retrovirol 1993;6(2):171–175.
37. Agostini C, Zambello R, Facco M, Perin A, Piazza F, Siviero M, et al: CD8 T-cell infiltration in extravascular tissues of patients with human immunodeficiency virus infection. Interleukin-15 upmodulates costimulatory pathways involved in the antigen-presenting cells-T-cell interaction. Blood 1999;93(4):1277–1286.
38. Agostini C, Poletti V, Zambello R, Trentin L, Siviero F, Spiga L, et al: Phenotypical and functional analysis of bronchoalveolar lavage lymphocytes in patients with HIV infection. Am Rev Respir Dis 1988;138(6): 1609–1615.
39. Sierra-Madero JG, Toossi Z, Hom DL, Finegan CK, Hoenig E, Rich EA: Relationship between load of virus in alveolar macrophages from human immunodeficiency virus type 1-infected persons, production of cytokines, and clinical status. J Infect Dis 1994;169(1):18–27.
40. Blanche S, Mayaux MJ, Rouzioux C, Teglas JP, Firtion G, Monpoux F, et al: Relation of the course of HIV infection in children to the severity of the disease in their mothers at delivery. N Engl J Med 1994;330(5): 308–312.
41. Martin R, Boyer P, Hammill H, Peavy H, Platzker A, Settlage R, et al: Incidence of premature birth and neonatal respiratory disease in infants of HIV-positive mothers. The Pediatric Pulmonary and Cardiovascular Complications of Vertically Transmitted Human Immunodeficiency Virus Infection Study Group. J Pediatr 1997;131(6):851–856.
42. Marolda J, Pace B, Bonforte RJ, Kotin NM, Rabinowitz J, Kattan M: Pulmonary manifestations of HIV infection in children. Pediatr Pulmonol 1991;10(4):231–235.
43. Lucas SB, Peacock CS, Hounnou A, Brattegaard K, Koffi K, Honde M, et al: Disease in children infected with HIV in Abidjan, Cote d'Ivoire. BMJ 1996;312(7027):335–338.
44. Kattan M, Platzker A, Mellins RB, Schluchter MD, Chen XC, Peavy H, et al: Respiratory diseases in the first year of life in children born to HIV-1-infected women. Pediatr Pulmonol 2001;31(4):267–276.
45. Spira R, Lepage P, Msellati P, Van De Perre P, Leroy V, Simonon A, et al: Natural history of human immunodeficiency virus type 1 infection in children. A five-year prospective study in Rwanda. Mother-to-Child HIV-1 Transmission Study Group. Pediatrics 1999;104(5):e56.
46. Diaz C, Hanson C, Cooper ER, Read JS, Watson J, Mendez HA, et al: Disease progression in a cohort of infants with vertically acquired HIV infection observed from birth. The Women and Infants Transmission Study (WITS). J Acquir Immune Defic Syndr Hum Retrovirol 1998;18(3): 221–228.
47. Mofenson LM, Yogev R, Korelitz J, Bethel J, Krasinski K, Moye J Jr, et al: Characteristics of acute pneumonia in human immunodeficiency virus-infected children and association with long term mortality risk. National Institute of Child Health and Human Development Intravenous Immunoglobulin Clinical Trial Study Group. Pediatr Infect Dis J 1998; 17(10):872–880.
48. Ikeogu MO, Wolf B, Mathe S: Pulmonary manifestations in HIV seropositivity and malnutrition in Zimbabwe. Arch Dis Child 1997;76(2): 124–128.
49. Chokephaibulkit K, Wanachiwanawin D, Chearskul S, Wanprapa N, Unganont K, Tantinikorn W, et al: Pneumocystis carinii severe pneumonia among human immunodeficiency virus-infected children in Thailand. The effect of a primary prophylaxis strategy. Pediatr Infect Dis J 1999;18(2): 147–152.
50. Adamson PC, Wu TC, Meade BD, Rubin M, Manclark CR, Pizzo PA: Pertussis in a previously immunized child with human immunodeficiency virus infection. J Pediatr 1989;115(4):589–592.
51. Mofenson LM, Moye J Jr, Bethel J, Hirschhorn R, Jordan C, Nugent R: Prophylactic intravenous immunoglobulin in HIV-infected children with $CD4^+$ counts of 0.20×10^9/L or more. Effect on viral, opportunistic, and bacterial infections. The National Institute of Child Health and Human Development Intravenous Immunoglobulin Clinical Trial Study Group. JAMA 1992;268(4):483–488.
52. Spector SA, Gelber RD, McGrath N, Wara D, Barzilai A, Abrams E, et al: A controlled trial of intravenous immune globulin for the prevention of serious bacterial infections in children receiving zidovudine for advanced human immunodeficiency virus infection. Pediatric AIDS Clinical Trials Group. N Engl J Med 1994;331(18):1181–1187.
53. American Academy of Pediatrics: Red Book. 2003 Report of the Committee on Infectious Diseases. Elk Grove Village, Ill: American Academy of Pediatrics, 2003.
54. Murray JF. Cursed duet. HIV infection and tuberculosis. Respiration 1990;57(3):210–220.
55. Luo C, Chintu C, Bhat G, Raviglione M, Diwan V, DuPont HL, et al: Human immunodeficiency virus type-1 infection in Zambian children with tuberculosis. Changing seroprevalence and evaluation of a thioacetazone-free regimen. Tuber Lung Dis 1994;75(2):110–115.
56. Moss WJ, Dedyo T, Suarez M, Nicholas SW, Abrams E: Tuberculosis in children infected with human immunodeficiency virus. A report of five cases. Pediatr Infect Dis J 1992;11(2):114–116.
57. Khouri YF, Mastrucci MT, Hutto C, Mitchell CD, Scott GB: Mycobacterium tuberculosis in children with human immunodeficiency virus type 1 infection. Pediatr Infect Dis J 1992;11(11):950–955.

58. American Thoracic Society: Diagnostic Standards and Classification of Tuberculosis in Adults and Children. Am J Respir Crit Care Med 2000;161(4 Part 1):1376–1395.
59. Abadco DL, Steiner P: Gastric lavage is better than bronchoalveolar lavage for isolation of *Mycobacterium tuberculosis* in childhood pulmonary tuberculosis. Pediatr Infect Dis J 1992;11(9):735–738.
60. Somu N, Swaminathan S, Paramasivan CN, Vijayasekaran D, Chandrabhooshanam A, Vijayan VK, et al: Value of bronchoalveolar lavage and gastric lavage in the diagnosis of pulmonary tuberculosis in children. Tuber Lung Dis 1995;76(4):295–299.
61. Zar HJ, Tannenbaum E, Apolles P, Roux P, Hanslo D, Hussey G: Sputum induction for the diagnosis of pulmonary tuberculosis in infants and young children in an urban setting in South Africa. Arch Dis Child 2000;82(4): 305–308.
62. Jeena PM, Mitha T, Bamber S, Wesley A, Coutsoudis A, Coovadia HM: Effects of the human immunodeficiency virus on tuberculosis in children. Tuber Lung Dis 1996;77(5):437–443.
63. Pape JW, Jean SS, Ho JL, Hafner A, Johnson WD Jr: Effect of isoniazid prophylaxis on incidence of active tuberculosis and progression of HIV infection. Lancet 1993;342(8866):268–272.
64. Kaplan JE, Masur H, Holmes KK: Guidelines for preventing opportunistic infections among HIV-infected persons—2002. Recommendations of the U.S. Public Health Service and the Infectious Diseases Society of America. MMWR Morb Mortal Wkly Rep 2002;51(RR-8):1–52.
65. Lewis LL, Butler KM, Husson RN, Mueller BU, Fowler CL, Steinberg SM, et al: Defining the population of human immunodeficiency virus-infected children at risk for *Mycobacterium avium–intracellulare* infection. J Pediatr 1992;121(5 Part 1):677–683.
66. Chaisson RE, Moore RD, Richman DD, Keruly J, Creagh T: Incidence and natural history of *Mycobacterium avium*–complex infections in patients with advanced human immunodeficiency virus disease treated with zidovudine. The Zidovudine Epidemiology Study Group. Am Rev Respir Dis 1992;146(2):285–289.
67. Langston C, Cooper ER, Goldfarb J, Easley KA, Husak S, Sunkle S, et al: Human immunodeficiency virus-related mortality in infants and children. Data from the pediatric pulmonary and cardiovascular complications of vertically transmitted HIV (P(2)C(2)) Study. Pediatrics 2001;107(2): 328–338.
68. Bye MR, Bernstein L, Shah K, Ellaurie M, Rubinstein A: Diagnostic bronchoalveolar lavage in children with AIDS. Pediatr Pulmonol 1987;3(6): 425–428.
69. Chandwani S, Borkowsky W, Krasinski K, Lawrence R, Welliver R: Respiratory syncytial virus infection in human immunodeficiency virus-infected children. J Pediatr 1990;117(2 Part 1):251–254.
70. Pahwa S, Biron K, Lim W, Swenson P, Kaplan MH, Sadick N, et al: Continuous varicella-zoster infection associated with acyclovir resistance in a child with AIDS. JAMA 1988;260(19):2879–2882.
71. Kovacs A, Schluchter M, Easley K, Demmler G, Shearer W, La Russa P, et al: Cytomegalovirus infection and HIV-1 disease progression in infants born to HIV-1-infected women. Pediatric Pulmonary and Cardiovascular Complications of Vertically Transmitted HIV Infection Study Group. N Engl J Med 1999;341(2):77–84.
72. Schooley RT: Cytomegalovirus in the setting of infection with human immunodeficiency virus. Rev Infect Dis 1990;12(Suppl 7):811–819.
73. Murray JF, Mills J: Pulmonary infectious complications of human immunodeficiency virus infection. Part I. Am Rev Respir Dis 1990;141(5 Part 1): 1356–1372.
74. Murray JF, Mills J: Pulmonary infectious complications of human immunodeficiency virus infection. Part II. Am Rev Respir Dis 1990;141(6): 1582–1598.
75. Miles PR, Baughman RP, Linnemann CC Jr: Cytomegalovirus in the bronchoalveolar lavage fluid of patients with AIDS. Chest 1990;97(5): 1072–1076.
76. Jacobson MA, Mills J, Rush J, Peiperl L, Seru V, Mohanty PK, et al: Morbidity and mortality of patients with AIDS and first-episode *Pneumocystis carinii* pneumonia unaffected by concomitant pulmonary cytomegalovirus infection. Am Rev Respir Dis 1991;144(1):6–9.
77. Glaser JH, Schuval S, Burstein O, Bye MR: Cytomegalovirus and Pneumocystis carinii pneumonia in children with acquired immunodeficiency syndrome. J Pediatr 1992;120(6):929–931.
78. Chadwick EG, Chang G, Decker MD, Yogev R, Dimichele D, Edwards KM: Serologic response to standard inactivated influenza vaccine in human immunodeficiency virus-infected children. Pediatr Infect Dis J 1994;13(3): 206–211.
79. Grant IH, Armstrong D: Fungal infections in AIDS. Cryptococcosis. Infect Dis Clin North Am 1988;2(2):457–464.
80. Johnson PC, Hamill RJ, Sarosi GA: Clinical review. Progressive disseminated histoplasmosis in the AIDS patient. Semin Respir Infect 1989;4(2):139–146.
81. Wang H, Abrahams C, Hart J, Johnson D, Wollmann RL: Disseminated histoplasmosis in an infant with acquired immunodeficiency syndrome. J Infect 1998;37(3):298–301.
82. Galgiani JN, Ampel NM: Coccidioidomycosis in human immunodeficiency virus-infected patients. J Infect Dis 1990;162(5):1165–1169.
83. Denning DW, Follansbee SE, Scolaro M, Norris S, Edelstein H, Stevens DA: Pulmonary aspergillosis in the acquired immunodeficiency syndrome. N Engl J Med 1991;324(10):654–662.
84. Asnis DS, Chitkara RK, Jacobson M, Goldstein JA: Invasive aspergillosis. An unusual manifestation of AIDS. NY State J Med 1988;88(12): 653–655.
85. Lombardo GT, Anandarao N, Lin CS, Abbate A, Becker WH: Fatal hemoptysis in a patient with AIDS-related complex and pulmonary aspergilloma. NY State J Med 1987;87(5):306–308.
86. Pervez NK, Kleinerman J, Kattan M, Freed JA, Harris MB, Rosen MJ, et al: Pseudomembranous necrotizing bronchial aspergillosis. A variant of invasive aspergillosis in a patient with hemophilia and acquired immune deficiency syndrome. Am Rev Respir Dis 1985;131:961–963.
87. Pixley FJ, Wakefield AE, Banerji S, Hopkin JM: Mitochondrial gene sequences show fungal homology for *Pneumocystis carinii*. Mol Microbiol 1991;5(6):1347–1351.
88. Edman JC, Kovacs JA, Masur H, Santi DV, Elwood HJ, Sogin ML: Ribosomal RNA sequence shows Pneumocystis carinii to be a member of the fungi. Nature 1988;334(6182):519–522.
89. Simonds RJ, Oxtoby MJ, Caldwell MB, Gwinn ML, Rogers MF: Pneumocystis carinii pneumonia among US children with perinatally acquired HIV infection. JAMA 1993;270(4):470–473.
90. Thea DM, Lambert G, Weedon J, Matheson PB, Abrams EJ, Bamji M, et al: Benefit of primary prophylaxis before 18 months of age in reducing the incidence of *Pneumocystis carinii* pneumonia and early death in a cohort of 112 human immunodeficiency virus-infected infants. New York City Perinatal HIV Transmission Collaborative Study Group. Pediatrics 1996;97(1):59–64.
91. Scott GB, Hutto C, Makuch RW, Mastrucci MT, O'Connor T, Mitchell CD, et al: Survival in children with perinatally acquired human immunodeficiency virus type 1 infection. N Engl J Med1989;321(26):1791–1796.
92. Simonds RJ, Lindegren ML, Thomas P, Hanson D, Caldwell B, Scott G, et al: Prophylaxis against *Pneumocystis carinii* pneumonia among children with perinatally acquired human immunodeficiency virus infection in the United States. Pneumocystis carinii Pneumonia Prophylaxis Evaluation Working Group. N Engl J Med 1995;332(12):786–790.
93. Leibovitz E, Rigaud M, Pollack H, Lawrence R, Chandwani S, Krasinski K, et al: *Pneumocystis carinii* pneumonia in infants infected with the human immunodeficiency virus with more than 450 CD4 T lymphocytes per cubic millimeter. N Engl J Med 1990;323(8):531–533.
94. Bernstein LJ, Bye MR, Rubinstein A: Prognostic factors and life expectancy in children with acquired immunodeficiency syndrome and *Pneumocystis carinii* pneumonia. Am J Dis Child 1989;143(7):775–778.
95. Marolda J, Pace B, Bonforte RJ, Kotin N, Kattan M: Outcome of mechanical ventilation in children with acquired immunodeficiency syndrome. Pediatr Pulmonol 1989;7(4):230–234.
96. Zar HJ, Dechaboon A, Hanslo D, Apolles P, Magnus KG, Hussey G: *Pneumocystis carinii* pneumonia in South African children infected with human immunodeficiency virus. Pediatr Infect Dis J 2000;19(7): 603–607.
97. Israel-Biet D, Cadranel J, Even P: Human immunodeficiency virus production by alveolar lymphocytes is increased during *Pneumocystis carinii* pneumonia. Am Rev Respir Dis 1993;148(5):1308–1312.
98. Ognibene FP, Gill VJ, Pizzo PA, Kovacs JA, Godwin C, Suffredini AF, et al: Induced sputum to diagnose *Pneumocystis carinii* pneumonia in immunosuppressed pediatric patients. J Pediatr 1989;115(3):430–433.
99. Zar HJ, Tannenbaum E, Hanslo D, Hussey G: Sputum induction as a diagnostic tool for community-acquired pneumonia in infants and young children from a high HIV prevalence area. Pediatr Pulmonol 2003;36(1): 58–62.
100. Graham SM, Mtitimila EI, Kamanga HS, Walsh AL, Hart CA, Molyneux ME: Clinical presentation and outcome of *Pneumocystis carinii* pneumonia in Malawian children. Lancet 2000;355(9201):369–373.
101. Martino AM, Visconti E, Zolfo M, Genovese O, Rendeli C, Mencarini P, et al: Noninvasive diagnosis of *P. carinii* pneumonia on oral washes in an HIV-infected child. Pediatr Pulmonol 1999;28(5):352–355.
102. Baughman RP, Liming JD: Diagnostic strategies in *Pneumocystis carinii* pneumonia. Front Biosci 1998;3:E1–E12.

103. National Institutes of Health: Consensus statement on the use of corticosteroids as adjunctive therapy for pneumocystis pneumonia in the acquired immunodeficiency syndrome. The National Institutes of Health-University of California Expert Panel for Corticosteroids as Adjunctive Therapy for Pneumocystis Pneumonia. N Engl J Med 1990;323(21):1500–1504.
104. Bye MR, Cairns-Bazarian AM, Ewig JM: Markedly reduced mortality associated with corticosteroid therapy of *Pneumocystis carinii* pneumonia in children with acquired immunodeficiency syndrome. Arch Pediatr Adolesc Med 1994;148(6):638–641.
105. Girard PM: Discontinuing *Pneumocystis carinii* prophylaxis. N Engl J Med 2001;344(3):222–223.
106. Norton KI, Kattan M, Rao JS, Cleveland R, Trautwein L, Mellins RB, et al: Chronic radiographic lung changes in children with vertically transmitted HIV-1 infection. AJR Am J Roentgenol 2001;176(6):1553–1558.
107. Jeena PM, Coovadia HM, Thula SA, Blythe D, Buckels NJ, Chetty R: Persistent and chronic lung disease in HIV-1 infected and uninfected African children. AIDS 1998;12(10):1185–1193.
108. Evlogias NE, Leonidas JC, Rooney J, Valderama E: Severe cystic pulmonary disease associated with chronic *Pneumocystis carinii* infection in a child with AIDS. Pediatr Radiol 1994;24(8):606–608.
109. Wassermann K, Pothoff G, Kirn E, Fatkenheuer G, Krueger GR: Chronic *Pneumocystis carinii* pneumonia in AIDS. Chest 1993;104(3):667–672.
110. Katz BZ, Berkman AB, Shapiro ED: Serologic evidence of active Epstein-Barr virus infection in Epstein-Barr virus-associated lymphoproliferative disorders of children with acquired immunodeficiency syndrome. J Pediatr 1992;120(2 Part 1):228–232.
111. Chayt KJ, Harper ME, Marselle LM, Lewin EB, Rose RM, Oleske JM, et al: Detection of HTLV-III RNA in lungs of patients with AIDS and pulmonary involvement. JAMA 1986;256(17):2356–2359.
112. Andiman WA, Eastman R, Martin K, Katz BZ, Rubinstein A, Pitt J, et al: Opportunistic lymphoproliferations associated with Epstein-Barr viral DNA in infants and children with AIDS. Lancet 1985;2(8469–70):1390–1393.
113. Sharland M, Gibb DM, Holland F: Respiratory morbidity from lymphocytic interstitial pneumonitis (LIP) in vertically acquired HIV infection. Arch Dis Child 1997;76(4):334–336.
114. Rubinstein A, Bernstein LJ, Charytan M, Krieger BZ, Ziprkowski M: Corticosteroid treatment for pulmonary lymphoid hyperplasia in children with the acquired immune deficiency syndrome. Pediatr Pulmonol 1988;4(1):13–17.
115. Joshi VV, Kauffman S, Oleske JM, Fikrig S, Denny T, Gadol C, et al: Polyclonal polymorphic B-cell lymphoproliferative disorder with prominent pulmonary involvement in children with acquired immune deficiency syndrome. Cancer 1987;59(8):1455–1462.
116. Amorosa JK, Miller RW, Laraya-Cuasay L, Gaur S, Marone R, Frenkel L, et al: Bronchiectasis in children with lymphocytic interstitial pneumonia and acquired immune deficiency syndrome. Plain film and CT observations. Pediatr Radiol 1992;22(8):603–607.
117. Buck BE, Scott GB, Valdes-Dapena M, Parks WP: Kaposi sarcoma in two infants with acquired immune deficiency syndrome. J Pediatr 1983;103(6):911–913.
118. Chadwick EG, Connor EJ, Hanson IC, Joshi VV, Abu-Farsakh H, Yogev R, et al: Tumors of smooth-muscle origin in HIV-infected children. JAMA 1990;263(23):3182–3184.
119. Bye MR, Palomba A, Bernstein L, Shah K: Clinical Candida supraglottitis in an infant with AIDS-related complex. Pediatr Pulmonol 1987;3(4):280–281.
120. Diamant EP, Dische RM, Barzilai A, Hodes DS, Peters VB: Chronic epiglottitis in a child with acquired immunodeficiency syndrome. Pediatr Infect Dis J 1992;11(9):770–771.
121. Tovo PA, de Martino M, Gabiano C, Cappello N, D'Elia R, Loy A, et al: Prognostic factors and survival in children with perinatal HIV-1 infection. The Italian Register for HIV Infections in Children. Lancet 1992;339(8804):1249–1253.
122. Luginbuhl LM, Orav EJ, McIntosh K, Lipshultz SE: Cardiac morbidity and related mortality in children with HIV infection. JAMA 1993;269(22):2869–2875.
123. Starc TJ, Lipshultz SE, Easley KA, Kaplan S, Bricker JT, Colan SD, et al: Incidence of cardiac abnormalities in children with human immunodeficiency virus infection. The prospective P2C2 HIV study. J Pediatr 2002;141(3):327–334.
124. Lipshultz SE, Easley KA, Orav EJ, Kaplan S, Starc TJ, Bricker JT, et al: Left ventricular structure and function in children infected with human immunodeficiency virus. The prospective P2C2 HIV Multicenter Study. Pediatric Pulmonary and Cardiac Complications of Vertically Transmitted HIV Infection (P2C2 HIV) Study Group. Circulation 1998;97(13):1246–1256.

Noninfectious Disorders of the Respiratory Tract

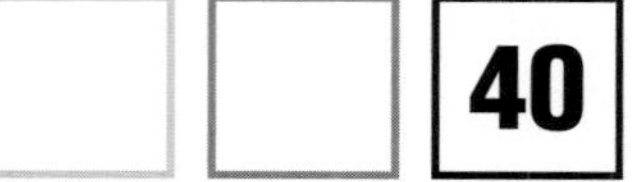

40 Gastroesophageal Reflux and Aspiration Syndromes

Arnold C.G. Platzker, MD

Aspiration constitutes one of the most serious challenges to the integrity of the developing airways. Pediatricians have long recognized that infants and children are particularly at risk for aspiration and contamination of the airways as a result of faulty or dysfunctional swallowing. Although aspiration is more common in newborn infants, especially premature neonates, it continues to be a major health hazard throughout infancy and early childhood. It was only in the late 1970s that disorders of the esophageal motility, cardiac sphincter tone, and gastric emptying became recognized as frequent causes of acute and chronic respiratory disease in infancy and childhood. Even in the 1967 *Pediatric Clinics of North America* edition dedicated to topics in pediatric gastroenterology, there was no mention of gastroesophageal reflux (GER). Subsequently, not only GER but also pediatric conditions heightening the risk for aspiration (e.g., congenital anomalies of the palate and upper respiratory tract and swallowing disorders) have become the focus of development of new diagnostic tests for measuring effectiveness of deglutition and gastroesophageal function in infants and children. Although the association between the disorders of gastrointestinal motility and acute and chronic respiratory disease in infants and children is now well accepted, the mechanism by which GER precipitates respiratory illness in infants and children still remains incompletely understood. In fact, at the present time, it is often difficult to document a relationship between GER-associated respiratory illness and aspiration. GER is common in pediatric patients, but it is not always associated with respiratory illness. Thus, we make a distinction between GER and the respiratory illness it precipitates, gastroesophageal reflux disease (GERD). GER is a passage of gastric contents cephalad into the esophagus, while GERD reflects GER in addition to symptoms of reflux and/or the esophageal and/or respiratory complications it induces. In adults, GER occurs in approximately one third of the population, but in only 10% of adults does GER ever result in respiratory symptoms. GER is probably an even more common occurrence in infants and children, although it may be a less frequent cause of significant symptoms or respiratory illness than in adults. However, because of the lack of extensive prospective studies, the incidence of GER and GERD in infants and children is unknown.

This chapter reviews the current understanding of the developmental and pathophysiologic aspects of aspiration in early childhood and focuses on the special relationship between GER and airways disease. The pathogenesis, current approach to the diagnosis, therapy, and prevention of aspiration and GERD are reviewed and discussed.

FUNCTIONAL DEVELOPMENTAL ANATOMY OF THE AIRWAY AND ITS PROTECTIVE APPARATUS

The airway is capped by the larynx, which acts to protect the airway from penetration from airway mucus, liquids, or swallowed food; participates in regulating the airway inlet resistance to respiration; and facilitates phonation. All three functions of the larynx are immature at birth. The development of swallow and the coordination between breathing and swallowing begins early in fetal life.[1] By 12 weeks of gestation the fetus commences sucking and swallowing movements, but it is not usually until after the 34th week of gestation that the prematurely delivered infant begins to achieve sufficient coordination of the sequence of sucking, swallowing, and breathing to permit feedings to be taken by nipple. At this point in neurologic development, sucking precedes and, in fact, facilitates swallowing, which, in turn, inhibits respiratory effort.[2] At birth the glottal apparatus is immature. The larynx is seated high in the airway and permits a nasolaryngeal connection by apposition of the epiglottis with the soft palate. This facilitates the cessation of breathing with the initiation of swallow. This process is complex and is easily fatigued in the premature or overwhelmed, resulting in penetration of oral contents to the level of the vocal cords. When the laryngeal protective mechanisms fail, aspiration into the airway occurs. Stimulation of the supraglottic or tracheal mucosa by solids or some liquids may invoke a vagally mediated protective response (i.e., apnea and an increase in airway tone). As growth and development progress, the larynx descends and attains a lower position in the neck,[3,4] and the anatomic protection against aspiration is lost in favor of potentiating and optimizing the phonation potential of the larynx. With attainment of anatomic maturity, functional development of the glottal protective mechanism evolves. The epiglottis attains a flat, shieldlike configuration, diverting fluids and foods laterally into the pyriform fossae, away from the midline laryngeal aperture.[3] Thus, food and fluids pass laterally into the airway opening in the gutters formed by the aryepiglottic folds and the lateral pharyngeal walls. Reinforcing the aryepiglottic folds are the corniculate and cuneiform cartilages, which add further stiffness to these folds, enhancing the protection of the airway. Later in childhood, through elevation of the soft palate and the larynx, in synchrony, swallowing proceeds with less risk for penetration of the airway by fluid or food.

The human larynx functions as a valve to protect the lower airway from penetration by fluids or solid matter. This valvelike function is based on the structural and functional relationships of the superior (ventricular) and inferior laryngeal folds, that is, the false and true cords, respectively. The ventricular folds act as the exit valve, preventing the escape of air from the lower respiratory tract. With increasing contraction of the supporting musculature, the adducted false cords seal the airway even more tightly as pressure from the lower airway increases. This action facilitates forceful expectoration, a function that is preserved even in the presence of bilateral vocal cord paralysis. In contrast, the true cords serve as a one-way valve in the opposite direction, restricting the passage of air or aspirated matter into the subglottic airway. In the adult, the valvelike resistance to inflow through the true vocal cords can effectively withstand a 140 mm Hg pressure from above.[3,4] This resistance is seen clinically as laryngospasm, which is occasionally observed in the operating room during induction of anesthesia, resulting in difficult intubation.

The control of upper airway and laryngeal function is mediated by sensory innervation to the larynx through the superior laryngeal nerve and motor function by the recurrent laryngeal nerve. The greatest density of sensory innervation is in the laryngeal inlet, consistent with its role in the protection of the lower airway. The nerve supply includes chemical and thermal receptors as well. These specialized receptors are confined to the supraglottic larynx. There is also a differential sensitivity to various noxious stimuli that vary in intensity with age and with the nature of the noxious challenge. While slowing of respiratory rate and an increase in tidal volume occur in the older child and adult with chemical stimulation of the epiglottic receptors, in the premature infant it has been hypothesized that there is decreased laryngeal sensitivity to mechanical stimulation of the larynx.[2,5–8] However, in the premature infant there is a heightened sensitivity to chemical stimulation of these receptors, precipitating reflex apnea and bradycardia. The full-term infant is less likely to experience apnea in response to saline stimulation of the laryngeal receptors.

The motor limb of deglutition and reflex protection of the airway resides in the intrinsic laryngeal musculature with neural innervation from the nucleus ambiguus. The right and left recurrent laryngeal nerves innervate ipsilateral muscles, except for the cricothyroid muscle, which is innervated by the external division of its ipsilateral superior laryngeal nerve. The interarytenoid muscle receives bilateral recurrent laryngeal nerve innervation. In total, there are five muscles that compose the intrinsic muscles of the larynx. These muscles are responsible for adduction and abduction of the larynx and vocal cords. Adduction of the vocal cords is controlled by the cricothyroid (superior laryngeal nerve), thyroarytenoid, lateral cricoarytenoid, and interarytenoid muscles (recurrent laryngeal nerve). The muscles making the major contribution to adducting the vocal folds are the thyroarytenoid and lateral cricoarytenoid. The posterior gap in the glottis is closed by the contraction of the interarytenoid muscle. Through the action of the cricothyroid muscle, the vocal cord adducts, resulting in an increase in its tone and a 30% passive lengthening. Abduction of the glottis and vocal cords occurs exclusively through the contraction of the posterior cricoarytenoid muscle (recurrent laryngeal nerve).

With aspiration, reflux or regurgitation to the level of the supraglottic space (proximal esophageal sphincter) or penetration of the larynx by foreign liquids or solids, stimulation of sensory afferent nerve endings in the supraglottic mucosa and subglottic mucosa (superior laryngeal nerve, recurrent laryngeal nerve) occurs. The motor response includes contraction of tracheal smooth muscle (narrowing the tracheal lumen) and stimulation of secretory elements in the tracheoesophageal mucosa, both mediated by the autonomic nervous system (nerve of Galen). The latter forms the secretory component of the glottic response; the motor component is the glottic closure reflex, which includes three levels of response. In the first level, the aryepiglottic folds approximate to cover the superior inlet of the larynx. The anterior gap is filled by the epiglottic tubercle with the posterior gap filled by the arytenoid cartilages.

Recurrent aspiration of foreign substances provokes and sustains inflammation of the respiratory tract. This inflammatory process results in impaired airway mechanics and mucociliary blanket function. A recent study has found that pulmonary surfactant proteins (Sp-A and Sp-D) are significantly reduced in the bronchoalveolar lavage (BAL) fluid of children with gastroesophageal reflux and respiratory disease compared with children with reflux but without associated respiratory illness.[9] This suggests that compromise in host defense mechanisms in the children with reflux and respiratory illness from aspiration may be due in part to the impact of aspiration suppressing either the secretion or increasing turnover of these surfactant apoproteins, which are thought to be important in airway host defense through the modulation of airway inflammation. Other consequences of continued aspiration include perpetuating the inflammatory process leading to peribronchial edema, hypertrophy of airway smooth muscle, narrowing of the airway, and progressive airway and interstitial fibrosis.

ASPIRATION FROM ABOVE

The principal causes of aspiration from above in infancy and childhood are listed in Box 40-1. In newborn infants, prematurity and incomplete development of the coordination between suck, swallow, and breathing constitute a major risk for aspiration. Generally, by 34 weeks' gestation the swallowing mechanism has developed to the point where the infant is usually able to begin a successful transition from gavage to feeding by nipple or at the breast. Lingering neonatal respiratory illness with or without

BOX 40-1 Aspiration from *Above*

- Congenital
  - Developmental
    - Prematurity
    - Fatigue aspiration
  - Dysfunctional swallow[95–99]
    - Anatomic
      - Congenital anomalies
        - Cleft palate[12,100]
        - Esophageal atresia/TEF[12,101–105]
        - Laryngotracheal cleft[100,102,105]
        - Choanal stenosis and/or atresia
        - Micrognathia syndromes (Pierre Robin, Goldenhar, Treacher Collins)
        - Macroglossia (Beckwith-Wiedemann syndrome, lingual hemangiomas and tumors)
        - Pharyngeal diverticulum
        - Pulmonary vascular ring or sling
        - Cysts or tumors (cystic hygroma [cavernous lymphangioma], neuroblastoma)
    - Neurologic/myotonic
      - Congenital
        - Postasphyxial brain damage[97]
        - Cerebral palsy
      - Bulbar paresis-post-traumatic
        - Vocal cord
        - Palate
      - Dysmorphia, e.g., de Lange syndrome
      - Conditions that may become symptomatic after the neonatal period
        - Familial dysautonomia
        - Möbius syndrome
        - Myopathies
        - Myotonic dystrophy
        - Werdnig-Hoffmann disease
- Acquired[106,107]
  - Anatomic
    - Palatopharyngeal incompetence
      - Cricopharyngeal achalasia[108]
    - Intubation of the trachea[13]
    - Tracheostomy[15–17]
  - Functional
    - Sinobronchitis
    - Exogenous lipids[109]
  - Pica, etc.
    - Volatile liquid aspiration[23,24,26]
    - Acidic liquids[7,53]
    - Foreign body aspiration[25,27,110–114]
  - Respiratory illness[8,115]

associated tachypnea may delay the achievement of competent swallow or limit the infant's ability to successfully integrate suck and swallow with breathing. However, even in the full-term newborn, compromised ventilation or tachypnea with increased work of breathing, following neonatal respiratory illness (e.g., perinatal asphyxia, meconium aspiration syndrome, sepsis with pneumonia), may result in difficulty establishing effective and efficient nipple feeding without invoking a significant risk for aspiration. A second problem leading to aspiration in early infancy is fatigue of the deglutition or swallowing mechanism. While this phenomena is most commonly seen in the premature infant, it is also noted in the premature or the full-term neonate recovering from respiratory illness, especially in those infants with tachypnea or increased work of breathing due to poor lung compliance. It is frequently seen at the end of a prolonged feeding when the infant is pushed to take all of the feeding by mouth rather than partially by gavage.

Dysfunctional swallow is seen in infants with anatomic defects in the naso- and oroposterior pharynx or trachea and in the infants with various neuromuscular disorders. Infants with a cleft palate may experience nasal reflux of feeding, precipitating a gasp, followed by micro- or frank aspiration of feeding. Infants with an H-type tracheoesophageal fistula (TEF) experience aspiration, most often when fed in the supine position due to the inclination of the fistulous tract in many infants with TEF (i.e., the tracheal opening of the fistulous tract cephalad to the esophageal opening). Thus, when infants with an H-type TEF are fed in a semi-upright (i.e., semi-Fowler) position, there is a lower risk for aspiration than when fed supine. Laryngotracheal cleft is an anomaly that occurs when there is incomplete development of the septation separating the trachea from the esophagus, due to failure of the interarytenoid tissues or cricoid cartilage to fuse at the end of the first month of gestation. This may occur in association with a TEF (all types) or may occur as an isolated defect. The type I laryngotracheal cleft[10] is difficult to diagnose, even on rigid bronchoscopic examination. The defect should be included in the differential diagnosis of aspiration, especially in the infant following TEF repair who continues to experience aspiration or frequent vigorous or paroxysmal coughing associated with feeding or with swallow of mucus.

The infant born with choanal atresia is usually identified and treated prior to feedings being initiated. However, in some cases of choanal stenosis rather than choanal atresia, respiratory distress is not apparent until feedings are attempted. These infants are at great risk for aspiration because they are often unable to successfully coordinate breathing with sucking and swallowing due to the markedly elevated nasal airways resistance. The small mandible that results in relative macroglossia in the Pierre Robin syndrome compromises the oral airway and often interrupts, impairs, or prevents successful oral feeding. In infants with this condition, tongue-lip adhesion surgery pulls the tongue sufficiently anterior in the oral cavity, opening the posterior pharynx in some infants, enabling them to grasp the nipple and to successfully suck and swallow and to experience unobstructed breathing as well. However, the infant with Pierre Robin syndrome may continue to aspirate intermittently due to the small size of the oropharynx or when there is an associated cleft palate. Similar problems are often seen in the infant with Beckwith-Weidemann syndrome.

Infants and children with neurologic or neuromuscular dysfunction (see Box 40-1) either fail to feed by nipple, are unable to coordinate breathing and swallow, or lack adequate bulbar muscle function to successfully feed. Often in the early stages of some of these disorders the first indication of neurologic or neuromuscular impairment is either a single episode or multiple episodes of aspiration. At birth, in addition to perinatal asphyxia, cranial nerve injury, such as recurrent laryngeal nerve paralysis following a difficult vaginal delivery (of the head), often leads to defective deglutition and aspiration. Recurrent laryngeal nerve injury occurs during delivery with extraction of the anterior shoulder. Vigorous traction on the head in the presence of fetal dystocia may lead to traction injury of the recurrent laryngeal nerve and transient or, less frequently, permanent complete or incomplete paralysis of the swallowing mechanism. The recurrent laryngeal nerve is particularly vulnerable as it loops around the ductus arteriosus, which is quite large at the time of birth. Feeding or swallowing dysfunction may also be seen following perinatal asphyxia and in association with congenital hydrocephalus, or neonatal intraventricular hemorrhage. Other less common congenital neuromuscular disorders that may present at birth with aspiration are Werdnig-Hoffmann disease (spinal muscular atrophy) and myotonic dystrophy. Cornelia de Lange syndrome infants, usually diagnosed by their characteristic dysmorphic features, have dysfunctional swallow. Familial dysautonomia is often not suspected until later in infancy and childhood. Diffuse autonomic dysfunction rather than aspiration alone is usually the precipitating factor in the diagnostic workup to confirm this diagnosis.

Causes of aspiration seen later in infancy and childhood fall into four categories: anatomic, functional, pica, and iatrogenic. Infants who have had an endotracheal tube for long periods of time following birth, for assisted ventilation during the neonatal period and beyond, are likely to experience remodeling of the palate[11] due to pressure of the endotracheal tube on the hard and soft palate. Following extubation, during nipple feedings, this may lead to both difficulty establishing a seal around the nipple during sucking and to a gap in the closure of the soft palate with the posterior pharyngeal wall during swallow. Either of these anatomic problems may result in aspiration due to nasal reflux of feedings and/or defective integration of the sucking and swallowing mechanism. Indeed, it is frequently difficult to weigh the importance of each factor (palatal deformity and the functional impediment) on the impaired swallow and the risk for aspiration. There are also infants who, although lacking overt defects or defective development of the hard or soft palate, are prone to aspirate.[12] Examples of infants in this category include those with submucous clefts, occult muscular deficiencies, congenital palatal fistulas, abnormality of the faucial pillars, or palatopharyngeal disproportion. The anatomic defects and/or neuromuscular dysfunction interfere with the normal swallowing mechanism, leading to either extrapharyngeal spillage or leakage of feedings, swallowing muscular dysfunction, cricopharyngeal achalasia, or palatopharyngeal insufficiency or incompetence. In addition, after prolonged mechanical ventilation, even in the absence of disordered anatomy or palatal remodeling, swallowing dysfunction may occur.[13] Finally, tracheostomy alone has been shown to interfere with the swallowing mechanism in adults and in pediatric patients.[14–17] Tracheostomy interferes with several important physiologic events in swallow, including preventing the subglottic rise in tracheal pressure and limiting the elevation of the larynx during swallow. In infants, intubated with an uncuffed endotracheal tube and receiving mechanical assisted ventilation, have been found to have an increased risk for aspiration of mucus or GER liquid around the tube. In these infants, studies using methylene blue dye placed in the distal esophagus have confirmed that the dye is later found in mucus suctioned from the endotracheal tube in 77% of neonates and 8% of older infants and children.[18] Recently, the utility of methylene blue dye study to detect pulmonary aspiration has been questioned.[19] Other studies, including the nuclide salivagram[20] and videoendoscopy,[21,22] have been proposed as more sensitive and specific for aspiration than the blue dye study of swallow.

Even normal infants and children have been documented to aspirate mucus during sleep. The aspirated mucus is then cleared from the airway by the mucociliary mechanism. However, with increased nasopharyngeal mucus drainage such as seen in sinusitis or nasopharyngitis (with purulent drainage into the posterior pharynx), there is a heightened risk with even small amounts of the infected mucus aspirated into the trachea during sleep to precipitate inflammation and airway infection, tracheitis, sinobronchitis, or pneumonia.

Iatrogenic aspiration occurs when infants or small children are fed or attempt to swallow mineral oil, vegetable oil–containing liquids, such as medium-chain triglyerides (Fig. 40-1). In addition, infants and small children who get into and/or attempt to swallow volatile liquids, such as furniture polish[23,24] or small objects such as peanuts[25] frequently become victims of pulmonary aspiration. With volatile liquids, rarely does a child swallow a large amount. Thus, while only a small amount of the fluid is aspirated, extensive airway mucosal and lung parenchymal inflammation and injury often occur (Fig. 40-2). The liquid, warmed to body temperature, vaporizes in the pharynx and leads to inhalation of the vapor into the lungs with each subsequent breath. Even small amounts of aspirated hydrocarbon-containing liquids are very toxic to the mucous membrane of the airway. In addition, inhalation of hydrocarbon vapor into the terminal units of the lung often results in devastating injury to the surface terminal airspaces, causing a severe life-threatening condition resembling acute respiratory distress syndrome (ARDS).[24] Pediatric patients surviving severe hydrocarbon aspiration pneumonia, even if apparently asymptomatic or mildly distressed, may experience chronic airway inflammation and eventual pulmonary parenchymal fibrosis and severe chronically compromised lung function.[26]

With foreign body aspiration in infancy and childhood, approximately 80% of the patients are 3 years of age or younger. In the vast majority of the reported cases (>80%),[25] symptomatic aspiration is the result of aspiration of peanuts. Here, the combination of the salt coating and the peanut oil results in a severe mucosal and parenchymal inflammatory reaction and an often rapidly evolving toxic pneumonitis. Most often, ingestion of the peanut is not observed and aspiration may not be suspected as

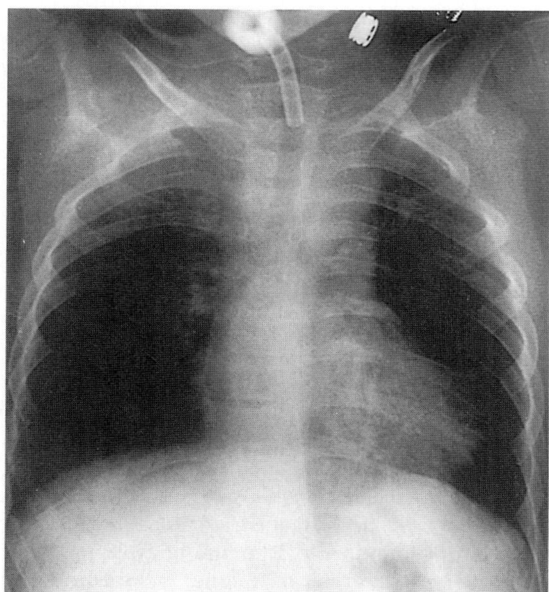

■ **FIGURE 40-1.** Chest roentgenogram, anterior posterior view, in a patient who was thought to have ingested and aspirated furniture polish. There are diffuse peribronchial thickening, interstitial infiltrates, and hyperlucency of the lung fields, suggesting residual obstruction of the airways.

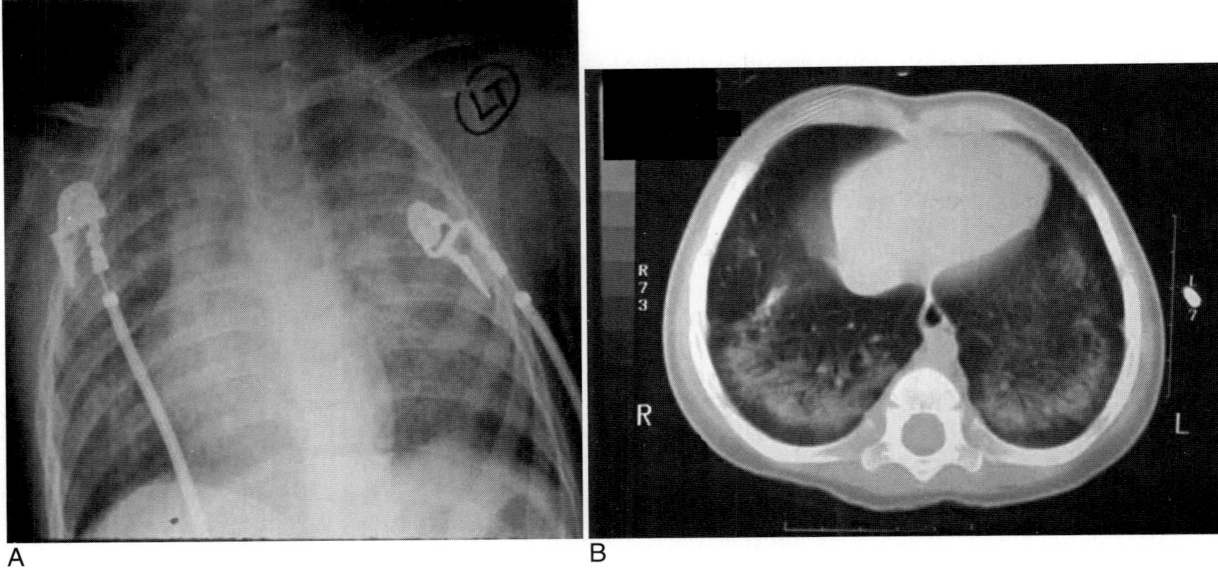

■ **FIGURE 40-2.** CT of chest in an infant who had aromatic lipid aspiration while lying supine. **A,** Chest (AP view): diffuse infiltrates bilaterally, more prominent in hilar areas. **B,** Chest (CT): dorsal alveolar density, consolidation with a small rim of peripheral lucency. Anterior hyperinflation is present.

the cause of the respiratory distress. The pneumonia is then treated symptomatically and with antibiotics. The symptoms may improve with time. However, the vegetable foreign body remaining in the airway may cause residual chronic airway obstruction, usually persisting atelectasis, and often localized recurrent pneumonia. In this instance, the long-term outcome may be the development of bronchiectasis. While the routine chest radiograph may not define a nonradiopaque foreign body such as a peanut, on careful examination of the lung fields an area of hyperlucency suggests that the airways leading into the region may be partially obstructed. In this case, a chest fluoroscopy should be performed. On this study the obstructed area becomes apparent during the respiratory cycle; the airway and vascular structures of the obstructed region do not become more dense as the surrounding airspaces decrease in volume during exhalation. Decubitus chest radiography may also identify hyperinflation of the obstructed segment or lung. Coins and other radiopaque foreign bodies are less often missed in the infant and child who presents with a sudden onset of respiratory distress and a segmental or lobar consolidation on chest radiography. Only in rare instances are other imaging techniques, such as computed tomography (CT) of the airways and lungs, indicated in the diagnosis of an aspirated foreign body.

ASPIRATION FROM ABOVE: THERAPEUTIC CONSIDERATIONS

When a foreign body has been identified in the airway of an infant or child, the removal of the foreign body should be by rigid, rather than flexible, bronchoscopy under general anaesthesia. In the infant and small child, the suction channel of a flexible fiberoptic bronchoscope is frequently inadequate to accommodate forceps for removal of the foreign body or for removal of the foreign body itself. Other techniques such as bronchodilator aerosols followed by percussion and drainage[27] have been studied and found to have a high incidence of cardiac arrhythmias from vagal stimulation associated with movement of the foreign body following chest physiotherapy and a significant incidence of incomplete or failure to clear the foreign body from the airway. This is not a procedure that can be recommended.

PULMONARY IMPACT OF GASTROESOPHAGEAL REFLUX: PATHOGENETIC CONSIDERATIONS

The prime reason for considering GERD in the same chapter with aspiration from above is the fact that GER when associated with respiratory symptoms appears to have a kinship with or a similar pathogenesis with aspiration syndromes from above. Although the pathophysiology of the respiratory symptoms associated with GERD has yet to be clarified, three mechanisms have been proposed based primarily on studies in animals and adult humans. Mendelson[28] was first to associate respiratory disease as a consequence of GER. He described an "asthma-like" syndrome following GER and aspiration of acidic gastric contents during the induction of obstetric anesthesia. Subsequent studies in animals have documented the esophageal and airway mucosal injury from GER and characterized the respiratory consequences of aspiration of various amounts of gastric juice. Aspiration of small amounts of gastric juice ($>$1.0 mL/kg of pH $<$2.5) can result acutely in marked respiratory embarrassment and pneumonia. Aspiration of less than 1.0 mL/kg of gastric juice results in significant, but less violent, clinical respiratory illness, characterized by an obstructive bronchitis or asthma-like syndrome. With chronic aspiration, the pathologic picture may evolve into chronic pulmonary interstitial inflammation, which radiologically may appear similar to interstitial pneumonitis. Over time, continued acid soiling of the airways and lungs results in interstitial thickening and fibrosis of the lungs. In pediatric patients, chronic respiratory symptoms, although frequently mild, are commonly associated with GERD. This has led to the proposal of a second hypothesis, that of "silent" or microaspiration to explain the respiratory symptoms and pathologic findings associated with GER. In this theory, a small amount of soiling of the upper airway by an aerosol of acidic gastric fluid provokes bronchospasm by stimulating the irritant receptors in the trachea and upper airway. The aspirate is isolated and confined to the upper airway through the normal protective mechanisms of cough and vagally mediated bronchospasm. The offending aspirate is removed from the respiratory tract by mucociliary clearance. Each episode of GER is followed by a swallow, although the exact role of the post-GER swallow has not been determined. It has been demonstrated, however, that after infusion of acid into the esophagus, esophageal pH rises toward neutral following a swallow. Successive swallows induce esophageal peristaltic waves that effectively clear the esophagus of acid and restore esophageal pH neutrality. Virtually all acid is cleared from the esophagus within two peristaltic sequences, and the remaining acid is effectively neutralized by swallowed saliva. Unfortunately, aspiration of saliva from the mouth arrests esophageal acid clearance.[29] More significant consequences of GER occur when gastric reflux is associated with defects in swallowing, cough, or mucosal clearance mechanisms. With defects in these "protective" mechanisms, aspiration of the contents of the oral cavity is frequent and the respiratory symptoms are likely to result as much from aspiration from above as from GER.

In the final mechanism proposed to explain the respiratory illness associated with GER, distal esophageal reflux of acidic gastric juice or distention of the esophagus stimulates esophageal stretch, pH, or thermal mucosal receptors, resulting in reflex bronchoconstriction. Interest in this hypothesis may be due to the difficulty and lack of success in documenting penetration of the airway by gastric contents in most patients with GER. Studies to test the hypothesis that distal esophageal reflux of gastric juice alone is sufficient to induce reflex bronchospasm in animal models of GER have been plagued with conflicting results. Investigations have focused on both animals with intact esophageal mucosa and on those with chronic acid reflux esophagitis. In the former, most studies have been unable to document a consistent temporal relationship between acid infused into the distal esophagus and changes in airway mechanics.[30] In one study, 0.1 N hydrochloric acid (HCl) infused into the distal esophagus of kittens appeared to stimulate only a mild increase in the bronchomotor tone. In this study, the induction of esophagitis provoked no greater increase in bronchomotor tone following infusion of acid into the distal esophagus than observed in kittens without esophagitis, although with esophagitis, lower esophageal sphincter tone was decreased. In infants referred for the diagnosis of GER and associated respiratory illness, our group has performed measurements of esophageal manometry and pH with concurrent measurement of airway mechanics and respiratory resistance. We have not been able to confirm any change in airway mechanics during or following distal esophageal acidification with 0.1 N HCl regardless of the state of injury of the esophageal mucosa. Significant respiratory illness was present in all of the patients selected for study, and clear clinical findings and positive imaging studies supported the diagnosis of GER.

DIAGNOSTIC CONSIDERATIONS

ASPIRATION FROM ABOVE

Establishing the diagnosis of GERD is often a very difficult task because this disorder must be distinguished from all other disorders that are associated with aspiration. The aspiration of nasal or sinus secretions and oropharyngeal contents is considered to be aspiration coming from above, as is aspiration of swallowed liquids or a foreign body, whereas aspiration of gastric contents (or esophageal-tracheal aspiration through an H-type TEF) is referred to as aspiration from below. Respiratory illness due to aspiration from above may be caused by a toxic reaction to the fluid aspirated or from an inflammatory response in the respiratory mucosa in response to infectious drainage from the sinuses or oral cavity gaining entry into the airway. This occurs most commonly during sleep and when airway clearance mechanisms are depressed. Thus, acute or chronic sinobronchitis may be misinterpreted as GERD. However, two conditions lead to aspiration from above: congenital craniofacial or upper airway malformations and neurologic or muscular disorders. These disorders are grouped together as oral and pharyngeal dysphagia-related aspiration (see Box 40-1). Aspiration in these conditions results from weakness or bulbar musculature dysfunction, resulting in aspiration during swallow. In craniofacial anomalies, the defect in swallowing is anatomic, and the congenital deformity of the face or cranium interferes with the swallowing process. A poor palatal seal with the posterior pharyngeal wall during swallow (e.g., cleft palate) and an abnormal communication between the respiratory and digestive tracts (e.g., TEF, larygotracheal cleft) are typical examples of this type of swallowing dysfunction, leading to a heightened risk of aspiration. Some of these disorders are also associated with a heightened risk for GER. Therefore, to formulate an appropriate and effective therapeutic plan, diagnostic studies must focus on whether one or both of these disorders are responsible for the patient's respiratory illness.

DISORDERS OF GASTROESOPHAGEAL MOTILITY AND SPHINCTER TONE

Although, as already discussed, the respiratory disease may not be the result of actual aspiration, GERD, or GER-related respiratory illness, is defined as aspiration from below. It comprises a complex of disorders with abnormalities of gastroesophageal motility. Although the overriding physiologic feature of GER is decreased lower esophageal sphincter (LES) pressure, the mean resting LES pressure is reduced in patients with GER, but there are also large swings in LES pressure rising as high as 60 cm H_2O. In pediatric patients with GER, only slightly greater than 10% of the episodes of GER occur while there is a continuous reduction in the resting LES pressure. More than half of the GER episodes occur during a transient increase in intra-abdominal pressure that exceeds the resting level of LES pressure. These transient episodes are thought to occur during wakefulness, when a patient's activity is sufficient to provoke a rise in intra-abdominal pressure, such as when straining, crying, coughing, or during a Valsalva maneuver when passing stool. Only a third of the episodes of GER occur during a brief period of complete relaxation of the LES. These episodes do not occur in association with swallowing or esophageal peristalsis. In normal infants and children, only 1% of GER episodes occur against a background of reduced LES pressure; the vast majority of GER episodes occur during a transient relaxation of the LES. Thus, these two factors—frequent spontaneous relaxation of the LES and frequent, sometimes unexplained, episodes in which intra-abdominal pressure exceeds LES pressure—differentiate abnormal GER from asymptomatic GER in normal infants and children. Finally, when pathologic GER occurs, the refluxate is more frequently acidic in patients (66% compared with 34% in normal individuals).

Surprisingly, the tone of the LES is affected only partially by neural blockade and to a different degree in each of the species studied. Cervical vagotomy has no effect on LES tone. However, LES relaxation is neurally mediated under normal conditions. It is probable that inappropriate relaxation of LES tone may be an important factor in the development of GER. Because LES tone decreases normally only in association with esophageal peristalsis, a decline in LES pressure in the absence of peristalsis is considered inappropriate and results in GER. Table 40-1 lists the agents responsible for modulating, positively or negatively, the tone of the LES.

A second mechanism protecting against GER and transit of esophageal reflux into the pediatric airway is the tone or the competence of the upper esophageal sphincter (UES). The UES, like the cardioesophageal sphincter, is another critical sphincter mechanism protecting against soiling of the airway from below. Little is known about UES function or the control of its tone in humans. There have been few studies of UES function in either normal infants and children, or in pediatric patients with GER. Our knowledge of the anatomy and function of this sphincter is derived largely from studies of animals and adult humans. Anatomically, the UES is formed by the cricopharyngeus and the inferior pharyngeal constrictor muscles, which maintain the tone of the sphincter by "firing" continuously under vagal control. The activity of this sphincter is directly proportional to upper esophageal intraluminal pressure. The tone of the UES increases with acidification of the lower esophagus and with distention of the esophagus. In addition, with either upper esophageal distention or lower esophageal acidification, a secondary esophageal peristalsis is initiated. This secondary peristalsis is a centrally mediated reflex affecting the striated portion of the esophageal musculature, with secondary peristalsis in the smooth muscle portions of the esophagus being initiated locally solely by esophageal distention and not requiring central input.

There are other considerations in this complex relationship between passage of food from the mouth through the esophagus and stomach into the small intestines and the protective mechanisms preventing contamination of the parallel respiratory tract during this process. These factors include swallowing, epiglottis/vocal cord function, and gastric emptying.

TABLE 40-1. Impact of drugs on lower esophageal sphincter tone and intestinal motility

Augmenting Tone/Motility	Lessening Tone/Motility
Gastrin	Methylxanthine compounds
Motilin	Caffeine
Substance P	Theophylline
Prostaglandin F_2	Aminophylline
Adrenergic agonists	Chocolate
Cholinergic agents	β-adrenergic agonists
Bethanechol	α-adrenergic antagonists
Methacholine	Glucagon
Histamine	Secretin
Gastric alkalinization	Cholecystokinin
Metoclopramide	Anticholinergic agents
Indomethacin	Gastric acidification
5-Hydroxytryptamine	Fatty meal
High-protein meal	Narcotic agents
Cisapride	Ethanol
Erythromycin	Diazepam (Valium)
	Peppermint
	Protaglandins E_1, E_2, A_2

Recently, it has been discovered that the tendency for pediatric patients to experience severe GERD is genetically mediated. This genetic predisposition locus (GERD1) has been identified at the 9–centi Morgan interval on chromosome 13q14.[31] However, the role of this gene in the pathophysiology of GERD is not yet clarified.

SYMPTOMS: ASPIRATION, MICROASPIRATION, AND GASTROESOPHAGEAL REFLUX

Infants and small children with aspiration may not exhibit overt findings of inability to swallow without contaminating their airway. Those infants and children with an absent or blunted cough reflex may have silent aspiration and have findings of only increased respiratory mucus, congestion and chronic wheeze or rhonchi, recurrent bronchitis, or recurrent pneumonia. Others with an active cough reflex may have cough associated with feeding and swallowing or sometimes only a chronic cough. When there is nasal reflux of feedings due to a cleft palate, palatal paralysis, or a defect in the palate-posterior pharyngeal wall seal with swallow, then chronic otitis and sinusitis may occur and the purulent drainage from these sites into the pharynx may provoke nighttime cough as well. Some of these patients may be misdiagnosed as having cough-variant asthma. However, this cough does not resolve with bronchodilator treatment as it would in cough-variant asthma.

The presenting gastrointestinal symptoms of GER are often not clearly defined in the history because they are frequently subtle. Even when patients are old enough to assist in providing a history, they may not localize the complaints to the gastrointestinal tract. It is uncommon for an infant or young child with this disorder to experience overt emesis, and when emesis does occur, this symptom may be overlooked and called a "wet burp." The gastrointestinal symptoms are often misinterpreted as behavioral[32] or associated with problems with other organ systems. For example, irritability in an infant as a result of retrosternal discomfort from reflux esophagitis may be misinterpreted as hunger if the irritability improves with feeding. Another important finding in reflux is gagging with or even after feeding, especially if preceded by cough. In the infant younger than 2 years, refusal to feed may be a finding associated with GER.[20,33] Rarely, the diagnosis of GER in such an infant may elude the pediatrician until the infant has a complete investigation for associated respiratory complaints or presents with clearly recognizable gastrointestinal findings such as hematemesis or melena.

On the other hand, the respiratory symptoms and findings are usually overt, but still may be confusing, and it may be difficult to document their relationship to GER. The respiratory symptoms and respiratory illness associated with GER must be differentiated from the respiratory illness due to aspiration from above. This is particularly true when GER and aspiration may coexist. A common theme in these disorders is muscle weakness or incoordination. That is, a small premature infant may experience both GER on a developmental basis and have a dyskinetic or dysfunctional swallow (more commonly termed oropharyngeal dysphagia, difficulty in initiating a swallow) also due to immaturity of the swallowing mechanism (common before 34 weeks' gestation) or resulting from perinatal injury to cranial nerves V, VII, X, and XII. These cranial nerves are involved in both the afferent and efferent limbs of the central nervous system control of swallow. In both premature and full-term infants, cranial nerves X and XII can be injured as a result of abnormal intrauterine head position or more commonly by excessive neck hyperextension in an effort to deliver the anterior shoulder. Swallowing may also be compromised in infants and children with anoxic encephalopathy (e.g., cerebral palsy), congenital myopathies, or failure to thrive. In addition, infants who are not fed orally for long periods of time after birth may have to receive oromotor training in order to achieve competence in sucking and the coordination of breathing and swallowing.

Perhaps the major reason for the apparent difficulty in identifying infants and children with GER is that GER is prevalent in patients suffering from preexisting respiratory illness (e.g., asthma and chronic lung disease of infancy). The symptoms of GER-related respiratory illness are similar to or masked by the symptoms of the patient's primary illness. For example, infants with apnea and GER may manifest only increased frequency of apneic episodes, whereas patients with asthma and GER may experience only more severe or unresponsive wheezing. Therefore, the awareness of a linkage between a particular illness and GER is key to the successful identification and treatment of this disorder. Box 40-2 lists the disorders with which GER may be associated.

The most common respiratory symptoms of GER are wheezing and nighttime coughing (Box 40-3). However, the particular presenting symptoms may be age dependent. Infants who in the early part of the first year have GER may also have dysphagia, gagging with feeding,[32] rejection of feedings,[20,33] stridor,[32,34] or, most troubling, intermittent or frequent apnea.[35] In some, apnea presents as an acute life-threatening event (ALTE, also known as near-miss sudden infant death syndrome [SIDS]) that may even require full resuscitation to reestablish spontaneous breathing. Although GER does not cause apnea, it may cause increased frequency of episodes of apnea in infants already at risk for apnea. In fact, the GER-related symptoms may be so prominent as to mask and delay the diagnosis of the underlying GER condition. Effective medical or surgical treatment of GER may be accompanied by reduction in the frequency of apneic episodes, but usually not their elimination. Wheezing and nighttime cough are common and are often unresponsive to treatment with bronchodilator medications. In infants and children with severe respiratory symptoms due to GERD, otitis media, sinusitis, recurrent illness with bronchitis, and pneumonia are common. Some infants and children present with stridor or hoarseness, suggesting that during episodes of reflux, gastric juice has risen to the level of the UES or vocal cords and has caused inflammation and edema of the pharynx and vocal cords. In these children, erosion, often severe, of posterior molar teeth may be present as a result of nighttime acid reflux bathing the posterior dentition.[36] However, studies have indicated that it might not be solely the level of the esophagus to which the gastric acid rises that results in airway hyperreactivity and wheeze. Distal esophageal acid reflux with or without esophageal mucosal inflammation may trigger bronchospasm. Less commonly, infants present with anemia and hemoptysis or melena, suggesting that GER has resulted in severe hemorrhagic esophagitis. In its most extreme presentation, GER may first come to the attention of a pediatrician when an infant is brought to the office for evaluation of failure to thrive, with GER worsened by inadequate caloric intake from difficulty in swallowing from chronic esophageal inflammation and odynophagia (painful swallowing). In the chronic, long-term respiratory illness of GER, diffuse pulmonary fibrosis may result from chronic soiling and inflammation of the airway and lung parenchyma.

In infants and small children there is a growing body of literature to suggest that some GER is obligatory, that is, the patient has obstruction to exhalation sufficiently severe that the mobilization of accessory muscles of ventilation is required to effect successful exhalation. The sudden, large rise in intra-abdominal pressure necessary to successfully overcome the airway obstruction forces the cardiac sphincter open, and a pulse of gastric acid is propelled into the distal esophagus. Recent studies have suggested that children younger than 2 years with upper airway obstruction undergoing adenoidectomy and ventilation tube placement have a high incidence of GER when compared

BOX 40-2 Disorders Associated with Gastroesophageal Reflux

- Anoxic encephalopathy
- Esophageal atresia/TEF
- Congenital diaphragmatic hernia (postsurgical repair)
- Bronchopulmonary dysplasia
- Infant apnea
- Failure to thrive
- Asthma
- Cystic fibrosis
- Achalasia
- Neuromuscular disorders
- Neurologic impairment
- Hiatal hernia

BOX 40-3 Clinical Findings in Gastroesophageal Reflux

Frequent

- Cough—nighttime
- Gagging
- Emesis
- Feeding resistance
- Wheezing
- Recurrent bronchitis/pneumonia
- Recurrent otitis media
- Upper airway obstruction
- Esophagitis
- Colic

Common

- Apnea[5]
- ALTE (acute life threatening event, i.e., near-miss sudden infant death syndrome)[35,116]
- Failure to thrive
- Stridor
- Dental erosion
- Abnormal head, neck, and thorax positioning

Uncommon

- Hoarseness
- Hemoptysis
- Anemia
- Pulmonary fibrosis

with children undergoing ventilation tube placement for serous otitis media.[37] There is a similar high incidence of GER in children with chronic lung disease of infancy.

■ DIAGNOSIS

The goal of the diagnostic evaluation of patients suspected of having respiratory illness resulting from GER and/or aspiration is the demonstration of GER or aspiration and time-related abnormalities in ventilatory function or penetration of the vocal cords by refluxate. Establishing the diagnosis of GER increasingly means ruling out other causes of aspiration. This goal of confirming aspiration in GER is rarely achieved. The diagnostic studies available have improved, but are frequently found to lack sufficient sensitivity, and few centers are equipped to perform the sophisticated measurements of gastroesophageal function and concurrent ventilatory function necessary to confirm the diagnosis of GER and to elucidate its relationship to the cause of an infant's or child's respiratory symptoms.

Box 40-4 lists the laboratory diagnostic studies that may be used for establishing or confirming the clinical diagnosis of GER and/or aspiration. An upper gastrointestinal (UGI) series of roentgenograms using barium sulfate as the contrast medium is the most often used, but not necessarily always the most definitive of the diagnostic studies. However, it is a widely available radiologic examination. With the use of fluoroscopy, the barium swallow provides the best imaging of swallow. This study is perhaps the best widely available method to study the competence of suck (in infants) and swallow (throughout infancy and childhood). In many hospitals, pediatric feeding therapists participate in these studies and improve the diagnostic reliability of the study. Videofluoroscopy also provides sufficient structural detail of the UGI tract to aid in the diagnosis of structural defects.

BOX 40-4 **Diagnostic Studies to Confirm the Diagnosis of Gastroesophageal Reflux (GER) and/or Aspiration**

GER

- Barium swallow (i.e., UGI series)[117]
- Gastric scintiscan[38,118–121]
- 24-hour esophageal pH monitoring[38,39,41,53,54,57,98,122–125]
- Ultrasound examination of the gastroesophageal junction[9,43]
- Sleep polysomnography[126]

Aspiration

- Chest radiograph (foreign body detection)
- Decubitus chest radiograph (unilateral hyperinflation)
- Fluoroscopy lungs (unilateral static hyperinflation)
- Videofluoroscopy (detection of dysphagic aspiration)[21,22,48]
- Blue dye test (aspiration)[16,22]
- Radionuclide salivagram (microaspiration)[127]
- Scintiscan (detection of lung uptake)[46,128]
- Carbohydrate analysis of tracheal secretions[46,27,128]
- Bronchoalveolar lavage (for presence of lactose or lipid-laden macrophages)[44–47,60]

Thus, lesions impinging on the esophagus, such as vascular rings or slings, may often be clearly defined on fluoroscopy as a pulsating narrowing or stricture of the esophageal barium column. Abnormal communication between the airway and esophagus may occasionally be defined with positive-contrast roentgenograms. An H-type TEF and laryngotracheal clefts are difficult to identify on a single UGI study even when performed by an experienced pediatric radiologist. Finally, the UGI series is helpful in the study of swallowing, esophageal motility, cardiac sphincter function, GER, and gastric emptying. The technique for performing this study varies widely. When evaluating an infant with this technique, it is important to feed the barium to the infant by nipple (infant) or cup (child) in order to look for the presence of oral or pharyngoesophageal dysphagia or swallowing dyskinesis. Some radiologists prefer to insert a feeding tube and infuse the barium into the distal esophagus. This practice should be discouraged if a complete study, including swallow, is to be obtained. During the study, if the patient cries vigorously, if excessive pressure is placed on the patient's abdomen, or if the patient is positioned in the head-down position, a positive result may be seen in a patient who normally does not have significant reflux. It is also possible that the extent of the reflux, if present, may be exaggerated.

The limitations of the barium swallow include the static nature of the study (i.e., only one swallow is studied) and the use of only a thickened swallowing medium (not thin liquids or solids). The barium swallow is also not sufficiently sensitive to detect microaspiration. The UGI is appropriate for the study of gastroesophageal function only during the wakeful state. Thus, the barium swallow is frequently not the final or the only diagnostic study used for confirming the diagnosis of GER in infants or children with respiratory illness, although it remains the mainstay for the diagnosis of swallowing disorders. With the UGI series for detection of GER the false-positive diagnostic rate for this study is in excess of 30% and the false-negative rate 14%. Finally, the barium swallow is not suitable for the combined study of ventilation and gastroesophageal function.

The gastric scintiscan may be used to complement or confirm the results of the barium swallow. It is more sensitive than the barium swallow and therefore occasionally yields false-positive results, but it is only rarely associated with false-negative results. This study is performed using a technetium 99m sulfur colloid-tagged meal. In this study, the isotope may be mixed with formula or a mixed fluid-solid meal. The isotopic meal is either ingested orally or administered by nasogastric tube into the lower esophagus or stomach. Detectors under the supine infant or child monitor the progress of the tagged meal through the esophagus into the stomach and its transit time in the stomach.[38–40] Reappearance of radioactivity in the esophagus[41] and its subsequent appearance in the peripheral lung fields is an indication that reflux and pulmonary aspiration have taken place. This study, when carefully performed, may allow discrimination between aspiration during deglutition and aspiration after GER. Reflux is confirmed when a vertical column of radioactivity reappears above the diaphragm. With the gastric scintiscan, continuous monitoring of the progress of the radioactive meal is critical to the sensitivity of the study. Ideally, accumulation and decay of radioactivity should be monitored by computer as well as the scintillation camera to permit second-to-second replay and quantization of the events. In this way, a continuous and uninterrupted picture of the passage of the radioactive meal through the UGI tract is possible. Prolonging the study time for at least

4 hours allows accurate measurement of gastric emptying time, allows recognition of the role of delayed gastric emptying or of gastric outlet obstruction in the patient's clinical problem, and increases the sensitivity of the study for the detection of pulmonary aspiration. To achieve the goal of detecting late reflux, gastric emptying times and detecting aspiration imaging of the patient should continue until complete emptying of the stomach has occurred. Disadvantages of this technique (Table 40-2) include the failure to provide high-quality resolution of the esophageal and gastric surface anatomy and the difficulties with interpretation in the presence of congenital anomalies affecting function of the UGI or upper respiratory tract or both. These anomalies and disorders include esophageal atresia and TEF, laryngotracheal clefts, rings, slings, hiatal hernia, or pyloric stenosis. In some patients with esophageal stricture or poor distal esophageal motility following surgical correction of congenital esophageal atresia and TEF, the abnormal distal esophageal transit time may be misinterpreted as GER.

Recently, ultrasonographic imaging of the gastroesophageal junction has been used in the diagnosis of GER.[42,43] Unfortunately, there are, as yet, no comparisons of the sensitivity and specificity of this test with other diagnostic tests for the diagnosis of GER.

Esophagoscopy and bronchoscopy alone are of little value in defining the cause of GER and respiratory illness or aspiration, but esophagoscopy may confirm the presence of GER by confirming the presence of acid reflux with thickening and inflammatory change in the mucous membrane of the lower esophagus. Microscopic examination of the mucosal biopsy specimen may reveal intraepithelial eosinophils, further supporting a diagnosis of esophagitis. However, this diagnostic technique does not provide confirmation of a linkage of GER and the respiratory illness experienced by the patient. Bronchoscopy and tracheal lavage, on the other hand, may reveal inflammatory change in the airway mucosa and the presence of lipid-laden macrophages in the lavage,[44–47] but this procedure, although confirming the presence or absence of pulmonary aspiration, contributes little information about the origin of the aspirate. The aspirate may result from dysphagia (aspiration from above), rather than from GER (aspiration from below). Finally, video-endoscopic swallow studies are reported to be an important adjunct to the diagnosis of aspiration due to defective swallow.[21,48] There are comparison studies in adult patients of this technique with other studies to detect aspiration, but pediatric studies have yet to confirm the place of videoendoscopy in the diagnosis of aspiration from defect in the mechanics of swallow.

As long ago as 1958, Tuttle[49] described a method for detecting incompetence of the gastrocardiac sphincter mechanism. He determined that the concurrent measurement of distal esophageal pressure and pH would be the most sensitive method for recognizing incompetence of the sphincter mechanism. In recent years, this test has been modified for use in infants and children. Arndorfer and colleagues[50] developed a double-lumen catheter that permits concurrent monitoring of upper and lower esophageal pressure at the LES and UES, as well as esophageal pH. This technique permits the detection of reflux, the determination of the height of reflux, and the competence of the UES as well as the LES. This study was initially performed with acid first introduced into the stomach through the catheter, which was then withdrawn into the distal esophagus to monitor the time course of esophageal pH after an initial clearance of residual acid from the esophagus by perfusion of a small amount of saline into the esophagus. The study technique has evolved, and the length of monitoring of esophageal manometry and pH has been increased. In 1985, at the American Thoracic Society Conference on Aspiration Hazards to the Developing Lung,[51] the panel on Swallowing and Upper Gastrointestinal Function proposed that the method be standardized to include the following:

1. Placement of the pH probe in the distal esophagus, using LES pressure determined manometrically as the landmark.[52]
2. Monitoring of pH for at least 6 hours, including one cycle of rapid eye movement (REM) sleep and feeding.
3. Standardized position (not in an infant seat) without medication.
4. Simultaneous monitoring of pharyngeal and esophageal function and possibly LES function to determine mechanisms of reflux clearance.
5. Standardized scoring methods; either the Euler[53,54] or Herbst[55] method could be used. Normal values should be more definitively established.

The panel further recommended that respiratory function should be monitored along with the manometric and pH monitoring to establish a temporal relationship between reflux and respiratory symptoms or alterations in respiratory function.[51] Table 40-3 lists the criteria separating physiologic from pathologic GER in infants (<1 year old), children (<1 year old), and adults.

With the availability of the portable esophageal pH probe with microprocessor recorder, the study of ambulatory esophageal

TABLE 40-2. Comparative features of gastroesophageal reflux (GER) diagnostic studies

Diagnostic Test	Advantages	Limitations
Upper GI series	Widely available Detects anatomic abnormalities	Does not discriminate physiologic from pathologic reflux
Gastric scintiscan	Detects acid, nonacidic reflux Quantifies timing of gastric emptying Detects aspiration	Requires specialized equipment No standardization of methodology Lacks normative data for each age group Lacks resolution of anatomic detail of esophagus, stomach, and airway
pH probe study (24-hour protocol)	Detects esophageal pH change (acid reflux) Identifies temporal relationship of acid reflux and symptoms Assesses effectiveness of antiacid therapy	Does not detect nonacidic reflux Probe location must be confirmed Alone, does not detect association of apnea and GER

GI, gastrointestinal.

TABLE 40-3. Physiologic gastroesophageal reflux (GER)

Reflux Episodes	<1 Year Old	>1 Year Old	Adults
No. of episodes daily	73	25	45
No. of episodes ≥ 5 min	9.7	6.8	3.2
% time pH < 4 (GER index)	11.7	5.4	6

From Rudolph CD, Mazur LJ, Liptak GS, et al: Pediatric GE reflux clinical practice guidelines. J Pediatr Gastroenterol Nutr 2001;32(Suppl):1–31.

pH monitoring is now standardized and should be performed over a 24-hour period. With the publication of the pediatric GER clinical practice guidelines, there is now consensus among pediatric gastroenterologists concerning the normal values for the 24-hour pH probe study in infants and children.[56] The data are reported as total time or percentage of the study time with pH less than 4.0, number of episodes of pH less than 4.0 in a 24-hour period, and the number of episodes lasting longer than 5 minutes.[56] Each of these values is also broken down into the supine or sleep time and the upright or awake time. If this study is performed using milk-containing feedings, the test may miss episodes of reflux because the milk entering the stomach acts to neutralize or partially neutralize the acidic gastric contents. Thus, if postprandial reflux takes place, esophageal pH will not fall below 4 and the episode of reflux will be missed.[38,41,57] The esophagus has an alkaline output, which may also mask some episodes of reflux.[58] To remedy this interference with the diagnostic value of the esophageal pH study, feeding of acidic liquids such as apple or cranberry juice is advisable, especially for infants who take a bottle feeding before bedtime. With the growing interest in rapid diagnosis of GER, the use of the sleep laboratory for nap studies to detect reflux during sleep has become fashionable. However, Graff and colleagues[59] have found that while it is possible to confirm the presence of GER during sleep with a nap study, this method significantly underestimates the incidence of reflux. That is, there is a high incidence of falsely negative studies with use of nap studies. Table 40-3 lists the normal values for infants, children, and adults. Figure 40-3 illustrates the radiologic confirmation of the placement of the esophageal probe for a 24-hour study of esophageal pH. The recording accompanying the roentgenogram illustrates the monitoring of upper and lower esophageal pH in an infant with GER and chronic lung disease. Note that shortly after the beginning of the tracing, there are two episodes of GER during which the pH of the lower esophagus falls below 2, but the upper esophagus remains above 6. Both of these episodes occurred immediately after feeding, and the esophageal pH gradually returned to baseline values during the postprandial period. After these two episodes are GER episodes with reflux of gastric juice to the level of the upper probe, causing a decrease in upper esophageal pH below 4.0. In this infant, reflux occurred for 23% of the time and occurred for almost one third of the time during meals when supine and for 20% of the time when held upright. However, with episodes of GER there was no temporally related change in lung mechanics. This infant had unexplained chronic lung disease and was oxygen dependent. A chest roentgenogram revealed chronic right upper and middle lobe infiltrates. Barium swallow failed to reveal a defect in swallowing. The gastric scintiscan failed to confirm delayed gastric emptying, but the scintiscan confirmed the presence of GER and aspiration. Six hours following the ^{99m}Tc feeding, a delayed scan detected a small amount of radioactivity over the right upper lung fields, suggesting that aspiration followed the episode of GER. In only a few patients will the diagnostic studies be as helpful or definitive. This illustrative case, however, is a fitting example of how each of the

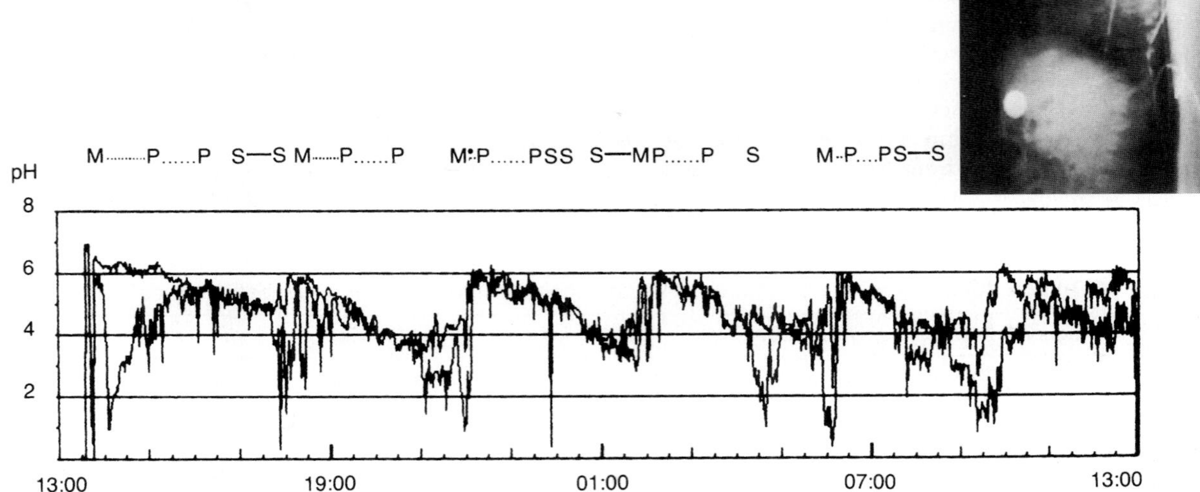

FIGURE 40-3. Chest roentgenogram, lateral view, showing the double-lumen pH probe with the lower sensor resting in the esophagus immediately cephalad to the level of the diaphragm and the upper lumen sensor at the level of the upper esophageal sphincter *(arrow)*. The pH tracing reveals multiple episodes of gastroesophageal reflux, resulting in the fall of the esophageal pH. Shortly after 1300 hours, only the lower esophageal reflux is recorded, with a fall in pH below 2. At 2330 hours another episode of reflux to the level of the upper esophageal sphincter is recorded beginning with (M) through the entire postprandial period (P....P) and during sleep in the supine position (SS). At 0900 a fall in both the lower and the upper esophageal pH below 4 is recorded, with the onset of the drop in pH associated with feeding, (M) beginning of the feeding through the postprandial period (P), and continuing during supine positioning (S) after feeding. No change was recorded in total respiratory resistance with any episode of reflux.

diagnostic studies may be used in evaluation of a patient in an attempt to confirm the diagnosis of GER and respiratory illness.

A comparison of the effectiveness and limitations of the UGI series, gastric scintiscan, and pH probe study in the diagnosis of GERD is listed in Table 40-2. Several other diagnostic studies are appropriate in some instances in which a diagnosis of GER is being considered. In an infant or child receiving assisted ventilation through an uncuffed endotracheal tube or a tracheostomy and experiencing frequent unexplained exacerbations of respiratory disease, GER is often a diagnostic consideration. Study of the tracheal aspirate for reducing substances (if the patient is receiving gastric feedings) or lipid-laden macrophages has been advocated.[60] In an older child with a tracheostomy, cytologic examination of the tracheal aspirate may contain vegetable fibers when aspiration has taken place. Each of these studies, if positive, merely confirms that aspiration is likely to have occurred. They do not rule out the possibility that contamination of the respiratory tract may be the result of a congenital or, rarely, an acquired abnormal connection between the upper respiratory and gastrointestinal tracts. When any of these test results are positive, further investigation with the imaging and respiratory function and UGI manometric and pH studies is indicated.

Diagnostic studies to detect aspiration (see Box 40-4) include a chest radiograph, both inspiratory and expiratory films, chest fluoroscopy or decubitus chest x-ray, the modified barium swallow, blue dye or radionuclide salivagram, and BAL. When swallow is intact (i.e., negative modified barium swallow and salivagram study results) and aspiration of a liquid in suspected, BAL is often helpful in confirming the diagnosis. Oil detected in lavage fluid suggests lipoid aspiration. The chest CT in patients with this diagnosis is very characteristic (see Figs. 40-2 and 40-4). These patients have dorsal consolidation and anterior hyperlucency when the oil aspiration occurred with the infant supine. Chest CT is helpful but rarely necessary for detection of a radiopaque foreign body.

THERAPY

MEDICAL

Aspiration

Although there are specific measures that should be taken to treat aspiration in order to manage the acute symptoms and to prevent damage to the airway and parenchyma, prevention of aspiration should be integrated into parent education in pediatric practice. Assuring that infants and small children are not offered peanuts and other small foods that might be accidentally aspirated and assuring that all volatile liquids have child-proofed closures and are well marked and placed in either locked cabinets or on high shelves should be a main objective in the pediatrician's discussions with each parent. However, even with heightened awareness of the importance of child proofing the home, aspiration does occur. Treatment of aspiration differs depending on the type of aspiration—solid object (i.e., foreign body) or liquid—and whether the aspiration is acute or chronic. With liquid aspiration, treatment varies depending on the nature of the liquid (e.g., gastric contents, infectious versus noninfectious, nonvolatile versus volatile liquids [such as furniture polish]). Foreign body aspiration is covered in a separate chapter. Acute liquid aspiration of gastric contents is likely to cause pneumonia (which may evolve into ARDS). Treatment should include monitoring vital signs (including oxygen saturation), providing supplemental oxygen to prevent severe hypoxemia, placing a nasogastric tube to drain the stomach (because an acute postaspiration ileus may occur), and placing a secure venous cannula for provision of hydration and intravenous medications such as antibiotics[61,62] and glucocorticoids.[63] Nonaerobic antibiotic coverage is indicated.

Aspiration of volatile liquid frequently precipitates a severe, persisting inflammatory reaction in the airway and lung parenchyma. Oxygen, intravenous fluids, antibiotics, and steroids are often administered during the acute period of treatment.

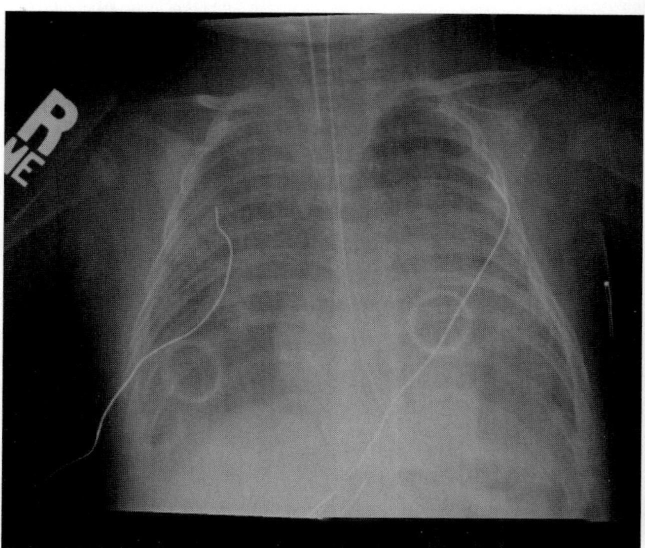

A

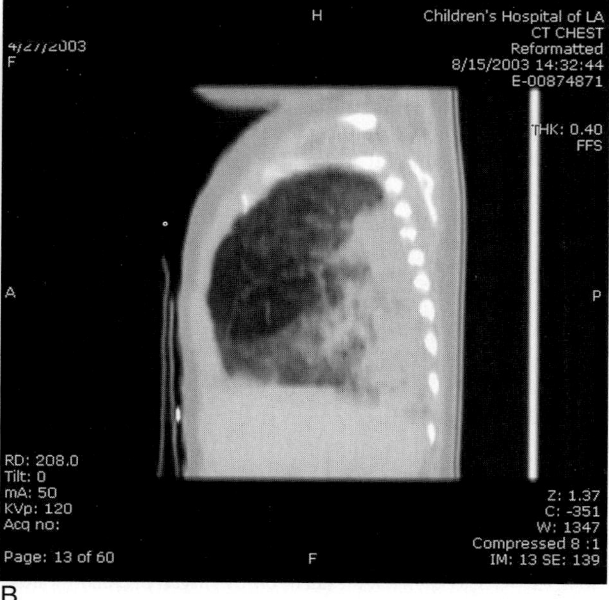

B

FIGURE 40-4. **A,** Chest radiograph (anteroposterior view) of an infant who had inadvertently been fed mineral oil by nipple while lying supine. Hazy lung fields with streaky densities most pronounced in the middle and lower lung fields with apical hyperlucency. **B,** Helical computed tomography image (3-D reconstruct) of the chest extensive dorsal, basilar consolidation bilaterally with apical hyperlucency.

The effectiveness of this therapy in preventing long-term damage to the airway and lung parenchyma has never been proven.

Aspiration of lipid-containing liquids, such as mineral oil, aromatic oils, or polyethylene glycol solution, provokes an often severe airway obstructive and pulmonary inflammatory syndrome. This form of aspiration requires treatment both of airway obstruction and of airway and pulmonary parenchymal inflammation. Immediate treatment following aspiration includes passing a nasogastric tube to empty the stomach of residual toxic liquid and starting intravenous hydration, supplemental oxygen, and monitoring of arterial carbon dioxide tension. Assisted ventilation is required when there is evidence of inability to maintain adequate oxygen saturation with oxygen supplementation alone and/or progressive deterioration in carbon dioxide exchange. Flexible fiberoptic bronchoscopy and BAL are indicated to document the aspiration and to clear the aspirated liquid from the airway.[64,65] This procedure has been advocated in instances in which the aspirated liquid is both toxic to the airway and lung and "nonabsorbable." However, due to the rarity of this form of aspiration, there have not been any controlled trials to critically assess the effectiveness and efficiency and efficacy of BAL. We have found that in patients with this form of aspiration, a beneficial response to glucocorticoid therapy is often followed by a long course of glucocorticoid therapy with increase in respiratory distress and a decline in lung function when weaning of steroid therapy is attempted. The long-term prognosis for complete recovery of lung function in this patient group is uncertain, although it is usually dependent on the extent of the initial illness after lipid aspiration.

Chronic aspiration is common, especially in infants and children with neurologic disability from perinatal asphyxia, traumatic birth injury, neuromuscular disorders, congenital anomalies of the upper airway, Down syndrome, and chronic lung disease (see Box 40-1). In these conditions, after documentation of the severity and chronicity of aspiration, a decision of treatment will depend on the extent of aspiration. If the modified barium swallow confirms inability to swallow liquids but competent swallow of thick liquids and solids, treatment might consist of changing the diet with the exclusion of clear and thin liquids. If fluid intake is not adequate, then gastrostomy tube placement will be required to assure adequate hydration. All patients with chronic aspiration from above will require a complete evaluation to rule out GER in order to rule out aspiration from below as well. Full recovery following treatment of aspiration from above depends on the cause of the aspiration, extent of impairment in swallow, duration following the onset of aspiration until effective treatment is implemented, and whether there is aspiration from below as well. When aspiration from below is also present, GERD therapy, as listed in the next section, should be included. In patients with an impairment in swallow so severe that there is chronic aspiration of saliva and nasopharyngeal drainage that impair ventilation, placement of a tracheostomy provides better access to the airway and permits improved tracheal toilet.

Gastroesophageal Reflux Management

Although medical therapy for GER has changed little in the past decade, it is still the initial therapy of choice in infants and children (Box 40-5). Infants have been found to respond favorably to positioning. When infants are placed prone with the head of the crib elevated, gravity aids esophageal motility and emptying of the stomach. The head-down supine position and the upright position in an infant seat encourage or increase reflux in an infant at high risk for GER. Thickening of the feedings is also indicated in small infants with GER. Although thickened feedings reduce the overt findings of GER such as emesis, it is not considered to be effective in reducing episodes of reflux. Recent studies suggest that thickened feedings reduce the frequency of nonacid (i.e., pH > 7.40) GER episodes due to the decrease in height of the esophageal reflux, although the occurrence of acid GER is not affected.[66] Those encouraging thickened feedings contend that for this therapy to be effective, rice cereal must be added to the formula until the formula is the consistency of raw honey. This usually requires 2 to 3 teaspoons of rice cereal per ounce of formula. Augmenting positioning of the infant by placing the infant in an infant seat during and after feeding and thickened feeding, changing to smaller volume but more frequent feeding, and withholding feedings for several hours before bedtime may improve the effectiveness of medical therapy by reducing postprandial stomach volume and minimizing the volume of the potential refluxate.

BOX 40-5 Therapy for Gastroesophageal Reflux Disease

Medical

- Thickened feedings[129,130]
- Positioning[66,120,131–133]
- Reduction of gastric acidity[134]
  - H_2 blockade
  - PPI[68–72]
- Prokinetic agents
  - Bethanechol[135]
  - Cisapride[73,74]
  - Metaclopramide[136–139]
  - Erythromycin[75,140,141]

Medical Compared to Surgical Therapy[142]

Surgical

- Fundoplication by laparotomy
  - Nissen procedure[81–83,93,143–146]
  - Thal procedure[88,147]
- Fundoplication by laparoscopy[85–87,91–93]

Three pharmacologic approaches have been used for the treatment of GER. Reduction in gastric acidity with either histamine (H_2) antagonists or proton pump inhibitors (PPIs) and prokinetic agents to accelerate emptying of the stomach are commonly prescribed in the treatment of GERD.

H_2 receptor antagonists[67] are used to reduce gastric acidity by decreasing the release of gastric juice. Ranitidine, cimetidine, and famotidine are the most frequently used medications in this class. When GER is complicated by esophagitis or UGI bleeding, the use of PPI medications is clearly superior to H_2 antagonists. Omeprazole[67,68] and lansoprazole are more potent and produce more sustained inhibition of acid secretion. In contrast to H_2 receptor antagonists, PPIs are especially beneficial in the treatment of erosive esophagitis. Previously documented to be effective in adults with reflux esophagitis, it is now clear that PPIs are effective in the treatment of reflux esophagitis in infants and children. Omeprazole in a dose of 0.7 to 3.3 mg/kg/dose once a day has proven very effective in the short-term control of reflux esophagitis in patients who failed to respond to other classes of gastric acid inhibitors. Subsequently, similar effectiveness has been shown for lansoprazole, 1.5 mg/kg/day (in children 3 months to 14 years of age).[69–71] Other medications in this class include rabeprazole, esomeprazole, and pantoprazole. These medications are all metabolized by cytochrome P450 isoenzyme in the liver.[71] For an in-depth review of the pharmacology of PPI medications, the reader is directed to Furuta and colleagues.[72]

Prokinetic medications may improve sphincter tone and increase esophageal motility, and they have been documented to accelerate gastric emptying . Agents with cholinergic activity, such as metoclopramide and bethanechol, were the first to be prescribed in the treatment of GERD. Bethanechol has the potential for causing increased bronchomotor tone and is not a useful drug in infants and children with GER in whom airway hyperreactivity is their major clinical finding. Metoclopramide (0.1–0.3 mg/kg three or four times daily) has been found to be effective in improving delayed gastric emptying and has been reported to be an effective medication for improving gastroesophageal motility and sphincter tone. This medication has been reported to cause extrapyramidal side effects manifested as acute dystonic reactions. However, this problem is rarely seen with the prescribed dosage. Benadryl is effective in the treatment of pediatric patients experiencing dystonic reaction from metaclopramide therapy. With the withdrawal of the motility agent cisapride[73,74] from use in the United States, besides metoclopramide, erythromycin is now the other available prokinetic agent. Low-dose erythromycin stimulates motility of the stomach and small intestines by binding to sensitive neural motilin receptors to induce antral migrating motor complexes.[75] The mechanism for this pharmacologic effect is different in premature infants, but it has been documented to occur as early as 34 weeks' gestation. Dosage for erythromycin as a prokinetic agent varies with the age of the patient. Premature infants respond to per gastrum dosages of 10 mg/kg administered every 8 hours,[76] and full-term infants have been treated effectively with dosages of 0.75 to 3 mg/kg twice a day.[77] Children have responded to erythromycin dosages of 10 to 20 mg/kg administered orally three to four times a day.[78] The effectiveness of erythromycin as a prokinetic agent may decrease over time in some patients, requiring increasing dosage to achieve continued effectiveness in promoting gastric emptying.

Other considerations in treating pediatric patients with GERD include the fact that in some patients GER is complicated by *Helicobacter pylori* infection. Infection with this organism is a particular risk in pediatric patients who are neurologically impaired.[79] Therefore, when treatment of GER is not effective, further workup might include UGI endoscopy to rule out esophagitis and to obtain cultures for *H. pylori*. In addition, baclofen, a GABA type B receptor agonist, has been reported to reduce gastroesophageal reflux in neurologically impaired children 2 months old to 16 years old in a dosage of 0.7 mg/kg/day administered orally or by nasogastric tube.[80]

SURGICAL

Surgery is indicated for the treatment of GER when medical therapy has not led to an improvement in the gastrointestinal and respiratory findings of GER (see Box 40-5). There are three conditions in which medical management frequently fails and surgical management should be considered. These disorders are esophageal atresia/TEF anomaly following complete surgical repair, profound (usually perinatal) neurologic injury, and severe chronic lung disease of infancy (i.e., bronchopulmonary dysplasia). Unfortunately, many of the infants with GER and severe respiratory illness who fail to respond to medical management are also quite malnourished. These infants are poor surgical candidates and are at risk for postoperative problems with wound healing, respiratory infection, and failure or slippage of the fundoplication and recurrence of GER. In this instance, surgery is best postponed. Patients should be treated with either a nasojejunal feeding tube or total parenteral nutrition, and all oral feedings should be discontinued. The goals of therapy in the preoperative period are to effect improvement in nutrition, prevent further GER and aspiration, and reduce or eliminate symptoms and findings of airway and parenchymal lung disease. Nasogastric drainage is maintained as an adjunct to keep the stomach empty and reduce the risk for GER and further aspiration.

In preparation for antireflux surgery, treatment of airway disease is very important. This may include antibiotics for treatment of pneumonia, chest percussion, postural drainage, and, in infants, pharyngeal suctioning, following chest physical therapy, to provoke cough and aid in the clearance of pulmonary secretions. Bronchodilator medications are better administered as an aerosol or metered-dose inhaler (MDI) rather than per gastrum. Both methylxanthine and β-adrenergic bronchodilator medications have the side effect of reducing distal esophageal pressure and encouraging esophageal reflux. With β-adrenergic agonist aerosol treatments, systemic absorption of the medications is minimized. In order to determine which infants or children with GERD require supplemental oxygen therapy, a number of diagnostic options are available. These include nap or overnight polysomnography with continuous monitoring of transcutaneous oxygen and carbon dioxide tension and oxygen saturation. Interval monitoring and chart recording of oxygen saturation by pulse oximetry is a less sensitive diagnostic study to define which infants will benefit from continuous or intermittent supplemental oxygen therapy.

The appropriate surgical procedure for the treatment of GER depends on the constellation of pathologic gastrointestinal findings.[81] With GER alone, a simple fundoplication is indicated. When the patient also has delayed gastric emptying, fundoplication and pyloroplasty should be considered. In 1987, Fonkalsrud and colleagues[82] reported that in more than 50% of infants and children who were younger than 18 years and were referred for fundoplication, GER was complicated by delayed gastric emptying. Subsequently, in 1995 Fonkalsrud and colleagues[83] reported a retrospective analysis of the use of a combined fundoplication and gastric emptying procedure (pyloroplasty) for the treatment of GER complicated by delayed gastric emptying. They concluded that the procedure was highly effective in relieving the symptoms of reflux and associated pulmonary disease, reversed poor weight gain, and was not associated with undue risk for complications. A final consideration is whether a gastrostomy should be placed: This procedure is indicated when GER is complicated by oral or pharyngeal dysphagia. In these patients, long-term gastrostomy feedings are advisable to avoid the risk for worsening respiratory disease from continued aspiration from above.

In the past 10 years, minimally invasive surgery has become clinically available.[82,84] It is now possible to perform antireflux surgery through laparascopy in appropriate patients. The benefits of this new technique include avoidance of a large laparotomy, fewer respiratory sequelae,[85,86] faster postoperative recovery, less incisional pain, and the option of converting from laparoscopic to open repair should the laparoscopic repair not be technically possible. There are the usual postoperative problems common to both the open and laparoscopic procedure. With the laparoscopic technique, the rare occurrence of gastric volvulus has been reported.[87] Infants and children with respiratory disease and those with neurologic and neurodevelopmental problems appear to be those who benefit most from this less invasive surgery.

In follow-up of infants and children receiving surgical treatment for GER, specific complications and long-term sequelae have been described. Although in adults nearly 50% experience continued symptoms after fundoplication, less than one third of the infants and children undergoing antireflux surgery experience side effects from the surgical procedure. The frequency of long-term problems includes the inability to vomit or even burp in 28%, gas bloating in approximately 36%, slow eating in 32%, and choking on some solids in 25%. In a large series of 335 infants and children treated surgically with a partial fundoplication procedure, Ashcraft and associates in 1981 reported that 9% required reoperation.[88] Of these, 10 patients experienced a "slipped" wrap or disrupted fundoplication, 6 an incisional hernia or dehiscence, 4 a hiatal hernia, and 3 a bowel obstruction. In this review of the literature studies on outcome of fundoplication, 15 series are reviewed comprising close to 10,000 antireflux procedures, including the Nissen, Nissen-Rossetti, Toupet, and Thal procedures.[89] While GERD recurrence varies from 0 to 7.1 in the largest study of 7467 patients, the length of the follow-up also varied from 1 year to 7.3 years in the largest study. Other significant complications included dysphagia in 1% to 19% in the 13 studies that recorded this problem, gas bloat syndrome in 2% to 50% in the 7 studies reporting this complication. Other less frequent complications reported included dumping syndrome, esophageal dysmotility and achalasia. Finally, in a worldwide survey conducted by Bettex and colleagues in 1979,[90] including 3917 operative procedures, a 1.3% fatality rate was reported.

The most recent innovation for repair of GER has been the development of percutaneous surgical techniques for repair of GER.[91] This technique employs a laparoscopic method for the Nissen fundoplication. The benefits are the avoidance of complications such as bowel obstruction secondary to adhesive bands, wound dehiscence, and postoperative pulmonary complications, and a rapid recovery, including early institution of feedings and a shorter hospitalization. Some complications have been reported.[92] These include gastric perforation and hepatic or pleural perforations. Occasionally, a laparoscopic surgery is unsuccessful and the surgeon must be prepared to convert the surgery to an open fundoplication. In a large study comparing the outcome of open versus laparoscopic Nissen repair, the two techniques were shown to have a similar outcome, although the open surgery took approximately 25% longer and the laparoscopic technique was associated with significantly shorter hospitalizations.[93] A newer approach to the treatment of GER in patients who are neurologically impaired is the use of percutaneous gastrostomy technique to place an anterograde percutaneous gastrojejunostomy (APGJ). This technique has been compared to the Nissen fundoplication[94] and was found to have a lower complication rate (33.3% for the Nissen versus 11.8% for the APGJ). In addition, 22.2% of the Nissen patients required reoperation. Thus, the APGJ technique may prove to be a very useful and low-risk procedure for GER patients who might not tolerate a major surgical procedure for correction of GER. Finally, if the APGJ is unsuccessful, percutaneous or open surgery for correction of GER is still an alternative.

The consensus now is that fundoplication is an appropriate treatment for pediatric patients with GER and respiratory illness unresponsive to an adequate course of appropriate medical therapy. The most favorable outcome and the lowest morbidity are achieved when surgery is postponed until the patient is adequately nourished. Surgery should be delayed in malnourished infants or children until patients have had adequate nutritional rehabilitation with total parenteral nutrition as determined by consistent weight gain and skinfold thickness. During this period of parenteral nutrition, patients should not be fed by mouth, and a program of respiratory care, as already outlined, should be undertaken.

REFERENCES

1. Wilson SL, Thach BT, Brouillette RT, Abu-Osba YK: Coordination of breathing and swallowing in human infants. J Appl Physiol 1981;50:851–858.
2. Harding R, Titchen DA: Chemosensitive vagal endings in the esophagus of the cat. J Physiol 1975;247:52P–53P.
3. Sasaki CT, Levine PA, Laitman JT, Crelin ES Jr: Postnatal descent of the epiglottis in man. A preliminary report. Arch Otolaryngol 1977;103:169–171.
4. Sasaki CT, Isaacson G: Functional anatomy of the larynx. Otolaryngol Clin North Am 1988;21:595–612.
5. Menon AP, Shefft GL, Thach BT: Apnea associated with regurgitation in infants. J Pediatr 1985;106:625–629.
6. Menon AP, Shefft GL, Thach BT: Airway protective and abdominal expulsive mechanisms in infantile regurgitation. J Appl Physiol 1985;59:716–721.
7. Davies AM, Koenig JS, Thach BT: Upper airway chemoreflex responses to saline and water aspiration in preterm infants. J Appl Physiol 1988; 64:1412–1420.
8. Pickens DL, Schefft GL, Thach BT: Pharyngeal fluid clearance and aspiration preventive mechanisms in sleeping infants. J Appl Physiol 1989;66: 1164–1171.
9. Griese M, Maderlechner N, Ahrens P, Kitz R: Surfactant proteins A and D in children with pulmonary disease due to gastroesophageal reflux. Am J Respir Crit Care Med 2002;165:1546–1550.
10. Platzker ACG: Congenital anomalies causing respiratory failure. Neonatal Pulmonary Care, 2nd ed. Reading, Mass: Addison-Wesley, 1984, pp 372–406.
11. Rotschild A, Dison PJ, Chitayat D, Solimano A: Mid-facial hypoplasia associated with long-term intubation for bronchopulmonary dysplasia. Am J Dis Child 1990;144:1302–1306.
12. Peterson-Falzone SJ: Velopharyngeal inadequacy in the absence of overt cleft palate. J Craniofacial Gen Devel Biol 1985;1(Suppl):97–124.
13. Tolep K, Getch C, Criner G: Swallowing dysfunction in patients receiving long term mechanical ventilation. Chest 1996;109:167–172.
14. Eibling DE, Gross RD: Subglottic air pressure. A key component of swallowing efficiency. Ann Otol Rhinol Laryngol 1996;105:253–258.
15. Gross RD, Mahlmann J, Grayhack JP: Physiologic effects of open and closed tracheostomy tubes on the pharyngeal swallow. Ann Otol Rhinol Laryngol 2003;112:143–152.
16. Abraham SS, Wolf EL: Swallowing physiology of toddlers with long-term tracheostomies. A preliminary study. Dysphagia 2000;15:206–212.
17. Finder JD, Yellow R, Charron M: Successful management of tracheostomized patients with chronic saliva aspiration by use of constant positive airway pressure. Pediatrics 2001;107:1343–1345.
18. Goodwin SR, Graves SA, Haberkern CM: Aspiration in intubated premature infants. Pediatrics 1985;75:85–88.
19. Belafsky PC, Blumenfeld L, LePage A, Nahrstedt K: The accuracy of the modified Evan's blue test in predicting aspiration. Laryngoscope 2003;113: 1969–1972.
20. Hyman PE: Gastroesophageal reflux. One reason why baby won't eat. J Pediatr 1994;125(Suppl):103–109.
21. Bastian RW: The videoendoscopic swallow study. An alternative and partner to the videofluoroscopic swallow study. Dysphagia 1993;8:359–367.
22. Brady SL, Hildner CD, Hutchins BF: Simultaneous videofluoroscopic swallow study and modified Evan's blue dye procedure: an evaluation of blue dye visualization in cases of known aspiration. Dysphagia 1999;14:146–149.

23. Arena JM: Hydrocarbon poisoning—Current management. Pediatr Ann 1987;16:879–883.
24. Bysani GK, Rucoba RJ, Noah ZL: Treatment of hydrocarbon pneumonitis. Chest 1994;106:300–303.
25. Wolach B, Raz A, Weinberg J, et al: Aspirated foreign bodies in the respiratory tract of children. 11 years experience with 127 patients. Int J Pediatr Otorhinol 1994;30:1–10.
26. Gurwitz D, Kattan M, Levison H, Culham JAG: Pulmonary function abnormalities in asymptomatic children after hydrocarbon pneumonitis. Pediatrics 1978;62:789–794.
27. Cotton EK, Abrams G, Vanhoutte J: Removal of aspirated foreign bodies by inhalation and postural drainage. Clin Pediatr 1973;12:270–276.
28. Mendelson CL: The aspiration of stomach contents into the lungs during obstetric anesthesia. Am J Obstet Gynecol 1946;52:191.
29. Helm JF, Dodds WJ, Pelc LR, et al: Effect of esophageal emptying and saliva on clearance of acid from the esophagus. N Engl J Med 1984; 310:284–288.
30. Boyle JT, Tuchman DN, Altschuler SM, et al: Mechanisms for the association of gastroesophageal reflux and bronchospasm. Am Rev Respir Dis 1985;131(Suppl):S16–S30.
31. Hu FZ, Donfack J, Ahmed A, et al: Fine mapping of a gene for pediatric gastroesophageal reflux on human chromosome 13q14. Hum Genet 2004;114:562–572.
32. Feranchak AP, Orenstein SR, Cohn JF: Behaviors associated with onset of gastroesophageal reflux episodes in infants. Clin Pediatr 1994;33:654–662.
33. Dellert SF, Hyams JS, Treem WR, Geertsman MA: Feeding resistance in gastroesophageal reflux in infancy. J Pediatr Gastroenterol Nutr 1993; 17:66–71.
34. Nielsen DW, Heldt GP, Tooley WH: Stridor and gastroesophageal reflux in infants. Pediatrics 1990;85:1034–1039.
35. Kahn A, Rebuffat E, Sottiaux M, et al: Sleep apneas and acid esophageal reflux in control infants and in infants with apparent life-threatening event. Biol Neonate 1990;57:144–149.
36. Dahshan A, Patel H, Delaney J, et al: Gastroesophageal reflux disease and dental erosion in children. J Pediatr 2002;140:474–478.
37. Carr MM, Poje CP, Ehrig D, Brodsky LS: Incidence of reflux in young children undergoing adenoidectomy. Laryngoscope 2001;111:2170–2172.
38. Orenstein SR, Klein HA, Rosenthal MS: Scintigraphy versus pH probe for quatification of pediatric gastroesophageal reflux. A study using concurrent multiplexed data and acid feedings. J Nucl Med 1993;34: 1228–1234.
39. Tolia V, Kuhns L, Kauffman RE: Comparison of simultaneous esophageal pH monitoring and scintigraphy in infants with gastroesophageal reflux. Am J Gastroenterol 1993;88:661–664.
40. Thomas EJ, Kumar R, Dasan J, et al: Prevalence of silent gastroesophageal reflux in association with recurrent lower respiratory tract infections. Clin Nucl Med 2003;28:476–479.
41. Shay S, Eggli S, Johnson L: Simultaneous esophageal pH monitoring and scintigraphy during postprandial period in patients with severe reflux esophagitis. Dig Dis Sci 1991;36:558–564.
42. Gomes H, Lallemand A, Lallemand P: Ultrasound of the gastroesophageal junction. Pediatr Radiol 1993;24:94–94.
43. Westra SJ, Derkx HHF, Taminiau JAJM: Symptomatic gastroesophageal reflux. Diagnosis with ultrasound. J Pediatr Gastroenterol Nutr 1994;19: 58–64.
44. Colombo JL, Hallberg TK: Recurrent aspiration in children. Lipid-laden alveolar macrophage quantification. Pediatr Pulmonol 1987;3:86–89.
45. Corwin RW, Irwin RS: The lipid-laden alveolar macrophage as a marker of aspiration in parenchymal lung disease. Am Rev Respir Dis 1985;132: 576–581.
46. Moran JR, Block SM, Lyerly AD, et al: Lipid-laden alveolar macrophage and lactose assay as markers of aspiration in neonates with lung disease. J Pediatr 1988;112:643–645.
47. Nussbaum E, Maggi JC, Manthis R, Galant SP: Association of lipid-laden alveolar macrophage and gastroesophageal reflux in children. J Pediatr 1987;110:190–194.
48. Langmore SE, Schatz K, Olson N: Endoscopic and videofluoroscopic evaluations of swallow and aspiration. Otol Rhinol Laryngol 1991;100: 678–681.
49. Tuttle SG, Grossman MI: Detection of gastro-esophageal reflux by simultaneous measurement of intraluminal pressure and pH. Proc Soc Exp Med Biol 1958;98:225–227.
50. Arndorfer RC, Steff JJ, Dodds WJ, et al: Improved infusion system for intraluminal esophageal manometry. Gastroenterology 1977;73:23–27.
51. American Thoracic Society Conference: Aspiration hazards to the developing lung. Am Rev Respir Dis 1985;131(Suppl):1–69.
52. Cohen SR: Cleft larynx. A report of seven cases. Ann Otol Rhinol Laryngol 1975;84:747–756.
53. Euler AR, Ament ME: Detection of gastroesophageal reflux in the pediatric age patient by esophageal intraluminal pH probe measurement (Tuttle test). Pediatrics 1977;60:65–68.
54. Euler AR, Byrne WJ: Twenty-four hour esophageal intraluminal pH probe testing. A comparative analysis. Gastroenterology 1981;80:957–961.
55. Herbst JJ, Book LS, Johnson DG, Jolly S: The lower esophageal sphincter in gastroesophageal reflux. J Clin Gastroenterol 1979;1:119–123.
56. Rudoph CD, Mazur LJ, Liptak GS, et al: Pediatric GE reflux clinical practice guidelines. J Pediatr Gastroenterol Nutr 2001;32(Suppl 2):1–31.
57. Tovar JA, Resti M, Fontana R, et al: Simultaneous esophageal pH monitoring and the diagnosis of alkaline reflux. J Pediatr Surg 1993;28: 1386–1392.
58. Brown CM, Snowdon CF, Slee B, et al: Measurement of bicarbonate output from the intact human esophagus. Gut 1993;34: 872–880.
59. Graff MA, Kashian F, Carter M, et al: Nap studies underestimate the incidence of gastroesophageal reflux. Pediatr Pulmonol 1994;18:258–260.
60. Ahrens P, Noll C, Kitz R, et al: Lipid-laden alveolar macrophages (LLAM). A useful marker of silent aspiration in children. Pediatr Pulmonol 1999;28: 83–88.
61. Allewelt M, Schuler P, Bolcskei PL, et al: Ampicillin + sublactam vs clindamycin ± cephalosporin for the treatment of aspiration pneumonia and primary lung abscess. Clin Microbiol Infect 2004;10:163–170.
62. Brook I, Finegold SM: Bacteriology of aspiration pneumonia in children. Pediatrics 1980;65:1115–1120.
63. Sukumaran M, Granada MJ, Berger HW, et al: Evaluation of corticosteroid treatment in aspiration of gastric contents. A controlled clinical trial. Mt Sinai J Med 1980;47:335–340.
64. Liangthanasarn P, Nemet D, Sufi R, Nussbaum E: Therapy for pulmonary aspiration of polyethylene glycol solution. J Pediatr Gastroenterol Nutr 2003;37:192–194.
65. Ciravegna B, Sacco, Moroni C, et al: Mineral oil lipoid pneumonia in a child with anoxic encephalopathy. Treatment by whole lung lavage. Pediatric Pulmonol 1997;23:233–237.
66. Wenzl TG, Schenider S, Scheele F, et al: Effects of thickened feedings on gastroesophageal reflux in infants. A placebo-controlled crossover study using intraluminal impedance. Pediatrics 2003;111:e355–e399.
67. Kelly DA: Do H2 receptor antagonists have a therapeutic role in childhood? J Pediatr Gastroenterol Nutr 1994;19:270–276.
68. Gunasekaran TS, Hassall EG: Efficacy and safety of omeprazole for severe gastroesophageal reflux in children. J Pediatr 1993;123:148–154.
69. Franco MT, Salvia G, Terrin G, et al: Lansoprazole in the treatment of gastroesophageal reflux disease in childhood. Dig Liver Dis 2000;32: 660–666.
70. Colleti RB, DiLorenzo C: Overview of pediatric gastroesophageal reflux disease and proton pump inhibitor therapy. J Pediatr Gastroenterol Nutr 2003;37(Suppl):7–11.
71. Li X-Q, Andersson TB, Ahlström M, Weidolf L: Comparison of inhibitory effects of the proton pump-inhibiting drugs omeprazole, esomeprazole, lansoprazole, pantoprazole and rabeprazole on human cytochrome P450 activities. Drug Metab Dispos 2004;32:821–827.
72. Furuta T, Shirai N, Sugimoto M, et al: Pharmacogenomics of proton pump inhibitors. Pharmacogenomics 2004;5:181–202.
73. Barone JA, Jessen LM, Colaizzi JL, Bierman RH: Cisapride. A gastrointestinal prokinetic agent. Ann Pharmacotherapy 1994;28:488–500.
74. Tucci F, Resti M, Fontana R, et al: Gastroesophageal reflux and bronchial asthma. Prevalence and effect of cisapride therapy. J Pediatr Gastroenterol Nutr 1993;17:265–270.
75. Tack J, Janssens J, Vantrappen G, et al: Dose-related effect of erythromycin on gastroduodenal motility and plasma motilin levels. Studies in healthy volunteers and in patients with diabetic gastroparesis. Gastroenterology 1992;103:72–79.
76. Costalos C, Gounaris A, Varhalama E, et al: Erythromycin as a prokinetic agent in preterm infants. J Pediatr Gastroenterol Nutr 2002;34:23–25.
77. Jadcherla SR, Berseth CL: Effect of gastroduodenal contractile activity in developing neonates. J Pediatr Gastroenterol Nutr 2002;34:16–22.
78. Takatomo C, ed: Pediatric Dosing Handbook and Formulary, 17th ed. Hudson, Ohio: Lexi-Comp, 2004.
79. Pollet S, Gottrand F, Vincent P, et al: Gastroesophageal reflux disease and Helicobacter pylori infection in neurologically impaired children. Inter-relations and therapeutic implications. J Pediatr Gastroenterol Nutrition 2004;38:70–74.

80. Kawai M, Kawahara H, Hirayama S, et al: Effect of Baclofen on emesis and 24 hour esophageal pH in neurologically impaired children with gastroesophageal reflux. J Pediatr Gastroenterol Nutr 2004;38:317–323.
81. Foglia RP, Fonkalsrud EW, Ament ME, et al: Gastroesophageal fundoplication for the management of chronic pulmonary disease in children. Am J Surg 1980;140:72.
82. Fonkalsrud EW, Berquist W, Vargas J, et al: Surgical treatment of gastroesophageal reflux syndrome in infants and children. Am J Surg 1987;154:111–118.
83. Fonkalsrud EW, Ellis DG, Shaw A, et al: A combined hospital experience with fundoplication and gastric emptying procedure for gastroesophageal reflux in children. J Am Coll Surg 1995;180:449–455.
84. Collins JB, Georgeson KE, Vincente Y, Hardin WD Jr: Comparison of open and laparoscopic gastrostomy and fundoplication in 120 patients. J Pediatr Surg 1995;30:1065–1071.
85. Tashjian DB, Tirabassi MV, Moriarty KP, Salva PS: Laparoscopic Nissen fundoplication for reactive airways disease. J Pediatr Surg 2002;37:1021–1023.
86. Powers CJ, Levitt MA, Tantoco J, et al: The respiratory advantage of laparoscopic Nissen fundoplication. J Pediatr Surg 2003;38:886–891.
87. Kuenzler KA, Wolfson PH, Murphy SG: Gastric volvulus after laparoscopic Nissen fundoplication with gastrostomy. J Pediatr Surg 2003;38:1241–1243.
88. Ashcraft KW, Holder TM, Amoury RA: Treatment of gastroesophageal reflux in children by Thal fundoplication. J Thorac Cardiovasc Surg 1981;82:706–712.
89. DiLorenzo C, Orenstein S: Fundoplication Friend or Foe? J Pediatr Gastroenterol Nutr 2002;34:117–124.
90. Bettex M, Oesch-Amrein I, Kuffer F: Mortality after operation for hiatus hernia. Prog Pediatr Surg 1979;13:245–252.
91. Lobe TE: Laparoscopic fundoplication. Semin Pediatr Surg 1993;2:178–181.
92. Cadière GB, Houben JJ, Bruyns J, et al: Laparoscopic Nissen fundoplication. Technique and preliminary results. Br J Surg 1994;81:400–403.
93. Peters JH, Heimbucher J, Kauer WKH, et al: Clinical and physiologic comparison of laparoscopic and open Nissen fundoplication. J Am Coll Surg 1995;180:385–393.
94. Albanese CT, Towbin RB, Ulman I, et al: Percutaneous gastrojejunostomy versus Nissen fundoplication for enteral feeding of the neurologically impaired child with gastroesophageal reflux. J Pediatr 1993;123:371–375.
95. Loughlin GM: Respiratory consequences of dysfunctional swallowing and aspiration. Dysphagia 1989;3:126–130.
96. Tuchman DN, Boyle JT, Pack AI, et al: Comparison of airway responses following tracheal or esophageal acidification in the cat. Gastroenterology 1984;87:872–881.
97. Arvedson J, Rogers B, Buck G, et al: Silent aspiration prominent in children with dysphagia. Int J Pediatr Otorhinolaryngol 1994;28:173–181.
98. Jolley SG, Herbst JJ, Johnson DG, et al: Esophageal pH monitoring during sleep identifies children with respiratory symptoms from gastroesophageal reflux. Gastroenterology 1981;80:1501–1506.
99. Logan WJ, Bosma JF: Oral and pharyngeal dysphagia in infancy. Pediatr Clin North Am 1967;14:47–61.
100. Evans JNG: Management of the cleft larynx and tracheoesophageal clefts. Ann Otol Rhinol Laryngol 1985;94:627–630.
101. Ashcraft KW, Goodwin C, Amoury RA, Holder TM: Early recognition and aggressive treatment of gastroesophageal reflux following repair of esophageal atresia. J Pediatr Surg 1977;12:317–321.
102. Benjamin B, Inglis A: Minor congenital laryngeal clefts. Diagnosis and classification. Ann Otolaryngol Rhinol Laryngol 1989;98:417–420.
103. Parker AF, Christie DL, Cahill JL: Incidence and significance of gastroesophageal reflux following repair of esophageal atresia and tracheoesophageal fistula and the need for antireflux procedures. J Pediatr Surg 1979;14:5–8.
104. Pieretti R, Shandling B, Stephens CA: Resistant esophageal stenosis associated with reflux after repair of esophageal atresia. A therapeutic approach. J Pediatr Surg 1974;9:355–357.
105. Cotton RT, Schreiber JT: Management of laryngotracheo-esophageal cleft. Ann Otol Rhinol Laryngol 1981;90:401–405.
106. Jolley SG, McClelland KK, Mosesso-Rousseau M: Pharyngeal and swallowing disorders in infants. Semin Pediatr Surg 1995;4:157–165.
107. Tuchman DN: Cough, choke, sputter. The evaluation of the child with dysfunctional swallowing. Dysphagia 1989;3:111–116.
108. Blank RH, Silbiger M: Cricopharyngeal achalasia as a cause of respiratory distress in infancy. J Pediatr 1972;81:95–98.
109. Furuya ME, Martinez I, Zuniga-Vasquez G, Hernandez-Contreras I: Lipoid pneumonia in children. Clinical and imagenological manifestations. Arch Med Res 2000;31:42–47.
110. O'Neill JA, Holcomb GW, Neblett WW: Management of tracheobronchial and esophageal foreign bodies in childhood. J Pediatr Surg 1983;18:475–479.
111. Steen K, Zimmerman T: Tracheo-bronchial aspiration of foreign bodies in children. A study of 94 cases. Laryngoscope 1990;100:525–529.
112. Hoeve LJ, Rombout J, Pot DJ: Foreign body aspiration in children. The diagnostic value of signs, symptoms and pre-operative examination. Clin Otolaryngol Allied Sci 1993;18:55–57.
113. Van Looij MA, Rood PP, Hoeve LJ, Borgstein JA: Aspirated foreign body in children. Why are they more commonly found on the left? Clin Otolaryngol Sci 2003;28:364–367.
114. McDonald JW, Roggli VL, Bradford WD: Co-existing endogenous exogenous lipoid pneumonia and pulmonary alveolar proteinosis in a patient with neurodevelopmental disease. Pediatr Pathol 1994;14:505–511.
115. Radford PJ, Stillwell PC, Blue B, Hertel G: Aspiration complicating bronchopulmonary dysplasia. Chest 1995;107:185–188.
116. Macfadyen UM, Hendry GMA, Simpson H: Gastro-oesophageal reflux in near-miss sudden infant death syndrome or suspected recurrent aspiration. Arch Dis Child 1983;58:87–91.
117. Darling DB, McCauley RGK, Leonidas JC, Schwartz AM: Gastroesophageal reflux in infants and children. Correlation of radiologic severity and pulmonary pathology. Radiology 1978;127:735–740.
118. Ghaed N, Stein MR: Assessment of a technique for scintographic monitoring of pulmonary aspiration of gastric contents in asthmatics with gastroesophageal reflux. Ann Allergy 1979;42:306–308.
119. Blumhagen JD, Rudd TG, Christie DL: Gastroesophageal reflux in children. Radionuclide gastroesophagography. Am J Roentgenol 1980;135:1001–1004.
120. Jona JZ, Sty JR, Glicklich M: Simplified radioisotope technique for assessing gastroesophageal reflux in children. J Pediatr Surg 1981;16:114–117.
121. Russell CO, Hill LD, Holmes ER III, et al: Radionuclide transit. A sensitive screening test of esophageal dysfunction. Gastroenterology 1981;80:887–892.
122. Johnson LF, Demeester TR: 24 hour pH monitoring in the study of gastroesophageal reflux. J Clin Gastroenterol 1974;62:325–337.
123. Fink SM, McCallum RW: The role of prolonged esophageal pH monitoring in the diagnosis of gastroesophageal reflux. JAMA 1984;252:1160–1164.
124. Sondheimer JM, Haase GA: Simultaneous pH recordings from multiple sites in children with and without distal gastroesophageal reflux. J Pediatr Gastroenterol Nutr 1988;7:46–51.
125. Vandeplas Y, Sacre-Smits L: Continuous 24-hour esophageal monitoring in 285 asymptomatic infants 0–15 months old. J Pediatr Gastroenterol Nutr 1987;6:220–224.
126. Berquist WE, Ament ME: Upper GI function in sleeping infants. Am Rev Respir Dis 1985;131(Suppl):S26–S29.
127. Boonyaprapa S, Alderson PO, Garfinkel DJ, et al: Detection of pulmonary aspiration in infants and children with respiratory disease. Concise communication. J Nucl Med 1980;21:314–318.
128. Hopper AO, Kwong LK, Stevenson DK, et al: Detection of gastric contents in tracheal fluid of infants by lactose assay. J Pediatr 1983;102:415–418.
129. Bailey DJ, Andres JM, Danek GD, Pinero-Carrero VM: Lack of efficacy of thickened feedings as treatment for gastroesophageal reflux. J Pediatr 1987;110:187–189.
130. Orenstein SR, Magill HL, Brooks P: Thickening of infant feedings for therapy of gastroesophageal reflux. J Pediatr 1987;110:181–186.
131. Myers WF, Herbst JJ: Effectiveness of positioning therapy for gastroesophageal reflux. Pediatrics 1982;69:768–772.
132. Orenstein SR, Whitington PF: Positioning for prevention of infant gastroesophageal reflux. J Pediatr 1983;103:534–537.
133. Orenstein SR, Whitington PF, Orenstein DM: The infant seat as treatment for gastroesophageal reflux. N Engl J Med 1983;309:760–763.
134. Higgs RH, Smyth RD, Castell DO: Gastric alkalinization. Effect on lower-esophageal sphincter pressure and serum gastrin. N Engl J Med 1974;291:486–490.
135. Euler AR: Use of bethanechol for the treatment of gastroesophageal reflux. J Pediatr 1980;96:321–324.
136. Harrington RA, Hamilton CW, Brogden RN, et al: Metoclopramide. An updated review of its pharmacological properties and clinical use. Drugs 1983;25:451–494.

137. Berquist WE, Rachelefsky GS, Rowshan N, et al: Quantitative gastroesophageal reflux and pulmonary function in asthmatic children and normal adults receiving placebo, theophylline, and metoclopramide sulfate therapy. J Allergy Clin Immunol 1984;73:253–258.
138. Hyams JS, Leichtner AM, Zamett LO, Walters JK: Effect of metoclopramide on prolonged intraesophageal pH testing in infants with gastroesophageal reflux. J Pediatr Gastroenterol Nutr 1986;5:716–720.
139. Machida HM, Forbes DA, Gall DG, Scott RB: Metoclopramide in gastroesophageal reflux. J Pediatr 1988;112:483–487.
140. Costalos C, Gounaris A, Varhalama E, et al: Erythromycin as a prokinetic agent in premature infants. J Pediatr Gastroenterol Nutr 2002;34:23–25.
141. Jadcherla SR, Berseth CL: Effect of erythromycin on gastroduodenal contractile activity in developing neonates. J Pediatric Gastroenterol Nutr 2002;34:16–22.
142. Wilkinson JD, Dudgeon DL, Sondheimer JM: A comparison of medical and surgical treatment of gastroesophageal reflux. J Pediatr 1981;99:202.
143. Nissen R: Gastropexy and "fundoplication" in surgical treatment of hiatal hernia. Am J Dig Dis 1961;6:954–961.
144. Harnsberger JK, Corey JJ, Johnson DG, Herbst JJ: Long-term follow-up of surgery for gastroesophageal reflux in infants and children. J Pediatr 1983;102:505–508.
145. Giuffre RM, Rubin S, Mitchell I: Antireflux surgery in infants with bronchopulmonary dysplasia. Am J Dis Child 1987;141:648–651.
146. Byrne WJ, Euler AR, Ashcraft E, et al: Gastroesophageal reflux in the severely retarded who vomit. Criteria for and results of surgical intervention. Surgery 1982;91:95–98.
147. Thal AP: A unified approach to surgical problems of the esophagastric junction. Ann Surg 1968;168:542–550.

SUGGESTED READING

Davies H, Gordon I, Matthews DJ: Long term follow up of inhalation of foreign body. Arch Dis Child 1990;65:619–621.

Hyman S, Respondek M: Detection of pulmonary aspiration in children by radionuclide "salivagram." J Nucl Med 1989;30:697–699.

Orenstein SR, Shalaby TM, Finch R, et al: Autosomal dominant infantile gastroesophageal reflux disease. Exclusion of a 13q14 locus in five well characterized families. Am J Gastroenterol 2002;97:2725–2732.

Spitzer AR, Boyle JT, Tuchman DN, Fox WW: Awake apnea associated with gastroesophageal reflux. A specific clinical syndrome. J Pediatr 1984; 104:200.

41 Foreign Body Aspiration

Robin T. Cotton, MD • Michael J. Rutter, MD

Inhalations and ingestions are common and potentially fatal pediatric accidents. In 1984, aspiration or ingestion of food or foreign objects accounted for 271 deaths in children younger than 5 years in the United States.[1] This has not changed substantively in recent decades.[2] Ninety percent of children who aspirate foreign bodies (FBs) are younger than 3 years and two thirds are boys.[3] There are several reasons for this: toddlers lack discretion concerning objects ingested, exploring the environment by oral tactile sensation; they lack molar teeth and thus chew food poorly; and they often engage in play while eating. Most foreign objects are coughed or regurgitated spontaneously via protective refluxes, or pass unimpeded through the alimentary tract. Some, however, become impacted within the upper aerodigestive tract. Food and toys account for approximately 90% of FB aspiration in children.[2] Nuts, and most especially peanuts, are the most common inhaled objects. In a survey of 103 food-related asphyxiation episodes in children, the hot dog impacted in the upper airway or upper esophagus was the single most common agent in this type of death.[4] In 1984, the National Safety Council identified FB aspiration or ingestion as the fourth leading cause of accidental death in this age group and as the third leading cause in infants younger than 1 year. Recently, fruit gel snacks have been reported as a serious cause of FB aspiration.[5]

Advances in radiology, anesthesia, and endoscopic instrumentation have improved patient care and lowered the complication rate associated with the treatment of upper aerodigestive tract FBs. Hopkins rod lens telescopes coupled to ventilating bronchoscopes, esophagoscopes, and grasping FB forceps provide superior visualization for inspection of the esophagus and tracheobronchial tree, making extraction of foreign objects more controlled than in decades past. Development of new anesthetic agents and the use of physiologic monitoring devices as a standard technique have resulted in improved safety for the delivery of general anesthesia to young children. In children, flexible bronchoscopy has a limited role in the diagnosis of FB of the upper aerodigestive tract and a minimal role in the extraction, which is performed using rigid endoscopes. However, prevention remains the benchmark for measurement of further improvements in childhood safety.[6]

PATIENT ASSESSMENT

HISTORY

FB location may be supraglottic, glottic, subglottic, tracheal, bronchial, or esophageal. The manifestations of aspiration depend on the size of the FB, its composition, its location, the degree of blockage, and the duration of obstruction. Except in the rare instance of impending asphyxia due to an impacted laryngeal FB, time exists for a careful history, physical examination, and radiologic examination. History is of paramount importance in the diagnosis of FB aspiration because the physical examination and radiographic study can be unremarkable as time passes after the acute event. The characteristic history of a choking or gagging episode, followed by a coughing spell, should be carefully considered from the caretakers.[7] Serious attention should be directed to such a history witnessed while the child was eating nuts, seeds, beans, or carrots, the primary culprits in FB aspiration in younger children. Nuts and vegetables account for approximately 80% of aspirated FBs, while plastic, wooden, or metal objects are aspirated much less often.[8]

Most inhaled FBs travel distally into the tracheobronchial tree, but laryngeal impaction occasionally occurs and accounts for the highest rate of mortality in the aerodigestive tract (45%).[9] Survivors of transient obstruction also carry a risk for hypoxic encephalopathy. Large objects such as hot dogs or balloons are apt to obstruct the glottic inlet and precipitate acute respiratory arrest (Fig. 41-1). These children may survive if resuscitated by caretakers, paramedics, or emergency physicians. In the rare instance in which the child is blue and apneic, the adult should quickly look into the back of the child's throat and remove any visible object that is identified. Blind finger sweeps in the pharynx, however, are discouraged, because the FB may easily be pushed further into the airway during such attempts. Mouth-to-mouth resuscitation is ineffective if the upper airway is completely blocked. Specific recommendations for the acute management of the choking child depends on his or her age.[10] The Heimlich maneuver is the preferred technique for pediatric FB airway obstruction in toddlers and older children, but a combination of chest thrusts and back blows is preferred for infants.

Fortunately, most smaller, nonobstructing objects bypass the supraglottis, glottis, and trachea and lodge most commonly in the right main stem bronchus. Depending on the size, location, and nature of the FB, local irritation produces complaints that include cough, inspiratory stridor, hoarseness, wheezing, shortness of breath, and fever, symptoms that mimic the more common diseases of the respiratory tract, including asthma, bronchiolitis, laryngitis, pharyngitis, and croup. Symptoms may occur within hours of the aspiration or weeks later. Thus, some aspirated FBs may go unrecognized for weeks or longer.

The absence of obvious symptoms after a witnessed choking episode does not exclude the presence of a retained FB. Following the initial episode of paroxysmal coughing, an asymptomatic lag period occurs as the surface sensory receptors of the respiratory tract undergo physiologic adaptation. This situation may falsely reassure the parent and the physician that the child has cleared the airway. Only two thirds of patients seek treatment within 1 week following aspiration.[11] Thus, the first symptoms prompting medical attention may represent a complication of FB impaction, such as chronic cough and fever due to recurrent or persistent pneumonia, bronchitis, or even bronchiectasis. Atypical asthma is a common misdiagnosis assigned to unsuspected airway FBs.[8] Physician-related factors still account for the largest portion of delay in diagnosis, with

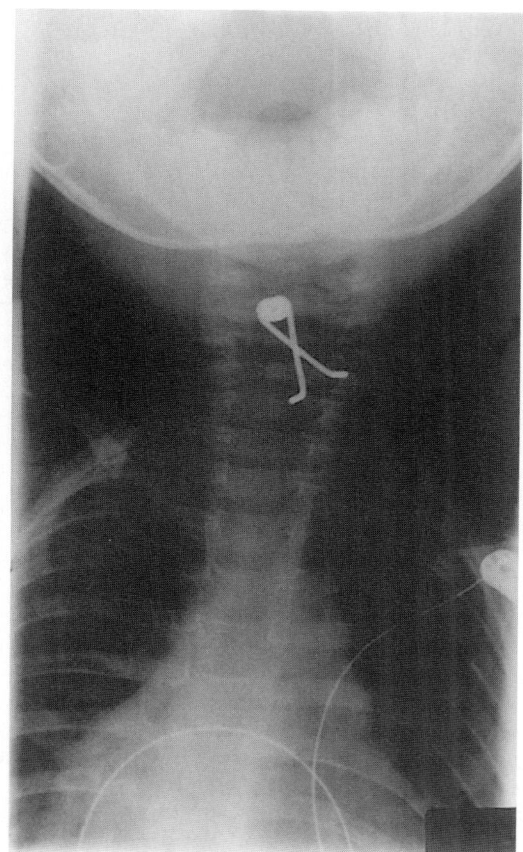

■ **FIGURE 41-1.** Metal spring from clothespin impacted in larynx.

reliance on a negative radiographic report being one of the most important factors.[2] Subglottic FBs present unique clinical challenges.[12] The majority of FBs in this location are delayed in diagnosis and may likely present as protracted episodes of stridor, croup, or hoarseness. Tracheobronchial FBs in the neonatal intensive care unit (almost always portions of a suction catheter) present very special diagnostic and management challenges.[13]

PHYSICAL EXAMINATION

Physical findings following aspiration are variable and dependent on the location and degree of luminal obstruction by the FB. The child may be quiet and comfortable or exhibit signs of respiratory distress ranging from mild tachypnea to severe stridor with retractions and cyanosis. Classic physical findings in case of FB aspiration consist of unilateral decreased breath sounds as a result of decreased aeration of the lung and unilateral rhonchi due to partial occlusion of the bronchus. The clinical triad of wheezing, coughing, and diminished or absent breath sounds is present in only about 40% of patients,[14] although 75% have one or more of these findings. Rapid changes in respiratory status may occur due to development of edema or change in location of the FB. Tracheal FBs are particularly treacherous in this regard, with patients alternating between periods of normality and severe obstruction due to a ball-valving effect.

Findings on physical examination will help to localize an airway FB. If there is significant obstruction to local air flow, FBs in the larynx or upper cervical trachea produce aphonia or hoarseness with inspiratory or biphasic stridor. A prolonged wheeze in the expiratory phase is suggestive of intrathoracic tracheal or bronchial obstruction. Stridor is frequently absent with smaller objects at any airway location. Careful auscultation of the neck and chest is an important part of an examination. A discrepancy in intensity of timing of breath sounds between sides of the chest and unilateral wheezing are findings of great significance, because the majority of aspirated objects impact in the right or left main stem bronchus. More complex physical findings occur if there are multiple FBs. In many cases, however, the signs are subtle, and it is important to appreciate that the physical examination may be normal.

Flexible nasolaryngoscopy may add valuable diagnostic information when inspiratory stridor is the sole physical finding and a laryngeal or hypopharyngeal FB is suspected by history. Laryngomalacia or inflammatory etiologies of stridor also may be identified. This examination should be performed using topical anesthesia in the awake, nonsedated, upright child. It should be performed with extreme caution in small children with severe obstruction or when supraglottitis is suspected, and should only be performed when airway resuscitative equipment is immediately available. When performed appropriately and correctly, this procedure is very safe.

RADIOGRAPHY

After a thorough history and physical examination, plain neck and chest radiographs should be obtained. About 10% of aspirated FBs are radiopaque, making the radiologic diagnosis easy (Fig. 41-2). However, the majority of FBs are not obvious, and changes seen are secondary to the obstruction of the airway by the object. Anteroposterior and lateral views of the neck and chest may reveal signs of a partially obliterated tracheobronchial air column (Fig. 41-3) or abnormal ventilation of the affected lung. Inspiratory and expiratory views are very important. The classic radiographic abnormality is unilateral hyperlucency on an expiratory film. A ball-valve effect of a partial occlusion of the bronchus allows air to enter the affected lobe or lung on inspiration but traps the air on expiration[15] (Fig. 41-4). Other studies that may demonstrate unilateral air trapping are decubitus views of the chest or chest fluoroscopy. Indirect radiologic signs include resorption atelectasis, compensatory emphysema of the contralateral lung, pneumonia, pneumothorax, and expiratory shift of the mediastinum. Late findings such as pulmonary abscess or bronchiectasis are still occasionally seen. Lobar or segmental pulmonary infiltrate from impaired clearance of respiratory secretions usually implies obstruction of days or weeks (Fig. 41-5). Although radiography is useful for confirmation and localization of FB aspiration, up to 25% of bronchial FBs, and over half of those in the trachea, yield no abnormalities on plain chest radiographs.[11] For this reason, FB aspiration can never be excluded on the basis of a chest radiograph alone. Operative intervention is based on history and physical examination, and should not be changed because of a negative radiographic study.[16,17] Fluoroscopy has a greater diagnostic sensitivity than inspiratory and expiratory radiographs and may be appropriate in some cases. Just as migration of the FB in the airways leads to changing clinical patterns, so do changes in radiographic findings occur.

A final diagnosis is only achieved at the time of bronchoscopic examination. Because the clinical and radiographic

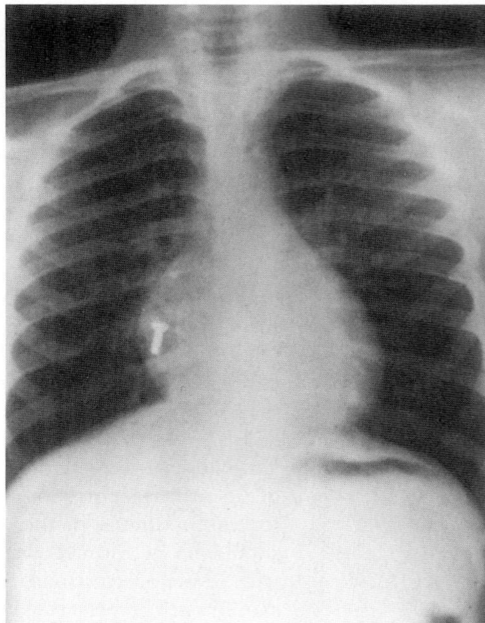
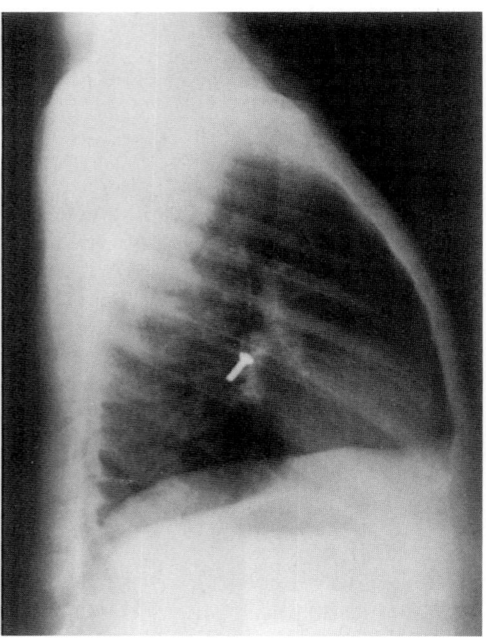

■ **FIGURE 41-2.** Posteroanterior and lateral roentgenograms of a screw aspirated into the right lower lobe of the lung.

findings can be variable and mimic so many different pulmonary conditions, it is inevitable that a proportion of endoscopic evaluations will be performed without finding an FB. It is certainly preferable to perform a negative endoscopic evaluation than to leave an FB undiagnosed.

■ MANAGEMENT

■ ANESTHESIA

Once the diagnosis of an aspirated FB is considered, it is the duty of the treating physician to confirm its presence and proceed with removal or to eliminate it from the differential diagnosis. Direct laryngoscopy and bronchoscopy in the pediatric population are most safely accomplished under general anesthesia with spontaneous ventilation, choosing from the state-of-the-art Hopkins rod lens telescopes presently available. In most cases, endoscopy should be undertaken expeditiously to decrease the hazard of complication, particularly in children with laryngeal obstruction or with suspected vegetable objects that swell in contact with respiratory secretions and become tightly impacted in the airway. A complete main stem bronchial obstruction causing unilateral pulmonary hypoventilation is a particularly dangerous situation, especially if it has been present for some hours or days; should the FB or a sizeable fragment migrate to the contralateral main stem bronchus, abrupt blockage of ventilation to the lung that has the only functional alveoli can lead to acute respiratory decompensation.

With the exception of impending death due to severe laryngeal obstruction, "crash" endoscopy is not recommended. The patient's status and the availability of medical personnel must be carefully assessed. If respiratory distress is not severe, it is appropriate to allow time for gastric emptying, which decreases the anesthetic risk. It is important to allow time to assemble the instruments, surgeon, anesthesiologist, and operative staff experienced in pediatric airway management. An inexperienced team is more likely not to have appropriate instruments, leading to a difficult extraction or even a major complication. Because there are no good alternative therapies, the patient's condition should be assessed carefully in this situation and transfer planned to a center capable of taking care of the problem.

There is no place for primarily medical therapy involving the inhalation of bronchodilators and chest physiotherapy.[18] This carries a significant risk for cardiopulmonary arrest associated with FB migration during therapy.

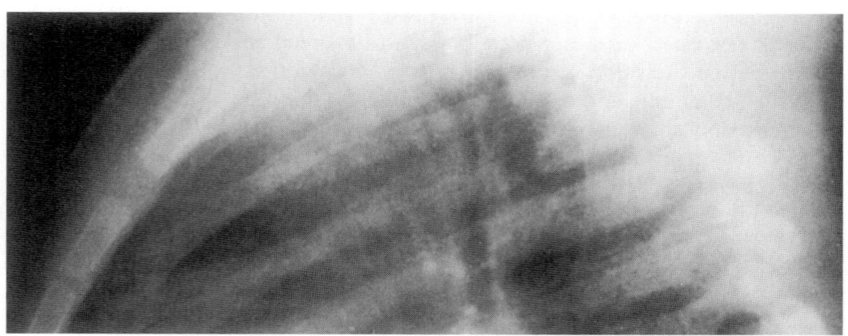

■ **FIGURE 41-3.** Lateral chest roentgenogram showing an aspirated peanut in the thoracic trachea just proximal to the carina.

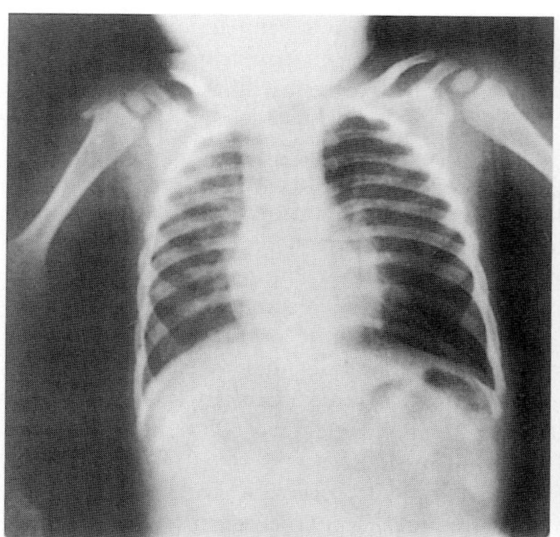
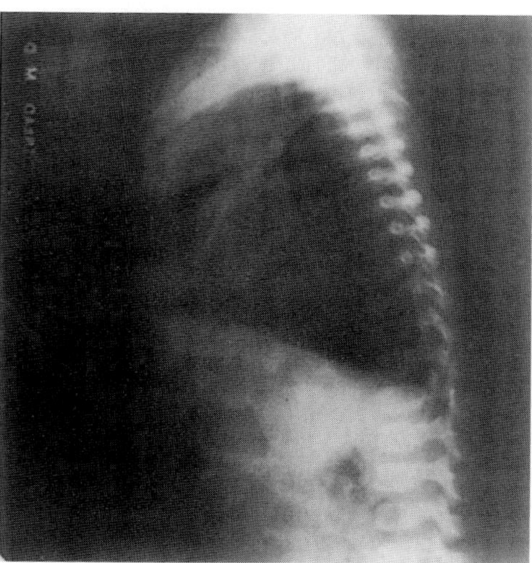

■ **FIGURE 41-4.** Air trapping of the left lower lobe of the lung due to an aspirated peanut.

The pediatric airway is small and, when compromised by an FB, the potential for sudden deterioration on induction of anesthesia should be uppermost in the minds of the treating medical personnel. A full complement of endoscopic equipment of size appropriate to the patient, including laryngoscopes, ventilating bronchoscopes, FB forceps with rod lens, suction devices, and light cables, must be selected, assembled, tested, and ready to use prior to the administration of any anesthetic agent. All efforts should be made to obtain a duplicate of the FB to allow the endoscopist to select the best extraction forceps and to practice the extraction technique prior to the actual procedure. A dress rehearsal should be routine.

Besides controlling ventilation, the anesthesiologist must continuously monitor the patient's oxygenation, cardiovascular parameters, and temperature. Perioperative steroids may help to decrease any edema associated with bronchoscopic manipulation. Maintenance of spontaneous ventilation is preferred via the bronchoscope, and intubation with an endotracheal tube is to be avoided. If the FB is impacted in the larynx or upper trachea, the surgeon should have a tracheotomy tray ready for instant use in the operating room in the rare circumstance that the anesthesiologist is unable to control the airway satisfactorily and ventilation is seriously impaired.

The majority opinion considers the use of flexible bronchoscopy in the management of airway FBs in children to be minor and restricted largely to diagnosis rather than extraction. Even those who advocate flexible bronchoscopy in the management of airway FBs caution that provisions for immediate rigid bronchoscopic management should be made if attempts at flexible bronchoscopic extraction fail.[19] Rigid bronchoscopy remains the standard of care for management of tracheobronchial FBs in children.[20]

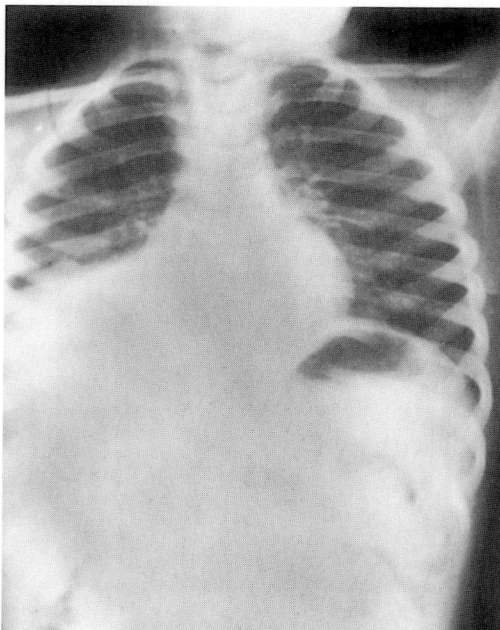
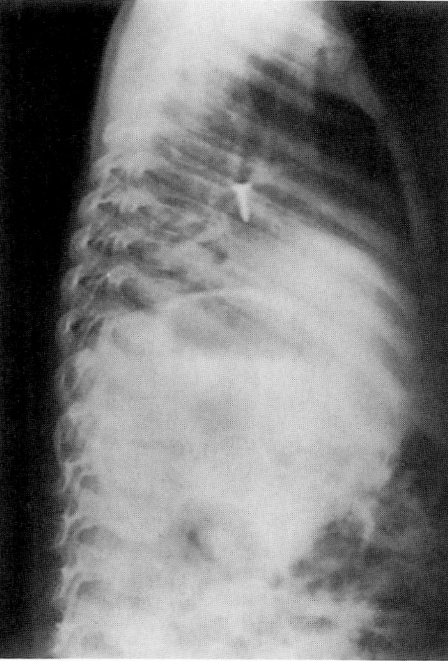

■ **FIGURE 41-5.** Atelectasis and pneumonia of the right lower lobe of the lung due to a screw aspirated into the right lower lobe approximately 96 hours before these roentgenograms were made.

ENDOSCOPY AND FOREIGN BODY REMOVAL

After topically anesthetizing the larynx and examining the larynx and hypopharynx for possible FBs, a ventilating bronchoscope of suitable size is inserted and spontaneous ventilation maintained. The bronchoscope is advanced to the point of FB impaction. Once the FB and its presentation have been identified and studied, the telescope is withdrawn, leaving the bronchoscopic sheath in place. An appropriate grasping forceps with its companion telescope is inserted via the sheath prior to FB removal. To help maintain ventilation, it may be necessary to place the bronchoscope in such a position that the ventilating ports are above the carina to maintain adequate ventilation of the patient via the unobstructed contralateral bronchus.

FB extraction requires considerable care to avoid traumatizing the mucosa or pushing the object peripherally out of reach of the forceps. Smaller objects or fragments can occasionally be withdrawn into the bronchoscope, but more commonly the object will be too big to enter the lumen of the bronchoscope. Under these circumstances, the object must be held close to the tip of the bronchoscope, and all is removed as a single unit. Continuous dialogue between the surgeon and the anesthesiologist increases the safety of the patient. Should the FB become dislodged during the extraction process, the bronchoscope must be reinserted to push the object distally far enough to establish controlled ventilation, and a further attempt at extraction is made. Under rare circumstances the object may be too big to be withdrawn through the glottis. Should this occur, a tracheostomy is performed over the bronchoscope and the FB retrieved through the tracheotomy site. After FB removal, repeat bronchoscopy should be performed, looking for multiple objects or fragments of the original object. In addition, thorough aspiration of the bronchial tree distal to the site of the FB impaction will aid postoperative reexpansion of collapsed lung parenchyma. Granulation tissue should be left untouched, since it will resolve quickly after FB removal.

The Fogarty catheter has been employed to remove an impacted FB.[21] This tool must be used with much caution, because the balloon tip may break and become a second FB.[22]

The extraction of sharp objects necessitates special attention, using techniques such as sheathing the point within the bronchoscope to protect the respiratory mucosa during the withdrawal. The vast majority of airway FBs are managed successfully by endoscopic techniques. In rare cases when there is major impaction or severe chronic inflammatory changes secondary to delay in diagnosis, endoscopic removal may be impossible and thoracostomy is indicated (Fig. 41-6).

Particularly dangerous for babies is the aspiration of baby powder, which requires urgent lavage of the bronchial system.[23]

POSTOPERATIVE MANAGEMENT

Antibiotics and humidification should be considered if the FB has been present long enough to cause significant pulmonary infection. Steroids may be indicated if there is significant inflammatory edema or edema caused endoscopic removal. Chest physiotherapy is indicated to mobilize retained secretions in an effort to avoid or manage pneumonia, the most common clinically significant complication. Segmental atelectasis may occur for a few days after endoscopy, and this should initially be treated with the above measures. Persistence of respiratory symptoms such as cough, wheezing, and fever or persistent radiographic changes more than a few days after FB removal should

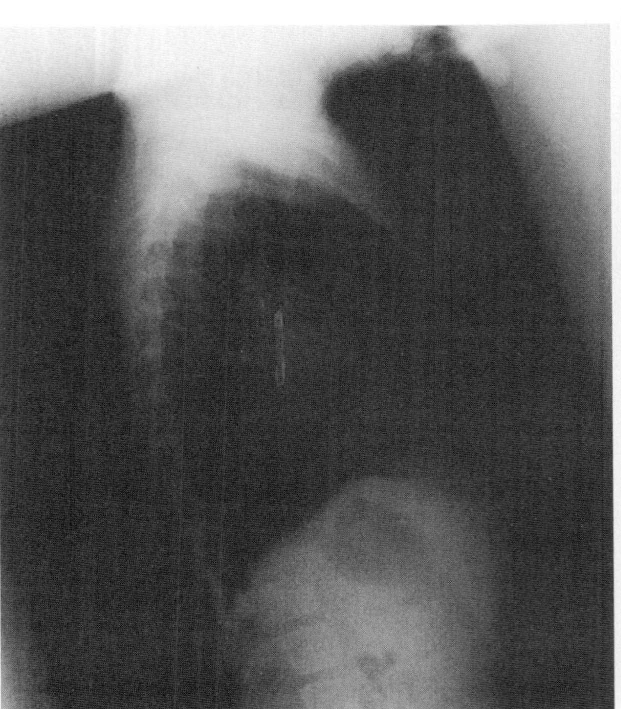

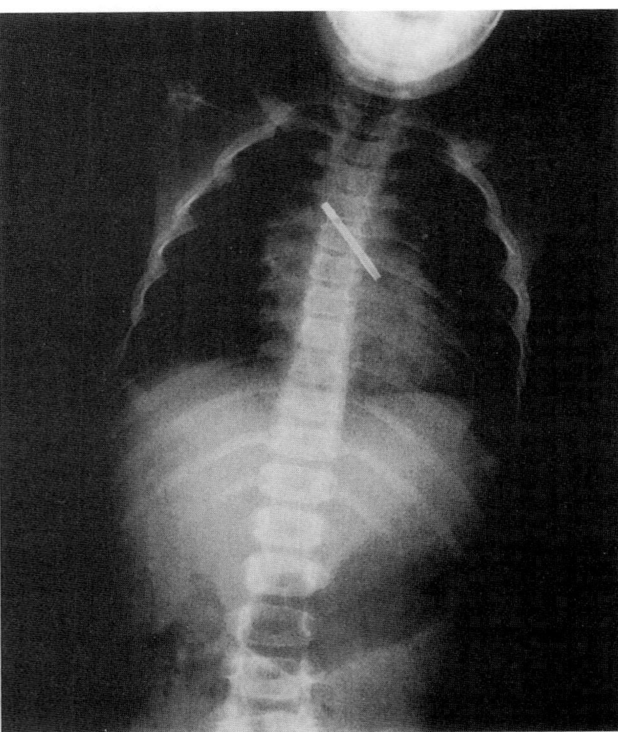

FIGURE 41-6. Pen top impacted in left bronchus requiring thoracotomy for removal.

lead the endoscopist to consider further retained material. Under these circumstances, repeat bronchoscopy is appropriate.

Postoperative radiographs may be obtained to ensure that full reexpansion of the lung has occurred and that no evidence of pneumothorax exists.

Pneumomediastinum and pneumothorax are unusual complications of FB removal and are managed in a similar manner to those arising from other etiologies. Major complications following FB removal are unusual.[2,16]

■ ESOPHAGEAL FOREIGN BODIES

Esophageal FBs in young children, particularly in infants, may present primarily with pulmonary symptoms. Symptoms common to FB aspiration such as a choking spell or cough are common and may raise an initial concern of aspiration rather than ingestion. The impacted object produces pressure on the anterior esophageal wall, which is transmitted to the membranous tracheal wall, compromising the airway lumen.

Infants with esophageal FB impaction exhibit subtle and nonspecific symptoms: a history of fussing, poor appetite, drooling, or emesis. Thus, many unsuspected FBs are initially diagnosed as viral, upper respiratory, or gastrointestinal illnesses and may be discovered incidentally on a chest radiograph intended to rule out a pulmonary process. When present, persistent neck extension is a selective sign. Fortunately, and in contrast to FB of the tracheobronchial tree, esophageal objects are frequently radiopaque and therefore easily identified from plain chest radiography. Coins are by far the most commonly ingested objects, and food products are the second most common. A child with a history of an anatomic or physiologic abnormality of the esophagus is at increased risk of FB impaction. Particularly at risk are children who have undergone repair for esophageal atresia. Esophageal FB impaction is also seen in eosinophilic esophagitis and may be the initial presentation.[24] Clues to the presence of radiolucent esophageal FBs are best seen on lateral neck and chest films, looking for a localized tracheal compression, tracheal deviation, and air within the esophagus.

As with FBs in the tracheobronchial tree, endoscopy is the gold standard for diagnosis of FBs in the digestive tract.

■ CONCLUSIONS

A relative lack of symptoms following a witnessed choking episode is not unusual following an FB aspiration and should not be used to exclude FB aspiration. Unilateral wheezing and decreased breath sounds are the most common and characteristic physical findings of a bronchial FB and should not be mistaken for atypical asthma. Subacute laryngeal FB impaction is often overlooked initially because its symptoms mimic the more common airway problems such as laryngitis and croup. Chest radiographs can be normal with either a tracheal or bronchial FB and do not rule out the diagnosis of an aspirated object.

Laryngoscopy and rigid bronchoscopy are the gold standard for removing tracheobronchial FBs in infants and children. Careful patient preparation and the assembly of an appropriately experienced medical team is recommended if the child is clinically stable. Ventilating bronchoscopes with all the necessary accessories should be assembled and tested prior to anesthesia being induced. Thorough dialogue between the endoscopist and the anesthesiologist and nursing personnel maximize the safety of FB removal in children. Further bronchoscopic examination of the airways is necessary following FB extraction to search for multiple objects or fragments. Impacted esophageal FB may present primarily as respiratory problems in infants and younger children.·

REFERENCES

1. National Safety Council: Accident Facts. Chicago: National Safety Council, 1987.
2. Tan HK, Brown K, McGill T, et al: Airway foreign bodies (FB). A 10-year review. Int J Pediatr Otorhinolaryngol 2000;56:91–99.
3. Black RE, Choi KJ, Syme WC, et al: Bronchoscopic removal of aspirated foreign bodies in children. Am J Surg 1984;148:778–781.
4. Harris CS, Baker SP, Smith GA, et al: Childhood asphyxiation by food. A national analysis and overview. JAMA 1984;251:2231–2235.
5. Qureshi S, Mink R: Aspiration of fruit gel snacks. Pediatrics 2003;111: 687–689.
6. Reilly JS: Prevention of aspiration in infants and young children. Federal regulations. Ann Otol Rhinol Laryngol 1990;99:273–276.
7. Wolach B, Raz A, Weinberg J, et al: Aspirated foreign bodies in the respiratory tract of children. Eleven years experience with 127 patients. Int J Pediatr Otorhinolaryngol 1994;30:1–10.
8. Steen KH, Zimmermann T: Tracheobronchial aspiration of foreign bodies in children. A study of 94 cases. Laryngoscope 1990;100:525–530.
9. Lima JA: Laryngeal foreign bodies in children. A persistent, life-threatening problem. Laryngoscope 1989;99:415–420.
10. American Academy of Pediatrics Committee on Accident and Poison Prevention: First aid for the choking child, 1988. Pediatrics 1988; 81:740–742.
11. Mu L, He P, Sun D: Inhalation of foreign bodies in Chinese children. A review of 400 cases. Laryngoscope 1991;101:657–660.
12. Halvorson DJ, Merritt RM, Mann C, et al: Management of subglottic foreign bodies. Ann Otol Rhinol Laryngol 1996;105:541–544.
13. Shapiro NL, Kaselonis GL: Tracheobronchial foreign body management in an acutely ill neonate. Int J Pediatr Otorhinolaryngol 2000;52:75–77.
14. Wiseman NE: The diagnosis of foreign body aspiration in childhood. J Pediatr Surg 1984;19:531–535.
15. Burton EM, Brick WG, Hall JD, et al: Tracheobronchial foreign body aspiration in children. South Med J 1996;89:195–198.
16. Zerella JT, Dimler M, McGill LC, et al: Foreign body aspiration in children. Value of radiography and complications of bronchoscopy. J Pediatr Surg 1998;33:1651–1654.
17. Silva AB, Muntz HR, Clary R: Utility of conventional radiography in the diagnosis and management of pediatric airway foreign bodies. Ann Otol Rhinol Laryngol 1998;107:834–838.
18. Burrington JD, Cotton EK: Removal of FB from the tracheobronchial tree. J Pediatr Surg 1972;7:119–122.
19. Swanson KL, Prakash UB, Midthun DE, et al: Flexible bronchoscopic management of airway FB in children. Chest 2002;121:1695–1700.
20. Gibson SE, Shott SR: Foreign Bodies of the Upper Aerodigestive Tract. Philadelphia: JB Lippincott, 1995, pp 195–222.
21. Kosloske A: Foreign Bodies in the Pediatric Airway. Philadelphia: WB Saunders, 1991, pp 168–180.
22. Cohen SR: Unusual presentations and problems created by mismanagement of foreign bodies in the aerodigestive tract of the pediatric patient. Ann Otol Rhinol Laryngol 1981;90:316–322.
23. Pfenninger J, D'Apuzzo V: Powder aspiration in children. Report of two cases. Arch Dis Child 1977;52:157–159.
24. Khan S, Orenstein SR, Di Lorenzo C, et al: Eosinophilic esophagitis: Strictures, impactions, dysphagia. Dig Dis Sci 2003;48:22–29.

42 Atelectasis

Michelle Duggan, MB •
Brian P. Kavanagh, MB

Atelectasis, the reversible loss of aerated lung, is a key component of many acute lung disease states. Although classically considered to be a depletion of lung volume through degassing of the alveoli, recent insights suggest an alternative explanation for atelectasis: that it represents accumulation of alveolar fluid. This chapter addresses a clinical diagnosis of atelectasis, effects of atelectasis and lung physiology, causes of atelectasis, new concepts about the nature of atelectasis, and its prevention or reversal.

WHAT IS ATELECTASIS?

This is a complex question. Characteristically, atelectasis represents a radiologically apparent volume loss in a segment or lobe of a lung, or sometimes the whole lung. This situation is associated with impaired gas exchange with potential impaired lung mechanics. Recent studies in animals have directly visualized atelectasis occurring in the subpleural alveoli and have demonstrated the opening and closing of alveoli with positive-pressure ventilation, and the collapse of alveoli in the absence of end-expiratory pressure.[1] Several studies using computed tomography (CT) have documented atelectasis related to general anesthesia and have categorized the densities, whose radiologic features suggest are closer to tissue than to water.[2,3] This suggests that atelectasis represents alveolar collapse, as opposed to fluid accumulation.

However, the nature of atelectasis may not be so simple. Based on a variety of arguments, Hubmayr suggests that instead of loss of alveolar volume, atelectasis may represent replacement of alveolar volume by airspaces being filled with edema fluid.[4] There are three cardinal lines of reasoning that support such a hypothesis.

PRESSURE-VOLUME CHARACTERISTICS

Convincing evidence for this is derived from the pressure-volume characteristics of different lung conditions. When fluid is injected into a fluid-filled lung, low pressures are required for inflation. Similarly, when air is injected into an air-filled lung, relatively low pressures are also required. However, when air is injected into a fluid-filled lung, the opening pressure is high, similar to that of the atelectatic lung, and not consistent with the traditional view of atelectasis.

WEIGHT OF THE LUNG

In addition, the idea that atelectasis represents simple compression from heavier lung has been refuted because the weight of the lung accounts for only approximately one fifth of the vertical pleural pressure radiant.

INTERPRETATION OF COMPUTED TOMOGRAPHY IMAGES

Conventionally, vertical gradients in the gray scale of pixels in a CT scan have been interpreted as evidence of steeper gradients in alveolar size. However, the correlation between gray scale and alveolar size holds only if the amount of water per alveolus is uniform. CT provides data on regional air content but not on regional volume or parenchymal strain, so it has limitations as a measurement tool of regional lung mechanics.

Thus, the exact nature of atelectasis remains a complex issue, and the answer appears to depend on the technique used.

WHY DOES ATELECTASIS OCCUR?

Theories of the development of atelectasis are traditionally based on the idea of maintenance of "opened lung" units, which are considered to reflect the balance of inward recoil of the lung tissue tending to collapse the lung countered by outward recoil of the chest wall tending to expand the lung. The exact balance of these forces at the end of expiration represents the functional residual capacity (FRC) of the lung. The loss of lung volume is conventionally thought to reflect an imbalance of forces that usually keep the lung open, thereby allowing lung tissue to contract around empty air spaces.

CLASSIFICATION OF ATELECTASIS

Atelectasis may be the result of one or more of the following mechanisms: inhibition of surfactant, resorption of alveolar gas, or compression of regional lung. It is possible that more than one of these influences is at play in any particular instance.

SURFACTANT INHIBITION

The composition of the surfactant includes phospholipids, natural lipids, and specific apoproteins as described elsewhere in this text. A major overall function is to stabilize the alveoli by reducing alveolar surface tension, thus preventing collapse. Many factors, including leakage of plasma proteins and vigorous ventilatory stretch, may alter the function of surfactant and its composition (e.g., may reduce the proportion of large aggregate fractions, tubular myelin, which are important for reducing surface tension). However, two factors make this an unlikely sole explanation for the development of atelectasis. First, the lungs have a large reserve of surfactant (surfactant pool) and are therefore unlikely to become deficient except over a protracted period. Second, surfactant has a long turnover time (12–14 hours). Thus, it is unlikely that atelectasis commonly occurs on the basis of changes in surfactant, in the absence of other factors, in an otherwise healthy lung.

GAS RESORPTION

There are two means whereby gas absorption may result in atelectasis. First, in the presence of a patent airway, regions that have low ventilation compared with perfusion will have low alveolar oxygen tensions when the fraction of inspired oxygen

(FIO_2) is low. When the FIO_2 is increased (i.e., with supplemental oxygen) the alveolar oxygen tension (i.e. PAO_2) increases, and thus the rate at which gas transfers from the alveolus to the capillary blood is increased. In addition, as PAO_2 increases, alveolar nitrogen tension (PAN_2) decreases. Because nitrogen is inert, any increased absorption of oxygen must result in loss of alveolar volume.

The second mechanism is thought to occur in the presence of an occluded airway. Here, ongoing gas uptake by the blood is not replenished by incoming gas from the airway, and the size of the lung unit becomes progressively smaller.

COMPRESSION ATELECTASIS

Compression atelectasis is defined as atelectasis that results when the forces causing the alveoli to collapse are exceeded by the transmural pressure that distends and maintains the alveoli in an open state (Fig. 42-1). The pleural pressure, which compresses the lung from the outside, is obviously greatest in the most dependent areas. During positive pressure ventilation, distention of the alveoli is enhanced, and during spontaneous ventilation it is dependent on the elastic recoil of the chest wall and the stability of the diaphragm. When in the supine position, the weight of the abdominal contents results in a net vector that tends to shift the dependent areas of the diaphragm into the chest.

During positive pressure ventilation, as in the operating room or intensive care unit, these changes may be compounded by several factors. First, use of sedation and neuromuscular blockade reduces the stability of the diaphragm, allowing its progressive shift into the chest. Second, positive pressure ventilation may result in a displacement of thoracic central blood from the chest into the abdomen, with further displacement of the diaphragm cephalad, which potentiates the development of atelectasis. These changes may account for the reduction in FRC associated with induction of general anaesthesia, or in the critically ill child, where sedation and paralysis are being employed in an effort to facilitate positive pressure ventilation.

CONSEQUENCES OF ATELECTASIS

Like many things, atelectasis is only as important as the consequences that are associated with it.

IMPAIRED GAS EXCHANGE

Impairment of gas exchange, often the most obvious effect of atelectasis, in the absence of supplemental oxygen will lead to worsened arterial oxygenation. This concept was recognized following general anesthesia in the classic studies of Bendixen and colleagues.[5] The basis for impaired gas exchange in atelectasis is the absence of ventilation in the collapsed or filled alveoli, coupled with the perfusion of such nonventilated lung units (Fig. 42-2). The latter issue results in shunting of intrapulmonary blood, and pronounced hypoxemia.

The consequences of impaired oxygenation are frequently unimportant in a healthy lung but in a diseased lung may necessitate the application of higher FIO_2 or, in mechanically ventilated children, greater elevations in either the inspiratory airway pressures or the pressure at end-expiration (i.e., positive end-expiratory pressure [PEEP]). The application of higher levels of FIO_2 can, as discussed above, paradoxically worsen the situation through development of absorption atelectasis. In this situation, although the partial pressure of oxygen in arterial blood (PaO_2) may be improved, with time, additional atelectasis develops and the PaO_2 will become lower relative to FIO_2. Thus, higher levels of FIO_2 will raise the PaO_2 (the immediate aim), but measures of oxygenation efficiency will be worsened (e.g., the alveolar-arterial oxygen gradient will be increased, or the ratio of PaO_2/FIO_2 will be decreased). The alternative therapies, increases in inflation pressure or PEEP, are associated with adverse effects of their own.

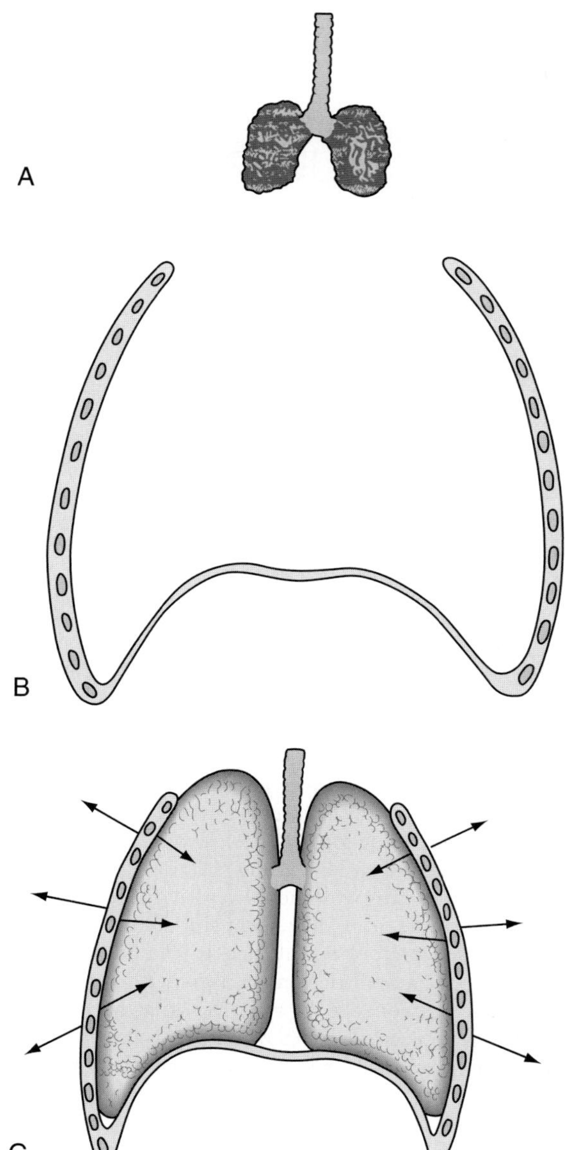

FIGURE 42-1. The balance of inward recoil of the lung tissue tending to collapse the lung countered by outward recoil of the chest wall tending to expand the lung. The exact balance of these forces at the end of expiration represents the functional residual capacity (FRC) of the lung. **A,** The resting state of the lungs when they are removed from the chest cavity, that is, total collapse. **B,** The resting state of the normal chest wall and diaphragm when open to the atmosphere and thoracic contents removed. **C,** The lung volume that exists at the end of expiration, the FRC. (From Shapiro BA, Harrison RA, Trout CA: The mechanics of ventilation. In: Clinical Applications of Respiratory Care, 3rd ed. Chicago: Year Book Medical, 1985, p 57.).

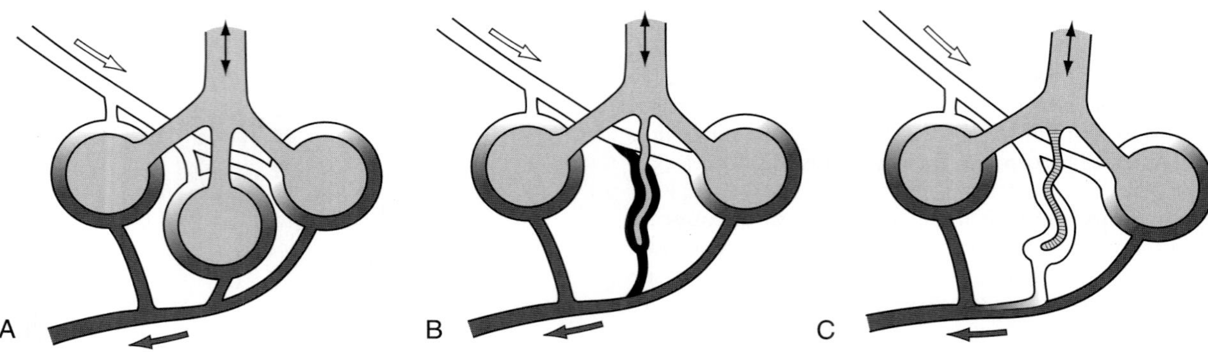

■ **FIGURE 42-2.** The basis for impaired gas exchange in atelectasis. The absence of ventilation in the collapsed or filled alveoli, coupled with the perfusion of such nonventilated lung units. This results in shunting of intrapulmonary blood, and pronounced hypoxemia. **A,** The ideal relationship between alveolar ventilation and pulmonary circulation (V/Q ratio) is an even distribution of adequate ventilation and perfusion of pulmonary vessels. **B,** If alveolar collapse occurs but those alveoli are not perfused, then the overall relationship between ventilation and perfusion will remain unchanged and all venous blood will be oxygenated. **C,** If capillary blood flow is maintained through collapsed alveoli, venous admixture will occur, leading to hypoxemia. (Figure 1 in Bendixen HH, Hedley-Whyte J, Chir B, Laver MB: Impaired oxygenation in surgical patients during general anesthesia with controlled ventilation. N Engl J Med 1963;269:991–997.)

IMPAIRED LUNG MECHANICS

A major consequence of atelectasis is impaired lung mechanics. This issue has been recognized since the 1950s,[6] before the effects on oxygenation were acknowledged. It was demonstrated that with spontaneous or mechanical breaths with the same tidal volume there was associated progressive impairment of the respiratory system compliance. Normal compliance could be restored by a large breath at intervals (three times normal tidal volume). This phenomenon has been explored in detail in the perioperative setting, where using fluoroscopy it has been demonstrated that lung volume decreases during general anesthesia.[7] Importantly, the decrement in compliance resulting from progressive atelectasis is related to the lung volume lost, and is reversed by recruitment maneuvers.

The major consequence of impaired lung mechanics is that compliance is worsened. This means that larger changes in transpulmonary pressure are required to generate a given tidal volume. Thus, for spontaneously breathing children, the work of breathing is increased, and for children on mechanical ventilation, increased ventilatory pressures are required.

INCREASED PULMONARY VASCULAR RESISTANCE

Another complication of atelectasis is associated with increased pulmonary vascular resistance. Early classic studies suggested that the pulmonary vascular resistance was minimal at ideal FRC, and whereas lung volume much above this notional value resulted in alveolar compression due to lung stretch, lung volume falling below the FRC was thought to result in compression of extra-alveolar vessels. Thus, this notion explained the changes in pulmonary vascular resistance on the basis of physical alteration of the pulmonary blood vessels—either stretching or narrowing because of increased lung volume, or compression because of decreased lung volume. Subsequent work has changed that notion, and has demonstrated that increases in pulmonary vascular resistance associated with atelectasis result not from physical compression of the vessels but rather from regional alveolar hypoxia with reduced alveolar and mixed venous oxygen tension, leading to local hypoxic pulmonary vasoconstriction.[8] Indeed, recent studies have demonstrated that this significant increase in vascular resistance can occur in previously normal lungs in an experimental setting, resulting in ventricular dysfunction and increased microvascular leakage.[9]

WORSENING OF LUNG INJURY

An important consequence of atelectasis is the potentiation of lung injury. While mechanical ventilation is designed as a supportive measure, its use can be associated with what is now termed ventilatory-associated lung injury. Most experimental studies have demonstrated that ventilator-induced lung injury occurs much more readily in the presence of low PEEP or low lung volume. Conversely, application of PEEP reduces or eliminates ventilator-associated lung injury in some situation, making it almost negligible.[10,11]

In experimental settings, this phenomenon is not restricted to ventilator-associated lung injury, and several studies have demonstrated that maintenance of lung volume (i.e., prevention of atelectasis) is associated with reduced injury secondary to reperfusion injury and possibly sepsis.[12–14] This may be because maintenance of lung volume reduces endothelial shear stress and optimizes vascular resistance, but the explanation is incompletely understood.

DIAGNOSIS

The diagnosis of atelectasis is most easily made bearing in mind the context of the patient, for example, a postoperative scenario, paralysis of a hemidiaphragm, known airway obstruction, or the presence of neuromuscular weakness.

CLINICAL FEATURES

In such a setting, the clinical findings include dyspnea or tachypnea, asymmetrical chest movement, and reduced breath sounds on the ipsilateral side. In cases of upper lobe atelectasis, instead of reduced or absent breath sounds, bronchial breath sounds may be heard, because of the proximity of the upper lobes to the major airways. Percussion of the affected lobes will demonstrate increased dullness.

RADIOLOGIC FEATURES

The standard radiologic approach is a plain portable radiographic study of the chest. Segmental or lobar atelectasis or atelectasis of the whole lung is associated with increased density (i.e., opacification) of the atelectatic area, and secondary signs of volume loss in adjacent regions. Indications of volume loss include hyperlucency of adjacent lung tissue and shift of adjoining structures. Hyperlucency occurs because the nonatelectatic lung is stretched to replace the lung volume that has become atelectatic. The shift of adjoining structures occurs because of the loss of lung volume inherent to the development of atelectasis. For example, atelectasis of a lower lobe can result in a downward shift of the ipsilateral horizontal fissure or hilum, or an upward shift of the ipsilateral diaphragm. In addition, the mediastinum can be displaced toward an atelectatic side.

The presence of atelectasis can also be noted in a specific lobe because of the relationship to the heart or diaphragm. Lower lobe atelectasis, resulting in dense opacification of that lobe, can obliterate the normal contour of the adjacent diaphragm. Similarly, the presence of atelectasis in the right middle lobe or in the lingula can obliterate the normally visible right or left heart borders, respectively. In addition, obstruction of a main stem bronchus, causing atelectasis, can sometimes be appreciated on the plain chest film.

Computed tomography (CT) can be used in the diagnosis of atelectasis with greater sensitivity than the plain radiograph. However, CT-based diagnosis of atelectasis is usually made when performed for another indication and CT is seldom indicated for the diagnosis of atelectasis per se. Nonetheless, atelectasis is an integral element of acute respiratory distress syndrome (ARDS), and some centers determine the distribution of atelectasis—usually in the dependent regions—through utilization of CT scans. In such cases, CT is important because it may assist in directing the optimal position for care of the ventilator-dependent patient (e.g., prone versus supine positioning). In addition to a response to prone positioning that can sometimes be predicted by CT, modern CT approaches can demonstrate relative overinflation of nonatelectatic areas induced by overly aggressive attempts to recruit atelectatic regions.[15]

A new approach is the use of ultrasonography. Several studies suggest that it is an extremely straightforward technique with higher sensitivity and ease of use than CT scanning in critically ill patients. The potential use for this technique is to distinguish between pleural fluid, consolidation, and atelectasis. Ultrasonography allows imaging without the use of ionizing radiation. In addition, it can be done at the bedside quickly and with less cost. It may become a new standard of care in the near future.

FACTORS MODIFYING THE DEVELOPMENT OF ATELECTASIS

Several important factors modify the development of atelectasis, resulting in worsening of the condition where initiating factors were already present.

POSTURE

Changing from the upright position to the supine position reduces the FRC substantially.[16] The basis for this is that the abdominal contents tend to exert pressure on the diaphragm, especially on its dependent (i.e., posterior) aspects (Fig. 42-3). The resultant diaphragmatic displacement coupled with the weight of the mediastinum, and to some extent the weight of the overlying nondependent lung, combine to compress the dependent lung, thereby potentiating the development of atelectasis. Turning patients to the prone position during mechanical ventilation appears to largely reverse these effects.[17]

The effects of the supine position on atelectasis are exaggerated in obese subjects,[18] because the influence of the mass of abdominal contents is significantly greater in obese compared with lean subjects.

DEVELOPMENTAL INFLUENCES

Young children, up to the age of 3 years, develop atelectasis more readily than older children. Several factors may contribute to this. The compliance of the thoracic rib cage is far higher in very young children. This results in less outward recoil of the chest wall, thereby causing less distending force on the lung and increasing the propensity of the lungs to develop atelectasis.[19] In addition to the reduced influence of the chest wall, young infants have an especially high closing volume (i.e., the lung volume at which the small airways begin to close). The greater closing volume means that airways, and subsequently lung units, become closed and set up conditions for development of atelectasis.

SUPPLEMENTAL OXYGEN

Use of supplemental oxygen, although sometimes necessary for treating the hypoxemia associated with atelectasis, can worsen the development of atelectasis per se (for reasons outlined above), despite augmenting the arterial oxygen tension. In this context, the arterial oxygen levels are increased but the efficiency of gas exchange in the lungs is worsened.

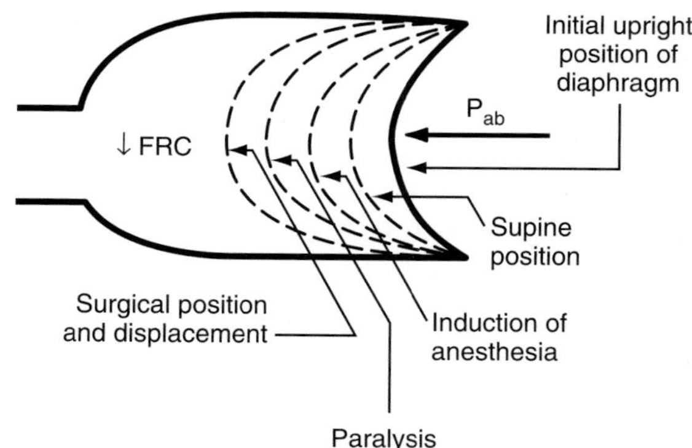

FIGURE 42-3. Several important factors modify the development of atelectasis. Anesthesia and surgery cause a cephalad displacement of the diaphragm, leading to a decreased functional residual capacity. The sequence of events includes assumption of the supine position, induction of anesthesia, muscle paralysis, surgical position, and displacement by surgical packs and retractors. Pab, pressure of the abdominal contents. (From Benumof JL: General respiratory physiology and respiratory function during anesthesia. In: Anesthesia for Thoracic Surgery. Philadelphia: WB Saunders, 1987, p 100, fig 3-44.)

PREEXISTING LUNG DISEASE

In addition, preexisting lung disease or acute lung disease will increased the likelihood of atelectasis formation, and if present, will worsen it.

TREATMENT FOR ATELECTASIS

Although there are no evidence-based studies that prove any outcome benefits associated with the treatment of atelectasis, common sense suggests that in the presence of significant hypoxemia, increased work of breathing, or respiratory distress, measures should be considered to reverse the effects of atelectasis. The feasibility of treating atelectasis depends on the balance between the physiologic burden caused by atelectasis, the risks of the intervention, and the potential for the therapy to work. The following approaches can be considered.

RECRUITMENT MANEUVERS

Recruitment maneuvers are designed to recruit atelectatic lung. In the setting of mechanical ventilation, such maneuvers usually take the form of either increases in end-expiratory pressure (PEEP) in the setting of ongoing positive-pressure ventilation, or the application of continuous positive airway pressure (CPAP). It is not clear whether either of these approaches is superior, and the major issues for the clinician are the likelihood of there being recruitable lung (i.e., what are the chances of success?) balanced against the potential adverse effects associated with the maneuver.

The probability of success is difficult to predict, but in the postoperative state, for example, positive pressure can be expected to readily reverse the atelectasis. The situation is quite different in lung injury, such as ARDS, where the presence of atelectasis may have far more impact in terms of oxygenation and potentially also for lung mechanics and pulmonary vascular resistance. In lung injury states, prediction of response may be possible on the basis of the topographic distribution of the lung injury, as evidenced by CT. In addition, the timing of the lung injury also appears to be important. For example, recruitment maneuvers undertaken in early (i.e., approximately 1 day's duration) ARDS have a far higher chance of success compared with those attempted at a later (i.e., approximately 7 days' duration) degree of maturation.[20] Finally, the cause of lung injury, for example, whether originating from a pulmonary (e.g., aspiration injury, lung trauma, pneumonia) versus a nonpulmonary (e.g., systemic sepsis, pancreatitis) etiology, has a major impact. Nonpulmonary types of ARDS demonstrate recruitable lung potential that is not apparent in pulmonary types of ARDS.[21]

CHEST PHYSIOTHERAPY

Although randomized controlled trials of chest physiotherapy for atelectasis are lacking, it is standard practice to attempt physiotherapy. For the older child, this involves deep breathing and coughing exercises, in addition to incentive spirometry. Percussion therapy is traditional and may be most effective in the context of coughing. In addition, vibration therapy can also be used. For younger children and infants, because of the lack of cooperation, the options are limited to percussion and vibration treatments. Techniques or devices that either encourage or force the patient to inspire deeply are of most clinical importance.[22]

REMOVAL OF ENDOBRONCHIAL OBSTRUCTION

Bronchoscopy and removal of an intraluminal obstruction (e.g., blood clot, inspissated secretions, etc.) are indicated in situations where atelectasis of a lobe or a whole lung is thought to be due to an obstruction that has not responded to conservative measures.

SUPPLEMENTAL OXYGEN

Although frequently necessary to overcome systemic hypoxemia in atelectasis, the use of supplemental oxygen may be associated with the development of absorption atelectasis, as discussed above.

SUMMARY

Atelectasis is generally a benign disease, although, in the presence of preexisting lung disease or limited cardiopulmonary reserve, it may have significant consequences. Increasing understanding of the underlying nature of atelectasis and its contribution to acute lung injury will hopefully improve our approach to the prevention and management of atelectasis.

REFERENCES

1. Halter JM, Steinberg JM, Schiller HJ, DaSilva M, Gatto LA, Landas S, Nieman GF: Positive end-expiratory pressure after a recruitment maneuver prevents both alveolar collapse and recruitment/derecruitment. Am J Respir Crit Care Med 2003;167:1620.
2. Brismar B, Hedenstierna G, Lundquist H, Strandberg A, Svensson L, Tokics L: Pulmonary densities during anesthesia with muscular relaxation—A proposal of atelectasis. Anesthesiology 1985;62:422.
3. Lundquist H, Hedenstierna G, Strandberg A, Tokics L, Brismar B: CT-assessment of dependent lung densities in man during general anaesthesia. Acta Radiol 1995;36:626.
4. Hubmayr RD: Perspective on lung injury and recruitment. A skeptical look at the opening and collapse story. Am J Respir Crit Care Med 2002; 165:1647.
5. Bendixen HH, Hedley-Whyte J, Chir B, Laver MB: Impaired oxygenation in surgical patients during general anesthesia with controlled ventilation. N Engl J Med 1963;269:991.
6. Mead J, Collier C: Relation of volume history of lungs to respiratory mechanics in anesthetized dogs. J Appl Physiol 1958;14:669.
7. Froese AB, Bryan AC: Effects of anesthesia and paralysis on diaphragmatic mechanics in man. Anesthesiology 1974;41:242.
8. Benumof JL, Pirlo AF, Johanson I, Trousdale FR: Interaction of PVO_2 with PAO_2 on hypoxic pulmonary vasoconstriction. J Appl Physiol 1981; 51:871.
9. Duggan M, McCaul CL, McNamara PJ, Engelberts D, Ackerley C, Kavanagh BP: Atelectasis causes vascular leak and lethal right ventricular failure in uninjured rat lungs. Am J Respir Crit Care Med 2003;167:1633.
10. Muscedere JG, Mullen JB, Gan K, Slutsky AS: Tidal ventilation at low airway pressures can augment lung injury. Am J Respir Crit Care Med 1994;149:1327.
11. Webb HH, Tierney DF: Experimental pulmonary edema due to intermittent positive pressure ventilation with high inflation pressures. Protection by positive end-expiratory pressure. Am Rev Respir Dis 1974;110:556.
12. DeCampos KN, Keshavjee S, Slutsky AS, Liu M: Alveolar recruitment prevents rapid-reperfusion-induced injury of lung transplants. J Heart Lung Transplant 1999;18:1096.
13. Hamvas A, Park CK, Palazzo R, Liptay M, Cooper J, Schuster DP: Modifying pulmonary ischemia-reperfusion injury by altering ventilatory strategies during ischemia. J Appl Physiol 1992;73:2112.
14. Veith FJ, Sinha SB, Graves JS, Boley SJ, Dougherty JC: Ischemic tolerance of the lung. The effect of ventilation and inflation. J Thorac Cardiovasc Surg 1971;61:804.
15. Rouby JJ, Puybasset L, Nieszkowska A, Lu Q: Acute respiratory distress syndrome. Lessons from computed tomography of the whole lung. Crit Care Med 2003;31(Suppl):285.

16. Nunn JF: Nunn's Applied Respiratory Physiology, 4th ed. London: Butterworth Heinemann, 1993.
17. Gattinoni L, Tognoni G, Pesenti A, Taccone P, Mascheroni D, Labarta V, Malacrida R, Di Giulio P, Fumagalli R, Pelosi P, Brazzi L, Latini R: Effect of prone positioning on the survival of patients with acute respiratory failure. N Engl J Med 2001;345:568.
18. Vaughan RW, Wise L: Intraoperative arterial oxygenation in obese patients. Ann Surg 1976;184:35.
19. Davis GM, Coates AL, Papageorgiou A, Bureau MA: Direct measurement of static chest wall compliance in animal and human neonates. J Appl Physiol 1988;65:1093.
20. Grasso S, Mascia L, Del Turco M, Malacarne P, Giunta F, Brochard L, Slutsky AS, Marco Ranieri V: Effects of recruiting maneuvers in patients with acute respiratory distress syndrome ventilated with protective ventilatory strategy. Anesthesiology 2002;96:795.
21. Gattinoni L, Pelosi P, Suter PM, Pedoto A, Vercesi P, Lissoni A: Acute respiratory distress syndrome caused by pulmonary and extrapulmonary disease. Different syndromes? Am J Respir Crit Care Med 1998; 158:3.
22. Bartlett RH, Gazzaniga AB, Geraghty TR: Respiratory maneuvers to prevent postoperative pulmonary complications. A critical review. JAMA 1973;224:1017.

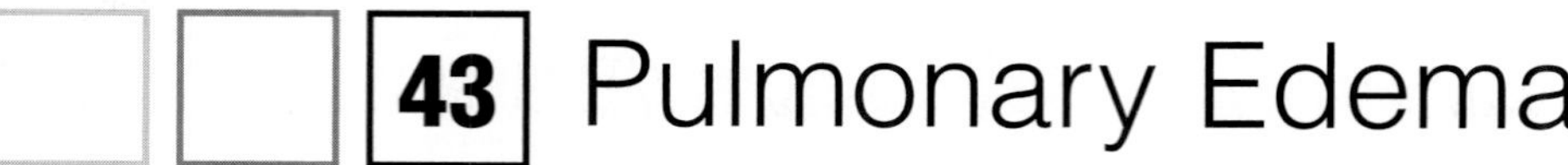

43 Pulmonary Edema

Hugh O'Brodovich, MD

Improvements in the intensive care and monitoring of patients with serious illnesses led to a greater appreciation of the significance of fluid movement into the lung as a complication of a variety of conditions. This, coupled with an improved understanding of the pathogenesis of pulmonary edema, has enhanced our ability to treat a variety of illnesses in which pulmonary edema develops.

■ ANATOMIC CONSIDERATIONS

Certain structural features of the lung are worth pointing out because they have a bearing on gas exchange during pulmonary edema. The capillaries are placed eccentrically within the alveolar septum (Fig. 43-1*A*). In some areas, the basement membranes of the capillary endothelium and the alveolar epithelium are fused with no additional space between them, even during edema formation. This situation would seem to be ideal for preserving gas exchange, at least until such time as the alveoli themselves are filled with liquid. In other areas, there is an interstitial space between the endothelial and epithelial basement membranes that contains secreted matrix. This matrix consists of structural proteins (e.g., collagens and elastin), attachment proteins for cells (e.g., laminin), and proteoglycans and glycosaminoglycans (e.g., hyaluronic acid, chrondroitins, and heparan sulfate). In addition to supplying support to the capillary network, this widened portion of the alveolar-capillary membrane provides a channel for water and protein en route to the lymphatics and larger interstitial fluid spaces (see Fig. 43-1*B*). As long as fluid can be confined to these channels, gas exchange can be preserved.

Pulmonary capillaries, like muscle capillaries, have a continuous endothelium with relatively tight intercellular junctions. The bronchial microvasculature, much like visceral capillaries, is discontinuous, with intercellular fenestrations or gaps. Whether these gaps account for the greater fluid movement across the bronchial, but not the pulmonary, capillaries remains to be determined. The role of the bronchial circulation in the genesis of pulmonary edema may have been underestimated, but it is certain that the bronchial circulation plays an important pathophysiologic role in inflammatory airway diseases such as asthma or inhalational lung injury.

At the ultrastructural level, the available evidence from tracer studies indicates that the alveolar epithelial membrane contains tighter cellular junctions than does the capillary endothelial membrane. These epithelial tight junctions (zonulae occludentes) are estimated by both morphologic and physiologic studies to have an effective molecular radius of approximately 4 Å. This has two implications. First, that they markedly restrict the movement of small ions, thereby making ions osmotically active across the epithelial membrane. Second, that fluid leaking from the vascular spaces is likely to be confined initially to the interstitial and lymphatic spaces; alveolar edema results only when the volume that can be handled by these is overwhelmed. In contrast to the epithelium, the pores between endothelial cells have an effective molecular radius of approximately 40 Å. This 10-fold difference in pore size allows the free movement of small ions and noncharged solutes, such as urea, but restricts the movement of larger macromolecules such as albumin and globulins. These large macromolecules move across the microvasculature, but the relative contributions of movement via pinocytotic vesicles (vesicular shuttle) versus across pores that can enlarge ("stretched pores"), especially when there is increased intravascular pressure or injury, are unclear.

Although the alveoli are often portrayed as spherical, a polyhedral model is closer to reality. Figure 43-2 shows that surfactant removed from the lung does indeed assume a polyhedral shape. From the point of view of fluid movement in the lung, the importance of this shape is that the walls of the alveolar septa are flat, except at the corners where the septa meet. Thus, it is only at the corners, where the alveolar air-liquid interface is curved, that the force exerted by surface tension can lower alveolar fluid and interstitial fluid pressures as predicted by the Laplace relationship (Fig. 43-3). The lower pressures at the corners favor movement of interstitial fluid that has traversed the alveolar capillary wall toward the corners of the alveolus. This is important from a lung fluid balance point of view. Alveolar type II epithelial cells are also predominately found in the corners of the alveoli, and since these cells actively transport Na^+, with Cl^- and water following, from the alveolar space (see later section on Clearance of Pulmonary Edema Fluid), the fluid can then be picked up by the terminal lymphatics and eventually returned to the systemic venous system.

Pulmonary blood vessels have been defined using anatomic and physiologic criteria. Anatomically, the vessels have been classified traditionally by their morphologic characteristics as arteries, arterioles, capillaries, venules, or veins. Physiologically, these divisions are included under two broad classifications based on their behavior relative to the hydrostatic pressures of the interstitium surrounding the vessels, the interstitial fluid pressure; specifically, alveolar and extra-alveolar vessels. Alveolar vessels are in the alveolar walls or septa and behave as if they were exposed to alveolar pressure. These vessels may collapse if airway pressures exceed vascular pressures, as is the case in zone I perfusion conditions. Extra-alveolar vessels lie in the larger interstitial spaces and behave as if surrounded by a pressure that is as negative as or more negative than pleural pressure and that tends to vary with pleural pressure. In addition, there are vessels lying in the intersections of alveolar septal walls (corner vessels) that are exposed to more negative pressures than the alveolar vessels, at least in part because of the acute radius of curvature found at the alveolar corners, as described above (see Fig. 43-3). The functional classification is important because it predicts the pressures surrounding the vessels participating in fluid exchange, and it is used in subsequent analyses of fluid movement and edema in this chapter. Unfortunately, there is no clear-cut correlation between the functional and the anatomic classifications. Although fluid movement occurs at the level of the arterioles and venules,[1] it is generally considered that the bulk of fluid

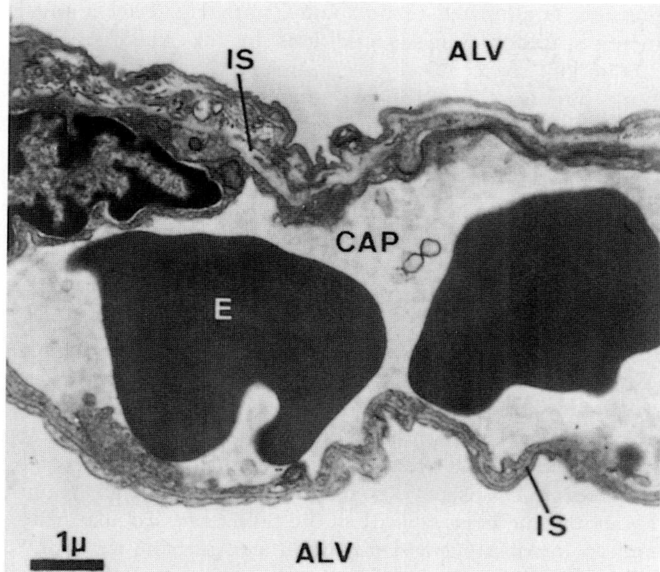

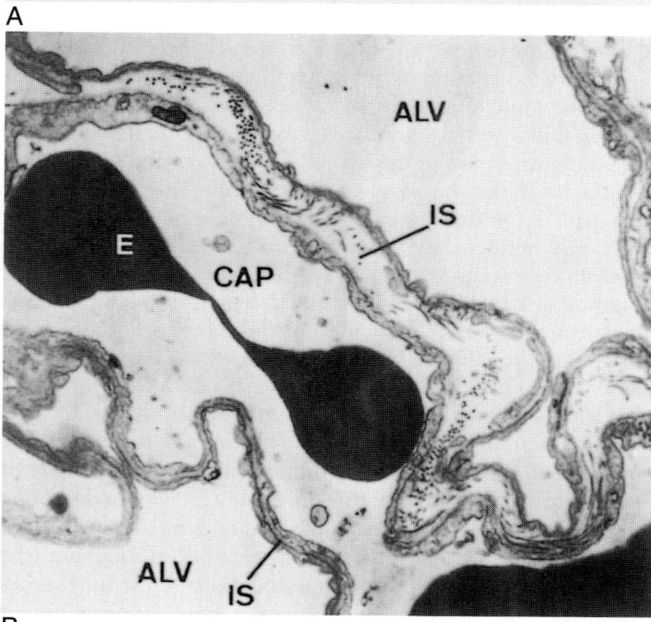

■ **FIGURE 43-1.** **A,** The normal alveolar septum in which the epithelial and endothelial basement membranes are fused in some areas and separated by an interstitial space of connective tissue in others. **B,** The alveolar septum in pulmonary edema. The areas where the basement membranes are fused remain thin; only the areas with a connective tissue interstitial space widen. ALV, alveolar lumen; CAP, capillary; E, erythrocyte; IS, interstitial space. (From Mellins RB, Levine OR, Skalak R, Fishman AP: Interstitial pressure of the lung. Circ Res 1969;24:197.)

movement occurs at the level of the capillaries, with approximately three fourths arising from the alveolar vessels.[2]

Anatomically, the lung has two main compartments, each possessing markedly different potential volumes, into which edema fluid can move. The interstitial spaces of the alveolar capillary septae and peribronchovascular compartment can only accommodate small amounts of fluid. When this small interstitial safety reservoir, estimated to be a few hundred milliliters in an adult lung,[3] is filled with edema fluid, subsequent

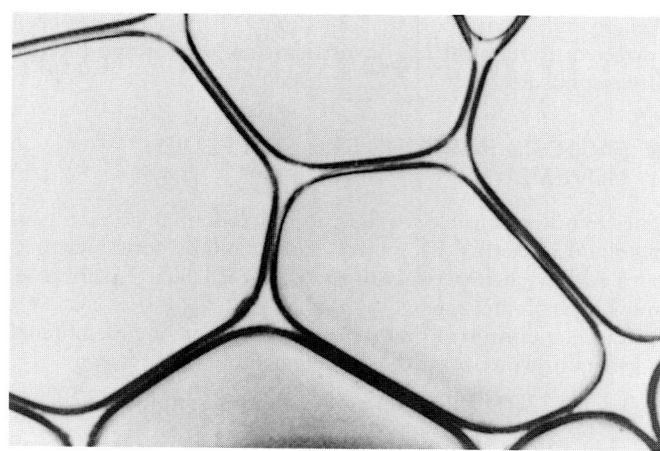

■ **FIGURE 43-2.** Surfactant foam obtained from the lung by bronchial rinsing assumes a polyhedral shape. (From Reifenrath R: The significance of alveolar geometry and surface tension in the respiratory mechanics of the lung. Respir Physiol 1975;24:115, with permission.)

accumulation must take place in the alveolar space, which at functional residual capacity (FRC) has a volume of approximately 30 mL/kg body weight or approximately 5000 mL in the adult lung. This anatomic difference, in part, explains why interstitial edema may resolve quickly whereas alveolar edema takes significantly longer periods of time.

Juxtacapillary (J) receptors are distributed throughout the lung's interstitium and are stimulated by the presence of edema. They induce an increase in respiratory rate and their continued activation is responsible, in large part, for the continued tachypnea

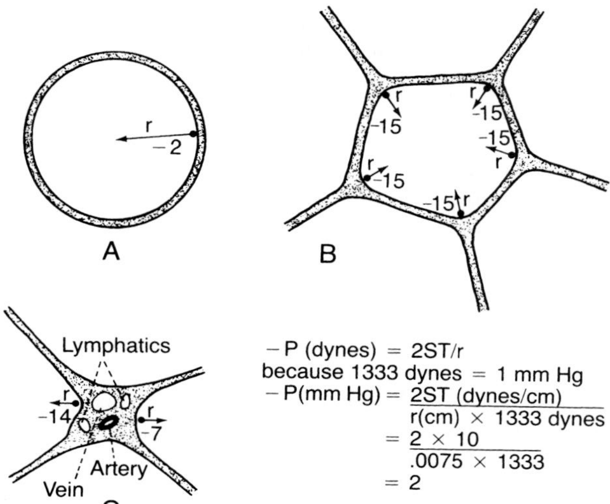

■ **FIGURE 43-3.** Effect of surface tension on the alveolar fluid and interstitial fluid pressure. **A,** Assuming a spherical model of the alveolus with a radius of 75 mm and a surface tension of 10 dynes/cm, we calculate that the fluid lining the alveolus would be pulled away with a pressure of −2 mm Hg. **B,** Assuming a polyhedral model with the radius of curvature at the corners of 10 mm, the negative pressure in the corners would be −15 mm Hg. The pressure at the angles (not shown) where the alveolar air-liquid interface is cylindrical and where $P = ST/r$ would be −7.5 mm Hg. **C,** Dynamics at alveolar angles adjacent to interstitial spaces surrounding larger blood vessels and lymphatics; pressures of −7 to −14 mm Hg can be calculated, depending on the radius of curvature at the angles. (Modified from Guyton AC, Taylor AE, Drake RE, Parker JC: Lung Liquids. Ciba Symposium 38. New York: American Elsevier, 1976.)

seen in pulmonary edema, even though hypoxemia has been corrected through the use of supplemental oxygen and positive airway pressure.

FACTORS RESPONSIBLE FOR FLUID MOVEMENT

The factors responsible for fluid accumulation include intravascular and interstitial hydrostatic and colloid osmotic pressures, permeability characteristics of the fluid-exchanging membrane, and lymphatic drainage.

The equilibrium of fluid across fluid-exchanging membranes is generally expressed as the Starling equation as follows:

$$Q_f = K_f((Pmv - Ppmv) - \sigma(\pi mv - \pi pmv))$$

wherein Q_f = the net transvascular flow; K_f = the filtration coefficient of the fluid-exchanging vessels and includes both the contribution of the permeability of the vessels and the surface area across which fluid exchange occurs; Pmv = microvascular hydrostatic pressure; Ppmv = perimicrovascular (interstitial fluid) hydrostatic pressure; πmv = colloid osmotic pressure in the microvasculature; πpmv = colloid osmotic pressure in the perimicrovasculature, the interstitial fluid colloid osmotic pressure; and σ = the reflection coefficient and is a measure of the resistance of the membrane to the movement of protein. Thus, it determines the "effective" osmotic pressure of the protein. If the endothelium were completely impermeant to protein ($\sigma_{protein}$ = 1) then the 5 g/dL of plasma would yield approximately 28 mm Hg oncotic pressure (each 1 mOsm/L of solute yields 19 mm Hg pressure).

Experiments have shown that the walls of the pulmonary circulation are not a perfect semipermeable membrane and that the normal pulmonary vasculature has $0 << \sigma < 1$. The endothelial membrane has "pores" that are larger than some protein molecules. Fluid filtering through a pore will drag some protein with it. The larger the protein relative to the size of the pore, the less protein will be dragged. When the protein is the same size as or larger than the pore, the reflection coefficient σ is 1. As the size of the protein becomes progressively smaller, σ approaches zero.[4]

The term *microvasculature* is used to describe the vessels from which fluid leaks because, as previously indicated above, fluid exchange is not limited to the capillaries alone. In the following discussion, each of the previously cited factors and the pathophysiologic influences on them are described in detail.

As discussed below, the absolute values for the variables within the Starling equation may change during health and disease. However, it should be emphasized that in the normal lung, Q_f is positive and there is a continuous movement of fluid from the vascular to interstitial spaces of the lung. Experimentally derived approximate values are Pmv = 20 cm H_2O, Ppmv = −2 cm H_2O, πmv = −33 cm H_2O, πpmv = 20 cm H_2O, and $0.7 < \sigma < 0.95$. There are significant technical difficulties in obtaining an accurate estimate of K_f within intact lungs and, dependent on the species and experimental approach, estimates have varied by more than three orders of magnitude.

VASCULAR FORCES

The pressure in the pulmonary microvasculature, Pmv, which is frequently, but not precisely, referred to as pulmonary capillary pressure, is estimated to be about 7 mm Hg. Pmv normally increases under exercise conditions in the adult, rising to 20 mm Hg. For technical reasons, this pressure is extremely difficult to measure in vivo. The pulmonary artery wedge pressure reflects the pressure in the first pulmonary veins where there is flow from nonobstructed vascular routes. This is usually minimally higher than left atrial (LA) pressure in lungs in zone III perfusion status. Pmv is believed to be higher than LA pressure by approximately 40% of the difference between LA pressure and pulmonary arterial (PA) pressure. The relative amounts of arterial and venular resistance within the pulmonary vasculature are altered during hypoxia, the infusion of vasoactive agents (e.g., catecholamines) or during disease (e.g., endotoxinemia). An increase in either PA or LA pressure will tend to increase the hydrostatic pressure, favoring movement out of the fluid-exchanging vessels. For example, Pmv may be increased by the elevation in LA pressures in left-sided heart failure or by increases in PA pressure as seen in large left-to-right shunts. Because of the large capacity of the pulmonary vascular bed to undergo recruitment and distention, considerable elevation in blood flow can occur (as in exercise, shunts, or pneumonectomy) without raising PA pressures appreciably or dramatically increasing movement of fluid into the lungs.[5,6] Despite the pulmonary vasculature of young children being more recruited relative to adults under resting conditions,[7] it still has a significant capability to accommodate increases in blood flow by either distending or recruiting vessels.

Because the pulmonary vascular membrane is only slightly permeable to proteins and freely permeable to ions and small uncharged solutes, the plasma proteins normally are responsible for osmotic pressure (πmv) well in excess of the pulmonary microvascular hydrostatic pressure. The plasma colloid osmotic pressure may be markedly reduced in clinical conditions in which the plasma proteins are low (e.g., malnutrition, nephrosis, and massive burns), and thus may facilitate edema formation.

It should also be emphasized that the rapid infusion of noncolloid-containing fluids not only raises vascular hydrostatic pressure but also lowers the colloid osmotic pressure because of hemodilution. In addition, the infusion of colloid-containing fluids may be of limited benefit. Colloid will raise microvascular hydrostatic pressure by absorption of fluid throughout the body yet pull little fluid out of the lung because the lung represents only 1% of the total body mass (see later section on Therapy).

INTERSTITIAL FORCES

The interstitial hydrostatic pressure throughout the lung is normally negative relative to alveolar pressure and appears to be maintained by a low effective microvascular pressure, lymphatic removal of interstitial fluid and protein, low microvascular permeability, and low filtration coefficient.[8,9]

Some studies on the manner in which pleural pressures are transmitted to the interstitium of the lung have special relevance to the development of pulmonary edema, especially in diseases that affect the lung nonuniformly. As indicated above, the pressure surrounding the corner and extra-alveolar vessels is believed to be less than pleural pressure and to become considerably more negative at high lung volumes. In disease, these negative pressures may be amplified manyfold because of "mechanical interdependence" of lung units.[10] When the expansion of some units of the lung lags behind surrounding lung units because of disease, the force per unit area distending the lagging unit is increased. Amplification of transpulmonary (distending) pressures by mechanical interdependence is seen in conditions characterized by increased respiratory resistance, decreased lung compliance, and expansion of the lung from the airless state. Mechanical interdependence can act on diseased areas of the lung to produce distending pressures that are exceedingly high. When transmitted to the interstitial space around blood vessels, these pressures can enhance edema formation and can cause the rupture of vessels. These considerations become especially important because various forms of constant distending pressures are used therapeutically. Although only 5 to 10 cm H_2O may be applied, if the pressure does not distend some areas of the lung as quickly as others, the pressure surrounding lagging units may be considerably greater because of amplification.

The interplay between maturation and surfactant on alveolar interstitial pressure has been demonstrated by studies in isolated lungs of mature and immature rabbits.[11] The pressure and alveolar wash phospholipids were lower in the immature lung but rose toward the higher levels of pressure of the mature lung following surfactant replacement.

MICROVASCULAR FILTRATION COEFFICIENT AND VASCULAR PERMEABILITY

Several groups of investigators have attempted to characterize the ease with which water crosses the pulmonary fluid-exchanging vessels by calculating K_f. K_f includes both the surface area of the membrane and its porosity. For the most part, the data to date indicate that K_f is in the range of 0.03 to 0.2 mL/min per mm Hg per 100 g.[4] Early experimental evidence suggested that the microvascular permeability to protein is greater in the young than in the adult animal; however, subsequent works showed that there was no difference in lung microvascular permeability to protein before and after birth and that the greater fluid likely results from a greater portion of the younger smaller lung being in West's zone III perfusion status.[12]

There are various mechanisms involved in increasing microvascular permeability (see later section on Increased Vascular Permeability in Fluid-Exchanging Vessels), and the list of clinical entities in which increased lung water content is secondary to increased permeability is growing. Because the only Starling force holding fluid in the vascular compartment is the osmotic pressure generated by the protein concentration gradient across the capillary membrane, even slight decreases in this gradient (consequent to movement of protein from inside to outside the vessel) have profound effects on net water balance. An increase in microvascular hydrostatic pressure or pulmonary blood flow produces a much greater outward flow of water when the protein gradient is reduced because of altered permeability,[5,13] so the combination of increased permeability and high LA pressures represents an especially difficult clinical challenge.

LYMPHATIC CLEARANCE

Whether there is fluid accumulation in the lung depends on the balance between fluid filtration into the lung and lymphatic clearance. Early in the onset of interstitial edema, lymphatic drainage of fluid is an important protective mechanism preventing alveolar flooding. Although early work had indicated that increased motion or ventilation of the lung increased the lymphatic fluid drainage, suggesting a passive milking action, it now appears that the contribution of active contractions of the smooth muscle of the lymphatics is significant and can be augmented by vasoactive agents. It has been shown that rhythmic inflation and deflation is not required for normal lymphatic function in lungs that are normal or have increased permeability.[14] Lung lymph flow can increase up to 10-fold acutely, and in chronic edema the maximal ability of the lymphatics to clear fluid may increase severalfold, presumably as the result of proliferation of the lymphatic vasculature. Because the lymphatics ultimately drain into the great veins, elevation of systemic venous pressure might be expected to increase fluid accumulation not only by raising pressure in the fluid-exchanging vessels but also by impairing lymphatic drainage. The concentration of protein in lymph is generally high. Although our focus is on pulmonary edema, a major role of the lymphatics is to return the interstitial protein back to the circulation.

SURFACE TENSION

Surface tension at the air-liquid interface on the inner surface of the alveolus tends to pull fluid away from the alveolar epithelium with a force of at least 2 mm Hg (see Fig. 43-3*A*). This figure is based on the assumption that the alveolar surface is spherical and that the surface tension is 10 dynes/cm, which is low presumably because of the presence of the surfactant. However, because the alveoli are polyhedral, there are many angles at which two alveoli come together and corners at which more than two alveoli abut. Although the shape of the alveolar air-liquid interface is spherical in the corners as well as in crypts in the alveolar walls, it is cylindrical at the angles, and therefore $P = ST/r$ would be the appropriate formula to use at the angles. Because the radii of curvature at the angles and corners of the alveoli are much smaller, the pressures are much more negative (see Fig. 43-3*B*). Surface tension at the alveolar air-liquid interface would be expected to expand the perivascular space and to lower perimicrovascular pressure, thus promoting the formation of interstitial edema. The effect of the change in radius of curvature of the alveolar air-liquid interface on surface forces is further illustrated in Figure 43-4. Initially, as fluid collects in the corners, the radius of curvature becomes greater and the pressure becomes less negative (see Fig. 43-4*B*). Once the fluid layer becomes spherical throughout the inner surface of the alveoli, additional fluid will decrease the radius, and the pressure will become more negative (see Fig. 43-4*C*). This process explains why the filling of an alveolus with fluid is self-accelerating once there is a critical amount of fluid in it.

Surface tension at the alveolar air-liquid interface opposes the transmission of alveolar pressure to the fluid-exchanging vessels.[8] Therefore, the beneficial effects of positive pressure breathing in the treatment of pulmonary edema probably do not relate to an increase in the pressure surrounding the fluid-exchanging vessels, but rather to (1) an increase in intrathoracic pressures, impeding venous return to the thorax, and thus lowering the hydrostatic pressures within the pulmonary vascular bed; (2) the prevention of airway collapse, thus enhancing blood gas exchange; and (3) an increase in lung volume through the recruitment (opening) of fluid-filled airspaces, which once partially filled with air can participate in gas exchange.

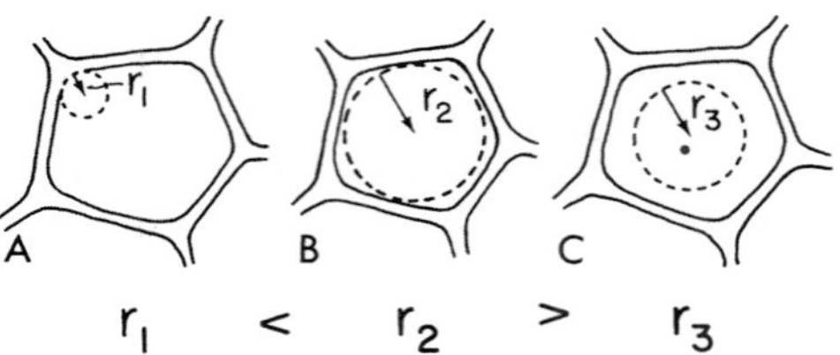

■ **FIGURE 43-4.** **A-C,** Effect of fluid accumulation on the radius of curvature at the alveolar air-liquid interface. See text for description.

■ "SAFETY FACTORS" THAT OPPOSE EDEMA FORMATION

A variety of clinical observations have indicated that vascular hydrostatic pressures must be raised by 15 to 20 mm Hg, or plasma colloid osmotic pressures must be reduced an equivalent amount, before edema develops. Several factors contribute to this protection against edema. The interstitial fluid pressure, which, as we have noted previously, is below alveolar pressure, is not a fixed value but will rise to approximately zero with minimal amounts of fluid filtration into the lung. With increased fluid filtration, it may increase further by 4 or 5 mm Hg and thus oppose fluid movement. At the same time, the filtered fluid will dilute the interstitial plasma protein, thus lowering the interstitial colloid osmotic pressure and diminishing the movement of fluid out of the microvasculature. Lymphatic drainage of fluid and protein also contributes to this "margin of safety." The ability of the lymphatics to concentrate protein by filtering fluid through their walls, although still an area of controversy, probably also contributes by keeping the interstitial osmotic pressure low. The interstitial space itself, especially around the bronchi and blood vessels (bronchovascular cuffs), can sequester fluid (as much as 500 mL in the adult) and thus can provide an additional safety factor before fluid floods the alveoli. In addition, surfactant, by keeping surface tension low, tends to prevent the lowering of alveolar interstitial pressure.

■ PATHOPHYSIOLOGIC CONSEQUENCES OF EDEMA

Edema accumulates within the lung in a stepwise fashion (Fig. 43-5). The gas volume of the alveolus decreases in a nonlinear relationship with the distending pressure, and the absolute size of the alveolus decreasing as it becomes fluid filled. Distal lung units in different regions of the lung, however, may be at different stages of fluid accumulation due to regional differences in pressure, alveolar-capillary integrity, and gravitationally dependent factors.

Increased pulmonary blood volumes may occur without associated pulmonary edema formation and will cause a small decrease in lung compliance (i.e., increased lung recoil) at normal or high lung volumes.[15] However, at low lung volumes there is a decrease in lung recoil. The concomitant presence of interstitial edema does not further reduce the compliance at high lung volumes until the extravascular fluid volumes increase at least threefold.[16] The pathophysiologic consequences and clinical findings in pulmonary edema are best understood by reviewing the sequence of events that lead from interstitial to airspace edema.

In humans, an increase in small airway resistance occurs early during the development of interstitial edema; however, this results from a vagally mediated reflex rather than from large increases in lung water content.[17] Although peribronchiolar cuffs of fluid would be expected to lead to increases in airway closure and airway resistance, morphometric studies provide no support for the notion that interstitial lung edema directly compresses the airways.[18] They suggest that alveolar or airway luminal edema may be responsible for the increase in resistance with edema. If the small airways contribute a relatively greater proportion of the total airway resistance in infants than in adults, one might expect edema to lead to a greater increase in airway resistance in infants. Indeed, small airway obstruction

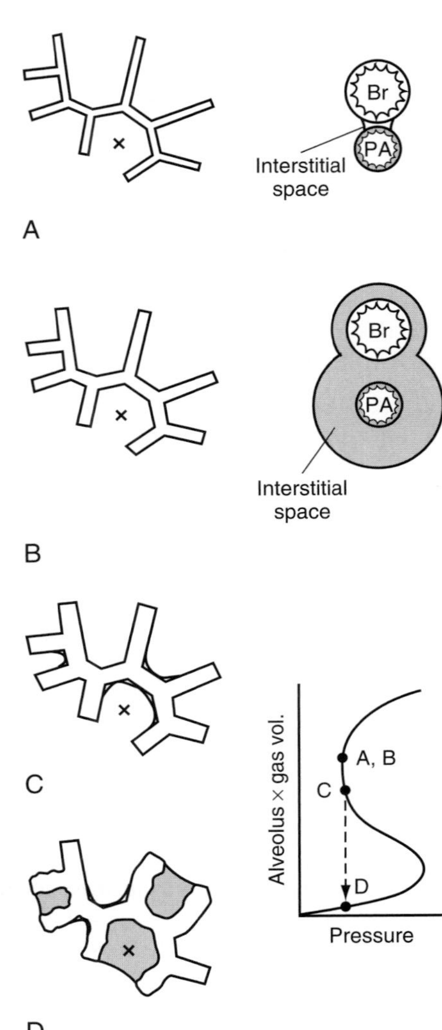

■ **FIGURE 43-5.** Schematic representation of the sequence of fluid accumulation during acute pulmonary edema. **A,** Normal alveolar walls and no excess fluid in perivascular connective tissue spaces. **B,** Initial fluid leak. Fluid flows to the interstitial space (at subatmospheric pressure) around the conducting vessels and airways. **C,** Tissue space fills, alveolar edema increases, and fluid begins to overflow into the alveoli, notably at the corners where curvature is pronounced. **D,** Quantal filling. Individual alveoli reach a critical configuration at which existing inflation pressure can no longer maintain stability. Alveolar gas volume rapidly passes to a new configuration with much reduced curvature (see graph insert). The volume deficit is absorbed by additional fluid filling or alveolar collapse, depending on associated conditions such as alveolar surface tension and availability of fluid. (From Staub NC, Nagano K, Pearce ML: Pulmonary edema in dogs, especially the sequence of fluid accumulation in lungs. J Appl Physiol 1967;22:227–240.)

has been a presenting sign of a group of infants with ventricular septal defects and left-to-right shunts.[19] In addition, some children with interstitial edema as a result of LA obstruction (e.g., cor triatriatum) have also presented with a history of recurrent asthmatic attacks. To minimize the markedly increased work of moving their stiff lungs, a pattern of rapid, shallow breathing is used. It is also believed that stimulation by edema of vagal juxta-alveolar receptors, or J receptors, within the interstitium contributes to the hyperventilation as well as the tachypnea and dyspnea so characteristic of early pulmonary edema. It is not clear whether increased ventilation enhances or impedes fluid accumulation. Increased ventilation is known to, at least transiently, promote the removal of excess water by the lymphatics. However, if there are inhomogeneities of disease within the lung, mechanical amplification of pressures could lead to enhanced edema formation, as we have already indicated.

Initially, edema fluid collects within the bronchovascular connective tissue sheath surrounding the larger blood vessels and airways. Airway resistance increases, perhaps as suggested previously because of vagally mediated bronchoconstriction or airway luminal edema. The airways are narrowed and more likely to close at higher than normal lung volumes. Alveolar gas exchange is impaired because of the resultant VA/Q ratio imbalance. At this stage, there is hypocapnia as the result of the J receptor vagally mediated reflex hyperventilation, whether or not there is hypoxemia. As edema worsens and alveolar flooding occurs, there is further hypoxemia as the blood shunts past nonventilating alveoli. Respiratory acidosis may supervene if the patient is depressed by sedation or if exhaustion develops. The extent to which bronchial mucosal edema intensifies the increase in airway resistance when pulmonary edema is accompanied by elevated systemic venous pressure is not known. With alveolar flooding and disruption of the normal alveolar lining, resistance to airflow increases, dynamic and static compliance are reduced, and there is increasing inhomogeneity of airflow. One can account for most of the clinical findings (e.g., crackles and diffuse wheezing) on the basis of interstitial, airway, and alveolar edema.

CLEARANCE OF PULMONARY EDEMA FLUID

How quickly pulmonary edema resolves once the basic condition producing the edema is reversed depends on whether the fluid is confined to the interstitium, from which it can be cleared in hours, or is also located in the alveolar space, from which it may take days to clear.

There are two potential routes for clearance of edema fluid from the lung's interstitial space. As discussed above, lymphatics play a major role in this clearance, although it is uncertain as to the absolute rate of lymph flow in normal and edematous human lungs. Experiments have shown that the normal adult sheep lung can increase its lymphatic flow rate from basal values of 5 to 10 mL/hour up to 30 to 50 mL/hour. It has also been demonstrated that the lymphatics can increase their capacity manyfold when there is pulmonary edema on a long-standing basis. The second route for interstitial fluid clearance is reabsorption in the venular end of the microvascular bed. Since Pmv has decreased in the venular region, the balance of Starling forces can favor reabsorption in downstream regions of the pulmonary and bronchial vessels. Recall that one of the major sites of fluid sequestration during interstitial edema is around the large airways.

Alveolar edema fluid may ultimately be returned to the circulation either by direct entry into the pulmonary microvasculature across the thin side of alveolar capillary membrane or by the lymphatics after it has been translocated back to the interstitial space. Both of these potential pathways, however, require water and solutes to have traversed the distal lung epithelium.

It had been assumed that the airspace fluid traversed the distal lung epithelium in response to hydrostatic and osmotic pressure gradients. However, in both high-pressure and high-permeability pulmonary edema, there are substantial amounts of protein within the alveolar fluid that would oppose osmotic reabsorption. Indeed, it was demonstrated that passive forces could not explain the clearance of alveolar fluid from the intact lung,[20] and long-term studies demonstrated that as edema fluid is reabsorbed, the protein concentration in the alveolar space actually increases above levels in the plasma. This suggested that an active transport of salt and water was involved in the clearance of airspace fluids. Numerous studies, as reviewed recently,[21–23] have now demonstrated that nonprimate mammalian and human distal lung epithelium actively transports Na^+, with Cl^- and water following (Fig. 43-6). Studies in the adult lung[24] have indicated that fluid clearance rates in the human are in the range of 25% per hour. The rate of airspace fluid clearance varies between different mammalian species: dogs approximately 5% per hour; sheep approximately 10% per hour; rabbits approximately 15% per hour; rats approximately 30% per hour; and mice 35% per hour.

This active Na^+ transport by the lung's epithelium plays an important role in the clearance of alveolar edema fluid. Indeed, as described in detail in the section on Augmentation of the Rate of Clearance of Airspace Fluid, it correlates with clinical outcome (Fig. 43-7) and survival from congestive heart failure (CHF)– and acute respiratory distress syndrome (ARDS)–induced pulmonary edema.

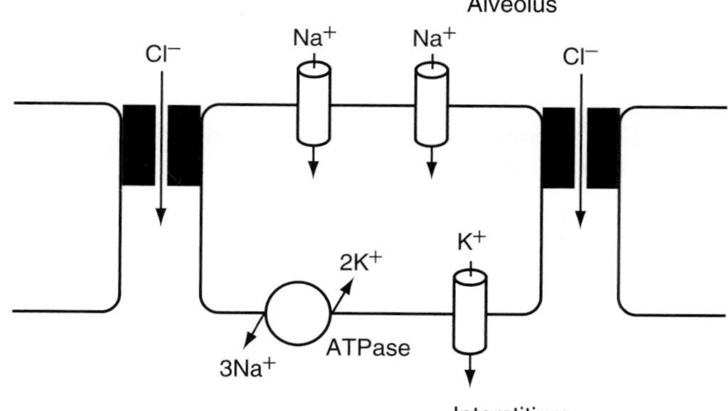

FIGURE 43-6. Model for Na^+ transport by the alveolar epithelium. The Na^+/K^+ ATPase located on the basolateral membrane is responsible for the creation of the marked intracellular/extracellular (10:150 mM) Na^+ concentration gradient. This chemical gradient along with the negative intracellular electrical potential arising from the permeability of the basolateral K^+ channels attracts Na^+ ions into the cell through Na^+-permeant ion channels located in the apical membrane to be extruded across the basolateral membrane. The activity of these Na^+-permeant ion channels represents the rate-limiting step in Na^+ transport. It is presumed that Cl^- follows via the paracellular pathway past the tight junctions, with water following in response to the osmotic gradient. It is uncertain whether water moves via the paracellular or intracellular pathway through water pores that have been identified in alveolar epithelium.

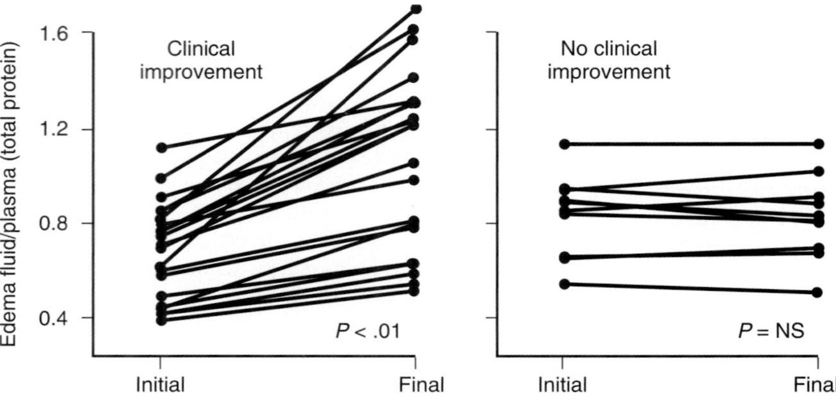

■ **FIGURE 43-7.** Individual data points are shown for the initial and final pulmonary edema fluid-to-plasma total protein concentration in the 24 patients with clinical improvement compared with 10 patients with no clinical improvement. The time intervals between the initial and final sample was 5.3 ± 3.9 hours for the clinical impairment group and 5.3 ± 4.7 hours for the no clinical improvement group. (From Matthay MA, Wiener-Kronish JP: Intact epithelial barrier function is critical for the resolution of alveolar edema in man. Am Rev Respir Dis 1990;142: 1250–1257.)

Protein clearance from the alveolar spaces is significantly slower than salt and water and in animals is in the range of 1% per hour.[20] The relative amount of protein cleared by metabolic degradation and macrophage ingestion versus active transport by the pulmonary epithelium is unknown, but it is clear that active transport is involved in the clearance of at least some proteins from the airspaces of the lungs.[25,26] Protein clearance from the interstitial space is believed to occur primarily by lymphatic clearance, but direct penetration into the circulation either before or after metabolic degradation has not been excluded as a potential mechanism.

The presence of protein in the alveolar and interstitial spaces may serve as a stimulant for the attraction of inflammatory cells, which can occur during the development of pulmonary edema, whether there has been lung injury and hence increased alveolar-capillary permeability. In acute lung injury syndromes there is marked leakage of plasma protein into the alveolar space, and resultant activation of the coagulation cascade results in fibrin formation. The coagulum opposes the efficient reabsorption of fluid, and fibrin and fibrin degradation products are potent stimuli for fibrosis within the lung. Circulating monocytes and alveolar macrophages likely play a major role in the clearance of inflammatory edema protein from the lung's airspaces (for further details see Chapter 44).

In summary, a wide variety of mechanisms and sites exist for protein and electrolyte clearance and fluid removal, including pulmonary and bronchial circulations, lymphatics, active transport of ions, macromolecular metabolism and degradation, and mononuclear cell activity.

■ MECHANISMS CAUSING PULMONARY EDEMA

There has been much effort to classify the different causes of pulmonary edema into cardiogenic and noncardiogenic pulmonary edema. Although this is useful to some degree, it should be remembered that both abnormal transvascular pressure gradients and increased permeability to solutes are present or subsequently develop in many lung diseases characterized by pulmonary edema. The various etiologies of pulmonary edema will be introduced by using the Starling equation as the basis for the discussion.

■ INCREASED HYDROSTATIC PRESSURE IN THE PULMONARY MICROVASCULATURE

This is the most common and perhaps most easily understood cause of pulmonary edema in the pediatric and adult population. A variety of clinical conditions are associated with increased hydrostatic pressures in the pulmonary microvasculature, either as the result of elevation of vascular pressures distal to the lung, increased blood flow, increased blood volume, or PA hypertension. In each case there would be an increase in the amount of water and solute leaving the microvasculature and entering the interstitium. Hypoxia increases PA pressures but does not increase vascular permeability to solutes.[3,27,28]

■ DECREASED PLASMA COLLOID OSMOTIC PRESSURE

If a patient has no other disorders, hypoproteinemia will not, by itself, cause pulmonary edema. Large pleural effusions may develop in diseases such as the nephrotic syndrome, but there is no evidence of lung edema as assessed by gas exchange and chest radiography. However, in patients where vascular pressure or alveolar capillary membrane permeability increases, pulmonary edema is more likely to develop and be more severe when the plasma proteins are low. This condition is seen with severe malnutrition, massive burns, protein-losing enteropathies, and nephrosis. Hypoproteinemia can also be seen in patients with a variety of other conditions when withdrawal of multiple blood samples for diagnostic purposes is coupled with the administration of large amounts of non-colloid-containing fluids.

■ DECREASED INTERSTITIAL HYDROSTATIC PRESSURE

As previously emphasized, because of mechanical interdependence of adjacent lung units, when inflation of some units lags behind that of others, large negative interstitial pressures can be generated around and within the lagging units. These negative pressures can be transmitted to the fluid-exchanging vessels (when there is airway closure), enhancing edema formation, especially in obstructive lung diseases such as asthma, bronchiolitis, and bronchopulmonary dysplasia (BPD), as well as in nonobstructive "stiff lung" disorders such as the respiratory distress syndrome (RDS).

■ INCREASED PULMONARY VASCULAR SURFACE AREA

The normal adult lung usually has approximately one third of its microvascular bed perfused under resting conditions. As discussed above (see section on Increased Hydrostatic Pressure in the Pulmonary Microvasculature), there are data indicating that infants (and young children) have a greater percentage of their vascular bed distended with blood. Regardless of the absolute percentage, the lungs of all age groups can undergo significant pulmonary vascular recruitment and distention. Although some reports suggest that various regions of the normal lung have different permeability to solutes, most studies suggest that lung fluid movement will increase in direct proportion to the increase in perfused pulmonary vascular surface area. Under normal conditions the lung lymphatics can easily accommodate the three- to fourfold increase in lung water and solute movement that is associated with full recruitment of the vasculature. However, when pulmonary vascular permeability is increased, similar amounts of recruitment can lead to marked increases in fluid movement as vessels with high permeability are recruited.[5,13]

INCREASED VASCULAR PERMEABILITY IN FLUID-EXCHANGING VESSELS

Increased alveolar-capillary membrane permeability to solutes can occur by several routes. Classic modeling of the pulmonary microvasculature has utilized the concept of various-sized "pores" through which various-sized solutes move under normal physiologic conditions. Thus, when permeability increases, the mechanisms could increase the total number of pores or the diameter of the pores. An example of this phenomenon would be an increase in the size of the interendothelial junctions from vasoactive agents. Alternatively, or in addition, direct and extensive damage to the alveolar epithelium or endothelium occurring during overventilation lung injury[29,30] or stress-induced endothelial injury[31] will open up large nonphysiologic pathways for fluid and solute movement.

A variety of clinical conditions are believed to alter the permeability of the alveolar capillary membrane, presumably by damage to epithelial or endothelial cells. The cellular mechanisms for this injury can be divided into two major categories: direct and inflammatory-mediated lung injury.

Direct lung injury can occur when a toxic substance directly causes cell injury without an associated inflammatory response. Direct lung injury is seen during the inhalation of a variety of noxious gases, many of which may be generated during fires, producing denaturation of proteins, cellular damage, and pulmonary edema. These include the oxides of sulfur and nitrogen, hydrocyanic acid, and several aldehydes. Similarly, the inhalation of gastric acid can directly damage lung epithelium.

Inflammatory-mediated lung injury (see Chapter 44) most frequently arises from leukocytes and their products. The unregulated release of leukocyte-derived toxic products occurs in response to direct injury or in response to various infective and inflammatory stimuli. These toxic products include reactive oxygen species (superoxide, hydrogen peroxide, hypochlorous acid, and the hydroxyl radical), proteolytic enzymes (elastase, collagenase, lysozyme), products of arachidonic acid (e.g., platelet-activating factor), and cationic proteins. Leukocytes have been implicated in animal models of acute lung injury induced by the administration of endotoxin, hyperoxia, microembolization, and mechanical ventilation. Non-leukocyte-derived vasoactive mediators can also increase vascular permeability. Examples include histamine, prostaglandins, cytokines, proteases, and reactive oxygen intermediates.

Increased permeability of the microvasculature also occurs in a variety of disorders characterized by aberrant regulation of the immune system. These include hypersensitivity pneumonitis (see Chapter 49) and pulmonary vasculitis, which can occur in various disorders such as systemic lupus erythematosus.

There are examples where the initial lung injury is mediated by a toxic substance but the secondary inflammatory response contributes significantly to the lung damage. Examples include hyperoxic lung injury and the inhalation of herbicides, such as paraquat, which results in the generation of reactive oxygen intermediates. These noxious agents cause pulmonary edema, presumably on the basis of a change in permeability. Even before morphologic evidence of alveolar injury is apparent, there is an increase in surface tension, presumably as the result of inactivation or impaired synthesis of pulmonary surfactant.[32]

CLINICAL EXAMINATION

In a general way, small increases in lung fluid are too subtle to detect by currently available clinical methods and only when the extravascular fluid volume has increased considerably is the condition obvious clinically. The patient will be tachpneic, not just when hypoxemia stimulates ventilation, but also because of the stimulation of the J receptors. This latter point explains, at least in part, the continuing tachypnea even after correction of arterial hypoxemia by supplemental oxygen therapy. On auscultation, crackles occur when edema fluid is present in the terminal airways and is produced by the sudden opening of peripheral lung units (alveolar ducts or terminal bronchioli). When the fluid moves up to larger airways, rhonchi and wheezes are to be expected. The relative contributions of bronchial wall edema and bronchoconstriction to rhonchi and wheezes is not known. Chest wall retractions will be observed as the spontaneously breathing patient must generate more negative pleural pressures to overcome the markedly decreased total respiratory system compliance and mild increases in airway resistance.

CLINICAL ASSESSMENT OF PULMONARY EDEMA

Although the distinction between cardiogenic or high-pressure edema and high-permeability or low-pressure edema has been based on the finding of a low pulmonary artery wedge pressure in the latter, it is now clear that Pmv may be elevated in the presence of a normal LA or wedge pressure and that there are limitations to using the wedge pressure to separate hemodynamic or cardiogenic edema from permeability or noncardiogenic edema.[33]

The double-indicator dilution technique depends on one tracer that is confined to the vascular space and another tracer that diffuses into the perfused tissue. The difference in the sum of the two time concentration curves has been used to calculate the lung water. Unfortunately, it can only measure that portion of the lung that is perfused and therefore may underestimate the total lung water. Measurements of thermal volume of the lung that also provide an estimate of lung water content have also been assessed and regrettably demonstrate the same limitations. Thus, neither of these measurements are satisfactory for the routine monitoring of lung water content in critically ill patients with pulmonary edema.

When patients with pulmonary edema have been intubated, one can collect airway fluid, which may reflect alveolar fluid. On this basis, investigators had attempted to differentiate high-pressure from increased permeability pulmonary edema[34,35] by comparing the concentration of the protein in the airspace fluid with the simultaneously measured plasma protein concentration. Although this ratio was statistically significantly different between the two groups, there was such significant scatter that it was found to be of little diagnostic utility for the individual patient. The reason for this variation and lack of clinical utility is now understood; the alveolar fluid's protein concentration not only depends on the leakiness of the alveolar-capillary membrane, but also on the efficiency and amount of time available to actively pump salt and water out of the airspace with the resultant concentration of the protein that remains in the distal lung unit (see earlier section on Clearance of Pulmonary Edema Fluid).

PULMONARY FUNCTION TESTS

Initially, vascular engorgement may lead to an increase in the diffusion capacity of the lung for carbon monoxide (DLCO) by increasing the amount of perfused vasculature within the gas-exchanging regions of the lung. As interstitial edema increases, there will be an increase in closing volume, a decrease in maximum expiratory flow, an increase in ventilation-perfusion inhomogeneity, and a decrease in arterial partial pressure of oxygen ($Pa{O_2}$). With alveolar flooding, there is further air trapping, increased vascular resistance, decreased lung volumes, decreased dynamic lung compliance, decreased DLCO, and progressive hypoxemia arising from the increased intrapulmonary right-to-left shunting and rising partial pressure of carbon dioxide in arterial blood ($Pa{CO_2}$), the latter further decreasing alveolar partial pressure of oxygen ($PA{O_2}$). In patients with a probe patent foramen ovale, there may be right-to-left shunting at the atrial level as a result of the associated pulmonary hypertension and concomitant increase in right ventricular end-diastolic pressure.

Under conditions of chronic edema formation, lymphatics and interstitial accumulations of fluid may be visible as Kerley lines (see later section on The Chest Radiograph). Because pulmonary edema can lead to airway obstruction in children, airway closure can occur and produce air trapping.[19] Thus, low diaphragms may be a useful sign of interstitial edema, provided there are no other reasons for airway obstruction. Other signs that are useful in following the severity of pulmonary engorgement and edema include the rapidity and shallowness of breathing, the magnitude of inspiratory intercostal retractions, and changes in body weight. Grunting, which maintains positive airway pressures, is a common accompaniment of pulmonary edema and represents a useful maneuver to prevent lung collapse.

IMAGING STUDIES

It has been shown that an infusion of 30 mL/kg of saline into healthy adult volunteers over 30 minutes would increase extracellular fluid volume by 15% without altering the density of the lungs on computed tomography (CT) or the amount of Compton scattering; the only change on chest radiography and CT studies was an increase in the size of the azygus vein.[36] To my knowledge, studies such as these have not been repeated in humans, so it is unknown whether modern imaging techniques might be more sensitive.

THE CHEST RADIOGRAPH

Studies have suggested that pulmonary edema can be detected in adult humans and dogs on a chest radiograph when extravascular lung water is increased by approximately 35%. Although most of the radiographic signs of pulmonary edema are nonspecific, improved radiographic techniques, in conjunction with improved understanding of the pathophysiology of pulmonary edema, have enhanced the usefulness of the chest roentgenogram in the diagnosis of pulmonary edema.

The Kerley A and B lines represent interlobular sheets of abnormally thickened or widened connective tissue that are tangential to the radiographic beam; the A lines are in the depths of the lung near the hilum, and the B lines are at the periphery or surface of the lung (Fig. 43-8). These are more properly referred to as septal lines. Although thickening may occur from a variety of processes, including fibrosis, pigment deposition, and pulmonary hemosiderosis, when they are transient these lines are usually caused by edema. These septal lines of edema are more clearly visible in older children and adults with chronic edema (see Fig. 43-8) than in infants, presumably because they are wider.

Perivascular and peribronchial cuffing are also radiographic signs of interstitial edema fluid. Another radiographic sign of early pulmonary edema is prominent upper lobe vessels, which appear in conjunction with basal interstitial edema. For hydrostatic reasons, perivascular edema is greatest in the gravitationally dependent regions, and the normal tethering action of the lung is therefore less in this region. With increased resistance to the lower lobe vessels, there is redistribution to the upper lobes. This sign is, of course, of limited value in infants because they are most likely to be in the supine position, and they have

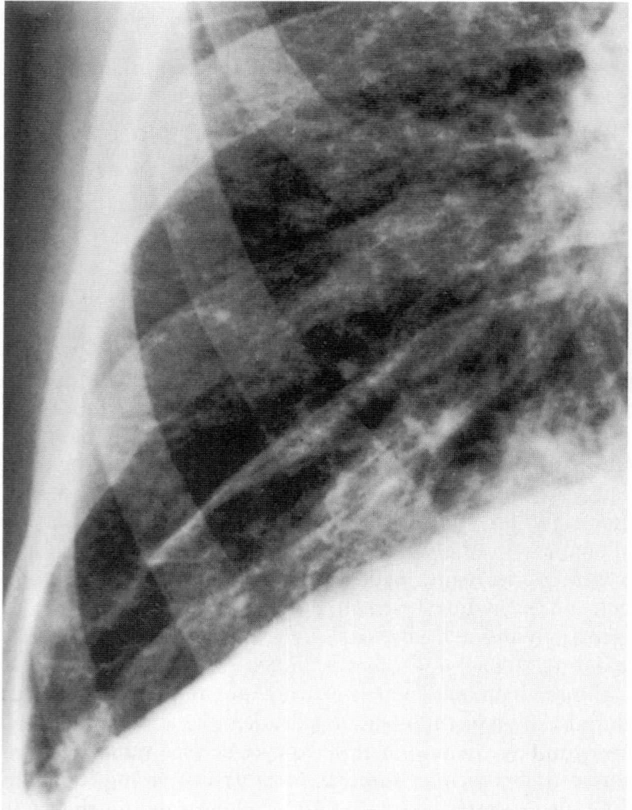

FIGURE 43-8. Chest roentgenogram of an 18-year-old with congenital mitral stenosis, demonstrating horizontal septal lines of edema (Kerley B lines) at the periphery of the lung.

smaller gravitationally induced differences due to their size and slightly increased PA pressures relative to children and adults.

More severe forms of pulmonary edema commonly produce a perihilar haze, presumably because the large perivascular and peribronchial collections of fluid are in this location. A reticular or lattice-like pattern may also be present and is more common at the base in an upright individual. Once the magnitude of pulmonary edema is sufficiently severe to lead to persistent airway closure or alveolar flooding, it is very difficult to separate edema, atelectasis, and inflammation on chest roentgenograms; air bronchograms indicate airless distal lung units and not the underlying cause.

Although studies in children are limited, a summary of findings that allow separation of cardiogenic or hemodynamic edema, renal or overhydration edema, and injury or ARDS edema has been provided in adults.[37] Thus, there is an inverted base-to-apex redistribution of blood flow in cardiac patients. The progressive recruitment of connective tissue spaces by edema fluid in both cardiac and renal disease gives rise to hilar blurring, peribronchial cuffing, and a hazy pattern of increasing lung density. In ARDS there is more likely to be a patchy peripheral distribution of edema and a paucity of such findings as septal lines and peribronchial cuffing.

One major difference between the chest radiograph of the young child as contrasted with the adult during early vascular engorgement and pulmonary edema is the increased lung volume (low diaphragm) in the child.[19] As discussed in the earlier section on Pathophysiologic Consequences of Edema, although this increased volume was originally attributed to compression of peripheral airways by interstitial edema and vascular engorgement (competition for space), morphometric studies in adult dogs offer little support for this mechanism.[18] Other potential mechanisms include transient bronchoconstriction mediated by vagal reflex[17] and increase in airway fluid and formation of bronchial froth.[38]

COMPUTED TOMOGRAPHY AND MAGNETIC RESONANCE IMAGING

Thin-section CT imaging of the thorax has provided new information regarding pulmonary edema. For example, studies in ARDS have shown that the lung densities, presumably representing regional edema and microatelectasis, are very heterogeneous and shift with the position of the patient, with densities appearing in the most gravitationally dependent lung regions.[39,40] The major limitation is that alterations in lung density have to be interpreted with caution. Increases in regional lung density can result from increases in extravascular lung water (i.e., edema); however, a decrease in regional gas volume will also increase density measurements.

Magnetic resonance imaging (MRI) to date has had limited use in management of patients with pulmonary edema but has the advantage that it does not require exposure to ionizing radiation. One major limitation is that, although one can obtain excellent imaging of the larger pulmonary vessels, MRI provides very poor resolution of the lung's parenchyma. The safe transport to and the management of the patient within the MRI suite is also a pragmatic limitation to this imaging modality. However, one center with an MRI apparatus within their critical care unit has utilized this approach to document that there is increased lung water content in premature babies with RDS.[41] These findings are consistent with earlier studies of gravimetric measurement of lung water content in postmortem infants and research studies in nonhuman primates (see later section on Neonatal Respiratory Distress Syndrome).

DETECTION OF LUNG INJURY

In order to differentiate high-pressure from high-permeability edema with certainty, it would be useful to have measurements that could detect damage to the alveolar-capillary membrane. It is impossible to directly measure Pmv in patients, and reliance on pulmonary artery wedge pressures has its limitations (see earlier section on Vascular Forces). Endothelial cell injury has been assessed by the removal and metabolism of a variety of substances; however, these tests are neither sufficiently sensitive nor specific. Similarly, the clearance rates of inhaled and deposited small solutes (e.g., ^{99m}Tc-DTPA) from the lungs provide an index of pulmonary epithelial integrity[42]; however, this approach is hampered by the inability to differentiate increased epithelial permeability from marked increases in regional lung volume.[43] Similarly, measurements of the relative concentrations of protein within the edema fluid and plasma are not helpful in proving increased permeability of the alveolar capillary membrane to protein (see earlier section on Clinical Assessment of Pulmonary Edema). Analysis of airspace fluid, however, may still be beneficial since a recent study utilizing a proteinomic analytic technique has shown that there are qualitative changes in the expression of some proteins; such analyses may provide new markers for lung injury.[44]

CLINICAL SYNDROMES ASSOCIATED WITH PULMONARY EDEMA

HIGH-PRESSURE (CARDIOGENIC) PULMONARY EDEMA

This diagnostic label refers to conditions where there is a demonstrable increase in the forces promoting fluid movement out of the microvasculature. By far the most common cause is left-sided heart disease, which results in marked elevations of pulmonary venous and hence microvasculature hydrostatic pressure.

Obstructive lesions such as cor triatriatum, mitral stenosis, congenital obstruction of pulmonary venous drainage, and pulmonary veno-occlusive disease directly cause pulmonary venous hypertension. In contrast, other obstructive lesions such as coarctation of the aorta and severe aortic stenosis only cause pulmonary edema once left ventricular failure has occurred.

Myocardial failure with subsequent pulmonary venous hypertension may arise from either congenital or acquired heart disease. Examples include hypoplastic left heart syndrome and intrinsic myocardial disease (e.g., cardiac glycogen storage diseases, endocardial fibroelastosis, viral and rheumatic myocarditis), and myocardial ischemia from anomalous left coronary artery or Kawasaki disease.

Markedly increased pulmonary blood flow occurs in patients with congenital arteriovenous fistulas or congenital heart defects that promote left-to-right shunting of blood (e.g., ventricular septal defect, patent ductus arteriosus). This leads to pulmonary vascular engorgement in the case of anatomic left-to-right shunting and in either case requires markedly increased left ventricular output. When the burden on the left ventricle becomes too great and left-sided heart failure supervenes, pulmonary vascular pressures are increased by both high-flow and increased LA pressures.

Marked increases in blood volume can result in pulmonary vascular engorgement and edema. Fluid retention rapidly occurs in acute renal disease as a result of the expansion of the extracellular fluid. Nephrosis and chronic renal disease may also predispose an individual to pulmonary edema by the associated hypoproteinemia. Perhaps the most common cause of increased pulmonary blood volume is the overzealous administration of fluids. This will intensify the development of pulmonary edema by raising hydrostatic pressures and diluting plasma proteins. Finally, to what extent the inappropriate secretion of antidiuretic hormone, which occurs in disorders such as pneumonia, asthma, and bronchopulmonary dysplasia, complicates and intensifies the development of pulmonary edema in disease is not known.

AIRWAY OBSTRUCTION

Croup and epiglottitis are associated with pulmonary edema.[45,46] Although there is some controversy whether severe large extrathoracic airway obstruction does indeed predispose the patient to pulmonary edema, it is possible that edema develops in those patients in whom there is airway closure so that very negative pressures are transmitted to the interstitium surrounding the fluid-exchanging vessels of the lung (see earlier section on Interstitial Forces).

Diffuse small airway obstruction can also promote the development of pulmonary edema as a result of a lag in the expansion of the lung in spite of the development of very negative intrathoracic pressures.[47] Although airway inflammation is recognized as an important part of the pathogenesis of asthma, it is not clear to what extent edema of the airways per se plays in the airway obstruction. Certainly, any inflammation-induced increase in permeability would dramatically increase the amount of fluid moving across the vascular bed in response to a more negative interstitial pressure. Clinically, it is not infrequent that significant improvements in gas exchange are seen in some patients with asthma and bronchiolitis following the use of diuretics. Because these diuretics could also change vascular compliance and pressures, the mechanism for the response is not clear. Nevertheless, this improved understanding of how airway obstruction can promote the development of pulmonary edema has led to the present therapeutic strategy of giving only maintenance fluids to patients after deficits have been replaced. In the past, it had been customary to advocate increased fluid intake for patients with asthma and bronchiolitis. The speculation that increased fluid intake will loosen secretions and facilitate their expectoration has never been established.

Cardiac failure and pulmonary edema is also rarely seen in obstructive sleep apnea; in children this condition is most frequently associated with hypertrophied tonsils and adenoids.[48,49] At the bedside, one cannot but be impressed with the severe intercostal retractions during inspiration. Indeed, this inspiratory pattern comes very close to simulating a Müller maneuver (i.e., a strong inspiration against a closed glottis or obstructed upper airway). The negative pressures surrounding and restraining the left ventricle are analogous to an afterload and would be expected to raise the pressures on the left side of the heart relative to pleural pressures. The large negative intrathoracic pressures may be at least partially responsible for the cardiomegaly, pulmonary vascular engorgement, and edema seen in severe cases. A dramatic example of the change in heart size following removal of the tonsils and adenoids is shown in Figure 43-9. Figure 43-9*A* shows the chest roentgenogram of a 3-year-old boy with chronic hypertrophied tonsils and adenoids at the time of presentation with clinical evidence of left-sided and right-sided heart failure. Figure 43-9*B* shows the improvement following removal of the tonsils and adenoids.

REEXPANSION PULMONARY EDEMA

Pulmonary edema is seen in some patients who have rapid lung reexpansion after drainage of a pneumothorax or pleural effusion.[50,51] The syndrome is associated with a sudden marked lowering of the interstitial fluid pressure, and this may be one

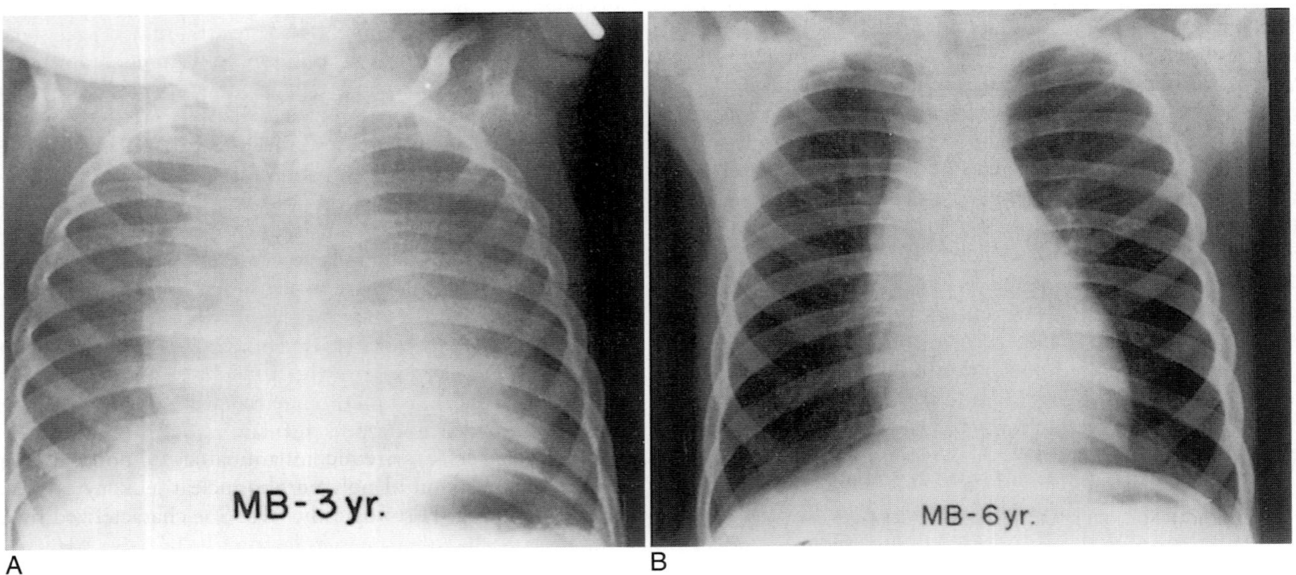

FIGURE 43-9. Chest roentgenogram before (**A**) and after (**B**) removal of tonsils and adenoids.

of the mechanisms responsible for edema. In most of the reported patients, lung collapse had been present for some time before reexpansion. Whether this factor alone restrains rapid expansion, as, for example, by a decrease in functional surfactant in the collapsed area, remains unclear. Regardless of the mechanism involved, this phenomenon highlights the caution that must be exercised when draining large collections of fluid from the pleural space when there is associated collapse of a lobe or lung. Rarely, reexpansion pulmonary edema can occur within the rapidly expanded lung and is associated with systemic hypovolemia and shock as large volumes of fluid move from the vascular to lobe airspace.

Experimental studies of reexpansion pulmonary edema in rabbits[52] provide evidence that increased vascular permeability to protein occurs. Although the mechanism for injury of the vascular membrane is not known, there are at least two possibilities. First, that there is increased and excessive stretch or tension of the alveolar septal walls during reexpansion of lungs that have been collapsed for several days. Stress-related pulmonary endothelial injury[31] has been described in other experimental conditions, and overexpansion of lungs during positive pressure ventilation is associated with increases in alveolar capillary permeability.[29,30] Other mechanisms, such as reperfusion lung injury from reactive oxygen intermediates, may also play a role in the increased alveolar-capillary membrane permeability. Indeed, it has been shown that collapsed lung tissue has decreased mitochondrial superoxide dismutase and cytochrome oxidase[53]; these changes could enhance oxygen free radical production.

NEONATAL RESPIRATORY DISTRESS SYNDROME

Studies in humans[41,54] and primates[55] prove that neonatal RDS (nRDS) in premature infants is associated with widespread airspace edema and that the well-described reduction in FRC results more from the excess fluid than from atelectasis.

A number of factors contribute to airspace fluid in patients with nRDS. First, there is the fluid that had been secreted into the developing lungs' airspaces; this is essential for normal lung development. However, this fluid must be cleared at birth so that effective gas exchange can occur and clearance of airspace fluid results from active transepithelial Na^+ transport (see Fig. 43-6). Impaired clearance of this fetal lung liquid combined with immaturity of the surfactant system results in nRDS.[23,56] Second, pulmonary edema fluid is generated during the course of nRDS by several mechanisms. These include the presence of excess fetal lung liquid at birth; high pulmonary vascular pressures and blood flow, especially if there is a ductus arteriosus; low interstitial pressures, in part the result of high alveolar surface tension; low plasma protein concentration (and hence low plasma osmotic pressure); increased epithelial permeability[14]; lung endothelial injury from inflammation and as a result of therapy; high airway pressures; and high inspired oxygen concentrations. The pulmonary edema that occurs after preterm birth as discussed in several reviews,[56,57] and RDS is discussed in greater detail in Chapter 18.

NEUROGENIC PULMONARY EDEMA

This condition is seen following head trauma, subarachnoid hemorrhage, brain tumors, and meningitis. The mechanism responsible for pulmonary edema following lesions of the brain is not fully understood but appears to result from a combination of hemodynamic and permeability-altering factors.[58] Neurogenic pulmonary edema may develop acutely over minutes to hours or may be delayed. Following acute head injury or sudden increases in intracerebral pressure, acute sympathetic discharge has been documented.[59] The discharge has the effect of acutely increasing left ventricular afterload. Cardiac output is maintained in this circumstance at the expense of increased left ventricular, and hence LA, filling pressures. This increase in pressure will lead to increased pulmonary microvascular hydrostatic pressure, which in turn will cause fluid to move into the lung interstitium.[60] Although this analysis favors microvascular hypertension as the primary cause of neurogenic pulmonary edema, studies of sheep in which lymph is collected and its protein content measured suggest that microvascular permeability is also increased[61]; high protein content has been noted in humans as well.[62] The more delayed forms of neurogenic pulmonary edema are characterized by normal pulmonary wedge and PA pressures and high protein content, suggesting that they result primarily from altered vascular permeability. Thus, factors raising pulmonary vascular pressure as well as factors altering vascular permeability are part of the pathogenesis. Ordinarily, neurogenic pulmonary edema may resolve with only supplemental oxygen. If positive ventilatory pressures, especially positive end-expiratory pressure (PEEP), are required, they should be administered cautiously, because they can interfere with cerebral venous return, thus leading to further cerebral edema.

UREMIA

Uremia may be associated with pulmonary edema as the result of overhydration, expansion of the blood volume, and elevation of the pulmonary microvascular pressures, compounded by anemia and reduced colloid osmotic pressures. In addition, vascular permeability may be altered as the result of increased metabolic products of uremia.

ACUTE LUNG INJURY AND THE ADULT RESPIRATORY DISTRESS SYNDROME

Conditions referred to as acute lung injury (ALI), and its most severe form, ARDS, frequently occur in critically ill patients. Regardless of the inciting event, the clinical and pathologic manifestations of ARDS are similar, indicating a final common pathway ultimately leading to severe endothelial and epithelial inflammatory injury. This causes a compromise of barrier and transport functions, which leads to high permeability pulmonary edema, which is often compounded by increases in microvascular pressure from concomitant pulmonary hypertension and pulmonary venoconstriction.

An initiating event, such as sepsis, shock, head injury, trauma, and other conditions outlined below (see later sections on High-Altitude Pulmonary Edema, Inhalation of Toxic Gases, Intravenous Agents, and Narcotic- and Drug-Induced Pulmonary Edema) triggers a systemic inflammatory response that promotes sequestration of polymorphonuclear leukocytes (PMNs) within the lung. Histologically, ARDS is characterized by large numbers of PMNs in the vascular, interstitial, and alveolar space in association with endothelial and epithelial injury. This, combined with the potential of PMNs to induce tissue injury in diverse experimental systems, has led to the widely held concept that these potent phagocytes are central to the pathogenesis of ARDS, a notion supported by numerous human and animal studies. The clinical presentation and pathogenic mechanisms and attempts at therapy are discussed in detail in Chapter 44.

HIGH-ALTITUDE PULMONARY EDEMA

It is well known that high-altitude pulmonary edema (HAPE) affects some sea level dwellers soon after arriving at a high altitude. However, it can also occur in some highlanders who return home after a brief stay at sea level. Much of our initial understanding of HAPE came from observations of Indian soldiers transported to high altitudes during the Indo-China war during the past century.[63] Subsequent work has shown that the incidence of HAPE and acute mountain sickness is increased when the rate of ascent is rapid and subjects have little opportunity for acclimatization, whereas gender or previous altitude exposure have no effect.[64] Of relevance to the above discussions regarding pulmonary vascular recruitment, the incidence of HAPE is increased in children and young adults,[65] and in subjects with only one pulmonary artery.[66] Fatigue, dyspnea, cough, and sleep disturbances are common and may progress rapidly to severe tachypnea, shock, and death unless rapid descent to a lower altitude or administration of oxygen occurs.

The mechanisms leading to HAPE are still incompletely understood. Experimental studies have shown that although hypoxia increases PA pressures, it does not by itself increase vascular permeability to solutes.[3,27,28] However, the best available evidence suggests that HAPE is initiated by an excessive increase in Pmv. The cause of the Pmv is unknown, although the two favored hypotheses are an unequal pulmonary vasoconstriction with resultant overperfusion of remaining lung microvessels or an abnormal vasoconstriction of the pulmonary venules. Prospective studies suggest that first there is a noninflammatory leakage of fluid across the alveolar-capillary membrane followed by a secondary inflammatory reaction[67] as the disease progresses.[68] Some researchers have assumed that, in addition to a constitutional predisposition of some individuals to pulmonary hypertension with hypoxia,[69] nonuniform increases in precapillary resistance are responsible for the very high pressures seen in at least some pulmonary capillaries. The observation that that prophylactic administration of the calcium channel blocker nifedipine can diminish the incidence of HAPE[70] and that inhalation of nitric oxide (NO) decreases PA pressures[71] and improves oxygenation[72] in such patients supports the speculation that an inappropriate pulmonary vasoconstrictive response causes HAPE. Observations that the amiloride-sensitive respiratory epithelial potential difference decreases in response to the decreased PO_2 at high altitude[73,74] suggest that the lung may not be able to clear the normal fluid lining its epithelium, thereby promoting the development of pulmonary edema or impairing the recovery from pulmonary edema (see earlier section on Clearance of Pulmonary Edema Fluid). The observation that salmeterol diminishes the frequency of HAPE[75] is intriguing, but the mechanism could include effects on vascular resistance and/or the augmentation of lung epithelial Na^+ transport.

INHALATION OF TOXIC GASES

Toxic lung injury can be induced by a wide variety of agents, and only two examples will be discussed. The most common agent is smoke from fires, the toxicity of which will vary with the nature of the combustible product (e.g., plastics versus wood). In victims of fires, the auscultatory evidence of pulmonary edema resulting from inhalation of smoke with damage to the distal lung unit, including the alveolar capillary membrane, always manifests within 24 hours and usually precedes roentgenographic changes.[76]

Chlorine gas inhalation is one example of a toxic gas that can cause severe lung injury. It is most frequently seen in industrial accidents, but can occur following exposure to fumes from liquid chlorine used in swimming pools. Pulmonary edema is frequently seen; however, if the patient survives there are no long-term sequelae.[77]

INTRAVENOUS AGENTS

Infusion of any compound that can act as a microembolic agent can result in high-permeability pulmonary edema in animal models of lung injury.[5] Clinical correlates in humans have been described where air microembolism[78] or infusion of lymphangiographic contrast material[79] has resulted in significant pulmonary edema.

NARCOTIC- AND DRUG-INDUCED PULMONARY EDEMA

Heroin and other narcotics have also been associated with pulmonary edema.[80,81] Pulmonary capillary wedge pressure has been elevated in some patients but has been normal in others. Whether hypoxia and acidosis or neurogenic pulmonary edema as the result of cerebral edema plays a role is not known. Clinical and roentgenographic signs of pulmonary edema have occurred following the intravenous administration of paraldehyde[82]; although a direct toxic action on the pulmonary vascular bed has been proposed, the cause remains obscure.

Salicylates have also been associated with the development of pulmonary edema.[83] Experimental studies in sheep indicate that salicylate pulmonary edema is due not to increased vascular pressure but rather to increased vascular permeability.[84] Insofar as these studies can be applied to the human, the researchers suggest that aspirin can cause pulmonary edema in doses considered therapeutic for some diseases. Although the mechanisms responsible for the altered vascular permeability remain unknown, at least two effects of salicylates could affect vascular integrity: alterations in platelet function and inhibition of prostaglandin synthesis.

THERAPY

REVERSAL OF HYPOXEMIA

The first step is to reverse the hypoxemia. If pulmonary edema is mild and predominantly interstitial in nature, then increasing the fraction of inspired oxygen (FIO_2) will be effective in correcting the low ventilation-perfusion (V/Q) ratios ($0 < V/Q < 1$) arising from airway dysfunction. However, most patients in acute pulmonary edema have significant airspace pulmonary edema and require increased transpulmonary pressures to hold the lung at a higher volume and recruit lung units, thereby decreasing shunt ($V/Q = 0$). Noninvasive and invasive approaches can be taken. Although out of favor in the recent past, several recent studies have demonstrated that noninvasive ventilation can be effective in cardiogenic pulmonary edema.[85,86] Most frequently, however, intubation and assisted ventilation are required both for efficacy and to minimize potential side effects such as overdistention of the stomach and potential aspiration. Mechanical aid not only reduces the oxygen consumption by reducing the work of breathing but also, when coupled with PEEP, improves oxygenation by preventing collapse of lung units and recruiting lung units. Numerous studies have shown that PEEP does not, on balance, directly decrease lung water content. Positive intrathoracic pressure generated by positive pressures at the mouth may reduce fluid filtration in the lung by impeding venous return and therefore decreasing pulmonary vascular volume and pressure. However, when vascular volume and pressures are maintained, positive pressure ventilation may actually enhance fluid accumulation in the lung.

REDUCTION OF THE RATE OF FLUID FILTRATION

The second step is to reduce the rate of fluid filtration into the lung. Treating the disorder creating the pulmonary edema, for example, CHF, is self-evident. Several therapeutic approaches are useful in treating CHF-induced elevation of pulmonary microvascular pressures, including measures that (1) improve cardiac contractility and allow the heart to achieve an increased stroke volume at a lower filling pressure (e.g., use of oxygen, digoxin, dopamine, dobutamine, etc.); (2) reduce preload, including the sitting position, rotating tourniquets, and positive-pressure ventilation; (3) reduce both preload and afterload primarily by relieving anxiety (e.g., use of morphine); (4) decrease plasma volumes and LA pressure and increase plasma colloid osmotic pressures (e.g., administration of diuretics); (5) decrease systemic or pulmonary vascular pressures or both using vasodilators such as prostacyclin, nitroprusside, or inhaled nitric oxide; and (6) reduce excessive salt and water intake. It should be noted that such measures are all very helpful in reducing the microvascular pressures in the lung regardless of whether the cause of the edema is hemodynamic or altered vascular permeability. As numerous studies have shown,[5,13,87] and as illustrated in Figure 43-10, small reductions in microvascular pressures can achieve large reductions in pulmonary edema when increased vascular permeability is the primary cause of the edema.

A reduction in the rate of fluid leakage from the vasculature could also be achieved using other strategies based on the Starling Equation (see earlier section on Factors Responsible for Fluid Movement). For patients suffering from ARDS and its associated high-permeability pulmonary edema, our goal is to return the permeability of the alveolar capillary membrane back to normal levels. Regrettably, despite decades of research, there is no proven way to modulate alveolar-capillary membrane permeability, although low-dose corticosteroids[88] or activated protein C in the subset of ARDS patients with sepsis[89] have been beneficial to some degree in altering the course of the overall disease.

Other strategies might include an increase in colloid osmotic pressure by an infusion of colloid; however, the concomitant rise in vascular pressure as vascular volume is increased secondary to the movement of water from the systemic tissues to the vascular compartment may undermine this effort. Lowering systemic vascular pressures by use of diuretics and drugs that reduce vascular resistance or afterload are both advantageous, as described above. It should be emphasized, however, that "diuretics" such

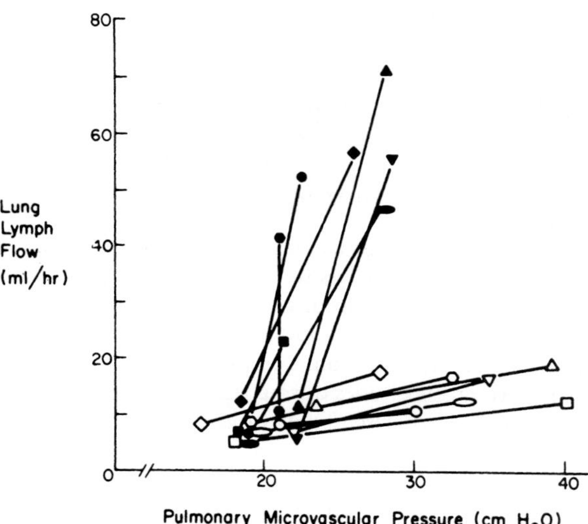

FIGURE 43-10. Relation of lung lymph flow to pulmonary microvascular pressures during hemodynamic edema *(open symbols)* and during permeability edema produced by infusion of *Pseudomonas (closed symbols)*. For a given reduction in vascular pressures, there is a much greater reduction in lung lymph flow in permeability edema than in hydrostatic edema. (From Brigham KL, Wolverton WC, Blake LH, Staub N: Increased sheep lung vascular permeability caused by *Pseudomonas* bacteremia. J Clin Invest 1974;54:792.)

as furosemide are beneficial in pulmonary edema because of their vascular effect of increasing systemic venous capacitance and not because of the induced diuresis. Improvement in the patient's status is usually seen within a few minutes after administering the diuretic, hence prior to the diuresis, and furosemide is helpful even in anuric patients. Since the lung represents only 1% of the total body weight, even a 3-L diuresis would only remove 30 mL from the lungs, with the remaining fluid coming from the remainder of the body. This 30 mL is trivial compared with the liters of fluid present in the airspaces of adult patients with florid alveolar edema (see earlier section on Anatomic Considerations).

MINIMIZATION OF TREATMENT-RELATED LUNG DAMAGE

The third step in therapy is to prevent or minimize treatment-related damage to the lung, whether this occurs through the inhalation of excessively high concentrations of oxygen or the suboptimal use of mechanical ventilation and overdistention of the lung, which induces damage to the lung's epithelium and endothelium,[29,30] thereby increasing the permeability of the alveolar-capillary membrane to water and solutes. Attention to treatment of the underlying condition combined with excellent supportive care using "lung-protective" ventilatory strategies to minimize treatment-related lung damage have contributed to successful clinical outcomes.[90] This subject is discussed in greater detail in Chapters 13, 18, and 44.

AUGMENTATION OF THE RATE OF CLEARANCE OF AIRSPACE FLUID

The fourth step is to augment the rate of clearance of the airspace fluid. It has now been demonstrated that intact active fluid absorption from the airspaces correlates with improved survival and various important clinical parameters such as the length of assisted ventilation and oxygen requirements, regardless of whether the patients suffer from acute CHF or ARDS-induced pulmonary edema.[24,91,92] Only 75% of patients with CHF-induced pulmonary edema have demonstrable alveolar fluid clearance, with only approximately 40% having maximal clearance rates (Fig. 43-11*A*).[24] The situation is even more grave for patients with ALI and ARDS because only 13% of these patients can achieve maximal rates of active airspace fluid clearance (see Fig. 43-11*B*).[92] Active clearance of airspace fluid was impaired more frequently in men and when there was associated sepsis.[92] Consistent with these observations suggesting the clinical importance of fluid clearance from the airspace by active Na transport mechanisms are the reports that the respiratory epithelium of adults who are susceptible to high altitude pulmonary edema have decreased Na^+ transport.[75] Together these studies and a recent report that pulmonary edema fluid itself can modulate Na and fluid transport by distal lung epithelium[93] suggest that increasing airspace epithelial active Na^+ transport will provide new treatment regimens for pulmonary edema.

Although studies in animals have shown that exogenous catecholamines can augment fluid clearance from the airspaces with experimentally elevated LA pressures,[94] studies in humans have not shown any correlation between the levels of circulating catecholamines and the rates of fluid clearance.[24,92] Other agents such as growth factors, cytokines, dopamine, and glucocorticoids are all capable of increasing pulmonary edema clearance in the normal lung.[21] The recent observation that pulmonary edema fluid itself, through previously unknown mechanisms, can increase active Na^+ and fluid transport by distal lung epithelium[93] suggests that there may be new therapeutic modalities for the treatment of CHF-induced pulmonary edema.

A recurrent theme throughout this chapter has been the potential role of vasoactive substances in the genesis or clearance of pulmonary edema by altering vascular pressures and permeability as well as active ion transport across the alveolar capillary membrane. Although the information about them is still limited, we have chosen to emphasize their importance because we believe that a more fundamental understanding of their role in the genesis of pulmonary edema is likely to lead to more specific forms of therapy.

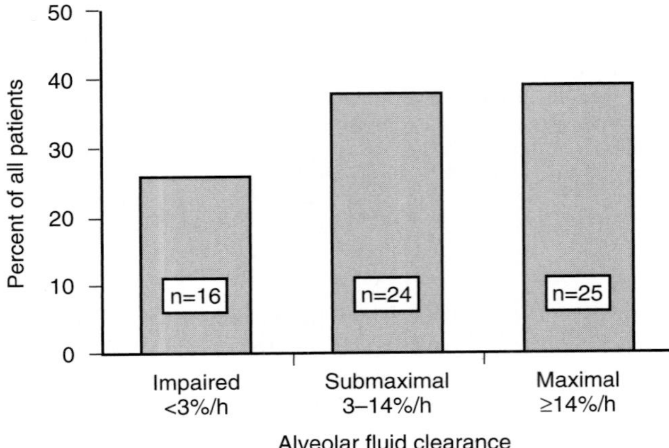

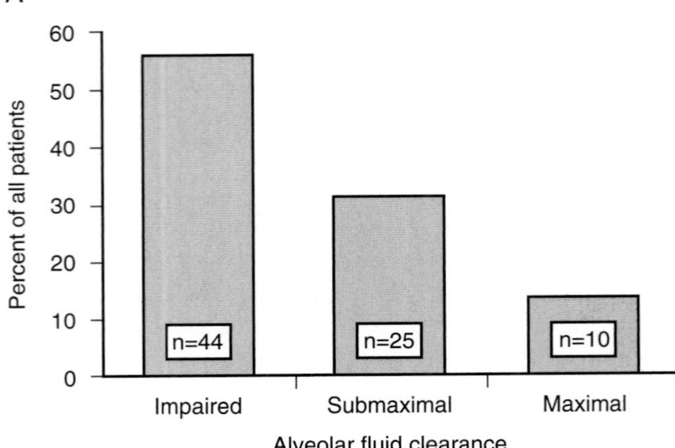

FIGURE 43-11. **A,** Rates of alveolar fluid clearance in 65 patients with severe hydrostatic pulmonary edema. *Solid bars* show percentage of 65 patients in each group. **B,** Percentage of patients with three categories of alveolar fluid clearance: impaired (<3%/hour), submaximal (>3%/hour, <14%/hour), or maximal (>14%/hour). Alveolar fluid clearance was measured during the first 4 hours after intubation and mechanical ventilation in 79 patients with acute lung injury or the acute respiratory distress syndrome. *Solid columns* show the percentage of 79 patients in each group (N = 5). (**A,** Reproduced from Verghese GM, Ware LB, Matthay BA, Matthay MA: Alveolar epithelial fluid transport and the resolution of clinically severe hydrostatic pulmonary edema. J Appl Physiol 1999;87(4):1301–1312; **B,** from Ware LB, Matthay MA: Alveolar fluid clearance is impaired in the majority of patients with acute lung injury and the acute respiratory distress syndrome. Am J Respir Crit Care Med 2001;163: 1376–1383.)

REFERENCES*

1. Iliff L: Extra-alveolar vessels and edema development in excised dog lungs. Circ Res 1971;28:524.
2. Gropper MA, Bhattacharya J, Staub NC: Filtration profile in isolated zone 1 and zone 3 dog lungs at constant high alveolar pressure. J Appl Physiol 1988;65:343.
3. Staub NC: Pulmonary edema. Physiol Rev 1974;54:678.
4. Drake RE, Laine GA: Pulmonary microvascular permeability to fluid and macromolecules. J Appl Physiol 1988;64:487.
5. O'Brodovich HM, Coates G: Effect of exercise on lung lymph flow in unanesthetized sheep with increased pulmonary vascular permeability. Am Rev Respir Dis 1986;134:862.
6. Stanek V, Widimsky J, Hurych J, Petrikova V: Pressure, flow, and volume changes during exercise within pulmonary vascular bed in patients after pneumonectomy. Clin Sci 1969;37:11.
7. O'Brodovich HM, Mellins RB, Mansell AL: Effects of growth on the diffusion constant for carbon monoxide. Am Rev Respir Dis 1982;125:670.
8. Mellins RB, Levine OR, Skalak R, Fishman AP: Interstitial pressure of the lung. Circ Res 1969;24:197.
9. Bhattacharya J, Staub NC: Interstitial fluid pressure gradient measured by micropuncture in the excised dog lung. J Appl Physiol 1984;56:271.
10. Macklem PT, Murphy B: The forces applied to the lung in health and disease. Am J Med 1974;57:371.
11. Raj JU: Alveolar liquid pressure measured by micropuncture in isolated lungs of mature and immature fetal rabbits. J Clin Invest 1987;79:1579.
12. Carlton DP, Cummings JJ, Scheerer RG, Bland RD: Lung vascular protein permeability in preterm fetal and mature newborn sheep. J Appl Physiol 1994;77:782.
13. Prewitt RM, McCarthy J, Wood LDH: Treatment of acute low pressure pulmonary edema in dogs. Relative effects of hydrostatic and oncotic pressure, nitroprusside, and positive end-expiratory pressure. J Clin Invest 1981;67:409.
14. Jefferies AL, Hamilton P, O'Brodovich HM: Effect of high-frequency oscillation on lung lymph flow. J Appl Physiol 1983;55:1373.
15. Levine OR, Mellins RB, Fishman AP: Quantitative assessment of pulmonary edema. Circ Res 1965;27:414.
16. Hauge A, Gunnar B, Waaler BA: Interrelations between pulmonary liquid volumes and lung compliance. J Appl Physiol 1975;38:608.

*The reader is referred to earlier editions of this book for references and review articles from the scientific literature up to the mid-1980s that underpin some of the comments within this chapter.

17. Goeree GW, Coates G, Powles ACP, Basalygo M: Mechanisms of changes in nitrogen washout and lung volumes after saline infusion in humans. Am Rev Respir Dis 1987;136:824.
18. Michel RP, Zocchi L, Rossi A, et al: Does interstitial lung edema compress airways and arteries. A morphometric study. J Appl Physiol 1987;62:108.
19. Hordof AJ, Mellins RB, Gersony WM, Steeg CN: Reversibility of chronic obstructive lung disease in infants following repair of ventricular septal defects. J Pediatr 1977;90:187.
20. Matthay MA, Landolt CC, Staub NC: Differential liquid and protein clearance from the alveoli of anesthetized sheep. J Appl Physiol 1982;53:96.
21. Matthay MA, Folkesson HG, Clerici C: Lung epithelial fluid transport and the resolution of pulmonary edema. Physiol Rev 2002;82:569.
22. Matalon S, O'Brodovich H: Sodium channels in alveolar epithelial cells. Molecular characterization, biophysical properties, physiological significance. Annu Rev Physiol 1999;61:627.
23. O'Brodovich H: Disorders of ion transport. In: Haddad G, Abman S, Chernick V, eds: The Basic Mechanisms of Pediatric Respiratory Disease, 2nd ed. New York: BC Dekker, 2002, p 294.
24. Verghese GM, Ware LB, Matthay BA, Matthay MA: Alveolar epithelial fluid transport and the resolution of clinically severe hydrostatic pulmonary edema. J Appl Physiol 1999;87(4):1301.
25. Kim KJ, LeBon TR, Shinbane JS, Crandall ED: Asymmetric [^{14}C] albumin transport across bullfrog alveolar epithelium. J Appl Physiol 1985;59:1290.
26. Kim KJ, Malik AB: Protein transport across the lung epithelial barrier. Am J Physiol Lung Cell Mol Physiol 2003;284:L247.
27. Hansen TN, Hazinski TA, Bland RD: Effects of asphyxia on lung fluid balance in baby lambs. J Clin Invest 1984;74:370.
28. Bland RD, Demling RH, Selinger SL, Staub NC: Effects of alveolar hypoxia on lung fluid and protein transport in unanesthetized sheep. Circ Res 1977;40:269.
29. Dreyfuss D, Soler P, Basset G, Saumon G: High inflation pressure pulmonary edema. Am Rev Respir Dis 1988;137:1159.
30. Carlton DP, Cummings JJ, Scheerer RG, et al: Lung overexpansion increases pulmonary microvascular protein permeability in young lambs. J Appl Physiol 1990;69:577.
31. West JB, Tsukimoto K, Mathieu-Costello O, Prediletto R: Stress failure in pulmonary capillaries. J Appl Physiol 1991;70:1731.
32. Robertson B: Paraquat poisoning as an experimental model of the idiopathic respiratory distress syndrome. Bull Physiopathol Respir (Nancy) 1973;9:1433.
33. Allen SJ, Drake RE, Williams JP, et al: Recent advances in pulmonary edema. Crit Care Med 1987;15:963.
34. Fein A, Grossman RE, Jones JG, et al: The value of edema fluid protein measurement in patients with pulmonary edema. Am J Med 1979;67:32.
35. Sprung CL, Long WM, Marcial EH, et al: Distribution of proteins in pulmonary edema. Am Rev Respir Dis 1987;136:957.
36. Coates G, Powles AC, Morrison SC, et al: The effects of intravenous infusion of saline on lung density, lung volumes, nitrogen washout, computed tomographic scans and chest radiographs in humans. Am Rev Respir Dis 1983;127:91.
37. Pistolesi M, Miniati M, Milne ENC, et al: The chest roentgenogram and pulmonary edema. Clin Chest Med 1985;6:315.
38. Ishii M, Matsumoto N, Fuyuki T: Effects of hemodynamics edema formation on peripheral vs. central airway dynamics. J Appl Physiol 1985; 59:1578.
39. Gattinoni L, Pelosi P, Vitale G, Pesenti A: Body position changes redistribute lung computed-tomographic density in patients with acute respiratory failure. Anesthesiology 1991;74:15.
40. Bombino M, Gattinoni L, Pesenti A, et al: The value of portable chest roentgenography in adult respiratory distress syndrome. Chest 1991;100:762.
41. Adams E, Counsell SJ, Hajnal JV, Cox PN, Kennea PL, Thornton ES, et al: Magnetic resonance imaging of lung water content and distribution in term and preterm infants. Am J Respir Crit Care Med 2002;166:397.
42. Jefferies AL, Coates G, O'Brodovich HM: Pulmonary epithelial permeability in hyaline membrane disease. N Engl J Med 1984;311:1075.
43. O'Brodovich HM, Coates G: Pulmonary clearance of ^{99m}Tc-DTPA. A noninvasive assessment of epithelial integrity. Lung 1987;165:1.
44. Bowler RP, Duda B, Chan ED, Enghild JJ, Ware LB, Matthay M, et al: A proteomic analysis of pulmonary edema fluid and plasma in patients with acute lung injury. Am J Physiol Lung Cell Mol Physiol 2004; 286: L1095.
45. Travis KW, Todres ID, Shannon DC: Pulmonary edema associated with croup and epiglottitis. Pediatrics 1977;59:695.
46. Kanter RK, Watchko JF: Pulmonary edema associated with upper airway obstruction. Am J Dis Child 1984;138:356.
47. Stalcup SA, Mellins RB: Mechanical forces producing pulmonary edema in acute asthma. N Engl J Med 1977;297:592.
48. Luke MJ, Mehrizi A, Folger GM Jr, Rowe RD: Chronic nasopharyngeal obstruction as a cause of cardiomegaly, cor pulmonale and pulmonary edema. Pediatrics 1966;37:762.
49. Cayler GG, Johnson EE, Lewis BE, et al: Heart failure due to enlarged tonsils and adenoids. Am J Dis Child 1969;118:708.
50. Childress ME, Moy G, Mottram M: Unilateral pulmonary edema resulting from treatment of spontaneous pneumothorax. Am Rev Respir Dis 1971;104:119.
51. Waqaruddin M, Bernstein A: Re-expansion pulmonary oedema. Thorax 1975;30:54.
52. Pavlin J, Nessly ML, Cheney FW: Increased pulmonary vascular permeability as a cause of re-expansion edema in rabbits. Am Rev Respir Dis 1981;124:422.
53. Jackson RM, Brannen AL, Vaal CF, Fulmer JD: Superoxide dismutase and cytochrome oxidase in collapsed lungs. Possible role in reexpansion edema. J Appl Physiol 1988;65:235.
54. deSa DJ: Pulmonary fluid content in infants with respiratory distress. J Pathol 1969;97:469.
55. Jackson C, Mackenzie A, Chi E, et al: Mechanisms for reduced total lung capacity at birth and during hyaline membrane disease in premature newborn monkeys. Am Rev Respir Dis 1990;142:413.
56. O'Brodovich H: Deficient Na^+ channel expression in newborn respiratory distress syndrome. Pediatr Pulmonol Suppl 2004;26:141.
57. Bland RD: Pathogenesis of pulmonary edema after birth. Adv Pediatr 1987;34:175.
58. Malik AB: Mechanisms of neurogenic pulmonary edema. Circ Res 1985;57:1.
59. Nathan MA, Reis DJ: Fulminating arterial hypertension with pulmonary edema from release of adrenomedullary catecholamines after lesions of the anterior hypothalamus in the rat. Circ Res 1975;37:226.
60 Theodore J, Robin ED: Speculations on neurogenic pulmonary edema (NPE). Am Rev Respir Dis 1976;113:405.
61. Bowers RE, McKeen CE, Park BE, Brigham KL: Increased pulmonary vascular permeability follows intracranial hypertension in sheep. Am Rev Respir Dis 1979;119:637.
62. Carlson RW, Schaeffer RC Jr, Michaels SG, et al: Pulmonary edema following intracranial hemorrhage. Chest 1979;75:731.
63. Singh I, Khanna PK, Srivastava MC, Lal M, Roy SB, et al: Acute mountain sickness. N Engl J Med 1969;280(4):175.
64. Hackett PH, Rennie D, Levine HD: The incidence, importance, and prophylaxis of acute mountain sickness. Lancet 1976;2:1149.
65. Scoggin CH, Hyers TM, Reeves JT, Grover RF: High-altitude pulmonary edema in the children and young adults of Leadville, Colorado. N Engl J Med 1977;297:1269.
66. Hackett PH, Creagh CE, Grover RF, et al: High-altitude pulmonary edema in persons without the right pulmonary artery. N Engl J Med 1980;302:1070.
67. Schoene RB, Swenson ER, Pizzo CJ, et al: The lung at high altitude. Bronchoalveolar lavage in acute mountain sickness and pulmonary edema. J Appl Physiol 1988;64:2605.
68. Bartsch P, Swenson ER, Maggiorini M: Update. High altitude pulmonary edema. Adv Exp Med Biol 2001;502:89.
69. Hultgren HN, Grover RF, Hartley LH: Abnormal circulatory response to high altitude in subjects with a history of high-altitude pulmonary edema. Circulation 1971;44:759.
70. Bartsch P, Maggiorini M, Ritter, et al: Prevention of high-altitude pulmonary edema by nifedipine. N Engl J Med 1991;325:1284.
71. Scherrer U, Vollenweider L, Delabays A, Savcic M, Eichenberger U, Kleger GR, Fikrle A, Ballmer PE, Nicod P, Bartsch P: Inhaled nitric oxide for high-altitude pulmonary edema. N Engl J Med 1996;334: 624.
72. Anand IS, Prasad BA, Chugh SS, Rao KR, Cornfield DN, Milla CE, et al: Effects of inhaled nitric oxide and oxygen in high-altitude pulmonary edema. Circulation 1998;98(22):2441.
73. Mairbaurl H, Schwobel F, Hoschele S, Maggiorini M, Gibbs S, Swenson ER, Bartsch P: Altered ion transporter expression in bronchial epithelium in mountaineers with high-altitude pulmonary edema. J Appl Physiol 2003; 95:1843.
74. Mason NP, Petersen M, Melot C, Imanow B, Matveykine O, Gautier MT, Sarybaev A, Aldashev A, Mirrakhimov MM, Brown BH, Leathard AD, Naeije R: Serial changes in nasal potential difference and lung electrical impedance. J Appl Physiol 2003;94:2043.

75. Sartori C, Allemann Y, Duplain H, Lepori M, Egli M, Lipp E, et al: Salmeterol for the prevention of high-altitude pulmonary edema. N Engl J Med 2002;346(21):1631.
76. Mellins R, Park S: Respiratory complications of smoke inhalation in victims of fires. J Pediatr 1975;87:1.
77. Jones RN, Hughes JM, Glindmeyer H, Weill H: Lung function after acute chlorine exposure. Am Rev Respir Dis 1986;134:1190.
78. Clark MC, Flick MR: Permeability pulmonary edema caused by venous air embolism. Am Rev Respir Dis 1984;129:633.
79. Silvestri RC, Huseby JS, Rughani I, et al: Respiratory distress syndrome from lymphangiography contrast medium. Am Rev Respir Dis 1980;122:543.
80. Paranthaman S, Khan F: Acute cardiomyopathy with recurrent pulmonary edema and hypotension following heroin overdosage. Chest 1976;69:117.
81. Katz S, Aberman A, Frand UI, et al: Heroin pulmonary edema. Am Rev Respir Dis 1972;106:472.
82. Sinal SH, Crowe JE: Cyanosis, cough and hypotension following intravenous administration of paraldehyde. Pediatrics 1976;57:158.
83. Heffner JE, Sahn SA: Salicylate-induced pulmonary edema. Ann Intern Med 1981;95:405.
84. Bowers RE, Brigham KL, Owen PJ: Salicylate pulmonary edema: the mechanism in sheep and review of the clinical literature. Am Rev Respir Dis 1977;115:261.
85. Masip J, Betbese AJ, Paez J, Vecilla F, Canizares R, Padro J, Paz MA, de Otero J, Ballus J: Non-invasive pressure support ventilation versus conventional oxygen therapy in acute cardiogenic pulmonary oedema. A randomised trial. Lancet 2000;356:2126.
86. Nava S, Carbone G, DiBattista N, Bellone A, Baiardi P, Cosentini R, et al: Noninvasive ventilation in cardiogenic pulmonary edema. A multicenter randomized trial. Am J Respir Crit Care Med 2003;168(12):1432.
87. Brigham KL, Woolverton WC, Blake LH, Staub N: Increased sheep lung vascular permeability caused by *Pseudomonas* bacteremia. J Clin Invest 1974;54:792.
88. Annane D, Sebille V, Charpentier C, Bollaert PE, Francois B, Korach JM, Capellier G, Cohen Y, Azoulay E, Troche G, Chaumet-Riffaut P, Bellissant E: Effect of treatment with low doses of hydrocortisone and fludrocortisone on mortality in patients with septic shock. JAMA 2002;288:862.
89. Bernard GR, Vincent JL, Laterre PF, LaRosa SP, Dhainaut JF, Lopez-Rodriguez A, Steingrub JS, Garber JE, Helterbrand JD, Ely EW, Fisher CJ Jr: Efficacy and safety of recombinant human activated protein C. N Eng J Med 2001;344:699.
90. The Acute Respiratory Distress Syndrome Network: Ventilation with lower tidal volumes as compared with traditional tidal volumes for acute lung injury and the acute respiratory distress syndrome. The Acute Respiratory Distress Syndrome Network. N Engl J Med 2000;342:1301.
91. Matthay MA, Wiener-Kronish JP: Intact epithelial barrier function is critical for the resolution of alveolar edema in man. Am Rev Respir Dis 1990;142:1250.
92. Ware LB, Matthay MA: Alveolar fluid clearance is impaired in the majority of patients with acute lung injury and the acute respiratory distress syndrome. Am J Respir Crit Care Med 2001;163:1376.
93. Rafii B, Gillie DJ, Sulowski C, Hannam V, Cheung T, Otulakowski G, et al: Pulmonary oedema fluid induces non-a-ENaC-dependent Na^+ transport and fluid absorption in the distal lung. J Physiol (Lond) 2002; 544(2):537.
94. Campbell AR, Folkesson HG, Berthiaume Y, Gutkowska J, Suzuki S, Matthay MA: Alveolar epithelial fluid clearance persists in the presence of moderate left atrial hypertension in sheep. J Appl Physiol 1999; 86(1):139.

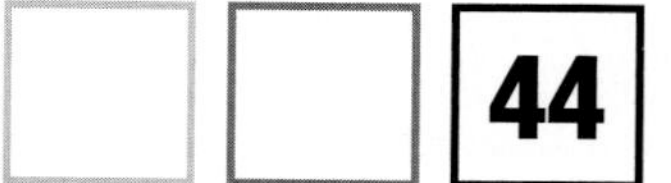

44 Acute Respiratory Distress Syndrome in the Pediatric Patient

Andrew H. Numa, MBBS •
Christopher J.L. Newth, MB

■ ACUTE RESPIRATORY DISTRESS SYNDROME

Acute respiratory distress syndrome (ARDS) is a syndrome of acute lung inflammation characterized by alveolar leukocyte infiltration and protein-rich pulmonary edema resulting in acute respiratory failure.[1] The first case series of ARDS was reported by Ashbaugh, Bigelow, Petty, and Devine in 1967.[2] These investigators described 12 patients, including one child of 11 years who suffered from "acute onset of tachypnea, hypoxemia and loss of compliance after a variety of stimuli" and "did not respond to usual and ordinary methods of respiratory therapy." The nomenclature was based on the observation that pathologic features closely resembled those seen in infants with respiratory distress. Numerous case series reports followed, but it was not until 1994 that a consensus view of diagnostic criteria was established.[3] The consensus committee defined two categories of acute lung disease: acute lung injury (ALI) and ARDS. Diagnostic criteria for both included acute onset, the presence of bilateral infiltrates on frontal chest radiograph, and a pulmonary artery wedge pressure less than or equal to 18 mm Hg (or no clinical evidence of left atrial hypertension). A ratio of partial pressure of oxygen in arterial blood to fraction of inspired oxygen (PaO_2/FIO_2) of less than or equal to 300 mm Hg was used to define ALI, whereas ARDS required a PaO_2/FIO_2 ratio of less than or equal to 200 mm Hg. Despite the limitations of these definitions (e.g., they do not allow for the effects of positive end-expiratory pressure [PEEP] on oxygenation), they remain a widely used standard. Another term, *acute hypoxemic respiratory failure* (AHRF) is also widely used in the literature to describe patients with acute severe lung disease who do not necessarily meet the strict diagnostic criteria for ARDS or ALI.

Although Ashbaugh's series included a solitary pediatric patient, it was not until the early 1980s that the first pediatric series of ARDS were reported.[4,5] These early case series were notable for high mortality and the use of ventilatory strategies that would now be regarded as highly injurious.

Despite significant advances in our understanding of the pathophysiology of acute lung disease, ARDS remains a substantial problem in the intensive care unit (ICU) and is overrepresented in both mortality and length of stay statistics.[6] Recent estimates of the incidence of ARDS as defined by the American-European consensus criteria in adult populations have ranged from 13.5 to 28 cases per 100,000 per annum in Scandinavia[7] and Australia,[8] respectively. Population-based studies have not been reported in pediatrics; however, Davis and colleagues estimated that 2.7% of ICU patients developed ARDS.[6]

■ PATHOPHYSIOLOGY

ARDS is an inflammatory disorder of the lungs that may arise as a result of a direct pulmonary disease or secondary to systemic disease elsewhere in the body. Almost any acute pulmonary disease or insult can cause ARDS, including aspiration, smoke inhalation, contusion, and bacterial, viral, or fungal infections. Systemic disorders commonly associated with ARDS include sepsis, trauma, near drowning, and massive transfusion.

Traditionally, ARDS has been divided into three phases: acute/exudative (characterized by interstitial and alveolar edema), fibroproliferative (cellular infiltrate with proliferation of fibroblasts), and fibrotic (fibrosis and ultimately healing of lung tissue). The early stages of ARDS are characterized by alveolar epithelial injury, with both type I and type II cells being affected, although type II cells appear to be relatively more resistant.[9] Both apoptosis and necrosis are responsible for epithelial cell death, the former largely mediated by accumulation of the natural ligand of a membrane surface receptor protein of the tumor necrosis factor (TNF) family (soluble *FasL*) in the alveolar spaces, the latter by ventilator-induced shear forces.[10,11] The loss of integrity of the alveolar epithelium increases the permeability of the alveolar-capillary barrier and leads to rapid accumulation of protein-rich edema in the interstitium and airspaces.[12] The quantity of protein in alveolar fluid is significantly higher than that seen in cardiogenic pulmonary edema.[13] Impaired surfactant production by type II cells unfavorably alters the mechanical properties of the lung and predisposes to atelectasis.

A number of inflammatory markers have been identified in the alveolar spaces in early ARDS, with interleukin-1 (IL-1) and TNF-α being responsible for the majority of proinflammatory activity.[12] Although both pro- and anti-inflammatory cytokines can be detected in the lungs, the net result favors inflammation.[14] These cytokines in turn induce release of IL-8 from endothelial and epithelial cells as well as alveolar macrophages. IL-8 is a powerful chemoattractant for neutrophils, which accumulate and are activated early in the course of ARDS, leading to further accumulation of proinflammatory cytokines.[15,16] Although the initial influx of cytokines is generated by the triggering insult (either pulmonary or systemic), further cytokine release occurs as a result of mechanical ventilation, particularly if injurious (high-volume, low-PEEP) strategies are used.[14,15,17–20] The large surface area and high blood flow of the lungs (they are the only organ to receive the entire cardiac output) facilitates migration of cytokines into the systemic circulation where they contribute to the development of the multiorgan failure that is a frequent feature of the disease.[21–23] There is an association between the levels of inflammatory mediators, including TNF-α, IL-1β, IL-6, and IL-8, in bronchoalveolar lavage (BAL) fluid and organ failure scores[15] and mortality.[23]

Proteases, including neutrophil elastase and matrix metalloproteinases released from neutrophils, lead to further increases in capillary permeability,[12,24] and there is good correlation between release of neutrophil elastase and serum levels of IL-6,[15] which in turn is implicated in the pathogenesis of multiorgan failure.[25] Persistent elevation of neutrophils in BAL fluid has been correlated with increased mortality.[26,27] Although neutrophil infiltration is clearly an important factor in the genesis of the disease, ARDS can develop in the absence of neutrophils.[28] Nevertheless, animal models indicate that neutrophil depletion favorably modifies the pathologic and clinical manifestations of ARDS.[29]

Abnormal activation of coagulation cascades also plays a significant role in the pathogenesis of ARDS. Microthrombi in pulmonary vasculature have long been recognized as a histologic feature of ARDS.[30,31] Patients with both early and unresolving ARDS demonstrate increased pulmonary sequestration of radiolabeled fibrinogen,[32] which accumulates both extravascularly, primarily in the alveolar spaces,[33] and intravascularly.[31] Alveolar fibrin impairs surfactant function[34] and forms the basis for the development of subsequent pulmonary fibrosis,[35] while intravascular thrombus formation causes pulmonary hypertension and ventilation-perfusion (V/Q) mismatch. Regulatory mechanisms are altered in ARDS, with elevated procoagulant activity and depressed fibrinolysis, comparable with that seen in severe sepsis.[33,36]

Early changes may resolve rapidly, with phagocytosis of apoptotic neutrophils by macrophage regeneration of alveolar epithelial cells and resorption of the alveolar exudates.[10] Alternately, progression into a more prolonged fibrotic phase may commence at around 1 week after the initial injury. This period is characterized by the accumulation of fibroblasts within the airspaces and interstitium together with neovascularization of the capillary bed.[9,37] Although fibrosis may represent a further step toward eventual recovery, progression to this stage is associated with a high rate of mortality.[38]

Although ARDS appears as a diffuse disease on plain chest radiographs, chest CT scans (Fig. 44-1) demonstrate areas of relatively normal lung interspersed with atelectatic and consolidated regions that are concentrated toward the dependent zones: dorsally in the supine patient and ventrally in the prone patient.[39] This observation, first made by Gattinoni,[40] has led to the development of the concept of ARDS as a heterogeneous disease with three zones of lung: a small healthy zone, a recruitable zone, and a diseased zone.

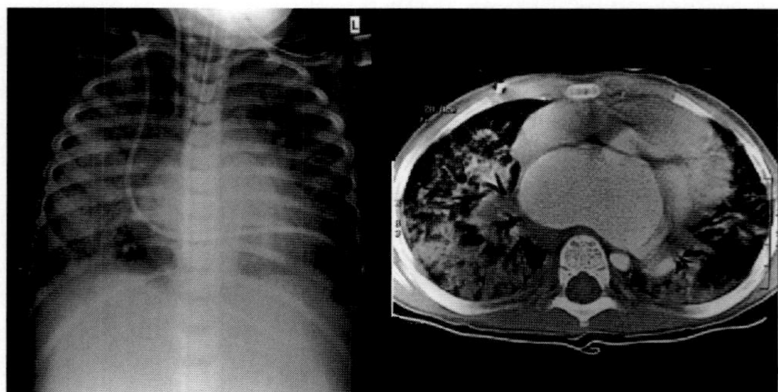

■ **FIGURE 44-1.** Although acute respiratory distress syndrome appears as a diffuse disease on plain chest radiographs *(left)*, chest CT scans *(right)* demonstrate areas of relatively normal lung interspersed with atelectatic and consolidated regions that are concentrated toward the dependent zones, that is, dorsally in the supine position (as in this patient) and ventrally in the prone patient.

Analysis of pressure-volume relationships is consistent with the presence of a volume of lung tissue that can be recruited with application of sufficient PEEP. This gives rise to a static pressure-volume relationship that in many (although not all) patients has a clearly defined lower inflection point where the pressure-volume relationship moves from a relatively flat (noncompliant) to a steeper more compliant slope.[41] An upper inflection point, where the curve passes from relatively steep (compliant) to flat (noncompliant), is also often observed, and occurs at low lung volumes in both adult and pediatric patients with ARDS.[42,43] There are relatively few reports of respiratory mechanics in pediatric patients with ARDS, but these confirm the existence of decreased lung volumes (total lung capacity and functional residual capacity) together with low compliance in the early (acute) stages of the disease.[43–47] The technique of low-flow inflation pressure-volume curves and subsequent fitting of a second-order polynomial equation appears to give a better measure of overdistention than does the C20/C ratio described by Fisher and colleagues.[48]

Long-term survivors of ARDS have good functional outcomes, but lung function testing demonstrates a high incidence of both reversible and nonreversible obstructive airways disease[49,50] and restrictive disease.[50,51] Total lung capacity is reduced in about one third of survivors, and between 12.5% and 80% have reduced values for diffusion capacity of the lung for carbon monoxide (DLCO).[49–51]

■ VENTILATORY MANAGEMENT OF ACUTE RESPIRATORY DISTRESS SYNDROME

Mechanical ventilation is the key supportive therapy for ARDS, but it must be used judiciously in order to maximize the chances for survival. There is little doubt that inappropriate use of mechanical ventilation can cause significant lung injury and significantly increase morbidity and mortality. There is a wealth of evidence from animal studies that ventilation which utilizes high FIO_2, high tidal volumes, and low PEEP is directly injurious to previously normal lungs. Injury can occur in as little as a few minutes in small animals, to a few hours in larger ones, and the histologic appearance of lungs injured in this way is indistinguishable from the changes observed in ARDS (Figs. 44-2 and 44-3).[18,52–54] Similarly, excessively high ventilatory settings can exacerbate the changes of ARDS in already injured lungs.[55] Good clinical evidence now exists to indicate that avoidance of high tidal volumes and judicious use of PEEP leads to lower mortality rates in adults with ARDS.[41,56,57] So called "protective ventilation" is in fact the only intervention proven to improve outcomes of ARDS in randomized controlled trials.[20,58] In the large ($n = 861$) multicenter study carried out by the Acute Respiratory Distress Syndrome Network, patients randomized to low (6 mL/kg) tidal volume ventilation had a mortality of 31.0% compared with 39.8% in those ventilated with a tidal volume of 12 mL/kg; a 22% reduction in mortality. There is a paucity of randomized controlled trial evidence to support this approach in pediatrics, but case series reporting good survival in recent years have invariably utilized protective ventilation.[59,60]

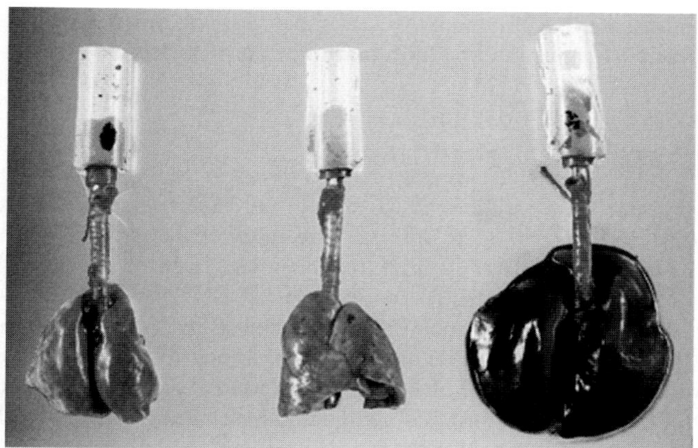

■ **FIGURE 44-2.** Macroscopic aspect of rat lungs after mechanical ventilation at 45 cm H_2O peak airway pressure. *Left,* Normal lungs. *Middle,* After 5 minutes of high airway pressure mechanical ventilation. Note the focal zones of atelectasis (in particular at the left lung apex). *Right,* After 20 minutes, the lungs were markedly enlarged and congested; edema fluid fills the tracheal cannula. (See Color Plate 35.) (From Dreyfuss D, Saumon G: Ventilator-induced lung injury. Lessons from experimental studies. Am Rev Respir Crit Care Med 1998;157:294–323.)

Given the high rate of death from noncardiorespiratory causes in adult patients with ARDS, it is perhaps surprising that respiratory manipulations alone can increase survival. However, it is increasingly recognized that multiorgan failure may be exacerbated by the release of inflammatory mediators from the lungs, and there is good evidence for this in both animal models and human studies as discussed above. In the large multicenter trial recently reported by the ARDS Network,[20] patients randomized to the low tidal volume group demonstrated significantly greater falls in plasma IL-6 concentration than those ventilated at higher tidal volumes by day 3 of their illness. Similarly, Ranieri and colleagues[19] reported decreased concentrations of inflammatory mediators IL-1β, IL-6, and TNF-α in BAL specimens, and in plasma concentrations of IL-6 and TNF-α in patients allocated to a protective ventilatory strategy. These patients had tidal volume and PEEP based on a volume-pressure curve, and were compared with those ventilated with the aim of normalizing partial pressure of carbon dioxide in arterial blood ($PaCO_2$).

Protective ventilation has three key features: generous use of PEEP, limitation of tidal volume or peak inspiratory pressure, and reduction in FIO_2 to around 0.60 or less. The beneficial effects of PEEP in the treatment of ARDS were recognized simultaneously with the description of the disease itself.[2] Increasing levels of PEEP recruit alveoli and improve oxygenation. In 1964, Faridy and colleagues demonstrated an inverse relationship between PEEP and loss of surfactant activity in mechanically ventilated dog lungs.[61] A decade later, Webb and Tierney demonstrated less lung injury in rat lungs ventilated at pressures of 45/10 cm H_2O compared with those ventilated at 45/0,[52] and other researchers have made similar observations.[53] The best method of determining the optimal level of PEEP is not clearly established. Optimal PEEP cannot simply be determined by titration against PaO_2 or pulse oximetry (SpO_2)—such an approach has not demonstrated any improvement in outcomes in clinical settings.[62] Amato's approach of determining the lower inflection point of the static pressure volume curve (P_{flex}) is relatively simple to apply but does not yield a result in all patients.[58] Furthermore, there is evidence that PEEP well beyond the value of P_{flex} may be necessary to prevent derecruitment.[40,63] It has been proposed that the deflation limb of the pressure volume curve may provide a more accurate reflection of the closing pressure of alveolar units and be a better guide to optimizing PEEP.[63,64] An alternative approach is to periodically use recruitment maneuvers (e.g., very high levels of PEEP up to 40 cm H_2O with prolonged inspiratory times of 3 seconds and low ventilator rates for a 2-minute period) to recruit atelectatic segments when oxygenation is compromised.[64] Similarly, a "safe" level of peak inspiratory pressure is difficult to determine, but a reasonable approach is to limit tidal volume to 6 mL/kg[20,58] and allow peak inspiratory pressures of no more than 40 cm H_2O[57,58] and preferably less than 30 to 35 cm H_2O.[57,60] Optimal FIO_2 is also an area where substantial doubt exists. Pulmonary oxygen toxicity appears to be species dependent,[65] and there is some evidence that inflammatory mediators present in the lungs of patients with ARDS protect against oxygen toxicity.[66] Of note is the finding in the ARDS network trial that patients in the 6 mL/kg group, who had significantly lower rates of mortality, received higher FIO_2 on days 1 and 3 than patients in the higher tidal volume group, suggesting that oxygen toxicity is less important than volutrauma in terms of mortality.[20]

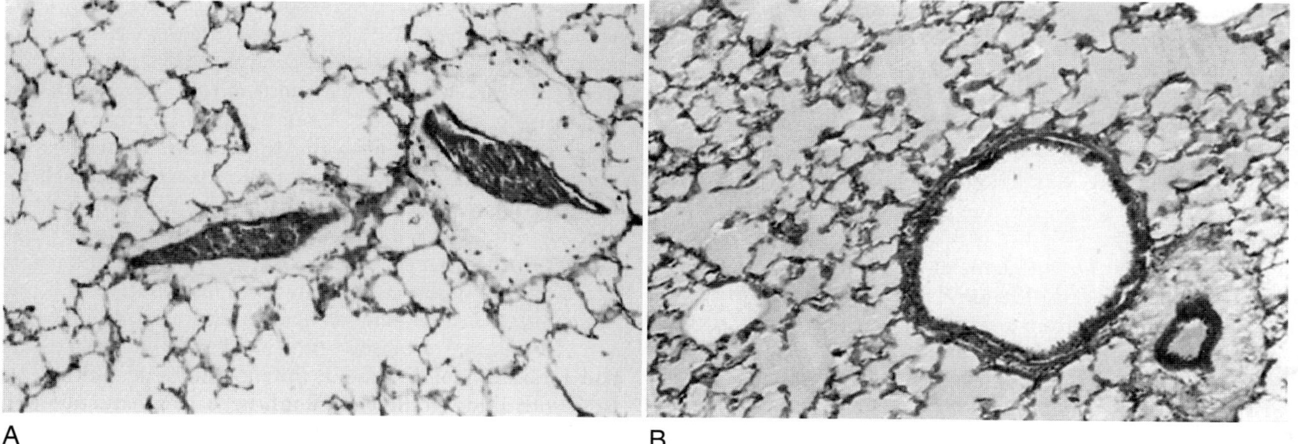

■ **FIGURE 44-3.** Light microscopic appearance of rat lungs after mechanical ventilation at 45 cm H_2O peak airway pressure. **A,** After 5 minutes of ventilation, interstitial edema is found in large perivascular cuffs. **B,** After 20 minutes of ventilation, there is widespread alveolar edema that fills nearly all the alveoli on this slide. (See Color Plate 36.) (From Dreyfuss D, Saumon G: Ventilator-induced lung injury. Lessons from experimental studies. Am Rev Respir Crit Care Med 1998;157:294–323.)

Apart from direct toxicity, high FIO_2 predisposes to resorption atelectasis, and the aim in management of ARDS should be to limit the FIO_2 as much as possible while maintaining acceptable oxygen saturations.

A more novel form of protective ventilation is high-frequency oscillatory ventilation (HFOV). In this mode of ventilation, first proposed by Bohn and colleagues[67] both inspiration and expiration are active and are driven as high rates, typically 5 to 15 Hz by an oscillating membrane that is essentially a modified loudspeaker. HFOV provides active inspiration and expiration around a mean airway pressure. In contrast to conventional ventilation, where gas exchange is achieved by bulk convection, tidal volumes in HFOV may be at or below the physiologic dead space, although at lower frequencies, tidal volumes may approach those of conventional ventilation.[68] The corollary is that ventilation may be achieved by means other than bulk convection, such as pendelluft movement of gas from areas of short- to long-time constants and molecular diffusion.

In animal studies, HFOV has been demonstrated to recruit atelectatic lung, improve respiratory compliance, and ameliorate the inflammatory response of ventilator-induced lung injury.[69,70] In premature infants, a number of studies have demonstrated reduction in the incidence of air leak and or chronic lung disease,[71,72] although this is not a universal observation.[73,74] However, no trial has demonstrated improved long-term survival, and there have been concerns raised regarding a possible increased incidence of intraventricular hemorrhage in premature infants receiving this mode of ventilation.[75] HFOV is a widely used ventilatory mode for pediatric patients with respiratory failure, being used in 2.9% of all ventilated patients and as many as one in three patients with ARDS.[70] Although the intervention is widely used, only a single study has prospectively evaluated the effectiveness of HFOV in children. Arnold and colleagues failed to demonstrate any reduction in mortality in a randomized crossover trial of HFOV versus conventional ventilation in 58 patients.[76] This result is disappointing, especially since the conventionally ventilated patients were exposed to relatively high peak inspiratory pressures and thus would be expected to have a higher rate of mortality than patients ventilated using current protective strategies. However, the results must be viewed in light of a prolonged period of conventional ventilation (mean of 80 hours) prior to randomization, which may have reduced the beneficial effects of HFOV. A larger adult study enrolling 148 patients similarly failed to show statistically significant improvements in survival, although there was a trend toward lower a mortality rate in patients randomized to HFOV.[77] Therefore, the place of HFOV in the treatment of ARDS is not well defined. While philosophically attractive, it may be that HFOV has little, if any, benefit over intelligently selected conventional protective ventilation settings in the majority of patients, and there is some experimental evidence to support this observation.[78]

Other variations on mechanical ventilation have been proposed. Tracheal gas insufflation (TGI) uses fresh gas flow directly into the trachea from a small catheter positioned at the end of the endotracheal tube to wash out CO_2-rich O_2-poor end-expiratory (alveolar) gas, thus reducing physiologic dead space. Care must be taken to not generate auto-PEEP and drying of secretions. Mucosal injury can be problematic.[79] A single study in premature infants with hyaline membrane disease demonstrated a reduced duration of mechanical ventilation in infants managed with TGI.[80] However, its use in older children and adults with ARDS is experimental at present and requires further investigation before it can be recommended for routine use.

ADJUNCTIVE THERAPIES

Over the past decade a plethora of novel therapies for patients with ARDS have been utilized. The ready availability of nitric oxide (NO), surfactant, high-frequency ventilation (HFV), and extracorporeal membrane oxygenation (ECMO) leads to a confusing array of treatments that can be offered to the patient with ARDS. In addition, more subtle but not necessarily less important variations on conventional ventilatory strategies may also offer real improvements in outcome. Finally, systemically administered therapies such as steroids are also appropriate in certain situations.

LIQUID VENTILATION

The potential for achieving satisfactory oxygenation in mammals using liquid ventilation was first demonstrated by Kylstra and colleagues[81] in a series of experiments in the 1960s. Early studies relied on hyperbarically oxygenated fluids due to the low solubility of oxygen in most physiologically compatible fluids. The recognition of a class of biologically inert, nonabsorbable liquid solvents known as perfluorocarbons with high O_2 and CO_2 solubility and relatively low viscosity and surface tension vastly improved the prospects of liquid ventilation. Although early studies of this modality relied on specially constructed ventilators that achieved ventilation by bulk convection of the liquid, a more common and simple technique of perfluorocarbon-assisted gas exchange (PAGE) utilizing a conventional ventilator to provide ventilation to perfluorocarbon-filled lungs has been shown to be highly effective. Recent evidence suggests that administration of as little as 1 mL/kg perfluorocarbon provides substantial improvements in lung recruitment and oxygenation.[82] Clearly, such small volumes of perfluorocarbon cannot act as oxygen carriers regardless of the excellent solubility of oxygen in this medium; it is more likely that their surface-active properties, particularly their effect on equilibrium surface tension, is responsible for the dramatic clinical response. Perfluorocarbons may also have intrinsic anti-inflammatory properties.[83]

Animal trials of liquid ventilation using various models of lung injury including hyaline membrane disease (HMD), meconium aspiration, diaphragmatic hernia, and lavage lung injury (ARDS) report improvements in PaO_2, $PaCO_2$, compliance, survival, and preservation of normal or near-normal lung histology.[84–87] A number of human studies have also shown encouraging results, including in children.[88,89] A pilot-randomized controlled trial involving 90 adult patients with ARDS reported no improvement in survival or number of ventilator-free days at 28 days. However, a preponderance of older patients in the treatment group may have adversely influenced the results in this study, because post-hoc analysis of the younger than 55 year subgroup demonstrated a significant reduction in ventilator-free days and a trend toward reduced mortality in patients treated with partial liquid ventilation.[90] In a large pediatric series in North America, "an unexplained substantial decrease in the mortality rate for the control group" resulted in the abandonment of a prospective trial of partial liquid ventilation (press release, Alliance Pharmaceutical Corporation, San Diego, April 14, 1997).

Perfluorocarbons have also been successfully combined with a number of other treatment modalities, including HFV,[91]

NO,[92] and exogenous surfactant.[86] There is evidence that the combination of partial liquid ventilation and administration of exogenous surfactant may be more efficacious than either agent in isolation.[86,93] The addition of perfluorocarbon may enhance delivery of surfactant to the alveoli and may also wash out proteinaceous exudates that might otherwise inactivate surfactant. Because surfactant and perfluorocarbon are immiscible, however, it is critical that the surfactant be administered first so that the higher density perfluorocarbon will then "push" the surfactant into the alveoli. Endogenous surfactant production may also be enhanced by the alveolar recruitment that occurs during PAGE.[94] The combination of HFV and PAGE has been demonstrated to be more effective than HFV alone in some studies.[91,95] Other researchers have compared PAGE plus HFV with PAGE plus conventional mechanical ventilation and found no additional benefit of HFV over and above conventional ventilation in the perfluorocarbon-filled lung.[96] The addition of NO to perfluorocarbon may offer additional improvements in oxygenation over perfluorocarbon alone.[92] At present, perfluorocarbons are not commercially available and their use is confined to research trials.

NITRIC OXIDE

Although a number of researchers have reported improvements in oxygenation and pulmonary vascular resistance in pediatric patients with ARDS treated with inhaled NO,[97–100] there has been no demonstrated improvement in survival with NO therapy. In a multicenter randomized controlled trial of NO versus placebo gas in 108 children with AHRF (defined as an oxygenation index of >0.15 in two blood gases within 6 hours), NO administration improved oxygenation but had no effect on mortality (42% for NO versus 43.4% for control patients).[99] Similar results have been reported from adult populations, including the recent publication of two large multicenter trials in Europe with a total of 471 patients.[101,102] A recent report[100] demonstrates greater improvements in oxygenation for patients treated with NO and high-frequency ventilation compared with the combination of NO and conventional ventilation; however, the lack of a demonstrable effect on outcomes suggests a limited role at best for NO in patients with ARDS.

PRONE POSITIONING

There is a wealth of evidence indicating that prone positioning is a useful means of improving oxygenation in neonatal, pediatric, and adult patients with acute lung injury.[39,103–105] Although it was initially proposed that prone positioning would improve oxygenation via an increase in functional residual capacity,[106] it is now accepted that improvements in oxygenation in the prone position probably arise as a result of reduced intrapulmonary shunting[107] secondary to favorable redistributions of both pulmonary blood flow[108] and ventilation.[107] Several studies have demonstrated a lack of significant improvement in either respiratory mechanics or lung volumes in the prone position.[109,110] Prone positioning has been demonstrated to generate more substantial improvements in oxygenation than NO at 11 ppm.[111] Recently, Stocker and colleagues[112] reported impressively high survival rates (88%) in adult patients with ARDS managed with pressure-limited (35 cm H_2O) low tidal volume ventilation and the use of prone positioning to improve oxygenation. However, the relative contributions of each strategy to the excellent outcome figures are not clear from this observational study. Evidence from animal studies suggests that in lung injury induced purely by high tidal volume (15 mL/kg) mechanical ventilation, prone positioning results in a reduction in pulmonary edema together with a less severe and more homogeneous distribution of histologic changes.[113]

A large prospective study in adults with acute lung injury that randomized patients to ventilation in the supine position or to a strategy that involved placing patients prone for 6 or more hours daily for 10 days failed to demonstrate any improvement in survival despite demonstrating significant improvements in oxygenation in the prone group.[114] An intriguing finding in this study was a post-hoc analysis indicating that the quartiles of patients with the worst PaO_2/FIO_2 ratio and highest simplified acute physiology score had statistically significant reductions in mortality (relative risk for death of 0.49 and 0.40, respectively). In the pediatric population, a number of studies have failed to demonstrate any survival benefit with regular use of prone positioning, although improvements in oxygenation have been observed in the majority of patients.[104,105,109,115] Pediatric studies to date have enrolled relatively small numbers of patients and are thus not adequately powered to detect even a moderate to large improvement in survival. Casado-Flores and colleagues in a study of 23 pediatric patients noted that survival in the 78% of patients classified as "responders" tended to be higher than in nonresponders (80% compared with 39%, $P = .095$), suggesting that the response to prone positioning may have prognostic implications.[115]

While the technique is not without potential complications, including pressure ulcers, corneal abrasions, and accidental extubation, it is generally safe and simple to apply in the majority of patients.[104] Given the widely reported benefits on oxygenation, together with convincing animal evidence of histologic improvement, prone positioning should at least be considered for all patients with ARDS. Gattinoni's work suggests there may be a survival advantage for the most severely affected patients, but this will need to be confirmed in prospective studies.[114]

SURFACTANT

ARDS is associated with decreased production, inactivation, and inhibition of endogenous surfactant[116,117]; thus, surfactant replacement therapy seems an ideal intervention. Surfactant has proven to be effective in animal models, preventing and reversing pulmonary changes in hyperoxic viral sepsis and chemically induced acute lung injury.[118–121] Human trials have demonstrated improvements in oxygenation but no decrease in mortality. The largest adult trial reported enrolled 725 patients with sepsis-induced ARDS who were administered aerosolized Exosurf (GlaxoSmithKline, Philadelphia, Pennsylvania) or placebo (0.45% saline) continuously for up to 5 days.[122] No beneficial effects were observed on 30-day survival, length of stay in the ICU, or duration of mechanical ventilation; however, there were several methodologic flaws in this trial. The method of delivery—nebulization—results in less than 5% of the administered dose reaching the lungs.[123] The choice of artificial surfactant—Exosurf—may also have resulted in suboptimal results. Exosurf is a protein-free preparation, but surfactant-associated proteins play an important role in overcoming the inactivation of surfactant caused by plasma proteins leaking into the alveolar space.[124] However, a large multicenter trial using a recombinant surfactant protein C–based surfactant in a placebo-controlled, double-blind trial failed to demonstrate any benefit in either 28-day mortality or duration of mechanical ventilation in a heterogeneous group of 448 adult patients with ARDS.[125] In this study, a post-hoc analysis suggested a lower rate of mortality in surfactant-treated patients with ARDS secondary to direct lung injury (30% versus 36% in the placebo group) but a higher mortality rate in surfactant-treated patients with ARDS secondary to indirect lung injury (41% versus 28%).

Smaller studies have suggested more positive results. Gregory and colleagues[126] administered bovine surfactant by endotracheal instillation in a maximum dose of 100 mg/kg in up to eight doses, demonstrating a significant improvement in oxygenation at day 5 in treated patients and a trend toward an improved mortality rate in this group—18.8% versus 43.8% ($P = .075$). Willson and colleagues[127] used 80 mL/m^2 of a bovine surfactant (Infasurf, Forest Pharmaceuticals, St. Louis, Missouri) in a multicenter trial involving 29 pediatric patients. The study was somewhat flawed by using a "convenience sample" and by enrolling some children with relatively mild lung disease; an oxygenation index of greater than 0.07 was used as an enrollment criteria, and only 9 of the 29 patients had ARDS. A positive response to the first dose of surfactant was observed in 24 of 29 patients, who demonstrated an improved oxygenation index. Less impressive responses were seen in patients eligible for second and subsequent doses, however. In a European multicenter randomized open study of pediatric patients with severe ARDS ($PaO_2/FIO_2 < 100$), a dose of 100 mg/kg bovine surfactant instilled as a bolus to the distal end of the ETT resulted in significant improvements in oxygenation (measured by PaO_2/FIO_2 and oxygenation index) at 2 hours and 48 hours after treatment when compared with a control group who received no surfactant.[117] In this relatively small cohort of 35 patients (20 surfactant treated, 15 controls) a trend toward decreased mortality rate was also observed—44% versus 60%—but it was not statistically significant. Post-hoc analysis demonstrated 100% mortality for both treatment and control groups with PaO_2/FIO_2 less than 65, suggesting that use of this expensive therapy might be more cost effective if targeted to the subgroup of patients with PaO_2/FIO_2 greater than 65. Similarly, patients with pneumonia were identified post-hoc as not responding to surfactant therapy, while those without underlying pneumonia responded well (provided the PaO_2/FIO_2 was >65).

It appears that surfactant is well tolerated and leads to improvements in oxygenation in the majority of patients, but larger trials will be needed to determine whether outcomes can be substantially improved with this drug. Clinicians also need to be aware that a minority of patients experience deterioration in oxygenation following surfactant therapy.

EXTRACORPOREAL MEMBRANE OXYGENATION

Despite widespread use of ECMO for children with ARDS over the past three decades, there is substantial doubt over the efficacy of this therapy. Although the concept of allowing the diseased lungs to recover while taking over their function with an extracorporeal circuit is superficially appealing, at least for the subset of patients with ARDS who are likely to succumb from respiratory causes, there is no compelling evidence to support the use of ECMO in ARDS—either in adults or children. Several randomized controlled trials in adults clearly demonstrate a lack of efficacy. Mortality in both ECMO and non-ECMO groups exceeded 90% in an early randomized controlled trial of this therapy.[128] Refinements in ECMO technology allowed improved survival in patients subjected to extracorporeal circuits, but parallel improvements in outcomes from patients treated with conventional ventilatory support have also occurred. In the mid-1980s, venovenous ECMO circuits were advocated. These circuits did away with the need to cannulate the carotid artery and provided good CO_2 clearance with some improvements in oxygenation. Survival rates significantly superior to those of retrospective controls were achieved; for example, Gattinoni and colleagues[129] reported survival of 50% in patients treated in this way, which was clearly superior to the commonly assumed mortality rate of 90% for similar patients. However, a randomized and carefully controlled trial of venovenous circuits subsequently failed to demonstrate a survival advantage over conventional ventilation.[130] No controlled trials have been reported in pediatric patients, although a number of researchers have reported "favorable" results for ECMO in ARDS and ALI.[131–137] Unfortunately, these reports all lack the inclusion of suitable controls, which is needed to prove a survival benefit. These studies generally report an enrollment criteria of patients judged "likely to die" with conventional treatment and attempt to justify benefit on the basis of an implied or assumed near 100% mortality rate in retrospectively derived controls. The dangers of this approach are perhaps best illustrated by Nading,[138] who reported a series of five neonates (obtained from retrospective chart review) who had met ECMO criteria, with a predicted mortality rate of 80% to 94%, and who had been conventionally ventilated. Five of five survived, none with neurologic handicap. Similarly, in a randomized controlled trial of ECMO in neonates with persistent pulmonary hypertension, a predicted mortality rate of 85% in the control group (based on historical data) was prospectively observed to be only 40% in the study.[139] Morris and colleagues[130] also noted a 38% survival rate in patients with a predicted survival rate of only 10% based on retrospectively derived criteria. Dworitz and colleagues[140] noted a reduction in mortality rate from 83% to 10% in infants meeting generally accepted ECMO criteria[141] when comparing infants admitted to their neonatal ICU in 1980–1981 with those admitted in 1986–1988. During this period, a change in ventilatory strategy for neonates with severe lung disease had occurred. Green and colleagues[136] attempted retrospectively to match controls from a large database of patients with acute respiratory failure. However, matches could not be found for 24% of the 38 ECMO patients, and of those that could be matched, 49% did not have the same diagnoses. Such flaws make truly accurate comparisons impossible and underscore the need for prospective randomized studies.

Many case series of patients treated with ECMO indicate pre-ECMO ventilatory strategies that are highly injurious. For example, Butt and colleagues, in a series of 18 patients with severe primary or secondary lung disease, reported pre-ECMO ventilation settings of peak inspiratory pressures as high as 64 cm H_2O with positive end-expiratory pressures as low as 5 cm H_2O.[131] Moler and colleagues[135] similarly reported a mean pre-ECMO peak inspiratory pressure of 57.9 cm H_2O in nonsurvivors and 43.1 cm H_2O in survivors, while Green and colleagues[136] reported mean highest peak inspiratory pressures of 51 cm H_2O in patients subjected to ECMO. Twenty patients were reported by Vats and colleagues, of whom four had mean airway pressures of more than 35 cm H_2O, which is inconsistent with current ventilatory practices.[137] Clearly, ECMO may offer some protection against such aggressive use of the mechanical ventilator. However, a large body of evidence exists to support the case that adoption of protective ventilatory strategies would be at least as efficacious in reducing mortality.

Survival rates in pediatric series range from 25%[134] to 80%.[137] However, several large series of patients with ARDS managed without ECMO report similar or superior results. Such data need to be considered in the light of ECMO not necessarily being offered to all patients with ARDS; that is, "hopeless" cases such as those with substantial neurologic injury or end-stage malignancies will probably be selected out,[136,137] whereas conventional support is generally offered to a much more inclusive group, a selection bias that is highly likely to favor ECMO outcomes. Furthermore, the use of ECMO is not confined to ARDS patients alone, because some centers offer this modality to patients with less severe lung disease, which of course further improves reported mortality. For example, Vats and colleagues[137] reported 2 patients in a series of 20 who were placed on ECMO as therapy for persistent air leak while having relatively mild lung disease and a further 3 who received ECMO for respiratory syncytial virus bronchiolitis, a condition where mortality rates from 0.3% to 1.1% have been reported in large series of patients managed without ECMO.[142,143]

Complications related to the use of extracorporeal circuits occur frequently—in 88% of patients in one series[135]—and include hemorrhagic complications related to the necessary anticoagulation, sepsis from cannulas, and cerebral injury related to carotid cannulation. In contrast, survivors of conventional ventilation rarely suffer long-term neurologic morbidity.[49] The significant cost of ECMO, both in equipment and labor, cannot be ignored. Morris and colleagues[130] estimated that supporting all adult ARDS patients in North America with venovenous extracorporeal CO_2 removal as opposed to conventional ventilation would increase intensive care costs for these patients by $295,000,000 per annum, while Vats and colleagues[137] estimated a cost of $199,096 per patient.

The recent advent of low-resistance membrane oxygenators has allowed development of a simplified extracorporeal circuit that relies on the patient's own blood pressure to generate flow through an extracorporeal membrane oxygenator via cannulation of the femoral artery and vein.[144] Such a circuit reduces some of the expense and complications of pump-driven circuits and allows for more conservative anticoagulation regimens. However, application of this device is limited to patients with good blood pressure and cardiac output, and at this stage it is limited to adults.

STEROIDS

It is possible that an overaggressive and protracted host defense response, rather than the etiologic condition precipitating respiratory failure, is the major factor influencing the outcome in ARDS.[37] Sustained inflammatory responses in the lungs are injurious, resulting in fibroproliferative changes that substantially impair lung function. Pulmonary fibrosis directly causes death in 15% to 40% of ARDS patients; most of the remainder die from multiorgan dysfunction or sepsis.[37] Glucocorticoids moderate the host defense response at virtually every level, and secretion of glucocorticoids is an important host response to the acute lung injury. However, cytokines can cause a concentration-dependent resistance to glucocorticoids by reducing receptor binding affinity,[145] and supraphysiologic levels may be required to overcome this problem.

Short course (<48 hours) of high-dose (e.g., 30 mg/kg methylprednisolone) intravenous steroid administered early in sepsis and ARDS offers no benefit compared with placebo,[146,147] although several groups have reported improved lung function during prolonged administration of glucocorticoids. Meduri and colleagues[148] administered intravenous methylprednisolone in a 6-week course beginning with doses of 2 to 3 mg/kg after a mean of 15 days of mechanical ventilation in 25 patients with unresolving ARDS and no evidence of active infection. Overall, 88% of patients improved—15 of 25 were classified as "rapid responders," showing improvement within 7 days; 7 of 25 were "delayed responders," improving within 14 days; and 3 of 25 did not respond. Only 6 patients died (mortality rate 24%), comprising all (3 of 3) of the nonresponders and 3 of 22 of the responders. Survivors had significantly greater reductions than nonsurvivors in cytokine levels by day 5 of prednisolone therapy, and reductions in cytokine levels paralleled improvement in lung injury scores.[149] Biffl and colleagues[150] reported a small series (n = 6) of patients treated with intravenous methylprednisolone 1 to 2 mg/kg every 6 hours, commencing after a mean of 16 days (range, 12–26) of mechanical ventilation. Steroids were continued for a mean of 21 days, with weaning from the initial high dose commencing at days 4 to 7. Lung injury scores improved significantly within 7 days in all those who survived (5 of 6). Steroid therapy was potentially associated with significant morbidity in this study, however, including stomach necrosis, staphylococcal lung abscess, prolonged polyneuropathy, urinary tract infection, and catheter-related sepsis. In a randomized double-blind placebo-controlled trial, 24 patients with ARDS who had failed to improve by day 7 of illness were treated with methylprednisolone commencing at 2 mg/kg/day for a total of 32 days, demonstrating marked improvements in lung injury score after 10 days of treatment and substantially better intensive care mortality (0 versus 62% in controls, P = .002).[38] A pathophysiologic correlate of the clinical improvement observed with steroids is the reduction in both serum and BAL levels of procollagen I and III observed in steroid-treated patients compared with those receiving placebo.[151]

Glucocorticoids are effective in reducing lung inflammatory responses provided treatment is prolonged, but short courses may have a deleterious effect. For example, limiting therapy to the first 6 days after acute lung injury enhances the accumulation of collagen after discontinuation of steroids,[37] while a similar duration of therapy commencing later in the illness (from days 7 to 12) has the desired result of reducing collagen formation.[152] Shorter courses of steroids may result in significant enhancement of cytokine responses for up to 6 days following drug administration.[153] Two studies demonstrate that premature discontinuation of steroid therapy in late ARDS was associated with deterioration in lung function that resolved with the reinstitution of treatment.[154,155] Hooper's group treated patients for 21 days,[155] while Meduri advocates 6 weeks. All studies that indicate potential benefits describe treatment commencing beyond the first week of mechanical ventilation.

There is no conclusive evidence to support the use of steroids in ARDS in children. If steroid therapy is used, it should probably be for refractory ARDS (e.g., >7 days of mechanical ventilation) and the course should be prolonged. Intercurrent infection should be excluded prior to embarking on a prolonged course of steroid therapy. Significant improvements in clinical parameters should be seen within 1 week in the majority of patients, but a smaller subgroup may require up to 2 weeks to demonstrate a response. Inhaled steroids may also have a role.

ANTICOAGULATION

Given the well-documented increase in procoagulant activity that accompanies ARDS,[32–34,36] it is reasonable to hypothesize that there may be a role for anticoagulation in this disorder. This is supported by the improved outcomes demonstrated from the use of activated protein C in sepsis,[156] the marked pathophysiologic similarities between the procoagulant states of ARDS and of sepsis, and the close clinical relationship between the two disorders.

Animal studies have demonstrated favorable effects of activated protein C,[157] tissue factor pathway inhibitor,[158] heparin,[159] antithrombin III,[160] and thrombomodulin[161] in models of acute lung injury and ARDS. While no agents have been specifically tested in humans with ARDS, there is some indirect evidence from studies of patients with sepsis that suggests a possible beneficial effect. Activated protein C (APC), which has both anticoagulant and anti-inflammatory actions, is an effective therapy for patients with sepsis, reducing mortality in the Protein C Worldwide Evaluation in Severe Sepsis (PROWESS) study.[156] There was some evidence in the PROWESS study that respiratory disease resolved more rapidly in patients treated with APC, with increased number of ventilator-free days and improved PaO_2/FIO_2 ratios. Despite promising early results in septic patients, including a statistically significant reduction in 28-day mortality rate for septic patients with ARDS (37% compared with 57% for the placebo group),[162] tissue factor pathway inhibitor has not lived up to its early promise either as a treatment for sepsis, or for the subgroup of septic patients with ARDS. A recent large multicenter trial of tissue factor pathway inhibitor for adult patients with sepsis demonstrated no improvement in mortality rate in the group as a whole or for a predetermined subset of patients with ALI.[163]

OTHER AGENTS OF INTEREST

Several other systemically administered drugs have been investigated as potential treatments in ARDS, including vitamin E,[164] prostaglandin E_1,[165] ibuprofen,[166] ketoconazole,[167] fluconazole,[168] and *N*-acetyl cysteine.[169] None of these agents has demonstrated clinically important positive results in human trials. Hemofiltration has been demonstrated to significantly reduce levels of circulating inflammatory mediators and histologic changes in an animal model of ARDS, but there are no data from human studies at the present time.[1] Recently, positive results have been obtained with an enteral feeding regimen consisting of a low-carbohydrate, high-fat, antioxidant-containing diet, with recipients demonstrating improved gas exchange, shorter duration of ventilation and ICU stay, and substantially reduced neutrophil counts in BAL specimens.[170]

OUTCOMES

Ashbaugh's first description of ARDS indicated a mortality rate of 58% (7 of 12 patients); subsequent pediatric series have reported mortality rates ranging from 9.5%[59] to 94%,[4] although since the publication of a consensus definition of ARDS in 1994[3] there has been greater consistency in reported mortality rates. Because ARDS is not a single disorder, it is likely that a large part of the variation in reported outcomes arises as a result of etiologic differences. For example, a strong relationship between the presence of immune compromise and outcome has been reported. In patients with acute respiratory failure treated with high-frequency ventilation, Arnold and colleagues[70] found that in patients without preexisting lung disease the presence of immune compromise was associated with an odds ratio of 5.28 for death. Similarly, Keenan and colleagues reported a survival of only 4% in children who required mechanical ventilation for respiratory failure after bone marrow transplantation.[171] A wide variety of management protocols and strategies further confuses the picture.

There has been a trend toward improved survival in case series over recent years, approximately coinciding with the widespread adoption of protective ventilatory strategies. Early studies reported mortality rates largely in the range of 40% to 60%,[5,172–176] while a number of studies in the last decade have reported mortality rates of 10% to 40%.[59,60,177] Several large adult series have also reported low mortality rates.[20,56,58,177,178] This apparent improvement in survival is usually attributed to adoption of protective ventilation, but other factors, including improved general care in the ICU or the more widespread use of interventions such as prone positioning and HFV, may have also played a role. It is also possible that the disease itself, or underlying conditions in affected patients, are changing. It should be noted that most pediatric studies reporting mortality rates less than 50% have not used American-European consensus criteria,[5,76,127,172,179,180] enrolled relatively few patients with immunodeficiency,[60,97] or excluded certain patients (e.g., those regarded as being "futile" or those with severe neurologic insult) from their analyses.[5,59,76,99,172,181] Similarly, investigators reporting higher mortality rates have often reported series with relatively large proportions of high-risk patients or using more stringent enrollment criteria. For example, DeBruin and colleagues[182] reported a mortality rate of 72%, but their cohort included numerous oncology patients as well as many with human immunodeficiency virus (HIV) infection and other causes of immune compromise (in total, 74% of patients had solid tumor, leukemia, HIV, or other causes of immune suppression, with a mortality rate for this subgroup of 78%) and used a definition of ARDS that required a PaO_2/FIO_2 ratio of less than 150 mm Hg rather than the 200 mm Hg used in the American-European consensus definition. Mortality in the 26 nonimmunocompromised patients in this series was only 54%. Conversely, some subgroups of ARDS such as those caused by respiratory syncytial virus have been reported as being associated with very low mortality rates.[44] Thus, true trends in mortality are difficult to discern. Nevertheless, two recent large series strongly suggest that low mortality rates are achievable.

Paulson and colleagues[59] excluded patients with "neurological futility" and reported survival in 57 of 63 patients fulfilling American-European consensus criteria (90.5%). Including the futile cases gives a survival rate of 77% (57 of 74), suggesting that the approach used by this group (ventilation at high frequencies and low tidal volume using a conventional pressure-controlled ventilator) is worthy of serious consideration despite the high incidence of air leak (51%) encountered with this ventilatory mode. Peters and colleagues[60] reported excellent outcomes from a prospective study of 118 children with acute hypoxemic respiratory failure, including 52 with ARDS managed with well-defined strategies—conventional ventilation with permissive hypercapnia and limiting of peak inspired pressure to a maximum of 35 cm H_2O, HFV being used if conventional techniques were unsuccessful, and ECMO being used in a minority (n = 4) of patients. Some patients also received surfactant and NO at the discretion of the treating physician. All deaths were included in the mortality statistics, including patients with brain death or elective withdrawal of support; nevertheless, the mortality rate was encouragingly low at 22% overall (36.5% for ARDS, 10.6% for non-ARDS). Both the Paulson[59] and Peters[60] articles indicate that mortality less than the traditionally quoted 40% to 60% is achievable in modern ICUs.

■ OUTCOME PREDICTION

A significant challenge facing investigators and clinicians in dealing with ARDS is the ability to accurately predict outcome. There are two principal areas of interest in outcome prediction. First, can the development of ARDS be accurately predicted in patients with ALI or even in those without ALI who suffer an insult recognized as a trigger for ARDS, and second, once ARDS develops, can the likelihood of death be accurately determined? Resolving the first question may allow early application of prophylactic strategies such as anti-inflammatory agents to patients at high risk for developing the disease. Resolving the second question is crucial in assessing the impact of new therapies and in appropriately allocating very high-risk patients to experimental or unconventional therapies.

A variety of respiratory indices have been investigated as possible mortality indicators. Given that many patients dying with ARDS succumb to nonrespiratory problems, it is not surprising that generally investigators have been unable to link respiratory indices with outcome. Simple indices such as lung injury scores are of no predictive value in the first 24 to 72 hours following the onset of ARDS,[9,183] and even more detailed measurements such as static[129] and dynamic[184] compliance do not discriminate between survivors and nonsurvivors. In pediatric studies, investigators have struggled to find significant relationships between mortality and respiratory indices obtained in the first 24 to 48 hours of illness. Only a few positive associations have been documented. Tamburro and colleagues[185] reported an alveolar to arterial oxygen gradient of greater than 450 mm Hg for any 16-hour period during the first 48 hours of AHRF as being 100% specific (and 86% sensitive) for death. Zobel and colleagues[176] reported that a respiratory severity index ([mean airway pressure × A-a PO_2/PaO_2] / 100) of greater than 0.75 at 48 hours after first meeting criteria for ARDS predicted death with 100% specificity and positive predictive value, with 77.7% sensitivity and 75% negative predictive value. Timmons and colleagues[181] attempted to overcome the problems inherent with single-institution studies by a retrospective survey involving 41 pediatric ICUs. A predictive algorithm was based on age, operative status, PRISM score, FIO_2, ventilator rate, peak inspiratory pressure, PEEP, PaO_2, and $PaCO_2$. This "PeRF" score generated areas under a receiver operating curve of 0.769 to 0.846 for variables scored at 12-hour intervals over the first 48 hours after meeting criteria for ARDS, with further improvements in accuracy up to 156 hours. The resulting PeRF algorithm is, however, complex, involving nine variables, and is yet to be validated prospectively. Arnold and colleagues found the oxygenation index at 24 hours to be one of two predictive parameters in patients treated with HFOV (the other predictor was the presence of immunocompromise). However, it was relatively weak, generating an odds ratio of only 1.05 for death in a multivariate model.[70] Sarnaik and colleagues found that a combination of an initial oxygenation index greater than 20 and a failure of the oxygenation index to fall by greater than 20% after 6 hours of HFV gave an odds ratio of 33 for death in a group of patients with severe respiratory failure treated with HFV.[186] Other researchers have been unable to identify significant associations between mortality and respiratory indices measured early in the course of illness.[6,60,76,180,187]

In recent years the focus in outcome prediction has shifted away from ventilatory indices, with encouraging results. Multiorgan failure has become increasingly recognized as a strong predictor of mortality in the ICU,[188,189] and it is a frequent occurrence in patients with ARDS,[21] suggesting a possible role for organ failure scores as predictive tools in this disorder. There is also a growing awareness of the important role of underlying disorders, particularly immunocompromise, in determining mortality.[70,171] In adults, outcome of ARDS is closely related to other organ involvement; the mortality rate rises with increasing numbers of failing organ systems.[57,129,184] Similar observations have been made in children.[5,60,180] Measurement of a variety of inflammatory markers in both plasma and BAL specimens appears to offer the opportunity to not only accurately predict the outcome of established ARDS but also to predict the development of ARDS in at-risk patients. Plasma levels of the soluble form of L-selectin (sL-selectin) are significantly decreased in patients at risk for developing ARDS (such as trauma patients) who go on to develop ARDS compared with those who do not. Plasma sL-selectin concentration is also significantly related to number of days of mechanical ventilation, worst values of PaO_2/FIO_2, organ failure score, and patient mortality in subsequent disease course.[190] Von Willebrand factor antigen (vWf-Ag) is a protein synthesized principally by vascular endothelial cells that has been shown to be a sensitive marker of cellular injury and is elevated in patients with acute respiratory failure.[191] Prospective data indicate that in a select group of patients at risk for developing ARDS (patients with nonpulmonary sepsis), vWf-Ag levels were substantially higher in patients who went on to develop ARDS than in those who did not.[192] Unfortunately, much of the predictive power is lost in less-selected populations.[193] In patients at risk for ARDS, serum ferritin levels are substantially higher in those that progress to ARDS compared with those who do not. Serum ferritin levels also correlate significantly with levels of sE-selectin and soluble intercellular adhesion molecule-1 (sICAM-1), but unfortunately do not allow accurate prediction of death or days of ventilation.[194] Clark and colleagues demonstrated that BAL procollagen III obtained on days 3 and 7 of the illness was substantially higher in patients with ARDS who died compared with survivors.[27] Subsequent studies have described elevations of procollagen III in alveolar edema fluid as early as day 1,[195] and there is prognostic value in serum procollagen III levels taken on day 7 of ARDS, with patients with higher values being more likely to die.[151] IL-8 levels measured in BAL fluid at hospital admission in patients at risk for developing ARDS are significantly higher in those who progress to ARDS compared with those who do not.[22] In patients with established ARDS, IL-8 in BAL on day 1 of ARDS is significantly higher in patients with a fatal outcome than in those who survive.[23] Other inflammatory mediators in BAL fluid, including TNF-α, IL-1β, and IL-6, are also significantly higher in nonsurvivors than survivors. Meduri's group reported an association between elevated TNF-α levels in the first 48 hours of ARDS and poor outcome[23]; however, there appears to be little value in either BAL or serum levels as predictors for the development of ARDS.[196] Both surfactant-associated proteins A and B (SP-A and SP-B) are found in decreased concentrations in BAL samples of patients with acute lung injury, and SP-A levels correlate well with severity of lung injury[197]; however, neither SP-A nor SP-B levels in BAL fluid are predictive of outcome, although SP-D has some predictive value in this regard on both days 1 and 3 of illness.[198] As well as being a useful marker in BAL fluid, surfactant proteins are measurable in serum, where elevated rather than decreased levels indicate lung injury. Serum SP-A and -B levels correlate well with severity of pulmonary dysfunction as indicated by static respiratory compliance and PaO_2/FIO_2 throughout the course of the illness.[199] SP-B is far less abundant than SP-A and is more difficult to measure in serum, but because of its relatively low molecular weight, it is hypothesized to leak into serum more readily and therefore to be a better marker of ARDS. Serum SP-B is markedly elevated on day 1 in patients with ARDS and is significantly different from that in normal controls, patients ventilated for nonrespiratory indications, and patients with acute pulmonary edema.[199] Day 1 serum SP-B levels are also higher in patients dying from ARDS compared with those who survive or die from nonrespiratory causes.[199] In addition to their outcome-predictive ability, surfactant proteins may also be useful in predicting the development of ARDS in at-risk patients. Greene and colleagues reported that in a patient population at risk for developing ARDS (principally patients with trauma or sepsis), SP-A in BAL fluid taken on day 1 of intubation was significantly lower in those that went on to develop ARDS compared with those who did not.[198]

CONCLUSIONS

ARDS remains a significant problem in the pediatric ICU. Interpretation of outcome data is hampered by poor study design and relatively small numbers reported in most series; however, recently published data suggest that mortality rates substantially less than 50% can be achieved in this disease. Several strategies have been established as effective in recent years. Adult data support the use of PEEP beyond the lower inflection point of the pressure-volume curve, and limiting peak inspiratory pressures to 30 to 35 cm H_2O or tidal volumes to 6 mL/kg. Ventilator-induced lung injury is ameliorated by prone positioning, and this simple technique, which has few if any serious deleterious effects, should be considered in most patients. There is good evidence that in chronic ARDS (persisting beyond 1 week) a course of steroids is likely to improve long-term survival. Neither surfactant nor NO have been demonstrated to be of proven benefit in large series, although surfactant is worthy of further investigation given that the largest trial probably used a suboptimal delivery method. Until the results of further surfactant trials are published, its use in individual patients outside a trial setting cannot be justified on evidence available at this time. Perfluorocarbons remain a potentially valuable agent in ARDS, having numerous favorable physical properties and spectacularly successful results in animal studies. The ability to predict outcomes accurately plays an important role in the assessment of the impact of new therapies. Adult and animal data suggest that improved prediction not only of the outcome of established ARDS but also of the development of ARDS in at-risk subjects may be obtained by measuring the concentrations of inflammatory mediators or surfactant-associated proteins in plasma BAL samples. As well as enhancing the ability to predict outcome, such data are also important in our understanding of the pathophysiology of ARDS. Our understanding of the influence of genetics on susceptibility to, and outcome of, ARDS is still in its infancy and is likely to add considerably to our knowledge of this disorder over coming years. Further refinements and improvements in techniques of mechanical ventilation are likely, and agents targeted to block specific proinflammatory cytokines will add to our understanding of pathophysiology and perhaps allow effective early therapy in some patients.

REFERENCES

1. Su X, Bai C, Hong Q, et al: Effect of continuous hemofiltration on hemodynamics, lung inflammation and pulmonary edema in a canine model of acute lung injury. Intensive Care Med 2003;29:2034–2042.
2. Ashbaugh DG, Bigelow DB, Petty TL, Levine BE: Acute respiratory distress in adults. Lancet 1967;2(7511):319–323.
3. Bernard GR, Artigas A, Brigham KL, et al: The American-European consensus committee on ARDS. Definition, mechanisms, relevant outcomes, and clinical trial coordination. Am J Respir Crit Care Med 1994; 149:818–824.
4. Holbrook PR, Taylor G, Pollack MM, Fields AI: Adult respiratory distress syndrome in children. Pediatr Clin North Am 1980;27:677–685.
5. Pfenniger J, Gerber A, Tschäppeler H, Zimmerman A: Adult respiratory distress syndrome in children. J Pediatr 1982;101:352–357.
6. Davis SL, Fuhrman BP, Costarino AT: Adult respiratory distress syndrome in children. Associated disease, clinical course, and predictors of death. J Pediatr 1993;123:35–45.
7. Luhr OR, Antonsen K, Karlsson M, et al: Incidence and mortality after acute respiratory distress syndrome in Sweden, Denmark and Iceland. Am J Respir Crit Care Med 1999;159:1849–1861.
8. Bersten AD, Edibam C, Hunt T, Moran J, The Australian and New Zealand Intensive Care Society Clinical Trials Group: Incidence and mortality of acute lung injury and the acute respiratory distress syndrome in three Australian States. Am J Respir Crit Care Med 2002;165:443–448.
9. Ware LB, Matthay MA: The acute respiratory distress syndrome. N Engl J Med 2000;342:1334–1349.
10. Martin TR, Nakamura M, Matute-Bello G: The role of apoptosis in acute lung injury. Crit Care Med 2003;31(Suppl):184–188.
11. Nakamura M, Matute-Bello G, Liles WC, et al: Differential response of human lung epithelial cells to Fas-induced apoptosis. Am J Pathol 2004; 164:1949–1958.
12. Pugin J, Verghesse G, Widmer MC, Matthay MA: The alveolar space is the site of intense inflammatory and profibrotic reactions in the early phase of acute respiratory distress syndrome. Crit Care Med 1999;27:304–312.
13. Pittet JF, Mackersie RC, Martin TR, Matthay MA: Biological markers of acute lung injury. Prognostic and pathogenetic significance. Am J Respir Crit Care Med 1997;155:1187–1205.
14. Tremblay L, Valenza F, Ribeiro SP, et al: Injurious ventilatory strategies increase cytokines and c-fos m-RNA expression in an isolated rat lung model. J Clin Invest 1997;99:944–952.
15. Zhang H, Downey GP, Suter PM, et al: Conventional mechanical ventilation is associated with bronchoalveolar lavage-induced activation of polymorphonuclear leukocytes. Anesthesiology 2002;97:1426–1433.
16. Abraham MB: Neutrophils and acute lung injury. Crit Care Med 2003; 31(Suppl):195–199.
17. Chu EK, Whitehead T, Slutsky AS: Effects of cyclic opening and closing at low- and high-volume ventilation on bronchoalveolar lavage cytokines. Crit Care Med 2004;32:168–174.
18. Dreyfuss D, Saumon G: Ventilator-induced lung injury. Lessons from experimental studies. Am Rev Respir Crit Care Med 1998;157:294–323.
19. Ranieri VM, Suter PM, Tortorella C, et al: Effect of mechanical ventilation on inflammatory mediators in patients with acute respiratory distress syndrome. A randomized controlled trial. JAMA 1999;282:54–61.
20. The Acute Respiratory Distress Syndrome Network: Ventilation with lower tidal volumes as compared with traditional tidal volumes for acute lung injury and the acute respiratory distress syndrome. N Engl J Med 2000;342: 1301–1308.
21. Slutsky AS, Tremblay LN: Multiple system organ failure. Is mechanical ventilation a contributing factor? Am J Respir Crit Care Med 1998;157: 1721–1725.
22. Donnelly SC, Streiter RM, Kunkel SL, et al: Interleukin-8 and the development of adult respiratory distress syndrome in at-risk patient groups. Lancet 1993;341:643–647.
23. Meduri GU, Kohler G, Headley S, et al: Inflammatory cytokines in the BAL of patients with ARDS. Persistent elevation over time predicts poor outcome. Chest 1995;108:1303–1314.
24. Moraes TJ, Chow CW, Downey GP: Proteases and lung injury. Crit Care Med 2003;31(Suppl):189–194.

25. Katsouyanni K, Sfyras D, Malagari K, Roussos C: The regional production of cytokines and lactate in sepsis-related multiple organ failure. Am J Respir Crit Care Med 1997;155:53–59.
26. Steinberg KP, Milberg JA, Martin TR, et al: Evolution of bronchoalveolar cell populations in the adult respiratory distress syndrome. Am J Respir Crit Care Med 1994;150:113–122.
27. Clark JG, Milberg JA, Steinberg KP, Hudson LD: Type III procollagen peptide in the adult respiratory distress syndrome. Association of increased peptide levels in bronchoalveolar lavage fluid with increased risk for death. Ann Intern Med 1995;122:17–23.
28. Sivan Y, Mor C, al-Jundi S, Newth CJL: Adult respiratory distress syndrome in severely neutropaenic children. Pediatr Pulmonol 1990;8:104–108.
29. Kawano T, Mori S, Cybulski M, et al: Effect of granulocyte depletion in a ventilated surfactant-depleted lung. J Appl Physiol 1987;62:27–33.
30. Bone RC, Francis PB, Pierce AK: Intravascular coagulation associated with the adult respiratory distress syndrome. Am J Med 1976;61:585–598.
31. Zapol WM, Jones R: Vascular components of ARDS. Clinical pulmonary hemodynamics and morphology. Am Rev Respir Dis 1987;136:471–474.
32. Quinn DA, Carvalho AC, Geller E, et al: 99mTc-fibrinogen scanning in adult respiratory distress syndrome. Am Rev Respir Dis 1987;135:100–106.
33. Idell S: Coagulation, fibrinolysis and fibrin deposition in acute lung injury. Crit Care Med 2003;31(Suppl):213–220.
34. Seeger W, Stohr G, Wolff HR, Neuhof H: Alteration of surfactant function due to protein leakage. Special interaction with fibrin monomer. J Appl Physiol 1985;58:326–328.
35. Marshall R, Bellingan G, Laurent G: The acute respiratory distress syndrome. Fibrosis in the fast lane. Thorax 1998;53:815–817.
36. Günther A, Mosavi P, Heinemann S, et al: Alveolar fibrin formation caused by enhanced procoagulant and depressed fibrinolytic capacities in severe pneumonia. Am J Respir Crit Care Med 2000;161:454–462.
37. Meduri GU: The role of the host defence response in the progression and outcome of ARDS. Pathophysiological correlations and response to glucocorticoid treatment. Eur Respir J 1996;9:2650–2670.
38. Meduri GU, Headley AS, Golden E, et al: Effect of prolonged methylprednisolone therapy in unresolving acute respiratory distress syndrome. A randomized controlled trial. JAMA 1998;280:159–165.
39. Gattinoni L, Pelosi P, Vitale G, et al: Body position changes redistribute lung computed tomographic density in patients with acute respiratory failure. Anesthesiology 1991;74:15–23.
40. Gattinoni L, Pesenti A, Avalli L, et al: Pressure-volume curve of total respiratory system in acute respiratory failure. Computed tomographic scan study. Am Rev Respir Dis 1987;136:730–736.
41. Amato MB, Barbas CS, Medeiros DM, et al: Beneficial effects of the "open lung approach" with low distending pressures in acute respiratory distress syndrome. A prospective randomized study on mechanical ventilation. Am J Respir Crit Care Med 1995;152:1835–1846.
42. Roupie E, Dambrosio M, Servillo G, et al: Titration of tidal volume and induced hypercapnia in acute respiratory distress syndrome. Am J Respir Crit Care Med 1995;152:121–128.
43. Nève V, de la Roque ED, Leclerc F, et al: Ventilator-induced overdistension in children—dynamic versus low-flow inflation volume-pressure curves. Am J Respir Crit Care Med 2000;162:139–147.
44. Hammer J, Numa A, Newth CJL: Acute respiratory distress syndrome caused by respiratory syncytial virus. Pediatr Pulmonol 1997;23:176–183.
45. Newth CJL, Stretton M, Deakers TW, Hammer J: Assessment of pulmonary function in the early phase of ARDS in pediatric patients. Pediatr Pulmonol 1997;23:169–175.
46. Hammer J, Numa A, Newth C: Total lung capacity by N_2 washout from high and low lung volumes in ventilated infants and children. Am J Respir Crit Care Med 1998;158:526–531.
47. Sivan Y, Deakers TW, Newth CJL: Functional residual capacity in ventilated infants and children. Pediatr Res 1990;28:451–454.
48. Fisher JB, Mammel MC, Coleman JM, et al: Identifying lung overdistention during mechanical ventilation by using volume-pressure loops. Pediatr Pulmonol 1988;5:10–14.
49. Weiss I, Ushay HM, DeBruin W, et al: Respiratory and cardiac function in children after acute hypoxemic respiratory failure. Crit Care Med 1996; 24:148–154.
50. Orme J, Romney JS, Hopkins RO, et al: Pulmonary function and health-related quality of life in survivors of acute respiratory distress syndrome. Am J Respir Crit Care Med 2002;167:690–694.
51. Neff TA, Stocker R, Frey HR, et al: Long-term assessment of lung function in survivors of severe ARDS. Chest 2003;123:845–853.
52. Webb HH, Tierney DF: Experimental pulmonary edema due to intermittent positive-pressure ventilation with high inflation pressures. Protection by positive end-expiratory pressure. Am Rev Respir Dis 1974;110:556–565.
53. Dreyfuss D, Soler P, Basset G, Saumon G: High inflation pressure pulmonary edema. Respective effects of high airway pressure, high tidal volume, and positive end-expiratory pressure. Am Rev Respir Dis 1988;139:1159–1164.
54. Hernandez LA, Peevy KJ, Moise AA, Parker JC: Chest wall restriction limits high airway pressure-induced lung injury in young rabbits. J Appl Physiol 1989;66:2364–2368.
55. Bowton DL, Kong DL: High tidal volume ventilation produces increased lung water in oleic acid-injured rabbit lungs. Crit Care Med 1989;17: 908–911.
56. Lewandowski K, Rossaint R, Pappert D, et al: High survival rate in 122 ARDS patients managed according to a clinical algorithm including extracorporeal membrane oxygenation. Intensive Care Med 1997;23:819–835.
57. Hickling KG, Walsh J, Henderson S, Jackson R: Low mortality rate in adult respiratory distress syndrome using low-volume pressure-limited ventilation with permissive hypercapnia. A prospective study. Crit Care Med 1994;22: 1568–1578.
58. Amato MBP, Barbas CSV, Medeiros DM, et al: Effect of a protective-ventilation strategy on mortality in the acute respiratory distress syndrome. N Engl J Med 1998;338:347–354.
59. Paulson TE, Spear RM, Silva PD, Peterson BM: High frequency pressure control ventilation with high positive end-expiratory pressure in children with acute respiratory distress syndrome. J Pediatr 1996;129:566–573.
60. Peters MJ, Tasker RC, Kiff KM, et al: Acute hypoxaemic respiratory failure in children. Case mix and the utility of respiratory severity indices. Intensive Care Med 1998;24:699–705.
61. Faridy EE, Permutt S, Riley RL: Effect of ventilation on surface forces in excised dog's lungs. J Appl Physiol 1966;21:1453–1462.
62. Stewart TE, Meade MO, Cook DJ, et al: Evaluation of a ventilation strategy to prevent barotrauma in patients at high risk for acute respiratory distress syndrome. N Engl J Med 1998;338:355–361.
63. Hickling KG: The pressure-volume curve is greatly modified by recruitment. Am J Respir Crit Care Med 1998;158:194–202.
64. Medoff BD, Harris RS, Kesselman H, et al: Use of recruitment maneuvers and high positive end-expiratory pressure in a patient with acute respiratory distress syndrome. Crit Care Med 2000;28:1210–1216.
65. Capellier G, Beuret P, Clement G, et al: Oxygen tolerance in patients with acute respiratory failure. Intensive Care Med 1998;24:422–428.
66. White C, Ghezzi P, Dinarello C, et al: Recombinant tumor necrosis factor/cachectin and interleukin 1 pretreatment decrease lung oxidized glutathione accumulation, lung injury and mortality in rats exposed to hyperoxia. J Clin Invest 1987;79:1868–1873.
67. Bohn DJ, Miyasaka K, Marchak BE, et al: Ventilation by high frequency oscillation. J Appl Physiol 1980;48:710–716.
68. Sedeek KA, Takeuchi M, Suchodolski K, Kacmarek RM: Determinants of tidal volume during high-frequency oscillation. Crit Care Med 2003;31: 227–231.
69. McCulloch PR, Forkert PG, Froese AB: Lung volume maintenance prevents lung injury during high frequency oscillatory ventilation. Am Rev Respir Dis 1988;137:1185–1192.
70. Arnold JH, Anas NG, Luckett P, et al: High-frequency oscillatory ventilation in pediatric respiratory failure. A multicenter experience. Crit Care Med 2000;28:3913–3919.
71. HiFO Study Group: Randomized study of high-frequency oscillatory ventilation in infants with severe respiratory distress syndrome. J Pediatr 1993;122:609–619.
72. Gerstmann DR, Minton SD, Stoddard RA, et al: The Provo multicenter early high-frequency oscillatory ventilation trial. Improved pulmonary and clinical outcome in respiratory distress syndrome. Pediatrics 1996;98: 1044–1057.
73. Rettwitz-Volk W, Veldman A, Roth B, et al: A prospective, randomized, multicenter trial of high-frequency oscillatory ventilation compared with conventional ventilation in preterm infants with respiratory distress syndrome receiving surfactant. J Pediatr 1998;132:249–254.
74. Bollen CW, Uiterwaal CS, van Vught AJ: Cumulative metaanalysis of high-frequency versus conventional ventilation in premature neonates. Am J Respir Crit Care Med 2003;168:1150–1155.
75. Clark RH, Dykes FD, Bachman TE, Ashurst JT: Intraventricular hemorrhage and high-frequency ventilation. A meta-analysis of prospective clinical trials. Pediatrics 1996;98:1058–1061.
76. Arnold JH, Hanson JH, Toro-Figuero LO, et al: Prospective randomized comparison of high-frequency oscillatory ventilation and conventional mechanical ventilation in pediatric respiratory failure. Crit Care Med 1994; 22:1530–1539.
77. Derdak S, Mehta S, Stewart TE, et al: High-frequency oscillatory ventilation for acute respiratory distress syndrome in adults. Am J Respir Crit Care Med 2003;166:801–808.

78. Sedeek KA, Takeuchi M, Suchodolski K, et al: Open-lung protective ventilation with pressure control ventilation, high-frequency oscillation and intratracheal pulmonary ventilation results in similar gas exchange, hemodynamics and lung mechanics. Anesthesiology 2003;99: 1102–1111.
79. Olarte JL, Gelvez J, Fakioglu H, et al: Tracheobronchial injury during intratracheal pulmonary ventilation in rabbits. Crit Care Med 2003;31: 916–923.
80. Dassieu G, Brochard L, Benani M, et al: Continuous tracheal gas insufflation in preterm infants with hyaline membrane disease. Am J Respir Crit Care Med 2000;162:826–831.
81. Kylstra JA, Paganelli CV, Lanphier EH: Pulmonary gas exchange in dogs ventilated with hyperbarically oxygenated liquid. J Appl Physiol 1966; 21:177–184.
82. Cox PN, Frndova H, Karlsson O, et al: Fluorocarbons facilitate lung recruitment. Intensive Care Med 2003;29:2297–2302.
83. Rotta AT, Gunnarsson B, Hernan LJ, et al: Partial liquid ventilation with perflubron attenuates in vivo oxidative damage to proteins and lipids. Crit Care Med 2000;28:202–208.
84. Leach CL, Holm B, Morin FC, et al: Partial liquid ventilation in premature lambs with respiratory distress syndrome. Efficacy and compatibility with exogenous surfactant. J Pediatr 1995;126:412–420.
85. Wilcox DT, Glick PL, Karamanoukian HL, et al: Partial liquid ventilation and nitric oxide in congenital diaphragmatic hernia. J Pediatr Surg 1997;32:1211–1215.
86. Mrozek JD, Smith KM, Bing DR, et al: Exogenous surfactant and partial liquid ventilation. Physiologic and pathologic effects. Am J Respir Crit Care Med 1997;156:1058–1065.
87. Houmes RJ, Verbrugge SJ, Hendrik ER, Lachmann B: Hemodynamic effects of partial liquid ventilation with perfluorocarbon in acute lung injury. Intensive Care Med 1995;21:966–972.
88. Leach CL, Greenspan JS, Rubenstein SD, et al: Partial liquid ventilation with perflubron in premature infants with severe respiratory distress syndrome. The LiquiVent Study Group. N Engl J Med 1996;335: 761–767.
89. Hirschl RB, Pranikoff T, Gauger P, et al: Liquid ventilation in adults, children and full-term neonates. Lancet 1995;346:1201–1202.
90. Hirschl RB, Croce M, Gore D, et al: Prospective, randomized, controlled pilot study of partial liquid ventilation in adult acute respiratory distress syndrome. Am J Respir Crit Care Med 2002;165: 781–787.
91. Sukumar M, Bommaraju M, Fisher JE, et al: High-frequency partial liquid ventilation in respiratory distress syndrome. Hemodynamics and gas exchange. J Appl Physiol 1998;84:327–334.
92. Houmes RJM, Hartog A, Verbrugge SJC, et al: Combining partial liquid ventilation with nitric oxide to improve gas exchange in acute lung injury. Intensive Care Med 1997;23:163–169.
93. Tarczy-Hornoch P, Hildebrandt J, Mates EA, et al: Effects of exogenous surfactant on lung pressure-volume characteristics during liquid ventilation. J Appl Physiol 1996;80:1764–1771.
94. Steinhorn DM, Leach CL, Fuhrman BP, Holm BA: Partial liquid ventilation enhances surfactant phospholipid production. Crit Care Med 1996;24:1252–1256.
95. Baden HP, Mellema JD, Bratton SL, et al: High frequency oscillatory ventilation with partial liquid ventilation in a model of acute respiratory failure. Crit Care Med 1997;25:299–302.
96. Smith KM, Bing DR, Meyers PA, et al: Partial liquid ventilation. A comparison using conventional and high frequency techniques in an animal model of acute respiratory failure. Crit Care Med 1997;25: 1179–1186.
97. Nakagawa TA, Morris A, Gomez RJ, et al: Dose response to inhaled nitric oxide in pediatric patients with pulmonary hypertension and acute respiratory distress syndrome. J Pediatr 1997;131:63–69.
98. Okamoto K, Hamaguchi M, Kukita I, et al: Efficacy of inhaled nitric oxide in children with ARDS. Chest 1998;114:827–833.
99. Dobyns EL, Cornfield DN, Anas NG, et al: Multicenter randomized controlled trial of the effects of inhaled nitric oxide therapy on gas exchange in children with acute hypoxemic respiratory failure. J Pediatr 1999;134:406–412.
100. Dobyns EL, Anas NG, Fortenberry JD, et al: Interactive effects of high-frequency oscillatory ventilation and inhaled nitric oxide in acute hypoxemic respiratory failure in pediatrics. Crit Care Med 2002;30: 2425–2429.
101. Payen D, Vallet B: Results of the French prospective multicentre randomized double-blind placebo-controlled trial of inhaled nitric oxide (NO) in ARDS. Intensive Care Med 1999;25(Suppl):166.
102. Lundin S, Mang H, Smithies M, et al, for the European Study Group of Inhaled Nitric Oxide: Inhalation of nitric oxide in acute lung injury. Results of a European multicentre study. Intensive Care Med 1999;25:911–919.
103. Murdoch IA, Storman MO: Improved arterial oxygenation in children with the adult respiratory distress syndrome. The prone position. Acta Pediatr 1994;83:1043–106.
104. Curley MA, Thompson JE, Arnold JH: The effects of early and repeated prone positioning in pediatric patients with acute lung injury. Chest 2000; 118:156–153.
105. Relvas MS, Silver PC, Sagy M: Prone positioning of pediatric patients with ARDS results in improvement in oxygenation if maintained > 12 h daily. Chest 2003;124:269–274.
106. Bryan AC: Comments of a devil's advocate. Am Rev Respir Dis 1974; 110(Suppl):143–144.
107. Lamm WJE, Graham MM, Albert RK: Mechanism by which the prone position improves oxygenation in acute lung injury. Am J Respir Crit Care Med 1994;150:184–193.
108. Hakim TS, Dean GW, Lisbona R: Effect of body posture on spatial distribution of pulmonary blood flow. J Appl Physiol 1988;23: 694–705.
109. Kornecki A, Frndova H, Coates AL, Shemie S: A randomized trial of prolonged prone positioning in children with acute respiratory failure. Chest 2001;119:211–218.
110. Numa A, Hammer J, Newth CJL: The effect of prone and supine positions on functional residual capacity, oxygenation, and respiratory mechanics in ventilated infants and children. Am J Respir Crit Care Med 1997; 156:1185–1189.
111. Dupont H, Mentec H, Cheval C, et al: Short-term effect of inhaled nitric oxide and prone positioning on gas exchange in patients with severe acute respiratory distress syndrome. Crit Care Med 2000;28:304–308.
112. Stocker R, Neff T, Stein S, et al: Prone positioning and low-volume pressure limited ventilation improve survival in patients with severe ARDS. Chest 1997;111:1008–1017.
113. Broccard A, Shapiro RS, Schmitz LL, et al: Prone positioning attenuates and redistributes ventilator induced lung injury in dogs. Crit Care Med 2000;28:295–303.
114. Gattinoni L, Tognoni G, Pesenti A, et al: Effect of prone positioning on the survival of patients with acute respiratory failure. N Engl J Med 2001;345:568–573.
115. Casado-Flores J, de Azagra AM, Ruiz-Lopez MJ, et al: Pediatric ARDS. Effect of supine-prone postural changes on oxygenation. Intensive Care Med 2002;28:1792–1796.
116. Gregory TJ, Longmore WJ, Moxley MA, et al: Surfactant chemical composition and biophysical activity in acute respiratory distress syndrome. J Clin Invest 1991;88:1976–1981.
117. Möller JC, Schaible T, Roll C, et al: Treatment with bovine surfactant in severe acute respiratory distress syndrome in children. A randomized multicenter study. Intensive Care Med 2003;29:437–466.
118. Matalon S, Holm BA, Notter RH: Mitigation of pulmonary hyperoxic injury by administration of exogenous surfactant. J Appl Physiol 1987;62: 756–761.
119. Lamm WJE, Albert RK: Surfactant replacement improves lung recoil in rabbit lungs after acid aspiration. Am Rev Respir Dis 1990;142: 1281–1283.
120. Lachmann B, Bergmann KC: Surfactant replacement improves thorax-lung compliance and survival rate in mice with influenza infection. Am Rev Respir Dis 1987;135:A6.
121. Lutz CJ, Picone A, Gatto LA, et al: Exogenous surfactant and positive end-expiratory pressure in the treatment of endotoxin-induced lung injury. Crit Care Med 1998;26:1379–1389.
122. Anzueto A, Baughman RP, Kalpalatha K, et al: Aerosolised surfactant in adults with sepsis-induced acute respiratory distress syndrome. N Engl J Med 1996;224:1417–1421.
123. MacIntyre NR, Coleman RE, Schuller FS, et al: Efficiency of the delivery of aerosolised artificial surfactant in intubated patients with the adult respiratory distress syndrome. Am J Respir Crit Care Med 1994; 149:A125.
124. Nicholas TE, Doyle IR, Bersten AD: Surfactant replacement therapy in ARDS. White knight or noise in the system? Thorax 1997;52:195–197.
125. Spragg RG, Lewis JF, Walmrath HD, et al: Effect of recombinant surfactant protein C-based surfactant on the acute respiratory distress syndrome. N Engl J Med 2004;351:884–892.
126. Gregory TJ, Steinberg KP, Spragg R, et al: Bovine surfactant therapy for patients with acute respiratory distress syndrome. Am J Respir Crit Care Med 1997;155:1309–1315.

127. Willson DF, Jiao JH, Bauman LA, et al: Calf's lung surfactant extract in acute hypoxemic respiratory failure in children. Crit Care Med 1996;24:1316–1322.
128. Zapol WM, Snider MT, Hill JD, et al: Extracorporeal membrane oxygenation in severe acute respiratory failure. A randomized prospective study. JAMA 1979;242:2193–2199.
129. Gattinoni L, Pesenti A, Mascheroni D, et al: Low-frequency positive-pressure ventilation with extracorporeal CO_2 removal in severe acute respiratory failure. JAMA 1986;256:881–886.
130. Morris AH, Wallace JC, Menlove RL, et al: Randomized clinical trial of pressure-controlled inverse ratio ventilation and extracorporeal CO_2 removal for adult respiratory distress syndrome. Am J Respir Crit Care Med 1994;149:295–305.
131. Butt W, Karl T, Horton A, et al: Experience with extracorporeal membrane oxygenation in children more than one month old. Anaesth Intensive Care 1992;20:308–310.
132. Morton A, Dalton H, Kochanek P, et al: Extracorporeal membrane oxygenation for pediatric respiratory failure. Five year experience at the University of Pittsburgh. Crit Care Med 1994;22:1659–1667.
133. Moler FW, Palmisano JM, Custer JR, et al: Alveolar-arterial oxygen gradients before extra-corporeal life support for severe pediatric respiratory failure. Improved outcome for extracorporeal life support-managed patients? Crit Care Med 1994;22:620–625.
134. Lillehei CW, O'Rourke PP, Vacanti JP, Crone RK: Role of extracorporeal membrane oxygenation in selected pediatric respiratory problems. J Thorac Cardiovasc Surg 1989;98:968–971.
135. Moler FW, Custer JR, Bartlett RH, et al: Extracorporeal life support for pediatric respiratory failure. Crit Care Med 1992;20: 1112–1118.
136. Green TP, Timmons OD, Fackler JC, et al: The impact of extracorporeal membrane oxygenation on survival in pediatric patients with acute respiratory failure. Crit Care Med 1996;24:323–329.
137. Vats A, Pettignano R, Culler S, Wright J: Cost of extracorporeal life support ion pediatric patients with acute respiratory failure. Crit Care Med 1998;26:1587–1592.
138. Nading JH: Historical controls for extracorporeal membrane oxygenation in neonates. Crit Care Med 1989;17:423–425.
139. O'Rourke PP, Crone RK, Vacanti JP, et al: Extracorporeal membrane oxygenation and conventional medical therapy in neonates with persistent pulmonary hypertension of the newborn. A prospective randomized study. Pediatrics 1989;84:957–963.
140. Dworitz AR, Moya FR, Sabo B, Gross I: Survival of infants with persistent pulmonary hypertension of the newborn without ECMO. Pediatrics 1989;84:1–6.
141. Bartlett RH, Roloff DW, Cornell RG, et al: Extracorporeal circulation in neonatal respiratory failure. A prospective randomized study. Pediatrics 1985;76:479–487.
142. Navas L, Wang E, deCarvalho V, Robinson J: RSV infection in high risk hospitalized children. J Pediatr 1992;121:348–354.
143. Numa AH: Outcome of respiratory syncytial virus infection and a cost-benefit analysis of prophylaxis. J Paediatr Child Health 2000;36: 422–427.
144. Liebold A, Reng CM, Phillip A, et al: Pumpless extracorporeal lung assist—experience with the first 20 cases. Eur J Cardiothoracic Surg 2000;17:608–613.
145. Kam JC, Szefler SJ, Surs W, et al: Combination IL-2 and IL-4 reduces glucocorticoid receptor-binding affinity and T cell response to glucocorticoids. J Immunol 1993;151:3460–3466.
146. Lefering R, Neugebauer EAM: Steroid controversy in sepsis and septic shock. A meta-analysis. Crit Care Med 1995;23:1294–1303.
147. Bernard GR, Luce JM, Sprung CL, et al: High dose corticosteroids in patients with the adult respiratory distress syndrome. N Engl J Med 1987;317:1565–1570.
148. Meduri GU, Chinn AJ, Leeper KV, et al: Corticosteroid rescue treatment of progressive fibroproliferation in late ARDS. Patterns of response and predictors of outcome. Chest 1994;105:1516–1527.
149. Meduri GU, Headley S, Tolley E, et al: Plasma and BAL cytokine response to corticosteroid rescue treatment in late ARDS. Chest 1995;108: 1315–1325.
150. Biffl WL, Moore FA, Moore EE, et al: Are corticosteroids salvage therapy for refractory acute respiratory distress syndrome? Am J Surg 1995; 170:591–596.
151. Meduri GU, Tolley EA, Chinn A, et al: Procollagen types I and III aminoterminal propeptide levels during acute respiratory distress syndrome and in response to methylprednisolone treatment. Am J Respir Crit Care Med 1998;158:1432–1441.
152. Hesterberg TW, Last JA: Ozone-induced acute pulmonary fibrosis in rats—prevention of increased rates of collagen synthesis by methylprednisolone. Am Rev Respir Dis 1981;123:47–52.
153. Barber AE, Coyle SM, Marano MA, et al: Glucocorticoid therapy alters hormonal and cytokine responses to endotoxin in man. J Immunol 1993; 150:1999–2006.
154. Ashbaugh DG, Maier RV: Idiopathic pulmonary fibrosis in adult respiratory distress syndrome. Diagnosis and treatment. Arch Surg 1985;120: 530–535.
155. Hooper RG, Kearl RA: Established ARDS treated with a sustained course of adrenocortical steroids. Chest 1990;97:138–143.
156. Bernard GR, Vincent JL, Laterre PF, et al: Efficacy and safety of recombinant human activated protein C for severe sepsis. N Engl J Med 2001;344:699–709.
157. Murakami K, Okajima K, Uchiba M, et al: Activated protein C prevents LPS-induced pulmonary vascular injury by inhibiting cytokine production. Am J Physiol 1997;272:L197–L202.
158. Enkhbaatar P, Okajima K, Murakami K, et al: Recombinant tissue factor pathway inhibitor reduces lipopolysaccharide induced pulmonary vascular injury by inhibiting leukocyte activation. Am J Respir Crit Care Med 2000;162:1752–1759.
159. Abubakar K, Schmidt B, Monkman S, et al: Heparin improves gas exchange during experimental acute lung injury in newborn piglets. Am J Respir Crit Care Med 1998;158:1620–1625.
160. Uchiba M, Okajima K, Murakami K: Effects of various doses of antithrombin III and endotoxin-induced endothelial cell injury and coagulation abnormalities in rats. Thromb Res 1998;89:233–241.
161. Uchiba M, Okajima K, Murakami K, et al: rhs-Tm prevents ET-induced increase in pulmonary vascular permeability through protein C activation. Am J Physiol 1997;273:L889–L894.
162. Abraham E, Reinhart K, Svoboda P, et al: Assessment of the safety of recombinant tissue factor pathway inhibitor in patients with severe sepsis. A multicenter, randomized, placebo-controlled, single-blind, dose escalation study. Crit Care Med 2001;29:2081–2089.
163. Abraham E, Reinhart K, Demeyer I, et al: Efficacy and safety of Tifacogin (recombinant tissue factor pathway inhibitor) in severe sepsis. A randomized controlled trial. JAMA 2003;290:238–247.
164. Wolff HRD, Seegert HW: Experimental and clinical results in shock lung treatment with vitamin E. Ann NY Acad Sci 1982;393:392–409.
165. Bone RC, Slotman GJ, Maunder RJ, et al: Randomized double-blind multi-centre study of prostaglandin E1 in patients with the adult respiratory distress syndrome. Chest 1989;96:114–119.
166. Bernard GR, Wheeler AP, Russell JA, et al: The effects of ibuprofen on the physiology and survival of patients with sepsis. N Engl J Med 1997;336: 912–918.
167. Yu M, Tomasa G: A double-blind, prospective, randomized trial of ketoconazole, a thromboxane synthetase inhibitor, in the prophylaxis of the adult respiratory distress syndrome. Crit Care Med 1993;21:1634–1642.
168. Tariq M, Moutaery AA, Arshaduddin M, et al: Fluconazole attenuates lung injury and mortality in a rat peritonitis model. Intensive Care Med 2003;29:2043–2049.
169. Bernard GR, Wheeler AP, Arons MM, et al: A trial of antioxidants N-acetyl cysteine and procysteine in ARDS. Chest 1997;112:164–172.
170. Gadek JE, DeMichele SJ, Karlstad MD, et al: Effect of enteral feeding with eicosapentaenoic acid, gamma-linolenic acid, and antioxidants in patients with acute respiratory distress syndrome. Crit Care Med 1999;27: 1646–1648.
171. Keenan HT, Bratton SL, Martin LD, et al: Outcome of children who require mechanical ventilatory support after bone marrow transplantation. Crit Care Med 2000;28:830–835.
172. Rivera RA, Butt W, Shann F: Predictors of mortality in children with respiratory failure. Possible indications for ECMO. Anaesth Intensive Care 1990;18:385–389.
173. Timmons OD, Dean MJ, Vernon DD: Mortality rates and prognostic variables in children with adult respiratory distress syndrome. J Pediatr 1991;119:896–899.
174. Lyrene RK, Truog WE: Adult respiratory distress syndrome in a pediatric intensive care unit. Predisposing conditions, clinical course, and outcome. Pediatrics 1981;67:790–795.
175. Effman EL, Merton DF, Kirks DR, et al: Adult respiratory distress syndrome in children. Radiology 1985;157:69–74.
176. Zobel G, Kuttnig M, Trop M: A respiratory severity index (RSI) for children with ARDS. Crit Care Med 1989;17(Suppl):110.
177. Abel SJC, Finney SJ, Brett SJ, et al: Reduced mortality in association with the acute respiratory distress syndrome (ARDS). Thorax 1998;53: 292–294.

178. Jardin F, Fellahi JL, Beauchet A, et al: Improved prognosis of acute respiratory distress syndrome 15 years on. Intensive Care Med 1999;25: 936–941.
179. Nussbaum E: Adult-type respiratory distress syndrome in children. Clin Pediatr 1983;22:401–406.
180. Möller JC, Raszynski A, Vardag A, et al: The usefulness of mortality predicting indices in paediatric ARDS. Eur Respir J 1991;4(Suppl):205.
181. Timmons OD, Havens PL, Fackler JC: Predicting death in pediatric patients with acute respiratory failure. Chest 1995;108:789–797.
182. DeBruin W, Notterman DA, Magid M, et al: Acute hypoxemic respiratory failure in infants and children. Clinical and pathologic characteristics. Crit Care Med 1992;20:1223–1234.
183. Krafft P, Fridrich P, Pernerstorfer T, et al: The acute respiratory distress syndrome. Definitions, severity and clinical outcome. An analysis of 101 investigations. Intensive Care Med 1996;22:519–529.
184. Bartlett RH, Morris AH, Fairley HB, et al: A prospective study of acute hypoxic respiratory failure. Chest 1986;89:684–689.
185. Tamburro RF, Bugnitz MC, Stidham GL: Alveolar-arterial oxygen gradient as a predictor of outcome in patients with non-neonatal paediatric respiratory failure. J Pediatr 1991;119:935–938.
186. Sarnaik AP, Meert KL, Pappas MD, et al: Predicting outcome in children with severe acute respiratory failure treated with high frequency ventilation. Crit Care Med 1996;24:1396–1402.
187. Paret G, Ziv T, Barzilai A, et al: Ventilation index and outcome in children with acute respiratory distress syndrome. Pediatr Pulmonol 1998;26: 125–128.
188. Proulx F, Gauthier M, Nadeau D, et al: Timing and predictors of death in pediatric patients with multiple organ system failure. Crit Care Med 1994;22:1025–1031.
189. Leteurtre S, Martinot A, Duhamel A, et al: Validation of the paediatric logistic organ dysfunction (PELOD) score. Prospective, observational, multicentre study. Lancet 2003;362:192–197.
190. Donnelly SC, Haslett C, Dransfield I, et al: Role of selectins in development of adult respiratory distress syndrome. Lancet 1994;344: 215–219.
191. Carvalho AC, Bellman SM, Saullo VJ, et al: Altered factor VIII in acute respiratory failure. N Engl J Med 1982;307:1113–1119.
192. Rubin DB, Weiner-Kronish JP, Murray JF, et al: Elevated von Willebrand factor antigen is an early plasma predictor of acute lung injury in nonpulmonary sepsis syndrome. J Clin Invest 1990;86:474–480.
193. Moss M, Ackerson L, Gillespie MK, et al: Von Willebrand factor antigen levels are not predictive for the adult respiratory distress syndrome. Am J Respir Crit Care Med 1995;151:15–20.
194. Sharkey RA, Donnelly SC, Connelly KG, et al: Initial serum ferritin levels in patients with multiple trauma and the subsequent development of acute respiratory distress syndrome. Am J Respir Crit Care Med 1999;159:1506–1509.
195. Chesnutt AN, Matthay MA, Clark JG: Type III procollagen peptide is present in pulmonary edema fluid on day one in patients with acute respiratory distress syndrome. Am J Respir Crit Care Med 1996;153:A11.
196. Hyers TM, Tricomi SM, Dettenmeier PA, Fowler AA: Tumour necrosis factor levels in serum and bronchoalveolar lavage fluid of patients with the adult respiratory distress syndrome. Am Rev Respir Dis 1991;144: 268–271.
197. Greene KE, Wright JR, Wong WB, et al: Serial SP-A levels in BAL and serum of patients with ARDS. Am J Respir Crit Care Med 1996; 153:A587.
198. Greene KE, Wright JR, Steinberg KP, et al: Serial changes in surfactant-associated proteins in lung and serum before and after the onset of ARDS. Am J Respir Crit Care Med 1999;160:1843–1850.
199. Doyle IR, Bersten AD, Nicholas TE: Surfactant proteins-A and -B are elevated in plasma of patients with acute respiratory failure. Am J Respir Crit Care Med 1997;156:1217–1229.

45 Lung Injury from Hydrocarbon Aspiration and Smoke Inhalation

Ada S. Lee, MD • Michael R. Bye, MD • Robert B. Mellins, MD

LUNG INJURY FROM HYDROCARBON ASPIRATION

Hydrocarbon toxicity resulting from the ingestion of petroleum solvents, dry-cleaning fluids, lighter fluids, kerosene, gasoline, and liquid polishes and waxes (mineral seal oil) continues to be a common occurrence in small children. In 1998, over 730,000 nonpharmaceutical exposures in children younger than 6 years were reported; of these, approximately 26,000 involved hydrocarbons and over 126,000 involved household cleaning products.[1] Kerosene heaters, cleaning fluids, furniture polishes, and liquid floor waxes in the home too frequently within the easy reach of toddlers help account for the persistence of hydrocarbon poisoning. In one series of hydrocarbon ingestions, the material was stored in a standard beverage container almost one third of the time.[2] The most commonly ingested materials are household cleaning products, solvents, and fuels; in some areas kerosene ingestion is once again common. Of 184 cases of hydrocarbon ingestion in Texas, 71% were under 2 years of age, with one death.[3] A lack of delayed-onset symptoms differs from other data.[4,5] In 1998, approximately 75% of the hydrocarbon exposures in children involved gasoline, kerosene, lighter fluid/naphtha, and mineral spirits/varsol. Of these, gasoline was most commonly involved; kerosene exposure resulted in the highest morbidity and two deaths occurred with lighter fluid/naphtha exposure.[6]

Although central nervous system (CNS) abnormalities (weakness, confusion, and coma), gastrointestinal irritation, cardiomyopathy, and renal toxicity all occur, the most common as well as the most serious complication is pneumonitis. Deaths from hydrocarbon poisoning are almost always from pneumonitis.

PATHOLOGY

Lung pathology in fatal cases includes necrosis of bronchial, bronchiolar, and alveolar tissue; atelectasis; interstitial inflammation; hemorrhagic pulmonary edema; vascular thromboses; necrotizing bronchopneumonia; and hyaline membrane formation.[7]

Experimental studies in rats reveal an acute alveolitis that is most severe at 3 days, subsides at 10 days, and is followed by a chronic proliferative phase that may take weeks to resolve.[8] Rats develop hyperemia and vascular engorgement of both large and small blood vessels within 1 hour of aspiration.[9] At 24 hours there is a focal bronchopneumonia with microabscess formation. By 2 weeks the process largely resolves, although some vascular engorgement and rare peribronchial inflammation persist. The observation in humans that the chest roentgenographic abnormalities persist for some time after the physical findings have cleared suggest a similar prolonged recovery.

Dogs show different responses,[10] which vary with the amount of kerosene ingested. A low dose causes destruction of alveolar cell linings and cells, resulting in emphysema but insignificant airway involvement. More intense airway obstruction is seen in a high-dose group. At 1 hour after high-dose ingestion, intraalveolar edema and hemorrhage occur most prominently in the subpleural air spaces and those adjacent to large bronchi, suggesting induced interstitial inflammation. By 24 hours after ingestion, many airways show severe destruction and desquamation of the lining epithelium, resulting in near complete obliteration of the airways. The lumina are filled with degenerating neutrophils and scattered macrophages and lymphocytes. The surrounding lung parenchyma and the interstitium of the blood vessels show intense infiltration by macrophages and neutrophils, with microabscesses in the lung parenchyma. While most of the findings resolve by 1 week, scattered bronchiolitis obliterans may still be seen. By 2 weeks, the lungs are almost normal, with rare areas of bronchiolitis obliterans. The severity of these dose-related changes can be explained by two characteristics of kerosene. First, it is a solvent that can dissolve the cell walls and/or the lipid linings of the lining layer resulting in the desquamation of cells and fluid into the airways. Second, acting as a foreign substance with access to the interstitium via its dissolving power, it may provoke an intense inflammatory reaction. Since there are not only dose-related responses to kerosene but also interspecies differences, one cannot accurately predict the changes in humans.

PATHOPHYSIOLOGY

The risk for aspiration varies with some inherent properties of the hydrocarbon. Aspiration is much more likely to occur with a substance that has low surface tension, low viscosity, and high volatility. Low surface tension allows the substance to spread throughout the tracheobronchial tree. Low viscosity allows the substance to spread more readily, and to seep deeper into the tissues. High volatility increases the likelihood of CNS involvement, presumably due to more rapid absorption across the mucosa and into the bloodstream; highly volatile substances may also rapidly spread to the alveoli and immediately interfere with gas exchange.

Hydrocarbons increase surface tension by altering surfactant,[11] predisposing to alveolar instability and atelectasis. The instillation of artificial surfactant into the trachea of sheep following kerosene exposure resulted in significant improvement in oxygenation and mortality.[12] There are no published human studies using artificial surfactant for the treatment of hydrocarbon aspiration.

In the past, considerable controversy centered on whether the toxicity resulted from direct aspiration or gastrointestinal absorption with subsequent transport to the lungs. It is now clear that the pulmonary lesions are caused by direct aspiration of the hydrocarbon into the airways. This may occur either during the initial ingestion or during subsequent emesis. Evidence that hydrocarbons are removed by the first capillary bed they encounter[13,14] reinforces the notion that pulmonary damage occurs from aspiration. Indeed, the liver and the lungs filter out sufficient amounts of kerosene to protect the brain from damage.[13]

Fatalities are rarely attributed to CNS involvement per se. Small amounts of aspirated hydrocarbons may produce more serious disease than larger amounts in the stomach.

CLINICAL FINDINGS

Intercostal retractions, grunting, cough, and fever may appear within 30 minutes of aspiration or may be delayed for hours. Initially, auscultation of the chest may reveal only coarse or decreased sounds. When severe injury occurs, hemoptysis and pulmonary edema develop rapidly and respiratory failure may occur within 24 hours. Radiographic signs of chemical pneumonitis, when present, will develop within 2 hours after ingestion in 88% of cases and within 6 to 12 hours in 98%.[15,16] The findings vary from punctate, mottled densities to pneumonitis and/or atelectasis and tend to predominate in dependent portions of the lung (Fig. 45-1*A*). Air trapping with overdistention of the lungs, pneumatoceles,[17] and pleural effusions may also develop (see Fig. 45-1*B*). The radiographic abnormalities reach their peak within 72 hours and then usually clear within days. A review of 16 children found that children whose chest radiographs were to become abnormal did so by 24 hours after the ingestion, and most cleared within 2 to 3 weeks.[5] Occasionally, the radiographic findings persist for several weeks. There is a poor correlation between clinical symptoms, physical findings, and radiographic abnormalities. In general, the radiographic changes are more prominent than the findings on physical examination and persist for a longer period. Pneumatoceles, when they occur, are likely to do so after a patient has become asymptomatic. They require several months for spontaneous resolution.

Blood gas studies reveal hypoxemia without hypercapnia, suggesting ventilation-perfusion mismatch or diffusion block. Destruction of the epithelium of the airways together with bronchospasm caused by surface irritation adds to the ventilation-perfusion abnormalities.

Long-term follow-up studies of pulmonary function in patients with hydrocarbon pneumonitis indicate residual injury to the peripheral airways. A study of 17 asymptomatic children 8 to 14 years after a hydrocarbon pneumonitis showed abnormal lung function in 14 (82%). The most common abnormalities were an elevated ratio of residual volume to total lung capacity, an increased slope of phase III, reduced forced expiratory volume in 1 second (FEV_1) and a high volume of isoflow[18]; these results indicate small airway obstruction and gas trapping. When radiographic changes accompany the ingestion of hydrocarbons, abnormal lung function is detected 10 years later in otherwise asymptomatic subjects; these included an elevated volume of isoflow and a low maximal expiratory flow at 50% vital capacity ($Vmax_{50}$), again indicative of airway obstruction. However, the frequency of airway reactivity appeared to be normal.[19]

MANAGEMENT

Initial management should comprise a history, physical examination, and chest radiograph. Because hydrocarbons do less damage when swallowed than when aspirated into the lungs, it is important to avoid emetics or gastric lavage. If the child had no symptoms at the scene or in the emergency room and has a normal chest radiograph, observation for 6 to 8 hours is important. If no symptoms develop, the child may be safely discharged home.[16] If an abnormality is detected by history, examination, or radiography, arterial blood gas analysis should be performed. Even if no symptoms develop, a repeat chest radiograph at 24 hours is a reasonable and prudent measure. If results of examination and radiography are normal at 24 hours and the child has no further symptoms, it is reasonable to discharge the child after providing education and reassurance.

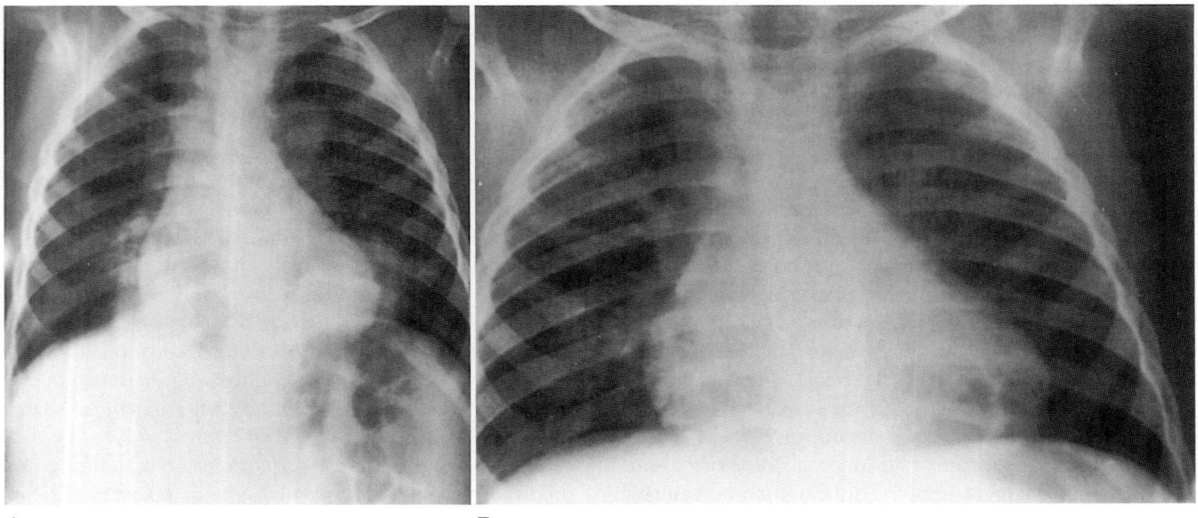

FIGURE 45-1. Hydrocarbon pneumonia. **A,** Confluent sequential infiltrate is present in the left lower lobe. **B,** Three weeks later, pneumatoceles are apparent; the large pneumatocele in the left lower lobe is at the site of the previous infiltrate. (From Felman AH: Radiology of the Pediatric Chest. New York: McGraw-Hill, 1987.)

Supplemental oxygen must be given if the child is hypoxemic. Adequate hydration should be maintained, but excessive fluid administration may be counterproductive as pulmonary pathology evolves. Hypoxemic respiratory failure should be treated with mechanical ventilation and positive end-expiratory pressure. If the child fails conventional mechanical ventilation, both extracorporeal membrane oxygenation (ECMO)[20] and high-frequency jet ventilation[21] have been successful in improving oxygenation and allowing survival.

Although superimposed bacterial infection is always of concern, there is no evidence that this is a common occurrence. Because leukocytosis and fever are common after hydrocarbon aspiration, it is often difficult to decide whether bacterial superinfection has occurred. One thoughtful review concluded that bacterial complications are rare.[22] Until there is further evidence on this subject, antimicrobial therapy should be reserved for patients who are severely compromised by malnutrition, debilitation, or underlying disease or in whom the pneumonia is especially severe. Nor should focusing on the possibility of infection obscure or delay initiation of other forms of therapy when pulmonary disease is severe. Because airway closure and collapse are a significant part of the disease, some form of continuous distending airway pressure seems desirable, especially to attempt to keep the concentration of inspired oxygen low, while maintaining an acceptable partial pressure of oxygen in arterial blood (PaO_2). Bronchodilators should be used to relieve bronchospasm. Studies in animals and humans fail to demonstrate either a therapeutic or prophylactic role for corticosteroids.[23–25]

Prevention of the accidental ingestion of products containing hydrocarbons is a high priority. Education of parents to keep potentially toxic materials out of the reach of young children seems obvious. Education about storage of such materials and avoiding containers that children associate with potable liquids must be stressed. If kerosene heaters are used in the home, the kerosene must be out of the reach of children.

HYDROCARBON “SNIFFING”

Deliberate inhalation of volatile hydrocarbons to induce a state of euphoria is common among adolescents. The euphoria of mild intoxication may be accompanied by mild nausea and vomiting. Prolonged exposure may lead to violent excitement followed by CNS depression, unconsciousness, and coma. Large doses of halogenated hydrocarbons, especially when combined with exertion, excitement, and hypercapnia, may be associated with dysrhythmias and death. Medullary depression and respiratory paralysis are generally accepted as the mechanism of death in most gasoline inhalation fatalities. Strong psychological dependence may develop in some sniffers. Lung injury per se from hydrocarbon sniffing has not been described. A toluene embryopathy has been described in infants born to mothers who sniffed toluene,[26] although the “polypharmacy” often used by the mothers may obscure some of the data.[27]

RESPIRATORY COMPLICATIONS OF SMOKE INHALATION

In the United States in 2001, the mortality rate from smoke inhalation was 1.42 per 100,000 in the age range 0 to 4 years; the mortality rate was 3.07 per 100,000 in the same age in African American subjects.[28] A great deal of the morbidity and mortality in victims of fires results from pulmonary injuries due to smoke inhalation.[29] The severity of the lung injury depends on (1) the nature of the material involved in the conflagration and the products of incomplete combustion that are generated and (2) whether the victim has been confined in a closed space. The subject’s minute ventilation also plays a role. The deeper and more rapidly the victim breathes, the greater the amount and degree of deposition of toxic materials into the airways and alveoli. Thus, there may be a teleologic explanation for the initial vagal-mediated bradypnea within two or three breaths in rats exposed to wood smoke.[30]

PATHOGENESIS

The pathogenesis of lung injury from smoke inhalation includes thermal and chemical factors. Because the upper air passage is such an effective heat exchanger, most of the heat from inhaled smoke is dissipated by the time the inhaled material reaches the carina. Direct thermal damage, then, primarily affects the supraglottic airways. Only with steam, which is very unusual in most fires, or with prolonged exposure to high ambient temperatures, will there be thermal injury to the intrathoracic airways.

Depending on the material involved in fires, a wide variety of noxious gases may be generated. These include the oxides of sulfur and nitrogen, acetaldehydes, hydrocyanic acid, and carbon monoxide (CO). Irritant gases such as nitrous oxide or sulfur dioxide may combine with lung water to form corrosive acids. Aldehydes from the combustion of furniture and cotton materials induce denaturation of protein, cellular damage, and pulmonary edema. The combustion of wood generates considerable quantities of CO and carbon dioxide. Plastics, if heated to sufficiently high temperatures, may be the source of very toxic vapors. Thus, chlorine and hydrochloric acid may be generated from polyvinyl chloride; hydrocarbons, aldehydes, ketones, and acids from polyethylene; and isocyanate and hydrogen cyanide from polyurethane.[31] Although the particulate matter carried in the smoke (soot) probably does not of itself produce injury, toxic gases may be absorbed on the surface of the particles and carried into the lungs; the soot particles may also be responsible for inducing reflex bronchoconstriction.

CARBON MONOXIDE POISONING

CO poisoning is an especially serious complication of smoke inhalation that occurs soon after exposure. The toxicity results from the combination of CO with hemoglobin to form carboxyhemoglobin (COHb), leading to severely impaired tissue oxygenation. It acts as a chemical asphyxiant by displacing oxygen from hemoglobin, thereby directly interfering with the delivery and utilization of oxygen. CO not only has a higher affinity for hemoglobin than oxygen but also shifts the oxyhemoglobin dissociation curve to the left.[32] For this reason, the toxicity of CO poisoning is greater at high altitude and in the presence of anemia. It is important to emphasize that although the oxygen content of the arterial blood is low in CO poisoning, the PaO_2 is not reduced. Because the carotid body responds to PaO_2, ventilation may not be stimulated until acidosis develops. This, together with the fact that COHb is bright red, makes the clinical diagnosis very difficult. The bright red color of the blood also makes the currently available oximeters unreliable. The reduction in hemoglobin available to oxygen in CO poisoning is much more serious than an equivalent anemia because there is a left shift as well as a change in the shape of the oxygen dissociation curve, which decreases oxygen delivery to the tissues. CO also binds to myoglobin, resulting in anoxia of muscle cells. With prolonged exposure, CO binds to cytochrome oxidase, impairing mitochondrial function and reducing production of adenosine triphosphate.

PATHOLOGY

Various pathologic lesions are described after smoke inhalation. Part of the variability in pathology may be attributed to differences in the toxic products generated in fires. However, many of the changes may not result simply from the direct chemical injury to the respiratory tract. Rather, they may reflect secondary circulatory, metabolic, or infectious complications of surface burns or may be induced by the administration of oxygen, the use of a mechanical ventilator, and the administration of excessive volumes of intravenous fluids.

The use of animal models to study the pathologic process was of limited value in older studies because steam rather than pure smoke was usually used, and the modifying effects of the upper air passages were eliminated by the use of tracheal cannulas. Recent experimental evaluation of the pathologic and pathophysiologic response to smoke exposure has been carried out in anesthetized and intubated sheep, kept light enough to breathe spontaneously. Smoke was generated by burning material such as dyed cotton toweling. The smoke was then insufflated into the lungs. In sheep a volume of 20 cc/kg for 12 breaths and an inspiratory time of 3 to 4 seconds produced physiologic effects similar to natural smoke inhalation, including mean COHb levels of 45%.[33]

This method shows that the initial pathologic changes are of a tracheobronchitis. The greater the tidal volume of the insufflated smoke, the more intense the tracheobronchitis. With sufficient smoke quantity, denudation of intact ciliated cells of the trachea occurred, most likely from disruption of the cell-cell and the cell–basal layer adhesions.[34] With much larger inspiratory challenges, an acute pulmonary edema due to increased pulmonary vascular permeability occurred within 30 minutes.[35] The next finding of atelectasis also correlated with the amount of smoke insufflated. Subsequent airway edema only occurred in those animals given large tidal volumes of smoke.[33] The degree of hypoxemia over the 24 hours studied did not correlate with the tidal breath size, but was constant for a given total smoke exposure. This suggests that the gas exchange deterioration was based more on the airway pathology than on the alveolar atelectasis or edema.

A group of infants carefully studied after exposure to smoke in a newborn nursery[36] were found to have necrosis of bronchial and bronchiolar epithelium with vascular engorgement and edema and with the formation of dense membranes or casts that partially obstructed the large and small airways. Bronchiolitis and bronchopneumonia were present in some, as were interstitial and alveolar edema. There was carbonaceous material in the alveoli, with alveolar hemorrhage.

Electron microscopic studies of 10 fatal cases of smoke inhalation following a hotel fire revealed interstitial and alveolar edema as well as engorgement of alveolar vessels.[37] Carbon particles were seen within alveolar macrophages. Type I pneumocytes showed greater injury than the pulmonary endothelial cells. Patients who died after severe surface burns have had necrotizing bronchitis and bronchiolitis with intra-alveolar hemorrhage and hyaline membrane formation and massive pulmonary edema. In these patients, it is difficult to know how much to attribute to direct pulmonary injury from smoke or to the complex metabolic, infectious, chest wall, and circulatory derangements that complicate surface burns. However, sheep exposed to surface burns plus smoke inhalation sufficient to raise the COHb levels to 25% to 30% fared much worse than those who received surface burns alone. The burn/inhalation group had greater amounts of lung lipid peroxidation products from bronchoalveolar lavage and lung lipid analysis at autopsy, even without evidence of pulmonary infection or the acute respiratory distress syndrome.[38]

PATHOPHYSIOLOGY

Severe damage to the upper air passages leads to stridor, with increased extrathoracic resistance. Bronchiolitis and alveolitis impair gas exchange, exaggerating the hypoxemia. Depending on the severity and distribution of the airway obstruction, there may be atelectasis or air trapping. The latter is especially likely with premature closure of small airways. Altered surfactant predisposes to atelectasis. Although reflex bronchoconstriction may contribute to the increase in airway resistance, it is difficult to assess the magnitude of its contribution because airway resistance is already high as a result of bronchial and bronchiolar edema and inflammation.

The toxic effects of smoke are primarily seen when animals are exposed to whole smoke. When the particle phase of the smoke was filtered out, there were neither acute nor delayed toxic effects on lung function or gas exchange.[39] Since many of the oxidants are in the gas phase as well in whole smoke, it is possible that only those toxins carried on the smoke particles remain in the airway long enough to elicit the abnormal response.

Pulmonary edema plays a prominent role in the pathophysiology of lung injury from smoke inhalation.[31] Studies in adults demonstrate increased extravascular lung water without a concomitant increase in pulmonary capillary wedge pressure. Studies in sheep reveal increased lung lymph flow and an increase in the lymph/plasma ratio of protein, suggesting increased permeability of the alveolar capillary membrane.[40] Increased bronchial circulation contributed to the pulmonary edema. Nitric oxide at extremely elevated levels acts as a free radical and potentiates the inflammatory response. Inhibition of inducible nitric oxide synthase reverses the loss of hypoxic pulmonary vasoconstriction and attenuates acute respiratory distress syndrome.[41,42]

In dogs, the addition of acrolein (an aldehyde generated from wood combustion) to pure smoke results in delayed-onset pulmonary edema. The edema was attenuated or eliminated by ligation of the ipsilateral bronchial artery, but not by ligation of the pulmonary artery. Pure smoke, and smoke with added hydrochloric acid, did not have the same effects.[43] The animal model showed increased pulmonary vascular resistance and decreased cardiac output concomitant with increased secretion of leukotrienes C4, D4, and E4. Pretreatment with a leukotriene antagonist markedly attenuated and delayed those cardiovascular changes.[44] Additional studies in sheep suggest that the acrolein-induced pulmonary edema and pulmonary hypertension are mediated by cyclo-oxygenase products, because pretreatment with cyclo-oxygenase inhibitors blocks the cardiorespiratory changes.[45] The acute pulmonary edema associated with very high-dose cotton smoke in sheep is blocked by a combined cyclo-oxygenase and leukotriene antagonist, but not by indomethacin, a cyclo-oxygenase inhibitor. Both agents block the elevated airway resistance and hypoxemia that occur presumably as a result of acute bronchoconstriction.[35] Acrolein is also a byproduct of prolonged cooking of vegetable oil. Prolonged exposure to acrolein in a kitchen resulted in severe respiratory distress in a previously healthy 27-month-old who developed bronchiectasis 18 months after the initial exposure.[46]

Oxidants directly from the products of combustion also contribute to airway damage, closure, and atelectasis.[47] Early therapy with aerosolized deferoxamine-pentastarch in sheep exposed to cotton smoke attenuated these findings.[48] It is not clear whether the deferoxamine was acting directly as an antioxidant or reducing the free iron released in the airway, which could have been causing local oxidant release.

Neutrophil-mediated proteolytic activity has been implicated in the airway pathology. Sheep treated intravenously with the synthetic protease inhibitor gabexate mesilate after insufflation with cotton smoke had a significant reduction in transvascular fluid and protein flux and were able to maintain better gas exchange than a vehicle-treated control group.[49] Impaired chemotactic and phagocytic function of the alveolar macrophage after smoke inhalation increases the risk for pulmonary infection several days after the acute event.

The cyanide that may be inhaled binds to the intracellular cytochrome system, inhibiting cell metabolism and the production of adenosine triphosphate. While all cells contain the enzyme rhodanese, which is capable of converting hydrocyanide to thiocyanate, this capability will be outstripped by continued or high levels of cyanide. The thiocyanate will be excreted in the urine, unless hypovolemia decreases renal blood flow and urine output.[50]

CLINICAL FINDINGS

The initial assessment of a victim of a fire should focus on CNS damage due to hypoxemia. Hypoxemia, whether the result of asphyxia or of CO poisoning, may produce irritability or depression. Oxygen should be administered while blood gas studies, including CO levels, are conducted. The clinical manifestations of CO poisoning vary with the level of COHb. Mild intoxication leads to headache, diminished visual acuity, irritability, and nausea. COHb levels in excess of 40% produce confusion, hallucination, ataxia, and coma. CO may increase cerebral blood flow, the permeability of cerebral capillaries, and the cerebrospinal fluid pressure. CO may have long-term effects on the CNS. Myocardial dysfunction and irritability can result directly from CO, as well as from hypoxemia.

Patients immediately assessed at the scene of a fire have elevated blood cyanide concentrations. The cyanide levels of victims who die as a result of the smoke inhalation are significantly higher than the levels of survivors. Blood cyanide levels correlate with CO levels, and plasma lactate levels were better correlated with cyanide levels than with CO level. A plasma lactate concentration above 10 mM in the emergency department is a sensitive indicator of cyanide poisoning.[51]

Maximum inspiratory and expiratory flow-volume curves and flexible fiberoptic nasopharyngoscopy or bronchoscopy have been helpful in the early assessment of the extent of supraglottic or tracheobronchial injury and the likelihood of subsequently developing airway obstruction.[52]

Although there may be some delay in the clinical evidence of respiratory tract injury resulting from smoke inhalation, manifestations of respiratory distress (including tachypnea, cough, hoarseness, and stridor) and auscultatory evidence of respiratory tract damage (including decreased breath sounds, wheezes, rhonchi, and rales) will usually develop within 12 to 24 hours. Absence of roentgenographic pulmonary disease is not very helpful in early diagnosis because abnormal findings may lag several hours or more behind auscultatory or physiologic evidence of damage.

Respiratory insufficiency may occur early in the course of smoke inhalation, not only as the result of asphyxia and CO poisoning, but also as the result of airway obstruction anywhere from the supraglottic airways to the alveoli. It may be difficult to localize the level of obstruction; therefore, whenever there is clinical evidence of severe obstruction, the upper airways should be assessed by direct laryngoscopy before swelling of the head, neck, or oropharynx and trismus make this examination difficult. Fiberoptic bronchoscopy may be very useful to evaluate the extent of mucosal damage, but intense vasoconstriction in hypovolemic patients may mask the findings.[53]

TREATMENT

As already indicated, the initial treatment should focus on reversing CO poisoning, if present, by the administration of high concentrations of humidified oxygen. CO levels may be reduced by half in about an hour when the patient breathes 100% oxygen. If severe CO poisoning is suspected, it is helpful to administer oxygen by nonrebreathing mask at flow rates higher than the victim's minute ventilation in order to achieve concentrations close to 100%. If results of clinical examination or arterial blood gas studies suggest alveolar hypoventilation, mechanical ventilation is necessary. Subsequently, the administration of oxygen may be important because of the hypoxemia resulting from bronchiolitis and alveolitis with premature closure of small airways. Constant positive distending airway pressure may also be necessary to maintain reasonable levels of PaO_2 without using excessively high and potentially toxic concentrations of inspired oxygen for prolonged periods of time.

Controversy exists regarding the importance of, and need for, hyperbaric oxygen in the management of CO poisoning. Hyperbaric oxygen at 2 to 3 atmospheres markedly hastens the decline of COHb levels, reducing the half-life of COHb to 20 to 25 minutes. However, the advantages of hyperbaric oxygen therapy may be offset by complications during transfer to the hyperbaric chamber. While some clinicians claim that all patients with significant COHb levels should be sent to a hyperbaric chamber, there is scant evidence for this approach.[50] One review suggests hyperbaric therapy for children with COHb levels of 25% or greater if symptomatic; and any with levels of 40% or higher.[54] The potential risks of the hyperbaric chamber include oxygen toxicity to the lung, the fact that patients are not amenable to appropriate observation and intervention while they are in the chamber, and the need for tympanotomy. More data are necessary to adequately assess the risks and benefits of hyperbaric oxygen in the therapy of CO poisoning in children related to fires.[55] The incidence of cognitive deficits at 6 weeks and 1 year following acute CO poisoning has been reported to be reduced in adults treated with hyperbaric oxygen therapy.[56] Its long-term benefits in children remain to be studied.

Intubation of the trachea may be necessary when there are (1) severe burns of the nose, face, or mouth, because of the likelihood that nasopharyngeal edema and obstruction will develop; (2) edema of the vocal cords with laryngeal obstruction; (3) difficulty handling secretions; (4) progressive respiratory insufficiency requiring mechanical assistance to ventilation; and (5) altered mental status that decreases minute ventilation and diminishes the protective reflexes of the airway. Regardless of whether the glottis is bypassed by endotracheal tube or tracheostomy tube, constant positive airway pressure or positive end-expiratory pressure helps minimize edema and improve oxygenation. Noninvasive positive pressure ventilation may be attempted in patients with acute respiratory decompensation who are otherwise hemodynamically stable, conscious, and without extensive and deep facial burns or trauma. This mode of ventilation has been reported to be effective in avoiding intubation/reintubation in a group of patients with burns with acute respiratory failure.[57]

In addition to the increased airway resistance resulting from edema in and around the walls of airways, it is likely that some reflex bronchoconstriction occurs from irritation of airway receptors. This is more likely to occur in subjects with preexisting lung disease such as asthma or cystic fibrosis, or in cigarette smokers. For this reason, it seems reasonable to administer inhaled bronchodilators.

As in many other conditions, the role of chest physiotherapy is poorly defined. Nevertheless, the encouragement of deep breathing and cough or gentle endotracheal suction in the presence of endotracheal intubation coupled with postural drainage would seem to be reasonable.

Although corticosteroids are frequently advocated in the hope of suppressing inflammation and edema, most controlled studies fail to demonstrate a significant effect. Thus, it is difficult to marshal strong support for their use. Furthermore, long-term steroid therapy in victims of fires increases the susceptibility to infection. Until further evidence is available, the empirical use of corticosteroids is discouraged. One review suggests using corticosteroids only for evidence of peripheral airway obstruction, other illnesses requiring steroids, or recent use of steroids.[54] At the experimental level, ibuprofen but not indomethacin when given immediately after smoke inhalation injury prevented the development of pulmonary edema.[58] As animal studies further elicit the basic mechanisms of the events occurring within the airways and the parenchyma, specific agents may become available to counteract the pathophysiology.

The available evidence indicates that antimicrobial agents do not prevent subsequent infection and may only predispose to infection with resistant organisms. Because fever, elevated white blood cell count, and increased erythrocyte sedimentation rate all may result from smoke inhalation, and because the chest roentgenogram may show nonspecific opacities that represent either atelectasis or edema, it may be extremely difficult to establish the presence of an infection in the absence of positive blood cultures or a positive Gram stain of airway secretions. It would seem preferable to reserve antimicrobial therapy for those patients in whom there is clinical deterioration despite supportive therapy. Changes in the amount, nature, or color of the secretions should raise the suspicion of a bacterial superinfection, confirmed by Gram stain and/or culture. Because the prevention of infection is clearly an important part of the therapy in victims of fires, aseptic care of the trachea and humidifying equipment is essential. In a retrospective analysis of children, high-frequency percussive ventilation was associated with a lower incidence of pneumonia.[59]

Nieman and colleagues[60] have shown that exogenous surfactant (Infasurf, Forest Pharmaceuticals, St. Louis, Missouri) administered immediately after wood smoke inhalation in dogs improved pulmonary function and gas exchange. To our knowledge, no such studies have been conducted in human subjects.

ECMO is used increasingly in infants and children with respiratory failure poorly responsive to conventional ventilation. Nonetheless, smoke-exposed sheep did worse with ECMO support than with conventional mechanical ventilation. The ECMO was associated with pulmonary sequestration of leukocytes, increased pulmonary thromboxane B_2, increased blood-free wet/dry lung weight ratios, and more significant hypoxemia at 24 hours after identical degrees of smoke exposure.[61] In spite of these shortcomings in animal studies, two children with inhalation injury and resultant respiratory failure refractory to conventional mechanical ventilation were successfully treated with ECMO.[62]

THE RELATION OF PULMONARY INJURY FROM SMOKE INHALATION TO THE PULMONARY COMPLICATIONS OF SURFACE BURNS

Pulmonary damage from smoke inhalation generally declares itself during the first 24 hours. Individuals with widespread surface burns may develop pulmonary complications after several days, but these late complications are not the result of direct chemical or thermal injury. It is more likely that late pulmonary injury is attributable to metabolic, infectious, or circulatory derangements complicating the surface burns.[52]

Surface burns may be directly and indirectly related to pulmonary pathophysiology. The large amounts of intravenous fluids usually given to counteract ongoing surface and "third-space" losses in the tissues may increase pulmonary disease through two mechanisms. First, there may be pulmonary vascular engorgement from diminished myocardial function due to CO poisoning, the initial hypoxia, and the other toxins involved in the fire. Second, the diffuse inflammation within the airways increases vascular permeability with fluid leak into the areas of gas exchange, worsening the hypoxemia and causing additional pulmonary edema. Careful monitoring of fluid balance is critical in these children.

A second indirect relationship between the surface burns and the lung is in the area of infection. Clearly, the postburn lung is at risk for pneumonia. Organisms may enter the body through the skin at the burn site. Scrupulous attention to the burn sites is necessary to reduce this possibility.

The skin surface and lung may be directly related with severe skin burns, especially if they are circumferential at the thorax and/or upper abdomen. Chest wall edema or eschar formation, in addition to the pain at the skin site, all increase the risk for hypoventilation and atelectasis.[63] Attention must be directed to the skin manifestations such as eschars, and to pain control. Pain control with narcotics may increase the risk for hypoventilation, but this can be easily monitored and adequate pain control is recommended for these children.

REFERENCES

1. American Association of Poison Control Centers. Available at http://www.aapcc.org/poison1.htm. Accessed July 1, 2004.
2. Truemper E, Reyes de la RS, Atkinson SD: Clinical characteristics, pathophysiology, and management of hydrocarbon ingestion. Case report and review of the literature. Pediatr Emerg Care 1987;3:187–193.

3. Machado B, Cross K, Snodgrass WR: Accidental hydrocarbon ingestion cases telephoned to a regional poison center. Ann Emerg Med 1988;17:804–807.
4. Victoria MS, Nangia BS: Hydrocarbon poisoning. A review. Pediatr Emerg Care 1987;3:184–186.
5. Cesaretti G, Di SG, Cioni C, Saggese G: Hydrocarbon poisoning in childhood. Minerva Pediatr 1991;43:583–585.
6. McGuigan ME: Poisoning potpourri. Pediatr Rev 2001;22:295–302.
7. Klein BL, Simon JE: Hydrocarbon poisonings. Pediatr Clin North Am 1986;33:411–419.
8. Gross P, McNerney JM, Babyak MA: Kerosene pneumonitis. An experimental study with small doses. Am Rev Respir Dis 1963;88:656–663.
9. Scharf SM, Heimer D, Goldstein J: Pathologic and physiologic effects of aspiration of hydrocarbons in the rat. Am Rev Respir Dis 1981;124:625–629.
10. Scharf SM, Prinsloo I: Pulmonary mechanics in dogs given different doses of kerosene intratracheally. Am Rev Respir Dis 1982;126:695–700.
11. Giammona ST: Effects of furniture polish on pulmonary surfactant. Am J Dis Child 1967;113:658–663.
12. Widner LR, Goodwin SR, Berman LS, Banner MJ, Freid EB, McKee TW: Artificial surfactant for therapy in hydrocarbon-induced lung injury in sheep. Crit Care Med 1996;24:1524–1529.
13. Bratton L, Haddow JE: Ingestion of charcoal lighter fluid. J Pediatr 1975; 87:633–636.
14. Wolfsdorf J, Paed D: Kerosene intoxication. An experimental approach to the etiology of the CNS manifestations in primates. J Pediatr 1976;88: 1037–1040.
15. Blattner RJ, Collins VP, Daeschner CW Jr: Hydrocarbon pneumonitis. Pediatr Clin North Am 1957;31:243–253.
16. Anas N, Namasonthi V, Ginsburg CM: Criteria for hospitalizing children who have ingested products containing hydrocarbons. JAMA 1981;246: 840–843.
17. Bergeson PS, Hales SW, Lustgarten MD, Lipow HW: Pneumatoceles following hydrocarbon ingestion. Report of three cases and review of the literature. Am J Dis Child 1975;129:49–54.
18. Gurwitz D, Kattan M, Levison H, Culham JA: Pulmonary function abnormalities in asymptomatic children after hydrocarbon pneumonitis. Pediatrics 1978;62:789–794.
19. Tal A, Aviram M, Bar-Ziv J, Scharf SM: Residual small airways lesions after kerosene pneumonitis in early childhood. Eur J Pediatr 1984;142: 117–120.
20. Scalzo AJ, Weber TR, Jaeger RW, Connors RH, Thompson MW: Extracorporeal membrane oxygenation for hydrocarbon aspiration. Am J Dis Child 1990;144:867–871.
21. Bysani GK, Rucoba RJ, Noah ZL: Treatment of hydrocarbon pneumonitis. High frequency jet ventilation as an alternative to extracorporeal membrane oxygenation. Chest 1994;106:300–303.
22. Eade NR, Taussig LM, Marks MI: Hydrocarbon pneumonitis. Pediatrics 1974;54:351–357.
23. Albert WC, Inkley SR: The efficacy of steroid therapy in the treatment of experimental kerosene pneumonitis. Am Rev Respir Dis 1968;98: 888–889.
24. Steele RW, Conklin RH, Mark HM: Corticosteroids and antibiotics for the treatment of fulminant hydrocarbon aspiration. JAMA 1972;219:1434–1437.
25. Marks MI, Chicoine L, Legere G, Hillman E: Adrenocorticosteroid treatment of hydrocarbon pneumonia in children—a cooperative study. J Pediatr 1972;81:366–369.
26. Arnold GL, Kirby RS, Langendoerfer S, Wilkins-Haug L: Toluene embryopathy. Clinical delineation and developmental follow-up. Pediatrics 1994;93:216–220.
27. Pearson MA, Hoyme HE, Seaver LH, Rimsza ME: Toluene embryopathy. Delineation of the phenotype and comparison with fetal alcohol syndrome. Pediatrics 1994;93:211–215.
28. Centers for Disease Control and Prevention, National Center for Injury Prevention and Control. Available at http://webappa.cdc.gov/cgi-bin/broker.exe. Accessed June 30, 2004.
29. Mellins RB: Respiratory complications of smoke inhalation in victims of fires. J Pediatr 1975;87:1–7.
30. Kou YR, Lai CJ: Reflex changes in breathing pattern evoked by inhalation of wood smoke in rats. J Appl Physiol 1994;76:2333–2341.
31. Witten ML, Quan SF, Sobonya RE, Lemen RJ: New developments in the pathogenesis of smoke inhalation-induced pulmonary edema. West J Med 1988;148:33–36.
32. Murray JF: Diffusion of gases, oxyhemoglobin equilibrium, and carbon dioxide equilibrium. In: The Normal Lung. Philadelphia: WB Saunders, 1986, pp 163–182.
33. Demling R, LaLonde C, Heron P, Picard L, Blanchard J, Brain J: Effect of increasing the tidal volume of smoke breaths on smoke-induced lung dysfunction. J Appl Physiol 1994;76:283–290.
34. Abdi S, Evans MJ, Cox RA, Lubbesmeyer H, Herndon DN, Traber DL: Inhalation injury to tracheal epithelium in an ovine model of cotton smoke exposure. Early phase (30 minutes). Am Rev Respir Dis 1990;142:1436–1439.
35. Hales CA, Musto S, Hutchison WG, Mahoney E: BW-755C diminishes smoke-induced pulmonary edema. J Appl Physiol 1995;78:64–69.
36. Cox ME, Heslop BF, Kempton JJ, Ratcliff RA: The Dellwood fire. BMJ 1955;4919:942–946.
37. Burns TR, Greenberg SD, Cartwright J, Jachimczyk JA: Smoke inhalation. An ultrastructural study of reaction to injury in the human alveolar wall. Environ Res 1986;41:447–457.
38. Demling RH, Knox J, Youn YK, LaLonde C: Oxygen consumption early postburn becomes oxygen delivery dependent with the addition of smoke inhalation injury. J Trauma 1992;32:593–598.
39. LaLonde C, Demling R, Brain J, Blanchard J: Smoke inhalation injury in sheep is caused by the particle phase, not the gas phase. J Appl Physiol 1994;77:15–22.
40. Traber DL, Herndon DN, Stein MD, Traber LD, Flynn JT, Niehaus GD: The pulmonary lesion of smoke inhalation in an ovine model. Circ Shock 1986;18:311–323.
41. Soejima K, Traber LD, Schmalstieg FC, Hawkins H, Jodoin JM, Szabo C, Szabo E, Varig L, Salzman A, Traber DL: Role of nitric oxide in vascular permeability after combined burns and smoke inhalation injury. Am J Respir Crit Care Med 2001;163:745–752.
42. Enkhbaatar P, Murakami K, Shimoda K, Mizutani A, Traber L, Phillips GB, Parkinson JF, Cox R, Hawkins H, Herndon D, Traber D: The inducible nitric oxide synthase inhibitor BBS-2 prevents acute lung injury in sheep after burn and smoke inhalation injury. Am J Respir Crit Care Med 2003;167:1021–1026.
43. Hales CA, Barkin P, Jung W, Quinn D, Lamborghini D, Burke J: Bronchial artery ligation modifies pulmonary edema after exposure to smoke with acrolein. J Appl Physiol 1989;67:1001–1006.
44. Quinn DA, Robinson D, Jung W, Hales CA: Role of sulfidopeptide leukotrienes in synthetic smoke inhalation injury in sheep. J Appl Physiol 1990;68:1962–1969.
45. Janssens SP, Musto SW, Hutchison WG, Spence C, Witten M, Jung W, Hales CA: Cyclooxygenase and lipoxygenase inhibition by BW-755C reduces acrolein smoke-induced acute lung injury. J Appl Physiol 1994;77:888–895.
46. Mahut B, Delacourt C, de Blic J, Mani TM, Scheinmann P: Bronchiectasis in a child after acrolein inhalation. Chest 1993;104:1286–1287.
47. Haponick E, Summer W: Respiratory complications in burned patients. Pathogenesis and spectrum of inhalation injury. J Crit Care 1987;2:49–54.
48. LaLonde C, Ikegami K, Demling R: Aerosolized deferoxamine prevents lung and systemic injury caused by smoke inhalation. J Appl Physiol 1994;77: 2057–2064.
49. Niehaus GD, Kimura R, Traber LD, Herndon DN, Flynn JT, Traber DL: Administration of a synthetic antiprotease reduces smoke-induced lung injury. J Appl Physiol 1990;69:694–699.
50. Demling RH: Smoke inhalation injury. New Horiz 1993;1:422–434.
51. Baud FJ, Barriot P, Toffis V, Riou B, Vicaut E, Lecarpentier Y, Bourdon R, Astier A, Bismuth C: Elevated blood cyanide concentrations in victims of smoke inhalation. N Engl J Med 1991;325:1761–1766.
52. Herndon DN, Langner F, Thompson P, Linares HA, Stein M, Traber DL: Pulmonary injury in burned patients. Surg Clin North Am 1987;67:31–46.
53. Shirani KZ, Moylan JA, Pruitt BA Jr: Diagnosis and treatment of inhalation injury in burn patients. In: Loke J, ed: Pathophysiology and Treatment of Inhalation Injuries. New York: Marcel Dekker, 1988, pp 239–348.
54. Ruddy RM: Smoke inhalation injury. Pediatr Clin North Am 1994;41: 317–336.
55. Liebelt EL: Hyperbaric oxygen therapy in childhood carbon monoxide poisoning. Curr Opin Pediatr 1999;11:259–264.
56. Weaver LK, Hopkins RO, Chan KJ, Churchill S, Elliott CG, Clemmer TP, Orme JF, Thomas FO, Morris, AH: Hyperbaric oxygen for acute carbon monoxide poisoning. N Engl J Med 2002;347:1057–1067.
57. Smailes ST: Noninvasive positive pressure ventilation in burns. Burns 2002;28:795–801.
58. Shinozawa Y, Hales C, Jung W, Burke J: Ibuprofen prevents synthetic smoke-induced pulmonary edema. Am Rev Respir Dis 1986;134: 1145–1148.
59. Cortiella J, Mlcak R, Herndon D: High frequency percussive ventilation in pediatric patients with inhalation injury. J Burn Care Rehabil 1999;20:232–235.

60. Nieman GF, Paskanik AM, Fluck RR, Clark WR: Comparison of exogenous surfactants in the treatment of wood smoke inhalation. Am J Respir Crit Care Med 1995;152:597–602.

61. Zwischenberger JB, Cox CS, Minifee PK, Traber DL, Traber LD, Flynn JT, Linares HA, Herndon DN: Pathophysiology of ovine smoke inhalation injury treated with extracorporeal membrane oxygenation. Chest 1993;103:1582–1586.

62. O'Toole G, Peek G, Jaffe W, Ward D, Henderson H, Firmin RK: Extracorporeal membrane oxygenation in the treatment of inhalation injuries. Burns 1998;24:562–565.

63. Quinby WC Jr: Restrictive effects of thoracic burns in children. J Trauma 1972;12:646–655.

46 Near-Drowning and Drowning

Andrew H. Numa, MBBS • Jürg Hammer, MD • Christopher J.L. Newth, MB

DEFINITIONS

Traditionally, the definition of drowning has been death within 24 hours of an immersion event, and near-drowning had been defined as any survival from such an event. A new uniform definition of drowning was agreed upon during the World Congress on Drowning in Amsterdam, The Netherlands, in 2002. Drowning is now defined as death by asphyxia due to submersion in a liquid medium, and near-drowning is defined as immediate survival after asphyxia due to submersion.

EPIDEMIOLOGY

Drowning occurs in all age groups and is responsible for approximately 4000 deaths per annum in the United States, with a mortality frequency of 12 to 18 deaths per million person-years.[1,2] The highest mortality rates of approximately 30 deaths per million person-years are observed in the 0- to 4-year and 15- to 19-year age groups.[1,2] In the first year of life, drowning mortality in the United States is 63 per 100,000 live births.[2] Worldwide, drowning is the 11th most frequent cause of death in the 0- to 4-year age group, the 3rd most frequent cause of death in children aged from 5 to 14 years,[3] and the 2nd leading cause of injury-related death in childhood.[4] The vast majority of drowning deaths occur in non-Western countries; in Bangladesh more children in the 1- to 4-year age group die from drowning than from diarrhea or respiratory infection.[5] Even in a well-developed country such as Australia, where drowning accounts for less than 1% of all reported deaths, there is a disproportionate rate of death in children. The rate of drowning is 4.6 per 100,000 per year for children under 5 years of age, three times the rate for adults.[1]

Near-drowning episodes are believed to occur around 3 to 10 times more frequently than drowning, worldwide.[6–10]

There is a strong male preponderance, with male-to-female incidence ratios ranging from 2:1 to 10:1, as with the majority of accidental deaths.[1,2,4,9] Children can and do drown in any receptacle containing water, from buckets to bathtubs to the ocean. The majority of drowning events occur in swimming pools (usually the child's home pool) for children aged under 4 years and in open water for older children.[1,8,11]

Drowning is most frequently a primary event. However, the presence of underlying disease such as epilepsy or cardiac arrhythmia should always be considered, along with the possibility of drug or alcohol intoxication in older children. Approximately 6% to 10% of drowning victims have a previous history of a seizure disorder,[1,12] and it has been estimated that children with epilepsy have a relative risk for drowning of 96 in the bathtub and 23.4 in a swimming pool compared with nonepileptic subjects.[12] A primary arrhythmia such as prolonged QT syndrome should always be considered, particularly in subjects who are capable swimmers.[13] Approximately 40% to 50% of adolescents who drown are intoxicated with drugs or alcohol.[11,14]

DROWNING SEQUENCE

According to studies in animals,[15] the sequence of events in drowning has been reported as: (1) immediate struggle, (2) suspension of movement with frequent swallowing, (3) violent struggle, (4) convulsions and spasmodic inspiratory efforts, and (5) death.

Some observers have reported human victims who stop moving suddenly after swimming under water, then float motionless on the surface of the water and subsequently quietly disappear.[6] The scenario of drowning without a struggle is probably due to a primary loss of consciousness secondary to other influences such as hypothermia[16] or cardiac arrhythmia.[8]

SEQUELAE OF SUBMERSION/IMMERSION EVENTS

Near-drowning has both pulmonary and nonpulmonary sequelae.

PULMONARY INJURY

The majority of drowning victims aspirate water (salt or fresh) at the time of drowning. However, in about 10% of cases, laryngospasm prevents the entry of water into the lungs.[9,17,18] The quantity of fluid aspirated is usually less than 22 mL/kg,[19] a volume that approximates the functional residual capacity. In cases wherein aspiration occurs, local insult arises secondary to infection, surfactant depletion, aspiration of debris, and fluid shifts that depend on the relative tonicity of body fluids and aspirated fluid. While radiologically evident pulmonary edema is the most common finding, the incidence and degree appears to be the same irrespective of saltwater or freshwater immersion. In addition to aspiration, pulmonary edema in submersion injuries has been ascribed to neurogenic causes, forced inspiration against a closed glottis, and altered surfactant or pulmonary capillary permeability.[20]

Sepsis may occur, sometimes with unusual and or atypical organisms,[21] and significant allergic reactions to aspirated materials have been described.[22] The incidence of pneumonia in adult patients requiring mechanical ventilation is around 50%, as deduced from a retrospective study in The Netherlands.[23]

Animal data suggest that 0.225% and 0.45% saline solutions are least injurious to the lungs in terms of gas exchange, possibly because they are rapidly absorbed from the alveolar spaces into the circulation along an osmotic gradient.[10] Fresh water will also be rapidly absorbed but causes rapid inactivation of surfactant and is probably the most injurious fluid to aspirate, followed closely by seawater, which is approximately 3% saline.[10,24–26] Hypertonic fluids will osmotically attract water into the lungs, further impairing gas exchange.[27,28] The presence of chlorine at 1 to 2 ppm in fresh water does not influence the pulmonary injury.[10]

Although it has been postulated that drowning in hypertonic fluid may lead to hypovolemia secondary to fluid shifts into the alveolar spaces, animal data indicate that hemodynamic changes following drowning are entirely attributable to hypoxia and are independent of the tonicity of the aspirated fluid.[10,26]

Pathologic findings are inconsistent and nonspecific. The most common finding in cases wherein the drowning medium has entered the lungs is the presence of reactive edema, with hyperinflation of the lungs and increase in lung weight (emphysema aquosum); however, these findings may also be seen in deaths from other causes including asphyxia and drug overdose.[29] Even where no water has been aspirated into the lungs, neurogenic pulmonary edema can occur.[30]

In severe cases of immersion/submersion accidents (with or without aspiration of fluid), some patients will develop pneumonia and acute respiratory distress syndrome. The management of this disorder is discussed elsewhere in this textbook (Chapter 44). However, in a database review of the 205 patients admitted to the intensive care unit at Children's Hospital Los Angeles over the past 17 years after near-drowning, only 21 (~10%) developed this serious complication. Figures 46-1 and 46-2 show the typical radiologic course of pulmonary injury in a near-drowning patient.

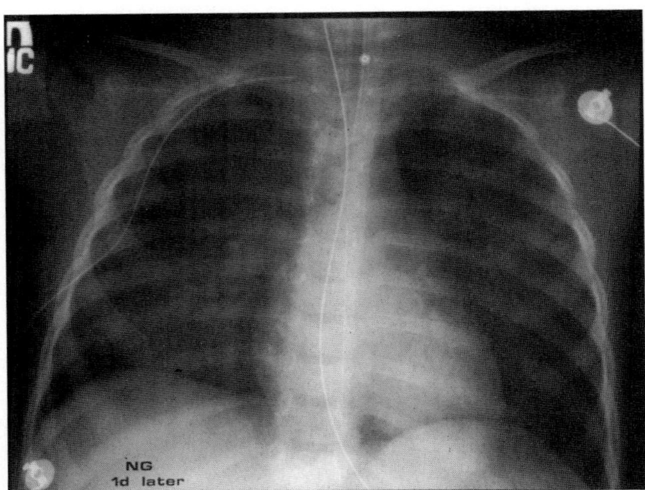

FIGURE 46-2. Chest radiograph of a near-drowning victim 1 week after the event. Patient is still intubated and has a nasogastric tube into the stomach. The lung fields are almost clear again, but there is a chest tube on the right side that has drained a pneumothorax subsequent to right-sided aspiration pneumonia.

NONPULMONARY SEQUELAE

Hypothermia

Hypothermia is a common manifestation of drowning in water of almost any temperature, and there is anecdotal evidence that rapid hypothermia in a submersion incident is neuroprotective, particularly in children. Conductive losses through the skin are compounded by rapid heat exchange across the pulmonary capillaries if a significant volume of water is inhaled. In a canine model, dogs breathing water at 4°C demonstrated a decrease in carotid artery blood temperature of 8°C within 5 minutes.[16] Cooling occurs most rapidly in small infants who have a relatively large surface area.[31] In cases of extreme hypothermia, rewarming will be essential to allow return of cardiac function.[32,33] Hypothermia can also play a major role in facilitating aspiration in immersion victims. As the core temperature drops below 35°C, muscular incoordination and weakness occur; these can interfere with swimming. As the core temperature decreases further, obtundation develops. At core temperatures below 30°C, unconsciousness can occur and the myocardium becomes irritable. Atrial fibrillation can occur, and at temperatures below 28°C, ventricular fibrillation is likely.

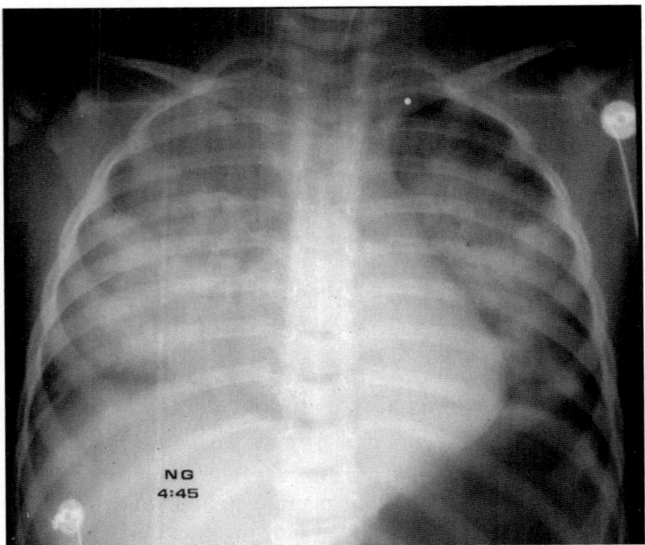

FIGURE 46-1. Initial chest radiograph of a near-drowning victim. The patient has an endotracheal tube in place and a right subclavian venous line going up into the internal jugular vein. Moderate pulmonary edema and some aspiration pneumonitis are seen, especially on the right.

Electrolyte Imbalances

Electrolyte imbalances may arise if a significant amount of nonisotonic water is aspirated, although this is unusual in regular seawater.[34] Although freshwater immersion victims have decreased serum sodium, and saltwater immersion victims have elevated serum sodium and chloride levels,[17] these are rarely substantial or clinically significant. Even in the Dead Sea, which has electrolyte concentrations approximately 10 times higher than seawater, immersion victims rarely have severe abnormalities of sodium or chloride, although hypercalcemia and hypermagnesemia are common.[35,36] Hemolysis due to aspiration of hypotonic or hypertonic fluids appears to be an extremely infrequent complication.

Trauma

Traumatic injuries resulting from a fall into water must be considered but are generally of lesser importance than the immersion itself. Cervical spine injuries are the most critical to consider but are uncommon, occurring in only 0.5% of all near-drowning cases, and only then in cases with a clear history of diving, motorized vehicle crash, or fall from a height.[37]

Hypoxic-Ischemic Damage

All organs are susceptible to hypoxic-ischemic injury following prolonged low cardiac output and inadequate oxygenation, and multiorgan failure is an almost inevitable consequence of severe submersion/immersion injury. Clinically, the brain is particularly susceptible, with the liver and the gastrointestinal tract being the most resistant.

■ MANAGEMENT

Management of the pulmonary injury will usually require supplemental oxygen, diuretic administration for pulmonary edema, and the most severe cases will require support with intubation and mechanical ventilation. In severe cases, the lung injury will comprise all the features of acute respiratory distress syndrome, and the management of this disorder is addressed elsewhere.

Instillation of surfactant has been reported[38,39] and is an appealing therapeutic intervention given that the majority of victims aspirate a quantity of fluid that will denature and wash out existing surfactant. However, the temptation to administer surfactant should be considered in the light of recent randomized controlled trials demonstrating a lack of efficacy of surfactant in acute respiratory distress syndrome.[40,41]

Broad-spectrum antibiotics should be administered to treat likely bacterial contamination of the lungs, such as after near-drowning in stagnant water.[42] The incidence of neurologic infection is stated to be high, with a number of case reports in children.[43]

Most drowning victims will be hypothermic at the time of presentation. In cases of extreme hypothermia, rewarming will be essential to allow return of cardiac function,[32,33] and if the core temperature is below 26°C to 28°C or the patient is in cardiac arrest, rewarming is probably best achieved using cardiopulmonary bypass.[44] Given the potential benefits of hypothermia on hypoxic central nervous system injury, it is our view that 24 to 48 hours of modest hypothermia (core temperature 32°C to 33°C) should be maintained immediately following the injury, regardless of the core temperature at presentation, if there is any suspicion of the patient having sustained a hypoxic brain injury. Several recent studies have highlighted the beneficial effects of hypothermia on a variety of hypoxic central nervous system injuries in humans, and there is a wealth of animal evidence to support these observations.[45,46] Excellent neurologic outcomes have been reported after prolonged immersion in very cold water, with several case reports indicating full neurologic recovery after periods of as long as 66 minutes in near-freezing water.[32,47,48] Children lose body heat more rapidly than adults, and if significant brain cooling occurs before cessation of circulation, then some degree of neuroprotection may occur. It has been estimated that brain temperature must fall by at least 3°C within the first 5 minutes of immersion if cerebral protection is to be effective.[31] However, a 1988 trial in Canada used hypothermia in near-drowned children to reduce intracranial pressure and limit brain injury.[49] The death rate in the hypothermic group was higher than in the normothermic group, with most deaths attributed to neutropenic sepsis. This complication may occur only in children.

Other management comprises support of multiorgan failure that is beyond the scope of a respiratory text.

■ OUTCOME OF PULMONARY INJURY

Routine tests of pulmonary function have been reported as normal in adults[50] following a near-drowning accident. However, in a series of 10 functionally normal children[51] studied 6 months to 8.5 years (mean, 3.3 years) after the submersion incident, only one had completely normal pulmonary function. Seven had abnormal methacholine challenges, demonstrating a high incidence of bronchial hyperreactivity, and five had clear evidence of peripheral airways disease. It is possible these children are at risk for developing chronic lung disease, especially if exposed to further airway or parenchymal irritants.

■ OUTCOME PREDICTION OF NEUROLOGIC INJURY

Biggart and Bohn[52] in Toronto conducted a retrospective review of 55 near-drowning victims (mean age, 4.75 years) admitted to the intensive care unit during a 5-year period, to determine the variables that may influence survival both before and after hospital admission. A total of 37 children survived and 18 died; 5 survivors had profound neurologic damage resulting in a persistent vegetative state, whereas the remaining 32 (58%) survived intact. The major variables that separated intact survivors from those who died and from survivors in a persistent vegetative state were the presence of a detectable heartbeat and hypothermia (less than 33°C) on initial examination in the emergency department.

In a subsequent review of 101 pediatric patients who had suffered an out-of-hospital respiratory or cardiac arrest over a 7.5-year span, Schindler and colleagues[53] confirmed these findings. Specifically, they noted that cardiac arrest as opposed to isolated respiratory arrest had a very poor prognosis, especially when efforts at resuscitation continued for more than 20 minutes and required more than two doses of epinephrine. They recorded nine patients with drowning, all of whom had cardiac arrest before reaching the emergency department and all of whom died.

Quan and co-workers[54] studied 77 children who nearly drowned or drowned in the Seattle area and concluded that advance life support resuscitation efforts that continued for longer than 25 minutes were associated with a bad neurologic outcome and were therefore not warranted.

At this point, the best outcome predictors are observed in the field. Good outcomes are associated with sinus rhythm, reactive pupils, and neurologic responsiveness at the scene.[55]

The prediction of the neurologic outcome of those children who survive the initial resuscitation event and arrive in the intensive care unit in a comatose state is highly relevant for parents and caregivers. It is difficult to provide early and accurate prognostic information on comatose children, especially if brain stem functions are intact. Severity of illness scores such as the Pediatric Index of Mortality (PIM2) and Pediatric Risk of Mortality (PRISM3) scores were developed to predict the risk of death in groups of patients, not individuals. However, PRISM has recently been applied to individuals, and it enables the prediction of either absence or presence of serious neurologic impairment or death in pediatric drowning patients, if they present at extreme values on this scale. However, in patients with intermediate PRISM scores, it is not possible to establish a reliable prognosis.[56] Electrophysiologic investigations, such as brainstem auditory evoked potentials and short-latency somatosensory evoked potentials

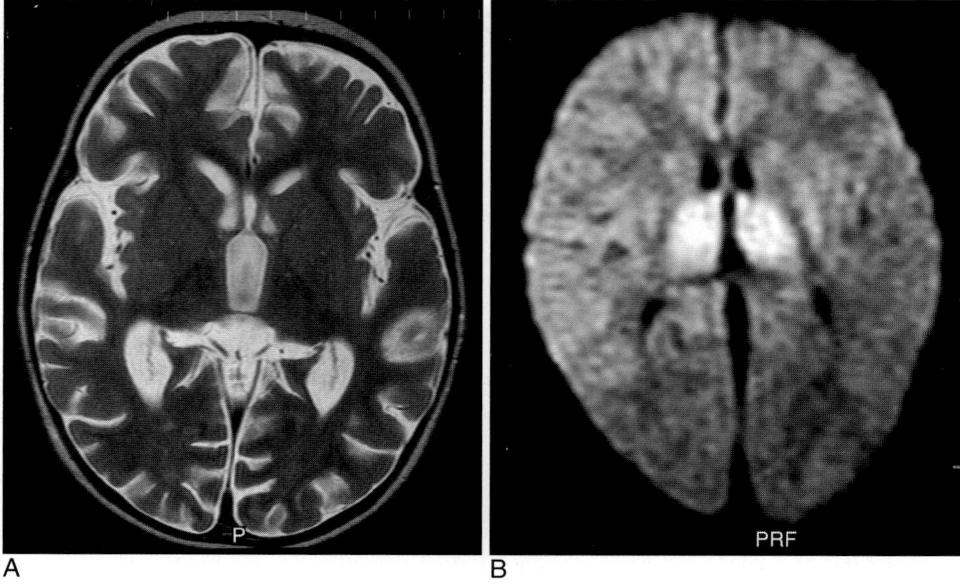

■ **FIGURE 46-3.** Magnetic resonance imaging (MRI) of the brain of a 3-year-old child 36 hours after a near-drowning accident. The child remained in a persistent vegetative state. **A,** The T2-weighted conventional MRI revealed no signs of hypoxia. **B,** Diffusion-weighted imaging shows hyperintensity bilaterally in the basal ganglia.

are helpful to assess the likelihood of a permanent vegetative state or a higher level of cognition. Until now, the bilateral absence of somatosensory evoked potentials is the only established predictor for a worse clinical outcome after cerebral hypoxia.[57,58] Today, diffusion-weighted magnetic resonance imaging (MRI) provides a quick and reliable tool to detect early tissue injury in acute cerebral ischemia, because it is sensitive to water shifts between the extra- and intracellular compartments that conventional MRI often cannot detect. Preliminary results suggest that the extent of diffusion-weighted MRI pathology may serve as a reliable predictor for neurologic outcome after cerebral hypoxia (Fig. 46-3).[59]

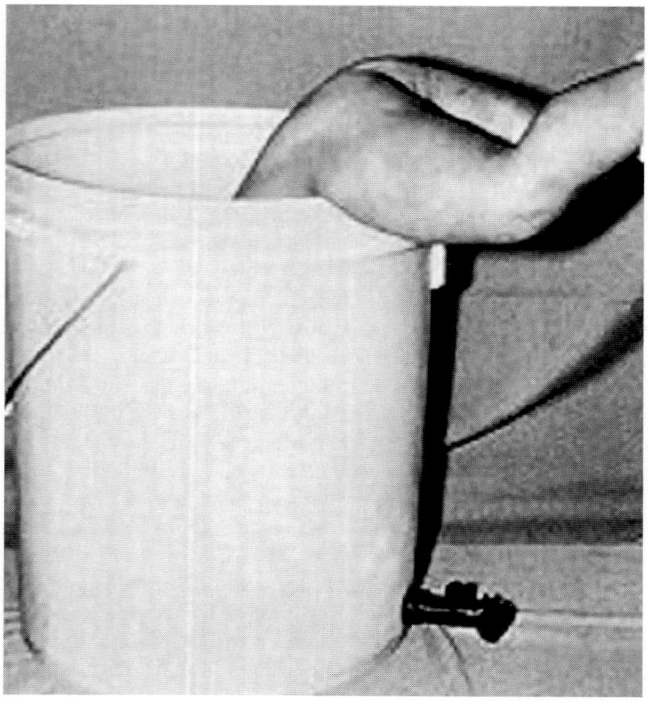

■ **FIGURE 46-4.** The body of a small child who had tipped head first into a bucket of water. The upper segment (torso and head) of a child are longer and heavier than the lower segment (unlike an older child or adult), and he could not extract himself. (From Moon RE, Long RJ: Drowning and near-drowning. Emergency Med 2002:14:378, Blackwell Publishing.)

■ PREVENTION

Drowning disproportionately affects children, and the majority of drownings are preventable. Drowning and near-drowning together create significant mortality and morbidity throughout the world, although modest decreases in the overall instances have been reported recently in the United States. Actions that appear to have reduced the number of those drowned each year are legislative and public health interventions, such as pool fencing, and public education campaigns that have improved awareness of the dangers of leaving children unattended in bathtubs and of large commercial-type buckets into which smaller children can fall but cannot extract themselves (Fig. 46-4). Improvements in postresuscitation care have thus far not been shown to alter outcome significantly if there has been an out-of-hospital cardiac arrest.

REFERENCES

1. Quan L, Cummings P: Characteristics of drowning by different age groups. Inj Prev 2003;9:163–168.
2. Kochanek KD, Murphy SL, Anderson RN, Scott C: Deaths. Final Data for 2002. Washington, DC: Centers for Disease Control and Prevention, October 12, 2004.
3. Krug EG: Injury surveillance is key to preventing injuries. Lancet 2004;364: 1563–1566.
4. O'Flaherty JE, Pirie PL: Prevention of pediatric drowning and near-drowning. A survey of members of the American Acadamy of Pediatrics. Pediatrics 1997;99:169–174.
5. Bierens JJ, Knape JT, Gelissen HP: Drowning. Curr Opin Crit Care 2002;8: 578–586.
6. Szpilman D: Near-Drowning and Drowning Classification. A proposal to stratify mortality based on the analysis of 1,831 cases. Chest 1997;112: 660–665.
7. Wintemute GJ: Childhood drowning and near-drowning in the United States. Am J Dis Child 1990;144:663–669.

8. Pearn JH, Wong RYK, Brown J, et al: Drowning and near-drowning involving children. A five-year total population study from the City and County of Honolulu. Am J Public Health 1979;69:450–454.
9. Levin DL, Morriss FC, Toro LO, et al: Drowning and near-drowning. Pediatr Clin North Am 1993;340:321–326.
10. Orlowski JP, Abulleil MM, Phillips JM: Effects of tonicities of saline solutions on pulmonary injury in drowning. Crit Care Med 1987;15:126–130.
11. Fields AI: Near drowning in the pediatric population. Crit Care Clin 1992;8:113–129.
12. Diekema DS, Quan L, Holt V: Epilepsy as a risk factor for submersion injury in children. Pediatrics 1993;91:612–616.
13. Ackerman MJ, Tester DJ, Porter CJ, Edwards WD: Molecular diagnosis of the inherited long-QT syndrome in a woman who died after near-drowning. N Engl J Med 1999;341:1121–1125.
14. Moon RE, Long RJ: Drowning and near-drowning. Emerg Med 2002;14: 377–386.
15. Karpovich PV: Water in the lungs of drowned animals. Arch Pathol Lab Med 1933;87:828–833.
16. Conn AW, Miyasaka K, Katayama M, et al: Canine study of cold water drowning in fresh versus salt water. Crit Care Med 1995;23:2029–2037.
17. Modell JH: Current concepts. Drowning. N Engl J Med 1993;328: 253–256.
18. DeNicola LK, Falk JL, Swanson ME, et al: Submersion injuries in children and adults. Crit Care Clin 1997;13:477–502.
19. Modell JH, Davis JH: Electrolyte changes in human drowning victims. Anesthesiology 1969;30:414–420.
20. Rumbak MJ: The etiology of pulmonary edema in fresh water near-drowning. Am J Emerg Med 1996;14:176–179.
21. Miyake M, Iga K, Izuma C, et al: Rapidly progressive pneumonia due to *Aeromonas hydrophila* shortly after near-drowning. Intern Med 2000;39: 1128–1130.
22. Mangge H, Plecko B, Grubbauer HM, et al: Late onset miliary pneumonitis after near drowning. Pediatr Pulmonol 1993;15:122–124.
23. van Berkel M, Bierens JJ, Lie RL, et al: Pulmonary oedema, pneumonia and mortality in submersion victims. A retrospective study in 125 patients. Intensive Care Med 1996;22:101–107.
24. Giammona ST, Modell JH: Drowning by total immersion. Effects on pulmonary surfactant of distilled water, isotonic saline, and sea water. Am J Dis Child 1967;114:612–616.
25. Scarpelli EM, Gabbay KH, Kochen JA: Lung surfactants, counter-ions, and hysteresis. Science 1965;148:1607–1609.
26. Kylstra JA: Drowning. The role of salts in the drowning fluid. Acta Physiol Pharmacol Neerl 1962;10:327–334.
27. Modell JH, Moya F, Newby EJ, et al: The effects of fluid volume in seawater drowning. Ann Intern Med 1967;67:68–80.
28. Orlowski JP, Abulleil MM, Phillips JM: The hemodynamic and cardiovascular effects of near-drowning in hypotonic, isotonic, or hypertonic solutions. Ann Emerg Med 1989;18:1044–1049.
29. Lunetta P, Penttilä A, Sajantila A: Circumstances and macropathologic findings in 1590 consecutive cases of bodies found in water. Am J Forensic Med Pathol 2002;23:371–376.
30. Rumbak MJ: The etiology of pulmonary edema in fresh water near-drowning. Am J Emerg Med 1996;14:176–179.
31. Xu X, Tikusis P, Giesbrecht G: A mathematical model for human brain cooling during cold water near drowning. J Appl Physiol 1999;86:265–272.
32. Antretter H, Dapunt OE, Mueller LC: Survival after prolonged hypothermia. N Engl J Med 1994;330:219.
33. Gilbert M, Busund R, Skagseth A, et al: Resuscitation from accidental hypothermia with circulatory arrest. Lancet 2000;355:375–376.
34. Ellis RJ: Severe hypernatremia from sea water ingestion during near-drowning in a hurricane. West J Med 1997;167:430–433.
35. Saidel-Odes LR, Almog Y: Near-drowning in the Dead Sea. A retrospective observational analysis of 69 patients. Isr Med Assoc J 2003;5:856–858.
36. Yagil Y, Stalnikowicz R, Michaeli J, Mogle P: Near-drowning in the Dead Sea. Electrolyte imbalances and therapeutic implications. Arch Intern Med 1985;145:50–53.
37. Watson RS: Cervical spine injuries among submersion victims. J Trauma 2001;51:658–662.
38. McBrien M, Katumba JJ, Mukhtar AI: Artificial surfactant in the treatment of near drowning. Lancet 1993;342:1485–1486.
39. Staudinger T, Bankier A, Strohmaier W, et al: Exogenous surfactant therapy in a patient with adult respiratory distress syndrome after near drowning. Resuscitation 1997;35:179–182.
40. Spragg RG, Lewis JF, Walmrath HD, et al: Effect of recombinant surfactant protein C–based surfactant on the acute respiratory distress syndrome. N Engl J Med 2004;351:884–892.
41. Anzueto A, Baughman RP, Kalpalatha K, et al: Aerosolised surfactant in adults with sepsis-induced acute respiratory distress syndrome. N Engl J Med 1996;224:1417–1421.
42. Ender PT, Dolan MJ: Pneumonia associated with near-drowning. Clin Infect Dis 1997;25:896–907.
43. Messori A, Lanza C, De Nicola M, et al: Mycotic aneurysms as lethal complication of brain pseudallescheriasis in a near-drowned child. A CT demonstration. Am J Neuroradiol 2002;23:1697–1699.
44. Walpoth BH, Walpoth-Aslan BN, Mattle HP, et al: Outcome of survivor of accidental deep hypothermia and circulatory arrest treated with extracorporeal blood warming. N Engl J Med 1997;337:1500–1505.
45. The Hypothermia after Cardiac Arrest Study Group: Mild therapeutic hypothermia to improve the neurologic outcome after cardiac arrest. N Engl J Med 2002;346:549–556.
46. Bernard SA, Gray TW, Buist MD, et al: Treatment of comatose survivors of out-of-hospital cardiac arrest with induced hypothermia. N Engl J Med 2002;346:557–563.
47. Perk L, Borger van de Burg F, et al: Full recovery after 45 min accidental submersion. Intensive Care Med 2002;28:524.
48. Bolte RG, Black PG, Bowers RS, et al: The use of extracorporeal rewarming in a child submerged for 66 minutes. JAMA 1988;260:377–379.
49. Bohn DJ, Biggar WD, Smith CR, et al: Influence of hypothermia, barbiturate therapy and intracranial pressure monitoring on morbidity and mortality after near drowning. Crit Care Med 1986;14:529–534.
50. Butt MP, Jalowayski A, Modell JH, Giammona ST: Pulmonary function after resuscitation from near-drowning. Anesthesiology 1970;32: 275–277.
51. Laughlin JJ, Eigen H: Pulmonary function abnormalities in survivors of near drowning. J Pediatr 1982;100:26–30.
52. Biggart MJ, Bohn DJ: Effect of hypothermia and cardiac arrest on outcome of near-drowning accidents in children. J Pediatr 1990;117: 179–183.
53. Schindler MB, Bohn D, Cox PN, et al: Outcome of out-of-hospital cardiac or respiratory arrest in children. N Engl J Med 1996;335:1473–1479.
54. Quan L, Kinder D: Pediatric submersions. Prehospital predictors of outcome. Pediatrics 1992;90:909–913.
55. Graf WD, Cummings P, Quan L, Brutocao D: Predicting outcome in pediatric submersion victims. Ann Emerg Med 1995;26:312–319.
56. Gonzalez-Luis G, Pons M, Cambra FJ, et al: Use of the Pediatric Risk of Mortality Score as predictor of death and serious neurologic damage in children after submersion. Pediatr Emerg Care 2001;17:405–409.
57. Young GB, Wang JT, Connolly JF: Prognostic determination in anoxic-ischemic and traumatic encephalopathies. J Clin Neurophysiol 2004;21: 379–390.
58. Zandbergen EGJ, de Haan RJ, Stoutenbeek CP, et al: Systematic review of early prediction of poor outcome in anoxic-ischemic coma. Lancet 1998;352:1808–1812.
59. Els T, Kassubek J, Kubalek R, Klisch J: Diffusion-weighted MRI during early global cerebral hypoxia. A predictor for clinical outcome? Acta Neurol Scand 2004;110:361–367.

47 Interstitial Lung Disease

Leland L. Fan, MD • Claire Langston, MD

The spectrum of interstitial lung disease (ILD) includes a large, heterogeneous group of mostly rare pulmonary conditions that cause derangements of the alveolar walls and loss of functional alveolar capillary units. Pediatric ILD (PILD) is uncommon and constitutes a small percentage of children seen by pediatric pulmonologists worldwide. The prevalence was estimated to be 0.36 per 100,000 in a recent study in the United Kingdom and Ireland.[1] It is difficult to define exactly which disorders should be included and which should be excluded within the spectrum of PILD. Therefore, it is probably better to think of PILD as a syndrome characterized by diffuse pulmonary infiltrates that result in tachypnea, crackles, and hypoxemia. Once the syndrome of PILD is recognized, a search for a more specific diagnosis should be undertaken.[2]

CLASSIFICATION

More than 100 different disorders of known and unknown etiology have been described within the spectrum of ILD in both adults and children. However, the distribution of diseases is different for children from what it is for adults, and there are conditions that are relatively unique to infants. Although no classification is entirely adequate, a classification for PILD of known and unknown etiologies and of conditions that are unique to infants is presented in Boxes 47-1 to 47-3.

PEDIATRIC INTERSTITIAL LUNG DISEASE OF KNOWN ETIOLOGY

Infection, either chronic or acute with long-term sequelae, accounts for many cases of ILD of known etiology. That acute adenovirus pneumonia can lead to permanent lung damage in the form of bronchiolitis obliterans has been well documented.[3] Chronic diffuse lung disease has also developed after influenza, *Mycoplasma*, and *Chlamydia* infections. In a prospective study of immunocompetent children with chronic diffuse infiltrates, an infectious agent was determined to be the underlying cause of ILD in 20% (10/51) of pediatric ILD cases.[4]

Aspiration from swallowing dysfunction and anatomic disorders such as tracheoesophageal fistula can cause chronic lung disease in children. While gastroesophageal reflux is frequently demonstrated in children with ILD and other chronic respiratory disorders, its role in the etiology of these disorders is often difficult to demonstrate. It may be caused by the lung disease and may exacerbate lung disease of other etiologies.

Hypersensitivity pneumonitis, an immunologic response to inhaled organic dusts, is a poorly recognized cause of PILD. In children, the most common cause is avian antigens, although some cases of pediatric hypersensitivity pneumonitis have been caused by mold exposure.[6] See Chapter 49 for more details on hypersensitivity pneumonitis.

Some patients have a known underlying systemic condition, such as immunodeficiency or malignancy, that predisposes to ILD. Diffuse infiltrates in a patient with malignancy may be the result of the primary malignancy, opportunistic infection, or therapeutic intervention, including chemotherapy and radiation injury.

PEDIATRIC INTERSTITIAL LUNG DISEASE OF UNKNOWN ETIOLOGY

In adults, the idiopathic pneumonias have recently been reclassified in an International Consensus Statement, based on the expert opinions of adult pulmonologists, radiologists, and pathologists.[7] This classification includes usual interstitial pneumonia (UIP), nonspecific interstitial pneumonia (NSIP), organizing pneumonia, acute interstitial pneumonia, respiratory bronchiolitis, desquamative interstitial pneumonia (DIP), and lymphoid interstitial pneumonia (LIP). With the exception of UIP (discussed later) and respiratory bronchiolitis, these entities are seen in children, although most are quite rare.

Usual Interstitial Pneumonia

The International Consensus Statement validates the concept that UIP is the pathologic pattern for patients with a clinical diagnosis of idiopathic pulmonary fibrosis or cryptogenic fibrosing alveolitis.[7] The key histologic features of UIP are architectural destruction, fibrosis often with honeycombing, scattered fibroblastic foci, patchy distribution, and involvement of the periphery of the acinus or lobule. Some authorities emphasize that the fibroblastic foci are the leading edge of the fibrotic process and their presence is essential to the diagnosis of UIP.[8]

To our knowledge, despite more than 100 reported cases of UIP (and its clinical equivalents, idiopathic pulmonary fibrosis and cryptogenic fibrosing alveolitis) in children (including two reported by L.L.F.), the diagnostic fibroblastic foci have not been described in any of these reports. A recent pathologic study of 25 pediatric ILD cases at the Royal Brompton Hospital in London uncovered no cases with the histologic features of UIP.[9] The prognosis of adults with UIP is poor, with the majority of patients succumbing within 5 years of diagnosis. In contrast, children given a diagnosis of idiopathic pulmonary fibrosis or

BOX 47-1 Interstitial Lung Disease of Known Etiology

- Aspiration syndromes
- Infectious or postinfectious lung disease
- Drug or radiation-induced lung disease
- Hypersensitivity pneumonitis
- Lysinuric protein intolerance
- Lysosomal storage disorders
- Neurocutaneous syndromes
- Surfactant dysfunction mutations

BOX 47-2 Interstitial Lung Disease of Unknown Etiology

Primary Pulmonary Disorders

- Desquamative interstitial pneumonia (DIP)
- Lymphoid interstitial pneumonia (LIP) and related disorders
- Nonspecific interstitial pneumonia (NSIP)
- Cryptogenic organizing pneumonia
- Acute interstitial pneumonia
- Alveolar hemorrhage syndromes
- Pulmonary infiltrates with eosinophilia
- Bronchiolitis obliterans
- Pulmonary alveolar proteinosis
- Pulmonary vascular disorders (proliferative and congenital)
- Pulmonary lymphatic disorders
- Pulmonary microlithiasis

Systemic Disorders with Pulmonary Involvement

- Connective tissue disease
- Malignancies
- Histiocytosis
- Sarcoidosis

cryptogenic fibrosing alveolitis often live much longer and have a nonprogressive course, suggesting that they do not have UIP. These findings have led authorities to doubt whether true UIP actually exists in children.[8]

Desquamative Interstitial Pneumonia

In contrast to UIP, DIP is a uniform and monotonous histologic process. It is characterized by hyperplasia of alveolar epithelial cells and by an abundance of large macrophages within airspaces.[7] It is these cells within airspaces, initially misidentified as desquamated epithelial cells, that give this condition its name.[10] Inflammatory cells (i.e., histiocytes, lymphocytes, plasma cells, and eosinophils) are present in the interstitium, but usually only in small numbers. Fibrosis is not a notable feature; there may be minimal, and generally uniform, widening of alveolar septa by increased connective tissue (Fig. 47-1). It is important to recognize that DIP-like reactions often occur in association with more specific lesions and may obscure the picture.

BOX 47-3 Unique Forms of Interstitial Lung Disease in Infancy

- Disorders of lung growth and development
- Neuroendocrine cell hyperplasia of infancy/persistent tachypnea of infancy
- Follicular bronchitis/bronchiolitis
- Infantile cellular interstitial pneumonitis/pulmonary interstitial glycogenosis
- Acute idiopathic pulmonary hemorrhage of infancy
- Chronic pneumonitis of infancy/genetic defects of surfactant function

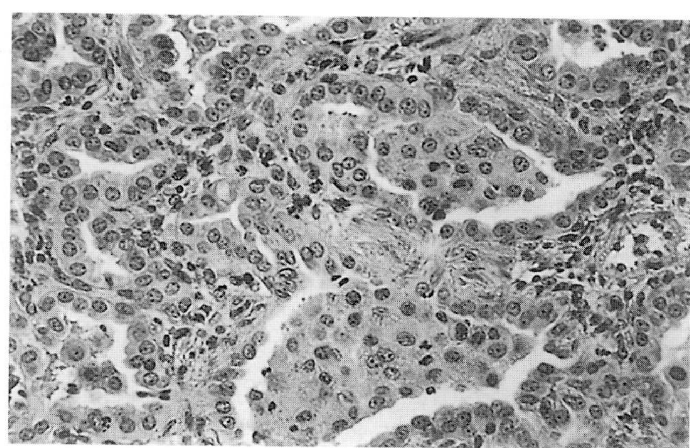

■ **FIGURE 47-1.** Desquamative interstitial pneumonitis (DIP) is characterized histologically by an intra-alveolar accumulation of large epithelioid histiocytes/macrophages. There is mild uniform alveolar epithelial hyperplasia and a minimal infiltrate of small lymphocytes (hematoxylin and eosin, original magnification ×100). This familial case of DIP has recently been discovered to be caused by surfactant protein C deficiency.

Desquamative interstitial pneumonia is largely disappearing as an entity in adults; this is thought to be related to changes in smoking patterns with decreasing use of unfiltered cigarettes. Also, the notion that DIP is a stage in the evolution of UIP is no longer tenable. It is clear that DIP in childhood is a different process from DIP in adults. It is not decreasing in incidence as is that in adults, and it is not linked to smoking. Recently, the highly lethal, familial form of DIP has been linked to genetic defects in surfactant function (see Fig. 47-1).

Lymphoid Interstitial Pneumonia

Although it is the most common of the classically described interstitial pneumonias in childhood,[10] LIP is not truly an interstitial pneumonitis but rather a form of pulmonary lymphoproliferative disease.[7] It is characterized histologically by a diffuse infiltrate of mature lymphocytes, with smaller numbers of plasma cells and histiocytes in the pulmonary interstitium, including the alveolar wall. The infiltrate also may be found along lymphatic pathways and thus is evident in bronchovascular bundles and interlobular septa, but usually spares the pleura (Fig. 47-2). The lymphocytes are small, noncleaved cells that may accumulate as small nodules, sometimes with germinal centers. Although a polyclonal and polymorphous process with both B and T lymphocytes is usually present, LIP, like other lymphoproliferative processes, may occasionally progress through oligo- and monoclonal changes to frank malignancy. Fibrosis is not a feature, nor is airspace disease significant.

Lymphoid interstitial pneumonia should be clearly distinguished from other benign lymphoid disorders of the lung, which include intraparenchymal lymph nodes, hyperplasia of the bronchial-associated lymphoid tissue (Fig. 47-3), nodular lymphoid hyperplasia, and angioimmunoblastic lymphadenopathy. Hyperplasia of the bronchial-associated lymphoid tissue and nodular lymphoid hyperplasia are often not clearly separated from LIP by clinicians or pathologists, many of whom assume that these are stages in the evolution of LIP. This, however, has not been clearly demonstrated, and the tendency to group these entities together may impair ongoing studies of the etiologies of these disease processes. LIP usually occurs in association with abnormalities of immune status including

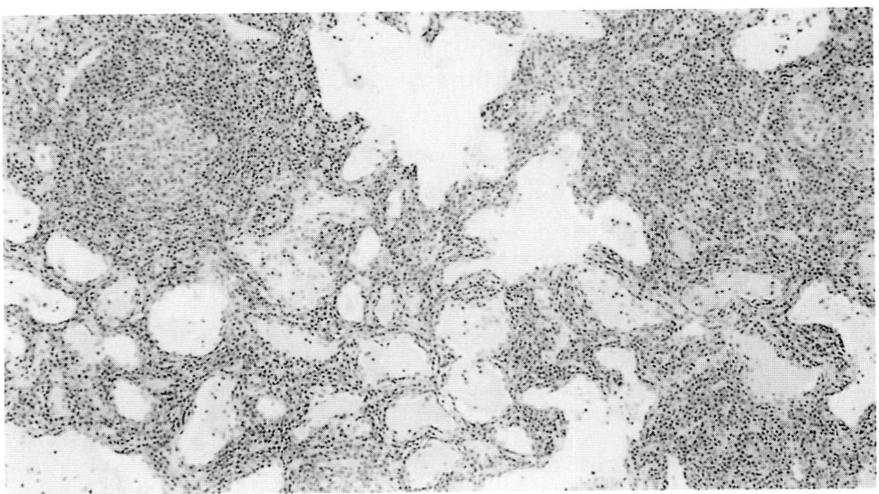

■ **FIGURE 47-2.** Lymphocytic interstitial pneumonitis (LIP) is characterized histologically by a diffuse infiltrate of small lymphocytes widening alveolar walls. It sometimes forms small nodules that may have a follicular appearance with geminal center formation (hematoxylin and eosin, original magnification ×25).

autoimmune disorders and immunodeficiency states, particularly solid-organ transplantation. It has been prominently associated with pediatric acquired immunodeficiency syndrome and is said to occur in 30% of children infected perinatally with human immunodeficiency virus 1. In this situation, it is often not separated from nodular lymphoid hyperplasia, or hyperplasia of the bronchial lymphoid tissue, and the diagnosis is often made without biopsy. The roles of Epstein-Barr virus, other viral agents, and human immunodeficiency virus 1 itself in the etiology of this process require clarification. LIP may also be familial.

Nonspecific Interstitial Pneumonia

In adults, NSIP has come to be recognized as a distinctive form of ILD that conveys a better prognosis than UIP.[11] It must be emphasized that NSIP is a histologic diagnosis that may be seen in a number of clinical settings and with various exposure histories, although most cases are of unknown etiology. Histologically, NSIP is a mixture of inflammation and fibrosis and has been subdivided into a cellular and a fibrosing pattern based on the relative prominence of these particular components (Fig. 47-4). It lacks the specific diagnostic features of other idiopathic interstitial pneumonias. In adults with NSIP, those with a cellular histologic pattern have a better response to steroid therapy and may resolve completely, while those with fibrosis are likely to progress to end-stage lung disease.[12] In a pathologic study of 25 children with ILD, 4 children had cellular NSIP and 3 had fibrotic NSIP.[9]

Acute Interstitial Pneumonia

Acute interstitial pneumonitis, sometimes known as rapidly progressive interstitial pneumonitis or Hamman-Rich syndrome, is distinct clinically and pathologically from the other forms of idiopathic interstitial pneumonitis (Fig. 47-5).[7] The histologic picture is that of diffuse alveolar damage, a nonspecific histologic pattern of acute lung injury with synchronous onset of injury. There is progression from an acute exudative process with hyaline membranes, and often hemorrhagic edema, through a diffuse proliferative process, affecting epithelial and interstitial compartments, to diffuse fibrosis. However, it occurs without known antecedent events leading to lung injury. This severe and rapidly progressive process has a fatality rate of about 50%, and it is impossible to predict from the biopsy findings which patients will progress and which will recover.

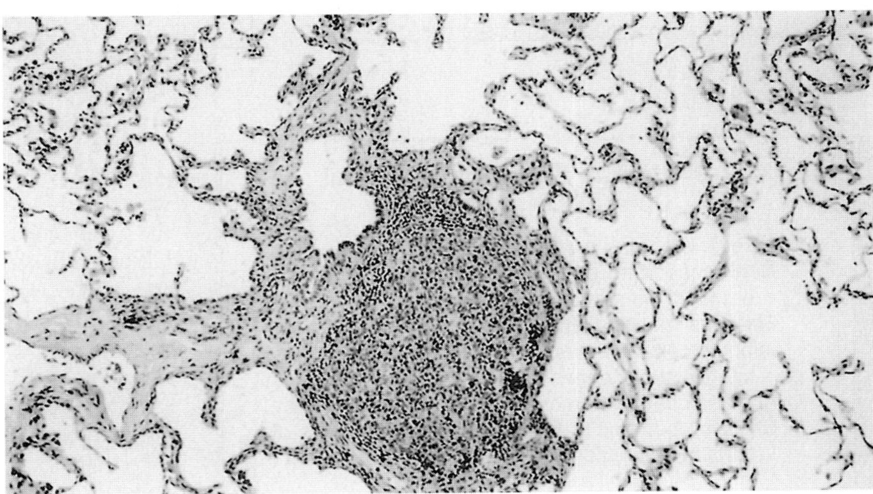

■ **FIGURE 47-3.** Hyperplasia of the bronchus-associated lymphoid tissue is characterized histologically by prominence of the normal pulmonary lymphoid tissue, both adjacent to airways, as seen here, and at the lobular periphery. This process does not extend significantly into adjacent alveolar walls (hematoxylin and eosin, original magnification ×25).

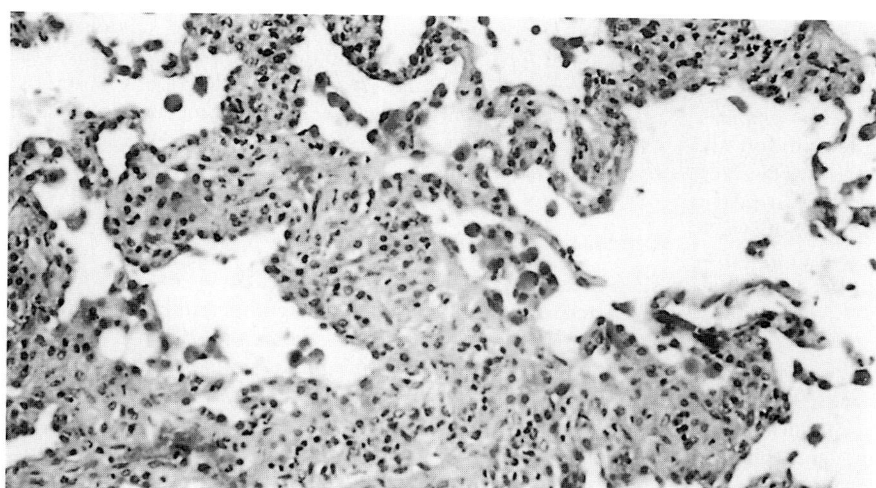

■ **FIGURE 47-4.** Nonspecific interstitial pneumonitis shows characteristic features of interstitial pneumonitis with an irregular lymphocytic infiltrate, variable widening of alveolar walls, and alveolar epithelial hyperplasia, without any specific characteristics histologically or clinically that imply a specific process or etiology (hematoxylin and eosin, original magnification ×50).

INTERSTITIAL LUNG DISEASE SYNDROMES UNIQUE TO INFANCY

In recent years, several "new" and unique forms of PILD have been described in neonates and infants.[2] It is quite likely that these entities are not new but rather are more precise descriptions of previously misidentified disorders.[13] For many years, pediatric lung specialists would try to fit their ILD cases into adult categories. Since many of these patients were infants, it is quite likely that a number of these cases called UIP, idiopathic pulmonary fibrosis, and cryptogenic fibrosing alveolitis were actually cases of these newly defined entities.

Persistent Tachypnea of Infancy/Neuroendocrine Cell Hyperplasia of Infancy

We have identified a group of infants who presented with persistent tachypnea, crackles, hypoxemia, and no evidence of an underlying disease to explain the symptoms.[14] Affected infants showed hyperinflation on chest radiographs, with hyperinflation and ground-glass opacities on high-resolution computed tomography (HRCT). Consistent with radiographic findings, infant pulmonary function testing demonstrated air trapping. Lung biopsies showed no interstitial involvement or inflammation and no identifiable disease process. Mild and nonspecific changes were found, including mild airway smooth muscle hyperplasia and increased numbers of alveolar macrophages. Interestingly, hyperplasia of neuroendocrine cells, as demonstrated by bombesin immunohistochemistry, was a consistent and significant finding in the distal airways. Aggregates of neuroendocrine cells, called neuroendocrine bodies, were also often increased within the lobular parenchyma. No infectious agents were recovered from the patients. Most striking was the discrepancy between the infants' ill appearance clinically and the lack of demonstrably significant abnormalities in the chest films, HRCT, and biopsy material.

No study has systematically evaluated the treatment of this condition, but clinical improvement with corticosteroids, bronchodilators, and other agents has been inconsistent. Although patients have been symptomatic and have often required oxygen for months to years, their clinical condition gradually improved over time. There have been no known pulmonary-related deaths. Many patients, followed for more than 5 years, still have occasional mild pulmonary symptoms associated with

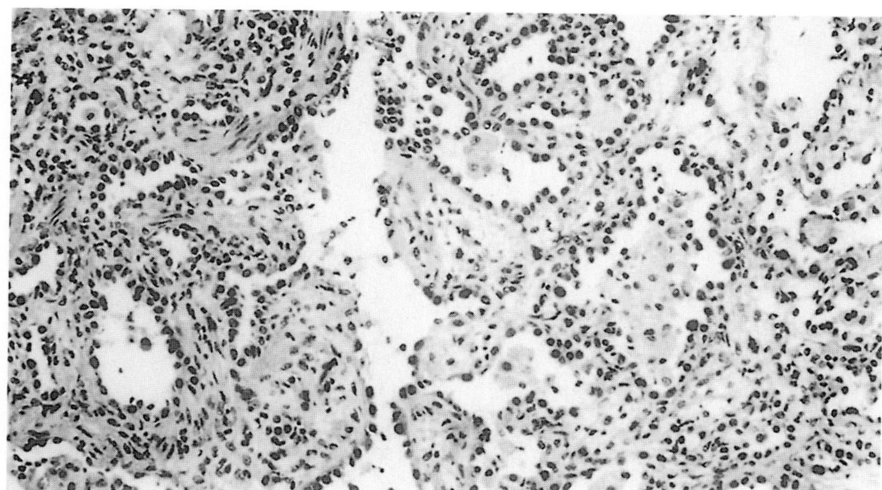

■ **FIGURE 47-5.** Acute interstitial pneumonitis, a rapidly progressive and diffuse process shows uniform alveolar epithelial hyperplasia and diffuse interstitial widening with fibroblastic proliferation and a minimal inflammatory infiltrate. All areas are uniformly involved (hematoxylin and eosin, original magnification ×50).

viral infections or exercise, and there is evidence in some of continued hyperinflation. Longitudinal studies will be required to determine the impact of this disorder on adult lung disease.

Originally, we used the term *persistent tachypnea of infancy* to describe this clinical condition, but with the recognition of neuroendocrine cell hyperplasia in the distal airways, we believe *neuroendocrine cell hyperplasia of infancy* is a better descriptive term. Although these infants have predominantly airway involvement on histopathology, their clinical presentation with ILD syndrome still suggests that this disorder best fits under the heading of PILD.

Follicular Bronchitis and Bronchiolitis

Kinane and colleagues[15] reported five infants with follicular bronchitis and bronchiolitis presenting with tachypnea, fine crackles, and chronic cough by 6 weeks of age. Lung biopsy revealed follicular lymphocytic infiltration surrounding and locally infiltrating the bronchial walls; no organisms were recovered. All patients improved gradually over several years. Similar features were reported more recently by Hull and co-workers,[16] who described chronic bronchiolitis in eight infants, although two had normal biopsy results. It is quite possible that neuroendocrine cell hyperplasia of infancy and follicular or chronic bronchiolitis are the same entity, although in our experience, airway inflammation is not a prominent or consistent feature of neuroendocrine cell hyperplasia of infancy.

Infantile Cellular Interstitial Pneumonitis/Pulmonary Interstitial Glycogenosis

Schroeder and colleagues[17] described five infants with tachypnea since birth and diffuse infiltrates of unknown etiology. Lung biopsy revealed interstitial proliferation of bland, nondescript histiocytic-type cells and minimal or no inflammation (Fig. 47-6). The authors called this new entity cellular interstitial pneumonitis. Although the patients remained tachypneic for prolonged periods of time (4 to 18 months after diagnosis), the overall clinical course was marked by general improvement in four of the five infants. The fifth infant died at 3½ years of age.

Recently, Canakis and co-workers[18] described seven infants whose lung biopsy material had the histologic appearance of infantile cellular interstitial pneumonitis. Utilizing electron microscopy, they demonstrated that the characteristic interstitial cells contained monoparticulate glycogen and postulated an abnormality of lung cytodifferentiation. The authors used the term *pulmonary interstitial glycogenosis* to describe this finding. Six of the seven infants had a favorable outcome, but one died of extreme prematurity and bronchopulmonary dysplasia. Thus, pulmonary interstitial glycogenosis is probably a more complete description of infantile cellular interstitial pneumonitis.

Chronic Pneumonitis of Infancy

Katzenstein and colleagues[19] described nine infants with ILD characterized by alveolar septal thickening, striking pneumocyte hyperplasia, and an alveolar exudate containing numerous macrophages, occasional eosinophilic globules, and rare cholesterol clefts. Since this pattern was markedly different from the previously described classic patterns of ILD (DIP, UIP, LIP) and from the cellular interstitial pneumonitis of infancy, they chose the term *chronic pneumonitis of infancy* to reflect the uniqueness of this entity. Of the six whose clinical course was known, two died and one required lung transplantation. Actually, Fisher and co-workers[20] had previously described a similar process in eight children, although the majority were much older. Typical chest radiograph findings include ground-glass densities, consolidation, volume loss, and hyperinflation.[21] An autopsy study of 12 cases of chronic pneumonitis of infancy revealed an age of onset of 1 to 9 months with an ultimate fatal outcome despite treatment.[22] Thus, it appears this condition carries a high mortality rate. Since these original reports, we have come to recognize that many cases with the histologic pattern of chronic pneumonitis of infancy have genetic abnormalities of surfactant function (unpublished data).

Genetic Abnormalities of Surfactant Function

Without a doubt, the most important advance in the field of PILD has been the discovery of genetic defects of surfactant function. These include mutations in surfactant proteins B and C genes and in the newly described *ABCA3* gene. Although the original histologic description of surfactant protein B deficiency was alveolar proteinosis, it is now known that surfactant mutations can present with a variety of histologic patterns (see Figures 47-1 and 47-7). Since surfactant dysfunction mutations have major genetic implications for families, physicians should consider looking for these in any young child with (1) severe unexplained lung disease in the newborn period, (2) diffuse disease

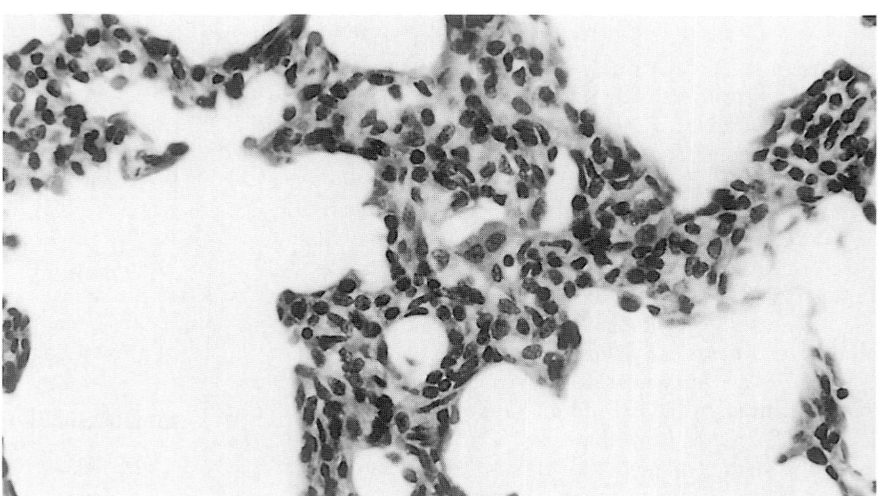

■ **FIGURE 47-6.** Infantile cellular interstitial pneumonitis, a nonspecific reactive change of the infant lung, is characterized by an interstitial proliferation of nondescript cells that are not inflammatory in character. There is usually mild alveolar epithelial cell prominence and no significant airspace exudate (hematoxylin and eosin, original magnification ×100).

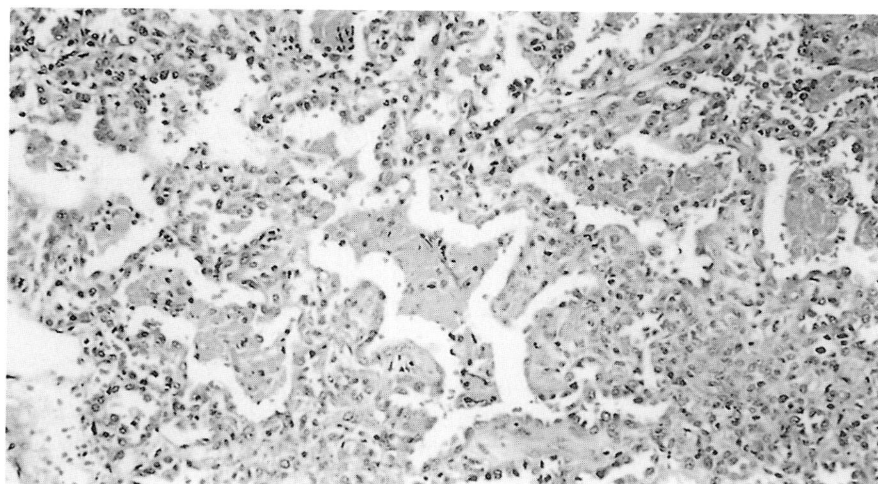

■ **FIGURE 47-7.** Surfactant protein B deficiency may appear as classic alveolar proteinosis but is more likely to have a less specific histologic appearance, as seen here with alveolar epithelial hyperplasia, irregular intra-alveolar exudates of periodic acid–Schiff-positive material intermixed with cellular debris, and a paucity of inflammatory cells (hematoxylin and eosin, original magnification ×50).

involving the entire lung on HRCT, (3) histopathology that demonstrates alveolar proteinosis, DIP, or chronic pneumonitis of infancy, or (4) electron microscopic findings of abnormal or absent lamellar bodies. The story of surfactant dysfunction mutations is evolving and worthy of continuing attention. For a complete description of these disorders, including known mutations to date, the reader is referred to Chapter 20.

■ PATHOGENESIS

Although the acute inflammatory process in the lung is critical for protection against infectious and other exogenous agents, an altered or overexuberant response can in itself cause significant damage. If the inflammatory process is controlled and orderly, then repair and healing can occur, with the lung returning to a normal or near-normal state. However, if the process of injury is severe, inflammation may persist or the reparative phase may become disordered and lead to the development of permanent scarring or fibrosis. Although this classical model of inflammation and repair has been used to explain the pathogenesis of ILD, recent evidence suggests that UIP may be more of a primarily fibrotic process rather than an inflammatory process that leads to fibrosis.[7] However, since UIP is not a pediatric disease and very little work has been done in children, the pathogenesis of PILD remains largely unknown.

Bronchoalveolar lavage (BAL) has been the main tool used to investigate PILD.[2] Clement and associates demonstrated that BAL fluid in children with ILD contained an increase in oxygen metabolites released by alveolar macrophages[23] and an increase in insulin-like growth factor–binding protein-2 as well.[24] In a similar pediatric group, Ronchetti and colleagues[25] reported increased numbers of foamy macrophages and increases in fibronectin, hyaluronic acid, and albumin in the early stages of disease and increased lymphocytes in long-standing disease. Taken together, these studies suggest that, in PILD, lung injury may be due to oxidant damage in part and that certain profibrotic constituents can be identified in BAL.

In children with sarcoidosis, Clement and associates found that BAL fluid contained more lymphocytes, with an elevated CD4/CD8 ratio, and an enhanced ability of alveolar macrophages to release hydrogen peroxide, an effect that diminished after corticosteroid treatment.[26] In a subsequent study, the same group found varying degrees of interleukin-1β, tumor necrosis factor-α, interleukin-6, and transforming growth factor-β expression not found in the control group.[27]

Finally, Ratjen and co-workers[28] found an increase in lymphocytes in children with hypersensitivity pneumonitis. Unlike adults, no differences were found in the CD4/CD8 ratios between children with hypersensitivity pneumonitis and those without lung disease, but there was increased expression of human leukocyte antigen-DR and elevation of natural killer cells in most subjects. These studies in pediatric sarcoidosis and hypersensitivity pneumonitis confirm the presence of a lymphocytic alveolitis and suggest that cellular and cytokine expression patterns in BAL fluid may help to evaluate disease activity and severity in these conditions. However, the prognostic significance of these BAL constituents needs further validation before they can be used to predict outcome in individual patients.

■ CLINICAL PRESENTATION

Children with ILD present with dyspnea, tachypnea, cough, exercise limitation, and frequent respiratory infections.[10] Symptoms are often insidious and may have been present for years before receiving medical attention.[29] A search for precipitating influences should include a careful history to rule out potential causes of aspiration, any previous acute or severe respiratory infections, and environmental exposures especially to birds or molds. Hemoptysis may indicate a pulmonary vascular disorder or alveolar hemorrhage syndrome. Joint disease or rash may indicate a systemic process such as a connective tissue disease. A family history of relatives or siblings with similar lung conditions would implicate a genetic mutation related to surfactant function.

On physical examination, tachypnea and retractions are often observed, and crackles are commonly heard, particularly at the bases. In severe cases, cyanosis, clubbing, an increased pulmonic component of the second heart sound, and evidence of growth failure will be present.

■ DIAGNOSTIC EVALUATION

A systematic approach to the evaluation of pediatric patients with ILD is essential, because the differential diagnosis is extensive.[2]

Diagnostic studies can be divided into those used to assess extent and severity of disease, to identify disorders that predispose to ILD, or to identify the primary ILD (Box 47-4). A systematic approach, utilizing a combination of history, physical examination, and both noninvasive and invasive studies, has been shown to be useful in the diagnosis of PILD, although invasive studies such as lung biopsy are the most helpful.[4,30]

PULMONARY FUNCTION TESTS

Conventional pulmonary function tests in older children typically show a pattern of restrictive lung disease with a reduced forced vital capacity (FVC) and forced expiratory volume in 1 second (FEV_1), and a normal or elevated FEV_1/FVC ratio.[2] However, although total lung capacity (TLC) may be reduced, functional residual capacity (FRC) and residual volume (RV) are often normal or elevated resulting in an increased FRC/TLC and RV/TLC. The latter finding suggests air trapping, and the composite picture may be one of mixed restrictive/obstructive disease.

Pressure-volume curves are typically shifted downward and to the right with an increase in elastic recoil pressure at maximum inspiration consistent with restrictive lung disease. Diffusion of carbon monoxide is low in absolute terms but normal when corrected for alveolar volume.

With recent advances, infant pulmonary function testing is proving useful in evaluating PILD syndromes. Preliminary studies suggest that these techniques can identify functional patterns that distinguish different disorders and correlate with radiologic and histologic findings (Chapter 10).

Most patients with mild disease are normoxic under all conditions, but they may desaturate with exercise or during sleep as the disease progresses and ventilation-perfusion mismatch ensues. Patients with more advanced disease will be hypoxemic at rest. The development of pulmonary hypertension is often indicative of a poor prognosis. A severity of illness classification based on these progressive changes has been shown to be a predictor of survival (Table 47-1) (see section on Outcome).[31]

BOX 47-4 Diagnostic Studies

To Assess Extent and Severity of Disease

- Chest films, high-resolution computed tomography
- Pulmonary function studies: Spirometry; pulse oximetry and arterial blood gases (resting, sleeping, and with exercise); diffusion, pressure-volume curve, infant studies
- Electrocardiogram, echocardiogram

To Identify Primary Disorders That Predispose to Interstitial Lung Disease

- Human immunodeficiency virus
- Immune studies: Immunoglobulins including IgE, skin tests for delayed hypersensitivity, response to immunizations, T and B subsets, complement, others as indicated
- Barium swallow, pH probe

To Identify Primary Interstitial Lung Disease

- Genetic studies for surfactant defects
- Serology: antinuclear antibodies, angiotensin-converting enzyme, antineutrophil cytoplasmic antibody, hypersensitivity pneumonitis screen
- Infectious disease evaluation: Cultures, titers, skin tests
- Cardiac catheterization in selected cases
- Bronchoalveolar lavage and transbronchial biopsy
- Transthoracic biopsy

TABLE 47-1. Severity-of-illness score for interstitial lung disease

Score	Symptoms	Saturation < 90% Exercise/ Sleep	Saturation < 90% Rest	Pulmonary Hypertension
1	No	No	No	No
2	Yes	No	No	No
3	Yes	Yes	No	No
4	Yes	Yes	Yes	No
5	Yes	Yes	Yes	Yes

HIGH-RESOLUTION COMPUTED TOMOGRAPHY

In PILD, HRCT is being utilized with greater frequency to provide precise detail about the extent and distribution of parenchymal disease and to select appropriate biopsy sites.[32] In addition, HRCT may increase the level of diagnostic confidence for the diagnosis of pediatric ILD, improve diagnostic accuracy, and provide a useful classification system.[33,34] Our limited experience with HRCT in children with surfactant protein C mutations suggests that they have diffuse involvement of most of the lung parenchyma with ground-glass opacities, or "fibrotic" changes with cystic lung disease.

In infants, the usefulness of HRCT has been previously limited by rapid breathing causing motion artifacts. This problem can be overcome by a method known as controlled-ventilation HRCT, recently described by Long and associates.[35,36] With this technique, a sedated child is hyperventilated by applying positive pressure through a facemask to produce a brief respiratory pause. As a result, motionless HRCT images can be obtained at either full inflation or resting end-expiration. This technique has been successfully used to obtain both infant lung function testing and HRCT in a single sedation period.

BRONCHOALVEOLAR LAVAGE

In children, as in adults, BAL is now routinely performed for sampling cellular and biochemical components of alveolar lining fluid.[37]

Recent reports, summarized by the European Respiratory Society Task Force on BAL in children, have established normal pediatric BAL indices with which abnormal values can be compared.[37] In most of these studies, the normal pediatric values for BAL fluid constituents were similar to those found in adults. The technique lacks standardization with respect to lavage fluid amount and temperature, dwell time, and whether or not to include the first aliquot. With respect to the aliquot volume, pediatric pulmonologists either calculate by size/body weight (e.g., 10% FRC or 1 mL/kg/aliquot times 3 aliquots), or use a fixed amount of lavage fluid regardless of size (e.g., 10 mL/aliquot times 2 aliquots). We favor the former approach, because a BAL protocol adjusted to body weight has been shown to yield constant fractions of epithelial lining fluid in children aged 3 to 15 years, facilitating the comparison of BAL fluid constituents in children of different age groups.

The most common indication for pediatric BAL has been to detect infection in the immunocompromised host.[10] The overall diagnostic yield for a specific infectious agent was 47% (117 of 249 patients) in eight studies of immunocompromised children without acquired immunodeficiency syndrome. The yield was 77% (134 of 174 patients) in five studies of children with acquired immunodeficiency syndrome. BAL has also been used to detect infection in immunocompetent hosts. However, it is often difficult to determine whether recovered organisms represent true infection, colonization, or contamination.

It has been suggested that the recovery of lipid-laden macrophages from BAL is an indicator of aspiration in children.[5] The presence of lipid-laden macrophages in BAL may be sensitive but not specific for aspiration, since any lung injury may result in the release of lipid from damaged cell membranes, limiting the value of this assessment. Although the detection of specific milk proteins in alveolar macrophages in BAL fluid was more sensitive and specific for aspiration in a mouse model,[38] the results were not as promising in a study of tracheal aspirates in neonates.[39]

The recovery of hemosiderin-laden macrophages has been used to detect alveolar hemorrhage. However, similar to lipid, hemosiderin in macrophages may be sensitive for blood within the lungs, but not specific for an alveolar hemorrhage syndrome.[40] In a murine model, Epstein and colleagues[41] have shown that hemosiderin-laden macrophages appear at 3 days, peak at 1 week, and persist in small numbers for 2 months following a single instillation of blood.

Bronchoalveolar lavage has also been used to diagnose alveolar proteinosis, lysosomal storage disorders, histiocytosis, and surfactant protein deficiency in children.[2]

As a diagnostic tool in immunocompetent children with ILD, Fan and co-workers[42] found that BAL, studied prospectively, was diagnostic of a primary disorder in only 5 of 29 patients; aspiration was detected in 3 and infection in 2. The presence of lymphocytosis, neutrophilia, or eosinophilia narrowed the differential diagnosis in 15 patients. A secondary disorder was uncovered in 8 patients. These results suggest that BAL provides useful information in children with ILD but that its ability to determine the primary cause is limited.

■ LUNG BIOPSY

A tissue diagnosis is required for most types of PILD. Although transbronchial or percutaneous needle biopsy has been successfully used in some cases, a transthoracic approach, either by open-lung biopsy or video-assisted thoracoscopic surgery, remains the gold standard for obtaining tissue adequate for diagnosis.

Lung biopsy material must be processed in a consistent manner to ensure optimal interpretation. This includes the preparation of imprints from biopsy tissue and the preservation of tissue using several modalities for optimum diagnostic yield. Tissue for light microscopy should be fixed in expansion by methods that have been previously reported.[43] Tissue should also be frozen for possible immunofluorescence and other studies, as well as preserved in glutaraldehyde for electron microscopy. It is critical that all biopsy specimens be interpreted by a pathologist with considerable expertise in pediatric lung disease, since the normal lung of an infant differs from that of an older child or adolescent, and any pathologic findings should be interpreted in light of the normal age-dependent variations of lung architecture.

As in adults, the use of video-assisted thoracoscopic surgery is rapidly becoming the method of choice for lung biopsy in children, and technical modifications have permitted it even in infants.[44] In a prospective study in a small group of immunocompetent children with ILD, Fan and colleagues[45] found that the diagnostic yield was comparable for open-lung biopsy (57%) and video-assisted thoracoscopic surgery (54%), but the morbidity from video-assisted thoracoscopic surgery was clearly lower with respect to duration of surgery, chest tube, and hospitalization. Overall, the diagnostic yield from transthoracic lung biopsy (open-lung biopsy and video-assisted thoracoscopic surgery) was disappointing, in large part because of an extremely low diagnostic yield in children younger than 2 years of age. Since this study was done before many of the recently defined ILD syndromes of infants were described, the diagnostic yield in infants is likely to be much higher in the future.

■ TREATMENT

Supportive care includes adequate nutrition, annual influenza vaccination, aggressive treatment of intercurrent infections, a carefully supervised fitness and exercise program, avoidance of inhalant hazards such as tobacco smoke, selective use of bronchodilators, and oxygen for chronic hypoxemia. Patients with underlying systemic disorders need primary treatment for that disorder, such as immunoglobulins for hypogammaglobulinemia. Obviously, specific therapy for primary ILD should be used when possible, such as anti-infective therapy for chronic infections, interferon-α for pulmonary hemangiomatosis, and lung lavage and possibly granulocyte-macrophage colony-stimulating factor therapy for alveolar proteinosis. When environmental agents such as bird antigens are causative, avoidance is critical.

In general, corticosteroids remain the treatment of choice for most patients with ILD on the presumption that suppression of inflammation might be beneficial.[46] Although controlled clinical studies are lacking, a trial of prednisone or equivalent corticosteroid, 1 to 2 mg/kg/day, for at least 6 to 8 weeks is usually warranted. Intravenous-pulse steroid therapy is becoming a common alternative to oral therapy, because it works at least as well or better, and it is associated with fewer side effects.[47] The recommended dose is methylprednisolone, 30 mg/kg, administered intravenously over 1 hour daily, for 3 consecutive days, and repeated monthly. Alternative, but unproven, therapy includes hydroxychloroquine, azathioprine, cyclophosphamide, methotrexate, cyclosporine, and intravenous gamma globulin. Of these, hydroxychloroquine has probably been used the most.[48]

The fact that many alternative pharmacologic approaches are considered for both children and adults with ILD implies that conventional therapy is often ineffective. Therefore, new strategies are being developed using animal models of pulmonary fibrosis and recent advances in the cellular and molecular biology of inflammatory reactions. Such therapies are directed against the action of certain cytokines, oxidants, and growth factors that may be involved in the fibrotic process. The potential to deliver specific inflammatory inhibitors, or inhibitors of collagen biosynthesis, directly to the lung via aerosolization suggests that disease processes in the lung may be more amenable to novel therapies than those in other internal organs.

More children are receiving lung transplantation for end-stage ILD.[49] For some lethal disorders, such as surfactant protein B deficiency and alveolar capillary dysplasia, lung transplantation is the only therapy available. The long-term survival of children transplanted for PILD is at least as good as for cystic fibrosis and pulmonary hypertension.

OUTCOME

The prognosis for children with ILD is variable.[2] Infants with neuroendocrine cell hyperplasia of infancy or pulmonary interstitial glycogenosis generally do well, although they may remain symptomatic and require oxygen for years. At the other end of the spectrum, neonates and infants with surfactant protein B and *ABCA3* mutations, as well as older children with PILD and growth failure, pulmonary hypertension, and severe fibrosis do poorly.

Fan and colleagues[31] reviewed the outcome of 99 children with a variety of PILDs seen in Denver, Colorado, over a 15-year period (1980–1994). There were 15 recorded deaths with a probability that a patient would survive to 24, 48, and 60 months after onset of symptoms of 83%, 72%, and 64%, respectively. With respect to the clinical features present at the time of initial evaluation, weight less than 5% , crackles, clubbing, family history of ILD, and symptom duration were not associated with decreased survival. In contrast, a severity-of-illness classification (see Table 47-1) appeared to be a useful measure of outcome, with an increased score at the time of initial evaluation associated with a higher probability of decreased survival.

REFERENCES

1. Dinwiddie R, Sharief N, Crawford O: Idiopathic interstitial pneumonitis in children. A national survey in the United Kingdom and Ireland. Pediatr Pulmonol 2002;34:23–29.
2. Fan LL, Deterding RR, Langston C: Pediatric interstitial lung disease revisited. Pediatr Pulmonol 2004;38:369–378.
3. Kim CK, Kim SW, Kim JS, Koh YY, Cohen AH, Deterding RR, et al: Bronchiolitis obliterans in the 1990s in Korea and the United States. Chest 2001;120:1101–1106.
4. Fan LL, Kozinetz CA, Deterding RR, Brugman SM: Evaluation of a diagnostic approach to pediatric interstitial lung disease. Pediatrics 1998;101:82–85.
5. Colombo JL: Assessment of aspiration syndromes in children. Clin Pulm Med 1998;5:300–306.
6. Fan LL: Hypersensitivity pneumonitis in children. Curr Opin Pediatr 2002; 14:323–326.
7. The Joint Statement of the American Thoracic Society (ATS), and the European Respiratory Society (ERS). American Thoracic Society/European Respiratory Society international multidisciplinary consensus classification of the idiopathic interstitial pneumonias. Am J Respir Crit Care Med 2002;165:277–304.
8. Katzenstein AL, Myers JL: Idiopathic pulmonary fibrosis—clinical relevance of pathologic classification. Am J Respir Crit Care Med 1998;157: 1301–1315.
9. Nicholson AG, Kim H, Corrin B, Bush A, du Bois RM, Rosenthal M, et al: The value of classifying interstitial pneumonitis in childhood according to defined histological patterns. Histopathology 1998;33:203–211.
10. Fan LL: Pediatric interstitial lung disease. In: Schwarz MI, King TE, eds: Interstitial lung disease, 4th ed. Hamilton, Ont: BC Decker, 2003, pp 134–151.
11. Katzenstein AL, Fiorelli RF: Nonspecific interstitial pneumonia/fibrosis—histologic features and clinical significance. Am J Surg Pathol 1994;18: 136–147.
12. Travis WD, Matsui K, Moss J, Ferrans VJ: Idiopathic nonspecific interstitial pneumonia. Prognostic significance of cellular and fibrosing patterns. Survival comparison with usual interstitial pneumoia and desquamative interstitial pneumonia. Am J Surg Pathol 2000;24:19–33.
13. Fan LL, Langston C: Pediatric interstitial lung disease—children are not small adults. Am J Respir Crit Care Med 2002;165:1466–1467.
14. Deterding RR, Fan LL, Morton R, Hay TC, Langston C: Persistent tachypnea of infancy (PTI)—a new entity. Pediatr Pulmonol 2001;S23:72–73.
15. Kinane BT, Mansell AL, Zwerdling RG, Lapey A, Shannon DC: Follicular bronchitis in the pediatric population. Chest 1993;104:1183–1186.
16. Hull J, Chow CF, Robertson CF: Chronic idiopathic bronchiolitis of infancy. Arch Dis Child 1997;77:512–515.
17. Schroeder SA, Shannon DC, Mark EJ: Cellular interstitial pneumonitis in infants—a clinicopathologic study. Chest 1992;101:1065–1069.
18. Canakis AM, Cutz E, Manson D, O'Brodovich H: Pulmonary interstitial glycogenosis. A new variant of neonatal interstitial lung disease. Am J Respir Crit Care Med 2002;165:1557–1565.
19. Katzenstein AL, Gordon LP, Oliphant M, Swender PT: Chronic pneumonitis of infancy—a unique form of interstitial lung disease occurring in early childhood. Am J Surg Pathol 1995;19:439–447.
20. Fisher M, Roggli V, Merten D, Mulvihill D, Spock A: Coexisting endogenous lipoid pneumonia, cholesterol granulomas, and pulmonary alveolar proteinosis in a pediatric population. A clinical, radiographic, and pathologic correlation. Pediatr Pathol 1992;12:365–383.
21. Abe K, Kamata N, Okazaki E, Moriyama S, Funata N, Takita J, et al: Chronic pneumonitis of infancy. Eur Radiol 2002;12:S155–S157.
22. Kavantzas N, Theocharsis S, Agapitos E, Davaris P: Chronic pneumonitis of infancy. An autopsy study of 12 cases. Clin Exp Pathol 1999;47:96–100.
23. Clement A, Chadelat K, Masliah J, Housset B, Sardet A, Grimfeld A, et al: A controlled study of oxygen metabolite release by alveolar macrophages from children with interstitial lung disease. Am Rev Resp Dis 1987;136: 1424–1428.
24. Chadelat K, Boule M, Corroyer S, Fauroux B, Delaisi B, Tournier G, et al: Expression of insulin-like growth factors and their binding proteins by bronchoalveolar lavage cells from children with and without interstitial lung disease. Eur Respir J 1998;11:1329–1336.
25. Ronchetti R, Midulla F, Sandstrom T, Bjermer L, Zebrak J, Pawlik J, et al: Bronchoalveolar lavage in children with chronic diffuse parenchymal lung disease. Pediatr Pulmonol 1999;27:395–402.
26. Chadelat K, Baculard A, Grimfeld A, Tournier G, Boule M, Boccon-Gibod L, et al: Pulmonary sarcoidosis in children. Serial evaluation of bronchoalveolar lavage cells during corticosteroid treatment. Pediatr Pulmonol 1993;16:41–47.
27. Tessier V, Chadelat K, Baculard A, Housset B, Clement A: BAL in children—a controlled study of different cytology and cytokine expresson profiles by alveolar cells in pediatric sarcoidosis. Chest 1996;109:1430–1438.
28. Ratjen F, Costabel U, Griese M, Paul K: Bronchoalveolar lavage fluid findings in children with hypersensitivity pneumonitis. Eur Respir J 2003;21:144–148.
29. Fan LL, Mullen ALW, Brugman SM, Inscore SC, Parks DP, White CW: Clinical spectrum of chronic interstitial lung disease in children. J Pediatr 1992;121:867–872.
30. Barbato A, Panizzolo C, Cracco A, de Blic J, Dinwiddie R, Zach M: Interstitial lung disease in children. A multicentre survey on diagnostic approach. Eur Respir J 2000;16:509–513.
31. Fan LL, Kozinetz CA: Factors influencing survival in children with chronic interstitial lung disease. Am J Respir Crit Care Med 1997;156:939–942.
32. Koh DM, Hansell DM: Computed tomography of diffuse interstitial lung disease in children. Clin Radiol 2000;55:659–667.
33. Lynch DA, Hay T, Newell JD, Divgi VD, Fan LL: Pediatric diffuse lung disease. Diagnosis and classification using high-resolution CT. AJR Am J Roengenol 1999;173:713–718.
34. Copley SJ, Coren M, Nicholson AG, Rubens MB, Bush A, Hansell DM: Diagnostic accuracy of thin-section CT and chest radiography of pediatric interstitial lung disease. AJR Am J Roengenol 2000;174:549–554.
35. Long FR, Castile RG, Brody AS, Hogan MJ, Flucke RL, Filbrun DA, et al: Lungs in infants and young children. Improved thin-section CT with a noninvasive controlled-ventilation technique—initial experience. Radiology 1999;212:588–593.
36. Long FR, Castile RG: Technique and clinical applications of full-inflation and end-exhalation controlled-ventilation chest CT in infants and young children. Pediatr Radiol 2001;31:413–422.
37. ERS Task Force on bronchoalveolar lavage in children. Bronchoalveolar lavage in children. Eur Respir J 2000;15:217–231.
38. Elidemir O, Fan LL, Colasurdo GN: A novel diagnostic method for pulmonary aspiration in a murine model—immunocytochemical staining of milk proteins in alveolar macrophages. Am J Respir Crit Care Med 2000; 161:622–626.
39. Miller J, Colasurdo GN, Khan AM, Jajoo C, Patel TJ, Fan LL, et al: Immunocytochemical detection of milk proteins in tracheal aspirates of ventilated infants. A pilot study. Pediatr Pulmonol 2002;34:369–374.
40. Epstein CE, Fan LL: Alveolar hemorrhage syndromes.Uupdate on pulmonary hemosiderosis. J Respir Dis Pediatrician 2001;3:49–56.

41. Epstein CE, Elidemir O, Colasurdo GN, Fan LL: Time course of hemosiderin production by alveolar macrophages in a murine model. Chest 2001;120:2013–2020.
42. Fan LL, Lum Lung MC, Wagener JS: The diagnostic value of bronchoalveolar lavage in immunocompetent children with chronic diffuse pulmonary infiltrates. Pediatr Pulmonol 1997;23:8–13.
43. Fan LL, Langston C: Chronic interstitial lung disease in children. Pediatr Pulmonol 1993;16:184–196.
44. Rothenberg SS, Wagener JS, Chang JHT, Fan LL: The safety and efficacy of thoracoscopic lung biopsy for diagnosis and treatment of infants and children. J Pediatr Surg 1996;31:100–104.
45. Fan LL, Kozinetz CA, Wojtczak HA, Chatfield BA, Cohen AH, Rothernberg SS: The diagnostic value of transbronchial, thoracoscopic, and open lung biopsy in immunocompetent children with chronic interstitial lung disease. J Pediatr 1997;131:565–569.
46. de Benedictis FM, Canny GJ, Levison H: The role of corticosteroids in respiratory disease in children. Pediatr Pulmonol 1996;22:44–57.
47. Desmarquest P, Tamalet A, Fauroux B, Boule M, Boccon-Gibod L, Tournier G, et al: Chronic interstitial lung disease in children. Response to high-dose intravenous methylprednisolone pulses. Pediatr Pulmonol 1998;26:332–338.
48. Avital A, Godfrey S, Maayan C, Diamnat Y, Springer C: Chloroquine treatment of interstitial lung disease in children. Pediatr Pulmonol 1994;18:356–360.
49. Mallory GB: The special challenges of pediatric lung transplantation. J Respir Dis Pediatrician 2001;3:105–114.

48 Pulmonary Hemorrhage and Hemoptysis

Thomas F. Boat, MD

Bleeding into the lungs and the conducting airways is encountered infrequently in children but is often life-threatening. Hemoptysis, the expectoration of blood, is an acute manifestation of this bleeding and provides a rough measure of the amount of pulmonary hemorrhage (PH). *Pulmonary hemosiderosis* is a term that is often used synonymously with PH. However, it denotes the presence of lung macrophages containing the degradation products of hemoglobin, the so-called hemosiderin-laden macrophages. Thus, pulmonary hemosiderosis is a pathologic state, diagnostic for bleeding of any type into the lungs. The use of the term *PH* is the most descriptive and is preferred.

Pulmonary hemorrhage may be diffuse or focal (Fig. 48-1). Diffuse PH has distinct causes that can be categorized by age: newborn, first year of life, and older children. Focal hemorrhage is classified by lung site: conducting airways or parenchyma. Diffuse alveolar hemorrhage frequently occurs as an isolated condition, but in children beyond infancy it is not infrequently associated with other organ system injury or dysfunction; PH may be entirely secondary to injurious agents or dysfunction of other organ systems. The bleeding may be subclinical and chronic, presenting as iron deficiency anemia, may be episodic and symptomatic, or may present as massive, life-threatening blood loss.

Figure 48-1 presents a useful taxonomy for the causes of PH. The major childhood etiologies will be described in this chapter, but it will not be possible to review exhaustively all of the causes and associated conditions.

■ PATHOLOGY AND PATHOPHYSIOLOGY

The presence of blood or hemosiderin in the lung historically has been a sine qua non for the definitive diagnosis of PH (Fig. 48-2). Following diffuse, fresh bleeding, many red cells can be seen, often in both intra-alveolar and interstitial sites. If the bleeding occurred at least 2 to 3 days earlier, there will be many macrophages, again in alveoli and interstitial areas, that are filled with hemosiderin. Diffuse alveolar hemorrhage may occur with pulmonary capillaritis (Box 48-1). In these cases, neutrophilic invasion of the interstitium followed by fibrinoid necrosis of the alveolar walls can be identified,[1] small thrombi may be present in capillaries and venules, and alveoli show evidence for injury including thickening of the epithelium and hyperplasia of type 2 pneumocytes. Staining for collagen early after the onset of PH will often demonstrate mild interstitial fibrosis. With chronic bleeding into the lung, fibrosis can become a prominent aspect of the pathology. Intra-alveolar organization of hemorrhage contributes to fibrosis. Lobular and lobar septa may be thickened.[2]

The conducting airways contain relatively large amounts of mucus after brisk bleeding. In vitro studies have demonstrated that large airway mucosa responds to the presence of blood with a brisk mucus secretory response.[3] With chronic PH, a bronchitic picture can develop, including goblet cell hyperplasia.

Diffuse alveolar bleeding is thought to occur under conditions of endothelial injury, allowing red blood cell leakage from intravascular spaces. Cell or molecular mechanisms are not understood in many cases. Some injury appears to be immune complex related. In Goodpasture's disease, the epithelial basement membrane may be the primary site of barrier dysfunction. Alveolar hemorrhage secondary to congestive heart failure may simply relate to mechanical injury of the endothelium as the result of high pulmonary capillary pressures. In some cases of idiopathic pulmonary hemosiderosis, electron microscopy has failed to demonstrate structural changes of the pulmonary endothelial barrier. In other cases focal interruptions, thickening, or vacuolation of endothelial cells have been described.

However, animal studies have shed new light on potential mechanisms of alveolar hemorrhage. Conditional transgenic mice overexpressing vascular endothelial growth factor starting on postnatal day 1 develop diffuse alveolar hemorrhage and 50% neonatal mortality by 2 weeks of age.[4] By 2 weeks of age an inflammatory response and lung remodeling were apparent. Electron microscopy demonstrated attenuated endothelial cells and a discontinuous endothelial barrier for alveolar capillaries. Animals surviving to adulthood displayed large numbers of alveolar and perivascular hemosiderin-laden macrophages as well as variable degrees of emphysema. This model approximates the pathologic findings in idiopathic pulmonary hemosiderosis. Vascular endothelial growth factor–induced PH in immature mice offers a possible mechanism for diffuse alveolar hemorrhage, episodic or chronic, in humans. It is likely that molecular factors other than vascular endothelial growth factor will ultimately be implicated in vascular injury and widespread hemorrhage.

On the basis of investigations of home environments of infants in Cleveland presenting with acute idiopathic pulmonary hemorrhage (AIPH) and severe respiratory distress or failure, it was proposed that a mycotoxin associated with *Stachybotrys chartarum*, growing on water-damaged walls of homes, was an associated if not causative factor in AIPH.[5] Subsequently, *S. chartarum* was recovered in airway lavage fluid from a child with primary PH.[6] On the basis of these findings, families have been encouraged to seek other housing, public buildings have been closed, and personal injury claims have been filed.

However, other studies of clustered (Chicago)[7] and isolated cases of AIPH[8] have not found this organism in homes of affected infants. Furthermore, a detailed study of the evidence by the Centers for Disease Control and Prevention found shortcomings in the original data gathering and analysis and led that institution to conclude that evidence is insufficient to support an association between *S. chartarum* and AIPH. Meticulous environmental

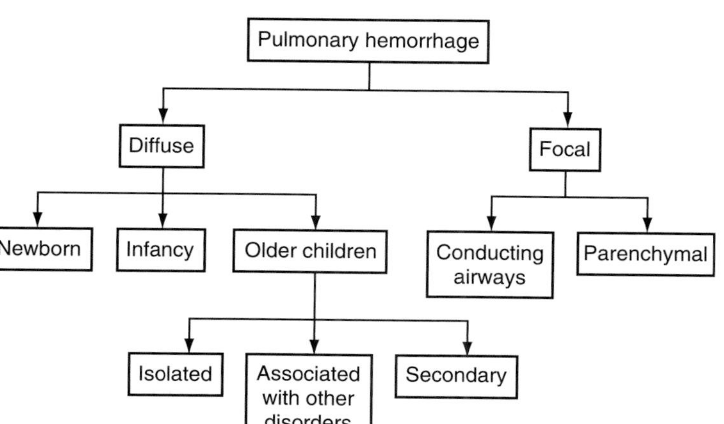

■ **FIGURE 48-1.** Taxonomy of PH in children.

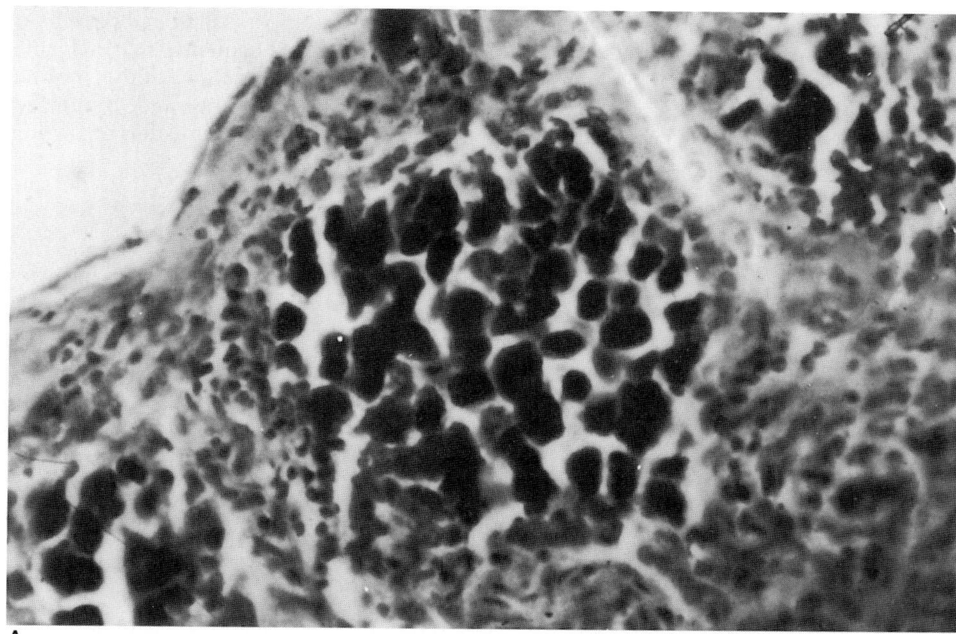

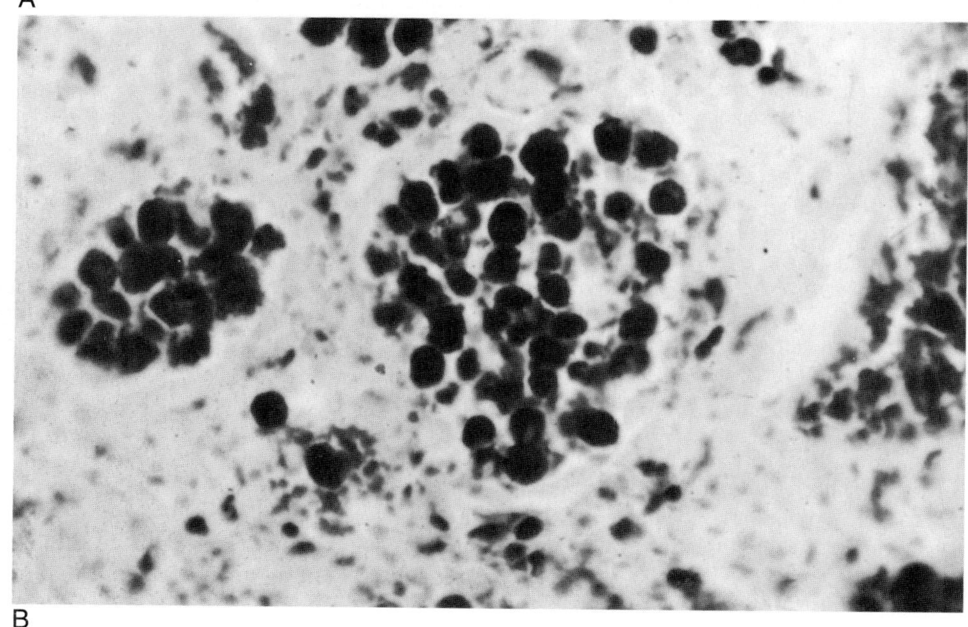

■ **FIGURE 48-2.** Microscopic sections of lung from a 3-year-old boy with PH who died several hours after a diagnostic needle biopsy of the lung. **A,** Hematoxylin and eosin stain showing iron-containing macrophages filling an alveolus, marked alveolar epithelial proliferation, fibrosis, and fresh intra-alveolar bleeding. **B,** Prussian blue stain showing hyperplastic alveolar walls and alveoli containing red blood cells and many deeply stained iron-laden macrophages (×500).

BOX 48-1 Causes of Diffuse Alveolar Hemorrhage with Pulmonary Capillaritis

Wegner's granulomatosis
Systemic necrotizing vasculitis (microscopic polyarteritis)
Mixed connective tissue disease
Behçet's syndrome
Anaphylactoid (Henoch-Schönlein) purpura
Goodpasture's syndrome
Nephritis with and without immune complexes

studies of future cases were recommended.[9] Other reported potential risk factors include household smokers and lack of breastfeeding. However, no evidence for cause and effect or insight into molecular mechanisms has been uncovered.

Hemoptysis associated with bronchiectasis involves the presence of dilated, tortuous bronchial arteries.[10] Destruction of structural elements in the airway wall leads to erosion of these high-flow vessels and large-volume hemoptysis.

DIAGNOSIS

PRESENTING MANIFESTATIONS

Expectoration of blood often, but by no means always, heralds diffuse or focal pulmonary hemorrhage. Hemoptysis, particularly in younger children, must be distinguished from hematemesis, or bleeding from the nasopharyngeal airway. Ability of the patient to localize a bubbling sensation to the right or left side suggests focal rather than diffuse hemorrhage. Extremes of hemoptysis range from massive losses of blood from the mouth and nose, to expectoration of blood-tinged mucus.

Massive blood loss presents with cardiovascular instability. Pallor and fatigue, symptomatic of iron deficiency anemia, occasionally may be the initial clinical observation. In these cases, subclinical bleeding has usually been present for a long time.

Symptoms of ongoing or episodic lung disease not infrequently constitute the presenting manifestations. These symptoms may include shortness of breath, chronic cough, wheezing, cyanosis, and decreased activity. If chronic and sufficiently severe, failure of the child to gain weight or grow may be noted.

Finally, a number of patients have presented with what is initially considered recurrent pneumonia. This diagnosis may be based on recurring pulmonary symptoms and the identification of infiltrates on the chest radiograph. These infiltrates may or may not clear up between exacerbations of disease. Conversely, it is possible to have symptomatic pulmonary hemorrhage with minimal roentgenographic findings.

PHYSICAL EXAMINATION

Children with chronic ongoing bleeding into the lung present with pallor, decreased activity, tachypnea, and signs of labored ventilation. Cyanosis may be prominent but will not be seen in severely anemic children. A productive or nonproductive cough may be present. The chest may be locally or diffusely dull to percussion, and breath sound intensity may be diminished. Course and fine crackles as well as wheezes are not infrequently heard. Children with chronic disease may display digital clubbing and nail bed cyanosis. Hepatosplenomegaly occasionally accompanies these findings.

LABORATORY EVALUATION

A complete blood count will demonstrate microcytic, hypochromic anemia unless hemorrhage has occurred only recently. Reticulocytosis is variable, depending on available iron stores. The total white blood cell count may be moderately elevated and occasionally is quite high with a shift to the left. Eosinophilia suggests cow's milk hyperreactivity or perhaps an autoimmune process.

During active bleeding, guaiac testing of stools may be positive. Urinalysis can rule out syndromes also involving nephritis. Hemoglobinuria may be detected with brisk lung hemorrhage that is diffuse.

Chest radiographs may show acute or chronic changes as demonstrated in Figure 48-3. Acutely, peribronchial or more extensive fluffy infiltrates may be seen. Chronically, nodular lesions and diminished aeration of the lungs are noted. Overinflation of the lungs is not uncommon, especially during

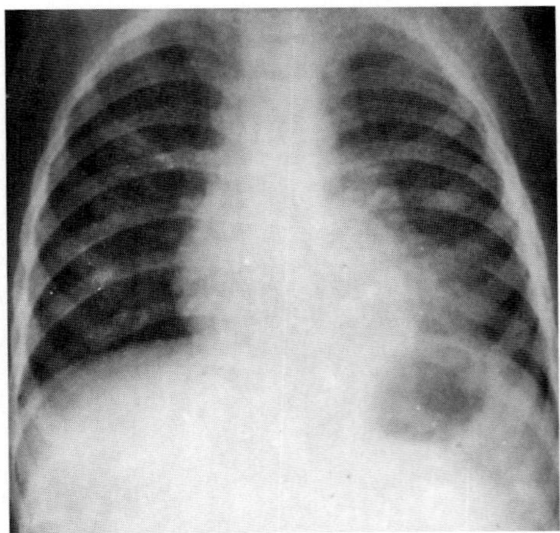

A

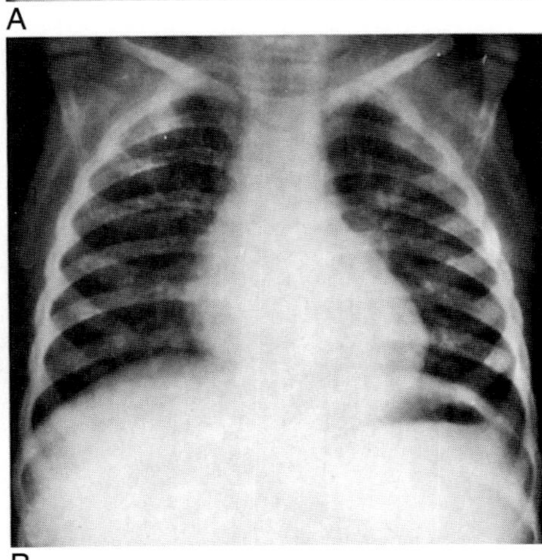

B

FIGURE 48-3. **A,** Chest radiograph of a boy with idiopathic pulmonary hemosiderosis of 2 years' duration during an exacerbation at 27 months of age. Note the soft perihilar infiltrates, most evident along the left cardiac border. **B,** The same patient 4 months later when asymptomatic. Note the decrease in soft infiltrates but a prominent bilateral reticulonodular pattern suggesting interstitial fibrosis.

acute exacerbations. The fissures may be thickened. Computed tomography scan may be helpful for assessing the extent of hemorrhage and for detecting underlying pathology (Fig. 48-4). Changes are often more striking in the lower than in the upper lobes. Serial chest radiographs may show progression, clearing, or even migratory infiltrates.

An immunologic work-up is only occasionally helpful. Serum immunoglobulin levels may all be increased, but in conditions such as hemosiderosis with cow's milk protein hyperreactivity, serum IgE levels may be very high, exceeding 2000 or 3000 units/mL. Heiner has reported deficiencies of IgA and IgG in approximately 15% of patients with hemosiderosis.[11] Low total complement levels suggest systemic lupus erythematosus. In pulmonary bleeding associated with autoimmune disease, antinuclear antibodies, rheumatoid factor, and erythrocyte sedimentation rate may be elevated, depending on the underlying condition.

The key laboratory finding for pulmonary hemorrhage is the hemosiderin-laden macrophage (see Fig. 48-2). The macrophages may be found in sputum and in gastric washings. However, the most direct and reliable method of recovering macrophages containing hemosiderin is by bronchial lavage at the time of bronchoscopy. An iron stain index for macrophages has been suggested,[12] scoring 100 alveolar macrophages for hemosiderin staining on a scale of 0 to 3. A score of greater than 20 out of a maximum 300 points suggests hemosiderosis. Immediately after an acute episode of bleeding into the lung, there may be no hemosiderin staining of macrophages. Animal studies as well as human studies have demonstrated that it takes between 2 and 3 days for hemosiderin to appear in macrophages after introduction of blood into the lungs.[12] Staining for hemosiderin is carried out by reaction with potassium ferrocyanide and hydrochloric acid (the Prussian blue reaction). Although other interstitial lung diseases may be accompanied by a minor degree of red cell loss from the intravascular space, the intensity of hemosiderin staining and the percentage of stained macrophages (<20%) are low.[13]

Demonstration of serum precipitating antibodies to cow's milk proteins suggests an association between PH and hyperreactivity to cow's milk protein.[14] Renal function testing as well as urinalysis should be carried out to look for evidence of nephritis that may occur in Goodpasture's syndrome, Wegner's granulomatosis, systemic lupus erythematosus, and Henoch-Schönlein purpura. Antibodies to basement membrane in serum would be consistent with the diagnosis of Goodpasture's syndrome. Antinuclear cytoplasmic antibodies in the serum suggest the presence of Wegner's granulomatosis. IgA antibodies to endomysium and tissue glutaminase are both sensitive and specific screening tests for celiac disease, which has been described repeatedly in association with PH. If these antibodies are present, further investigation of the gastrointestinal tract, including documentation of steatorrhea and intestinal biopsy, are warranted.

Evaluation of pulmonary function is important to establish the extent of involvement. In small children, oxygen saturation recordings or arterial blood gas results may suggest problems with oxygenation or even ventilation. Pulmonary function testing in older children often demonstrates an obstructive as well as restrictive component. The former is undoubtedly due to irritative bronchitis, while the latter suggests chronicity and lung fibrosis. After an acute bleeding episode, gas diffusion is impaired and lung compliance is decreased. However, with the presence of red blood cells in the lung, single-breath carbon monoxide uptake is enhanced as a result of binding of the carbon monoxide to hemoglobin in extravasated red blood cells.[15]

In conditions that appear to be secondary to cardiovascular problems, a thorough cardiac evaluation including electrocardiogram, echocardiogram, and, in selected cases, catheterization will be indicated.

In the past, lung biopsy and direct demonstration of bleeding into the peripheral lung was the sine qua non for the diagnosis of diffuse PH. Routine hematoxylin and eosin stains, as well as staining for hemosiderin, are mandatory. Additional studies such as immunofluorescent staining for immune complexes or basement membrane antibodies can be helpful to demonstrate specific associated conditions. If focal lung bleeding is suspected, immediate bronchoscopy will occasionally demonstrate the area or region of lung from which the bleeding is emanating. However, most often acute bleeding has stopped

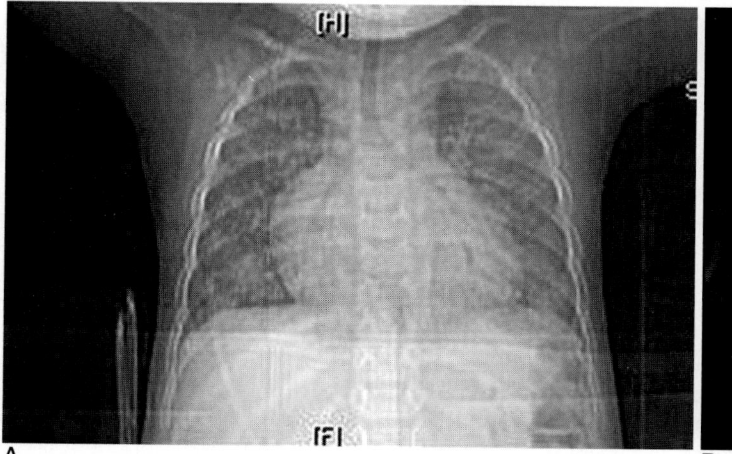

A

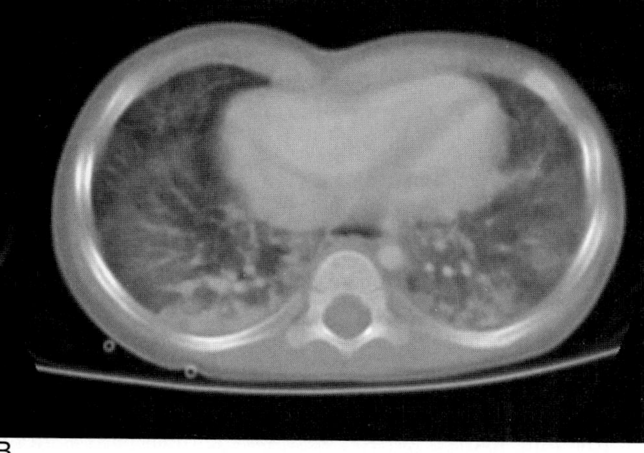
B

■ **FIGURE 48-4.** **A,** Posteroanterior chest radiograph of a 1-year-old boy at the time of diagnosis of idiopathic diffuse PH. Symptoms had been present for several months. Note the diffuse nodular pattern of parenchymal disease superimposed on poorly aerated lungs. **B,** Computed tomography scan of the lower chest from the same patient on the same day. Dense opacification is prominent in dependent areas of the lungs and in a bilateral nodular distribution. Diffusely opacified areas of both lungs are interspersed with regions of aerated and even hyperaerated lung.

by the time bronchoscopy can be performed. A thorough evaluation of the airways by fiberoptic bronchoscopy, looking for lesions such as hemangiomas, is required when recurrent bleeding is encountered in the absence of chronic lung disease. The combination of lung lavage and imaging techniques may be sufficient to make a firm diagnosis of PH.

TREATMENT

Whenever possible, the treatment of PH should address the cause of the disorder or pathologic process. However, in the face of life-threatening bleeding, empirical therapy is required. In these cases, blood or other volume expanders may be needed to treat or prevent shock. Short-term ventilatory support or even extracorporeal membrane oxygenation has been lifesaving. In the face of suspected diffuse PH, most caretakers would treat with large doses of corticosteroids until the bleeding is under control. Chronic corticosteroid therapy seems not to be helpful, and other immunosuppressive agents are used for extended therapy of ongoing hemorrhage. Children with chronic bleeding into the lung and iron deficiency anemia will respond to administration of iron, unless the severity of chronic illness has suppressed hemoglobin synthesis. With bronchiectasis, severe and nonremitting bleeding may require embolization of bronchial arteries. Clotting disorders should be treated vigorously. Details of therapy will be discussed under specific conditions.

PROGNOSIS

The outcome for PH depends on the nature of the underlying process and its severity. Bleeding may be isolated and never recur. Repetitive bleeding into the lungs causes progressive pulmonary injury and dysfunction. Massive pulmonary bleeding may be life threatening because of acute blood loss or interference with gas exchange. In general, prognosis will depend on expert management of acute bleeding, knowledgeable evaluation and management of the various causes of chronic or repetitive bleeding, and the presence or absence of systemic or other severe organ system involvement.

CAUSES OF PULMONARY HEMORRHAGE IN CHILDREN

NEONATAL PULMONARY HEMORRHAGE

Pulmonary hemorrhage in the newborn is a relatively frequent and sometimes fatal event, occurring more often in very low birth weight infants than in term newborns. The cause of PH is not always immediately discernible. Several conditions are associated with PH of the newborn (Box 48-2).

The more premature the child, the higher the likelihood for diffuse PH. This linkage, at least in part, relates to an immature vascular system and endothelial barrier. Onset of bleeding from the lungs may occur almost immediately after birth, or any time in the first several weeks of life. In the face of other lung diseases such as respiratory distress syndrome, bleeding into the lung may go undetected for some time. Pathologically, the bleeding may be into the airspaces, or both alveolar and interstitial.

Pulmonary edema may accompany frank bleeding into the lung in many neonates. The basis for this claim lies in the fact that airway liquids recovered from newborns with PH have a much lower hematocrit level and protein content than that of the blood.[16] Conditions frequently contributing to pulmonary edema include increased blood flow, either from left-to-right shunting or overtransfusion/overhydration. Patent ductus arteriosus is increasingly cited in the literature as an underlying influence.[17] A number of conditions obstructing flow through the left heart are reported in association with PH. For a number of infants, left ventricular failure may be a major contributor to pulmonary edema. Congenital heart lesions that obstruct the flow of blood from the lungs to the left ventricle also contribute.

BOX 48-2 Neonatal Conditions Associated with Pulmonary Hemorrhage

1. Very low birth weight
2. Respiratory distress syndrome
3. Other chronic lung disorders
4. Mechanical ventilation
5. Persistent pulmonary hypertension
6. Left-to-right cardiac shunts
7. Left-sided obstructive cardiac lesions
8. Veno-occlusive disease
9. Cardiac failure
10. Coagulation defects: thrombocytopenia, disseminated intravascular coagulation
11. Instrumentation of the nasopharynx or airway (e.g., intubation, nasogastric feeding tubes)
12. Congenital anomalies
13. Central nervous system disorders
    - Intracranial hemorrhage
    - Kernicterus
    - Perinatal asphyxia
14. Hypothermia

Lung disorders may promote bleeding into the lung. Among these are the respiratory distress syndrome, chronic lung disease of infancy, and pneumonia of various etiologies. In surveys of newborns with lung disease and subsequent PH, bleeding is associated with lack of treatment with antenatal corticosteroids or postnatal surfactant delivery, emphasizing the contribution that severe respiratory distress syndrome can make to PH.

Several pathologists have noted that infants dying of massive PH also have central nervous system edema. Based on these findings, there have been claims that an increase in intracranial pressure may play a primary etiologic role in the development of PH. Along these lines, perinatal asphyxia, kernicterus, and intracranial hemorrhage have all been associated with the occurrence of newborn PH.

Other contributory conditions include hypothermia, coagulation defects such as those occurring in infants with sepsis and disseminated intravascular coagulation, and metabolic disorders leading to hyperammonemia. Treatment of other lung conditions, including mechanical ventilation and exposure to high concentrations of oxygen, are also linked to PH.

Treatment usually includes assisted ventilation. Other symptomatic or supportive therapies may be needed, including replacement of red blood cells, treatment of left heart failure, and correction of hypothermia or acidosis.

PULMONARY HEMORRHAGE IN INFANCY

Acute Idiopathic Pulmonary Hemorrhage

Sudden, unexpected, and life-threatening diffuse PH, at times occurring in clusters, has been described in the first year of life, usually beyond the neonatal period. These children, in general, present with cough, pallor, irritability, decreased activity, hemoptysis, and respiratory distress with grunting. On physical examination, cyanosis is usually noted, and crackles are heard on auscultation. Between 1993 and 2000, 30 infants with this presentation were treated in a pediatric hospital in Cleveland, Ohio.[18] Most required intensive support; 73% needed ventilatory assistance. During the same period of time, seven infants were seen in Chicago hospitals with the same presentation.[7] All of these were admitted to a pediatric intensive care unit and given respiratory support by mechanical ventilation. Little evidence for lung infection was found in either series. All but two infants recovered fully from the first bleeding episode. Six infants from Cleveland and one from Chicago apparently experienced recurrent PH, resulting in three subsequent deaths. The clustering of these cases suggests that environmental etiologic factors are at work. Reports from Cleveland suggested an association with the toxigenic fungus *S. chartarum*, found in the infants' homes.[5] This association is no longer accepted according to the epidemiologic studies conducted. A search for additional environmental or genetic contributing variables has been recommended.[9] Many of the infants from the Cleveland AIPH series had bronchoscopic evidence of low-grade bleeding for longer than 4 months after diagnosis.[18] This finding raises the question of how these cases differ from idiopathic pulmonary hemosiderosis, other than early onset of PH.

Pulmonary Hemorrhage with Cow's Milk Hyperreactivity

In 1962 Heiner described infants and small children with evidence of bleeding into the lungs on a persistent or recurring basis.[11] These patients all shared the feature of high titers of serum precipitins to multiple proteins in cow's milk. Additional patients were reported by Boat and colleagues.[14] Evidence for persistent upper respiratory tract symptoms, including rhinorrhea and failure to thrive, were consistent and prominent features. In addition, approximately half of the patients eventually developed lymphoid hypertrophy in the upper airway and experienced airway obstruction sufficiently severe to cause cor pulmonale. Prominent laboratory features included a striking eosinophilia and impressively elevated levels of IgE. Chest roentgenograms showed fluffy and sometimes evanescent infiltrates. All of the children dramatically improved on a diet free of cow's milk. Early return to cow's milk feedings in one study subject was associated with brisk bleeding and death. All of the pulmonary and secondary cardiovascular symptoms disappeared with time on proper dietary control. Reintroduction of cow's milk feedings was possible after 1 or 2 years.

Extensive immunologic evaluation of a subgroup of these children revealed no consistent abnormality.[19] Speculation that reflux and aspiration of milk contributes to the onset of the PH has never been confirmed. What relationship might exist among this group of children, infants with idiopathic PH, and AIPH in infants is uncertain.

PULMONARY HEMORRHAGE IN OLDER CHILDREN

Idiopathic Pulmonary Hemosiderosis

Idiopathic PH (hemosiderosis) occurs at any age. It is defined by an absence of identifiable causation or associated disease. Symptoms tend to be episodic, although evidence for ongoing subclinical bleeding is present in some patients. Symptoms include cough, shortness of breath, and wheezing. Pallor, cyanosis, diminished intensity of breath sounds, crackles, and overinflation of the chest may be noted on physical examination (Box 48-3).

Leukocytosis is often a prominent feature during an exacerbation of bleeding. Reticulocytosis is a response to acute bleeding, but with prolonged hemorrhage, findings of an iron deficiency anemia are common. Immunologic abnormalities, including

BOX 48-3 Conditions Associated with Pulmonary Hemorrhage in Older Children

A. Diffuse
  1. Isolated
    a. Idiopathic pulmonary hemosiderosis
    b. Pulmonary capillary hemangiomatosis
    c. Lymphangioleiomyomatosis
  2. Associated with other organ dysfunction
    a. Kidney
      - Goodpasture's syndrome
      - Nephritis with immune complexes
      - Nephritis without immune complexes
      - Wegner's granulomatosis
      - Collagen vascular disease (systemic lupus erythematosus)
      - Henoch-Schönlein purpura
    b. Other
      - Celiac disease
      - Myocarditis
  3. Secondary
      - Obstruction to flow through the left side of the heart
      - High pulmonary flow (e.g., left-to-right shunt)
      - Heart failure
      - Clotting disorders
      - Malignancy and immunosuppressive therapy
      - Bone and marrow transplant
      - Diffuse alveolar injury

B. Focal
  1. Conducting airways
    a. Bronchitis
    b. Bronchiectasis (especially cystic fibrosis)
    c. Airway anomalies
    d. Vascular malformations
    e. Foreign bodies
  2. Parenchymal
    a. Trauma
    b. Pneumonia
    c. Infection
    d. Infarction
    e. Neoplasms (e.g., in tuberous sclerosis)
    f. Cavitary lesions
    g. Disseminated endometriosis (catamenial)

a positive direct Coombs' test, serum cold hemagglutinins, increased serum levels of immunoglobulins, and low levels of complement component C4 have been described, each in a few patients. No consistent pattern has emerged. Representative chest roentgenograms are shown in Figures 48-3 and 48-4.

Stool guiaic tests frequently are positive, undoubtedly because of swallowed blood. Hemosiderin-laden macrophages can be identified with potassium ferrocyanide staining of gastric aspirates or lung lavage fluid. These macrophages are also diagnostic when biopsy of the lung is performed. Immunofluorescent and electron microscopic studies of the lung have revealed no specific pathophysiologic clues.[20] Type I alveolar cells may be disrupted with exposure of the basement membrane. The alveolar endothelial layer and its basement membrane may display discontinuities or thickening.[21,22]

Therapy during an acute exacerbation should be supportive. The administration of blood may be lifesaving. Generally, patients who are symptomatic are treated with high doses of corticosteroids. Anecdotally, use of this therapy is associated with cessation of bleeding. Many patients are continued on corticosteroids for long periods of time. There is no convincing evidence that maintenance corticosteroid therapy prevents recurrent bleeding episodes. Patients who experience repeated life-threatening episodes, or who experience progression of pulmonary dysfunction over time, may be candidates for immunosuppressive drug therapy. Azathioprine (Imuran) has been used most frequently.[23] Response to cyclophosphamide has also been reported.[24] If the patient is doing well, an attempt should be made to discontinue all therapy within 1 year, but reinstitution of pharmacologic intervention may be required. Inhaled steroids have also been used, but no trials have been conducted.[25] Two children with life-threatening idiopathic hemorrhage appeared to respond to chloroquine.[26]

Initiation of a hypoallergenic diet has been suggested, but no reports of efficacy in systematic studies have been published. A trial of a cow's milk–free diet may distinguish milk-related from idiopathic hemorrhage. A gluten-free diet has been associated with improvement of lung symptoms when celiac disease also is present. The use of an iron-chelating drug (deferoxamine) has been suggested, but its effects are largely undocumented. The prognosis for idiopathic PH varies from complete resolution to death during an acute exacerbation of hemorrhage. Chronic disabling lung disease is a common outcome.

Pulmonary Capillary Hemangiomatosis

A few cases of pulmonary capillary hemangiomatosis have been reported in children and young adults.[27] In one family, three siblings developed this disorder. The condition is characterized by a proliferation of capillaries that infiltrate the interstitium and infringe on alveolar spaces. The capillaries also invade the walls of pulmonary veins and produce a form of veno-occlusive disease. Significant alveolar hemorrhage and hemosiderosis result. Pulmonary hypertension is a prominent finding in these patients. Lung biopsy is required to make this diagnosis. The prognosis is poor, although in one case, treatment with recombinant interferon-$\alpha 2$ was followed by considerable improvement.

Pulmonary Hemorrhage Associated with Nephritis

Goodpasture's syndrome occurs occasionally in children and more often in adults. It was first reported in 1919 in an 18-year-old man who was found to have diffuse alveolar hemorrhage, glomerulonephritis, peritonitis, splenic infarcts, and vasculitis of the small intestine.[28] In 1965, antibodies to glomerular basement membrane were identified in the kidneys and lungs of patients with both PH and glomerulonephritis.[29] Now the diagnosis of Goodpasture's syndrome is defined by the detection of circulating antibodies to basement membrane and linear immunofluorescence in alveolar walls as well as kidneys. In the majority of cases, lung and renal disease appear simultaneously. In some cases only the kidney is involved. Occasionally, only lung symptoms are noted. In these cases, a renal biopsy will still reveal staining of the basement membrane with antibody directed against IgG and complement, even though renal function tests are normal. Diffuse alveolar hemorrhage is more likely to occur in those patients who smoke. The standard histologic appearance of the lungs in Goodpasture's syndrome is similar to that in idiopathic PH. Goodpasture's syndrome can be distinguished by the demonstration of an uninterrupted linear deposit of immunoglobin and complement along the alveolar wall basement membrane. Symptoms most often consist of hemoptysis, cough, and dyspnea. Fatigue may occur secondary to iron deficiency anemia. The chest roentgenogram reveals patchy or diffusely dense alveolar infiltrates. After active bleeding, regression of infiltrates leaves a residual reticulonodular change. The patient with symptomatic lung but not renal disease often responds to corticosteroids. However, disease with glomerulonephritis is treated with a combination of plasmapheresis, corticosteroids, and cytotoxic drugs. Dialysis may be required for some patients. A 2-year survival rate is approximately 50% for all treated patients.[30]

Other forms of diffuse PH with nephritis (pulmonary-renal syndrome) are unusual in children. Several cases of alveolar hemorrhage with crescentic glomerulonephritis accompanied by immune complex deposits in the kidneys, but not the lungs, have been described.[31] Glomerulonephritis and alveolar hemorrhage without immune complex deposition may represent microseptic polyangitis. Antinuclear cytoplasmic antibodies are present in the serum as in Wegner's granulomatosis. The absence of antibodies to glomerular basement membrane differentiates these conditions from Goodpasture's syndrome. The treatment of these conditions is usually corticosteroid drugs plus immunosuppressive therapy.

Diffuse PH has been described with myocarditis, celiac disease, diabetes, and several collagen vascular diseases such as systemic lupus erythematosus and juvenile rheumatoid arthritis. In general, the pathogenesis of these disorders and specifically the cause of PH are not understood.

Several conditions characterized pathologically by systemic vasculitis may cause diffuse PH (see Box 48-3). These include Wegner's granulomatosis, systemic necrotizing vasculitis, and, perhaps most commonly in children, anaphylactoid or Henoch-Schönlein purpura. The finding of antibodies to cytoplasmic components of neutrophils (antinuclear cytoplasmic antibodies) is characteristic. A definitive diagnosis requires histopathologic confirmation. In anaphylactoid purpura, the joints and gastrointestinal tract are commonly involved. Pulmonary disease is rare. However, there are many well-described cases of Henoch-Schönlein purpura with diffuse PH in the literature. Corticosteroids are the recommended form of treatment.

Lymphangioleiomyomatosis and tuberous sclerosis may be pathologically identical. Intermittent hemoptysis occurs as a result of pulmonary venous obstruction and capillary rupture.

BOX 48-4 Pulmonary Hemorrhage due to Diffuse Alveolar Injury

A. Drug toxicity
   1. Penicillamine
   2. Nitrofurantoin
   3. Cytotoxic agents
   4. Other immunosuppressive agents
   5. Trimellitic anhydride
B. Insecticide exposure
   • Paraquat
C. Smoke inhalation
D. Acid aspiration
E. Radiation
F. Oxygen toxicity
G. Mechanical ventilation

Tuberous sclerosis, which begins in childhood, is accompanied by pulmonary disease in approximately 1% of cases.[32]

Pulmonary Hemorrhage Secondary to Other Disease Processes

Many cases of acute PH have occurred in patients with malignancies, especially during chemotherapy. In some instances, secondary lung infection, at times associated with unusual organisms such as *Legionella* and *Micrococcus* have been reported. PH occurs fairly frequently as a complication of blood and marrow transplantation in adults, less commonly in children. In one series of 138 children undergoing blood and marrow transplantation, 6 (4.3%) developed fulminant bleeding into the lung.[33] Only 1 survived.

It is well known that mitral stenosis or congestive heart failure can result in bleeding into the lungs. The mechanism is thought to be largely if not purely mechanical. Treatment is that of the underlying condition. Veno-occlusive disease occurs rarely, but most cases are in children. This disease is a cause of primary pulmonary hypertension.[34] Patients present with dyspnea and syncope, and physical findings suggest cor pulmonale. Veno-occlusive disease is a postcapillary form of pulmonary hypertension, resulting from intimal fibrosis and obstruction of small veins and venules. Immunosuppressant therapy seems to have been effective in ameliorating symptoms in several patients. Anticoagulation may be temporarily effective. Chronic vasodilator therapy may also improve symptoms.

A lengthy list of drugs, environmental agents, and trauma has been associated with diffuse PH (Box 48-4). Discontinuation of exposure is mandatory when pulmonary bleeding occurs.

HEMOPTYSIS

Hemoptysis, as pointed out in the first paragraph of this chapter, is the expectoration of blood. It may be a manifestation of diffuse PH. However, this section will concentrate on focal lesions in the airways that lead to expectoration of blood. As outlined in Figure 48-1, focal lesions can occur either at conducting airways or parenchymal levels in the lung. Hemoptysis may be associated with chronic lung disease (Box 48-5) or may occur in the absence of any known lung lesions (Box 48-6).

BOX 48-5 Chronic Airways Disease of Childhood Causing Hemoptysis

1. Bronchiectasis
   • Cystic fibrosis
   • Bronchopulmonary aspergillosis
   • Primary ciliary dyskinesia
2. Tuberculosis
3. Nontuberculous cavitary lung lesions including abscess
4. Metastatic neoplasms
5. Retained foreign bodies
6. Extended tracheostomy with tracheal wall erosion
7. Direct and repeated suctioning of airways

CAUSES

By far, the most common nontraumatic pediatric cause of hemoptysis in the United States and most European countries is cystic fibrosis (CF). Children and young adults with CF frequently experience small-volume hemoptysis (e.g., blood streaking of sputum). Expectoration of a "mouthful" of blood is not uncommon. These events are episodic and tend to occur during exacerbations of lung disease. Large-volume (massive) hemoptysis is an unusual but life-threatening event. Although some have attempted to define massive hemoptysis by volume (e.g., 200–500 mL/24 hr), a functional definition such as loss of a volume of blood that causes cardiovascular instability may be more useful clinically with CF and other causes of bronchiectasis; the bronchial arteries and their branches are large, tortuous, and easily eroded, presumably by the same processes that injure the bronchial walls.[35] Small-volume hemoptysis may occur when the mucosal/submucosal integrity is lost, resulting in capillary or small vein bleeding. A second reason for hemoptysis in individuals with CF is a coagulopathy secondary to vitamin K deficiency.

BOX 48-6 Causes of Large-Volume Hemoptysis in Asymptomatic Children and Young Adults with No Known Lung Disease

1. Airway hemangioma
2. Pulmonary sequestration and foregut duplication
3. Congenital arteriovenous malformation and hereditary hemorrhagic telangiectasia
4. Bronchial adenoma
5. Mild hemophilia
6. Unilateral pulmonary artery agenesis
7. Catamenial hemoptysis (teenage girls)
8. Bronchial artery aneurysm
9. Congenital absence of a segment of the inferior vena cava
10. Ehlers-Danlos syndrome
11. Idiopathic

For those patients not taking vitamin K supplements, hemoptysis should trigger the investigation of clotting status by ordering a prothrombin time test. An occasional individual with CF will have severe liver disease and an inability to synthesize coagulation factors.

Other nontraumatic chronic lung diseases infrequently cause hemoptysis (see Box 48-5). On the other hand, traumatic injury to the central airways by endotracheal or tracheostomy tubes frequently causes some expectoration of blood. Minor bleeding is most often associated with deep (beyond the end of the tube) and vigorous suctioning that injures the mucosal/submucosal airway layers. Massive hemoptysis can occur when an airway tube erodes into a larger vessel in the tracheal wall or mediastinum. Exsanguination is a well-documented complication of long-term tracheostomy.

Large-volume hemoptysis occasionally occurs in children with no history of lung disease, acute or chronic (see Box 48-6). Lesions of the lung vasculature such as a hemangioma, arteriovenous malformation, or unilateral absence of a pulmonary artery should be considered. Pediatric endobronchial lesions that bleed are unusual to rare; they may include an adenoma, papillomatous carcinoid, malignant neoplasm, or bronchial artery aneurysm. Several individuals with mild, undetected hemophilia have presented with hemoptysis. Teenage girls with periodic hemoptysis could have ectopic endometrial tissue in the lungs (catamenial hemoptysis).

DIAGNOSIS

For small children, it is essential, though at times quite difficult, to determine that the blood is indeed coming from the lungs rather than from the upper airway or the gastrointestinal tract. Direct observation generally will distinguish between these possibilities. Occasionally, bronchoscopy or gastrointestinal endoscopy is required to locate the bleeding source.

Most children with large-volume hemoptysis of unknown cause get a chest roentgenogram. Only occasionally will an etiology be suggested by this procedure. In the absence of obvious cause, bronchoscopy may be the first diagnostic test. Bronchoscopy serves to: (1) determine whether the bleeding is coming from right or left, (2) locate the specific site, and (3) identify the cause of bleeding.[36] If active bleeding persists, therapy also can be initiated via the bronchoscope (see next section on Treatment). However, usually bleeding has stopped and no evidence implicating a site or a specific lesion is found. The airways should be thoroughly inspected for a related lesion. The choice of rigid versus fiberoptic bronchoscopy has been debated. The former affords superior suctioning capability, but the latter can evaluate more distal airways.

Recurrent or massive bleeding may suggest the need for additional imaging studies, namely a computed tomography scan or magnetic resonance imaging to identify lung abnormalities (e.g., a sequestered lobe or a large-vessel anomaly such as unilateral pulmonary artery aneurysm or agenesis) or pulmonary angiography to identify an arteriovenous malfunction. Systemic angiography may be useful for suspected bronchial artery anomalies.

TREATMENT

Most hemoptysis is self-limiting and not life threatening. In these instances, there is time to evaluate the patient thoroughly and to institute therapy as indicated. However, massive hemoptysis is a life-threatening event and requires an emergent response. Stabilization of intravascular volume is paramount. Blood should be available for immediate transfusion if necessary. Easily remedied contributory conditions such as a coagulation factor or platelet deficiency should be identified and treated. Oxygen should be administered for any evidence of hypoxemia; sedation should be used sparingly, even though anxiety and agitation are likely to complicate management.

The use of intravenous vasopressin has appeared to be effective in controlling massive hemoptysis, presumably by constricting systemic vessels.[37] This treatment at best is a stabilizing maneuver until more definitive therapy can be provided.

If bleeding is brisk and unilateral, endobronchial tamponade or unilateral intubation of the nonbleeding lung may be lifesaving. Double-lumen tubes have been used as a temporizing measure to ventilate the healthy lung and tamponade the bleeding lung.[38] Endobronchial thrombin applications may also be helpful.[39]

Continuing bleeding is an indication for arteriography of bronchial vessels. While the site of bleeding may be identified using this approach, rapid assessment of the bronchial artery anatomy, including identification of collaterals to spinal arteries, and embolization of vessels thought to be contributing is perhaps the most direct and effective therapy. This approach is not only indicated for massive hemoptysis but is often used for recurrent moderate-volume hemoptysis, as in patients with CF.[40] Embolization in these patients frequently controls bleeding for prolonged periods. Bronchial stenosis is an infrequent long-term complication.

The last resort for uncontrolled massive hemoptysis is lung resection. Previously, surgical resection was the procedure of choice. However, improved diagnostic strategies and alternative therapeutic approaches have made surgery, with its attending complications and long-term consequences, an only infrequently invoked option. Persistent bleeding secondary to vascular anomalies such as unilateral absence of a pulmonary artery may require surgical resection of involved lung.[41] The definitive treatment of hemoptysis, of course, is that of the underlying lesion or process. Every attempt should be made to thoroughly investigate and characterize the underlying structural or functional abnormality, and to definitively treat this abnormality.

REFERENCES

1. Mark EJ, Ramierez JF: Pulmonary capillaritis and hemorrhage in patients with systemic vasculitis. Arch Pathol Lab Med 1985;109:413–418.
2. Travis WD, Colby TV, Lomard C, Carpenter HA: A clinicopathologic study of 34 cases of diffuse pulmonary hemorrhage with lung biopsy confirmation. Am J Surg 1990;14:1112–1125.
3. Boat TF, Polony I, Cheng PW: Mucin release from rabbit tracheal epithelium in response to sera from normal and cystic fibrosis subjects. Pediatr Res 1982;16:792–797.
4. LeCras TD, Spitzmiller RE, Albertine KH, et al: VEGF causes pulmonary hemorrhage, hemosiderosis and airspace enlargement in neonatal mice. Am J Physiol Lung Cell Mol Physiol 2004;287:L134–L142.
5. Etzel RA, Montana E, Sorenson WG, et al: Acute pulmonary hemorrhage in infants associated with exposure to *Stachybotrys atra* and other fungi. Arch Pediatr Adolesc Med 1998;152:757–762.
6. Elidemir O, Colasurdo GN, Rossman SN, Fan LL: Isolation of *Stachybotrys* from the lung of a child with pulmonary hemosiderosis. Pediatrics 1999;104: 964–966.
7. Centers for Disease Control and Prevention: Acute pulmonary hemorrhage among infants—Chicago, April 1992–November 1994. MMWR Morb Mortal Wkly Rep 1995;44:67–74.

8. Norotny WE, Dixit A: Pulmonary hemorrhage in an infant following 2 weeks of fungal exposure. Archiv Pediatr Adol Med 2000;154:271–275.
9. Centers for Disease Control and Prevention: Acute idiopathic pulmonary hemorrhage among infants. Recommendation from the Working Group for Investigation and Surveillance. MMWR Morb Mortal Wkly Rep 2004; 53:1–12.
10. Mack JF, Moss AF, Harper WW, O'Loughlin BJ: The bronchial arteries in cystic fibrosis. Br J Radiol 1965;38:422–429.
11. Heiner DC, Sears JW, Kniker WT: Multiple precipitins to cow's milk in chronic respiratory disease. Am J Dis Child 1962;103:40–60.
12. Sherman JM, Winnie G, Thomassen MJ, et al: Time course of hemosiderin production and clearance by human pulmonary macrophages. Chest 1984;86:409–411.
13. Pere-Arellano JL, Losa-Garcia JE, Garcia Macias MC, et al: Hemosiderin-laden macrophages in bronchoalveolar lavage fluid. Acta Cytologica 1992;36:26–30.
14. Boat TF, Polmar SH, Whitman V, et al: Hyperreactivity to cow milk in young children with pulmonary hemosiderosis and cor pulmonale secondary to nasopharyngeal obstruction. J Pediatr 1975;87:23–39.
15. Ewan PW, Jones HA, Rhodes CG, Hughes JMB: Detection of intrapulmonary hemorrhage with carbon monoxide uptake. Application in Goodpasture's syndrome. N Engl J Med 1976;295:1391–1396.
16. Cole VA, Normand ICS, Reynolds EOR, Rivers RPA: Pathogenesis of hemorrhagic pulmonary edema and massive pulmonary hemorrhage in the newborn. Pediatrics 1973;51:175–187.
17. Kluckow M, Evans N: Ductal shunting, high pulmonary blood flow, and pulmonary hemorrhage. J Pediatr 2000;137:68–72.
18. Dearborn DG, Smith PG, Dahms BB, et al: Clinical profile of 30 infants with acute pulmonary hemorrhage in Cleveland. Pediatrics 2002;110: 627–637.
19. Stafford HA, Polmar SH, Boat TF: Immunologic studies in cow's milk–induced pulmonary hemosiderosis. Pediatr Res 1977;11:898–903.
20. Irwin RS, Cotrell TS, Hsu KC, et al: Idiopathic pulmonary hemosiderosis. An electron microscopic and immunofluorescent study. Chest 1974;65: 41–45.
21. Elliot ML, Kuhn C: Idiopathic pulmonary hemosiderosis—ultrastructure abnormalities in capillary walls. Am Rev Respir Dis 1970;102:895–904.
22. Gonzales-Crussi F, Hull MT, Crosfeld JL: Idiopathic pulmonary hemosiderosis. Evidence of capillary basement membrane abnormality. Am Rev Respir Dis 1976;114:689–698.
23. Byrd RB, Gracey DR: Immunosuppressive treatment of idiopathic pulmonary hemosiderosis. JAMA 1973;226:458–459.
24. Columbo JR, Stol SM: Treatment of life-threatening primary pulmonary hemosiderosis with cyclophosphamide. Chest 1992;102:959–960.
25. Tutor JD, Eid NS: Treatment of idiopathic pulmonary hemosiderosis with inhaled flunisolide. South Med J 1995;88:984–986.
26. Bush A, Sheppard MN, Warner J: Chloroquin in idiopathic pulmonary hemosiderosis. Arch Dis Child 1992;67:625–627.
27. Faber CH, Yousem SA, Dauber JH, et al: Pulmonary capillary hemangiomatosis. A report of three cases and review of the literature. Am Rev Respir Dis 1989;140:808–813.
28. Goodpasture EW: The significance of certain pulmonary lesions in relation to the etiology of influenza. Am J Med Sci 1919;158:863–870.
29. Duncan DA, Drummond KN, Michael AF, Vernier RL: Pulmonary hemorrhage and glomerulonephritis. Report of six cases and study of the renal lesion by fluorescent antibody technique and electron microscopy. Ann Intern Med 1965;62:920–938.
30. Schwartz MI, Cherniack RM, King TE: Diffuse alveolar hemorrhage and other rare infiltrative disorders. In: Murray J, Nadel J, eds: Textbook of Respiratory Medicine. Philadelphia: WB Saunders, 1994, pp 1889–1912.
31. Lewis EJ, Schur PH, Busch GJ, et al: Immunopathologic features of a patient with glomerulonephritis and pulmonary hemorrhage. Am J Med 1973;54:507–513.
32. Liberman BA, Chamberlain DW, Goldstein RS: Tuberous sclerosis with pulmonary involvement. Can Med Assoc J 1984;130:287–289.
33. Ben Abraham R, Paret G, Cohen R, et al: Diffuse alveolar hemorrhage following allogeneic bone marrow transplantation in children. Chest 2003; 124:660–664.
34. Wagenvoort CA, Wagenvoort TN, Takahashi T: Pulmonary veno-occlusive disease. Involvement of pulmonary arteries and review of the literature. Hum Pathol 1985;16:1033–1041.
35. Schidlow DV, Taussig LM, Knowles MR: Cystic Fibrosis Foundation consensus conference report on pulmonary complications of cystic fibrosis. Pediatr Pulmonol 1993;15:187–198.
36. Cahill BC, Ingbar, DH: Massive hemoptysis assessment and management. Clin Chest Med 1994;15:147–167.
37. Pea L, Roda L, Boussard V, Lonjon B: Desmopressin therapy for massive hemoptysis associated with leptospirosis. Am J Respir Crit Care Med 2003;167:726–728.
38. Freitag L, Tekolf E, Stamatis G, Montag M: Three years' experience with a new balloon catheter for the management of hemoptysis. Eur Respir J 1994;7:2033–2037.
39. Tsukamoto T, Sasaki H, Nakamura H: Treatment of hemoptysis by thrombin and fibrinogen-thrombin infusion therapy using a fiberoptic bronchoscope. Chest 1989;96:473–476.
40. Cipolli M, Perini S, Valetta EA, Mastella G: Bronchial artery embolization in the management of hemoptysis in cystic fibrosis. Pediatr Pulmonol 1995; 19:344–347.
41. Bekoe S, Pellegrini RV, DiMarco RF, et al: Pneumonectomy for unremitting hemoptysis in unilateral absence of pulmonary artery. Ann Thorac Surg 1993;55:1553–1554.

49 Hypersensitivity Pneumonitis and Eosinophilic Pulmonary Diseases

Alan P. Knutsen, MD • Raouf S. Amin, MD • James Temprano, MD • Robert W. Wilmott, MD

HYPERSENSITIVITY PNEUMONITIS

The terms *hypersensitivity pneumonitis* (HP) and *extrinsic allergic alveolitis* are used to describe a wide group of interstitial and alveolar diseases that develop as a result of repeated exposure to a variety of inhaled organic dusts and occupational antigens. Two common forms are farmer's lung and pigeon breeder's disease. Farmer's lung was the first occupationally related form of HP to be clearly described, and it is the most widely recognized. One of the earliest descriptions was by Ramazzini in his book *Diseases of Workers*: "Almost all who make a living by sifting or measuring grain are short of breath and cachectic and rarely reach old age."[1]

In 1932 Campbell described pulmonary symptoms of five farmers exposed to dense clouds of "white" or hay dust after a heavy rainy season: "The onset was very similar in each case: a noticeable shortness of breath for some weeks whilst carrying out the normal routine, including work with hay, until a climax was reached by some specific act (for example, clearing out the remainder of the hay from a barn) and within thirty-six hours the man was extremely dyspneic—a step or two being impossible—distressed, and cyanosed, and appeared almost in extremis."[2]

The early studies of pigeon breeder's lung, caused by avian antigens, were described in adults by Reed and Barbee in the United States[3] and by Hargreave and colleagues in the United Kingdom.[4] The initial study of HP caused by avian antigens in children was the 1967 study by Stiehm and co-workers,[5] and several other cases have since been reported.

CLINICAL FEATURES

Hypersensitivity pneumonitis presents as a syndrome of respiratory symptoms with or without systemic features. The symptoms are similar in the various diseases despite the diversity of inducing agents, suggesting that the mechanism(s) involved and the pulmonary responses are the same. The form of the disease in a specific patient is affected by the nature of the biologic dust inhaled, the intensity and frequency of exposure, the severity of the immune inflammatory response, and the sequelae of the inflammatory response. The symptoms resulting from sensitization and repeated inhalation of the organic dust take several forms.

Acute Form

Typically, patients with acute disease present with a history of multiple bouts of fever and respiratory distress. They often receive a presumptive diagnosis of atypical, viral, or bacterial pneumonia. It is, therefore, important to consider HP in the differential diagnosis for patients who have recurrent bouts of pneumonia in the absence of immune deficiency. The episodes are explosive in nature, often resembling a flulike illness, and they occur 4 to 6 hours after exposure to the offending agent. Typically, the patient develops acute cough, dyspnea, and fever as high as 40°C with chills and malaise that may persist for as long as 18 hours. Patients usually recover spontaneously within 2 to 5 days, and episodes recur with every exposure. In one report a child with the acute form of HP presented with the unusual problem of reversible pulmonary hypertension.[6]

Physical examination usually reveals an ill-appearing patient with rapid respiration. Weight loss is a common finding in children with HP that is probably due to anorexia and progressive dyspnea. Fine inspiratory crackles are usually heard at the lung bases, and they may persist for several weeks after the acute episode. Wheezing is uncommon, since most patients exposed to organic dusts do not develop HP and asthma. However, laboratory studies have shown that some patients have a dual response: An initial obstructive phase followed by a late-onset, restrictive response. Studies of these patients, using methacholine challenge, demonstrate that 60% of them may have airway hyperreactivity.[7] Occasionally, the lungs are clear to auscultation.

Subacute Form

More continuous exposure to the antigen may cause subacute pneumonitis, an insidious but usually reversible disorder. The symptoms are usually milder and extend over a 10- to 14-day period. Typical symptoms are malaise, low-grade fever, cough, chills, and progressive dyspnea, often associated with anorexia and weight loss.

Chronic Form

Exposure to small amounts of antigen for a long period, which sometimes happens with people exposed to animal antigens, or to a contaminated home air humidifier, may lead to the development of chronic disease with minimal reversibility. These patients usually have dyspnea, chronic cough, fatigue, anorexia, and weight loss.

The division of the clinical manifestations into three forms does not presume that the syndromes are stages of a single disease process, since patients with acute HP usually do not progress to chronic disease, and patients with chronic disease may not have the acute episodes.[8]

RADIOGRAPHIC STUDIES

The sensitivity of chest radiography for the detection of HP has been decreasing, because the proportion of normal chest radiographs in patients with HP has increased from 0% in the past to more that 80% today.[9] This apparent decline is due to several influences, such as a higher index of suspicion for the disease leading to earlier diagnosis, and the increased sensitivity of other diagnostic techniques. Therefore, abnormal findings on a chest radiograph should no longer be regarded as a major diagnostic criterion for the disease. Cook and colleagues separated the radiographic abnormalities of HP into acute, subacute, and chronic forms.[10] Patients with isolated acute disease had radiographic abnormalities that were more severe in the lower zones of the lung, whereas the patient with chronic disease had more severe disease in the upper zones of the lung. Patients with subacute disease have mixed features, some having disease that is more severe in the lower zones and some having more disease in the upper zones of the lung. Typical changes on the chest radiograph are fine nodules and reticular shadowing (Fig. 49-1); localized patchy opacities also occur. Atelectasis, cavities, and calcification have not been reported. Hilar adenopathy is rare in HP, and pleural effusion or thickening is usually absent.

High-resolution computed tomography (HRCT) is more sensitive for the detection of HP than chest radiography.[11] The most common abnormalities are an increase in the density of the lungs, poorly defined centrilobular nodules, and linear opacities. The centrilobular nodules on HRCT correlate with the presence of granulomas on lung biopsy, and linear opacities usually indicate lung fibrosis. Although HRCT is more sensitive than chest radiography in detecting early stages of pneumonitis, false-negative examinations may be a problem, as with chest radiography. Lynch and colleagues reported a sensitivity of 45% for the detection of HP.[12] In a comparison between HRCT and magnetic resonance imaging in the evaluation of chronic infiltrative lung diseases, HRCT was superior to magnetic resonance imaging in the anatomic assessment of the lung parenchyma and in showing fibrosis. However, areas of airspace opacification were seen equally well on magnetic resonance imaging and HRCT.[13] Diffuse pulmonary uptake of gallium-67 has been demonstrated in HP. However, it is a nonspecific finding and has been described in a variety of disorders, such as *Pneumocystis carinii* pneumonia, sarcoidosis, and pulmonary fibrosis.

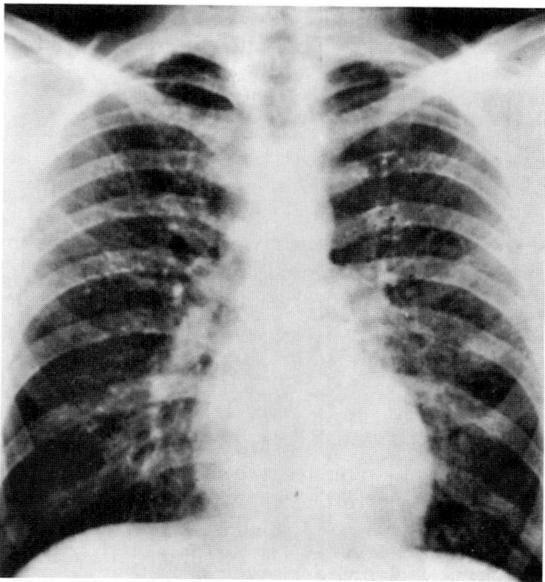

FIGURE 49-1. Chest radiograph of a patient with hypersensitivity pneumonitis. Note fine reticulonodular infiltrates of both lungs. (From Warren CPW, Tse KS: Extrinsic allergic alveolitis owing to hypersensitivity to chickens. Am Rev Respir Dis 1974;109:672.)

IMMUNOPATHOGENESIS

The immunopathogenesis of HP appears to involve both type III antigen-antibody complex and type IV cell-mediated delayed hypersensitivity responses.[14] The initial event in the pathogenesis in HP is sensitization to an inhaled antigen in the distal airway. After repeat antigen challenge, an acute alveolitis develops, with an influx of polymorphonuclear cells into the alveoli.[15] This is transient and is followed by an influx of $CD8^+$ T cells. Although several aspects of the disease, such as time course of clinical symptoms after exposure and presence of precipitating antibodies against the offending agent, support a type III hypersensitivity immune reaction, other aspects of the disease are contradictory. For instance, precipitating antibodies to the offending antigen can be found in a high percentage of individuals who have a history of exposure but lack clinical disease. In a study by Reyes and co-workers,[16] 60 patients with farmer's lung underwent pulmonary biopsy. The most common features identified were interstitial pneumonitis (100%), unresolved pneumonias (65%), granulomas (70%), interstitial fibrosis (65%), and bronchiolitis obliterans (50%). However, there were no cases of vascultic, immune complex–mediated disorder observed.

Type III Hypersensitivity Response

Serum precipitating antibodies specific to the inciting antigen can be found in most patients; however, serum precipitins can be found in the majority of healthy, exposed individuals.[17,18] The precipitating antibodies are usually IgG, but can be IgM or IgA.[19] Immune complex formation in the lungs may lead to activation of the complement cascade and to the production of interleukin-1 (IL-1) and tumor necrosis factor-α (TNF-α) by pulmonary macrophages.[20] Activation of the complement cascade could lead to enhanced vascular permeability through C3a and chemoattraction of neutrophils and macrophages via C5a.[21] Secretion of IL-1 and TNF-α may lead to adhesion molecule expression on leukocytes and endothelial cells, thus promoting adherence before leukocyte migration into the alveolar interstitium.[22] Additionally, pulmonary macrophages secrete IL-8, monocyte chemoattractant protein 1 (MCP-1), macrophage inflammatory protein 1α (MIP-1α), and RANTES (released on activation, normal T cell expressed and secreted), which act as chemotactic factors for a variety of cells.[23] IL-8 is a chemotactic factor for neutrophils, and MIP-1α is a chemotactic factor for $CD8^+$ T cells.[23] MCP-1 is a chemotactic factor for lymphocytes.[24] MIP-1α also promotes polarization of $CD4^+$ Th0 cells to Th1 cells, which produce interferon-γ (IFN-γ). IFN-γ has been shown to be essential for the expression of granulomatous reactions in a mouse model of hypersensitivity pneumonitis.[25]

Treatment of acute HP patients with antigen avoidance and corticosteroids has been shown to decrease the synthesis of both MIP-1α and IL-8 in alveolar macrophages, further implicating their role in the pathogenesis of this disorder.[23]

Type IV Hypersensitivity Response

Type IV cell-mediated immune responses are thought to predominate with continued antigen exposure. Activated pulmonary macrophages secrete several cytokines, such as IL-1, TNF-α, IL-6, IL-12, and MIP-1α, and have increased expression of CD80/CD86 as well.[16,25,26] IL-12 and MIP-1α secretion by alveolar macrophages promotes polarization of $CD4^+$ Th0 cells to the Th1 phenotype.[19,27,28] Secretion of IL-1 and TNF-α cause fever and acute-phase reactions and stimulate Th1 cells to produce IFN-γ.[19] IFN-γ production by Th1 cells causes alveolar macrophages to secrete more IL-1 and TNF-α, thus creating a positive-feedback loop. Gudmundsson and colleagues found that IFN-γ is essential for the development of HP in mice.[25] The authors demonstrated that IFN-γ knockout mice developed only minimal inflammation and no granulomas after exposure to *Saccharopolyspora rectivirgula*, the causative agent in farmer's lung disease. Additionally, these mice developed inflammation and granulomas when given replacement IFN-γ. Other chemokines that are inducible by IFN-γ, such as IP-10, Mig, and I-TAC, have been found to be increased in the lungs of wild-type mice during development of HP after exposure to *S. rectivirgula*; however, IFN-γ knockout mice had reduced levels of these chemokines in the lungs after *S. rectivirgula* exposure. The production of IP-10, Mig, and I-TAC correlated with the presence of $CXCR3^+CD4^+$ T cells in wild-type mice exposed to *S. rectivirgula* compared with IFN-γ knockout mice.

Th1/Th2 Polarization

Th1 and Th2 cytokine profiles have been analyzed from bronchoalveolar lavage (BAL) and peripheral blood (PB) T cells in patients with HP.[29] Although there was no difference in IL-12 production between BAL and PB T cells, there was an increase in high-affinity IL-12R in BAL T cells and an increase in production of IFN-γ when recombinant IL-12 was added in the BAL T-cell group only. Additional support for the role of Th1 cytokines was shown in a study by Schuyler and co-workers.[30] The authors in this study showed that only Th1 $CD4^+$ T-cell lines were able to adoptively transfer experimental HP in mice exposed to *Micropolyspora faeni*. Additionally, Butler and colleagues showed that in mice susceptible to HP with a Th1 bias (C57BL/6 mice), Th2 cytokine messenger RNA was less stable than in Th2-biased mice (DBA/2 mice).[31] $CD8^+$ T cells are the most predominant T cell found in the BAL fluid and the lung tissue of patients with HP. These cells may produce Th1 or Th2 cytokines and modulate granuloma formation. Tc1 and Tc2 designate Th1- and Th2-like cytokine profiles produced by $CD8^+$ T cells.[32] These $CD8^+$ T cells are probably cytotoxic T cells, since suppressor function is decreased. The anti-inflammatory cytokine IL-10 appears to be necessary in preventing a severe granulomatous response in mice with HP.[33] Production of IL-10 was found to be decreased when BAL cells of patients with HP were stimulated compared with the patient's stimulated PB cells, thus suggesting a role for decreased IL-10 production in human HP.[29] Several chemokines also play a role in HP.[28] IL-8 is a chemotactic factor for $CD8^+$ T cells and neutrophils. IL-6 is also a chemoattractant for $CD8^+$ T cells and has been found to be increased in the BAL fluid of HP patients.

Costimulatory and Adhesion Molecules

An up-regulation of CD80/CD86 (B7-1/B7-2) on alveolar macrophages has been demonstrated in patients with HP.[26] These costimulatory molecules are involved in the differentiation and activation of T cells. Antigen-presenting cells present foreign antigen to the T cell via major histocompatibility complex and T-cell receptor interactions. CD80/CD86 on the antigen-presenting cell interacts with either CD28 or CTLA-4 during this process. CD28 is expressed on resting or activated T cells and promotes T-cell differentiation, while CTLA-4 negatively regulates T-cell proliferation. CTLA4-immunoglobulin treatment in mice exposed to intranasal *S. rectivirgula* has been shown to decrease inflammatory cell numbers in both BAL and lung tissue, and also to decrease the production of IL-4, IL-10, and IFN-γ in IL-2-stimulated pulmonary T cells.[34] The B7-CD28 costimulatory pathway has also been implicated as a cause for the accumulation of lymphocytes in the lungs of HP patients.[35] The expression of Bcl-xL, an antiapoptotic product of the *Bcl-2* gene family, and IL-2, which can inhibit apoptosis of inflammatory cells, are both increased through CD28 stimulation.[36] It has been demonstrated that patients with HP have increased levels of soluble Fas and an increased quantity of intracellular, inducible antiapoptotic gene Bcl-xL product in BAL fluid compared with normal patients. An increase in soluble Fas would prevent cross-linking between Fas antigen (CD95) and Fas ligand (FasL, CD95L), thus inhibiting apoptosis.[32,35]

Adhesion molecules may also play a role in the pathogenesis of HP. TNF-α induces the expression of adhesion molecules and chemoattractants, thus promoting the adhesion, activation, and migration of circulating leukocytes.[37] It has been demonstrated that HP patients have elevated levels of L-selectin in BAL fluid, and increased levels of E-selectin and P-selectin in PB compared with controls.[38] L-selectin, which is normally expressed on leukocytes, and E-selectin, which is normally expressed on endothelial cells, actively participate in leukocyte–endothelial cell interactions. P-selectins are involved in neutrophil migration at endothelial borders. In a study by Pan and colleagues, inhibition of E- and P-selectins in a murine model of HP, secondary to *S. rectivirgula*, led to decreased numbers of lymphocytes in BAL fluid and a decrease in the inflammatory response.[39]

Surfactant

Other factors that may play a role in the pathogenesis of HP are surfactant properties, properties of the extracellular matrix, and free-radical formation. Normal surfactant has been shown to inhibit the release of inflammatory cytokines by macrophages. Surfactant from HP patients has been shown in some studies to have a higher content of surfactant protein A, which stimulates inflammatory cytokine release, immunoglobulin production, and mitogen-induced proliferation.[40] Israel-Assayag and Cormier reported that surfactant was isolated from normal individuals and in patients with HP and were added to alveolar macrophage–PB monocyte cell cocultures and stimulated with phytohemagglutinin. This study demonstrated that surfactant from control subjects inhibited alveolar macrophage-induced lymphocyte proliferation in patients with HP, while surfactant from HP patients had a lower inhibitory effect on alveolar macrophage-induced lymphocyte proliferation.[41] This may indicate that changes in surfactant composition may lead to decreased suppressive activity of alveolar macrophages in patients with HP. However, another study detected a decrease in the surfactant protein A concentration in the BAL fluid from patients with HP.[42] Fatty acid composition of lung surfactant in patients with HP has not been shown to be significantly different from that in control patients.[43]

Free radicals may play a role in the inflammation of lung parenchyma through the oxidative action of lung neutrophils. Glutathione is an antioxidant normally found in the lungs, and it has been shown to be decreased in the BAL fluid of patients with farmer's lung compared with asymptomatic farmers after a standardized hay challenge.[44] Manganese superoxide dismutase and catalase are two intracellular antioxidant enzymes that are involved in lung defense.[45] Catalase was found to be constitutively expressed, but not up-regulated, in patients with a variety of interstitial lung diseases, including HP. Manganese superoxide dismutase, however, was found to be markedly up-regulated in patients with interstitial lung disease, including those with HP. This would suggest that these antioxidants are involved in protecting the lung from the progression of interstitial lung disease. Variants in the promoter region of tissue inhibitor of metalloproteinases-3 (TIMP-3) have been shown to decrease the susceptibility of patients to pigeon breeders' disease.[46] Matrix metalloproteinases are zinc-dependent proteinases that are involved in the degradation and turnover of extracellular matrix, and TIMPs are inhibitory to these proteinases. Therefore, TIMPs exert a regulatory role over the turnover of the extracellular matrix. TIMP-3 has been implicated as a fibrosis-promoting factor in mice.[47] Deposition of the proteoglycan versican in the extracellular matrix has also been shown to be specific for the early remodeling process in granulomatous lung diseases such as HP.[48]

TNF-α Polymorphisms

Genetic predisposition may also play a role, either through TNF-α polymorphisms or through HLA haplotypes. In a mouse model of HP, TNF-α has been shown to be elevated in the BAL fluid after challenge with *S. rectivirgula*, and an polyclonal antibody specific to TNF-α was demonstrated to abolish disease.[20] Schaaf and colleagues[49] demonstrated that patients with farmer's lung had an increased frequency of the *TNFA2* allele (polymorphism of the TNF-α gene promoter at position–308), which is associated with high TNF-α production, compared with controls and those with pigeon breeder's disease. Another study in Mexican patients with pigeon breeder's disease revealed an increase in this polymorphism compared with controls; however, there was no increase in the levels of TNF-α compared to those without the polymorphism, but there was an increase in BAL lymphocytosis.[50]

HLA Haplotypes

Patients with pigeon breeder's disease were shown to have a relative increase in the frequency of the alleles *HLA-DRB1*1305* and *HLA-DQB1*0501* and a decrease in *HLA-DQB1*0402* as well.[50] Other studies have shown a correlation between *HLA-DR3* and pigeon breeder's disease[51]; a correlation between *HLA-DR7* and haplotype *HLA-B35, DR4,* in a Mexican population (thought to be a Hispanic equivalent of Caucasian *HLA-B8, DR3*) and pigeon breeder's disease[52,53]; and a nonsignificant increase in *HLA-B8-DR3* in patients with pigeon breeder's disease.[54] *HLA-DR2* was found to be overrepresented among patients with farmer's lung, although the increase was not statistically significant.[55] In Japanese summer-type HP, a significant relationship was found among patients and *HLA-DQw3* compared with normal subjects.[56]

PATHOPHYSIOLOGY

All the disorders that comprise the HPs are due to the inhalation of organic antigens. The size of the protein complex is extremely small (1–2 μm) and always less than 5 μm in diameter. In general, particles greater than 5 μm in size are filtered by the tracheobronchial tree and removed by mucociliary clearance. The particle distribution in the lungs parallels the distribution of ventilation. It has demonstrated[57] that ventilation is greater in the dependent lung bases than it is in the apices of the lung. Therefore, the majority of organic antigens deposit in the dependent regions of the lung. However, as a result of regional differences in pulmonary artery pressure, lymphatic clearance of particulate material from the upper zones of the lung is slower than that in the lower zones of the lung. Therefore, antigen concentration depends on the balance between deposition and clearance. With chronic exposure, the upper zones of the lungs are more severely affected as a result of chronic retention of particles in this region of the lung. Seal and colleagues studied the biopsy and necropsy findings in five patients with acute HP and six with chronic HP. The upper lobes were more severely involved by fibrosis or cystic changes in patients with chronic disease, while patients with acute disease had more involvement of the lower lobes.[58]

HISTOPATHOLOGY

The histopathologic changes seen in patients with HP vary according to whether the disease is acute or chronic. Lung biopsy specimens from patients with acute hypersensitivity show alveolar and interstitial inflammation with marked prominence of lymphocytes, increased numbers of plasma cells, and activated macrophages with foamy cytoplasm (Fig. 49-2). Obstructive bronchiolitis with destruction of the airway wall has been reported. The classic triad of HP, mononuclear cell bronchiolitis, mononuclear cell interstitial infiltrates, and scattered nonnecrotizing granulomas is better identified in biopsy specimens from patients with the chronic form of HP. Reyes and co-workers reviewed the pathologic findings in 60 biopsy specimens from patients with farmer's lung. Prominent findings included interstitial fibrosis (65%), bronchiolitis obliterans (50%), foamy histiocytes (65%), granulomas that contained giant cells (70%), and mild pleural fibrosis (~50%).[16] The presence of noncaseating granulomas and a lymphocytic alveolitis is reminiscent of sarcoidosis, which has a similar pathologic presentation. Several characteristics help to distinguish between the two disorders. The granulomas in sarcoidosis are generally observed in bronchial wall, subpleural, and perivascular locations in contrast to their location in hypersensitivity pneumonitis, in which the granulomas are most frequently found in alveolar walls in a centrilobular distribution. The granulomas of sarcoidosis are usually demarcated either by a fibrous capsule or by surrounding normal lung. In HP, the granulomas are less well defined, and, frequently, the surrounding lung is abnormal because of lymphocytic infiltration.

LABORATORY FINDINGS

Bronchoalveolar Lavage

Sampling of the alveolar milieu by repeated BAL has become an important tool in understanding the mechanisms of inflammatory

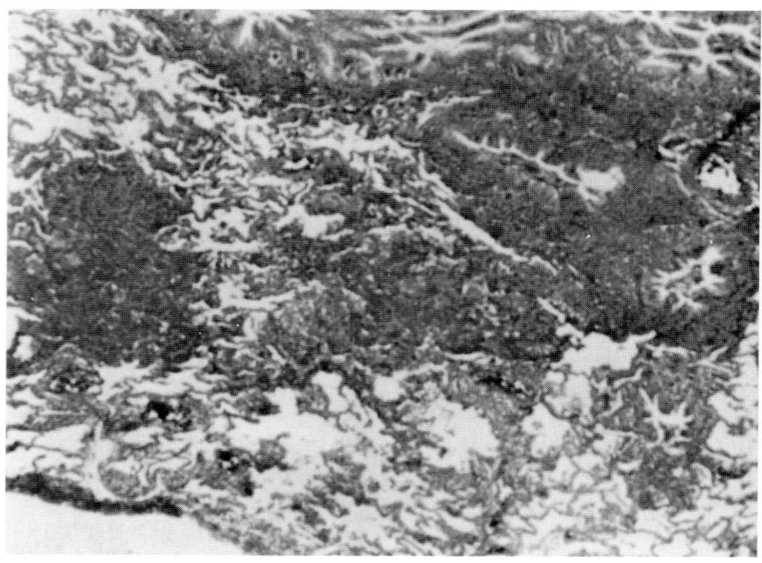

■ **FIGURE 49-2.** Appearance of a typical section of lung obtained by biopsy from a patient with "pigeon fancier's disease." Note the diffuse involvement as well as the large nodular cellular aggregates. At higher magnification, these were seen to contain chronic inflammatory cells, including plasma cells, lymphocytes, rare multinucleated giant cells, and large sheets of finely vacuolated histiocytes. Most of the alveolar septa were thickened by similar cells. (From Van Arsdel PP Jr, Thune R: Infiltrative lung disease and hypersensitivity to organic dusts. Yale J Biol Med 1967;40:501.)

lung disease. In the normal lung, macrophages represent about 90% of the cells, lymphocytes represent about 6% to 8%, and polymorphonuclear leukocytes represent 1% to 2% (see Chapter 7). The lymphocyte subpopulation is similar to that seen in PB, with the T cell being the predominant lymphocyte present in lavage fluid. The ratio of T cells to B cells is about 7:1, while the $CD4^+/CD8^+$ T-cell ratio is about 1.5:1.8. Results of BAL performed on patients with subacute and chronic forms of HP showed a significant increase in the percentage of lymphocytes ranging from 60% to 70%. The percentage of suppressor cytotoxic $CD8^+$ cells is greater than 40%, and that of the helper $CD4^+$ cells is 30% or less (with a reversal of the $CD4^+/CD8^+$ ratio to a value less than 1).[59] The soluble form of the CD8 molecule ($_s$CD8) was measured in the BAL fluid in Japanese summer-type HP and found to be significantly increased compared with healthy controls. The increased levels of $_s$CD8 correlated with the numbers of $CD8^+$ T cells in the BAL fluid.[60] In sarcoidosis, another systemic disease associated with lymphocytic alveolitis, the percentage of lymphocytes obtained from BAL fluid is usually close to 50%, and the $CD4^+/CD8^+$ ratio is usually 5:1 or higher. The increase in percentage of lymphocytes in the BAL fluid from patients with HP does not, however, correlate with the disease activity, since suppressor $CD8^+$ cells have also been shown to be present in BAL fluid of asymptomatic subjects exposed to a relevant antigen. $CD4^+$ and $CD8^+$ cells obtained from BAL fluids have been shown to be markedly activated, as determined by the presence of class II histocompatibility antigen (HLA-DR) and markers of activated T cells. It is, therefore, likely that the presence of activated cells in BAL fluid reflects a local ongoing T-cell-dependent process rather than a marker of disease activity. BAL studies in patients with HP have been used to examine sequential changes in the alveolar lining fluid after antigen exposure. Drent and colleagues studied 67 BAL fluid samples from 59 patients with HP due to bird exposure.[61] Patients were divided into four categories, based on the time period between the presumed termination of antigen exposure and the BAL:

Group 1: less than 24 hours
Group 2: 2 to 7 days
Group 3: 8 to 30 days
Group 4: 1 to 12 months

The early changes seen in the BAL fluid consisted of an increase in the percentage of polymorphonuclear neutrophils and total lymphocytes. The total lymphocyte count in the BAL fluid remained significantly elevated above control levels in group 4 (1–12 months following exposure), even when clinical symptoms subsided, while the polymorphonuclear cell count returned to baseline levels after the first week following antigen exposure. The increase in T-cell count was predominantly due to an increase in $CD8^+$ T cells.

The appearance of the alveolar macrophages in HP is distinctive. Large cells with excessive cytoplasmic vacuoles (foamy macrophages) constitute about 10% of the macrophage population. Although eosinophils are not increased, basophils and mast cells are present in increased numbers. Total protein content in lavage fluid is increased as well as IgG, IgA, and IgM.

Pulmonary Function Tests

Since 1966, almost 40 reports of respiratory function tests in children with HP have been published. The objective of those reports was to identify the typical physiologic abnormality, the rate of recovery after cessation of exposure, and the risk factors for permanent functional abnormalities. The most common abnormalities are decreased lung volume, decreased compliance, and diminished carbon monoxide diffusion. Several reports have shown evidence of small airway obstruction, consistent with the pathologic findings of bronchiolitis. However, it is difficult to document even severe small airway obstruction in the presence of severe interstitial disease, because the increased elastic recoil pressures produce normal or increased flow rates. In some patients with HP, a two-stage reaction may occur following inhalation of the offending dust. A bronchospastic response with a decrease in forced vital capacity, forced expiratory volume in 1 second, and forced expiratory flow occurs within minutes, followed by the late 5- to 6-hour response.

In 1984 Chiron and colleagues studied 12 children with HP aged 4 to 15 years and followed their pulmonary functions for several months after cessation of exposure to the relevant antigen.[62]

The pulmonary function results were grouped according to the length of the follow-up period: short term (<2 months), midterm (2–8 months), and long term (>8 months). During the short-term period, there was initial hypoxemia that gradually improved by the end of 2 months. The vital capacity, dynamic compliance, and carbon monoxide diffusion were significantly reduced. During the midterm period, the mean arterial oxygen tension (PaO_2) was normal; however, lung volumes, compliance, and diffusion capacity remained low. During the long-term period, all pulmonary functions were within normal limits, except for one patient who had reduced diffusion capacity and two patients who had a decrease in PaO_2 with exercise. For prognostic evaluation in children, total length of exposure to the antigen and severity of the initial respiratory symptoms had no influence on the pattern of pulmonary function or on the rate of recovery. In a longitudinal study of pulmonary function changes over a period of 18 years in 15 adults with pigeon breeder's disease, Schmidt and colleagues showed that, compared with the normal changes in pulmonary function expected with increasing age, the rates of decline in forced viral capacity, forced expiratory volume in 1 second, and diffusion capacity were four times greater in the symptomatic group.[63] Similar studies have not been reported in children; however, the vast majority of the case reports in children showed normal pulmonary function tests at the end of the follow-up period that ranged from less than 15 days to 2 years.

Immunologic Studies

A leukocytosis of up to 25,000/mm^3, with predominance of segmented neutrophils and eosinophilia up to 10%, may be seen during the acute phase of HP. In the chronic form the blood count is usually normal. Immunoglobulin levels, except for IgE, are often increased. Rheumatoid factor is present during the acute illness but disappears after cessation of exposure. Most patients with HP have precipitating antibodies to the offending antigen; for example, precipitating antibodies to pigeon serum and crude extracts of pigeon droppings have been reported in pigeon breeder's disease. Similarly, precipitating antibodies to thermophilic actinomycetes are common in patients with farmer's lung disease. Precipitating antibodies do not correlate with disease activity and are, therefore, not diagnostic but simply a marker for environmental exposure. Several techniques are available to detect hypersensitivity. The conventional Ouchterlony double-diffusion test is relatively insensitive and can also give a false-positive reaction. More sensitive methods, such as counterimmunoelectrophoresis, enzyme-linked immunosorbent assay, or radioimmunoassay, are also available. Reports from commercial laboratories are sometimes inaccurate, and selection of a special laboratory experienced in performing assays for the diagnosis of HP is important. Several in vitro tests to demonstrate cellular immune responses have been studied in the evaluation of HP; however, they are not routinely used in clinical practice. Skin tests with crude preparations of different antigens cause nonspecific irritation of the skin and give a positive reaction in 40% to 60% of exposed asymptomatic individuals.

Inhalation Challenge Studies

To establish a diagnosis and identify the offending antigen in HP, it is sometimes important to perform inhalation challenge testing. Patients are exposed to the suspected environment after being away from it for at least 72 hours and then monitored for 24 hours. Challenge can be carried out in the laboratory with close monitoring and should only be performed at centers well versed in inhalational challenges. Patients usually have baseline pulmonary function tests, blood studies, and chest radiography. They are then exposed to an extract of the suspected antigen via a nebulizer, and clinical and laboratory parameters are monitored for 24 hours. A typical response occurs between 4 and 6 hours after the challenge. This method is the only way to show a direct relationship between a suspected antigen and the disease process. A false-positive reaction can develop in normal individuals because of endotoxin present in the crude extracts. Another disadvantage of this method is the potential risk of having an exaggerated response to the antigen when delivered in high concentration by nebulizer.

ETIOLOGY

There are numerous causes of HP. The majority of the causes of HP in adult patients are related to occupational exposure. However, the majority of the causes of HP in children are related to environmental exposure at home; exposure to avian antigens is the most commonly reported cause in children.

A classification of the currently recognized diseases that occur with the inhalation of organic dusts is shown in Table 49-1.

SPECIFIC SYNDROMES

Bird Fancier's Lung

Hypersensitivity pneumonitis has been reported after longstanding exposure to avian antigens from pigeons, parrots, doves, parakeets, and chickens (Fig. 49-3). Proteins derived from feathers, serum, and excrement of several avian species have been shown to cause HP. Immunoelectrophoresis of pigeon droppings yielded four major antigens, two of which seem to be derived from pigeon.

Hypersensitivity pneumonitis is a rare diagnosis in pediatric respiratory diseases, with most of the cases reported due to exposure to avian proteins. Hendrick and colleagues estimated in 1978 that the prevalence of parakeet fancier's lung was between 0.5% and 7.5% among parakeet fanciers in the United Kingdom.[64] Thus, between 65 and 900 persons per 100,000 were likely to be affected by HP on the basis of statistics showing that 12% of the population was exposed to parakeets. At that time there were only two cases of parakeet hypersensitivity in children reported in the literature. The reasons for the relative infrequency of all forms of HP in children, compared with adults, are not understood. A difference in the intensity of exposure to environmental antigens, in individual susceptibility, and in the immune response to the antigens might explain this observation. However, misdiagnosis of this condition as recurrent pulmonary infections or atypical pneumonia might also be important. In fact, the majority of the reports of bird fancier's lung in children show that patients were initially treated for pulmonary infection before the diagnosis of HP was contemplated. There is usually an insidious onset with a prolonged course. The diagnosis should be considered in any child with persistent unexplained respiratory symptoms. Therapy consists of elimination of the birds and a course of corticosteroids. However, bird removal and environmental cleanup do not guarantee complete elimination of the bird's antigen. Craig and co-workers showed that bird antigens could be detected at high levels as long as 18 months after bird elimination, despite extensive environmental controls.[65]

TABLE 49-1. Classification of hypersensitivity pneumonitis

Type of Exposure	Disease	Source	Antigen
Environment	Humidifier lung	Home or work humidifiers, vaporizers, air-conditioning systems	*Amoeba proteus*, bacterial endotoxin, *Candida albicans*, *Acremonium*, *Flavobacterium*, *Klebsiella oxytoca*, *Pseudomonas*, thermophilic actinomycetes
	Home	Wood decay	*Leucogyrophana pinastri*
		Wet flooring	*Penicillium* and various fungi
		Contaminated basement (sewage)	*Acremonium*
		Residential composter's lung	*Streptomyces albus*
Hobbies and pets	Bird fancier's lung	Parakeet, pigeon droppings	Avian antigens
	Pigeon breeder's disease		Altered pigeon serum (IgA)
Vegetable products	Farmer's lung disease	Moldy hay	Thermophilic actinomycetes, *Micropolyspora faeni*, *Thermoactinomyces vulgaris*, *Aspergillus* sp.
	Bagassosis	Moldy pressed sugar cane	*Thermophilic actinomycetes*, *Thermoactinomyces sacchari*, *T. vulgaris*
	Cheese worker's disease	Cheese mold spores	*Penicillium casei*
	Coffee worker's lung	Green coffee	Unknown
	Detergent worker's disease	Detergent	*Bacillus subtilis* enzyme
	Enzyme worker's lung	Bacterial products	*B. subtilis* enzyme
	Familial hypersensitivity pneumonitis	Contaminated wood dust in walls	*B. subtilis*
	Mushroom worker's disease	Moldy compost	Thermophilic actinomycetes, *M. faeni*, *T. vulgaris*
	Malt worker's lung	Contaminated barley	*Aspergillus clavatus*
	Maple bark disease	Contaminated maple logs	*Cryptostroma corticale*
	Paprika splitter's lung	Paprika dust	*Mucor stolonifer*
	Sauna taker's disease	Sauna water	*Pullularia* sp.
	Sequoiosis	Moldy redwood sawdust	*Graphium* sp., *Pullularia* sp.
	Suberosis	Moldy cork	*Penicillium* sp.
	Tea grower's disease	Tea plants	Unknown
Animal products	Duck fever	Duck feathers	Duck proteins
	Turkey handler's disease	Turkey products	Turkey proteins
	Laboratory worker's hypersensitivity pneumonitis	Rat fur	Male rat urine
Insect products	Mill worker's disease	Mill dust, wheat flour	*Sitophilus granarius*
Chemicals	TDI hypersensitivity pneumonitis	TDI	Altered proteins (albumin, others)
	Plastic worker's lung	Trimellitic anhydride	Altered proteins
	Porcelain refinisher's lung	Diphenylmethane diisocyanate	Altered proteins
	Epoxy resin lung	Heated epoxy resin	Phthalic anhydride
Medications		Acebutolol	
		Acetaminophen	
		Amiodarone	
		Bleomycin	
		Ceftazidime	
		Chlorambucil	
		D-penicillamine	
		Fluoxetine hydrochloride (Prozac)	
		Gold	
		Hydroxyurea	
		INH	
		Minocycline	
		Nalidixic acid	
		Naproxen	
		Procarbazine	
		Propranolol	
		Trimethoprim	
	Pancreatic extract lung	Pancreatic enzymes (inhalation)	Pig pancreatic protein
	Pituitary snuff taker's lung	Pituitary powder (inhalation)	Ox or pig protein

INH, isoniazid; TDI, toluene diisocyanate.

Hypersensitivity Related to Home Environment

Hypersensitivity pneumonitis in office workers exposed to a contaminated humidifier or air-conditioning system was first reported by Banaszak and colleagues.[66] Subsequently, several cases of HP from exposure to contaminated water from humidifiers or vaporizers have been reported. The water in humidifiers is warm and may be grossly contaminated with a variety of microorganisms. In most cases thermophilic actinomycetes have been isolated from the humidifier water. Recently, there has been an increased use of ultrasonic humidifiers in homes. The water in the ultrasonic humidifiers can be contaminated with different microorganisms, such as fungi or bacteria, if the humidifiers are not cleaned completely. Thermophilic actinomycetes have rarely been isolated from ultrasonic humidifiers,

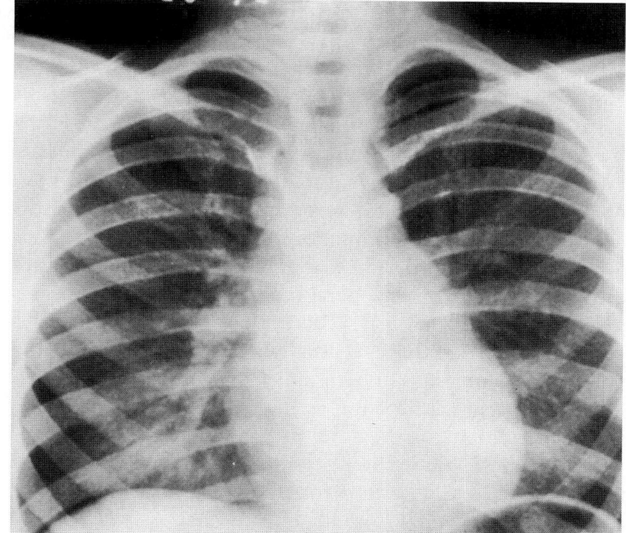

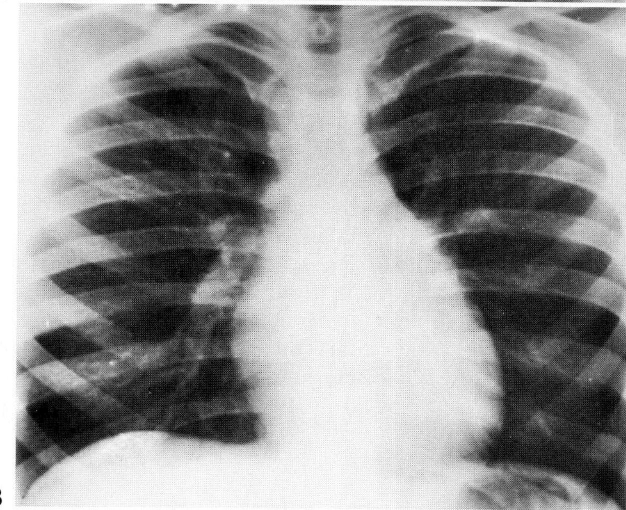

■ **FIGURE 49-3.** Chest radiographs of a child with hypersensitivity pneumonitis due to exposure to doves in the home taken during the acute (**A**) and convalescent (**B**) periods. (From Cunningham AS, Fink JN, Schlueter DP: Childhood hypersensitivity pneumonitis due to dove antigens. Pediatrics 1976;58:436.)

probably because of the absence of the heated environment suitable for their growth. The ultrasonic humidifiers disperse the causative antigens in droplets ranging in size from 0.5 to 3 μm that easily reach the distal airway. The inhalation of these antigens by sensitized individuals can therefore result in HP. The different etiologic antigens identified as cause for humidifier lung are listed in Table 49-1.

■ DIAGNOSIS

The diagnosis of HP depends on a high index of suspicion and a thorough history, with particular attention to the patient's home environment, hobbies, and work. The key to the diagnosis of HP lies in the identification of an etiologic agent and in the establishment of a relationship between exposure to the antigen and the development of symptoms. The laboratory results, namely chest radiographs showing fine nodular and reticular densities, pulmonary function tests with restrictive patterns, serum precipitins, BAL fluid showing an elevated lymphocyte count, and lung biopsy showing noncaseating granulomas in the alveolar walls, greatly aid in the diagnosis of HP.

■ THERAPY

Avoidance of re-exposure to causative antigens usually yields a complete remission of symptoms and normalization of pulmonary function, provided that chronic, irreversible, fibrotic changes have not developed. Among drug therapies, corticosteroids inhibit the pathologic lesions of HP and usually lead to remission of the acute form of the disease. Steroid therapy is given as prednisone at a dose of 40 to 60 mg/day, or 1.5 mg/kg body weight, in divided doses until there is significant clinical improvement, normalization of the roentgenogram, and return of pulmonary function tests to normal, at which point the steroids might be slowly tapered over a period of 6 weeks. Inhaled budesonide, 1000 μg four times daily, has been used successfully in a 12-year-old child with bird fancier's lung following a 5-day course of oral steroids.[67] The long-term use of steroids does not alter the respiratory symptoms or lung function in the chronic form of HP. In a double-blind, placebo-controlled study on the effects of corticosteroid treatment on farmer's lung, Kokkarinen and colleagues demonstrated that steroid therapy hastened the recovery from the acute phase, but there was no long-term beneficial effect.[68] Bronchodilators and antihistamines are not useful unless there is significant airway obstruction. Cromolyn sodium has been tried to prevent acute episodes, but the effect is variable. To prevent the permanent pulmonary parenchymal changes seen with the chronic form of HP, it is essential to make an early diagnosis and undertake the necessary measures to reduce the ongoing or recurrent pulmonary inflammatory process.

■ EOSINOPHILIC LUNG DISEASES

The eosinophilic lung diseases are a diverse group of lung disorders for which the common finding is an increase in circulating or tissue eosinophils. The early description of this group of diseases included illness associated with pulmonary symptoms or chest radiographic abnormalities and PB eosinophilia. However, the introduction of fiberoptic bronchoscopy in the early 1970s led to a substantial expansion of the list of eosinophilic lung diseases by identifying disorders characterized by an increase in BAL eosinophil number but not necessarily blood eosinophils. Although the term *eosinophilic lung diseases* implies that the inflammatory changes consist only of eosinophilic infiltrates, the lung injury is the net result of the recruitment of eosinophils, alveolar macrophages, lymphocytes, and neutrophils. The rapid expansion in the understanding of eosinophil cell biology and biochemistry; the role of different cytokines important for eosinophil generation, localization, and function; and finally the interaction between the eosinophil and other inflammatory cells have contributed to a better understanding of the development and outcome of pulmonary eosinophilic disease. In fact, eosinophilic lung diseases bear little clinical relationship to one another. Some affect the airways predominantly, some affect the lung parenchyma, and others affect predominantly the lung vasculature. Eosinophilic lung diseases also differ in their clinical course and outcome. While some diseases present with subtle symptoms and are self-limited, others present with respiratory failure and have a fatal outcome. Thus, the general concepts of eosinophilic lung diseases have changed since 1932 when Löffler initially described simple pulmonary eosinophilia.[69]

CLASSIFICATION

The term *pulmonary infiltrates with eosinophilia* was first described in 1952 by Reeder and Goodrich.[70] This led to the initial classification proposed by Croften and associates, who divided the eosinophilic lung diseases into five groups: Group I, Löffler syndrome or simple pulmonary eosinophilia; group II, prolonged pulmonary eosinophilia; group III, Weingarten's syndrome or tropical eosinophilia; group IV, pulmonary eosinophilia with asthma; and group V, polyarteritis nodosa.[71]

In 1969, Liebow and Carrington revised Croften's classification and included the term *chronic eosinophilic pneumonia*.[72] In 1973, McCarthy and Pepys classified eosinophilic pulmonary disorders as allergic bronchopulmonary aspergillosis and cryptogenic pulmonary eosinophilia.[73]

There is currently no optimal classification given the diversity of the diseases included under the term *eosinophilic lung disease*. However, the identification of the different immunopathologic mechanisms for the different entities might allow a more comprehensive classification in the future. In this chapter we will review a limited number of diseases in which eosinophils play a major role in lung inflammation.[74]

SIMPLE PULMONARY EOSINOPHILIA (LÖFFLER'S SYNDROME)

Simple pulmonary eosinophilia, as originally described by Löffler in 1932, is a transient illness characterized by migratory pulmonary infiltrates and increased PB eosinophil counts.[69] In the original description of the disease, most patients with simple pulmonary eosinophilia had *Ascaris* infection. Parasitic infection and drug reactions are currently an important etiology of this illness; however, in some reports no cause could be found for as many as one third of patients.

Patients usually have minimal or no pulmonary symptoms. Symptomatic patients have a mild febrile illness with myalgias, nonproductive cough, and dyspnea. There are usually no abnormalities on physical examination, but sometimes a few crackles or wheezes are heard. The chest radiograph abnormalities are usually bilateral and peripheral in nature, and may appear to be pleural based (Fig. 49-4). There are opacities that vary from patient to patient, that are usually a few centimeters in diameter, and that migrate and disappear within 2 weeks; in some cases they may last as long as 4 weeks. Parasites and ova are sometimes found in the stool after the resolution of the pulmonary illness. Since the disease is self-limited, asymptomatic patients do not require therapy. In patients with a severe illness, corticosteroid therapy is highly effective.

TROPICAL EOSINOPHILIA

In 1943 Weingarten assigned the term *tropical eosinophilia* to a syndrome characterized by severe spasmodic cough, massive peripheral eosinophilia, diffuse mottling in both lungs, and an excellent clinical response to neoarsphenamine. Neoarsphenamine was discovered accidentally when a patient with concurrent syphilis was given the drug and was cured of his tropical eosinophilia. The syndrome is endemic in India, Sri Lanka, and Southeast Asia (particularly Singapore) and has also been reported from endemic filarial regions worldwide. Immigration or travel from endemic to nonendemic zones has resulted in the syndrome being observed in North America and Europe.

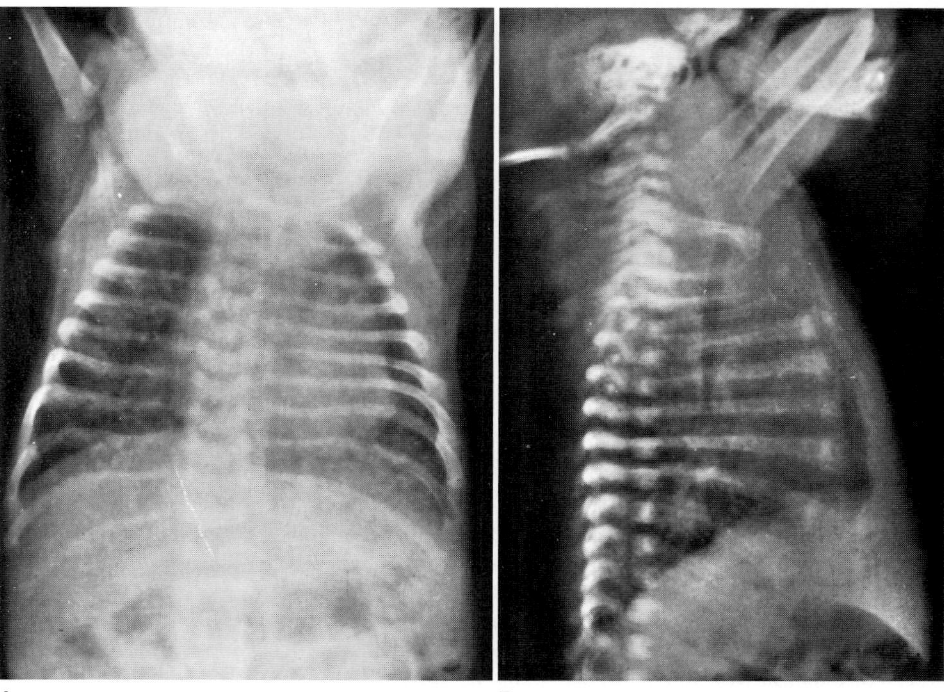

FIGURE 49-4. **A** and **B**, Radiograph, on admission, of a child with Löffler's syndrome. There is increased density at the base of the right lung. (Courtesy of the late John Kirkpatrick, MD, Boston Children's Hospital and Harvard University.)

Human filarial parasites, *Wuchereria bancrofti* or *Brugia malayi*, cause the vast majority of cases of tropical pulmonary eosinophilia syndrome.[75] The clinical features of tropical pulmonary eosinophilia syndrome result from an immunologic hyperresponsiveness to infection with the filaria parasites.[76] The pathogenesis of tropical pulmonary eosinophilia syndrome appears to be that microfilariae are released into the circulation from adult worms dwelling in lymphatics and are rapidly opsonized with antibody to filariae. They are then cleared in the pulmonary bed, where the parasites degenerate and release their antigenic components, initiating a local inflammatory response. The early pathologic findings are those of an alveolitis with a dense eosinophilic exudate. Lung biopsy specimens show eosinophilic pneumonia, bronchopneumonia, microabscesses, and granulomas. Six months to 2 years after the onset of symptoms, the eosinophilic exudate becomes a mixed-cell exudate consisting of eosinophils, mononuclear cells, and histiocytes. Persistent alveolitis leads to progressive interstitial fibrosis in many untreated or inadequately treated patients.

In the early stages of the disease, patients may have few localizing signs or symptoms, and they may present only with marked peripheral eosinophilia (>3000/mm^3). Very soon, the characteristic pulmonary involvement is seen with bouts of cough (classically nocturnal), dyspnea, and nocturnal wheezing. These symptoms are often accompanied by systemic manifestations such as low-grade fever, weight loss, and fatigue. Radiographs of the chest show increased bronchovascular markings with diffuse interstitial lesions, 1 to 3 mm in size, or mottled opacities involving primarily the middle and the basal regions of the lungs. The most common pulmonary function abnormalities are restrictive defects with reduced total lung capacity, vital capacity, residual volume, and diffusion capacity. In some patients there are superimposed obstructive abnormalities with decreased forced expiratory flow rates. In the PB, in addition to eosinophilia, levels of IgE are markedly increased (>1000 U/mL), and filarial antibodies can be detected. The presence of antibodies is diagnostically useful. Microfilariae can be found in biopsy specimens of lymph nodes or lung tissue, but histologic identification is not necessary for clinical diagnosis.

Periods of temporary remission occur even in untreated patients; however, in the absence of appropriate treatment, the pulmonary abnormalities become progressively worse. There is usually prompt symptomatic improvement following administration of the antifilarial drug diethylcarbamazine in doses of 6 to 12 mg/kg/day in three divided daily doses for 3 weeks. However, coughing, wheezing, dyspnea, PB eosinophilia, chest radiograph changes, and pulmonary function abnormalities may persist after treatment, secondary to the development of chronic interstitial lung disease. New therapies for tropical pulmonary eosinophilia include the microcline antibiotic ivermectin, which clears the microfilariae, and corticosteroids for their anti-inflammatory action.

PARASITIC INFECTIONS

Many parasites can cause pulmonary infiltrates with blood or pulmonary eosinophilia (Box 49-1 and Chapter 38). *Strongyloides*, *Ascaris*, *Toxocara*, and *Ancylostoma* are frequently the cause of infections in the United States. Patients could be infected with more than one parasite; therefore, persistence of pulmonary symptoms, despite treatment for one parasite, should prompt a search for other parasites.

Strongyloides stercoralis infection can cause transient pulmonary infiltrates, rash, and PB eosinophilia. The larvae enter the host through exposed skin and migrate to the lung. Then the larvae migrate up the airway and are swallowed into the gastrointestinal tract, where they develop into adult worms. Pulmonary infiltrates occur before the adult worms develop and consequently before ova can be found in the stool. *Strongyloides* can remain in the host indefinitely; therefore, patients could become symptomatic long after the initial infection. An enzyme-linked immunosorbent assay is available from commercial laboratories. The treatment is thiabendazole, 50 mg/kg/day in two divided doses for 2 days.

In developing countries *Ascaris lumbricoides* is the most common cause of PB eosinophilia with pulmonary infiltrates. After ingestion of eggs, the larvae hatch in the small intestine, pass through the intestinal wall, and migrate to the lungs. In the lungs the larvae mature into adult worms that move up the airway to be swallowed and to return to the gastrointestinal tract where they remain.

Patients with *Ascaris* infection are usually febrile with a nonproductive cough and chest pain. In severe cases hemoptysis occurs. Crackles and wheezes are heard on lung auscultation. The chest radiograph reveals bilateral densities that often involve the perihilar regions. Pulmonary function abnormalities are usually restrictive; however, mild airway obstruction can also develop. The pulmonary syndrome occurs before the adult worms mature; therefore, the stool examination for ova is usually negative for as long as 8 weeks after the onset of respiratory symptoms. During the pneumonic stage, the larvae can be isolated from gastric aspirates or sputum. The pig tapeworm *Ascaris suum* has been reported to cause pulmonary eosinophilic disease in humans. The intestinal infection is usually treated with oral mebendazole, 100 mg twice a day for 3 days.

Toxocara canis (the dog roundworm) is the cause of visceral larva migrans (see Chapter 38). The ingested eggs hatch in the intestine and then migrate via the blood to the liver, lungs, and other organs. Since mature worms do not develop in humans, stool examination for ova is usually negative. The syndrome is associated with pica, and neurodevelopmentally impaired children are at particular risk. Pulmonary symptoms, such as coughing and wheezing, are usually present in 80% of patients with visceral larva migrans, and crackles are sometimes heard

BOX 49-1 Parasites That Cause Eosinophilic Lung Disease

Ancylostoma sp.
Ascaris sp.
Brugia malayi
Opisthorchis sinensis
Dirofilaria immitis
Echinococcus sp.
Opisthorchis sp.
Paragonimus westermani
Schistosoma sp.
Strongyloides stercoralis
Toxocara sp.
Trichinella spiralis
Wuchereria bancrofti

on auscultation. Patients usually have increased levels of IgE and increased numbers of eosinophils in the blood. The diagnosis is made serologically. The infection is usually self-limited; however, treatment with thiabendazole or mebendazole may relieve the symptoms.

DRUG-INDUCED EOSINOPHILIA

Many different drugs have been associated with the development of pulmonary eosinophilia. In fact, drug reactions are one of the most commonly reported causes of pulmonary infiltrates with blood or pulmonary eosinophilia. Sulfonamides, including sulfasalazine, were the first recognized cause of this reaction, but more recently it has been described with the structurally similar drugs, sulfonylurea and chlorpropamide, and the antituberculous drug *p*-aminosalicylic acid. The tricyclic compounds imipramine and carbamazepine may also cause pulmonary eosinophilia. Of the hydantoins (nitrofurantoin, dantrolene, and phenytoin), nitrofurantoin is most likely to cause an adverse pulmonary reaction. The reaction may be seen within days of starting treatment.

Other drugs that have been implicated in pulmonary eosinophilia are listed in Box 49-2. Drug reactions may be associated with the simple form of pulmonary eosinophilia-like syndrome or the fulminant acute eosinophilic pneumonia-like syndrome, or may follow a more chronic course. Symptoms normally start within a month of starting the drug and include cough, dyspnea, and fever. Histologically, there is pulmonary interstitial edema with a lymphocytic and eosinophilic infiltrate, and the alveoli contain eosinophils and histiocytes. Peripheral eosinophilia, though common, is not an invariable finding. Chest radiographs show interstitial or alveolar infiltrates and often demonstrate Kerley B lines.

Confirmation of the adverse reactions may be carried out by challenging the patient with a single dose of the drug. Skin testing with either patch or prick tests is usually negative. In vitro lymphocyte transformation tests have been positive with some drugs, such as nitrofurantoin and carbamazepine. When the offending drug is discontinued, there is usually resolution of the symptoms and the eosinophilia, together with clearing of the chest radiograph. When resolution is slow, corticosteroid drugs may hasten the recovery, though not invariably.

ACUTE EOSINOPHILIC PNEUMONIA

Idiopathic acute eosinophilic pneumonia was first described in adults,[77–79] and in 1992 the first pediatric case was reported.[80] Patients usually present with an acute febrile illness of 1 to 5 days, associated with generalized myalgias, pleuritic chest pain, and severe hypoxemia. Patients rapidly develop hypoxemic respiratory failure, and the majority require mechanical ventilation. Pertinent findings on physical examination are high fever, respiratory distress, and basilar or diffuse crackles on auscultation. Wheezing may be noted. The initial chest radiograph may show mild interstitial infiltrates; however, within a few hours diffuse alveolar infiltrates involving all lobes are seen. Small to moderate-sized pleural effusions are common. The effusions have a high percentage of eosinophils (42% in one series) and usually have a high pH, consistent with the release of eosinophilic cationic protein. The percentage of eosinophils in the PB is usually normal. Serum IgE levels have been elevated in some patients. Lung biopsy specimens show alveolar edema and eosinophilic infiltrates in the interstitium, alveoli, and airway walls. There is a dramatic response to corticosteroids, usually within 24 to 48 hours. Usually therapy with steroids is prescribed for 4 to 8 weeks, and there has been no relapse of the disease after the discontinuation of treatment.[81] The diagnosis of acute eosinophilic pneumonia is one of exclusion, and every effort should be made to exclude an infectious etiology even after corticosteroid therapy is begun.

BOX 49-2 **Drugs That Cause Eosinophilic Lung Disease**

Ampicillin
Aspirin
Beclomethasone dipropionate (inhaled)
Bleomycin
Captopril
Carbamazepine
Chlorpromazine
Clarithromycin
Chlorpropamide
Clofibrate
Cocaine (inhaled)
Cromolyn (inhaled)
Desipramine
Diclofenac
Febarbamate
Fenbufen
Glafenine
GM-CSF
Gold
Ibuprofen
Imipramine
IL-2
IL-3
Iodinated contrast dye
L-Tryptophan
Mephenesin carbamate
Methotrexate
Minocycline
Naproxen
Nickel
Nitrofurantoin
p-Aminosalicylic acid
Penicillamine
Penicillin
Pentamidine (inhaled)
Phenytoin
Pyrimethamine
Rapeseed oil
Sulfadimethoxine
Sulfadoxine
Sulfasalazine
Sulindac
Tamoxifen
Tetracycline
Tolazamide
Tolfenamic acid
Vaginal sulfonamide cream

GM-CSF, granulocyte-macrophage colony-stimulating factor; IL-2, interleukin-2; IL-3, interleukin-3.

CHRONIC EOSINOPHILIC PNEUMONIA

Chronic eosinophilic pneumonia is an illness occurring predominantly in middle-aged women,[82,83] but it can occur at any age and in either sex. Its onset is usually insidious with profound systemic symptoms including fever, night sweats, weight loss, and anorexia, together with localized pulmonary manifestations such as cough, dyspnea, and wheezing. Asthma is present in 50% of cases. Patients may also have lymphadenopathy and hepatomegaly. Peripheral blood eosinophilia is typical, although it is not always present. Eosinophils can be found in the sputum, and they are nearly always found in BAL fluid. The erythrocyte sedimentation rate is usually elevated, and serum IgE is elevated in two thirds of the patients. The radiographic finding of extensive, dense, bilateral, peripheral infiltrates (the so-called negative image of pulmonary edema) is said to be diagnostic of chronic eosinophilic pneumonia.[84] CT images show peripheral airspace disease and may show hilar lymphadenopathy. Lung biopsy samples display accumulation of eosinophils and lymphocytes in the alveoli and the interstitium with thickened alveolar walls. Interstitial fibrosis has been reported in 50% of patients, and 25% show evidence of bronchiolitis obliterans. Corticosteroids cause a dramatic resolution of symptoms within 24 to 48 hours, and disappearance of chest radiograph abnormalities within 10 to 21 days. Most patients have a relapse of their symptoms if corticosteroids are discontinued in the first 6 months. If not treated, fewer than 10% of the patients have spontaneous resolution of their symptoms.

ALLERGIC ANGIITIS AND GRANULOMATOSIS

Allergic angiitis and granulomatosis was first described in 1951 by Churg and Strauss.[85] The clinical picture is one of systemic vasculitis, which is usually preceded for several years by allergies in the form of allergic rhinitis and asthma.[86] Patients develop peripheral eosinophilia with values up to 80%, and they gradually develop vasculitis involving small and medium-sized arteries and veins. Several organs are involved in Churg-Strauss syndrome: Eosinophilic infiltration of the upper airways presents with sinusitis, rhinitis, and nasal polyps; gastrointestinal symptoms include abdominal pain, diarrhea, bleeding, and obstruction; cardiovascular involvement presents with hypertension, pericarditis, and heart failure. Cardiac involvement is a common cause of death. Renal disease occurs in 49% of cases, and the central nervous system is involved in 27% of cases. Chest radiographs show pulmonary infiltrates that are patchy and transient. Eosinophilic pleural effusions and hilar adenopathy have been reported. Pulmonary function tests show obstructive defects, and lung histology demonstrates necrotizing giant cell vasculitis with interstitial and perivascular granulomas. Approximately 50% of affected people die within 3 months of the onset of vasculitis; however, those treated with corticosteroids have a mean survival time of 9 years. Therapy is usually continued for as long as 1 year.

IDIOPATHIC HYPEREOSINOPHILIC SYNDROME

Idiopathic hypereosinophilic syndromes (HESs) comprise diverse disorders that are characterized by elevated blood eosinophils (>1500 eosinophils/mm^3). HES typically involves the skin, heart, and lung. Skin lesions occur in more than 50% of patients. Cardiac disease is characterized by eosinophilic endocardial myelofibrosis, cardiomyopathy, valvular disease, and/or mural thrombus formation, and is life threatening. The diagnosis is established when there is elevated eosinophila for 6 months or longer, or for less than 6 months with evidence of organ damage. There is lack of evidence for parasitic, allergic, or other recognized causes of eosinophilia. Although HES is most common in adults 20 to 50 years old and shows a male preponderance, pediatric patients have also been identified. Investigators have recognized heterogeneity among patients with HES and have classified subtypes: myeloproliferative, lymphoproliferative, and unclassified.

The myeloproliferative or "classic" HES affects young male adults with eosinophilic endomyocardial disease and mucosal ulcers. Eosinophilic granules and mediators are deposited on the endocardium, resulting in myocardial degeneration and fibrosis. In addition, there are elevated serum tryptase levels, tissue fibrosis, and splenomegaly. Bone marrow biopsy specimens reveal increased numbers of CD25$^+$ atypical spindle-shaped mast cells. The majority of patients have been identified with a novel fusion gene, *FIP1L1-PDGFRA*. *FIP1L1-PDGFRA* is the result of an 800-kilobase deletion on chromosome 4 that brings together the *FIP1L1* and the gene for the cytoplasmic domain of the PDGFRα receptor. This results in a novel kinase protein. Importantly, most patients with this genetic cause of HES are responsive to the Bcr-Abl kinase inhibitor imatinib mesylate.[87]

The lymphoproliferative subtype of HES is characterized by T-cell clones producing Th2 cytokines, such as IL-5. The unclassified subtype comprises necrotizing eosinophilic vasculitis, episodic angioedema with eosinophilia, and nodules, eosinophilia, rheumatism, dermatitis, and swelling syndrome. Control of the eosinophilia is important to prevent organ damage from deposition of eosinophilic mediators. Typically, corticosteroids have been the mainstay of treatment. Other drugs have often been recommended in conjunction with corticosteroids, especially hydroxyurea, but also busulfan, cyclophosphamide, azathioprine, cyclosporine A, and vincristine. More recently, immunomodulatory therapy with IFN-α and monoclonal antibody to IL-5 has been described. In a recent report four patients with HES were treated with three doses of antibody to IL-5 (10 mg/kg; maximum 750 mg). Blood eosinophils declined by 10-fold and were sustained for 12 weeks after the last dose of antibody to IL-5.[88]

ALLERGIC BRONCHOPULMONARY ASPERGILLOSIS

Allergic bronchopulmonary aspergillosis (ABPA) is a Th2 hypersensitivity pulmonary disease caused by bronchial colonization with *Aspergillus* sp. that affects approximately 1% to 2% of asthmatics and 7% to 9% of individuals with cystic fibrosis (CF). It is relatively uncommon in childhood, although it has been reported in children with CF from England and the United States.[89–91]

Allergic bronchopulmonary aspergillosis is characterized by transient pulmonary infiltrates with eosinophilia in the PB and sputum. It was first described in adults in 1952 in England.[92] The disease is most commonly caused by *Aspergillus fumigatus*. This is a ubiquitous mold that is commonly encountered around farm buildings, barns, stables, silos, and compost heaps. Human disease has been reported from most countries of the world.

Allergic bronchopulmonary aspergillosis should be distinguished from other lung diseases caused by *A. fumigatus*, such as invasive aspergillosis, aspergilloma, IgE-mediated asthma from *A. fumigatus* sensitivity, and HP due to *A. fumigatus* or *A. clavus* (malt worker's disease).

PATHOLOGY

The gross pathology of ABPA demonstrates cylindrical bronchiectasis of the central airways, particularly those to the upper lobes. These airways may be occluded by "mucoid impaction," a condition in which large airways are occluded by impacted mucus and hyphae (Fig. 49-5). Airway occlusion may lead to atelectasis of a segment or lobe and, if the atelectasis is long-standing, saccular bronchiectasis may result. Typically, ABPA is worse in the upper lobes than in the lower lobes.

Microscopic examination of the airways shows infiltration of the airway wall with eosinophils, lymphocytes, and plasma cells. The airway lumen may be occluded by mucus containing hyphal elements and inflammatory cells, especially eosinophils. Squamous metaplasia of the bronchial mucosa commonly develops, and sometimes granulomas forms. Rarely, bronchiolitis obliterans or bronchocentric granulomatosis develops.

PATHOGENESIS

In the pathogenesis of ABPA, *A. fumigatus* spores 3 to 5 μm in size are inhaled and germinate deep within the bronchi into hyphae. In addition, fragments of the hyphae can be identified within the interstitia of the pulmonary parenchyma. The implication of this is that there is the potential for high concentrations of *A. fumigatus* allergens exposed to the respiratory epithelium and immune system. *Aspergillus fumigatus* releases a variety of proteins, including superoxide dismutases, catalases, proteases, ribotoxin, phospholipases, hemolysin, gliotoxin, phthioic acid, and other toxins.

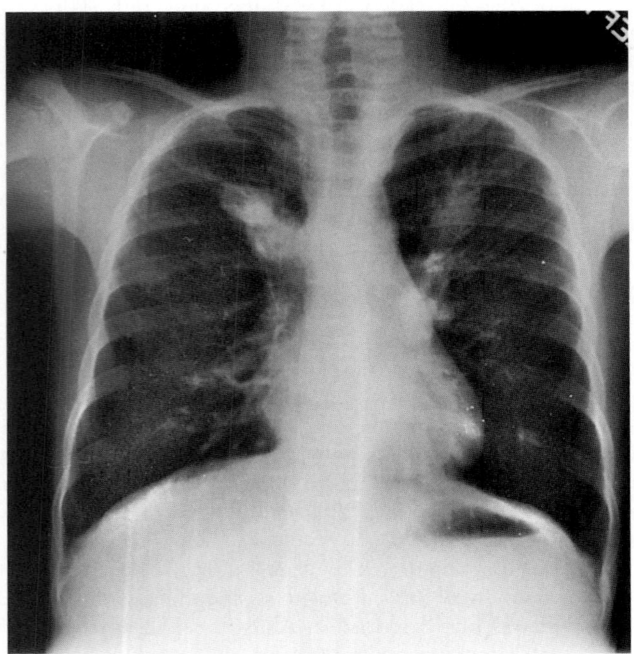

FIGURE 49-5. The chest radiograph of a 9-year-old girl with cystic fibrosis and allergic bronchopulmonary aspergillosis shows the radiologic features of mucoid impaction in dilated large airways. (Courtesy of Donald R. Kirks, MD. From Wilmott RW, Kravitz RM: Allergic bronchopulmonary aspergillosis. In: Hilman BC, ed: Pediatric Respiratory Disease. Philadelphia: WB Saunders, 1994.)

The first line of defense against *Aspergillus* colonization in the lungs is macrophage and neutrophil killing of the conidia and the hyphae. In the development of ABPA, Kauffman's group proposed that *Aspergillus* proteins have a direct effect on the pulmonary epithelia and macrophage inflammation. They demonstrated that *Aspergillus* proteases induce epithelial cell detachment.[93,94] In addition, protease-containing culture filtrates of *Aspergillus* induce human bronchial cell lines to produce proinflammatory chemokines and cytokines, such as IL-8, IL-6, and MCP-1. Thus, various *Aspergillus* proteins have significant biologic activity that disrupts the epithelial integrity and induces a monokine inflammatory response. This protease activity allows for enhanced allergen exposure to the bronchoalveolar lymphoid tissue immune system. This is evident by the bronchoalveolar lymphoid tissue synthesis of *Aspergillus*-specific IgE and IgA antibodies.

Recently, two genetic susceptibility factors have been proposed in the development of ABPA. Chauhan and colleagues[95–97] observed that asthmatic and CF patients who expressed *HLA-DR2* and/or *DR5* and lacked *HLA-DQ2* were at increased risk to develop ABPA after exposure to *A. fumigatus*. Furthermore, within *HLA-DR2* and *HLA-DR5*, there are restricted genotypes. In particular, *HLA-DRB1*1501* and *HLA-DRB1*1503* were reported to produce high relative risk. On the other hand, 40% to 44% of non-ABPA atopic *Aspergillus*-sensitive individuals have the *HLA-DR2* and/or *HLA-DR5* genotype. Additional studies indicated that the presence of *HLA-DQ2* (especially *HLA-DQB1*0201*) provided protection from the development of ABPA. Recently, increased sensitivity to in vitro IL-4 stimulation as measured by enhanced expression of the low-affinity IgE receptor, CD23, on B cells was observed in ABPA patients.[98,99] This was associated with single-nucleotide polymorphisms of the IL-4 receptor alpha chain (IL-4Rα) in 92% of ABPA subjects, principally the IL-4-binding single-nucleotide polymorphism Ile75Val.[100]

This increased sensitivity to IL-4 is demonstrated by increased expression of CD23 and CD86 on B cells of ABPA subjects and CD23 expression increased during flares of ABPA.[99] CD23 is expressed on a variety of cells, including B cells, natural killer cells, subpopulations of T cells, and a subpopulation of dendritic cells. T-cell CD23 and B-cell CD21 form a costimulatory pathway. T-cell CD28 and B-cells CD80 and CD86 costimulatory pathways activate both T and B cells, and CD28:CD86 is important in IgE synthesis. CD86 is also found on dendritic cells that have the histamine receptor 2, which skews antigen-specific T cells to a Th2 response. In a murine model of ABPA, Kurup and colleagues have found that CD86 expression is up-regulated in the lung tissue (V.P. Kurup, Medical College of Wisconsin, personal communication). Recently, we have also observed increased CD86 expression on monocyte-derived dendritic cells of ABPA subjects. Thus, antigen-presenting cells such as monocytes and dendritic cells bearing *HLA-DR2* and/or *HLA-DR5* and increased sensitivity to IL-4 stimulation probably play a critical role in skewing *A. fumigatus*–specific Th2 responses in ABPA.

Brouard and co-workers recently reported a third genetic risk, the association of the *−1082GG* genotype of the IL-10 promoter with colonization with *A. fumigatus* and the development of ABPA in CF.[101] The *−1082GG* polymorphism has been associated with increased IL-10 synthesis; whereas the *−1082A* allele has lower IL-10 synthesis. Thus, dendritic cells expressing HLA-DR2/DR5 that have an HR2 phenotype, increased IL-10 synthesis, and increased sensitivity to IL-4 stimulation due to IL-4Rα polymorphisms, may be responsible for skewing *Aspergillus*-specific Th2 responses in ABPA. In summary, there are probably three genetic risks in the development of ABPA: (1) HLA-DR2/DR5 restriction, (2) IL-4Rα single-nucleotide polymorphisms, and (3) IL-10 promoter mutations that result in increased B-cell activity, increased HR2 monocyte–dendritic cell phenotype, and increased *Aspergillus*-specific Th2 responses.

Recent studies in asthma have also implicated the role of bronchial epithelia and mesenchymal cells forming the epithelial-mesenchymal trophic unit in airway remodeling.[102] It was reported that the epithelial-mesenchymal trophic unit in asthma responded to IL-4 and allergens, such as Der p1, with a profibrotic response. In ABPA subjects with IL-4Rα single-nucleotide polymorphisms and with increased sensitivity to IL-4 stimulation, this may result in increased bronchial epithelial secretion of IL-8, granulocyte-macrophage colony-stimulating factor, and transforming growth factor (TFG-α), the ligand for epidermal growth factor, and stimulation by *Aspergillus* proteases augment this activity. Thus, the genetic risk factors that result in increased allergic *Aspergillus*-specific Th2-mediated responses, in conjunction with increased reactivity to *Aspergillus* proteins in the epithelial-mesenchymal trophic unit, lead to bronchial destruction and fibrosis.

CLINICAL MANIFESTATIONS

Clinical symptoms of ABPA include increased coughing, episodes of wheezing, anorexia, malaise, fever, and expectoration of brown plugs. ABPA can present acutely with acute symptoms and signs associated with transient pulmonary infiltrates and eosinophilia or with mucoid impaction; it may also present as an exacerbation of a chronic disease characterized by proximal bronchiectasis. It is thought that the chronic form of the disease develops following the acute process and that it can be prevented by effective therapy. In chronic ABPA, the acute episodes are superimposed on a background of chronic cough and sputum production.

In adults, ABPA usually affects the younger age group of adult asthmatics, and most cases occur before 40 years of age. In pediatrics, ABPA rarely affects children with asthma, and it is usually seen in children with CF, who may simply appear to have a worsening of their pulmonary status or an acute pulmonary exacerbation of CF. ABPA does sometimes affect children with asthma, and there is a report of three children who developed it before 2 years of age.[103]

Physical examination shows the signs of chronic lung disease from CF or asthma, such as hyperaeration of the lungs, expiratory wheezing, a chronic productive cough, and crackles or wheezes. The chronically ill patient with bronchiectasis may have coarse crackles, weight loss, and digital clubbing.

The clinical criteria for the diagnosis of ABPA developed at a recent Cystic Fibrosis Foundation consensus conference are shown in Box 49-3. It has been suggested that a certain number of these criteria should be present to make the diagnosis of ABPA, although this approach has not been validated in childhood. A problem with applying the criteria in children is that usually ABPA occurs in children with CF in whom many of the criteria could be due to the underlying disease. Some children with CF appear to have a clinical variant of ABPA without having all the typical criteria, and they may respond clinically to corticosteroids. Patients being considered for this diagnosis should have skin testing with *A. fumigatus* antigen. The simple skin-prick test is a useful screening test, as ABPA is very unlikely in patients with a negative reaction. If the skin-prick test is negative but the diagnosis appears likely, serum should be studied for the presence of specific IgE and IgG antibodies. A dual-reaction skin test with an immediate (10–15 minutes) and a late (4–8 hours) reaction occurs in one third of patients with ABPA.

BOX 49-3 Criteria for Diagnosis of Allergic Bronchopulmonary Aspergillosis in Cystic Fibrosis

Classic Case

1. Acute or subacute clinical deterioration not attributable to another etiology
2. Total serum IgE concentration greater than 1000 IU/mL unless patient is receiving corticosteroid therapy
3. Immediate cutaneous reactivity to *Aspergillus fumigatus* while the patient is not being treated with antihistamines or in vitro presence of serum IgE antibody to *A. fumigatus*
4. Precipitating antibodies or serum IgG antibody to *A. fumigatus*
5. New or recent abnormalities on chest radiography or chest CT that have not cleared with antibiotics and standard physiotherapy

Minimal Diagnostic Criteria

1. Acute or subacute clinical deterioration not attributable to another etiology
2. Total serum IgE concentration greater than 500 IU/mL unless patient is receiving corticosteroid therapy. If ABPA is suspected and the total level is 200 to 500 IU/mL, repeat testing in 1 to 3 months is recommended. If patient is taking steroids, repeat when steroid treatment is discontinued.
3. Immediate cutaneous reactivity to *Aspergillus fumigatus* while the patient is not being treated with antihistamines or in vitro presence of serum IgE antibody to *A. fumigatus*
4. One of the following: (a) precipitins to *A. fumigatus* or in vitro documentation of IgG antibody to *A. fumigatus;* or (b) new or recent abnormalities on chest radiography or chest CT that have not cleared with antibiotics and standard physiotherapy

Modified from Stevens DA, Moss RB, Kurup VP, et al: Allergic bronchopulmonary aspergillosis in cystic fibrosis—state of the art. Cystic Fibrosis Foundation Consensus Conference. Clin Infect Dis 2003;37(Suppl 3):S225–S264.

DIFFERENTIAL DIAGNOSIS

Several diseases cause pulmonary infiltrates in children with asthma or CF. The differential diagnosis of ABPA should include the following: viral or bacterial pneumonia, poorly controlled asthma with mucoid impaction or atelectasis, inhaled foreign body, CF (with or without ABPA), immotile cilia syndrome, tuberculosis with eosinophilia, sarcoidosis, pulmonary infiltrates with eosinophilia syndrome, HP, and pulmonary neoplasm.

CLINICAL STAGING

The spectrum of ABPA varies widely, from individuals with mild asthma and occasional episodes of pulmonary eosinophilia (with no long-term sequelae), to patients with fibrosis, honeycomb lung, and respiratory failure. Patterson and colleagues have suggested a clinical classification with five clinical stages.[104] Stage I is the acute stage of ABPA with many of the typical features of the disease. If this stage goes into remission, the infiltrates clear, symptoms reduce, and the serum IgE value will decline by up to 35% within 6 weeks. Stage II is remission. Stage III is an exacerbation associated with the recurrence of the initial symptoms and a twofold increase in serum IgE level. Stage IV is reached when patients need continuous corticosteroids either to control their asthma or to prevent a recurrence of ABPA. Stage V is the fibrotic stage, which is present when there is severe upper lobe fibrosis present on the chest radiograph, and it may be associated with honeycombing. The stage V lesions may not respond to corticosteroids, although steroids are often necessary to maintain a bronchodilator response, and severe wheezing may develop if steroids are discontinued. Pulmonary fibrosis is an advanced complication that can lead to pulmonary hypertension and cor pulmonale.

BOX 49-4 The Radiologic Features of Allergic Bronchopulmonary Aspergillosis

- Homogeneous consolidation—patchy, segmental, triangular, or oblong
- Air-fluid levels in proximal bronchi
- "Tram-line" shadows—two parallel hairline shadows radiating from a hilum
- "Toothpaste" shadows—secretions in ectatic bronchi
- "Gloved-finger" shadows-secretions in a dilated bronchus with an occluded blunt end
- Ring shadows—small, circular lesions representing bronchiectasis
- Atelectasis—affecting a segment, lobe, or whole lung
- Contracted upper lobes with honeycomb lung—advanced irreversible lung disease

RADIOGRAPHIC FINDINGS

There are several characteristic radiographic abnormalities associated with ABPA (Box 49-4). The most common lesion is a large, homogeneous shadow in one of the upper lobes with no change in volume (Fig. 49-6). The shadow may be triangular, lobar, or patchy, and it frequently moves to another site. "Tram line"

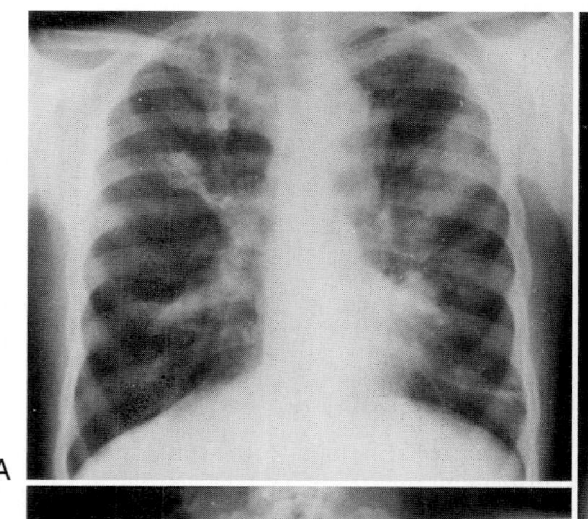

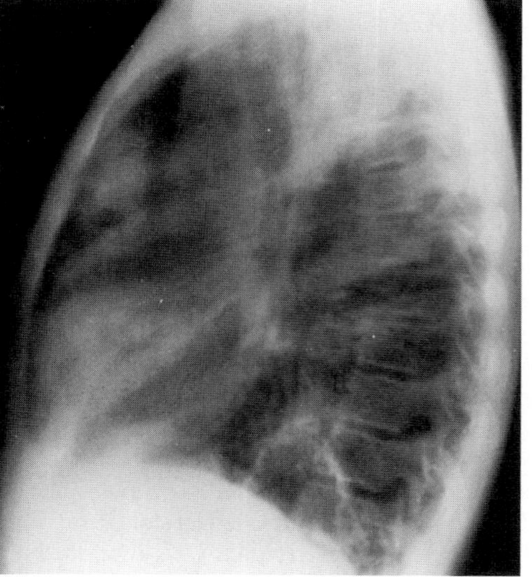

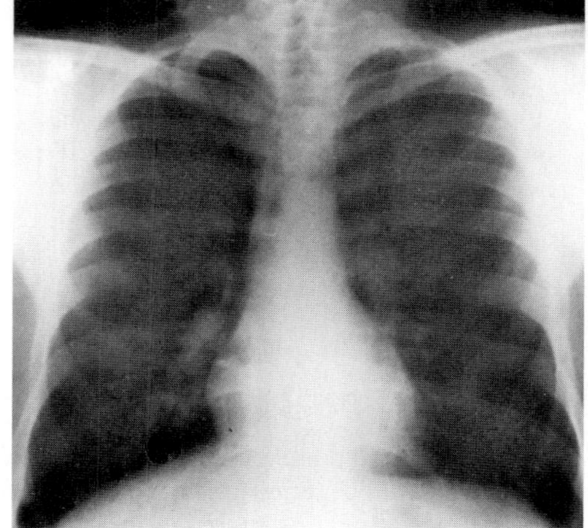

FIGURE 49-6. A and **B,** Roentgenograms of a 13-year-old boy with allergic bronchopulmonary aspergillosis. Note atelectasis in the left base and the left lingula. There is consolidation of the right upper lobe and both mid-lungs with dilated bronchi in apical segments of both upper lobes. Note bullous lesion of right suprahilar area. **C,** In same patient at age 19 years, lungs are clear except for the right hilar density and linear streaking (probable fibrosis) in the left lower lobe.

shadows are fine parallel lines radiating from the hila that represent inflammation of airway walls. Mucoid impaction causes toothpaste shadows or gloved-finger shadows (see Fig. 49-5). Several adult patients have been reported with normal chest radiographs, so radiographic abnormalities are not invariably present. In these individuals, cylindrical bronchiectasis was demonstrated by tomography or CT scan.

LABORATORY INVESTIGATIONS

Laboratory tests that support the diagnosis of ABPA are those that demonstrate allergy to the mold, such as a positive specific IgE test and positive *Aspergillus* precipitins. The precipitins are only weakly positive compared with the strong reactions seen in patients with mycetomas. Culture of *A. fumigatus* from the sputum is only a secondary criterion for the diagnosis of ABPA, because a large proportion of individuals with CF without ABPA have *Aspergillus* on sputum cultures. Some normal individuals and many individuals with lung diseases have small numbers of spores in their sputum; these are probably present because of passive inhalation. The presence of hyphae is more specific, and the presence of eosinophils in association with hyphal elements is suggestive of the diagnosis. The presence of eosinophilia in sputum or blood is suggestive of ABPA and is a primary diagnostic criterion. The PB eosinophil count is usually greater than $1000/mm^3$, and values greater than $3000/mm^3$ are common.

An increased serum IgE value is very characteristic of ABPA, and values may reach as high as 30,000 IU/mL. Usually, the value is greater than 1000 IU/mL. Much of the IgE is not specific to *Aspergillus* but is the result of polyclonal B-cell activation.[105] The IgE level is a very useful marker of disease activity, and it can be used to follow outpatients for "flares."

The usual pattern of serum precipitins is that immunoelectrophoresis shows one to three precipitin lines, often to only one extract. Patients with aspergilloma will have multiple precipitin lines to all antigen extracts. Extracts of *A. fumigatus* contain a complex mixture of proteins that are mainly derived from the hyphae. Antigenic composition varies between batches according to the culture conditions, even within the same laboratory. There is, therefore, a lack of standardization that makes it difficult to compare results between laboratories. However, there has been some success with purification of the major antigenic components that may lead eventually to improved diagnosis. We find it best to send all our testing to one central laboratory that has well-established methods for the characterization of the serologic responses to *A. fumigatus*.

THERAPY

Treatment is designed first to control the acute episodes and then to limit the development of chronic lung disease. Most cases of ABPA require treatment with systemic corticosteroids, and the treatment of choice is oral prednisone. Steroid therapy rapidly clears the eosinophilic infiltrates and the associated symptoms, although it is less effective at treating mucus impaction. The usual starting dose is 0.5 mg/kg/day, taken each morning, and this dose is maintained for 2 to 4 weeks while following the patient clinically and checking the chest radiograph for resolution of the acute process. After this induction treatment, the dose of prednisone should be reduced to 0.5 mg/kg given on alternate days. If mucus impaction persists and is associated with atelectasis, bronchoscopy should be performed to confirm the diagnosis and to attempt to remove the mucus plugs.

Following resolution of the acute process, the dose of prednisone should be reduced over 1 to 3 months. Chronic treatment with corticosteroids is controversial, especially in adults, because only a minority of patients with ABPA are at risk of chronic lung disease. The relationship between acute episodes and lung damage is unclear, and the precise dose of prednisone is not certain, since acute exacerbations may continue while the patients are on low doses of steroids. However, children with ABPA usually have CF and may need treatment with long-term corticosteroids to prevent progressive lung damage. Therefore, we usually maintain therapy with a dose of 0.5 mg/kg on alternate days for 3 months and then, after 3 months, the dose of prednisone is tapered over a further 3 months while checking the chest radiograph and the serum IgE level for evidence of relapse. Initially, the serum IgE level should be checked at every visit and, if the level increases by twofold or more, the steroid dose should be increased. We recommend that patients are followed with serum IgE levels and chest radiographs every 6 months for the first 1 to 2 years, and then, if the child remains in remission, it should be possible to reduce the frequency of these studies.

In recent years, the antifungal agent itraconazole has been used as adjunctive therapy in an attempt to reduce the doses of steroids that are required. Itraconazole should not be used as a sole agent. Initially, there were only open nonrandomized studies that indicated that itraconazole is a useful adjunct to systemic corticosteroid therapy. More recently a double-blind, randomized, placebo-controlled trial of itraconazole 200 mg twice daily for 16 weeks has demonstrated a reduction in corticosteroid dose and IgE level with an increase in pulmonary function and exercise tolerance.[106] A more recent randomized, controlled trial showed that treatment of stable ABPA in adults with 400 mg/day itraconazole resulted in a significant reduction in sputum eosinophil count, sputum eosinophilic cationic protein levels, serum IgE concentrations, and *Aspergillus*-specific IgG. There was also a reduction in episodes of exacerbation requiring treatment with systemic steroids.[107] In the treatment of children with ABPA, we have used a dose of 10 mg/kg/day of itraconazole.[108]

There is no place for immunotherapy in children with ABPA, since it is ineffective and potentially dangerous. Inhaled anti-inflammatory agents, such as cromoglycate and beclomethasone are not generally thought to be effective. The role of inhaled spores in the pathogenesis of ABPA is unclear, but there is a seasonal incidence of ABPA that is probably related to seasonal changes in mold spore counts. Therefore, it is reasonable to advise patients with ABPA to avoid exposure to places with high spore counts, such as damp basements, barns, and compost heaps.

PROGNOSIS

The prognosis for children with ABPA is good if the disease is detected early and treatment started promptly. It is important that the diagnosis is made and treatment commenced before there is permanent lung damage from bronchiectasis. In such patients, there should be no progression of the disease, although relapses can occur many years later, and long-term follow-up is recommended. In children with CF, the relapses seem to be more frequent than they are in people with asthma, and careful surveillance is necessary to ensure resolution of the disease process. In some CF patients, it is difficult to wean the steroids without an increase in symptoms, such as dyspnea and wheezing; whether this is due to the underlying CF lung disease or due to patients going from stage II to stage III ABPA on withdrawal of steroids is unclear. Symptoms are not a reliable guide to therapy; therefore, it is important to reevaluate the chest radiograph and the serum IgE at regular intervals until a long-term remission is established.

CLINICAL APPROACH TO EOSINOPHILIC PULMONARY DISEASES

The diagnosis of eosinophilic lung disease should be considered when peripheral eosinophilia occurs in conjunction with lung disease or when there are increased numbers of eosinophils in lung tissue or BAL fluid. Several pulmonary diseases that do not fall in the classification of an eosinophilic lung disease are associated with some degree of PB eosinophilia or increased eosinophil count in BAL fluid. For example, interstitial lung diseases, such as idiopathic pulmonary fibrosis and HP, are associated with increased PB eosinophil counts. In idiopathic pulmonary fibrosis and bronchiolitis obliterans with organizing pneumonia, there is an increased eosinophil count in the BAL fluid. An increase in BAL and PB eosinophils has also been reported in Hodgkin's disease. Fungal infections with coccidioidomycosis and *P. carinii* are associated with BAL eosinophilia.

The most valuable information is derived from the history and physical examination. A history of asthma may suggest ABPA or Churg-Strauss syndrome. Travel history may raise the suspicion of parasitic infection and tropical eosinophilia. Remote travel history should be elicited, since *Strongyloides stercoralis* and *Opisthorchis sinensis* can persist for several decades before clinical presentation. Contact with dogs may suggest *Toxocara* or *Ancylostoma* infection. A detailed history of the use of prescription and nonprescription drugs should be obtained. A white blood cell count and differential cell count might help to distinguish between the diseases associated with low PB eosinophil counts with increased eosinophil counts in BAL fluid and diseases with both peripheral and tissue eosinophilia. Acute eosinophilic pneumonia, *P. carinii* pneumonia, and some drug-induced lung diseases have eosinophilia in the BAL fluid. Simple pulmonary eosinophilia, chronic eosinophilic pneumonia, ABPA, Churg-Strauss syndrome, idiopathic hypereosinophilic syndrome, and parasitic infection typically have increased numbers of blood eosinophils. Stools should be examined on multiple occasions for evidence of parasitic infection. Certain parasites such as *Trichinella*, *Paragonimus*, *Ancylostoma*, *Toxocara*, and *Filaria* cannot be diagnosed by stool examination. Serologic tests can help to make a diagnosis of ABPA. Pulmonary function tests help to categorize eosinophilic lung diseases into those that are usually accompanied by restrictive ventilatory defects and those that are accompanied by an obstructive ventilatory defect. Acute eosinophilic pneumonia, chronic eosinophilic pneumonia, interstitial lung diseases, and tropical eosinophilia usually lead to a restrictive defect, whereas asthma, bronchiolitis obliterans, ABPA, and Churg-Strauss syndrome are associated with an obstructive defect. BAL can provide the first indication of an eosinophilic lung disease. A very high percentage of eosinophils in BAL cell counts (>20%) suggests acute eosinophilic pneumonia, chronic eosinophilic pneumonia, hypereosinophilic syndrome, parasitic infections, Churg-Strauss syndrome, or drug reactions. Parasitic and fungal infections could be diagnosed if the organism were identified in the BAL fluid. Finally, lung biopsy may be indicated to diagnose interstitial diseases, vasculitis, or fungal infections.

Eosinophilia serves as a marker for a group of diverse lung diseases. It is hoped that, with understanding of the immunopathology and the factors that regulate eosinophil traffic, a comprehensive, systematic classification will become a reality.

REFERENCES

1. Ramazzini B: De Morbis Artificum Diatriba (Diseases of Workers). Modena, Italy, 1700.
2. Campbell JM: Acute symptoms following working with hay. BMJ 1932;2: 1143–1144.
3. Reed CE, Barbee RA: Pigeon-breeders' lung. A newly observed interstitial pulmonary disease. JAMA 1965;193:261–265.
4. Hargreave FE, Pepys J, Longbottom JL, Wraith DG: Bird breeder's (fancier's) lung. Lancet 1966;1:445–449.
5. Stiehm ER, Reed CE, Tooley WH: Pigeon breeder's lung in children. Pediatrics 1967;39:904–915.
6. Ostergaard JR: Reversible pulmonary arterial hypertension in a 6-year-old girl with extrinsic allergic alveolitis. Acta Paediatr Scand 1989;78:145–148.
7. Fink JN: Hypersensitivity pneumonitis. Clin Chest Med 1992;13:303–309.
8. Bourke SJ, Banham SW, Carter R, et al: Longitudinal course of extrinsic allergic alveolitis in pigeon breeders. Thorax 1989;44:415–418.
9. Hodgson MJ, Parkinson DK, Karpf M: Chest X-rays in hypersensitivity pneumonitis. A metaanalysis of secular trend. Am J Ind Med 1989;16:45–53.
10. Cook PG, Wells IP, McGavin CR: The distribution of pulmonary shadowing in farmer's lung. Clin Radiol 1988;39:21–27.
11. Hansell DM: High resolution computed tomography in sarcoidosis and extrinsic allergic alveolitis. Imaging insights. Sarcoidosis 1992;9:21–28.
12. Lynch DA, Rose CS, Way D, King TE Jr: Hypersensitivity pneumonitis. Sensitivity of high-resolution CT in a population-based study. AJR Am J Roentgenol 1992;159:469–472.
13. Muller NL, Mayo JR, Zwirewich CV: Value of MR imaging in the evaluation of chronic infiltrative lung diseases. Comparison with CT. AJR Am J Roentgenol 1992;158:1205–1209.
14. Gurney JW: Hypersensitivity pneumonitis. Radiol Clin North Am 1992;30:1219–1230.
15. Agostini C, Trentin L, Facco M, Semenzato G: New aspects of hypersensitivity pneumonitis. Curr Opin Pulm Med 2004;10:378–382.
16. Reyes CN, Wenzel FJ, Lawton BR, Emanuel DA: The pulmonary pathology of farmer's lung disease. Chest 1982;81:142–146.
17. Wild LG, Lopez M: Hypersensitivity pneumonitis. A comprehensive review. J Investig Allergol Clin Immunol 2001;11:3–15.
18. Fink JN, Schlueter DP, Sosman AJ, et al: Clinical survey of pigeon breeders. Chest 1972;62:277–281.
19. Mohr LC: Hypersensitivity pneumonitis. Curr Opin Pulm Med 2004;10: 401–411.
20. Denis M, Cormier Y, Tardif J, et al: Hypersensitivity pneumonitis. Whole *Micropolyspora faeni* or antigens thereof stimulate the release of proinflammatory cytokines from macrophages. Am J Respir Cell Mol Biol 1991;5: 198–203.
21. Yoshizawa Y, Nomura A, Ohdama S, et al: The significance of complement activation in the pathogenesis of hypersensitivity pneumonitis. Sequential changes of complement components and chemotactic activities in bronchoalveolar lavage fluids. Int Arch Allergy Appl Immunol 1988;87:417–423.
22. Kaltreider HB: Hypersensitivity pneumonitis. West J Med 1993;159:570–578.
23. Denis M: Proinflammatory cytokines in hypersensitivity pneumonitis. Am J Respir Crit Care Med 1995;151:164–169.
24. Schuyler M, Gott K, Cherne A: Experimental hypersensitivity pneumonitis. Role of MCP-1. J Lab Clin Med 2003;142:187–195.
25. Gudmundsson G, Hunninghake GW: Interferon-gamma is necessary for the expression of hypersensitivity pneumonitis. J Clin Invest 1997;99:2386–2390.
26. Israel-Assayag E, Dakhama A, Lavigne S, et al: Expression of costimulatory molecules on alveolar macrophages in hypersensitivity pneumonitis. Am J Respir Crit Care Med 1999;159:1830–1834.
27. Schuyler M, Gott K, Cherne A: Mediators of hypersensitivity pneumonitis. J Lab Clin Med 2000;136:29–38.
28. Girard M, Israel-Assayag E, Cormier Y: Pathogenesis of hypersensitivity pneumonitis. Curr Opin Allergy Clin Immunol 2004;4:93–98.

29. Yamasaki H, Ando M, Brazer W, et al: Polarized type 1 cytokine profile in bronchoalveolar lavage T cells of patients with hypersensitivity pneumonitis. J Immunol 1999;163:3516–3523.
30. Schuyler M, Gott K, Cherne A, Edwards B: Th1 CD4+ cells adoptively transfer experimental hypersensitivity pneumonitis. Cell Immunol 1997;177:169–175.
31. Butler NS, Monick MM, Yarovinsky TO, et al: Altered IL-4 mRNA stability correlates with Th1 and Th2 bias and susceptibility to hypersensitivity pneumonitis in two inbred strains of mice. J Immunol 2002;169: 3700–3709.
32. Ando M, Suga M, Kohrogi H: A new look at hypersensitivity pneumonitis. Curr Opin Pulm Med 1999;5:299–304.
33. Gudmundsson G, Bosch A, Davidson BL, et al: Interleukin-10 modulates the severity of hypersensitivity pneumonitis in mice. Am J Respir Cell Mol Biol 1998;19:812–818.
34. Israel-Assayag E, Fournier M, Cormier Y: Blockade of T cell costimulation by CTLA4-Ig inhibits lung inflammation in murine hypersensitivity pneumonitis. J Immunol 1999;163:6794–6799.
35. Laflamme C, Israel-Assayag E, Cormier Y: Apoptosis of bronchoalveolar lavage lymphocytes in hypersensitivity pneumonitis. Eur Respir J 2003;21: 225–231.
36. Boise LH, Minn AJ, Noel PJ, et al: CD28 costimulation can promote T cell survival by enhancing the expression of Bcl-XL. Immunity 1995;3: 87–98.
37. Popper HH, Pailer S, Wurzinger G, et al: Expression of adhesion molecules in allergic lung diseases. Virchows Arch 2002;440:172–180.
38. Navarro C, Mendoza F, Barrera L, et al: Up-regulation of L-selectin and E-selectin in hypersensitivity pneumonitis. Chest 2002;121:354–360.
39. Pan LH, Yamauchi K, Sawai T, et al: Inhibition of binding of E- and P-selectin to sialyl-Lewis X molecule suppresses the inflammatory response in hypersensitivity pneumonitis in mice. Am J Respir Crit Care Med 2000;161:1689–1697.
40. Kremlev SG, Phelps DS: Surfactant protein A stimulation of inflammatory cytokine and immunoglobulin production. Am J Physiol 1994;267:L712–L719.
41. Israel-Assayag E, Cormier Y: Surfactant modifies the lymphoproliferative activity of macrophages in hypersensitivity pneumonitis. Am J Physiol 1997;273:L1258–L1264.
42. Gunther A, Schmidt R, Nix F, et al: Surfactant abnormalities in idiopathic pulmonary fibrosis, hypersensitivity pneumonitis and sarcoidosis. Eur Respir J 1999;14:565–573.
43. Schmidt R, Meier U, Markart P, et al: Altered fatty acid composition of lung surfactant phospholipids in interstitial lung disease. Am J Physiol Lung Cell Mol Physiol 2002;283:L1079–L1085.
44. Behr J, Degenkolb B, Beinert T, et al: Pulmonary glutathione levels in acute episodes of farmer's lung. Am J Respir Crit Care Med 2000;161:1968–1971.
45. Lakari E, Paakko P, Pietarinen-Runtti P, Kinnula VL: Manganese superoxide dismutase and catalase are coordinately expressed in the alveolar region in chronic interstitial pneumonias and granulomatous diseases of the lung. Am J Respir Crit Care Med 2000;161:615–621.
46. Hill MR, Briggs L, Montano MM, et al: Promoter variants in tissue inhibitor of metalloproteinase-3 (TIMP-3) protect against susceptibility in pigeon breeders' disease. Thorax 2004;59:586–590.
47. Leco KJ, Waterhouse P, Sanchez OH, et al: Spontaneous air space enlargement in the lungs of mice lacking tissue inhibitor of metalloproteinases-3 (TIMP-3). J Clin Invest 2001;108:817–829.
48. Bensadoun ES, Burke AK, Hogg JC, Roberts CR: Proteoglycans in granulomatous lung diseases. Eur Respir J 1997;10:2731–2737.
49. Schaaf BM, Seitzer U, Pravica V, et al: Tumor necrosis factor-alpha -308 promoter gene polymorphism and increased tumor necrosis factor serum bioactivity in farmer's lung patients. Am J Respir Crit Care Med 2001; 163:379–382.
50. Camarena A, Juarez A, Mejia M, et al: Major histocompatibility complex and tumor necrosis factor-alpha polymorphisms in pigeon breeder's disease. Am J Respir Crit Care Med 2001;163:1528–1533.
51. Rittner C, Sennekamp J, Mollenhauer E, et al: Pigeon breeder's lung: association with HLA-DR 3. Tissue Antigens 1983;21:374–379.
52. Selman M, Teran L, Mendoza A, et al: Increase of HLA-DR7 in pigeon breeder's lung in a Mexican population. Clin Immunol Immunopathol 1987;44:63–70.
53. Saltini C, Amicosante M, Franchi A, et al: Immunogenetic basis of environmental lung disease. Lessons from the beryllіosis model. Eur Respir J 1998; 12:1463–1475.
54. Muers MF, Faux JA, Ting A, Morris PJ: HLA-A, B, C and HLA-DR antigens in extrinsic allergic alveolitis (budgerigar fancier's lung disease). Clin Allergy 1982;12:47–53.
55. Wahlstrom J, Berlin M, Lundgren R, et al: Lung and blood T-cell receptor repertoire in extrinsic allergic alveolitis. Eur Respir J 1997;10:772–779.
56. Ando M, Hirayama K, Soda K, et al: HLA-DQw3 in Japanese summer-type hypersensitivity pneumonitis induced by *Trichosporon cutaneum*. Am Rev Respir Dis 1989;140:948–950.
57. Milic-Emili J, Henderson JA, Dolovich MB, et al: Regional distribution of inspired gas in the lung. J Appl Physiol 1996;21(3):749–759.
58. Seal RM, Hapke EJ, Thomas GO, et al: The pathology of the acute and chronic stages of farmer's lung. Thorax 1968;23:469–489.
59. Leatherman JW, Michael AF, Schwartz BA, Hoidal JR: Lung T cells in hypersensitivity pneumonitis. Ann Intern Med 1984;100:390–392.
60. Hamagami S, Miyagawa T, Ochi T, et al: A raised level of soluble CD8 in bronchoalveolar lavage fluid in summer-type hypersensitivity pneumonitis in Japan. Chest 1992;101:1044–1049.
61. Drent M, van Velzen-Blad H, Diamant M, et al: Bronchoalveolar lavage in extrinsic allergic alveolitis. Effect of time elapsed since antigen exposure. Eur Respir J 1993;6:1276–1281.
62. Chiron C, Gaultier C, Boule M, et al: Lung function in children with hypersensitivity pneumonitis. Eur J Respir Dis 1984;65:79–91.
63. Schmidt CD, Jensen RL, Christensen LT, et al: Longitudinal pulmonary function changes in pigeon breeders. Chest 1988;93:359–363.
64. Hendrick DJ, Faux JA, Marshall R: Budgerigar-fancier's lung. The commonest variety of allergic alveolitis in Britain. BMJ 1978;2:81–84.
65. Craig TJ, Hershey J, Engler RJ, et al: Bird antigen persistence in the home environment after removal of the bird. Ann Allergy 1992;69:510–512.
66. Banaszak EF, Thiede WH, Fink JN: Hypersensitivity pneumonitis due to contamination of an air conditioner. N Engl J Med 1970;283:271–276.
67. Carlsen KH, Leegaard J, Lund OD, Skjaervik H: Allergic alveolitis in a 12-year-old boy. Treatment with budesonide nebulizing solution. Pediatr Pulmonol 1992;12:257–259.
68. Kokkarinen J, Tukiainen H, Terho EO: Mortality due to farmer's lung in Finland. Chest 1994;106:509–512.
69. Löffler W: Zur differential-diagnose der Lungeninfiltrierungen, II Über fluchtige Succedan-infiltrate (mit Eosinophilie). Beitr Klin Tuberk 1932; 79:368–392.
70. Reeder WH, Goodrich BE: Pulmonary infiltration with eosinophilia (PIE syndrome). Ann Intern Med 1952;36:1217–1240.
71. Croften JW, Livingstone JL, Oswald NC, Roberts ATM: Pulmonary eosinophilia. Thorax 1952;7:1–35.
72. Liebow AA, Carrington CB: The eosinophilic pneumonias. Medicine (Baltimore) 1969;48:251–285.
73. McCarthy DS, Pepys J: Cryptogenic pulmonary eosinophilias. Clin Allergy 1973;3:339–351.
74. Sharma OP, Bethlem EP: The pulmonary infiltration with eosinophilia syndrome. Curr Opin Pulm Med 1996;2:380–389.
75. Udwadia FE: Tropical eosinophilia. A review. Respir Med 1993;87:17–21.
76. Ong RK, Doyle RL: Tropical pulmonary eosinophilia. Chest 1998;113: 1673–1679.
77. Badesch DB, King TE Jr, Schwarz MI: Acute eosinophilic pneumonia. A hypersensitivity phenomenon? Am Rev Respir Dis 1989;139:249–252.
78. Allen JN, Pacht ER, Gadek JE, Davis WB: Acute eosinophilic pneumonia as a reversible cause of noninfectious respiratory failure. N Engl J Med 1989;321:569–574.
79. Pope-Harman AL, Davis WB, Allen ED, et al: Acute eosinophilic pneumonia. A summary of 15 cases and review of the literature. Medicine (Baltimore) 1996;75:334–342.
80. Buchheit J, Eid N, Rodgers G Jr, et al: Acute eosinophilic pneumonia with respiratory failure. A new syndrome? Am Rev Respir Dis 1992;145:716–718.
81. St John RC, Allen JN, Pacht ER: Postoperative respiratory failure due to acute eosinophilic pneumonia. Intensive Care Med 1990;16:408–410.
82. Fox B, Seed WA: Chronic eosinophilic pneumonia. Thorax 1980;35: 570–580.
83. Jederlinic PJ, Sicilian L, Gaensler EA: Chronic eosinophilic pneumonia. A report of 19 cases and a review of the literature. Medicine (Baltimore) 1988;67:154–162.
84. Gaensler EA, Carrington CB: Peripheral opacities in chronic eosinophilic pneumonia. The photographic negative of pulmonary edema. AJR Am J Roentgenol 1977;128:1–13.
85. Churg J, Strauss L: Allergic granulomatosis, allergic angiitis, and periarteritis nodosa. Am J Pathol 1951;27:277–301.

86. Katzenstein AL: Diagnostic features and differential diagnosis of Churg-Strauss syndrome in the lung. A review. Am J Clin Pathol 2000;114: 767–772.
87. Leiferman KM, Gleich GJ: Hypereosinophilic syndrome. Case presentation and update. J Allergy Clin Immunol 2004;113:50–58.
88. Garrett JK, Jameson SC, Thomson B, et al: Anti-interleukin-5 (mepolizumab) therapy for hypereosinophilic syndromes. J Allergy Clin Immunol 2004; 113:115–119.
89. Laufer P, Fink JN, Bruns WT, et al: Allergic bronchopulmonary aspergillosis in cystic fibrosis. J Allergy Clin Immunol 1984;73:44–48.
90. Knutsen AP, Slavin RG: Allergic bronchopulmonary aspergillosis in patients with cystic fibrosis. Clin Rev Allergy 1991;9:103–118.
91. Murali PS, Pathial K, Saff RH, et al: Immune responses to *Aspergillus fumigatus* and *Pseudomonas aeruginosa* antigens in cystic fibrosis and allergic bronchopulmonary aspergillosis. Chest 1994;106:513–519.
92. Hinson KF, Moon AJ, Plummer NS: Broncho-pulmonary aspergillosis. A review and a report of eight new cases. Thorax 1952;7:317–333.
93. Kauffman HF, Tomee JF, van de Riet MA, et al: Protease-dependent activation of epithelial cells by fungal allergens leads to morphologic changes and cytokine production. J Allergy Clin Immunol 2000;105:1185–1193.
94. Tomee JF, Kauffman HF, Klimp AH, et al: Immunologic significance of a collagen-derived culture filtrate containing proteolytic activity in *Aspergillus*-related diseases. J Allergy Clin Immunol 1994;93:768–778.
95. Chauhan B, Santiago L, Kirschmann DA, et al: The association of HLA-DR alleles and T cell activation with allergic bronchopulmonary aspergillosis. J Immunol 1997;159:4072–4076.
96. Chauhan B, Knutsen A, Hutcheson PS, et al: T cell subsets, epitope mapping, and HLA-restriction in patients with allergic bronchopulmonary aspergillosis. J Clin Invest 1996;97:2324–2331.
97. Chauhan B, Santiago L, Hutcheson PS, et al: Evidence for the involvement of two different MHC class II regions in susceptibility or protection in allergic bronchopulmonary aspergillosis. J Allergy Clin Immunol 2000;106: 723–729.
98. Khan S, McClellan JS, Knutsen AP: Increased sensitivity to IL-4 in patients with allergic bronchopulmonary aspergillosis. Int Arch Allergy Immunol 2000;123:319–326.
99. Knutsen AP, Hutchinson PS, Albers GM, et al: Increased sensitivity to IL-4 in cystic fibrosis patients with allergic bronchopulmonary aspergillosis. Allergy 2004;59:81–87.
100. Knutsen AP: Immune responses in allergic bronchopulmonary aspergillosis and fungal allergy. In: Kurup VP, ed: Mold Allergy, Biology and Pathogenesis. Kerala, India: Research Signpost, 2005, pp 209–235.
101. Brourad J, Knauer N, Boelle P-Y, et al: Influence of interleukin-10 on airways colonization by Aspergillus fumigatus in cystic fibrosis patients. J Infect Dis 2005;191:1988–1991.
102. Davies DE, Wicks J, Powell RM, et al: Airway remodeling in asthma. New insights. J Allergy Clin Immunol 2003;111:215–226.
103. Imbeau SA, Cohen M, Reed CE: Allergic bronchopulmonary aspergillosis in infants. Am J Dis Child 1977;131:1127–1130.
104. Patterson R, Greenberger PA, Radin RC, Roberts M: Allergic bronchopulmonary aspergillosis. Staging as an aid to management. Ann Intern Med 1982;96:286–291.
105. Slavin RG: Allergic bronchopulmonary aspergillosis. Clin Rev Allergy 1985;3:167–182.
106. Stevens DA, Schwartz HJ, Lee JY, et al: A randomized trial of itraconazole in allergic bronchopulmonary aspergillosis. N Engl J Med 2000;342:756–762.
107. Wark PA, Hensley MJ, Saltos N, et al: Anti-inflammatory effect of itraconazole in stable allergic bronchopulmonary aspergillosis. A randomized controlled trial. J Allergy Clin Immunol 2003;111:952–957.
108. Wark PA, Gibson PG, Wilson AJ: Azoles for allergic bronchopulmonary aspergillosis associated with asthma. Cochrane Database Syst Rev 2004: CD001108.

50 Tumors of the Chest

James W. Brooks, MD •
Thomas M. Krummel, MD

■ DIAGNOSIS OF PULMONARY OR MEDIASTINAL TUMOR

Infants or children who have respiratory symptoms that do not disappear promptly when treated in the usual manner by expectorants, bronchodilators, and antibiotics must be suspected of having a space-occupying lesion. Posteroanterior and lateral chest radiographs are essential whenever symptoms persist.

Indeed, it might seem logical for all children to have a routine chest roentgenogram within the first 6 months of life. Certainly a physical examination in an adult patient is no longer considered complete without a chest radiograph. Why should children be excluded from this adjunctive diagnostic test? Without such refinement, how can we expect to help those with potentially curable lesions? Only by such techniques can obstructive emphysema (Fig. 50-1), atelectasis (Fig. 50-2), and actual solid masses be seen at a stage of development when a resectional operation may offer some hope of cure (Figs. 50-3 to 50-7). The increasingly routine use of prenatal ultrasound may represent a start.

In addition to having a probing history and complete physical examination, children with respiratory symptoms should have other studies.

It is impossible to obtain sputum voluntarily from an infant, but swabs from the posterior portion of the pharynx may be studied. In older children, however, sputum can be collected. A small catheter placed through the nose and adjusted into the trachea, thereby producing cough, will allow one to collect sputum through the catheter (Fig. 50-8). Any sputum thus collected should be studied by smear and culture for routine bacteria, acid-fast bacilli, and fungi; bacteria should be tested for antibiotic sensitivity. Cytologic analysis for tumor cells may be carried out, based on suspicion.

The tuberculin (purified protein derivative or tine) skin test should be applied. Coccidioidin, blastomycin, and histoplasmin skin tests may be applied, although they are not as accurate as complement-fixation studies.

Protein electrophoresis may show hypogammaglobulinemia to be primary or secondary in the etiology of recurrent pulmonary infectious processes. Complement fixation blood studies for fungal infections are generally more reliable than skin tests. Pulmonary complications of hematologic disorders, such as leukemia, Hodgkin's disease, and lymphosarcoma, may be properly identified by examination of the peripheral blood smear.

Examination of the bone marrow may give diagnostic evidence of blood dyscrasia, such as leukemia or myeloma, or even metastatic malignancy.

Cystic fibrosis as a cause of chronic recurrent pulmonary inflammatory disease may be suggested or ruled out by sweat chloride determination, and more precisely by genetic testing (see Section VIII, Cystic Fibrosis).

Radiographic examination of the chest with fluoroscopy and cinefluoroscopy, special views such as apical lordotic and right and left oblique, and computed tomography (CT) scans may be necessary for final definition. Cinefluoroscopy allows repeated examination of the thoracic organs in motion (function) without subjecting an infant to excessive radiation exposure. During this examination and at the time of fluoroscopy, studies with barium in the esophagus will aid in determining any displacement of the posterior mediastinum. Ultrasonography is useful in locating and assisting in the needle aspiration of pleural fluid collections (Fig. 50-9). Mediastinal, pulmonary, and diaphragmatic densities are best detailed with axial CT of the thorax, which has added greatly to the accurate study of all these areas (Figs. 50-10 to 50-12).

Magnetic resonance imaging (MRI) has had a substantial impact on thoracic diagnostic work-up in the last 5 years. It can discriminate masses in the mediastinum from vascular structures better than CT and is more sensitive in detecting intraspinal extension. The two studies may be complementary, since CT demonstrates calcifications and bronchial abnormalities that are not seen on MRI. Thoughtful use and sequencing of these studies should be based on location of the abnormality and a provisional working diagnosis.

Diagnostic pneumoperitoneum (introduction of air into the peritoneal cavity, thereby outlining and crossing the diaphragm) may aid in the diagnosis of abnormalities adjacent to the diaphragm; congenital diaphragmatic hernias may also be visualized (Fig. 50-13). Its use is less frequent now, given the sensitivity of CT and MRI.

Echocardiography and, occasionally, cardiac catheterization will demonstrate any displacement of the heart due to masses in the lung, mediastinum, or pericardium. The use of aortograms will assist in ruling out such vascular causes of symptoms as vascular ring, congenital aneurysm, congenital vascular malformations of the pulmonary tree, and sequestration. Aortograms are used to define bronchial arteries in patients with massive hemoptysis. Once a bleeding vessel has been identified, selective embolization often successfully stops the hemorrhage.

Bronchoscopy is an essential procedure for the study of tracheobronchial tree and pulmonary disease. This procedure permits visual study of the vocal cords, larynx, trachea, and major bronchi and their segmental orifices. Congenital anatomic abnormalities may be visualized; biopsy of lesions within the lumen can be performed for a definitive diagnosis; prognosis in extensive lesions is evaluated by study of the carina and trachea. Aspiration of secretions is an important therapeutic contribution. Study of secretions and washings must include cytologic studies for malignant cells, routine bacterial smear, culture and sensitivity studies, acid-fast smear and cultures, and fungal smear and cultures (see discussion of bronchoscopy in Chapter 7).

Biopsy of palpable lymph nodes may aid in the diagnosis of abnormal processes in the lung. Most important are the scalene lymph nodes, which drain the pulmonary parenchyma. Scalene lymph node biopsy, mediastinoscopy, or thoracoscopy with biopsy of available mediastinal nodes as distal as the carina are of great help in the diagnosis of sarcoidosis, in lymphatic malignancies such as Hodgkin's disease and lymphosarcoma, and in primary

■ **FIGURE 50-1.** Chest radiograph revealing obstructive emphysema of the left lower lobe bronchus caused by partial occlusion of the lumen. **A,** Posteroanterior view. **B,** Lateral view. The left diaphragm is flattened, mediastinal and cardiac shadows are displaced toward the right, the left upper lobe is compressed, and there is increased radiolucency of the left lower lobe.

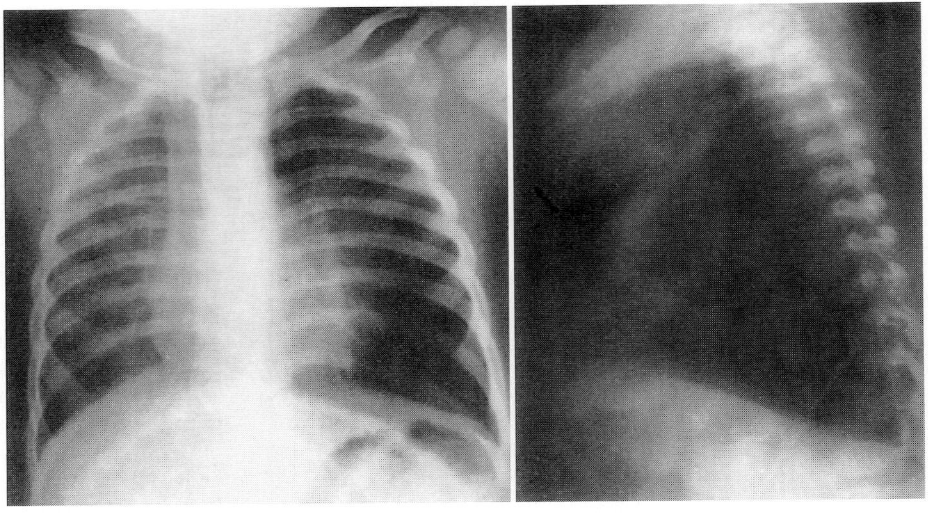

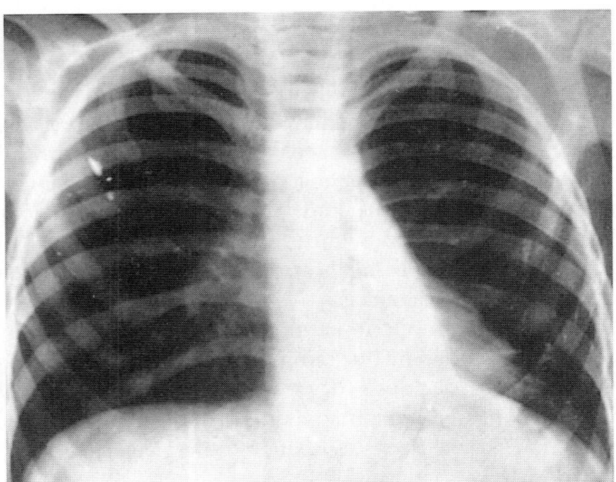

■ **FIGURE 50-2.** Chest radiograph revealing total atelectasis of the left lower lobe secondary to an inflammatory stricture of the left lower lobe bronchus. A retrocardiac position tends to confuse diagnosis in some cases.

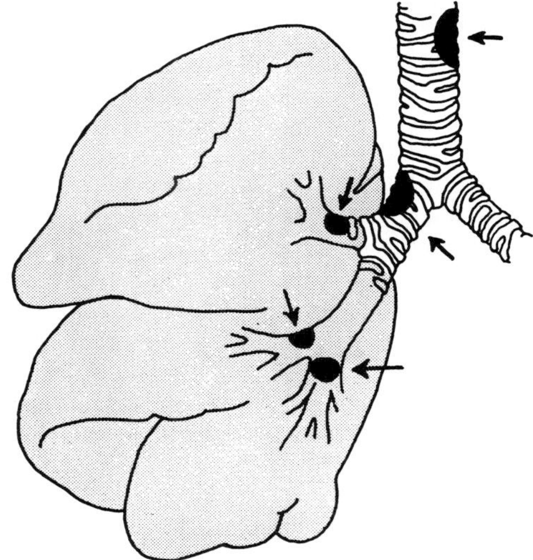

■ **FIGURE 50-3.** A diagram illustrating locations of lesions within the lumens of the major bronchi. The location of such lesions dictates the area of pulmonary involvement, unilaterality or bilaterality, and the extent of signs and symptoms.

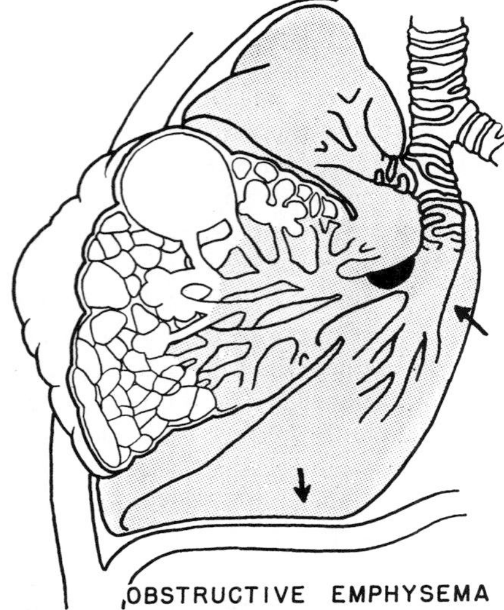

■ **FIGURE 50-4.** A diagram of obstructive emphysema. A partial obstruction leads to the retention of air in the pulmonary parenchyma distal to the obstructed bronchus. Retention of air will cause an ipsilateral compression of the adjacent, normally aerated lung tissue, widening of intercostal spaces, descent of the diaphragm, a shift of the mediastinum away from the lung with the partially obstructing lesion, and a wheeze accompanied by decreased breath sounds over the affected lung.

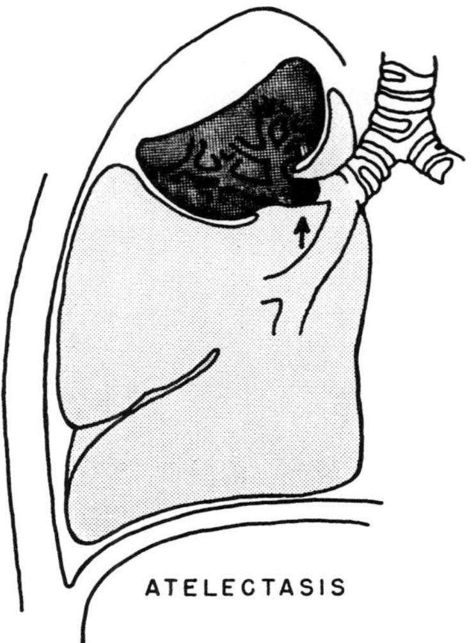

■ **FIGURE 50-5.** Diagram showing that persistence of the lesion with ultimate total obstruction gives rise to atelectasis, an absence of breath sounds over the affected lung tissue, an overexpansion of the surrounding lung tissue, and a shift of the diaphragm to a more normal position, with a return of the mediastinum to midline. Bronchial secretions may actually decrease in amount.

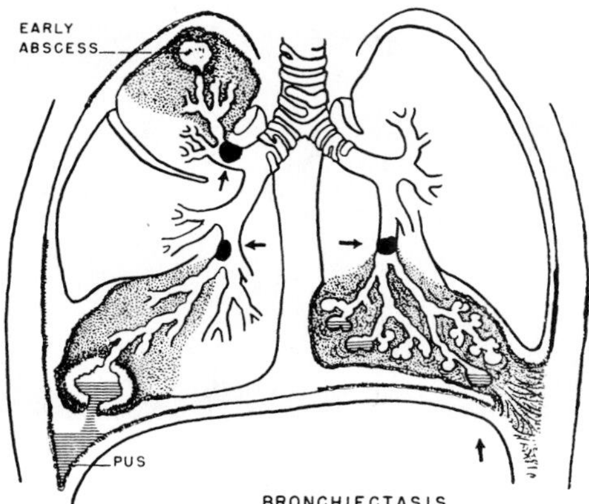

■ **FIGURE 50-6.** Diagram showing that the persistence of an obstructing lesion leads to permanent destructive changes in the pulmonary parenchyma distal to the lesion, such as abscess formation, chronic pneumonitis with fibrosis, pleurisy, empyema, and bronchiectasis with parenchymal contracture secondary to fibrosis.

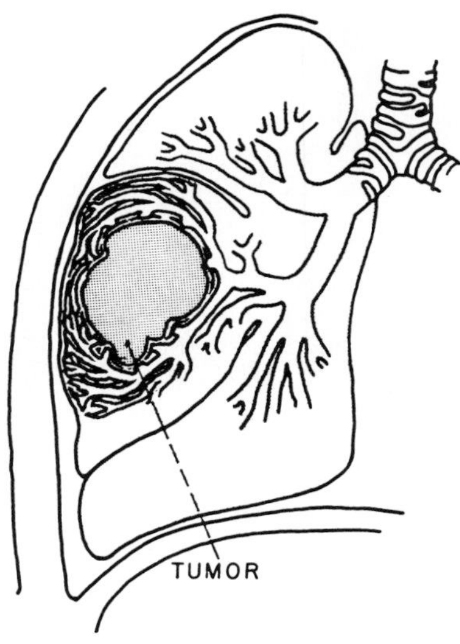

■ **FIGURE 50-7.** Diagram showing that if the tumor is within the pulmonary parenchyma, pressure on the adjacent lung and bronchi will give rise to a surrounding zone of pneumonitis that may actually show incomplete, temporary improvement with antibiotic therapy.

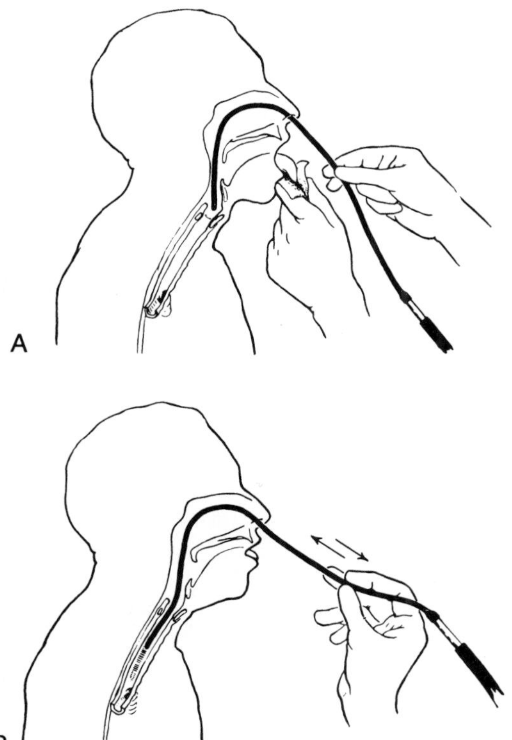

■ **FIGURE 50-8.** A diagram illustrating the placement of a rubber catheter through the nose into the posterior pharynx **(A),** followed by its insertion into the trachea **(B)** through the opened epiglottis at a time of deep inspiration or cough to obtain bronchial secretions.

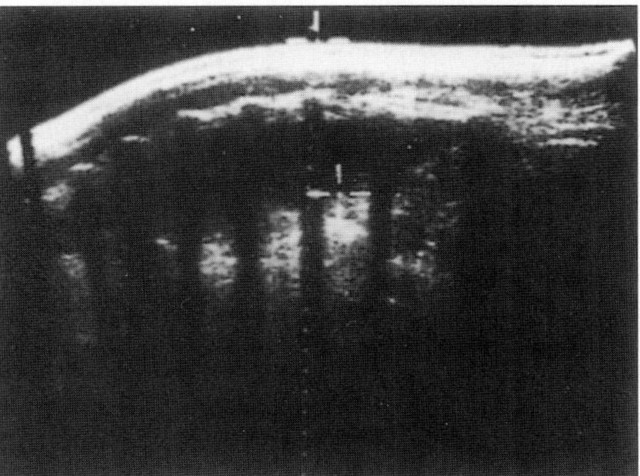

■ **FIGURE 50-9.** A typical ultrasonogram of pleural fluid. With such accurate localization, needle aspiration is easily carried out.

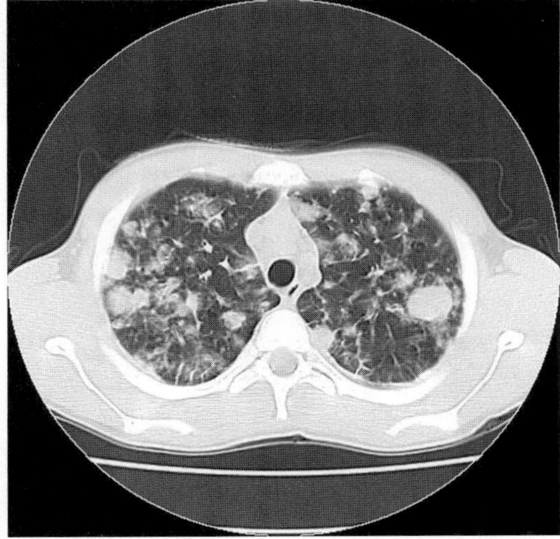

■ **FIGURE 50-10.** CT study of the chest showing metastatic pulmonary disease in a 14-year-old boy with testicular rhabdomyosarcoma.

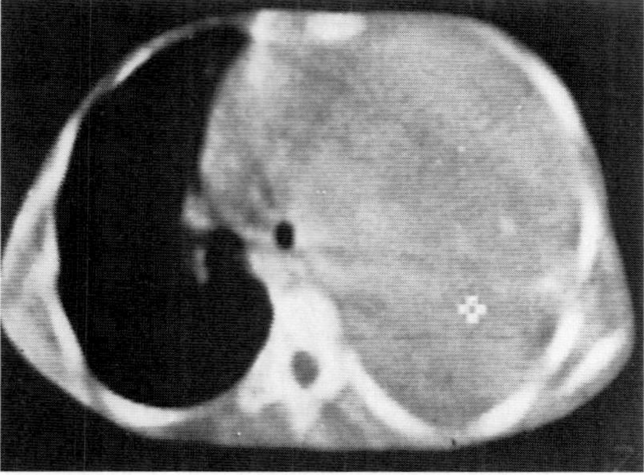

■ **FIGURE 50-11.** A CT scan of a child with small-cell carcinoma.

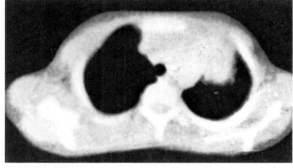

■ **FIGURE 50-12.** A CT scan of the mediastinum and lung in a child with Hodgkin's disease.

neoplasms of the lung and mediastinum. CT-guided fine-needle percutaneous needle biopsy of intrapulmonic and mediastinal masses is an excellent approach in selected cases, though sometimes limited by sample size. The use of a thoracoscope to obtain biopsy specimens of lesions on the mediastinal, pleural, or diaphragmatic surfaces can satisfactorily avoid thoracotomy in almost all cases.

Lymph nodes obtained at the time of biopsy should be subjected to histologic study, and a portion should be sent to the bacteriology laboratory for routine bacterial smear and culture, studies for sensitivity of the organism to antibiotics, acid-fast smear and culture, and fungal smear and culture (Fig. 50-14).

Air bronchograms may show sufficient detail of the bronchial tree to dispense with any other diagnostic test for anatomy identifications (Fig. 50-15).

When all other methods have failed to produce a definitive diagnosis, thoracotomy should be considered. A limited incision may first be made, and biopsy can be performed. The use of single-lung anesthetic techniques (selective bronchial intubation, or the use of balloon occlusion catheters) and preoperative placement of a radiologically guided blood patch can greatly facilitate the pursuit of tiny lesions. If the situation seems to present an inoperable problem, biopsy may afford useful information (Fig. 50-16).

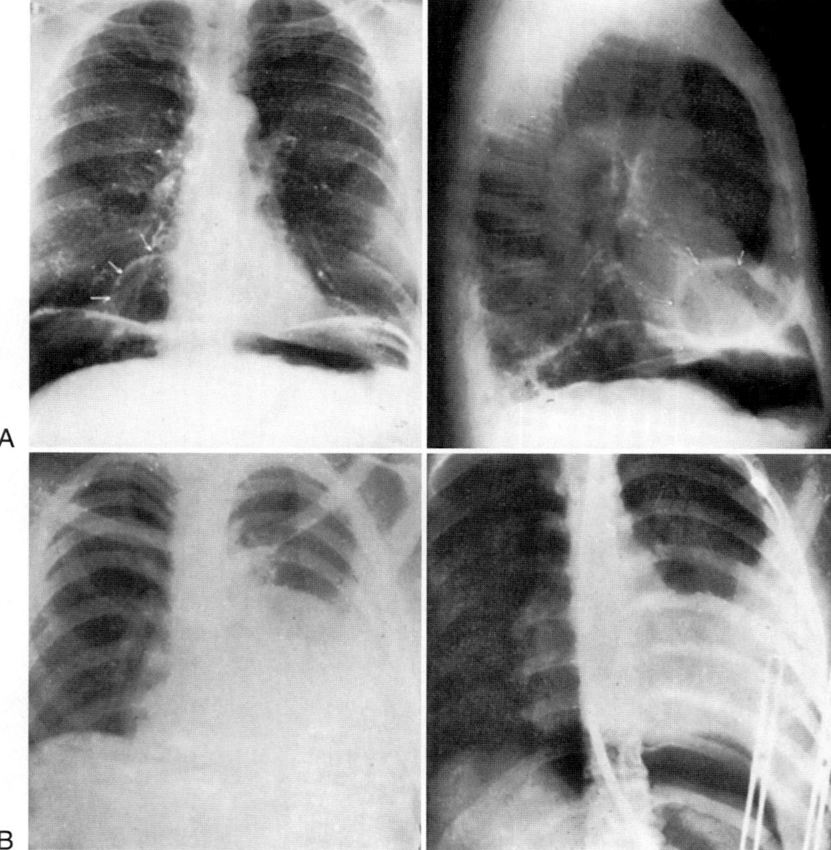

■ **FIGURE 50-13.** **A,** Diagnostic pneumoperitoneum showing congenital diaphragmatic Morgagni hernia. **B,** An outline of a normal diaphragm with intrapleural or pneumonic density above.

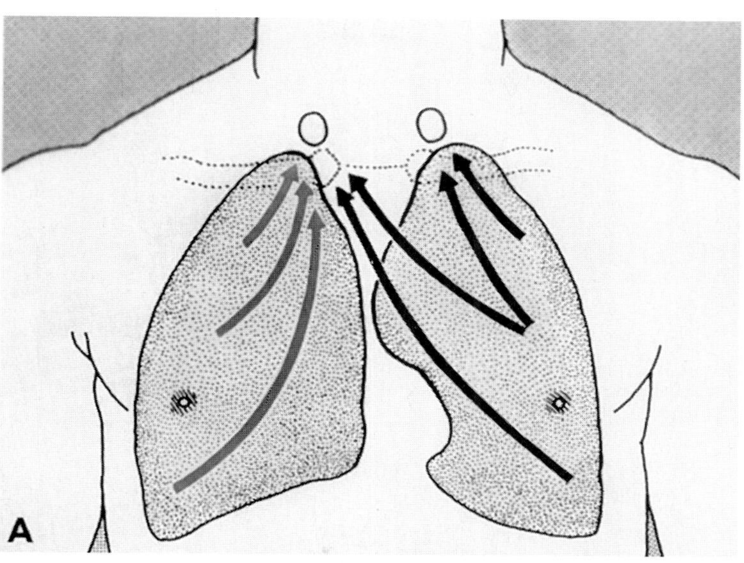

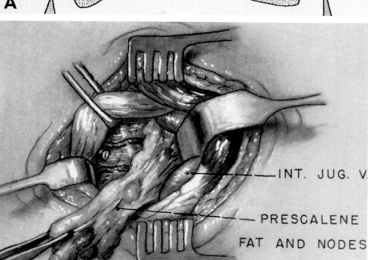

■ **FIGURE 50-14. A,** Disease within the right lung usually drains into the right scalene lymph node group. Disease within the left lung may drain to either scalene node group in a pattern similar to that indicated on the illustration. Generally, left lung disease requires bilateral scalene node biopsy, whereas right lung disease requires only right scalene node biopsy. Regardless of the side of lung disease, all palpable nodes in the scalene node area should be examined by biopsy. **B,** The scalene group of nodes is contained in the fat pad bounded medially by the internal jugular vein, inferiorly by the subclavian vein, and superiorly by the posterior belly of the omohyoid muscle. The base of the triangle is formed by the anterior scalene muscle. Retraction of the internal jugular vein is essential to obtain access to all nodes in this group.

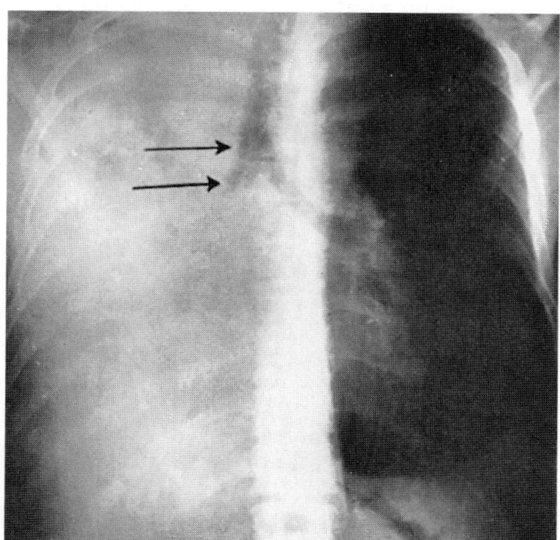

■ **FIGURE 50-15.** An air bronchogram showing a complete block of the right main bronchus in a patient with total right lung atelectasis.

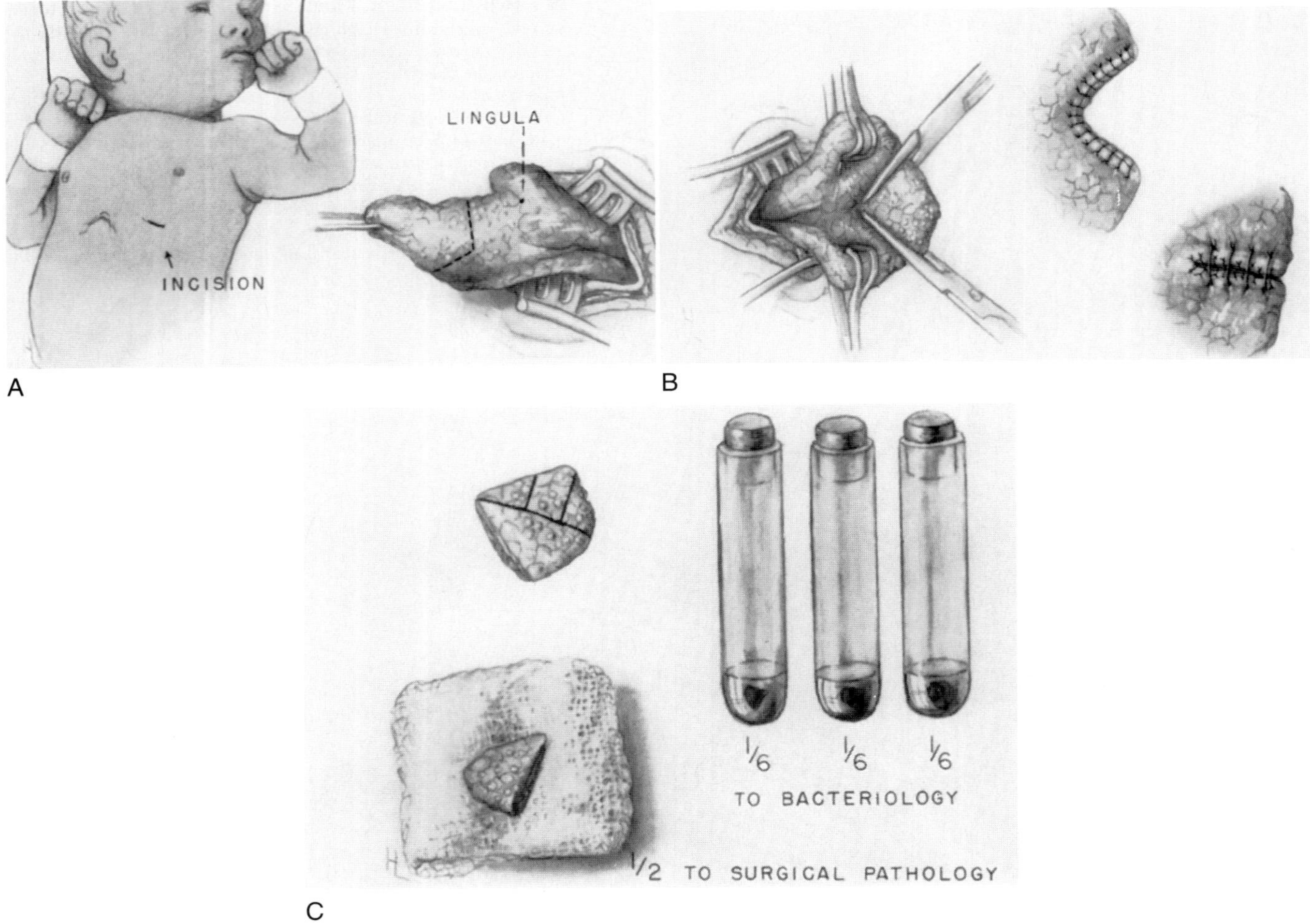

FIGURE 50-16. **A–C,** An adequate lung biopsy with specimens for bacteriology and pathology laboratories is essential. In general, a small open thoracotomy has many advantages over the blind needle biopsy technique.

Finally, prenatal ultrasound, now routine, has led to a greater understanding of the natural history of those lesions presenting in the fetus. Previously undiagnosed lesions are now seen with increasing frequency. Perhaps such imaging will supplant the notion of a neonatal chest radiograph.

PULMONARY TUMORS

IN THE PEDIATRIC AGE GROUP, ALL FORMS OF PRIMARY PULMONARY TUMORS ARE UNUSUAL

Benign Pulmonary Tumors

Hamartoma

The term *hamartoma* was coined in 1904 by Albrecht, who defined it as a tumor-like malformation formed by an abnormal mixing of the normal components of the organ. Hamartomas of the lung consist largely of cartilage and also include variable quantities of epithelium, fat, and muscle (Fig. 50-17). They are usually located in the periphery of the lung, but involvement of intermediate and primary bronchi has been reported. Developmental derangement is apparently responsible for their occurrence. Popcorn-like calcification is pathognomonic.

The incidence of hamartoma is 0.25% among all patients,[1] but only six have been reported in children; four of these were discovered at autopsy, and two were successfully removed.

Unlike hamartomas in adults, which are usually asymptomatic and small, the rare tumor found in infancy has been large and symptomatic and has contributed to the death of the infant (prematurity combined with respiratory inadequacy). At least four of the six reported hamartomas showed obvious progressive intrauterine development and had attained considerable size at the time of birth. Recognition and prompt removal of such large intrapulmonic tumors are necessary for survival.

In 1964, Holder and Christy[2] first collected from the literature 32 cases of cystic adenomatoid malformation of the lung in newborn infants. These authors suggest that the entity be designated adenomatoid hamartoma; although this is a form of congenital cystic disease of the lung resulting from abnormal growth of normal lung components, it is not a true hamartoma.

Nomenclature now refers to such a lesion as congenital cystic adenomatoid malformation (CCAM). It may be macrocystic or microcystic; the latter appear as solid echo-dense masses.

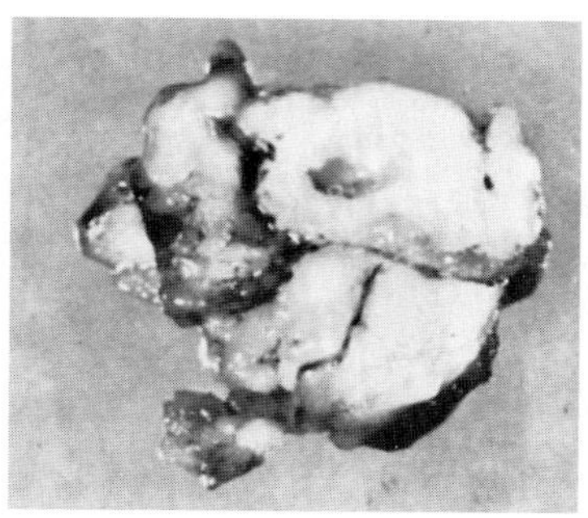

■ **FIGURE 50-17.** A hamartoma removed from the right upper lobe of an adult. Note the predominance of cartilage.

Mesodermal Tumors

Benign Parenchymal Tumors. Plasma cell granuloma (inflammatory pseudotumor) of the lung has been reported infrequently in pediatric patients, with the greatest number between 8 and 12 years of age. Many patients are asymptomatic; others show signs of antecedent pulmonary infection. Radiographic appearance is typically that of a peripherally based lesion that may extend beyond the pulmonary parenchyma. The diagnosis is usually made histologically; lung-conserving resection should be performed if the diagnosis is suspected; however, gross resection is essential.

Bronchial Adenoma. Bronchial adenoma is a neoplasm arising from either the cells of the mucous glands of the bronchi or the cells lining the excretory ducts of these glands.

Two histologic types are defined. The carcinoid type (90%) has histologic resemblance to carcinoid tumor of the small bowel; it is composed of somewhat oval cells filled almost entirely by nucleus. The cells, which have barely detectable lumina, are arranged in a quasiacinar fashion and are piled up in several layers. The tumor is very vascular and is surrounded by a thin capsule of fibrous tissue that is not invaded by the tumor cells. Metaplastic epithelium of the bronchial mucosa covers the intrabronchial component. The tumor is frequently shaped like a dumbbell, with the smaller component intrabronchial and the larger one intrapulmonic. Though considered benign, bronchial adenomas have a definite malignant potential; lymph node metastasis is more frequent (15%) than distant blood-borne metastasis. The cylindromatous type (10%) is made up of cuboidal or flattened epithelial cells, arranged in two layers, which form corelike structures of the cylinders. Histologically, it closely resembles mixed tumor of the salivary glands and basal cell carcinoma of the skin. There is a 40% incidence of malignancy.

More than 100 cases of bronchial adenoma, all apparently of the carcinoid type, have been reported in the pediatric age group. There were metastases in 10% of the cases, and one case of carcinoid syndrome has been described.

The most prominent symptoms and signs are recurrent and refractory pneumonitis, elevated temperature, cough, and chest pain due to bronchial obstruction with associated distal infection. Hemoptysis and wheeze are not as common in children as in adults. The right main bronchus is most commonly involved, and the diagnosis can usually be made by biopsy performed at bronchoscopy. The tumor occurs five times more commonly in males. The youngest recorded patient was a 10-month-old infant; all the other pediatric tumors were seen in children at least 4 years of age (Fig. 50-18).

Resection of a segment, lobe, or total lung, according to the degree of involvement, is indicated. Depending on the skills and experience of the surgeon and surgical team, and the location and extent of the lesion, this may be done thoracoscopically or via open thoracotomy. Treatment by bronchoscopy is not effective, because it does not permit complete removal of the tumor. Rarely, a bronchial adenoma can be removed by bronchial or sleeve resection, followed by airway reconstruction.

Tracheal Tumors

Papilloma of the Trachea and Bronchi. These lesions may be single but are more frequently multiple and often misdiagnosed as vocal cord nodules. Thought to be caused by the human papillomaviruses HPV-6 and HPV-11, these lesions are seen predominantly in the larynx; tracheobronchial and pulmonary seeding has been reported.

Symptoms depend on the location and size of the tumor. The lesions may be attached by a pedicle and may oscillate in and out of orifices during inspiration and expiration (flutter valve). Single, slow-growing, high lesions within the trachea may be asymptomatic for years. Dyspnea, hoarseness, and stridor are the most common symptoms, occurring in two thirds of the cases. Cough, at first dry and later productive, is another common symptom.

Wheeze, audible at the open mouth, is the earliest sign of papilloma of the trachea. This eventually develops into stridor and is associated with slowly increasing dyspnea. Such secondary changes as obstructive emphysema, atelectasis, pneumonia, lung abscess, and bronchiectasis may occur in the distal parts of the tracheobronchial tree; empyema may also occur.

These tumors should be removed because of their tendency to obstruct. Distal pulmonary infection or death from asphyxia may result. Additionally, Ogilvie[3] reported in 1953 two instances of malignancy arising from tracheobronchial papillomas.

Since papillomata are confined to the mucosal layer, surface destruction rather than full-thickness excision is warranted. Laser (CO_2) ablation is now used; interferon-α2a, retinoic acid, and indole-3-carbinol/diindolylmethane have been used as adjuvant therapies to expand the intervals between endoscopic laser treatments. Cidofovir has been used with success in selected patients. Future therapies hinge on the development of a safe, effective vaccine.

Fibroma of the Trachea. Nine cases of primary fibroma of the trachea have been recorded in infants,[4] none since 1953.

Hemangioma of the Trachea. Six children with benign hemangioma have been first reported by Gilbert and colleagues.[4] Seikaly[5] more recently reviewed this problem. Congenital hemangioma of the trachea may cause death by the compromise of the airway, bleeding complications, intractable cardiac failure from atrioventricular shunting of blood within the tumor, or malignant change. In infants and children, these tumors are usually below the vocal cords, sessile, flat, and associated with dyspnea. Among the recorded patients, 90% have been 6 months of age at the time of the onset of symptoms, and females predominate over males two to one. More than half of the infants have hemangiomas elsewhere.

The onset is insidious, with symptoms of respiratory obstruction such as stridor, retraction, dyspnea, wheezing, and sometimes cyanosis and cough. The symptoms tend to be intermittent and labile. Fever and leukocytosis are usually absent, but superimposed infection may produce fever and an elevated white blood

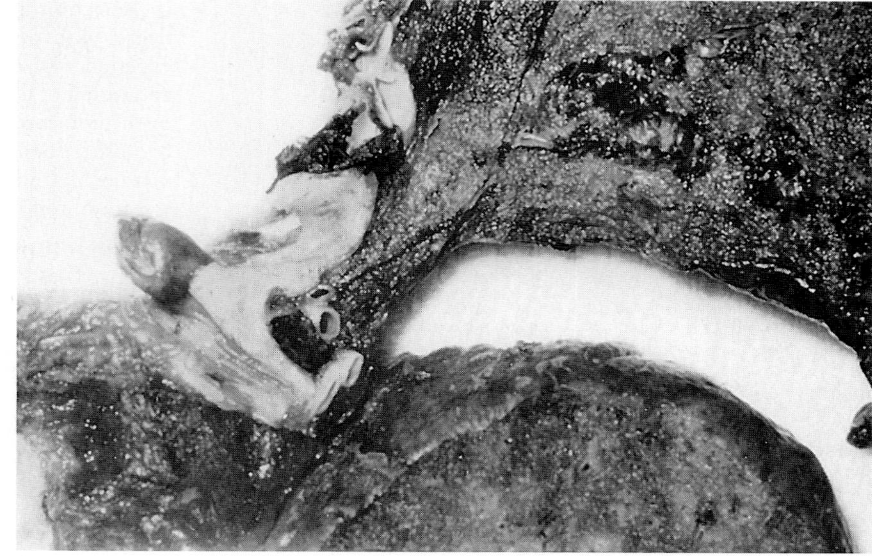

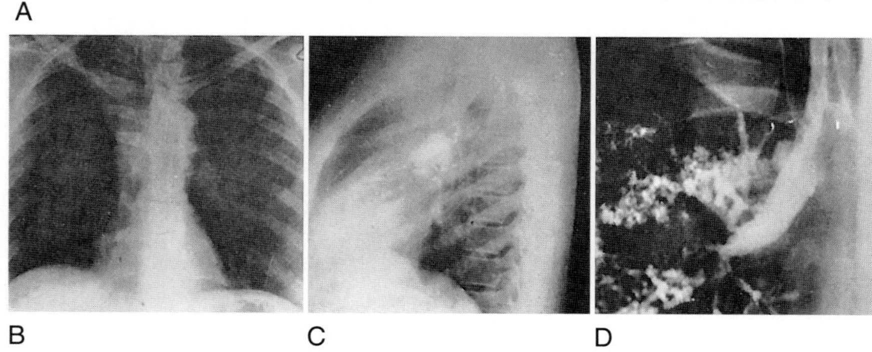

■ **FIGURE 50-18.** A bronchial adenoma (carcinoid type) (**A**) and total obstruction of the right upper lobe bronchus with resultant distal atelectasis (**B** and **C**). Recurrent pneumonitis, cough, and hemoptysis had occurred. Diagnostic biopsy at the time of bronchoscopy. **D,** Obstruction of the right upper lobe bronchus is demonstrated with bronchograms. Treated by performing a right upper lobectomy.

cell count. The best diagnostic tool is bronchoscopy. Biopsy is not advisable at the time of endoscopy, because bleeding may cause asphyxia or an exsanguinating hemorrhage. Tracheostomy is necessary for severe obstructions. Since many hemangiomas involute, observation can be undertaken once the airway is secure. Corticosteroids, both systemic and intralesional, have their champions and their skeptics. Antiangiogenesis therapies are under investigation.

Leiomyoma of the Lung

Grossly, these tumors cannot be differentiated from other benign tumors of the lung. Leiomyomas of the lung are usually asymptomatic unless there is partial or complete bronchial obstruction. In a review of the world literature, Guida and co-workers[6] found only one case in a child. This 6-year-old had a tumor in the right lower lobe; it was successfully treated by lobectomy. Since then, five additional cases have been reported.

Lipoma

Review of the literature reveals no cases of lipoma of the bronchus or lung in the pediatric age group.

Neurogenic Tumors

Of the more than 50 patients with proven primary intrapulmonic neurogenic tumors recorded in the world literature, 9 were seen in children. Neurofibroma, schwannoma, and neurilemomas have been described.

MALIGNANT PULMONARY TUMORS

Bronchogenic Carcinoma

Primary tumors of the lung are rare in the pediatric age group. Forty-nine cases of bronchogenic carcinoma are reported in children.[7] The youngest patient was a 5-month-old girl with cystic lung disease and malignancy in the left lung. Every cell type except alveolar cell carcinoma, giant cell carcinoma, and carcinosarcoma has been seen in the pediatric age group. Interestingly, squamous cell carcinoma is rare. Most cases present late, with mortality approaching 90% and mean duration of survival of 7 months.

Despite the rarity of primary pulmonary neoplasms in children, this diagnosis should be considered in young patients with solitary pulmonary masses or persistent, atypical pulmonary symptoms. Localized lesions should be completely excised.

Fibrosarcoma of the Bronchus

Review of the literature reveals 28 cases of primary fibrosarcoma of the bronchus in the pediatric age group. Fever, probably due to bronchial obstruction and distal infection, is the most common symptom; hemoptysis is relatively uncommon. Diagnosis in these cases can be established by bronchoscopy. Resection is the treatment of choice, because recurrence is common when any other mode of therapy is used. As a rule, metastasis is hematogenous.

Leiomyosarcoma

Eleven cases of primary leiomyosarcoma[8,9] and six cases of nonspecific primary sarcoma of the lung have been reported in children. Cough, dyspnea, and signs of obstructive pneumonitis are usually present. Surgical excision is indicated (Fig. 50-19).

Multiple Myeloma

Multiple myeloma is usually limited to the medullary space. Extramedullary plasma cell tumors are relatively uncommon (myeloma or solitary plasmacytoma of the lung parenchyma). In a 1965 review of the literature, Sekulich and co-workers[10] found only 19 cases since 1911; one of these was a plasmacytoma in a 3-year-old girl. Cytologic examination of sputum may be diagnostic.

Chorioepithelioma

A case of chorioepithelioma of the lung in a 7-month-old white girl was reported in 1953 by Kay and Reed.[11] The presenting symptoms were fever, dyspnea, and anorexia; massive hemoptysis then occurred. Roentgenogram showed almost complete opacity of the right side of the chest. Pneumonectomy was performed, but the child died several hours postoperatively. This rare lesion has other scattered case reports in the literature.

Systemic Neoplasms Affecting the Lung

Myeloid and lymphatic leukemia may have a pulmonary component, but isolated pulmonary disease has not been recorded. Similarly, Hodgkin's disease and lymphosarcoma may involve the lung during the course of the disease, but neither occurs as an isolated pulmonary lesion.

METASTATIC PULMONARY TUMORS

Primary pulmonary malignancies in children are rare; the majority of malignant lung lesions are metastatic. The principles of evaluation are standard. Surgical therapy should be based on the primary tumor, the characteristics of the metastatic lesion, and a full metastatic work-up. Pulmonary metastases should only be resected after the primary site is eradicated and other sites are confirmed to be disease free. Primary tumors most amenable to excision of pulmonary metastases include soft tissue sarcomas and osteogenic sarcomas.

Beyond the general principles outlined, there are disease-specific guidelines. With osteogenic sarcoma, survival is considerably better in those with four or fewer lesions. Even in those with many nodules, complete resection of all lesions correlates with survival; pleural invasion is ominous.

Since soft tissue sarcomas encompass a broad spectrum of sites of origin and cell type, rational resectional therapy of pulmonary metastases depends on both site and histology. Rarely does rhabdomyosarcoma come to metastatic resection, and resection has not shown increased survival in Ewing's sarcoma.

Resection of metastatic Wilms' tumor has shown no advantage compared to systemic therapy and radiotherapy.

Overall, resection of other lesions, single or multiple, unilateral or bilateral, has increased survival by 10% to 20%. Surgical approaches have been historically via thoracotomy, bilateral thoracotomy, or sternotomy; minimal access via the thoracoscopy is now a selected option. Preoperative mapping by CT scan, tattooing of small lesions by a blood patch, and single-lung anesthesia all facilitate precise localization and wedge resection.

MEDIASTINAL TUMORS

The mediastinum, the portion of the body that lies between the lungs, is bounded anteriorly by the sternum and posteriorly by the vertebrae. It extends superiorly from the suprasternal notch and terminates inferiorly at the diaphragm. Cysts or tumors that arise within the mediastinum may originate from any of the structures contained therein or may be the result of developmental abnormalities. The mediastinum is lined on both sides by parietal pleura and contains all structures of the thoracic cavity except the lungs.

For ease of definition of sites of disease, the mediastinum may be thought of as divided into four compartments (Fig. 50-20): (1) the superior mediastinum (the portion of the mediastinum above a hypothetical line drawn from the junction of the manubrium and gladiolus of the sternum (angle) to the intervertebral disk between the fourth and fifth thoracic vertebrae); (2) the anterior mediastinum (the portion of the mediastinum that lies anterior to the anterior plane of the trachea); (3) the middle mediastinum (the portion containing the heart and pericardium, the ascending aorta, the lower segment of the superior vena cava bifurcation of the pulmonary artery, the trachea, the two main bronchi, and the bronchial lymph nodes); and (4) the posterior mediastinum (the portion that lies posterior to the anterior plane of the trachea).

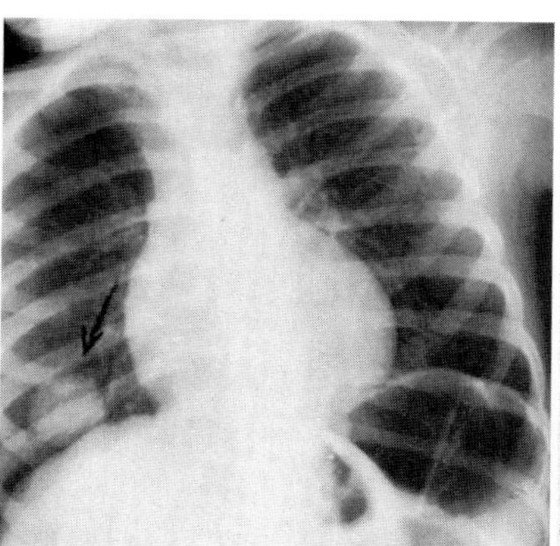
A

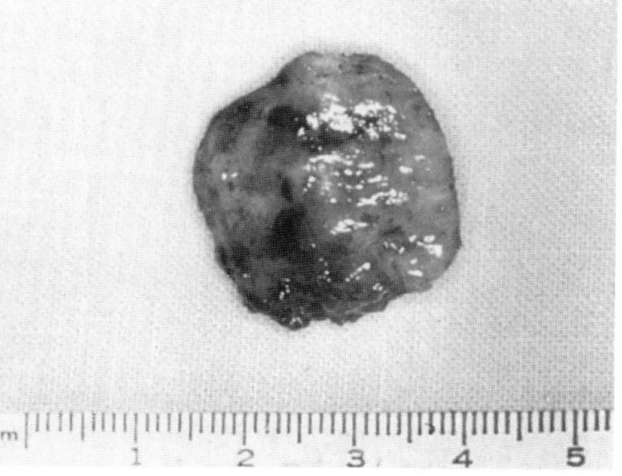

B

FIGURE 50-19. **A,** A 3-year-old white male with an increasing mass in the right lower lobe of the lung. **B,** The shelled-out leiomyosarcoma after a lower lobectomy. No recurrence after 1 year.

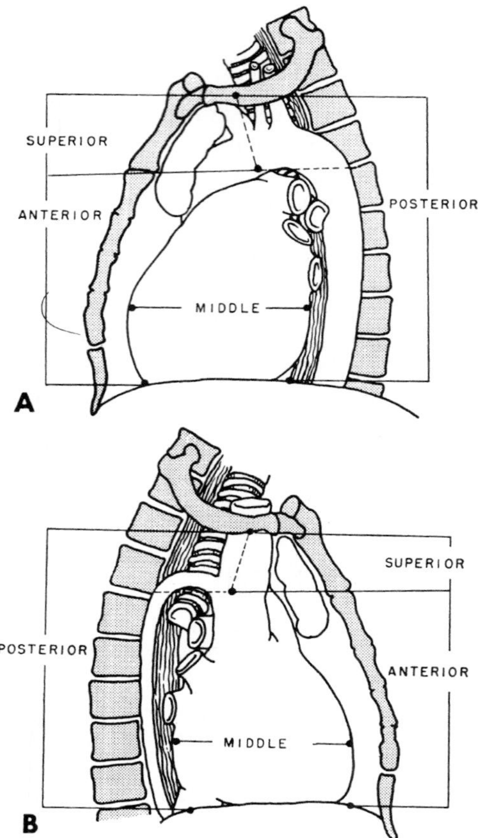

■ **FIGURE 50-20.** **A,** The mediastinal compartment as seen from the left hemithorax. **B,** Mediastinal compartments as seen from the right hemithorax.

SIGNS AND SYMPTOMS OF MEDIASTINAL TUMOR

A great number of lesions (even very large ones) in the mediastinum remain asymptomatic for a considerable period. The patient becomes aware of lesions within the mediastinum only when pressure is exerted on sensitive structures of the mediastinum or when the structures are displaced; therefore, the severity of symptoms depends on the size and location of the tumor, the rapidity of its growth, and the presence or absence of actual invasion of organs. Symptoms resulting from mediastinal lesions may become manifest according to the degree of functional disturbance of the various organs in the mediastinum.

Respiratory Symptoms

In a mediastinal lesion in a child, respiratory symptoms are the most important. They are the result of direct pressure on some portion of the respiratory tract. This pressure causes narrowing of the trachea or bronchi or compression of the lung parenchyma (Fig. 50-21). Dry cough may be present; stridor or wheeze may occur at the same time or may precede it. The compression may be sufficient to produce enough occlusion to cause distal obstructive emphysema or atelectasis, pneumonitis, or chronic recurrent lower respiratory tract infections with associated fever and leukocytosis. The dry cough may be replaced by a productive one with mucoid sputum; if infection occurs, the secretion will become purulent. The unilateral nature of the wheezing and respiratory complaints serves to rule out asthma, bronchiolitis, and chronic recurrent infections secondary to cystic fibrosis or hypogammaglobulinemia but will not eliminate the possibility of endobronchial or endotracheal lesions; nor can the possibility of a foreign body in the tracheobronchial tree be discarded. Bronchoscopy is necessary to make this differentiation.

If the lesion in the mediastinum exerts pressure on the recurrent laryngeal nerve, hoarseness and a brassy cough result. Dyspnea, which may be progressive, is a common symptom of mediastinal tumors. Acute episodes of dyspnea with associated pneumonitis may occur when there is tracheal or bronchial obstruction, leading to distal infection. Hemoptysis occurs in fewer than 10% of mediastinal tumors in children.

Gastrointestinal Symptoms

Symptoms referable to the gastrointestinal tract result primarily from pressure on the esophagus. Regurgitation of food and dysphagia with a slight sensation of sticking in the lower esophagus are common. Displacement of the esophagus usually does not cause dysphagia; however, if there is fixation of the mass secondary to infection, hemorrhage, or malignant degeneration, thereby causing interference with the peristaltic activity of the esophagus, dysphagia will occur.

Neurologic Symptoms

Older children often describe a feeling of vague intrathoracic discomfort, fullness, or ache caused by pressure on the sensitive intercostal nerves. Such pain may be mild or severe and is common in tumors of neurogenic origin. The appearance of herpes zoster may indicate involvement of an intercostal nerve, but this is not common in the pediatric age group. When lesions impinge on the pleura, the pain may be pleuritic. Erosion of vertebrae causes a boring pain located in the interscapular area. A malignant lesion that invades the brachial plexus causes severe pain in the upper extremities; the presence of Horner syndrome indicates involvement of the cervical sympathetic nerves. Inflammation, intracystic hemorrhage, or malignant degeneration causing pressure on the phrenic nerve may result in hiccups. Certain dumbbell tumors of the spinal cord and mediastinum may result in symptoms referable to spinal cord pressure.

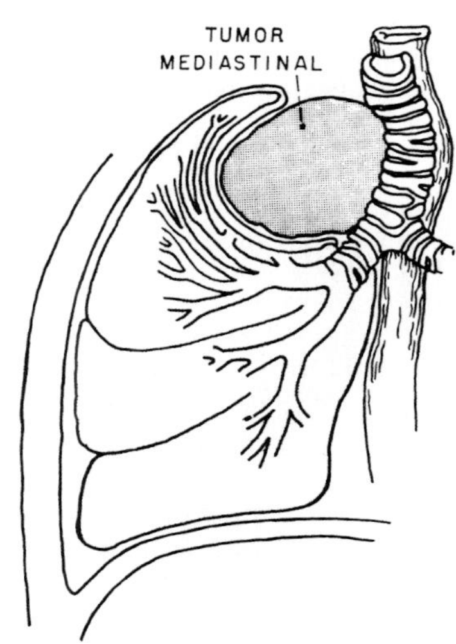

■ **FIGURE 50-21.** A diagram illustrating a large mediastinal tumor or cyst with pressure on the tracheobronchial tree as well as on the pulmonary parenchyma. Such a condition might possibly give rise to pulmonary symptoms.

Vascular Symptoms

Benign lesions of the mediastinum rarely cause obstruction of the great vessels in the mediastinum; however, obstruction is a common finding in malignant mediastinal tumors and carries a poor prognosis. Superior vena caval involvement gives rise to a dilatation of veins in the upper extremity, head, and neck. As the obstruction progresses, cyanosis of the head and neck area occurs in association with headaches and tinnitus. Either innominate vein may be involved, causing unilateral venous distention and edema of the ipsilateral upper extremity, head, and neck. Obstruction on the inferior vena cava is less common, but when it is present there may be associated edema of the lower extremities.

Miscellaneous Symptoms

Fever is uncommon in mediastinal lesions unless there is secondary infection in the tracheobronchial tree; it is also seen with Hodgkin's disease, lymphosarcoma, and degeneration of malignant disease. Weight loss, malaise, anemia, and anorexia are uncommon unless there is malignancy.

Physical Findings

Often, there are no unusual physical findings; wheeze, rhonchi, or rales may occasionally be present. There may be dullness to percussion over the area of mediastinal enlargement, extending laterally from each sternal border or posteriorly between the scapulas and above the diaphragm. Occasionally, there is tenderness over the chest wall, when a mediastinal tumor exerts pressure on the parietal pleura in that area.

DIAGNOSTIC PROCEDURES

The diagnostic procedures used for suspected lung lesions also apply for mediastinal tumors. However, the widespread use of and rapid improvements in CT scan and MRI have greatly aided the understanding of lesions and adjacent mediastinal structures. Certain situations unique to mediastinal tumors will be mentioned.

A tumor or lesion of the mediastinum should not be aspirated preoperatively if an operation is clearly indicated. Needle aspiration should be reserved for inoperable tumors and for emergencies in which tremendous cystic enlargement may jeopardize the child's life or may interfere with the induction of anesthesia.

Hydatid disease is not common in the United States, and only when it is present in the lung adjacent to the mediastinum can mediastinal tumor be simulated. The precipitin and skin test results are positive with an active hydatid cyst. Hooklets have been found in the sputum of patients so affected.

Mediastinal abscess is rarely confused with a neoplasm of the mediastinum. With abscess there is usually a history of trauma, foreign body in the esophagus, or use of surgical or gastroscopic instruments in the area. High fever, tachycardia, dyspnea, extreme weakness, and prostration usually develop rapidly; thus, the signs and symptoms of acute infection are paramount. The development of an air-fluid level in the mediastinum is diagnostic of mediastinal abscess if the preceding physical findings are also present. Intensive antibiotic therapy and prompt surgical drainage are indicated. There may be masses in the neck secondary to extension from lesions within the mediastinum.

PRIMARY MEDIASTINAL CYSTS

Lesions occurring within the mediastinum may be predominantly cystic or predominantly solid. Cystic lesions are usually benign, and solid lesions have higher malignant potential.

Primary mediastinal cysts probably represent abnormalities in embryologic development at the site of the foregut just when separation of esophageal and lung beds occurs (Fig. 50-22).

Structures that arise from the foregut are the pharynx, thyroid, parathyroid, thymus, respiratory tract, esophagus, stomach, upper part of the duodenum, liver, and pancreas; thus, abnormal development at this stage may give rise to bronchogenic cysts, esophageal duplication cysts, and gastroenteric cysts.

Bronchogenic Cysts

Maier[12] classified bronchogenic cysts according to location (Fig. 50-23) as tracheal, hilar (Fig. 50-24), carinal (Fig. 50-25), esophageal, and miscellaneous (Fig. 50-26). This classification remains useful. Modern nomenclature also uses the term *foregut duplication cysts,* a correct embryologic description of their developmental origin.

Bronchogenic cysts are usually located in the middle mediastinum but have been described in all mediastinal locations. Under microscopic examination, bronchogenic cysts may contain any or all of the tissues normally present in the trachea and bronchi (fibrous connective tissue, mucous glands, cartilage, smooth muscle, and a lining formed by ciliated pseudostratified columnar epithelium or stratified squamous epithelium). The fluid inside the cyst is either clear water-like liquid or viscous gelatinous material.

Bronchogenic cysts are usually asymptomatic. There may, however, be frequent upper respiratory tract infections, vague feelings of substernal discomfort, and respiratory difficulty (cough, noisy breathing, dyspnea, and possibly cyanosis). Bronchogenic cysts may communicate with the tracheobronchial tree and show varying air-fluid levels accompanied by the expectoration of purulent material. If communication with the tracheobronchial tree is present, it may be visualized using bronchoscopy.

On radiologic examination, the bronchogenic cyst is usually a single, smooth-bordered, spherical mass (Fig. 50-27). It has a uniform density similar to that of the cardiac shadow. Calcification is unusual. Fluoroscopic examination of the cyst may demonstrate that it moves with respiration (it is attached to the tracheobronchial tree); its shape may alter during the

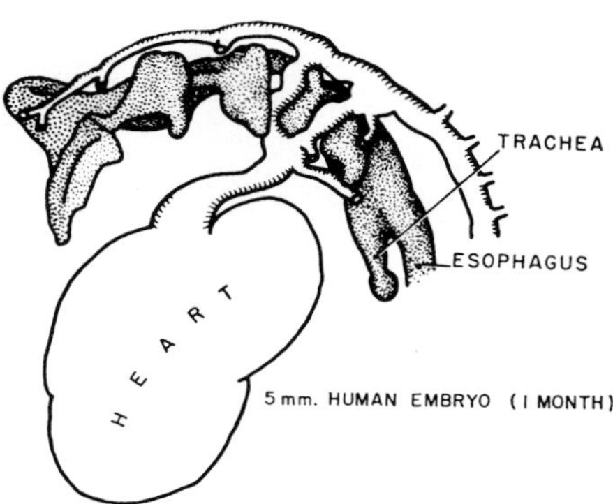

FIGURE 50-22. The foregut, lying between the tracheal and esophageal buds, is the probable site of embryologic maldevelopment, which gives rise to the growth of foregut cysts.

■ **FIGURE 50-23.** A diagram of the location of bronchogenic cysts, as suggested by Maier.[12] Sites B and C are the ones most commonly recorded.

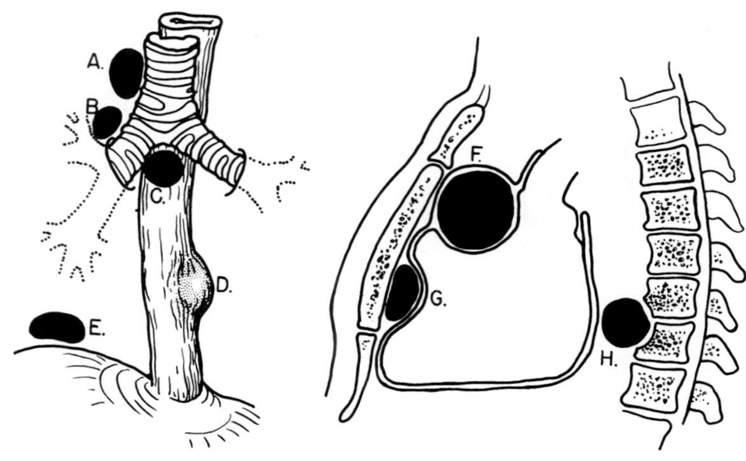

cycles of respiration. These lesions are occasionally identified on prenatal ultrasound.

When the bronchogenic cyst is located just below the carina, it may cause severe respiratory distress due to compression of either one or both major bronchi (Fig. 50-28). Early diagnosis and prompt removal are necessary.

There are no meticulous population-based studies, so incidence is conjecture. Phillipart and Farmer assembled perhaps the best composite review of all mediastinal masses; some 7% of mediastinal tumors were bronchogenic cysts.[13]

Bronchogenic cysts should be treated by surgical removal. Like most discrete lesions, most of these can be handled with

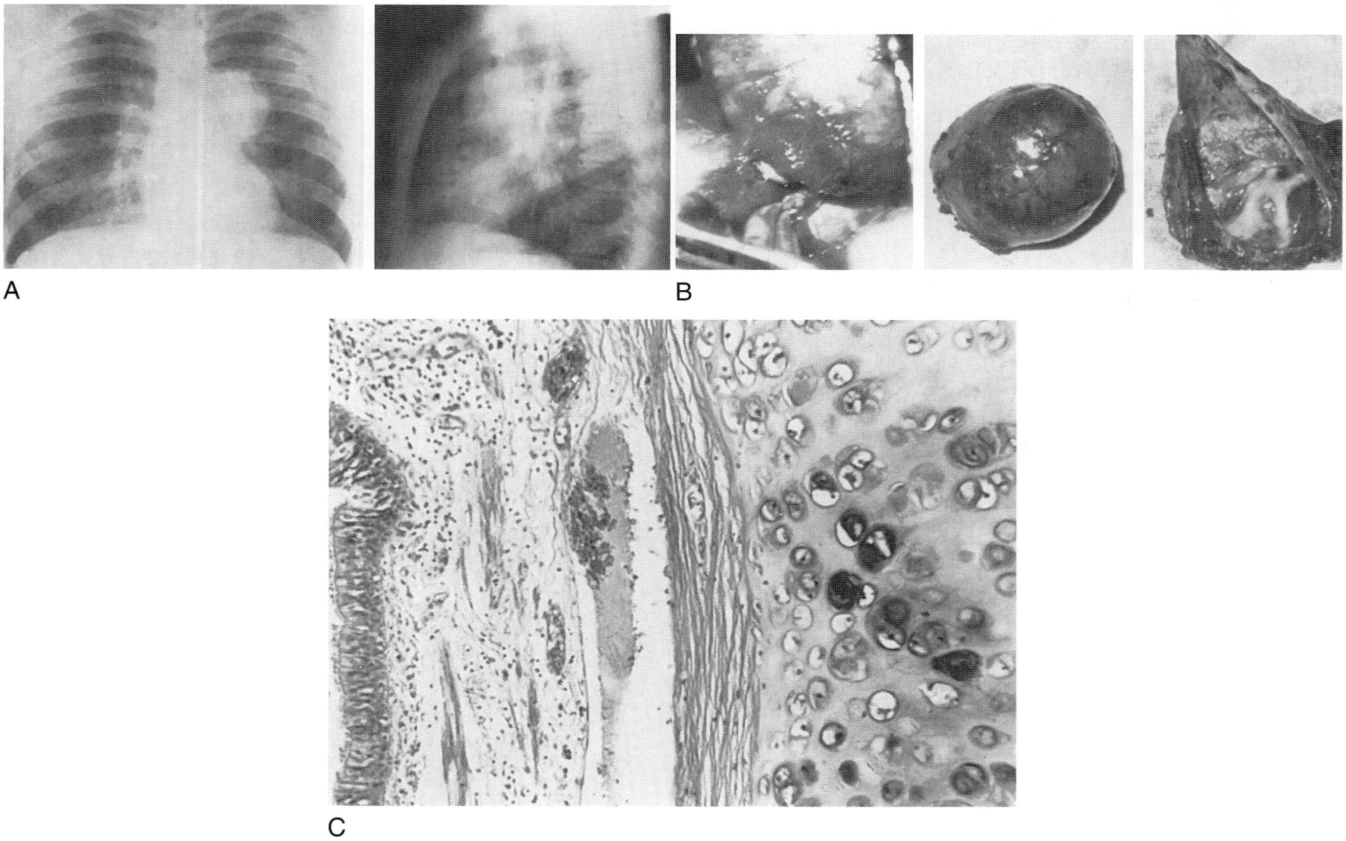

A

B

C

■ **FIGURE 50-24.** **A,** Typical left hilar bronchogenic cyst with a rounded, smooth border, and a density similar to cardiac density. **B,** At the time of thoracotomy, a solid stalk was found attached to the left main bronchus. The cyst was unilocular and contained thick, yellowish mucoid material. The wall was thin with typical trabeculations. **C,** Microscopic study revealed cartilage, smooth muscle, and pseudostratified, ciliated, columnar epithelium.

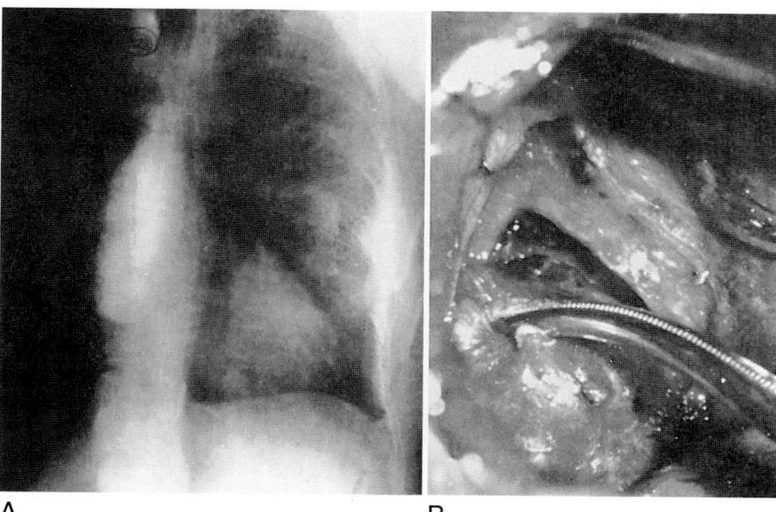

■ **FIGURE 50-25.** **A,** An overexposed posteroanterior chest radiograph shows a carinal bronchogenic cyst. **B,** At the operation, the location is clearly seen at the carina. A solid fibrous stalk is attached at the carina and is separated just beneath the instrument dissector.

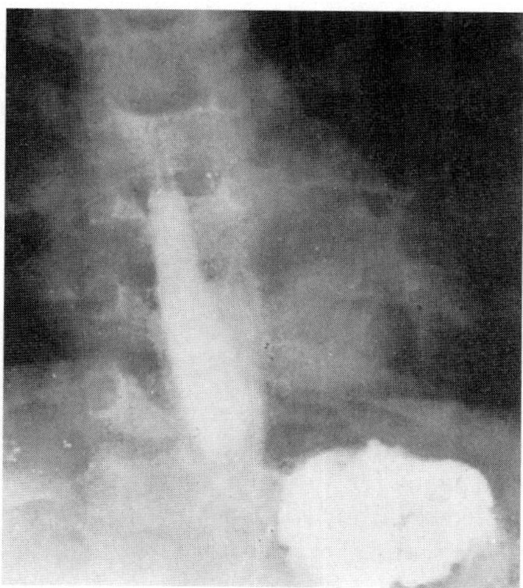

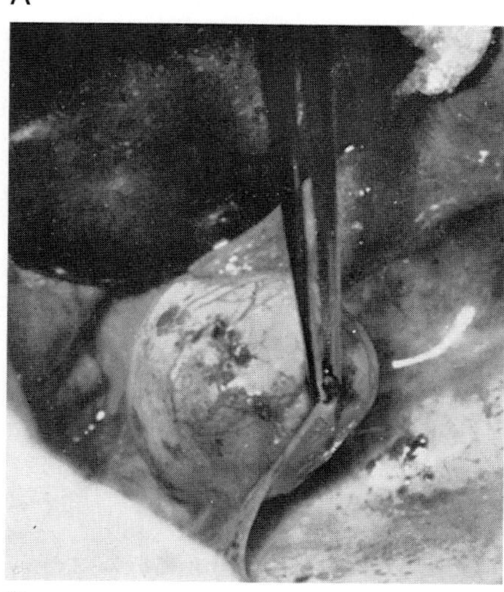

■ **FIGURE 50-26.** A bronchogenic cyst in a child. **A,** Radiograph. **B,** Photograph at surgery. The cyst is located retropleurally, overlying the distal thoracic aorta, and not attached to the respiratory tract or esophagus.

thoracoscopic techniques. Regardless of approach, care must be taken when these lesions share a common wall with either the airway or the esophagus. Resection is complicated, and tissue planes may be obliterated if there has been antecedent infection.

Esophageal Cysts (Duplication)

Esophageal cysts are located in the posterior mediastinum; they are usually on the right side and are intimately associated in the wall of the esophagus (Fig. 50-29). They occur more frequently in males than in females.

There are two types of esophageal cysts; the more characteristic type resembles adult esophagus with the cyst lined by noncornified stratified squamous epithelium having a well-defined muscularis mucosae and striated muscle in the wall. Intimate association in the muscular wall of the esophagus is not, however, accompanied by communication with the lumen of the esophagus.

The second type is lined by ciliated mucosa, thus resembling the fetal esophagus. Esophageal cysts may be associated with mild dysphagia and regurgitation but most frequently are asymptomatic. Barium esophagogram shows smooth indentation of the esophagus. On esophagoscopy there is indentation of the

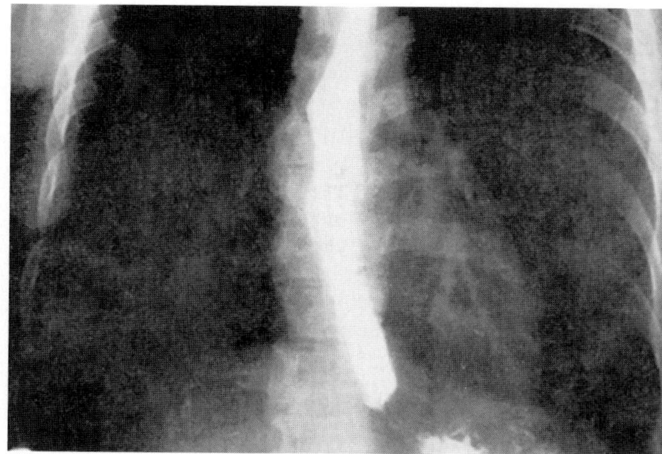

■ **FIGURE 50-27.** An esophagogram of a hilar bronchogenic cyst with an esophageal indentation.

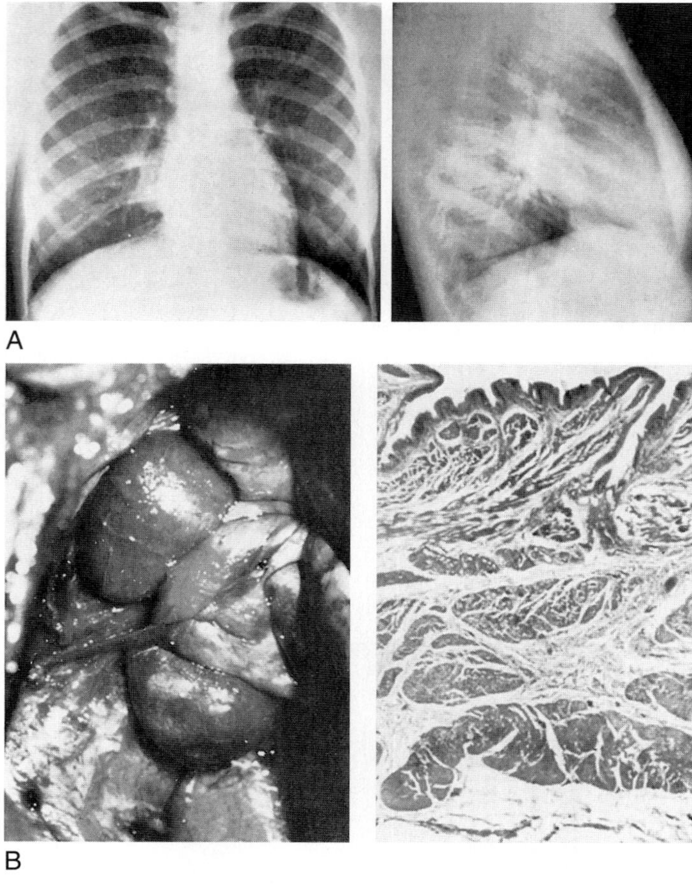

■ **FIGURE 50-28.** **A,** A bronchogenic cyst in a child whose mother had tuberculosis. The child was treated with antituberculous drugs for 1 year without change. **B,** A dumbbell-shaped bronchogenic cyst was found in the region of the inferior pulmonary vein during an operation. The microscopic section shows a wall with ciliated epithelium, no cartilage, and a smooth muscle wall of two layers.

normal mucosa by a pliable, movable, soft extramucosal mass. Removal is indicated for the same reasons as noted in discussion of the therapy of bronchogenic cysts; techniques are similar. Technically, these lesions may be more difficult to excise, especially if they are extensive or cross the diaphragm.

Gastroenteric Cysts

The third type of cyst arising from the foregut is the gastroenteric. This lies against the vertebrae, posterior or lateral to and usually free of the esophagus, and usually in the posterior mediastinum with the main attachment posterior. It may be recalled that the fetal esophagus is lined by columnar epithelium, much of which is ciliated, and this is only gradually converted to the stratified epithelium of the definitive organ. The change is generally complete or almost complete at birth.[14] Thus, if a cyst arises from the embryonic esophagus, it has a ciliated lining.

The enteric nature of a posterior mediastinal cyst is presumably certain if microscopic examination reveals a frank gastric or intestinal type of epithelium, but in general a better index of the nature and origin of such a cyst is the presence of well-developed muscularis mucosae, and two or even three main muscle coats. Gastric glands are most common, but esophageal, duodenal, or small-intestinal glands may be found. At operation, the cyst sometimes seems grossly "stomach-like" or "bowel-like." Cysts encountered in the posterior mediastinum show a highly developed mesodermal wall and even the presence of Meissner's and Auerbach's plexuses, whereas the lining epithelium varies in type from case to case, from columnar ciliated to typical small intestinal.

Two types of gastroenteric cysts have been described: (1) acid-secreting cysts, which are functionally active, and (2) cysts in which the mucosa has no functional activity.

Males are predominantly affected with this abnormality. Unlike other foregut cysts, posterior gastroenteric cysts are usually symptomatic. The symptoms are usually due to pressure on thoracic structures or rupture into bronchi with massive hemoptysis and death. Actual peptic perforation of the lung with hemorrhage has been recorded.

Hemoptysis in young infants is difficult to distinguish from hematemesis; it may follow ulceration of a gastroenteric cyst (with gastric lining) of the mediastinum, with subsequent erosion into the lung. Gastric epithelium associated with intestinal or respiratory epithelium is apparently less secretory. Many functional cysts may lose their functional activity when the secretory areas of the mucosa are destroyed. Renin, pepsin, chlorides, and free hydrochloric acid have been demonstrated in the contents of some of the cysts.

Posterior gastroenteric foregut cysts of the mediastinum are frequently associated with two other types of congenital anomalies: mesenteric abnormalities and vertebral abnormalities. When these are suspected, an MRI scan is the preferred diagnostic test. Both types may occur in the same case. In the embryo, the notochord and the entoderm are at one time in intimate contact; thus, this combined developmental anomaly may result from abnormal embryonic development.

Penetration of the diaphragm by a cyst arising primarily from the thorax may occur; conversely, penetration of the diaphragm

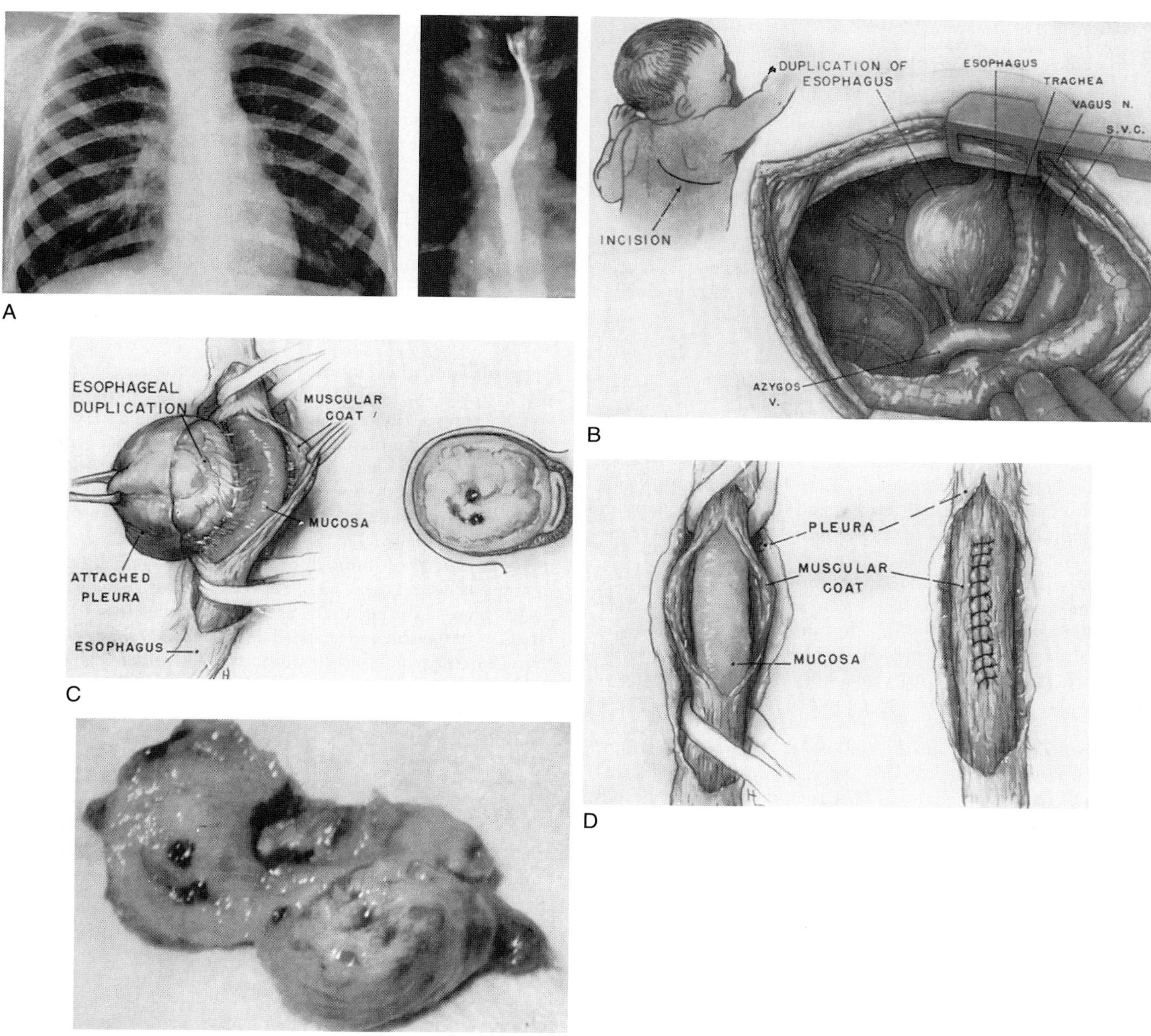

■ **FIGURE 50-29. A,** A posteroanterior chest roentgenogram taken of a child with an upper respiratory tract infection. A mass is seen in the posterior superior mediastinum presenting into the right hemithorax. At the time of an esophagogram, the esophagus is seen displaced toward the left by a smooth mass. **B–D,** Drawings of findings at the operation. Note the plane of separation from the mucosa of the esophagus and the lack of communication with the esophageal lumen. **E,** An opened operative specimen, the cavity of which was filled with mucoid fluid. The lining of the duplication was typical squamous cell.

by the free end of an intramesenteric intestinal duplication is also possible.

A survey of the literature confirms that as many as two thirds of patients with mediastinal cysts have vertebral anomalies including hemivertebra, spina bifida anterior, or infantile scoliosis. Most of these vertebral lesions involve the upper thoracic and lower cervical vertebrae, and the cyst tends to be caudad to the vertebral lesion. MRI may be helpful in demonstrating these lesions and the cyst.

The presence of spina bifida anterior, congenital scoliosis, Klippel-Feil syndrome, or similar but less well-defined lesions in the cervical or dorsal vertebrae suggests enteric cysts in the mediastinum or in the abdomen.

Pericardial Coelomic Cysts

These mesothelial cysts are developmental in origin, and persistence is related to the pericardial coelom. The primitive pericardial cavity forms by the fusion of coelomic spaces on each side of the embryo. During the process, dorsal and ventral parietal recesses are formed. Dorsal recesses communicate with the pleuroperitoneal coelom, and the ventral recesses end blindly at the septum transversum. Persistence of segments of the ventral parietal recess accounts for most pericardial coelomic cysts.

The cysts are usually located anteriorly in the cardiophrenic angles, more frequently on the right, and occasionally on or in the diaphragm (Fig. 50-30). They are usually asymptomatic and are discovered on routine chest roentgenogram. Rarely do they reach sufficient size to cause displacement of the heart or to produce pressure on the pulmonary tissue. Infection is unusual.

Pericardial cysts are usually unilocular. The walls are thin, and the intersurfaces are smooth and glistening, lined by a single layer of flat mesothelial cells. The mesothelium is supported by fibrous tissue with attached adipose tissue.

These cysts are very rare; two have been reported in children. Because these cysts are benign, observation may be warranted. Alternatively, thoracoscopic excision can be undertaken.

Intrathoracic Meningoceles

Intrathoracic meningoceles are not true mediastinal tumors or cysts; they are diverticuli of the spinal meninges that protrude through the neuroforamen adjacent to an intercostal nerve and manifest beneath the pleura in the posterior medial thoracic gutter. The wall represents an extension of the leptomeninges, and the content is cerebrospinal fluid. Enlargement of the intervertebral foramen is common; vertebral or rib anomalies adjacent to the meningocele are also frequent. The most commonly associated anomalies are kyphosis, scoliosis, and bone erosion or destruction. The wall of these cysts is formed by two distinct components, the dura mater and the arachnoidea spinalis, with small nerve trunks and ganglia occasionally incorporated in it.

A syndrome of generalized neurofibromatosis (von Recklinghausen's disease), kyphoscoliosis, and intrathoracic meningocele may occur, but thoracic meningocele as an isolated defect is much less frequent; four pediatric cases have been reported. This lesion is usually asymptomatic; it occurs on the right side approximately three times more often than on the left. Rarely, the lesion may be bilateral. In patients with neurofibromatosis, posterior sulcus tumors are usually meningoceles and rarely neurofibromas.

On x-ray examination, the lesion is a regular, well-demarcated intrathoracic density located in the posterior sulcus; associated congenital anomalies of the spine and thorax may be noted. On fluoroscopic examination, pulsations may be noted in the sac. Diagnosis may be confirmed by myelograms and/or MRI.

When diagnosis is securely established, no therapy is indicated unless the lesion is symptomatic. Operative complications such as empyema, meningitis, and spinal fluid fistula have been greatly reduced since the advent of antibiotic therapy.

TUMORS OF THE THYMUS

Normally, the thymus is located in the anterior superior mediastinum, but abnormalities of the thymus have been reported in all areas of the mediastinum. Abnormalities of the thymus in children are: (1) hyperplasia, (2) neoplasms, (3) benign thymomas, (4) cysts, (5) teratoma, and (6) tuberculosis.

Hyperplasia of the Thymus. Hyperplasia of the thymus is the most frequent of the thymic lesions.

The normal thymus varies greatly in size, and with age. Thus, thymic hyperplasia is seldom clear-cut. Steroids, infection, androgens, and irradiation may make the thymus smaller; those stimuli that cause hyperplasia are not well understood. As in other ductless glands, variations in size are probably related to patient individuality.

In a review of normal chest roentgenograms, Ellis and colleagues[15] found that a recognizable thymic shadow was almost always present during the first month of life; there was great variation in the size and shape. The mediastinal shadow in these young infants seemed to be proportionally wider than in older children and adults because of the proportionally larger heart and thymic shadow between 1 and 12 months, the thymic shadow was still present if it had been seen earlier. Between 1 and 3 years, very little of the thymic shadow remained. Among children older than 4 years of age, 2% still have a recognizable thymus on x-ray examination. It does not contain calcium, and there are transmitted pulsations on fluoroscopy. Cervical extension of the thymus gland is common. If the thymus is located in the superior thoracic inlet, its enlargement may cause tracheal compression (Fig. 50-31).

In the unusual situation where an enlarged thymus causes respiratory obstruction, treatment may be carried out in one of three ways. First, the thymus does respond rapidly to small doses (70–150 cGy) of irradiation; however, the clear carcinogenic effect has caused this method of treatment to be abandoned. Second, corticosteroids cause a rapid decrease in the size of the thymus, usually within 5 to 7 days. However, after cessation of corticosteroid therapy, the gland may reach a size greater than that before treatment was instituted. Such a response may also be used in distinguishing between a physiologic enlargement of the thymus and a neoplasm (Fig. 50-32). Third, excision may be indicated both for the treatment of respiratory obstruction and for diagnosis.

Neoplasm of the Thymus. Malignant thymic tumors in children are quite rare. Lymphosarcoma is more frequent; primary Hodgkin's disease of the thymus and carcinoma have both been described. In only one 19-year-old has there been an associated myasthenia gravis syndrome.

Benign Thymoma. Rarely, benign thymic tumors have been reported in children (Fig. 50-33).

Thymic Cysts. Multiple small cysts of the thymus are frequently observed in necropsy material, but large thymic cysts are rare (Fig. 50-34). Fridjon[16] described a large cyst in the thymus of

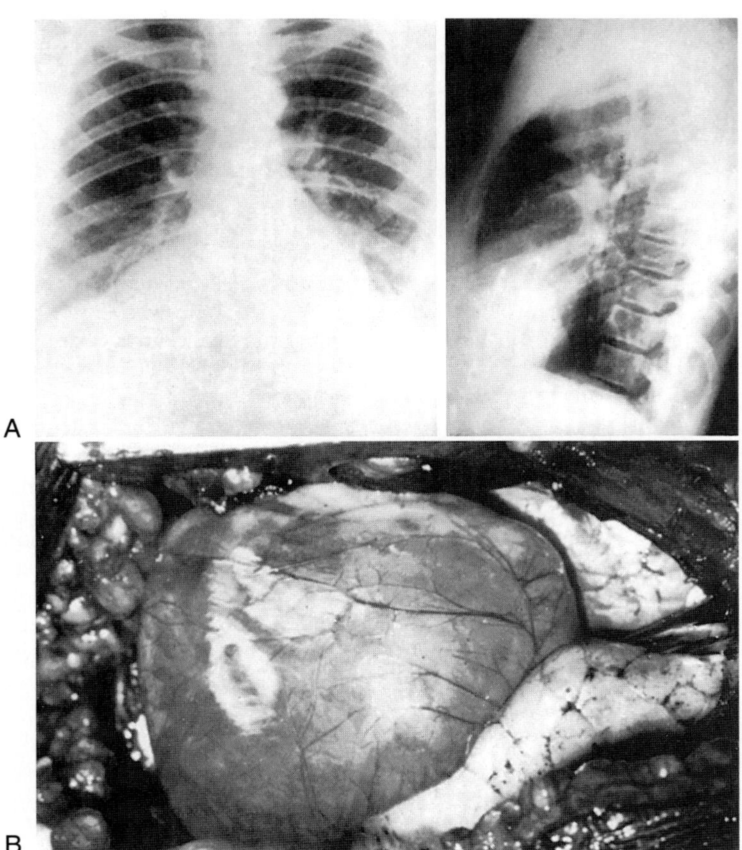

■ **FIGURE 50-30. A,** The typical location of a pericardial cyst in posteroanterior and lateral chest films at the right cardiophrenic angle. **B,** A large cyst seen at the time of a thoracotomy.

a 1-day-old infant. Thymic cysts have been resected from the neck (Fig. 50-35).

Teratoma of the Thymus. A teratoma of the thymus in a 2-day-old infant was described by Sealy and colleagues[17]; she suffered progressive respiratory distress and underwent operation at 7 weeks of age.

Tuberculosis of the Thymus Gland. A single case of tuberculosis involving only the thymus gland has been described in a stillborn infant.

TERATOID MEDIASTINAL TUMORS

Teratoid tumors of the mediastinum may be classified as: (1) benign cystic teratomas, (2) benign teratoids (solid), or (3) teratoids (carcinoma).

Benign Cystic Teratoma

Teratoma of the anterior mediastinum probably results from faulty embryogenesis of the thymus or from local dislocation of tissue during embryogenesis.

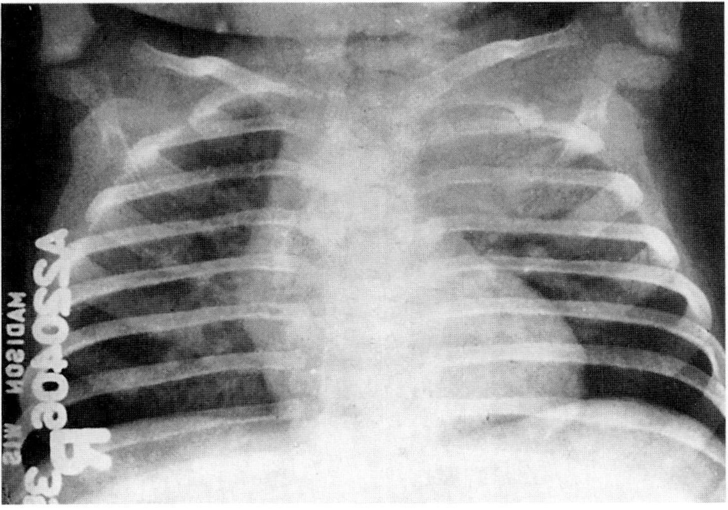

■ **FIGURE 50-31.** Mild respiratory distress in an infant with an enlarged thymus. Gradual improvement occurred with age and no specific therapy.

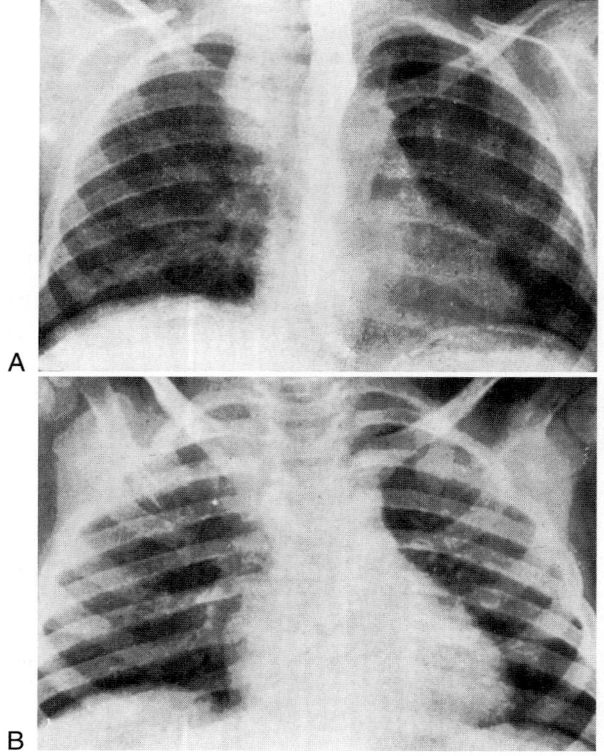

■ **FIGURE 50-32.** **A,** An enlarged thymus in an infant. **B,** A reduction in size can be seen after 7 days of steroid therapy.

Benign cystic teratoma (mediastinal dermoid cyst) contains such elements of ectodermal tissue as hair, sweat glands, sebaceous cysts, and teeth. Other elements, including mesodermal and entodermal tissue, may also be found when benign cystic teratoid lesions are subjected to comprehensive examination; thus, such tumors are more properly classified as teratoid than dermoid cysts.

Cystic teratomas are more common than solid ones. These lesions are predominantly located in the anterior mediastinum and may project into either hemithorax, more commonly the right. In children, females are affected more often than males. Malignant degeneration is less common than in the solid form of teratoid tumor.

It seems reasonable to assume that most, perhaps all, mediastinal teratomas are present at birth; however, Edge and Glennie[18] reported two adult patients from whom large teratoid tumors were removed 2 years and 4 years after routine chest roentgenograms were normal.

These cystic masses usually cause symptoms because of pressure on or erosion into the adjacent respiratory structures. Symptoms usually include vague chest discomfort associated with cough, dyspnea, and pneumonitis. Infection may cause a sudden exacerbation of symptoms, and rupture into the lung may occur with expectoration of hair; rupture into the pleura or pericardium may also occur.

The lesion is usually in the anterior mediastinum. On x-ray film, the lesion is well outlined, with sharp borders; definite diagnosis is not possible unless teeth can be demonstrated in the mass. Calcification, which is not unusual, appears as scattered

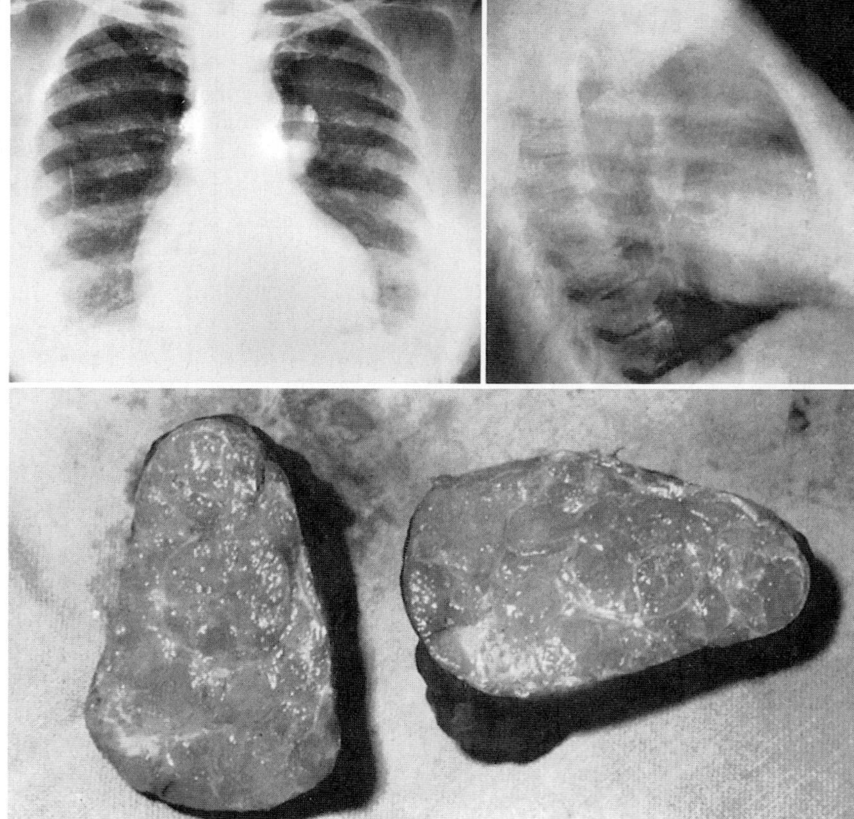

■ **FIGURE 50-33.** A benign thymoma located in the anterior superior mediastinum. **A,** Posteroanterior and lateral radiographs before surgery. **B,** Photograph of thymoma after excision.

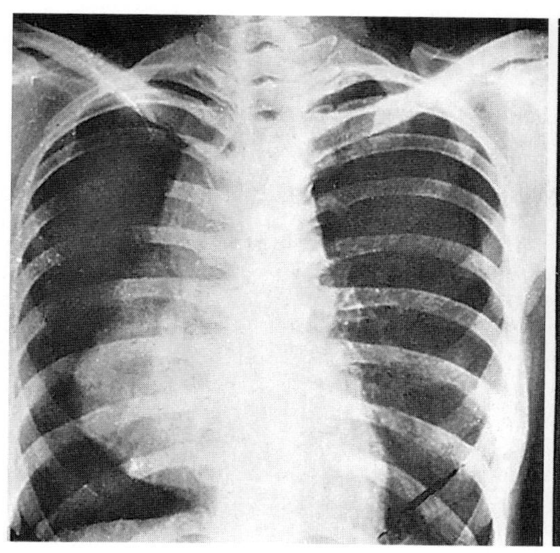
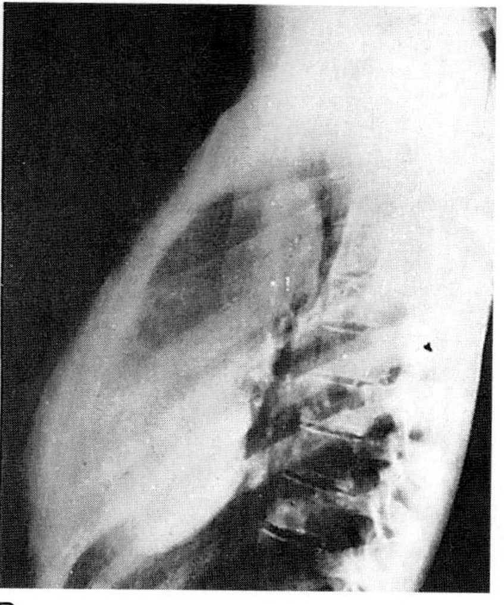

■ **FIGURE 50-34.** A large thymic cyst located near the diaphragm in an adult. Posteroanterior **(A)** and left lateral **(B)** radiographs.

masses rather than as diffuse, small densities. Cystic swelling in the suprasternal notch may occur.

Benign cystic teratomas should be removed. In cases in which infection, perforation, intracystic hemorrhage, or malignant degeneration has occurred, complete removal may be difficult or impossible, owing to adherence to surrounding vital structures.

Benign Solid Teratoid Tumors and Malignant Teratoid Tumors

Teratoma is the most common tumor occurring in the anterior mediastinum of infants and children (Fig. 50-36), and the mediastinum is the second most common location. The solid tumors in the teratoid group are much more complex and have a greater propensity for malignant change (Fig. 50-37). The incidence of malignancy has been reported from 10% to 25%. In addition to standard imaging studies, preoperative serum studies should include serum alpha fetoprotein, carcinoembryonic antigen, and β-human chorionic gonadotropin, both as diagnostic markers and as baseline values to monitor disease burden.

Benign solid teratoid tumors have well-differentiated structures that are rarely observed in malignant tumors. The connective tissue stroma of malignant teratoma is usually poorly arranged, but that of benign teratoma is dense and of the adult type. In the benign type, nerve tissue, skin, and teeth may be found.

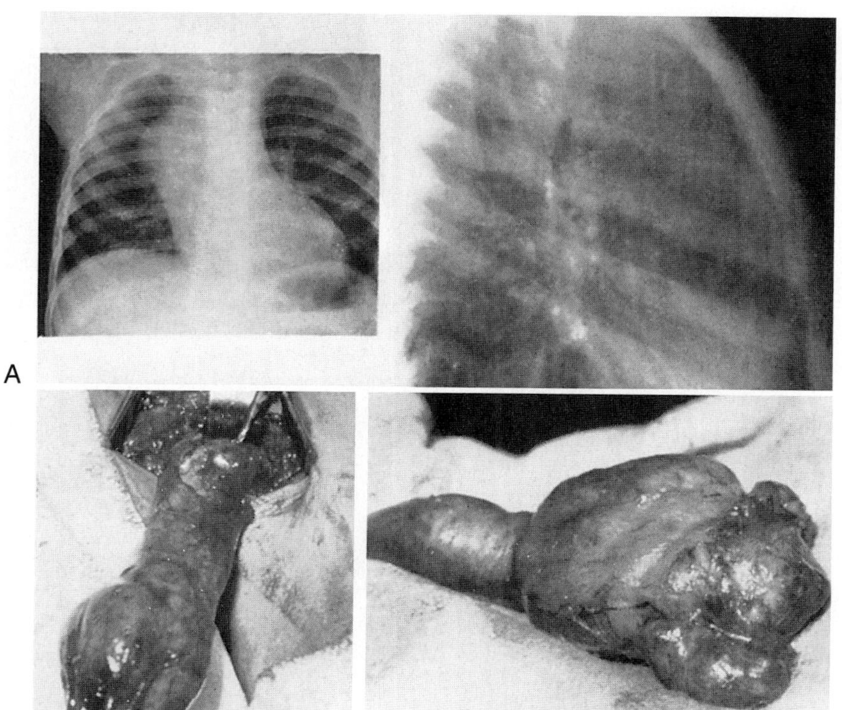

■ **FIGURE 50-35. A,** A large thymic cyst in a 4-year-old boy that was evident as a mass in the right side of the neck clinically as well as on a chest roentgenogram. Removal required a thoracotomy and a supraclavicular incision. **B,** A thymic cyst as seen after a thoracotomy and at the time of removal through a neck incision.

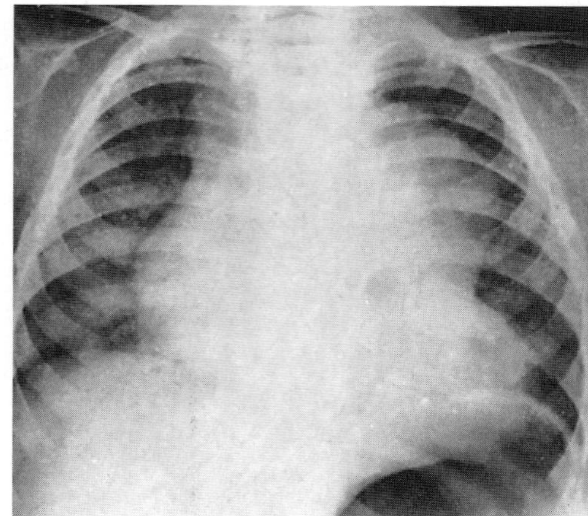

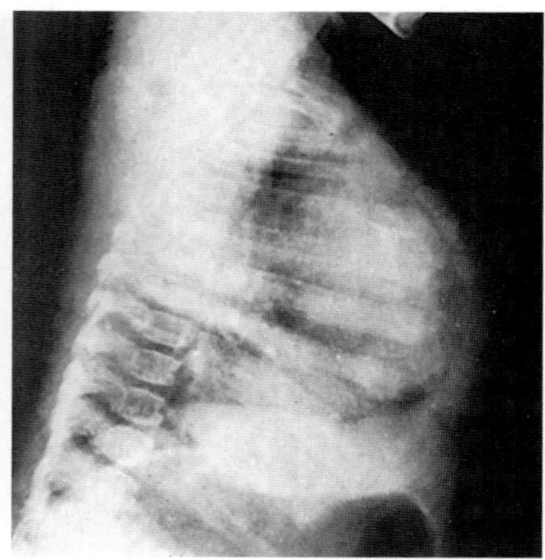

■ **FIGURE 50-36.** A large, solid, benign teratoma in an infant. Note the anterior mediastinal position and the forward displacement of the sternum.

Skin and its appendages are usually present and remarkably well formed. Hair follicles preserve their normal slightly oblique position relative to the free surface and are always accompanied by well-developed sebaceous glands. Sweat glands, often of the apocrine type, are frequently located near the sebaceous glands. Smooth muscle closely resembling arrectores pilorum is occasionally encountered.

Mesodermal derivatives, such as connective tissue, bone, cartilage, and muscle arranged in organoid pattern, are frequently found. When present, hematopoietic tissue is found only in association with cancellous bone. Smooth muscle is most often observed as longitudinal or circular bundles in organoid alimentary structures. Occasionally, it is also seen in bronchial walls. Entodermal derivatives representing such structures as intestine and respiratory and pancreatic tissue are also present.

The final diagnosis of malignancy can be determined only after removal and histologic study of the tumor. Malignant degeneration usually involves only one of the cellular components. In general, the outcome is poor with malignant teratomas, chemotherapy and radiotherapy notwithstanding.

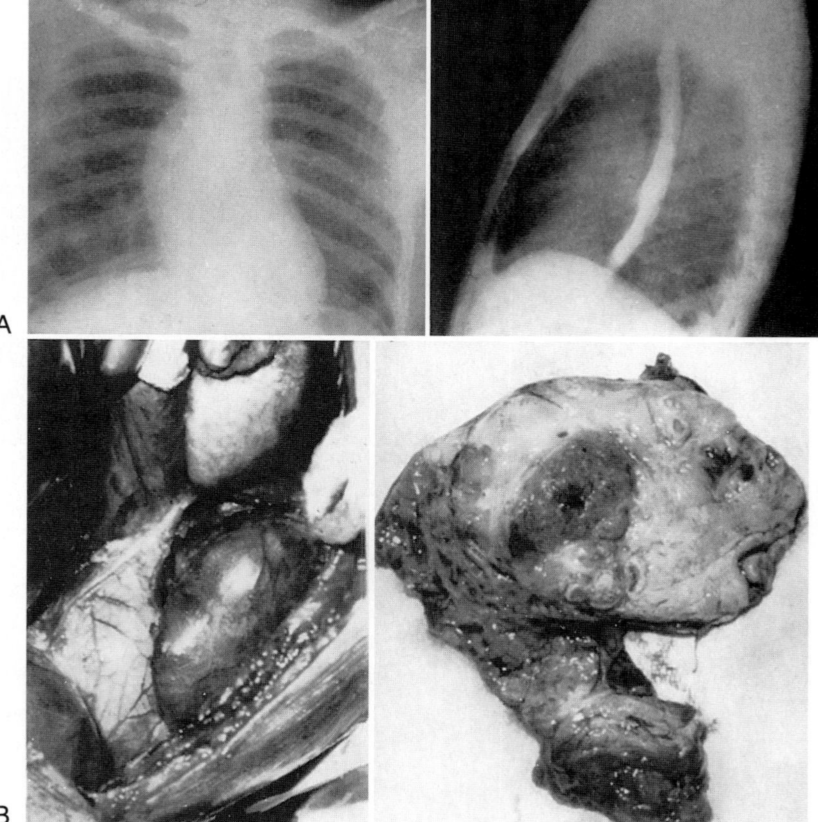

■ **FIGURE 50-37.** **A,** Posteroanterior and lateral radiographs of an anterior malignant teratoma in an older child. **B,** Note the anterior mediastinal position, with the teratoma wedged between the heart and the sternum.

NEUROGENIC MEDIASTINAL TUMORS

Neurogenic tumors, by far the most common tumors with posterior mediastinal origin, may be classified as follows:

1. Neurofibroma and neurilemoma
   - Malignant schwannoma
2. Tumors of sympathetic origin
   - Neuroblastoma
   - Ganglioneuroma
   - Ganglioneuroblastoma
   - Pheochromocytoma
3. Chemodectoma

Benign neurofibromas, neurilemomas, and malignant schwannomas are extremely unusual in the pediatric age group and when present are most often asymptomatic (Fig. 50-38).

A neuroblastoma is a malignant tumor arising from a neural crest origin; typically the site is the adrenal medulla, but these may occur anywhere along the ganglia of the sympathetic nervous system from neck to pelvis. Although a primary neuroblastoma may cause the first clinical signs or symptoms, metastases in the bone, skin, or lymph nodes may be the first indication of its presence. While most other childhood cancers have shown marked improvement in survival over the last 20 years, neuroblastoma has not.

The ganglioneuroma is a benign tumor made up of mature ganglion cells, few or many, in a stroma of nerve fibers. Ganglioneuroblastoma is a tumor composed of various proportions of neuroblastoma and ganglioneuroma.

Ganglioneuroma and ganglioneuroblastoma are more likely to present after the age of 2 years. The more malignant forms, such as neuroblastoma, frequently become manifest before the age of 2 years. Ganglioneuroma is more common in children than in adults; respiratory symptoms are rare (Fig. 50-39).

Most of these tumors usually occur in the upper two thirds of the hemithorax and tend to extend locally. They may grow into the lower part of the neck and across the midline through the posterior mediastinum to the opposite hemithorax, descend through the diaphragm into the upper part of the abdomen or into the intercostal spaces posteriorly, and involve one or several of the vertebral foramina.

A large number of neurogenic tumors, more often the benign type, may be asymptomatic. Symptoms such as radicular pain, paraplegia, motor disturbances, and Horner syndrome may occur.

Upper respiratory tract infections, dyspnea, elevated temperature, and weight loss may occur. Neurogenic tumors of the neuroblastoma group usually occur in younger children, and respiratory symptoms, thoracic pain, and fever are more common (Fig. 50-40).

On x-ray examination, neurogenic tumors are round, oval, or spindle-shaped and are characteristically located posteriorly in the paravertebral gutter. On thoracic radiographs, a ganglioneuroma appears as an elongated lesion and may extend over a distance of several vertebrae. Typically, a neurofibroma tends to be more rounded in outline. Calcifications within the tumor may be seen, more commonly in the malignant forms. Even though not demonstrated on radiologic examination, calcification may be found at the time of histologic examination. Bone lesions, such as intercostal space widening, costal deformation, vertebral involvement, and metastatic bone disease, are not uncommon.

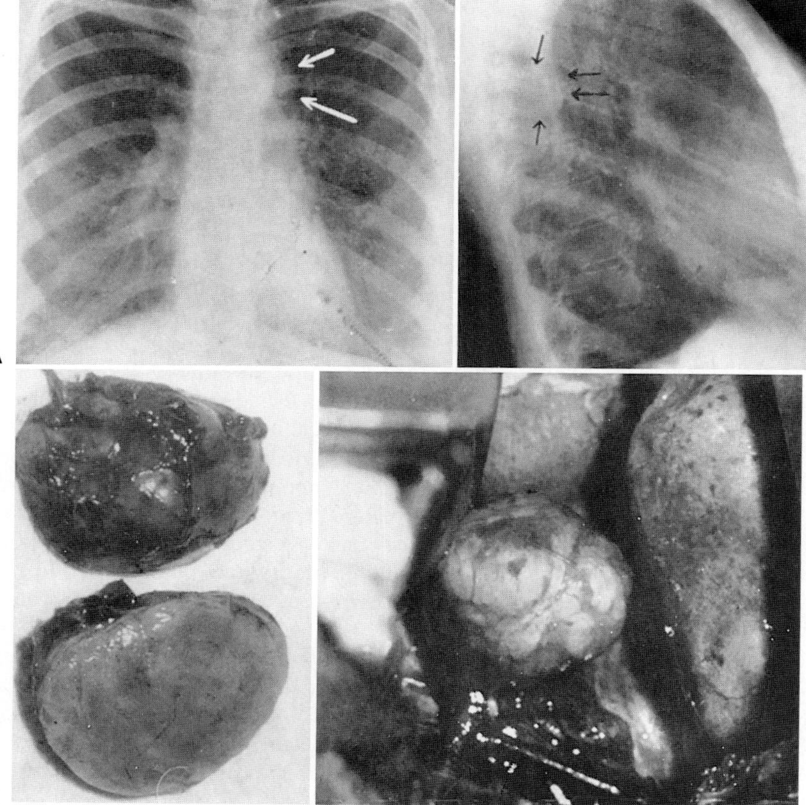

FIGURE 50-38. **A,** Neurofibroma seen posteriorly located in posteroanterior and lateral radiographs. **B,** Note the solid nature of the lesion, its round smooth outline, and its attachment to the intercostal nerve.

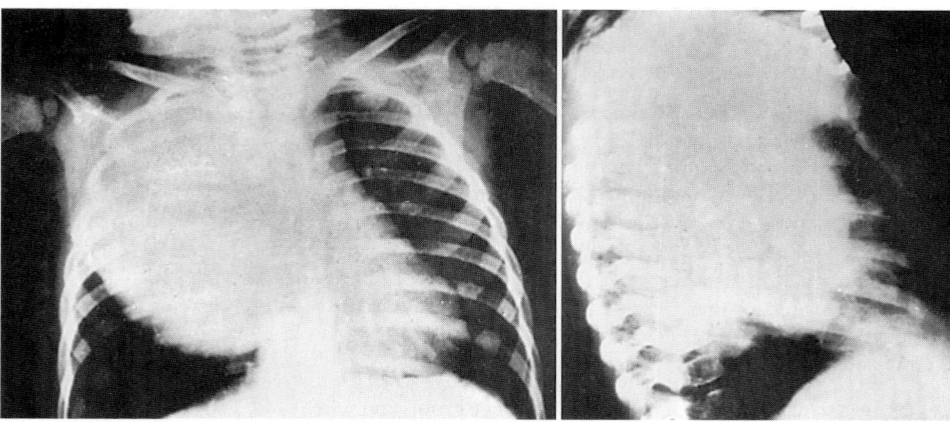

■ **FIGURE 50-39.** A large ganglioneuroma in an infant. The benign lesion was removed, with a good follow-up result.

The primary therapy for localized thoracic neurogenic tumors is surgical excision. Every case of ganglioneuroma (benign) reported in a study by Schweisguth and co-workers[19] was amenable to resection. In malignant neurogenic tumors, all possible tumor should be excised and postoperative irradiation therapy initiated. Radiotherapy must be given judiciously, because growth disturbances, pulmonary fibrosis, and other sequelae may develop. In the hourglass type of tumor, with intravertebral foramina extension, diagnostic CT myelogram is followed by laminectomy and excision of the extradural tumor to relieve spinal cord compression. Excision of the mediastinal component may be delayed for several days.

Mediastinal chemodectomas are usually located anteriorly; they are likely to be associated with similar tumors in the carotid body and elsewhere. There is a tendency for these tumors to be multiple. Mediastinal pheochromocytomas are extremely rare and have not been recorded in the pediatric age group.

In Heimburger and Battersby's[20] series of mediastinal tumors in childhood, 25% of 36 tumors were of the neurogenic type. Ellis and DuShane[21] reported 32% neurogenic tumors in a review of primary mediastinal cysts and neoplasms in infants. More recently, a persistent incidence of 33% was demonstrated in Phillipart and Farmer's collected series.[13]

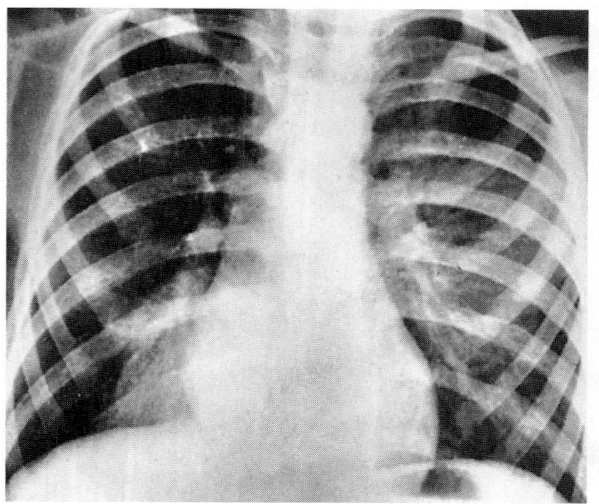

■ **FIGURE 50-40.** A neuroblastoma in a 6-year-old boy.

MEDIASTINAL LYMPH NODE ABNORMALITIES

Abnormalities of the lymph nodes in the mediastinum may be classified as follows:

1. Leukemia
2. Hodgkin's disease
3. Lymphosarcoma
4. Sarcoidosis
5. Inflammatory disorders
    - Fungus
    - Nonspecific

Any lymph node enlargement in a child should be viewed with suspicion, since lymphatic tumors are one of the more frequently observed malignant growths in childhood. The diagnosis is made by biopsy. Hodgkin's disease, lymphosarcoma, and reticulum cell sarcoma group are found primarily in children more than 3 years of age, with a peak incidence from 8 to 14 years. More than 95% of children with primary lymphatic malignancy have lymph node enlargement as the presenting sign. Tonsillar hypertrophy and adenoidal hyperplasia, pulmonary hilar enlargement, splenomegaly, bone pain, unexplained fever, anemia, infiltrative skin lesions, and, rarely, central nervous system symptoms may also be present. The diagnosis should be sought through the study of peripheral blood smears, lymph node biopsy, pleural fluid examination, or bone marrow examination.

If all other diagnostic studies are negative, the mediastinal node can be biopsied. Fine needle aspiration is usually not satisfactory, thus Tru-cut biopsy, thoracoscopy, or anterior thoracotomy is frequently required. Anesthetic management is complicated if there is greater than 50% tracheal luminal compression.

In most cases of mediastinal malignancy, bilateral hilar nodal involvement is present. The lymph node enlargement may rarely be unilateral and relatively localized. In such cases, routine study of the blood smear, bone marrow studies may not provide the diagnosis, and thoracoscopic biopsy may be necessary. In such localized cases, complete lymph node removal should be carried out if technically feasible.

Surgical excision has limited value in lymphosarcoma, because the disease is usually widespread. However, when the lesions are apparently isolated in the neck, axilla, mediastinum, or gastrointestinal tract, removal makes sense. With few exceptions, all the tumors in this group are radiosensitive; however, they are not curable by x-ray therapy.

Inflammatory Disorders

Lymph node enlargement in the hilus of the lung or mediastinum may be secondary to tuberculous, fungal, or bacterial lung disease. Diagnosis is usually confirmed by means of sputum culture, examination of washings from the tracheobronchial tree taken at the time of bronchoscopy, scalene node biopsy, and skin tests correlated with the general clinical picture. The same is true in sarcoidosis. In sarcoidosis there may be involvement of the eye, skin, peripheral lymph nodes, mediastinal or hilar lymph nodes, and the lung parenchyma. Although nonspecific symptomatic or asymptomatic enlargement of the mediastinal lymph nodes may occur, a cause can usually be found.

Castleman disease, or giant lymph node hyperplasia, was first described in 1954. Although this rare, benign, localized lymph node enlargement may occur in extrathoracic locations, it most often occurs as an isolated asymptomatic mediastinal or pulmonary hilar tumor. Grossly, the tumors are moderately firm and usually well encapsulated. Calcification may occur but is unusual. On microscopic examination, the two main features of these lymphoid masses are a diffuse follicular replacement of the lymph node architecture and much follicular and interfollicular vascular proliferation. Sixty percent of patients with this entity are asymptomatic. When symptoms occur, they may include cough, fatigue, chest pain, and fever. Surgical excision is the treatment of choice and is usually curative.

VASCULAR LYMPHATIC ABNORMALITIES OF THE MEDIASTINUM

Vascular-lymphatic abnormalities of the mediastinum may be classified as: (1) cavernous hemangioma, (2) hemangiopericytoma, (3) angiosarcoma, or (4) lymphangioma.

Vascular tumors isolated to the mediastinum in children are rare. Vascular tumors may occur at any level in the mediastinum but are more frequent in the upper portion of the thorax and in the anterior mediastinum. They are uniformly rounded in appearance and are moderately dense. Calcification within the tumor is unusual. They are usually asymptomatic.

Isolated mediastinal lymphangiomas are relatively rare but occur more often in infants and children than in adults. These tumors consist of masses of dilated lymphatic channels containing lymph; they are lined with flat endothelium and are usually multilocular. They may appear to be isolated in the mediastinum (Fig. 50-41) but much more often have an associated cervical component. They may be rather large and unilateral, with lateral masses in the superior mediastinum. In 1948, Gross and Hurwitt[22] reported 21 cases of cervical mediastinal hygromas and only 8 cases of isolated mediastinal hygromas.

Diagnosis of a cervicomediastinal lymphangiomas is made by physical examination of the cervical swelling and radiographic examination of the chest. Periodic fluctuation in size frequently occurs in the cervical location. This is even more characteristic of the combined cervicomediastinal lesions; in these, the cervical component may increase in size during inspiratory movements. Radiographic and fluoroscopic examination may show descent of the mass into the mediastinum on inspiration with prominence in the neck during expiration.

Cystic hygroma confined to the mediastinum is usually discovered as an unanticipated finding on radiographic examination. The soft and yielding nature of the cysts allows them to attain considerable size without producing symptoms. On radiograph there is a somewhat lobulated, smoothly outlined mass; however, it is usually not possible to distinguish lymphangiomas from other benign tumors or cysts of the mediastinum by this method.

When respiratory infections occur, lymphangiomas may become infected. Such infections are usually controlled by antibiotics or by drainage. Infection may be followed by local fibrosis and the disappearance of the mass. Spontaneous or posttraumatic hemorrhage into a cyst may result in extension of the cyst; this may cause sudden tracheal compression, a surgical emergency. Malignant change in lymphangiomas has not been reported.

Surgical excision is the treatment of choice for localized lesions. Extensive disease remains an unsolved problem; for macrocystic variants, intralesional sclerotherapy has had some utility. Chylothorax may result when there is involvement of the thoracic duct.

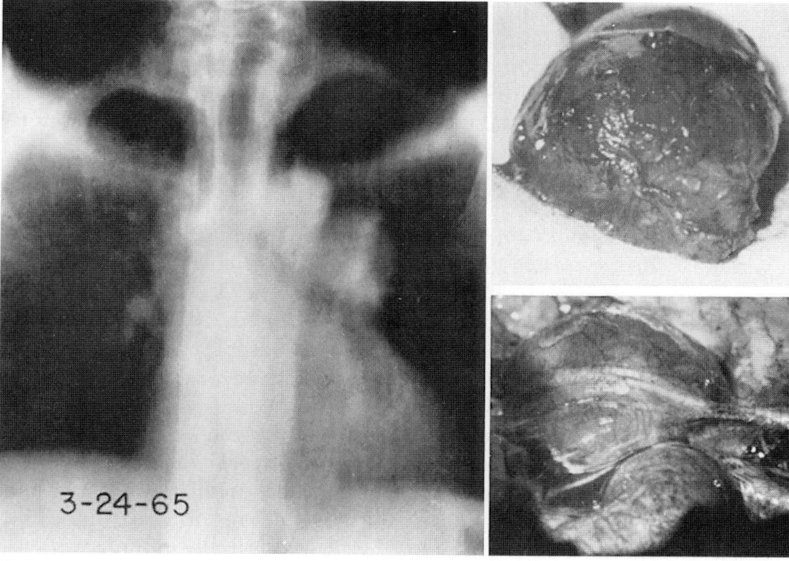

FIGURE 50-41. A large lymphatic cyst in the anterior mediastinum. **A,** Posteroanterior radiograph. **B,** Photographs.

MEDIASTINAL LIPOMA AND LIPOSARCOMA

Intrathoracic lipoma is rare in children. Lipomas of the mediastinum have been divided into three groups according to their location and form: (1) tumors confined within the thoracic cage, (2) intrathoracic lipomas that extend upward into the neck, and (3) intrathoracic lipomas with an extrathoracic extension forming a dumbbell configuration.

Of the lipomas reported in the world literature, 76% were intrathoracic, 10% were cervicomediastinal, and 14% were of the dumbbell type. Only 15 occurred in the pediatric age group, and these were intrathoracic. Four cases of liposarcoma of the mediastinum in children have been reported. Although these tumors usually do not metastasize, their invasiveness and tendency to recur locally place them in the malignant group.

Lipoblastoma is a rare benign tumor occurring in children and arising from fetal embryonal fat. Five cases have been reported in the world literature and 90% of the tumors are detected in children younger than 3 years. Seventy percent of them occur in the extremities. At surgery the lipoblastoma appears as a soft, yellow-gray or white-gray mass that can be easily removed.

In general, lipomas of the subcutaneous tissue are benign, whereas those of the retroperitoneal area and deep somatic soft tissue are usually malignant. The tumors of the mediastinum seem to have an incidence and behavior similar to those of lipomas in the peritoneal region.

Radical surgical excision is the procedure of choice. Repeated surgical attacks may serve as a method of extended control, and x-ray therapy may be added for palliative purposes.

THYROID DISORDERS

Substernal thyroid is a common anterior superior mediastinal tumor in the adult age group but apparently does not occur before puberty. Ectopic thyroid in the mediastinum does occur in children, and in such cases blood supply is derived from a mediastinal vessel.

PRIMARY CARDIAC AND PERICARDIAL TUMORS

Primary tumors of the heart in infants may cause cardiac enlargement or enlargement of the cardiac silhouette, giving rise to symptoms in the lungs or esophagus. Most frequently, the signs and symptoms of congestive heart failure are much more prominent than those of tumors of the respiratory system or esophagus.

Rhabdomyoma appears to be the only cardiac tumor showing a definite predilection for the younger age groups. This is particularly true of children with tuberous sclerosis, in whom rhabdomyoma of the heart is prone to occur. Such tumors are not considered true neoplasms and probably represent an area of developmental arrest in the fetal myocardium. It is not unusual for rhabdomyoma to regress spontaneously without having caused any appreciable impairment of cardiac function.

Myxoma is by far the most common primary tumor of the heart, accounting for slightly more than 50% of all primary cardiac tumors. It may be encountered at almost any age. The signs and symptoms vary widely but ultimately lead to cardiac failure that does not respond to the usual medical management. Most myxomas are located in the atria, more frequently on the left than on the right. They tend to proliferate and project into the chambers of the heart, preventing normal cardiac filling by obstruction to the mitral or tricuspid valve. The origin appears to be in the atrial septa.

Primary sarcoma of the heart is less common than myxoma but may occur at any age. It does not, as a rule, proliferate into the lumina of the heart; it infiltrates the wall of the myocardium and frequently extends into the pericardial cavity. Other primary tumors of the heart are angioma, fibroma, lipoma, and hamartoma. All are rare and usually produce prominent circulatory symptoms. Aggressive surgical approach is advised in the management of cardiac tumors using present surgical techniques ranging from hypothermic circulatory arrest, cardiac bypass surgery, and even cardiac autotransplantation.

Primary neoplasms of the pericardium are rare. On histologic examination, the predominant tumors are mesotheliomas (endotheliomas) and sarcomas, but leiomyomas, hemangiomas, and lipomas occasionally occur. A single instance of a large cavernous hemangioma of the pericardium has been described in an 8-year-old girl; it was successfully removed.

TUMORS OF THE DIAPHRAGM

Tumors involving the diaphragm may cause chest pain and discomfort or pulmonary compression; thus, they may simulate mediastinal or primary pulmonary neoplasms. Primary tumors of the diaphragm are extremely rare in the pediatric age group.

Benign tumors of the diaphragm that have been reported, though not necessarily in children, are lipoma, fibroma, chondroma, angiofibroma, lymphangioma, neurofibroma, rhabdomyofibroma, fibromyoma, and primary diaphragmatic cyst.

Malignant tumors of the diaphragm that have been reported are fibrosarcoma, rhabdomyosarcoma, myosarcoma, leiomyosarcoma, and fibromyosarcoma. None of these tumors appears to have been reported in children.

PRIMARY TUMORS OF THE CHEST WALL

Figures 50-42 and 50-43 illustrate findings seen in two forms of chest wall tumors.

Lipoma of the chest wall is seen in adults but rare in the pediatric age group. As noted previously, these may be dumbbell in shape, presenting on the chest wall with a large intrathoracic component. Chest radiographs, followed by CT scan, aid in its definition.

Extensive cavernous hemangiomas of the thoracic wall are seen in infancy or childhood. They may be isolated or associated with similar lesions in other tissues, including the lung. In these cases, the diagnosis of Osler-Weber-Rendu syndrome is suggested. Intrathoracic extension of these lesions may occur.

In von Recklinghausen's disease, multiple cutaneous and subcutaneous nodules are present. Patients with this disease should be carefully studied for the possible coexistence of mediastinal neurofibromas or intrathoracic meningocele.

Chondroma and chondrosarcoma are the principal bony tumors of the chest wall; 80% of these occur in the ribs or sternum, usually in the anterior extremity of a rib near the costochondral junction. They may also occur in the sternum, scapula, clavicle, or vertebral bodies. There may be few, if any, symptoms.

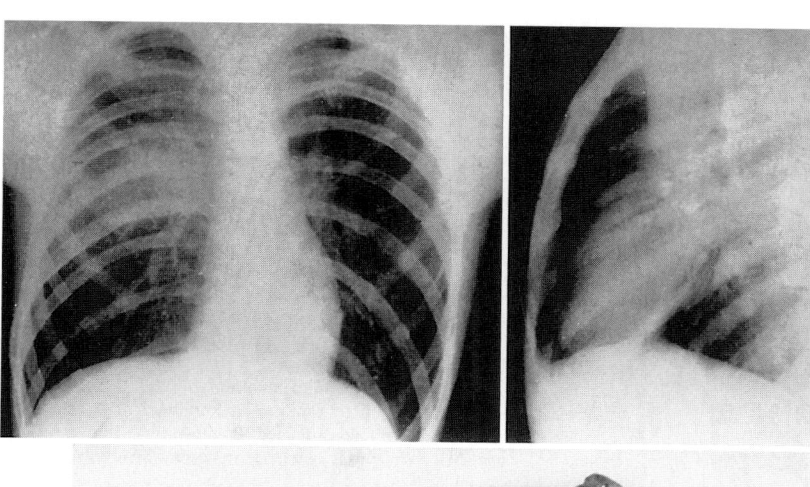

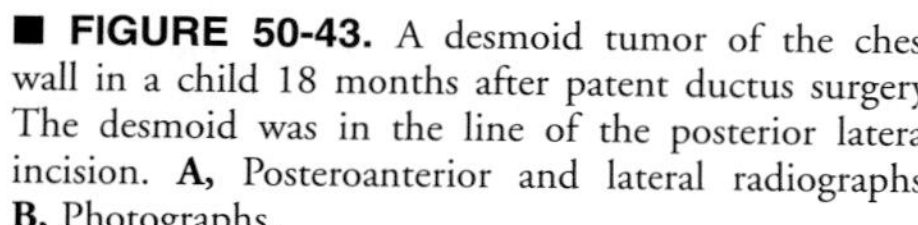

■ **FIGURE 50-42.** Reticulum cell sarcoma in the chest wall of an 8-year-old white boy. He survived for more than 18 months.

■ **FIGURE 50-43.** A desmoid tumor of the chest wall in a child 18 months after patent ductus surgery. The desmoid was in the line of the posterior lateral incision. **A,** Posteroanterior and lateral radiographs. **B,** Photographs.

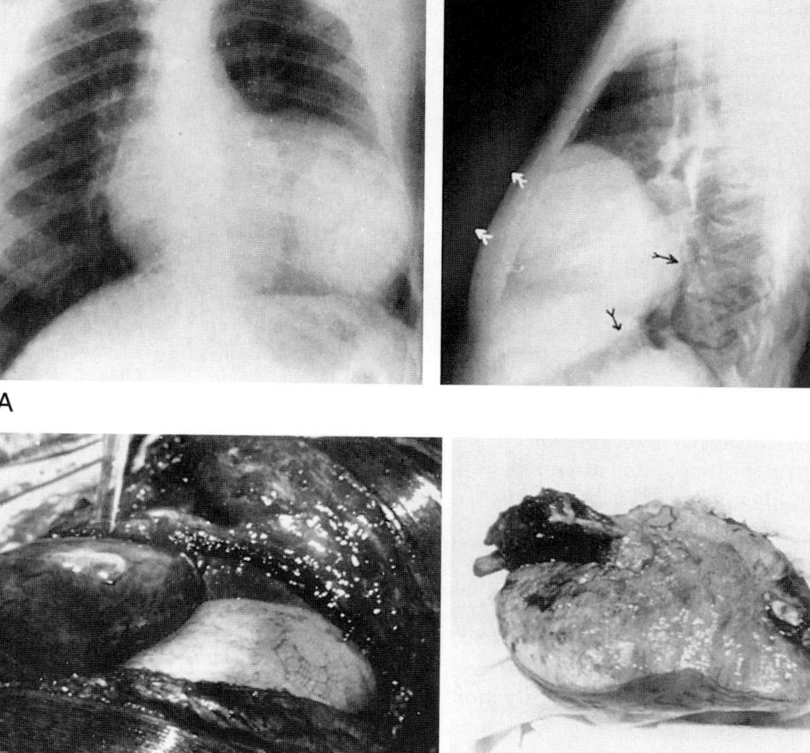

Radiographic examination reveals a discrete expansion of the bone with an intact, thinned-out cortex.

Chondrosarcoma of the rib occurs more frequently in males; it is usually seen in the posterior half and paravertebral portion of the rib, but it sometimes involves the transverse process and the vertebral body either primarily or secondarily. The direction of growth occasionally appears to be entirely internal, thus simulating the radiologic appearance of a primary pleural or mediastinal tumor. However, there usually is an externally visible and palpable tumefaction. This usually occurs during the middle decades of life.

Solitary plasmacytoma, a lesion histologically similar to multiple myeloma but localized to a single bone, may involve any part of the thoracic cage; it may involve the vertebrae, rarely attacks the ribs, and may involve the lung itself. In solitary plasmacytoma, the bone is thinned and may be greatly expanded.

Ewing's sarcoma with a primary location in a rib is unusual before the second decade of life.

REFERENCES

1. Lindskog GE, Liebow AA: Thoracic and Cardiovascular Surgery, 3rd ed. New York: Appleton-Century-Crofts, 1962.
2. Holder TM, Christy MG: Cystic adenomatoid malformation of the lung. J Thorac Surg 1964;47:590.
3. Ogilvie OE: Multiple papillomas of the trachea with malignant degeneration. Arch Otolaryngol 1953;58:10.
4. Gilbert JG, Mazzarella LA, Feit EJ: Primary tracheal tumors in the infant and adult. Arch Otolaryngol 1953;58:1.
5. Seikaly H, Cuyler JP: Infantile subglottic hemangioma. Otolaryngology 1994;23:135.
6. Guida PN, Fultcher T, Moore SW: Leiomyoma of the lung. J Thorac Surg 1965;49:1058.
7. Shochat S: Tumors of the lung. In: O'Neill JA, Rowe MI, Grosfeld JL, et al, eds: Pediatric Surgery, 5th ed. St. Louis: Mosby, 1998, p 921.
8. Jimenez JF, Uthman EO, Townsend JW, et al: Primary bronchopulmonary leiomyosarcoma in childhood. Arch Pathol Lab Med 1986; 110:348.
9. Hancock BJ, Di Lorenzo M, Youssef S, et al: Childhood primary pulmonary neoplasms. J Pediatr Surg 1993;28:1133.
10. Sekulich M, Pandola G, Simon T: A solitary pulmonary mass in multiple myeloma. Report of a case. Dis Chest 1965;48:100.
11. Kay S, Reed WG: Chorioepithelioma of the lung in a female infant seven months old. Am J Pathol 1953;29:555.
12. Maier HC: Bronchogenic cysts of the mediastinum. Ann Surg 1948; 127:476.
13. Phillipart AI, Farmer DL: Benign mediastinal cysts and tumors. In: O'Neill JA, Rowe MI, Grosfeld JL, et al, eds: Pediatric Surgery, 5th ed. St. Louis: Mosby, 1998, p 839.
14. Arey LB: Developmental Anatomy, rev. 7th ed. Philadelphia: WB Saunders, 1974.
15. Ellis FH Jr, Kirklin JW, Hodgson JR, et al: Surgical implications of the mediastinal shadow in thoracic roentgenograms of infants and children. Surg Gynecol Obstet 1955;100:532.
16. Fridjon MH: Cysts of the thymus in a newborn baby. BMJ 1943;2: 553.
17. Sealy WC, Weaver WL, Young WG Jr: Severe airway obstruction in infancy due to the thymus gland. Ann Thorac Surg 1965;1:389.
18. Edge JR, Glennie JS: Teratoid tumors of the mediastinum found despite previous normal chest radiography. J Thorac Cardiovasc Surg 1960; 40:172.
19. Schweisguth O, Mathey J, Renault P, Binet JP: Intrathoracic neurogenic tumors in infants and children. A study of forty cases. Ann Surg 1959; 150:29.
20. Heimburger IL, Battersby JS: Primary mediastinal tumors of childhood. J Thorac Cardiovasc Surg 1965;50:92.
21. Ellis FH Jr, DuShane JW: Primary mediastinal cysts and neoplasms in infants and children. Am Rev Tuberc Pulm Dis 1956;74:940.
22. Gross RE, Hurwitt ES: Cervical mediastinal cystic hygromas. Surg Gynecol Obstet 1948;87:599.

SUGGESTED READING

General

Adzick NS, Flake AW, Crombleholme TM: Management of congenital lung lesions. Semin Pediatr Surg 2003;12(1):10.

Adzick NS, Harrison MR, Crombleholme TM, et al: Fetal lung lesions. Management and outcome. Am J Obstet Gynecol 1998;179(4):884.

Azizkhan RG, Caty MG: Subglottic airway. In: Oldham KT, Colombani PM, Foglia RP, eds: Surgery of Infants and Children—Scientific Principles and Practice. Philadelphia: Lippincott-Raven, 1997, p 897.

Batra P, Brown K, Collins JD, et al: Mediastinal masses. Magnetic resonance imaging in comparison with computed tomography. J Natl Med Assoc 1991; 83:969.

Bromley B, Parad R, Estroff JA, Benacerraf BR: Fetal lung masses. Prenatal course and outcome. J Ultrasound Med 1995;14:927.

Cohen MC, Kashula RO: Primary pulmonary tumors in childhood. A review of 31 years experience and the literature. Pediatr Pulmonol 1992;14:222.

DeLorimier AA: Respiratory problems related to the airway and lung. In: O'Neill JA, Rowe MI, Grosfeld JL, et al, eds: Pediatric Surgery, 5th ed. St. Louis: Mosby, 1998, p 873.

Dillon PW, Cilley RE, Krummel TM: Video-assisted thoracoscopic excision of intrathoracic masses in children. Report of two cases. Surg Laparosc Endosc 1993;3:433.

Eggli KD, Newman B: Nodules, masses and pseudomasses in the pediatric lung. Radiol Clin North Am 1993;31:651.

Fellows KE, Stigol L, Shuster S, et al: Selective bronchial arteriography in patients with cystic fibrosis and massive hemoptysis. Radiology 1975;114:551.

Gushiken BD, Filly RA: Sonography for fetal thoracic intervention. In: Harrison MR, Evans MI, Adzick NS, Hoizegreve W, ed: The Unborn Patient. Philadelphia: WB Saunders, 2001, p 95.

Harrison MR, Evans MI, Adzick NS, Hoizegreve W, eds: The Unborn Patient. Philadelphia: WB Saunders, 2001.

Hebra A, Othersen HD, Tagge EP: Bronchopulmonary malformations. In: Ashcroft KW, ed: Pediatric Surgery. New York: WB Saunders, 2000, p 273.

Holcomb GW III, Tomita SS, Haase GM, et al: Minimally invasive surgery in children with cancer. Cancer 1995;76:121.

Hubbard AM, Adzick NS, Crombleholme TM, et al: Congenital chest lesions. Diagnosis and characterization with prenatal MR imaging. Radiology 1999; 212(1):43.

Ivancev K, Halldorsdottir A, Laurin S, et al: Computed tomography in the diagnosis and treatment of mediastinal abnormalities in children. Acta Radiol 1988;29:115.

Kern JA, Daniel TM, Tribble CG, et al. Thoracoscopic diagnosis and treatment of mediastinal masses. Ann Thorac Surg 1993;56:92.

Lemoine G, Montupet P: Mediastinal tumors in infancy and childhood. In: Fallis JC, Filler PM, Lemoine G, eds: Pediatric Thoracic Surgery. New York: Elsevier, 1991.

Lobe TE: Pediatric thoracoscopy. Semin Thorac Cardiovasc Surg 1993;5:298.

McGahren ED, Kern JA, Rodgers BM: Anesthetic techniques for pediatric thoracoscopy. Ann Thorac Surg 1995;60:927.

Meizner I, Levy A: A survey of non-cardiac fetal intrathoracic malformations diagnosed by ultrasound. Arch Gynecol Obstet 1994;255:31.

Merten DF: Diagnostic imaging of mediastinal masses in children. AJR Am J Roentgenol 1992;158:825.

Naidich DP, Zerhouni EA, Siegelman SS: Computed Tomography and Magnetic Resonance of the Thorax, 2nd ed. New York: Raven, 1991, p 321.

Oldham KT, Colombani PM, Foglia RP (eds): Surgery of Infants and Children—Scientific Principles and Practice. Philadelphia: Lippincott-Raven, 1997.

O'Neill JA, Rowe MI, Grosfeld JL, Fonkalsrud EW, Coran AG (eds): Pediatric Surgery, 5th ed. St. Louis: Mosby, 1998.

Phillipart AI, Farmer DL: Benign mediastinal cysts and tumors. In: O'Neill JA, Rowe MI, Grosfeld JL, et al, eds: Pediatric Surgery. Philadelphia: Mosby, 1998, p 839.

Reynolds M: Disorders of the thoracic cavity and pleura and infections of the lung, pleura and mediastinum. In: O'Neill JA, Rowe MI, Grosfeld JL, et al, eds: Pediatric Surgery, 5th ed. St. Louis: Mosby, 1998, p 899.

Rodgers BM: Thoracoscopy. In: Holcomb GR, ed: Pediatric Endoscopic Surgery. Norwalk, Conn: Appleton & Lange, 1993.

Rodgers BM, McGahren ED: Mediastinum and pleura. In: Oldham KT, Colombani PM, Foglia R, eds: Surgery of Infants and Children—Scientific Principles and Practice. Philadelphia: Lippincott-Raven, 1997, p 915.

Rodgers BM, McGahren ED: Laryngoscopy, bronchoscopy, and thoracoscopy. In: O'Neill JA, Rowe MI, Grosfeld JL, et al, eds: Pediatric Surgery, 5th ed. St. Louis: Mosby, 1998, p 853.

Rothenberg SS: Thoracoscopic lung resection in children. J Pediatr Surg 2000;35:271.

Rothenberg SS: Experience with thoracoscopic lobectomy in infants and children. J Pediatr Surg 2003;38:102.

Ryckman FC, Rodgers BM: Thoracoscopy for intrathoracic neoplasia in children. J Pediatr Surg 1982;17:521.

Skandalakis JE, Gray SW (eds): Embryology for Surgeons. Philadelphia: WB Saunders, 1994.

Sylvester KG, Albanese CT: Bronchopulmonary malformation. In: Ashcraft K, Murphy P, Holcomb GW, eds: Pediatric Surgery, 4th ed. Philadelphia: WB Saunders, 2004.

Tsao K, Albanese CT, Harrison MR: Prenatal therapy for thoracic and mediastinal lesions. World J Surg 2003;27:77.

Benign Pulmonary Tumors

Abramson AL, Shikowitz MJ, Mullooly VM, et al: Variable light-dose effect on photodynamic therapy on recurrent laryngeal papillomas. Arch Otolaryngol Head Neck Surg 1994;120:852.

Archer FL, Harrison RW, Moulder PV: Granular cell myoblastoma of the trachea and carina treated by resection and reconstruction. J Thorac Surg 1963; 45:539.

Baker DC Jr, Pemington CL: Congenital hemangioma of the larynx. Laryngoscope 1956;66:696.

Borkowsky W, Martin D, Lawrence HS: Juvenile laryngeal papillomatosis with pulmonary spread. Regression following transfer factor therapy. Am J Dis Child 1984;138:667.

Campbell JS, Wiglesworth FW, Latarroca R, Wilde H: Congenital subglottic hemangiomas of the larynx and trachea in infants. Pediatrics 1958;22:727.

Daudi FA, Lees GM, Higa TE: Inflammatory pseudotumors of the lung. Two cases and a review. Can J Surg 1991;34:461.

Doyle DJ, Henderson LA, LeJeune FE Jr, Miller RH: Changes in human papillomavirus typing of recurrent respiratory papillomatosis progressing to malignant neoplasm. Arch Otolaryngol Head Neck Surg 1994;104:1273.

Endres DR, Bauman NM, Burke D, Smith RJ: Acyclovir in the treatment of recurrent respiratory papillomatosis. Ann Otol Rhinol Laryngol 1994;103:301.

Eraklis AJ, Griscom NT, McGovern JB: Bronchogenic cysts of the mediastinum in infancy. N Engl J Med 1969;218:1150.

Filler RM, Forte V: Lesions of the larynx and trachea. In: O'Neill JA, Rowe MI, Grosfeld JL, et al, eds: Pediatric Surgery, 5th ed. St. Louis: Mosby, 1998, p 863.

Gaissert HA, Mathisen DJ, Grillo HC, et al: Tracheobronchial sleeve resection in children and adolescents. J Pediatr Surg 1994;29:192.

Kashima H, Mounts P, Levanthal B, Hruban RH: Sites of predilection in recurrent respiratory papillomatosis. Ann Otol Rhinol Laryngol 1993;102: 580.

Littler ER: Asphyxia due to hemangioma in the trachea. J Thorac Cardiovasc Surg 1963;45:552.

Moran CA, Suster S: Mediastinal hemangiomas. A study of 18 cases with emphasis on the spectrum of morphological features. Hum Pathol 1995; 26:416.

Pearl M, Woolley MW: Pulmonary xanthomatous postinflammatory pseudotumors in children. J Pediatr Surg 1973;8:255.

Rohrlich P, Peuchmaur M, Cocci SN: Interleukin-6 and Interleukin-1 beta production in a pediatric plasma cell granuloma of the lung. Am J Surg Pathol 1995;19:590.

Taylor TL, Miller DR: Leiomyoma of the bronchus. J Thorac Cardiovasc Surg 1969;57:284.

Verska JJ, Connolly JE: Bronchial adenomas in children. J Thorac Cardiovasc Surg 1968;55:411.

Vujanic GM, Dojcinov D: Inflammatory pseudotumor of the lung in children. Pediatr Hematol Oncol 1991;8:121.

Primary and Metastatic Malignant Pulmonary Tumors

Archer RL, Grogg SE, Sanders SP: Mucoepidermoid bronchial adenoma in a 6 year old girl. A case report and review of the literature. J Thorac Cardiovasc Surg 1987;94:452.

Beardsley JM: Primary carcinoma of the lung in a child. Can Med Assoc J 1933;29:257.

Beattie EJ Jr: Surgical treatment of pulmonary metastases. Cancer 1984; 54:2729.

Benjamin DR, Cahil JL: Bronchoalveolar carcinoma of the lung and congenital cystic adenomatoid malformation. Am J Pathol 1991;95:889.

Brandt B III, Heintz SE, Rose EF, Ehrenhaft JL: Bronchial carcinoid tumors. Ann Thorac Surg 1984;39:63.

Calabria R, Srikanth MS, Chamberlin K, et al: Management of pulmonary blastoma in children. Am Surg 1993;59:192.

Carter SR, Grimer RJ, Sneath RS, Matthews HR: Results in thoracotomy in osteogenic sarcoma with pulmonary metastases. Thorax 1991;46:727.

Cayley CK, Mersheimer W, Caez HJ: Primary bronchogenic carcinoma of the lung in children. J Dis Child 1951;82:49.

D'Agnostino S, Bonoldi E, Dante S: Embryonal rhabdomyosarcoma of the lung arising in cystic adenomatoid malformation. J Pediatr Surg 1997;32:1381.

Davis SD: CT evaluation for pulmonary metastases in patients with extrathoracic malignancy. Radiology 1991;180:1.

de Parades CG, Pierce WS, Groff DB, Waldhausen JA: Bronchogenic tumors in children. Arch Surg 1970;100:574.

Dehner LP: Germ cell tumors of the mediastinum. Semin Diagn Pathol 1990;7:266.

Dehner LP: Pleuropulmonary blastoma is the pulmonary blastoma of childhood. Semin Diagn Pathol 1994;11:144.

Dowell AR: Primary pulmonary leiomyosarcoma. Ann Thorac Surg 1974;17:384.

Dulmet EM, Macchiarini P, Suc B, et al: Germ cell tumor of the mediastinum. Cancer 1993;72:1984.

Giritsky AS, Etcubanas E, Mark JBD: Pulmonary resection in children with metastatic osteogenic sarcoma. J Thorac Cardiovasc Surg 1978;75:354.

Goorin AM, Delorcy MJ, Lack EE, et al: Prognostic significance of complete surgical resection of pulmonary metastases in patients with osteogenic sarcoma. Analyses of 32 patients. J Clin Oncol 1984;2:425.

Green DM, Breslow NE, Ii Y, et al: The role of surgical excision in the management of relapsed Wilms' tumor patients with pulmonary metastases. A report from the national Wilms' tumor study. J Pediatr Surg 1991;26:728.

Harris M, et al: Treatment of metastatic osteosarcoma at diagnosis. A pediatric oncology group study. J Clin Oncol 1995;14:445.

Hartman GE, Shochat SJ: Primary pulmonary neoplasms of childhood. A review. Ann Thorac Surg 1983;36:108.

Heij HA, Vos A, de Kraker J, Voute PA: Prognostic factors in surgery for pulmonary metastases in children. Surgery 1994;115:687.

Hollinger PH, Johnston KC, Gosswiller N, Hirsch EC: Primary fibrosarcoma of the bronchus. Dis Chest 1960;37:137.

Jimenez JF: Pulmonary blastoma in childhood. J Surg Oncol 1987;34:87.

Kyriakos M, Webber B: Cancer of the lung in young men. J Thorac Cardiovasc Surg 1974;67:634.

Lack EE, Harris GB, Eraklis AJ, Vawterg F: Primary bronchial tumors in childhood. A clinicopathologic study of six cases. Cancer 1983;51:492.

LaQuaglia MP: The surgical management of metastases in pediatric cancer. Semin Pediatr Surg 1993;2:75.

Marina NM, Pratt CB, Rao BN, et al: Improved prognosis of children with osteosarcoma metastatic to the lung(s) at the time of diagnosis. Cancer 1992;70:2722.

McNamara JJ, Paulson DL, Kinglsey WB, et al: Primary leiomyosarcoma of the lung. J Thorac Cardiovasc Surg 1969;57:635.

Murphy JJ, Blair GK, Fraser GC: Rhabdomyosarcome arising within congenital pulmonary cysts. Reports of three cases. J Pediatr Surg 1992;27:1364.

Roth JA, Putnam JB Jr, Wesley MN, Rosenberg SA: Differing determinants of prognosis following resection of pulmonary metastases from osteogenic and soft tissue sarcoma patients. Cancer 1985;55:1361.

Mediastinal Tumors

Agrawal D, Suri A, Mahapatra AK, Sharma MC: Intramedullary neurenteric cyst presenting as infantile paraplegia. A case and review [Comment]. Pediatr Neurosurg 2002;37(2):93.

Azarow KS, Pearl RH, Zurcher R, et al: Primary mediastinal masses. J Thorac Cardiovasc Surg 1993;106:67.

Azizkhan RG, Dudgeon DL, Buck JR, et al: Life threatening airway obstruction as a complication to the management of mediastinal masses in children. J Pediatr Surg 1985;20:816.

Bale PM: A congenital intraspinal gastroenterogenous cyst in diastematomyelia. J Neurol Neurosurg Psychiatry 1973;36:1011.

Beardmore HE, Wigglesworth FW: Vertebral anomalies and alimentary duplication. Pediatr Clin North Am 1958;5:457.

Boothroyd AE, Hall-Craggs MA, Dicks-Mireaux C, Shaw DG: The magnetic resonance appearances of the normal thymus in children. Clin Radiol 1992;45:378.

Bower RJ, Kiesewetter WB: Mediastinal masses in infants and children. Arch Surg 1977;112:1003.

Boyle LM, Drake DP: Mediastinal teratomas. Review of 15 pediatric cases. J Pediatr Surg 1993;28:1162.

Bunin NJ, Hvizdala E, Link M, et al: Mediastinal nonlymphoblastic lymphomas in children. A clinicopathologic study. J Clin Oncol 1986;4:154.

Caffey J, Silbey R: Regrowth and overgrowth of the thymus after atrophy induced by oral administration of adrenocorticosteroids to human infants. Pediatrics 1960;26:762.

Castleberry RP, Kelly DR, Wilson ER, et al: Childhood liposarcoma. Report of a case and review of the literature. Cancer 1984;54:579.

Cavett C: Mediastinal tumors. In: O'Neill JA, Rowe MI, Grosfeld JL, et al, eds: Pediatric Surgery, 5th ed. St. Louis: Mosby, 1998, p 318.

Cicciarelli EH, Soule EH, McGoon DC: Lipoma and liposarcoma of the mediastinum, a report of fourteen tumors including one lipoma of the thymus. J Thorac Surg 1964;47:411.

Cohen AJ, Thompson L, Edwards FH, Bellamy RF: Primary cysts and tumors of the mediastinum. Ann Thorac Surg 1991;51:378.

Cohn SR, Geller KA, Birns JW, et al: Foregut cysts in infants and children. Diagnosis and management. Ann Otol Rhinol Laryngol 1982;91:622.

Copper JD: Current therapy for thymoma. Chest 1993;103:3345.

Duprez A, Corlier R, Schmidt P: Tuberculoma of the thymus. J Thorac Cardiovasc Surg 1962;44:115.

Ferrari LR, Bedford RF: General anesthesia prior to treatment of anterior mediastinal masses in pediatric cancer patients. Anesthesiology 1990;72:991.

Flege JB Jr, Valencia AG, Zimmerman G: Obstruction of a child's trachea by polypoid hemangioendothelioma. J Thorac Cardiovasc Surg 1968;56:144.

Folkman J, Mulliken JB, Ezekowitz RA: Angiogenesis and hemangiomas. In: Oldham KT, Colombani PM, Foglia RP, eds: Surgery of Infants and Children—Scientific Principles and Practice. Philadelphia: Lippincott-Raven, 1997, p 569.

Griffiths SP, Levine OR, Baker DH, Blumenthal S: Evaluation of an enlarged cardiothymic image in infancy. Thymolytic effect of steroid administration. Am J Cardiol 1961;8:311.

Grosfeld JL: Neuroblastoma. In: O'Neill JA, Rowe MI, Grosfeld JL, et al, eds: Pediatric Surgery, 5th ed. St. Louis: Mosby, 1998, p 405.

Grosfeld JL, Skinner MA, Rescorla FJ, et al: Mediastinal tumors in children. Experience with 196 cases. Ann Surg Oncol 1994;1:121.

Grosfeld JL, Weber TR, Vane DW: One-stage resection for massive cervicomediastinal hygroma. Surgery 1982;92:693.

Halpern S, Chatten J, Meadows AT, et al: Anterior mediastinal masses. Anesthesia hazards and other problems. J Pediatr 1983;102:407.

Hancock JP, St-Vil D, Luka FI, et al: Complications of lymphangiomas in children. J Pediatr Surg 1992;27:220.

Handorf CR: Intrathoracic lipoma in children. South Med J 1982;75:1403.

Holcomb GW III, Gheissari A, O'Neill JA Jr, et al: Surgical management of alimentary tract duplication. Ann Surg 1989;209:167.

Ingram L, Rivera GK, Shapiro DN: Superior vena cava syndrome associated with childhood malignancy. Analysis of 24 cases. Med Pediatr Oncol 1990; 18:476.

Kern JA, Daniel TM, Tribble CG, et al: Thoracoscopic diagnosis and treatment of mediastinal masses. Ann Thorac Surg 1993;56:92.

Kessel AWL: Intrathoracic meningocele, spinal deformity and multiple neurofibromatosis. J Bone Joint Surg Br 1951;33:87.

Kirwan WO, Walbaum PR, McCormack RJM: Cystic intrathoracic derivatives of the pregut and their complications. Thorax 1973;28:424.

Kostopoulos GK, Fessatidis JT, Hevas AL, et al: Mediastinal cystic hygroma. Report of a case with review of the literature. Eur J Cardiothorac Surg 1993; 7:166.

Lack EE, Weinstein HJ, Welch KJ: Mediastinal germ cell tumors in childhood. A clinical and pathological study of 21 cases. J Thorac Cardiovasc Surg 1985;89:826.

Lakhoo K, Boyle M, Drake DP: Mediastinal teratomas. Review of 15 pediatric cases. J Pediatr Surg 1993;28:1161.

LeGolvan DP, Abell MR: Thymomas. Cancer 1977;39:2142.

Linegar AG, Odell JA, Fennell WM, et al: Massive thymic hyperplasia. Ann Thorac Surg 1993;55:1197.

Marsten JL, Cooper AG, Ankeney JL: Acute cardiac tamponade due to perforation of a benign mediastinal teratoma into the pericardial sac. J Thorac Cardiovasc Surg 1966;51:700.

Mauch PM, Lakish LA, Kaden M, et al: Patterns of presentation of Hodgkin disease. Implication for etiology and pathogenesis. Cancer 1993;71:2062.

Moran CA, Suster S: Mediastinal hemangiomas. A study of 18 cases with emphasis on the spectrum of morphologic features. Hum Pathol 1995;26:416.

Muraskas JK, Gianopoulos JG, Husain A, Black PR: Mediastinal cystic hygroma. Prenatal decompression with neonatal resection and recurrence at 19 months of age. J Perinatol 1993;13:381.

Nagabuchi E, Ziegler MM: Neuroblastoma. In: Oldham KT, Colombani PM, Foglia RP, eds: Surgery of Infants and Children—Scientific Principles and Practice. Philadelphia: Lippincott-Raven, 1997, p 593.

Ogita S, Tsuto T, Deguchi E, et al: OK-432 therapy for unresectable lymphangiomas in children. J Pediatr Surg 1991;26:263.

Okada A, Kubota A, Fukuzawa M, et al: Injection of bleomycin as a primary therapy of cystic lymphangioma. J Pediatr Surg 1992;27:440.

Patcher MR: Mediastinal non-chromaffin paraganglioma. J Thorac Surg 1963;45:152.

Pirawoon AM, Abbassioun K: Mediastinal enterogenous cyst with spinal cord compression. J Pediatr Surg 1974;9:543.

Pokorny WJ, Goldstein IR: Enteric thoracoabdominal duplications in children. J Thorac Cardiovasc Surg 1984;87:821.

Ramon Y, Cajal S, Suster S: Primary thymic epithelial neoplasms in children. Am J Surg Pathol 1991;15:466.

Rendina EA, Venuto F, De Giacomo T, et al: Comparative merits of thoracoscopy, mediastinoscopy, and mediastinotomy, and mediastinotomy for mediastinal biopsy. Ann Thorac Surg 1994;57:992.

Rizk T, Lahoud GA, Maarrawi J, et al: Acute paraplegia revealing an intraspinal neurenteric cyst in a child. Childs Nerv Syst 2001;17(12):754.

Robie DK, Gursoy MH, Pokorny WJ: Mediastinal tumors—airway obstruction and management. Semin Pediatr Surg 1994;3:259.

Rubush JL, Gardner IR, Boyd WC, Ehrenhaft JL: Mediastinal tumors. A review of 186 cases. J Thorac Cardiovasc Surg 1973;65:216.

Saini VK, Wahi PL: Hour glass transmural type of intrathoracic lipoma. J Thorac Surg 1964;47:600.

Salyer WR, Eggleston JC: Thymoma. A clinical and pathological study of 65 cases. Cancer 1976;37:229.

Schwartz H II, Williams CS: Thoracic gastric cysts, report of two cases with review of the literature. J Thorac Surg 1942;12:117.

Seybold WD, McDonald JR, Clagget OT, Harrington SW: Mediastinal tumors of blood vascular origin. J Thorac Surg 1949;18:503.

Seydel GN, Valle ER, White ML Jr: Thoracic gastric cysts. Ann Surg 1946; 123:377.

Shamberger RC, Holzman RS, Griscom NT, et al: CT quantitation of tracheal cross-sectional area as a guide to the surgical and anesthetic management of children with anterior mediastinal masses. J Pediatr Surg 1991;26:138.

Touroff ASW, Sealey HP: Chronic chylothorax associated with hygroma of the mediastinum. J Thorac Surg 1953;26:318.

Weimann RB, Hallman GL, Bahar D, Greenberg SD: Intrathoracic meningocele. A case report and review of the literature. J Thorac Surg 1963;46:40.

Welch CS, Ettinger A, Hecht PL: Recklinghausen's neurofibromatosis associated with intrathoracic meningocele. Report of case. N Engl J Med 1948; 238:622.

Williams KR, Burgord TH: Surgical treatment of granulomatous paratracheal lymphadenopathy. J Thorac Surg 1964;48:13.

Willis RA: An intrapericardial teratoma in an infant. J Pathol Bacteriol 1946; 58:284.

Ya Deau RE, Clagett OT, Divertie MB: Intrathoracic meningocele. J Thorac Surg 1965;49:202.

Cardiac Tumors

Arciniegas E, Hakimi M, Farooki ZQ, et al: Primary cardiac tumors in children. J Thorac Cardiovasc Surg 1980;79:582.

DeBusatmante TD, Azpeitia J, Mirailes M, et al: Prenatal sonographic detection of pericardial teratoma. J Clin Ultrasound 2000;28:194.

Murphy MC, Sweeney MS, Putman JB, et al: Surgical treatment of cardiac tumors. A 25-year experience. Ann Thorac Surg 1990;49:612.

Diaphragm and Chest Wall Tumors

Anderson LS, Forrest JV: Tumors of the diaphragm. Am J Roentgenol 1973; 119:259.

Ayala AG, Ro JY, Bolio-Solis A, et al: Mesenchymal hamartoma of the chest wall in infants and children. A clinicopathological study of five patients. Skeletal Radiol 1993;22:569.

Bolanowski PJP, Groff DB: Thoracic wall desmoid tumor in a child. Ann Thorac Surg 1973;15:632.

Grundy GW, Miller RW: Malignant mesothelioma in childhood. Report of 13 cases. Cancer 1972;30:1216.

Hopkins SM, Freitas EL: Bilateral osteochondroma of the ribs in an infant, an unusual cause of cyanosis. J Thorac Surg 1965;49:247.

Ochsner A Jr, Lucas GL, McFarland GB Jr: Tumors of the thoracic skeleton, review of 134 cases. J Thorac Cardiovasc Surg 1966;52:311.

Perry TM, Smith WA: Rhabdomyosarcoma of the diaphragm, a case report. Am J Cancer 1939;35:416.

Weinstein EC, Payne WS, Soule EH: Surgical treatment of desmoid tumor of the chest wall. J Thorac Surg 1963;46:242.

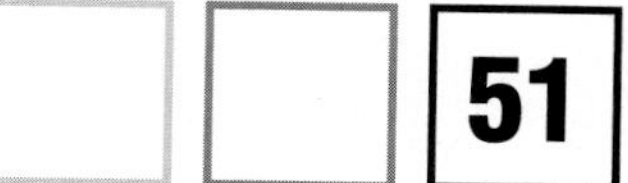

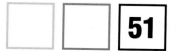

51 Chest Wall Function and Dysfunction

Jean-Paul Praud, MD • Emmanuel Canet, MD

GENERAL CONSIDERATIONS

Since Lavoisier's stipulation in 1791 that respiration is essentially a phenomenon of oxygen (O_2) consumption and carbon dioxide (CO_2) production, the chest wall has been recognized as the vital pump responsible for the movement of gases between the atmosphere and the lungs. Today much is known regarding the adaptability of this vital pump to satisfy the changing metabolic needs under various physiologic and pathologic conditions (e.g., rest, exercise, and hyperthermia). Patients must overcome adverse conditions affecting chest wall function, conditions ranging from the cartilaginous, pliable rib cage of the preterm infant to the scoliotic thorax of the adolescent, and from the weak chest wall in neuromuscular disease to the stiff rib cage in asphyxiating thoracic dystrophy or obesity. The vital pump also participates in numerous functions such as singing, talking, wind instrument playing, coughing, sneezing, parturition, and hiccupping.

In normal resting conditions, the diaphragm is the principal muscle used for inspiration, the accessory inspiratory muscles fixating the rib cage in a stable condition. When the inspiratory workload is increased, additional accessory inspiratory muscles are recruited, thereby producing an upward motion of the ribs, resulting in a more pronounced thoracic expansion. Conversely, even during resting breathing, failure to fixate the rib cage would result, as it does in the case of chest wall muscle weakness, in an inward motion of the rib cage (i.e., rib cage paradoxic breathing). In normal resting conditions, expiratory muscles are inactive. During increased demands for air pumping, the expiratory muscles become activated during the second phase of expiration and decrease the end-expiratory volume below functional residual capacity (FRC). Any decrease in the force of the expiratory muscles leads to a decreased vital capacity.

Sleep is responsible for significant modifications in lung mechanics and respiratory muscle control. The passage to the supine position alone leads to a decrease in FRC and sleep leads to a decrease in tonic activity of intercostal muscles and upper airway muscles, a phenomenon further pronounced in REM sleep. These changes are responsible for paradoxic inward rib cage movement in neonates due to their compliant rib cage and in patients with neuromuscular disorders. Nocturnal hypoventilation with alteration of blood gases is often the first sign of chronic respiratory failure in progressive neuromuscular disorders such as Duchenne's muscular dystrophy (DMD).

RESPIRATORY MUSCLE FATIGUE

The respiratory muscles may become fatigued when an imbalance develops between the energy supply to the inspiratory muscles and the demand of work to be accomplished. Loss of energy supply to the muscles results from a severe decrease in systemic arterial pressure and/or arterial O_2 tension. Alternatively, amyotrophy, rib cage deformity, and/or increased work to move the chest wall may lead to muscular fatigue and precipitate respiratory failure (Fig. 51-1). In an attempt to avoid fatigue, a patient may opt to use less force per breath, thereby reducing tidal volume and compensating by taking more breaths per minute. Clinical and laboratory evaluation of the chest wall can provide essential information with regard to chest wall function in a particular patient (Box 51-1), and lead to recognition of respiratory muscle fatigue and/or respiratory insufficiency. Acute respiratory muscle fatigue is characterized by progressive exhaustion of the respiratory muscles, leading to respiratory failure within minutes or hours. Careful bedside observation of the at-risk patient usually allows the recognition of signs indicating progression of fatigue. These include loss of nonbreathing functions of the respiratory apparatus, inappropriate respiratory rate and pattern of breathing, as well as other warning signs reported in Box 51-2. Chronic respiratory muscle fatigue is not as easily identified as the acute form, and respiratory symptoms may not correlate well with the degree of respiratory muscle fatigue. General fatigue and dyspnea on exertion can be the first alleged symptoms of chronic respiratory impairment. However, the first manifestations of chronic respiratory muscle impairment often are symptoms of sleep hypoventilation, either nocturnal (parasomnias, enuresis, hypersudation) or daytime symptoms (morning headaches, hypersomnolence, chronic fatigue, decreased attention span, shortness of breath, right ventricular failure). Unfortunately, even a specific questionnaire fails to predict sleep disordered breathing in children with advanced neuromuscular disorders.[1]

LABORATORY ASSESSMENT OF RESPIRATORY FUNCTION IN CHILDREN WITH CHEST WALL DYSFUNCTION

Longitudinal assessment of respiratory function should be repeated from 6 to 7 years of age. Routine measurements of lung function include static lung volumes, forced spirometry, and blood gases. Respiratory muscle strength can also be assessed by measuring maximal inspiratory and expiratory pressures at the mouth, while cough efficacy can be assessed by measuring peak cough flow (PCF) using a simple peak flowmeter. Overnight assessment of respiratory function can be performed through pulse oximetry, transcutaneous or end-tidal CO_2, or polysomnography. Other measurements such as muscle electromyography or measurement of esophageal pressure or occlusion pressure may be of interest in research, but are not used in clinical practice. The following international guidelines have

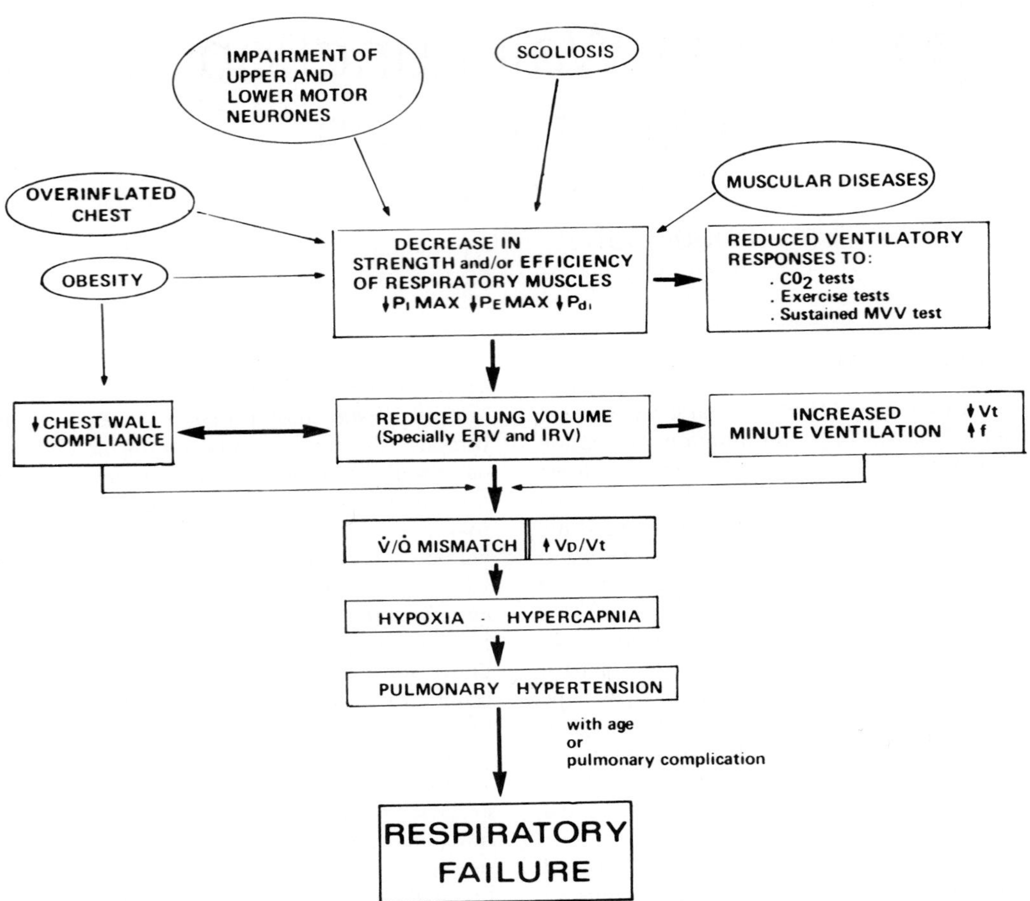

FIGURE 51-1. Schematic representation of the pathogenesis of respiratory failure in diseases with chest wall dysfunction.

recently been developed under the auspices of the European Neuromuscular Center for patients with congenital neuromuscular disorders.[2] It is recommended that forced vital capacity (FVC) be measured annually in the sitting position. When abnormal (FVC < 80%), FVC should also be measured in the supine position, to investigate for diaphragm weakness (decrease in FVC > 20% from the sitting position). While FVC of less than 60% indicates a low risk for nocturnal hypoventilation, FVC of less than 40% or diaphragm weakness indicates a significant risk for nocturnal hypoventilation. Continuous overnight pulse oximetry (and end-tidal or transcutaneous CO_2, if available) should be performed annually in children too young for FVC assessment or when FVC is less than 60% and even more often when FVC is less than 40%. Full overnight polysomnography should be performed when overnight pulse oximetry is not diagnostic in the presence of symptoms suggestive of sleep-disordered breathing. Arterial blood gas analysis should be performed in patients with clinical signs of respiratory failure, recurrent or current lower respiratory infection, abnormal overnight pulse oximetry and/or capnometry findings, or FVC less than 40%. Peak cough flow should be measured annually during a steady state and at any episode of respiratory infection; values under 160 to 200 L/min may indicate that cough is ineffective and could place patients at risk for recurrent respiratory infections and respiratory failure.

MANAGEMENT OF CHILDREN WITH CHEST WALL DYSFUNCTION

Adequate nutrition is essential for ensuring adequate functioning of the respiratory muscles.[3] Patients with a chronic condition (e.g., cystic fibrosis, severe asthma, severe DMD) are commonly malnourished, a state that can lead to muscle atrophy and loss of respiratory muscle capacity to perform the work of breathing. An adequate O_2 supply and the correction of electrolytic imbalance (hypophosphatemia, hypocalcemia, hypokalemia, acidosis) are also needed for muscles to perform their work. Associated nonrelated respiratory problems, such as asthma, allergic rhinitis, or enlarged adenoids and/or tonsils causing sleep-disordered breathing, must be carefully treated, if present. Prevention of respiratory infections must be implemented by ensuring an optimal environment (e.g., avoidance of passive smoking and large daycare centers) and by providing pneumococcal and annual flu vaccination. Respiratory physiotherapy is essential in the management of chest wall dysfunction. Assisted cough techniques, either manually or through the use of equipment such as mechanical insufflator-exsufflator devices (Cough-assist, Emerson, Cambridge, Massachusetts), are of paramount importance in the management of patients with neuromuscular problems, especially during respiratory infections. In addition, respiratory muscle training has been shown to yield encouraging results in patients with neuromuscular disorders such as DMD or type II spinal muscular amyotrophy.

Impaired muscles can indeed be trained, leading to increased muscle strength and decreased respiratory load perception, at least in the less severely affected patients. Further studies are needed, however, to establish whether respiratory training programs are effectively associated with favorable outcomes in the long term (i.e., for decreasing respiratory morbidity and mortality).[4] Of note, respiratory muscle training is clearly beneficial in specific conditions where respiratory muscles are intact, such as in quadriplegic patients, following spinal cord injury. Ventilatory support has finally become an essential tool for increasing quality of life and prolonging life in the most severely affected patients with neuromuscular disorders, by resting weakened respiratory muscles.[5] The development of noninvasive intermittent positive pressure using bilevel positive airway pressure (BiPAP) ventilation via nasal mask during nocturnal sleep has been especially instrumental in this regard. Recent international guidelines suggest that noninvasive nocturnal ventilatory support is clearly indicated for patients with symptomatic daytime hypercapnia and probably helpful for patients with nocturnal hypercapnia (arterial partial pressure of carbon dioxide [Pa_{CO_2}] > 50 mm Hg for 50% of sleep time), even in the absence of daytime hypercapnia. Indeed, repeated nocturnal hypercapnia may blunt central respiratory drive, which probably leads to daytime respiratory insufficiency. Noninvasive ventilatory support should also be considered in patients with symptomatic sleep hypopneas, because of the anticipated progression toward nocturnal hypercapnia. Moreover, the presence of failure to thrive or recurrent chest infections (more than three per year) should be considered in the decision to recommend ventilatory support. A tracheostomy for ventilatory support should be considered in patients with bulbar involvement, severe retention of secretions despite noninvasive assisted cough techniques, extreme ventilator dependency, or ineffective noninvasive ventilation.[2]

BOX 51-1 Guidelines for Assessment of Chest Wall Function

Clinical Evaluation

- Chest wall configuration (e.g., scoliosis, overdistention)
- Pattern of spontaneous breathing:
  - Rate and amplitude of breathing
  - Thoracic and/or abdominal breathing
  - Coordination or paradoxic thoracic and abdominal expansion
- Specific maneuvers:
  - Maximal variation in thoracic circumference
  - Maximal excursion of diaphragm (inspection and percussion)
  - Cough maneuver—feeble or strong?

Laboratory Evaluation

- Electromyographic studies of various respiratory muscles
- Roentgenograms (in supine position):
  - Cinefluoroscopic studies of diaphragmatic and rib cage movements
  - Plain roentgenograms in full expiration and inspiration
- Real-time ultrasonography
- Pulmonary function tests:
  - Pressures: maximal inspiratory pressure (PI max), maximal expiratory pressure (PE max), transdiaphragmatic pressure (Pdi)
  - Lung volumes
  - Coordination of breathing (respiratory inductance plethysmography)

BOX 51-2 Clinical Signs and Symptoms of Respiratory Muscle Failure

Inability to Perform Nonventilatory Functions

Inability to eat/drink/cry
Reluctance to pause breathing voluntarily

Major Use of Accessory Muscles

Sternocleidomastoid muscles, pectoral

Increase in Respiratory Rate to Critical Level

Adolescents	55 breaths/min
Children, 4–10 years	70–75 breaths/min
Infants, 1–3 years	90 breaths/min
Neonates	120 breaths/min

Signs Reflecting Options Taken to Relieve Fatigue

Reduced inspiratory time (TI) and decreased Pdi: very shallow breathing
Deep breaths with a brief pause to rest the muscles
Respiratory alternans

Signs Indicating Pending Respiratory Arrest

Cyanotic spell
Cyanosis with brief cough or brief pause
Inappropriate pause
Sustained paradoxic thoracic/abdominal movement
Drooling in absence of airway obstruction (cannot pause to swallow)
Central nervous system signs (confusion)

CAUSES OF CHEST WALL DYSFUNCTION

Chest wall movements should be envisioned as the result of a chain of effectors that successively transmit the drive to breathe from the respiratory centers to the upper motor neurons of the central nervous system, the lower motor neurons, and finally the respiratory muscle fibers.[3] The central drive to breathe is transformed into a mechanical force resulting from contractions of respiratory muscles, which move the chest wall and generate inspiratory and expiratory pressures responsible for air movement into and out of the lungs. Table 51-1 illustrates the systemic conditions that cause disturbances at these various levels. Neurologic diseases at the level of the central nervous system (upper motor neurons) or at the level of peripheral innervation of the chest wall (lower motor neurons) may lead to secondary dysfunction of the muscular components of the chest wall. The best examples of these entities are hemiplegia, quadriplegia, infantile spinal muscular atrophy, and polyradiculitis (Guillain-Barré syndrome). Muscular diseases from various types of muscular dystrophy and myasthenia gravis result in failure of the respiratory muscles to produce an adequate contraction. In addition, systemic diseases associated with severe malnutrition may lead to a loss in respiratory muscle mass and force.

Malformation of the chest wall architecture, such as scoliosis, asphyxiating thoracic dystrophy, or advanced cystic fibrosis impairs the transformation of respiratory muscle contraction into adequate pressure due to malpositioning of these muscles. Finally, obesity causes an additional mechanical load on both the thoracic and abdominal components of the chest wall and limits its performance capacity.

Despite their major differences in pathogenesis, the various entities that cause chest wall dysfunction share some clinical and physiologic features. Chest wall dysfunction leads to restrictive pulmonary disease with reduced lung volume, reduced absolute flow rate values, normal forced expiratory volume in 1 second (FEV_1)/forced vital capacity (FVC) ratio, reduced strength of respiratory muscles, and decreased ventilatory performance in response to exercise. Residual volume can be normal or augmented, depending on normal or decreased strength of the expiratory muscles, respectively (Fig. 51-2). With respiratory muscle strength less than 50% predicted, the decrease in vital capacity is greater than expected, due to decreased lung compliance (atelectasis) and rib cage (costovertebral and costosternal joint ankylosis) compliance. Hypercapnia is usually present when respiratory muscle strength is less than 25% predicted. Even with less severe diseases, affected patients are at risk for ventilatory failure during critical periods of their lives, such as in the neonatal period, during respiratory infections, following general anesthesia, and during the last trimester of pregnancy.

Finally, diagnosis of the cause of chest wall dysfunction in the floppy newborn/infant can be especially challenging, as underlined in a recent review.[6]

TABLE 51-1. Causes of chest wall dysfuction

Site of Defect	Causes
Central Drive of Breathing	Congenital or acquired
Upper Motor Neuron	Hemiplegia
	Cerebral palsy
	Quadriplegia
Lower Motor Neuron	Poliomyelitis
	Spinal muscular atrophies
	Guillain-Barré syndrome
	Tetanus
	Friedreich's ataxia
	Traumatic nerve lesions
	Phrenic nerve paralysis
Neuromuscular Junction	Myasthenia gravis
	Congenital myasthenic syndromes
	Botulism
	Drugs
Respiratory Muscles	Muscular dystrophies
	Congenital myopathies
	Metabolic myopathies
	Steroid myopathy
	Connective tissue disease
	Diaphragmatic malformation
Nonmuscular, Chest Wall Structures	Scoliosis
	Congenital rib cage abnormality
	Overinflated rib cage in COPD
	Connective tissue disease
	Thoracic burns
	Obesity
	Giant exomphalos

COPD, chronic obstructive pulmonary disease.

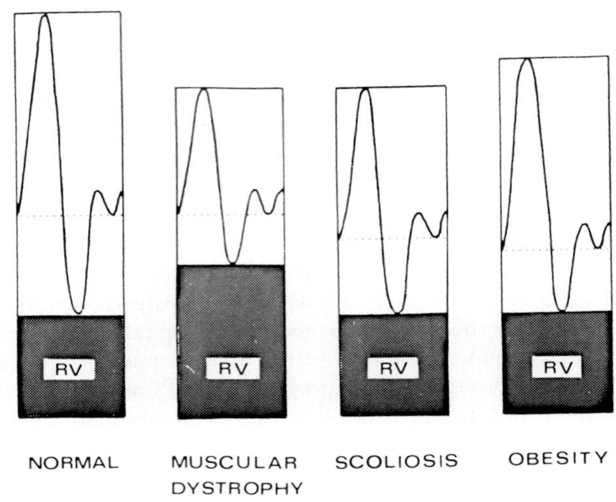

FIGURE 51-2. Changes in lung volume in diseases characterized by chest wall dysfunction.

DISEASES OF THE MOTOR NEURONS

SPINAL CORD INJURY AND CEREBRAL PALSY

Spinal Cord Injury

Spinal cord injury resulting in quadriplegia can occur at any age, including at birth or after cervical trauma in later childhood. Respiratory complications continue to be the major cause of morbidity and mortality in patients with cervical spinal cord injury.[3,7] The importance of respiratory impairment largely depends on the level of the spinal lesion and associated cerebral injuries, especially brainstem lesions leading to central hypoventilation. Ventilatory support is usually needed during the acute phase of cervical spine injury. Thereafter, patients with high cervical lesions (C1–C3) almost invariably require long-term continuous ventilatory support. Younger patients are usually managed by positive pressure ventilation via tracheostomy, sometimes with bilateral diaphragm pacing for daytime ventilatory support, to free the child from the ventilator. In older patients, alternative methods of ventilatory support have been described. Noninvasive positive pressure ventilation via the nose or mouth has become the first choice for nocturnal ventilatory support when possible, while daytime ventilation can be provided either continuously by abdominal displacement ventilator (pneumobelt) or up to several hours by glossopharyngeal breathing. Nocturnal negative pressure ventilation is currently less frequently used. On the other hand, patients with lower (C5–C6) spinal lesions can usually be weaned from the ventilator and do not have severe, long-term respiratory impairment, despite alterations of intercostal and abdominal muscle function. Patients with C3–C5 lesions (at the site of phrenic nerve emergence) will have variable respiratory dysfunction. Many patients can eventually be weaned from the ventilator. Breathing exercise programs have also been shown to be of crucial importance in the respiratory rehabilitation of these quadriplegic patients. In addition, cough assist techniques are an essential addition in the management of quadriplegic patients, especially during respiratory infections.

Cerebral Palsy

The consequences of cerebral palsy on respiratory function are variable, depending on the extent of the cerebral lesions, and can include respiratory muscle dysfunction and dystonia, abnormal breathing patterns, lung aspiration, and scoliosis. They are sometimes intermingled with abnormalities related to concomitant bronchopulmonary dysplasia. Upper airway muscle dysfunction can also be responsible for obstructive sleep disordered breathing and swallowing disorders. Therapeutic options should be tailored to each patient and guided by ethical considerations, in close collaboration with the family.

FRIEDREICH'S ATAXIA

Hereditary ataxias are very heterogeneous disorders. Friedreich's ataxia, the most common form of recessive ataxias, is a neurodegenerative disorder with autosomal-recessive inheritance. The gene has been localized on the long arm of chromosome 9, where the X25 gene codes for the protein frataxin. Friedreich's ataxia is characterized by onset usually between the ages of 8 and 15 years, progressive cerebellar ataxia, dysarthria, areflexia, sensory loss in lower limbs, pyramidal weakness, and Babinski signs. In addition, patients with Friedreich's ataxia suffer from respiratory muscle weakness and progressive scoliosis, responsible for a restrictive syndrome, as well as frequently from cardiomyopathy. This progressive cardiorespiratory impairment leads to early death. Unfortunately, there is no specific therapy for this disease, and physicians must aim at minimizing the development of scoliosis and treat recurrent pulmonary complications with physiotherapy, antibiotics, and noninvasive ventilatory support as required.

SPINAL MUSCULAR ATROPHIES

Childhood spinal muscular atrophies (SMAs) are a group of autosomal-recessive neurodegenerative disorders classified as type I (Werdnig-Hoffman disease), type II, and type III (Kugelberg-Welander disease), based on the age of onset of muscle weakness and clinical severity. SMAs are due to a mutation of the survival motor neuron gene located on chromosome 5q13.[6] This mutation is responsible for primary degeneration of the anterior horn cells of the spinal cord and often of the bulbar motor nuclei, which leads to skeletal muscle paralysis and atrophy.

Werdnig-Hoffman disease is the most common monogenic cause of death in infancy and the most common severe neuromuscular childhood disorder after DMD. Clinical manifestations are apparent in the first 6 months of life, sometimes even at birth when the disease has begun in utero, which is recognized in retrospect by a reduction in fetal breathing movements. Infants with Werdnig-Hoffman disease are nearly always unable to sit and rapidly adopt a frog leg position. Intercostal muscle weakness is responsible for paradoxic inward rib cage movement with each inspiration, the diaphragm being relatively spared. Roentgenograms of the chest show a reduced intrathoracic volume and a bell-shaped thorax. These patients suffer from swallowing disorders and aspirations and are at risk for recurrent respiratory failure with viral respiratory infections. The prognosis is poor, with 95% of infants dying from respiratory failure by the age of 18 months. While most patients with this disease are still denied any mechanical ventilatory support, management of Werdnig-Hoffman disease raises great ethical concerns, currently giving rise to lively discussions.[8] These have been triggered by the publication, in 2000, of a case series showing that an aggressive management program directed at preventing and treating respiratory failure increases life expectancy significantly. Elements of this management include permanent nocturnal, noninvasive mask ventilation, recognition of impeding respiratory failure by using pulse oximetry at home, use of cough-assisted devices (insufflator-exsufflator), and early endotracheal intubation for ventilatory support as needed during respiratory infections. Interestingly, respiratory failure with intercurrent viral infections appear to be self-limited with age.[9]

SMA type II is an intermediate form and represents the largest group of SMA patients. Patients usually present with abnormal muscle weakness between the ages of 6 months to 1 year of life. They are able to sit, but are not capable of ambulation. Swallowing disorders, recurrent atelectasis, and respiratory infections vary in their degree of severity and carry the risk for respiratory failure. With adequate respiratory management tailored to respiratory involvement, as described above for patients with Werdnig-Hoffman disease, life span is expected to extend to adulthood for most patients. Patients with Kugelberg-Welander disease have onset of muscle weakness after 18 months. Respiratory involvement is usually minimal, and a normal life span is expected in most cases.

Finally, an unusual variant of SMA (SMA with respiratory distress type 1 [SMARD1]) has been reported, usually presenting at a few weeks of life with acute life-threatening respiratory distress caused by diaphragmatic paralysis.[10] SMARD1 has been retrospectively identified to be responsible for cases of sudden infant death syndrome in consanguineous parents. Peripheral weakness in SMARD1 patients is initially limited to distal lower limb muscles and is not the presenting symptom. Cranial involvement also appears later in the evolution. SMARD1 has been linked to mutations in the gene encoding for the immunoglobulin μ binding protein 2 on chromosome 11q13. This allows prenatal diagnosis and helps in decision making for initiating chronic ventilatory support, knowing the fatal issue of the disease.

POLIOMYELITIS

The acute disease induced by a poliovirus infection typically occurs in very young children. Destruction of the motor neurons of the spinal cord can result in irreversible paralysis/paresis of thoracic muscles, with the risk for acute respiratory insufficiency. In addition, bulbar poliomyelitis can result in upper airway obstruction, aspiration, and/or respiratory failure. Various permanent sequelae, including scoliosis, restrictive pulmonary disease, and respiratory insufficiency, can occur. Treatment is only supportive.

DIAPHRAGMATIC PARALYSIS

Diaphragm dysfunction can be due to a wide variety of disorders (Box 51-3), many of which are dealt with in other sections of the present chapter or in other chapters of this textbook. The present section will focus on diaphragmatic paralysis caused by phrenic nerve impairment.

Diaphragmatic paralysis generally results from injury to the phrenic nerve during thoracic or neck surgery. Tumors of the mediastinum, peripheral neuropathy, and agenesis of the phrenic

BOX 51-3 Classification of Diaphragmatic Disorders

Disorders of Innervation

- Traumatic injury to the head or brainstem, cerebral stroke
- Spinal cord disorders: spinal cord injury, syringomyelia, anterior horn disease (e.g., spinal muscle atrophy, poliomyelitis)
- Phrenic nerve injury: birth traumatism, neck and thoracic surgery or traumatism, demyelinating disease (e.g., Guillain-Barré syndrome), neoplasm, infectious neuropathies (e.g., tetanus, typhoid, diphtheria, measles, West Nile virus, cytomegalovirus), radiotherapy

Neuromuscular Junction

- Myasthenia gravis, congenital myasthenic syndromes
- Botulism

Muscle Disorders

- Myotonic dystrophies, Duchenne's muscular dystrophy, congenital muscular dystrophy
- Congenital and metabolic myopathies
- Polymyositis

Disorders of Anatomy

- Congenital: congenital diaphragmatic hernia, congenital diaphragmatic eventration, diaphragmatic agenesis
- Acquired: traumatic rupture

Idiopathic

nerve are other less likely causes. In the newborn, stretching of the root C3–C5 during breech delivery is a frequent cause, most often in association with brachial plexus injuries (Erb's paralysis). Most diaphragmatic paralyses are on the right side, with bilateral paralysis occurring in only 10% of cases. Diaphragmatic paralysis is responsible for abnormal elevation of the hemidiaphragm and decrease in the space available for the ipsilateral lung. It frequently causes respiratory failure in neonates, whereas it can be asymptomatic in older children. Prominent clinical features are unexplained tachypnea, hypoxia, respiratory distress, or failure to wean from ventilatory support after surgery. In less severe cases, recurrent atelectasis and infections and failure to thrive can be observed. On chest x-ray, unilateral paralysis of the right hemidiaphragm should be suspected if it is more than two rib spaces higher than the left hemidiaphragm; on the left side, it results in an elevation of the hemidiaphragm of at least one rib space above the right hemidiaphragm. Contralateral mediastinal shift can also be observed in severe cases. Fluoroscopy and ultrasonography performed in a spontaneously breathing patient show a paradoxic inspiratory upward motion of the hemidiaphragm. Electromyography in association with percutaneous stimulation of the phrenic nerve can confirm the paralysis. Repeated evaluations by fluoroscopy, ultrasonography, and/or electromyography can aid in the search for improving diaphragmatic function.

Treatment depends mainly on the presence of respiratory symptoms. Asymptomatic diaphragmatic paralysis does not require any therapy. Treatment for symptomatic cases first consists of ventilatory support, when needed. Surgical plication is generally indicated in the presence of persistent or recurrent respiratory symptoms. Optimal timing for surgery in the neonate or child with diaphragmatic paralysis is controversial. Waiting for spontaneous recovery in symptomatic patients can be associated with significant morbidity, especially in high-risk patients on ventilatory support. Recommendations for such patients vary from immediate repair to waiting 2 to 4 weeks for signs of spontaneous recovery. The possibility of use of video-assisted thoracoscopic surgery for diaphragm plication decreases the morbidity associated with traditional open thoracotomy.[11]

GUILLAIN-BARRÉ SYNDROME

Guillain-Barré syndrome (GBS) is an acute, inflammatory demyelinating disease of the peripheral nerves.[12] Median annual incidence of GBS is about 1.3 per 100,000 population, with 30% of cases occurring in the under-20 age group. It is considered to be an autoimmune disease triggered by a preceding viral or bacterial infection, including cytomegalovirus, Epstein-Barr virus, *Mycoplasma pneumoniae,* and *Campylobacter jejuni.* Diagnosis is mainly based on clinical criteria. Progressive muscle weakness develops over several days to 4 weeks, followed by a plateau period of 2 to 4 weeks and then progressive recovery. Polyradiculitis can involve various levels of lower motor neurons, including to the diaphragm and to other thoracoabdominal muscles, and cranial nerves. Respiratory failure due to respiratory muscle weakness, aspiration pneumonia, and cough impairment can develop. Repeated measurements of vital capacity and blood gases are essential for appropriate decisions as to the need of mechanical ventilatory support, which is required in 15% to 20% of affected children. Decrease in vital capacity to 50% of the predicted tidal volume and/or dysphagia are indications for intubation. While the duration of mechanical ventilation varies widely, recovery of adequate respiratory function is the rule. Early use of high-dose intravenous (IV) immunoglobulins or plasma exchange induces a more rapid resolution of the disease. There is, as of yet, insufficient evidence for the use of corticosteroids.

MUSCLE DISEASES AFFECTING THE CHEST WALL

MUSCULAR DYSTROPHIES

Muscular dystrophies are a group of genetically determined diseases that primarily affect skeletal muscle and are characterized by progressive muscle wasting and weakness. Two types of muscular dystrophies commonly lead to respiratory insufficiency before adulthood: DMD and myotonic dystrophy. In addition, pulmonary function abnormalities and respiratory failure may occur in the childhood form of limb girdle muscle dystrophy, facioscapulohumeral dystrophy, and Emery-Dreifuss syndrome, and in congenital muscular dystrophy.

Duchenne's Muscular Dystrophy

DMD is the most common and severe form of muscular dystrophy that afflicts humans. Inherited as an X-linked recessive trait, it has an incidence of approximately 1 in 3500 male births. Almost one third of cases result from new mutations. The gene responsible for DMD and Becker's muscular dystrophy has been localized within the dystrophin gene located on the short arm of the X chromosome (Xp21). The dystrophin gene regulates the expression of dystrophin, a protein that links the normal contractile apparatus to the sarcolemma in skeletal muscle. Dystrophin gene mutation results in either a lack of dystrophin (usually DMD) or the expression of mutant forms of dystrophin (usually Becker's muscular dystrophy). DMD presents in boys with proximal muscle weakness at 2 to 4 years of age. The progression is fairly rapid, with the patient becoming confined to a wheelchair at around 10 to 12 years of age and dying prematurely before the age of 30. Death is due to respiratory failure in 80% of cases or to cardiac failure in 10% to 20% of cases. In the early phases of the disease, when gait is still preserved, respiratory function is essentially normal, although a loss in the strength of the respiratory muscles can be readily shown by measuring inspiratory and expiratory pressures. Impairment of respiratory function is accelerated by loss of ambulation. DMD patients present a restrictive syndrome due to muscle weakness and contractures, spinal deformity, vertebrocostal joint ankylosis, and frequent obesity (see Fig. 51-2). Serial assessment of lung function (FVC, maximal inspiratory and expiratory pressures, peak cough flow, arterial blood gases, and overnight pulse oximetry) are essential in evaluating progression of the respiratory system disability (see earlier section on Laboratory Assessment of Respiratory Function in Children with Chest Wall Dysfunction). Serial measurements of vital capacity reported in absolute value have been found especially useful in DMD patients. Indeed, every DMD patient experiences a maximum plateau in absolute vital capacity between the ages of 10 and 12 years and a progressive decrease thereafter. Until the 1990s, before the regular use of nocturnal ventilatory support, the maximal vital capacity recorded and its rate of decline thereafter predicted survival time. Age when vital capacity was less than 1 L reliably indicated a greater risk for dying in the next 3 years. Currently, the use of nocturnal ventilatory support, together with early, aggressive management of respiratory infections, can prolong life beyond the age of 30 for many DMD patients, while usually ensuring a seemingly appreciable quality of life.

Management

In most DMD patients, death is related to respiratory insufficiency. Management of DMD patients should therefore be directed at slowing down the progression of respiratory insufficiency, while ensuring a good quality of life. In the first decade, general physiotherapy and surgery should aim at prolonging ambulation. Loss of ambulation coincides with the onset of progressively increasing respiratory problems. Scoliosis is responsible for back pain and difficulty in positioning, and contributes to the decrease in vital capacity. Management of DMD should therefore also focus on preventing spinal curve progression. Early surgical correction is the treatment of choice, because spinal bracing is not effective in DMD patients and may further reduce vital capacity. Surgery should be performed in DMD patients with a Cobb angle of 30 degrees and a vital capacity of at least 40% of predicted values, to avoid postoperative respiratory failure. However, a recent study has shown that surgery should not be refused in more severely affected patients, when appropriate perioperative care is implemented.[13] Of note, although surgery improves the quality of life of DMD patients, it does not slow down the progression of respiratory impairment.

Respiratory infection is a serious complication in patients with DMD, because expiratory muscle weakness impairs both the ability to breathe and to clear airway secretions. Afflicted children should avoid contact with individuals with respiratory infections, and preventive immunization (influenza, pneumococcal pneumonia) should be performed. If respiratory impairment increases during respiratory infection, patients with DMD should be hospitalized for early appropriate antibiotic treatment, assisted cough techniques, and noninvasive nasal ventilatory support by BiPAP as required.

Obesity is frequent in patients with DMD after loss of ambulation, and all obese patients should undergo a controlled weight reduction program. Obesity in these patients increases the work of breathing and further compromises chest wall disability. Conversely, patients with end-stage disease may suffer from severe weight loss with important amyotrophy and bedsores, secondary to bulbar weakness (mastication and swallowing difficulties) and inability to feed themselves. Specialized dietary management must be implemented, and the use of gastrostomy for enteral feeding should be discussed with such patients and their family.

Until the 1990s, long-term ventilatory support was often not advocated for DMD patients with chronic respiratory failure. Some patients were chronically treated by tracheostomy and positive pressure ventilation, often following acute respiratory deterioration with subsequent impossible weaning from the ventilator. This raised enormous ethical concerns; indeed, the decision to perform the tracheostomy had to be made in the context of a life-threatening episode without the necessary time for decision making by the patient and his family. The development of nasal interfaces for noninvasive, intermittent positive pressure ventilation, together with the recognition that nocturnal ventilation corrects daytime blood gas abnormalities and symptoms, has led to a major change in the management of chronic respiratory failure in DMD patients.[5,8] Indications for noninvasive intermittent positive pressure ventilation have already been discussed (see earlier section on Management of Children with Chest Wall Dysfunction).[2] However, the use of home nocturnal positive pressure ventilation should not obliterate the fact that progression of respiratory muscle weakness in DMD patients is not slowed by nocturnal noninvasive ventilatory support, which will eventually become insufficient. Available alternatives in end-stage disease are 24-hour use of intermittent positive pressure ventilation via oral/nasal interface or via tracheostomy. Although many patients seem to enjoy an appreciable quality of life even at this stage of the disease, this should be discussed with the patient before initiating noninvasive nocturnal mechanical ventilation.

DMD still remains an untreatable disease in humans. However, several therapeutic approaches are worth mentioning. Gene- and cell (myoblast)-based therapy have yielded encouraging results in preclinical studies in animals and are currently under investigation in a few pilot studies in humans.[14] Pharmacologic candidate treatments include aminoglycoside antibiotics to promote read-through of nonsense mutations (animal studies), oral albuterol to improve skeletal muscle mass (human study in progress[15]), and corticosteroids for limiting muscle inflammation associated with DMD. Treatment by prednisone has been shown to increase muscle strength and function in DMD patients, but at the expense of too many side effects. Deflazacort, a prednisolone derivative, currently attracts a great deal of interest, since it may have fewer side effects than prednisone while preserving gross motor and pulmonary function in DMD patients.[16] However, further randomized trials are necessary to confirm the efficacy and safety of deflazacort.[17]

Congenital Muscular Dystrophy

The term *congenital muscular dystrophy* refers to a group of rare genetic disorders in which weakness and an abnormal muscle biopsy are present at birth.[6] While muscle weakness tends to be stable over time, complications become more severe over the long run. Diagnosis is established from an observed increase in serum creatine kinase and dystrophic or myopathic pattern on muscle biopsy. Abnormality in muscle immunostaining and abnormalities in brain magnetic resonance imaging can aid in distinguishing some subtypes. Several forms of congenital muscular dystrophy, especially rigid spine muscular dystrophy and Ullrich's congenital muscular dystrophy, bring about frequent respiratory failure despite patients being ambulant, due to early diaphragm weakness.[2]

Myotonic Dystrophy

Myotonic diseases are divided into nondystrophic types (hyperkalemic periodic paralysis, paramyotonia congenita, myotonia congenita) and dystrophic types such as myotonic dystrophy (Steinert's disease).[18]

Myotonic dystrophy is an autosomal-dominant, inherited, and progressive disease occurring at a frequency of 1 in 7500 to 1 in 18,500 individuals. The mutation responsible is an expansion of an unstable trinucleotide (CTG) in the region of the myotonic dystrophy protein kinase (DMPK) gene, on the long arm of chromosome 19. The degree of expression of this disorder is quite variable, leading to marked variation in clinical severity and age of onset. Myotonia and muscle weakness are the prominent clinical features, but many other organ systems can be affected (cataracts, cardiac dysrhythmias, hypersomnia, frontal balding, and endocrine disorders). Involvement of the respiratory system is the major factor contributing to morbidity and mortality.

Congenital Myotonic Dystrophy

Ten percent to 15% of patients with myotonic dystrophy have a severe congenital form, which presents as generalized hypotonia without myotonia, along with respiratory and feeding difficulties.[6] Thin ribs and right diaphragmatic elevation can be observed on chest radiography. Diagnostic suspicion is increased by examining the mother, who most often carries the mutation. Indeed, mild weakness of eyelid closure and grip myotonia are often present in the mother. DNA-based diagnostic tests confirm the diagnosis. Polyhydramnios, prematurity, hydrops fetalis with pleural effusions, and pulmonary hypoplasia can increase respiratory difficulties due to diaphragmatic weakness at birth. Fifty percent of neonates with congenital myotonic dystrophy need respiratory support at birth. The condition usually improves in early childhood but deteriorates in late childhood or adolescence, when features of the classic disease gradually appear. However, if ventilatory support is needed beyond 4 weeks of life in the neonatal period, prognosis is poor, with risk of sudden death in survivors, even without apparent respiratory exacerbation.

Classic Myotonic Dystrophy

It is unclear whether congenital myotonic dystrophy with neonatal onset differs from the classic disease that begins in childhood. Although clinical signs of weakness of the expiratory muscles have been shown in children with myotonic dystrophy, a true restrictive syndrome is commonly reported in adult patients only, and respiratory failure is rare before late adulthood. However, weakness of the respiratory muscles and the muscles of deglutition render myotonic dystrophy patients prone to postanesthetic failure, repeated aspiration pneumonias, and pulmonary infections. In addition, subjects with myotonic dystrophy are prone to sleep-disordered breathing, which may be either obstructive or central. Obesity can be an aggravating factor. Death in adults usually results from respiratory failure, and less commonly from heart failure.

OTHER HERITABLE MYOPATHIES

Aside from muscular dystrophies, several other rare inherited myopathies can also be responsible for respiratory function abnormalities of variable expression, from a severe neonatal form with acute bulbar weakness and respiratory failure to a more benign adult form.[6] A remarkable feature of these diseases is that the respiratory muscles are occasionally severely impaired, up to respiratory failure, while the other skeletal muscles are relatively spared by the myopathy. Abnormal respiratory control can also participate in causing respiratory failure in some cases. Nemaline myopathy can present as a severe neonatal form requiring full-time ventilation or as a typical nemaline myopathy with progressive onset of respiratory insufficiency in later childhood. Severe respiratory insufficiency is also frequent in the neonatal period in myotubular myopathy. Respiratory failure has been reported in most patients with multicore disease, despite being ambulant, due to important diaphragmatic weakness. Conversely, respiratory impairment is observed more rarely in central core disease. Patients with nonprogressive respiratory abnormalities can be managed with intermittent positive pressure ventilation via nasal mask or tracheostomy. The decision to begin continuous mechanical ventilatory support in the most severe neonatal forms must be thoroughly discussed in each case with the parents, taking into account ethical considerations and the frequent lack of reliable prognostic factors.[2]

Hereditary metabolic myopathies[6] constitute a heterogeneous group of muscular diseases, which can present with respiratory failure. Glycogenosis type II (Pompe's disease) is characterized by infiltration of all organs by glycogen, due to an inherited deficiency in acid maltase. While the neonatal form is fatal through cardiorespiratory failure, a milder form with primary alveolar hypoventilation due to respiratory muscle involvement has been reported in adolescence. Mitochondrial myopathies, a group of rare disorders with accumulation of abnormal mitochondria in skeletal muscle fibers, can affect both the peripheral and central nervous systems. Some forms present from infancy to young adulthood with respiratory insufficiency due to skeletal muscle weakness and/or respiratory control abnormality. Periodic paralysis is characterized by recurrent attacks of weakness due to severe respiratory muscle paralysis in the hypokalemic form. Management of the latter includes IV administration of potassium during attacks and prevention of recurrences by dietary modifications.

NEUROMUSCULAR JUNCTION DISEASES

MYASTHENIA GRAVIS

Myasthenia gravis and the myasthenic syndromes, disorders of neuromuscular transmission associated with muscle weakness and fatigability, are attributed to various recognized pathologic mechanisms.

Juvenile Myasthenia Gravis

Similar to the adult form, juvenile myasthenia gravis is an acquired autoimmune disorder of neuromuscular transmission associated with circulating autoantibodies against acetylcholine receptors (AchR) in 80% to 90% of cases. The juvenile form accounts for 10% of all cases of myasthenia gravis and may present at any age during childhood, even as early as 6 months of age.[19] Myasthenia gravis can remain focal (ocular, facial, and neck muscles) or progress to a more generalized form, consisting of generalized progressive weakness in all muscles and abnormal fatigability on exertion, which improves with rest. Severe generalized disease can cause a progressive decrease in respiratory muscle strength, leading to a restrictive lung pattern. Myasthenia gravis crisis with life-threatening respiratory involvement can also be triggered by infections, stress, or certain drugs.

Diagnosis of juvenile myasthenia gravis relies on clinical symptoms, electrophysiologic studies, a positive finding of circulating AchR autoantibodies, and a transient improvement with anticholinesterase medication (edrophonium chloride, children <35 kg, 1 mg IV, titrated up to 5 mg, given in increments of 1 mg every 35 seconds if there is no response. The dose is doubled for children >35 kg). Management is primarily based on anticholinesterase medication (pyridostigmine bromide). However, improvement with anticholinesterase medication is usually incomplete, and most patients require further therapeutic measures, namely thymectomy and immunosuppressive drugs (prednisone, azathioprine, or cyclosporine). During acute exacerbation of the disease or in the course of respiratory complications, respiratory support may be required for various lengths of time (a few days to several weeks), in association with short-term immunotherapy, including plasmapheresis and IV immune globulins. Corticosteroids and/or plasmapheresis may also be used to improve respiratory function prior to surgery for thymectomy, in order to allow for independent respiration in the postoperative period.

Neonatal Myasthenia Gravis

This transient disorder affects 10% to 30% of infants born to mothers with autoimmune myasthenia gravis.[6] It results, at least partly, from passively transmitted maternal AchR autoantibodies, even if the mother has shown no clinical symptoms. Clinical features are usually noted within hours of birth and include feeding and respiratory difficulties, hypotonia, weak cry, facial weakness, and palpebral ptosis. Respiratory difficulties are related to feeding problems causing aspiration pneumonia, upper airway obstruction due to inability to handle pharyngeal secretions, and/or respiratory muscle weakness and fatigability. Antenatal onset of the disease with polyhydramnios, joint retractions, hypoplasia of the lung, and respiratory distress at birth has also been reported. Diagnosis is made on the presence of myasthenia gravis in the mother, a transient improvement in clinical symptoms after administration of anticholinesterase medication and the presence of circulating antibodies against AchR. Management relies on anticholinesterase medication (pyridostigmine) as well as adequate feeding and respiratory support until spontaneous remittance of muscle weakness. If the response to anticholinesterase medication is negative, exchange transfusion or plasmapheresis should be proposed. Total and definitive resolution occurs with adequate treatment within 2 to 8 weeks.

Congenital Myasthenic Syndromes

Congenital myasthenic syndromes refer to a group of genetic disorders resulting from various defects in neuromuscular transmission.[20] Congenital myasthenic syndromes are usually characterized by an autosomal-recessive (less often dominant) inheritance, absence of myasthenia gravis in the mother, occurrence among siblings, and a wide spectrum in the age of onset. With early neonatal onset, clinical features can mimic neonatal myasthenia gravis and lead to respiratory failure with sudden apnea. Other types beginning after the neonatal period are characterized by usually mild symptoms but sudden exacerbations of muscle weakness and respiratory failure, which can be triggered by infections or stress. Diagnosis relies on family history, clinical myasthenic findings, electromyographic studies, absence of circulating AchR antibodies, and a positive response to the anticholinesterase medication test in some forms of congenital myasthenic syndrome. As in neonatal myasthenia gravis, antenatal onset of congenital myasthenic syndrome has been reported. Management is based on either anticholinesterase medication, 3,4-diaminopyridine, or quinidine, depending on the specific type of congenital myasthenic syndrome. Feeding and respiratory support are used as needed. Plasmapheresis, exchange transfusion, thymectomy, and immunosuppressive drugs are not indicated in congenital myasthenic syndromes, which are not immunologically mediated.

BOTULISM

Botulism is a rare cause of neuromuscular transmission blockade in the pediatric population. The toxins produced by *Clostridium botulinum* are responsible for the impaired release of acetylcholine at the neuromuscular junction.

In classical food-borne botulism, the disease is related to the ingestion of the botulism toxin. The first symptoms usually occur 16 to 60 hours after toxin ingestion and are related to autonomic involvement; progressive generalized muscle weakness then develops and can result in respiratory failure. Careful monitoring of clinical symptoms, lung function tests, and arterial blood gases is useful for assessing the need for ventilatory support. The duration of the disease varies considerably, but as long as appropriate respiratory support is provided, full recovery is the rule and normal pulmonary function testing at 1 year has been reported for adults. Although specific and prompt antitoxin therapy can be valuable in neutralizing the toxin before the bulk of it is bound to the axon terminals, hypersensitivity reactions are frequent.

A specific entity, infantile botulism, has been described in infants 1 to 12 months of age. *C. botulinum* colonizes the infant's intestine and produces the endogenous toxin that is responsible for the clinical syndrome. Constipation is usually the first symptom; thereafter, neuromuscular dysfunction results in progressive descending muscle weakness, with early bulbar involvement and hypotonia. Diagnosis can be made by electrophysiologic studies showing a presynaptic block of neuromuscular transmission.[6] Acute or progressive respiratory failure is reported in 50% to 90% of affected infants. Respiratory failure results from (1) respiratory muscle weakness and paralysis, causing hypoventilation; (2) bulbar palsy and upper airway muscle weakness, leading to aspiration pneumonia and/or upper airway obstruction; and (3) inability to clear pulmonary secretions, resulting in pneumonia and atelectasis. Endotracheal intubation should be performed whenever significant depression of the gag reflex is noted, and ventilatory support should be offered if needed. The duration of ventilatory support is variable, but affected infants usually recover fully if treated properly. In infantile botulism, antitoxins have no benefit, and as in other forms of the disease, it is recommended that aminoglycoside antibiotics be avoided.

SKELETAL ANOMALIES

SCOLIOSIS

Scoliosis is the result of an underlying pathologic process leading to lateral curvature of the spine. The curvature of the spine causes a rotation of the vertebral bodies and distortion of all attached structures. The effects of scoliosis on pulmonary disability and reduced life expectancy have resulted in the development of screening programs in school-aged children. The goal of such programs is to detect scoliosis and implement proper therapy early enough to avoid curve progression, subsequent chest wall deformity, and cardiopulmonary dysfunction.

Classification and Natural History

Etiology determines the basis for the most commonly used classification of scoliosis (Box 51-4). Idiopathic scoliosis is defined as a structural scoliosis for which no specific cause can be established. Current population studies suggest that it is a single-gene disease with variable penetrance and heterogeneity.[21] Idiopathic scoliosis, which accounts for 80% to 85% of cases, is further categorized into three types, according to the age at which the deformity is first noted: infantile, juvenile, and adolescent. Since numerous factors are known to cause scoliosis, the diagnosis of idiopathic scoliosis can be made only after exclusion of a primary etiology, such as Marfan's syndrome, neuromuscular disease, or vertebral anomaly. Congenital scoliosis is due to the presence of vertebral anomalies, which cause an imbalance in the longitudinal growth of the spine. While congenital scoliosis is often recognized at birth, diagnosis can be delayed until adolescence, when more subtle vertebral anomalies are present. Another classification uses radiographic measurement of the severity of the curve (Cobb angle), as well as the level of the apex of the spinal curvature (cervical, high thoracic, thoracic, thoracolumbar, lumbar), and the number of curves (single or double) to allow for comparison, prognostication, and development of treatment guidelines.

BOX 51-4 Classification of Scoliosis

Idiopathic (85% of All Scoliosis)

- Infantile (<3 years old)
- Juvenile (3–9 years old)
- Adolescent (10 years old to skeletal maturity)

Congenital (5% of All Scoliosis)

- Failure of formation (hemivertebra)
- Failure of segmentation
- Mixed

Neuromuscular (5% of All Scoliosis)

- Neuropathic
- Lower motor neuron (e.g., poliomyelitis)
- Upper motor neuron (e.g., cerebral palsy)
- Other (e.g., syringomyelia)
- Myopathic
- Progressive (e.g., muscular dystrophy)
- Static (e.g., amyotonia)
- Others (e.g., Friedreich's ataxia)

Associated with Neurofibromatosis (Von Recklinghausen Disease)

Mesenchymal

- Congenital (e.g., Marfan's syndrome)
- Acquired (e.g., rheumatoid disease)
- Others (e.g., juvenile apophysitis)

Traumatic

- Vertebral (e.g., fracture, radiation, surgery)
- Extravertebral (e.g., burns, thoracoplasty)
- Secondary to irritative phenomenon (e.g., spinal cord tumor)

In the general population, the prevalence of a scoliosis of 10 degrees or more is 2% to 3%, dropping to 0.5% and 0.2% for curve magnitudes greater than 20 degrees and 30 degrees, respectively. Although the natural history of scoliosis is associated with curve progression, cardiopulmonary impairment, back pain, cosmetic deformity, and neurologic compromise, it varies greatly, depending on specific etiology, age of onset, genetic background, and curve pattern. Untreated adolescents with severe idiopathic scoliosis followed over a 50-year period were shown to have a mortality rate 2.2 times greater than controls. These deaths generally occurred in the fourth or fifth decade of life, due to cardiopulmonary insufficiency. Most of the survivors showed significant physical disability characterized by dyspnea, back pain, and exercise limitation. Untreated children with infantile scoliosis followed to maturity are often found to have severe and crippling deformities, with a spinal curvature usually exceeding 70 degrees; spontaneous regression of the scoliosis, however, has been reported in 10% to 60% of patients. Congenital scoliosis is usually progressive and, if untreated, results in severe spinal deformity. The ultimate severity of the curve depends on both the type of anomaly and the site at which it occurs. The most progressive of all anomalies is a unilateral unsegmented bar combined with single or multiple convex hemivertebrae on the contralateral side. In untreated infantile and congenital scoliosis, death may occur before adulthood as a result of cardiopulmonary insufficiency. However, the vast majority of individuals with scoliosis never develop cardiorespiratory failure.

Pulmonary Function in Scoliosis

At an early stage of the disease, scoliosis is generally painless and asymptomatic. The impairment of pulmonary function due to scoliosis has been studied by numerous investigators, all of whom generally agree that (1) a Cobb angle greater than 90 degrees greatly predisposes to cardiorespiratory failure, (2) lung function abnormalities are detectable when the Cobb angle is greater than 50 to 60 degrees, (3) lung function abnormalities are of the restrictive type, and (4) the duration of the scoliosis correlates with the patient's degree of disability.

Lung Volumes

The degree of restrictive lung disease is related to the severity of the scoliosis. In patients with moderate to severe scoliosis, a negative linear correlation has been established between the magnitude of the curve and FVC. In adolescent idiopathic scoliosis, the features of the spinal deformity (Cobb angle, number of vertebrae involved, cephalad location of the curve, and loss of the normal thoracic kyphosis) are the major determinants of reduced percentage of FVC. In some subjects with mild scoliosis (e.g., Cobb angle less than 35 degrees), a reduction of lung volume was also reported, although no correlation between the magnitude of the curve and lung volume was clearly established. Total lung capacity (TLC) decreases in proportion to the fall in FVC, although residual volume (RV) remains more or less within the predicted normal values, unless the scoliosis has progressed to a severe degree, in which case RV declines slightly. The functional residual capacity (FRC) is also slightly diminished, and both the RV/TLC and FRC/TLC ratios are increased, due to the relative decrease in TLC with almost normal RV and FRC (see Fig. 51-2). In addition, although the absolute values of anatomic and alveolar dead space are believed to remain normal, the ratio of dead space to tidal volume (V_D/V_T) is increased, which plays a major role in the development of alveolar hypoventilation. It is generally agreed that reduction of chest wall compliance, impaired lung growth, and/or impaired respiratory muscle strength account for the effects of scoliosis on lung volumes. Patients with mild to moderate idiopathic scoliosis have been reported to exhibit a correlation between the decrease in maximum inspiratory pressure and the fall in FVC, whereas maximum expiratory pressure is normal. This finding suggests that in scoliotic patients with chest deformity, inspiratory muscles work at a mechanical disadvantage, thereby accounting for the reduction in lung volume.

Respiratory Flow Rate and Airway Resistance

Expiratory flows are decreased in proportion to the restricted lung volume, while the FEV_1/FVC ratio is normal. Reduction of peak flow, which is effort dependent, has been attributed to the disadvantageous working conditions of the respiratory muscles. Airway resistance may be normal or slightly increased, due to airway distortion associated with chest deformity.

Elastic Properties

Decreased chest wall compliance plays an important role in the impairment of lung volumes. Associated mild reduction of lung compliance may be attributed to compression of the lung, reorientation of surface tension forces, and/or alteration of elastic properties of the lung. Decreased compliance of the respiratory system may account for the increased work of breathing as well as the increased O_2 cost of ventilation reported in scoliotic patients.

Chest Wall Movements

Little information is available on breathing strategies and the susceptibility of scoliotic patients to respiratory muscle fatigue. A few radiologic studies have shown that movements of the diaphragm are greater on the side of the convex spinal curve. In addition, rib cage expansion is reported to vary considerably, from almost no expansion of the chest to normal thoracic movement.

Regional Ventilation and Perfusion

Studies using xenon 133 have shown that the lung on the convex side (the larger lung) receives a greater volume of alveolar ventilation than the lung on the (smaller) concave side. In fact, alveolar gas "maldistribution" is correlated with both the angulation of the spine and age of the patient. Hence, near normal values of ventilation have been found in young subjects despite rather severe scoliosis, while air maldistribution is more often observed in older patients.

Blood Gases

Scoliotic individuals commonly exhibit mild hypoxemia with normocapnia, presumably due to the mismatch in ventilation-perfusion ratio ($\dot{V}/\dot{Q}$). In severe scoliosis, hypoxemia may also be attributed to diffusion limitation and/or alveolar hypoventilation and, as a consequence, be linked to CO_2 retention. The elevated V_D/V_T ratio contributes to alveolar hypoventilation.

Response to Exercise and to CO_2 Inhalation

Resting ventilation is increased in scoliotic patients, who maintain a normal $Pa{CO_2}$ despite an increased V_D/V_T ratio and an abnormal $\dot{V}/\dot{Q}$. During exercise testing or CO_2 inhalation, the magnitude of the ventilatory response is lower in scoliotic patients than in normal subjects. The strategy of breathing adopted by scoliotic patients during hypercapnia or exercise combines a reduced V_T and increased breathing frequency in order to minimize the increase in the work of breathing. Decreased exercise tolerance in individuals with mild to moderate scoliosis may be the first evidence of respiratory impairment. Reduced respiratory system compliance, increased work of breathing, and perhaps a defective respiratory drive presumably account for their lower ventilatory performances. In addition, with a Cobb angle greater than 100 degrees, pulmonary hypertension may contribute to decreased exercise capacity. However, in contrast to normal individuals, exercise tolerance in scoliotic patients is limited rather by ventilation than circulatory factors. Finally, physical and cardiovascular deconditioning are probably important factors influencing exercise tolerance in patients with moderate idiopathic scoliosis.

Cardiorespiratory Failure in Scoliosis

In a long-term follow-up study of patients with untreated scoliosis, vital capacity expressed as percentage predicted value was the strongest predictor of subsequent development of cardiorespiratory failure, followed by the Cobb angle. In practice, cardiorespiratory failure usually develops in patients with a Cobb angle greater than 90 degrees, and is more likely in those patients with an upper thoracic curve, associated thoracic lordosis, structural vertebral anomaly, or respiratory muscle weakness. Severe scoliosis leads to respiratory failure through alveolar hypoventilation and to circulatory failure through pulmonary arterial hypertension and cor pulmonale. Alveolar hypoventilation first occurs at night, especially during REM sleep, and probably plays a major role in the development of pulmonary hypertension. Patients with moderate to severe scoliosis should therefore be evaluated for respiratory impairment during sleep and, if needed, overnight noninvasive ventilatory support should be proposed.

Lung Growth

The consequences of scoliosis on lung growth remain unclear. Nevertheless, postmortem quantitative studies suggest that alveolar multiplication is decreased in congenital or infantile scoliosis, whereas the alveoli may not enlarge normally in idiopathic juvenile or adolescent scoliosis. The number of pulmonary

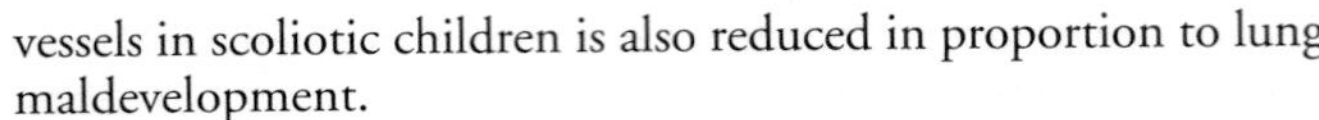

vessels in scoliotic children is also reduced in proportion to lung maldevelopment.

Management

Management of scoliosis depends on the age of the child and the degree of scoliosis, as well as the underlying condition that led to the scoliosis.

Adolescent Idiopathic Scoliosis

Management of adolescent scoliosis should start with early detection, based on school screening programs before onset of the adolescent growth spurt. In skeletally immature patients with curves of less than 25 degrees, the risk for progression is low and a close follow-up may be sufficient. In patients with progressive curves greater than 25 degrees, bracing is used to stop spinal curve progression. Such orthotic management is cumbersome and limits chest wall expansion, and is usually based on a full-time (20–23 hours per day) treatment regimen. The weaning period begins when spine growth stops. Electrostimulation has been used in some cases of mild scoliosis, but most studies have now reported that outcomes are no better than simple observation in stopping progression. Uncontrolled curve progression despite orthotic treatment, or curves greater than 50 degrees, require surgical treatment, which are based on fusion of several vertebrae and spinal instrumentation to maintain the spine in a corrected position. The traditional Harrington rod has been gradually replaced by new surgical methods, which allow three-dimensional correction of spinal deformity (e.g., segmental pedicle screw fixation with direct vertebral rotation).[22] In addition, a more complex surgical procedure, combining an anterior, thoracic approach for discoidectomy to a posterior instrumentation must often be used to obtain a satisfactory correction of the most severe cases. Video-assisted thoracoscopy is increasingly used for this anterior surgical approach.

Juvenile Scoliosis

Children with nonprogressive spinal curves of less than 20 degrees usually require no other intervention than a close follow-up, especially at the time of the adolescent growth spurt. Children with a progressive spinal curve should be treated with a brace; those whose curve progression has not stopped or who have spinal curves greater than 40 degrees will require surgical treatment. Whenever possible, spinal fusion should be delayed until the onset of the adolescent growth spurt.

Congenital and Infantile Scoliosis

Both congenital and infantile scoliosis should be considered to be very serious conditions. Indeed, it is difficult to stop the progression of the spinal curve in young children and the consequences of a severely deformed and rigid chest can be catastrophic on a rapidly growing lung. Most cases of congenital scoliosis are rapidly progressive and do not respond to bracing. Surgical treatment for most patients is based on spinal fusion and instrumentation performed before severe deformity occurs, and before chronic respiratory failure is established. However, spinal fusion in young children can be responsible for important inhibition of spinal growth leading to a short trunk and restrictive lung function, which can be severe. A totally different surgical approach, an expansion thoracoplasty on the concave side of the scoliosis by means of a vertical, expandable titanium prosthetic rib, without spinal surgery, has been recently proposed in the most severe cases. Preliminary results obtained a few years after surgery suggest that this procedure allows the spine to continue to grow, with no increase in curve amplitude.[23] However, improvement in lung function has yet to be shown.

Patients with nonprogressive juvenile scoliosis should be followed closely until skeletal maturity is attained. Active treatment is mandatory for progressive scoliosis. Failure to control the curve by bracing warrants surgery involving spinal fusion and instrumentation. Pre- and postoperative halo gravity traction has been used in the past few years as an adjunct to surgery to improve correction of severe congenital and infantile scoliosis.[24]

Scoliosis in Neuromuscular Diseases

The problems in patients with neuromuscular diseases are more complex (severity of deformity, involvement of the pelvis, associated nutritional, neurologic, and cardiopulmonary problems). Although surgery provides significant benefit with regard to quality of life, the consequences on long-term pulmonary function depend on the underlying disease. In particular, surgical correction of scoliosis in DMD patients does not halt progressive deterioration of lung function.

Postoperative Pulmonary Function in Scoliosis

Pulmonary complications are the principal cause of morbidity and mortality in the immediate period following surgery for scoliosis. Preoperative assessment of pulmonary function, including overnight oximetry, should therefore be performed as a guide to prevent postoperative complications. The most frequent respiratory problems reported in the immediate postoperative course of surgery for scoliosis include atelectasis, hemo/pneumothorax, pneumonia, pulmonary edema, upper airway obstruction, pulmonary fat emboli, and, consequently, respiratory failure. These complications require preventive measures pre- and postoperatively and, when present, require specific treatments such as nasotracheal intubation, mechanical ventilation, and chest tube insertion with drainage and/or antibiotic therapy. Immediate pulmonary complications result from multiple factors such as the surgical procedure itself, the degree of preoperative pulmonary disability, and the transient limitation of chest wall expansion as a result of pain and effects of anesthetics and analgesics. After surgery, a transient reduction of between 10% and 30% of lung volume and flow rates usually occurs and contributes to postoperative respiratory failure in any patient with severe preoperative pulmonary function impairment. The underlying pathologic conditions associated with scoliosis also contribute to the immediate postoperative course. In neuromuscular diseases, respiratory muscle weakness, cough impairment, and swallowing disorders increase the risk for immediate postoperative pulmonary complications.

Surgical intervention corrects the spinal curvature, but its effect on lung volume and arterial oxygenation only becomes apparent late after surgery. Improvement may not be measurable for 2 years or more after surgery. In some cases, especially when an anterior fusion is added to posterior instrumented fusion and thoracoplasty, surgery can cause a deterioration of lung function.[25]

ASPHYXIATING THORACIC DYSTROPHY

Asphyxiating thoracic dystrophy, also known as Jeune's syndrome or thoracic-pelvic-phalangeal dystrophy, is an autosomal-recessive disorder characterized by a narrow, constricted rib cage and generalized chondrodystrophy with short limb dwarfism. Pelvic and phalangeal abnormalities, polydactyly, renal and hepatic disorders, thrombocytopenia, as well as the Schwachman syndrome have also been reported in conjunction with asphyxiating thoracic dystrophy. Estimates suggest that about 600 patients per year are born worldwide with this disease. Asphyxiating thoracic dystrophy is usually diagnosed immediately after birth when the thoracic circumference is found to be much smaller than that of the head. Characteristic chest radiographic findings reveal a narrow and bell-shaped chest cage, with high positioned clavicles, short horizontal ribs, and flaring of the costochondral junctions. The hypoplastic ribs result in a fixed chest with a very small volume and poorly inflated lungs. If untreated, most infants with asphyxiating thoracic dystrophy die soon after birth as a result of respiratory failure. Less severe variants have been reported with clinical courses that vary from respiratory failure in infancy to few or no respiratory symptoms at all. In those patients who survive the neonatal period, respiratory failure may occur during infancy and childhood because of chest constriction, impairment of lung growth, recurrent pneumonia, or atelectasis. Improvement in bone abnormalities may occur with age, however, thereby justifying life-support procedures in early life, such as long-term mechanical ventilation. In addition, surgery for thoracic expansion has been attempted with various degrees of success, such as the lateral thoracic expansion procedure, using multiple costal osteotomies and titanium plates in such a way that new bone formation enlarges rib cage dimensions.[26]

Similar severe respiratory distress leading to death in infancy or early childhood has been reported as well in other non-asphyxiating thoracic dystrophy patients with severe rib cage deformities such as thanatophoric dwarfism, achondroplasia, chondroectodermal dysplasia, and giant exomphalos.

MISCELLANEOUS DISORDERS CAUSING CHEST WALL DYSFUNCTION

THE CHEST WALL IN OBSTRUCTIVE PULMONARY DISEASE

In obstructive pulmonary disease, overinflation of the chest wall places the diaphragm and the other breathing muscles in a position disadvantageous for breathing. The diaphragm is flattened and the inspiratory force generated by contraction of muscle fibers is lower than that generated by the diaphragm when it is in its usual upward position with a normal dome. Because the ribs are in a more horizontal position, the inspiratory force generated by the intercostal muscles is also lower than that found with ribs in their normal oblique position. As a result, the maximal inspiratory and expiratory pressures generated in patients with severe forms of bronchopulmonary dysplasia, asthma, or cystic fibrosis are lower than in normal individuals. In addition, dysfunction of the chest wall may also be due to reduction in the mass of the respiratory muscles, due to malnutrition and weight loss commonly found in patients with an advanced form of chronic obstructive pulmonary disease.

OBESITY

Obesity in children is becoming epidemic in developed countries. Consequences of obesity on pulmonary function in children have been examined in only a few studies, and results are controversial. While some studies have reported normal pulmonary function, others have either found bronchial obstruction, decreased diffusion capacity of the lung for carbon monoxide (DLCO) or decreased lung volumes (FVC, expiratory reserve volume, and/or FRC). Preferential decrease in vital capacity in males has been explained by the preferential distribution of fat in the abdominal area, conversely to females. Abnormalities of pulmonary function were noted in a few reports to be correlated to the degree of obesity. While the potential association between asthma and obesity has been underlined in recent years, the results of recent studies are controversial.[27–29] Some experts suggest that fat accumulation triggers reactive airways; however, others think that asthma can be misdiagnosed due to the increased effort required for breathing during physical activity.

In addition, physical performance is decreased in obese children and adolescents. Compared with controls, obese children and adolescents have similar ventilatory efficiency (minute ventilation/CO_2 production), but a higher absolute metabolic cost of exercise, an increased awareness of fatigue,[30] and increased exercise-induced bronchospasm, even in nonasthmatic individuals.[31] Physical performance has been shown to be amenable to improvement, at least in the short term, by an intense management program, including dietary restriction, psychological support, and physical activity.[32] Moreover, abnormalities during sleep have been found in obese children and even in obese infants, with an increased number of obstructive apneas comparatively to controls. Finally, although an abnormal CO_2 response has also been reported in some obese children, the syndrome of obesity with hypoventilation syndrome (the so-called pickwickian syndrome) seems to be less frequent than in obese adults, and most obese children behave like adults with simple obesity.

The Willi-Prader syndrome is a specific condition due to either paternal deletion of 15q11-13 or maternal disomy for chromosome 15. It is characterized by neonatal hypotonia, early childhood obesity, characteristic facial appearance, mental deficiency, hypogonadism, short stature, and behavioral disorders with increased appetite. Restrictive ventilatory impairment resulting primarily from respiratory muscle weakness has been reported. Furthermore, REM sleep-related O_2 desaturations with or without apneas are common, at times with hypercapnia. Typical obesity hypoventilation syndrome has also been reported. Hypothalamic dysfunction is probably partly responsible for sleep abnormalities.

THE CHEST WALL OF THE NEWBORN

The diaphragm and chest wall are immature at birth, especially in the preterm newborn. The insertion of the diaphragm to the rib cage is more perpendicular, which favors inward displacement of the lower ribs with any forceful diaphragmatic contraction. Moreover, the whole rib cage of the newborn is a highly pliable structure. This results in an inward movement of the ribs and the sternum with deep inspirations, such as with crying, hiccupping, or sighing. In the absence of intercostal muscle activity to stiffen the rib cage (e.g., during REM sleep or in conditions with abnormal muscle weakness), even a normal inspiration causes inward movement of the rib cage with a proportional reduction of the inspired tidal volume. Excessive diaphragm contraction therefore has to be used to produce an adequate tidal volume. In addition, respiratory muscle mass and the proportion of fatigue-resistant fibers in the diaphragm are lower, resulting in less resistance to fatigue. This can be further amplified by nutritional difficulties and/or hypoglycemia, hypocalcemia, hypophosphatemia, or acidosis. To cope with all of the above difficulties, the newborn in resting conditions breathes rapidly, with limited excursion of the diaphragm. In disease conditions, rather than increasing the depth of each breath, the newborn further increases respiratory rate, thereby preventing diaphragmatic fatigue by decreasing duration of the inspiratory contraction. In addition, the newborn often prevents respiratory failure by increasing his resting alveolar gas stores (i.e., the end-expiratory lung volume). This is accomplished by increasing respiratory rate, hence decreasing the time devoted to lung deflation, or by breaking the expiratory flow, through active glottal closure and progressive postinspiratory decontraction of the diaphragm. However, newborns are prone to respiratory muscle fatigue, sometimes even in resting, normal conditions, in situations of extreme prematurity. Respiratory muscle fatigue is more often the cause of respiratory failure in the newborn than at any other time in life.

Acknowledgments

The authors acknowledge the helpful review of the manuscript by Drs. Mario-Eddy Dumas and Chantal Thoéret. Jean-Paul Praud is supported by the Fonds de la recherche en santé du Québec and the Canadian Institutes for Health Research.

REFERENCES

1. Mellies U, Ragette R, Schwake C, Boehm H, Voit T: Daytime predictors of sleep disordered breathing in children and adolescents with neuromuscular disorders. Neuromusc Disord 2003;13:123–128.
2. Wallgren-Pettersson C, Bushby K, Mellies U, Simonds A: 117th ENMC Workshop: Ventilatory Support in Congenital Neuromuscular Disorders-Congenital Myopathies, Congenital Muscular Dystrophies, Congenital Myotonic Dystrophy and SMA (II). Neuromusc Disord 2004;14:56–69.
3. Laghi F, Tobin M: Disorders of the respiratory muscles. Am J Respir Crit Care Med 2003;168:10–48.
4. Gozal D: Pulmonary manifestations of neuromuscular disease with special reference to Duchenne muscular dystrophy and spinal muscular dystrophy. Pediatr Pulmonol 2000;29:141–150.
5. Shneerson JM, Simonds AK: Noninvasive ventilation for chest wall and neuromuscular disorders. Eur Respir J 2002;20:480–487.
6. Prasad AN, Prasad C: The floppy infant. Contribution of genetic and metabolic disorders. Brain Dev 2003;27:457–476.
7. Agency for Healthcare Research and Quality: Treatment of pulmonary disease following cervical spinal cord injury. Summary, Evidence/Report/Technology Assessment: Number 27. AHRQ Publication No. 01-E013, June 2001. Available at http://www.ahrq.gov/clinic/epcsums/spinalsum.htm.
8. Mallory G: Pulmonary complications of neuromuscular disease. Pediatr Pulmonol 2004;(Suppl 26):138–140.
9. Bach JR, Niranjan V, Weaver B: Spinal muscular atrophy type I. A noninvasive respiratory management approach. Chest 2000;117:1100–1105.
10. Grohmann K, Varon R, Stolz P, Schuelke M, Janetzki C, Bertini E, et al: Infantile spinal muscular atrophy with respiratory distress type 1 (SMARD1). Ann Neurol 2003;54:719–724.
11. Hines MH. Video-assisted diaphragm plication in children. Ann Thorac Surg 2003;76:234–236.
12. Hughes RA, Wijdicks EF, Barohn R, Benson E, Cornblath DR, Hahn AF, et al: Practice parameter. Immunotherapy for Guillain-Barré syndrome. Neurology 2003;61:736–740.
13. Marsh A, Edge G, Lehovsky J: Spinal fusion in patients with Duchenne's muscular dystrophy and a low forced vital capacity. Eur Spine J 2003;12: 507–512.
14. Bogdanovich S, Perkins KJ, Krag TO, Khurana TS: Therapeutics for Duchenne muscular dystrophy. Current approaches and future directions. J Mol Med 2004;82:102–115.
15. Fowler EG, Graves MC, Wetzel GT, Spencer MJ: Pilot trial of albuterol in Duchenne and Becker muscular dystrophy. Neurology 2004;62:1006–1008.
16. Biggar WD, Gingras M, Fehlings DL, Harris VA, Steele CA: Deflazacort treatment of Duchenne muscular dystrophy. J Pediatr 2001;138:45–50.
17. Campbell C, Jacob P: Deflazacort for treatment of Duchenne dystrophy. A systematic review. BMC Neurol 2003;3:7.
18. Mankodi A, Thornton CA: Myotonic syndromes. Curr Opin Neurol 2002;15:545–552.
19. Anlar B: Juvenile myasthenia. Diagnosis and treatment. Paediatr Drugs 2000;2:161–169.
20. Engel AG, Ohno K, Sine SM: Congenital myasthenic syndromes. Progress over the past decade. Muscle Nerve 2003;27:4–25.
21. Sarwark JF: What's new in pediatric orthopaedics? J Bone Joint Surg Am 2002;84:887–893.
22. Lee SM, Suk SI, Chung ER: Direct vertebral rotation. A new technique of three-dimensional deformity correction with segmental pedicle screw fixation in adolescent idiopathic scoliosis. Spine 2004;29:343–349.
23. Campbell RM Jr, Smith MD, Hell-Vocke AK: Expansion thoracoplasty. The surgical technique of opening-wedge thoracostomy. Surgical technique. J Bone Joint Surg Am 2004;86(Suppl 1):51–64.
24. Sink EL, Karol LA, Sanders J, Birch JG, Johnston CE, Herring JA: Efficacy of perioperative halo-gravity traction in the treatment of severe scoliosis in children. J Pediatr Orthop 2001;21:519–524.
25. Chen SH, Huang TJ, Lee YY, Hsu RW: Pulmonary function after thoracoplasty in adolescent idiopathic scoliosis. Clin Orthop 2002;399: 152–161.
26. Davis T: Chest wall surgery for asphyxiating thoracic dystrophy. Pediatr Pulmonol 2004;(Suppl 26):136–137.
27. Gilliland FD, Berhane K, Islam T, McConnell R, Gauderman J, Gilliland SS et al: Obesity and the risk of newly diagnosed asthma in school-age children. Am J Epidemiol 2003;158:406–415.
28. Sin DD, Jones RL, Man SF: Obesity is a risk factor for dyspnea but not for airflow obstruction. Arch Intern Med 2002;162:1477–1481.
29. To T, Vydykhan TN, Dell S, Tassoudji M, Harris JK: Is obesity associated with asthma in young children? J Pediatr 2004;144:162–168.
30. Marinov B, Kostaniev S, Turnovska T: Ventilatory efficiency and rate of perceived exertion in obese and non-obese children performing standardized exercise. Clin Physiol Funct Imaging 2002;22:254–260.
31. Gokbel H, Atas S: Exercise-induced bronchospasm in nonasthmatic obese and nonobese boys. J Sports Med Phys Fitness 1999;39:361–364.
32. Deforche B, De Bourdeaudhuij I, Debode P, Vinaimont F, Hills AP, Verstraete S, et al: Changes in fat mass, fat-free mass and aerobic fitness in severely obese children and adolescents following a residential treatment program. Eur J Pediatr 2003;162:616–622.

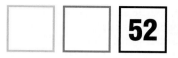

52 Rare Childhood Lung Disorders: α_1-Antitrypsin Deficiency, Pulmonary Alveolar Proteinosis, and Pulmonary Alveolar Microlithiasis

Pierre-Yves Berclaz, MD •
Bruce C. Trapnell, MD

This chapter describes a collection of rare lung diseases that generally occur in either neonates or adults but that also can affect children and adolescents. For most, recent basic and clinical research has improved our ability to recognize and accurately diagnose these diseases and has significantly improved our understanding of the pathogenic mechanisms involved. For some, studies have also elucidated important mechanisms underlying lung function in health and disease. One important example is the identification of a critical role for the hematologic growth factor granulocyte-macrophage colony-stimulating factor (GM-CSF) in surfactant homeostasis and lung host defense.

α_1-ANTITRYPSIN DEFICIENCY

Alpha-1 antitrypsin (AAT) is a member of the serine proteinase inhibitor (SERPIN) family and functions to inhibit the activity of proteolytic enzymes with a serine residue within the active site.[1] AAT deficiency is an autosomal-recessive disorder involving mutations of the gene encoding AAT, *SERPINA1*. The association between serum AAT deficiency and severe emphysema in adults was first recognized by Laurell and Eriksson in 1963.[2] While children with AAT deficiency can also develop emphysema, it is rare in individuals before the third to fourth decade of life, unless a history of significant tobacco use is also present. More commonly, infants and children develop manifestations in the liver that range from asymptomatic elevation of liver enzymes in the blood to clinically apparent liver disease that can progress to cirrhosis and liver failure.[3] The pathogenesis of the liver disease is different from that of the lung disease. Although AAT deficiency is one of the most common inherited disorders, it is severely underrecognized and diagnosed. The mean interval between onset of symptoms and diagnosis is 7 years, suggesting that lack of awareness by health care workers is a significant problem. Patient advocacy groups such as the Alpha-1 Foundation and Alpha-1 Association have raised awareness of this condition by conducting educational programs for the medical community and the general public, as well as providing funds for research and interacting with various health care and government organizations. Recently, a joint commission of the American Thoracic Society (ATS) and the European Respiratory Society (ERS) issued standards for the diagnosis and management of individuals with AAT deficiency.[4] The Alpha-1 Foundation also provides information for treating physicians, patients, families, and the general public through its website (http://www.alphaone.org).

MOLECULAR BIOLOGY

AAT is a 52-kd glycoprotein and is the major α_1 globulin present in serum. It has a globular shape of 6.7 nm by 3.2 nm and consists of a single polypeptide chain with three carbohydrate side chains, attached to amino acid residues 46, 83, and 247. Structurally, these chains consist of a short carbohydrate core terminating in mannose and "antennae" (composed of *N*-acetylglucosamine-galactose-sialic acid) attached to the terminal mannose, resulting in biantennary or triantennary structures. The side chains at residues 46 and 247 are predominantly biantennary, whereas at residue 83 the side chains are 65% biantennary and 35% triantennary. Several salt bridges are present within the molecule—between Lys290 and Glu343 and between Glu264 and Lys387—and are important in maintaining its structural integrity.

More than 100 AAT variants have been identified, most of which are due to single amino acid substitutions. AAT variants are classified according to the protease inhibitor (Pi) system of nomenclature, which is based on the banding pattern of AAT on polyacrylamide isoelectric focusing (IEF) gel electrophoresis. Variants are assigned a letter to indicate the class, corresponding to the rate at which the variant migrates toward the anode (i.e., "F" for fast, "M" for medium, "S" for slow, and "Z" for very slow). Some variants are also assigned a number or a name subscript (indicating the city in which the variant was first identified) when multiple subtypes are present in a given class.

AAT is synthesized primarily by liver hepatocytes and then secreted into the blood. The normal AAT level in serum is 20 to 48 μM. Its half-life is 4 to 6 days and is determined in part by the carbohydrate structure. Removal of the side chains from Pi M AAT dramatically shortens the half-life. Pi Z AAT has a shorter half-life than Pi M AAT. About 34 mg of AAT per kg body weight is produced per day, of which approximately 40% is present in the plasma while the remainder is found in the interstitium, along epithelial surfaces, on the surfaces of circulating cells and platelets, and in bodily secretions. A small amount of AAT is secreted locally by macrophages, monocytes, and various tissues, including intestinal, kidney, and respiratory epithelium.[1,5] AAT diffuses from the blood into tissues, where interstitial concentrations are lower due to the presence of tissue barriers to diffusion. AAT is only minimally transported across the placenta, and the Pi type of the cord serum is that of the fetus rather than the mother. AAT is an acute phase reactant, and its concentration increases by two- to threefold in inflammatory processes, pregnancy, smoking, cancer, surgical stress, or administration of certain drugs, including estrogens, steroids, and vaccines. The increase occurs due to elevated production and is mediated during inflammation by interleukin-6. In AAT deficiency states, the increase in AAT levels during an acute phase response is blunted.

AAT functions as the major protease inhibitor in human plasma, where it comprises 95% of the total trypsin inhibitory capacity. Despite this nomenclature, maintained primarily for historical purposes, AAT also inhibits neutrophil elastase, collagenase, macrophage cathepsin, plasmin, plasminogen, tissue kallikrein, thrombin, factor IX, cathepsin G, pancreatic elastase, renin, and chymotrypsin. During its interaction with neutrophil elastase, AAT binds with such a high affinity and low dissociation rate that binding is essentially irreversible.[1] Thus, the interaction is a "suicide" interaction limiting the neutralizing capacity of each AAT molecule to one protease molecule. The crystal structure of AAT has been determined (Fig. 52-1). The active site of AAT (Met358-Ser359) is centered at the tip of a mobile external loop that protrudes from the otherwise globular AAT protein. The high-affinity binding of AAT is mediated by the external loop, which acts as pseudosubstrate "bait" for neutrophil elastase; docking occurs by insertion of the external loop of AAT into a cleft in the protease containing the active site. Concurrently, the protease is inactivated by a mousetrap action that swings the mobile reactive loop (and the protease) from the upper to the lower pole of the AAT molecule (see Fig. 52-1). The molecular complex of AAT and protease is recognized by hepatic receptors and is rapidly cleared from the circulation. In addition to its role as the major protease inhibitor, AAT has been reported to have a number of other immunomodulatory activities, including an anti-inflammatory effect and modulation of T- and B-lymphocyte functions.

The *SERPINA1* gene comprises 6 exons occupying 12.2 kilobases located at 14q32.1. The upstream 3 exons (IA, IB, IC) are noncoding and represent alternative transcriptional initiation sites, and the remaining exons (II, III, IV, and V) encode the entire primary amino acid sequence of AAT. The normal gene encodes a 418–amino acid precursor protein, including a 24-residue N-terminal secretion peptide cleaved before secretion of the mature 394–amino acid protein. The active site of AAT (Met358-Ser359) is located within exon V. The gene is differentially transcribed into messenger RNA (mRNA) 1.6 and 1.9 nucleotides in length. Hepatocytes express only the shorter transcripts, initiated from exon 1C, while mononuclear phagocytes also express the longer transcripts, initiated from exons 1A and 1B. The transcription initiation start site utilized in lung epithelial cells has not yet been defined.

AAT mRNA is translated on ribosomes attached to the membrane of the endoplasmic reticulum (ER). The nascent AAT molecule is secreted directly into the ER lumen and glycosylated during synthesis. It then undergoes a complex series of posttranslational modifications by physically interacting with molecular chaperones and various carbohydrate-modifying enzymes that alter the side chains in specific ways. This system simultaneously promotes the correct folding of the AAT molecule and provides a means to recognize and remove AAT molecules that

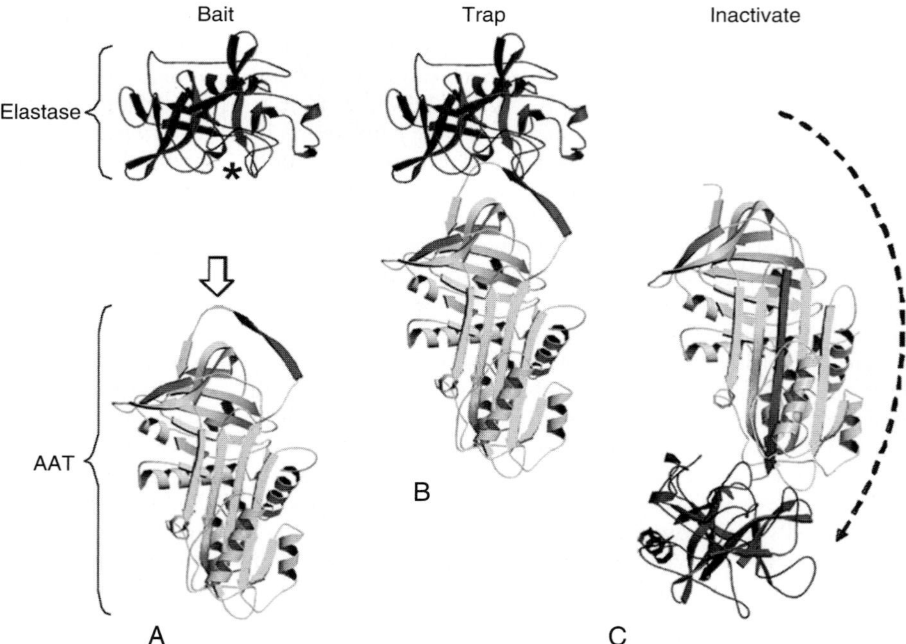

FIGURE 52-1. Alpha-1 antitrypsin "baits," traps, and irreversibly inactivates neutrophil elastase using a mousetrap-like action. AAT is a globular protein with a reactive external loop *(open arrow)* (the loop is shown in *red* on the color plate) that acts as bait for neutrophil elastase by virtue of its ability to bind the active site of the protease *(asterisk)* (**A**). Docking of neutrophil elastase on the reactive external loop of AAT (*red* on the color plate) (**B**) is associated with movement of the reactive external loop from the upper pole to the lower pole of AAT, its insertion into β-sheet A (shown in *green* on the color plate) of AAT, and inactivation of the protease (**C**). (See Color Plate 37.) (From Lomas DA, Parfrey H: Alpha1-antitrypsin deficiency. 4: Molecular pathophysiology. Thorax 2004;59[6]: 529–535.)

do not mature properly; a process known as glycoprotein ER-associated degradation (GERAD). The molecular mechanism has now been partially elucidated[6,7] and depends on three basic steps: (1) an initial discrimination of non-native glycoprotein structure mediated by UDP-glucose-glycoprotein glucosyltransferase (UGGT); (2) "marking" of the misfolded protein with a glycan-based GERAD signal by ER manosidase I (ER Man I); and (3) recognition of the GERAD signal followed by recruitment of the marked protein for degradation, primarily by cytosolic proteosomes.

Reduced or slowed protein folding prolongs retention in the ER, which in turn increases GERAD marking by ER Man I and intracellular degradation, and thus reduces secretion of AAT. Conversely, correctly folded glycoproteins traverse the ER rapidly and receive little GERAD marking (and degradation), resulting in a greater proportion of the protein that is secreted.

GENETICS

Serum AAT levels are determined by a codominant pattern of expression of both alleles. Serum levels are 20 to 40 μM in individuals with the common (Pi MM) AAT phenotype (Table 52-1). Serum AAT levels are mildly reduced (15–33 μM) in Pi SS individuals, severely reduced (2.5–7 μM) in Pi ZZ individuals, and absent in Pi Null individuals. Heterozygosity for different AAT alleles results in intermediate reductions in plasma AAT levels according to resultant Pi phenotype (see Table 52-1). The concept of "deficient" levels of AAT derives from the observation that serum levels of AAT below a threshold level (11 μM) are associated with an increased risk for development of emphysema.[8] At least one AAT variant (Pi Pittsburgh) is associated with altered function. Thus, AAT variants can be classified based on the serum level and functional activity into four groups[9]: normal, deficient, null, and dysfunctional.

Normal Variants

All normal variants are associated with normal serum AAT levels and antiprotease activity and most migrate in the M region on polyacrylamide isoelectric focusing gels.[9–11] Although at least 47 normal variants have been identified, 4 are disproportionately represented at increased frequency in the general population (see Table 52-1). These include $M_{1\text{-Val}}{}^{213}$, which has a valine substitution at position 213; $M_{1\text{-Ala}}{}^{213}$, which has an alanine at position 213; M_2, which has a histidine at position 101; and M_3, which has an aspartic acid substitution at position 376. The allelic frequencies of these M family subtypes in the United States are 0.44 to 0.49, 0.20 to 0.23, 0.14 to 0.19, and 0.10 to 0.11, respectively.

Deficient Variants

Deficient variants are associated with reduced AAT levels in serum and slower migration on IEF gels, and may or may not have impaired antiprotease activity.[9–11] S and Z variants are the most frequent deficient alleles, although at least 11 deficient variants have been reported.

The S variant is the most common allele associated with AAT deficiency and has a frequency of 0.02 to 0.03 in the United States and a slightly higher frequency (0.13) in Spain and Portugal. It arises due to a single nucleotide substitution (A to T) in exon III, resulting in a single amino acid substitution (glutamine to valine) at position 265 of the mature AAT molecule. Except for this change, the sequence of the S AAT gene is identical to that of the $M_{1\text{-Val}}{}^{213}$ AAT gene. This single amino acid change is sufficient to increase the proportion of nascent protein that is degraded intracellularly before secretion. This occurs because the protein is misfolded during posttranslational modification.[1] The net result is a mild reduction in secretion of S AAT and a corresponding mild reduction in serum AAT levels to 15 to 33 μM in homozygous individuals. The antiprotease activity of S AAT is normal.

The Z variant is the most important of the deficient AAT variants, clinically, and has been the subject of extensive basic and clinical research.[1,10,12,13] The frequency of the Z allele is 0.01 to 0.02 among whites in the United States, slightly higher (0.026) in Scandinavia, and is rare in individuals of Asian or African origin. The Z variant is caused by a single nucleotide substitution (G to A) in exon V, resulting in a single amino acid substitution (glutamine to lysine) at position 342. The sequence of the Z AAT is otherwise identical to that of the $M_{1\text{-Ala}}{}^{213}$ AAT gene. This amino acid change blocks the formation of a critical salt bridge between positions 290 and 342, thus altering the folding pattern of the nascent protein in the rough ER, and slows its translocation to the Golgi. Thus, like the S variant, misfolded Z AAT protein is subjected to increased intracellular degradation. However, the posttranslational modification Z AAT is further complicated by the tendency of Z AAT to form long polymers, a phenomenon linked to the pathogenesis of both the liver and lung disease associated with this variant. Polymerization occurs because aberrant folding creates a novel "cleft" in the Z molecule that permits the external loop of one molecule to insert tightly into the cleft of another AAT molecule (Fig. 52-2). Thus, the remarkable mousetrap-like action of the AAT, so important in protease inhibition, in the case of Z and some other variants (Pi S_{iiyama}, Pi M_{malton}, Pi S, Pi I), paradoxically causes AAT polymer formation.[1] The polymerized Z AAT accumulates within the rough ER, resulting in the formation of endoplasmic globules that are visible on light microscopy. Together,

TABLE 52-1. AAT common variants, serum levels, and risk for organ involvement

Phenotype	Serum Levels (mg/dL)	Serum Levels (μM)	Allelic Frequency	RISK FOR INVOLVEMENT In Lung	In Liver
MM	150–350	20–48	0.1–0.49	—	—
MZ	90–210	17–33		—	—
SS	100–200	15–33	0.02–0.04	—	—
SZ	75–120	8–16		Minimal risk	Minimal risk
ZZ	20–45	2.5–7	0.01–0.02	Yes	Yes
Pi(-)	0	0	Rare	Yes	Negligible

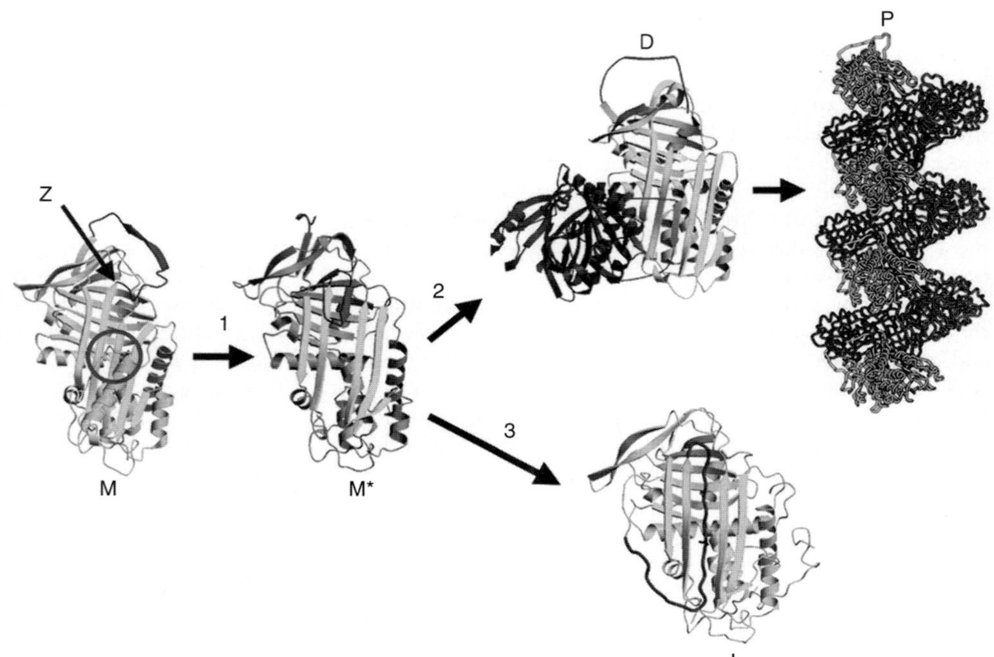

■ **FIGURE 52-2.** Abnormal folding of Z-type α1-antitrypsin molecules creates a cleft that leads to polymerization into long chains. The structure of AAT *(M)* is centered on β-sheet A (shown in *green* on the color plate) and the mobile reactive external loop (shown in *red* on the color plate). Polymer formation results from the Z variant of AAT *(arrow)* or the S_{iiyama}, M_{malton}, S, or I mutations in the shutter domain (*circle* [shown in *blue* on the color plate]) that open β-sheet A to favor partial insertion (step 1) and the formation of an unstable intermediate *(M*)*. The patent β-sheet A can either accept the loop of another molecule (step 2) to form dimer *(D)*, which then extends into polymers *(P)* or its own loop (step 3) to form a latent conformation *(L)*. The individual molecules of AAT within the polymer are shown in various colors on the color plate. (See Color Plate 38.) (From Lomas DA, Parfrey H: Alpha1-antitrypsin deficiency. 4: Molecular pathophysiology. Thorax 2004;59[6]:529–535.)

increased intracellular protein degradation and accumulation of Z AAT in the ER results in severely reduced serum AAT concentrations (2.5–7 μM) in homozygous individuals. The mature Z protein is also functionally impaired and is unable to irreversibly inhibit neutrophil elastase.

At least nine other deficient alleles are associated with severely reduced serum AAT levels in the same range as the Z allele. All are rare and increase intracellular degradation of the protein before secretion.[1]

Null Variants

Null AAT variants are rare, and each occurs due to a mutation in the *SERPINA1* gene, resulting in the absence of detectable AAT in the serum. Some null alleles are associated with base changes that lead to formation of premature stop codons and prevent normal protein synthesis (Pi $Null_{Bellingham}$, Pi $Null_{Granite\ Falls}$) or disrupt the tertiary structure of the molecule ($PiNull_{QOludwigshafen}$).

Dysfunctional Variants

An interesting rare variant (Pi Pittsburgh) is associated with normal serum AAT levels but has a significantly altered substrate specificity. This variant has a mutation in the active site of AAT (arginine is substituted for methionine at position 358), which reduces its ability to inhibit neutrophil elastase while dramatically increasing its ability to inhibit thrombin. The phenotypic result is a bleeding diathesis.

EPIDEMIOLOGY

Genetic studies demonstrate that the prevalence of individuals homozygous for the common deficient AAT allele (Z) is 70,000 to 100,000 in the United States and more than 1 million worldwide, making AAT deficiency one of the most common inherited disorders known.[10] Severe AAT deficiency caused by the Z allele is more common in individuals of Northern and Western European descent, while mild deficiency caused by the S allele is more prevalent in individuals of Southern European descent. Despite its prevalence, AAT deficiency is significantly underrecognized, and only about 5% of Pi ZZ individuals with severe deficiency have been identified. Our knowledge of the clinical manifestations is therefore incomplete and subject to ascertainment bias.

The risk for development of emphysema varies inversely with the serum AAT level.[12] Emphysema develops in all Pi Null-Null individuals in whom AAT is undetectable and in 85% of Pi ZZ individuals. Emphysema may develop in individuals with Pi SZ, MZ, and SS in whom the serum AAT levels are approximately 37%, 55%, and 40% to 60% of normal, respectively. However, the risk for development of emphysema in these individuals is only slightly increased over the general population. Pi MS individuals are not at increased risk for emphysema and have AAT levels that are 80% of normal.

A smaller proportion of Pi ZZ individuals develop clinical manifestations in the liver.[12] In one longitudinal study of 127 Pi ZZ infants,[14] 22 had biochemical or clinical liver abnormalities and 2 died in early life from cirrhosis. The overall incidence of abnormal liver function tests at age 18 was 12% in Pi ZZ individuals, but none were found to have clinical liver disease. AAT deficiency accounts for a high proportion of liver transplants in children with chronic liver disease, when biliary atresia is excluded. Chronic liver abnormalities including fibrosis and cirrhosis also occur in Pi ZZ individuals, especially with advanced age. Hepatocellular carcinoma also occurs at increased frequency in Pi ZZ individuals, especially in association with cirrhosis.

LABORATORY EVALUATION AND DIAGNOSIS

AAT deficiency should be considered in the differential diagnosis of neonates with prolonged jaundice; infants, children, adolescents, and adults with liver disease; and adults with emphysema and other forms of chronic obstructive pulmonary disease (COPD), bronchitis, and late-onset asthma.[4] Diagnostic laboratory tests include serum electrophoresis, gene identification, and functional evaluations.[15] In cases of clinically suspected disease, routine serum electrophoresis is the first test ordered and can be done in most hospitals. This test can be used to examine the relative abundance of the serum globulins (albumin, α_1 [AAT], α_2, β, and γ), and commonly is used to determine their concentration. This is sufficient to identify Pi ZZ and Pi Null-Null individuals, who are at the greatest risk for emphysema and liver disease.

Serum AAT levels lower than normal (150–350 mg/dL; 20–48 μm) suggest the presence of one or more deficient or null alleles and should be further evaluated to accurately determine the serum AAT concentration and the AAT phenotype. Various tests are available for these purposes. The serum levels of AAT can be quantified by radial immunodiffusion or nephelometry. However, some commercially available standards used for these tests tend to overestimate the AAT concentration.[9] When interpreting borderline serum AAT concentrations, it is important to remember that AAT concentrations can increase by up to threefold in conditions associated with inflammation (e.g., during a pulmonary exacerbation in an individual with AAT deficiency–related lung disease). AAT variants can usually be identified (phenotyped) by their characteristic patterns of major and minor bands on thin layer IEF gel electrophoresis. While this test in not universally available, IEF performed by a reliable laboratory is the accepted gold standard for diagnosing AAT deficiency.[4] Several approaches are available to definitively identify AAT variants based on detection of gene sequences for the specific alleles. These involve isolation of DNA, which is then subjected to polymerase chain reaction amplification with allele-specific oligonucleotides or by oligonucleotide hybridization. The older technique of isolating and sequencing the entire AAT gene (or its exons) is seldom used except when evaluating a previously unidentified AAT variant.

Serum is routinely used for all evaluations except gene-based testing, which is generally done with DNA extracted from blood mononuclear cells or cells obtained by buccal swabs. Most of these tests, including genetic tests, can now be done using "dried blood spot" samples collected on special absorbent paper in dedicated testing facilities such as the Central Genetics Laboratory of the Alpha-1 Foundation (www.alphaone.org).

PATHOGENESIS

Several lines of evidence support the concept that the cause of emphysema in individuals who are severely deficient in AAT is a reduction in the amount of antiprotease in the lungs relative to the amount of protease present, the protease-antiprotease imbalance theory. First, the risk for disease development varies with the degree of AAT deficiency: emphysema develops in 100% of individuals with no detectable AAT, in 60% to 85% of individuals with severe AAT deficiency, and at a frequency slightly above that of the general population in individuals with mild AAT deficiency. Second, AAT levels in the lung interstitium and epithelial lining fluid are normally approximately 80% and 10% that of plasma levels, respectively, due to tissue barriers that slow AAT diffusion down a concentration gradient from the higher concentrations present in blood. AAT levels in the lungs of Pi ZZ and Pi Null-Null individuals are reduced even further. Consistent with this, the antineutrophil elastase capacity of the lower respiratory tract fluid in such patients is also markedly reduced. Third, the normal lower respiratory tract is constantly exposed to neutrophil elastase from aging neutrophils that release their contents, including elastase and other proteases, into the lung tissue. The neutrophil elastase burden is increased in AAT-deficient individuals because neutrophils accumulate to greater numbers in lungs of Pi Z individuals compared with controls. This is due in part to the release of leukotriene B_4 and other chemotactic factors from alveolar macrophages. Another recently identified mechanism of neutrophil recruitment is the polymerized Z AAT, which is itself directly chemotactic for neutrophils. AAT is expressed by lung epithelial cells and also alveolar macrophages.[5] If polymerization of Z AAT occurs in the ER of airway cells (or macrophages) as it does in hepatocytes,[1] it may elicit a stress response in lung epithelial cells, resulting in increased inflammation. Thus, polymerization of an otherwise anti-inflammatory protein converts it into an inflammatory protein. Fourth, purified neutrophil elastase has been shown to degrade elastin in the alveolar septa after intratracheal instillation into the lungs of rodents. Furthermore, several well-studied rodent models have demonstrated that emphysema is induced in several hours after intratracheal instillation of any one of a variety of proteases, including papain, or pancreatic elastase. Importantly, intratracheal, but not intravascular, coadministration of human AAT can prevent the development of emphysema. Since AAT functions to inhibit proteases and is particularly effective at inhibiting neutrophil elastase, these observations strongly support the concept that unchecked neutrophil elastase present in the absence of the necessary antiprotease protection damages the lung by degrading interstitial proteins.

Smoking is an independent risk factor for development of emphysema and hastens the onset and accelerates the rate at which severely AAT-deficient individuals develop disease. Smoking appears to act via several distinct mechanisms, including (1) an increase in the recruitment and accumulation of neutrophils and macrophages in the lungs; (2) stimulation of the release of elastase and other proteases from neutrophils and macrophages; and (3) reduction of the antiprotease activity of AAT due to oxidation of a methionine residue in the active site of AAT. The latter reduces the ability of AAT to inhibit neutrophil elastase by 2000-fold. AAT activity is also similarly reduced by cellular oxidants. Finally, a number of proteolytic enzymes released from neutrophils and macrophages are capable of cleaving AAT near the active site, rendering it inactive.

While severe AAT deficiency is clearly an important risk factor for development of emphysema, other factors are involved, since not all at-risk individuals develop disease. Smoking is the most important environmental factor for development of emphysema in AAT-deficient individuals. Evidence also suggests that modifier genes may alter the risk for development of emphysema. One approach to identifying such genes under way in the United States and Europe is the use of genome-wide linkage-based approaches in Pi ZZ siblings discordant for emphysema. Notwithstanding, it is important to recognize that our current understanding of the association of AAT deficiency with emphysema is derived from only a small proportion (~5%) of the individuals who are homozygous for Z AAT. Thus, our current understanding may be confounded by ascertainment bias. It is currently unclear whether the remaining 95% of Pi ZZ individuals are asymptomatic or are symptomatic and diagnosed with COPD but without the AAT risk factor having been identified.

CLINICAL PRESENTATION

Most individuals with symptomatic familial emphysema and AAT deficiency present with dyspnea in the third or fourth decade of life.[13] However, symptoms and signs of emphysema can appear a decade earlier in those who smoke. Other common presenting symptoms can include cough, sputum production (even in nonsmokers), wheeze (with and without lung infection), and fatigue. Typically, there is a prolonged period of progressive dyspnea that began with an insidious onset years earlier, unrecognized by the patient. Notwithstanding, long delays (up to 7 years in one study) can occur between the onset of symptoms and the time a diagnosis is made. Such delays have important implications for patients who smoke because smoking greatly accelerates the rate of disease progression.

Although symptoms and signs of emphysema are rare in Pi ZZ individuals younger than 25 years, a handful of case reports have demonstrated the presence of emphysema in association with severe AAT deficiency in children. One such case was reported in a 13-year-old with a Pi ZZ phenotype. Although rare, reports have clearly documented the occurrence of emphysema in Pi Null-Null individuals in their twenties.

Children, adolescents, and adults with severe AAT deficiency may also have a history of asthma. In the Swedish cohort of 127 Pi ZZ infants, follow-up evaluation at 22 years of age showed no clinical, radiographic, or pulmonary function abnormalities consistent with emphysema.[16] However, 15% of subjects had been diagnosed with asthma, and 29% of subjects reported recurrent wheezing. This is consistent with the U.S. National Heart Lung and Blood Registry data, in which 21% of the total group and 12.5% of individuals with a normal forced expiratory volume in 1 second (FEV_1) had asthma as defined by reversible airflow obstruction, recurrent wheezing, and a reported diagnosis of asthma or allergy with or without elevated IgE levels. Increasingly, AAT-deficient individuals are being identified through family screening of an index case or other types of state or national screening programs, such as the National Targeted Detection Program of the Alpha-1 Foundation in the United States. Thus, children with AAT deficiency may have a greater risk for asthma, and by the second decade of life, especially if smoking is initiated early, they may develop subtle symptoms of reversible airflow obstruction.

The physical examination in AAT-deficient individuals is frequently unremarkable. However, in advanced cases, the examination may show dyspnea, tachypnea, hyperexpansion and hyperresonance of the chest, diminished breath sounds, wheeze, and other signs of COPD.

The plain chest radiograph may show evidence of hyperinflation with reduced interstitial markings. Diaphragmatic flattening occurs as the disease progresses, and in severe cases, hyperlucency suggestive of emphysema is apparent in a basilar distribution and may be associated with formation of bullae. High-resolution computed tomography (HRCT) scanning of the chest is more sensitive than plain chest radiography in demonstrating the presence of emphysema and may detect changes before abnormalities are apparent on pulmonary function testing.[17] HRCT is the most reliable tool with which to detect the presence of bronchiectasis in individuals with severe AAT deficiency.

Pulmonary function tests may be normal in asymptomatic patients or may show evidence of mild airflow obstruction and air trapping. Tests performed on symptomatic patients often show evidence of COPD, including a scooped appearance of the flow-volume loop, a reduced FEV_1, a reduced FEV_1/forced vital capacity (FVC) ratio, increased residual volume, increased total lung capacity (consistent with increased air trapping and hyperinflation, respectively), and a reduced carbon monoxide diffusion capacity.

Routine laboratory tests are usually within the normal range unless infection is also present or the disease is far advanced. Blood gases are usually affected only in the later stages of the disease.

Importantly, radiographic changes or pulmonary function abnormalities that are suggestive of COPD in a young individual or that are out of proportion to the smoking history should prompt an evaluation of serum AAT levels to determine if AAT deficiency is present. Although lung biopsies are not commonly necessary, the histopathologic appearance of the lung in patients with severe AAT deficiency is quite characteristic and shows panacinar emphysema in contrast to centrilobular emphysema that is seen in smokers who develop emphysema in the absence of AAT deficiency. In AAT deficiency, emphysema usually begins in the basal lung segments in contrast to emphysema in nondeficient individuals, where it more commonly occurs in the apical lung segments.

NATURAL HISTORY

The clinical course of the lung disease in individuals with AAT deficiency is quite variable among individuals with the same severely deficient phenotype. This is even true for siblings with the same severe deficiency phenotype, strongly implicating other environmental and/or genetic modifiers in the mechanism underlying the variability in disease progression.

Frequent pulmonary exacerbations occur in more than 50% of patients and occur more frequently in individuals with chronic bronchitis than in individuals without this pulmonary manifestation. Exacerbations are frequently triggered by upper respiratory infections and can last up to 2 weeks. For reasons that are unclear, exacerbations are associated with more lung inflammation than pulmonary exacerbations in COPD patients who do not have severe AAT deficiency.

Active smoking is the most important risk factor for development of emphysema in AAT-deficient individuals and dramatically alters disease progression. In normal adults, the annual decline in FEV_1 is about 30 mL. In one study of individuals with severe AAT deficiency, individuals who never smoked had an annual decline in FEV_1 of 47 mL.[13] In this same study, active smokers had an increased annual rate of FEV_1 decline of 70 mL, which was reduced to 41 mL in ex-smokers. AAT-deficient patients who do not smoke live 10 to 20 years longer than those who do.

Other environmental factors include domiciliary use of kerosene heaters and prolonged exposure to agricultural work. A variety of other self-reported exposures may be important, including exposure to gas, fumes, and dust. However, too little data are available for such exposures to reach a conclusion regarding the actual risk for disease progression.

As the lung disease progresses, recurrent infections develop and bronchitis and bronchiectasis develop and progressively worsen. Eventually, very severe impairment due to progressive obstruction to airflow and loss of gas exchange units leads to progressive hypoxia, oxygen dependence, polycythemia, and cor pulmonale. Only 16% of severely AAT-deficient patients survive to age 62.

LIVER MANIFESTATIONS

Clinical manifestations of AAT deficiency in the liver are primarily found in individuals with the Z variant. They include jaundice and acute liver injury in neonates and infants, and chronic liver disease in children, adolescents, and adults, and hepatocellular carcinoma. For Pi ZZ infants in Sweden followed for 25 years,[16] biochemical evidence of liver dysfunction (elevated transaminases) occurred in only 6% in the neonatal period. By 6 months of age, liver function abnormalities were present in 60% and thereafter declined to 12% of individuals at 18 years of age. Notwithstanding this high incidence of biochemical abnormalities, prolonged obstructive jaundice occurred in only 11%, and only two of the children (1.6%) died in early life with cirrhosis. The overall incidence of cirrhosis was 10% to 15%. Others have reported higher rates of severe liver complications. The liver disease appears frequently as neonatal hepatitis syndrome with delayed jaundice, failure to thrive, hepatosplenomegaly, severe portal hypertension, and conjugated hyperbilirubinemia. Up to 30% of infants with neonatal hepatitis syndrome have been reported to have a Pi ZZ AAT phenotype. A Pi ZZ phenotype is the strongest genetic risk factor for neonatal liver disease, excluding extrahepatic biliary atresia and the most common reason for liver transplantation in children.

THERAPY

An important concept underlying many of the approaches for both prevention and treatment of the lung disease associated with AAT deficiency is that reduction of the neutrophil burden in the lungs and airways will be beneficial to minimize the protease-antiprotease imbalance, the destruction of lung parenchyma, and thus the decline in FEV_1. Although no studies have adequately explored the impact on neutrophilic inflammation on lung function, an aggressive approach appears justified in the context of our current understanding of the disease pathogenesis in AAT deficiency. A recent Joint Statement of the ATS/ERS[4] has reviewed the various treatment approaches for AAT deficiency–related lung disease and has grouped them into four categories: (1) prevention; (2) nonspecific medical treatment; (3) augmentation therapy; and (4) surgical procedures. The discussion that follows is consistent with the ATS/ERS recommendations.

Prevention

Behavior and lifestyle modification are the first priorities in strategies aimed at prevention of emphysema in children known to be AAT deficient. Such strategies are dependent on the success of efforts to avoid cigarette smoking and environmental exposure to pollutants/irritants that cause airway irritation or inflammation. Avoidance or early cessation of smoking is particularly important in individuals with severe deficiency or absence of AAT (Pi ZZ, or Pi Null-Null, respectively). Pharmacologic aids to quitting are available and should be used when appropriate. Exposure to respiratory irritants such as second-hand tobacco smoke, dusts, and fumes should be minimized or avoided. Unless contraindicated, AAT-deficient individuals should receive vaccinations for influenza yearly and for *Pneumococcus* every 5 to 6 years. Individuals with severe AAT deficiency with overt liver disease should be vaccinated against hepatitis B.

Nonspecific Medical Treatment

The guidelines for therapy of patients with COPD not related to AAT deficiency have been well documented and are applicable to the treatment of lung disease associated with AAT deficiency.

Most patients with AAT deficiency and COPD benefit from bronchodilators even when objective evidence of a bronchodilator response is lacking. Patients with evidence of bronchial hyperreactivity may also benefit from an inhaled steroid on the theoretical grounds that it will reduce airway inflammation and thus reduce the decline of FEV_1 over time. Oral steroids are useful in AAT-deficient patients with significant asthma. However, caution should be used because long-term use is associated with osteopenia, which ultimately contributes to reduced spine height, loss of lung volume, and bone pain.

Control of respiratory infections and bronchial hyperreactivity is theoretically advantageous in lessening neutrophil burden in the lungs and airways. Consequently, antibiotic therapy should be used in patients with evidence of bronchitis or upper respiratory infection. Macrolides may be useful in reducing neutrophilic inflammation; however, development of bacterial resistance can occur and may necessitate use of alternative agents. Individuals with bronchiectasis usually require a longer duration of therapy and microbiological culture with antibiotic sensitivities to tailor therapy.

Oxygen therapy should be used in patients with desaturation during exercise. While supplemental oxygen increases exercise capacity in these individuals, it has not been shown to improve their quality of life or conditioning over that obtained from pulmonary rehabilitation. Oxygen therapy in these individuals when traveling by air may be helpful because the drop in cabin pressure reduces the partial pressure of oxygen in the inhaled air. Long-term oxygen therapy should be used in individuals with significant resting hypoxemia.

Augmentation Therapy

A specific therapy for AAT-deficient individuals is available and currently consists of AAT protein replacement.[4] This approach has been a major focus of therapy for individuals with emphysema due to severe AAT deficiency for several decades and is based on the concept that if the deficiency could be abolished, further lung destruction might be prevented and the disease stabilized. Clinical studies demonstrated that intravenous administration of purified human AAT concentrate to AAT-deficient individuals can increase the level of AAT and antineutrophil elastase capacity in the lung epithelial lining fluid to a value 60% to 70% that of individuals without AAT deficiency.[4] Based on such findings, AAT concentrate was manufactured from fractionated plasma, shown to be biologically effective, and then approved for use in AAT deficiency by the U.S. Food and Drug Administration. It was subsequently approved for use by the regulatory agencies in Canada, Germany, Spain, and Italy. The recommended dose for individuals with emphysema due to severe AAT deficiency is 60 mg/kg once weekly administered by intravenous infusion.

The clinical efficacy of AAT augmentation therapy has been addressed in two nonrandomized, concurrently controlled observational studies: the German-Danish study and the National Heart, Lung, and Blood Institute (NHLBI) Registry in the United States.[4] The former compared the decline in FEV_1 in German patients treated with weekly infusions of AAT with Danish patients who had never received augmentation therapy. Although there were differences among the two groups in gender and initial FEV_1, the study found a significantly lower annual rate of decline in FEV_1 in the treatment group (–53 mL/yr) compared with the control group (–75 mL/yr) ($P = .02$). Subgroup analysis showed that a significant treatment effect was demonstrated only in individuals with an initial FEV_1 of 31% to 65% predicted. The researchers concluded that weekly infusion of human AAT in patients with moderately reduced lung function may slow the annual decline in FEV_1.

In the NHLBI Registry, 1129 individuals with severe AAT-deficiency were followed for 3.5 to 7 years.[4] The 5-year mortality rate was 19%. Multivariate analysis showed that mortality was lower in those receiving augmentation therapy compared with those who did not ($P = .02$). However, there was no overall difference in the annual decline of FEV_1 (−54 mL/yr) between individuals on augmentation therapy compared with untreated individuals. As for the German-Danish study, subgroup analysis showed a significantly reduced rate of decline in FEV_1 in individuals with moderate emphysema (FEV_1 of 35%–49% of predicted).

These studies suggest that intravenous AAT augmentation therapy in individuals with severe AAT deficiency (<11μM) may slow the progression of emphysema in patients with moderate obstruction (FEV_1 of 35%–49% of predicted) and may reduce mortality in this subgroup of patients.

AAT infusion therapy is well tolerated in most patients.[4] In one study conducted between 1989 and 1995, administration of 58,000 infusions to 443 patients was associated with only 124 mild adverse reactions (fever, chills, dyspnea) in 65 patients. Three individuals terminated therapy because of repeated chills and fever immediately after infusion and 4 had anaphylactic reactions but recovered completely. No viral transmission has been observed.

Several formulations of human AAT have been developed, including human plasma–derived protein and recombinant AAT produced in yeast or purified from the milk of sheep transgenic for the human AAT complementary DNA. Aerosol delivery of AAT is under development and may be useful because it may permit a reduction in the amount of protein needed. Another treatment approach that has been developed is recombinant secretory leukoprotease inhibitor, a potent inhibitor of neutrophil elastase. Gene therapy approaches to augment AAT production have also been developed. A phase I trial of gene therapy using an adeno-associated viral vector to express human AAT in AAT-deficient individuals is currently under way.[18] Synthetic antineutrophil elastase inhibitors represent a potential alternative to protein replacement therapy and have been developed. Another novel approach employs a small peptide that fits into the abnormal cleft of Z AAT to block polymerization of the protein.

Surgical Procedures

Lung transplantation is an option for AAT patients with end-stage lung disease, and transplantation in this group represents 12% of all lung transplantation procedures performed.[4] Most transplantations in this group are performed as single-lung transplantations due to the lack of donor organs, although double-lung transplantation offers a better functional outcome. The actuarial 5-year survival rate following lung transplantation is 50%, and bronchiolitis obliterans remains the major cause of death. The need for posttransplantation augmentation therapy is currently debated but has not been generally recommended in this setting. However, it may be useful during episodes of respiratory tract inflammation and possibly during chronic rejection because of the presence of chronic inflammation in these individuals.

Lung volume reduction surgery (LVRS) involving the resection of 20% to 30% of the most severely involved areas of emphysema with poor perfusion may be helpful in some patients. However, the usefulness of the procedure is controversial and requires careful selection of patients who may be likely to benefit.

Liver transplantation is the only specific therapy that is effective for the liver disease associated with severe AAT deficiency. Three percent of individuals with severe AAT deficiency will develop cirrhosis before adolescence, and in these individuals liver transplantation can be effective. AAT deficiency–related liver disease, which progresses to end-stage liver disease requiring liver transplantation, accounts for 14% to 46% of liver transplantation in children when extrahepatic biliary atresia is excluded as a cause.[4]

PULMONARY ALVEOLAR PROTEINOSIS AND OTHER DISORDERS OF DISRUPTED SURFACTANT HOMEOSTASIS

Our understanding of the structure, function, and metabolism of pulmonary surfactant has advanced considerably over the past decade in parallel with identification of a group of specific diseases that are associated with abnormalities in either the production or clearance of surfactant. Although some similarities exist, it is now clear that each disease has distinct clinical manifestations, lung histopathology, pathogenesis, and natural history.

Surfactant is a complex mixture of phospholipids and proteins produced by alveolar epithelial cells and functions by reducing surface tension at the alveolar wall-liquid-air interface to prevent alveolar collapse. Surfactant is composed of 90% lipids, predominantly phosphatidylcholine and phosphatidylglycerol, and 10% proteins, including surfactant protein A (SP-A), SP-B, SP-C, and SP-D. SP-B and SP-C are hydrophobic surfactant proteins necessary to maintain surfactant homeostasis and normal pulmonary function. SP-A and SP-D are hydrophilic surfactant proteins belonging to the collectin family and have important roles in lung host defense.

Pulmonary alveolar proteinosis (PAP) (also referred to as alveolar proteinosis, alveolar lipoproteinosis, alveolar phospholipidosis, and pulmonary alveolar lipoproteinosis) is a rare syndrome that is characterized pathologically by intra-alveolar filling with surfactant lipids and proteins. The syndrome occurs in three clinically recognized forms: primary or idiopathic, secondary, and congenital. The pathogenesis is due to acquired or genetic dysfunction of alveolar macrophages that impairs catabolism of surfactant lipids and proteins, thereby reducing clearance of surfactant from the lungs.

Specific pulmonary diseases also occur in association with altered surfactant production due to hereditary deficiency of SP-B, SP-C, or the lipid transporter protein ABCA3. While these three disorders share some features in common with PAP, the pulmonary histopathology, clinical presentation, and natural history are distinct. Thus, hereditary SP-B, SP-C, and ABCA3 deficiency are more usefully considered as specific diseases of surfactant production rather than congenital forms of PAP.

Animal models of PAP have provided critical insights regarding the pathogenesis of PAP in humans and have identified GM-CSF as a critical factor in pulmonary surfactant homeostasis and innate immune host defense.[19] Animal models of genetic SP-B and SP-C deficiency have also been helpful in delineating the pathogenesis of their respective human disease counterparts.

EPIDEMIOLOGY AND GENETIC ASSOCIATIONS

PAP has an estimated annual incidence and prevalence of 0.36 and 3.7 cases per million individuals, respectively.[20] A meta-analysis of published reports of PAP by Seymour in 2002 identified 410 separate cases, representing most if not all reported cases of idiopathic PAP.[21] More than 90% of cases of PAP are idiopathic and are not associated with any familial predisposition or genetic mutations.[21] The overall incidence of secondary PAP in hematologic malignancies is 5.3%, although it is higher in neutropenic patients (8.8%) and in those with acute myeloid leukemia (10%).[22]

Severe respiratory diseases have been identified in association with mutations within the genes encoding SP-B, SP-C, and ABCA3, although the incidence and prevalence of each have not been well established.

In contrast, human lung diseases have not been identified in association with mutations in either SP-A or SP-D. Hereditary SP-B deficiency has an estimated incidence of approximately 0.66 cases per million births.[23] The incidence and prevalence of hereditary SP-C deficiency and ABCA3 deficiency are not known. In one study conducted from July 1995 until April 2003, 337 infants were identified with severe respiratory disease as part of a study to identify abnormalities of surfactant metabolism. Among these individuals, the molecular basis of the lung disease was determined to be SP-B deficiency in 47 (14%), ABCA3 deficiency in 16 (4.7%), and SP-C deficiency in 6 (1.8%), as defined by the presence of loss-of-function mutations on both alleles of the respective genes.

IDIOPATHIC PULMONARY ALVEOLAR PROTEINOSIS

Clinical Presentation

Idiopathic PAP usually presents in adult male smokers, although it occurs without a gender bias in nonsmokers and children. The major presenting symptom in children and adults is progressive exertional dyspnea of insidious onset. A mild cough occurs in some cases and can be accompanied by expectoration of airway secretions containing white solid material. Fever, chest pain, and hemoptysis are rare and only occur in the context of secondary infection. Significant pulmonary exposure is not a feature in most cases.

The physical examination is frequently unremarkable but may show tachypnea and fine basilar crackles when alveolar filling is extensive. Cyanosis and digital clubbing occur in advanced cases.

The plain chest radiograph reveals a patchy bilateral airspace disease often similar in appearance to pulmonary edema but without other radiographic signs of left heart failure (Fig. 52-3). High-resolution computed tomography shows patchy ground-glass opacifications with superimposed interlobular septal and intralobular thickening that are typical but not diagnostic of PAP. The extent of the radiographic abnormalities is usually disproportionately greater than expected based on the clinical findings.

Routine laboratory tests are frequently within the normal range; however, when present, an isolated elevation of serum lactate dehydrogenase correlates with the degree of pulmonary impairment[21] and can be a useful marker of disease severity or exacerbation. Arterial partial pressure of oxygen (PO_2) and oxygen saturation are lowered in proportion to disease severity and are accompanied by an elevated partial pressure of carbon dioxide (PCO_2) with a normal pH in advanced cases due to hypoxic ventilatory stimulus. On pulmonary function testing, the most common pattern seen is that of a restrictive defect, with a disproportionate reduction in diffusing capacity for carbon monoxide.

Diagnosis

PAP is suspected based on clinical features and its characteristic radiographic appearance. Infection may be the initial consideration, especially in cases where the symptoms have been insidious and acute secondary infection is the reason for the evaluation. Occasionally, PAP patients present with secondary lung infection. In such cases, evaluation of the immune status may be warranted because PAP has been linked to immunodeficiency states.

A diagnosis of PAP can be made definitively by open lung biopsy and demonstration of the unique pathologic findings (see Fig. 52-3). However, the diagnosis can also be established by bronchoscopy and lavage in approximately 75% of clinically suspected cases.[24] The lavage fluid is milky in appearance and forms a waxy sediment upon standing. Light microscopic examination of the sediment reveals amorphous debris; large "foamy" macrophages may also be seen, and both macrophages and debris stain intensely with periodic acid-Schiff (PAS). Detection of increased concentrations of surfactant proteins is confirmatory, although such testing is generally available only in specialized centers. Light microscopic evaluation reveals parenchymal architecture that is relatively preserved unless secondary infection is present. Alveoli are filled with acellular granular material that is eosinophilic and stains strongly with PAS. If inflammatory cells are present, infection or other reasons for an inflammatory response should be considered. Electron microscopy reveals the presence of lamellar bodies and tubular myelin, but is seldom needed to confirm the diagnosis.

Recently, idiopathic PAP was shown to be specifically and strongly associated with anti-GM-CSF autoantibodies, which has provided an additional diagnostic approach.[25] Detection of such antibodies in the blood or lung lavage fluid now provides a convenient and accurate means for diagnosing idiopathic PAP with a sensitivity and specificity approaching 100%.

Natural History

The clinical course of idiopathic PAP falls into one of three categories: stable but with persistent symptoms, progressive deterioration, or spontaneous improvement.[19] Most affected individuals have persistent, albeit variable, symptoms; however, a small proportion (~8%) show spontaneous improvement while others progressively deteriorate. The overall 5-year survival rate in untreated individuals is 85%.[21] The majority of PAP deaths result directly from respiratory failure (~72%), while a smaller proportion are the result of uncontrolled infection (~20%).

Patients with idiopathic PAP are at risk for secondary infections from a variety of pathogens. Organisms include those commonly seen in community- and hospital-acquired lung infections (e.g., *Streptococcus, Klebsiella, Haemophilus, Staphylococcus, Pseudomonas, Proteus,* and *Escherichia*). However, an unexpected proportion of secondary infections in these patients involve unusual or opportunistic organisms (e.g., *Nocardia, Mycobacterium, Pneumocystis, Aspergillus, Cryptococcus*). The relative frequency of secondary infections that occur outside the lungs suggests a possible defect in systemic host defense.[19,21] Although a molecular mechanism responsible for the increased frequency of secondary infections in PAP has not yet been identified,

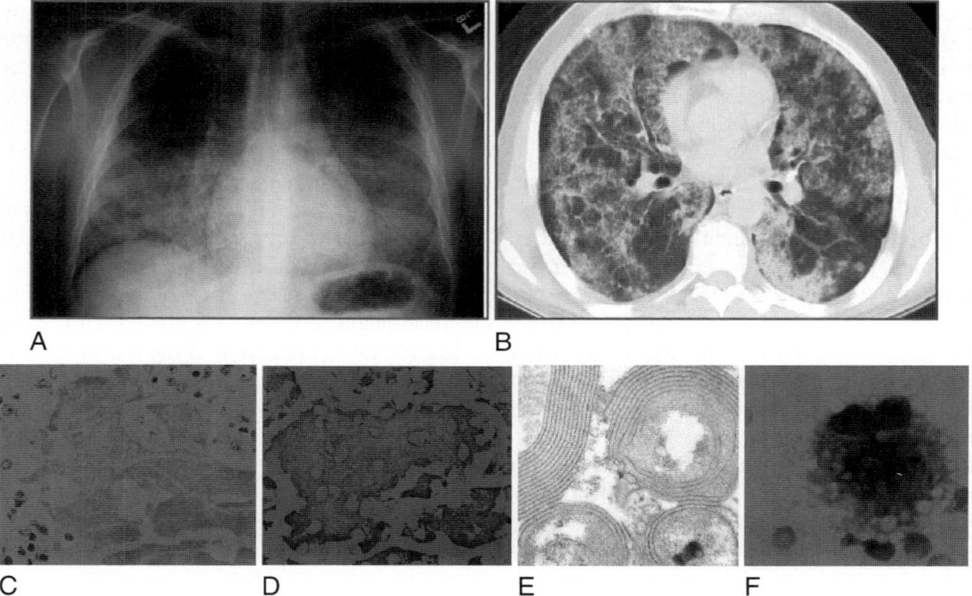

■ **FIGURE 52-3.** Radiographic, histologic, and ultrastructural features of pulmonary alveolar proteinosis. **A,** Posteroanterior chest radiograph showing the typical features of pulmonary alveolar proteinosis, including diffuse, patchy, bilateral airspace disease unaccompanied by evidence of cardiac failure, adenopathy, or effusion. **B,** High-resolution computed tomographic scan of the chest showing patchy ground-glass opacification and interlobular septal thickening. This pattern, commonly referred to as "crazy paving," is characteristic, but not diagnostic, of the disease. **C,** Lung biopsy specimen showing intra-alveolar material that stains positively with periodic acid-Schiff reagent. **D,** Immunohistochemical staining of a lung biopsy specimen showing abundant intra-alveolar accumulation of surfactant protein A. **E,** Ultrastructural examination of the bronchoalveolar lavage sediment showing the characteristic features of pulmonary surfactant including laminated membrane structures and amorphous debris. **F,** Cytologic appearance of a "foamy" alveolar macrophage present in bronchoalveolar fluid. (See Color Plate 39.) (From Trapnell BC, Whitsett JA, Nakata K: Pulmonary alveolar proteinosis. N Engl J Med 2003;349(26):2527–2539.)

the observation that anti-GM-CSF autoantibodies completely eliminate GM-CSF bioactivity in vivo, systemically, suggests a potential role for GM-CSF.

Pathogenesis

The initial description of PAP in 1958 established that the intra-alveolar material was composed primarily of phospholipids and proteins.[26] Subsequent studies confirmed that this material was pulmonary surfactant but failed to determine if the abnormality was due to increased production, decreased clearance, or the expression of abnormal surfactant lipids or proteins. A prolonged search over three decades to identify a presumed "irritant" (i.e., silica or an infectious agent) believed to stimulate increased surfactant production was fruitless. Notwithstanding, a number of abnormalities in alveolar macrophages were identified, including the presence of surfactant inclusion bodies responsible for the foamy appearance of these cells in PAP. Functional abnormalities included defects in chemotaxis, adhesion, phagocytosis, microbicidal activity, and phagolysosome fusion.

A serendipitous but important clue came from studies involving genetically altered mice in which expression of GM-CSF or the GM-CSF receptor β chain (GM-CSF Rβc) was abolished by gene targeting. Mice with such defects developed a pulmonary phenotype consisting of intra-alveolar surfactant accumulation that was biochemically, histologically, and ultrastructurally identical to idiopathic PAP in humans.[27] Synthesis of mRNA for surfactant proteins was not altered in these mice, and subsequent studies demonstrated that pulmonary surfactant accumulation was due to defective catabolism of surfactant by alveolar macrophages rather than an increase in surfactant production. Reconstitution of pulmonary GM-CSF expression from a second, lung-specific transgene in GM-CSF-/- mice prevented development of PAP and strengthened the concept that GM-CSF acts within the lung to maintain surfactant homeostasis. A study in which PAP was corrected in GM-CSF Rβc-/- mice by transplantation of bone marrow from wild-type mice supported the concept that surfactant accumulation was due to defective catabolism in alveolar macrophages and that GM-CSF acted within the lung to maintain surfactant homeostasis.

GM-CSF-/- mice also have increased susceptibility to microbial lung infection and decreased pulmonary clearance of bacterial, fungal, and viral pathogens.[19] Their alveolar macrophages display numerous abnormalities including a foamy appearance from accumulated surfactant and defects in cell adhesion and cytoskeletal organization, pathogen recognition receptor expression, phagocytosis, microbial killing, Fc receptor signaling, proinflammatory cytokine release in response to lipopolysaccharide, as well as other defects. This diversity of alveolar macrophage defects in GM-CSF-/- mice suggested the possibility that maturation of alveolar macrophages may be arrested in the absence of GM-CSF. This hypothesis was supported by the observation that pulmonary GM-CSF regulates expression of the macrophage differentiation-inducing transcription factor PU.1 levels in alveolar macrophages.[28] Further support came from studies in which retrovirally mediated replacement of PU.1 in alveolar macrophages from GM-CSF-/- mice restored all of the abnormal alveolar macrophage immune functions described above as well as the defective surfactant catabolism. In summary, the numerous and diverse defects observed in alveolar macrophages from GM-CSF-/- mice, all of which are coordinately corrected by either pulmonary GM-CSF expression in vivo or PU.1 expression in the absence of GM-CSF in vitro, strongly suggest that GM-CSF, via PU.1, stimulates the terminal differentiation of alveolar macrophages in mice.

The discovery of the critical role of GM-CSF in pulmonary surfactant homeostasis in mice prompted a reevaluation of the pathogenesis of idiopathic PAP in humans as a disorder of GM-CSF deficiency. To date, no mutations have been found in the genes encoding GM-CSF or its receptor in individuals with idiopathic PAP. Furthermore, GM-CSF levels are increased in idiopathic PAP, not decreased as would be predicted based on the mouse findings.

Nakata and colleagues made an important observation linking the pathogenesis of human idiopathic PAP to GM-CSF[25] through a series of experiments that reexamined a previously identified "immunoinhibitory" activity present in lungs and sera of these patients. They demonstrated the presence of high levels of circulating anti-GM-CSF autoantibody in idiopathic PAP patients that were not present in individuals with congenital PAP, secondary PAP, other lung diseases, or normal individuals. These autoantibodies are polyclonal, present at very high levels in blood and lungs, bind GM-CSF with very high affinity, and virtually eliminate GM-CSF bioactivity from the lung: the neutralizing capacity in the serum can exceed the serum concentration of GM-CSF by 25,000-fold or more.[29] These findings show that while GM-CSF itself is not absent in acquired PAP, it is biologically inactivated by neutralizing antibody. Thus, idiopathic PAP is equivalent to a functional knockout of GM-CSF in humans.

The pattern of alveolar macrophage defects is similar in idiopathic PAP in humans and in PAP in GM-CSF-deficient mice. This suggests that GM-CSF may be important in promoting terminal differentiation of alveolar macrophages in humans as well as mice and that the pathogenesis of idiopathic PAP in humans may be due to deficiency of GM-CSF bioactivity. This hypothesis is supported by other studies demonstrating that PU.1 levels are reduced in alveolar macrophages from idiopathic PAP patients and can be restored by GM-CSF immunotherapy.[30]

Therapy

The treatment of choice for PAP depends on the clinical context and clinical subtype. Standard therapy in cases of idiopathic PAP is whole lung lavage, and this improves symptoms in most or all patients. The procedure involves placement of a double-lumen endotracheal tube under general anesthesia. With the patient in a lateral supine position, the nondependent lung is mechanically ventilated while the dependent lung is "washed" with up to 20 L of warmed normal saline. Subsequently, the process is repeated in reverse to treat the other lung. While not documented in prospective, randomized trials, whole-lung lavage improves clinical, physiologic, and radiographic findings and improves survival in acquired PAP (5-year survival rate 94% ± 2% with lavage vs. 85% ± 5% without lavage; $n = 146$, $P = .04$).[21] In patients requiring repeated lavage, the median duration of clinical benefit from lavage has been reported to be 15 months.[21]

Several experimental therapies for idiopathic PAP are also currently under evaluation in clinical trials. One approach that has been under evaluation for the past decade involves daily administration of GM-CSF. Seymour and colleagues first evaluated subcutaneous GM-CSF in a single patient and then in 14 PAP patients. They found an overall improvement rate of 43%.[31] An ongoing study in the United States is also evaluating subcutaneous GM-CSF therapy in acquired PAP.[32] In Japan, a network of investigators is evaluating the effectiveness of aerosolized GM-CSF in idiopathic PAP. Although the early results from these trials are encouraging, no firm conclusions can yet be drawn regarding the effectiveness of GM-CSF therapy for idiopathic PAP. Other potential therapeutic approaches include plasmapheresis, immune globulin administration, and anti-B-lymphocyte immunotherapy. As for many of the rare diseases, the low prevalence has hampered the development of potential new therapies.

SECONDARY PULMONARY ALVEOLAR PROTEINOSIS

Although rare in children, secondary PAP can occur after exposure to a definite etiologic agent or in association with other diseases that result in either a functional impairment or reduced numbers of alveolar macrophages. Secondary PAP has been reported following heavy inhalation exposure to silica, titanium, or aluminum dusts, or fibrous insulation material. A variety of hematologic and oncologic disorders are also associated with secondary PAP, including chronic myeloid leukemia, myelomonocytic leukemia, acute myeloid leukemia, acute lymphoid leukemia, hairy cell leukemia, lymphoma, myelofibrosis, aplastic anemia, myelodysplasia, thrombocythemia, polycythemia vera, idiopathic thrombocytopenic purpura, myeloma, macroglobulinemia, Fanconi's anemia, and glioblastoma.[33] In cancer patients, secondary PAP can develop following a period of neutropenia or bone marrow aplasia when alveolar macrophage numbers are decreased. Secondary PAP may be distinguished from idiopathic PAP on the basis of the clinical context. However, the pattern of surfactant protein immunostaining in histologic specimens of lung tissues obtained by transbronchial biopsy can be helpful. Idiopathic PAP is associated with a more homogeneous staining pattern, while secondary PAP is associated with a patchy, focal staining pattern.[21] The recent availability of a blood test to detect the high levels of anti-GM-CSF autoantibodies that are present in idiopathic PAP now offers an additional, convenient approach to exclude a diagnosis of this clinical form. Although a common pathogenic pathway has not been described for PAP in all of these illnesses or exposures, interference with the role played by alveolar macrophages in surfactant clearance is a likely general explanation. Secondary PAP generally resolves with treatment of the underlying condition (e.g., chemotherapy for hematologic malignancy).[33]

CONGENITAL PULMONARY ALVEOLAR PROTEINOSIS

PAP has been reported in infants with no demonstrable disturbance of SP-B expression where impaired expression of GM-CSF Rβc was implicated. In one report, peripheral blood mononuclear cells of four of seven infants had dramatically reduced GM-CSF Rβc expression, binding of GM-CSF, and impaired in vitro responsiveness to both GM-CSF and interleukin-3.[34] To date, these results have not been confirmed by other investigators.

HEREDITARY SURFACTANT PROTEIN B DEFICIENCY

Hereditary SP-B deficiency is an autosomal-recessive disorder involving mutations within the gene encoding SP-B. Affected individuals present with respiratory insufficiency within 12 to 24 hours after birth. Evidence of infection or congenital heart disease is absent, but there may be a family history of siblings who died in infancy of respiratory failure or of unknown cause.

The chest radiograph generally shows a diffuse alveolar filling process, reduced lung volumes, and air bronchograms. HRCT scans demonstrate ground-glass opacification and geometric interlobular septal thickening. Laboratory analysis of tracheal aspirates demonstrating the absence of SP-B strongly suggests SP-B deficiency but is not diagnostic. Definitive diagnosis requires the demonstration of disease-causing mutations on both SP-B alleles. Over 30 mutations of the SP-B gene have been described to date. In two thirds of cases, an insertional frameshift mutation causes replacement of a single nucleotide at codon 121 in exon 4 by a trinucleotide (designated 131ins2). This mutation is present as a homozygous mutation in 60% of cases and as a heterozygous mutation in 25% of cases. Prenatal diagnosis of hereditary SP-B deficiency has been achieved by chorionic villus sampling and the absence of SP-B protein in amniotic fluid.

While the histopathologic appearance of SP-B deficiency has features in common with PAP, important differences exist. In SP-B deficiency, the alveoli are filled with eosinophilic granular material, macrophages, and desquamated alveolar epithelial cells. Alveolar type II cells are hyperplastic, and the alveolar septa are markedly thickened and fibrotic.

The natural history of hereditary SP-B is progressive respiratory failure unless acute intervention with mechanical ventilation is instituted. Corticosteroids, surfactant replacement therapy, and cardiopulmonary bypass have not been shown to alter the clinical course, and most infants die within 6 months. Lung transplantation is the only definitive therapy and has been used successfully in at least three infants at the time of this writing.

SURFACTANT PROTEIN C DEFICIENCY

Abnormalities in SP-C expression have been linked to lung disease in older children and adults, although the disease pathogenesis is incompletely understood. Complete absence of SP-C in the lungs was initially identified in one family with an autosomal-dominant pattern of inheritance, but no mutations within the gene encoding SP-C could be found. Subsequently, mutations in the gene encoding SP-C have been clearly associated with interstitial lung disease.[23]

The age of onset and clinical presentation vary widely. In one large kindred with familial pulmonary fibrosis, a missense mutation was identified in the SP-C gene (L188Q) that segregated with disease. The onset of lung disease in the affected individuals ranged from early infancy to the fifth decade of life. Furthermore, some individuals carrying the mutation were symptom free, suggesting the possibility of incomplete penetrance of the mutation. The natural history of SP-C deficiency has not been well studied; however, individuals manifest varying degrees of pulmonary fibrosis and restrictive lung impairment.

The lung histopathology of individuals carrying the SP-C mutation L188Q varied, including elements of both nonspecific interstitial pneumonitis and usual interstitial pneumonitis and pulmonary fibrosis.[23] Interestingly, genetically altered mice deficient in SP-C due to gene ablation develop subtle pulmonary abnormalities consisting of progressive airspace enlargement, macrophage infiltration and pulmonary fibrosis on some but not other genetic backgrounds, suggesting that modifier genes may be important in the pathophysiology of the lung disease. Collectively, studies to date suggest that SP-C mutations may cause lung disease due to chronic cellular stress and injury resulting from an accumulation of the misfolded SP-C precursor, pro-SP-C.

No specific therapy is currently available for the treatment of individuals with SP-C deficiency.

HEREDITARY ABCA3 DEFICIENCY

Hereditary ABCA3 deficiency is an autosomal-recessive disorder involving mutations within the gene encoding the adenosine triphosphate (ATP)-binding cassette (ABC) transporter protein, *ABCA3*.[35] ABC transporters belong to a family of proteins, the individual members of which utilize ATP hydrolysis to drive the transport of various specific compounds across biologic membranes. Transported materials include lipids, ions, amino acids, peptides, sugars, vitamins, hormones, drugs, and toxins. ABCA3 belongs to the ABC protein subfamily A, which includes lipid transporters, multidrug resistance membrane-associated transporters, the cystic fibrosis transmembrane conductance regulator, and adrenoleukodystrophy proteins. The *ABCA3* gene encodes a 1704–amino acid protein that is highly expressed in lung and is specifically localized to the limiting membrane of lamellar bodies within type II alveolar epithelial cells. The role of ABCA3 appears to involve lipid transport and may have a role in surfactant phospholipid metabolism.

While the epidemiology has not been established, affected individuals can be of Northern and Southern European, African American, Asian, and Middle Eastern origin. Affected infants are born after a gestation of at least 36 weeks and develop severe respiratory insufficiency within hours after birth. All individuals have clinical and/or radiographic findings of surfactant deficiency. The chest radiogram demonstrates a diffuse alveolar filling process with ground-glass opacifications, reduced lung volumes, and air bronchograms.

ABCA3 deficiency is uniformly fatal; most individuals die within 1 month of birth. Lung histopathology shows accumulation of proteinaceous material and macrophages within alveolar spaces, widening of the interstitium, and alveolar type II cell hyperplasia. Ultrastructural analysis of type II alveolar epithelial cells demonstrates that lamellar bodies are either absent or morphologically abnormal with tightly packed membranes and dense eccentric inclusion bodies.

PULMONARY ALVEOLAR MICROLITHIASIS

Pulmonary alveolar microlithiasis (PAM) is a rare idiopathic lung disease characterized by the presence of innumerable tiny calculi (microliths) composed primarily of calcium phosphate within alveolar air spaces. PAM was identified and described macroscopically in 1668 by Malpighi and evaluated radiographically in 1918, but it was not well characterized until the 1950s. Since then, interest in the disease (and the number of reports) has increased; in 1957 one report described 26 cases, and by 1997, 300 cases had been reported in the literature. The disease can occur in individuals of any age and has been reported in stillborn twins and an 80-year-old woman. However, it occurs most often in adults between the ages of 30 and 50. PAM must be differentiated from diffuse pulmonary calcinosis, which can be seen in hyperthyroidism, chronic renal disease, and vitamin D intoxication. PAM must also be differentiated from miliary tuberculosis and from healed disseminated histoplasmosis.

EPIDEMIOLOGY AND GENETIC AND OTHER ASSOCIATIONS

The incidence and prevalence of PAM are unknown. Less than 450 cases have been reported,[36] of which approximately 50 occurred in children. PAM has been reported to occur throughout the world; however, 100 of the reported cases occurred in Turkey and Italy, suggesting a clustering in these regions. Most reports have not found a predilection for either men or women. Two different patterns have been described, familial and sporadic. Familial transmission occurs in half of the cases and appears to follow an autosomal-recessive inheritance, but environmental and dietetic factors may play a role and are difficult to exclude. PAM has been reported in association with mitral stenosis, milk alkali syndrome, pericardial cyst, renal transplantation, Waardenburg anophthalmia syndrome, diaphyseal aclasia and lymphocytic interstitial pneumonitis, and nephrolithiasis. The relationship between PAM and these disorders, if any, is unclear.

CLINICAL PRESENTATION

Children with PAM are usually asymptomatic, although chronic cough may be present and one case was reported to occur with hemoptysis. Many adult patients are also asymptomatic when the disease is first discovered. Symptoms may be absent even when the plain chest radiograph reveals involvement throughout both lungs with little air-containing parenchyma visible. When symptoms are present, dyspnea on exertion is the most common finding. Cough develops in some patients and is usually nonproductive, but sputum may be present and can contain microliths. Chest pain is uncommon and hemoptysis is rare even in adults with advanced disease. A number of cases have been identified by radiologic evaluation of asymptomatic relatives of an index case.

The physical examination is usually unremarkable in children and even in adults unless the disease is very advanced. In the late stages, tachypnea may be present and auscultation of the chest may reveal diminished breath sounds, particularly at the bases. Clubbing, cyanosis, and signs of pulmonary hypertension may be present in such cases.

The plain chest radiograph in PAM has a "sandstorm" appearance, which has been said to be a more characteristic and diagnostic pattern than the chest radiograph in any other pulmonary disease.[37] Of diagnostic importance, the radiographic findings are usually significantly out of proportion compared with the more mild clinical findings. Although considerable variation occurs among patients depending on the severity of the disease, the fundamental pattern is one of a very fine micronodulation diffusely involving both lungs (Fig. 52-4). Individual microliths are identifiable as very sharply defined nodules measuring less than 1 mm in diameter. The opacities are more prominent in the lower lung zones and can be seen regardless of superimposition or summation of shadows. In more advanced cases, they may be so numerous so as to appear confluent; the normally exposed radiograph may show a "white out" of the lungs that can totally obliterate the mediastinal and diaphragmatic contours. In such cases, use of an overexposed radiographic technique usually reveals the underlying pattern of sharply defined micronodules. Occasionally, the radiographic changes include a superimposed reticular pattern of septal lines. Less frequent findings include apical bullae, a zone of increased lucency between the lung parenchyma and the ribs (known as a black pleural line), and pleural and pericardial calcification.

HRCT of the chest reveals diffusely distributed calcific nodules measuring 1 mm or less in diameter (see Fig. 52-4). Nodules are sometimes distributed predominantly along the cardiac borders and dorsal portions of the lower lung zones. The high dorsal attenuation persists when scans are obtained with the patient in the prone position. Calcific interlobular septal thickening is commonly seen[38] and is due to the high concentration of microliths in the periphery of the secondary lobules, rather than calcification of the septa themselves. Other findings include apical bullae, thin-walled subpleural cysts, and pleural and pericardial calcification.

Routine laboratory tests in individuals with PAM are frequently within the normal range and are generally not helpful. In most cases, serum calcium and phosphorus levels are normal.

Results of pulmonary function tests vary considerably among cases, depending on the extent of disease and the presence or absence of interstitial fibrosis. When abnormalities are present, a decrease in residual volume may be an early finding and is likely due to physical displacement of air by calculi within the intra-alveolar space. Other findings may include decreased vital capacity and diffusing capacity. Arterial blood gases may show mild hypoxemia and an increased alveolar-arterial oxygen gradient, but only in more advanced cases.

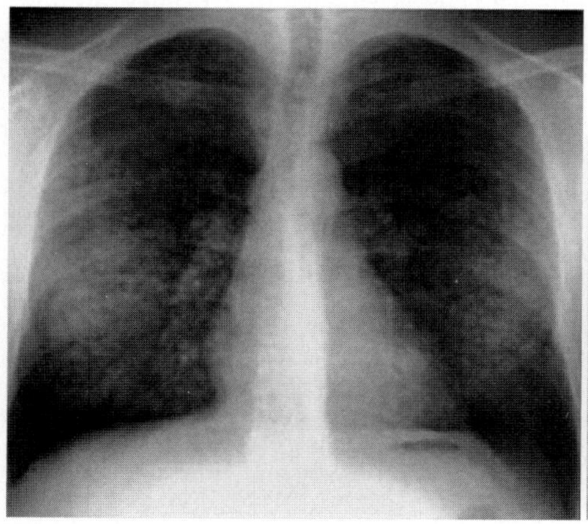

A

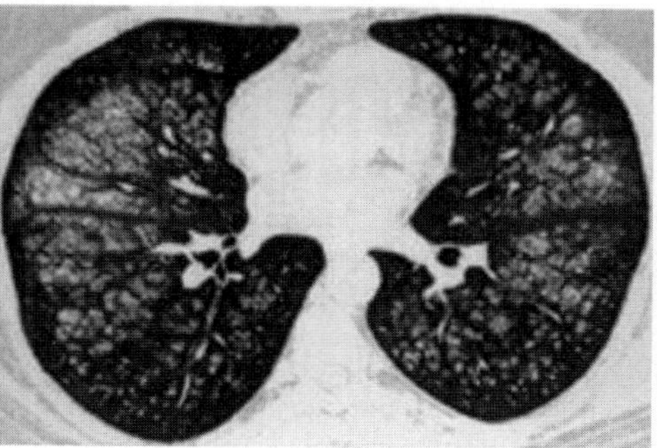

B

FIGURE 52-4. Radiographic features of pulmonary alveolar microlithiasis. **A,** Posteroanterior chest radiograph showing the classic "sandstorm" appearance of pulmonary alveolar microlithiasis, including diffuse, patchy, bilateral sharp micronodular disease. **B,** High-resolution computed tomographic scan of the chest showing micronodular densities. (From Brandenburg VM, Schubert H: Images in clinical medicine. Pulmonary alveolar microlithiasis. N Engl J Med 2003;348 [16]:1555.)

DIAGNOSIS

The diagnosis of PAM can usually be confidently made by the characteristic appearance of the plain chest radiograph and the striking radiologic-clinical dissociation. The HRCT can be helpful when the extent of disease is minimal. Occasionally, microliths may be observed in sputum. Bronchoscopy with bronchoalveolar lavage may reveal the presence of microliths in the lavage fluid that stain pink with Papanicolaou dye or PAS reagent. Transbronchial biopsy reveals characteristic microliths that measure in diameter from 50 to 750 μm and are located almost invariably within alveolar air spaces. The alveolar walls are usually normal in the early stages of the disease but show interstitial fibrosis in the later stages. Open lung biopsy is definitive but is seldom necessary or indicated. Occasionally, microliths are present in the bronchial wall or interstitium and, rarely, in extrapulmonary sites (e.g., in the seminal vesicles, sympathetic ganglia, or gonads).

Individual microliths vary in shape and can be round, oval, or irregular and have a distinctive concentric laminated appearance. They are composed primarily of calcium phosphate and often have a PAS-positive central core. Some reports have described evidence of a noncalcified stage that presumably occurs before the development of dense calcification. Microliths must be differentiated from corpora amylacea, which are round, laminated bodies that can be present in the alveolar airspaces in individuals without PAM. Copora amylacea are round, laminated bodies that measure in diameter from 50 to 250 μm, usually contain a central birefringent core, and are surrounded by one or more macrophages. They are strongly PAS positive and contain little or no calcium. Corpora amylacea are present in up to 0.5% to 4% of autopsies.

NATURAL HISTORY

Typically, affected individuals are asymptomatic or mildly symptomatic at the time of diagnosis, depending on ascertainment. The low incidence of the disease has precluded detailed natural history studies, and much of our knowledge regarding the course of disease comes from small studies involving several affected family members. Such reports suggest that the disease begins with involvement of the lung bases and progresses slowly, albeit inexorably, toward involvement of a progressively larger fraction of the lungs, leading ultimately to death from respiratory failure, usually in early adult life. In contrast, the disease can be stable for long periods (up to 30 years in some patients), even when extensive radiographic changes are present initially. Pneumothorax can occur, presumably from bullae and subpleural cysts, and can be recurrent in some patients.

PATHOGENESIS

Some evidence suggests that microliths may be formed in the alveolar walls, possibly in type II alveolar epithelial cells, and then extruded into the adjacent airspaces. The concentric laminar deposits suggest that they grow by surface deposition; microliths are believed to form and increase in size as the disease progresses.[39]

The etiology and pathogenesis of PAM are unknown. Hypothetical mechanisms that have been postulated include an inborn error of metabolism, a response to a pulmonary insult or inhaled agent, and an acquired abnormality of calcium or phosphorous metabolism.[39] While roughly half of cases of PAM occur in families, usually a common environmental factor cannot be eliminated. For example, in one family of seven siblings, PAM developed in four siblings who lived together and not in three who left home at an early age. PAM has been reported in association with inhalation of various materials (e.g., mica, calcium-containing snuff, or sand); however, a history of occupational exposure is generally lacking in most patients. Theoretically, calcareous salts could precipitate on the alveolar surfaces that could become alkalinized by the action of carbonic anhydrase.[40] Most PAM patients have normal serum calcium and phosphorus levels and no known disorder of calcium metabolism. The observation of increased expression of BAX and bcl-2 proteins in two siblings with PAM suggested that an abnormality of apoptosis of lung cells might play a role.[41]

A lung phenotype similar to that observed in PAM patients has been reported to occur in *nackt* mice.[42] These mice have a recessive mutation on chromosome 13 and also develop skin defects and $CD4^+$ T-cell deficiency. Only a small number of *nackt* mice develop PAM, suggesting that in this model, the pathogenesis is likely multifactorial.

THERAPY

There is no specific therapy available for PAM. A variety of approaches have been tried, albeit without clear success. These include the use of systemic corticosteroids, chelator therapy with disodium etidronate, and bronchoalveolar lavage. Lung transplantation has been used successfully to treat PAM.

REFERENCES

Alpha-1 Antitrypsin Deficiency

1. Lomas DA, Parfrey H: Alpha1-antitrypsin deficiency. 4. Molecular pathophysiology. Thorax 2004;59(6):529–535.
2. Laurell CB, Eriksson S: The electrophoretic α1-globulin pattern of serum in α1-antitrypsin deficiency. Scand J Clin Lab Invest 1963;15:132–140.
3. Sharp HL, Bridges RA, Krivit W, Freier EF: Cirrhosis associated with alpha-1-antitrypsin deficiency. A previously unrecognized inherited disorder. J Lab Clin Med 1969;73(6):934–939.
4. American Thoracic Society/European Respiratory Society Statement: Standards for the diagnosis and management of individuals with alpha-1 antitrypsin deficiency. Am J Respir Crit Care Med 2003;168(7):818–900.
5. Mulgrew AT, Taggart CC, Lawless MW, et al: Z alpha1-antitrypsin polymerizes in the lung and acts as a neutrophil chemoattractant. Chest 2004;125(5):1952–1957.
6. Sifers RN: Insights into checkpoint capacity. Nat Struct Mol Biol 2004;11(2):108–109.
7. Wu Y, Swulius MT, Moremen KW, Sifers RN: Elucidation of the molecular logic by which misfolded alpha 1-antitrypsin is preferentially selected for degradation. Proc Natl Acad Sci U S A 2003;100(14):8229–8234.
8. Blank CA, Brantly M: Clinical features and molecular characteristics of alpha 1-antitrypsin deficiency. Ann Allergy 1994;72(2):105–122.
9. Brantly ML, Wittes JT, Vogelmeier CF, et al: Use of a highly purified alpha 1-antitrypsin standard to establish ranges for the common normal and deficient alpha 1-antitrypsin phenotypes. Chest 1991;100(3):703–708.
10. DeMeo DL, Silverman EK: Alpha1-antitrypsin deficiency. 2. Genetic aspects of alpha(1)-antitrypsin deficiency. Phenotypes and genetic modifiers of emphysema risk. Thorax 2004;59(3):259–264.
11. Fagerhol MK, Laurell CB: The Pi system-inherited variants of serum alpha 1-antitrypsin. Prog Med Genet 1970;7:96–111.
12. Luisetti M, Seersholm N: Alpha1-antitrypsin deficiency. 1: Epidemiology of alpha1-antitrypsin deficiency. Thorax 2004;59(2):164–169.
13. Needham M, Stockley RA: Alpha 1-antitrypsin deficiency. 3. Clinical manifestations and natural history. Thorax 2004;59(5):441–445.
14. Sveger T: Liver disease in alpha1-antitrypsin deficiency detected by screening of 200,000 infants. N Engl J Med 1976;294(24):1316–1321.

15. Brantly ML: Laboratory diagnosis of α1-antitrypsin deficiency. In: Crystal RG, ed: Alpha-1-Antitrypsin Deficiency. New York: Marcel Dekker, 1995, pp 45–60.
16. Piitulainen E, Sveger T: Respiratory symptoms and lung function in young adults with severe alpha(1)-antitrypsin deficiency (PiZZ). Thorax 2002; 57(8):705–708.
17. Newell JD Jr, Hogg JC, Snider GL: Report of a workshop: quantitative computed tomography scanning in longitudinal studies of emphysema. Eur Respir J 2004;23(5):769–775.
18. Flotte TR, Brantly ML, Spencer LT, et al: Phase I trial of intramuscular injection of a recombinant adeno-associated virus alpha 1-antitrypsin (rAAV2-CB-hAAT) gene vector to AAT-deficient adults. Hum Gene Ther 2004;15(1):93–128.

Pulmonary Alveolar Proteinosis, SP-B Deficiency, SP-C Deficiency, ABCA3 Deficiency

19. Trapnell BC, Whitsett JA, Nakata K: Pulmonary alveolar proteinosis. N Engl J Med 2003;349(26):2527–2539.
20. Ben-Dov I, Kishinevski Y, Roznman J, et al: Pulmonary alveolar proteinosis in Israel. Ethnic clustering. Isr Med Assoc J 1999;1(2):75–78.
21. Seymour JF, Presneill JJ: Pulmonary alveolar proteinosis. Progress in the first 44 years. Am J Respir Crit Care Med 2002;166(2):215–235.
22. Shah PL, Hansell D, Lawson PR, et al: Pulmonary alveolar proteinosis. Clinical aspects and current concepts on pathogenesis. Thorax 2000; 55(1):67–77.
23. Nogee LM: Alterations in SP-B and SP-C expression in neonatal lung disease. Annu Rev Physiol 2004;66:601–623.
24. Schoch OD, Schanz U, Koller M, et al: BAL findings in a patient with pulmonary alveolar proteinosis successfully treated with GM-CSF. Thorax 2002;57(3):277–280.
25. Kitamura T, Tanaka N, Watanabe J, et al: Idiopathic pulmonary alveolar proteinosis as an autoimmune disease with neutralizing antibody against granulocyte/macrophage colony-stimulating factor. J Exp Med 1999; 190(6):875–880.
26. Rosen SG, Castleman B, Liebow AA: Pulmonary alveolar proteinosis. N Engl J Med 1958;258:1123–1142.
27. Dranoff G, Crawford AD, Sadelain M, et al: Involvement of granulocyte-macrophage colony-stimulating factor in pulmonary homeostasis. Science 1994;264(5159):713–716.
28. Shibata Y, Berclaz P-Y, Chroneos Z, et al: GM-CSF regulates alveolar macrophage differentiation and innate immunity in the lung through PU.1. Immunity 2001;15:557–567.
29. Uchida K, Nakata K, Trapnell BC, et al: High-affinity autoantibodies specifically eliminate granulocyte-macrophage colony-stimulating factor activity in the lungs of patients with idiopathic pulmonary alveolar proteinosis. Blood 2004;103(3):1089–1098.
30. Bonfield TL, Raychaudhuri B, Malur A, et al: PU.1 regulation of human alveolar macrophage differentiation requires granulocyte-macrophage colony-stimulating factor. Am J Physiol Lung Cell Mol Physiol 2003; 285(5):L1132–L1136.
31. Seymour JF, Presneill JJ, Schoch OD, et al: Therapeutic efficacy of granulocyte-macrophage colony-stimulating factor in patients with idiopathic acquired alveolar proteinosis. Am J Respir Crit Care Med 2001;163(2): 524–531.
32. Kavuru MS, Sullivan EJ, Piccin R, et al: Exogenous granulocyte-macrophage colony-stimulating factor administration for pulmonary alveolar proteinosis. Am J Respir Crit Care Med 2000;161(4 Part 1):1143–1148.
33. Ladeb S, Fleury-Feith J, Escudier E, et al: Secondary alveolar proteinosis in cancer patients. Support Care Cancer 1996;4(6):420–426.
34. Dirksen U, Nishinakamura R, Groneck P, et al: Human pulmonary alveolar proteinosis associated with a defect in GM- CSF/IL-3/IL-5 receptor common beta chain expression. J Clin Invest 1997;100(9): 2211–22217.
35. Shulenin S, Nogee LM, Annilo T, et al: ABCA3 gene mutations in newborns with fatal surfactant deficiency. N Engl J Med 2004;350(13): 1296–1303.

Pulmonary Alveolar Microlithiasis

36. Castellana G, Castellana R, Fanelli C, et al: [Pulmonary alveolar microlithiasis. Clinical and radiological course of three cases according to conventional radiology and HRCT. A hypothesis for radiological classification]. Radiol Med (Torino) 2003;106(3):160–168.
37. Brandenburg VM, Schubert H: Images in clinical medicine. Pulmonary alveolar microlithiasis. N Engl J Med 2003;348(16):1555.
38. Gasparetto EL, Tazoniero P, Escuissato DL, et al: Pulmonary alveolar microlithiasis presenting with crazy-paving pattern on high resolution CT. Br J Radiol 2004;77(923):974–976.
39. Fraser RS, Mulligan RC, Colman N, Pare PD: Pulmonary alveolar microlithiasis. In: Fraser and Pare's Diagnosis of Diseases of the Chest, 4th ed. Philadelphia: WB Saunders, 1999, pp 2719–2723.
40. Lopez-Areal L, Zumarraga R, Gil Turner C, et al: [Infantile familial pulmonary alveolar microlithiasis. Description of 5 cases in 2 families]. Rev Clin Esp 1965;97(6):389–395.
41. Barbolini G, Rossi G, Bisetti A: Pulmonary alveolar microlithiasis. N Engl J Med 2002;347(1):69–70.
42. Starost MF, Benavides F, Conti CJ: A variant of pulmonary alveolar microlithiasis in nackt mice. Vet Pathol 2002;39(3):390–392.

Asthma

53 Epidemiology of Asthma

M. Innes Asher, MD • Cameron Grant, FRACP

Studies of the epidemiology of asthma have burgeoned in the past two decades. This reflects worldwide concern that asthma is increasing in prevalence and is an important cause of morbidity not only in developed countries, but also in developing countries.[1] The hope of finding factors influencing asthma in populations that are amenable to interventions has not yet been fulfilled. This chapter gives an overview of the key advances in the epidemiologic knowledge that have public health and clinical relevance.

DEFINITION AND MEASUREMENT IN EPIDEMIOLOGIC STUDIES

When a child presents to a clinician, the diagnosis of asthma is made in clinical practice by characteristic findings on history of episodic wheeze, cough, or breathlessness, and usually a normal physical examination in the interval phase. Wheeze is the most frequent symptom of the variable airway obstruction that occurs in asthma. Clinical definitions are described in all pediatric asthma guidelines. For example, the British guidelines[2] and Global Initiative for Asthma (GINA) guidelines.[3] These guidelines emphasize the exclusion of other conditions causing wheeze, cough, or breathlessness, especially in the very young child. There are, however, difficulties in defining and measuring asthma, because children most commonly have intermittent symptoms.

Epidemiologic studies investigate populations rather than individuals, and thus the methods of assessment need to be appropriate for this task. Measurements are made in individuals from which the presence or absence of asthma is determined, and thus the population prevalence or incidence is estimated, sometimes with characterization by severity or some other parameter. Where comparisons are made between populations, and within populations at different points in time, it is vital that the same standardized methods are used, so that there can be confidence in the estimates obtained.

The most common approach in epidemiologic studies is the use of written questionnaires completed by the parent for younger age groups and self-reported by adolescents. The latter may report a higher rate of symptoms than reported by the parent for the same adolescents.[4] This may be due to greater awareness in the adolescent of milder symptoms, or symptoms occurring when the parent is not present. An asthma symptoms video questionnaire was developed in 1992 in response to possible translation problems with written questionnaires used between populations who speak different languages, some of whom have no word for "wheeze." The video shows scenes of young people with asthma, thereby avoiding the need to describe symptoms verbally. The validity of the video has been investigated by comparison with bronchial hyperresponsiveness (BHR)[5–9] and shows a close relationship. Its relationship to the written questionnaire is close between populations,[10] but its relationship within individuals is not clear-cut.[7,11,12]

Questions about more recent symptoms (in the past 12 months) are more reliable than questions about symptoms in the past, because they reduce errors of recall. The most commonly used standard question is "Have you (has your child) had wheezing or whistling in the chest in the past 12 months?" Parental report of wheeze over the past 12 months has been shown to have a sensitivity of 0.81 and a specificity of 0.85 for physician diagnosis of childhood asthma.[13] Provided that the information has been collected in a standardized manner, any information biases are expected to be in both directions, thus enabling reliable comparisons between populations.[14]

In view of some of the potential limitations of questionnaires, there has been a search for an objective "asthma test" from which the diagnosis can be made with certainty. In the late 1970s a test of nonspecific airway hyperresponsiveness (AHR) or BHR was suggested as an objective test for diagnosing asthma and assessing its severity.[15,16] AHR is measured using a nonspecific inhaled challenge such as methacholine, histamine or hypertonic saline challenge, or a standardized exercise test.[17] Its usefulness in children is limited, because the test cannot be reliably performed in epidemiologic studies in the field with children younger than 6 years.

The initial inclusion of BHR as a diagnostic test for asthma was based on subjects who were attending hospital clinics, and were not representative of the community at large. In 1990 Pattemore and colleagues reported a study of an unbiased community sample in which they found that the level of BHR was a poorer predictor of doctor diagnosis of asthma than responses to the question "Has your child had wheezing in the past 12 months?" on written questionnaires.[18] Although there was a trend for greater BHR among children with more severe symptoms, the confidence intervals showed a large overlap between groups. Similar observations have been made in subsequent population-based studies. Thus, AHR, while related to asthma, is not equivalent to asthma.

STUDY DESIGNS

Several basic designs are commonly used in studies of asthma epidemiology. The randomized trial has been rarely used. Care must be taken in the interpretation of study findings because of the many factors that may influence asthma.[14] Cross-sectional studies are most suitable for estimating the prevalence of asthma symptoms, diagnosis, and severity, relating these to other measured factors and generating hypotheses. Most such studies have been within populations, but in 1985 the first study between centers in different countries was completed.[19] This was followed by several other comparisons between populations, and then in 1992 the International Study of Asthma and Allergies (ISAAC) was established, a multiphase cross-sectional study that became the largest epidemiologic study of asthma in children ever undertaken.[20] ISAAC uses simple standardized methodology with written and video questionnaires about asthma symptoms. In Phase One of ISAAC, 156 centers in 56 countries participated.[10] ISAAC Phase One used a conventional cross-sectional study design and has been followed by Phase Two, which uses more intensive standardized modules[21] to make comparisons between populations (centers) using objective measures of disease, environmental exposures, lifestyle, and clinical management. Populations that are potentially informative were chosen, such as those with contrasting prevalence of disease, environmental exposures, management, or genetic characteristics.[22] The sample sizes for ISAAC Phase Two are smaller than those in Phase One, reflecting the more intensive nature of the studies, and the age group (9–10 years) is more appropriate for procedures requiring cooperation of subjects.

Ecologic studies can be used to compare cross-sectional population data with environmental data, but they have recognized limitations compared with individual level studies.[23,24] In particular, the estimated ecologic effect may not reflect the biologic effect at the individual level. However, ecologic analyses are appropriate for attempting to explain why prevalence varies between populations and for putting the results of individual level epidemiologic studies within populations in context.[25] Ecologic studies have therefore been used by ISAAC to identify associations that may be worthy of further investigation.

Longitudinal studies (cohort studies) involve repeated observation of participants over time, and may also include a series of cross-sectional measurements. Studies measuring the incidence of asthma (number of new cases per year) involve long periods of time and especially large resources.

Case-control studies identify children with asthma and a control group of children without asthma, followed by comparison of exposure of cases and controls to factors of interest such as environmental tobacco smoke.

VARIATION IN THE PREVALENCE OF ASTHMA IN DIFFERENT LOCATIONS

VARIATION BETWEEN COUNTRIES

Until the mid-1980s most studies of asthma had been undertaken within developed countries whose populations originated from the British Isles, and thus the global distribution of asthma was largely unknown. From the mid-1980s to the mid-1990s there were a few studies of asthma in children between regions of the world.[19,26–33] ISAAC developed a standardized and coordinated approach with simple methodology that enabled the collection of comparable data from children throughout the world, including non–English language populations, and countries in the developing world.[34–38]

ISAAC Phase One collected information concerning symptoms of asthma on more than 700,000 children (6–7 years) and adolescents (13–14 years) in 156 centers located in 56 countries around the world.[34,39] Wide variation in the prevalence of asthma was found around the world with up to 15-fold differences between countries (Figs. 53-1 and 53-2). Although countries with English as the main language predominated among those with the highest prevalence, high prevalences were also found in some Latin American centers. An analysis of ISAAC data for the Latin America region showed that large differences in prevalence existed for centers in this developing region and that in some cases prevalence was as high as that experienced in centers in industrialized countries.[40] The lowest prevalences, less than 5%, were found mainly in Asia and in Eastern and Southern Europe. Some centers with people of similar ancestry had different prevalences, for example, Guangzhou and Hong Kong in China, Portugal and Brazil, and Spain and Spanish-speaking Latin America. The size and location of these differences suggests that environmental factors are the most likely explanation for the global variations. However, environmental factors that are known to be important in some individuals who have established asthma, such as outdoor air pollution, house dust mite (HDM), and tobacco exposure, do not seem likely to be the explanation for this worldwide pattern.

There were large international variations in the prevalence of more clinically important symptoms—frequent, sleep-disturbing, or speech-limiting attacks of wheeze that are measures of severity (Fig. 53-3). The proportion of wheezy children with severe asthma symptoms changed little with increasing prevalence of wheeze. Thus, the high prevalences of asthma symptoms found in some centers are not explained by excessive inclusion of children with mild wheeze.

DIFFERENCES BETWEEN RURAL AND URBAN SETTINGS

Comparisons between urban and rural areas in the same country, with most reports coming from Africa, have shown consistent differences, with asthma prevalence being higher in the urban locations. For example, in Ghanaian children, exercise-induced bronchospasm was found more commonly in urban rich than in urban poor or rural children.[41] In Zimbabwean children, urban living and higher material standards were associated with higher prevalence of reversible airways obstruction.[42] In Kenyan children, exercise-induced bronchospasm and symptoms of asthma were found more commonly in urban than rural children.[43,44] Wheeze and asthma are especially rare in rural subsistence areas in Ethiopia.[45] The investigators in these studies suggest that wealth, lifestyle, housing, and urban environmental exposures may contribute to increasing asthma prevalences. Subsequent studies of the effect of the farming environment on the occurrence of asthma, especially in European settings, suggest that the potentially protective effect of microbial exposure may be a factor that contains asthma prevalences to low levels in rural environments (see later section on Microbial Exposure).

CHANGES WITH MIGRATION

Studies of migration have provided further evidence of powerful environmental influences on the occurrence of asthma, demonstrating an increase in prevalence when children migrate from low- to high-prevalence areas. In 1975 to 1976, the first of these studies, Tokelauan children were observed in two environments. Asthma was more than twice as common among Tokelauan children in New Zealand than in Tokelau. There was no significant difference in the prevalence of asthma between those born in New Zealand and those born in Tokelau.[46] Among Asian immigrants from Pakistan, India, and East Africa in Blackburn, United Kingdom, there was an increasing rate of asthma symptoms with increasing duration of stay in the United Kingdom.[47] In Australia the prevalence of asthma has been studied in Asian immigrants of Chinese origin in Melbourne. The prevalence of wheeze was higher in Australian-born Asians and non-Asians than in Asian immigrants. The prevalence of asthma was also strongly associated with length of stay in Australia.[28] In the ISAAC Australia study, asthma prevalence was higher among Australian-born children than among those born elsewhere.[48] In teenagers in Melbourne, Australia, there was an effect of length of residence on the prevalence of symptoms in subjects born outside Australia and now living in Melbourne.[49]

IS THE PREVALENCE OF ASTHMA INCREASING?

Many studies show that asthma prevalence increased during the 1990s in Great Britain,[50–54] Australia,[55,56] New Zealand,[57,58] and Japan.[59] These large increases in prevalence over short periods of time cannot be explained by any genetic variation, and therefore are most likely to be due to environmental factors. These time trend studies have been undertaken in only a limited number of countries, and do not necessarily reflect the situation in other countries and regions.

ISAAC Phase Three has undertaken an extensive study of time trends in asthma prevalence in over 100 centers in over 50 countries after a period of at least 5 years.[60] The first ISAAC time trends report from Münster, Germany, showed an increase in asthma symptoms in two age groups of children from 1994–1995 to 1999–2000.[61,62] However in the United Kingdom[63] and

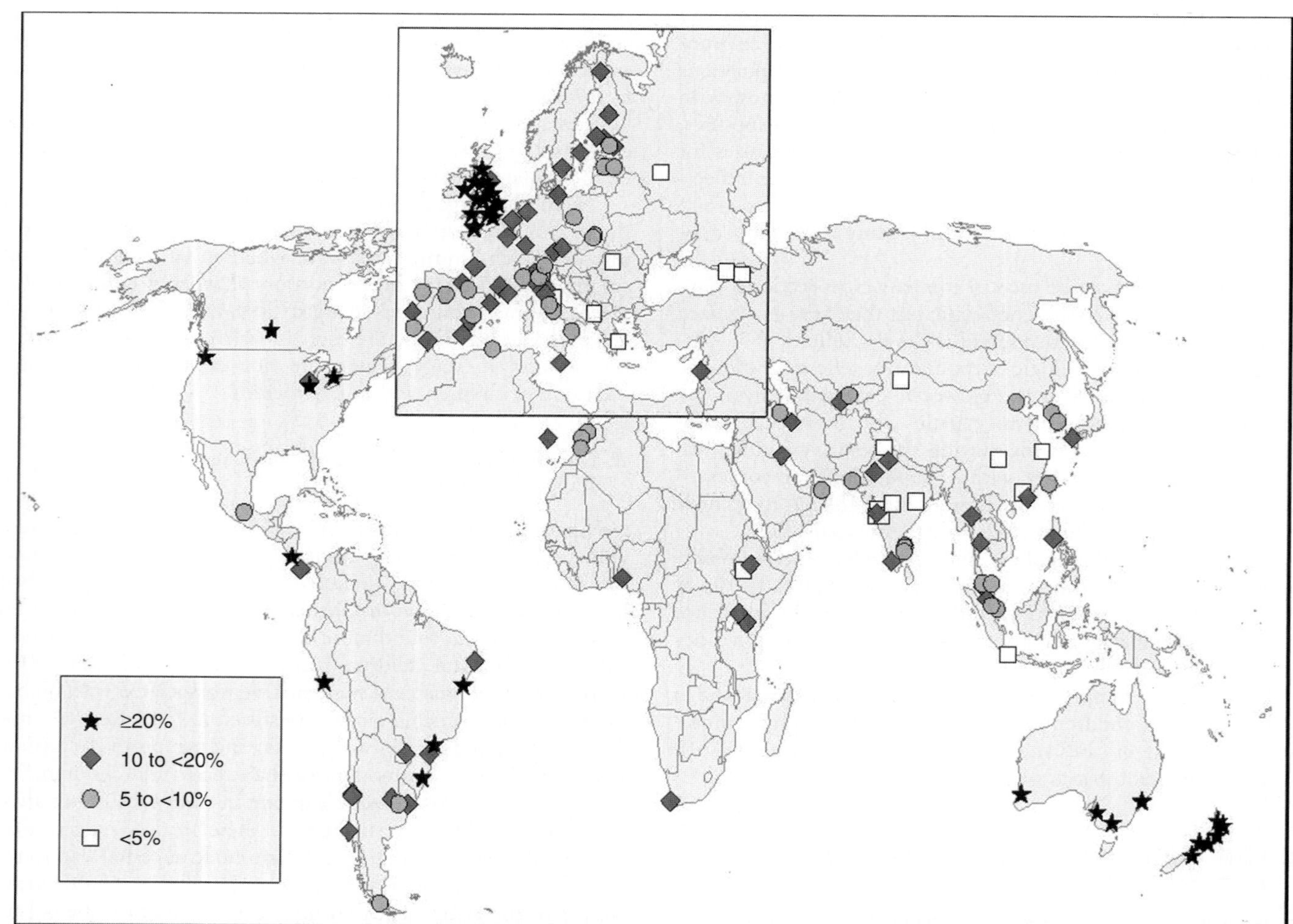

FIGURE 53-1. World map for the 13- to 14-year-old age group, showing the percentage of children who answered yes to the written question "Have you had wheezing or whistling in the chest in the past 12 months?" Each point represents the prevalence for one collaborating center, with distinct symbols used for different prevalence ranges. (From ISAAC Steering Committee: Worldwide variations in the prevalence of asthma symptoms. The International Study of Asthma and Allergies in Childhood (ISAAC). Eur Respir J 1998;12[2]:321.)

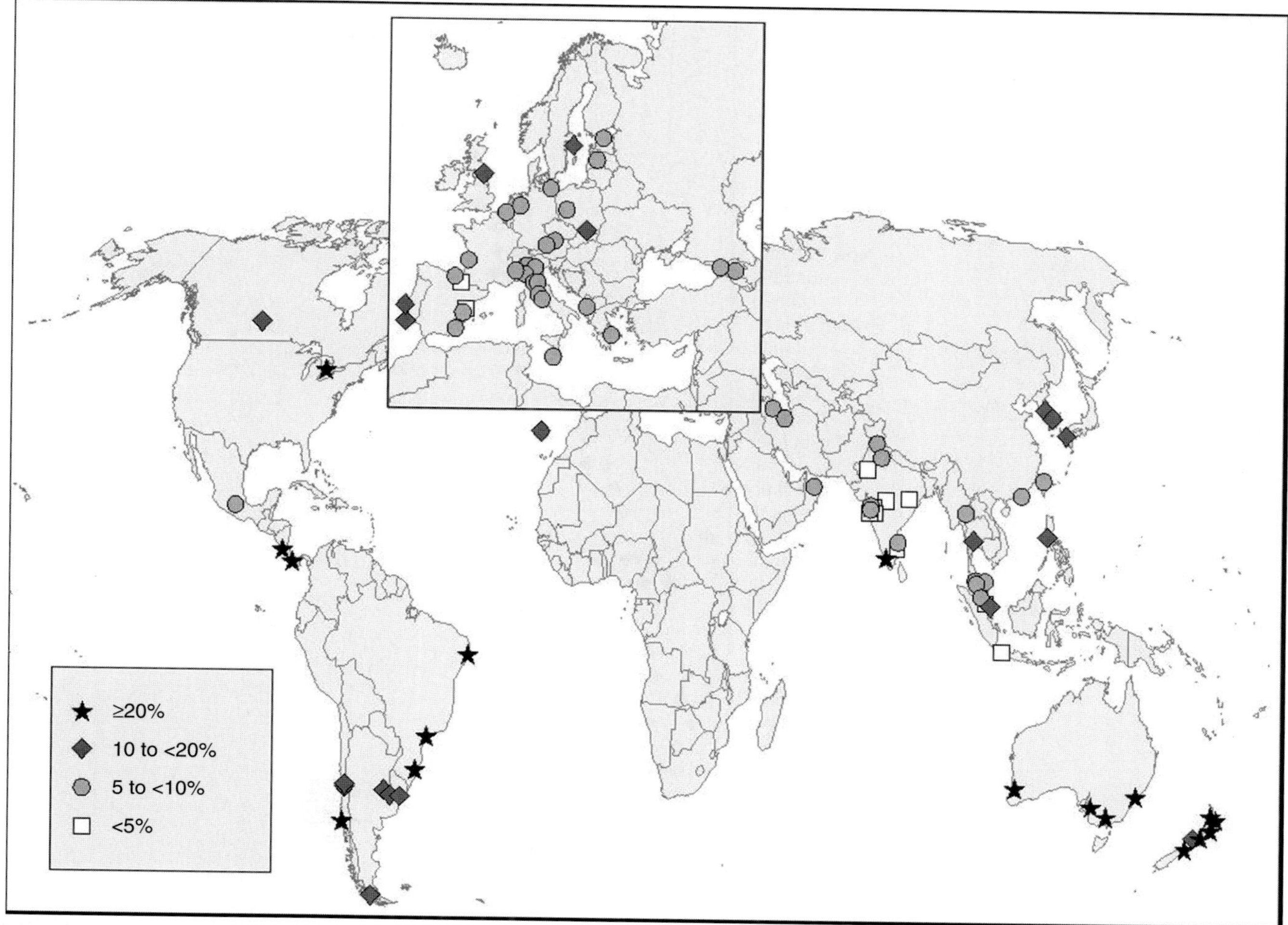

■ **FIGURE 53-2.** World map for the 6- to 7-year-old age group, showing the percentage of parents of children who answered yes to the written question "Has your child had wheezing or whistling in the chest in the past 12 months?" Each point represents the prevalence for one collaborating center, with distinct symbols used for different prevalence ranges. (From ISAAC Steering Committee: Worldwide variations in the prevalence of asthma symptoms. The International Study of Asthma and Allergies in Childhood (ISAAC). Eur Respir J 1998;12[2]:325.)

Australia[64] the time trends analyses have shown that the prevalence is now lower than it was 8 years previously. The full results of the worldwide ISAAC Phase Three are awaited with interest.

■ THE BURDEN OF ASTHMA

The numbers of children with asthma symptoms, especially severe symptoms, hospital admissions, and deaths from asthma, contribute to the personal, health care service, and economic burden of asthma. The costs of asthma to the children, their families, and society[65] are both medical and nonmedical, including days off work, premature disability, and death. ISAAC found that the prevalence of wheeze in the previous 12 months in centers studied ranged from 0.8% to 36.7%. Among 6- to 7-year-olds and 13- to 14-year-olds, the prevalence in the previous 12 months of four or more attacks of wheezing ranged from 0.1% to 10.2% and 0.3% to 12.8%; of wheeze-disturbing sleep from 0.2% to 10% and 0 to 5.9%; and of severe wheeze-limiting speech from 0.3% to 11.3% and 0.4% to 13.5%, respectively.[10]

The global burden of asthma has recently been estimated to include 300 million symptomatic people.[66] Asthma is emerging as an important public health problem in developing countries, albeit secondary in importance to infectious diseases such as malaria, pneumonia, and tuberculosis (TB). If the low prevalence in the most populous countries rose to the higher levels in countries like New Zealand, there would be tens of millions more people with asthma, a huge health burden for the world.

■ HOSPITALIZATION WITH ASTHMA

Admission to hospital with asthma is commonly used as a measure of asthma severity and morbidity. While hospital admissions clearly have an impact on health services, children, and their families, how should they be interpreted?

■ LIMITATIONS IN ESTIMATES OF ASTHMA HOSPITALIZATIONS AS A MEASURE OF ASTHMA MORBIDITY

Asthma is one of the frequent reasons for children requiring inpatient care in the developed world. Asthma hospital admission rates vary considerably between hospitals within the same city, regionally within a country, and between neighboring countries.[67–69] Although some of this variability is due to differences

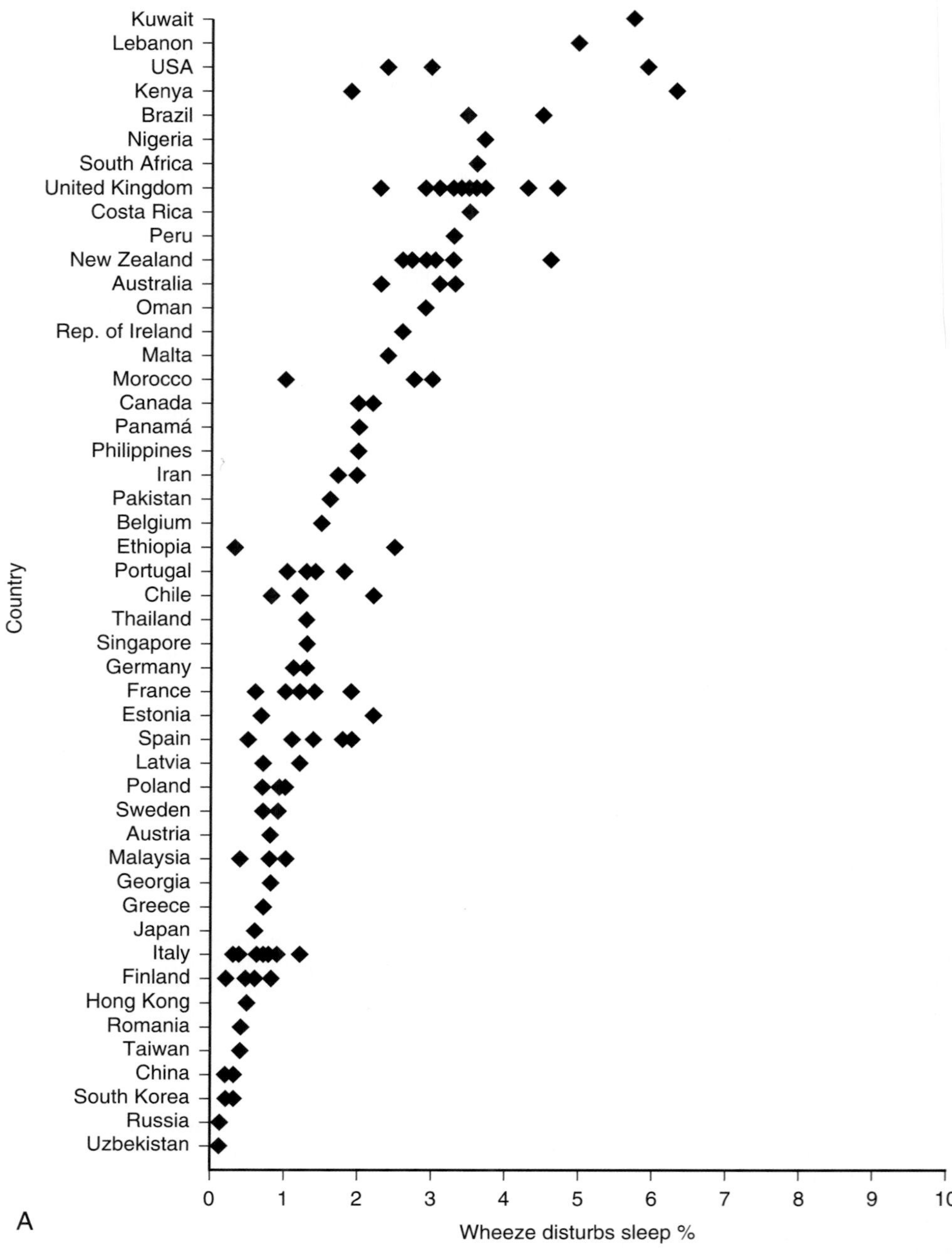

■ **FIGURE 53-3.** Ranking of the participating countries for the percentage who answered positively to the question "In the past 12 months, how often, on average, has your (child's) sleep been disturbed due to wheezing: one or more nights per week?" for the 13- to 14-year-olds (**A**) and the 6- to 7-year-olds (**B**). From ISAAC Steering Committee: Worldwide variations in the prevalence of asthma symptoms. The International Study of Asthma and Allergies in Childhood (ISAAC). Eur Respir J 1998;12[2]:322.)

in disease prevalence and severity, other factors including variability in primary care, admitting practices, and the organization of acute inpatient facilities also contribute.

■ TRENDS OVER TIME IN ASTHMA HOSPITALIZATIONS

Asthma hospital admission rates increased dramatically from the middle to late 1960s through the 1980s. These increases were evident in several countries, including Australia, Canada, England and Wales, New Zealand, and the United States.[70,71] In the United States, the hospitalization rate continued to increase until the mid-1990s.[72] The size of the increase was significant, ranging from a threefold increase in the United States to a tenfold increase in New Zealand over an approximately 15-year time period.[71] In New Zealand, admission rates increased in both the 0- to 4-year-old and 5- to 14-year-old age groups.[71] In England, Wales, and the United States, the largest increase in hospitalization rates occurred in children younger than 5 years.[73,74]

Potential explanations for these trends have been examined in several countries. An increase in the number of children hospitalized and, to a lesser extent, the number of hospitalizations per child contributed to the increase in asthma hospitalization rates in England and Wales and New Zealand from the 1960s to the 1980s.[75,76] Neither diagnostic transfer nor an increase in admissions for less severe asthma were contributory.[71,75,77]

Increase in both prevalence and severity of asthma were thought to be the main contributing factors to the increase in

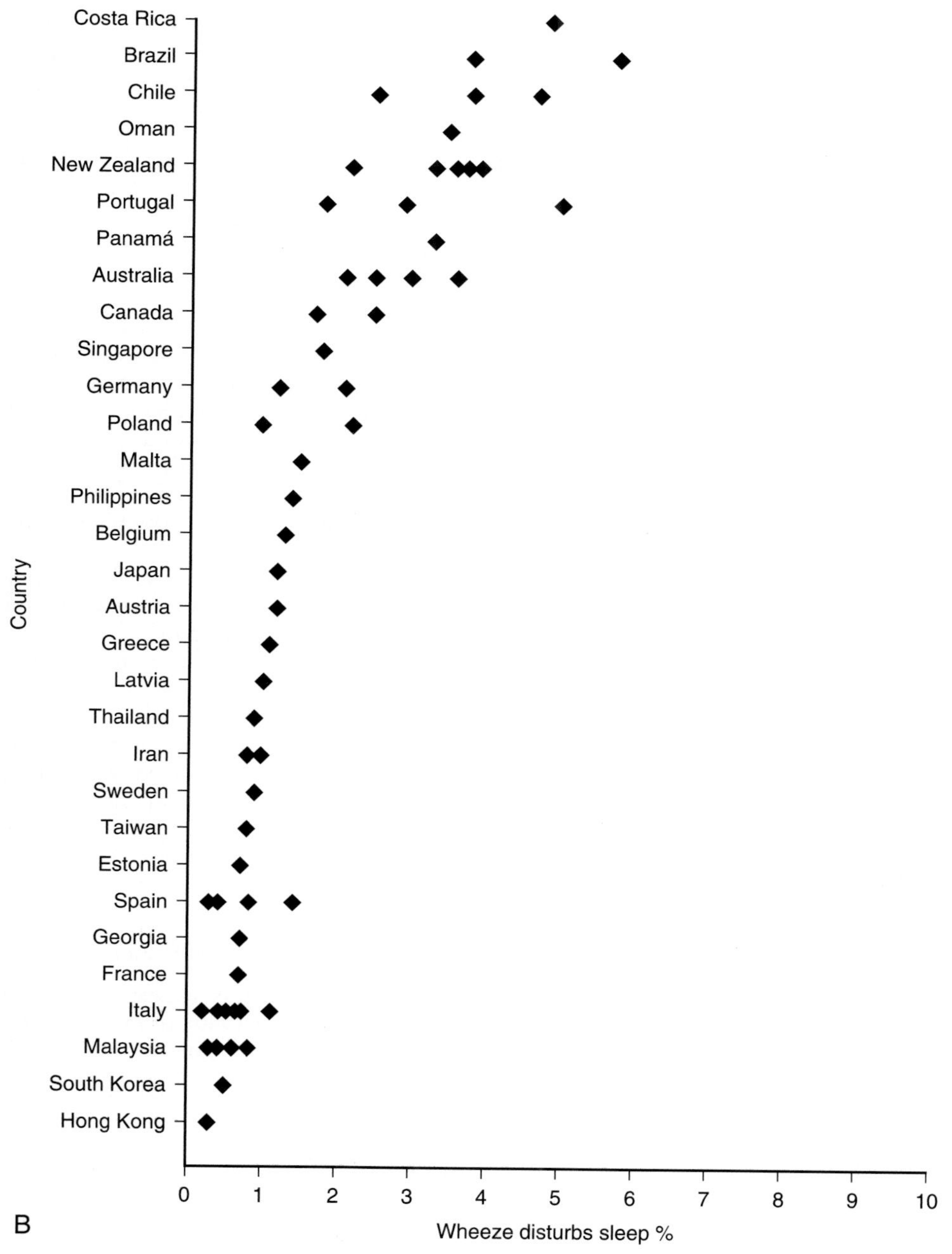

■ **FIGURE 53-3, cont'd**

hospitalization rates.[51,77] Evidence of an increase in severity includes an increase in the proportion of patients hospitalized with asthma who then required intubation.[77] The increase in hospital admission rates in New Zealand was substantially greater than the twofold increase in asthma prevalence over this time period.[71]

Pediatric asthma hospital admission rates stabilized or decreased during the 1990s in several countries, including England, Wales, New Zealand, and the United States.[72,73,78–81] In England, the decrease in number of hospital admissions for wheeze or asthma in children in 2000 to 2001 compared with 1993 to 1994 was approximately 44% for children 0 to 4 years old and 30% for children 5 to 14 years old.[78] The decreases that occurred in New Zealand were thought unlikely to be due to a single cause. Reduced use of fenoterol, a potent and relatively nonselective β_2 agonist, increased use of inhaled corticosteroids, improved asthma education, and greater use of asthma management plans were all considered likely contributors.[80]

CONTEXT OF ASTHMA ADMISSIONS

Primary Care

Asthma hospitalizations are sensitive to the quality of primary and ambulatory care. In the United States, regional differences in the frequency of use of inhaled preventive therapy and appropriate acute therapy are associated with regional differences in hospitalization rates. In addition, receipt of ambulatory care of lower quality is associated with more severe asthma on hospital admission.[82]

Poverty

Living in poverty remains one of the major factors that increase the likelihood of a child being hospitalized with asthma. The adverse effects of poverty are multiple. Poor and ethnic minority children with asthma receive primary care that is of poorer quality, with less continuity.[83,84] The adverse indoor environment to which these children are exposed also increases the likelihood that their asthma will be symptomatic.[85]

Season

Asthma hospitalization rates vary with season. Autumn is the peak season in both hemispheres.[86–88] In England and Wales, a second asthma hospitalization peak in spring is described for children 5 to 14 years of age.[88]

RISK FACTORS FOR HOSPITALIZATION WITH ASTHMA

AGE AND GENDER

The largest proportion of hospital admissions for asthma occur in earlier childhood. An earlier age of onset of symptoms is associated with an increased risk for hospitalization.[89] Gender differences in asthma hospitalization rates vary with age. In the 5- to 14-year-old age group, boys are more likely to be hospitalized with asthma than girls, and in the 15- to 24-year-old age group, girls are twice as likely to be hospitalized with asthma as boys.[74]

ETHNICITY

Asthma hospital admission rates vary with ethnicity. In the United States, the hospitalization rate for African American children is more than three times greater than for white children. A substantial proportion of this difference is attributable to poverty.[90] The decrease in hospitalization rate in the United States from 1995–1996 to 1998–1999 was more marked for African American than for white children.[72]

DISEASE SEVERITY

Children with more severe asthma are at increased risk for hospital admission. This has been demonstrated using a variety of measures of disease severity, including frequency of respiratory symptoms, medication use, lung function, and AHR. In a child with asthma, the presence of atopy increases the risk for hospitalization.[89]

RISK FACTORS FOR ADMISSION TO INTENSIVE CARE

Among children hospitalized with asthma, risk factors for admission to an intensive care unit include multiple emergency department visits in the preceding 12 months, longer duration of symptoms prior to admission, hypoxia on presentation, and an elevated serum immunoglobulin E (IgE).[91]

ASTHMA MORTALITY

Asthma is an infrequent cause of death during childhood. For example, the death rate from asthma in the United States in 2000 for children 5 to 14 years old was 0.3 per 100,000. Although this was the sixth most frequent cause, it accounted for less than 2% of total deaths in this age group. The five leading causes—accidents, malignant neoplasms, homicide, major cardiovascular disease, and suicide—together result in an annual death rate of 12.7 per 100,000. In this same age group in the United States, however, asthma is a more frequent cause of death than pneumonia, other diseases of the respiratory system, or septicemia.[92]

LIMITATIONS IN ESTIMATES OF ASTHMA MORTALITY

The case fatality rate from asthma among the population of children with asthma is not easy to determine. This is because accurate determination of the denominator is necessary. This depends on prevalence studies, which may not have been done for the population of interest. The large world coverage of ISAAC using standard methodology has provided the opportunity for comparable denominators in the calculations. However, a standardized international approach to case definitions of the deaths has been difficult to achieve.

Although changes in asthma mortality rates have been reported in all ages, epidemiologic studies have focused on the 5- to 34-year-old age group, where the diagnosis of asthma, as distinct from other chronic respiratory diseases, is more readily made.[79]

Implementation of revisions of the International Classification of Diseases has made the interpretation of temporal trends more difficult, although this effect has been less marked for children than for adults. For example, in the United States, introduction of the 10th revision in 1998 was estimated to have accounted for approximately 25% of the decrease in asthma deaths that occurred from 1998 to 1999.[92]

TRENDS OVER TIME IN ASTHMA MORTALITY

Data from Australia, England and Wales, New Zealand, and the United States show that from 1910 to 1940, asthma mortality rates were low (less than 1 per 100,000 in persons 5 to 34 years of age) and relatively stable. Death rates increased gradually in Australia and New Zealand in the 1950s.[93]

ASTHMA EPIDEMICS

In the 1960s, asthma mortality rates increased two- to tenfold within a 2- to 5-year period in Australia, England and Wales, New Zealand, Norway, and Scotland, but no increase was observed in Canada, Denmark, Germany, or the United States. Peak mortality rates during these epidemics were from 2 to 3 per 100,000 persons 5 to 34 years of age, lasting 10 to 15 years in affected countries.[93] An increase in the case fatality rate was the most likely explanation for the epidemic of deaths among asthmatics. The use of isoprenaline forte inhalers was a major, but probably not the only, causal factor.[93]

A further epidemic of asthma deaths occurred in New Zealand from 1976 to 1989. During this period, the asthma mortality rate in New Zealand was the highest in the world, peaking in 1979 at 4.1 per 100,000 persons 5 to 34 years of age.[94,95] An increased case fatality rate was again thought to be the most important causal factor.[96] The use of the potent and less selective β_2 agonist fenoterol was considered the major factor. Asthma mortality rates fell rapidly in New Zealand following warnings and subsequent restrictions of the sale of fenoterol.[97]

INCREASE IN ENDEMIC ASTHMA MORTALITY DURING THE 1970S AND 1980S

During these decades there was a gradual increase in asthma mortality rates in many countries, including those that were affected by the earlier epidemics. These increases were substantial, with a median increase in mortality of 45% in 15 developed countries from 1975–1977 to 1985–1987.[93] The increases occurred in a wide range of countries with differing lifestyles, and were variable in countries with similar lifestyles. A wide range of age groups were affected. For example, in the United States, from 1980 to 1993, increases were evident in the 0- to 4-, 5- to 14-, and 15- to 24-year-old age groups.[98]

Unlike the epidemics of the 1960s and 1970s, the increase in endemic asthma mortality rates did not appear to be due to a single predominant factor and were not due to an increased case fatality rate. Mortality, hospitalization, and incidence rates all increased over this same time period.[93]

Although the trend across developed countries for asthma mortality to increase was consistent, there was considerable variability between countries in pediatric asthma mortality rates. For example, from 1981 to 1990, in the 5- to 14-year-old age group, mortality rates ranged from 0.38 per 100,000 per year in Sweden to 1.75 per 100,000 per year in New Zealand.[98] Mortality rates were higher in countries with higher proportions of 12-year-old children who had a history of asthma.

DECREASE IN ASTHMA MORTALITY SINCE THE 1990S

Since the late 1980s in New Zealand, Australia, Canada, England and Wales, and West Germany, and since the mid-1990s in the United States, asthma mortality rates have decreased in children and adults.[72,92,93,99,100]

Over the same time period as this decrease in asthma mortality, asthma prevalence and severity has increased. This suggests that improved management of asthma has contributed to the reduced mortality. In Australia, Israel, and the United States, the development of consensus guidelines for the diagnosis and management of asthma and increased sales of inhaled corticosteroids were thought to be important contributors.[92,101,102] The association between increased use of inhaled corticosteroids and decreased risk for fatal or near-fatal asthma was demonstrated in a Canadian case-control study of children and adults with at least one hospitalization for asthma in the preceding 2 years.[103]

RISK FACTORS FOR FATAL ASTHMA IN CHILDREN

In response to the increase in asthma mortality in many countries during the 1970s and 1980s, studies sought to determine the epidemiologic features of fatal asthma in children. Two patterns have been described. The most frequent is one of delayed presentation in someone known to have severe asthma, but in whom the severity of the fatal attack is underestimated or escalation in treatment is delayed. The alternative pattern is rapid unexpected deterioration and death. Such precipitous deaths have been reported to occur in children with mild asthma.[104,105] Sensitization to a specific aeroallergen accounts for some of the seasonal and regional clusters of sudden, life-threatening asthma.[106]

In the 5- to 34-year-old age group, asthma mortality is highest in summer, in contrast with the winter peak in older age groups. This seasonal mortality pattern is at variance with hospitalization rates, which in the 5- to 34-year-old age group are highest in early winter. These seasonal patterns have been demonstrated in England and Wales, France, New Zealand, and the United States.[86–88,93,107] In the United States, a disproportionate number of summer deaths in this age group occur out of hospital, implying either seasonally specific rapidly progressive asthma or acute asthma occurring in a time or place with reduced hospital access.[87]

RISK FACTORS FOR FATAL ASTHMA IN A CHILD KNOWN TO HAVE SEVERE ASTHMA

Age

Within pediatric and adolescent age groups, those younger than 10 years are at lower risk and those 15 to 24 years of age at higher risk for death from asthma.[108] The increased risk for fatal asthma in adolescent age groups is thought to be due to poor compliance, impaired recognition of disease severity, and rejection of parental supervision of treatment.

Gender

Male gender is associated with a 1.5-fold increased risk for fatal asthma.[98] The associations between gender and fatal asthma appear to vary with age. In Australia, males predominate in asthma fatalities in those younger than 15 years and females in later adolescence and early adulthood.[109]

Disease Severity

Children with more severe asthma are at increased risk for death. Cohort studies of children with a near-fatal asthma episode have demonstrated that such children are at increased risk for subsequent fatal episodes. When compared with children seen in the same asthma clinic who did not have a life-threatening episode, those with a life-threatening episode had a more than 1000-fold increased risk for a subsequent fatal episode.[110]

Psychological factors appear to make a significant contribution to the risk for death in children with severe asthma. A case-control study compared children hospitalized with severe asthma who died over the subsequent months to years with a control group of children with asthma of similar severity. Factors apparent during the hospital admission that were associated with an increased risk for subsequent fatal asthma included conflict about asthma management between parents and hospital staff, age-inappropriate self-care of asthma, depressive symptoms, and disregard of asthma symptoms.[111]

Poverty and Ethnicity

The risk for fatal asthma is greatest among children from the lowest socioeconomic households. In the United States, the increased risk for fatal asthma associated with poverty appears to be primarily an urban phenomenon, and among the urban poor, the increased risk affects African American children disproportionately.[112] African American ethnicity is associated with a four- to fivefold increased risk for fatal asthma. The size of the increased risk for both hospitalization and death from asthma associated with African American ethnicity is greater than the ethnic difference in prevalence.[72]

The increased risk for fatal asthma associated with African American ethnicity appears to be primarily due to poverty rather than being genetically determined. As for hospitalization, poverty mediates its adverse effect both through increased environment exposures and reduced access to optimal health care.[72,112]

Genetic Determinants on Mortality

Genetic polymorphisms have been described that are associated with variable responses to β_2-adrenergic agonists.[113] The RANTES (regulated upon activation normal T cell expressed and secreted) gene on chromosome 17q11.2-q12 produces chemotaxis and activation of several cell types involved in the asthmatic airway inflammatory response, including eosinophils, monocytes, basophils, and T cells. A polymorphism for this gene has been described that is present at increased frequency in Taiwanese children with near-fatal asthma compared to those with mild to moderate asthma and compared with Taiwanese nonasthmatic children.[114] The gene polymorphism was also more frequent in those with moderate compared with mild asthma. Its presence was associated with an increased eosinophil count and a higher degree of BHR. It is unclear how much polymorphisms like these, which affect the extent of response to drugs used in the treatment of acute asthma, contribute to childhood deaths.

GENETIC DETERMINANTS OF ASTHMA

The genetic contribution to asthma is large. Twin studies have estimated that genetic factors account for between 36% and 75% of the variance in risk of asthma between individuals.[115] There is a growing list of asthma susceptibility genes but limited data as yet on how or to what extent they determine the clinical presentation of asthma.[116] Several genetic locations have been linked to asthma and atopy.[117] Genetic locations associated with variance in response to bronchodilators have also been identified.[113]

The majority of children developing asthma during the first years of life are born into families without any manifestation of the atopic constitution. The majority of prospectively affected children will not be identified at birth by consideration of family history alone.[118] However, asthma does aggregate in families. The familial determinants are likely polygenic, with multiple factors then influencing phenotypic expression. For example, although total serum IgE levels are inherited and are strongly associated with the risk for developing asthma,[119] children with asthma have higher total IgE levels than would be predicted from the IgE levels of their parents. However, the relationship between IgE and asthma is not clear-cut (see later section on The Relationship between Asthma and Atopy).

Maternal influences on asthma appear to be stronger than paternal influences.[120] The risk for asthma is greater for a child whose mother has asthma compared with one whose father has asthma. Although potentially due to respondent bias (most caregiver interviews are with mothers, who are likely to be more familiar with their own past medical history that that of the child's father), it may also be due to the maternal immune influences on the development of the fetal immune system.

Maternal influences are likely to be via antigen exposure both directly across the placenta and via amniotic fluid. Antigen transfer across the placenta occurs mostly in complexes with immunoglobulin G (IgG) and therefore is thought to happen predominantly during the third trimester, when there is active IgG cross-placental transport. The presence of IgG antibodies to inhalant allergens in cord blood samples is independent of a maternal history of atopy.[121] However, the concentrations of food and inhalant allergen-specific IgG antibodies are higher in cord blood from infants of atopic compared with nonatopic mothers.[122] Antigens in amniotic fluid are swallowed by the fetus, with the relative maturity of the fetal gut immune system then enabling sensitization (antigen presenting cells are detectable within the fetal gut from as early as 11 to 12 weeks' gestation).[123] The major HDM antigen, Der p 1, is present in amniotic fluid from 16 to 17 weeks' gestation and in cord blood.[124] Amniotic fluid IgE concentrations are proportional to maternal serum IgE concentrations. Therefore, although IgE cannot cross the placenta, fetuses of mothers with high IgE concentrations will have greater IgE exposure in utero. Maternal IgG may also have a modulating effect on fetal immune responses. High maternal IgG antibody titers may suppress IgE responses in newborns.[124] Thus, high allergen exposure in the mother during pregnancy may have a protective effect against the development of allergy in the child. For example, there is an inverse relationship between cat IgE antibody concentrations at age 8 years and cat IgG antibodies concentrations at birth. Higher cord blood IgG antibody concentrations to aeroallegens are associated with fewer atopic symptoms at school age.[123]

THE RELATIONSHIP BETWEEN ASTHMA AND ATOPY

Atopy (from Greek "strangeness") is defined as "a personal, and/or familial tendency to produce IgE antibodies in response to ordinary exposure to allergens, usually proteins."[125] Asthma in children is commonly described as an allergic, IgE-mediated, atopic disease. The proposed process is that allergen exposure produces allergic sensitization and that continual exposure leads to clinical asthma through the development of airways inflammation, BHR, and reversible airflow obstruction. Various measures of atopy (positive skin test results, elevated serum IgE levels, parental history of asthma) are associated with an increased risk for developing asthma.[126] For example, in the Tucson Children's Respiratory Study (Arizona), when compared with children who had not wheezed, a larger proportion of children with persistent wheezing were more likely to have mothers with a history of asthma, elevated serum IgE levels at age 9 months, or positive skin test results for aeroallergens. Positive skin test results for aeroallergens were also associated with an increased risk for later onset wheezing.[126] Atopy causes an increased risk for persistence and severity of asthma, and this is discussed later in the section on The Natural History of Asthma.

However, atopy does not explain the many children with asthma who do not have an atopic constitution. Pearce and colleagues have challenged the closeness of the relationship between asthma and atopy.[127] The epidemiologic evidence suggests that only 50% of the adult population with asthma have IgE-mediated disease (allergies or asthma). Comparisons across populations or time periods show only a weak and inconsistent association between the prevalence of atopy and asthma. Nonallergic asthma may be a separate entity from allergic asthma, and a different set of preventive strategies may be required for this type of asthma. The etiology of and risk factors for non-IgE-mediated asthma therefore need to be explored further.[127] Comparatively little research has been done in this direction.

ISAAC confirmed a strong correlation between symptoms of asthma and allergic rhinoconjunctivitis, as well as atopic eczema, which is not surprising.[35] However, in this cross-sectional study most children had symptoms of only one condition, and fewer than 1 in 10 symptomatic children had symptoms of all three diseases. Some of this lack of concurrent symptoms may be explainable by the "allergic march," with eczema occurring in the youngest children, followed by asthma, and later by allergic rhinitis, but the lack of overlap even for "symptoms ever" is less than expected if the explanatory mechanism were the same for all three conditions. Thus, the relationship between atopy and asthma is important, but may have been overemphasized to the detriment of exploration of the nonallergic mechanisms of asthma.

The World Allergy Organization has articulated the distinction between allergic and nonallergic asthma in its recent recommendations on nomenclature.[128] In their summary and guideline on the prevention of allergy and allergic asthma, Johansson and Haahtela state that individuals with a family history of atopy have an increased risk for allergic sensitization, and that this represents a high risk for allergic asthma.[129] However, the distinction between allergic and nonallergic asthma may be difficult in clinical practice, especially since the measurement of total serum IgE and skin prick testing is not routine in many countries, and in much of the world it is unavailable to most of the population due to cost.

ENVIRONMENTAL FACTORS

Evidence from population studies over time, between countries and regions of the world, and of migrants suggests that variations in prevalences of asthma are too large to be explained by genetic variation, and are therefore likely to be due to environmental factors. But which are the important environmental factors? Do some protect against asthma starting up in the first place, and some increase risk? Finding factors that are the key to primary prevention of asthma in populations would give the maximum chance of reducing the population burden of asthma.

In a recent extensive review of this topic, Asher and Dagli presented an approach to seeking environmental factors that may prevent asthma.[130] One theoretically ideal outcome of research would be to find environmental factors that are sufficiently potent in "causing" asthma that their removal would eliminate asthma in those who already have it. It seems unlikely that one environmental factor could be the sole explanation for the observations. However, all the research to date has failed to identify any such factors. Therefore, the search must include the identification of factors that reduce the number of people with asthma in populations, and a less radical approach would be sensible. If environmental factors could be found for which a small change in relative risk (preventive or causative) applied to a large number of people could bring a large absolute benefit to the population, this would be worth having. Rose labeled this the prevention paradox: "a preventive measure that brings large benefits to the community but offers little to each participating individual."[131] "When many people receive a little benefit, the total benefit may be large."[131] It follows that if the benefit to the individual is small, we are looking for factors that can be translated into interventions that are not inconvenient or hazardous, but rather are safe, low cost, and easy to implement.

Using the vast worldwide ISAAC Phase One data, environmental factors that may contribute to the population prevalence of asthma have been explored using ecologic analyses to identify hypotheses that warrant further investigation. The Phase One symptom prevalence of asthma was examined with country level environmental data to identify possible risk factors. A weak positive relationship was found between gross national product (GNP) per capita and symptoms,[132] and this was adjusted for in all subsequent ecologic analyses. The ISAAC dietary analysis showed a consistent inverse relationship between symptoms and levels of intake of food of plant origin, suggesting a potential protective effect,[133] a new finding. The strongest relationship was for the consumption of calories from cereal and rice and country symptom prevalence of asthma. ISAAC found a weak negative association with TB notifications in the population.[134] Measles immunization and diphtheria, tetanus, and pertussis (DTP) vaccines were reassuringly slightly protective.[135] There were associations between indoor and outdoor climatic factors and symptoms of asthma.[136] There were no clear associations between variations in asthma prevalence and pollen exposure,[137] tobacco sales,[138] or antibiotic sales.[139] What have other studies found about these and other environmental factors?

DIET

It is not surprising that diet may be linked to asthma as it has been for many noncommunicable diseases. Over the past few decades, "westernization" has seen many countries moving away from the traditional diet of locally grown foods to a more Western diet. Rapid changes have occurred in association with westernization, including changes to the production and availability of food, changing food preferences, increased supply of processed foods for consumption, as well as supplies for food aid, use of fertilizers and pesticides, reduced land availability, increased prices of staple foods, urbanization, migration, economic factors, and market fluctuations. Most of the dietary studies to date have a cross-sectional design, and therefore they are more suited for raising questions and hypotheses than in proving causative relationships. The ISAAC ecologic diet analyses support the earlier migration studies showing that when a population adopts a new lifestyle, symptoms prevalence increases. This needs fuller exploration.

FISH

The low prevalence of asthma among populations with high fish intake[46] has suggested that there may be a protective factor. Oily fish is rich in omega-3 fatty acids, which potentially reduce the synthesis of proinflammatory cytokines, and it is speculated that they could either prevent the development of asthma or reduce its severity by altering airway inflammation and AHR. Regular consumption of fresh, oily fish was observed to be associated with reduced risk of asthma symptoms in Australian children.[140] Clinical trials of fish oil or omega-3 and omega-6 fatty acid supplements have shown no effect,[141–143] an increase in fatty acid levels,[144,145] a positive effect on forced expiratory volume in 1 second (FEV_1),[146] a decrease in AHR,[145] and a reduction in the occurrence of cough in atopic children at 3 years and of wheeze at 18 months but not 3 years.[147] Further studies of the long-term effectiveness of these supplements are awaited with interest.

VEGETABLES, FRUIT, AND ANTIOXIDANTS

Several cross-sectional studies suggest that fresh vegetables and fruit may be protective against the development of asthma in children, possibly through the antioxidant properties of vitamins

A, C, E, and β-carotene.[147–149] Ecologic analysis of ISAAC Phase One data found an inverse association between asthma symptoms and food of plant origin.[133] The possible protective value of antioxidants is supported by an ecologic study of exposure to paracetamol (which depletes the antioxidant glutathione), which was associated with an increase of asthma symptoms.[150] In a large cross-sectional study of youth (NHANES III), serum vitamin C and β-carotene but not vitamin E were inversely associated with asthma.[151] Interventions with antioxidants have not been shown to be effective, and further studies are needed in this area. Other potential constituents of fresh fruit and vegetables that may be protective also need consideration.

CEREALS AND RICE

Many of the protective compounds in whole grains (wheat, rice, and corn) are also found in fruit and vegetables, but some plant compounds are more concentrated in whole grains. The ISAAC analysis showed a consistent, negative association between calories from cereal, rice, and protein from cereal and nuts, and symptoms. It was speculated that if the daily per capita amount of calories from cereal and rice consumed were to be increased by 10% of total energy consumption, it may be possible to achieve a 3.2% decrease in the prevalence of current wheeze, and a 0.4% decrease in severe wheeze.[133]

POLYUNSATURATED FAT

As intake of saturated fats and cholesterol is reduced in Western societies, more polyunsaturated fatty acid (PUFA) is consumed. Increased consumption of linoleic acid, found in PUFA, is thought to be linked to asthma,[152] and this was supported by observations in a cross-sectional study in Germany.[153] However, PUFA derived from vegetables in the ISAAC analysis was associated with decreased symptom prevalence, supporting the hypothesis that it is industrially derived PUFA that is responsible, rather than naturally derived PUFA from vegetables.

TRANS FATTY ACIDS

Trans fatty acids are found in industrially hydrogenated fats used in spreads and are also found in dairy products and in the fat of ruminant animals. These *trans* fatty acids may influence the desaturation and chain elongation of n-6 and n-3 fatty acids into precursors of inflammatory mediators, such as leukotrienes. A European ISAAC investigation found a significantly positive association between *trans* fatty acids and the prevalence of childhood asthma, and the hypothesis that they may play a part in the development of childhood asthma seems worth pursuing.[154]

CHEMICALS AND TRACE ELEMENTS

Several studies have investigated the relationship between sodium intake and asthma, demonstrating a small adverse effect of increased sodium intake on bronchial reactivity, but no significant effect on clinical symptoms of asthma.[143] Selenium is an essential component of the antioxidant enzyme glutathione peroxidase, but examination of a possible relationship between low selenium levels and asthma has yielded inconsistent results, and no beneficial effect of selenium supplementation on asthma has been shown.[143] Although intravenous magnesium may have a minimal role in the treatment of acute severe asthma by enhancing bronchial smooth muscle relaxation, magnesium deficiency has not been shown in asthma patients.[143]

FOOD PRESERVATIVES AND ADDITIVES

The changes of dietary habits with migration include the addition of preservatives, traces of pesticides, and food additives such as metabisulphates, benzoate, and tartrazine, which have also been implicated in asthma exacerbations.[155] There have been no studies of the separate effect of food preservatives and additives on asthma and allergy.

BREASTFEEDING

Patterns of breastfeeding have changed in the past few decades, particularly in affluent countries, where the rates became particularly low three to four decades ago, but have gradually increased since.[156] The relationship between breastfeeding and the development of asthma is unclear because of the conflicting outcomes of longitudinal studies. These show either no beneficial effect,[157–160] a beneficial effect,[161–163] or even an increased risk for asthma in those breastfed.[164] The lack of consistency of research findings makes it difficult to make any recommendations. Controversy about the interpretation of the evidence has recently been appraised.[165,166] However, breastfeeding has other child health benefits, and thus its encouragement until 4 to 6 months of age is recommended.

Would some high-risk infants benefit from modulation of maternal diet during lactation? A few studies indicate that the preventive effect of breastfeeding on development of "atopic eczema" may be enhanced by maternal avoidance of potential food allergens (milk, egg, fish) during the lactation period, but other studies do not confirm this finding.[157,167,168] The effects on the infant of other variations in the diet of a breastfeeding mother have not been studied, such as increased antioxidant intake. Currently, no special diet for the lactating mother is recommended.[129]

MATERNAL DIET IN PREGNANCY

The intrauterine environment is thought to play an important part in the development of chronic disease in later life,[169] although there is no documented direct effect of maternal diet during pregnancy on asthma.[157] Diet during pregnancy could potentially influence asthma protectively (e.g., through antioxidant intake) or alternatively adversely, with antigens passing through the placenta and amniotic fluid leading to programming of the developing immune system by stimulating T cells and cytokines. No advantages were found in a randomized controlled trial eliminating cow's milk and eggs in the last trimester.[170,171]

GROWTH

In a prospective British cohort, low birth weight was found to be a risk factor for early childhood wheezing, independent of maternal smoking.[160] This may be mediated through intrauterine undernutrition causing small airways. In a study from Israel, 17-year-olds had a higher risk for asthma if they had birth weights less than 2500 g. This may be mediated through lung function.[172] The relationship between low birth weight and asthma could be explored further, especially with studies from developing countries.

OBESITY

The prevalence of obesity among children and adolescents has increased in Western countries due to changes in diet and physical activity. Several single cross-sectional studies have reported an association between asthma and obesity, and in several longitudinal studies, an increased incidence of asthma has also been reported in subjects who are overweight. Repeated cross-sectional studies in the United Kingdom[173] and New Zealand[174] found little difference in the odds ratios (ORs) for BMI. However, the more recent studies found a stronger relationship than the earlier studies. In a recent report of a cross-sectional study, increased BMI was found to influence asthma prevalence.[175] If there is an association, its maximally predicted effect would explain only a small amount of the increase in asthma.[176] The nature of the association has yet to be clarified, and it cannot be concluded that obesity has contributed to the rise in asthma.[177]

Does physical fitness have a role? In a prospective community-based study of Danish children, there was a weak correlation between physical fitness and reduced risk for the development of asthma.[178] In a cross-sectional Norwegian study, children with asthma who exercised less had more BHR than those who exercised more, but the cause of this relationship is not clear.[179] The relationship between physical fitness and possible protection from the development of asthma may be worthy of further exploration.

INFECTION

The relationship between infection and asthma symptoms has intrigued clinicians and epidemiologists for decades. The "hygiene hypothesis" was first proposed by Strachan in 1989: that allergic diseases could be prevented by infection in early childhood.[180] This hypothesis was suggested by the observation that hay fever (but not asthma) at 11 and 23 years of age was inversely related to the number of children in the household at age 11 years, with the number of older children being more influential than birth order. Strachan proposed that allergic diseases could be "prevented by infection in early childhood transmitted by unhygienic contact with older siblings or acquired prenatally from a mother infected by contact with her older children. Later infection or reinfection by younger siblings might confer additional protection against hay fever."[180] The first decade of the hygiene hypothesis has recently been carefully reviewed by Strachan.[181] The hypothesis that was proposed about hay fever has been widely applied to asthma, with little evidence.

A 1995 review suggests that infants with wheeze fall into two groups: infants with viral infection–associated wheeze who have lower than normal lung function shortly after birth, who will become symptom free during the preschool years, and children who will continue to wheeze. The factors that determine which group will be persistent wheezers are not well understood, but viral infections are unlikely to play a major part.[182] A recent comprehensive review of asthma and respiratory infections is unable to provide a clear answer to the central question of whether respiratory viral illness causes asthma, exacerbates underlying asthma, or both, due to limitations in the existing literature.[183]

A recent prospective cohort study in Germany showed that children with two or more episodes of runny nose before 1 year of age were less likely to have been diagnosed as asthmatic by a doctor or have wheeze by 7 years, and were less likely to be atopic by 5 years. One or more viral infections of the herpes type before 3 years of age were also inversely associated with asthma at age 7. Conversely, repeated lower respiratory tract infections in the first 3 years was associated with increased risk of wheeze at age 7.[184]

Notwithstanding these studies, in his recent review, Strachan states that "the totality of current evidence from cross-sectional and longitudinal studies, of common specific and non-specific infectious illness in infancy and childhood, offers no support for the hygiene hypothesis."[185]

Respiratory syncytial virus has warranted special consideration because it is the most common cause of bronchiolitis, an acute wheezy illness of infants. A study of children enrolled in the longitudinal cohort study, the Tucson Children's Respiratory Study (Arizona), showed that respiratory syncytial virus lower respiratory tract infections before 3 years of age were associated with an increased risk for infrequent wheeze and frequent wheeze at age 6. Risk decreased with age and was not observable at age 13. Respiratory syncytial virus lower respiratory tract infections were also associated with lower forced expiratory volumes, but there was no difference after inhalation of salbutamol.[186]

A further analysis of the Tucson study showed that daycare attendance in children younger than 6 months was protective against the development of asthma. Daycare attendance during the first 6 months also increased the risk for frequent wheeze (more than three episodes in the previous year) at age 2 years, but decreased the risk for frequent wheeze at ages 6 to 13 years.[187]

Although a cross-sectional study in Finland showed a positive association between measles infection and asthma,[188] this finding has not been replicated.

In an Italian population, a history of pertussis or pneumonia was not associated with asthma.[189] In a randomized double-blind controlled trial of pertussis vaccine in Sweden, there was a positive association between whooping cough disease and asthma by 2$^{1}/_{2}$ years of age.[190]

There has been interest in the relationship between parasitic infections, IgE, and asthma. It has been suggested that high degrees of parasitic infections could prevent asthma symptoms in atopic individuals in Ethiopia in a comparison of urban and rural areas.[191] However, studies in Latin America demonstrate high prevalence of asthma symptoms in areas with higher endemic parasite load.[40]

Recent experimental evidence suggests that exposure to *Mycobacterium tuberculosis* may reduce the risk for developing asthma. In a partly longitudinal study of children in Japan, an inverse relationship was found between tuberculin skin response and symptoms of asthma. However, it is unclear whether bacillus Calmette-Guérin (BCG) vaccination, primary TB infection in childhood, or sensitization to harmless environmental mycobacteria were responsible.[192] (BCG vaccination is discussed further in the later section on Immunization).

An ecologic analysis of ISAAC Phase One data has shown an inverse association between TB notification rates and the lifetime prevalence of wheeze and asthma and the 12-month prevalence of wheeze assessed from a video questionnaire, adjusted for GNP. A decrease in TB notifications of 25 cases per 100,000 was associated with a 4.7% increase in the prevalence of wheeze ever,[134] and this was confirmed in a larger group of ISAAC centers.[193]

IMMUNIZATION

It has been postulated that immunization in early life may either promote or protect against asthma. The balance of evidence from studies to date suggests no effect. In a small cross-sectional study carried out in London, England, asthma was found more commonly in immunized than unimmunized children.[194] A large cross-sectional study in United States found that DTP or measles vaccine appeared to increase the risk for asthma ever, but not wheezing in the past 12 months.[195] Other studies have found that immunization has no effect or even a protective effect on IgE-mediated disease. In a large prospective cohort study in the United Kingdom, there was no increased risk for wheezing illnesses in pertussis-vaccinated children.[196] In a randomized double-blind controlled trial of the pertussis vaccine in Sweden, the cumulative incidence of IgE-mediated disease was similar in the three vaccination and placebo groups.[187]

An ecologic analysis of the ISAAC Phase One data using immunization rates for the year of birth of the ISAAC participants, adjusted for GNP, showed no association between symptoms of asthma and national immunization rates for DTP, measles, and BCG.[135] However, for local immunization rates in 13- to 14-year-olds, there were significant negative associations of symptoms of all three conditions and DTP and measles, but BCG had no effect. No associations were seen in the 6- to 7-year-old age group between any symptoms and any of the three vaccines. This large worldwide ecologic study is reassuring for population immunization programs.

MICROBIAL EXPOSURE

The concept that live microbial food constituents may have a beneficial effect on human health was first proposed in the early 1900s by Metchnikoff.[197] In the past century, a striking alteration in the early immune exposures of infants has been the change in initial gut colonization. The dominance of *Bifidobacteria* and *Lactobacillus* in the initial flora of the developing world infant has been increasingly replaced by a variety of other organisms in the developed world, and this has been an intriguing area for further exploration.[198–200] However, in two double-blind randomized placebo-controlled trials in Finland there was no difference in the prevalence of asthma symptoms following *Lactobacillus* administered in pregnancy and for 6 months after birth.[201,202]

Does antibiotic usage have any effect through the unwanted effects of antibiotics causing major depletion of the commensal microflora of the gut? Most of the relevant studies are retrospective, and potentially one of the largest problems is the concept of self-selection. For children who wheeze with lower respiratory infections, prescription of antibiotic treatment may be a marker for children who are more likely to wheeze in the first place. ISAAC Phase One found no relationship between antibiotic sales and the prevalence of asthma.[139] The Boston birth cohort study[203] followed infants at high risk for atopy, from birth to 5 years, excluding children who were treated with antibiotics for wheezing. No association was seen between antibiotic use and asthma at age 5.

The role of the farm environment and animal contact associated with the development of asthma has captured a lot of interest.[204,205] Although the first report from Switzerland showed no protective effect,[206] the next cross-sectional study of Finnish children showed that the childhood farm environment reduced the risk for asthma and wheezing.[207] Among Austrian children living in a rural area, children living on a farm had less asthma than those in a nonfarming environment.[208] In Bavaria, Germany, farmers' children had lower prevalences of asthma and wheeze than their peers that did not live in an agricultural environment.[204]

In a subsequent study of Austrian, German, and Swiss farmers' children, current wheeze was lower among children who spent time in the stables. This effect was stronger for children who spent time during the first year of life in the stables (OR 0.36 and 0.33, respectively) than for those who spent time in the stables from 2 to 5 years of age (OR 0.73 and 0.87), compared with nonfarming children. Similar reductions were found with those who drank unpasteurized farm milk. Time spent in the stables and consumption of farm milk in the first year were independently associated with health outcome. Among farmers' children who spent time in the stables in the first year of life, drank farm milk, and whose mother spent time in the stables while pregnant, there was only one case of asthma (expected 19 cases).[209] These results suggest that exposure to the farming environment influences the development of asthma and IgE sensitization in a potently protective way. A protective effect of the farm environment has since also been found in Finland,[210] four European centers and New Zealand in the ECRHS study,[211] Nepal,[212] Crete,[213] Canada,[214] and Australia,[215] but not in a further New Zealand study.[216]

Influences on a farm, such as increased exposure to bacterial compounds in stables where livestock is kept, may prevent the development of allergic disorders in children. The consumption of "raw" unpasteurized milk may contain a higher microbial load, particularly of *Lactobacillus*, than industrial processed skim milk. Increased concentrations of bacterial compounds such as endotoxin and its purified derivative lipopolysaccharide have been found in stables where livestock has been kept.[217] Endotoxin levels are also high in stables of farming families in the European Alps, and in the dust from their kitchen floors and children's mattresses compared with nonfarming families.[218]

Endotoxin levels are also likely to be particularly high in developing countries where poultry and livestock are kept in close proximity to human housing. One study from Africa has found a significantly decreased development of IgE-sensitization in children in whose homes pigs were kept.[219] Bacterial endotoxin is known to induce production of T-helper 1 (Th1)-associated cytokines, interferon-γ, and interleukin-12, and therefore has the potential to decrease allergen sensitization. Reductions in allergen sensitization and IgE-mediated disease have been found in children of farmers, children with pigs, dogs, or cats in their homes, children raised in daycare from an early age, and children of large families.

An intriguing notion for further exploration is whether endotoxin could reduce the clinical expression of atopy. To date there is no evidence to support this, but observational studies and randomized trials to test this hypothesis would be of interest.[220]

In the Boston Home Allergens and Asthma Study,[221] a longitudinal analysis of wheezing in young children, and the independent effects of early life exposures to house dust endotoxin, allergens, and pets, suggests that the timing, dose, and other environmental factors may be important. In this study, the investigators found that higher levels of endotoxin were associated with increased risk for wheezing initially, but this risk rapidly decreased with time. The protective effects of cat and dog ownership were independent of the endotoxin level.

ALLERGENS

The concept of allergen exposure causing asthma dates back to the 17th century, and clinical studies date back to the first part of the 20th century.[222] The major airborne allergens associated with the risk for asthma differ within and between communities, and may alter with climate, season, housing, and hygiene. How important then are they in the cause of asthma and its maintenance? Are they triggers that just exacerbate asthma or are they a cause?

Many studies show that persistent asthma is associated with exposure to allergens in the indoor environment. Also, typical outdoor allergens like pollens are also regularly found indoors. Pollen allergy is associated with acute hospital admissions[223] but is rarely an independent risk factor for persistent asthma.[224]

In many temperate and humid regions the greatest risk for asthma has been associated with allergy to HDM.[225] In Australia, the association between exposure to HDM, sensitization, and asthma is very strong. Increased use of nonfeather pillows which have less tightly woven encasements and more allergens appeared to explain a modest rise in prevalence of wheeze over a 13-year period in London, United Kingdom.[226] In some dry climates the strongest risk factor is allergy to the fungus *Alternaria*.[227,228] In other urban communities, allergy to cockroach appears to be the dominant allergen and is strongly associated with asthma risk.[229,230]

It is not clear whether household pets influence the occurrence and severity of clinical asthma and in what direction. Allergy to cats and dogs appears to be important in many places.[231] In a study of children in the Netherlands, pet ownership (cats, dogs, birds, and/or rodents in the home) was associated with lower prevalence of respiratory allergy and symptoms. However, past, but not current, pet ownership was associated with a higher prevalence of symptoms and pet allergy. These results suggest that selective avoidance and removal of pets leads to distortion of cross-sectional associations of pet ownership and respiratory allergy and disease among children.[232] In adolescents in Norway, sensitization to pet allergens (cat, dog, and horse) was associated with increased AHR in children with asthma. The risk of being sensitized to cat allergens was significantly reduced in those who had kept cats, compared with those who had never kept them. Keeping dogs or horses did not influence the risk of being sensitized to the respective allergens. Therefore, keeping pets did not increase the risk for being sensitized to pet allergens.[233] In Sweden, early exposure to cats and dogs appeared to have a protective effect on the development of IgE sensitization.[234] However, in a study in New Delhi, India, dogs and cats at home were significant risk factors associated with the symptoms of asthma in schoolchildren.[235]

Numerous studies demonstrate a relationship between risk for sensitization and the level of exposure to allergen.[222] The relationship between the incidence of sensitization to HDM and cat allergens during the first 3 years of life has been clearly demonstrated by the West German study conducted by Wahn and colleagues.[236] Increasing exposure, both in a group of infants with atopic parents and in a group with nonatopic parents, was associated with increasing incidence of sensitization, and Wahn and colleagues concluded that allergen intervention needs to begin in early life.

If allergen exposure is important in the etiology of asthma, it seems probable that it will be involved in its persistence rather than its initial occurrence. This hypothesis is supported by a cohort study in Scandinavia in which children with positive skin test results to HDM allergen, who became negative over a period of 24 years, were exposed to a low level of HDM allergens, whereas those whose skin test responses remained positive had a higher level in their environment. Furthermore, in the setting of occupational asthma, continuing exposure to the relevant occupational allergen is associated with a higher risk for persisting asthma.

Recent recommendations have been made that for young children already sensitized to HDM, pets, or cockroaches, exposure should be reduced to prevent the onset of allergic disease. Patients with asthma who are allergic to indoor allergens such as HDM, cockroaches, and animal danders should eliminate or reduce the exposure to improve symptoms and control and prevent exacerbations.[129]

Despite all that has been researched and written about allergen avoidance, the recent Cochrane Review found no significant clinical benefit on the tertiary prevention of asthma and recommended larger and more rigorous trials with more careful monitoring of exposure and clinical outcomes.[237] This suggests that reducing allergen exposure is unlikely to make an important impact on the burden of asthma in populations.

ENVIRONMENTAL TOBACCO SMOKE

Tobacco smoke exposure is undoubtedly an important risk factor for asthma. Both active smokers and nonsmokers exposed to environmental tobacco smoke (ETS) have been found to be affected adversely. ETS—consisting of mainstream smoke that has been inhaled and exhaled by the primary smoker and sidestream smoke that arises directly from a burning cigarette—contains many agents that have pathologic effects on human tissues.[130]

Children can be exposed to tobacco smoke before or after birth. It has been difficult to isolate intrauterine exposure per se, because postnatal exposure continues in many instances. Does prenatal ETS cause allergic sensitization? No correlation was found between cord blood IgE of newborns and an active smoking history of either mothers or fathers.[238,239] However, cord blood eosinophil counts were found to correlate with the urinary cotinine levels of mothers.[240]

Exposure to ETS during childhood, and intrauterine exposure to maternal smoking, are also associated with adverse effects on lung growth and development. In a cross-sectional study of schoolchildren in Southern California, intrauterine exposure to maternal smoking was associated with reduced maximal expiratory flow rates, but not FEV_1, and was independently associated with decreased lung function in children of school age, especially for small airway flow rates.[241] In the Tucson Children's Respiratory Study (Arizona), maternal prenatal but not postnatal smoking was associated with current wheeze at 3 years only.[242]

What about the effects of postnatal exposure? In a large meta-analysis of 21 studies of school-aged children, the percentage reduction in FEV_1 in children exposed to parental smoking, compared with those not exposed, was 1.4%.[243] Effects were greater on mid-expiratory flow rates (5.0% reduction) and end-expiratory flow rates (4.3% reduction).

The effect of tobacco smoke on BHR and asthma, apart from lung size and lung function, has also been studied. In a large meta-analysis, the pooled OR for maternal smoking was 1.29. However, in five further studies of 3531 children, there was a weak effect but none were statistically significant. Four studies of circadian variation in peak expiratory flow found increased variation in children exposed to ETS. A clear effect of exposure to ETS on BHR in the general population has not been established. While the meta-analysis suggests a small but real increase in BHR in school-aged children, limited evidence suggests greater variation in peak expiratory flow in children of smoking parents.[244]

In investigating the effects of ETS on asthma,[245] the relationship of parental smoking to wheezing and asthma occurring after the first year of life has been assessed. Maternal smoking was associated with an increased incidence of wheezing illness up to age 6 (pooled OR 1.31), but less strongly thereafter (pooled OR 1.13). The pooled OR for asthma prevalence from 14 case-control studies was 1.37 if either parent smoked. Four studies suggest that parental smoking is more strongly associated with wheezing among "nonatopic" children. Indicators of disease severity, including symptom scores, attack frequency, medication use, hospital attendance, and life-threatening bronchospasm, were, in general, positively related to household smoke exposure. The excess incidence of wheezing in smoking households appears to be largely early wheezers with a relatively benign prognosis, but among children with established asthma, parental smoking is associated with more severe disease. These studies suggest that ETS is a cofactor provoking wheezing attacks, rather than a cause of the underlying asthmatic tendency.[245]

In a cohort study of 6000 children that investigated the effect of maternal smoking together with socioeconomic status (SES) and low birth order on the risk of allergic disease, maternal smoking was found to be an additional risk factor for wheeze primarily in low-SES groups.[246,247] Similarly, the asthma severity in children whose mothers stopped smoking was found to decrease.[248] In a subsequent study investigating the effect of intrauterine and postnatal ETS exposure in high-risk infants in the first 3 years of life, ETS exposure increased the risk for wheezing in the first year of life, but had little effect on the development of atopy.[249]

About half the world's children may be exposed to ETS, exacerbating symptoms in 20% of children with asthma. However, it is reassuring that favorable health outcomes can be attained with reduced exposure. Community opinion may need to shift further in favor of protecting children and others from ETS before minimal interventions can be successful. This will require continued efforts by the medical and public health establishments, combined with legislation mandating tobacco-free public places and ETS-related media campaigns.[250]

What about adolescents who take up smoking? Asthma and active cigarette smoking interact to cause more severe symptoms, decline in lung function, and impaired short-term therapeutic response to corticosteroids. Clinical and public health programs should encourage asthmatics who smoke to quit.[251]

DAMP AND MOLD

There is a common belief that damp housing is bad for respiratory health, including asthma. Cross-sectional and longitudinal cohort studies that have been conducted in children show a small increased risk of having asthma symptoms if the home has damp or mold. However, the potential benefits of reducing mold in the home have not been investigated. In a study in the Netherlands, sensitization to HDM and possibly mold allergen is related to living in a damp home and childhood respiratory symptoms.[252] In a study in children in the United States, dampness in the home was common and a predictor of wheeze and asthma.[253] In a population study in Israel, viable molds were common, but IgE sensitization to molds was a poor predictor of development of allergic symptoms. However, allergy to molds in atopic subjects increases the risk for symptomatic allergic disease.[254] In a study in children in London, England, there was no significant difference in the degree of bronchospasm measured from children in homes with or without mold, but wheeze in the last year was associated with reported dampness and mold.[255] However, simultaneous estimation of relative humidity in bedrooms and recordings of ambient temperature and humidity showed no association with respiratory symptoms.[256] Nevertheless, it seems prudent to reduce or avoid damp housing conditions.[129]

OTHER INDOOR FACTORS

Exposure to nitrogen dioxide (NO_2) through the use of unvented gas cookers in homes is associated with respiratory symptoms. In addition, NO_2 may aggravate respiratory symptoms in the presence of coexistent infection.[257] A study of children in Victoria, Australia, showed that NO_2 was a marginal risk factor for respiratory symptoms, with a dose-response association present. Gas stove exposure was a significant risk factor, even after controlling for personal NO_2 exposure, suggesting an additional risk. No difference was noted between atopic and nonatopic children.[258] A study of asthmatics in Port Adelaide, Australia, demonstrated associations between personal NO_2 exposure measured by lapel sensors and asthmatic symptoms such as chest tightness, breathlessness on exertion, and day- and nighttime asthma attacks in children.[259]

In a study in Bavaria, Germany, coal or wood heating in children's homes reduced the risk for becoming sensitized to pollen and developing hay fever, BHR, and asthma.[260]

Indoor exposure to mixtures and single components of volatile organic compounds can be related to asthma symptoms, but there is no evidence that increasing exposure of a population to these compounds initiates asthma and allergic disease. Although gasoline is a common volatile organic compound, and can contaminate the indoor environment in motor vehicles and buildings, there is no evidence to link this to asthma.[261]

Formaldehyde is one of several volatile organic compounds now commonly found indoors in homes in Western environments. Sources are particle board, plywood, fiber board, paneling, urea formaldehyde foam insulation, and some carpets and furniture, as well as some household chemicals. Formaldehyde exposure may increase the risk for IgE sensitization to common aeroallergens.[262] Frequent use of chemical-based products is associated with persistent wheezing in preschool children.[263]

In Kenya, the higher prevalence of asthma symptoms in urban than rural localities has been related to the home environment.[44] Urban homes tend to have a higher number of windows than rural homes, and carpets are exclusively found in the urban setting. Urban homes use gas and electricity as the major domestic fuel, also using kerosene and charcoal, whereas rural homes use firewood as the major domestic fuel. In Germany, wood and coal heating and feather bedding were negatively associated with symptoms, whereas exposures such as truck traffic in a residential street and active smoking were positively associated with symptoms.[32]

OUTDOOR AIR POLLUTION

There is a great deal of interest in the relationship of air pollution and asthma that needs clarification.[264] Urban air pollution comprises several factors that may affect respiratory illness: ozone (O_3),

NO_2, sulphur dioxide (SO_2), acid aerosols, and particulates. Many children with established asthma experience deterioration of their symptoms associated with an increase in outdoor air pollution.[265] However, there is no evidence for increased air pollution contributing to increased prevalence of asthma.[266] In ISAAC Phase One, countries with low ambient air pollution such as New Zealand were among those with the highest prevalence of asthma symptoms. In contrast, regions such as China and eastern Europe, which experience some of the highest levels of air pollutants such as particulate matter and SO_2, generally had low rates of asthma prevalence. Regions such as western Europe and the United States, with high degrees of air pollutants such as O_3, had intermediate levels.[10] Thus, there is no evidence that outdoor air pollution increases the risk for development of asthma and allergy.

To the contrary, studies in Germany have found lower rates of the prevalence of asthma in the more polluted East Germany compared with the West. During 1989 to 1991, there was a lower prevalence of asthma in Leipzig in the former East Germany compared with Munich (former West Germany).[31,152] A study of children in Dresden, Germany, using the ISAAC Phase Two protocol[22] showed that benzene, NO_2, and carbon monoxide were associated with increased prevalence of morning cough and bronchitis. However, IgE sensitization, symptoms of IgE-mediated diseases, and BHR were not associated with these pollutants.[267] In a study in Swiss schoolchildren, there was no association between long-term exposure to air pollution and asthmatic and allergic symptoms.[268] However, in Latin America, a high prevalence of asthma was found in heavily polluted São Paulo, Brazil, with symptom rates comparable with less polluted cities in Australia and New Zealand, indicating that urban air pollution is not always protective.[40]

A cohort study of children in Japan identified increasing prevalence of bronchitis, wheeze, and asthma, with increasing indoor NO_2 exposure among girls, but not boys. Increased incidence of asthma was also identified among children living in areas with high outdoor NO_2 concentrations.[269]

Motor vehicle traffic has increased greatly in recent decades, and its role in the development of asthma has been studied. A positive association between self-reported truck traffic in the street of residence and reported asthma symptoms in adolescents was observed in German cities.[270,271] There were similar findings in the Netherlands. Diesel exhaust may have a particularly strong influence.[272,273] In Italy, exposure to exhaust from heavy vehicular traffic in metropolitan areas increased the occurrence of wheezing.[274] In Kenya, children from an urban area were exposed more frequently to motor vehicle fumes on the way to school than rural children, and this partially explained observed differences in prevalence.[44] In asthmatic children in the Netherlands, black smoke, particulates, and O_3 were associated with acute respiratory symptoms and medication use.[273] A study of children younger than 5 years in Birmingham, United Kingdom, showed an increased risk for hospitalization for asthma in children living in areas with high traffic flow.[275] Recent reports for Germany found no association with traffic pollution and BHR.[276] Society is experiencing a transition from classical pollution, dominated by SO_2 and particulates generated by coal and oil combustion, with the effects primarily on cough and bronchitis, to pollution mixtures dominated by traffic exhausts represented by NO_2, with effects on wheeze.[277] The potential effect on asthma prevalence requires further study.

ECONOMIC FACTORS

It is tempting to hypothesize that asthma is associated with the economic development occurring with westernization. This hypothesis was explored in an ecological analysis of ISAAC Phase One data from 52 countries using GNP as a marker of economic development of countries. A weak positive association was found between GNP and symptoms of asthma; an increase of US$10,000 per capita was associated with a 3% increase in the prevalence of wheeze.[132] However, within Latin America, ISAAC suggested a reverse trend, with prevalence of symptoms of asthma tending to be higher in poorer areas.[40]

Some studies have shown that severe asthma symptoms in developed countries are more frequent in poorer sections of society.[278] In a prospective British cohort, high SES was related to persistence of wheeze at 16 years.[160] In a national birth cohort study from England, Wales, and Scotland, the prevalence of asthma showed no social class gradient.[279] In Cardiff, Wales, social deprivation was not related to asthma prevalence, but was related to admission to hospital.[280] A South African study had a similar finding with severity measured by high symptoms occurrence.[281] In a cross-sectional study in Italy, socioeconomic conditions were associated with hospitalization for asthma and severity and weakly associated with prevalence, with the association being strongest for individual indicators (parental education) rather than area-based indicators.[282] Poorer disease management is the postulated mechanism.

In Auckland, New Zealand, there was no association between SES and asthma diagnosis and BHR, but there were higher lifetime and current prevalence rates of wheeze in children in lower SES groups. The use of bronchodilators and asthma prophylactic drugs was less frequent in the lower SES groups of children with wheeze in the past 12 months both with concurrent BHR or irrespective of BHR than in those in higher SES groups.[283] Greater severity among Maori and Pacific children suggested poorer disease management.[284] This is borne out by a recent cross-sectional survey of caregivers of children with asthma, which showed that Maori and Pacific children had higher levels of asthma morbidity, and higher primary practitioner usage, but received less education about asthma and its management, and in the severe morbidity group were less likely to receive preventive medication (S. Crengle, personal communication).

CLIMATE AND WEATHER

A potential role of climatic conditions in the etiology of asthma and allergy has often been suspected. Most studies on the effects of climate have looked at short periods of variations in the occurrence or severity of symptoms. Little is known about the effect of long-term climatic conditions on the prevalence of asthma symptoms. Studies on the long-term effect of climate have been limited to comparisons of areas within countries.[285] A study in Bermuda related emergency department acute asthma visits with weather parameters.[286] In a comparative study in the United Kingdom, Australia, and New Zealand, the prevalence of asthma among children was greater in the warmer regions.[287] In London, England, new episodes of asthma in adults during a 2-day thunderstorm were associated with a fall in air temperature and a rise in grass pollen concentration.[223] A larger study in England of the effect of thunderstorms and airborne grass pollen over a 4-year period showed that thunderstorm-associated rises in hospital admissions for acute asthma were amplified after a run of high pollen counts.[288] An inverse association between the prevalence of BHR and altitude of the study area has been observed in mountaineering expeditions in Italy and Nepal.[289]

Because climate affects whole populations, ecologic studies are ideally suited to examine the relationship between prevalence of diseases and climatic conditions between populations. The association between climate and asthma was studied using ISAAC Phase One worldwide data from 146 centers.[136] In Western Europe (57 centers in 12 countries), the prevalence of asthma symptoms increased by 2.7%, with an increase in estimated annual mean indoor relative humidity of 10%. Altitude and the annual variation of temperature and relative humidity outdoors were negatively associated with asthma symptoms. Worldwide data showed similar trends, suggesting that climate may affect the prevalence of asthma in children.

SUMMARY OF ENVIRONMENTAL FACTORS

As countries develop and change their lifestyles, environmental factors that protect against asthma and allergic diseases may be lost. At the same time, environmental factors that may initiate and aggravate asthma and allergic disease may be being added. Much of the research efforts until 2000 have been focused on classical risk factors, such as allergen exposure, and it is only in the past 5 years that the focus has moved to the identification of potentially protective factors. Examples of this are the potentially protective effects of the plant content of diet, and microbial exposure on the occurrence of asthma.

The case for ETS in causing wheeze in infancy and aggravating asthma is well proven. A multifaceted approach is required by governments to reduce tobacco consumption and ETS exposure. This will have benefits for many diseases as well as asthma.

Unfortunately, efforts aimed at prevention of allergic sensitization through avoidance of allergen exposure have been largely unsuccessful because they are very difficult to implement, and any beneficial effects are small and not sustained. This may not be an important mechanism in many children with asthma.

An increasing body of evidence suggests that within populations those with socioeconomic disadvantage have more problematic asthma, and this disparity should be addressed with improved management strategies for these children.

THE NATURAL HISTORY OF ASTHMA

Wheeze is a prevalent symptom of asthma in both children and adults. Birth cohort studies from the United Kingdom and New Zealand have shown that between 43% and 73% of people wheeze at some time between birth and early to mid adulthood.[290,291]

Different patterns of wheezing in childhood are associated with differing risks of subsequent asthma. Wheeze was present by age 6 years in 48% of children enrolled into a birth cohort in Tucson, Arizona, from 1980 to 1984.[126] Three patterns of wheezing were evident: wheeze during the first 3 years of life but not subsequently (~40% of those with wheeze), wheeze during the first 3 years of life that continued (~30%), and wheeze at age 6 years but not before age 3 years (~30%).

Between 30% and 70% of children with asthma or wheezing illness in childhood enter remission during the transition to adult life.[291] In approximately two thirds of children with asthma, the disease becomes asymptomatic prior to adulthood.[292–294] However, between 40% and 50% of asthmatic children with apparent remission will again become symptomatic by early adulthood.[291]

FACTORS ASSOCIATED WITH PERSISTENCE OF ASTHMA

Factors associated with an increased risk for childhood asthma persisting or recurring during adulthood include female gender, parental history of asthma, more severe asthma as measured by earlier onset, more attacks and lower peak flow rates during childhood, AHR, and positive skin test responses to HDM antigen during childhood.[291–294] The earlier the age of onset of wheeze, the greater the risk for relapse.[291,295]

GENDER

The association between gender and asthma varies with age. During earlier childhood, asthma and wheeze occurs more frequently in boys than in girls. During adolescence, asthma symptoms tend to remit more frequently in boys.[296] ISAAC demonstrated that this is a consistent worldwide observation, occurring not only in Western countries. In the younger age group, there were more boys than girls with asthma, consistent in all centers and countries. However, in the older age group, asthma symptoms occurred equally in boys and girls.[39] Thus, although less common in girls during childhood, in those with asthma, female gender is associated with an increased risk for asthma as an adult.[294,297]

ATOPY

A personal or family history of allergy is one of the most consistent risk factors for persistent asthma in childhood.[292] In the Tucson Children's Respiratory Study among children who wheeze in the first 3 years of life, the risk for symptomatic asthma at age 6 to 13 years is increased four- to tenfold if the child also has eczema, or a parental history of asthma, or if two or more of allergic rhinitis, eosinophilia, or wheezing other than with upper respiratory infections are present.[126,298,299] Atopy is associated with more severe asthma.[300–302]

AIRWAY HYPERRESPONSIVENESS

The magnitude of the risk of asthma during adolescence or early adulthood associated with wheeze, atopy, and AHR in early childhood has been estimated from cohort studies performed in Australia, Great Britain, Denmark, Japan, Italy, New Zealand, and the United States.[126,294,297,303–308] These risks are best expressed as likelihood ratios (the true-positive rate as a proportion of the false-positive rate).[309] The likelihood ratios for asthma associated with wheeze before age 8 years range from 1.0 to 1.7, for atopy at age 8 to 10 years from 1.5 to 2.5, and for AHR from age 5 to 17 years between 2.5 and 4.5.[303]

CONCLUSION

In the past 10 to 20 years, epidemiological studies have provided advances in knowledge about the worldwide prevalence and variation in asthma and its natural history. Wide scale analyses have suggested that there has been an emphasis on atopy in the explanation of the occurrence of asthma, and it is now time to focus more on the nonatopic causes. Evidence suggests that the search for environmental contributors to asthma should shift away from commonly cited risk factors such as allergens to consideration of potentially protective factors such as components of the diet, and the human microbial environment.

Acknowledgment

The authors thank the following department colleagues for their assistance with the preparation of the manuscript: Tadd Clayton, Philippa Ellwood, and Va Strong.

REFERENCES

1. Zar HJ, Mulholland K: Global burden of pediatric respiratory illness and the implications for management and prevention. Pediatric Pulmonology 2003;36(6):457–461.
2. British Thoracic Society (BTS), Scottish Intercollegiate Guidelines Network (SIGN): British Guideline on the Management of Asthma. British Thoracic Society, 2004.
3. Global Initiative for Asthma (GINA): Pocket Guide for Asthma Management and Prevention in Children. Global Initiative for Asthma, 2003.
4. Braun-Fahrlander C, Gassner M, Grize L, Minder C, Varonier H, Vuille J, et al: Comparison of responses to an asthma symptom questionnaire (ISAAC core questions) completed by adolescents and their parents. SCARPOL-Team. Swiss Study on Childhood Allergy and Respiratory Symptoms with respect to Air Pollution. Pediatr Pulmonol 1998;25(3):159–166.
5. Shaw RA, Crane J, O'Donnell TV, Lewis ME, Stewart B, Beasley R: The use of a videotaped questionnaire for studying asthma prevalence. A pilot study among New Zealand adolescents. Med J Aust 1992;157(5):311–314.
6. Ponsonby A, Couper D, Dwyer T, Carmichael A, Wood-Baker R: Exercise-induced bronchial hyperresponsiveness and parental ISAAC questionnaire responses. Eur Respir J 1996;9(7):1356–1362.
7. Lai CKW, Chan JKW, Chan A, Wong G, Ho A, Choy D, et al: Comparison of the ISAAC video questionnaire (AVQ3.0) with the ISAAC written questionnaire for estimating asthma associated with bronchial hyperreactivity. Clin Exp Allergy 1997;27(5):540–545.
8. Gibson PG, Henry R, Shah S, Toneguzzi R, Francis JL, Norzila MZ, et al: Validation of the ISAAC video questionnaire (AVQ3.0) in adolescents from a mixed ethnic background. Clin Exp Allergy 2000;30(8):1181–1187.
9. Chan HH, Pei A, Van Krevel C, Wong GW, Lai CK: Validation of the Chinese translated version of ISAAC core questions for atopic eczema. Clin Exp Allergy 2001;31(6):903–907.
10. ISAAC Steering Committee: Worldwide variations in the prevalence of asthma symptoms. The International Study of Asthma and Allergies in Childhood (ISAAC). Eur Respir J 1998;12(2):315–335.
11. Crane J, Mallol J, Beasley R, Stewart A, Asher MI, International Study of Asthma and Allergies in Childhood Phase I study group: Agreement between written and video questions for comparing asthma symptoms in ISAAC. Eur Respir J 2003;21(3):455–461.
12. Shaw R, Woodman K, Ayson M, Dibdin S, Winkelmann R, Crane J, et al: Measuring the prevalence of bronchial hyper-responsiveness in children. Int J Epidemiol 1995;24(3):597–602.
13. Jenkins M, Clarke J, Carlin J, Robertson C, Hopper J, Dalton M, et al: Validation of questionnaire and bronchial hyperresponsiveness against respiratory physician assessment in the diagnosis of asthma. Int J Epidemiol 1996;25(3):609–616.
14. Pearce N, Beasley R, Burgess C, Crane J: Asthma Epidemiology. Principles and Methods. New York: Oxford University Press, 1998.
15. Cockcroft DW, Killian DN, Mellon JJ, Hargreave FE: Bronchial reactivity to inhaled histamine. A method and clinical survey. Clin Allergy 1977;7(3):235–243.
16. Hopp RJ, Bewtra AK, Nair NM, Townley RG: Specificity and sensitivity of methacholine inhalation challenge in normal and asthmatic children. J Allergy Clin Immunol 1984;74(2):154–158.
17. Joos GF, O'Connor B, Anderson SD, Chung F, Cockcroft DW, Dahlen B, et al: Indirect airway challenges. Eur Respir J 2003;21(6):1050–1068.
18. Pattemore PK, Asher MI, Harrison AC, Mitchell EA, Rea HH, Stewart AW: The interrelationship among bronchial hyperresponsiveness, the diagnosis of asthma, and asthma symptoms. Am Rev Respir Dis 1990;142(3):549–554.
19. Asher MI, Pattemore PK, Harrison AC, Mitchell EA, Rea HH, Stewart AW, et al: International comparison of the prevalence of asthma symptoms and bronchial hyperresponsiveness. Am Rev Respir Dis 1988;138(3):524–529.
20. Guinness World Records. London: Guinness World Records, 2004.
21. ISAAC Steering Committee: International Study of Asthma and Allergies in Childhood Phase II Modules. Münster, Germany: ISAAC Steering Committee, 1998, p 68.
22. Weiland SK, Bjorksten B, Brunekreef B, Cookson WO, von Mutius E, Strachan DP, et al: Phase II of the International Study of Asthma and Allergies in Childhood (ISAAC II). Rationale and methods. Eur Respir J 2004;24(3):406–412.
23. Greenland S, Morgenstern H: Ecological bias, confounding, and effect modification. Int J Epidemiol 1989;18(1):269–274.
24. Morgenstern H: Ecological studies. In: Rothman KJ, Greenland S, eds: Modern Epidemiology. Boston: Lippincott-Raven, 1998, pp 459–480.
25. Marmot MG: Improvement of social environment to improve health. Lancet 1998;351(9095):57–60.
26. Robertson CF, Bishop J, Sennhauser FH, Mallol J: International comparison of asthma prevalence in children. Australia, Switzerland, Chile. Pediatr Pulmonol 1993;16(4):219–226.
27. Burr ML, Limb ES, Andrae S, Barry DM, Nagel F: Childhood asthma in four countries. A comparative survey. Int J Epidemiol 1994;23(2):341–347.
28. Leung R, Ho P: Asthma, allergy, and atopy in three south-east Asian populations. Thorax 1994;49(12):1205–1210.
29. Barry DM, Burr ML, Limb ES: Prevalence of asthma among 12 year old children in New Zealand and South Wales. A comparative survey. Thorax 1991;46(6):405–409.
30. Ring J, Kramer U, Schafer T, Abeck D, Vieluf D, Behrendt H: Environmental risk factors for respiratory and skin atopy. Results from epidemiological studies in former East and West Germany. Int Arch Allergy Immunol 1999;118(2–4):403–407.
31. von Mutius E, Fritzsch C, Weiland SK, Roll G, Magnussen H: Prevalence of asthma and allergic disorders among children in united Germany. A descriptive comparison. BMJ 1992;305(6866):1395–1399.
32. Duhme H, Weiland SK, Rudolph P, Wienke A, Kramer A, Keil U: Asthma and allergies among children in West and East Germany. A comparison between Münster and Greifswald using the ISAAC phase I protocol. International Study of Asthma and Allergies in Childhood. Eur Respir J 1998;11(4):840–847.
33. Weiland SK, von Mutius E, Hirsch T, Duhme H, Fritzsch C, Werner B, et al: Prevalence of respiratory and atopic disorders among children in the East and West of Germany five years after unification. Eur Respir J 1999;14(4):862–870.
34. Asher MI, Keil U, Anderson HR, Beasley R, Crane J, Martinez F, et al: International Study of Asthma and Allergies in Childhood (ISAAC). Rationale and methods. Eur Respir J 1995;8(3):483–491.
35. Anonymous: Worldwide variation in prevalence of symptoms of asthma, allergic rhinoconjunctivitis, and atopic eczema: ISAAC. The International Study of Asthma and Allergies in Childhood (ISAAC) Steering Committee. Lancet 1998;351(9111):1225–1232.
36. Anonymous: Worldwide variations in the prevalence of asthma symptoms. The International Study of Asthma and Allergies in Childhood (ISAAC). Eur Respir J 1998;12(2):315–335.
37. Strachan D, Sibbald B, Weiland S, Ait-Khaled N, Anabwani G, Anderson HR, et al: Worldwide variations in prevalence of symptoms of allergic rhinoconjunctivitis in children. The International Study of Asthma and Allergies in Childhood (ISAAC). Pediatr Allergy Immunol 1997;8(4):161–176.
38. Williams H, Robertson C, Stewart A, Ait-Khaled N, Anabwani G, Anderson R, et al: Worldwide variations in the prevalence of symptoms of atopic eczema in the International Study of Asthma and Allergies in Childhood. J Allergy Clin Immunol 1999;103(1 Part 1):125–138.
39. Asher M, Weiland S: The International Study of Asthma and Allergies in Childhood (ISAAC). Clin Exp Allergy 1998;28(Suppl 5):52–66, 90–91.
40. Mallol J, Sole D, Asher I, Clayton T, Stein R, Soto-Quiroz M: Prevalence of asthma symptoms in Latin America. The International Study of Asthma and Allergies in Childhood (ISAAC). Pediatr Pulmonol 2000;30(6):439–444.
41. Addo Yobo EO, Custovic A, Taggart SC, Asafo-Agyei AP, Woodcock A: Exercise induced bronchospasm in Ghana. Differences in prevalence between urban and rural schoolchildren. Thorax 1997;52(2):161–165.
42. Keeley DJ, Neill P, Gallivan S: Comparison of the prevalence of reversible airways obstruction in rural and urban Zimbabwean children. Thorax 1991;46(8):549–553.
43. Ng'ang'a LW, Odhiambo JA, Mungai MW, Gicheha CM, Nderitu P, Maingi B, et al: Prevalence of exercise induced bronchospasm in Kenyan school children. An urban-rural comparison. Thorax 1998;53(11):919–926.
44. Odhiambo JA, Ng'ang'a LW, Mungai MW, Gicheha CM, Nyamwaya JK, Karimi F, et al: Urban-rural differences in questionnaire-derived markers of asthma in Kenyan school children. Eur Respir J 1998;12(5):1105–1112.

45. Yemaneberhan H, Bekele Z, Venn A, Lewis S, Parry E, Britton J: Prevalence of wheeze and asthma and relation to atopy in urban and rural Ethiopia [see comments]. Lancet 1997;350(9071):85–90.
46. Waite DA, Eyles EF, Tonkin SL, O'Donnell TV: Asthma prevalence in Tokelauan children in two environments. Clin Allergy 1980;10(1):71–75.
47. Ormerod LP, Myers P, Prescott RJ: Prevalence of asthma and "probable" asthma in the Asian population in Blackburn, U.K. Respir Med 1999; 93(1):16–20.
48. Robertson CF, Dalton MF, Peat JK, Haby MM, Bauman A, Kennedy JD, et al: Asthma and other atopic diseases in Australian children. Australian arm of the International Study of Asthma and Allergy in Childhood. Med J Aust 1998;168(9):434–438.
49. Powell CV, Nolan TM, Carlin JB, Bennett CM, Johnson PD: Respiratory symptoms and duration of residence in immigrant teenagers living in Melbourne, Australia. Arch Dis Child 1999;81(2):159–162.
50. Burr ML, Butland BK, King S, Vaughan-Williams E: Changes in asthma prevalence. Two surveys 15 years apart [see comments]. Arch Dis Child 1989;64(10):1452–1456.
51. Burney PG, Chinn S, Rona RJ: Has the prevalence of asthma increased in children? Evidence from the national study of health and growth 1973–86. BMJ 1990;300(6735):1306–1310.
52. Anderson HR, Butland BK, Strachan DP: Trends in prevalence and severity of childhood asthma. BMJ 1994;308:1600–1604.
53. Rona RJ, Chinn S, Burney PG: Trends in the prevalence of asthma in Scottish and English primary school children 1982–92. Thorax 1995;50(9): 992–993.
54. Omran M, Russell G: Continuing increase in respiratory symptoms and atopy in Aberdeen schoolchildren. BMJ 1996;312(7022):34.
55. Robertson CF, Heycock E, Bishop J, Nolan T, Olinsky A, Phelan PD: Prevalence of asthma in Melbourne schoolchildren. Changes over 26 years [see comments]. BMJ 1991;302(6785):1116–1118.
56. Peat JK, van den Berg RH, Green WF, Mellis CM, Leeder SR, Woolcock AJ: Changing prevalence of asthma in Australian children [see comments]. BMJ 1994;308(6944):1591–1596.
57. Mitchell EA: Increasing prevalence of asthma in children. N Z Med J 1983; 96(734):463–464.
58. Mitchell EA, Asher MI: Prevalence, severity and medical management of asthma in European school children in 1985 and 1991. J Paediatr Child Health 1994;30(5):398–402.
59. Nakagomi T, Itaya H, Tominaga T, Yamaki M, Hisamatsu S, Nakagomi O: Is atopy increasing? Lancet 1994;343(8889):121–122.
60. Ellwood P, Asher MI, Beasley R, Clayton TO, Stewart AW, and the ISAAC Steering Committee: The International Study of Asthma and Allergies in Childhood (ISAAC). Phase three rationale and methods. Int J Tuberculosis Lung Dis 2005;9(1):10–16.
61. Rzehak P, Maziak W, Duhme H, Keil U, Weiland S: Time trends in the prevalence of asthma and allergies among children in Münster, West Germany: 1994/95–1999/2000. Epidemiology 2001;12(4):480.
62. Maziak W, Behrens T, Brasky TM, Duhme H, Rzehak P, Weiland SK, et al: Are asthma and allergies in children and adolescents increasing? Results from ISAAC phase I and phase III surveys in Munster, Germany. Allergy 2003;58(7):572–579.
63. Anderson HR, Ruggles R, Strachan DP, Austin JB, Burr M, Jeffs D, et al: Trends in prevalence of symptoms of asthma, hay fever, and eczema in 12–14 year olds in the British Isles, 1995–2002. Questionnaire survey. BMJ 2004;328(7447):1052–1053.
64. Robertson CF, Roberts MF, Kappers JH: Asthma prevalence in Melbourne schoolchildren. Have we reached the peak? [see comment]. Med J Aust 2004;180(6):273–276.
65. Stevens CA, Turner D, Kuehni CE, Couriel JM, Silverman M: The economic impact of preschool asthma and wheeze. Eur Respir J 2003;21(6): 1000–1006.
66. Masoli M, Fabian D, Holt S, Beasley R: Global Burden of Asthma. Global Initiative for Asthma, 2004.
67. Payne SM, Donahue C, Rappo P, McNamara JJ, Bass J, First L, et al: Variations in pediatric pneumonia and bronchitis/asthma admission rates. Is appropriateness a factor? Arch Pediatr Adolesc Med 1995;149(2): 162–169.
68. Ford JB, Henry RL, Sullivan EA: Comparison of selected reasons for hospitalization of children among children's/tertiary hospitals, Australia, 1996–97 and 1997–98. J Paediatr Child Health 2004;40(7):374–379.
69. Kocevar VS, Bisgaard H, Jonsson L, Valovirta E, Kristensen F, Yin DD, et al: Variations in pediatric asthma hospitalization rates and costs between and within Nordic countries. Chest 2004;125(5):1680–1684.
70. Jackson RT, Mitchell EA: Trends in hospital admission rates and drug treatment of asthma in New Zealand. N Z Med J 1983;96(740):728–730.
71. Mitchell EA: International trends in hospital admission rates for asthma. Arch Dis Child 1985;60(4):376–378.
72. Akinbami LJ, Schoendorf KC: Trends in childhood asthma. Prevalence, health care utilization, and mortality. Pediatrics 2002;110(2 Part 1):315–322.
73. Hyndman SJ, Williams DR, Merrill SL, Lipscombe JM, Palmer CR: Rates of admission to hospital for asthma. BMJ 1994;308(6944):1596–1600.
74. Anonymous: Asthma mortality and hospitalization among children and young adults—United States, 1980–1993. MMWR Morb Mortal Wkly Rep 1996;45(17):350–353.
75. Anderson HR: Increase in hospitalisation for childhood asthma. Arch Dis Child 1978;53(4):295–300.
76. Mitchell EA, Cutler DR: Paediatric admissions to Auckland Hospital for asthma from 1970-1980. N Z Med J 1984;97(749):67–70.
77. Gergen PJ, Weiss KB: Changing patterns of asthma hospitalization among children. 1979 to 1987. JAMA 1990;264(13):1688–1692.
78. MacFaul R: Trends in asthma hospitalisation. Is this related to prevention inhaler usage? Arch Dis Child 2004;89(12):1158–1160.
79. Beasley R: The burden of asthma with specific reference to the United States. J Allergy Clin Immunol 2002;109(5 Suppl).
80. Kemp T, Pearce N: The decline in asthma hospitalisations in persons aged 0–34 years in New Zealand. Aust N Z J Med 1997;27(5):578–581.
81. Sears MR: Changing patterns in asthma morbidity and mortality. J Invest Allergol Clin Immunol 1995;5(2):66–72.
82. Homer CJ, Szilagyi P, Rodewald L, Bloom SR, Greenspan P, Yazdgerdi S, et al: Does quality of care affect rates of hospitalization for childhood asthma? Pediatrics 1996;98(1):18–23.
83. Halfon N, Newacheck PW: Childhood asthma and poverty. Differential impacts and utilization of health services. Pediatrics 1993;91(1):56–61.
84. Finkelstein JA, Brown RW, Schneider LC, Weiss ST, Quintana JM, Goldmann DA, et al: Quality of care for preschool children with asthma. The role of social factors and practice setting. Pediatrics 1995;95(3):389–394.
85. Kattan M, Mitchell H, Eggleston P, Gergen P, Crain E, Redline S, et al: Characteristics of inner-city children with asthma. The National Cooperative Inner-City Asthma Study. Pediatr Pulmonol 1997;24(4):253–262.
86. Kimbell-Dunn M, Pearce N, Beasley R: Seasonal variation in asthma hospitalizations and death rates in New Zealand. Respirology 2000;5(3): 241–246.
87. Weiss KB: Seasonal trends in US asthma hospitalizations and mortality. JAMA 1990;263(17):2323–2328.
88. Khot A, Burn R, Evans N, Lenney C, Lenney W: Seasonal variation and time trends in childhood asthma in England and Wales 1975–81. BMJ 1984;289(6439):235–237.
89. Rasmussen F, Taylor DR, Flannery EM, Cowan JO, Greene JM, Herbison GP, et al: Risk factors for hospital admission for asthma from childhood to young adulthood. A longitudinal population study. J Allergy Clin Immunol 2002;110(2):220–227.
90. Wissow LS, Gittelsohn AM, Szklo M, Starfield B, Mussman M: Poverty, race, and hospitalization for childhood asthma. Am J Public Health 1988; 78(7):777–782.
91. Belessis Y, Dixon S, Thomsen A, Duffy B, Rawlinson W, Henry R, et al: Risk factors for an intensive care unit admission in children with asthma. Pediatr Pulmonol 2004;37(3):201–209.
92. Sly RM: Continuing decreases in asthma mortality in the United States. Ann Allergy Asthma Immunol 2004;92(3):313–318.
93. Beasley CR, Peare NE, Crane J: Worldwide trends in asthma mortality during the twentieth century. In: Sheffer AL, Busse WW, Eggleston PA, Platts-Mills TA, Sears MR, Weiss KB, eds: Fatal Asthma. New York: Marcel Dekker, 1998, pp 13–30.
94. Crane J, Pearce N, Flatt A, Burgess C, Jackson R, Kwong T, et al: Prescribed fenoterol and death from asthma in New Zealand, 1981–83. Case-control study [see comment]. Lancet 1989;1(8644):917–922.
95. Garrett J, Kolbe J, Richards G, Whitlock T, Rea H: Major reduction in asthma morbidity and continued reduction in asthma mortality in New Zealand. What lessons have been learned? [see comment]. Thorax 1995;50(3):303–311.
96. Jackson RT, Beaglehole R, Rea HH, Sutherland DC: Mortality from asthma. A new epidemic in New Zealand. BMJ 1982;285(6344): 771–774.
97. Pearce N, Beasley R, Crane J, Burgess C, Jackson R: End of the New Zealand asthma mortality epidemic [see comment]. Lancet 1995;345(8941): 41–44.
98. Lemanske RF, Larsen GL: Fatal asthma in children. In: Sheffer AL, Busse WW, Eggleston PA, Platts-Mills TA, Sears MR, Weiss KB, eds: Fatal Asthma. New York: Marcel Dekker, 1998, pp 347–362.
99. Comino EJ, Bauman A: Trends in asthma mortality in Australia, 1960–1996. Med J Aust 1998;168(10):525, 527.

100. Campbell MJ, Cogman GR, Holgate ST, Johnston SL: Age specific trends in asthma mortality in England and Wales, 1983–95. Results of an observational study [see comment]. BMJ 1997;314(7092):1439–1441.
101. Comino EJ, Mitchell CA, Bauman A, Henry RL, Robertson CF, Abramson MJ, et al: Asthma management in eastern Australia, 1990 and 1993. Med J Aust 1996;164(7):403–406.
102. Goldman M, Rachmiel M, Gendler L, Katz Y: Decrease in asthma mortality rate in Israel from 1991–1995. Is it related to increased use of inhaled corticosteroids? J Allergy Clin Immunol 2000;105(1 Part 1):71–74.
103. Ernst P, Spitzer WO, Suissa S, Cockcroft D, Habbick B, Horwitz RI, et al: Risk of fatal and near-fatal asthma in relation to inhaled corticosteroid use. JAMA 1992;268(24):3462–3464.
104. Robertson CF, Rubinfeld AR, Bowes G: Pediatric asthma deaths in Victoria. The mild are at risk. Pediatr Pulmonol 1992;13(2):95–100.
105. Fletcher HJ, Ibrahim SA, Speight N: Survey of asthma deaths in the Northern region, 1970–85. Arch Dis Child 1990;65(2):163–167.
106. O'Hollaren MT, Yunginger JW, Offord KP, Somers MJ, O'Connell EJ, Ballard DJ, et al: Exposure to an aeroallergen as a possible precipitating factor in respiratory arrest in young patients with asthma. N Engl J Med 1991;324(6):359–363.
107. Khot A, Burn R: Seasonal variation and time trends of deaths from asthma in England and Wales 1960–82. BMJ 1984;289(6439):233–234.
108. Lanier B: Who is dying of asthma and why? [see comment]. J Pediatrics 1989;115(5 Part 2):838–840.
109. Woolcock AJ: Learning from asthma deaths [comment]. BMJ 1997; 314(7092):1427–1428.
110. Strunk RC, Nicklas RA, Milgrom H, Davis ML, Ikle DN: Risk factors for fatal asthma. In: Sheffer AL, Busse WW, Eggleston PA, Platts-Mills TA, Sears MR, Weiss KB, eds: Fatal Asthma. New York: Marcel Dekker, 1998, pp 31–44.
111. Strunk RC, Mrazek DA, Fuhrmann GS, LaBrecque JF: Physiologic and psychological characteristics associated with deaths due to asthma in childhood. A case-controlled study. JAMA 1985;254(9):1193–1198.
112. Lang DM, Polansky M: Patterns of asthma mortality in Philadelphia from 1969 to 1991. N Engl J Med 1994;331(23):1542–1546.
113. Martinez FD, Graves PE, Baldini M, Solomon S, Erickson R: Association between genetic polymorphisms of the beta2-adrenoceptor and response to albuterol in children with and without a history of wheezing. J Clin Invest 1997;100(12):3184–3188.
114. Yao TC, Kuo ML, See LC, Chen LC, Yan DC, Ou LS, et al: The RANTES promoter polymorphism. A genetic risk factor for near-fatal asthma in Chinese children. J Allergy Clin Immunol 2003;111(6):1285–1292.
115. Koppelman GH, Los H, Postma DS: Genetic and environment in asthma. The answer of twin studies. Eur Respir J 1999;13(1):2–4.
116. Cookson W, Moffatt M: Making sense of asthma genes. N Engl J Med 2004;351(17):1794–1796.
117. Daniels SE, Bhattacharrya S, James A, Leaves NI, Young A, Hill MR, et al: A genome-wide search for quantitative trait loci underlying asthma. Nature 1996;383(6597):247–250.
118. Wahn U, Chuchalin A, Kowalski ML: Prediction and early diagnosis. In: Prevention of Allergy and Allergic Asthma. World Allergy Organization Project Report and Guidelines. Basel, Switzerland: Karger, 2004, pp 128–134.
119. Burrows B, Martinez FD, Halonen M, Barbee RA, Cline MG: Association of asthma with serum IgE levels and skin-test reactivity to allergens. N Engl J Med 1989;320(5):271–277.
120. von Mutius E, Nicolai T: Familial aggregation of asthma in a South Bavarian population. Am J Respir Crit Care Med 1996;153(4 Part 1):1266–1272.
121. Casas R, Bjorksten B: Detection of Fel d 1-immunoglobulin G immune complexes in cord blood and sera from allergic and non-allergic mothers. Pediatr Allergy Immunol 2001;12(2):59–64.
122. Jenmalm MC, Bjorksten B: Cord blood levels of immunoglobulin G subclass antibodies to food and inhalant allergens in relation to maternal atopy and the development of atopic disease during the first 8 years of life. Clin Exp Allergy 2000;30(1):34–40.
123. Warner JO: The early life origins of asthma and related allergic disorders. Arch Dis Child 2004;89(2):97–102.
124. Holloway JA, Warner JO, Vance GH, Diaper ND, Warner JA, Jones CA: Detection of house-dust-mite allergen in amniotic fluid and umbilical-cord blood. Lancet 2000;356(9245):1900–1902.
125. Holloway JW, Holgate ST: Genetics. In: Prevention of Allergy and Allergic Asthma: World Allergy Organization Project Report and Guidelines. Basel, Switzerland: Karger, 2004, pp 1–35.
126. Martinez FD, Wright AL, Taussig LM, Holberg CJ, Halonen M, Morgan WJ: Asthma and wheezing in the first six years of life. The Group Health Medical Associates. N Engl J Med 1995;332(3):133–138.
127. Pearce N, Pekkanen J, Beasley R: How much asthma is really attributable to atopy? Thorax 1999;54(3):268–272.
128. Johansson SG, Bieber T, Dahl R, Friedmann PS, Lanier BQ, Lockey RF, et al: Revised nomenclature for allergy for global use: Report of the Nomenclature Review Committee of the World Allergy Organization, October 2003. J Allergy Clin Immunol 2004;113(5):832–836.
129. Johansson SGO, Haahtela T: Summary and guidelines. In: Prevention of Allergy and Allergic Asthma. World Allergy Organization Project Report and Guidelines. Basel, Switzerland: Karger, 2004, pp 193–199.
130. Asher MI, Dagli E: Environmental influences on asthma and allergy. In: Prevention of Allergy and Allergic Asthma. World Allergy Organization Project Report and Guidelines. Basel, Switzerland: Karger, 2004, pp 36–101.
131. Rose G: The Strategy of Preventive Medicine. Oxford, UK: Oxford University Press, 1992.
132. Stewart AW, Mitchell EA, Pearce N, Strachan DP, Weiland SK, on behalf of the Isaac Steering Committee: The relationship of per capita gross national product to the prevalence of symptoms of asthma and other atopic diseases in children (ISAAC) [see comments]. Int J Epidemiol 2001;30(1):173–179.
133. Ellwood P, Asher MI, Björkstén B, Burr M, Pearce N, Robertson CF, et al: Diet and asthma, allergic rhinoconjunctivitis and atopic eczema symptom prevalence. An ecological analysis of the International Study of Asthma and Allergies in Childhood (ISAAC) data. Eur Respir J 2001;17(3): 436–443.
134. von Mutius E, Pearce N, Beasley R, Cheng S, von Ehrenstein O, Bjorksten B, et al: International patterns of tuberculosis and the prevalence of symptoms of asthma, rhinitis, and eczema [see comments]. Thorax 2000;55(6):449–453.
135. Anderson HR, Poloniecki JD, Strachan DP, Beasley R, Björkstén B, Asher MI, et al: Immunization and symptoms of atopic disease in children: Results from the International Study of Asthma and Allergies in Childhood. Am J Public Health 2001;91(7):1126–1129.
136. Weiland SK, Husing A, Strachan DP, Rzehak P, Pearce N, Group IPOS: Climate and the prevalence of symptoms of asthma, allergic rhinitis, and atopic eczema in children. Occup Environ Med 2004;61(7):609–615.
137. Burr M, Emberlin J, Treu R, Cheng S, Pearce N, ISAAC Phase One Study Group: Pollen counts in relation to the prevalence of allergic rhinoconjunctivitis, asthma and atopic eczema in the International Study of Asthma and Allergies in Childhood (ISAAC). Clin Exp Allergy 2003; 33(12):1675–1680.
138. Mitchell EA, Stewart AW, on behalf of the Isaac Phase One Study Group: The ecological relationship of tobacco smoking to the prevalence of symptoms of asthma and other atopic diseases in children. The International Study of Asthma and Allergies in Childhood (ISAAC). Eur J Epidemiol 2001;17(7):667–673.
139. Foliaki S, Nielsen SK, Bjorksten B, Von Mutius E, Cheng S, Pearce N: Antibiotic sales and the prevalence of symptoms of asthma, rhinitis, and eczema: The International Study of Asthma and Allergies in Childhood (ISAAC). Int J Epidemiol 2004;33(3):558–563.
140. Hodge L, Salome CM, Peat JK, Haby MM, Xuan W, Woolcock AJ: Consumption of oily fish and childhood asthma risk. Med J Aust 1996; 164(3):137–140.
141. Stenius-Aarniala B, Aro A, Hakulinen A, Ahola I, Seppala E, Vapaatalo H: Evening primose oil and fish oil are ineffective as supplementary treatment of bronchial asthma. Ann Allergy 1989;62(6):534–537.
142. Schwartz J, Weiss ST: The relationship of dietary fish intake to level of pulmonary function in the first National Health and Nutrition Survey (NHANES I). Eur Respir J 1994;7(10):1821–1824.
143. Monteleone CA, Sherman AR: Nutrition and asthma. Arch Intern Med 1997;157(1):23–34.
144. Hodge L, Salome CM, Hughes JM, Liu-Brennan D, Rimmer J, Allman M, et al: Effect of dietary intake of omega-3 and omega-6 fatty acids on severity of asthma in children. Eur Respir J 1998;11(2):361–365.
145. Nagakura T, Matsuda S, Shichijyo K, Sugimoto H, Hata K: Dietary supplementation with fish oil rich in omega-3 polyunsaturated fatty acids in children with bronchial asthma. Eur Respir J 2000;16(5):861–865.
146. Dry J, Vincent D: Effect of a fish oil diet on asthma. Results of a 1-year double-blind study. Int Arch Allergy Appl Immunol 1991;95(2–3): 156–157.
147. Hijazi N, Abalkhail B, Seaton A: Diet and childhood asthma in a society in transition. A study in urban and rural Saudi Arabia. Thorax 2000;55(9): 775–779.
148. Seaton A, Godden DJ, Brown K: Increase in asthma. A more toxic environment or a more susceptible population? Thorax 1994;49(2):171–174.
149. Forastiere F, Pistelli R, Sestini P, Fortes C, Renzoni E, Rusconi F, et al: Consumption of fresh fruit rich in vitamin C and wheezing symptoms

in children. SIDRIA Collaborative Group, Italy (Italian Studies on Respiratory Disorders in Children and the Environment). Thorax 2000; 55(4):283–288.

150. Newson RB, Shaheen SO, Chinn S, Burney PG: Paracetamol sales and atopic disease in children and adults. An ecological analysis. Eur Respir J 2000;16(5):817–823.
151. Rubin RN, Navon L, Cassano PA: Relationship of serum antioxidants to asthma prevalence in youth. Am J Respir Crit Care Med 2004;169(3): 393–398.
152. von Mutius E, Weiland SK, Fritzsch C, Duhme H, Keil U: Increasing prevalence of hay fever and atopy among children in Leipzig, East Germany. Lancet 1998;351(9106):862–866.
153. Bolte G, Frye C, Hoelscher B, Meyer I, Wjst M, Heinrich J: Margarine consumption and allergy in children. Am J Respir Crit Care Med 2001; 163(1):277–279.
154. Weiland SK, von Mutius E, Husing A, Asher MI: Intake of trans fatty acids and prevalence of childhood asthma and allergies in Europe. ISAAC Steering Committee. Lancet 1999;353(9169):2040–2041.
155. Leung RC, Carlin JB, Burdon JG, Czarny D: Asthma, allergy and atopy in Asian immigrants in Melbourne. Med J Aust 1994;161(7):418–425.
156. Peat JK, Allen J, Oddy W: Beyond breast-feeding. J Allergy Clin Immunol 1999;104(3 Part 1):526–529.
157. Halken S, Jacobsen HP, Host A, Holmenlund D: The effect of hypo-allergenic formulas in infants at risk of allergic disease. Eur J Clin Nutr 1995;49(Suppl 1):77–83.
158. Fergusson DM, Horwood LJ, Shannon FT: Asthma and infant diet. Arch Dis Child 1983;58(1):48–51.
159. Lucas A, Brooke OG, Morley R, Cole TJ, Bamford MF: Early diet of preterm infants and development of allergic or atopic disease. Randomised prospective study. BMJ 1990;300(6728):837–840.
160. Lewis S, Richards D, Bynner J, Butler N, Britton J: Prospective study of risk factors for early and persistent wheezing in childhood. Eur Respir J 1995;8(3):349–356.
161. Saarinen UM, Kajosaari M: Breastfeeding as prophylaxis against atopic disease. Prospective follow-up study until 17 years old. Lancet 1995; 346(8982):1065–1069.
162. Oddy WH, Holt PG, Sly PD, Read AW, Landau LI, Stanley FJ, et al: Association between breast feeding and asthma in 6 year old children. Findings of a prospective birth cohort study. BMJ 1999;319(7213):815–819.
163. Chandra RK, Singh G, Shridhara B: Effect of feeding whey hydrolysate, soy and conventional cow milk formulas on incidence of atopic disease in high risk infants. Ann Allergy 1989;63(2):102–106.
164. Sears MR, Greene JM, Willan AR, Taylor DR, Flannery EM, Cowan JO, et al: Long-term relation between breastfeeding and development of atopy and asthma in children and young adults. A longitudinal study. Lancet 2002;360(9337):901–907.
165. Peat JK, Allen J, Oddy W, Webb K: Breastfeeding and asthma. Appraising the controversy. Pediatr Pulmonol 2003;35(5):331–334.
166. Sears MR, Taylor DR, Poulton R: Breastfeeding and asthma. Appraising the controversy—A rebuttal [comment]. Pediatr Pulmonol 2003;36(5): 366–368.
167. Sigurs N, Hattevig G, Kjellman B: Maternal avoidance of eggs, cow's milk, and fish during lactation. Effect on allergic manifestations, skin-prick tests, and specific IgE antibodies in children at age 4 years. Pediatrics 1992;89(4 Part 2):735–739.
168. Chandra RK: Prospective studies of the effect of breast feeding on incidence of infection and allergy. Acta Paediatr Scand 1979;68(5):691–694.
169. Barker DJ, Godfrey KM, Fall C, Osmond C, Winter PD, Shaheen SO: Relation of birth weight and childhood respiratory infection to adult lung function and death from chronic obstructive airways disease. BMJ 1991;303(6804):671–675.
170. Falth-Magnusson K, Kjellman NI: Allergy prevention by maternal elimination diet during late pregnancy—a 5-year follow-up of a randomized study. J Allergy Clin Immunol 1992;89(3):709–713.
171. Lilja G, Dannaeus A, Foucard T, Graff-Lonnevig V, Johansson SG, Oman H: Effects of maternal diet during late pregnancy and lactation on the development of atopic diseases in infants up to 18 months of age—in-vivo results. Clin Exp Allergy 1989;19(4):473–479.
172. Seidman DS, Laor A, Gale R, Stevenson DK, Danon YL: Is low birth weight a risk factor for asthma during adolescence? Arch Dis Child 1991; 66(5):584–587.
173. Chinn S, Rona RJ: Can the increase in body mass index explain the rising trend in asthma in children? Thorax 2001;56(11):845–850.
174. Wickens K, Barry D, Friezema A, Rhodius R, Bone N, Purdie G, et al: Obesity and asthma in 11–12 year old New Zealand children in 1989 and 2000. Thorax 2005;60(1):7–12.
175. Romieu I, Mannino DM, Redd SC, McGeehin MA: Dietary intake, physical activity, body mass index, and childhood asthma in the Third National Health and Nutrition Survey (NHANES III). Pediatr Pulmonol 2004;38(1):31–42.
176. Chinn S: Concurrent trends in asthma and obesity. Thorax 2005;60(1):3–4.
177. Shaheen SO: Obesity and asthma. Cause for concern? [editorial; comment]. Clin Exp Allergy 1999;29(3):291–293.
178. Rasmussen F, Lambrechtsen J, Siersted HC, Hansen HS, Hansen NC: Low physical fitness in childhood is associated with the development of asthma in young adulthood. The Odense schoolchild study. Eur Respir J 2000;16(5):866–870.
179. Nystad W, Stigum H, Carlsen KH: Increased level of bronchial responsiveness in inactive children with asthma. Respir Med 2001;95(10):806–810.
180. Strachan DP: Hay fever, hygiene, and household size. BMJ 1989;299 (6710):1259–1260.
181. Strachan DP: Family size, infection and atopy. The first decade of the "hygiene hypothesis." Thorax 2000;55(Suppl 1):2–10.
182. Martinez FD: Viral infections and the development of asthma. Am J Respir Crit Care Med 1995;151(5):1644–1648.
183. Skoner DP, ed. Asthma and Respiratory Infections. New York: Marcel Dekker, 2001.
184. Illi S, von Mutius E, Lau S, Bergmann R, Niggemann B, Sommerfeld C, et al: Early childhood infectious diseases and the development of asthma up to school age. A birth cohort study [see comment]. BMJ 2001;322 (7283):390–395.
185. Strachan DP: The role of environmental factors in asthma. Br Med Bull 2000;56(4):865–882.
186. Stein RT, Sherrill D, Morgan WJ, Holberg CJ, Halonen M, Taussig LM, et al: Respiratory syncytial virus in early life and risk of wheeze and allergy by age 13 years. Lancet 1999;354(9178):541–545.
187. Ball TM, Castro-Rodriguez JA, Griffith KA, Holberg CJ, Martinez FD, Wright AL: Siblings, day-care attendance, and the risk of asthma and wheezing during childhood [see comments]. N Engl J Med 2000;343(8): 538–543.
188. Paunio M, Heinonen OP, Virtanen M, Leinikki P, Patja A, Peltola H: Measles history and atopic diseases. A population-based cross-sectional study. JAMA 2000;283(3):343–346.
189. Forastiere F, Agabiti N, Corbo GM, Dell'Orco V, Porta D, Pistelli R, et al: Socioeconomic status, number of siblings, and respiratory infections in early life as determinants of atopy in children. Epidemiology 1997;8(5): 566–570.
190. Nilsson L, Kjellman NI, Bjorksten B: A randomized controlled trial of the effect of pertussis vaccines on atopic disease. Arch Pediatr Adolesc Med 1998;152(8):734–738.
191. Scrivener S, Yemaneberhan H, Zebenigus M, Tilahun D, Girma S, Ali S, et al: Independent effects of intestinal parasite infection and domestic allergen exposure on risk of wheeze in Ethiopia. A nested case-control study. Lancet 2001;358(9292):1493–1499.
192. Shirakawa T, Enomoto T, Shimazu S, Hopkin JM: The inverse association between tuberculin responses and atopic disorder. Science 1997;275(5296): 77–79.
193. Shirtcliffe P, Weatherall M, Beasley R, International Study of Asthma and Allergies in Childhood: An inverse correlation between estimated tuberculosis notification rates and asthma symptoms. Respirology 2002;7(2):153–155.
194. Odent MR, Culpin EE, Kimmel T: Pertussis vaccination and asthma. Is there a link? [letter; comment]. JAMA 1994;272(8):592–593.
195. Hurwitz EL, Morgenstern H: Effects of diphtheria-tetanus-pertussis or tetanus vaccination on allergies and allergy-related respiratory symptoms among children and adolescents in the United States. J Manipulative Physiol Ther 2000;23(2):81–90.
196. Henderson J, North K, Griffiths M, Harvey I, Golding J: Pertussis vaccination and wheezing illnesses in young children. Prospective cohort study. The Longitudinal Study of Pregnancy and Childhood Team. BMJ 1999;318(7192):1173–1176.
197. Larkin M. Probiotics strain for credibility. Lancet 1999;354(9193):1884.
198. Fang H, Elina T, Heikki A, Seppo S: Modulation of humoral immune response through probiotic intake. FEMS Immunol Med Microbiol 2000;29(1):47–52.
199. Bjorksten B: Allergy priming early in life. Lancet 1999;353(9148): 167–168.
200. Bjorksten B, Naaber P, Sepp E, Mikelsaar M: The intestinal microflora in allergic Estonian and Swedish 2-year-old children. Clin Exp Allergy 1999;29(3):342–346.
201. Kalliomaki M, Salminen S, Arvilommi H, Kero P, Koskinen P, Isolauri E: Probiotics in primary prevention of atopic disease. A randomised placebo-controlled trial. Lancet 2001;357(9262):1076–1079.

202. Helin T, Haahtela S, Haahtela T: No effect of oral treatment with an intestinal bacterial strain, Lactobacillus rhamnosus (ATCC 53103), on birch-pollen allergy. A placebo-controlled double-blind study. Allergy 2002; 57(3):243–246.
203. Celedon JC, Litonjua AA, Ryan L, Weiss ST, Gold DR: Lack of association between antibiotic use in the first year of life and asthma, allergic rhinitis, or eczema at age 5 years. Am J Respir Crit Care Med 2002;166(1):72–75.
204. von Mutius E: Environmental factors influencing the development and progression of pediatric asthma. J Allergy Clin Immunol 2002;109(6 Suppl).
205. Braback L: Does farming provide protection from asthma and allergies? [comment]. Acta Paediatr 2002;91(11):1147–1149.
206. Braun-Fahrlander C, Gassner M, Grize L, Neu U, Sennhauser FH, Varonier HS, et al: Prevalence of hay fever and allergic sensitization in farmer's children and their peers living in the same rural community. SCARPOL team. Swiss Study on Childhood Allergy and Respiratory Symptoms with Respect to Air Pollution. Clin Exp Allergy 1999;29(1): 28–34.
207. Kilpelainen M, Terho EO, Helenius H, Koskenvuo M: Farm environment in childhood prevents the development of allergies. Clin Exp Allergy 2000;30(2):201–208.
208. Riedler J, Eder W, Oberfeld G, Schreuer M: Austrian children living on a farm have less hay fever, asthma and allergic sensitization. Clin Exp Allergy 2000;30(2):194–200.
209. Riedler J, Braun-Fahrlander C, Eder W, Schreuer M, Waser M, Maisch S, et al: Exposure to farming in early life and development of asthma and allergy. A cross-sectional survey. Lancet 2001;358(9288):1129–1133.
210. Remes ST, Pekkanen J, Soininen L, Kajosaari M, Husman T, Koivikko A: Does heredity modify the association between farming and allergy in children? [see comment]. Acta Paediatr 2002;91(11):1163–1169.
211. Leynaert B, Neukirch C, Jarvis D, Chinn S, Burney P, Neukirch F, et al: Does living on a farm during childhood protect against asthma, allergic rhinitis, and atopy in adulthood? Am J Respir Crit Care Med 2001;164(10 Part 1):1829–1834.
212. Melsom T, Brinch L, Hessen JO, Schei MA, Kolstrup N, Jacobsen BK, et al: Asthma and indoor environment in Nepal. Thorax 2001;56(6):477–481.
213. Barnes M, Cullinan P, Athanasaki P, MacNeill S, Hole AM, Harris J, et al: Crete. Does farming explain urban and rural differences in atopy? Clin Exp Allergy 2001;31(12):1822–1828.
214. Ernst P, Cormier Y: Relative scarcity of asthma and atopy among rural adolescents raised on a farm. Am J Respir Crit Care Med 2000;161(5): 1563–1566.
215. Downs SH, Marks GB, Mitakakis TZ, Leuppi JD, Car NG, Peat JK: Having lived on a farm and protection against allergic diseases in Australia. Clin Exp Allergy 2001;31(4):570–575.
216. Wickens K, Lane JM, Fitzharris P, Siebers R, Riley G, Douwes J, et al: Farm residence and exposures and the risk of allergic diseases in New Zealand children. Allergy 2002;57(12):1171–1179.
217. Von Ehrenstein OS, Von Mutius E, Illi S, Baumann L, Bohm O, von Kries R: Reduced risk of hay fever and asthma among children of farmers [see comments]. Clin Exp Allergy 2000;30(2):187–193.
218. von Mutius E, Braun-Fahrlander C, Schierl R, Riedler J, Ehlermann S, Maisch S, et al: Exposure to endotoxin or other bacterial components might protect against the development of atopy. Clin Exp Allergy 2000; 30(9):1230–1234.
219. Shaheen SO, Aaby P, Hall AJ, Barker DJ, Heyes CB, Shiell AW, et al: Measles and atopy in Guinea-Bissau [see comments]. Lancet 1996;347 (9018):1792–1796.
220. Douwes J, Le Gros G, Gibson P, Pearce N: Can bacterial endotoxin exposure reverse atopy and atopic disease? J Allergy Clin Immunol 2004;114(5):1051–1054.
221. Litonjua AA, Milton DK, Celedon JC, Ryan L, Weiss ST, Gold DR: A longitudinal analysis of wheezing in young children. The independent effects of early life exposure to house dust endotoxin, allergens, and pets. J Allergy Clin Immunol 2002;110(5):736–742.
222. Tovey E, Marks G: Methods and effectiveness of environmental control. J Allergy Clin Immunol 1999;103(2 Part 1):179–191.
223. Celenza A, Fothergill J, Kupek E, Shaw RJ: Thunderstorm associated asthma. A detailed analysis of environmental factors. BMJ 1996;312(7031): 604–607.
224. Sears MR, Herbison GP, Holdaway MD, Hewitt CJ, Flannery EM, Silva PA: The relative risks of sensitivity to grass pollen, house dust mite and cat dander in the development of childhood asthma. Clin Exp Allergy 1989;19(4):419–424.
225. Platts-Mills TA, Thomas WR, Aalberse RC, Vervloet D, Champman MD: Dust mite allergens and asthma. Report of a second international workshop. J Allergy Clin Immunol 1992;89(5):1046–1060.
226. Butland BK, Strachan DP, Anderson HR: The home environment and asthma symptoms in childhood. Two population based case-control studies 13 years apart. Thorax 1997;52(7):618–624.
227. Perzanowski MS, Sporik R, Squillace SP, Gelber LE, Call R, Carter M, et al: Association of sensitization to Alternaria allergens with asthma among school-age children. J Allergy Clin Immunol 1998;101(5):626–632.
228. Halonen M, Stern DA, Wright AL, Taussig LM, Martinez FD: Alternaria as a major allergen for asthma in children raised in a desert environment. Am J Respir Crit Care Med 1997;155(4):1356–1361.
229. Rosenstreich DL, Eggleston P, Kattan M, Baker D, Slavin RG, Gergen P, et al: The role of cockroach allergy and exposure to cockroach allergen in causing morbidity among inner-city children with asthma. N Engl J Med 1997;336(19):1356–1363.
230. Sarpong SB, Wood RA, Karrison T, Eggleston PA: Cockroach allergen (Bla g 1) in school dust. J Allergy Clin Immunol 1997;99(4):486–492.
231. Custovic A, Simpson A, Pahdi H, Green RM, Chapman MD, Woodcock A: Distribution, aerodynamic characteristics, and removal of the major cat allergen Fel d 1 in British homes. Thorax 1998;53(1):33–38.
232. Brunekreef B, Groot B, Hoek G: Pets, allergy and respiratory symptoms in children. Int J Epidemiol 1992;21(2):338–342.
233. Henriksen AH, Holmen TL, Bjermer L: Sensitization and exposure to pet allergens in asthmatics versus non-asthmatics with allergic rhinitis. Respir Med 2001;95(2):122–129.
234. Hesselmar B, Aberg N, Aberg B, Eriksson B, Bjorksten B: Does early exposure to cat or dog protect against later allergy development? Clin Exp Allergy 1999;29(5):611–617.
235. Pokharel PK, Kabra SK, Kapoor SK, Pandey RM: Risk factors associated with bronchial asthma in school going children of rural Haryana. Indian J Pediatr 2001;68(2):103–106.
236. Wahn U, Lau S, Bergmann R, Kulig M, Forster J, Bergmann K, et al: Indoor allergen exposure is a risk factor for sensitization during the first three years of life. J Allergy Clin Immunol 1997;99(6 Part 1):763–769.
237. Gøtzsche PC, Johansen HK, Hammarquist C, Burr ML: House dust mite control measures for asthma (Cochrane Review). In: The Cochrane Library, Issue 2. Oxford, UK: Update Software, 2001.
238. Oryszczyn MP, Godin J, Annesi I, Hellier G, Kauffmann F: In utero exposure to parental smoking, cotinine measurements, and cord blood IgE. J Allergy Clin Immunol 1991;87(6):1169–1174.
239. Ownby DR, Johnson CC, Peterson EL: Maternal smoking does not influence cord serum IgE or IgD concentrations. J Allergy Clin Immunol 1991;88(4):555–560.
240. Berrak GS, Ozek E, Cebeci D, Karakoc F, Yusufoglu C, Basaran M, et al: Effects of active and/or passive smoking on cord blood cotinine, IgE concentrations and eosinophil count (abstract). Eur Respir J 1997;10(Suppl):334.
241. Gilliland FD, Berhane K, McConnell R, Gauderman WJ, Vora H, Rappaport EB, et al: Maternal smoking during pregnancy, environmental tobacco smoke exposure and childhood lung function. Thorax 2000; 55(4):271–276.
242. Stein RT, Holberg CJ, Sherrill D, Wright AL, Morgan WJ, Taussig L, et al: Influence of parental smoking on respiratory symptoms during the first decade of life. The Tucson Children's Respiratory Study. Am J Epidemiol 1999;149(11):1030–1037.
243. Cook DG, Strachan DP, Carey IM: Health effects of passive smoking. 9. Parental smoking and spirometric indices in children [see comments]. Thorax 1998;53(10):884–893.
244. Cook DG, Strachan DP: Parental smoking, bronchial reactivity and peak flow variability in children. Thorax 1998;53(4):295–301.
245. Strachan DP, Cook DG: Health effects of passive smoking. 6. Parental smoking and childhood asthma. Longitudinal and case-control studies. Thorax 1998;53(3):204–212.
246. Lewis SA, Britton JR: Consistent effects of high socioeconomic status and low birth order, and the modifying effect of maternal smoking on the risk of allergic disease during childhood. Respir Med 1998;92(10):1237–1244.
247. Evans D, Levison MJ, Feldman CH, Clark NM, Wasilewski Y, Levin B, et al: The impact of passive smoking on emergency room visits of urban children with asthma. Am Rev Respir Dis 1987;135(3):567–572.
248. Murray AB, Morrison BJ: The decrease in severity of asthma in children of parents who smoke since the parents have been exposing them to less cigarette smoke. J Allergy Clin Immunol 1993;91(1 Part 1):102–110.
249. Murray CS, Woodcock A, Smillie FI, Cain G, Kissen P, Custovic A, et al: Tobacco smoke exposure, wheeze, and atopy. Pediatr Pulmonol 2004; 37(6):492–498.
250. Wahlgren DR, Hovell MF, Meltzer EO, Meltzer SB: Involuntary smoking and asthma. Curr Opin Pulm Med 2000;6(1):31–36.
251. Thomson NC, Chaudhuri R, Livingston E: Asthma and cigarette smoking. Eur Respir J 2004;24(5):822–833.

252. Verhoeff AP, van Strien RT, van Wijnen JH, Brunekreef B: Damp housing and childhood respiratory symptoms. The role of sensitization to dust mites and molds. Am J Epidemiol 1995;141(2):103–110.
253. Brunekreef B, Dockery DW, Speizer FE, Ware JH, Spengler JD, Ferris BG: Home dampness and respiratory morbidity in children. Am Rev Respir Dis 1989;140(5):1363–1367.
254. Katz Y, Verleger H, Barr J, Rachmiel M, Kiviti S, Kuttin ES: Indoor survey of moulds and prevalence of mould atopy in Israel. Clin Exp Allergy 1999;29(2):186–192.
255. Strachan DP: Damp housing and childhood asthma. Validation of reporting of symptoms. BMJ 1988;297(6658):1223–1226.
256. Strachan DP, Sanders CH: Damp housing and childhood asthma. Respiratory effects of indoor air temperature and relative humidity. J Epidemiol Commun Health 1989;43(1):7–14.
257. Chauhan AJ, Krishna MT, Frew AJ, Holgate ST: Exposure to nitrogen dioxide (NO_2) and respiratory disease risk. Rev Environ Health 1998; 13(1–2):73–90.
258. Garrett MH, Hooper MA, Hooper BM, Abramson MJ: Respiratory symptoms in children and indoor exposure to nitrogen dioxide and gas stoves. Am J Respir Crit Care Med 1998;158(3):891–895.
259. Smith BJ, Nitschke M, Pilotto LS, Ruffin RE, Pisaniello DL, Willson KJ: Health effects of daily indoor nitrogen dioxide exposure in people with asthma. Eur Respir J 2000;16(5):879–885.
260. von Mutius E, Illi S, Nicolai T, Martinez FD: Relation of indoor heating with asthma, allergic sensitisation, and bronchial responsiveness. Survey of children in south Bavaria. BMJ 1996;312(7044):1448–1450.
261. Becher R, Hongslo JK, Jantunen MJ, Dybing E: Environmental chemicals relevant for respiratory hypersensitivity. The indoor environment. Toxicol Lett 1996;86(2–3):155–162.
262. Garrett MH, Hooper MA, Hooper BM, Rayment PR, Abramson MJ: Increased risk of allergy in children due to formaldehyde exposure in homes. Allergy 1999;54(4):330–337.
263. Sherriff A, Farrow A, Golding J, Henderson J: Frequent use of chemical household products is associated with persistent wheezing in pre-school age children. Thorax 2005;60(1):45–49.
264. Stevens E, Cullinan P, Colvile R: Urban air pollution and children's asthma. What do parents and health professionals think? Pediatr Pulmonol 2004;37(6):530–536.
265. Migliaretti G, Cavallo F: Urban air pollution and asthma in children. Pediatr Pulmonol 2004;38(3):198–203.
266. Anto JM, Sunyer J: Nitrogen dioxide and allergic asthma. Starting to clarify an obscure association. Lancet 1995;345(8947):402–403.
267. Hirsch T, Range U, Walther KU, Hederer B, Lassig S, Frey G, et al: Prevalence and determinants of house dust mite allergen in East German homes. Clin Exp Allergy 1998;28(8):956–964.
268. Braun-Fahrlander C, Vuille JC, Sennhauser FH, Neu U, Kunzle T, Grize L, et al: Respiratory health and long-term exposure to air pollutants in Swiss schoolchildren. SCARPOL Team. Swiss Study on Childhood Allergy and Respiratory Symptoms with Respect to Air Pollution, Climate and Pollen. Am J Respir Crit Care Med 1997;155(3):1042–1049.
269. Shima M, Adachi M: Effect of outdoor and indoor nitrogen dioxide on respiratory symptoms in schoolchildren. Int J Epidemiol 2000;29(5):862–870.
270. Weiland SK, Mundt KA, Ruckmann A, Keil U: Self-reported wheezing and allergic rhinitis in children and traffic density on street of residence. Ann Epidemiol 1994;4(3):243–247.
271. Duhme H, Weiland SK, Keil U: Epidemiological analyses of the relationship between environmental pollution and asthma. Toxicol Lett 1998;102–103:307–316.
272. Brunekreef B, Janssen NA, de Hartog J, Harssema H, Knape M, van Vliet P: Air pollution from truck traffic and lung function in children living near motorways. Epidemiology 1997;8(3):298–303.
273. Gielen MH, van der Zee SC, van Wijnen JH, van Steen CJ, Brunekreef B: Acute effects of summer air pollution on respiratory health of asthmatic children. Am J Respir Crit Care Med 1997;155(6):2105–2108.
274. Ciccone G, Forastiere F, Agabiti N, Biggeri A, Bisanti L, Chellini E, et al: Road traffic and adverse respiratory effects in children. SIDRIA Collaborative Group. Occup Environ Med 1998;55(11):771–778.
275. Edwards J, Walters S, Griffiths RK: Hospital admissions for asthma in preschool children. Relationship to major roads in Birmingham, United Kingdom. Arch Environ Health 1994;49(4):223–227.
276. Nicolai T, Carr D, Weiland SK, Duhme H, von Ehrenstein O, Wagner C, et al: Urban traffic and pollutant exposure related to respiratory outcomes and atopy in a large sample of children [see comment]. Eur Respir J 2003;21(6):956–963.
277. Brunekreef B, Sunyer J: Asthma, rhinitis and air pollution. Is traffic to blame? [comment]. Eur Respir J 2003;21(6):913–915.
278. Duran-Tauleria E, Rona RJ: Geographical and socioeconomic variation in the prevalence of asthma symptoms in English and Scottish children [see comment]. Thorax 1999;54(6):476–481.
279. Williams HC, Strachan DP, Hay RJ: Childhood eczema. Disease of the advantaged? BMJ 1994;308(6937):1132–1135.
280. Burr ML, Verrall C, Kaur B: Social deprivation and asthma. Respir Med 1997;91(10):603–608.
281. Poyser MA, Nelson H, Ehrlich RI, Bateman ED, Parnell S, Puterman A, et al: Socioeconomic deprivation and asthma prevalence and severity in young adolescents. Eur Respir J 2002;19(5):892–898.
282. Cesaroni G, Farchi S, Davoli M, Forastiere F, Perucci CA: Individual and area-based indicators of socioeconomic status and childhood asthma. Eur Respir J 2003;22(4):619–624.
283. Mitchell EA, Stewart AW, Pattemore PK, Asher MI, Harrison AC, Rea HH: Socioeconomic status in childhood asthma. Int J Epidemiol 1989; 18(4):888–890.
284. Pattemore PK, Ellison-Loschmann L, Asher MI, Barry DM, Clayton TO, Crane J, et al: Asthma prevalence in European, Maori, and Pacific children in New Zealand. ISAAC study. Pediatr Pulmonol 2004;37(5): 433–442.
285. Hales S, Lewis S, Slater T, Crane J, Pearce N: Prevalence of adult asthma symptoms in relation to climate in New Zealand. Environ Health Perspect 1998;106(9):607–610.
286. Carey MJ, Cordon I: Asthma and climatic conditions. Experience from Bermuda, an isolated island community. BMJ 1986;293(6551):843–844.
287. Cullen KJ: Climate and chest disorders in schoolchildren. BMJ 1972; 4(832):65–67.
288. Newson R, Strachan D, Archibald E, Emberlin J, Hardaker P, Collier C: Effect of thunderstorms and airborne grass pollen on the incidence of acute asthma in England, 1990–94. Thorax 1997;52(8):680–685.
289. Allegra L, Cogo A, Legnani D, Diano PL, Fasano V, Negretto GG: High altitude exposure reduces bronchial responsiveness to hypo-osmolar aerosol in lowland asthmatics. Eur Respir J 1995;8(11):1842–1846.
290. Strachan DP, Butland BK, Anderson HR: Incidence and prognosis of asthma and wheezing illness from early childhood to age 33 in a national British cohort. BMJ 1996;312(7040):1195–1199.
291. Sears MR, Greene JM, Willan AR, Wiecek EM, Taylor DR, Flannery EM, et al: A longitudinal, population-based, cohort study of childhood asthma followed to adulthood [see comment]. N Engl J Med 2003;349(15): 1414–1422.
292. Sears MR: Growing up with asthma. BMJ 1994;309(6947):72–73.
293. Oswald H, Phelan PD, Lanigan A, Hibbert M, Bowes G, Olinsky A: Outcome of childhood asthma in mid-adult life. BMJ 1994;309(6947): 95–96.
294. Jenkins MA, Hopper JL, Bowes G, Carlin JB, Flander LB, Giles GG: Factors in childhood as predictors of asthma in adult life. BMJ 1994; 309(6947):90–93.
295. Martin AJ, McLennan LA, Landau LI, Phelan PD: The natural history of childhood asthma to adult life. BMJ 1980;280(6229):1397–1400.
296. Clifford RD, Radford M, Howell JB, Holgate ST: Prevalence of respiratory symptoms among 7 and 11 year old schoolchildren and association with asthma. Arch Dis Child 1989;64(8):1118–1125.
297. Anderson HR, Pottier AC, Strachan DP: Asthma from birth to age 23. Incidence and relation to prior and concurrent atopic disease. Thorax 1992;47(7):537–542.
298. Guill MF: Asthma update. Epidemiology and pathophysiology. Pediatr Rev 2004;25(9):299–305.
299. Castro-Rodriguez JA, Holberg CJ, Wright AL, Martinez FD: A clinical index to define risk of asthma in young children with recurrent wheezing. Am J Respir Crit Care Med 2000;162(4 Part 1):1403–1406.
300. Peat JK, Tovey E, Gray EJ, Mellis CM, Woolcock AJ: Asthma severity and morbidity in a population sample of Sydney schoolchildren. Part II—Importance of house dust mite allergens. Aust N Z J Med 1994;24(3): 270–276.
301. Nelson HS: The importance of allergens in the development of asthma and the persistence of symptoms. J Allergy Clin Immunol 2000;105(6 Part 2; Suppl):628–632.
302. Ponsonby AL, Gatenby P, Glasgow N, Mullins R, McDonald T, Hurwitz M: Which clinical subgroups within the spectrum of child asthma are attributable to atopy? [see comment]. Chest 2002;121(1):135–142.
303. Peat JK, Toelle BG, Mellis CM: Problems and possibilities in understanding the natural history of asthma. J Allergy Clin Immunol 2000;106(3 Suppl): 144–152.
304. Burrows B, Sears MR, Flannery EM, Herbison GP, Holdaway MD, Silva PA: Relation of the course of bronchial responsiveness from age 9 to age 15 to allergy. Am J Respir Crit Care Med 1995;152(4 Part 1):1302–1308.

305. Kagamimori S, Naruse Y, Kakiuchi H, Yamagami T, Sokejima S, Matsubara I, et al: Does an allergy skin test on school-children predict respiratory symptoms in adulthood? Clin Exp Allergy 1996;26(3):262–269.
306. Sherrill D, Stein R, Kurzius-Spencer M, Martinez F: On early sensitization to allergens and development of respiratory symptoms. Clin Exp Allergy 1999;29(7):905–911.
307. Forastiere F, Corbo GM, Dell'Orco V, Pistelli R, Agabiti N, Kriebel D: A longitudinal evaluation of bronchial responsiveness to methacholine in children. Role of baseline lung function, gender, and change in atopic status. Am J Respir Crit Care Med 1996;153(3):1098–1104.
308. Ulrik CS, Backer V: Increased bronchial responsiveness to exercise as a risk factor for symptomatic asthma. Findings from a longitudinal population study of children and adolescents. Eur Respir J 1996;9(8):1696–1700.
309. Sackett DL: On some clinically useful measures of the effects of treatment. Evidence-Based Med 1996;1:37–38.

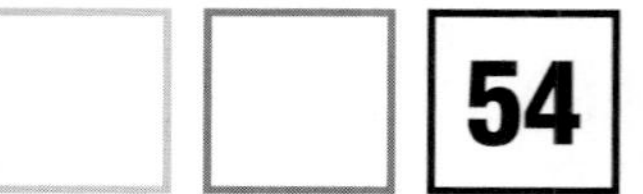

54 Immunopathogenesis of Asthma

Thomas A.E. Platts-Mills, MD •
Peter W. Heymann, MD

Wheezing in childhood has become progressively more common as a cause for visits to physicians, emergency rooms, or hospital.[1–3] Some of the increase may reflect misdiagnoses, overanxious parents, or shortage of breath in unfit children. However, the large majority of children receiving treatment have objective evidence of asthma: audible wheezing on chest examination, reversible changes in expiratory flow, or bronchial hyperreactivity (BHR). A large proportion of these children also have indirect evidence of inflammation, which includes elevated exhaled nitric oxide (NO), lowered pH of lung condensate, and peripheral blood eosinophilia, as well as evidence of allergic sensitization.[4–7] The general acceptance that asthma is an inflammatory disease came partly from biopsy studies but, more significantly, from the evidence that steroid treatment is effective, and the reversibility of BHR with prolonged allergen avoidance.[8,9] The fact that lung inflammation and attacks of asthma can be caused by allergen exposure is undoubted. Many children are aware of acute episodes related to visiting a house with an animal. In addition, bronchial challenge can induce both eosinophil infiltration of the lungs and prolonged increases in BHR as well as acute changes in forced expiratory volume in 1 second (FEV_1). Indeed, the only consistent method of inducing "inflammation" in the lungs is to put allergen into the lungs of an allergic subject. However, bronchial challenge or segmental challenge is not the same as natural exposure. Not only is the quantity of allergen inhaled much greater, but the number of particles and the size of particles is dramatically different. The natural form of exposure to allergens is as a relatively small number of particles that are 2 to 20 μm in diameter. These are inhaled over prolonged periods (i.e., months or all year round). Only a small proportion of naturally occurring attacks of asthma appear to be directly related to increased exposure. It appears more likely that allergen exposure plays a chronic role in maintaining bronchial inflammation and reactivity.

Although many different foreign proteins can give rise to sensitization, a select group dominates the epidemiology of asthma. This group includes mites, cat, dog, cockroach, and the fungus *Alternaria*. The main characteristic of these protein sources may be the fact that exposure is perennial. However, recent evidence suggests that the allergens are not equal; either the properties of the protein or the nature of the particles may influence the immune response sufficiently to influence both the prevalence and titer of immunoglobulin E (IgE) antibody responses.

Understanding the immunopathogenesis of asthma is important intellectually because it has to be taken into account in hypotheses about the increase in asthma. In addition, understanding the immunopathogenesis is important as part of the rationale for allergen-specific treatment and pharmacologic anti-inflammatory treatment. Although short-term increases in allergen exposure are not thought to be an important precipitant of acute episodes of asthma, there is a very strong association between immediate hypersensitivity and acute episodes. In part, this may reflect the increased BHR associated with elevated IgE and IgE antibodies. More significant may be recent evidence that the impact of rhinovirus infections on the lungs is strongly related to elevated IgE and elevated IgE antibodies.[10,11]

■ THE RELATIONSHIP BETWEEN ALLERGENS, ALLERGEN SENSITIZATION, AND ASTHMA

The evidence that allergens play a causal role in asthma comes from a wide variety of experiments (Box 54-1).[12] However, the primary evidence concerns the association between sensitization and asthma. These studies are case control, population based, and prospective, but in all cases the evidence for sensitization comes from measurement of IgE antibodies or immediate responses to skin testing. Although the implication of these studies is that allergen entering the lungs plays an important role in lung inflammation, only a minority of studies show a clear dose response between exposure and asthma symptoms. On the other hand, there are no studies showing a relationship between inhaled allergens and asthma in nonallergic individuals. The most likely explanation of dose-response data (i.e., lack of simple dose response to relationship) comes from (1) the effect of sensitization, (2) the inaccuracy of the measurements of allergen exposure, (3) differences between allergen sources, and (4) the fact that most acute episodes, and probably most episodes of wheezing, are triggered by one of the many nonspecific factors that can contribute to symptoms (Fig. 54-1).

■ THE ALLERGENS ASSOCIATED WITH ASTHMA

Dozens if not hundreds of sources of allergens have been associated with asthma. However, there are only a few that are common enough to play a role in epidemiologic studies, and most of these are either perennial indoor allergens or have a long season (Table 54-1). The first studies used "house dust" to skin test, but because it was impossible to define what was in the extract, it was difficult to take the results seriously.[13] The discovery or definition of house dust mites was a critical event in understanding the pathogenesis of asthma. Voorhorst and Spieksmah identified *Dermatophagoides pteronyssinus* in dust and developed skin test reagents. It rapidly became obvious that dust mites were an extraordinarily important cause of sensitization in all countries where the humidity was high enough to support their growth.[9,14] The reasons why dust mites are so important are still not clear. It could reflect their presence in bedding; the nature of the particles that become airborne; the biochemical/immunologic nature of the allergens; or some other factor present in the particles (e.g., endotoxin).[15,16]

BOX 54-1 Hill's Criteria for Causality and the Evidence Supporting a Causal Link between Mite Allergen Exposure of a Sensitive Person and the Development of Asthma

1. The strength of the association is large and has been supported by:
   A. Population studies
   B. Control studies
   C. Prospective studies
2. Repeated observations in different populations have consistent findings: Europe, United States, Australia, New Zealand, and Japan.
3. A cause leads to a specific effect: asthma is the only lung disease that has been associated with sensitivity to inhalant allergens.
4. A cause precedes an effect.
5. There is a dose-response gradient: good evidence for dust mite and cockroach allergens.
6. There is experimental evidence from:
   A. Avoidance studies
   B. Challenge studies
7. The mechanism is biologically plausible.

The other allergens that appear to play an important role in asthma include cats, dogs, rodents, and cockroaches, all of which are predominantly inside the house. Although pollens are an important source of sensitization and can cause asthma, seasonal asthma is generally less severe and is often not consistent from one year to the next. Sensitization to fungi is also observed in children with asthma. However, there are great problems with the consistency of the fungal extracts, and there is no consistent method for measuring mold allergens indoors. The only molds that are thought to play an important role in childhood asthma are *Alternaria* and *Aspergillus*.[17,18]

The obvious common feature of the allergens listed in Table 54-1 is that they are perennial. While in most cases this means indoor, it may not be true for the fungi. Inhalation of dust mite and cockroach allergens is thought to be largely in the patients' house. For many years it was assumed that all significant exposure to the indoor allergens occurred at home. This concept has had to be revised, because it is now clear that significant exposure to cat and mite allergens can and does occur outside the child's home. For cat and dog, significant allergen is present in schools and also most houses that do not have a cat. Furthermore, there is extensive evidence that the quantities found away from animals are sufficient to sensitize.[19,20] Indeed, in a recent study, 80% of the children who were skin test positive to cat allergen had never lived in a house with a cat. The message is that preventing primary exposure to animal dander is not possible. Dust mite allergens are not widely distributed away from the sites of mite growth, but children may get high exposure in daycare centers or in Granny's house.[21] The effects of exposure to mite outside the child's house for a week or two, or of exposure in daycare 3 days a week, are not known. However, one explanation of the lack of success of primary avoidance studies is that sensitization can occur outside the house. Some of the recent studies suggest that avoidance measures at home can prevent the lung effects of sensitization even if they cannot prevent sensitization.[21]

The importance of cockroaches as a source of allergen in the United States has become obvious.[5,22] Most of the published data relate to cockroach-derived allergens in the patients' home or own bedroom.[23] On the other hand, it is well recognized that many children spend time living in the houses of friends or relatives, and this is particularly common among children in the cities. The implication is that exposure outside the child's normal home could be relevant to both sensitization and ongoing symptoms.

■ ALLERGEN PROTEINS

Over the past 20 years, a large number of proteins have been identified and cloned. In many cases the proteins show sequence

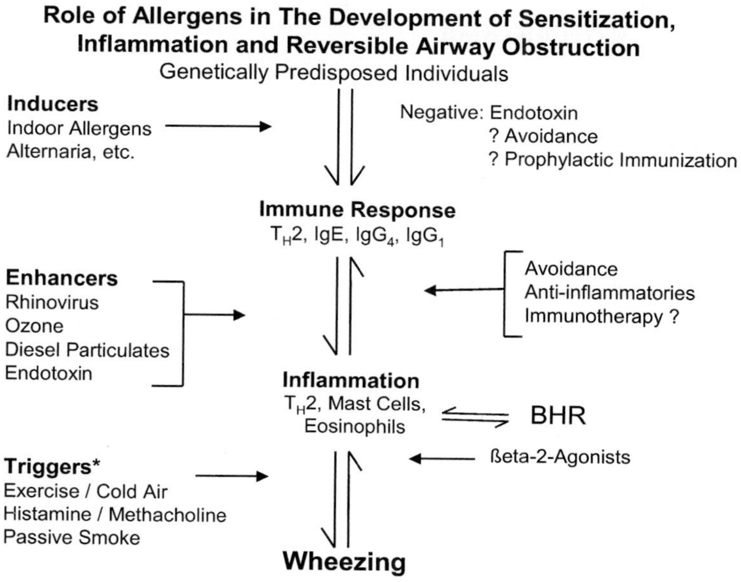

■ **FIGURE 54-1.** The immune response to allergens requires exposure, but the time course and the dose response are variable. On its own, this response is asymptomatic. Continued exposure to allergen gives rise to inflammation, and this response can be enhanced by diesel particulates, endotoxin, or rhinovirus infection. Inflammation is not necessarily associated with symptoms, but most of the patients have increased BHR, so that bronchospasm can easily be triggered.

■ **TABLE 54-1.** Properties of indoor allergens: 2005

Source	Airborne Particles	Size	Allergen		Function/Homology
Dust mite *Dermatophagoides pteronyssinus*	Feces	10–40 μm	Der p 1	25 kd	Cysteine protease
			Der p 2	13 kd	Epididymal protein
German cockroach *Blattella germanica*	Frass saliva	>5 μm	Bla g 2	36 kd	Aspartic protease
			Bla g 5	23 kd	GST
Cat *Felis domesticus*	Dander particles		Fel d 1	36 kd	Uteroglobin
Dog *Canis familiaris*		2–15 μm	Can f 1	21 kd	Lipocalin
Mouse *Mus domesticus*	Urine on bedding, etc.	2–20 μm	Mus m 1	22 kd	MUP
Rat *Rattus norwegicus*			Rat n 1	19 kd	Pheromone binding
Grass	Pollen	30 μm	Lol p 1	29 kd	Cysteine proteinase

For details of properties of allergens, see www.allergen.org.

homology with other proteins that have a defined function (e.g., proteinases, transport proteins, and profilins).[24,25] It is important to remember that sequence homology does not define function: enzymic activity in particular can be completely lost with minor changes in structure.[26] On the other hand, the mite allergen Der p1 is a cysteine protease, and can act on many proteins including CD-25 and CD-23.[25] Although this protein can cleave biologically relevant surface antigens and can open up tight junctions in vitro, it is much more difficult to establish that these activities are relevant to its allergenicity.[24] Certainly, enzymic activity is not a necessary property of allergens since many major allergens are not enzymes (e.g., Fel d 1, Der p 2, Bla g 2). The recent evidence about mechanisms of tolerance to cat allergens suggest that the structure of the allergen is significant. However, it is not clear whether this reflects the primary structure, the tertiary structure, or the biologic properties of the allergens. The allergen proteins do have some physical properties in common. In particular, the molecular weight is generally between 15 and 40 kd. In addition, the proteins are almost all freely soluble in aqueous solution and are antigenically foreign. Thus, the simple view had been that all proteins that were soluble and were inhaled could give rise to an IgE antibody response in children and thus could become an allergen. In the past 5 years it has become clear that all allergens are not "created equal."

■ AIRBORNE PARTICLES CARRYING FOREIGN PROTEINS, RELEVANCE TO EXPOSURE, AND DEPOSITION IN THE CHEST

The saturated vapor pressure of molecules the size of allergens is close to zero. Thus, airborne exposure to allergens is only in the form of particles, and these are dramatically different from one source to another. In the outdoor air, most particles can be identified under a microscope (e.g., pollen grains and fungal spores). Most areas have regular counts of pollen grains and mold spores reported to the public. By contrast, the particles on which mite, cat, dog, and cockroach allergens become airborne cannot be reliably identified microscopically (Fig. 54-2). Because of this, the science of indoor allergens is dependent on sensitive assays for the major allergens (see Table 54-1). The situation is made more difficult because the particles that have been defined for two of the major indoor allergens are only airborne transiently after disturbance. Airborne behavior, particle size, and allergen content have been estimated for many allergens (Table 54-2).

The aerodynamic size of particles not only defines the speed at which the particles fall in still air (i.e., indoors) but is also relevant to the deposition of particles in the respiratory tract. Traditionally, it was considered that particles larger than 5 μm in diameter were "nonrespirable." However, that term came out of research in the mining industry, and "nonrespirable" meant that particles would not reach the alveoli. For many inorganic particles, it is thought that deposition in the alveoli causes the maximum damage. By contrast, larger particles can reach the tracheobronchial tree. Here the situation is complex because the size of particles is inversely related to the proportion of the particles that enters the lungs; on the other hand, the quantity of allergen per particle increases by the cube of the diameter. Thus, although only 5% of particles of 20 μm in diameter enter the lungs, this may be a more effective method of delivering protein to the bronchi. For a particle of 1 μm, approximately 30% will enter the lungs, but the volume and thus the quantity of protein is only 0.05% of a particle of 20 μm. Thus, although mite fecal particles and pollen grains are large, they may be an effective method of delivering allergen to the lungs, particularly during quiet mouth breathing.

Although mold spores are generally considered to be "outdoor" allergens, indoor exposure may also be relevant because of the long periods of time spent indoors—on average, 23 hours per day. Thus, 200 spores/m^3 indoors may be more significant than 2000 spores/m^3 outdoors. And, again, particle size may be important. Strikingly, *Alternaria* spores are larger than most other fungal spores and have been associated strongly with asthma in the Southwest and Midwest of the United States.[17,18] Mold spores are different from pollen grains, mite fecal particles, cat dander, or cockroach debris in that they have a firm outer surface that is designed to resist desiccation. As a result, they do not release proteins rapidly. Indeed, some of the major allergens of *Aspergillus* are not expressed until the spores germinate. The importance of these differences in particles can be appreciated by comparing (1) mite fecal particles, (2) cat dander, and (3) *Aspergillus* spores (see Table 54-2).

The characteristics of the particles carrying allergens dictate not only the total quantity inhaled, but also the speed of release locally and the quantity of allergen released at each site of deposition. Whether these properties contribute to differences of

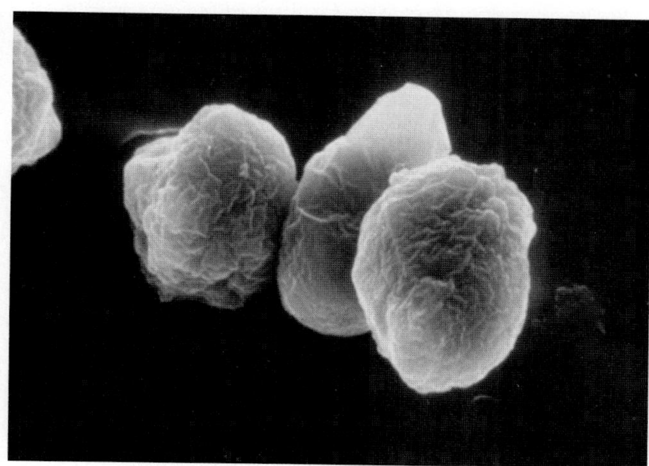

A

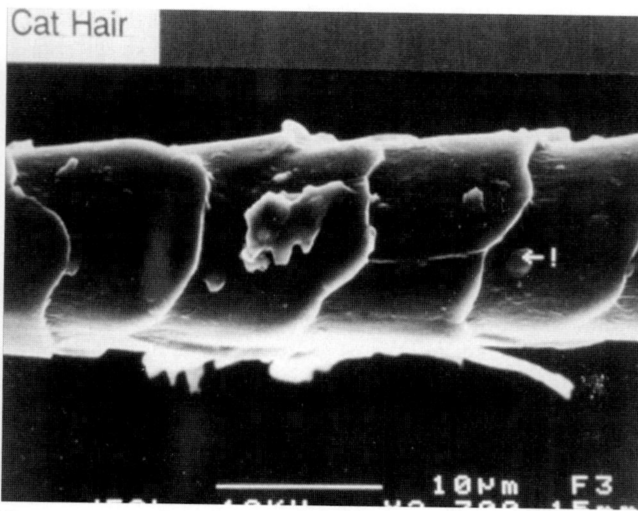

B

C

■ **FIGURE 54-2.** **A,** Mite fecal particles seen with scanning electron microscopy, approximate size 25 µm in diameter. **B,** Cat hair showing pattern of hair and dander particles. **C,** *Aspergillus* sporing bodies with multiple spores forming on the endospore.

immune response remains to be determined. However, there are major differences between the allergens that are relevant to (1) the prevalence of sensitization and (2) the nature of symptoms.

■ THE PARADOXICAL EFFECTS OF CAT OWNERSHIP

Children raised in a house with a cat are not at increased risk for sensitization and, indeed, in many studies the presence of a cat in the house leads to a decreased risk for sensitization to cat allergens. This can be seen in case-control studies or by comparing population-based studies.[27–30] The studies on populations show that children raised in countries with the highest percentage of cat ownership have a lower prevalence of skin sensitivity or IgE antibody to cats. This becomes particularly obvious when comparing IgE antibody to cat with IgE antibody to mite.[31] On the other hand, in countries where cat sensitization is the most important correlation with asthma, cat ownership can decrease the risk for asthma.[32]

There are important differences between studies in relation to cat ownership that may reflect differences in dose or timing of exposure. However, there may also be more complex issues of the relationship between different allergens and the concomitant effects of endotoxin exposure.[33,34] There have been three major proposals to explain the cat paradox:

1. That the effect is due to reverse causation (i.e., that allergic families avoid owning cats).
2. That the presence of cats or dogs or both increases levels of bacterial contamination in the house and that this can be measured as endotoxin.[33,34]

■ **TABLE 54-2.** Contrast between different allergens

	Dust Mites	Cats	Aspergillus
Species	*D. pteronyssinus*	*F. domesticus*	*A. fumigatus*
Particles	Fecal pellets	Dander	Spores
Size	15–30 µm	2–20 µm	1–4 µm
Airborne	10 min post disturbance	Many hours	Fall slowly outdoors
Allergens	Der p 1, Der p 2	Fel d 1	Asp f 1 – Asp f 6
Mass per particle	0.2 ng	0.01 ng	<0.001 ng
Mass inhaled per day	~10 ng	0.5 µg	No estimates

3. That high-dose exposure to the cat allergen Fel d 1 (i.e., the presence of a cat in the house) can induce an allergen-specific form of immunologic tolerance.[27,35]

Investigation of the cat paradox has been carried out in countries with different climates, housing conditions, and furnishing. The extremes may be the most instructive. In northern Scandinavia, cat allergen is the most important cause of sensitization and there is virtually no sensitization to mites or cockroaches. Most of the children who become allergic to cats and become asthmatic have never lived in a house with a cat. In this environment, cat ownership leads to decreased allergy, decreased prevalence of asthma, and decreased incidence of asthma.[32,36] By contrast, in an environment with high concentrations of mite allergen in most houses (i.e., the United Kingdom, Australia, New Zealand, or southeastern United States), sensitization to dust mites dominates other forms of sensitization in childhood.[4,6,27,31,37,38] As a result, the presence of a cat has no effect on the prevalence of asthma. In addition, the presence of a cat has no effect on the prevalence of sensitization to dust mite. Thus, cat exposure can induce a specific form of tolerance. The implications of this phenomenon go beyond the relevance of cats in the house:

1. That allergens are distinct not only in their ability to sensitize but also in their ability to tolerize at high dose.
2. That producing IgG and IgG4 antibodies to the cat allergen Fel d 1 does not create a risk for symptoms on exposure to cat allergen; this argues very strongly that IgE antibodies are essential for the response that gives rise to asthma (Fig. 54-3).
3. That the effects of cat ownership cannot be ascribed to a nonspecific effect on sensitization or IgE antibody production, because cat ownership does not decrease IgE antibody to dust mites.

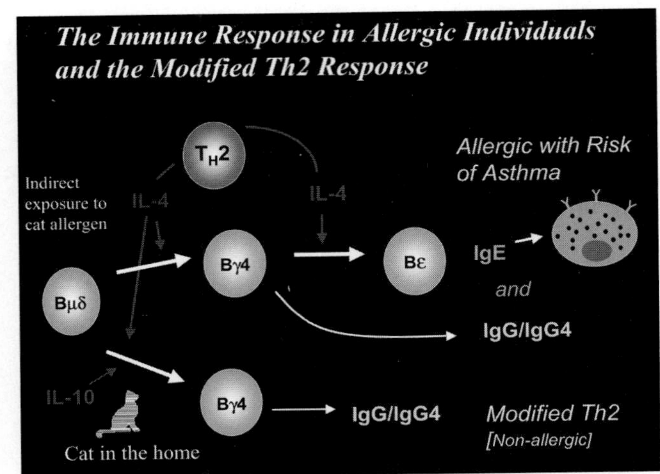

■ **FIGURE 54-3.** The immune response to cat allergens may take a traditional T-helper 2 (Th2) response with immunoglobulin G4 (IgG4) and IgE antibodies. Alternatively, among children living with a cat a significant number produce IgG1 and IgG4 antibodies to Fel d 1 without IgE (modified Th2 response). The T cells are thought to control IgE production both in nonallergic and allergic children. (See Color Plate 40.)

■ RELEVANCE OF DIFFERENT ALLERGENS TO TOTAL SERUM IGE AND THE ASSOCIATED RISK FOR ACUTE ASTHMA

When comparing IgE antibody responses to dust mite and cat, not only is the prevalence of IgE antibody to mite higher, but the titer of IgE antibody to mite can be much higher. In addition, the mean total IgE is higher in some cohorts of children. This raises the question of whether specific IgE responses can increase the total. At present, the evidence is unclear but the prevalence of wheezing children with a total IgE greater than 200 IU/mL is far higher in countries where dust mite is the dominant source of allergens. The relevance of an elevated total IgE is clear from prospective studies, emergency room, and hospitalization data.[5,11] In several different studies, increased risk for acute episodes of asthma can be seen with either total serum IgE or elevated specific IgE antibody greater than 10 IU/mL.

■ THE INTERACTION BETWEEN VIRAL INFECTION AND ALLERGIC RESPONSES IN CHILDREN WITH ACUTE EPISODES OF ASTHMA

Viral infection can be seen as a precipitant of asthma either in a prospective study on wheezing children or in case-control studies in an emergency room or in a hospital.[5,11,39] The results show unequivocally that viral infections are an important precipitant of acute episodes. However, the data for children younger than 3 years is strikingly different from the data on older children. Younger than 3 years, it is possible to identify one or more viruses in a very large proportion of children presenting with, or admitted to hospital with, acute episodes of asthma or bronchiolitis (Fig. 54-4). This includes not only respiratory syncytial virus (RSV), influenza, and coronavirus, but also rhinovirus and the newly described metapneumovirus.[11,40] At this age, the symptomatic children are no more allergic than age-matched children without respiratory symptoms admitted to the same emergency room or hospital. Indeed, in one study the mean total IgE of children admitted to hospital was 8 IU/mL. Among children older than 2 (or 3) years, and also in young adults, the data are completely different because rhinovirus is the only virus that has been shown to be associated with acute episodes and the children are highly allergic.[11,39,40] Indeed, the mean total IgE of children admitted to hospital for asthma 3 to 11 years of age was approximately 330 IU/mL, while the value for controls was approximately 35 IU/mL. Very similar data have been seen from a study in the United Kingdom.[40] The question is how does rhinovirus precipitate acute episodes of wheezing and why is this response so strongly associated with allergy?

Understanding of the mechanisms by which rhinovirus induces acute episodes of asthma in allergic children has been obtained from observational studies or challenge studies. The evidence from emergency room studies is that when the children present, they have elevated peripheral blood and nasal eosinophils, as well as elevated exhaled nitric oxide and lower pH of exhaled condensates.[7,10,11,40] All of these features can be induced to some degree with rhinovirus challenge of a nonsymptomatic asthmatic.[10,41] These studies are done in children using the NIH definition of children (i.e., up to 21 years). However, what is striking is that the response to rhinovirus challenge is much more marked among asthmatics with total IgE of greater than 200 IU/mL.[10] Rhinovirus challenge has been investigated experimentally for approximately 20 years, primarily in nonallergic or nonasthmatic individuals. The results are absolutely clear that this virus does not induce asthma in a

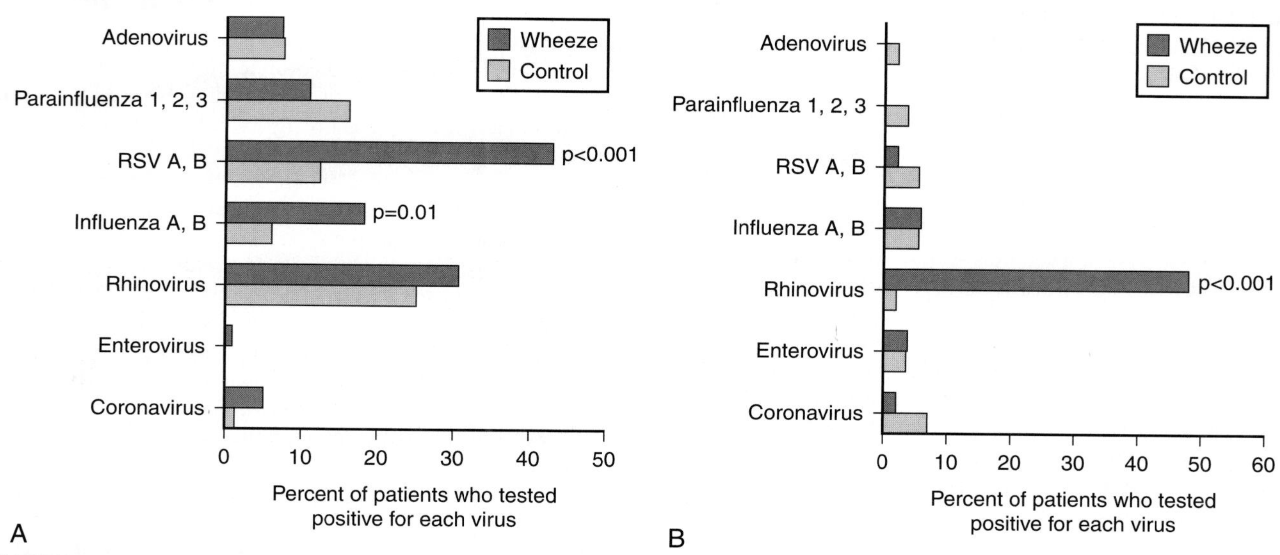

■ FIGURE 54-4. Evidence of recent viral infection was obtained from nasal secretions on children admitted to hospital with or without wheezing. The results are shown for children younger than 3 years (**A**) and children age 3–18 (**B**). (From Heymann PW, Carper HT, Murphy DD, Platts-Mills TA, Patrie J, McLaughlin AP, Erwin EA, Shaker MS, Hellems M, Peerzada J, Hayden FG, Hatley TK, Chamberlain R: Viral infections in relation to age, atopy, and season of admission among children hospitalized for wheezing. J Allergy Clin Immunol 2004;114:239–247, fig 4, p 244.)

nonasthmatic individual. Of course, the rhinovirus is primarily a pathogen of the nose and is an extremely unusual cause of pneumonia. Thus, there are two possible explanations. The first is that rhinovirus does enter the lungs sufficiently to cause increased symptoms and pathology in allergic individuals or second that events in the nose can trigger events in the lungs by a neurologic, cellular, or cytokine-mediated effect. The studies of Dr. Busse's group in Madison have established beyond doubt that a rhinovirus infection can alter response of the lungs to an allergen challenge.[41,42] They have also argued that the virus can be identified in the lung using reverse transcriptase polymerase chain reaction.[43] Surprisingly, repeated nasal allergen challenge prior to rhinovirus challenge did not increase either the severity of the "cold" or the lung response.[44]

Given the apparent effect of total IgE on the risk for asthma and the different effect of some allergens on total IgE, we could ask whether these allergens increase the risk for acute episodes. Preliminary evidence suggests that acute episodes and hospitalization for asthma are less common in countries where the houses do not have dust mite allergens. Equally, those children who make an IgG and IgG4 antibody response without IgE antibody have very low mean levels of total IgE (i.e., ~25 IU/mL) and no associated risk for wheezing.

■ MECHANISMS OF INFLAMMATION IN THE RESPIRATORY TRACT

There is little doubt that inflammation in the lungs contributes to asthma symptoms and to reversible changes in lung function. Indeed, it has been shown that prolonged allergen avoidance, or steroid treatment, can decrease inflammation of the lungs in parallel with improvement of asthma. Thus, both allergen avoidance and steroids can decrease symptoms, improve lung function, and decrease bronchial hyperreactivity (BHR). What is not clear is how much different elements of the predominantly allergen-induced inflammation contribute to BHR or changes in lung function. The most convincing association with symptoms is the presence of peripheral blood eosinophils and the presence of eosinophils in the nose. Given the evidence that eosinophil granule contents (e.g., major basic protein [MBP] or eosinophil cationic protein [ECP]) are toxic to bronchial epithelium, it seemed logical that eosinophils played a major role in the inflammation of asthma. Surprisingly, treatment with anti-interleukin-5 (anti-IL-5), which successfully reduced peripheral blood eosinophil counts, did not improve asthma symptoms.[45] Considerable attention has been focused on the sequence of events that leads to deposition of collagen below the basement membrane in children with asthma. This and other changes have been associated with the term *remodeling*; however, this term should be avoided because it is widely misinterpreted. Remodeling has been used to imply (1) progressive decline in lung function; (2) collagen deposition, increase in goblet cells, and fibroblast activity; and (3) changes in the elasticity of the lung. Unfortunately, there are no clear studies that connect any of the inflammatory changes with decreases in lung function. Furthermore, there is little evidence that progressive decline in lung function is an important feature of asthma in childhood. In most studies those patients who present with lower than average lung function will maintain decreased lung function over long periods of time. In the Childhood Asthma Management Program study there was little evidence for decline in lung function over 4 years. Furthermore, the beneficial effects of inhaled steroids in controlling the disease that were highly significant did not result in any significant difference in lung function 1 month after stopping treatment. Thus, the evidence that inflammatory changes can lead to progressive changes in lung function is not clear, and the term *remodeling* should be avoided. On the other hand, the fact that inhaled steroids provide effective control for mild or moderate asthma argues strongly that inflammation plays an ongoing role in the symptoms. However, steroids have such a wide range of actions that their efficacy does not provide evidence about which part of the inflammatory response is relevant.

RELATIONSHIP BETWEEN IMMUNE RESPONSES, INFLAMMATION, AND SYMPTOMS

The primary epidemiologic evidence linking allergens to asthma relates to skin tests or serum IgE antibodies. However, IgE antibody production is T-cell dependent and the immune response to allergens also includes IgG, IgG4, and IgA antibodies. It could be argued that the association with IgE is seen most clearly because this form of sensitization is easy to detect (i.e., radioallergosorbent test [RAST] in vitro or skin tests in vivo). There are many studies, however, in which T-cell responses or IgG antibodies to allergens have been found in nonallergic and nonwheezing children. Thus, there are good reasons to focus on the role of immediate (i.e., IgE-mediated) hypersensitivity. Allergen challenge of the lungs of an allergic subject produces immediate (i.e., within 15 minutes) declines in FEV_1, late responses, eosinophil infiltration, and prolonged increases in BHR. Mast cells can release not only histamine, cystinyl leukotrienes, and platelet activating factor (PAF), but also cytokines including IL-5 and chemokines. There are several recent developments that relate directly to understanding the role of the immune response in inflammation and symptoms:

1. The response of the lungs to intradermal injections of allergen derived peptides that will react directly with T cells.
2. The clinical efficacy of anti-IgE treatment in patients with moderate to severe asthma.
3. The evidence that children who make IgG and IgG4 antibodies to cat allergen without IgE antibodies do not have an increased risk for asthma.

T-CELL PEPTIDE RESPONSES

Although not currently available as a treatment, there is extensive evidence that injections of peptides derived from Fel d 1 can induce a delayed (i.e., within hours) response in the lung and can have a beneficial effect on symptoms.[46,47] These results strongly support the view that T cells in the lung can contribute to the pathology of asthma. However, to date the studies have all been conducted in allergic subjects. Thus, there are two questions: First, are the quantities of peptides reaching the lungs a realistic model of what could happen during natural exposure; and second, how do the T cells get to the lungs? Lymphocytes are recruited to sites of local "inflammation" following the presence of a foreign antigen. Thus, an attractive argument is that in children with IgE antibody, the local deposition of an allergen particle can trigger mast cell degranulation, which leads to the recruitment of a variety of cells, including lymphocytes. Most of these cells are short lived in the tissues. However, T cells recruited to the tissues may persist locally. The presence of T cells in the lungs of allergic patients could explain many features of the chronicity of asthma. However, the hypothesis is that these cells will only accumulate locally in children who already have immediate hypersensitivity.

TREATMENT WITH MONOCLONAL ANTIBODIES TO IMMUNOGLOBULIN E

Injecting polyclonal anti-IgE into the skin produces a wheal and flare reaction in all subjects except the very small number of IgE-deficient patients, most of whom have hypogammaglobulinemia. Thus, treatment with anti-IgE that binds the main epitopes on the epsilon heavy chain is not possible. However, antibodies to the site that binds to the receptor for IgE (Fc-ε-R1) will only bind IgE that is not bound to a mast cell or basophil. Treatment with monoclonal antibodies to IgE would seem to be a logical treatment for allergic disease. However, there are some reasons why it should not succeed. First, other monoclonal antibodies that are in use clinically act on cytokines or interleukins that are present in much smaller quantities. Second, the short half-life of IgE means that these antibodies pass rapidly through the circulation but remain for much longer periods (i.e., up to 6 weeks) on mast cells in the skin. Third, as discussed above, it seems likely that at least part of the inflammatory response in the lungs is mediated by T cells (i.e., not dependent on IgE antibodies). Given the potential problems, the success of anti-IgE treatment in clinical trials has been encouraging.[48] Indeed, some children derive major benefit from this form of treatment. The implication is that IgE antibodies play a role in the persistence of inflammation and BHR in the lungs. This finding is not only significant clinically but also because it provides proof of the concept that IgE antibodies play a direct role in asthma.

A MODIFIED TH2 RESPONSE TO CAT ALLERGEN IS NOT ASSOCIATED WITH SYMPTOMS OF ASTHMA OR INFLAMMATION IN THE LUNGS

Children raised in a house with a cat are less likely to develop IgE antibody to cat allergens, but as many as 50% of these children have made an IgG antibody response to the cat allergen Fel d 1 without IgE antibody.[9,32] What is relevant to the present discussion is that this IgG antibody response on its own does not create a risk for wheezing. Thus, children living in a house with a cat with very high exposure to cat allergen do not develop symptoms unless the immune response includes IgE antibody. Furthermore, the nonallergic subjects mount a T-cell response that is similar to the response observed in allergic children. The implication is that T cells only play a role if there is also an IgE antibody response, which could mean either that the T cells have a subtle difference or that IgE antibody is necessary for T cells to be recruited to the lungs.

Changes in the lungs of children with asthma include a cellular infiltrate, excess mucus production, collagen deposition, and irritability of smooth muscle. The mechanism of this response includes a cascade of leukotrienes, prostaglandins, cytokines, and chemokines. Many of these have been identified as potential targets for treatment. However, given the number of molecules identified, it has been difficult to establish their role in the lung response. Many different approaches have been used, including measurement of cytokines, in samples obtained from the lungs, gene expression studies, detailed studies in murine models, and the development of antagonists or monoclonal antibodies suitable for clinical trials. Ultimately, it is clinical trials that provide the most convincing evidence. Thus, the efficacy of leukotriene antagonists strongly supports a role for these molecules in asthma. The results of the studies with anti-IL-4 or IL-4 receptor antagonists have been positive in moderate to severe asthma but were unconvincing in mild persistent asthma. Some years ago, the results with antagonists for PAF were consistently negative. Several other targets have been investigated and abandoned by the pharmaceutical industry. The continuing success of corticosteroids either as a local or a systemic drug may reflect the fact that they influence the expression of multiple genes as well as dramatically reducing circulating and tissue eosinophils. If, as seems obvious, corticosteroids are clinically effective because they have multiple actions, other agents may need to be combined (e.g., anti-IL-5 and an IL-4 antagonist). However, experiments of that kind would be difficult to carry out as clinical trials.

CONCLUSIONS

The treatment of asthma in children older than 3 years is focused on long-term anti-inflammatory treatment. This strategy recognizes that the large majority of these children have inflammation in their medium and large bronchi, and that this response is a major cause of reversible airflow obstruction. In addition, many or most of these children are allergic to one or more of the allergens that are found in homes in the area where they live. It is well established that inhaling allergen in an allergen challenge can induce an eosinophil-rich cellular infiltrate and prolonged increases in nonspecific BHR. Thus, there is a logical case that inhaling allergens is a cause not only of sensitization but also of the disease. This view is supported by some but not all results of allergen avoidance studies.[9,49] On the other hand, it is difficult to establish a simple dose response between allergen exposure and the prevalence or severity of asthma. However, the complexity of the relationship between allergens and asthma (see Fig. 54-1) would tend to obscure the dose response. Simple relationships between exposure in the patient's home and wheezing could be obscured by (1) genetics, (2) the inaccuracy of floor dust assays as a measurement of inhaled exposure, (3) exposure to "indoor" allergens in buildings other than the child's home, and (4) tolerance to allergens at high dose.

Virus infection plays an important role in bronchiolitis/wheezing/asthma throughout childhood. In children younger than 3 years, many different viruses can induce bronchiolitis. At this age, RSV, influenza, metapneumovirus, and rhinovirus may all play a role. The major defined risk factor for viral-induced wheezing episodes in children younger than 3 years is small lung size at birth, and at this age, allergy does not play a significant role. Many of the children who have early viral-induced episodes will go on to have persistent asthma. However, early episodes are common, and it is not clear whether the early infections influence the subsequent development of allergy or persistence of asthma. After age 3 years, the role of viral infections changes completely. Presumably, because of lung growth, viral infection of nonallergic children is no longer a cause of emergency room or hospital visits. At this age, the only virus that appears to play an important role is rhinovirus, and this effect is only seen in allergic children. More significantly, these children are not simply skin test positive, but they have major elevations of total serum IgE (geometric mean value for 53 children age 3–18 years was 390 IU/mL).[11] This result is consistent with other studies and suggests that conditions that increase total IgE could be a risk factor for severe episodes of asthma.

Elevated total IgE is strongly associated with asthma. Burrows and colleagues[50] reported that the higher the total IgE, the greater the prevalence of asthma. It has been clearly shown that total IgE is strongly influenced by genetics; however, recent studies suggest that some allergens can contribute more than others. In particular, dust mite, cockroach, grass pollens, and the fungus *Alternaria* have been shown to induce high-titer IgE antibody (i.e., 10 IU/mL) and in some instances to increase total serum IgE. In contrast, with cat and dog allergens, not only are positive skin tests less common, but the titer of IgE antibody is generally lower. Thus, some allergens, but not others, can increase total IgE to a level that is associated with acute episodes. This effect may contribute to the higher prevalence and severity of asthma in some communities (e.g., New Zealand, United Kingdom, and the North American inner city) compared with others (e.g., Scandinavia).

The relevance of immunopathogenesis to treatment can be seen in three ways. First, controlling the inflammatory response has become a mainstay of treatment using inhaled steroids, leukotriene antagonists, and, in a small number of cases, anti-IgE. Second, allergen-specific treatment using avoidance or immunotherapy can influence inflammation in the lungs. Third, some future approaches to therapy could focus on altering the immune response using peptides or recombinant molecules that can influence T-cell responses and IgE antibody production. Given the complexity of the immune response to allergens and its relationship to symptoms, it is no surprise that analysis of the genetics of asthma has provided inconsistent results. Presumably, environmental effects related to both the time course and the dose of different allergens as well as the modulating effects of endotoxin exposure can alter the association with different genes. In addition, the effects of many different changes in lifestyle may also influence these relationships. The implication is that we should focus on interpreting and altering the inflammatory response to the environment.

REFERENCES

1. Woolcock AJ, Peat JK: Evidence for the increase in asthma worldwide. Ciba Found Symp 1997;206:122–134.
2. Beasley R, Ellwood P, Asher I: International patterns of the prevalence of pediatric asthma. The ISAAC program. Pediatr Clin North Am 2003;50:539–553.
3. Crater DD, Heise S, Perzanowski M, Herbert R, Morse CG, Hulsey TC, Platts-Mills T: Asthma hospitalization trends in Charleston, South Carolina, 1956 to 1997. Twenty-fold increase among black children during a 30-year period. Pediatrics 2001;108:E97.
4. Sporik R, Holgate ST, Platts-Mills TA, Cogswell JJ: Exposure to house-dust mite allergen (Der p I) and the development of asthma in childhood. A prospective study. N Engl J Med 1990;323:502–507.
5. Call RS, Smith TF, Morris E, Chapman MD, Platts-Mills TA: Risk factors for asthma in inner city children. J Pediatr 1992;121:862–866.
6. Sears MR, Greene JM, Willan AR, Wiecek EM, Taylor DR, Flannery EM, Cowan JO, Herbison GP, Silva PA, Poulton R: A longitudinal, population-based, cohort study of childhood asthma followed in adulthood. N Engl J Med 2003;349:1414–1422.
7. Hunt JF, Erwin E, Palmer L, Vaughan J, Malhotra N, Platts-Mills TA, Gaston B: Expression and activity of pH-regulatory glutaminase in the human airway epithelium. Am J Respir Crit Care Med 2002;165:101–107.
8. Boner AL, Bodini A, Piacentini GL: Environmental allergens and childhood asthma. Clin Exp Allergy 1998;28:76–81.
9. Platts-Mills TA, Vervloet D, Thomas WR, Aalberse RC, Chapman MD: Indoor allergens and asthma. Report of the Third International Workshop. J Allergy Clin Immunol 1997;100(Suppl):2–24.
10. Zambrano JC, Carper HT, Rakes GP, Patrie J, Murphy DD, Platts-Mills TA, Hayden FG, Gwaltney JM Jr, Hatley TK, Owens AM, Heymann PW: Experimental rhinovirus challenges in adults with mild asthma. Response to infection in relation to IgE. J Allergy Clin Immunol 2003;111:1008–1016.
11. Heymann PW, Carper HT, Murphy DD, Platts-Mills TA, Patrie J, McLaughlin AP, Erwin EA, Shaker MS, Hellems M, Peerzada J, Hayden FG, Hatley TK, Chamberlain R: Viral infections in relation to age, atopy, and season of admission among children hospitalized for wheezing. J Allergy Clin Immunol 2004;114:239–247.
12. Sporik R, Chapman MD, Platts-Mills TA: House dust mite exposure as a cause of asthma. Clin Exp Allergy 1992;22:897–906.
13. Kern RA: Dust sensitization in bronchial asthma. Med Clin North Am 1921;5:571.

14. Voorhorst R, Spieksma FTM, Varekamp H, Leupen MJ, Lyklema AW: The house dust mite *(Dermatophagoides pteronyssinus)* and the allergens it produces. Identity with the house dust allergens. J Allergy 1967;39:325–332.
15. Braun-Fahrlander C, Riedler J, Herz U, Eder W, Waser M, Grize L, Maisch S, Carr D, Gerlach F, Bufe A, Lauener RP, Schierl R, Renz H, Nowak D, von Mutius E, Allergy and Endotoxin Study Team: Environmental exposure to endotoxin and its relation to asthma in school-age children. N Engl J Med 2002;347:869–877.
16. Gereda JE, Leung DY, Thatayatikom A, Strieb JE, Price MR, Klinnert MD, Liu AH: Relation between house-dust endotoxin exposure, type 1 T-cell development, and allergen sensitization in infants at high risk of asthma. Lancet 2000;355:1680–1683.
17. Halonen M, Stern DA, Wright AL, Taussig LM, Martinez FD: Alternaria as a major allergen for asthma in children raised in a desert environment. Am J Respir Crit Care Med 1997;155:1356–1361.
18. Perzanowski MS, Sporik R, Squillace Sp, Gelber LE, Call R, Carter M, Platts-Mills TA: Association of sensitization to Alternaria allergens with asthma among school-age children. J Allergy Clin Immunol 1998;101: 626–632.
19. Wickman M: Indirect exposure to cats at school and worsening of asthma in children. Monaldi Arch Chest Dis 2002;57:113–114.
20. Perzanowski MS, Ronmark E, Nold B, Lundback B, Platts-Mills TA: Relevance of allergens from cats and dogs to asthma in the northernmost province of Sweden. Schools as a major site of exposure. J Allergy Clin Immunol 1999;103:1018–1024.
21. Simpson A, Custovic A: Allergen avoidance in the primary prevention of asthma. Curr Opin Allergy Clin Immunol 2004;4:45–51.
22. Rosenstreich DL, Eggleston P, Kattan M, Baker D, Slavin RG, Gergen P, Mitchell H, McNiff-Mortimer K, Lynn H, Ownby D, Malveaux F: The role of cockroach allergy and exposure to cockroach allergen in causing morbidity among inner-city children with asthma. N Engl J Med 1997;336: 1356–1363.
23. Eggleston, PA Rosenstreich D, Lynn H, Gergen P, Baker D, Kattan M, Mortimer KM, Mitchell H, Ownby D, Slavin R, Malveaux F: Relationship of indoor allergen exposure to skin test sensitivity in inner-city children with asthma. J Allergy Clin Immunol 1998;102:563–570.
24. Wan H, Winton HL, Soeller C, Tovey ER, Gruenert DC, Thompson PJ, Stewart GA, Taylor GW, Garrod DR, Cannell MB, Robinson C: Der p 1 facilitates transepithelial allergen delivery by disruption of tight junctions. J Clin Invest 1999;104:123–133.
25. Gough L, Schulz O, Sewell HF, Shakib F: The cysteine protease activity of the major dust mite allergen Dr p 1 selectively enhances the immunoglobulin E antibody response. J Exp Med 1999;190:1897–1902.
26. Pomes A, Chapman MD, Vailes LD, Blundell TL, Dhanaraj V: Cockroach allergen Bla g 2: structure, function, and implication of allergic sensitization. Am J Respir Crit Care Med 2002;165:391–397.
27. Platts-Mills T, Vaughan J, Squillace S, Woodfolk J, Sporik R: Sensitisation, asthma, and a modified Th2 response in children exposed to cat allergen. A population-based cross-sectional study. Lancet 2001;357:752–756.
28. Ownby Dr, Johnson CC, Peterson EL: Exposure to dogs and cats in the first year of life and risk of allergic sensitization at 6 to 7 years of age. JAMA 2002;288:963–972.
29. Hesselmar B, Aberg N, Aberg B, Eriksson B, Bjorksten B: Dose early exposure to cat or dog protect against later allergy development? Clin Exp Allergy 1999;29:611–617.
30. Roost HP, Kunzli N, Schindler C, Jarvis D, Chinn S, Perruchoud AP, Ackermann-Liebrich U, Burney P, Wuthrich B: Role of current and childhood exposure to cat and atopic sensitization. J Allergy Clin Immunol 1999;104:941–947.
31. Erwin EA, Wickens K, Custis NJ, Siebers R, Woodfolk J, Barry D, Crane J, Platts-Mills TA: Cat and dust mite sensitivity and tolerance in relation to wheezing among children raised with high exposure to both allergens. J Allergy Clin Immunol 2005;115:74–79.
32. Perzanowski MS, Ronmark E, Platts-Mills TA, Lundback B: Effect of cat and dog ownership on sensitization and development of asthma among preteenage children. Am J Respir Crit Care Med 2002;166:696–702.
33. Litonjua AA, Milton DK, Celedon JC, Ryan L, Weiss ST, Gold DR: A longitudinal analysis of wheezing in young children. The independent effects of early life exposure to house dust endotoxin, allergens, and pets. J Allergy Clin Immunol 2002;110:736–742.
34. Gereda JE, Leung DY, Liu AH: Levels of environmental endotoxin and prevalence of atopic disease. JAMA 2000;284:1652–1653.
35. Reefer AJ, Carneiro RM, Custis NJ, Platts-Mills TA, Sungs SS, Hammer J, Woodfolk JA: A role of IL-10-mediated HLA-DR7-restricted T cell-dependent events in development of the modified Th2 response to cat allergen. J Immunol 2004;172:2763–2772.
36. Platts-Mills TA: Paradoxical effect of domestic animals on asthma and allergic sensitization. JAMA 2002;288:1012–1014.
37. Peat JK, Tovey E, Mellis CM, Leeder SR, Woolcock AJ: Importance of house dust mite and Alternaria allergens in childhood asthma. Epidemiological study in two climatic regions of Australia. Clin Exp Allergy 1993;23:812–820.
38. Woodcock A, Lowe LA, Murray CS, Simpson BM, Pipis SD, Kissen P, Simpson A, Custovic A, NAC Manchester Asthma and Allergy Study Group: Early life environmental control. Effect on symptoms, sensitization, and lung function at age 3 years. Am J Respir Crit Care Med 2004;170: 433–439.
39. Johnston SL, Pattemore PK, Sanderson G, Smith S, Lampe F, Josephs L, Symington P, O'Toole S, Myint SH, Tyrrell DA: Community study of role of viral infections in exacerbations of asthma in 9-year old children. BMJ 1995;310:1225–1229.
40. Green RM, Custovic A, Sanderson G, Hunter J, Johnston SL, Woodcock A: Synergism between allergens and viruses and risk of hospital admission with asthma. Case-control study. BMJ 2002;324:763–770.
41. Lemanske RF Jr, Dick EC, Swenson CA, Vrtis RF, Busse WW: Rhinovirus upper respiratory infection increases airway hyperreactivity and asthmatic reactions. J Clin Invest 1989;83:1–10.
42. Calhoun WJ, Swenson CA, Dick EC, Schwartz LB, Lemanske RF Jr, Busse WW: Experimental rhinovirus 16 infection potentiates histamine release after antigen bronchoprovocation in allergic subjects. Am Rev Respir Dis 1991;144:1267–1273.
43. Gern JE, Calhoun W, Swenson C, Shen G, Busse WW: Rhinovirus infection preferentially increases lower airway responsiveness in allergic subjects. Am J Respir Crit Care Med 1997;155:1872–1876.
44. Avila PC, Abisheganaden JA, Wong H, Liu J, Yagi S, Schmurr D, Kishiyama JL, Boushey HA: Effects of allergic inflammation of the nasal mucosa on the severity of rhinovirus 16 cold. J Allergy Clin Immunol 2000;105:923–932.
45. Leckie MJ, ten Brinke A, Khan J, Diamant Z, O'Connor BJ, Walls CM, Mathur AK, Cowley HC, Chung KF, Djukanovic R, Hansel TT, Holgate ST, Sterk PF, Barnes PJ: Effects of an interleukin-5 blocking monoclonal antibody on eosinophils, airway hyper-responsiveness, and the late asthmatic response. Lancet 2000;356:2144–2148.
46. Haselden BM, Kay AB, Larche M: Immunoglobulin E-independent major histocompatibility complex-restricted T cell peptide epitope-induced late asthmatic reactions. J Exp Med 1999;189:1885–1894.
47. Oldfield WL, Larche M, Kay AB: Effect of T-cell peptides derived from Fel d 1 on allergic reactions and cytokine production in patients sensitive to cats. A randomised controlled trial. Lancet 2002;360: 47–53.
48. Milgrom H, Fick RB Jr, Su JQ, Reimann JD, Bush RK, Watrous ML, Metzger WJ: Treatment of allergic asthma with monoclonal anti-IgE antibody. rhuMAb-E25 Study Group. N Engl J Med 1999;341:1966–1973.
49. Morgan WJ, Crain EF, Gruchalla RS, O'Connor GT, Kattan M, Evans R 3rd, Stout J, Malindzak G, Smartt E, Plaut M, Walter M, Vaughn B, Mitchell H, Inner-City Asthma Study Group: Results of a home-based environmental intervention among urban children with asthma. N Engl J Med 2004;351:1068–1080.
50. Burrows B, Martinez F, Halonen M, Barbee RA, Cline MG: Association of asthma with serum IgE levels and skin test reactivity to allergens. N Engl J Med 1989;320:271–277.

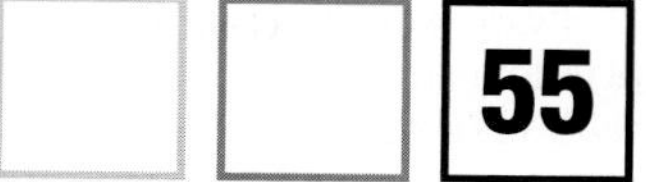

55 Asthma in the Preschool Child

Miles Weinberger, MD •
Mutasim N. Abu-Hasan, MD

■ ASTHMA—WHAT IS IT?

What is asthma? This question is of particular importance in evaluating respiratory disease in the young child where euphemisms for asthma have been common, including reactive airway disease (RAD), wheezy bronchitis, obstructive bronchitis, recurrent bronchiolitis, and so forth. Sometimes describing or defining asthma is like the parable of the blind men describing the elephant who felt it was like a tree, a snake, or a rope depending on whether they were feeling a leg, the trunk, or the tail. Like the blind men examining only one part of the elephant, asthma is sufficiently diverse in its presentation that its perception depends on the experience of the observer. Some have suggested that, like love, it cannot be defined, but it is recognizable when confronted.[1]

The complexity and challenge of defining asthma has been discussed extensively by Sears.[2] In examining the 12 definitions and references in his review, a common theme to all is the presence of airway disease that varies over time either spontaneously or as a result of treatment. A committee of the American Thoracic Society agreed on the definition that "Asthma is a disease characterized by an increased responsiveness of the trachea and bronchi to various stimuli and manifested by a widespread narrowing of the airways that change in severity either spontaneously or as a result of therapy."[3] This definition was expanded by a subsequent committee of the American Thoracic Society to include "The major symptoms of asthma are paroxysms of dyspnea, wheezing and cough, which may vary from mild and almost undetectable to severe and unremitting . . ."[4] That definition and others, most notably that of Simon Godfrey, added to the definition that the airflow obstruction and clinical symptoms are largely or completely reversed by treatment with bronchodilators or corticosteroids.[5]

Inflammation was introduced into the definition by Hargreave[6] and subsequently incorporated into the National Asthma Education Program Expert Panel Reports from the U.S. National Institute of Health.[7,8] However, a definition based on inflammation is not helpful in differential diagnosis or early disease identification since noninvasive measures of inflammation are neither readily available nor well validated. This is especially true for young children, in whom even the ability to make physiologic measurements is limited. For a definition of a disease to be useful, it should provide a basis for making the diagnosis. While airway inflammation is certainly a component of asthma, the value of including this as a major component of the definition has also been challenged by McFadden and Gilbert, who commented, "Airway inflammation and hyperresponsiveness . . . are not unique to this illness. The usefulness of these characteristics in defining asthma is unclear."[9] This issue is discussed further by Brusasco and colleagues, who argued that airway narrowing in asthma is not necessarily related to airway inflammation.[10] Asthma has thus proved challenging to define because of the diversity in its clinical presentation, variability of its clinical course, and absence of any specific diagnostic test.

The ability to define asthma is essential for both study of the disease and diagnosis. The reported prevalence of asthma varies greatly depending on how asthma is defined for the purpose of diagnosis in epidemiologic studies.[11,12] Similarly, researchers attempting to study the genetics of asthma have struggled with the definition.[13–15] The challenge of defining asthma becomes greatest in the very young child. While there is an absence of an internationally accepted criteria for the definition of asthma in early childhood, birth cohort studies have nonetheless been attempted using various criteria to define asthma or potential asthma.[16] Martinez has emphasized the heterogeneity of asthma and the identification of specific phenotypes based on patterns of natural history and presence of early allergic sensitization.[17]

■ EPIDEMIOLOGY OF EARLY CHILDHOOD ASTHMA

■ WHEN DOES IT START?

While asthma can begin at almost any age, it most commonly begins in infancy with a viral respiratory infection that causes the lower airway inflammatory disease with consequent wheezing and coughing that is commonly known as bronchiolitis. The most common cause of this initial wheezing episode is respiratory syncytial virus (RSV). As many as 3% of infants in the United States have been hospitalized annually because of lower respiratory illness from this infection.[18] While it is premature to call the first episode of such symptoms asthma, this initial viral respiratory infection–induced lower airway obstruction in infancy is often the harbinger of more to come, consistent with a diagnosis of asthma. In fact, when the onset of symptoms consistent with asthma was examined in an epidemiologic study of the population in the vicinity of Rochester Minnesota by investigators at Mayo Clinic, the predominance of children with asthma had their onset during the first year of life (Fig. 55-1).[19]

Thus, when a healthy baby becomes infected with RSV, as virtually all of them eventually do, most get only the symptoms of a common cold with coryza. A substantial minority suffer from bronchiolitis, the most common cause of hospitalization during the first year of life. Of those who experience bronchiolitis, about 25% to 50% subsequently have symptoms of an intermittent pattern of asthma manifested by recurrent wheezing only in association with subsequent viral respiratory infections.[20,21] While clinical experience and natural history

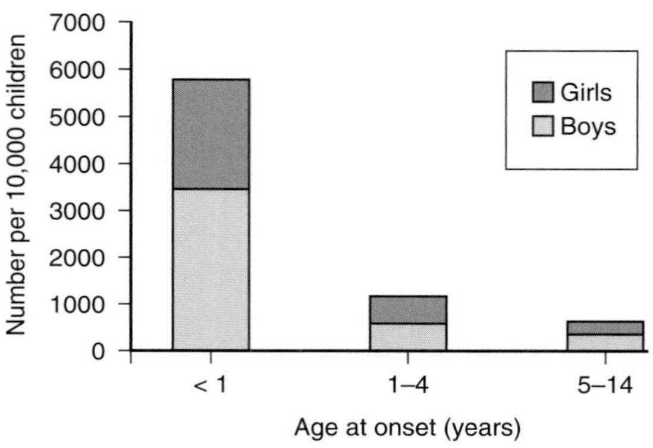

■ **FIGURE 55-1.** Annual age- and sex-adjusted incidence of asthma onset in a population-based epidemiologic study in Rochester, Minnesota.

studies suggest that the majority of such children remit later in childhood, some continue to have recurrent or chronic symptoms consistent with a diagnosis of asthma throughout childhood, and some also continue into adult life[22] (Fig. 55-2).[23]

WHO GETS ASTHMA?

An asthma phenotype is present in approximately 25% of the offspring of a parent with asthma.[24] Further evidence for a genetic influence on the asthma phenotype is seen in twin studies where there is a higher concordance in monozygotic twins compared with dizygotic twins, even though both twins share the same environment.[25,26] But the concordance even in identical twins is not much over 50%. Both genetics and environment therefore appear to contribute to asthma.

The genetics are complex, with apparently separate contributions to airway hyperresponsiveness and immunoglobulin E (IgE)–mediated sensitivity to inhalant allergens.[27] Airway reactivity or hyperresponsiveness is considered a hallmark of asthma.[28] Persistence of asthma beyond the preschool years has been found to be associated with increased airway responsiveness in early life.[29]

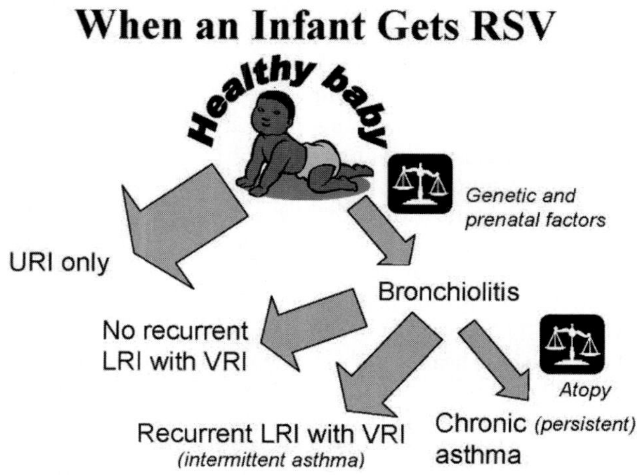

When an Infant Gets RSV

Healthy baby

Genetic and prenatal factors

URI only

Bronchiolitis

No recurrent LRI with VRI

Atopy

Recurrent LRI with VRI (intermittent asthma)

Chronic (persistent) asthma

■ **FIGURE 55-2.** Clinical consequences of initial infection following respiratory syncytial virus in infancy. LRI, lower respiratory illness; URI, upper respiratory illness; VRI, viral respiratory infection. (From Weinberger M: Clinical patterns and natural history of asthma. J Pediatr 2003;142[Suppl]: 15–20.)

However, airway hyperresponsiveness is not diagnostic of asthma. Airway hyperresponsiveness to a cholinergic stimulus is found with increased frequency in nonasthmatic parents of children with asthma at a frequency suggestive that such responsiveness is transmitted as an autosomal-dominant trait that is a necessary but not sufficient biologic variable to cause clinical asthma.[30,31] Total IgE production appears to have strong genetic determination based on the observations of very high concordance in monozygotic twins and lesser concordance in dizygotic twins, both of whom should have similar environmental exposures.[32] However, less well studied is the genetics of antigen-specific IgE. Other genetic variables that can affect the phenotypic manifestations of atopic sensitization include the affinity of IgE receptors on target cells, the interaction of IgE with the receptors, IgE-induced release of mediators, and end-organ responsiveness. Despite their clinical usefulness as an aid to the assessment of diseases affected by atopic sensitization, neither the size of allergy skin tests nor the titer of antigen-specific IgE on in vitro tests reliably predicts either disease or severity.

Although inhalant sensitivity tends to develop later than ingestant sensitivity in early childhood, Wilson and colleagues found cockroach sensitivity in 29%, dust mite in 10%, cat in 10%, and *Alternaria* in 4% among 49 asthmatic infants under 1 year of age.[33] Arshad and Hide examined the development of atopic related findings in a prospective study of 1167 infants.[34] They found that dust mite–positive skin test results were more prevalent in formula-fed infants. While skin test results positive for animal danders were more prevalent among infants exposed to the respective animals, they did not find that exposure to animal dander influenced the prevalence of clinical disorders. However, Lindfors and colleagues, in a case-control study of 193 children with asthma who were 1 to 4 years of age, did find that high-dose exposure to cats and/or dogs resulted in an increased risk for asthma, with indoor dampness and exposure to environmental tobacco smoke having an apparent synergistic effect.[35] In a subsequent report, they described a dose-response relationship between cat exposure and sensitization to cats but not to dogs.[36] Sears and colleagues found a relationship between children born in winter and sensitization to cats and house dust mites.[37] Sherrill and colleagues, in a prospective longitudinal study in Tucson, found an association between sensitization before age 8, as determined by skin testing, and symptoms of asthma, whereas those who developed positive skin test results only after age 8 did not differ in frequency of asthmatic symptoms from those never sensitized.[38] While Nelson and colleagues found an association of many positive skin test results among 1041 school-aged children with "mild to moderate" asthma, these investigators found that only exposure to dogs, cats, and *Alternaria* mold correlated independently with increased lower airway hyperresponsiveness as measured by methacholine challenge, although not with decreased pulmonary function.[39] Although this latter study did not involve preschool-aged children, it indicates that some inhalant allergens are more asthmagenic than others.

Thus, getting asthma is a function of genetic and environmental variables, not all of which are known. While those with a viral respiratory infection–induced intermittent pattern appear to have a familial predisposition, the genetics of that pattern are not well studied. Both airway hyperresponsiveness and IgE-mediated sensitivity to inhalant allergens in infancy appear to be predictors of those who eventually have persistent symptoms.

PATHOPHYSIOLOGY OF EARLY CHILDHOOD ASTHMA

Characterizing the pathophysiology of asthma in preschool children has been complicated by the limited studies in this age group. Such studies are obviously hindered by the ethical dilemma of subjecting nonconsenting and vulnerable children to intrusive pathologic and physiologic assessment procedures.[40] Autopsy and bronchial biopsy data confirming the presence of the typical pathologic changes found in the airways of adult asthmatics, such as smooth muscle hyperplasia and hypertrophy, mucous cell hyperplasia and mucus hypersecretion, eosinophil and neutrophil infiltrate, epithelial sloughing, and subepithelial deposition, are rare in infants and young children due to the rare occurrence of death in this age group and the evident difficulty of obtaining transbronchial biopsies in children.[41–43]

Because of the paucity of data, there has been a tendency to discuss the pathophysiology of asthma as if it were a homogeneous entity across age groups. However, concepts and models of asthma derived from adult studies may not be applicable to common phenotypes of asthma in the young child.[44] This is particularly evident for the nonatopic intermittent viral respiratory infection–induced asthma that predominates in infants and children, which seems to be distinct from the chronic atopic asthma more commonly found in older children and adults.[23,45,46] Recent bronchoalveolar lavage studies, for instance, show no evidence of airway inflammation in children with a history of intermittent nonatopic asthma during their symptom-free periods while airway inflammation seems to persist in patients with atopic asthma even when they are asymptomatic.[47,48] If symptomatic, on the other hand, nonatopic asthmatic children and wheezy infants seem to have predominantly noneosinophilic airway inflammation as compared with the eosinophilic airway inflammation characteristic of atopic children with asthma, suggesting different inflammatory mechanisms between these asthma phenotypes.[49–54]

Airway inflammation in atopic asthma is well characterized in adults and to some extent in children by studies using induced sputum, lavage, transbronchial biopsy, and from animal models of allergen-induced sensitization. These studies determine a strong association of atopic asthma with dysregulation of T-helper (Th) cell subset response in which there is overproliferation and overactivity of the Th2 cell subtype. This selectively overexpresses certain proinflammatory cytokines, including interleukin-4 (IL-4), IL-5, and IL-13, resulting in activation and recruitment of eosinophils and neutrophils to the airways with consequent airway hyperactivity.[55–62] The pathogenesis of this Th cell dysregulation in atopic asthmatics is poorly understood but hypothesized to be due to abnormal maturation of the immune cells caused by timely complex interaction of certain infectious and environmental factors (some inductive and some protective) in genetically predisposed subjects.[63–65] The potential effect of prenatal versus postnatal or early versus late childhood exposure to certain inhaled and ingested allergens on the development of atopic asthma is not decisively determined by the current epidemiologic data.[66–68] There are intriguing data leading to speculation that certain early bacterial, mycobacterial, and parasitic infections during early childhood are protective against the development of atopic asthma.[69–72]

For nonatopic viral-induced asthma, the most common asthma phenotype in young children, there is reason to question the assumption that airway inflammation is mainly of the Th2 type.[73–76] In one study conducted during acute asthma exacerbations, eosinophil count in sputum and nasal swab was found to be lower in infants than older children.[77] In another study where cytokine profile in bronchoalveolar lavage fluid was measured, Th2 type response (high IL-4 and low interferon-γ) was found in children presenting with frequent asthma symptoms, while a Th1-type response (low IL-4 and high interferon-γ) was found in children with less frequent symptoms.[78] These studies and others demonstrate the great degree of heterogeneity present in the airway inflammation in young children diagnosed with asthma and indicate that while a predominantly Th2 response is most prominent in atopic asthma, a predominantly Th1 inflammatory type response is more common in nonatopic asthma. This suggests different immune and inflammatory mechanisms for viral respiratory infection–induced and atopic asthma.[79–81]

Since severe RSV bronchiolitis is associated with a higher incidence of subsequent wheezing and asthma later in life,[82–84] it may be that RSV bronchiolitis can potentially alter airway immune and neurochemical responses to subsequent infectious or environmental triggers.[85,86] Such alterations, which include Th2 enhancement, up-regulation of neurogenic inflammation, and abrogation of the inhibitory nonadrenergic noncholinergic system, are extensively demonstrated in studies of animal models of RSV infection.[87–91] The association between severe RSV bronchiolitis and asthma, however, could equally indicate that symptoms with RSV infection manifests more severely in patients who are already predisposed for asthma without necessarily implying a cause-effect relationship. This later hypothesis is supported by the heterogeneity of airway inflammation found during RSV infection and the fact that subsequent development of asthma symptoms in RSV-infected individuals is more likely to occur in atopic subjects and in subjects with a predominantly Th2 response to RSV infection.[21,92–97] This heterogeneity found in children with RSV infection undermines further the assumption that all viral-induced asthma symptoms are due to triggering of a dormant chronic Th2-type airway inflammation.

When compared with older children, infants and young children have small and rapidly declining airway resistance due to smaller total airway cross-sectional area as related to the growing alveolar volume.[98,99] In addition, infants also have increased airway responsiveness to nonspecific stimuli and to viral infection.[100–102] Therefore, viral infections in infants and young children can understandably result in severe airway obstruction, whether through direct inflammation of their small airways or through triggering of airway hyperresponsiveness. In one large prospective epidemiologic study of healthy full-term neonates, mean flow rate at functional residual capacity at time of recruitment was lower in subjects who later developed wheezing in the first 3 years of life than the subjects who did not.[103,104] Compared with older children, infants have decreased chest wall compliance and higher lung elastic recoil, leading to a lower residual volume, which gives them a greater propensity to being symptomatic during infections due to atelectasis and to increased work of breathing from chest wall distortion.[105–108] Finally, infants are obligatory nose breathers, and the nose accounts for large portion of their total airway resistance, which means that even upper airway infection can produce more severe symptoms in this age group.[109]

Thus, the apparent heterogeneity in the clinical manifestations of asthma in infants and young children is probably due to underlying complex interaction among multiple factors, including genetic, immunologic, environmental, infectious, and physiologic. Current evidence is increasingly supportive of the presence of different pathophysiologic paradigms that correspond to the two distinct clinical patterns in this age group: nonatopic viral respiratory infection–induced asthma and atopic asthma with persistent symptoms. While the latter typically starts at this age, it is the less common of the two in preschool-aged children. Exhaled nitric oxide is a marker of airway inflammation that correlates with atopic airway inflammation.[110–113] Once better standardized and made applicable for young children, it might be useful to confirm the presence or absence of airway inflammation during symptom-free periods. This could potentially provide a noninvasive pathophysiologic marker to differentiate between these two patterns of asthma.[114–118]

NATURAL HISTORY OF EARLY CHILDHOOD ASTHMA

Viral respiratory infections are a major cause of asthma exacerbations at all ages[97,119–122] and appear to be the major risk factor for the large increase in hospital admissions for asthma that occurs every autumn.[123] Preschool-aged children have a particularly high frequency of viral respiratory infections, with most getting three to eight infections per year and 10% to 15% getting 12 or more per year.[124] This is the likely explanation for a frequency of asthma hospitalization in the preschool-aged group that far exceeds that of older children and adults. The rate of hospitalization for asthma among children 1 to 4 years of age has been about 1 in 200 children compared with 1 in 500 children 5 to 14 years of age, and 1 in 1000 for individuals 15 to 24 years of age (Fig. 55-3).[125]

The long-term clinical course of asthma in young children has been examined in a prospective study with repeated evaluations for up to 35 years.[126] In 1963, all children entering first grade in Melbourne, Australia, had a medical examination that included a short questionnaire and interview. As part of that questionnaire, parents were asked if their children had experienced episodes of wheezing or asthma during their preschool years and whether that had been associated with a viral respiratory infection. Based on that survey, an overall community prevalence for asthma symptoms in childhood was estimated to be about 20%, a rate similar to that described more recently in the United States.[127–129] A stratified sample was then randomly selected the following year from the approximately 30,000 7-year-old children previously surveyed. This included 105 second-graders who had never wheezed to serve as controls, 75 with fewer than five episodes of wheezing with viral respiratory infections, 104 with five or more episodes of wheezing with viral respiratory infections, and 113 with recurrent wheezing not limited to association with viral respiratory infections. Three years later, the investigators entered 83 children from the same population who had chronic asthma. These children with severe chronic asthma, now 10 years old, had a history of onset before age 3 years with persistent symptoms at the time of entry with barrel chest deformity and/or forced expiratory volume in 1 second (FEV_1) that was 50% or less than the forced vital capacity. All of the groups of children were reevaluated at ages 14, 21, 28, 35, and 42 years.[130–133]

The subsequent spot prevalence of continued wheezing episodes was 12% at ages 14 and 21. However, 75% of the stratified samples followed longitudinally, an estimated 15% of all children, had infrequent episodes, while 25%, an estimated 5% of all children, had frequent episodes. Only an estimated 0.5% of all children had chronic or persistent asthma based on their survey. Forty percent of the initial children followed were free of respiratory symptoms by age 10, and 50% were asymptomatic by age 14. The remainder continued into adult life, but symptoms were rarely troublesome, usually only present with viral respiratory infections or exercise. However, 10% who had ceased wheezing in childhood had recurrences as young adults, and some of those had troublesome symptoms. Those with chronic or persistent wheezing had growth failure and delayed puberty but eventually attained normal adult height. While 50% of this group improved considerably at puberty, most did not become totally asymptomatic.

When the subjects were examined at 42 years of age, a correlation between the nature of the symptoms in childhood and the subsequent outcome was apparent (Fig. 55-4). Over half of those with symptoms of asthma limited to an association with viral respiratory infection prior to age 7 were asymptomatic at age 42. A substantial number were still having episodic asthma, and a few had developed persistent asthma. Nevertheless, the frequency of all patterns of active asthma at age 42 years was greater among those in whom wheezing without viral respiratory infection had been reported in childhood. About half of those with chronic asthma as children continued to have

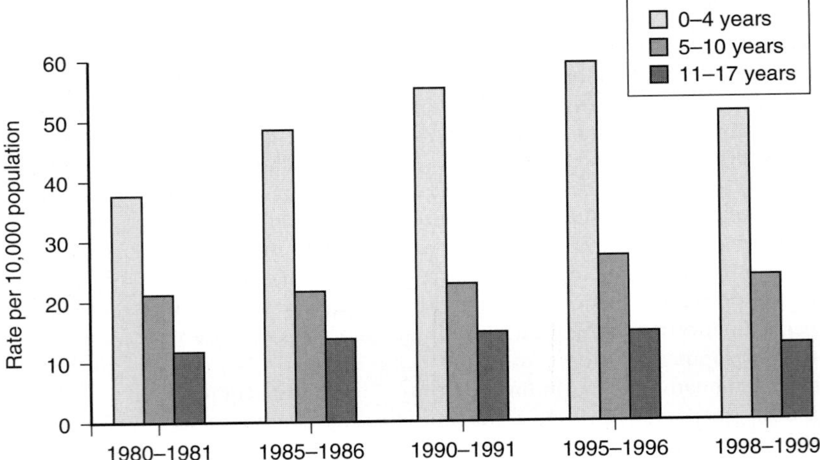

FIGURE 55-3. Hospital discharge rates for asthma as the first listed, by age group and year, in the United States, 1980–1999. (Data from the National Center for Health Statistics, Centers for Disease Control and Prevention; adapted from Akinbami LJ, Schoendorf KC: Trends in childhood asthma. Prevalence, health care utilization, and mortality. Pediatrics 2002;110:315–322.)

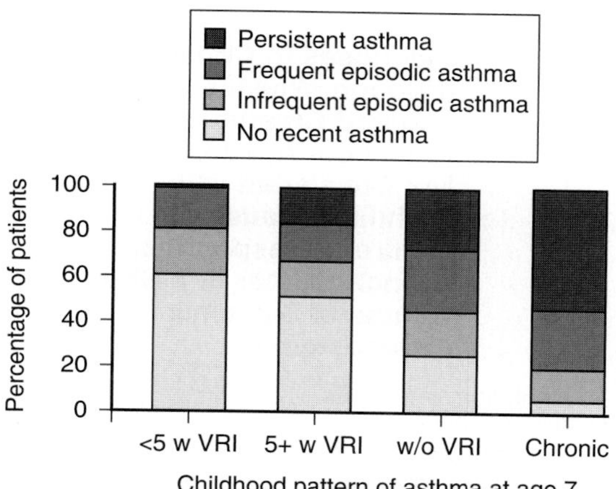

■ **FIGURE 55-4.** Clinical expression of childhood asthma at age 42 years among a stratified random sample from a population of 30,000 children surveyed at entry to first grade, about 20% of whom had symptoms consistent with asthma. The sample included 105 second-graders who never wheezed, 75 with fewer than 5 episodes of wheezing with viral respiratory infections (<5 w VRI), 104 with 5 or more episodes of wheezing with viral respiratory infections (5+ w VRI), 113 with recurrent wheezing not associated with viral respiratory infections (w/o VRI), and 83 children from the same population who had severe chronic asthma (chronic). (Adapted from Phelan PD, Robertson CF, Olinsky A: The Melbourne asthma study: 1965–1999. J Allergy Clin Immunol 2002;109: 189–194.)

persistent symptoms at age 42, with only 11% reporting no recent asthma. Repeated measurements of FEV_1 to age 42 did not differ significantly from controls among the two groups of children who had only wheezing with viral respiratory infection. Those with chronic asthma generally had significant decrements in the FEV_1 that persisted but were not progressive (Fig. 55-5).

It is notable that the patients in this 35-year study who began with asthma in their preschool years had, for the most part, little in the way of what today would be considered optimal treatment. The initial identification of these patients occurred prior to the introduction of inhaled corticosteroids, cromolyn, or even optimal use of oral theophylline. The investigators did not intervene in the patients' care, limiting their involvement to the interval assessments and recommendations communicated only to the patients' physicians. However, the researchers commented that the recommendations were rarely followed. This longitudinal study therefore provides unique data regarding the natural history of asthma, beginning in the preschool years, that is generally untreated by current standards.

■ DIAGNOSIS AND ASSESSMENT

■ CLINICAL PRESENTATION

The typical symptoms of asthma include cough, expiratory wheezing, and dyspnea. Wheezing, the classical finding associated with asthma, is defined as musical, continuous sounds that originate from oscillations in narrowed airways. However, parents reporting of wheezing is confounded by their conceptual understanding of the term.[134] In a survey of parents whose infants had noisy breathing, 59% initially used *wheeze* to describe the respiratory noise their infant made. However, after being shown video clips illustrating wheezing and an upper airway rattle (*ruttle* is the British term), only 36% still described the respiratory sound of their infant as wheezing, whereas the use of the word *ruttle* doubled.[135] In another report using video clips, 30% of parents labeled other sounds as wheeze, while 30% used other words to describe wheezing.[136] Confusion regarding terminology for respiratory sounds is also seen among health care professionals.[137]

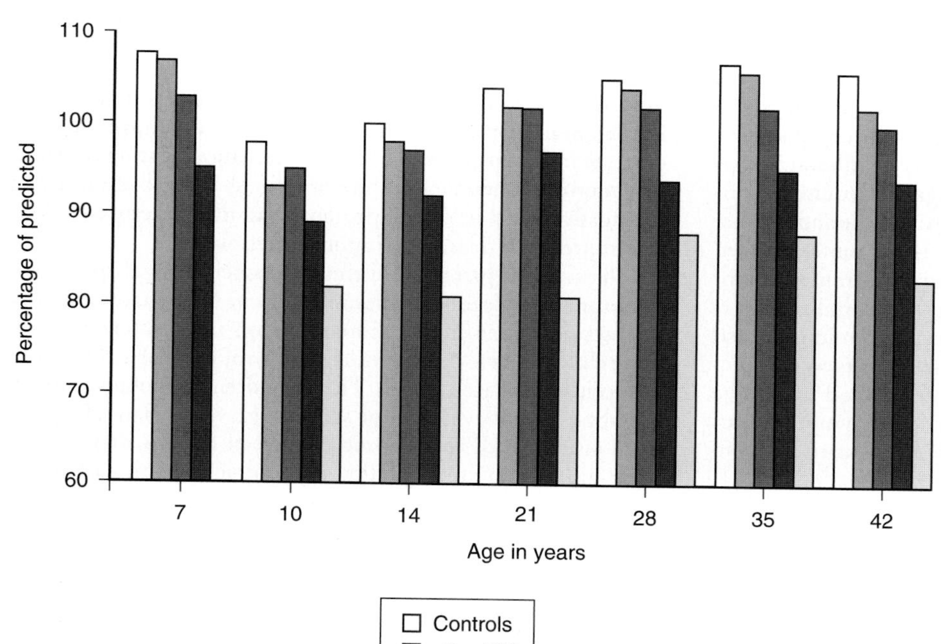

■ **FIGURE 55-5.** One-second forced expiratory volume (FEV_1 expressed as percentage of predicted) for children over time by classification of childhood asthma at the time of recruitment. The categories of asthma at the time of entry into the study included those with fewer than 5 wheezing episodes with viral respiratory infections (<5 w VRI), those with at least 5 episodes with VRI (5+ w VRI), those with episodic wheezing without VRI (w/o VRI), and those with severe persistent asthma (chronic), and controls from the same cohort. (Adapted from Phelan PD, Robertson CF, Olinsky A: The Melbourne asthma study: 1965–1999. J Allergy Clin Immunol 2002;109:189–194.)

Troublesome cough is a characteristic of asthma,[138] and in our own experience, cough is as frequent a symptom as is wheezing. In one report where children with chronic cough as the only symptoms were followed for 3 years, 75% were subsequently diagnosed with classic asthma as the cause of the cough.[139] Shortness of breath and recurrent dyspnea, especially with exertion, are other typical symptoms of asthma but are rarely present alone in the absence of wheezing or cough.

During an acute severe exacerbation of asthma, labored breathing with intercostal and supra- and substernal retractions may be present. Physical findings commonly include polyphonic expiratory wheezing as a manifestation of diffusely narrowed small airways. Course crackles can be present from mucus in the larger airways. Hypoxemia from ventilation-perfusion mismatching is common early in the course of acute asthma with a somewhat decreased partial pressure of carbon dioxide (pCO_2) resulting from the increased hypoxemic ventilatory drive. A rising pCO_2 is an indication of impending respiratory failure. At other times, physical signs of asthma may be absent. This may mean that the asthma is quiescent at the time, but symptoms present hours before, and a nightly cough may still be occurring in the absence of any physical signs when seen by the physician.

Chest x-rays of infants and young children with asthma often show varying patterns of opacification. Common observations include areas of atelectasis from mucous plugging of airways. Peribronchial thickening by inflammation may appear as "rings" and "tram tracks" when airways are cut on cross-section or linearly, respectively. These radiologic abnormalities are the likely explanation for the diagnoses of pneumonia associated with infants and young children with asthma.[140,141] In our own survey of school-aged children with unequivocal asthma referred to our clinic, 30% had prior diagnoses of pneumonia associated with symptoms identical to those subsequently associated with diagnoses of asthma.

Therefore, in the preschool child not symptomatic at the time seen, the diagnosis is dependent on a careful history of previous symptoms consistent with the definition of asthma. Specifically, children with recurrent lower airway symptoms manifested by wheezing, cough, or labored breathing should be considered to potentially have asthma. A family history of asthma or recurrent lower respiratory disease in early childhood is supportive evidence. Confirmation of the diagnosis requires a convincing history of completely symptom-free periods either spontaneously or as a result of treatment. If encountered when symptomatic, a complete response to an inhaled bronchodilator is strong supportive evidence. However, commonly a short course of a relatively high-dose systemic corticosteroid is needed to reverse the inflammation contributing to the airway obstruction. This is a particularly efficient and safe method to test the reversibility of the airway disease. Persistence of symptoms not responsive to such a diagnostic trial of systemic corticosteroid requires consideration of alternative diagnoses (Box 55-1).

BOX 55-1 Diagnoses to Consider if Cough, Wheeze, and/or Labored Breathing in the Preschool-Aged Child Is Not Consistent with Asthma Because of Failure to Respond to Bronchodilator or a Short Course of Systemic Corticosteroid

Aspiration syndromes
Bronchomalacia
Bronchopulmonary dysplasia
Chronic idiopathic purulent bronchitis
Compression of the airway from aberrancy of the great vessels (e.g., vascular ring)
Cystic fibrosis
Foreign body in airway
Foreign body in esophagus (compressing airway)
Primary ciliary dyskinesia
Pertussis
Tracheal polyps
Tracheomalacia

CLINICAL PATTERNS OF ASTHMA

Three rather distinct clinical patterns of asthma can be seen. By far the most common, particularly in the preschool child, is an intermittent pattern where symptoms occur exclusively following the viruses that cause the common cold; these children are completely free of symptoms during the intercurrent periods. Although an intermittent pattern, these symptoms are not necessarily mild and are the major contributors to the high hospitalization rate in this age group (see Fig. 55-3).[125] Since children in this age group have a particularly high frequency of acquiring viral respiratory infections, especially if they are in daycare or have older siblings in school, it can be difficult at the peak times of the seasonal viral respiratory illnesses to distinguish this pattern from the less common chronic pattern of asthma. Moreover, children with persistent symptoms also experience exacerbations from viral respiratory infections, which compounds the diagnostic difficulty. An absence of specific IgE to inhalant allergens is generally predictive of a child in this age group whose pattern will most likely be this viral respiratory infection–induced pattern.[142] When the pattern is unclear during the peak of the viral respiratory disease season, the marked decrease in the frequency of acute exacerbations during the summer months, when viral respiratory illness is less common, can eventually make it more apparent that the pattern is indeed intermittent from viral respiratory infections.[123]

The chronic pattern of asthma is associated with persistent symptoms. While exacerbations may occur with viral respiratory illnesses as is seen in the more common intermittent pattern, these children have daily or near daily symptoms of asthma even between such exacerbations. These children commonly, though not always, have evidence for specific IgE to inhalant allergens. Demonstration of the chronic pattern of asthma may require close clinical monitoring following complete clearing of symptoms with a short course of systemic corticosteroid to determine if symptoms return spontaneously shortly after discontinuation of the systemic corticosteroid. If the patient remains well until a future clinically apparent viral respiratory illness, this is consistent with an intermittent pattern of asthma.

Less common in this age group but nonetheless important to recognize are those children with a seasonal allergic pattern to their asthma. Diagnosis of this pattern requires demonstration of specific IgE to seasonal inhalant allergens associated with asthma in patients whose symptoms occur in association with the presence of those seasonal inhalant allergens. These vary with the region and therefore require some knowledge of the aerobiology of the region where the child lives. Examples of major allergens that contribute to seasonal allergic asthma are grass pollen that peaks in May and June in the California and Pacific Northwest valley areas[143] and *Alternaria* in the Midwest farm country that is variably present throughout the growing season but peaks when the farmers are stirring up the decaying vegetation on which *Alternaria* thrives during harvest time.[144]

EVALUATION OF THE PRESCHOOL CHILD WITH ASTHMA

A detailed history is the major tool for evaluating asthma, and this is particularly true for the preschool child. Recurring lower respiratory symptoms consisting of cough, labored breathing, and expiratory wheezing are consistent with a diagnosis of asthma. Since the major event preceding these symptoms is commonly that of a viral respiratory infection, sometimes with an initial fever at the onset of the illness, diagnoses of bronchitis or pneumonia might have been made previously for these symptoms. It therefore becomes essential in the history to query the specific symptoms that have occurred rather than to accept prior diagnoses of bronchitis or pneumonia uncritically. The history is essential for both diagnosing asthma and identifying the clinical pattern. When the history is unclear or the duration of symptoms has been brief, a prospective history can be useful by utilizing parental maintained diaries of symptoms and response to bronchodilators and/or corticosteroids.

The physical examination in the preschool child with asthma may be normal at the time seen since an intermittent pattern is most common at this age. If symptomatic at the time of the examination, physical findings may include varying degrees of respiratory distress with retractions, tachypnea, and use of accessory muscles of respiration. Even if such findings are present, a diagnosis of asthma can only be made if there have been recurrences of lower respiratory symptoms, since a single episode may be an isolated event; in infancy, the first episode would be called bronchiolitis. While such an initial presentation identifies a child at risk for having recurrences consistent with a diagnosis of asthma, it is the pattern of recurrences that characterizes asthma.

A chest x-ray is not generally helpful in evaluating asthma but may be useful if the diagnosis of asthma is questionable and other diagnoses need to be considered. Pulse oximetry provides a useful screen for oxygenation. Oxygen saturation that is low justifies blood gases to determine if the pCO_2 is low or elevated, which identifies whether the desaturation is a manifestation of ventilation-perfusion mismatching or a sign of respiratory failure that requires prompt admission to an intensive care unit capable of providing assisted ventilation. Pulmonary function testing, so valuable in the evaluation of asthma, is not readily obtainable in the preschool-aged child. However, carefully and patiently instructed older preschoolers have the potential to perform spirometry, and the effort can be rewarded with useful information.[145]

The evaluation to confirm the diagnosis sometimes requires a therapeutic trial. When a child is seen with expiratory wheezing and increased work of breathing who has impressive response to a bronchodilator, this is obviously supportive of the diagnosis. But particularly with viral respiratory infection–induced symptoms, where the inflammatory component of airway obstruction with mucous secretion and mucosal edema predominate, a therapeutic trial of a systemic corticosteroid becomes an effective means to provide support for the diagnosis.

Allergy skin testing is a quick and useful evaluative means of assessing the potential role for specific IgE to inhalant allergens in a child with asthma. There is a common belief that allergy skin testing is not useful in this age group. However, there is extensive documentation of the presence of allergic antibody demonstrable with allergy skin testing in the preschool child and even in infancy.[33–38] The presence of specific IgE to inhalant allergens can identify the young child with asthma who has a potential for an allergic component to his or her disease (see Fig. 56-7). Even when not correlating with symptoms in a child with the common pattern of viral respiratory infection–induced asthma at the time initially evaluated, the presence or absence of specific IgE to inhalant allergens provides prognostic information regarding those children at greater risk for developing persistent symptoms.[146,147]

From the history, physical findings, response to treatment, and allergy skin testing, the diagnosis can be confirmed, the pattern of asthma identified, and the prognosis for continued symptoms reasonably predicted. When the findings raise doubts about the diagnosis of asthma, alternative diagnoses can be considered and appropriate diagnostic tests undertaken.

TREATMENT

There have been many therapeutic options available for asthma.[148] Epinephrine was introduced for treatment of asthma by injection in the early 20th century. Ephedrine, an oral agent with epinephrine-like properties, was isolated from the ancient Chinese herb, Ma Huang, in the 1920s. Subsequent evolution of pharmaceutical development led to inhalational adrenergic bronchodilators with progressively more β_2-specific agonist activity and longer duration of action. Theophylline had been used as a bronchodilator for the relief of acute asthmatic symptoms since the 1930s, initially in patients unresponsive to injected epinephrine,[149] and subsequently as an oral agent in fixed-dose combination with a weak sympathomimetic bronchodilator, ephedrine.[150] Its most important use eventually became maintenance therapy for controlling the symptoms of chronic asthma.[151] Studies of the pharmacodynamic and pharmacokinetic characteristics of theophylline, the development of reliably absorbed slow-release formulations, and the availability of rapid, specific serum assays improved both the efficacy and safety of this drug. Identification of anti-inflammatory effects for theophylline has increased current interest in this venerable medication.[152] Corticosteroids were introduced for treatment of asthma in the 1950s, initially for systemic use and in the 1970s as inhalational agents. Cromolyn, a mast cell stabilizer, also became available in the 1970s. Leukotriene modifiers are the newest class of medications available for the treatment of asthma. Other agents described in the medical literature as having a role for asthma treatment are anticholinergic bronchodilators, magnesium sulfate, and nedocromil. Injections of allergenic extracts have been used for many years as treatment for inhalant allergen-induced asthma, and an anti-IgE monoclonal antibody is available as another means of treating allergic asthma. Environmental manipulation has long been a nonpharmaceutical approach to treatment. The availability of so-called alternative therapy and folk remedies further confound choices by both physician and patient.

Consideration of strategies for treatment selection allows a more focused selection of therapeutic options. Essentially, treatment can be divided into intervention, those measures used to stop acute symptoms of asthma, and maintenance medication, those measures used to prevent symptoms of asthma.

INTERVENTION MEASURES

Acute symptoms generally can be relieved by an inhaled β_2 agonist. Infants, toddlers, and preschool-aged children can receive this bronchodilator effectively from a metered-dose inhaler (MDI) when combined with a valved holding chamber (Fig. 55-6). Efficacy generally matches or exceeds that from a nebulizer with more rapid delivery and convenience for home care.[153–155] The addition of theophylline to vigorous use of an inhaled β_2 agonist such as albuterol is not routinely beneficial in children.[156] However, studies concluding lack of benefit from added theophylline have excluded children in respiratory failure. The potential for theophylline added to children requiring intensive care should not therefore be discounted. The addition of ipratropium to albuterol, while not routinely of benefit, has clinically important additive effects for those with more severe airway obstruction.[157] The limitation of any bronchodilator is the failure to affect the inflammatory component of asthma, which during acute asthma is the predominant reason for continuation of symptoms and eventual hospitalization.

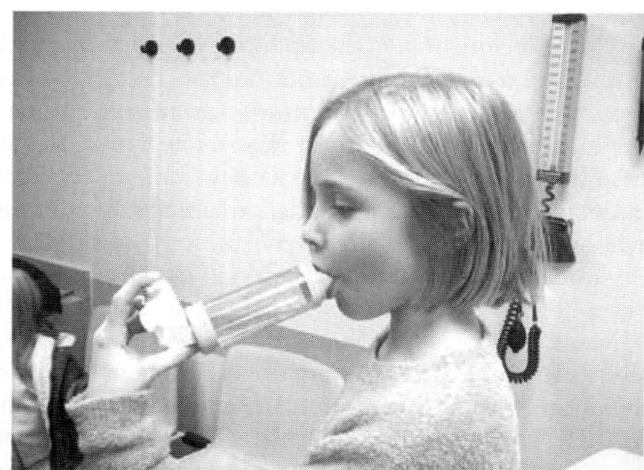

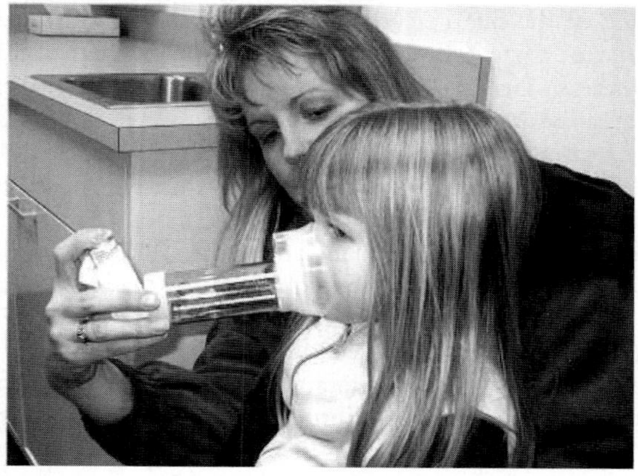

FIGURE 55-6. Demonstration of inhaled medication from a metered dose inhaler (MDI) with a valved holding chamber in a preschool-aged child **(A)** and with a face mask in a toddler **(B).** The MDI injects aerosol into the chamber with one-way valves that permit inhalation of the medication from the chamber while exhalation is into the ambient air. Three to six actuations of albuterol (90 μg/actuation) in this manner with at least three to four breaths after each actuation to evacuate the chamber provides bronchodilator effectiveness equivalent to 2.5 mg of albuterol by open nebulizer with greater convenience and lower cost.

Systemic corticosteroids are potent anti-inflammatory agents for asthma and have long been recognized as being effective for treating acute exacerbations. However, the tradition for many years was to use them only when it was apparent that more conservative measures had failed. Several studies over the past 15 years have demonstrated that earlier aggressive use of systemic steroids in children having an acute exacerbation of asthma decreases the likelihood of requiring urgent care and hospitalization.[158] While there is concern that the high frequency of viral respiratory infection–induced asthma in the preschool child will, at least for periods of time, result in an excessive frequency of oral corticosteroid use, the risks of this effective strategy appear minimal.[159]

Storr and colleagues examined the effect of oral prednisolone in children hospitalized with acute asthma.[160] In a randomized, double-blind, placebo-controlled trial, 67 children received prednisolone and 73 received placebo shortly after admission. Mean age of the children was 5 years. Those younger than 5 years received 30 mg of prednisolone and those 5 or older received 60 mg. At a 5-hour decision time, about 20% of those who received prednisolone could be discharged compared with only about 2% of those who received placebo. Among those not discharged at 5 hours, more rapid improvement and earlier discharge occurred in the prednisolone-treated patients than in those who received placebo.

Tal and colleagues examined the value of systemic corticosteroids in children ranging from 0.5 to 5 years of age seen in an emergency room for acute asthma.[161] Using 4 mg/kg of intramuscular methylprednisolone or normal saline in a double-blind, placebo-controlled trial, decision to admit to hospital at 3 hours after medication administration was reduced from over 40% of the 35 given the placebo to about 20% of the 39 given the methylprednisolone.

Scarfone and colleagues examined the effect of oral prednisone in children with a mean age of 5 years seen in an emergency room.[162] In a randomized, double-blind trial, 36 received 2 mg/kg of prednisone and 39 received placebo. No differences were seen in a mock decision to admit at 2 hours, but at 4 hours, about 50% of the placebo-treated children were admitted compared with only about 30% of the prednisone-treated children. The differences were substantially larger for a subgroup judged most sick, in which over 70% of the placebo-treated children were admitted compared with less than half of the prednisone-treated children.

Even bronchiolitis, often the first viral respiratory infection–induced episode of lower airway obstruction in children who subsequently have asthma exacerbations from the same viruses, has been shown to respond to corticosteroids if a sufficient dose is used early in the course.[163] Although previous studies at lower doses resulted in equivocal benefit at best, the study by Schuh and colleagues demonstrated 57% fewer hospitalizations (19% versus 44%) in blinded decisions to hospitalize infants with bronchiolitis seen in the emergency department by 4 hours after administration of 1 mg/kg of dexamethasone or placebo.[163] Another study involving treatment in the emergency department using more modest doses of corticosteroid was associated with a decrease in duration of illness.[164] In an attempt to reconcile the conflicting data regarding corticosteroids for very young children with an initial episode of viral respiratory infection–induced wheezing (i.e., bronchiolitis), a review of the existing studies suggested that high doses early in the course but not later after hospitalization had the potential to favorably influence the clinical course.[165]

The use of inhaled corticosteroids for intervention of acute symptoms has been examined in the emergency department and at the onset of an exacerbation at home. Such attempts have been at best marginally successful with some amelioration of symptoms at very high doses but no significant effect on the need for subsequent emergency care, hospitalization, or decisions to use an oral corticosteroid.[166]

MAINTENANCE THERAPY

Maintenance medication, sometimes called controller therapy, has evolved considerably over the years. These are medications used to prevent daily or frequently recurring symptoms. Cromolyn sodium, nedocromil, theophylline, montelukast, and the various inhaled corticosteroids have been the major maintenance medications. Cromolyn and nedocromil generally have become of historical interest only. They are weakly potent, require frequent administration, and if an aerosol medication is to be given, low doses of inhaled corticosteroids are more effective and equally safe. Theophylline, while more effective than cromolyn and nedocromil, has a narrow therapeutic index and is still less effective than a low-dose inhaled corticosteroid.[151] Montelukast appears to be no more effective than cromolyn or nedocromil but has the convenience factor of being a once daily oral medication with no known adverse effects.

Inhaled corticosteroids have become the maintenance medication with the greatest degree of efficacy. In preschool-aged children with persistent asthma, these agents can be effectively delivered, by both MDI via a valved holding chamber and by nebulizer, with efficacy in decreasing asthmatic symptoms.[167–169] Although there is evidence for dose-related systemic effects,[170] conventional low doses have an established safety record.[171,172] A minimal degree of hypothalamic-pituitary axis suppression and a small degree of transient growth suppression is detectable at modest doses, but neither clinically detectable adverse effects nor sustained effect on growth are apparent except at higher doses.[173]

LIMITATION OF MAINTENANCE MEDICATION

There is considerable emphasis currently on maintenance medication, with inhaled corticosteroids demonstrably and unequivocally the most effective medication for eliminating the daily symptoms and signs of chronic (persistent) asthma. However, convincing data have demonstrated that these agents, at least in conventional doses, do not prevent exacerbations of asthma from viral respiratory infections.[174–176] Nor are there any other currently available therapeutic measures that can, as safe maintenance therapy, prevent viral respiratory infection–induced asthma.[177] Since viral respiratory infections are the major contributors to acute care requirements for asthma,[97,119–123] especially in young children who have an especially high frequency of these common cold viruses,[124] providing effective intervention measures to treat viral respiratory infection–induced asthma is critically important in current efforts to stem the endemic tide of asthma morbidity.

ENVIRONMENTAL ASPECTS OF TREATMENT

Environmental factors that influence the course of asthma in young children include both irritant and immunologic (i.e., allergic) stimuli. By far the most important well-documented factor that worsens asthma and increases the risk for emergency care requirements and hospitalizations is environmental tobacco smoke.[178–180] The greatest effect appears to be in younger children, although many asthmatic children readily relate an increase in symptoms from even casual exposure to cigarette smoke. While parents may state that they do not smoke around the child, such partial measures appear to have little effect in decreasing exposure to the young child. In a cross-sectional survey, only banning smoking from the home was found to be associated with reduction in urinary cotinine in infants.[181] Particulate-producing indoor burning such as from wood-burning stoves and fireplaces are potential offenders. Strong odors such as perfume, incense, and other airway irritants such as burning leaves can also act as environmental triggers for asthma.[182] Leaf burning, with its release of toxic and irritating smoke, can cause considerable problems in those communities that continue to permit that practice in populated areas.[183]

Questions have been raised about other environmental substances and their role in asthma. Natural gas from range-top burners or nonventilated room heaters releases substances that have the potential to be airway irritants and have been associated with some increase in the frequency of respiratory illness in children.[184] Areas of controversy relate to low levels of naturally occurring chemicals. Formaldehyde has been a topic of concern. While formaldehyde (and many other chemicals) has potentially toxic effects on the airway at high concentrations as may occur during occupational exposure,[185] it is not apparent that normal household exposure of trace amounts of formaldehyde that leach from some manufactured products actually causes problems.[186,187] Since asthma is commonly triggered by multiple factors with common cold viruses causing some of the most severe symptoms in children and accounting for the majority of emergency room visits and hospitalizations,[97] the mere presence of low levels of chemical substances, such as formaldehyde, does not necessarily imply an etiologic role.

Of environmental allergic factors that have a high rate of increasing asthma symptoms once children are identified with the disease, dust mites have been identified as a major factor in humid areas such as the southeastern United States but probably are a less major problem in dry climates or cold northern climates where central heating results in very low humidity during the winter. Airborne particles from cockroaches have been identified as an environmental factor triggering asthma in northeastern inner city areas.[188] Indoor molds can be a major trigger for asthma depending on the indoor environment. Indoor molds thrive in high-humidity situations and particularly when there is water seepage, such as in basements or bathrooms.[35] Outdoor molds that grow on decaying vegetation are a major seasonal allergic trigger for asthma in many parts of the country, particularly in the U.S. farm belt.[144] Animal danders can be triggers for asthma in sensitized children.[36]

Environmental manipulation as treatment of asthma in young children therefore requires identification of the major offenders. Tobacco smoke and other indoor lung irritants should obviously be avoided. Traditional environmental control measures for allergens requires documentation that the child has specific IgE to those factors. Removing pets or compulsive housecleaning in the case of a nonallergic child with predominantly viral respiratory infection–induced asthma is not advisable. When specific IgE to a household inhalant is found, measures to decrease exposure should be undertaken if the history supports those inhalants as risk factors for worsening the disease currently or in the future. There are no rigid guidelines for making these decisions, which require a clinical judgment that is complicated by the multiple factors that can worsen asthma. Placing dust-proof casings on the mattress and pillow, the major sources of exposure to dust mites, is a prudent measure for those with large positive skin test results to dust mites, as is using a vacuum cleaner with a high-efficiency particulate air filter. These and other dust mite measures have the potential to be effective for selected patients.[189–191] Reducing humidity in the home to below 60% has the potential to decrease indoor molds and thereby potentially decrease symptoms for those demonstrated to be clinically sensitive to these common aeroallergens.

IMMUNOTHERAPY (ALLERGY SHOTS) FOR ENVIRONMENTAL AEROALLERGENS

There has long been controversy regarding the potential of injections of allergenic extracts to ameliorate the clinical course of asthma. The issue is not whether or not injections of some allergenic extracts can reduce symptoms of inhalant allergy; that evidence is well supported with controlled clinical trials.[143] The problem relates to the complexity of asthma, the multiple factors that contribute to symptoms, not all of which are allergic, and the limitations of evidence from controlled clinical trials. The major precipitants for asthma in young children are viral respiratory infections, for which there is little reason to expect benefit from immunotherapy with allergenic extracts even among those with some positive allergy skin test results. Even for those where aeroallergens are judged to contribute to the asthma of a young child, some of the most potent asthmagenic aeroallergens such as the molds have little supportive evidence for efficacy of immunotherapy.[192] In contrast, injection of allergenic extracts for pollen-induced asthma is highly effective.[143] Thus, while the indications for injections of allergenic extracts are extremely limited for asthma, especially for preschool children, there will be occasional exceptions where it should be considered as an option (Fig. 55-7).

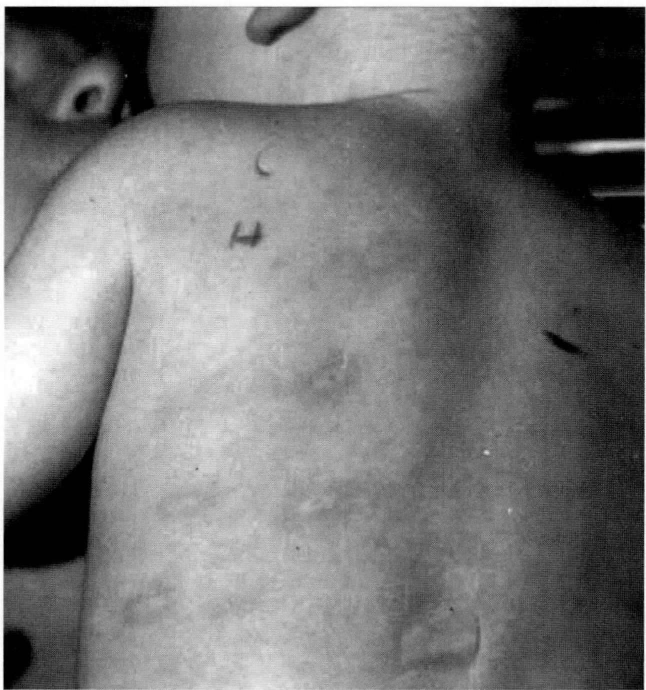

FIGURE 55-7. This 11-month-old infant was hospitalized at 9 months of age with severe acute asthma preceded by rhinoconjunctivitis during the peak of the grass pollen season in a northern California valley area. The typical wheal and flare of the multiple related species of grass pollen native to that area are seen on the left side of the infant's back. They are much larger than the histamine control (*H*) with no reactivity to the diluent control (*C*). Skin tests on the right side of the back to other common inhalant allergens were all negative. While immunotherapy using injections of allergenic extracts is rarely indicated at this age, this infant illustrates a striking exception where benefit could reasonably be expected. (See Color Plate 41.)

FAMILY EDUCATION

Many families who have young children with asthma lack knowledge of their disease[193,194] and fail to recognize and respond appropriately to symptoms and signs that precede severe attacks.[195,196] The recognition that patient self-management skills needed to be upgraded led to the development of several self-management programs.[197] Most cover similar topics: discrimination of symptoms, explanations of how different medications work and when to use them, recognition of situations that require emergency care, discussions of asthma triggers and how to avoid them, and the importance of effective communication between the patient or family and health care workers.[198] These programs are based on social and behavioral theories that suggest education can improve understanding of asthma and thereby provide motivation to take an active part in their own asthma management.[199] Social learning theory suggests that cognitive factors, memory or retention, motivation, and self-efficacy are crucial links between initial training and subsequent performance of the desired tasks in asthma self-management programs.[200] However, the results of these programs has often been equivocal at best.[198,201,202]

Since asthma is a heterogeneous disease with various clinical patterns, generic family education has limited value. Once the diagnosis is made and the asthma in the individual child is characterized regarding clinical pattern and precipitating factors, the information should be shared with the family. Since the most common pattern of asthma in young children is viral respiratory infection induced, an explanation of that mechanism and the frequency of viral respiratory infections in the preschool age group prepares the family for anticipated events. Whether or not maintenance medication is used for an element of persistent symptoms unrelated to viral respiratory infections, an explanation that exacerbations are likely to occur with colds prepares the family for the need to utilize intervention measures at those times. Further explaining the limitation of bronchodilators with regard to the inflammatory component of airway disease in asthma prepares them for the need to recognize bronchodilator subresponsiveness as a sign of progressive airway inflammation and the need to intervene with an oral corticosteroid. These principles should be outlined in a very simple written action plan (Box 55-2).

SUMMARY

The controversies and confusion regarding defining asthma are greater in the preschool child than later in childhood. This is due, at least in part, to the varying clinical patterns of asthma with the predominance of viral respiratory infection–induced asthma in the early years. While the persistent pattern of asthma in later childhood typically has its origins in the early years, spontaneous improvement with age is typical of the intermittent

BOX 55-2 Patient Instruction Intervention Action Plan for Acute Symptoms of Asthma

Asthma symptoms include cough, wheeze, or shortness of breath. They are particularly likely with a viral respiratory infection *(common cold)*. Increasing cough is often the first sign of asthma triggered by a viral respiratory infection.

When asthma symptoms are observed in your child, follow these steps:

First, use the inhaled bronchodilator.

If symptoms stop completely, repeat use of the inhaled bronchodilator when necessary.

If symptoms are not completely relieved, repeat use of the inhaled bronchodilator.

If symptoms are still not completely relieved, or if a third dose for acute symptoms is needed within 8 hours, or if more than 4 doses are needed in 24 hours, a short course of oral corticosteroids may be needed—call for advice if you have questions, or give the first dose and then call so that the frequency of courses and response can be monitored.

viral respiratory infection–induced pattern. The genetics of asthma in young children is complex, with components of both airway hyperresponsiveness and atopic allergy for those who eventually develop persistent asthma, but even the intermittent viral respiratory infection–induced pattern appears to have a familial tendency, although this has been less well studied. The inflammatory component of asthma is different for asthma associated exclusively with viral respiratory infections than that seen in the allergic model of asthma. The natural history of asthma in the preschool years has been well studied. While over half of those with the common viral respiratory infection–induced pattern remit, most with severe chronic asthma continue into adult life. Despite the benign course of the intermittent pattern in the early years, this age group has the greatest frequency of hospitalizations as a result of the frequency of viral respiratory infections in this age group. Maintenance therapy, even with inhaled corticosteroids, does not prevent viral respiratory infection–induced exacerbations in these patients. Early intervention with a short course of relatively high-dose oral corticosteroids is essential to minimize the need for urgent care and hospitalization for acute exacerbations from viral respiratory infections. Inhaled corticosteroids are the most effective agents for maintenance in those with persistent asthma, and can be effective when given by nebulizer or more conveniently by MDI with a valved holding chamber in infants and young children. Allergic evaluation may provide information for therapeutic environmental elimination measures but often in this age group is primarily of prognostic value, with the absence of specific IgE to common inhalant allergens predictive of less likelihood for persistent symptoms later in childhood.

REFERENCES

1. Gross NJ: What is this thing called love?—or, defining asthma. Am Rev Respir Dis 1980;121:203–204.
2. Sears MR: The definition and diagnosis of asthma. Allergy 1993;48:12–16.
3. Meneely GR, Renzetti AD, Steele JD, Wyatt JP, Harris HW: Chronic bronchitis, asthma and pulmonary emphysema. A statement by the committee on diagnostic standards for nontuberculous respiratory disease. Am Rev Respir Dis 1962;85:762–768.
4. Dantzker DR, Pingleton SK, Pierce JA, Niewoehner DE, Thurlbeck WM, Buist AS: Standards for the diagnosis and care of patients with chronic obstructive pulmonary disease and asthma. Am Rev Respir Dis 1987; 136(Part 2):225–243.
5. Godfrey S: What is asthma? Arch Dis Child 1985;60:997–1000.
6. Hargreave FE, Gibson PG, Ramsdale EH: Airway hyperresponsiveness, airway inflammation, and asthma. Immunol Allergy Clin North Am 1990; 10:439–448.
7. U.S. Department of Health and Human Services, National Institutes of Health: Guidelines for the diagnosis and management of asthma. In: National Asthma Education Program Expert Panel Report. Publication no. 91-3042. Washington, DC: U.S. Department of Health and Human Services, National Institutes of Health, 1991.
8. National Heart, Lung, and Blood Institute, National Institutes of Health: Guidelines for the Diagnosis and Management of Asthma. Publication no. 97-4051. Washington, DC: U.S. Government Printing Office, 1997, pp 7–8.
9. McFadden ER, Gilbert IA: Asthma. N Engl J Med 1992;327:1928–1937.
10. Brusasco V, Crimi E, Pellegrino R: Airway hyperresponsiveness in asthma. Not just a matter of airway inflammation. Thorax 1998;53:992–998.
11. Joseph CL, Foxman B, Leickly FE, Peterson E, Ownby D: Prevalence of possible undiagnosed asthma and associated morbidity among urban schoolchildren. J Pediatr 1996;129:735–742.
12. Yeatts K, Shy C, Sotir M, Music S, Herget C: Health consequences for children with undiagnosed asthma-like symptoms. Arch Pediatr Adolesc Med 2003;157:540–544.
13. Postma DS, Meijer GG, Koppelman GH: Definition of asthma. Possible approaches in genetic studies. Clin Exp Allergy 1998;28(Suppl 1):62–64.
14. Blumenthal MN, Rich SS, King R, Weber J: Approaches and issues in defining asthma and associated phenotypes map to chromosome susceptibility areas in large Minnesota families. Clin Exp Allergy 1998;28(Suppl 1): 51–55.
15. Kauppi P, Laitinen LA, Laitinen H, Kere J, Laitinen T: Phenotyping asthma patients for a gene mapping study in Finland. Clin Exp Allergy 1998; 28(Suppl 1):40–42.
16. Koopman LP, Brunekreef B, deJongste JC, Neijens HJ: Definition of respiratory symptoms and disease in early childhood in large prospective birth cohort studies that predict the development of asthma. Pediatr Allergy Immunol 2001;12:118–124.
17. Martinez FD: Development of wheezing disorders and asthma in preschool children. Pediatrics 2002;109:362–367.
18. Shay DK, Holman RC, Newman RD, Liu LL, Stout JW, Anderson LJ: Bronchiolitis-associated hospitalizations among US children, 1980–1996. JAMA 1999;282:1440–1446.
19. Yunginger JW, Reed CE, O'Connell EJ, Melton LJ III, O'Fallon WM, Silverstein MD: A community-based study of the epidemiology of asthma. Incidence rates, 1964–1983. Am Rev Respir Dis 1992;146:888–894.
20. Welliver RC, Sun M, Rinaldo D, Ogra PL: Predictive value of respiratory syncytial virus-specific IgE responses for recurrent wheezing following bronchiolitis. J Pediatr 1986;109:776–780.
21. Sigurs N, Bjarnason R, Sigurbergsson F, Kjellman B, Bjorksten B: Asthma and immunoglobulin E antibodies after respiratory syncytial virus bronchiolitis. A prospective cohort study with matched controls. Pediatrics 1995;95:500–505.
22. von Mutius E: Paediatric origins of adult lung disease. Thorax 2001;56: 153–157.
23. Weinberger M: Clinical patterns and natural history of asthma. J Pediatr 2003;142(Suppl):15–20.
24. Panhuysen CI, Bleecker ER, Koeter GH, Meyers DA, Postma DS: Characterization of obstructive airway disease in family members of probands with asthma. An algorithm for the diagnosis of asthma. Am J Respir Crit Care Med 1998;157:1734–1742.
25. Edfors-Lubs ML: Allergy in 7000 twin pairs. Acta Allergol 1971;26:249–285.
26. Duffy DL, Nicholas MG, Battistutta D, Hopper JL, Mathews JD: Genetics of asthma and hay fever in Australian twins. Am Rev Respir Dis 1990;142: 1351–1358.
27. Wiesch DG, Meyers DA, Bleecker ER: Genetics of asthma. J Allergy Clin Immunol 1999;104:895–901.
28. Weinberger MM: Mechanisms and management of reactive airways in children. Curr Opin Pediatr 1991;3:399–407.
29. Palmer LJ, Rye PJ, Gibson NA, Burton PR, Landau LI, LeSouëf PN: Airway responsiveness in early infancy predicts asthma, lung function, and

respiratory symptoms by school age. Am J Rev Respir Crit Care Med 2001;163:37–42.

30. Longo G, Strinati R, Poli F, Fumi F: Genetic factors in nonspecific bronchial hyperreactivity. Am J Dis Child 1987;141:331–334.
31. Hopp RJ, Bewtra AK, Biven R, Nair NM, Townley RG: Bronchial reactivity pattern in nonasthmatic parents of asthmatics. Ann Allergy 1988;61: 184–186.
32. Hopp RJ, Bewtra AK, Watt GD, Nair NM, Townley RG: Genetic analysis of allergic disease in twins. J Allergy Clin Immunol 1984;73:265–270.
33. Wilson NW, Robinson NP, Hogan MB: Cockroach and other inhalant allergies in infantile asthma. Ann Allergy Asthma Immunol 1999;83:27–30.
34. Arshad SH, Hide DW: Effect of environmental factors on the development of allergic disorders in infancy. J Allergy Clin Immunol 1992;90:235–241.
35. Lindfors A, Wickman M, Hedlin G, Pershagen G, Rietz H, Nordvall SL: Indoor environmental risk factors in young asthmatics. A case-control study. Arch Dis Child 1995;73:408–412.
36. Lindfors A, van Hage-Hamsten M, Rietz H, Wickman M, Nordvall SL: Influence of interaction of environmental risk factors and sensitization in young asthmatic children. J Allergy Clin Immunol 1999;104:755–762.
37. Sears MR, Holdaway MD, Flannery EM, Herbison BG, Silva PA: Parental and neonatal risk factors for atopy, airway hyper-responsiveness, and asthma. Arch Dis Child 1996;75:392–398.
38. Sherrill D, Stein R, Kurzius-Spencer M, Martinez F: On early sensitization to allergens and development of respiratory symptoms. Clin Exp Allergy 1999;29:905–911.
39. Nelson HS, Szefler SJ, Jacobs J, Huss K, Shapiro G, Sternberg AL: The relationships among environmental allergen sensitization, allergen exposure, pulmonary function, and bronchial hyperresponsiveness in the Childhood Asthma Management Program. J Allergy Clin Immunol 1999;104:775–785.
40. Payne D, McKenzie SA, Stacey S, Misra D, Haxby E, Bush A: Safety and ethics of bronchoscopy and endobronchial biopsy in difficult asthma. Arch Dis Child 2001;84:423–426.
41. Jorgensen IM, Bulow S, Jensen VB, Dahm TL, Prahl P, Juel K: Asthma mortality in Danish children and young adults, 1973–1994. Epidemiology and validity of death certificates. Eur Respir J 2000;15:844–848.
42. Weitzman JB, Kanarek NF, Smialek JE: Medical examiner asthma death autopsies. A distinct subgroup of asthma deaths with implications for public health preventive strategies. Arch Pathol Lab Med 1998;122:691–699.
43. Cutz E, Levison H, Cooper DM: Ultrastructure of airways in children with asthma. Histopathology 1978;2:407–401.
44. McKay KO, Hogg JC: The contribution of airway structure to early childhood asthma. Med J Aust 2002;177(Suppl):45–47.
45. Shields MD, Brown V, Stevenson EC, Fitch PS, Schock BC, Turner G, Taylor R, Ennis M:. Serum eosinophilic cationic protein and blood eosinophil counts for the prediction of the presence of airways inflammation in children with wheezing. Clin Exp Allergy 1999;29:1382–1389.
46. Kurukulaaratchy RJ, Fenn MH, Waterhouse LM, Matthews SM, Holgate ST, Arshad SH: Characterization of wheezing phenotypes in the first 10 years of life. Clin Exp Allergy 2003;33:573–578.
47. Stevenson EC, Turner G, Heaney LG, Schock BC, Taylor R, Gallagher T, Ennis M, Shields MD: Bronchoalveolar lavage findings suggest two different forms of childhood asthma. Clin Exp Allergy 1997;27:1027–1035.
48. Ennis M, Turner G, Schock BC, Stevenson EC, Brown V, Fitch PS, Heaney LG, Taylor R, Shields MD: Inflammatory mediators in bronchoalveolar lavage samples from children with and without asthma. Clin Exp Allergy 1999;29:362–366.
49. Oh JW, Lee HB, Yum MK, Kim CR, Kang JO, Park IK: ECP level in nasopharyngeal secretions and serum from children with respiratory virus infections and asthmatic children. Allergy Asthma Proc 2000;21:97–100.
50. Najafi N, Demanet C, Dab I, De Waele M, Malfroot A: Differential cytology of bronchoalveolar lavage fluid in asthmatic children. Pediatr Pulmonol 2003;35:302–308.
51. Cai Y, Carty K, Henry RL, Gibson PG: Persistence of sputum eosinophilia in children with controlled asthma when compared with healthy children. Eur Respir J 1998;11:848–853.
52. Marguet C, Jouen-Boedes F, Dean TP, Warner JO: Bronchoalveolar cell profiles in children with asthma, infantile wheeze, chronic cough, or cystic fibrosis. Am J Respir Crit Care Med 1999;159:1533–1540.
53. Azevedo I, de Blic J, Vargaftig BB, Bachelet M, Scheinmann P: Increased eosinophil cationic protein levels in bronchoalveolar lavage from wheezy infants. Pediatr Allergy Immunol 2001;12:65–72.
54. Oymar K: High levels of urinary eosinophil protein X in young asthmatic children predict persistent atopic asthma. Pediatr Allergy Immunol 2001;12:312–317.
55. Pizzichini E, Pizzichini MM, Kidney JC, Efthimiadis A, Hussack P, Popov T, Cox G, Dolovich J, O'Byrne P, Hargreave FE: Induced sputum, bronchoalveolar lavage and blood from mild asthmatics. Inflammatory cells, lymphocyte subsets and soluble markers compared. Eur Respir J 1998;11:828–834.
56. Bodey KJ, Semper AE, Redington AE, Madden J, Teran LM, Holgate ST, Frew AJ: Cytokine profiles of BAL T cells and T-cell clones obtained from human asthmatic airways after local allergen challenge. Allergy 1999;54:1083–1093.
57. Kraft M, Djukanovic R, Torvik J, Cunningham L, Henson J, Wilson S, Holgate ST, Hyde D, Martin R: Evaluation of airway inflammation by endobronchial and transbronchial biopsy in nocturnal and nonnocturnal asthma. Chest 1995;107(Suppl):162S.
58. Tillie-Leblond I, Hammad H, Desurmont S, Pugin J, Wallaert B, Tonnel AB, Gosset P: CC chemokines and interleukin-5 in bronchial lavage fluid from patients with status asthmaticus. Potential implication in eosinophil recruitment. Am J Respir Crit Care Med 2000;162:586–592.
59. Magnan AO, Mely LG, Camilla CA, Badier MM, Montero-Julian FA, Guillot CM, Casano BB, Prato SJ, Fert V, Bongrand P, Vervloet D: Assessment of the Th1/Th2 paradigm in whole blood in atopy and asthma. Increased IFN-gamma-producing CD8(+) T cells in asthma. Am J Respir Crit Care Med 2000;161:1790–1796.
60. Kips JC, Anderson GP, Fredberg JJ, Herz U, Inman MD, Jordana M, Kemeny DM, Lotvall J, Pauwels RA, Plopper CG, Schmidt D Sterk PJ, Van Oosterhout AJ, Vargaftig BB, Chung KF: Murine models of asthma. Eur Respir J 2003;22:374–382.
61. Foster PS, Mould AW, Yang M, Mackenzie J, Mattes J, Hogan SP, Mahalingam S, Mckenzie AN, Rothenberg ME, Young IG, Matthaei KJ, Webb DC: Elemental signals regulating eosinophil accumulation in the lung. Immunol Rev 2001;179:173–181.
62. Webb DC, McKenzie AN, Koskinen AM, Yang M, Mattes J, Foster PS: Integrated signals between IL-13, IL-4, and IL-5 regulate airways hyperreactivity. J Immunol 2000;165:108–113.
63. Wilson NM. Virus infections, wheeze and asthma. Paediatr Respir Rev 2003;4:184–192.
64. Fitch PS, Brown V, Schock BC, Ennis M, Shields MD: Interleukin-4 and interleukin-4 soluble receptor alpha levels in bronchoalveolar lavage from children with asthma. Ann Allergy Asthma Immunol 2003;90: 429–433.
65. Juntti H, Kokkonen J, Dunder T, Renko M, Niinimaki A, Uhari M: Association of an early respiratory syncytial virus infection and atopic allergy. Allergy 2003;58:878–884.
66. Zeiger RS, Heller S, Mellon MH, Forsythe AB, O'Connor RD, Hamburger RN, Schatz M: Effect of combined maternal and infant food-allergen avoidance on development of atopy in early infancy. A randomized study. J Allergy Clin Immunol 1989;84:72–89.
67. Hattevig G, Sigurs N, Kjellman B: Effects of maternal dietary avoidance during lactation on allergy in children at 10 years of age. Acta Paediatr 1999;88:7–12.
68. Ring J, Kramer U, Schafer T, Abeck D, Vieluf D, Behrendt H: Environmental risk factors for respiratory and skin atopy. Results from epidemiological studies in former East and West Germany. Int Arch Allergy Immunol 1999;118:403–407.
69. Shirtcliffe P, Weatherall M, Beasley R: An inverse correlation between estimated tuberculosis notification rates and asthma symptoms. Respirology 2002;7:153–155.
70. Jones PD: The cause of Th2 to Th1 imbalance in asthma: a function of exposure to typhoid and tuberculosis? J Pediatr Gastroenterol Nutr 2002;34(Suppl 1):31–32.
71. Marks GB, Ng K, Zhou J, Toelle BG, Xuan W, Belousova EG, Britton WJ: The effect of neonatal BCG vaccination on atopy and asthma at age 7 to 14 years. An historical cohort study in a community with a very low prevalence of tuberculosis infection and a high prevalence of atopic disease. J Allergy Clin Immunol 2003;111:541–549.
72. Bager P, Rostgaard K, Nielsen NM, Melbye M, Westergaard T: Age at bacille Calmette-Guerin vaccination and risk of allergy and asthma. Clin Exp Allergy 2003;33:1512–1517.
73. Pizzichini MM, Pizzichini E, Efthimiadis A, Chauhan AJ, Johnston SL, Hussack P, Mahony J, Dolovich J, Hargreave FE: Asthma and natural colds. Inflammatory indices in induced sputum. A feasibility study. Am J Respir Crit Care Med 1998;158:1178–1184.
74. Teran LM, Johnston SL, Schroder JM, Church MK, Holgate ST: Role of nasal interleukin-8 in neutrophil recruitment and activation in children with virus-induced asthma. Am J Respir Crit Care Med 1997;155: 1362–1366.
75. Teran LM, Seminario MC, Shute JK, Papi A, Compton SJ, Low JL, Gleich GJ, Johnston SL: RANTES, macrophage-inhibitory protein 1alpha, and the eosinophil product major basic protein are released into upper

respiratory secretions during virus-induced asthma exacerbations in children. J Infect Dis 1999;179:677–681.
76. Twaddell SH, Gibson PG, Carty K, Woolley KL, Henry RL: Assessment of airway inflammation in children with acute asthma using induced sputum. Eur Respir J 1996;9:2104–2108.
77. Nagayama Y, Odazima Y, Nakayama S, Toba T, Funabashi S: Eosinophils and basophilic cells in sputum and nasal smears taken from infants and young children during acute asthma. Pediatr Allergy Immunol 1995;6: 204–208.
78. de Blic J, Tillie-Leblond I, Tonnel AB, Jaubert F, Scheinmann P, Gosset P: Difficult asthma in children. An analysis of airway inflammation. J Allergy Clin Immunol 2004;113:94–100.
79. Marguet C, Dean TP, Basuyau JP, Warner JO: Eosinophil cationic protein and interleukin-8 levels in bronchial lavage fluid from children with asthma and infantile wheeze. Pediatr Allergy Immunol 2001;12:27–33.
80. Gibson PG, Norzila MZ, Fakes K, Simpson J, Henry RL: Pattern of airway inflammation and its determinants in children with acute severe asthma. Pediatr Pulmonol 1999;28:261–270.
81. Miranda C, Busacker A, Balzar S, Trudeau J, Wenzel SE: Distinguishing severe asthma phenotypes. Role of age at onset and eosinophilic inflammation. J Allergy Clin Immunol 2004;113:101–108.
82. Sigurs N: Epidemiologic and clinical evidence of a respiratory syncytial virus-reactive airway disease link. Am J Respir Crit Care Med 2001; 163(Suppl):2–6.
83. Sigurs N: A cohort of children hospitalised with acute RSV bronchiolitis. Impact on later respiratory disease. Paediatr Respir Rev 2002;3:177–183.
84. Stein RT, Sherrill D, Morgan WJ, Holberg CJ, Halonen M, Taussig LM, Wright AL, Martinez FD: Respiratory syncytial virus in early life and risk of wheeze and allergy by age 13 years. Diminished lung function as a predisposing factor for wheezing respiratory illness in infants. Lancet 1999;354:541–545.
85. Oymar K, Elsayed S, Bjerknes R: Serum eosinophil cationic protein and interleukin-5 in children with bronchial asthma and acute bronchiolitis. Pediatr Allergy Immunol 1996;7:180–186.
86. Pala P, Bjarnason R, Sigurbergsson F, Metcalfe C, Sigurs N, Openshaw PJ: Enhanced IL-4 responses in children with a history of respiratory syncytial virus bronchiolitis in infancy. Eur Respir J 2002;20:376–382.
87. Randolph DA, Stephens R, Carruthers CJ, Chaplin DD: Cooperation between Th1 and Th2 cells in a murine model of eosinophilic airway inflammation. J Clin Invest 1999;104:1021–1029.
88. King KA, Hu C, Rodriguez MM, Romaguera R, Jiang X, Piedimonte G: Exaggerated neurogenic inflammation and substance P receptor upregulation in RSV-infected weanling rats. Am J Respir Cell Mol Biol 2001;24: 101–107.
89. Auais A, Adkins B, Napchan G, Piedimonte G: Immunomodulatory effects of sensory nerves during respiratory syncytial virus infection in rats. Am J Physiol Lung Cell Mol Physiol 2003;285:L105–L113.
90. Hu C, Wedde-Beer K, Auais A, Rodriguez MM, Piedimonte G: Nerve growth factor and nerve growth factor receptors in respiratory syncytial virus-infected lungs. Am J Physiol Lung Cell Mol Physiol 2002;283:L494–L502.
91. Colasurdo GN, Hemming VG, Prince GA, Gelfand AS, Loader JE, Larsen GL: Human respiratory syncytial virus produces prolonged alterations of neural control in airways of developing ferrets. Am J Respir Crit Care Med 1998;157:1506–1511.
92. Pifferi M, Ragazzo V, Caramella D, Baldini G: Eosinophil cationic protein in infants with respiratory syncytial virus bronchiolitis. Predictive value for subsequent development of persistent wheezing. Pediatr Pulmonol 2001;31:419–424.
93. Oh JW, Lee HB, Park IK, Kang JO: Interleukin-6, interleukin-8, interleukin-11, and interferon-gamma levels in nasopharyngeal aspirates from wheezing children with respiratory syncytial virus or influenza A virus infection. Pediatr Allergy Immunol 2002;13:350–356.
94. Oymar K, Havnen J, Halvorsen T, Bjerknes R: Eosinophil counts and urinary eosinophil protein X in children hospitalized for wheezing during the first year of life. Prediction of recurrent wheezing. Acta Paediatr 2001;90: 843–849.
95. Kim CK, Kim SW, Park CS, Kim BI, Kang H, Koh YY: Bronchoalveolar lavage cytokine profiles in acute asthma and acute bronchiolitis. J Allergy Clin Immunol 2003;112:64–71.
96. Zhao J, Takamura M, Yamaoka A, Odajima Y, Iikura Y: Altered eosinophil levels as a result of viral infection in asthma exacerbation in childhood. Pediatr Allergy Immunol 2002;13:47–50.
97. Rakes GP, Arruda E, Ingram JM, Hoover GE, Zambrano JC, Hayden FG, Platts-Mills TA, Heymann PW: Rhinovirus and respiratory syncytial virus in wheezing children requiring emergency care. IgE and eosinophil analyses. Am J Respir Crit Care Med 1999;159:785–790.
98. Beydon N, Pin I, Matran R, Chaussain M, Boule M, Alain B, Bellet M, Amsallem F, Alberti C, Denjean A, Gaultier C: Pulmonary function tests in preschool children with asthma. Am J Respir Crit Care Med 2003;168: 640–644.
99. Tepper RS, Jones M, Davis S, Kisling J, Castile R: Rate constant for forced expiration decreases with lung growth during infancy. Am J Respir Crit Care Med 1999;160:835–838.
100. Chitano P, Murphy TM: Maturational changes in airway smooth muscle shortening and relaxation. Implications for asthma. Respir Physiol Neurobiol 2003;137:347–359.
101. Redline S, Tager IB, Segal MR, Gold D, Speizer FE, Weiss ST: The relationship between longitudinal change in pulmonary function and nonspecific airway responsiveness in children and young adults. Am Rev Respir Dis 1989;140:179–184.
102. Tepper RS, Rosenberg D, Eigen H: Airway responsiveness in infants following bronchiolitis. Pediatr Pulmonol 1992;13:6–10.
103. Martinez FD, Morgan WJ, Wright AL, Holberg CJ, Taussig LM: Diminished lung function as a predisposing factor for wheezing respiratory illness in infants. N Engl J Med 1988;319:1112–1117.
104. Hopp RJ: Recurrent wheezing in infants and young children and bronchial hyperresponsiveness. A perspective. Clin Rev Allergy Immunol 2003;24:7–18.
105. Papastamelos C, Panitch HB, England SE, Allen JL: Developmental changes in chest wall compliance in infancy and early childhood. J Appl Physiol 1995;78:179–184.
106. Allen JL, Greenspan JS, Deoras KS, Keklikian E, Wolfson MR, Shaffer TH: Interaction between chest wall motion and lung mechanics in normal infants and infants with bronchopulmonary dysplasia. Pediatr Pulmonol 1991;11:37–43.
107. Silva Neto G, Gerhardt TO, Claure N, Duara S, Bancalari E: Influence of chest wall distortion and esophageal catheter position on esophageal manometry in preterm infants. Pediatr Res 1995;37:617–622.
108. LeSouef PN, Lopes JM, England SJ, Bryan MH, Bryan AC: Influence of chest wall distortion on esophageal pressure. J Appl Physiol 1983;55: 353–358.
109. Lacourt G, Polgar G: Interaction between nasal and pulmonary resistance in newborn infants. J Appl Physiol 1971;30:870–873.
110. Piacentini GL, Bodini A, Costella S, Suzuki Y, Zerman L, Peterson CG, Boner AL: Exhaled nitric oxide, serum ECP and airway responsiveness in mild asthmatic children. Eur Respir J 2000;15:839–843.
111. Mattes J, Storm van's Gravesande K, Reining U, Alving K, Ihorst G, Henschen M, Kuehr J: NO in exhaled air is correlated with markers of eosinophilic airway inflammation in corticosteroid-dependent childhood asthma. Eur Respir J 1999;13:1391–1395.
112. Warke TJ, Fitch PS, Brown V, Taylor R, Lyons JD, Ennis M, Shields MD: Exhaled nitric oxide correlates with airway eosinophils in childhood asthma. Thorax 2002;57:383–387.
113. Lanz MJ, Leung DY, White CW: Comparison of exhaled nitric oxide to spirometry during emergency treatment of asthma exacerbations with glucocorticoids in children. Ann Allergy Asthma Immunol 1999;82: 161–164.
114. Spallarossa D, Battistini E, Silvestri M, Sabatini F, Fregonese L, Brazzola G, Rossi GA: Steroid-naive adolescents with mild intermittent allergic asthma have airway hyperresponsiveness and elevated exhaled nitric oxide levels. J Asthma 2003;40:301–310.
115. Baraldi E, Dario C, Ongaro R, Scollo M, Azzolin NM, Panza N, Paganini N, Zacchello F: Exhaled nitric oxide concentrations during treatment of wheezing exacerbation in infants and young children. Am J Respir Crit Care Med 1999;159:1284–1288.
116. Zambrano JC, Carper HT, Rakes GP, Patrie J, Murphy DD, Platts-Mills TA, Hayden FG, Gwaltney JM, Hatley TK, Owens AM, Heymann PW: Experimental rhinovirus challenges in adults with mild asthma. Response to infection in relation to IgE. J Allergy Clin Immunol 2003;111: 1008–1016.
117. Silvestri M, Spallarossa D, Battistini E, Brusasco V, Rossi GA: Dissociation between exhaled nitric oxide and hyperresponsiveness in children with mild intermittent asthma. Thorax 2000;55:484–488.
118. Silvestri M, Sabatini F, Spallarossa D, Fregonese L, Battistini E, Biraghi MG, Rossi GA: Exhaled nitric oxide levels in non-allergic and allergic mono- or polysensitised children with asthma. Thorax 2001;56:857–862.
119. McIntosh K, Ellis EF, Hoffman LS, Lybass TG, Eller JJ, Fulginiti VA: The association of viral and bacterial respiratory infections with exacerbations of wheezing in young asthmatic children. J Pediatr 1973;82:578–590.
120. Minor TE, Dick EC, DeMeo AN, Ouellette JJ, Cohen M, Reed CE: Viruses as precipitants of asthmatic attacks in children. JAMA 1974;227: 292–298.

121. Nicholson KG, Kent J, Ireland DC: Respiratory viruses and exacerbations of asthma in adults. BMJ 1993;307:982–986.
122. Johnston SL, Pattemore PK, Sanderson G, Smith S, Lampe F, Josephs, L, Symington P, O'Toole S, Myint SH, Tyrrell AJ, Holgate ST: Community study of role of viral infections in exacerbations of asthma in 9–11 year old children. BMJ 1995;310:1225–1229.
123. Dales RE, Schweitzer I, Toogood JH, Drouin M, Yang W, Dolovich J, Boulet J: Respiratory infections and the autumn increase in asthma morbidity. Eur Respir J 1996;9:72–77.
124. Rosenstein N, Phillips WR, Gerber MA, Marcy SM, Schwartz B, Dowell SF: The common cold—Principles of judicious use of antimicrobial agents. Pediatrics 1998;101:181–184.
125. Akinbami LJ, Schoendorf KC: Trends in childhood asthma. Prevalence health care utilization, and mortality. Pediatrics 2002;110:315–322.
126. Phelan PD, Robertson CF, Olinsky A: The Melbourne asthma study: 1965–1999. J Allergy Clin Immunol 2002;109:189–194.
127. Joseph CL, Foxman B, Leickly FE, Peterson E, Ownby D: Prevalence of possible undiagnosed asthma and associated morbidity among urban schoolchildren. J Pediatr 1996;129:735–742.
128. Grant EN, Daugherty SR, Moy JN, Nelson SG, Piorkowski JM, Weiss KB: Prevalence and burden of illness for asthma and related symptoms among kindergartners in Chicago public schools. Ann Allergy Asthma Immunol 1999;83:113–120.
129. Yawn BP, Wollan P, Kurland M, Scanlon P: A longitudinal study of the prevalence of asthma in a community population of school-age children. J Pediatr 2002;140:576–581.
130. Williams HE, McNicol KN: Prevalence, natural history and relationship of wheezy bronchitis and asthma in children. An epidemiological study. BMJ 1969;4:321–325.
131. McNicol KN, Williams HE, Gillam GL: Chest deformity, residual airway obstruction and hyperinflation and growth in children with asthma. I. Prevalence findings from an epidemiological study. Arch Dis Child 1970;45:783–788.
132. McNicol KN, Williams HB: Spectrum of asthma in children. I. Clinical and physiological components. BMJ 1973;4:7–11.
133. Martin AJ, McLennan LA, Landau LI, Phelan PD: Natural history of childhood asthma to adult life. BMJ 1980;280:1397–1400.
134. Cane RS, Ranganathan SC, McKenzie SA: What do parents of wheezy children understand by "wheeze"? Arch Dis Child 2000;82:327–332.
135. Elphick HE, Sherlock P, Foxall G, Simpson EJ, Shiell NA, Primhak RA, Everard ML: Survey of respiratory sounds in infants. Arch Dis Child 2001;84:35–39.
136. Cane RS, McKenzie SA: Parents' interpretations of children's respiratory symptoms on video. Arch Dis Child 2001;84:31–34.
137. Elphick HE, Ritson S, Rodgers H, Everard ML: When a "wheeze" is not a wheeze. Acoustic analysis of breath sounds in infants. Eur Respir J 2000;16:593–597.
138. Li AM, Lex C, Zacharasiewicz A, Wong E, Erin E, Hansel T, Wilson NM, Bush A: Cough frequency in children with stable asthma. Correlation with lung function, exhaled nitric oxide, and sputum eosinophil count. Thorax 2003;58:974–978.
139. Todokoro M, Mochizuki H, Tokuyama K, Morikawa A: Childhood cough variant asthma and its relationship to classic asthma. Ann Allergy Asthma Immunol 2003;90:652–659.
140. Castro-Rodriquez JA, Holberg CJ, Wright AL, Halonen M, Taussig LM, Morgan WJ, Martinez FD: Association of radiologically ascertained pneumonia before age 3 years with asthmalike symptoms and pulmonary function during childhood. A prospective study. Am J Respir Crit Care Med 1999;159:1891–1897.
141. Mahabee-Gittens EM, Bachman DT, Shapiro ED, Dowd MD: Chest radiographs in the pediatric emergency department for children < or = 18 months of age with wheezing. Clin Pediatr 1999;38:395–399.
142. Castro-Rodriguez JA, Holberg CJ, Wright AL, Martinez FD: A clinical index to define risk of asthma in young children with recurrent wheezing. Am J Respir Crit Care Med 2000;162:1403–1406.
143. Reid MJ, Moss RB, Hsu YP, Kwasnicki JM, Commerford TM, Nelson BL: Seasonal asthma in northern California. Allergic causes and efficacy of immunotherapy. J Allergy Clin Immunol 1986;78:590–600.
144. Bush RK, Prochnau JJ: Alternaria-induced asthma. J Allergy Clin Immunol 2004;113:227–234.
145. Marostica PJ, Weist AD, Eigen H, Angelicchio C, Christoph K, Savage J, Grant D, Tepper RS: Spirometry in 3- to 6-year-old children with cystic fibrosis. Am J Respir Crit Care Med 2002;166:67–71.
146. Clough JB, Keeping KA, Edwards LC, Freeman WM, Warner JA, Warner JO: Can we predict which wheezy infants will continue to wheeze? Am J Respir Crit Care Med 1999;160:1473–1480.
147. Kotaniemi-Syrjänen A, Reijonen TM, Romppanen J, Korhonen K, Sabolainen K, Korppi M: Allergen-specific immunoglobulin E antibodies in wheezing infants. The risk for asthma in later childhood. Pediatrics 2003;111:e255–e261.
148. Weinberger M: Innovative therapies for asthma—Where we've been and where we're going. Innovative approaches of the past, present, and future. Pediatr Respir Rev 2004;5(Suppl):113–114.
149. Herrmann G, Aynesworth MB: Successful treatment of persistent extreme dyspnea "status asthmaticus." J Lab Clin Med 1937;23:135–148.
150. Brown EA: New type of medication to be used in bronchial asthma and other allergic conditions. N Engl J Med 1940;223:843–846.
151. Weinberger M, Hendeles L: Theophylline in asthma. N Engl J Med 1996;334:1384–1388.
152. Barnes PJ: Theophylline. New perspectives for an old drug. Am J Respir Crit Care Med 2003;167:813–818.
153. Chou KJ, Cunningham SJ, Crain EF: Metered-dose inhalers with spacers vs nebulizers for pediatric asthma. Arch Pediatr Adolesc Med 1995;149: 201–205.
154. Wildhaber JH, Devadason SG, Hayden MJ, Eber E, Summers QA, LeSouef PN: Aerosol delivery to wheezy infants. A comparison between a nebulizer and two small volume spacers. Pediatr Pulmonol 1997;23: 212–216.
155. Dewar AL, Stewart A, Cogswell JJ, Connett GJ: A randomised controlled trial to assess the relative benefits of large volume spacers and nebulisers to treat acute asthma in hospital. Arch Dis Child 1999;80:421–423.
156. Carter E, Cruz M, Chesrown S, Shieh G, Reilly K, Hendeles L: Efficacy of intravenous theophylline in children hospitalized with severe asthma. J Pediatr 1993;122:470–476.
157. Schuh S, Johnson DW, Callahan S, Canny G, Levison H: Efficacy of frequent nebulized ipratropium bromide added to frequent high-dose albuterol therapy in severe childhood asthma. J Pediatr 1995;126:639–645.
158. Weinberger M: Treatment strategies for viral respiratory infection induced asthma. J Pediatr 2003;142(Suppl):34–39.
159. Ducharme FM, Chabot G, Polychronakos C, Glorieux F, Mazer B: Safety profile of frequent short courses of oral glucocorticoids in acute pediatric asthma. Impact on bone metabolism, bone density, and adrenal function. Pediatrics 2003;111:376–383.
160. Storr J, Barrell E, Barry W, Lenney W, Hatcher G: Effect of a single oral dose of prednisolone in acute childhood asthma. Lancet 1987;1:879–882.
161. Tal A, Levy N, Bearman JE: Methylprednisolone therapy for acute asthma in infants and toddlers. A controlled clinical trial. Pediatrics 1990;86: 350–356.
162. Scarfone RJ, Fuchs SM, Nager AL, Shane SA: Controlled trial of oral prednisone in the emergency department treatment of children with acute asthma. Pediatrics 1993;92:513–518.
163. Schuh S, Coates AL, Binnie R, Allin T, Goia C, Corey M, Dick PT: Efficacy of oral dexamethasone in outpatients with acute bronchiolitis. J Pediatr 2002;140:27–32.
164. Csonka P, Kaila, Pekka M, Laippala P, Iso-Mustajärvi P, Vesikari T, Ashorn P: Oral prednisolone in the acute management of children age 6 to 35 months with viral respiratory infection-induced lower airway disease. A randomized, placebo-controlled trial. J Pediatr 2003;143:725–730.
165. Weinberger M: Corticosteroids for first time young wheezers: current status of the controversy. J Pediatr 2003;143:700–702.
166. Hendeles L, Sherman J: Are inhaled corticosteroids effective for acute exacerbations of asthma in children? J Pediatr 2003;142(Suppl):26–33.
167. Baker JW, Mellon M, Wald J, Welch M, Cruz-Rivera M, Walton-Bowen K: A multiple-dosing placebo-controlled study of budesonide inhalation suspension given once or twice daily for treatment of persistent asthma in young children and infants. Pediatrics 1999;103:414–421.
168. Nielsen KG, Bisgaard H: The effect of inhaled budesonide on symptoms, lung function, and cold air and methacholine responsiveness in 2- to 5-year old asthmatic children. Am J Respir Crit Care Med 2000;162: 1500–1506.
169. Chavasse RJ, Bastian-Lee Y, Richter H, Hilliard T, Seddon P: Persistent wheezing in infants with an atopic tendency responds to inhaled fluticasone. Arch Dis Child 2001;85:143–148.
170. Eid N, Morton R, Olds B, Clark P, Sheikh S, Looney S: Decreased morning serum cortisol levels in children with asthma treated with inhaled fluticasone propionate. Pediatrics 2002;109:217–221.
171. Allen DB: Inhaled corticosteroid therapy for asthma in preschool children. Growth issues. Pediatrics 2002;109:373–380.
172. Kelly HW: Potential adverse effects of the inhaled corticosteroids. J Allergy Clin Immunol 2003;112:469–478.
173. Doull IJ: The effect of asthma and its treatment on growth. Arch Dis Child 2004;89:60–63.

174. Wilson N, Sloper K, Silverman M: Effect of continuous treatment with topical corticosteroid on episodic viral wheezing in preschool children. Arch Dis Child 1995;72:317–320.
175. Stick SM, Burton PR, Clough JB, Cox M, LeSouef PN, Sly PD: The effects of inhaled beclomethasone dipropionate on lung function and histamine responsiveness in recurrently wheezy infants. Arch Dis Child 1995;73:327–332.
176. Doull IJ, Lampe FC, Smith S, Schreiber J, Freezer NJ, Holgate ST: Effect of inhaled corticosteroids on episodes of wheezing associated with viral infection in school age children. Randomized double blind placebo controlled trial. BMJ 1997;315:858–862.
177. Doull IJ: Limitations of maintenance therapy for viral respiratory infection-induced asthma. J Pediatr 2003;142:21–25
178. Cook DG, Strachan DP: Health effects of passive smoking. 3. Parental smoking and prevalence of respiratory symptoms and asthma in school age children. Thorax 1997;52:1081–1094.
179. Feoreani AA, Rennard SI: The role of cigarette smoke in the pathogenesis of asthma and as a trigger for acute symptoms. Curr Opin Pulm Med 1999;5:38–46.
180. Joad JP: Smoking and pediatric respiratory health. Clin Chest Med 2000;21:37–46, vii–viii.
181. Blackburn C, Spencer N, Bonas S, Coe C, Dolan A, Moy R: Effect of strategies to reduce exposure of infants to environmental tobacco smoke in the home. Cross sectional survey. BMJ 2003;327:257–261.
182. From LJ, Bergen LG, Humlie CJ: The effects of open leaf burning on spirometric measurements in asthma. Chest 1992;101:1236–1239.
183. Friedman L, Calabrese EJ: The health implications of open leaf burning. Rev Environ Health 1977;2:257–283.
184. Ekwo E, Weinberger M, Lachenbruch PA, Huntley WH: Relationship of parental smoking and gas cooking to respiratory disease in children. Chest 1983;84:662–668.
185. Bardana EJ, Andrach RH: Occupational asthma secondary to low molecular weight agents used in the plastic and resin industries. Eur J Respir Dis 1983;64:241–251.
186. Frigas E, Filley WV, Reed CE: Bronchial challenge with formaldehyde gas. Lack of bronchoconstriction in 13 patients suspected of having formaldehyde-induced asthma. Mayo Clin Proc 1984;59:295–299.
187. Harving H, Korsgaard J, Pedersen OF, Molhave L, Dahl R: Pulmonary function and bronchial reactivity in asthmatics during low-level formaldehyde exposure. Lung 1990;168:15–21.
188. Eggleston PA, Rosenstreich D, Lynn H, Gergen P, Baker D, Kattan M, Mortimer KM, Mitchell H, Ownby D, Slavin R, Malveaux F: Relationship of indoor allergen exposure to skin test sensitivity in inner-city children with asthma. J Allergy Clin Immunol 1998;102:563–570.
189. Murray AB, Ferguson AG: Dust-free bedrooms in the treatment of asthmatic children with house dust or house dust mite allergy. A controlled trial. Pediatrics 1983;71:418–422.
190. Halken S, Høst A, Niklassen U, Hansen LG, Nielsen F, Pedersen S, Østerballe O, Veggerby C, Pousen LK: Effect of mattress and pillow encasings on children with asthma and house dust mite allergy. J Allergy Clin Immunol 2003;111:169–176.
191. Weinberger M: Allergen-impermeable bedding covers for asthma. N Engl J Med 2003;349:1669–1670.
192. Dhillon M: Current status of mold immunotherapy. Ann Allergy 1991;66:385–392.
193. Spykerboer JE, Donnelly WJ, Thong YH: Parental knowledge and misconceptions about asthma. A controlled study. Soc Sci Med 1986;22:553–558.
194. Sinclair BL, Clark DW, Sears MR: How well do New Zealand patients understand and manage their asthma? A community study. N Z Med J 1987;100:674–677.
195. Burdon JG, Juniper EF, Killian KJ, Hargreave FE, Campbell EJ: The perception of breathlessness in asthma. Am Rev Respir Dis 1982;126: 825–826.
196. Rubinfeld AR, Pain MC: Perception of asthma. Lancet 1976;1:882–885.
197. Feldman CH: Asthma education. General aspects of childhood programs. J Allergy Clin Immunol 1987;80:494–497.
198. Clark NM: Asthma self-management education. Research and implications for clinical practice. Chest 1989;95:1110–1113.
199. Hindi-Alexander MC: Asthma education programs. Their role in asthma morbidity and mortality. J Allergy Clin Immunol 1987;80:492–494.
200. Creer TL: Self-management in the treatment of childhood asthma. J Allergy Clin Immunol 1987;80:500–505.
201. Hilton S, Anderson HR, Sibbald B, Freeling P: Controlled evaluation of the effects of patient education on asthma morbidity in general practice. Health Education. Lancet 1986;1:26–29.
202. Howland J, Bauchner H, Adai R: The impact of pediatric asthma education on morbidity. Assessing the evidence. Chest 1988;94:964–969.

56 Wheezing in Older Children: Asthma

Carolyn M. Kercsmar, MD

Wheezing, a musical, high-pitched, largely expiratory sound made through the partially obstructed larger airways, is most commonly caused by asthma in school-aged children. A number of other conditions can cause both acute and chronic wheezing in children, but many causes are associated with other symptoms that generally distinguish them from asthma (Box 56-1). Even when the diagnosis is indeed asthma, many children are considered to have recurrent pneumonia, chronic bronchitis, or recurrent colds with chest congestion. Although there has been an increased awareness of the prevalence of childhood asthma, substantial physical, psychological, and socioeconomic morbidity continue to occur. The annual direct and indirect health care costs for treatment of asthma were recently estimated at nearly $14 billion per year in the United States. The major focus of this chapter will be on the diagnosis and treatment of asthma.

Asthma is the predominant cause of wheezing in older children. As defined in the National Heart, Lung, and Blood Institute (NHLBI) guidelines, asthma is characterized by variable, reversible obstruction of airflow (but not completely so in some patients), which may improve spontaneously or may subside only after specific therapy.[1] Airway hyperreactivity, defined as the inherent tendency of the trachea and bronchi to narrow in response to a variety of stimuli, such as allergens, nonspecific irritants, or infection, is also a prominent feature. Both the airway obstruction and hyperreactivity may be caused by chronic airway inflammation that involves many cell types (eosinophils, lymphocytes, neutrophils, epithelial cells) and mediators (cytokines, chemokines, enzymes). Symptoms of wheeze, cough, and shortness of breath are generally episodic in most patients but may occur daily in some.

Morbidity due to asthma is extraordinarily high. It is estimated that more than 10 million school days are lost, 3 million sick visits to a health care provider occur, and 200,000 hospitalizations take place because of asthma each year.[2] Poor, disadvantaged minority-group children who reside in central urban areas have both the highest prevalence and greatest morbidity. Recently estimated health care costs for children under the age of 17 years in the United States were almost $2 billion.

PATHOLOGY

Examination of postmortem lung specimens of patients who died of asthma shows marked hyperinflation with smooth muscle hyperplasia of bronchial and bronchiolar walls, thick tenacious mucous plugs often completely occluding the airways, markedly thickened basement membrane, and variable degrees of mucosal edema and denudation of bronchial and bronchiolar epithelium[3] (Fig. 56-1). Eosinophilia of the submucosa and secretions is prominent whether or not allergic (immunoglobulin E [IgE]–mediated) mechanisms are present. Mucous plugs contain layers of shed epithelial cells and eosinophils, and may also contain neutrophils and lymphocytes. Although the exact role of airway eosinophils in causing and perpetuating the asthma phenotype remains controversial, eosinophil products, such as major basic protein and other proteases, may play an important role in the destructive changes observed. The mucosal edema with separated columnar cells and stratified nonciliated epithelium, which replaces ciliated epithelium, results in abnormal mucociliary clearance. Mast cells often are absent, possibly reflecting degranulation and discharge of the chemical mediators. Submucosa gland hypertrophy and increased goblet cell size are not constant features of asthma, being more characteristic of chronic bronchitis. The thickened basement membrane due to submucosal deposition of type IV collagen and various other materials is a striking feature of asthma and has been reported even in mild asthmatics. Basement membrane thickening is thought to occur early in the disease, but its pathogenetic significance remains to be determined. All of these findings have been observed in symptom-free asthmatic individuals who died accidental deaths as well as in transbronchial biopsy specimens taken from research subjects (Fig. 56-2). Such observations have called into question the role and significance of so-called "airway remodeling" typified in part by basement membrane abnormalities. Although an occasional patient may show localized bronchiectasis and small focal areas of alveolar destruction, these are not characteristic of asthma, and there is little evidence that asthma leads to destructive emphysema. However, the incomplete reversibility of airflow limitation seen in some asthmatics suggests that a phenotype exists that may be considered a form of chronic obstructive pulmonary disease.

PATHOPHYSIOLOGY

Airflow limitation in asthma results from a combination of obstructive processes, principally mucosal edema, bronchospasm, and mucous plugging. The relative roles these processes play in producing obstruction may differ, however, according to the age of the child, the size and anatomy of various portions of the airway, the type of agent precipitating obstruction, and the duration and severity of asthma.

Airway obstruction results in increased resistance to airflow through the trachea and bronchi and in decreased flow rates due to narrowing and premature closure of the smaller airways. These changes lead to a decreased ability to expel air and result in hyperinflation. Although pulmonary overdistention benefits respiration by helping to maintain airway patency, the work of breathing increases because of the altered pulmonary mechanics. To a certain extent, increasing lung volumes can compensate for pulmonary obstruction, but compensation is limited as tidal volume approaches the volume of pulmonary dead space, with resultant alveolar hypoventilation.

Changes in resistance to airflow are not uniform throughout the tracheobronchial tree, and because of regional differences in this resistance, the distribution of inspired air is uneven, more

BOX 56-1 Causes of Wheezing in Older Children

Acute Wheezing

- Asthma
- Exercise-induced asthma
- Angioedema
- Vocal cord adduction/dysfunction syndrome
- Infection
  - Mycoplasma
  - Virus (adenovirus, RSV, metapneumovirus, parainfluenza, influenza)
  - Pertussis
- Inflammation
  - Irritant inhalation (smoke, illicit drugs, cocaine)
  - Hypersensitivity pneumonitis
  - Aspiration/gastric reflux
- Foreign body aspiration

Recurrent or Chronic Wheezing

- Asthma
- Angioedema
- Exercise-induced asthma
- Vocal cord dysfunction
- Anatomic lesion or airway compression
  - Tumor (carcinoid, lymphoma)
  - Granulation tissue
  - Lymph nodes (mediastinal, paratracheal)
  - Bronchogenic or pulmonary cyst
  - Vascular ring
- Postinfectious
  - Adenovirus
  - Mycoplasma
  - Bronchiectasis
- Inflammatory
  - Cystic fibrosis
  - Dyskinetic cilia syndrome
  - Immune deficiency
  - Sarcoid
  - Vasculitis (Wegener's granulomatosis, other)
  - α_1-antiprotease deficiency (adolescent, young adult)
  - Eosinophilic bronchitis
  - Congestive heart failure

air flowing to the less resistant portions. In most patients with asthma, both larger and smaller airways are obstructed, but some patients may have small airway obstruction primarily or even exclusively. The pulmonary circulation also is affected by hyperinflation, which induces increased intrapleural and intra-alveolar pressures and uneven circulation to the alveoli. The increased intra-alveolar pressure, decreased ventilation, and decreased perfusion (the last through hypoxic vasoconstriction) lead to variable and uneven ventilation-perfusion relationships within different lung units. The ultimate result is early reduction in blood oxygenation, even though carbon dioxide is eliminated effectively because of its ready diffusibility across alveolar

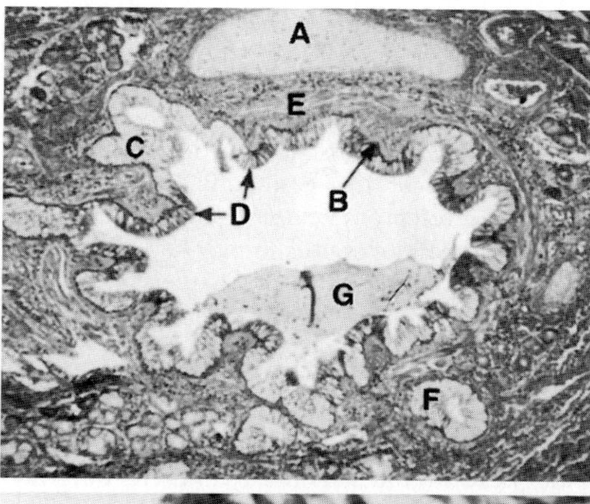

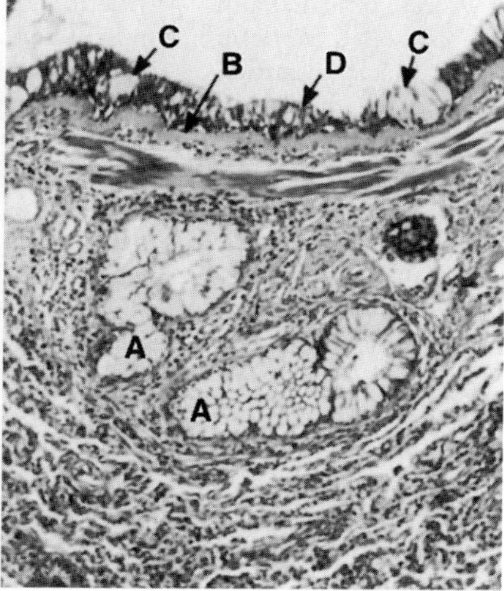

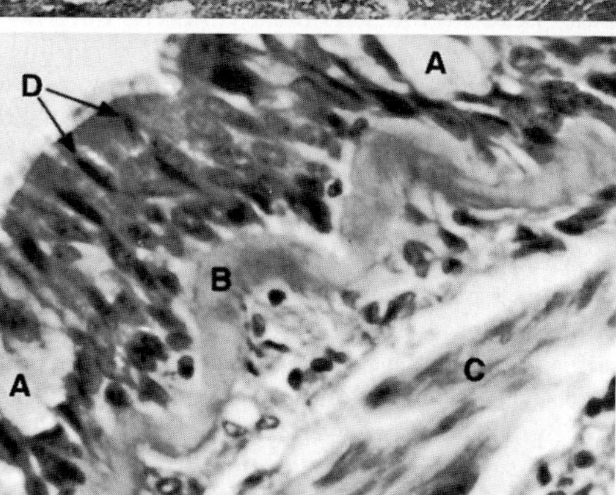

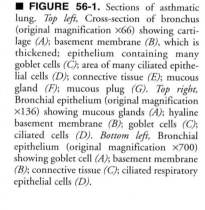

■ **FIGURE 56-1.** Sections of asthmatic lung. *Top left,* Cross-section of bronchus (original magnification ×66) showing cartilage *(A)*; basement membrane *(B)*, which is thickened; epithelium containing many goblet cells *(C)*; area of many ciliated epithelial cells *(D)*; connective tissue *(E)*; mucous gland *(F)*; mucous plug *(G)*. *Top right,* Bronchial epithelium (original magnification ×136) showing mucous glands *(A)*; hyaline basement membrane *(B)*; goblet cells *(C)*; ciliated cells *(D)*. *Bottom left,* Bronchial epithelium (original magnification ×700) showing goblet cell *(A)*; basement membrane *(B)*; connective tissue *(C)*; ciliated respiratory epithelial cells *(D)*.

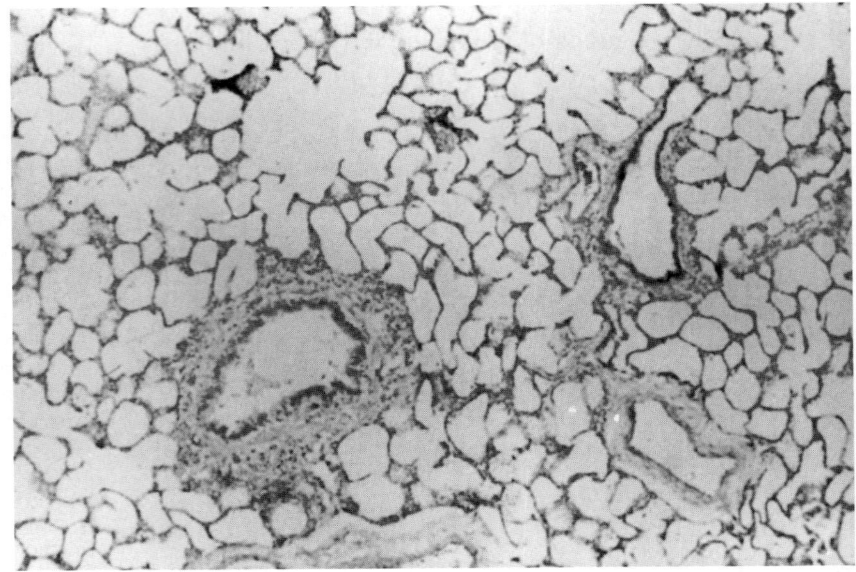

■ **FIGURE 56-2.** Autopsy specimen from asthmatic child who died from toxic ingestion. Note the infiltration of cells around the bronchus with sloughing of epithelial cells into the bronchial lumen. The alveoli all appear normal.

capillary membranes. Thus, early in acute asthma, hypoxemia occurs in the absence of CO_2 retention. The hyperventilation resulting from the hypoxemic drive causes a fall in partial pressure of carbon dioxide in alveolar gas ($PACO_2$). However, as the obstruction becomes more severe and the number of alveoli being adequately ventilated and perfused decreases, a point is reached at which CO_2 retention occurs.

Alterations in pH homeostasis result from respiratory and metabolic factors. Early in the course of acute asthma, respiratory alkalosis may occur because of hyperventilation. Coincidentally, metabolic acidosis occurs because of the increased work of breathing, increased oxygen consumption, and increased cardiac output. When respiratory failure is superimposed, respiratory acidosis may result in a precipitous fall in pH.

In short attacks of acute asthma, bronchospasm, mucosal edema, or both can occur. In a minority of asthmatics, acute severe episodes are characterized by neutrophilic, not eosinophilic infiltration; and bronchospasm occurs with little mucus secretion. These episodes may have an abrupt onset and cause severe or life-threatening symptoms. Mucous secretions become far more important as a cause of obstruction as the inflammation becomes more intense and prolonged, and when damage to and sloughing of epithelial cells impairs mucociliary function and increases reflex bronchoconstriction.

■ INFLAMMATORY CELL BIOLOGY AND ASTHMA ETIOLOGY AND PATHOPHYSIOLOGY

Although tremendous strides have been made in the cellular and molecular biology of asthma in the past decade, a complete understanding of the causative factors and those responsible for perpetuating the asthmatic state remain inadequately explained. Current data support the hypothesis that inflammation underlies the pathophysiology of asthma, and airway eosinophilic infiltration, an almost universal finding, is considered a major marker of the inflammatory activity of the disease. The mechanisms producing the inflammation are legion and the roles for each only partially understood. Certain processes appear to initiate inflammatory cascades, others perpetuate the response, and some do both. Recruitment of leukocytes from the microvasculature to the airways, their activation, and subsequent release and/or synthesis of inflammatory substances may be a primary means for initiating the asthmatic state. The persistence and chronic activation of mast cells, eosinophils, and lymphocytes in the airways as a result of cytokine-mediated events, such as interruption of apoptosis, may be important in producing chronic asthma. Prolonged inflammation probably results in progressive structural and functional changes in the airway epithelium, musculature, and connective tissue. The continued dysregulation of the cytokine networks perpetuates inflammation in what now may be the structurally altered airways of chronic asthma. Several specific effector mechanisms, such as IgE, arachidonic acid metabolites, mast cell proteases, eosinophil products, nitric oxide, the β-adrenergic receptor, neutral endopeptidase, and intrinsic muscular abnormalities appear to play key roles in airway inflammation are discussed further in Chapter 54.

■ NATURAL HISTORY AND PROGNOSIS

Knowledge of the natural history of asthma remains incompletely defined, but several longitudinal studies have added substantial insight. The widespread notion that most children "outgrow" their asthma in adolescence is only partially true. Between 30% and 70% of children with asthma have less severe or absent symptoms by late adolescence, and some features of childhood presentation and course seem to predict clinical outcome. Several studies indicate that disease severity in childhood usually determines disease severity in adolescence and adulthood. Data from the Melbourne Asthma Study suggested that mild asthma or infrequent wheezing associated with viral infections in childhood were not likely to progress to severe disease in adulthood. In this longitudinal cohort of approximately 500 subjects, data have been collected on the symptoms, growth, and lung function for almost 40 years.[4] Subjects were entered in the study at age 7 and were classified as never wheezed (controls), mild wheezy bronchitis, wheezy bronchitis, and asthma; a cohort with more severe asthma was added a few years later. The loss of lung function seen in the groups with asthma and severe asthma by age 14 years did not worsen over time. Asthma exacerbations and symptoms did continue in over half the patients.

Careful studies of children with asthma based both on history and on assessment of pulmonary function indicate that many children who lose overt symptoms have persistent airway obstruction. Nonspecific airway hyperreactivity, associated with asthma, is present in formerly asthmatic patients who are free from clinical asthma.[5] Individuals who had asthma as children have significantly lower forced expiratory volume in 1 second (FEV_1), more airway reactivity, and more frequent persistence of symptoms than those with infection-induced wheezing or the controls. In addition, 88% of the adults with childhood asthma who had persistent symptoms had positive methacholine challenge test results, as did 42% of the asymptomatic former asthmatics. The recurrence of overt asthma after years of freedom from symptoms is not unusual. Thus, asthma is often a lifelong disease with periodic exacerbations and remissions, although laboratory evidence of decreased pulmonary function and airway hyperresponsiveness may persist.

In children and adolescents, asthma frequently is a completely reversible obstructive airways disease, and indeed no abnormalities in pulmonary functions can be detected in many asthmatic patients when they become symptom free. However, recent studies that examine not only symptoms and pulmonary function, but also indices of airway inflammation and bronchial hyperresponsiveness, suggest that airway inflammation may persist in the absence of symptoms. In a study of 54 young adults (age 18–25 years) with atopic asthma or asthma in clinical remission (absence of symptoms for at least 12 months, median duration 5 years), subjects in remission were found to have evidence of airway inflammation and remodeling.[5] When compared with normal healthy controls, the subjects in remission had increased epithelial and subepithelial major basic protein and reticular basement membrane thickness; values were close to those of subjects with active asthma. Peripheral eosinophil counts were also elevated in the remission patients, and there was a significant correlation between basement membrane thickness, exhaled nitric oxide, and hyperresponsiveness to adenosine monophosphate (AMP). These findings indicate that the airways of asymptomatic asthmatics, seemingly in clinical remission, still show significant abnormalities and evidence of active inflammation. Such changes could result in disease reactivation later in life and may have implications for continued treatment in the face of absent symptoms.

Asthma does progress to chronic obstructive disease in some, but not all, individuals. The functional and structural causes of this irreversible airway obstruction variant of asthma are not understood. A process referred to as airway remodeling is often suggested as the cause of chronic obstruction and severe asthma, but data to conclusively support this hypothesis are lacking. It is believed that chronic mucous plugging, tracheobronchial ciliary dysfunction, smooth muscle and goblet cell hyperplasia, and collagen deposition in the lamina reticularis of the basement membrane occur as a consequence of persistent inflammation. Genetically determined dysregulation of inflammatory mediator production with or without repeated exposure to certain environmental stimuli may also play a role. As mentioned earlier, some of these pathologic changes can be seen in the airways of children with mild asthma and reversible obstruction. In addition, data from animal models demonstrate that even when inflammation is suppressed and changes consistent with remodeling are reduced markedly, airway hyperresponsiveness persists.[6] Taken together, these data suggest that airway remodeling alone may not be responsible for severe, irreversible airway obstruction or bronchial hyperresponsiveness.

The natural history of childhood asthma and the effects of aggressive long-term management on outcomes remains incompletely understood, but a great deal of data have accumulated over the past decade. Much of the knowledge regarding the disease progression and treatment has come from the Childhood Asthma Management Program (CAMP).[7] CAMP was a well-designed comprehensive longitudinal study in which the primary objective was to compare the effects of long-term treatment (4 years) with an inhaled steroid (budesonide [BUD]) and a nonsteroidal treatment (nedocromil) to placebo in school-aged children (n = 1041) with mild to moderate asthma. The hypothesis was that treatment with an inhaled steroid would result in better lung growth than no or lesser treatment. Primary outcome was postbronchodilator FEV_1, but a wealth of other data on atopy, airway reactivity, symptoms, exacerbations, and linear growth was obtained. Surprisingly, after a brief improvement in FEV_1 in the BUD group, there was no difference in FEV_1 among the groups over the last 3 years of the study (Table 56-1). However, patients in the BUD group had decreased hospitalizations and urgent care visits compared with the placebo group. Patients in the nedocromil group also had fewer emergency visits but not hospitalizations, and both groups had less oral prednisone use. There was a small, transient decrease in growth velocity in the budesonide group compared to the placebo and nedocromil groups. These data suggest that long-term treatment with inhaled steroids in school-aged asthmatics does not alter pulmonary function over time, even though the symptom control improved. This may be because the treatment was started too late after the onset of the disease. Other data obtained as part of the CAMP study found an association between duration of asthma and diminished lung function, airway hyperreactivity, and symptoms. A multicenter trial of inhaled steroid treatment in younger children (age 2 years) who have recurrent wheezing and are at very high risk for developing asthma is currently under way and may help elucidate whether early aggressive treatment helps preserve lung function and growth in asthmatic children.

ASTHMA MORTALITY

Despite the relatively high prevalence of asthma, mortality rates for asthma in childhood fortunately are extremely low. Overall, approximately 5000 people, about 300 of whom are children, die of asthma in the United States each year. The mortality rate

TABLE 56-1. Select primary and secondary outcomes from the CAMP study[7]

	Budesonide	Nedocromil	Placebo
FEV_1 (% predicted)	0.6	–0.5	–0.1
AHR	3.0*	1.8	1.9
Height change (cm)	22.7†	23.7	23.8

Note: Values are means of data obtained at last follow-up visit, which occurred approximately 4 years after study entry. FEV_1 is postbronchodilator. AHR is airway hyperreactivity measured by methacholine challenge; ratio of follow-up to baseline value.

*$P < .001$, budesonide compared with placebo.
†$P < .005$, budesonide compared with placebo.

has stabilized over the past decade.[2] However, death rates are higher in African Americans of all ages. Analyses of causes of death in children with asthma suggest that the major causes are the failure of the physician, parent, or patient to appreciate the severity of asthma, which results in inadequate or delayed treatment, poor access to health care, and the use of inappropriate medications, such as overreliance on β-adrenergic agonists and avoidance of use of corticosteroids.[8] Labile asthma, regardless of severity, also is a risk factor, as are respiratory infections, nocturnal asthma, history of respiratory failure, and marked diurnal variation in airflow limitation. Some patients cannot perceive severe airflow obstruction, especially when it occurs gradually, and a small number may have sudden profound bronchospasm, which is fatal. Other factors, such as exposure to allergens (mold), psychosocial disturbance, poverty, previous episodes of respiratory failure, history of hypoxic seizure, previous admission to an intensive care unit, and psychological factors in both the patient and family have been implicated in deaths from asthma.

DIAGNOSIS OF ASTHMA

Although patients with asthma may present in a variety of ways, most have certain common historical features. Most patients will come with a complaint of intermittent wheezing, an expiratory, musically high-pitched, whistling sound produced by airflow turbulence in the large airways below the thoracic inlet. Many parents and even older children cannot accurately describe wheezing and may actually report stridor (from upper airway obstruction), snoring, or rhonchorous breathing. Careful explanation or even demonstration of wheezing is often necessary to obtain an accurate history. Wheezing can also be generated by adduction of the vocal cords and forceful inspiration and expiration. Inspiratory wheezing per se is not characteristic of asthma and suggests obstruction in the laryngeal area, such as that induced by croup or vocal cord dysfunction. However, wheezing also occurs during inspiration when asthma worsens and may disappear altogether as obstruction becomes more severe and airflow is limited. Asthma can occur without wheezing if the obstruction involves small airways predominantly. Occasionally, coughing or shortness of breath may be the only complaint. So-called "cough-equivalent asthma" may be overdiagnosed. Probably no more than 5% of asthmatic children have cough as the only or primary symptom. Older children often complain of a "tight" chest with colds, recurrent "chest congestion," or bronchitis. Usually, symptoms are more severe at night or in the early morning and improve through the day. A history of symptomatic improvement after treatment with a bronchodilator suggests the diagnosis of asthma, but a failure of response does not rule out asthma.

Family history is often positive for asthma or allergy (allergic rhinitis, eczema) in a first-degree relative. A history of personal allergy is commonly found in children with asthma.

Physical Examination

The physical examination should focus on overall growth and development; on the condition of the entire respiratory tract including the upper airway, ears, and paranasal sinuses as well as the chest; and on other associated signs of allergic disease. Weight and height should be recorded and plotted on a growth grid. Although severe asthma can adversely affect linear growth, it is not a common feature.

Examination of the lungs frequently reveals coarse crackles or unequal breath sounds, which may clear at least partly on changing position or coughing. Although wheezing can be elicited frequently with a forced expiratory maneuver, occasionally there is only prolongation of expiration without wheezing. The older child or adolescent may resist exhaling forcefully to induce latent wheezes, because such a maneuver may induce coughing that can increase bronchospasm. Some patients with severe asthma do not wheeze because too little air is exchanged to generate the sound. Wheezing from the lower respiratory tract should be differentiated from similar sounds that can emanate from the laryngeal area in (normal) children with sufficient forced expiration.

A variety of extrapulmonary signs indicating the presence of complicating factors, such as allergy or cystic fibrosis, should be sought in all children being evaluated for asthma. Nasal polyps occur rarely in the child with uncomplicated asthma, and their presence suggests cystic fibrosis. Digital clubbing is not a feature of asthma; although clubbing may be a nonpathologic familial trait, its presence suggests cystic fibrosis, congenital heart disease, or other chronic lung problems. The conjunctivae should be examined for edema, inflammation, and tearing, suggesting allergy. Flexor creases and other areas of skin should be examined for active or healed atopic dermatitis.

Hyperventilation and/or vocal cord dysfunction (VCD) syndrome should be considered in the differential diagnosis of the child with asthma apparently refractory to all therapy. Both conditions are more likely to occur in adolescence or later childhood, and may be mistaken for asthma or may coexist with it. Typically, the patient with hyperventilation is anxious and complains of marked dyspnea and difficulty getting enough air to breathe in spite of excellent air exchange on auscultation and an absence of wheezing. Often, there are associated complaints of headache and tingling of the fingers and toes. Pulmonary function tests are helpful in differentiating hyperventilation syndrome from asthma; a normal spirogram during or around the time of symptoms is inconsistent with asthma. Immediate therapy consists of giving reassurance and having the patient rebreathe into a paper bag to elevate $Pa\text{CO}_2$. Long-term therapy involves evaluation of the cause of anxiety and psychotherapy if appropriate.

VCD is another condition that must be differentiated from true asthma.[9] In these patients, wheezing is often a prominent feature, may occur on inspiration and expiration, and is typically loudest over the trachea or central, anterior chest. This condition is more common in older children and adolescents, and may also be seen in elite athletes. The mechanism involves holding the vocal cords in a position of relative adduction during inspiration, but also in expiration. The result is loud wheezing in a patient who appears quite comfortable, has normal oxygen saturation, and responds poorly to inhalation of a bronchodilating aerosol. Pulmonary function testing may reveal a pronounced flattening of the inspiratory loop; however, since most patients with VCD also have true asthma, there may be some evidence of large and/or small airway obstruction on the expiratory loop as well (Fig. 56-3). An increase in the mid–vital capacity expiratory/inspiratory flow ratio from the normal value of about 0.9 to a value of greater than 2 indicates extrathoracic obstruction, consistent with VCD. The diagnosis is confirmed by direct observation of paradoxical vocal cord movement via flexible laryngoscopy during an acute episode. Most patients with VCD cannot voluntarily induce an episode, although in

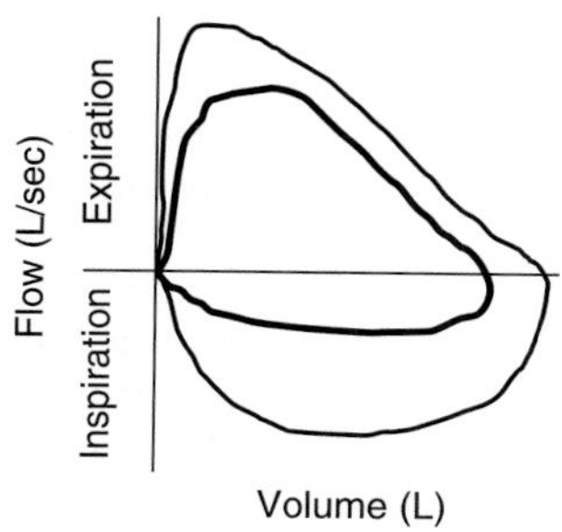

■ **FIGURE 56-3.** Flow volume curve from patient with vocal cord dysfunction. Thin line represents flow at normal baseline. Thick line represents flow during obstructive episode, depicting slight decrease in expiratory flow and marked decrease in and flattening of inspiratory loop.

some patients, including highly trained athletes, exercise can precipitate an attack. Older children with both VCD and asthma often can distinguish the "site" of the wheezing when the source of the problem is explained to them. Although VCD was originally described in adults with psychiatric disorders, this condition in children is less frequently associated with serious psychological disturbances and should not be labeled as such. The etiology in children remains poorly understood. Effective treatment consists of appropriate asthma medication and referral to a speech therapist or psychologist specializing in behavior modification in order to learn relaxation techniques.

Asthma Triggers

Most older children will identify more than one precipitating factor responsible for asthma. Moreover, patterns of reactivity may change. Thus, exercise-induced asthma may not be viewed as a problem in many adults with asthma who have learned in childhood that exercise induces symptoms and consequently have developed a lifestyle that avoids exercise. Allergic factors that precipitated asthma in childhood may no longer cause symptoms in adolescence or adulthood even though the patient continues to have asthma. Patterns also may change with treatment or the institution of environmental control measures. The use of quality of life questionnaires can help uncover latent symptoms and provide information that may be useful in identifying more subtle triggers and then customizing a treatment plan to match the patient's symptoms and lifestyle.

Allergens

In the majority of children with asthma, it is possible to induce an asthmatic reaction to substances in which IgE can be demonstrated. Allergic reactions may induce bronchoconstriction directly, may increase tracheobronchial sensitivity in general, or may be obvious or subtle precipitating factors. Bronchoconstrictor responses to allergens via IgE antibody–induced mediator release from mast cells generally occur within minutes of exposure, last for a relatively short period of time (20–30 minutes), and resolve; such reactions are often termed early antigen or asthmatic response. It is the so-called "late asthmatic response" (which occur 4–12 hours after antigen contact) that result in more severe and protracted symptoms (lasting hours) and ultimately contribute to the chronicity and severity of the disease. The early response is largely triggered by allergen or other exposure, while the late response is due to inflammatory cell infiltration and release of multiple mediators, as discussed in a previous section. Such allergen-induced dual responses can only be demonstrated in approximately half of all asthmatics challenged in a laboratory setting. It is unclear why mast cell degranulation that should induce an inflammatory infiltration in all patients does not induce late symptoms in all patients.

Allergens that can induce asthma include animal allergens, mold spores, pollens, insects (cockroach), infectious agents (especially fungi), and, occasionally, drugs and foods. Cockroach allergen appears to be a potent factor, particularly in inner city children, and has been associated with increased health care utilization in those children both sensitized and exposed to allergen.

Irritants

Numerous upper and lower respiratory irritants have been implicated as precipitants of asthma. These include paint odors, hair sprays, perfumes, chemicals, air pollutants, tobacco smoke, cold air, cold water, and cough. Some allergens may act as irritants (e.g., molds). Some irritants such as ozone and industrial chemicals also may initiate bronchial hyperresponsiveness by inducing inflammation, yet do not produce a late-phase response. Active and passive exposure to tobacco smoke, in addition to acting as precipitants and aggravators of asthma, also can be associated with an accelerated irreversible loss of pulmonary function.

Weather Changes

Atmospheric changes commonly are associated with an increase in asthmatic activity. The mechanism of this effect has not been defined but may be related to changes in barometric pressure and alterations in the allergen or irritant content of the air.

Infections

By far, the most common infectious agents responsible for precipitating or aggravating asthma are viral respiratory pathogens. It is estimated that up to 85% of asthma exacerbations in school-aged children are due to viral infections, and rhinovirus has emerged as a prominent pathogen in causing acute asthma. In some instances bacterial infections (e.g., pertussis or mycoplasma), and, more rarely, fungal infections or colonization (e.g., bronchopulmonary aspergillosis) and parasitic infestations (e.g., toxocariasis and ascariasis) can be triggers. Various mechanisms have been implicated to explain the role of viruses in asthma and other allergic diseases, including IgE-mediated mechanisms and imbalance of T-lymphocyte responses. The mechanisms of viral-induced exacerbations are incompletely understood, but probably involve some direct respiratory epithelial injury due to infection, host inflammatorily responses driven by the infection, and influence of other cofactors (concomitant allergen exposure or mediator production).

Exercise

Strenuous exercise ordinarily associated with breathlessness, such as running or bicycle riding, may induce bronchial obstruction in as many as 80% of individuals with asthma. Exercise can be a subtle though significant problem associated with only cough or excessive breathlessness. Symptoms typically begin after 5 to 10 minutes of vigorous activity and are most prominent after activity ceases. The mechanisms underlying exercise-induced asthma remain somewhat uncertain. Hyperventilation of cold, dry air may cause heat and water loss from the airways, produce a hyperosmolar lining fluid, and result in mediator release (e.g., histamine from mast cells).[10] Cooling of the airways has also been described to result in vascular congestion and dilatation in the bronchial circulation. This phenomenon may be particularly prominent during the rewarming phases after exercise, and the changes are magnified if the ambient air breathed during recovery is warm rather than cool. The subsequent mucosal swelling as a result of vascular congestion and edema produces airway narrowing.

Emotional Factors

Emotional upsets clearly aggravate asthma in some individuals; however, there is no evidence that psychological factors are the basis for asthma. Coping styles of patients, their families, and their physicians can intensify or lead to more rapid amelioration of asthma. Conversely, denial of asthma by patients, parents, or physicians may delay therapy to the point that reversibility of obstruction is more difficult. Psychological factors have been implicated in deaths from asthma in children. The influence of psychosocial factors on compliance is yet another important factor related to treatment failure or success. Asthma itself can strongly influence the emotional state of the patient, of the family, and of other individuals associated with the patient.

Gastroesophageal Reflux

Reflux of gastric contents into the tracheobronchial tree can aggravate asthma in children and is one of the causes of nocturnal asthma. Typical symptoms of reflux—heartburn, chest pain, regurgitation, sour brash—may be absent in many children with asthma; estimates are that reflux may be "silent" in over 50% of asthmatic patients.[11] Although the exact extent to which reflux exacerbates asthma remains controversial, it is clear that acid (or even nonacid) reflux of gastric contents into the distal esophagus can lead to cough and bronchospasm, presumably via increased vagal activity. Aspiration of gastric contents in even micro amounts is also presumed to cause bronchial irritation and bronchospasm.

Allergic Rhinitis and Sinusitis

Acute or chronic sinusitis can be associated with aggravation of asthma and can be a cause of recalcitrant asthma. In some patients, asthma and sinusitis occur at the same time; the nasal symptoms from the sinusitis may make cough and other symptoms of asthma worse and less responsive to bronchodilator therapy alone. The upper airway may be viewed to some extent as a continuum of the lower airway; inflammatory mediator release in the lower airway may be triggered as a response to infection in the sinuses.

Nonallergic Hypersensitivity to Drugs and Chemicals

Aspirin and nonsteroidal anti-inflammatory drugs (NSAIDs), such as indomethacin and ibuprofen, can exacerbate asthma in selected individuals by increasing production of 5-lipoxygenase metabolites, including leukotrienes. Aspirin ingestion may diminish pulmonary function, produce wheeze, cough, rhinitis, conjunctivitis, urticaria, and angioedema in 10% to 15% of individuals with asthma. Aspirin is more common as a cause of symptom production after the third decade of life. As a general rule, it is wise to restrict aspirin and other NSAIDs for all asthmatics; aspirin in particular is contraindicated in children and adolescents due to the risk of Reye's syndrome. High-dose acetaminophen may also cause wheezing in a small portion of aspirin-sensitive asthmatics. Thoughtful use of all analgesic and antipyretic agents is recommended.

Metabisulfite can be an important precipitant or aggravator of asthma, both by allergic and nonallergic mechanisms. Sensitive individuals should avoid foods containing or preserved using sulfites, such as shrimp, dried fruit, beer, and wine.

Endocrine Factors

Aggravation of asthma and increased peak flow variability occurs in some patients in relation to the menstrual cycle, beginning shortly before menstruation and ending at the onset of menses. Whether this reflects changes in water and salt balance, irritability of bronchial smooth muscle, or other factors is unknown. The use of birth control pills occasionally also aggravates asthma. Hyperthyroidism has been reported to worsen or precipitate asthma severely in an occasional patient. Treatment of hyperthyroidism usually ameliorates the asthma.

Sleep or Nocturnal Asthma

There is a circadian variation in airway function and bronchial hyperresponsiveness in most patients with asthma; the worst peak expiratory flow rate (PEFR) and most pronounced reactivity occur at approximately 4 AM and the best at 4 PM in individuals with a normal sleep-wake cycle. Sleep or nocturnal asthma is a risk factor for asthma severity and even death in some asthmatics. Although nocturnal asthma may result from late-phase reactions to earlier allergen exposure, gastroesophageal reflux, or sinusitis in some patients, these conditions are not present in most patients with severe nocturnal asthma. Another explanation is an increase in inflammatory cell infiltrate as an exaggerated normal circadian variation. Abnormalities in central nervous system control of respiratory drive, particularly with defective hypoxic drive and obstructive sleep apnea, as well as enhanced melatonin release resulting in increased inflammation, also may be present in some patients with nocturnal asthma.

LABORATORY DIAGNOSIS

A number of laboratory studies may be useful in confirming the diagnosis of asthma, and objective measures of pulmonary function are among the most important.

LUNG FUNCTION TESTS

Pulmonary function tests (PFTs) are objective, noninvasive, and extremely helpful in the diagnosis and follow-up of patients with asthma. A PFT should be attempted on all older children when considering the diagnosis of asthma. Results are then compared with normal standards for age, gender, and race. Measurement of PEFR or FEV_1 alone may miss small airway obstruction in some patients; the forced expiratory flow rate over 25% to 75% of the forced vital capacity (FEF_{25-75}) has been proposed as a more sensitive indicator of obstruction, particularly in children with milder disease. Patients may have an FEF_{25-75} more than 2 SD below predicted normal values even in the presence of no clinical symptoms.

Documentation of reversibility of airflow obstruction following inhalation of a bronchodilator is central to the definition of asthma. Examination of the forced vital capacity (FVC), FEV_1, and FEF_{25-75} is a reliable way to detect baseline airway obstruction. Examination of the volume-time curve and shape of the flow-volume loop provides an estimate of the adequacy of the patient effort in performing the test. If obstruction is demonstrated on a baseline PFT, a bronchodilating aerosol (albuterol) should be administered and the PFT repeated in 10 to 20 minutes. An improvement of at least 12% and 200 mL in the FEV_1 is considered a positive response and is consistent with a diagnosis of asthma. The FEV_1 can also be used to monitor response to therapy and disease progression. Data also indicate that the FEV_1 in asthmatics is inversely correlated with the occurrence of acute exacerbations. In a large retrospective study examining the data from the Six Cities Study, an FEV_1 less than 60% of the predicted value was associated with a significantly increased risk (odds ratio [OR] 2.2), independent of age or sex in a group of school-aged children. Over 60% of the group with an FEV_1 of less than 60% reported an exacerbation in the next year compared to 24.5% of those with an FEV_1 of greater than 80%. When a more liberal definition of reduced FEV_1 was used ($FEV_1 < 80\%$ predicted), the relationship between FEV_1 and risk of attack was similar, but the risk was lower.[12] These data strongly support the use of pulmonary function and particularly the FEV_1 as a monitoring tool to guide asthma therapy and help prevent acute attacks.

Although the FEV_1 has long been considered the gold standard for use in diagnosing and monitoring change in airway function in patients with asthma and other obstructive airway diseases, other modalities are now also available and may have particular application in both younger and older children. Impulse oscillometry capitalizes on the resonant oscillation properties of the airways to measure conductance and reactance and, indirectly, airway resistance.[13] The technique requires only tidal breathing on a mouthpiece for 30 seconds in order to obtain a measurement. Response to the bronchodilator can also be detected.

Use of a peak flow meter in the office setting may provide some useful information about obstruction in the large central airways, but the test should not be used to diagnose asthma. PEFR is extremely effort dependent and is reflective of obstruction only in the large central airways. The latest National Asthma Education and Prevention Program (NAEPP) guidelines no longer recommend PEFR monitoring for all patients, but rather suggest considering use in those with moderate to severe asthma. The best efficacy of PEFR is probably to follow trends, measured as day-to-day variability or the mean PEFR over several weeks as treatment is adjusted.[14] Moreover, PEFR can be used to provide the patient and physician with objective data on airflow that may be particularly useful for children and parents who have difficulty perceiving symptoms. Nevertheless, PEFR has serious limitations in that it provides no information on small airways function, which may be significantly reduced in patients with normal or near normal PEFR. PEFR may also be easily "adjusted" by operator technique; spitting into the meter can artificially elevate the test while a less than maximal effort will lower it. Finally, PEFR, like other measures of pulmonary function, may not have a direct correlation with symptoms. Therefore, reported symptoms should not be ignored even if the PEFR appears to be in an acceptable range.

BRONCHIAL CHALLENGE TESTS

Airway hyperreactivity to substances such as methacholine, histamine, hypertonic saline, or AMP forms the basis of a diagnostic test for asthma. Methacholine and histamine responsiveness are similar when tested in the same individual, but methacholine is the more commonly used drug. FEV_1 is the primary measure used to assess response, and a 20% fall in FEV_1 induced by a concentration of methacholine of less than 4 mg/mL is considered a positive test result.

Methacholine challenge testing has a better negative than positive predictive value and as such may be more helpful in excluding than diagnosing asthma.[15] A number of disease states, such as cystic fibrosis, chronic obstructive pulmonary disease, chronic bronchitis, and allergic rhinitis all have airway hyperreactivity to methacholine as a common finding. Inhalation challenge with AMP has been suggested to be a more realistic stimulus for assessing hyperreactivity, since it indirectly causes release of inflammatory mediators (e.g., histamine) from airway mast cells. Methacholine challenge has also been suggested as a surrogate marker for persistent airway inflammation and has been used clinically as a guide to adjust therapy.[16] Although improved asthma control has been reported using decreased sensitivity to methacholine challenge as a guide to treatment level, the routine use of such testing is cumbersome and expensive.

Mild transient adverse effects (cough, wheezing, chest tightness, dizziness) are uncommon and occur in less than 20% of patients receiving either histamine or methacholine challenge. Delayed or prolonged reactions are extremely rare, and fatalities after methacholine have not been reported. Other agents such as allergens and occupational sensitizers have been used for inhalation challenge tests, but such challenges may pose significant risk and should only be performed by experienced physicians and investigators in the context of specific clinical or research settings. Indeed, bronchial challenge tests with methacholine, saline, adenosine, or histamine should only be performed in certified pulmonary function laboratories and under the direct supervision of a trained specialist.

EXERCISE TOLERANCE TEST

In children 6 years of age through adulthood, a treadmill exercise test provides useful information about the individual's ability to exercise and to participate in sports. It also measures functionally how well drugs have controlled the asthma. In addition, the exercise test can be useful in diagnosing asthma in children with histories suggestive of exercise-induced bronchospasm; in such patients, an exercise challenge test is a more useful diagnostic aid than a methacholine challenge test. A cold air inhalation challenge test is another alternative; for this study the child hyperventilates (20–25 times the FEV_1) subfreezing (–4°C) dry air for at least 4 minutes (CO_2 must be added to the circuit and end-tidal CO_2 monitored to prevent hypocarbia). In order to ensure hyperventilation, this test should be performed while the patient is exercising or with the use of a continuously evacuating target balloon.

Pulmonary function should be measured 5 minutes before exercise. Following exercise, serial pulmonary function measurements should be obtained for at least 20 minutes (at 5, 10, and 20 minutes postexercise) to determine the severity of exercise-induced asthma. A decrease of more than 10% in peak expiratory flow rate, of more than 12% in FEV_1, or of more than 25% in FEF_{25-75} is diagnostic of exercise-induced asthma.

OTHER TESTS

Complete Blood Cell Count

Often the complete blood cell count is normal and offers little information in the diagnosis or management of asthma. However, eosinophilia, if present, most commonly suggests asthma, allergy, or both. Although there are other causes of peripheral eosinophilia in children (parasitic infection, malignancy, human

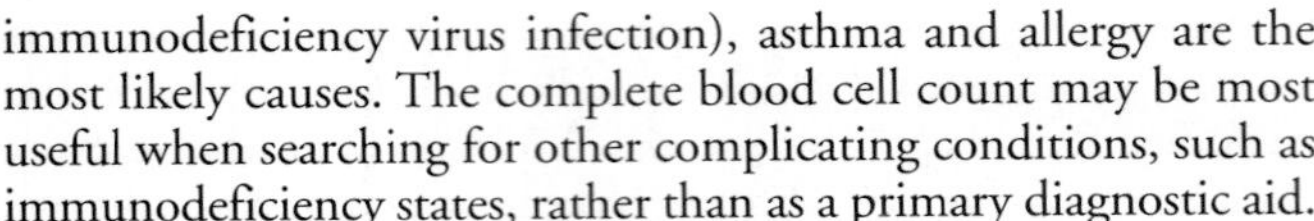

immunodeficiency virus infection), asthma and allergy are the most likely causes. The complete blood cell count may be most useful when searching for other complicating conditions, such as immunodeficiency states, rather than as a primary diagnostic aid.

Cytologic Examination of Sputum

Obtaining induced sputum by inhaling hypertonic saline aerosols generated by an ultrasonic nebulizer has become a popular and useful technique for helping identify active inflammation in the airways characteristic of asthma.[17] The presence and number of eosinophils and other inflammatory cells can provide useful information about disease activity and response to therapy. Improved asthma control and reduced exacerbations were noted when there was less than 3% eosinophils in the induced sputum of adult asthmatics.[18] Although the technique of obtaining induced sputum is relatively simple, it does require trained personnel, use of an established protocol, and subjects that are at least 10 years of age.

Exhaled Nitric Oxide

Nitric oxide is an important and widespread regulatory molecule that has diverse biological functions, such as smooth muscle relaxation, immune reaction, neural transmission, and regulation of peripheral blood flow. NO is synthesized from L-arginine by three different forms of the enzyme NO synthase (NOS): constitutive forms—exhaled NOS (eNOS) found in endothelial cells and nNOS in neuronal tissue—and an inducible form, iNOS. NO can be measured in exhaled breath (eNO) and is elevated in the exhaled breath of asthmatics. These elevated levels of NO are correlated with increases in airway inflammation and are reduced when asthma is treated with inhaled corticosteroids (ICS) and other anti-inflammatory medications, such as leukotriene receptor antagonists. Commercial devices are now available that permit the rapid, noninvasive and easy measure of eNO. Although it is still somewhat controversial, eNO may be a useful adjunctive marker for asthma control, and has been found to correlate with other measures of asthma disease activity such as bronchial hyperresponsiveness, bronchodilator use, and nocturnal symptoms.[19] Measure of eNO may also be a useful adjunct diagnostic tool for asthma. Unfortunately, the currently available technology is quite expensive and its use is most likely to be in specialized pulmonary function laboratories and in the research setting for the next few years.

Exhaled Breath Condensate

A number of studies have demonstrated the presence of a variety of inflammatory mediators in the liquid condensate from cooled exhaled air collected over a number of minutes. Cytokines, leukotrienes, nitrates, and other substances have all been reported in exhaled breath condensate (EBC), and some may correlate with asthma disease activity.[20] In addition, an acid pH in the EBC has also been reported to be a marker of airway inflammation. However, there is still great controversy over standardization of the technique, the derivation of the measured substances (sampling of airway lining fluid rather than volatilized molecules), and measurement of mediators. Although EBC may prove useful as another noninvasive measure of airway inflammation in the future, it is currently a research tool.

Serum Tests

Determining quantitative levels of immunoglobulin G (and subclasses), M, and A is useful only to rule out immunodeficiency syndromes in children with recurrent or chronic infection. In children with asthma, IgG levels usually are normal, IgA levels occasionally are low, and IgM levels may be elevated. Systemic steroids, however, can depress IgG and perhaps IgA levels. IgE is likely to be elevated in the child with asthma, atopy, or both; however, a normal IgE does not rule out asthma as a cause of symptoms. In addition, in the child with shifting pulmonary infiltrates, a marked elevation of serum IgE (>1000 IU) should prompt tests for both IgG and specific IgE antibody to *Aspergillus*.

Sweat Test

A sweat test should be performed on children with chronic respiratory symptoms, including recurrent wheezing, to rule out cystic fibrosis; associated signs and symptoms that should prompt a sweat test include poor weight gain and short stature, steatorrhea, nasal polyps, pansinusitis, hemotypsis, and digital clubbing. Although most cases of cystic fibrosis are diagnosed in the preschool years, mutations conferring pancreatic sufficiency are typically associated with milder pulmonary disease and may present much later.

Radiograms

All children with asthma should have a chest radiogram at some time to rule out parenchymal disease, congenital a nomaly, and (direct or indirect) evidence of a foreign body. A chest radiogram should be considered for every child admitted to a hospital with asthma, particularly if there are localized findings on physical examination (crackles, egophony, diminished breath sounds). Radiographic findings in asthma may range from normal to hyperinflation with peribronchial interstitial infiltrates and atelectasis. The following abnormalities are those most commonly seen in hospitalized children with asthma: hyperinflation with increased bronchial markings (Fig. 56-4*A*); infiltrates, atelectasis, pneumonia, or a combination of the three (see Fig. 56-4*B*); and pneumomediastinum (see Fig. 56-4*C*), often with infiltrates. Pneumothorax occurs rarely (see Fig. 56-4*D*).

Paranasal sinus radiograms also should be considered for children with persistent nocturnal coughing, nasal symptoms, and headaches. Screening sinus computed tomography cuts are a more desirable study because they provide a more thorough examination of the paranasal sinuses than do plain films, for a similar cost and radiation exposure.

Allergy Testing

Allergy testing—skin testing or in vitro serum measures—is indicated in patients in whom specific allergic factors are believed to be important and probably in all children with severe asthma to rule out allergic factors that might contribute significantly to the asthma (e.g., pollen, mold, dust mite, cockroach, or danders from domestic animals in the home or in school). After a detailed environmental history is taken, skin testing (usually percutaneous or scratch), limited to most likely allergens as suggested by the history, should be performed.

Skin test results may vary with age, drug therapy, and inherent skin factors. Drugs affecting skin test results include antihistamines (which may inhibit skin reactions for up to 72 hours or longer), tricyclic antidepressants, and some histamine (H_2) blockers. Topical and systemic corticosteroids or montelukast do not affect skin reactions. Positive (histamine) and negative (saline) control tests should be included to detect inherent skin factors that may affect the reaction to allergen, such as dermatographism and extensive dryness or eczema.

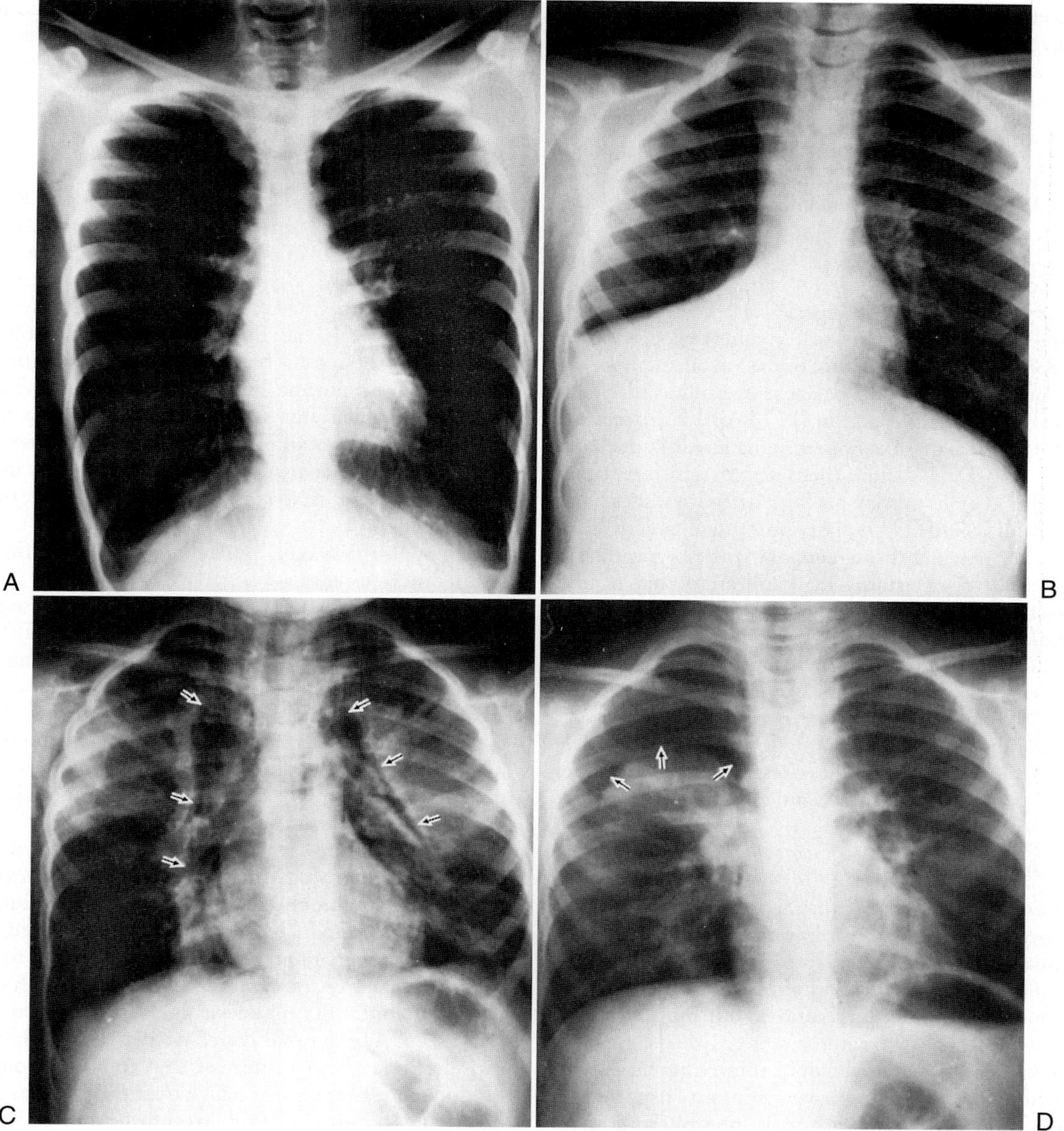

■ **FIGURE 56-4.** Radiographic findings in asthma. **A,** Hyperinflation with increased bronchial markings. **B,** Atelectasis involving a complete lobe. **C,** Massive pneumomediastinum complicating asthma. **D,** Pneumothorax secondary to paroxysmal coughing in asthma. *Arrows* mark air in **C,** lung margin in **D.**

The in vitro radioallergosorbent test (RAST) makes use of the affinity of serum IgE antibody for antigen that has been bound to a cellulose disk. A radio-tagged or enzyme-linked anti-IgE detects the quantity of specific IgE bound to the disk. The RAST is no more specific than the antigen employed (hence, not more specific than a skin test), is significantly more expensive, is less sensitive, and should be reserved for special situations in which skin tests are impractical, as in the patient with generalized dermatitis, and the rare patient who is too ill for direct testing or must continue to receive medications with antihistaminic activity (e.g., tricyclic antidepressants).

■ THERAPEUTIC CONSIDERATIONS

The goals of asthma management are to prevent both daytime and nighttime symptoms, to prevent acute episodes and minimize the need for emergency department treatment or hospitalization, to maintain normal or near normal pulmonary function as measured by spirometry, to avoid functional morbidity and maintain normal activities of daily living (attending school, exercising), to provide effective pharmacologic treatment with minimal or no adverse effects, and to meet the parent's and child's expectations of satisfactory asthma care.[1] As more insight into the nature of the inflammatory process in the asthmatic airway is obtained, and newer noninvasive monitoring techniques are developed, control of airway inflammation and prevention of airway remodeling and chronic obstructive pulmonary disease may also become a realistic goal of asthma management. Psychosocial factors such as the child's behavior, social adjustments in the family, school, and attitudes toward managing asthma should also be addressed. Parents should understand that asthma is a chronic disease with acute exacerbations that with currently available treatments can be controlled, but not cured; it is best managed in a continuous fashion by forming a partnership with a knowledgeable physician. The concept of expecting a near symptom-free life style (for all but the most severely affected patients) should be instilled in the patients and their families. Unnecessary restrictions of the child's and family's lifestyles should be avoided. Participation in recreational activities, sports, and school attendance should all be expected.

CLASSIFICATION OF ASTHMA

It is useful to stage asthma into categories, based on symptoms (cough, wheeze, shortness of breath), frequency of episodes (number of episodes per week), functional impairment (sleep disturbances, play disruption, school absenteeism), and objective measures of pulmonary function (PEFR or FEV_1) that are typically present if the patient is not receiving any (or adequate) treatment (Table 56-2). Although these designations are somewhat arbitrary and there is overlap between categories, such staging may be helpful in order to design appropriate and effective management strategies, which are coupled with severity levels. The degree of severity of asthma may appear to change in a given individual with time, reflecting growth, the development of newly acquired allergic sensitivities, change in exposure to recognized factors, or therapy. It is important to remember that asthma is a chronic disorder that may become clinically obvious only periodically, one in which the severity of airway obstruction is frequently underestimated by physician and patient alike.

The most recent NHLBI guidelines classify asthma as either intermittent or persistent; and then as mild, moderate, or severe (see Table 56-2).[1]

Intermittent Asthma

When symptoms are mild, easily controlled, and occur no more often than twice per week, and baseline pulmonary function is normal, asthma is classified as mild intermittent. In addition, patients with intermittent asthma do not require chronic administration of anti-inflammatory medications, but may be treated with a short-acting inhaled β agonist alone. Exercise-induced asthma (EIA) may also be considered mild or intermittent disease. Individuals with only EIA rarely have symptoms triggered by other agents. Although children with mild intermittent asthma have little daily morbidity due to asthma, it is important to remember that severe attacks can occur, particularly in response to certain viral infections or profound allergen exposure.

Mild Persistent Asthma

Children with mild persistent asthma have cough or wheeze more than twice per week, but less than daily. Nocturnal symptoms of cough or wheeze occur no more often than twice per month, and pulmonary function (PEFR or FEV_1) is normal. Peak flow variability (day to day) is not greater than 20%. Airway obstruction and overt asthmatic symptoms may occur within minutes and resolve more or less completely in a similar time. There are relatively few of these brief episodes (more than two per week, but less than daily), with no symptoms or functional impairment between episodes. This form of asthma probably represents at least one half of all cases of childhood asthma.

Moderate Persistent Asthma

There is evidence of mild airway obstruction, with some functional impairment and noticeable asthmatic symptoms between overt episodes. Patients have symptoms most to all days, nocturnal symptoms at least weekly, and may report frequent slowed play and missed days at school. PEFR varies by at least 30% from day to day, and FEV_1 measures are often in the range of mild obstructive lung disease (60%–80% of predicted).

Severe Persistent Asthma

These children have overt symptoms that occur more or less constantly, and have obvious functional impairment most days. Exercise tolerance is impaired regularly due to the frequency of asthma symptoms. Night awakenings occur most nights, and school attendance may be poor (>20 days missed per year). Spirometry reveals the FEV_1 to be less than 60% predicted for age and there may be greater than 30% diurnal variation in PEFR measurement. This pattern is typical of no more than 5% to 10% of children with asthma. Children with life-threatening asthma may exhibit most or all of the above symptoms, but in addition, have experienced an extremely severe asthma episode or event that places them at risk for death due to asthma.

Although the NHLBI guidelines may be useful in a clinical setting, more recent data suggest that relying on symptoms and simple pulmonary function testing may not provide adequate information for optimum asthma management. Patients often underreport symptoms, and patient recall during a telephone call or office visit may be colored by recent events (i.e., an exacerbation) and may not be accurately reflective of chronic symptoms at baseline. Use of a prospective symptom diary may provide a more accurate picture of daily symptoms, but many patients fail to record data without a reminder. Physicians may not gather appropriate historical data during an office visit or may fail to accurately interpret the data and misclassify the severity. Relying on pulmonary function and symptoms may not portray an accurate picture of asthma morbidity. In a multicenter trial conducted by the Asthma Clinical Research Network, patients previously well controlled on treatment with triamcinolone were randomized to treatment with either an ICS (triamcinolone 400 μg twice daily), a long-acting β agonist (salmeterol 42 μg twice daily), or placebo for 16 weeks. Both active treatments were superior to placebo. Although there was no difference between the active treatment groups in the typical outcomes of morning PEFR, symptom score, or bronchodilator use, the group treated with salmeterol had significantly more treatment failures (24% vs. 6%) and acute exacerbations (20% vs. 7%) than the steroid group.[21] Relying on the level of pulmonary function alone would have misclassified the response to treatment in the two groups. Finally, there may be other measures of airway function or inflammation that are more indicative of the need for treatment. Sont and co-workers compared a strategy of using guidelines alone (symptoms and pulmonary function) compared with guidelines and airway hyperresponsiveness measured by methacholine challenge to adjust asthma treatment.[16] Patients treated using the hyperresponsiveness strategy received a higher dose of ICS throughout the course of the study, but also achieved better pulmonary function and had fewer exacerbations than those treated using the guideline strategy alone. Finally, Green and colleagues demonstrated that using the number of eosinophils found in induced sputum sample to adjust level of treatment resulted in fewer acute exacerbations and hospitalizations than reliance on symptoms and pulmonary function alone.[18] These data suggest that more in-depth monitoring strategies that include biomarkers reflective of

TABLE 56-2. Criteria for determining asthma severity or control level and recommended medications for treatment

Classify Severity: Clinical Features Before Treatment or Adequate Control			Medications Required To Maintain Long-Term Control
	Symptoms/Day / *Symptoms/Night*	*PEF or FEV$_1$* / *PEF Variablility*	*Daily Medications*
Step 4: Severe Persistent	Continued / Frequent	≤ 60% / > 30%	■ Preferred treatment: High-close inhaled corticosteroids AND Long-acting inhaled beta$_2$-agonists AND, if needed. Corticosteroid tablets or syrup long term (2 mg/kg/day, generally do not exceed 60 mg per day). (Make repeat attempts to reduce systemic corticosteroids and maintain control with high-dose inhaled corticosteroids.
Step 3: Moderate Persistent	Daily / > 1 night/week	> 60% – < 90% / > 30%	■ Preferred treatment Low-to-medium dose inhaled corticosteroids and long-acting inhaled beta$_2$-agonists. ■ Alternative treatment (listed alphabetically) Increase inhaled corticosteroids within medium-dose range OR ■ Low-tomedium dose inhaled corticosteroids and either leukotriene modifier or theophylline. If needed (particularly in patients with recurring severe exacerbations): ■ Preferred treatment: Increase inhaled corticosteroids within medium-dose range and add long-acting inhaled beta$_2$-agonists. ■ Alternative Treatment: Increase inhaled corticosteroids within medium-dose range and add either leukotriene modifier or theophylline.
Step 2: Mild Persistent	>2/week but <1/day / >2 nights/month	> 90% / 20–30%	■ Preferred treatment: Low-dose inhaled corticosteroids. ■ Alternative treatment (listed aplphabetically): cromolyn, leukotriene modifier, nedocromil, OR sustained release theophylline to serum concentration of 5–15 mcg/mL.
Step 1: Mild Intermittent	< 2 days/week / < 2 nights/month	>90% / <20%	■ No daily medication needed. ■ Severe exacerbations may occur, separated by long periods of normal lung function and no symptoms. A course of systemic corticosteroids is recommended.
Quick Relief: All Patients	■ Short-acting bronchodilator: 2-4 puffs short-acting inhaled beta$_2$-agonists as needed for symptoms. ■ Intensity of treatment will depend on severity of exacerbation: up to 3 treatments at 20- minute intervals or a single nebulizer treatment as needed. Course of systemic corticosteroids may be needed. ■ Use of short-acting beta$_2$-agonists >2 times a week in intermittent asthma (daily, or increasing use in persistent asthma) may indicate the need to initiate (increase) long-term control therapy.		
Step Down Review treatment every 1 to 6 months: a gradual stepwise reduction in treatment may be possible. Step up If control is not maintained, consider step up, First, review patient medication technique, adherence, and environmental control.	Note ■ The stepwise approach is meant to assist, not critical discrimating required to most individuals patient needs. ■ Classify severity, assign patients to most severe step in which any feature occurs (PEF is % of personal best; FEV1 is % predicated. ■ Gain control as quickly as possible (consider a short course of systemic corticosteroids% than step down to the least medication necessary to maintain control. ■ Provide education on self-management and controlling environmental factors that make asthma worse (e.g. allergens and irritants.) ■ Refer to an asthma specialist if there are difficulties controlling asthma or if step 4 care is required. Referral may be considered if step 3 care is required.		
Goals of Therapy: Asthma control	■ Minimal or no chronic symptoms day or night ■ Minimal or no exacerbations ■ No limitations on activities; no alcohol /week missed. ■ Maintain (near) normal pulmonary function ■ Minimal use of short-acting inhaled beta$_2$-agonist (< lz per day, <1 canister/month) ■ Minimal or no adverse effects from medications		

From National Institutes of Health: Guidelines for the diagnosis and management of asthma—update on selected topics 2002. In: National Asthma Education and Prevention Program. Expert Panel Report. Publication no. 02-5074. Bethesda, Md: National Institutes of Health, 2002.

airway inflammation may provide better guidance for classifying asthma severity and adjusting medications than symptoms and spirometry.

PHARMACOLOGIC MANAGEMENT OF ASTHMA IN CHILDREN OLDER THAN 5 YEARS

Asthma medical treatment involves the chronic administration of controller medications designed to prevent asthma symptoms and the use of rapid-acting reliever medications that act quickly to abort acute exacerbations. Controller medications are administered to all asthmatics other than those with mild intermittent disease and are typically, but not uniformly, anti-inflammatory in nature (Table 56-3). Reliever medications are short-acting β_2 agonists or anticholinergics. Several new classes of immunomodulatory drugs are under development, and one, anti-IgE, is currently available for treatment of severe persistent asthma.

RELIEVER MEDICATIONS: SHORT-ACTING β AGONISTS

β_2-adrenergic agonists constitute the most potent bronchodilators currently available for treatment of asthma[1] and are used to relieve bronchospasm and its attendant symptoms of cough, wheeze, and shortness of breath. Adrenergic agents bind to the widely distributed β receptors, primarily those located on the bronchial smooth muscle, airway epithelial cell, or mast cell, and result in the intracellular conversion of adenosine triphosphate (ATP) to adenosine 3',5' cyclic monophosphate. The result is relaxation of airway smooth muscle and improved airflow. Onset of action is generally within a few minutes, peak action occurring at approximately 30 minutes, and duration of action from 4 to 6 hours.[1] Preferred route of administration is via inhalation, because this method results in the most rapid onset of action and offers excellent duration of action as well, while minimizing adverse effects. Inhalation of short-acting β agonists can be accomplished with use of a small-volume jet nebulizer, metered-dose inhaler (MDI), or dry powder inhaler (not currently available in the United States).

There are several β-adrenergic agonists available for use in treating acute asthma. Isoetharine and metaproterenol have largely been replaced in clinical use by the highly selective β_2 agonists, such as terbutaline, pirbuterol, and albuterol. The predominant bronchodilator in current use, racemic albuterol, is a 50:50 mixture of (R)- and (S)-enantiomers. Levalbuterol, the (R)-albuterol isomer, has 100-fold more potent β_2 receptor binding than (S)-albuterol, and is responsible for the bronchodilator effects of the racemate. The ability to separate the isomers of β_2 agonists has challenged previous assumptions that (S)-albuterol is inert. In vitro, (S)-albuterol has been demonstrated to increase intracellular Ca^{2+} and to stimulate eosinophil recruitment and degranulation. (S)-albuterol has essentially no bronchodilator activity, but does have a prolonged plasma half-life, and in vitro it can increase intracellular calcium and activate and recruit inflammatory cells. The in vivo effects of (S)-albuterol are more controversial and require more study to substantiate clinical effects. Racemic albuterol and levalbuterol have an onset of action within minutes and duration of action of 4 to 6 hours. Racemic albuterol is available as tablets and solution for oral administration as well as a nebulizer solution and MDI; levalbuterol is currently available only as an inhalant solution. Terbutaline, available in tablets, an MDI, and a solution for parenteral use in the United States, is similar to albuterol in duration and specificity. Other β_2-specific agents and doses are listed in Table 56-3.

Systemic administration of these relatively specific β_2 agents may produce side effects, such as muscular tremor and some cardiovascular effects, in addition to bronchodilation, whereas administration by aerosol in the usual dose induces bronchodilation with minimal tremor and cardiovascular effects. Skeletal muscle tremor invariably accompanies systemic administration of moderate doses of β_2 agents. Tremor tends to decrease with chronic use.

The occurrence of serious adverse events following the chronic administration of inhaled β agonists remains controversial. The increase in asthma deaths reported in the United Kingdom in the late 1960s was initially related to overuse of high-dose isoproterenol inhalers, and the rise in asthma deaths reported in New Zealand was believed to be associated with the use of inhaled fenoterol, a drug never available in the United States. A retrospective review of prescription records to track medication use in patients in Canada found an increased risk for asthma death or near-death in patients who used more than one canister of a β agonist per month. However, an association with the use of a number of other asthma medications was also noted, suggesting that disease severity might actually be more causative than overuse of β agonists alone.

Other reports have suggested that repeated use of β agonists may result in an increase in airway hyperresponsiveness or decrease in protection from allergen-induced bronchospasm. The reduction in beneficial effects of β agonists following chronic use may result in part from receptor desensitization, a known phenomenon that results from continuous agonist application to target cells. The decrease in response may be the result of uncoupling of the receptor from its signaling (G protein), inactivation of receptors, or decreased receptor number due to increased degradation or decreased synthesis. Although these actions occur in vitro, the in vivo biological correlates are somewhat more controversial. In at least some patients, following chronic administration of β agonists, the ability of acute premedication with a short-acting β agonist to block an allergen or other challenge is diminished but not abolished. The clinical significance of this decreased effect is questionable. A well-designed randomized double-blind placebo-controlled study performed in adults with mild asthma examined the effects of regularly administered albuterol versus intermittent administration compared with placebo.[22] There was no significant difference in any outcome measures between the groups, including exacerbations, treatment failures, lung function, symptoms, or methacholine responsiveness. However, regular use of albuterol was also not beneficial to the patients. The current recommendation is for the as-needed use of short-acting β agonists for relief of symptoms or protection against exercise-induced asthma.

Finally, there may be specific subgroups of patients who are at risk for developing adverse effects as measured by worsening pulmonary function with chronic use of β agonists, and this may be related to genetic variability in the β-adrenergic receptor. Nine polymorphisms in the β-adrenergic receptor gene have been described, and several of the more frequent types may have biological significance. One of interest involves the β2AR-16 region, with replacement of arginine (Arg16) for glycine (Gly16). In a study involving bronchodilator response in children, those with the Arg/Arg polymorphism had the highest prevalence (60%) of bronchodilator response to albuterol, whereas fewer than 30% of those with the Arg/Gly responded and only 13% of those with Gly/Gly were responders. In contrast, a retrospective

TABLE 56-3. Usual dosages for long-term control medications

Medication	Dosage Form	Adult	Child Dose
Inhaled Corticosteroids (See Estimated Comparative Daily Dosages for Inhaled Corticosteroids)			
Systemic Corticosteroids		*(Applies to all three Corticosteroids)*	
Methylprednisolone Prednisolone Prednisone	2, 4, 8, 16, 32 mg tablets 5 mg tablets, 5 mg/5 cc 15 mg/5 cc 1, 2.5, 5, 10, 20, 50 mg tablets; 5 mg/cc, 5 mg/5 cc	■ 7.5–60 mg daily in a single dose in a.m or qod as needed for control ■ Short-course "burst" to achieve control: 40–60 mg per day as single or 2 divided single doses for 3–10 days.	■ 0.25–2 mg/kg dialy in single dose in a.m. or qod as needed for control ■ Short-course "burst" : 1–2 mg/kg/day, maximum 60 mg/day for 3–10 days.
Long-Acting Inhaled Beta$_2$-Agonists (Should not be used for symptom relief or for exacerbations. Use with inhaled corcosteroids.)			
Salmeterol	DPI 50 mcg/blister	1 blister q 12 hours	1 blister q 12 hours
Formoterol	DPI 12 mcg/singl-use capsule	1 capsule q 12 hours	1 capsule q 12 hours
Combined Medication			
Fluticasone/Salmeterol	DPI 100, 250, or 500 mcg/50 mcg	1 inhalation bid; dose depends on severity of asthma	1 inhalation bid; dose depends on severity of asthma
Cromolyn and Nedocromil			
Cromolyn	MDI 1 mg/puff Nebulizer 20 mg/ampule	2–4 puffs tid-qid 1 ampule tid-qid	1–2 puffs tid-qid 1 ampule tid-qid
Nedocromil	MDI 1.75 mg/puff	2–4 puffs bid-qid	1–2 puffs bid-qid
Leukotriene Modifiers			
Montelukast Zafirlukast	4 or 5 mg chewable tablet 10 mg tablet	10 mg qhs	4 mg qhs (2-5 yrs) 5 mg qhs (6-14 yrs) 10 mg qhs (>14 yrs) 20 mg daily (7–11 yrs) (10 mg tablet bid)
Zileuton	10 or 20 mg tablet 300 or 600 mg tablet	40 mg daily (20 mg tablet bid 2400 mg daily (give tablets qid)	
Methylxanthines (Serum monitoring is important (serum concentration of 5–15 mcg/mL at steady state)			
Theophylline	Liquids, sustained-release tablets, and capsules	Starting dose 10 mg/kg/day up to 300 mg max; usual max 800 mg/day	Starting dose 10 mg/kg/day; usual max: ■ <1 year of age: 0.2 (age in weeks) + 5 = mg/kg/day ■ ≥1 year of age: 16 mg/kg/day

look at patients who participated in the study comparing regular to intermittent use of albuterol found that those with the Arg16 homozygous polymorphism who were treated chronically with albuterol had steadily declining PEFR as compared with those receiving intermittent treatment.[23] These data suggest that in the future, knowing a patient's β-receptor genotype may aid in prescribing β agonist use in the most effective and safe manner.

CONTROLLER MEDICATIONS

METHYLXANTHINES: THEOPHYLLINE

Although methylxanthines have been used for the treatment of asthma since the early part of the 20th century, their role in managing acute and chronic asthma remains somewhat controversial. Theophylline is now considered a second- or third-line medication, largely because it is a poor acute bronchodilator, it has a narrow therapeutic index and significant adverse effects, and other anti-inflammatory drugs have replaced it.[1]

The action of theophylline is largely thought to be as a smooth muscle relaxant and bronchodilator. However, theophylline can also act centrally as a respiratory stimulant and may also increase diaphragmatic contractility and help prevent diaphragmatic fatigue.

Although a serum concentration of 10 to 15 mg/mL is required for significant effectiveness, clinically apparent therapeutic effects can be achieved at blood levels lower than 10 mg/mL in many children. If the concentration is near or above 20 mg/mL, the likelihood of significant drug toxicity is greatly increased. However, adverse effects may occur at levels substantially lower. Careful monitoring of serum concentration in relation to clinical effectiveness (symptom control, need for rescue medication) is mandatory.

Theophylline overdose results in gastric irritation, gastrointestinal hemorrhage in rare instances, and central nervous system symptoms, such as agitation, convulsions, coma, respiratory failure, and vasomotor collapse.

CROMOLYN SODIUM

Cromolyn was believed to be effective in asthma prophylaxis in children and adolescents with mild to moderate asthma. However, its activity has recently been called into question. Comparative studies and reanalysis of previous data suggest that cromolyn has minimal to no effect on controlling chronic asthma, particularly in younger children. These data, coupled with the fact that cromolyn is relatively expensive and must be inhaled four times per day, suggest that cromolyn is not likely to be used as a controller medication for asthma in the future. Cromolyn is effective in preventing exercise-induced bronchospasm, but less so than a short-acting adrenergic bronchodilator.

NEDOCROMIL

Nedocromil sodium is another NSAID effective for the treatment of chronic asthma. Although its in vitro potency is sevenfold that of cromolyn, clinical trials indicate that nedocromil is most beneficial for patients with mild asthma. Nedocromil has been shown to be as effective as cromolyn in reducing exercise-induced symptoms, and also reduces airway hyperresponsiveness to allergen challenge. Nedocromil was compared to placebo and inhaled BUD in the CAMP study and was found to be effective in reducing symptoms and exacerbations compared with placebo, but less so than BUD.[7] Nedocromil appears to be quite safe, with no significant adverse effects following long-term administration. The most common adverse effect is an unpleasant, bitter taste, reported by 20% to 30% of patients. In addition, some patients cough with nedocromil administration; use of a spacer device or holding chamber can minimize both of these problems.

INHALED CORTICOSTEROIDS

The anti-inflammatory action of the adrenal corticosteroids was discovered in 1948; thereafter both acute asthma and chronic asthma were found to respond well to cortisone. The most commonly used ICS have a high topical potency and relatively low systemic effects, either as a result of poor absorption and/or rapid and effective metabolism to inactive compounds. However, other factors, such as pharmacologic properties of the drugs (receptor affinity, lipophilicity, delivery device) can all affect therapeutic efficacy and adverse effect profile. There are six ICS preparations currently available in the United States market, and others that are in clinical trials.

Fluticasone Propionate

Fluticasone propionate (FP) is a potent and poorly absorbed topically active corticosteroid that is extensively metabolized in the liver to an inactive compound. This highly lipophilic drug demonstrates an extremely high affinity for lung glucocorticoid receptors (GRs) compared with beclomethasone (BDP; parent compound beclomethasone dipropionate) and shows a slow rate of dissociation from its receptor. In vivo, it appears at least twice as potent as BDP and BUD on a milligram per milligram basis. As a result, FP has negligible oral bioavailability, and the topical to systemic activity ratio is exceptionally favorable and better than currently available ICS. However, FP is readily absorbed through the respiratory mucosa and can enter the systemic circulation in this fashion (without hepatic metabolism). It is currently available in an MDI in three strengths, and may soon be available in a dry powder inhaler (see Table 56-4).

Budesonide

BUD has been widely studied and used clinically for many years. It has moderate potency in vitro and in vivo with well-documented clinical efficacy and safety. In addition, the presence of a free C21 hydroxy group on the BUD molecule results in formation of esters with long-chain fatty acids. This results in an inactive depot of drug within the airway cells that is released slowly into an active state. This property of BUD may be partially responsible for its efficacy in once-a-day dosing. BUD is currently available in a dry powder inhaler and a nebulizer suspension.

Beclomethasone

Although clearly less potent than FP and slightly less so than BUD, BDP is effective in reducing symptoms and improving pulmonary function. However, BDP is readily absorbed from the gastrointestinal tract, and the parent compound beclomethasone dipropionate is metabolized to the more potent monopropionate. As a result, BDP has a less favorable topical to systemic potency ratio, and concerns remain about its ability to cause adverse effects. BDP is currently available as a fine-particle aerosol dispensed by a hydrofluoroalkene propellant. This propellant system permits greater deposition into the lower and smaller airways and a reduction in the effective dose. The clinical advantage of these properties remains to be clarified.

Others

Triamcinolone and flunisolide are relatively less potent steroids that while effective are less commonly used. Both must be given in fairly high microgram amounts, resulting in a bitter unpleasant taste. Mometasone is a potent, highly topically active steroid that is currently used to treat allergic rhinitis and dermatologic disorders. It was recently approved for treatment of asthma in the United States. It has the advantage of poor systemic absorption and is likely to cause little significant growth suppression.

Ciclesonide is a prodrug that must be metabolized to active form in the lung, where its metabolite has approximately 100 times greater receptor affinity. It has essentially no oral bioavailability and is tightly bound to plasma proteins. Efficacy in reducing bronchial hyperresponsiveness has been demonstrated, and further clinical trials are under way.

Mechanism of Action and Clinical Use

The action of corticosteroids begins as passive diffusion across the cell membrane and into the cytoplasm where binding to the GR occurs. The unliganded GR exists in the cytoplasm as a large heterodimeric complex that includes two 90-kd heat shock protein molecules. After hormone binding, the heat shock proteins are shed. The complex is then translocated to the nucleus and as a dimer binds to a glucocorticoid response element (GRE) on steroid-responsive genes.

The GR acts to regulate transcription of target genes either directly or indirectly by interaction with other transcription factors. The binding of GR to GRE results in either induction or repression of the gene. The number of GREs and the proximity to transcriptional start sites results in increased steroid inducibility of the gene. GRs may also act independently of binding to GRE by acting as a coactivator of other transcription factors (e.g., STAT5) or by modulating chromatin structure by recruiting histone deacetylase and effecting gene silencing.[24]

A major target of GRs is the transcription factor, NF-κB. The actions of NF-κB results in increased synthesis of proinflammatory cytokines. GRs may block NF-κB signaling by one of two mechanisms. Through direct protein-protein interactions, the GR may bind to the p65 subunit of NF-κB and prevent it from binding to DNA and enhancing transcription. Corticosteroids may also inhibit NF-κB by directly increasing inhibitory (I)–κB production. I-κB proteins bind to NF-κB and keep it anchored in the cytoplasm. Steroid-induced inhibition of cytokine production is likely a significant anti-inflammatory feature. Corticosteroids inhibit the transcription of a number of cytokines and chemokines implicated in the pathogenesis of asthma, such as interleukin-1 (IL-1) through IL-6, tumor necrosis factor-α, granulocyte-macrophage colony-stimulating factor, IL-13, IL-8, RANTES (released on activation, normal T cell expressed and secreted), and eotaxin. Steroids may also inhibit the synthesis of some cytokine receptors, such as the IL-4 receptor, intracellular adhesion molecule (ICAM), and vascular cell adhesion molecule (VCAM). In addition to the action on cytokines, steroids also inhibit the inducible form of nitric oxide synthase, cyclo-oxygenase, phospholipase A2, and endothelin, all important factors in the inflammatory cascade relevant to asthma. Corticosteroids also increase the synthesis of β-adrenergic receptors by increasing gene transcription.

ICS are currently recommended as first-line therapy for children over the age of 5 years and adults with other than mild intermittent asthma. ICS reduce airway reactivity, reduce acute symptoms and exacerbations, and decrease the need for rescue bronchodilators. When administered chronically, ICS can also lead to attenuation of late allergen responses. In addition, ICS decrease deposition of collagen and tenascin in the subepithelial basement membrane. Withdrawal of ICS treatment is usually accompanied by a rapid return of airway hyperresponsiveness and decreased symptom control. Although ICS are the most effective chronic treatment for chronic persistent asthma, some questions regarding the optimum dose, method of delivery, timing and duration of therapy, and long-term safety in children remain. In addition, a small but substantial proportion of patients do not have a significant response to ICS, and the mechanisms of this relative steroid resistance is not yet fully understood.[25] However, currently available data provide acceptable guidelines for the safe and effective use of inhaled steroids in older children.

It was long assumed that a dose-response effect would occur during treatment with ICS. Several studies suggested that there was indeed a dose response when outcomes such as pulmonary function measures (PEFR or FEV_1) were used. However, it appeared that the dose-response curve reached a plateau at a fairly low dose and little added benefit was seen when doses were as much as quadrupled. A recent study performed in adults and designed to evaluate the relative efficacy and safety of escalating doses of inhaled steroids demonstrated that for the majority of patients, maximal benefit as measured by improvement in FEV_1 and methacholine responsiveness occurred at low to moderate doses of FP and BDP.[26] However, at doses greater than the lowest effective, a substantial increase in adverse effect, measured by cortisol suppression was seen. Although similar studies need to be repeated in children, it is likely that most of the clinical benefit with the least risk will occur at low doses. Nevertheless, some patients may not show improvement at conventional steroid doses and will require more tailored dosing and careful monitoring for both response to therapy and emergence of systemic side effects.

The actual incidence and clinical significance of the adverse effects of long-term use of ICS in children remains uncertain. Local adverse effects, such as oral candidiasis and dysphonia, are the most common but least severe complications of treatment, are dose-related, and only occur in a small minority of patients. Reducing the dose, using a spacer device, and rinsing the mouth out with water after use may minimize both these symptoms. Cough and/or throat irritation is reported by approximately 10% of children treated with inhaled steroids and often responds to use of a spacer device, inhalation of a bronchodilator prior to steroid inhalation, slowing the inhalation technique, or switching to a dry powder inhaler.

The more serious systemic adverse effects for children include adrenal suppression and effects on bone and linear growth. Adrenal suppression has been extensively studied, although the results are often difficult to interpret owing to lack of an appropriate control group, previous use of oral corticosteroids, or inappropriate tests used to assess adrenal function. Nonetheless, a number of studies indicate that adrenal suppression is unlikely in children receiving less than 400 μg/day of either inhaled BUD or fluticasone 200 μg/day even after long-term use.[7,14] Adrenal suppression can be measured in children receiving higher doses, as indicated by impaired adrenocorticotropic hormone stimulation tests or decreased urinary cortisol excretion. However, in most patients, even these impairments are of no or uncertain clinical significance when the patient is well. A significant stress (major illness, surgery) could warrant administration of exogenous corticosteroid to prevent an addisonian response.

The effect of ICS on linear growth also remains somewhat controversial, but more recent studies point to a minimal effect of long-term administration of low-dose inhaled steroids on linear growth. Most earlier studies on the effect of inhaled steroids on growth focused on short-term growth rate assessed by knemometry, a sensitive method to measure growth velocity of the lower leg. In such short-term studies, there was a dose-dependent growth suppression with the use of 200 to 800 μg/day of BUD for 6 weeks. Studies in which children were treated with inhaled BDP at doses of 400 to 800 μg/day for up to 1 year showed a significant growth suppression with growth decreasing by 0.28 standard deviation scores in the steroid group compared with 0.03 scores in the β-agonist group or as much as 1.3 cm difference in height in the steroid versus β-agonist group.[27] Moreover, most of the decrease in growth velocity appeared in the first few months after initiating steroid treatment. Although initially feared that each year of treatment even with low-dose inhaled steroids would result in over a centimeter of lost height, longer-term studies have not confirmed this. The CAMP study was a placebo-controlled comparison of the effect of nedocromil and BUD on pulmonary function in school-aged asthmatic children. Data on the growth of children in this 4-year long trial demonstrated that there was indeed a significant decline in growth velocity over the first year of the study, but the growth rate returned to normal thereafter. Children in the BUD group were on average 1.1 cm shorter than those children in the placebo and nedocromil groups at the end of the 4-year treatment period.[7] In addition, Agertoft and Pedersen showed that there was no reduction in final predicted adult height in a group of 142 children treated with a mean dose of 400 μg/day of BUD for an average of 9.2 years.[28] These longer-term studies of chronic low-dose inhaled steroids point to an excellent safety profile and potential to reach final predicted adult height, in spite of short-term decline in height velocity. Since there is also likely to be interindividual variability in response to corticosteroids and predisposition to develop adverse effects, careful monitoring of individual patients growth during treatment with ICS should be performed and the dose adjusted to the lowest necessary to achieve good symptom control.

SYSTEMIC CORTICOSTEROIDS

The therapeutic benefits of systemic corticosteroids are marred by their potential adverse effects, which include excessive weight gain, hypertension, osteoporosis, decreased linear growth, metabolic derangement, and cataracts. Adverse effects from long-term steroid therapy may be reduced, but not eliminated, by using steroids with shorter half-lives (prednisone, prednisolone, methylprednisolone) at the lowest possible dose administered in the morning in a single dose and given every other day (see Table 56-3).

LONG-ACTING β AGONISTS

β-adrenergic agonists that have a prolonged (>12 hours) duration of action occupy a unique niche in the asthma treatment armamentarium, somewhat between that of a controller and reliever medication. There are currently two long-acting β-agonists (LABAs) available on the U.S. market and approved for use in children: salmeterol (approved for ages 4 years and older) and formoterol (approved for age 12 years and older). The two agents differ in structure, potency, efficacy, and selectivity for the β receptor. Salmeterol is a partial agonist, has a relatively slow onset of action (10–20 minutes), and has extremely high selectivity for the β_2 receptor. It is currently available as a dry powder inhaler in a Diskus device (GlaxoSmithKline, Research Triangle, North Carolina) that contains a 30-day supply of drug. Formoterol is a full agonist with a very different molecular structure than salmeterol. It has a rapid onset of action (<5 minutes) like albuterol, but a duration of activity of 12 hours. Formoterol is also dispensed in a dry powder inhaler (Aerolizer, Schering-Plough, Kenilworth, New Jersey), with each dose contained in a capsule that must be inserted separately. Following a single dose of salmeterol (25–50 μg), there is sustained improvement in bronchodilation for at least 12 hours, as well as a bronchoprotective effect to both methacholine and exercise. However, after repeated doses, within a few days or weeks there is loss in degree of bronchodilation, bronchoprotection to methacholine, and exercise. For methacholine, there is a smaller increase in doubling doses, but it is unclear if this is clinically significant. When used as monotherapy, protection from exercise-induced bronchospasm persists after daily dosing for 2 to 4 weeks, but in several studies the duration of action decreases from 9 to 12 hours to as little as 1 hour. Although mechanisms of action of this tolerance to the bronchoprotective effect are unclear, down-regulation of β-receptor number or lack of receptor sensitivity are possibilities. Formoterol is likely to behave in a fashion similar to salmeterol.

The LABAs are not generally considered anti-inflammatory agents, but studies show that salmeterol has either no effect on airway inflammation or reduces inflammatory cells in the airway mucosa. It has also been proposed that LABAs may enhance the actions of ICS, although the mechanisms are controversial.

Past and recent concerns about the use of LABAs as monotherapy persist. A study performed by the Asthma Clinical Research Network demonstrated that the combination of triamcinolone and salmeterol was effective in controlling asthma in patients 12 to 65 years of age.[21] However, complete withdrawal of the inhaled steroid and continuation of the LABA resulted in significant deterioration in asthma control as measured by asthma exacerbations, deterioration in pulmonary function, and need for oral corticosteroid treatment. These data and those from similar studies all suggest that LABAs should not be used as monotherapy for treatment of chronic asthma.

Deaths have also been reported in patients chronically using inhaled salmeterol. It remains uncertain if there is a direct link between medication use and death or if the increase in deaths is a reflection of inappropriate use of a LABA (e.g., attempt to use as an acute bronchodilator and/or in place of a preventative medication). A recent large, unpublished trial (>25,000 enrollees) compared the safety of daily salmeterol or placebo added to usual treatment for chronic asthma over a 28-week period. The trial was stopped early when an interim analysis showed an association between salmeterol use and severe or fatal asthma. The risk for death, albeit small (13 of 13,174) in the salmeterol group was significantly greater than that in the placebo group (4 of 13,179). Importantly, the increased risk for death was only found in African American subjects, and there was no significant difference in the endpoints of death or severe respiratory events in the total study population. Although there were a number of flaws in this trial, the data resulted in a warning being placed on the salmeterol package insert advising of the study results. These data are also consistent with the recommendation not to use salmeterol as monotherapy.

The major benefit of LABAs is probably with use in combination with an ICS to improve asthma control and permit reduction of the steroid dose. A number of studies that included older children and adults have demonstrated that the addition of a LABA to a regimen that includes an ICS results in improved asthma control and improved pulmonary function.[29] More importantly, the dose of inhaled steroid can often be reduced by as much as 50% and still maintain asthma control when the LABA is added. Although the data are striking and consistent in studies on adults, the few pediatric studies have not been as convincing. A study performed in 177 schoolchildren 6 to 16 years of age compared 400 μg/day of BDP alone to 400 μg BDP plus salmeterol 50 μg/day to 800 μg/day BDP. All patients improved with respect to pulmonary function, symptom score, and airway reactivity, with no significant differences among the groups during the 1 year of treatment.[30] These data suggest that addition of a LABA to an ICS in pediatric patients may not have the same steroid-sparing effect or enhancement of steroid effect as that seen in adults. However, it is also possible that the relatively mild asthmatics studied in this trial reached maximum treatment benefit at even the lowest dose of BDP tested, and that addition of a LABA or higher dose steroid conferred no further benefit. Further studies in children are necessary to better understand the role of addition of LABAs to ICS.

There are currently two fixed-dose combination inhaled steroid and LABA medications available. Salmeterol is combined with fluticasone in a dry powder inhaler; the dose of salmeterol is fixed at 50 μg per inhalation, while the fluticasone component is available in either 100, 250, or 500 μg per inhalation. Typical dosing regimen is one puff given every 12 hours. In order to increase the dose of steroid, a separate inhaler is necessary, in order to avoid excessive dosing of salmeterol that could occur if the number of inhalations were increased. A combination of formoterol and BUD is also available in a dry powder inhaler, but this is currently not available in the United States. It is also possible to administer each medication separately from individual inhalers; this is less convenient for the patient, may be more expensive, but does allow more flexibility in adjusting the dose of inhaled steroid.

ANTICHOLINERGIC AGENTS

Ipratropium bromide is a quaternary ammonium congener of atropine and is an anticholinergic compound approved for use as a bronchodilator. Anticholinergic agents produce bronchodilation by antagonizing the activity of acetylcholine at the level of its receptor, particularly those found on airway smooth muscle located in the large, central airways. The onset of action of ipratropium is relatively slow (~20 minutes) and the peak effect occurs at 60 minutes.[14] Ipratropium, unlike atropine, is poorly absorbed across mucous membranes and has little toxicity at the stated dose. In particular, ipratropium does not inhibit mucociliary clearance. Data from several studies conducted in children presenting to the emergency department for treatment of acute asthma indicates that when combined with a β-adrenergic agonist, ipratropium improves pulmonary function and relieves symptoms better than either drug alone.[14] The effect is modest, and appears to be most evident in those who present with the most severe airway obstruction, as measured by PEFR; this may be a marker for patients who have increased cholinergic tone in the large central airways. Ipratropium has not been shown to be effective in the treatment of children hospitalized with acute asthma.[31] It is also not recommended for chronic use or acute use at home for relief of bronchospasm.

LEUKOTRIENE ANTAGONISTS

Therapeutic agents aimed at inhibiting lipoxygenase products can also be effective treatment, particularly for mild persistent asthma or as an adjunct therapy in combination with an inhaled steroid. Leukotrienes are lipid mediators that are produced by the catabolism of arachidonic acid via the action of phospholipase A2. The enzyme 5-lipoxygenase produces leukotrienes: LTB4 and the cysteinyl members LTC4, LTD4, and LTE4. LTC4 is metabolized to LTD4, and LTE4 is the final metabolic product, which is excreted via the urine. Arachidonic acid can also be a precursor for the cyclo-oxygenase pathway and results in production of prostaglandins and thromboxane. However, it is the cysteinyl leukotrienes (cysLTs) that are the more potent mediators capable of inducing the asthma phenotype. Actions of cysLTs include smooth muscle constriction, increased vascular permeability, mucus hypersecretion, edema formation, and inflammatory cell recruitment into the airways. Furthermore, elevated levels of cysLTs are recovered from the bronchoalveolar lavage fluid, and urinary LTE4 levels are elevated following airway allergen challenge in atopic asthmatics. Application of exogenous cysLTs to the airways of experimental animals and human subjects causes bronchoconstriction. CysLTs are produced by a number of cell types found in the airways, including mast cells, eosinophils, basophils, macrophages, and neutrophils. Corticosteroids do not directly inhibit the synthesis or block the action of leukotrienes.

Two basic strategies targeting cysLTs have been most commonly employed: inhibition of 5-lipoxygenase and leukotriene receptor antagonism. Because of the nature of the lipoxygenase synthetic cascade (Fig. 56-5), interruption at an early level (e.g., at the 5-lipoxygenase) could diminish overall cysteinyl LT and LTB production, both of which are generally elevated in biological fluids (blood, bronchoalveolar lavage fluid, urine) from symptomatic asthmatics. The 5-lipoxygenase inhibitor Zileuton (Critical Therapeutics, Inc., Lexington, Massachusetts) blocks the bronchoconstrictor response to inhaled allergen or cold air challenge, exercise, and aspirin ingestion in sensitive individuals. However, since the drug must be given four times per day and reversible elevation of liver function tests are noted in some patients, it has been replaced by safer leukotriene receptor antagonists.

The leukotriene effect in asthma can also be blocked with receptor antagonists. When administered orally, 40 mg twice daily of the LTD receptor antagonist zafiruklast resulted in significant reduction in daytime and nighttime symptoms and the need for β-agonist inhalation compared with placebo. Zafirlukast has modest efficacy at best, must be given twice daily, and in some patients also results in elevated hepatic enzymes. Montelukast is an effective LTD4 receptor antagonist and is administered once a day. It has been shown in a number of studies to decrease urinary excretion of LTE4, reduce both circulating and sputum eosinophil counts, and decrease exhaled nitric oxide.[14] Clinical effects include improvement in FEV_1 and protection from exercise- and allergen-induced bronchospasm. Improvement in pulmonary function can be detected after a first dose and reaches a peak after a few weeks of treatment. However, montelukast does not result in as much improvement in asthma control as does treatment with inhaled steroid, as measured by improvement in FEV_1, symptom control, and

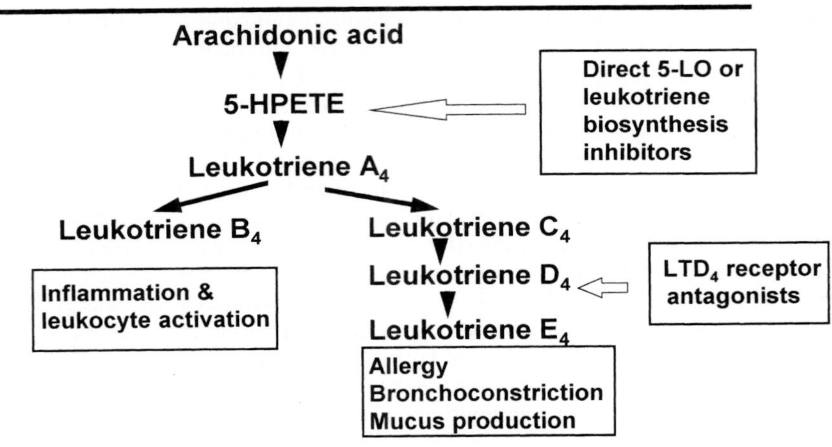

FIGURE 56-5. Metabolic pathways and functions of leukotrienes. 5-HPETE, 5S-hydroperoxy-6,8,11,14-eicosatetraenoate; 5-LO, 5-lipoxygenase LTD_4, leukotriene D_4.

reduction in inflammatory markers.[14,25] In addition, perhaps a third of patients do not respond well or at all to montelukast.[25] Although certain genetic polymorphisms have been associated with a poor response to LTRA, at present detection of these markers is still a research tool. Montelukast may also provide improved asthma control when combined with other controller medications, such as inhaled steroids. Although study results are somewhat conflicting, most show that the addition of montelukast to an inhaled steroid results in modest improvement that is not quite as efficacious as adding an LABA, particularly on pulmonary function outcomes. One pediatric trial demonstrated a small improvement in FEV_1 (6.0% montelukast, 4.1% placebo, $P = .01$) and in the need for rescue bronchodilator (1.65 puffs/day montelukast, 1.98 puffs/day placebo, $P = .013$) use when montelukast was added to a regimen of low-dose BUD.[32] Adverse effects of montelukast have been relatively minor and mainly consist of headache, abdominal pain, and vivid dreams. There are several case reports of adults who developed Churgg-Strauss syndrome when treatment with montelukast was instituted and oral corticosteroid treatment withdrawn. Since the majority of these patients had what was considered to be severe, steroid-dependent asthma, it is believed that the development of systemic vasculitis was actually emergence of underlying disease as a result of steroid withdrawal and less likely due to a direct action of montelukast. Care should be taken, however, if montelukast is used in an attempt to decrease or discontinue oral steroids in a patient with presumed severe asthma.

OTHER DRUGS

A number of medications currently used for other indications have been utilized in the treatment of severe, refractory asthma with varying degrees of success. Gold salts, methotrexate, and cyclosporine all have anti-inflammatory properties and have had some efficacy in ameliorating severe, steroid-resistant asthma. However, these medications have significant untoward effects, limited efficacy, or both and are rarely used.

Several other novel approaches to asthma therapy involve immune modulation. Use of a humanized monoclonal anti-IgE antibody (omalizumab) to complex with and lower the circulating concentration of IgE has shown some promise. This drug has recently obtained approval from the U.S. Food and Drug Administration for use in patients ages 12 years and up. When administered subcutaneously every 2 to 4 weeks to patients with moderate elevations of serum IgE (<750 IU), an improvement in symptoms, decrease in exacerbations, and reduced need for inhaled or oral corticosteroid dose is demonstrated. In one series, nearly 40% of omalizumab-treated patients were able to discontinue use of inhaled steroids compared with less than 20% in the placebo group.[33] Adverse effects have been mild and comparable with those receiving placebo. Treatment is extremely expensive and thus far reserved for patients with severe asthma that remains poorly controlled with use of high-dose inhaled and oral steroids.

Trials using other antibodies targeting important proinflammatory cytokines have also been conducted with disappointing results. Administration of anti-IL-5 antibodies resulted in significant reduction in circulating and airway eosinophils without significant improvement in asthma symptoms or pulmonary function. However, the study may have been underpowered and also may not have succeeded in reducing eosinophils in the airway mucosa. Use of an anti-IL-4 receptor as a "decoy" to bind and inactivate IL-4 may hold some promise, but more studies are needed. IL-13 appears to be an important molecule to target in future studies.

Immunotherapy for asthma may afford some promise, particularly with the use of newer antigens, such as immunostimulatory DNA sequences and CpG DNA vaccines.

MANAGEMENT OF CHRONIC ASTHMA

The effective management of chronic asthma should focus on (1) identification and elimination of exacerbating or aggravating factors, (2) pharmacologic therapy, and (3) education of the patient and family about the disease and the management skills necessary to avoid and treat acute exacerbations. The goals of effective management of chronic asthma in children include minimizing symptoms and exacerbations, maintaining normal activities of daily living, maintaining normal or near normal pulmonary function, and avoiding adverse effects from asthma medications. To achieve these goals, a combination of pharmacologic and nonpharmacologic modalities must be utilized.

Successful asthma management requires appropriate grading of disease severity as either intermittent, or mild, moderate, or severe persistent (see Table 56-2). These categories refer to the characteristics of patients prior to receiving any medications, but are typically also applied to patients currently receiving treatment. It may be argued that asthma severity should be distinguished from asthma control. Patients may have relatively mild asthma that is poorly controlled due to multiple factors, such as inadequate treatment, impaired adherence to treatment, or excessive exposure to allergens or irritants. Once appropriate medical and environmental measures are instituted, the asthma may become "mild" in terms of absence of symptoms and normalization of pulmonary function while taking low doses of medication. Features such as progressive decline in pulmonary function leading to frequent exacerbations and increasing symptoms may be more important identifiers of disease severity. Future studies may identify other biomarkers of airway inflammation (eNO, sputum eosinophils, markers of oxidative stress in exhaled breath condensate) that may add more useful data for grading asthma severity and modifying treatment. Use of the current guidelines can still offer a reasonable infrastructure upon which to initiate and modify asthma therapy.

MILD INTERMITTENT ASTHMA: STEP 1 THERAPY

Children with mild intermittent or exercise-induced asthma have brief episodes of wheeze or cough that are easily relieved with treatment and occur no more frequently than once or twice per week. Treatment is with the as-needed use of an inhaled β agonist. Exercise-induced asthma may be prevented to large extent with inhalation of albuterol (or formoterol) 5 to 20 minutes before exercise or salmeterol 30 to 60 minutes before exercise. Oral administration is not generally recommended, because the inhaled route is safer and more effective, and has more rapid onset of action, good duration of action, and fewer adverse reactions.[1] The usual dose of nebulized racemic albuterol is two puffs every 3 to 4 hours or 0.15 mg/kg (usual dose 2.5 mg) in 2 mL of saline. Although most dose-response studies have been conducted using a per-kilogram basis, there is little physiologic reason to do so. Most patients will achieve significant benefit and suffer no adverse effect if given 2.5 mg of nebulized solution, since much of the dose never leaves the nebulizer cup and deposition in the airways depends in part on the patient's tidal volume and respiratory rate. Other β agonists, such as pirbuterol, levalbuterol, and terbutaline, may also be used, but it remains uncertain if there is any significant difference in efficacy among the drugs. Numerous studies have demonstrated that administration of albuterol by MDI is equally effective as that given by nebulizer.[14] Moreover, use of an MDI by older children is far more convenient and less expensive than a nebulizer.

MILD PERSISTENT ASTHMA: STEP 2 THERAPY

The majority of asthmatics will be classified as having mild persistent asthma, based on symptoms that occur several times per week, but not daily; infrequent nocturnal symptoms; and normal pulmonary function. Current recommendations for treatment of mild persistent asthma stress the importance of use of low-dose ICS. Data from multiple studies support the superior efficacy of inhaled steroids in improving pulmonary function, reducing symptoms and need for rescue medications, and improving bronchial hyperreactivity compared with other treatments. As outlined previously, the safety profile for inhaled steroids given at low dose is excellent. There are few data to suggest that one type of inhaled steroid will offer significantly better benefit than the others, but both fluticasone and BUD have been extensively studied in children, are available in easy-to-use devices (MDIs and/or dry powder inhalers), and are well-tolerated by most patients. The dose considered to be "low" has been fairly well defined for both drugs (Table 56-4), and the adverse event profile is well understood. Every attempt should be made to use inhaled steroids at doses in the low range in order to avoid adverse systemic effects.

An alternative treatment is a leukotriene receptor antagonist, such as montelukast. This drug has the advantage of once-a-day oral administration and only uncommon mild adverse effects (nausea, headache, vivid dreams). These features may enhance compliance. However, numerous comparative studies indicate that inhaled steroids provide superior asthma control. Although the current NAEPP guidelines still list cromolyn, nedocromil, and theophylline as alternative treatments, the use of all of these drugs is cumbersome, expensive (cromolyn, nedocromil), or less well tolerated (theophylline).

MODERATE PERSISTENT ASTHMA: STEP 3 THERAPY

Children who have daily symptoms, nocturnal symptoms more than weekly, and mild obstruction on pulmonary function have moderate persistent asthma. Current recommendations for

TABLE 56-4. Comparative daily dosages for inhaled corticosteroids

	LOW DAILY DOSE		MEDIUM DAILY DOSE		HIGH DAILY DOSE	
Drug	**Adult**	**Child***	**Adult**	**Child***	**Adult**	**Child***
Mometasone 220 mcg/puff	220 mcg		220–440 mcg		440–880 mcg	
Beclomethasone HFA 40 or 80 mcg/puff	90–240 mcg	90–160 mcg	240–480 mcg	160–320 mcg	>490 mcg	320
Budesonide DPI 200 mcg/inhalation	200–600 mcg	200–400 mcg	600–1200 mcg	400–800 mcg	>1200 mcg	800 mcg
Inhalation suspension for nebulization (child dose)		0.5 mg		1.0 mg		2.0 mg
Flunisolide 250 mcg/puff	500–1000 mcg	500–750 mcg	1000–2000 mcg	1000–1250 mcg	>2000 mcg	>1250 mcg
Fluticasone MDI: 44, 110, or 220 mcg/puff	88–264 mcg	88–176 mcg	264–660 mcg	176–440 mcg		
DPI: 50, 100, or 250 mcg/inhalation	100–300mcg	100–200 mcg			>660 mcg	>440 mcg
Triamcinolone acetonide 100 mcg/puff	400–1000 mcg	400–800 mcg	1000–2000 mcg	800–1200 mcg	>2000 mcg	>1200 mcg

Note: For inhaled steroids, the low-medium doses reflect findings, from dose-ranging studies that show incremental efficacy within the low- to medium-dose ranges; however, the dose response curves are relatively flat at the moderate level. Doses at the high level are those at or beyond the point at which it is likely there will be further efficacy, but adverse effects on the hypothalamic-pituitary axis (and possibly on other systems) are likely.

*Children ≤ 12 years of age.

From National Institutes of Health: Guidelines for the diagnosis and management of asthma—update on selected topics 2002. In: National Asthma Education and Prevention Program. Expert Panel Publication no. 02-5474. Bethesda, Md: National Institutes of Health, 2002.

treatment include continuing low-dose inhaled steroid and adding a second drug with a complimentary action. LABAs are the current add-on drugs of choice, due to the large body of evidence from randomized controlled trials that indicate efficacy. In older children and adults, the addition of a LABA to low- or medium-dose inhaled steroids results in greater improvement in pulmonary function and reduction in symptoms than a further increase in steroid dose. In addition, some patients who are receiving medium-dose inhaled steroid may be able to reduce the dose without change in asthma control. The availability of fixed-dose combination of fluticasone and salmeterol or BUD and formoterol in a single dry powder inhaler make this combination attractive. An alternative is to raise the dose of the inhaled steroid alone to the medium range or add a leukotriene receptor antagonist or low-dose theophylline. Data indicate that the latter two add-on medicines are also effective in improving asthma control, but less so than with the addition of the LABA. Use of theophylline as a single daily dose of a time-release preparation can be well tolerated and is typically less expensive than using a LABA or LTRA. Long-term use of β agonists may be detrimental in some patients, such as those with the Arg16 polymorphism. Any patient who has deterioration of lung function while using a LABA chronically should have an alternative medication prescribed. Whatever combination of medications is used, attempts should be made at regular intervals to decrease the dose of inhaled steroid to the lowest level that adequately controls symptoms and maintains normal pulmonary function. Children in this category will benefit from referral to a pulmonologist and may also require ongoing specialty care.

SEVERE PERSISTENT ASTHMA: STEP 4 THERAPY

Approximately 10% of patients will have severe persistent asthma as described by persistent daily symptoms, frequent nocturnal awakenings, and a moderate or severe obstructive pattern on pulmonary function testing. These symptoms may occur in spite of treatment with moderate-dose inhaled steroids, LABAs, and/or an LTRA. Patients with the most severe disease have inadequate response to even high doses of inhaled steroid in combination with other available controller medications. This is not surprising, since it is clear from a number of studies that the dose-response curve for inhaled steroids is relatively flat even at doses currently considered below the maximum recommended levels. Nevertheless, patients with severe disease may respond to high-dose inhaled steroids in combination with other controllers. If there is no response, oral corticosteroids are the next recommended treatment step. It may be necessary to administer a short course (<10 days) of everyday dosing (40–60 mg/day) and then a longer every-other-day course at the lowest effective dose (0.5 mg/kg every other day). Before instituting such therapy, a thorough search for remediable exacerbating factors (e.g., sinusitis, persistent allergen exposure, poor compliance, gastroesophageal reflux, vocal cord dysfunction) should be sought. As soon as symptoms are controlled, the lowest possible dose at which symptom control is maintained should be administered. Although a single morning dose is generally preferred in order to minimize systemic side effects, some patients with severe or refractory symptoms may benefit from twice-daily dosing. Children receiving chronic oral corticosteroid therapy should be carefully monitored for development of adverse effects, such as hypertension, cataract formation, hyperglycemia, loss of bone mineral content, and impaired linear growth. Systemic corticosteroids may be given in the presence of acute viral infections, otitis media, or pneumonia and will not result in worsening infections. Certain precautions must be taken when there is a history of varicella exposure or if active disease develops. Although the vast majority of children with varicella who are taking systemic corticosteroids do quite well, there have been reports of disseminated and even fatal disease, especially when the drug is administered during the varicella incubation period. Patients who develop varicella while taking corticosteroids or take the medication during the incubation period should have the steroid dose reduced to the minimum tolerable to control the asthma and be provided adrenal replacement. In addition, consideration should be given to administering acyclovir (20 mg/kg given four times daily, maximum dose 800 mg four times daily) for 5 to 7 days. The patient should also be carefully observed for signs of severe or disseminated disease. If there has been a significant exposure to varicella identified within the previous 96 hours, passive immunization with varicella zoster immune globulin can be offered. Children with persistent asthma should receive varicella vaccine if they have not contracted the disease. All children with persistent asthma should also receive influenza vaccine yearly.

A proportion of severe asthmatics may be steroid resistant; in one series of patients with refractory asthma, 25% were determined to be steroid resistant. Such patients may have altered steroid metabolism or receptor dysfunction. A careful evaluation and specialized pharmacokinetic and cellular studies may be needed to ascertain the etiology of the defect. Patients deemed to be severely steroid resistant may be candidates for alternative therapies, such as omalizumab or other immunosuppressants.

Children with severe asthma should receive routine care from a specialist. Frequent monitoring of patients with moderate/severe disease is vital to successful management. Routine visits to assess symptom control, pulmonary function testing, quality of life, patterns of medication use, and adherence to treatment regimen are essential. Medical treatment should be increased during allergen or respiratory virus seasons and scaled down to the least necessary as symptoms remit.

HOLDING CHAMBERS AND SPACER DEVICES

A number of studies indicate that as many as 80% of patients use MDIs incorrectly even after appropriate instruction, and many residents, physicians, and nurses are unable to teach patients correctly. Proper steps are given in Table 56-5. Although there is a relatively small difference in the amount of medication that reaches the lower respiratory tract from a properly used MDI alone compared with an MDI plus spacer (10% for MDI alone, 15% for MDI plus spacer), spacer use helps ensure that the maximum possible dose reaches its target. The holding chamber also minimizes deposition of the medication in the mouth and oropharynx, a particularly important feature when ICS are prescribed. There are several important points to remember when using a spacer device. The child should take a slow deep inspiration and try to hold his or her breath for 5 to 10 seconds. Only one medication should be dispensed into the chamber at a time, although the same chamber may be used for other medications. A holding chamber that accommodates the MDI canister in its original boot is preferable to one that requires the canister to be inserted into an adapter. The latter chambers may not result in accurate dispensing of medication due to mismatch between the adapter and the actuator.

PEAK EXPIRATORY FLOW RATE MONITORING

Home monitoring of PEFR has been advocated for the optimal management of the patient with moderate to severe persistent asthma, but the utility remains uncertain. Use of these small portable hand-held devices provides an objective measure of lung function that can serve as an indicator of airway hyperresponsiveness, an early warning system for impending asthma exacerbation, and facilitate communication between patient and physician regarding the severity of disease activity. Patients may use the PEFR reading to alter medications according to a predetermined plan. Patients and families must know when and how to use the PEFR meter, how to interpret the measurement and respond to the reading, and when to communicate with their physician. Some of these steps can be obviated with the use of a commercial system that uses a recording PEFR meter capable of transmitting via phone line or the Internet, a longitudinal collection of readings synthesized into a report to the managing physician. Several recent studies suggest that routine use of PEFR monitoring is more likely to be of benefit to those with more severe, unstable disease and is more likely to be used intermittently rather than continuously.[1,14]

Normal PEFR ranges are determined by the patient's age, gender, and height; and are readily available. Some patients have PEFR readings well above, or in some cases below published standards. For this reason, an individual patient's personal best reading is often used as a target. It is important that the personal best be determined only when efforts have been made to ensure that asthma is optimally managed at the time the measure is made; this may require short courses of oral corticosteroids and other anti-inflammatory medications. After determining the target, normal, or personal best PEFR reading, a care plan incorporating the measure can be made. The most common model incorporates the traffic light analogy of green, yellow, and red zones, corresponding to all clear, caution, and emergency.[1] Sample plans may be obtained in readily available sources (Fig. 56-6).[1]

The zones are generally defined as follows:

Green: PEFR 80% to 100% predicted; all clear, no symptoms.

Yellow: PEFR 50% to 80% predicted; indicates worsening airway obstruction or an impending attack. Symptoms include slowed play, intermittent cough, wheeze, and dyspnea.

Red: PEFR less than 50% predicted; indicates significant airway obstruction and need for immediate medical attention. Symptoms include severe dyspnea, retractions, continuous wheeze, and/or cough.

Although PEFR monitoring is widely recommended, there are limitations to its efficacy. The PEFR is quite effort dependent; some children learn how to deliberately adjust the reading by the effort used. In addition, PEFR only measures obstruction in the large central airways; many asthmatics have normal or near normal PEFR, but significant obstruction in the small airways; in this case, the PEFR reading provides misleading information. Moreover, it is unclear that long-term PEFR use results in better outcomes than monitoring symptoms without PEFR and adjusting therapy accordingly.[14] In fact, recent studies have questioned the utility of asthma action plans with or without PEFR use.[14] Nevertheless, asthma treatment often involves several medications given at different times, and written instructions in some form should be provided.

NONPHARMACOLOGIC MEASURES

Nonpharmacologic interventions necessary for successful management include formation of an effective partnership with a knowledgeable health care provider, frequent monitoring of asthma symptoms and response to therapy, objective measures of pulmonary function, and avoidance of asthma triggers. Trigger avoidance is extremely important, yet patients are often unaware of how effective this modality can be. Contrary to popular belief, the indoor environment probably contains more hazards than the outdoor air. Most notably, dust mite, cat and dog dander, mold, and, in the inner city, cockroach antigen have all been strongly linked to asthma exacerbations and morbidity.[34] Removal of these allergens can result in reduced symptoms and airway hyperresponsiveness. The use of room air filters and special cleaning agents have some appeal, but are not as effective as keeping ambient humidity low (30%–40%), putting plasticized covers on pillows and mattresses, washing bedding weekly in hot water, and removing carpeting. A recent study suggested that application of dust covers alone is not effective in improving airway function. Removing pets from the bedroom and ideally from the household is also desirable. Exterminating roaches is difficult, but use of integrated pest management strategies can be effective. For all asthmatics, avoidance of passive exposure to cigarette smoke is of paramount importance.

Table 56-5. Directions for use of a metered dose inhaler, with and without a spacer

MDI Use Without Spacer Device	MDI Use with Spacer Device
1. Shake canister for 5 seconds.	1. Shake canister for 5 seconds.
2. Position finger on top of canister for support.	2. Attach canister to spacer.
3. Patient exhales normally (to FRC).	3. Patient exhales normally (to FRC).
4. Place mouthpiece 2 cm in front of open mouth (may place in mouth if coordination is a problem)	4. Place mouthpiece in mouth and close lips around the tube.
5. Begin slow inspiration.	5. Activate canister.
6. Activate canister.	6. Begin slow inspiration.
7. Complete inhalation over several seconds.	7. Complete inhalation over several seconds.
8. Hold breath for 10 seconds.	8. Hold breath for 10 seconds.
9. Wait 30–60 seconds and repeat steps 2–8 for prescribed number of inhalation.	9. Wait 30–60 seconds and repeat steps 2–8 for prescribed number of inhalations.

ASTHMA ACTION PLAN

PLAN FOR: ____________ **Date:** ________ **Nurse:** **Doctor:** Dr.

Hospital/Emergency Phone Number:_xxx-xxx-xxxx/ 911 **Doctor's Phone:_xxx-xxx-xxxx** (weekdays) / xxx-xxx-xxxx (night and weekend)

GREEN ZONE: Doing Well

- **No cough, wheeze, chest tightness, or shortness of breath during day or night**
- **Can do usual activities**

PEAK FLOW between ______ **and** ______

(80%–100% of my best)

Take these control medicines every single day. They work to keep your lungs healthy and prevent asthma symptoms.

Medicine	How much to take	When to take it

Before running or sports:

☐ ____________ ☐ 2 puffs ☐ 4 puffs ☐ 1 aerosol ☐ 5 to 20 minutes ☐ 60 minutes before exercise

YELLOW ZONE: Asthma Getting Worse

- **Cough, wheeze, chest tightness, or shortness of breath, or**
- **Waking at night due to asthma, or**
- **Can do some, but NOT all activities**

PEAK FLOW between ______ **and** ______

(50%–80% of my best)

First: Add quick-relief medicine: Albuterol, ventolin, proventil, maxair, or xopenx
Inhaler ☐ 2 to 4 puffs **OR** ☐ **aerosol machine** (1 vial) once

Next: AFTER 1 hour

- IF your symptoms return to the GREEN ZONE:
  - ☐ Take the quick-relief medicine every 6–8 hours for 1–2 days
- IF your symptoms **DO NOT** return to the GREEN ZONE:
  - ☐ Repeat quick-relief medication NOW and then every 4–6 hours for 1–2 days
  - ☐ ADD/DOUBLE inhaled steroid: __________ puffs/vial twice daily for 7–10 days
  - ☐ **Advair**: stop 100/50 and start higher strength preparation: 250/50 or 500/50
  - ☐ Add ______________
  - ☐ Call doctor for more advice

Remember: Continue all green zone medications.

RED ZONE: Medical Alert!

- **Very short of breath, or**
- **Quick-relief medicines have not helped, or**
- **Cannot do usual activities, or**
- **Symptoms are the same or worse after 24 hours in the yellow zone**

PEAK FLOW less than ______

(less than 50% of my best)

Add this medicine (In addition to green and yellow zone medicines):
☐ **Albuterol or** ____________ ☐ 4 puffs or ☐ aerosol machine

☐ **Repeat albuterol or** __________ **in 20 minutes if NOT better**

☐ **Oral steroid: one dose a day for 3–5 days**
Take ______ pills (______mg) prednisone **OR** Take ______ cc/mL Prelone or Orapred

Then: • **Call your asthma doctor (xxx-xxx-xxxx) or pediatrician *NOW*.**
• Go to the hospital or call an ambulance if your child is still in the RED ZONE after 20 minutes **AND** you have not reached the doctor.

■ **FIGURE 56-6.** Sample treatment plan form for management of chronic asthma. Instructions may use peak expiratory flow rate monitoring in addition to symptoms to assess need for additional treatment.

BOX 56-2 Constructs for Facilitating Patient Adherence

I. Establishing a relationship with the patient and family
   A. Demonstrate verbal and nonverbal attentiveness.
      1. Address the child and parent by name.
      2. Sit down; speak to the child and parent directly.
   B. Listen attentively to and show concern for the parent and child.
   C. Offer praise for doing a good job.
II. Promotion of health care
   A. Identify and address at least one *real concern* of the parent.
      1. Ask directly, "Is there anything else that is concerning you that we haven't talked about?"
   B. Ask the parent if he or she thinks the child is getting better.
   C. Set a short-term goal for asthma management.
III. Educating the patient and family and improving adherence
   A. Use simple diagrams and drawings to present pathophysiology.
      1. Give these to the patient to take home.
   B. Identify *risks* of the disease (limitation of play, absence from school and work, discomfort, hospitalization).
   C. Review long-term goals and plans.
      1. Assure the parent that the child should be able to sleep, play, learn.
   D. Ask about *and* suggest solutions for barriers to complying with care.
      1. Ask the parent and child about problems.
      2. Solicit their opinions about possible solutions.
      3. Reach an agreement on the management plan.
   E. Help the patient use criteria for making decisions about asthma management.
   F. Tailor the treatment schedule to the family's daily routine.
   G. Be proactive in discussing adverse effects.
   H. Provide simple, *written* instructions.
   I. Facilitate a telephone follow-up whenever possible.
      1. Facilitate both acute and nonacute advice calls; refill prescriptions.

Development of patient and parent asthma management skills, including use of an asthma exacerbation management plan, is also likely to improve asthma control. Impaired maternal mental health, lack of social supports, and child behavior problems may all contribute to poor adherence and asthma control. Use of ancillary personnel, such as a social worker, may be of great benefit in improving asthma control.[35]

Adherence to a treatment regimen is key to successful asthma management. Adherence differs from compliance, in that adherence stresses the role of the patient and family in helping to develop a treatment program and contributing to the strategies necessary to utilize the treatment plan. Compliance implies that a patient must utilize a plan derived by the physician; failure to do so indicates that the patient is at fault and irresponsible. The factors that contribute to adherence are complex and incompletely understood. It is difficult to predict which patients will have good adherence, and it is not well correlated with race, gender, and intelligence. Moreover, many patients overreport good adherence in an attempt to please the physician. Adherence to suggested medical treatment for asthma often ranges from 30% to 70% use of prescribed medicine. Families should be encouraged to identify areas of a treatment regimen that might offer difficulty, concerns they have about medications, and lifestyle issues that might impair compliance. Physicians must be willing to provide suitable alternatives (medications, dose schedules). Regularly scheduled office visits should be conducted to evaluate the success of the treatment plan and offer the patient the opportunity to voice concerns and ask for help. When a child or the parents fail to adhere, the physician should try to find out the reasons and to work out a practical solution acceptable to the patient and the family. Suggested constructs for conducting office visits that promote adherence are in Box 56-2.

Patients must be given ready access to medical advice, for example, over the telephone, including how to deal with school-related asthma management and behavior problems. Most importantly, parents and patients must learn that frequent symptoms and limitation of lifestyle due to illness should not be accepted; a symptom-free existence should be the goal.

MANAGEMENT OF AN ACUTE EPISODE

Acute asthma in children can occur as a mild illness that responds promptly to bronchodilators, or it can develop into a medical emergency over a matter of a few hours or days. Failure to respond to aggressive home treatment mandates further evaluation and treatment in the physician's office or a hospital emergency room. Use of treatment algorithms and guidelines provide useful infrastructure on which to base treatment, referral, and admission decisions (Fig. 56-7).

For mild acute asthma (cough, wheeze without dyspnea; PEFR >50% <80%) treatment can begin at home or in the physician's office, and the drug of choice is an inhaled β-adrenergic agonist, most commonly albuterol, 0.15 to 0.3 mg/kg/dose (or 2.5–5.0 mg) given once or the preferred route for older children, two to four puffs (90 μg/puff) of albuterol (using a holding chamber if necessary) every 20 minutes for one hour (see Figs. 56-6 and 56-7). If symptoms resolve, PEFR improves, and the patient remains well for 3 to 4 hours, the albuterol can be repeated as necessary, routine medications continued, and contact with the physician considered. The recommendation to double or initiate the dose of inhaled steroids for the next 7 to 10 days is sometimes made in these circumstances, with the intent of avoiding progression of symptoms and obviating the need for oral steroids. This recommendation has been called into question recently, because some studies have not found a clear benefit. However, one negative study was flawed by patient selection, which included predominantly elderly women who had required several courses of oral steroids in the previous year, thereby making the results less generalizable to the broader population of mild asthmatics. Some authorities recommend even higher (quadruple) doses of inhaled steroids for acute exacerbations. Although this may benefit some patients, the relatively flat dose-response curve for inhaled steroids suggests this too may be inadequate.[26] If symptoms persist and PEFR improves little, the

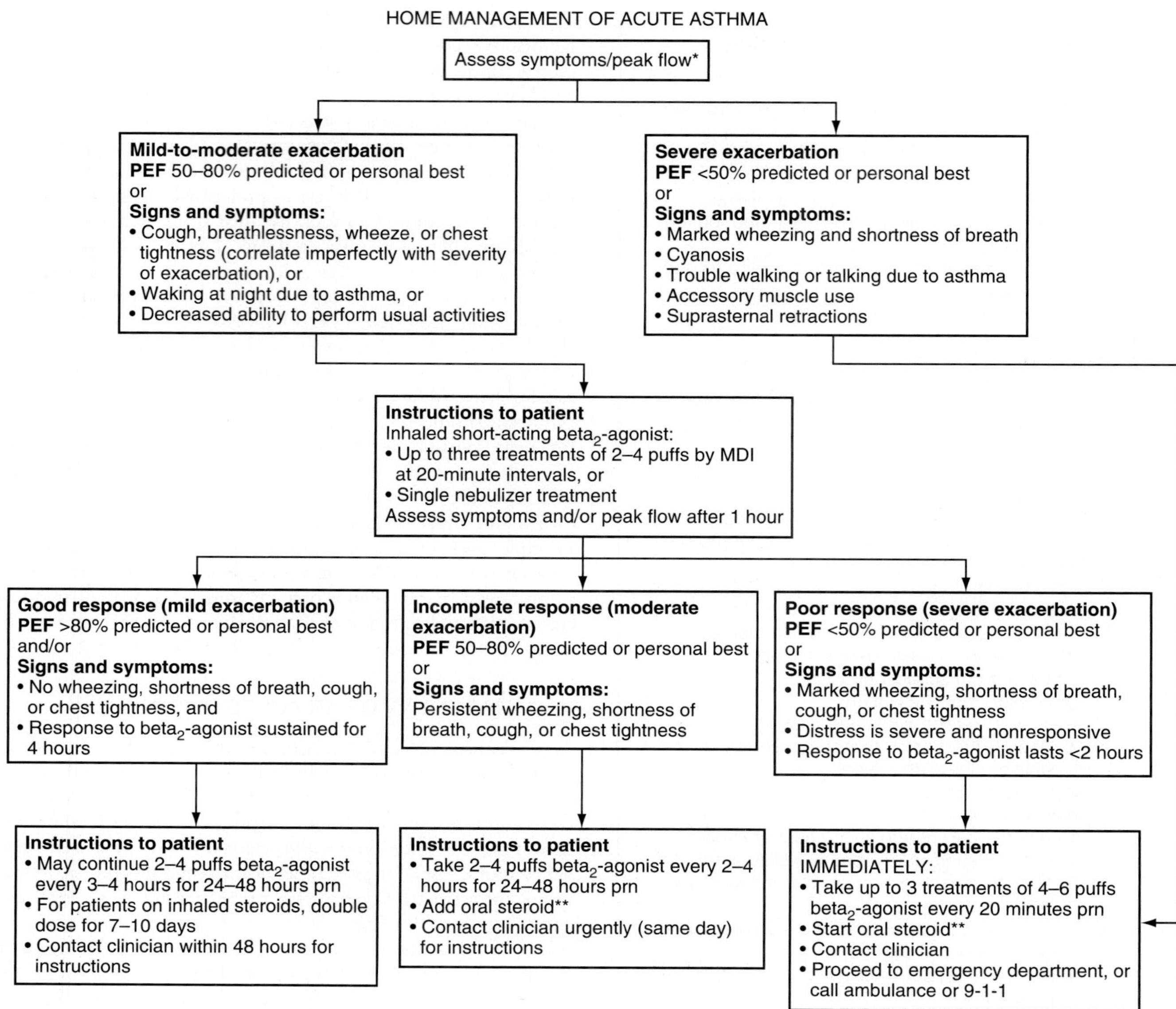

FIGURE 56-7. Treatment algorithm for home and hospital management of acute asthma.

dose of inhaled albuterol should be repeated and a dose of oral steroid (2 mg/kg, maximum 60 mg prednisone) should be given. Physician contact is necessary at this point.

For the patient with progressive symptoms in spite of all of the listed measures, care should be sought in a medical facility. In the emergency department, further administration of nebulized albuterol (2.5–5.0 mg) or four to six puffs every 20 minutes may be continued for another hour, oral corticosteroid dose given if not done earlier. There is no benefit to giving intravenous steroids unless the patient cannot tolerate or will not take the oral form. Levalbuterol 1.25 mg may be considered as an alternative treatment, in place of racemic albuterol. A recent prospective, double-blind, randomized study demonstrated almost 10% fewer hospital admissions in the group treated with levalbuterol compared with the group receiving racemic albuterol using a standardized emergency department care path.[36] Ipratropium (250 or 500 μg) should also be given every 20 to 30 minutes by nebulizer for three doses as well. Alternatively, a subcutaneous injection of epinephrine (or terbutaline) can be given if the patient is in severe distress and unable to comply with aerosol therapy. Studies of continuous albuterol nebulization (10–15 mg/hour) have yielded mixed results, although most favor continuous nebulization. Significant adverse side effects during continuous nebulization protocols in severe acute pediatric asthma are rare, suggesting that this mode of delivery is safe, if not necessarily more effective, and may be more convenient for patient and staff.

Other treatments that may be used in the acute hospital setting include intravenous magnesium sulfate and heliox. Magnesium sulfate ($MgSO_4$) can act as a smooth muscle relaxant, possibly

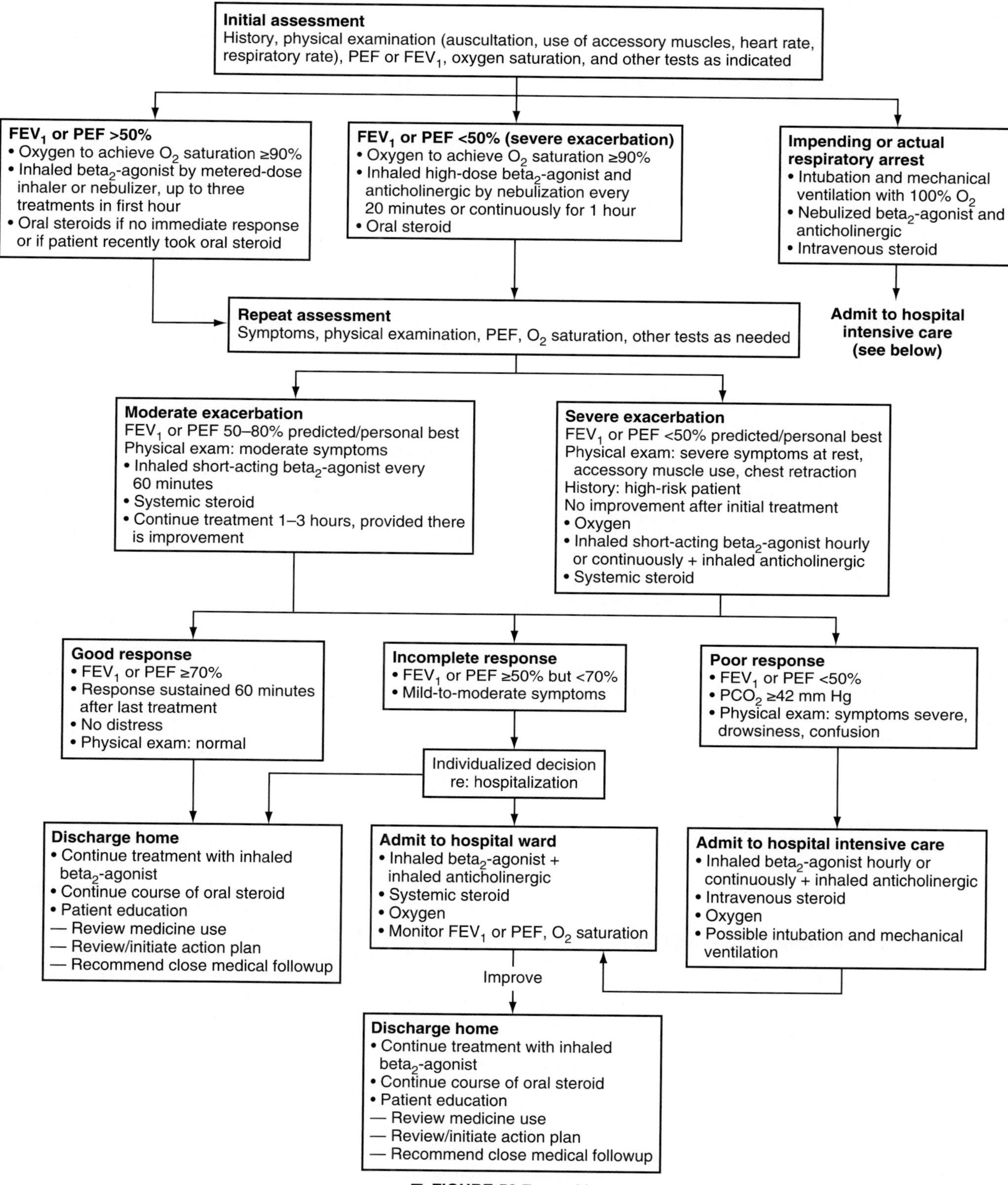
HOME MANAGEMENT OF ACUTE ASTHMA
MANAGEMENT OF ASTHMA EXACERBATIONS: EMERGENCY DEPARTMENT AND HOSPITAL-BASED CARE
Initial assessment
History, physical examination (auscultation, use of accessory muscles, heart rate, respiratory rate), PEF or FEV_1, oxygen saturation, and other tests as indicated
FEV_1 or PEF >50%
• Oxygen to achieve O_2 saturation ≥90%
• Inhaled $beta_2$-agonist by metered-dose inhaler or nebulizer, up to three treatments in first hour
• Oral steroids if no immediate response or if patient recently took oral steroid
FEV_1 or PEF <50% (severe exacerbation)
• Oxygen to achieve O_2 saturation ≥90%
• Inhaled high-dose $beta_2$-agonist and anticholinergic by nebulization every 20 minutes or continuously for 1 hour
• Oral steroid
Impending or actual respiratory arrest
• Intubation and mechanical ventilation with 100% O_2
• Nebulized $beta_2$-agonist and anticholinergic
• Intravenous steroid
Admit to hospital intensive care (see below)
Repeat assessment
Symptoms, physical examination, PEF, O_2 saturation, other tests as needed
Moderate exacerbation
FEV_1 or PEF 50–80% predicted/personal best
Physical exam: moderate symptoms
• Inhaled short-acting $beta_2$-agonist every 60 minutes
• Systemic steroid
• Continue treatment 1–3 hours, provided there is improvement
Severe exacerbation
FEV_1 or PEF <50% predicted/personal best
Physical exam: severe symptoms at rest, accessory muscle use, chest retraction
History: high-risk patient
No improvement after initial treatment
• Oxygen
• Inhaled short-acting $beta_2$-agonist hourly or continuously + inhaled anticholinergic
• Systemic steroid
Good response
• FEV_1 or PEF ≥70%
• Response sustained 60 minutes after last treatment
• No distress
• Physical exam: normal
Incomplete response
• FEV_1 or PEF ≥50% but <70%
• Mild-to-moderate symptoms
Poor response
• FEV_1 or PEF <50%
• PCO_2 ≥42 mm Hg
• Physical exam: symptoms severe, drowsiness, confusion
Individualized decision re: hospitalization
Discharge home
• Continue treatment with inhaled $beta_2$-agonist
• Continue course of oral steroid
• Patient education
— Review medicine use
— Review/initiate action plan
— Recommend close medical followup
Admit to hospital ward
• Inhaled $beta_2$-agonist + inhaled anticholinergic
• Systemic steroid
• Oxygen
• Monitor FEV_1 or PEF, O_2 saturation
Admit to hospital intensive care
• Inhaled $beta_2$-agonist hourly or continuously + inhaled anticholinergic
• Intravenous steroid
• Oxygen
• Possible intubation and mechanical ventilation
Improve
Discharge home
• Continue treatment with inhaled $beta_2$-agonist
• Continue course of oral steroid
• Patient education
— Review medicine use
— Review/initiate action plan
— Recommend close medical followup

■ **FIGURE 56-7, cont'd**

by blocking calcium-mediated contraction, decreasing acetylcholine release from neuromuscular junctions, and reducing histamine-induced airway spasm. $MgSO_4$ has been utilized for patients who fail to improve significantly following administration of inhaled β agonists and systemic corticosteroids. There are several reports of improved pulmonary function and decreased symptoms following a single infusion of 40 mg/kg (maximum 2 g) over a 20-minute period. However, in another study no difference from placebo was seen after a dose of 75 mg/kg was given.[37] Although still controversial, $MgSO_4$ can be considered in severely ill patients who are in a monitored unit and are failing conventional therapy. Adverse events include flushing, headache, decreased blood pressure, and weakness; the more significant effects are infrequent unless the serum magnesium level rises above twice normal.

Heliox, a mixture of helium (80%) and oxygen (20%), is a specialty gas that is less dense than nitrogen. When administered to the acutely ill asthmatic, heliox can decrease airway resistance by restoring laminar flow in obstructed airways where flow has become more turbulent. Work of breathing is decreased and the patient is less likely to fatigue. However, there is no direct curative action of helox and its effect occurs only while in use. It may also be used to drive a small-volume nebulizer to deliver albuterol, but this requires a specialized closed delivery system. Such systems are expensive, require higher than normal flow rates, and should not be considered for routine treatment of all asthmatics. Current data do not support the routine use of heliox in the emergency department. Heliox may be a useful bridge therapy for the severely ill patient in the intensive care unit who is tiring. It becomes less effective if concentrations lower than 70% helium are used, making it less useful in significantly hypoxemic patients.

Montelukast administered intravenously may also help improve status asthmaticus when added to conventional therapy for patients treated in the emergency department.[38] Further studies in children are needed to confirm the utility of this treatment.

Failure to clear symptoms, particularly dyspnea, chest wall retractions or use of accessory muscles, reverse persistent hypoxemia (O_2 saturation less than 92% while breathing room air), and improve air exchange and, if measured, PEFR to above 40% to 50% predicted are some indicators for hospital admission (see Fig. 56-7).

HOSPITAL MANAGEMENT OF ASTHMA

Status asthmaticus, or acute severe asthma that is resistant to appropriate outpatient therapy, is a significant medical emergency that requires prompt, systematic, and aggressive management in the hospital. The initiation of early, appropriate therapy shortens hospitalization and reduces complications. In spite of improved efforts at diagnosing and treating asthma, status asthmaticus continues to be the single most common discharge diagnosis from children's hospitals, accounting for 15% to 30% of all admissions. The increase in hospitalizations for asthma reported in all age groups during the previous decade now appears to have stopped.

GENERAL TREATMENT

A physician, nurse, respiratory therapist, and consultant pulmonologist team should manage the child with status asthmaticus in a closely monitored inpatient unit. Although the management of each child with status asthmaticus must be individualized, certain general principles apply to all patients with this disease.

Humidified oxygen should be administered (2–3 L/min by nasal cannula or 30% fraction of inspired oxygen [FIO_2] by face mask) to maintain partial pressure of oxygen in arterial blood (PaO_2) of 80 to 100 mm Hg or oxygen saturation in arterial blood (SaO_2) greater than 93% at sea level. The appropriate use of oxygen helps relieve dyspnea, aids in bronchodilation, supports the myocardium, and helps to prevent arrhythmias. Failure of improvement in hypoxemia with modest amounts of oxygen suggests either severe airway obstruction and impending respiratory failure or a complicating factor, such as pneumonia, atelectasis, or another diagnosis besides asthma. Intravenous infusion is generally not required unless the patient is unable to take or tolerate oral fluids, steroids, or, if needed for concomitant infection, antibiotics. Pulmonary function tests (FEV_1 or PEFR) may be performed at the bedside if the child can cooperate. Pulse oximetry (or arterial blood gas if hypercarbia or acidosis is suspected) should be measured as soon as possible and repeated as the patient's condition warrants. A chest radiogram, although not needed on all asthmatics, provides information on other pulmonary problems, such as pneumonia, atelectasis, pneumomediastinum, or pneumothorax, that might complicate management on those patients not responding rapidly to treatment.

Details about the acute illness—its duration, progression, manifestations, and initiating factors—as well as information on the duration of asthma and the reports of previous acute episodes, and level of functional morbidity and medication use at the patient's stable baseline should be noted. The patient's medication (including the names, dosages, and exact time of all medications administered within 24 hours) and any systemic corticosteroid drugs administered within 12 months should be documented. These data will be useful in constructing a treatment plan upon hospital discharge.

On physical examination, the general appearance and level of activity, respiratory effort, presence or absence of wheezing, tachycardia, tachypnea, air exchange, adventitious breath sounds, use of accessory muscles, dyspnea, and color are important clinical parameters that provide information about pulmonary dysfunction.

Although the number of pharmacologic agents for treatment of status asthmaticus is relatively limited, management strategies are inconsistent among and within institutions. Evidence-based practice is often replaced by physician personal experience and preference. Elimination of treatment that adds risk and cost but does not improve quality of care should be a primary goal. Status asthmaticus readily lends itself to treatment by the standardized clinical pathway, and several published studies have demonstrated shortened hospital stays using such care paths.[39]

Medical management of the hospitalized asthmatic should include aggressive use of inhaled bronchodilators, most commonly albuterol and systemic corticosteroids. The frequency of treatment should be guided by the patient's condition. In most inpatient, non–intensive care unit settings, inhalations may be administered as frequently as every 1 to 2 hours. In some settings, where careful monitoring is available outside the intensive care unit, consideration may be given to administering albuterol continuously (10–15 mg/hour) for short time periods (1–4 hours). If the patient cannot tolerate oral therapy, intravenous administration of corticosteroids should be ordered. Solumedrol, 1 to 2 mg/kg (maximum 125 mg) may be given daily. Failure to improve significantly after a maximum of 12 hours of such therapy should prompt a search for other complicating factors, impending respiratory failure, and need for more aggressive monitoring and treatment. If at any time the patient's condition deteriorates, consideration should be given to administering an immediate intensified treatment, such as subcutaneous epinephrine (0.01 mL/kg, maximum 0.3 mL) or terbutaline, or 500 μg aerosolized ipratropium with 5 mg albuterol. If a favorable response is observed, the aerosol treatment may be repeated every 20 minutes over the next hour. Patients who fail to sustain improvement after such treatment should be transferred to the intensive care unit.

The asthmatic child requiring intensive care should be monitored carefully for the development of respiratory failure; physical findings, such as severe dyspnea, inability to lie flat, poor air exchange, severe wheezing, and use of accessory muscles of respiration are all indicators of impending respiratory failure. Continuous cardiorespiratory monitoring and pulse oximetry with intermittent determination of arterial or venous blood gas measurement to assess oxygenation, ventilation, serum electrolyte, and acid-base status is necessary. Treatment should consist of continuously nebulized albuterol (0.15 mg/kg/hour), ipratropium 500 μg nebulized every 4 to 6 hours, and solumedrol 1 to 2 mg/kg every 6 hours. Consideration should be given to administering aminophylline to maintain serum concentration of 8 to 15 μg/mL; however, the efficacy of this therapy is uncertain. A recent report suggests that aminophylline may result in more rapid resolution of symptoms compared with placebo, although overall intensive care length of stay was not affected. In this setting, aminophylline may function more as a respiratory stimulant and help restore diaphragmatic contractility rather than acting as a bronchodilator. Careful monitoring for adverse effects due to elevated serum concentrations, and the protean drug interaction with other commonly administered medications (e.g., antibiotics) is imperative. Serum potassium concentration should also be closely monitored because frequent β agonist administration may deplete levels. For the patient who fails to respond, treatment with a bolus and possible continuous intravenous infusion of a β-adrenergic agonist, such as terbutaline, can be considered (intravenous albuterol or salbutamol is not available in the United States). Delivery of the medication via the circulation may provide relief of bronchospasm in areas not receiving medication via the inhaled route due to severe airway obstruction. However, most studies do not report significant improvement compared with use of continuous nebulized β-agonist treatment, and some studies suggest that aminophylline infusion may be superior to a β agonist. The starting dose of terbutaline is 5 μg/kg, followed by a continuous infusion of 0.4 μg/kg/min. The dose is increased by 0.2 μg/kg/min to a maximum dose of 12 to 16 μg/kg/min, although higher doses may be necessary. Baseline and twice-daily cardiac isoenzymes and continuous electrocardiograms must be monitored, since myocardial toxicity has been reported.

Although every effort should be made to avoid intubation and mechanical ventilation, a small percentage of severely ill patients (~10%) may require invasive ventilatory support. It is difficult to mechanically ventilate an asthmatic, and the complication rate may exceed 30%. Indications for intubation have become more conservative and should be reserved for patients who have (near) apnea, unstable vital signs, impaired consciousness, severe acidosis, extreme fatigue, and failure of noninvasive ventilation. A trial of noninvasive ventilation using continuous positive airway pressure (CPAP) or bilevel positive airway pressure (Bi-Pap) may be successful in some patients. Low levels of pressure 5 to 10 cm may be helpful in reducing work of breathing and improving oxygenation over a several hour trial. Some patients become anxious using the tight-fitting face mask necessary for effective CPAP and may require a modest dose of a short-acting benzodiazepine to comply with treatment. Risks include gastric distention, vomiting, aspiration, or air leak.

A skilled intensivist or anesthesiologist using rapid sequence induction anesthesia should perform intubation. Orotracheal intubation with as large a size tube as possible should be used in order to minimize air leak and maximize ability for secretion removal. It is important to make certain the patient is adequately hydrated prior to intubation and not given excessive positive pressure bag ventilation immediately after. Asthmatic patients are at risk for significant hypotension following intubation due to extreme hyperventilation impeding cardiac venous return with further exacerbation by volume depletion and application of aggressive positive pressure ventilation. Continuous sedation and paralysis will be required during mechanical ventilation. High peak inspiratory pressure is often noted, and efforts should be made to reduce it to less than 45 mm Hg. Use of selective hypoventilation must be practiced, and attempts to immediately normalize ventilation should be avoided. Relief of hypoxemia, respiratory distress, and muscle fatigue are the goals. Volume ventilation with a square wave form and the lowest volume and flow to minimize peak pressure and volume damage while maximizing expiratory time is vital. Relatively low respiratory rates (8–10/min) and low tidal volumes (6–10 mL/kg) should be tried. Decreasing the minute ventilation can maximize expiratory time; this can be best accomplished by using a lower respiratory rate or tidal volume. Shortening the inspiratory time by increasing the inspiratory flow rate can work, but may be less effective and contribute to airway injury due to high shear forces. As long as metabolic acidosis is not present, a pH as low as 7.2 should be tolerated. Intravenous infusion of sodium bicarbonate for more profound acidosis is controversial and generally not recommended. All medications should be continued while the patient is mechanically ventilated. Delivery of aerosolized bronchodilators through the endotracheal tube using an MDI and spacer device should be continued as well. Extubation should be considered and attempted using standard criteria, such as normoxemia with an FIO_2 of less than 0.40, spontaneous tidal volume greater than 5 mL/kg, vital capacity greater than 15 mL/kg, maximum inspiratory pressure greater than –25 cm, and ability to protect the airway and handle secretions. Most patients can be successfully weaned and extubated within 72 hours.

Several other therapies for the severely ill asthmatic have been tried, but are still considered unproven or experimental. As mentioned in an earlier section, intravenous $MgSO_4$ has been tried, but may be of little added value in the face of continuously aerosolized and intravenous β agonists. Heliox has been reported to decrease pulsus paradoxus and improve airflow in acutely ill, nonintubated asthmatic children and can also be administered during mechanical ventilation. However, this therapy is unproven, and the less dense gas alters ventilator function, requiring careful adjustment and a knowledgeable respiratory therapist. Administration of inhaled general anesthetic agents, such as enflurane and sevoflurane, which are bronchodilators, has also been used with some success; however, reports are anecdotal and no controlled trials have been conducted. These agents are also myocardial irritants and may precipitate serious arrhythmias in the acidotic, hypoxemic asthmatic. Ketamine infusions can be considered for sedation of the intubated patient, since the drug also has some bronchodilator properties. However, the psychoactive adverse effects of ketamine can be problematic in older children and may only be partially obviated by the concomitant administration of a benzodiazepine.

REFERENCES

1. National Institutes of Health: Guidelines for the Diagnosis and Management of Asthma. Expert panel report 2. Publication no. 97-4051. Bethesda, MD: National Institutes of Health, 1997.
2. Mannino DM, Homa DM, Akinbami LJ, Moorman JE, Gwynn C, Redd SC: Surveillance for asthma—United States, 1980–1999. MMWR Morb Mortal Wkly Rep 2002;51(1):1–13.
3. Jenkins HA, Cool C, Szefler SJ, Covar R, Brugman S, Gelfand EW, et al: Histopathology of severe childhood asthma. A case series. Chest 2003;124:32–41.
4. Phelan PD, Robertson CF, Olinsky A: The Melbourne asthma study: 1964–1999. J Allergy Clin Immunol 2002;109:189–194.
5. Van den Toorn LM, Overbeek SE, De Jongste JC, Leman K, Hoogsteden HC, Prins J: Airway inflammation is present during clinical remission of atopic asthma. Am J Respir Crit Care Med 2001;164:2107–2113.
6. Henderson WR Jr, Tang L-Q, Chu SJ, Tsao SM, Chiang GKS, Jones F, et al: A role for cysteinyl leukotrienes in airway remodeling in a mouse asthma model. Am J Respir Crit Care Med 2002;165:108–116.
7. Childhood Asthma Management Program Research Group: Long-term effects of budesonide or nedocromil in children with asthma. N Engl J Med 2000;343:1054–1063.
8. Abramson MJ, Bailey MJ, Couper FJ, Driver JS, Drummer OH, Forbes AB, et al: Are asthma medications and management related to deaths from asthma? Am J Respir Crit Care Med 2001;163:12–18.
9. McFadden ER, Zawadski DK: Vocal cord dysfunction masquerading as exercise-induced asthma. Am J Respir Crit Care Med 1996;153:942–947.
10. Hashimoto S, Gon Y, Matsumoto K, Takeshita I, Maruoka S, Horie T: Inhalant corticosteroids inhibit hyperosmolarity-induced, and cooling and rewarming-induced interleukin-8 and RANTES production by human bronchial epithelial cells. Am J Respir Crit Care Med 2000;162(3, pt 1): 1075–1089.
11. Harding SM, Guzzo MR, Richter JE: The prevalence of gastroesophageal reflux in asthma patients without reflux symptoms. Am J Respir Crit Care Med 2000;162:34.
12. Fuhlbrigge A, Kitch BT, Paltiel AD, Kuntz KM, Neumann PJ, Dockery DW, et al: FEV_1 is associated with risk of asthma attacks in a pediatric population. J Allergy Clin Immunol 2001;107:61–67.
13. Vink GR, Arets HG, van der Laag J, van der Ent CK: Impulse oscillometry. A measure for airway obstruction. Pediatr Pulmonol 2003;35(3):214–219.
14. National Institutes of Health: Guidelines for the diagnosis and management of asthma—update on selected topics 2002. In: National Asthma Education and Prevention Program. Expert Panel Report. Publication no. 02-5074. Bethesda, Md: National Institutes of Health, 2002.
15. American Thoracic Society, Committee on Proficiency Standards for Clinical Pulmonary Function Laboratories: Guidelines for methacholine and exercise challenge testing—1999. Am J Respir Crit Care Med 2000; 161:309–329.
16. Sont JK, Willems LNA, Bel EH, van Krieken JHJM, Vandenbroucke JP, Sterk PJ, et al: Clinical control and histopathologic outcome of asthma when using airway hyperresponsiveness as an additional guide to long-term treatment. Am J Respir Crit Care Med 1999;159:1043–1051.
17. Fahy JV, Boushey HA, Lazarus SC, Mauger EA, Cherniack RM, Chinchilli VM, et al: Safety and reproducibility of sputum induction in asthmatic subjects in a multicenter study. Am J Respir Crit Care Med 2001;163:1470–1475.
18. Green RH, Brightling CE, McKenna S, Hargadon B, Parker D, Bradding P, et al: Asthma exacerbations and sputum eosinophil counts. A randomized controlled trial. Lancet 2002;360:1715–1721.
19. Covar R, Szefler SJ, Martin RJ, Sundstrom DA, Silkoff PE, Murphy J, et al: Relations between exhaled nitric oxide and measures of disease activity among children with mild-to-moderate asthma. J Pediatr 2003;142:469–475.
20. Hunt J: Exhaled breath condensate. An evolving tool for noninvasive evaluation of lung disease. J Allergy Clin Immunol 2002;110:28–34.
21. Lemanske RF Jr, Sorkness CA, Mauger EA, Lazarus SC, Boushey HA, Fahy JV, et al: Asthma Clinical Research Network for the National Heart, Lung, and Blood Institute. Inhaled corticosteroid reduction and elimination in patients with persistent asthma receiving salmeterol. A randomized controlled trial. JAMA 2001;285:2594–2603.
22. Drazen JM, Israel E, Boushey HA, Chinchilli VM, Fahy JV, Fish JE, et al: Comparison of regularly scheduled with as-needed use of albuterol in mild asthma. N Engl J Med 1996;335:841–847.
23. Israel E, Drazen JM, Liggett SB, Boushey HA, Cherniack RM, Chinchilli VM, et al: The effect of polymorphisms of the beta(2)-adrenergic receptor on the response to regular use of albuterol in asthma. Am J Respir Crit Care Med 2000;162:75–80.
24. Leung DYM, Bloom JW: Update on glucocorticoid action and resistance. J Allergy Clin Immunol 2003;111:3–22.
25. Malmstrom K, Rodriguez-Gomez G, Guerra J, Villaran C, Pineiro A, Wei LX, et al: Oral montelukast, inhaled beclomethasone, and placebo for chronic asthma. A randomized, controlled trial. Montelukast/Beclomethasone Study Group. Ann Intern Med 1999;130:487–495.
26. Szefler SJ, Martin RJ, King TS, Boushey HA, Cherniack RM, Chinchilli VM, et al: Significant variability in response to inhaled corticosteroids for persistent asthma. J Allergy Clin Immunol 2002;109:410–418.
27. Wolthers OD, Pedersen S: Growth of asthmatic children during treatment with budesonide. A double blind trial. BMJ 1991;303:163–165.
28. Agertoft L, Pederson S: Effect of long-term treatment with inhaled budesonide on adult height in children with asthma. N Engl J Med 2000;343: 1064–1069.
29. Kavuru M, Melamed J, Gross G, Laforce C, House K, Prillaman B, et al: Salmeterol and fluticasone propionate combined in a new powder inhalation device for the treatment of asthma. A randomized, double-blind, placebo-controlled trial. J Allergy Clin Immunol 2000;105:1108–1116.
30. Verberne AA, Frost C, Duiverman EJ, Grol MH, Kerrebijn KF: Addition of salmeterol versus doubling the dose of beclomethasone in children with asthma. Am J Respir Crit Care Med 1998;158:213–219.
31. Craven D, Kercsmar CM, Myers TR, O'Riordan MA, Golonka G, Moore S: Ipratropium bromide plus nebulized albuterol for the treatment of hospitalized children with acute asthma. J Pediatr 2001;138:51–58.
32. Simons FER, Villa JR, Lee BW, Teper AM, Lyttle B, Aristizabal G, et al: Montelukast added to budesonide in children with persistent asthma. A randomized, double-blind, crossover study. J Pediatr 2001;138:694–698.
33. Busse W, Corren J, Lanier BQ, McAlary M, Fowler-Taylor A, Cioppa GD, et al: Omalizumab, anti-IgE recombinant humanized monoclonal antibody, for the treatment of severe allergic asthma. J Allergy Clin Immunol 2001; 108:184–190.
34. Rosenstreich DL, Eggleston P, Kattan M, Baker D, Slavin R, Gergen P, et al: The role of cockroach allergy and exposure to cockroach allergen in causing morbidity among inner-city children with asthma. N Engl J Med 1997;336:1356–1363.
35. Evans R, Gergen P, Mitchell, H, Kattan M, Kercsmar C, Crain E, et al, for the National Cooperative Inner City Asthma Study: An intervention to reduce asthma morbidity among inner-city children. Results of the National Cooperative Inner City Asthma Study (NCICAS). J Pediatr 1999;135: 332–338.
36. Carl JC, Myers TR, Kirchner HL, Kercsmar CM: Racemic albuterol is less effective than levalbuterol for treatment of acute asthma in children. J Pediatr 2003;143:731–736.
37. Scarfone RJ, Loiselle JM, Joffe MD, Mull CC, Stiller S, Thompson K, et al: A randomized trial of magnesium in the emergency department treatment of children with asthma. Ann Emerg Med 2000;36:572–578.
38. Camargo CA Jr, Smithline HA, Malice M-P, Green SA, Reiss TF: A randomized controlled trial of intravenous montelukast in acute asthma. Am J Respir Crit Care Med 2003;167:528–533.
39. Kercsmar CM, Myers TR: Clinical pathways in treatment of asthma. Curr Opin Allergy Clin Immunol 2002;2:183–187.

57 The Influence of Upper Airway Disease on the Lower Airway

Jonathan Corren, MD

During the past century, practicing clinicians have frequently observed that allergic rhinitis, sinusitis, and asthma coexist in the same patients. Despite a wealth of data supporting an association between the upper and lower airways, not until recently have reliable data emerged that suggest that upper airway disease is a risk factor for the development of asthma and that experimentally induced nasal dysfunction causes asthma to worsen. In addition, there is a growing body of literature demonstrating that appropriate treatment of nasal allergy and chronic sinus disease results in improvements in asthma symptoms and lower airway function. In this review, data from a variety of epidemiologic, clinical, and laboratory studies will be highlighted to help clarify our understanding of these complex and important relationships.

■ ALLERGIC RHINITIS AND ASTHMA

■ EPIDEMIOLOGIC RELATIONSHIP BETWEEN ALLERGIC RHINITIS AND ASTHMA

Cross-sectional Studies

Many cross-sectional studies have demonstrated that rhinitis and asthma commonly occur together. Many studies have reported that nasal symptoms occur in 28% to 78% of patients with asthma[1] as compared with approximately 5% to 20% of the general population.[2] Generally, these data were drawn from a variety of epidemiologic studies and clinical settings in which patients were not interviewed in a standardized fashion and insensitive instruments were used for detecting rhinitis. A more recent study, which utilized a standardized questionnaire in 478 patients across all age groups, demonstrated that rhinitis is a nearly universal phenomenon in patients with allergic asthma, occurring in 99% of adults and 93% of adolescents.[3] Conversely, asthma has been shown to affect up to 38% of patients with allergic rhinitis,[1] which is substantially higher than the 3% to 5% prevalence noted in the general population.

Temporal Connection between Onset of Rhinitis and Asthma

The onset of rhinitis and asthma appears to be temporally related; a number of studies in children, adolescents, and adults have shown that upper airway symptoms either preceded or started at the same time as asthma in 59% to 85% of patients with both diseases.[3] Although these studies suggest that rhinitis often begins before the onset of lower airway symptoms, prospective studies are required to accurately assess the actual risk for developing asthma in patients with rhinitis alone. Settipane and colleagues[4] published the results of a prospective, 23-year follow-up study of 690 adolescents who had no evidence of bronchial asthma. Students who reported nasal symptoms in 1961 developed asthma three times more often (10.5%) than individuals without rhinitis (3.6%).

In younger children, it has been more difficult to prospectively assess the progression of allergic rhinitis to asthma, in part due to the high prevalence of viral upper respiratory tract infections. In studies of children younger than 2 years,[5] chronic allergic rhinitis has often been shown to develop after the onset of persistent or recurrent wheezing. Japanese investigators have recently reported that 82.2% of 107 asthmatic children (mean age 7.9 years) had persistent nasal symptoms, with the mean age of onset of asthma and nasal symptoms being 3.2 and 4 years, respectively.[6]

Role of Bronchial Hyperresponsiveness

Although patients with rhinitis appear to be more likely to develop asthma, it has not been possible to predict which patients are at greatest risk for manifesting lower airway symptoms. Patients with allergic rhinitis and no clinical evidence of asthma frequently exhibit bronchial hyperresponsiveness to bronchoconstrictor agents such as methacholine or histamine.[7] This high incidence of hyperresponsiveness has caused some investigators to postulate that bronchial hyperreactivity may represent an intermediate phase between nasal allergy and symptomatic asthma. Although some small investigations suggested that lower airway hyperresponsiveness conferred a higher risk for developing symptoms and signs of asthma,[8] future large-scale, prospective studies will be needed to confirm these findings.

Pharmacoeconomic Studies

Recent pharmacoeconomic studies have attempted to correlate the presence of rhinitis with asthma severity and health care costs attributable to asthma. In an analysis of a database of 1261 children with asthma, Huse and colleagues[9] compared patients with significant nasal allergy with those who had mild or no symptoms of nasal disease. These investigators noted that patients with more severe rhinitis were much more likely to have nocturnal awakening due to asthma (19.6% vs. 11.8%, respectively), "moderate to severe asthma" as defined by the National Asthma Education Program (60.2% vs. 51.2%, respectively), or work loss related to asthma (24.1% vs. 21.1%, respectively). Similarly, Halpern and co-workers[10] observed that patients with symptomatic rhinitis used more asthma medications, particularly more inhaled and supplemental oral corticosteroids. Judging from these recent investigations, one can postulate that allergic rhinitis may also be related to increased asthma severity and the use of more potent antiasthma medications. Although these data suggest that rhinitis may be contributing to asthma, an alternative explanation for this association may be that nasal inflammation is a marker for increasing dysfunction of the entire respiratory tract. The possibility of a cause-and-effect relationship is better addressed by therapeutic studies of rhinitis therapy in patients with asthma.

COMMON IMMUNOPATHOLOGY OF ALLERGIC RHINITIS AND ASTHMA

During the past decade, we have learned that the immunologic processes leading to allergic rhinitis and atopic asthma are the same. A large number of studies have examined the composition of inflammatory cell infiltrates in the nasal and bronchial mucosa of patients with allergic rhinitis and asthma. Critical cells that have been consistently identified in both upper and lower respiratory tissue include eosinophils, mast cells,[11] and T-helper (Th) lymphocytes expressing the Th2 type.[12]

Allergen provocation studies have also demonstrated striking similarities between immunopathologic processes in the nasal and bronchial mucosa, including allergen-induced infiltration by inflammatory cells, cellular activation, and cytokine and chemokine expression or production.[13] In addition, the development of early- and late-phase reactions and the acquisition of airway hyperresponsiveness have been convincingly demonstrated in both the nasal and the lower airways after allergen provocation.[14]

Histologic studies of individuals with allergic rhinitis and no evidence of clinical asthma consistently demonstrate abnormalities of the bronchial mucosa, including thickening of the lamina reticularis and mucosa eosinophilia. These abnormalities are generally less pronounced than those of asthmatic patients,[15] but sometimes the findings in subjects with rhinitis are indistinguishable from those in subjects with mild asthma.[16] These findings are compatible with the above-mentioned studies of bronchial responsiveness in patients with allergic rhinitis, and suggest that both the upper and lower airways are histologically and functionally abnormal in patients with rhinitis and no asthma.

EFFECTS OF RHINITIS THERAPY ON ASTHMA

Physicians often note anecdotally that treatment of allergic nasal disease results in improvements in asthma symptoms and pulmonary function. However, there have been relatively few well-controlled, large-scale clinical trials that have attempted to quantify this effect.

Intranasal Corticosteroids

Several small studies have examined the efficacy of topical intranasal corticosteroids in patients with allergic rhinitis and mild asthma. Two of these trials addressed the role of prophylactic, preseasonal treatment with nasal corticosteroids in patients with primarily seasonal symptoms. Welsh and co-workers[17] compared the effects of intranasal beclomethasone dipropionate, flunisolide, and cromolyn versus placebo in adolescent and adult patients with ragweed-induced rhinitis. Both of the topical corticosteroids were significantly more effective in reducing nasal symptoms than was either cromolyn or placebo. Unexpectedly, in 58 of the subjects who also had mild ragweed asthma, lower airway symptoms were also significantly improved in the patients receiving intranasal corticosteroids. Corren and co-workers[18] later examined the effects of seasonal administration of intranasal beclomethasone dipropionate on bronchial hyperresponsiveness in adolescent and adult patients with fall rhinitis and mild asthma. Compared with baseline values, bronchial responsiveness to inhaled methacholine worsened significantly in the placebo group but did not change in the group using active treatment. Together, these two small trials suggest that prevention of seasonal nasal inflammation with topical corticosteroids reduces subsequent exacerbations of allergic asthma.

Other studies have examined the effects of intranasal corticosteroids in patients with chronic perennial allergic rhinitis and mild asthma. The first study to document these effects used intranasal budesonide in children with severe allergic rhinitis and concomitant asthma.[19] Four weeks of active therapy significantly reduced the objective measures of nasal obstruction as well as daily asthma symptoms and exercise-induced bronchospasm. In a subsequent study of children with perennial rhinitis and asthma, Watson and colleagues[20] evaluated the effects of intranasal beclomethasone dipropionate on chest symptoms and bronchial responsiveness to methacholine. After 4 weeks of active treatment, asthma symptoms were significantly reduced, as was airway reactivity to methacholine. As an adjunct to this study, the investigators performed a radiolabeled deposition study of the beclomethasone aerosol and found that less than 2% of the drug was deposited into the chest area. These studies demonstrate that intranasal corticosteroids are effective in improving lower airway symptoms and bronchial hyperresponsiveness in patients with chronic, established nasal disease, and asthma. In view of the fact that the corticosteroid spray did not penetrate into the lungs, the study by Watson and colleagues[20] also asserts that the reduction observed in asthma was due to improvements in nasal function rather than direct effects of the medication on the lower airways.

Antihistamines

The presence of histamine in the lower airways has been correlated with bronchial obstruction,[21] and histamine has long been thought to play a role in bronchial asthma. However, early studies of first-generation antihistamines in adolescents and adults showed minimal improvements in bronchial asthma, and initial small trials of second-generation antihistamines yielded mixed results.[22,23] However, two recent large-scale clinical studies using an antihistamine alone and an antihistamine-decongestant combination both resulted in significant improvements in asthma control. Grant and colleagues[24] demonstrated that seasonal symptoms of rhinitis and asthma were significantly attenuated in patients treated with cetirizine 10 mg once daily in a large group of adolescents and adult patients. In a second study using loratadine 5 mg plus pseudoephedrine 120 mg twice daily in patients with seasonal allergic rhinitis and asthma, Corren and colleagues[25] demonstrated that asthma symptoms, peak expiratory flow rates, and forced expiratory volume in 1 second (FEV_1) were all significantly improved in patients taking active therapy. In reviewing data from these and similar trials, it is difficult to determine whether the salutory effects of antihistamines in asthma can be attributed to direct effects on lower airway physiology or are due to improvements in rhinitis. Because many of the currently available agents appear to have weak or transient effects on resting airway tone, benefits to the lower airway may in fact be due to modulation of upper airway function.

The above studies have shown that treatment of rhinitis may result in improvements in asthma symptoms, lower airway caliber, and bronchial hyperresponsiveness and suggest that nasal disease contributes to the pathophysiology of asthma.

Based on the above data, treatment of rhinitis may reduce symptoms of mild asthma to such an extent that the requirement for asthma therapy may be reduced. It is uncertain whether these findings are applicable to patients with more severe asthma.

PATHOPHYSIOLOGIC CONNECTIONS BETWEEN ALLERGIC RHINITIS AND ASTHMA

Although there is increasing evidence that allergic rhinitis may influence the clinical course of asthma, the mechanisms connecting upper and lower airway dysfunction are not entirely understood. A variety of theories have been invoked, including both direct and indirect effects of nasal dysfunction on the lower airways.

Systemic Effects of Nasal Inflammation on the Lower Airways

Research over the past few years has demonstrated that several inflammatory substances produced during allergic reactions may enter the systemic circulation. Experimental nasal allergen challenge has been shown to induce both peripheral blood eosinophilia[26] and activation of peripheral blood leukocytes.[27] It has been postulated that the net result of these various factors on the systemic circulation is the promulgation of inflammation in other sites. Clinical research that supports this hypothesis was recently completed by Braunstahl and colleagues,[26] in which nasal allergen provocation was performed in subjects with allergic rhinitis. Prior to and 24 hours after the nasal challenge, bronchial mucosa biopsies were performed which demonstrated that the number of eosinophils in the lower airway mucosa, as well as the expression of adhesion molecules, increased after nasal allergen challenge. Further supporting this interaction between the upper and lower airways, Braunstahl and colleagues[28] also found increased inflammatory markers in the nasal mucosa following the instillation of allergen into the lower airways of subjects with allergic rhinitis. Given this emerging evidence, it is likely that systemic factors do play a critical role in the interaction between the upper and lower airways.

Nasal-Bronchial Reflex

Early mechanistic studies investigated the effects of several mucosal irritants on lower airway function in normal human subjects. In 1969, Kaufman and Wright[29] applied silica particles onto the nasal mucosa of individuals without lower airway disease and noted significant, immediate increases in lower airway resistance. Bronchospasm induced by nasal silica was blocked by both resection of the trigeminal nerve[30] and systemic administration of atropine. Fontanari and co-workers[31] recently reevaluated the possibility of a neural connection between the upper and lower airways by using cold, dry air as the nasal stimulus. These investigators demonstrated that nasal exposure to very cold air caused an immediate and profound increase in pulmonary resistance that was prevented by both topical nasal anesthesia and cholinergic blockade induced by inhalation of ipratropium bromide. Both these studies strongly suggest the presence of a reflex involving irritant receptors in the upper airway (afferent limb) and cholinergic nerves in the lower airway (efferent limb).

Subsequent studies used challenge materials considered to be more biologically relevant to allergic rhinitis, including histamine, whole pollen particles, and allergen extracts. Yan and Salome[32] performed nasal histamine challenges in subjects with perennial rhinitis and stable asthma and observed that FEV_1 was reduced by 10% or more immediately after provocation in 8 of 12 subjects. Importantly, radiolabeling studies were performed as part of this study that demonstrated that histamine was not deposited into the lower airways. However, other studies that used histamine[33] or allergen[34] failed to demonstrate bronchoconstriction after nasal provocation. This discrepancy in results may be partly explained by the type of patients who participated in these studies. Whereas Yan and Salome investigated subjects with perennial, symptomatic nasal disease, the majority of other studies examined asymptomatic patients outside their pollen season. Certainly, a substantial degree of heterogeneity exists between patients in their lower airway response to nasal stimulation.

In addition to neurally mediated bronchospasm, it has also been postulated that a nasal allergic reaction might result in an alteration in lower airway responsiveness. Corren and colleagues[34] investigated the effects of nasal allergen provocation on nonspecific bronchial responsiveness to methacholine. Ten subjects with seasonal allergic rhinitis and asthma were selected for study; all patients related worsening of their asthma to the onset of hay fever symptoms. Nonspecific bronchial responsiveness was significantly increased 30 minutes after nasal challenge and persisted for 4 hours.

Because radionuclide studies demonstrated no evidence of allergen deposition into the lungs, it seems unlikely that these increases in airway reactivity can be attributed to direct effects of allergen. In addition, the rapidity with which these changes occurred suggests the possibility of a reflex mechanism.

Mouth Breathing Caused by Nasal Obstruction

Nasal blockage resulting from tissue swelling and secretions may cause a shift from the normal pattern of nasal breathing to predominantly mouth breathing. Previous work has shown that mouth breathing associated with nasal obstruction resulted in worsening of exercise-induced bronchospasm, whereas exclusive nasal breathing significantly reduced asthma after exercise.[35] Improvements in asthma associated with nasal breathing may be the result of superior humidification and warming of inspired air before it reaches the lower airways.[36] Similarly, it would be expected that airborne allergens and pollutants would also be less likely to enter the lungs during periods of normal nasal function.

Postnasal Drip of Inflammatory Material

Patients frequently complain that postnasal drip triggers episodes of coughing and wheezing. Early studies investigating the possibility of aspiration of nasal secretions demonstrated that substances placed in the upper respiratory tract could later be recovered from the tracheobronchial tree.[37] More recently, Huxley and colleagues[38] investigated pharyngeal aspiration during sleep both in healthy subjects and in patients with depressed sensorium. With the use of a radiolabeled marker that was intermittently released into the nose, pulmonary aspiration was detected in a significant number of both the normal and the ill subjects. In a more recent and definitive investigation, however, Bardin and colleagues[39] were unable to document significant aspiration of radionuclide in a study of 13 patients with chronic rhinosinusitis and asthma.

It is difficult to determine which of these experimental mechanisms is most important in linking the nose to the lower airways. In all likelihood, however, several of these phenomena may contribute in some way to alterations in lung physiology in patients with allergic rhinitis and asthma.

DIAGNOSTIC AND THERAPEUTIC IMPLICATIONS

Diagnosis

The above data suggest that all patients with asthma should be evaluated for probable concomitant allergic rhinitis. The patient should be questioned regarding types of symptoms, focusing on the presence of nasal congestion, sneezing, itching, discharge, and postnasal drip. Other associated symptoms (e.g., snoring, poor sleep quality, and ear congestion or popping) should also be investigated and kept in mind when choosing therapy. The upper airway should then be carefully examined, with an emphasis on the size and vascularity of the nasal turbinates, type and presence of nasal secretions, tonsillar size, and color and elasticity of the tympanic membranes.

With regard to diagnostic testing in patients with persistent rhinitis and asthma, allergy skin tests or in vitro measures of specific IgE should be performed using a panel of common airborne allergens. At a minimum, these should include house dust mite (*Dermatophagoides farinae* and *D. pterynissinus*), cockroach, animal danders (cat and dog), indoor and outdoor molds (*Penicillium, Aspergillus, Cladosporium,* and *Alternaria*), and regional pollens. This information is critical in establishing an appropriate program of environmental control measures. Other tests, including total serum IgE level, microscopic analysis for nasal cytology, and total circulating blood eosinophils, have not proven helpful in either differentiating allergic rhinitis from other nasal disorders or in assessing the severity of the problem.

BOX 57-1 Allergen Avoidance Strategies

House Dust Mites

- Weekly washing of all bedding in hot water (>130° F)
- Weekly vacuum cleaning of all floor surfaces, using HEPA-type vacuum cleaner or standard vacuum-cleaner with double-thickness reservoir bag
- Removal of carpeting or treatment of carpeting every 2 to 3 months with acaricidal spray or powder

Animal Danders (Any Furry Pet)

- Optimal—removal of the animal from indoor environment, followed by replacement of carpeting and aggressive house cleaning
- Possibly effective—keeping the cat indoors and instituting the following measures:
  - Noncarpeted floors
  - Plastic or leather furniture
  - Frequent vacuum cleaning of floors
  - High-flow air filtration
  - Frequent cat bathing

Indoor Mold

- Thorough eradication of infestation
- Repair of source of water intrusion

Cockroach

- Appropriate handling and storage of food and garbage

Allergen Avoidance

Once allergy testing is complete, the physician may devise a comprehensive program of allergen avoidance. The effects of environmental control strategies have been most heavily studied with regard to dust mites and furry pets (Box 57-1).[40] Compliance with these measures may be difficult but will certainly be helpful in many patients with hypersensitivity to these allergens.

Pharmacotherapy

While carefully designed allergen avoidance strategies may reduce symptoms to varying degrees, most patients will still require pharmacotherapy. In patients with persistent symptoms, particularly if nasal congestion is present, intranasal corticosteroids should be considered as first-line therapy. A large number of studies have established that there are no differences in efficacy between all of the available compounds,[41] and most (including budesonide, mometasone furoate, and fluticasone propionate) have been shown to have no significant effects on linear growth velocity in young children. These drugs should be used on a regular basis in patients with daily symptoms, or as long as symptoms dictate in children with intermittent problems.

Oral H_1 antihistamines have long been a mainstay of therapy for allergic rhinitis and are most effective in relieving sneezing, itching, and rhinorrhea, with minimal effects on nasal congestion. For this reason, they are often combined with oral decongestants, such as pseudoephedrine. A number of newer oral antihistamines that cause minimal or no sedation have been approved for use in young children, including cetirizine, fexofenadine, and loratadine.[42] Because they are available in a number of different formulations (tablets, rapidly dissolving pills, and liquids), patient preference may dictate choice of medication.

Recently, montelukast, a leukotriene D4 receptor antagonist, has gained approval as treatment for allergic rhinitis in children.[43] Montelukast has been shown to reduce all of the symptoms of rhinitis, including nasal congestion. Because montelukast has been shown to also be effective in treating concomitant asthma, this medication may be very effective as a solo treatment for children with mild persistent allergic rhinitis and concomitant asthma.

Specific Allergen Immunotherapy

Many children will continue to have persistent symptoms of rhinitis despite employing environmental control measures for indoor allergens and a combination of drugs, often including an intranasal corticosteroid with an antihistamine or montelukast. Occasionally, children may experience adverse effects that necessitate discontinuation of some or all of their rhinitis medications. In these children, specific allergen immunotherapy should be strongly considered. Studies performed over the past decade have demonstrated that specific allergen immunotherapy to a wide range of allergens, including dust mites, cat dander, selected outdoor molds, and numerous grass, tree, and weed pollens, had a high rate of clinical efficacy, with approximately 75% of children manifesting a good clinical response. Other studies have documented multiple salutary immunologic effects of immunotherapy, including a reduction in allergen-induced early- and late-phase allergic responses and attenuation of cytokine (e.g., interleukin-4) production. An important potential benefit of immunotherapy is its effect on progression of allergic airway disease. A recent large, prospective study in children with seasonal allergic rhinitis demonstrated that a 3-year course of immunotherapy reduced the development of asthma symptoms and improved bronchial responsiveness compared with an open control group.[44] Regarding duration of treatment, once initiated, immunotherapy should be continued for at least 3 years.

SUMMARY

Allergic rhinitis is virtually ubiquitous in children with asthma. In adolescents, allergic rhinitis may in fact serve as a risk factor for developing asthma. Intranasal corticosteroids appear to significantly modulate lower airway reactivity, and have been shown in a number of small studies to have beneficial effects on mild asthma. Current research suggests that the upper and lower airways are most importantly connected via the systemic circulation, which likely distributes products of inflammation throughout the respiratory tree. Allergic rhinitis should always be considered in patients with asthma, and treated aggressively once it has been identified. Immunotherapy may be particularly useful in children with allergic rhinitis and new-onset asthma, because it may modify the long-term prognosis of their airway disease.

CHRONIC SINUSITIS AND ASTHMA

EPIDEMIOLOGIC RELATIONSHIP BETWEEN CHRONIC SINUSITIS AND ASTHMA

Since early in the 20th century, physicians have noted that chronic sinus disease and asthma frequently coexist in the same patients. In 1925, Gottlieb[45] noted that 31 of 117 adolescent and adult patients with asthma suffered from severe symptoms of sinusitis. Other investigators reported similar findings in both children and adults during the next decade, with an incidence of symptomatic sinusitis as high as 72% in patients with asthma.[46] Conversely, a large retrospective study of pediatric, adolescent, and adult patients with chronic sinusitis noted a 12% incidence of asthma.[47] Only one third of the patients with both sinus disease and asthma in this study reported that sinusitis preceded their lower airway symptoms.

Attempts to define the incidence of sinus disease in patients with asthma again lay dormant until the early 1970s. These more recent reports have emphasized the role of radiography in diagnosing sinusitis. Several studies have demonstrated that between 31% and 53% of asthmatics across all age groups have abnormal sinus radiographs, with 21% to 31% of patients demonstrating significant findings (defined as opacification of one or both maxillary sinuses, air-fluid levels, or mucosal thickening greater than 5 mm).[48–51] In a more recent study that examined the utility of sinus computed tomography (CT) scanning in children with asthma, it was noted that 58% of the children had varying abnormalities of all of the sinuses[52] (Table 57-1).

Although the incidence of radiographic sinus abnormalities is universally high in asthmatics, others have questioned whether these changes have clinical significance. Fascenalli[53] prospectively performed sinus radiography on 411 asymptomatic adolescent

TABLE 57-1. Prevalence of radiographic sinusitis in asthmatics

Study	Sample Size	Age Range (Yr)	Total Abnormalities (%)	Significant Abnormalities (%)*
Berman et al.[48†]	52	19–80	62	NA
Rachelefsky et al.[49†]	70	3–16	52	27
Schwartz et al.[50†]	217	9–70	47	21
Zimmerman et al.[51†]	138	6–19	31	31
Chen et al.[52‡]	53	4–14	58	NA

*Opacification, air-fluid level, or >5 mm mucosal thickening.
†Plain films only.
‡Plain films and computed tomography.

NA, not assessed.

and adult male volunteers and noted a 28% incidence of maxillary sinus abnormalities. Most of these changes, however, consisted of minimal thickening, and only 5% of the group demonstrated significant thickening (>5 mm) of the maxillary antrum. In a similar prospective study of young children, Kovatch and colleagues[54] noted that 8 of 22 (36%) asymptomatic children younger than 1 year demonstrated either thickening greater than 4 mm or opacification of the maxillary sinuses. Only 2 of 31 (6%) children older than 1 year, however, demonstrated these same changes. These two studies demonstrate that it is unusual to detect significant radiographic abnormalities of the maxillary sinuses in normal, healthy individuals older than 1 year. Significant abnormalities of sinus x-ray films are much more common in patients with asthma than in healthy, nonasthmatic individuals, suggesting that these radiographic findings most likely reflect pathologic changes of the sinus tissue rather than radiologic artifact.

UNIQUE FEATURES OF CHRONIC SINUSITIS IN ASTHMATICS

Although a large proportion of asthmatics have abnormal sinus radiographs, it remains controversial whether these changes are caused by bacterial infection or represent chronic, noninfectious inflammation or both. Clinical and histologic studies suggest that the paranasal sinuses of these patients may be affected by a process that is clinically and pathogenetically distinct from sinusitis in nonasthmatics.

Clinical Features

Chronic sinusitis in children is often an indolent illness, usually characterized by one or more of the following symptoms: nasal congestion, purulent anterior or posterior nasal drainage, or cough.[55] Although headache may also be a prominent complaint in adolescents and adults, it is uncommon in children with chronic sinusitis. Additionally, fever is most unusual. Because cough may be the most prominent presenting symptom of chronic sinusitis in children, the physician must maintain a high index of suspicion regarding this possibility. Therefore, any child with symptomatic asthma and cough who has responded poorly to conventional asthma treatment (e.g., inhaled corticosteroid plus a long-acting β_2 agonist, a leukotriene D4 receptor antagonist, or both), should be evaluated thoroughly for chronic sinus disease, particularly if nasal congestion or postnasal drip are present.

Histopathology

More than 60 years ago, Hansel[56] studied the histology of nasal and sinus mucosa in patients with asthma, allergic rhinitis, or both conditions. Pathologic examination of sinus tissue in these patients revealed infiltration with a large number of eosinophils, hyperplasia of mucus-producing cells, and stromal edema. Moreover, these findings were remarkably similar to the pathologic features of bronchial asthma.

More recently, Harlin and colleagues[57] explored the role of the eosinophil and eosinophilic granular proteins in chronic sinusitis by assessing sinus tissue specimens obtained at surgery from 26 patients ranging in age from 13 to 74 years. Sinus tissue was examined by routine histology as well as immunofluorescent staining for major basic protein, a principal granule-stored protein of the eosinophil. All 13 sinus specimens from patients with asthma (allergic and nonallergic) and 6 of 7 specimens from patients with allergic rhinitis demonstrated significant numbers of eosinophils and tissue deposition of major basic protein. In six patients with chronic sinusitis and no history of asthma or nasal allergy, however, none demonstrated significant sinus tissue eosinophilia, and only one of six showed significant tissue staining for major basic protein. In a study limited to children (mean age 9 years), Baroody and colleagues characterized the histopathology of chronic sinusitis in patients with and without asthma.[58] Sinus tissue in all patients with chronic sinusitis contained large numbers of eosinophils, and was highest in those children with concomitant asthma. Additionally, the presence of allergy was not predictive of sinus eosinophilia in these patients.

While the above studies the reveal the nature of the inflammatory infiltrate in chronic sinusitis, Hisamatsu and colleagues[59] examined the effect of eosinophilic proteins on the ciliary activity of sinus mucosa in vitro. The investigators found that eosinophil-derived major basic protein damaged the mucosal epithelium and caused ciliostasis at concentrations that may be achieved in vivo. These findings have great clinical importance, because ciliary dysfunction may be one of the key factors contributing to persistent bacterial infection of the paranasal sinuses.

The above studies indicate that there is significant eosinophil invasion and deposition of eosinophilic granule-derived proteins into the tissues of the paranasal sinuses in both children and adolescents with concomitant sinusitis and asthma. Additionally, eosinophil infiltration of sinus mucosa causes epithelial alterations, which may predispose to recurrent or chronic infection.

Microbiology

In 1974, Berman and colleagues[48] studied 21 adolescent and adult patients with asthma and radiographic abnormalities of the maxillary sinuses. Bacterial cultures of sinus aspirates demonstrated positive bacterial growth in only 5 of 25 aspirates. Eighty percent of the subjects in this study, however, had minimal evidence of sinusitis (mucosal swelling >2 mm or sinus polyps). Therefore, conclusions from this study are most relevant to patients with mild sinusitis and may not be applicable to individuals with evidence of more severe disease. In children with asthma and chronic sinusitis, several bacteriologic studies have been conducted. In 1983, Adinoff and colleagues[60] published a report regarding 42 asthmatic children with sinusitis. Only 12% of maxillary sinus aspirates grew positive bacterial cultures; however, many of the studies involving children showed only mild radiographic abnormalities with less than 5 mm mucosal thickening. Friedman and colleagues[61] in 1984 and Goldenhersh and colleagues[62] in 1990 performed maxillary aspirates in groups of 8 and 12 asthmatic children, respectively, with significant radiographic evidence of sinusitis (opacification, air-fluid levels, or mucosal thickening >5 mm). The two groups of researchers demonstrated that 60% and 75% of these children, respectively, had positive bacterial cultures, and the organisms were the same as those found in acute sinusitis, including *Streptococcus pneumoniae, Haemophilus influenzae,* and *Moraxella catarrhalis.* Taken together, the above studies demonstrate that the majority of children with sinusitis and asthma appear to have a chronic inflammatory disease of the sinus mucosa that is prone to persistent infection with predominantly aerobic bacteria. Data from the radiographic studies also suggest that minor degrees of mucosal inflammation observed on sinus radiograph are usually not associated with active bacterial infection.

EFFECTS OF SINUS THERAPY ON ASTHMA

For the past century, otolargyngologists have catalogued the effects of sinus therapy on asthma symptoms. Because most of the earliest data were based on postsurgical observations, we will review those studies first.

Surgical Treatment

Early in the 20th century, physicians observed that surgical treatment of nasal and sinus disease resulted in variable improvements in asthma symptoms. In 1936, Weille[63] published his study of 500 asthmatic patients of varying ages, 72% of whom had chronic sinus disease. Following sinus surgery in 100 of the patients, 56 reported that their chest symptoms were improved, and 10 experienced complete resolution of asthma. Improvement in asthma symptoms, however, also occurred in 40% of the patients who did not undergo sinus surgery. In 1969, Davison[64] reported that 23 of 24 adolescent and adult patients with chronic sinusitis and asthma experienced a 75% or greater improvement in asthma symptoms after surgical drainage of the sinuses. Werth[65] presented the results of sinus surgery in children, noting that 20 of 22 pediatric patients with severe asthma and sinusitis experienced a marked improvement in asthma after sinus surgery.

To date, there have been no randomized, controlled trials examining the effects of sinus surgery on lower airway symptoms or function. The study by Weille does indicate that asthma symptoms may improve spontaneously in the absence of surgical intervention. Collectively, however, these reports suggest that long-term control of asthma symptoms may improve after surgical sinus procedures.

Medical Treatment

During the past decade, multiple investigators have studied the effect of medical therapy on asthma symptoms, primarily in children. In 1981, Businco and colleagues[66] reported that 10 of 12 children with chronic asthma had an improvement in lower airway symptoms after medical therapy, although no objective measures of pulmonary function were performed. In 1983, Cummings and colleagues[67] performed a double-blind, placebo-controlled study of sinus therapy in asthma. Active treatment (antibiotics, nasal steroids, and oral decongestants) of children with opacification or marked thickening of the maxillary sinuses resulted in significantly fewer asthma symptoms and a reduced requirement for inhaled bronchodilator and oral steroid therapy. Neither pulmonary function results nor measures of bronchial reactivity were significantly improved with active treatment.

In 1984, Rachelefsky and colleagues[68] studied 48 children with a 3-month or longer history of sinusitis and wheezing. After 2 to 4 weeks of antibiotics with or without antral lavage, 38 of the patients were able to discontinue daily bronchodilator therapy, and 20 of 30 demonstrated normalization of pulmonary function tests. During that same year, Friedman and colleagues[61] studied eight children experiencing asthma exacerbations associated with sinusitis. After 2 to 4 weeks of antimicrobial therapy, seven of eight patients reported improvement in lower airway symptoms. Although baseline indices of pulmonary function were not changed after the completion of antibiotics, there was a mean twofold improvement in FEV_1 following inhaled bronchodilator therapy.

Similar to the surgical observations, these studies suggest that medical treatment of sinusitis may result in improvement of bronchial asthma. Although only one randomized, placebo-controlled trial has been done, both chest symptoms and lower airway function do appear to improve significantly after aggressive medical therapy.

PATHOPHYSIOLOGIC LINKS BETWEEN CHRONIC SINUSITIS AND ASTHMA

As noted above in the section regarding allergic rhinitis and asthma, a number of potential mechanisms may help explain the connection between upper and lower airway dysfunction. Specifically, with respect to the relationship between sinus inflammation and asthma, an animal model has provided some promising insights into this interaction. Brugman and colleagues[69] created an experimental model of sinus inflammation in rabbits using complement fragment C5a. Although induction of sterile sinus inflammation in rabbits caused no changes in baseline lung function, bronchial responsiveness to inhaled histamine was significantly increased. Because these changes could be prevented by strategies that blocked drainage of inflammatory exudates beyond the larynx, the researchers postulated that postnasal drip was most likely responsible for the alteration in airway reactivity. Importantly, however, there was no evidence of lower airway inflammation by either histologic examination or bronchoalveolar lavage. This association of hyperresponsiveness with morphologically normal airways is difficult to explain but again suggests the possibility of neurally mediated response.

DIAGNOSTIC AND THERAPEUTIC IMPLICATIONS

In children with moderate to severe asthma, we believe that chronic sinusitis should always be considered as a possible provocative factor. The clinical history and physical examination, however, are neither sensitive nor specific for chronic sinus disease. Therefore, we evaluate all children with poorly controlled or steroid-requiring asthma with a Waters' view (occipitomental) sinus radiograph, which is primarily useful for examining the maxillary sinuses. Although CT of the paranasal sinuses has proven to be considerably more sensitive than plain films in detecting subtle mucosal disease,[70] we believe that plain film examination has an important role as an initial imaging study. First, plain films are simple, convenient, and relatively inexpensive to perform. Second, in contrast to CT imaging, plain films do not require sedation in infants or young children. Finally, the significance of subtle sinus CT changes is unclear because such abnormalities may be present in up to 50% of children[71] who have no clinical evidence of either sinusitis or asthma. We reserve CT imaging of the sinuses for patients with clinical histories strongly suggestive of sinusitis who have normal plain films and patients with persistent, severe sinus disease before surgical intervention.

Flexible fiberoptic rhinoscopy has been suggested as an alternative to plain radiographic films because purulent drainage may be visualized in the vicinity of the middle and superior meatus.[72] In our experience, however, the absence of pus does not rule out active infection because sinus drainage may be obstructed by ostial edema or obstructing lesions of the nasal airway. Additionally, rhinoscopy will not detect significant hyperplastic changes in the sinuses, which may play an important pathogenic role in asthma. In the context of sinus disease, we generally use rhinoscopy for identifying anatomic lesions (e.g., adenoidal hypertrophy) that may predispose the patient to sinusitis.

Patients who demonstrate significant radiographic abnormalities of the maxillary sinuses (opacification, air-fluid levels, or thickening greater than 5 mm, or more than 50% of the maxillary antrum) are treated with medical therapy. We classify medical treatment modalities for chronic sinusitis into three categories: antibiotics to eliminate possible concomitant infection, medications to reduce swelling, and measures to thin and evacuate secretions (Box 57-2).

Because up to 25% of the bacterial isolates found in chronic sinusitis are β-lactamase producers, we prescribe amoxicillin-clavulanate potassium as a first-line antibiotic for a period of no less than 3 weeks. In children who are allergic to penicillin, clarithromycin is employed as an alternative agent. For nasal swelling, we often use topical decongestants (e.g., oxymetolazine) for the initial 3 days of therapy and continue oral decongestants (either phenylpropanolamine or pseudoephedrine) for an additional 7 to 10 days. If nasal swelling does not respond to these

BOX 57-2 Medical Treatment of Chronic Sinusitis in Asthmatics

Antibiotics

- Amoxicillin-clavulanate potassium for a minimum of 21 days (or clarithromycin in penicillin-allergic patients)
- If the patient does not respond, alternative use of β-lactamase-resistant antibiotic (e.g., cefuroxime) for 21 additional days

Medications to Reduce Swelling

- For severe swelling, topical oxymetolazine for 3 days
- If swelling persists, continue with oral pseudoephedrine on a regular basis for 7 to 10 days or longer if needed
- Use of intranasal corticosteroid spray for 3 to 6 weeks
- If swelling does not respond, use of prednisone 0.5 mg/kg body weight, tapered over 5 to 7 days

Measures to Enhance Evacuation of Secretions

- Use of saline irrigations
- Use of hot steam inhalations

measures, we prescribe a 5- to 7-day tapering course of oral corticosteroids. All patients are also started on a topical nasal corticosteroid, which is usually continued on a long-term basis. We have found that evacuation of secretions is enhanced by performing nasal irrigations with saline or increasing humidification using a free-standing humidifier or hot shower. Although these measures have not been tested in controlled trials, we are impressed that they help to reduce patient discomfort and facilitate resolution of the chronic infection in selected patients. If no improvement in nasal symptoms occurs and the patient's asthma remains poorly controlled, we institute a second 3-week course of another β-lactamase-resistant antibiotic (e.g., cefuroxime axetil). If a patient fails to respond adequately to the aforementioned regimen, we consider sinus CT and refer them to an otolaryngologist for consideration of endoscopic sinus surgery.

SUMMARY

A great deal of data support an association between chronic sinusitis and asthma. We have developed a better understanding of the pathogenesis of sinus disease in asthmatic patients and now realize that eosinophilic sinus infiltration plays a direct role in chronic mucosal inflammation that may predispose the paranasal sinuses to recurrent or chronic bacterial infection. Long-term, blinded, placebo-controlled trials need to be completed before we can reliably predict the effect of sinus therapy on clinical asthma. Until then, we recommend that sinus disease be considered in all patients with moderate to severe asthma and treated aggressively when it is identified.

REFERENCES

1. Smith JM: Epidemiology and natural history of asthma, allergic rhinitis and atopic dermatitis (eczema). In: Middleton E, ed: Allergy, Principles and Practice, 3rd ed. St. Louis, Mo: CV Mosby, 1988.
2. Settipane GA: Allergic rhinitis-update. Otolaryngol Head Neck Surg 1986; 94:470–475.
3. Kapsali T, Horowitz E, Diemer F, Togias A: Rhinitis is ubiquitous in allergic asthmatics [Abstract]. J Allergy Clin Immunol 1997;99(Suppl):138.
4. Settipane RJ, Hagy GW, Settipane GA: Long-term risk factors for developing asthma and allergic rhinitis. A 23-year follow-up study of college students. Allergy Proc 1994;15:21–25.
5. Bergmann R, Bergmann K, Lau-Schadendorf S, Wahn U: Atopic diseases in infancy. The German Multicenter Atopy study (MAS-90). Pediatr Allergy Immunol 1994;5:19–25.
6. Masuda S, Fujisawa T, Katsumata H, Atsuta J, Iguchi K, Kamiya H: Nasal symptoms in children with bronchial asthma [Abstract]. J Allergy Clin Immunol 2003;111(Suppl):138.
7. Madonini E, Briatico-Vangosa G, Pappacoda A, Maccagni G, Cardani A, Saporiti F: Seasonal increase of bronchial reactivity in allergic rhinitis. J Allergy Clin Immunol 1987;79:358–363.
8. Braman SS, Barrows AA, DeCotiis BA, Settipane GA, Corrao WM: Airway hyperresponsiveness in allergic rhinitis. A risk factor for asthma. Chest 1987;91:671–674.
9. Huse DM, Harte SC, Russel MW, Piercey G, Weiss S: Allergic rhinitis may worsen asthma symptoms in children. The International Asthma Outcomes Registry [Abstract]. Am J Respir Crit Care Med 1996;153:A860.
10. Halpern M, Richner R, Togias A, et al: Allergic rhinitis may increase asthma costs [Abstract]. Am J Respir Crit Care Med 1996;153:A860.
11. Pipkorn U, Karlsson G, Enerback L: The cellular response of the human allergic mucosa to natural allergen exposure. J Allergy Clin Immunol 1988; 82:1046–1054.
12. Robinson D, Hamid Q, Ying S, Tsicopoulos A, Barkans J, Bentley A, et al: Predominant TH2 like bronchoalveolar T-lymphocyte population in atopic asthma. N Engl J Med 1992;326:298–304.
13. Durham S, Ying S, Varney V, Jacobson M, Sudderick R, Mackay I, et al: Cytokine messenger RNA expression for IL-3, IL-4, IL-5, and granulocyte/macrophage-colony-stimulating factor in the nasal mucosa after local allergen provocation. Relationship to tissue eosinophilia. J Immunol 1992; 148:2390–2394.
14. Naclerio R, Meier H, Kagey-Sobotka A, Adkinson N, Meyers D, Norman P, et al: Mediator release after nasal airway challenge with allergen. Am Rev Respir Dis 1983;128:597–602.
15. Djukanovic R, Lai C, Wilson J, Britten K, Wilson S, Roche W, et al: Bronchial mucosa manifestations of atopy. A comparison of markers of inflammation between atopic asthmatics, atopic nonasthmatics and healthy controls. Eur Respir J 1992;5:538–544.
16. Crimi E, Milanese M, Oddera S, Mereu C, Rossi GA, Riccio A, et al: Inflammatory and mechanical factors of allergen-induced bronchoconstriction in mild asthma and rhinitis. J Appl Physiol 2001;91:1029–1034.
17. Welsh PW, Stricker EW, Chu-Pin C, Naessens JM, Reese ME, Reed CE, et al: Efficacy of beclomethasone nasal solution, flunisolide and cromolyn in relieving symptoms of ragweed allergy. Mayo Clin Proc 1987;62:125–134.
18. Corren J, Adinoff AD, Buchmeier AD, Irvin CG: Nasal beclomethasone prevents the seasonal increase in bronchial responsiveness in patients with allergic rhinitis and asthma. J Allergy Clin Immunol 1992;90:250–256.
19. Henriksen JW, Wenzel A: Effect of an intranasally administered corticosteroid (budesonide) on nasal obstruction, mouth breathing and asthma. Am Rev Respir Dis 1984;130:1014–1018.
20. Watson WTA, Becker AB, Simons FER: Treatment of allergic rhinitis with intranasal corticosteroids in patients with mild asthma. Effect on lower airway responsiveness. J Allergy Clin Immunol 1993;91:97–101.
21. Casale TB, Wood D, Richerson HB, Trapp S, Metzger WJ, Zavala D, et al: Elevated bronchoalveolar lavage fluid histamine levels in allergic asthmatics are associated with methacholine bronchial hyperresponsiveness. J Clin Invest 1987;79:1197–1203.
22. Wood-Baker R, Smith R, Holgate ST: A double-blind, placebo controlled study of the effect of the specific histamine H_1-antagonist, terfenadine, in chronic severe asthma. Br J Clin Pharmacol 1995;39:671–675.
23. Bruttman G, Pedraii P, Arendt C, Rihoux JP: Protective effect of cetirizine in patients suffering from pollen asthma. Ann Allergy 1990;64:224–228.
24. Grant JA, Nicodemus CF, Findlay SR, Glovsky MM, Grossman J, Kaiser H, et al: Cetirizine in patients with seasonal allergic rhinitis and concomitant asthma. Prospective, randomized, placebo-controlled trial. J Allergy Clin Immunol 1995;95:923–932.
25. Corren J, Harris A, Aaronson D, Beaucher W, Berkowitz R, Bronsky E, et al: Efficacy and safety of loratadine plus pseudoephedrine in patients with seasonal allergic rhinitis and mild asthma. J Allergy Clin Immunol 1997; 100:781–789.
26. Braunstahl G-J, Overbeek S, Kleinjan A, Prins J-B, Hoogsteden H, Fokkens W: Nasal allergen provocation induces adhesion molecules expression and tissue eosinophilia in upper and lower airways. J Allergy Clin Immunol 2001;107: 469–476.
27. Togias A, Bieneman A, Bloom D, Schleimer R, Iezzoni D, Harris A: Changes in blood leukocyte cytokine expression following repeated nasal allergen provocation. Evidence for systemic manifestations [Abstract]. J Allergy Clin Immunol 2002;109(Suppl):262.
28. Braunstahl G-J, Kleinjan A, Overbeek S, Prins J-B, Hoogsteden H, Fokkens W: Segmental bronchial provocation induces nasal inflammation in allergic rhinitis patients. Am J Respir Crit Care Med 2000;161:2051–2057.
29. Kaufman J, Wright GW: The effect of nasal and nasopharyngeal irritation on airway resistance in man. Am Rev Respir Dis 1969;100:626–630.
30. Kaufman J, Chen JC, Wright GW: The effect of trigeminal resection on reflex bronchoconstriction after nasal and nasopharyngeal irritation in man. Am Rev Respir Dis 1970;101:768–769.
31. Fontanari P, Burnet H, Zattara-Harmann MC, Jammes Y: Changes in airway resistance induced by nasal inhalation of cold dry, dry, or moist air in normal individuals. J Appl Physiol 1996;81:1739–1743.
32. Yan K, Salome C: The response of the airways to nasal stimulation in asthmatics with rhinitis. Eur J Respir Dis 1983;64:105–108.
33. Littell NT, Carlisle CC, Millman RP, Braman SS: Changes in airway resistance following nasal provocation. Am Rev Respir Dis 1990;141:580–583.
34. Corren J, Adinoff AD, Irvin CG: Changes in bronchial responsiveness following nasal provocation with allergen. J Allergy Clin Immunol 1992; 89:611–618.
35. Shturman-Ellstein R, Zeballos RJ, Buckley JM, Souhrada JF: The beneficial effect of nasal breathing on exercise-induced bronchoconstriction. Am Rev Respir Dis 1978;118:65–73.
36. Griffin MP, McFadden ER, Ingram RH: Airway cooling in asthmatic and nonasthmatic subjects during nasal and oral breathing. J Allergy Clin Immunol 1982;69:354–359.
37. McLaurin JG: Chest complications of sinus disease. Ann Otol Rhinol Laryngol 1932;41:780.

38. Huxley EJ, Viroslav J, Gray WR, Pierce AK: Pharyngeal aspiration in normal adults and patients with depressed consciousness. Am J Med 1978;64:564–568.
39. Bardin PG, Van Heerden BB, Joubert JR: Absence of pulmonary aspiration of sinus contents in patients with asthma and sinusitis. J Allergy Clin Immunol 1990;86:82–88.
40. Platts-Mills TA: Allergen avoidance. J Allergy Clin Immunol 2004;113: 388–391.
41. Corren J: Intranasal corticosteroids for allergic rhinitis. How do different agents compare? J Allergy Clin Immunol 1999;104(Suppl):144–149.
42. Howarth PH: Assessment of antihistamine efficacy and potency. Clin Exp Allergy 1999;29:87–97.
43. Wilson AM, O'Byrne PM, Parameswaran K: Leukotriene receptor antagonists for allergic rhinitis. A systematic review and meta-analysis. Am J Med 2004;116:338–344.
44. Moller C, Dreborg S, Ferdousi HA, Halken S, Host A, Jacobsen L, et al: Pollen immunotherapy reduces the development of asthma in children with seasonal rhinoconjunctivitis (the PAT-study). J Allergy Clin Immunol 2002;109:251–256.
45. Gottlieb MJ: Relation of intranasal disease in the production of bronchial asthma. JAMA 1925;95:105.
46. Chobot R: The incidence of sinusitis in asthmatic children. Am J Dis Child 1930;39:257.
47. Bullen SS: Incidence of asthma in 400 cases of chronic sinusitis. J Allergy 1932;4:402
48. Berman SZ, Mathison DA, Stevenson DD, Tan EM, Vaughan JH: Maxillary sinusitis and bronchial asthma. Correlation of roentgenograms, cultures, and thermograms. J Allergy Clin Immunol 1974;53:311–317.
49. Rachelefsky GS, Goldberg M, Katz RM, Boris G, Gyepes MT, Shapiro MJ, et al: Sinus disease in children with respiratory allergy. J Allergy Clin Immunol 1978;61:310–314.
50. Schwartz HJ, Thompson JS, Sher TH, Ross RJ: Occult sinus abnormalities in the asthmatic patient. Arch Intern Med 1987;147:2194–2196.
51. Zimmerman B, Stringer D, Feanny S, Reisman J, Hale H, Rashed N, et al: Prevalence of abnormalities found by sinus x-rays in childhood asthma. Lack of relation to severity of asthma. J Allergy Clin Immunol 1987;88:268–273.
52. Chen LC, Huang JL, Wang CR, Yeh KW, Lin SJ: Use of standard radiography to diagnose paranasal sinus disease of asthmatic children in Taiwan. Comparison with computed tomography. Asian Pac J Allergy Immunol 1999;17:69–76.
53. Fascenelli FW: Maxillary sinus abnormalities. Radiographic evidence in an asymptomatic population. Arch Otolaryngol 1969;90:190–193.
54. Kovatch AL, Wald ER, Ledesma-Medina J, et al: Maxillary sinus radiographs in children with nonrespiratory complaints. Pediatrics 1984;73:306–308.
55. Shapiro G. Rachelefsky GS: Introduction and definition of sinusitis. J Allergy Clin Immunol 1992;90(Suppl):417–418.
56. Hansel FK: Clinical and histopathologic studies of the nose and sinuses in allergy. J Allergy 1929;1:43.
57. Harlin SL, Ansel DG, Lane SR, Myers J, Kephart GM, Gleich GJ: A clinical and pathologic study of chronic sinusitis. The role of the eosinophil. J Allergy Clin Immunol 1988;81:867–875.
58. Baroody FM, Hughes CA, McDowell P, Hruban R, Zinreich SJ, Naclerio RM: Eosinophilia in chronic childhood sinusitis. Arch Otolaryngol Head Neck Surg 1995;121;1396–1402.
59. Hisamatsu K, Ganbo I, Nakazawa T, Murakami Y, Gleich GJ, Makiyama K, et al: Cytotoxicity of human eosinophil granule major basic protein to human nasal mucosa in vitro. J Allergy Clin Immunol 1990;86:52–63.
60. Adinoff AD, Wood RW, Buschman D: Chronic sinusitis in childhood asthma. Correlations of symptoms, x-rays, culture and response to treatment. Pediatr Res 1983;17:64.
61. Friedman R, Ackerman M, Wald E, Casselbrant M, Friday G, Fireman P: Asthma and bacterial sinusitis in children. J Allergy Clin Immunol 1984; 74:185–189.
62. Goldenhersh MJ, Rachelefsky GS, Dudley J, Brill J, Katz RM, Rohr AS, et al: The microbiology of chronic sinus disease in children with respiratory allergy. J Allergy Clin Immunol 1990;85:1030–1039.
63. Weille FL: Studies in asthma. Nose and throat in 500 cases of asthma. N Engl J Med 1936;215:235.
64. Davison FW: Chronic sinusitis and infectious asthma. Arch Otolaryngol 1969;90:202–207.
65. Werth G: The role of sinusitis in severe asthma. Immunol Allergy Proc 1984;45.
66. Businco L, Fiore L, Frediani T, Artuso A, Di Fazio A, Bellioni P: Clinical and therapeutic aspects of sinusitis in children with bronchial asthma. Int J Pediatr Otorhinolaryngol 1981;3:287–294.
67. Cummings NP, Wood RW, Lere JL: Effect of treatment of rhinitis/sinusitis on asthma. Results of a double-blind study [Abstract]. Pediatr Res 1983;17:373a.
68. Rachelefsky GS, Katz RM, Siegel SC: Chronic sinus disease with associated reactive airway disease in children. Pediatrics 1984;73:526–529.
69. Brugman SM, Larsen GL, Henson PM, Honor J, Irvin CG: Increased lower airways responsiveness associated with sinusitis in a rabbit model. Am Rev Respir Dis 1993;147:314–320.
70. McAlister WH, Lusk R, Mutz HR: Comparison of plain radiographs and coronal CT scans infants and children with recurrent sinusitis. Am J Roentgenol 1989;153:1259–1264.
71. Diament MJ, Senac MO, Gilsanz V, Baker S, Gillespie T, Larsson S: Prevalence of incidental paranasal sinuses opacification in pediatric patients. A CT study. J Comput Assist Tomogr 1987;11:426–431.
72. Castellanos J, Axelrod D: Flexible fiberoptic rhinoscopy in the diagnosis of sinusitis. J Allergy Clin Immunol 1989;83:91–94.

Cystic Fibrosis

58 Genetics and Pathophysiology of Cystic Fibrosis

Garry R. Cutting, MD • Pamela L. Zeitlin, MD

Since the 1940s the genetic basis of cystic fibrosis (CF) has been recognized by the medical community.[1] A genetic etiology and autosomal-recessive inheritance was suggested by the recurrence of CF in siblings and the absence of the illness in parents. Genetic linkage analysis confirmed that a single locus was responsible for classic CF.[2,3] In 1989 technical breakthroughs, allowing identification of disease-causing genes on the basis of position rather than function, enabled Tsui and colleagues to clone the gene responsible for this disorder.[4] The identified gene was aptly named the cystic fibrosis transmembrane conductance regulator (*CFTR*).[5] During the past 15 years, our understanding of the molecular basis of CF has exploded. We now recognize that mutations in *CFTR* give rise to a range of phenotypes that includes classic CF and reaches to single-organ pathologies at the other end of the spectrum. The consequences of many mutations on the function of the encoded protein have been determined, allowing correlation of altered function of CFTR with CF pathophysiology.

■ *CFTR* GENE

■ STRUCTURE

The *CFTR* gene resides on the long arm of human chromosome 7 and encompasses approximately 189,000 base pairs of DNA.[6] The coding portion of the gene is divided into 27 exons that are transcribed into a messenger RNA (mRNA) of approximately 6500 base pairs.[5] The exon and intron structure of the *CFTR* gene is well conserved among mammals and evolutionarily distant species such as amphibians (*Xenopus*) and fish (killifish and dogfish).[7]

Transcription of the *CFTR* gene is initiated 80 base pairs upstream from the start site of translation.[8,9] Minor start sites for transcription have also been identified.[5,10] The *CFTR* gene demonstrates exquisite temporal and spatial differences in expression. For example, specific cell types within the human lung express high levels of CFTR, while surface epithelial cells have a very low level of CFTR expression.[11] CFTR expression is also regulated during development, as detailed in studies of the mouse.[12,13] Despite considerable evidence that the expression of CFTR is highly regulated, the *cis-* and *trans-*acting elements that regulate CFTR expression have not been identified. Sequences immediately upstream of the transcriptional start site of *CFTR* generate low-level expression in most tissues. This pattern of expression is consistent with the presence of basal promoter elements.[8,10] A cyclic adenosine monophosphate (cAMP) response element has been identified within this region of *CFTR*, but this element does not appear to account for the spatial and temporal expression patterns.[14] Assays that search for binding of protein to DNA have identified several regions elsewhere in the *CFTR* gene that may be involved in transcriptional regulation.[15–17] Furthermore, cross-species analysis has identified regions of the *CFTR* gene that are highly conserved, suggesting a possible role in regulation of gene expression.[7] Finally, strain-specific differences in CFTR expression in mice have been mapped to sequences about 700 base pairs upstream of the *CFTR* gene, indicating the existence of regulatory elements in this region.[18] Thus, despite extensive efforts to locate transcriptional elements, the molecular mechanisms regulating CFTR expression are poorly understood.

■ SPLICING

Numerous variations in *CFTR* splicing patterns have been identified by the reverse transcription–polymerase chain reaction technique.[19,20] Only two appear to be alternatively spliced transcripts that create functional isoforms of *CFTR*. RNA transcripts missing exon 5 encode a functional form of CFTR in the rabbit heart.[21–23] However, RNA transcripts resulting from alternative splicing of exon 5 CFTR have not been identified in other species or in other tissues. Transcripts missing a portion of exons 13 and 14a encode a functional isoform of CFTR expressed in mouse and human kidney.[24] Neither the heart nor the kidney appears to be primarily involved in CF pathophysiology, thus the role of these alternatively spliced forms of CFTR is unclear.

In contrast to alternative splicing, many aberrantly spliced versions of CFTR have been identified. Aberrantly spliced CFTR RNA transcripts do not produce functional CFTR. Aberrant splicing occurs as a result of variation in intronic or exonic sequences required for normal splicing of CFTR. The aberrant splicing of exon 9 is a notable example.[25,26] Variation in the length of the polythymidine tract, an element in the 3′ splice site of intron 8 is correlated with the amount of properly spliced CFTR mRNA.[27] Longer versions of this tract called 9T and 7T are common in the population and are associated with high levels of normally spliced CFTR mRNA. A shorter version of this tract called 5T is associated with a substantial reduction in full-length CFTR RNA.[28] While abbreviated polythymidine tracts in 3′ splice sites do not usually cause missplicing of the subsequent exon, it appears that a special situation occurs in the *CFTR* gene. Sequence surrounding exon 9, including unusual variation in splice sites surrounding exon 9 and splice-silencing sequences in intron 9, appear to make exon 9 vulnerable to missplicing.[29–31] Thus, alterations in secondary splicing signals of this exon such as the polythymidine tract have an exaggerated effect on splicing. The splicing efficiency of *CFTR* genes bearing 5T also varies by tissue. The vas deferens splices *CFTR* genes bearing the 5T variant less efficiently than respiratory epithelia.[32,33]

Individuals carrying the 5T mutation in their other *CFTR* gene manifest a variety of phenotypes ranging from healthy to nonclassic CF (see later). The latter phenomenon is due to the variable effect that 5T has on splicing of *CFTR* exon 9. This splicing variability is caused by variation in the number of TG dinucleotides adjacent to the polythymidine tract.[34] The role of the TG tract in splicing of 5T alleles is controversial. It may serve as a site for binding of a splicing repressor, or the RNA may form a secondary structure such as a hairpin.[35,36] Either way, there is a robust correlation between the length of the TG tract and the phenotypes associated with a 5T variant.[37]

Many other CFTR transcripts derived from aberrant splicing of exons 9 through 12 have been reported, yet none appear to be correlated with phenotype.[20,38–41] Another example of aberrant CFTR splicing involves exons 23 and 24, resulting in a prematurely truncated CFTR protein that is nonfunctional.[42] The many mutations that affect CFTR splicing and result in disease are summarized in the following section.

■ MUTATIONS

More than 1100 mutations in the *CFTR* gene associated with disease have been reported to the Cystic Fibrosis Genetic Analysis Consortium (http://www.genet.sickkids.on.ca/cftr/). The vast majority of mutations involve only one or a few nucleotides. Nearly 50% of mutations change an amino acid, while mutations that affect splicing or introduce a nonsense codon account for approximately 28%. Deletion and insertion mutations that alter the reading frame and usually result in the introduction of a premature termination codon account for about 20%. Deletions and insertions involving multiples of three nucleotides are much less common (2%). The latter mutations do not shift the reading frame, so a protein missing one or more amino acids is usually produced (e.g., CFTR with the ΔF508 mutation). Most of the remaining disease-associated mutations (2.7%) involve the deletion of larger regions of DNA involving hundreds to thousands of base pairs. Finally, a few mutations (0.7%) have been purported to have occurred in sequences thought to be involved in transcriptional regulation of the *CFTR* gene, although a convincing case has been made in only a few cases.[43]

In addition to the disease-associated mutations, there are almost 200 mutations in *CFTR* that have not been associated with disease. These mutations have been termed as benign, or as polymorphisms. However, there are some polymorphisms in the *CFTR* gene (e.g., M470V) wherein an effect on phenotype has been suggested.[34,44] Mutations that are "silent" (that do not change an encoded amino acid or known splicing signal) are not predicted to alter CFTR function. However, the elucidation of intronic and exonic signals that enhance or repress exon splicing raises the possibility that some "silent" changes may affect CFTR splicing.[45,46]

The distribution of disease-associated mutations in the *CFTR* gene among human populations has been extensively reviewed.[47,48] One mutation, a deletion of three nucleotides that leads to loss of a single phenylalanine residue at codon 508 (ΔF508), accounts for approximately 70% of CF alleles in northern European whites. The frequency of the ΔF508 mutation varies on the European continent from lower than 50% of CF alleles in southern Europe to as high as 88% of CF alleles in Denmark. The ΔF508 mutation is quite rare in native Africans and native Asians. However, the ΔF508 mutation is found in racially admixed populations. For example, 30% of the *CFTR* genes in American CF patients of African descent have the ΔF508 mutation.[49] On the other hand, the second most common mutation in African Americans with CF (3120 + 1G→A) appears to be a common CF allele in native Africans.[50,51] Deleterious CF alleles have also been found in CF patients of Asian ancestry.[52,53] These mutations have not been observed in white or native African populations. Thus, rare deleterious mutations in the *CFTR* gene occur in all human populations. However, it is the commonness of the ΔF508 mutation in Europeans that accounts for the high incidence of CF in whites.

In addition to ΔF508, about 25 other mutations occur with a frequency of 0.1% or greater in the white CF population.[49,54] Other mutations are seen with some frequency in African Americans.[50] Finally, some ethnic groups have one or several mutations that reach a frequency of 1% or greater that are rare in the general population. The higher frequency of the latter mutations is probably the consequence of a founder effect.[55] The remainder of the reported mutations (~1000) have been reported in only a small number of individuals. Screening for the ΔF508 mutation and the 25 mutations that have a frequency of 0.1% detects about 85% of mutations in white CF patients.[56] Mutation screens involving 50 to 100 CF mutations produce a minimal increase in detection rate in the general CF population (1% to 3%). Since there are so many rare mutations, in order to achieve a detection rate for classic CF over 95%, screening of the entire coding region of the *CFTR* gene is required.[57,58]

■ CFTR PROTEIN

■ CHARACTERISTICS

The CFTR protein is composed of a linear stretch of 1480 amino acids that form an integral membrane glycoprotein.

A comparison of the nucleotide sequence across available databases places this protein as a member of the ABC transporter superfamily. The topology of the protein contains the common features of twofold symmetry with six transmembrane domains and an intracellular nucleotide-binding fold. The CFTR is unique in the presence of a central intracellular R domain enriched in phosphorylation sites utilized by the protein kinases A and C. Although most members of the superfamily are transporters (e.g., the multi-drug resistance transporter MDR transports chemotherapy agents), the CFTR is a cAMP-regulated chloride channel that must function for the outwardly rectifying chloride channel (ORCC) to transport chloride. Functional CFTR also down-regulates the epithelial sodium channel (ENaC) in those cells in which both reside. More controversial functions have been reported, including transport of nucleotides or fatty acids.

BIOGENESIS

The CFTR polypeptide is translated from the mRNA in the endoplasmic reticulum (ER) as a linear chain of amino acids with hydrophilic (water-soluble) and hydrophobic (lipid-soluble) domains. The nascent polypeptide is assisted by interactions with chaperone proteins within and outside the ER to assume a tertiary or folded structure that buries the membrane-spanning domains in the ER membrane. The process is relatively slow, taking approximately 10 to 15 minutes to complete, and is followed by two different fates. Depending on the cell type making the CFTR, the wild-type chain could be ubiquitinated and sent to the proteasome for degradation or it could continue along the trafficking pathway to the Golgi apparatus. Chloride transport through the CFTR can be detected in the ER using patch-clamping techniques, but it is not known whether the immature functional channel is the one protected from proteasomal degradation. The successful CFTR is packaged into vesicles for transport via a CopI ER exit machinery.[59]

FUNCTION

The three-dimensional topology of CFTR is under investigation. The two nucleotide binding domains (NBDs) and the R domain probably interact such that phosphorylation of the R domain is required for chloride channel opening and probably affects the affinity of the NBDs for adenosine triphosphate (ATP).[60] ATP hydrolysis at NBD1 is associated with opening the channel, but hydrolysis at NBD2 is associated with closure. The chloride pore is formed by transmembrane domains, and the single-channel conductance is low at 6 to 10 picoSiemens. The current-voltage relationship is linear, meaning that it is just as easy for chloride to leave as to enter the cell, depending on the direction of the voltage applied across the membrane. This bidirectionality is possible because ATP is the ligand that is hydrolyzed to gate the channel.

The most common mutation in *CFTR*, the ΔF508 deletion of the code for phenylalanine at position 508, has two consequences. First, the channel has a low open time for chloride—about 10% of normal.[61,62] Second, the newly translated CFTR is unstable in the ER, leading to premature proteolysis and a reduced half-life in the cell. The mutation appears to affect intermolecular interactions within *CFTR* rather than NBD1 folding.[63]

CELLULAR DISTRIBUTION AND FUNCTION

DEVELOPMENTAL EXPRESSION AND FUNCTION

CFTR mRNA is detectable in many fetal tissues in the first trimester. Data have been collected for fetal lung, intestine, pancreas, and kidney from humans, rats, rabbits, and mice. During early mammalian embryonic tissue development, CFTR may be more important as a regulator of other ion channels rather than as a pathway for chloride transport.[64] CFTR protein becomes detectable in the second trimester, still quite early in development. CFTR expression declines in postnatal lung, and this decline begins even earlier in rat in the last trimester. There is a bronchial centrifugal expression gradient and a developmental shift from apolar localization to apical localization, with a timing that matches that of CFTR regulation of the ENaC. Since ENaC function is required to resorb fetal lung fluid at birth, CFTR expression, a down-regulator of ENaC function, declines and ENaC expression increases.

POSTNATAL EXPRESSION AND FUNCTION

Regulated airway fluid and ion composition becomes more important for the air-breathing mammal than it was during lung development. CF lungs are morphologically normal at birth, in part because there are sufficient alternative chloride transport pathways in fetal lung to support tissue expansion and differentiation.[13,64] After birth, airway mucociliary clearance is affected by the depth and characteristics of the periciliary fluid layer, which in turn is dependent on ENaC function.[65–67] Over time, the human infant with pancreatic-insufficient CF is increasingly vulnerable to infection and inflammation in the airways, which lead to the classic lung phenotype of airways obstruction.

TISSUE DISTRIBUTION

Absent or reduced function of CFTR can be measured quantitatively in the sweat duct, where the reabsorptive coil is designed to conserve chloride, sodium, and water to protect the mammal from dehydration. The diagnostic sweat test takes advantage of the cholinergic pathway for generation of sweat by the sweat gland coil. Since CFTR is only responsible for at most 1% of sweat generation but is required for chloride reabsorption in the duct, the sweat can be collected and analyzed chemically to determine the sweat electrolyte concentration.

CFTR plays a vital role in several other organs, tissues where epithelial proteins are secreted along with electrolytes. The most important organs are the airways, bile ducts, pancreatic ducts, and vas deferens. Interestingly, although CFTR is highly expressed in the kidney, its absence is not detrimental. The simplified scheme in which CFTR plays an electrophysiologic role to control the ion and water content of luminal secretions is insufficient to explain the nature of CF lung disease. In CF lungs, additional abnormalities of fluid are associated with chronic inflammation and infection.

GENOTYPE-PHENOTYPE CORRELATIONS

MOLECULAR CONSEQUENCES OF MUTATIONS

The effect of disease-associated mutations on CFTR function has been investigated for a small fraction of CF alleles.

Mutations that have been studied include those that are common in CF patients (e.g., ΔF508, G551D), those that occur in patients with mild forms of the disease (e.g., A455E), and those that occur in known or putative functional domains of CFTR (e.g., R347H and R347P). The functional consequences of these mutations can be grouped into five classes.[68] Mutations that have consequences that do not fall into one of the five classes will be discussed at the end of this section.

Class I mutations cause changes in the synthesis of CFTR by affecting CFTR transcription. These mutations manifest their effect within the nucleus and usually involve the processing of transcripts with pancreatic termination mutations. In most cases, the introduction of a premature termination codon, whether by a change of a codon to a nonsense mutation or by frameshift, results in degradation of the transcript by a nonsense-mediated mRNA decay mechanism.[69] G542X is an example of this type of mutation.[70] In some cases, the premature termination codon does not lead to nonsense-mediated decay, and a truncated but nonfunctional protein is produced. R1162X is one such example.[71,72] A third consequence of nonsense mutations is that they can cause skipping of the exon in which they occur.[73] An example of this phenomenon is seen with the R553X mutation.[74] Mutations in the highly conserved splicing signals 5′ and 3′ of exons invariably lead to a loss of full-length transcript due to exon skipping.[75] Loss of exons can also cause a shift in the reading frame leading to the introduction of a premature termination codon and subsequent RNA degradation. In each case, these types of mutations lead to complete, or almost complete, loss of functional CFTR protein and produce a classic form of CF (Fig. 58-1).

The second class of mutations involves those that affect the processing of CFTR[76] (see Fig. 58-1). A prime example of a class II mutation is ΔF508. Loss of the phenylalanine residue at codon 508 within the first nucleotide-binding fold leads to a misfolding of CFTR.[77] Misfolded CFTR is recognized by chaperones that shunt the misfolded protein to degradation pathways.[78] The folding defect can be partially overcome by reduction in temperature. Cells grown at 21°C instead of 37°C can produce properly folded CFTR.[79] Folded CFTR bearing ΔF508 is functional in the cell membrane, but it is not stable and is more rapidly removed from the membrane than its wild-type counterpart.[80] Since ΔF508 is found in at least 70% of CF patients, the mechanisms underlying CFTR degradation have been studied intensively in hopes of finding approaches that permit CFTR bearing the ΔF508 mutation to evade degradation (see the Experimental Genetic-Based Therapies section in this chapter). Other class II mutations have been found that reduce folding efficiency, resulting in a small amount of properly folded functional CFTR at the cell membrane.[81,82]

Disease-associated mutations in class III affect the regulation of CFTR (see Fig. 58-1). Binding of ATP to the NBDs is required to activate CFTR. Mutations that affect CFTR interaction with ATP have been shown to alter its function.[61,83] An example is the G551D mutation in which the glycine (G) at codon 551 is substituted with aspartic acid (D). This glycine residue occurs in the C-motif of the first NBD within the ATP-binding pocket. The G551D mutation severely affects interaction with ATP, creating a form of CFTR that is properly folded and inserted in the cell membrane, yet unable to be activated.[77,84] Intriguingly, a second mutation has been reported to the same residue in which serine replaces glycine. This substitution reduces but does not eliminate function, so a mild CF phenotype is created.[85]

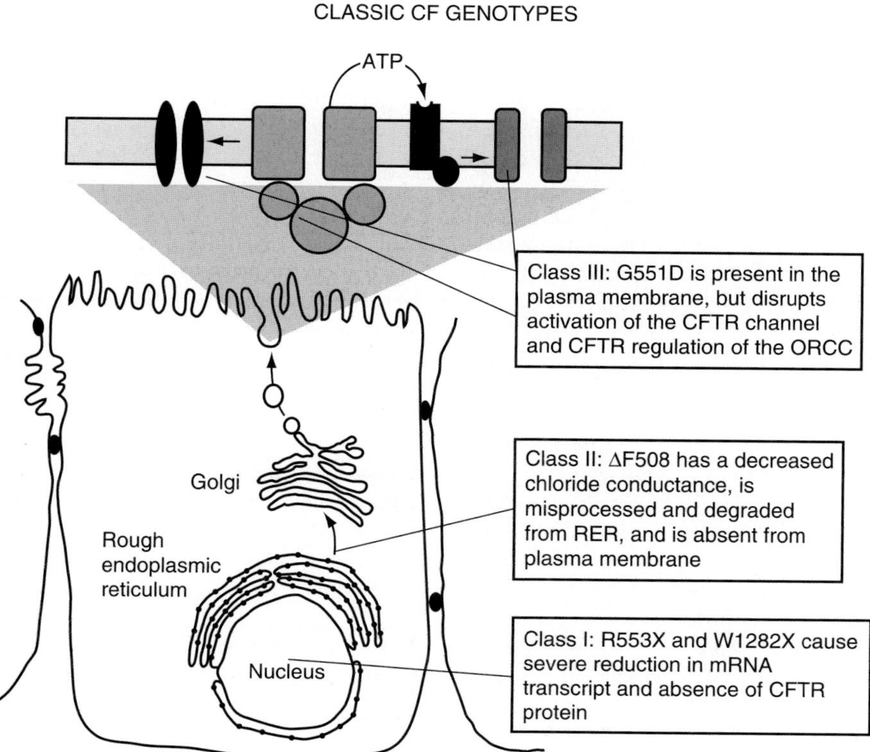
CLASSIC CF GENOTYPES
ATP
Class III: G551D is present in the plasma membrane, but disrupts activation of the CFTR channel and CFTR regulation of the ORCC
Golgi
Class II: ΔF508 has a decreased chloride conductance, is misprocessed and degraded from RER, and is absent from plasma membrane
Rough endoplasmic reticulum
Nucleus
Class I: R553X and W1282X cause severe reduction in mRNA transcript and absence of CFTR protein

■ **FIGURE 58-1.** Functional consequences of severe classic mutations leading to pancreatic insufficiency. ORCC, outwardly rectifying chloride channel; RER, rough endoplasmic reticulum.

Class IV mutations alter the chloride conduction properties of CFTR, and in some cases affect the magnitude and the ion selectivity of the channel pore.[86,87] Most class IV mutations occur in the transmembrane domains. Since class IV mutations may reduce but not eliminate the flow of ions, some CFTR function is preserved (Fig. 58-2), which in turn leads to a milder phenotype or a nonclassic form of CF. However, by the same token, it is recognized that altering this property of CFTR produces CF. Thus, loss or alteration of the chloride channel function of CFTR is key to the development of the CF phenotype, demonstrating that a defect in chloride transport is the primary abnormality in cells of CF patients.

Class V mutations are also associated with a milder form of CF, because they can also result in the production of a reduced amount of normally functional protein (see Fig. 58-2). An example of the latter type of mutation is 3849 + 10 kbC→T. This mutation occurs within intron 19, approximately 10 kilobases from the nearest splice site of exon 19, and leads to the aberrant splicing of CFTR, which produces a nonfunctional protein.[88] However, the aberrant splicing mechanism is incomplete, and a small amount of normally spliced CFTR transcript is made, leading to the synthesis of some normal CFTR that produces a CF phenotype that is moderate in severity.

Cystic fibrosis–causing mutations have been shown to affect other functions of CFTR. CFTR regulates other ion channels such as the ENaC and the ORCC.[89] Mutations in the first NBD have been shown to variably affect CFTR regulation of these channels.[90,91] Mutations in the N terminus or in the C terminus of CFTR can affect the trafficking, membrane insertion, or stability of CFTR.[92,93] These genotypes are sometimes classified as class VIA or VIB.

CLINICAL CONSEQUENCES OF MUTATIONS

Correlation of *CFTR* genotype with CF phenotype has been investigated using three methods. In genotype-driven studies, patients are grouped according to genotype and clinical features are compared. When patients who were homozygous for the ΔF508 mutation were compared to patients who carry one copy of ΔF508 and a different CF mutation, it was shown that a number of the less common mutations produce the same degree of disease severity as the ΔF508 mutation.[94] Some mutations cause less severe organ disease, or disease in a subset of organ systems affected in classic CF, resulting in a "nonclassic" CF phenotype.[95] *CFTR* genotype demonstrates a consistent association with the severity of pancreatic disease.[96] A less consistent correlation has been noted with abnormalities in sweat chloride concentration.[97] However, only one mutation, A455E, has been unequivocally correlated with severity of lung disease.[98,99] A few other mutations, particularly those in class IV, may associate with less severe lung disease.[100] In the phenotype-driven method, *CFTR* mutations are identified in patients grouped according to disease severity. This approach has identified relatively uncommon mutations that are associated with nonclassic forms of disease.[101–104] A third approach has been to correlate the class of mutation with the severity of disease. Those who carry mutations that cause a complete or nearly complete loss of function, such as class I and class II mutations, usually manifest classic CF. Mutations that permit some residual function, such as those in class III and class IV, have been associated with milder phenotypes.[97,100,105] However, it is important to recognize that many exceptions exist. For example, CFTR bearing G551D, a class III mutation, is associated with the classic form of CF.[106]

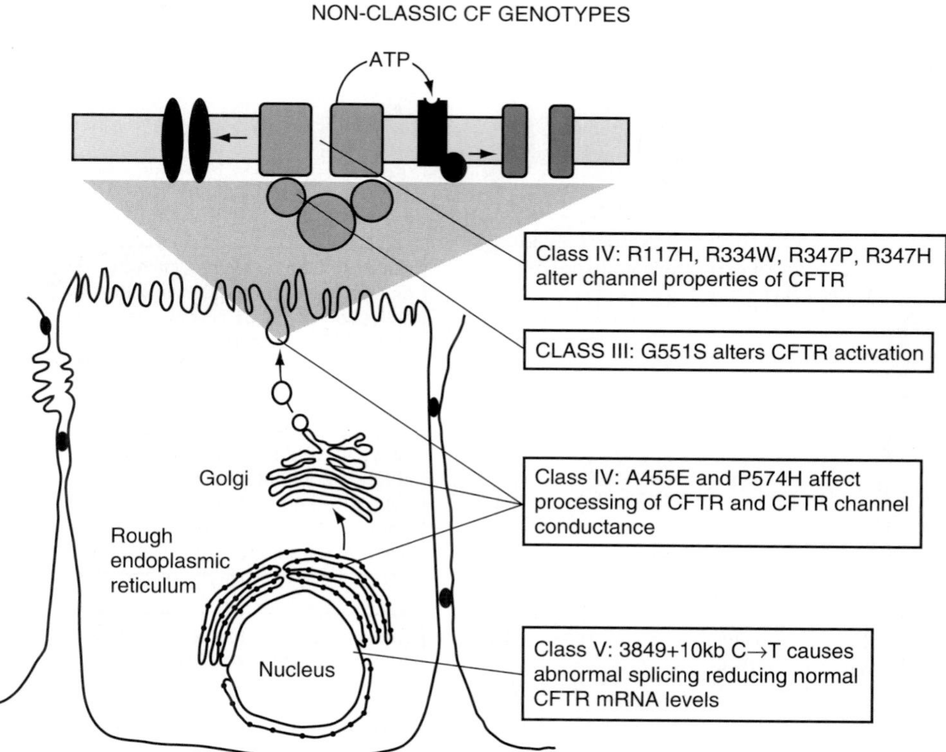
NON-CLASSIC CF GENOTYPES
ATP
Class IV: R117H, R334W, R347P, R347H alter channel properties of CFTR
CLASS III: G551S alters CFTR activation
Golgi
Rough endoplasmic reticulum
Nucleus
Class IV: A455E and P574H affect processing of CFTR and CFTR channel conductance
Class V: 3849+10kb C→T causes abnormal splicing reducing normal CFTR mRNA levels

■ **FIGURE 58-2.** Functional consequences of mutations leading to nonclassic (mild) forms of CF.

Another problem with utilizing mutation class is that some mutations have more than one effect on CFTR function. For example, A455E affects processing of CFTR (class II) and channel activity (class IV).[81,82]

■ CHARACTERISTICS OF SYSTEMIC DISEASE

AIRWAYS, UPPER AND LOWER

Lung disease remains the major expression of morbidity and mortality in CF. Infants with CF are born with normal lungs, and pulmonary disease develops over a variable time course. The earliest lesion is obstruction of the small airways by abnormally viscous airway mucus. A secondary bronchiolitis with plugging of the airways invariably follows and develops into bronchiectasis as the respiratory epithelium becomes chronically infected. It is a striking feature of CF lungs that the parenchyma is virtually untouched for much of the course, while the airways are severely afflicted. The airways become a reservoir for chronically infected mucopurulent secretions, first by *Staphylococcus aureus* and *Haemophilus influenzae*, and later by a distinctive mucoid form of *Pseudomonas aeruginosa*. Once mucoid *P. aeruginosa* colonizes the lungs, it is literally impossible to eradicate. Respiratory failure is the major cause of death, with the median life span now increased to 32 years.

The respiratory disease is usually progressive, with superimposed acute exacerbations. Cough is an early symptom and may be nonproductive and mistaken for reactive airways disease. Production of sputum develops and is an indicator of chronic inflammation and infection. A typical course is characterized by intermittent acute pulmonary exacerbations in which there is an increased volume of sputum, a change in the color of sputum, decreased exercise tolerance, and weight loss. Digital clubbing is a universal finding with progression of the lung disease. The chest radiograph becomes abnormal early in the course of the disease and demonstrates hyperinflation (Fig. 58-3) and patchy atelectasis (Fig. 58-4). The chest computed tomography (CT) scan is even more sensitive to changes (Fig. 58-5) and may be preferred over the chest radiograph for a quantitative assessment of progression of lung disease.[107] Bronchiectasis develops from progressive chronic infection and destruction of the airways (Fig. 58-6). Pulmonary function tests early in the disease reflect small airways obstruction but then progress toward a decrease in the FEV_1 (forced expiratory volume in 1 second) and increases in residual volume, functional residual capacity, and the ratio of residual volume to total lung capacity. The vital capacity is eventually reduced. With treatment of the acute exacerbations, small improvements in some of these lung functions can be documented.

The upper airway is also severely affected in CF. Chronic pansinusitis is found in more than 99% of patients with CF due in part to mucus gland hyperplasia, abnormal chloride ion transport by the sinus epithelial cells, and colonization with bacteria. Chronic sinusitis may contribute to infection of the lower respiratory tract by acting as a reservoir of infection. CT scans of the sinuses are useful in assessing the extent of sinus involvement and in the selection of patients who might benefit from a surgical drainage procedure.

Sinus involvement is complicated by nasal polyposis in 6% to 40% of patients. Nasal polyps should be suspected if nasal air flow is obstructed, the nasal bridge widens, or there is persistent epistaxis or loss of taste and appetite. Polyps appear in childhood and can recur after initial resection. If the disease is left untreated, serious bony erosions can occur. Medical management consists of topical glucocorticoids, macrolide antibiotics for anti-inflammatory action, antibiotics to cover the organisms in the sinuses, and surgical approaches.[108]

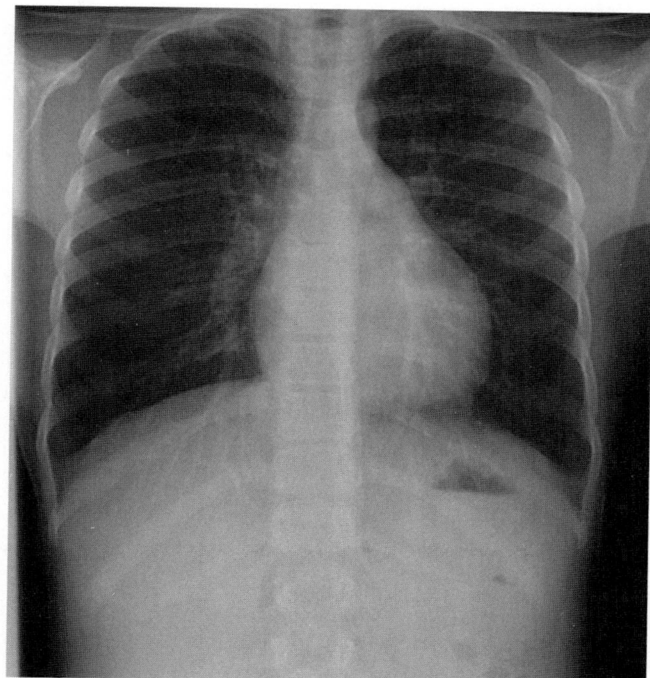

■ **FIGURE 58-3.** Chest radiograph of a 10-year-old female with CF (genotype ΔF508 homozygous) who complained of increasing cough and sputum production. Both lung fields are hyperinflated, and there are increased lung markings. Expectorated sputum culture grew nonmucoid *P. aeruginosa*.

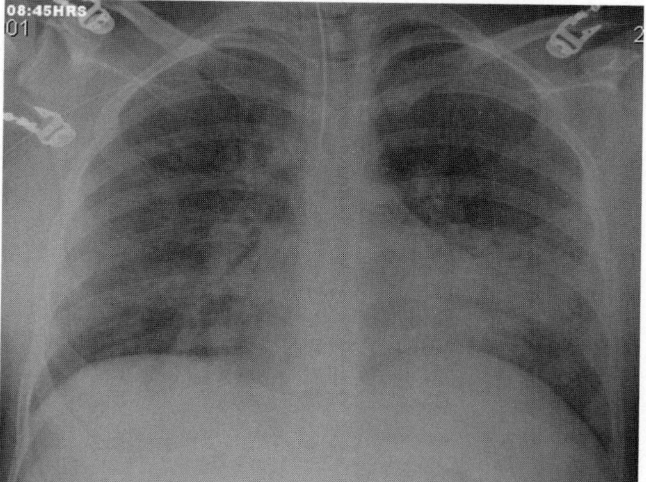

■ **FIGURE 58-4.** Chest radiograph at bronchoscopy of an adolescent female with CF (genotype ΔF508/621 + 1G) who complained of sudden and transient chest pain on the left side, followed by an increase in cough. There are lingular, right lower, and right middle lobe infiltrates and atelectasis. Lung fields improved after 14 days of intravenous antibiotics directed against the *S. aureus* and mucoid *P. aeruginosa* that grew from bronchoalveolar lavage cultures.

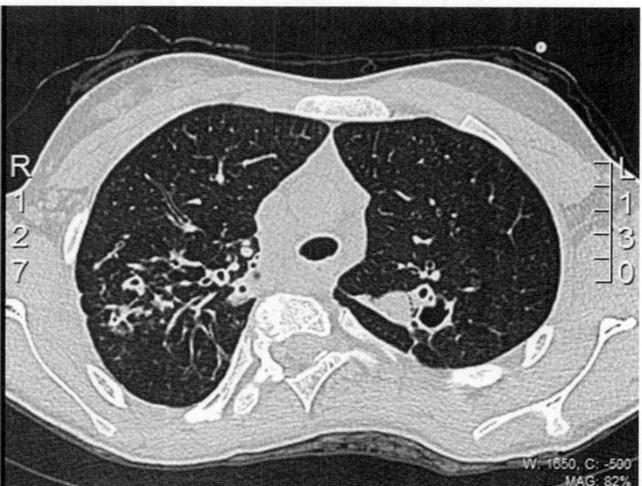

■ **FIGURE 58-5.** Spiral chest CT scan of an adolescent female with CF (genotype ΔF508 homozygous) and a slight decline in forced expiratory volume in 1 second. There is bilateral upper lobe bronchiectasis. Her sputum cultures grew *P. aeruginosa* and methicillin-resistant *S. aureus*.

Inflammation

A particularly intense inflammatory state appears early in the CF lung. Konstan and colleagues[109] demonstrated that the inflammatory infiltrate is predominantly neutrophilic. Bronchoalveolar lavage studies in infants suggest that inflammation may even precede colonization with bacteria, although this is controversial.[110,111]

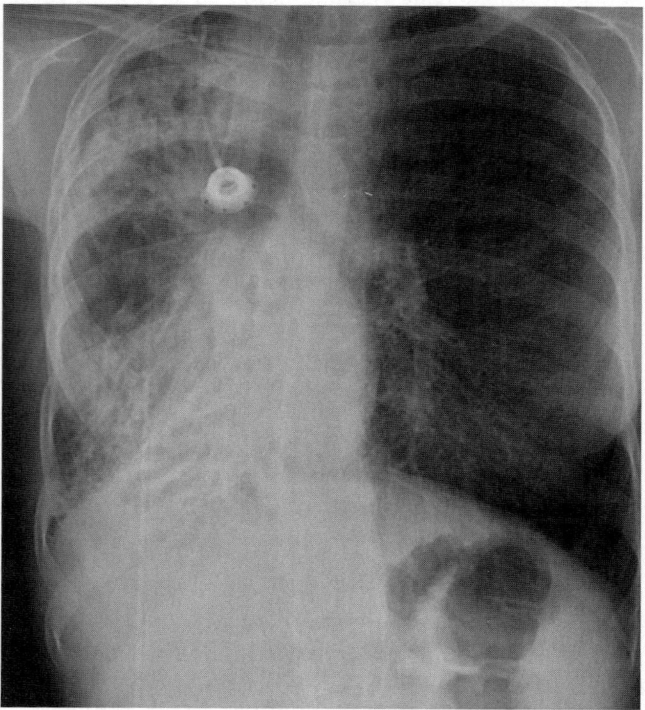

■ **FIGURE 58-6.** Chest radiograph of a 16-year-old female with CF (genotype ΔF508 homozygous) and recurrent pulmonary exacerbations. The left lung shows hyperaeration and bronchial wall thickening. The right lung shows decrease in volume, bronchial wall thickening, and bronchiectasis. Sputum cultures grew *Achromobacter xylosoxidans*.

If inflammation is both a primary defect related to dysfunctional CFTR and a result of infection, then anti-inflammatory therapy may be helpful.

Immune-mediated inflammation contributes significantly to the lung damage present in patients with CF. Specific antipseudomonal antibiotics do not eradicate the organism permanently. Despite aggressive intravenous therapy with large doses of increasingly more potent agents, colonization proceeds. Chronic infection then elicits recruitment and activation of neutrophils in the airways. The neutrophils release proteases such as granulocyte elastase and cathepsin G. This protease burden has been associated with both destruction of the lung matrix and cleavage and inactivation of a variety of opsonins. There is also evidence of immune complex formation in CF patients that correlates with disease severity and prognosis.

Infection

Nonencapsulated *H. influenzae* often colonizes the oropharynx of the young child with CF. Although it is not considered a serious pathogen, rising antibody titers to *H. influenzae* have been detected.[112] *Staphylococcus aureus* is the most frequent organism detected initially on oropharyngeal cultures, and it is still debated whether chronic antibiotic prophylaxis against this organism is useful. The acquisition of methicillin-resistant *S. aureus* is increasing and emerging as a potential pathogen in communities of healthy children as well as the CF clinics. *Pseudomonas aeruginosa*, nonmucoid, is acquired at varying times after birth, and transformation to a mucoid phenotype is associated with increased inflammatory burden and sputum volume. Early intervention strategies as well as chronic antibiotic protocols are aimed at eradicating or reducing the infection for as long as possible. *Burkholderia cepacia* complex (composed of nine different species) is particularly feared. Genomovar III is highly virulent and transmissible and can be associated with a sepsis-like condition that markedly reduces survival. Transient colonization with a *B. cepacia* species is becoming more common.

With more aggressive antibiotic strategies in place as well as frequent sputum and oropharyngeal cultures, a number of multiply resistant organisms are being identified. *Stenotrophomonas maltophilia*, *Alcaligenes xylosoxidans*, and nontuberculous mycobacteria alone or in combination with *P. aeruginosa* or *S. aureus* are challenging clinicians.

Additional details pertaining to bacterial, viral, and fungal pathogens in CF are discussed in Chapter 61. An extremely important message to learn from this work is that infection control strategies in the acute care setting, ambulatory clinics, and the home are mandatory if we are to contain the spread of transmissible organisms.[113]

■ GASTROINTESTINAL DISEASE

Gastrointestinal disease begins in utero in the pancreas, where dysfunctional CFTR produces a deficiency in exocrine pancreatic secretions because of progressive plugging of the pancreatic ducts by viscous secretions. The combination of the in utero deficiency of proteolytic enzymes with secretion of abnormal mucoproteins by the goblet cells of the small intestine leads to obstruction of the distal ileum by inspissated, tenacious meconium. About 15% of infants with CF are born with intestinal obstruction called meconium ileus. There are associated intestinal complications including small bowel atresia, volvulus, perforation, and peritonitis; alternately, there may simply be delayed passage of meconium and distal colonic obstruction secondary to the meconium plug syndrome.

The loss of pancreatic enzyme activity leads to intestinal malabsorption of fats and proteins and, to a lesser extent, carbohydrates, after birth. Pancreatic function is lost incrementally until complete loss is seen in 85% of patients. Infants manifest poor or absent weight gain, chronic abdominal distention, absence of subcutaneous fat and muscle tissue, steatorrhea, and rectal prolapse. Paradoxically, the untreated child is said to have a voracious appetite, but the caloric intake is insufficient to meet daily needs.

In older individuals, intestinal mucous gland hyperplasia is associated with abnormal mucins and slowing of intestinal transit time. If pancreatic enzyme replacement is inadequate, fecal impaction or distal intestinal obstruction syndrome can result.

Children, adolescents, and adults with residual pancreatic function may develop recurrent episodes of pancreatitis. Serum and urine amylase and serum lipase are elevated. Attacks can be precipitated by a fatty meal, alcohol, or tetracycline. Patients with one or more class IV or V mutations tend to have residual pancreatic function.

SWEAT GLAND EFFECTS

The gold standard for diagnosis of CF for many years has been the demonstration of elevated Cl^- and Na^+ in sweat collected by quantitative pilocarpine iontophoresis. Although no histopathologic changes can be found in the CF sweat gland, the function is abnormal as a result of inadequate reabsorption of salt by the distal collecting duct. The CF sweat is hypertonic, and the skin of affected infants has been described as tasting "salty." Heavy exercise in hot, humid climates can lead to increased salt losses and profound clinically significant dehydration.

Sweat production occurs in all individuals primarily by cholinergic stimulation. Cyclic AMP-mediated sweat secretion is present but insignificant. That is why sweat can be produced in CF individuals using the cholinergic pathway. Sweat chloride concentrations can sometimes be normal or borderline in people with a mild *CFTR* mutation. Thus, genetic mutation analysis or nasal potential difference testing may be required to make the diagnosis of CF.

REPRODUCTIVE TISSUES

The male reproductive tract is exquisitely sensitive to defects in CFTR function. Even carriers of one CF gene can present with isolated male infertility. Azoospermia results from an atretic or absent vas deferens that begins in utero. Most males with CF are infertile by this mechanism.

DISORDERS RELATED TO THE CYSTIC FIBROSIS TRANSMEMBRANE CONDUCTANCE REGULATOR

CONGENITAL BILATERAL ABSENCE OF THE VAS DEFERENS

Male infertility due to obstructive azoospermia is a consistent feature of CF. It has been estimated that 98% of all males with CF have this condition.[114] One notable exception has been males who carry the 3849 + 10 kbC→T mutation, where a substantial fraction are fertile.[88] Male infertility is due to malformation of structures derived from the Wolffian duct reproductive tract manifesting as atrophy of the vas deferens. The seminal vesicles and associated structures can also be involved.[115] Abnormal development of the male reproductive tract begins in utero and continues in the first year of life.[114] On occasion, only one of the vas deferens is destroyed while the other remains patent. This reduced-fertility condition is termed unilateral absence of the vas deferens. Males with CF produce sperm, although spermatic morphologic abnormalities have been reported.

Congenital bilateral absence of the vas deferens (CBAVD) has also been reported in healthy males as an isolated cause of male infertility.[116] It has been estimated that approximately 1 in 5000 males are affected with this condition. Because of the phenotypic overlap between CBAVD and male infertility seen in CF males, investigators analyzed the *CFTR* genes in males with isolated CBAVD and discovered that a high proportion carried CF mutations.[117] More recent studies with extensive analysis of the *CFTR* gene indicate that approximately 86% of CBAVD patients carry at least one deleterious mutation.[118] ΔF508 is the most common mutation occurring in approximately 44% of the cases.[118] The second most common *CFTR* mutation in CBAVD males (32%) is the 5T polymorphism of the intron 8 splice acceptor.[119] The frequency of 5T in the general population (10% carrier rate) posed a question as to how it could be associated with male infertility. Pedigree studies revealed that 5T is inconsistently associated with CBAVD, suggesting that other variables contribute to the disease. The dinucleotide TG tract immediately adjacent to the T tract (see earlier) determines whether the 5T variant produces male infertility in an individual who carries a mutation in his other *CFTR* gene.[34,37] The mutation R117H is also quite common in males with CBAVD. Approximately 10% of CBAVD males carry this mutation, yet less than 1% of CF patients carry this mutation. The 5T variant in intron 8 also plays a role in this phenomenon. The R117H mutation has occurred at least twice in human evolution—once in association with the 5T variant and once in association with the more common 7T variant.[120] Males and females who have a CF mutation paired with R117H and the 5T variant invariably have a CF phenotype, while those males who have R117H with the 7T variant usually develop CBAVD, although some cases of CF have been observed.[118,120] Notably, females with this combination of mutations have presented with pancreatitis and with a normal phenotype.[121,122]

PANCREATITIS

Pancreatitis is a rare presenting sign of CF in patients with residual pancreatic function.[123] Isolated pancreatitis does not present with similar clinical features to CF. However, the concept that CFTR dysfunction may play a role in idiopathic pancreatitis is supported by two observations. First, sweat electrolyte concentrations have been found to be elevated in a subset of chronic pancreatitis patients.[124] Second, CFTR is known to be expressed in pancreatic ducts, a major site of disease in pancreatitis. In 1998, two studies of patients with idiopathic pancreatitis found an increased frequency of mutations in the *CFTR* gene.[121,125] In both studies, the frequency of CFTR mutations in the pancreatitis patients was significantly higher than in the control population and higher than the expected frequency in the general population. Several other reports have since confirmed that CF mutations occur at a higher frequency in patients with isolated pancreatitis.[126–129] However, it appears that additional genetic or environmental influences are required for the development of pancreatitis.[130] Mutations in other genes known to give rise to monogenic forms of pancreatitis such as the secretory trypsinogen inhibitor gene *ST8SIA4* (*PST1*) can combine with *CFTR* mutations to increase the risk of developing pancreatitis.[126,127] While nonalcoholic chronic pancreatitis has been associated with CF mutations, it is not clear that the risk of developing pancreatitis in the case of alcohol abuse is increased in the presence of *CFTR* mutations.[131]

SINUSITIS

Chronic sinusitis is a consistent feature of CF, including mild forms of the disease.[123] In addition, some males with CBAVD and *CFTR* mutations also have chronic rhinosinusitis[132,133] Since the sinus epithelium is reliant on CFTR function for fluid and electrolyte transport, alterations in CFTR could play a role in isolated cases of chronic rhinosinusitis. Indeed, patients who presented with chronic rhinosinusitis to an otorhinolaryngology clinic were found to have a higher frequency of CF mutations than disease-free control populations, suggesting that deleterious mutations in *CFTR* predispose to the development of sinusitis.[44] Two other studies have found that patients with chronic rhinosinusitis have an increased frequency of CF mutations,[134,135] while one study did not find this association.[136] More recently it has been demonstrated that the prevalence of chronic rhinosinusitis in CF carriers is approximately twice the population prevalence.[137] Thus, reduction of CFTR function by approximately 50% appears to increase the risk of developing chronic forms of sinus disease.

THERAPY

CURRENT INTERVENTIONS

The standard therapeutic regimens in CF consist of: pancreatic enzymes; fat-soluble vitamins; inhaled recombinant human DNase; intravenous, oral, or inhaled antibiotics (aminoglycosides, macrolides, penicillins, fluoroquinolones, cephalosporins, antifungals); mucolytics; chest physiotherapy devices; anti-inflammatory drugs (inhaled or systemic steroids, nonsteroidal agents); and H2 or proton pump blockers. None of these therapies treats the fundamental defect in CF, the dysfunctional CFTR. Linking the absence of the CFTR ion channel to the CF phenotype has been a complex undertaking for many researchers around the world. It is predicted that a better understanding of the properties of CFTR should lead to novel, and perhaps multiple, therapeutic targets.

EXPERIMENTAL GENETIC-BASED THERAPIES

There are more than 1000 different disease-causing mutations reported for the *CFTR* gene. Some occur more frequently among certain ethnic groups or with certain geographic origins. The classification scheme based on the molecular consequences of the mutation presents opportunities for novel therapeutic intervestions (see Figs. 58-1 and 58-2).[68] The ΔF508 deletion of a phenylalanine at position 508 has a 70% allelic frequency and a 48% homozygous frequency.[94] This missense mutation produces a full-length protein in the ER that is unstable and preferentially targeted for proteolytic degradation in the proteosome.[76,78,138–140] The ΔF508 protein is absent from the Golgi cisternae, the plasma membrane, and the intervening vesicular pathways between ER and Golgi and between Golgi and the plasma membrane. The ΔF508 mutation and others such as N1303K or P574H mutations[141] that also are misprocessed in the ER have been grouped together as class II mutations in *CFTR*.[142] Pharmacologic restoration of ΔF508 to the biosynthetic pathway is a logical goal, because measurements of chloride channel function in ΔF508 suggest impairment but not complete absence of chloride conductance.[143,144] Phase I and II clinical trials of low molecular weight investigational drugs such as phenylbutyrate[145,146] and curcumin[147] have not fully restored the normal phenotype, perhaps because the channel is only partially functional and is unstable at the plasma membrane.

Class I mutations are associated with absent CFTR function because of an unstable mRNA species that is prematurely degraded before a full-length protein can be generated by the ribosome. The mRNA levels for these mutations are extremely low. Examples in this class include the G542X, W1282X, R553X, and 621 + 1G→T. The premature stop codon mutations in this class present an opportunity for correction at the level of the interaction between the ribosome and transfer RNA. Phase I and II clinical trials of topical aminoglycoside to restore readthrough of the premature stop codon have suggested biologic efficacy.[148–150]

Class III mutations produce full-length mRNA and protein that is delivered in normal quantities to the plasma membrane. Yet function is undetectable, because the protein is defective for cAMP regulation of chloride transport. This group includes G551D and G551S. A lead compound has already been identified that is capable of activating the G551D channel to near–wild type levels, offering the greatest hope for pharmacologic correction.[151–154]

Class IV mutations are also present on the plasma membrane and retain a partial conductance to chloride. The R117H, R334W, and R347P mutations are examples that appear to yield a milder clinical phenotype (pancreatic sufficiency) even when in combination with a more severe allele. This dominant feature of the class IV mutations leads to additional optimism, since even partial restoration of chloride conductance to a patient with homozygous ΔF508 alleles should be of significant therapeutic benefit.

Class V mutations lead to reduced levels of a normally functioning CFTR by splicing errors during the production of mRNA. Examples of class V mutations include 3849 + 10 kB C→T, A455E, or 2789 + 5G→A. Such mutations lead to alternative splicing of CFTR by inefficient alternative processes that are incomplete, so that some proportion of CFTR mRNA remains full length. Other forms of mutations in this class are located in the promoter region of the gene and reduce the amount of normal mRNA for CFTR. Thus, genetic methods to up-regulate CFTR mRNA may be sufficient to have real impact on this group of patients.

Recently, newer classifications of mutants have been proposed to describe versions of CFTR that are unable to interact properly with other ion channels or unable to be moved between subapical vesicles and the plasma membrane.[155,156] These have been labeled classes 6A and 6B.

With better understanding of the functional consequences of specific mutations in *CFTR*, future therapies for CF may be much more targeted to what is unique about an individual. This will mandate full genotyping of every CF patient. Class I mutations with absent or low levels of CFTR mRNA might respond to enhancement of transcription of mRNA and stabilization of the mRNA. For class I mutations that produce a truncated CFTR protein because of early stop codons, mechanisms to read through the stop may be used. Class II mutant proteins that are unstable in the ER and removed for degradation might be amenable to modulation of ER and ER-associated chaperones and chaperone-CFTR interactions. The mutations that are inefficient at escape from the Golgi, or transport through the cytoplasmic matrix to the plasma membrane, could be responsive to modulation of the cytoskeleton or CFTR-interacting proteins. Class III mutants with disrupted ion conductance may be overcome by compounds that interact directly with CFTR to stimulate conductance through non-cAMP-mediated processes. In all situations, augmentation of alternative chloride channels could be partially effective at ameliorating the CF phenotype. Gene therapy to add excess wild-type CFTR proteins (while theoretically most desirable, since carriers of *CFTR* mutations who have 50% of normal wild-type CFTR function do not suffer from the consequences of the mutant allele) will only be completely effective if the mutant *CFTR* that remains within the cell does not continue to trigger pathways that promote injury or inflammation. The adeno-associated virus appears to deliver wild-type CFTR to the airways for a limited life span and with minimal toxicities.[157–159] Non-viral carriers such as cationic liposomes or compacted DNA are similarly nontoxic, with transient biologic effect.[160] Targeting these genetic therapies to the affected tissues and possibly stem cells within these tissues is under intensive investigation.

REFERENCES

1. Andersen DH, Hodges RG: Celiac syndrome. Am J Dis Child 1946;72: 62–80.
2. Knowlton RG, Cohen-Haguenauer O, Van Cong N, et al: A polymorphic DNA marker linked to cystic fibrosis is located on chromosome 7. Nature 1985;318:380–382.
3. Tsui LC, Buchwald M, Barker D, et al: Cystic fibrosis locus defined by a genetically linked polymorphic DNA marker. Science 1985;239:1054–1057.
4. Rommens JM, Iannuzzi MC, Kerem B, et al: Identification of the cystic fibrosis gene. Chromosome walking and jumping. Science 1989;245: 1059–1065.
5. Riordan JR, Rommens JM, Kerem B, et al: Identification of the cystic fibrosis gene. Cloning and characterization of complementary DNA. Science 1989;245:1066–1073.
6. Ellsworth RE, Jamison DC, Touchman JW, et al: Comparative genomic sequence analysis of the human and mouse cystic fibrosis transmembrane conductance regulator genes. Proc Natl Acad Sci USA 2000;97:1172–1177.
7. Thomas JW, Touchman JW, Blakesley RW, et al: Comparative analyses of multi-species sequences from targeted genomic regions. Nature 2003; 424:788–793.
8. Chou J-L, Rozmahel R, Tsui LC: Characterization of the promoter region of the cystic fibrosis transmembrane conductance regulator gene. J Biol Chem 1991;266:24471–24476.
9. Koh J, Sferra TJ, Collins FS: Characterization of the cystic fibrosis transmembrane conductance regulator promoter region. J Biol Chem 1993;268: 15912–15921.
10. Yoshimura K, Nakamura H, Trapnell BC, et al: The cystic fibrosis gene has a "housekeeping"-type promoter and is expressed at low levels in cells of epithelial origin. J Biol Chem 1991;266:9140–9144.
11. Engelhardt JF, Yankaskas JR, Ernst SA, et al: Submucosal glands are the predominant site of CFTR expression in the human bronchus. Nat Genet 1992;2:240–247.
12. Tizzano EF, Chitayat D, Buchwald M: Cell-specific localization of CFTR mRNA shows developmentally regulated expression in human fetal tissues. Hum Mol Genet 1993;2:219–224.
13. Trezise AEO, Chambers JA, Wardle CJ, et al: Expression of the cystic fibrosis gene in human foetal tissues. Hum Mol Genet 1993;2(3):213–218.
14. Matthews RP, McKnight GS: Characterization of the cAMP response element of the cystic fibrosis transmembrane conductance regulator gene promoter. J Biol Chem 1996;271:31869–31877.
15. Moulin DS, Manson AL, Nuthall HN, et al: In vivo analysis of DNase I hypersensitive sites in the human CFTR gene. Mol Med 1999;5:211–223.
16. Nuthall HN, Vassaux G, Huxley C, Harris A: Analysis of a DNase I hypersensitive site located −20.9 kb upstream of the CFTR gene. Eur J Biochem 1999;266:431–443.
17. Smith DJ, Nuthall HN, Majetti ME, Harris A: Multiple potential intragenic regulatory elements in the CFTR gene. Genomics 2000;64:90–96.
18. Ulatowski LM, Whitmore KL, Romigh T, et al: Strain-specific variants of the mouse Cftr promoter region reveal transcriptional regulatory elements. Hum Mol Genet 2004;13:1933–1941.
19. Cutting GR: Splicing of the CFTR gene. In: Dodge JA, Brock DJH, Widdicombe JH, eds: Current Topics in Cystic Fibrosis, Vol. II. Chichester: Wiley & Sons, 1994, pp 55–74.
20. Hull J, Shackleton S, Harris A: Analysis of mutations and alternative splicing patterns in the CFTR gene using mRNA derived from nasal epithelial cells. Hum Mol Genet 1994;3:1141–1146.
21. Horowitz B, Tsung SS, Hart P, et al: Alternative splicing of CFTR Cl^- channels in the heart. Am J Physiol 1993;264(6, pt. 2):H2214–H2220.
22. Hart P, Warth JD, Levesque PC, et al: Cystic fibrosis gene encodes a cAMP-dependent chloride channel in heart. Proc Natl Acad Sci USA 1996; 93:6343–6348.
23. Xie J, Drumm ML, Zhao J, et al: Human epithelial cystic fibrosis transmembrane conductance regulator without exon 5 maintains partial chloride channel function in intracellular membranes. Biophys J 1996;71: 3148–3156.
24. Morelos MM, Carroll TP, Morita T, et al: Both the wild type and a functional isoform of CFTR are expressed in kidney. Am J Physiol 1996; 270:F1038–F1048.
25. Chu C-S, Trapnell BC, Murtagh JJ, et al: Variable deletion of exon 9 coding sequences in cystic fibrosis transmembrane conductance regulator gene mRNA transcripts in normal bronchial epithelium. EMBO J 1991; 10:1355–1363.
26. Strong TV, Wilkinson DJ, Mansoura MK, et al: Expression of an abundantly alternatively spliced form of the cystic fibrosis transmembrane conductance regulator (CFTR) gene is not associated with a cAMP-activated chloride conductance. Hum Mol Genet 1993;2:225–230.
27. Chu C-S, Trapnell BC, Curristin S, et al: Genetic basis of variable exon 9 skipping in cystic fibrosis transmembrane conductance regulator mRNA. Nat Genet 1993;3:151–156.
28. Chu C-S, Trapnell BC, Curristin SM, et al: Extensive post-translational deletion of the coding sequences for part of nucleotide-binding fold 1 in respiratory epithelial mRNA transcripts of the cystic fibrosis transmembrane conductance regulator gene is not associated with the clinical manifestations of cystic fibrosis. J Clin Invest 1992;90:785–790.
29. Niksic M, Romano M, Buratti E, et al: Functional analysis of *cis*-acting elements regulating the alternative splicing of human CFTR exon 9. Hum Mol Genet 1999;8:2339–2349.
30. Pagani F, Buratti E, Stuani C, et al: Splicing factors induce cystic fibrosis transmembrane regulator exon 9 skipping through a nonevolutionarily conserved intronic element. J Biol Chem 2000;275:21041–21047.
31. Hefferon TW, Broackes-Carter FC, Harris A, Cutting GR: Atypical 5' splice sites cause CFTR exon 9 to be vulnerable to skipping. Am J Hum Genet 2002;71:294–303.
32. Mak V, Jarvi K, Zielenski J, et al: Higher proportion of intact exon 9 CFTR MRNA in nasal epithelium compared with vas deferens. Hum Mol Genet 1997;6:2099–2107.
33. Teng H, Jorissen M, Poppel H, et al: Increased proportion of exon 9 alternatively spliced CFTR transcripts in vas deferens compared with nasal epithelial cells. Hum Mol Genet 1997;6:85–90.
34. Cuppens H, Lin W, Jaspers M, et al: Polyvariant mutant cystic fibrosis transmembrane conductance regulator genes. The polymorphic (TG)m locus explains the partial penetrance of the 5T polymorphism as a disease mutation. J Clin Invest 1998;101:487–496.
35. Buratti E, Dork T, Zuccato E, et al: Nuclear factor TDP-43 and SR proteins promote in vitro and in vivo CFTR exon 9 skipping. EMBO J 2001;20:1774–1784.
36. Hefferon TW, Groman JD, Yurk CE, Cutting GR: A variable dinucleotide repeat in the CFTR gene contributes to phenotype diversity by forming RNA secondary structures that alter splicing. Proc Natl Acad Sci USA 2004;101:3504–3509.
37. Groman JD, Hefferon TW, Casals T, et al: Variation in a repeat sequence determines whether a common variant of the cystic fibrosis transmembrane conductance regulator gene is pathogenic or benign. Am J Hum Genet 2004;74:176–179.

38. Will K, Stuhrmann M, Dean M, Schmidtke J: Alternative splicing in the first nucleotide binding fold of CFTR. Hum Mol Genet 1993;2:231–235.
39. Melo CA, Serra C, Stoyanova V, et al: Alternative splicing of a previously unidentified CFTR exon introduces an in-frame stop codon 5' of the R region. FEBS Lett 1993;329(1,2):159–162.
40. Delaney SJ, Rich DP, Thomson SA, et al: Cystic fibrosis transmembrane conductance regulator splice variants are not conserved and fail to produce chloride channels. Nat Genet 1993;4:426–430.
41. Slomski R, Schloesser M, Berg LP: et al: Omission of exon 12 in cystic fibrosis transmembrane conductance regulator (CFTR) gene transcripts. Hum Genet 1992;89:615–619.
42. Yoshimura K, Chu CS, Crystal RG: Alternative splicing of intron 23 of the human cystic fibrosis transmembrane conductance regulator gene resulting in a novel exon and transcript coding for a shortened intracytoplasmic C terminus. J Biol Chem 1993;268:686–690.
43. Romey MC, Guittard C, Chazalette JP, et al: Complex allele [−102T > A + S549R(T > G)] is associated with milder forms of cystic fibrosis than allele S549R(T > G) alone. Hum Genet 1999;105:145–150.
44. Wang X, Moylan B, Leopold DA, et al: Mutation in the gene responsible for cystic fibrosis and predisposition to chronic rhinosinusitis in the general population. JAMA 2000;284:1814–1819.
45. Aznarez I, Chan EM, Zielenski J, et al: Characterization of disease-associated mutations affecting an exonic splicing enhancer and two cryptic splice sites in exon 13 of the cystic fibrosis transmembrane conductance regulator gene. Hum Mol Genet 2003;12:2031–2040.
46. Steiner B, Truninger K, Sanz J, et al: The role of common single-nucleotide polymorphisms on exon 9 and exon 12 skipping in nonmutated CFTR alleles. Hum Mutat 2004;24:120–129.
47. Bobadilla JL, Macek M, Fine JP, Farrell PM: Cystic fibrosis. A worldwide analysis of CFTR mutations—correlation with incidence data and application to screening. Hum Mutat 2002;19:575–606.
48. WHO/ECFTN/ICF(M)A/ECFS: The molecular genetic epidemiology of cystic fibrosis. Report of a joint meeting of WHO/ECFTN/ICF(M)A/ECFS, Genoa, Italy, 19 June 2002. 6-19-2002. WHO.
49. Cutting GR, Curristin SM, Nash E, et al: Analysis of four diverse population groups indicates that a subset of cystic fibrosis mutations occur in common among Caucasians. Am J Hum Genet 1992;50:1185–1194.
50. Macek M Jr, Macoková A, Hamosh A, et al: Identification of common CF mutations in African-Americans with cystic fibrosis increases the detection rate to 75%. Am J Hum Genet 1997;60:1122–1127.
51. Carles S, Desgeorges M, Goldman A, et al: First report of CFTR mutations in black cystic fibrosis patients of southern African origin. J Med Genet 1996;33:802–804.
52. Macek M Jr, Hamosh A, Kiesewetter S, et al: Identification of a novel nonsense mutation (L88X) in exon 3 of the CFTR gene on a native Korean cystic fibrosis chromosome. Hum Mutat 1992;1:501–502.
53. Macek M Jr, Mercier B, Macková A, et al: Sensitivity of the denaturing gradient gel electrophoresis technique in detection of known mutations and novel Asian mutations in the CFTR gene. Hum Mutat 1997;9: 136–147.
54. Estivill X, Bancells C, Ramos C: Geographic distribution and regional origin of 272 cystic fibrosis mutations in European populations. The Biomed CF Mutation Analysis Consortium. Hum Mutat 1997;10:135–154.
55. Zielenski J, Fujiwara TM, Markiewicz D, et al: Identification of the M1101K mutation in the cystic fibrosis transmembrane conductance regulator (CFTR) gene and complete detection of cystic fibrosis mutations in the Hutterite population. Am J Med Genet 1993;52:609–615.
56. Grody WW, Cutting GR, Klinger KW, et al: Laboratory standards and guidelines for population-based cystic fibrosis carrier screening. Genet Med 2001;3:149–154.
57. Cheadle JP, Goodchild MC, Meredith AL: Direct sequencing of the complete CFTR gene. The molecular characterisation of 99.5% of CF chromosomes in Wales. Hum Mol Genet 1993;2:1551–1556.
58. Girodon-Boulandet E, Cazeneuve C, Goossens M: Screening practices for mutations in the CFTR gene ABCC7. Hum Mutat 2000;15:135–149.
59. Riordan JR: Assembly of functional CFTR chloride channels. Annu Rev Physiol 2005;67:701–718.
60. Nilius B, Droogmans G: Amazing chloride channels. An overview. Acta Physiol Scand 2003;177:119–147.
61. Drumm ML, Wilkinson DJ, Smit LS, et al: Chloride conductance expressed by delta F508 and other mutant CFTRs in *Xenopus* oocytes. Science 1991;254:1797–1799.
62. Hwang TC, Lu L, Zeitlin PL, et al: Cl^- channels in CF. Lack of activation by protein kinase C and cAMP-dependent protein kinase. Science 1989;244:1351–1353.
63. Lewis HA, Zhao X, Wang C, et al: Impact of the ΔF508 mutation in first nucleotide-binding domain of human cystic fibrosis transmembrane conductance regulator on domain folding and structure. J Biol Chem 2005; 280:1346–1353.
64. Horster M: Embryonic epithelial membrane transporters. Am J Physiol Renal Physiol 2000;279:F982–F996.
65. Barker PM, Boucher RC, Yankaskas JR: Bioelectric properties of cultured monolayers from epithelium of distal human fetal lung. Am J Physiol 1995;268:L270–L277.
66. Boucher RC, Stutts MJ, Knowles MR, et al: Na^+ transport in cystic fibrosis respiratory epithelia. Abnormal basal rate and response to adenylate cyclase activation. J Clin Invest 1986;78:1245–1252.
67. Gabriel SE, Clarke LL, Boucher RC, Stutts MJ: CFTR and outward rectifying chloride channels are distinct proteins with a regulatory relationship. Nature 1993;363:263–268.
68. Welsh MJ, Smith AE: Molecular mechanisms of CFTR chloride channel dysfunction in cystic fibrosis. Cell 1993;73:1251–1254.
69. Frischmeyer PA, Dietz HC: Nonsense-mediated mRNA decay in health and disease. Hum Mol Genet 1999;8:1893–1900.
70. Hamosh A, Trapnell BC, Zeitlin PL, et al: Severe deficiency of CFTR mRNA carrying nonsense mutations R553X and W1316X in respiratory epithelial cells of patients with cystic fibrosis. J Clin Invest 1991;88:1880–1885.
71. Rolfini R, Cabrini G: Nonsense mutation R1162X of the cystic fibrosis transmembrane conductance regulator gene does not reduce messenger RNA expression in nasal epithelial tissue. J Clin Invest 1993;92: 2683–2687.
72. Will K, Dörk T, Stuhrmann M, et al: Transcript analysis of CFTR nonsense mutations in lymphocytes and nasal epithelial cells from cystic fibrosis patients. Hum Mutat 1995;5:210–220.
73. Dietz HC, Valle D, Francomano CA, et al: The skipping of constitutive exons in vivo induced by nonsense mutations. Science 1993;259:680–683.
74. Hull J, Shackleton S, Harris A: The stop mutation R553X in the CFTR gene results in exon skipping. Genomics 1994;19:362–364.
75. Zielenski J, Bozon D, Markiewicz D, et al: Analysis of CFTR transcripts in nasal epithelial cells and lymphoblasts of a cystic fibrosis patient with 621 + 1G→T and 711 + 1G→T mutations. Hum Mol Genet 1993;2:683–687.
76. Cheng SH, Gregory RJ, Marshall J, et al: Defective intracellular transport and processing of CFTR is the molecular basis of most cystic fibrosis. Cell 1990;63:827–834.
77. Kartner N, Augustinas O, Jensen TJ, et al: Mislocalization of ΔF508 CFTR in cystic fibrosis sweat gland. Nat Genet 1992;1:321–327.
78. Jensen TJ, Loo MA, Pind S, et al: Multiple proteolytic systems, including the proteasome, contribute to CFTR processing. Cell 1995;83:129–135.
79. Denning GM, Anderson MP, Amara JF, et al: Processing of mutant cystic fibrosis transmembrane conductance regulator is temperature-sensitive. Nature 1992;358:761–764.
80. Lukacs GL, Chang X-B, Bear C, et al: The ΔF508 mutation decreases the stability of cystic fibrosis transmembrane conductance regulator in the plasma membrane. J Biol Chem 1993;268(29):21592–21598.
81. Champigny G, Imler J-L, Puchelle E, et al: A change in gating mode leading to increased intrinsic Cl^- channel activity compensates for defective processing in a mild form of the disease. EMBO J 1995;14:2417–2423.
82. Sheppard DN, Ostedgaard LS, Winter MC, Welsh MJ: Mechanism of dysfunction of two nucleotide binding domain mutations in cystic fibrosis transmembrane conductance regulator that are associated with pancreatic sufficiency. EMBO J 1995;14:876–883.
83. Anderson MP, Welsh MJ: Regulation by ATP and ADP of CFTR chloride channels that contain mutant nucleotide-binding domains. Science 1992;257:1701–1704.
84. Logan J, Hiestand D, Daram P, et al: Cystic fibrosis transmembrane conductance regulator mutations that disrupt nucleotide binding. J Clin Invest 1994;94:228–236.
85. Strong TV, Smit LS, Turpin SV, et al: Cystic fibrosis gene mutation in two sisters with mild disease and normal sweat electrolyte levels. N Engl J Med 1991;325:1630–1634.
86. Sheppard DN, Rich DP, Ostedgaard LS, et al: Mutations in CFTR associated with mild-disease-form Cl^- channels with altered pore properties. Nature 1993;362:160–164.
87. Tabcharani JA, Rommens JM, Hou Y-X, et al: Multi-ion pore behavior in the CFTR chloride channel. Nature 1993;366(4):79–82.
88. Highsmith WE Jr, Burch LH, Zhou Z, et al: A novel mutation in the cystic fibrosis gene in patients with pulmonary disease but normal sweat chloride concentrations. N Engl J Med 1994;331:974–980.
89. Schwiebert EM, Benos DJ, Egan ME, et al: CFTR is a conductance regulator as well as a chloride channel. Physiol Rev 1999;79:S145–S166.

90. Fulmer SB, Schwiebert EM, Morales MM, et al: Two cystic fibrosis transmembrane conductance regulator mutations have different effects on both pulmonary phenotype and regulation of outwardly rectified chloride currents. Proc Natl Acad Sci USA 1995;92:6832–6836.
91. Ismailov II, Awayda MS, Jovov B, et al: Regulation of epithelial sodium channels by the cystic fibrosis transmembrane conductance regulator. J Biol Chem 1996;271:4725–4732.
92. Moyer BD, Denton J, Karlson KH, et al: A PDZ-interacting domain in CFTR is an apical membrane polarization signal. J Clin Invest 1999; 104:1353–1361.
93. Fu J, Ji HL, Naren AP, Kirk KL: A cluster of negative charges at the amino terminal tail of CFTR regulates ATP-dependent channel gating. J Physiol 2001;536:459–470.
94. Cystic Fibrosis Genotype/Phenotype Consortium: Correlation between genotype and phenotype in cystic fibrosis. N Engl J Med 1993;329: 1308–1313.
95. Knowles MR, Durie PR: What is cystic fibrosis? N Engl J Med 2002;347: 439–442.
96. Kristidis P, Bozon D, Corey M, et al: Genetic determination of exocrine pancreatic function in cystic fibrosis. Am J Hum Genet 1992;50:1178–1184.
97. Wilschanski M, Zielenski J, Markiewicz D, et al: Correlation of sweat chloride concentration with classes of the cystic fibrosis transmembrane conductance regulator gene mutations. J Pediatr 1995;127:705–710.
98. Gan K-H, Veeze HJ, Van den Ouweland, et al: A cystic fibrosis mutation associated with mild lung disease. N Engl J Med 1995;333:95–99.
99. De Braekeleer M, Allard C, Leblanc J-P, et al: Genotype-phenotype correlation in cystic fibrosis patients compound heterozygous for the A455E mutation. Hum Genet 1997;101:208–211.
100. Koch C, Cuppens H, Rainisio M, et al: European Epidemiologic Registry of Cystic Fibrosis (ERCF). Comparison of major disease manifestations between patients with different classes of mutations. Pediatr Pulmonol 2001;31:1–12.
101. Ferec C, Verlingue C, Guillermit H, et al: Genotype analysis of adult cystic fibrosis patients. Hum Mol Genet 1993;2:1557–1560.
102. Brancolini V, Cremonesi L, Belloni E, et al: Search for mutations in pancreatic sufficient cystic fibrosis Italian patients. Detection of 90% of molecular defects and identification of three novel mutations. Hum Genet 1995;96:312–318.
103. Lebecque P, Leal T, De Boeck C, et al: Mutations of the cystic fibrosis gene and intermediate sweat chloride levels in children. Am J Respir Crit Care Med 2002;165:757–761.
104. Feldmann D, Coudere R, Audrezet MP, et al: CFTR genotypes in patients with normal or borderline sweat chloride levels. Hum Mutat 2003;22:340.
105. McKone EF, Emerson SS, Edwards KL, Aitken ML: Effect of genotype on phenotype and mortality in cystic fibrosis. A retrospective cohort study. Lancet 2003;361:1671–1676.
106. Hamosh A, King TM, Rosenstein BJ, et al: Cystic fibrosis patients bearing the common missense mutation Gly→Asp at codon 551 and the ΔF508 are indistinguishable from ΔF508 homozygotes except for decreased risk of meconium ileus. Am J Hum Genet 1992;51:245–250.
107. Goris ML, Zhu HJ, Blankenberg F, et al: An automated approach to quantitative air trapping measurements in mild cystic fibrosis. Chest 2003; 123:1655–1663.
108. Tandon R, Derkay C: Contemporary management of rhinosinusitis and cystic fibrosis. Curr Opin Otolaryngol Head Neck Surg 2003;11: 41–44.
109. Konstan MW, Hilliard KA, Norvell TM, Berger M: Bronchoalveolar lavage findings in cystic fibrosis patients with stable, clinically mild lung disease suggest ongoing infection and inflammation. Am J Respir Crit Care Med 1994;150:448–454.
110. Khan TZ, Wagner JS, Bost T, et al: Early pulmonary inflammation in infants with cystic fibrosis. Am J Respir Crit Care Med 1995;151: 1075–1082.
111. Armstrong DS, Grimwood K, Carlin JB, et al: Lower airway inflammation in infants and young children with cystic fibrosis. Am J Respir Crit Care Med 1997;156:1197–1204.
112. Doring G, Hoiby N: Early intervention and prevention of lung disease in cystic fibrosis. A European consensus. J Cyst Fibros 2004;3:67–91.
113. Saiman L, Siegel J: Infection control in cystic fibrosis. Clin Microbiol Rev 2004;17:57–71.
114. Kaplan E, Schwachman H, Perlmutter AD, et al: Reproductive failure in males with cystic fibrosis. N Engl J Med 1968;279:65–69.
115. Wilschanski M, Corey M, Durie P, et al: Diversity of reproductive tract abnormalities in men with cystic fibrosis. JAMA 1996;276:607–608.
116. McKusick VA: Online Mendelian Inheritance in Man [abstract]. Johns Hopkins Institute for Genetic Medicine, Johns Hopkins University. Available at http://www.ncbi.nlm.nih.gov/entrez/query.fcgi?db=OMIM.
117. Anguiano A, Oates RD, Amos JA, et al: Congenital bilateral absence of the vas deferens—a primarily genital form of cystic fibrosis. JAMA 1992; 267:1794–1797.
118. Claustres M, Guittard C, Bozon D, et al: Spectrum of CFTR mutations in cystic fibrosis and in congenital absence of the vas deferens in France. Hum Mutat 2000;16:143–156.
119. Chillón M, Casals T, Mercier B, et al: Mutations in the cystic fibrosis gene in patients with congenital absence of the vas deferens. N Engl J Med 1995;332:1475–1480.
120. Kiesewetter S, Macek M Jr, Davis C, et al: A mutation in the cystic fibrosis transmembrane conductance regulator gene produces different phenotypes depending on chromosomal background. Nat Genet 1993; 5:274–278.
121. Cohn JA, Friedman KJ, Noone PG, et al: Relation between mutations of the cystic fibrosis gene and idiopathic pancreatitis. N Engl J Med 1998; 339:653–658.
122. Witt DR, Hallam P, Wi S, et al: Cystic fibrosis heterozygote screening in 5,161 pregnant women. Am J Hum Genet 1996;58:823–835.
123. Welsh MJ, Ramsey BW, Accurso FJ, Cutting GR: Cystic fibrosis. In: Scriver CR, Beaudet AL, Valle D, Sly WS, eds: The Metabolic and Molecular Bases of Inherited Disease. New York: McGraw-Hill, 2001, pp 5121–5188.
124. Bank S, Marks IN, Novis B: Sweat electrolytes in chronic pancreatitis. Am J Dig Dis 1978;23:178–181.
125. Sharer NS, Schwarz M, Malone G, et al: Mutations of the cystic fibrosis gene in patients with chronic pancreatitis. N Engl J Med 1998;339: 645–652.
126. Noone PG, Zhou Z, Silverman LM, et al: Cystic fibrosis gene mutations and pancreatitis risk. Relation to epithelial ion transport and trypsin inhibitor gene mutations. Gastroenterology 2001;121:1310–1319.
127. Audrezet MP, Chen JM, Le Marechal C, et al: Determination of the relative contribution of three genes—the cystic fibrosis transmembrane conductance regulator gene, the cationic trypsinogen gene, and the pancreatic secretory trypsin inhibitor gene—to the etiology of idiopathic chronic pancreatitis. Eur J Hum Genet 2002;10:100–106.
128. Choudari CP, Imperiale TF, Sherman S, et al: Risk of pancreatitis with mutation of the cystic fibrosis gene. Am J Gastroenterol 2004;99: 1358–1363.
129. Gaia E, Salacone P, Gallo M, et al: Germline mutations in CFTR and PSTI genes in chronic pancreatitis patients. Dig Dis Sci 2002;47:2416–2421.
130. Malats N, Casals T, Porta M, et al: Cystic fibrosis transmembrane regulator (CFTR) ΔF508 mutation and 5T allele in patients with chronic pancreatitis and exocrine pancreatic cancer. Gut 2001;48:70–74.
131. Perri F, Piepoli A, Stanziale P, et al: Mutation analysis of the cystic fibrosis transmembrane conductance regulator (CFTR) gene, the cationic trypsinogen (PRSS1) gene, and the serine protease inhibitor, Kazal type 1 (SPINK1) gene in patients with alcoholic chronic pancreatitis. Eur J Hum Genet 2003;11:687–692.
132. Pradal U, Castellani C, Delmarco A, Mastella G: Nasal potential difference in congenital bilateral absence of the vas deferens. Am J Respir Crit Care Med 1998;158:896–901.
133. Castellani C, Bonizzato A, Pradal U, et al: Evidence of mild respiratory disease in men with congenital absence of the vas deferens. Respir Med 1999;93:869–875.
134. Raman V, Clary R, Siegrist KL, et al: Increased prevalence of mutations in the cystic fibrosis transmembrane conductance regulator in children with chronic rhinosinusitis. Pediatrics 2002;109:E13.
135. Coste A, Girodon E, Louis S, et al: Atypical sinusitis in adults must lead to looking for cystic fibrosis and primary ciliary dyskinesia. Laryngoscope 2004;114:839–843.
136. Hytonen M, Patjas M, Vento SI, et al: Cystic fibrosis gene mutations ΔF508 and 394delTT in patients with chronic sinusitis in Finland. Acta Otolaryngol 2001;121:945–947.
137. Wang XJ, Kim J, McWilliams R, Cutting GR: Increased prevalence of chronic rhinosinusitis in carriers of a cystic fibrosis mutation. Arch Otolaryngol Head Neck Surg 2005;131:237–240.
138. Cheng SH, Fang SL, Zabner J, et al: Functional activation of the cystic fibrosis trafficking mutant delta F508-CFTR by overexpression. Am J Physiol 1995;268:L615–L624.
139. Loo MA, Jensen TJ, Cui L, et al: Perturbation of Hsp90 interaction with nascent CFTR prevents its maturation and accelerates its degradation by the proteasome. EMBO J 1998;17:6879–6887.

140. Ward CL, Omura S, Kopito RR: Degradation of CFTR by the ubiquitin-proteasome pathway. Cell 1995;83:121–127.
141. Ostedgaard LS, Zeiher B, Welsh MJ: Processing of CFTR bearing the P574H mutation differs from wild-type and ΔF508-CFTR. J Cell Sci 1999;112:2091–2098.
142. Choo-Kang LR, Zeitlin PL: Type I, II, III, IV, and V cystic fibrosis transmembrane conductance regulator defects and opportunities for therapy. Curr Opin Pulm Med 2000;6:521–529.
143. Li C, Ramjeesingh M, Reyes E, et al: The cystic fibrosis mutation (ΔF508) does not influence the chloride channel activity of CFTR. Nat Genet 1993;3:311–316.
144. Pasyk EA, Foskett JK: Mutant (ΔF508) cystic fibrosis transmembrane conductance regulator Cl^- channel is functional when retained in endoplasmic reticulum of mammalian cells. J Biol Chem 1995;270:12347–12350.
145. Rubenstein RC, Zeitlin PL: A pilot clinical trial of sodium 4-phenylbutyrate (Buphenyl) in ΔF508-homozygous cystic fibrosis patients. Evidence of restoration of nasal epithelial CFTR function. Am J Respir Crit Care Med 1998;157:484–490.
146. Zeitlin PL, Diener-West M, Rubenstein RC, et al: Evidence of CFTR function in cystic fibrosis after systemic administration of 4-phenylbutyrate. Mol Ther 2002;6:119–126.
147. Egan ME, Pearson M, Weiner SA, et al: Curcumin, a major constituent of turmeric, corrects cystic fibrosis defects. Science 2004;304:600–602.
148. Clancy JP, Bebok Z, Jones J, et al: A controlled trial of gentamicin to suppress premature stop codons in CF patients [abstract]. Pediatr Pulmonol 1999;239–240.
149. Wilschanski M, Famini C, Blau H, et al: A pilot study of the effect of gentamicin on nasal potential difference measurements in cystic fibrosis patients carrying stop mutations. Am J Respir Crit Care Med 2000;161: 860–865.
150. Wilschanski M, Yahav Y, Yaacov Y, et al: Gentamicin-induced correction of CFTR function in patients with cystic fibrosis and CFTR stop mutations. N Engl J Med 2003;349:1433–1441.
151. Fischer H, Illek B: Effects of genistein on disease-causing mutant CFTRs [abstract]. Pediatr Pulmonol 1998;S17:239.
152. Gondor M, Nixon PA, Devor DC, et al: Genistein stimulates chloride secretion in normal volunteers and CF patients with a G551D mutation [abstract]. Pediatr Pulmonol 1998;S17:253.
153. Hwang TC, Wang F, Yang IC, Reenstra WW: Genistein potentiates wild-type and ΔF508-CFTR channel activity. Am J Physiol 1997;273: C988–C998.
154. Illek B, Fischer H, Santos GF, et al: cAMP-independent activation of CFTR Cl channels by the tyrosine kinase inhibitor genistein. Am J Physiol 1995;268:C886–C893.
155. Mickle JE, Cutting GR: Clinical implications of cystic fibrosis transmembrane conductance regulator mutations. Clin Chest Med 1998;19: 443–458, v.
156. Haardt M, Benharouga M, Lechardeur D, et al: C-terminal truncations destabilize the cystic fibrosis transmembrane conductance regulator without impairing its biogenesis. A novel class of mutation. J Biol Chem 1999;274:21873–21877.
157. Aitken ML, Moss RB, Waltz DA, et al: A phase I study of aerosolized administration of tgAAVCF to cystic fibrosis subjects with mild lung disease. Hum Gene Ther 2001;12:1907–1916.
158. Flotte TR, Zeitlin PL, Reynolds TC, et al: Phase I trial of intranasal and endobronchial administration of a recombinant adeno-associated virus serotype 2 (rAAV2)-CFTR vector in adult cystic fibrosis patients. A two-part clinical study. Hum Gene Ther 2003;14:1079–1088.
159. Moss RB, Rodman D, Spencer LT, et al: Repeated adeno-associated virus serotype 2 aerosol-mediated cystic fibrosis transmembrane regulator gene transfer to the lungs of patients with cystic fibrosis. A multicenter, double-blind, placebo-controlled trial. Chest 2004;125:509–521.
160. Konstan MW, Davis PB, Wagener JS, et al: Compacted DNA nanoparticles administered to the nasal mucosa of cystic fibrosis subjects are safe and demonstrate partial to complete cystic fibrosis transmembrane regulator reconstitution. Hum Gene Ther 2004;15:1255–1269.

59 Neonatal Screening for Cystic Fibrosis

Michael J. Rock, MD • Philip M. Farrell, MD

PRINCIPLES OF POPULATION-BASED SCREENING

HISTORY AND PRINCIPLES OF NEWBORN SCREENING

Screening, by definition, detects disorders in individuals before the onset of clinical symptoms. The prototypical disorder for newborn screening is phenylketonuria, which results from a lack of the enzyme phenylalanine hydroxylase to catalyze the conversion of phenylalanine to tyrosine. Serum levels of phenylalanine, phenylethylamine, and phenylpyruvic acid increase early in life with the feeding of standard formula or breast milk. The mental retardation that results from this enzyme deficiency can be prevented by the early initiation of a low-phenylalanine formula. In 1963, Robert Guthrie demonstrated that the growth of *Bacillus subtilis* (ATCC6051) is inhibited by beta-2-thienylalanine in a minimal culture medium. This inhibition of growth is prevented by phenylalanine, phenylpyruvic acid, and phenyllactic acid. A simple method to detect phenylketonuria was developed using dried blood spots on filter paper cards. These cards are now also known as Guthrie cards in honor of Dr. Guthrie and this landmark discovery.[1]

NEWBORN SCREENING FOR CYSTIC FIBROSIS

The first demonstration of a potential benefit of early diagnosis of cystic fibrosis (CF) was made in 1970 by Harry Shwachman.[2] In his study of 103 neonates younger than 3 months of age who were diagnosed during a 20-year period, those newborns who were sufficiently ill to be diagnosed during a hospitalization had a decreased survival rate compared with those diagnosed before the development of symptoms or with only mild symptoms. The effect of early diagnosis and treatment in CF was further suggested by a retrospective, observational 7-year study of 16 sibling pairs in which the younger sibling demonstrated better scores on chest radiography, better total clinical scores, better residual volumes, and significantly lower ratios of residual volume to total lung capacity.[3]

Early attempts at CF neonatal screening consisted of measuring increased protein (mainly albumin) in meconium. The BM-test strip (Boehringer-Mannheim Corporation) was used for this test, but it was fraught with multiple difficulties, including the use of a substance that is not traditionally obtained and transported to a centralized testing laboratory. Additionally, CF patients with pancreatic exocrine sufficiency will be missed, and there were many cases of false-positive and false-negative results. Therefore, this test was abandoned. Newborn screening for CF became practical in 1979 with the first description of the elevation of immunoreactive trypsinogen (IRT) in the blood of newborns with CF.[4] This elevation of serum IRT was confirmed from dried blood spots on Guthrie cards, and mass newborn screening for CF became practical. The Cystic Fibrosis Foundation convened a task force in 1983 to consider issues surrounding neonatal screening for CF, and Box 59-1 presents the recommendations from this task force.[5] In addition to confirming the positive effect of early treatment on prognosis, the committee also identified a need for more research on the IRT method and for elucidation of the sensitivity, specificity, and age-related decline of IRT.

The initial screening strategy for CF was measurement of IRT from Guthrie cards obtained in the first 24 to 72 hours of life. If the IRT concentration was higher than the cutoff value, then a second IRT measurement was done at 2 to 4 weeks of age. If this second IRT reading was also high, then a sweat test was recommended to rule out a diagnosis of CF. This screening strategy assumes that infants with CF have a persistent elevation of IRT at 2 to 4 weeks of age, whereas infants without CF have a decline in their IRT levels in the first few weeks of life. However, a disadvantage of the IRT/IRT screening methodology is that infants with CF can have a decline of IRT values in the first few weeks of life.[6] Additionally, the IRT/IRT combination necessitates choosing a high cutoff value, such as the highest 1% of IRT results, so as to have a practical number of infants with positive newborn screens. However, newborn infants with CF can have IRT values that are not above the 99th percentile of IRT values. The discovery of the CF gene[7] in 1989 allowed the development of a two-tier screen. The first tier is IRT measurement, and if this result is above the cutoff value, then the DNA on the original Guthrie card is analyzed for CF mutations. The IRT/DNA screening methodology allows for decreasing the cutoff value of the original IRT to a lower decision point (such as the 94th to 96th percentile), without generating a tremendously increased number of infants with a positive newborn screen. There are several advantages[8] of two-tier IRT/DNA analysis over IRT/IRT testing:

1. Infants can be identified earlier by demonstration of two mutations from the newborn screening.
2. There is better sensitivity, specificity, and positive predictive value with IRT/DNA testing than with IRT testing alone.
3. The IRT/DNA analysis reduces the disproportionate number of positive screens among African American infants or newborns with low Apgar scores.
4. The two-tier strategy avoids the need to arrange for collection of a second specimen as in IRT/IRT screening.
5. There is a genetic counseling benefit for families in which an infant is identified as a CF carrier.

When IRT/DNA screening methodology was first developed, ΔF508 was the only mutation on the second tier of the screen. Screening with ΔF508 allowed identification of CF infants who were homozygous for this mutation and those infants who had one ΔF508 mutation. However, this screening strategy would miss infants who had two non-ΔF508 CF mutations. More recently, CF newborn screening programs have expanded the screening

BOX 59-1 Recommendations from Cystic Fibrosis Foundation Ad Hoc Committee Task Force on Neonatal Screening (1983)

1. Determine the value of early treatment on prognosis and what forms of treatment are best.
2. Determine the benefits and risks of early detection.
3. Determine the reliability and validity of the screening method.
4. Define the incidence and preventability of stigmatization in families with false positive and true positive tests.
5. Determine the cost effectiveness of mass screening.
6. Define the availability of competent counseling for families with false negative, false positive, and true positive tests.

methodology to IRT/*CFTR* multiple-mutation analysis. This results in a substantial increase of the detection sensitivity (to ~99%) and leads to an increase in the direct diagnosis of CF from the newborn screening specimen. Regions of the world that are contemplating the addition of CF newborn screening will need to examine the prevalence of CF mutations in their population and will need to formulate a mutation panel that is relevant for their racial and ethnic mix. Mutations that should be included are those that occur with a prevalence of greater than 0.1%. A panel of 50 suggested mutations has been recommended by Bobadilla and colleagues.[9] With future advances in DNA testing technology, it should be possible to customize mutation panels by region and/or increase the number of mutations for which there is screening without a significant increase in cost.

Sweat testing is necessary in CF newborn screening programs for neonates who have one mutation identified or have two different mutations identified. In the latter case, these newborns could have two mutations on the same chromosome and thus not have CF. In the former case, these newborns are either normal heterozygote carriers or have CF. Although there has been concern that adequate quantities of sweat cannot be obtained from young neonates, this concern has not been substantiated in recent studies. Adequate quantities of sweat can be obtained from young neonates and it is reasonable to proceed with sweat testing in newborns as young as 2 or 3 weeks of age.[10] The interpretation of sweat chloride results in infants, however, is different from that for older children and adults. The traditional interpretation of a sweat chloride value of less than 40 mmol/L as normal and one of 40 to 60 mmol/L as borderline does not apply to infants. Studies have confirmed that, in infants, a sweat chloride value of more than 40 mmol/L is almost invariably associated with a diagnosis of CF, and a sweat chloride value of 30 to 40 mmol/L generates a strong possibility of CF.[11]

COST OF CYSTIC FIBROSIS NEWBORN SCREENING

The traditional method for diagnosing CF is to order sweat tests on newborns with characteristic clinical features such as meconium ileus, diarrhea, failure to thrive, or chronic cough, or when there is a positive family history (which occurs in approximately 15% of cases). However, many normal sweat test results are obtained for every patient with CF diagnosed by this traditional method. There have been estimates of approximately 100 sweat tests done on newborns to diagnose one CF patient.

Newborn screening can potentially reduce costs compared with the traditional method of diagnosis of CF. A survey of hospital laboratories in Wisconsin between the years 1991 and 2000 demonstrated that the number of laboratories performing sweat tests decreased from 44 to 15 and the total number of annual sweat tests decreased from 1670 to 804 during that period.[12] The estimated annual cost of Wisconsin CF newborn screening and diagnosis (IRT/DNA and sweat testing) was $4.58 per newborn infant; this compared favorably to the annual cost per newly diagnosed CF infant using the traditional method of $4.97 per newborn infant. If no additional sweat tests were ordered outside the newborn screening program, then the annual cost of CF neonatal screening in Wisconsin was estimated as $2.66 per newborn. The projected cost of a national CF newborn screening program to the entire United States is estimated as $2.47 per newborn. This is similar to the costs for other screening tests such as that for phenylketonuria.

OUTCOMES OF CLINICAL INVESTIGATIONS

COLORADO

The first newborn screening program to use IRT measurement in the United States was established in Colorado beginning in 1982. Investigators in Colorado have contributed importantly to our knowledge of nutritional deficits in asymptomatic newborns with CF. In their earliest study, Reardon and colleagues demonstrated that 50% of children had poor weight gain at diagnosis at a mean of 5.5 weeks of age.[13] Low serum albumin occurred in 5 of 17 patients, and low prealbumin concentrations were present in 13 of 16 patients. The Colorado investigators extended their previous observations by examining the correction of low serum albumin levels on initiation of pancreatic enzyme therapy after newborn screening.[14] In this follow-up study, hypoalbuminemia was corrected in all children within 2 weeks. In addition to low levels of serum albumin at diagnosis in neonates with CF, it has been shown that low serum concentrations of retinol and α-tocopherol are common at the initial evaluation of neonates diagnosed by newborn screening.[15] One of the early clinical manifestations of CF that can lead to significant morbidity and mortality is the clinical syndrome of protein-calorie malnutrition that is characterized by the triad of hypoproteinemia, edema, and anemia. Newborn screening presents the opportunity to intervene early during this window of opportunity and to avoid the development of kwashiorkor and other conditions of nutritional deficiency.

WISCONSIN

In Wisconsin, a randomized controlled trial of newborn screening was conducted for neonates born between 1985 and 1994. In this study, half of the newborns were randomized to an early-diagnosis group in which the results of the newborn screening test were reported to the study investigators. These newborns underwent a sweat test at approximately 6 weeks of age and were entered into the study if they were diagnosed with CF and the parents consented. The newborn screening tests for the other half of the population were stored on computer, and these newborns presented conventionally with symptoms or a positive family history. To completely identify neonates in both study groups, a unique unblinding protocol was used at 4 years of age. Patients in both study groups were treated with a similar evaluation and treatment protocol at one of the two CF centers in Wisconsin. In the Wisconsin study, there is indisputable evidence of nutritional benefit from screening in the early-diagnosis group.[16] Compared with the conventionally diagnosed patients, this group of patients has improved height and weight that extends into the late teen years. Previously, the dogma was that there is potential for catch-up growth in CF patients diagnosed conventionally. The Wisconsin randomized controlled trial has demonstrated that there is probably a permanent stunting of growth with a delayed diagnosis of CF. Additionally, early diagnosis allows for the immediate institution of vitamin supplementation including fat-soluble vitamins. Patients diagnosed conventionally have a longer period of vitamin E deficiency compared with patients diagnosed by newborn screening. Administration of a cognitive skills index test to these study populations demonstrated that patients diagnosed conventionally with low vitamin E levels have cognitive dysfunction compared with patients diagnosed by newborn screening.[17] This evidence suggests that early supplementation with vitamin E and the prevention of prolonged malnutrition by early diagnosis are associated with better cognitive functioning in children with CF. In the Wisconsin trial, the pulmonary benefits of CF neonatal screening have been more difficult to establish. Lung disease in CF has a variable pattern and age of onset, the methods for quantifying pediatric lung disease are relatively insensitive, and there is variability in genotype and environmental exposures that strongly influences CF lung disease. The Wisconsin trial has shown that both early-diagnosis and conventionally diagnosed patients have very mild lung disease as reflected by a ratio of forced expiratory volume in 1 second to forced vital capacity of greater than 0.8. Quantitative scoring of chest radiographs has revealed significantly better scores in the early-diagnosis group at the time of diagnosis, but these scores become worse after *Pseudomonas aeruginosa* infection develops in these screened patients.[18]

BRITTANY, FRANCE

A study in France compared the outcomes of infants born between January 1, 1989, and December 31, 1998, diagnosed by newborn screening in Brittany, with the outcomes of patients diagnosed conventionally in Loire-Atlantique.[19] Excluding patients with meconium ileus, false-negative screens, deaths independent of CF, and nonclassic CF patients, there were 77 patients diagnosed by neonatal screening in Brittany compared to 36 patients diagnosed conventionally in Loire-Atlantique. There was no significant difference between the two groups in gestational age, birth weight, frequency of ΔF508 mutation, or frequency of ΔF508 homozygotes. However, there was a significant difference in the age of diagnosis, with the newborn-screened patients diagnosed at an average of 38 days of age compared with conventionally diagnosed patients at 472 days of age. Similar to the findings in the Wisconsin study, there were significant differences for weight and height in the screened patients compared with those not screened. The frequencies of the first hospitalization were also lower in the screened population of Brittany. During the entire time of the study, the Shwachman-Kulczycki and Brasfield scores were significantly better in the screened CF patients compared with those not screened. Similar to the Wisconsin study, there were no significant differences between both populations in pulmonary function tests.

THE NETHERLANDS

In the Netherlands there has been long-term observation of patients diagnosed with CF who were in one of three birth cohorts.[20,21] Between March 1973 and March 1979, there was in the northern part of the Netherlands an experimental newborn screening program for CF using albumin content of meconium. There were 19 patients diagnosed by screening during this period versus 25 patients born during this same time and diagnosed conventionally. The third birth cohort consisted of patients with CF born in the same region between 1979 and 1986 and diagnosed conventionally (postscreening group). Patients in the screened group maintained stable values of forced expiratory volume in 1 second during the observation period, while patients in the unscreened and postscreened groups showed a statistically significant decrease in lung function with increasing age. Up to the age of 12 years, 52% of the unscreened patients were chronically colonized with *P. aeruginosa* compared with 15% of the screened patients. Survival curves were strikingly different between patients in the screened group versus the unscreened group, with 94% survival for the screened patients at age 11 years compared with 65% for the unscreened patients.

ITALY

A study in Italy has demonstrated the nutritional and survival benefits of CF neonatal screening.[22] Comparison was made for CF patients born between July 1983 and June 1992 in two Italian regions. In Veneto, there was a CF newborn screening program established using IRT measurement. In Sicily, patients were diagnosed by symptoms. The 126 CF patients diagnosed by screening in Veneto were compared to 152 patients diagnosed by symptoms in Sicily. The prevalence of class I and II mutations was similar in the two regions, as was the ratio of those who were pancreatic sufficient to those who were pancreatic insufficient. As expected, patients were diagnosed at a much earlier age in Veneto (1 month) compared with Sicily (6–9 months). There was a significant difference in weight and height z scores in the newborn screen group in Veneto compared with conventionally diagnosed patients in Sicily. Growth was nearly normal for the newborn screen patients, with z scores very close to zero. Significantly, there was a difference in patient survival as analyzed by Kaplan-Meier curves. There were 2 deaths in the Veneto cohort (1.6%), compared with 18 in the Sicily cohort (11.8%).

NEW SOUTH WALES, AUSTRALIA

The state of New South Wales in Australia has conducted CF newborn screening using IRT measurement since July 1981. Investigators studied a historical cohort, in which they compared a group of 57 patients born with CF in the 3 years immediately before the newborn screening program was introduced (July 1978 to July 1981, "nonscreened") with 60 infants born during the first 3 years of the newborn screening program (July 1981 to July 1984, "screened").[23] The median age at diagnosis was significantly lower in screened patients (1.8 months) compared with nonscreened patients (5.7 months). Height and weight z scores were significantly lower in the nonscreened patients compared with the screened patients at diagnosis. At 1 year of age, screened patients had significantly better weights than nonscreened patients. At 5 years of age, screened patients were significantly taller than nonscreened patients. Pulmonary function parameters were significantly higher in the screened cohort at 5 years of age, and by 10 years of age, there was an average difference of 9.4% in the predicted value of forced expiratory volume in 1 second and of 8.4% in the predicted value of forced vital capacity. The Shwachman-Kulczycki score was 5.3 points higher in the screened group at 10 years of age compared with the nonscreened group.

WALES/WEST MIDLANDS, UNITED KINGDOM

A clinical study of newborn screening was done in the Wales and the West Midlands regions of the United Kingdom. Between January 1985 and December 1989, neonates born in these regions were screened for CF by IRT measurement on alternate weeks (those born in the non-IRT weeks were diagnosed conventionally), thus generating a screened and a nonscreened group of CF patients. In the initial analysis of these two groups, there were 65 infants with CF detected after positive screening and 66 infants diagnosed conventionally.[24] Analysis of data excluded infants with meconium ileus and infants identified because of an older sibling with CF, yielding 58 infants detected by screening and 34 infants detected clinically. The mean age of diagnosis of the screened neonates was 9.1 ± 3.1 weeks versus 50.7 ± 60.5 weeks for infants diagnosed clinically ($P < .001$). These investigators found no significant differences in the weight and height standard deviation scores between the two groups, nor did they find a difference in the Shwachman-Kulczycki scores and Chrispin-Norman scores. However, the screened group had fewer hospital admissions and length of time spent in the hospital in the first year of life than did the clinically diagnosed patients. The mean number of hospital admissions for the screened patients was 1.3 ± 1.9 versus 3.2 ± 2.7 for clinically diagnosed patients, and the length of time spent in the hospital for the screened patients was 19.2 ± 42.9 days versus 27 ± 22.7 days for the clinically diagnosed infants ($P < .001$). In a more recent analysis of these two cohorts, death from CF in childhood was examined for the first 5 years of life.[25] There were five deaths in unscreened children, with age at death ranging from 6 weeks to 22 months of age. There were two deaths in the screened group of neonates, both of whom were premature and had meconium ileus. The investigators concluded that newborn screening has the potential to decrease deaths in newborns with CF.

BENEFITS OF NEWBORN SCREENING

From the studies just described, it is clear that there are many benefits of CF newborn screening. Nutritional deficits occur very early in CF and can lead to possible permanent stunting of growth. Protein-calorie malnutrition and hyponatremic dehydration are potentially fatal in neonates with CF. Early identification of CF patients before the onset of symptoms allows for the immediate administration of pancreatic enzymes and avoidance of this morbidity. CF newborn screening also provides the opportunity to intervene early and avoid a prolonged vitamin E deficiency, which appears to lead to cognitive dysfunction. Newborn screening also provides the opportunity to diagnose patients before colonization with *P. aeruginosa* and to provide the opportunity to intervene early and delay the onset of chronic colonization with this bacterium. CF newborn screening also helps to eliminate the disparities that arise from a lower index of suspicion in non-Caucasians. Using the IRT/DNA technique, carriers are identified. Although there is short-term anxiety and grief in these families, CF newborn screening also provides an opportunity to provide genetic counseling.[26] Newborn screening for CF is favored by both families in which an infant is identified with disease[27] and families in which their infant was identified as a carrier.[26]

IMPLEMENTATION CHALLENGES: ENSURING MORE GOOD THAN HARM

Box 59-2 demonstrates the opportunities to achieve more good than harm through CF neonatal screening.[28] There are implementation challenges of instituting CF newborn screening. Additionally, screening itself does not automatically lead to more good than harm. Two opportunities to ensure benefit are optimized communication and the delivery of improved medical care. After the newborn screening laboratory generates a positive report, the first major opportunity occurs for the provision of effective communication among the newborn screening laboratory, the primary care provider, and the CF center. Within CF centers, there is the necessity for high-quality sweat testing and the provision of genetic counseling. Additionally, CF care physicians will require a new paradigm of aggressive treatment of young infants with CF who are initially asymptomatic. These challenges, though significant, are not insurmountable. There now exist effective methods for aggressive nutritional therapy and for early intervention before the onset of irreversible lung disease. Improved respiratory therapies

BOX 59-2 Opportunities to Achieve More Good than Harm through Cystic Fibrosis Neonatal Screening

Opportunity to eliminate disparities associated with sex, race, and access associated with recognition deficiencies, economic limitations, and geographic forces

Opportunity to take advantage of informed reproduction after genetic risk communication and counseling

Opportunity to prevent potentially fatal salt depletion

Opportunity to prevent malnutrition after diagnosing pancreatic insufficiency
- Appropriate use of pancreatic enzyme supplements
- High-calorie diet with abundant essential fatty acids
- Fat-soluble vitamin supplements

Opportunity to prevent progressive lung disease
- Frequent, careful evaluation of pulmonary status
- Judicious use of oral antibiotics
- Protection from exposure to *Pseudomonas aeruginosa*
- Serologic and microbiologic monitoring for *P. aeruginosa* acquisition and infection
- Aggressive antimicrobial therapy for *P. aeruginosa*, as indicated, in an effort to prevent bronchopulmonary disease

From Farrell MH, Farrell PM: Newborn screening for cystic fibrosis. Ensuring more good than harm. J Pediatr 2003; 143:707–712.

will probably be developed that will provide even greater benefit in delaying bronchopulmonary disease. Newborn screening coupled to optimal follow-up care will lead to less morbidity and improved survival in CF.

REFERENCES

1. Guthrie R, Susi A: A simple phenylalanine method for detecting phenylketonuria in large populations of newborn infants. Pediatrics 1963;32: 338–343.
2. Shwachman H, Redmond A, Khaw K-T: Studies in cystic fibrosis. Report of 130 patients diagnosed under 3 months of age over a 20-year period. Pediatrics 1970;46:335–343.
3. Orenstein DM, Boat TF, Stern RC, Tucker AS, Charnock EL, Matthews LW, Doershuk CF: The effect of early diagnosis and treatment in cystic fibrosis. A seven-year study of 16 sibling pairs. Am J Dis Child 1977;131:973–975.
4. Crossley JR, Elliott RB, Smith PA: Dried-blood spot screening for cystic fibrosis in the newborn. Lancet 1979;1:472–474.
5. Ad hoc committee task force on neonatal screening, Cystic Fibrosis Foundation: Neonatal screening for cystic fibrosis. Position paper. Pediatrics 1983;72:741–745.
6. Rock MJ, Mischler EH, Farrell PM, Bruns WT, Hassemer DJ, Laessig RH: Immunoreactive trypsinogen screening for cystic fibrosis. Characterization of infants with a false positive screening test. Pediatr Pulmonol 1989;6:42–48.
7. Rommens JM, Iannuzzi MC, Kerem B-S, Drumm ML, Melmer G, Dean M, Rozmahel R, Cole JL, Kennedy D, Hidaka N, Zsiga M, Buchwald M, Riordan JR, Tsui L-C, Collins FS: Identification of the cystic fibrosis gene. Chromosome walking and jumping. Science 1989;245:1059–1065.
8. Gregg RG, Simantel A, Farrell PM, Koscik R, Kosorok MR, Laxova A, Laessig R, Hoffman G, Hassemer D, Mischler EH, Splaingard M: Newborn screening for cystic fibrosis in Wisconsin. Comparison of biochemical and molecular methods. Pediatrics 1997;99:819–824.
9. Bobadilla JL, Macek M, Fine JP, Farrell PM: Cystic fibrosis. A worldwide analysis of CFTR mutations—correlation with incidence data and application to screening. Hum Mutat 2002;19:575–606.
10. Rock MJ, Hoffman G, Laessig RH, Kopish GJ, Litsheim TJ, Farrell PM: Newborn screening for cystic fibrosis in Wisconsin. Nine years experience with routine trypsinogen/DNA testing. J Pediatr 2005;147(Suppl):S73–S77.
11. Padoan R, Bassotti A, Seia M, Corbetta C: Negative sweat test in hypertrypsinaemic infants with cystic fibrosis carrying rare CFTR mutations. Eur J Pediatr 2002;161:212–215.
12. Lee DS, Rosenberg MA, Peterson A, Makholm L, Hoffman G, Laessig RH, Farrell PM: Analysis of the costs of diagnosing cystic fibrosis with a newborn screening program. J Pediatr 2003;142:617–623.
13. Reardon MC, Hammond KB, Accurso FJ, Fisher CD, McCabe ERB, Cotton EK, Bowman CM: Nutritional deficits exist before 2 months of age in some infants with cystic fibrosis identified by screening test. J Pediatr 1984;105:271–274.
14. Abman SH, Reardon MC, Accurso FJ, Hammond KB, Sokol RJ: Hypoalbuminemia at diagnosis as a marker for severe respiratory course in infants with cystic fibrosis identified by newborn screening. J Pediatr 1985;107:933–935.
15. Sokol RJ, Reardon MC, Accurson FJ, Stall C, Narkewicz M, Abman SH, Hammond KB: Fat-soluble-vitamin status during the first year of life in infants with cystic fibrosis identified by screening of newborns. Am J Clin Nutr 1989;50:1064–1071.
16. Farrell PM, Kosorok MR, Rock MJ, Laxova A, Zeng L, Lai H-C, Hoffman G, Laessig RH, Splaingard ML: Early diagnosis of cystic fibrosis through neonatal screening prevents severe malnutrition and improves long-term growth. Pediatrics 2001;107:1–13.
17. Koscik RL, Farrell PM, Kosorok MR, Zaremba KM, Laxova A, Lai H-C, Douglas JA, Rock MJ, Splaingard ML: Cognitive function of children with cystic fibrosis. Deleterious effect of early malnutrition. Pediatrics 2004;113: 1549–1558.
18. Farrell PM, Li Z, Kosorok MR, Laxova A, Green CG, Collins J, Lai H-C, Rock MJ, Splaingard ML: Bronchopulmonary disease in children with cystic fibrosis after early or delayed diagnosis. Am J Respir Crit Care Med 2003;168:1100–1108.
19. Siret D, Bretaudea G, Branger B, Dabadie A, Dagorne M, David V, de Braekeleer M, Moisan-Petit V, Picherot G, Rault G, Storni V, Roussey M: Comparing the clinical evolution of cystic fibrosis screened neonatally to that of cystic fibrosis diagnosed from clinical symptoms. A 10-year retrospective study in a French region (Brittany). Pediatr Pulmonol 2003;35:342–349.
20. Dankert-Roelse JE, te Meerman GJ: Long term prognosis of patients with cystic fibrosis in relation to early detection by neonatal screening and treatment in a cystic fibrosis centre. Thorax 1995;50:712–718.
21. Merelle ME, Schouten JP, Gerritsen J, Dankert-Roelse JE: Influence of neonatal screening and centralized treatment on long-term clinical outcome and survival of CF patients. Eur Respir J 2001;18:306–315.
22. Mastella G, Zanolla L, Castellani C, Altieri S, Furnari M, Giglio L, Lombardo M, Miano A, Sciuto C, Pardo F, Magazzu G: Neonatal screening for cystic fibrosis. Long-term clinical balance. Pancreatology 2001; 1:531–537.
23. Waters DL, Wilcken B, Irwig L, Van Asperen P, Mellis C, Simpson JM, Brown J, Gaskin KJ: Clinical outcomes of newborn screening for cystic fibrosis. Arch Dis Child Fetal Neonatal Ed 1999;80:F1–F7.
24. Chatfield S, Owen G, Ryley HC, Williams J, Alfaham M, Goodchild MC, Weller P: Neonatal screening for cystic fibrosis in Wales and the West Midlands. Clinical assessment after 5 years of screening. Arch Dis Child 1991;66:29–33.
25. Doull IJM, Ryley HC, Weller P, Goodchild MC: Cystic fibrosis-related deaths in infancy and the effect of newborn screening. Pediatr Pulmonol 2001;31:363–366.
26. Ciske DJ, Haavisto A, Laxova A, Zeng L, Rock M, Farrell PM: Genetic counseling and neonatal screening for cystic fibrosis. An assessment of the communication process. Pediatrics 2001;107:699–705.
27. Merelle ME, Huisman J, Alderden-van der Vecht A, Taat F, Bezemer D, Griffioen RW, Brinkhorst G, Dankert-Roelse JE: Early versus late diagnosis. Psychological impact on parents of children with cystic fibrosis. Pediatrics 2003;111:346–350.
28. Farrell MH, Farrell PM: Newborn screening for cystic fibrosis. Ensuring more good than harm. J Pediatr 2003;143:707–712.

60 Diagnosis and Presentation of Cystic Fibrosis

Colin Wallis, MD

A diagnosis of cystic fibrosis (CF) has lifelong implications for the affected individuals, their families, and their acquaintances. This important designation must be made accurately and early. A late diagnosis is often preceded by a catalogue of doctor's visits, family anguish, and anger with a delay in the initiation of treatment that may have an impact on long-term outcome. Equally disturbing is an infrequent but increasingly documented experience involving children who are diagnosed as having CF but on review, often years later, are found to be normal.

For the great majority of children the diagnosis is easy. A clinical suspicion of CF is confirmed by a positive sweat test, and additional support is provided by the identification of two disease-causing mutations in the gene on chromosome 7 that encodes the cystic fibrosis transmembrane regulator (CFTR). A classic phenotype is either obvious at the time of diagnosis or presents soon thereafter, and a relatively predictable clinical course unfolds.

During the last decade, several developments have led to the question: "What makes a diagnosis of CF?"[1–4] These developments include: (1) the recognition of an ever-widening phenotype for an individual with two *CFTR* mutations ranging from completely normal to a classical CF phenotype; (2) the development of screening programs whereby a newborn or fetus, on the basis of genetic information alone, could be given the CF label without necessarily developing clinical disease; (3) the recognition that a CF phenotype can emerge over time presenting de novo in adulthood; (4) the development of sophisticated clinical investigations that allow detection of subtle changes in end organs that hitherto would have gone undetected (e.g., detailed computed tomography scanning and the measurement of epithelial potential difference or PD).

■ DIAGNOSTIC CRITERIA FOR CYSTIC FIBROSIS

A possible definition for the disease CF could involve the following sequence of pathologic events:

- Disease usually arises from two disease-causing mutations in the gene encoding CFTR.
- Mutations result in changes to the fluid and electrolytes on cell surfaces.
- Changes may lead to abnormal secretions and inflammatory responses.
- These manifestations may predispose to obstruction and infection.
- Obstruction and infection may produce end-organ disease in tubular structures such as the upper and lower airways, vas deferens, gut, liver, and pancreas, with secondary impact on growth and nutrition.

In more than 90% of cases, CF is diagnosed from a clinical suspicion supported by a positive sweat test and genetic confirmation.[5] A Cystic Fibrosis Foundation Consensus Panel (USA) synthesized diagnostic criteria for CF.[6] The key features are summarized in Box 60-1. The basic premise of the consensus statement is that CF is a clinical and not a genetic diagnosis, though acknowledging that genetic testing may have a role in sorting out atypical clinical situations. Any such document must be considered a work in progress to accommodate new developments and acknowledged shortcomings.[7]

■ MAKING THE DIAGNOSIS OF CYSTIC FIBROSIS

A clinician may have to confirm a diagnosis of CF in various situations, such as when (1) a patient has one or more suspicious clinical features, (2) a postnatal screening program has identified a child as at a high risk for CF, (3) an individual is being examined after the diagnosis of CF in a family member, or (4) postnatal confirmation is required when an antenatal test has led to a suspicion of CF. Evidence for the diagnosis of CF can be accumulated from several sources.

■ CLINICAL SUSPICION

The majority of children with CF present with a history of bulky offensive fatty stools, failure to thrive, and recurrent chest infections.[8] Shortly after birth, 10% to 15% will present with meconium ileus. However, there is a wide range of less common presenting features, as highlighted in Box 60-2. Any child or adult presenting with the stigmata of CF should be investigated further. The diagnosis in a child with clinical findings suggesting CF should not be discounted just because the child appears too well or is thought to be too old. Although the diagnosis is established in most children by the age of 1 year,[9] in approximately 10% of children the diagnosis is delayed until after 7 years.[8,10] Patients with pancreatic sufficiency and non-Caucasian patients are vulnerable to delays in diagnosis.[11,12]

■ THE SWEAT TEST

The sweat test was first described in 1959 and remains a gold standard for the diagnosis of CF.[13] In the appropriate clinical setting, a positive sweat test is diagnostic of CF. There are a number of other rare conditions (sometimes single case reports) that have been associated with a positive sweat test, but these are usually clearly distinguishable by their clinical features. Examples are listed in Box 60-3.

The standard sweat test (Gibson and Cooke technique) requires skill and care and should be undertaken by accredited laboratories. Localized sweating is stimulated by the iontophoresis of pilocarpine into the skin. Sweat is collected on filter paper or gauze, or in microduct tubing over a specific period of time to ensure that the rate of sweating and the total amount collected are

BOX 60-1 Diagnostic Criteria for Cystic Fibrosis (CF Foundation Consensus Panel)

One or more characteristic phenotypic features consistent with CF:

- Chronic sinopulmonary disease
- Gastrointestinal and nutritional abnormalities
- Salt loss syndromes
- Male urogenital abnormalities resulting in obstructive azoospermia

OR

A history of CF in a sibling

OR

A positive newborn screening test result

AND

An increased sweat chloride concentration

Or identification of two CF mutations

Or demonstration of abnormal nasal epithelial ion transport

sufficient and standardized. Guidelines for sweat testing procedures and precautions are available in published[14,15] and electronic format (http://acb.org.uk/site/guidelines.asp).

Chloride is the analyte of choice.[16,17] A sweat chloride concentration of more than 60 mmol/L is considered positive, and concentrations below 40 mmol/L are probably in the normal range; however, a normal sweat test does not exclude CF. Intermediate levels between 40 and 60 mmol/L may be associated with atypical forms of CF and should be interpreted with caution. Some healthy adults can have values in the intermediate range. A false-positive sweat test in the severely malnourished child, or the critically ill child in intensive care should have cautious interpretation and follow-up. Initial intermediate or high-normal chloride readings may also occur in the affected premature infant or newborn and may merit repeating.[18] Case reports also describe a nonsense mutation in the *CFTR* gene associated with elevated sweat chloride in the absence of clinical features of CF.[19] The sodium levels and osmolality of sweat are less reliable and should never be used in isolation.

Researchers continue to explore the development of a more efficient sweat test. Collecting systems such as the macroduct[20] and nanoduct[21] are achieving credibility, and the role of sweat conductivity as a diagnostic tool in CF is also gaining credence.[22] In one large trial the best conductivity cutoff value to diagnose CF was 90 mmol/L or higher, and the best conductivity cutoff value to exclude CF was less than 75 mmol/L.[23] Many clinicians and laboratories will now choose to confirm a positive sweat conductivity result with a formal measurement of chloride concentration.

■ MUTATION ANALYSIS

The 1989 identification of the CF gene[24] and the characterization of its protein product (CFTR) held the promise that the diagnostic dilemmas for the condition were over. If a person had two *CFTR* mutations, he or she had CF; in the absence of these, the diagnosis did not apply. Unfortunately, it has not worked out that simply.

BOX 60-2 Clinical Features of Cystic Fibrosis at Diagnosis in Unscreened Populations, Grouped according to Age and Approximate Order of Frequency

0–2 Years

Failure to thrive
Steatorrhea
Recurrent chest infections including bronchiolitis/bronchitis
Meconium ileus
Rectal proplapse
Edema/hypoproteinemia/dermatitis
Severe pneumonia/empyema
Salt depletion syndrome
Prolonged neonatal jaundice
Vitamin K deficiency with bleeding diathesis

3–16 Years

Recurrent chest infections or “asthma”
Clubbing and “idiopathic” bronchiectasis
Steatorrhea
Nasal polyps and sinusitis
Chronic intestinal obstruction, intussusception
Heat exhaustion with hyponatremia
CF diagnosis in a relative, usually a younger sibling

Adulthood (Often Atypical CF)

Azoospermia/congenital absence of the vas deferens
Bronchiectasis
Chronic sinusitis
Acute or chronic pancreatitis
Allergic bronchopulmonary aspergillosis
Focal biliary cirrhosis
Abnormal glucose tolerance
Portal hypertension
Cholestasis/gallstones

BOX 60-3 Examples of Non-Cystic Fibrosis Causes of a Positive Sweat Test

- Adrenal insufficiency or stress
- Anorexia nervosa
- Ectodermal dysplasia
- Eczema
- Fucosidosis
- Glucose 6-phosphate dehydrogenase deficiency
- Glycogen storage disease type 1
- Human immunodeficiency viral infection
- Hypoparathyroidism
- Hypothyroidism
- Malnutrition from various causes
- Nephrogenic diabetes insipidus
- Pseudohypoaldosteronism

First, there are over a thousand different CF gene mutations associated with CF disease. Techniques now available do not allow a full screen of the entire CF genome, and most laboratories will only search routinely for the most common mutations within their region. Examples of CFTR mutations are listed in Table 60-1, highlighting the dominance of the ΔF508 mutation (present in >70% of CF alleles in Caucasian populations).[8] Customizing mutation panels to match the patient's ethnic background and clinical presentation can enhance the sensitivity of DNA testing in CF.

Second, there is a range of mutation types that have been classified according to the functional impact on the CFTR.[25] The final protein product may be either incomplete or complete but incorrectly packaged and processed; alternatively, the final CFTR molecule produced may be unstable or incapable of reaching the cell surface in sufficient numbers to be physiologically effective. In addition to the "disease-causing" mutations, there are also recognizable polymorphisms that do not necessarily result in a clinical phenotype but may influence the structure of the final protein product when associated with another mild mutation. The thymidine run in intron 8 is a well-described example wherein the 5T allele leads to a substantial reduction in functional protein compared with the 9T allele; the 7T allele is intermediate in its effect.

Even though the presence of two mutations strongly supports the diagnosis of CF in the appropriate clinical setting, two alterations in the gene that encodes CFTR do not necessarily mean that the patient will develop classic CF disease. The clinical phenotype associated with two *CFTR* mutations is far broader than could ever have been anticipated.[26] Examples are listed in Box 60-4.

BOX 60-4 Examples from the Range of Clinical Features That Can Be Associated with Two Mutations in the Cystic Fibrosis Gene

- "Classic CF" with pancreatic insufficiency
- Sinopulmonary disease, pancreatic sufficiency, and positive sweat test
- Sinopulmonary disease and male fertility with a normal sweat test
- Severe sinusitis and congenial bilateral absence of the vas deferens
- Male infertility only
- Chronic pancreatitis only
- Allergic bronchopulmonary aspergillosis
- Sclerosing cholangitis
- Positive sweat test only
- No clinical features including normal sweat chloride

Failure to find two CF mutations from a selective or extended search does not exclude the diagnosis of CF. To exclude a patient with symptoms of CF and a positive sweat test from potentially beneficial treatment because the laboratory cannot detect two CF mutations would clearly be misguided. There are also rare reports of patients with classic CF symptoms and signs and a positive sweat test who do not appear to have any mutations in the *CFTR* gene—even when the entire gene has been sequenced, with screening of all 27 exons and the intron-exon boundaries.[27] These findings suggest that, on these rare occasions, CF may be caused by mutations within the promoter region of the *CFTR* gene, in one of the introns, or even in a distant controlling gene from an unrelated locus.[28]

TABLE 60-1. Common mutations that cause cystic fibrosis listed according to frequency*

Mutation	Frequency (%)
ΔF508	75.0
G551D	3.4
G542X	1.8
R117H	1.3
621 + 1G→T	1.3
ΔI507	0.5
N1303K	0.5
R560T	0.4
Q493X	0.3
R1162X	0.3
R533X	0.3
W1282X	0.3
3659delC	0.3
1154insTC	0.3
E60X	0.2
G85E	0.2
P67L	0.2
R347P	0.2
V520F	0.2
1078delT	0.1
2184delA	0.1
A455E	0.1
R334W	0.1
S549N	0.1
2789 + 5G→A	0.1
3849 + 10kb C→T	0.1
711 + 1G→T	0.1
1717 + 1G→T	0.6
1898 + 1G→T	0.6

*In Caucasian populations; variations in frequency occur between different ethnic groups and geographic regions.

ASSESSMENT FOR END-ORGAN INVOLVEMENT

To determine the presence of end-organ disease in a patient with the genetic predisposition to develop CF disease but in whom there are few clinical indicators, a more detailed end-organ assessment is sometimes suggested. Examples include the following:

1. Computed tomography scanning can be used to evaluate subtle pulmonary changes not readily visible on plain radiography.
2. Computed tomography can also be used to evaluate the sinuses.
3. Testing for pancreatic function can involve sophisticated tests or timed stool collections for fecal fat analysis. A simple test for quantification of fecal elastase 1[29,30] has shown considerable sensitivity and reliability and is not contaminated by exogenous enzyme administration. Caution is required in the interpretation of early stool samples, especially in the premature infant or newborn within the first few days of life.[31]

4. Sputum, bronchoalveolar lavage fluid, oropharyngeal swabs, or sinus aspirates can be cultured for known CF pathogens. If a child with "idiopathic" bronchiectasis is found to be infected with typical CF pathogens such as *Staphylococcus aureus* or mucoid *Pseudomonas aeruginosa*, then reevaluation of the possibility of a CF diagnosis is necessary.
5. Postpubertal males can have semen analysis, or younger males can be assessed with ultrasound for congenital bilateral absence of the vas deferens.[32]
6. Valuable information can be obtained from lung function testing, including assessment of the small airways even in young children and using such newer techniques as the multiple breath washout.[33]

TRANSEPITHELIAL POTENTIAL DIFFERENCE MEASUREMENTS

In rare instances wherein the diagnosis of CF remains unclear or the evidence is equivocal, additional evidence of CFTR dysfunction is sometimes sought. Patients with CF show a more negative PD across respiratory epithelium than normal individuals.[34] Nasal PD can be measured in the mucosa of the inferior turbinates, and additional diagnostic accuracy is assured by documenting a bioelectric profile of change to the basal reading in the presence of amiloride perfusion with the subsequent addition of a chloride-free solution and isoproterenol (Fig. 60-1).[35] PD measurements are difficult to do, especially in young children, and the technique is generally confined to specialist centers.[36] Results are influenced

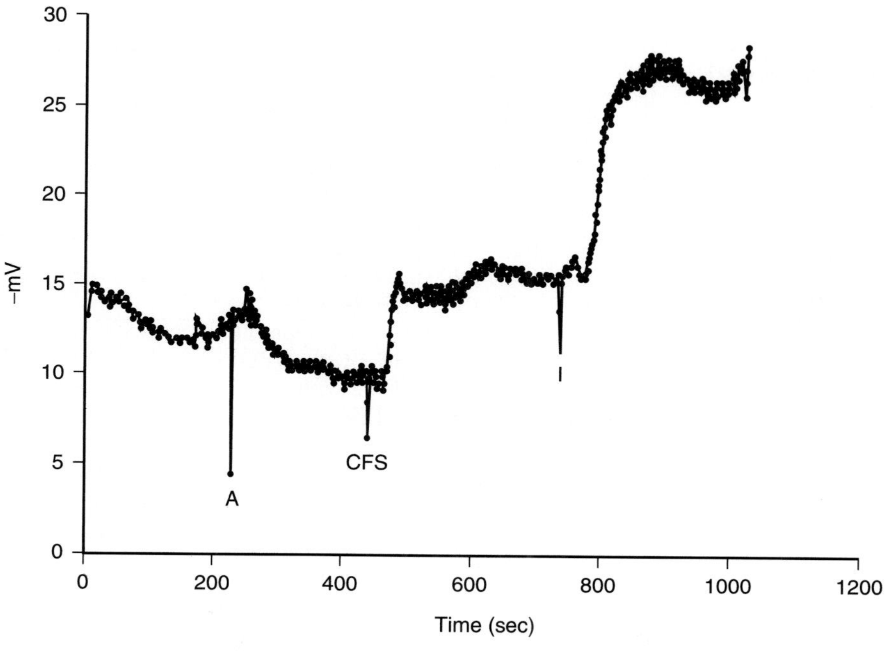

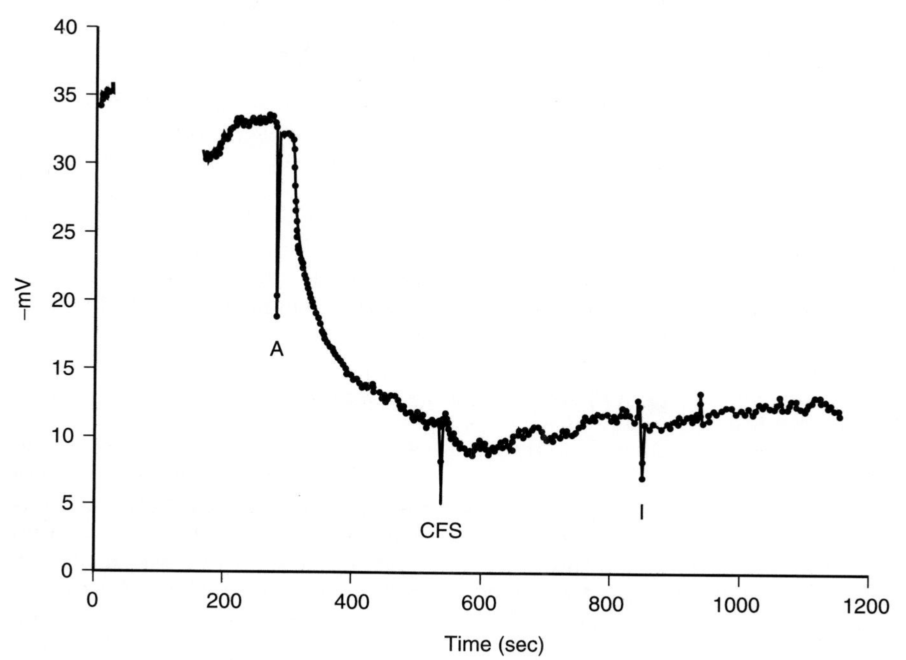

FIGURE 60-1. Nasal PD in a normal subject *(top)* and a CF patient *(bottom)*, illustrating the response to perfusion with amiloride (*A*), followed by the addition of a chloride-free solution (*CFS*) and then isoproterenol (*I*).

by recent viral infections, the presence of rhinitis, the precise anatomic localization of the measuring catheter, as well as polyps and the genotype. Not infrequently, atypical forms of CF with borderline sweat chloride levels produce a nasal PD that is also equivocal.[37]

Recent publications on the diagnostic value of rectal PD done either in vivo or on biopsy specimens have considered the advantages in assessing CFTR function in gut epithelium.[38,39] These techniques are not yet widely available.

ANTENATAL TESTING FOR CYSTIC FIBROSIS

Parents with an increased risk of having a child with CF, because either their own carrier status is known or they already have an affected child, may request antenatal testing. The diagnosis can be confirmed or excluded with a high degree of accuracy by direct mutation analysis done on fetal cells obtained by chorionic villus sampling (10 weeks' gestation) or occasionally from cultured amniotic fluid cells (15–18 weeks' gestation).

Preimplantation diagnosis is an alternative for couples at risk. After in vitro fertilization, a cleavage-stage biopsy is carried out on day 2 or 3, and normal or carrier embryos are then transferred to establish pregnancy. Further postnatal confirmation is still recommended.

Occasionally, routine fetal anomaly scans may detect evidence of meconium ileus by abnormal bowel echogenicity or evidence of perforation. Although such findings are usually available too far into the second trimester to permit decisions on the fate of the pregnancy, a positive scan will help in providing optimal facilities for the delivery and subsequent medical and surgical care. Hyperechoic bowel often occurs as a benign variant and is distinguished by spontaneous resolution usually before the third trimester.[40]

GENOTYPE-PHENOTYPE CORRELATIONS

Although an abnormal CF genotype will probably give a positive sweat test and result in end-organ disease, the road from genotype to phenotype is highly unpredictable. There may be mild and severe mutations, and mild mutations may be dominant over severe ones, but the final effect on the phenotype is far more complex.[26,41,42] Authors do propose a few possible exceptions to the general disappointment:

1. Pancreatic sufficiency has been linked to certain mutations such as R117H and A445E, although insufficiency may emerge with time.
2. Homozygosity for the ΔF508 mutation generally (but not exclusively) produces a more severe phenotype in all affected organs when compared with CF patients carrying one ΔF508 mutation or none.[43]
3. Mutations carrying a milder pancreatic phenotype (e.g., R117H, R334W, 3849 + 10kb C→T) may be associated with more mildly abnormal sweat tests[44] and perhaps a similarly mild effect on nasal PD responses.[45]
4. The male reproductive tract appears to have a high demand for fully functioning CFTR, but splice mutations such as 3849 + 10kb C→T allows for the production of enough CFTR to make fertility possible (though not guaranteed).[46]

There are four major contributing influences on the path from genotype to end-organ involvement and an individual's eventual phenotype[47]:

1. The severity of the individual *CFTR* mutations: "Mild" mutations may cause milder phenotypic effects, but when there is a mixture of mild and severe mutations the final impact is unpredictable. Sometimes mild mutations may have a dominant effect on severe mutations with a "corrective" effect. Similarly, coexistent polymorphisms hitchhiking within the *CFTR* gene may influence the final protein product.
2. Modifying genes (genes lying elsewhere in the genome that can have significant influence on the behavior of the CFTR protein) and their protein products can correct or exacerbate influential pathologic processes such as the biochemistry of the cell surface liquid, and the innate and acquired immunity of the lungs. Such genes may even influence the predisposition to meconium ileus.[48] Each individual with CF probably has an immense orchestra of modifying genes and proteins that are unique to themselves and influential in their clinical outcome.
3. The environment in which patients with CF live and grow has central bearing on the outcome of their disease.[49] Treatment and adherence to therapy, social circumstances and diet, exposure to infections such as *Pseudomonas*,[50] or viral infections in infancy can produce a sustained negative influence on the clinical course.
4. The passage of time is an important influence on outcome. CF is not necessarily an all-or-nothing disease. A clinical phenotype can emerge with time, especially in some of the atypical forms. Effective therapies and adherence to treatment can help stall the disease progression. Patients with documented pancreatic sufficiency in childhood can become pancreatic insufficient in later life. Some patients with CF, but not all, will develop diabetes, liver disease, and osteoporosis.

CYSTIC FIBROSIS PHENOTYPES

CLASSICAL CYSTIC FIBROSIS

The diagnosis of classic CF must be made early and confidently. No racial group is exempt, and children of ethnic minorities or mixed heritage are at greatest risk of a delayed or missed diagnosis. The clinical features of recurrent chest infections, malabsorption with pancreatic insufficiency in the majority (but not all), or an infant presenting with meconium ileus or rectal prolapse require investigation. A positive sweat test and/or two *CFTR* mutations is diagnostic. Appropriate therapy should be introduced without delay.

ATYPICAL CYSTIC FIBROSIS

There is a growing number of children and adults who do not present with the full spectrum of clinical features associated with classic CF. The terms *equivocal CF* or *CF-related disorders* or *variant CF* have also been used to describe these atypical forms. Frequently, there is single-organ involvement. Sweat testing can be normal, equivocal, or positive, and mutation analysis can reveal two, one, or no mutations. Examples of such conditions are listed in Box 60-5. Recent reviews have recognized that it is

BOX 60-5 Conditions That May Be Associated with an Increased Incidence of *CFTR* Mutations but Insufficient Evidence to Fulfill a Cystic Fibrosis Diagnosis

- Pancreatitis, acute or recurrent
- Disseminated bronchiectasis
- Isolated obstructive azoospermia
- Allergic bronchopulmonary aspergillosis
- Diffuse panbronchiolitis
- Sclerosing cholangitis
- Neonatal hypertrypsinogenemia
- Rhinosinusitis
- Heat exhaustion

inappropriate to label individuals with these atypical forms as having classic CF.[4] Both the diagnostic labeling and the management must be tailored to the patient's individual phenotype and requirements. The introduction of arduous therapies aimed at the patient with classic CF does not seem appropriate or beneficial. The negative connotations of a CF label can be avoided with a more considered approach to diagnostic categorization. It was with these considerations in mind that a joint workshop considered the current International Classification of Diseases entry for CF and proposed a new, broader, and more flexible classification that will hopefully be included in the next edition acknowledging the entity of atypical CF.[51]

GENETIC CYSTIC FIBROSIS

There is at present no satisfactory term to describe a very small but important group of individuals with the genetic potential to develop CF (i.e., two mutations in the *CFTR* gene) but in whom, on careful and detailed clinical assessment, there is no evidence of end-organ CF disease. Some authors have considered the term *pre-CF*.[3] There is the potential that clinical features will emerge with the passing of time, but there is insufficient clinical evidence to label the carrier of the gene mutations with a disease. Most clinicians would advise a program of surveillance in these cases and reserve therapy for a time when early changes occur. The role of prophylactic therapy in this situation (such as physiotherapy or antibiotics) is unclear.

REFERENCES

1. Wilmott RW: Making the diagnosis of cystic fibrosis. J Pediatr JID - 0375410 1998;132:563–565.
2. Knowles MR, Durie PR: What is cystic fibrosis? N Engl J Med JID - 0255562 2002;347:439–442.
3. Bush A, Wallis C: Time to think again. Cystic fibrosis is not an "all or nothing" disease. Pediatr Pulmonol 2000;30:139–144.
4. Dodge JA: CF or not CF? That is the question. J Cyst Fibros 2002;1(1):3–4.
5. Wallis C: Diagnosing cystic fibrosis. Blood, sweat, and tears. Arch Dis Child JID - 0372434 1997;76:85–88.
6. Rosenstein BJ, Cutting GR: The diagnosis of cystic fibrosis. A consensus statement. Cystic Fibrosis Foundation Consensus Panel. J Pediatr JID - 0375410 1998;132:589–595.
7. Rosenstein BJ: Cystic fibrosis diagnosis. New dilemmas for an old disorder. Pediatr Pulmonol JID - 8510590 2002;33:83–84.
8. McCormick J, Green MW, Mehta G, Culross F, Mehta A: Demographics of the UK cystic fibrosis population. Implications for neonatal screening. Eur J Hum Genet JID - 9302235 2002;10:583–590.
9. Fitzsimmons SC: The changing epidemiology of cystic fibrosis. J Pediatr 1993;122:1–9.
10. Gan KH, Geus WP, Bakker W, Lamers CB, Heijerman HG: Genetic and clinical features of patients with cystic fibrosis diagnosed after the age of 16 years. Thorax JID - 0417353 1995;50:1301–1304.
11. Gaskin K, Gurwitz D, Durie P, Corey M, Levison H, Forstner G: Improved respiratory prognosis in patients with cystic fibrosis with normal fat absorption. J Pediatr JID - 0375410 1982;100:857–862.
12. Spencer DA, Venkataraman M, Weller PH: Delayed diagnosis of cystic fibrosis in children from ethnic minorities. Lancet JID - 2985213R 1993; 342:238.
13. Gibson LE, Cooke RE: A test for concentration of electrolytes in sweat in cystic fibrosis of the pancreas utilizing pilocarpine by iontophoresis. Pediatrics JID - 0376422 1959;23:545–549.
14. Baumer JH: Evidence based guidelines for the performance of the sweat test for the investigation of cystic fibrosis in the UK. Arch Dis Child JID - 0372434 2003;88:1126–1127.
15. LeGrys VA: Sweat testing for the diagnosis of cystic fibrosis: practical considerations. J Pediatr JID - 0375410 1996;129:892–897.
16. Gleeson M, Henry RL: Sweat sodium or chloride? Clin Chem JID – 9421549 1991;37:112.
17. Green A, Dodds P, Pennock C: A study of sweat sodium and chloride. Criteria for the diagnosis of cystic fibrosis. Ann Clin Biochem JID - 0324055 1985;22(Pt 2):171–174.
18. Massie J, Gaskin K, Van Asperen P, Wilcken B: Sweat testing following newborn screening for cystic fibrosis. Pediatr Pulmonol JID - 8510590 2000;29:452–456.
19. Mickle JE, Macek MJ, Fulmer-Smentek SB, Egan MM, Schwiebert E, Guggino W, et al: A mutation in the cystic fibrosis transmembrane conductance regulator gene associated with elevated sweat chloride concentrations in the absence of cystic fibrosis. Hum Mol Genet JID - 9208958 1998; 7:729–735.
20. Mastella G, Di Cesare G, Borruso A, Menin L, Zanolla L: Reliability of sweat-testing by the Macroduct collection method combined with conductivity analysis in comparison with the classic Gibson and Cooke technique. Acta Paediatr JID - 9205968 2000;89:933–937.
21. Webster HL, Quirante CG: Micro-flowcell conductometric sweat analysis for cystic fibrosis diagnosis. Ann Clin Biochem JID - 0324055 2000;37 (Pt 3):399–407.
22. Heeley ME, Woolf DA, Heeley AF: Indirect measurements of sweat electrolyte concentration in the laboratory diagnosis of cystic fibrosis. Arch Dis Child JID - 0372434 2000;82:420–424.
23. Lezana, JL, Vargas MH, Karam-Bechara J, Aldana, RS, Furuya MEY: Sweat conductivity and chloride titration for cystic fibrosis diagnosis in 3834 subjects. J Cyst Fibros 2003;2:1–7.
24. Kerem BS, Rommens JM, Buchana JA, Markiewicz D, Cox TK, Chakravati A, et al: Identification of the cystic fibrosis gene. Genetic analysis. Science 1989;245:1073–1079.
25. Welsh MJ, Smith AE: Molecular mechanisms of CFTR chloride channel dysfunction in cystic fibrosis. Cell JID - 0413066 1993;73:1251–1254.
26. Cutting G: Phenotype-genotype relationships. In: Hodson M, Geddes D, eds: Cystic Fibrosis. London: Arnold, 2000, pp 49–60.
27. Mekus F, Ballmann M, Bronsveld I, Dork T, Bijman J, Tummler B, et al: Cystic-fibrosis-like disease unrelated to the cystic fibrosis transmembrane conductance regulator. Hum Genetics 1998;102:582–586.
28. Groman JD, Meyer ME, Wilmott RW, Zeitlin PL, Cutting GR: Variant cystic fibrosis phenotypes in the absence of CFTR mutations. N Engl J Med JID - 0255562 2002;347:401–407.
29. Wallis C, Leung T, Cubitt D, Reynolds A: Stool elastase as a diagnostic test for pancreatic function in children with cystic fibrosis. Lancet JID - 2985213R 1997;350:1001–1002.
30. Stein J, Jung M, Sziegoleit A, Zeuzem S, Caspary WF, Lembcke B: Immunoreactive elastase I. Clinical evaluation of a new noninvasive test of pancreatic function. Clin Chem JID - 9421549 1996;42:222–226.
31. Kori M, Maayan-Metzger A, Shamir R, Sirota L, Dinari G: Faecal elastase 1 levels in premature and full term infants. Arch Dis Child Fetal Neonatal Ed JID - 9501297 2003;88:F106–F108.
32. Blau H, Freud E, Mussaffi H, Werner M, Konen O, Rathaus V: Urogenital abnormalities in male children with cystic fibrosis. Arch Dis Child JID - 0372434 2002;87:135–138.
33. Gustafsson PM, Aurora P, Lindblad A: Evaluation of ventilation maldistribution as an early indicator of lung disease in children with cystic fibrosis. Eur Respir J JID - 8803460 2003;22:972–979.

34. Knowles MR, Paradiso AM, Boucher RC: In vivo nasal potential difference. Techniques and protocols for assessing efficacy of gene transfer in cystic fibrosis. Hum Gene Ther JID - 9008950 1995;6:445–455.
35. Middleton PG, Geddes DM, Alton EW: Protocols for in vivo measurement of the ion transport defects in cystic fibrosis nasal epithelium. Eur Respir J JID - 8803460 1994;7:2050–2056.
36. Standaert TA, Boitano L, Emerson J, Milgram LJ, Konstan MW, Hunter J, et al: Standardized procedure for measurement of nasal potential difference. An outcome measure in multicenter cystic fibrosis clinical trials. Pediatr Pulmonol JID - 8510590 2004;37:385–392.
37. Wilson DC, Ellis L, Zielenski J, Corey M, Ip WF, Tsui LC, et al: Uncertainty in the diagnosis of cystic fibrosis. Possible role of in vivo nasal potential difference measurements. J Pediatr JID - 0375410 1998;132: 596–599.
38. Greger R: Role of CFTR in the colon. Annu Rev Physiol JID - 0370600 2000;62:467–491.
39. Mall M, Kreda SM, Mengos A, Jensen TJ, Hirtz S, Seydewitz HH, et al: The DeltaF508 mutation results in loss of CFTR function and mature protein in native human colon. Gastroenterology JID - 0374630 2004;126:32–41.
40. Muller F, Dommergues M, Aubry MC, Simon-Bouy B, Gautier E, Oury JF, et al: Hyperechogenic fetal bowel. An ultrasonographic marker for adverse fetal and neonatal outcome. Am J Obstet Gynecol JID - 0370476 1995; 173:508–513.
41. Correlation between genotype and phenotype in patients with cystic fibrosis. The Cystic Fibrosis Genotype-Phenotype Consortium. N Engl J Med JID - 0255562 1993;329:1308–1313.
42. Zielenski J: Genotype and phenotype in cystic fibrosis. Respiration JID - 0137356 2000;67:117–133.
43. Kerem E, Corey M, Kerem BS, Rommens J, Markiewicz D, Levison H, et al: The relation between genotype and phenotype in cystic fibrosis—analysis of the most common mutation (ΔF508). N Engl J Med 1990;323:1517–1522.
44. Stewart B, Zabner J, Shuber AP, Welsh MJ, McCray PBJ: Normal sweat chloride values do not exclude the diagnosis of cystic fibrosis. Am J Respir Crit Care Med JID - 9421642 1995;151:899–903.
45. Lebecque P, Leal T, De Boeck C, Jaspers M, Cuppens H, Cassiman JJ: Mutations of the cystic fibrosis gene and intermediate sweat chloride levels in children. Am J Respir Crit Care Med JID - 9421642 2002;165: 757–761.
46. Dreyfus DH, Bethel R, Gelfand EW: Cystic fibrosis 3849 + 10kb C → T mutation associated with severe pulmonary disease and male fertility. Am J Respir Crit Care Med JID - 9421642 1996;153:858–860.
47. Wallis C: Atypical cystic fibrosis—diagnostic and management dilemmas. J R Soc Med JID - 7802879 1904;96 (Suppl 43):2–10.
48. Zielenski J, Corey M, Rozmahel R, Markiewicz D, Aznarez I, Casals T, et al: Detection of a cystic fibrosis modifier locus for meconium ileus on human chromosome 19q13. Nat Genet JID - 9216904 1999;22:128–129.
49. Schechter MS: Non-genetic influences on CF lung disease. The role of sociodemographic characteristics, environmental exposures and healthcare interventions. Pediatr Pulmonol Suppl JID - 9014095 2004;26:82–85.
50. Kosorok MR, Zeng L, West SE, Rock MJ, Splaingard ML, Laxova A, et al: Acceleration of lung disease in children with cystic fibrosis after *Pseudomonas aeruginosa* acquisition. Pediatr Pulmonol JID - 8510590 2001;32:277–287.
51. WHO/ICF(M)A/ECFTN: Classification of cystic fibrosis and related disorders. J Cyst Fibros 2002;1(1):5–8.

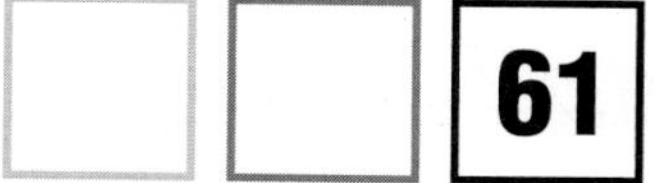

61 Pulmonary Disease in Cystic Fibrosis

Pamela B. Davis, MD

■ HOW DO MUTATIONS IN *CFTR* LEAD TO LUNG DISEASE?

Cystic fibrosis (CF) arises from defects in the CF gene, which encodes the cystic fibrosis transmembrane conductance regulator (CFTR). This cyclic adenosine monophosphate–regulated chloride channel is expressed on the apical surface of airway epithelial cells and the serous cells of the submucosal glands, and possibly in alveoli as well. Chloride is transported down its electrochemical gradient; in the airway, this is usually in the direction of chloride secretion, and secretion is often stimulated by airway irritants such as are continuously present in the CF airway. Another chloride channel, the outwardly rectifying chloride channel, depends on active CFTR for its own activity, and does not transport chloride ion in the absence of active CFTR. CFTR also regulates the epithelial sodium channel, which contributes to reabsorption of sodium ion in the airways. Lack of CFTR activity releases the normal CFTR down-regulation of the epithelial sodium channel, so activity of that channel is consistently increased. All these abnormalities combine to reduce the water content of airway surface liquid (Fig. 61-1).[1–4] In both cell and animal models, the electrolyte content of the airway surface liquid (sodium, chloride, osmolality) is maintained at normal levels in CF. However, at least in human cell models, there is less fluid volume. This causes reduction in depth of the periciliary fluid, dysfunction of ciliary clearance, and possibly reduced mucus hydration as well. All of these conditions combine to increase airway obstruction. This situation can be mimicked in animal models by overexpression of the epithelial sodium channel; thus, much of the disordered fluid balance may be due to poor regulation of sodium transport.

In this setting, bacteria, when they impact on the airway, are not efficiently cleared. In addition, some of the innate immune killing mechanisms are impaired in the CF lung. For example, epithelial release of nitric oxide, which assists in killing small quantities of surface bacteria, is impaired in CF, since nitric oxide synthase-2 expression is down-regulated.[5] Moreover, bacteria provoke intense inflammatory responses (i.e., exaggerated compared to normal) in the CF airway epithelial cell and probably the macrophage as well. Excess chemokines are released, recruiting excess neutrophils to the airway, where their apoptosis is delayed by reduced interleukin-10 (IL-10) and increased granulocyte-macrophage colony-stimulating factor and granulocyte colony-stimulating factor in airway secretions. Neutrophils secrete chemokines such as IL-8 and lipid mediators such as leukotriene B_4 (LTB_4) that sustain ongoing neutrophil recruitment. In addition to the initial increase in the inflammatory response in CF, inflammation fails to resolve promptly, even if the initiating stimulus (e.g., bacteria) is removed. Persistence of neutrophils allows prolonged secretion of enzymes that digest the structural proteins of the airway wall (Fig. 61-2). Neutrophil elastase is especially noxious. Not only does it degrade elastin, but it is also a potent secretogogue for macromolecules and IL-8 from airway epithelial cells. Elastase also cripples opsonophagocytic defenses against *Pseudomonas aeruginosa* by cleaving IgG, the opsonin utilized by macrophages for *P. aeruginosa*, at the hinge region, and destroying the complement system used by neutrophils to opsonize *P. aeruginosa*. Complement opsonization occurs via binding of C3b to its receptor CR1 and binding of C3bi to its receptor CR3 on neutrophils. Elastase cleaves CR1 and C3bi, the receptor of one pair and the ligand of the other, thus neutrophil phagocytosis of *P. aeruginosa* is also impaired.[6,7] These effects combine to assure persistence of *P. aeruginosa* in the airways of patients with CF. With ongoing stimulus, the inflammatory response is sustained, and persistence of live neutrophils assures continuing damage to the airway walls. Bronchiectasis occurs and eventually progresses to respiratory failure (Fig. 61-3).

■ PATHOLOGY OF THE CYSTIC FIBROSIS LUNG DISEASE

The histology of the lung in CF infants who die of meconium ileus without evidence of lung infection is normal, except possibly for widened mouths of the submucosal glands (as if they were already plugged). However, once lung infection occurs, the inflammatory response appears to reverberate even after the stimulus can no longer be detected. Once established, the CF lung disease involves the airways, sparing the alveoli until late in the course. Acute inflammation (i.e., neutrophilic infiltration) persists, although there is lymphocytic infiltration of the submucosa. Neutrophils persist in and around the airways throughout life, damaging the airway walls. Hence, bronchiectasis is the most prominent feature.

At postmortem examination, the airways are filled with thick secretions, pus, and colonies of bacteria, often surrounded by a mucoid coat. The lung is dense and airless, with hemorrhagic pneumonitis in some areas (Fig. 61-4). Usually, with infection by *P. aeruginosa*, bacteria are found almost entirely within the airway lumen, but with some infecting organisms, such as *Burkholderia cepacia*, tissue invasion is sometimes seen. Despite the name of the disease, fibrosis is not a prominent feature of its pathology. Bronchiectasis is the dominant feature. Airways that are enlarged and lack appropriate support to remain open and are prone to develop saccular outpouchings or varicosities, which soon become repositories for pus, mucus, and bacteria. Enlarged airways, airspaces, blebs, and bronchiectatic cysts are common. Bronchial arteries are often enlarged and tortuous. Muscular hypertrophy is prominent in the pulmonary arteries, and muscularization extends well into the smaller arteries. Consistent with the relative alveolar sparing, emphysema, defined as alveolar simplification, is not prominent. The older the patient at the time of death, the larger the volume of the lung that is subsumed by emphysematous changes, but this area is only about 10% even in adults.[8]

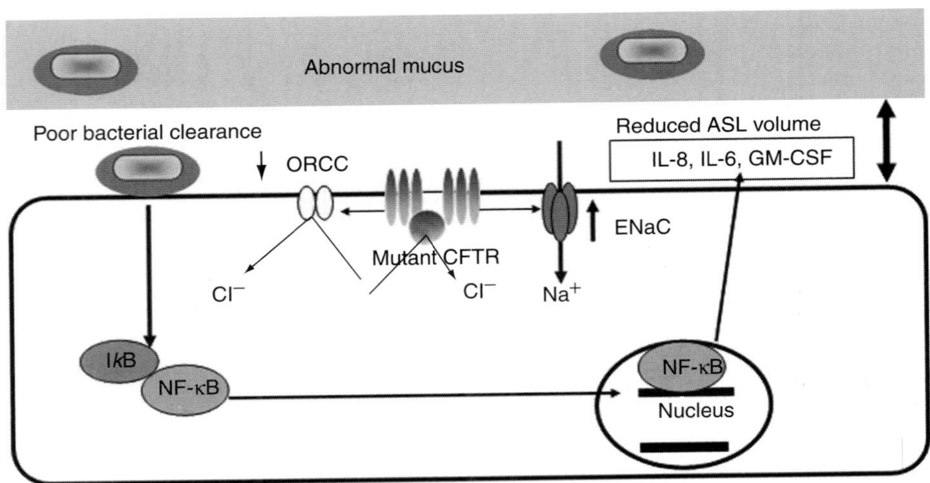

■ **FIGURE 61-1.** Conditions associated with the CF defect in the airway. Reduced function of CFTR affects the regulation of other channels, including the epithelial sodium channel (ENaC) and other chloride channels such as the outwardly rectifying chloride channel (ORCC). These abnormalities in ion transport result in reduced volume of airway surface liquid and reduced hydration of mucins with abnormal carbohydrate composition, so that bacteria are trapped and mucociliary clearance is impaired. Bacteria or their products interact with the cell surface to stimulate an inflammatory response, in large measure acting through the transcription factor NF-κB, which promotes transcription of proinflammatory cytokines and mucin. ASL, airway surface liquid; GM-CSF, granulocyte-macrophage colony-stimulating factor; IkB, inhibitor of kappa B.

■ INFECTING AGENTS

Cystic Fibrosis National Patient Registry data from 2002 show that among 1000 infants younger than 2 years of age, the first bacterial pathogens detected are *Haemophilus influenzae* (seen in 19%), *Staphylococcus aureus* (42%), and *P. aeruginosa* (29%). In addition, even at this age 7% display *Stenotrophomonas maltophilia*, but fewer than 1% harbor *B. cepacia* complex. The prevalence of *S. aureus* infection increases to 60% among 6- to 10-year-old patients, then falls to 30% in patients over 45 years of age. The overall reported prevalence of *S. aureus* infection has increased markedly over the last decade, from 29.1% in 1991 to 49.7% in 2002; about 35% are methicillin resistant.

In the first year of life, the prevalence of *P. aeruginosa* infection is only about 30%, but by age 10 years it has become the dominant pathogen, and by age 25, its prevalence has reached 80% (Fig. 61-5). About 18 months after *P. aeruginosa* becomes established in the lung, it acquires a mucoid phenotype, an event that marks acceleration of the decline of pulmonary function. Antibiotic-resistant strains of *P. aeruginosa* occur in patients with CF with increasing frequency: About 11% are resistant to tobramycin, 12% to ciprofloxacin, and 5% to meropenem. Although it was originally thought that *P. aeruginosa* is not transmitted from one person to another, distinct clusters of particular strains of *P. aeruginosa* are reported from some centers.[9] Thus, infection containment policies that prevent close contact between patients with CF have become the norm. Such policies have changed the psychosocial dynamic of the disease, precluding patient support groups, gatherings for fund raising, and even social commerce among affected families. As bronchiectasis becomes

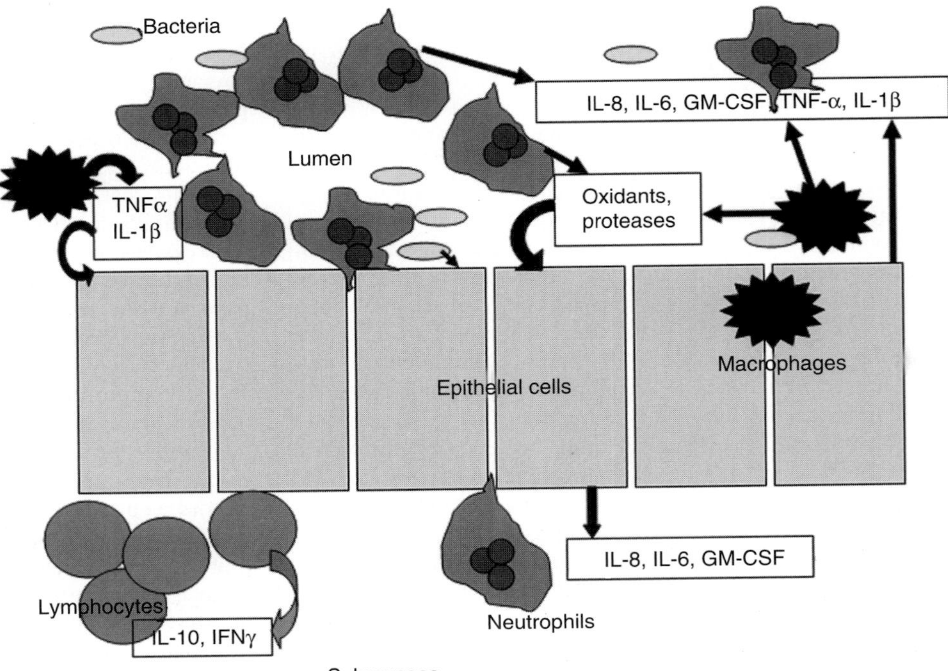

■ **FIGURE 61-2.** Development of inflammatory response in the CF airway. Through interaction either directly with bacteria or with their products, or stimulation by the products of activated macrophages, TNF-α and IL-1β, epithelial cells produce IL-8, which attracts neutrophils, and GM-CSF, which helps prolong their survival in the airway. CF lymphocytes produce less IL-10 and thus neither promote apoptosis of neutrophils nor modulate the inflammatory response appropriately. Large numbers of neutrophils accumulate, which, together with activated macrophages, release oxidants and proteases that in turn damage the airway, interact with epithelial cells to drive chemokine production and secretion, and cleave defensive molecules such as antibodies and complement opsonins, allowing bacteria to persist in the airways.

established and the disease progresses, other antibiotic-resistant organisms are sometimes observed. Acquisition of some of these organisms may also be associated with more frequent medical care, hospitalizations, and exposure to other, sicker patients. One of the most dangerous is *B. cepacia.* This organism can clearly be transmitted from one person to another, particularly genomavar III (now called *B. cenocepacia,* a so-called epidemic strain),[4,10,11] but transmission of other genomavars, including I (or *B. multivorans*) or *B. dolosa*, has also been reported.[12] Therefore, infection control policies are of paramount importance in limiting its spread. Limiting the acquisition of *B. cepacia* is critical, since it is associated with significantly higher mortality (about fourfold) than is observed in otherwise comparable patients who are not infected.[13] Moreover, this organism has been associated with a rapidly progressive syndrome of fever, progression of lung disease to necrotizing pneumonia, and sometimes sepsis, both as an initial presentation of *B. cepacia* infection and spontaneously, after colonization has been present for some time (so-called *cepacia* syndrome). Prevalence of *B. cepacia* varies from center to center, from 0 to 30% in 2002, with a prevalence overall in the entire United States CF population of about 3%. Other highly resistant organisms, which are not associated with rapid decline or even significant impact on the course of disease, such as *Alcaligenes* or *Achromobacter xylosidans* (prevalence 5.2%) and *S. maltophilia* (prevalence 9.4% in 2002, more than four times the prevalence reported in 1992), are also recovered from the CF airway (see Fig. 61-5).

Many patients also harbor fungi such as *Aspergillus* or yeast in their airways either intermittently or persistently. Occasionally, these organisms can be implicated as invasive pathogens, but usually there is not sufficient evidence to warrant specific therapy. Allergic sensitization to *Aspergillus*, however, gives rise to a syndrome of allergic bronchopulmonary aspergillosis, which is

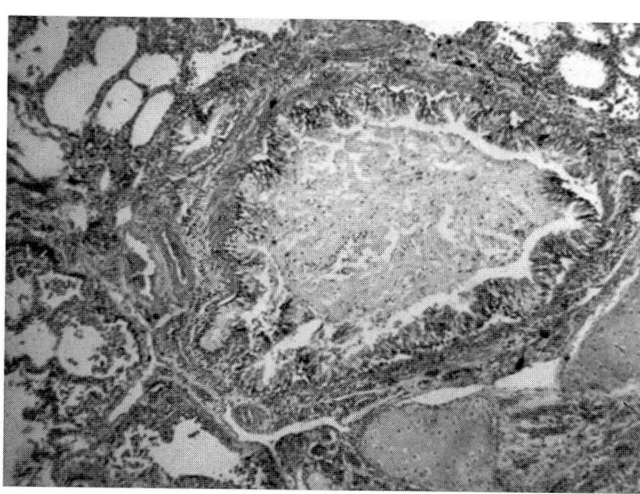

■ **FIGURE 61-4.** Photomicrograph of a section of CF lung taken at postmortem examination. This section illustrates the intense inflammation about the airways with relative alveolar sparing, and the plugging of airways with pus, bacteria, and mucus.

described further below. About 13% of patients nationwide, but with large variation from center to center, harbor atypical mycobacteria, usually *M. avium-intracellulare* complex or *M. abscessus.*[14] Prevalence is higher in older patients and in coastal states. When these organisms are recovered regularly from the sputum, and especially if the patient does not improve with treatment of the more usual bacteria recovered from the airway, specific therapy must be considered.

Although in CF the picture is dominated by bacterial infection, viral infections are common and likely to be more symptomatic and prolonged than they are in control populations. In the past, acquisition of measles pneumonia was a grim prognostic sign. With immunization against this virus, such infections occur only rarely, if at all. Influenza may have serious consequences in the CF lung, but immunization and chemoprophylaxis with amantidine or rimantidine, or treatment after the fact if necessary, has mitigated its impact. However, the greater the number of respiratory viral infections that occur each year, the more rapid is the downhill course.[15]

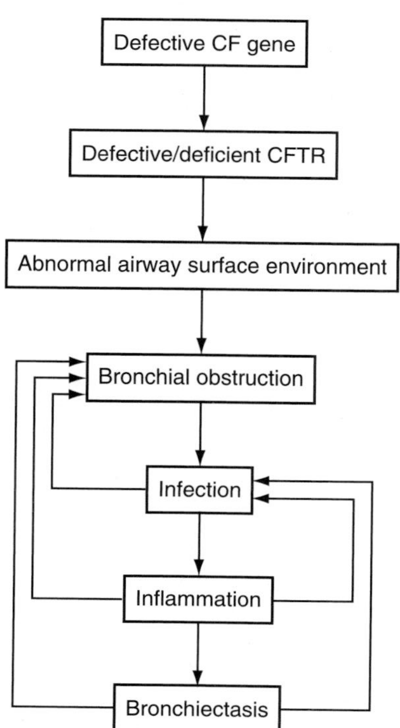

■ **FIGURE 61-3.** Pathophysiologic cascade leading from mutant CFTR to bronchiectasis in the CF lung.

■ INFLAMMATORY RESPONSE

When CF lung disease was first described, the inflammatory response to infection was thought to be an appropriate and necessary response to control bacterial load. Later, it became clear that patients who had lower blood concentrations of IgG had a better prognosis than those with high IgG concentrations, and the idea took hold that the host response contributed to the progression of the disease.[16] Although initially it was thought that the increased IgG presaged the formation of immune complexes that initiated independent inflammatory responses, later it became clear that the increases in IgG indicate greater antigenic exposure from the systemic presentation of bacterial antigens through the damaged airway. Moreover, the inflammatory response in CF airways appears to be excessive relative to the stimulus. Comparison of infants with CF with bacterial infection and infants who do not have CF but who also have bacterial infection showed that the CF infants had increased neutrophils and IL-8 in the bronchoalveolar lavage (BAL) fluid, even when adjusted for the bacterial burden or

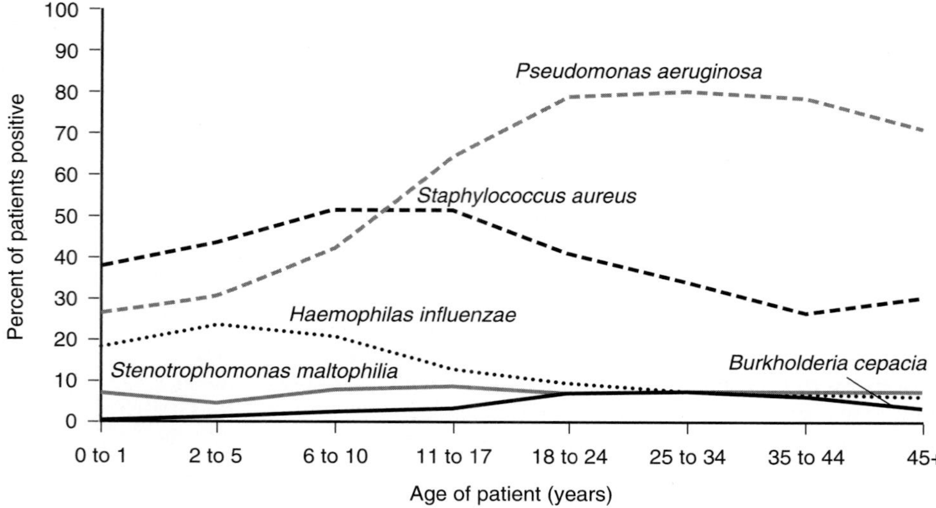

■ **FIGURE 61-5.** Prevalence of recovery of indicated bacteria from patients with CF in the illustrated age groups. (Data are taken from the Cystic Fibrosis Foundation Data Registry of 2002.)

endotoxin concentration.[17] Infants with CF who have no evidence of active lung infection often still have increased IL-8 and neutrophils in their BAL fluid.[18] It may be that these children were infected at an earlier time, but the inflammatory response failed to resolve once the bacteria were no longer present. Gradually, infection becomes permanent, and the persistent neutrophil response leads to continuous release of neutrophil proteases and airway damage. By the age of 1 year, in patients with CF, the amount of neutrophil elastase in the airways has overwhelmed the antiprotease defenses, and free elastase is regularly detected in BAL fluid.[19] Excess free elastase contributes to the persistence of bacteria in the airway in CF by reducing opsonophagocytosis of *P. aeruginosa,* acting as a potent airway secretogogue, and stimulating synthesis of the chemokine IL-8 by epithelial cells, thus both exacerbating airway obstruction and maintaining the infection and the neutrophilic inflammatory response (Fig. 61-6).

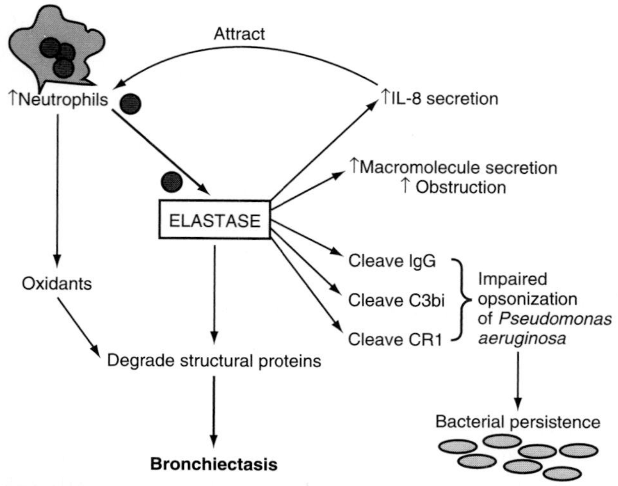

■ **FIGURE 61-6.** Multifaceted damage to the lung and its defenses is mediated by neutrophil elastase, including stimulation of secretion of macromolecules and IL-8, cleavage of all relevant opsonins for *Pseudomonas*, and destruction of structural proteins in the airway wall.

It is probable that both the epithelial cells that line the airways and the lung macrophages contribute to the excess inflammatory response in the CF airways. The bulk of the data suggests that airway epithelial cells of CF phenotype respond in excess to bacterial stimulation with production of IL-8, a potent chemokine, and granulocyte-macrophage colony-stimulating factor, a cytokine that allows prolonged survival of neutrophils in the airway lumen.[20] A few studies indicate that airway macrophages from CF patients may respond with increased tumor necrosis factor-α (TNF-α) to bacterial challenge. TNF-α drives many other inflammatory responses, including those of epithelial cells, may contribute to systemic illness with appetite suppression, and is markedly increased in the CF airway. The hypothesis that inflammation contributes independently to progression of the CF lung disease was supported by the findings of clinical trials of the anti-inflammatory agents corticosteroids and high-dose ibuprofen, both of which retarded the progression of the disease.

■ EVALUATION OF THE CYSTIC FIBROSIS LUNG DISEASE

Assessment of the CF lung disease and its progression not only contributes to prognosis but also serves as an indicator for initiating, intensifying, reducing, or stopping therapy. Several global scoring systems have been proposed, but none has emerged to dominate as an outcome measure for clinical trials or even for prognostication for clinical purposes.

Standard chest radiographs may be normal early in life or show only hyperinflation. However, eventually, peribronchial thickening indicative of edema and infiltration about the airways is observed. As bronchiectasis progresses, "tram tracks" and ring shadows may be seen. Hyperinflation may cause the heart to appear vertical, and as disease progresses, the pulmonary arteries seem prominent. Sometimes large blebs or cysts are identified. During an exacerbation, there may be generalized increase in the markings, localized infiltrate, or very little change in the chest radiograph at all. Various scoring systems have been devised to grade chest radiographs for group comparisons or to assess progression of the radiographic abnormalities.[21] Such scoring systems tend to be more useful for following progression of disease over time than they are for an acute episode of deterioration. Chest radiography may be an insensitive indicator of exacerbation or progression.

High-resolution computed tomography of the chest is more sensitive.[22,23] High-resolution computed tomography demonstrates thickening of airway walls, mucus plugging, and development of bronchiectasis well before they are detected on plain film, and it demonstrates disease progression in children when the pulmonary function has not worsened or has even improved. Localized disease is also easily detected. Chest tomography can be performed even on infants and small children. In older children, an index derived from the combination of pulmonary function testing and high-resolution chest tomography may be the most sensitive measure of disease progression.

Pulmonary function testing is the most frequently used assessment for CF lung disease in older children and adults. In most centers, children can be introduced to conventional pulmonary function testing between the ages of 5 and 6 years, and after about 6 months' practice, the results become reliable. Both spirometry and plethysmography contribute to the assessment. Often, air trapping is the initial manifestation of disease, signaled by an increased ratio of the residual volume to total lung capacity (RV/TLC), but as disease becomes more severe, this becomes an insensitive indicator of change. The small airways display the earliest abnormalities in the spirogram, so the forced expiratory flow rate between 25% and 75% of total lung capacity ($FEF_{25\%-75\%}$) is reduced well before other flows or volumes. However, eventually the forced expiratory volume in 1 second (FEV_1) becomes the parameter of choice to follow, as both an index of airway obstruction and an index of overall disease severity. Many centers also follow the forced vital capacity, which is preserved until much later in the disease course than the FEV_1. (Note that the slow vital capacity deteriorates even more slowly.)

Evaluation of pulmonary function in young children who are not able to cooperate with conventional spirometry has become much more routine and standardized in recent years. The most common approach is to sedate the infant and place him or her in a plethysmograph with a tight-fitting facemask and a jacket that can be rapidly inflated, forcing rapid expiration, and allowing flow rates to be measured. Infant pulmonary function testing has been conducted in patients with CF but has not become a mainstay of clinical evaluation, partly because it requires that patients be sedated, and partly because it is still highly variable. Usually, the critical parameter is the $FEV_{0.5}$ (the volume of air expelled in the first 0.5 second), since the infant can empty the lung much more rapidly than older patients. However, when patients with CF have been followed over time, some improve and some decline, sometimes dramatically, but the predictive value of these infant pulmonary function tests for later measures of disease severity has not been clearly demonstrated, except at the extremes (all tests normal or all tests showing severe impairment). Increased experience with such testing as well as better standardization may improve the value of this test.[24]

Blood gases may be surprisingly well preserved until late in the course of disease. Eventually, however, the matching of ventilation and perfusion can no longer be sustained, and hypoxemia occurs. Initial manifestations of the failure to match ventilation and perfusion may be oxygen desaturation during exercise, accompanied by the sensation of dyspnea on exertion. Often, oxygenation is maintained by increasing minute ventilation, but eventually, it is not possible to sustain the effort, even at rest, and hypoventilation, manifested by an increase in the partial pressure of alveolar carbon dioxide (PA_{CO_2}), supervenes. It is not possible to predict from spirometric measures when this will occur. Hypoventilation occurs in most individuals during sleep, and nocturnal hypoxemia may be manifest before hypoxemia at rest. No properly powered study has investigated whether provision of nocturnal supplemental oxygen improves the course of the disease in CF.

Evaluation of respiratory secretions for inflammatory parameters has received renewed attention in the last few years. Collection of sputum for assessment of bacterial flora, content of neutrophils or neutrophil products, or inflammatory mediators is limited to those patients who produce sputum (often those later in the course of the disease, and older) and runs the risk of sampling error. BAL requires the invasive bronchoscopy procedure and also samples only the areas that were wedged and washed, but is very useful in evaluating progression of lung disease.[24,25] Recently, investigators have capitalized on the ability of aerosolized hypertonic saline to provoke secretions that can be expectorated. Results from this so-called induced sputum correspond well to values from BAL, and the method of collection is much less invasive.[26] The values most often measured are neutrophil counts, IL-8, and uninhibited elastase. Concentrations of other cytokines (e.g., TNF-α, IL-1β, IL-6) and lipid mediators (e.g., prostaglandin E_2, LTB_4) are shown to be markedly elevated in BAL of CF patients compared with normal controls, but this may not be surprising given the chronic infection in the patients with CF.[27–29] Clear demonstration of association of any of these markers or any combination of them with disease initiation or progression is lacking, however.

Evaluation of inflammatory parameters in blood (such as cytokines, C-reactive protein, white blood cell counts) has not been helpful so far in defining the progression of the lung disease over time, although proteomic analysis may eventually reveal a protein that is more closely linked with disease progression. For some exacerbations, however, the C-reactive protein increases, along with the erythrocyte sedimentation rate and, sometimes, the white blood cell count, and these values return to the normal range after therapy. However, some exacerbations can occur without such increases, and without fever or other signs of systemic inflammatory response, yet the exacerbation responds to treatment with antibiotics. A proteomic investigation of serum and BAL fluid is under way in an attempt to detect proteins that can be used as markers of disease.

Clinical evaluation is also important. Weight loss, anorexia, irritability, exercise tolerance, ability to conduct the affairs of daily living, capacity to work or attend school, ability to leave the house for shopping and recreation, and recovery time after exertion, all contribute to the evaluation of the disease. Some of these parameters may be represented in a 6-minute walk test (distance walked in 6 minutes) or more formal exercise testing in which heart rate is monitored as the patient progressively increases exercise stress.

■ PROGRESSION OF THE DISEASE

Except for widened mouths of the submucosal glands, patients with CF are born with normal lungs, and, early in life, the lung function of patients with CF may also be perfectly normal. Over time, however, one can expect lung function to deteriorate. Indeed, at the earliest age at which reliable conventional pulmonary function tests can be obtained, about 5 to 6 years, the mean FEV_1 is about 95% of predicted normal, within the normal range. However, bronchiectasis may be developing even in children with normal pulmonary function,[30] and considerable disease may lurk in the small airways. Early changes in pulmonary function demonstrate air trapping, as shown by increase in the RV/TLC, and other evidence of small airways disease, manifest by reduced flow rates at mid-lung volumes (e.g., $FEF_{25\%-75\%}$ and scooping of the flow-volume loop). Later, flow in the larger airways is compromised, and the FEV_1 is reduced. This measure is of particular importance, since it, of all the pulmonary function tests, correlates best with mortality. As the FEV_1 declines, the $FEF_{25\%-75\%}$ simply remains very low and can no longer be used to detect further impairment. The FEV_1 can certainly improve with therapy or remain stable for long periods; but over time, decline is evident. When the FEV_1 reaches about 30% of predicted normal, 2-year mortality is 50%, according to some investigators.[31] However, other centers find that 7 years are required to reach 50% mortality from this point.[32] This difference is important, since if the patient wishes to be considered for transplantation, there must be time for thoughtful evaluation as well as to wait for donor lungs, so evaluation is usually undertaken about 2 years before anticipated demise. However, younger patients with severe disease may decline more quickly. Those with compromised oxygenation or carbon dioxide retention, or on a rapid downhill course, also decline more rapidly.[33]

Patterns of deterioration vary widely among patients, with some maintaining excellent pulmonary function for extended periods of time, then suffering decline. In 2002, nearly half of the CF patients in the United States who were younger than 18 years of age had FEV_1, in the normal range, but fewer than 20% of those older than 18 years of age had such excellent values. On the average, there is a gradual, steady decline throughout life, averaging 2% to 2.5% predicted FEV_1 per year. Some patients have a dramatic drop at some point, followed by a relatively slow decline; others show a steady drop, and still others do well until a precipitous drop to death. Because steady declines can be slowed and patients can be stabilized even after rapid and profound decline, aggressive treatment is administered at all stages of the disease.

Survival of patients with CF has improved dramatically over the 65 years since the disease was first described (Fig. 61-7). Initially, death in infancy, often from malnutrition or staphylococcal septicemia, was the rule. In the 1950s after the sweat test came into use, identification of milder cases was possible; moreover, antibiotics became widely available. At that time the median survival age was estimated at 4 to 5 years. In the mid-1950s, patients began to gather into centers for care, and physicians had the opportunity to learn from a larger spectrum of patients. Aggressive application of symptomatic therapies proved remarkably effective, and survival increased dramatically with the institution of comprehensive care programs. In the 1990s several new therapies were introduced that have the potential to prolong life. By the end of the 20th century, median predicted survival age for a newborn with CF was hovering about 31 years, with the actual median age of death in 2002 about 25 years. However, the range of age at death is broad, and some patients succumb early in childhood, while others survive into their sixth, seventh, or even eighth decade.

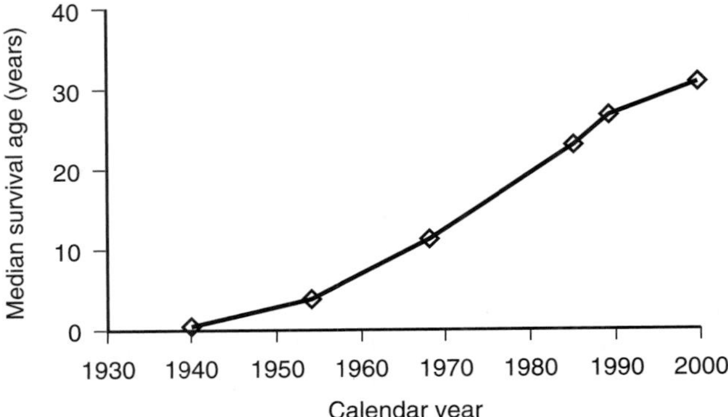

FIGURE 61-7. Median survival age in CF patients over time since first report of the disease in 1936.

Some of this wide variation in the severity of disease and its rate of progression can be attributed to the nature of the CF gene defect itself. More than 1000 individual mutations in the CF gene have been described. Most are "severe" mutations that are associated with full-blown CF, including both lung disease and pancreatic insufficiency. The "mild" mutations are associated with pancreatic sufficiency, although impairment of pancreatic function may develop later. Examples of mild mutations are R117H, A455E, or the splice mutation 3849 + 10 kB C→T. Patients with CF who have at least one mild mutation have, in addition to milder pancreatic disease, milder lung disease, lower sweat chloride concentrations (some in the normal range), and longer survival. At the extreme end of the spectrum of mild mutations are lesions in the CF gene that lead only to congenital bilateral absence of the vas deferens in men, without evidence of lung disease, pancreatic disease, or sweat duct involvement. One genotype associated with this phenotype is the 5T variant in intron 8. In intron 8, a run of thymidine residues may be five, seven, or nine residues long, and the number profoundly influences the proportion of CFTR mRNA that is alternatively spliced to give inactive product. The more inactive product there is, the less normal CFTR mRNA is transcribed. A run of nine thymidines results in little alternative splicing and the full complement of CFTR mRNA; seven thymidines give only 35% of the full complement of normal CFTR mRNA, and five thymidines give only about 10% of the normal CFTR mRNA. Men with the 5T allele on both chromosomes may have congenital bilateral absence of the vas deferens and no other manifestation of CF. Other than infertility, these individuals have normal phenotype and presumably normal life expectancy. Women with such genotypes are phenotypically normal. Other genotypes that can lead to reduced but not absent CFTR function can also give rise to such a phenotype. The amount of CFTR transcribed can influence the impact of amino acid substitutions, as well. For example, the R117H mutation, which causes modest diminution of chloride transport through CFTR, occurs on either the 5T or the 7T background. Individuals with R117H on a 5T background can be considered to have a disease-causing allele (i.e., they have too little of a defective protein), whereas the R117H/7T allele may have little clinical impact, even in the presence of a severe allele on the opposite chromosome (i.e., even the defective function, if present in sufficient quantity, may protect the patient against severe disease).[34] Other genetic alterations, such as the M470V substitution, may also have an impact on the quantity of CFTR that is produced, as well as affecting the impact of other mutations in the coding sequence. Thus, severity of disease can be strongly influenced by the nature of the mutations in CFTR.

However, even among patients with the same CF mutations, such as patients homozygous for the ΔF508 mutation, there is wide variation in disease severity.[35] Male patients do better than female patients, at least from ages 1 through 20, for reasons that are unclear.[36] Patients who acquire *B. cepacia* infection have a significantly poorer prognosis than those with disease of comparable severity who do not become infected.[13] Patients who acquire *P. aeruginosa* infection before the age of 6 years have significantly higher mortality than those who acquire the infection after that age.[37] In addition, environmental influences contribute to this variation. Exposure to tobacco smoke, the accidental acquisition of viral respiratory infections, and environmental pollutants all have negative effects on the disease. Variations in medical care may also contribute: Survival varies from center to center, even after controlling for population characteristics. There is some suggestion that greater use of all treatment modalities is associated with better outcomes. There is a strong influence of socioeconomic status on the survival of patients with CF. The adjusted risk of death for patients covered by public assistance was 3.65 (confidence interval 3.03–4.40) times higher than for those not covered by public assistance in one analysis of Cystic Fibrosis Foundation Registry data (1986–1994). However, the number of outpatient clinic visits was the same for those covered or not covered by public assistance. The poorer outcomes of patients with public assistance are incompletely explained.[38]

To some extent, variability in disease progression may derive from variations in other genes that could influence outcome, that is, modifier genes.[39] Minor variations in amino acid sequence of a protein, or in the nucleotide sequence of the promoter region of a gene, could lead to a protein that is reduced (or increased) in quantity or function. Some of these variants are of no consequence in normal individuals under ordinary circumstances, but when they occur in the setting of disease that arises from another source, such as the CF lung disease, they may have profound consequences. So, for example, a protein that helps defend against bacterial infection in the airways, if increased, may delay colonization in patients with CF and so prolong life. Genes that exacerbate the lung inflammatory response are likely to accelerate the rate of decline of pulmonary function in CF, whereas those that tend to reduce the inflammatory response could retard disease progression. Several extensive studies are now under way to identify modifier genes for CF and, from them, to identify new therapeutic targets.

TREATMENT

The treatment of the lung disease rests on the pillars of attention to nutrition, vigorous airway clearance, aggressive infection control, and anti-inflammatory therapy. Since the progression of the disease occurs because inflammatory cells, enzymes, and oxidants are retained in the airway and renewed as a result of ongoing infection and the inflammatory response to it, these are logical areas to attack. However, prevention of disease, initial colonization, and host response is also fundamental.

PROPHYLAXIS

Forestalling the complications of CF has been a high priority. Nutritional prophylaxis (maintaining nutrition from the outset rather than treating malnutrition after it develops) may allow better initial defenses against colonization and infection. Children with better nutrition in the first 3 years of life have better pulmonary function at age 6 years, suggesting that good nutrition may indeed prevent progression of disease, although association may not prove causation.[40] Immunization has also contributed considerably to improved survival. Particularly, infection with measles or influenza virus can be devastating to patients with CF, and these diseases can be prevented by immunization. In the case of influenza, immunization can be supplemented with antiviral agents such as amantidine, rimantidine, or ostelamavir, which can shorten the duration and modulate the severity of disease. It is not clear whether immunization against type B *H. influenzae* has altered the course of the disease, because the role of that pathogen in disease progression is not clear.

Since survival has improved so dramatically in the last 65 years as a result of aggressive treatment, it makes sense that the earlier intervention can be instituted, the better the outcome is likely to be. However, this has been clearly proven only for nutritional parameters in controlled trials,[41] and the association of better nutrition with better survival, though highly suggestive, may not be causal. Several studies of early, presymptomatic identification of patients with CF using neonatal and prenatal screening show benefit in pulmonary function, but these studies use historical controls.[42] Because of both cohort effects and continuous improvement in therapeutic strategies for CF, such controls are unsatisfactory. One study that used concomitant controls suggests little advantage in pulmonary disease to patients identified by screening and not by symptoms. However, in one of the clinics in this study, rigorous infection control practices were not in place. It is, therefore, possible that infection was transmitted from older, infected patients to infants in a hospital or clinic setting, resulting in earlier colonization and initiation of pulmonary decline. Therefore, assiduous infection control policies are absolutely required if the full potential benefits of neonatal screening are to be realized.[43]

STRATEGIES OF ANTIBIOTIC THERAPY

The bacterial infection so characteristic of the CF lung disease is not evident at birth but rather occurs with time, as bacteria impact on the airway mucus, are trapped, overwhelm the host's innate defenses and later the specific defenses, and begin to colonize the airway. Thus, there is a time early in life in which chronic colonization has not yet occurred. If this window could be extended, both symptomatic and longevity benefits might accrue, although this hypothesis remains to be proven. The best way to maintain airways in the uncolonized state has not been established. Since *S. aureus* is often the initial pathogen in the airways, continuous anti-staphylococcal prophylaxis has been proposed for infants with CF, but the benefits could not be proven in clinical trials, and this strategy is not widely used in U.S. CF centers. Moreover, the association of many of the early colonizing organisms with disease progression is unclear, and so the benefits to be expected from treatment or prevention are similarly uncertain. However, the acquisition of *P. aeruginosa* is associated with poorer prognosis, especially once the mucoid phenotype is established in the lung.[36] Thus, attention has focused on whether the onset or progression of lung disease can be prevented or delayed by prevention of colonization with *P. aeruginosa*. In Denmark, every culture positive for *P. aeruginosa* is aggressively treated; permanent acquisition of the organism is delayed, and so is the associated decline in pulmonary function.[44] However, the comparison in the Danish report is to historical controls, so other variables might also have contributed.

Once colonization of the airways has occurred, it has been proposed that suppressive antibiotic therapy may result in better outcomes. The rationale is that the less intense the bacterial stimulus, the less the host response, and the less likely symptomatic exacerbation and/or lung damage. Although continuous oral antibiotic coverage of patients with CF has not become a standard of care in the last decade, continuous or regularly scheduled intermittent therapy with suppressive inhaled antibiotics has become common. The approach subjected to large clinical trials is administration of tobramycin, 300 mg twice daily by aerosol for 1 month, followed by a month without treatment, followed by a month on treatment to patients infected with *P. aeruginosa*. This strategy results in an increase in FEV_1, which gradually declines in the "off month" but is reclaimed as soon as the drug regimen is resumed. The rate of acquisition of tobramycin resistance is reported to be low, although the results of intravenous antibiotic therapy with tobramycin when required in those on intermittent inhaled therapy have not been studied systematically.[45] Some centers also use other drugs in aerosol form, even if they are not specially formulated for this route of administration, with good success.

Symptomatic exacerbations of the lung disease (increased cough, sputum production, fever, dyspnea, fatigue, anorexia, or weight loss) are treated with intensification of the bronchial drainage regimen and antibiotic therapy directed at the organisms recovered in sputum cultures or deep throat swabs. However, whether it is appropriate to treat the chronic infection with *P. aeruginosa* or other organisms with intravenous antibiotics at regular intervals or only when symptoms increase is not established. The Danish Cystic Fibrosis Center reports that regular intensive antibiotic therapy prolongs life, but the study compares current therapy with historical controls.[44] Many centers in the United States mix therapy for symptoms with regular intensification of antibiotic therapy and airway clearance. Therapy may be occasioned by a gradual, asymptomatic decline in pulmonary function. This strategy represents an attempt to restore the best baseline of pulmonary function regardless of the symptomatic indications for treatment. Many centers treat with an intensified antibiotic and airway clearance regimen, even in the absence of symptoms, if the pulmonary function (FEV_1) has declined by 10% from the best baseline value in patients whose FEV_1 is outside the normal range, and if the RV/TLC has increased or the $FEF_{25\%-75\%}$ has decreased by more than 25% in patients whose FEV_1 is in the normal range. Analysis of registry data indicates that intensity of therapy, gauged by use of all modalities of pulmonary therapy, is associated with better outcomes.

Antibiotics are a mainstay of treatment of CF lung disease (Table 61-1). Antibiotics are usually selected on the basis of culture and antibiotic susceptibility of the organisms recovered in deep throat or sputum culture. Although in older children and

TABLE 61-1. Appropriate antibiotics for treatment of cystic fibrosis pathogens

Prevalent Bacteria	Antibiotic Options	Pediatric Dose*	Adult Dose*	Notes
Staphylococcus aureus	Cefazolin	30 mg/kg IV q8h	1 g IV q8h	
	Nafcillin	25–50 mg/kg IV q6h	2 g IV q6h	
Methicillin-resistant *S. aureus*	Vancomycin	15 mg/kg IV q6h	500 mg IV q6h OR 1 g IV q12h	Administer slowly to avoid histamine release
	Linezolide	10 mg/kg q12h		
Pseudomonas aeruginosa	**Beta-lactam**			
	Ceftazidime	50 mg/kg IV q8h	2–4 g IV q8h	Usual strategy is one beta-lactam and one aminoglycoside or colistin
	Ticarcillin	100 mg/kg IV q6h	3 g IV q6h	
	Piperacillin	100 mg/kg IV q6h	3 g IV q6h	
	Imipenem	15–25 mg/kg IV q6h	500 mg–1 g IV q6h	
	Meropenem	40 mg/kg IV q8h	1–2 g IV q8h	
	Aztreonam	50 mg/kg IV q8h	2 g IV q8h	
	Aminoglycoside			
	Tobramycin	3 mg/kg IV q8h	3–4 mg/kg IV q8h OR 9–10 mg/kg q24h	Serum concentration peak 8–12 μg/mL, trough <2 μg/mL are sought
	Amikacin	5–7.5 mg/kg IV q8h	5–7.5 mg/kg IV q8h	Serum levels peak 20–30 μg/mL, trough <10 μg/mL are sought
	Colistin	1 mg/kg IV q8h	50–80 mg IV q8h	
Burkholderia cepacia	Meropenem	40 mg/kg IV q8h	1–2 g IV q8h	
	Minocycline	2 mg/kg IV or PO q12h	100 mg IV or PO q12h	Should not be given to those <8 years of age
	Amikacin	5–7.5 mg/kg IV q8h	5–7.5 mg/kg IV q8h	
	Ceftazidime	50 mg/kg IV q8h	2 g IV q8h	
	Chloramphenicol	15–20 mg/kg IV q6h	15–20 mg/kg IV q6h	Serum level peak 15–25 μg/mL, trough <5–15 mg/mL are sought
	Trimethoprim/ Sulfamethoxazole	4–5 mg/kg of trimethoprim component IV q12h	4–5 mg/kg of trimethoprim component IV q12h	
Stenotrophomonas maltophilia	Ticarcillin/clavulanate	100 mg/kg of ticarcillin component IV q6h	3 g of ticarcillin component IV q6h	
	Trimethoprim/ Sulfamethoxazole	4–5 mg/kg of trimethoprim component IV q12h	4–5 mg/kg of trimethoprim component IV q12h	
	Aztreonam	50 mg/kg IV q8h	2 g IV q8h	
Achromobacter xylosoxidans	Chloramphenicol	15–20 mg/kg IV q6h	15–20 mg/kg q6h	Serum level peak 15–25 μg/mL, trough <5–15 μg/mL are sought
	Minocycline	2 mg/kg IV or PO q12h	100 mg IV or PO q12h	Should not be given to those <8 years old
	Ciprofloxacin	15 mg/kg IV or PO q12h	400 mg IV or 500–750 mg PO q12h	
	Imipenem	15–25 mg/kg IV q6h	500 mg–1 g IV q6h	
	Meropenem	40 mg/kg IV q8h	1–2 g IV q8h	

*Most doses are expressed as milligrams per kilogram of body weight. The dose given to children should not exceed that for adults.

adults such cultures reflect the lower airway flora quite accurately, in infants the correspondence is not as good, and BAL may be of great assistance in microbiologic diagnosis. Most clinicians administer antibiotics if the patient has an increase in symptoms or a fall in pulmonary function (i.e., for a *pulmonary exacerbation*). This term is used for an increase in cough, sputum production, dyspnea, hemoptysis, pneumothorax, often accompanied by weight loss and sometimes by fever, or for a fall in FEV_1 of 10% or more from best recent baseline value. If the exacerbation is severe, or the patient is perceived to be in danger, or requires treatment with drugs that are difficult to administer at home, treatment is begun in the hospital. For milder exacerbations, patients can be treated at home with oral or intravenous antibiotics and intensification of the airway clearance program. The doses of antibiotics required for CF patients are often greater than those required by non-CF patients to achieve comparable levels in the blood. The precise explanation for this difference is not clear. Therapy must be continued for a sufficient time for symptoms to resolve, the pulmonary function to recover to best baseline or to a new plateau value, and for the organisms harbored to be suppressed, and to avoid selection of resistant organisms. For all these reasons, a minimum course of antibiotics is usually 10 days for a mild exacerbation in a relatively mild patient, and 2 weeks for one that is more severe. However, in older, sicker patients, much longer periods of intensive antibiotic therapy may be required to restore best baseline. For the typical exacerbation, there are no good data to determine whether treatment for an arbitrary time course or until pulmonary function returns to best baseline is superior for long-term results. Unlike courses of antibiotic therapy in non-CF patients, the therapeutic goal cannot be eradication of the organism, for in most cases, the infection cannot be eradicated no matter how long or intensive the treatment.

To treat the most common infecting organism, *P. aeruginosa*, aminoglycoside antibiotics are often used in combination with a semisynthetic penicillin or cephalosporin for intravenous therapy (see Table 61-1). If there is hypersensitivity to penicillin or cephalosporins, or bacterial antibiotic resistance, other classes of drugs such as meropenem or aztreonam may be used. When the organisms are resistant to aminoglycosides, colistin may be available, although it is quite toxic and blood levels cannot be obtained. Quinolones such as ciprofloxacin or levofloxacin are effective orally, but resistance develops rapidly in a substantial number of patients. For *S. aureus*, nafcillin or cefazolin is a good choice, and if methicillin resistance is present, vancomycin or linezolide is required. To fight other organisms, antibiotics are often selected on the basis of drug sensitivities. Sometimes the spectrum of available antibiotics is quite limited, and in such cases, synergy testing with two or more drugs in combination may identify appropriate therapeutic strategies. Such testing is available at particular reference laboratories in the United States and Canada for mailed-in cultures. Although most centers determine the susceptibilities of the organisms and treat accordingly, some studies find no benefit to culture-specific therapy over empirical therapy with tobramycin and ceftazidime. However, combination therapy has been shown to be superior to monotherapy with either tobramycin or a cephalosporin or semisynthetic penicillin alone. Careful monitoring for drug toxicities is required to avoid permanent damage. For example, the aminoglycosides are toxic for the kidneys and eighth nerve, and semisynthetic penicillins can result in neutropenia. Intensive antibiotic therapy with any drugs may be complicated by the acquisition of *Clostridium difficile*, which may lead to intractable diarrhea, sometimes bloody. Sometimes treatment is ineffective, and colectomy is required.

AIRWAY CLEARANCE

Airway clearance is critical in the treatment of CF. Besides being an important maintenance therapy, intensification of airway clearance regimens appears to contribute substantially to improvement during hospitalization for pulmonary exacerbations.[46] Airway clearance measures are clearly synergistic with antibiotic treatment, and one is unlikely to succeed without the other. Several pathophysiologic problems impede clearance. Early in the course of the disease, airway obstruction is probably the result of the impaired mucociliary clearance as well as the abnormal mucins secreted by patients with CF. Later in the course of the disease, much of the difficulty is caused by the viscosity contributed by DNA from dead neutrophils in the airway. As the disease advances further, the floppiness of the airway in bronchiectasis contributes to impaired clearance, and when saccular bronchiectasis occurs, these pockets of pus off the airway are very difficult to clear. The traditional method of postural drainage and clapping is still the method of choice for infants and for site-directed clearance, and most patients find the human hand superior to mechanical percussors. However, some clinicians are cautious about prescribing postural draining and clapping for all infants on a regular basis, however, for fear of exacerbating the tendency toward gastroesophageal reflux disease by the head-down postures and the stimulation of cough in that position. However, a vest that claps the chest with high frequency by changes in air pressure has proven useful for clearance, allows the patient to perform clearance without an assistant, and reaches all areas of the lung. Other hand-held devices are most useful in dislodging and carrying mucus upward toward the mouth, by applying high-frequency oscillations to the airway wall. Such devices are efficient and, when properly used, result in more sputum expectoration in a timed session in trained subjects than either directed coughing alone or postural drainage. For example, the Flutter device (Axcam Scandipharm, Birmingham, Alabama) resembles a plastic pipe. In the bowl of the pipe is a steel ball, which vibrates up and down as the patient expires, applying end-expiratory pressure and vibrating the airway, dislodging mucus and keeping the airway open so that it can be cleared. Although patients must be trained to use the device, it is convenient, portable, and versatile. Other variations are now available. In addition, controlled breathing patterns, called autogenic drainage, can be of great assistance, but when compared directly to the Flutter device lack the device's ability to alter sputum viscoelastic properties. Application of positive end-expiratory pressure is recommended by some authorities and can be achieved with an Acappella device (DHD Healthcare, Wampsville, New York). Many clinicians recommend an exercise regimen, because it enforces a period of time in which deep breathing occurs, the most distal segments of the lung are ventilated, and a period of directed coughing afterward is very beneficial. Moreover, prescription of an exercise program can seem an investment in wellness rather than the drudgery of treatment. Because of the continuous bronchorrhea, it is rare that physical removal of mucus by suction or at bronchoscopy serves any useful purpose beyond the acute, and sometimes no immediate benefit accrues. Lavage of large sections of the lung may compromise ventilation and upset the ventilation-perfusion relationship, and is often unsuccessful in improving gas exchange, even if much mucus is removed.

Drugs may assist in airway clearance. Bronchodilators are useful to keep the airways open and facilitate mucus removal. Both β-adrenergic agonists and anticholinergics can be effective, but β-adrenergic agonists reportedly increase ciliary beat frequency and may assist clearance independent of their relaxant effects on smooth muscle. Anticholinergic agents may reduce secretion and risk further drying of the airway. *N*-acetylcysteine is an effective mucolytic but is often poorly tolerated because of its smell and its propensity to act as a bronchial irritant. Hypertonic saline has attracted interest in assisting airway clearance, but its effects are short lived and of modest magnitude. The newest entry into this class of drugs is recombinant human DNase, which cleaves the DNA in sputum (mostly derived from necrotic neutrophils) into smaller pieces, reducing its viscosity and increasing its ability to be cleared. Patients who take recombinant human DNase have, on an average, a 5% to 7% increase in FEV_1, as well as an improved sense of well-being, although its long-term effects are still being evaluated.[47]

ANTI-INFLAMMATORY THERAPY

Specific anti-inflammatory therapy is useful in patients with CF, particularly those who are relatively young and have only mild disease. Although oral corticosteroids are effective in slowing the decline of the FEV_1, the complications of steroids in CF (marked increase in diabetes, cataracts, and growth failure, the latter persisting for years after the drug was discontinued, especially in the younger boys) make them unsuitable for long-term use.[48] High-dose ibuprofen is highly effective in reducing the rate of decline of pulmonary function.[49] However, this drug increases the already-elevated incidence of gastrointestinal hemorrhage in patients with CF (from about 0.22% per year to 0.4% per year, still a very low rate of complications for an effective therapy). This adverse event is so dramatic, however, that the drug has lost favor because of it. Other available anti-inflammatory agents, such as inhaled steroids, have not yet been subjected to rigorous clinical trial. Whether a new therapy for CF, continuous administration of macrolide antibiotics such as azithromycin, should be classified as anti-inflammatory or anti-infectious has not been clearly established. Although patients enrolled in the clinical trials usually did not harbor organisms sensitive to this antibiotic on routine sensitivity testing, it is possible that azithromycin inhibits *P. aeruginosa* in its stationary phase of growth, as it probably is in the CF lung. However, macrolides have also been reported to have anti-inflammatory properties, and when given to patients with CF result in increase in FEV_1 of 5% to 6% predicted, and also fewer exacerbations.[50,51] Anti-inflammatory therapy is an area of active research, since it has been proven that such therapy alters the course of the disease, and safer alternatives are urgently needed.[52]

TRANSPLANTATION

Despite the best efforts of CF clinicians, patients with CF eventually reach the point of respiratory insufficiency, and the lungs can no longer sustain life. In these patients, transplantation offers the best hope of life extension. In 1988, only 5 transplants were performed in patients with CF, but in 1995, 146 were performed. That number has held relatively steady ever since. The limited supply of organs and the slightly poorer results for patients with CF compared with those suffering from other types of lung disease make it difficult for every patient with interest in this option to take advantage of it. In 2002, for example, 592 patients were evaluated for transplant and 388 were accepted: 53 were declined and 156 deferred. However, only 147 transplants were performed. The 1-year survival is about 80%, and 5-year survival 50% to 59% for patients with CF after lung transplantation in the United States.[53] Those infected with *B. cepacia* have poorer post-transplant survival than those who are not so infected. Other organisms harbored by CF patients are also highly resistant to antibiotic therapy, and some, like *Aspergillus fumigatus*, may thrive under conditions of immunosuppression. Since the patient's upper airway is left intact after transplantation, the upper trachea may remain infected after it is transected and reattached, and sinusitis is nearly universal in CF. Thus, seeding of the transplanted lungs with the patient's own organisms from the sinuses or upper airway may complicate the postoperative course, especially in the face of the immunosuppression that is required to sustain the transplant. Some centers have advocated sinus surgery and regular irrigation and clearance both pre- and postoperatively, and some report fewer infections after transplant with this strategy. Since in CF patients, the main cause of death after transplant is infection, this approach has the potential to improve outcome. CF patients also have the disadvantage of multisystem disease, so the nutritional deficits, abnormalities in drug metabolism, gastrointestinal and hepatic complications, and other problems progress unabated in the face of transplant and can complicate administration of antirejection regimens.

The timing of transplant is optimal if it occurs just before life with the disease becomes unbearable. Since there is usually an extensive pretransplant work-up and a wait for a suitable lung, referral for transplantation usually occurs when the patient's life expectancy is about 2 years. However, making this projection is challenging. According to data from the Toronto center, many clinicians consider referrals for transplantation when the FEV_1 falls to 30% predicted or below,[31] but the inadequacies of universal adherence to such a criterion have also been documented. Other issues, such as the frequency of respiratory exacerbations requiring intravenous antibiotics, age, rate of decline, and respiratory microbiology, contribute to the downward course, but a complex regression model including these variables is reportedly no better at predicting survival than simple FEV_1. Therefore, although the simple criterion of FEV_1 is inadequate to determine timing of listing for transplant, a better algorithm has not been proven. Some recommend that once the FEV_1 is less than 30% predicted, a rapid rate of decline or age younger than 15 years should prompt referral for transplantation, but others suggest that clinical judgment, taking into account all the variables of the case, remains paramount.

FUTURE THERAPIES DIRECTED AT THE BASIC DEFECT

A great hope for the future of patients with CF is the treatment of the basic defect.[54] Three basic strategies are being explored. The first is to activate or inhibit non-CFTR ion transporters to achieve the appropriate ion and fluid balance in the airway. This may involve activation of non-CFTR chloride conductance, combined with inhibition of the excessive epithelial sodium transport. Several such drugs have reached clinical trial, but none have thus far proven to be of striking benefit. However, other chloride transporters have kinetic properties different from those of CFTR and thus may not mimic the sustained chloride transport needed to keep the airway hydrated. Moreover, the complications of lack of CFTR function may extend beyond ion transport. Abnormal cell signaling may allow excessive inflammatory responses, and there may be reduced bacterial killing in the CF airway. These defects may not be readily corrected by activating other transporters. Inhibiting the activity of the amiloride-sensitive sodium transporter seems logical as a therapeutic approach, but a large trial of amiloride was unsuccessful in slowing the rate of decline, despite promising results in a pilot study.

A second strategy is to discover small molecules capable of activating mutant forms of CFTR. This strategy has the advantage that CFTR is already present in the correct cells and regulated under its own promoter, and, by correcting the lack of CFTR function, it might well correct most of the downstream effects. These therapeutic agents may be allele-specific or at least specific for the class of mutation. For example, gentamicin in high doses can cause readthrough of single "stop" codons and may be therapeutic for patients with genotypes such as W1282X or G542X, but not for amino acid substitutions. Clearly, the most important mutation to be activated is ΔF508, since it is the most common mutation and occurs in at least 92% of CF patients in the United States. Many studies are in progress to identify the right drug. For ΔF508, however, three problems must be corrected: This mutant fails to exit the endoplasmic reticulum in the synthetic pathway and is degraded there, but it also has poorer chloride transport activity than does wild type and is retrieved from the plasma membrane much more rapidly than is wild type. More than one drug may be needed to address all of these issues. Recently, a mix of curcuminoid compounds has been reported to activate this mutant both in vitro and in vivo, but the extent of correction and the bioavailability and toxicity of the drug remain to be determined, and other laboratories have been unable to confirm the initial promising results in CF mice bearing the ΔF508 mutation.

The third strategy is to provide a normal copy of the CF gene to the appropriate cells (i.e., gene therapy). This approach should theoretically correct all the downstream effects of CFTR deficiency. However, gene therapy has not been easy. Adenoviral vectors initially had great appeal because of their tropism for the lung, but these vectors failed to enter airway epithelial cells from the apical surface. Moreover, they produced acute inflammatory responses and provoked antibody formation that interfered with repetitive dosing. Lipid-mediated gene transfer efficiently delivers genes to cells but not to the nuclei of nondividing cells. Since most airway epithelial cells are not dividing, and genes must reach the nucleus to be transcribed, this proved problematic for lipid vectors. When the dose was increased to overcome this inefficiency, inflammatory responses occurred. The adeno-associated virus provokes little or no inflammatory response, but it also fails to enter airway cells efficiently from the apical surface and is immunogenic as well. However, strains of adeno-associated virus other than those used initially may enter the airway cells with greater efficiency. Recently, compacted DNA that has been coated with polyethylene glycol has been used to deliver genes to the airways of mice and humans. These nanoparticles can gain access to the nucleus of nondividing cells. This vector is not immunogenic, so repetitive dosing is feasible. Although compacted DNA is efficacious, it is not efficient, and more efficient ways of delivering the cargo are under development.

COMPLICATIONS

Multiple complications of the CF lung disease can occur. One of the most regular complications is the involvement of the upper airway, in the form of pansinusitis, which is nearly universal. In fact, its absence in an American CF patient may be cause to question the diagnosis. Patients with CF may have underdeveloped sinuses as well. Sinusitis is ordinarily not treated unless it is symptomatic, although some clinicians believe that this may be a reservoir of infection that should be cleared before lung transplantation. If symptoms occur, antibiotic treatment is required. With persistence of symptoms, surgical drainage may be helpful. Often, the organisms are the same as those recovered from the lower airways, and therefore intensive anti-pseudomonal antibiotic coverage is required. About 15% of children and 20% to 35% of adults develop nasal polyps. There is some clinical impression that this complication is reduced in the era of nasal corticosteroid preparations, but this has not been proven. Surgical management is usually successful, but polyps often recur and repeated resections may be required.

Bronchiectasis is the end result of the CF lung disease. The bronchial wall is weakened and the lumen widened. In the early stages of cylindrical bronchiectasis, the lesions may be reversible, but in the later stages, when saccular bronchiectasis supervenes and there are outpouchings of the bronchial wall filled with purulent secretions and bacteria, the lesions cannot be reversed. Many of the additional complications of the CF airways disease are complications of bronchiectasis. The treatment of bronchiectasis is really the treatment for the CF lung disease, described earlier. However, occasionally, resection is suggested when bronchiectasis is localized and perceived to be seeding the remainder of the lung with infectious material, or if hemoptysis unresponsive to the usual therapies (or for which the usual therapies are contraindicated) is persistent, severe, and localized. For patients with CF, resection is undertaken only as a last resort, because the disease will ultimately progress to involve all lobes, progression cannot be prevented by resection, and eventually all viable lung will be needed to sustain gas exchange.

Atelectasis is a common complication of bronchiectasis. Lobar atelectasis is reported in 4.1% of patients and segmental atelectasis in another 0.8% of patients. Collapse occurs more often on the right, and the upper and middle lobes are more common sites than the lower lobes. Often, the patient presents with increased pulmonary symptoms, pain from traction on the pleura, and increase in dyspnea, but occasionally the complication is identified incidentally on chest radiography. Ordinarily, therapy is instituted with intensification of the airway clearance regimen (with intensified postural drainage to the affected lobe), antibiotics, recombinant human DNase, and bronchodilators, and resolution is expected. Bronchoscopy with instillation of mucolytics was not helpful in the early case series, but later reports suggest that bronchoscopic instillation of recombinant human DNase may be helpful.

Pneumothorax occurs usually by rupture of bronchiectatic cysts into the pleural space. The incidence in the 2002 Cystic Fibrosis Foundation Data Registry[55] is about 1% per year, but the lifetime probability of occurrence is about 6% to 8%. The older the patient, the more probable is the complication. Patients at age 18 years have a 16% to 20% probability of having a pneumothorax at some point in their lives. One study that recorded the FEV_1 in the year before an episode of pneumothorax found a mean of 58% predicted and a range of 33% to 70% predicted.[56] Thus, this is a complication associated with more advanced disease in older patients. It is also a marker of poor prognosis: Median survival from the first pneumothorax was 29.9 months in one large series.[57] Episodes may themselves be associated with fatalities. The right and left sides seem equally affected, and both sexes are equally vulnerable. Initial therapy is usually tube drainage. For very small pneumothoraxes (<10%), watchful waiting may be the preferred course, but usually a small "pigtail" catheter is used to drain the air and reexpand the lung. Larger pneumothoraxes demand prompt tube drainage, and because of prior episodes of pleural disease, the pneumothorax may be loculated and the location of the chest tube critical for drainage. Without specific intervention and only tube drainage, the probability of recurrence is very high (>50%), and even if sclerosing agents are applied to the pleura via chest tube (a painful form of therapy), recurrence is common. Therefore, surgical pleurodesis or partial pleurectomy is often recommended as first-line therapy, since it is definitive and results in a very low rate of recurrence of pneumothorax. All forms of chemical pleurodesis have substantial rates of recurrence, although they may be used if the patient is too ill for surgery. Specific therapy for pneumothorax must also be accompanied by therapy for pulmonary exacerbation. However, in the current era of lung transplantation, it has been suggested that more conservative therapies be used if the pneumothorax is small and not life threatening, since sclerosing the pleura may vastly complicate removal of the lungs for transplantation and even lead to death from intractable oozing in the divided pleura. Pneumothorax is a late and ominous complication of the CF lung disease.

Blood streaking of the sputum is common in patients with CF, particularly adults, in whom more than two thirds report such a symptom at one time or another. As bronchiectasis progresses, the bronchial arteries become enlarged and tortuous, and, in the face of inflammation and pressure changes due to coughing, may rupture, producing massive hemoptysis (usually defined as more than 500 mL in 24 hours). Although the incidence is much greater in older patients (1.5% of those older than 18 years of age report this complication each year, compared with only 0.2% of those younger than 18 years of age), even children as young as 4 years of age have suffered this complication. Patients who have had massive hemoptysis tend to be sicker than age-matched controls, but overall mortality in patients with hemoptysis is similar to patients matched for FEV_1. Occasionally, the episode is rapidly fatal, usually by exsanguination (but sometimes by drowning), but often the patient survives to receive treatment. Patients with massive hemoptysis who present promptly for therapy can often be stabilized with intravenous vasopressin. The more definitive treatment of choice is embolization of the bleeding vessels.[58] After angiography of the bronchial circulation has been performed, the bleeding site is located and expanding gel particles injected to tamponade the tear. Sometimes the site is located only by inference, if bleeding has slowed or stopped; in this case, large, tortuous vessels are sought for embolization. This procedure is 95% effective in stopping the acute episode, but about half the patients bleed again, months or years later, and require a second procedure. Embolization has also been reported to be effective in patients with lesser degrees of hemoptysis that is recurrent, persistent, and annoying. However, there are risks with the procedure. For example, if a spinal artery arises distal to the point of embolization, the procedure is contraindicated for fear of spinal cord infarction. Complications include chest pain and bleeding at the site of the arteriographic puncture. To control the increase in inflammation that probably led to the episode in the first place, it is important to treat the patient for a pulmonary exacerbation, even if the acute episode is controlled by embolization.

Clubbing of the digits is nearly universal in patients with CF. Although its origins are not entirely certain, recent reports that it disappears after lung transplantation confirm that at least a major association is with the CF lung disease. Another detailed study correlating the degree of clubbing with lung disease parameters concluded that clubbing is related to hypoxemia, airways obstruction, hyperinflation, and nonuniformity of ventilation. A few patients progress to hypertrophic pulmonary osteoarthropathy with elevation of the periosteum, pain in the distal long bones, and disability.

Airway reactivity, defined as reversible airways obstruction, is thought to be common in CF but is difficult to define. At any given time about 40% to 60% of patients respond to β-adrenergic agonists with an increase in FEV_1 of more than 10%. However, if the study is repeated at another time, the same proportion of patients is responsive but not necessarily the same individuals. It is difficult to use such criteria to define airway reactivity in patients with CF, because there is considerable variability in pulmonary function testing from test to test, even on the same day. In addition, about 20% to 60% of CF patients respond to histamine, methacholine, or cold air inhalation with bronchoconstriction, to a degree typical of that required for diagnosing asthma. Often, the pattern of response differs from that seen in asthma, with the response occurring at higher doses of methacholine or histamine, and resolution taking much longer to occur. In exercise testing, the flows often increase markedly during exercise in patients with CF. These observations suggest that the mechanisms of reduction of airflow following inhalation of such agents or cold air may be different from the mechanisms that cause reduced airflow in asthma. However, patients in whom reduced flows are observed after challenge tend to have a more severe course for CF in the subsequent 2 years. Asthma-like symptoms are also associated with poorer pulmonary function. When β-adrenergic agents are administered, there may be a paradoxical decrement in FEV_1 among patients with CF. Presumably, these are the patients for whom bronchial smooth muscle tone is required to maintain the patency of airway walls that are badly damaged in the progression of bronchiectasis. More than 40% of patients with CF have positive skin tests to common airborne allergens, and although this may indicate atopy, it is also the case that if the responses to fungi are disregarded, then the incidence of positive skin tests is no greater than that of the general population. It may be that the CF patient is exposed to fungal antigens because of failure to achieve good clearance of inhaled particles from the lung, and that this eventually provokes immune response.

Clinicians have struggled to identify CF patients with concomitant asthma and airway reactivity, because they will benefit from bronchodilators and anti-inflammatory therapy. Although few controlled studies of β-adrenergic agents have been performed in patients with CF, most patients both in the United States and in Great Britain are treated with these agents. In recent years, the use of inhaled corticosteroids has increased as well, although it is difficult to discern whether the therapeutic intent is control of asthmatic symptoms or anti-inflammatory therapy directed at the CF disease process itself. Some studies suggest that such treatment is beneficial, but one small trial was halted when several of the treated patients had new acquisition of *P. aeruginosa*. Clear conclusions cannot be drawn about this therapy from current literature. Other bronchodilators have been used in patients with CF, including theophylline and LT antagonists, but there are few well-controlled efficacy studies reported.

Allergic bronchopulmonary aspergillosis (ABPA) occurs in 1% to 15% of patients with CF in various series, with the incidence and prevalence varying with geographic location.[59] ABPA is an immunologic response to surface colonization with the fungus *A. fumigatus*. In response to mycelial fungal antigens, CD4$^+$ Th2 cells are activated and excess IgE and IgG1 are produced, all of which combine to drive an inflammatory response in the airways. In non-CF patients, classic ABPA is defined by asthma with infiltrates on chest radiography, immediate cutaneous reactivity to *Aspergillus,* elevated total serum IgE above 417 IU/mL or greater than 1000 ng/mL, serum precipitating antibodies to *A. fumigatus,* central bronchiectasis on chest computed tomography, peripheral blood eosinophilia, and elevated serum IgE and/or IgA directed against *A. fumigatus*. However, among CF patients, airway reactivity is common and so are infiltrates on chest radiograph. Moreover, immediate cutaneous reactivity to *A. fumigatus* is present in more than half of the CF patients in most series. Therefore, a recent conference recommended the following minimal diagnostic criteria for ABPA in patients with CF:

1. Acute or subacute clinical deterioration that is not explained by other etiologies.
2. Total serum IgE greater than 500 IU/mL (or 1200 ng/mL), unless the patient is taking corticosteroids. In this case, the test should be repeated when steroids have been discontinued. If the total serum IgE is 200 to 500 IU/mL, retesting in 1 to 3 months is recommended.
3. Immediate cutaneous reactivity to *Aspergillus* or in vitro demonstration of IgE antibody to *A. fumigatus*.
4. One of the following: (a) precipitins to *A. fumigatus* or IgG antibody to *A. fumigatus* demonstrated in vitro, or (b) new or recent abnormalities on chest radiography that are not responsive to conventional CF antibiotic therapy and chest physiotherapy.

This conference also recommended that a high index of suspicion be maintained for the diagnosis of ABPA in children with CF older than 6 years of age, and that annual determinations of serum IgE be made. If levels above 500 IU/mL are obtained, immediate cutaneous reactivity to *Aspergillus* or an in vitro test for IgE against *A. fumigatus* should be determined promptly. For values of 200 to 500 IU/mL, more frequent follow-up, within 1 to 3 months, is indicated, and the patient should be monitored closely for clinical deterioration. Once the diagnosis has been established, treatment with high-dosage (2 mg/kg/day) prednisone is initiated. After 1 week the dosage can be reduced to 1 mg/kg/day for another week and then a gradual taper undertaken. The entire clinical picture must be taken into account as treatment is altered, but some authorities recommend monitoring of the serum IgE, which correlates with disease activity. The steroids control the immunologic response to *A. fumigatus* but do not reduce the antigen burden. For this reason, many clinicians add itraconazole (200–400 mg/day) to the regimen to allow more rapid reduction in the steroid dose and suppress the antigenic burden. Because of the negative effects of high-dose steroids in CF, including impaired glucose tolerance and growth suppression, minimizing the duration of treatment and the number of episodes of treatment is highly desirable.

Gastroesophageal reflux disease is surprisingly common in patients with CF, from infancy onward. In adults, the prevalence may be as high as 94% by symptoms and 80% by manometry and other objective measurements.[60] The prevalence is reportedly about 25% in children older than 5 years of age.[61] In infants, prevalence was reported as 20% by pH monitoring.[62] The contribution of gastroesophageal reflux disease to the lung disease is unclear. However, there is an association of severity of gastroesophageal reflux disease and severity of lung disease. The mechanism of gastroesophageal reflux disease in CF seems to be predominantly transient inappropriate lower esophageal sphincter relaxation rather than low steady-state basal lower esophageal sphincter pressure. This may be aggravated by cough, bronchodilators, and positioning for clapping and postural drainage. Because reflux has been associated with airway irritation and asthma, its treatment is prudent if symptoms are present. Ordinarily, treatment with antacids, histamine, or proton pump blockers, and the device of eating multiple small meals will control symptoms. Gastric motility agents are also of use in about half of the patients with such symptoms.

Cor pulmonale is a complication of hypoxemia, and thus usually occurs late in the course of the disease. However, since intermittent hypoxemia is as effective in developing pulmonary hypertension as continuous hypoxemia, reduced oxygen saturation measured awake and at rest may not be a good indicator for cardiac risk. Patients with CF may display significant desaturation on exercise or during sleep. The primary means of therapy for cor pulmonale is vigorous treatment of the underlying pulmonary disease. Early pulmonary hypertension can be reversed by administration of oxygen. Some studies indicate that diltiazam, but not nifedipine, may also be beneficial in reducing pulmonary hypertension. However, once established, the fluid overload and complications of cor pulmonale are managed by diuresis and maintenance of oxygenation. As the pressure in the right side of the heart rises, some patients with a patent foramen ovale may experience sudden hypoxemic episodes due to shunting. These patients may be protected against overt right-sided heart failure yet have a complicated course due to severe and largely intractable hypoxemia.

REFERENCES

1. Boucher RC: Regulation of airway surface liquid volume by human airway epithelia. Pflugers Arch 2003;445(4)495–498.
2. Boucher RC: An overview of the pathogenesis of cystic fibrosis lung disease. Adv Drug Deliv Rev 2002;54(11):1359–1371.
3. Kunzelmann K: CFTR. Interacting with everything? News Physiol Sci 2001;16:167–170.
4. Verkman AS, Song Y, Thiagarajah JR: Role of airway surface liquid and submucosal glands in cystic fibrosis lung disease. Am J Physiol Cell Physiol 2003;284(1):C2–C15.
5. Steagall WK, Elmer HL, Brady KG, Kelley TJ: Cystic fibrosis transmembrane conductance regulator-dependent regulation of epithelial inducible nitric oxide synthase expression. Am J Respir Cell Mol Biol 2000;22(1): 45–50.
6. Berger M: Inflammation in the lung in cystic fibrosis. A vicious cycle that does more harm than good? Clin Rev Allergy 1991;9(1–2):119–142.
7. Berger M: Lung inflammation early in cystic fibrosis: Bugs are indicted, but the defense is guilty. Am J Respir Crit Care Med 2002;165(7): 857–858.
8. Bedrossian CW, Greenberg SD, Singer DB, et al: The lung in cystic fibrosis. A quantitative study including prevalence of pathologic findings among different age groups. Hum Pathol 1976;7(2):195–204.
9. Saiman L, Marshall BC, Mayer-Hamblett N, et al: Macrolide Study Group. Azithromycin in patients with cystic fibrosis chronically infected with *Pseudomonas aeruginosa*. A randomized controlled trial. JAMA 2003; 290(13):1749–1756.
10. Vandamme P, Holmes B, Coenye T, et al: *Burkholderia cenocepacia* sp. nov.—a new twist to an old story. Res Microbiol 2003;154(2):91–96.
11. Coenye T, LiPuma JJ: Molecular epidemiology of *Burkholderia* species. Front Biosci 2003;8:e55–e67.
12. Biddick R, Spilker T, Martin A, LiPuma JJ: Evidence of transmission of *Burkholderia cepacia, Burkholderia multivorans* and *Burkholderia dolosa* among persons with cystic fibrosis. FEMS Microbiol Lett 2003;228(1): 57–62.

13. Lewin LO, Byard PJ, Davis PB: Effect of *Pseudomonas cepacia* colonization on survival and pulmonary function of cystic fibrosis patients. J Clin Epidemiol 1990;43(2):125–131.
14. Maiz-Carro L, Navas-Elorza E: Nontuberculous mycobacterial pulmonary infection in patients with cystic fibrosis. Diagnosis and treatment. Am J Respir Med 2002;1(2):107–117.
15. Wang EE, Prober CG, Manson B, et al: Association of respiratory viral infections with pulmonary deterioration in patients with cystic fibrosis. N Engl J Med 1984;311(26):1653–1658.
16. Wheeler WB, Williams M, Matthews WJ Jr, Colten HR: Progression of cystic fibrosis lung disease as a function of serum immunoglobulin G levels. A 5-year longitudinal study. J Pediatr 1984;104(5):695–699.
17. Muhlebach MS, Noah TL: Endotoxin activity and inflammatory markers in the airways of young patients with cystic fibrosis. Am J Respir Crit Care Med 2002;165(7):911–915.
18. Khan TZ, Wagener JS, Bost T, et al: Early pulmonary inflammation in infants with cystic fibrosis. Am J Respir Crit Care Med 1995;151(4): 1075–1082.
19. Birrer P, McElvaney NG, Rudeberg A, et al: Protease-antiprotease imbalance in the lungs of children with cystic fibrosis. Am J Respir Crit Care Med 1994;150(1):207–213.
20. Chmiel JF, Davis PB: State of the art: Why do the lungs of patients with cystic fibrosis become infected and why can't they clear the infection? Respir Res 2003;4(1):8.
21. Koscik RE, Kosorok MR, Farrell PM, et al: Wisconsin cystic fibrosis chest radiograph scoring system. Validation and standardization for application to longitudinal studies. Pediatr Pulmonol 2000;29(6):457–467.
22. Demirkazik FB, Ariyurek OM, Ozcelik U, et al: High resolution CT in children with cystic fibrosis. Correlation with pulmonary functions and radiographic scores. Eur J Radiol 2001;37(1):54–59.
23. Marchant JM, Masel JP, Dickinson FL, et al: Application of chest high-resolution computer tomography in young children with cystic fibrosis. Pediatr Pulmonol 2001;31(1):24–29.
24. Ranganathan SC, Bush A, Dezateux C, et al: Relative ability of full and partial forced expiratory maneuvers to identify diminished airway function in infants with cystic fibrosis. Am J Respir Crit Care Med 2002;166(10): 1350–1357.
25. Konstan MW, Walenga RW, Hilliard KA, Hilliard JB: Leukotriene B4 markedly elevated in the epithelial lining fluid of patients with cystic fibrosis. Am Rev Respir Dis 1993;148(4 Pt 1):896–901.
26. Ordonez CL, Henig NR, Mayer-Hamblett N, et al: Inflammatory and microbiologic markers in induced sputum after intravenous antibiotics in cystic fibrosis. Am J Respir Crit Care Med 2003;168(12):1471–1475.
27. Bonfield TL, Panuska JR, Konstan MW, et al: Inflammatory cytokines in cystic fibrosis lungs. Am J Respir Crit Care Med 1995;152(6 Pt 1): 2111–2118.
28. Noah TL, Black HR, Cheng PW, et al: Nasal and bronchoalveolar lavage fluid cytokines in early cystic fibrosis. J Infect Dis 1997;175(3):638–647.
29. Konstan MW, Hilliard KA, Norvell TM, Berger M: Bronchoalveolar lavage findings in cystic fibrosis patients with stable, clinically mild lung disease suggest ongoing infection and inflammation. Am J Respir Crit Care Med 1994;150(2):448–454.
30. Farrell PM, Li Z, Kosorok MR, et al: Longitudinal evaluation of bronchopulmonary disease in children with cystic fibrosis. Pediatr Pulmonol 2003;36(3):230–240.
31. Kerem E, Reisman J, Corey M, et al: Prediction of mortality in patients with cystic fibrosis. N Engl J Med 1992;326:1187–1191.
32. Doershuk CF, Stern RC: Timing of referral for lung transplantation for cystic fibrosis. Overemphasis on FEV_1 may adversely affect overall survival. Chest 1999;115(3):782–787.
33. Augarten A, Akons H, Aviram M, et al: Prediction of mortality and timing of referral for lung transplantation in cystic fibrosis patients. Pediatr Transplant 2001;5(5):339–342.
34. Groman JD, Hefferon TW, Casals T, et al: Variation in a repeat sequence determines whether a common variant of the cystic fibrosis transmembrane conductance regulator gene is pathogenic or benign. Am J Hum Genet 2004; 74(1):176–179.
35. Navarro J, Rainisio M, Harms HK, et al: Factors associated with poor pulmonary function. Cross-sectional analysis of data from the ERCF. European Epidemiologic Registry of Cystic Fibrosis. Eur Respir J 2001;18(2):298–305.
36. Davis PB: The gender gap in cystic fibrosis survival. J Gend Specif Med 1999;2(2):47–51.
37. Demko CA, Byard PJ, Davis PB: Gender differences in cystic fibrosis. *Pseudomonas aeruginosa* infection. J Clin Epidemiol 1995;48(8): 1041–1049.
38. Schechter MS, Shelton BJ, Margolis PA, Fitzsimmons SC: The association of socioeconomic status with outcomes in cystic fibrosis patients in the United States. Am J Respir Crit Care Med 2001;163(6):1331–1337.
39. Drumm ML: Modifier genes and variation in cystic fibrosis. Respir Res 2001;2(3):125–128.
40. Konstan MW, Butler SM, Wohl ME, et al: Investigators and Coordinators of the Epidemiologic Study of Cystic Fibrosis. Growth and nutritional indexes in early life predict pulmonary function in cystic fibrosis. J Pediatr 2003;6:624–630.
41. Farrell PM, Kosorok MR, Laxova A, et al: Nutritional benefits of neonatal screening for cystic fibrosis. Wisconsin Cystic Fibrosis Neonatal Screening Study Group. N Engl J Med 1997;337(14):963–969.
42. Merelle ME, Schouten JP, Gerritsen J, Dankert-Roelse JE: Influence of neonatal screening and centralized treatment on long-term clinical outcome and survival of CF patients. Eur Respir J 2001;18(2):306–315.
43. Farrell PM, Li Z, Kosorok MR, et al: Bronchopulmonary disease in children with cystic fibrosis after early or delayed diagnosis. Am J Respir Crit Care Med 2003;168(9):1100–1182.
44. Hoiby N: Antibiotic therapy for chronic infection of *Pseudomonas* in the lung. Annu Rev Med 1993;44:1–10.
45. Cheer SM, Waugh J, Noble S: Inhaled tobramycin (TOBI). A review of its use in the management of *Pseudomonas aeruginosa* infections in patients with cystic fibrosis. Drugs 2003;63(22):2501–2520.
46. Regelmann WE, Elliott GR, Warwick WJ, Clawson CC: Reduction of sputum *Pseudomonas aeruginosa* density by antibiotics improves lung function in cystic fibrosis more than do bronchodilators and chest physiotherapy alone. Am Rev Respir Dis 1990;141(4 Pt 1):914–921.
47. Jones AP, Wallis CE: Recombinant human deoxyribonuclease for cystic fibrosis. Cochrane Database Syst Rev 2003;3:CD001127.
48. Eigen H, Rosenstein BJ, FitzSimmons S, Schidlow DV: A multicenter study of alternate-day prednisone therapy in patients with cystic fibrosis. Cystic Fibrosis Foundation Prednisone Trial Group. J Pediatr 1995; 126(4):515–523.
49. Konstan MW, Byard PJ, Hoppel CL, Davis PB: Effect of high-dose ibuprofen in patients with cystic fibrosis. N Engl J Med 1995;332(13):848–854.
50. Southern K, Barker P, Solis A: Macrolide antibiotics for cystic fibrosis. Cochrane Database Syst Rev 2004;2:CD002203.
51. Saiman L, Siegel J: Infection control in cystic fibrosis. Clin Microbiol Rev 2004;17(1):57–71.
52. Cantin AM: Novel approaches to inflammation and infection in the cystic fibrosis lung. Pediatr Pulmonol 2001;Suppl 23:94–96.
53. Egan TM, Detterbeck FC, Mill MR, et al: Long term results of lung transplantation for cystic fibrosis. Eur J Cardiothorac Surg 2002;22(4):602–609.
54. Davis PB, Drumm M, Konstan MW: Cystic fibrosis. Am J Respir Crit Care Med 1996;154(5):1229–1256.
55. Cystic Fibrosis Foundation: Patient Registry 2002 Annual Data Report to the Center Directors. Bethesda, Md: Cystic Fibrosis Foundation, 2003.
56. Flume PA: Pneumothorax in cystic fibrosis. Chest 2003;123(1):217–221.
57. Schidlow DV, Taussig LM, Knowles MR: Cystic Fibrosis Foundation consensus conference report on pulmonary complications of cystic fibrosis. Pediatr Pulmonol 1993;15(3):187–198.
58. Brinson GM, Noone PG, Mauro MA, et al: Bronchial artery embolization for the treatment of hemoptysis in patients with cystic fibrosis. Am J Respir Crit Care Med 1998;157(6 Pt 1):1951–1958.
59. Stevens DA, Moss RB, Kurup VP, et al: and participants in the Cystic Fibrosis Foundation Consensus Conference: Allergic bronchopulmonary *Aspergillosis* in cystic fibrosis—state of the art. Cystic Fibrosis Foundation Consensus Conference. CID 2003;37(Suppl 3):S225–S264.
60. Ledson MJ, Tran J, Walshaw MJ: Prevalence and mechanisms of gastro-oesophageal reflux in adult cystic fibrosis patients. JR Soc Med 1998; 91(1):7–9.
61. Malfroot A, Dab I: New insights on gastro-oesophageal reflux in cystic fibrosis by longitudinal follow-up. Arch Dis Child 1991;66(11):1339–1345.
62. Heine RG, Button BM, Olinsky A, et al: Gastro-oesophageal reflux in infants under 6 months with cystic fibrosis. Arch Dis Child 1998;78(1): 44–48.

62 Nonpulmonary Manifestations of Cystic Fibrosis

Najma N. Ahmed, MD • Peter R. Durie, MD

Cystic fibrosis (CF) is characterized by the abnormal secretion of fluid, electrolytes, and macromolecules by exocrine glands. In 1989, Tsui and colleagues isolated the CF gene on chromosome 7, and this led to the discovery of its gene product, the cystic fibrosis transmembrane conductance regulator (CFTR), which functions as a cyclic adenosine monophate (cAMP)-dependent chloride channel.[1] The pathophysiologic basis of CF centers on the defective function of this protein in various tissues. In the gastrointestinal tract, CFTR is expressed in the crypt and villous cells of the intestine, the apical membrane of cholangiocytes, and the apical membrane of the pancreatic ductal epithelium. CFTR is also expressed in the reproductive tract, resulting in altered fertility in patients with CF. The absence or dysfunction of CFTR in various tissues results in a broad spectrum of disease manifestations involving the bronchopulmonary tree, exocrine pancreas, and hepatobiliary system, as well as the male reproductive system. The spectrum of clinical manifestation is summarized in Box 62-1.

PANCREATIC DISEASE

PATHOBIOLOGY

Quantitative pancreatic stimulation testing shows that patients with CF have abnormal ductal chloride and bicarbonate secretion.[2] The impaired electrolyte transport results in a reduction in fluid secretion, which leads in turn to protein hyperconcentration and ductal obstruction by viscous secretions (Fig. 62-1).[3] Impaired ductal secretion of Cl^- by dysfunctional or absent CFTR was proposed to reduce the amount of Cl^- available for transport via the ductal apical Cl^-/HCO_3^- exchanger, and thus to result in low levels of pancreatic HCO_3^- secretion.[4] However, it is now understood that pancreatic HCO_3^- secretion can also occur in the absence of luminal chloride.[5] CFTR-mediated Cl^- transport results in the depolarization of the ductal epithelial cell, stimulating entry of HCO_3^- via basolateral electrogenic Na/HCO_3^- cotransporters. Bicarbonate is then secreted via a predominantly conductive pathway.[6] CFTR also appears to be directly involved in HCO_3^- transport.

In its most severe form, pancreatic disease begins in utero. There is rapid progression of acinar damage within the first year of life in patients with pancreatic insufficiency. Morphologic evaluation of the pancreas in infants dying with CF has shown a marked lack of development of acinar tissue. Duct obstruction by proteinaceous secretions is thought to lead to duct dilatation and acinar loss. Histologically, there is extensive destruction of pancreatic acini, with replacement by fat and fibrous tissue. It is important to note that to develop pancreatic insufficiency, more than 95% of pancreatic function must be lost.

PANCREATIC PHENOTYPE

Cross-sectional data indicate that approximately 85% of CF patients are pancreatic insufficient (PI) and require enzyme supplementation. The remaining patients have adequate pancreatic reserve to allow for adequate nutrient digestion and do not require enzymes. This group of patients is termed pancreatic sufficient (PS). Studies have shown that PS patients are diagnosed at a later age and have lower mean sweat chloride concentrations and better pulmonary function than patients with pancreatic insufficiency. Moreover, the PS patients, as a group, have better survival. In contrast, PI patients are more likely to have meconium ileus, distal intestinal obstruction syndrome (DIOS), and severe liver disease.

Newborn screening programs have shown that approximately 60% of patients are PI at diagnosis. PI infants have high serum trypsinogen levels at diagnosis that decline to undetectable levels by 7 years of age. The majority of the PS infants progress to PI within the first 2 to 3 years of life. Such patients show a progressive but delayed decline in serum trypsinogen levels. As we will describe later, the remaining PS patients show prolonged retention of their PS status.

GENOTYPE-PHENOTYPE CORRELATIONS

More than 1200 different mutations or putative mutations have been identified in the *CFTR* gene, most of which are rare. Genotype-phenotype studies have shown that the strongest association between the CFTR genotype and the clinical phenotype is in the exocrine pancreas. The PI and PS phenotypes are associated with distinct "severe" or "mild" mutations in the *CFTR* gene, respectively. Patients who are PI at diagnosis, or who progress to PI, carry severe mutations on both alleles, while patients who are PS carry at least one mild mutation. The mild allele confers a dominant effect over the severe allele. This subject is covered in more detail in Chapter 58.

The pancreatic phenotype has been shown to correlate with the functional consequences of CFTR mutations. Over 95% of patients with severe class I, II, and III mutations were PI or progressed to pancreatic insufficiency after diagnosis. In contrast, most patients with mild class IV and V mutations were consistently PS.[7]

CLINICAL PRESENTATION

Pancreatic Insufficiency

The vast majority of patients who present with the "classic" PI form of CF present in infancy or early childhood with classical

BOX 62-1 Clinical Manifestations of Cystic Fibrosis

Systemic

- Failure to thrive
- Malnutrition/kwashiorkor
- Micronutrient deficiencies

Esophagus

- Gastroesophageal reflux
- Esophagitis/stricture
- Esophageal varices

Pancreas

- Pancreatic insufficiency
- Pancreatitis
- CF-related diabetes

Intestine

- Meconium ileus
- DIOS
- Constipation
- Rectal prolapse
- Fibrosing colonopathy

Hepatobiliary

Extrahepatic

- Microgallbladder
- Distended gallbladder
- Cholelithiasis
- Common bile duct stenosis
- Cholangiocarcinoma
- Sclerosing cholangitis

Intrahepatic

- Neonatal cholestasis
- Steatosis
- Focal biliary cirrhosis
- Multilobular cirrhosis

Reproductive

- Infertility due to obstructive azoospermia in men
- Impaired fertility in women

manifestations of CF such as meconium ileus, malnutrition/growth failure, steatorrhea, and rectal prolapse. Even patients diagnosed by newborn screening at 6 to 8 weeks of age may have signs and symptoms of malnutrition. They may or may not have respiratory symptoms. Laboratory testing shows microscopic evidence of undigested triglyceride, increased fecal fat losses after a 72-hour balance study, or low fecal enzymes (elastase-1 or chymotrypsin). There may be biochemical evidence of fat-soluble vitamin deficiencies. Some patients may present with hemolysis secondary to vitamin E deficiency or with bleeding due to vitamin K deficiency. At presentation, up to 50% of conventionally diagnosed patients may be hypoalbuminemic. Patients may present with severe protein calorie malnutrition and evidence of kwashiorkor. Infants can present with hypoproteinemia, edema, growth failure, and ascites.[8,9] A small minority of CF patients who are PI are not diagnosed until later childhood and rarely adolescence.

Pancreatic Sufficiency

Patients with the "nonclassic" PS phenotype usually present later in childhood and early adulthood. Clinical manifestations are frequently quite subtle, usually involving a single organ, and unlike patients with the classic form of CF, patients usually grow relatively normally and do not have symptoms of impaired digestion.

Adolescents and adults presenting with sinopulmonary disease, such as chronic sinusitis, recurrent nasal polyps, recurrent chest infections, or bronchiectasis, should undergo further investigation for CF. A significant subgroup of these patients will in fact carry a diagnosis of CF. However, the diagnosis of CF may be more difficult to establish or exclude. Sweat chloride measurements are, on average, lower in PS patients than those observed in the classic CF patient population, and in many cases individual values may be within the normal or borderline range.

Cross-sectional data from our center indicate that approximately one fifth of nonclassic CF patients develop pancreatitis, and in one third of PS patients, the diagnosis of pancreatitis preceded the diagnosis of CF. More recently, it has been shown that otherwise healthy patients with idiopathic recurrent acute pancreatitis or chronic pancreatitis have a higher incidence of *CFTR* gene mutations.[10–12] In a subgroup of patients with nonclassic CF who present with idiopathic pancreatitis in the absence of other symptoms, the diagnosis is confirmed by demonstrating abnormalities of ion transport, such as sweat chloride and nasal potential difference testing, or by genotype analysis. Liver disease may also be an isolated presenting feature of CF disease, although this is extremely uncommon.

As will be described in more detail later, otherwise healthy men with infertility due to obstructive azoospermia carry a much higher frequency of *CFTR* gene mutations than the general population. Approximately 20% of men with the severest form of obstructive azoospermia, congenital bilateral absence of the vas deferens, have the PI form of CF on the basis of current diagnostic criteria. While a small percentage of these men have clinical evidence of bronchopulmonary disease at the time of diagnosis, the long-term risk of developing significant bronchopulmonary disease with advancing age remains to be determined.

ASSESSMENT OF PANCREATIC FUNCTION

Pancreatic function should be objectively assessed at the time of diagnosis. Also, patients who are PS should be monitored regularly for evidence of progression to pancreatic insufficiency. Pancreatic function may be assessed using several methods. Most commonly, 72-hour fecal fat balance studies are used to identify patients with the PI phenotype. Accurate measurement of fat intake is critical in obtaining a valid result. Pancreatic insufficiency is defined by fat losses of more than 15% of intake in newborns younger than 6 months of age, whereas in older infants a cutoff of more than 7% of intake is used. Serum trypsinogen measurement can also be used to distinguish between PI and PS patients who are older than 7 years of age. At birth serum levels are usually elevated, but then they decline to low or undetectable levels in PI patients by 5 to 7 years of age. In contrast, PS patients show fluctuating levels both within and above the normal range at all ages. In patients who are PS at diagnosis and progress to PI, there is a delayed decline in serum trypsinogen levels.

Fecal pancreatic elastase-1 is a good alternative test for the assessment of pancreatic function, although it does have

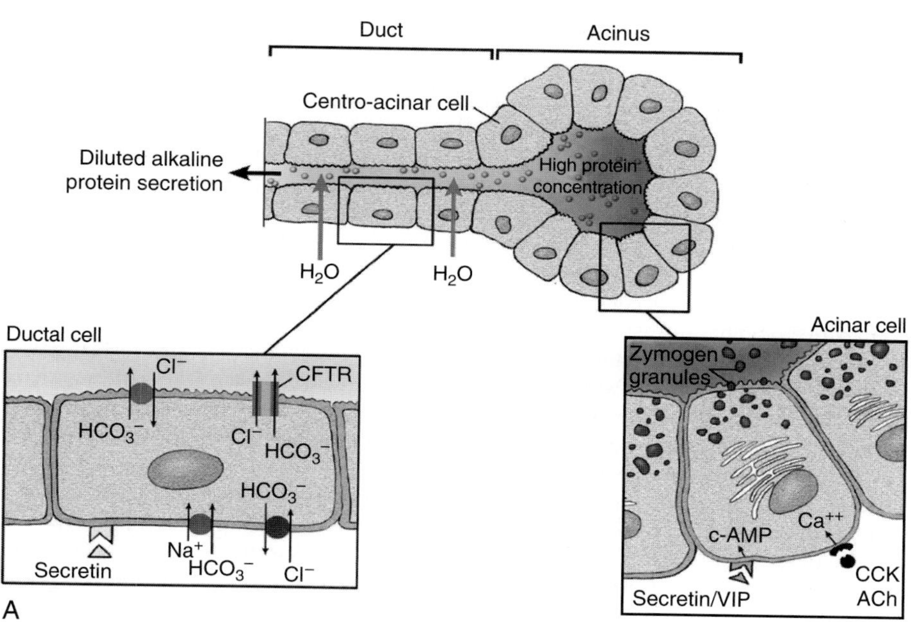

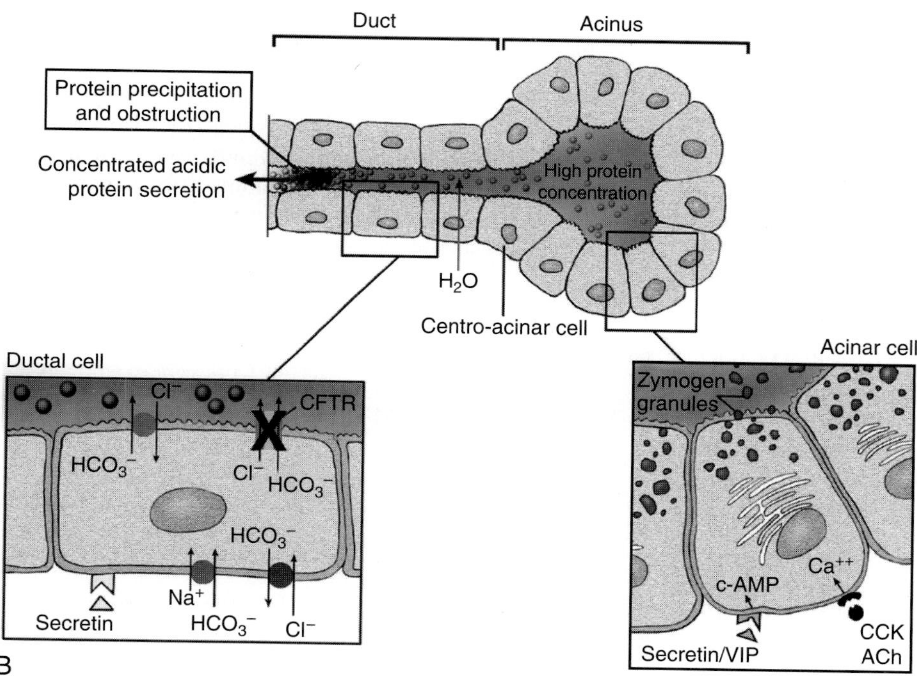

■ **FIGURE 62-1.** Pathophysiology of pancreatic disease in CF. Under normal circumstances (**A**), Cl^- and HCO_3^- secretion provides a driving force for the movement of fluid into the lumen of the duct, which maintains the solubility of secreted proteins in a dilute, alkaline solution. In CF (**B**), impaired anion transport results in decreased secretion of more acidic fluid, which leads to precipitation of secreted proteins. Intraluminal obstruction of the ducts then causes progressive pancreatic damage and atrophy. ACh, acetylcholine; cAMP, cyclic adenosine monophosphate; CCK, cholecystokinin; VIP, vasoactive intestinal polypeptide.

some limitations. The test is not influenced by the concurrent ingestion of pancreatic enzymes. In a recent study a negative test result (>100 μg/g stool) had a 99% predictive value for ruling out pancreatic insufficiency. In patients with CF, the sensitivity and specificity were 100%. However, in other conditions causing steatorrhea, including short gut and Shwachman-Diamond syndrome, fecal elastase-1 measurements had a lower specificity.[13]

Quantitative pancreatic function testing, using duodenal intubation and a marker perfusion technique, is useful to quantify pancreatic reserve as well as fluid and anion secretion. However, this test is limited by its invasive nature, cost, and complexity. Quantitative exocrine pancreatic function correlates with the functional consequences of *CFTR* gene mutations. Patients with class I, II, or III mutations have severely impaired acinar and ductular function, as compared with controls. In contrast, those with class IV or V mutations have a wide range of enzyme output extending from just above the threshold for developing pancreatic insufficiency into the normal range.

MANAGEMENT OF PANCREATIC INSUFFICIENCY

Only patients who have documented pancreatic insufficiency should receive pancreatic enzyme supplementation. Enzymes are available in tablet, powdered, or microencapsulated forms. Most clinics use some form of pH-resistant, enteric-coated microsphere preparation. These preparations were developed to protect the enzymes from degradation by acid and pepsin in the stomach. They allow for release of the enzymes at a pH of 5.5 to 6, and in theory, the enteric coating of the microspheres should dissolve in the proximal small intestine. Ideally, the dose of enzyme should be determined by nutrient intake of fat, protein, and carbohydrate. However, a simplified approach has been established that is based on the patient's age and weight (Table 62-1). Usually, half the standard dose is used for snacks. The dose should be started at 1000 lipase units/kg/meal for children under the age of 4 years, or at 500 lipase units/kg/meal for children older than 4 years of age. The total daily dose should reflect three meals a day and two to three snacks per day. Patients should be maintained on a high-energy diet that is rich in fat, and their growth should be monitored closely.

The response to pancreatic enzymes is extremely variable among patients, and consequently dosing requirements may vary. If there is a poor response to enzyme therapy, or there are persistent symptoms or poor growth, the patient should be reevaluated for other contributing influences (Box 62-2). Patients should not arbitrarily increase enzymes dosing without consulting their CF team. The dose should not exceed 2500 lipase units/kg/meal because of the increased risk of fibrosing colonopathy, as discussed later.[14] Children who are unable to swallow whole capsules may open the capsule and mix the contents with a small amount of applesauce or other acidic food. The microspheres should not be crushed or allowed to remain in food not being consumed immediately. Enzymes should be stored in a cool dark place and expiration dates should be observed.

One condition that can interfere with the efficacy of pancreatic enzymes is the inability of the CF pancreas to produce the normal alkaline secretions that help to neutralize acidic gastric contents entering the small bowel. The lower intestinal pH results in impaired enzyme release, and/or reduced enzyme activity. Acid suppression therapy may, therefore, be useful to raise the intestinal pH. Furthermore, severe cholestatic hepatobiliary disease can contribute to malabsorption in CF. Patients who do not respond to therapy should have thorough investigation to identify other comorbid conditions. A poor response to therapy may also result from a concomitant gastrointestinal disorder, including chronic giardiasis, celiac disease, inflammatory bowel disease, and bacterial overgrowth.

TABLE 62-1. Dosing guidelines for pancreatic enzymes

Age	Dose of Enzymes
Infant	2000–4000 units lipase/120 mL formula or breastfeeding
<4 yr	1000–2500 units lipase/kg/meal
>4 yr	500–2500 units lipase/kg/meal

COMPLICATIONS OF THERAPY

Fibrosing Colonopathy

The first description of colonic strictures in CF patients occurred in 1994. In fibrosing colonopathy, there is colonic narrowing with circular intramural fibrosis that may be limited to the ascending colon or may extend to involve the entire colon. Barium enema may demonstrate a localized apple core–like lesion in the ascending colon, or the entire colon may appear contracted and featureless. Bowel wall thickness is increased on two-dimensional imaging. However, evidence of bowel wall thickening should be interpreted with caution, since unaffected patients with CF have colonic wall thickening on ultrasound.[15,16] Histology may show evidence of severe fibrosis in the lamina propria, and superficial inflammation with eosinophils, cryptitis, or apoptosis (Fig. 62-2).

Although the precise cause is unknown, retrospective case-control studies showed a strong risk association with high-dose pancreatic enzyme use. Patients at higher risk for this complication include children younger than 12 years of age who have been taking enzymes, with lipase intake exceeding 6000 units/kg/meal for longer than 6 months. Other risk factors may be a history of DIOS or meconium ileus, or prior intestinal surgery.[17] Clinically, patients may have symptoms of obstruction, abdominal pain, bloody diarrhea, or poor weight gain.

A significant subgroup of patients with fibrosing colonopathy has required surgical intervention. Patients with this condition must be monitored closely, since they may develop strictures. Management of patients with fibrosing colonopathy also includes immediate reduction of the dose of enzyme supplements to within the recommended range.[14] The long-term prognosis for patients with this condition remains unclear.

Allergy

Immediate hypersensitivity reactions to pancreatic extracts have been reported in patients, caregivers, and parents of patients with CF. Clinical symptoms often mimic asthma, but severe anaphylactic reactions have been reported. This reaction is an IgE-mediated phenomenon and occurs rarely.[18,19]

BOX 62-2 **Factors Affecting Response to Enzyme Supplements**

Enzyme supplements
- Inappropriate storage
- Expiration of product

Poor compliance
- Refusal of medication
- Incorrect administration
- Desire to lose weight

Dietary issues
- Excessive juice intake (carbohydrate malabsorption)
- Inappropriate eating behavior (i.e., frequent small meals)
- High-fat "fast foods"

Low intestinal pH
- Inadequate breakdown of enteric coating
- Contents released all at once

Concurrent gastrointestinal disorder

Adapted from Borowitz D, Baker RD, Stallings V: Consensus report on nutrition for pediatric patients with cystic fibrosis. J Pediatr Gastroenterol Nutr 2002;35(3):246–259.

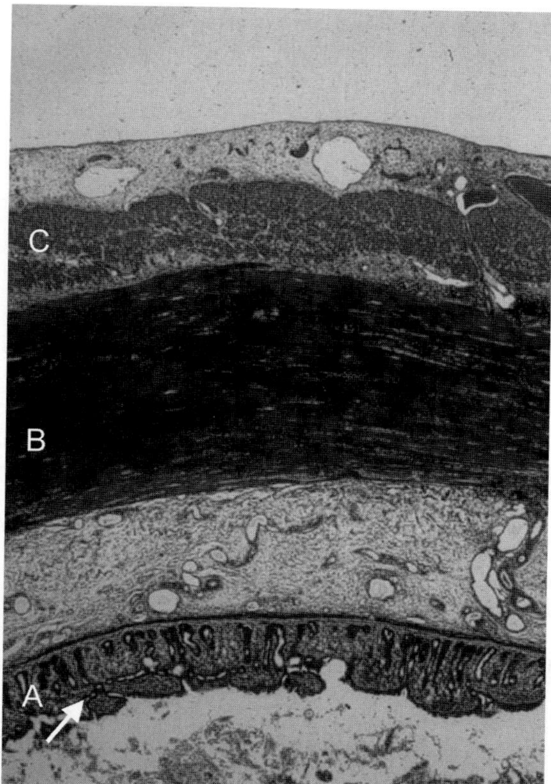

■ **FIGURE 62-2.** Histologic findings in fibrosing colonopathy. Intestinal cross-section from a patient with fibrosing colonopathy illustrating nonspecific acute and chronic inflammation in the mucosa *(A [arrow])*, hypertrophy of the muscularis mucosa *(B)*, and a ring of fibrous tissue *(C)*. (See Color Plate 42.)

CYSTIC FIBROSIS–RELATED DIABETES MELLITUS

PATHOBIOLOGY

Glucose intolerance in CF was first described by Andersen.[20] However, it was not until 1962 that diabetes mellitus was established as a secondary complication of CF. Only patients with pancreatic insufficiency are at risk for this complication. The prevalence of CF-related diabetes mellitus (CFRD) ranges from 12% to 34%; it varies according to the age and ethnicity of the population and is also dependent on the rigor of screening. Children with CF who are younger than 10 years of age seem to have a risk of insulin-requiring diabetes mellitus that is similar to that of the general population. During adolescence and adulthood, there is a progressive increase in the incidence of CFRD, with the median age of onset being 20 years of age. In patients older than 30 years of age, impaired glucose tolerance and CFRD occur with a prevalence of 43% and 27%, respectively. Unlike type 1 and 2 diabetes mellitus, a family history of diabetes mellitus is much less common in CFRD.

The pathogenesis of CFRD is unclear but was initially thought to be a result of fibrosis resulting in strangulation of the islets of Langerhans by fibrous tissue. However, subsequent studies have shown a reduction in islets in patients with CFRD. Amyloid deposits have also been described in CFRD. Basal insulin secretion appears to be maintained in CF patients with or without CFRD. However, there is a reduction in insulin secretion in response to stimulation. Initially, insulin sensitivity is increased, but after a period of time insulin resistance may develop.

There has been some debate about the impact of CFRD on morbidity and mortality. However, a recent multicenter study showed that patients with CFRD had worse lung function and nutritional status and concluded that CFRD reduces survival. Treatment with insulin seems to reverse the decline in pulmonary function and restore nutritional status. Long-term morbidity from microvascular complications was initially thought to be low, but recent studies have shown high incidence that appears to be similar to type 2 diabetes mellitus. Wilson and colleagues[21] demonstrated a 23% incidence of microvascular complications among patients with CFRD, including diabetic retinopathy and nephropathy. In contrast, macrovascular complications seem to be rare, probably because of steatorrhea and loss of lipoproteins.

DIAGNOSIS

Rarely, patients may present with overt symptoms such as polydipsia and polyuria. More frequently patients are asymptomatic or present with subtle symptoms such as impaired growth or delayed puberty. There may also be an unexplained decline in lung function. CFRD may be intermittent at first and occur in association with physical stress such as infection, nocturnal enteral feedings, or steroid treatment.

The 1999 CF Diabetes Consensus Conference proposed a classification system for CFRD that is shown in Table 62-2. Studies have shown that a subgroup of CF patients may have diabetic glucose tolerance as illustrated by an oral glucose tolerance test without fasting hyperglycemia. Moreover, there is no consensus on whether such patients should be treated with insulin. Diagnostic criteria for CFRD were also established, with the understanding that this entity can exist with or without fasting hyperglycemia (Box 62-3). In types 1 and 2 diabetes mellitus, fasting glucose is the diagnostic test of choice; however, numerous patients with CFRD will be missed if this is used as the sole screening test, and thus an oral glucose tolerance test may be required. Hemoglobin A1C is not a reliable diagnostic screening test.

MANAGEMENT

Nutritional management of CFRD is aimed at maintaining normal nutritional status. A multidisciplinary approach including members of the CF and endocrine teams is essential. Strong evidence-based data for the management of CFRD is lacking, and therefore current management is based on extrapolation from standard CF and diabetes care. It is vitally important to

■ **TABLE 62-2.** Classification of glucose intolerance in cystic fibrosis

Glucose Tolerance	Fasting Blood Glucose (mmol/L)	2-Hr Blood Glucose (mmol/L)
CFRD with fasting hyperglycemia	≥7.0	N/A
CFRD without fasting hyperglycemia	<7.0	AND ≥11.1
Impaired glucose tolerance	<7.0	AND 7.8–11.1
Normal glucose tolerance	<7.0	AND <7.8

CFRD, cystic fibrosis–related diabetes mellitus.

BOX 62-3 Diagnosis of Cystic Fibrosis–Related Diabetes

Fasting plasma glucose ≥ 7.0 mmol/L on two occasions
Fasting plasma glucose ≥ 7.0 mmol/L plus casual glucose ≥ 11.1 mmol/L
Casual glucose level ≥ 11.1 mmol/L on two or more occasions with symptoms
2-hour plasma glucose ≥ 11.0 mmol/L during a 75-hr oral glucose tolerance test

maintain normal growth in adolescents or to maintain an acceptable body mass index (20–25 kg/m^2) in adults. Therefore, instead of adjusting nutrient intake to maintain euglycemia, insulin therapy should be adjusted to permit an appropriate energy intake for the CF patient. As with all patients with CF, 35% to 40% of calories should be derived from fat. Carbohydrate intake should not be excessively restricted, and patients should follow a daily diet consisting of three meals and three snacks.

Patients with CFRD and fasting hyperglycemia will require insulin therapy. At the present time there is no evidence of a defined role for oral hypoglycemic agents. Insulin therapy is tailored on an individual basis, since there are no data on specific insulin regimens in patients with CFRD. Most regimens combine a basal bolus schedule with intermittent doses of short-acting insulin at mealtimes. Hemoglobin A1C measurements should be done to monitor long-term glycemic control. Patients should also be screened annually for the development of microvascular complications, with an eye examination and urinalysis for microalbuminuria.

Patients with CFRD without fasting hyperglycemia are at risk of progression to fasting hyperglycemia and should be carefully monitored. At the present time there are no data to guide whether treatment with insulin should be initiated for such patients. Similarly, patients with impaired glucose tolerance should also be closely monitored for progression and the development of clinical symptoms.

INTESTINAL DISEASE

PATHOBIOLOGY

CFTR is localized to the apical surface of intestinal crypt and villous cells. At the cellular level, mutations give rise to impaired Cl^- and HCO_3^- secretion by epithelial cells and, consequently, decreased fluid content in the intestinal lumen. In the CF intestine, the consequences of impaired fluid and electrolyte transport are demonstrated clinically by meconium ileus in the infant and DIOS in the older child and adult. CF meconium has lower water content and a high protein concentration, which is thought to result in more viscous, adherent meconium on the ileal surface, leading to luminal obstruction.

Meconium ileus occurs in about 15% to 20% of patients and is almost exclusively seen in individuals who carry two severe mutations (class I, II, or III). Concordance studies have shown that there is an increased risk of developing meconium ileus in affected siblings if the index case has this condition, and, conversely, there is a decreased risk if the index case does not have the condition. Given that only a small subgroup of patients develops meconium ileus, the effect of secondary genetic variables on intestinal disease has been evaluated. A modifier locus for the intestinal phenotype was identified on murine chromosome 7, using a CF mouse model.[22] A modifier locus for meconium ileus was identified on human chromosome 19q13 subsequently,[23] in a region that is syntenic to the murine locus. However, a correlation between specific alleles and the intestinal phenotype has not yet been shown. While CFTR plays a major role in fluid and electrolyte transport in the intestine, recently it was suggested that other Cl^- channels also play a role and may, therefore, have an impact on disease manifestations.[24,25]

CLINICAL MANIFESTATIONS OF INTESTINAL DISEASE

Intestinal disease in CF can present with various manifestations, and it appears that there are genetic factors other than CFTR, as well as environmental variables, that contribute to a specific phenotype.

CFTR-Related Intestinal Diseases

Meconium Ileus

Meconium ileus may be the earliest clinical manifestation of CF. In patients with this condition, one should strongly suspect CF. However, patients without CF may also present with meconium ileus, especially premature infants, thus additional diagnostic testing is required to confirm the diagnosis.[26] Meconium ileus can be simple, in which there is bowel obstruction, or complicated, wherein intrauterine complications as well as bowel obstruction occur. Approximately 50% of patients with meconium ileus develop complications that include ileal atresia, necrosis, intestinal volvulus, or meconium peritonitis secondary to bowel perforation.

Clinically, the neonate presents with signs and symptoms suggestive of intestinal obstruction, including abdominal distention, and bilious vomiting without the passage of meconium. Roentgenograms may show multiple dilated bowel loops with a ground-glass appearance, with or without calcification, in the right lower quadrant. Contrast studies with nonionic contrast material, which should be avoided in patients with suspected perforation, show an unused microcolon and ileal obstruction (Fig. 62-3).

In simple meconium ileus, nonsurgical intervention using a hypertonic contrast medium such as gastrograffin[27] will often relieve the obstruction by allowing for dissolution and subsequent passage of the inspissated meconium. Since the hypertonicity of these agents may induce dehydration or fluid and electrolyte disturbances, intravenous fluid and electrolyte therapy is recommended. Failure of enema therapy, or complicated meconium ileus is an indication for surgical intervention. In some cases, the inspissated material can be manually dislodged or irrigated and removed. A T-tube ileostomy may be placed for instillation of *N*-acetylcysteine or gastrograffin. Surgical resection is rarely required in cases with simple meconium ileus, but it is common in those with the complicated form. Patients with complicated meconium ileus have a higher incidence of surgical complications. A recent evaluation in an animal model suggests that surfactant may be considered as an alternative therapy for the treatment of meconium ileus.[28] Survival of patients with meconium ileus is higher than 90%, and long-term survival is similar to CF patients without this complication.[29]

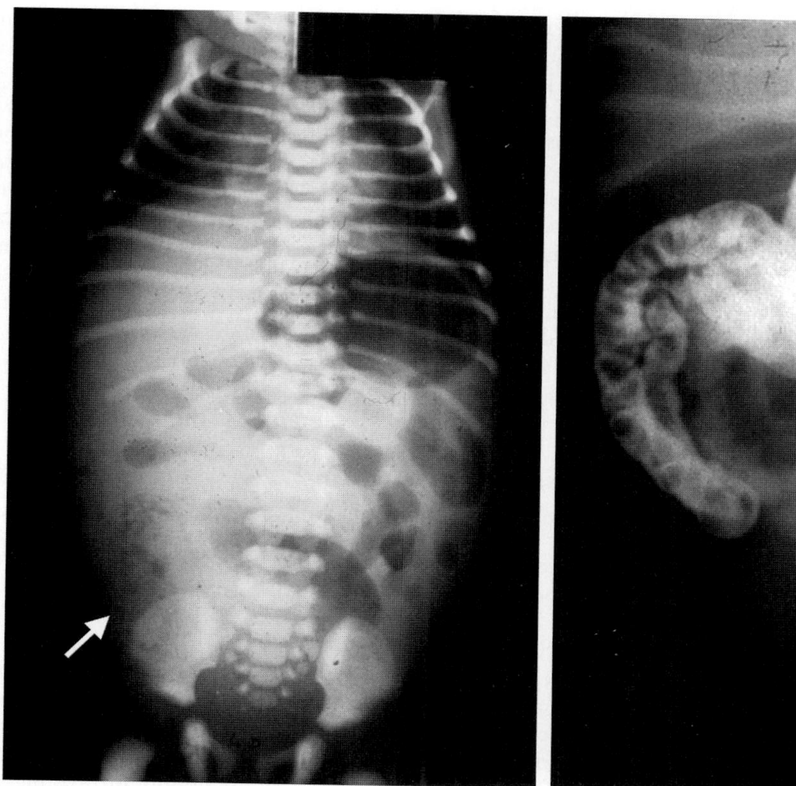

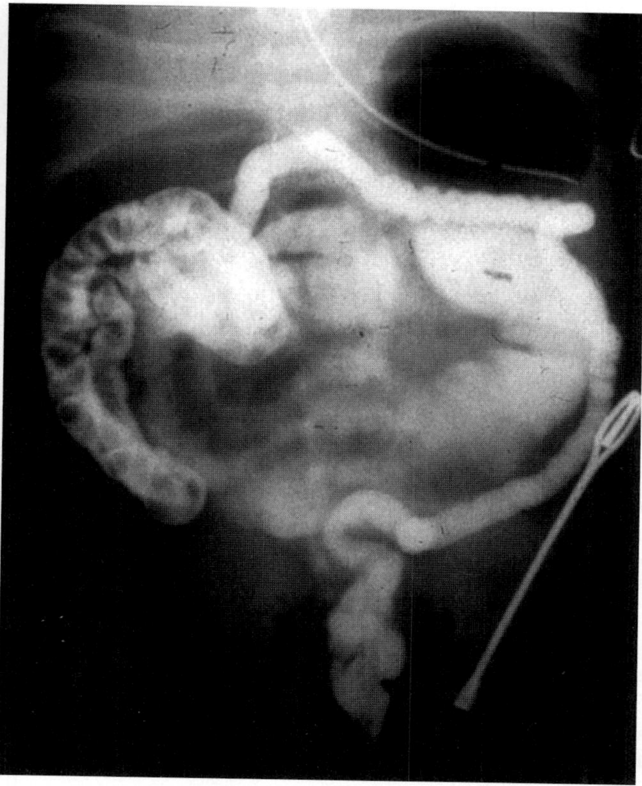

■ **FIGURE 62-3.** Meconium ileus. **A,** Abdominal roentgenogram showing air-fluid levels in the small bowel and granular material in the right lower quadrant with an absence of air in the colon. **B,** Barium enema showing the presence of inspissated material in the small bowel and a microcolon.

Distal Intestinal Obstruction Syndrome

Because of the viscous nature of intestinal contents, some CF patients develop symptoms of partial or complete bowel obstruction at an older age. This is a result of inspissated material in the ileum, cecum, and proximal colon. Previously, this condition was termed meconium ileus equivalent; however, it has been renamed DIOS. Approximately 4% to 5% of patients with CF will develop this complication, most of whom are PI. DIOS is uncommon in infancy, and the incidence appears to increase with age, occurring most commonly in adolescents and adults.

Clinically, patients present with abdominal pain that may be associated with a palpable fecal mass in the right lower quadrant. In most cases there is no associated vomiting. However, on the rare occasion that there is vomiting, complete bowel obstruction should be suspected. It is important to consider other entities that may present with similar features, including appendicitis, appendiceal abscess, intussusception, Crohn's disease, and fibrosing colonopathy. Plain roentgenograms are helpful if they demonstrate a fecal mass in the right lower quadrant, with or without evidence of obstruction. Sonography or computed tomography may be important to rule out other causes for the patient's symptoms.

There are several options for managing DIOS that can be tailored to the severity of symptoms. In milder cases, mineral oil or other laxatives may be of benefit. Patients who do not respond to mineral oil treatment should be considered for oral or nasogastric lavage using a balanced electrolyte and polyethylene glycol solution.[30] The lavage solution is usually administered at a rate of 750 to 1000 mL/hr (20 mL/kg/hr for younger children) to a total volume of 4 to 6 L. Contraindications to lavage include complete obstruction or signs of peritonitis. Gastrograffin enemas, or enemas with other hyperosmolar contrast media, may also be useful both to provide additional imaging and to help relieve the obstruction, particularly if complete bowel obstruction is suspected. Adequate volumes of contrast are required to enter the ileum. Gastrograffin should not be used if the patient is dehydrated or has symptoms and signs of peritonitis. *N*-acetylcysteine, a mucolytic agent, may also be of benefit. Patients with recurrent DIOS can be considered for the placement of a button gastrostomy or gastrostomy button in the appendix to allow for regular irrigation.[31]

Constipation

Patients with CF are much more likely to have constipation than true DIOS. The history is often helpful in distinguishing the two problems, since patients with DIOS usually have normal stool frequency and consistency. In contrast, patients with constipation may have abdominal cramping, altered frequency of bowel movements, and difficulty passing stool. Unlike the findings in DIOS, roentgenograms show diffuse distribution of fecal material throughout the colon. Patients with constipation should be evaluated for evidence of a poor compliance or inadequate response to enzyme therapy. Treatment involves long-term laxative use, such as mineral oil. Severe cases may require colonic lavage with a balanced electrolyte solution.

Rectal Prolapse

Rectal prolapse occurs in approximately a fifth of patients with CF, and in about 50% of cases it may be the presenting feature of CF disease. Most patients present at a young age between

1 month and 3 years of age. Rectal prolapse is more common in PI patients, and may be related to the bulky stools. In most cases, it resolves spontaneously after the age of 3 years. In patients for whom this is the presenting feature of CF, the institution of enzyme supplementation may result in improvement, but some patients will continue for some time to suffer from prolapse. In patients with constipation, treatment of this symptom is also of benefit. Surgical intervention is rarely indicated.

Appendicitis

Appendicitis is often difficult to diagnose in patients with CF. Symptoms may be mild, and other diagnoses such as DIOS are often considered first. It is, therefore, important to strongly suspect this condition to avoid a delay in diagnosis and an increased risk of complications, which include abscess formation, perforation, and portal vein thrombosis. The incidence of acute appendicitis is reported to be lower in patients with CF than in the general population (1% vs. 7%). Clinical symptoms may be mild or severe, and the milder presentation may be tempered by concurrent antibiotic use. The presence of peritoneal signs or fever should lead to further evaluation either by ultrasound or computed tomography. Data from our center covering a 10-year period show that 9 of 803 patients with CF underwent an appendectomy. In all patients, an initial diagnosis of DIOS had been made. Of the 9 patients, 5 had surgery within 3 days of symptom onset. In the remaining patients the diagnosis was delayed, and all developed appendiceal abscesses.[32]

Intussusception

Intussusception occurs in patients with CF with an estimated prevalence of 1%. Patients may present with classical colicky abdominal pain, vomiting, and a palpable mass with rectal bleeding.[33] However, the symptoms can be quite nonspecific and may resemble DIOS. Most intussusceptions are ileoileal or ileocolic, and the lead point for the intussusception is thought to be mucoid fecal material that is adherent to the intestinal mucosa. The diagnosis is made by ultrasound, single-contrast enema, or air enema. The latter two interventions can be used to reduce the intussusception.[34] Surgical intervention for manual reduction or resection is rarely required.

Secondary Intestinal Complications

Pseudomembranous Colitis

As many as 50% of patients with CF are colonized with *Clostridium difficile*.[35] This high colonization rate may be related to chronic antibiotic use. However, pseudomembranous colitis is considered to be rare, according to case report data.[35–37] Despite its rare occurrence, *C. difficile*–related colitis has been fatal in patients with CF.[37] In our experience, CF patients with *C. difficile* colitis may not present clinically with diarrhea or bloody diarrhea but may present dramatically with toxic megacolon. Other patients may have subtle symptoms that mimic other clinical diagnoses. Stools should be tested for *C. difficile* toxin if the clinical diagnosis is unclear. Treatment should be instituted with metronidazole or oral vancomycin if indicated. Patients with toxic megacolon may need emergency subtotal colectomy as a lifesaving intervention.[37]

Gastroesophageal Reflux Disease

Gastroesophageal reflux is common in both children and adults with CF. The etiology is probably multifactorial and may be related to respiratory disease, physiotherapy, and transient relaxation of the lower esophageal sphincter. pH monitoring has indicated that there is an estimated 20% incidence of gastroesophageal reflux in infants with CF.[38] In some patients with CF, postural drainage may exacerbate symptoms, and alteration of the physiotherapy technique may be beneficial. Some reports suggest that gastroesophageal reflux is more frequent in patients with severe lung disease.[39] There have been several case reports of complications including esophageal stricture and Barrett's esophagus.[40]

The diagnosis is usually established by symptoms such as heartburn, regurgitation, dysphagia, or anorexia. Esophagogastroscopy and esophageal biopsy may be useful if the diagnosis is in doubt or if the response to therapy is poor. Treatment with histamine (H2) receptor antagonists or proton pump inhibitors usually results in symptomatic improvement.

Associated Conditions

Inflammatory Bowel Disease

Crohn's disease has been reported in patients with CF.[41,42] In one study, the prevalence of Crohn's disease has been shown to be 11 times that observed in a non-CF population.[43] Symptoms of inflammatory bowel disease may mimic CF-associated symptoms, such as DIOS. Investigations should be initiated if, despite appropriate management of CF, there is continued abdominal pain, anemia, hypoalbuminemia, and poor weight gain or growth disturbance. Furthermore, any extraintestinal features that suggest inflammatory bowel disease should prompt further investigation.

Gastrointestinal Malignancies

There are reports of an increased risk of gastrointestinal malignancy in patients with CF. This trend is becoming more evident as patient survival increases. A large population-based study has shown an approximately sevenfold increased risk of gastrointestinally related malignancy. Cholangiocarcinoma has been reported,[44,45] as well as early-onset colon cancer,[46] pancreatic adenocarcinoma,[47] and intestinal adenocarcinoma.[48] Furthermore, patients undergoing transplantation may be at even higher risk of malignancy as a result of the immunosuppressive medications they must take. It is thus important to be vigilant for these complications, since the symptoms may mimic other CF-associated manifestations.

HEPATOBILIARY DISEASE

Liver disease was described in the earliest reports of CF by Andersen.[20] The presence of bile duct plugging in the livers of CF patients led to the hypothesis that bile duct obstruction by viscous secretions was the trigger for progressive liver damage. Liver disease in CF is characterized by abnormalities of the intrahepatic and extrahepatic biliary tracts. There is a spectrum of liver abnormalities ranging from mild elevation of liver enzymes to focal biliary cirrhosis, multilobular biliary cirrhosis with portal hypertension, and rarely, liver failure. The development of liver disease is in many cases not accompanied by clinical symptoms, and, therefore, early identification of CF-associated liver disease is difficult.

PATHOBIOLOGY

Cystic fibrosis transmembrane conductance regulator is expressed at the apical surface of cholangiocytes and the epithelium of the

TABLE 62-3. Hepatobiliary manifestations of cystic fibrosis

Disease	Incidence (%)
Extrahepatic	
Micro-gallbladder	30
Distended gallbladder	20
Cholelithiasis	1–10
Common bile duct stenosis	Rare
Cholangiocarcinoma	Rare
Sclerosing cholangitis	Rare
Intrahepatic	
Neonatal cholestasis	<2
Steatosis	20–60
Focal biliary cirrhosis	11–70
Multilobular cirrhosis	5–15

gallbladder but not in hepatocytes. It functions in ductal secretion by creating both osmotic and electrogenic driving forces for the passive movement of sodium and water. The apical Cl^- gradient is also thought to facilitate HCO_3^- secretion via CFTR and the Cl^-/HCO_3^- exchanger. CFTR may also be involved in the regulation of other ion channels in bile duct epithelium. Dysfunction of CFTR leads to an alteration in bile composition, with increased concentrations of bile acids and other biliary constituents, resulting in inspissation and obstruction of small bile ducts. The mechanisms by which this leads to hepatic fibrosis are not clear, but there are probably several pathways, culminating in the recruitment and activation of hepatic stellate cells.

Almost all patients with CF have minor focal hepatobiliary manifestations of disease.[49] Progression to multilobular cirrhosis, which occurs in a small group of CF patients, is probably attributable to the influence of *CFTR* gene mutations, modifier genes, and/or environmental influences. While severe liver disease is more frequently encountered in patients who carry class I, II, or III mutations on both alleles, it has also been described in PS patients with class IV or V mutations.[50] There are no specific genotypes that correlate with more severe liver disease. Given the variability of liver disease in CF, research studies are now examining other genetic factors that may contribute. While individual candidate genes have been proposed as potential modifiers of the hepatic phenotype, including alpha1-proteinase inhibitor and transforming growth factor-β1,[49,51,52] it appears that several secondary genetic factors contribute to the development of severe CF-associated liver disease.

Because CF-associated liver disease is primarily biliary in nature, progression from multilobular cirrhosis to end-stage liver failure frequently takes decades to occur.

Many patients with CF also develop hepatic steatosis, which is probably the result of several influences, including malnutrition, deficiency of essential fatty acids, and the presence of proinflammatory cytokines. It is unclear whether this entity progresses to fibrosis.

CLINICAL PRESENTATION

A wide variety of intrahepatic and extrahepatic manifestations of disease have been described in CF patients (Table 62-3). The prevalence of liver disease in children with CF is not entirely clear, although 5% to 10% of patients are estimated to develop clinically relevant CF-associated liver disease, defined by evidence of multilobular cirrhosis, portal hypertension, and hypersplenism.[53] The median age at diagnosis is 9 to 10 years. Since there are no reliable biochemical markers available that can identify patients with severe liver disease, each clinic visit should include careful physical examination to monitor for the development of hepatosplenomegaly. The presence of a firm liver, which may be enlarged, and/or splenomegaly indicates the presence of significant liver disease. With disease progression, the liver may shrink and no longer be palpable.

There is no reliable marker for the early detection of liver disease in patients with CF. Annual blood tests, such as those listed in Table 62-4, are often done in patients with CF, and in our experience approximately 40% of patients have biochemical abnormalities that are generally one- to twofold higher than the upper reference limits. These values tend to fluctuate with time in each individual. Monitoring of coagulation and albumin should be done to assess liver synthetic function. There is no association between elevated transaminases and the severity or progression of liver disease. However, if biochemical tests are greatly elevated, it is important to consider biliary tract obstruction with stones or sludge or other causes of liver disease. Other etiologies include viral hepatitis, metabolic liver disease, autoimmune liver disease, drug toxicity, structural abnormalities, and hepatic congestion secondary to right-sided heart failure. It should also be noted that normal biochemical hepatic tests do not exclude severe CF-associated liver disease.[53,54]

Ultrasound is a useful monitoring tool for assessing CF patients in whom liver disease is suspected. It can permit visualization of extrahepatic abnormalities (gallbladder abnormalities, cholelithiasis, and bile duct dilation) and define the size and texture of the liver and spleen. In more advanced liver disease, Doppler studies can document the direction of flow in the

TABLE 62-4. Assessment for liver disease

History	Physical Examination	Laboratory Investigation
Jaundice (including neonatal history)	Liver span, texture	AST, ALT, GGT, ALP
Pruritus	Splenomegaly	Bilirubin (total and direct)
Hematemesis/melena	Ascites	Albumin
Bruising/bleeding	Chronic liver disease	INR, PTT
Medication use	Nutritional status	CBC, differential, platelets
Alcohol intake		Screen for other causes of liver disease if indicated
Family history of liver disease		

ALP, alkaline phosphatase; ALT, alanine transaminase; AST, aspartate transaminase; CBC, complete blood count; GGT, γ-glutamyltransferase; INR, international normalized ratio; PTT, partial thromboplastin time.

portal vein and sometimes detect varices. Sonography may also be useful in documenting hepatic abnormalities in the absence of biochemical abnormalities.

Liver biopsy is not recommended as a routine procedure for the evaluation of CF-associated liver disease. It may be helpful if a diagnosis of liver disease not related to CF is suspected, or it may be useful to assess whether there is predominantly steatosis or focal biliary cirrhosis. Because of its focal nature, a normal biopsy result does not exclude the presence of CF-associated liver disease. From a technical perspective, if a biopsy is to be performed, it should only be done after ultrasound evaluation to determine a safe location, since the lungs may be hyperinflated. Ultrasound guidance can also be useful to target an affected region of the liver. Contraindications to percutaneous liver biopsy include an uncorrectable coagulopathy, thrombocytopenia (<80,000 platelets/µL), dilated intrahepatic ducts or hepatic veins, significant ascites, or concerns regarding patient cooperation. If a biopsy is warranted in such patients, a transjugular or laparoscopic approach should be considered.

DISEASE MANIFESTATIONS

Extrahepatic Complications

Micro-gallbladder

Micro-gallbladder is present in as many as 30% of patients with CF of all ages. Among CF patients younger than 5 years of age, 20% have gallbladder anomalies; this proportion increases to 40% between the ages of 5 and 10 years, and to 60% of patients between the ages of 15 and 20 years. Gallbladder dysfunction has also been reported. The underlying cause of these abnormalities is unclear.

Cholelithiasis

The incidence of gallstones in patients with CF seems to be decreasing. Early studies indicated that between 8% and 12% of children with CF had gallstones. The incidence seems to increase with age, and a separate study showed that among adults, 24% to 33% had gallstones. However, recent studies suggest that prevalence figures may be as low as 1%.

The development of cholelithiasis is probably related to the presence of lithogenic bile secondary to increased losses of bile acids.[55] Patients with pancreatic insufficiency have increased bile acid losses in the stool, which does not appear to occur in PS patients. There are several mechanisms by which malabsorption leads to the development of gallstones, including interference with the binding of bile salts to ileal receptors as well as bile acid precipitation. Defective chloride transport by biliary epithelium may also contribute by altering the viscosity of bile and allowing for stone formation.

Patients may be asymptomatic or may present with biliary colic. Laboratory investigations may show elevation of γ-glutamyltransferase, alkaline phosphatase, and bilirubin. If symptoms are persistent or recurrent, a laparoscopic or open cholecystectomy should be considered. At the time of cholecystectomy, an intraoperative cholangiogram and liver biopsy should also be performed.[56] Ursodeoxycholic acid (UDCA) is not useful in the management of gallstones in CF patients.[57]

Abnormalities of the Biliary Tree

Biliary tree abnormalities, which were first described at autopsy in CF adults, identified focal dilatation and fibrosis of the biliary tree, cholelithiasis, and solitary paraductal mucous cysts. Subsequently, it has become apparent that the intrahepatic and extrahepatic bile ducts can be obstructed with sludge or mucus. Cholangiopancreatography or percutaneous transhepatic cholangiograms often reveal images that appear identical to sclerosing cholangitis. Distal common bile duct stenosis was first described in case reports, which identified extrinsic compression of the distal common bile duct by the fibrotic head of the pancreas.[58,59] A prospective study using hepatobiliary scintigraphy and transhepatic cholangiography suggested that as many as 48 of 50 patients with CF-related liver disease had bile duct stenosis.[54] However, other studies using endoscopic retrograde cholangiopancreatography[60,61] suggest that the prevalence of this complication is less than 10% among patients with CF-associated liver disease.

Patients with common bile duct stenosis or intrinsic common bile duct obstruction with stones or sludge may present with right upper quadrant pain and/or jaundice.[54] These patients also seem to have more severe steatorrhea. If this condition is suspected, abdominal ultrasonography and hepatobiliary scintigraphy should be done. If these test results suggest biliary obstruction, more detailed imaging by cholangiopancreatography or percutaneous transhepatic cholangiograms should be performed. Such procedures can be diagnostic as well as therapeutic, because sludge or stones can be removed, strictures can be dilated, biliary stents can be placed, or a sphincterotomy can be performed. If the problem is persistent or recurrent, surgical intervention may be required to relieve the obstruction.

Cholangiocarcinoma

Cholangiocarcinoma has been reported rarely in adult patients with CF.[45,62] This complication, though rare, should be considered in adult CF patients who present with obstructive jaundice, abdominal pain, or weight loss.[62]

Intrahepatic Complications

Neonatal Cholestasis

The exact incidence of neonatal cholestasis in CF infants is unclear. Some believe that this complication is rare, while other studies have shown that as many as 68% of infants may have evidence of cholestasis.[63] An association between the presence of meconium ileus and the development of neonatal cholestasis has been suggested,[64] although this has not been confirmed.[53]

Infants may present clinically with jaundice and/or acholic stools, before the diagnosis of CF. Consequently, CF should always be considered in the differential diagnosis of neonatal cholestasis. The clinical picture can sometimes be difficult to distinguish from extrahepatic biliary atresia. Hepatobiliary scintigraphy may not distinguish between CF and extrahepatic biliary atresia. Similarly, the histologic findings in bile duct proliferation and plugging may be similar in both conditions. Characteristic inspissated, eosinophilic material within the bile ducts of CF liver biopsy samples is not a feature of extrahepatic biliary atresia. It is important to differentiate between CF and extrahepatic biliary atresia, since most infants with CF have spontaneous resolution of their cholestasis, while those with biliary atresia should undergo a Kasai portoenterostomy in a timely fashion. There have been occasional reports of patients with both CF and extrahepatic biliary atresia.

The long-term prognosis of patients with neonatal cholestasis is not well defined, but it seems that most of these patients do well.[65] While the occasional infant with neonatal cholestasis has developed multilobular cirrhosis at an older age, there is no clear association between the two entities.

Hepatic Steatosis

Steatosis is a common finding in patients with CF. Autopsy studies have documented steatosis in 60% of liver biopsy specimens. Steatosis may be focal or involve the entire liver. It may occur in isolation or in association with fibrosis and cirrhosis. While the pathogenesis of CF-associated steatosis is not understood, it may be related to malnutrition, fatty acid deficiency, cytokines, and concomitant medication use. It remains to be determined whether steatohepatitis progresses to cirrhosis.

Clinically, patients may or may not have an enlarged, soft liver. Ultrasound can also be helpful to determine the presence of steatosis. A careful nutritional assessment should be done, documenting dietary intake and enzyme use. A thorough history should also be taken, specifically concerning alcohol and medication use. Diabetes mellitus can also be associated with steatosis, and oral glucose tolerance testing should be done if clinically indicated.[56]

Focal Biliary Cirrhosis

Focal biliary cirrhosis is the pathognomonic hepatic lesion of CF. It occurs with a variable frequency, but the incidence seems to increase with age. One autopsy study indicated that 72% of patients who died after the age of 24 had focal biliary changes.[66] Some patients with focal biliary cirrhosis may progress to multilobular biliary cirrhosis. Grossly, the liver may show fibrotic changes that may be superficial or may create a furrowed appearance. Histologically, there are varying degrees of focal portal fibrosis and bile duct obstruction with bile duct proliferation, and adjacent areas may appear normal. Periodic acid–Schiff-positive material can be seen obstructing the ducts. Most patients with focal biliary cirrhosis are asymptomatic and do not develop any significant hepatic complications. Liver enzymes may be normal or moderately elevated.

Multilobular Biliary Cirrhosis

Multilobular biliary cirrhosis is the most severe form of CF-related liver disease. The time frame for this progression is variable, but the median age of diagnosis is 9 years. The primary complications are related to portal hypertension and hypersplenism. Hepatocellular dysfunction is usually not a problem, and most patients do not progress to liver failure for decades.

On examination, a nodular liver may be evident, often on palpation of the left lobe. Splenomegaly, which can be massive, is an indication of the development of portal hypertension. Abdominal distention, with dilated abdominal wall veins, spider nevi, and palmar erythema may become evident with progressive liver disease. Deterioration in nutritional status may also be noted as liver function worsens, and fat-soluble vitamin concentrations may be inadequate. The development of jaundice, hypoalbuminemia, and coagulopathy are usually late and ominous signs, indicative of hepatic failure. Evidence of hypersplenism can be seen on laboratory testing with thrombocytopenia and/or anemia or neutropenia. With the development of cirrhosis and portal hypertension, patients may present with secondary complications including variceal hemorrhage. Ultrasonography may suggest fibrosis and cirrhosis but is not very sensitive. However, it can help document the direction of portal venous flow and may reveal the presence of varices, although it is not a reliable diagnostic tool.

MANAGEMENT OF LIVER DISEASE

Pharmacologic interventions

No specific therapy has been shown to alter the course of cirrhosis in CF. UDCA has been shown to improve bile flow.[67] It may also displace toxic bile acids[68] and improve HCO_3^- secretion by cholangiocytes.[68] Treatment does result in improvement of routine biochemical tests,[69,70] but there is no evidence that it alters the long-term outcome. Furthermore, there does not appear to be any beneficial effect on nutritional status or when advanced liver disease is already present.[71] In theory, if there were a method to identify which patients with CF were at risk for severe biliary cirrhosis, it would be possible to assess the long-term prophylactic potential of UDCA. Pharmacokinetic studies indicate that the correct dose of UDCA is 20 to 25 mg/kg/day divided twice daily.[69]

Taurine therapy has been recommended for patients with CF-associated liver disease, either alone or in addition to UDCA. CF patients with liver disease may be deficient in taurine secondary to bile acid malabsorption. UDCA may also increase the taurine required for bile acid conjugation.[72] However, a randomized controlled trial has not shown any significant effect on liver function or fecal fat excretion.[70] At present, there is no evidence to support the routine use of this agent.

Nutrition

Because of an increased risk of malnutrition, special attention should be given to the nutritional status of patients with liver disease. Energy requirements may be higher because of increased intestinal fat losses. Protein intake should not be restricted unless encephalopathy develops. Fat-soluble vitamin levels should be monitored closely and doses increased as necessary. Guidelines for vitamin supplementation in the setting of liver disease are shown in Table 62-5. Following a change in dose, levels should be repeated in 1 to 2 months.[56]

Portal Hypertension and Hypersplenism

Patients with portal hypertension should be counseled about the risk for variceal bleeding. Appropriate precautions should be taken to prevent blunt abdominal trauma, which could lead to splenic rupture. Gastrointestinal bleeding can also occur as a result of portal gastropathy or portal colopathy. Patients are also at increased risk of bleeding due to thrombocytopenia related to hypersplenism.

At the present time, there is insufficient evidence for prophylactic treatment of portal hypertension in patients with CF, before the first variceal bleeding episode. Studies in adults with

TABLE 62-5. Fat-soluble vitamin dosage in patients with liver disease

	Dose	Lab Monitoring
Vitamin E	15–25 IU/kg/day	Vitamin E levels
Vitamin D	800–1600 IU/day vitamin D_2 or D_3	25-hydroxyvitamin D
Vitamin K	2.5 mg/day (infants) 10 mg/day (adolescents/adults)	INR
Vitamin A	Optimal dose not clear (2–4 × RDA)	Retinol, retinol-binding protein

INR, International Normalized Ratio; RDA, recommended daily allowance.

known varices have shown that beta blockade is useful in the prevention of initial variceal hemorrhage.[73] However, there have not been any randomized controlled trials in children. Furthermore, the possibility of bronchospasm as a side effect makes these agents less appealing for patients with CF.

The treatment of variceal bleeding is not any different from that given to patients with other causes of portal hypertension. Emergent treatment with packed red blood cells and platelets, as well as fresh frozen plasma to correct the coagulopathy may be required. Adjuvant treatment with intravenous octreotide and proton pump inhibitors should also be instituted.[74] Endoscopy should be deferred until the patient has been stabilized; interventional endoscopy should be undertaken if the bleeding does not respond to conservative measures. Endoscopic intervention with sclerotherapy or variceal band ligation may be required depending on the age of the patient and/or size and nature of the varices. These procedures are usually performed serially until varices are ablated. Annual follow-up should then be done to screen for recurrence. Some patients may require a transjugular intrahepatic portosystemic shunt or a surgical shunt procedure if bleeding cannot be controlled with endoscopic therapy.

Liver Failure

Liver failure is a rare complication of CF-related liver disease, but with an increase in survival of patients with chronic liver disease, it will probably become more common. Initial treatment is supportive, including: correction of the coagulopathy, treatment of ascites, management of hypoglycemia and fluid and electrolytes, and management of hepatic encephalopathy. Treatment of ascites often results in symptomatic improvement, and maintenance therapy with spironolactone may be useful in managing fluid retention. If hepatic encephalopathy develops, treatment with lactulose should be instituted along with dietary protein restriction. Early referral to a transplant center is important, given the long waiting times for cadaveric donors. Five-year survival rate after liver transplant approaches 80% and is similar to that of patients undergoing liver transplantation for other reasons.[75] There is no evidence that immunosuppressive therapy has an adverse effect on pulmonary disease. A few patients have undergone successful combined transplants of the lung and liver.

NUTRITION

PATHOBIOLOGY

Malnutrition has been an important concern in CF since early descriptions of the disease. Both impaired weight gain and linear growth are seen in CF patients; however, over the past decade, aggressive nutritional support has improved nutritional status and survival. Nutritional support is an integral part of comprehensive care of individuals with CF, with the goal of maintaining normal growth.

The impact of nutritional support on survival is most strikingly shown by a comparative study of two CF clinics (Boston and Toronto). The major difference between these two clinics at the time of the study was the approach to nutrition, with the Toronto clinic having a more aggressive approach to nutritional intervention. The patients attending the Toronto clinic were taller, and the Toronto male patients were also heavier. In this study, Corey and colleagues[76] showed marked differences in patient survival despite no other differences in the patient population and their pulmonary function. This study, therefore, suggested that improved survival was linked to better nutritional status.

The pathogenesis of malnutrition in CF is complex. It is probably the result of a number of influences that ultimately lead to energy imbalance (Fig. 62-4). First, there are increased energy losses in CF patients with pancreatic insufficiency because of poor digestion and malabsorption. Despite adequate enzyme supplementation, persistent fat and protein maldigestion occurs, as a result of several influences (see Box 62-2). Furthermore, increased energy losses can occur in the setting of CF-related diabetes and CF-related liver disease. Energy intake also plays a role in the development of the energy imbalance in CF. Oral intake may be limited for many reasons, including anorexia secondary to respiratory disease, gastroesophageal reflux, DIOS, and advanced liver disease. There are variable reports about energy intake in CF patients; some studies show increased intake in those with normal growth compared with those with growth retardation. However, other studies have found nutrient intakes to be close to the normal range. Resting energy expenditure in CF patients is increased and this correlates with worsening pulmonary status. The precise basis for the increase in resting energy expenditure in patients with CF is not clear, but the relationship to the severity of lung disease suggests that it is due to inflammation and/or increased work of breathing. While it has been suggested that a component of increased resting energy expenditure is a result of the underlying CF defect, not all studies have demonstrated evidence that the primary CF defect results in increased cellular energy expenditure.

Ultimately, it is the imbalance among energy needs, losses, and intake that results in an energy deficit in patients with CF. Furthermore, over time, with progression of lung disease, there may be an increasing energy deficit and weight loss. Loss of muscle mass in turn affects respiratory status, resulting in a vicious cycle involving progressive nutritional and pulmonary deterioration. It is important to emphasize that this imbalance can be corrected with adequate caloric intake.

NUTRITIONAL MANAGEMENT

A multidisciplinary approach to nutritional therapy is imperative. Patients should have anthropometrics done at diagnosis and at each visit, and should have their diet and enzyme intake reviewed. Patients with CF should follow a high-energy diet with 35% to 40% of the energy in the form of fat. This diet reflects an attempt to optimize caloric intake and prevent an energy deficit. Because of impaired fat absorption, PI patients do not seem to be at risk of hyperlipidemia. However, if there

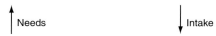

Needs
Intake
• Increased intestinal losses
• Pancreatic insufficiency
• Bile salt metabolism
• Hepatobiliary disease
• Gastroesophageal reflux
• Increased energy expenditure
• Pulmonary disease
• Increased energy losses
• CF related diabetes
• Anorexia (due to severe lung disease)
• Cytokine release (due to inflammation)
• Esophagitis
• Iatrogenic fat restriction
• Distal intestinal obstruction syndrome
• Psychosocial issues
• Feeding disorders
• Depression

FIGURE 62-4. Model for the development of energy imbalance in CF.

are concerns about a family history of hyperlipidemia, lipid levels should be monitored, particularly in PS patients.

When CF patients are losing weight, it is important to review all aspects that contribute to energy balance—that is, intake, losses, and expenditure. Dietary records can be used to assess intake, and fat absorption can be assessed using 72-hour fat balance studies. If available, indirect calorimetry can be used to estimate energy expenditure. Alternatively, energy requirements can be estimated using the following equation: Basal metabolic rate × 1.1 (for malabsorption) × activity factor (1.5 to 1.7) + 200 to 400 kcal/day. Intervention is then targeted appropriately to increase caloric intake and optimize enzyme supplementation.

In some patients, nutritional therapy with nasogastric or gastrostomy feedings is needed to improve nutritional status. A number of studies have looked at the benefit of enteral feeding in patients with CF. Short-term supplementation is of no long-term benefit. Although there is an initial improvement in nutritional status with supplementation, this effect is lost when supplementation is ceased. However, studies have shown that long-term nocturnal enteral supplementation results in an improvement in growth and body composition. While there is no direct evidence that nutritional intervention results in improved long-term survival, several studies have shown a decrease in the rate of deterioration of pulmonary function subsequent to improvement in nutritional status.

VITAMIN SUPPLEMENTATION

Fat-soluble vitamin deficiency is common in patients with CF because of their pancreatic insufficiency and hepatobiliary dysfunction. A prospective study of patients identified by newborn screening indicated that 35% of patients had vitamin A, D, or E deficiency.[77] Follow-up of these patients showed that although vitamin A and D deficiency resolved with supplementation, vitamin E deficiency was still common. Vitamin E deficiency can lead to hemolysis and, if prolonged, to peripheral neuropathy. Vitamin A deficiency can result in night blindness, keratomalacia, pigmentary retinopathy, and/or permanent corneal damage. Vitamin A deficiency may also result in immune dysfunction and predispose to infection. Prepubertal children with CF do not appear to have osteopenia, although this has been well documented in adolescents and adults.[78] Osteopenia in patients with CF is probably multifactorial in etiology. Vitamin D supplementation is important to maintain normal bone mineralization, since it has been shown that bone demineralization occurs in these patients. Adults with CF are at a high risk for complications secondary to vitamin D deficiency, including the development of fractures. This deficiency is even more important for patients living in areas with reduced exposure to sunlight.

Subclinical vitamin K deficiency, measured by serum PIVKA-II (prothrombin induced in vitamin K absence) has been shown to be almost universal in PI patients with CF who do not receive supplementation.[79] However, supplementation does not appear to return serum PIVKA-II levels to normal in all patients.[80] This may be in fact related to inadequate dosing, since there is little evidence regarding appropriate dosing of vitamin K. Subclinical vitamin K deficiency may be important in the development of metabolic bone disease in patients with CF, because of its role in the carboxylation of the bone matrix protein osteocalcin. Fat-soluble vitamin levels should be serially monitored in PI patients, and doses of supplements should be adjusted if necessary (Table 62-6).

TABLE 62-6. Recommended dosage of fat-soluble vitamins for cystic fibrosis patients with pancreatic insufficiency

	AGE			
	0–12 Mo	**1–3 Yr**	**3–8 Yr**	**>8 Yr**
Vitamin A (IU)	1500	5000	5000–10,000	10,000
Vitamin D (IU)	400	400–800	400–800	400–800
Vitamin E (IU)	40–50	80–150	100–200	200–400
Vitamin K (mg)*	0.3–0.5	0.3–0.5	0.3–0.5	0.3–0.5

*Objectively determined dosing guidelines are not available for vitamin K, and dosage should be adjusted according to coagulation parameters and serum prothrombin levels induced in vitamin K absence (PIVKA-II).

Adapted from Borowitz D, Baker RD, Stallings V: Consensus report on nutrition for pediatric patients with cystic fibrosis. J Pediatr Gastroenterol Nutr 2002;35(3):246–259.

MALE INFERTILITY

PATHOBIOLOGY

The vast majority of adult men with CF are infertile because of obstructive azoospermia.[81,82] Whereas earlier studies had attributed CF male infertility to congenital bilateral agenesis of the vas deferens, more detailed evaluation of the reproductive tract of men by careful genital examination, hormone and semen analysis, testicular and transrectal ultrasound, as well as genotyping, has revealed a variety of obstructive anatomic abnormalities.[83] Among 23 men with an established diagnosis of CF (14 were PI), secondary sexual characteristics and testicular size were normal in all cases. Only one patient, who was PS, had semen findings compatible with possible fertility, but sperm motility was reduced. However, 45% of the men had a palpable vas deferens. Transrectal sonography revealed numerous testicular and extratesticular abnormalities that suggested obstruction. We have since demonstrated that many of these patients in fact have isolated areas of obstruction, which cannot always be detected by clinical palpation or sonography.

It is also recognized that 1% to 2% of otherwise healthy males who are infertile also have obstructive azoospermia. Phenotype evaluation of these men reveal that more than two thirds of them carry at least one *CFTR* gene mutation, and on extensive mutation analysis as many as 50% carry *CFTR* gene alterations on both alleles.[84,85] All have at least one mild class IV or class V mutation on at least one allele. Some of these patients carry a diagnosis of CF based on abnormal ion channel function and/or the presence of CF-causing mutations on both alleles. These findings suggest that the male genital tract is exquisitely sensitive to even minor losses of CFTR function, because the majority of healthy men with congenital bilateral agenesis of the vas deferens do not appear to have any evidence of clinically significant CF-associated disease in other organs.

CLINICAL ASSESSMENT

At the time of diagnosis, it is important to inform families that approximately 99% of men with CF are infertile. If patients are diagnosed in infancy, it is advisable to communicate factual information about the nature of infertility at an older age, ideally in adolescence or young adulthood. In our clinical experience, parents are reticent about communicating this information to their sons, and a surprisingly high percentage of affected patients remain unaware of this information until they reach the stage of planning to have children. Adolescents are usually too self-conscious to be considered for detailed fertility testing. Therefore, the potential need for fertility testing should be broached when CF men are in their third decade of life, particularly in individuals considering conceiving offspring. Men who are interested in further evaluation should be referred to an andrologist who has expertise in CF-related infertility. Testing usually includes careful genital examination, hormone analysis (prolactin, follicle-stimulating hormone, luteinizing hormone, and testosterone), semen analysis, as well as testicular and transrectal sonography. If the individual is considering conception using his own aspirated sperm, the patient and his female partner should undergo careful genetic counseling. Furthermore, the female partner should undergo genetic testing for CF even in situations where there is a negative family history. Extensive genotyping of the healthy population show that approximately 20% of individuals without a family history of CF carry *CFTR* gene mutations and/or variants on at one chromosome.

CONCLUSIONS

The discovery of the *CFTR* gene has provided great insight into the pathogenesis of CF. However, it has become clear that it is a complex disease and that there are probably several genetic and environmental contributors to the development of disease heterogeneity. With continuing improvement in survival, many other complications are now becoming evident, such as gastrointestinal malignancies and CFRD, as well as issues concerning infertility and procreation. Comprehensive care addressing all the aspects of CF, in childhood and adulthood, continues to be central to optimizing the health and well-being of these patients.

REFERENCES

1. Kerem B, Rommens JM, Buchanan JA, et al: Identification of the cystic fibrosis gene. Genetic analysis. Science 1989;245(4922):1073–1080.
2. Kopelman H, Corey M, Gaskin K, et al: Impaired chloride secretion, as well as bicarbonate secretion, underlies the fluid secretory defect in the cystic fibrosis pancreas. Gastroenterology 1988;95(2):349–355.
3. Kopelman H, Durie P, Gaskin K, et al: Pancreatic fluid secretion and protein hyperconcentration in cystic fibrosis. N Engl J Med 1985;312(6): 329–334.
4. Go L, ed: Pancreatic Duct Cell Secretion. Control and Mechanisms of Secretion. New York: Raven Press, 1993.
5. Ishiguro H, Steward MC, Wilson RW, Case RM: Bicarbonate secretion in interlobular ducts from guinea-pig pancreas. J Physiol 1996;495(Pt 1): 179–191.
6. Shumaker H, Amlal H, Frizzell R, et al: CFTR drives Na^+-$nHCO_3^-$ cotransport in pancreatic duct cells. A basis for defective HCO_3^- secretion in CF. Am J Physiol 1999;276(1 Pt 1):C16–C25.
7. Ahmed N, Corey M, Forstner G, et al: Molecular consequences of cystic fibrosis transmembrane regulator (CFTR) gene mutations in the exocrine pancreas. Gut 2003;52(8):1159–1164.
8. Phillips RJ, Crock CM, Dillon MJ, et al: Cystic fibrosis presenting as kwashiorkor with florid skin rash. Arch Dis Child 1993;69(4):446–448.
9. Reisman J, Petrou C, Corey M, et al: Hypoalbuminemia at initial examination in patients with cystic fibrosis. J Pediatr 1989;115(5 Pt 1):755–758.
10. Cohn JA, Friedman KJ, Noone PG, et al: Relation between mutations of the cystic fibrosis gene and idiopathic pancreatitis. N Engl J Med 1998; 339(10):653–658.
11. Sharer N, Schwarz M, Malone G, et al: Mutations of the cystic fibrosis gene in patients with chronic pancreatitis. N Engl J Med 1998;339(10):645–652.
12. Noone PG, Zhou Z, Silverman LM, et al: Cystic fibrosis gene mutations and pancreatitis risk. Relation to epithelial ion transport and trypsin inhibitor gene mutations. Gastroenterology 2001;121(6):1310–1319.
13. Beharry S, Ellis L, Corey M, et al: How useful is fecal pancreatic elastase 1 as a marker of exocrine pancreatic disease? J Pediatr 2002;141(1):84–90.
14. Borowitz DS, Grand RJ, Durie PR: Use of pancreatic enzyme supplements for patients with cystic fibrosis in the context of fibrosing colonopathy. Consensus Committee. J Pediatr 1995;127(5):681–684.
15. Haber HP, Benda N, Fitzke G, et al: Colonic wall thickness measured by ultrasound. Striking differences in patients with cystic fibrosis versus healthy controls. Gut 1997;40(3):406–411.
16. Ramsden WH, Moya EF, Littlewood JM: Colonic wall thickness, pancreatic enzyme dose and type of preparation in cystic fibrosis. Arch Dis Child 1998;79(4):339–343.
17. Freiman JP, FitzSimmons SC: Colonic strictures in patients with cystic fibrosis. Results of a survey of 114 cystic fibrosis care centers in the United States. J Pediatr Gastroenterol Nutr 1996;22(2):153–156.
18. Allan JD, Moss AD, Wallwork JC, McFarlane H: Immediate hypersensitivity in patients with cystic fibrosis. Clin Allergy 1975;5(3):255–261.
19. Lipkin GW, Vickers DW: Allergy in cystic fibrosis nurses to pancreatic extract. Lancet 1987;1(8529):392.
20. Andersen D: Cystic fibrosis of the pancreas and its relation to celiac disease. Am Dis Child 1938;56:344–399.
21. Wilson DC, Kalnins D, Stewart C, et al: Challenges in the dietary treatment of cystic fibrosis related diabetes mellitus. Clin Nutr 2000;19(2): 87–93.
22. Rozmahel R, Wilschanski M, Matin A, et al: Modulation of disease severity in cystic fibrosis transmembrane conductance regulator deficient mice by a secondary genetic factor. Nat Genet 1996;12(3):280–287.
23. Zielenski J, Corey M, Rozmahel R, et al: Detection of a cystic fibrosis modifier locus for meconium ileus on human chromosome 19q13. Nat Genet 1999;22(2):128–129.
24. Gyomorey K, Garami E, Galley K, et al: Non-CFTR chloride channels likely contribute to secretion in the murine small intestine. Pflugers Arch 2001;443(Suppl 1):S103–S106.
25. Mohammad-Panah R, Gyomorey K, Rommens J, et al: ClC-2 contributes to native chloride secretion by a human intestinal cell line, Caco-2. J Biol Chem 2001;276(11):8306–8313.
26. Fakhoury K, Durie PR, Levison H, Canny GJ: Meconium ileus in the absence of cystic fibrosis. Arch Dis Child 1992;67(10 Spec No): 1204–1206.
27. Noblett HR: Treatment of uncomplicated meconium ileus by Gastrografin enema. A preliminary report. J Pediatr Surg 1969;4(2):190–197.
28. Burke MS, Ragi JM, Karamanoukian HL, et al: New strategies in nonoperative management of meconium ileus. J Pediatr Surg 2002;37(5): 760–764.
29. Fuchs JR, Langer JC: Long-term outcome after neonatal meconium obstruction. Pediatrics 1998;101(4):E7.
30. Koletzko S, Stringer DA, Cleghorn GJ, Durie PR: Lavage treatment of distal intestinal obstruction syndrome in children with cystic fibrosis. Pediatrics 1989;83(5):727–733.
31. Redel CA, Motil KJ, Bloss RS, et al: Intestinal button implantation for obstipation and fecal impaction in children. J Pediatr Surg 1992; 27(5):654–656.
32. Shields MD, Levison H, Reisman JJ, et al: Appendicitis in cystic fibrosis. Arch Dis Child 1991;66(3):307–310.
33. Holsclaw DS, Rocmans C, Shwachman H: Intussusception in patients with cystic fibrosis. Pediatrics 1971;48(1):51–58.
34. Stringer DA, Ein SH: Pneumatic reduction. Advantages, risks and indications. Pediatr Radiol 1990;20(6):475–477.
35. Pokorny CS, Bye PT, MacLeod C, Selby WS: Antibiotic-associated colitis and cystic fibrosis. Dig Dis Sci 1992;37(9):1464–1468.
36. Welkon CJ, Long SS, Thompson CM Jr, Gilligan PH: *Clostridium difficile* in patients with cystic fibrosis. Am J Dis Child 1985;139(8): 805–808.
37. Rivlin J, Lerner A, Augarten A, et al: Severe *Clostridium difficile*–associated colitis in young patients with cystic fibrosis. J Pediatr 1998;132(1): 177–179.
38. Heine RG, Button BM, Olinsky A, et al: Gastro-oesophageal reflux in infants under 6 months with cystic fibrosis. Arch Dis Child 1998;78(1): 44–48.
39. Gustafsson PM, Fransson SG, Kjellman NI, Tibbling L: Gastro-oesophageal reflux and severity of pulmonary disease in cystic fibrosis. Scand J Gastroenterol 1991;26(5):449–456.
40. Hassall E, Israel DM, Davidson AG, Wong LT: Barrett's esophagus in children with cystic fibrosis: not a coincidental association. Am J Gastroenterol 1993;88(11):1934–1938.
41. O'Connor J, Lawson J: Fibrocystic disease of pancreas and Crohn's disease. Br Med J 1972;4(840):610.
42. Lloyd-Still JD: Crohn's disease and cystic fibrosis. Dig Dis Sci 1994;39(4): 880–885.

43. Lloyd-Still JD: Crohn's accounts for increased prevalence of inflammatory bowel disease in CF. Pediatr Pulmonol 1992;(8 Suppl):307–308.
44. Abdul-Karim FW, King TA, Dahms BB, et al: Carcinoma of extrahepatic biliary system in an adult with cystic fibrosis. Gastroenterology 1982; 82:758–762.
45. Tesluk H, McCauley K, Kurland G, Ruebner BH: Cholangiocarcinoma in an adult with cystic fibrosis. J Clin Gastroenterol 1991;13(4):485–487.
46. Chaun H, Paty B, Nakielna EM, et al: Colonic carcinoma in two adult cystic fibrosis patients. Can J Gastroenterol 1996;10(7):440–442.
47. Tsongalis GJ, Faber G, Dalldorf FG, et al: Association of pancreatic adenocarcinoma, mild lung disease, and delta F508 mutation in a cystic fibrosis patient. Clin Chem 1994;40(10):1972–1974.
48. Samuels LE, Amrom G, Kerstein MD: Adenocarcinoma of the ileum in a patient with cystic fibrosis. Dig Dis Sci 1995;40(1):107–108.
49. Lewindon PJ, Pereira TN, Hoskins AC, et al: The role of hepatic stellate cells and transforming growth factor-beta(1) in cystic fibrosis liver disease. Am J Pathol 2002;160(5):1705–1715.
50. Waters DL, Dorney SF, Gruca MA, et al: Hepatobiliary disease in cystic fibrosis patients with pancreatic sufficiency. Hepatology 1995;21(4):963–969.
51. Gabolde M, Hubert D, Guilloud-Bataille M, et al: The mannose binding lectin gene influences the severity of chronic liver disease in cystic fibrosis. J Med Genet 2001;38(5):310–311.
52. Rohlfs EM, Shaheen NJ, Silverman LM: Is the hemochromatosis gene a modifier locus for cystic fibrosis? Genet Test 1998;2(1):85–88.
53. Scott-Jupp R, Lama M, Tanner MS: Prevalence of liver disease in cystic fibrosis. Arch Dis Child 1991;66(6):698–701.
54. Gaskin KJ, Waters DL, Howman-Giles R, et al: Liver disease and common-bile-duct stenosis in cystic fibrosis. N Engl J Med 1988;318(6):340–346.
55. Roy CC, Weber AM, Morin CL, et al: Abnormal biliary lipid composition in cystic fibrosis. Effect of pancreatic enzymes. N Engl J Med 1977; 297(24):1301–1305.
56. Sokol RJ, Durie PR: Recommendations for management of liver and biliary tract disease in cystic fibrosis. Cystic Fibrosis Foundation Hepatobiliary Disease Consensus Group. J Pediatr Gastroenterol Nutr 1999;28(Suppl 1):S1–S13.
57. Colombo C, Bertolini E, Assaisso ML, et al: Failure of ursodeoxycholic acid to dissolve radiolucent gallstones in patients with cystic fibrosis. Acta Paediatr 1993;82(6–7):562–565.
58. Lambert JR, Cole M, Crozier DN, Connon JJ: Intrapancreatic common bile duct compression causing jaundice in an adult with cystic fibrosis. Gastroenterology. 1981;80(1):169–172.
59. Vitullo BB, Rochon L, Seemayer TA, et al: Intrapancreatic compression of the common bile duct in cystic fibrosis. J Pediatr 1978;93(6):1060–1061.
60. Nagel RA, Westaby D, Javaid A, et al: Liver disease and bile duct abnormalities in adults with cystic fibrosis. Lancet 1989;2(8677):1422–1425.
61. O'Brien S, Keogan M, Casey M, et al: Biliary complications of cystic fibrosis. Gut 1992;33(3):387–391.
62. Neglia JP, FitzSimmons SC, Maisonneuve P, et al: The risk of cancer among patients with cystic fibrosis. Cystic Fibrosis and Cancer Study Group. N Engl J Med 1995;332(8):494–499.
63. Oppenheimer EH, Esterly JR: Hepatic changes in young infants with cystic fibrosis. Possible relation to focal biliary cirrhosis. J Pediatr 1975; 86(5):683–689.
64. Maurage C, Lenaerts C, Weber A, et al: Meconium ileus and its equivalent as a risk factor for the development of cirrhosis. An autopsy study in cystic fibrosis. J Pediatr Gastroenterol Nutr 1989;9(1):17–20.
65. Shapira R, Hadzic N, Francavilla R, et al: Retrospective review of cystic fibrosis presenting as infantile liver disease. Arch Dis Child 1999;81(2): 125–128.
66. Vawter GF, Shwachman H: Cystic fibrosis in adults. An autopsy study. Pathol Annu. 1979;14(Pt 2):357–382.
67. Colombo C, Castellani MR, Balistreri WF, et al: Scintigraphic documentation of an improvement in hepatobiliary excretory function after treatment with ursodeoxycholic acid in patients with cystic fibrosis and associated liver disease. Hepatology 1992;15(4):677–684.
68. Heuman DM: Hepatoprotective properties of ursodeoxycholic acid. Gastroenterology 1993;104(6):1865–1870.
69. Colombo C, Crosignani A, Assaisso M, et al: Ursodeoxycholic acid therapy in cystic fibrosis-associated liver disease. A dose-response study. Hepatology 1992;16(4):924–930.
70. Colombo C, Battezzati PM, Podda M, et al: Ursodeoxycholic acid for liver disease associated with cystic fibrosis. A double-blind multicenter trial. The Italian Group for the Study of Ursodeoxycholic Acid in Cystic Fibrosis. Hepatology 1996;23(6):1484–1490.
71. Cotting J, Lentze MJ, Reichen J: Effects of ursodeoxycholic acid treatment on nutrition and liver function in patients with cystic fibrosis and longstanding cholestasis. Gut 1990;31(8):918–921.
72. Colombo C, Battezzati PM, Crosignani A, et al: Effects of taurine and ursodeoxycholic acid on liver function tests in patients with cystic fibrosis. Acta Univ Carol [Med] (Praha) 1990;36(1–4):148–151.
73. Teran JC, Imperiale TF, Mullen KD, et al: Primary prophylaxis of variceal bleeding in cirrhosis. A cost-effectiveness analysis. Gastroenterology 1997; 112(2):473–482.
74. Erstad BL: Octreotide for acute variceal bleeding. Ann Pharmacother 2001;35(5):618–626.
75. Mack DR, Traystman MD, Colombo JL, et al: Clinical denouement and mutation analysis of patients with cystic fibrosis undergoing liver transplantation for biliary cirrhosis. J Pediatr 1995;127(6):881–887.
76. Corey M, McLaughlin FJ, Williams M, Levison H: A comparison of survival, growth, and pulmonary function in patients with cystic fibrosis in Boston and Toronto. J Clin Epidemiol 1988;41(6):583–591.
77. Feranchak AP, Sontag MK, Wagener JS, et al: Prospective, long-term study of fat-soluble vitamin status in children with cystic fibrosis identified by newborn screen. J Pediatr 1999;135(5):601–610.
78. Conway SP, Morton AM, Oldroyd B, et al: Osteoporosis and osteopenia in adults and adolescents with cystic fibrosis. Prevalence and associated factors. Thorax 2000;55(9):798–804.
79. Rashid M, Durie P, Andrew M, et al: Prevalence of vitamin K deficiency in cystic fibrosis. Am J Clin Nutr 1999;70(3):378–382.
80. Wilson DC, Rashid M, Durie PR, et al: Treatment of vitamin K deficiency in cystic fibrosis. Effectiveness of a daily fat-soluble vitamin combination. J Pediatr 2001;138(6):851–855.
81. Kaplan E, Shwachman H, Perlmutter AD, et al: Reproductive failure in males with cystic fibrosis. N Engl J Med 1968;279(2):65–69.
82. Stern RC, Boat TF, Doershuk CF: Obstructive azoospermia as a diagnostic criterion for the cystic fibrosis syndrome. Lancet 1982;1(8286): 1401–1404.
83. Wilschanski M, Corey M, Durie P, et al: Diversity of reproductive tract abnormalities in men with cystic fibrosis. JAMA 1996;276(8):607–608.
84. Chillon M, Casals T, Mercier B, et al: Infertility due to congenital absence of the vas deferens is mainly caused by variable exon 9 skipping of the *CFTR* gene in heterozygote males for cystic fibrosis mutations. Am J Hum Genet 1994;55(Suppl):A217.
85. Jarvi K, Zielenski J, Wilschanski M, et al: Cystic fibrosis transmembrane conductance regulator and obstructive azoospermia. Lancet 1995; 345(8964):1578.

Other Diseases with a Prominent Respiratory Component

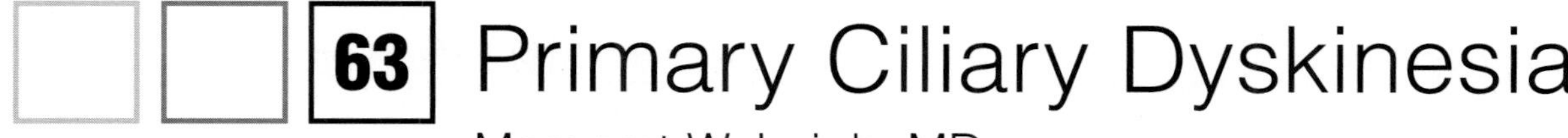

63 Primary Ciliary Dyskinesia

Margaret W. Leigh, MD

Primary ciliary dyskinesia (PCD) is an inherited disorder characterized by specific ultrastructural defects of cilia that are associated with impaired ciliary motion and mucociliary clearance. The basic biochemical defect has not been defined; however, molecular genetic studies have identified mutations involving different dynein genes in several PCD families. In PCD, impaired ciliary function results in ineffective clearance of mucous secretions and inhaled particles, including bacteria. Consequently, recurrent or persistent rhinitis, sinusitis, otitis media, and bronchitis are characteristic clinical features of PCD. Bronchiectasis is the predominant pulmonary complication.

■ HISTORICAL BACKGROUND AND NOMENCLATURE

In the 1930s, Kartagener described a clinical syndrome (previously identified by others) manifested by the triad of situs inversus, chronic sinusitis, and bronchiectasis[1] that later was defined as Kartagener's syndrome. Several decades later, patients with Kartagener's syndrome as well as other patients with chronic sinusitis and bronchiectasis were noted to have defects in the ultrastructural organization of cilia.[2–4] Initially, the term *immotile cilia syndrome* was used to describe this disorder. Subsequent studies demonstrated that cilia are often motile but their beat is uncoordinated and ineffective. The name was changed to PCD to more appropriately describe the spectrum of ciliary dysfunction and to distinguish genetic ciliary defects from those acquired following epithelial injury from insults such as viral respiratory tract infections or exposure to toxic agents.

■ CILIA: STRUCTURE AND FUNCTION

The large airways and contiguous structures, such as nares, paranasal sinuses, and middle ear, are lined by a ciliated, pseudostratified columnar epithelium that is important for mucociliary clearance. The cells on the luminal surface of this epithelium are predominantly ciliated cells with interspersed goblet cells. Other epithelia containing motile ciliated cells are found in the ependyma of the brain and the fallopian tubes. Flagella (e.g., tails of spermatozoa) have a core structure similar to that of cilia with the same fundamental motility characteristics.

Mature respiratory ciliated cells contain approximately 200 cilia of uniform size with an average length of 6 μm and diameter of 0.2 μm. Each normal cilium contains an array of longitudinal microtubules, consisting of nine doublets arranged in an outer circle around a central pair (Fig. 63-1). The microtubules are anchored by a basal body in the apical cytoplasm of the cell. Several different proteins contribute to ciliary structure and function. Tubulin, a dimeric molecule with distinct α and β subunits, is the principal protein of microtubules. A network of structural proteins provide intertubular linkages to maintain the 9 + 2 pattern of microtubules in healthy cilia. The protein nexin links the outer microtubular doublets, creating a circumferential network, and radial spokes connect the outer microtubular doublets with a central sheath of protein that surrounds the central tubules. Dynein is attached to the microtubules as distinct inner and outer "arms," recognizable on electron micrographs of ciliary cross-sections, and is thought to participate in the provision of energy for microtubule sliding through adenosine triphosphatase (ATPase) activity. Inner and outer dynein arms are attached to each microtubule doublet at distinct intervals—approximately 25 nm for outer dynein arms and approximately 100 nm for inner dynein arms. The outer dynein arms (closer to the cell membrane) are longer and form a hook, while the inner dynein arms (closer to the central pair of microtubules) are short and straight. Each dynein arm is a multimer of two to three heavy chains (400–500 kd), two to four intermediate chains (45–110 kd), and at least eight light chains (8–55 kd).[5,6] The dynein heavy chains contain the ATPase that provides the energy for ciliary movement.

Ciliary bending results from the longitudinal displacement of adjacent microtubular doublets. Because nexin links maintain the axonemal relationships and the basal bodies anchor the microtubules, the sliding of the outer microtubules is converted

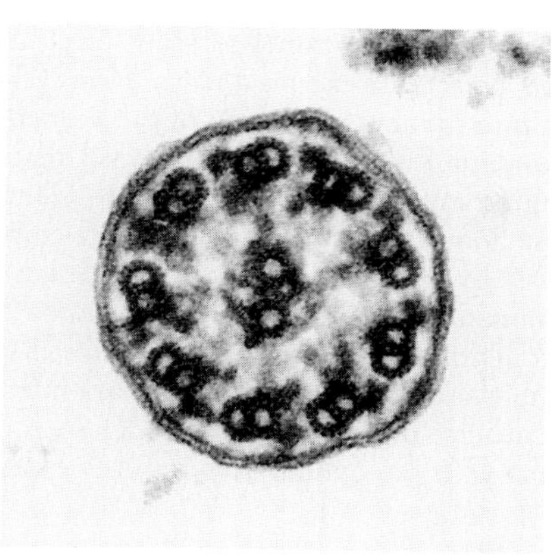

A

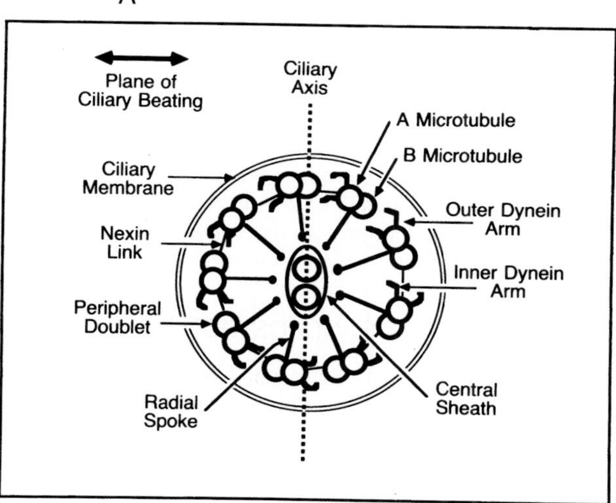

B

FIGURE 63-1. **A,** Ultrastructure of a normal cilium in cross-section. **B,** A diagrammatic representation illustrating the major structural components. The nine outer doublet tubules and two central singlet tubules are interconnected by nexin and radial spoke linkages. Outer and inner dynein arms are attached to A subunits of the outer doublets. The plane of ciliary beating is perpendicular to the ciliary axis, determined by the alignment of the central tubules. (**A,** Courtesy of J.L. Carson. **B,** From Rutland J, deIongh RU: Random ciliary orientation—a cause of respiratory tract disease. N Engl J Med 1990; 323[24]:1681–1684.)

into a bending movement of the cilia. Ciliary motion takes place within an aqueous layer of airway surface liquids and is divided into two phases: an effective stroke phase that sweeps forward and a recovery phase during which the cilia bend "backward" and extend into the starting position for the stroke phase. Typically, the tips of cilia contact the overlying mucous layer during the stroke phase to propel mucous secretions forward, but during the recovery phase, cilia lose contact with the mucus. Normal human cilia bend in a rapid, rhythmic, wave-like motion. The ciliary beat frequency is faster in the proximal airways than in the distal airways (~12 beats/second in the nose and trachea vs. 8 beats/second in the bronchioles) and is faster in children than in adults (nasal ciliary beat frequency is close to 13 beats/second in young children vs. 11.5 beats/second in adults).[7] In healthy epithelium, cilia are aligned spatially with parallel orientation of the central pair of tubules in adjacent cilia (Fig. 63-2*A*); therefore, ciliary motility is maintained in the same plane along the length of airways. Normal mucociliary transport rates may be as rapid as 20 to 30 mm/min. Although the regulation of ciliary actions is complex and not fully understood, it is clear that several signaling mechanisms, including intracellular Ca^{2+}, cyclic adenosine monophosphate, extracellular nucleotides such as adenosine triphosphate, and airway nitric oxide play key roles in regulating ciliary beat frequency.[8–11]

ULTRASTRUCTURAL CILIARY DEFECTS IN PRIMARY CILIARY DYSKINESIA

By routine light microscopy, the ciliated epithelium of patients with PCD appears normal. Examination of the ultrastructural organization of cilia by transmission electron microscopy has identified a number of distinct ciliary defects in patients with PCD, including defects in the dynein arms, radial spokes, and nexin links as well as microtubular transpositions (Box 63-1, Fig. 63-3). These distinct ultrastructural defects are generally apparent in cilia throughout the airways, middle ear, and oviduct, as well as in sperm tails, providing evidence that PCD is a generalized disorder of genetic origin.

DYNEIN ARM DEFECTS

Dynein defects that have been described in patients with PCD include complete absence of both inner and outer dynein arms[2,12] as well as complete or partial absence of either the inner or the outer dynein arms.[13] In some cases, a portion of the inner or outer dynein arm may remain attached to the microtubular doublet. Outer dynein arms are easy to identify because the

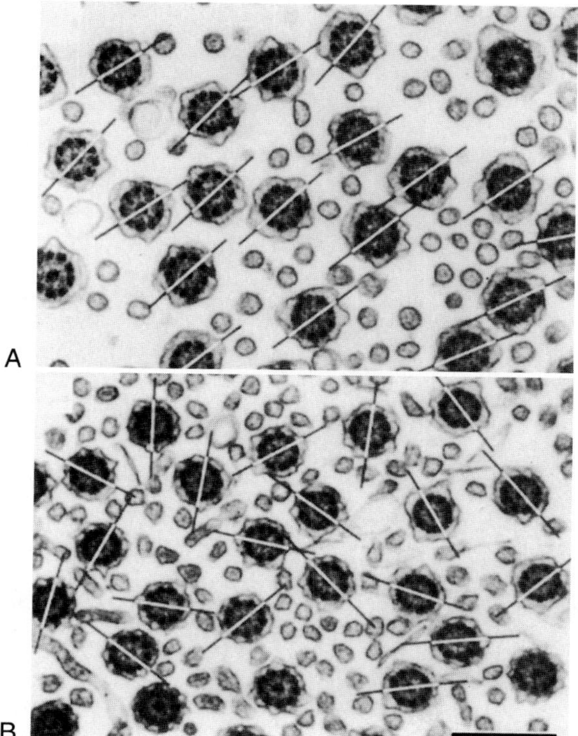

FIGURE 63-2. Ciliary orientation determined by the alignment of the central tubules is almost parallel in normal subjects **(A),** but can be random in patients with primary ciliary dyskinesia **(B),** resulting in uncoordinated and ineffective ciliary beating. (From Rutland J, deIongh RU: Random ciliary orientation—a cause of respiratory tract disease. N Engl J Med 1990;323[24]: 1681–1684.)

BOX 63-1 Ultrastructural Defects in Primary Ciliary Dyskinesia

Dynein Arm Defects

- Total or partial absence of inner and outer dynein arms
- Total or partial absence of inner dynein arms
- Total or partial absence of outer dynein arms
- Shortening of dynein arms

Radial Spoke Defects

- Total absence of radial spokes
- Absence of radial spoke heads

Microtubular Transposition

- Absence of the central pair of tubules with transposition of outer doublet to the center

Other

- Ciliary disorientation
- Ciliary aplasia
- Absence of nexin links
- Basal body anomalies
- Central microtubular agenesis
- Normal ultrastructure but impaired function

periphery of the axoneme contains scant electron-dense material; therefore, defects are easy to discern. However, inner dynein arms project into the central portion of the axoneme where there is more abundant overlying electron-dense material that can obscure margins and confound the ability to identify ultrastructural defects. Some investigators have used computer-assisted image analysis to improve visualization of inner dynein arms, thereby enhancing the ability to detect inner arm defects.[14] Because partial absence of inner dynein arms may be observed in normal subjects without recent respiratory infections or other identifiable insults, the diagnosis of PCD in individuals with partial absence of inner dynein arms can be challenging.

RADIAL SPOKE DEFECTS

A number of defects in radial spokes have been associated with ciliary dysmotility, including total absence of radial spokes and absence of radial spoke heads.[15] These defects are easily recognized by an eccentric position of the central pair of microtubules that are normally stabilized in a central position by the radial spokes. Central displacement of one of the outer microtubular doublets may also occur. The radial spoke is composed of numerous polypeptides; the distinct protein defects underlying these radial spoke abnormalities has not been identified.

MICROTUBULAR TRANSPOSITION DEFECT

A characteristic alteration in the 9 + 2 configuration of axonemal microtubules has been described in some families with PCD.

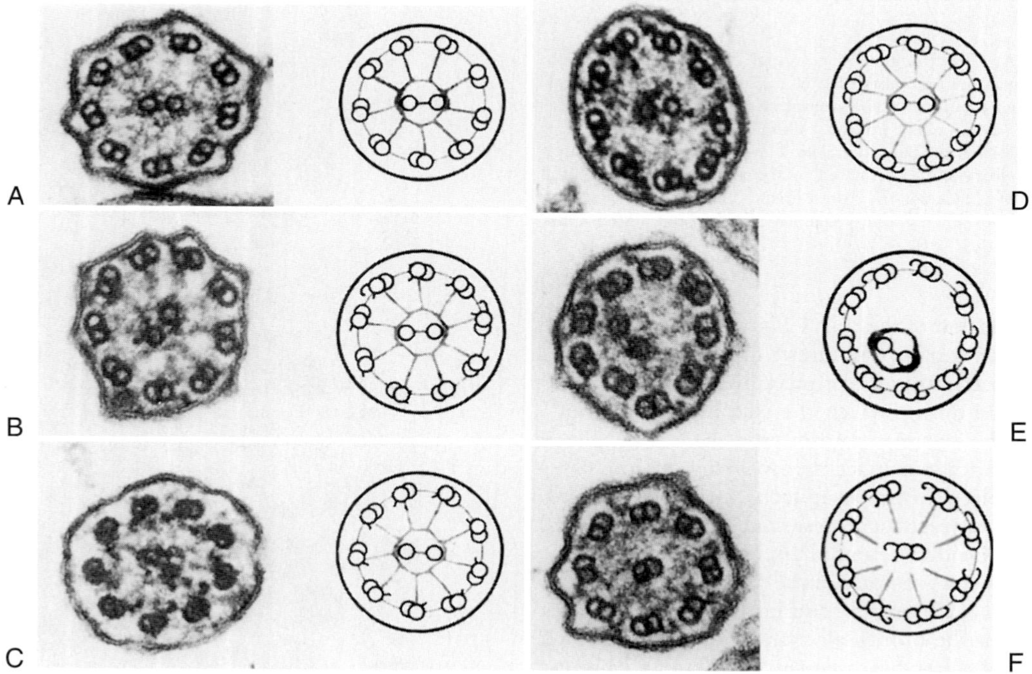

FIGURE 63-3. Specific ciliary defects that cause primary ciliary dyskinesia cross-sections with corresponding diagrammatic representations (*right*). **A,** Dynein arm defect: total absence of outer and inner dynein arms. **B,** Dynein arm defect: partial absence of outer and inner dynein arms (>60% of dynein arms are absent). **C,** Dynein arm defect: absence of outer dynein arms. **D,** Dynein arm defect: absence of inner dynein arms. **E,** Radial spoke defect: absence of radial spokes with eccentric central core. **F,** Microtubular transposition defect: absence of central tubules with transposition of one doublet to the central axis of the cilium. (**A, B,** and **D,** Original magnification ×106,000; **C,** original magnification ×104,000; **E,** original magnification ×140,000; **F,** original magnification ×110,000.) (Photomicrographs courtesy of J.M. Sturgess and J.A.P. Turner.)

Typically, the central pair of tubules is missing and one of the outer microtubular doublets is transposed to the center in both cilia and flagellae.[16]

OTHER DEFECTS

A number of other defects have been identified in patients with ciliary dysmotility, including ciliary aplasia (no cilia and no apparent ciliogenesis), ciliary disorientation (the central pairs of microtubules in adjacent cilia are not aligned as shown in Fig. 63-2*B*),[17] absence of nexin links,[18] basal body anomalies, and central microtubular agenesis.[19] All of these defects may be apparent to some degree following insults such as viral infections; therefore, it is not clear whether these are primary or secondary defects. One approach to discern whether defects are acquired or congenital is to examine ciliary ultrastructure after a prolonged period in cell culture during which cells dedifferentiate and then reciliate. If the defect does not persist after reciliation, then the defect is more likely an acquired defect as shown for ciliary disorientation.[20] In some patients with typical clinical manifestations of PCD and ciliary dysmotility, ciliary ultrastructure appears normal, suggesting other defects that affect function but not structure. Isolation and development of probes for the numerous components of cilia or their genes are needed to further define primary defects in cilia and to understand the steps in ciliogenesis that are interrupted to create secondary ciliary defects.

FUNCTIONAL CILIARY DEFECTS IN PRIMARY CILIARY DYSKINESIA

Ciliary motion may be assessed by videomicroscopy of freshly excised ciliated epithelium obtained by scrape or brush biopsy of the inferior surface of the nasal turbinate, or by bronchial brush biopsy. Freshly excised ciliated cells maintain ciliary beat for several hours if placed in appropriate culture media. In PCD, the cilia may be immotile or dyskinetic. Recent studies have shown that certain beat patterns are associated with specific ultrastructural defects; specifically, absence of outer dynein arms is associated with immotility or a slightly flickering beat pattern; isolated inner dynein arm defects or radial spoke defects are associated with a slow, stiff motion; and ciliary transposition defects are associated with a circular beat pattern that may have a normal beat frequency but lacks the directional bend.[21] At this time, assessment of ciliary beat pattern and ciliary beat frequency has not been sufficiently standardized for screening or diagnosis of PCD.

Effectiveness of ciliary beat can be evaluated by measuring mucociliary clearance. As a screening assessment of mucociliary clearance, some clinicians apply saccharin particles to the anterior nares and measure the time interval until the bitter saccharin is tasted (saccharin test).[22] This procedure has limited usefulness in children because the patient must lie still with no sneezing, sniffing, or coughing for up to 1 hour. In specialized centers, nasal or lung mucociliary clearance is determined by using a gamma counter to measure the rate of removal of inhaled radiolabeled particles.[23,24] When cough is suppressed, patients with PCD have no (or little) clearance of isotope from the lung.[23–27] Unlike in cystic fibrosis, cough clearance in PCD is preserved and serves as a compensatory clearance mechanism.[27]

NASAL NITRIC OXIDE IN PRIMARY CILIARY DYSKINESIA

In 1994, Lundberg and colleagues reported that children with Kartagener's syndrome (situs inversus, sinusitis, and bronchiectasis) produced very little nasal nitric oxide (NO).[28] Subsequent studies have demonstrated that nasal NO is extremely low (10%–20% of normal) in PCD patients,[29–32] and hence may be useful for screening for PCD. NO is formed by the nitric oxide synthase (NOS) enzyme system, in the presence of appropriate substrate (L-arginine and oxygen) and cofactors including tetrahydrobiopterin. In normal adults, production of NO from the nose (primarily from paranasal sinuses) is 10- to 50-fold greater than from the lower airways. Therefore, accurate assessment of nasal NO production requires maneuvers for palate closure, breath holding, or intubation to exclude contaminating gases from the lower airway that have much lower NO concentrations. The mechanism for altered nasal NO production in PCD has not been defined. Interestingly, patients with cystic fibrosis also have low nasal NO, but not as low as in PCD.[29]

GENETICS

PCD has been reported in many ethnic groups without apparent racial or gender predilection. In most families, PCD appears to be transmitted by an autosomal-recessive pattern of inheritance; however, rare instances of autosomal-dominant or X-linked inheritance patterns have been reported.[33,34] Parents of affected children are normal and have no evidence of impaired ciliary function. The incidence of PCD is 1 in 15,000 to 1 in 20,000 births. The specific type of ultrastructural ciliary defects appears to be genetically determined because of their consistency within individual families. The incidence of situs inversus is random within affected families, suggesting that this phenotype is not genetically determined. Further support comes from a case report of twins with PCD who were genetically identical. One twin had situs inversus totalis and the other had situs solitus.[35] Presently, probes for prenatal diagnosis of PCD are not readily available; however, recent advances in molecular genetics have identified mutations that can be tracked in certain families.

The numerous ultrastructural phenotypes suggest genetic heterogeneity,[36] and this has been confirmed in a recent genome-wide linkage search.[37] Molecular genetic studies have focused primarily on dyneins and other ciliary proteins. The axoneme of cilia and flagellae is conserved phylogenetically with remarkably high sequence conservation between flagellar proteins in unicellular organisms (e.g., *Chlamydomonas*, a flagellate alga) and mammalian ciliary proteins. Consequently, information obtained from studies in normal and mutant dysmotile strains of *Chlamydomonas* has provided clues about mammalian dyneins and other ciliary proteins (and their respective genes).[6] The outer dynein arm in *Chlamydomonas* is composed of three heavy chains, two intermediate chains, and at least eight light chains. Several human homologues of outer arm dyneins in *Chlamydomonas* are likely candidate genes for PCD. To date, mutations in two outer dynein arm genes have been identified in patients with PCD: DNAH5 (γ heavy chain) and DNAI1 (intermediate chain IC78).[6,38–41] Several other outer dynein arm genes and inner dynein arm genes are candidate genes. For the subset of PCD patients with normal dynein arms, genes under investigation include radial spoke genes and central apparatus genes.

CLINICAL FEATURES OF PRIMARY CILIARY DYSKINESIA IN CHILDHOOD

Patients with different ultrastructural defects manifest similar clinical features. Children present with a history of chronic, productive cough and a combination of chronic and recurrent respiratory infections, including rhinitis, sinusitis, otitis media, bronchitis, and pneumonia.[32,42,43] The majority of PCD patients have a history of respiratory problems (tachypnea, cough, hypoxemia) in the newborn period attributed to neonatal pneumonia, transient tachypnea of the newborn, or aspiration pneumonitis; however, the possibility of PCD is rarely considered except in patients with situs inversus, persistent atelectasis, persistent pneumonia, or a family history of PCD.[32,44] More typically, the diagnosis is made in children and young adults who have chronic cough, sinusitis, and otitis media. The clinical and radiographic findings in childhood are summarized in Boxes 63-2 and 63-3.

LOWER RESPIRATORY TRACT MANIFESTATIONS

Chronic cough is an almost universal feature of PCD. Typically, the cough is productive and most apparent in the early morning but may also occur at night or in association with exercise. Sputum may be mucoid or purulent. Most patients describe yellow or yellow-green sputum that clears with antibiotic therapy. In many children, exercise tolerance is normal but becomes impaired with advancing obstructive airways disease in older children and young adults. Findings on chest examination are variable. Some patients have localized crackles that may or may not clear following forceful cough, and some may have hyperinflation of the chest. Wheezing is relatively uncommon. Digital clubbing may be apparent in the older patients with bronchiectasis.

BOX 63-2 Primary Ciliary Dyskinesia: Clinical Findings in Childhood

Frequent (in >60% of Patients)

- Respiratory distress during the neonatal period
- Chronic productive cough
- Recurrent pneumonia
- Airflow obstruction
- Chronic rhinitis and rhinorrhea
- Chronic otitis media
- Chronic sinusitis
- Male sterility

Common (in 20%–60% of Patients)

- Situs inversus
- Nasal polyps
- Conductive hearing loss
- Tympanic membrane perforation
- Digital clubbing (more prevalent in adults than in children)

BOX 63-3 Primary Ciliary Dyskinesia: Radiographic Findings in Childhood

Frequent (in >60% of Patients)

- Hyperinflation
- Bronchial wall thickening
- Segmental atelectasis
- Mucosal thickening of the paranasal sinuses

Common (in 20%–60% of Patients)

- Situs inversus
- Bronchiectasis
- Opacification of paranasal sinuses

Bacterial cultures of bronchoscopic aspirates yield a number of organisms, such as nontypable *Haemophilus influenzae, Staphylococcus aureus, Streptococcus viridans,* and *Streptococcus pneumoniae,* that may be inhaled or aspirated from the upper respiratory tract. Older patients with long-standing disease may be colonized with *Pseudomonas aeruginosa.*[32,45] Chest radiographic findings, in order of frequency, include hyperinflation, bronchial wall thickening, segmental atelectasis/consolidation, situs inversus, and bronchiectasis.[46] Typically, radiographic findings are most apparent in the middle lobe and lingula. With the exception of situs inversus, these radiographic features may be apparent in other chronic disorders, including cystic fibrosis, immunodeficiency, and chronic aspiration.

Pulmonary function tests may be normal during early childhood but more typically demonstrate obstructive airway disease that becomes more severe in adulthood. Typical findings include decreased flow rates (forced expiratory flow between 25% and 75% of vital capacity [$FEF_{25\%-75\%}$] and forced expiratory volume in 1 second [FEV_1]), increased residual volume (RV), and increased ratio of residual volume to total lung capacity (RV/TLC). Bronchodilator responsiveness is variable. Longitudinal analyses of children with PCD suggest that lung function may remain stable over relatively long periods of time.[47,48]

NOSE AND PARANASAL SINUSES

Nasal congestion, a common presenting feature, often is present since early infancy, with little to no seasonal variation. Most patients describe chronic mucopurulent nasal drainage. Typically, sinus radiographs or computed tomograms demonstrate mucosal thickening, cloudiness, and/or opacification of all paranasal sinuses, even in the absence of sinus symptoms. Nasal polyps occur in approximately one third of patients and may be apparent in early childhood. Anosmia, hyponasal speech, and halitosis are more apparent in severely affected patients.

MIDDLE EAR

Chronic otitis media of variable severity is present in almost all patients with PCD. At the time of diagnosis, most patients have either chronic tympanic membrane perforations or have had multiple tympanostomies with insertion of ventilation tubes in the tympanic membranes. Many have conductive hearing loss. Middle ear findings may be most helpful in distinguishing PCD from cystic fibrosis or other causes of chronic lung disease.

SITUS INVERSUS TOTALIS

Situs inversus occurs in approximately 50% of patients with PCD. Typically, all viscera in the chest and abdomen are transposed (i.e., situs inversus totalis). Bronchoscopic evaluation of patients with situs inversus demonstrates transposition of the right and left bronchial configuration, consistent with transposition of the right and left lungs. The underlying basis for situs inversus has not been completely defined. According to the most widely accepted hypothesis, normal rotation of viscera depends on functioning embryonic cilia. With disruption of normal ciliary movement, as in PCD, rotation becomes a chance occurrence; 50% have normal rotation and 50% have dextrorotation or situs inversus.[38,40,49] This randomness of laterality in PCD has been demonstrated in genetically identical twins with PCD: one with situs solitus and one with situs inversus[35] as well as in dynein knockout mouse models.[38,40,50]

GENITOURINARY SYSTEM

Male infertility is common and attributable to impaired sperm motility. The ultrastructural and functional defects in cilia are mirrored in sperm flagellae in some but not all PCD patients.[12,51] The occurrence of ultrastructural ciliary defects in ciliated cells lining fallopian tubes[52,53] has led to speculation that infertility and ectopic pregnancies could be increased in women with primary ciliary defects, but this association has not been examined systematically.

OTHER

Hydrocephalus has been reported in a few patients with PCD[54–56] and in some knockout mouse models for PCD; ultrastructural and functional defects in ventricular ependymal cilia provide a theoretical basis for this association. Defective leukocyte migration has been reported in a few PCD patients, suggesting that the cytoplasmic microtubules of leukocytes may be altered, but specific defects in neutrophil chemotaxis have not been defined.[57,58]

DIAGNOSIS OF THE IMMOTILE CILIA SYNDROME

Definitive diagnosis of PCD requires demonstration of abnormal ciliary motility and ultrastructure. Suitable samples for examination include nasal biopsies obtained by brushing or curettage of the inferior surface of the nasal turbinates, or bronchial brush biopsy. Identification of impaired motility and one of the specific ultrastructural defects in a patient with chronic cough, sinusitis, and otitis media provides solid evidence for the diagnosis. Airway insults such as exposure to pollutants and respiratory viral infections may be accompanied by nonspecific ultrastructural changes in cilia that impair motility. Therefore, analysis of ciliary ultrastructure should be performed by an electron microscopist who has extensive experience examining ciliated cells. Despite expert review, the ultrastructural analysis may be inconclusive in some cases because of uncertainty in distinguishing primary from secondary ciliary defects; long-term follow-up and repeat biopsies may be needed before a firm diagnosis can be made. The role of nasal NO measurement in the diagnostic evaluation has not been defined; however, recent studies suggest that this assay may be a useful screening test for PCD or serve as an adjunctive diagnostic test in individuals with "uncertain" ciliary ultrastructural studies.[29–32]

TREATMENT

At present, no specific therapeutic modalities are available to correct the ciliary dysfunction. Management should include aggressive measures to enhance clearance of mucus, prevent respiratory infections, and treat bacterial superinfections.[42]

Approaches to enhance mucus clearance in PCD are similar to those used in the management of cystic fibrosis. Chest percussion and postural drainage facilitate clearance of distal airways. Because cough is an effective clearance mechanism, patients are encouraged to cough and to engage in activities such as vigorous exercise that stimulate cough. All patients and families should be counseled about the importance of cough and instructed to avoid cough suppressants. Bronchodilators such as albuterol may aid mucus clearance in patients who are bronchodilator responsive. As in cystic fibrosis, anti-inflammatory agents and deoxyribonuclease may be beneficial; however, specific indications and utility in PCD have not been defined.

A number of measures to prevent respiratory tract infection and irritation should be considered. PCD patients should receive routine immunizations that provide protection against a number of respiratory pathogens, including pertussis, measles, and *Haemophilus influenzae* type b, as well as the pneumococcal vaccine and a yearly influenza virus vaccine. Preventive counseling should include avoidance of exposure to respiratory pathogens, tobacco smoke, and other pollutants and irritants that may damage airway mucosa and stimulate mucus secretion.

Prompt institution of antibiotic therapy for bacterial superinfections (bronchitis, sinusitis, and otitis media) is crucial for preventing irreversible damage. Sputum Gram stain and culture results may be used to direct appropriate choice of antimicrobial therapy. In some patients, symptoms recur within days to weeks after completing a course of antibiotics. This subgroup may benefit from extended use of a broad-spectrum antibiotic such as trimethoprim-sulfamethoxazole.

Surgical intervention may be indicated for specific complications. Tympanostomy with ventilation tube placement may be necessary to control chronic serous otitis media that persists despite antibiotic therapy. Nasal polypectomy and/or sinus drainage may benefit patients with severe sinusitis that does not respond to antibiotic therapy. Lobectomy may be considered in patients with localized bronchiectasis or atelectasis that is thought to be a nidus for chronic infection. However, lobectomy should be approached cautiously, recognizing that removal of any functioning lung tissue in patients with progressive lung disease could have long-term adverse consequences. Lung transplantation (including heart-lung, bilateral lung, and living related bilateral lung transplantation) has been performed successfully in PCD patients with end-stage lung disease (with surgical modifications for patients with situs inversus).

PROGNOSIS

Chronic lung disease with bronchiectasis and some degree of pulmonary disability has been the usual outcome. Progression of lung disease is quite variable, and a number of individuals have experienced a normal or near-normal life span. Little is known about the impact that current symptomatic therapy may have on the course of lung disease.

REFERENCES

1. Kartagener M: Zur pathogenese der bronkiectasien. Bronkiectasien bei situs viscerum inversus. Beitr Klin Tuberk 1933;82:489–501.
2. Afzelius BA: A human syndrome caused by immotile cilia. Science 1976;193: 317–319.
3. Pedersen M, Mygind N: Absence of axonemal arms in nasal mucosal cilia in Kartagener's syndrome. Nature 1976;62:494–495.
4. Eliasson R, Mossberg B, Camner P, Afzelius BA: The immotile cilia syndrome. A congenital ciliary abnormality as an etiologic factor in chronic airways infections and male sterility. N Engl J Med 1977;297:1–6.
5. Holwill MEJ: Dynein motor activity during ciliary beating. In: Salathe M, Adler KB, Boucher RC, Satir P, eds: Cilia and Mucus. From Development to Respiratory Defense. New York: Marcel Dekker, 2001, pp 19–26.
6. Ibanez-Tallon I, Heintz N, Omran H: To beat or not to beat. Roles of cilia in development and disease. Hum Mol Genet 2003;12:R27–R35.
7. Chilvers MA, Rutman A, O'Callaghan C: Functional analysis of cilia and ciliated epithelial ultrastructure in healthy children and young adults. Thorax 2003;58:333–338.
8. Sanderson MJ, Lansley AB, Evans JH: The regulation of airway ciliary beat frequency by intracellular calcium. In: Salathe M, Adler KB, Boucher RC, Satir P, eds: Cilia and Mucus. From Development to Respiratory Defense. New York: Marcel Dekker, 2001, pp 39–58.
9. Braiman A, Uzlaner N, Priel Z: Enhancement of CBF is dominantly controlled by PKG and/or PKA. In: Salathe M, Adler KB, Boucher RC, Satir P, eds: Cilia and Mucus. From Development to Respiratory Defense. New York: Marcel Dekker, 2001, pp 67–80.
10. Jain B, Rubenstein I, Robbins RA, et al: Modulation of airway epithelial cell ciliary beat frequency by nitric oxide. Biochem Biophys Res Commun 1993;191:83–88.
11. Li D, Shirakami G, Zhan X, Johns RA: Regulation of ciliary beat frequency by the nitric oxide-cyclic guanosine monophosphate signaling pathway in rat airway epithelial cells. Am J Respir Cell Mol Biol 2000;23:175–181.
12. Afzelius BA, Eliasson R: Flagellar mutants in man. On the heterogeneity of the immotile cilia syndrome. J Ultrastruct Res 1979;69:43–52.
13. Sturgess JM, Chao J, Turner JAP: Genetic heterogeneity among dynein deficient cilia. Am Rev Respir Dis 1982;126:302–305.
14. Escudier E, Couprie M, Duriez B, et al: Computer-assisted analysis helps detect inner dynein arm abnormalities. Am J Respir Crit Care Med 2002; 166:1257–1262.
15. Sturgess JM, Chao J, Wong J et al: Cilia with defective radial spokes. A cause of human respiratory disease. N Engl J Med 1979;300:53–56.
16. Sturgess JM, Chao J, Turner JAP: Transposition of ciliary microtubules. Another cause of impaired ciliary motility. N Engl J Med 1980;303:318–322.
17. Rutland J, delongh RU: Random ciliary orientation—a cause of respiratory tract disease. N Engl J Med 1990;323:1681–1684.
18. Carlen B, Lindberg S, Stenram U: Absence of nexin links as a possible cause of primary ciliary dyskinesia. Ultrastruct Pathol 2003;27:123–126.
19. Stannard W, Rutman A, Wallis C, O'Callaghan C: Central microtubular agenesis causing primary ciliary dyskinesia. Am J Respir Crit Care Med 2004;169:634–637.
20. Jorissen M, Willems T: The secondary nature of ciliary (dis)orientation in secondary and primary ciliary dyskinesia. Acta Otolaryngol 2004;124:527–531.
21. Chilvers MA, Rutman A, O'Callaghan C: Ciliary beat pattern is associated with specific ultrastructural defects in primary ciliary dyskinesia. J Allergy Clin Immunol 2003;112:518–524.
22. Canciani M, Barlocco EG, Mastella G, et al: The saccharin method for testing mucociliary function in patients suspected of having primary ciliary dyskinesia. Pediatr Pulmonol 1988;5:210–214.
23. Camner P, Mossberg B, Afzelius BA: Measurements of tracheobronchial clearance in patients with immotile-cilia syndrome and its value in differential diagnosis. Eur J Respir Dis Suppl 1983;64(Suppl 127):57–63.
24. van der Baan S, Veerman AJ, Heidendahl GA, et al: Primary ciliary dyskinesia and nasal mucociliary clearance. Respiration 1987;52:69–75.
25. Ruusa J, Svartengren M, Philipson K, Camner P: Tracheobronchial particle deposition and clearance in immotile cilia patients. J Aerosol Med 1993;6: 89–98.
26. Noone PG, Bennett WD, Regnis JA, et al: Effect of aerosolized uridine-5′-triphosphate on airway clearance with cough in patients with primary ciliary dyskinesia. Am J Respir Crit Care Med 1999;160:144–149.
27. Regnis JA, Zeman KL, Noone PG, et al: Prolonged airway retention of insoluble particles in cystic fibrosis versus primary ciliary dyskinesia. Exp Lung Res 2000;26:149–162.
28. Lundberg JON, Weitzberg E, Nordvall SL, et al: Primarily nasal origin of exhaled nitric oxide and absence in Kartagener's syndrome. Eur Respir J 1994;7:1501–1504.
29. Wodehouse T, Kharitonov SA, Mackay IS, et al: Nasal nitric oxide measurements for the screening of primary ciliary dyskinesia. Eur Respir J 2003;21:43–47.
30. Corbelli R, Bringolf-Isler B, Amacher A, et al: Nasal nitric oxide measurements to screen children for primary ciliary dyskinesia. Chest 2004;126: 1054–1059.
31. Narang I, Ersu R, Wilson NM, Bush A: Nitric oxide in chronic airway inflammation in children: diagnostic use and pathophysiological significance. Thorax 2002;57:586–589.
32. Noone PG, Leigh MW, Sannuti A, et al: Primary ciliary dyskinesia. Diagnostic and phenotypic features. Am J Respir Crit Care Med 2004;169: 459–467.
33. Narayan D, Krishnan SN, Upender M, et al: Unusual inheritance of primary ciliary dyskinesia (Kartagener's syndrome). J Med Genet 1994;31: 493–496.
34. van Dorp DB, Wright AF, Carothers AD, Bleeker-Wagemakers EM: A family with RP3 type X-linked retinitis pigmentosa. An association with ciliary abnormalities. Hum Genet 1992;88:331–334.
35. Noone PG, Bali D, Carson JL, et al: Discordant organ laterality in monozygotic twins with primary ciliary dyskinesia. Am J Med Genet 1999;82: 155–160.
36. Chao J, Turner JAP, Sturgess JM: Genetic heterogeneity of dynein-deficiency in cilia from patients with respiratory disease. Am Rev Respir Dis 1982; 126:302–305.
37. Blouin JL, Meeks M, Radhakrishna, et al: Primary ciliary dyskinesia. A genome-wide linkage analysis reveals extensive locus heterogeneity. Eur J Hum Genet 2000;8:109–118.
38. Olbrich H, Haffner K, Kispert A, et al: Mutations in DNAH5 cause primary ciliary dyskinesia and randomization of left-right asymmetry. Nat Genet 2002;30:43–44.
39. Ibanez-Tallon I, Gorokhova S, Heintz N: Loss of function of axonemal dynein *Mdnah5* causes primary ciliary dyskinesia and hydrocephalus. Hum Mol Genet 2002;11:715–721.
40. Guichard C, Harricane MC, Lafitte JJ, et al: Axonemal dynein intermediate-chain gene (DNAI1) mutations result in situs inversus and primary ciliary dyskinesia (Kartagener syndrome). Am J Hum Genet 2001;68: 1030–1035.
41. Zariwala M, Noone PG, Sannuti A, et al: Germline mutations in an intermediate chain dynein cause primary ciliary dyskinesia. Am J Respir Cell Mol Biol 2001;25:577–583.
42. Bush A, Cole P, Hariri M, et al: Primary ciliary dyskinesia. Diagnosis and standards of care. Eur Respir J 1998;12:982–988.
43. Coren ME, Meeks M, Morrison I, et al: Primary ciliary dyskinesia. Age at diagnosis and symptom history. Acta Paediatr 2002;91:667–669.
44. Holzmann D, Felix H: Neonatal respiratory distress syndrome—a sign of primary ciliary dyskinesia? Eur J Pediatr 2000;159:857–860.
45. Turner JAP, Corkey CWB, Lee JYC, et al: Clinical expressions of immotile cilia syndrome. Pediatrics 1981;67:805–810.
46. Nadel HR, Stringer DA, Levison H, et al: The immotile cilia syndrome. Radiological manifestations. Radiology 1985;154:651–655.
47. Corkey CWB, Levison H, Turner JAP: The immotile cilia syndrome—a longitudinal survey. Am Rev Respir Dis 1981;124:544–548.
48. Ellerman A, Bisgaard H: Longitudinal study of lung function in a cohort of primary ciliary dyskinesia. Eur Respir J 1997;10:2376–2379.
49. Brueckner M: Cilia propel the embryo in the right direction. Am J Med Genet 2001;101:339–344.
50. Schneider H, Brueckner M: Of mice and men. Dissecting the genetic pathway that controls left-right asymmetry in mice and humans. Am J Med Genet 2000;97:258–270.
51. Munro NC, Currie DC, Lindsay KS, et al: Fertility in men with primary ciliary dyskinesia presenting with respiratory infection. Thorax 1994;49: 684–687.
52. Bleau G, Richer CL, Bousquet D: Absence of dynein arms in cilia of endocervical cells in a fertile woman. Fertil Steril 1978;30:362–363.
53. Halbert SA, Patton DL, Zarutskie PW, Soules MR: Function and structure of cilia in the fallopian tube of an infertile woman with Kartagener's syndrome. Hum Reprod 1997;12:55–58.
54. Greenstone MA, Jones RW, Dewar A, et al: Hydrocephalus and primary ciliary dyskinesia. Arch Dis Child 1984;59:481–482.

55. deSanti MM, Magni A, Valleta EA, et al: Hydrocephalus, bronchiectasis and ciliary dyskinesia. Arch Dis Child 1990;65:543–544.
56. Al-Shroof M, Karnik AM, Karnik AA, et al: Ciliary dyskinesia associated with hydrocephalus and mental retardation in a Jordanian family. Mayo Clin Proc 2001;76:1219–1224.
57. Corkey CWB, Minta JO, Turner JAP, Biggar WD: Neutrophil function in the immotile cilia syndrome. J Lab Clin Med 1982;99:838–844.
58. Fiorini R, Littarru GP, Coppa GV, Kantar A: Plasma membrane polarity of polymorphonuclear leucocytes from children with primary ciliary dyskinesia. Eur J Clin Invest 2000;30:519–525.

64 Childhood Pulmonary Arterial Hypertension

Erika Berman Rosenzweig, MD • Robyn J. Barst, MD

Pulmonary arterial hypertension (PAH) is a serious progressive condition with a poor prognosis if not identified and treated early. Until recently the diagnosis of idiopathic pulmonary arterial hypertension (IPAH, previously primary pulmonary hypertension [PPH]) was virtually a death sentence, particularly for children, with a median survival of less than a year. The data in the Primary Pulmonary Hypertension National Institutes of Health Registry illustrate the worse prognosis for children than adults.[1] In this registry, the median survival for all of the 194 patients was 2.8 years, whereas it was only 0.8 years for children. Fortunately, there has been significant progress in the field of PAH over the past several decades, with significant advances in the treatment that can improve quality of life, exercise capacity, hemodynamics, and survival.[2–4] Nevertheless, extrapolation from adults to children is not straightforward. This chapter reviews PAH in children with an emphasis on the latest therapeutic advances, which have dramatically improved the prognosis for children with this condition.

■ DEFINITION AND CLASSIFICATION

The definition of PAH in children is the same as for adult patients. It is defined as a mean pulmonary artery pressure of greater than or equal to 25 mm Hg at rest or greater than or equal to 30 mm Hg during exercise, with a normal pulmonary artery wedge pressure (i.e., ≤15 mm Hg) and an increased pulmonary vascular resistance (PVR) index of greater than or equal to 3 Wood units × m^2. PAH occurs in the "precapillary" pulmonary vascular bed and therefore excludes causes of pulmonary venous hypertension (e.g., mitral stenosis). The inclusion of exercise hemodynamic abnormalities in the definition of PAH is important, since children with PAH often have an exaggerated response of the pulmonary vascular bed to exercise. Children also often have a greater vasoreactive response to hypoventilation compared with adults. Not uncommonly, children with a history of recurrent exertional or nocturnal syncope have a resting mean pulmonary artery pressure that markedly increases with exercise as well as with modest systemic arterial oxygen desaturation during sleep.

In 1998, at the Primary Pulmonary Hypertension World Symposium, clinical scientists from around the world proposed a new diagnostic classification system; this classification system categorizes pulmonary vascular disease by common clinical features. This classification reflected the recent advances in the understanding of pulmonary hypertensive diseases and recognized the similarity between IPAH and PAH of certain other causes. At the 2003 World Pulmonary Hypertension Symposium, the term *primary pulmonary hypertension* was officially changed to *idiopathic pulmonary arterial hypertension*, reflecting the fact that this is a diagnosis of exclusion with exact causes yet unknown (Box 64-1). Thus, in addition to IPAH (both sporadic and familial), PAH related to congenital heart disease, connective tissue disease, portal hypertension, human immunodeficiency virus (HIV) infection, drugs and toxins (including anorexigens), and persistent pulmonary hypertension of the newborn (PPHN) is classified along with IPAH as PAH. This classification separates these types of PAH from pulmonary venous hypertension, pulmonary hypertension associated with disorders of the respiratory system and/or hypoxemia, pulmonary hypertension due to chronic thrombotic and/or embolic disease, as well as pulmonary hypertension due to disorders directly affecting the pulmonary vasculature. The diagnostic classification also provides rationale for considering many of the therapeutic modalities that have been demonstrated to be efficacious for IPAH for children who have PAH related to these other conditions.

PAH may be further classified into three clinical entities by physiologic characteristics. First, there is PAH associated with a large congenital systemic to pulmonary shunt that causes pulmonary vascular disease from increased shear stress (increased pulmonary blood flow). Ultimately, there is reversal of shunting leading to cyanosis. Right ventricular function is usually preserved because of decompression of the right ventricle at the expense of right-to-left shunting. Second, there is classic IPAH in which a vasculopathy occurs within the pulmonary arterioles leading to right heart pressure overload. Patients who have pulmonary vascular disease and subsequently undergo closure of a congenital systemic to pulmonary shunt will behave just as an IPAH patient with increased pressure load to the right ventricle and the absence of cyanosis. Last, there is the group of patients who have PAH from infancy in whom the PVR remains elevated (e.g., PPHN). This may resolve in the neonatal period or persist well beyond infancy. There may be overlap between these entities for, for example, a congenital heart defect (CHD) and elevated PVR from birth in which there was never left-to-right shunting leading to shear stress, but rather, right-to-left shunting and the absence of congestive heart failure symptoms from the beginning. While the classification helps in understanding the pathophysiologic basis of PAH patients, it also has implications for the natural history, which will be discussed later. Despite the different physiologic classifications of PAH, the histopathologic changes are similar, and thus similar treatment strategies have evolved. As insight is advanced into the mechanisms responsible for the development of PAH, the introduction of novel therapeutic modalities will hopefully increase the overall efficacy of therapeutic interventions for PAH.

BOX 64-1 Diagnostic Classification of Pulmonary Hypertension

- Pulmonary arterial hypertension (PAH)
  - Sporadic (IPAH)
  - Familial (FPAH)
  - Related to:
    - Connective tissue disease
    - Congenital heart disease
    - Portal hypertension
    - HIV infection
    - Drugs and toxins
    - Other: type I glycogen storage disease, Gaucher's disease, hemoglobinopathies, myeloproliferative disorders, hereditary hemorrhagic helangiectasia (Rendu-Osler-Weber disease)
- PAH with significant venule and/or capillary involvement
  - Pulmonary veno-occlusive disease
    - Sporadic
    - Familial
  - Pulmonary capillary hemangiomatosis
  - Persistent fetal circulation (persistent pulmonary hypertension of the newborn)
- Pulmonary venous hypertension
  - Pulmonary venous obstruction (discrete)
  - Left-sided heart disease
- Pulmonary hypertension associated with disorders of the respiratory system or hypoxemia
  - Hyaline membrane disease
  - Bronchopulmonary dysplasia
  - Congenital diaphragmatic hernia
  - Pulmonary hypoplasia
  - Alveolar capillary dysplasia
  - Cystic fibrosis
  - Chronic obstructive pulmonary disease
  - Interstitial lung disease
  - Sleep-disordered breathing
  - Alveolar hypoventilation disorders
  - Chronic exposure to high altitude
- Pulmonary hypertension due to chronic thrombotic and/or embolic disease
  - Thromboembolic obstruction of proximal pulmonary arteries
  - Thromboembolic obstruction of distal pulmonary arteries
  - Pulmonary embolism (tumor, parasites, foreign material)
- Miscellaneous
  - Sarcoidosis
  - Histiocytosis X
  - Fibrosing mediastinitis
  - Adenopathy and tumors
  - Lymphangiomatosis

From Third World Symposium on Pulmonary Arterial Hypertension, 2003.

NEONATAL PULMONARY HYPERTENSION

PERSISTENT PULMONARY HYPERTENSION OF THE NEWBORN

PPHN is a unique form of PAH, which most often resolves completely with proper intervention. PPHN is a syndrome characterized by increased PVR, right-to-left shunting (at the atrial and/or ductal level), and severe hypoxemia.[5] PPHN is frequently associated with pulmonary parenchymal abnormalities (e.g., meconium aspiration, pneumonia, or sepsis), or may occur when there is pulmonary hypoplasia, maladaptation of the pulmonary vascular bed postnatally as a result of perinatal stress, or maladaptation of the pulmonary vascular bed in utero from unknown causes. In some instances there is no evidence of pulmonary parenchymal disease, and the "injury" that is the "trigger" of PAH is unknown. Although some children die during the neonatal period despite maximal cardiopulmonary therapeutic interventions, PPHN is almost always transient,[6] with infants recovering completely without requiring long-term medical therapy. In contrast to these infants, patients with IPAH as well as PAH related to the other conditions discussed above appear to require treatment indefinitely. It is possible that in some neonates the PVR does not fall normally after birth, and goes unrecognized during the neonatal period; the patient is diagnosed with PAH at a later date as the pulmonary vascular disease progresses. Pathologic studies examining the elastic pattern of the main pulmonary artery[7,8] suggest that IPAH is present from birth in some patients, although it is acquired later in life in others. The histopathologic changes have also illustrated increased muscularity of the peripheral pulmonary arteries, similar to IPAH.[9]

Although misalignment of the pulmonary veins with alveolar capillary dysplasia is often diagnosed as PPHN, it is a separate entity, that is, a rare disorder of the pulmonary vascular development that most often is diagnosed only after an infant has died from fulminant PAH.[10] Features that should raise a clinician's suspicion of the possibility of alveolar capillary dysplasia include association with other nonlethal congenital malformations, late onset of presentation (i.e., after 12–24 hours of age), and severe hypoxemia refractory to medical therapy. Infants most often present with severe PAH with transient responses to inhaled nitric oxide, as well as transient responses after intravenous epoprostenol is added to the inhaled nitric oxide, and virtually all infants subsequently die within the first several weeks of life. There may be a heterogeneous involvement in the pulmonary parenchyma that delays presentation. This variability in clinical severity and histopathology is consistent with the marked biologic variability that occurs in many forms of PAH. When pulmonary hypertension results from neonatal lung disease such as meconium aspiration, the pulmonary vascular changes are most severe in the regions of the lung showing the greatest parenchymal damage.

PULMONARY ARTERIAL HYPERTENSION IN CHILDHOOD

The remainder of this review will focus on pulmonary hypertension beyond the neonatal period. Whether pulmonary hypertension is due to increased flow or resistance depends on the cause of the pulmonary hypertension. By definition, hyperkinetic pulmonary hypertension refers to PAH from congenital systemic to pulmonary communications with increased pulmonary blood flow (e.g., ventricular septal defect or patent ductus arteriosus). Pulmonary venous hypertension is caused by disorders of left heart filling (e.g., pulmonary venous obstruction, mitral stenosis, or left ventricular failure). Unless left heart obstruction or dysfunction is causing pulmonary venous hypertension, the pulmonary artery wedge pressure is normal. Pulmonary vascular disease related to congenital heart disease (Eisenmenger syndrome) is thought to develop after exposure to hyperkinetic shear stress following a period of normal PVR and increased pulmonary blood flow. With pulmonary venous hypertension as seen with mitral stenosis or left ventricular dysfunction, pulmonary arterial pressure may vary from one child to another with the same elevations of pulmonary venous pressure because of differences in pulmonary arterial vasoreactivity. If secondary to a structural abnormality (e.g., mitral stenosis), this form of hypertension is most often reversible with surgical correction of the left-sided defect. Several types of congenital heart defects are associated with an increased risk for the development of pulmonary vascular disease. Approximately one third of patients with uncorrected congenital heart disease will die from pulmonary vascular disease.[11] It is not known why some children with the same underlying congenital heart defect develop irreversible pulmonary vascular obstructive disease in the first year of life and others maintain "operable" levels of PVR into the second decade and beyond. In children whose congenital heart disease is diagnosed later in life, one needs to determine whether the patient is "operable" or has "irreversible" pulmonary vascular disease. In the past, the evaluation of operability included anatomic criteria based on microscopic findings from lung biopsies to aid in the determination.[12] Lung biopsies, however, carry a significant risk for morbidity and mortality in this population. The current approach is to use acute pulmonary vasodilator testing during cardiac catheterization to evaluate operability. The assessment of surgical operability requires an accurate evaluation of the degree of pulmonary vasoreactivity or reversibility. It is important to determine whether the elevated PVR index responds favorably to pharmacologic vasodilatation (i.e., with a fall into the near normal range of ≤ 3 Wood units $\times$ m^2. In the past several years, studies with inhaled nitric oxide and intravenous epoprostenol have been useful in both the preoperative evaluations as well as in the treatment of postoperative patients with elevated PVR.[13–19] The availability of pulmonary vasodilators such as inhaled nitric oxide for perioperative management of pulmonary hypertension have allowed for surgical "corrections" in select patients who present later in life with borderline elevated PVR (e.g., 3–5 Wood units $\times$ m^2). If a patient with elevated PVR is being considered for surgery, there is an increased risk for postoperative pulmonary hypertensive crises. Thus, knowing if the pulmonary circulation will respond favorably to inhaled nitric oxide or intravenous prostacyclin will help guide the management of this potentially life-threatening postoperative complication.[14,20] For patients with elevated PVR (i.e., at least 3 Wood units $\times$ m^2, and particularly > 6 Wood units $\times$ m^2), surgical closure of a systemic to pulmonary communication can be catastrophic and lead to severe right heart failure since the "pop-off" valve for the right ventricle is suddenly removed.

Pulmonary venous hypertension has several causes and is also a clinically distinct entity from PAH and will be discussed briefly in this section. Congenital heart disease is the most common cause of pulmonary venous hypertension in children and is most often due to total anomalous pulmonary venous return with obstruction, left heart obstruction, or severe left ventricular failure. The lungs of those born with left inflow obstruction show pronounced thickening in the walls of both the pulmonary arteries and the pulmonary veins; and the outcome depends on the results of the surgical intervention. Pulmonary veno-occlusive disease has a distinct pathologic feature of uniform fibrotic occlusion of peripheral small venules.[21] Although rare, it does occur early in childhood and has been reported in familial cases.[22] It is important to be aware that in pulmonary veno-occlusive disease, the pulmonary capillary wedge pressure is often normal with a hemodynamic profile similar to that of IPAH patients. Progressive long segment pulmonary vein hypoplasia leading to pulmonary venous atresia is another uniformly fatal condition presenting in infancy with severe pulmonary venous hypertension.

EPIDEMIOLOGY

The frequency of PAH in children as well as in adults remains unknown. Estimates of the incidence of IPAH ranges from one to two new cases per million people in the general population.[23] Although the disease is rare, with improved diagnostics and awareness it appears that more patients (both children and adults) have PAH than had been previously recognized. On occasion, infants who have died with the presumed diagnosis of sudden infant death syndrome have had IPAH diagnosed at the time of postmortem examination. The sex incidence in adult patients with IPAH is approximately 1.7:1 females:males,[24] similar to the incidence in children (1.8:1), with no significant difference in younger children compared with older children.

NATURAL HISTORY

Historically, untreated IPAH exhibits a course of progressive right heart failure and early death. Several large survival studies of primarily adult patients with IPAH were conducted in the 1980s prior the modern treatment era. These retrospective and prospective studies have yielded quite uniform results: adult patients with IPAH who have not undergone lung or heart/lung transplantation had actuarial survival rates at 1, 3, and 5 years of 68% to 77%, 40% to 56%, and 22% to 38%, respectively.[1,25,26] In the era before the use of continuous intravenous epoprostenol, the 1-, 3-, and 5-year survival rates in children who were nonresponsive to conventional therapy (including anticongestive medications and oral calcium channel blockade) were 66%, 52%, and 35%, respectively.[27] In a more recent treatment era using epoprostenol treatment for nonresponders, and calcium channel blockade for responders, the 10-year survival for children is estimated at 78%.[28] However, there is significant biologic variability in the natural history of the disease in both adults and children, with some patients having a rapidly progressive downhill course resulting in death within several weeks after diagnosis as well as instances of survival for at least several decades. In contrast, the long-term natural history for patients with PAH and associated congenital heart disease is much more favorable, with survival often into the fourth and fifth decades of life. The natural history of the Eisenmenger syndrome also demonstrates a wide spectrum of variability, with the overall survival significantly better than for patients with IPAH.[26] For a classic Eisenmenger syndrome patient, death in childhood is unusual, with most patients surviving into their mid-twenties to thirties. There have even been patients found to survive to the seventh decade of life, although this is rare. The better prognosis for Eisenmenger syndrome patients is likely due to the presence of a "pop-off" valve. For Eisenmenger syndrome patients or patients with a CHD and elevated PVR greater than or equal to 3 to 5 U × m^2, closing the heart defect can change the natural history from an Eisenmenger syndrome patient to the worse prognosis of an IPAH patient. Therefore, operability needs to be assessed carefully if considering closure. For borderline patients, one may consider closure of the CHD, leaving a smaller residual defect or creating an atrial septal defect. There is also debate as to whether an atrial communication is as effective as a "pop-off" as a shunt at the ventricular level since shunting at the atrial level would require significant right ventricular failure.

PATHOBIOLOGY

Vasoconstriction

There have been many recent advances in the understanding of the pathobiology of PAH. Most importantly, pulmonary vascular disease is a multifactorial disease with several causes that lead to a final common histopathologic vasculopathy. Recent investigations in the basic science arena have uncovered several different biochemical/mechanistic features of pulmonary vascular obstructive disease that lead to novel treatments. These include abnormalities of the endothelin system, nitric oxide production/availability, and so forth. In 1977, Wagenvoort and Wagenvoort hypothesized that "primary pulmonary hypertension (IPAH) is a disease of individuals with hyperreactive lung vessels in whom various stimuli initiate vasoconstriction, with subsequent development of the characteristic vascular lesions."[29] While the early focus for treatment of this disease stemmed from this hypothesis (i.e., finding the ideal pulmonary vasodilator), more recent evidence has pointed to other vasoproliferative abnormalities. In young children, the pathobiology suggests failure of the neonatal vasculature to relax, in addition to a striking reduction in arterial number/surface area. However, with time the changes become fixed with a vasodilator-unresponsive component that appears to be temporally related to the development of thickened vascular media and adventitia with dramatic increases in the deposition of structural matrix proteins such as collagen and elastin in the pulmonary arterial wall.[30] In older children, intimal hyperplasia and occlusive changes as well as the presence of plexiform lesions is found in the pulmonary arterioles. Despite significant advances in the understanding of the pathobiology of IPAH, the mechanisms that initiate and perpetuate this disease process remain speculative. Adults with IPAH often have severe plexiform lesions and what appears to be "fixed" pulmonary vascular changes. In contrast, children with IPAH have more pulmonary vascular medial hypertrophy and less intimal fibrosis and fewer plexiform lesions. In the classic studies by Wagenvoort and Wagenvoort in 1970,[31] medial hypertrophy was severe in patients younger than 15 years, and it was usually the only abnormality seen in infants. Among the 11 children younger than 1 year at the time of death, all had severe medial hypertrophy, yet only three had intimal fibrosis—two with minimal intimal fibrosis and one with moderate intimal fibrosis—and none had plexiform lesions. With increasing age, intimal fibrosis and plexiform lesions were seen more frequently. These postmortem studies suggested that pulmonary vasoconstriction, leading to medial hypertrophy, may occur early in the course of the disease and may precede the development of plexiform lesions and other fixed pulmonary vascular changes. Furthermore, these observations may offer clues to the observed differences in the natural history and factors influencing survival in children with IPAH compared with adult patients. In general, younger children appear to have a more reactive pulmonary vascular bed relative to both vasodilatation and vasoconstriction. Severe acute pulmonary hypertensive crises occur in response to pulmonary vasoconstrictor "triggers" more often in young children than in older children or adults. Thus, based on these early pathologic studies, the most widely proposed mechanism for IPAH until the late 1980s and early 1990s was pulmonary vasoconstriction.[30–35]

Endothelial Dysfunction

Endothelial dysfunction appears to be a key factor in mediating the structural changes that occur in the pulmonary vasculature. The integrity of the pulmonary vascular endothelium is critical for maintaining vascular tone, homeostasis, leukocyte trafficking, transduction of luminal signals to abluminal vascular tissues, production of growth factors, and cell signals with autocrine and paracrine effects and barrier function.[36] In addition, abnormalities in vasoactive mediators contribute to the pathobiology of PAH. Whether these perturbations are a cause or consequence of the disease process remains to be elucidated.[37–44]

One theory is that there may be a "trigger" for endothelial activation in "genetically susceptible patients" (Fig. 64-1). Endothelial activation then leads to apoptosis of quiescent cells, destabilization of the pulmonary vascular intima, and uncontrolled proliferation of endothelial cells, leading to the classic plexiform lesions. Once the vascular wall is damaged, proliferative mediators may cross into the matrix and lead to degradation of matrix and proliferation of smooth muscle.

The vascular endothelium is now recognized as an important source of locally active mediators that contribute to the control of vasomotor tone and structural remodeling, and appears to play a crucial role in the pathogenesis of IPAH.[45] A number of studies have suggested that imbalances in the production or metabolism of several vasoactive mediators produced in the lungs as well as substances involving control of pulmonary vascular growth may be important in the pathogenesis of IPAH. These may include increased thromboxane, endothelin, and serotonin, and decreased prostacyclin[37,38] and nitric oxide,[39–41,44] as well as vascular endothelial growth factor and xanthine oxidoreductase.[37–41,44,46] The endothelial cell dysfunction seen in association with PAH leads to the release of vasoproliferative substances in addition to vasoconstrictive agents that ultimately result in progression of pulmonary vascular remodeling and progressive vascular obstruction and obliteration. For example, Stewart and colleagues[40] and Giaid and colleagues[47] reported elevated circulating levels of endothelin, a potent vasoconstrictor and mitogen, in patients with PAH. Increased local production of endothelin by the pulmonary arterial endothelium in patients with PAH has also been demonstrated.[40] Endothelial dysfunction also likely results in the release of chemotactic agents, leading to the migration of smooth muscle cells into the vascular wall, which may lead to the characteristic pulmonary arteriolar medial hypertrophy and hyperplasia. In addition, this endothelial dysfunction, coupled with the excessive release of locally active thrombogenic mediators, promotes a procoagulant state, leading to further vascular obstruction. The process is

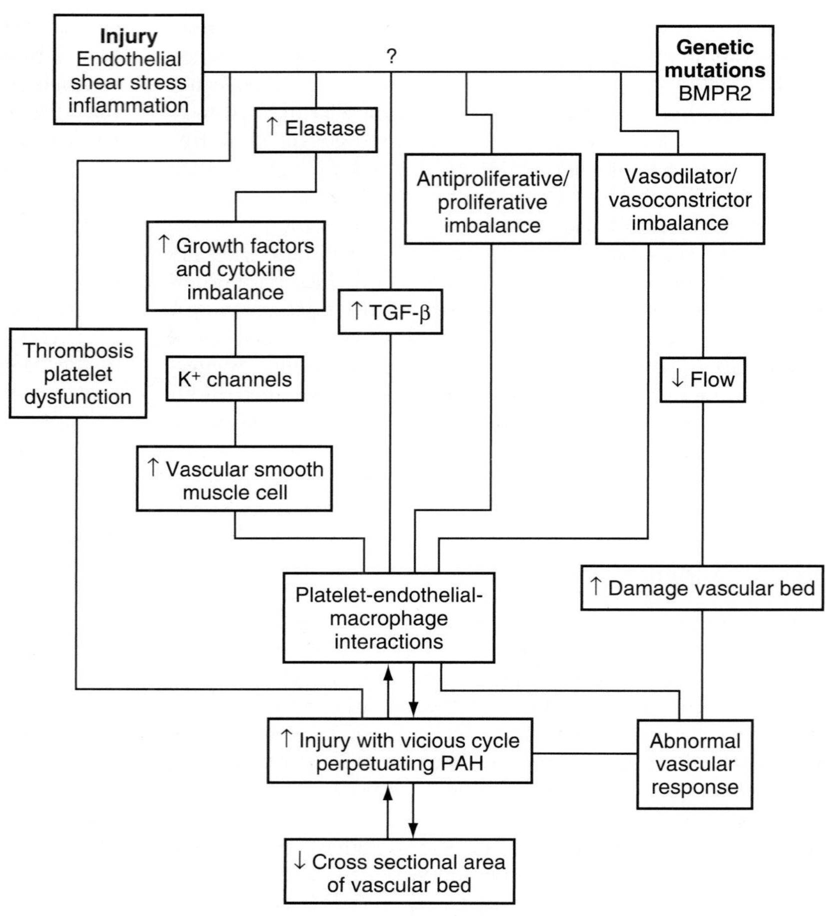

■ **FIGURE 64-1.** Possible pathogenesis of primary pulmonary hypertension. BMPR2, bone morphogenetic protein receptor-2; PAH, pulmonary arterial hypertension; TGF, transforming growth factor. (Adapted from Barst RJ: Medical therapy of pulmonary hypertension. An overview of treatment and goals. Clin Chest Med 2001;22:509–515.)

characterized, therefore, by an inexorable cycle of endothelial dysfunction leading to the release of vasoconstrictive, vasoproliferative, and prothrombotic substances, ultimately progressing to vascular remodeling and progressive vascular obstruction and obliteration. Thus, despite our lack of complete understanding of the pathogenesis of PAH, these imbalances and abnormalities have changed the focus of clinical investigations from looking purely at chronic vasodilator therapy, to the evaluation of medical agents that may reverse the vasoproliferation, and ultimately result in pulmonary vascular regression and remodeling. Although various studies have demonstrated endothelial dysfunction in patients with PAH, whether the dysfunction is the primary problem or secondary to another insult remains unknown.

The theory that certain individuals are genetically susceptible has led to more genetically oriented research. It is now clear that gene expression in pulmonary vascular cells responds to environmental factors, growth factors, receptors, signaling pathways, and genetic influences that can interact with each other. The molecular processes behind the complex vascular changes associated with IPAH include phenotypic changes in endothelial and smooth muscle cells in hypertensive pulmonary arteries, the recognition that cell proliferation contributes to the structural changes associated with the initiation and progression of IPAH, the role of matrix proteins and matrix turnover in vascular remodeling, and the importance of hemodynamic influences on the disease process. Examples of effector systems controlled by gene expression include transmembrane transporters, ion channels, transcription factors, modulators of apoptosis, kinases, cell-to-cell interactive factors (e.g., integrins and membrane receptors), mechanotransducers, extracellular matrix turnover and growth factors/cytokines, and chemokine networks.

In addition, defects in the potassium channels of pulmonary vascular smooth muscle cells may also be involved in the initiation and/or progression of IPAH. Inhibition of the voltage-regulated (Kv) potassium channels in pulmonary artery smooth muscle cells from patients with IPAH has been reported.[48] Whether a genetic defect related to potassium channels leading to vasoconstriction is relevant to the development of IPAH in some patients remains unknown. However, these studies suggest that IPAH is a disease of "predisposed" individuals, in whom various "stimuli" may initiate the pulmonary vascular disease process. By identifying causes of molecular processes that are linked to epidemiologic risk factors as well as developing molecular, genetic, biochemical, and physiologic tests to monitor and diagnose IPAH, novel treatment strategies will increase the overall efficacy of therapeutic interventions for IPAH. There may be different subsets of patients in whom vasoconstriction is the predominant feature, and those in whom vascular injury/endothelial dysfunction is the primary problem. Even so, these components appear closely intertwined. And, whether these physiologic processes (i.e., vasoconstriction vs. vascular injury) are a cause or a consequence of the disease remains unclear.

Recent studies have suggested a genetic predisposition for developing PAH in up to 10% of individuals affected. Mutations of the BMPR2 gene were first described in individuals with familial IPAH,[49–52] with a decrease in the alveolar density of BMPR expression in patients with pulmonary hypertension. Other candidate genes such as ALK-1, which encodes transforming growth factor-β (TGF-β) receptor, and angiopoietin-1 (Ang-1, an inducer of angiogenesis, endothelial cell survival, and vessel stabilization) have been recently described. Future investigations will focus on these genetic influences on the pathogenesis of PAH.

The endothelium also has a key role in maintaining normal coagulation through elaborating various factors (e.g., heparan sulfates, urokinase type plasminogen activator, and von Willebrand factor). Therefore, endothelial dysfunction may cause abnormalities of coagulation, leading to the prothrombotic state seen in pulmonary hypertension patients. In addition to these changes, there may be a physiologic effect from pulmonary arteriole lumen narrowing, which leads to stasis and thrombosis.[53] Coagulation abnormalities may also coexist, initiating or further exacerbating the pulmonary vascular disease.[54,55] The interactions between the humoral and cellular elements of the blood on an injured endothelial cell surface result in remodeling of the pulmonary vascular bed and contribute to the process of pulmonary vascular injury.[56,57] Endothelial cell damage can also result in thrombosis in situ, transforming the pulmonary vascular bed from its usual anticoagulant state (owing to the release of prostacyclin and plasminogen activator inhibitors) to a procoagulant state.[58] Elevated fibrinopeptide-A levels and P-selectin in IPAH patients also suggests that in situ thrombosis occurs.[59] A reduction in thrombomodulin (which activates the anticoagulant protein C) has also been documented.[60,61] Further support for the role of coagulation abnormalities at the endothelial cell surface comes from the reports of improved survival in patients treated with chronic anticoagulation.[2,23,62]

PATHOPHYSIOLOGY

Although the histopathology in children with IPAH is often similar to that seen in adult patients, there may be differences in the pathophysiology that alters the clinical presentation, natural history, and factors influencing survival in children. For example, children appear to have differences in their hemodynamic parameters at the time of diagnosis compared with adult patients.[63] Children with IPAH have a normal cardiac index (as opposed to adults, who most often present with a low cardiac index). This may reflect an earlier diagnosis and why children tend to have a greater acute vasodilator response rate with acute vasodilator testing than do adults.

A brief review of the normal physiology of the pulmonary circulation will enable a better understanding of the pathophysiology of the pulmonary vascular bed. The normal fall in PVR occurs soon after birth and reaches normal adult levels by the first 4 to 6 weeks of life. The normal pulmonary vascular bed is a low-pressure, low-resistance, highly distensible system that can accommodate large increases in pulmonary blood flow with minimal elevations in pulmonary arterial pressure. In PAH, however, this capacity to accommodate increases in pulmonary blood flow is lost due to the increase in PVR, leading to increases in pulmonary artery pressure at rest and further elevations in pulmonary artery pressure with exercise. The right ventricle becomes hypertrophied in response to the increase in afterload. If there has been a gradual exposure over time, the right ventricle has the ability to remodel and adapt to the pressure load by recruitment of sarcomeres and hypertrophy of myocytes. The adaptation of the right ventricle to increased afterload such as in IPAH or CHDs with increased right ventricular afterload (e.g., pulmonic stenosis) is a double-edged sword. The right ventricular hypertrophy will assist the right ventricle in pumping against increased afterload; however, this occurs at a cost to left ventricular integrity. Under normal conditions the right ventricle is crescentic or pancake shaped, with the right ventricular free wall and interventricular septum concave around the left ventricle at both end diastole and end systole. During systole, the left ventricle contracts toward a central axis, while the right ventricular free wall and septum contract in parallel. With right ventricular hypertrophy, the interventricular septal orientation flattens and ultimately commits to the right ventricle in severe cases. This may lead to a vicious cycle of left ventricular diastolic dysfunction and subsequent worsening of right heart failure in severe cases.[64,65] In the early stages, the right ventricle is capable of sustaining normal cardiac output at rest, but the ability to increase cardiac output with exercise is impaired. As pulmonary vascular disease progresses, the right ventricle fails, and resting cardiac output decreases. As right ventricular dysfunction progresses, right ventricular diastolic pressure increases and evidence of right ventricular failure manifests, the most ominous sign of pulmonary vascular disease. Dyspnea is the most frequent presenting complaint in adults as well as in some children with IPAH, and it is due to impaired oxygen delivery during physical activity as a result of an inability to increase cardiac output in the presence of increased oxygen demands. Syncopal episodes, which occur more frequently with children than with adults, are often exertional or postexertional, and imply a severely limited cardiac output, leading to diminished cerebral blood flow. Peripheral vasodilatation during physical exertion can exacerbate this condition.

The two most frequent mechanisms of death are progressive right ventricular failure and sudden death, with the former occurring more often.[1] Progressive right ventricular failure leads to dyspnea, hypoxemia, and a progressive decrease in cardiac output. Complicating illnesses including pneumonia may be fatal as a result of alveolar hypoxia causing further pulmonary vasoconstriction and an inability to maintain adequate cardiac output, resulting in cardiogenic shock and death. When arterial hypoxemia and acidosis occur, life-threatening arrhythmias may develop. Postulated mechanisms for sudden death include bradyarrhythmias and tachyarrhythmias, acute pulmonary emboli, massive pulmonary hemorrhage, and sudden right ventricular ischemia. Hemoptysis appears to be due to pulmonary infarcts with secondary arterial thromboses.

DIAGNOSIS AND ASSESSMENT

The diagnosis of IPAH is one of exclusion. It is critical to exclude all likely related or associated conditions that might be treated differently. A detailed history and physical examination, as well as appropriate tests, must be performed to uncover potential causative or contributing factors, many of which may not be readily apparent. A family history of pulmonary hypertension, connective tissue diseases, congenital heart disease, other congenital anomalies, and early unexplained deaths may be contributory. If the family history suggests familial IPAH, careful screening of all first-degree relatives is recommended. Genetic testing is also available in select centers. Additional issues to address include a carefully detailed birth/neonatal history; drug usage history; medication history including psychotropic drugs, appetite suppressants, and all over-the-counter drugs;

exposure to high altitude or to toxic cooking oil[66,67]; travel history; and any history of frequent respiratory tract infections or venous or arterial thrombi. The answers to these questions may offer clues to a possible "trigger" for the development of the PAH.

The diagnostic evaluation in children suspected of having IPAH is similar to that of adult patients (Fig. 64-2), with the exception of certain conditions that rarely occur in children (e.g., chronic thromboembolic pulmonary hypertension). Serial World Health Organization (WHO) functional class assessments are also helpful using the WHO functional classification for patients with pulmonary hypertension (Box 64-2).[68]

HEMODYNAMICS/CARDIAC CATHETERIZATION

Despite advances in noninvasive technology, cardiac catheterization remains the gold standard for the diagnosing and determining the severity of PAH, assessing the prognosis, and selecting appropriate treatment. As shown in the treatment algorithm guidelines (Fig. 64-3), all children should undergo acute pulmonary vasodilator testing at the time of the diagnostic right heart catheterization with a short-acting vasodilator to determine vascular responsiveness. The younger the child is at the time of diagnosis, the more likely it is that the child will respond to acute testing, but there is wide variability.[27] Unfortunately, there are no additional hemodynamic or demographic variables that accurately predict whether or not a child will respond to acute vasodilator testing. Previous studies suggest that up to 40% of children with symptoms for several years suggestive of severe pulmonary vascular compromise may manifest near complete reversibility with chronic oral calcium channel blockade therapy, while others with only recent symptoms may have what appears to be irreversible disease. These observations underscore the marked biologic variability in the time course of IPAH and serve to emphasize the need to individualize the therapeutic approach. The vasodilators recommended for acute vasodilator drug testing include intravenous epoprostenol, inhaled nitric oxide, intravenous adenosine, and/or inhaled iloprost. Patients who are responsive to acute vasodilator testing are likely to have a favorable response with acute calcium channel blocker testing and subsequent long-term chronic oral calcium channel blockade treatment.[2,27] A significant response to acute pulmonary vasodilator testing is considered a reduction in mean pulmonary artery pressure of at least 20%, with no change or an increase in cardiac output. Patients who do not manifest a response to acute vasodilator challenge are unlikely to have clinical benefit from chronic oral calcium channel blockade therapy. Furthermore, acute deterioration and decompensation may occur with empiric calcium channel blockade therapy in patients who are not acutely responsive,[69,70] particularly in children with underlying lung disease.

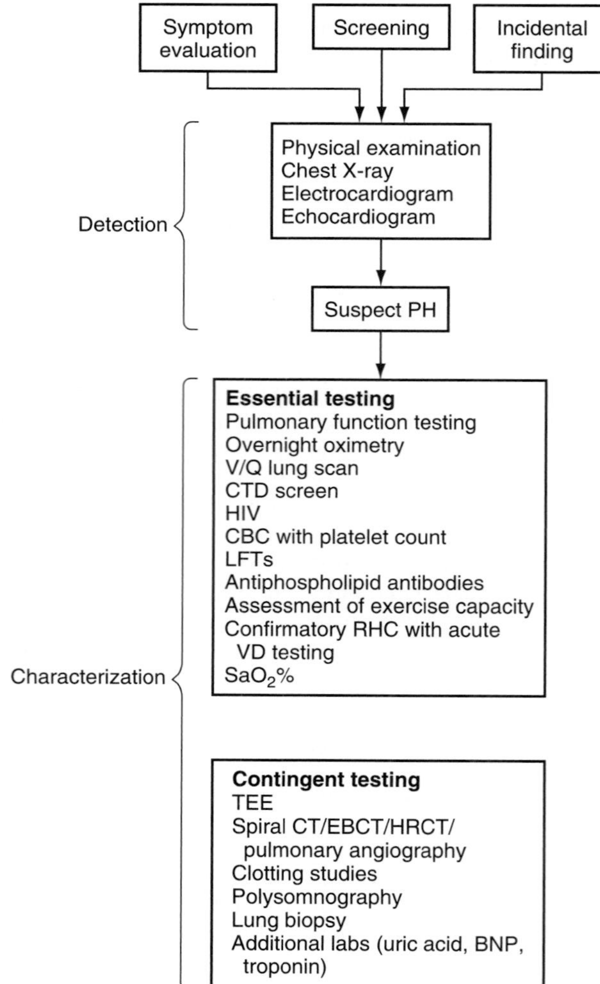

FIGURE 64-2. Diagnostic workup for patients with suspected pulmonary arterial hypertension. BNP, brain natriuretic peptide; CTD, connective tissue disease; PH, pulmonary hypertension; RHC, right heart cardiac catheterization; SaO_2, arterial saturation; TEE, transesophageal echocardiogram; VD, vasodilator. (Adapted from Berman Rosenzweig E, Widlitz AC, Barst RJ: Pulmonary arterial hypertension in children. State of the art. Pediatr Pulmonol 2004;38[1]:2–22.)

BOX 64-2 WHO Functional Classification

Class I: Patients with pulmonary hypertension but without resulting limitations of physical activity. Ordinary physical activity does not cause undue dyspnea or fatigue, chest pain, or near syncope.

Class II: Patients with pulmonary hypertension resulting in slight limitation of physical activity. They are comfortable at rest. Ordinary physical activity causes undue dyspnea or fatigue, chest pain, or near syncope.

Class III: Patients with pulmonary hypertension resulting in marked limitation of physical activity. They are comfortable at rest. Less than ordinary activity causes undue dyspnea or fatigue, chest pain, or near syncope.

Class IV: Patients with pulmonary hypertension with inability to carry out any physical activity without symptoms. These patients manifest signs of right heart failure. Dyspnea and/or fatigue may even be present at rest. Discomfort is increased by any physical activity.

Modified from the NYHA functional classification, Second World Symposium on Pulmonary Arterial Hypertension, 1998.

CLINICAL PRESENTATION

The presenting symptoms in children with PAH are highly variable. Infants with PAH often present with signs of low cardiac output (e.g., tachypnea, tachycardia, poor appetite, failure to thrive, lethargy, diaphoresis, and irritability). Some infants have crying spells, presumably as a result of chest pain that cannot be otherwise verbalized. In addition, infants and older children may develop cyanosis with exertion, due to right-to-left shunting through a patent foramen ovale or CHD. The patent foramen ovale serves as a "pop-off" valve for the hypertensive right heart in children without other systemic to pulmonary communications. Children without adequate shunting through a patent foramen ovale or CHD may present with syncope due to the inability to achieve an adequate cardiac output with exertion. After early childhood, children present with symptoms similar to those of adults. In the older children, the most common symptoms are exertional dyspnea and, occasionally, chest pain. Chest pain, or angina, results from right ventricular ischemia and is often underappreciated. Clinical right ventricular failure is rare in young children, occurring most often in children older than 10 years with severe long-standing PAH. Peripheral edema is generally a reflection of right ventricular failure and is more likely to be associated with advanced pulmonary vascular disease.

The interval between onset of symptoms and time of diagnosis is usually shorter in children than in adults, particularly in those children who present with syncope. In addition to exertional or postexertional syncope, children also may present with hypoxic seizures resulting from exertional syncope as well as exaggerated pulmonary vasoconstriction due to systemic arterial oxygen desaturation during sleep (particularly in the early morning hours).

PHYSICAL EXAMINATION

Physical Signs

Many of the physical findings in children with PAH are similar for those of children with IPAH as well as PAH related to other conditions (see Box 64-1). On physical examination, signs differ for children with and without an intracardiac or extracardiac shunt. In patients who have undergone "corrective" surgery for their congenital heart defects, the physical findings may be identical to patients with IPAH or other types of PAH. Careful attention should be directed to the cardiac examination and other signs of systemic venous congestion related to right "pump" failure. The cardiac signs of elevated right ventricular systolic pressure include a loud single P2, murmur of tricuspid

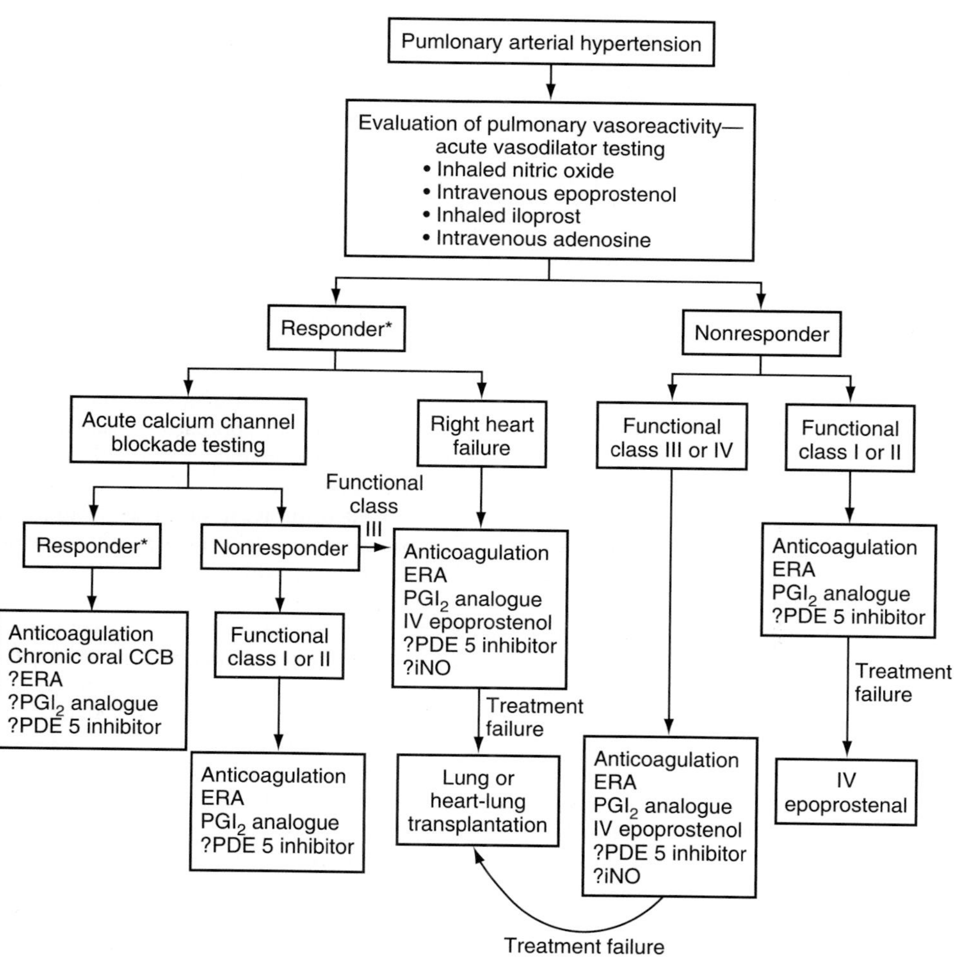

FIGURE 64-3. Algorithm for treating pulmonary arterial hypertension, including novel agents. CCB, calcium channel blockade; ERA, endothelin receptor antagonist; PGI_2, prostacyclin; iNO, inhaled nitric oxide; PDE 5, phosphodiesterase type 5; PGI_2 analog, subcutaneous treprostinil, inhaled iloprost or oral beraprost; ?, not demonstrated in randomized controlled trials to date. (Adapted from Widlitz A, Barst RJ: Pulmonary arterial hypertension in children. Eur Respir J 2003;21:155–176.)

insufficiency, and/or murmur of pulmonary insufficiency. A pansystolic murmur of tricuspid regurgitation is common. The high-pitched diastolic murmur of pulmonary insufficiency may also be heard and usually relates to the high pulmonary arterial pressures and dilatation of the main pulmonary artery. In addition, there may be an S3 or S4 right ventricular gallop. An increase in the pulmonic component of the second heart sound and a right-sided fourth heart sound are early findings. When heard, a right ventricular third heart sound generally reflects advanced disease. Jugular venous distention, although rare in children, may be present with a prominent *a* wave. Hepatomegaly may also be present. Because the liver capsule is more distensible in children, the size of the liver is a good marker of the degree of right heart failure and response to therapy. Ascites and peripheral edema can also occur in severe cases. Other findings may implicate a systemic cause for the PAH (e.g., rash of systemic lupus erythematosus). Clubbing and cyanosis may be present in children with underlying lung disease or Eisenmenger syndrome. Clubbing is not a typical feature of IPAH, although on rare occasions it has been observed in patients with long-standing disease who develop chronic hypoxemia secondary to right-to-left shunting via a patent foramen ovale. Clubbing of the digits is rare following early complete surgical repair of a CHD unless there is underlying pulmonary disease, since these patients are no longer cyanotic.

TREATMENT

Although there is no cure for PAH, nor a single therapeutic approach that is uniformly successful, therapy has dramatically improved over the past several decades, resulting in sustained clinical and hemodynamic improvement as well as increased survival in children with various types of PAH.[27] An overview of our current approach and guidelines for treatment are shown in Figure 64-3. Noninvasive studies obtained prior to initiating therapy, as well as periodically thereafter, are useful in guiding changes in therapeutic regimens, particularly in light of recent advances with various novel therapeutic agents.

GENERAL MEASURES

The pediatrician plays an invaluable role in the care of children with PAH. Since children often have a more reactive pulmonary vascular bed than adult patients do, any respiratory tract infection that results in ventilation-perfusion mismatching from alveolar hypoxia can result in a catastrophic event if not treated aggressively. Annual influenza vaccination as well as pneumococcal vaccination is recommended unless there are contraindications. Antipyretics should be administered for temperature elevations greater than 101°F (38°C) to minimize the consequences of increased metabolic demands on an already compromised cardiorespiratory system. Children may also require aggressive therapy (e.g., inhaled nitric oxide) for acute pulmonary hypertensive crises occurring with episodes of pneumonia or other infectious diseases. Patients may also require antitussive medications during upper respiratory tract infections. Decongestants with pseudephedrine should be avoided because they may exacerbate the pulmonary hypertension. Diet and/or medical therapy should be used to prevent constipation, since Valsalva maneuvers transiently decrease venous return to the right side of the heart and may precipitate syncopal episodes.

ANTICOAGULATION

Consideration of chronic anticoagulation in children with PAH is based on studies in adults with IPAH.[2,25,62] The lung histopathology often demonstrates thrombotic lesions in small pulmonary arteries of adult patients with IPAH. Some patients have an underlying coagulopathy (e.g., antiphospholipid syndrome, or protein C/S deficiency). And for patients with poor right ventricular function, thrombi can form within the ventricle. In addition, postmortem examinations of patients with pulmonary vascular disease who have died suddenly often demonstrate fresh clot in the pulmonary vascular bed. Whether or not secondary thrombosis in situ is a significant exacerbating factor in patients with a normal resting cardiac output is unknown. In addition, even a small pulmonary embolus can be life threatening in patients who cannot vasodilate or recruit additional pulmonary vessels. Clinical data supporting the chronic use of anticoagulation are limited but supportive. Warfarin has been shown to be associated with improved survival in two retrospective studies and one prospective study; all three studies were in adult patients.[2,25,62] The dosage of anticoagulation that is usually recommended is to achieve an international normalized ratio (INR) of 1.5 to 2; however, certain clinical circumstances (e.g., positive lupus anticoagulant, positive anticardiolipin antibodies, factor V Leiden, and/or factor II 20210A variant[71–74]), as well as documented chronic thromboembolic disease may require dose adjustment to maintain a higher INR. For patients at a higher risk for bleeding (e.g., patients with significant thrombocytopenia), the dosage should be adjusted to maintain a lower INR. Whether or not chronic anticoagulation is efficacious as well as safe with a low risk-benefit profile for children with pulmonary hypertension remains to be determined. Our approach has been to anticoagulate children who are hypercoagulable or in right heart failure, similar to the approach for adult patients. In children who are extremely active, particularly toddlers, unless there is severe pulmonary vascular disease, we recommend maintaining an INR of less than 1.5. Antiplatelet therapy with aspirin or dipyridamole does not appear to be effective in areas of low flow, where thrombosis in situ is known to occur. Parents should be advised to avoid administering other medications that could interact with the warfarin unless the drug-drug interactions are known and the dose of the warfarin is adjusted as needed. Similar to our approach with adult pulmonary hypertension patients, if anticoagulation with warfarin is contraindicated or dose adjustments are difficult, low molecular weight heparin at a dose of 0.50 mg/kg to 0.75 mg/kg by subcutaneous administration twice daily may be a reasonable alternative. However, the long-term side effects of heparin, such as osteopenia and thrombocytopenia, are of concern. To date there are no studies comparing the safety and efficacy of anticoagulation with warfarin to heparin. There may be additional benefits of heparin on the pulmonary vascular bed. Experimental studies by Thompson and colleagues in vivo[75] and Benitz and colleagues in vitro[76] suggest that vascular smooth muscle growth inhibitors, such as heparin, may be useful in preventing progression of pulmonary vascular disease.

CALCIUM CHANNEL BLOCKADE

Calcium channel blockers are a chemically heterogeneous group of compounds that inhibit calcium influx through the slow channel into cardiac and smooth muscle cells. Their usefulness for select patients with PAH is based on the ability to cause pulmonary vasodilation. Acute vasodilator testing during right heart cardiac catheterization is a critical part of the initial assessment of patients with PAH to determine the appropriate treatment course. Chronic calcium channel blockade is efficacious for patients (responders) who demonstrate an acute response to vasodilator testing (i.e., fall in mean pulmonary arterial pressure by ≥ 20% from baseline with no decrease in cardiac output),[77] although not all acute "responders" have a sustained response long term.[27] In contrast, patients who do not respond acutely fail to respond to long-term calcium channel blockade.[2,27] In general, these patients (e.g., "nonresponders") will respond to long-term treatment with intravenous prostacyclin (i.e., epoprostenol) and may respond to other novel treatments (see Fig. 64-3).[78]

Fewer than 20% of adult patients with IPAH will respond to chronic oral calcium channel blockade,[2] as documented by improvement in symptoms, exercise tolerance, hemodynamics, and survival. A significantly greater percentage of children than adults are acute "responders" (40%), and can be effectively treated with chronic oral calcium channel blockade.[27] For acute responders, most studies have used calcium channel blockers at relatively high doses (e.g., long-acting nifedipine 120–240 mg daily or amlodipine 20–40 mg daily); however, the optimal dosing for both children and adults with IPAH is uncertain. Because of the frequent occurrence of significant adverse effects with calcium channel blockade therapy in nonresponders, including systemic hypotension, pulmonary edema, right ventricular failure, and death, treatment with calcium channel blockers is not recommended for patients in whom acute effectiveness has not been demonstrated. This supports the importance of an initial assessment with acute vasodilator therapy before prescribing a long-term pulmonary vasodilator.

Serial reevaluations, including repeat acute vasodilator testing, to maintain an "optimal" chronic therapeutic regimen is essential to the care of children with PAH. In our experience, acute "responders" who are treated with chronic oral calcium channel blockade therapy continue to do exceedingly well as long as they remain acutely reactive to vasodilator testing on repeat cardiac catheterizations. In contrast, children who were initially acute "responders" and were treated with chronic calcium channel blockade, and who no longer demonstrate active vasoreactivity on repeat testing, usually deteriorate clinically and hemodynamically despite continuation of chronic calcium channel blockade therapy. If they are then treated with continuous intravenous epoprostenol, they will likely demonstrate improvement with chronic epoprostenol therapy similar to the experience with children who are "nonresponders" and are initiated on epoprostenol at their initial evaluation. Other novel therapeutic agents, as discussed below, may also be considered for these patients.

PROSTAGLANDINS

Epoprostenol (prostacyclin) has been used for almost two decades for the treatment of PAH with great success. Epoprostenol has been shown to improve hemodynamics, quality of life, and exercise capacity in patients with IPAH and PAH associated with other conditions such as congenital heart disease, connective tissue disease, HIV infection, and portal hypertension. In the mid-1990s epoprostenol became the gold standard for treatment of IPAH in patients who were not responsive to acute vasodilator testing and therefore would not benefit from chronic oral calcium channel blockade. The use of prostacyclin or a prostacyclin analog for the treatment of IPAH is supported by the demonstration of an imbalance in the thromboxane to prostacyclin metabolites in patients with IPAH,[38] as well as the demonstration of a reduction in prostacyclin synthase in the pulmonary arteries of patients with IPAH.[43] Although chronic intravenous epoprostenol does improve exercise tolerance, hemodynamics, and survival in patients with IPAH, its mechanisms of action remain unclear.[3,4,79–81] Epoprostenol lowers pulmonary artery pressure, increases cardiac output, and increases oxygen transport. These effects occur with long-term use even if there is no acute response to vasodilator testing, which supports the idea that epoprostenol has additional properties that cause pulmonary vascular remodeling in addition to its vasodilator properties.[27] The development of tolerance to the effects of intravenous epoprostenol is possible; some children appear to need periodic dose "escalation," which may represent "tolerance" and/or disease progression. In addition, the optimal dose of intravenous epoprostenol is unclear. The dose (ng/kg/min) is titrated incrementally, with the most rapid increases during the first several months of epoprostenol use. Although a mean dosage at 1 year in adult patients is approximately 20 to 40 ng/kg/min, the mean dosage at 1 year in children, particularly young children, is closer to 50 to 80 ng/kg/min, but there is a significant patient variability of the "optimal" dose.

Because epoprostenol is chemically unstable at neutral pH/room temperature, and has a short half-life (1–2 minutes), chronic epoprostenol treatment requires a continuous intravenous delivery system with cold packs to maintain stability. Permanent central venous access is required to administer the medication. Thus, serious complications are associated with its use, which include line sepsis, local infection, and catheter dislodgment. In addition, pump malfunction may rarely lead to a sudden bolus of epoprostenol or interruption of the medication, which can cause severe rebound PAH. Therefore, a search for alternate routes of drug delivery has led to the clinical investigation of oral, inhaled, and subcutaneous prostacyclin analog. Thus far, none have been proven as efficacious as intravenous epoprostenol.

PROSTACYCLIN ANALOGS

Oral Prostacyclin Analog

Beraprost sodium is an oral prostacyclin analog.[82] It is chemically stable and an orally active prostaglandin I_2 derivative with a substantially longer half-life than epoprostenol (peak concentration is reached after 30 minutes and elimination half-life is 35–40 minutes after oral administration).[83] The drug has properties similar to those of epoprostenol; for example, it produces vasodilatation and decreases platelet adherence to the endothelium, disaggregates platelets that have already clumped, increases red blood cell flexibility, decreases blood viscosity, and inhibits platelet aggregation. Its potency is approximately 50% that of epoprostenol. A number of small open-label uncontrolled studies from Japan have reported improved hemodynamics, functional class, and survival in patients with IPAH.[82,84,85] Although these studies were open-label uncontrolled clinical trials, they provided "proof of concept" for further clinical investigation. Subsequently, a double-blind, placebo-controlled study (ALPHABET Trial) was performed in Europe with 130 PAH patients, including children older than 8 years, who were randomized to receive the maximum tolerated dose of beraprost (median dosage 80 μg four times daily) or placebo for 12 weeks.[86] Patients treated with beraprost had improved exercise capacity, as measured by the 6-minute walk test, and symptoms. Patients with IPAH fared better than those with PAH related to other conditions. There was no significant change in hemodynamics or New York Heart Association (NYHA) functional class.

A longer (12-month) multicenter double-blind, placebo-controlled, randomized study was performed in 116 patients to evaluate the effects of beraprost compared with placebo on disease progression in patients (including children older than 8 years) with symptom-limiting NYHA functional class II/III PAH. This study demonstrated that patients treated with beraprost showed less evidence of disease progression at 6 months. However, this effect was not evident at shorter or longer intervals of follow-up. In addition, exercise capacity (assessed by the 6-minute walk test) improved at 3 and 6 months but not at 9 or 12 months. Side effects (e.g., nausea, headache, dizziness) often limited dose increases.[87] Beraprost is approved for PAH treatment in Japan but is not approved for use in the United States.

Inhaled Prostacyclin Analog

Iloprost, an inhaled prostacyclin analog, has recently gained attention as a long-term therapeutic agent for PAH because of the potential benefits of inhaled delivery, which may avoid some of the systemic side effects including hypotension that may accompany epoprostenol use. Iloprost is a more stable synthetic analog of prostacyclin.[88] It has a molecular structure similar to that of prostacyclin and acts through prostacyclin receptors on vascular endothelial cells.[89,90] Iloprost has both vasodilator and platelet aggregation inhibition properties similar to prostacyclin.[88] Unfortunately, it has a short biologic half-life (i.e., 20–25 minutes) in humans.[91]

Iloprost is a potent pulmonary vasodilator with more pronounced short-term hemodynamic effects than inhaled nitric oxide in patients with IPAH.[92] While several preliminary studies demonstrate clinical, hemodynamic, and exercise capacity improvements from intermittent short-term use of iloprost,[93] more recent studies demonstrate the benefits of long-term iloprost administered over 1 year in adult patients with IPAH.[94,95] In a long-term study, WHO functional class III/IV patients refractory to conventional medical treatment, including the use of oral calcium channel blockers, had improved exercise capacity and hemodynamics following 1 year of inhaled iloprost treatment with minimal side effects.[94] The 24 of 31 patients who completed this study were tested acutely in the cardiac catheterization laboratory to determine the maximal short-term effect and onset of hemodynamic response. Patients were then started on a daily dose of 100 μg of aerosolized iloprost per day divided into six to eight inhalations every 2 to 3 hours while awake. Both acute "responders" and "nonresponders" were treated with iloprost, although acute "responders" (defined by a fall in PVR of > 20%), were treated eight times per day and "nonresponders" six times per day. However, patients with PAH who respond to acute pulmonary vasodilator testing usually respond favorably to long-term treatment with oral calcium channel blocker therapy that can be administered once daily as opposed to an inhalation eight times per day. Nevertheless, both "nonresponders" and "responders" improved clinically as well as hemodynamically while on chronic iloprost therapy consistent with pulmonary vascular remodeling similar to previous observations with epoprostenol.

In another large randomized placebo-controlled study, 203 patients with selected forms of severe PAH and chronic thromboembolic pulmonary hypertension (WHO functional class III and IV) were randomized to receive aerosolized iloprost six to nine times a day (median dose 30 μg/day) or inhalation of placebo.[96] The primary endpoint was met if after week 12 the functional class improved by one class and distance walked in 6 minutes improved by at least 10%, in the absence of clinical deterioration and death. The combined clinical endpoint was met by 17% of the patients receiving iloprost versus 5% of the placebo patients. Hemodynamic improvements at the week 12 follow-up were only present when measured after iloprost inhalation.

A recent report comparing the acute effects of inhaled nitric oxide with aerosolized iloprost for children with pulmonary hypertension and congenital heart defects found them equally efficacious.[97] When used together, there were no additive or synergistic effects. Iloprost is now FDA approved in the United States. Although most of the studies have been performed in adult patients, this drug shows promise for patients of all ages. The noninvasive delivery system makes this drug appealing, but the need for six to nine treatments a day of iloprost (each lasting 5–15 minutes) may be a burden for some patients, particularly children. Randomized treatment trials of iloprost versus epoprostenol are warranted, although the feasibility of a comparison trial is problematic.

Subcutaneous Prostacyclin Analog

Treprostinil sodium is a chemically stable prostacyclin analog that also shares the same pharmacologic actions as epoprostenol. Previous studies have demonstrated acute hemodynamic effects similar to those of intravenous epoprostenol in patients with IPAH; however, treprostinil is stable at room temperature and neutral pH and has a longer half-life (i.e., ~3 hours) when delivered subcutaneously.[98] Similar to epoprostenol, treprostinil is infused continuously by a portable pump, but it is administered subcutaneously. Double-blind, randomized, placebo-controlled trials demonstrated improved exercise capacity and clinical signs and symptoms as well as hemodynamic measurements in patients with PAH including children.[99] The risk for central venous line infection is eliminated when treprostinil is used subcutaneously. Although no serious adverse events related to treprostinil or its delivery system have been reported, discomfort at the infusion site is common and may not be well tolerated by young children.[100] Intravenous treprostinil is also FDA approved for the treatment of PAH.

ENDOTHELIN RECEPTOR ANTAGONISTS

Endothelin-1, one of the most potent vasoconstrictors identified to date,[101] has been implicated in the pathobiology of PAH. Plasma endothelin-1 levels are increased in patients with IPAH and correlate inversely with prognosis.[102] Thus, endothelin receptor antagonists are promising drugs for the treatment of PAH. There are at least two different receptor subtypes: ET_A receptors are localized on smooth muscle cells and mediate vasoconstriction and proliferation,[103] while ET_B receptors are found predominantly on endothelial cells and are associated with (1) endothelium-dependent vasorelaxation through the release of vasodilators (i.e., prostacyclin and nitric oxide), (2) clearance of endothelin, and (3) vasoconstriction (on smooth muscle cells) and bronchoconstriction.[104,105] The oral dual endothelin receptor antagonist bosentan has been shown to improve exercise capacity, quality of life, and cardiopulmonary hemodynamics in patients with PAH.[106,107] Additionally, a small, two-center, open-label study of 19 pediatric patients with IPAH or pulmonary hypertension associated with CHDs and WHO functional class II and III was performed with measurements of pharmacokinetic and hemodynamic parameters at baseline and 12-week follow-up.[108] Exercise capacity was measured in children at least 8 years of age. Patients weighing 10 to 20 kg, 20 to 40 kg, and greater than or equal to 40 kg received 31.25 mg once daily, 31.25 mg twice daily, and 62.5 mg twice daily, respectively, for 1 month and then 31.25 mg twice daily, 62.5 mg twice daily, and 125 mg twice daily, respectively, for the remainder of the study. Hemodynamic improvement was demonstrated at 12 weeks (e.g., decrease in pulmonary arterial pressure and PVR). Bosentan appeared to be well tolerated in the dosing regimens used and is now approved by the U.S. Food and Drug Administration for the treatment of PAH.[109]

Sitaxsentan, a highly selective ET_A receptor antagonist, has also been studied. The rationale for selective ET_A receptor blockade is that it may benefit patients by blocking the vasoconstrictor effects of the ET_A receptor while maintaining the vasodilator and clearance effects of the ET_B receptor. In a 12-week open-label study of 20 patients (children and adults) with IPAH or PAH related to CHDs or connective tissue disease, the selective ET_A receptor antagonist sitaxsentan improved exercise capacity and hemodynamics.[110] Subsequently, the effects of sitaxsentan on exercise capacity were studied in a double-blind, randomized, placebo-controlled study in patients with symptomatic IPAH or PAH related to connective tissue disease or congenital heart disease.[111] Similar to the bosentan trials, sitaxsentan improved 6-minute walk distance, NYHA functional class, cardiac index, and PVR. Pharmacokinetic studies with sitaxsentan are currently in progress. Risks associated with endothelin receptor antagonists include acute hepatotoxicity (dose related), teratogenicity, and possibly male infertility. In addition, in patients treated with sitaxsentan, significantly lower doses of warfarin are needed to maintain a therapeutic INR.

Future use of endothelin receptor antagonists, both dual receptor and selective ET_A receptor, seems very promising for patients with PAH. For patients who do not have an acute response to vasodilator testing or have failed treatment with oral calcium channel blockade, endothelin receptor antagonists may offer a viable treatment option. Furthermore, in the future, the addition of endothelin receptor antagonists to chronic calcium channel blockade therapy or to epoprostenol or a prostacyclin analog therapy may increase the overall efficacy of the treatment for PAH.

NITRIC OXIDE

Nitric oxide is an inhaled vasodilator that exerts selective effects on the pulmonary circulation.[112] Nitric oxide activates guanylate cyclase in pulmonary vascular smooth muscle cells, which increases cyclic guanosine monophosphate (cGMP) and decreases intracellular calcium concentration, thereby leading to smooth muscle relaxation. When inhaled, the rapid combination of nitric oxide and hemoglobin inactivates any nitric oxide diffusing into the blood, preventing systemic vasodilatation. Nitric oxide is therefore a potent and selective pulmonary vasodilator when administered by inhalation. Nitric oxide may also have antiproliferative effects on smooth muscle and inhibit platelet adhesion. Inhaled nitric oxide has been demonstrated to be safe and efficacious in the treatment of PPHN.[113,114] Inhaled nitric oxide has also been useful for determining operability of patients with CHD. It has been used for the treatment of IPAH exacerbations, perioperative pulmonary hypertension following cardiac surgery, and other forms of PAH. Although there is considerable experience with the use of inhaled nitric oxide as a short-term treatment for PAH in a variety of clinical situations, the role of inhaled nitric oxide as a chronic therapy for PAH remains under clinical investigation.[115] It is possible that in some children, a low-dose inhalation of nitric oxide may become a useful agent in the treatment of PAH, both by reversing the vasoconstrictor component when present as well as stimulating the regression of remodeling that obliterates the pulmonary vascular bed. Despite this rationale, clinical trials are needed to evaluate the safety and efficacy of chronic inhaled nitric oxide.

PHOSPHODIESTERASE INHIBITORS

Additional investigations evaluating nitric oxide–potentiating compounds, such as phosphodiesterase type 5 inhibitors (e.g., sildenafil), have been studied.[116,117] Phosphodiesterase type 5 inhibitors prevent the breakdown of cGMP, thereby raising cGMP levels. This effect should potentiate the pulmonary vasodilatation with nitric oxide. Phosphodiesterase type 5 inhibitors may be particularly beneficial in conjunction with chronic inhaled nitric oxide, where withdrawal of nitric oxide may lead to rebound PAH. Intravenous, long-acting oral or aerosolized forms of phosphodiesterase type 5 inhibitors all have therapeutic appeal. A recent study compared the effects of intravenous sildenafil with inhaled nitric oxide in preoperative and postoperative patients with congenital heart disease and elevated PVR.[118] In this study, intravenous sildenafil was as effective as inhaled nitric oxide in children with congenital heart disease. A recent randomized double-blind crossover design study of patients with IPAH compared the efficacy of sildenafil with placebo. Twenty-two patients completed the study. Exercise on treadmill increased by 44% from the end of the placebo phase to the end of the treatment phase. There was also an increase in cardiac index despite no significant change in systolic pulmonary arterial pressure, and improvement in dyspnea and fatigue components of a quality of life questionnaire.[119] Carefully designed short- and long-term studies of the possible therapeutic usefulness of phosphodiesterase type 5 inhibitors alone, and in combination with inhaled nitric oxide, are warranted. Preliminary safety and efficacy trials are under way in the pediatric population.

ELASTASE INHIBITORS

Rabinovitch and colleagues have suggested that increased activity of an elastolytic enzyme may be important in the pathophysiology of pulmonary vascular disease.[120,121] A cause and effect relationship between elastase and pulmonary vascular disease is supported by studies showing the reversal of advanced pulmonary vascular disease in the monocrotaline rat model. Part of the novelty of these observations is the complete regression of pathophysiologic findings in the treatment group even though treatment began after the disease was developed. The presumed mechanism of an apoptotic cascade with regression of smooth muscle hypertrophy and neointimal proliferation has exciting therapeutic implications; human trials are being considered. However, one must bear in mind that the monocrotaline model does not exhibit identical vascular pathology to the human condition and rodent models of successful treatment of vascular disease have not always borne similar success in analogous human diseases.

The 3-hydroxy-3-methylglutaryl-coenzyme A (HMG-CoA) reductase inhibitors (statins) have been shown to exert numerous effects on vascular wall function, independent of their cholesterol-lowering effect, which prompted recent investigation in an animal model of PAH.[122] In this study using a rat model of hypoxic PAH, simvastatin treatment potently attenuated chronic hypoxic pulmonary hypertension in rats and inhibited vascular remodeling.[123] Further investigation in humans is warranted.

GENE THERAPY

With the identification of an IPAH gene in selected families, which codes for the BMPR2 protein, attention has focused on gene replacement therapy linked to the mutated 2q33 chromosome. An alternative therapeutic approach has been to induce the overexpression of vasodilator genes, notably endothelial nitric oxide synthase and prostacyclin synthase, since patients with IPAH have been shown to have deficiencies in both prostacyclin synthase and nitric oxide synthase. Given the preliminary clinical observations that exogenous administration of chronic nitric oxide or epoprostenol may have salutary effects on even advanced forms of the disease, it seems worthwhile to pursue these alternative modes of "drug delivery." Advances in our understanding of the genetic predisposition associated with at least some, if not all, patients with PAH, suggest that gene delivery treatment(s) may be possible in the future.

OXYGEN

Some children who remain fully saturated while awake demonstrate modest systemic arterial oxygen desaturation with sleep, which appears to be due to mild hypoventilation.[124] During these episodes, children with pulmonary hypertension may experience severe dyspnea, as well as syncope with or without hypoxic seizures. Desaturation during sleep usually occurs during the early morning hours and can be eliminated by using supplemental oxygen. We also recommend that children have supplemental oxygen available at home for emergency use. Children with PAH should also be treated with supplemental oxygen during any significant upper respiratory tract infections if systemic arterial oxygen desaturation occurs. Children with desaturation due to right to left shunting through a patent foramen ovale usually do not improve their oxygen saturation with supplemental oxygen, although oxygen supplementation may reduce the degree of polycythemia in these children. A small study of children with Eisenmenger syndrome demonstrated improved long-term survival with supplemental oxygen.[125] In contrast, in a more recent report of 23 adult patients with Eisenmenger syndrome, there was no significant improvement in survival with nocturnal oxygen.[126] Similar to the experience with adult patients, some children experience arterial blood oxygen desaturation with exercise as a result of increased oxygen extraction in the face of fixed oxygen delivery and may benefit from ambulatory supplemental oxygen. In addition, children with severe right ventricular failure and resting hypoxemia, resulting from a markedly increased oxygen extraction, should also be treated with chronic supplemental oxygen therapy. Furthermore, supplemental oxygen is recommended for air travel to avoid alveolar hypoxia and exacerbation of the pulmonary hypertension.

ADDITIONAL PHARMACOTHERAPY: CARDIAC GLYCOSIDES, DIURETICS, ANTIARRHYTHMIC THERAPY, INOTROPIC AGENTS, AND NITRATES

Although controversy persists regarding the value of digitalis in IPAH,[127] children with right-sided heart failure may benefit from digitalis, in addition to diuretic therapy. Diuretic therapy must be initiated cautiously, since these patients are preload dependent to maintain optimal cardiac output. Despite this, relatively high doses of diuretic therapy are often needed. Although malignant arrhythmias are rare in pulmonary hypertension, treatment is appropriate for documented cases. Atrial flutter or fibrillation often precipitates an abrupt decrease in cardiac output and clinical deterioration due to the loss of the atrial component. As opposed to healthy children, in whom atrial systole accounts for approximately 25% of the cardiac output, atrial systole in children with IPAH often contributes as much as 70% of the cardiac output. Therefore, aggressive treatment of atrial flutter or fibrillation is advised.

Although there are no studies on the usefulness of intermittent or continuous treatment with inotropic agents, dobutamine can be used for additional inotropic support in conjunction with continuous intravenous epoprostenol in children with severe right ventricular dysfunction, as a bridge to transplantation. Children have also benefited from short-term inotropic support during acute pulmonary hypertensive crises to augment cardiac output during a period of increased metabolic demand.

Oral and sublingual nitrates have been used to treat chest pain in some children with IPAH, although the experience with these agents remains limited. Children who complain of chest tightness, pressure, or vague discomfort that is responsive to sublingual nitroglycerin should be treated with chronic oral nitrates as well as sublingual nitroglycerin.

ATRIAL SEPTOSTOMY

Children with recurrent syncope in severe right heart failure have a poor prognosis.[1,128] Exercise-induced syncope is due to systemic vasodilation, with an inability to augment cardiac output (through a fixed pulmonary vascular bed) to maintain adequate cerebral perfusion. If right-to-left shunting through an interatrial or interventricular communication is present, cardiac output can be maintained or increased if necessary. In addition, right-to-left shunting at the atrial level alleviates signs and symptoms of right heart failure by decompression of the right atrium and right ventricle. Increased survival has been reported in patients with IPAH with a patent foramen ovale, although this remains controversial.[129] Patency of the foramen ovale may improve survival if it allows sufficient right-to-left shunting to occur to maintain cardiac output. Successful palliation of symptoms with atrial septostomy has been reported in several series.[130–134] In our experience, patients with PAH with recurrent syncope or right heart failure significantly improve clinically as well as hemodynamically following atrial septostomy; that is, patients experience no further syncope, and signs and symptoms of right-sided heart failure improve. Although systemic arterial oxygen saturation decreases, overall cardiac output and oxygen delivery improve despite the right-to-left shunting at the atrial level. In our experience, atrial septostomy results in a survival benefit (i.e., survival rates at 1 and 2 years are 87% and 76%, respectively) compared with conventional therapy (64% and 42% at 1 and 2 years, respectively).[133] Thus, although atrial septostomy does not alter the underlying disease process, it may improve quality of life and represent an alternative for selected patients with severe IPAH. However, this invasive procedure is not without risk; our indications for the procedure include recurrent syncope or right ventricular failure despite maximal medical therapy, as well as a bridge to transplantation. Although there is a worldwide experience in over 100 patients, with atrial septostomy the procedure should still be considered investigational. Closure of the atrial septal defect can be performed at the time of transplantation.

TRANSPLANTATION

While successful heart-lung transplantation as well as single- and double-lung transplantation with repair of CHDs have been available for over 20 years, there are several limitations to these procedures. A limited number of centers perform the procedures in children, and the availability of suitable donors is limited. Furthermore, the high incidence of chronic allograft rejection or bronchiolitis obliterans in the transplanted organs of these patients (25%–50%) and the potential consequences of life-long immunosuppression are of great concern.[135] Both single and bilateral lung transplantation have been performed in pediatric patients with pulmonary vascular obstructive disease, including patients with severe right ventricular failure.[136] Currently, the overall 1-year, 5-year, and 10-year survival rates for lung transplantation in PAH patients are 64%, 44%, and 20%, respectively.[135,137,138] There has been no significant improvement in survival in more recent years (e.g., 1998–2001 vs. 1992–1998). For untreated Eisenmenger syndrome patients, the natural history is much more favorable. The 5-year and 25-year survival rates are greater than 80% and 40%, respectively, for untreated Eisenmenger syndrome patients, as opposed to following lung transplantation,[138] with 1-year and 5-year survival rates of 52% and 39%, respectively.[135] Thus, transplantation should be reserved for WHO functional class III and IV patients with PAH who have progressed despite optimal medical therapy. As progress is made in the medical management of PAH, the indications for transplantation will change. The course of the disease and the waiting time must be taken into account when referring for transplantation. Ideally, children should be listed for transplant when their probability of 2-year survival without transplantation is 50% or less. While there are advantages and disadvantages to each operation (i.e., single- or double-lung vs. heart-lung transplantation), there is currently no consensus regarding the optimal procedure. The availability of donor organs often influences the choice of procedure. It is possible that data on long-term survival will demonstrate a survival advantage of one procedure over another. Although lung and heart-lung transplantation are imperfect therapies for PAH, when offered to an appropriately selected population, transplantation may improve survival with an improved quality of life.

Early referral to a center with expertise in pediatric lung and heart-lung transplantation will decrease pretransplantation mortality and allow families to have adequate time to make an informed and thoughtful choice about this therapy. Living related donor transplantation remains controversial; although it has been successful, there is limited experience.[139,140]

CONCLUSIONS

Recent therapeutic advances have significantly improved the prognosis for children with PAH. However, PAH continues to be a serious condition that is extremely challenging to manage. Chronic vasodilator therapy with calcium channel blockade in "acute responders" to vasodilator testing and continuous intravenous epoprostenol in "nonresponders" appear to be effective in children and improve survival, hemodynamics, and symptoms.[2–4,81,141–143] This is an exciting time for the treatment of PAH, with the introduction of promising new drugs such as prostacyclin analog, endothelin receptor antagonists, phosphodiesterase 5 inhibitors, inhaled iloprost, and inhaled nitric oxide. There will undoubtedly be more treatment options for patients with PAH. However, in the early stages of use, and without controlled studies for comparison, the newer agents should be used cautiously with close monitoring for treatment failure. Based on distinct mechanisms, a role for combination therapy may further improve the overall efficacy in treating a child's PAH. Future developments in vascular biology will improve our understanding of its etiologies and pathobiology, as well as provide rationale for more specific medical therapies. The treatment algorithm will continue to evolve as newer agents become available (see Fig. 64-3).[144,145] Whether these new agents will prove to be as effective as intravenous epoprostenol in selected children remains unknown. We hope that by increasing our understanding of the pathobiology of PAH, novel treatment strategies will continue to evolve and we will be able to prevent or cure this disease in the future.

REFERENCES

1. D'Alonzo GE, Barst RJ, Ayres SM, Bergofsky EH, Detre KM, Fishman AP, et al: Survival in patients with primary pulmonary hypertension. Results from a national prospective registry. Ann Intern Med 1991;115:343–349.
2. Rich S, Kaufmann E, Levy PS: The effect of high doses of calcium-channel blockers on survival in primary pulmonary hypertension [see comments]. N Engl J Med 1992;327:76–81.
3. Higenbottam T, Wheeldon P, Wells F, Wallwork J: Long-term treatment of primary pulmonary hypertension with continuous intravenous epoprostenol (prostacyclin). Lancet 1984;1:1046–1047.
4. Barst, RJ, Rubin LJ, McGoon MD, Caldwell EJ, Long WA, Levy PS: Survival in primary pulmonary hypertension with long-term continuous intravenous prostacyclin. Ann Intern Med 1994;121:409–415.
5. Gersony WM, Duc GV, Sinclair JC: "PFC" syndrome (persistence of the fetal circulation). Circulation 1969;40(Suppl III):87.
6. Long WA: Persistent pulmonary hypertension of the newborn syndrome. In: Long WA, ed: Fetal and Neonatal Cardiology. Philadelphia: WB Saunders, 1989, pp 627–655.
7. Heath D, Edwards JE: Configuration of elastic tissue of pulmonary trunk in idiopathic pulmonary hypertension. Circulation 1960;21:59.
8. Roberts WC: The histologic structure of the pulmonary trunk in patients with "primary" pulmonary hypertension. Am Heart J 1963;65:230.
9. Raine J, Hislop AA, Redington AN: Fatal persistent pulmonary hypertension presenting late in the neonatal period. Arch Dis Child 1991;66:398–402.
10. Wagenvoort CA: Misalignment of lung vessels. A syndrome causing persistent neonatal pulmonary hypertension. Hum Pathol 1986;17:727–730.
11. Friedman WF: Proceedings of National Heart, Lung, and Blood Institute pediatric cardiology workshop. Pulmonary hypertension. Pediatr Res 1986; 20(9):811–824.

12. Yamaki S, Mohri H, Haneda K, Endo M, Akimoto H: Indications for surgery based on lung biopsy in cases of ventricular septal defect and/or patent ductus arteriosus with severe pulmonary hypertension. Chest 1989;96(1):31–39.
13. Atz AM, Adatia I, Jonas RA, Wessel DL: Inhaled nitric oxide in children with pulmonary hypertension and congenital mitral stenosis. Am J Cardiol 1996;77(4):316–319.
14. Beghetti M, Habre W, Friedli B, Berner M: Continuous low dose inhaled nitric oxide for treatment of severe pulmonary hypertension after cardiac surgery in pediatric patients. Br Heart J 1995;73:65–68.
15. Berner M, Beghetti M, Spahr-Schopfer I, Oberhansli I, Friedli B: Inhaled nitric oxide to test the vasodilator capacity of the pulmonary vascular bed in children with long-standing pulmonary hypertension and congenital heart disease. Am J Cardiol 1996;77(7):532–535.
16. Bush A, Busst C, Knight WB, Shinebourne EA: Modification of pulmonary hypertension secondary to congenital heart disease by prostacyclin therapy. Am Rev Respir Dis 1987;136(3):767–769.
17. Cremona G, Higenbottam T: Role of prostacyclin in the treatment of primary pulmonary hypertension. Am J Cardiol 1995;75(3):67A–71A.
18. Miller OI, Celermajer DS, Deanfield JE, Macrae DJ: Very-low-dose inhaled nitric oxide. A selective pulmonary vasodilator after operations for congenital heart disease. J Thorac Cardiovasc Surg 1994;108:487–494.
19. Roberts JD Jr, Lang P, Bigatello LM, Vlahakes GJ, Zapol WM: Inhaled nitric oxide in congenital heart disease. Circulation 1993;87:447–453.
20. Hopkins RA, Bull C, Haworth SG, de Leval MR, Stark J: Pulmonary hypertensive crises following surgery for congenital heart defects in young children. Eur J Cardiothorac Surg 1991;5:628–634.
21. Holcomb BW Jr, Loyd JE, Ely EW, Johnson J, Robbins IM: Pulmonary veno-occlusive disease. A case series and new observations. Chest 2000; 118(6):1671–1679.
22. Davies P, Reid L: Pulmonary veno-occlusive disease in siblings. Case reports and morphometric study. Hum Pathol 1982;13:911–915.
23. Rubin LJ: Primary pulmonary hypertension. N Engl J Med 1997;336(2): 111–117.
24. Rich S, Dantzker DR, Ayres SM, Bergofsky EH, Brundage BH, Detre KM, et al: Primary pulmonary hypertension. A national prospective study. Ann Intern Med 1987;107:216–223.
25. Fuster V, Steele PM, Edwards WD, Gersh BJ, McGoon MD, Frye RL: Primary pulmonary hypertension. Natural history and the importance of thrombosis. Circulation 1984;70:580–587.
26. Hopkins WE, Ochoa LL, Richardson GW, Trulock EP: Comparison of the hemodynamics and survival of adults with severe primary pulmonary hypertension or Eisenmenger syndrome. J Heart Lung Transplant 1996;15: 100–105.
27. Barst RJ, Maislin G, Fishman AP: Vasodilator therapy for primary pulmonary hypertension in children. Circulation 1999;99:1197–1208.
28. Yung, D, Maislin G, Widlitz, AC, Rosenzweig EB, Schmitt, K, Brady D, et al: Outcomes in children with idiopathic pulmonary arterial hypertension. Circulation 2004;110:660–665.
29. Wagenvoort CA, Wagenvoort N: Primary Pulmonary Hypertension. New York: Wiley & Sons, 1977.
30. Durmowicz AG, Stenmark KR: Mechanisms of structural remodeling in chronic pulmonary hypertension. Pediatr Rev 1999;20(11):e9–e102.
31. Wagenvoort CA, Wagenvoort N: Primary pulmonary hypertension. A pathological study of the lung vessels in 156 clinically diagnosed cases. Circulation 1970;42:1163–1184.
32. Yamaki S, Wagenvoort CA: Comparison of primary plexogenic arteriopathy in adults and children. A morphometric study in 40 patients. Br Heart J 1985;54:428–434.
33. Barst RJ: Pharmacologically induced pulmonary vasodilatation in children and young adults with primary pulmonary hypertension. Chest 1986;89: 497–503.
34. Edwards WD, Edwards KE: Clinical primary pulmonary hypertension. Three pathologic types. Circulation 1977;56:884–888.
35. Rich S, Brundage BH: High-dose calcium channel-blocking therapy for primary pulmonary hypertension. Evidence for long-term reduction in pulmonary arterial pressure and regression of right ventricular hypertrophy. Circulation 1987;76:135–141.
36. Budhiraja R, Tuder RM, Hassoun PM: Endothelial dysfunction in pulmonary hypertension. Circulation 2004;109(2):159–165.
37. Barst RJ, Stalcup SA, Steeg CN, Hall JC, Frosolono MF, Cato AE, et al: Relation of arachidonate metabolites in abnormal control of the pulmonary circulation in a child. Am Rev Respir Dis 1985;131:171–177.
38. Christman BW, McPherson CD, Newman JH, King GA, Bernard GR, Groves BM, et al: An imbalance between the excretion of thromboxane and prostacyclin metabolites in pulmonary hypertension. N Engl J Med 1991;327:70–75.
39. Yoshibayashi M, Nishioka K, Nakao K, Saito Y, Matsumura M, Ueda T, et al: Plasma endothelin concentrations in patients with pulmonary hypertension associated with congenital heart defects. Circulation 1991;84: 2280–2295.
40. Stewart DJ, Levy RD, Cernacek P, Langleben D: Increased plasma endothelin-1 in pulmonary hypertension. Marker or mediator of disease? Ann Intern Med 1991;114:464–469.
41. Giaid A: Nitric oxide and endothelin-1 in pulmonary hypertension. Chest 1998;114(Suppl):208–212.
42. Christman BW: Lipid mediator disregulation in primary pulmonary hypertension. Chest 1998;114(Suppl):205–207.
43. Tuder RM, Cool CD, Geraci MW, Wang J, Abman SH, Wright L, et al: Prostacyclin synthase expression is decreased in lungs from patients with severe pulmonary hypertension. Am J Respir Crit Care Med 1999;159: 1925–1932.
44. Giaid A, Saleh D: Reduced expression of nitric oxide synthase in the lungs of patients with pulmonary hypertension. N Engl J Med 1995;333: 214–221.
45. Umetsu T, Murata T, Nishio S: Studies on the antiplatelet effect of the stable epoprostenol analogue beraprost sodium and its mechanism of action in rats. Arzneimittelforschung 1989;39:68–73.
46. Eddahibi S, Humbert M, Fadel E, Raffestin B, Darmon M, Capron F, et al: Serotonin transporter overexpression is responsible for pulmonary artery smooth muscle hyperplasia in primary pulmonary hypertension. J Clin Invest 2001;108:1109–1111.
47. Giaid A, Yanagisa WAM, Langleben D, Michel RP, Levy R, Shennib H, et al: Expression of endothelin-1 in the lungs of patients with pulmonary hypertension. N Engl J Med 1993;328:1732–1739.
48. Yuan JX, Aldinger AM, Juhaszova M, Wang J, Conte JV Jr, Gaine SP, et al: Dysfunctional voltage gated K^+ channels in pulmonary artery smooth muscle cells of patients with primary pulmonary hypertension. Circulation 1998;98:1400–1406.
49. Deng Z, Morse JH, Slager SL, Cuervo N, Moore KJ, Venetos G, et al: Familial primary pulmonary hypertension (gene PPH 1) is caused by mutations in the bone morphogenetic protein-receptor-II gene. Am J Hum Genet 2000;67:737–744.
50. Lane KB, Machado RD, Pauciulo MW, Thomson JR, Phillips JA III, Loyd JE, et al: Heterozygous germline mutations in BMPR2, encoding a TGF-B receptor, causes familial primary pulmonary hypertension. Nat Genet 2000;26(1):81–84.
51. Morse JH, Deng Z, Knowles JA: Genetic aspects of pulmonary arterial hypertension. Ann Med 2001;33(9):596–603.
52. Atkinson C, Stewart S, Upton PD, Machado R, Thomson JR, Trembath RC, et al: Primary pulmonary hypertension is associated with reduced pulmonary vascular expression of type II bone morphogenetic protein receptor. Circulation 2002;105(14):1672–1678.
53. Cool CD, Stewart JS, Werahera P, Miller GJ, Williams RL, Voelkel NF, et al: Three-dimensional reconstruction of pulmonary arteries in plexiform pulmonary hypertension using cell-specific markers. Evidence for a dynamic and heterogeneous process of pulmonary endothelial cell growth. Am J Pathol 1999;155(2):411–419.
54. Rabinovitch M, Andrew M, Thom H, Trusler GA, Williams WG, Rowe RD, et al: Abnormal endothelial factor VIII associated with pulmonary hypertension and congenital heart defects. Circulation 1987;76: 1043–1052.
55. Geggel RL, Carvalho AC, Hoyer LW, Reid LM: von Willebrand factor abnormalities in primary pulmonary hypertension. Am Rev Respir Dis 1987;135:294–299.
56. Rosenberg HC, Rabinovitch M: Endothelial injury and vascular reactivity in monocrotaline pulmonary hypertension. Am J Physiol 1988;255: JH1484–JH1491.
57. Todorovich-Hunter L, Johnson DJ, Ranger P, Keeley FW, Rabinovitch M: Altered elastin and collagen synthesis associated with progressive pulmonary hypertension induced by monocrotaline. A biochemical and ultrastructural study. Lab Invest 1988;58:184–195.
58. Ryan US: The endothelial surface and responses to injury. Fed Proc 1986;45:101–108.
59. Eisenberg PR, Lucore C, Kaufman L, Sobel BE, Jaffe AS, Rich S: Fibrinopeptide A levels indicative of pulmonary vascular thrombosis in patients with primary pulmonary hypertension. Circulation 1990;82: 841–847.
60. Sakamaki F: Coagulation and fibrinolytic abnormality related to endothelial injury in pulmonary arterial hypertension. Nippon Rinsho 2001;59(6): 1053–1058.
61. Cella G, Bellotto F, Tona F, Sbarai A, Mazzaro G, Motta G, et al: Chest 2001;120(4):1226–1230.

62. Frank H, Mlczoch J, Huber K, Schuster E, Gurtner HP, Kneussl M: The effect of anticoagulant therapy in primary and anorectic drug- induced pulmonary hypertension. Chest 1997;112(3):714–721.
63. Barst RJ: Primary pulmonary hypertension in children. In: Rubin LJ, Rich S, eds: Primary Pulmonary Hypertension (Lung Biology in Health and Disease). New York: Marcel Dekker, 1976, pp 179–225.
64. Boxt LM, Katz FJ, Kolb T: Direct quantitation of right and left ventricular volumes with nuclear magnetic resonance imaging in patients with primary pulmonary hypertension. J Am Coll Cardiol 1992;19:1508–1515.
65. Tanaka H, Tei C, Nakao S, Tahara M, Sakurai S, Kashima T, et al: Diastolic bulging of the interventricular septum toward the left ventricle. An echocardiographic manifestation of negative interventricular pressure gradient between left and right ventricles during diastole. Circulation 1980; 62(3): 558–563.
66. Gomez-Sanchez MA, Mestre de Juan MJ, Gomez-Pajuelo C, Lopez JI, Diaz de Atauri MJ, Martinez-Tello FJ: Pulmonary hypertension due to toxic oil syndrome. A clinicopathologic study. Chest 1989;95:325–331.
67. Gomez-Sanchez MA, Saenz de la Calzada C, Gomez-Pajuelo C, Martinez-Tello FJ, Mestre de Juan MJ, James TN: Clinical and pathologic manifestation of pulmonary vascular disease in the toxic oil syndrome. J Am Coll Cardiol 1991;18:1539–1545.
68. Rich S, ed: Primary Pulmonary Hypertension: Executive Summary from the World Symposium-Primary Pulmonary Hypertension 1998. Available from the World Health Organization at http://www.who.int/ncd/dvd/pph.html.
69. Packer M, Greenberg B, Massie B, Dash H: Deleterious effects of hydralazine in patients with pulmonary hypertension. N Engl J Med 1982;306(22): 1326–1331.
70. Packer M, Medina N, Yushak M, Weiner I: Detrimental effects of verapamil in patients with primary pulmonary hypertension. Br Heart J 1984;52(1): 106–111.
71. Lockshin MD: Antiphospholipid antibody syndrome. JAMA 1992;268: 1451–1453.
72. Luchi ME, Asherson RA, Lahita RG: Primary idiopathic pulmonary hypertension complicated by pulmonary arterial thrombosis. Association with antiphospholipid antibodies. Arthritis Rheum 1992;35:700–705.
73. Liu XY, Nelson D, Grant C, Morthland V, Goodnight SH, Press RD: Molecular detection of a common mutation in coagulation factor V causing thrombosis via hereditary resistance to activated protein C. Diagn Mol Pathol 1995;4(3):191–197.
74. Poort SR, Rosendaal FR, Reitsma PH, Bertina RM: A common genetic variation in the 3'-untranslated region of the prothrombin gene is associated with elevated plasma prothrombin levels and an increase in venous thrombosis. Blood 1996;88(10):3698–3703.
75. Thompson BT, Spence CR, Janssens SP, Joseph PM, Hales CA: Inhibition of hypoxic pulmonary hypertension by heparins of differing antiproliferative potency. Am J Respir Crit Care Med 1994;149:1512–1517.
76. Benitz WE, Lessler DS, Coulson JD, Bernfield M: Heparin inhibits proliferation of fetal vascular smooth muscle cells in the absence of platelet derived growth factor. J Cell Physiol 1986;127:1–7.
77. Sitbon O, Humbert M, Ioos et al: Who benefits from long-term calcium-channel blocker (CCB) therapy in primary pulmonary hypertension (PPH)? Am J Respir Crit Care Med 2003;167:A440.
78. Barst RJ: Pulmonary hypertension. In: Goldman L, Ausielo D, eds: Cecil Textbook of Medicine, 22nd ed. Philadelphia, PA: WB Saunders, Elsevier Science, 2003, pp 363–370.
79. Barst RJ, Rubin LJ, Long WA, McGoon MD, Rich S, Badesch DB, et al: A comparison of continuous intravenous epoprostenol (prostacyclin) with conventional therapy for primary pulmonary hypertension. The Primary Pulmonary Hypertension Study Group. N Engl J Med 1996; 334(5):296–302.
80. Shapiro SM, Oudiz RJ, Cao T, Romano MA, Beckmann XJ, Georgiou D, et al: Primary pulmonary hypertension. Improved long-term effects and survival with continuous intravenous epoprostenol infusion. J Am Coll Cardiol 1997;30(2):343–349.
81. McLaughlin VV, Genthner DE, Panella MM, Rich S: Reduction in pulmonary vascular resistance with long-term epoprostenol (prostacyclin) therapy in primary pulmonary hypertension [see comments]. N Engl J Med 1998;338(5):273–277.
82. Okano Y, Yoshioka T, Shimouchi A, Satoh T, Kunieda T: Orally active prostacyclin analogue in primary pulmonary. Lancet 1997;349:1365.
83. Galie N, Manes A, Branzi A: The new clinical trials on pharmacological treatment in pulmonary arterial hypertension. Eur Respir J 2002;20:1037–1049.
84. Saji T, Ozawa Y, Ishikita T, Matsuura H, Matsuo N: Short-term hemodynamic effect of a new oral PGI2 analogue, beraprost, in primary and secondary pulmonary hypertension. Am J Cardiol 1996;78:244–247.
85. Nagaya N, Uematsu M, Okano Y, Satoh T, Kyotani S, Sakamaki F, et al: Effect of orally active prostacyclin analogue on survival of outpatients with primary pulmonary hypertension. J Am Coll Cardiol 1999;4:1188–1192.
86. Galie N, Humbert M, Vachiery JL, et al: Arterial Pulmonary Hypertension and Beraprost European (ALPHABET) Study Group. Effects of beraprost sodium, an oral prostacyclin analogue, in patients with pulmonary arterial hypertension. A randomized, double-blind, placebo-controlled trial. J Am Coll Cardiol 2002;39:496–502.
87. Barst RJ, McGoon M, McLaughlin V, Tapson V, Rich S, Rubin L, et al, for the Beraprost Study Group: Beraprost therapy for pulmonary arterial hypertension. J Am Coll Cardiol 2003;41(12):2119–2125.
88. Kaukinen S, Ylitalo P, Pessi T, Vapaatalo H: Hemodynamic effects of Iloprost, a prostacyclin analogue. Clin Pharm Ther 1984;36:464–469.
89. Schror K, Darius H, Matzky R, Ohlendorf R: The anti-platelet and cardiovascular actions of a new carbacyclin derivative (ZK36374)—equipotent to PGI2 in vitro. Arch Pharmacol 1981;316:252–255.
90. Bugiardini R, Galvani M, Ferrini D, Gridelli C, Mari L, Puddu P, et al: Effects of Iloprost, a stable prostacyclin analogue, on exercise capacity and platelet aggregation in stable angina pectoris. Am J Cardiol 1986;58: 453–459.
91. Skuballa W, Raduchel B, Vorbruggen H: Chemistry of stable prostacyclin analogues; synthesis of Iloprost. In: Gryglewski RS, Stock G, eds: Prostacyclin and Its Stable Analogue Iloprost. Berlin, Germany: Springer, 1987, pp 17–24.
92. Hoeper MM, Olschewski H, Ghofrani HA, Wilkens H, Winkler J, Borst MM, et al: A comparison of the acute hemodynamic effects of inhaled nitric oxide and aerosolized iloprost in primary pulmonary hypertension. J Am Coll Cardiol 2000;35:176–182.
93. Olschewski H, Ghofrani HA, Schmehl T, Winkler J, Wilkens H, Hoper MM, et al: inhaled iloprost to treat severe pulmonary hypertension. An uncontrolled trial. German PPH Study Group. Ann Intern Med 2000; 132:435–443.
94. Hoeper MM, Schwarze M, Ehlerding S, Adler-Schuermeyer A, Spiekerkoetter E, Niedermeyer J, et al: Long-term treatment of primary pulmonary hypertension with aerosolized iloprost, a prostacyclin analogue. N Engl J Med 2000;342:1866–1870.
95. Wensel R, Opitz CF, Ewer R, Bruch L, Kleber FX: Effects of iloprost inhalation on exercise capacity and ventilatory efficiency in patients with primary pulmonary hypertension. Circulation 2000;101:2388–2892.
96. Olschewski H, Simonneau G, Galie N, Higenbottam T, Naeije R, Rubin LJ, et al: Aerosolized Iloprost Randomized Study Group: Inhaled iloprost for severe pulmonary hypertension. N Engl J Med 2002;347: 322–329.
97. Rimensberger PC, Spahr-Schopfer I, Berner M, Jaeggi E, Kalangos A, Friedli B, et al: NO versus aerosolized iloprost in secondary pulmonary hypertension in children with congenital heart disease. Vasodilator capacity and cellular mechanisms. Circulation 2001;103:544–548.
98. Gaine SP, Barst RJ, Rich S, Brundage BH, Bourge R, Rubin LJ, et al: Acute hemodynamic effects of subcutaneous UT-15 in primary pulmonary hypertension. Am J Respir Crit Care Med 1999;159:A161.
99. Barst RJ, Simonneau G, Rich S, Blackburn SD, Naeije R, Galie N, et al, for the Uniprost PAH Study Group: Efficacy and safety of chronic subcutaneous infusion of UT-15 (Uniprost) in pulmonary arterial hypertension (PAH). Circulation 2000;102:100–101.
100. Barst RJ, Horn EM, Widlitz AC, Goudie SM, Kerstein D, Berman-Rosenzweig E: Efficacy of long-term subcutaneous infusion of UT-15 in primary pulmonary hypertension. Eur Heart J 2000;21:315.
101. Yanagisawa M, Kurihara H, Kimura S, Tomobe Y, Kobayashi M, Mitsui Y, et al: A novel potent vasoconstrictor peptide produced by vascular endothelial cells. Nature 1988;332:411–415.
102. Galie N, Grigioni F, Bacchi-Reggiani L, et al: Relation of endothelin-1 to survival in patients with primary pulmonary hypertension. Eur J Clin Invest 1996;26:273.
103. Ohlstein EH, Douglas SA: Endothelin-1 modulates vascular smooth muscle structure and vasomotion. Implications in cardiovascular pathology. Drug Dev Res 1993;29:108–128.
104. Fukuroda T, Fujikawa T, Ozaki S, Ishikawa K, Yano M, Nishikibe M: Clearance of circulating endothelin-1 by ET_B receptors in rats. Biochem Biophys Res Commun 1994;199:1461–1465.
105. Ozaki S, Ohwaki K, Ihara M, Fukuroda T, Ishikawa K, Yano M: ET_B-mediated regulation of extracellular levels of endothelin-1 in cultured endothelial cells. Biochem Biophys Res Commun 1995;209:483–489.
106. Channick RN, Simonneau G, Sitbon O, Robbins IM, Frost A, Tapson VF, et al: Effects of the dual endothelin-receptor antagonist bosentan in patients with pulmonary hypertension. A randomised placebo-controlled study. Lancet 2001;358:1119–1123.

107. Rubin LJ, Badesch DB, Barst RJ, Galie N, Black CM, Keogh A, et al: Bosentan therapy for pulmonary arterial hypertension. N Engl J Med 2002;346:896–903.
108. Barst RJ, Ivy D, Dingemanse J, et al: Pharmacokinetics, safety, and efficacy of bosentan in pediatric patients with pulmonary arterial hypertension. Clin Pharm Ther 2003;73:37–82.
109. Roux S, Breu V, Ertel S, Clozel M: Endothelin antagonism with bosentan. A review of potential applications. J Mol Med 1999;77:364–376.
110. Barst RJ, Rich S, Widlitz A, Horn EM, McLaughlin V, McFarlin J: Clinical efficacy of sitaxsentan, an endothelin A receptor antagonist, in patients with pulmonary arterial hypertension. Open label pilot study. Chest 2002; 121:1860–1868.
111. Barst RJ, Langleben D, Frost A, et al, for the STRIDE Study Group: Sitaxsentan, a selective ET-A receptor antagonist, improves exercise capacity and NYHA functional class in pulmonary arterial hypertension (PAH). Am J Respir Crit Care Med 2004;164(4):441–447.
112. Frostell C, Fratacci MD, Wain JC, Jones R, Zapol WM: Inhaled nitric oxide. A selective pulmonary vasodilator reversing hypoxic pulmonary vasoconstriction. Circulation 1991;83:2038–2047.
113. The Neonatal Inhaled Nitric Oxide Study Group: Inhaled nitric oxide in full-term and nearly full-term infants with hypoxic respiratory failure. N Engl J Med 1997;336:597–604.
114. Clark RH, Kueser TJ, Walker MW, Southgate WM, Huckaby JL, Perez JA, et al: Low-dose nitric oxide therapy for persistent pulmonary hypertension of the newborn. Clinical Inhaled Nitric Oxide Research Group. N Engl J Med 2000;342:469–474.
115. Channick RN, Newhart JW, Johnson FW, Williams PJ, Auger WR, Fedullo PF, et al: Pulsed delivery of inhaled nitric oxide to patients with primary pulmonary hypertension. An ambulatory delivery system and initial clinical tests. Chest 1996;109:1545–1559.
116. Abrams D, Schulze-Neick I, Magee AG: Sildenafil as a selective pulmonary vasodilator in childhood primary pulmonary hypertension. Heart 2000; 84:E4.
117. Prasad S, Wilkinson J, Gatzoulis MA: Sildenafil in primary pulmonary hypertension. N Engl J Med 2000;343:1342.
118. Schulze-Neick I, Hartenstein P, Li J: Intravenous sildenafil is a potent pulmonary vasodilator in children with congenital heart disease. Circulation 2003;108:II-167–II-173.
119. Sastry BKS, Narasimhan C, Krishna Reddy N, Soma Raju B: Clinical efficacy of sildenafil in primary pulmonary hypertension. J Am Coll Cardiol 2004;43(7):1149–1153.
120. Cowan KN, Heilbut A, Humpl T, Lam C, Ito S, Rabinovitch M: Complete reversal of fatal pulmonary hypertension in rats by a serine elastase inhibitor. Nat Med 2000;6(6):698–702.
121. Cowan KN, Jones PL, Rabinovitch M: Elastase and matrix metalloproteinase inhibitors induce regression, and tenascin-C antisense prevents progression of vascular disease. J Clin Invest 2000;105:21–34.
122. Takemoto M, Liao JK: Pleiotropic effects of 3-hydroxy-3-methylglutaryl coenzyme a reductase inhibitor. Arterioscler Thromb Vasc Biol 2001;21: 1712–1719.
123. Girgis RE, Li D, Zhan X, Garcia JG, Tuder RM, Hassoun PM, et al: Attenuation of chronic hypoxic pulmonary hypertension by simvastatin. Am J Heart Circ Physiol 2003;10:H938–H945.
124. Ngai P, Basner RC, Yoney AM, Jelic S, Koumbourlis AC, Barst RJ: Nocturnal oxygen desaturation predicts poorer pulmonary hemodynamics in children with primary pulmonary hypertension. Am J Respir Crit Care Med 2002;165:A99.
125. Boyer JJ, et al: Effect of long-term oxygen treatment at home in children with pulmonary vascular disease. Br Heart J 1985;55:385–390.
126. Sandoval J, Aguirre JS, Pulido T, Martinez-Guerra ML, Santos E, Alvarado P, et al: Nocturnal oxygen therapy in patients with Eisenmenger syndrome. Am J Respir Crit Care Med 2001;164:1682–1687.
127. Rich S, Seidlitz M, Dodin E, Osimani D, Judd D, Genthner D, et al: The short-term effects of digoxin in patients with right ventricular dysfunction from pulmonary hypertension. Chest 1998;114:787–792.
128. Thilenius OG, Nadas AS, Jockin H: Primary pulmonary vascular obstruction in children. Pediatrics 1965;36:75–87.
129. Rozkovec A, Montanes P, Oakley CM: Factors that influence the outcome of primary pulmonary hypertension. Br Heart J 1986;55:449–458.
130. Rich S, Lam W: Atrial septostomy as palliative therapy for refractory primary pulmonary hypertension. Am J Cardiol 1983;51:1560–1561.
131. Nihill MR, O'Laughlin MP, Mullins CE: Blade balloon atrial septostomy is effective palliation for terminal cor pulmonary. Am J Cardiol 1987;60:1.
132. Hausknecht MJ, Sims RE, Nihill MR, Cashion WR: Successful palliation of primary pulmonary hypertension by atrial septostomy. Am J Cardiol 1990;65:1045–1046.
133. Kerstein D, Levy PS, Hsu DT, Hordof AJ, Gersony WM, Barst RJ: Blade balloon atrial septostomy in patients with severe primary pulmonary hypertension. Circulation 1995;91:2028–2035.
134. Sandoval J, Gaspar J, Pulido T, Bautista E, Martinez-Guerra ML, Zeballos M, et al: Graded balloon dilation atrial septostomy in severe primary pulmonary hypertension. A therapeutic alternative for patients nonresponsive to vasodilator treatment. J Am Coll Cardiol 1998;32:297–304.
135. Trulock EP: Lung transplantation for primary pulmonary hypertension. Clin Chest Med 2001;22:583–593.
136. Boucek MM, Novick RJ, Bennett LE, Fiol B, Keck BM, Hosenpud JD: The Registry of the International Society for Heart and Lung Transplantation. Sixth official pediatric report—2003. J Heart Lung Transplant 2003;22:636–652.
137. Trulock EP, Edwards LB, Taylor DO, Boucek MM, Mohacsi PJ, Keck BM, et al: The Registry of the International Society for Heart and Lung Transplantation. Twentieth official adult lung and heart-lung transplant report—2003. J Heart Lung Transplant 2003;22(6):625–635.
138. Clarkson PM, Frye RL, DuShane JW, Burchell HB, Wood EH, Weidman WH: Prognosis for patients with ventricular septal defect and severe pulmonary vascular obstructive disease. Circulation 1968;38:129.
139. Starnes VA, Barr ML, Schenkel FA, Horn MV, Cohen RG, Hagen JA, et al: Experience with living-donor lobar transplantation for indications other than cystic fibrosis. J Thorac Cardiovasc Surg 1997;114:917–922.
140. Starnes VA, Woo MS, MacLaughlin EF, Horn MV, Wong PC, Rowland JM, et al: Comparison of outcomes between living donor and cadaveric lung transplantation in children. Ann Thoracic Surg 1999;68:2279–2283.
141. Sandoval J, Bauerle O, Gomez A, Palomar A, Martinez Guerra ML, Furuya ME: Primary pulmonary hypertension in children. Clinical characterization and survival. J Am Coll Cardiol 1995;25:466–474.
142. Houde C, Bohn DJ, Freedom RM, Rabinovitch M: Profile of paediatric patients with pulmonary hypertension judged by responsiveness to vasodilator. Br Heart J 1993;70:461–468.
143. Clabby ML, Canter CE, Moller JH, Bridges ND: Hemodynamic data and survival in children with pulmonary hypertension. J Am Coll Cardiol 1997;30:554–560.
144. Barst RJ: Medical therapy of pulmonary hypertension. An overview of treatment and goals. Clin Chest Med 2001;22:509–515.
145. Berman Rosenzweig E, Widlitz AC, Barst RJ: Pulmonary arterial hypertension in children. State of the art. Pediatr Pulmonol 2004;38(1):2–22.

65 Sarcoidosis

Marianna M. Henry, MD • Terry L. Noah, MD

Since initial descriptions of dermatologic features more than a century ago, a coherent view of sarcoidosis has emerged that synthesizes recognition of multisystem involvement with granulomatous inflammation as a pathologic hallmark.[1,2] Granulomatous inflammation of sarcoidosis can involve virtually any organ, but typically involves the lung, eyes, skin, and lymph nodes. Young and middle-aged adults are most commonly affected, but the disorder occurs in children of any age. Clinical presentation is variable, ranging from asymptomatic individuals with hilar adenopathy to those with insidious or more acute onset of malaise, fever, cough, visual disturbances, skin rash, or other symptoms. Course of disease can be acute and self-limited, but can be chronic and, rarely, life threatening. The etiology of this multifaceted disorder remains unknown. Progress in understanding the pathogenesis of granuloma formation, including immunologic, genetic, and environmental influences, provides new insights to guide investigation and opportunity for more targeted therapy in the future.

EPIDEMIOLOGY

Investigation of the epidemiology of sarcoidosis has been challenging, related in part to the absence of precise criteria for case definition, variable disease presentation, different methods of case ascertainment, and lack of sensitive and specific diagnostic tests.[2,3] Available data demonstrate that incidence varies by age, race, and geographic location and identify other factors that relate to occurrence of disease.

INCIDENCE

In a recent population-based study in the United States, the incidence of sarcoidosis was 10.9 and 35.5 cases per 100,000 adults per year in whites and African Americans, respectively.[4] Sarcoidosis occurs less commonly in children. More than 500 cases have been reported among children; however, data concerning incidence are limited. The incidence of sarcoidosis among Danish children younger than or equal to 15 years has been reported as 0.29 per 100,000 person-years. This incidence was low compared with an incidence of 7.2 per 100,000 person-years among Danes of all ages.[5–7]

AGE

The highest incidence of sarcoidosis is in adults 20 to 50 years of age[8]; however, the disease occurs at any age, with a 2-month-old being the youngest biopsy-proven case.[9] Among children, most sarcoidosis is diagnosed in the school-age and adolescent years. In the two largest pediatric series, approximately 70% of 129 children were 8 to 15 years of age at diagnosis.[10,11] In Danish children, the incidence has been reported as 0.06 per 100,000 person-years in children younger than or equal to 4 years, with a gradual increase to 1.02 per 100,000 person-years in children 14 to 15 years of age.[7]

GENDER

Among adults, risk of disease is modestly greater for women than men.[8] Proportions of boys and girls in most pediatric series are approximately equal.

RACE

Differences in incidence based on race vary by geographic location. In the United States, studies in military populations suggest that African American adults are affected 10 to 17 times more frequently than whites,[8] although a recent population-based study conducted in a health maintenance organization demonstrated only a threefold increase in incidence in African Americans.[4] In the three largest pediatric series in the United States, approximately 75% of children were African American.[12] Wide variation by ethnicity has been reported in a London borough, where the annual incidence was 4 per 100,000 in British-born persons, 21 per 100,000 among Irish immigrants, and 58 per 100,000 in those of West Indian background.[13] In many other countries, the disease occurs most commonly in the predominant race.[14] In Scandinavian countries where the incidence of sarcoidosis is relatively high, disease occurs primarily in the white population.[15]

GEOGRAPHY

Sarcoidosis occurs worldwide, with the highest prevalence in Norway, Sweden, and Ireland, and among African Americans.[3] In the United States, studies of birthplace and residence of military personnel demonstrate the highest prevalence in South Atlantic and Gulf states,[16–19] particularly along the coastal plains.[16] Similarly, more than 70% of pediatric cases in the United States have been reported from Virginia, the Carolinas, and Arkansas,[20] and, in the largest series, 88% resided in the coastal plain of North Carolina.[10] When rates of hospitalization for sarcoidosis in South Carolina have been used as a geographic indicator, higher rates have been observed in counties located along the coastline, a finding not explained by socioeconomic status or several health care indicators.[21] Rural residence has been observed to confer increased risk for disease.[16,19] Studies of rural exposures have been inconclusive,[3,22,23] although a recent case-control study demonstrated increased risk associated with use of wood stoves, fireplaces, nonpublic water sources, and farm life.[24]

TIME-SPACE/ENVIRONMENTAL FACTORS AND FAMILIAL CLUSTERING

Evidence for a time-space association was identified in a cluster analysis of data from the Isle of Man.[25,26] A greater than expected number of "case pairs" (i.e., pairs of affected individuals) lived or worked in close proximity or were diagnosed within a 3-year period. Eighteen percent of case pairs were blood relatives. These data support potential person-to-person transmission or a common exposure, but also suggest an underlying hereditary risk.[8] A recent case-control study involving Navy personnel has demonstrated that having had only "clean ship" assignments (i.e., occupations with less exposure to dusty, manual labor) was associated with a decreased risk for diagnosis of sarcoidosis as compared with "industrial-like" assignments. This protective effect was greater for African Americans than for whites and has lessened in recent decades as practices to reduce potential toxic exposures have been implemented.[27] Recent focus on genetic factors has followed numerous reports of familial clustering. Fourteen percent of adults with sarcoidosis had an affected first- or second-degree relative in a survey conducted in Michigan.[28] In a large multicenter case-control study, first- or second-degree relatives with a history of sarcoidosis were approximately four times more likely to be related to a case than to a control.[29] It is commonly hypothesized that an interaction of hereditary and environmental factors underlies pathogenesis.

PATHOGENESIS/IMMUNOPATHOLOGY

Sarcoidosis is the result of a granulomatous immune response in the lung, lymphatics, and other tissues. The histopathologic hallmark of sarcoidosis is the presence in multiple organs of noncaseating granulomas that do not stain for acid-fast bacilli or fungi.[2] The granulomas consist of organized collections of predominantly $CD4^+$ T lymphocytes and mononuclear phagocytes (epithelioid cells and giant cells). In the lung, most are located in perilymphatic areas, including near bronchioles, in the subpleural space, and in perilobular spaces (Fig. 65-1). Sarcoid granulomas in the lung may resolve or progress to fibrosis. While tightly organized, non-necrotizing granulomas are typical, there are case reports in children of a rare "necrotizing sarcoid granulomatosis" usually associated with vasculitis and presenting with multiple nodular lung opacities.[30,31]

GRANULOMA FORMATION

The pathogenesis of granuloma formation in sarcoidosis is probably similar to that in other granulomatous disorders such as mycobacterial infection or berylliosis. The key initial event is the presentation of antigen, in the context of class II major histocompatibility complex (MHC) molecules to T-cell receptor (TCR)–expressing T lymphocytes. In the genetically susceptible host, this interaction triggers local proliferation of T cells and mononuclear phagocytes to form granulomas, a process promoted by T-helper 1 (Th1) cytokines such as interferon-γ (IFN-γ), interleukin-2 (IL-2), and IL-18. There is some evidence that clearing of antigen and resolution of the process is dependent on humoral immunity driven by Th2 cytokines (IL-4, IL-5, IL-13), while a predominantly Th1 immune response may favor antigenic persistence and the establishment of chronic disease.[32]

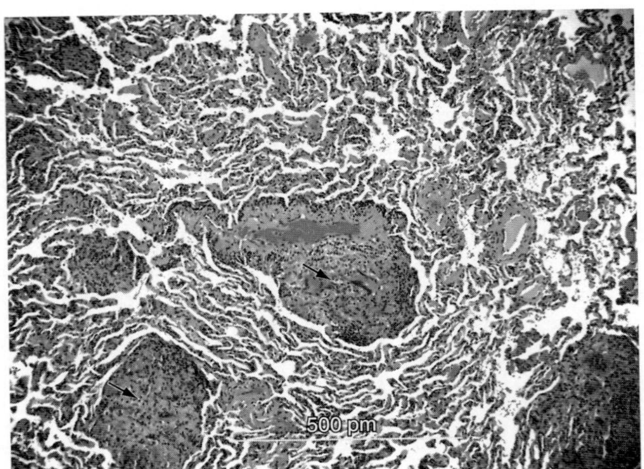

FIGURE 65-1. Biopsy of the apex of the left lung from a 15-year-old African American boy with a history of skin lesions, bilateral ankle swelling, a painful red eye, and lung infiltrate (see Fig. 65-2). Biopsy shows non-necrotizing interstitial granulomas *(arrows)*. Special stains for acid-fast bacillus and fungi were negative, as were stains for vasculitis. Similar results were found on biopsy of axillary lymph nodes. (See Color Plate 43.)

IMMUNOLOGIC FACTORS

Factors influencing granuloma formation that have been investigated in relation to sarcoidosis include alveolar macrophage function, T-lymphocyte recruitment and activation, and patterns of cytokine and chemokine expression. Sarcoid bronchoalveolar lavage fluid (BALF) contains a relative predominance of $CD4^+$ lymphocytes, which are activated as evidenced by increased expression of the Th1-promoting cytokines IL-2 and IFN-γ, and surface activation markers HLA-DR and very late antigen-1 (VLA-1).[33] Most of these studies have been carried out in adult patients. However, children with symptomatic sarcoidosis have been noted to have lymphocytosis with an elevated $CD4^+/CD8^+$ ratio in BALF.[34] A study in 11 children 4 to 16 years of age with sarcoidosis showed 25% to 30% lymphocytes in BALF, compared with an average of 9% in controls.[35] In this study, increased transcripts for IL-1β, IL-6, tumor necrosis factor-α (TNF-α), and transforming growth factor-β (TGF-β) were noted in BALF cells, but only IL-6 and TGF-β appeared to correlate with lymphocyte numbers. Katchar and colleagues[36] in Sweden noted expansion of BALF T cells bearing the TCR AV2S3 in adult patients with active sarcoidosis and reduction of this clone with recovery.[37] While studies generally indicate increased T cell–dominated inflammation in sarcoid lung disease, peripheral lymphopenia and decreased delayed cutaneous hypersensitivity test wheals to nonsarcoid antigens have been reported in active versus asymptomatic sarcoid patients,[38] suggesting that T-cell activation is antigen specific and organ specific in sarcoidosis.

Although a characteristic feature of BALF in sarcoidosis is lymphocytosis, numbers of alveolar macrophages are also increased and appear to overproduce certain matrix metalloproteinases and proinflammatory cytokines, including IL-1, TNF-α, and IL-12.[33,39] Another Th1 cytokine, IL-18, is strongly expressed in $CD68^+$ macrophages in muscle granulomas from sarcoid patients.[40] Chemokines capable of recruiting and activating T cells, such as RANTES (released on activation, normal T cell expressed and secreted), macrophage chemoattractant protein-1 (MCP-1), and macrophage inflammatory protein-1α (MIP-1α) have also been shown to be spontaneously released by BALF alveolar macrophages from sarcoid but not control patients.[41]

GENETIC FACTORS

A genetic predisposition to sarcoidosis has long been suspected because of racial and familial clustering of cases. No single gene conferring susceptibility to the disease has yet been identified. It is instead likely that susceptibility to sarcoidosis depends on multiple genes. This topic has been reviewed recently by Moller and Chen[32] and Ianuzzi and colleagues.[42] Evidence supports some impact on disease severity for specific gene polymorphisms, many but not all affecting the MHC region on chromosome 6.[43] Many studies suggesting an association between MHC molecules and sarcoidosis have focused on the class II factors, HLA-DP, -DQ, and -DR. Whether a particular MHC molecule allele has an effect on sarcoid lung disease appears to depend on the race or geographic location of the population studied. For example, in Dutch and British sarcoid patients, the HLA-DQB1*0201 allele appears to have protective effects, while HLA-DQB1*0602[44] has a negative impact. In African Americans, DQB1*0201 has no effect, while DQB1*0602 is associated with radiographic disease progression.[45] In Scandinavia, HLA-DR17$^+$ sarcoid patients appear to have a significantly better prognosis compared to HLA-DR17$^-$ patients.[46]

Associations between specific gene polymorphisms and clinical outcomes have also been investigated for cytokines or chemokines and their receptors. Polymorphisms in CCR5, TNF-β, RANTES, MCP-1, and IL-18[47–51] have all been associated with either sarcoidosis itself or, more frequently, with altered prognosis or laboratory results among populations of sarcoid patients. In aggregate, these reports support the concept that regulation of immunity is central to the pathogenesis of sarcoidosis and that there are multiple genetic influences.

ENVIRONMENTAL FACTORS

Granulomatous diseases are generally felt to represent immunologic responses to persistent or poorly degraded antigen, but the specific triggering agent for sarcoidosis remains unknown. A variety of noninfectious (pine pollen, clay soil, talc, beryllium, zirconium) and infectious (mycobacteria, propionibacterium, rickettsiae, viruses) agents have been implicated by serologic, tissue culture, and molecular techniques, but no single factor has yet been proven to be the universal cause. This topic was recently reviewed by Du Bois and colleagues.[52] Circumstantial evidence includes the study of Navy personnel that suggests that military occupations involving greater exposure to industrial dusts and fumes confer higher risks for sarcoidosis.[27]

Due to the histopathologic similarity between sarcoid and mycobacterial granulomas, mycobacterial infection has long been suspected to cause sarcoidosis. However, experimental evidence for a mycobacterial etiology is not strong. Inoculation of rabbits with BALF from sarcoid patients caused noncaseating granulomatous disease in half the animals, but polymerase chain reaction (PCR) analysis did not reveal evidence for mycobacterial infection.[53] Mycobacterial cell wall–deficient forms (CWDF) have been postulated to explain the lack of evidence for mycobacteria in sarcoid lesions using typical staining methods. CWDF have been recovered from the blood of sarcoid patients, but not in higher numbers than in controls.[54] Thus, a search for mycobacteria or their products in sarcoidosis lesions has yielded only inconsistent results. Perhaps the most compelling recent evidence for a microbial trigger for sarcoidosis is for *Propionibacterium*, a bacterial skin and intestinal commensal in normal humans. *P. acnes* and *P. granulosum* DNA has been isolated from a high proportion of lymph nodes, using quantitative PCR, in Japanese sarcoid patients.[55] This result was duplicated in an international study involving both Japanese and European patients.[56] While these sequences were also isolated fairly frequently in lymph nodes from control patients, the quantities of DNA were much higher in sarcoid patients, leading investigators to conclude that these bacteria may be an etiologic factor in sarcoidosis.

CLINICAL MANIFESTATIONS

Clinical manifestations of this multisystem disease are varied and relate to organ systems involved. Any organ can be affected. Seventy-five percent of children in the series from North Carolina had involvement of at least five areas.[10] Patterns of organ involvement may be age related, with lungs, lymph nodes, and eyes being affected more commonly in older children, while involvement of eyes, skin, and joints predominates in those younger than 5 years. Signs and symptoms result primarily from tissue infiltration and injury by pressure and displacement by granulomas.[9]

Most children are symptomatic at presentation. Common nonspecific symptoms are weight loss, cough, fatigue or lethargy, anorexia, and fever. Other symptoms related to specific organ involvement may include bone or joint pain, visual abnormalities, dyspnea, chest pain, skin rash, nausea, or abdominal pain, and those related to lymph node or parotid enlargement.[10]

LUNGS/UPPER AIRWAY

Lung involvement was documented in 80% to 100% of the largest pediatric series,[12] but is less common in young children. Chest symptoms are often limited to a dry, hacking cough with or without dyspnea[9] or chest pain. Chest examination may reveal wheezing, crackles, or diminished breath sounds, but typically is normal.

By convention, abnormalities of chest radiographs are classified as: stage 0, no intrathoracic findings; stage I, bilateral hilar lymphadenopathy with or without paratracheal adenopathy; stage II, bilateral hilar adenopathy with parenchymal infiltrate; stage III, parenchymal infiltrate without hilar adenopathy (Fig. 65-2); and stage IV, advanced fibrosis with evidence of honeycombing, hilar retraction, bullae, cysts, and emphysema.[2] Although no infiltrates are observable on plain chest radiographs in stage I disease, parenchymal granulomas are often found in lung biopsies.[2] Radiographic parenchymal abnormalities are described as small irregular interstitial, small nodular, alveolar, and fibrotic.[57]

Bilateral hilar lymph node enlargement with or without parenchymal involvement is the most frequent chest radiographic finding. Ninety percent of 128 children from the two largest series had hilar adenopathy (50% also with parenchymal abnormality), 6% had parenchymal abnormalities alone, and 4% had normal radiographs.[58] Pleural effusion and pneumothorax have been reported.[57]

Functional abnormalities consistent with restrictive lung disease (e.g., reduced forced vital capacity and total lung capacity) were documented in 50% of children from one large series.[59] Fifteen percent of these children had evidence of obstruction. Obstruction may be related to airway hyperreactivity, nodal compression, or endobronchial granuloma.

No comprehensive description of bronchoscopic findings of lower airways of affected children has been reported. In adults, mucosal nodularity (with nodules typically 2–4 mm in diameter), hypervascularity, erythema, friability, plaques and/or edema, and bronchial stenosis (related to a concentrated area of endobronchial granulomas or external lymph node compression) have been described as principal abnormalities.[60–62]

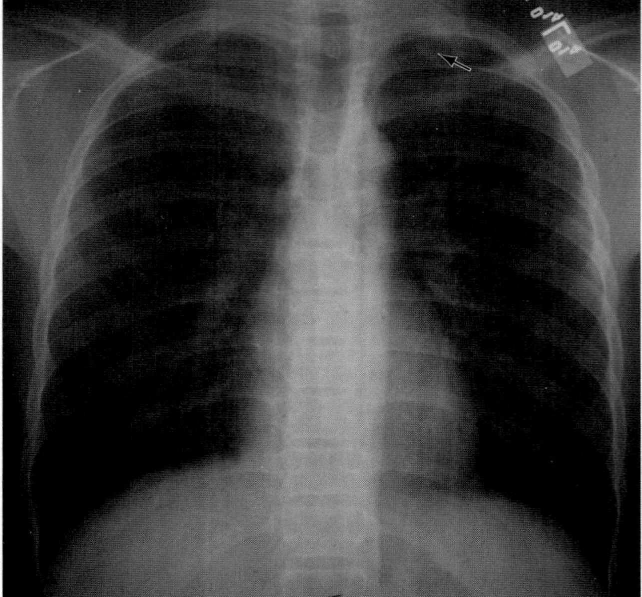

A

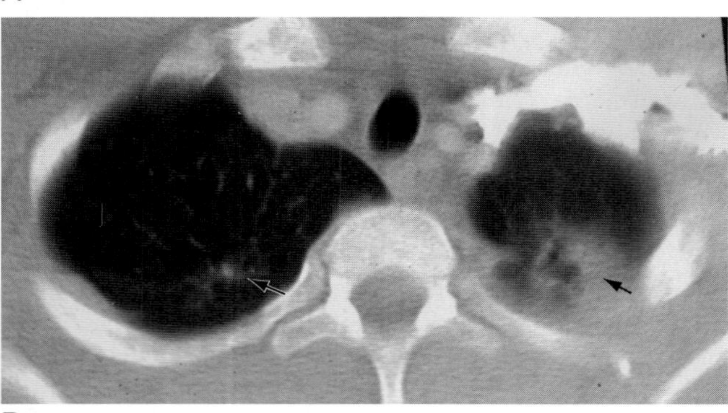

B

■ **FIGURE 65-2.** Chest radiograph **(A)** from the adolescent described in Figure 65-1 that shows an 8-mm density in the left lung apex *(arrow)*. Chest computed tomography image **(B)** shows parenchymal opacifications in the lung apices *(arrows)* and axillary adenopathy on the right (not shown). The patient was diagnosed with sarcoidosis after lung and axillary lymph node biopsies revealed typical sarcoid granulomas (see Fig. 65-1).

Sarcoidosis of the upper airway has been reported in approximately 20 children, primarily during adolescence, including several with isolated laryngeal involvement.[63–69] Signs and symptoms include hoarseness, stridor, nasal obstruction, obstructive sleep apnea, dyspnea on exertion, cough, and dysphagia. Endoscopic findings of diffuse edema with mucosal pallor of the epiglottis, arytenoids or aryepiglottic folds, laryngeal mass lesions, tonsillar and/or adenoidal hypertrophy, and swelling of nasal turbinates have been associated with noncaseating granuloma on biopsy at each site.

LYMPHATICS

Peripheral lymphadenopathy is identified in 40% to 60% of children. Cervical, axillary, epitrochlear, and inguinal nodes are most frequently enlarged.[2] Nodes are discrete, painless, and freely movable.[9]

EYES

Ocular involvement is reported in approximately 25% to 40% of children 8 to 15 years of age; however, limited data suggest that more than 60% of preschoolers have eye disease.[70–73] Symptoms include redness, pain, reduced visual acuity, and photophobia, although eye involvement is often asymptomatic in children. Because of the frequent absence of symptoms and potential for ocular complications including blindness, children with sarcoidosis must undergo complete ophthalmologic examination at diagnosis and during follow-up. Ophthalmic manifestations are classified as anterior segment, posterior segment, and orbit/lid disease.[74] Anterior segment disease is most frequently identified with anterior uveitis specifically, being the most common ocular manifestation in children.[70] Anterior uveitis is typically granulomatous, with "mutton-fat" keratic precipitates.[74,75] Iris nodules on the papillary margin or surface of the iris may be present. Detailed pediatric data are limited; however, anterior uveitis is acute and self-limited in 50% of adults, while the remaining patients have recurrent or chronic disease, potentially complicated by synechiae, glaucoma, cataract formation, and other sequelae. Conjunctival nodules constitute the most common manifestation of conjunctival involvement and provide an accessible site for biopsy. Involvement of the posterior segment is less common and may coexist with anterior disease or be present alone, and among adults is associated with increased risk for involvement of the central nervous system. Posterior segment disease includes uveitis (with findings of vitritis, chorioretinitis, retinal periphlebitis, and retinal neovascularization) and optic nerve disease, including edema of the optic disk and granulomas. Lesions characteristic of vitreous inflammation are grayish white globoid bodies (or "snowballs") often occurring in chains, while retinal lesions are typically yellow, discrete retinal and choroidal infiltrates around retinal veins described as "candle wax drippings."[74] Macular edema may develop consequent to retinal and choroidal inflammation and result in diminished visual acuity.[76] Orbital involvement is uncommon. Lacrimal gland involvement may interfere with tearing and present with enlargement identifiable on examination or by gallium or computed tomography (CT) scan. Rarely, inflammation of orbital tissue is manifested as pain, reduced vision and extraocular movement, and proptosis.[74]

SKIN

Skin involvement occurs in 25% to 40% of older children and 80% of preschoolers and may be present at diagnosis or later in the course of disease. Lesions likely to demonstrate characteristic noncaseating granulomas on biopsy include small papules, nodules, plaques, changes in old scars, subcutaneous nodules, and, rarely, icthyosis and erythematous scaly patches.[77] Small papules, red to yellowish brown or violaceous in color, that occur on eyelids, nasolabial folds, and other areas of the face are among the most common lesions. Plaques tend to be larger, round to oval, brownish red or hypopigmented, indurated lesions that occur on the face, trunk, buttocks, and extremities.[78,79] Lupus pernio, a distinctive violaceous plaque occurring primarily on the nose, lips, cheeks, ears, and fingers, is described primarily in African American women and is associated with involvement of nasal mucosa, pulmonary fibrosis, and bone cysts.[2,77] Plaques, lupus pernio, and granulomatous infiltrations of old scars have been associated with chronic disease in adults.[79,80] Subcutaneous nodules are painless, round to oval, mobile lesions found on the trunk and extremities. Erythema nodosum, a lesion consisting of erythematous, raised, tender nodules on the anterior aspects of the legs without granuloma on biopsy, is a nonspecific but common feature of acute disease in adults often associated with painful swelling of adjacent joints. Although considered rare in childhood, this lesion has been reported in well-documented cases in young children.[71,81]

KIDNEYS/CALCIUM METABOLISM

Renal involvement includes calcemic nephropathy, granulomatous interstitial nephritis, glomerulopathy, and hypertension related to chronic renal failure.[82–84] Abnormal calcium metabolism is the most common cause of renal dysfunction. Extrarenal production of 1,25-hydroxyvitamin D (calcitriol) by macrophages leads to hypercalcemia, an abnormality reported in 30% of children. Hypercalciuria with or without hypercalcemia is less well documented, but was identified in 67% of children in one series.[10] Nephrolithiasis and nephrocalcinosis are consequences of the increased renal load of calcium. Renal granulomas are relatively common (found in 15%–40% of adults) and often do not affect renal function, but may be associated with renal failure. Glomerular disease, reported as membranous nephropathy in children, occurs rarely.[85]

BONES/JOINTS

Musculoskeletal manifestations are reported in approximately 20% of children overall,[10] but they are much more common among preschool children.[86] In a registry established by pediatric rheumatologists comprising 53 children, 38 children (72%) had persistent arthritis that was apparent at presentation in 42%. Seventy-two percent of children in this registry were younger than or equal to 5 years. The arthritis is typically polyarticular, involving the knees, ankles, and wrists and other joints less commonly, and often presents with synovial hypertrophy and large effusions. Pain and restricted motion may be absent Although differences in severity are reported, morning stiffness, symmetric small joint involvement, and joint destruction with restriction may develop over time.[72,73,87,88] Lytic bone lesions of the hands or feet (often accompanying skin manifestations), osteoporosis, and muscle involvement (myopathy or myositis) occur uncommonly.[78,89,90]

LIVER/SPLEEN

Enlargement of the liver or spleen occurs in 20% to 40% of affected children. Mild elevations of liver function tests (alkaline phosphatase, transaminases, and bilirubin) are frequent; however, severe symptomatic disease with cirrhosis or portal hypertension is rare. Low-attenuation nodules in the liver and/or spleen, possibly related to coalescence of microscopic granulomas, have been identified infrequently on abdominal CT scan.[91] Hepatic granulomas located commonly in the portal/periportal areas are reported in greater than 50% of liver biopsy specimens from patients with clinical evidence of liver disease, including three other categories of abnormalities: cholestatic (58%), necroinflammatory or hepatitis-like (41%), and vascular (20%).[20,92]

HEART/BLOOD VESSELS

Granulomatous involvement of the heart has been identified at autopsy in 27% of 84 consecutive examinations in adults with sarcoidosis; however, clinically apparent involvement of the heart has been estimated to occur in 5% of adults.[93,94] Cardiac involvement appears to be rare in children.[95–97] Complete heart block and ventricular dysrhythmias related to granulomatous infiltration are the most common manifestations and may precipitate sudden death, an outcome reported in a substantial proportion of adults with cardiac involvement. Cardiomyopathy, papillary muscle dysfunction, ventricular aneurysm, and pericardial effusion are also reported.

Vasculitis involving small, medium, and large vessels is well-documented in adults but reported infrequently in children.[98–102]

PAROTID GLAND

Unilateral or bilateral parotid enlargement is relatively common, identified in 20% to 40% of children in large series.[10] Uveoparotid fever or Heerfordt's syndrome (parotid enlargement with fever, anterior uveitis, and cranial nerve palsy) is rarely reported in children.[2] The enlarged parotid is nontender and smooth. Hyposialia is reported to be frequent and may be associated with dry mouth and xerostomia.[103]

NERVOUS SYSTEM/ENDOCRINE GLANDS

Neurologic involvement is estimated to occur in 5% to 10% of adults with sarcoidosis and is considered rare in children.[104,105] Neurologic manifestations include cranial nerve abnormalities, particularly involving the facial nerve, granulomatous meningitis, space-occupying masses, communicating or obstructive hydrocephalus, peripheral neuropathy, spinal cord involvement, psychiatric symptoms, and hypothalamic and/or pituitary lesions.[78,106,107] In a recent literature review of 29 children with neurologic involvement (48% of whom were younger than 13 years, range 3 months to 18 years), seizures were the most common presentation (38% but occurring in 75% of children younger than 13 years) followed by intracranial mass lesions (24%), cranial nerve involvement (21%, all older than 11 years), and hypothalamic dysfunction (21%).[105] Patterns of presentation, dominated by seizures in prepubertal children and cranial nerve involvement in older children, were suggested. Hypothalamic and/or pituitary involvement may present as diabetes insipidus, secondary amenorrhea, or growth hormone deficiency.[108–111]

SARCOIDOSIS IN YOUNG CHILDREN

Children younger than 5 years present with a constellation of symptoms that appear to be relatively distinct from those of older children and adolescents. Young children are typically white and often present with rash (>80%), uveitis (>60%), and arthritis (>60%). Most (~75%) do not have evidence of pulmonary disease.[71,72,112] Symptoms and signs at presentation may cause diagnostic confusion with juvenile rheumatoid arthritis, although features of rash, arthritis, and uveitis facilitate differentiation.[88,113–115] Prognosis may be worse in the early-onset form, with complications of blindness, growth failure, cardiac involvement, and renal failure.[112]

SARCOIDOSIS AND HUMAN IMMUNODEFICIENCY VIRUS

Sarcoidosis has been described in approximately 20 adults pre- and/or postdiagnosis of human immunodeficiency virus (HIV) infection. Some cases are thought to be related to the immune restoration syndrome, occurring following treatment with highly active antiretroviral therapy and consequent increase in $CD4^+$ T lymphocytes.[116]

DIAGNOSIS

Diagnostic criteria for sarcoidosis were reviewed in the 1999 American Thoracic Society's consensus statement[2] and do not differ between children and adults. Diagnosis requires (1) a compatible clinical picture, (2) histologic evidence of noncaseating granulomas, and (3) exclusion of other conditions with similar histologic or clinical features.

In children, sarcoidosis is suspected based on clinical features such as symptoms (e.g., fevers, rashes, peripheral lymphadenopathy) or radiologic findings (e.g., hilar adenopathy). Laboratory studies are then typically obtained, including blood for complete blood count with differential, erythrocyte sedimentation rate (ESR), angiotensin-converting enzyme (ACE), immunoglobulin levels, calcium, creatinine, and liver function tests. Anemia and/or leukopenia are present in 30% to 40%, and eosinophilia is identified in 40% to 50% of affected children. Elevation of ESR and hypergammaglobulinemia are common, being present in 60% to 80% of children with sarcoidosis.[10] ACE is produced by the epithelioid cells of granulomas and is elevated in the serum of up to 80% of children[117]; however, elevated serum ACE alone is not diagnostic, since it may also be elevated in primary biliary cirrhosis, tuberculosis, diabetes, pulmonary neoplasm, and lymphoma.[15,118] While none of these tests is specific, results may increase or decrease the level of suspicion for sarcoidosis. Early in the evaluation, it is also appropriate to obtain ophthalmologic evaluation, and a tuberculin skin test should be done to exclude tuberculosis. A purified protein derivative test should be interpreted in relation to a control skin test, because impaired delayed hypersensitivity is typical. Flexible bronchoscopy may reveal abnormalities in the appearance of the airways[60–62] or a relative lymphocytosis in BALF, but is most useful in ruling out infectious causes of pulmonary manifestations.

In adults, some reports have suggested clinical or laboratory features that support a diagnosis of sarcoidosis. For example, clinical and radiographic features alone are reliable in radiographic stage I or stage II disease, and a BALF $CD4^+/CD8^+$ ratio of greater than 3.5 has been reported to be 94% specific for sarcoidosis, although relatively insensitive (53%).[119] On high-resolution chest CT, peripheral distribution of nodules, an increased number of thickened interlobular septae, and thickening of interlobar fissures were reported to differentiate sarcoidosis from other nodular lung diseases.[120] However, there are insufficient data to define the diagnostic value of these tests in children.

Biopsy is necessary to confirm the diagnosis in suspected cases. In children, a reasonable approach is to choose a biopsy site based on clinical manifestations and start with the least invasive sites, such as skin,[121] conjunctiva,[70] or superficial lymph nodes. In a series of sarcoidosis patients in Turkey, minor salivary gland biopsy of the lip yielded noncaseating granulomas in 48% of patients with proven sarcoidosis, compared with no positives in tuberculosis patients.[122] Muscle biopsy may prove useful as well. Gastrocnemius muscle biopsy was reported to be diagnostic for sarcoidosis in 22 adult patients with hilar adenopathy,[123] and a 10-year-old presenting with muscle weakness was diagnosed with sarcoidosis after muscle biopsy showed noncaseating granulomas.[90] In patients with evidence of liver disease, liver biopsy may be diagnostic.[115] In children with pulmonary manifestations of sarcoidosis but without appropriate superficial sites for tissue procurement, biopsy of lung or mediastinal nodes should be considered. In adult patients, transbronchial biopsy has a high diagnostic yield,[60–62] but this procedure is not feasible in most younger children. Biopsy of mucosal lesions in the lower airways has also added to diagnostic yield in adult patients.[60–62] If no easily accessible biopsy sites are identified and mediastinal adenopathy is present, biopsy of mediastinal nodes by mediastinoscopy should be considered. Fine-needle aspiration biopsy of hilar lymph nodes has been reported to accurately diagnose sarcoid granulomas, as confirmed by subsequent excisional biopsy, in patients as young as 12 years.[124] Biopsy of the larynx,[69] tonsils,[125] and lung[30,126] have been reported as diagnostic for sarcoidosis in children with clinical findings localized to those organs.

Once diagnosis is made, additional evaluations are indicated to assess the severity and need for therapy of lung disease, diagnose disease of other organ systems, and monitor course of disease. Serial determination of lung function may be helpful in assessing effects of corticosteroid treatment. Chest CT may be useful for defining the presence and type of interstitial changes; patterns of fibrosis have been correlated with lung function abnormalities in adult patients.[127] Repeated bronchoscopy for monitoring BALF lymphocytosis did not appear to be helpful in a prospective follow-up study of children with sarcoidosis.[128] Additional studies to detect and monitor extrapulmonary disease include a urinalysis, 24-hour urine collection for calcium and creatinine clearance, serial screening studies such as ESR, ACE, renal and liver function, repeated ophthalmologic examination, and electrocardiography.[73,84,97,102,129] Twenty-four-hour Holter monitoring, echocardiography, exercise testing, cardiac catheterization with endomyocardial biopsy, electrophysiologic studies, cardiac MRI, and radionuclide imaging with thallium 201 and gallium 67 should be considered in evaluation of children with suspected cardiac involvement.[130] Because of the potential for sudden death, aggressive evaluation and treatment with cardiology consultation are required. Evaluation by cranial MRI has been advocated, even in children without neurologic symptoms, because significant central nervous system involvement may be asymptomatic.[131] Other testing may be indicated depending on specific organ involvement.

TREATMENT

Decisions concerning treatment of pulmonary disease are complex, requiring consideration of extent and severity of disease, probability of spontaneous resolution, and risks of therapy. Radiographic staging has been used to guide therapy of adults based on recognition that spontaneous remissions occur in 60% to 90% of patients with stage I, 40% to 70% with stage II, 10% to 20% with stage III, and 0% with stage IV disease.[132] Although formal consensus data are limited, similar principles of therapy have been applied to children. Asymptomatic children with hilar adenopathy alone do not generally require therapy. Therapy should be considered for children with severe cough, dyspnea, progressive reduction in lung function, or significant or worsening radiographic findings.[5,58]

Indications for treatment of extrapulmonary disease include ophthalmologic involvement not treatable with topical therapy, neurologic disease, myocardial involvement, hypercalcemia, hypercalciuria and potentially other rare renal manifestations, severe cutaneous lesions, and prolonged constitutional symptoms. Joint disease and significant hepatic disease may also require therapy.[2,5,58,132]

The objective of therapy is reduction of inflammation and granuloma formation to limit development of progressive fibrosis and organ dysfunction. Although progress in understanding the pathogenesis of granuloma formation offers potential for targeted immunosuppression, nonspecific anti-inflammatory therapy with systemic corticosteroids is currently used most frequently to attempt to reverse disease or prevent progression.[133]

Although corticosteroid therapy has been widely observed to alleviate symptoms and improve disease manifestations, efficacy of corticosteroid therapy for lung disease remains controversial. A meta-analysis of a modest number of randomized controlled trials of treatment with oral corticosteroids found greater improvement in chest radiographs in treated versus control adults with stage II and III disease.[134] Data concerning lung function could not be combined and were inconsistent. Available data did not suggest that corticosteroid therapy alters long-term progression of disease. Clinical efficacy of inhaled corticosteroids administered alone or in combination with oral corticosteroids has not been demonstrated consistently.[2,134] Interpretation of these studies is complicated by differences in study populations, treatment protocols, and lack of a gold standard for disease activity.[132] No randomized controlled trials of corticosteroid therapy have been reported in children. Small studies report improvement in radiographs and spirometry among children treated with combined oral/inhaled[135] or oral[34] corticosteroids alone, although serial bronchoalveolar lavage performed in a small group showed persistence of an elevated proportion of T lymphocytes and $CD4^+/CD8^+$ ratios despite oral therapy.[34]

The optimal dose and length of corticosteroid therapy have not been evaluated in randomized, controlled trials. Treatment protocols for children vary modestly, but most suggest initiating treatment with 1 mg/kg/day of prednisone or prednisolone. Gradual reduction to a maintenance dose should begin when symptoms or manifestations have improved, typically after 4 to 8 weeks. This maintenance dose is the lowest dose that controls symptoms, often in the range of 10 to 15 mg given daily or, if possible, every other day.[5,58] Depending on the organs involved and response, maintenance therapy should be continued for 3 to 6 months and then tapered. Total duration of therapy is typically at least 6 months. Relapses that occur during tapering or following completion of therapy may require reinitiation of treatment using a similar regimen. Corticosteroid therapy requires individualization and monitoring for side effects.

Alternatives to steroid therapy have been used in adults for progressive disease poorly responsive to corticosteroids or as steroid-sparing agents. These include methotrexate, antimalarial agents (chloroquine and hydroxchloroquine), azathioprine, cyclophosphamide, thalidomide, and infliximab.[132,133,136] Use of low-dose methotrexate has been reported in a small number of children.[20,137,138]

Organ transplantation (heart and/or lung, kidney, liver) has been performed in adults with organ failure related to sarcoidosis. Complication rates and survival have been comparable with those undergoing transplantation for other indications, although development of granulomas in transplanted lungs has been reported.[139,140]

■ PROGNOSIS

In older children and adults, the overall prognosis of sarcoidosis is good. Spontaneous remission occurs in two thirds of patients, while only 10% to 20% of patients have long-term pulmonary or extrapulmonary sequelae. Increased risk for developing chronic or progressive disease among adults is associated with lupus pernio, uveitis, chronic hypercalcemia, nephrocalcinosis, African American race, cystic bone lesions, neurosarcoidosis, and radiographic stage III or stage IV lung disease.[2] The proportion of patients progressing from one stage of lung disease to another appears to be small.[141] Prognosis of eye disease is apparently unrelated to the extent of extraocular disease at onset.[142] Sarcoidosis is fatal in 1% to 5% of patients due to cardiac, pulmonary, or neurologic complications. Children younger than 5 years who present with involvement of eyes, skin, and joints may have a poorer long-term prognosis than older children, who typically present with lung disease and have a similar prognosis as young adults.[5] However, Roy and colleagues[81] reported a case of sarcoidosis presenting at age 3 months with a good long-term outcome.

Acknowledgment

The authors thank Lynn A. Fordham, MD (Pediatric Radiology), and William K. Funkhouser Jr, MD, PhD (Pathology), University of North Carolina, Chapel Hill, for their assistance with the preparation of figures.

REFERENCES

1. James DG, Sharma OP: From Hutchinson to now. A historical glimpse. Curr Opin Pulm Med 2002;8:416–423.
2. Statement on sarcoidosis. Joint Statement of the American Thoracic Society (ATS), the European Respiratory Society (ERS) and the World Association of Sarcoidosis and Other Granulomatous Disorders (WASOG) adopted by the ATS Board of Directors and by the ERS Executive Committee, February 1999. Am J Respir Crit Care Med 1999;160:736–755.
3. Bresnitz EA, Strom BL: Epidemiology of sarcoidosis. Epidemiol Rev 1983; 5:124–156.
4. Rybicki BA, Major M, Popovich J Jr, Maliarik MJ, Iannuzzi MC: Racial differences in sarcoidosis incidence. A 5-year study in a health maintenance organization. Am J Epidemiol 1997;145:234–241.
5. Milman N, Hoffmann AL, Byg K-E: Sarcoidosis in children. Epidemiology in Danes, clinical features, diagnosis, treatment and prognosis. Acta Paediatr 1998;87:871–878.
6. Byg KE, Milman N, Hansen S: Sarcoidosis in Denmark 1980–1994. A registry-based incidence study comprising 5536 patients. Sarcoidosis Vasc Diffuse Lung Dis 2003;20:46–52.
7. Hoffman AL, Milman N, Byg K-E: Childhood sarcoidosis in Denmark 1979–1994. Incidence, clinical features and laboratory results at presentation in 48 children. Acta Paediatr 2004;93:30–36.
8. Rybicki BA, Maliarik MJ, Major M, Popovich H Jr, Iannuzzi MC: Epidemiology, demographics, and genetics of sarcoidosis. Semin Respir Infect 1998;13:166–173.
9. McGovern JP, Merritt DM: Sarcoidosis in childhood. Adv Pediatr 1956;8:97–135.
10. Pattishall EN, Strope GL, Spinola SM, Denny FW: Childhood sarcoidosis. J Pediatr 1986;108:169–177.
11. Kendig EL Jr: Sarcoidosis in children. Personal observations on age distribution. Pediatr Pulmonol 1989;6:69–70.
12. Pattishall EN, Kendig EL Jr: Sarcoidosis in children. In: James DG, ed: Sarcoidosis and Other Granulomatous Disorders. New York: Marcel Dekker, 1994, pp 387–400.

13. McNicol MW, Luce PJ: Sarcoidosis in a racially mixed community. J R Coll Physicians Lond 1985;19:179–183.
14. Pattishall EN, Kendig EL Jr: Sarcoidosis in children. Pediatr Pulmonol 1996;22:195–203.
15. Sharma OP: Sarcoidosis. Dis Mon 1990;36:469–535.
16. Gentry JT, Nitowski HM, Michael M Jr: Studies on the epidemiology of sarcoidosis in the United States. Relationship to soil area and to urban-rural residence. J Clin Invest 1955;34:1839–1856.
17. Cummings MM, Dunner E, Schmidt RH Jr, Barnwell JB: Concepts of epidemiology of sarcoidosis. Postgrad Med 1956;19:437–446.
18. Cooch JW: Sarcoidosis in the United States army, 1952–1956. Am Rev Respir Dis 1961;84:103–108.
19. Sartwell PE, Edwards LB: Epidemiology of sarcoidosis in the U.S. Navy. Am J Epidemiol 1974;99:250–257.
20. Shetty AK, Gedalia A: Sarcoidosis in children. Curr Probl Pediatr 2000;30: 153–176.
21. Kajdasz DK, Judson MA, Mohr LC Jr, Lackland DT: Geographic variation in sarcoidosis in South Carolina. Its relation to socioeconomic status and health care indicators. Am J Epidemiol 1999;150:271–278.
22. Buck AA, Sartwell PE: Epidemiologic investigations of sarcoidosis. II. Skin sensitivity and environmental factors. Am J Hyg 1961;74:152–173.
23. Terris M, Chaves AD: An epidemiologic study of sarcoidosis. Am Rev Respir Dis 1966;94:50–55.
24. Kajdasz DK, Lackland DT, Mohr LC Jr, Judson MA: A current assessment of rurally linked exposures as potential risk factors for sarcoidosis. Ann Epidemiol 2001;11:111–117.
25. Parkes SA Baker SB, Bourdillon RE, Murray CRH, Rakshit M: Epidemiology of sarcoidosis in the Isle of Man - 1. A case controlled study. Thorax 1987;42:420–426.
26. Hills SE, Parkes SA, Baker SB: Epidemiology of sarcoidosis in the Isle of Man - 2. Evidence for space-time clustering. Thorax 1987;42:427–430.
27. Jajosky P: Sarcoidosis diagnoses among U.S. military personnel. Trends and ship assignment associations. Am J Prev Med 1998;14:176–183.
28. Harrington DW, Major M, Rybicki B, Popovich J, Maliarik M, Iannuzzi MC: Familial sarcoidosis. Analysis of 91 families. Sarcoidosis 1994;11:240–243.
29. Rybicki BA, Iannuzzi MC, Frederick MM, Thompson BW, Rossman MD, Bresnitz EA, et al: Familial aggregation of sarcoidosis. A case-control etiologic study of sarcoidosis (ACCESS). Am J Respir Crit Care Med 2001;164: 2085–2091.
30. Tauber E, Wojnarowski C, Horcher E, Dekan G, Frischer T: Necrotizing sarcoid granulomatosis in a 14-year-old female. Eur Respir J 1999;13:703–705.
31. Heinrich D, Gordjani N, Trusen A, Marx A, Hebestreit H: Necrotizing sarcoid granulomatosis. A rarity in childhood. Pediatr Pulmonol 2003;35: 407–411.
32. Moller R, Chen ES: Genetic basis of remitting sarcoidosis. Triumph of the trimolecular complex? Am J Respir Cell Mol Biol 2002;27:391–395.
33. Conron M, DuBois RM: Immunological mechanisms in sarcoidosis. Clin Exp Allergy 2001;31:543–554.
34. Chadelat K, Baculard A, Grimfeld A, Tournier G, Boule M, Boccon-Gibod L, et al: Pulmonary sarcoidosis in children. Serial evaluation of bronchoalveolar lavage cells during corticosteroid treatment. Pediatr Pulmonol 1993;16: 41–47.
35. Tessier V, Chadelat K, Baculard A, Housset B, Clement A: BAL in children. A controlled study of differential cytology and cytokine expression profiles by alveolar cells in pediatric sarcoidosis. Chest 1996;109:1430–1438.
36. Katchar K, Wahlstromo J, Eklund A, Grunewald J: Highly activated T-cell receptor AV2S3(=) CD4(+) lung T-cell expansions in pulmonary sarcoidosis. Am J Respir Crit Care Med 2001;163:1540–1545.
37. Grunewald I, Eklund A: Specific bronchoalveolar lavage fluid T cells associate with disease in a pair of monozygotic twins discordant for sarcoidosis. J Intern Med 2001;250:535–539.
38. Morell F, Levy G, Orriols R, Ferrer J, De Gracia J, Sampol G: Delayed cutaneous hypersensitivity tests and lymphopenia as activity markers in sarcoidosis. Chest 2002;121:1239–1244.
39. John M, Oltmanns U, Fietze I, Witt C, Jung K: Increased production of matrix metalloproteinase-2 in alveolar macrophages and regulation by interleukin-10 in patients with acute pulmonary sarcoidosis. Exp Lung Res 2002;28:55–68.
40. Fukami T, Miyazaki E, Matsumoto T, Kumamoto T, Tsuda T: Elevated expression of interleukin-18 in the granulomatous lesions of muscular sarcoidosis. Clin Immunol 2001;101:12–20.
41. Ziegenhagen MW, Muller-Quernheim J: The cytokine network in sarcoidosis and its clinical relevance. J Intern Med 2003;253:18–30.
42. Iannuzzi MC, Maliarik M, Rybicki BA: Nomination of a candidate susceptibility gene in sarcoidosis. The complement receptor 1 gene. Am J Respir Cell Mol Biol 2002;27:3–7.
43. Schurmann M, Reicehl P, Muller-Myhsok B, Schlaak M, Muller-Quernheim J, Schwinger E: Results from a genome-wide search for predisposing genes in sarcoidosis. Am J Respir Crit Care Med 2001;164:840–846.
44. Sato H, Grutters JC, Pantelidis P, Mizzon AN, Ahmad T, Van Houte AJ, et al: HLA-DQB1*0201. A marker for good prognosis in British and Dutch patients with sarcoidosis. Am J Respir Cell Mol Biol 2002;27: 406–412.
45. Iannuzzi MC: The major histocompatibility complex gene region and sarcoidosis susceptibility in African Americans. Am J Respir Crit Care Med 2003;167:444–449.
46. Planck A, Eklund A, Grunewald J: Markers of activity in clinically recovered human *leukocyte antigen-DR17-positive sarcoidosis patients. Eur Respir J 2003;21:52–57.
47. Petrek M, Drabek J, Kolek V, Zlamal J, Welsh KI, Bunce M, et al: CC chemokine receptor gene polymorphisms in Czech patients with pulmonary sarcoidosis. Am J Respir Crit Care Med 2000;162:1000–1003.
48. Yamaguchi E, Itoh A, Hizawa N, Kawakami Y: The gene polymorphism of tumor necrosis factor-beta, but not that of tumor necrosis factor-alpha, is associated with the prognosis of sarcoidosis. Chest 2001;119:753–761.
49. Takada T, Suzuki E, Ishida T, Moriyama H, Ooi H, Hasegawa T, et al: Polymorphism in RANTES chemokine promoter affects extent of sarcoidosis in a Japanese population. Tissue Antigens 2001;58:293–298.
50. Takada T, Suzuki E, Morohashi K, Geyjo F: Association of single nucleotide polymorphisms in the IL18 gene with sarcoidosis in a Japanese population. Tissue Antigens 2002;60:36–42.
51. Takada T, Suzuki E, Morohashi K, Omori K, Geyjo F: MCP-1 and MIP-1A gene polymorphisms in Japanese patients with sarcoidosis. Intern Med 2002;41:813–818.
52. Du Bois RM, Goh N, McGrath D, Cullinan P: Is there a role for microorganisms in the pathogenesis of sarcoidosis? J Intern Med 2003;253: 4–17.
53. Ikonomopoulos JA, Gorgoulis VG, Kastrinakis NG, Galanos AA, Karameris A, Kittas C: Experimental inoculation of laboratory animals with samples collected from sarcoidal patients and molecular diagnostic evaluation of the results. In Vivo 2000;14:761–765.
54. Brown ST, Brett I, Almenoff PL, Lesser M, Terrin M, Teirstein AS, et al: Recovery of cell wall–deficient organisms from blood does not distinguish between patients with sarcoidosis and control subjects. Chest 2003;123: 413–417.
55. Ishige I, Usui Y, Takemura T, Eishi Y: Quantitative PCR of mycobacterial and propionibacterial DNA in lymph modes of Japanese patients with sarcoidosis. Lancet 1999;354:120–123.
56. Eishi Y, Suga M, Ishige I, Kobayashi D, Yamada T, Takemura T, et al: Quantitative analysis of mycobacterial and propionibacterial DNA in lymph nodes of Japanese and European patients with sarcoidosis. J Clin Microbiol 2002;40:198–204.
57. Merten DF, Kirks DR, Grossman H: Pulmonary sarcoidosis in childhood. AJR Am J Roentgenol 1980;135:673–679.
58. Pattishall EN, Denny FW Jr, Kendig EL Jr: Sarcoidosis. In: Chernick V, Boat TF, Kendig EL Jr, eds: Kendig's Disorders of the Respiratory Tract in Children. Philadelphia: WB Saunders, 1998, pp 934–946.
59. Pattishall EN, Strope GL, Denny FW: Pulmonary function in children with sarcoidosis. Am Rev Respir Dis 1986;133:94–96.
60. Armstrong JR, Radke JR, Eichenhorn MS, Kvale PA, Popovich J Jr: Endoscopic findings in sarcoidosis. Characteristics and correlations with radiographic staging and bronchial mucosal biopsy yield. Ann Otol Rhinol Laryngol 1981;90:339–342.
61. Torrington KG, Shorr AF, Parker JW: Endobronchial disease and racial differences in pulmonary sarcoidosis. Chest 1997;111:619–622.
62. Chapman JT, Mehta AC: Bronchoscopy in sarcoidosis. Diagnostic and therapeutic interventions. Curr Opin Pulm Med 2003;9:402–407.
63. Kirschner BS, Holinger PH: Laryngeal obstruction in childhood sarcoidosis. J Pediatr 1976;88:263–265.
64. Neel HB, McDonald TJ: Laryngeal sarcoidosis. Ann Otol Rhinol Laryngol 1982;91:359–362.
65. Leahy F, Mina M, deSa D: Sarcoidosis of the larynx of a child. J Otolaryngol 1985;14:372–374.
66. Rybak LP, Falconer R: Pediatric laryngeal sarcoidosis. Ann Otol Rhinol Laryngol 1987;96:670–673.
67. McHugh K, deSilva M, Kilham HA: Epiglottic enlargement secondary to laryngeal sarcoidosis. Pediatr Radiol 1993;23:71.
68. Roger G, Gallas D, Tashjian G, Baculard A, Tournier G, Garabedian EN: Sarcoidosis of the upper respiratory tract in children. Int J Pediatr Otorhinolaryngol 1994;30:233–240.
69. Kenny TJ, Werkhaven J, Netterville JL: Sarcoidosis of the pediatric airway. Arch Otolaryngol Head Neck Surg 2000;126:536–539.

70. Hoover DL, Khan JA, Giangiacomo J: Pediatric ocular sarcoidosis. Surv Ophthalmol 1986;30:215–227.
71. Hetherington S: Sarcoidosis in young children. Am J Dis Child 1982;136: 13–15.
72. Hafner R, Vogel P: Sarcoidosis of early onset. A challenge for the pediatric rheumatologist. Clin Exp Rheumatol 1993;11:685–691.
73. Lindsley CB, Petty RE: Overview and report on international registry of sarcoid arthritis in childhood. Curr Rheumatol Rep 2000;2: 343–348.
74. Hunter DG, Foster CS: Ocular manifestations of sarcoidosis. In: Albert DM, Jakobiec FA, eds: Principles and Practice of Ophthalmology. Philadelphia: WB Saunders, 2000, pp 1217–1225.
75. Constantino T, Kigre K, Zimmerman P: Neuro-ophthalmic complications of sarcoidosis. Semin Neurol 2000;20:123–137.
76. Kataria S, Trevathan GE, Holland JE, Kateria YP: Ocular presentation of sarcoidosis in children. Clin Pediatr 1983;22:793–797.
77. Elgart ML: Cutaneous sarcoidosis. Definitions and types of lesions. Clin Dermatol 1986;4:35–45.
78. Lynch JP III, Sharma OP, Baughman RP: Extrapulmonary sarcoidosis. Semin Respir Infect 1998;13:229–254.
79. Mana J, Marcoval J, Graells J, Salazar A, Peyri J, Rujol R: Cutaneous involvement in sarcoidosis. Arch Dermatol 1997;133:882–888.
80. Veien NK, Stahl D, Brodthagen H: Cutaneous sarcoidosis in Caucasions. J Am Acad Dermatol 1987;16:534–540.
81. Roy M, Sharma OP, Chan K: Sarcoidosis presenting in infancy. A rare occurrence. Sarcoidosis Vasc Diffuse Lung Disease 1999;16:224–227.
82. Casella FJ, Allon M: The kidney in sarcoidosis. J Am Soc Nephrol 1993;3: 1555–1562.
83. Nocton JJ, Stork JE, Jacobs G, Newman AJ: Sarcoidosis associated with nephrocalcinosis in young children. J Pediatr 1992;121:937–940.
84. Coutant R, Leroy B, Niaudet P, Loirat C, Dommergues JP, Andre JL, et al: Renal granulomatous sarcoidosis in childhood. A report of 11 cases and a review of the literature. Eur J Pediatr 1999;158:154–159.
85. Dimitriades C, Shetty AK, Vahaskari M, Craver RD, Gedalia A: Membranous nephropathy associated with childhood sarcoidosis. Pediatr Nephrol 1999;13:444–447.
86. Rosenberg AM, Yee EH, MacKenzie JW: Arthritis in childhood sarcoidosis. J Rheumatol 1983;10:989–990.
87. Torralba KD, Quismorio P Jr: Sarcoid arthritis. A review of clinical features, pathology and therapy. Sarcoidosis Vasc Diffuse Lung Dis 2003;20: 95–103.
88. Cimaz R, Ansell BM: Sarcoidosis in the pediatric age. Clin Exp Rheumatol 2002;20:231–237.
89. Mallory SB, Paller AS, Ginsburg BC, McCrossin ID, Abernathy R: Sarcoidosis in children. Differentiation from juvenile rheumatoid arthritis. Pediatr Dermatol 1987;4:313–319.
90. Ramanan AV, Thimmarayappa AD, Baildam EM: Muscle involvement in childhood sarcoidosis and need for muscle biopsy. Ann Rheum Dis 2002;61:376–377.
91. Warshauer DM, Molina PL, Hamman SM, Koehler RE, Paulson EK, Bechtold RE, et al: Nodular sarcoidosis of the liver and spleen: analysis of 32 cases. Radiology 1995;195:757–762.
92. Devaney K, Goodman ZD, Epstein MS, Zimmerman HJ, Ishak KG: Hepatic sarcoidosis. Clinicopathologic features in 100 patients. Am J Surg Pathol 1993;17:1272–1280.
93. Silverman KJ, Hutchins GM, Bulkley BH: Cardiac sarcoid. A clinicopathologic study of 84 unselected patients with systemic sarcoidosis. Circulation 1978;58:1204–1211.
94. Swanton RH: Sarcoidosis of the heart. Eur Heart J 1988;9(Suppl G): 169–174.
95. Serwer GA, Edwards SB, Benson DW Jr, Anderson PAW, Spach M: Ventricular tachyarrhythmia due to cardiac sarcoidosis in a child. Pediatrics 1978;62:332–335.
96. Burton DA, Kapur S, Shapiro SR, Leatherbury L, Scott LP III: Fulminant cardiac sarcoidosis in childhood. Am J Cardiol 1986;58:177–178.
97. Duke C, Rosenthal E: Sudden death caused by cardiac sarcoidosis in childhood. J Cardiovasc Electrophysiol 2002;13:939–942.
98. Gross KR, Malleson PN, Culham G, Lirenman DS, McCormick AQ, Petty RE: Vasculopathy with renal artery stenosis in a child with sarcoidosis. J Pediatr 1986;108:724–726.
99. Rose CD, Eichenfield AH, Goldsmith DP, Athreya BH: Early onset sarcoidosis with aortitis—"juvenile systemic granulomatosis?" J Rheumatol 1990;17:102–106.
100. Kwong T, Valderrama E, Paley C, Ilowite N: Systemic necrotizing vasculitis associated with childhood sarcoidosis. Semin Arthritis Rheum 1994;23: 388–395.
101. Gedalia A, Shetty AK, Ward K, Correa H, Venters CL, Loe WA: Abdominal aortic aneurysm associated with childhood sarcoidosis. J Rheumatol 1996; 23:757–759.
102. Fernandes SRM, Singsen BH, Hoffman GS: Sarcoidosis and systemic vasculitis. Semin Arthritis Rheum 2002;30:33–46.
103. Olivieri D, Marvisi M: Parotid involvement in sarcoidosis. Semin Respir Med 1992;13:520–524.
104. Weinberg S, Bennett H, Weinstock I: Central nervous system manifestations of sarcoidosis in children. Clin Pediatr 1983;22:477–481.
105. Baumann RJ, Robertson WC Jr: Neurosarcoid presents differently in children than in adults. Pediatrics 2003;112:e480–e486.
106. Kidd D, Beynon HLC: The neurological complications of systemic sarcoidosis. Sarcoidosis Vasc Diffuse Lung Dis 2003;20:85–94.
107. Smith JK, Matheus MG, Castillo M: Imaging manifestations of neurosarcoidosis. AJR Am J Roentgenol 2004;182:289–295.
108. Lipnick RN, Hung W, Pandian MR: Neurosarcoidosis presenting as secondary amenorrhea in a teenager. J Adolesc Health 1993;14: 464–467.
109. Basdemir D, Clarke W, Rogol AD: Growth hormone deficiency in a child with sarcoidosis. Clin Pediatr 1999;38:315–316.
110. Konrad D, Gartenmann M, Martin E, Schoenle EJ: Central diabetes insipidus as the first manifestation of neurosarcoidosis in a 10-year-old girl. Horm Res 2000;54:98–100.
111. Murialdo G, Tamagno G: Endocrine aspects of neurosarcoidosis. J Endocrinol Invest 2002;25:650–662.
112. Fink CW, Cimaz R: Early onset sarcoidosis. Not a benign disease. J Rheumatol 1997;24:174–177.
113. Mallory SB, Paller AS, Ginsburg BC, McCrossin ID, Abernathy R: Sarcoidosis in children. Differentiation from juvenile rheumatoid arthritis. Pediatr Dermatol 1987;4:313–319.
114. Sahn EE, Hampton MT, Garen PD, Warrick J, Smith D, Silver RM: Preschool sarcoidosis masquerading as juvenile rheumatoid arthritis. Two case reports and a review of the literature. Pediatr Dermatol 1990;7: 208–213.
115. Sarigol SS, Kay MH, Wyllie R: Sarcoidosis in preschool children with hepatic involvement mimicking juvenile rheumatoid arthritis. J Pediatr Gastroenterol 1999;28:510–512.
116. Trevenzoli M, Cattelan AM, Marino F, Marchioro U, Cadrobbi P: Sarcoidosis and HIV infection. A case report and a review of the literature. Postgrad Med J 2003;70:535–538.
117. Rodriguez GE, Shin BC, Abernathy RS, Kendig EL: Serum angiotensin-converting enzyme activity in normal children and in those with sarcoidosis. J Pediatr 1981;99:68–72.
118. Saboor SA: Sarcoidosis. Br J Hosp Med 1992;48:293–302.
119. Costabel U: Sensitivity and specificity of BAL findings in sarcoidosis. Sarcoidosis 1992;9(Suppl 1):211–214.
120. Voloudaki AE, Tritou IN, Magkanas EG, Chalkiadakis GE, Siafakas NM, Gourtsoyiannis NC: HRCT in miliary lung disease. Acta Radiol 1999;40: 451–456.
121. Hunt SJ, O'toole E, Philips W, Hardman C, Wakelin SH, Walters S: A case of childhood sarcoidosis. Clin Exp Dermatol 2002;27:448–450.
122. Rybicki BA, Maliarik MJ, Posson LM, Sheffer R, Chen KM, Major M, et al: The value of labial biopsy in the differentiation of sarcoidosis from tuberculosis. Sarcoidosis Vasc Diffuse Lung Dis 2001;18:191–195.
123. Andonopoulos AP, Papadimitriou C, Melachrinou M, Meimaris N, Vlahanastasi C, Bounas A, et al: Asymptomatic gastrocnemius muscle biopsy. An extremely sensitive and specific test in the pathologic confirmation of sarcoidosis presenting with hilar adenopathy. Clin Exp Rheumatol 2001;19:569–572.
124. Tambouret R, Geisinger KR, Powers CN, Khurama KK, Silverman JF, Bardales R, et al: The clinical application and cost analysis of fine-needle aspiration biopsy in the diagnosis of mass lesions in sarcoidosis. Chest 2000;117:1004–1011.
125. Kardon DE, Thompson LD: A clinicopathologic series of 22 cases of tonsillar granulomas. Laryngoscope 2000;110:476–481.
126. Tsagris VA, Liapi-Adamidou G: Sarcoidosis in infancy. A case with pulmonary involvement as a cardinal manifestation. Eur J Pediatr 1999;158: 258–260.
127. Abehsara M, Valeyre D, Grenier P, Jailliet H, Battesti JP, Brauner MW: Sarcoidosis with pulmonary fibrosis. CT patterns and correlation with pulmonary function. AJR Am J Roentgenol 2000;174:1751–1757.
128. Baculard A, Blanc N, Boule M, Fauroux B, Chadelat K, Boccon-Gibod I, et al: Pulmonary sarcoidosis in children. A follow-up study. Eur Respir J 2001;17:628–635.
129. Amarapurkar DN, Patel ND, Amarapurkar AD: Hepatic sarcoidosis. Indian J Gastroenterol 2003;22:98–100.

130. Sharma OP: Cardiac and neurologic dysfunction in sarcoidosis. Clin Chest Med 1997;18:813–825.
131. Kone-Paut I, Portas M, Wechsler B, Girard N, Raybaud C: The pitfall of silent neurosarcoidosis. Pediatr Neurol 1999;20:215–218.
132. Baughman RP, Sharma OP, Lynch JP III: Sarcoidosis. Is therapy effective? Semin Respir Infect 1998;13:255–273.
133. Moller DR: Treatment of sarcoidosis—from a basic science point of view. J Intern Med 2003;253:31–40.
134. Paramothayan S, Jones PW: Corticosteroid therapy in pulmonary sarcoidosis. JAMA 2002;287:1301–1307.
135. Kipper N, Anadol D, Ozcelik U, Gocmen A: Inhaled corticosteroids for maintenance treatment in childhood pulmonary sarcoidosis. Acta Paediatr 2001;90:953–956.
136. Baughman PR: Therapeutic options for sarcoidosis. New and old. Curr Opin Pulm Med 2002;8:464–469.
137. Gedalia A, Molina JF, Ellis GS Jr, Galen W, Moore C, Espinoza LR: Low-dose methotrexate therapy for childhood sarcoidosis. J Pediatr 1997;130:25–29.
138. Shetty AK, Zganjar BE, Ellis GS Jr, Ludwig IH, Gedalia A: Low-dose methotrexate in the treatment of severe juvenile rheumatoid arthritis and sarcoid iritis. J Pediatr Ophthalmol Strabismus 1999;36:125–128.
139. Padilla ML, Schilero GJ, Teirstein AS: Sarcoidosis and transplantation. Sarcoidosis Vasc Diffuse Lung Dis 1997;14:16–22.
140. Martinez FJ, Orens JB, Deeb M, Brunsting LA, Flint A, Lynch JP III: Recurrence of sarcoidosis following bilateral allogeneic lung transplantion. Chest 1994;106:1597–1599.
141. Chappell AG, Cheung WY, Hutchings HA: Sarcoidosis. A long-term follow up study. Sarcoidosis Vasc Diffuse Lung Dis 2000;17:167–173.
142. Edelsten C, Pearson A, Joynes E, Stanford MR, Graham EM: The ocular and systemic prognosis of patients presenting with sarcoid uveitis. Eye 1999;13:748–753.

66 Histiocytic Disorders of the Lung

Robert J. Arceci, MD • Amir H. Shahlaee, MD

The histiocytoses are a group of rare hematopoietic disorders characterized by the clonal proliferation and pathologic accumulation of cells of the mononuclear phagocyte system (MPS) in tissues. Our understanding of this family of diseases has significantly improved since the original description by Alfred Hand in 1893. We now recognize that this family includes a spectrum of diseases ranging from Langerhans cell histiocytosis (LCH) and other disorders of the dendritic cells to disorders of macrophage/monocyte development and frank monocytic leukemia (French-American-British [FAB] M5 classification). In this chapter we will describe normal function and development of the cells of the MPS in addition to their capacity for aberrant proliferation, pathologic tissue involvement, and eventual clinical development of histiocytosis. The modern classification of these disorders, as described by the Histiocyte Society, will be utilized to describe each syndrome, its clinical presentation, and therapeutic options. Emphasis will be placed on the involvement of the pulmonary system. We also will bring attention to our increased molecular understanding of these disorders. Unfortunately, therapeutic options remain limited, and patients with extensive disease continue to have poor outcomes. Improved awareness of these syndromes hopefully will lead to increased collaborative efforts in clinical, basic, and translational research, with the ultimate goal of better care and outcomes.

MONONUCLEAR PHAGOCYTE SYSTEM

DENDRITIC CELLS AND MACROPHAGES

The MPS is a system of cells whose primary functions consist of phagocytosis of foreign material, antigen processing and antigen presentation to lymphocytes. This system was originally recognized by Ludwig Aschoff in the early part of the 20th century and termed the reticuloendothelial system. The effector cell of this system, the mononuclear phagocyte or histiocyte, represents a group of anatomically and functionally distinct cells. Histiocytosis is by definition an abnormal proliferation of cells comprising the MPS.

Cells of the MPS have a wide range of morphologic, anatomic, and functional characteristics that makes classification of this system difficult. As our knowledge of the molecular biology governing basic hematopoiesis has improved, we have been able to identify characteristics enabling us to classify and subclassify cells of the MPS. Mononuclear phagocytes are subclassified into two major classes, macrophages and dendritic cells, based on (1) phagocytic and antigen-presenting abilities, (2) morphologic and ultrastructural appearance, (3) expression of common enzymes, (4) presence of common cell surface antigens, and (5) common regulatory cytokine and transcription factor networks.

Tissue macrophages are the primary class of cells in the MPS. These cells are derived from bone marrow hematopoietic precursors and arise directly from circulating peripheral blood monocytes. Monocytes and macrophages typically have a single bean-shaped nucleus and finely granular, vacuolated cytoplasm. These cells enter different tissues and assume tissue-appropriate morphology based on the local cytokine microenvironment. Note has to be made that regardless of the location of tissue macrophages and the local cytokine stimuli, all cells of this lineage are dependent on the presence of macrophage colony-stimulating factor (M-CSF). Cells of the MPS express receptors to granulocyte-macrophage colony-stimulating factor (GM-CSF) and M-CSF, cytokines critical to the development, differentiation, and function of this system. The M-CSF receptor is a product of the *c-fms* proto-oncogene and is expressed by most members of the MPS. When bound by M-CSF, this receptor dimerizes, leading to the activation of its kinase domain and initiation of downstream signal transduction cascades. The signaling cascade initiated by the binding of M-CSF to its receptor is essential for the proliferation of progenitor cells of the monocyte-macrophage lineage, their differentiation, and their long-term survival. Most of our knowledge regarding the role of M-CSF arises from studies of the *op/op* knockout mice which are deficient in M-CSF.[1] Interestingly, despite their severe monocyte-macrophage deficiencies, *op/op* mice maintain normal levels of dendritic cells in their spleens and skin.[2,3] The GM-CSF receptor can also be found on most members of the MPS and plays a critical role in normal cellular homeostasis, differentiation, and function.[2] Macrophages have significant tissue-based differences in their morphology. For example, they can develop large amounts of cytoplasm or, alternatively, fuse to form multinucleated giant cells.[4] Peritoneal and soft tissue macrophages, Kupffer cells, foam cells, synovial cells, osteoclasts, and microglial cells are all members of this class. The tissue-dependent functional heterogeneity of macrophages is attributed to location-specific cytokine stimulation of the multipotent monocyte. More recent studies have also pointed to local proliferation of macrophages, independent of monocytic replenishment, as a potential source of macrophage diversity. This process, however, is believed to play a minor role in macrophage proliferation.[5]

Macrophages are ubiquitously distributed in the body and are heavily represented in mucosal tissues and other potential portals of entry for microorganisms where they function in both innate and adaptive immunity. They have the capacity to phagocytose foreign organisms and release inflammatory cytokines that in turn recruit other cells to the site of insult. They also maintain the ability to process and present antigenic portions of foreign organisms to T cells. Tissue macrophages have significant functional variability depending on their location within the body. In the bones as well as in the lungs these cells play a critical role in tissue growth, repair, and remodeling. Macrophages typically express lysosyme, α_1-antitrypsin, α_1-antichymotrypsin, aminopeptidase, peroxidase, alkaline phosphatase, α-naphtol-chloroacetate esterase, and β-glucouronidase.

The second class of mononuclear phagocytes, the dendritic cells, consist of dendritic cells of the lymphoid follicle, the interdigitating dendritic cell of the paracortical regions of lymph nodes, and Langerhans cells of the skin and other organs. Langerhans cells, originally identified by Paul Langerhans in 1868, are mononuclear cells with little cytoplasmic vacuolization and a folded or indented nucleus. The membranous, and often spinous tree-like, cytoplasmic aberrations from which their name is derived, are the distinguishing morphologic characteristic of dendritic cells. Electron microscopic observation of Langerhans cells reveals the presence of Birbeck granules, a distinguishing characteristic of these cells. Birbeck granules or X bodies are rod-shaped, pentalaminar, cytoplasmic structures with a central striated line, typically ending in a vesicular structure. These structures arise as a result of receptor-mediated endocytosis.

In contrast to macrophages, dendritic cells are only weakly phagocytic but play an essential role in antigen presentation. These cells are located in skin, mucosa, bone marrow, spleen, thymus, lymph nodes, and other organs. Langerhans cells and the interdigitating dendritic cells primarily present antigens to T lymphocytes. It is well established that the precursor to dendritic cells is bone marrow derived; however, the exact cell of origin and the sequence of development remain undetermined. Although dendritic cells have poor phagocytic activity, they express high levels of class II major histocompatibility complex (MHC) antigens and costimulatory receptors, making them excellent effector cells in antigen presentation. Langerhans cells express adenosine triphosphatase and higher concentrations of α-mannosidase than macrophages. These cells also have a distinguishable paranuclear and cell surface–staining pattern with peanut agglutinin that contrasts with the diffuse staining pattern demonstrated by macrophages.[4,6]

The development of monoclonal antibody technology in the 1980s significantly enhanced our knowledge of the MPS. The F4/80 antibody, a murine pan-macrophage antibody, was the first well-recognized marker of the MPS. This antibody recognizes members of a gene family that includes the human epidermal growth factor (EGF) module containing mucin-like hormone receptor 1 and CD97. The presence of this antigen on the surface of tissue macrophages and dendritic cells helped confirm the hypothesis that these cells defined the polar extremes of a continuum of cellular phenotypes that can be grouped together in one system. This proposal was subsequently confirmed with the use of transgenic mice expressing M-CSF receptor-green florescent protein.[5,7] Other markers used clinically to distinguish between these cells include S-100β subunit and CD1a, both of which are found on Langerhans cells, but usually absent on macrophages. Conversely, monocytes and macrophages express nonspecific carcinoembryonic cross-reacting antigen, CD4 antigen, nonspecific esterase, and the cell surface marker CD11c (Leu-M5). Both types of cells, however, express class II MHC molecules and T-lymphocyte costimulatory receptors.

The development and differentiation of the cells of the MPS, much like other hematopoietic lineages, has a tightly regulated gene expression pattern. More specifically, cells of the MPS have a distinctive set of transcription factors that appear to regulate their growth and differentiation in a time-sequential, developmental stage-appropriate manner. The main transcription factor families implicated in the development of this system include the *myb* family, the *Ets* family, and the C/EBP family. PU.1, a member of the *Ets* family, plays a central role in monocyte-macrophage lineage as demonstrated by PU.1 knockout mice, which lack functional monocytes and tissue macrophages and display significant dendritic cell abnormalities.[8–10] This has become clearer recently as it was shown that PU.1 regulates the expression of *c-fms,* the gene coding for the M-CSF receptor, in addition to other critical genes such as FcγRI, FcγRIIIA, scavenger receptors type 1 and 2, CD11b, CD18, and CD14.[8]

The MPS represents a variable continuum of functionally distinct cell types that arise from common bone marrow progenitors and differentiate depending on the appropriate environmental stimuli. These cells develop under the control of common genetic programs, respond to similar cytokines, and share many essential functions. The differences are the result of functional adaptation within a biologic system and variable microenvironment after arising from a common progenitor.

MONONUCLEAR PHAGOCYTES IN THE LUNG

In the lungs, much like the remainder of the body, the primary function of innate and adaptive immunity falls on the members of the MPS. In addition, these cells play critical roles in modulating the inflammatory response and tissue remodeling. The most common, and most widely studied, pulmonary phagocytes are the alveolar and the airway macrophages. With the exception of their location within the respiratory tract, alveolar and airway macrophages are indistinguishable. These cells are primarily responsible for the sequestering and disposal of inhaled particles and pulmonary surfactant. They are able to produce large amounts of reactive oxygen species and play an active role in the maintenance and remodeling of the extracellular connective tissue matrix through the secretion of cytokines that regulate matrix production and degradation. Aberrations in this function can lead to a wide range of emphysematous or fibrotic disorders.

A less well recognized but important function of these cells is their ability to control adaptive immunity. Under normal conditions, pulmonary macrophages suppress T-cell and antigen-presenting cell functions. Under conditions where an inflammatory response is essential, such as in overwhelming infection, the immunosuppressive activity of pulmonary macrophages is suppressed and an adaptive immune response is initiated.

Interstitial macrophages are the second class of pulmonary macrophages that differ from the aforementioned class of macrophages by their improved antigen-presenting capability in the face of inferior phagocytic abilities.[11] These cells express higher levels of MHC class II and CD54 necessary for their superior antigen-presenting abilities.[12] Much like the airway macrophages, interstitial macrophages can multiply and undergo functional changes in the presence of inflammation. Interestingly, these cells, unlike their airway counterparts, can interact with pulmonary dendritic cells.[13] Pulmonary dendritic cells are located both within the airways and in the lung parenchyma, where their primary role is in antigen presentation. As noted above, the ability of airway dendritic cells in antigen presentation appears to be suppressed by airway macrophages under normal conditions. However, during periods of acute inflammation or overwhelming infection, this suppressive effect is overcome by cytokines and direct interaction with invading organisms.[14] Another group of cells, the pulmonary intravascular macrophages, has also been described in certain animal models, but appear to be absent from the human pulmonary system. A review of these cells is beyond the scope of this chapter.

In the pulmonary system, members of the MPS function in ways similar to their function elsewhere in the body. Their involvement in innate and adaptive immunity, in addition to their role in tissue remodeling, is critical for normal lung function. Later in this chapter we will review the consequences of overproliferation of these cells and its effects on normal physiology, both in the lungs and in other organ systems.

DISORDERS OF DENDRITIC CELLS AND MACROPHAGES

The histiocytic disorders have historically been a source of significant confusion and clinical dilemma for clinicians.[15] These disorders are characterized by the abnormal proliferation and accumulation of macrophage-like or dendritic cell–like cells in tissues. The variability of clinical presentation, pathologic appearance, and therapeutic response as well as the rarity of this family of diseases has rendered a full understanding of these disorders particularly difficult. Our improved knowledge of the molecular and cellular basis of hematopoiesis, and more specifically the MPS, in addition to successful clinical group trials has significantly advanced our current understanding and treatment of these disorders.

The histiocytic disorders, as proposed in 1987, can be classified into three classes based on the pathologic cells present within the lesions: class 1, dendritic cell histiocytoses; class II, non–dendritic cell histiocytosis, primarily consisting of hemophagocytic lymphohistiocytosis (HLH); and class III, malignant histiocytosis (Box 66-1). The remainder of this chapter will be devoted to the description of the pathophysiology, clinical presentation, and treatment of these disorders, with particular emphasis on LCH and histiocytic disorders involving the lung. A more detailed discussion of class II and III disorders can be found in several available reviews.[6,15]

BOX 66-1 Classification of the Histiocytic Disorders

Class I: Dendritic Cell Histiocytoses

- Langerhans cell histiocytosis
- Secondary dendritic cell processes
- Juvenile xanthogranuloma and related disorders
- Erdheim-Chester disease
- Solitary histiocytomas of various dendritic cell phenotypes

Class II: Non–dendritic Cell Histiocytoses

- Primary hemophagocytic lymphohistiocytosis
- Familial hemophagocytic lymphohistiocytosis
- Secondary hemophagocytic lymphohistiocytosis
  - Infection associated
  - Malignancy associated
- Rosai-Dorfman disease (sinus histiocytosis with massive lymphadenopathy)
- Solitary histiocytoma with macrophage phenotype

Class III: Malignant Histiocytoses

- Monocyte related
  - Leukemias (FAB and revised FAB classification)
  - Monocytic leukemia M5A and M5B
  - Acute myelomonocytic leukemias M4
  - Chronic myelomonocytic leukemias
- Extramedullary monocytic tumor or sarcoma
- Dendritic cell–related histiocytic sarcoma
- Macrophage-related histiocytic sarcoma

CLASS I: DENDRITIC CELL HISTIOCYTOSES

LCH is the most common member of this class of histiocytic disorders. *LCH* is the term used to describe the compendium of syndromes formerly identified as eosinophilic granuloma, Abt-Letterer-Siwe syndrome, and Hand-Schüller-Christian syndrome. As the name implies, all of these disorders are characterized by the abnormal proliferation and accumulation of clonally derived Langerhans cells, resulting in the replacement and destruction of normal tissue. These cells are typically diploid, have a normal proliferative index, and do not exhibit the degree of atypia seen in highly malignant processes.[15] Genetic, immunodysregulatory, and neoplastic mechanisms have all been postulated to play a role in LCH, but no definitive evidence is currently available to clearly delineate the etiologic role of these processes.[15] However, evidence indicates that excessive local release of inflammatory cytokines contributes to the pathophysiology of LCH. LCH cells accumulate in tissues and release cytokines that recruit other immune system cells such as lymphocytes, granulocytes, eosinophils, and macrophages.[16] In addition to the architectural damage to normal tissue from the accumulation of LCH cells, cytokines released by these cells can further cause local tissue damage or systemic symptoms such as fever, skin rashes, and hypotension. Although local proinflammatory cytokine production has been shown to be present, unlike HLH, there is no clear-cut evidence for a major role for systemic cytokine overproduction in most cases of LCH.[15,17]

As mentioned earlier, the term *LCH* is now applied to a wide variety of different clinical entities recognized to be pathologically identical. Sidney Farber first noted the pathologic similarity of these disorders in 1941, and by the 1950s, as a result of the work of Lichtenstein, these disorders were collectively referred to as histiocytosis X.[15] The term *LCH* has since replaced the more historical terminology. The diagnosis of LCH still requires a biopsy with the typical pathologic features of Langerhans cell infiltrates and confirmatory positive staining for CD1a and S-100 (Fig. 66-1). Alternatively, the demonstration of Birbeck granules by electron microscopy has been used for confirmation of this diagnosis.

In light of the pathologic basis of the diagnosis of LCH and the variable nature of clinical presentations, LCH is now further subclassified by the degree of organ involvement: localized single-system disease, multifocal single-system disease, and multisystem disease. The location of involvement has also been shown to be of prognostic importance, with bone marrow, pulmonary, spleen, and liver involvement denoted as "risk organs," while involvement of facial bones or spine with extradural soft tissue extension considered to be central nervous system (CNS) risk.[18,19] This classification currently serves as the basis for all modern LCH treatment protocols.

At the time of diagnosis, a complete workup should be performed to establish the full extent of disease and delineate risk-based therapy (Box 66-2). The workup should include detailed history and physical examination, complete and differential blood count, metabolic panel including liver and renal function tests, bone scan, skeletal survey, and chest radiograph. Urinalysis should also be performed to assess for diabetes insipidus

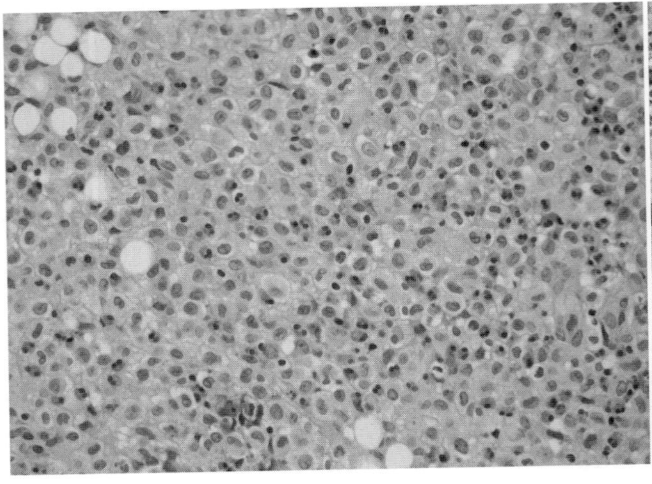

A

B

■ **FIGURE 66-1.** **A,** Langerhans cell histiocytosis in bone, showing mixture of eosinophils and Langerhans cells. The eosinophils contain bilobed nuclei and prominent eosinophilic, granular cytoplasm. The Langerhans cells are the larger cells with variable eosinophilic to clear cytoplasm and indented, cerebriform-like nuclei (hematoxylin and eosin stain, original magnification ×400). Immunostains for S-100 protein (**B**) and CD1a (**C**) highlight Langerhans cells. (See Color Plate 44.) (Courtesy of Dr. John D. Reith, Department of Orthopaedic Pathology, University of Florida School of Medicine, Gainesville.)

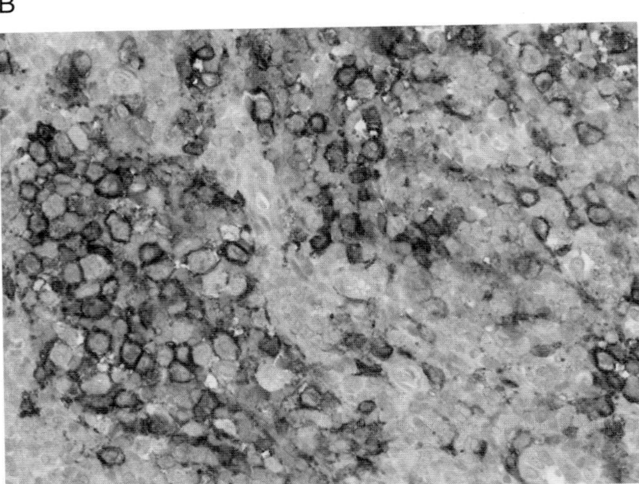

C

and pituitary involvement. Additional studies such as water deprivation test, antidiuretic hormone (ADH) levels, or other endocrinologic examinations evaluating pituitary/hypothalamic function may be necessary depending on the clinical presentation. Magnetic resonance imaging (MRI) of the brain is becoming a more common part of the staging work up of "CNS risk" patients because of the recognition of significant incidence of CNS involvement. Bone marrow studies, computed tomography (CT) scan of the chest, and pulmonary function tests (PFTs) should also be performed as clinically indicated to assess for risk of organ involvement (Box 66-3).

Localized LCH, involving skin, lymph node, or bones, usually carries a good prognosis. Lesions of bone, a condition formerly referred to as eosinophilic granuloma, usually present as a painful swelling. Radiographically these lesions appear as "punched out" sites and most commonly affect the calvarium, although they can involve any part of the skeleton (Fig. 66-2). Vertebra plana or collapsed vertebrae are a common presentation of this disease process in the spine. Single bone lesions rarely need therapy beyond biopsy or curettage except in the case of severe symptoms or danger of organ dysfunction, such as spinal cord compression or loss of vision. Treatment options in these cases include nonsteroidal anti-inflammatory agents or local steroid injections and, rarely, local low-dose radiation therapy of 400 to 800 cGy. Alternatively, 1200 cGy given as six 200-cGy fractions has been commonly used by many radiation therapists. Skin disease typically involves the scalp, retroauricular area, neck, upper chest, axilla, and groin. This rash can vary from maculopapular to more eruptive and nodular in appearance. In some cases the rash can be quite erosive and predisposes to serious superinfection. Therapy for isolated skin disease typically involves topical steroids, or in some steroid-refractory cases, topical nitrogen mustard or psoralen plus ultraviolet-A light (PUVA). Systemic steroids and vinblastine are reserved for extensive single-system or skin disease, usually with relatively good responses.[20]

In contrast to localized LCH, systemic therapy is indicated in patients with multisystem LCH. The most common presentation of multifocal LCH includes diffuse skin and multifocal bone involvement. The oral cavity, lymph nodes, and, to a lesser extent, lungs (see Fig. 66-2), liver, and brain are common sites of involvement in this disease. Diabetes insipidus is the most common manifestation of CNS involvement in LCH and is reported in 5% to 30% of patients. The triad of lytic skull lesions, exophthalmos, and diabetes insipidus has historically been referred to as Hand-Schüller-Christian syndrome. In addition to acute CNS involvement, patients with LCH can develop a severe neurodegenerative process involving loss of motor functions and cognition. Interestingly, the clinical severity of this disease can be independent of radiologic involvement. There are currently

BOX 66-2 Diagnostic and Staging Laboratory and Radiologic Interventions

Langerhans Cell Histiocytosis*

Minimum Baseline Studies

- Biopsy (skin/bone/lymph node/reticuloendothelial system)
- Complete blood count and differential
- Liver function tests
- Electrolytes/renal function tests
- Prothrombin time/INR
- Activated partial thromboplastin time
- Serum and urine osmolality
- Urine analysis/specific gravity
- Skeletal radiographic survey

Supplementary Studies†

- Bone scan
- MRI of brain with gadolineum contrast
- MRI/CT of specific bone lesions
- Panoramic dental radiograph
- Water deprivation test

Pulmonary Langerhans Cell Histiocytosis*,‡

- Biopsy
- Chest radiography (posteroanterior and lateral)
- High-resolution pulmonary CT
- PFT
- BAL
- Echocardiography

*All staging studies should be repeated every 2 to 3 months as clinically indicated for 1 to 2 years.
†Supplementary studies are only indicated as clinically relevant.
‡HIV, mycobacterial infection, Wegener's granulomatous disease, lung carcinoma or other metastatic carcinomas, alveolar carcinoma, sarcoidosis, septic emboli, and lymphangiomyomatosis in women should all be ruled out as part of the differential diagnosis.

no effective means of ameliorating the progression of this process. Liver involvement is another commonly seen complication of LCH that portends a poor prognosis. Transaminitis and hyperbilirubinemia are the hallmarks of acute liver involvement in LCH. Patients with hepatic LCH run the risk for developing sclerosing cholangitis that can in turn lead to hepatic fibrosis and liver failure.

In addition to site of involvement, age has been thought to be a significant prognostic factor in LCH, with younger patients having a significantly higher mortality rate. However, more recent clinical trial data have shown the response to the initial (6–12 weeks) therapy with vinblastine and steroids to be the best prognostic sign, outweighing the value of age. Abt-Letterrer-Siwe syndrome is a historical eponym used to describe systemic LCH characterized by extensive skin, bone marrow, spleen, and liver involvement, usually observed in children younger than 2 years. Oral cavity, gastrointestinal, and pulmonary involvement are other commonly seen manifestations of this severe form of LCH. Patients typically suffer from intractable fevers and failure to thrive, and in later phases of the disease have significant pancytopenia and hepatic failure leading to hemorrhage and sepsis. Abt-Letterrer-Siwe disease carries a particularly poor prognosis in patients with advanced hematopoietic involvement who do not show a good response to initial therapy.[6] Patients with Abt-Letterer-Siwe disease should undergo a full evaluation for congenital and acquired immunodeficiency syndromes in addition to infectious etiologies as part of their diagnostic workup. It should be noted that although LCH is historically considered to be a pediatric disease, it is now clear that similar presentations, including Abt-Letterer-Siwe type disease, are also seen in adults.

As mentioned above, patients with multisystem LCH have been demonstrated to benefit from systemic chemotherapy. The current therapeutic regimens have evolved from work originally performed in the 1970s and 1980s. Multiple small studies during that time period demonstrated that single-agent therapy with agents such as methotrexate, vincristine, vinblastine, etoposide, 6-mercaptopurine, and prednisone was effective treatment for LCH. These trials were subsequently followed by the larger AIEOP-CNR-HX and DAL-HX 83/90 studies, all of which utilized regimens with multiple agents. These studies demonstrated response rates of 60% to 90% utilizing combinations of vinblastine, etoposide, and prednisone. In these studies it was

BOX 66-3 Risk Groups as Defined by the Langerhans Cell Histiocytosis-III Protocol

Group 1: Multisystem "Risk" Patients

Multisystem patients with involvement of one or more "risk" organs (i.e., hematopoietic system, liver, spleen, or lungs). Patients with single-system lung involvement are not eligible for randomization.

Group 2: Multisystem "Low-Risk" Patients

Multisystem patients with multiple organs involved but without involvement of "risk" organs.

Group 3: Single-System "Multifocal Bone Disease" and Localized "Special Site" Involvement

Patients with multifocal bone disease; that is, lesions in two or more different bones. Patients with localized special site involvement, such as "central nervous system risk" lesions with intracranial soft tissue extension or vertebral lesions with intraspinal soft tissue extension.

Adapted from Arceci RJ, Longley BJ, Emanuel PD: Atypical cellular disorders. Hematology 2002;297–314.

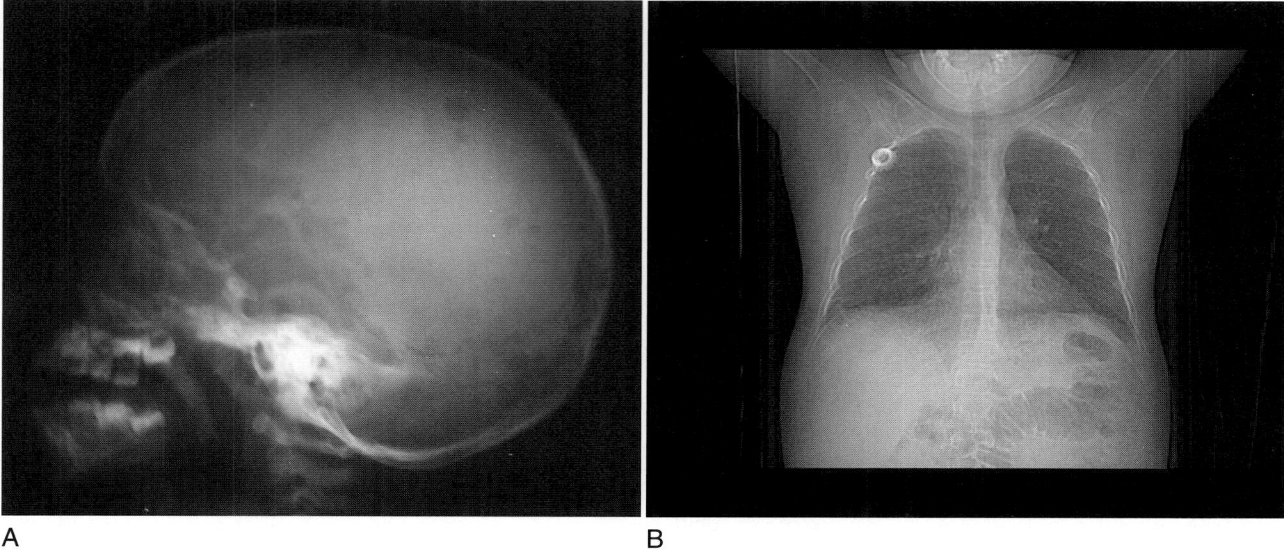

■ **FIGURE 66-2.** Skull and chest radiograph from a 2-year-old with Langerhans cell histiocytosis (LCH). **A,** Multiple "punched out" lytic skull lesions are apparent. **B,** Chest radiograph from the same patient demonstrates nonspecific findings of early LCH. (Courtesy of Dr. William Cummings, Department of Pediatric Radiology, University of Florida School of Medicine, Gainesville.)

also noted that patients with extensive disease and organ dysfunction had significantly higher mortality and recurrence rates.[21,22]

These studies were then followed by the first international, prospective, randomized study, LCH-I. This trial was crucial to our understanding of therapeutic response in LCH and represented the first international clinical trial of the Histiocyte Society. The results of this study demonstrated that patients treated with etoposide did not have a better outcome than those treated with vinblastine. In addition, this study revealed that response to the 6-week induction phase of therapy was strongly predictive of overall outcome: patients without a response to therapy after 6 weeks had a survival rate of less than 40% at 5 years. Another critical outcome of this study was the confirmation of earlier work of Lahey that patients older than 2 years and without pulmonary, hepatosplenic, or hematopoietic involvement had an excellent prognosis with a response rate of 90% and survival of 100% at 6-year follow-up.[23] In comparison to the AIEOP-CNR-HX and DAL-HX 83/90 trials, which used multidrug regimens, LCH-I showed a higher recurrence rate and higher frequency of diabetes insipidus. This raised the question of whether more aggressive therapy in patients with high-risk disease would provide a therapeutic advantage.

The second Histiocyte Society Protocol, LCH-II, attempted to answer this question in a randomized fashion. The results of this study are still under analysis, although preliminary evaluations have confirmed three important observations: (1) response to therapy by 12 weeks of therapy is an important prognostic sign; (2) etoposide does not confer any benefit over therapy with vinblastine when used in combination with prednisone, and (3) prolonged therapy may decrease the reactivation rate of LCH. In light of the risk for therapy-associated acute myelogenous leukemia/myelodysplastic syndrome (AML/MDS) in patients treated with epidopophylotoxins (i.e., etoposide or VP-16), this study obviated the use of etoposide in uncomplicated LCH. This trial also confirmed that age less than 2 years without risk for organ involvement is not an independent prognostic factor.

The current Histiocyte Society Protocol, LCH-III, attempts to determine in a randomized design whether (1) intensified induction, with the addition of intermediate dose methotrexate, improves induction rates in risk patients, and (2) whether prolonging continuation therapy reduces the rate of disease reactivation (see Box 66-2). Based on the results of the previous studies, etoposide is no longer recommended as initial therapy.

Despite the recent successes in the treatment of LCH, the treatment of refractory disease remains problematic. Experience with immunosuppressive agents such as cyclosporin A and antithymocyte globulin is limited and responses most commonly transient. There is, however, significant experience with the nucleoside analog 2-chlorodeoxyadenosine (2-CDA), independently or in combination with cytosine arabinoside. Although significantly more toxic than routine LCH therapy, 2-CDA has shown a sustained remission rate in more than a third of patients with refractory disease in an international phase II study. The response rate was even better in patients with a good initial response to treatment.[20,24–26] 2-CDA has also shown anecdotal efficacy in the treatment of parenchymal CNS disease, although no agent has been shown to be effective in halting the progression of the neurodegenerative disease. Other recent approaches that have been tried to treat the neurodegenerative disease associated with LCH include the use of drugs that decrease inflammatory responses, such as thalidomide and tumor necrosis factor (TNF) inhibitors such as infliximab (Remicaid, Centocor, Malvern, Pennsylvania) and etanercept (Enbrel, Immunex Corporation, Thousand Oaks, California.)[27,28] Alemtuzumab (Campath, Genzyme, Cambridge, Massachusetts), an anti-CD52 antibody, also may have promise in the treatment of LCH, especially in patients with advanced disease, and should be tested in prospective clinical trials. There are case reports of hematopoietic stem cell transplantation in patients with refractory LCH, but the role of this therapeutic approach remains unclear in part due to difficulty in identifying matched donors, and the high mortality rate in patients with significant disease-related organ dysfunction.

There remains a significant need for more effective agents in the treatment of patients with significant organ involvement and dysfunction, including patients with progressive CNS, hepatic, and pulmonary disease. Several new agents including antibodies to CD1a and antifibrosis agents are currently in preclinical/early clinical phases of development.

Erdheim-Chester disease (ECD) is a less common member of the class I histiocytoses. This disease is extremely rare in the pediatric age group, with patients typically older than 50 years. The histologic hallmark of this disease is a collagenized fibrous infiltrate with interspersed foamy histiocytes and Touton giant cells and, to a lesser extent, lymphocytes and plasma cells. The etiology of these foamy histiocytes is unclear because they are CD1a and S-100 negative, but CD68 positive. Only 20% of these histiocytes have Birbeck granules.[29,30] Clinically, this disease presents with xanthoma-like skin nodules and bilateral lower extremity bone pain. Radiography shows symmetric sclerosing bone lesions typically affecting the lower extremity bones. Patients with disseminated disease may have severe cardiopulmonary insufficiency from parenchymal involvement of heart and lung tissues, in addition to CNS involvement with ataxia, diabetes insipidus, and confusion.[29] Pulmonary manifestations consist of parenchymal, pleural, and interlobular involvement with fibrosis and inflammation. Currently, no definitive treatment is available for ECD, although case reports for therapeutic success using steroids alone, or in combination with other chemotherapeutic agents, can be found.[31]

CLASS II: NON–DENDRITIC CELL HISTIOCYTOSES

Class II histiocytic disorders are all characterized by the abnormal accumulation of activated macrophages, as opposed to Langerhans cells, in tissues. The predominant member of the class II histiocytoses is HLH, a disorder that can be further subdivided into primary HLH (familial erythrophagocytic lymphohistiocytosis [FEL]) and secondary HLH (infection-associated hemophagocytic syndrome [IAHS]). These two disorders are clinically indistinguishable with the exception of a positive family history in the case of primary HLH. The presentation of these disorders is typically fulminant and consists of cytopenias, hepatosplenomegaly, hyperlipidemia, and/or hypofibrinogenemia, fever, and hemophagocytosis.[32] Family history of consanguinity and age of less than 2 years at time of onset are highly suggestive of primary HLH.

It is been shown that patients with primary HLH have low or absent natural killer (NK) cell and cytotoxic T-cell function, in addition to significant hypercytokinemia. The abnormalities in the activity of NK cells have been shown to be secondary to a deficiency in perforin expression or function. Mutations in two well-defined genes, PRF1 (perforin) and Munc13-4, both of which affect cytolytic granule function, have been shown to be present in patients with primary HLH. Mutations in the perforin gene are thought to account for 20% to 40% of cases of primary HLH.[33–35] Interestingly, Munc13-4 is a member of the munc13 family of proteins involved in vesicle priming. Munc13-4 mutations cause a defect in cytolytic granule exocytosis, effectively blocking the release of active enzymes into target cells.[36]

HLH is fatal if appropriate therapy is not instituted rapidly. Current therapy, based on the HLH-2004 protocol of the histiocyte society, consists of dexamethasone, etoposide, and cyclosporin A in combination with intrathecal methotrexate when indicated by positive cerebrospinal fluid findings. Cases of primary HLH tend to be recurrent and do not permanently respond to chemotherapy, necessitating stem cell transplantation for cure.[37,38] IAHS, however, with the exception of refractory cases, can be treated with chemotherapy alone with good outcomes. Because these disorders are clinically identical and family history is not always reliable, all patients are similarly treated unless strong evidence for primary HLH is available. The current international protocol, HLH-2004, is for the most part identical to the HLH-94 protocol with only minor modifications.[36]

Other members of class II histiocytoses, rarely seen in the pediatric age group, tend to have a more indolent course than HLH. Sinus histiocytosis with massive lymphadenopathy (SHML, also known as Rosai-Dorfman disease) is characterized by a lymphohistiocytic accumulation in the sinuses of lymph nodes without architectural effacement.[39] The proliferative macrophages seen in this disorder are typically S-100 positive but CD1a negative and can be seen engulfing intact lymphocytes or other cells, a process known as emperipolesis. SHML has a predilection for lymph nodes of the head and neck but can be seen elsewhere, including extranodal tissue.[40] SHML is more commonly seen in patients of African ancestry and is not responsive to most therapeutic approaches.[41] Recent reports have documented response to therapy with high-dose dexamethasone.[42] This experience needs to be further verified in a prospective manner. Although SHML can be potentially disfiguring, it is only rarely life threatening.

CLASS III: MALIGNANT HISTIOCYTOSES

This class of disorders consists of malignant histiocytosis, histiocytic sarcoma, and acute monocytic leukemia. For the most part, these disorders can be characterized by malignant transformation of cells of the MPS with significant cellular atypia. The wide variety of these conditions, the rarity of occurrence, and the lack of significant direct pulmonary involvement preclude a more detailed discussion in this chapter.

PULMONARY INVOLVEMENT IN HISTIOCYTOSIS

EPIDEMIOLOGY

Primary pulmonary LCH (PLCH) is a disease that most frequently affects young adults. There is a strong association with smoking. This disease primarily affects whites, and less commonly, African Americans.[43,44] Contrary to original reports suggesting a male predilection, more recent reports show equal rates of involvement in both sexes, but with women having a later presentation.[45–48] The differences in the patient populations are thought to be in part secondary to an association with smoking.[49] In contrast to PLCH, pulmonary involvement can be part of multisystem LCH. The relationship between isolated pulmonary histiocytosis (PLCH) and involvement as part of a systemic disease is not clear, but it has been reported that up to 20% of patients presenting with PLCH have skeletal involvement.[50] Although PLCH can occur at any age, it is rarely seen in patients younger than 15 years.[51] Pulmonary involvement as part of systemic LCH, however, is a common feature of multisystem LCH, seen in up to one third of patients. The progression of pulmonary symptoms in multisystem LCH mirrors the disease

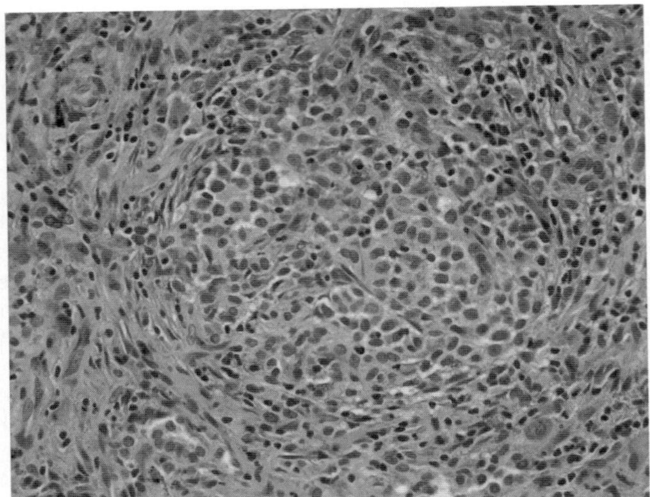

■ **FIGURE 66-3.** The typical low-power appearance of pulmonary Langerhans cell histiocytosis is of a multiple nodular interstitial infiltrate with a stellate border. At high magnification the cellular infiltrate consists of sheets of Langerhans cells characterized by abundant eosinophilic cytoplasm and prominent nuclear indentation (grooves). Scattered eosinophils are often present. Lymphocytes, macrophages, and fibroblasts may also be present. (See Color Plate 45.) (Courtesy of Dr. Li Lu, Department of Pathology, University of Florida School of Medicine, Gainesville.)

progression in other organ systems. It is generally believed that pulmonary involvement as part of multisystem LCH, although histopathologically similar to PLCH, represents a more aggressive clinical process than PLCH. For the sake of this review we will distinguish between these presentations when relevant.

ETIOLOGY AND PATHOGENESIS

The pathogenesis underlying PLCH, much like systemic LCH, is not well defined but thought to be the result of an abnormal immune reaction to a stimulant (i.e., smoke). As mentioned above, a strong association between PLCH and tobacco use has been demonstrated, with up to 100% of patients in some series reported to be smokers.[45,46,49,52,53] Interestingly, this disease is more common in patients with recent heavy smoking.[49] Although the exact role of smoking in the pathogenesis of PLCH remains to be defined, several lines of evidence point to smoking as a major etiologic factor: (1) the peribronchiolar location of pulmonary histiocytosis matches the distribution of smoke-induced small airway disease,[53] (2) the presence of relatively large numbers of Langerhans cells in bronchoalveolar lavage (BAL) fluid of smokers as compared to nonsmokers,[54] (3) peripheral blood lymphocytes of patients with pulmonary LCH have an attenuated T-cell proliferative response to tobacco constituents.[55,56]

Langerhans cells, alveolar macrophages, and lymphocytes are all believed to play an active role in the tissue damage seen in PLCH. LCH cells from patients with pulmonary disease have been demonstrated to have a phenotype consistent with activated Langerhans cells in vitro (Fig. 66-3). These cells have an increased number of Birbeck granules, higher expression levels of CD1a, and expression of CD1c, CD4, CD24, and CD32.[57,58] Furthermore, these cells also express the leukocyte markers CD54 and CD58 in addition to other adhesion molecules.[57,59,60] The close interaction of LCH cells with $CD4^+$ T lymphocytes,[57] the elevated level of blood and tissue immune complexes in active LCH,[61] and the elevated level of immunoglobulins in the BAL fluid of PLCH patients all point to an active role for lymphocytes in the pathogenesis of PLCH.[62] PLCH is known to be associated with significant pulmonary fibrosis, a process typically involving alveolar macrophages. In addition, much like other interstitial lung diseases, fibroblast proliferation and collagen deposition is thought to be secondary to platelet-derived growth factor, while tissue damage may be due to increases in plasminogen activator, both of which are released by alveolar macrophages.[63,64] Active inflammatory PLCH lesions have also been shown to contain TGF-β_1 and GM-CSF. These cytokines, in addition to TNF-α, are expressed by alveolar macrophages and other cells in the proximity of the pulmonary dendritic cells and are believed to directly contribute to the pathogenesis of PLCH.[65,66]

CLINICAL FEATURES

PLCH is mostly seen in young adults, typically in the third or fourth decade of life.[50] Twenty percent to 25% of patients are asymptomatic at the time of diagnosis, with the disease being identified on a screening chest radiograph.[45] Physical examination is typically unremarkable.[52] One third of symptomatic patients report constitutional symptoms for 6 months or more, while the remainder have respiratory symptoms. Respiratory symptoms can manifest as dry cough and dyspnea and, more rarely, as hemoptysis or chest pain. Chest pain can be due to pneumothoraces or rib lesions.[45] Pneumothoraces are significantly less common in pediatric patients than in adults, where 15% of patients present with this complication.[60] Patients may have recurrent pneumothoraces requiring surgical management.[60] PLCH in adults tends to present as single system disease, although 4% to 20% (Table 66-1) of patients may have skeletal lesions and, less commonly, other organ involvement.[50,56] Advanced pulmonary disease may be associated with clubbing or cor pulmonale.[45,50,52]

Many patients with PLCH are found to initially have normal pulmonary function.[67] Reductions in diffusing capacity are typically the first abnormality noted in PLCH, while advanced disease can be manifested by a restrictive, obstructive, or mixed pattern.[50,68] One study of 18 patients demonstrated that increases in airflow limitation correlated with disease progression.[69] Exercise intolerance is a common feature of PLCH. Vascular involvement can consist of intimal fibrosis, medial hypertrophy, or destruction of the vessel lumen with infiltrating inflammatory cells such as lymphocytes, eosinophils, and Langerhans cells into the vessel wall. Pulmonary vasculopathy is a prominent part of PLCH, particularly in late-stage disease, and is considered to

■ **TABLE 66-1.** Clinical features of pulmonary Langerhans cell histiocytosis in adults

Features	%
Asympotomatic	14
Cough	58
Dyspnea	38
Chest pain	21
Fever	15
Weight loss	20
Fatigue	33
Hemoptysis	7
Pneumothorax	14
Diabetes insipidus	7
Bone lesions	8

Adapted from Marcy T, Reynolds H: Pulmonary histiocytosis X. Lung 1985;163:129.

be responsible for elevated pulmonary hypertension, cor pulmonale, and eventual cardiac failure seen in these patients.[70]

Chest radiography typically reveals a symmetric, nodular to reticulonodular pattern in the middle and upper lobes of the lung early in the course of PLCH (Fig. 66-4). Lung volumes are initially well preserved or increased.[48,50] The costophrenic angles are typically spared, a finding considered by some to carry a good prognosis.[46] Hilar and mediastinal lymphadenopathy are rarely seen in adult patients but are more common in pediatric cases.[71–75] Nodular findings on chest radiography are eventually replaced by cystic lesions. Chest CT findings are variable depending on the stage of the disease but are typically diagnostic. Approximately 80% of patients with PLCH have cysts and 60% to 80% have nodules present on chest CT.[50,56] Early-stage PLCH is characterized by a centrilobular pattern, with nodules typically measuring 1 to 5 mm.[76] These nodules progress by undergoing cavitation, leading to variably sized cystic lesions. The typical CT finding in PLCH patients is a mixture of nodular and cystic lesions in addition to reticulation and ground-glass opacities in the upper and middle areas of the lung (see Fig. 66-4).[76] Eventually, there is worsening with the appearance of fibrosis and honeycombing secondary to confluent cysts.[77] The CT findings of PLCH, particularly high-resolution CT, are quite characteristic and result in limited interobserver variability.[50] Pathologically, the presentation and progression of the disease mimics its appearance as depicted by CT: centrilobular micronodules to cavitated micronodules to thick-walled cysts to thin-walled cysts and eventual fibrosis with honeycombing (Fig. 66-5).

TREATMENT

The optimal therapy for PLCH remains undefined. Smoking cessation is typically recommended, although limited data exist to support long-term improvement in outcome after smoking cessation.[56,78] The use of steroids and other immunosuppressive regimens remains unproven, although prospective trials are ongoing.[79,80] Cytotoxic and immunosuppressive agents with efficacy in multisystem disease, such as 2-CDA, may potentially be of benefit in PLCH but need further clinical trial testing. Therapy for multisystem LCH with lung involvement should be attempted with standard LCH regimens prior to the development of cystic lesions and fibrosis, because these changes are less likely to be reversible. Colchicine has in the past been proposed as a potential antifibrotic agent based on its efficacy in some cases of cirrhosis of the liver, although newer and more effective agents are needed.[81] Lung transplantation has been attempted in patients with progressive PLCH with some success, although recurrences have been noted with and without smoking.[82,83] New therapeutic trials should be initiated through the multi-institutional groups in order to evaluate novel therapies or appropriately investigate traditional therapies for this disease.[80]

PLCH, much like other types of LCH, has a variable clinical course characterized by intermittent symptomatology, spontaneous remissions, reactivation, and progression to end-stage pulmonary disease.[45,48] Although no prospective data for long-term outcome of adults with PLCH is available, occurrence of respiratory failure, pulmonary hypertension, and cor pulmonale in this patient population necessitates long-term follow-up.[66,79] Furthermore, adequate clinical markers to identify subpopulations of patients for early intervention have not been determined.[66] It is generally recommended that patients undergo PFTs, high resolution CT, and chest radiography on a 3-month basis during the first year after diagnosis. Follow-up after the initial phase and stabilization of patient disease should be individualized and guided by patient symptomatology. In the absence of obvious functional deterioration and in light of the asymptomatic nature of some pulmonary changes detected by high-resolution CT, clinical follow-up consisting of careful history, physical examination, and chest radiography with occasional PFTs remains the standard of care.[66] Patients with worsening symptoms should

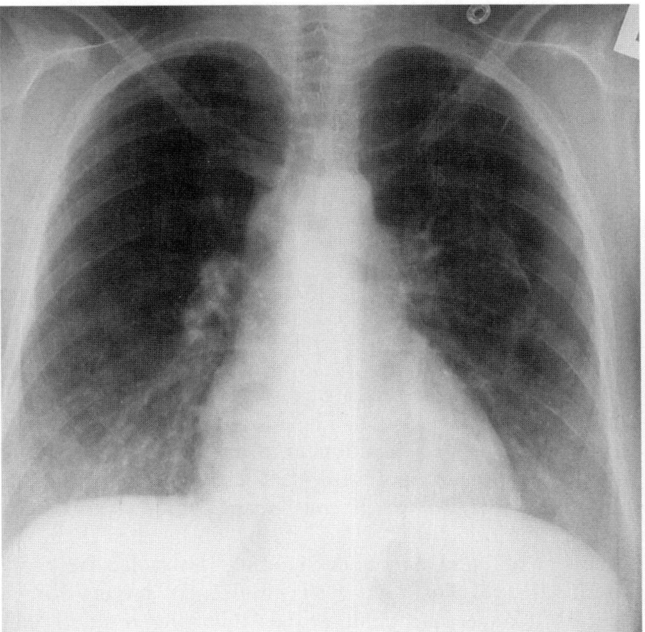

A

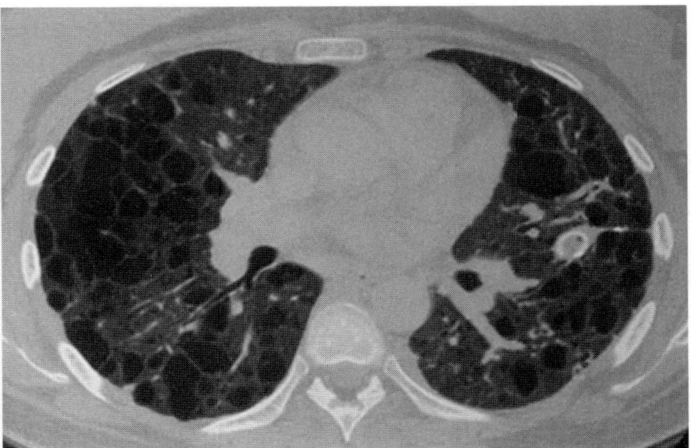

B

■ **FIGURE 66-4.** Chest radiograph **(A)** and computed tomography (CT) scan **(B)** from a 21-year-old patient with pulmonary Langerhans cell histiocytosis (PLCH). CT scan demonstrates cystic changes, fibrosis, and emphesyma. **B,** Comparison with the chest radiograph reveals the ability of CT scans to detect considerably more disease involvement compared with radiography in patients with PLCH.

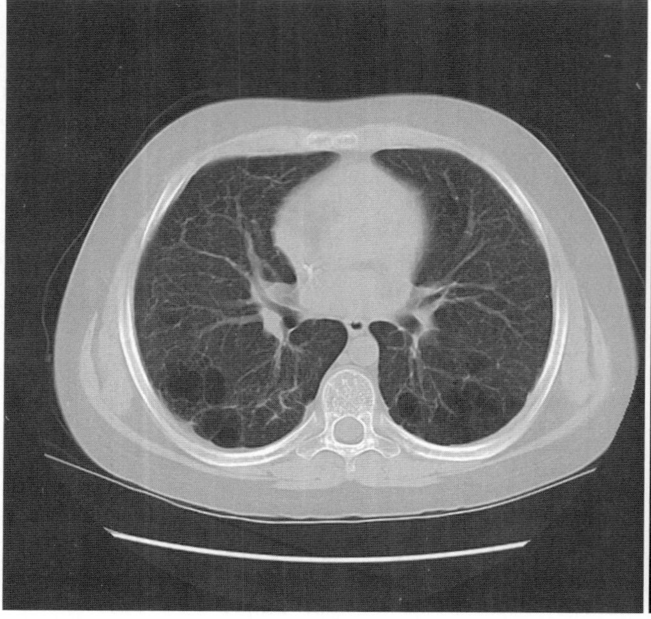

A

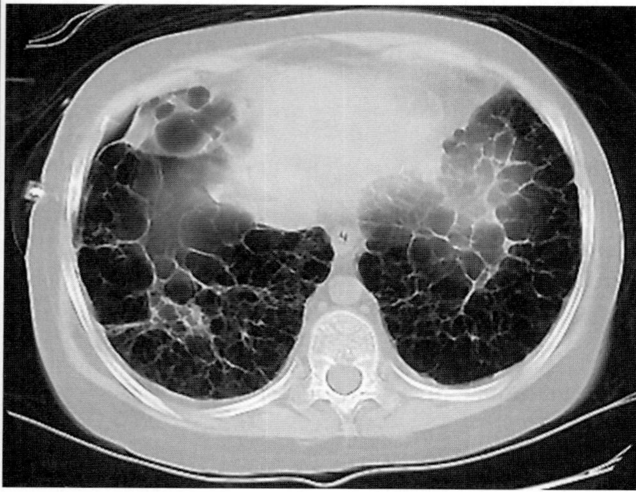

B

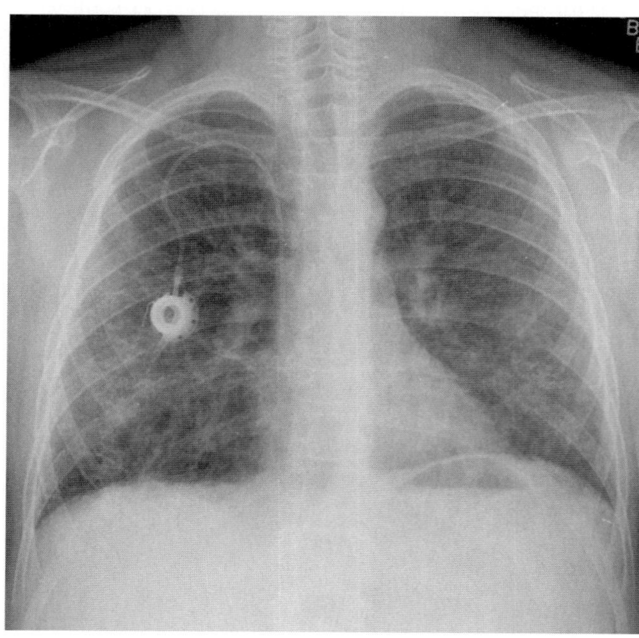

C

FIGURE 66-5. Early **(A)** and late **(B)** computed tomography (CT) scans from a 12-year-old patient with pulmonary Langerhans cell histiocytosis demonstrate the rapid progression of cystic changes over a short time interval to end-stage disease. Chest radiography **(C)** demonstrates findings from the time of the final CT. (Courtesy of Dr. William Cummings, Department of Pediatric Radiology, University of Florida School of Medicine, Gainesville.)

also be evaluated for potential pulmonary hypertension and cor pulmonale using echocardiography and electrocardiography as indicated.[66,80] The guidelines for the follow-up of patients with multisystem disease and pulmonary involvement are similar and should be based primarily on patient symptomatology.

FUTURE DIRECTIONS

Important landmarks have been reached in our understanding of LCH since the first descriptions in the 1800s. We have a better understanding of the normal and abnormal responses of the cells belonging to the MPS as well as to the etiology, presentation, natural history, and treatment of LCH. Nevertheless, large numbers of patients remain undiagnosed, inadequately treated, or simply do not respond to current therapies. The morbidity and mortality of LCH, particularly when refractory to therapy and involving organs such as the bone marrow, liver, and lung, remains poor. The rarity of the histiocytoses has historically been an impediment to the study of these disorders. The formation of the Histiocyte Society has helped establish a framework within which collaborative studies can be undertaken. Future efforts should focus on further defining the etiology of LCH and understanding the molecular pathways with the goal of identifying molecular targets for novel agents. Cooperative clinical trials involving multidisciplinary approaches, particularly involving pulmonologists and oncologists, should help establish future improvements in outcome for patients with LCH.

REFERENCES

1. Wiktor-Jedrzejczak W, Bartocci A, Ferrante AW Jr, et al: Total absence of colony-stimulating factor 1 in the macrophage-deficient osteopetrotic (op/op) mouse. Proc Natl Acad Sci U S A 1990;87:4828–4832.
2. Riches DWH: Monocytes, macrophages, and dendritic cells of the lung. In: Murray JF, Nadel JA, eds: Textbook of Respiratory Medicine, 3rd ed. Philadelphia: WB Saunders, 2000, pp 385–412.
3. Takahashi K, Naito M, Shultz LD, et al: Differentiation of dendritic cell populations in macrophage colony-stimulating factor deficient mice homozygous for the osteopetrosis (op) mutation. J Leukoc Biol 1993;53:19–28.
4. Abbas AK, Lichtman AH, Jordan SP: Cells and tissues of the immune system. In: Abbas AK, Lichtman AH, Jordan SP, eds: Cellular and Molecular Immunology, 4th ed. Philadelphia: WB Saunders, 2000, pp 17–38.
5. Hume DA, Ross IL, Himes SR, et al: The mononuclear phagocyte system revisited. J Leukoc Biol 2002;72:621–627.
6. Arceci RJ, Grabowski G: Histiocytoses and disorders of the reticuloendothelial system. In: Handin RI, Stossel TP, Lux SE, eds: Blood: Principles and Practice of Hematology, 2nd ed. Philadelphia: JB Lippincott, 2003, 921–957.
7. Sasmono RT, Oceandy D, Pollard JW, et al: A macrophage colony-stimulating factor receptor-green fluorescent protein transgene is expressed throughout the mononuclear phagocyte system of the mouse. Blood 2003;101(3):1155–1163.
8. Valledor AF, Borras FE, Cullel-Young M, Celada A: Transcription factors that regulate monocyte/macrophage differentiation. J Leukoc Biol 1998; 63:405–417.
9. Anderson KL, Perkin H, Surh CD, et al: Transcription factor PU.1 is necessary for development of thymic and myeloid progenitor-derived dendritic cells. J Immunol 2000;15;164(4):1855–1861.
10. Guerriero A, Langmuir PB, Spain LM, Scott EW: PU.1 is required for myeloid-derived but not lymphoid-derived dendritic cells. Blood 2000; 95(3):879–885.
11. Prokhorova S, Lavnikova N, Laskin DL: Functional characterization of interstitial macrophages and subpopulations of alveolar macrophages from rat lung. J Leukoc Biol 1994;55:141–146.
12. Masten BJ, Yates JL, Pollard-Koga AM, Lipscomb MF: Characterization of accessory molecules in murine lung dendritic cell function. Roles for CD80, CD86, CD54, and CD40L. Am J Respir Cell Mol Biol 1997; 16:335–342.
13. Gong JL, McCarthy KM, Rogers RA, Schneeberger EE: Interstitial lung macrophages interact with dendritic cells to present antigenic peptides derived from particulate antigens to T cells. Immunology 1994;81:343–351.
14. MacLean JA, Xia W, Pinto CE: Sequestration of inhaled particulate antigens by lung phagocytes. Am J Pathol 1996;148:657–666.
15. Arceci RJ: The histiocytoses. The fall of the Tower of Babel. Eur J Cancer 1999;35(5):747–769.
16. Banchereau J, Steinman RM: Dendritic cells and the control of immunity. Nature 1998;392:245–252.
17. Kannourakis G, Abbas A: The role of cytokines in the pathogenesis of Langerhans cell histiocytosis. Br J Cancer 1994;23(Suppl):37–40.
18. Gadner H et al: LCH III. Treatment protocol of the Third International Study for Langerhans Cell Histiocytosis, 2nd version. January 2002.
19. Lahey ME: Histiocytosis-X. An analysis of prognostic factors. J Pediatr 1975;87:179–183.
20. Arceci RJ, Longley BJ, Emanuel PD: Atypical cellular disorders. Hematology (Am Soc Hematol Educ Program) 2002;297–314.
21. Ceci A, de Terlizzi M, Colella R, et al: Langerhans cell histiocytosis in childhood. Results from the Italian Cooperative AIEOP-CNR-H.X'83 study. Med Pediatr Oncol 1993;21:259–264.
22. Gadner H, Heitger A, Grois N, et al: Treatment strategy for disseminated Langerhans cell histiocytosis. DAL HX-83 Study Group. Med Pediatr Oncol 1994;23:72–80.
23. Ladisch S, Gadner H, Arico M, et al: LCH-I. A randomized trial of etoposide vs vinblastine in disseminated Langerhans cell histiocytosis. The Histiocyte Society. Med Pediatr Oncol 1994;23:107–110.
24. Weitzman S, Wayne AS, Arceci R, et al: Nucleoside analogues in the therapy of Langerhans cell histiocytosis. A survey of members of the histiocyte society and review of the literature. Med Pediatr Oncol 1999;33:476–481.
25. Saven A, Piro LD: 2-chlorodeoxyadenosine. A potent antimetabolite with major activity in the treatment of indolent lymphoproliferative disorders. Hematol Cell Ther 1996;38(Suppl 2):93–101.
26. Stine KC, Saylors RL, Williams LL, Becton DL: 2-chlorodeoxyadenosine (2-CDA) for the treatment of refractory or recurrent Langerhans cell histiocytosis (LCH) in pediatric patients. Med Pediatr Oncol 1997;29:288–292.
27. Thomas L, Ducros B, Secchi T, et al: Successful treatment of adult's Langerhans cell histiocytosis with thalidomide. Report of two cases and literature review. Arch Dermatol 1993;129:1261–1264.
28. Henter J-I, Karlen J, Calming U, et al: Successful treatment of Langerhans'-cell histiocytosis with etanercept. N Engl J Med 2001;345:1577–1578.
29. Veyssier-Belot C, Cacoub P, Caparros-Lefebvre D, et al: Erdheim-Chester disease. Clinical and radiologic characteristics of 59 cases. Medicine (Baltimore) 1996;75(3):157–169.
30. Opie KM, Kaye J, Vinciullo C: Erdheim-Chester disease. Aust J Dermatol 2003;44(3):194–198.
31. Bourke SC, Nicholson AG, Gibson GJ: Erdheim-Chester disease. Pulmonary infiltration responding to cyclophosphamide and prednisolone. Thorax 2003;58(11):1004–1005.
32. Henter J-I, Elinder G, Öst Å, the FHL Study Group of the Histiocyte Society: Diagnostic guidelines for hemophagocytic lymphohistiocytosis. Semin Oncol 1991;18(1):29–33.
33. Trapani JA, Davis J, Sutton VR, Smyth MJ: Pro-apoptotic functions of cytotoxic lymphocyte granule constituents in vitro and in vivo. Curr Opin Immunol 2000;12:323–329.
34. Stepp SE, Dufourcq-Lagelouse R, Le Deist F, et al: Perforin gene defects in familial hemophagocytic lymphohistiocytosis. Science 1999;286: 1957–1959.
35. Ericson K et al: Spectrum of perforin gene mutations in familial hemophagocytic lymphohistiocytosis. Am J Hum Genet 2000;68:590–597.
36. Feldmann J, Callebaut I, Raposo G, et al: Munc13-4 is essential for cytolytic granules fusion and is mutated in a form of familial hemophagocytic lymphohistiocytosis (FHL3). Cell 2003;115:461–473.
37. Henter J-I, Arico M, Egeler M, et al: HLH-94. A treatment protocol for hemophagocytic lymphohistiocytosis. Med Pediatr Oncol 1997;28: 342–347.
38. Arico M, Janka G, Fisher A, et al: Hemophagocytic lymphohistiocytosis. Report of 122 children from the International Registry. FHL Study Group of the Histiocyte Society. Leukemia 1996;10:197–203.
39. Foucar E, Rosai J, Dorfman R: Sinus histiocytosis with massive lymphadenopathy (Rosai-Dorfman disease). Review of the entity. Semin Diagn Pathol 1990;7:19–73.
40. Rodriguez-Galindo C, Helton KJ, Sanchez ND, et al: Extranodal Rosai-Dorfman disease in children. J Pediatr Hematol Oncol 2004;26(1):19–24.
41. Pulsoni A, Anghel G, Falcucci P, et al: Treatment of sinus histiocytosis with massive lymphadenopathy (Rosai-Dorfman disease). Report of case and literature review. Am J Hematol 2002;69:67–71.
42. Stein KC, Westfall C: Sinus histiocytosis with massive lymphadenopathy (SHML) prednisone resistant but dexamethasone sensitive. Pediatr Blood Cancer 2005;44(1):92–94.
43. Dunmore LA Jr, El-Khoury SA: Eosinophilic granuloma of the lung. A report of three cases in Negro patients. Am Rev Respir Dis 1964; 90:789–791.
44. Morley TF, Silverstein SD, Giudice JC, et al: Multifocal eosinophilic granuloma. Respiration 1988;54:89–93.
45. Friedman P, Liebow AA, Sokoloff J: Eosinophilic granuloma of lung. Medicine 1981;60:385–396.
46. Colby T, Lombard C: Histiocytosis X in the lung. Hum Pathol 1983;14: 847–856.
47. Malpas JS, Norton AJ: Langerhans' cell Histiocytosis in the adult. Med Pediatr Oncol 1996;27:540–546.
48. Lacronique J, Roth C, Battesti J-P, et al: Chest radiological features of pulmonary histiocytosis X: A report based on 50 adult cases. Thorax 1982; 37:104–109.
49. Hance A, Basset F, Saumon G, et al: Smoking and interstitial lung disease. The effect of cigarette smoking on the incidence of pulmonary histiocytosis X and sarcoidosis. Ann NY Acad Sci 1986;465:643–656.
50. Sundar KM, Gosselin MV, Hannah LC, Cahill BC: Pulmonary Langerhans cell histiocytosis. Emerging concepts in pathobiology, radiology, and clinical evolution of disease. Chest 2003;123(5):1673–1683.
51. Nondahl S, Finlay JL, Farrell PM, et al: A case report and literature review of "primary" pulmonary histiocytosis X of childhood. Med Pediatr Oncol 1986;14:57–62.
52. Marcy T, Reynolds H: Pulmonary histiocytosis X. Lung 1985;163:129–150.
53. Travis WD, Borok Z, Roum JH, et al: Pulmonary Langerhans' cell granulomatosis (histiocytosis X). A clinicopathologic study of 48 cases. Am J Surg Pathol 1993;17:971–986.
54. Casolaro MA, Bernaudin JF, Saltini C, et al: Accumulation of Langerhans' cells on the epithelial surface of the lower respiratory tract in normal subjects in association with cigarette smoking. Am Rev Respir Dis 1988; 137:406–411.

55. Youkeles LH, Grizaanti JN, Liao Z, et al: Decreased tobacco-glycoprotein-induced lymphocyte proliferation in vitro in pulmonary eosinophilic granuloma. Am J Respir Crit Care Med 1995;151:145–150.
56. Fraser RS, Muller NL, Coleman N, Pare PD: Langerhans cell histiocytosis. In: Fraser and Pare's Diagnosis of Diseases of the Chest, 4th ed. Philadelphia: WB Saunders, 1999, pp 1627–1640.
57. Tzi A, Bonay M, Grandsaigne M, et al: Surface phenotype of Langerhans' cells and lymphocytes in granulomatous lesions from patients with pulmonary histiocytosis X. Am Rev Respir Dis 1993;147:1531–1536.
58. Emile JF, Fraitag S, Leborgne M, et al: Langerhans' cell histiocytosis cells are activated Langerhans' cells. J Pathol 1994;174:71–76.
59. de Graff JH, Tamminga RY, Kamps WA, et al: Langerhans cell histiocytosis: Expression of leukocyte cellular adhesion molecules suggests abnormal homing and differentiation. Am J Pathol 1994;144:466–472.
60. Ruco LP, Stoppacciaro A, Vitolo D, et al: Expression of adhesion molecules in Langerhans' cell histiocytosis. Histopathology 1993;23:29–37.
61. King TE Jr, Schwarz MI, Dreisin RE, et al: Circulating immune complexes in pulmonary osinophilic granuloma. Ann Intern Med 1979;91:397–399.
62. Weinberger SE, Kelman JA, Elson NA, et al: Bronchoalveolar lavage in interstitial lung disease. Ann Intern Med 1978;89:459–466.
63. Uebelhoer M, Bewig B, Kreipe H, et al: Modulation of fibroblast activity in histiocytosis X by platelet-derived growth factor. Chest 1995;107:701–705.
64. Robinson BW: Production of plasminogen activator by alveolar macrophages in normal subjects and patients with interstitial lung disease. Thorax 1988; 43:508–515.
65. Asakura S, Colby TV, Limper AH: Tissue localization of transforming growth factor-beta$_1$ in pulmonary eosinophilic granuloma. Am J Respir Crit Care Med 1996;154:1525–1530.
66. Vassallo R, Ryu JH: Pulmonary Langerhans' cell histiocytosis. Clin Chest Med 2004;25(3):561–571, vii.
67. Bates DV: Respiratory Function in Disease, 3rd ed. Philadelphia: WB Saunders, 1989.
68. Schonfeld N, Frank W, Wenig S, et al: Clinical and radiologic features, lung function and therapeutic results in pulmonary histiocytosis X. Respiration 1993;60:38–44.
69. Basset F, Corrin B, Spencer H, et al: Pulmonary histiocytosis X. Am Rev Respir Dis 1978;118:811–820.
70. Fartoukh M, Humbert M, Capron F, et al: Severe pulmonary hypertension in histiocytosis X. Am J Respir Crit Care Med 2000;161:216–223.
71. Takahashi M, Martel W, Oberman HA: The variable roentgenographic appearance of idiopathic histiocytosis. Clin Radiol 1966;17:48–53.
72. Carlson RA, Hattery RR, O'Connell EJ, et al: Pulmonary involvement by histiocytosis X in the pediatric age group. Mayo Clin Proc 1976;51: 542–547.
73. Tittel PW, Winkler CF: Chronic recurrent pleural effusion in adult histiocytosis X. Br J Radiol 1981;54:68–69.
74. Guardia J, Pedreira J-D, Esteban R, et al: Early pleural effusion in histiocytosis X. Arch Intern Med 1979;139:934–936.
75. Matlin AH, Young LW, Klemperer MR: Pleural effusion in two children with histiocytosis X. Chest 1972;61:33–36.
76. Moore ADA, Godwin JD, Muller NL, et al: Pulmonary histiocytosis X. Comparison of radiographic and CT findings. Radiology 1989;172:249–254.
77. Brauner MW, Grenier P, Tijani K, et al: Pulmonary Langerhans cell histiocytosis. Evolution of lesions of CT scans. Radiology 1997;204:497–502.
78. Von Essen S, West W, Sitorius M, et al: Complete resolution of roentgenographic changes in a patient with pulmonary histiocytosis X. Chest 1990;98:765–767.
79. Vassallo R, Ryu JH, Schroeder DR, et al: Clinical outcomes of pulmonary Langerhans' cell histiocytosis in adults. N Engl J Med 2002;346:484–490.
80. Arico M, et al: LCH-A1. First International Study for Langerhans Cell Histiocytosis in Adults. Histiocyte Society, October 2004.
81. Kobrinsky NL, Gritter HL, Shuckett B: Langerhans cell histiocytosis. In: Chernick VC, Boat TF, eds: Kendig's Disorders of the Respiratory Tract in Children, 6th ed. Philadelphia: WB Saunders, 1998, pp 1058–1071.
82. Etienne B, Bertocchi M, Gamondes JP, et al: Relapsing pulmonary Langerhans cell histiocytosis after lung transplantation. Am J Respir Crit Care Med 1998;157(1):288–291.
83. Habib SB, Congleton J, Carr D, et al: Recurrence of recipient Langerhans' cell histiocytosis following bilateral lung transplantation. Thorax 1998; 53(4):323–325.

67 Pulmonary Involvement in Rheumatoid Disorders of Childhood

Arnold C.G. Platzker, MD

Rheumatoid disorders of childhood have both traditional and unusual presentations. While these conditions are systemic, clinical evidence of pulmonary involvement is not uniform and onset of pulmonary illness is often insidious. The etiology of these conditions is still not completely understood. The disease manifestations are primarily immunologically mediated, although there is already evidence of a genetic predisposition for some of these disorders. The clinical manifestations may be triggered by infectious or environmental influences. While these disorders are usually progressive, their course is also unpredictable. The same may be said for the lung involvement in these conditions.

In these conditions, an immune-mediated acute inflammation results in associated tissue injury leading to the following cascade:

1. Mediators are released into the circulation, accompanied by alteration of the vascular basement membrane, extravascular leakage of fluid, accumulation of phagocytic cells, and activation of the coagulation pathway.
2. This precipitates an exudative stage, with release of chemoatractants, proinflammatory lymphokines, and attraction of neutrophils and macrophages in an attempt to remove damaged cellular debris. This process may invoke antigen release and processing.
3. The final phase of tissue repair involves activation of fibroblasts and deposition of collagen, leading to scarring rather than resolution of the tissue injury.

This cycle of immune-mediated inflammation, vascular leakage, and attempts at repair recurs with progressive organ damage leading to loss of organ function. Available pharmacologic therapies directed at mitigating the inflammation in these disorders merely inhibit but do not yet arrest the inflammatory process sufficiently to prevent further organ damage. There are instances, though, in which the process goes into remission, although remission is unpredictable and the influences responsible are not known.

The serologic hallmark of rheumatoid disorders is the presence and persistence of antinuclear antibodies (ANAs) in the peripheral circulation. ANA is found in the circulation of patients with systemic lupus erythematosus (SLE); however, this finding is not diagnostic, because ANA and rheumatoid factor (RF) are also found in the blood in other disorders, which are listed in Table 67-1. Similarly, the major finding in juvenile rheumatoid arthritis (JRA) of joint swelling and synovitis is not unique to JRA, although the conditions can be classified into those associated with destructive joint changes and those that are nondestructive. However, it is still possible to specifically diagnose the form of the rheumatoid condition. The list of childhood rheumatologic conditions is long and is shown in Box 67-1, in which the conditions discussed in this chapter are italicized.

SYSTEMIC LUPUS ERYTHEMATOSUS

Systemic lupus erythematosus is the first of the collagen vascular diseases to be discussed, because 20% of all SLE cases have their onset before 18 years of age.[1] Males tend to be more commonly affected with this illness than females until adolescence. Diagnosis is suggested by malar rash, photosensitivity, arthritis, nephropathy, and fever; it is confirmed by a positive ANA titer (>1:100).[2] High titers of antibodies to double-stranded DNA (anti-dsDNA) are reported in 85% of pediatric SLE patients, similar to that found in adult SLE patients.[3] Approximately 65% of children and adolescent SLE patients have antiphospholipid antibodies,[4,5] and IgG anticardiolipin antibodies (ACLAs) have been noted in 29% of these children.[3] Lung disease is seen in approximately 6% of children upon diagnosis of SLE (Table 67-2).[6–29] In addition, heart and lung involvement is relatively common during the course of pediatric SLE, with pericarditis occurring in 45%, pleurisy with or without effusion in 35%, and pulmonary hemorrhage in 5%. Other findings including acute SLE pneumonitis, chronic interstitial lung disease (ILD), bronchiolitis obliterans (BO) with organizing pneumonia (BOOP), pulmonary hypertension (PH), and diaphragm and laryngeal dysfunction complete the spectrum of respiratory tract involvement in SLE.[8,30,31] There is also a significant incidence of lung disease characterized by abnormal pulmonary function tests (PFTs) in asymptomatic SLE patients and in adult nonsmoking SLE patients even when chest roentgenograms are normal. Abnormal PFTs are found in 67% of SLE patients.[32] The diffusion capacity for carbon monoxide (DLCO) was reduced in 31% of the patients, whereas midmaximal (forced) expiratory flow ($FEF_{25\%-75\%}$) was reduced to 25% predicted in 24% of the patient group, consistent with obstruction of middle sized and

TABLE 67-1. Rheumatoid factor and antinuclear antibodies in childhood disorders

Diagnosis	No. of Patients	RF (% positive)	ANA (% positive)
Systemic lupus erythematosus	108	5	95
Juvenile rheumatoid arthritis	110	25	28
Dermatomyositis	20	0	55
Scleroderma	19	25	47
Ulcerative colitis	34	11	23
Mixed connective tissue disease	14	64	100
Controls	49	0	6

BOX 67-1 The Rheumatic Diseases of Childhood*

Systemic lupus erythematosus (SLE)
Scleroderma and CREST syndrome (calcinosis, Raynaud's phenomenon, esophageal dysfunction, sclerodactyly, and telangiectasia)
Dermatomyositis
Juvenile rheumatoid arthritis (JRA)
Sjögren's syndrome (SS)
Mixed connective tissue disease (MCTD)
Wegener's granulomatosis (WG)
Systemic vasculitis
- *Henoch-Schönlein purpura*
- *Stevens-Johnson syndrome*
- *Churg-Strauss vasculitis*
- *Periarteritis nodosa*
- Kawasaki syndrome

Postinfectious reactive arthritis
Ankylosing spondylitis
Ulcerative colitis
Regional enteritis
Lyme disease
Reiter syndrome
Psoriatic arthritis
Familial Mediterranean fever (FMF)
Acute rheumatic fever
Sarcoidosis

*Diseases discussed in this chapter are shown in italics.

small airways. Normal PFT results are found in only 35% of adult SLE patients with reduced total lung capacity (TLC) or vital capacity (VC) in one third of the patients and abnormal DLCO in 16% with abnormal PFT results.[33] Exercise stress testing is the best way to detect the presence and assess the magnitude of the airway, interstitial, and pulmonary vascular involvement in SLE. However, exercise testing is often not feasible because of the other SLE systemic manifestations such as fever, arthritis, polyserositis, muscle discomfort, and renal and neurologic involvement in SLE.

In SLE patients at the Childrens Hospital Los Angeles (CHLA), PFTs carried out during long-term follow-up in SLE patients (mean age of 16 years) without obvious respiratory symptoms and with a normal chest roentgenogram, revealed a reduced DLCO in 25% of SLE patients, reduced TLC in 35% of the patients, and a reduced partial pressure of oxygen, arterial (PaO_2) in 10%. A subsequent autopsy study of SLE patients, including some in the pulmonary function study group, revealed diffuse interstitial pneumonitis in all of the patients, acute pneumonitis in 77%, evidence of present or past pulmonary hemorrhage in 70%, small vessel lesions in 58%, BO in 35%, and mild interstitial fibrosis in 46% of the patients.[34] In a small study of chest roentgenogram and pulmonary function conducted in a group of SLE patients during the course of 2 years, all but one child were without pulmonary symptoms or physical findings of lung disease.[35] However, slightly more than half were found to have an abnormal chest roentgenogram, forced vital capacity (FVC) was reduced in 67%, and DLCO was reduced in 22%. In a 6-year study of 22 children with SLE, 36% at diagnosis of SLE, and 59% of the entire group had abnormal chest roentgenograms, 18% had dyspnea, 46% had restriction, and 67% had reduced DLCO.[36]

While pleural disease is the most common diagnosed respiratory complication of SLE, it may result from extrapulmonary SLE-associated problems, such as renal nephrosis, cirrhosis, and congestive heart failure. Vasculitis and pulmonary infection can also result in pleural fluid collection. Therefore, when pleural effusion is noted in SLE, diagnostic thoracentesis for pleural fluid aspiration and analysis is indicated. The presence of LE cells or ANA-positive pleural fluid suggest that the pleural effusion is a result of SLE. This complication is treated with nonsteroidal anti-inflammatory drugs (NSAIDs) to relieve discomfort. Drainage of pleural fluid is rarely necessary and is reserved for those instances in which large pleural effusion results in respiratory embarrassment.

TABLE 67-2. Frequency of pulmonary disease in collagen vascular disorders

Pulmonary Disorder	SLE	JRA	PSS	Dermatomyositis	SS	MCTD	Wegener's
Pleuritis*	++	++	+	–	+	++	+
UIP	+	++	++	++	+	++	–
IP	+	+	++++	++++	+	+++	–
DAD	++	+	+	+ (ref. 22)	+	–	+
BOOP	+ (ref. 6)	Rare	+	++ (ref. 23)	+	–	+ (ref. 29)
LIP	–	(refs. 15,16)	–	–	+++	+	–
Vasculitis	++ (refs. 7–9)	–	+	–	–		+++ Granulomatous
PHN	++	Rare	+ (refs. 19,20)	Rare	+	+	
Hemorrhage†	++ (refs. 10,11)	Rare	–	–	–	+	+++
Air leak‡	12	++	–	+ (refs. 24,25)	– (ref. 28)	Rare	
Airway disease	–	++	–	–	++	–	+++ Stenoses
Other§	++ (refs. 13,14)	++ (refs. 17,18)	++ (ref. 21)	++ (refs. 26,27)	++ Cysts, nodules	+	+++ Nodules

*With or without effusion.
†Pulmonary hemorrhage.
‡Pneumothorax.
§Includes phrenic palsy, muscle weakness, pulmonary vasculitis.

BOOP, bronchiolitis obliterans organizing pneumonia; DAD, diffuse alveolar damage; IP, nonspecific interstitial pneumonia; JRA, juvenile rheumatoid arthritis; LIP, lymphocytic interstitial pneumonia; MCTD, mixed connective tissue disease; PHN, pulmonary hypertension; PSS, progressive systemic sclerosis; SLE, systemic lupus erythematosus; SS, Sjögren's syndrome; UIP, usual interstitial pneumonia; + to ++++, frequency of the finding; –, finding not reported in this disorder.

Pulmonary parenchymal infiltrates that appear suddenly and are associated with respiratory distress and/or oxygen desaturation may indicate pulmonary hemorrhage, especially when there is anemia in the peripheral blood. In acute SLE, pneumonitis can present with fever, cough, dyspnea, and chest pain; chest roentgenograms show densities (commonly in the lower lobe), atelectasis, and elevation of the diaphragms.

Chronic interstitial lung disease (CHILD) in SLE is thought to have a 1% to 6% incidence.[13] It is probably underreported, since CHILD may cause few symptoms early in the course of this SLE complication. Children with SLE also limit their exercise because of other organ involvement or arthritis, so that tachypnea may not be recognized and cough may be attributed to allergy or an upper respiratory tract infection. In addition to the few findings early in the course of ILD, the plain chest roentgenogram is usually insufficiently sensitive for detection of ILD. The clinical findings of CHILD include nonproductive cough, tachypnea, and crackles on auscultation of the chest. When present on plain chest roentgenogram, CHILD appears as reticular nodular densities scattered throughout the lung fields. However, thin-cut high-resolution computed tomography (HRCT) of the lung area in SLE may present with one of three radiologic patterns (Table 67-3).[37]

Pulmonary alveolar hemorrhage has been reported in 5% to 10% of children with SLE, but it is generally uncommon.[38,39] Although it is rare, of those who experience pulmonary hemorrhage, in 23% it is the presenting clinical manifestation of SLE.[40] Pulmonary hemorrhage is most often experienced by patients who have high anti-dsDNA titers and active extrapulmonary organ involvement. It may mimic or occur in association with acute pneumonitis.[10] Pulmonary hemorrhage occurs five times more often in female than in male SLE patients and has been characterized as the result of a small pulmonary vessel angiitis.[7] Dyspnea, fever, and pulmonary infiltrates are the usual presenting symptom. Frank hemoptysis occurs in only one half of the patients.[10] Pulmonary hemorrhage can be catastrophic. Only 12% to 20% of the reported cases had unilateral presentation. While usually bilateral and diffuse, pulmonary hemorrhage may also be seen in association with pleural effusion in about 30% of the cases. Lung densities clear as the hemorrhage abates, and complete clearing of alveolar hemorrhage may take 1 to 2 weeks. Histology of the lung tissue reveals alveolar fibrin and red blood cell deposition, diffuse injury to the pulmonary microcirculation with focal alveolar septal necrosis, and, depending on the length of time that has passed since the acute hemorrhage, an influx of neutrophils with hemosiderin-laden alveolar macrophages.[7] Treatment is generally supportive, normalizing gas exchange with supplemental oxygen and assisted ventilation when severe hypercapnia is present. With assisted ventilation, the addition of positive end-expiratory pressure should theoretically be beneficial, impeding alveolar bleeding and maintaining expansion of the alveoli. Although high-dose intravenous steroids, immunosuppressive medications, and plasmapheresis have been used in the treatment of pulmonary hemorrhage, their effectiveness has not been confirmed.

Bronchiolitis obliterans may occur as a very rare complication of SLE in which there is chronic inflammation of small airways with an influx of inflammatory cells, neutrophils, and plasma cells.[6] Fibroblasts attracted to the site of the inflammation deposit fibrin, and there is obliteration of small airways. Over time this evolves into a chronic progressive destructive process in association with an organizing pneumonia, so-called BOOP. Plain chest roentgenograms are rarely suggestive of this condition, and HRCT provides better images of this process. However, the final confirmation of this disorder comes through lung biopsy. PFT confirms the extent of lung dysfunction, with small airway obstruction, nonuniform distribution of ventilation, and reduction in TLC. High-dose glucocorticoid treatment is the usual treatment, but proof of efficacy is lacking.

Pulmonary hypertension occurs in SLE usually late in the course of the illness and may occur without previously recognized ILD or pulmonary thromboembolism.[33,41] It also occurs in SLE patients with long-standing ILD. There are no reports of successful treatment of PH in SLE with pulmonary vasodilator medications (prostacyclins) or nitric oxide. However, there is some support for cyclophosphoramide therapy and low-dose glucocorticoid treatment.[33] While there are few reports of SLE-associated PH, the outcome and prognosis for survival in reported cases has been poor.

Neuromuscular disease associated with SLE may result in impaired lung function. Diaphragm elevation on chest roentgenogram, an indication of shrinking lung, is often seen. This finding may be present even when there is no evidence of parenchymal or pleural disease.[42] In such cases, this finding has been attributed to diaphragmatic and intercostal muscle weakness. Laryngeal dysfunction has been reported in SLE patients and is probably more frequent than the 30% incidence reported.[43] In this disorder, swallowing is compromised because of mucosal edema, mild mucosal ulceration, inflammation of the epiglottis, and vocal cord paralysis. Airway obstruction results from vocal cord paralysis or necrotizing vasculitis. Laryngoscopy, bronchoscopy, and CT scan of the upper airway assist in confirming the clinical diagnosis. Long-term consequences reported include tracheal stenosis. Steroid administration often leads to improvement in this condition.

TABLE 67-3. Histologic appearance and chest radiographic and HRCT evidence of lung effects in SLE

Histologic Pattern	Chest Roentgenogram	HRCT
Usual interstitial pneumonia	Reticular abnormalities with basilar volume loss	Irregular linear hyperattenuated areas, honeycombing, traction bronchiectasis, or bronchiolectasia (peripheral, subpleural, basilar)
Nonspecific interstitial pneumonia	Ground-glass and reticular opacities, most prominent in the basilar portions of lung	Ground-glass attenuation, irregular linear hyperattenuated areas, consolidation (peripheral, subpleural, basilar, symmetrical)
Bronchiolitis obliterans with organizing pneumonia	Patchy bilateral consolidation	Patchy consolidation or nodularity (subpleural, peribronchovascular)

After Kim EA, Lee KS, Johkoh T, et al: Interstitial lung diseases associated with collagen vascular diseases. Radiologic and histopathologic findings. Radiographics 2002;22:S151–S165.

Patients with SLE have immune compromise, placing them at risk for respiratory tract infection, often with opportunistic organisms.[44] Compromised immune responsiveness in SLE is a result of:

1. Abnormalities of complement and/or cell-mediated immunity
2. Depressed pulmonary macrophage function, reduced neutrophil chemotaxis, and impaired phagocytosis
3. Treatment with medications (e.g., steroids and immunosuppressive agents) that suppress the immune response
4. Compromised airway clearance mechanisms resulting from airway inflammation, weak cough (respiratory muscle weakness)

In a 15-year period at CHLA in 130 patients with SLE there were 21 deaths. Almost 60% of these patients suffered from bronchopneumonia. After 15 of the 21 deaths, an autopsy was performed. The most common organisms responsible for respiratory infection were bacterial, including *Klebsiella aerobacter*, *Escherichia coli*, and β-streptococcus. However, *Candida albicans*, *Aspergillus* sp., *Pneumocystis carinii*, cytomegalovirus, and *Cryptococcus neoformans* were also cultured from the lungs of these patients. In other series, *Nocardia*, mycobacteria, herpes simplex, and *Legionella* have been reported.[45] Patients with immune dysfunction and those receiving immunosuppressive therapy should receive routine trimethoprim-sulfamethoxazole prophylaxis.

DRUG-INDUCED SYSTEMIC LUPUS ERYTHEMATOSUS

For many years it has been well documented that medications may induce a SLE-like condition that may affect joints, the kidneys, lungs, and pleural cavities, as well as the central nervous system.[46] The list of drugs responsible for lupus-like disease continues to expand as new therapeutic agents enter the marketplace. While hydralazine and procainamide are the most common medications incriminated (accounting for as much as one quarter to one half of this complication), nitrofurantoin, methyldopa, quinidine, pronestyl, and quinolones are also known to cause a lupus-like condition. High ANA titers, LE cells, and reduced complement (in pleural effusions) have been reported. Prompt recognition of this complication and immediate discontinuation of the suspected medication are essential for reversal of this condition. However, while the acute clinical findings appear to improve rapidly with discontinuation of the medication responsible for precipitating the SLE-like condition, weeks may elapse before all of the findings resolve completely. The ANA titer may remain elevated for many months after resolution of the clinical findings.

Case 1. A 4-year-old girl presented with a 3-month history of arthralgia, malaise, fever, and a malar rash. Physical examination revealed arthritis of the elbows, wrists, and knees. An erythematous maculopapular rash covered the trunk and thighs. Moderate lymphadenopathy and hepatosplenomegaly were also noted. The lungs were clear on auscultation, but tachypnea was present. There was a regular cardiac rhythm and normal rate, but a grade 2/6 systolic ejection murmur was audible.

Laboratory findings included white blood cell count of 11,800 cells/mm^3, hemoglobin of 8.8 g/dL, erythrocyte sedimentation rate (ESR) of 130 mm/hr, and a positive direct and indirect Coombs' test. Serum albumin was 2.9 g/dL and globulin was 5.2 g/dL. There was an ANA titer of 1:2560, RF of 1:160. IgG was 3525 mg/dL (normal, 550–1100 mg/dL), C3 was less than 10 mg/dL (normal, 60–140 mg/dL). Creatinine clearance was 47 mL/min/1.73m^2. Urinalysis revealed glucosuria, 25 to 30 white blood cells per high-power field, 75 to 100 erythrocytes per high-power field, and there were granular and hyaline casts. Chest radiography revealed moderate cardiomegaly with slightly increased pulmonary vascularity. An electrocardiogram and echocardiogram were normal.

Systemic lupus erythematosus with renal disease and mild myocarditis was diagnosed, and initial treatment with prednisone 35 mg/day and hydroxychloroquine 100 mg was prescribed. Renal biopsy revealed diffuse, chronic interstitial nephritis and severe proliferative glomerulonephritis. Diuretic treatment was started for progressive hypertension and edema. Within 3 months, C3 had fallen to 133 mg/dL, ANA had fallen to 1:160. During the next 18 months, an episode of pneumonia was treated with oral ampicillin therapy, and there was active nephritis, intermittent rash, and arthritis. Despite prednisone administration in dosages of 15 to 40 mg every other day, serum C3 progressively fell to 30 mg/dL.

At 6.5 years of age, she developed fever and headaches. The cerebrospinal fluid protein was 30 mg/dL, but an electroencephalogram revealed mild, diffuse cerebral dysfunction. Renal biopsy revealed diffuse proliferative lupus nephritis with positive immunofluorescence for IgG, IgM, IgA, C3, and fibrin. Urine protein rose to 4.1 g/24 hr. Cyclophosphoramide therapy (50 mg/day) was begun, and prednisolone dosage was increased to 30 mg/day. Serum C3 and ANA titers slowly normalized.

She was rehospitalized twice in the next 6 months because of fever and pneumonia. Serum C3, C4, and ANA titers remained normal during these hospitalizations. Cyclophosphoramide administration was discontinued, and with administration of intravenous cephalothin her clinical status and chest radiography infiltrates improved, although her ANA titer became positive again within 4 months and never became negative again during the course of her SLE illness. Renal disease, proteinuria, and hypertension became more persistent, and serum C3 and C4 fluctuated.

At 8 years of age, the patient developed fever and a left lower lobe pneumonia that responded to intravenous antibiotic therapy. However, 3 months later she developed pericarditis, chorea, and *Haemophilus influenzae* cellulitis of her left arm. Intravenous therapy with antibiotics and dexamethasone brought about clinical and radiographic improvement, although serum blood urea nitrogen and creatinine rose to 66 mg/dL and 1.5 mg/dL, respectively.

Several weeks later she had fever, cough, and chest pain, with mild cardiomegaly on chest radiography. Electrocardiography revealed changes

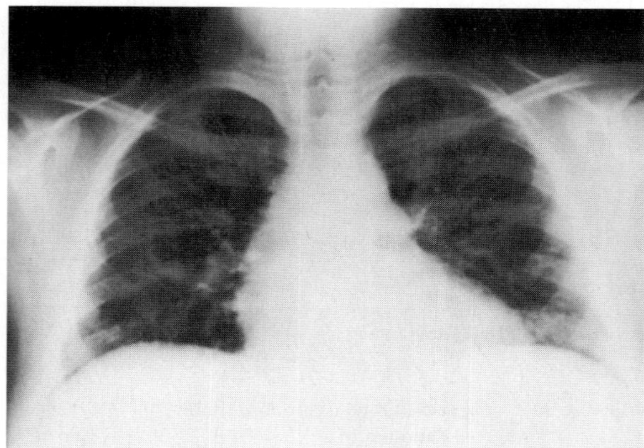

FIGURE 67-1. Case 2. A chest roentgenogram showing a poor inspiratory effort with resultant prominent cardiac silhouette. The lungs show diffuse reticular changes suggestive of chronic pulmonary fibrosis. There are no pleural effusions or acute infiltrates.

■ **TABLE 67-4.** Case 2. Pulmonary function test

Parameter	Percentage Predicted*
VC	64
FEV_1	61
FEV_1/FVC	87
$FEF_{25\%-75\%}$	57
RV	69
TLC	65
RV/TLC	22
DLCO	64
pH	7.40
$PaCO_2$ (mm Hg)	30
PaO_2 (mm Hg)	82

*All values are percentage predicted except FEV_1/FVC and RV/TLC, which are recorded as percentage.

consistent with myocarditis. Her dexamethasone dosage was increased to 2 mg every 6 hours, and treatment with diuretics and an antibiotic was begun. Tachypnea, nasal flaring, blood-tinged sputum, and diffuse bilateral infiltrates on chest roentgenogram suggested worsening congestive heart failure, pneumonia, and/or pulmonary hemorrhage. The patient did not respond to intravenous, high-dose methylprednisolone and antibiotic therapy. Fulminant cardiorespiratory failure did not respond to endotracheal intubation, assisted ventilation, and intravenous inotropic medications, and she died shortly thereafter. Postmortem examination revealed focal vasculitis of the heart and histologic changes consistent with hypertension, myocardial edema, and pericarditis. There was massive alveolar hemorrhage with focal necrotizing pneumonitis, interstitial pulmonary inflammatory cell infiltration, panacinar edema, and arteriolar edema with fibrinoid deposition obstructing arteriolar lumina.

This case is an example of SLE with the rapid onset and persistence of primary lupus pneumonitis, complicated by nephritis, hypertension, and myocarditis, and ending with fulminant pneumonitis, pulmonary hemorrhage, and worsening congestive heart failure. Treatment for SLE and the attendant complications only slowed but did not alter the fatal outcome.

Case 2. A 9-year-old girl developed SLE with typical malar rash, spiking fevers, malaise, arthralgias, nephritis, myocarditis, and congestive heart failure. Treatment included digitalis and diuretics. She had a positive ANA, reduced C3, anti-dsDNA antibodies, and an active urinary sediment. There were no clinical or radiographic findings of lung involvement. During therapy she had persisting low C3 and C4 and malar rash. Within 5 months, nephritis improved and resolved. She experienced the onset and frequent exacerbations of severe headache, mood swings, episodes of psychosis, and deterioration of fine motor coordination. Cerebrospinal fluid protein rose to 76 mg/dL.

Episodes of severe oropharyngeal vasculitis along with the neurologic manifestations were treated with intermittent cyclophosphoramide and continuous prednisone therapy with dosages adjusted to the response to therapy. She appeared to tolerate this therapy. On chest radiography there was only slight prominence of bronchovascular markings, but no infiltrates were noted (Fig. 67-1).

Pulmonary function tests were done 5 years after the initial chest radiography findings just described (Table 67-4). VC and its subdivision were only mildly reduced. Functional residual capacity (FRC), residual volume (RV), and TLC reflected similar reduction in predicted volumes. Forced expiratory volume in 1 second (FEV_1) was reduced in proportion to the reduction in VC, and was normal when expressed as a percentage of the FVC (i.e., FEV_1/FVC). The maximal expiratory flow-volume curve was convex, suggesting normal expiratory flow at all lung volumes. The single-breath oxygen test to assess uniformity of distribution of ventilation was normal. The single-breath DLCO was reduced. PaO_2 was within the low end of the normal range for age, and partial pressure of carbon dioxide, arterial ($PaCO_2$) and pH showed a compensated respiratory alkalosis. Therefore, pulmonary function was measured during exercise stress testing with bicycle ergometry (Table 67-5). Oxygen consumption at rest ($\dot{V}O_2$) was normal, but the ratio of carbon dioxide production to oxygen consumption (CO_2/O_2) was increased. Minute respiratory volume increased as a function of respiratory rate, while wasted ventilation (ratio of dead space volume to tidal volume, V_D/V_T) remained in the normal range. With increasing exercise loads, there was increasing hypoxemia and a threefold increase in oxygen consumption after 6 minutes at the initial exercise level, but the V_D/V_T was unchanged. Six minutes after a stepwise increase in exercise load, her heart rate was 178 beats/min and she was exhausted and unable to continue exercise. The PaO_2 had fallen farther to 64 mm Hg, and oxygen consumption had risen more than fourfold above pre-exercise levels with a 20% further increase in respiratory rate, but the carbon dioxide production and oxygen consumption remained balanced and V_D/V_T was again unchanged. After 4 minutes of rest, her tachypnea continued and hypocapnia persisted ($PaCO_2$ 29 mm Hg), but the PaO_2 had returned to the normal range, suggesting a reduction of oxygen consumption.

This patient has moderately severe restrictive lung disease with chronic tachypnea and hypocapnia. The DLCO was decreased, reflecting reduction in the pulmonary capillary blood volume consistent with moderate restrictive disease and/or pulmonary vascular disease. The magnitude of the physiologic dysfunction was characterized with even low loads of exercise, and there was inability to improve wasted ventilation during exercise with increasing tidal volume as well as respiratory rate.

This patient had slowly progressive chronic respiratory insufficiency with parenchymal fibrosis due to SLE without documented prior pulmonary infection or lupus pneumonitis.

Case 3. This 15-year-old adolescent girl developed progressive weight loss, anorexia, fatigue, anemia, and 1 month of frequent epistaxis. She was a thin adolescent with arthritis, no rash, and clear lungs.

■ **TABLE 67-5.** Case 2. Pulmonary function during exercise

Parameter	Rest	Exercise Load 150 kg-m/min	Exercise Load 250 kg-m/min	Recovery
Time	*Rest*	*6 Min*	*6 Min*	*4 Min*
PaO_2 (mm Hg)	86	72	64	88
$PaCO_2$ (mm Hg)	32	29	Not recorded	29
pH	7.43	7.42	7.41	7.41
$\dot{V}O_2$ (O_2 consumption, L/min)	0.129	0.415	0.550	
Ratio (CO_2/O_2)	1.03	0.87	0.98	
$\dot{V}_E$ (expired volume, L/min)	11.9	32.9	45.3	
Respiratory rate (breaths/min)	28.3	48	58	
Heart rate (beats/min)	99	148	178	
V_D/V_T	0.41	0.41	0.38	

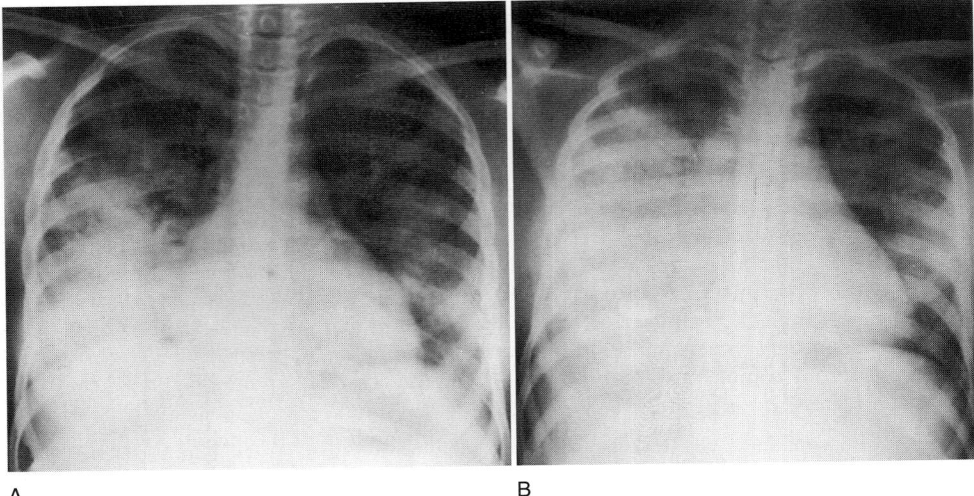

■ **FIGURE 67-2.** Case 3. **A,** The heart is slightly enlarged in the transverse diameter. There is a diffuse, bilateral alveolar process, which is more pronounced on the right. This pattern is not etiologically specific and may reflect hemorrhage, edema, or infection. **B,** There is no appreciable change in heart size. The bilateral alveolar infiltrates have progressed and the right diaphragm is obscured, despite the clinical evidence of improvement.

Her blood pressure was 100/70, her hemoglobin value was 8.1 g/dL, and her white blood cell count was 7200 cells/mm^3. The ESR was 152 mm/hr, and ANA and anti-dsDNA antibodies were present. Serum C3 was less than 10 mg/dL, blood urea nitrogen was elevated at 67 mg/dL, and creatinine was 1.9 mg/dL, with urinalysis revealing 1 to 3 white blood cells per high-power field and 15 to 20 erythrocytes per high-power field. A 24-hour urine collection contained 2.5 g protein.

With the onset of fever, tachypnea, and documented pericarditis, but a clear chest radiograph, initial therapy for SLE consisted of prednisone 15 mg every 6 hours. Renal biopsy confirmed diffuse lupus glomerulonephritis. Prednisone was increased to 25 mg every 6 hours.

Two weeks after diagnosis, the patient developed dyspnea, orthopnea, and severe chest pain but remained afebrile. Respiratory rate was 60 breaths/min and heart rate 160 beats/min. Breath sounds were diminished over the right hemithorax, and bilateral crackles were present. Cardiac examination was normal, but the liver was 5 cm below the right costal margin and the chest radiograph revealed cardiomegaly and a diffuse alveolar process with prominence on the right and dorsally (Fig. 67-2*A*). Blood and sputum cultures were obtained. Oxygen was administered by facemask to relieve marked oxygen desaturation. Treatment included intravenous antibiotics and hydrocortisone 150 mg every 6 hours, and digitalis and diuretics for treatment of congestive heart failure precipitated by severe pneumonitis.

Within 3 days after initiation of therapy, tachypnea and tachycardia were improved. Sputum was negative for *P. carinii.* Over the next 4 days, her condition continued to improve, although improvement in the chest radiograph infiltrates was minimal (see Fig 67-2*B*). Prednisone, 25 mg every 6 hours, was substituted for hydrocortisone; oxygen and antibiotic therapy were discontinued. The illness appeared to be severe primary lupus pneumonitis responding to high-dose corticosteroid treatment.

Shortly thereafter, severe peripheral neuropathy, diffuse lupus nephritis, recurrent arthralgias, rash, and fatigue prompted the initiation of cyclophosphoramide treatment, which brought about complete remission of the nephritis. However, she developed severe hemorrhagic cystitis, apparently attributable to the cyclophosphoramide treatment. A positive ANA, anti-dsDNA antibodies, and hypocomplementemia persisted, though without other clinical finding of SLE. She did not experience any additional pulmonary symptoms.

Five years later, PFTs were conducted (Table 67-6). The patient admitted to smoking cigarettes, two to three packs per day for 4 years and, incredibly, seven packs per day during the previous year. VC and its subdivisions were within the normal range, as were the RV and TLC. Maximal expiratory flow measured at all lung volumes was within the normal range. However, the single-breath DLCO was reduced but was still within one standard deviation below the predicted mean value. Arterial oxygen tension was normal, and there was a mild, uncompensated metabolic acidosis and an acute respiratory alkalosis. At this point, while lung volumes and the distribution and mechanics of ventilation were within the predicted range, this patient did have a reduced DLCO even when corrected for alveolar volume. Complicating the interpretation of these findings was the 4-year history of cigarette smoking, since the contour of her maximal expiratory flow-volume curve was flattened over the lower lung volumes, suggesting small airway obstruction. Her arterial blood gas analysis revealed marked hyperventilation, but the oxygen tension was normal (at rest) and the A-a dO_2 was also normal. Therefore, at this point, V_D/V_T at rest and during graded exercise should have been measured to determine the extent of impaired ventilation and gas exchange. Then, graded exercise should have been added to the pulmonary function measurements obtained at regular follow-up evaluations, since it should prove to be the most sensitive method for assessment of the progression of the SLE lung involvement.

DIAGNOSTIC AND THERAPEUTIC CONSIDERATIONS

Patients with SLE may present with a wide variety of symptoms and findings. However, the pulmonary presentation may be divided into three major clinical patterns of pulmonary disease seen in pediatric SLE:

1. Mild to moderately impaired pulmonary function without significant clinical or radiologic findings (Case 2)

■ **TABLE 67-6.** Case 3. Pulmonary function test

Parameter	Value	Percentage Predicted*
VC (L)	2.2	84
FEV_1 (L)	1.9	77
FEV_1/FVC (%)	91	
$FEF_{25\%-75\%}$ (L/sec)	2.58	82
RV (L)	0.7	90
TLC (L)	2.8	86
RV/TLC		22
DLCO (mL/min/mm Hg)	12.7	68
pH	7.42	
$PaCO_2$ (mm Hg)	28.0	
PaO_2 (mm Hg)	114	

*All values are percentage predicted except FEV_1/FVC and RV/TLC, which are recorded as percentages.

2. Slow progression of respiratory symptoms with radiologic findings, most often chest CT findings
3. Rapid onset of severe pulmonary clinical findings and impaired lung function

Therefore, careful periodic screening of lung function is required after the diagnosis of SLE and during the course of this disease on which to predicate appropriate treatment of SLE and slow the progression of the pulmonary disease. Since these patients are immune compromised, the finding of clinical and/or pulmonary functional impairment should prompt a diagnostic evaluation to rule out infection rather than assuming that these changes are caused by SLE lung disease. Screening for changes in serum complement or in ANA and antibodies to dsDNA titers, or increasing fatigue, rash, and arthralgias should also be included in the evaluation of these symptoms and/or those suggesting worsening pulmonary disease.

The sudden onset of fever, cough, and tachypnea is almost invariably a result of infection, and after conducting the appropriate bacterial, fungal, and viral cultures, the clinician should begin treatment with broad-spectrum antibiotics. There are three rapid-onset SLE complications that are an exception to this rule:

1. Spontaneous hemothorax is a rare complication of primary SLE lung disease[47]; with this complication, ACLAs and the antibodies to the lupus anticoagulant should be assessed.
2. The presence of frothy, blood-tinged sputum suggests alveolar hemorrhage due to SLE (Case 1). Intravenous methylprednisolone pulse therapy, 30 mg/kg/day (maximum of 1.0 g/day) for 3 days, and/or immunosuppressive drugs or plasmapheresis may be effective in containing and treating this SLE pulmonary complication. Mortality rates with pulmonary hemorrhage may exceed 50%, however.[8]
3. If dyspnea and chest pain are prominent, primary SLE pneumonia (Case 3) should be considered. This requires an aggressive diagnostic evaluation that should include bronchoscopy for bronchoalveolar lavage (BAL), respiratory and blood cultures (bacterial, fungal, mycobacterial, and other opportunistic organisms). When these diagnostic studies are not definitive, a lung biopsy should be considered.[48] Recently, lung biopsy by video-assisted thoracoscopic surgery has proven to be as effective as open-lung biopsy. Video-assisted thoracoscopic surgery is also much less invasive and is associated with a more rapid recovery than open-lung biopsy. In SLE pneumonitis, treatment with high-dose corticosteroids and antibiotics together is appropriate. Some children have been observed to respond to combined therapy with an immunosuppressive agent and plasmapheresis.[49] However, the potential for secondary infection is great, and the patient undergoing this form of therapy must be monitored carefully to avoid infections, which often result from opportunistic agents.

Those children with a rapid onset of respiratory symptoms who do not respond rapidly to antibiotic therapy present a difficult diagnostic dilemma, as do the children who have both very slowly progressive respiratory effects and chest radiologic findings. Results of blood and sputum cultures from these patients may be negative or inconclusive. When there are major pulmonary abnormalities (e.g., tachypnea, oxygen desaturation, pleuritis, infiltrates, pneumonia) in association with renal disease (e.g., impaired renal function, uremia) and cardiomegaly (e.g., myocarditis, pericarditis), interpretation of the radiologic lung findings is difficult, because the impact of the impaired renal and cardiac function on the clinical and radiologic pulmonary findings must be taken into account. In this situation, a broad diagnostic approach is required, and HRCT[50] and radionuclide lung scans may be helpful. BAL and lung biopsy are often required to rule out infectious agents and to assess the microscopic pulmonary pathology.

The temptation to change or continue antibiotics, to markedly increase corticosteroid doses, or to add immunosuppressive agents should be tempered by the knowledge that any course may lead to pulmonary or systemic superinfection. Flexible fiberoptic bronchoscopy for BAL is valuable for diagnosis of pulmonary opportunistic infections, such as *Candida* and *P. carinii* in the immunocompromised patient. This diagnostic technique has an advantage that it can be carried out without general anesthesia. Though not without risk, many now strongly prefer thoracoscopic over open-lung biopsy to obtain tissue for microscopic examination.

In SLE, it is important to recognize many possible causes of protracted bleeding. Thrombocytopenia, circulating anticoagulants, ACLAs, and other abnormalities of prothrombin time and partial thromboplastin time are common in SLE. Additionally, template bleeding times may be prolonged even when coagulation parameters are normal. Therefore, complete evaluation of coagulation status should be obtained before performing BAL or biopsy of lung or kidney.

■ SCLERODERMA

Scleroderma (systemic sclerosis) is the rheumatic disease in which severe pulmonary involvement is frequently observed. Although the prevalence of pulmonary disease is lower in children than adults, the spectrum of pulmonary findings in pediatric scleroderma is different from that in adult patients. Scleroderma is usually divided into two major categories: (1) progressive systemic sclerosis (PSS) and (2) "localized" scleroderma. Morphea and linear scleroderma are the major subdivisions of localized scleroderma. PSS is more prevalent than localized forms of scleroderma in adults,[51,52] while the opposite is true for children.[53,54] In one large 15-year experience with 48 children with scleroderma,[55] 27% had PSS, 40% had predominantly linear scleroderma, and 33% developed morphea.

The course of PSS in children closely parallels that in adults; there is a slow but relentless progression of major internal organ involvement, most predominantly affecting the heart, intestines, kidneys, and lungs. Raynaud's phenomenon, severe skin changes, and articular disability also occur later in the course of scleroderma and are not life threatening.[56,57]

The typical microscopic finding on biopsy in childhood scleroderma is extensive fibrosis with hyperplasia of connective tissue, from overproduction of collagen. Impressive vascular and inflammatory lesions may also be evident.[58] Microvascular damage occurs because of the presence of abnormal endothelial cells with vaso-dysregulation, coagulation, and thrombosis. RF, elevated ANA titers, antibodies to dsDNA, and elevated immunoglobulin levels are present in about one half of the children with scleroderma.[55] A broad spectrum of nuclear, nucleolar, and mitochondrial autoantibodies are also found in adults with PSS[59] and are thought to be related to the disease pathogenesis.

Pulmonary manifestations of childhood PSS have received little attention, because the findings are generally considered identical with those found in adults. Even early in the course of PSS, there may be an increase in inflammatory cells and fibroblasts in the interstitium of the lung.[60] At autopsy, the lungs are affected in almost 90% of adults with PSS.[56] The predominant pulmonary microscopic changes are subpleural cysts, pleural thickening, and peribronchial and interstitial fibrosis.[56]

The lungs rank behind only the skin, peripheral vasculature, and esophagus in frequency of organ involvement in scleroderma. Pulmonary disease is now a leading cause of death, because of improvement in the renal prognosis resulting from early and aggressive antihypertensive therapy. However, lung involvement in PSS is often remarkable for the dissociation between the clinical, radiologic, pulmonary function, and pulmonary microscopic findings.[19] Pulmonary disease is often present before the classical rawhide skin findings on which a diagnosis of scleroderma is often based.

The histopathology of the lung includes features of interstitial pneumonitis with alveolar wall hypercellularity, interstitial edema, and alveolar septal fibrosis. There is airway epithelial cell morphologic transformation from columnar to cuboidal, airway smooth muscle fibrosis, bronchiectasis, and bronchiolectasia. Vascular lesions may be prominent, with pulmonary small artery and arteriolar intimal proliferation along with medial hypertrophy. In early lesions, acid mucopolysaccharides are increased in the intima of small muscular arteries. Small vessel change is an early component of PSS, but later in the course of PSS it may be difficult to distinguish from chronic pulmonary fibrosis. Clinically pulmonary and/or systemic hypertension are found at this late stage of scleroderma. The use of BAL documents alveolitis in 49% of scleroderma patients, as evidenced by increases in BAL alveolar macrophage, neutrophil and eosinophil counts, and higher levels of IgG and immune complexes in the BAL fluid.[61] While these findings may occur early in the disease course, they usually persist, but treatment may lead to improved BAL and pulmonary function findings.

It has been well documented in PSS that the extent of the interstitial pulmonary fibrosis and the severity of vascular lesions often are not correlated. Fibrosis is not a constant finding. Pulmonary arterial involvement correlates better with the presence of severe right ventricular hypertrophy. On cardiac catheterization, up to 32% of adults with PSS have PH and marked vascular disease.[62] When present, these findings are associated with rapidly progressive respiratory failure, extensive vascular sclerosis, cor pulmonale, and death.

The pathogenesis of the vascular abnormalities in PSS have been postulated to be related to Raynaud's phenomenon, because renal vascular changes can be detected in response to peripheral cold challenge.[63] Decreased pulmonary perfusion, measured by krypton Kr 81m scan, occurs following cold challenge to the hands.[64] In patients with scleroderma, the DLCO has been found to decrease during winter, and DLCO is also acutely decreased in cold-induced Raynaud's phenomenon in scleroderma, although the magnitude of DLCO change is small.[19] Conversely, others were not able to confirm the occurrence of either pulmonary vasospasm or transient PH during episodes of Raynaud's phenomenon in PSS.[65] Both severe Raynaud's phenomenon and smoking increase susceptibility to rapid deterioration in lung function in scleroderma.[66]

It is useful to recognize three types of pulmonary disease in PSS:

1. Predominant lung fibrosis, with insidious, progressive destruction of the pulmonary microcirculation and eventual cor pulmonale
2. Combined pulmonary parenchymal and vascular lesions
3. Predominantly pulmonary vascular involvement associated with rapidly lethal right ventricular failure

Impaired DLCO is usually the earliest physiologic abnormality and often can be found before there is clinical or radiographic evidence of pulmonary disease.[67] Decreased lung compliance and reduced VC usually develop as PSS progresses. Restrictive lung dysfunction reflects the extent of the peribronchial and interstitial fibrosis. When classified by type of their pulmonary function abnormality, 29% of PSS patients had restrictive disease, 27% had obstructive disease, and 42% had small airways disease.[63] One patient (2%) had abnormal DLCO alone. It has been suggested that small airways disease precedes the gas diffusion abnormality in PSS.[63] Others believe that reduced elastic recoil is the most sensitive index of the lung involvement in PSS. Some report difficulty, even with sensitive exercise studies, in detecting gas exchange abnormalities in PSS patients documented to have pulmonary vasculitis.[68] However, this apparent conflict may be a result of the difficulty PSS patients have in performing exercise studies.

Obstructive lung disease with hyperinflation (e.g., reduced maximal breathing capacity and increased RV) may become prominent late in the disease course. Exertional dyspnea is the most common respiratory complaint in PSS (47% to 80% of cases). It is rarely the presenting complaint. Tightness of skin of the chest is not a cause of dyspnea. Rather, decreased lung compliance and increased work of breathing resulting from pulmonary fibrosis are the most common cause of dyspnea. Chest pain due to PSS lung disease is very rare, and cough is not common unless PSS is complicated by respiratory tract infection and pleurisy. Fine, bibasilar inspiratory crackles are the most frequent auscultatory finding; clubbing is less frequently seen than with other causes of interstitial fibrosis.

Lung cancer (adenocarcinoma and squamous cell carcinoma) is another late complication of scleroderma,[69] but alveolar cell carcinoma has not been documented in PSS. Reported increases of lung cancer (relative risk up to 16.5:1) in scleroderma may be attributed to the following:

1. Impaired clearance of carcinogens due to abnormal lung architecture
2. Defects in host immunity
3. Susceptibility to malignant transformation due to epithelial hyperplasia

Chest roentgenograms are abnormal in 25% to 64% of patients with scleroderma. CT of the chest is a more sensitive method for detecting pulmonary involvement, and CT provides more elegant and fine detail of the lung pathology. The most prominent CT findings are fine interstitial, reticulonodular, or linear changes, with accentuation at the lung bases.[19] In the late stages of PSS lung disease there is diffuse fibrosis, honeycomb lung, and decreased lung volume. Vascular congestion, pleural thickening, and cardiomegaly are also observed. Spontaneous pneumothorax is rare, usually arising from rupture of a cyst on the pleural surface of the lung with reexpansion occurring slowly. Evidence of pulmonary fibrosis does not uniformly correlate with respiratory symptoms, skin changes, or involvement of other organ systems.

From the foregoing it is clear that HRCT scan of the lungs is appropriate for use in the early detection of scleroderma ILD. In one report, abnormalities were found in 21 of 23 cases, including 14 patients of the 21 patients with positive HRCT who had had normal routine chest roentgenograms.[70] However, the prognostic value, correlation with PFT, and the therapeutic implications of these HRCT findings have not yet been clearly defined. Although theoretically useful for detection of inflammation, Gallium Ga 67 citrate lung scans have not received wide use, and the findings of these studies have not been shown to correlate well with clinical, functional, or radiographic findings.

Pulmonary disease in PSS has been very difficult to treat, although discontinuation of cigarette smoking in adults and reducing the frequency and severity of Raynaud's phenomenon may be helpful. Vasodilators, steroids, aspirin, NSAIDs, colchicine, griseofulvin, chlorambucil, and extracorporeal photochemotherapy have all been shown to be ineffective in treating PSS, while total lymphoid irradiation appears to adversely affect the lung, with acceleration of the progression of lung disease.[71] In a preliminary study, D-penicillamine treatment resulted in significant improvement in the DLCO, blunting progression of dyspnea and/or parenchymal fibrosis, and reduction of skin thickening in scleroderma.[72] In another study a regimen of daily oral cyclophosphamide (1–2 mg/kg) and low-dose prednisone (5–40 mg/day) in adults with PSS resulted in maintenance or improvement in FVC for 12 to 24 months.[73] DLCO was not improved, but it did not decline significantly. Patients with early PSS and active inflammatory alveolitis may be the best treatment candidates. The following is an illustrative case.

Case 4. This 18-year-old girl developed "arthritis" at 4 years of age and had the onset of progressive systemic sclerosis at 6 years. The initial skin involvement, Raynaud's phenomenon, and dysphagia were treated unsuccessfully with prednisone, 2.5 mg three times per day for 2 months. Growth failure noted before steroid therapy persisted after steroid therapy was discontinued. At age 10 years she underwent a skin biopsy that revealed increased fibrosis with reduced cellularity of the dermis and atrophic sweat glands surrounded by "constricting collagen fibers." A chest radiograph revealed very little subcutaneous tissue, marked emphysema, and severe interstitial fibrosis. Cystic changes were present in the lower lung fields bilaterally.

By age 18, the patient experienced shortness of breath, moderate dyspnea on exertion, alternating constipation and diarrhea, and severe Raynaud's phenomenon. Examination revealed generalized atrophic skin with variable hypopigmentation and hyperpigmentation. She had mild nasal flaring, poor chest expansion, intercostal and supracostal retractions, and fine crackles at both lung bases. The cardiac and abdominal findings were not remarkable. Generalized muscle wasting and severe joint flexion contractures were evident. Laboratory studies revealed negative ANA and RF, normal complete blood count, blood urea nitrogen, and creatinine. Barium enema revealed severely abnormal motility. Chest roentgenograms revealed advanced pulmonary parenchymal fibrosis. Serial PFTs were performed during the final 2 years of her disease.

D-Penicillamine and corticosteroids were administered without success. Her course was marked by tachypnea, progressive cough, shortness of breath, and dyspnea on exertion. By 20 years of age she required continuous oxygen supplementation. Oxygen supplementation was maintained at a fraction of inspired oxygen of 0.30 to prevent hypoxemia. Arterial blood gases analysis revealed pH 7.37, Pa_{CO_2} 55 mm Hg, and Pa_{O_2} of 75 mm Hg. The patient developed pneumonia, precipitating cor pulmonale and congestive heart failure, which responded favorably to intravenous gentamicin and methicillin, diuretics, and oral digoxin.

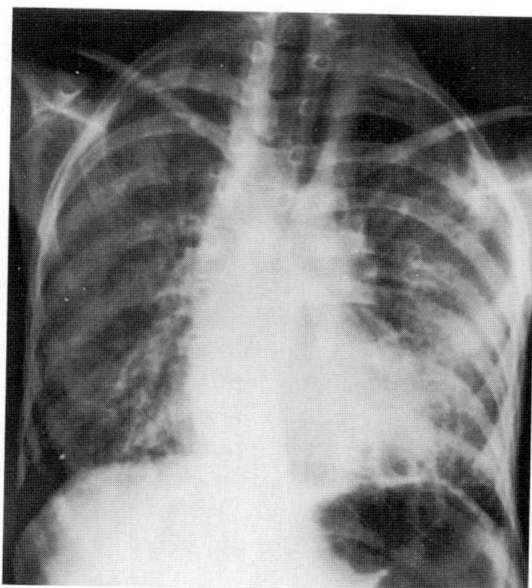

FIGURE 67-3. Case 4. An advanced case of scleroderma lung with chronic pulmonary fibrosis in a reticulated honeycomb pattern more prominent in the lower lobes. The heart is minimally enlarged, gaseous distention of the proximal and distal thirds of the esophagus is present, and there is a moderate right convex scoliosis.

Chest roentgenogram revealed progressive fibrosis (Fig. 67-3). She subsequently developed severe hypoxia and hypercapnia.

She was rehospitalized after diagnosis of a spontaneous right pneumothorax. Insertion of a chest tube resulted in only partial lung expansion. During the next 2 months the pneumothorax failed to resolve and there was reaccumulation of air in the right pleural cavity. She developed a right-sided empyema, progressive weakness, and severe decubitus ulcers occurred due to immobility. She showed advanced psychiatric pathology with disassociation. She became progressively weaker, and respiratory status continued to deteriorate. However, there was no cardiomegaly on chest radiography, and only a 10% right pneumothorax persisted. The patient had a sudden cardiorespiratory arrest and died at the age of 20.

Results of the PFTs performed before her terminal admission to the hospital are listed in Table 67-7. The FVC and its subdivisions are severely reduced. The RV and TLC were markedly reduced, reflecting the reduction in FVC. The FEV_1 was moderately reduced, but it appeared within the normal range when expressed as a percentage of the FVC. Maximal expiratory flow, measured over all lung volumes, was within the normal range when corrected for the reduction in FVC. The DLCO (corrected for hemoglobin) was markedly reduced. This patient had severe restrictive lung dysfunction and reduced pulmonary capillary blood volume as a result of severe pulmonary vascular disease

TABLE 67-7. Case 4. Pulmonary values

Parameter	Value	Percentage Predicted
FVC (L)	0.6	21
FEV_1 (L)	0.5	20
FEV_1/FVC (%)	83	
$FEF_{25\%-75\%}$ (L/sec)	1.05	35
TLC (L)	1.0	30
RV (L)	0.5	64
RV/TLC	0.5	
DLCO (mL/min/mm Hg)	2.7	14.9
pH	7.39	
Pa_{CO_2} (mm Hg)	30.5	
Pa_{O_2} (mm Hg)	57.9	

resulting in a severe reduction in carbon monoxide uptake into the alveolar capillary blood.

CREST SYNDROME

The CREST syndrome variant of scleroderma consists of calcinosis, Raynaud's phenomenon, esophageal dysfunction, sclerodactyly, and telangiectasia.[51] Initial reports of the CREST syndrome stressed its benign prognosis in comparison with PSS, but prolonged evaluation reveals slowly developing gastrointestinal involvement, PH, Sjögren's syndrome (SS), and biliary cirrhosis. Thus, its distinguishing features are onset with Raynaud's phenomenon, extensive calcinosis, and profuse telangiectasia. CREST syndrome has not been specifically reported in children, but its features are similar to "acrosclerosis" and to some forms of focal scleroderma of childhood.[53,58]

In a study of lung involvement in 120 patients, 10 had PH, exertional dyspnea, and tricuspid regurgitation with enlarged pulmonary arteries, and congestive heart failure.[74] Of the 10 patients, 6 died of PH. Chest roentgenograms and postmortem studies did not confirm interstitial pulmonary fibrosis, but late in the course of the disease, the DLCO was diminished in 5 of the 10 patients studied. PFTs in 88 adults with the CREST syndrome showed that only 28% had no abnormalities.[72] Pulmonary fibrosis was noted on chest imaging in 37% of patients, and calcified pulmonary granulomas were also detected in 67% of these patients.

DERMATOMYOSITIS

Childhood or juvenile dermatomyositis (JDM) is a chronic inflammatory disease of skin and muscle, but it may affect other organs as well. JDM presents as a systemic angiopathy, which distinguishes it from adult dermatomyositis.[75] This angiopathy (also called vasculopathy or vasculitis) is marked early in the course of the disease, while acute and chronic lymphocytic inflammation of skeletal muscle and skin) progressing to the development of calcinosis is found in the later course of JDM.[76] This results in proximal muscle weakness and a characteristic erythematous or violaceous rash around the eyes and over the malar eminences, the extensor surfaces of the elbows and knees, and the metacarpal-phalangeal and proximal interphalangeal joints are common presenting features.[77] Laboratory findings include elevated serum muscle enzymes and characteristic electromyographic changes. Recent studies suggest that a unique gene expression profile *HLA-DQA1*0501* may be present in 85% of JDM patients.[78] The initial immune response with this profile is an interferon-α/β-induced cascade with secondary stimulation of interferon-γ. There is increased synthesis of tumor necrosis factor-α (TNF-α), with TNF-α-308A allele. Thus, histologic changes on muscle biopsy include muscle fiber degeneration, sarcolemmic nuclear proliferation, mononuclear cell infiltrates around muscle fibers; vascular changes include prominent perivascular infiltrates and the occlusion of small vessels by intimal proliferation and fibrin thrombi. Recent research suggests that muscle fibers may regulate local inflammation by production of TNF-α, interleukin-15, interleukin-1α, and transforming growth factor-β.[76,78]

Prognosis of childhood dermatomyositis has significantly improved in the past three decades[75,79,80] because of continuation of corticosteroid therapy for as long as there is persistence of clinical or serologic evidence of muscle disease. Addition of therapy with aspirin and/or hydroxychloroquine (as steroid-sparing agents) has been effective as well. Low-dose methotrexate (MTX) therapy has proven beneficial when steroid resistance is present. Strict attention to affected areas of calcinosis has also been important in care of JDM. JDM is a systemic vasculopathy, and the potential for life-threatening internal organ involvement, particularly in the gastrointestinal tract[75] and heart and lungs, may occur at any time during the course of the disease.[24,81]

Diffuse interstitial pulmonary fibrosis is a well-documented complication of adult polymyositis and dermatomyositis. The clinical onset may be acute with fever, dyspnea, and cough, or may be insidious with initially mild, but slowly progressive nonproductive cough and dyspnea on exertion. Bibasilar crackles are a common physical finding, but clubbing is usually not present. Chest roentgenograms usually reveal the appearance and slow progression of diffuse interstitial fibrosis. This is occasionally noted incidentally in adults with dermatomyositis who have no symptoms to suggest pulmonary involvement. There are other infrequent radiologic findings that include patchy alveolar infiltrates, pneumomediastinum, spontaneous pneumothorax, or decreased lung volumes. A retrospective analysis of 105 adults with dermatomyositis found that 10% had radiologic evidence of interstitial pulmonary disease. Eight of these dermatomyositis patients had PFT results that were abnormal, with the mean TLC equal to 67% predicted and a mean VC equal to 60% predicted.[82] Restrictive defects and diminished DLCO were typical PFT abnormalities in most of the dermatomyositis patients studied. The findings were stable over time with only infrequent progression.

In 65 adults with polymyositis/dermatomyositis who came to autopsy, 66% were found to have pulmonary symptoms (including dyspnea in 48% and cough in 35%).[83] Interstitial lung disease was found in 42% and bronchopneumonia in 54%, while pulmonary vasculitis was noted in 7.5%.

In a study of lung biopsy findings from 15 adults with dermatomyositis and clinical lung disease,[22] three histopathologic patterns were identified:

1. There were six cases of BOOP, including reactive pneumocytes, and granulation tissue–filling bronchioles and alveolar ducts.
2. Five patients had usual interstitial pneumonia, showing interstitial scarring and honeycombing, bronchiectasis, and moderately cellular interstitial inflammation.
3. Diffuse alveolar damage was found in four cases and included damaged alveolar lining cells, hyaline membranes, intra-alveolar edema, and focal hemorrhage.

Vasculitis of the lung is usually not a feature in polymyositis/dermatomyositis, but lung cyst formation may be observed. The antibody to Jo-1 has been associated with ILD and pulmonary fibrosis in polymyositis/dermatomyositis.[84]

Corticosteroids are the mainstay for treating pulmonary disease in dermatopolymyositis, particularly with an acute onset or early chronic fibrosis.[83,85] In patients whose lung disease responds to steroids, the histologic features often include interstitial round cell infiltrates, alveolar epithelial hyperplasia, desquamation, and fibrosis. Patients who are unresponsive have demonstrated predominantly fibrosis.[82] Some clinicians add low-dose oral MTX for resistant lung involvement, and there are also reports of improvement with azathioprine,[86] cyclophosphamide,[87] and cyclosporine.[88]

In childhood dermatomyositis, radiographic evidence of pulmonary fibrosis has been reported in four cases,[89,90] with histologic confirmation in two. Spontaneous pneumothorax has been reported in three cases, in one case as a terminal event.[24,26] Pneumothorax may be a complication of the basic angiopathic and inflammatory disease process. One case of alveolar lipoproteinosis in a 9-year-old boy with JDM was successfully treated with BAL.[91] The subtypes of myositis associated with antibodies to t-His-RNA synthetase, Jo-1, and PM/Scl-70 are rare in children, but when they occur, they may be associated with marked dyspnea on exertion, pulmonary perfusion defects, and early radiologic and histologic evidence of pulmonary fibrosis.[27,92]

The most common forms of respiratory involvement are respiratory muscle weakness, impaired swallowing, and impaired airway mucus clearance in children with active early dermatomyositis, or rarely, in those with end-stage JDM. In these cases, aspiration pneumonia and hypoventilation with secondary hypostatic pneumonia may occur. In patients with acute JDM and active muscle disease, vigorous corticosteroid therapy should be pursued to improve strength. MTX has been found to be an effective treatment for steroid-resistant dermatomyositis, but MTX therapy increased the risk of opportunistic infections or, rarely, drug-induced pneumonia.[93]

Case 5. This 21-year-old woman was well until age 12, when she developed a red and scaly rash over the metacarpal phalangeal and proximal interphalangeal joints, anorexia, and weight loss; her upper eyelids showed a violaceous discoloration. The initial 6 months were marked by progressive weakness of the quadriceps, neck, and abdominal flexors. A muscle biopsy revealed fiber degeneration, sarcolemmic proliferation of nuclei, and vascular intimal thickening with perivascular infiltration of chronic inflammatory cells. Serum muscle enzyme levels were elevated.

Treatment with prednisone led to almost complete resolution of the rash and muscle weakness over 4 months. Prednisone doses, varying from 5 to 15 mg/day, were required during the next 4 years to maintain control of the dermatomyositis. Numerous complications occurred during her disease course, including vasculitis of the fingertips and progressive Raynaud's phenomenon, which began when she was 14 and resulted in the autoamputation of several fingertips. Progressive generalized calcinosis was first detected at age 15 years. At age 18 years, perforation of the nasal septum occurred; a biopsy of the adjacent mucosa revealed vasculitis, fibrosis, and chronic inflammatory infiltrates.

At age 18 years, she developed a nonproductive cough; chest examination revealed fine, bibasilar crackles. Serial chest roentgenograms from 14 to 18 years were reviewed and showed "progressive interstitial markings" suggestive of slowly increasing pulmonary fibrosis. A spontaneous left pneumothorax occurred at age 19 years, in association with exacerbation of the Raynaud's phenomenon and worsening vasculitis of the fingertips. The patient was not receiving corticosteroids at this time. Thoracotomy, chest tube placement, and open-lung biopsy were performed. The lungs revealed histologic evidence of pleural and interstitial fibrosis with focal, subpleural chronic pneumonitis. Irregular patterns of aeration, centrolobular emphysema, and perivascular fibrosis were present, but no obliterative vascular lesions were observed. Prednisone treatment (5 mg four times per day) was begun, and resolution of the pneumothorax and decrease in the vasculitis of the fingertips were observed over the next 6 weeks.

The last 2 years of her illness included numerous complications, including severe muscle atrophy and flexion contractures, limited exercise tolerance, recurrent pneumonia and pneumothoraxes, and an unexplained bout of abdominal pain, without evidence of gastrointestinal involvement. Depression and withdrawal from reality occurred; several episodes of psychosis responded poorly to medication and psychotherapy. An elevated cerebrospinal fluid protein level and an electroencephalogram showing diffuse slowing were suggestive of cerebral dysfunction, perhaps due to dermatomyositis. However, the patient resisted further hospitalization or corticosteroid therapy. The pulmonary fibrosis slowly advanced, as can be seen on a chest roentgenogram taken when she was 21 (Fig. 67-4). The following month, the patient died at home from cardiorespiratory failure. No postmortem examination was done.

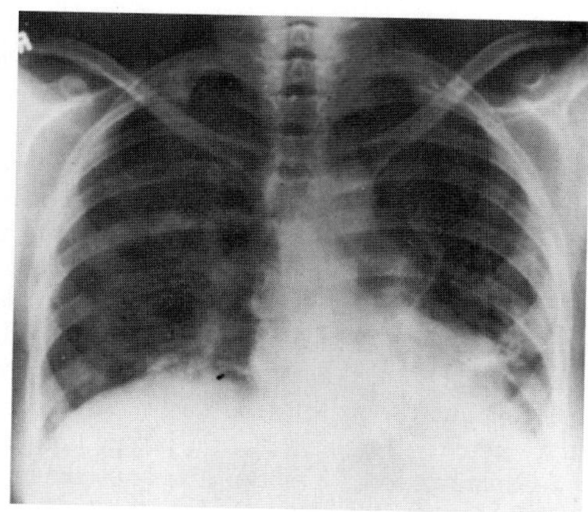

■ **FIGURE 67-4.** Case 5. Dermatomyositis with chronic pulmonary fibrosis of 2 years' duration. The heart is normal in size, and soft tissue calcifications are present in both axillae. Interstitial thickening and cystic changes are bilateral and most pronounced at the bases.

Pulmonary function data are shown in Table 67-8. The FVC and its subdivisions are severely reduced. RV and TLC are within 1 SD of the mean, with the RV equal to the mean predicted value. The FEV_1, expressed as a percentage of the FVC, is normal, as is the maximal expiratory flow measured at all lung volumes. Distribution of ventilation is in the normal range. The DLCO, measured by the steady-state method, is less than 50% of predicted, even when corrected for alveolar volume. There is moderate arterial hypoxemia, an enlarged alveolar-arterial oxygen difference, and a marked acute and chronic alveolar hyperventilation in the face of a mild metabolic acidosis.

This patient had a severe restrictive lung disorder, compromised alveolar volume and alveolar surface area, and reduced alveolar capillary blood volume resulting in hypoxia.

■ **TABLE 67-8.** Case 5: Pulmonary values

Parameter	Value	Percentage Predicted
FVC (L)	1.3	38
FEV_1 (L)	1.2	38
FEV_1/FVC (%)	87	
$FEF_{25\%-75\%}$ (L/sec)	1.3	33
TLC (L)	2.3	55
RV (L)	1.1	116
RV/TLC	0.48	
DLCO (mL/min/mm Hg)	8.1	35
pH	7.45	
PCO_2 (mm Hg)	25.0	
PO_2 (mm Hg)	62.0	

■ JUVENILE RHEUMATOID ARTHRITIS

There are at least 110 medical conditions associated with arthritis in children, of which JRA is the most well known. JRA afflicts approximately 175,000 children in the United States alone.[94] The terms *Still's disease* and *JRA* are often used interchangeably by physicians, but Still's disease should be reserved for the acute systemic-onset juvenile rheumatoid illness that presents with spiking fever, typical rash, polyserositis, and organomegaly. There are two other presentations of JRA: (1) polyarticular (five or more joints) and (2) pauciarticular (four or fewer joints). The JRA type is confirmed only after an observation period of at least 3 months. Until the etiology and subtle differential diagnostic points of JRA are better understood, some children with arthritis and associated inflammatory bowel disease, ankylosing spondylitis, psoriatic arthritis, Reiter syndrome, or the postinfectious reactive arthropathies will undoubtedly continue to be included in surveys of children with JRA.[95] The interested reader is referred to several excellent monographs covering these disorders.[96–101]

Lung involvement is rare in JRA. It is largely limited to children with a systemic onset, in whom it may present before the appearance of joint findings, leading to misdiagnosis.[15,17,102] Interstitial pneumonitis and pleural effusions may accompany early systemic manifestations and are frequently associated with myocarditis or pericarditis. Rarely, asymptomatic pleural involvement will be an incidental finding on chest imaging studies. A child with symptomatic pleural effusions, improving following thoracentesis, has been reported.[103] In one series only 4% of 191 cases of JRA had pleuropulmonary manifestations: 75% had systemic onset.[104] Respiratory complaints included cough, chest pain, and dyspnea and/or tachypnea. All had both pericardial and pleural effusions. Only 2.5% had interstitial pulmonary disease, and spirometry revealed a decrease in FVC. There is one report of acute hypoxic respiratory failure in an 8-year-old girl, heralding the onset of systemic JRA, with a severe respiratory relapse occurring 16 months later.[102] Both episodes responded to intravenous pulsed methylprednisolone therapy. Additionally confirming the rarity of overt pulmonary disease in JRA, other reports of pulmonary involvement are only contained in individual case reports.[105–107]

Other reported pulmonary complications of JRA include rheumatoid nodules, obliterative bronchiolitis, lymphoid bronchiolitis, fatal pulmonary amyloidosis,[108] recurrent pneumonitis,[109] lymphoid interstitial pneumonia,[16] and primary pulmonary hypertension (PPH) in systemic JRA.[110] BO has been observed in a 22-year-old with a 9-year history of JRA treated with penicillamine for 6 years,[111] and in a 12-year-old with polyarticular JRA treated with a 6-month course of intramuscular gold.[112]

Pulmonary function in JRA may still be abnormal despite the absence of prominent respiratory complaints. Pulmonary function in 16 children with JRA, younger than 18 years old,[113] revealed 10 with abnormal PFTs, including 5 who had reduced forced expiratory flow at 75% of FVC ($FEF_{75\%}$), suggesting small airways disease.[113] In another study that evaluated lung function in 34 children with JRA, there were no abnormalities in FRC or $FEF_{25\%-75\%}$ compared to controls, but in 6 of 20 with active JRA, significant reduction in FVC was noted, and 6 of 15 also had significant decreases in DLCO.[114] These studies did not assess the response to therapy.

Rheumatoid arthritis (RA) in adults is recognized as a systemic disorder, with lung involvement being the second most common cause of death (18%) after infection (27%).[115] In summary, the nine types of pulmonary involvement documented in RA include the following:

1. Pleural effusion
2. Pleuroparenchymal rheumatoid nodules
3. ILD
4. Interstitial pulmonary fibrosis
5. BOOP or BO
6. Bronchiectasis
7. Drug-induced lung disease
8. Caplan's syndrome (modified pneumoconiosis in RA)
9. Pulmonary vasculitis (rare)

Although the reported prevalence of pleural involvement in RA may be only 5%, 20% of RA patients have findings suggestive of pleural disease, and in autopsy studies pleural disease has been found associated with RA in 40% to 75% of cases. Pleural effusion may be transient and asymptomatic. However, pleural effusion is frequently found during periods of active arthritis and can be associated with subpleural nodules or parenchymal disease.[116] A chest roentgenogram is the best means of diagnosing the presence of pleural fluid. Only symptomatic patients require treatment, usually thoracentesis to relieve respiratory distress. Rheumatoid lung nodules are found in only 1% of chest imaging studies in adults with RA. Lung nodules are most often located at the periphery of the right middle or both upper lobes, and in these patients there is frequently a high RF titer.[117] The early detection of lung nodules in RA is improved with CT, while the course of lung nodules is highly variable.[118] Lung nodules are the most common histologic finding in lung biopsy samples from patients with RA. Caplan's syndrome is an RA lung complication consisting of an association of rheumatoid nodules and pneumoconiosis.[119]

In 1948 interstitial lung disease in RA was first described.[120] ILD occurs in RA in adults commonly as the disease progresses. Decreased DLCO is the hallmark. ILD may occur as an expected complication or be associated with chemotherapeutic agents. On HRCT, ILD was found in 47% of 91 patients with RA, but with chest roentgenograms alone only half of these ILD cases were detected.[121] However, using BAL criteria, ILD was found in 72% of 58 nonsmoking RA patients.[122] In a study of unselected patients with RA, lung biopsy revealed interstitial lesions in 80% of cases, while only half were symptomatic at the time of lung biopsy.[123]

The prevalence of interstitial pulmonary fibrosis in RA depends on the diagnostic criteria and detection methods used to detect it. Interstitial pulmonary fibrosis in RA ranges in frequency from 1% to 5% by chest radiograph, 40% by PFT, and 80% by pulmonary biopsy.[115] The history and physical examination are of limited value in diagnosing early rheumatoid ILD, although dyspnea, cough, clubbing, and bibasilar rales may accompany advanced disease; in 90% of cases, arthritis precedes lung involvement. The classic presentation on radiography is of a reticular, reticulonodular, or honeycomb pattern at the lung bases. While PFTs reveal a restrictive pattern with decreased lung volumes and impaired DLCO, and decreased FEV_1 and VC.

The pattern of ILD in RA seems to resemble that of idiopathic pulmonary fibrosis with the overproduction of local immunoglobulin, immune complex deposition, and neutrophil-mediated oxidant injury. RA-independent variables include smoking, and certain α_1-antitrypsin phenotypes,[116] while RA-associated variables include production of TNF by alveolar macrophages and the presence of HLA-B40 and HLA-DRB1 as susceptibility markers. An association has been noted between the B-cell alloantigen HLA-DR4 and significant reductions in FEV_1/FVC in patients with RA, appearing to develop irrespective of smoking status.[124] Upon pulmonary lavage of patients with RA, an active neutrophil collagenase that could have contributed to the development of ILD has been isolated.[125]

The course of interstitial pulmonary fibrosis in RA is variable; it is usually slowly progressive and severe loss of lung function is rare, although PH may develop as a result of progressive pulmonary fibrosis. However, once RA patients are hospitalized for diffuse interstitial fibrosis, the prognosis is poor, with a median survival of 3.5 years and a 39% 5-year survival rate.[126]

Bronchiolitis obliterans with organizing pneumonia is equally common in women and men in the general population. Although there have been fewer than 30 cases of BOOP reported in patients with RA, BOOP is now widely recognized in RA. It seems to occur more often in women and may respond favorably to steroid therapy.[127]

It is preceded by a flulike febrile illness in about 30% of cases, and the presentation often includes cough, dyspnea, and crackles.[126] The ESR is elevated. Chest radiographs often reveal a peripheral patchy, linear, or acinar pattern. PFTs may demonstrate a restrictive pattern with reduced DLCO. BAL may suggest a lymphocytic alveolitis.[115] However, infection must first be ruled out. Antibiotic therapy is usually prescribed initially. The progression of symptoms should prompt further diagnostic evaluation including an open-lung biopsy. Anti-inflammatory therapy with steroids is often prescribed, but its effectiveness in halting the progression of BOOP in RA has not been documented.[128]

Bronchiectasis may occur in RA as a product of fibrotic ILD. In 18 of 23 patients with bronchiectasis, the active arthritis preceded the diagnosis of bronchiectasis.[129] The majority of these patients were women with seropositive nodular disease. The most frequent roentgenographic findings were increased bibasilar interstitial markings and focal infiltrates. However, HRCT is required to diagose and assess effectively the extent of disease and to monitor the progression of bronchiectasis.

Bronchiolitis obliterans in RA may be part of the primary disease, although some report BO as a consequence of treatment, with many early cases suspected of being associated with D-penicillamine therapy.[130] Clinically, the onset of BO is usually acute heralded by cough, shortness of breath, and exercise limitation. Chest radiographs may reveal patchy infiltrates and/or hyperinflation. PFTs reveal airway obstruction, but without reduced DLCO. Histopathology of the lung usually consists of acute and chronic cellular bronchiolitis, with relatively little scarring, or constrictive bronchiolitis with inflammation, fibrosis, or complete luminal loss. The prognosis for BO is poor, and thus aggressive therapy is indicated in an attempt to slow the progression of this complication.

Pulmonary function in RA has been studied by many investigators. However, risk factors such as antecedent or current pack-year smoking history, α_1-antitrypsin status, prior pulmonary infections, and use of medications known to induce lung abnormalities have often not been quantified. Additionally, study populations were sometimes small or not controlled, results might not be correlated with biopsy findings, and imaging or histologic evaluation often revealed several processes taking place simultaneously, or over time. Thus, most RA patients with pulmonary involvement have abnormal PFTs, but correlation of specific functional changes with the nine forms of lung disease listed earlier is difficult.

In a study of 100 unselected RA patients and 50 controls, matched for atopy and smoking history, there were significant increases in both airflow obstruction and bronchial reactivity in the RA group.[131] PFTs were done in a group of 342 patients with RA and 265 controls regardless of their lung disease status.[132] Abnormal PFTs were often associated with nonrheumatoid conditions, frequently associated with and exacerbated by cigarette smoking. Tobacco use, not the rheumatoid process, was the most common cause of abnormal lung function in RA.

Drug-induced pulmonary disease is documented in both JRA and RA, as well as in many other rheumatic disorders, and is discussed in Chapter 71.

One additional form of progressive, severe pulmonary impairment occurs in JRA as a result of chest wall and spine involvement. In both adults and children, marked thoracolumbar spine and sternoclavicular joint disease may lead to severe thoracic cage deformities and restrictive pulmonary defects.

Case 6. This 6-year-old girl had a 3-year history of polyarticular JRA. Despite aggressive medical therapy, she had become nonambulatory as a result of severe lower extremity joint disease. She had poor weight gain, and cricoarytenoid joint involvement was associated with partial vocal cord paralysis. Chest radiography revealed moderate dextroscoliosis, dorsal kyphosis, and a bell-shaped rib cage (Fig. 67-5).

Because of very active synovitis, marked muscle wasting, severe flexion contractures, and respiratory insufficiency, she received intensive inpatient rehabilitation for 8 months. Efforts to achieve ambulation were successful, but progressive weight bearing was associated with progression of the thoracic curvature from 10 degrees to 85 degrees. Respiratory symptoms, tachypnea, and poor exercise tolerance, thought to be associated with chest wall disease, persisted. Harrington rod placement to arrest the progression of scoliosis was considered, but the patient was judged an unacceptable operative risk and her osteoporotic spine appeared too frail to retain the rod.

D-Penicillamine was substituted for intramuscular gold therapy, without success. However, a Milwaukee brace arrested progression of the kyphoscoliosis. The addition of oral chlorambucil led to a marked reduction in joint disease activity, increased exercise tolerance, and improved pulmonary function.

Results of pulmonary function studies are listed in Table 67-9. The FVC and its subdivisions are greater than 2 SD below the predicted mean. The FEV_1/FVC is normal, as are the maximal expiratory rates taken from the flow-volume curve, after correction for the reduction in FVC. A resting arterial blood sample reveals mild reduction in the PaO_2 and a compensated respiratory alkalosis.

This girl has severe restrictive lung disease but normal airway function. Her maximal expiratory flow rates at all lung volumes are reduced, but they are normal when corrected for the degree of lung restriction due to the chest wall disease. The restrictive lung disease is so severe that alveolar volume and pulmonary ventilation-perfusion

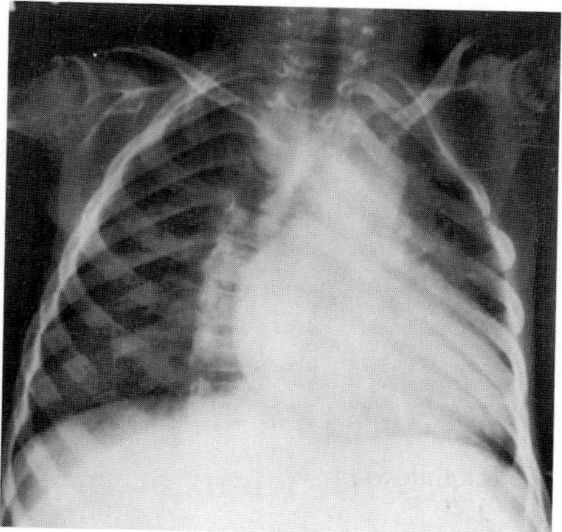

■ **FIGURE 67-5.** Case 6. The bones are severely demineralized. Right convex scoliosis is present, and the heart is moderately enlarged and projected to the left. The rib cage is noticeably bell shaped. A severe pectus carinatum cannot be appreciated in this view. The lung fields are clear.

TABLE 67-9. Case 6: Pulmonary values

Parameter	Value	Percentage Predicted
FVC (L)	0.35	35
FEV_1 (L)	0.30	42
FEV_1/FVC (%)	86	Normal
$FEF_{25\%-75\%}$ (L/sec)	0.78	56
pH	7.39	
PCO_2 (mm Hg)	34.0	
PO_2 (mm Hg)	69.0	

matching are impaired. Thus, the patient has mild hypoxemia despite sustained alveolar hyperventilation. These findings are all attributed to the severe chest wall deformity and scoliosis resulting from the arthritis.

ANKYLOSING SPONDYLITIS

Ankylosing spondylitis (AS) and related spondyloarthropathies in children are increasingly being recognized. These disorders often manifest asymmetrical, large joint, and predominantly lower extremity involvement with enthesitis, including Achilles tenosynovitis, heel spurs, and arthritis of the great toe. The prevalence of this condition is greater in boys, who usually are of the HLA-827 haplotype (40% to 90% of cases). The diagnostic criteria for adult AS do not apply, because children (1) have late or asymptomatic development of sacroiliac joint disease by either clinical or radiologic evaluation, (2) limited chest expansion is infrequent, and (3) obvious spinal involvement is rare, even after long-term follow-up.[133]

Pulmonary involvement in children with AS has not been described, but lung disease in adults with AS is well known; the reported incidence ranges from 0 to 30%. The most common initial finding is upper lobe fibrosis, but this may progress from spotty linear apical shadows to nodules that coalesce or cavitate (nontuberculous fibrocavitary disease).[134]

In a series of 2080 adults with AS, 28 (1.3%) had pleuropulmonary manifestations, including 5 who developed pulmonary aspergillomas.[135] Pleural effusion was rare, but thickening of the apical and nonapical pleura, and rarely calcification, were observed. In none of these cases did pulmonary disease precede arthritis. Apical fibrobullous disease usually began unilaterally, but eventually it was noted bilaterally. There were few clinical findings of lung disease; cough, pain, dyspnea, or hemoptysis did not usually occur. Nail bed clubbing was rare. Pneumothorax and bronchopleural fistula following thoracotomy were also rare.

Chest wall restriction due to arthritis or ankylosis of sternocostal or costovertebral joints may occur. PFTs in 32 asymptomatic adults with AS who had had normal chest radiographs revealed a decreased FVC and TLC, but normal FRC, RV, DLCO, static compliance, and maximal elastic recoil pressure.[136] The use of NSAIDs does not improve VC by reducing arthritis of the chest wall joints, but patients with AS and no more than 75% reduction in VC do not show reductions in maximal exercise performance.[46]

MIXED CONNECTIVE TISSUE DISEASE

Rheumatologists have long recognized unusual overlap syndromes, those that include features of several of the rheumatic disorders. Mixed connective tissue disease (MCTD) was described in 1972 as a unique overlap entity in which there were high titers of speckled ANAs, antibody against a ribonucleoprotein antigen (RNP), arthritis, frequent Raynaud's phenomenon, sausage-shaped fingers, and clinical features suggestive of SLE, scleroderma, and dermatomyositis.[137]

Mixed connective tissue disease may include one or more of the following clinical findings: RA, renal disease (15% to 40% of patients), or thyroiditis. Pulmonary involvement has been reported in 20% to 85% of the cases, but a complete description of the clinical features of the interstitial lung involvement has yet to be fully described.[138,139] In MCTD, study of the lung with HRCT and lung biopsy reveals a diffuse alveolar inflammatory process that progresses to fibrosis, and honeycomb lung, which is most advanced in those patients having scleroderma features as part of the MCTD. Lung biopsy reveals alveolar septal lymphocytic and plasma cell infiltration, with the collagen staining for type III collagen.[140] In those patients experiencing progressive scleroderma-like skin changes, lung disease is most common, most rapidly progressive, and most resistant to therapy.[141]

The first child with MCTD was reported in 1973. In 1977, 14 children with MCTD with a median age of 10.5 years were described, and their serologic findings were compared with those from 127 children with other rheumatic diseases.[142] MCTD findings are usually sequential in children, often beginning with Raynaud's phenomenon (85%), then developing features of JRA, SLE, dermatomyositis, and/or scleroderma. Approximately 85 children with MCTD have now been reported. In pediatric cases the findings are generally similar to those of their adult counterparts. However, polyarthritis (95% of cases) is more frequent in children, along with significant cardiac involvement in 41%, renal involvement in 43%, and severe thrombocytopenia in 20% of cases.[137] Antibodies directed against extractable nuclear antigens or ribonucleoprotein alone are insufficient to make a diagnosis of MCTD.

About half of children with MCTD have keratoconjunctivitis sicca, xerostomia, or parotitis (SS).[143] In addition, 65% have chest radiographic or PFT abnormalities and 30% develop PH.[144] High-dose steroid therapy of long duration may be required in children with MCTD. Unfortunately, when MCTD is complicated by hemorrhage or septicemia, a guarded prognosis prevails.

The prominent findings on biopsy of organs involved in MCTD are consistent. Histology of skin and muscle biopsy in MCTD reveals widespread proliferative vascular disease.[145] Silent involvement of other organs is likely, with pulmonary disease among the most common and severe late complications of MCTD.

In the early stages of MCTD, pulmonary dysfunction is often silent and obvious clinical respiratory symptoms are absent. Harmon and colleagues reported that 80% of adults with MCTD had pulmonary involvement (unexplained dyspnea and abnormal physical examination, chest roentgenograms, or PFTs).[146] The symptomatic patients had abnormal pulmonary function, with restrictive lung disease in 50% and evidence of pulmonary vascular disease (i.e., reduced DLCO) in 67%. Chest imaging revealed alveolar infiltrates and honeycombing in the advanced cases. As mentioned earlier, pulmonary fibrosis was most severe in those patients with scleroderma-like skin changes. Some of the patients had chest roentgenograms suggestive of volume loss and/or pleural disease. On HRCT of MCTD patients studied within a year of diagnosis, ground-glass attenuation and nonseptal linear opacities with peripheral and lower lobe predominence were found.[147] Later in the course of MCTD, subpleural micronodules were found in 94%, honeycombing in 51.4%, pleural thickening in 65.7%, and septal thickening in 100% of 73 adult Japanese MCTD patients, with two thirds of the patients having normal PFTs.[148]

In a prospective evaluation of pulmonary disease in 34 patients with MCTD, 58% developed dyspnea, 42% had evidence of pleural disease, and 24% had cough.[138] While only 33% were asymptomatic, in these patients 73% had abnormal PFTs and/or chest roentgenograms. Overall, 85% had pulmonary involvement (confirmed by PFT). Cardiac catheterization showed PH in 73% of the 15 patients studied. The presence of early PH could not be predicted by PFTs, gallium scanning, or exercise testing, but nail fold capillary microscopy correlated well with the presence of PH, as it does in JDM.[149–151]

Pulmonary hypertension also occurs in children with MCTD.[144,152] PH may be a clinical reflection of proliferative vascular changes and/or thrombus formation in the pulmonary microcirculation and may respond to steroids or immunosuppressive agents.[140] However, recovery from PH in MCTD of childhood occurs only rarely.[153]

Case 7. A 15-year-old girl had a 7-month history of swelling of the hands, arthralgias, malar rash, substernal chest pain, shortness of breath, malaise, and a 20-pound weight loss. She was thought to have SLE, and she was treated with prednisone, 5 mg three times per day. Further history revealed Raynaud's phenomenon, dysphagia, and chronic constipation. On examination her skin was clear; arthritis of the wrists, knees, and ankles was present, and "sausage fingers" and mild digital vasospasm were noted. The lungs and heart were normal on physical examination.

Laboratory data included a white blood cell count of 4200 cells/mm^3. Serum creatinine phosphokinase was 464 IU (normal, 0–100); a speckled ANA (titer 1:256) was detected. Antibody against ribonucleoprotein was present in a titer of 1×10^1:2.0×10^7. An upper gastrointestinal series using barium as the contrast agent revealed diminished peristalsis and dilation of the distal third of the small bowel. Barium enema revealed pseudo-diverticula at the hepatic and splenic flexures. A chest roentgenogram and ventilation-perfusion lung scan were both normal. A diagnosis of MCTD was confirmed because of overlapping clinical and laboratory features of SLE, dermatomyositis, and scleroderma.

Therapy with hydroxychloroquine, 400 mg/day, and prednisone, 40 mg/day, were effective in controlling the disease activity. Seven months later the patient was being treated with only prednisone, 15 mg/day. She had no respiratory or articular complaints. She continued to have Raynaud's phenomenon, intermittent myalgias, and dysphagia.

Results of PFTs are listed in Table 67-10. The FVC and its subdivisions, though reduced from predicted values, fall within 1 SD of the mean. The RV approximates the mean predicted value. The TLC is reduced but is within 1 SD of the predicted mean. The FEV_1/FVC is normal, as is the maximal expiratory flow rate at all lung volumes. The distribution of ventilation, measured by the single-breath oxygen test and 40-breath nitrogen washout test results, is normal. The DLCO is reduced. A resting arterial blood sample has normal oxygen tension and alveolar-arterial oxygen difference and reveals a partially compensated respiratory alkalosis.

This patient has mild restrictive lung disease and evidence of interstitial disease. The shortness of breath is thought to result mostly from the interstitial rather than the restrictive component. Thus, measurement of ventilation and blood gases during exercise would be valuable for assessment of the pulmonary response to therapy.

Treatment of MCTD includes NSAIDs or other anti-inflammatory agents for arthritis. Steroid therapy may be effective for other early inflammatory features of MCTD. However, in many cases of MCTD immunosuppressive medications are required to arrest the progression of the clinical findings.

TABLE 67-10. Case 7: Pulmonary values

Parameter	Value	Percentage Predicted
FVC (L)	2.5	78
FEV_1 (L)	2.2	72
FEV_1/FVC (%)	93	
$FEF_{25\%-75\%}$ (L/sec)	3.76	98
TLC (L)	3.2	76
RV (L)	0.6	70
RV/TLC	0.18	
DLCO (mL/min/mm Hg)	14.3	63
pH	7.45	
$PaCO_2$ (mm Hg)	32.0	
PaO_2 (mm Hg)	106.0	

SJÖGREN'S SYNDROME

Sjogren's syndrome is a disease of unknown etiology characterized by lymphocyte-mediated destruction of exocrine glands. SS primarily affects adult women and is the second most common autoimmune disorder after RA.[154] SS has been defined as an autoimmune epithelitis characterized by lymphocytic infiltration of exocrine glands and epithelia in multiple sites (i.e., sicca).The involvement of salivary glands produces the typical features of dry eyes and salivary dysfunction, but approximately one third of the patients have extraglandular manifestations as well.[155,156] Thus, SS may occur alone (primary) or in combination with almost any other rheumatic disorder (secondary). Both the primary and secondary forms are extremely immunoreactive. Clinical manifestations include dry eyes, dry mouth with oral ulcerations, dental caries, salivary gland swelling, difficulty swallowing, vulvovaginitis, and gastrointestinal abnormalities. Schirmer's test for tear production and a lip biopsy for accessory salivary glands are both helpful in establishing the diagnosis. In 25% of adults with SS, the lymphoproliterative process involves extraglandular sites, such as muscles, kidneys, lungs, and nervous system. Lymphoma and pseudo-lymphomatous transformation are complications seen in SS.

The majority of children who develop SS present with parotitis, sicca symptoms, and multiple autoantibodies.[157] The occurrence of "recurrent mumps" in children, and recurrent benign parotitis of adolescence should prompt consideration of an early manifestation of sicca syndrome. The suggested criteria for diagnosing SS in children include the following:

- Keratoconjunctivitis sicca evidenced by positive Schirmer's and/or quantitative rose bengal tests
- Xerostomia with decreased basal and stimulated salivary flow
- Lymphocytic infiltration in a minor salivary gland biopsy specimen
- Laboratory evidence of a systemic autoimmune disorder[158]

In a series of 35 children with SS, the mean age of onset was 7.8 years, with 77% female.[159] Half of the SS patients had at least one extraglandular manifestation, including two with pulmonary findings.

Cough, dyspnea, recurrent pneumonitis, and pleural effusion are the most common pulmonary features of SS in adults.[160] Pulmonary involvement was found in 9%, with diffuse infiltrates observed to be the most common roentgenographic pattern, followed by pleural effusion. Pulmonary pathology in SS includes desiccation and infiltration of bronchial glands, peribronchial lymphocytic infiltrates, lymphocytic interstitial pneumonitis, and interstitial fibrosis. PFT in SS may reveal a restrictive ventilatory pattern and/or a low DLCO. Diffuse interstitial fibrosis is a frequent late finding on chest imaging. Diffuse ILD develops in 38% of primary SS patients and in 12% of secondary SS patients. However, the clinical findings are often confined to dry cough or mild dyspnea, with these symptoms only slightly greater than found in normal control subjects.[161–163] In a series of 150 adults with SS, 16 complained of dyspnea, and PFT abnormalities were found in 69% of these dyspneic SS patients.[164] Among the 16 dyspneic patients, 6 had evidence of interstitial fibrosis, 5 had peribronchial lymphocytic infiltration, and 3 had pleural thickening, suggesting that progressive pulmonary disease is common in primary SS. When BAL was performed in primary SS patients who did not have pulmonary symptoms (normal PFT and chest roentgenograms), 55% of 29 patients had either lymphocytic or neutrophilic alveolitis. These patients also had clinical and biologic indices of more severe SS.[165] The clinical relevance of these findings is not yet clear.[166] In 20 patients with recently diagnosed SS[167] (90% with respiratory complaints), half had radiologic findings of ILD, and gallium scanning was positive in the lungs of 75% of the patients. On BAL, increase in lymphocytes and/or neutrophils was present. Lung biopsy in 60% of the patients revealed ILD, follicular bronchiolitis, or lymphocytic interstitial pneumonitis. Fibrosis and honeycomb lung was reported, and one patient had associated sarcoid granuloma. Azothiaprine-treated patients had a better outcome.

■ BEHÇET'S DISEASE

Behçet's syndrome is a clinical triad of relapsing iritis, ulcers of the mouth, and genital ulcers, but that may also manifest systemic features including arthritis, thrombophlebitis migrans, erythema nodosum, meningoencephalitis, and arterial aneurysms.[168] It has few serologic markers, and responses to all forms of treatment have been inconsistent. Immunosuppressive medications and corticosteroids are most often prescribed in an effort to treat this disorder. Behçet's disease has a peak incidence of onset in the third decade. It is rare in children, but males and younger patients tend to have a more severe disease course. There are 37 reported pediatric cases in the English language literature, and, notably, there is a lower incidence of ocular disease in children and an absence of lung involvement.[169]

In contrast, adults with Behçet's syndrome have recurrent episodes of dyspnea, cough, pleuritic chest pain, and hemoptysis that appear a mean of 3.6 years after disease onset.[170] Pulmonary findings are often noted during disease exacerbation in other organs. Fatal pulmonary hemorrhage is common, as are pulmonary artery aneurysms and PH. Vasculature involvement is noted in 25% of Behçet's syndrome cases, leading to aneurysms, thrombophlebitis, superior vena cava thrombosis, and pulmonary emboli. Histologic study of the lungs reveals a predominantly lymphocytic pulmonary vasculitis, destruction of the elastic lamina, aneurysms, fibrosis, intimal sclerosis, and aphthous lesions resulting in arteriobronchial fistulas.

Chest roentgenograms are abnormal in 90% of cases, pleural effusion in 70%, diffuse bilateral infiltrates in 37%, right lower lobe infiltration in 28%, hilar vascular prominence in 14%, and round densities in 10% of cases.[170] PFTs are rarely performed in Behçet's disease. Successful treatment of pulmonary complications with steroids was observed in 23 cases. While cytotoxic agents have been used in a few cases, the results have been inconclusive.

■ WEGENER'S GRANULOMATOSIS

Wegener's granulomatosis (WG) is a necrotizing, granulomatous vasculitis with a broad spectrum of findings and progression varying from indolent and limited to a rapidly progressive and life-threatening syndrome. WG appears to be a continuum, which begins with localized involvement eventually progressing to include the upper and lower respiratory tract, skin, kidneys, and other organs.[171,172] The etiology of WG is unknown, and it does not have unique genetic markers. The similarity of many clinical, laboratory, and histologic features of WG to other vasculitic, granulomatous, or infectious disorders, including benign lymphocytic angiitis and lymphomatoid granulomatosis, may cause difficulty in establishing the diagnosis.

Rhinorrhea, sinus pain, fever, arthralgias or arthritis, cough, hemoptysis, and skin rashes or ulceration are among the most common signs and symptoms of WG. Renal involvement may occur early or late in the course and, when present, it requires aggressive management to avoid rapid progession to end-stage renal disease. CT scans of the sinuses and of the lungs (Fig. 67-6) are helpful for diagnosis. CT virtual bronchoscopy (i.e., thin-cut helical HRCT with three-dimensional reconstruction) allows exceptional visualization of central airway stenoses (high specificity, but sensitivity of only 55% to 60%), thus it does not yet eliminate the need for bronchoscopy.[173] c-Antineutrophil cytoplasmic autoantibodies or antibodies to proteinase-3 are highly specific (90% to 97%) for WG but have limited value for following the disease progression or the response to therapy, or to assess prognosis.[174] Confirmation of the WG diagnosis and occasionally assessment of the response to therapy requires lung biopsy.[175–177] Lung biopsy reveals necrotizing granulomas with or without vasculitis (Fig. 67-7). However, as noted in Table 67-11, there is a wide scope of lung involvement in WG that may be divided into acute, subacute, and chronic stages.[29,173,177–180] The findings are specific for each stage, with the most extensive and varied lung pathology seen in the chronic stage. Almost all organ systems can be involved, although the

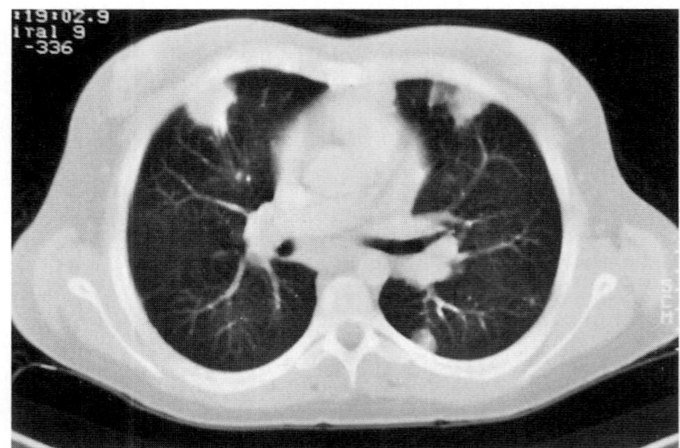

■ **FIGURE 67-6.** This CT scan is from a 14-year-old girl with WG who presented with nasal congestion, chest pain, mild hemoptysis, and a small purpuric vasculitic rash. Her chest radiograph revealed minimal diffuse infiltrate, but the CT scan reveals multiple nodules in a typical peripheral (pleural) distribution anteriorly, and posteriorly on the left.

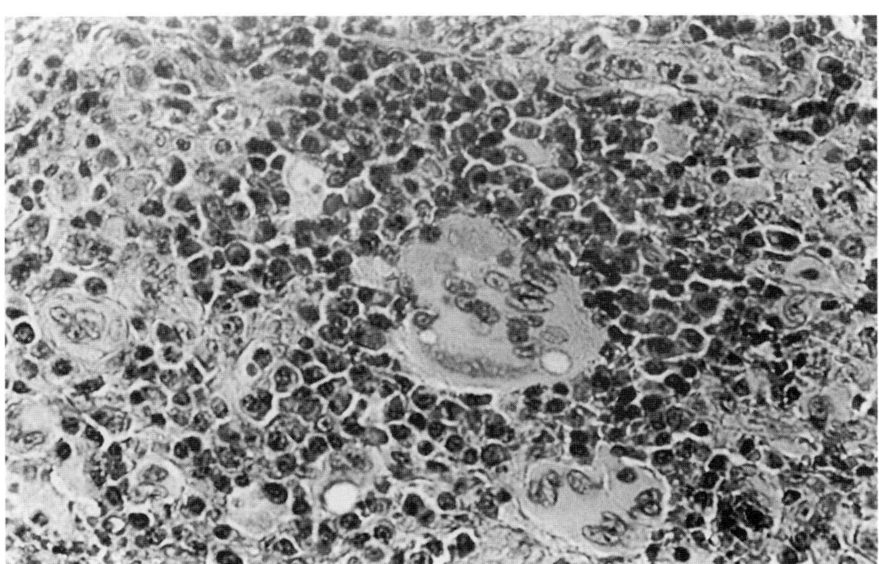

■ **FIGURE 67-7.** Photomicrograph of a lung biopsy from a patient with WG showing a dense pleomorphic infiltrate, numerous mononuclear cells, scattered neutrophils, and several giant cells. This aggregate of cells would be considered a granuloma.

nasopharynx, sinuses, lungs, kidneys, skin, and joints are the organs predominantly attacked in this disorder.

Wegener's granulomatosis is rare in children. In a series of 23 children there was a mean follow-up of 7.6 years, with permanent morbidity observed in 86% of cases, although only 2 patients died.[181] Major clinical features at onset and during the disease course are shown in Table 67-12.

Children with WG were twice as likely to have nasal deformity as adults (48%), and subglottic stenosis was found in 48% (five times more frequent than in adults with WG). Patients experiencing an airway stenosis may require laryngotracheoplasty (Fig. 67-8).[182] Main stem bronchial stenosis has also been reported.[179] Approximately 35 other cases in children have been described in retrospective case reports or in small series. Four children with WG presented with Henoch-Schönlein purpura-like vasculitis, including gastrointestinal involvement.[183]

The clinical spectrum of pulmonary involvement in WG includes cough, sinusitis, chest pain, pleuritis, or hemoptysis. However, in children, densities on the chest roentgenogram of the asymptomatic patient may be the first sign of disease. One third of all abnormal chest radiographs in children with WG are not associated with pulmonary symptoms. Roentgenographic findings commonly include fleeting or persistent densities (67%) and nodules (58%), while focal atelectasis, pleural effusion, pulmonary hemorrhage, and mediastinal or hilar lymph node enlargement are less frequent. Nodules may be unilateral or bilateral, multiple or solitary, may vary in size from less than 1 cm to more than 10 cm, can have vague or sharply demarcated borders, may cavitate, and often are transient and fleeting. It should be emphasized that the diagnostic yield of lung biopsies depends on an adquate sample size. Thus, transbronchial biopsies are rarely diagnostic (7%), while open-lung biopsies reveal vasculitis, necrosis, or granulomas in 90% of cases.[184] Assessment of the WG disease activity is daunting. The usual indices for monitoring WG disease activity include the following: clinical findings; c-antineutrophil cytoplasmic autoantibodies (ANCA, immunofluorescence), proteinase-3 antibodies (enzyme-linked immunoabsorbent assay), inflammatory markers (ESR,

■ **TABLE 67-11.** Clinical and lung pathology in wegener's granulomatosis

Acute Disease	Subacute	Chronic
Vascular Lesions		
Necrotizing arteritis Capillaritis Fulminant pulmonary hemorrhage[178]	Granulomatous arteritis Phlebitis	Segmental mural scarring Fibrous occlusion Hemosiderosis
Extra-vascular Lesions		
Microabscesses Necrotizing bronchiolitis Palisading granuloma	Granulomatous bronchiolitis Fibrosing bronchiolitis Palisading granuloma	Necrosis with palisading histiocytosis[177] Inflammatory tumor Lipoid pneumonia Interstitial pneumonitis Cavitation/fibrosis Bronchial stenoses[173,179] Tracheal stenosis, subglottic[180] Bronchiolitis obliterans organizing pneumonia-like (BOOP-like)[29]

Modified from Cases of the Massachusetts General Hospital. N Engl J Med 2002;346:1899.

TABLE 67-12. Wegener's granulomatosis, frequency of findings

Finding	At Diagnosis (%)	Later in course (%)
Fever	22	43
Rash	9	52
Arthritis/arthralgias	30	78
Eye disease	13	48
Sinusitis	61	83
Lung disease	22–45	74–87
Glomerulonephritis	6	61

From Summers RM, Aggarwal NR, Sneller MC: CT virtual bronchoscopy of the central airways in patients with Wegener's granulomatosis. Chest 2002;121:242–250; and Rottem M, Fauci AS, Hallahan CW, et al: Wegener granulomatosis in children and adolescents. Clinical presentation and outcome. J Pediatr 1993;122:26.

c-reactive protein, gallium Ga 67 citrate scintigraphy), CT scanning, BAL, biopsy of a lesion (usually cutaneous lesions), indices of renal function, and PFTs.[185]

Wegener's granulomatosis shows significant pulmonary morbidity. PFTs may reveal obstructive defects in up to 55% of cases; such defects are often caused by endobronchial lesions and scarring, while restrictive defects and reduced lung volumes and/or DLCO may be found in 30% to 40% of cases. Polymicrobial sinus or lung infections may mask the diagnosis or be found at the time of the initial evaluation. Similar findings often occur during treatment, so that pneumonia accounts for 40% of serious infections and is associated with 16% of WG mortality. Prophylaxis with trimethoprim-sulfamethoxazole is now commonly prescribed for pediatric WG patients. Late in the course of WG, pulmonary insufficiency develops in 17% of patients, probably because of end-stage pulmonary fibrosis from active or unremitting lung disease or, not infrequently, as a result of pulmonary disease secondary to medications used to arrest WG.

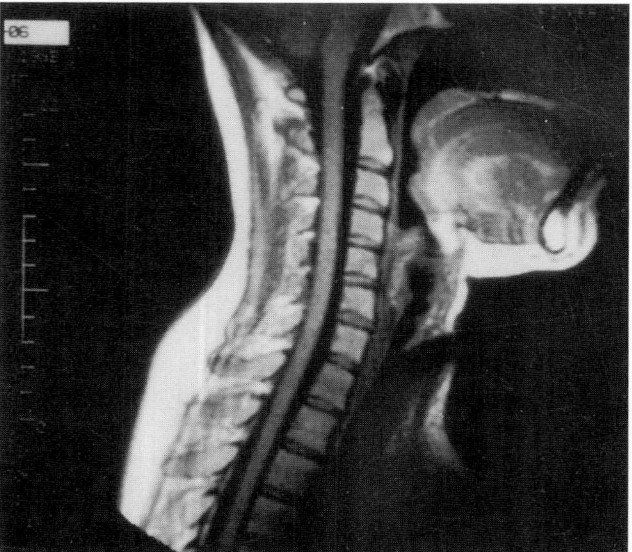

FIGURE 67-8. This T1-weighted magnetic resonance image demonstrates two foci of subglottic stenosis above a tracheostomy site. These ring lesions substantially reduced airway diameter. Failure of dilations to restore adequate airway led to tracheal reconstructive surgery, which was only partially successful. (From Hoffman GS, Kerr GS, Leavitt RY, et al: Wegener granulomatosis. An analysis of 158 patients. Ann Intern Med 1992;116:488.)

The prognosis for WG has dramatically improved in recent decades, but effective management requires early diagnosis, careful patient follow-up, and meticulous attention to treatment complications. Combination therapy is usually initiated with high-dose prednisone (≥1 mg/kg/day) and oral daily cyclophosphamide (2 mg/kg/day).[172] High-dose prednisone is maintained until active disease manifestations have abated (usually about 1 month), and then tapered, depending on disease activity. Cyclophosphamide therapy is continued for at least 1 year after achieving complete remission, and is then tapered. Although complete remission occurs in most patients with this regimen, 53% of all patients and 38% of those followed for more than 5 years had at least one relapse that required retreatment.[181] Rates of remission and relapse in childhood-onset patients are not significantly different from those of adult-onset patients. Permanent morbidity caused only by treatment (mean duration 28 months) was observed in 22% of children, including cystitis in 50% and infertility in at least 28%. Malignancies were not observed during a median follow-up of 8.3 years. Because of its toxicity, cyclophosphamide should be used only by those experienced in its administration. Recently, intravenous immunoglobulin has been successfully used in some treatment-resistant cases of WG.[182,186] Chlorambucil may occasionally be indicated as a first cytotoxic drug because of its fewer short-term side effects. Azathioprine often does not provide sufficient or lasting disease suppression. There have been no controlled studies of cyclosporine or FK-506 in WG. An open-label trial of weekly, low-dose oral MTX (15–20 mg/week) with prednisone (~1 mg/kg/day) has been used in 42 adults with WG.[187] Remission occurred in 71% of patients over a median of 4.2 months. However, four patients developed *P. carinii* pneumonia, emphasizing the need for vigilance in monitoring for infectious complications. In addition, three cases of MTX pneumonitis were noted. Weekly low-dose MTX may be an acceptable alternative therapy for selected patients with mild WG or for those who have developed serious toxicity due to cyclophosphamide. Combination therapy with cyclophosphoramide and prednisolone is frequently prescribed for remission-induction therapy. Following remission, a recent study has found that azathioprine may be successfully substituted for cyclophosphoramide to reduce the exposure to cyclophosphoramide and reduce the incidence of toxicity from this medication.[186] Other drug substitutions for cyclophosphoramide are presently in open-label trials.[188] When cyclophosphoramide therapy is continued, it is recommended that once-daily administration be accompanied by large fluid intake, weekly complete blood counts (to assess neutropenia), *P. carinii* prophylaxis, and cystoscopy assessment for nonglomerular hematuria.[188] Recently, there has been interest in treatment with anti-TNF agents. Etanercept was used in a multicenter trial of 20 adult WG patients who had an incomplete response to prednisone (100%) alone or in combination with one of the following medications: MTX (80%), cyclophosphoramide (60%), azathioprine (40%), and cyclosporine (5% patients).[189] While 80% of the patients had upper respiratory tract involvement, only 10% suffered from pulmonary nodules; 5% had experienced either alveolar hemorrhage or endobronchial disease. The drug was well tolerated with only minor injection site reactions. The patients experienced improvement in their Birmingham Vasculitis Activity Score for WG.[189,190]

The following case illustrates the protean nature of WG, an excellent response to cyclophosphamide, and late findings of PFTs.

Case 8. This 12-year-old female had a 5-month history of fatigue, weight loss, gingival inflammation, and a slowly enlarging submandibular mass. There was progressive cough but no dyspnea or hemoptysis. Physical examination revealed diffuse granulomatous inflammation of the oral cavity, obstruction of the left nostril by a mass, and a 7-cm by 7-cm mass in the right submandibular area. She also occasionally had small nodules on her legs. Her lungs were clear to percussion and auscultation.

A chest radiograph was free of densities and consolidation. She had absent serum ANAs and RF. Serum creatinine, blood urea nitrogen, quantitative immunoglobulin levels, and a 24-hour urine determination for protein and creatinine clearance were normal.

A skin biopsy from the left leg revealed a necrotizing dermal granuloma consistent with WG. There was no evidence of vasculitis on this biopsy. One month later she experienced the onset of hematuria and diminished creatinine clearance. A percutaneous renal biopsy revealed extracapillary proliferative and necrotizing glomerulonephritis without evidence of granulomas or vasculitis. Cultures of all biopsy specimens were negative for tuberculosis and other pathogens.

Therapy with prednisone and cyclophosphamide was begun when increasing respiratory distress occurred due to upper airway obstruction. Serial chest roentgenograms revealed progressive hilar prominences, perihilar infiltrates, and diffuse enlarging pulmonary nodules. Several weeks later, the appearance of lung consolidation was thought to reflect pneumonia. Antibiotic administration was begun, and cyclophosphamide and prednisone therapy was discontinued. After clearing of the pulmonary infilrates and lung consolidation, cyclophosphamide therapy was reinstituted without further complications. One year later, the patient was in total remission except for residual bronchial stenosis, which required repeated dilations.

After the patient had been free of disease and receiving no medications for 2 years, a chest roentgenogram demonstrated multiple cavitations with accompanying densities of the left perihilar and midlung zones. Lingular and right middle lobe densities were also present (Fig. 67-9). Pulmonary function studies were also performed (Table 67-13). The FVC and its subdivisions were moderately reduced, as were the RV and TLC. However, the helium gas dilution method was used to measure lung volume. This method may significantly underestimate the size of both RV and RLC in WG patients with obstructive airways disease. The FEV_1 was reduced to a larger degree than the FVC. Thus, the FEV_1 expressed as a percentage of the FVC was reduced.

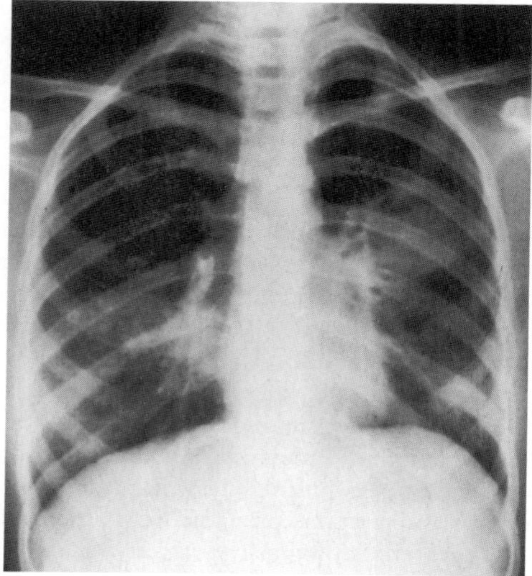

FIGURE 67-9. Case 8. The heart is small, and the left border is obscured by a lingular, segmental infiltrate. Patchy infiltrates are also present in the left upper and right middle lung zones, where cystic pneumatoceles or cavities are seen.

TABLE 67-13. Case 8: Pulmonary values

Parameter	Value	Percentage Predicted
FVC (L)	2.3	66
FEV_1 (L)	1.7	51
FEV_1/FVC (%)	68	
$FEV_{25\%-75\%}$ (L/sec)	1.53	38
TLC (L)	3.1	69
RV (L)	0.8	83
RV/TLC	0.26	
DLCO (mL/min/mm Hg)	19.0	78
pH	7.43	
P_{CO_2} (mm Hg)	30.0	
P_{O_2} (mm Hg)	97.0	

There was a marked reduction in the $FEF_{25\%-75\%}$ and the expiratory flow rates measured at all lung volumes consistent with large, medium-sized, and small airway obstruction. The single-breath DLCO was within the normal range when corrected for the reduction in alveolar volume and the hemoglobin. Arterial blood gas analyses revealed compensated respiratory alkalosis and a normal arterial oxygen tension. After bronchodilator inhalation, there was moderate improvement in the FVC and the FEV_1/FVC. Midmaximal end-expiratory flow rates and the maximal expiratory flow rates measured at all lung volumes also improved, suggesting at least partially reversible expiratory airway obstruction. There was no PFT finding suggestive of ILD, although exercise testing was not performed.

This girl had mild to moderate restrictive lung disease and partially reversible airways obstruction. Although the restrictive component was consistent with WG, the reversible airway obstructive disease is unusual and might not be related to WG. There was no evidence from this study of pulmonary vascular disease, which might be demonstrable only with measurement of ventilation, ventilatory dead space, and arterial blood gases during exercise.

PULMONARY HYPERTENSION

Primary PH in children is rare, but some evidence suggests that it may have an immunologic etiology.[191–193] The most common presenting symptoms in adults that assist in definitive diagnosis are dyspnea (60%), fatigue (19%), and near syncope (13%) leading to progressive right-sided heart failure.[194] Known causes of potentially treatable PH include chronic respiratory insufficiency, sleep apnea, recurrent pulmonary emboli, rheumatic diseases (including vasculitis), and a rare familial form.[195] PH in rheumatologic conditions may be due to irreversible obstruction or obliteration of the pulmonary vascular bed, and thus pharmacologic therapy at this stage in the disease has been of limited benefit, because PPH is a result of pulmonary fibrosis and/or end-stage lung disease.

A rapidly fatal case of PPH in a 17-year-old male without evidence of a rheumatic disorder but with an ANA titer of 1:80, a weakly positive IgG ACLA of 3.7 SD (normal, <2.0 SD), and a negative IgM and IgA has been reported.[196] Fifty-four percent of adults experiencing pulmonary thromboembolism or deep vein thrombosis also have ACLAs, but without an underlying autoimmune disorder.[197] However, PPH is far less common in the antiphospholipid antibody syndrome. ACLAs have been found in many pediatric rheumatic disorders, and are a well-known cause of idiopathic stroke in children, but the prevalence and clinical significance of ACLAs in children are not known. Rheumatic disorders having associated PH include scleroderma, SLE, and vasculitis syndromes. PH may occur in children with rheumatic diseases who experience ILD progressing to interstitial pulmonary fibrosis or BOOP.

Recent therapeutic advances have included trials of prostacyclin[198–201] and prostacyclin analog[202] in patients with rheumatologic conditions. There are no studies of the effectiveness and efficacy of sildanafil, which stabilizes the second messenger of endogenous nitric oxide (cyclic guanosine monophosphate), or of bosentan, an oral dual endothelin receptor antagonist in rheumatologic conditions complicated by PH. Both of these medications have proven effective and efficacious in treatment of PPH. In SLE, intermittent intravenous pulsed cyclophosphoramide has been documented to be superior to oral enalapril in reducing systolic pulmonary artery pressure in patients with either mild or moderate PH.[203] Cyclophosphoramide was twice as effective as enalapril in reducing systemic pulmonary artery pressure in both mild and moderate PH but was most effective in reducing systolic pulmonary artery pressure in moderate PH, while enalapril was not effective in this group. There was improvement in the New York Heart Association functional class only in the cyclophosphoramide-treated group. Unfortunately, the use of cyclophosphoramide was associated with an increased risk of side effects, principally infection (risk ratio [RR] = 1.6) and gastrointestinal (*RR* = 14.6). Another therapy to be considered in rheumatologic patients with PH is oxygen supplementation, especially during sleep to sustain the daytime level of oxygen saturation. Oxygen supplementation should be considered if an overnight sleep study documents increased oxygen desaturation during sleep resulting from hypopnea or other forms of disordered breathing during sleep. Inhaled bronchodilator medications have been found to improve maximal expiratory flow rates in PPH in pediatric patients.[204]

VASCULITIS SYNDROMES

The pulmonary vasculitides are a heterogeneous group of diseases, either primary or secondary, in which there is inflammation that may lead to progressive destruction of the pulmonary microcirculation.[205] Pulmonary involvement may develop because (1) the lung has an extensive vascular and microvascular network, (2) sensitizing antigens can easily reach the lung through the respiratory tract, and (3) there are large numbers of vasoactive and activated immune cells in the lung.[195] Acute pulmonary vasculitis syndromes may be initiated through immune complex deposition and complement activation, since the chronic vasculitic and granulomatous syndromes are often associated with alterations in cell-mediated immunity. The disease patterns represent a continuum of pathologic changes ranging from various forms of angiitis to necrosis and granuloma formation. The clinical presentation is related to the size and location of affected vessels. Administration of glucocorticoids, with or without immunosuppressive agents, has been the most effective therapy for these rare diseases.[206,207] Table 67-14 is an extensive but by no means all-inclusive list of the vasculitides and references.[208–238] Goodpasture's syndrome and idiopathic pulmonary hemosiderosis are discussed in Chapter 48.

Animal models of hypersensitivity pneumonitis suggest a disturbance in cellular immunoregulatory mechanisms.[239] Only rarely, such as in serum sickness and Stevens-Johnson syndrome, can a specific etiologic agent be identified. However, several postinfectious "reactive arthropathies" have been associated with clinical manifestations of vasculitis. These disorders may follow hepatitis, as well as infections with *Mycoplasma*, *Streptococcus*, *Shigella*, *Salmonella*, meningococcus, and *Yersinia*. In our experience, affected patients are often ill but usually recover rapidly without sequelae, often after steroid therapy. We have studied lung function in several children with Stevens-Johnson syndrome and detected severe impairment of gas exchange during the acute illness, with the subsequent development of pulmonary interstitial fibrosis and chronic obstructive lung disease.

TABLE 67-14. The major vasculitides

Vasculitis	References
Periarteritis nodosa	208–214
Henoch-Schönlein purpura	205,215,216
Pulmonary vasculitis	195,205,217–220
Stevens-Johnson syndrome	222
Erythema nodosum	223
Takayasu arteritis	224,225
Churg-Strauss vasculitis	226–232
Goodpasture's syndrome	See Chapter 48
Idiopathic pulmonary hemosiderosis	See Chapter 48
Temporal arteritis (giant cell arteritis)	233
Hypersensitivity angiitis (systemic vasculitits)	234
Serum sickness	235
Cryoglobulinemia	236
Kawasaki disease	237,238

Other than WG, polyarteritis, idiopathic pulmonary hemosiderosis, and Kawasaki, Löffler's, and Goodpasture's syndromes, pulmonary involvement has only rarely been associated with the pediatric primary vasculitides. The character of the histopathologic changes in the primary vasculitides suggests that pulmonary involvement might occur, but in our experience, in children primary pulmonary vasculitis is quite rare.

POLYARTERITIS NODOSA

As a diagnosis, polyarteritis nodosa (PAN) has evolved and is now usually only considered when hypersensitivity angiitis, WG, allergic granulomatosis, and Kawasaki disease have been excluded. PAN is a disease of inflammation and necrosis of medium and small muscular arteries. Initially, leukocytic infiltration and fibrinoid change involve the intima. The process is often longitudinal and may skip areas of an affected vessel. Subsequently, there is intimal proliferation, destruction of the elastic layer, secondary thromboses, aneurysm formation, and infarction of target organs may occur. Although well described, PAN is one of the least common vasculitides in children.[208–210] Until recently there have been only isolated case reports of pulmonary involvement in children with PAN.[208,211] Clinical features of PAN include fever, hypertension, weight loss, muscle pain, and cutaneous features such as livido, painful nodules, ulcers, or gangrene. Myocarditis and/or coronary artery involvement occurs, while necrotizing glomerulitis is not uncommon. The liver, spleen, gastrointestinal tract, adrenal glands, testes, brain, and peripheral nerves are less commonly affected. Differentiation from other rheumatic disorders may be difficult. When diagnostic biopsies are not definitive, then diagnosis is occasionally not made until autopsy. The prognosis is guarded, with death occurring when there is progressive cardiac, renal, central nervous system, gastrointestinal, or multiorgan failure. PAN has been reported after intravenous drug abuse and hepatitis B,[240] and in some cases streptococcal infection may have an etiologic role. There have been many recent advances in treatment.[172,207]

Adult criteria for PAN are not appropriate in pediatrics.[241] In children there are four basic patterns of PAN[217]:

1. A cutaneous variant is seen in 30% of pediatric cases. C-reactive protein and ESR are elevated. Treatment usually includes steroids, cyclophosphoramide, and azathioprine with good response. Often patients are also treated with prophylactic antibiotics (one third of cases);
2. Classic PAN associated with hepatitis B surface antigen occurs in 4.6% of cases, with a high incidence of hypertension, myalgia, and gastrointestinal involvement. Aneurysm of the renal arteries is demonstrable on angiograms. Myeloperoxidase–antineutrophil cytoplasmic antibody (MPO-ANCA) is usually negative. Treatment has included antiviral medications, corticosteroids, and cyclophosphoramide.
3. Microscopic polyarteritis in children, as in adults, is ANCA positive and occurs in 8.1% of children, almost all of whom have renal disease and a high risk of progression to end-stage renal disease. Lung involvement is also very common. A preceding history of upper respiratory tract infection is present in almost half the patients in this category. Elevated MPO-ANCA (enzyme-linked immunosorbent assay) and/or strong p-ANCA staining by immunoglobulin immunofluorescence is very common. Treatment includes pulsed or oral corticosteroids and azathioprine subsequent to a course of cyclophosphoramide. The course of disease in this group can be fatal.
4. Systemic PAN in 57% of cases with all having elevated acute-phase reactants (ESR and C-reactive protein). Cutaneous lesions are noted in 90% and hypertension in 43%. Musculoskeletal complaints are noted in 71%. About 30% have abnormal urinalysis, with one third of these patients eventually developing impaired renal function. Pulmonary and cardiac involvement occurs in 11% and 13%, respectively. Diagnosis is by angiography in one half of the cases (i.e., aneurysm formation or change consistent with mid-size arterial vasculitis). In the remaining cases diagnosis is made through renal, liver, muscle, skin, or testicular biopsy. ANCA is positive in 11% of cases, none with elevated MPO-ANCA. Associated infections are diagnosed in 37% of cases. Treatment included corticosteroids in all patients, and two thirds received cyclophosphoramide treatment, with half of these patients eventually transferred to therapy with azothioprine. A few of the patients in this group received MTX therapy, while 10% were treated with intravenous immunoglobulin. After successful treatment, relapse was uncommon, with an adjusted mortality of only 1%.

Although the range of age of the affected pediatric patients is between 1 and 16 years, the mean in a large series of 110 patients was 9.01 ± 3.57 years old.[217] Clinical findings vary with the disease pattern. Constitutional symptoms are reported in 64% to 100% of pediatric cases. The clinical findings may include high fever (40% to 60%), weight loss (0 to 15%), arthralgias (20% to 40%), myalgias (15% to 46%), and tender subcutaneous nodules (33% to 97%). Less frequent organ involvement includes gastrointestinal (0 to 40%), central nervous system (0 to 22%), cardiac (0 to 6%), testes (0 to 6.3%), while pulmonary findings in PAN are confined to the microscopic PAN (56%) and the systemic (1.6%) groups. Pulmonary involvement in PAN varies from 0 to 65%, with the variation due to the varying lung involvement between patterns of PAN disease.[242]

Polyarteritis in infants is very rare. Several studies have found that the histopathology of infantile PAN and Kawasaki syndrome are very similar and that the two illnesses are closely linked.[243,244]

■ KAWASAKI SYNDROME

Kawasaki syndrome is an acute-onset systemic vasculopathy occurring in infants and young children. This illness is characterized by fever, polymorphous exanthema, conjunctivitis, strawberry tongue, erythematous cracked lips, desquamation of the skin, cervical lymphadenopathy, arthritis, and coronary artery aneurysms in 15% to 25% of untreated cases. Involvement of essentially all organs has been described.[245]

A review of chest roentgenograms from 129 children with Kawasaki syndrome (mean age 1.8 years; range 2 months to 12.8 years) found abnormalities in 19 patients (14.7%) of cases.[246] The most frequent finding was a reticulogranular pattern noted in 90%, while peribronchial cuffing (21%), pleural effusion (16%), atelectasis (11%), and air trapping (5%) were also observed. Radiographic changes always appeared within 10 days of disease onset. Biopsies were not done, but the causes for the chest radiographic changes were believed to be lower respiratory tract inflammation and/or pulmonary arteritis. In autopsy series of Kawasaki disease, interstitial pneumonia has been reported in 30% to 90% of cases, while pulmonary arteritis is noted in 45% to 71% of cases.[237] While rare, unresolving pneumonia has recently been reported at the main manifestation of Kawasaki disease in two young children. In each case, persisting lobar consolidation was found on chest radiography along with unrelenting fever and leukocytosis, and only later did other typical symptoms and findings lead to the diagnosis of Kawasaki disease and rapid defervescence with intravenous immunoglobulin or prednisone therapy.[238]

A recent Clinical Report from the American Academy of Pediatrics and the American Heart Association endorses a new diagnostic algorithm in which fever for 5 days or longer and four or fewer of the classical criteria are indications for electrocardiography to confirm the diagnosis. Present therapy includes initial treatment with intravenous immunoglobulin and in cases of persisting or recrudescent fever retreatment with intravenous immunoglobulin and use of corticosteroids, TNF-α antagonists, and abciximab.[247]

■ RHEUMATIC PNEUMONIA

The incidence of acute rheumatic fever (ARF) in children continues to decline in both developed and less developed countries, although it has not been entirely conquered.[248] Outbreaks in the United States may be related to increased "rheumatogenicity" of specific streptococcal serotypes. The Jones criteria were updated in 1992[249] and should further reduce both overdiagnosis and misdiagnosis.

Since there are no pathognomonic findings or test for rheumatic pneumonia, diagnosis and treatment remain controversial. Indeed, many major texts make no mention of lung involvement in rheumatic fever. The pulmonary findings in 87 children who died between 1919 and 1954 during an active attack of ARF have been described.[250] There were 54 cases of rheumatic pneumonia, an overall incidence of 62%. Of these rheumatic pneumonia patients, 39% had only mild pulmonary involvement, while 54% had pulmonary disease of moederate severity. Older reports of rheumatic pneumonia had an 11.3% and 12.7% incidence.[251,252]

Thus rheumatic pneumonia is rare, difficult to differentiate from congestive heart failure, and may on occasion be impossible to confirm without microscopic examination of a lung biopsy sample. Indeed, pulmonary edema and rheumatic pneumonia may coexist and may be distinguishable only at autopsy.[253] The first histologic description of rheumatic pneumonia was made in 1928, and the lungs were described as enlarged with dark red areas due to scattered hemorrhages.[254] The lungs were elastic and resilient on palpation and had a rubbery consistency. Microscopic examination revealed hemorrhage, necrosis of alveolar walls, arteriolitis, and vasculitis with occasional thrombosis, hyaline membrane lining of alveoli and alveolar ducts, and alveolar proliferation of mononuclear fibroblast cells. Examination of the pleura may reveal a fibrinous exudate, usually without effusion. Unfortunately, none of the lesions just described is pathognomonic for rheumatic pneumonia. However, pathologists have attempted to define rheumatic pneumonitis. One pathologic study suggested that the best diagnostic criterion was a focal mononuclear, fibrinous, intra-alveolar or intraductal exudate containing protein-rich fluid.[250] Another investigator observed unusual bronchiolar changes involved desquamation of the epithelial cells, which were stripped completely from the bronchi, and an eosinophilic granular necrosis of the lamina.[255]

Explanations of the etiology of lung damage in ARF have included a hypersensitivity phenomenon leading to arteriolar damage or an allergic basis in which there is capillary endothelial injury with a hyaline membrane developing due to seepage of fibrinogen from the pulmonary capillaries into the alveoli[256] (Fig. 67-10).

In a series of 24 patients dying of ARF between 1949 and 1970, arteriolitis that was present in 4 patients was associated in 3 of these cases with an acute pneumonitis.[257] In lung sections from one third of the patients (3–25 years old) there were arterial and arteriolar thrombi, and, in some, thromboembolism was detected. In only two patients was there evidence of nonrheumatic lung disease. Influenza virus was cultured from one patient, and in another cytomegalic inclusion disease was identified. Finally, chronic interstitial pulmonary fibrosis is reported in some ARF cases, developing late in the course of rheumatic fever. Recently, rheumatogenic *Streptococcus pyogenes* binding to collagen and the presence of collagen-reactive autoantibodies in the serum of ARF patients has been reported.[258] This might explain the late findings of pulmonary interstitial fibrosis in some patients who have had ARF pneumonia.

The predominant pulmonary symptoms in ARF are dyspnea, tachypnea, tachycardia (usually out of proportion to fever and the degree of illness), persistent cough, and blood-streaked sputum. Pleuritic chest pain, restlessness, and cyanosis may develop. The presence, degree, and duration of fever are variable. The onset of pneumonia may be insidious, simulating an upper respiratory tract infection, or occasionally it may be heralded as an acute attack of dyspnea. Rheumatic pneumonia may rarely occur before there are other signs of ARF.[259,260] A case of an 18-year-old male with fever, malaise, and cough, and a history of suspected ARF with carditis 11 years previously has recently been reported.[260] Chest roentgenograms over several days revealed normal-sized cardiac silhouette but progressive lung densities initially in the left lower lobe progressing to consolidation of the lobe despite aggressive intravenous antibiotic therapy for suspected community-acquired pneumonitis. Extensive clinical and laboratory evaluation, including chest CT, echocardiography, bronchoscopy, and BAL, as well as microbiologic and serologic testing for *Mycobacterium pneumoniae*, *Chlamydia pneumoniae*, *Legionella* spp., cytomegalovirus, and Epstein-Barr virus were negative, as were ANA and serum angiotensin-converting enzyme. The onset of arthritis of the knee occurred 24 days after the initial symptoms and 10 days after hospitalization and continued fever. Thoracoscopic lung

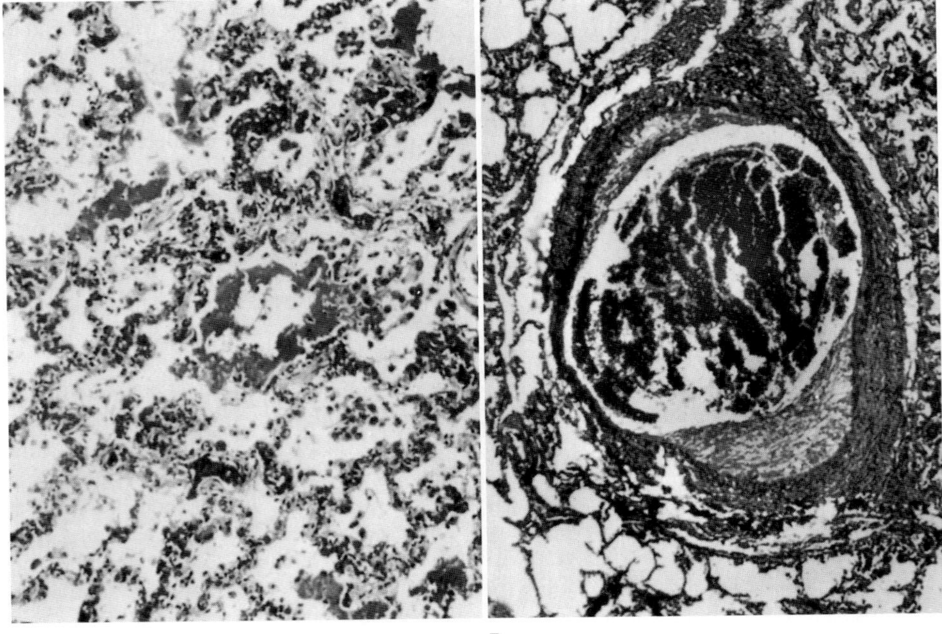

■ **FIGURE 67-10.** A 4-year-old girl was admitted to the hospital with acute arthritis and active carditis. She was treated with digitalis and salicylates, and her condition improved. Three months later, fever, substernal pain, and pericarditis developed. Crackles were also heard in the chest. She was in acute respiratory distress and died 4 months after admission. The lungs showed some pathologic features described in rheumatic pneumonia. **A,** Hyaline membranes and congestion (×150). **B,** Arterial thrombus, organized (×30).

biopsy revealed parenchymal lung inflammation with thickened alveolar septae and fibrosis with nodular aggregates of lymphocytes. Arthritis and pulmonary infiltrates resolved, and antistreptolysin O antibody and C-reactive protein titers fell rapidly after corticosteroid therapy.

A clinical classification has been suggested[251]: (1) primary acute pneumonitis as an initial manifestation of ARF, (2) secondary acute pneumonitis occurring during the polycyclic course of ARF, and (3) subclinical pneumonitis, in which lung involvement may remain undiagnosed. There may be few symptoms or clinical signs of pneumonia. For example, a history of pneumonia of unknown etiology was significantly more common in 279 Denver schoolchildren who had had ARF than in 556 control subjects who had not.[261]

A

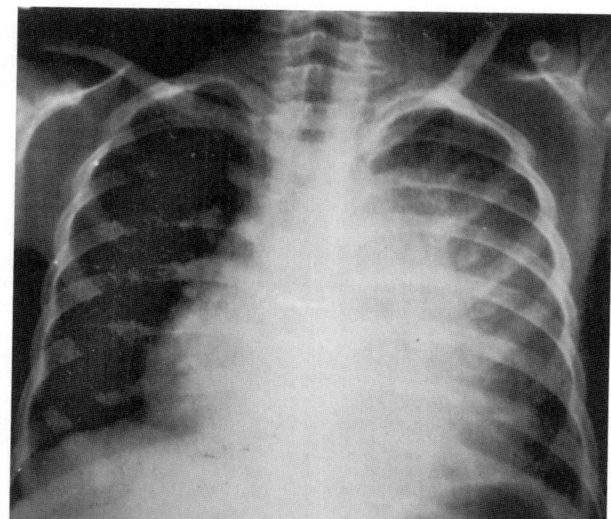

B

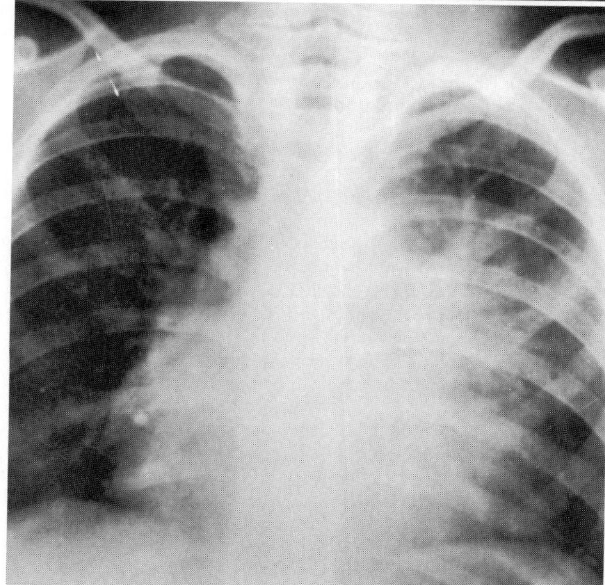

■ **FIGURE 67-11.** **A,** A chest roentgenogram, taken 24 hours after the onset of symptoms, shows a fuzzy-edged, homogeneous, nonsegmental infiltrate in the middle third of the lung. The cardiac silhouette is enlarged. **B,** The right diaphragm and costophrenic angle are clear 20 days later. The infiltrate in the left midlung shows some clearing at the periphery. The cardiac silhouette is smaller, but the left border remains obscured by a mottled infiltrate with increased bronchovascular markings.

Chest roentgenograms in ARF may reveal the sudden appearance and, then, resolution of hazy-edged densities, which are reported as peripheral, central, in the left mid-lung, in the right upper lobe, or, more commonly, bilateral. Pleurisy is frequently transient. Chest roentgenograms may also have increased bronchovascular markings, homogeneous segmental densities, or even small, soft, mottled densities. Lobar involvement is rare and usually of short duration. The lung apices and bases are usually clear.

The list of diseases simulating rheumatic pneumonitis is long, including congestive heart failure, viral or bacterial pneumonia, and Löffler's pneumonia (reacting to antigens other than *S. pyogenes*). Great diagnostic difficulty lies in distinguishing between viral pneumonitis and pulmonary edema, especially when there is active ARF carditis. There are few published reports of testing for cytomegalovirus or *P. carinii* in these cases. Figure 67-11 is an example of rheumatic pneumonitis as the initial manifestation of ARF.

Although the existence of rheumatic pneumonitis remains hotly debated, this complication of ARF has continued to be the subject of case reports.[260,262,263] When it occurs, ARF pneumonitis may have a guarded prognosis, particularly during the initial attack, when it presents as diffuse pulmonary disease. However, rapid clearing of rheumatic pneumonitis following treatment with steroids has been described.[264]

■ PNEUMONITIS DUE TO ANTIRHEUMATIC THERAPY

Though uncommon, medication-induced lung disease is an important consideration in the care and treatment of children with rheumatic disorders. Not only are there no specific markers to warn of potential pulmonary complications of antirheumatic drug therapy, there are few clear-cut risk factors and almost no clinical predictors of disease onset. Adverse pulmonary reactions to drugs have been reported with azathioprine, chlorambucil, colchicine, cyclophosphamide, D-penicillamine, gold, MTX, NSAIDs, salicylates, sulfasalazine, and others.[178,265]

The spectrum of drug-induced pulmonary disease ranges from asymptomatic radiographic findings to mild dyspnea to fatal pulmonary disease. Common symptoms are nonspecific and include shortness of breath, nonproductive cough, and chest pain. Fever and symmetrical crackles audible at the bases of the lungs are the most frequent physical findings.

Diagnosis of medication-related lung disease can only be made after exclusion of other common and uncommon etiologies such as aspiration; gastroesophageal reflux disease with microaspiration; community-associated pneumonitis; bacterial, fungal, mycobacterial, and opportunistic infections; congestive heart failure; pulmonary embolism; neoplasia; pulmonary vasculitis; and pulmonary edema. Since these conditions may also involve rheumatoid-related lung disease, these disorders must be differentiated from medication-induced lung disease. Finally, since treatment of most rheumatic conditions involves combination drug therapies either simultaneously or sequentially, these often complicate establishing a firm diagnosis for the etiology of the lung disease in these patients.

There are five major clinical syndromes associated with exposure to antirheumatic medications[265]:

1. Hypersensitivity pneumonitis (NSAIDs, MTX, penicillamine, gold)

2. Chronic alveolitis and fibrosis (MTX, NSAIDs, penicillamine, gold)
3. Pulmonary-renal syndrome similar to Goodpasture's syndrome (penicillamine)
4. BO (gold, penicillamine)
5. Noncardiogenic pulmonary edema (NSAIDs, salicylates, colchicine)

Mechanisms of action for these lung complications of drug therapy include: (1) immediate and/or delayed hypersensitivity, (2) bronchospasm, (3) prior lung disease, (4) direct cytotoxic activity, (5) immune aberrations due to abnormal lymphocyte function or alterations in lymphokine activity, (6) increased vascular permeability related to altered platelet and/or prostaglandin function (aspirin), (7) association with HLA-B35 and HLA-B40 (gold).[266]

Approaches to diagnosis include drug withdrawal, analysis of lung lavage from BAL, and transbronchial, thoracoscopic, or open-lung biopsy. Treatment includes withdrawal of the drug and supportive care. If active inflammation is present, corticosteroids are indicated, and impaired gas exchange may require oxygen supplementation and/or assisted ventilation. Both plasmapheresis and immunosuppressive therapy have been recommended in refractory cases, but these approaches are based only on isolated case reports. Recently, prophylaxis for *P. carinii* infection with trimethoprim-sulfamethoxazole has been advocated when high-dose immunosuppressive therapy is used.[267]

Methotrexate-related pulmonary complications are of particular interest in rheumatology because MTX is now widely used to treat RA, JRA, psoriatic arthritis, dermatomyositis, Behçet's syndrome, SS, WG, resistant arthritis in SLE, and other vasculitides. A cumulative prevalence of MTX pulmonary toxicity from 16 published prospective and retrospective reports is 3%. Possible causal mechanisms include hypersensitivity, idiosyncratic reactions, and specific cellular immune responses. Age, sex, disease duration, cumulative drug dose, and route of administration are not risk factors; however, renal function impairment and concomitant use of aspirin or NSAIDs have been suggested to increase the risk in some studies but not confirmed by others.[268] Smoking, preexisting lung disease, and/or abnormal pre-MTX radiographs may be predisposing influences.

Chest imaging most often reveals interstitial pneumonitis, alveolar infiltrates, or fibrosis, commonly at the lung bases.[269] Treatment of MTX lung disease includes discontinuation of MTX and use of high-dose intravenous corticosteroid therapy until improvement is evident. Neither steroids nor folic acid appear to prevent MTX-induced lung disease. Although the outcome is usually favorable, fatalities have been reported. In JRA, MTX-induced pulmonary toxicity is very rare. Study of 40 children receiving MTX therapy and in whom chest radiographs and PFTs were obtained before, during, and following MTX therapy failed to identify any radiologic or lung function abnormalities during therapy or subsequently.[267,270] No large-scale evaluation of JRA patients or those with other rheumatologic conditions treated with MTX or other antimetabolites has been reported.

■ SUMMARY

A majority of rhe rheumatic diseases can and do involve the pulmonary system at some time during their course. The most common initial events seem to be pleural inflammation, vasculitis, or granulomatous parenchymal involvement, frequently resulting in slowly progressive interstitial fibrosis. However, pulmonary function studies in adults with various rheumatic diseases frequently suggest that initial pulmonary impairment may occur silently, without obvious antecedent respiratory system events. The same is probably true for the childhood rheumatic diseases.

Most childhood rheumatic diseases are associated with, or are suspected to cause, defects in humoral or cell-mediated immunity. In addition, many patients are receiving steroids or immunosuppressive agents. Thus, it is imperative that infection be the first consideration when any sudden change in respiratory status occurs. Complete cultures should always be taken and appropriate antimicrobial therapy begun before the addition to the regimen, or change thereof, of corticosteroids or immunosuppressive drugs.

It is not clear what role chronic pulmonary impairment plays in the apparently increased incidence of lung infections in children with rheumatic diseases. Detailed serial pulmonary function studies and correlation with immune and pulmonary infectious status, and medications in use in the childhood rheumatic diseases are important areas for further study.

REFERENCES

1. Silverman ED, Eddy A: Systemic lupus erythematosis in childhood and adolescence. In: Maddison PJ, Isenberg DA, Woo P, Glass D, eds: Oxford Textbook of Rheumatology. New York: Oxford University Press, 1993, pp 756–771.
2. Tan EM, Cohen AS, Fries JF, et al: The 1982 revised criteria for the classification of systemic lupus erythematosus. Arthritis Rheum 1982;25:1271–1277.
3. Font J, Cervera R, Espinosa G, et al: Systemic lupus erythematosis (SLE) in childhood. Analysis of clinical and immunological findings in 34 patients and comparison with SLE characteristics in adults. Ann Rheum Dis 1998; 57:456–459.
4. Seaman DE, Londino V, Kwoh CK, et al: Antiphospholipid antibodies in paediatric systemic lupus erythematosus. Pediatrics 1995;96:1040–1045.
5. Berube C, Mitchell L, Silverman E, et al. The relationship of antiphopholipid antibodies to thromboembolic events in pediatric patients with systemic lupus erythematosis. A cross-sectional study. Pediatric Res 1998;44:351–356.
6. Gammon RB, Bridges TA, Al-Nezir H, et al: Bronchiolitis obliterans organizing pneumonia associated with systemic lupus erythematosus. Chest 1992;102:1171–1174.
7. Myers JL, Katzenstein AA: Microangiitis in lupus-induced hemorrhage. Am J Pathol 1985;85:552–556.
8. Orens JB, Martinez FJ, Lynch JP: Pleuropulmonary manifestations of systemic lupus erythematosus. Rheum Dis Clin North Am 1994;20:159–193.
9. Groen H, Bootsma H, Postma DS, Kallenberg CG: Primary pulmonary hypertension in systemic lupus erythematosis. Partial improvement with cyclophosphoramide. J Rheum 1993;20:1055–1057.
10. Santos-Ocampo AS, Mandell BF, Fessler BJ: Alveolar hemorrhage in systemic lupus erythematosis. Chest 2000;118:1083–1090.
11. Sanad AS, Lindsley CB: Treatment of pulmonary hemorrhage in childhood systemic lupus erythematosus with mycopholate mofetil. South Med J 2003;96:705–707.
12. Wilhelm M, Van Why SK: Pneumothoraces complicating systemic lupus erythematosis with nephritis. Pediatr Nephrol 2002;17:261–263.
13. Weinrib L, Sharma OP, Quismorio FP: A long-term study of interstitial lung disease in systemic lupus erythematosus. Semin Arthritis Rheum 1990;20:48–56.
14. Hardy K, Herry I, Attali V, et al: Bilateral phrenic paralysis in a patient with systemic lupus erythematosis. Chest 2001;119:1274–1277.
15. Uziel Y, Hen B, Cordoba M, Wolach B: Lymphocytic interstitial pneumonitis preceding polyarticular juvenile rheumatoid arthritis. Clin Exp Rheumatol 1998;16:617–619.
16. Lovell D, Lindsley C, Langston C: Lymphoid interstitial pneumonia in juvenile rheumatoid arthritis. J Pediatr 1984;105:947–950.
17. Noyes BE, Albers GM, deMello DE, et al: Early onset of pulmonary parenchymal disease associated with juvenile rheumatoid arthritis. Pediatr Pulmonol 1997;24:444–446.

18. Schultz R, Mattila J, Gappa M, Verronen P: Development of progressive interstitial and intra-alveolar cholesterol granulomas (PICG) associated with therapy-resistant chronic systemic juvenile arthritis (CJA). Pediatr Pulmonol 2001;32:397–402.
19. Arroliga AC, Podell DN, Matthay RA: Pulmonary manifestations of scleroderma. J Thorac Imaging 1992;7:30–45.
20. Schachna L, Wigley F, Chang B, et al: Age and risk of pulmonary arterial hypertension in scleroderma. Chest 2003;124:2098–2104.
21. Witt C, Borges AC, John M, et al: Pulmonary involvement in diffuse cutaneous systemic sclerosis. Bronchoalveolar fluid granulocytosis predicts progression of fibrosing alveolitis. Ann Rheum Dis 1999;58:635–640.
22. Tazelaar HD, Viggiano RW, Pickersgill J, Colby TV: Interstitial lung disease in polymyositis and dermatomyositis. Clinical features and prognosis as correlated with histologic findings. Am Rev Respir Dis 1990;141:727–733.
23. Kobayashi I, Yamada M, Takahashi Y, et al: Interstitial lung disease associated with juvenile dermatomyositis. Clinical features and efficacy of cyclosporin A. Rheumatology 2003;43:371–374.
24. Singsen BH, Tedford JS, Platzker ACG, Hanson V: Spontaneous pneumothorax. A complication of juvenile dermatomyositis. J Pediatr 1978; 92:771–774.
25. Al-Mayouf SM, Al-Eid W, Bahabri S, Al-Mofada S: Interstitial pneumonitis and air leakage in juvenile dermatomyositis. Rheumatology 2001;40: 588–590.
26. Park S, Nyhan WL: Fatal pulmonary involvement in dermatomyositis. Am J Dis Child 1975;129:723–726.
27. Chmiel JF, Wessel HU, Targoff IN, Pachnan LM: Pulmonary fibrosis and myositis in a child with anti-Jo-1 autoantibody. J Rheumatol 1995;22:762–765.
28. Kono H, Inokuma S: Visualization and functional consequences of pulmonary vascular impairment in patients with rheumatic diseases. Chest 2003;124:255–261.
29. Uner AH, Rozum-Slota B, Katzenstein A-L: Bronchiolitis obliterans-organizing pneumonia (BOOP)-like variant of Wegener's granulomatosis. A clinicopathological study of 16 cases. Am J Surg Pathol 1996;20: 794–801.
30. Segal AM, Calabrese LH, Ahmad M, et al: The pulmonary manifestations of systemic lupus erythematosus. Semin Arthritis Rheum 1985;14:202–224.
31. Weidemann HP, Matthay RA: Pulmonary manifestations of systemic lupus erythematosus. J Thorac Imaging 1992;7:1–18.
32. Andonopoulos AP, Constantopoulos SH, Galanopoulou V, et al: Pulmonary function of nonsmoking patients with systemic lupus erythematosus. Chest 1988;94:312–315.
33. Groen H, TerBorg EJ, Postma DS, et al: Pulmonary function in systemic lupus erythematosus is related to distinct clinical, serologic, and nail-fold capillary patterns. Am J Med 1992;93:619–627.
34. Nadorra RL, Landing BH: Pulmonary lesions in childhood onset systemic lupus erythematosus. Analysis of 26 cases and summary of the literature. Pediatr Pathol 1987;7:1–18.
35. Miller RW, Magilavy DB, Bock GH, et al: Pulmonary function abnormalities in pediatric patients with systemic lupus erythernatosus. Immunol Allergy Pract 1988;10:143.
36. Delgado EA, Malleson PN, Pirie GE, Petty RE: The pulmonary manifestations of childhood onset systemic lupus erythematosis. Semin Arthritis Rheum 1990;19:285–293.
37. Kim EA, Lee KS, Johkoh T, et al: Interstitial lung diseases associated with collagen vascular diseases. Radiologic and histopathologic findings. Radiographics 2002;22:S151–S165.
38. Ramirez RE, Glasier C, Kirks D, et al: Pulmonary hemorrhage associated with systemic lupus erythematosus in children. Radiology 1984;152:409– 412.
39. Miller RW, Salcedo JR, Fink RJ, et al: Pulmonary hemorrhage in pediatric patients with systemic lupus erythematosus. J Pediatr 1986;108: 576–579.
40. Zamora MR, Warner ML, Tuder R, Schwartz MI: Diffuse alveolar hemorrhage and systemic lupus erythematosus. Clinical presentation, histology, survival and outcome. Medicine 1997;76:192–202.
41. Asherson RA, Higenbottam TW, Dinh Xuan AT, et al: Pulmonary hypertension in a lupus clinic. Experience with twenty-four patients. J Rheumatol 1990;17:1292–1298.
42. Laroche CM, Mulvey DA, Hawkins, PN, et al: Diaphragmatic strength in the shrinking lung syndrome of systemic lupus erythematosus. Q J Med 1989;71:429–439.
43. Teitel AD, MacKenzie CR, Stern R, Paget SA: Laryngeal involvement in systemic lupus erythematosus. Semin Arthritis Rheum 1992;22:203–214.
44. Hellmann DB, Petri M, Whiting-O'Keefe Q: Fatal infections in systemic lupus erythematosus. The role of opportunistic organisms. Medicine 1987; 66:341–348.
45. Nived O, Sturfelt G, Wollheim F: Systemic lupus erythematosus and infection. A controlled and prospective study including an epidemiologic group. Q J Med 1985;55:271–287.
46. Wiedemann HP, Matthay RA: Pulmonary manifestation of the collagen vascular diseases. Clin Chest Med 1989;10:677–722.
47. Mulkey D, Hudson L: Massive spontaneous unilateral hemothorax in systemic lupus erythematosus. Am J Med 1974;56:570–574.
48. Grubben MJ, Kerstens PJ, Wiersma JM, et al: Pleuropulmonary involvement in patients with connective tissue disease. The role of open lung biopsy. Neth J Med 1993;43:269–276.
49. Isbister JP, Ralston M, Hayes JM, Wright R: Fulminant lupus pneumonitis with acute renal failure and RBC aplasia. Successful management with plasmapheresis and immunosuppression. Arch Intern Med 1981;141:1081–1083.
50. Nishimura K, Kitaichi M, Izumi T, et al: Usual interstitial pneumonia. Histologic correlation with high-resolution CT. Radiology 1992;182: 337–342.
51. Medsger TA: Systemic sclerosis (scleroderma), localized forms of scleroderma, and calcinosis. In: McCarty DJ, ed: Arthritis and Allied Conditions. I2th ed. Philadelphia: Lea & Febiger, 1993.
52. LeRoy EC, ed: Scleroderma. Rheum Dis Clin North Am 1990;16:1–249.
53. Singsen BH: Scleroderma in childhood. Pediatr Clin North Am 1986;33: 1119–1139.
54. Cassidy JT, Petty RE: Textbook of Pediatric Rheumatology, 3rd ed. New York: Wiley, 1995.
55. Kornreich HK, King KK, Bernstein BH, et al: Scleroderma in childhood. Arthritis Rheum 1977;20(Suppl 2):343–350.
56. D'Angelo WA, Fries JF, Masi AT, Shulman LE: Pathologic observations in systemic sclerosis (scleroderma). A study of fifty-eight autopsy cases and fifty-eight matched controls. Am J Med 1969;46:428–440.
57. Seibold JR: Scleroderma. In: Kelley WN, Hams ED, Ruddy S, Sledge CB, eds: Textbook of Rheumatology. Philadelphia, WB Saunders, 1993.
58. Hanson V: Systemic lupus erythematosus, dermatomyositis, scleroderma and vasculitides in childhood. In: Kelley WN, Harris ED, Ruddy S, Sledge CB, eds: Textbook of Rheumatology, 2nd ed. Philadelphia: WB Saunders, 1985.
59. Reimer G: Autoantibodies against nuclear, nucleolar, and mitochondrial antigens in systemic sclerosis (scleroderma). Rheum Dis Clin North Am 1990;16:169–183.
60. Rossi GA, Bitterman PB, Rennard SI, et al: Evidence for chronic inflammation as a component of the interstitial lung disease associated with progressive systemic sclerosis. Am Rev Respir Dis 1985;131:612–617.
61. Silver RM, Miller KS, Kinsella MB, et al: Evaluation and management of scleroderma lung disease using bronchoalveolar lavage. Am J Med 1990; 88:470–476.
62. Ungerer RG, Tashkin DP, Furst D, et al: Prevalence and clinical correlates of pulmonary arterial hypertension in progressive systemic sclerosis. Am J Med 1983;75:65–74.
63. Guttadauria M, Eliman H, Kaplan D: Progressive systemic sclerosis. Pulmonary involvement. Clin Rheum Dis 1979;5:151–167.
64. Furst DE, David JA, Clements PJ, et al: Abnormalities of pulmonary vascular dynamics and inflammation in early progressive systemic sclerosis. Arthritis Rheum 1981;24:1403.
65. Shuck JW, Oetgen WJ, Tesar JT: Pulmonary vascular response during Raynaud's phenomenon in progressive systemic sclerosis. Am J Med 1985; 78:221–227.
66. Peters-Golden M, Wise RA, Schneider P, et al: Clinical and demographic predictors of loss of pulmonary function in systemic sclerosis. Medicine 1984;63:221–231.
67. Greenwald GI, Tashkin DP, Gong H, et al: Longitudinal changes in lung function and respiratory symptoms in progressive systemic sclerosis. Am J Med 1987;83:83–92.
68. Mohsenifar Z, Tashkin DP, Levy SE, et al: Lack of sensitivity of measurements on Vd/Vt at rest and during exercise in detection of hemodynamically significant pulmonary vascular abnormalities in collagen vascular disease. Am Rev Respir Dis 1981;123:508–512.
69. Roumm AD, Medsger TA Jr: Cancer and systemic sclerosis. An epidemiologic study. Arthritis Rheum 1985;28:1336–1340.
70. Schurawitzki H, Stiglbauer R, Grainger W, et al: Interstitial lung disease in progressive systemic sclerosis. High resolution CT versus radiography. Radiology 1990;176:755–759.
71. Wigley FM, Wise RA: The management of pulmonary involvement in systemic sclerosis. In: Klippel JH, Dieppe PA, eds: Rheumatology. Baltimore: Mosby–Year Book Europe Ltd, 1994.
72. Steen VD, Owens GR, Redmond C, et al: The effect of D-penicillamine on pulmonary findings in systemic sclerosis. Arthritis Rheum 1985;28:882–888.
73. Silver RM, Warrick JH, Kinsella MB, et al: Cyclophosphamide and low-dose prednisone therapy in patients with systemic sclerosis (scleroderma) with interstitial lung disease. J Rheumatol 1993;20:838–844.
74. Salerni R, Rodnan GP, Leon DF, Shaver JA: Pulmonary hypertension in the CREST syndrome variant of progressive systemic sclerosis (scleroderma). Ann Intern Med 1977;86:394–399.

75. Pachman LM: Juvenile dermatomyositis. Pathophysiology and disease expression. Pediatr Clin North Am 1995;42:1071–1098.
76. Reed AM, Lopez M: Juvenile dermatomyositis. Recognition and treatment. Paediatr Drugs 2002;4:315–321.
77. Ansell BM, Rudge S, Schaller JG: Color Atlas of Pediatric Rheumatology. St. Louis: Mosby-Wolfe, 1991.
78. Uzel G, Pachman LM: Cytokines in juvenile dermatomyositis pathophysiology. Potential and challenge. Curr Opin Rheumatol 2003;15: 691–697.
79. Spencer CH, Hanson V, Singsen BH, et al: Course of created juvenile dermatomyositis. J Pediatr 1984;105:399–408.
80. Miller LC, Sisson BA, Tucker LB, et al: Methotrexate treatment of recalcitrant childhood dermatomyositis. Arthritis Rheum 1992;3:1143–1149.
81. Singsen BH, Goldreyer B, Stanton R, Hanson V: Childhood polymyositis with cardiac conduction defects. Am J Dis Child 1976;130:72.
82. Salmeron G, Greenberg SD, Lidsky MD: Polymyositis and diffuse interstitial lung disease. A review of the pulmonary histopathologic findings. Arch Intern Med 1981;141:1005–1010.
83. Lakhanpal S, Lie JT, Conn DL, Martin WJ: Pulmonary disease in polymyosins/dermatomyosins. A clinicopathological analysis of 65 cases. Ann Rheum Dis 1987;46:23–29.
84. Love LA, Leff RL, Fraser DD, et al: A new approach to the classification of idiopathic inflammatory myopathy. Myositis specific autoantibodies define useful homogeneous patient groups. Medicine 1991;70:360–374.
85. Hunninghake GW, Fauci AS: Pulmonary involvement in the collagen vascular diseases. Am Rev Respir Dis 1979;119:471–503.
86. Rowen AJ, Reichel J: Dermatomyositis with lung involvement, successfully treated with azathioprine. Respiration 1983;44:143–146.
87. Plowman PN, Stableforth DE: Dermatomyositis with fibrosing alveolitis. Response to treatment with cyclophosphamide. Proc Soc Med 1977; 70:738–740.
88. Gruhn WB, Diaz-Buxo JA: Cyclosponne treatment of steroid resistant interstitial pneumonitis associated with dermatomyositis/polymyositis. J Rheumatol 1987;14:1045–1047.
89. Dubowitz LM, Dubowitz V: Acute dermatomyositis presenting with pulmonary manifestations. Arch Dis Child 1964;39:293–296.
90. Gwinn JL, Lee FA: Radiological case of the month. Dermatomyositis with interstitial lung disease and soft tissue calcification. Am J Dis Child 1975; 129:703–704.
91. Samuels MP, Warner JO: Pulmonarv alveolar lipoproteinosis complicating juvenile dermatomyositis. Thorax 1988;43:939–940.
92. Rider LG, Miller FW, Targoff IN, et al: A broadened spectrum of juvenile myositis. Myositis-specific auto antibodies in children. Arthritis Rheum 1994;37:1534–1538.
93. Batist G, Andrews JL: Pulmonary toxicity of antineoplastic drugs. JAMA 1981;246:1449–1453.
94. Singsen BH: Epidemiology of the rheumatic diseases of childhood. In: Hochberg MC, ed: Epidemiology of the Rheumatic Diseases. Rheum Dis Clin North Am 1990;16:581–599.
95. Brewer E: Pitfalls in the diagnosis of juvenile rheumatoid arthritis. Pediatr Clin North Am 1986;33:1015–1032.
96. Miller JJ III, ed: Juvenile Rheumatoid Arthritis. Littleton, Mass: PSG Publishing, 1979.
97. Ansell BM: Rheumatic Diseases in Childhood. Boston: Butterworth's, 1930.
98. Jacobs JC: Pediatric Rheumatology for the Practitioner. New York: Springer-Verlag, 1982.
99. Cassidy JT: Miscellaneous conditions associated with arthritis in children. Pediatric Clin North Am 1986;33:1033–1152.
100. Bywaters EGL, White P, Petty RE, et al: Juvenile chronic arthritis. In: Klippel JH, Deippe PA, eds: Rheumatology. St. Louis: Mosby–Yearbook Europe Ltd, 1994.
101. Johnson K, Gardner-Medwin J: Childhood arthritis. Classification and radiology. Clin Radiol 2002;57:47–58.
102. Rochat I, Sayegh Y, Gervaix A, et al: Acute hypoxic respiratory failure as the first manifestation of systemic-onset juvenile rheumatoid arthiris in a child. Pediatr Pulmonol 2004;38(6):483–487.
103. Gewanter HL, Baum J: The use of tolmetin sodium in systemic onset juvenile rheumatoid arthritis. Arthritis Rheum 1981;24:1316–1319.
104. Athreya BH, Doughty RA, Bookspan M, et al: Pulmonary manifestations of juvenile rheumatoid arthritis. A report of eight cases and review. Clin Chest Med 1980;1:361–374.
105. Brinkman GL, Chaikof L: Rheumatoid lung disease. Report of a case which developed in childhood. Am Rev Respir Dis 1959;80:732–737.
106. Jordan JD, Snyder CH: Rheumatoid disease of the lung and cor pulmonale. Am J Dis Child 1964;108:174–180.
107. Smith BS: Idiopathic pulmonary haemosiderosis and rheumatoid arthritis. BMJ 1966;1:1403–1404.
108. Romicka A, Maldyk E: Pulmonary lesions in the course of rheumatoid arthritis in children. Bull Polish Med Sci 1975;15:263–268.
109. Yousefzadeh DK, Fishman PA: The triad of pneumonitis, pleuritis, and pericarditis in juvenile rheumatoid arthritis. Pediatr Radiol 1979;8:147–150.
110. Padeh S, Laxer RM, Silver MM, Silverman ED: Primary pulmonary hypertension in a patient with systemic-onset juvenile arthritis. Arthritis Rheum 1991;34:1575–1579.
111. Porter DR, Stevenson RD, Sturrock RD: Obliterative bronchiolitis in juvenile chronic arthritis. J Rheumatol 1992;19:476–477.
112. Pegg SJ, Lang BA, Mikhail EL, Hughes DM: Fatal bronchiolitis obliterans in a patient with juvenile rheumatoid arthritis receiving chrysotherapy. J Rheumatol 1994;21:549–551.
113. Wagener JS, Taussig LM, DeBenedetti C, et al: Pulmonary function in juvenile rheumatoid arthritis. J Pediatr 1981;99:108–110.
114. Cerveri I, Bruschi C, Ravelli A, et al: Pulmonary function in childhood connective tissue diseases. Eur Respir J 1992;5:733–738.
115. Anaya JM, Diethelm L, Ortiz LA, et al: Pulmonary involvement in rheumatoid arthritis. Semin Arthritis Rheum 1995;24:242–254.
116. Kelly CA: Rheumatoid arthritis. Classical rheumatoid lung disease. Bailliere's Clin Rheumatol 1993;7:1–16.
117. Shannon TM, Gale E: Noncardiac manifestations of rheumatoid arthritis in the thorax. J Thorac Imaging 1992;7:19–29.
118. Remy-Jardin M, Remy J, Wallaert B, et al: Pulmonary involvement in progressive systemic sclerosis. Sequential evaluation with CT, pulmonary function tests, and bronchoalveolar lavage. Radiology 1993;188:495–506.
119. Caplan A: Certain unusual radiological appearances in the chest of coal miners suffering from rheumatoid arthritis. Thorax 1953;8:29–37.
120. Ellmann P, Ball RE: Rheumatoid disease with joint and pulmonary manifestations. BMJ 1948;2:816–820.
121. Fujii M, Adachi S, Shimizu T, et al: Interstitial lung disease in rheumatoid arthritis. Assessment with high resolution computed tomography. J Thorac Imaging 1993;8:54–62.
122. Popp W, Raucher H, Ritschka L, et al. Prediction of interstitial lung involvement in rheumatoid arthritis. The value of clinical data, chest roentgenogram, lung function, and serologic parameters. Chest 1992; 102:391–394.
123. Cervantes-Perez P, Toro-Perez AM, Rodriguez Jurado P: Pulmonary involvement in rheumatoid arthritis. JAMA 1980;243:1715–1719.
124. Scott TE, Wise RA, Hochberg MA, Wigley FM: HLA-DR-4 and pulmonary dysfunction in rheumatoid arthritis. Am J Med 1987;82:765–771.
125. Weiland JE, Garcia JGN, Davis WB, Gadek JE: Neutrophil collagenase in juvenile rheumatoid interstitial lung disease. J Appl Physiol 1987;62:628–633.
126. Hakala M: Poor prognosis in patients with rheumatoid arthritis hospitalized for interstitial lung fibrosis. Chest 1988;93:114–118.
127. Ippolito JA, Palmer L, Spector S, et al: Bronchiolitis obliterans organizing pneumonia and rheumatoid arthritis. Semin Arthritis Rheum 1993;23: 70–78.
128. Remy-Jardin M, Remy J, Cortet B, et al: Lung changes in rheumatoid arthritis. CT findings. Radiology 1994;193:375–382.
129. Shadick NA, Fanta CH, Wemblatt ME, et al: Bronchiectasis. A late feature of severe rheumatoid arthritis. Medicine 1994;73:161–170.
130. Yam LY, Wong R: Bronchiolitis obliterans and rheumatoid arthritis. Report of a case in a Chinese patient on D-penicillamine and review of the literature. Ann Acad Med Singapore 1993;22:365–368.
131. Hassan WU, Keaney NP, Holland CD, Kelly CA: Bronchial reactivity and airflow obstruction in rheumatoid arthritis. Ann Rheum Dis 1994; 53:511–514.
132. Banks J, Banks C, Cheong B, et al: An epidemiological and clinical investigation of pulmonary function and respiratory symptoms in patients with rheumatoid arthritis. Q J Med 1992;85:795–811.
133. Cabral DA, Malleson PN, Petty RE: Spondyloarthropathies of childhood. Pediatr Clin North Am 1995;42:1051–1070.
134. Appelrouth D, Gottlieb NL: Pulmonary manifestations of ankylosing spondylitis. J Rheumatol 1975;2:446–453.
135. Rosenow EC, Strimlan CV, Muhm JR, Ferguson RH: Pleuropulmonary manifestations of ankylosing spondylitis. Mayo Clin Proc 1977;52:641–649.
136. Feltelius N, Hedenstrom H, Hillerdal G, Hallgren R: Pulmonary involvement in ankylosing spondylitis. Ann Rheum Dis 1986;45:736–740.
137. Sharp GC, Singsen BH: Mixed connective tissue disease. In: McCarty DJ, ed: Arthritis and Allied Conditions, 12th ed. Philadelphia: Lea & Febiger, 1993, pp 92–107.
138. Sullivan WD, Hurst DJ, Harmon CE, et al: A prospective evaluation emphasizing pulmonary involvement in patients with mixed connective tissue disease. Medicine 1984;63:92–107.

139. Izumiyama T, Hida W, Ichinose M, Inoue H, et al: Small airways involvement in mixed connective tissue disease. Tohoku J Exp Med 1993;170:273–283.
140. Wiener-Kronish JP, Solinger AM, Warnock ML, et al: Severe pulmonary involvement in mixed connective tissue disease. Am Rev Respir Dis 1981; 124:499–503.
141. Prakash UBS: Pulmonary manifestations in mixed connective tissue disease. Semin Resp Med 1988;9:318–324.
142. Singsen BH, Bernstein BH, Kornreich HK, et al: Mixed connective tissue disease (MCTD) in childhood. A clinical and serological survey. J Pediatr 1977;90:893–900.
143. Fraga A, Gudino J, Ramos-Niembro F, Alarcon-Segovia D: Mixed connective tissue disease in childhood. Relationship with Sjögren syndrome. Am J Dis Child 1978;132:263–265.
144. Rosenberg AM, Petty RE, Cumming GR, Koehler BE: Pulmonary hypertension in a child with mixed connective tissue disease. J Rheumatol 1979;6:700–704.
145. Singsen BH, Swanson VL, Bernstein BH, et al: A histological evaluation of mixed connective tissue disease in childhood. Am J Med 1980;68:710–714.
146. Sullivan WD, Hurst DJ, Harmon CE, et al: A prospective evaluation of pulmonary involvement in patients with mixed connective tissue disease. Medicine 1984;63:92–107.
147. Kozuka T, Johkoh T, Honda O, et al: Pulmonary involvement in mixed connective tissue disease. High-resolution CT findings in 41 patients. J Thorac Imag 2001;16:94–98.
148. Saito Y, Terada M, Takada T, et al: Pulmonary involvement in mixed connective tissue disease. Comparison with other collagen vascular diseases using high resolution CT. J Comput Assist Tomogr 2002;26:349–357.
149. Scheja A, Elborgh R, Wildt M: Decreased capillary density in juvenile dermatomyositis and in mixed connective tissue disease. J Rheumatol 1999;26:1377–1381.
150. Prakash UBS, Luthra HS, Divertie MB: Intrathoracic manifestations of mixed connective tissue disease. Mayo Clin Proc 1985;60:813–821.
151. Derderian SS, Tellis CJ, Abbrecht PH, et al: Pulmonary involvement in mixed connective tissue disease. Chest 1985;88:45–48.
152. Jones MB, Osterholm RK, Wilson RB, et al: Fatal pulmonary hypertension and resolving immune-complex glomerulonephritis in mixed connective tissue disease. Am J Med 1978;65:855–863.
153. Friedman DM, Mitnick HJ, Danilowicz D: Recovery from pulmonary hypertension in an adolescent with mixed connective tissue disease. Ann Rheum Dis 1992;51:1001–1004.
154. Talal N: Sjogren's syndrome. Historical overview and clinical spectrum of disease. In: Fox RI, ed: Sjogren's syndrome. Rheum Dis Clin North Am 1992;18:507–515.
155. Fries JF, Hochberg MC, Medsger TA, et al: Criteria for rheumatic diseases. Different types and functions. Arthritis Rheum 1994;37:454–462.
156. Vitali C, Bombardieri S, Jonsson R, et al: Classification criteria for Sjögren's syndrome. A revised version of the European criteria proposed by the American-European Consensus Group. Ann Rheum Dis 2002;61: 554–558.
157. Kraus A, Alarcon-Segovia D: Primary juvenile Sjogren's syndrome. J Rheumatol 1988;15:803–806.
158. Deprettere AJ, Van Acker KJ, De Cleck LS, et al: Diagnosis of Sjögren's syndrome in children. Am J Dis Child 1988;142:1185–1187.
159. Anaya JM, Ogawa N, Talal N: Sjögren's syndrome in childhood. J Rheumatol 1995;22:1152–1158.
160. Strimlan CV, Rosenow EC, Divertie MB, Harrison EG: Pulmonary manifestations of Sjogren's syndrome. Chest 1976;70:354–361.
161. Kelly C, Gardiner P, Pal E, Griffiths I: Lung function in primary Sjögren's syndrome. A cross sectional and longitudinal study. Thorax 1991;46: 180–183.
162. Linstow M, Kriegbaum NJ, Backer V, et al: Follow-up study of pulmonary function in patients with primary Sjögren's syndrome. Rheumatol Int 1990;10:47–49.
163. Papathanasiou MP, Constantopoulos SH, Tsampoulas C, et al: Reappraisal of respiratory abnormalities in primary and secondary Sjögren's syndrome. A controlled study. Chest 1986;90:370–374.
164. Gardiner P, Ward C, Allison A, et al: Pleuropulmonary abnormalities in primary Sjogren's syndrome. J Rheumatol 1993;20:831–837.
165. Hatron P-Y, Wallaert B, Gosset D, et al: Subclinical lung inflammation in primary Sjögren syndrome. Arthritis Rheum 1987;30:1226–1231.
166. Dalavanga YA, Constantopoulos SH, Galanopoulou V, et al: Alveolitis correlates with clinical pulmonary involvement in primary Sjögren's syndrome. Chest 1991;99:1394–1397.
167. Deheinzelin D, Capelozzi VL, Kairalla RA, et al: Interstitial lung disease in primary Sjögren's syndrome. Clinical-pathological evaluation and response to treatment. Am J Respir Crit Care Med 1996;154:794–799.
168. Yazici H: Behcet syndrome. In: Klippel JH, Dieppe PA, eds: Rheumatology. Baltimore: Mosby–Year Book Europe Ltd, 1994.
169. Lang BA, Laxer RM, Thorner P, et al: Pediatric onset of Behcet's syndrome with myositis. Case report and literature review illustrating unusual features. Arthritis Rheum 1990;33:418–425.
170. Raz I, Okon E, Chajek-Shaul T: Pulmonary manifestations in Behcet's syndrome. Chest 1989;95:585–589.
171. Fauci AS, Haynes BF, Katz P, Wolff SM: Wegener's granulomatosis. Prospective clinical and therapeutic experience with 85 patients for 21 years. Ann Intern Med 1983;98:76–85.
172. Duna GF, Gaiperin C, Hoffman GS: Wegener's granulomatosis. Rheum Dis Clin North Am 1995;21:949–986.
173. Summers RM, Aggarwal NR, Sneller MC: CT virtual bronchoscopy of the central airways in patients with Wegener's granulomatosis. Chest 2002;121:242–250.
174. Kerr GS, Fleisher TA, Hallahan CW, et al: Limited prognostic value of changes in antineutrophil cytoplasmic antibody titer in patients with Wegener's granulomatosis. Arthritis Rheum 1993;36:365–371.
175. Mark EJ, Matsubara O, Tan-Lui NS, Fienberg R: The pulmonary biopsy in the early diagnosis of Wegener's (pathergic) granulomatosis. A study based on 35 open lung biopsies. Hum Pathol 1988;19:1065–1071.
176. Travis WD, Hoffman GS, Leavitt RY, et al: Surgical pathology of the lung in Wegener's granulomatosis. Review of 87 open lung biopsies from 67 patients. Am J Surg Pathol 1991;15:315–333.
177. Mark EJ, Flieder DB, Matsubara O: Treated Wegener's granulomatosis. Distinctive pathological findings in the lungs of 20 patients and what they tell us about the natural history of the disease. Hum Pathol 1997;28:450–458.
178. Cannon GW: Pulmonary complications of antirheumatic drug therapy. Semin Arthritis Rheum 1990;19:353–364.
179. Stavngaard T, Mortensen J: Wegener's granulomatosis causing main stem bronchial stenosis and large perfusion-ventilation defects. Clin Nucl Med 2002;27:440–441.
180. Lebovics, RS, Hoffman GS, Leavitt RY, et al: The management of subglottic stenosis in patients with Wegener's granulomatosis. Laryngoscope 1992;102:1341–1345.
181. Rottem M, Fauci AS, Hallahan CW, et al: Wegener granulomatosis in children and adolescents. Clinical presentation and outcome. J Pediatr 1993;122:26–31.
182. Adlakha A, Rao K, Adlakha K, Ryu JH: A case of pediatric Wegener's granulomatosis with recurrent venous thromboses treated with intravenous immunoglobulin and laryngotracheoplasty. Pediatr Pulmonol 1995;20: 265–268.
183. Hall SL, Miller LC, Duggan E, et al: Wegener granulomatosis in pediatric patients. J Pediatr 1985;106:739–744.
184. Hoffman GS, Kerr GS, Leavitt RY, et al: Wegener's granulomatosis. An analysis of 158 patients. Ann Intern Med 1992;116:488–498.
185. Slart RHJA, Jager PL, Poot L, et al: Clinical value of gallium-67 scintography in assessment of disease activity in Wegener's granulomatosis. Ann Rheum Dis 2003;62:659–662.
186. Jayne DRW, Davies MJ, Fox CJV, et al: Treatment of systemic vasculitis with pooled intravenous immunoglobulin. Lancet 1991;337:1137–1139.
187. Sneller MC, Hoffman OS, Talar-Williams C, et al: An analysis of forty-two Wegener's granulomatosis patients created with methotrexate and prednisone. Arthritis Rheum 1995;38:608–613.
188. Langford CA: Treatment of ANCA-associated vasculitis. N Engl J Med 2003;34:3–4.
189. Stone JH, Hoffman GS, Merkel PA, et al: A disease-specific activity index for Wegener's granulomatosis. Modification of the Birmingham Vasculitis Activity Score. Arthritis Rheum 2001;44:912–920.
190. Leavitt RY, Fauci AS, Bloch DA, et al: The American College of Rheumatology 1990 criteria for the classification of Wegener's granulomatosis. Arthritis Rheum 1990;33:1101–1107.
191. Barst RJ, Morse JH, Fotino M: Immunogenetic studies of childhood pulmonary hypertension [Abstract]. Arthritis Rheum 1990;33:S120.
192. Rosenzweig EB, Widlitz AC, Barst RJ: Pulmonary arterial hypertension in children. Pediatr Pulmonol 2004;38:2–22.
193. Farber HW, Loscalzo J: Pulmonary arterial hypertension. N Engl J Med 2004;351:1655–1665.
194. Rich S, Dantzker D: Baseline characteristics of the population in the registry. Abstracts of the International Conference on Primary Pulmonary Hypertension (sponsored by the National Institutes of Health), Philadelphia, 1987.
195. Leavitt RY, Fauci AS: Pulmonary vasculitis. Am Rev Respir Dis 1986; 134:149–166.
196. Rider LG, Clarke WR, Rutiedge J: Pulmonary hypertension in a seventeen-year-old boy. J Pediatr 1992;120:149–159.

197. Asherson RA, Khamashta MA, Ordi-Ros J, et al: The "primary" antiphospholipid syndrome. Major clinical and serological features. Medicine 1989;63:366–374.
198. Humbert M, Sanchez O, Fartoukh M, et al: Treatment of severe pulmonary hypertension secondary to connective tissue diseases with continuous IV epoprostenol (prostacyclin). Chest 1998;114:80S–82S.
199. Klings ES, Hill NS, Ieong MH, et al: Systemic sclerosis-associated pulmonary hypertension. Short- and long-term effects of epoprostenol (prostacyclin). Arthritis Rheum 1999;42:2638–2645.
200. Robbins IM, Gaine SP, Schilz R, et al: Epoprostenol for treatment of pulmonary hypertension in patients with systemic lupus erythematosus. Chest 2000;117:14–18.
201. Humbert M, Sitbon O, Simonneau G: Treatment of pulmonary hypertension. N Engl J Med 2004;351:1425–1436.
202. Oudiz RJ, Schilz RJ, Barst RJ, et al: Treprostinil, a prostaclyclin analog, in pulmonary arterial hypertension associated with connective tissue disease. Chest 2004;126:420–427.
203. Gonzalez-Lopez L, Cardona-Munoz EG, Celis A, et al: Therapy with intermittent pulse cyclophosphoramide for pulmonary hypertension associated with systemic lupus erythematosis. Lupus 2004;13:105–112.
204. Rastogi D, Hgai P, Barst RJ, Koumbourlis AC: Lower airway obstruction, bronchial hyperresponsiveness, and primary pulmonary hypertension in children. Pediatr Pulmonol 2004;37:50–55.
205. Chandler DB, Fulmer JD: Pulmonary vasculitis. Lung 1985;163:257–273.
206. Duna GF, Hoffman GS: Immunosuppression. New perspectives in the treatment of the systemic vasculitides. Ann Med Interne (Paris) 1994;145:581–594.
207. Calabrese LH, Hoffman GS, Guillevin L: Therapy of resistant systemic necrotizing vasculitis. pPolyarteritis, Churg-Strauss syndrome, Wegener's granulomatosis, and hypersensitivity vasculitis group disorders. Rheum Dis Clin North Am 1995;21:41–57.
208. Reimold EW, Weinberg AG, Fink CW, Battles ND: Polyarteritis in children. Am J Dis Child 1976;130:534–541.
209. Magilavy DB, Petty RE, Cassidy JT, Sullivan DB: A syndrome of childhood polyarteritis. J Pediatr 1977;91:25–30.
210. Athreya BH: Vasculitis in children. Pediatr Clin North Am 1995;42: 1239–1261.
211. Melam H, Patterson R: Periarteritis nodosa. A remission achieved with combined prednisone and azathioprine therapy Am J Dis Child 1971; 121:424–427.
212. Savage COS, Winearls CG, Evans DJ, et al: Microscopic polyarteritis. Presentation, pathology, and prognosis. Q J Med 1985;56:467–483.
213. Guillevin L, Lhote F: Distinguishing polyartentis nodosa from microscopic polyangiitis and implications for treatment. Curr Opin Rheumatol 1995; 7:20–24.
214. Stone JH: Polyarteritis nodosa. JAMA 2002;288:1632–1639.
215. Emery H: Henoch-Schonlein purpura. In: Hicks RV, ed: Vasculopathies of Childhood. Littleton, Mass: PSG Publishing, 1988.
216. Niaudet P, Habib R: Schonlein-Henoch purpura nephritis. Prognostic factors and therapy. Ann Med Interne (Paris) 1994;145:577–580.
217. Ozen S, Anton J, Arisoy N, et al: Juvenile polyarteritis. Results of a multicenter survey of 110 children. J Pediatrics 2004;145:517–522.
218. Churg A: Vasculitis and mimics of vasculitis involving the lung. In: Churg A, Churg J, eds: Systemic Vasculitides. New York: Igaku-Shoin Publishing, 1991.
219. Nash MC, Dillon MJ: Antineutrophil cytoplasm antibodies and vasculitis. Arch Dis Child 1997;77:261–264.
220. Schwartz MI, Brown KK: Small vessel vasculitis of the lung. Thorax 2000;55:502–510.
221. Stone JH: Current status of tumor necrosis factor inhibition in the treatment of vasculitis. Kidney Blood Press Res 2003;26:240–248.
222. Prendiville JS, Hebert AA, Greenwald MJ, Esterly NB: Management of Stevens-Johnson syndrome and toxic epidermal necrolysis in children. J Pediatr 1989;115:881–887.
223. Gorin L: Erythema nodosum. In: Hicks RV, ed: Vasculopathies of Childhood. Littleton, Mass: PSG Publishing, 1988.
224. Vanoli M, Castellani M, Bacchiani G, et al: Non-invasive assessment of pulmonary artery involvement in Takayasu's arteritis. Clin Exp Rheumatol 1999;17:213–218.
225. Cilli A, Osdemir T, Ogus C: Takayasu's arteritis presenting with bilateral parencymal consolidations and severe respiratory failure. Respiration 2001;68:628–630.
226. Wishnick MM, Valensi Q, Doyle EF, et al: Churg-Strauss syndrome. Development of cardiomyopathy during corticosteroid treatment. Am J Dis Child 1982;136:339–344.
227. Hamilos DL, Christensen J: Treatment of Churg-Strauss syndrome with high-dose intravenous immunoglobulin. J Allergy Clin Immunol 1991;88:823–824.
228. Oermann CM, Panesar KS, Langston C, et al: Pulmonary infiltrates with eosinophilia in children. J Pediatr 2000;136:351–358.
229. Richeldi L, Rossi G, Ruggieri MP, et al: Churg-Strauss syndrome in a case of asthma. Allergy 2002;57:647–654.
230. Abril A, Calamia KT, Cohen MD: The Churg Strauss syndrome (allergic granulomatous angiitis). Review and update. Semin Arthritis Rheum 2003;33:106–114.
231. Tomac N, Yuksek M, Kunak B, et al: Churg-Strauss syndrome. A patient report in infancy. Clin Pediatr 2003;42:367–370.
232. Kobayashi S, Ishizuka S, Tamura N, et al: Churg-Strauss syndrome (CCS) in a patient receiving pranlukast. Clin Rheumatol 2003;22:494–492.
233. Healy LA: Polymyalgia rheumatica and giant celi arteritis. In: McCarty DJ, ed: Arthritis and Allied Conditions, 11th ed. Philadelphia: Lea & Febiger, 1989.
234. Swerlick RA, Lawley TJ: Small-vessel vasculiris and cutaneous vasculitis. In: Churg A, Churg J, eds: Systemic Vasculitides. New York: Igaku-Shoin Publishing, 1991.
235. Haber MM, Marboe CC, Fenogho JJ: Vasculitis in drug reactions and serum sickness. In: Churg A, Churg J, eds: Systemic Vasculitides, New York: Igaku-Shoin Publishing, 1991.
236. Bambardieri S, Paoletti P, Ferri C, et al: Lung involvement in essential mixed cryoglobulinemia. Am J Med 1979;66:748–756.
237. Freeman AF, Crawford SE, Finn LS, et al: Inflammatory pulmonary nodules in Kawasaki disease. Pediatr Pulmonol 2003;36:102–106.
238. Uziel Y, Hashkes PJ, Kassem G, et al: Unresolving pneumonia as the main manifestation of atypical Kawasaki disease. Arch Dis Child 2003;88:940–942.
239. Schuyler M, Subrarnanyan S, Hassan MO: Experimental hypersensitivity pneumonitis. Transfer with cultured cells. J Lab Clin Med 1987;109:623–630.
240. Guillevin L, Lhote F, Cohen P, et al: Polyarteritis nodosa related to hepatitis B virus. A prospective study with long-term observation of 42 patients. Medicine 1995;74:238–253.
241. Ozen S, Besbas N Saatci U, Bakkaloglu A: Diagnostic criteria for polyarteritis nodosa in childhood. J Pediatr 1992;120:206–209.
242. Rosen S, Falk RJ, Jennette JC: Polyarteritis nodosa, including microscopic form and renal vasculitis. In: Churg A, Churg J, eds: Systemic Vasculitides. New York: Igaku-Shoin Publishing, 1991.
243. Landing BH, Larson EJ: Are infantile periarteritis nodosa with coronary artery involvement and fatal mucocutaneous lymph node syndrome the same? Comparison of 20 patients from North America with patients from Hawaii and Japan. Pediatrics 1977;59:651–662.
244. Hicks RV, Melish ME: Kawasaki disease. Pediatric Clin North Am 1986;33:1151–1175.
245. Gersony WM: Diagnosis and management of Kawasaki disease. JAMA 1991;265:2699–2703.
246. Umezawa T, Saji T, Matsuo N, Odagire K: Chest x-ray findings in the acute phase of Kawasaki disease. Pediatr Radiol 1989;20:48–51.
247. Newburger JW, Takahashi M, Gerber MA, et al: Diagnosis, treatment, and long-term management of Kawasaki disease. A statement for health professionals from the Committee on Rheumatic Fever, Endocarditis, and Kawasaki Disease, Council on Cardiovascular Disease in the Young, American Heart Association. Pediatrics 2004;114:1708–1733.
248. Homer C, Shulman ST: Clinical aspects of acute rheumatic fever. J Rheumatol 1991;(Suppl 29):2–13.
249. Special Writing Group of the Committee on Rheumatic Fever, Endocarditis, and Kawasaki Disease of the Council on Cardiovascular Diseases in the Young of the American Heart Association: Guidelines for the diagnosis of rheumatic fever. Jones criteria, 1992 update. JAMA 1992;268:2069–2073.
250. Scott RF, Thomas WA, Kissane JM: Rheumatic pneumonitis. Pathologic features. J Pediatr 1959;54:60–67.
251. Griffith GC, Phillips AW, Asher C: Pneumonitis occurring in rheumatic fever. Am J Med Sci 1946;212:22–25.
252. Neubuerger KT, Geever EF, Rutledge EK: Rheumatic pneumonia. Arch Pathol 1944;37:1–10.
253. Mahajan CM, Bidwai PS, Walia BNS, Berry JN: Some uncommon manifestations of rheumatic fever. Indian J Pediatr 1973;40:103–105.
254. Naish AE: The rheumatic lung. Lancet 1928;2:10.
255. Lustock MJ, Kuzrna JF: Rheumatic fever pneumonitis. A clinical and pathological study of 35 cases. Ann Intern Med 1956;44:337–357.
256. Van Wijk E: Rheumatic pneumonia. Acta Paediatr 1948;35:108–112.
257. Grunow WA, Esterly JR: Rheumatic pneumonitis. Chest 1972;61:298–301.
258. Dinkla K, Rohde M, Wouter TMJ, et al: Rheumatic fever-associated *Streptococcus pyogenes* isolates aggregate collagen. 2003;111:1905–1912.

259. Brown G, Goldring D, Behrer MR: Rheumatic pneumonia. Pediatrics 1958;52:598–619.
260. De La Fuente J, Nodar A, Sopeña B, et al: Rheumatic pneumonia. Ann Rheum Dis 2001;60:990–991.
261. Wedum BG: Rheumatic fever in school children of Denver, Colorado. Public Health Rep 1981;96:157–161.
262. Serlen SP, Rimsza ME, Gay JH: Rheumatic pneumonia. The need for a new approach. Pediatrics 1975;56:1075–1078.
263. Yamamoto LG, Seto DSY, Reddy V: Pneumonia associated with acute rheumatic fever. Clin Pediatr 1987;26:198–200.
264. Raz I, Fisher J, Israeli A, et al: An unusual case of rheumatic pneumonia. Arch Intern Med 1985;145:1130–1131.
265. Zitnik RJ, Cooper JAD: Pulmonary disease due to anti-rheumatic agents. Clin Chest Med 1990;11:139–150.
266. Partanen J, van Assendelft AHW, Koskimies S, et al: Patients with rheumatoid arthritis and gold-induced pneumonias express two high-risk major histocompatibility complex patterns. Chest 1987;92:277–281.
267. Rose CD, Singsen BH, Eichenfield AJ, et al: Safety and efficacy of methotrexate therapy for juvenile rheumatoid arthritis. J Pediatr 1990;117:653–659.
268. Barrera P, Laan RF, van Riel PL, et al: Methotrexate-related pulmonary complications in rheumatoid arthritis. Am Rheum Dis 1994;53:434–439.
269. Carroll KI, Thomas R, Phatouros CC, et al: Incidence, prevalence and possible risk factors for pneumonitis in patients with rheumatoid arthritis receiving methotrexate. J Rheumatol 1994;21:51–54.
270. Graham LD, Myones BL, Rivas-Chacon RF, Pachman LM: Morbidity associated with long-term methotrexate therapy in juvenile rheumatoid arthritis. J Pediatr 1992;120:468–473.

SUGGESTED READING

ACCP: Diagnosis and management of pulmonary arterial hypertension. ACCP evidence-based clinical practice guidelines. Chest 2004;126(Suppl 1):1S–92S.

Alarcon-Segovia D, Villarreal M: Classification and diagnostic criteria for mixed connective tissue diesase. In: Kasukawa R, Sharp GC, eds: Mixed Connective Tissue Disease and Anti-nuclear Antibodies. Amsterdam: Exerpta Medica, International Congress Series 719, 1987, pp 33–40.

Brentjens JR, Andres GA: The pathogenesis of extra-renal lesions in systemic lupus erythematosus. Arthritis Rheum 1982;25:880–886.

Brentjens JR, O'Connell DW, Pawlowski IB, et al: Experimental immune complex disease of the lung. The pathogenesis of a laboratory model resembling certain human interstitial lung diseases. J Exp Med 1974;140:105–125.

Brown G, Goldring D, Behrer MR: Rheumatic pneumonia. J Pediatr 1958;52:598–619.

Burgert SJ, Classen DC, Burke JP, Veasy LG: Rheumatic pneumonia. Reappearance of a previously recognized complication of acute rheumatic fever. Clin Infect Dis 1995;21:1020–1022.

Cairns D, Shelley L, Burke WMJ, et al: The differing patterns of interstitial lung involvement in connective tissue diseases, J Rheumatol 1992;19:1089–1095.

Caro I, Zembowicz A: Case 5-2003. A 16-year old girl with a rash and chest pain. N Engl J Med 2003;348:630–637.

Clausen KP, Bronstein H: Granulomatous pulmonary arteritis. A hypereosinophilic syndrome. Am J Clin Pathol 1974;62:82–87.

Emery H: Clinical aspects of systemic lupus erythematosus in childhood. Pediatr Clin North Am 1986;33:1177–1190.

Haworth SJ, Savage COS, Carr D, et al: Pulmonary hemorrhage complicating Wegener's granulomatosis and micoscopic polyarteritis. BMJ 1985;290:1775–1778.

Hyun BH, Diggs CL, Toone EC: Dermatomyositis with cystic fibrosis honeycombing of the lung. Dis Chest 1962;42:449–453.

Komocsi A, Reuter M, Heller M, et al: Active disease and residual damage in treated Wegener's granulomatosis. An observational study using pulmonary high-resolution computed tomography. Eur Radiol 2003;13:36–42.

Koyama M, Johkoh T, Honda O, et al: Pulmonary involvement in primary Sjögren's syndrome spectrum of pulmonary abnormalities and computed tomography findings in 60 patients. J Thorac Imaging 2001;16:290–296.

Lang BA, Shore A: A review of current concepts on the pathogenesis of juvenile rheumatoid arthritis. J Rheumatol 1990;17(Suppl 21):1–15.

Murin S, Wiedemann HP, Matthay RA: Pulmonary manifestations of systemic lupus erythematosus. Clin Chest Med 1998;19:6422–6465.

Schaller J: Lupus in childhood. Clin Rheum Dis 1982;51:45–51.

Stokes TC, McCann BG, Rees RT, et al: Acute fulminating intrapulmonary hemorrhage in Wegener's granulomatosis.Thorax 1982;37:315–316.

Wilhelm M, Van Why SK: Pneumothoraces complicating systemic lupus erythematosis with nephritis. Pediatr Nephrol 2002;17:261–263.

68 Familial Dysautonomia

Robert Dinwiddie, FRCPCH •
Samatha Sonnappa, FRCPCH

Familial dysautonomia (FD; also known as Riley-Day syndrome) is the best recognized and most frequent of a group of hereditary sensory and autonomic neuropathies seen in clinical practice. Originally described by Riley and colleagues in 1949, it is an autosomal-recessive disorder, almost exclusively occurring in Ashkenazi Jewish (AJ) individuals and is characterized by widespread sensory and variable autonomic dysfunction.[1,2]

■ GENETICS

FD is caused by mutations in the IKBKAP gene, which encodes the IκB kinase complex-associated protein (IKAP). The defective genes have been mapped to a 0.5-centimorgan region on chromosome 9q31. Two IKBKAP mutations, IVS20 (+6T → C) and R696P, have been identified.[3,4] A third deficient gene has also been described in one case. By far the most common is a splice mutation that results in the production of aberrant tissue-specific messenger RNA (mRNA), resulting in a truncated form of IKAP.[5,6] This splice site mutation IVS20 (+6T → C) is responsible for greater than 99.5% of known AJ patients with FD, and in these patients haplotype analyses were consistent with a common ancestral founder. In contrast, the R696P mutation has been identified in only a few AJ patients.[7] Tissues from individuals homozygous for the major mutation contains both mutant and wild-type IKAP transcripts. In the AJ population, the carrier rate has been estimated to be 1 in 30, with a disease frequency of 1 in 3600 live births.[8] Although penetrance appears to be complete, there is marked variability in clinical expression of the disease.

A single polymerase chain reaction and allele-specific oligonucleotide hybridization assay has been developed to facilitate the detection of both the IVS20 (+6T → C) and R696P mutations. This sensitive and specific assay facilitates carrier screening for FD mutations in the AJ community, as well as prenatal and postnatal diagnostic testing.[3–7]

■ PATHOPHYSIOLOGY

Pathologic findings indicate that within the peripheral sensory and autonomic nervous systems, individuals affected with FD have incomplete neuronal development as well as progressive neuronal degeneration. The autonomic nervous system (ANS) subserves many nonvolitional body functions and controls internal body homeostasis, including regulation of blood pressure, fluid, temperature, and electrolyte balance. The ANS is composed of parasympathetic and sympathetic nerve fibers, each of which has components in the central and peripheral nervous systems. FD is characterized by an initial reduction, and a progressive decrease, in the number of preganglionic sympathetic neurons in the cervical sympathetic ganglia, sensory neurons in the lateral columns of the spinal cord, and parasympathetic neurons in the parasympathetic ganglia.[9] The sensory abnormalities involve primarily functions transmitted by the unmyelinated neuronal population. Pain and temperature sensations are decreased, but not absent. Studies have shown a marked reduction in unmyelinated neuronal populations as well as in small-diameter myelinated axons. This reduction seems to indicate a developmental arrest in the sensory and autonomic systems and, in the latter, principally in the sympathetic fibers. Sympathetic ganglia have been found to be one third of the normal size, and the neuronal population has been found to be one tenth of the normal number.[9–11]

The fungiform and circumvallate papillae on the tongue, in which the taste buds are found, are sparse and rudimentary. The transverse fascicular area of the sural nerves in patients of all ages is reduced because of diminution of small-caliber myelinated axons, severe depletion in unmyelinated axons, and absence of catecholamine-containing fibers.[11–13]

Pathologic involvement of the kidneys is common even in the young, progressing in severity with age. Glomerulosclerosis, abnormalities of the capillary basement membrane, and associated tubular atrophy are most prominent. Repeated incidents of postural hypotension or vasoconstriction of renal vessels as a result of poor sympathetic control and renal hypoperfusion secondary to cardiovascular instability are postulated mechanisms. Renal function is, however, generally well preserved throughout childhood.

Hypersensitivity to sympathomimetic and parasympathomimetic drugs occurs. Norepinephrine synthesis is diminished, while dopamine products are excreted in normal amounts. During physical and emotional stress, plasma norepinephrine and dopamine are elevated and autonomic storms or crises may develop.[9–13]

Abnormalities of sucking and swallowing, often associated with gastroesophageal reflux, occur in almost all patients. These problems result in recurrent aspiration of fluids into the lungs, which is a major potential cause of pathology, including the development of bronchiectasis, throughout life.

■ CLINICAL FEATURES AND DIAGNOSIS

The diagnosis of FD is suspected by clinical findings and established by molecular genetic testing for the defective IKBKAP gene. Prior to the discovery of the molecular genetic basis of FD and the introduction of molecular genetic testing, the diagnosis of FD relied on the clinical recognition of both sensory and autonomic dysfunction and the presence of AJ ancestry. It was necessary for the following six cardinal features to be present in each affected individual:

1. Decreased taste sensation and absence of fungiform papillae of the tongue, giving it a smooth, pale appearance.
2. Absence of axon flare response after intradermal histamine injection. In a normal child, intradermal injection of 1:1000 histamine produces intense pain and erythema followed within minutes by the development of a central wheal surrounded by an axon flare, which is maintained

for more than 10 minutes. In FD patients, the pain is greatly reduced and there is no axon flare.

3. Decreased or absent deep tendon reflexes.
4. Hypotonia in infancy.
5. Absence of overflow tears with emotional crying (alacrima). Either the history or the Schirmer test can be used to demonstrate this sign. The Schirmer test can be performed after 6 months of age, because newborns do not cry with tears. In this test, the end of a filter paper 5 mm wide and 3 mm long is placed in the lateral portion of a lower eyelid. Less than 10 mm of wetting of the filter paper after 5 minutes indicates diminished baseline and reflex tear secretion.
6. Pupillary hypersensitivity to parasympathomimetic agents. Topical administration of methacholine 2.5% or pilocarpine 0.0625% has no observable effect on the normal pupil, but causes miosis after about 20 minutes in almost all patients with FD.[11,14–16]

■ RESPIRATORY PROBLEMS

In babies with FD there is a high prevalence of breech presentation births, poor muscle tone, and meconium stained liquor.[17] This can lead to an increased risk of meconium aspiration pneumonitis in the presence of coexisting fetal distress. In the neonatal period the problems encountered may be delayed initiation of breathing and difficulty in coordination of sucking and swallowing, which can result in subsequent aspiration of feeds. Individuals with FD usually develop a number of pulmonary disorders, including recurrent wheezing and pneumonia secondary to aspiration, due to impaired swallowing, and severe gastroesophageal reflux. Recurrent lobar collapse and subsequently bronchiectasis caused by repeated episodes of aspiration are major presenting features and potential complications of the illness (Fig. 68-1). Insensitivity to pain and poor cough reflex contribute to the inability of the patient to mobilize aspirated material and to clear excessive lung secretions. Because oropharyngeal incoordination is prominent, concomitant use of gastrostomy and Nissen's fundoplication results in a significant improvement in the quality of life for the majority of patients, by preventing development of severe respiratory disease.[18,19] The oral intake of fluid and food that is permissible and safe in order to avoid recurrent aspiration damage varies from one case to another and has to be decided on an individual basis. Atelectasis, spontaneous pneumothorax, and air trapping can occur. In addition, kyphoscoliosis in later childhood can contribute to reduced pulmonary function.[20]

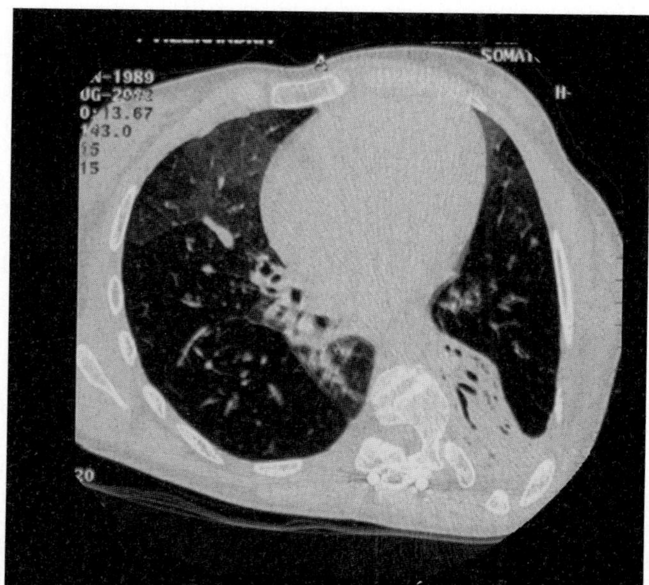

■ **FIGURE 68-1.** Computed tomographic image of the chest showing bilateral bronchiectasis and lobar collapse due to recurrent aspiration.

Diminished responses to hypoxia and hypercarbia are often seen and are caused by abnormalities in central control of breathing. These can result in breath-holding spells with syncope and nonresponsiveness to hypoxic stimuli. This can be a particular problem during air travel and when undertaking certain sports such as swimming and underwater diving, where fatalities have occurred due to the inability to respond appropriately to hypoxia and hypercarbia. If there is any doubt about a patients' ability to undertake air travel, a "fitness to fly test" should be performed in a suitably equipped respiratory function laboratory to assess oxygen requirement. Overnight sleep study monitoring should be part of the regular review of FD patients, because irregular breathing patterns, apneic spells, hypoxia, and hypercarbia can occur during sleep.[11,21,22] The frequency of these assessments is determined on an individual basis. When these studies demonstrate significant hypoventilation and hypoxia, overnight oxygen supplementation and noninvasive ventilation should be considered.

■ CHEST WALL DISORDERS AND KYPHOSCOLIOSIS

The development of kyphoscoliosis is a major complication of the illness. It is estimated that progressive scoliosis develops in as many as 95% and kyphosis in 53% of patients.[10] The onset generally occurs in mid-childhood but accelerates during puberty and adolescence. Early referral to a scoliosis clinic is recommended. A significant number of affected children will need spinal fusion surgery to control this problem (Figs. 68-2 and 68-3). This may be complicated by the development of osteoporosis, which is increasingly being recognized in the adolescent FD population. The presence of significant spinal osteoporosis makes the placement and retention of orthopedic screws more challenging. Routine monitoring of spinal curvature on an annual basis is recommended. This should be combined with yearly bone density (dual-energy x-ray absorptiometry) scans. Dietary supplementation with calcium, phosphate, and vitamin D is recommended. Where there is continuing evidence of decreased bone density with age, therapy with agents such as pamidronate is indicated.[20] Respiratory function is compromised by an increased spinal curvature due to compression of lung tissue, resulting in reduced vital capacity and restrictive lung disease. This is especially relevant if there has been previous atelectasis due to recurrent aspiration in early childhood.

■ COMMON NONRESPIRATORY COMPLICATIONS

■ AUTONOMIC CRISES

One of the most major complications of the disease is that of autonomic crises. These are induced by stress of any type such

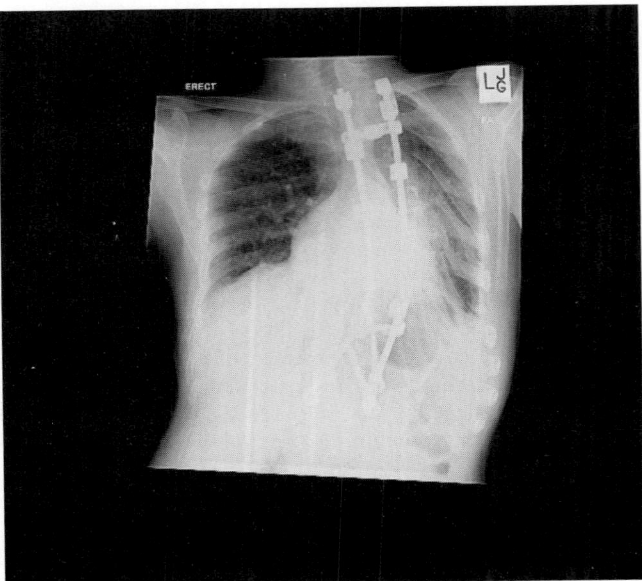

■ **FIGURE 68-2.** Chest radiograph (posteroanterior view) showing thoracic scoliosis with spinal fixation rods and loss of volume in the left lung.

as infection, tiredness, anxiety, sibling rivalry, or pressures at school. They are manifested by vomiting, or retching in those who have had a fundoplication, ineffective coughing resulting in difficulty in clearing upper and lower airway secretions, excessive drooling or salivation, and major instability of blood pressure with either hypotension or more commonly hypertension. The child is emotionally labile with anxiety and irritability being common features. Skin perfusion is often poor with cold extremities and blotching present.

The frequency of crises varies greatly from one child to another. Most children exhibit these at least once or twice per month. Others, however, have them several times per week or even daily.

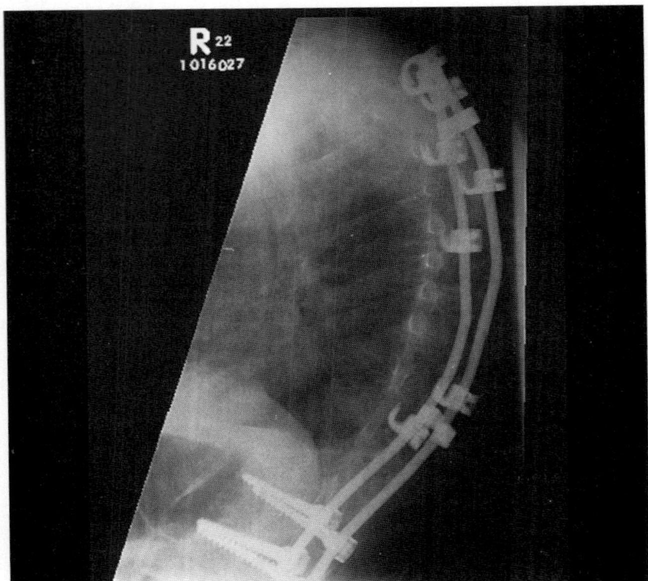

■ **FIGURE 68-3.** Spine radiograph (lateral view) after spinal surgery for severe thoracic and lumbar scoliosis. Also note the osteoporosis.

If the crises are of such frequency a search should be made for triggering factors. Recurrent subtle pulmonary aspiration is a common cause and particular attention should be directed to the assessment of swallowing, especially of liquids and semi-solids. Because most children are fed by gastrostomy, this problem is easily remediable. Diazepam is the drug of choice to treat the dysautonomic crises.[22]

CARDIOVASCULAR IRREGULARITIES

Patients with FD exhibit profound orthostatic hypotension without compensatory tachycardia as well as recumbent hypertension. Orthostatic hypotension in FD is thought primarily to be due to a lack of sympathetically mediated vasoconstriction without evidence of abnormally large shifts in blood volume toward the legs during orthostasis.[23] This clinically manifests as episodes of light-headedness or dizzy spells and some patients complain of weak legs. General anesthesia has the potential for inducing severe hypotension.[22] First-line therapy for orthostatic hypotension should be with fludrocortisone, midodrine, or a combination of both.[12] In addition, during dysautonomic crises, patients have hypertension that is presumed to be secondary to episodic vasoconstriction, as well as swollen hands thought to be secondary to vasodilatation. This discrepancy in vascular control is poorly understood, yet provides an insight into the pathophysiology of autonomic crises. The reduced limb perfusion and the dysfunctional end-organ blood supply in FD patients are likely to be major contributors to the vasomotor instability observed in these subjects, particularly during periods of stress.[24] Hypertension also can exist without any other symptoms. Because blood pressure is so labile in individuals with FD, asymptomatic hypertension is not specifically treated because it is most often transitory and appears to be better tolerated than hypotension. When necessary, clonidine is used for treatment of episodic hypertension.

CENTRAL NERVOUS SYSTEM DYSFUNCTION

Emotional lability and behavioral abnormalities have been considered one of the prominent features of FD. They are now acknowledged as part of the crisis constellation and may be secondary to periodic catecholamine imbalance. Most affected individuals are of normal intelligence. About 25% of patients with FD have abnormal electroencephalograms, but fewer than 10% actually have a true seizure disorder. Prolonged breath holding with crying can be severe enough to result in cyanosis, syncope, and decerebrate posturing. Breath holding is frequent in the early years, occurring at least one time in 63% of patients. This phenomenon is probably a manifestation of diminished sensitivity to hypoxia and hypercapnia.[22]

TREATMENT

The treatment is aimed at being supportive, symptomatic, and preventative. The regimen for each patient needs to be determined on an individual basis. The most important issues from the respiratory point of view relate to the prevention and control of recurrent aspiration leading to chronic pulmonary suppuration and bronchiectasis in the longer term. Speech and language therapists play a vital role in the initial assessment and ongoing management of these patients. The use of gastrostomy and fundoplication has already been outlined. In our experience, prophylactic antibiotic therapy against common respiratory pathogens using broad-spectrum antibiotics and nebulized aminoglycosides in patients chronically colonized with *Pseudomonas aeruginosa* has been found to be beneficial. Administration of pneumococcal and influenza vaccines prevents further morbidity. Chest physiotherapy, inhaled bronchodilators, and other relevant age-appropriate methods of clearance of secretions from the lungs are helpful as a daily routine, particularly in children with residual effects from aspiration or infection.

General anesthesia for surgical procedures requires careful monitoring for hypoxia and hypercapnia, in addition to heart rate and blood pressure. Specific attention to hydration and control of fluid balance is important in order to avoid perioperative autonomic crises.

Control of the other aspects of the condition—including the avoidance and treatment of autonomic crises, seizures, and blood pressure lability resulting in syncopal attacks, and the prevention of nighttime hypoxia—will all result in a decrease in respiratory-related morbidity and mortality.

■ PROGNOSIS

FD is a potentially life-threatening disorder with a high morbidity and mortality. The cause of death is usually from respiratory failure due to chronic lung damage secondary to recurrent aspiration, unexplained sudden deaths, or renal failure. However, early diagnosis and better understanding of the pathophysiology have led to modification of treatment measures, including surgery, to cope with the gastrointestinal and cardiovascular irregularities. This has significantly improved survival rates and quality of life among the FD patients. The majority of patients are now surviving into adulthood and early middle age and many of them function independently.[25,26]

■ RECENT ADVANCES

With the recent discovery of the genetic defect, definitive treatments are anticipated. The FD mutation found on greater than 99.5% of FD chromosomes does not cause complete loss of function. Instead, it results in a tissue-specific decrease in splicing efficiency of the IKBKAP transcript; cells from patients retain some capacity to produce normal mRNA and protein.[27] Various laboratory studies and clinical trials are being conducted, treating cells with compounds that modulate the splicing of IKAP, resulting in an up-regulation of IKBKAP transcription and elevation of cellular levels of functional IKAP protein.[28,29] However, effective management for FD is still not available, making preimplantation genetic diagnosis a useful option for at-risk couples to establish an FD-free pregnancy from the outset. This provides an alternative for those at-risk couples who cannot accept prenatal diagnosis and termination of pregnancy as an option for avoiding FD.[30]

REFERENCES

1. Riley CM, Day RL, Greely DM, Langford WS: Central autonomic dysfunction with defective lacrimation. Report of five cases. Pediatrics 1949;3:468–478.
2. Slaugenhaupt SA, Blumenfeld A, Gill SP, Leyne M, Mull J, Cuajungco MP, et al: Tissue-specific expression of a splicing mutation in the IKBKAP gene causes familial dysautonomia. Am J Hum Genet 2001;68:598–605.
3. Anderson SL, Coli R, Daly IW, Kichula EA, Rork MJ, Volpi SA, et al: Familial dysautonomia is caused by mutations of the IKAP gene. Am J Hum Genet 2001;68:753–758.
4. Eng CM, Slaugenhaupt SA, Blumenfeld A, Axelrod FB, Gusella JF, Desnick RJ: Prenatal diagnosis of familial dysautonomia by analysis of linked CA-repeat polymorphisms on chromosome 9q31-q33. Am J Med Genet 1995;59:349–355.
5. Anderson SL, Qiu J, Rubin BY: Tocotrienols induce IKBKAP expression. A possible therapy for familial dysautonomia. Biochem Biophys Res Commun 2003;306:303–309.
6. Slaugenhaupt SA, Gusella JF: Familial dysautonomia. Curr Opin Genet Dev 2002;12:307–311.
7. Dong J, Edelmann L, Bajwa AM, Kornreich R, Desnick RJ: Familial dysautonomia. Detection of the IKBKAP IVS20 (+6T → C) and R696P mutations and frequencies among Ashkenazi Jews. Am J Med Genet 2002;110:253–257.
8. Maayan C, Kaplan E, Shachar C, Peleg O, Godfrey S: Incidence of familial dysautonomia in Israel 1977–1981. Clin Genet 1987;32:106–108.
9. Laplaza FJ, Turajane T, Axelrod FB, Burke SW: Nonspinal orthopaedic problems in familial dysautonomia (Riley-Day syndrome). J Pediatr Orthop 2001;21:229–232.
10. Rubery PT, Spielman JH, Hester P, Axelrod F, Burke SW, Levine DB: Scoliosis in familial dysautonomia. Operative treatment. J Bone Joint Surg Am 1995;77:1362–1369.
11. Dancis J: Familial dysautonomia. In: Mathias CJ, Bannister R, eds: Autonomic Failure: A Textbook of Clinical Disorders of the Autonomic Nervous System. New York: Oxford University Press, 1992, pp 615–639.
12. Donofrio PD, Caress JB: Autonomic disorders. Neurologist 2001;7:220–233.
13. Aguayo AJ, Nair CP, Bray GM: Peripheral nerve abnormalities in the Riley-Day syndrome. Findings in a sural nerve biopsy. Arch Neurol 1971;24: 106–116.
14. Wright JC, Meger GE: A review of the Schirmer test for tear production. Arch Ophthalmol 1962;67:564–565.
15. Goldberg MF, Payne JW, Brunt PW: Ophthalmologic studies of familial dysautonomia. The Riley-Day syndrome. Arch Ophthalmol 1968;80: 732–743.
16. Fernhoff PM: No pains, many gains [Editorial]. J Pediatr 2002;141:470–471.
17. Axelrod FB, Gouge TH, Ginsburg HB, Bangaru BS, Hazzi C: Fundoplication and gastrostomy in familial dysautonomia. J Pediatr 1991;118:388–394.
18. Udassin R, Seror D, Vinograd I, Zamir O, Godfrey S, Nissan S: Nissen's fundoplication in the treatment of children with familial dysautonomia. Am J Surg 1992;164:332–336.
19. Inselman LS: Pulmonary manifestations of systemic disorders. In: Taussig LM, Landau LI, eds: Pediatric Respiratory Medicine. St. Louis: CV Mosby, 1999, pp 1254–1255.
20. Maayan C, Bar-On E, Foldes AJ, Gesundheit B, Dresner P: Bone mineral density and metabolism in familial dysautonomia. Osteoporos Int 2002;13:429–433.
21. Axelrod FB, Porges RF, Sein ME: Neonatal recognition of familial dysautonomia. J Pediatr 1987;110:946–948.
22. Axelrod FB, Maayan C: Familial dysautonomia. In: Burg FD, Ingelfinger JR, Wald ER, Polin RA, eds: Gellis and Kagan's Current Pediatric Therapy. Philadelphia: WB Saunders, 1999, pp 466–469.
23. Brown CM, Stemper B, Welsch G, Brys M, Axelrod FB, Hilz MJ: Orthostatic challenge reveals impaired vascular resistance control, but normal venous pooling and capillary filtration in familial dysautonomia. Clin Sci (Lond) 2003;104:163–169.
24. Stemper B, Axelrod FB, Marthol H, Brown C, Brys M, Welsch G, et al: Terminal vessel hyperperfusion despite organ hypoperfusion in familial dysautonomia. Clin Sci (Lond) 2003;105:295–301.
25. Axelrod FB, Goldberg JD, Ye XY, Maayan C: Survival in familial dysautonomia. Impact of early intervention. J Pediatr 2002;141:518–523.
26. Axelrod FB: Familial dysautonomia. Muscle Nerve 2004;29:352–363.
27. Mezey E, Parmalee A, Szalayova I, Gill SP, Cuajungco MP, Leyne M, et al: Of splice and men. What does the distribution of IKAP mRNA in the rat tell us about the pathogenesis of familial dysautonomia? Brain Res 2003; 983:209–214.
28. Anderson SL, Qiu J, Rubin BY: EGCG corrects aberrant splicing of IKAP mRNA in cells from patients with familial dysautonomia. Biochem Biophys Res Commun 2003;310:627–633.
29. Slaugenhaupt SA, Mull J, Leyne M, Cuajungco MP, Gill SP, Hims MM, et al: Rescue of a human mRNA splicing defect by the plant cytokinin kinetin. Hum Mol Genet 2004;13:429–436.
30. Rechitsky S, Verlinsky O, Kuliev A, Ozen RS, Masciangelo C, Lifchez A, et al: Preimplantation genetic diagnosis for familial dysautonomia. Reprod Biomed Online 2003;6:488–493.

69 Chronic Granulomatous Disease of Childhood

Daniel R. Ambruso, MD •
Richard B. Johnston, Jr., MD

Chronic granulomatous disease of childhood was first described by Berendes and colleagues[1] and by Landing and Shirkey[2] as a distinct clinical entity of unknown cause.[3] This disease is characterized by recurrent infections with usually low-grade pathogens, formation of suppurative granulomas, and normal humoral and cellular immunity. The usual onset of symptoms is early in life (most in the first 2 years of life), the disease is generally chronic, and, unless diagnosed and treated, the outcome is commonly death as the result of overwhelming infection.

After the original patients, similar cases were reported using various names.[4–7] *Chronic granulomatous disease* (CGD) is now the generally accepted term for this syndrome. Quie and colleagues[8] defined the basic step in pathophysiology as an inability of phagocytic cells to kill ingested bacteria; and Baehner and Nathan[6] showed that CGD neutrophils did not undergo the phagocytosis-associated "respiratory burst" of oxygen consumption and hydrogen peroxide (H_2O_2) production that characterizes phagocytic cells.

Although most of the cases initially documented were in males, two reports described females, suggesting the possibility of autosomal-recessive variants.[9,10] In the 1970s, progress was made in elucidating the nature of the basic biochemical defect, decreased oxidase activity, a process by which oxygen (O_2) is reduced to superoxide anion (O_2^-) using NADPH as the electron source.[11–13] In 1978 Segal and Jones reported the association of a *b*-type cytochrome and the NADPH oxidase, as well as its deficiency in CGD. Continued studies firmly defined the relationship between X-linked CGD and deficiency of cytochrome b_{558}.[14] In the late 1980s, the gene that is abnormal in X-linked CGD was cloned and subsequently shown to produce the heavy-chain component of the cytochrome b_{558} heterodimer (gp91phox).[15–17] Subsequently, the light chain (p22phox) was described and found to be the basis for the autosomal-recessive form of cytochrome b–deficient CGD.[18]

In the late 1980s and early 1990s, the molecular basis for other forms of autosomal-recessive CGD were defined. Cytosolic components, p47phox and p67phox, were identified, linked to distinct variants of CGD, and sequenced; and their genes were cloned.[19–22]

Thus, 84 years after Metchnikoff published his theory that phagocytosis is essential in fighting infection (in 1883), studies in patients with CGD documented that a defect in phagocyte function is a major breach in host defense resulting in predisposition to severe infections. Since 1967, the biochemistry of the oxidase enzyme system has been elucidated, the major components defined, and the molecular and genetic basis for the most common variants of CGD described. The understanding of this syndrome as an "experiment of nature" has greatly expanded our knowledge of the role of the phagocyte in host defense.

■ CLINICAL FEATURES

The hallmark of this disease is the occurrence of purulent inflammation due to catalase-positive, low-grade pyogenic bacteria. This syndrome should be considered in any individual with recurrent catalase-positive bacterial or fungal infections. Table 69-1 summarizes the relative frequencies of the most common clinical findings in patients with CGD in the earliest reported cases, before the general use of prophylactic antimicrobial therapy. A more recent analysis of infections in 368 patients enrolled in a registry for CGD[23,24] shows a general decline in most types of infection, with the notable exception of pneumonia (Table 69-2).

Of the 368 registry patients, 76% had the X-linked recessive form of CGD. The mean age at diagnosis in the registry patients was 3.0 years with the X-linked form and 7.8 years with an autosomal-recessive form.[23] These ages are much higher than they should be for the sake of the patient. In rare instances, the initial diagnosis has been made in adulthood. Several investigators have suggested that these clinically milder patients have an autosomal-recessive variant.[24,25] Testing of chorionic villous samples, fetal blood cells, or amniocytes can document the condition prenatally.[26]

Although any organ may be involved with infections, two patterns emerge (see Tables 69-1 and 69-2).[23,24,27] First, the inability of phagocytic cells to effect microbicidal activity at the interface between the host and the environment leads to infections such as pneumonitis, infectious dermatitis, and perianal abscesses. With the involvement of the mononuclear phagocyte system, deep-seated infections result in purulent lymphadenitis, hepatomegaly, splenomegaly, and hepatic and perihepatic abscesses. At all sites of infection, microbes may be sequestered and protected from intracellular killing mechanisms and antibiotics. Unable to destroy the microbes, the phagocytes die and release the organisms. Further microbial proliferation and leukocyte accumulation leads to the abscesses and granulomas that characterize the disorder. Septicemia may also occur because of the inability of phagocytes to localize microbial invasion.

Purulent rhinitis and otitis are common clinical features of this disease. With adequate antibiotic therapy, rhinitis clears up slowly, only to recur within a few days after the treatment is discontinued. The oropharynx and gastrointestinal tract are frequently infected, with ulcerative stomatitis, gingivitis, esophagitis, rectal abscesses, perianal abscesses, and fissures being common. Urinary tract infections and glomerulonephritis, renal abscesses, and cystitis have all been reported. Gonadal infections are rare, but have been described. Osteomyelitis is common: the most frequent sites include metacarpals, metatarsals, spine, and ribs.

■ **TABLE 69-1.** Clinical findings in the 168 earliest reported patients with chronic granulomatous disease

Finding	Percentage of Patients Involved
Marked lymphadenopathy	82
Pneumonitis	80
Dermatitis	71
Hepatomegaly	68
Onset by age 1 year	65
Suppuration of nodes	62
Splenomegaly	57
Hepatic-perihepatic abscess	41
Osteomyelitis	32
Onset with dermatitis	25
Onset with lymphadenitis	23
Facial periorificial dermatitis	21
Persistent diarrhea	20
Septicemia or meningitis	17
Perianal abscess	17
Conjunctivitis	16
Death from pneumonitis	15
Persistent rhinitis	15
Ulcerative stomatitis	15

Adapted from Johnston RB Jr, Newman SL: Chronic granulomatous disease. Pediatr Clin North Am 1977;24:365.

Lymphadenitis, a characteristic clinical feature, occurs in the majority of patients during the course of the disease. It is typically chronic, suppurative, and granulomatous and very often requires surgical drainage. Cervical, axillary, and inguinal nodes are usually involved, but hilar and mesenteric lymph nodes are also commonly enlarged.

Skin lesions include impetiginous eruptions that progress slowly to suppuration. The healing process can be slow, resulting in granulomatous nodules that persist for months. These lesions may be found in any part of the body, the face and neck being the most frequent sites. Furunculosis and subcutaneous abscesses may be chronic problems. Eczematoid dermatitis can be seen early in the diagnosis. Discoid lupus has been diagnosed in patients with autosomal-recessive variants of CGD and carriers of X-linked CGD.

While the major problems of patients with CGD are related to infections, these individuals can also be afflicted with a number of conditions reflecting a vigorous inflammatory response without a clear infectious cause.[25,27] Pyloric stenosis is common, and sterile granulomas can be found in the pyloric antrum. Similar lesions in the small and large bowel may be associated with diarrhea, malabsorption, or obstruction.[28] Some of the gut lesions have been described as eosinophilic gastroenteritis, gastrointestinal dysmotility, or inflammatory bowel disease. Granulomas in the urinary bladder can result in obstructive uropathy. Pericarditis and pleuritis have been noted. Chorioretinitis was detected in 9 of 30 boys with X-linked CGD and in 3 of 15 related carriers in one clinic.[29] The mechanism for these inflammatory lesions is not well understood, but the response of pyloric and bladder granulomas to steroids is well documented.

■ **TABLE 69-2.** Most common infections in 368 patients enrolled in a registry for chronic granulomatous disease

Infection	Percentage of Patients
Pneumonia	79
Abscess (any)	68
Subcutaneous	42
Liver	27
Lung	16
Perirectal	15
Brain	3
Suppurative adenitis	53
Osteomyelitis	25
Bacteremia/fungemia	18
Cellulitis or impetigo	10

Data from Winkelstein, JA, Marino MC, Johnston RB Jr, et al: Chronic granulomatous disease. Report on a national registry of 368 patients. Medicine 2000;79:155.

■ PULMONARY COMPLICATIONS

Both Tables 69-1 and 69-2 show that pneumonia continues to be one of the most common types of infection, occurring in about 80% of patients with CGD. Pulmonary disease has also become a major cause of mortality in this disease.[23] The onset of lower respiratory tract infection may be heralded by the usual clinical presentation of fever, cough, tachypnea, pleuritic pain, and abnormal auscultatory findings. In some patients, few, if any, signs or symptoms have been noted in the presence of marked infiltration on radiography. Chronic granulomatous infiltrations, pulmonary fibrosis, and interstitial lung disease have been noted in both pediatric and adult patients.[30,31]

The range of microbial agents causing pulmonary infections is shown in Table 69-3. Since the 1970s, the use of daily antimicrobial therapy in CGD has reduced the rate of infections due to *Staphylococcus aureus* and enteric bacteria,[32,33] but *Aspergillus* species has become a particularly troublesome offender.[23,34] Fungi now cause a large percentage of infections in CGD, and

■ **TABLE 69-3.** Most common infecting organisms in the 368 patients in the chronic granulomatous disease registry

Type of Infection	Organism	Percentage of Patients*
Pneumonia	*Aspergillus* species	33
	Staphylococcus species	9
	Burkholderia cepacia	7
	Nocardia species	6
	Serratia species	4
Abscess—subcutaneous, liver, and/or perirectal	*Staphylococcus* species	26
	Serratia species	3
	Aspergilllus species	3
Abscess—lung	*Aspergillus* species	4
Abscess—brain	*Aspergillus* species	2
Suppurative adenitis	*Staphylococcus* species	14
	Serratia species	5
Osteomyelitis	*Serratia* species	7
	Aspergillus species	5
Bacteremia/fungemia	*Salmonella* species	3
	Burkholderia cepacia	2
	Candida species	2

*Percentage of the 368 patients who had this organism isolated at least once from the infection shown.

Data from Winkelstein JA, Merino MC, Johnston RB Jr, et al: Chronic granulomatous disease. Report on a national registry of 368 patients. Medicine 2000;79:155.

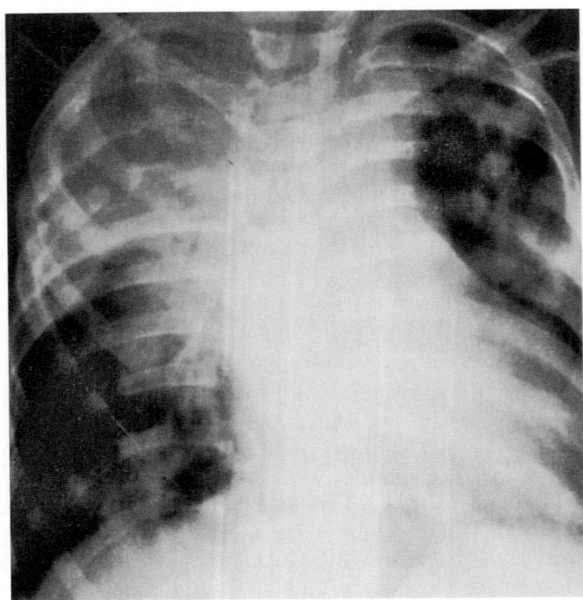

■ **FIGURE 69-1.** A chest roentgenogram from a patient with chronic granulomatous disease, showing extensive involvement of the right lung. This patient died of the overwhelming infection.

lung involvement may spread to the pleura and adjacent bone and soft tissues of the chest wall.[35,36] Although *Aspergillus* accounts for most of the fungal agents (>80%), other agents such as *Acremonium striatum, Candida albicans, Pneumocystis carinii,* and *Paecilomyces* species may also be isolated from infected lungs.[23,27,34] *Aspergillus* pneumonia, with or without dissemination, was the leading cause of death in the 368 registry patients (23 of 65 total deaths). *Nocardia,* atypical mycobacteria, and the bacillus Calmette-Guérin vaccine strain of mycobacteria can also cause pulmonary disease.

The most prominent pulmonary lesions include an extensive infiltration of the lung parenchyma and prominent hilar adenopathy demonstrable on roentgenogram (Fig. 69-1). In addition, bronchopneumonia, often combined with lobar pneumonia, pleural effusion, pleural thickening, pulmonary abscess, and atelectasis (especially of the right middle lobe), may be present. A process characterized by extensive reticulonodular infiltration often leads to pulmonary insufficiency and death.

The pneumonia may begin as hilar infiltration; it is peribronchial, either unilateral or bilateral, or it is basilar. Despite extensive antibiotic treatment, these lesions regress slowly over a period of weeks to months or frequently progress to involve an entire lobe (Figs. 69-2 and 69-3). An unusual manifestation of pulmonary involvement observed in these patients is so-called encapsulated pneumonia.[37] This pneumonia is characteristically seen on roentgenography as a homogeneous, discrete, relatively round lesion; it may occur singly or in groups of two to three infiltrates (see Fig. 69-2*A*). The size and contour of the lesions may change within a few days or remain unchanged for weeks

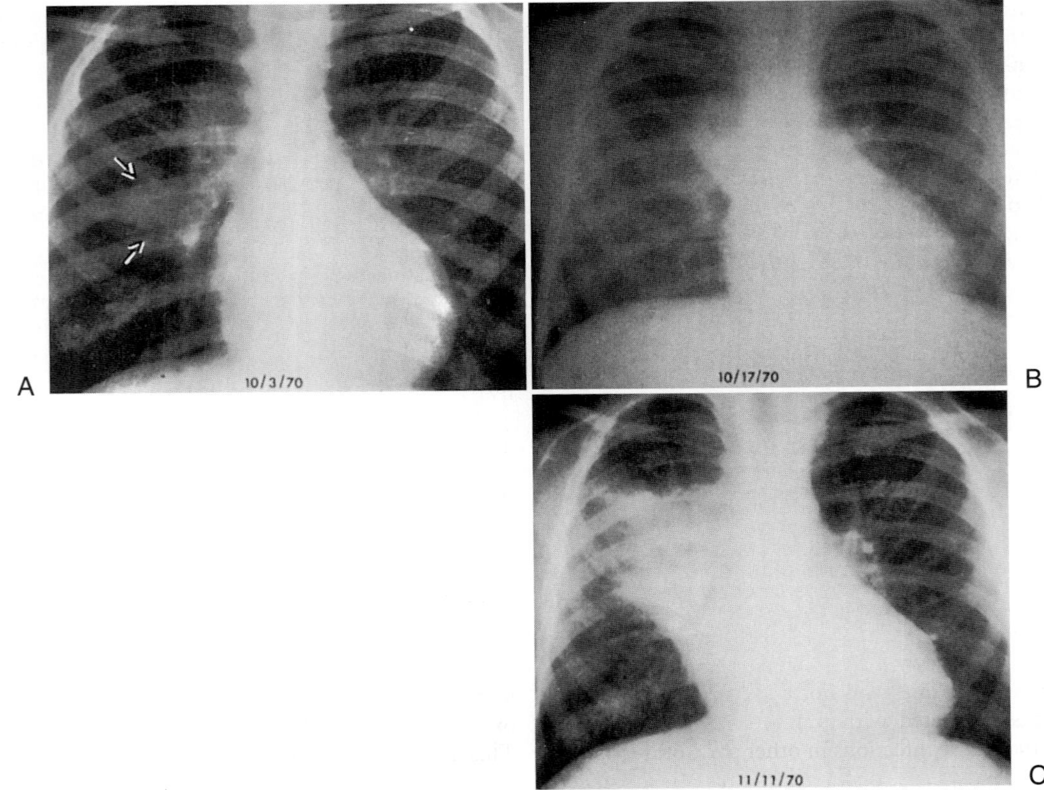

■ **FIGURE 69-2.** Chronic progressive infiltration of the right lung despite intensive antibiotic therapy. The right upper lobe was resected to control the infection. **A,** An early stage of infiltration with typical "encapsulated pneumonia" *(arrows)*. **B** and **C,** Progression of the lesion.

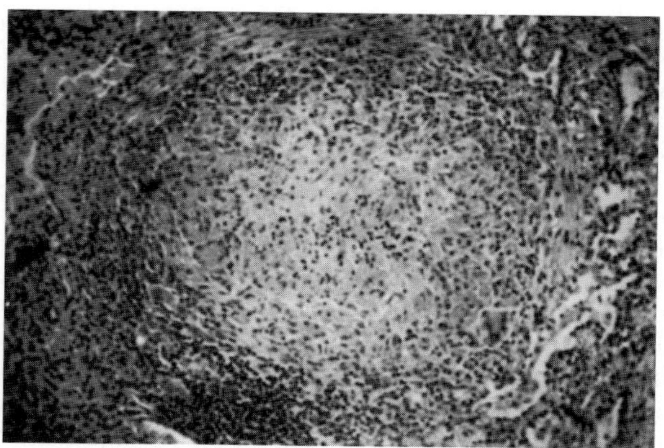

■ **FIGURE 69-3.** A typical granuloma of lung tissue removed from the patient shown in Figure 69-2 (original magnification approximately ×400).

or months. A homogeneous distribution of small granulomatous lesions can occur, which gives the radiographic appearance of miliary tuberculosis. Discoid atelectasis, thickening of the bronchi, air bronchograms, "honeycombing," and loss of lobar volume and bronchiectasis associated with hemoptysis are occasionally observed. When underlying reticulation of the lungs persists, the pulmonary function may be correspondingly impaired.

■ LABORATORY FINDINGS AND DIAGNOSIS

Except for abnormalities of phagocyte function, clinical laboratory findings reflect acute or chronic infection and inflammation. Leukocytosis with a neutrophilia, elevated erythrocyte sedimentation rate, and the anemia of chronic inflammation are commonly seen during infections. The anemia is usually not due to a deficiency of iron stores but to a decrease in iron release from the mononuclear phagocyte system and diminished utilization by the marrow.[38] It will not usually respond to iron administration but improves with resolution of infection. Evidence of hemolytic anemia with acanthocytosis suggests the absence of the K_x antigen on red blood cells, a trait close to the gp91phox gene on the x chromosome.

Screening evaluations of various aspects of immune function are usually normal, including complement, cellular immunity, and antibody production in response to immunization.[27] Polyclonal hypergammaglobulinemia is often present. A deficiency of microbicidal activity against catalase-positive bacteria and a diminished or absent respiratory burst by neutrophils and monocytes are the critical functional and biochemical findings for CGD.

Patients with CGD have a predisposition to infections with a variety of bacteria and fungi, as summarized in Table 69-3. The most common organisms are *S. aureus*, enteric bacteria, and *Aspergillus*.[23,33,39] Unusual pathogens may cause disease in patients with CGD. Recent studies have focused on *Burkholderia cepacia* as a significant pathogen, particularly in the lung.[25,40,41] Infection by this organism was the second leading cause of death in patients in the CGD registry. Its propensity to infect patients with either CGD or cystic fibrosis is not understood.

Microbial agents associated with pulmonary infections are the same as those that cause infections in other parts of the body. Of importance is the frequency of fungal pneumonitis, which, especially in the case of *Aspergillus*, can spread to the tissues of the chest wall. Other pathogens include *Nocardia* species, *P. carinii*, and mycobacteria. Infections due to pneumococci, streptococci, and *Haemophilus* species are no more common in children with CGD than in normal children, presumably because these organisms do not produce catalase and cannot protect against their own H_2O_2 production.

Tissue from infected sites shows granulomas like those typically seen with intracellular parasites such as mycobacteria. Granulomas in CGD patients include mononuclear phagocytes that can contain a tan or yellow pigmented material.[42] Granulomas in the presence of the pathogens noted above strongly suggests the diagnosis of CGD.

Simple screening tests for CGD are currently available. The histochemical nitroblue tetrazolium (NBT) test[43,44] remains a reliable screening measure. Stimulation of microbicidal activity and the respiratory burst results in the reduction of O_2 to O_2^-; NBT dye is reduced by the extra electron in O_2^- and converted from a yellow, water-soluble dye to a purple insoluble substance. In normal individuals, 95% or more of phagocytic cells reduce NBT. The phagocytes from most patients with the common variants of CGD do not reduce NBT. Carriers of the X-linked form, the most common type of CGD, exhibit two populations of cells: those that are normal and those that do not reduce NBT.

Fluorescence-based assays using flow cytometry provide an additional group of screening tests. Compounds such as dihydrorhodamine-123 can be readily loaded into neutrophils or monocytes. These compounds interact with oxygen metabolites produced during the respiratory burst to generate products with increased fluorescence.[45] Patients and X-linked carriers can be determined by the presence of cells that do not shift fluorescence after stimulation. Additionally, those variants distinguished by low but significant oxidase activity in all cells, particularly p47phox deficiency, can be easily defined by these techniques. These assays are more accurate than the NBT test. Other screening tests for CGD include microassays for hexose monophosphate shunt activity or luminol-enhanced chemiluminescence.

Positive screening test results should be confirmed with one or more quantitative tests. Bactericidal assays with *Eschericia coli* or *S. aureus* may be helpful in establishing the diagnosis.[8] Quantitative assays of O_2 consumption, O_2^- production, or generation of H_2O_2 can be used to further evaluate the patient.[46,47] Finally, an analysis of the various oxidase components will be important to define the molecular variant of CGD. Cytochrome b_{558} can be quantitated spectroscopically, and the individual oxidase components can be analyzed by Western blot. Identification of the mutation responsible for the protein defect may be helpful for genetic counseling and prenatal studies.

Prenatal diagnosis may be achieved with screening tests on fetal neutrophils obtained by percutaneous umbilical blood sampling.[48–50] The diagnosis for some CGD variants can be made from chorionic villus or amniocyte samples using restriction fragment length polymorphism or gene analysis without the risk of fetal blood sampling.[26,50]

■ NADPH OXIDASE

Initial investigations confirmed that the oxidase enzyme resided in the plasma membrane of stimulated cells and through the oxidation of NADPH catalyzed the reduction of O_2 to O_2^-. This represents the first step in a sequence that produces a number of toxic oxygen metabolites with the capacity to kill microbes. It is now known that the oxidase activity is the result of the interaction between several components that form an enzyme complex. In resting cells, these components reside in different compartments. With stimulation of the cell, these components are assembled in the plasma membrane and specific granules, and oxidase activity is expressed[27,51–53] (Fig. 69-4).

The main catalytic component of the oxidase is the cytochrome b_{558}. In resting cells, 10% to 20% of total cellular cytochrome b_{558} is located in plasma membrane, and 80% to 90% is in the membranes of specific granules. This protein is a heterodimer composed of an α (p22phox) subunit and a β (gp91phox) subunit.[54–57] Cytochrome b_{558} has a flavin binding site and a heme moiety, both of which are critical to shuttling electrons between NADPH and O_2.[58–60] In addition, this protein binds NADPH. The cytochrome b_{558} in specific granules serves as a mobilizable reserve for the oxidase. With stimulation, there is fusion of specific granule membranes with plasma membrane and translocation of more cytochrome b_{558} to the plasma membrane. In addition, cytosolic oxidase components translocate to the membrane of specific granules, providing an active oxidase complex that may also move to the plasma membrane.[52] A low molecular weight G protein, Rap1a, is associated with cytochrome b_{558} and may be important in assembly and activation of the oxidase complex.[27,61]

The cytosolic oxidase components include p47phox, p67phox, and p40phox.[21,22,62–66] A cytosolic low molecular weight guanosine triphosphate (GTP)–binding protein, p21rac2, is also involved and there may be other proteins that control GTP binding to the rac2 protein.[67–69] These latter elements are important links with receptors on the plasma membrane and help transmit and/or amplify biochemical signals from outside the cell-regulating assembly and activation of the oxidase.

The p47phox and p67phox probably exist as a complex in cytosol of resting cells.[70] Interactions between this complex, plasma membrane, and the cytoskeletal elements may be critical for activation of the oxidase.[71–73] Although these components do not contain critical redox elements for the oxidase function, their presence in the oxidase complex may be important for the transfer of electrons through flavin and heme elements that exist in cytochrome b_{558} to oxygen.[74,75] The gene for p40phox has been cloned, but its function is not well defined.[65,66] Initially, it was identified as binding very strongly to p67phox. Recently, an additional protein closely associated with p67phox has been described.[76] Identified by its binding to p67phox, this 29-kd protein is categorized as a peroxiredoxin by its sequence and activity. Peroxiredoxins are a class of peroxidases that oxidize H_2O_2 with sulfur groups on cysteine residues.[77] Neutrophil p29 peroxiredoxin enhances O_2^- production in subcellular systems of oxidase activity and translocates to plasma membrane after stimulation of the respiratory burst.[78] The p29 peroxiredoxin may protect the oxidase from its own toxic products or play a role in signaling.

The precise structural orientation and relevant domains of the various proteins in creating the complex is under intense investigation. Some details are known, however. For instance, the SH-3 domain in p67phox is critical, since cells that contain a protein mutated at this site do not exhibit a respiratory burst.[73] With the formation of the active oxidase complex, NADPH binds and donates electrons to the flavin domain, then through the heme moiety to O_2, reducing it to O_2^-. Several cell-free systems have been developed that can reproduce the assembly and activation of the oxidase in whole cells with the use of subcellular

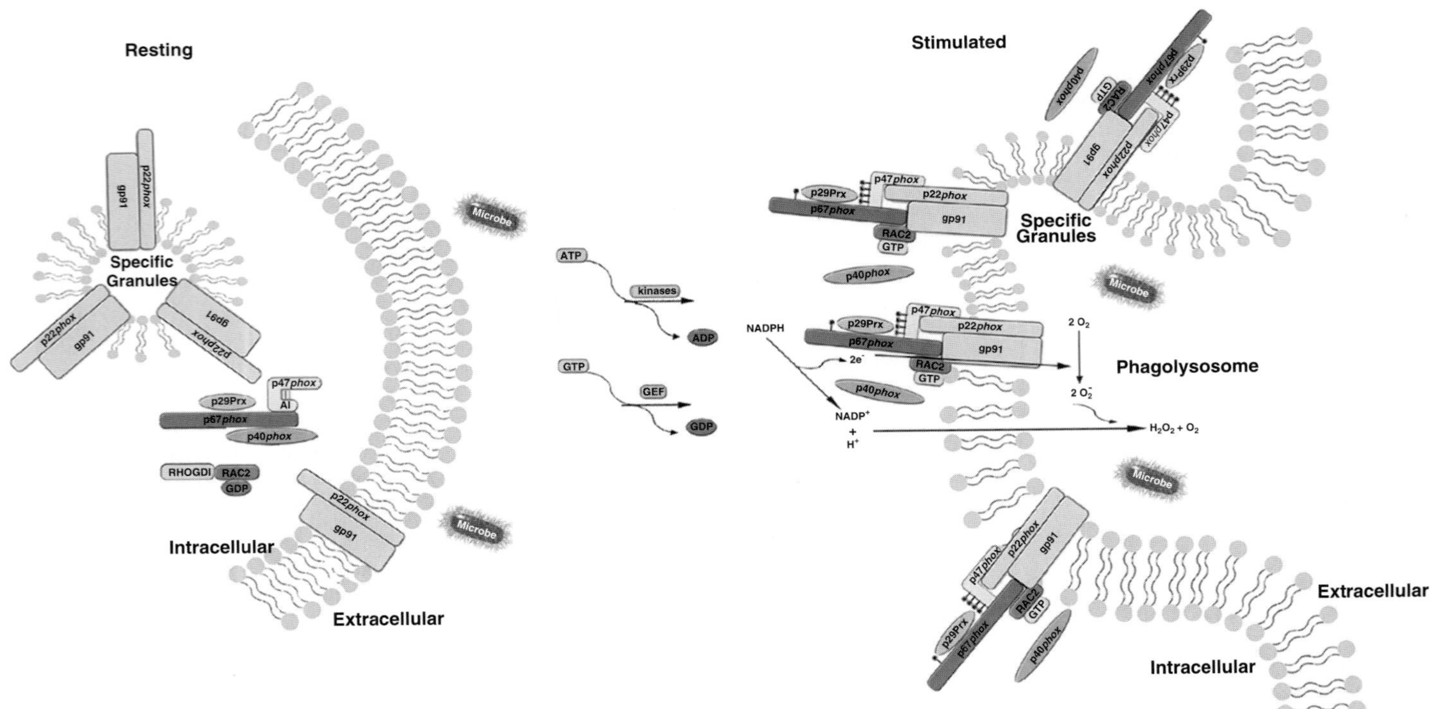

■ **FIGURE 69-4.** Schematic diagram of the NADPH oxidase enzyme system, its components, and its activation. In resting neutrophils, membrane components (gp91phox and p22phox) reside in plasma membrane and specific granules. With stimulation, degranulation of specific granules expands the amount of cytochrome b_{558} in plasma membrane and translocation of cytosolic components (rac2, p47phox, p67phox, and p40phox) and p29 peroxiredoxin (p29Prx) to the plasma membrane results in assembly of an active oxidase enzyme system that uses electrons from NADPH to reduce O_2 to form O_2^-.

fractions and/or recombinant oxidase components.[79,80] These systems are important for the investigation of complex biochemical processes subserving oxidase activity as well as approaches to define the clinical variants of CGD.

■ MOLECULAR DEFECTS AND INHERITANCE

Since the first case reports appeared in the literature, CGD has presented itself as a syndrome composed of a heterogeneity of clinical patterns. With the discovery of the various oxidase components over the past 15 years, the molecular basis of CGD has come into focus. Most patients express genetic or molecular abnormalities in one of the four major components of the oxidase: gp91phox, p22phox, p47phox, or p67phox (Table 69-4).[27,81–84] One patient has been reported with a mutation in Rac2 but no patients have been described with an abnormality of rap-1. Although p40phox is reported to be diminished in individuals with p67phox deficiency, no patients have been described with a primary deficiency in this component.

The most common molecular defects in CGD are related to gp91phox and account for 67% to 75% of all cases of this syndrome.[24,27] Located on the short arm of the X chromosome (Xp21.1), defects in the gene for gp91phox are inherited as X-linked recessive. In the most common variety, mutations in the gene result in the lack of a gp91phox protein due to instability of messenger RNA (mRNA) or of the protein in affected males. NADPH oxidase activity is totally absent in these patients, no cytochrome b_{558} is seen spectrophotometrically, and no gp91phox is detected on Western blot. A defect in the membrane contribution to oxidase activity is documented with analysis in cell-free systems. Cytosol and its components are normal. Deletions; insertions; and splice site, missense, and nonsense mutations have all been described and reviewed in detail.[27,81–85]

Other variants of gp91phox deficiency have been described. Some mutations have resulted in partial loss of protein expression and diminished oxidase activity in proportion to the decrease in protein content. In some, a truncated protein is expressed. Defects are found in exons, introns, intron/exon junctions, and promotors. A few cases have been described with normal gp91phox protein expression but nearly complete absence of oxidase activity. Additional variants have been reported with the inability to interact with NADPH or with p47phox and p67phox or to bind flavin adenine dinucleotide (FAD). Severity of disease in genetic variants correlates with the level of cytochrome b expression and superoxide production.

Patients who lack both the respiratory burst and cytochrome b_{558} and exhibit an autosomal-recessive mode of inheritance have a deficiency in p22phox. The gene for this oxidase component is found on chromosome 16 (16q24). These patients account for less than 5% of all cases. In the usual form, the deficiency in membrane contribution of oxidase activity is accompanied by absence of the cytochrome b_{558} spectrum and both gp91phox and p22phox by Western blot. Analysis of cytosolic components is normal. Although fewer genetic analyses have been completed, deletion, insertion, missense, and splice site mutations have been described.[27,81] A homozygous missense mutation affecting the area of interaction between p22phox and p47phox resulting in a normal cytochrome b_{558} that cannot form an oxidase complex completes the abnormalities of this type of CGD.

Patients who exhibit an autosomal-recessive mode of inheritance but whose neutrophils contain normal amounts of cytochrome b_{558} may have a deficiency of either p47phox or p67phox. Genes for these two components fall on chromosome 7 (7q11.23) and chromosome 1 (1q25) and account for approximately 25% to 30% and less than 5% of CGD cases, respectively. Absent or nearly absent oxidase in whole cells is coupled

■ TABLE 69-4. Molecular and genetic classification of chronic granulomatous disease

Affected Component*	Chromosome Location	Gene*	Inheritance*	Subtype Class*	NBT/DHR (% Positive)	Cytochrome b_{558} Spectrum	Western Blot Analysis†	Approximate Frequency
					O_2^- Production			
gp91phox	Xp21.1	CYBB	XL	X91°	0/0	0	Absent gp91phox Markedly decreased or absent p22phox	67%–75%
				X91⁻	80%–100%/3%–30% (weak)	3%–30%	Decreased gp91 and p22phox	
				X91⁻	5%–10%/5%–10%	5%–10%	Decreased gp91 and p22phox	
				X91⁺	0/0	100%	Normal gp91 and p22phox	
p22phox	16p24	CYBA	AR	A22°	0/0	0	Absent p22 and gp91phox	<5%
				A22⁺	0/0	100%	Normal p22 and gp91phox	
p47phox	7q11.23	NCF-1	AR	A47°	0/0–1%	100%	Absent p47phox	25%–30%
p67phox	1q25	NCF-2	AR	A67°	0/1–1%	100%	Absent	<5%

* Oxidase components expressed as gp91phox, p22phox, p47phox, p67phox, and their genes as CYBB, CYBA, NCF-1, and NCF-2, respectively. Subtypes represented by letter designating type of inheritance. The superscript designates detection of protein in patient samples. A, autosomal; AR, autosomal-recessive inheritance; O, absent; X, X-linked; XL, X-linked inheritance; –, diminished, +, present.

† For Western blot analyis, abnormalities in specific phox proteins are noted. Other components not described are normal with this technique.

Activity measurements may be made in the cell-free system of activation.[79,80] In this system, activity is defined by both cytosol (and associated components) and membrane. Deficiencies in gp91phox and p22phox exhibit diminished or absent membrane contribution, and deficiencies of p47phox and p67phox exhibit diminished or absent cytosol contribution.

Data from references 27 and 81–89.

with deficient cytosol contribution in the cell-free systems and deficiency of either of these proteins on Western blot. There appears to be much less heterogeneity in genetic mutations causing deficiency of p47phox.[27,81] Patients studied to date are either homozygous for a GT dinucleotide deletion in exon 2 of the NCF-1 gene or are compound heterozygotes with GT deletion on one allele and a point mutation on the second allele. GT deletion (ΔGT) results from recombination events between the NCF-1 gene and its highly homologous pseudogene in which the GT deletion originates.[86,87] In addition to heterozygous GT changes, missense and splice junction changes were described in several patients.[86] In all patients studied, normal amounts of mRNA are found in neutrophils with complete absence of p47phox, suggesting translation of an unstable protein.

Few mutations in patients with p67phox deficiency have been characterized. As with p47phox deficiency, mRNA for p67phox is usually present, but no protein is detected. With the few patients studied so far, nonsense, missense, homozygous point, splice site, insertion, and deletion mutations as well as one duplication have been documented, suggesting a heterogeneity of genetic abnormalities for p67phox compared with p47phox.[27,81,88,89]

Recently, a mutation in *rac*2 was described.[90,91] The patient presented with severe, recurrent perirectal abscesses and pyoderma; omphalitis; and poor wound healing. Neutrophils from this subject exhibited a unique pattern of functional abnormalities, including markedly diminished random and directed migration, decreased ingestion and bactericidal activity, and absent degranulation of azurophilic granules. Expression of CD11b and degranulation of specific granules was normal. Production of O_2^- in response to *N*-formyl-methionyl-leucyl-phenylalanine (fMLP) and platelet-activating factor (PAF)/fMLP was absent, to opsonized zymosan was decreased, but to phorbol myristate acetate (PMA) was normal. *Rac*2 was 30% of control, and all other oxidase components were normal. A mutation in one nucleotide of codon 57 for one *rac*2 allele resulted in a substitution of asparagine for aspartic acid. Although both the wild-type and mutant alleles were expressed, the mutant protein had a defect in the GTP binding site, could only bind guanosine diphosphate, and had a dominant-negative effect on the wild-type *rac*2 as well as other low molecular weight GTPases.[90,92] Because of this, the oxidase, as well as other neutrophil functions, was affected. The patient was cured by a bone marrow transplant from his human leukocyte antigen (HLA)–identical sibling.

Deficiency of glucose-6-phosphate dehydrogenase (G6PD) in leukocytes, which occurs in a small number of patients with erythrocytes deficient in this enzyme, has been considered a variant of CGD.[93–95] Patients whose neutrophils contain less than 5% of normal activity suffer from recurrent, sometimes fatal, infections. Their neutrophils do not exhibit a respiratory burst and exhibit a microbicidal defect against catalase-positive organisms. Deficiency of NADPH as the efficient electron donor to the oxidase may explain this disorder.

TREATMENT

The hallmark of management of CGD remains at this time preventive and supportive therapy.[32,33,96–98] This approach begins with prophylactic daily doses of trimethoprim-sulfamethoxazole (4–5 mg/kg trimethoprim, 20–25 mg/kg sulfamethoxazole), which will reduce the incidence of severe bacterial infections by 70%. Ciprofloxacin may be used as an alternative. Interferon-γ given at a dose of 1.5 μg/kg (surface area ≤0.5 m^2) or 50 μg/m^2 (surface area >0.5 m^2) three times weekly by subcutaneous injection also reduces the incidence and severity of infections.[99,100] Daily itraconazole at 100 to 300 mg/day (4–5 mg/kg in two doses) taken with food has been advocated as fungal prophylaxis.[101] Care should be taken to avoid environmental conditions that present a high risk for exposure to fungus (e.g., garden mulch, construction sites, leaves, and marijuana).

When infections develop, aggressive attempts should be made at obtaining material for culture and identification of organisms from localized areas. Surgical drainage is also critical to treatment, since antibiotics required to resolve infection do not penetrate well into abscesses.[102,103] The infected site should be aggressively débrided with prolonged drainage to prevent loculation and sequestration of infected areas.

In patients with fever but no definite locus for an infection, an empiric trial of parenteral antibiotics may be necessary. During the initiation of this therapy, definition of the infected area should be approached with routine radiographs, computed tomography or magnetic resonance imaging studies, or radionucleotide scans.

Identification of the infected site may provide clues to initial antibiotic coverage. For example, the vast majority of liver abscesses are caused by staphylococci (see Table 69-3), and vancomycin and levofloxacin might be used initially. *Burkholderia cepacia* is found in a higher incidence in the lung and *Serratia* in soft tissue and bones. For these latter infections, increasing the trimethoprim-sulfamethoxazole to a full therapeutic dose and adding a cephalosporin, meropenem, or levofloxacin could be considered. If microbes are recovered, antibiotic sensitivities will help define the most appropriate antibiotic coverage. Treatment for weeks or months may be required to resolve the infection.

If fungus is suspected or defined, vigorous antifungal therapy should be instituted. Although amphotericin has been advocated in the past, other agents such as itraconazole and voriconazole may be required.[104,105] Fungal infection of the lung may present as nodular discreet involvement or miliary and pan-lobular. Recent studies suggest voriconazole is appropriate at 5 to 6 mg/kg/day given in two doses. Prednisone may be considered for miliary involvement. Although not proved efficacious, daily granulocyte transfusions (≥10^{10} granulocytes per transfusion) have been used as a supplement to aggressive surgical and antibiotic therapy[25,27,106] and may be required for up to several weeks to support resolution of the infection.

Bone marrow transplantation has been attempted with mixed results.[27,107–109] Long-term engraftment and reversal of the defect has been documented. Sources of stem cells include bone marrow, mobilized peripheral blood, and umbilical cord blood. Although unrelated donors have been used, the vast majority of successful transplants have been completed with HLA-identical siblings. The majority of patients have had a myeloablative preparative regimen. While engraftment occurs in a high percentage of patients, the presence of concurrent infection presents a significant risk for severe complications, and death has been a common outcome. Recently, Horwitz and colleagues published the National Institutes of Health experience using a nonmyeloablative preparative regimen for transplantation with T cell–depleted peripheral blood stem cells from HLA-identical siblings.[109] After a median follow-up of 17 months, 8 of 10 patients had a significant enough percentage of normal neutrophils to provide normal host defense with resolution of granulomatous lesions. While this approach presents a hopeful solution to barriers for transplantation, the risks and management of infections, graft rejection, and graft-versus-host disease remain major impediments to this and other regimens.

Some patients with CGD inherit, as a closely associated X-linked allele, a deficiency in the K_x antigen affecting both erythrocytes and leukocytes.[27] This results in the lack of Kell antigens on the surface of the red cells, which can be associated with a chronic hemolytic anemia. In addition, transfusion of these patients can result in true isoimmunization for Kell antigens and the risk for immediate or delayed transfusion reactions.

Inflammatory conditions or obstructive lesions of the gastrointestinal tract (seen in up to 50% of the patients) or genitourinary tract (in up to 70% of the patients) usually respond to treatment with steroids.[28,110,111] The response may be prompt, but relapses can occur.

GENE THERAPY

Since CGD arises from defects in genes defining a finite group of proteins expressed in myeloid cells, transfer of a normally functioning gene into the pluripotent stem cell would, theoretically, constitute definitive treatment. The groundwork for this approach was laid with experiments in which Epstein-Barr virus–transformed B-lymphocyte cell lines from CGD patients with various molecular defects were transfected with complementary DNA (cDNA) for the missing oxidase component. Partial correction of protein expression and oxidase activity was obtained.[21,112–116] Similar results were obtained with myelomonoblastic cell lines.[117] These results, however, are not directly relevant to reconstitution in vivo, which would require transfection of normal genes into pluripotent stem cells. Recent studies, however, have demonstrated transduction of $CD34^+$ peripheral blood hematopoietic progenitor cells with cDNA for p47phox, p22phox, or gp91phox.[118,119] The development of murine models of CGD and their use in gene therapy protocols will provide useful information for successful application and advancement of human trials in gene therapy.[120,121]

Malech and co-workers have developed a model process for gene therapy in CGD, and have enrolled five patients with p47phox-deficient CGD.[122] $CD34^+$ progenitor cells were mobilized by granulocyte colony-stimulating factor (G-CSF) infusion, harvested by apheresis, and purified by an immunomagnetic bead separation. Cells were cultured ex vivo and expanded in the presence of interleukin-3/granulocyte-macrophage colony-stimulating factor fusion protein and G-CSF. Expanded $CD34^+$ cells were transfected with cDNA for normal p47phox in a retroviral vector. The patients received 0.1 to 4.7×10^6 transfected cells per kilogram. After 3 to 5 weeks, neutrophils with normal ability to oxidize dihydrorhodamine were detected in the peripheral circulation ranging from 1 per 1500 to 1 per 30,000 peripheral blood neutrophils. These cells declined to undetectable numbers over 3 to 6 months. Although the numbers of normal cells were too small to reconstitute the defect and the effect was not long lasting, the general principles of this approach have been demonstrated. Many problems remain to be solved before this can be considered a standard approach. Not the least of these is the recent occurrence of two cases of leukemia in gene therapy recipients caused by insertion of retroviral vectors in or near an oncogene.[123] Continued work with patients and knockout animal models will be of crucial importance for safe, effective gene therapy.

REFERENCES

1. Berendes H, Bridges RA, Good RA: A fatal granulomatosis of childhood. Minn Med 1957;40:309.
2. Landing BH, Shirkey HS: Syndrome of recurrent infection and infiltration of viscera by pigmented lipid histiocytes. Pediatrics 1957;20:431.
3. Bridges RA, Berendes H, Good RA: A fatal granulomatous disease of childhood. Am J Dis Child 1959;97:387.
4. Carson JM, Chadwick DL, Brubacker CA, et al: Thirteen boys with progressive septic granulomatosis. Pediatrics 1965;35:405.
5. Johnston RB Jr, McMurry JS: Chronic familial granulomatosis. Report of five cases and review of the literature. Am J Dis Child 1967;114:370.
6. Baehner RL, Nathan DG: Leukocyte oxidase. Science 1967;155:835.
7. Macfarlane PS, Speirs AL, Sommerville RG: Fatal granulomatous disease of childhood and benign lymphocytic infiltration of the skin (congenital dysphagocytosis). Lancet 1968;1:844.
8. Quie PG, White JC, Holmes D, Good RA: In vitro bactericidal capacity of human polymorphonuclear leukocytes. Diminished activity in chronic granulomatous disease of childhood. J Clin Invest 1968;46:668.
9. Baehner RL, Nathan DG: Quantitative nitroblue tetrazolium test in chronic granulomatous disease. N Engl J Med 1968;278:971.
10. Quie PG, Kaplan EL, Page AR, et al: Defective polymorphonuclear leukocyte function and chronic granulomatous disease in two female children. N Engl J Med 1968;279:967 and 1968:278;976.
11. Curnutte JT, Kipnes RS, Babior BM: Defect in pyridine nucleotide-dependent superoxide production by a particulate fraction from the granulocytes of patients with chronic granulomatous disease. N Engl J Med 1975;293:628.
12. McPhail LC, Dechatelet LR, Shirley PS, et al: Deficiency of NADPH oxidase activity in chronic granulomatous disease. J Pediatr 1977;90:213.
13. Segal AW, Jones OTG: Novel cytochrome b system in phagocytic vacuoles of human granulocytes. Nature 1978;276:515.
14. Segal AW, Cross AR, Garcia RC, et al: Absence of cytochrome b_{-245} in chronic granulomatous disease. A multicenter European evaluation of its incidence and relevance. N Engl J Med 1983;308:245.
15. Royer-Pokora B, Kunkel LM, Monaco AP, et al: Cloning the gene for an inherited human disorder—chronic granulomatous disease—on the basis of its chromosomal location. Nature 1986;322:32.
16. Dinauer MC, Orkin SH, Brown R, et al: The glycoprotein encoded by the X-linked chronic granulomatous disease locus is a component of the neutrophil cytochrome b complex. Nature 1987;327:717.
17. Teahan C, Rowe P, Parker P, et al: The X-linked chronic granulomatous disease gene codes for the β-chain of cytochrome b_{-245}. Nature 1987;327:720.
18. Dinauer MC, Pierce EA, Bruns GAP, et al: Human neutrophil cytochrome b light chain (p22-phox): gene structure, chromosomal location, and mutation in cytochrome-negative autosomal recessive chronic granulomatous disease. J Clin Invest 1990;86:1729.
19. Nunoi H, Rotrosen D, Gallin JI, Malech HL: Two forms of autosomal chronic granulomatous disease lack distinct neutrophil cytosol factors. Science 1988;242:1298.
20. Volpp BD, Nauseef WM, Clark RA: Two cytosolic neutrophil NADPH oxidase components absent in autosomal chronic granulomatous disease. Science 1988;242:1295.
21. Volpp BD, Nauseef WM, Donelson JE, et al: Cloning of the cDNA and functional expression of the 47-kilodalton cytosolic component of human neutrophil respiratory burst oxidase. Proc Natl Acad Sci U S A 1989;86:7195 (Erratum: Proc Natl Acad Sci U S A 1989;86:9563).
22. Leto TL, Lomax KJ, Volpp BD, et al: Cloning of a 67-kD neutrophil oxidase factor with similarity to a non-catalytic region of $p60_{c\text{-}src}$. Science 1990;248:727.
23. Winkelstein JA, Marino MC, Johnston RB Jr, et al: Chronic granulomatous disease. Report on a national registry of 368 patients. Medicine 2000;79:155.
24. Johnston RB Jr: Clinical aspects of chronic granulomatous disease. Curr Opin Hematol 2001;8:17.
25. Segal BH, Leto TL, Gallin JI, et al: Genetic, biochemical, and clinical features of chronic granulomatous disease. Medicine 2000;79:170.
26. DeBoer M, Bolscher BGJM, Sijmons RH, et al: Prenatal diagnosis in a family with X-linked chronic granulomatous disease with the use of the polymerase chain reaction. Prenat Diagn 1992;12:773.
27. Forehand JR, Nauseef WM, Curnutte JT, Johnston RB Jr: Inherited disorders of phagocyte killing. In: Scriver CR, Beaudet AL, Sly WS, Valle D, eds: The Metabolic and Molecular Bases of Inherited Disease. New York: McGraw-Hill, 1995.
28. Marciano BE, Rosenzweig SD, Kleiner DE, et al: Gastrointestinal involvement in chronic granulomatous disease. Pediatrics 2004;114:462.

29. Goldblatt D, Butcher J, Thrasher AJ, et al: Chorioretinal lesions in patients and carriers of chronic granulomatous disease. J Pediatr 1999;134:780.
30. Fleming GM, Kleinerman J, Doershuk CF, Perrin EV: Chronic granulomatous disease of childhood. An unusual case of honeycomb lung. Chest 1975;68:834.
31. Dilworth JA, Mandell GL: Adults with chronic granulomatous disease of "childhood." Am J Med 1977;63:233.
32. Cale CM, Jones AM, Goldblatt D: Follow up of patients with chronic granulomatous disease diagnosed since 1990. Clin Exp Immunol 2000;120:351.
33. Forrest CB, Forehand JR, Axtell RA, et al: Clinical features and current management of chronic granulomatous disease. Hematol Oncol Clin North Am 1988;2:253.
34. Segal BH, DeCarlo ES, Kwon-Chung KJ, et al: *Aspergillus nidulans* infection in chronic granulomatous disease. Medicine 1998;77:345.
35. White CJ, Kwon-Chung KJ, Gallin JI: Chronic granulomatous disease of childhood. An unusual case of infection with *Aspergillus nidulans* var. *echinulatus*. Am J Clin Pathol 1988;90:312.
36. Kawashima A, Kuhlman JE, Fishman EK, et al: Pulmonary *Aspergillus* chest wall involvement in chronic granulomatous disease. CT and MRI findings. Skeletal Radiol 1991;20:487.
37. Wolfson JJ, Quie PG, Laxdal SD, Good RA: Roentgenologic manifestations of children with a genetic defect of polymorphonuclear leukocyte function. Chronic granulomatous disease of childhood. Radiology 1968; 91:37–48.
38. Ambruso DR: The anemias of chronic diseases. In: Gross S, Roath S, eds: Hematology: A Problem-Oriented Approach. Baltimore: Williams & Wilkins, 1996, pp 179–186.
39. Johnston RB Jr, Newman SL: Chronic granulomatous disease. Pediatr Clin North Am 1977;24:365.
40. O'Neil KM, Herman JH, Modlin JF, et al: *Pseudomonas cepacia*. An emerging pathogen in chronic granulomatous disease. J Pediatr 1986;108:940.
41. Lacy DE, Spencer DA, Goldstein A et al: Chronic granulomatous disease presenting in childhood with *Pseudomonas cepacia* septicemia. J Infect 1993;27:301.
42. Johnston RB Jr: Unusual forms of an uncommon disease (chronic granulomatous disease). J Pediatr 1976;88:172.
43. Ochs HD, Igo RP: The NBT slide test. A simple screening method for detecting chronic granulomatous disease and female carriers. J Pediatr 1973; 83:77.
44. Meerhof J, Roos D: Heterogeneity in chronic granulomatous disease detected with an improved nitroblue tetrazolium slide test. J Leukoc Biol 1986; 39:699.
45. Vowells SJ, Sekhsaria S, Malech HL, et al: Flow cytometric analysis of the granulocyte respiratory burst. A comparison study of fluorescent probes. J Immunol Meth 1995;178:89.
46. Johnston RB Jr, Keele BB, Misra HP, et al: The role of superoxide anion generation in phagocytic bactericidal activity. Studies with normal and chronic granulomatous disease leukocytes. J Clin Invest 1975;55:1357.
47. Verhoeven AJ, Van Schaik MLJ, Roos D, Weening RS: Detection of carriers of the autosomal form of chronic granulomatous disease. Blood 1988; 71:505.
48. Huu TP, Dumez Y, Marquetty C, et al: Prenatal diagnosis of chronic granulomatous disease (CGD) in four high risk male fetuses. Prenat Diagn 1987;7:253.
49. Levinsky R, Harvey B, Nicolaides K, Rodeck C: Antental diagnosis of chronic granulomatous disease. Lancet 1986;1:50.
50. Pelham A, O'Reilly M-AJ, Malcolm S, et al: RFLP and deletion analysis for X-linked chronic granulomatous disease using the cDNA probe. Potential for improved prenatal diagnosis and carrier determination. Blood 1990;76:820.
51. Ambruso DR, Bolscher BGJM, Stokman PM, et al: Assembly and activation of the NADPH:O_2 oxidoreductase in human neutrophils after stimulation with phorbol-myristate acetate. J Biol Chem 1990;265:924 (Erratum: J Biol Chem 1990;265:19370).
52. Ambruso DR, Cusack N, Thurman G: NADPH oxidase activity of neutrophil specific granules. Requirements for cytosolic components and evidence of assembly during cell activation. Mol Genet Metab 2004;81:313.
53. Clark RA, Volpp BD, Leidal KG, Nauseef WM: Two cytosolic components of the human neutrophil respiratory burst oxidase translocate to the plasma membrane during cell activation. J Clin Invest 1990;85:714.
54. Segal AW, Jones OTG: Subcellular distribution and some properties of the cytochrome b component of the microbicidal oxidase system of human neutrophils. Biochem J 1979;182:181.
55. Borregaard N, Heiple JM, Simons ER, Clark RA: Subcellular localization of the b-cytochrome component of the human neutrophil microbicidal oxidase. Translocation during activation. J Cell Biol 1983;97:52.
56. Parkos CA, Allen RA, Cochrane CG, Jesaitis AJ: Purified cytochrome b from human granulocyte plasma membrane is comprised of two polypeptides with relative molecular weights of 91,000 and 22,000. J Clin Invest 1987; 80:732.
57. Segal AW: Absence of both cytochrome b_{-245} subunits from neutrophils in X-linked chronic granulomatous disease. Nature 1987;326:88.
58. Segal AW, West I, Wientjes F, et al: Cytochrome b_{-245} is a flavo-cytochrome containing FAD and the NADPH-binding site of the microbicidal oxidase of phagocytes. Biochem J 1992;284:781.
59. Gabig TG: The NADPH-dependent O_2^- generating oxidase from human neutrophils. Identification of a flavoprotein component that is deficient in a patient with chronic granulomatous disease. J Biol Chem 1983;258: 6352.
60. Quinn MT, Mullen ML, Jesaitis AJ: Human neutrophil cytochrome b contains multiple hemes. Evidence for heme associated with both subunits. J Biol Chem 1992;267:7303.
61. Quinn MT, Mullen ML, Jesaitis AJ, Linner JG: Subcellular distribution of the Rap1A protein in human neutrophils. Colocalization and cotranslocation with cytochrome b_{558}. Blood 1992;79:1563.
62. Lomax KR, Leto TL, Nunoi H, et al: Recombinant 47-kilodalton cytosol factor restores NADPH oxidase in chronic granulomatous disease. Science 1989;245:409 (Erratum: Science 1989;246:987).
63. Bolscher BGJM, van Zwieten R, Kramer IJM, et al: A phospho-protein of Mr 47,000. defective in autosomal chronic granulomatous disease, copurifies with one of two soluble components required for NADPH:O_2 oxidoreductase activity in human neutrophils. J Clin Invest 1989;83:757.
64. Clark RA, Malech HL, Gallin JI, et al: Genetic variants of chronic granulomatous disease. Prevalence of deficiencies of two cytosolic components of the NADPH oxidase system. N Engl J Med 1989;321:647.
65. Abo A, Boyhan A, West I, et al: Reconstitution of neutrophil NADPH oxidase activity in the cell-free system by four components: p67-phox, p47-phox, p21rac1 and cytochrome b_{-245}. J Biol Chem 1992;267:16767.
66. Wientjes FB, Hsuan JJ, Totty NF, Segal AW: p40-phox, a third cytosolic component of the activation complex of the NADPH oxidase to contain src homology 3 domains. Biochem J 1993;296:557.
67. Abo A, Pick E, Hall A, et al: Activation of the NADPH oxidase involves the small GTP-binding protein p21rac1. Nature 1991;353:668.
68. Knaus UG, Heyworth PG, Evans T, et al: Regulation of phagocyte oxygen radical production by the GTP-binding protein Rac 2. Science 1991; 254:1512.
69. Kwong CH, Malech HL, Rotrosen D, Leto TL: Regulation of human neutrophil NADPH oxidase by *rho*-related G-proteins. Biochemistry 1993; 32:5711.
70. Park JW, El Benna J, Scott KE, et al: Isolation of a complex of respiratory burst oxidase components from resting neutrophil cytosol. Biochemistry 1994;33:2907.
71. Finan P, Shimizu Y, Gout I, et al: An SH3 domain and proline-rich sequence mediate an interaction between two components of the phagocyte NADPH oxidase complex. J Biol Chem 1994;269:13752.
72. Sumimoto H, Kage Y, Nunoi H, et al: Role of src homology 3 domains in assembly and activation of the phagocyte NADPH oxidase. Proc Natl Acad Sci U S A 1994;91:5345.
73. de Mendez I, Garrett MC, Adams AG, Leto TL: Role of p67-phox SH3 domains in assembly of the NADPH oxidase system. J Biol Chem 1994; 269:16326.
74. Cross AR, Yarchover JL, Curnutte JT: The superoxide-generating system of human neutrophils possesses a novel diaphorase activity. Evidence for distinct regulation of electron flow within NADPH oxidase by p67-phox and p47-phox. J Biol Chem 1994;269:21448.
75. Cross AR, Curnutte JT: The cytosolic activating factors p47-phox and p67-phox have distinct roles in the regulation of electron flow in NADPH oxidase. J Biol Chem 1995;270:6543.
76. Leavey PJ, Gonzalez-Aller C, Thurman G, et al: A 29-kDa protein associated with p67phox expresses both peroxiredoxin and phospholipase A_2 activity and enhances superoxide anion production by a cell-free system of NADPH oxidase activity. J Biol Chem 2002;277:45181.
77. Rhee SG, Kang SW, Chang TS, et al: Peroxiredoxin, a novel family of peroxidases. IUBMB Life 2002;52:35.
78. Ambruso DR, Thurman G, Gonzalez-Aller C, Pabst M: Neutrophil (PMN) p29 peroxiredoxin translocates to the plasma membrane after stimulation with PMA and increases the vmax for superoxide anion (O_2^-) production by the NADPH oxidase enzyme system. Blood 2003;102:273a.
79. McPhail LC, Shirley PS, Clayton CC, Snyderman R: Activation of the respiratory burst enzyme from human neutrophils in a cell-free system. Evidence for a soluble cofactor. J Clin Invest 1985;75:1735.

80. Curnutte JT: Activation of human neutrophil nicotinamide adenine dinucleotide phosphate, reduced (triphospyridine nucleotide, reduced) oxidase by arachidonic acid in a cell-free system. J Clin Invest 1985;75:1740.
81. Roos D, de Boer M, Kuribayashi F, et al: Mutations in the X-linked and autosomal recessive forms of chronic granulomatous disease. Blood 1996; 87:1663.
82. Cross AR, Noack D, Rae J, et al: Hematologically important mutations. The autosomal recessive forms of chronic granulomatous disease (first update). Blood Cells Mol Dis 2000;26:561.
83. Heyworth PG, Curnutte JT, Rae J, et al: Hematologically important mutations. X-linked chronic granulomatous disease (second update). Blood Cells Mol Dis 2001;27:16.
84. Heyworth PG, Cross AR, Curnutte JT: Chronic granulomatous disease. Curr Opin Immunol 2003;15:578.
85. Rae J, Newburger PE, Dinauer MC, et al: X-linked chronic granulomatous disease. Mutations in the CYBB gene encoding the gp91-phox component of respiratory-burst oxidase. Am J Hum Genet 1998;62:1320.
86. Noack D, Rae J, Cross AR, et al: Autosomal recessive chronic granulomatous disease caused by defects in NCF-1, the gene encoding the phagocyte p47-phox. Mutations not arising in the NCF-1 pseudogenes. Blood 2001; 97:305.
87. Roesler J, Curnutte JT, Rae J, et al: Recombination events between the p47-phox gene and its highly homologous pseudogenes are the main cause of autosomal recessive chronic granulomatous disease. Blood 2000;95:2150.
88. Noack D, Rae J, Cross AR, et al: Autosomal recessive chronic granulomatous disease caused by novel mutations in NCF-2, the gene encoding the p67-phox component of phagocyte NADAPH oxidase. Hum Genet 1999; 105:460.
89. Borgato L, Bonizzato A, Lunardi C, et al: A 1.1-kb duplication in the p67-phox gene causes chronic granulomatous disease. Hum Genet 2001; 108:504.
90. Ambruso DR, Knall C, Abell AN, et al: Human neutrophil immunodeficiency syndrome is associated with an inhibitory Rac2 mutation. Proc Natl Acad Sci U S A 2000;97:4654.
91. Kurkchubasche AG, Panepinto JA, Tracy TF Jr, et al: Clinical features of a human Rac2 mutation. A complex neutrophil dysfunction disease. J Pediatr 2001;139:141.
92. Williams DA, Tao W, Kim C, et al: A dominant negative mutation of the hematopoietic-specific RhoGTPase, Rac2, is associated with a human phagocyte immunodeficiency. Blood 2000;96:1646.
93. Baehner RL, Johnston RB Jr, Nathan DG: Comparative study of the metabolic and bactericidal characteristics of severely glucose-6-phosphate dehydrogenase deficient polymorpho-nuclear leukocytes from children with chronic granulomatous disease. J Reticuloendothel Soc 1972;12:150.
94. Gray GR, Klebanoff SJ, Stamatayannopoulos G, et al: Neutrophil dysfunction, chronic granulomatous disease and non-spherocytic haemolytic anaemia caused by complete deficiency of glucose-6-phosphate dehydrogenase. Lancet 1973;2:530.
95. Mamlok RJ, Mamlok V, Mills GC, et al: Glucose-6-phosphate dehydrogenase deficiency, neutrophil dysfunction and *Chromobacterium violaceum* sepsis. J Pediatr 1987;111:852.
96. Fischer A, Segal AW, Seger R, Weening RS: The management of chronic granulomatous disease. Eur J Pediatr 1993;152:896.
97. Margolis DM, Melnick DA, Alling DW, Gallin JI: Trimethoprim-sulfamethoxazole prophylaxis in the management of chronic granulomatous disease. J Infect Dis 1990;162:723.
98. Mouy R, Fischer A, Vilmer E, et al: Incidence, severity, and prevention of infections in chronic granulomatous disease. J Pediatr 1989;114:555.
99. International Chronic Granulomatous Disease Study Group: A controlled trial of interferon gamma to prevent infection in chronic granulomatous disease. N Engl J Med 1991;324:509.
100. Mouy R, Seger R, Bourquin JP, et al: Interferon gamma for chronic granulomatous disease. N Engl J Med 1991;325:1516.
101. Gallin JI, Alling DW, Malech HL, et al: Itraconazole to prevent fungal infections in chronic granulomatous disease. N Engl J Med 2003;348:2416.
102. Pogrebniak HW, Gallin JI, Malech HL, et al: Surgical management of pulmonary infections in chronic granulomatous disease of childhood. Ann Thorac Surg 1993;55:844.
103. Sponseller PD, Malech HL, McCarthy EF Jr, et al: Skeletal involvement in children who have chronic granulomatous disease. J Bone Joint Surg Am 1991;73:37.
104. Spencer DA, John P, Ferryman SR, et al: Successful treatment of invasive pulmonary aspergillosis in chronic granulomatous disease with orally administered itraconazole suspension. Am J Respir Crit Care Med 1994; 149:239.
105. Donnelly JP, DePauw BE: Voriconazole—a new therapeutic agent with an extended spectrum of antifungal activity. Clin Microbiol Infect 2004; 10:107.
106. Ambruso DR, Johnston RB Jr: Chronic granulomatous disease. In: Hilman BC, ed: Pediatric Respiratory Disease: Diagnosis and Treatment. Philadelphia: WB Saunders, 1993, pp 697–702.
107. Seger RA, Gungor T, Belohradsky BH, et al: Treatment of chronic granulomatous disease with myeloablative conditioning and an unmodified hemopoietic allograft. A survey of the European experience, 1985–2000. Blood 2002;100:4344.
108. Del Giudice I, Iori AP, Mengarelli A, et al: Allogeneic stem cell transplant from HLA-identical sibling for chronic granulomatous disease and review of the literature. Ann Hematol 2003;82:189.
109. Horwitz ME, Barrett AJ, Brown MR, et al: Treatment of chronic granulomatous disease with nonmyeloablative conditioning and a T-cell-depleted hematopoietic allograft. N Engl J Med 2001;344:881.
110. Chin TW, Steim ER, Falloon J, Gallin JI: Corticosteroids in treatment of obstructive lesions of chronic granulomatous disease. J Pediatr 1987; 111:349.
111. Danziger RN, Goren AT, Becker J, et al: Outpatient management with oral corticosteroid therapy for obstructive conditions in chronic granulomatous disease. J Pediatr 1993;122:303.
112. Chanock SJ, Faust L-RP, Barrett D, et al: O_2^- production by B lymphocytes lacking the respiratory burst oxidase subunit p47-phox after transfection with an expression vector containing a p47-phox cDNA. Proc Natl Acad Sci U S A 1992;89:10174.
113. Cobbs CS, Malech HL, Leto TL, et al: Retroviral expression of recombinant p47-phox protein by Epstein-Barr virus-transformed B lymphocytes from a patient with autosomal chronic granulomatous disease. Blood 1992;79:1829.
114. Maly FE, Schuerer-Maly CC, Quilliam L, et al: Restitution of superoxide generation in autosomal cytochrome-negative chronic granulomatous disease (A22° CGD)-derived B lymphocyte cell lines by transfection with p22-phox cDNA. J Exp Med 1993;178:2047.
115. Porter CD, Parkar MH, Levinsky RJ, et al: X-linked chronic granulomatous disease. Correction of NADPH oxidase defect by retrovirus-mediated expression of gp91-phox. Blood 1993;82:2196.
116. Thrasher A, Chetty M, Casimir C, Segal AW: Restoration of superoxide generation to a chronic granulomatous disease-derived B-cell line by retrovirus mediated gene transfer. Blood 1992;80:1125.
117. Zhen L, King AAJ, Xiao Y, et al: Gene targeting of X chromosome-linked chronic granulomatous disease locus in a human myeloid leukemia cell line and rescue by expression of recombinant gp91-phox. Proc Natl Acad Sci U S A 1993;90:9832.
118. Li F, Linton GF, Sekhsaria S, et al: $CD34^+$ peripheral blood progenitors as a target for genetic correction of the two flavocytochrome b_{558} defective forms of chronic granulomatous disease. Blood 1994;84:53.
119. Sekhsaria S, Gallin JI, Linton GF, et al: Peripheral blood progenitors as a target for genetic correction of p47-phox deficient chronic granulomatous disease. Proc Natl Acad Sci U S A 1993;90:7446.
120. Goebel WS, Dinauer MC: Retroviral-mediated gene transfer and nonmyeloablative conditioning. Studies in a murine X-linked chronic granulomatous disease model. J Pediatr Hematol Oncol 2002;24:787.
121. Dinauer MC, Gifford MA, Pech N, et al: Variable correction of host defense following gene transfer and bone marrow transplantation in murine X-linked chronic granulomatous disease. Blood 2001;97:3738.
122. Malech HL, Maples PB, Whiting-Theobald N, et al: Prolonged production of NADPH oxidase-corrected granulocytes after gene therapy of chronic granulomatous disease. Proc Natl Acad Sci U S A 1997;94:12133.
123. Chinen J, Puck JM: Successes and risks of gene therapy in primary immunodeficiencies. J Allergy Clin Immunol 2004;113:595.

70 The Lung in Sickle Cell Disease

Thomas M. Murphy, MD •
Jennifer Knight-Madden, MBBS

Sickle cell disease (SCD) is a group of genetic disorders characterized by a predominance of hemoglobin S (HbS).[1] These are the most common genetic disorders of African Americans and occur less frequently in other ethnic groups.[2] Included in SCD are sickle cell anemia (SCA; HbSS, the homozygous state for the beta S globin gene), HbSC disease (HbS and HbC), sickle beta thalassemia syndrome (either $Hb\beta^0$ thalassemia or $Hb\beta^+$ thalassemia in combination with HbS), and other combinations of HbS and abnormal hemoglobins. SCD presents as a complex of disorders of anemia and intravascular obstruction owing to the genetically inherited abnormality of sickle hemoglobin (hemoglobin S) that confers rigidity to red blood cells and predisposes to their reduced half-life from splenic elimination early in life, elimination by macrophages throughout the body, and sickling (assumption of the collapsed sickle-shaped conformation) and intravascular coagulation. The complications of SCD follow from various physical attributes of the abnormal hemoglobin and include hemolytic anemia, vaso-occlusive pain crisis (VOC), splenic sequestration syndrome, functional asplenia with recurrent infections, dactylitis, priapism, avascular necrosis of the femoral head, cholelithiasis with bilirubin stones, stroke, acute chest syndrome (ACS), chronic sickle lung disease (SLD), pulmonary hypertension (PH), and cor pulmonale.[3]

Despite the failure to transform knowledge gleaned in the 1950s of the exact amino acid substitution in HbS (valine for glutamic acid in the sixth position of the beta globin chain) to a specific curative therapy, improvements in supportive care have advanced the median life expectancy from a few years in the 1960s to the current level of 42 years for men and 48 years for women.[4] Key features of supportive care responsible for this dramatic improvement in survival are improved access to health care, the creation of a network of comprehensive sickle cell care centers, the introduction of newborn screening, and prophylaxis of the young against bacterial sepsis with penicillin and immunizations.

■ EPIDEMIOLOGY

Some 60,000 persons in the United States, 10,000 in the United Kingdom, 1 in 60 in West Africa, and 1 in 250 persons in Jamaica are burdened with SCD.[5,6] Two thirds of cases of SCD are caused by the homozygous inheritance of HbSS.[2,3] Other important variants of SCD include sickle hemoglobin C and sickle β^+ thalassemia. Disease expression is usually less severe with these variants. Sickle cell trait (the combination of HbS and HbA) is not a disease, because HbA predominates. The prevalence of HbSS SCD is 0.14% among African Americans, while the sickle cell trait (HbAS) prevalence is 8.6%.[1]

■ PATHOPHYSIOLOGY

■ FACTORS THAT PREDISPOSE TO VASCULOPATHY

The most common complication of SCD is VOC and is the leading cause for hospitalization.[2] VOC is a pain syndrome resulting primarily from vascular obstruction in the marrow associated with bony infarcts. The second most common events are the pulmonary complications of SCD, which include ACS and chronic SLD, which are the most common causes of death.[7] Death in young adults is often related to sudden episodes of hypoxia and pulmonary hypertension.[2,8]

The vasculopathy of SCD is related to erythrocyte sickling; alteration of adhesion factors in the sickle erythrocyte membrane and their interactions with a number of clotting factors; and impaired antioxidant defenses and auto-oxidation in the sickle erythrocyte and the lung. The amino acid substitution of HbS in the beta globin chain alters the quaternary structure of sickle hemoglobin and reduces the solubility of deoxy-HbS to approximately 10% of that of the normal deoxy-HbA.[9] Deoxy-HbS forms a viscous solution within the erythrocyte that facilitates the formation of polymers and crystals. As the concentration of HbS increases, the erythrocyte collapses into a sickle shape, either reversibly or irreversibly. With repeated sickling this state becomes progressively irreversible. Sickling is also known to increase with dehydration, acidemia, hypoxia, and an increased intracellular concentration of HbS.

Vascular obstruction in SCD is also facilitated by the persistent expression of adhesion factors in the membranes of sickle reticulocytes (Fig. 70-1).[10] These factors, which are expressed in bone marrow–erythrocyte prescursors, normally lose their expression in reticulocytes as well as mature erythrocytes. These adhesion molecules are similar to those found on the membranes of leukocytes and function to facilitate adherence of the sickle erythrocytes to the vascular endothelium and to promote inflammation. Very late antigen-4 (VLA-4) is expressed on approximately 25% of sickle erythrocyte membranes.[10,11] The VLA-4 binds specifically to vascular cell adhesion molecules (VCAM) expressed on the endothelial surface. The VCAM expression is in turn regulated by inflammatory cytokines such as interleukin-1 (IL-1), IL-4, and tumor necrosis factor-α (TNF-α). Serum levels of TNF-α and IL-1 are known to be increased during steady state and during VOC in some SCD patients.[12] Increased concentrations of these cytokines promote increased adherence of sickle erythrocytes to vascular endothelium in vitro.

The interaction of sickle erythrocytes and the vascular endothelium is modified by a number of clotting factors,

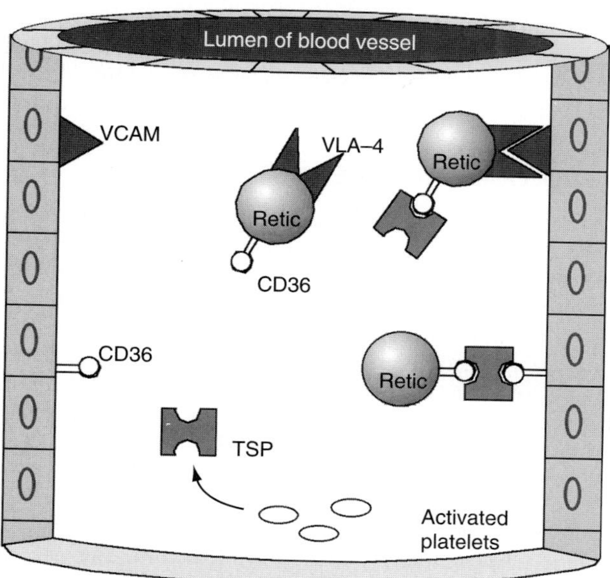

■ **FIGURE 70-1.** Sickle reticulocyte adherence via adhesion molecules. Erythrocyte adhesion factors that promote vascular obstruction. For details and an explanation of symbols, see text. (Adapted from Knight J, Murphy TM, Browning I: The lung in sickle cell disease. Pediatr Pulmonol 1999;28:205.)

including multimers of von Willebrand factor (vWF), thrombospondin (TSP), fibrinogen, and fibronectin. Sickle erythrocytes express the β-3 integrin GPIIb/IIIa, which binds to large multimers of vWF. The resulting complex binds to the endothelium through its vitronectin receptor (VNR).[13] This vWF binding is also facilitated by inflammatory cytokines that increase endothelial VNR expression and increase the release of vWF multimers. Sickle erythrocytes also express on their membranes the adhesion molecule platelet glycoprotein 36 (known as CD36), which is a receptor for TSP. Stimulated platelets release TSP, which then facilitates the adhesion of sickle erythrocytes to vascular endothelium via VNR and CD36. Inflammatory cytokines thus augment the complex process of the vascular endothelial adhesion of sickle erythrocytes, which in turn further promotes the inflammatory process and the participation of multiple clotting factors.[10]

A parallel inflammatory process caused by sickle erythrocytes is the facilitation of oxidative stress. The abnormal structure of HbS facilitates the participation of its heme moiety in a number of oxidative processes. Elements necessary for the generation of a variety of toxic reactive oxygen species (ROS) by the sickle erythrocyte are abundant—oxygen, iron, and unsaturated membrane lipid. The HbS is oxidized to methemoglobin S (met-HbS) along with the elaboration of a number of ROS. The met-HbS, unlike met-HbA, becomes irreversibly denatured and forms clumps on the erythrocyte membrane surface called hemichromes.[14] The iron in hemichromes is readily available to promote oxidation of oxygen to water with the elaboration of superoxide, peroxide, and hydroxyl radicals. The oxidative process also involves oxides of nitrogen and the production of toxic nitrogen metabolites, such as peroxynitrites, as well as toxic lipid oxides. The hemichromes also reduce membrane deformability, perhaps through interaction with structural membrane proteins such as spectrin, as well as membrane lipids. The reduced deformability is thought to predispose to hemolysis. The hemichromes cluster about an ion channel known as band 3. Since band 3 promotes the accumulation of surface immunoglobulins, this association and process is thought to promote erythrophagocytosis and thus hemolytic anemia.[14]

■ IMPACT ON OXYGEN TRANSPORT

Alterations in the quaternary structure of hemoglobin critically affect the uptake and off-loading of oxygen by erythrocytes in the lungs and throughout the body. Oxygen is bound less tightly to HbS than to normal HbA. Sickle erythrocyte levels of 2,3-diphosphoglycerate are greater than in normal erythrocytes. This causes the binding of oxygen to be even less in HbS than in HbA.[15] At any given partial pressure of oxygen in arterial blood (Pa_{O_2}) the HbS is less saturated than HbA. Greater concentrations of the fetal hemoglobin (HbF) lessen the difference. The impact of this physiologic feature of HbS is that normal Pa_{O_2} levels may be associated with oxygen desaturation in SCD patients who are clinically stable. Those with low Pa_{O_2} levels may have oxygen saturations that are substantially lower than expected in nonaffected persons. While the total amount of oxygen that is available per gram of Hb is reduced in SCD, a partial compensatory mechanism is that oxygen is off-loaded more readily by HbS at relatively high levels of Pa_{O_2}. Other compensatory mechanisms are at play. High levels of tissue extraction of oxygen would be predicted to generate low levels of mixed venous oxygen, which would then predispose to increased sickling. The anemia and inflammation-induced stress of SCD produce secondary tachycardia, increased stroke volume, and decreased peripheral vascular resistance that serve to decrease erythrocyte transit time through most tissues and reduce oxygen extraction, so that mixed venous oxygen levels in SCD are relatively close to normal.[2]

A technical consequence of the altered Hb-O_2 dissociation curve for HbS is that the values of oxygen saturation produced by automated blood gas analyzers, which calculate this value based on normal values of P_{50} (the oxygen tension Pa_{O_2} that produces an oxygen saturation of 50%) generate oxygen saturation values for HbS that are falsely elevated. The performance of the noninvasive method of pulse oximetry is variable. In many SCD patients the measured values of oxygen saturation are appropriate, but in some the measurements are problematic. Two factors are at play. The proportion of hemoglobin saturated with carbon monoxide (COHb) is increased in some SCD patients. Pulse oximeters do not distinguish between oxy-Hb and COHb. Greater levels of COHb would result in overestimation of oxygen saturation. The pigmentation of darker skin may interfere with the absorption of selective light waves important for calibration. The patterns of light absorption of HbS and HbF differ from those of HbA, which is the standard for calibration of pulse oximeters. Carbon monoxide oximeters (CO-oximeters) measure the saturation of oxygen spectrophotometrically, a method that distinguishes COHb and oxy-Hb and is not affected by skin pigmentation. In addition it does not assume a normal P_{50}. CO-oximeters provide measurements of oxygen saturation in SCD that are consistently more accurate. However, in most patients with SCD, the readings from pulse oximetry suffice.[16] Most sickle cell clinics perform initial assessments of oxygen saturation with pulse oximetry, while CO-oximetry is reserved for confirmation in patients who are ill or in those for whom the pulse oximetry measurements do not match the clinical presentation.

CONSEQUENCES OF VASCULOPATHY

The vascular consequences of increased erythrocyte sickling and adhesion and the activated function of clotting factors are endothelial damage and increased adherence of the erythrocytes to one another, leading to clot formation and vascular obstruction.[10] Endothelial cells in direct contact with sickle erythrocytes demonstrate effacement, loss of nuclei, and edema, with increased numbers of microfilaments and microvesicles. There is also microscopic evidence of vascular remodeling, with increased numbers of fibroblasts, myocytes, and collagen. These features may be mediated by ROS, which diffuse freely across the erythrocyte membrane.

The adherence of sickle erythrocytes to one another is likely facilitated by a reduction in SCD of natural anticoagulants such as proteins S and C and an increase in procoagulant proteins such as thrombin-antithrombin complexes (a marker of in vivo thrombin production) and D-dimers.[17] The most common site for vascular obstruction is the microvasculature, presumably because the slow velocity of the traversing sickle erythrocytes facilitates endothelial attachment. Older, less deformable, and sickled erythrocytes then become trapped, the clots propagate, and obstruction results. This phenomenon is not limited to small vessels, however. Branch points promote turbulence that causes intimal hyperplasia. Partial and complete obstruction of large arteries, including cerebral arteries that have caused strokes, has been well documented. Pathologic examination reveals not just clot formation and adherence of sickle erythrocytes to the endothelium, but extensive remodeling, including intimal proliferation (sometimes extensive), medial fibrosis, and segmental arterial wall thickening. Elevated hemoglobin levels (presumably as a result of the associated hypercoagulability) predispose to VOC and ACS. Because the vascular obstruction and remodeling in SCD are dispersed throughout the body, a wide variety of end-organ complications results. Following VOC, the next most frequent clinical presentation of SCD are the pulmonary complications.[7] The complications are both acute (ACS) and chronic (SLD).

ACUTE CHEST SYNDROME

DEFINITION

ACS is a clinical pulmonary exacerbation of SCD manifested usually by fever, a new chest radiographic infiltrate, and either the corresponding symptoms or signs.[2,18–23] The symptoms include cough, dyspnea, and chest pain. As with pneumonias in children without SCD, the initial radiograph may not demonstrate a new infiltrate. The most frequently presenting signs are fever, cough, tachypnea, crackles, and hypoxemia. Fever is more common in children with ACS and pain more common in adults. ACS is the second leading reason for hospitalization (behind VOC) and the leading cause of death. Sudden death in the setting of ACS may be associated with acute exacerbations of pulmonary hypertension.

EPIDEMIOLOGY

Approximately half of children with homozygous SS disease have had at least one episode of ACS by the age of 10 years. ACS is more common in children than adults and is more frequent in those patients with SCA (HbSS). The risk is decreased with greater levels of HbF and is increased with the magnitude of the anemia and with elevated steady-state white blood cell counts.

ETIOLOGIES AND THERAPIES

The etiology of ACS is complex and heterogeneous. In addition to the expected intravascular pulmonary thrombosis, ACS is marked by the co-occurrence of infection, fat embolism (presumably from bony infarcts), hypoventilation, edema, and reactive airways disease (RAD), and by the secondary problems of mucus hypersecretion and atelectasis (Box 70-1). Because multiple etiologic factors are usually involved, the diagnostic label of ACS is strongly preferred to the diagnostic label of pneumonia.

CLINICAL PRESENTATION

The clinical presentation of ACS is similar to that of pneumonia with the cardinal features being fever, a new radiographic pulmonary infiltrate, symptoms (cough, shortness of breath, chest pain) and/or signs (tachypnea, crackles, hypoxia), and a greater frequency of pain (Table 70-1). The presenting chest radiograph may be normal, as it may be with clinical pneumonia, so the study should be repeated as indicated by clinical suspicion. As with pneumonia, atelectasis and pleural effusions are also common complications. ACS is the second leading cause of hospitalization in SCD and the most common cause of death.

INTRAVASCULAR THROMBOSIS

Although long presumed to be a major cause of ACS, intravascular thrombosis has not been consistently demonstrated premortem. Part of the challenge is that ventilation-perfusion scans are difficult to interpret without a prior baseline study, something rarely available in asymptomatic patients. Angiography is not routinely performed because of concern that instillation of a hypertonic contrast agent might precipitate sickling. However, spiral computerized axial tomographic scans have demonstrated microvascular occlusion, which can be found on postmortem examinations.[24] Large pulmonary emboli are uncommon outside of pregnancy and the postpartum period.

INFECTION

Since the clinical presentation of ACS overlaps greatly with the signs, symptoms, and laboratory expression of pneumonia (see Table 70-1), one would expect infection to play a major role. Indeed, because of these similarities, pneumonia usually cannot be ruled out as a cause. Direct culture of lower airway secretions or serology is required for specific diagnosis. Concomitant infection and other causes, such as fat embolism, are common. In children with SCD, infections are more commonly documented, as are associated bacteremias. The most common agents are viruses such as respiratory syncytial virus, parvovirus, and rhinovirus, particularly during winter months.[22] These can be diagnosed through the immunofluorescent assessment of nasal secretions or by serial measurement of specific antibody titers. Bacterial infections are caused mostly by atypical bacteria, such as *Mycoplasma* and *Chlamydia*. Pneumonia from these agents is more severe in SCD than in normal children. In the era of chronic antibiotic prophylaxis and immunizations for *Streptococcus pneumoniae* and *Haemophilus influenzae*, these latter bacteria are less commonly responsible for ACS than previously, and other causes of community-acquired pneumonias have risen in prevalence.

The vasculopathy of SCD progresses in the first few years of life to render the spleen incapable of performing its immune functions, including the generation of antibodies to encapsulated organisms. In addition to this "functional asplenia," there are abnormalities of the complement defense system. Together these deficits predispose patients, especially children, to blood-borne infections with encapsulated organisms. Antimicrobial prophylaxis with penicillin and immunization for these organisms (*S. pneumoniae* and *H. influenzae*) are important strategies to limit episodes of bacterial sepsis and recurrences of ACS. After the age of 6 months, annual immunizations for influenza virus are recommended.

Empirical broad-spectrum antibiotic therapy is recommended in cases of ACS. This should include therapy directed against atypical bacteria. A typical regimen would be a combination of erythromycin or azithromycin with a second-generation cephalosporin.[2]

TABLE 70-1. Frequency of presenting symptoms and signs in acute chest syndrome

Symptom or Sign	Frequency (%)
Fever	80
Cough	74
Chest pain	57
Tachypnea	41
Extremity pain	37
Abdominal pain	31
Shortness of breath	28
Rib/sternal pain	23
Wheezing	11
Hemoptysis	2

Adapted from Vichinsky EP, Styles LA, Colangelo LH: Acute chest syndrome in sickle cell diseases. Clinical presentation and course. Blood 1997;89:1787.

BOX 70-1 Etiologies of Acute Chest Syndrome

Intravascular Thrombosis

Sickling
Erythrocyte-endothelial adhesion
Hypercoagulable state
Damaged endothelium
Vascular remodeling

Infection

Viruses
Atypical bacteria
Bacteria

Fat Embolism

Acute inflammation
Mechanical obstruction

Hypoventilation

Splinting secondary to pain
Excessive sedation

Dehydration

Fever
Tachypnea
Anorexia

Edema

Iatrogenic overhydration
Vascular leak
Inflammation

Reactive Airways Disease

Inflammation
Edema
Mucus hypersecretion
Hypoxia

Secondary Problems

Mucus hypersecretion
Atelectasis

Adapted from Knight J, Murphy TM, Browning I: The lung in sickle cell disease. Pediatr Pulmonol 1999;28:205.

FAT EMBOLISM

Among ACS patients who undergo diagnostic bronchoalveolar lavage, fat embolism (FE) (presumably from bony infarcts) appears to be the most commonly identified cause.[7,25] Since patients without ACS with FE usually develop their symptoms and signs a few days following bone trauma, it is noteworthy that one third of patients with ACS present initially with VOC and then develop their ACS syndrome 1 to 3 days later. The index of suspicion for this etiology should be increased in the event of mental status changes, thrombocytopenia, or petechiae, features that are uncommon with pneumonia.

When fat is released from bone marrow and circulates, it is thought to form aggregates with serum lipoprotein which are then trapped in the pulmonary microcirculation. Serum lipase then cleaves these aggregates in part to increase free fatty acids (FFAs). The FFAs serve to augment platelet aggregation and activate coagulation, promoting pulmonary vascular thrombosis. The FFAs are directly toxic to endothelium, promote inflammation by activation of the complement cascade, and inactivate surfactant. The result is acute lung injury and, in its more toxic presentation, acute respiratory distress syndrome (ARDS). While evidence is lacking for specific therapies for FE in ACS, the orthopedic surgery literature suggests that the early administration of corticosteroids may be of some benefit.[26] While a clinical trial of corticosteroid administration reported a shorter hospital stay for ACS patients receiving the drug, it was accompanied by a greater readmission rate for SCD events.[27] More study is needed.

HYPOVENTILATION

Hypoventilation may be a complication of VOC or other pain syndrome in ACS. Chest splinting may result in atelectasis, pneumonia, and/or ACS. The use of incentive spirometers in patients admitted with VOC has been demonstrated to reduce the risk for developing ACS.[28] Excessive sedation from narcotics may also predispose to this complication. In the event of respiratory failure, ventilatory support is required with supplemental oxygen and, if necessary, conventional mechanical ventilation (CMV). If CMV proves inadequate, both high-frequency oscillatory ventilation (HFOV) and extracorporeal membrane oxygenation (ECMO) therapy have been used with success.[29]

REACTIVE AIRWAYS DISEASE

Evidence is mounting that RAD may play a role both as a cause and consequence of ACS.[30–34] The prevalence of RAD in SCD may occur in half of SCD patients and appears to be a risk factor for the development of ACS and pulmonary hypertension.[35] The concomitant expression of asthma and ACS is associated with a more severe exacerbation of ACS and prolongation of the hospitalization. RAD is associated with the production of a wider variety of inflammatory mediators and cytokines than with ACS alone and is also associated with airway edema and mucus hypersecretion, factors known to worsen the course of ACS. Therapy of RAD exacerbations in the context of ACS is similar to routine asthma care.[30,31]

DEHYDRATION

Dehydration predisposes both to VOC and ACS and commonly follows episodes of fever, tachypnea, and/or anorexia. The renal lesion of SCD predisposes to diuresis. Adequate hydration is therefore an emphasis of prospective care, but at the same time overhydration poses risks. Correction of dehydration is often accomplished by the administration of fluids at a rate of 1.25 to 1.50 times maintenance and then reduced to maintenance when the patient is euvolemic.[6]

EDEMA

Lung and airway edema predispose to ACS and worsen its expression. The inflammation of ACS, especially if associated with FE, predisposes to vascular leak and edema and once established is difficult to remedy. In severe cases the florid vascular leak syndrome of ARDS results. While dehydration frequently occurs, the predisposition of the inflammatory process to edema causes the therapeutic window for fluid replacement to be narrow and challenging.

SECONDARY COMPLICATIONS

As with community-acquired pneumonias, ACS is frequently associated with atelectasis and/or pleural effusions. The pleural fluid is usually sterile and exudative (like most parapneumonic effusions) but may develop an empyema. The atelectasis may or may not be associated with retained airway mucus secretions. In some cases the mucus strings are extensive and dehydrated and may form bronchial casts (Fig. 70-2). Because of their firmness, the syndrome has been referred to as plastic bronchitis.[36] In these cases, fiberoptic bronchoscopy with washes of saline or *N*-acetyl cysteine may be useful in clearing the airway obstruction and expediting the resolution of the atelectasis.

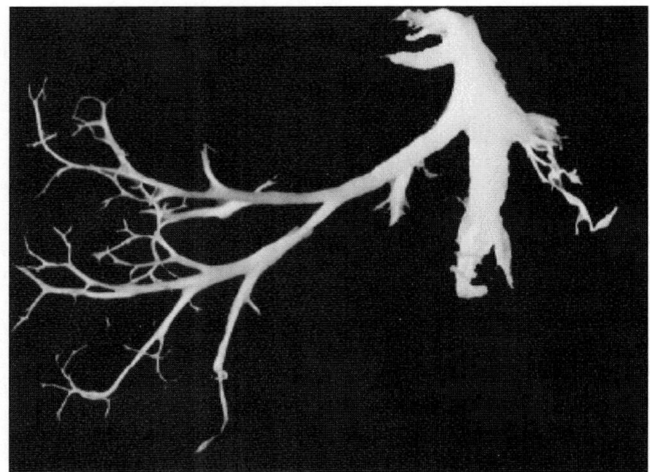

FIGURE 70-2. Extensive mucus cast seen following bronchoscopic removal from an 8-year-old boy with acute chest syndrome and right lung atelectasis.

CHRONIC SICKLE CELL LUNG DISEASE

SLD is a progressive disorder that is insidious in onset during childhood and may be asymptomatic in the absence of frequent exacerbations of ACS. The end stage of progression is characterized by persistent hypoxemia, radiographic evidence of interstitial fibrosis, restricted lung volumes on assessment by pulmonary function testing,[37] pulmonary hypertension, and cor pulmonale (Table 70-2). Pulmonary hypertension in patients with SCD has been associated with worsened survival.[38] Close pulmonary and cardiac follow-up are essential to monitor the progression of SLD and to introduce a growing list of supportive therapies that serve to retard the progression of this disorder.

PULMONARY HYPERTENSION

The obliterative vasculopathy of pulmonary hypertension (PH) is evident in one third of autopsies of patients with SCD.[8] Retrospective studies suggest that approximately 60% of SCD

TABLE 70-2. Clinical progression of sickle cell lung disease

	PROGRESSION	
Clinical Marker	**Mild**	**Severe**
Chest pain	None/recurrent	Severe persistent
Blood gas	Normaly	Hypoxemia at rest
Chest radiograph	Normal/mildly decreased vascularity	Severe pulmonary fibrosis
Pulmonary function	Mild restriction	Severe restriction
Electro cardiography/ Echo cardiography	Left ventricle predominant	Severe right ventricular and right atrial hypertrophy
Pulmonary artery pressure	Normal	Markedly elevated

From Knight J, Murphy TM, Browning I: The lung in sickle cell disease. Pediatr Pulmonol 1999;28:205.

patients may suffer from the disorder, but the true prevalence is unknown. The disorder is most frequently recognized in adults but doubtless originates earlier in life. While a worsened prognosis for SLD and PH is associated with recurrent episodes of ACS, the prevalence of PH is also high in patients without a history of ACS. This pathophysiologic predisposition is related to the combination of hemolytic anemia and functional asplenia.[35] Hemolysis in combination with inadequate splenic clearance results in the accumulation of iron-rich hemoglobin, which functions as a scavenger of nitric oxide (NO) and catalyzes the formation of ROS. Arginase is simultaneously released from erythrocytes and serves to limit the supply of arginine to nitric oxide synthase, limiting the synthesis of NO. The NO serves a critical function in promoting pulmonary vasodilation and limiting the impact of the many factors contributing to the vascular remodeling of PH. The functional asplenia contributes to the remodeling by the failure to clear platelet-derived mediators and cytokines that promote adherence of erythrocytes to the endothelium and cause microthrombosis.

Many patients with PH have minimal or no cardiopulmonary symptoms until their course is advanced. The diagnosis of PH in SCD is ominous, with a 10-fold increase in the risk for death[8] and survival less than 50% at 4 years. The recent validation of echocardiography as a diagnostic tool for PH in SCD should promote earlier detection.[38] Although there are brief studies and anecdotes suggesting a potential role for oxygen therapy, red cell transfusions, inhaled nitric oxide, intravenous L-arginine,[39] prostacyclin, and the newer vasodilators, controlled longer-term outcome studies are needed to demonstrate the effectiveness of these and other therapies with the potential to prevent or reverse the vascular remodeling. Retrospective analysis of monotherapy with hydroxyurea has failed to demonstrate a modification of the course of PH, strongly suggesting the need for additional therapies.[35]

THERAPY

GENERAL CARE

Much of the improved life span of patients with SCD is attributable to enhanced access to health care and attention to the details of preventive health care. Because the spleen is a victim of sickle cell vasculopathy in the first few years of life (functional asplenia), functional immunity to encapsulated organisms is impaired and the risk for sepsis from these organisms is increased. Protective strategies include penicillin prophylaxis and immunizations to *H. influenzae* and *S. pneumoniae.* A typical approach is as follows. Penicillin (or erythromycin) is administered twice daily from early infancy to age 5 years in those with the more severe hemoglobinopathies (HbSS and HbS/β^0 thalassemia) and through age 3 years in those with the less severe variants of SCD, such as HbSC. Prophylactic antibiotics are given permanently to patients who have undergone surgical splenectomy or have experienced pneumococcal sepsis. The 7-valent pneumococcal vaccine is administered to newborns beginning at 2 months of age with four doses administered by the age of 15 months, and the 23-valent vaccine is administered at ages 2 and 5 years and then every 5 to 7 years thereafter. The usual childhood schedule is followed for *H. influenzae* B immunizations. Immunizations to influenza virus are administered annually after the age of 6 months. The usual childhood immunization schedule for hepatitis B is emphasized to prevent this potential complication of recurrent red cell transfusions. Other components of general care include attention to nutrition and maintenance of adequate hydration. Transfusions with red blood cells are not administered routinely for anemia, but are usually selectively reserved for severe or recurrent cases of VOC or ACS, worsening anemia, or stroke prevention for those at increased risk.[42]

SPECIFIC CARE

Therapies to correct the basic genetic or beta globin protein defect of SCD and therapies to prevent the progression of SLD do not yet exist. The major current therapeutic strategies are designed to reduce the proportion of erythrocytes carrying predominantly sickle hemoglobin (HbS) and to retard the progression of pulmonary hypertension (Table 70-3).

HYDROXYUREA

Hydroxyurea is the cornerstone of therapies designed to increase the erythrocyte expression of HbF. This increase in HbF and a concomitant increase in red cell volume effectively reduce the intracellular concentration of HbS and result in decreased sickling. Hydroxyurea also reduces the expression of the VLA-4 and CD36 adhesion molecules on sickle erythrocytes. Trials of increasing length of hydroxyurea therapy in adults and children have demonstrated safety and clinical efficacy, including a reduction in the incidence of ACS.[40–42] While there are not long-term safety and efficacy data, these studies have generated increasing enthusiasm for this therapy. Since ACS is the most important predictor of the progression of SLD,[43] the studies hold out the hope that hydroxyurea may be disease modifying. Additional studies are under way.

ERYTHROPOIETIN

Therapy with erythropoietin also serves to increase HbF, but its effectiveness has been less than desired. Because of this and its substantial expense, its use has been limited. Its primary use is as adjunctive therapy for patients whose response to hydroxyurea is suboptimal or for patients with religious objections to blood transfusions.

TRANSFUSION THERAPY

Transfusion of normal erythrocytes serves to depress the bone marrow production of erythrocytes expressing sickle hemoglobin. The timing of transfusions may be acute, intermittent, or chronic. Many of the historical uses of this therapy are controversial. Adverse side effects of recurrent transfusions include iron

TABLE 70-3. Management of sickle cell lung disease

Treatment Objective	Specific Therapy
Increase hemoglobin F	Hydroxyurea Erythropoietin
Decrease hemoglobin S	Chronic transfusion
Alter bone marrow source of hemoglobin	Bone marrow transplantation
Manage pulmonary hypertension	Oxygen Vasodilators

Adapted from Knight J, Murphy TM, Browning I: The lung in sickle cell disease. Pediatr Pulmonol 1999;28:205.

overload, blood-borne infections, and alloimmunization, complications that can be reduced by erythrocytapheresis, highly specific cross-matching, and the newer iron-chelating therapies. Current indications of red cell transfusion therapy in SCD include severe cases of VOC, recurrent or severe ACS, severe or worsening anemia, and primary and secondary stroke prevention in patients at increased risk.[35]

BONE MARROW TRANSPLANTATION

Because of the potentially serious complications of bone marrow transplantation (BMT), in the United States it is offered primarily to those patients who have suffered serious complications, such as stroke or recurrent ACS, and to those with HLA-matched sibling donors. Its greatest benefit, however, is to those who have neither experienced significant complications nor have developed significant SLD, an approach that has been successfully used in Europe. Indeed, morbidity and mortality from BMT appear to be significantly less in younger, healthier patients. The challenge of determining the best application of BMT is the highly variable clinical expression of SCD.[2] Longer-term studies are necessary to accurately assess its risks and benefits.

GENE THERAPY

Efforts to develop effective gene therapy or beta globin substitution have so far failed. The technical impediments to gene therapy in SCD are similar to those encountered in other genetic disorders such as cystic fibrosis. The primary impediment has been the development of a vector suitable for the delivery of the replacement of beta globin–deoxyribonucleic acid to bone marrow erythrocyte precursors. Because of the potential disease-modifying impact of effective gene therapy, molecular research into the genetic origins, gene modification, and gene therapy continues. Important insights are expected from the development of a genetic mouse model of SCD.

CONCLUSION

Greatly improved clinical outcomes of the morbidity and mortality of SCD have resulted from the recognition and careful therapy of the multiple elements of the complex etiologies of VOC, ACS, and chronic sickle cell lung disease. Encouraging results have accumulated from improved experience with hydroxyurea therapy and from BMT. Further improvements will likely result from research to determine new etiologies and the best therapies for the complex interplay of the abnormal oxygen transport, coagulopathies, inflammation, and resulting lung and pulmonary vascular remodeling. Research in these areas promises progress toward corrective molecular therapies of the fundamental defects.

Acknowledgment

The authors wish to thank Thomas R. Kinney, MD, Sherri Zimmerman, MD, and Russell Ware, MD, for their helpful suggestions and editorial comments.

REFERENCES

1. Jandl JH: Abnormal hemoglobin and hemoglobinopathies. In: Jandl JH, ed: Blood: Pathophysiology. Boston: Blackwell Scientific, 1991, pp 182–191.
2. Knight J, Murphy TM, Browning I: The lung in sickle cell disease. Pediatr Pulmonol 1999;28:205.
3. Lane PA: Sickle cell disease. Pediatr Clin North Am 1996;43:639.
4. Platt OS, Brambilla DJ, Rosse WF, Milner PF, Castro O: Mortality in sickle cell disease. Life expectancy and risk factors for early death. N Engl J Med 1994;30:1639.
5. Farber MD, Koshy M, Kinney TR: Demographic and socioeconomic characteristics of patients and families with sickle cell disease. J Chronic Dis 1985;38:495.
6. Knight-Madden JM: Acute chest syndrome in sickle cell disease. Postgrad Doctor-Caribbean 2002;18(4):105.
7. Vichinsky E, Williams R, Das M, Earles AN, Lewis N, Adler A, et al: Pulmonary fat embolism. A distinct cause of severe acute chest syndrome in sickle cell anemia. Blood 1994;83:3107.
8. Gladwin MT, Sachdev V, Jison ML, Shizukuda Y, Plehn JF, Minter K, et al: Pulmonary hypertension as a risk factor for death in patients with sickle cell disease. N Engl J Med 2004;350:886.
9. Noguchi CT, Schechter AN, Rodgers GP: Sickle cell disease pathophysiology. Bailliere Clin Haematol 1993;6:57.
10. Moore CM, Ehlayel M, Leiva LE, Sorenson RU: New concepts in the immunology of sickle cell disease. Ann Allergy Asthma Immunol 1996;76:385.
11. Joneckis CC, Ackley RL, Orringer EP, Wayner EA, Parise LV: Integrin alpha 4 beta 1 and glycoprotein IV (CD36) are expressed on circulating reticulocytes in sickle cell anemia. Blood 1993;82:3548.
12. Francis RB Jr, Haywood LJ: Elevated tumor necrosis factor and interleukin-1 in sickle cell disease. J Natl Med Assoc 1992;84:611.
13. Wick TM, Moake JL, Udden MM, McIntire LV: Unusually large von Willebrand factor multimers preferentially promote young sickle and nonsickle erythrocyte adhesion to endothelial cells. Am J Hematol 1993;42:284.
14. Hebbel RP: Membrane-associated iron. In: Embury SH, Hebbel RP, Mohandas N, Steinberg, eds: Sickle Cell Disease; Basic Principles and Clinical Practice. New York: Raven, 1994, pp 163–172.
15. Fan LL: Evaluation and therapy of chronic interstitial pneumonitis in children. Curr Opin Pediatr 1994;6:248.
16. Rackoff WR, Kunkel N, Silber JH, Asakura T, Ohene-Frempong K: Pulse oximetry and factors associated with hemoglobin oxygen desaturation in children with sickle cell disease. Blood 1993;81:3422.
17. Hagger D, Wolff S, Owen J, Samson D: Changes in coagulation and fibrinolysis in patients with sickle cell disease compared with healthy black controls. Blood Coagul Fibrinolysis 1995;6:93.
18. Castro O, Brambilla DJ, Thorington B, Reindorf CA, Scott RB, Gillette P, et al: The acute chest syndrome in sickle cell disease. Incidence and risk factors. Blood 1994;84:643.
19. Quinn CT, Buchanan GR: The acute chest syndrome of sickle cell disease. J Pediatr 205;135:205.
20. Rucknagel DL: Progress and prospects for the acute chest syndrome. J Pediatr 2001;138:160.
21. Vichinsky EP, Neumayr LD, Earles AN, Williams R, Lennette E, Dean D, et al: Causes and outcomes of the acute chest syndrome in sickle cell disease. N Engl J Med 2000;342:1855.
22. Vichinsky EP, Styles LA, Colangelo LH: Acute chest syndrome in sickle cell diseases. Clinical presentation and course. Blood 1997;89:1787.
23. Golden C, Styles L, Vichinsky E: Acute chest syndrome and sickle cell disease. Curr Opin Hematol 1998;5:80.
24. Bhalla M, Abboud MR, McLoud TC, Shepard JA, Munden MM, Jackson SM, et al: Acute chest syndrome in sickle cell disease: CT evidence of microvascular occlusion. Radiology 1993;187:45.
25. Godeau B, Schaeffer A, Bachir D, Fleury-Feith J, Galacteros F, Verra F, et al: Bronchoalveolar lavage in sickle cell disease patients with acute chest syndrome. Value for diagnostic assessment of fat embolism. Am J Respir Crit Care Med 1996;153:1691.
26. Schonfeld SA, Ploysonsang Y, DiLisio R, Crissman JD, Miller E, Hammerschmidt DE, et al: Fat embolism prophylaxis with corticosteroids. Ann Intern Med 1983;99:438.
27. Bernini JC, Rogers ZR, Sandler ES, Reisch JS, Quinn CT, Buchanan GR: Beneficial effects of intravenous dexamethasone in children with mild to moderately severe acute chest syndrome complicate sickle cell disease. Blood 1998;92:3082.
28. Bellet PS, Kalinyak KA, Shukla R, Gelfand MJ, Rucknagel DL: Incentive spirometry to prevent acute pulmonary complications in sickle cell diseases. N Engl J Med 1995;333:699.
29. Wratney AT, Gentile MA, Hamel DS, Cheifetz IM: Successful treatment of acute chest syndrome with high frequency oscillatory ventilation in pediatric patients. Respir Care 2004;49:263.

30. Knight-Madden JM, Forrester TS, Lewis NA, Greenough A: Asthma in children with sickle cell disease and the association with acute chest syndrome. Thorax 2005;60:206.
31. Knight-Madden JM, Hambleton IR: Inhaled bronchodilators for acute chest syndrome in people with sickle cell disease. Cochrane Database Syst Rev 2003;3:CD003733.
32. Koumbourlis AC, Zar HJ, Hurlet-Jensen A, Goldberg MR: Prevalence and reversibility of lower airway obstruction in children with sickle cell disease. J Pediatr 2001;138:188.
33. Leong MA, Dampier C, Varlotta L, Allen JL: Airway hyperreactivity in children with sickle cell disease. J Pediatr 1997;131:278.
34. Boyd JH, Moinuddin A, Strunk RC, DeBaun MR: Asthma and acute chest in sickle-cell disease. Pediatr Pulmonol 2005;38:229.
35. Vichinsky EP: Perspective. Pulmonary hypertension in sickle cell disease. N Engl J Med 2004;350(9):857.
36. Raghuram N, Pettignano R, Gal AA, Harsch A, Adamkiewicz TV: Plastic bronchitis; an unusual complication associated with sickle cell disease and the acute chest syndrome. Pediatrics 1997;100:139.
37. Sylvester KP, Patey RA, Milligan P, Dick M, Rafferty GF, Rees D, et al: Pulmonary function abnormalities in children with sickle cell disease. Thorax 2004;59:67.
38. Castro O, Hoque M, Brown BD: Pulmonary hypertension in sickle cell disease. Cardiac catheterization results and survival. Blood 2003; 101:1257.
39. Morris CR, Morris SM Jr, Hagar W, van Warmerdam J, Claster S, Kepka-Lenhart D, et al: Arginine therapy—a new treatment for pulmonary hypertension in sickle cell disease? Am J Respir Crit Care Med 2003; 168:63.
40. Steinberg MH, Barton F, Castro O, Pegelow CH, Ballas SK, Kutlar A, et al: Effect of hydroxyurea on mortality and morbidity in adult sickle cell anemia. Risks and benefits up to 9 years of treatment. JAMA 2003;289:1645.
41. Zimmerman SA, Schultz WH, Davis JS, Pickens CV, Mortier MA, Howard TA, Ware RE: Sustained long-term hematologic efficacy of hydroxyurea at maximum tolerated dose in children with sickle cell disease. Blood 2004;103(6):2039.
42. Miller ST, Wright E, Abboud M, Berman B, Files B, Scher CD, et al: Impact of chronic transfusion on incidence of pain and acute chest syndrome during the stroke prevention trial (STOP) in sickle-cell anemia. J Pediatr 2001;139:785.
43. Powars D, Weidman JA, Odom-Maryon T, Niland JC, Johnson C: Sickle cell chronic lung disease. Prior morbidity and the risk of pulmonary failure. Medicine (Baltimore) 1988;67:66.

71 Lung Injury Caused by Pharmacologic Agents

Marianna M. Henry, MD •
Terry L. Noah, MD

Numerous drugs can cause pulmonary or pleural reactions in children. The most frequent offenders are certain chemotherapeutic agents used in the treatment of childhood neoplasms (Table 71-1), although the toxic effects of other agents are increasingly recognized (Table 71-2).[1,2] Diffuse interstitial pneumonitis and fibrosis constitute the most frequent clinical syndrome. Hypersensitivity lung disease, noncardiogenic pulmonary edema, pleural effusion, bronchiolitis obliterans, and alveolar hemorrhage are also encountered.

Although some drug-induced pulmonary damage is reversible, persistent and even fatal dysfunction may occur. Lung reactions occasionally are temporally remote from exposure to chemotherapeutic agents. Depending on the agent involved, the reaction may or may not be dose related. The mechanism of toxicity is thought to be direct injury to lung cells in most cases, but immunologic and central nervous system–mediated mechanisms seem to play a role in the toxicity of certain agents. Identified risk factors associated with cytotoxic drug therapy vary, but in general include cumulative dose, age of the patient, prior or concurrent radiation, oxygen therapy, and use of other toxic drugs. Most reactions to noncytotoxic drugs appear to develop idiosyncratically. When patients are treated with several potentially toxic drugs or with a toxic drug plus irradiation to the chest or high concentrations of oxygen, specific offenders often cannot be identified. There is little if any evidence that children are more susceptible to drug-related pulmonary injury, and in fact they may be less susceptible to some agents such as bleomycin.

The clinical presentation of drug-induced lung disease often includes fever, malaise, dyspnea, and a nonproductive cough. Radiologic studies almost always demonstrate diffuse alveolar and/or interstitial involvement. Segmental or lobar disease, particularly if unilateral, should suggest another diagnosis. Abnormal pulmonary function values, indicative of restrictive or obstructive disease, may be found before appearance of roentgenographic lesions. Chest computed tomography (CT) may also provide early evidence of parenchymal abnormalities. Hypoxemia is an early and clinically important functional consequence. Pathologic features do not distinguish among most drugs and most often consist of interstitial thickening with chronic inflammatory cell infiltrate in the interstitial or alveolar compartment, fibroblast proliferation, fibrosis, and hyperplasia of type II pneumocytes, which contain enlarged hyperchromatic nuclei.[3] With hypersensitivity reactions, the interstitial infiltrate includes substantial numbers of eosinophils. Other diagnoses, such as infection, pulmonary hemorrhage, lung disease related to an underlying disorder, and radiation damage must be considered in patients with suspected drug-induced lung injury. Bronchoalveolar lavage (BAL) is being increasingly utilized to provide microbiologic and cytologic information essential to differential diagnosis and as a tool to begin to identify disease markers and potential pathogenetic mechanisms.[4]

Practical criteria for diagnosing drug-induced lung disease have been suggested by Allen.[5] These include (1) no other likely cause of lung disease; (2) symptoms consistent with the suspect drug; (3) time course compatible with drug-induced lung disease; (4) compatible tissue or BAL findings; and (5) improvement after the drug is discontinued.

■ CYTOTOXIC DRUGS

■ ANTIBIOTICS

Bleomycin

Bleomycin is a mixture of peptide antibiotics obtained from *Streptomyces verticillus.* Although the drug is active against squamous cell carcinoma and testicular tumors, its major use in children is in the treatment of Hodgkin's disease and other lymphomas. Because of the high frequency of pulmonary reactions and the utility of bleomycin for generating animal models of lung fibrosis, this agent has been studied more thoroughly than others. Pulmonary damage develops in two distinct patterns, most commonly progressive fibrosis and uncommonly an acute hypersensitivity reaction.

Pulmonary disease secondary to bleomycin occurs in approximately 4% to 7% of all patients receiving the drug, although the reported incidence is as great as 40%.[6,7] The frequency of reactions in children is not well documented because relatively few children receive this agent. However, multivariate analyses of follow-up data from the multicenter Childhood Cancer Survivor Study indicated that use of bleomycin is significantly associated with lung fibrosis (relative risk [RR] 1.7), bronchitis (RR 1.4), and chronic cough (RR 1.9) at 5 years postdiagnosis.[8] Risk for lung disease depends largely on cumulative dose. Significant lung damage rarely occurs in adults at cumulative doses less than 400 to 500 units. At cumulative doses greater than 500 units, risk of toxicity apparently increases in adults.[9] Pulmonary damage is more severe in elderly than in young patients and in those with reduced glomerular filtration rate, but gender does not appear to influence toxicity.[7] Slow intravenous administration results in less lung disease than intramuscular injection or intravenous bolus. The combination of radiotherapy or high inspired oxygen concentrations and bleomycin produces more lung injury than either alone. Pulmonary toxicity to relatively small quantities of bleomycin has been reported during combination drug therapy.[10]

Pulmonary injury due to bleomycin occurs by direct injury to cells as well as by secondary immunologic reactions. Direct toxicity may be mediated by oxidant injury, either through the production of reactive oxygen metabolites or through inactivation

■ **TABLE 71-1.** Cytotoxic drugs

	Incidence (%)	Mortality (%)	Clinical Syndromes
Antibiotics			
Bleomycin	2–40	1–10	IP/PF, H, P Eff
Mitomycin	2–38	50 (90 in PE)	IP/PF, PE, P Eff
Alkylating agents			
Cyclophosphamide	≤1	40	IP/PF, PE, B
Chlorambucil	*	≤50	IP/PF
Busulfan	2–43	†	IP/PF, P Eff
Melphalan	*	≤60	IP/PF
Nitrosoureas			
Carmustine	20–30	15–90	PF
Antimetabolites			
Methotrexate	8	1	IP/PF, H, PE, P Eff
Azathioprine	*	†	IP/PF
6-Mercaptopurine	*	†	IP/PF
Cytosine arabinoside	13–28	50	IP/PF, PE, BOOP
Gemcitabine	*	*	PE
Other			
Hydroxyurea	*	*	H
Paclitaxel	4–9	0	H

*Infrequent case reports.
†Unknown.

B, bronchospasm; BOOP, bronchiolitis obliterans organizing pneumonia; H, hypersensitivity lung reaction; IP/PF, interstitial pneumonitis/pulmonary fibrosis; PE, pulmonary edema (noncardiogenic); P Eff, pleural effusion; PF, pulmonary fibrosis.

of antioxidants.[11,12] Data supporting this mechanism include the findings that pretreatment of rodents with antioxidants such as taurine, niacin, vitamin A, thioredoxin, or *N*-acetylcysteine can reduce subsequent bleomycin-induced pulmonary fibrosis.[12–14] Additionally, bleomycin may directly induce senescence of type II epithelium.[15] Bleomycin generates factors such as leukotriene B_4, platelet-activating factor, and cytokines such as monocyte chemoattractant protein-1, interleukin-1 (IL-1), transforming growth factor-β, and tumor necrosis factor-α (TNF-α), which are chemotactic for or activate leukocytes.[16–19] These inflammatory cells may participate in oxidant and perhaps proteolytic damage to lung cells.[20] Specific roles for eosinophils and T lymphocytes have been suggested by data from transgenic models overexpressing IL-5.[21] Bleomycin promptly increases collagen synthesis by fibroblasts, an effect that may be mediated in part by transforming growth factor-β.[22] Regenerative epithelial proliferation mediated by epithelial growth factor may be important in minimizing or resolving bleomycin-induced pulmonary fibrosis.[23] Gunther and colleagues[24] have reported complete abrogation of bleomycin-induced pulmonary fibrosis in rabbits using nebulized heparin or urokinase.

Bleomycin-induced lung disease can begin insidiously. Asymptomatic patients may have decreases in arterial oxygen saturation and carbon monoxide diffusing capacity (DLCO). As the illness progresses, there is a decline in vital capacity and total lung capacity, characteristic of restrictive lung disease. In both interstitial pneumonitis and hypersensitivity lung reactions, patients typically present with a dry hacking cough and dyspnea; these signs occur only on exertion in mild cases, but profound respiratory distress accompanies advanced illness. Fever suggests a hypersensitivity reaction. Physical examination reveals tachypnea and fine crackles. Chest roentgenograms in symptomatic patients most commonly demonstrate diffuse linear densities. A widespread reticulonodular or alveolar pattern may also be seen. Chest CT is more sensitive for detection of early interstitial disease, and in animal models chest CT findings correlate well with pathologic changes.[25,26] Biopsy specimens usually reveal interstitial pneumonitis and fibrosis and extensive alveolar damage. There is a decrease in type I pneumocytes and a subsequent hyperplasia of type II cells. In contrast to lesions caused by alkylating agents, this lesion is most prominent in subpleural and basilar regions.

Patients receiving bleomycin should be monitored by serial determinations of DLCO. Chest CT may also be useful for monitoring progression of disease.[26] Therapy of bleomycin-induced pneumonitis consists largely of supportive measures. Withdrawal of the drug at the onset of toxicity must be considered. Careful monitoring of oxygen therapy to avoid excessive exposure is imperative.[27] Although a portion of the cellular inflammatory element resolves with cessation of therapy, much of the fibrotic damage is irreversible. Treatment with bleomycin is a significant predictor of long-term respiratory symptomatology and pulmonary function decrements in survivors of Hodgkin's disease.[28] The use of steroids is controversial, but reversal of severe toxicity has been documented in some patients after use of high-dose steroids.[29] In the few patients exhibiting hypersensitivity reactions, corticosteroids have a definite role. Amifostine, an organic thiophosphate that acts as a cytoprotective oxidant scavenger, is selectively taken up by normal tissues and has been shown to protect against bleomycin-induced lung disease in animal models.[30] While it may reduce nephrotoxicity and mucositis in bone marrow transplant recipients,[31] its efficacy in preventing lung disease in patients is not yet known.

Granulocyte colony-stimulating factor (G-CSF) has been increasingly used in chemotherapy regimens to limit neutropenia.

■ **TABLE 71-2.** Noncytotoxic drugs

	Recorded Cases or Incidence	Mortality	Clinical Syndromes
Nitrofurantoin	>500 adult 8 pediatric	8%	H, IP/PF, B, AH, P Eff, BOOP
Sulfasalazine	26 adult	2 cases	H, BOOP, FA, B
Diphenylhydantoin	6 adult 4 pediatric	0	H, B, BOOP
Carbamazepine	7 adult 6 pediatric	0	H, B, BOOP
Pencillamine	32 adult 1 pediatric	50% (AH, BO)	H, DA, BOOP, AH
Gold	>140 adult 2 pediatric	12%	H, IP/PF, BOOP
Amiodarone	5%–15% 3 pediatric	5%–10%	H, IP/PF, BOOP
Interleukin-2	>50%	0	PE, P Eff
All-*trans* retinoic acid (ATRA)	5%–27%	5%–29%	IP, P Eff, PE, AH

AH, alveolar hemorrhage; B, bronchospasm; BO, bronchiolitis obliterans; BOOP, bronchiolitis obliterans organizing pneumonia; DA, diffuse alveolitis; FA, fibrosing alveolitis; H, hypersensitivity lung reaction; IP/PF, interstitial pneumonitis/pulmonary fibrosis; P Eff, pleural effusion; PE, pulmonary edema.

Studies in rats have suggested that coadministration of G-CSF with bleomycin increases both accumulation of neutrophils in the lung and the severity of direct bleomycin toxicity.[32] However, a retrospective analysis of patients with germ cell tumors receiving bleomycin did not suggest increased incidence of pulmonary toxicity in those who also received G-CSF.[33]

Mitomycin

Mitomycin is an antibiotic that is metabolized to an alkylating agent. Its major uses are in treatment of carcinomas of the cervix, colon, rectum, pancreas, and bladder. Although it is useful in treating some lymphomas and leukemias, mitomycin is rarely used in pediatrics. Two percent to 38% of patients receiving mitomycin develop lung disease.[34] Most cases develop within 6 months of institution of therapy. Suspected risk factors for mitomycin lung toxicity include frequent dosing (every 3–4 weeks vs. every 6–8 weeks), prior chest irradiation, concomitant vinca alkaloid therapy, and a cumulative dose of ≥20 mg/m.[2,34]

Clinical manifestations of mitomycin pulmonary toxicity are generally of two types. Rarely, a syndrome of acute dyspnea develops when mitomycin is given concomitantly with vinca alkaloids (e.g., vindesine or vinblastine). After a few doses of mitomycin, dyspnea develops within minutes after the subsequent dose of the vinca alkaloid and can lead to acute respiratory failure.[35] The more usual presentation involves slowly progressive dyspnea, dyspnea on exertion, and dry cough with or without fever. A restrictive ventilatory defect with fibrosis is most common, but noncardiogenic pulmonary edema may occur. Chest roentgenograms are normal or demonstrate a fine reticulonodular pattern. Pleural effusion occurs infrequently.[36] Lung biopsies show interstitial fibrosis, mononuclear cell infiltration, hyperplasia of type II alveolar epithelium, and occasional arterial wall muscular proliferation.[37] Mortality of mitomycin-associated pulmonary toxicity approaches 50%, but disease may improve after withdrawal of the drug or treatment with corticosteroids.[34]

ALKYLATING AGENTS

Cyclophosphamide

Cyclophosphamide is widely used in the treatment of leukemias, lymphomas, and nonmalignant illnesses. It frequently produces severe alopecia and hemorrhagic cystitis. Although pulmonary toxicity is uncommon, it does produce severe and even fatal lung damage.[38,39] Data from the Childhood Cancer Survivor Study indicate a significantly increased long-term risk for supplemental oxygen requirement, recurrent pneumonia, chronic cough, dyspnea on exertion, and bronchitis after cyclophosphamide use.[8] Frankovich and colleagues[40] reported a series of 34 children who underwent autologous bone marrow transplant for relapsing Hodgkin's disease and were treated with cyclophosphamide in combination with etoposide and either carmustine, chloroethylcyclohexylnitrosurea, or irradiation. Fifteen of these patients developed lung injury syndromes including interstitial pneumonitis ($n = 8$), acute alveolitis ($n = 2$), diffuse alveolar hemorrhage ($n = 2$), acute respiratory distress syndrome (ARDS) ($n = 2$), and bronchiolitis obliterans ($n = 1$). Four of the patients died of pulmonary complications. In this series, a history of atopy was highly predictive of pulmonary complications.

One documented mechanism of pulmonary injury is cytotoxicity mediated by oxidative processes. Experiments in rodents indicate that cyclophosphamide exposure results in leak of proteins across damaged endothelium, as well as a reduction in lung antioxidant levels.[41,42] These changes can be partly prevented by treatment with antioxidants.[43,44] A second potential mechanism of injury is activation and recruitment of immunocompetent cells with presumed immunotoxicity. Acute immunoglobulin E (IgE)–mediated systemic reactions have been reported, including angioedema and bronchospasm.

Little is known about the relationship of dose, duration, and frequency of administration to the appearance of parenchymal disease in humans, though cytotoxicity appears to be dose related in rats.[42] Pulmonary reactions have occurred following total doses between 0.15 and 50 g. Pulmonary disease may begin during, weeks after, or years after cyclophosphamide therapy.[45] Remote interstitial pneumonitis and fibrosis have been observed in two adolescents who were treated with the drug in early childhood.[46] The most striking feature in these cases was chest wall deformity secondary to failure of lung growth during the adolescent growth spurt.

Onset of pulmonary toxicity is usually subacute rather than insidious as with other alkylating agents. Dry cough and dyspnea herald the onset; malaise, anorexia, and weight loss follow.[45,47] Physical examination reveals tachypnea and diffusely diminished breath sounds. Adventitious breath sounds are uncommon. Chest roentgenograms may show diffuse bilateral infiltrates, sometimes with pleural thickening. Pulmonary function testing reveals hypoxemia and restrictive lung disease. Biopsy and postmortem specimens show interstitial fibrosis, alveolar exudates, and atypical alveolar epithelial cells.[45,47] Withdrawal of the drug, supportive therapy, and corticosteroids are recommended treatment. The disease may be progressive and even fatal despite therapeutic interventions.[37] Cyclophosphamide also may predispose to toxicity when medications such as bleomycin, azathioprine, and carmustine are used subsequently.

Chlorambucil

Chlorambucil is used in the treatment of leukemias, some lymphomas, nephrosis, and inflammatory conditions such as sarcoidosis.[48] Several well-documented reports indicate that the drug produces pulmonary toxicity, albeit rarely. Little is known concerning the dose or duration of therapy necessary to produce lung damage. Patients who develop lung disease have received the drug both intermittently and continuously. Duration of therapy before onset of disease ranges from months to several years.[49,50]

Patients develop cough, dyspnea, fatigue, and weight loss that appears 6 months to 3 years after initiation of therapy and progressively worsens. Physical examination reveals tachypnea and fine bibasilar crackles. Chest roentgenograms demonstrate a diffuse interstitial infiltrate. Pulmonary function tests indicate restrictive lung disease accompanied by a defect in DLCO. Histopathologic findings are similar to those associated with busulfan and cyclophosphamide therapy, including type II pneumocyte dysplasia, extensive fibrosis, and a scattered interstitial mononuclear infiltrate.[49,50] Although improvement with discontinuation of the drug and corticosteroid therapy has been reported,[51] progression of disease may occur despite this approach.[49]

Other Alkylating Agents

Busulfan (Myleran, GlaxoSmithKline, Research Triangle Park, North Carolina) is used to treat chronic myelogenous leukemia, which occurs occasionally in childhood, and in some preparative regimens for bone marrow transplantation. Four percent of adult patients undergoing long-term treatment with this drug develop interstitial pneumonitis and fibrosis.[52] Subclinical pulmonary changes are noted at autopsy in up to one half. One child died secondary to pulmonary toxicity. Mertens and colleagues[8] reported increased long-term risk for supplemental oxygen requirement and pleurisy after busulfan treatment. As with chlorambucil, pulmonary injury is usually not evident for many months after initiation of treatment. Radiation and previous cytotoxic therapy are risk factors.[53] The clinical syndrome is similar to that produced by the other alkylating agents.[52] Treatment consists of discontinuation of busulfan and a carefully monitored course of corticosteroids. Efficacy of corticosteroids is unproven, but a trial is indicated because of the poor prognosis.

An increase in incidence of alveolar hemorrhage has been reported when etoposide (VP-16) was added to a regimen of busulfan and cyclophosphamide for bone marrow transplantation; toxicity in this study was largely confined to patients who had been given prior chest radiotherapy.[54] However, Quigley and colleagues[55] found that in children, preparative regimens for bone marrow transplantation that included busulfan were associated with preservation of pulmonary function compared with regimens using other combination high-dose chemotherapeutic regimens or total body irradiation.

Melphalan is used primarily in the treatment of multiple myelomas and hence is employed infrequently in pediatrics. Although overt toxicity is unusual, the frequency of epithelial changes and fibrosis at autopsy may be as high as 50%.[56] Bronchial epithelial cell proliferation has been an unusual finding. Otherwise, the pathologic changes are typical for alkylating agents and may be reversible with discontinuation of the drug.[57] One variation in presentation is the occurrence of a productive rather than a dry cough.

NITROSUREAS

Carmustine

Carmustine (bischloroethylnitrosourea, or BCNU) is a synthetic antineoplastic compound. Its major use is in the therapy of lymphomas and gliomas. The incidence of BCNU pulmonary toxicity is quite variable; 20% to 30% of treated patients develop some lung disease.[58,59] The total dose administered, duration of therapy, and preexistence of lung disease are the most accurate predictors of pulmonary toxicity. Most patients with symptomatic respiratory disease have received large cumulative doses (>777 mg/m^2). When the cumulative dose exceeds 1500 mg/m^2, there is a 50% probability of lung disease. Patients with toxicity also appear to have received the drug over a shorter period, irrespective of the total dose given. The onset of pulmonary symptoms has been noted between 30 and 371 days after institution of therapy, sometimes after BCNU has been discontinued. Young patients reportedly are at greater risk, but this may be the result of relatively higher doses and increased numbers of therapy cycles because of greater general tolerance. Mertens and colleagues[8] reported a significant risk for supplemental oxygen requirement among children at least 5 years after BCNU or lomustine (chloroethylcyclohexlnitrosourea, or CCNU) treatment. Race and tumor type have no obvious predisposing effect. Radiation therapy may be synergistic. In two studies involving adult patients, female gender and combination with cyclophosphamide were identified as risk factors for pulmonary complications.[59,60]

Patients with BCNU pulmonary toxicity exhibit much the same clinical picture as that described for bleomycin.[58] Histologic findings are also similar, with alveolar exudates, dysplasia of alveolar epithelium, interstitial fibrosis, and pleural thickening. In a histopathologic study of eight patients who underwent lung biopsy 12 to 17 years after treatment with BCNU, there was electron microscopic evidence of ongoing endothelial and epithelial damage, suggesting long-term toxic effects of the drug.[61] One of these patients died with pulmonary hypertension due to interstitial fibrosis. The disease is fatal in approximately 15% of those affected.

Therapy is essentially supportive. Corticosteroids are often administered concomitantly with BCNU for brain tumors and afford no protection from subsequent pulmonary toxicity. However, corticosteroids may offer some benefit in the treatment of early stages of acute disease. Thymidine has been used as a biomodulator to protect from BCNU pulmonary toxicity in patients with malignant melanoma and may act via modulation of DNA repair enzymes in normal tissue.[62] Substitution of CCNU for BCNU in combination therapy for autologous marrow transplant did not reduce the incidence of interstitial pneumonitis in a phase II trial.[63]

ANTIMETABOLITES

Methotrexate

Methotrexate (4-aminopteroylglutamic acid) is a folic acid antagonist used in the treatment of several childhood malignancies, notably leukemias and osteogenic sarcoma, as well as nonmalignant conditions such as juvenile rheumatoid arthritis and psoriasis.[64,65] Unlike most other chemotherapeutic agents, methotrexate causes mild and most often reversible lung disease.

Prevalence rates between 0.3% and 11.6% have been reported for pulmonary toxicity due to methotrexate, but ascertainment of its effects is complicated by the frequent use of combination therapy and the tendency of underlying diseases such as rheumatoid arthritis to also cause lung disease.[65] No correlation has been found between lung toxicity and dose of methotrexate, and pneumonitis may occur long after discontinuation of therapy.

The clinical features of methotrexate lung toxicity are consistent with a hypersensitivity pneumonitis.[66] Disease usually begins slowly with a prodrome of headache and malaise, followed by dyspnea and dry cough. Pleuritic pain may be present but is rare. Fever may also occur. Physical examination reveals tachypnea, diffuse crackles, cyanosis, and occasionally skin eruptions. Hypoxemia is observed in 90% to 95% of patients, and mild eosinophilia has been reported in 41% of patients.[65] Few reports have documented pulmonary function changes, but decreased DLCO may occur.[67] Lung function testing in a series of children with juvenile rheumatoid arthritis who received methotrexate showed no increased incidence of abnormal function, including DLCO, compared with a similar population not receiving methotrexate.[68] The most common abnormalities on chest radiographs are bilateral interstitial infiltrates or mixed interstitial and alveolar infiltrates. Lung biopsy in adults reveals interstitial pneumonitis with lymphocytic and sometimes eosinophilic infiltrates, bronchiolitis, and granuloma formation consistent with a hypersensitivity reaction, although type II alveolar cell hyperplasia typical of cytotoxicity has also been found.[69,70] BAL fluids typically show hypercellularity, lymphocytosis with variable CD4/CD8 ratios, and moderate neutrophilia.[71,72]

Diagnosis of methotrexate-induced pneumonitis is difficult because this condition may mimic other diseases. Pulmonary infection must be excluded, particularly if high-dose methotrexate is used or if the underlying disease is associated with immunosuppression.

Therapy consists of withdrawal of the drug and administration of corticosteroids, but this approach has not been analyzed in controlled trials. Treatment with folinic acid (leucovorin rescue) does not prevent methotrexate lung toxicity.[65] Outcome is usually favorable with clinical improvement preceding radiographic and pulmonary function improvement.[65,73] Two fatal outcomes in a series of arthritis patients with lung toxicity suggest that caution be exercised when considering retreatment with this agent after recovery from methotrexate lung injury.[74]

Azathioprine

Azathioprine is an immunosuppressive agent that is used in a variety of pediatric clinical situations including renal transplantation, inflammatory bowel disease, autoimmune disorders, idiopathic pulmonary hemosiderosis, and fibrosing alveolitis.[75] A small number of cases of dose-related toxicity have been reported in adults, largely after renal transplantation.[76] Fever and hypoxemia are major presenting manifestations. Lung biopsy specimens reveal diffuse alveolar damage, including hyaline membranes and interstitial pneumonitis with fibrosis.[76] Eosinophilia and immune deposits have not been found; however, a hypersensitivity-like reaction including fever and hemoptysis was reported in a 21-year-old treated with azathioprine for end-stage glomerulonephritis.[77] Improvement has been reported following withdrawal of the drug or treatment with corticosteroids or Cytoxan (Bristol-Myers Squibb Company, Princeton, New Jersey). Progressive deterioration and death have occurred in about one half of patients.

6-Mercaptopurine, Cytosine Arabinoside, and Gemcitabine

Scattered case reports have linked pulmonary dysfunction to 6-mercaptopurine and cytosine arabinoside (Ara-C). In addition, an autopsy study of patients who had leukemia and who received Ara-C within 30 days of death demonstrated significant pulmonary edema for which there was no obvious other explanation in most instances. An adult patient receiving low-dose Ara-C (20 mg/m^2/day) and recombinant human granulocyte-macrophage colony-stimulating factor (GM-CSF) developed ARDS on day 12 and died 40 days after initiation of therapy.[78] It has recently been reported that 5 of 22 pediatric patients receiving Ara-C (1.0–1.5 g/m^2/day) for treatment of acute myelogenous leukemia developed pulmonary insufficiency secondary to noncardiogenic pulmonary edema. The outcome was fatal in 3 of 5 patients.[79] Bronchiolitis obliterans organizing pneumonia (BOOP) developed in an adult patient with chronic myelogenous leukemia after treatment with Ara-C in combination with interferon-α; the condition resolved after discontinuation of these agents.[80] Gemcitabine, a drug similar in structure and metabolism to Ara-C, has been associated with ARDS in three patients.[81] These researchers reported that corticosteroids and diuretics were helpful, but two of the three patients died.

Other Cytotoxic Agents

Procarbazine, VM-26, and vinca alkaloids (vinblastine and vindesine) have been associated with pulmonary injury, but in all cases other agents may have contributed. Three of five young adults treated with a regimen of vinblastine, doxorubicin, bleomycin, and dacarbazine for Hodgkin's disease, and G-CSF to increase neutrophil counts, developed pulmonary toxicity in one report.[10] G-CSF may thus potentiate the lung toxicity of these agents. Reactions to procarbazine have been of the hypersensitivity type. Hydoxyurea has been reported to induce severe, corticosteroid-responsive, hypersensitivity pneumonitis.[82] Paclitaxel is a plant-derived taxane agent that causes irreversible microtubule aggregation, hence disrupting cell division. It has been used against a broad range of tumors, including breast, ovarian, lung, head, and neck cancers. It has been associated with a high frequency of hypersensitivity pneumonitis reactions of unknown etiology. Lung biopsy has shown interstitial pneumonitis, and BAL fluid has shown eosinophilia and lymphocytosis with a depressed CD4/CD8 ratio.[83] In a 5-year review of a series of cancer patients who received monthly paclitaxel infusions, the incidence of hypersensitivity reactions was 4%, and pretreatment with dexamethasone, diphenydramine, and histamine (H_2)-blockers was effective in preventing recurrence.[84] Docetaxel, a semisynthetic taxane, has been proposed as a safer alternative but has also occasionally been associated with severe hypersensitivity reactions.[85,86]

Gefitinib is an inhibitor of the tyrosine kinase activity of the epidermal growth factor receptor (EGFR). It was found to inhibit the growth of human cancer cell lines expressing EGFR in preclinical studies. In clinical trials in patients with non–small cell lung cancer, gefitinib was associated with development of interstitial lung disease in about 1% of patients. Patients presented with acute dyspnea with or without cough or fever at a median of 24 to 42 days after starting treatment. About one third of cases of gefitinib-associated interstitital lung disease have been fatal.[87,88]

NONCYTOTOXIC DRUGS

NITROFURANTOIN

Nitrofurantoin is an antimicrobial agent used in the prophylaxis of urinary tract infections. Significant pulmonary reactions are relatively common; more than 500 cases have been reported, including scattered reports in children (see Table 71-2).[89–94] Pulmonary reactions occur in two distinct clinical patterns. In the more common acute presentation, patients report the abrupt onset of fever, cough, and dyspnea usually within hours to 2 weeks after initiation of therapy. Rash and flulike symptoms may occur. Diffuse fine crackles and, rarely, wheezes are noted on chest examination. Bilateral interstitial or alveolar infiltrates with or without pleural effusion are characteristically present on chest radiographs; however, chest radiographs may be normal. Physiologic abnormalities include hypoxemia, evidence of a restrictive ventilatory defect, and a reduced DLCO. Eosinophilia, leukocytosis, and an elevated sedimentation rate may accompany the reaction. Symptoms and chest radiographic abnormalities usually resolve within several days after withdrawal of the drug. Pulmonary histopathology associated with the acute syndrome has not been well defined, as patients improve rapidly after withdrawal of nitrofurantoin, making biopsy unnecessary. Alveolar hemorrhage has been described in two patients with the atypical symptom of hemoptysis.[95,96]

In the less common chronic presentation, patients develop the insidious onset of cough, dyspnea, and fatigue after months to years of nitrofurantoin therapy. Fever may be present. A lupus-like syndrome has also been reported.[93] Crackles are heard, and diffuse, usually interstitial infiltrates are present on chest radiographs. Pleural effusion is less common than in the acute reaction. Physiologic abnormalities are similar to those found in the acute reaction, but are often more severe. Eosinophilia, elevated gamma globulin and hepatic enzymes, and positive reactions for antinuclear antibodies are often found. Pulmonary histopathology typically reveals an interstitial pneumonitis with a variable amount of fibrosis. Desquamative interstitial pneumonia and BOOP have also been reported in several adults on long-term nitrofurantoin therapy.[97,98] Treatment includes permanent withdrawal of the drug and supportive measures. Corticosteroids have been used with apparent benefit in some patients; however, controlled studies to evaluate efficacy are not available. Resolution of symptoms, physiologic dysfunction, and radiographic abnormalities requires weeks to months and may be incomplete. Approximately 8% of adult cases with the chronic syndrome are fatal.

Nitrofurantoin may injure the lungs by several mechanisms. The findings of eosinophilia, elevation of sedimentation rate, positive antinuclear antibodies, and an enhanced blastogenic response of lymphocytes from some patients in the presence of nitrofurantoin support a role for a hypersensitivity reaction.[99] The drug may also damage the lungs by promoting production of toxic oxygen species. Nitrofurantoin induces production of superoxide and hydrogen peroxide in aerobic cultures of rat lung microsomes and is cytotoxic to rat lung parenchymal cells.[100,101] Parenchymal cell injury is reduced by antioxidants and accelerated by hyperoxia, supporting a role for oxidant mechanisms.[101] Modulation of lung injury by antioxidants has also been described in an in vivo rat model.[102]

SULFASALAZINE

Sulfasalazine, a combination of sulfapyridine and 5-aminosalicylic acid, is used primarily in the treatment of ulcerative colitis. Adverse reactions occur in approximately 20% of recipients and include fever, nausea, vomiting, rash, and blood dyscrasias. Pulmonary reactions are uncommon; 50 cases were identified in a recent literature review.[103–123] Diagnosis of drug-related lung disease may be particularly troublesome, because ulcerative colitis can be associated with various lung disorders including bronchitis, BOOP, bronchiectasis, and interstitial pneumonitis.[124–126] Patients experiencing drug-related illness typically report acute onset of fever, cough, dyspnea, and chest pain 1 to 6 months into therapy. Fine crackles are usually present. Chest radiographs reveal bilateral alveolar densities. Eosinophilia is often present. Pulmonary function tests reveal hypoxemia and evidence of obstructive and occasionally restrictive lung disease. Cytology from BAL has been reported infrequently and has not shown a consistent pattern of cell predominance. Histopathologic lesions include interstitial pneumonitis with fibrosis, fibrosing alveolitis, and bronchiolitis obliterans with or without a component of organizing pneumonia. Discontinuation of the drug usually results in resolution of symptoms and radiographic abnormalities in several weeks to months. Corticosteroids may accelerate improvement, although their effectiveness is not well established. Two fatalities have been reported.[115] Mechanism of toxicity is unknown.[123]

DIPHENYLHYDANTOIN AND CARBAMAZEPINE

The anticonvulsant agents diphenylhydantoin and carbamazepine have been associated rarely with acute pulmonary disease as part of a generalized hypersensitivity reaction.[127–143] Clinical manifestations include fever, cough, dyspnea, and rash occurring 2 to 6 weeks (14 months in 1 patient) after initiation of therapy. Crackles and, rarely, wheezes are heard, and bilateral interstitial or alveolar infiltrate with hilar adenopathy in some instances is seen on chest radiographs. Associated findings include eosinophilia, elevated liver enzymes, hypoxemia with a restrictive pattern of lung function, and reduced DLCO. Cell counts from BAL reveal a lymphocyte predominance, and lung biopsy typically shows an interstitial pneumonitis possibly with mild fibrosis, although both drugs have been associated rarely with BOOP.[144,145] Ventilatory failure has been described in two patients.[136,143] Rapid improvement over days to weeks follows discontinuation of the drug. Resolution may be hastened by corticosteroid administration.

PENICILLAMINE

Penicillamine, a chelating agent, is commonly used to treat Wilson's disease, cystinuria, and lead poisoning and, occasionally, in the management of rheumatoid arthritis and primary biliary cirrhosis. Nonpulmonary toxic reactions are sufficiently severe in 25% of patients to require discontinuation of therapy. A conclusive association between this agent and lung disease is problematic because of the occurrence of similar lung disorders in the underlying diseases.[146] At least 37 cases of well-documented penicillamine-associated lung disease are reported, primarily in patients with rheumatoid arthritis.[147–165] Several patterns have been described: diffuse alveolitis; hypersensitivity pneumonitis; alveolar hemorrhage with or without associated acute glomerulonephritis, similar to Goodpasture's syndrome; and obstructive airway disease characterized pathologically as bronchiolitis obliterans. Duration of therapy before the onset of symptoms tends to be short in patients with hypersensitivity reactions (<2 months), intermediate in those with diffuse alveolitis and bronchiolitis obliterans (3–19 months), and prolonged in patients with alveolar hemorrhage (7 months to 20 years, but typically 2–7 years). Cough and dyspnea develop progressively over several weeks but may begin abruptly in hypersensitivity reactions and with hemoptysis. Crackles and, occasionally, wheezes are present. Elevation of sedimentation rate, increased serum IgE, and eosinophilia may be noted. Chest x-ray films show diffuse alveolar or interstitial infiltrate, hyperinflation alone, or no changes. Hypoxemia and severe obstructive lung disease in patients with bronchiolitis obliterans or restrictive disease in those with alveolitis or hypersensitivity disease are usually identified. Discontinuation of the drug and corticosteroid therapy are warranted in most cases. Diffuse alveolitis and hypersensitivity pneumonitis generally improve using this approach, although some patients have residual lung disease. Response to corticosteroids alone has been disappointing in most cases of bronchiolitis obliterans and alveolar hemorrhage. The addition of azathioprine or cyclophosphamide in combination with plasmapheresis in some cases has been beneficial in several patients with Goodpasture-like syndrome and in a single patient with broncholitis obliterans.[147,149,151,156,157,163,165]

GOLD

Gold compounds are used chiefly in the therapy of rheumatoid arthritis. Pulmonary reactions are uncommon, and diagnosis is difficult because of the occurrence of lung disease in rheumatoid arthritis. Pulmonary reactions to gold do occur in patients treated for other disorders not associated with lung disease such as other arthritides and pemphigus foliaceus. The predominant clinical syndrome is a hypersensitivity pneumonitis.[166–173] At least 140 well-documented cases have been reviewed.[171,173] Cough and progressive shortness of breath develop over days to weeks. Symptoms begin after 1 to 4 months of therapy. Crackles are present, and chest radiographs show diffuse interstitial and/or alveolar infiltrates. Eosinophilia is found in approximately 40% of patients, and the sedimentation rate is usually elevated. Lung function tests reveal hypoxemia, a reduced DLCO, and restrictive lung disease. Lung histopathology reveals widened alveolar septa, interstitial infiltrate with lymphocytes and plasma cells, and a variable amount of fibrosis. Proliferation of type II pneumocytes may be a prominent feature. An increase in total cell count and percentage of lymphocytes and reduction in helper to suppressor lymphocyte ratio has been found in BAL fluid from several patients.[171,173,174] Withdrawal of gold therapy is associated with improvement or resolution of lung disease over weeks to months. Improvement appears to be hastened by the addition of corticosteroid therapy and may be dramatic early in the course of illness. The prognosis for survival is good; however, a substantial number of patients have residual restrictive lung disease.

The mechanism of gold-induced lung injury is unknown. Some evidence suggests that the process may be related to a cell-mediated immune reaction, including eosinophilia, lymphocyte predominance and inverted $CD4^+/CD8^+$ lymphocyte ratios in BAL fluid (as often occurs in hypersensitivity pneumonitis), positive lymphocyte stimulation tests using lymphocytes from blood and fluid from BAL (though not consistently observed), and in vitro lymphokine release from peripheral mononuclear cells with gold exposure.[166,171,173]

Several cases of BOOP associated temporally with gold therapy have been reported, including a child with a fatal outcome.[175–179] All patients had rheumatoid arthritis, a disease associated with bronchiolitis obliterans, and none had received penicillamine. While further description is needed to definitively establish a link between gold therapy and bronchiolitis obliterans, available data support immediate discontinuation of the drug in patients with dyspnea, cough, and/or abnormal pulmonary function followed by comprehensive evaluation. Cyclophosphamide in conjunction with corticosteroids was beneficial in one case.[175]

AMIODARONE

Amiodarone, a benzofurane derivative with class III antiarrhythmic activity, is used in the treatment of serious cardiac rhythm disturbances.[180] Pulmonary toxicity is the most serious complication of therapy.[181–183] Risk of lung toxicity appears to be dose related. Approximately 5% to 15% of patients who take at least 500 mg/day and 0.1% to 0.5% of those who take up to 200 mg/day develop drug-related lung disease.[184] Most affected patients have been adults; however, evidence of lung toxicity has now been reported in at least three children.[185–187] Exposure to elevated concentrations of oxygen may represent another risk factor. The majority of patients insidiously develop cough, dyspnea with exertion, weight loss, weakness, and, in some instances, pleuritic chest pain and fever during the first year of therapy. Approximately one third of patients have an acute onset of symptoms, more consistent with a hypersensitivity pneumonitis. Chest examination reveals tachypnea, crackles, and occasionally a pleural friction rub. Diffuse or asymmetric interstitial and/or alveolar infiltrate is typically present on chest x-ray films. Pleural effusion is uncommon. High-resolution chest CT shows bilateral involvement with ground-glass opacities in a mosaic distribution accompanied by a crazy-paving pattern with or without subpleural consolidation and bronchial wall thickening or dilatation.[188] Laboratory findings include leukocytosis, elevated hepatic enzymes, and a high sedimentation rate. Physiologic abnormalities include hypoxemia, restrictive lung disease, and impairment of diffusion. Lung biopsy reveals infiltration of alveolar septa with lymphocytes, plasma cells and histiocytes, patchy fibrosis, hyperplasia of type II pneumocytes, and intra-alveolar foamy macrophages representing lysosomal accumulation of phospholipids.[189,190] Foamy macrophages can also be recovered in BAL fluid. Although their presence is not pathognomonic of drug-induced injury, it has been suggested that their absence makes the diagnosis unlikely. Discontinuation of the drug results in immediate symptomatic improvement in most patients and resolution of physiologic and radiographic abnormalities over several months. The role of corticosteroid therapy is not defined, although clinical evidence supports treatment. Recurrence of symptoms has been observed in some patients as steroid doses are tapered, potentially related to the extended storage of the drug in the lung. Alternative drug therapies are preferred. Reinstitution of amiodarone therapy at lower doses after resolution of pulmonary disease, alone or in combination with low-dose corticosteroid therapy, has been successful in a few patients.[191]

The mechanism by which amiodarone causes lung injury is unknown. The most striking morphologic alterations that require explanation are the accumulation of multilamellar bodies in the cytoplasm of various cells and inflammation. Direct toxicity is supported by the finding that amiodarone injures cultured pulmonary arterial endothelial cells at concentrations equivalent to those reported in lung tissues of toxic patients.[192] Cellular accumulation of phospholipid was also observed in these drug-exposed cultured endothelial cells, an event that may cause cell injury. The mechanism of phospholipid accumulation is thought to be related, at least in part, to inhibition of phospholipid degradation secondary to reduction in activity of lysosomal phospholipases A_1 and A_2 induced by the drug.[193,194] Acute administration of amiodarone to cultured alveolar macrophages inhibited degradation of surfactant protein A and caused release of lysosomal enzymes.[194] Oxidant-mediated lung injury has been proposed; however, study results are conflicting.[195,196] Apoptosis of human pulmonary epithelial cells induced by amiodarone has been demonstrated in vitro.[197] An indirect, immune-mediated mechanism has been suggested by the finding of increased polymorphonuclear leukocytes and/or lymphocytes and a marked reduction in the normal ratio of helper to suppressor T lymphocytes in BAL fluid from some patients.[198–200] Amiodarone can alter patterns of cytokine secretion by alveolar macrophages and activate natural killer cells, but it is unclear whether these changes are initiating events or the consequence of injury.[194] Regardless of mechanism, injury of lung cells can initiate a reparative process that leads to fibrosis.

INTERLEUKIN-2

IL-2 has been used in the treatment of certain cancers as an antitumor factor that stimulates lymphokine-activated killer (LAK) cell and natural killer cell activity. It is sometimes given in combination with LAK cells. Although a number of systemic side effects such as fever and hypotension are seen, the major toxicity of IL-2 therapy appears to be a vascular leak syndrome characterized by fluid retention, peripheral edema, ascites, pleural effusion, and pulmonary edema.[201] This syndrome has been described in children with acute lymphocytic leukemia treated with IL-2.[202] Infusion of IL-2 in cancer patients has resulted in increased alveolar-arterial oxygen difference and decreased forced vital capacity, forced expiratory volume in 1 second, and DLCO.[203,204] A retrospective review of chest radiographic abnormalities in 54 patients with metastatic cancer receiving IL-2 revealed that 52% developed pleural effusion, 41% developed pulmonary edema, and 22% developed focal infiltrates. While most changes resolved by 4 weeks after therapy, residual pleural effusion was sometimes seen primarily in patients receiving IL-2 by intravenous bolus rather than by continuous infusion.[205] Lung histopathologic studies in rodents show widespread mononuclear and eosinophilic infiltration of pulmonary parenchyma, increased lung weight, and endothelial damage.[206] Mechanisms implicated in this process are increased generation of oxygen free radicals, activation of complement by IL-2, and injury mediated by TNF-α.[207–209] Rapid recovery from the toxic effects of IL-2 appears to follow withholding of treatment in most cases.[204]

OTHER AGENTS

The parenteral administration of lipid emulsions to infants has been associated with lipid accumulation in pulmonary capillaries and small muscular arteries.[210,211] Physiologic alterations in clinical and experimental studies include transient hypoxemia, decreased diffusing capacity, and pulmonary hypertension.[212,213] Several experimental studies suggest that functional alterations may be greater in injured lungs.[214,215] Although hypertriglyceridemia has been implicated as a potential mechanism, further studies suggest that increased ventilation-perfusion inequalities secondary to prostaglandin-mediated alterations in pulmonary vasomotor tone may explain the hypoxemia.[215,216] Although adverse cardiopulmonary responses to lipid administration are recognized infrequently in clinical practice, early administration of fat emulsions in the first week of life has been associated with greater mortality in 600- to 800-g infants.[217] Administration of lipid emulsion to adult patients with ARDS has been associated with alteration in BAL fluid consistent with worsening of alveolar membrane permeability, abnormalities of pulmonary surfactants, and inflammation of lung tissue compared to ARDS patients who did not receive lipids or to those without acute lung injury who were treated with lipids. Worsening oxygenation and respiratory compliance and increased pulmonary vascular resistance occurred in ARDS patients treated with lipids but not in either control group.[218]

Acute respiratory deterioration has been observed when the antifungal agent amphotericin B is administered to potentially septic, neutropenic patients being given leukocyte transfusions. Patients develop the acute onset of cough, hemoptysis, dyspnea, and hypoxemia in association with the appearance of new infiltrates on chest radiographs. In one study, this syndrome developed in 64% of courses of combined therapy compared with 6% of courses of leukocyte transfusions alone.[219] Subsequent studies have questioned the role of a specific interaction between amphotericin B and granulocyte transfusions in episodes of respiratory deterioration.[220] Approximately 20 pulmonary reactions to amphotericin B or to the newer lipidic formulations without leukocyte transfusion have been reported, including two children.[221] Symptoms tend to resolve relatively quickly when the infusion is stopped. Pathophysiology of these reactions is unclear, although development of pulmonary hypertension may be an important component. The mechanism for these reactions is not understood. Amphotericin has been found to injure endothelial cells directly, cause neutrophil-independent injury, and release cyclo-oxygenase products of arachidonic acid metabolism.[221]

A number of other drugs have been implicated sporadically in the development of hypersensitivity/eosinophilic lung disease. Table 71-3 shows a representative list of medications implicated, with focus on medications that may be given to children or adolescents.[222–235] An extensive compilation has been published recently by Allen.[5] Drugs producing a clinical syndrome consistent with noncardiogenic pulmonary edema are listed in Table 71-4,[236–255] as reviewed recently by Lee-Chiong and Matthay.[255] Some are associated with this clinical syndrome only after an overdose. Intravenous drug abuse with methylphenidate and methadone has been associated with the development of panlobular emphysema, possibly related to injected talc.[256–259]

TABLE 71-3. Additional drugs associated with hypersensitivity/eosinophilic lung disease

Penicillin	Para-aminosalicylic acid	Cocaine
Ampicillin	Isoniazid	Heroin
Tetracycline	Cromolyn sodium	Dantrolene
Minocycline	Zafirlukast*	Chlorpropamide
Erythromycin	Montelukast*	Hydralazine
Clarithromycin	Methylphenidate	Enalapril
Cephalosporins	Imipramine	Captopril
Sulfa-containing antibiotics	Nonsteroidal anti-inflammatory agents‡	Ranitidine
	Trazodone‡	Mesalamine

*Associated with Churg-Strauss syndrome.
‡Includes naproxen, sulindac, piroxicam, fenbufen, diclofenac, and ibuprofen.
‡With overdose.

TABLE 71-4. Noncytotoxic drugs associated with noncardiogenic pulmonary edema

Aspirin*	Naloxone	Haloperidol
Propoxyphene*	Nitric oxide	Phenothiazines
Calcium channel blockers*	Morphine	Ethchlorvynol*
Propranolol	Heroin*	Tricyclic antidepressants*
Epinephrine	Methadone*	Hydrochlorothiazide
Phenylephrine	Cocaine	Acetazolamide
Lidocaine	Tocolytic agents	Radiographic contrast media

*Pulmonary edema associated with overdose.

■ **TABLE 71-5.** Drugs associated with impairment of mucociliary clearance

Aspirin	General anesthetics
Opiates	*N*-acetylcysteine
Ethanol	Anticholinergic agents

A number of drugs impair airway mucociliary clearance (Table 71-5).[260–267] One of these agents, *N*-acetylcysteine, has been used as an aerosolized mucolytic agent in the treatment of cystic fibrosis and in the bronchoscopic lavage of tenacious mucous plugs. Although its effects on mucociliary clearance after acute administration appear to be transient, repeated use of this agent is potentially deleterious. Contrary to the effects of other anticholinergic agents, the atropine analog ipratropium has not been found to impair mucociliary clearance.[268]

All-*trans* retinoic acid (ATRA), a vitamin A derivative with multiple regulatory activities in the lung, has been found to be effective as induction and maintenance chemotherapy for acute promyelocytic leukemia (APL). Its major toxicity is a syndrome including fever, weight gain and peripheral edema, respiratory distress, interstitial infiltrates, pleural and pericardial effusions, hyperleukocytosis, intermittent hypotension, and acute renal failure. Chest CT shows small, irregular parenchymal lung nodules and pleural effusions.[269] The incidence of ATRA syndrome was 26% in a large series of APL patients followed prospectively in a treatment protocol.[270] Among patients developing ATRA syndrome, mortality was 2%, including a 4-year-old child. Mean duration of therapy before the syndrome appeared was 11 days, with a range of 2 to 47 days. Nicolls and colleagues[271] reported an 18-year-old with APL who developed diffuse alveolar hemorrhage 15 days after starting ATRA. Lung histology in patients who died of ATRA syndrome shows differentiation of APL cells, endothelial cell damage, and leukocyte infiltration, consistent with the hypothesis that ATRA alters the adhesive properties of APL cells, leading to extravasation.[270] The mechanism of this is unclear, but recent work has suggested that ATRA up-regulates TNF receptors on lung cell lines.[272] In a murine model of APL, ATRA increased lung and heart expression of the chemokines macrophage inflammatory protein-2 and KC, suggesting that proinflammatory cytokines play a role. The syndrome was prevented by dexamethasone.[273] Treatment for ATRA syndrome consists of prompt initiation of corticosteroids. Tallman and colleagues[270] used dexamethasone 10 mg/day and found that the syndrome resolved rapidly in most patients, even if ATRA was continued. These researchers suggested that ATRA may be safely restarted in most patients once the syndrome has resolved.

■ CONCLUSION

Lung injury caused by pharmacologic agents is recognized increasingly as a significant clinical problem. Lung disease caused by cytotoxic agents is particularly troublesome in that chronicity is the rule and death is a frequent outcome. Precise information about risk factors, including genetic susceptibilities to specific drug toxicities, is required to bolster predictive capabilities for patients using these drugs. Additional information is needed about mechanisms of injury in order to develop more specific interventions. Finally, more sensitive and widely available diagnostic and monitoring approaches are important if early intervention is to be of value.

REFERENCES

1. Rosenow EC, Limper AH: Drug-induced pulmonary disease. Semin Respir Infect 1995;10:86–95.
2. Erasmus JJ, McAdams HP, Rossi SE: Drug-induced lung injury. Semin Roentgenol 2002;37:72–81.
3. Flieder DB, Travis WD: Pathologic characteristics of drug-induced lung disease. Clin Chest Med 2004;25:37–45.
4. Costabel U, Uzaslan E, Guzman J: Bronchoalveolar lavage in drug-induced lung disease. Clin Chest Med 2004;25:25–35.
5. Allen JN: Drug-induced eosinophilic lung disease. Clin Chest Med 2004; 25:77–88.
6. De Lena M, Guzzon A, Monfardini S, et al: Clinical, radiologic, and histopathologic studies on pulmonary toxicity induced by treatment with bleomycin (NSC-125066). Cancer Chemother Rep 1972;56:343–356.
7. O'Sullivan JM, Huddart RA, Norman AR, et al: Predicting the risk of bleomycin lung toxicity in patients with germ-cell tumours. Ann Oncol 2003;14:91–96.
8. Mertens AC, Yasui Y, Liu Y, et al: Pulmonary complications in survivors of childhood and adolescent cancer. Cancer 2002;95:2431–2441.
9. Ginsberg SJ, Comis RL: The pulmonary toxicity of antineoplastic agents. Semin Oncol 1982;9:34–51.
10. Matthews JH: Pulmonary toxicity of ABVD chemotherapy and G-CSF in Hodgkin's disease. Possible synergy. Lancet 1993;342:988.
11. Tarnell EB, Oliver BL, Johnson GM, et al: Superoxide anion production by rat neutrophils at various stages of bleomycin-induced lung injury. Lung 1992;170:41–50.
12. O'Neill CA, Giri SN: Biochemical mechanisms for the attenuation of bleomycin-induced lung fibrosis by treatment with niacin in hamsters. The role of NAD and ATP. Exp Lung Res 1994;20:41–56.
13. Serrano-Mollar A, Closa D, Prats N, et al: In vivo antioxidant protects against bleomycin-induced lung damage in rats. Br J Pharmacol 2003;138: 1037–1048.
14. Hoshino T, Nakamura H, Okamoto M, et al: Redox-active protein thioredoxin prevents proinflammatory cytokine- or bleomycin-induced lung injury. Am J Respir Crit Care Med 2003;168:1027–1028.
15. Aoshiba K, Tsuji T, Nagai A: Bleomycin induces cellular senescence in alveolar epithelial cells. Eur Respir J 2003;22:436–443.
16. Phan SH, Kunkel SL: Lung cytokine production in bleomycin-induced pulmonary fibrosis. Exp Lung Res 1992;18:29–32.
17. Giri SN, Sharma AK, Hyde DM, et al: Amelioration of bleomycin-induced lung fibrosis by treatment with the platelet activating factor receptor antagonist WEB 2086 in hamsters. Exp Lung Res 1994;21:287–307.
18. Zhang K, Gharaee-Kermani M, Jones ML, et al: Lung monocyte chemoattractant protein-1 gene expression in bleomycin-induced pulmonary fibrosis. J Immunol 1994;153:4733–4741.
19. Cui T, Kusunose M, Hamada A, et al: Relationship between the eosinophilia of bronchoalveolar lavage fluid (BALF) and the severity of pulmonary fibrosis induced by bleomycin in rats. Biol Pharm Bull 2003;26:959–963.
20. Koslowski R, Knoch K, Kuhlisch E, et al: Cathepsins in bleomycin-induced lung injury in rat. Eur Respir J 2003;22:427–435.
21. Huaux F, Liu T, McGarry B, et al: Eosinophils and T lymphocytes possess distinct roles in bleomycin-induced lung injury and fibrosis. J Immunol 2003;171:5470–5481.
22. Teder P, Nettelbadt O, Heldin P: Characterization of the mechanism involved in bleomycin-induced increased hyaluranon production in rat lung. Am J Respir Cell Mol Biol 1995;12:181–189.
23. Suzuki H, Aoshiba K, Yokohori N, et al: Epidermal growth factor receptor tyrosine kinase inhibition augments a murine model of pulmonary fibrosis. Cancer Res 2003;63:5054–5059.
24. Gunther A, Lubke N, Ermert M, et al: Prevention of bleomycin-induced lung fibrosis by aerosolization of heparin or urokinase in rabbits. Am J Respir Crit Care Med 2003;168:1358–1365.
25. Balazs G, Noma S, Khan A, et al: Bleomycin-induced fibrosis in pigs. Evaluation with CT. Radiology 1994;191:269–272.
26. Kuhlman JE: The role of chest computed tomography in the diagnosis of drug-related reactions. J Thorac Imaging 1991;6:52–61.
27. Comis RL: Bleomycin pulmonary toxicity. Current status and future directions. Semin Oncol 1992;19:64–70.
28. Lund MB, Kongerud J, Nome O, et al: Lung function impairment in long-term survivors of Hodgkin's disease. Ann Oncol 1995;6:495–501.

29. Maher J, Daly PA: Severe bleomycin lung toxicity. Reversal with high dose corticosteroids. Thorax 1993;48:92–94.
30. Capizzi RL: The preclinical basis for broad-spectrum selective cytoprotection of normal tissues from cytotoxic therapies by amifostine. Semin Oncol 1999;26(Suppl 7):3–21.
31. Cronin S, Uberti JP, Ayash LJ, et al: Use of amifostine as a chemoprotectant during high-dose chemotherapy in autologous peripheral blood stem cell transplantation. Bone Marrow Transplant 2000;26:1247–1249.
32. Adachi K, Suzuki M, Sugimoto T, et al: Effects of granulocyte colony-stimulating factor on the kinetics of inflammatory cells in the peripheral blood and pulmonary lesions during the development of bleomycin-induced lung injury in rats. Exp Toxicol Pathol 2003;55:21–32.
33. Saxman SB, Nichols CR, Einhorn LH: Pulmonary toxicity in patients with advanced stage germ cell tumors receiving bleomycin with and without granulocyte colony stimulating factor. Chest 1997;111:657–660.
34. Linette DC, McGee KH, McFarland JA: Mitomycin-induced pulmonary toxicity. Case report and review of the literature. Ann Pharmacother 1992;26:481–484.
35. Rivera MP, Kris MG, Gralla RJ, et al: Syndrome of acute dyspnea related to combined mitomycin plus vinca alkaloid chemotherapy. Am J Clin Oncol 1995;18:245–250.
36. Gunstream SR, Seidenfeld JJ, Sobonya RE, et al: Mitomycin-associated lung disease. Cancer Treat Rep 1983;67:301–304.
37. Orwoll ES, Kiessling PJ, Patterson JR: Interstitial pneumonia from mitomycin. Ann Intern Med 1978;89:352–355.
38. Queffeulou G, Ducloux D, Faucher C, et al: Fatal cyclophosphamide-induced interstitial pneumonitis in a renal transplant patient. Nephrol Dial Transplant 1994;9:1655–1657.
39. Hamada K, Nagai S, Kitaichi M, et al: Cyclophosphamide-induced late-onset lung disease. Intern Med 2003;42:82–87.
40. Frankovich J, Donaldson SS, Lee Y, et al: High-dose therapy and autologous hematopoietic cell transplantation in children with primary refractory and relapsed Hodgkin's disease. Atopy predicts idiopathic diffuse lung injury syndromes. Biol Blood Marrow Transplant 2001;7:49–57.
41. Kachel DL, Martin WJ: Cyclophosphamide-induced lung toxicity. Mechanism of endothelial cell injury. J Pharmacol Exp Ther 1994;268:42–46.
42. Venkatesan N, Chandrakasan G: Cyclophosphamide induced early biochemical changes in lung lavage fluid and alterations in lavage cell function. Lung 1994;172:147–158.
43. Venkatesan N, Chandrakasan G: In vivo administration of taurine and niacin modulate cyclophosphamide-induced lung injury. Eur J Pharmacol 1994;292:75–80.
44. Venkatesan N, Chandrakasan G: Modulation of cyclophosphamide-induced early lung injury by curcumin, an anti-inflammatory antioxidant. Mol Cell Biochem 1995;142:79–87.
45. Topilow AA, Rothenberg SP, Cottrell TS: Interstitial pneumonia after prolonged treatment with cyclophosphamide. Am Rev Respir Dis 1973;108:114–117.
46. Alvarado CS, Boat TF, Newman AJ: Late-onset pulmonary fibrosis and chest deformity in two children treated with cyclophosphamide. J Pediatr 1978;92:443–446.
47. Spector JI, Zimbler H, Ross JS: Cyclophosphamide and interstitial pneumonitis. JAMA 1980;243:1133.
48. Israel HL, McComb BL: Chlorambucil treatment of sarcoidosis. Sarcoidosis 1991;8:35–41.
49. Cole SR, Myers TJ, Klatsky AU: Pulmonary disease with chlorambucil therapy. Cancer 1978;41:455–459.
50. Godard P, Marty JP, Michel FB: Interstitial pneumonia and chlorambucil. Chest 1979;76:471–473.
51. Khong HT, McCarthy J: Chlorambucil-induced pulmonary disease. A case report and review of the literature. Ann Hematol 1998;77:85–87.
52. Burns WA, McFarland W, Matthews MJ: Busulfan-induced pulmonary disease. Am Rev Respir Dis 1970;101:408–413.
53. Soble AP, Perry H: Fatal radiation pneumonia following subclinical busulfan injury. AJR Am J Roentgenol 1977;128:15–18.
54. Crilley P, Topolsky D, Styler MJ, et al: Extramedullary toxicity of a conditioning regimen containing busulphan, cyclophosphamide and etoposide in 84 patients undergoing autologous and allogenic bone marrow transplantation. Bone Marrrow Transplant 1995;15:361–365.
55. Quigley PM, Yeager AM, Loughlin GM: The effects of bone marrow transplantation on pulmonary function in children. Pediatr Pulmonol 1994;18:361–367.
56. Taetle R, Dickman PS, Feldman PS: Pulmonary histopathologic changes associated with melphalan therapy. Cancer 1978;42:1239–1245.
57. Goucher G, Rowland V, Hawkins J: Melphalan-induced pulmonary interstitial fibrosis. Chest 1980;77:805–806.
58. Aronin PA, Mahaley MS, Rudnick SA, et al: Prediction of BCNU pulmonary toxicity in patients with malignant gliomas. N Engl J Med 1980;303:183–188.
59. Alessandrino EP, Bernasconi P, Colombo A, et al: Pulmonary toxicity following carmustine-based preparative regimens and autologous peripheral blood progenitor cell transplantation in hematological malignancies. Bone Marrow Transplant 2000;25:309–313.
60. Rubio C, Hill ME, Milan S, et al: Idiopathic pneumonia syndrome after high-dose chemotherapy for relapsed Hodgkin's disease. Br J Cancer 1997;75:1044–1048.
61. Hasleton PS, O'Driscoll BR, Lynch P, et al: Late BCNU lung. A light and ultrastructural study on the delayed effect of BCNU on the lung parenchyma. J Pathol 1991;164:31–36.
62. Hwu WJ, Mozdziesz DE: Molecular basis for thymidine modulation of the efficacy and toxicity of alkylating agents. Pharmacol Ther 1997;76:101–116.
63. Stuart MJ, Chao NS, Horning SJ, et al: Efficacy and toxicity of a CCNU-containing high-dose chemotherapy regimen followed by autologous hematopoietic cell transplantation in relapsed or refractory Hodgkin's disease. Biol Blood Marrow Transplant 2001;7:552–560.
64. Olsen EA: The pharmacology of methotrexate. J Am Acad Dermatol 1991;25:306–318.
65. Barrera P, Laan RFJM, van Riel PLCM, et al: Methotrexate-related pulmonary complications in rheumatoid arthritis. Ann Rheum Dis 1994;53:434–439.
66. Sostman HD, Matthay RA, Putman CE, et al: Methotrexate-induced pneumonitis. Medicine 1976;55:371–388
67. Gillespie AM, Lorigan PC, Radstone CR, et al: Pulmonary function in patients with trophoblastic disease treated with low-dose methotrexate. Br J Cancer 1997;76:1382–1386.
68. Schmeling H, Stephan V, Burdach S, et al: Pulmonary function in children with juvenile idiopathic arthritis and effects of methotrexate therapy. J Rheumatol 2002;61:168–172.
69. St Clair EW, Rice JR, Snyderman R: Pneumonitis complicating low-dose methotrexate therapy in rheumatoid arthritis. Arch Intern Med 1985;145:2035–2038.
70. Imokawa S, Colby TV, Leslie KO, et al: Methotrexate pneumonitis. Review of the literature and histopathological findings in nine patients. Eur Respir J 2000;15:373–381.
71. Salaffi F, Manganelli P, Carotti M, et al: Methotrexate-induced pneumonitis in patients with rheumatoid arthritis and psoriatic arthritis. Report of five cases and review of the literature. Clin Rheumatol 1997;16:296–304.
72. Fuhrman C, Parrot A, Wislez M, et al: Spectrum of CD4 to CD8 T-cell ratios in lymphocytic alveolitis associated with methotrexate-induced pneumonitis. Am J Respir Crit Care Med 2001;164:1186–1191.
73. Hargreaves MR, Mowat AG, Benson MK: Acute pneumonitis associated with low dose methotrexate therapy for rheumatoid arthritis. Report of five cases and review of published reports. Thorax 1992;47:628–633.
74. Kremer JM, Alarcon GS, Weinblatt ME, et al: Clinical, laboratory, radiographic, and histopathologic features of methotrexate-associated lung injury in patients with rheumatoid arthritis. A multicenter study with literature review. Arthritis Rheum 1998;41:1327–1328.
75. Riedler J, Golser A, Huttegger I: Fibrosing alveolitis in an infant. Eur Respir J 1992;5:359–361.
76. Carmichael DJS, Hamilton DV, Evans DB, et al: Interstitial pneumonitis secondary to azathioprine in a renal transplant patient. Thorax 1983;38:951–952.
77. Stetter M, Schmidl M, Krapf R: Azathioprine hypersensitivity mimicking Goodpasture's syndrome. Am J Kidney Dis 1994;23:874–877.
78. Verhoef G, Boogaerts M: Treatment with granulocyte-macrophage colony stimulating factor and the adult respiratory distress syndrome. Am J Hematol 1991;36:285–287.
79. Shearer P, Katz J, Bozeman P, et al: Pulmonary insufficiency complicating therapy with high dose cytosine arabinoside in five pediatric patients with relapsed acute myelogenous leukemia. Cancer 1994;74:1953–1958.
80. Patel M, Ezzat W, Pauw KL, et al: Bronchiolitis obliterans organizing pneumonia in a patient with chronic myelogenous leukemia developing after initiation of interferon and cytosine arabinoside. Eur J Haematol 2001;67:318–321.
81. Pavlakis N, Bell DR, Millward MJ, et al: Fatal pulmonary toxicity resulting from treatment with gemcitabine. Cancer 1997;80:286–291.
82. Sandhu HS, Barnes PJ, Hernandez P: Hydroxyurea-induced hypersensitivity pneumonitis. A case report and literature review. Can Respir J 2000;7:491–495.

83. Fujimori K, Yokoyama A, Kurita Y, et al: Paclitaxel-induced cell-mediated hypersensitivity pneumonitis. Diagnosis using leukocyte migration test, bronchoalveolar lavage and transbronchial biopsy. Oncology 1998;55:340–344.
84. Quock J, Dea G, Tanaka M, et al: Premedication strategy for weekly paclitaxel. Cancer Invest 2002;20:666–672.
85. Bernstein BJ: Docetaxel as an alternative to paclitaxel after acute hypersensitivity reactions. Ann Pharmacother 2000;34:1332–1335.
86. Wang GS, Yang KY, Perng RP: Life-threatening hypersensitivity pneumonitis induced by docatexel (taxotere). Br J Cancer 2001;85:1247–1250.
87. Cohen MH, Williams GA, Sridhara R, et al: FDA drug approval summary. Gefitinib (ZD1839) (Iressa) tablets. Oncologist 2003;8:303–306.
88. Rabinowits G, Herchenhorn D, Rabinowits M, et al: Fatal pulmonary toxicity in a patient treated with gefitinib for non–small cell lung cancer after previous hemolytic-uremic syndrome due to gemcitabine. Anticancer Drugs 2003;14:665–668.
89. Mullick FG, Drake RM, Irey NS: Morphologic changes in adverse drug reactions in infants and children. Hum Pathol 1977;8:361–378.
90. Sovijarvi ARA, Lemola M, Stenius B, et al: Nitrofurantoin-induced acute, subacute and chronic pulmonary reactions. Scand J Respir Dis 1977;58:41–50.
91. Rantala H, Kirvela O, Anttolainen I: Nitrofurantoin lung in a child. Lancet 1979;2:799–800.
92. Holmberg L, Boman G: Pulmonary reactions to nitrofurantoin: 447 cases reported to the Swedish Adverse Drug Reaction Committee 1966–1976. Eur J Respir Dis 1981;62:180–189.
93. Broughton RA, Wilson HD: Nitrofurantoin pulmonary toxicity in a child. Pediatr Infect Dis 1986;5:466–469.
94. Cooper JAD Jr, White DA, Matthay RA: Drug induced pulmonary disease I. Cytotoxic drugs. II. Noncytotoxic drugs. Am Rev Respir Dis 1986;133:321–340, 488–505.
95. Averbuch SD, Yungbluth P: Fatal pulmonary hemorrhage due to nitrofurantoin. Ann Intern Med 1980;140:271–273.
96. Bucknall CE, Adamson MR, Banham SW: Nonfatal pulmonary haemorrhage associated with nitrofurantoin. Thorax 1987;42:475–476.
97. Cameron RJ, Kolbe J, Wilsher ML, et al: Bronchiolitis obliterans organizing pneumonia associated with the use of nitrofurantoin. Thorax 2000;55:249–251.
98. Fawcett IW: BOOP associated with nitrofurantoin. Thorax 2001;56:161.
99. Back O, Liden S, Ahlstedt S: Adverse reactions to nitrofurantoin in relation to cellular and humoral immune responses. Clin Exp Immunol 1977;28:400–406.
100. Sasame HA, Boyd MR: Superoxide and hydrogen peroxide production and NADPH oxidation stimulated by nitrofurantoin in lung microsomes. Possible implications for toxicity. Life Sci 1979;24:1091–1096.
101. Martin WJ II: Nitrofurantoin. Evidence for the oxidant injury of lung parenchymal cells. Am Rev Respir Dis 1983;127:482–486.
102. Boyd MR, Catignani GL, Sasame HA, et al: Acute pulmonary injury in rats by nitrofurantoin and modification by vitamin E, dietary fat, and oxygen. Am Rev Respir Dis 1979;120:93–99.
103. Berliner S, Neeman A, Shoenfeld Y, et al: Salazopyrin-induced eosinophilic pneumonia. Respiration 1980;39:119–120.
104. Williams T, Eidus L, Thomas P: Fibrosing alveolitis, bronchiolitis obliterans, and sulfasalazine therapy. Chest 1982;81:766–768.
105. Sigvaldason A, Sorenson S: Interstitial pneumonia due to sulfasalazine. Eur J Respir Dis 1983;64:229–233.
106. Yaffe BH, Korelitz BI: Sulfasalazine pneumonitis. Am J Gastroenterol 1983;78:493–494.
107. Wang KK, Bowyer BA, Fleming CR, et al: Pulmonary infiltrates and eosinophilia associated with sulfasalazine. Mayo Clin Proc 1984;59:343–346.
108. Averbuch M, Halpern Z, Hallak A, et al: Sulfasalazine pneumonitis. Am J Gastroenterol 1985;80:343–345.
109. Cazzadori A, Braggio P, Bontempini L: Salazoprin-induced eosinophilic pneumonia. Respiration 1985;47:158–160.
110. Moseley RH, Barwick KW, Dobuler K, et al: Sulfasalazine-induced pulmonary disease. Dig Dis Sci 1985;30:901–904.
111. Sullivan SN: Sulfasalazine lung. J Clin Gastroenterol 1987;9:461–463.
112. Valcke Y, Pauwels R, Van Der Straeten M: Bronchoalveolar lavage in acute hypersensitivity pneumonitis caused by sulfasalazine. Chest 1987;92:572–573.
113. Jordan A, Cowan RE: Reversible pulmonary disease and eosinophilia associated with sulphasalazine. J R Soc Med 1988;81:233–235.
114. Boyd O, Gibbs AR, Smith AP: Fibrosing alveolitis due to sulphasalazine in a patient with rheumatoid arthritis. Br J Rheumatol 1990;29:222–224.
115. Leino R, Liippo K, Ekfors T: Sulphasalazine-induced reversible hypersensitivity pneumonitis and fatal fibrosing alveolitis. Report of two cases. J Intern Med 1991;229:553–556.
116. Moss SF, Ind PW: Time course of recovery of lung function in sulphasalazine-induced alveolitis. Respir Med 1991;85:73–75.
117. Panayiotou BN: Pulmonary infiltrates and eosinophilia associated with sulphasalazine administration. Aust N Z J Med 1991;21:348–349.
118. Gabazza EC, Taguchi O, Yamakami T, et al: Pulmonary infiltrates and skin pigmentation associated with sulfasalazine. Am J Gastroentol 1992;87:1654–1657.
119. Hamadeh MA, Atkinson J, Smith LJ: Sulfasalazine-induced pulmonary disease. Chest 1992;101:1033–1037.
120. Case records of the Massachusetts General Hospital: Case 12-1993. A 44-year-old man with pulmonary disease and proctitis. N Engl J Med 1993;328:869–876.
121. Kolbe J, Caughey D, Rainer S: Sulphasalazine-induced subacute hypersensitivity pneumonitis. Respir Med 1994;88:149–152.
122. Salero SM, Ormseth EJ, Roth BJ, et al: Sulfasalazine pulmonary toxicity in ulcerative colitis mimicking clinical features of Wegener's granulomatosis. Chest 1996;110:556–559.
123. Parry SD, Barbatzas C, Peel ET, et al: Sulphasalazine and lung toxicity. Eur Respir J 2002;19:756–764.
124. Camus P, Piard F, Ashcroft T, et al: The lung in inflammatory bowel disease. Medicine 1993;72:151–183.
125. Mazer BD, Eigen H, Gelfand EW, et al: Remission of interstitial lung disease following therapy of associated ulcerative colitis. Pediatr Pulmonol 1993;15:555–559.
126. Teague WG, Sutphen JL, Fechner RE: Desquamative interstitial pneumonitis complicating inflammatory bowel disease of childhood. J Pediatr Gastroenterol Nutr 1985;4:663–637.
127. Fruchter L, Laptook A: Diphenylhydantoin hypersensitivity reaction associated with interstitial pulmonary infiltrates and hypereosinophilia. Ann Allergy 1981;47:453–455.
128. Lee T, Cochrane GM: Pulmonary eosinophilia and asthma associated with carbamazepine. BMJ 1981;282:440.
129. Michael JR, Rudin ML: Acute pulmonary disease caused by phenytoin. Ann Intern Med 1981;95:452–454.
130. Taylor MW, Smith CC, Hern JEC: An unexpected reaction to carbamazepine. Practitioner 1981;225:219–220.
131. Lewis IJ, Rosenbloom L: Glandular fever-like syndrome, pulmonary eosinophilia and asthma associated with carbamazepine. Postgrad Med J 1982;58:100–101.
132. Tolmie J, Steer CR, Edmunds AT: Pulmonary eosinophilia associated with carbamazepine. Arch Dis Child 1983;58:833–834.
133. De Swert LF, Ceuppens JL, Teuwen D, et al: Acute interstitial pneumonitis and carbamazepine therapy. Acta Paediatr Scand 1984;73:285–288.
134. Munn NJ, Baughman RP, Ploysongsang Y, et al: Bronchoalveolar lavage in acute drug-hypersensitivity pneumonitis probably caused by phenytoin. South Med J 1984;77:1594–1596.
135. Chamberlain DW, Hyland RJ, Ross DJ: Diphenylhydantoin-induced lymphocytic interstitial pneumonia. Chest 1986;90:458–459.
136. Mahatma M, Haponik EF, Nelson S, et al: Phenytoin-induced acute respiratory failure with pulmonary eosinophilia. Am J Med 1989;87:93–94.
137. Barreiro B, Manresa F, Valldeperas J: Carbamazepine and the lung. Eur Respir J 1990;3:930–931.
138. Katzin WE, Julius CJ, Tubbs RR, et al: Lymphoproliferative disorders associated with carbamazepine. Arch Pathol Lab Med 1990;114:1244–1248.
139. Takahashi N, Aizawa H, Takata S, et al: Acute interstitial pneumonitis induced by carbamazepine. Eur Respir J 1993;6:1409–1411.
140. Khan AS, Dadparvar S, Brown SJ, et al: The role of gallium-67-citrate in the detection of phenytoin-induced pneumonitis. J Nucl Med 1994;35:471–473.
141. King GG, Barnes DJ, Hayes MJ: Carbamazepine-induced pneumonitis. Med J Aust 1994;160:126–127.
142. De Vriese ASP, Philippe J, Van Renterghem DM, et al: Carbamazepine hypersensitivity syndrome. Report of 4 cases and review of the literature. Medicine 1995;74:144–151.
143. Murphy D, Kronick JB, Rieder MJ: Acute respiratory failure mediated by reactive drug metabolites. Biol Neonate 1995;67:223–229.
144. Angle P, Thomas P, Chiu B, et al: Bronchiolitis obliterans with organizing pneumonia and cold agglutinin disease associated with phenytoin hypersensitivity syndrome. Chest 1997;112:1697–1699.
145. Milesi AM, Schmidt J, Aumaitre O, et al: Lupus and pulmonary nodules consistent with bronchiolitis obliterans organizing pneumonia induced by carbamazepine. Mayo Clin Proc 1997;72:1145–1147.

146. Anaya J-M, Diethelm L, Ortiz LA, et al: Pulmonary involvement in rheumatoid arthritis. Semin Arthritis Rheum 1995;24:242–254.
147. Gibson T, Burry HC, Ogg C: Goodpasture syndrome and D-penicillamine. Ann Intern Med 1976;84:100.
148. Davies D, Jones JKL: Pulmonary eosinophilia caused by penicillamine. Thorax 1980;35:957–958.
149. Matloff DS, Kaplan MM: D-penicillamine-induced Goodpasture's-like syndrome in primary biliary cirrhosis—Successful treatment with plasmapheresis and immunosuppressives. Gastroenterology 1980;78:1046–1049.
150. Stein HB, Patterson AC, Offer RC, et al: Adverse effects of D-penicillamine in rheumatoid arthritis. Ann Intern Med 1980;92:24–29.
151. Gavaghan TE, McNaught PJ, Ralson M, et al: Penicillamine-induced "Goodpasture's syndrome." Successful treatment of a fulminant case. Aust N Z J Med 1981;11:261–265.
152. Murphy KC, Atkins CJ, Offer RC, et al: Obliterative bronchiolitis in two rheumatoid arthritis patients treated with penicillamine. Arthritis Rheum 1981;24:557–560.
153. Scott DL, Bradby GVH, Aitman TJ, et al: Relationship of gold and penicillamine therapy to diffuse interstitial lung disease. Ann Rheum Dis 1981;40:136–141.
154. Camus P, Degat OR, Justrabo E, et al: D-penicillamine-induced severe pneumonitis. Chest 1982;81:376–378.
155. Jansen HM, Elema JD, Hylkema BS, et al: Progressive obliterative bronchiolitis in a patient with rheumatoid arthritis. Eur J Respir Dis 1982; 63(Suppl 121):43–52.
156. Penny WJ, Knight RK, Rees AM, et al: Obliterative bronchiolitis in rheumatoid arthritis. Ann Rheum Dis 1982;41:469–472.
157. Swainson CP, Thomson D, Short AIK, et al: Plasma exchange in the successful treatment of drug induced renal disease. Nephron 1982;30:244–249.
158. Wolfe F, Schurle DR, Lin JJ, et al: Upper and lower airway disease in penicillamine treated patients with rheumatoid arthritis. J Rheumatol 1983;10:406–410.
159. Shettar SP, Chattopadhyay C, Wolstenholme RJ, et al: Diffuse alveolitis on a small dose of penicillamine. Br J Rheumatol 1984;23:220-224.
160. Kumar A, Bhat A, Gupta DK, et al: D-penicillamine-induced acute hypersensitivity pneumonitis and cholestatic hepatitis in a patient with rheumatoid arthritis. Clin Exp Rheumatol 1985;3:337–339.
161. van der Laar MAFJ, Westermann CJJ, Wagenaar SS, et al: Beneficial effect of intravenous cyclophosphamide and oral prednisone on D-penicillamine-associated bronchiolitis obliterans. Arthritis Rheum 1985;28:93–97.
162. Louie S, Gamble CN, Cross CE: Penicillamine associated pulmonary hemorrhage. J Rheumatol 1986;3:963–966.
163. Peces R, Riera JR, Arboleya LR, et al: Goodpasture's syndrome in a patient receiving penicillamine and carbimazole. Nephron 1987;45:316–320.
164. Zitnik RJ, Cooper JAD Jr: Pulmonary disease due to antirheumatic agents. Clin Chest Med 1990;11:139–150.
165. Derk C, Jimenez SA: Goodpasture-like syndrome induced by a D-penicillamine in a patient with systemic sclerosis. Report and review of the literature. J Rheumatol 2003;30:1616–1620.
166. McCormick J, Cole S, Lahirir B, et al: Pneumonitis caused by gold salt therapy. Evidence for the role of cell-mediated immunity in its pathogenesis. Am Rev Respir Dis 1980;122:145–152.
167. Smith W, Ball GV: Lung injury due to gold treatment. Arthritis Rheum 1980;23:351–354.
168. Levinson ML, Lynch JP III, Bower JS: Reversal of progressive, life-threatening gold hypersensitivity pneumonitis by corticosteroids. Am J Med 1981;71:908–912.
169. Morley TF, Komansky HJ, Adelizzi RA, et al: Pulmonary gold toxicity. Eur J Respir Dis 1984;65:627–632.
170. Akoun GM, Herman DP, Mayaud CM, et al: Bronchoalveolar T-cell subsets in gold lung [Letter]. Chest 1985;87:135.
171. Evans RB, Ettensohn DB, Fawaz-Estrup F, et al: Gold lung. Recent developments in the pathogenesis, diagnosis, and therapy. Semin Arthritis Rheum 1987;16:196–205.
172. Zitnik RJ, Cooper JAD Jr: Pulmonary disease due to antirheumatic agents. Clin Chest Med 1990;11:139–150.
173. Tomioka H, King TE Jr: Gold-induced pulmonary disease. Clinical features, outcome, and differentiation from rheumatoid lung disease. Am J Respir Crit Care Med 1997;155:1011–1020.
174. Costabel U, Schmitz-Schumann M, Matthys H: Bronchoalveolar T-cell subsets in gold lung [Letter]. Chest 1985;87:135.
175. Fort JG, Scovern H, Arbruzzo JL: Intravenous cyclophosphamide and methylprednisolone for the treatment of bronchiolitis obliterans and interstitial fibrosis associated with crysotherapy. J Rheumatol 1988;15: 850–854.
176. Holness L, Tenenbaum J, Cooter NBE, et al: Fatal bronchiolitis obliterans associated with chrysotherapy. Ann Rheum Dis 1983;42:593–596.
177. O'Duffy JD, Luthra HS, Unni KK, et al: Bronchiolitis in a rheumatoid arthritis patient receiving auranofin. Arthritis Rheum 1986;29:556–559.
178. Pegg SJ, Lang BA, Mikhail EL, et al: Fatal bronchiolitis obliterans in a patient with juvenile rheumatoid arthritis receiving chrysotherapy. J Rheumatol 1994;21:549–551.
179. Epler GR: Drug-induced bronchiolitis obliterans organizing pneumonia. Clin Chest Med 2004;25:89–94.
180. Paul T, Guccione P: New antiarrhythmic drugs in pediatric use. Amiodarone. Pediatr Cardiol 1994;15:132–138.
181. Martin WJ II, Rosenow EC III: Amiodarone pulmonary toxicity—Recognition and pathogenesis (parts 1 and 2). Chest 1988;93:1067–1075, 1242–1248.
182. Dusman RE, Stanton MS, Miles WM, et al: Clinical features of amiodarone-induced pulmonary toxicity. Circulation 1990;82:51–59.
183. Kennedy JI Jr: Clinical aspects of amiodarone pulmonary toxicity. Clin Chest Med 1990;11:119–129.
184. Camus P, Martin WJ II, Rosenow EC III: Amiodarone pulmonary toxicity. Clin Chest Med 2004;25:65–75.
185. Daniels CJ, Schutte DA, Hammond S, et al: Acute pulmonary toxicity in an infant from intravenous amiodarone. Am J Cardiol 1997;80:1113–1116.
186. Kothari SS, Balijepally S, Taneja K: Amiodarone-induced pulmonary toxicity in an adolescent. Cardiol Young 1999;9:194–196.
187. Bowers PN, Fields J, Schwartz D, et al: Amiodarone induced pulmonary fibrosis in infancy. PACE 1998;21:1665–1667.
188. Vernhet H, Bousquet C, Durand G, et al: Reversible amiodarone-induced lung disease. HRCT findings. Eur Radiol 2001;11:1697–1703.
189. Myers JL, Kennedy JI, Plumb VJ: Amiodarone lung. Pathologic findings in clinically toxic patients. Hum Pathol 1987;18:349–354.
190. Bedrossian CWM, Warren CJ, Ohar J, et al: Amiodarone pulmonary toxicity. Cytopathology, ultrastructure, and immunocytochemistry. Ann Diagn Pathol 1997;1:47–56.
191. Zaher C, Hamer A, Peter T, et al: Low dose steroid therapy for prophylaxis of amiodarone-induced pulmonary infiltrates. N Engl J Med 1983;308:779.
192. Martin WJ II, Howard DM: Amiodarone-induced lung toxicity. In vitro evidence for the direct toxicity of the drug. Am J Pathol 1985;120:344–350.
193. Hostetler KY, Reasor MJ, Walker ER, et al: Role of phospholipase A inhibition in amiodarone pulmonary toxicity in rats. Biochim Biophys Acta 1986;875:400–405.
194. Baritussio A, Marzini S, Agostini M, et al: Amiodarone inhibits lung degradation of SP-A and perturbs the distribution of lysosomal enzymes. Am J Physiol Lung Cell Mol Physiol 2001;281:L1189–L1199.
195. Leeder RG, Brien JF, Massey TE: Investigation of the role of oxidative stress in amiodarone-induced pulmonary toxicity in the hamster. Can J Physiol Pharmacol 1994;72:613–621.
196. Zitnik RJ, Cooper JAD Jr, Rankin JA, et al: Effects of in vitro amiodarone exposure on alveolar macrophage inflammatory mediator production. Am J Med Sci 1992;304:352–356.
197. Choi IS, Kim BS, Cho KS, et al: Amiodarone induces apoptosis in L-132 human lung epithelial cell line. Toxicol Lett 2002;132:47–55.
198. Israel-Biet D, Venet A, Caubarrere I, et al: Bronchoalveolar lavage in amiodarone pneumonitis. Cellular abnormalities and their relevance to pathogenesis. Chest 1987;91:214–221.
199. Akoun GM, Cadranel JL, Blanchette G, et al: Bronchoalveolar lavage cell data in amiodarone-associated pneumonitis. Chest 1991;99:1177–1182.
200. Coudert B, Bailly F, Lombard JN, et al: Amiodarone pneumonitis. Bronchoalveolar lavage findings in 15 patients and review of the literature. Chest 1992;102:1005–1012.
201. Fujita S, Puri RK, Yu Z-X, et al: An ultrastructural study of in vivo interactions between lymphocytes and endothelial cells in the pathogenesis of the vascular leak syndrome induced by interleukin-2. Cancer 1991;68:2169–2174.
202. Faroux B, Meyer-Milsztain A, Borcon-Gibod L, et al: Cytotoxic drug-induced pulmonary disease in infants and children. Pediatr Pulmonol 1994;18:347–355.
203. Villani F, Galimberti M, Rizzi M, et al: Pulmonary toxicity of recombinant interleukin-2 plus lymphokine-activated killer cell therapy. Eur Respir J 1993;6:828–833.
204. Ardizzoni A, Bonavia M, Viale M, et al: Biologic and clinical effects of continuous infusion interleukin-2 in patients with non-small cell lung cancer. Cancer 1994;73:1353–1360.
205. Vogelzang PJ, Bloom SM, Mier JW, et al: Chest roentgenographic abnormalities in IL-2 recipients. Incidence and correlation with clinical parameters. Chest 1992;101:746–752.

206. Cesario TC, Vaziri ND, Ulich TR, et al: Functional, biochemical, and histopathologic consequences of high-dose interleukin-2 administration in rats. J Lab Clin Med 1991;118:81–88.
207. Klausner JM, Paterson IS, Goldman G, et al: Interleukin-2-induced lung injury is mediated by oxygen free radicals. Surgery 1991;109:169–175.
208. Rabinovici R, Sofronski MD, Borboroglu P, et al: Interleukin-2-induced lung injury. The role of complement. Circ Res 1994;74:329–335.
209. Rabinovici R, Feuerstein G, Abdullah F, et al: Locally produced tumor necrosis factor-α mediates interleukin-2 induced lung injury. Circ Res 1996;78:3329–3336.
210. Levene MI, Batisti O, Wigglesworth JS, et al: A prospective study of intrapulmonary fat accumulation in the newborn lung following intralipid infusion. Acta Paediatr Scand 1984;73:454–460.
211. Puntis JWL, Rushton DI: Pulmonary intravascular lipid in neonatal necropsy specimens. Arch Dis Child 1991;66:26–28.
212. Pereira GR, Fox WW, Stanley CA, et al: Decreased oxygenation and hyperlipemia during intravenous fat infusion in premature infants. Pediatrics 1980;66:26–30.
213. Hageman JR, Hunt CE: Fat emulsions and lung function. Clin Chest Med 1986;7:69–77.
214. Inwood RJ, Gora P, Hunt CE: Indomethacin inhibition of intralipid-induced lung dysfunction. Prostaglandins Med 1981;6:503–514.
215. Hageman JR, McCulloch K, Gora P, et al: Intralipid alterations in pulmonary prostaglandin metabolism and gas exchange. Crit Care Med 1983;11:794–798.
216. McKeen CR, Brigham KL, Bowers RE, et al: Pulmonary vascular effects of fat emulsion infusion in unanesthetized sheep. J Clin Invest 1978;61: 1291–1297.
217. Sosenko IRS, Rodriguez-Pierce M, Bancalari E: Effect of early initiation of intravenous lipid administration on the incidence and severity of chronic lung disease in premature infants. J Pediatr 1993;123:975–982.
218. Lekka ME, Liokatis S, Nathanail C, et al: The impact of intravenous fat emulsion administration in acute lung injury. Am J Respir Crit Care Med 2004;169:638–644.
219. Wright DG, Robichaud KJ, Pizzo PA, et al: Lethal pulmonary reactions associated with the combined use of amphotericin B and leukocyte transfusions. N Engl J Med 1981;304:1185–1189.
220. Dutcher JP, Kendall J, Norris D, et al: Granulocyte transfusion therapy and amphotericin B. Adverse reactions? Am J Hematol 1989;31:102–108.
221. Collazos J, Martinez E, Mayo J, Ibarra S: Pulmonary reactions during treatment with amphotericin B. Review of published cases and guidelines for management. Clin Infect Dis 2001;33:e75–e82.
222. Bell RJM: Pulmonary infiltration with eosinophilia caused by chlorpropamide. Lancet 1964;286:1249–1250.
223. Demeter SL, Ahmad M, Tomashefski JF: Drug-induced pulmonary disease. Part I. Patterns of response. Cleve Clin Q 1979;46:89–99.
224. Ho D, Tashkin DP, Bein ME, et al: Pulmonary infiltrates with eosinophilia associated with tetracycline. Chest 1979;76:33–36.
225. Poe RH, Condemi JJ, Weinstein SS, et al: Adult respiratory distress syndrome related to ampicillin sensitivity. Chest 1980;77:449–451.
226. Bedrossian CWM: Pathology of drug-induced lung diseases. Semin Respir Med 1982;4:98–105.
227. Kissner DG, Lawrence WD, Selis JE, et al: Crack lung. Pulmonary disease caused by cocaine abuse. Am Rev Respir Dis 1987;136:1250–1252.
228. Goodwin SD, Glenny RW: Nonsteroidal anti-inflammatory drug-associated pulmonary infiltrates with eosinophilia. Arch Intern Med 1992;152: 1521–1524.
229. Allen JN, Davis WB: Eosinophilic lung disease. Am J Respir Crit Care Med 1994;150:1423–1438.
230. Pfitzenmeyer P, Meier M, Zuck P, et al: Piroxicam induced pulmonary infiltrates and eosinophilia. J Rheumatol 1994;21:1573–1577.
231. Dykhuizen RS, Zaidi AM, Godden DJ, et al: Minocycline and pulmonary eosinophilia. BMJ 1995;310:1520–1521.
232. Salerno SM, Strong JS, Roth BJ, et al: Eosinophilic pneumonia and respiratory failure associated with a trazodone overdose. Am J Respir Crit Care Med 1995;152:2170–2172.
233. Franco J, Artes MJ: Pulmonary eosinophilia associated with montelukast. Thorax 1999;54:558–560.
234. Ohnishi H, Abe M, Yokoyama A, et al: Clarithromycin-induced eosinophilic pneumonia. Intern Med 2004;43:231–235.
235. Wolff AJ, O'Donnell AE: Pulmonary effects of illicit drug use. Clin Chest Med 2004;25:203–216.
236. Heffner JE, Harley RA, Schabel SI: Pulmonary reactions from illicit substance abuse. Clin Chest Med 1990;11:151–162.
237. Howard JJ, Mohsenifar Z, Simons SM: Adult respiratory distress syndrome following administration of lidocaine. Chest 1982;81:644–645.
238. Mahutte CK, Nakasato SK, Light RW: Haloperidol and sudden death due to pulmonary edema. Arch Intern Med 1982;142:1951–1952.
239. Borish L, Matloff SM, Findlay SR: Radiographic contrast media-induced noncardiogenic pulmonary edema. Case report and review of the literature. J Allergy Clin Immunol 1984;74:104–107.
240. Prough DS, Roy R, Bumgarner J, et al: Acute pulmonary edema in healthy teenagers following conservative doses of intravenous naloxone. Anesthesiology 1984;60:485–486.
241. Conces DJ Jr, Kreipke DL, Tarver RD: Pulmonary edema induced by intravenous ethchlorvynol. Am J Emerg Med 1986;4:549–551.
242. Glassroth J, Adams GD, Schnoll S: The impact of substance abuse on the respiratory system. Chest 1987;91:596–602.
243. Pisani RJ, Rosenow EC III: Pulmonary edema associated with tocolytic therapy. Ann Intern Med 1989;110:714–718.
244. Kavaru MS, Ahmad M, Amirthalingam KN: Hydrochlorothiazide-induced acute pulmonary edema. Cleve Clin J Med 1990;57:181–184.
245. Heffner JE, Sahn SA: Salicylate-induced pulmonary edema. Ann Intern Med 1981;95:405–409.
246. Wells TG, Graham CJ, Moss M, et al: Nifedipine poisoning in a child. Pediatrics 1990;86:91–94.
247. Humbert VH Jr, Munn NJ, Hawkins RF: Noncardiogenic pulmonary edema complicating massive diltiazem overdose. Chest 1991;99:258–260.
248. Reed CR, Glauser FL: Drug-induced noncardiogenic pulmonary edema. Chest 1991;100:1120–1124.
249. Prigogine T, Waterlot Y, Gottignies P, et al: Acute nonhemodynamic pulmonary edema with nifedipine in primary pulmonary hypertension. Chest 1991;100:563–564.
250. Batlle MA, Wilcox WD: Pulmonary edema in an infant following passive inhalation of free-base ("crack") cocaine. Clin Pediatr 1993;32:105–106.
251. Laposata EA, Mayo GL: A review of pulmonary pathology and mechanisms associated with inhalation of freebase cocaine ("crack"). Am J Forensic Med Pathol 1993;14:1–9.
252. Zuckerman GB, Conway EE Jr: Pulmonary complications following tricyclic antidepressant overdose in an adolescent. Ann Pharmacother 1993;27:572–574.
253. Leesar MA, Martyn R, Talley JD, et al: Noncardiogenic pulmonary edema complicating massive verapamil overdose. Chest 1994;105:606–607.
254. Parsons PE: Respiratory failure as a result of drugs, overdoses, and poisonings. Clin Chest Med 1994;15:93–102.
255. Lee-Chiong T Jr, Matthay RA: Drug-induced pulmonary edema and acute respiratory distress syndrome. Clin Chest Med 2004;25:95–104.
256. Sherman CB, Hudson LD, Pierson DJ: Severe precocious emphysema in intravenous methylphenidate (Ritalin) abusers. Chest 1987;92:1085–1087.
257. Pare JP, Cote G, Fraser RS: Long-term follow-up of drug abusers with intravenous talcosis. Am Rev Respir Dis 1989;139:233–241.
258. Schmidt RA, Glenny RW, Godwin JD, et al: Panlobular emphysema in young intravenous Ritalin abusers. Am Rev Respir Dis 1991;143:649–656.
259. Stern EJ, Frank MS, Schmutz JF, et al: Panlobular pulmonary emphysema caused by IV injection of methylphenidate (Ritalin). Findings on chest radiographs and CT scans. AJR Am J Roentgenol 1994;162:555–560.
260. Gerrity TR, Cotromanes E, Garrard CS, et al: The effect of aspirin on lung mucociliary clearance. N Engl J Med 1983;308:139–141.
261. Leitch GJ, Frid LH, Phoenix D: The effects of ethanol on mucociliary clearance. Alcohol Clin Exp Res 1985;9:277–280.
262. Stafanger G, Bisgaard H, Pedersen M, et al: Effect of N-acetylcysteine on the human nasal ciliary activity in vitro. Eur J Respir Dis 1987;70:157–162.
263. Groth ML, Langenback EG, Foster WM: Influence of inhaled atropine on lung mucociliary function in humans. Am Rev Respir Dis 1991;144: 1042–1047.
264. O'Callaghan C, Atherton M, Karim K, et al: The effect of halothane on neonatal ciliary beat frequency. J Paediatr Child Health 1994;30: 429–431.
265. Rusznak C, Devalia JL, Lozewicz S, et al: The assessment of nasal mucociliary clearance and the effect of drugs. Respir Med 1994;88:89–101.
266. Cervin A, Lindberg S, Mercke U: Effects of halothane on mucociliary activity in vivo. Otolaryngol Head Neck Surg 1995;112:714–722.
267. Houtmeyers C, Gosselink R, Gayan-Ramirez G, Decramer M: Effects of drugs on mucus clearance. Eur Respir J 1999;14:452–467.
268. Matthys H, Hundenborn J, Daikeler G, et al: Influence of 0.2 mg ipratropium bromide on mucociliary clearance in patients with chronic bronchitis. Respiration 1985;48:329–339.
269. Davis BA, Cervi P, Amin Z, et al: Retinoic acid syndrome. Pulmonary computed tomography (CT) findings. Leuk Lymphoma 1996;23:113–117.
270. Tallman MS, Andersen JW, Schiffer CA, et al: Clinical description of 44 patients with acute promyelocytic leukemia who developed the retinoic acid syndrome. Blood 2000;95:90–95.

271. Nicolls MR, Terada LS, Tuder RM, et al: Diffuse alveolar hemorrhage with underlying pulmonary capillaritis in the retinoic acid syndrome. Am J Respir Crit Care Med 1998;158:1302–1305.
272. Manna SK, Aggarwal BB: All-trans-retinoic acid upregulates TNF receptors and potentiates TNF-induced activation of nuclear factors-kappaB, activated protein-1 and apoptosis in luman lung cancer cells. Oncogene 2000;19:2110–2119.
273. Ninomiya M, Kiyoi H, Ito M, et al: Retinoic acid syndrome in NOD/scid mice induced by injecting an acute promyelocytic leukemia cell line. Leukemia 2004;18:442–448.

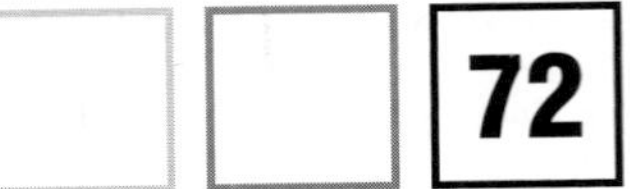

72 Disorders of the Respiratory Tract Due to Trauma

James W. Brooks, MD •
Thomas M. Krummel, MD

The occurrence of thoracic trauma in infants and children is exceedingly rare and is usually confined to automobile accidents, the battered-child syndrome, and falls from a considerable height. Stab and bullet wounds are rare. Nevertheless, the complete spectrum of chest trauma has been recorded, including pneumothorax, hemothorax, destruction of the integrity of the chest wall and diaphragm, thoracic visceral damage, and combined thoracoabdominal injuries (Fig. 72-1).

Thoracic trauma is frequently associated with head and abdominal trauma, making the mortality rate higher in this combined scenario. The mortality rate from thoracic trauma has been reported to be 26%.

As in adults, the significance of thoracic trauma parallels the pulmonary, cardiac, and systemic dysfunction that follows, and in the pediatric age group, because of chest wall resiliency, physiologic aberrations can occur with trauma that does not fracture or penetrate. The interruption of satisfactory respiration and circulation secondary to chest injury is frequently complicated by blood loss and hypotension, and all three factors must be quickly reversed for survival. Shock from hemorrhage can usually be managed through intelligent, arithmetic specific replacement, which is monitored by serial determination of blood pressures, hematocrit, central venous pressure, blood gases, and, if necessary, blood volume. Pulmonary artery catheterization with a Swan-Ganz catheter gives more precise information relating to pulmonary capillary wedge pressures and cardiac output. Restoration of the normal cardiopulmonary function fundamentally depends on a clean airway, intact chest and diaphragm, and unrestricted heart-lung dynamics. This condition can in most instances be accomplished by maneuvers other than thoracotomy.

Computed tomography (CT) of blunt chest trauma in the pediatric age group, with the exception of aortic injury where aortography is the diagnostic procedure of choice, should be strongly considered as a routine measure for the findings that may significantly alter the clinical approach to treatment.

■ STERNAL FRACTURES

Fractures of the sternum in infancy and childhood follow high-compression crush injuries and are usually associated with other thoracic and orthopedic problems elsewhere.

On physical examination there is local tenderness, ecchymosis, and sometimes a peculiar concavity or paradoxical respiratory movement, but the sternal segments usually are well aligned, without much displacement. Dyspnea, cyanosis, tachycardia (or arrhythmia), and hypotension may be evidence of an underlying contusion of the heart.

Cardiac tamponade and acute traumatic myocardial damage must be ruled out by various studies, including serial electrocardiography, echocardiography, sonography, and careful monitoring of venous blood pressure. If the bony deformity is minimal, appropriate posture will suffice. Markedly displaced fragments are reduced under general anesthesia by the closed or open technique in order to prevent a traumatic pectus excavatum. Violent paradoxical respirations can be controlled by operative fixation or, preferably, by assisted mechanical respiration through an artifical airway.

■ RIB FRACTURES

Rib fractures are unusual in children because of the extreme flexibility of the osseous and cartilaginous framework of the thorax. Crush and direct-blow injuries are the usual etiologic factors. In addition, manual compression of the lateral chest wall, rickets, tumors, and osteogenesis imperfecta have been incriminated. Multiple fractures of the middle ribs can be seen in the battered-child syndrome (Fig. 72-2). The upper ribs are protected by the scapula and related muscles, and the lower ones are quite resilient.

Violence to the chest wall may produce pulmonary and cardiac lacerations and contusions, various pneumothoraces, and hemothorax. Critical respiratory distress may also follow multiple anterior rib fractures, in which the integrity of the thoracic cabe is destroyed and the involved chest becomes flail (Fig. 72-3). The unsupported area of the chest wall moves inward with inspiration and outward with expiration, and these paradoxical respiratory excursions inexorably lead to dyspnea (Fig. 72-4). The explosive expiration of coughing is dissipated and made ineffectual by the paradoxical movement and intercostal pain. In effect, the ideal preparation for acute respiratory distress syndrome—airway obstruction, atelectasis, and pneumonia—has been established.

The clinical picture includes local pain that is aggravated by motion. Tenderness is elicited by pressure applied directly over the fracture or elsewhere on the same rib. The fracture site may be edematous and ecchymotic. The clinical manifestations may range from these minimal findings with simple, restricted fractures to the severest form of ventilatory distress with a flail chest and lung injury.

Chest roentgenograms demonstrate the extent and displacement of the fractures and underlying visceral damage.

Treatment of the uncomplicated fracture involves control of pain in order to permit unrestricted respiration. Displacement requires no therapy. With severe fractures, alleviation of pain and restoration of cough are important and can be provided by

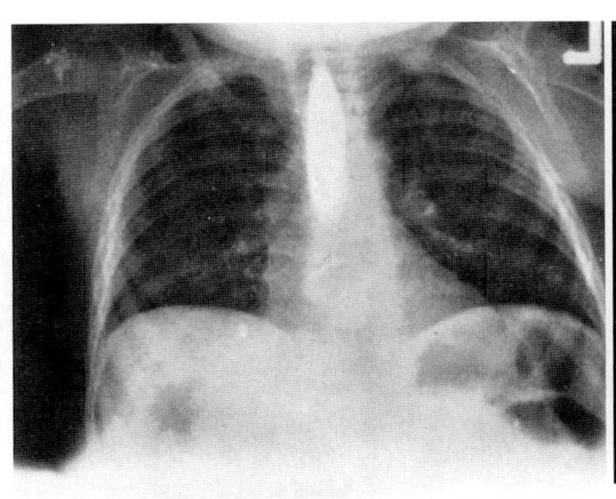

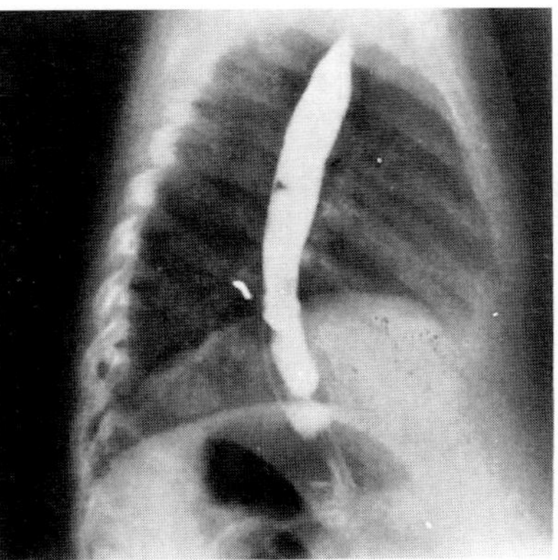

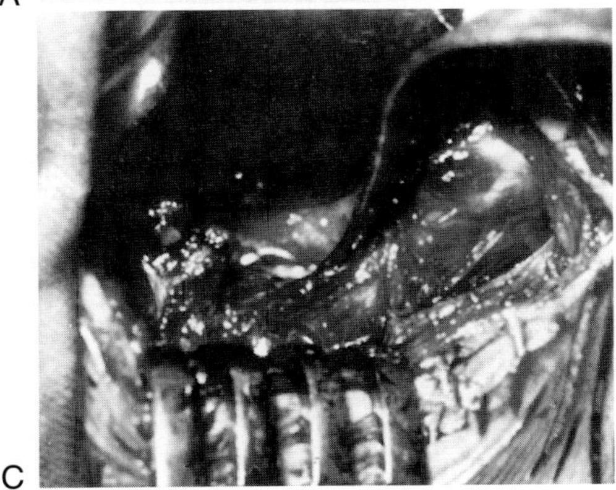

■ **FIGURE 72-1.** The posterior chest wall of this 8-year-old boy was penetrated by an object that was apparently accelerated by a power mower operating 8 feet away. **A** and **B,** Posteroanterior and lateral chest films with barium in the esophagus demonstrate an opaque foreign body in the posterior mediastinum. **C,** Through an extrapleural approach, a curved nail, seen just below the stump of the resected rib and lying on the aorta, was removed from the posterior mediastinum.

analgesics, physiotherapy, and intermittent positive-pressure breathing. Thoracentesis and insertion of intercostal tubes should be done promptly for pneumothorax and hemothorax, and shock should be managed by appropriate replacement therapy and oxygen (Figs. 72-5 and 72-6).

Paradoxical respiratory excursions with flail chest must be promptly brought under control to help prevent respiratory distress syndrome, which may be the morbid pulmonary complication (Fig. 72-7).

■ TRACHEOSTOMY IN CHEST WALL INJURY

Controlled mechanical respiration through an endotracheal tube has been used for paradox and respiratory insufficiency. In spite of vigorous therapy, secretions cannot be avoided, and they are managed using intermittent transnasal tracheal suctioning and bronchoscopy. Tracheostomy, then, becomes useful in providing

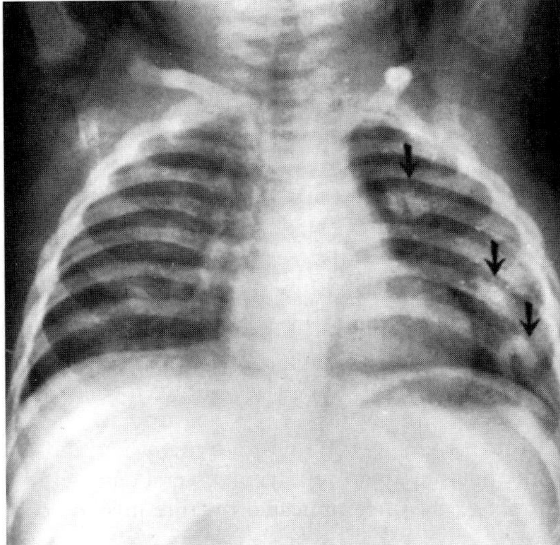

■ **FIGURE 72-2.** Multiple fractures of the left fourth and fifth ribs and fracture of the left clavicle in a battered child.

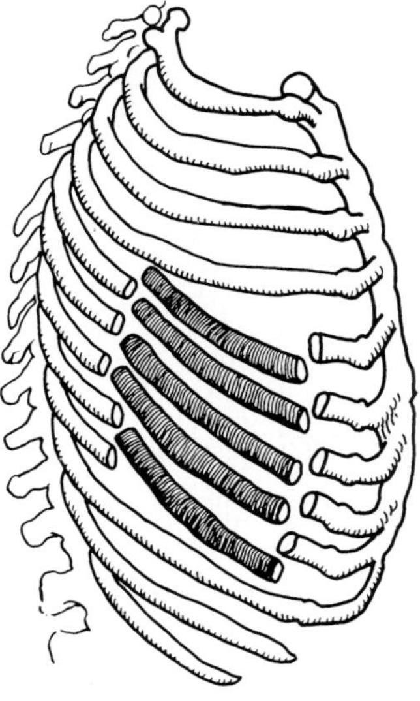

■ **FIGURE 72-3.** An illustration of five ribs broken in two places, with loss of chest wall stability and resultant paradoxical or "flail chest" wall.

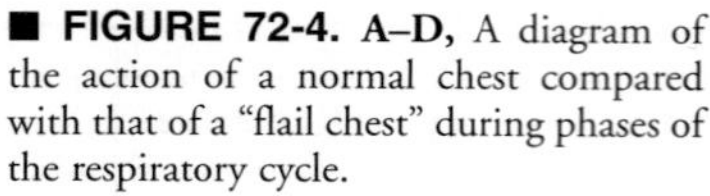

■ **FIGURE 72-4.** **A–D,** A diagram of the action of a normal chest compared with that of a "flail chest" during phases of the respiratory cycle.

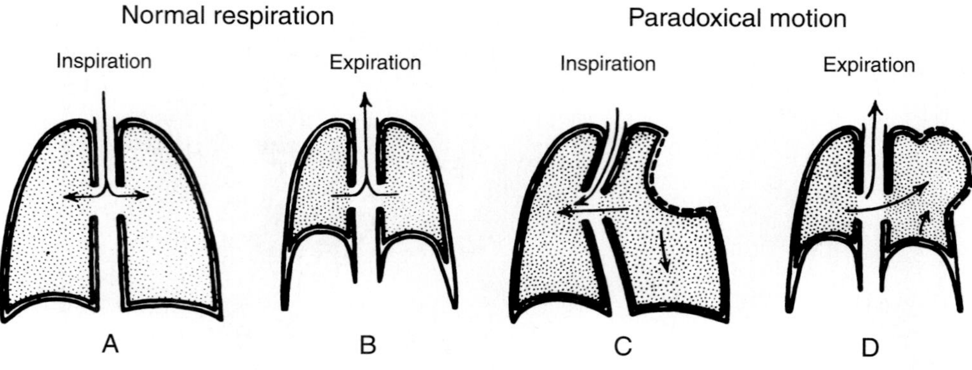

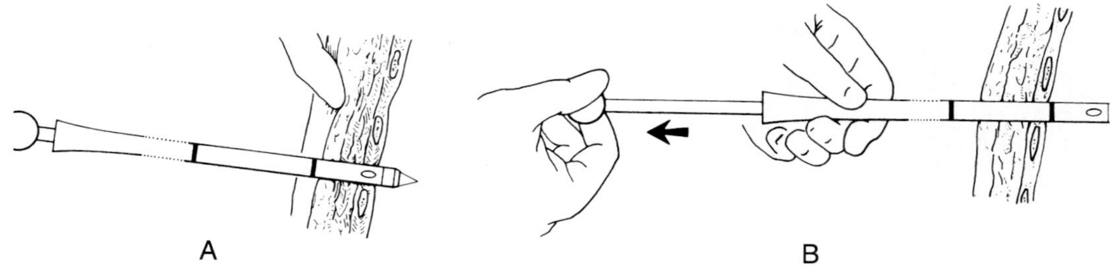

■ **FIGURE 72-5.** **A** and **B,** The trocar technique of chest tube insertion.

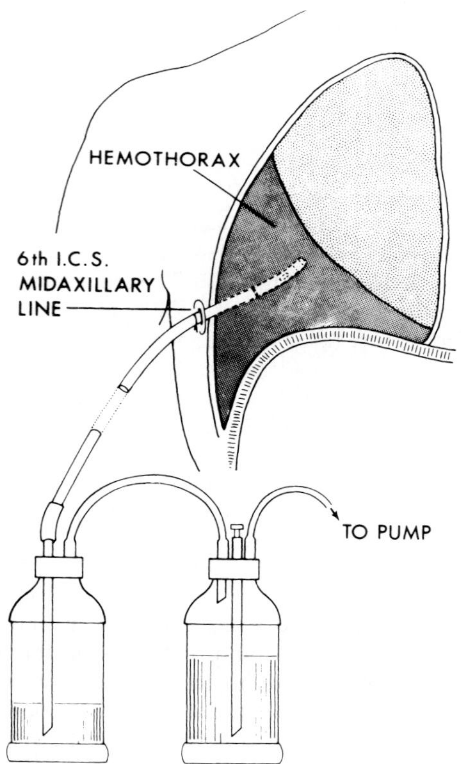

■ **FIGURE 72-6.** The classic setup for closed drainage of pleural space.

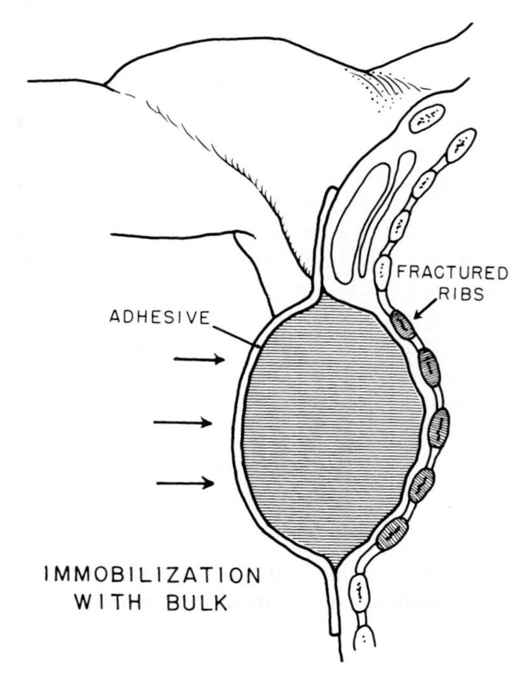

■ **FIGURE 72-7.** Bulky dressings applied as temporary stabilization for "flail chest" wall.

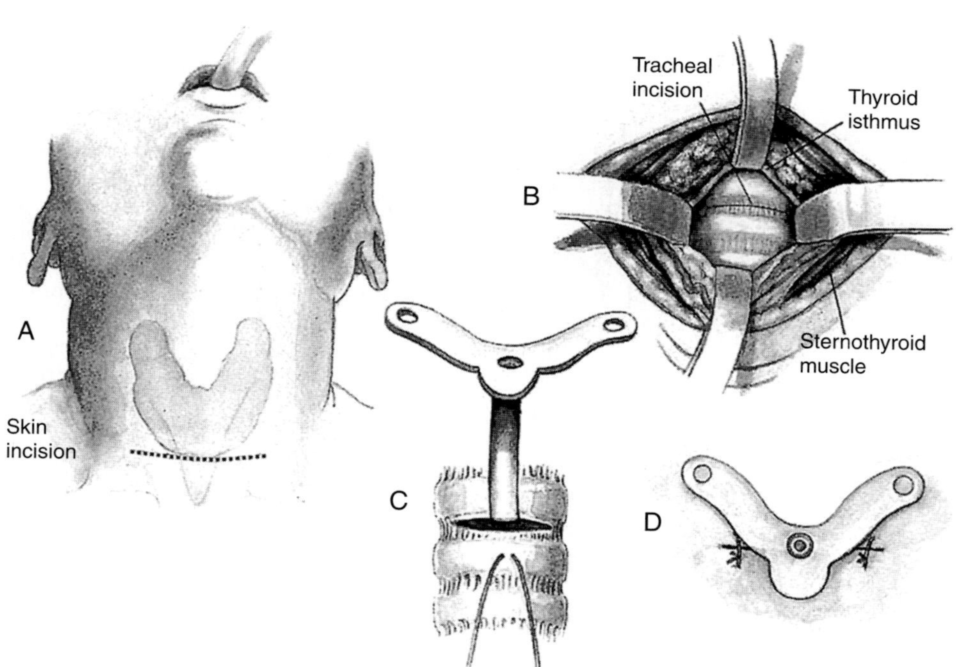

■ **FIGURE 72-8.** Techniques of tracheostomy performed over an oral endotracheal tube. Note the transverse skin incision **(A)** and the suture on the lower tracheal flaps to facilitate subsequent tube changes **(C)**. **B,** The anatomy of the area. **D,** The tube in place.

an avenue for the control of profuse secretions, diminishing the dead space, and bypassing an obstructed airway (Fig. 72-8). Mechanical respiration can be applied and maintained through the tracheotomy for several weeks.

During the first year of life, however, tracheostomy is a morbid operation and should be avoided if possible. Secretions may be difficult to aspirate, and the small tracheostomy tube easily becomes plugged; distal infection, often with staphylococci, is poorly handled by such young patients, and withdrawal of the tracheostomy tube at times is a precarious and unpredictable endeavor. Nevertheless, even in this age group, and certainly later, tracheostomy can be mandatory and life saving in specific instances of chest trauma.

The decision for tracheostomy in cases of chest injury can often be made if there is (1) a mechanically obstructed airway that cannot be managed more conservatively and (2) flail chest. The unstable, paradoxical chest wall movement can be controlled for long periods by assisted positive pressure respirations through a short, uncuffed Silastic tracheostomy tube.

Often, however, the decision for tracheostomy is first considered in the presence of minimal dyspnea. In this situation, use of blood gas studies can augment the clinical impression and intercept clinical respiratory failure. Serial measurements of pH and arterial carbon dioxide tension are a satisfactory chemical guide to imminent ventilatory distress and the need for and efficiency of assisted or controlled mechanical respiration, because the finding of normal values rules out the presence of significant hypoxemia.

■ TRAUMATIC PNEUMOTHORAX

Traumatic, simple, tension and open pneumothorax are rare in infants and children, in whom a very mobile mediastinum would compound the cardiorespiratory distress usually encountered in such injuries. The injuries are formidable and require specific maneuvers to reverse a malignant chain of events.

The creation of a tension pneumothorax in which intrapleural pressure is at or exceeds atmospheric pressures requires a valvular mechanism through which the amount of air entering the pleural space exceeds the amount escaping it. The positive intrapleural pressure is dissipated by a mediastinal shift, which compresses the opposite lung in the presence of ipsilateral pulmonary collapse and angulates the great vessels entering and leaving the heart. Intrapleural tension can be increased by traumatic hemothorax, and respiratory exchange and cardiac output are critically diminished by this form of mediastinal tamponade.

The etiologic possibilities, in addition to chest wall and lung trauma, include rupture of the esophagus, pulmonary cyst, emphysematous lobe, and postoperative bronchial fistula. These latter sources of tension pneumothorax almost always require thoracotomy for control.

The clinical findings may include external evidence of a wound, tachypnea, dyspnea, cyanosis with hyperresonance, absence or transmission of breath sounds, and dislocation of the trachea and apical cardiac impulse. The hemithoraces may be asymmetric, the involved side being the larger.

A confirmatory radiograph is comforting but often cannot be afforded in this thoracic emergency. Fiberoptic transillumination may be helpful. Chest tube insertion is indicated for a tension or simple pneumothorax. Prompt relief and pulmonary expansion can be anticipated if the source of the intrapleural air has been controlled. Obviously, a traumatic valvular defect in the chest wall can be occluded. If the pulmonary air leak persists or recurs, the possibility of tension pneumothorax is circumvented by the insertion of one or more intercostal tubes connected to water-seal drainage with mild suction. Most instances of traumatic tension pneumothorax require tube drainage for permanent decompression, although needle aspiration is indispensable for emergency management. Stubborn bronchopleural fistulas that continue to remain widely patent despite adequate intercostal tube deflation may close after a therapeutic pneumoperitoneum. If this fails, thoracotomy may be required.

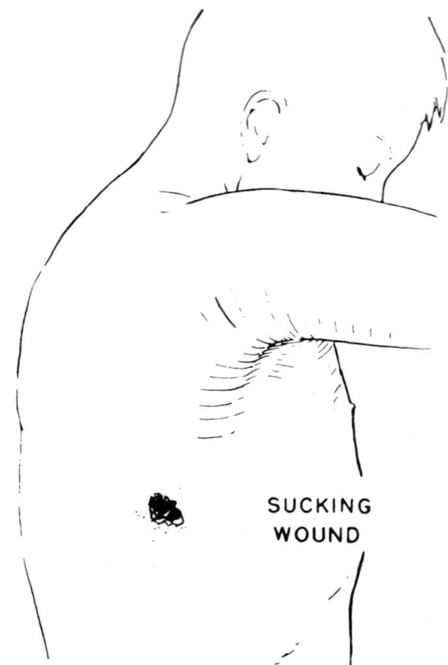

■ **FIGURE 72-9.** An open pneumothorax due to a traumatic chest wall defect allowing ingress and egress of air into and from the pleural cavity.

An open, sucking pneumothorax in which atmospheric air has direct, unimpeded entrance into and exit from a relatively free pleural space is a second, equally urgent thoracic emergency (Fig. 72-9). This access is almost invariably accomplished through a large traumatic hole in the chest wall. Ingress of air during inspiration and egress during expiration produce an extreme degree of paradoxical respiration and mediastinal flutter, which is partially regulated by the size of the chest wall defect in comparison with the circumference of the trachea. If a considerable segment of chest wall is absent, more air is exchanged at this site than through the trachea, because the pressures are similar. Inspiration collapses the ipsilateral lung and drives its alveolar air into the opposite side. During expiration, the air returns across the carina. In addition, the mediastinum becomes a widely swinging pendulum compressing the uninjured lung on inspiration and the lung on the injured side during expiration (Fig. 72-10). Obviously, under these circumstances, little effective ventilation is taking place because of the tremendous increase in the pulmonary dead space and the decrease in tidal exchange. A totally ineffective cough completes the clinical picture.

The diagnosis is readily made by inspection of the thoracic wound and the peculiar sound of air going into and coming out of the chest.

The emergency management of this critical situation is prompt occlusion of the chest wall defect by bulky sterile dressings (Fig. 72-11) and measures to prevent conversion of this open pneumothorax into an equally aggravating tension pneumothorax that can occur if the underlying lung has been traumatized. Simultaneous pleural decompression by closed intercostal tube drainage is essential. After systemic stabilization, more formal surgical débridement, reconstruction, and closure can be done in the operating room.

Subcutaneous emphysema usually results from injury to the pulmonary ventilatory system (Fig. 72-12). The possibility of gastrointestinal tract injury or gas-forming bacilli must not be overlooked.

■ HEMOTHORAX

Blood in the pleural cavity is perhaps the most common sequela of thoracic trauma, regardless of type. The source of the bleeding is either systemic (high pressure) from the chest wall or pulmonary (low pressure). Hemorrhage from pulmonary vessels is usually self-limiting unless major tributaries have been transected.

Intrapleural blood eventually clots and becomes organized fibrous tissue (fibrothorax) (Fig. 72-13). Before this development, pulmonary compression and mediastinal displacement with reduced vital capacity and atrial filling can occur. With the development of a fibrothorax, the changes in cardiorespiratory dynamics become chronic as the lung becomes incarcerated and the chest wall is immobilized. Empyema from secondary contamination is always a threat when the pleural space is filled with blood.

The immediate findings are those of blood loss compounded by respiratory distress and perhaps hemoptysis. The trachea and apical impulse are dislocated, the percussion note is flat, and the breath sounds are indistinct. The actual diagnosis is confirmed by thoracentesis after adequate radiographic studies, if time allows.

It has been established that aspiration of a hemothorax and expansion of the underlying lung do not instigate additional bleeding. Accordingly, the local management of hemothorax is prompt, continuous, and total evacuation without air replacement. The dead space is abolished, and without it empyema

■ **FIGURE 72-10.** **A–D,** Changes in the normal respiratory pattern brought about by an open, sucking thoracic wall injury.

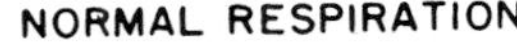

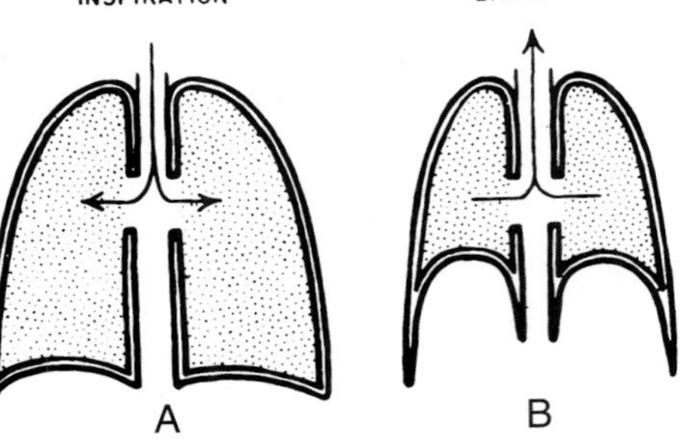

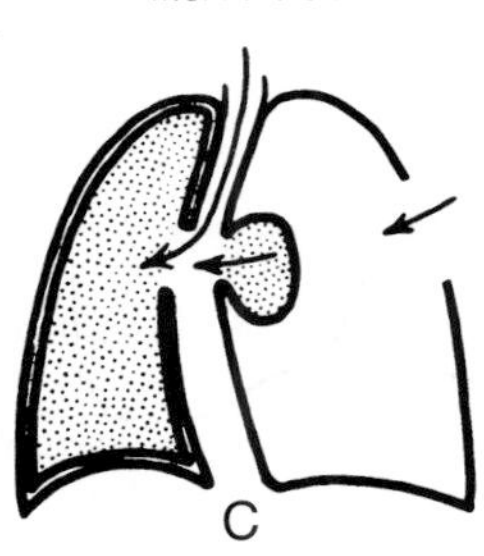

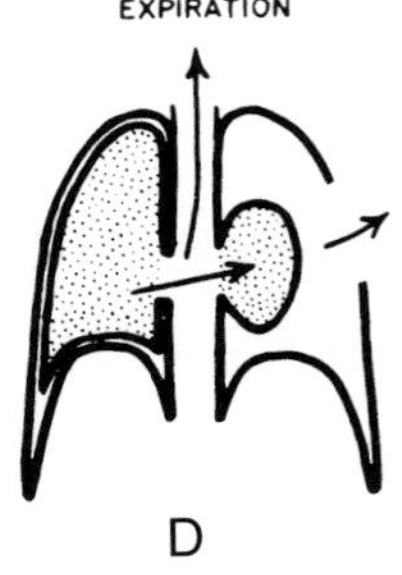

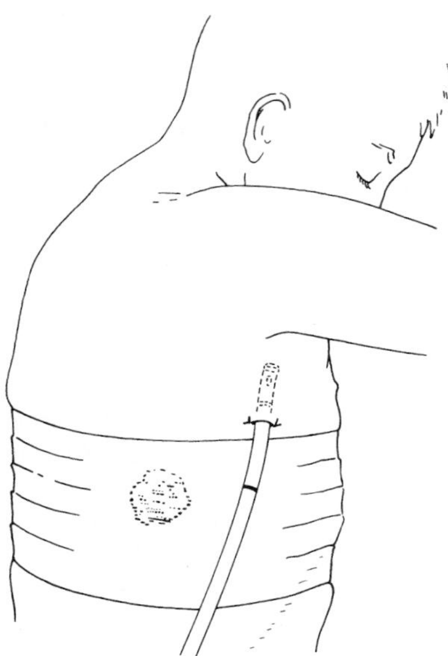

■ **FIGURE 72-11.** A temporary occlusive chest wall dressing applied to a sucking wound with underwater intercostal chest tube drainage. Once the period of emergency is over, operative débridement and closure of the chest wound is necessary.

cannot occur. Such evacuation is best accomplished by insertion of a chest tube (see Fig. 72-6). Clotting is circumvented, and pulmonary function is restored by pulmonary expansion. Further extensive bleeding must be controlled by operation. Obviously, systemic resuscitation has not been overlooked.

Clotting, loculation, and infection may supervene despite vigorous initial therapy. A rare patient eventually requires decortication.

■ TRACHEOBRONCHIAL TRAUMA

Rupture of the trachea or bronchus in infants and children is usually preceded by a severe compression injury of the chest or a sharp blow to the anterior part of the neck. This discontinuity of a major airway is characterized by intrathoracic tension phenomena; later, stricture at the site of rupture leads to loss of lung function by sepsis and atelectasis.

Rapidly progressive interstitial emphysema, pneumomediastinum, tension pneumothorax, and hemoptysis are fairly specific. Upper rib fractures usually occur on the involved side but certainly are not constant in children with partial tracheal or bronchial transection.

Conventional chest roentgenograms and the air tracheobronchogram can suggest the diagnosis in the presence of a compatible clinical picture, but bronchoscopic demonstration of the rupture is always necessary. The diagnosis may not be suspected during the acute phase of smaller transections of major or minor bronchi but becomes obvious when late stricture with distal atelectasis and chronic pneumonitis is related retrospectively to a history of fairly severe chest trauma.

The initial management of bronchial rupture is concerned with the maintenance of a patent airway and decompression of the pleura and mediastinum by one or more intercostal tubes connected to closed drainage. Confirmatory endoscopy and bronchoplasty are followed by little or no loss of pulmonary functions distal to the narrowed segment. Emergency bronchoscopy and immediate repair of the defect are preferred to a course of delayed recognition and repair, because morbidity can thus be circumvented.

Severe lacerations of the trachea can be immeasurably helped by bypassing the glottis with an artificial airway during the acute phase while preparing the patient for emergency tracheal repair. Smaller tears may heal spontaneously with tracheostomy alone; others result in stricture and require later tracheorrhaphy.

■ PULMONARY COMPRESSION INJURY (TRAUMATIC ASPHYXIA)

Explosive blasts compress a child's flexible ribs, sternum, and cartilages against the lungs with a sudden, violent increase in intra-alveolar pressure. Alveolar disruption, interstitial emphysema, and pneumothorax may follow if the glottis is closed when the

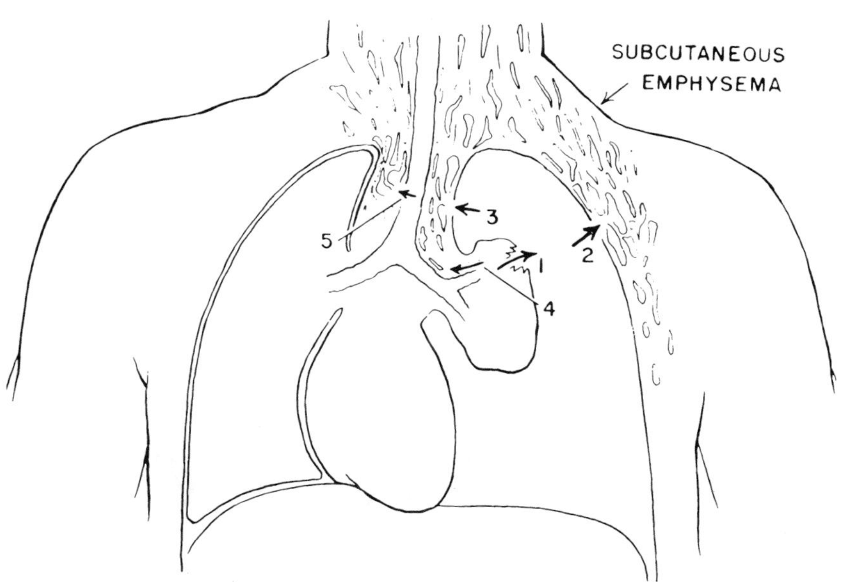

■ **FIGURE 72-12.** Subcutaneous emphysema resulting from an injury to the pulmonary system.

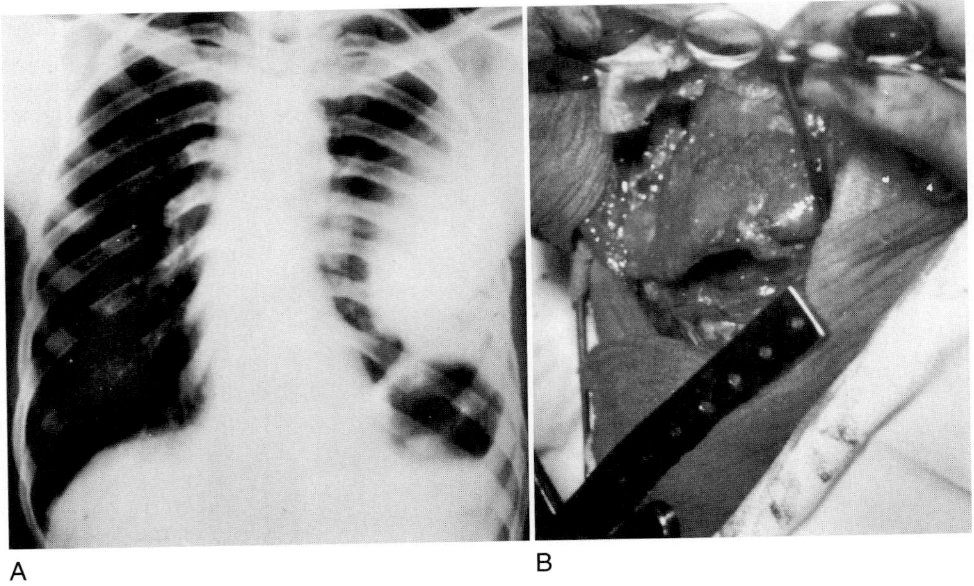

■ **FIGURE 72-13.** **A,** A clotted hemothorax. **B,** Operative decortication of the pleural peel of an improperly treated hemothorax.

compression occurs. Distribution of this force to the great, valveless veins of the mediastinum and jugular system leads to venous distention; extravasation of blood, purplish edema of the head, neck, and upper extremities; and possible central nervous system changes, due to intracerebral edema and petechial hemorrhages (traumatic asphyxia). The pulmonary contusion is represented pathologically by edema, hemorrhage, and atelectasis.

Clinically, there may be dyspnea, cough, chest pain, hemoptysis, hypoxia, hypercarbia, and mental confusion. The face and the neck can be grotesquely swollen, with crepitus and submucous and subconjunctival hemorrhage (Fig. 72-14). There need not be evidence of external trauma or fractured ribs in a child, and accordingly, the indication for chest roentgenogram is merely the possible history of a blast, acceleration (fall), or deceleration (automobile) injury. Unilateral or bilateral pulmonary hematoma, hemothorax, pneumothorax, and pneumomediastinum can be encountered.

With mild injuries, the subcutaneous emphysema and purplish hue gradually and spontaneously disappear over several days. Patients with more serious blast injuries are treated initially for anoxia and hypotension, and attention is then directed to the wet lung, atelectasis, and pleural complications. Rapid progression of the mediastinal and subcutaneous emphysema indicates a serious disruption of the trachea, bronchi, or lungs and may require intercostal tube drainage or even thoracotomy.

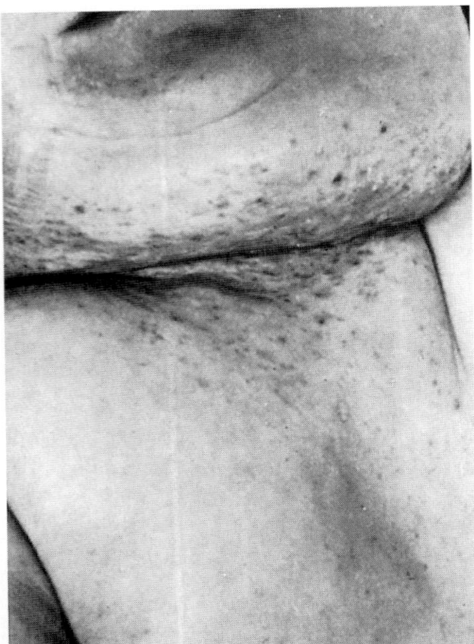

■ **FIGURE 72-14.** Subcutaneous hemorrhage and emphysema of the face and chest in an infant involved in an automobile accident. There were bilateral pulmonary contusions but not fractured ribs.

■ POSTTRAUMATIC ATELECTASIS (WET LUNG)

With pulmonary contusion from any source, production of tracheobronchial secretions is stimulated, but elimination is impeded by airway obstruction, pain, and depression of cough. The addition of hemorrhage to these accumulated secretions produce atelectasis in the damaged lung and inevitable infection, a syndrome aptly called wet lung.

The clinical findings are dyspnea and cyanosis, an incessant, unproductive cough with wheezing and audible rattling, and gross rhonchi and rales. Chest roentgenograms show varying degrees of unilateral and bilateral atelectasis.

The syndrome demands vigorous treatment to prevent morbidity and mortality. Such preventive treatment should be started, in all instances of chest trauma, by frequent changes of position, insistence on coughing, small amounts of depressant drugs, oxygen, humidification, antibiotics, mechanical ventilation, diuretics, intravenous colloid, and minimal hydration. If a child with chest trauma will not cough, tracheal catheterization, might be instituted before the appearance of early signs of the wet lung syndrome. Failure of this step should be followed in quick succession by bronchoscopy and an endotracheal tube insertion or tracheostomy if endoscopic aspiration is required too frequently.

The adult respiratory distress syndrome that occurs after critical illness, surgery, or trauma with congestion, edema, hemorrhage, pneumonia, and pulmonary fibrosis is rarely encountered in pediatric practice.

■ CARDIAC TRAUMA

Cardiac wounds should be suspected after penetration of any part of the chest, lower part of the neck, or upper part of the abdomen. The possibility of heart injury also exists in the presence of blunt trauma to the anterior or left hemithorax with laceration by fractured sternum or ribs, or severe compression between the sternum and the vertebral column. Blood loss with perforation varies between exsanguination, either internal or external, and minimal bleeding with or without acute cardiac tamponade. Tamponade usually follows trauma to the myocardium with both pleura intact. The hemopericardium cannot decompress into the pleura or externally, because the pericardial wound is dislocated from the soft tissue wound of entrance by the pericardial blood. The resulting increase in intrapericardial pressure constricts the heart and great veins, and the venous return and cardiac output are critically impaired.

The physical findings with acute tamponade are often classic. The veins of the neck and upper extremity may be distended. The heart sounds are distant and perhaps inaudible. The systolic pressure is depressed, the pulse pressure is narrow, and the pulse rate is relatively slow in spite of the lowered blood pressure.

The elevation of venous pressure is a valuable laboratory finding. Fluoroscopy demonstrates an inactive cardiac silhouette whose margins may not be widened. Sonography may be helpful.

With this clinical picture, emergency needle aspiration of the pericardial sac through a subxiphoid approach should be performed in addition to systemic resuscitation while the operating suite is being prepared. Aspiration of small amounts of blood can restore cardiopulmonary dynamics (Fig. 72-15).

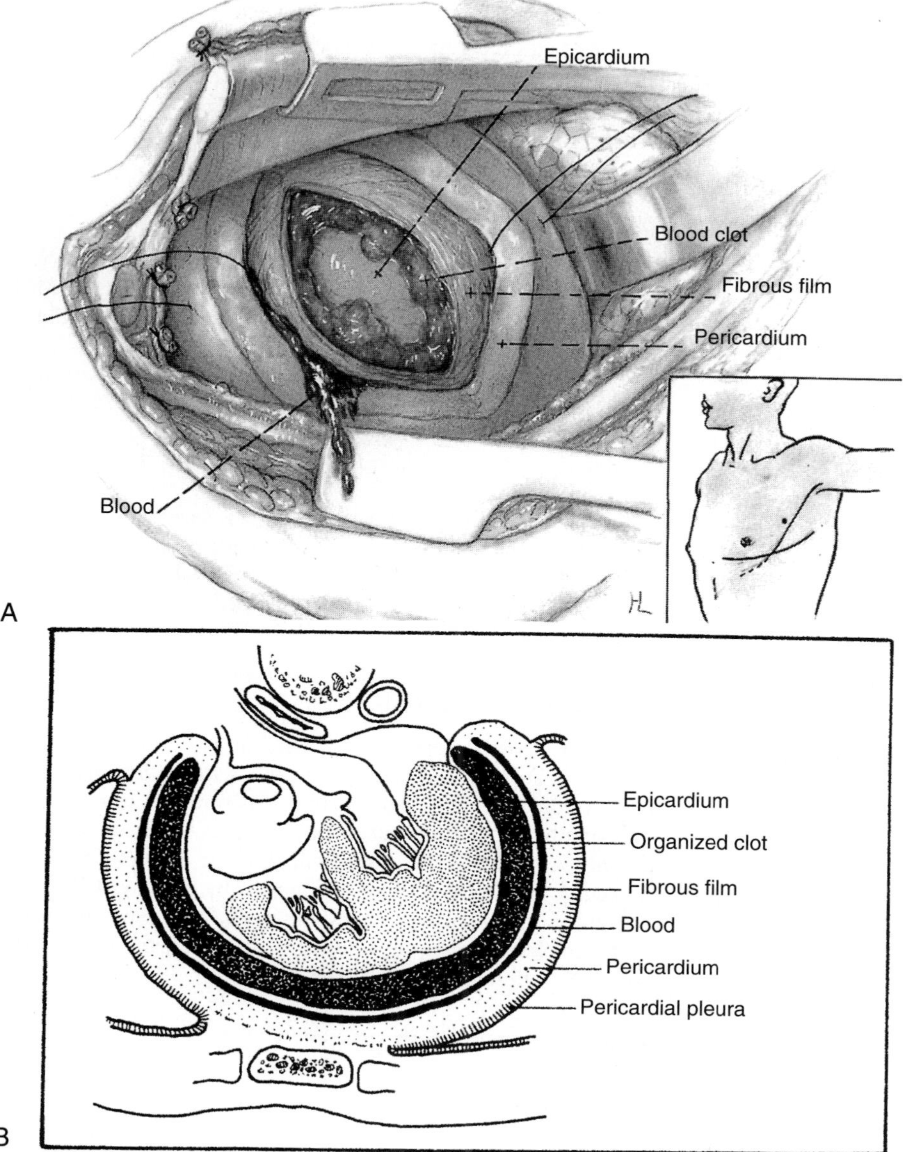

■ **FIGURE 72-15.** **A** and **B,** A traumatic cardiac tamponade relieved by an open thoracotomy 5 days following trauma and after two partially relieving pericardiocenteses.

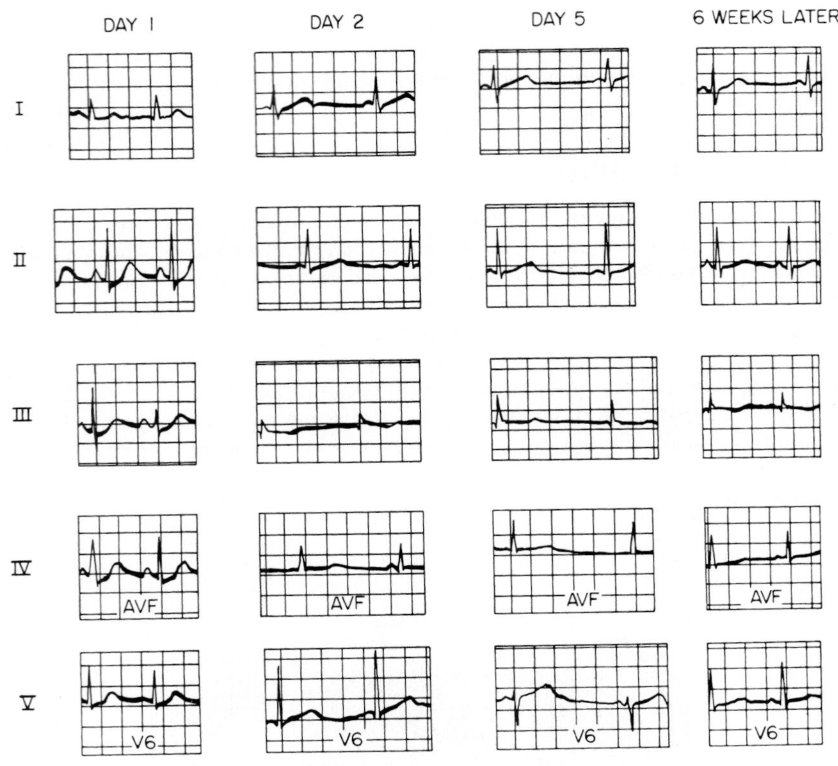

FIGURE 72-16. An electrocardiogram of a 15-year-old boy admitted for blunt chest wall trauma after an automobile accident. Note the progressive ST and T changes with marked depression immediately after the accident. There was an improvement in the ST segment and a flattening of the T waves on day 2 and a reversal to normal in later tracings. (Courtesy of Dr. C. McCue.)

Nonpenetrating trauma can produce various degrees of myocardial contusions ranging from a small area of edema to a ruptured chamber. The chest pain and tachycardia may be difficult to evaluate without evidence of cardiac failure. Serial electrocardiograms and cardiac enzyme determinations are essential for the diagnosis of myocardial damage secondary to trauma (Fig. 72-16).

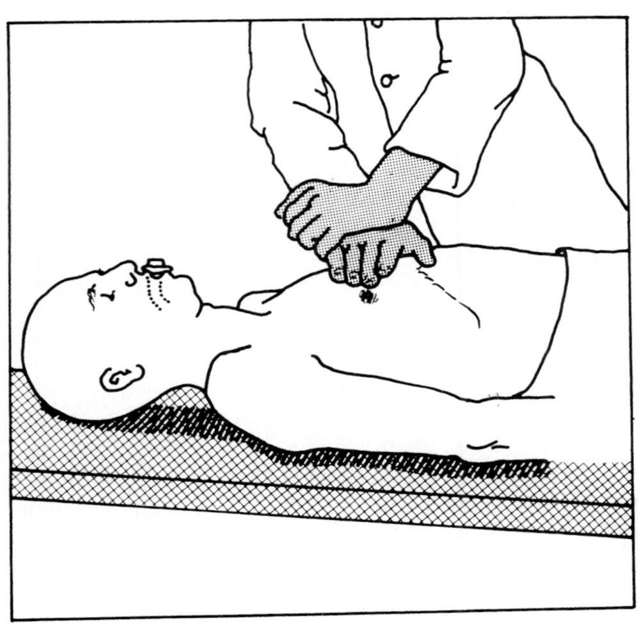

FIGURE 72-17. External cardiac massage.

Penetrating trauma may injure myocardial chambers or coronary arteries and may require closure of the myocardial chambers or even coronary bypass surgery in pediatric patients.

The treatment can follow the standard regimen for coronary occlusion, with the exclusion of anticoagulants, and complete rehabilitation can be anticipated. Late complications include chronic constrictive pericarditis, congestive heart failure, and ventricular aneurysm.

In this regard, physicians attending an acutely injured child in the emergency ward must be prepared to institute prompt external cardiac massage (Fig. 72-17), internal cardiac massage (Figs. 72-18 and 72-19), or cardiac defibrillation (Fig. 72-20).

TRAUMATIC RUPTURE OF THE THORACIC AORTA

Blunt chest trauma in the pediatric patient resulted in aortic rupture in 7.4% of thoracic injuries in a series of 54 consecutive chest trauma patients. Mediastinal widening on routine chest radiography with a distorted aortic contour is the most significant diagnostic study. When suspected, thoracic aortography is the procedure of choice. Delay in diagnosis by utilizing CT is not warranted in most cases. Many injuries of this type are associated with life-threatening injuries in other organs such as the abdomen and head.

INJURIES TO THE ESOPHAGUS

Perforation of the esophagus in the pediatric age group can occur in the delivery room from extreme positive pressure resuscitation or aspiration with a stiff catheter. In later infancy and

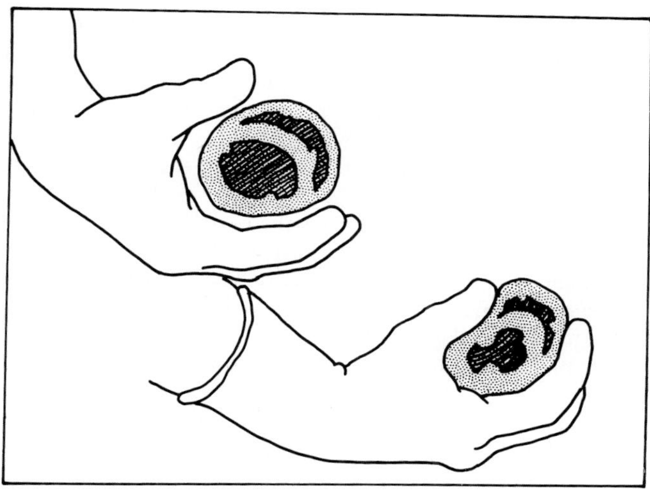

■ **FIGURE 72-18.** Internal cardiac massage: one-handed technique for neonates and infants.

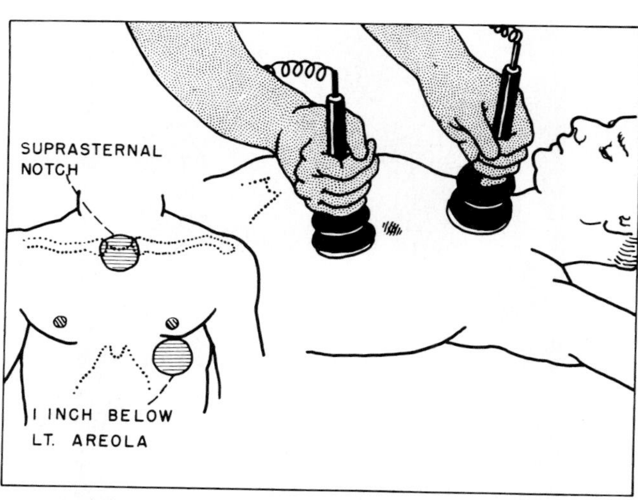

■ **FIGURE 72-20.** Electrode application for external cardiac defibrillation.

childhood, rupture can follow ingestion of lye or a solid foreign body, esophagoscopy, or dilation. Spontaneous rupture proximal to an esophageal web has been described. As in adults, stab and gunshot wounds can perforate the esophagus.

Clinically, hyperthermia, hypotension, and chest and neck pain mirror the mediastinitis. Pneumomediastinum, tension pneumothorax, subcutaneous emphysema, and hematemesis may be encountered.

Plain chest roentgenograms followed by a contrast esophagram and thoracentesis may demonstrate the tension sequelae, esophageal defect, and perhaps high-acid fluid.

The tension pneumothorax must quickly undergo decompression followed promptly by closure of the esophageal defect, mediastinal drainage, and massive doses of antibiotics.

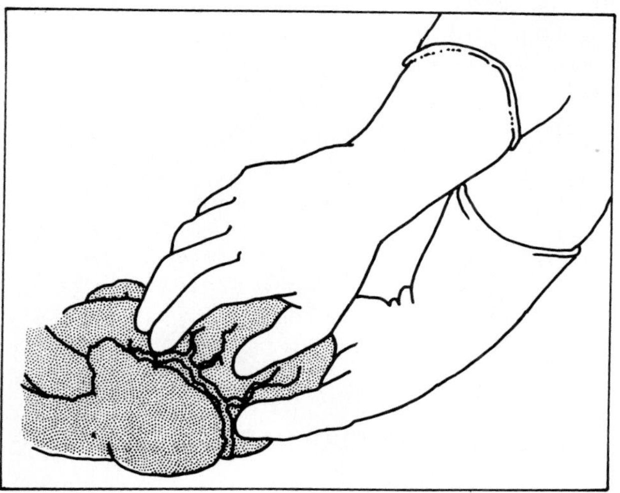

■ **FIGURE 72-19.** Internal cardiac massage: bimanual technique for older children and adults.

■ TRAUMATIC BLUNT RUPTURE OF THE DIAPHRAGM

Blunt trauma rupture of the diaphragm may occur with severe trauma. It is more common on the left (90%) than on the right.

The most significant study to arouse suspicion is routine chest radiography, which will frequently show an abnormal diaphragmatic contour. Initially, the herniation may not be present or suspected. Serial radiographs are important to determine later herniation. Significant cardiorespiratory abnormalities may occur in the early stages. If the rupture is not initially diagnosed, intestinal obstruction may be the leading symptom at the time of late diagnosis. Many significant injuries in other organ systems may confuse the early diagnosis. A contrast swallow of Gastrografin or barium will help confirm the presence of intestines in the hemithorax. A diagnostic pneumoperitoneum can prove such a rupture by the production of an ipsilateral pneumothorax.

■ THORACOABDOMINAL INJURIES

In infants and children, combined injury to the thorax and abdomen, including diaphragm rupture, is usually preceded by a violent traffic accident or other form of sudden, jolting impact. Splenic and hepatic lacerations commonly occur with minimal external evidence of injury and need not be associated with fractured ribs or soft tissue mutilation.

The clinical signs of upper abdominal tenderness, rigidity, and rebound tenderness almost uniformly accompany lower chest trauma and are explained by the abdominal distribution of the intercostal nerves. Therefore, peritoneal irritation, of itself, is not conclusive evidence of a combined or abdominal injury. Careful repeated examinations correlated with laboratory data are necessary for the diagnosis of intra-abdominal perforation or hemorrhage in the presence of chest trauma. Aspiration of the peritoneum may have a place and perhaps should be used more often.

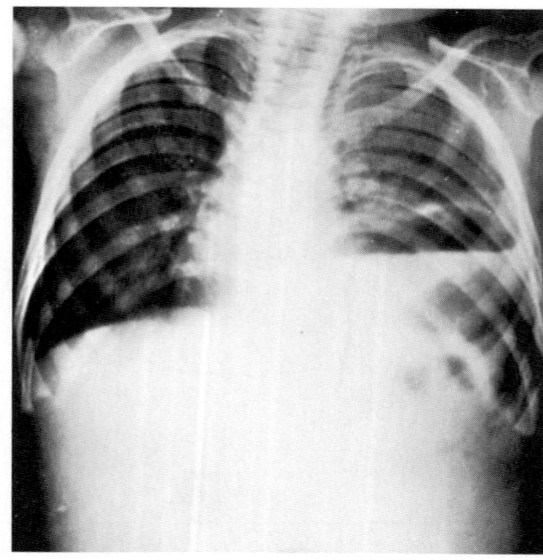

■ **FIGURE 72-21.** A blunt traumatic rupture of the left hemidiaphragm that went unrecognized. Death occurred 1 hour later from acute gastric dilation of the intrathoracic stomach (same physiologic effects as tension pneumothorax).

Diaphragm rupture can occur with minimal soft tissue injury, and there may be chest pain, dyspnea, and hypotension. On inspection, the involved chest wall lags during inspiration, and percussion can be dull or hyperresonant (Fig. 72-21). Chest roentgenograms may not show fractured ribs but almost invariably demonstrate abnormality or absence of the diaphragmatic shadow on the affected side. There is usually mediastinal shift to the right, because in 90% of cases the posterolateral left leaf of the diaphragm is torn in a radial manner (Fig. 72-22). At times a spontaneous pneumoperitoneum is seen. Diagnostic pneumoperitoneum may improve the radiologic diagnoses of rupture of the diaphragm (Fig. 72-23).

The preliminary management of combined thoracoabdominal injuries must provide an adequate airway and circulation, gastric decompression, and evaluation and control of other injuries. Intra-abdominal hemorrhage and perforation with thoracic and abdominal soiling is an obvious indication for

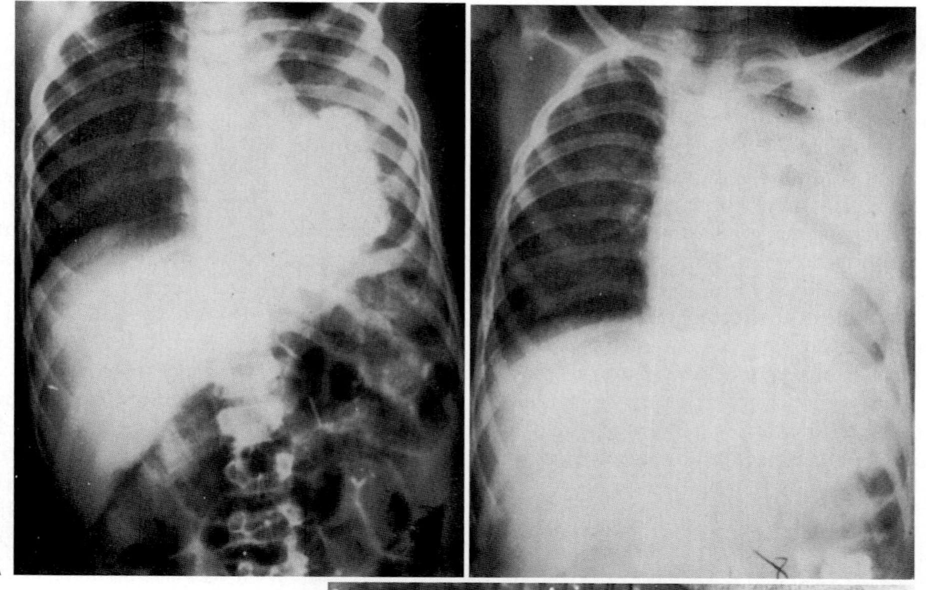

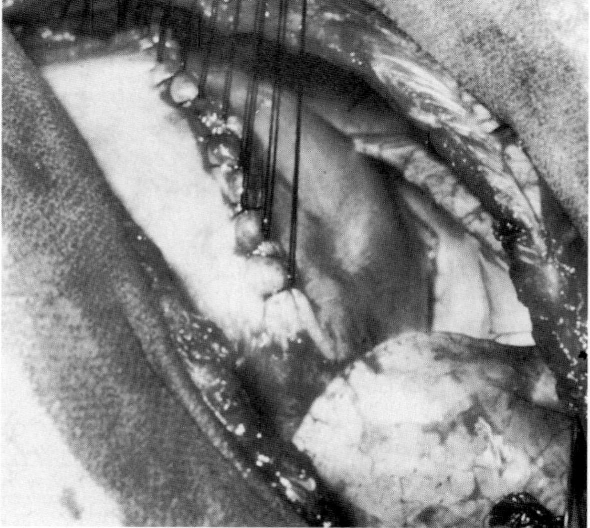

■ **FIGURE 72-22.** A blunt traumatic rupture of the left hemidiaphragm **(A)**, with barium swallow confirmation **(B)** and final closure at operation **(C)**.

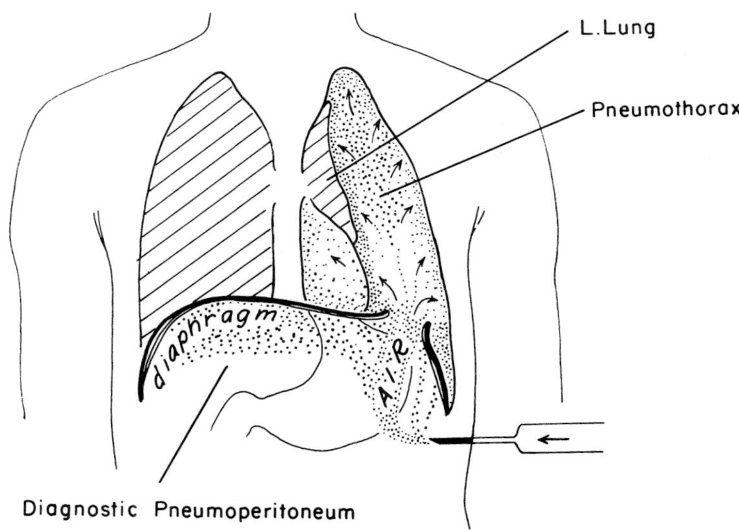

■ **FIGURE 72-23.** Diagnostic pneumoperitoneum in a suspected rupture of the diaphragm.

immediate exploration. Ideally, a ruptured diaphragm should be repaired as soon as systemic stabilization has been achieved.

SUGGESTED READING

Allen GS, Cox CS Jr: Pulmonary contusion in children. Diagnosis and management [Review]. South Med J 1998;91(12):1099–1106.

Azizkhan RG: Congenital pulmonary lesions in childhood. Chest Surg Clin North Am 1993;3:547–568.

Becmeur F, Donato L, Horta-Geraud P, Fraysse P, Schwaab C, Carrenard C, Sliman MA, Sauvage P: Rupture of the airways after blunt chest trauma in two children. Eur J Pediatr Surg 2000;10(2):133–135.

Bliss DW, Newth CJ, Stein JE: Blunt traumatic injury to the coronary arteries and pulmonary artery in a child. J Trauma 2000;49(3):550–552.

Brandt ML, Luks FI, Spigland NA, DiLorenzo M, Laberge JM, Ouimet A: Diaphragmatic injury in children. J Trauma 1992;32:298–301.

Coleman DM, Cox PN, Dyck J, Razzouk AJ, Rebeyka IM: Pediatric transesophageal echocardiography in the evaluation of acute disruption of the mitral valve following blunt thoracic trauma. Case report [Review]. J Trauma 1994;36(1):135–136.

Cooper A: Thoracic injuries [Review]. Semin Pediatr Surg 1995;4(2):109–115.

Cox CS Jr, Black CT, Duke JH, Cocanour CS, Moore FA, Lally KP, Andrassy RJ: Operative treatment of truncal vascular injuries in children and adolescents. J Pediatr Surg 1998;33(3):462–467.

Crankson SJ, Fischer JD, Al-Rabecah AA, Al-Jaddan SA: Pediatric thoracic trauma. Saudi Med J 2001;22(2):117–120.

Daughtry DC: Thoracic Trauma. Boston: Little, Brown, 1980.

Eddy AC, Rusch VW, Fligner CL, Reay DT, Rice CL: The epidemiology of traumatic rupture of the thoracic aorta in children. A 13-year review. J Trauma 1990;30:989–991 (discussion, 991–992).

Fernandez LG, Radhakrishnan J, Gordon RT, Shah MR, Lain KY, Messersmith RN, Roettger RH, Norwood SH: Thoracic BB injuries in pediatric patients. J Trauma 1995;38(3):384–389.

Gittelman MA, Gonzalez-del-Rey J, Brody AS, DiGiulio GA: Clinical predictors for the selective use of chest radiographs in pediatric blunt trauma evaluations. J Trauma 2003;55(4):670–676.

Grant WJ, Meyers RL, Jaffe RL, Johnson DG: Tracheobronchial injuries after blunt chest trauma in children—Hidden pathology. J Pediatr Surg 1998;33(11):11707–11711.

Grasso SN, Keller MS: Diagnostic imaging in pediatric trauma [Review]. Curr Opin Pediatr 1998;10(3):299–302.

Haller JA: Thoracic injuries. In: Welch KJ, Randolph JG, Ravitch M, O'Neill JA, Rowe MI, eds: Pediatric Surgery, 4th ed, Vol 1. Chicago: Year Book Medical Publishers, 1986, pp 143–154.

Holmes JF, Brant WE, Bogren HG, London KL, Kuppermann N: Prevalence and importance of pneumothoraces visualized on abdominal computed tomographic scan in children with blunt trauma. J Trauma 2001;50(3):516–520.

Holmes JF, Sokolove PE, Brant WE, Kuppermann N: A clinical decision rule for identifying children with thoracic injuries after blunt torso trauma. Ann Emerg Med 2002;39(5):492–499.

Karnak I, Senocak ME, Tanyel FC, Buyukpamukeu N: Diaphragmatic injuries in childhood. Surg Today 2001;31(1):5–11

Manson D, Babyn PS, Palder S, Bergman K: CT of blunt chest trauma in children. Pediatr Radiol 1993;23:1–5.

Melzig EP, Swank M, Salzberg AM: Acute blunt traumatic rupture of the diaphragm in children. Arch Surg 1976;111:1009–1011.

Ozdulger A, Cetin G, Erkmen Gulhan S, Topcu S, Tastepe I, Kaya S: A review of 24 patients with bronchial ruptures. Is delay in diagnosis more common in children? Eur J Cardiothorac Surg 2003;23(3):379–383.

Pearl M, Milstein M, Rook GD: Pseudocyst of the lung due to traumatic nonpenetrating lung injury. J Pediatr Surg 1973;8:967–968.

Peclet MH, Newman KD, Eichelberger MR, Gotschall CS, Garcia VF, Bowman LM: Patterns of injury in children. J Pediatr Surg 1990;25:85.

Peclet MH, Newman KD, Eichelberger MR, Gotschall CS, Garcia VF, Bowman LM: Thoracic trauma in children. An indicator of increased mortality. J Pediatr Surg 1990;25:961–965.

Peterson RJ, Tiwary AD, Kissoon N, Tepas JJ III, Ceithaml EL, Pieper P: Pediatric penetrating thoracic trauma. A five-year experience. Pediatr Emerg Care 1994;10(3);129–131.

Pilcher RS: Trachea, bronchi, lungs and pleura. In: Brown JJM, ed: Surgery of Childhood. Baltimore: Williams & Wilkins, 1963, pp 650–696.

Reilly JP, Brandt ML, Mattox KL, Pokorny WJ: Thoracic trauma in children. J Trauma 1993;34:329.

Rouse TM, Eichelberger MR: Trends in pediatric trauma management. Surg Clin North Am 1992;72(6)1347–1364.

Roux P, Fisher RM: Chest injuries in children. An analysis of 100 cases of blunt trauma from motor vehicle accidents. J Pediatr Surg 1992;27:551–555.

Sivit CT, Taylor GA, Eichelberger MR: Chest injury in children with blunt abdominal trauma. Evaluation with CT. Radiology 1989;717:815–818.

Slimane MA, Becmeur F, Aubert D, Bachy B, Varlet F, Chavrier Y, Daoud S, Fremond B, Guys JM, de Lagausie P, Algrain Y, Reinberg O, Sauvage P: Tracheobronchial ruptures from blunt thoracic trauma in children. J Pediatr Surg 1999;34(12):1847–1850.

Smyth BT: Chest trauma in children. J Pediatr Surg 1979;14:41–47.

Spouge AB, Burroughs PE, Armstrong D, Daneman A: Traumatic aortic rupture in the pediatric population. Role of plain film, CT and angiography in the diagnosis. Pediatr Radiol 1991;21:324–328.

Stylianos S, Eichelberger MR: Pediatric trauma. Preventive strategies. Pediatr Clin North Am 1993;40:1359–1368.

Taylor MW, Garber JC, Boswell WC, Boyd CR: Delayed hemopericardium and associated pericardial mass after blunt chest trauma. Am Surg 2003;69(4): 343–345.

Tiao GM, Griffith PM, Szmuszkovicz JR, Mahour GH: Cardiac and great vessel injuries in children after blunt trauma. An institutional review. J Pediatr Surg 2000;35(11):1656–1660.

Trachiotis GD, Sell JE, Pearson GD, Martin GR, Midgley FM: Traumatic thoracic aortic rupture in the pediatric patient. Ann Thorac Surg. 1996; 62(3):724–732.

Wesson DE: Trauma of the chest in children. Chest Surg Clin North Am 1992;3.

73 Sudden Infant Death Syndrome and Acute Life-Threatening Events

James S. Kemp, MD • Bradley T. Thach, MD

Infants experiencing an acute life-threatening event (ALTE) and premature infants with apnea may later die suddenly and unexpectedly, with a diagnosis of sudden infant death syndrome (SIDS). However, because about 80% of victims dying suddenly and unexpectedly were born at term and were never known to be apneic until they died, discussing ALTE, apnea of prematurity (AOP), and SIDS together has become controversial, particularly when the issue of apnea monitoring is raised.

Since the last edition of this textbook there has been a change in the focus of physiologic investigations into why infants die suddenly. The reason for this shift is that straightforward changes in sleep practices[1] have led to a marked reduction in infants dying during sleep (Fig. 73-1).[2] Through experiments based on death scene and epidemiologic data, much progress has been made in understanding the physiologic bases for the greater risk of sudden death of infants in the prone position (Table 73-1).

Whether or not increased risk is sufficient to justify apnea monitoring,[3,4] premature infants and those experiencing ALTE do die unexpectedly more often. We will discuss ALTE, AOP, and SIDS as separate entities but will point out common physiologic and epidemiologic characteristics. We will emphasize possible mechanisms for sudden and unexpected deaths that are attracting renewed interest during a time when sleep practices are reducing risk for death.

■ ACUTE LIFE-THREATENING EVENTS IN INFANTS AND APNEA IN PREMATURE INFANTS

■ ACUTE LIFE-THREATENING EVENTS

Definitions

An apparent life-threatening event is defined as "an episode that is frightening to the observer" and has one or more of the following characteristics: (1) apnea, usually central (less commonly obstructive); (2) color change, usually to blue or pale (less often to red and plethoric); (3) sudden limpness; (4) choking or gagging.

Apnea of infancy, by definition idiopathic or unexplained, is a type of ALTE because it frightens parents. Infants are beyond the term postconceptional age when apnea is first noted. The components of an ALTE are usually present, except perhaps the choking or gagging. (In our experience, caretakers will often describe gasping, also.)

These two definitions have remained standard for the past 20 years.[3]

Acute Life-Threatening Events and Recommendations for Home Cardiorespiratory Monitoring

The American Academy of Pediatrics (AAP) has recently published a new review and guidelines for home monitors.[3] The AAP recommends monitoring in two specific circumstances: (1) Monitoring "may be warranted" in selected premature infants until "43 weeks postmenstrual age," or until "extreme episodes" of apnea, bradycardia, and hypoxemia stop; (2) infants who are usually supported at home by mechanical ventilation through a tracheotomy should be monitored.

Routine monitoring is not recommended by the AAP for infants with an ALTE or among siblings of SIDS victims. In a list of instructions, the AAP states: (1) "Home cardiorespiratory monitoring should not be prescribed to prevent SIDS"; (2) "Parents should be advised that … monitoring has not been proven to prevent sudden unexpected deaths…."[3]

The AAP's recommendations reflect an accurate interpretation of published reports but also reflect compromises that are believed by some to be too generous toward[4] or restrictive of monitoring. One expert,[5] apparently in disagreement, has written that "[p]atients with ALTE represent perhaps the group in which the indication for monitoring is least ambiguous, not as much with regard to SIDS prevention…," but to understand the cause of unexplained apnea. In our opinion, approaches to monitoring that are dogmatic, either pro or con, and not sympathetic to parents' concerns, should not be the norm.[6]

Thus, although it is the official recommendation of the AAP that ALTE patients not be monitored, this appears to be a common practice.

Evaluation of an Infant with an Acute Life-Threatening Event

A clinical approach to the differential diagnosis is presented in Box 73-1.[7–11] In the next section, we discuss gastroesophageal reflux (GER) and upper airway protective reflexes, which may cause an infant to have an ALTE.[12]

The approach to infants with an ALTE will be influenced by one's understanding of the association between ALTE and eventual sudden death. Among infants with ALTEs requiring repeated resuscitation, 13% died in one series,[13] and in other studies, 7% to 9% of SIDS infants had a history of an ALTE.[14] Though representing a minority of infants dying, these percentages are similar to other high-risk problems such as the percentage of children dying from asthma who have a history of respiratory failure,[15]

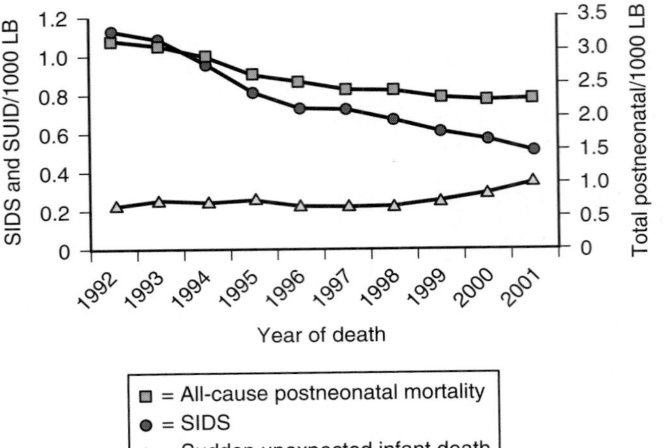

FIGURE 73-1. There has been a 53% fall in the rate of SIDS in the United States since 1992, from 1.20 to 0.56 deaths per 1000 live births (LB). SUID, sudden unexpected infant death. (From American Academy of Pediatrics Task Force on Sudden Infant Death Syndrome: The changing concept of sudden infant death syndrome. Diagnostic coding shifts, controversies regarding the sleeping environment, and new variables to consider in reducing risk. Pediatrics, published online October 10, 2005 [doi: 10.1542/peds.2005-1499].)

and are not insignificant. This does not suggest that monitoring is mandatory but rather that such infants are at a measurable risk of suddenly dying that far exceeds their age peers.

The clinical approach should also be based on one's assessment of the validity of the caregivers' observations; "benign physiological events in babies may sometimes cause an overreaction by parents, particularly those who are anxious, are attention-seeking, or suffer a personality disorder."[16,17]

The usefulness (positive predictive value) of any series of tests in identifying a cause for ALTEs is difficult to identify in the absence of protocols for evaluation that are consistently followed, and because patient identification often depends on the degree of parental concern. Not surprisingly, nearly 50% of ALTE cases[18] remain unexplained or idiopathic, and by default such idiopathic ALTEs are attributed to apnea of infancy.

To begin to allay parental concern, and to observe and monitor the infant, hospital admission for 2 to 3 days is often indicated after an ALTE.[17] The history is critical in beginning to understand an ALTE, and the attending physician supervising the evaluation should make every effort to obtain the history himself or herself, including the duration of the event, time of day, adequacy of lighting, infant's position within his or her surroundings, and whether the episode began while awake or asleep. The infant's color, tone, and the need for and type of resuscitation must be noted. Was blood or pink froth coming from the infant's mouth or nose? The appropriateness of the caregivers' concern should be noted. Family history of sudden death, or serious illness with coma among young people, must be ascertained. Was the infant in the early stages of a respiratory illness, or was he or she having coughing paroxysms? (It is surprising how often typical pertussis will evolve in infants presenting with an ALTE!)

Physical examination should focus on tone, alertness, evidence of bruising or scalp swelling or disuse of extremities, and fundoscopic evidence for retinal hemorrhages. Evidence of stridor, stertor, chest wall retractions, poor skin perfusion, and cardiac murmurs or dysrhythmias should be sought. Neonates younger than 2 months of age should be considered at risk for bacteremic sepsis when they present with apnea or hypotonia, and should be treated accordingly (see Box 73-1).

Initial laboratory evaluation should include measurement of hemoglobin and white blood cell count with differential cell count, culture of blood and urine, nasal swabs for respiratory syncytial virus (RSV) and pertussis, a chest radiograph, and serum glucose, sodium, potassium, chloride, and bicarbonate. The child should be admitted to a unit where cardiorespiratory monitoring is available, so that abnormalities in cardiac or respiratory rate can be detected in recorded data. If the infant continues to be limp, or apnea recurs, one should measure arterial blood gases, serum lactate, and ammonia, as well as screening the urine for abnormal levels of amino and organic acids and drugs. In children who continue to appear ill or who have altered mental status with no other cause detected, video electroencephalography (EEG)

TABLE 73-1. Selected traditional epidemiologic characteristics and risk factors for SIDS[9] and the possible effects of changes in sleep practices

Characteristic or Risk Factor	After Sleep Position Intervention
Preterm birth <37 weeks	Still significant[7]
Male sex	Still significant[8]
Black race	Probably more important
Maternal parity more than two	Still significant[8]
Late or no prenatal care	Less significant[7]
Mother <20 years old	Still significant
Smoking during pregnancy	More important
Never breastfed	Significance less
Upper respiratory infection	Significance less[7]
Winter peak	Results variable, sometimes absent[9]
Age at death (89% >2 but <23 weeks)[9]	Relatively fewer >1 month vs <1 month
	Little change[10]
	Younger[11]

BOX 73-1 Selected Causes in the Differential Diagnosis of an Acute Life-Threatening Event

- Respiratory syncytial virus, pertussis
- Sepsis with apnea
- Syndromes compromising the upper airway (e.g., Pierre Robin sequence)
- Breath-holding spells
- Seizures
- Intracranial hemorrhages, vascular malformations, child abuse, vitamin K deficiency
- Exaggerated laryngeal chemoreflex with or without gastroesophageal reflux
- Drugs (e.g., phenothiazines)
- Tachyarrhythmias (e.g., Wolfe-Parkinson-White, prolonged QT syndrome)
- Inborn errors of metabolism (e.g., MCAD deficiencies)
- Hypoventilation during bed sharing or because nose and mouth become covered with bedding

should be conducted and imaging of the central nervous system (CNS) by computed tomography or, preferably, magnetic resonance imaging, should be carried out.[19]

A Potential Mechanism for Acute Life-Threatening Events after Gastroesophageal Reflux or Respiratory Syncytial Virus Infection

We discuss laryngeal chemoreflex apnea (LCRA) at length because it may be a mechanism of life-threatening apnea in many conditions. Furthermore, we want to emphasize that what is usually pathologic when considering GER in this context is the severity of the reflex apnea, not the reflux per se.

Because it can be prolonged and fatal, LCRA has continued to interest many investigators.[20–24] Given the ubiquity of GER in young infants[25] and its vague link to apnea, a reflex such as LCRA elicited during GER that also may cause breathing to stop is of obvious importance. Inability to modulate LCRA has also been proposed as a mechanism for sudden death in the prone position.[20]

Relevant Epidemiology and Physiology of Gastroesophageal Reflux

The role of GER in infant apnea remains controversial, although in a recent series, 40% of ALTEs were attributed to it.[19] For more than 25 years, GER has been linked to ALTE.[26] Despite the relative thinness of the evidence, the majority of pediatricians in the United States believe that GER plays a key role in many ALTEs.

Acid reflux seems to be common even in normal infants.[25] Vandenplas and co-workers used the pH probe to study 509 normal, healthy infants younger than 12 months of age. Infants treated for GER had been excluded from their study. Among healthy neonates without apnea or undue irritability, the 95th percentile was 13% of the time with the pH less than 4 in the distal esophagus, and, at 1 year, 8% of the time. The average of the 95th percentile for reflux index for each of the first 12 months of life was 10%. Vandenplas and co-workers believe that "reflux is a phenomenon occurring to some extent in every human being."[25] It has even been speculated that, because GER might provoke or be associated with arousal from sleep,[27] it may be "protective" against sudden infant death, rather than causative.[28] Though provocative, this speculation reminds us that GER is more common, and SIDS less common, when infants sleep in the supine position.

Gastroesophageal reflux is common and ALTEs relatively rare, and there are few data linking duration of acid reflux to frequency of apnea. Nevertheless, we believe that reflex apnea may be elicited during GER in susceptible infants,[29] particularly when reflux reaches the pharynx, and this apnea may put these infants at risk for an ALTE if not sudden death.[29–31]

It is not necessary, however, for refluxed fluid to be acidic to elicit LCRA. Furthermore, the usefulness of conventional esophageal pH monitoring in identifying GER in infants has been questioned.[32] In studies of preterm infants who were fed every 2, 3, or 4 hours, the pH in the stomach approximately 2 hours after feedings was greater than 4, the pH threshold for detecting reflux into the esophagus. In all infants, gastric pH was less than 4 for only 24.5% of the time (range, 0.6% to 69.1%). The percentage of time with gastric pH greater than 4 may be even higher in older term infants. A pH-independent technique for diagnosing fluid reflux into the esophagus and pharynx has, therefore, been developed (Fig. 73-2).[33,34] Using this technique in 19 preterm infants studied for 6 hours, Peter and co-workers showed that apnea was no more common during reflux than during "reflux-free epochs" (see Fig. 73-2).[35] The time interval used to analyze for a temporal link was 20 seconds. Although reflux reached the pharynx in the majority of episodes (345 of 524, 65.8%), apnea occurring within 20 seconds of reflux into the pharynx was no more common than during "reflux-free epochs." The preterm subjects had very frequent apnea of longer than 4 seconds, on average approximately 20 apnea episodes per hour. Thus, in infants having frequent apnea, the temporal link of apnea with GER, even into the pharynx, is unclear. However, their findings were somewhat inconclusive, because reflux to the pharynx was more likely to occur within 20 seconds before apnea than within 20 seconds after, a sequence that would support a causal role.

The situation in term infants with less frequent apnea may be different. Among 22 term infants studied using the same technique, apnea was six times more likely to occur during GER than when GER was not occurring.[33] Again, the majority of reflux episodes extended to the pharynx (71.4%). During the 6-hour recordings, apnea was relatively infrequent in the term infants (1.2 per hour vs. nearly 20 per hour among preterm subjects).[35]

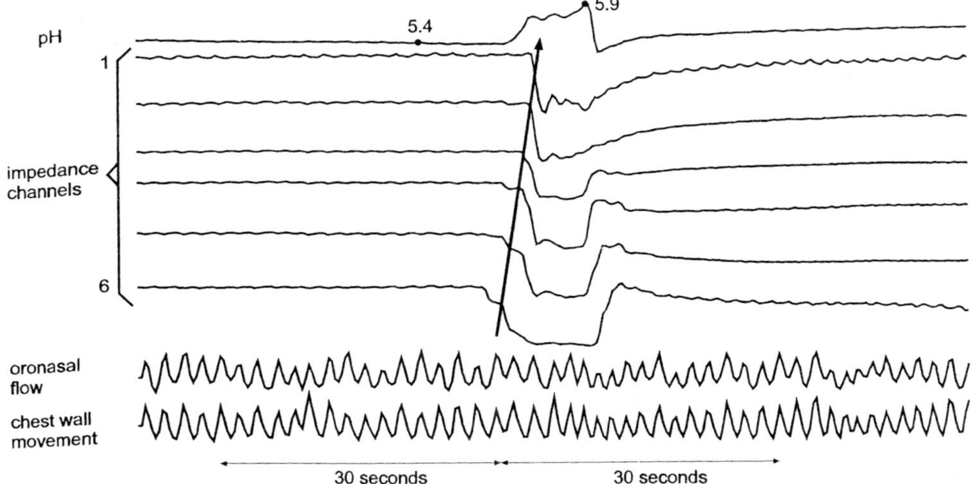

■ **FIGURE 73-2.** Sequential changes in electrical impedance between pairs were recorded for six electrodes positioned every 1.5 cm within a catheter from the pharynx to the gastric cardia.[28] During normal swallowing, impedance changes sequentially from the pharynx toward the stomach. During reflux, shown here, the sequence of impedance changes is reversed, beginning in the stomach and extending proximally to the pharynx *(channel 1)*. In this figure, pH increases in the esophagus during nonacid reflux. pH probe is at level of impedance *channel 5*. (From Wenzl TG, Schenke S, Peschgens T, Silny J, Heimann G, Skopnik H: Association of apnea and nonacid gastroesophageal reflux in infants. Investigations with intraluminal impedance technique. Pediatr Pulmonol 2001;31:144–149.)

To summarize these two studies using pH-independent methods to detect reflux, apnea temporally associated with reflux is common among term infants having relatively infrequent and brief apneic episodes. Among preterm infants having frequent apnea, the temporal link with GER is much less clear.

Finally, there seems to be no obvious mechanism for reflux to elicit apnea, if it extends only to the distal esophagus. There are no known receptors modulating respiration in the distal esophagus. As described later, the most potent reflexes are elicited only if the refluxed liquid passes the supraesophageal sphincter, which is rare with passive reflux.

Characteristics of Laryngeal Chemoreflex Apnea

In experimental animals, prolonged apnea, bradycardia, and marked increases in central venous and arterial blood pressure are caused by electrical stimulation of unmyelinated nerve fibers arising in the laryngeal epithelium and traveling in the superior laryngeal nerve. These unencapsulated nerve endings giving rise to afferent signals are most numerous in the mucosal epithelium of the epiglottis, aryepiglottic folds, and interarytenoid space.[36] The sequence of response after single-fiber stimulation of these nerves is dramatic and is most marked in younger animals (piglets, lambs, puppies). Apnea beginning within 0.25 seconds of the stimulus may last 20 to 90 seconds and be fatal in the laboratory.[22,23]

In young animals, LCRA is very robust, in that water applied to the larynx in minute quantities almost always elicits prolonged apnea with bradycardia (76 of 76 trials in puppies, 29 of 30 in piglets). The chloride concentration in fluids contacting laryngeal nerves seems critical in eliciting the reflex.[23] Apnea is more pronounced with water as a stimulus than normal saline. Cow's milk and dog's milk, each low in chloride, will elicit prolonged apnea when applied to the larynx of puppies, piglets, and lambs. If even small quantities of water or milk (e.g., 0.2 mL) remain on the larynx and are not removed by swallowing, the associated apnea has often been fatal in experimental animals.[22] Thus, LCRA, if elicited in humans, could cause an ALTE.

Human infants attempt to clear fluid that elicits LCRA by swallowing during a central apneic episode (Fig. 73-3).[21] After the central apneic event, any breaths attempted are obstructed so long as upper airway closure persists. When swallowing presumably clears the fluid, the upper airway is opened with a return to eupneic breathing. Less commonly, when elicited during sleep, LCRA is terminated by cough and arousal.[37] As in experimental animals, among human preterm infants water is more potent than normal saline in eliciting severe LCRA. In infants, should swallowing be delayed or fail to occur, the apneic phase of the laryngeal chemoreflex can be prolonged, extending over 20 seconds and causing hypoxemia.[21,30] These findings suggest that airway protection from aspiration takes precedence over ventilation in some circumstances when even small quantities of fluids (~0.1 mL), including water, come in contact with the larynx.

In older infants and older experimental animals, apnea occurs as part of the laryngeal chemoreflex, but it is shorter than in preterm infants and newborn animals. Maturation is associated with reduction in central respiratory inhibition. Cough and

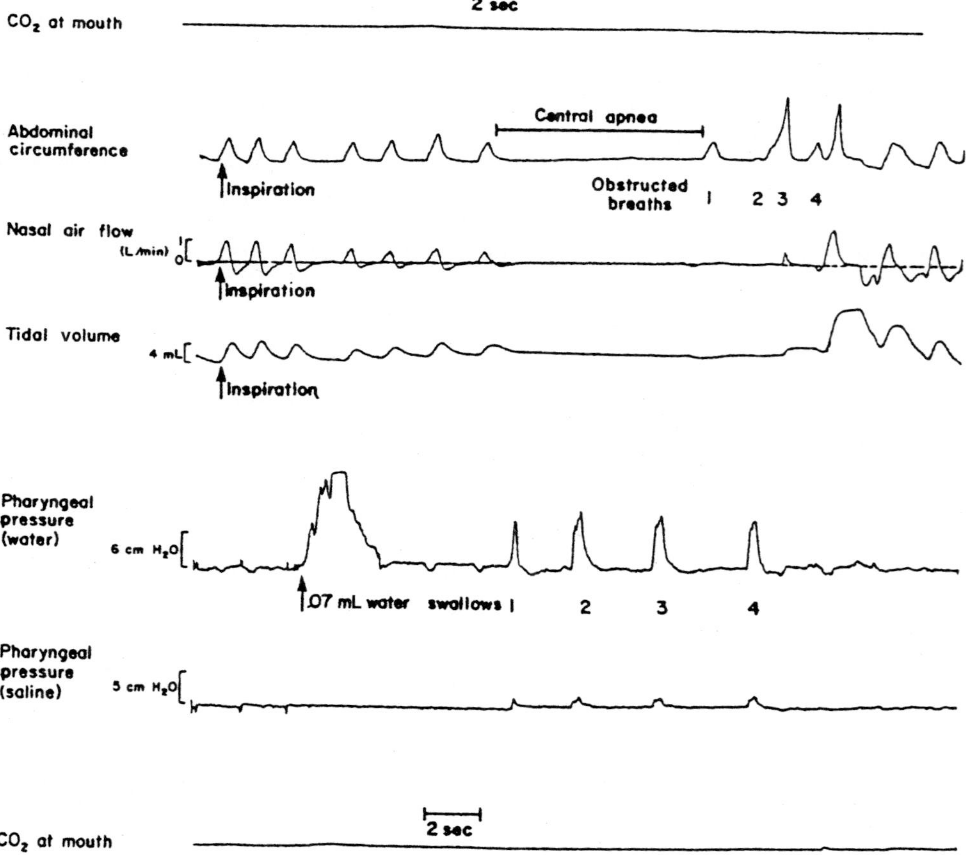

■ **FIGURE 73-3.** Sequence of response representing laryngeal chemoreflex apnea in an infant. Upward deflections on pharyngeal pressure tracing reflect swallows. Application of less than 0.1 mL of water onto the larynx leads to swallows and central apnea, followed by obstructive apnea and restoration of eupnea after water has been cleared by swallows. (From Davies AM, Koenig JS, Thach BT: Upper airway chemoreflex responses to saline and water in preterm infants. J Appl Physiol 1988;64:1412–1420.)

arousal from sleep are also more likely to occur among mature subjects when water, acid, or milk comes in contact with the larynx.[36] Nevertheless, in susceptible infants, delays in maturational influences could put them at risk for prolonged apnea as part of the laryngeal chemoreflex.[24]

Some risk factor for SIDS and ALTE may be explained by LCRA.

Laryngeal Chemoreflex Apnea and Nicotine Exposure

Prenatal and postnatal exposure to cigarette smoke consistently and powerfully increases risk for sudden unexpected infant death.[38,39] Lambs exposed to intravenous nicotine from birth, compared with controls, had longer bradycardias and LCRA (8–14 seconds longer) when 1 mL of water was placed on their larynx. Some nicotine-exposed lambs "developed ... a sudden loss of muscle tone and were unresponsive to external stimuli."[40] This series of events resembles the definition of an ALTE.

Laryngeal Chemoreflex Apnea and Respiratory Syncytial Virus Infections

Acute infection with RSV has been associated with apnea, particularly among prone infants.[41] Evidence of a recent RSV infection also markedly increases risk for SIDS among prone infants.[42] When studied in detail in a premature infant and a term infant, each experiencing apnea while infected with RSV, the spontaneous apneic events resemble LCRA (Fig. 73-4).[43] Duration of apnea in the RSV-infected infants was often longer than 30 seconds. Apnea was first central and then obstructed (i.e., mixed) and was usually terminated after a series of swallows, less often with a cough. Upper airway secretions, which are increased during acute RSV infection, might elicit prolonged LCRA, unless cleared efficiently by swallowing.

In addition to provoking more secretions, other aspects of infection with RSV could prolong LCRA. Inflammatory cytokines (interleukins IL-1β, IL-6) produced during the infection but acting within the CNS may prolong LCRA.[44]

Summary

The laryngeal chemoreflex is robust and the apnea produced profound, particularly in developmentally susceptible subjects. LCRA may help explain many types of ALTE. Reflux of acid to the larynx may elicit LCRA, but milk, water, and nonacid secretions are quite capable of eliciting profound apnea. The link between GER, which is common, and apnea, which is rare, may best be understood by asking why some infants have pathologic LCRA.

■ APNEA IN PREMATURE INFANTS

■ DEFINITION AND DIFFERENTIAL DIAGNOSIS

During their initial hospitalization, 50% to 100% of premature infants born weighing less than 1500 g will require mechanical or pharmacologic interventions because of apnea.[45,46] AOP is defined as cessation of airflow for 10 to 20 seconds or longer. Shorter pauses in respiration associated with falls in SpO_2%

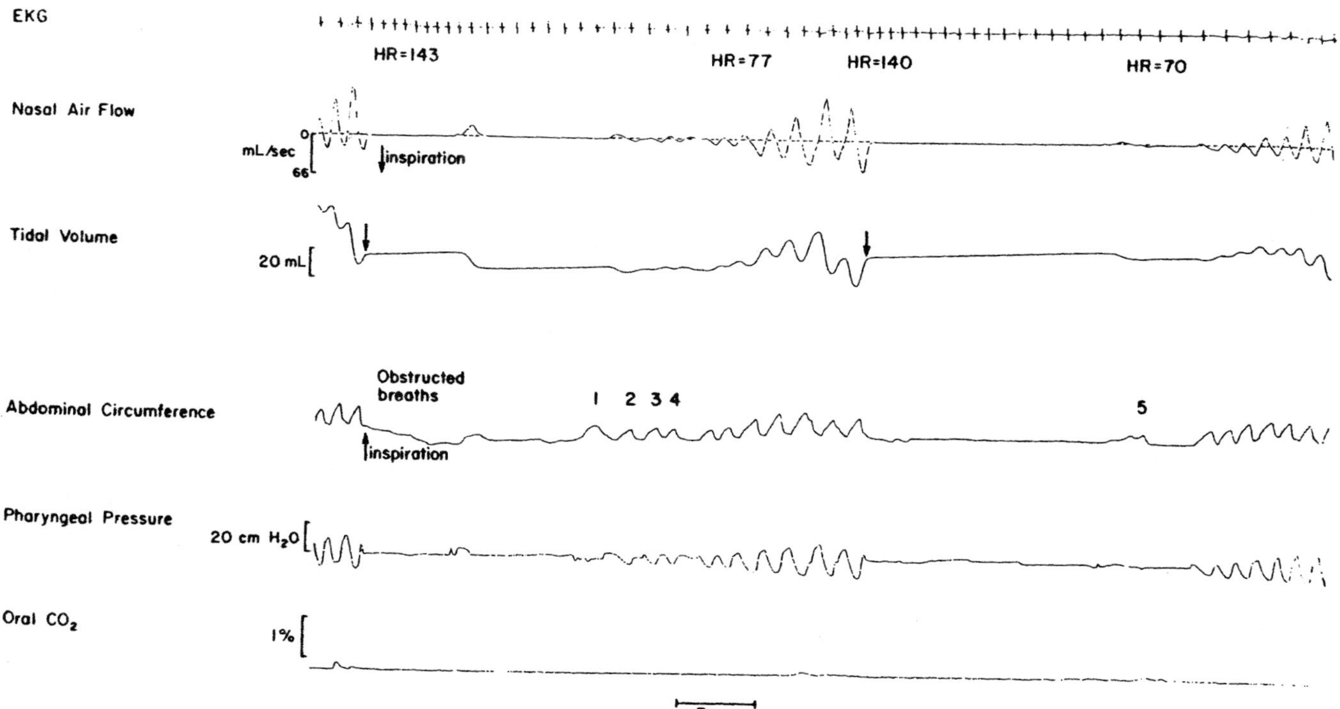

■ **FIGURE 73-4.** Spontaneous mixed apnea, resembling LCRA, in a preterm neonate at 37 weeks after conception, infected with RSV. The assumption is that fluid secretions from the infected nasopharynx drained onto the larynx (*arrow*, tidal volume tracing). The secretions elicited central and obstructive apnea (1–4 on abdominal circumference tracing), followed by swallows (pharyngeal pressure signal). The swallows cleared the secretions, and after a second period of central apnea, eupnea was restored. HR, heart rate (beats/min). (From Pickens DL, Schefft GL, Storch GA, Thach BT: Characterization of prolonged apneic episodes associated with respiratory syncytial virus infection. Pediatr Pulmonol 1989;6:195–201.)

(e.g., to <90%) or in heart rate (e.g., to <100 beats/min) also are seen as important episodes of apnea in most neonatal intensive care units (NICUs).[45,47]

Other possibilities in the differential diagnosis of apnea due to immaturity of ventilatory control include: intracranial hemorrhage, sedation crossing the placenta, sepsis with or without meningitis, heat or cold stress,[48] a patent ductus arteriosus, hypoglycemia, electrolyte abnormalities (particularly, hyponatremia), anemia, necrotizing enterocolitis, feeding-related apnea,[49] heart block or heart failure lowering cerebral perfusion, and excessive sedation given to the infant directly.

The majority of apnea among premature infants is "idiopathic."

HYPOTHESES FOR PATHOGENESIS OF APNEA OF PREMATURITY

Ventilatory control among premature infants is sufficiently unstable that apnea, even prolonged, is provoked by problems (e.g., hyponatremia, heart failure) that would not be sufficient explanations beyond term postconceptional age (PCA). Thus, the primary instability of ventilatory pattern and drive among premature infants, even when they are "well," is important.

It is simplistic to state that most apnea among premature infants is central, although most episodes can be prevented with stimulants whose primary action is central. Indeed, it is probable that the majority of apneic events in premature infants have both obstructive and central components (i.e., they are mixed[50]) and often respond to continuous positive airway pressure.

There is little recent published work that describes the prevalence of the various types of apnea (central, obstructive, or mixed) or the impact of sleep state, or that explores critically the continued relevance of what has become "cribside" dogma. Most detailed physiologic studies of apnea among premature infants were done 20 or more years ago, before the introduction of artificial surfactant.[51] Moreover, clinical rules have often been based on few observations; for example, the dogma that apnea is much more common in active than in quiet sleep is based on studies done on nine term infants.[52]

It was observed in the 1980s that the majority of central apneic episodes were either preceded or followed by evidence of upper airway obstruction (Fig. 73-5).[53,54] During apnea in premature infants, respiratory effort often continues, or resumes, before airflow returns, with phasic contraction of the diaphragm (electromyogram) associated with generation of progressively more negative intrathoracic pressures (P_{esoph}). Near the end of a typical mixed apnea, genioglossus contraction (submental electromyogram) opens the airway and flow resumes.[55] It was thus recognized that apneic episodes in premature neonates could also present as bradycardia with desaturation, because impedance chest movement monitors would correctly indicate that respiratory efforts continued.

During quiet sleep, premature neonates with frequent apnea are less able than nonapneic controls to compensate for progressive increases in upper airway resistance. Neonates with apnea have much shorter and weaker inspiratory efforts in response to end-expiratory occlusion. Premature neonates with apnea also have a higher Pa_{CO_2} (~9 mm Hg) and a much flatter ventilatory response to breathing 4% CO_2 (V_E/min/kg) compared with controls.[56,57] In addition, infants in general have a flatter CO_2 response when breathing progressively more hypoxic gas mixtures.[58]

A series of explanations for the most common type of apnea among premature infants—mixed apnea—can be constructed from these classic studies:

1. Upper airway obstruction, for which the infant has shorter and weaker "load compensation," is preceded by brief central apnea, or leads to longer central apnea.
2. Infants with a lower minute volume response to increasing CO_2 become progressively more hypercarbic and hypoxemic.

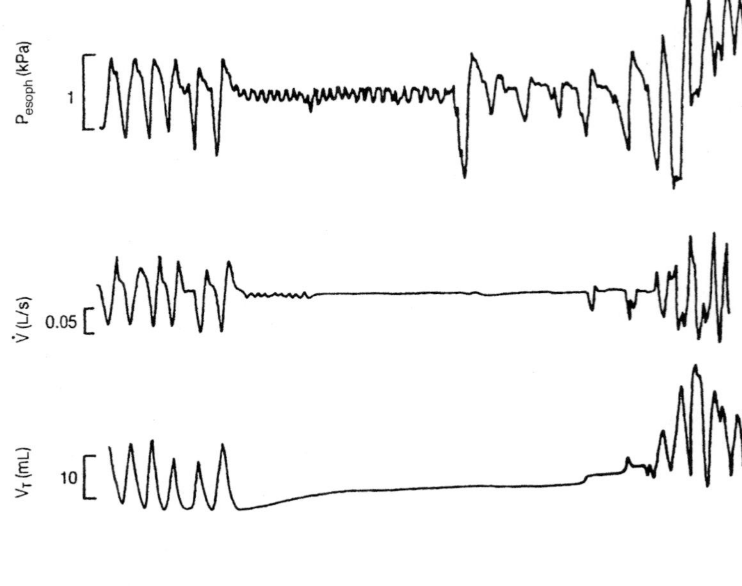

FIGURE 73-5. Spontaneous apnea in a premature infant. Esophageal pressure tracing, with cardiogenic artifact, demonstrates first central apnea, then respiratory efforts. Flow and volume tracings show that the first four or five efforts after central apnea are obstructed. Such mixed apneas are the most common type of apnea of prematurity. P_{esoph}, intrathoracic pressure; V_T, tidal volume; $\dot{V}$, airflow. (From Milner AD, Greenough A: The role of the upper airway in neonatal apnea. Semin Neonatol 2004;9:213–220.)

3. The development of hypoxemia further blunts CO_2 response, and the increasing CO_2 makes the activities of the diaphragm and genioglossus asynchronous,[59] perpetuating the cycle of obstructive and central (i.e., mixed) apneas.

Other "classic" studies from the mid-1980s suggested additional physiologic mechanisms to explain why premature infants might be more at risk for mixed apnea and its complications during active sleep:

1. The inspiratory "load" for which premature infants are unable to "compensate" is due to upper airway narrowing,[51,52] which usually occurs at the pharynx.[50]
2. Loss of intercostal tone[60] during active sleep would increase wasted "distortional" work[61] during the paradoxical breathing caused by pharyngeal airway narrowing.[50,62]
3. Loss of intercostal tone would also diminish functional residual capacity and thus worsen hypoxemia during compromised breathing.[60]

Furthermore, LCRA may also play a role in AOP. Swallowing interrupts LCRA. Premature infants swallow more frequently during apnea than during eupneic breathing. This suggests that exaggerated LCRA, such as that caused by spontaneous pooling of saliva, may explain some apneic episodes.[63] LCRA is, in fact, mixed apnea, and similar to the most frequent type of AOP.

Although it may be simplistic to describe AOP as "primarily central," inadequate responses to upper airway obstruction do reflect a significant "central immaturity" among premature infants. Other evidence of the "central immaturity" of younger infants is the marked increase in periodic breathing particularly during active sleep.[52] After the onset of periodic breathing, transient upper airway obstruction at the pharynx is common during the first inspiratory effort after the apneic pause. Thus, excessive periodic breathing, which is considered pathognomonic for "central immaturity" of respiratory control, frequently has both central and obstructive (i.e., mixed) apnea components.

Premature infants also have more active sleep than quiet sleep, with the attendant irregularity in tidal volume (V_T) and ventilatory frequency (V_f), and increase in apnea. In the episodes of apnea when obstruction is not found (<50%), irregularities in respiratory pattern (V_f, V_T, periodic breathing) often explain a propensity for apnea that is "primarily central."

Updated descriptive studies of the link to sleep state and the prevalence of pure central apneic episodes versus mixed or obstructive apneic episodes are needed to help understand why nearly all infants with birth weights less than 1500 g have significant apnea.

THE NATURAL HISTORY OF APNEA OF PREMATURITY

The natural history of AOP is unclear because interventions to treat it, and thus alter its natural history, have been tried ever since it was first described in detail.

Apneic pauses longer than 5 seconds are common on the first day of life among premature infants without respiratory distress syndrome and can increase to 25 per day by the third day.[64] One large study describing the incidence and age of cessation of apnea[51] showed that nearly all premature infants stopped having apnea of "clinical significance" by 40 weeks PCA. However, this study of more than 25,000 infants from the early 1980s included only 19 infants born before 28 weeks PCA (0.08%). By contrast, during a 5-year period (1989–1994), one NICU in the United States discharged 457 infants born at 24 to 28 weeks PCA.[46] All infants enrolled in the latter study were treated because all had apnea lasting longer than 20 seconds. In general, infants born earlier had apnea and bradycardia events that persisted until an older PCA (Fig. 73-6).

In the study by Eichenwald and co-workers,[46] apnea was diagnosed when chest wall movement was not detected by

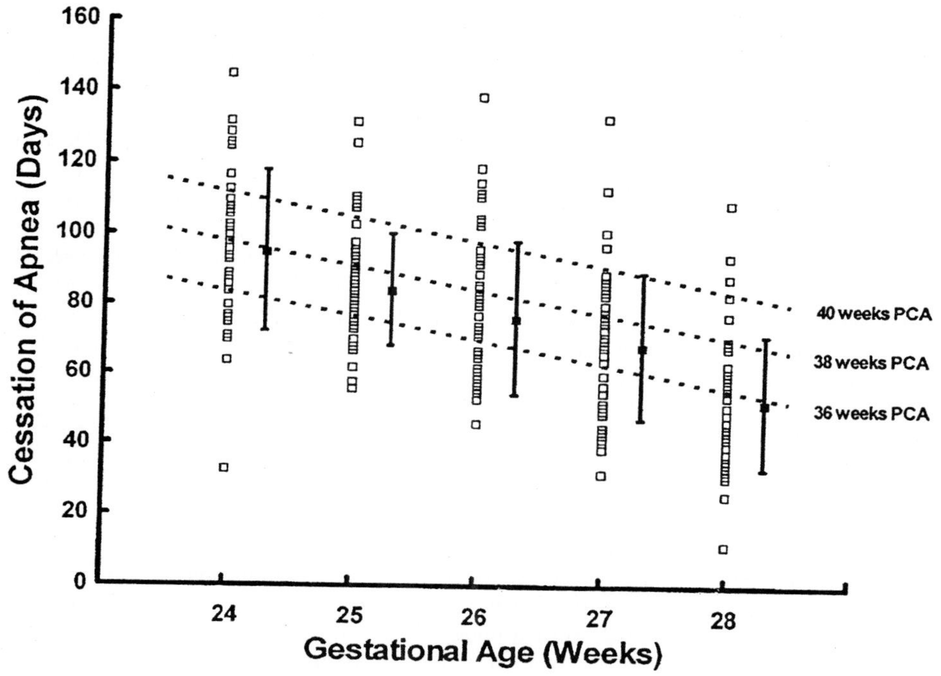

■ **FIGURE 73-6.** Infants born at earlier gestational ages, on average, have their last apneic event on a later postnatal day, even when correcting for PCA. Day of life is shown on y-axis. *Open squares,* individuals born at corresponding gestational age on x-axis. *Closed squares,* mean postnatal age (± SD) for last apnea episode at corresponding gestational age. (From Eichenwald EC, Abimbola A, Stark AR: Apnea frequently persists beyond term gestation in infants delivered at 24 to 28 weeks. Pediatrics 1997;100:354–359.)

impedance monitoring. The last events to disappear with maturation were bradycardia episodes without associated central apneic episodes. As noted earlier and as recognized by the authors, the explanation may be that obstructive apneic episodes with bradycardia continued until the age that the bradycardia episodes ceased. Additional evidence for persistence of undetected mixed apneas is suggested by studies of the maturation of upper airway–stabilizing mechanisms.[65] There seems to be a growth- and age-dependent threshold for improvement in upper airway stability beginning at about 36 weeks PCA.

THERAPIES FOR APNEA OF PREMATURITY AND MONITORING PREMATURE INFANTS AT HOME

The first-line treatment for AOP remains methylxanthines.[47,66,67] Approximately 75% of premature infants will respond to progressive increases in theophylline doses, with therapeutic levels ranging from 4.2 mg/L to 15.3 mg/L.[67]

Infants who fail to respond to methylxanthines will often respond to nasal continuous positive airway pressure (NCPAP) or nasal intermittent positive pressure ventilation.[68] Recently, high-flow nasal cannulas that deliver air to cause distending pressures comparable to NCPAP have been used (at flows up to 2.5 L/min).[69] These catheters have been shown to be as effective as NCPAP in reducing apnea, bradycardia, and episodes of desaturation. Concerns about toxicity from methylxanthines and mucosal injury from NCPAP have led to some enthusiasm for early use of high-flow nasal cannulas.

Another intervention for apnea, transfusion, though fairly well justified in published reports, remains "controversial."[47,70] A threshold for hematocrit below which transfusion is indicated is not established, but the authors of one study speculated that "relieving the (anemic) hypoxia may stabilize the respiratory pattern."

In a study of 132 premature infants, treatment of GER with promotility agents (cisapride and metaclopramide) seemed not to affect the frequency of apnea.[71] As discussed earlier, these findings are not surprising given the problematic relationship of GER (acidic or nonacidic) to apnea.

Pediatric pulmonologists who are not based in NICUs should be reminded that premature infants are at much greater risk for serious apnea after general anesthesia.[72] After anesthesia, increased frequency of apnea and bradycardia can continue to beyond 46 weeks PCA, particularly among infants who required prolonged ventilatory support just after birth, or who have significant residual lung injury. Pulmonologists should be aware of the policies of local pediatric anesthesiologists with respect to perioperative monitoring, even for semielective surgery such as herniorrhaphy.[73] At Cardinal Glennon Children's Hospital, former premature neonates are observed and monitored overnight if they are younger than 3 months of age, weigh less than 3.0 kg, or require home monitoring for continuing apnea.

In a large multicenter study[69,74] of neonates born at less than 34 weeks PCA and discharged home at 34 to 38 weeks PCA, 11% (1588 newborns) used apnea monitors at home. The range of percentage of monitor use among more than 20 NICUs was 0 to 57%. Infants with a history of apnea and those receiving methylxanthines were more likely to be prescribed monitors. Those on monitors were not sent home earlier or later.

Other studies evaluating compliance with apnea monitor use suggest high rates of compliance among infants with AOP, particularly during the first month at home.[75] Abuses because of self-interest among those prescribing monitors not withstanding,[4,6] the promise or potential of monitors, when used to prevent deaths among "nursery graduates," should not be discounted. Infants born at 24 to 36 weeks PCA are from 2.1 to 3.3 times as likely to die of SIDS as infants born at greater than 37 weeks.[76]

The issue of monitor use is complex, however. In their review of more than 37,000 deaths and 3.8 million linked births, Malloy and Hoffman[76] also showed that, depending on the estimated gestational age, the age of SIDS deaths among premature infants was, on average, 44.2 weeks to 47.8 weeks PCA (range, 32–85 weeks). On the basis of these data and those of the CHIMES study,[77] wherein "extreme" apneic spells among premature infants "disappeared once the infants were 43 weeks post-conceptional age," according to one editorial writer the usefulness of prescribing monitors to detect extreme apneic spells and to prevent sudden death among premature infants and the "physiological basis for such a practice are more in doubt than ever."[4] However, another possible scenario is that the time course of apnea activity among those premature infants dying is different from those having apnea and not dying. The vexing problem becomes whether it is possible to select candidates who will benefit most from monitoring.

For the time being, we are in agreement with the AAP recommendations for monitoring premature infants having apnea until they are 43 weeks PCA.[3,4] Because the average time course until cessation of apnea among those infants dying must be different from that for the premature infants in the CHIMES study, monitoring infants past 43 weeks PCA who have frequent apnea lasting longer than 20 seconds, especially with reductions in heart rate, also seems prudent in our estimation.

SUDDEN INFANT DEATH SYNDROME: NEW EXPLANATIONS WITHIN A NEW DEFINITION

TRIPLE-RISK MODEL AND NEW INFANT VARIABLES

The definition for SIDS during the first 20 years after the syndrome was recognized was "the sudden death of an infant or young child, which is unexpected by history, and in which a thorough postmortem examination fails to demonstrate an adequate cause of death."[78]

Because of the recognition of important variables related to sleep practices, the definition was broadened in 1991 to "the sudden death of an infant under one year of age which remains unexplained after a thorough case investigation, including performance of a complete autopsy, examination of the death scene, and review of the clinical history."[79,80] For a complete discussion of issues surrounding the definition of SIDS, categorization when investigations are incomplete, and the importance of alternative definitions with subtle changes in emphasis, the reader can refer to reviews by Rognum and by Krous and co-workers.[80,81]

The "SIDS era" arose from the recognition in the late 1960s that most sudden infant deaths occurred without sufficient pathologic findings to explain them.[82,83] Explanations were required beyond otitis media or mild interstitial pneumonia found at autopsy. This fundamental insight led to much research into reflexes, ventilatory control, and brain stem neurochemistry to clarify what was defined as "unexplained" based on conventional histopathology. While serving to stimulate new thinking about why infants die, the definitions just cited have led to nosologic uncertainty. Accepting an explanation for some deaths from a group defined because they "remain unexplained" presents an obvious conundrum.

For example, once empirical data became available[84–88] that suggested how infants diagnosed as having died from SIDS might have subtly suffocated while face down on soft bedding, it was claimed that these deaths were not due to SIDS (a mystery) as they were originally diagnosed, but, in fact, due to suffocation (Fig. 73-7). The diagnostic shifting described[89] is understandable in the context of a definition that, while useful in stimulating research, assured a nosologic conundrum if progress was made and some of the deaths became explicable.

A framework that, in our opinion, has stood the test of time as a way to study sudden unexpected infant deaths is the triple-risk model (Fig. 73-8).[90] Susceptible infants at a vulnerable physiologic and developmental stage are exposed to more-or-less potent environmental stressors that lead to death. In a given infant or group of infants the relative importance of each influence may vary. Investigations into sleep practices over the past 15 years have increased the understanding of exogenous stressors.[91,92] Some would argue that these deaths should not be categorized as SIDS because they have had partial, new explanations,[86] even though the triple-risk model for SIDS encompasses them perfectly. This is also likely to be the case, and the conundrum, as more inborn metabolic defects[93,94] and developmental anomalies[95,96] are identified that explain, at least partially, the previously inexplicable.

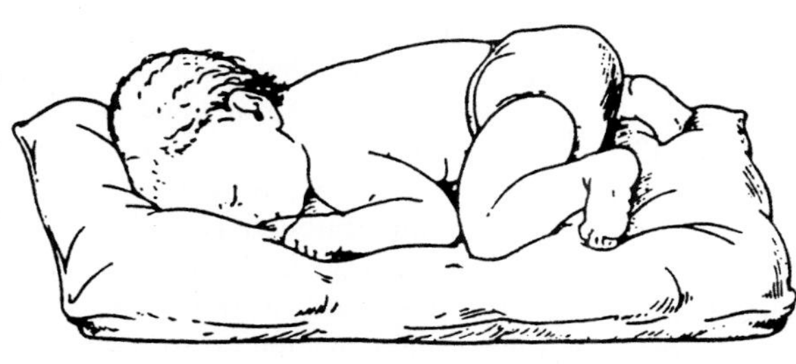

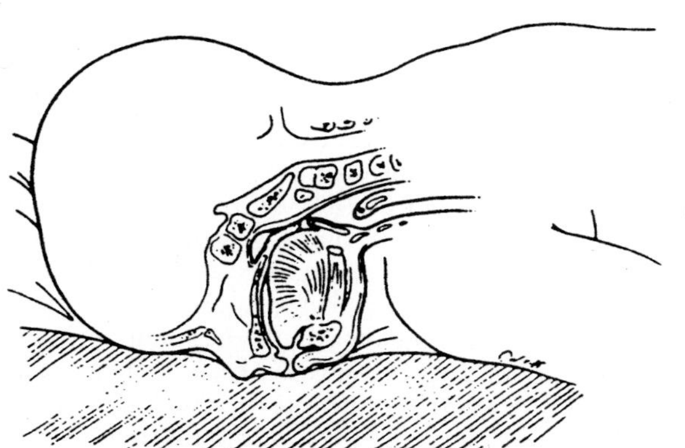

■ **FIGURE 73-7.** Infants placed prone to sleep on soft items may turn their nose and mouth down into the underlying bedding. Before sleep position interventions, 20% to 50% of sudden deaths diagnosed as SIDS occurred in this position. (From Gilbert-Barness E, Barness LA: Cause of death. SIDS or something else? Contemp Pediatr 1992;9:13–29.)

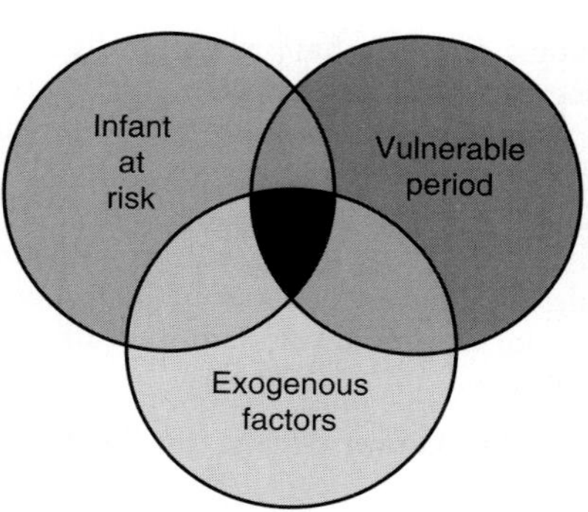

■ **FIGURE 73-8.** The triple-risk model, developed to address the problem of SIDS. It emphasizes the likelihood that most deaths have several partial explanations, within a causal sequence. It remains relevant when death scene investigations have caused diagnostic shifting among the diagnoses of SIDS, unexpected suffocation, and cause of death undetermined. (From Filiano JJ, Kinney HC: A perspective on neuropathologic findings in victims of the sudden infant death syndrome. The triple risk model. Biol Neonate 1994;65: 194–197.)

MULTIFACTORIAL EXPLANATIONS NOT SINGLE CAUSE

Although theoretically problematic, practical approaches to understanding related types of sudden unexpected infant deaths are possible under the rubric of SIDS. It is essential, however, to consider that there is little to be gained by an exclusionary definition of "true SIDS."[80,81]

Within the triple-risk model, for a given infant it is more helpful to think of a causal sequence. For example, we might consider a hypothetical infant with a sluggish arousal response to sleep environment threats while prone[97] who comes to lie prone on bedding that covers the nose and mouth.[98–100] The infant also has a respiratory infection[42] and is at a vulnerable age when the skills at gaining access to fresh air are poor.[95] In a given infant, each of these variables could be critical in leading to sudden death. Moreover, the amelioration of one or more of the seven risk factors present in this example would reduce the risk for death. The success of supine sleep interventions in many countries suggests that the prone position is critical in several hypothetical causal sequences, at least among infants sleeping alone.[100–103]

NEWER APPROACHES TO PATHOLOGY OF THE SUDDEN INFANT DEATH SYNDROME

By definition, conventional gross or microscopic necropsy materials do not explain a SIDS death. Consequently, studies of its pathology have usually described subtle quantitative abnormalities in groups of SIDS victims that distinguish them from controls dying of identified causes.[81,104,105] Alternatively, investigations relying on novel techniques that have been developed since SIDS was defined have been used to begin to understand lethal mechanisms that work quickly and do not yield abnormalities visible with light microscopy (e.g., autoradiography of neuroligands or markers for apoptosis). Studies of specimens from SIDS victims using the newest techniques have attempted to piece together its pathophysiology, rather than attempting to describe findings that are, by consensus, sufficient to explain death.

Epidemiologic findings have always influenced studies of SIDS pathology. In particular, for the past 15 years, many deaths diagnosed as SIDS have involved sleep practices that increase risk for death.[101] For this reason, pathogenetic models based on dysfunctional responses to stressors arising from sleep practices will be the focus of our review of newer approaches to pathology. In these models, the ultrastructural uniqueness of SIDS victims could cause abnormalities of ventilation, ventilatory control, or airway protection.

Programmed Cell Death within the Central Nervous System

Apoptosis, triggered presumably by CNS hypoxia within the previous 24 to 48 hours, has been studied in 29 SIDS victims.[106] Unlike nine controls, none of whom had positive findings, 80% of the SIDS victims had markers of apoptosis in the brain stem or "hypoxia-sensitive subregions of the hippocampus," or both locations. In the medulla, markers were found in the dorsal, rather than ventral, nuclei. Dorsal nuclei involved included those serving the spinal trigeminal tract and vestibular function of the eighth cranial nerve. Although areas studied were limited to the hippocampus and 17 medullary nuclei, these preliminary findings are intriguing. They are relevant to sleep practice data because, as the authors speculate, the head and neck positioning (eighth nerve) and facial sensation (fifth nerve) may be altered in these infants, so that "suffocation may occur."

Neural Receptors and Sudden Infant Death Syndrome

Extensive investigations using carefully chosen controls seem to have established that specific receptors within the CNS are reduced in number among SIDS victims. These receptors are needed for the excitatory function of serotonergic networks within the brain stem, across sleep and wake cycles. A less well-known body of work, also discussed later, suggests that airway inflammation causing peripheral chemoreceptor dysfunction could also lead to SIDS.

During the past 15 years, Filiano and Kinney[90] have compared the brain stems of SIDS victims to brain stems from infants dying acutely from a known cause, or from chronic diseases causing hypoxia. Their approaches show that attempts to explain abnormal function, rather than only histologic neuropathology, are critical to understanding SIDS. Highlights of their work, for our purposes, can be summarized as follows:

1. These authors contend that structures in the human brain stem are "anatomically homologous" to chemosensitive areas in animals,[107] and two SIDS victims they studied had hypoplasia of the arcuate nucleus, a prime "candidate" site for human brain stem chemosensitivity.
2. SIDS victims have less functional activity of receptors binding radiolabeled cholinergic transmitters within the arcuate nucleus in vitro, compared with acute and chronic controls.[108]
3. Serotonin binding by serotonin receptors in the brain stems of SIDS victims compared with controls is reduced not only in the arcuate nucleus, but also in four other brain stem structures derived from the embryonic "rhombic lip" and the intermediate reticular zone.[93]
4. The differences they describe occur within a serotonergic neural network involved with arousal, respiratory patterns, thermoregulation, chemoreception, and upper airway patency.[109] These findings are particularly relevant to asphyxia and hypercarbia that might occur but not be sensed by infants dying prone or supine with their nose and mouth covered.
5. The activity of receptors binding serotonin seems to be developmentally regulated, at least between 35 and 70 weeks after conception.[93]

Thus, this group of researchers has shown, with respect to key receptor networks, that SIDS victims seem to have the substrate for underlying susceptibilities that change with development. Taken together, their findings complete a triple-risk model (see Fig. 73-8) that might include exogenous stressors within the sleep environment.

Others have addressed the availability of serotonin to its receptors within the brain stems of SIDS victims. Polymorphisms occur in the promoter region for a gene controlling the reuptake of serotonin within the CNS. The number of repeats within the promoter region determines promoter activity. The majority of humans have either 14 or 16 repetitive elements—the S or L promoter alleles, respectively. In studies by Narita and co-workers,[110] genomic DNA in frontal cortex samples from SIDS victims ($n = 27$) was more likely to have 18 or 20 repetitive elements ($n = 3$, 11.1%) within the promoter alleles than was genomic DNA taken from peripheral blood of controls ($n = 115$, 0.9%). The effect of this promoter region difference on serotonin activity within the CNS is unclear, but the existence of polymorphisms that distinguish SIDS victims is probably significant. Other studies suggest distinctive polymorphisms among SIDS victims for genes controlling autonomic nervous system development.[111]

Cutz and colleagues have studied the role of peripheral receptors arising in the lung. Their studies offer one explanation using neural receptors for a classic finding,[112,113] namely, the association of SIDS deaths with findings of nonlethal airways inflammation.[42,83] Cutz and co-workers have shown marked increases in numbers of inflammatory cells in the airway epithelium and alveolar septa of SIDS victims.[113] They have also demonstrated RSV in similar sites by immunostaining, and RSV, parainfluenza types 2 and 3, and cytomegalovirus have been found in bronchoalveolar lavage fluid from lungs at postmortem examination. The model developed by Cutz and co-workers rests on the consistent finding in SIDS victims of greater numbers of pulmonary neuroendocrine cells (PNECs) and neuroendocrine bodies (NEBs) found in the intrapulmonary airways, near branchpoints.[114] PNECs and NEBs are composed of clusters of cells[115] containing serotonin and peptide neurotransmitters (bombesin, calcitonin, enkephalin, and others). They are detected using scanning electron microscopy near nerve endings whose afferent fibers ultimately reach the CNS via the vagus. The primary function of PNECs and NEBs is theorized to be that they are sensors of airway hypoxia during the first months of extrauterine life.[116] In animals, airway hypoxia leads to local secretion of serotonin by NEBs, presumably the beginning of a message to the CNS that local gas exchange has been compromised.

The numbers of NEBs increase in the lungs of animals breathing hypoxic gases.[116] However, the function of NEBs as O_2 sensors can be reduced in the presence of irritants and products of inflammation within the lung: H_2O_2, cytokines, and nicotine. In response to hypoxia, afferent signals to the brain stem and to the carotid nerve, via the vagus, are reduced after respiratory infection or smoke exposure.[117]

The models based on the work by Cutz and co-workers postulate that the peripheral hypoxia-sensing function of PNECs and NEBs may be a critical complement to carotid body chemoreception. Receptors within inflamed and tobacco smoke–exposed airways may have blunted responses to hypoxia during a time in infancy when carotid body sensitivity is down-regulated. Their model, though complex, is based on increasing empirical evidence, especially findings showing increases in PNECs and NEBs in SIDS victims,[114] whose airways are more likely to be exposed to cigarette smoke and to be infected. Again, the findings of Cutz and co-workers are consistent with the tenets of the triple-risk model: hypoxia due to sleep environment plus developmental down-regulation of carotid body chemosensitivity plus susceptibility due to PNECs and NEBs dysfunction caused by known risk factors for SIDS (infection and smoke exposure).[38,42]

Fatty Acid Oxidation Deficiencies and the Contribution of Genetic Diseases of Metabolism to Sudden Infant Death Syndrome

The last two topics in our discussion of new pathology do not primarily involve respiration. However, a pulmonologist dealing with the sudden death of an infant will need a working familiarity with them.

Under the wide umbrella of SIDS, and related causes of death, there has been much recent interest in heritable diseases affecting energy metabolism.[80] It is not clear whether the diseases are similar to SIDS in that they can be lethal in 2 hours or less in previously healthy infants, or whether the age of death from inherited metabolic disease overlaps classic SIDS ages (peak rate at 3 months, 95% of deaths by age 6 months).[9]

The epidemiologic features of sudden deaths due to inborn errors of energy metabolism are not well established. Furthermore, although techniques such as tandem mass spectroscopy can be used on neonatal blood spots to screen for many inborn errors, the ratios of false positive to true positive may be 8:1 or greater. It is unclear whether the public health commitment exists to address with new parents the problems of false-positive tests, or unpredictable prognosis of many diseases.[118] Nevertheless, it is certain that some deaths once called SIDS, or attributed to parental neglect, can now be explained by deranged energy metabolism. We will discuss two important examples, without further considering the complex issue of newborn screening.[94,118]

During significant fasting, beta oxidation of fatty acids occurs in mitochondria to provide energy substrates as alternatives to dietary sources of energy. There are 11 proteins controlling the 20 steps leading to beta oxidation, and, ultimately, the tricarboxylic acid cycle and flavoprotein electron transport cycle.[94] Disorders may disrupt any step in the process, from substrate uptake to actual beta oxidation, and have their primary effects on the liver, the CNS, or the heart. The disorders are manifest during fasting, either very shortly after birth, or, in particular, associated with anorexia caused by a viral illness.

The most well-known defects are those causing pediatric cardiomyopathies. Newborns need the relevant enzyme, VLCAD (very long chain acyl-CoA dehydrogenase) to meet the extreme demands on their heart during the transition to extrauterine life. Infants with VLCAD deficiency may die suddenly but usually present in heart failure with a cardiomyopathy that is often familial and that responds to low-fat diets and avoidance of fasting.[119]

Altogether, recognized disorders of fatty acid beta oxidation may be more common (1:10,000 live births) than phenylketonuria (1:15,000). The most common inborn error of beta oxidation is a deficiency in medium-chain acyl-CoA dehydrogenase (MCAD). After periods of inadequate oral intake, infants present with hypoglycemia, neonatal apnea, and, in as many as one third of cases, sudden death.[120] However, their most frequent presentation is profound encephalopathy with cerebral edema, hypoketotic hypoglycemia, elevation of liver transaminases, and hyperammonemia. Because MCAD deficiency was not recognized until the early 1980s, it is probable, in retrospect, that some cases of Reye's syndrome were crises occurring in children with MCAD deficiency.[94,121]

It is also probable that infants with MCAD deficiency have been included in series of infants diagnosed as having died of SIDS.[122,123] For one large series of SIDS deaths in Maryland, the authors suggest that as many as 5% actually died of fatty acid oxidation disorders, although the very high frequency in this series of an otherwise very rare disorder is not explained (carnitine uptake deficiency).[122] Details about age at death, sleep practices, and prevalence of other SIDS risk factors have not been provided in the largest published series of infants with beta-oxidation defects, although there may be some age overlap with SIDS.[122] Two of three infants with MCAD or VLCAD deficiencies from Oregon died within the first 48 hours of life, and two of three were sharing a bed when found dead.[124]

The most common genetic defect leading to MCAD deficiency is homozygous A985G (A to G replacement within nucleotide 985). However, genetic testing after death may either underestimate or overestimate MCAD deficiency as a cause: Affected compound heterozygotes with only one A985G allele have been described. Alternatively, the infants' demise, particularly in the absence of fasting, could have been associated with a "coincidental" abnormality in MCAD.[125–127]

Improved postmortem approaches to the diagnosis of MCAD deficiency, once dependent on first identifying hepatic steatosis and then performing tissue culture analyses, have been made affordable by the availability of tandem mass spectroscopy. The protocol used in Oregon involves creating acyl-carnitine profiles using tandem mass spectroscopy on blood spots from postmortem cardiac puncture.[124] Markedly abnormal profiles of acyl-carnitine–fatty acid compounds—for example, abnormal levels of octanoyl-carnitine (C8)—suggest deranged beta oxidation for some period before death. Such findings are very suggestive of death due to MCAD and related disorders.[127] Infants dying suddenly and unexpectedly with a family history of a similar death, dying after fasting, or whose autopsy shows hepatic steatosis, should most certainly be evaluated using acyl-carnitine profiles from tandem mass spectroscopy. In St. Louis, the medical examiner orders this test through a commercial provider (NeoGen Screening, Pittsburgh, PA) on all children dying unexpectedly before reaching 5 years of age.

In Oregon, from 1996 through 2002, deaths due to disorders of beta oxidation occurred in an estimated 1.3 per 100,000 live births, and constituted 1.2% of deaths occurring suddenly and unexpectedly among infants younger than 1 year old. To understand whether these deaths fit within the context of established SIDS epidemiology (see Table 73-1),[124] future reports on these types of deaths should emphasize how the infants compare to other infants dying, for example, with problematic sleep practices, in terms of age at death, birth weight, history of maternal smoking, and other factors known to be associated with higher risk for sudden death.

Prolonged Electrocardiogram QT Intervals and Lethal Cardiac Arrhythmias

Schwartz and co-workers, in Italy, have been the most consistent proponents of the theory that cardiac arrhythmias can be lethal in SIDS victims with normal cardiac autopsy results. Arguments against this theory were as difficult to envision as were even partial proofs in empirical, population-based studies. Nevertheless, by recording more than 33,000 electrocardiograms on days 3 or 4 of life, Schwartz and co-workers[128] reported that the mean corrected QT (QT_C) interval was longer in the 24 infants eventually dying of SIDS (435 ± 45 vs. 400 ± 20 msec) than in survivors. None of the thousands of survivors had QT_C intervals greater than 440 msec, but 12 of 24 SIDS victims did. The prolonged QT_C interval is believed to be fatal because of a malignant arrhythmia (torsade de pointes).

Subsequently, Ackerman and co-workers[129] showed that 2 of 93 infants diagnosed as SIDS in Arkansas had mutations causing cardiac sodium channel dysfunction, as compared with none of 400 controls. The SCN5A mutation they studied is estimated to cause up to 10% of cases of long QT_C interval syndrome.

The theories of Schwartz and co-workers now seem well established as causes for a small percentage (~2%) of deaths that might meet the criteria for SIDS. The impact of potent SIDS risk factors (e.g., prone sleep, maternal smoking) on the risk for lethal outcomes in infants who are homozygous for mutations such as SCN5A has not been calculated, so it is not yet possible to use this information to understand clearly how it fits into the classic epidemiology of sudden death in infancy.

Will infants with MCAD deficiency or SCN5A be outliers in terms of age, or their risk of dying be relatively unaffected by sleep practices? Also, it is becoming less clear where the pathologic investigation of SIDS or other sudden unexpected infant death should stop,[80,130] as more causes for sudden death are discovered that were not known when SIDS was defined. Should molecular genetic mechanisms be pursued in all deaths? Alternatively, should they only be considered when there is a family history of SIDS, or only when sleep practices are not clearly implicated?

NEW UNDERSTANDING BASED ON INVESTIGATIONS OF THE SCENE AND CIRCUMSTANCES OF DEATH

After discussing high-technology tools, it is important to remember that major reductions in rates of sudden infant death in many countries have resulted from low-tech observations and rigorous epidemiology.[1]

Protocols for observing and documenting the circumstances of sudden infant death have existed for decades.[131,132] How useful these protocols might become, however, is determined by some understanding of what to focus on and what is germane to the sudden death of an infant. For example, in 1978, Beal called attention to the probable importance of sleep position when infants die at night.[133] Her scene observations were viewed as unimportant[134] for more than 10 years, until there was widespread acceptance of the risk from prone positioning on soft bedding.

One type of sudden unexpected death for which scene investigations have always been crucial is infanticide. The perceived importance of infanticide as a frequent cause of death has waxed and waned. Dramatic series of cases[6,135] remind us that infanticide, with or without antecedent Munchausen syndrome by proxy, cannot be ignored. Gross and, occasionally, microscopic autopsy findings are of obvious importance when diagnosing nonaccidental trauma as a cause of death. However, it is less clear by autopsy how to prove intentional but subtle suffocation (e.g., with a pillow).[136] Southall and co-workers[135] used covert video surveillance in the hospital to document that 30 of 39 very high-risk infants were subjected to intentional suffocation. Twelve had siblings who had died suddenly and unexpectedly. Although bloody froth about the nose and mouth is common among SIDS victims, 11 of 38 subjects in Southall's study had a history of an ALTE associated with frank bleeding from the nose and mouth, compared with none of 46 controls.

It seems probable that the percentage of sudden unexpected infant deaths that will be proven to be intentional will increase as the overall number of sudden deaths declines.[112] Before the Back-to-Sleep campaign in the United States, based on serial cross-checks of data from social and law enforcement agencies, it was estimated that about 5% of SIDS deaths were likely to be due to maltreatment.[137] Certainly, multiple deaths within families after genetic causes have been ruled out, and simultaneous deaths of twins should raise cautious suspicion. Nevertheless, the best evidence suggests that foul play is unlikely in the vast majority of second-infant deaths within a family.[138,139]

SLEEP PRACTICES AND THE DECLINE IN RATES OF SUDDEN INFANT DEATH SYNDROME—THE CHANGING EPIDEMIOLOGY

SUCCESS STORY FOR EPIDEMIOLOGY

Supine sleep was recommended routinely in pediatric textbooks until the 20th century. However, in developed countries by the late 20th century, 40% to 80% of infants were placed prone.[39]

In 1978, Susan Beal and colleagues published findings emphasizing the position in which the infant was found at the time of death.[133] Beal carried out home visits and death scene investigations for the 35 to 40 deaths per year in South Australia. Seventy-five percent of victims were found prone, and more than half of all victims were face down. Beal's findings triggered case-control studies in Australia and New Zealand, where in the mid-1980s the rates of SIDS were among the highest in the world. For example, in New Zealand the rate was 3.5 per 1000 births, and it was more than 6 per 1000 in the southern (Otago) district.[140,141]

In the New Zealand Cot Death Study, carried out from November 1987 through October 1990, the sleep practices and circumstances of death were reported for 485 SIDS victims and 1800 controls. The study emphasized four variables that increased risk that were also believed to be "modifiable"[142]: prone sleeping by infant (odds ratio, 3.70), maternal smoking, bed sharing, and never having been breastfed. Similar results that also implicated prone sleep were obtained in case-control studies in Australia and England.[143,144] Furthermore, several items of bedding were identified in these case-control studies that increased risk for dying among prone infants: sheepskins,[8] mattresses filled with bark and other natural fibers,[145] and duvets or comforters.[146] Subsequent interventions[7,144,147] in New Zealand, England, and Australia to reduce the prevalence of prone sleeping (from ~40% to <5%) were followed by reductions of 50% or more in deaths diagnosed as SIDS. Case-control studies in Seattle[148] and Chicago[149] have confirmed that prone sleep position and soft bedding[149] increase risk among infants in the United States.[150] The number of deaths appears to have fallen in the United States after the Back-to-Sleep program (1994; see Fig. 73-1), although no postintervention case-control studies have been published.

A formal argument has been made that prone sleeping, or some factors strongly linked to prone sleeping, are causal for SIDS.[103] The findings of increased risk associated with prone sleep have been reproducible,[39] the odds ratios large, and the temporal sequence (prone before death) correct; there appears to be a dose effect, and reducing prone prevalence has reduced SIDS rates. Although the reduction in SIDS rates is a "success story" based largely in epidemiology, the mechanisms giving the prone position "biologic plausibility" as a cause for SIDS have been vigorously debated.[91,151,152] Before discussing mechanisms, however, we will first review "classic" SIDS epidemiology (before Back-to-Sleep) and how avoiding the prone position has changed the epidemiology of sudden unexpected infant deaths.

EPIDEMIOLOGY OF SUDDEN INFANT DEATH SYNDROME BEFORE AND AFTER BACK-TO-SLEEP INTERVENTIONS

As it was defined before the current emphasis on knowledge of the circumstances of death,[79,80] infants dying of SIDS were often ill, but not ominously.[14] Their dispositions may have been placid, but their development was not worrisome. Complete autopsies showed groups of infants with minor abnormalities, but by definition, nothing per se that would explain death.

Those who sought to solve the mystery of SIDS, the most common diagnosis when infants died beyond the neonatal period, were reminded that their hypothesis must deal with and account for certain epidemiologic realities. For the United States, these epidemiologic variables were defined by an National Institute of Child Health and Human Development Collaborative study and are summarized in Table 73-1.

The epidemiology of SIDS and sudden unexpected infant deaths is changing after successful sleep position interventions and because of diagnostic shifting that has occurred with greater knowledge of the circumstances of death.[89]

THE IMPACT OF SCENE INVESTIGATIONS ON THE UNDERSTANDING OF SUDDEN DEATH AND DIAGNOSTIC SHIFTING

During the first 20 years after SIDS was recognized, the definition and most of the research into its causes did not consider where the infant died. Nevertheless, the epidemiologic success story leading to SIDS reduction was based on careful descriptions of what was near the infant and how the infant was lying. Much of this information was collected before and around the introduction of a new definition for SIDS that required a death scene investigation.

However, it is not clear, even now, that the majority of sudden unexpected infant deaths in the United States are diagnosed after a careful scene investigation. It is also disappointing that reports used to set intervention agendas in high-risk populations do not include direct observations of the death scene or scene data on all deaths.[153,154] Nevertheless, it seems that sleep practices that increase risk, and can be modified, are still common and present in more than 80% of deaths.[101]

When the rubric for SIDS was introduced in 1973, "most of the deaths previously assigned strangulation or suffocation diagnoses ... were called SIDS."[155] Beginning in 1973, and for most of the 20 years thereafter, in the absence of information about how an infant was found, the majority of post-neonatal deaths were considered unexplained and diagnosed as SIDS. However, by the early 1990s, as many 56% of deaths diagnosed as SIDS were shown to have occurred prone and face down on soft bedding, or with the head covered.[99,133] New hypothetical models suggested that thermal stress would be greater for those prone infants using soft bedding and comforters.[151,156] Furthermore, physiologic death scene re-creations showed that subtle but profound suffocation could have occurred in the infant's microenvironment within the death scene,[85–87,92,138,150,157] as the infant depleted the air near its nose of O_2 and enriched it with CO_2. Without scene information, deaths with negative autopsies alone met criteria used for SIDS before 1991. The addition of scene data and the appreciation of the potential for thermal stress and lethal rebreathing have led to diagnostic shifting: Very similar deaths that had been called unexplained (SIDS) before death scene data became available are now being diagnosed as accidental suffocation or positional asphyxia (Fig. 73-9). This evolution in designation of manner and cause of death reflects the increase in information available to forensics teams. The prevalence of risks created within the sleep environment, especially for prone infants, is also more broadly realized.

Thus, for the time being, two factors will have marked effects on the apparent epidemiology of SIDS: (1) Fewer sudden deaths

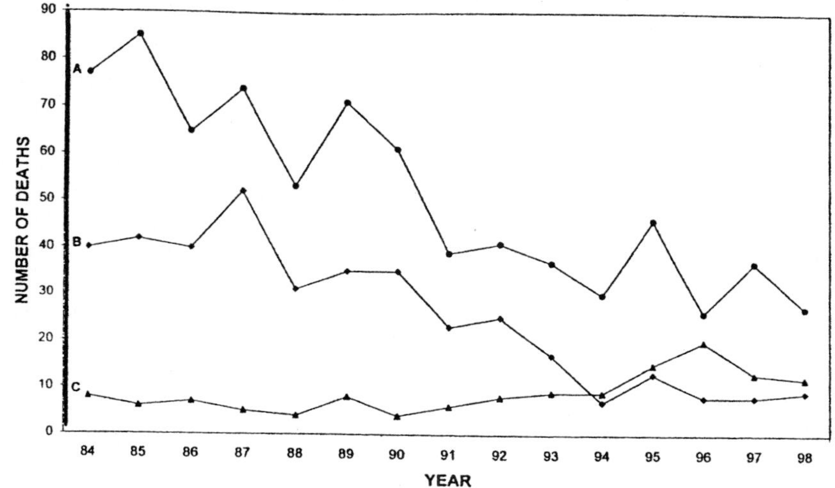

■ **FIGURE 73-9.** The conundrum arising because SIDS is defined as unexplained. Shown is the effect of greater knowledge of circumstances of death on what sudden infant deaths are attributed to in South Australia. *A,* all postneonatal deaths. *B,* All SIDS. *C,* All unexpected, non-SIDS deaths. Note the steady increase in *C,* many of which were attributed to accidents, against the backdrop of reduction in all deaths, and deaths called SIDS, since interventions began, about 1989. (From Mitchell E, Krous HF, Donald T, Byard RW: Changing trends in the diagnosis of sudden infant death. Am J Forensic Med Pathol 2000;21:311–314.)

are occurring when fewer infants are prone; (2) fewer deaths will be seen as unexplained, not because of arbitrary decisions, but because "previously unsuspected sleeping accidents are now being detected."[89]

PHYSIOLOGY RELATED TO SLEEP POSITION THAT MAY MAKE INFANTS MORE VULNERABLE

Infants at increased risk for SIDS have been postulated and shown to have abnormal arousal, hypoxic drive, and airway protective reflexes, among other physiologic aberrations.[158,159] These abnormalities are reviewed below, and in light of the risk associated with prone sleep position.

ABNORMAL AROUSAL AND THE IMPACT OF SLEEP POSITION

Arousal during sleep is defined as full awakenings with eyes opened, or as a change to a lower sleep stage by electroencephalogram (EEG) criteria, or by a constellation of EEG, electromyographic, and airflow changes. Arousal has been assessed experimentally in response to airway obstruction[160,161] and central apnea,[160] breathing hypercarbic[162] or hypoxic[163] gas mixtures, laryngeal stimulation with fluid,[37,164] sound,[165] and jets of air hitting the face.[166] Changes in sleep state or awakening "may produce a fundamental change in the nature of the ventilatory response to a respiratory stimulus."[164] Arousal is often associated with the termination of obstructive apnea[161] and is the probable cause of sleep fragmentation leading to daytime sleepiness with obstructive sleep apnea.

Infants and adults exposed to external threats to their airways will often change their sleep state and awaken.[95,167] However, arousal is not always apparently needed. Infants sleeping face down[168] and premature infants with central apnea[169] may also change position or resume breathing without awakening or showing changes in their cortical EEG.[160,169] These alternative strategies would preserve sleep while ending the threat to ventilation.

Infants at greater statistical risk for SIDS compared with controls may have diminished arousal to breathing hypoxic and hypercarbic gases[159,162] and longer obstructive apnea before arousal and resumption of eupneic breathing.[170] Cigarette smoke exposure in utero, which markedly increases risk for SIDS, is also associated with higher auditory arousal thresholds during non–rapid eye movement sleep.[171] Consistent with the notion that thermal stress is a mechanism for SIDS, higher ambient temperature (28°C vs. 24°C) increases arousal threshold to sound in infants about 3 months of age.[172] To summarize, then, in response to sound stimuli and air jets applied to the face, arousal from sleep is both altered and more difficult to elicit among prone-sleeping term and premature infants,[173] and among prone infants with obstructive apnea.[167,170]

Although full arousal may lessen the danger of threats to ventilation during sleep in infants, the reliability of arousal from sleep in interrupting threats due to sleep in risky environments is uncertain. For example, infants dying beneath bedclothes have often pulled them over their face, or moved beneath them.[174] Although these infants died while unobserved, it is conceivable that they suffocated while awake and not asleep, and that arousal played little role, except possibly to cause the awakening that got them into trouble in the first place. It has also been shown that the normal arousal sequence to having the nose and mouth covered—sigh, startle, arm thrashing, head lift, and turn—can actually worsen the infant's predicament within the sleep microenvironment, by pulling bedclothes farther over the head or by placing the infant face down into soft bedding.[84,95] Finally, infants may gain access to fresh air and end the threat to effective ventilation by subtle head (nose and mouth) repositioning without apparent awakening or EEG changes.[168]

In any event, whether or not an infant arouses to compromised ventilation, and how much ventilation is improved as a result of movements during an arousal, may together define a developmental vulnerability for specific infants exposed to threats within their sleep environment.

ABNORMALITIES IN VENTILATORY RESPONSE AND THREATS WITHIN THE SLEEP ENVIRONMENT

In addition to blunted arousal, infants at particular risk for SIDS may have blunted ventilatory responses. Minute volume increases while breathing hypercarbic or hypoxic air are less than controls,[57,58,163] and the ventilatory responses of normal infants may be less when prone than when supine.[175] Sleep environments that lead to trapping of exhaled air, and creation of relatively hypoxic and CO_2-rich environments would be of particular relevance in this regard. As noted earlier, those areas in the brain stem with diminished cholinergic and serotonergic receptor activity among SIDS victims may be chemosensitive areas, particularly for changes in CO_2 and pH.

Thus, lines of investigation within respiratory physiology and neuropathology have merged to provide insight into mechanisms pertinent to epidemiologic studies implicating prone sleep position.

SOFT BEDDING AS AN EFFECT MODIFIER: PHYSIOLOGIC IMPLICATIONS

Arousal and ventilatory responses to challenges may be less in prone than in supine sleeping infants. What gives rise to the "challenge" that must be responded to is suggested by studies of factors within the sleep environment that increase risk in the prone position.

It has been known for 40 years, for example, that soft bedding use increases risk for "cot death."[176] Items of bedding that dramatically increase risk when used by prone infants have been shown using quantitative criteria[150] to be much softer than items not associated with increased prone risk. Soft, natural-fiber mattresses[145] and sheepskins[141,145] are not associated with increased risk of sudden unexpected death among supine infants. However, in Australia, for example, sleeping prone on a mattress filled with natural fibers increased risk by 20-fold.[145]

Items of bedding sharing similar physical properties[150] (soft, with porous covers) have been identified in other case series and case-control studies of sudden, unexpected infant deaths.[146,149] The bedding includes polystyrene bead–filled cushions,[86] comforters or duvets, pillows,[99] and various forms of "ordinary bedding."[138]

Anywhere from 20% to 70% of infants[98,176,177] dying suddenly and unexpectedly will be both prone and face down when found (see Fig. 73-7). Using soft bedding increases the risk that an infant dying will be found face down into the underlying bedding.[99] It has been possible to show with mechanical and animal models, and human infants, that assuming the prone and

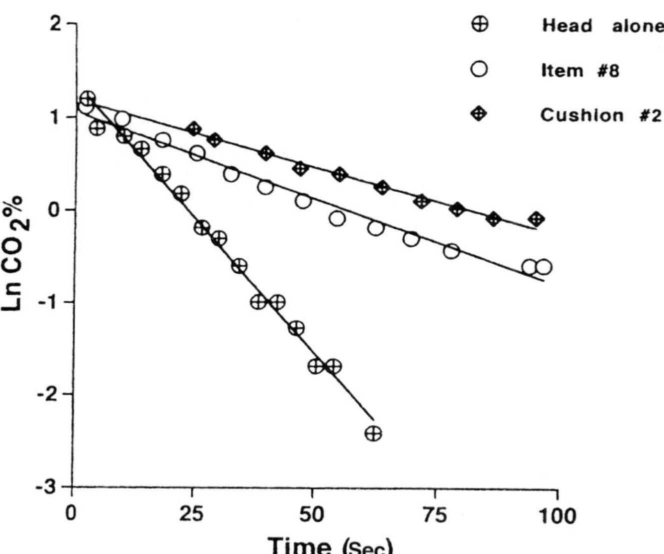

■ **FIGURE 73-10.** Results from studies done to quantify the rate of disappearance of exhaled CO_2. The mechanical model included the head from an infant mannequin, a syringe filled with 5% CO_2 attached to the mannequin's "airway" used to simulate ventilation, and an infrared CO_2 analyzer. The steepest line reflects the mannequin being ventilated without nose or mouth encumbered; the other two are with nose and mouth covered by soft "ordinary" bedding from death scene investigations. The rate constant for the time course of CO_2 dispersal correlates with the ability of the sleep environment to be asphyxiating. (From Kemp JS, Thach BT: Quantifying the potential of infant bedding to limit CO_2 dispersal and factors affecting rebreathing in bedding. J Appl Physiol 1995;78:740–745.)

face-down position on items of soft bedding can markedly increase CO_2 concentration and decrease O_2 concentration near the face of an infant so positioned (Figs. 73-10 and 73-11). This environment can be lethal in experimental animals and has been shown to cause hypercarbia and hypoxemia in living infants.[178]

Waters and co-workers[84] have also shown that this scenario occurs spontaneously. In a study done using home recordings of Sp_{O_2}, transcutaneous (P_{CO_2}), respiratory effort, and videos, they showed that an infant sleeping prone, without adults present, assumed the face-down position on a mattress pad. Although the infant escaped this position, her Ptc_{CO_2} rose from 50 to 87 mm Hg. The danger of such a scenario would be obvious for an otherwise healthy infant with blunted responses to hypoxemia or CO_2 concentration, or inefficient airway-protective behaviors.

In addition to preventing the ingress of fresh air, soft bedding, particularly comforters (duvets), provides much thermal insulation and has the potential to cause thermal stress.[146,151] The thermal stress theory as a mechanism for prone death has been discussed in detail elsewhere.[91] Increases in thermal insulation around infants (quantified in tog units) are associated with increased risk of sudden death, particularly if an infant is prone and has a respiratory illness such as RSV infection.[42] Infants who are prone with forehead covered have about 20% less surface for heat radiation than supine infants.[91]

The mechanism proposed is not heat stroke with multiorgan injury.[91,152] Rather, an abnormality in cardiorespiratory pattern may be elicited by their response to thermal stress and is suggested by preliminary studies in newborns. What the mechanism or resultant cardiorespiratory abnormality is, particularly beyond the first month of life, is a question of great interest. Infants do seem to be able to thermoregulate when exposed to environments that had been presumed to cause thermal stress,[179] and success with Back-to-Sleep occurred without reduction in thermal stress.[7,144,147]

SHARING BEDS AND RACIAL DISPARITIES IN RATES OF SUDDEN UNEXPECTED INFANT DEATHS

Among infants sleeping alone in cribs, staying supine and avoiding their heads being covered by blankets should lead to further reductions in sudden death during sleep. Sharing an adult sleep surface, however, has been and remains a factor that increases risks for sudden death.[14,149,176,180–184] In some multivariate analyses, risks associated with bed sharing have been "clouded," and rendered statistically insignificant, by very high rates (~90%)[182] of maternal cigarette smoking among infants dying while sharing a bed. More recent studies,[149,183,184] while noting an increased risk for infant death while sharing a bed if the mother smokes, have also found sharing a bed to be an important independent risk factor for sudden death (odds ratio [OR] 2.4 to 4.1).

In the United States, there are disparities in the rates of sudden unexpected infant deaths among African American infants. African American infants do sleep prone twice as often as other infants.[185] Thus, interventions to reduce racial disparities in SIDS should continue to foster supine sleep. Nevertheless, reducing rates of prone sleeping among African American infants may have only a small effect on disparities because of high rates of bed sharing among African American infants.[102] Supine sleep has never been shown to be protective while sharing a bed.[39]

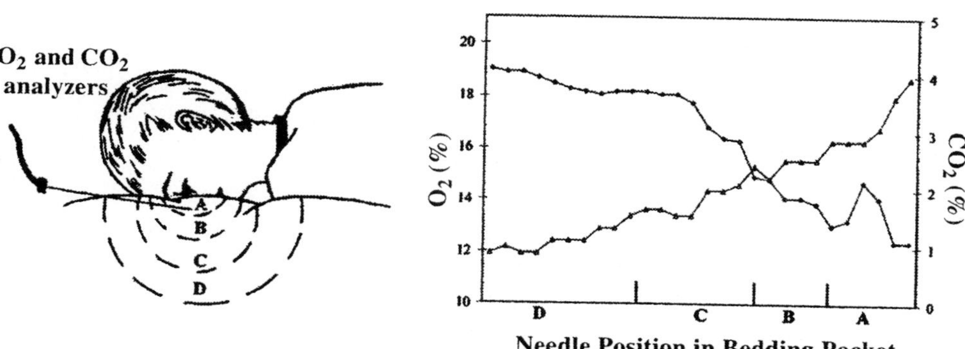

■ **FIGURE 73-11.** Inspired O_2 and CO_2 sampled at four different distances from the nose and mouth of an infant breathing into a comforter. The graph demonstrates the gradients of O_2 depletion and CO_2 accumulation. It is likely that hypoxemia is the more serious acute threat to vulnerable infants. (From Patel AL, Harris K, Thach BT: Inspired CO_2 and O_2 in sleeping infants rebreathing from bedding. Relevance for sudden infant death syndrome. J Appl Physiol 2001;91:2537–2545.)

For example, in New Zealand, among Maori infants, 29% of whom shared beds in a case-control study,[186] dramatic reductions in rates of prone sleeping occurred (43% to <5%) with little impact on the Maoris' rates of SIDS or infant mortality.[187] In the United States, since Back-to-Sleep began, rates of SIDS and sudden unexpected infant deaths have fallen among both white and African American infants, but the rate of fall has been much steeper among non–African American infants.

Bed-sharing rates may be increasing among all infants in the United States.[188] Given the above findings, one must consider whether bed sharing, either to enhance nurturing behaviors or to foster breastfeeding, can be done safely.[189] It is not clear that it can. Sleep arrangements for infants who are bed sharing are softer[190] and much more likely to be associated with suffocation deaths.[191] In Norway, recommendations to increase rates of breastfeeding that included bed sharing were followed by an increase in the rate of bed sharing in sudden deaths from 2% to 34%.[11] In Canada bed sharing has been officially discouraged,[192] and the AAP has developed a similar recommendation.

SUMMARY AND CONCLUSION

It was estimated in 1967 that in industrialized countries 25,000 infants per year died suddenly and unexpectedly.[82] Most children who died suddenly and unexpectedly do not have pathologic findings to explain their demise and, after 1967, their deaths were diagnosed as SIDS.[155] A triple-risk model can be used to explore explanations for sudden death: Infant susceptibility, developmental vulnerability, and exogenous stressors of varying magnitude. Abnormalities in ventilatory control or reflexes, and in behavioral or minute volume responses can usually be implicated. These abnormalities may be nonlethal when most infants sleep supine on their own sleep surface. Newer approaches to the pathology of cardiorespiratory control and energy metabolism, and continued emphasis on safe sleeping practices should lead to further reductions in the number of infants dying suddenly and unexpectedly each year.

REFERENCES

1. Dwyer T, Ponsonby A-L: The decline of SIDS. A success story for epidemiology. Epidemiology 1996;7:323–325.
2. American Academy of Pediatrics Task Force on Sudden Infant Death Syndrome: The changing concept of sudden infant death syndrome. Diagnostic coding shifts, controversies regarding the sleep environment, and new variables to consider in reducing risk. Pediatrics 2005;116:1245–1255.
3. American Academy of Pediatrics Committee on Fetus and Newborn: Apnea, sudden infant death syndrome, and home monitoring. Pediatrics 2003;111:914–917.
4. Jobe AH: What do home monitors contribute to the SIDS problem? JAMA 2001;285:2244–2245.
5. Poets CF: The role of monitoring. In: Byard RW, Krous HF, eds: Sudden Infant Death Syndrome—Problems, Progress and Possibilities. London: Edward Arnold, 2001, pp 243–257.
6. Firstman R, Talan J: SIDS and infanticide. In: Byard RW, Krous HF, eds: Sudden Infant Death Syndrome—Problems, Progress and Possibilities. London: Edward Arnold, 2001, pp 291–300.
7. Dwyer T, Ponsonby A-L, Blizzard L, Newman NM, Cochrane JA: The contribution of changes in the prevalence of prone sleeping position to the decline of sudden infant death syndrome in Tasmania. JAMA 1995;273:783–789.
8. Mitchell EA: The changing epidemiology of SIDS following the national risk reduction campaigns. Pediatr Pulmonol 1997;16(Suppl):117–119.
9. Malloy MH, Freeman DH: Age at death, season, and day of death as indicators of the effect of the back to sleep program on sudden infant death syndrome in the United States, 1992–1999. Arch Pediatr Adolesc Med 2004;158:359–365.
10. Skadberg BT, Morild I, Markestad T: Abandoning prone sleeping. Effect on risk of sudden infant death syndrome. J Pediatr 1998;132:340–343.
11. Arnestad M, Anderson M, Bege A, Rognum TO: Changes in the epidemiological pattern of sudden infant death syndrome in southeast Norway, 1993–1998. Implications for future prevention and research. Arch Dis Child 2001;85:108–115.
12. Brooks JG: Apparent life-threatening events. Pediatr Rev 1996;17:257–259.
13. Oren J, Kelly D, Shannon DC: Identification of a high risk group for sudden infant death syndrome among infants who were resuscitated for sleep apnea. Pediatrics 1986;77:495–499.
14. Hoffman HJ, Damus K, Hillman L, Krongrad E: Risk factors for SIDS. Results of the National Institute of Child Health and Human Development SIDS Cooperative Epidemiological study. Ann N Y Acad Sci 1988;533: 13–30.
15. Benatar SR: Fatal asthma. N Engl J Med 1986;314:423–428.
16. Samuels MP: Apparent life-threatening events. Pathogenesis and management. In: Loughlin GM, Carroll JL, Marcus CL, eds: Sleep and Breathing in Children. New York: Marcel Dekker, 2001, p 424.
17. Stratton SJ, Taves A, Lewis RJ, Clements H, Henderson D, McCollough M: Apparent life-threatening events in infants. High risk in the out-of-hospital environment. Ann Emerg Med 2004;43:711–717.
18. Kahn A, Groswasser J, Sottiaux M, Rebuffat E, Franco P: Clinical problems in relation to apparent life-threatening events in infants. Acta Pediatr Suppl 1993;389:107–110.
19. Piletti RD, Maffei F, Chang K, Hickey R, Berger R, Pierce MC: Prevalence of retinal hemorrhages and child abuse in children who present with an apparent life-threatening event. Pediatrics 2002;110:557–563.
20. Jeffery HE, Megevand A, Page M: Why the prone position is a risk factor for the sudden infant death syndrome. Pediatrics 1999;104:263–269.
21. Davies AM, Koenig JS, Thach BT: Upper airway chemoreflex responses to saline and water in preterm infants. J Appl Physiol 1988;64:1412–1420.
22. Downing SE, Lee JC: Laryngeal chemosensitivity. A possible mechanism for sudden infant death. Pediatrics 1975;55:640–649.
23. Boggs DF, Bartlett D: Chemical specificity of a laryngeal apneic reflex in puppies. J Appl Physiol 1982;53:455–462.
24. Abu-Shaweesh JM: Maturation of respiratory reflex responses in the fetus and neonate. Semin Neonatol 2004;9:169–180.
25. Vandenplas Y, Goyvaerts H, Helven R, Sacre L: Gastroesophageal reflux, as measured by 24-hour pH monitoring, in 509 healthy infants screened for risk of sudden infant death syndrome. Pediatrics 1991;88:834–840.
26. Herbst JJ, Minton SD, Book LS: Gastroesophageal reflux causing respiratory distress and apnea in newborn infants. J Pediatr 1979;95:763–768.
27. Kahn A, Rebuffat E, Sottiaux M, Dulfour D, Cadranel S, Reiterer F: Arousals induced by proximal esophageal reflux in infants. Sleep 1991;140:39–42.
28. Vandenplas Y, Hauser B: Gastro-oesophageal reflux, sleep pattern, apparent life threatening event, and sudden infant death. The point of view of a gastro-enterologist. Eur J Pediatr 2000;159:726–729.
29. Thach BT: Sudden infant death syndrome. Can gastroesophageal reflux cause sudden infant death? Am J Med 2000;108:144S–148S.
30. Menon AP, Schefft GL, Thach BT: Apnea associated with regurgitation in infants. J Pediatr 1985;106:625–629.
31. Ariagno RL, Guilleminault C, Baldwin R, Boeddiker MO: Movement and gastroesophageal reflux in awake term infants with "near miss" SIDS, unrelated to apnea. J Pediatr 1982;100:894–897.
32. Mitchell DJ, McClure BG, Tubman TRJ: Simultaneous monitoring of gastric and oesphageal pH reveals limitations of conventional oesophageal pH monitoring in milk fed infants. Arch Dis Child 2001;84:273–276.
33. Wenzl TG, Schenke S, Peschgens T, Silny J, Heimann G, Skopnik H: Association of apnea and nonacid gastroesophageal reflux in infants. Investigations with intraluminal impedance technique. Pediatr Pulmonol 2001;31:144–149.
34. Walsh JK, Farrell MK, Keenan WJ, Lucas M, Kramer M: Gastroesophageal reflux in infants. Relation to apnea. J Pediatr 1981;99:197–201.
35. Peter CS, Sprodowski N, Bohnhorst B, Silny J, Poets CF: Gastroesophageal reflux and apnea of prematurity. No temporal relationship. Pediatrics 2002; 109:8–11.
36. Thach BT: Maturation and transformation of reflexes that protect the laryngeal airway from liquid aspiration from fetal to adult life. Am J Med 2001; 111:S69–S70.
37. Sullivan CE, Murphy E, Kozar LF, Phillipson EA: Waking and ventilatory responses to laryngeal stimulation in sleeping dogs. J Appl Physiol 1978;45: 681–689.
38. Blair PS, Fleming PJ, Bensley D, Smith J, Taylor E, Berry J, et al: Smoking and the sudden infant death syndrome. Results from results from 1193-5 case-control study for confidential inquiry into stillbirths and deaths in infancy. BMJ 1996;313:195–198.
39. Hauck FR, Moore CM, Herman SM, Donovan M, Kalekar M, Christoffel KK, et al: The contribution of prone sleeping position to the

racial disparity in Sudden Infant Death Syndrome. The Chicago infant mortality study. Pediatrics 2002;110:772–780.
40. Sundell HW, Karmo H, Milerad J: Impaired cardiorespiratory recovery after laryngeal stimulation in nicotine-exposed young lambs. Pediatr Res 2002;53:104–112.
41. Anas N, Boettrich C, Hall CB, Brooks JG: The association of apnea and respiratory syncytial virus infections. J Pediatr 1982;101:65–68.
42. Gilbert R, Rudd P, Berry PJ, Fleming PJ, Hall E, White DG, et al: Combined effect of infection and heavy wrapping on the risk of sudden unexpected infant death. Arch Dis Child 1992;67:171–177.
43. Pickens DL, Schefft GL, Storch GA, Thach BT: Characterization of prolonged apneic episodes associated with respiratory syncytial virus infection. Pediatr Pulmonol 1989;6:195–201.
44. Vege A, Rognum TO, Anestad G: IL-6 cerebrospinal fluid levels are related to laryngeal IgA and epithelial HLA-DR response in sudden infant death syndrome. Pediatr Red 1999;45:803–809.
45. Miller MJ, Martin RJ: Apnea of prematurity. Clin Perinatol 1992;19: 789–797.
46. Eichenwald EC, Abimbola A, Stark AR: Apnea frequently persists beyond term gestation in infants delivered at 24 to 28 weeks. Pediatrics 1997;100: 354–359.
47. Gomella TL: Apnea and bradycardia. In: Gomella TL, ed: Neonatology. Management, Procedures, on-Call Problems, Diseases, and Drugs, 5th edition. New York: Lange Medical Books, 2004, pp 208–211.
48. Perlstein PH, Edwards NK, Sutherland JM: Apnea in premature infants and incubator-air temperature changes. N Engl J Med 1970;282:461–466.
49. Miller MJ, Kiatchoosakun P: Relationship between respiratory control and feeding in the developing infant. Semin Neonatol 2004;9:221–228.
50. Mathew OP, Roberts JL, Thach BT: Pharyngeal airway obstruction in preterm infants during mixed and obstructive apnea. J Pediatr 1982;100: 964–968.
51. Henderson-Smart DJ: The effect of gestational age on the incidence and duration of recurrent apnoea in newborn babies. Aust Paediatr J 1981;17: 273–276.
52. Hoppenbrowers T, Hodgeman JE, Harper RM, Hofman E, Sterman MB, McGinty DJ: Polygraphic studies of infants during the first six months of life. III. Incidence of apnea and periodic breathing. Pediatrics 1977;60:418–425.
53. Miller MJ, Carlo WA, Martin RJ: Continuous positive pressure selectively reduces obstructive apnea in preterm infants. J Pediatr 1985;106:91–96.
54. Milner AD, Greenough A: The role of the upper airway in neonatal apnea. Semin Neonatol 2004;9:213–220.
55. Gauda EB, Miller MJ, Carlo WA, Difiore JM, Johnsen DC, Martin R: Genioglossus response to airway occlusion in apneic versus nonapneic infants. Pediatr Res 1987;22:683–687.
56. Gerhardt T, Bancalari E: Apnea of prematurity. I. Lung function and regulation of breathing. Pediatrics 1984;74:58–62.
57. Gerhardt T, Bancalari E: Apnea of prematurity. II. Respiratory reflexes. Pediatrics 1984;74:63–66.
58. Rigatto H, Kalapesi Z, Leahy E, MacCallum M, Cates D: Ventilatory responses to 100% and 15% O_2 during wakefulness and sleep in preterm infants. Early Hum Dev 1982;7:1–10.
59. Carlo WA, DiFiore JM: Respiratory muscle responses to changes in chemoreceptor drive in infants. J Appl Physiol 1990;68:1041–1047.
60. Henderson-Smart DJ, Read DJC: Reduced lung volume during behavior active sleep in the newborn. J Appl Physiol 1979;46:1081–1085.
61. Heldt GP, McIrroy MB: Distortion of the chest wall and work of the diaphragm in preterm infants. J Appl Physiol 1987;62:164–169.
62. Stark AR, Thach BT: Mechanisms of airway obstruction leading to apnea in newborn infants. J Pediatr 1976;89:982–985.
63. Campbell K: Possible role of saliva in the sudden infant death syndrome. Lancet 1971;2:1314–1315.
64. Carlo WA, Martin RJ, Versteegh FG, Goldman MD, Robertson SS, Fanaroff AA: The effect of respiratory distress syndrome on chest wall movements and respiratory pauses in preterm infants. Am Rev Respir Dis 1982;126:103–107.
65. Duara S, Neto GS, Claure N, Gerhardt T, Bancalari E: Effect of maturation on the extrathoracic airway stability of infants. J Appl Physiol 1992;73:2368–2372.
66. Von Poblotzki M, Fackeldey ER, Schulze A: Effects of theophylline on the pattern of spontaneous breathing in preterm infants less than 1000 g of birth weight. Early Hum Dev 2003;72:47–55.
67. Mutitt SC, Tierney AJ, Finer NN: The dose response of theophylline in the treatment of apnea of prematurity. J Pediatr 1988;112:115–121.
68. DePaoli AG, Davis PG, Lemyre B: Nasal continuous positive airway pressure versus nasal intermittent positive pressure ventilation for preterm neonates. A systemic review and meta-analysis. Acta Pediatr 2003;92:70–75.
69. Sreenan C, Lemke RP, Mason AH, Osiovich H: High-flow nasal cannulae in the management of apnea of prematurity. A comparison with conventional nasal continuous positive airway pressure. Pediatrics 2001;107:1081–1083.
70. Joshi A, Gerhardt T, Shandloff P, Bancalari E: Blood transfusion effect on the respiratory pattern of preterm infants. Pediatrics 1987;80:79–84.
71. Kimball AL, Carlton DP: Gastroesophageal reflux medications in the treatment of apnea in premature infants. J Pediatr 2001;138:355–360.
72. Kurth CD, Spitzer AR, Broennle AM, Downes JJ: Postoperative apnea in preterm infants. Anesthesiology 1987;66:483–488.
73. Williams JM, Stoddart PA, Williams SAR, Wolf AR: Post-operative recovery after inguinal herniotomy in ex-premature infants. Comparison between sevoflurane and spinal anesthesia. Br J Anaesth 2001;86:366–371.
74. Sychowski SP, Dodd E, Thomas P, Peabody J, Clark R: Home apnea monitor use in preterm infants discharged from newborn intensive care units. J Pediatr 2001;139:245–248.
75. Carbone T, Ostfeld BM, Gutter D, Hegyi T: Parental compliance with home cardiorespiratory monitoring. Arch Dis Child 2001;84:270–272.
76. Malloy MH, Hoffman HJ: Prematurity, sudden infant death syndrome, and age of death. Pediatrics 1995;96:464–471.
77. Ramanathan R, Corwin MJ, Hunt CE, Lister G, Tinsley LR, Baird T, et al: Cardiorespiratory events recorded on home monitors: comparison of healthy infants to those at risk for SIDS. JAMA 2001;285:2199–2207.
78. Beckwith JB: Discussion of terminology and definition of the sudden infant death syndrome. In: Bergman AB, Beckwith JB, Ray CG, eds: Sudden Infant Death Syndrome. Seattle: University of Washington Press, 1970, pp 14–22.
79. Willinger M, James LS, Catz C: Defining the sudden infant death syndrome. Pediatr Pathol 1991;11:677–684.
80. Krous HF, Beckwith JB, Byard RW, Rognum TO, Bajanowski T, Corey T, et al: Sudden infant death syndrome and unclassified sudden infant deaths. A definitional and diagnostic approach. Pediatrics 2004;114:234–238.
81. Rognum TO: Definition and pathologic features. In: Byard RW, Krous HF, eds: Sudden Infant Death Syndrome—Problems, Progress and Possibilities. London: Edward Arnold, 2001, pp 4–30.
82. Valdes-Dapena MA: Sudden and unexpected death in infancy. A review of the world literature 1954–1966. Pediatrics 1967;39:123–138.
83. Kemp JS: Fifty years ago in The Journal of Pediatrics. Sudden death in infants. J Pediatr 2004;145:321–322.
84. Waters KA, Gonzalez A, Jean C, Morielli A, Brouillette RT: Face-straight-down and face-near-straight-down in healthy, prone-sleeping infants. J Pediatr 1996;128:616–625.
85. Carleton JN, Donoghue AM, Porter WK: Mechanical model testing of rebreathing potential in infant bedding materials. Arch Dis Child 1998;78: 323–328.
86. Kemp JS, Thach BT: Sudden death in infants sleeping on polystyrene-filled cushions. N Engl J Med 1991;423:1858–1864.
87. Kemp JS, Thach BT: Quantifying the potential of infant bedding to limit CO_2 dispersal and factors affecting rebreathing in bedding. J Appl Physiol 1995;78:740–745.
88. Gilbert-Barness E, Barness LA: Cause of death. SIDS or something else? Contemp Pediatr 1992;9:13–29.
89. Mitchell E, Krous HF, Donald T, Byard RW: Changing trends in the diagnosis of sudden infant death. Am J Forensic Med Pathol 2000;21:311–314.
90. Filiano JJ, Kinney HC: A perspective on neuropathologic findings in victims of the sudden infant death syndrome. The triple risk model. Biol Neonate 1994;65:194–197.
91. Kemp JS: Environmental stressors and sudden unexpected infant death. In: Loughlin GM, Carroll JL, Marcus CL, eds: Sleep and Breathing in Children. New York: Marcel Dekker, 2000, pp 465–488.
92. Patel AL, Harris K, Thach BT: Inspired CO_2 and O_2 in sleeping infants rebreathing from bedding. Relevance for sudden infant death syndrome. J Appl Physiol 2001;91:2537–2545.
93. Panigraphy A, Filiano J, Sleeper LA, Mandell F, Valdes-Dapena M, Krous HF, et al: Decreased serotonergic receptor binding in rhombic lip derived regions of the medulla oblongata in the sudden infant death syndrome. J Neuropathol Exp Neurol 2000;59:377–384.
94. Roe Cr, Ding J: Mitochondrial fatty acid disorders. In: Scriver CR, Beaudet AL, Sly WS, Valle D, eds: The Metabolic and Molecular Bases of Inherited Disease. New York: McGraw-Hill, 2001, pp 2297–2319.
95. Lijowska AS, Reed NW, Mertins-Chiodini BA, Thach BT: Sequential arousal and airway-defense behavior of infants in asyphyxial sleep environments. J Appl Physiol 1997;83:219–228.
96. Burns B, Lipsitt LP: Behavioral factors in crib death. Toward an understanding of the sudden infant death syndrome. J Appl Dev Psychol 1991;12:159–184.
97. Patel AL, Paluszynska D, Harris KA, Thach BT: Occurrence and mechanism of sudden oxygen desaturation in infants who sleep face down. Pediatrics 2003;111:e328–e332.

98. Mitchell EA, Thach BT, Thompson JMD, Williams S: Changing infants' sleep position increases risk of sudden death. Arch Pediatr Adolesc Med 1999;153:1136–1141.
99. Scheers NJ, Dayton CM, Kemp JS: Sudden infant death with external airways covered. Case comparison study of 206 deaths in the United States. Arch Pediatr Adolesc Med 1998;152:540–547.
100. Kemp JS, Thach BT: Rebreathing of exhaled air. In: Byard RW, Krous HF, eds: Sudden Infant Death Syndrome—Problems, Progress and Possibilities. London: Edward Arnold, 2001, pp 138–155.
101. Kemp JS, Unger B, Wilkins D, Psara RM, Ledbetter TL, Graham MA, et al: Unsafe sleep practices among infants dying suddenly and unexpectedly. Results of a four year, population-based, death-scene investigation study of SIDS and related deaths. Pediatrics 2000;106(3):e41. Available at http://www.pediatrics.org/cgi/content/full/106/3/e41.
102. Unger B, Kemp JS, Wilkins D, Psara R, Ledbetter T, Graham M, et al: Racial disparity and modifiable risk factors among infants dying suddenly and unexpectedly. Pediatrics 2003;111:e127–e131. Available at http://www.pediatrics.org/cgi/content/full/111/2/e127.
103. Mitchell EA, Ford RPK, Taylor BJ, Stewart AW, Becroft DMO, Scragg R, et al: Further evidence supporting a causal relationship between prone sleeping position and SIDS. J Paediatr Child Health 1992;28:S9–S12.
104. Valdes-Dapena M: The sudden infant death syndrome. Pathologic findings. Clin Perinatol 1992;17:701–715.
105. Beech DJ, Sibbons PD, Howard CV, Van Delzen D: Lung development. Number of terminal bronchiolar duct endings and gas exchange surface area in victims of sudden infant death syndrome. Pediatr Pulmonol 2001; 31:39–343.
106. Waters KA, Meehan B, Huang JQ, Gravel RA, Michaud J, Cote A: Neuronal apoptosis in sudden infant death syndrome. Pediatr Res 1999; 45:166–172.
107. Filiano JJ, Kinney HC: Arcuate nucleus hypoplasia in the sudden infant death syndrome. J Neuropathol Exp Neurol 1992;51:394–403.
108. Panigraphy A, Filiano JJ, Sleeper LA, Mandell F, Valdes-Dapena M, Krous HF, et al: Decreased kainate receptor binding in the arcuate nucleus of the sudden infant death syndrome. J Neuropathol Exp Neurol 1997;56: 1253–1261.
109. Gozal D, Harper RM: New insights into maturation of central components in cardiovascular and respiratory control. In: Loughlin GM, Carroll JL, Marcus CL, eds: Sleep and Breathing in Children. A Developmental Approach. New York: Marcel Dekker, 2000, pp 207–230.
110. Narita N, Narita M, Takashima S, Nakayama M, Nagai T, Okado N: Serotonin transporter gene variation is a risk factor for sudden infant death syndrome in the Japanese population. Pediatrics 2001;107:690–692.
111. Weese-Mayer DE, Berry-Kravis EM, Zhou L, Maher BS, Curran ME, Silvestri JM, et al: Sudden infant death syndrome: case-control frequency differences at genes pertinent to early autonomic nervous system embryologic development. Pediatr Res 2004;56:391–395.
112. Krous HF, Nadeau JM, Silva PD, Blackbourne BD: A comparison of respiratory symptoms and inflammation in sudden infant death syndrome and in accidental or inflicted infant death. Am J Forensic Med Pathol 2003;24:1–8.
113. Cutz E, Jackson A: Airway inflammation and peripheral chemoreceptors. In: Byard RW, Krous HF, eds: Sudden Infant Death Syndrome—Problems, Progress and Possibilities. London: Edward Arnold, 2001, pp 156–181.
114. Gillan JE, Curran C, O'Reilly E, Cahalane SF, Unwin AR: Abnormal patterns of pulmonary neuroendocrine cells in victims of sudden infant death syndrome. Pediatrics 1989;84:828–834.
115. Perrin DG, McDonald TJ, Cutz E: Hyperplasia of bombesin-immunoreactive pulmonary neuroendocrine cells and neuroepithelial bodies in sudden infant death syndrome. Pediatr Pathol 1991;11:431–447.
116. Cutz E, Jackson A: Neuroepithelial bodies as airway oxygen sensors. Respir Physiol 199;115:201–214.
117. Cutz E, Perrin DG, Hackman R, Czegledy-Nagy EN: Maternal smoking and pulmonary neuroendocrine cells in sudden infant death syndrome. Pediatrics 1996;98:668–672.
118. Schoen EJ, Baker JC, Colby CJ, To TT: Cost-benefit analysis of universal tandem mass spectroscopy for newborn screening. Pediatrics 2002;110: 781–786.
119. Mathur A, Sims HF, Gopalakrishnan D, Gibson B, Rinaldo P, Vockley J, et al: Molecular heterogeneity in very-long-chain acyl-CoA dehydrogenase deficiency causing pediatric cardiomyopathy and sudden death. Circulation 1999;99:1337–1343.
120. Pourfarzam M, Morris A, Appleton M, Craft M, Bartlett K: Neonatal screening for medium-chain acyl-CoA dehydrogenase deficiency. Lancet 2001;358:1063–1064.
121. Bove KE: The metabolic crisis. A diagnostic challenge. J Pediatr 1997;131: 181–182.
122. Boles RG, Buck EA, Blitzer MG, Platt MS, Cowan TM, Martin SK, et al: Retrospective biochemical screening of fatty acid oxidation disorders in postmortem livers in 418 cases of sudden death in the first year of life. J Pediatr 1998;132:924–933.
123. Lundemose JB, Kolvraa S, Gregersen N, Christensen E, Gregersen M: Fatty acid oxidation disorders as primary cause of sudden and unexpected death in infants and young children. An investigation performed on cultured fibroblasts from 79 children who died aged between 0–4 years. Mol Pathol 1997;50:212–217.
124. Wilcox RL, Nelson CC, Stenzel P, Steiner RD: Postmortem screening for fatty oxidation disorders by analysis of Guthrie cards with tandem mass spectroscopy in sudden unexpected death in infancy. J Pediatr 2002;141: 833–836.
125. Arens R, Gozal D, Jain K, Muscati S, Heuser ET, Williams JC, et al: Prevalence of medium-chain acyl-coenzyme A dehydrogenase deficiency in the sudden infant death syndrome. J Pediatr 1993;122:715–718.
126. Morbidity and Mortality Weekly Report: Contribution of selected metabolic diseases to early childhood deaths—Virginia, 1996–2001. MMWR Morb Mortal Wkly Rep 2003;52:677–679.
127. Rinaldo P, Tortorelli S, Matern D: Recent developments and new applications of tandem mass spectroscopy in newborn screening. Curr Opin Pediatr 2004;16:427–433.
128. Schwartz PJ, Badiale MS, Segantini A, Austoni P, Bosi G, Giorgetti R, et al: Prolongation of the QT interval and the sudden infant death syndrome. N Engl J Med 1998;338:1709–1714.
129. Ackerman MJ, Siu BL, Sturner WQ, Tester DJ, Valdivia CR, Makielski JC, et al: Postmortem molecular analysis of SCN5A defects in sudden infant death syndrome. JAMA 2001;286:2264–2269.
130. Mitchell E, Krous HF, Donald T, Byard RW: An analysis of the usefulness of specific stages in the pathologic investigation of sudden infant death. Am J Forensic Med Pathol 2000;21:395–400.
131. Jones AM, Weston JT: Examination of the sudden infant death syndrome infant. Investigative and autopsy protocols. J Forensic Sci 1976;21:833–841.
132. Iyasu S, Hanzlick R, Rowley D, Willinger M: Proceedings of Workshop on Guidelines for Scene Investigation of Sudden Unexplained Infant Deaths–1993. J Forensic Sci 1994;39:1126–1136.
133. Beal SM, Blundell H: Sudden infant death syndrome related to position in the cot. Med J Aust 1978;2:217–218.
134. Guntheroth WG: Epidemiology of SIDS. In: Guntheroth WG, ed: Crib Death. The Sudden Infant Death Syndrome. Mount Kisco, NY: Futura Publishing Co., 1989, pp 89–90.
135. Southall DP, Plunkett MCB, Banks MW, Falkov AF, Samuels MP: Covert video recordings of life-threatening child abuse. Lessons from child protection. Pediatrics 1997;100:735–760.
136. Gordon I, Shapiro HA: Forensic Medicine. A Guide to Principles. Edinburgh: Churchill Livingstone, 1982, p 31.
137. Ewigman B, Kivlahan C, Land G: The Missouri child fatality study. Underreporting of maltreatment among children younger than 5 years of age, 1983 through 1986. Pediatrics 1993;91:330–337.
138. Kemp JS, Kowalski RM, Burch PM, Graham MA, Thach BT: Unintentional suffocation by rebreathing. A death scene and physiological investigation of a possible cause of sudden infant death. J Pediatr 1993;122:874–880.
139. Carpenter RG, Waite A, Coombs RC, Caman-Willems C, McKenzie A, Huber J, et al: Repeat sudden and unexpected and unexplained infant deaths: natural or unnatural? Lancet 2005;365:29–35.
140. Mitchell EA, Scragg R, Stewart AW, Becroft DMO, Taylor BJ, Hassall IB, et al: Results from the first year of the New Zealand cot death study. NZ Med J 1991;104:71–76.
141. Nelson EAS, Taylor BJ, Mackay SC: Child care practices and the sudden infant death syndrome. Aust Paediatr J 1989;25:202–204.
142. Mitchell EA, Taylor BJ, Ford RPK, Stewart AW, Becroft DMO, Thomppson JMD, et al: Four modifiable and other major risk factors for cot death. The New Zealand study. J Paediatr Child Health 1992;28:S3–S8.
143. Dwyer T, Ponsonby A-L, Newman NM, Gibbons LE: Prospective cohort study of prone sleeping position and the sudden infant death syndrome. Lancet 1991;337:1244–1247.
144. Wigfield RE, Fleming PJ, Berry PJ, Rudd PT, Golding J: Can the fall in Avon's sudden infant death rate be explained by changes in sleeping position? BMJ 1992;304:281–283.
145. Ponsonby A-L, Dwyer T, Gibbons LE, Cochrane JA, Wang Y-G: Factors potentiating the risk of sudden infant death syndrome associated with the prone position. N Engl J Med 1993;329:377–382.

146. Fleming PJ, Gilbert R, Azaz Y, Berry PJ, Rudd PT, Stewart A, et al: Interaction between bedding and sleep position in the sudden infant death syndrome. A population based case-control study. BMJ 1990;301: 85–89.
147. Mitchell EA, Brunt JM, Everard C: Reduction in mortality from sudden infant death syndrome in New Zealand, 1986–92. Arch Dis Child 1994;70: 291–294.
148. Taylor JA, Krieger JW, Reay DT, Davis RL, Harruff R, Cheney LK: Prone sleep position and the sudden infant death syndrome in King County, Washington. A case-control study. J Pediatr 1996;128:626–630.
149. Hauck FR, Herman SM, Donovan M, Iyasu S, Merrick Moore C, Donoghue E, et al: Sleep environment and the risk of sudden infant death syndrome in an urban population. The Chicago infant mortality study. Pediatrics 2003;111:1207–1214.
150. Kemp JS, Nelson VE, Thach BT: Physical properties of bedding that may increase risk of sudden infant death syndrome in prone-sleeping infants. Pediatr Res 1994;36:7–11.
151. Nelson EAS, Taylor BJ, Weatherall IL: Sleeping position and infant bedding may predispose to hyperthermia and the sudden infant death syndrome. Lancet 1989;1:199–200.
152. Scheers-Masters JR, Schootman M, Thach BT: Heat stress and sudden infant death syndrome incidence. A United States population epidemiologic study. Pediatrics 2004;113:e586–e592.
153. Fleming PJ, Blair PS, Bacon C, Bensley D, Smith I, Taylor E, et al: Environment of infants during sleep and risk of the sudden infant death syndrome. Results of the 1993-5 case-control study for confidential inquiry into stillbirths and deaths in infancy. BMJ 1996;313:191–195.
154. Iyasu S, Randall L, Welty TK, Hsia J, Kinney HC, Mandell F, et al: Risk factors for sudden infant death syndrome among northern plains Indians. JAMA 2002;288:2717–2723.
155. Kraus JF: Effectiveness of measures to prevent unintentional deaths of infants and children from suffocation and strangulation. Public Health Rep 1985;100:231–240.
156. Fleming PJ, Levine MR, Azaz Y, Wigfield R, Stewart AJ: Interactions between thermoregulation and the control of respiration in infants. Possible relationship to sudden infant death. Act Paediatr Scand 1993;389: S57–S59.
157. Bolton DPG, Taylor BJ, Campbell AJ, Galland BC, Cresswell CA: A potential danger for prone sleeping babies. Rebreathing of expired gases when face down into soft bedding. Arch Dis Child 1993;69:187–190.
158. Kahn A, Groswasser J, Sottiaux M, Rebuffat E, Franco P, Dramaix M: Prone or supine body position and sleep characteristics in infants. Pediatrics 1993;91:1112–1115.
159. Van der Hal AL, Rodriguez AM, Sargent CW, Platzker ACG, Keens TG: Hypoxic and hypercapneic arousal responses and prediction of subsequent apnea in apnea of infancy. Pediatrics 1985;75:848–854.
160. McNamara F, Issa FG, Sullivan CE: Arousal pattern following central and obstructive breathing abnormalities in infants and children. J Appl Physiol 1996;81:2651–2657.
161. Gugger JM, Molloy J, Gould GA, Whyte KF, Raab GM, Shapiro CM, et al: Ventilatory and arousal responses to added inspiratory resistance during sleep. Am Rev Respir Dis 1989;140:1301–1307.
162. McCulloch K, Brouillette RT, Guzzetta AJ, Hunt CE: Arousal responses in near-miss sudden infant death syndrome and in normal infants. J Pediatr 1982;101:911–917.
163. Davidson-Ward SL, Bautista DB, Woo MS, Chang M, Schuetz S, Wachsman L, et al: Responses to hypoxia and hypercapnia in infants of substance-abusing mothers. J Pediatr 1992;121:704–709.
164. Phillipson EA, Sullivan CE: Arousal. The forgotten response to respiratory stimuli. Am Rev Respir Dis 1978;118:807–809.
165. Franco P, Pardou A, Hassid S, Lurquin P, Groswasser J, Kahn A: Auditory arousal thresholds are higher when infants sleep in the prone position. J Pediatr 1998;132:240–243.
166. Horne RS, Parslow PM, Ferens D, Watts AM, Adamson TM: Comparison of evoked arousability in breast and formula fed infants. Arch Dis Child 2004;89:22–25.
167. Thach BT: Sleep, sleep position, and the sudden infant death syndrome. To sleep or not to sleep? J Pediatr 2001;138:793–795.
168. Mograss MA, Ducharme FM, Brouillette RT: Movement/arousals. Description, classification, and relationship to sleep apnea in children. Am J Respir Crit Care Med 1994;150:1690–1696.
169. Thoppil CK, Belan MA, Cowen CP, Mathew OP: Behavioral arousal in newborn infants and its association with termination of apnea. J Appl Physiol 1991;70:2479–2484.
170. Groswasser J, Simon T, Scaillet S, Franco P, Kahn A: Reduced arousals following obstructive apneas in infants sleeping prone. Pediatr Res 2001; 49:402–406.
171. Chang AB, Wilson SJ, Masters IB, Yuill M, Williams J, Hubbard M: Altered arousal response in infants exposed to cigarette smoke. Arch Dis Child 2003;88:30–33.
172. Franco P, Scaillet S, Valente F, Chabanski S, Groswasser J, Kahn A: Ambient temperature is associated with changes in infants' arousability from sleep. Sleep 2001;24:325–329.
173. Goto K, Mirmiran M, Adams MM, Longford RV, Baldwin RB, Boeddiker MA, et al: More awakenings and heart rate variability during supine sleep in preterm infants. Pediatrics 1999;103:603–609.
174. Skadberg BT, Markestad T: Consequences of getting the head covered during sleep in infancy. Pediatrics 1997;100(2):E6. Available at http://www.pediatrics.org/cgi/content/full/100/2/e6.
175. Galland BC, Bolton DPG, Taylor BJ, Sayers RM, Williams SM: Ventilatory sensitivity to mild asphyxia. Prone versus supine sleep. Arch Dis Child 2000;83:423–428.
176. Carpenter RG, Shaddick CW: Role of infection, suffocation, and bottle feeding in cot death. An analysis of some factors in the histories of 110 cases and their controls. Br J Prev Soc Med 1965;19:1–7.
177. L'Hoir MP, Engelberts AC, Van Well GTJ, McClelland S, Westers P, Dandachll T, et al: Risk and preventive factors for cot death in the Netherlands, a low-incidence country. Eur J Pediatr 1998;157:681–688.
178. Chiodini BA, Thach BT: Impaired ventilation in infants sleeping facedown. Potential significance for sudden infant death syndrome. J Pediatr 1993;123: 686–692.
179. Petersen SA, Anderson ES, Lodemore M, Rawson D, Wailoo MP: Sleeping position and rectal temperature. Arch Dis Child 1991;66:976–979.
180. Luke JL: Sleeping arrangements of sudden infant death syndrome victims in the District of Columbia—a preliminary report. J Forensic Sci 1978;23: 379–383.
181. Scragg R, Mitchell EA, Taylor BJ, Stewart AW, Ford RPK, Thompson JMD, et al: Bed sharing, smoking, and alcohol in the sudden infant death syndrome. BMJ 1993;307:1312–1318.
182. Blair PS, Fleming PJ, Smith IJ, Platt MW, Young J, Nadin P, et al: Babies sleeping with parents. Case-control study of factors influencing the risk of the sudden infant death syndrome. BMJ 1999;319:1457–1462.
183. Carpenter RG, Irgens LM, Blair PS, England PD, Fleming P, Huber J, et al: Sudden unexplained infant death in 20 regions in Europe. Lancet 2004;363:185–191.
184. Tappin D, Ecob R, Brooke H: Bedsharing and sudden infant death syndrome in Scotland. A case-control study. J Pediatr 2005;147:32–37.
185. National infant sleep position public access website. Available at http://dccwww.bumc.bu.edu/Chime Nisp/Main_Nisp.asp.
186. Mitchell EA, Scragg R: Observations on ethnic differences in SIDS mortality in New Zealand. Early Hum Dev 1994;38:151–157.
187. Tipene-Leach D, Everard C, Haretuku R: Taking a strategic approach to SIDS prevention in Maori communities—an indigenous perspective. In: Byard RW, Krous HF, eds: Sudden Infant Death Syndrome—Problems, Progress and Possibilities. London: Edward Arnold, 2001, pp 275–282.
188. Willinger M, Ko C, Hoffman HJ, Kessler RC, Corwin MJ: Trends in infant bedsharing in the United States, 1993–2000. Arch Pediatr Adolesc Med 2003;157:43–47.
189. Quillin SI, Glenn LL: Interaction between feeding method and co-sleeping on maternal-newborn sleep. J Obstet Gynecol Neonatal Nurs 2004;33: 580–588.
190. Flick L, White DK, Vemulapalli C, Stulac B, Kemp JS: Sleep position and the use of soft bedding during bedsharing among 218 African-American infants at increased risk for sudden infant death syndrome. J Pediatr 2001; 138:338–343.
191. Scheers NJ, Rutherford GW, Kemp JS: Where should infants sleep? A comparison of risk for suffocation of sleeping in cribs, adult beds, and other sleeping locations. Pediatrics 2003;112:883–889.
192. Leduc D, Cote A, Woods S: Canadian Paediatric Society. Recommendations for safe sleeping environments for infants and children. Paediatr Child Health 2004;9:659–663.

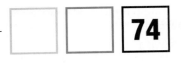

74 Disorders of Breathing during Sleep

David Gozal, MD • Leila Kheirandish, MD

BASIC MECHANISMS AND ARCHITECTURE OF NORMAL SLEEP

NEURAL CIRCUITRY OF SLEEP AND WAKING

Sleep is a global and dynamically regulated state, the control mechanisms of which are manifested at every level of biologic organization, from genes and intracellular mechanisms to networks of cell populations, and to all central neuronal systems at the organismal level, including those that control movement, arousal, autonomic functions, behavior, and cognition. In mammals, sleep states can be readily differentiated into two major types, namely rapid eye movement (REM) and non–rapid eye movement (NREM) sleep. These two distinctive sleep states are defined in terms of their electroencephalographic (EEG) and electromyographic (EMG) characteristics. NREM sleep involves high-voltage, low-frequency "synchronized" wave activity with relatively preserved skeletal muscle tonic activity, whereas REM sleep is characterized by wakelike high-frequency, low-amplitude "desynchronized" activity in the EEG along with a typical attenuation of skeletal muscle tonic activity (i.e., REM atonia). Bursts of 12- to 14-Hz sleep spindles are characteristic of NREM sleep in adults and children, although such bursts may also occur during REM sleep; maximal development of phasic spindle activity emerges after approximately 16 weeks postnatally.

The neural sites underlying the onset, maintenance, and function of NREM and REM sleep continue to be the object of intensive research; however, sufficient insights are now available to link certain breathing patterns with the neural properties and activity patterns of state-related regulatory structures. Areas within the basal forebrain, including regions within the preoptic region, have long been implicated in initiating NREM sleep, with local stimulation eliciting the typical NREM sleep state and lesion studies resulting in pronounced loss of sleep. Single-cell studies assessing the discharge patterns of neurons within these neural regions conclusively demonstrate the existence of neurons that selectively fire with the onset of NREM sleep in this area. Certain features of NREM sleep, such as the large synchronous slow waves (delta waves) and bursts of 12- to 14-Hz sleep spindles, are critically dependent on the integrity of the thalamocortical circuitry, even if these characteristic neural activity patterns can be generated under certain pharmacologic conditions, such as subsequent to atropine administration during waking states. Furthermore, recent work has implicated adenosine and its cognate receptors as an important mechanism of NREM sleep regulation, such that this neurotransmitter is currently believed to regulate metabolic and recovery aspects of NREM sleep within the basal forebrain and thalamocortical regions.[1,2] It should also be stressed that thermoregulatory areas of the anterior hypothalamus closely interact with sleep-associated regions in the brain and dictate the generation of close relationships between warming, discharge of thermoregulatory neurons, and induction of sleep. Indeed, higher temperatures, whether externally applied or through localized warming of hypothalamic structures, will lead to increased sleepiness and NREM sleep duration.

Since the principal physiologic characteristics of REM sleep persist even after separation of the forebrain from the pons, it has been suggested that mechanisms underlying this unique sleep state lie caudal to the diencephalon within specific and spatially restricted brain stem regions such as the locus coeruleus and several pontine nuclei; notably, areas within the dorsal lateral pons have been particularly implicated in eliciting some of the characteristics of REM sleep state. For example, the atonia of REM sleep can be abolished by lesions in the dorsal pons, ventral to the locus coeruleus, and phasic somatic events can be terminated by lesions in the pedunculopontine tegmentum. Certain phasic elements, such as the variation of sympathetic and parasympathetic outflow during REM sleep, are dependent on the integrity of vestibular nuclei, while phasic eye movements, a hallmark of REM sleep, will persist even in the presence of lesions in the vestibular sites. A number of brain stem regions, namely the dorsal and caudal raphe, locus coeruleus, and ventral medullary surface, show declines in neural activity during REM sleep; however, most of the brain will manifest substantial increases in neural cell activity and glucose consumption during REM sleep, sometimes exceeding levels seen during wakefulness. Brain regions that decrease their discharge patterns during REM sleep play important roles in blood pressure regulation; however, it is unclear whether the state-related cell patterns in these regions bear a relationship to blood pressure control (and indirectly to breathing patterns) during REM sleep.

DEVELOPMENTAL ASPECTS OF SLEEP

Sleep state organization undergoes rapid development during the first 6 months of life. Neonates and young infants spend a disproportionate amount of time in REM sleep; indeed infants exhibit REM sleep at sleep onset, an event that is considered abnormal in the adult. NREM sleep (also termed quiet sleep) is poorly developed in newborns, since the slow oscillatory EEG patterns that define this state are not as readily apparent during early postnatal life and may manifest as intermittent slow and faster EEG patterns (e.g., tracé alternans). However, the relative amount of quiet sleep increases over the first 3 months of life, with K-complexes and sleep spindles becoming increasingly evident. Therefore, scoring of sleep using adult criteria is not applicable before 3 to 6 months of age, and a more simplistic categorization of sleep states into awake, quiet sleep, active sleep (equivalent to REM sleep), and indeterminate sleep is normally used during the first year of life.[3–9] The total duration of sleep decreases relative to the 24-hour period, the relative proportion of NREM sleep increases, and that of REM sleep decreases with advancing age. At the age of 1 year, children will typically require

12 to 13 hours of sleep primarily during the night, with one or two naps during the day. At this age, well-defined NREM sleep alternates with REM sleep, the latter accounting for 30% of total sleep time in recurring 90-minute cycles very similar to those found in the adult. At approximately 2 years of age, the relative proportion of REM sleep will stabilize at approximately 20% to 25% of total sleep time and will remain somewhat constant until old age, despite gradual reductions in total sleep duration with advancing age. NREM sleep acquires its maximal expression in duration and depth during the first decade of life. Indeed, the depth of sleep in childhood is quite remarkable considering how difficult it is to arouse a child during the first cycle of slow-wave sleep. During the second decade of life, slow-wave sleep gradually decreases by approximately 40%, continuing its gradual decline until old age. It is during slow-wave sleep that growth hormone is secreted in large amounts, and thus either sleep deprivation or disorders of sleep may interfere with the secretion and regulation of growth hormone, with potential and rather immediate clinical consequences.

RESPIRATORY CONTROL MECHANISMS

Our understanding of respiratory control has undergone multiple evolutionary waves in the last century. Obviously, breathing is an important and vital function. Nevertheless, despite the critical functions of respiration, it is undeniable that the respiratory control system undergoes substantial maturation during the first few years of life. There is no doubt that the relative uncertainty about the anatomic and functional aspects pertaining to the neural respiratory pathways, the complexities of neuronal firing activities, the multitude of neurotransmitters within each brain stem nucleus, and the frequently nucleus-dependent opposing roles played by these neurotransmitters in respiratory function can be quite overwhelming and difficult to comprehend. Despite such problems, the field of respiratory control has evolved tremendously in recent years, and we are now witnessing the initial discovery of several of the genes that control the development and maturation of multiple neurally controlled respiratory functions.[10]

THE RESPIRATORY RHYTHM GENERATOR

The putative neural center responsible for generation of respiratory rhythmic activity has now been identified,[11] and specific markers such as neurokinin and opioid receptors in these neurons have yielded estimates that this uniquely important neural center is a cluster of 150 to 200 neurons in the brain stem region designated as Pre-Botzinger complex.[12] This small number of rhythmically firing neurons appears both necessary and sufficient to generate most of the complex normal respiratory behaviors that we know such as eupnea, sigh, and gasping.[13–15] The development of several elegant models ranging from highly reductionistic (brain stem slice) to less reductionistic approaches (whole brain stem–heart-lung preparation) will undoubtedly permit extensive characterization of the network configuration responses, the functional neurotransmitters involved in generation of respiratory rhythm, and permit a thorough understanding of the electrophysiologic properties of these unique cells both during development as well as during disease. Several genes, such as *PHOX2A, HOX* paralogs, and *HOX*-regulating genes *MAFB* (formerly "Kreisler [mouse] maf-related leucine zipper homolog") and *EGR2* (formerly *Krox20*), have been recently identified as important players in the embryonic generation of respiratory centers and their intrinsic connectivities.[16,17] These and other yet unknown genes that regulate the ontogeny of brain stem development may provide initial insights into the regulation of the initial phases involved in the normal and abnormal formation of the respiratory network.

SLEEP AND BREATHING DURING DEVELOPMENT

The cyclic activity of respiratory rhythm generation is further modulated by suprapontine sites that include important efferent projections to areas mediating the sleep-wake cycle, thermoregulation, and circadian rhythm rhythmicity. Respiratory control areas also receive afferent inputs from central and peripheral chemoreceptors and from other receptors within the respiratory pump (upper airways, chest wall, and lungs). During fetal life, breathing is discontinuous and coincides with REM-like sleep. After birth, respiratory rhythm is established as a continuous activity to maintain cellular O_2 and CO_2 homeostasis. Respiratory pattern instability during sleep is typically present during early life such that short apneic episodes lasting less than 5 seconds are extremely common in preterm neonates, and their frequency is reduced in full-term newborns. These episodes occur predominantly during REM sleep as a result of the greater respiratory instability in this state. Several developmental differences between the neonate and the adult respiratory systems may further account for the emergence of sleep-associated disruption of normal gas exchange in early postnatal life, and include the following:

- Neonates have greater difficulty switching from the nasal to the oral route of breathing, and the majority of younger neonates can be considered as obligatory or near-obligatory nasal breathers.
- In neonates, reflexes originating in the upper airway (laryngeal chemoreflex) are potentiated and can induce profound apnea and bradycardia. This respiratory depressant component of the laryngeal chemoreflex decreases with maturation, such that prolonged apnea induced by stimulation of the laryngeal chemoreflex is more prominent in preterm than in full-term neonates.[18]
- The chest wall compliance is increased in neonates, thereby requiring dynamic, rather than passive, maintenance of the functional residual capacity of the lungs. Furthermore, neonates have "barrel-shaped" rib cages, and the rib cage contribution to tidal breathing is smaller than in older children and adults. Thus, any condition whereby the ability to maintain functional residual capacity is compromised, as in REM sleep, will lead to increased susceptibility.
- Paradoxical breathing (i.e., asynchronous or out of phase motion of the chest and abdomen), especially during REM sleep, is common in newborns because of uncoordinated interactions between chest and abdominal respiratory musculature. The duration of paradoxical breathing during sleep decreases as postnatal age increases. Paradoxical breathing is rare or absent after 3 years of age.[19]
- The respiratory rate is high in the neonatal period and decreases during infancy and early childhood. Respiratory rate decreases exponentially with increasing body weight and parallels changes in overall metabolic rates. Notably, respiratory rate is higher during REM sleep than it is in NREM sleep.
- Apneas of short duration (less than 10 seconds) are extremely common during the early period of life. Apneic episodes are

more frequent in REM sleep than during NREM sleep. Apneic episodes are mostly central and will decrease in number with advancing postnatal age. Obstructive and mixed apneic episodes are more frequently seen in preterm than in full-term neonates, possibly reflecting developmental changes in pharyngeal, laryngeal, and central airway collapsibility.

- Periodic breathing, defined as three episodes of apnea lasting longer than 3 seconds and separated by continued respiration over a period of 20 seconds or less, is a common respiratory pattern in preterm neonates, and may also be highly prevalent in full-term newborns.[20,21] However, periodic breathing decreases in frequency during the first year of life and is usually not considered to be of any specific pathologic significance. Notwithstanding such considerations, environmental variables such as sleep state transitions, arousals, hypoxia, and hyperthermia can enhance the frequency and magnitude of periodic breathing in newborns, and ultimately lead to destabilization of cardiorespiratory homeostasis.
- Apneic episodes during sleep in neonates are associated with a fall in heart rate, particularly during NREM sleep. The presence of hypoxemia will enhance this reflex bradycardia during apnea.
- Arousal from sleep is thought to be a major determinant for termination of apnea, and therefore arousal deficits have been implicated in the pathophysiology of the sudden infant death syndrome (SIDS). However, fewer than 10% of apneic episodes will be terminated by a full-fledged EEG arousal in neonates. Autonomic arousals are nevertheless quite frequent during the period surrounding the termination of an apneic event. Moreover, while hypercapnia is a potent stimulus of arousal, hypoxia, and particularly rapidly developing hypoxia, is much less effective in inducing arousal. Finally, prone position, sleep deprivation, and prenatal-postnatal exposure to cigarette smoking are all accompanied by decreased arousability in neonates.
- Healthy full-term newborns will usually maintain oxyhemoglobin saturation values of 92% to 100% during sleep in the first 4 weeks of life. Blood O_2 levels are lowest during the first week of life and increase over the next 1 to 3 months, such that all newborns will have values of 97% to 100% after the age of 2 months. Basal values for arterial CO_2 tension during sleep are generally between 36 and 42 mm Hg in newborns and infants.

As delineated earlier, the implications of REM sleep on breathing are substantial, and as discussed later, the loss of muscle tone during REM sleep is particularly important to the upper airway muscles and airway patency. An important aspect of breathing control is the close interaction of breathing and blood pressure regulation. The respiratory system, using primarily somatic musculature, exerts substantial influence on moment-to-moment blood pressure; conversely, transient elevation of blood pressure can cease breathing efforts, while lowering of blood pressure can increase them. The interactions between the systems can be observed readily in breathing influences on heart rate (a classic example being respiratory sinus arrhythmia). Inspiratory efforts normally are associated with accelerated heart rate and expiratory efforts with deceleration, the result of reflex activity from pulmonary afferents and vagal outflow; the resulting coupling between breathing and heart rate is particularly prominent during NREM sleep, and measures of the interaction can provide a useful indication of state.[22] In addition, phasic activity during REM sleep induces substantial parasympathetic and sympathetic outflow, resulting in larger but typically slower variation in heart rate. Plots of cardiac beat-to-beat intervals demonstrate the substantial influences exerted normally during each state, with NREM sleep exerting a highly cyclic effect on heart rate variation and REM sleep showing a lesser extent of modulation by breathing but larger slower sources of variation. Waking shows a large variation in heart rate changes; typically very active periods are accompanied by high heart rates with little variation. The cyclic nature of cardiac rate variation has led to a variety of procedures to measure the sympathetic and parasympathetic influences. Particular syndromes exert unique patterns of respiration-related variation; for example, children with congenital central hypoventilation syndrome (CCHS) show a relative absence of variation of respiratory modulation of heart rate, and infants who later succumb to SIDS also show reduced variation to breathing.

CENTRAL CHEMORECEPTORS AND THEIR DEVELOPMENT

The chemoreflexes exert powerful influences over breathing as well as cardiac and vascular control. Chemoreflex physiology is complex, and the exact molecular mechanisms by which the chemoreflexes are activated remain unclear. The traditional and classic theory formulated during the late 1950s proposed that the central chemoreceptors were located in the ventrolateral medullary surface of the brain stem and responded to hypercapnia and pH changes, whereas the peripheral chemoreceptors were located in the carotid bodies and primarily responded to changes in blood O_2 tension. While this concept has now evolved (see later), it is worthwhile to mention that hypercapnia (particularly transient changes in CO_2 tension above the apneic threshold) can also activate the peripheral chemoreceptors, and may account for as much as one-third of peripheral chemoreceptor activity. Activation of either central or peripheral chemoreflexes exerts powerful effects on sympathetic activity in both health and disease and may be an important contributor to pathophysiology of obstructive sleep apnea (OSA).

MULTIPLICITY OF CENTRAL CHEMOSENSITIVE CENTERS

A critically important advance in the field of respiratory control involved discarding the classic concept of central chemosensitive sites as being located in restricted areas of the ventral medullary surface. Indeed, several lines of evidence have now clearly established that neurons showing intrinsic chemosensitive properties (i.e., the ability to sense changes in extracellular pH and contribute to the ventilatory response) are diffusely located in the central nervous system, and that regions such as the posterior hypothalamus, cerebellum, locus coeruleus, raphé, and multiple nuclei within the brain stem all contribute to the well-characterized hypercapnic ventilatory response.[23–25] Why is this important? One reason is that the phenotypic manifestations of conditions such as central alveolar hypoventilation, particularly when occurring secondary to other disorders (e.g., myelomeningocele, tumors, stroke) are not adequately explained by either the location or the magnitude of the brain lesions in these patients. Second, it is very possible that the normal developmental processes of the ventilatory response to elevations of CO_2 are not only important to long-term stability of the homeostatic system but may be even more important to the preservation of respiratory stability during respiratory transients, particularly during sleep. Conditions such as apparent life-threatening events or even SIDS may originate from dysfunctional development of either the respiratory rhythm controllers or, alternatively, that of the neural networks underlying hypoxic and hypercapnic chemosensitivities as well as those mediating arousal from sleep.[26,27]

The neurotransmitters involved in the intrinsic sensory pathways associated with central chemoreception are currently unknown. The presence of cholinergic muscarinic receptors in those brain stem areas traditionally associated with CO_2 chemosensitivity appears to play a major role in the neuronal excitation associated with the enhanced ventilatory response to hypercapnia, although additional neurotransmitters are also clearly involved. It must be emphasized that the central CO_2 chemosensory mechanisms may not be fully functional or mature at birth. Indeed, animal models in various species show that hypercapnic ventilatory responses will increase with advancing age. Hypercapnia elicits a relatively sustained ventilatory increase in term infants that is almost entirely due to an increase in tidal volume without consistent change in respiratory frequency. In contrast, the ventilatory response to hypercapnia in premature infants is attenuated and can even become inhibitory at higher concentrations of inhaled CO_2, with CO_2 overall respiratory responses increasing with postconceptional age. In preterm neonates, the ventilatory increase to hypercapnia is accompanied by a progressive increase in expiratory duration and a consequent reduction in frequency over time, both of which appear to be associated with diaphragmatic recruitment during expiration (respiratory braking or grunting). This unique mechanism appears to preserve a high end-expiratory lung volume such as to optimize gas exchange and promote respiratory stability. Little is known about the development of central chemoreceptor function beyond infancy. In awake prepubertal children there appears to be an enhanced ventilatory response to hypercapnia compared with adults, and these differences may underlie differences in metabolic rate.[28] Similarly, significant developmental differences in CO_2 responses emerge when the CO_2 stimulus is presented in either a step (sudden increase) or ramp (slow progressive increase) fashion.[29] These findings in older children suggest that at some time during transition from infancy to childhood and on to adulthood, major changes occur in the relative contributions and integration of peripheral and central chemoreceptor activity. The cascades of genes, receptors, and neurotransmitters that mediate these developmental changes are unknown at the present time. Similarly, the elements involved in the integrated coordination of the developmental changes at the level of the carotid body, neural transmission, or central nervous system remain unclear.

PERIPHERAL CHEMOREFLEXES

The ventilatory responses related to changes in blood O_2 levels are a complex interaction of a variety of peripheral and central responses. Nevertheless, the rapidity of the peripheral chemoreceptor responses to blood oxygenation changes allows for assessment of the initial stimulatory effect elicited by activation of these peripherally located chemosensory cells, of which the most important are glomus cells within the carotid bodies. Peripheral chemoreceptor activity is typically assessed by monitoring the fast transient increase in minute ventilation after inhalation of gases containing low concentrations of O_2. Isocapnic hypoxic responses (over a period of 2–3 minutes) or five tidal breaths of pure N_2 are among the strategies that have been used.[30–32] Alternatively, the ventilatory decline subsequent to inhalation of 100% O_2 is also considered as a reliable indicator of peripheral chemoreceptor gain (Dejours test). However, it is important to indicate that the ventilatory decrease to acute hyperoxia is ultimately followed by an increase in ventilation that is centrally mediated.[33] More sophisticated paradigms using random alternations of N_2 and O_2 in a computerized setting have recently permitted the development of reproducible and consistent findings in infants and children suspected at risk for chemoreceptor dysfunction.[34–37] Independent of the test selected, substantial attention to sleep state is required when assessing respiratory chemoreceptor drives in infants and in the interpretation of such tests, such that these tests are best reserved for specialized laboratories, in which specific normative values have been developed, and therefore allow for more reliable clinical assessment of individual patients presenting with symptoms suggestive of chemosensory dysfunction.

A typical phenomenon associated with more sustained exposure to hypoxic gas mixtures consists in the emergence of a relative ventilatory decline after 5 to 6 minutes of hypoxic exposure. This hypoxic ventilatory decline has also been termed hypoxic ventilatory roll-off. This phenomenon is particularly prominent during infancy, such that with sustained hypoxia in neonates there is a well-characterized increase in breathing followed by a reduction in ventilation that will usually reach levels below normoxic breathing. In more mature children and in adults, the reduction in ventilation will usually reach levels that are below peak but still higher than the ventilation measured during baseline, room air breathing. A study of premature neonates showed that this biphasic response will persist into the second month of postnatal life, but this only represented a postconceptional age of about 35 weeks.[38] Even term neonates may retain the biphasic response characteristic for at least 2 months when tested with normal bedding at room temperature of 24°C during NREM sleep. In addition, very small preterm neonates may show only a decrease in ventilation with hypoxia. The apparent differences between preterm and term neonates may be partially accounted for by developmental status in relation to postnatal age; indeed, premature but not term lambs or piglets also exhibit an attenuated hypercapnic response. Thus, prematurity and/or factors delaying normal maturation emerge as important contributors to the attenuated hypercapnic and hypoxic responses in newborns.

Studies suggest that a relatively high ventilatory drive exists during wakefulness in children, and that this drive decreases during adolescence and stabilizes during adulthood; the reason for this transition is currently unknown. Marcus and colleagues[28] studied hypercapnic and hypoxic ventilatory responses in a group of subjects aged 4 to 49 years and found significant correlations between both the awake hypercapnic and hypoxic ventilatory responses when corrected for age and body size.

THE UPPER AIRWAY

UPPER AIRWAY CONTROL

Since both snoring and OSA are opposite ends of a spectrum of increased upper airway resistance, it is important to review the anatomic and physiologic mechanisms that underlie the maintenance of upper airway patency during sleep.[39] The upper airway comprises the nose, pharynx, larynx, and extrathoracic trachea, and is designed for vocalization, ingestion, airway protection, and respiration. Maintenance of a rigid and patent upper airway is mandatory for achieving adequate respiration and is the result of a balance between forces that promote airway closure and dilatation. Thus, the inherent collapsibility of the pharynx predisposes to impaired respiration when the regulation of the pharyngeal muscles is impaired, such as may occur during sleep.

Anatomically, it is clear that a smaller cross-sectional area of the upper airway is associated with decreased ability to maintain upper airway patency, and in adults the upper airway behaves as predicted by the Starling resistor model, a model that has been well characterized in biologic systems. This model describes the major determinants of airflow in terms of the mechanical properties of collapsible tubes and predicts that, under conditions of flow limitation, maximal inspiratory flow will be determined by the pressure changes upstream (nasal) to a collapsible site of the upper airway, and flow will be independent of downstream (tracheal) pressure generated by the diaphragm. Collapse occurs when the pressure surrounding the collapsible segment of the upper airway becomes greater than the pressure within the collapsible segment of the airway. Pressures at which collapse of the airway occurs have been termed critical closing pressure (P_{crit}).[40,41] In normal subjects with low upstream resistance, pressures downstream never approach P_{crit} and airflow is not limited. This model explains why snoring and obstructive apnea worsen during a common cold (increased nasal upstream resistance). Marcus and colleagues[42] further demonstrated the validity of this model in children and found that the upper airway collapsibility in children is reduced compared with the adult. Notably, and as predicted by the Starling model, the collapsible segment of the upper airway in children displayed less negative (higher and thus more collapsible) pressures in children with OSA. It follows that components that affect the upstream segment pressures or increase P_{crit} will be of major consequence to the ability to maintain airway patency. The contribution of the various anatomic nasopharyngeal structures to P_{crit} and the interactions between these structures that will lead to upper airway patency or obstruction during sleep are thus of clear importance in increasing our understanding of the pathophysiology of childhood OSA.

Although the overall ventilatory drive appears to be normal in children with OSA, it is possible that central augmentation of upper airway neuromotor function is abnormal. During sleep, upper airway tone is diminished even though the same structural factors are present during wake and sleep, and OSA occurs only during sleep. It is unknown whether children with OSA become obstructed because of a relatively larger decrease in airway tone during sleep in comparison to controls, or whether the decrease in tone is similar but subjects with OSA have an increased structural load. The upper airway muscles are accessory muscles of respiration and, as such, are activated by stimuli such as hypoxemia, hypercapnia, and upper airway subatmospheric pressure. Previous studies have shown that, when upper airway muscle function is decreased or absent, as in postmortem preparations, the airway is prone to collapse.[43] Conversely, stimulation of the upper airway muscles with hypercapnia[44,45] or electrical stimulation[46] results in decreased collapsibility. These studies confirm that the tendency of the upper airway to collapse is inversely related to the level of activity of the upper airway dilator muscles. Therefore, increased upper airway neuromotor tone may be one way that patients can compensate for a narrow upper airway. Indeed, this has been shown in adults. Mezzanotte and colleagues demonstrated that adult patients with OSA compensated for their narrow upper airway during wakefulness by increasing their upper airway muscle tone.[47] This compensatory mechanism was lost during sleep.[48] Recent studies in children have shown that children with OSA have greater genioglossal EMG activity during the awake state than control children and a greater decline in EMG activity during sleep onset.[49] Furthermore, upper airway dynamic responses are decreased in children with OSA but appear to recover after treatment. Thus, pharyngeal airway neuromotor responses are present in normal children and serve as a compensatory response for a relatively narrow upper airway compared with adults. However, this compensatory neuromotor response is lacking in children with OSA, probably as a result of habituation to chronic respiratory abnormalities during sleep, mechanical damage to the upper airway, or genetically determined differences in these upper airway protective reflexes.[50–52]

Ventilatory control in patients with OSA is the subject of intense study. In adults with OSA, it is suggested that there is a high-gain ventilatory control system that results in ventilatory instability and apnea.[53] However, studies in children have shown overall normal ventilatory responses to hypoxia and hypercapnia during wakefulness and during sleep when using standard tests.[28,29,54] Indeed, ventilatory responses to rebreathing hyperoxic hypercapnia were measured in 20 children and adolescents with OSA, and the mean slopes of the hypercapnic response were similar to those measured in age- and sex-matched controls.[55] Furthermore, no differences were found in the slopes calculated from plotting minute ventilation against O_2 saturation during isocapnic hypoxia. Nevertheless, other investigators have found some degree of blunting in central chemosensitivity of children with OSA undergoing surgery.[56,57] Despite such findings, central chemosensitivity during sleep was similar in children with OSA and matched controls. However, arousal to acutely induced hypercapnia was blunted during sleep in children with OSA, suggesting that subtle alterations in the central chemosensitive-arousal network have occurred in these patients. These subtle changes have been further substantiated by examination of the ventilatory responses to repetitive hypercapnic challenges during wakefulness, whereby reciprocal changes in respiratory frequency and tidal volume do occur.[58] In the study by Gozal and colleagues,[59] repeated CO_2 challenges were given in the early morning to children with OSA who were hypercapnic (as a result of obstructive alveolar hypoventilation) during sleep. These children showed a respiratory response to the CO_2 challenge but did not show the same adaptive changes in respiratory pattern that would be anticipated over the course of several CO_2 challenges as elicited from children without OSA. However, when children with OSA were studied later in the day (i.e., a few hours after awakening and resolution of sleep-associated alveolar hypoventilation) or after treatment of OSA, a similar respiratory pattern to that seen in controls emerged, suggesting that such deficits may be related to habituation to nocturnal hypercapnia. Additional evidence in support of this comes from Marcus and collegues,[28] who found an inverse correlation between the duration of hypercapnia during the night and the awake hypercapnic ventilatory responses. In addition, children with OSA demonstrate impaired arousal responses to inspiratory loads during REM and non-REM sleep compared with control children.[60] This arousal threshold was particularly high during REM sleep, a time when most obstructive apneic events occur, and suggests that neuromotor influences play a key role. The absence or delayed arousal in children during an obstructive respiratory event and the presumed lack of ventilatory compensation to upper airway loading may contribute to the development of the prolonged periods of obstructive alveolar hypoventilation that uniquely characterize OSA in children. Furthermore, diminished laryngeal reflexes to mechanoreceptor and chemoreceptor stimulation with reduced afferent inputs into central neural regions underlying inspiratory inputs could be present. For example, chemoreceptor stimuli such as increased $PaCO_2$ or decreased PaO_2 stimulate the airway dilating muscles in a preferential mode; that is, upper airway musculature is more stimulated than the diaphragm.[61] This preferential recruitment tends to correct an imbalance of forces acting on the airway and therefore maintain airway patency. Similarly, stimuli resulting from suction pressures in the nose, pharynx, or larynx rapidly stimulate the activity of upper airway dilators, and this effect is also preferential to the upper airway, causing some degree of diaphragmatic inhibition and thus compensating for increase in upstream resistance. The function of these upper airway receptors in children with adenotonsillar hypertrophy with and without OSA is currently unknown.

While dynamic factors such as those just discussed have been implicated in the pathophysiology of upper airway obstruction during sleep in children, we should not omit the contribution of either anatomic elements or genetic factors to this complex equation. In otherwise normal children, Arens and colleagues have shown that the mandibular dimensions of children with OSA are similar to those of controls.[62] However, regional analysis of the upper airway using magnetic resonance imaging techniques further suggested that the upper airway in children with OSA is most restricted where adenoids and tonsils overlap. Furthermore, the upper airway is narrowed throughout the initial two thirds of its length in pediatric patients with OSA, and this narrowing is not in a discrete region adjacent to either the adenoids or tonsils, but rather emerges in a continuous fashion along both lymphadenoid structures.[63,64] It should be emphasized that, contrary to the previous conceptual framework whereby the higher prevalence of OSA in children during the age period from 2 to 8 years was attributed to the increased growth rate of lymphadenoid tissue within the upper airway compared with other upper airway structures,[65,66] the recent evidence refutes this concept and shows that all tissues within the upper airway including adenoids and tonsils grow proportionally and thus that stimuli leading to enhanced proliferation of lymphadenoid tissues within the airway are probably implicated in the pathophysiology of OSA.[67,68]

UPPER AIRWAY DYSFUNCTION

In infancy, abnormalities that reduce the patency of the upper airway are frequently associated with OSA. The upper airway has decreased muscle tone, there is high nasal resistance, and the chest wall is highly compliant. The exact prevalence of OSA in infants is not well documented, since most epidemiologic studies have concentrated on older children. However, OSA has been shown to occur in as many as 10% of infants, is more frequent in preterm infants, and is associated with hypoxemia. OSA occurs more frequently in male infants than in females, and this may be attributable to sex-related differences in the anatomy of the upper airway or to a protective role of female hormones. The main risk factors for OSA in this age group include: (1) craniofacial abnormalities (e.g., micrognathia, cleft palate, Pierre Robin syndrome, Treacher Collins syndrome, choanal atresia, mucopolysaccharidoses, Down syndrome); (2) soft tissue infiltration, which may result from infection, inflammation, laryngomalacia, subglottic stenosis, and adenotonsillar hypertrophy. Indeed, the latter has been found to contribute significantly to the generation of OSA in infants younger than 1 year old[69,70]; (3) neurologic disorders that induce pharyngeal hypotonia such as Arnold-Chiari malformation, cerebral palsy, and poliomyelitis are also associated with an increased risk for obstructed breathing. Although the anatomic site of obstruction in infants is widely believed to be the retroglossal region,[71] recent evidence using magnetic resonance imaging and airway manometry suggests that upper airway obstruction with clinically significant OSA occurs in the retropalatal region 80% of the time and only 20% of the time in the retroglossal region.[72] Other influences may alter breathing characteristics and predispose infants to OSA, including upper airway reflexes such as the laryngeal chemoreflex. This unique defense reflex that aims to prevent aspiration of food is enhanced by upper airway infection, and indeed, respiratory syncytial virus infection, which potentiates the laryngeal chemoreflex, has also been shown to facilitate the occurrence of both central and obstructive apneic episodes.[73] Similarly, prenatal exposure to maternal smoking, which potentiates the laryngeal chemoreflex, also increases the frequency of OSA in infants.[74,75]

To determine the region of maximal airway narrowing in children with OSA, the static pressure/area relationships of the passive pharynx were endoscopically measured in 14 children with OSA and 13 normal children under general anesthesia with complete paralysis.[76,77] The minimum cross-sectional area was found to be at the level of the adenoid and the soft palate. Thus, children with OSA closed their airways at the level of enlarged tonsils and adenoids at low positive pressures, whereas normal children required subatmospheric pressures to induce upper airway closure. The cross-sectional area of the narrowest segment was significantly smaller in children with OSA, and particularly involved at the retropalatal and retroglossal segments, such that it becomes clear that anatomic factors, both congenital and acquired, play a significant role in the pathogenesis of pediatric OSA.[78,79] Furthermore, as mentioned earlier, airway narrowing in children with OSA occurs along the upper two thirds of the airway and is maximal where the adenoids and tonsils overlap.[64,80]

In summary, several potential mechanisms have been identified in the maintenance of upper airway patency during sleep and wakefulness. Each of these mechanisms or a combination thereof probably plays a role in the causation of respiratory compromise in the normal child during sleep or in children with clinical problems that predispose to OSA. A systematic approach to identification and modification of these mechanisms may lead to improved therapeutic approaches and unnecessary morbidities in these patients.

APNEA

CENTRAL APNEA OR HYPOVENTILATION SYNDROMES

Unrelated to upper airway obstruction, insufficient central respiratory drive can also be a cause of hypoventilation. The presence of a hypoventilation syndrome is suggested by the medical history as well as examination of the patient during wakefulness and sleep. All disorders that could explain the hypoventilation must be excluded, and to confirm the diagnosis, a polysomnographic evaluation, including measurements of tidal volume, should be conducted. The measurement of spontaneous resting tidal volumes and noninvasive blood gas values across all sleep states should be sufficient to establish the presence and severity of alveolar hypoventilation. The most important objective is the inability to increase respiratory frequency, tidal volume, or both, regardless of the severity of the progressive asphyxia that occurs.

CONGENITAL CENTRAL HYPOVENTILATION SYNDROME

Central hypoventilation syndromes can be primary (congenital CHS [CCHS] and late-onset CHS) or secondary (Box 74-1). Primary CCHS is a rare entity, with approximately 300 cases worldwide. It was originally described in 1970 by Mellins and colleagues[81] and is traditionally defined as the idiopathic failure of automatic control of breathing.[81,82] CCHS is a life-threatening disorder primarily manifesting as sleep-associated respiratory insufficiency and markedly impaired ventilatory responses to hypercapnia and hypoxemia.[83] Ventilation is most severely affected during quiet sleep, a state during which automatic neural control is predominant. Abnormal respiratory patterns also occur during active sleep and even during wakefulness, though to a milder degree. The spectrum of disease in CCHS cases is wide, ranging from relatively mild hypoventilation during quiet sleep with fairly good alveolar ventilation during wakefulness, to complete apnea during sleep with severe hypoventilation during waking. Progress in the recognition and clinical management of CCHS patients has revealed the presence of broader structural and functional impairments of the autonomic nervous system.[84–86] In particular, Hirschsprung's disease[84] and tumors of autonomic neural crest derivatives such as neuroblastoma, ganglioneuroblastoma, and ganglioneuroma[87,88] are noted in 20% and in 5% to 10% of CCHS patients, respectively. In recent years, three major, clinically relevant advances have developed with respect to the pathophysiology and treatment of CCHS: (1) the identification of putative genes underlying CCHS; (2) the functional assessment of neural structures in patients with CCHS to provide insights into the respiratory and autonomic disturbances that characterize the syndrome; (3) the successful transition of many patients to noninvasive mechanical ventilatory support.

BOX 74-1 Causes of Central Hypoventilation in Children

Primary

- Congenital (CCHS/Ondine's curse)
- Late-onset CHS
- Idiopathic hypothalamic dysfunction
- Arnold-Chiari malformation

Secondary

- Trauma
- Infection
- Tumor
- Central nervous system infarct
- Asphyxia
- Increased intracranial pressure
- Metabolic

A genetic origin has been hypothesized for CCHS because of (1) its early manifestation in the newborn period; (2) published reports of familial recurrence of CCHS, including one case each of monozygotic female twins, female siblings, and male-female half-siblings[89,90]; (3) its association with Hirschsprung's disease, an autosomal-recessive disorder of neural crest origin.[91] Furthermore, a genetic segregation analysis among families of 50 probands with CCHS also indicated that CCHS was consistent with familial transmission.[92] Importantly, vertical transmission of CCHS has been reported, and among infants born to women with CCHS without Hirschsprung's disease.[93,94] The association of CCHS and Hirschsprung's disease suggests that both disorders may be related to abnormal development and/or migration of the neural crest cells; indeed, mutations of genes (e.g., the *RET* proto-oncogene) that are involved in neural crest development and/or migration have been found in patients with Hirschsprung's disease.[95–97]

The putative gene, paired-like homeobox 2B (*PHOX2B*), underlying CCHS has recently been described in exciting work by Amiel and colleagues in France.[98] The *PHOX2B* gene mutation, consisting primarily of polyalanine expansions, has been identified with an autosomal-dominant mode of inheritance and de novo mutation at the first generation. This gene is necessary for autonomic nervous system embryologic development, and *Phox2b*$^{-/-}$ mice die in utero with absent autonomic nervous system circuits, since neurons either fail to form or degenerate.[99–102] Furthermore, the same team has subsequently shown that heterozygous mutations of *PHOX2B* may account for several combined or isolated disorders of autonomic nervous system development, namely late-onset CHS,[103] Hirschsprung's disease,[104] and tumors of the sympathetic nervous system such as neuroblastoma.[105] The identification of *PHOX2B* mutations in most patients with CCHS is an important landmark in the pursuit of pathophysiologic mechanisms of this condition. Furthermore, the finding of de novo *PHOX2B* polyalanine expansion in the majority of patients with CCHS allows genetic counseling for a disease with an unexpected autosomal-dominant mode of inheritance. Future research into the genetic basis of CCHS may improve our understanding of early breathing control disturbances such as SIDS. The prevalence of SIDS is high in CCHS families, suggesting that these two disorders may share developmental breathing control abnormalities.[106]

Taken together, the genetic data strongly suggest a diffuse alteration in autonomic nervous system function in patients with CCHS. This concept includes major disruption of brain regions underlying autonomic functions, in particular those sites mediating respiratory and cardiovascular regulation, as evidenced from recent studies using functional magnetic resonance imaging approaches.[107–109] Decreased heart rate beat-to-beat variability is consistently found in Holter recordings, and the circadian patterning of such variability further suggests an imbalance in sympathetic/parasympathetic regulation in patients with CCHS.[110–113] As additional testament to such an assumption, alterations in blood pressure regulation during simple daily maneuvers or during sleep further support the presence of predominantly vagal dysfunction with signs of vagal withdrawal and baroreflex failure, and relative preservation of the cardiac and vascular sympathetic function.[114–116] In addition, the frequent neuro-ocular findings in children with CCHS[117] and the marked reduction in the size of arterial chemoreceptors, carotid bodies, and neuroepithelial bodies with decreased staining for tyrosine hydroxylase and serotonin[118] can all be construed as evidence for a more diffuse autonomic nervous system involvement. Putative models aiming to dissect the specific contributions of the various components of cardiorespiratory control have been recently proposed and provide a comprehensive and structured approach to the evaluation of patients with CCHS.[119]

Diagnosis and Clinical Management

The clinical presentation of CCHS varies greatly depending on the severity of the disorder. Some infants will not breathe at birth and will require assisted ventilation in the newborn nursery. Such infants may mature to a pattern of adequate breathing during wakefulness over time. However, apnea or hypoventilation will persist during sleep. The apparent improvement over the first few months of life most likely results from normal maturation of the respiratory system and does not represent a true change in the severity of the disorder.[120] Other infants may present at a later age with cyanosis, edema, and signs of right-sided heart failure and may be mistaken for patients with cyanotic congenital heart disease. However, cardiac catheterization reveals only pulmonary hypertension. Infants with even less severe CCHS may present with tachycardia, diaphoresis, and/or cyanosis during sleep, and others may present with unexplained apnea or an apparent life-threatening events. Thus, the wide spectrum of severity in clinical manifestations determines the age at which recognition of CCHS takes place. Increased awareness of this unusual clinical entity and a comprehensive evaluation of every patient are critical for early diagnosis and appropriate intervention.

Although other symptoms indicative of brain stem or autonomic nervous system dysfunction may be present, the criteria for diagnosis of CCHS usually include: (1) persistent evidence of sleep hypoventilation ($Pa{CO_2} > 60$ mm Hg), particularly during quiet sleep (best achieved by overnight polysomnography); (2) presentation of symptoms during the first year of life; (3) absence of cardiac, pulmonary, or neuromuscular dysfunction that could explain the hypoventilation.[83,121] Furthermore, hypercapnic ventilatory challenges are an important component for the diagnosis of CCHS. Steady-state or rebreathing incremental CO_2 challenges are similarly valid and will usually reveal an absent or near-absent response. Confounding variables, including asphyxia, infection, trauma, tumor, and infarction, must be discarded from CCHS by appropriate assessments. At this point in time, there are no specific guidelines regarding the usefulness of genetic testing for CCHS. However, identification of mutations in genes such as *RET*, *HASH*, *BDNF*, *GDNF*, the endothelin gene family, and more particularly in *PHOX2B* in the context of clinical manifestations supporting central alveolar hypoventilation should support the diagnosis of CCHS.[122,123]

Congenital CHS is a lifelong condition, and depending on the severity of clinical manifestations, patients may require ventilatory support while asleep or as much as 24 hours a day. As such, a multidisciplinary approach to provide for comprehensive care and support of every child is needed. The treatment of CCHS should aim to ensure adequate ventilation when the patient is unable to achieve adequate gas exchange while breathing spontaneously. Since CCHS does not resolve spontaneously, chronic ventilatory support is required, such as positive pressure ventilation, bilevel positive airway pressure, or negative pressure ventilation. The majority of children with CCHS use positive pressure ventilation through a permanent tracheotomy, although successful transition to noninvasive ventilation has now been extensively reported,[83] with a trend toward earlier intervention (sometimes even during infancy) and more widespread transition to noninvasive ventilation (typically mask ventilation).[124–129] Several families have opted to use negative pressure ventilation. Daytime diaphragm pacing in children with CCHS who exhibit 24-hour mechanical ventilation dependency provides greater mobility compared with mechanical ventilation. Thus, potential candidates for diaphragm pacing will be ambulatory patients who require ventilatory support 24 hours per day by means of tracheotomy and do not exhibit significant ventilator-related lung damage. Diaphragm pacer settings must provide adequate alveolar ventilation and oxygenation during rest as well as during daily activities such as exercise. Major disadvantages of diaphragm pacing include cost, discomfort associated with surgical implantation, and potential need for repeated surgical revisions due to pacer malfunction.[130,131] Despite such potential limitations, parental reports of their experience are favorable in the vast majority. Recent development of a quadripolar electrode offers several advantages, which primarily include greater durations of pacer support at diminished risk of phrenic nerve damage and diaphragmatic fatigue, and optimization of pacing requirements during exercise.[132,133]

SECONDARY CENTRAL HYPOVENTILATION SYNDROMES

Patients with myelomeningocele and/or Arnold-Chiari type II malformation frequently exhibit sleep-disordered breathing, and such respiratory control disturbances are frequently suspected as causative mechanisms in the sudden unexpected deaths that occur in this population. Moderate or severe breathing disturbances occur in approximately 20% of cases.[134,135] The largest proportion of patients exhibit central apnea, while others show obstructed breathing; patients with obstruction are seldom helped by surgical intervention for tonsillectomy, suggesting that the primary dysfunction is of neural origin. The possible damage to vermis cerebelli structures from foramen magnum herniation in Chiari type II malformation has the potential to interfere with both blood pressure and breathing regulation, particularly under extreme challenges of hypotension or prolonged apnea. Compression of ventral neural surfaces is also a concern. The presence of thoracic or thoracolumbar myelomeningocele or the addition of severe brain stem malformations has been shown to enhance the potential for manifesting sleep-disordered breathing. Support for affected patients with Chiari II syndrome must consider the needs for recovery from pronounced hypotension during sleep, the overall respiratory disturbances that are present, and the surgical interventions required for decompression of neural structures. As such, a multidisciplinary approach is necessary to yield optimal outcomes.[136]

Patients with Prader-Willi syndrome (PWS) present a unique combination of sleep- and breathing-related manifestations. Excessive daytime sleepiness and increased frequency of REM sleep periods occurs some PWS patients, while others show disturbances in circadian rhythmicity with a tendency for multiple microsleep periods. In addition, the combination of obesity and hypotonia favors the occurrence of OSA. Patients with PWS also display significant alterations in central and peripheral elements of respiratory control that, though not immediately related to the obesity, can be severely affected by the mechanical consequences of increased adiposity and that ultimately lead to ventilatory failure. A unique and almost universal feature of these patients is the absence of ventilatory responses to peripheral chemoreceptor stimulation; this deficiency leads to abnormal arousal patterns during sleep.[137–140] When untreated, obesity progressively reduces central chemosensitivity as well, with the latter being ameliorated by growth hormone therapy and increased muscle mass.[141,142]

The condition termed late-onset central hypoventilation has been observed in some children. Although an underlying congenital brain stem abnormality is probable, significant hypoventilation becomes evident only as a consequence of an intercurrent illness such as pneumonia, with the development of severe obesity, or as a consequence of cor pulmonale. A recognizable entity consisting of hypothalamic dysfunction and late onset of central hypoventilation is now well established.[143] Alveolar hypoventilation can also develop in a child with previously normal control of breathing subsequent to an event resulting in brain stem injury, such as severe asphyxia, encephalitis, and infectious encephalopathies.

APNEA OF PREMATURITY

Apnea in newborns has been defined as a pause in breathing of longer than 20 seconds or an apneic event of shorter than 20 seconds associated with either bradycardia and/or cyanosis. Recurrent episodes of apnea are common in preterm neonates, and the incidence and severity increases with earlier gestational age. Reduced respiratory drive and impaired pulmonary function due to lung immaturity as well as a variety of mechanical variables impinging on respiratory mechanics predispose the premature neonate to apnea and hypoventilation, which, in turn, may precipitate oxyhemoglobin desaturation and/or bradycardia. Although they can occur spontaneously and be attributable to prematurity alone, such events can also be provoked or worsened if there is some additional insult such as infection, underlying hypoxemia, hyperthermia, or any evolving intracranial pathology. Although most apneic events are self-resolving and do not prompt medical recognition or intervention, apneic events associated with hypoxemia and reflex bradycardia may require active resuscitative efforts to reverse this condition.

Idiopathic apnea of prematurity (AOP) is a common, albeit often unsuspected problem in the clinical setting,[144] and appears to be primarily due to immaturity of the neonate neurologic and respiratory systems. The preterm neonate breathes irregularly during sleep and, in comparison to both the full-term neonate and the adult, there is much greater breath-to-breath variability. Both central and obstructive apneic episodes are frequently reported in preterm neonates, although the most common form is mixed apnea. Mixed apnea typically accounts for more than half of all clinically relevant apneic episodes, followed in decreasing frequency by central and obstructive apnea. By definition, there are no obstructions in central apnea, although some reports have suggested that the central airways will frequently close during the course of central apnea, with a rule of thumb indicating that such airway occlusion will be more likely to occur with increased duration of such events.[145–148] Thus, these apneic events have also been termed silent obstruction because of the lack of respiratory effort. AOP generally resolves by about 36 to 40 weeks' postconceptional age. However, in the most premature infants (24–28 weeks' gestation) apnea may frequently persist beyond 40 weeks' postconceptional age, finally resolving at 43 to 44 weeks' postconceptional age.[149,150] Beyond this time, the incidence of cardiorespiratory events in preterm neonates does not appear to markedly exceed that of term newborns.

Pathophysiology

Immaturity of central respiratory control of the various ventilatory muscles is a key factor in the pathogenesis of AOP. The breathing pattern is more disorganized during REM sleep, which is the predominant mode of sleep in preterm neonates. Indeed, apneic episodes are more common, longer, and more frequently associated with profound bradycardia during active or REM sleep than during quiet or NREM sleep.[151,152] Although the pathogenesis of AOP has not been fully delineated, it is related to both neurologic and cardiorespiratory immaturity.[153,154] In particular, preterm neonates have an altered response to increased CO_2 and decreased O_2, in that they respond to increased CO_2 by diminished rather than increased inspiratory effort.[155,156] This unique response of respiratory timing during hypercapnic exposure is associated with prolongation of expiratory duration,[157,158] and animal models have revealed that this prolongation of expiration associated with hypercapnia is centrally mediated at the brain stem level.[159] Furthermore, the inhibitory neurotransmitter γ-aminobutyric acid (GABA) appears to be implicated.[160,161] It is well known that premature neonates exhibit a biphasic ventilatory response to a decrease in inspired O_2 concentration. Initially, there is a rapid increase in minute ventilation due to peripheral chemoreceptor stimulation; this is followed by a decline in ventilation to baseline or below. The decrease in ventilation, also termed hypoxic ventilatory depression,[162,163] may persist for several weeks postnatally. Several theories have been postulated to explain hypoxic ventilatory depression, including a decrease in $Pa{CO_2}$ secondary to the initial hyperventilation and accompanying decrease in cerebral blood flow, a decrease in metabolic rate with hypoxia, hypoxia-mediated central depression of ventilation, and activation of receptors such as GABA-ergic, adenosinergic, and/or platelet-derived growth factor β receptors.[164–166]

There has been speculation that the hypoxic ventilatory depression may predispose preterm neonates to additional episodes of apnea. In other words, neonates experiencing more apneic episodes would have less initial increase in ventilation and subsequent greater depression of ventilation in response to hypoxia. However, this speculation has been recently challenged by Nock and colleagues,[167] who documented increased initial ventilation but attenuated ventilatory depression during the hypoxic challenge in premature neonates who developed more frequent and severe apnea. The speculation is that neonates with more severe and/or prolonged apnea have greater peripheral chemoreceptor sensitivity and possibly increased central respiratory network gain due to the repetitive periods of intermittent hypoxia,[168] and that it is the resultant instability of respiratory control that may predispose preterm neonates to additional apneic episodes.[166]

The site of obstruction during either mixed or obstructive apneic events in the upper airways is mostly within the pharynx; however, it may also occur at the level of the larynx, and possibly at both sites. The mechanisms by which apnea may occur may be initiated by sleep-related decrease of pharyngeal airway dilation.[169–172] Integration of pharyngeal muscle function is reduced during sleep, resulting in collapse and subsequent apnea in susceptible infants. In addition, the airway may be compromised by postural changes, although spontaneous obstructive apnea in the absence of a positional problem is probably uncommon. Reflexes originating in the upper airway may alter the pattern of respiration and play a role in the initiation and termination of episodes of apnea.[173] Stimulation of the laryngeal mucosa, by either chemical or mechanical stimuli, may induce reflex inhibition of breathing and apnea in humans and animals, and is mediated through activation of the superior laryngeal nerve. There seems to be a maturational change in reflex-induced apnea,[73] since chemical stimulation of the larynx in newborn piglets causes respiratory arrest, which is not seen in older piglets. Preterm neonates have an exaggerated laryngeal inhibitory reflex, which may elicit prolonged apnea in response to instilling saline in the oropharynx, to gastroesophageal reflux (GER), or during the course of respiratory syncytial virus infection.[174–177]

Diagnosis

Although apnea typically results from immaturity of the respiratory control system, it also may constitute the presenting sign of other unrelated diseases or pathophysiologic states frequently affecting preterm neonates.[178] Thus, AOP is diagnosed after a thorough evaluation has been conducted and other potential influences have been excluded (Box 74-2). Particular caution must also be exercised when attributing apnea to GER.[179,180] Indeed, despite the frequent coexistence of apnea and GER in preterm neonates, investigations into the timing of reflux in relation to apneic events do not support a common temporal association.[181–183] Although physiologic experiments in animal models reveal that reflux of gastric contents to the larynx induces reflex apnea, there is no clear evidence that treatment of GER will affect frequency of apnea in most preterm neonates. Therefore, diagnosis of sleep-disordered breathing secondary to GER is not simple and can be easily missed or overinterpreted during polygraphic recordings. On the other hand, even the presence of GER as shown by esophageal pH monitoring or other techniques in an infant with polygraphically proven apnea does not necessarily demonstrate that GER is the cause of the respiratory disturbance during sleep. Hence, simultaneous recording of sleep measures and of esophageal pH is usually necessary to allow detection of tentative associations between GER and apnea, and may allow for formulation of more effective management in these infants.

Notably, hypoventilation, O_2 desaturation, frank apnea, and bradycardia have also been documented during nutritive sucking and ascribed to the immaturity of the normal mechanisms that coordinate breathing, sucking, and swallowing. In the normal healthy infant, as fluid enters the pharynx or larynx, breathing ceases. This normal response protects the airway and prevents aspiration. However, this protective reflex is excessive in some infants because of the immaturity of the nervous system, resulting in prolonged apnea. With advancing maturation, feeding-related episodes of apnea become less frequent and eventually disappear.[184]

BOX 74-2 Conditions Associated with Apnea in Infants

- Prematurity
- Infection
- Impaired oxygenation
- Central nervous system problems (intracranial hemorrhage; asphyxic episode; malformation of the brain)
- Gastroesophageal reflux
- Metabolic disorders (hypoglycemia, electrolyte imbalance, fatty acid disorders, metabolic acidosis)
- Temperature instability (hyperthermia, hypothermia)
- Drugs (e.g., narcotics, anticonvulsants)

Treatment

Treatment is usually with pharmacologic therapy or continuous positive airway pressure (CPAP) ventilation, although other measures such as placing the infant with the head in the midline and the neck in the neutral position to minimize upper airway obstruction are also important. Methylxanthines have been the mainstay of pharmacologic treatment of AOP.[185] Both theophylline and caffeine citrate are effective, possibly through multiple physiologic and pharmacologic mechanisms of action. A probable major mechanism of action for xanthine therapy is through competitive antagonism of adenosine receptors, since adenosine acts as an inhibitory neuroregulator in the central nervous system.

It is important to rule out systemic conditions (sepsis), seizure disorders, and GER before instituting methylxanthine therapy, since these agents have been known to lower the seizure threshold and decrease muscle tone of the esophageal sphincter.[186] Methylxanthines stimulate the central nervous system and rapidly decrease the frequency of all types of apnea. Xanthine therapy has been shown to increase minute ventilation, improve CO_2 sensitivity, decrease hypoxic depression of breathing, enhance diaphragmatic activity, and decrease periodic breathing. REM sleep may also be acutely decreased even if long-term therapy with xanthines does not seem to alter overall sleep architecture.[187] Caffeine has some advantages over theophylline, since it is considered to be more effective in stimulating the central nervous and respiratory systems. In addition, because caffeine has a higher therapeutic index, central nervous system toxicity is not as problematic. A recent Cochrane review on the use of methylxanthines concluded that both theophylline and caffeine are effective in reducing the frequency and severity of apneic episodes, and are also of value in reducing the need for mechanical ventilation in preterm neonates with AOP.[188] Elimination of methylxanthines is prolonged in infants in comparison with children or adults, and it is particularly prolonged in preterm neonates. The metabolic pathways for the elimination of theophylline are underdeveloped in the premature neonate, and thus serum measurement of theophylline should be monitored whenever aminophylline or theophylline is used. Caffeine levels are less critical but should also be followed at least during the beginning of treatment.

The decision to discontinue xanthine therapy is largely empirical, although it is to be encouraged at least 1 to 2 weeks before discharge, and this is especially relevant for caffeine with its longer half-life. Toxic levels may produce tachycardia, cardiac dysrhythmias, feeding intolerance, diuresis, and, infrequently, seizures, although these side effects are less commonly seen with caffeine at the usual therapeutic doses. However, recent concerns about potential long-term side effects of methylxanthines on the neurodevelopmental outcomes of low birth weight infants have led to an increased interest in alternate methods of treating AOP.[189]

Role of Continuous Positive Airway Pressure

Among nonpharmacologic strategies widely used in the treatment of apnea, CPAP is relatively safe and effective. Nasal CPAP (NCPAP) has also been shown to be effective in AOP,[190,191] with a therapeutic range usually within 3 to 6 cm H_2O. Since longer episodes of apnea frequently involve an obstructive component, CPAP seems to be effective through its effect in splinting the upper airway with positive pressure and decreasing the risk of pharyngeal or laryngeal obstruction. CPAP is also probably beneficial in AOP by increasing functional residual capacity and thereby improving oxygenation. Studies have also compared NCPAP to nasal intermittent positive pressure ventilation (NIPPV) in the treatment of AOP and found that NIPPV is potentially a beneficial treatment for AOP, particularly when apnea is frequent or severe.[192] NIPPV seems to reduce the frequency of apneic episodes more effectively than NCPAP.[193] Nonetheless, additional safety and efficacy data are required before recommending NIPPV as standard therapy for apnea. In addition, high-flow nasal cannula therapy has recently been suggested as an equivalent treatment modality to NCPAP while enhancing mobility of the infant for parents and caretakers.[194,195] Despite these noninvasive treatment options, endotracheal intubation and artificial ventilation may be needed for severe or refractory episodes.

The effect of supplemental O_2 on cardiorespiratory events and sleep architecture in premature neonates has also been explored; studies show that AOP and periodic breathing resolve when O_2 concentration is increased to a threshold level.[196,197] Rigatto and colleagues further reported that inhalation of 100% O_2 is associated with a decrease in periodic breathing and an increase in minute ventilation.[198] In fact, a modest increase in inspired O_2 concentration decreased apnea and periodicity in preterm neonates, not via an increase in alveolar ventilation but through a decrease in breath-to-breath variability instead.[199] Simakajornboon and colleagues have further demonstrated that in otherwise healthy premature neonates, unsuspected adverse cardiorespiratory events, including apnea and bradycardia, occur very frequently.[200] Moreover, administration of low-flow supplemental O_2 improves respiratory stability, as shown by a decrease in the frequency of respiratory and bradycardic events, a reduction in periodic breathing density, and an increase in overall O_2 saturation without adverse effects on alveolar ventilation. In addition, supplemental O_2 administration modified sleep architecture by increasing NREM sleep density and reciprocal decreases in REM sleep density.

As mentioned before, AOP generally resolves by 36 to 40 weeks' postconceptional age, and beyond 43 to 44 weeks' postconceptional age the incidence of cardiorespiratory events in preterm neonates is similar to that of term newborns. Thus, the majority of preterm neonates will have their AOP resolved by the time they are ready for home discharge.[201] In this context, a retrospective review of patient records by Darnall and colleagues[202] to determine the minimum apnea-free observation period before discharge suggested that 8 apnea-free days was probably safe. However, close monitoring in the neonatal intensive care unit is essential, since several reports have highlighted the observation that clinically significant apneas with resultant bradycardia and/or desaturation go unnoticed in the majority of cases.[203–205]

The clinical significance and long-term consequences of persistent apnea, bradycardia, or desaturation remain a subject of considerable debate. Although it is reasonable to be concerned about episodes that cause prolonged anoxia and acidosis, such events are unlikely to occur as a result of AOP in the closely monitored environment of modern neonatal intensive care units. Attempts to quantify any prognostic risk that may be attributable to AOP have produced conflicting results. Because idiopathic apnea is most often seen in high-risk preterm neonates, separating the global consequences of premature birth from the specific effects of AOP has proven difficult. Premature newborns often have many problems during their stay in the neonatal intensive care unit, and many of these conditions—particularly periventricular leukomalacia and intraventricular hemorrhage—may contribute to poor neurodevelopmental outcomes. Additionally, only a few studies have assessed improvement in long-term outcome as a result of treating AOP, and these studies have been confounded by these same problems. Reports of long-term follow-up of at-risk infants have attempted to address this issue.[206,207] In preterm infants followed to early school age, variables that predicted poor neurodevelopmental outcomes included AOP; however, these are by no means uniform findings and thus additional studies will be necessary. It is possible that the recurrent hypoxia accompanying AOP is the detrimental contributor to neurobehavioral outcome.

OBSTRUCTIVE SLEEP APNEA

The spectrum of sleep-disordered breathing, which includes OSA and upper airway resistance syndrome, occurs in children of all ages, from neonates to adolescents. OSA is characterized by repeated events of partial or complete upper airway obstruction during sleep, resulting in disruption of normal gas exchange and sleep patterns (Figs. 74-1 to 74-5).[208] Nighttime symptoms and signs include snoring, paradoxical chest and abdomen motion, retractions, witnessed apnea, snorting episodes, difficulty breathing, cyanosis, sweating, and disturbed sleep. Daytime symptoms can include mouth breathing, difficulty to wake up, moodiness, nasal obstruction, daytime sleepiness, hyperactivity, and cognitive problems, with severe cases of OSA associated with cor pulmonale, failure-to-thrive, developmental delay, or even death. This complex and relatively frequent disorder is only now being recognized as a major public health problem, despite being initially described more than a century ago[209] and rediscovered in children in 1976 by Guilleminault and colleagues.[210] It is clear that the classic clinical syndrome of OSA in children is a distinct disorder from the condition that occurs in adults, in particular with respect to gender distribution, clinical manifestations, polysomnographic findings, and treatment approaches.[211,212] As discussed before, childhood OSA is frequently diagnosed in association with adenotonsillar hypertrophy, and is also common in children with craniofacial abnormalities and neurologic disorders affecting upper airway patency.

Epidemiology

Obstructive sleep apnea occurs in all pediatric age groups including infancy. Accurate prevalence information is particularly missing in infants, since most epidemiologic studies have thus far concentrated on older children. OSA is particularly common in young children (preschool and early school years), with a peak prevalence around 2 to 8 years, and subsequent declines in frequency,[213] that are possibly related to reductions in viral loads associated with adenotonsillar lymphoid tissue proliferation.[214,215] Habitual snoring during sleep, the hallmark indicator of increased upper airway resistance, is an extremely frequent occurrence and affects as many as 27% of children.[216–223] While the exact clinical polysomnographically defined thresholds associated with morbidity in snoring children are only now being defined, the diagnosis of OSA based on consensus criteria[224] is currently estimated to affect approximately 2% to 3% of young children.[225] Thus, the ratio between habitual snoring and OSA is between 4:1 and 6:1,

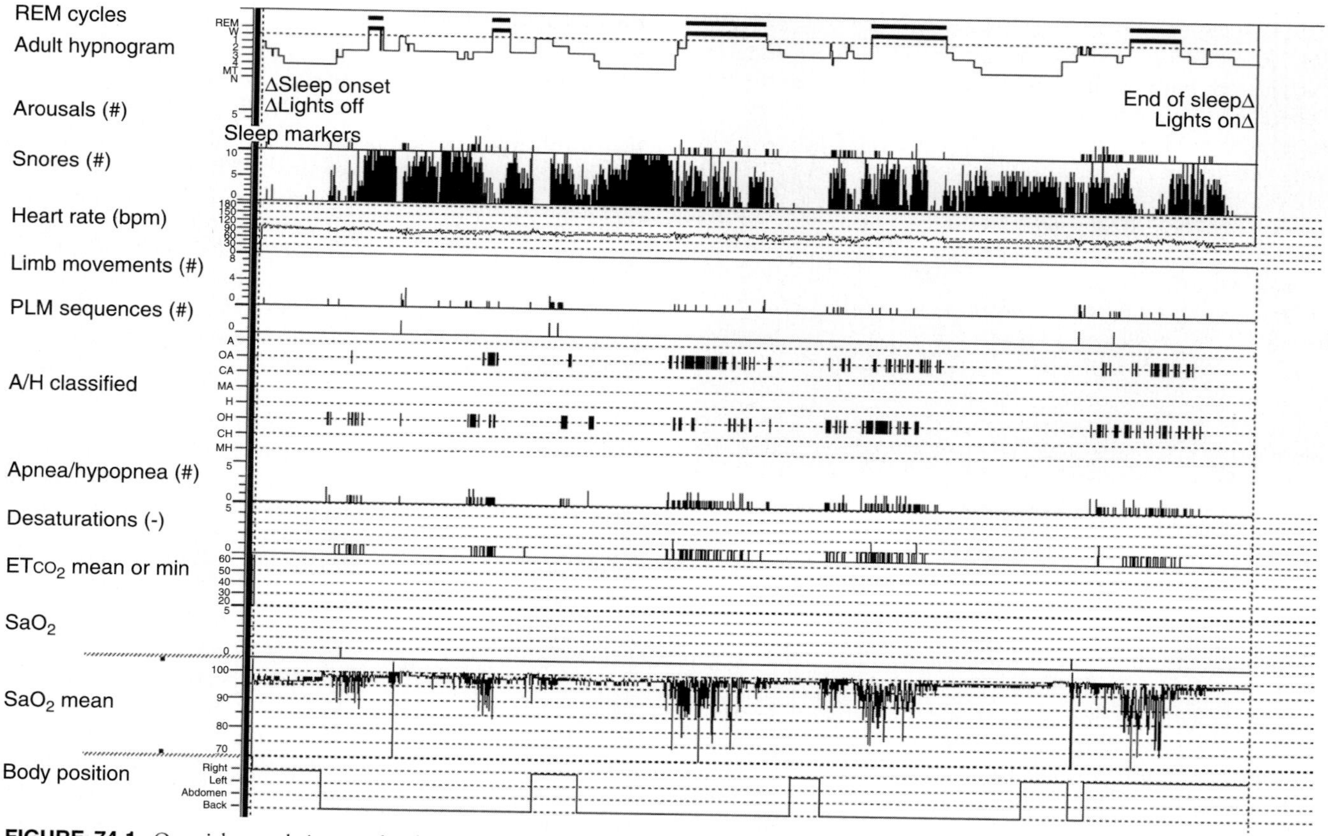

■ **FIGURE 74-1.** Overnight trends in several polysomnographic measures in a 7-year-old child with moderately severe OSA. Note REM sleep clustering of respiratory events. A, apnea; H, hypopnea.

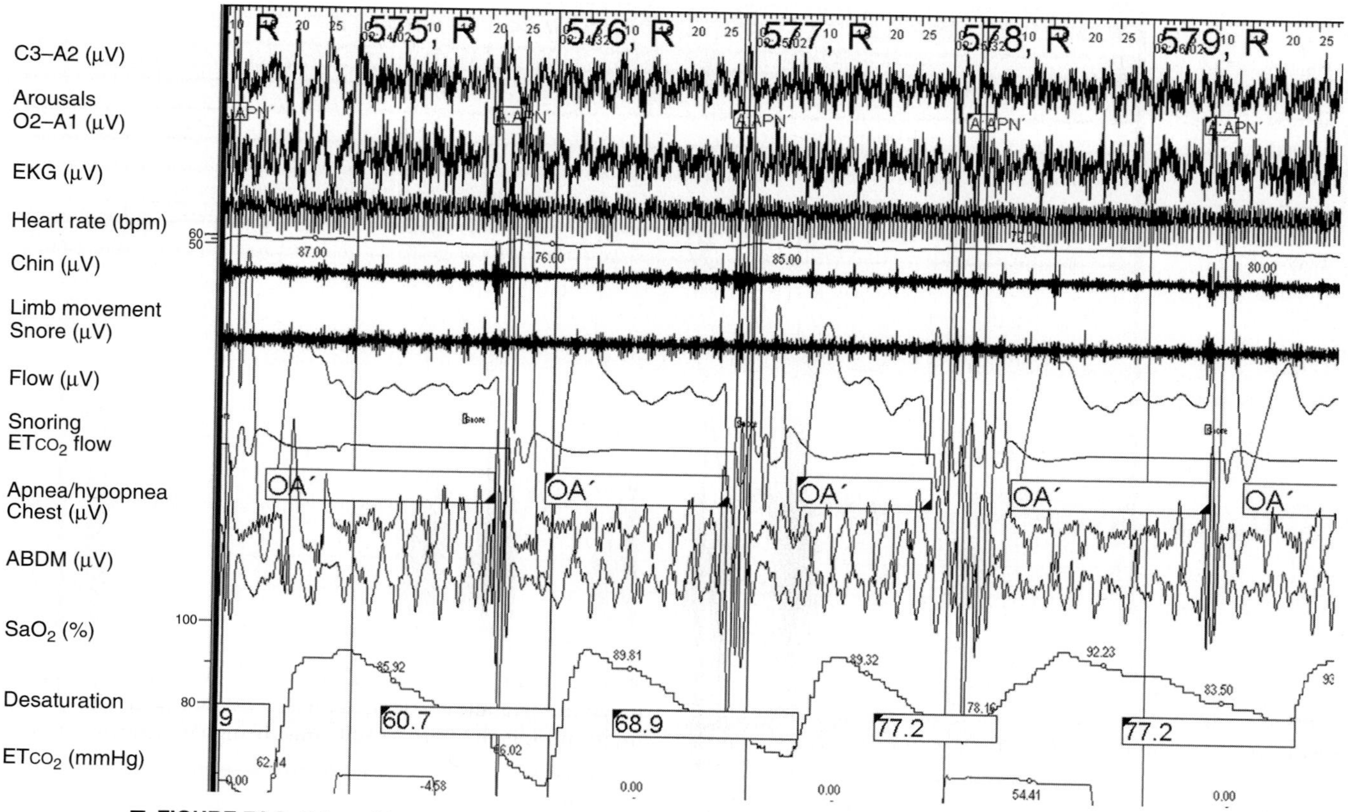

■ **FIGURE 74-2.** Polygraphic tracing in a child with REM-associated obstructive apneic events. ABDM, abdominal excursion.

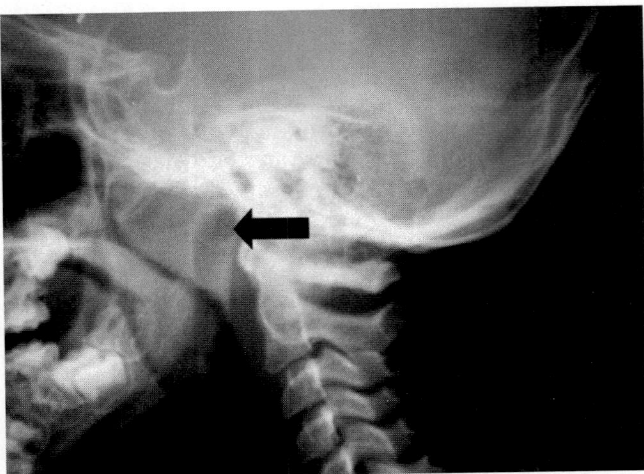

■ **FIGURE 74-3.** Lateral roentgenogram of the neck in a child with enlarged adenoid tissue and OSA.

and accurate identification of habitually snoring children who have OSA is particularly challenging, considering that clinical history and physical examination are poor predictors of disease,[226] and that—except for the onerous, yet thus far essential overnight polygraphic recordings—effective screening tools are not yet available; thus any attempt to perform an overnight polysomnographic study on every snoring child would be prohibitively expensive.

Pathophysiology

The pathophysiology of childhood OSA remains poorly understood. As discussed earlier, OSA occurs when the upper airway collapses during inspiration. Such collapse is a dynamic process that involves interaction between sleep state, pressure-flow airway mechanics, and respiratory drive. When resistance to inspiratory flow increases or when activation of the pharyngeal dilator muscle decreases, negative inspiratory pressure may collapse the airway.[43] Both functional and anatomic variables may tilt the balance toward airway collapse. Indeed, it has been determined that the site of upper airway closure in children with OSA is at the level of the tonsils and adenoids, whereas in normal children it is at the level of the soft palate.[76] The size of the tonsils and adenoids increases from birth to approximately 12 years of age, with the greatest increase being in the first few years of life, albeit proportionately to the growth of other upper airway structures.[39] However, lymphadenoid tissue will grow especially large in children exposed to cigarette smoking,[218,227] children with allergic rhinitis,[228,229] in children with asthma,[230] and obviously in children exposed to a variety of upper airway respiratory infections, particularly viruses.

Although childhood OSA is associated with adenotonsillar hypertrophy, it is not caused by large tonsils and adenoids alone. Several lines of evidence suggest that OSA is the combined result of structural and neuromuscular variables within the upper airway. Indeed, patients with OSA do not obstruct their upper airway during wakefulness, and thus structural factors alone cannot be fully responsible for this condition. In addition, several studies have failed to show a definitive correlation between upper airway adenotonsillar size and OSA, even if the latter accounts for a

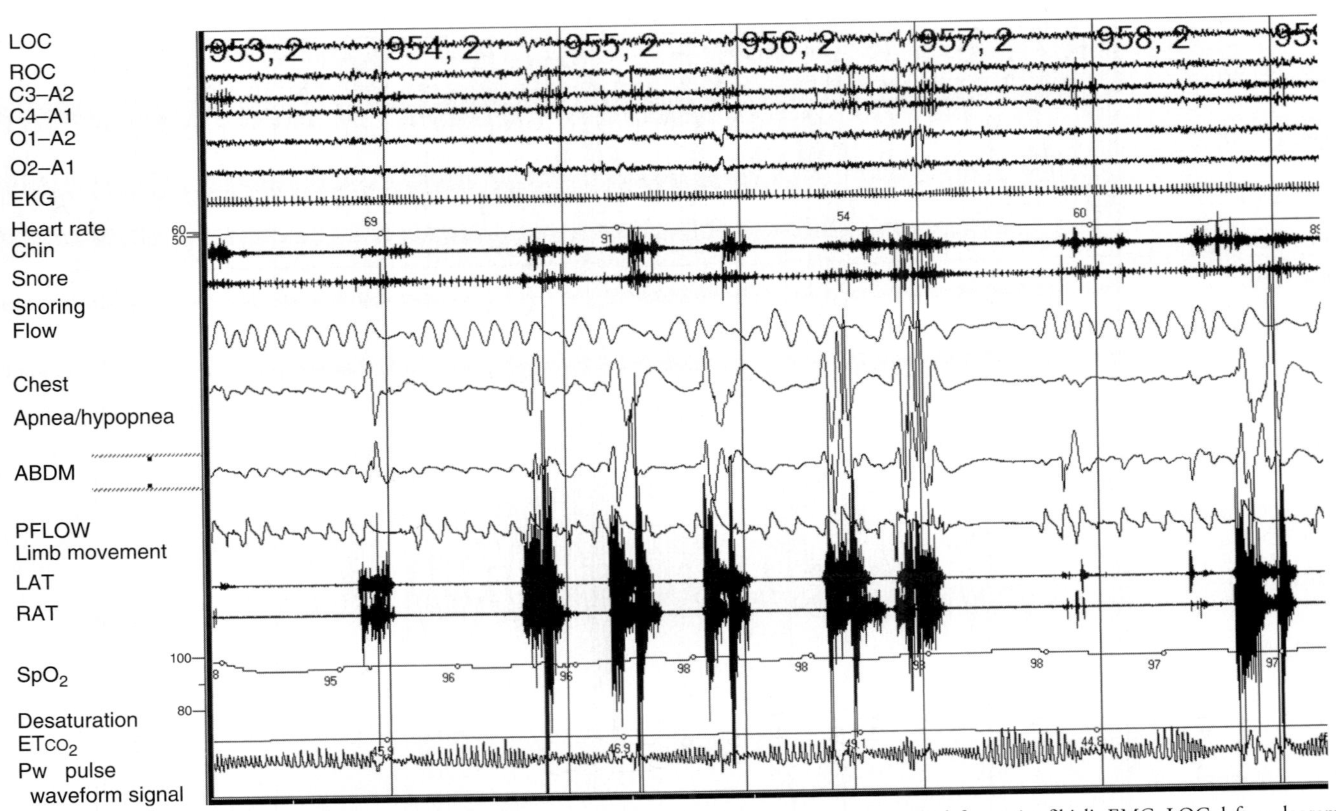

■ **FIGURE 74-4.** Bruxism in a child with mild sleep-disordered breathing. ABDM, abdominal excursion; LAT, left anterior fibialis EMG; LOC, left oculogram; PFLOW, nasal pressure–derived flow; RAT, right anterior fibialis EMG; ROC, right oculogram.

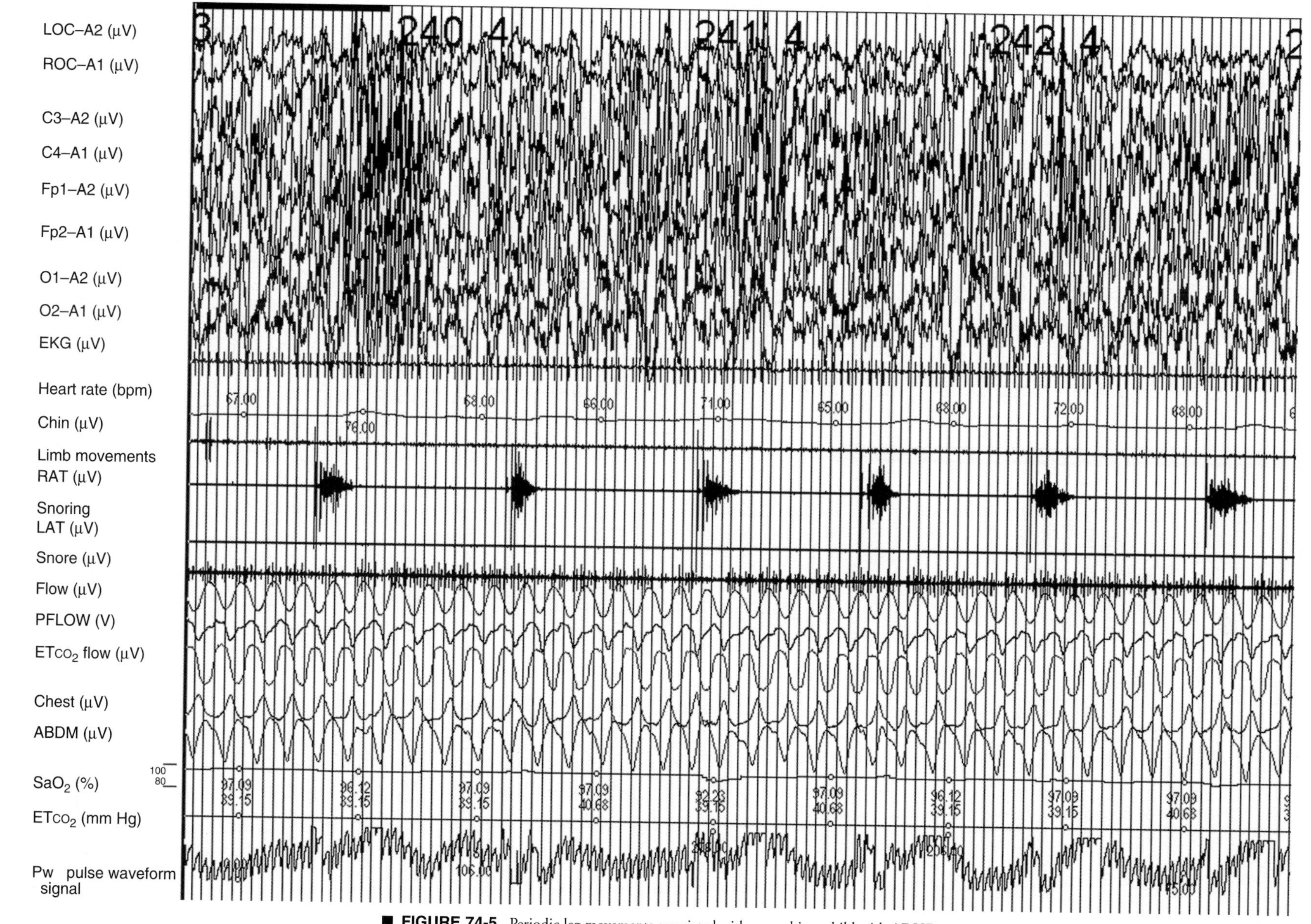

■ **FIGURE 74-5.** Periodic leg movements associated with arousal in a child with ADHD.

great proportion of the variance in the prediction of upper airway dysfunction during sleep. Furthermore, a small percentage of children with adenotonsillar hypertrophy but no other known risk factors for OSA are not cured by surgical removal of tonsils and adenoids. Finally, Guilleminault and colleagues reported a cohort of children whose OSA temporarily resolved after surgery but in whom OSA recurred during adolescence.[231,232] Thus, it appears that childhood OSA is a dynamic process resulting from a combination of structural and neuromotor abnormalities rather than from structural abnormalities alone. These predisposing factors occur as part of a spectrum: In some children (e.g., those with craniofacial anomalies), structural abnormalities predominate, whereas in others (e.g., those with cerebral palsy), neuromuscular factors predominate. In otherwise healthy children with adenotonsillar hypertrophy, neuromuscular abnormalities are probably subtle.

Conditions Associated with OSA

Obstructive sleep apnea also occurs in children with upper airway narrowing due to craniofacial anomalies, or those with neuromuscular abnormalities such as hypotonia (e.g., muscular dystrophy) or muscular lack of coordination (e.g., cerebral palsy). In addition to craniofacial anomalies and abnormalities of the central nervous system, altered soft tissue size may result from infection of the airways, allergy, supraglottic edema, adenotonsillar hypertrophy, mucopolysaccharide storage disease, laryngomalacia, subglottic stenosis, neck tumor, or hypothyroidism. In recent years, the epidemic increase in obesity seems to be leading to substantial changes in the cross-sectional demographic and anthropometric characteristics of the children being referred for evaluation of evaluation of OSA. Indeed, while fewer than 15% of all children were obese (i.e., <95th percentile for body mass index adjusted for age and gender) in the early 1990s, more than 50% meet the criteria for obesity in the last 2 years in our Sleep Center (D.G., unpublished observation, 2004). Genetic factors also play a role in the pathophysiology of OSA, as demonstrated by studies of family cohorts.[233,234] It is unclear whether the influence stems from the modulating effect of genetic factors on ventilatory drive, anatomic features, or both. Ethnicity is also important, with OSA occurring more commonly in African Americans.[222] Box 74-3 lists the major conditions associated with OSA in children.

BOX 74-3 Conditions Associated with Obstructive Sleep Apnea in Children

- Adenotonsillar hypertrophy
- Obesity
- African American race
- Allergic rhinitis
- Asthma
- Micrognathia
- Down syndrome
- Craniofacial syndromes (Treacher Collins syndrome, midfacial hypoplasia, Crouzon's syndrome, Apert's syndrome, Pierre Robin sequence, etc.)
- Achondroplasia
- Mucopolysaccharidoses
- Macroglossia
- Sickle cell disease
- Myelomeningocele
- Cerebral palsy
- Neuromuscular disorders (Duchenne's muscular dystrophy, spinal muscular atrophy, etc.)
- Cleft palate repair and velopharyngeal flap
- Foreign body

Clinical Evaluation and Diagnosis of Obstructive Sleep Apnea

It is clear that several potential mechanisms, including those genetically determined, are involved in the maintenance of upper airway patency during sleep and wakefulness. Each of these mechanisms or a combination thereof can, therefore, be implicated in the causation of respiratory compromise during sleep in the otherwise normal child with enlarged tonsils and/or adenoids, as well as in those children with clinical problems that predispose to OSA. The clinical presentation of a child with OSA syndrome is usually very nonspecific, requiring increased awareness on the part of the primary care professional, since the current number of children being referred for evaluation of sleep-disordered breathing may in fact represent only the tip of the iceberg. A thorough history should include detailed information pertaining to the sleep environment (Box 74-4). In the otherwise normal child, the principal parental complaint will be snoring during sleep. Nevertheless, even when the diagnostic interview is conducted by a sleep specialist, the accuracy of OSA prediction based on history alone is poor, such that an overnight polysomnographic evaluation is required as the more definitive diagnostic tool. The routine clinical evaluation of a snoring child is usually not likely to demonstrate significant and obvious findings. Attention should be directed to the size of the tonsils,[235,236] with careful documentation of their position and relative intrusion into the retropalatal space. In addition, the presence of allergic rhinitis, nasal polyps, nasal septum deviation, or any other condition likely to increase nasal airflow resistance should be sought. The relative size (i.e., micrognathia) and positioning of the mandible (e.g., retrognathia) should also be documented when present. Finally, attention should be paid to blood pressure values and to the presence of auscultatory findings suggestive of increased pulmonary artery pressures.

Polysomnography

An overnight polysomnographic evaluation is, at least presently, the only definitive diagnostic approach for OSA.[208,237,238] The American Academy of Pediatrics has published a consensus statement outlining the requirements for pediatric polysomnography.[224] Box 74-5 shows the currently recommended channels usually used in the laboratory evaluation of snoring children. Available reference values in children are clearly lower than the thresholds defined for adults.[239–246] While the reasons are not completely understood, the relative resistance of the upper airway of children to collapse may underscore that complete obstructive events are less likely and that instead prolonged periods of heightened upper airway resistance associated with alveolar hypoventilation (also termed obstructive hypoventilation) are more readily apparent in children.[247] It should also be mentioned that, unlike adults, children with OSA often will not develop EEG arousals following obstructive apneas,[248,249] and as a result, sleep architecture is relatively preserved in children with OSA.[250] This reduced propensity to manifest arousals (based on the 3-second EEG criteria developed for adults) has led to the assumption that excessive daytime sleepiness, the cardinal symptom of OSA syndrome in adults, is an uncommon feature in children with OSA. Indeed, in parental surveys, only 7% of parents indicated that excessive sleepiness was a problem.[226] Furthermore, more objective measurement of excessive daytime sleepiness using the multiple sleep latency test in snoring children revealed that, although linear relationships existed between the severity of OSA (as measured by the obstructive apnea-hypopnea index) and the mean sleep latency measured during the multiple sleep latency test, manifest excessive daytime sleepiness occurred in only 13% of children.[251] More elaborate examination of the patterns of arousal among snoring children further showed that as respiratory-related arousals increase in frequency with increasing OSA disease severity, the opposite phenomenon (i.e., decreases in spontaneous arousal index) occurs,[252] suggesting a very powerful attempt by these children to preserve sleep homeostasis. On the basis of the mutual interdependencies of these two types of arousal, a model was developed that allows for sensitive assessment of the resulting sleep pressure derived from disrupted sleep using polysomnographic data.[252] This approach has thus far permitted assessment of the independent contribution of sleep fragmentation to neurobehavioral morbidity in snoring children.[253] Thus, more subtle manifestations of arousal may be present in children, even if apnea-related EEG arousals are less common in children than in adults. For example, subcortical arousals, as demonstrated by movement, or autonomic changes, occur frequently in children.[254,255] It is also possible that subtle disturbances in sleep architecture are present that go undetected by routine polysomnography but are detectable through spectral analysis of EEG frequency domains,[256] and may contribute to neurobehavioral and autonomic complications of OSA (see later).

Notably, the role of ambulatory sleep studies, whether abbreviated (home video or sound recordings or nocturnal oximetry) is now being intensively explored.[257–262]

BOX 74-4 Pertinent Clinical Findings in Pediatric Obstructive Sleep Apnea

During Sleep

- Habitual snoring
- Difficulty breathing during sleep with snorting episodes
- Restless sleep and frequent awakenings
- Excessive sweating
- Night terrors
- Enuresis
- Breathing pauses reported by parents

During Daytime

- Mouth breathing and limited nasal airflow
- Chronic rhinorrhea
- Adenoid facies
- Recurrent ear infections
- Difficulty swallowing
- Pectus excavatum
- Retrognathia
- Enlarged neck circumference
- Truncal obesity
- Frequent visits to primary care physician for respiratory-related symptoms

Sequelae

- Neurobehavioral deficits (poor school performance, learning deficits, aggressive behavior, moodiness, shyness, and social withdrawal)
- ADHD-like behaviors
- Depression and low self-esteem
- Excessive daytime sleepiness
- Systemic hypertension
- Left ventricular hypertrophy
- Pulmonary hypertension and cor pulmonale
- Failure to thrive
- Reduced quality of life

BOX 74-5 Usual Polysomnographic Montage in Children Evaluated for Suspected Sleep-Disordered Breathing*

- Electroencephalogram: minimum two channels (central and occipital leads); usually four to eight channels
- Chin EMG
- Anterior tibial EMG, left and right
- Electro-oculogram, left and right
- Electrocardiogram
- Pulse oximeter and pulse waveform
- Oronasal airflow thermistor
- Nasal pressure catheter†
- End-tidal capnography and waveform
- Chest and abdominal respiratory inductance plethysmography
- Body position sensor
- Tracheal sound sensor or microphone
- Time-synchronized video

*In younger children, consider transcutaneous CO_2 tension measurements.
†Esophageal catheters are used in some laboratories instead of nasal pressure catheters to assess respiratory effort.

Short-Term and Long-Term Morbidity of Obstructive Sleep Apnea

One of the major drives to treat any medical condition is the prevention of morbidity and mortality. Indeed, the consequences of untreated OSA in young children can be serious.

Early reports of children with severe OSA were often associated with failure to thrive, although currently only a minority of children with OSA will present with this problem, most probably because of earlier recognition and referral for evaluation and treatment. The mechanisms mediating reductions in growth velocity most likely represent a combination of increased energy expenditure during sleep,[263,264] and disruption of the growth hormone and insulin growth factor and binding proteins.[265,266] Tonsillectomy and adenoidectomy (T&A) and complete resolution of OSA in children with failure to thrive will result in catch-up growth and will also increase the height and weight velocities even in children with normal growth and OSA. Interestingly, even obese children with OSA will demonstrate weight gain following surgery.[267]

Frequent O_2 desaturations during sleep are common in children with OSA. Elevation of pulmonary artery pressure due to hypoxia-induced pulmonary vasoconstriction is a serious consequence of OSA in children, and can lead to cor pulmonale. While pulmonary hypertension is probably more frequent than predicted from clinical assessment, the exact prevalence of this complication is unknown and may be more frequent than anticipated. In addition, while treatment of OSA will result in normalization of pulmonary artery pressures, it remains unclear whether untreated OSA will result in persistent vascular remodeling of the pulmonary circulation. Indeed, evidence from animal models exposed to hypoxia for a short period of time during early postnatal life reveals that pulmonary hypertension is increased when exposed to hypoxia later in infancy, suggesting that some remodeling may have occurred.[268–270] Furthermore, intermittent hypoxia may also affect left ventricular function through both direct and indirect effects on myocardial contractility.[271] In the context of OSA, systemic hypertension has emerged as a major cardiovascular consequence in adult patients. Although the pathophysiologic mechanisms of such elevation in arterial tension are still under intense investigation, it appears that intermittent hypoxemia is the major contributor to this serious consequence of OSA, with lesser roles being played by sleep fragmentation and episodic hypercapnia. It is now thought that intermittent hypoxia during the night will lead to increased sympathetic neural activity, and that the latter will be sustained and induce changes in baroreceptor function leading to hypertension.[272] While the data pertaining to pediatric patients are still scant, increased surges in sympathetic activity have been reported in children with OSA,[273,274] and elevation of arterial blood pressure will occur.[275–277] It is also probable that episodic nocturnal hypoxia will induce changes in the physical properties of resistance vessels and contribute to the overall elevation of blood pressure.[278,279] Furthermore, preliminary evidence suggests that OSA-induced disruption of baroreceptor function may not resolve after treatment and in fact may be lifelong.[280] Thus, early childhood perturbations may lead to lifelong consequences, or in other words, certain types of adult cardiovascular disease may represent at least in part, sequelae from a priori "unrelated events" during childhood. Therefore, early identification of children with alterations of baroreceptor and autonomic nervous system function in the context of pediatric OSA may lead to detection of a population potentially at risk for ulterior development of hypertension and its cardiovascular-associated morbidity. However, accurate assessment of the long-term implications of the cardiovascular morbidity found in pediatric OSA has yet to be pursued.

Another potentially very serious consequence of intermittent hypoxia may involve its long-term deleterious effects on neuronal and intellectual functions. Reports of decreased intellectual function in children with tonsillar and adenoidal hypertrophy date back to 1889, when Hill reported on "some causes of backwardness and stupidity in children."[281] Schooling problems have been repeatedly reported in case series of children with OSA, and in fact may underlie more extensive behavioral disturbances such as restlessness, aggressive behavior, excessive daytime sleepiness, and poor test performances.[282–295] Moreover, habitual snoring in the absence of OSA has also been demonstrated to be associated with neurocognitive deficits.[296]

There is increasing evidence to support an association between OSA and attention deficit–hyperactivity disorder (ADHD) in children, particularly with the hyperactive-impulsive subtype.[290] Several subjective studies have documented that children with habitual snoring and with OSA often have problems with attention and behavior similar to those observed in children with ADHD. In addition, several survey studies encompassing almost 8000 children have documented daytime sleepiness, hyperactivity, and aggressive behavior in children who snored. In a recent study from our laboratory, both subjective and objective sleep measures were obtained, and showed that objectively measured sleep and respiratory disturbances are relatively frequent among children with ADHD, albeit not as frequent as anticipated from parental reports.[218] In this study, the prevalence of OSA in a cohort of children with ADHD, verified by neuropsychologic testing, did not seem to differ from the prevalence found in the general population. However, an unusually high frequency of OSA was found among children with mild-to-moderate increases in hyperactivity, as opposed to those children with true ADHD. This suggests that while OSA can induce significant behavioral effects manifesting as increased hyperactivity and inattention, it will not overlap with true clinical ADHD when the latter is assessed by more objective tools than just parental perception.[218] Therefore, in a child presenting with parental complaints of hyperactivity and who does not meet the diagnostic criteria of ADHD after undergoing a thorough evaluation as recently recommended by the American Academy of Pediatrics,[224] a careful sleep history should be taken and if snoring is present, an overnight polysomnographic evaluation should be performed.

The mechanism(s) by which OSA may contribute to hyperactivity remain unknown. It is possible that both the sleep fragmentation and episodic hypoxia that characterize OSA will lead to alterations within the neurochemical substrate of the prefrontal cortex, with resultant executive dysfunction.[297,298] Notwithstanding these considerations, sleep disturbances are frequently reported by parents of ADHD children, even when snoring is excluded. According to the available literature, the comorbidity of OSA and ADHD could be shared by a substantial number of hyperactive children, and in fact, it has been suggested that as many as 25% of children with a diagnosis of ADHD may actually have OSA.[286] However, such rather extensive overlap may be less prominent than previously estimated if medication status and psychiatric comorbidity are accounted for in the analysis.

Inverse relationships between memory, learning, and OSA have also been documented. In addition, improvements in learning and behavior have been reported subsequent to treatment for OSA in children,[283,298–301] suggesting that the neurocognitive deficits are at least partially reversible. In a large cohort of first graders whose academic performance was in the lowest (10th) percentile of their class, a six- to ninefold increase in the expected incidence of OSA was found. More importantly, however, a significant improvement in school grades following T&A and resolution of OSA occurred in these children.[283] Since the optimal learning potential for these children is unknown, it is possible that long-term residual deficits may occur even after treatment. Indeed, children who snored frequently and loudly during their early childhood were at greater risk for poor academic performance in later years, well after snoring had resolved.[302] These findings suggest, therefore, that even if a component of the OSA-induced learning deficits is reversible, there may be a long-lasting residual deficit in learning capability, and that the latter may represent a "learning debt"; in other words, the decreased learning capacity during OSA may have led to such a delay in learned skills that recuperation is only possible with additional teaching assistance. Alternatively, the processes underlying the learning deficit during OSA may have irreversibly altered the performance characteristics of the neuronal circuitry responsible for learning particular skills.

As mentioned before, overt excessive daytime sleepiness is not immediately apparent in children with OSA, yet morbidity that could be construed as related to sleepiness is indeed detectable in children with OSA. More recent studies clearly support a role for sleepiness (measured as sleep pressure) in the cognitive and behavioral disturbances occurring in children with OSA.[253]

In animal models, we found that intermittent hypoxia during sleep is associated with significant increases in neuronal cell loss and adverse effects on spatial memory tasks in the absence of significant sleep fragmentation or deprivation. Furthermore, when this model was applied to developing rodents, a unique period of neuronal susceptibility to episodic hypoxia during sleep emerged and coincides with ages at which OSA prevalence peaks in children.[303–305] Since this age coincides with that of a critical period for brain development, it is possible that during a critical time for brain development delayed diagnosis and treatment of OSA will impose a greater burden on vulnerable brain structures and ultimately hamper the overall neurocognitive potential of children with OSA. More recently, evidence suggestive of adverse effects of sleep-disordered breathing on quality of life,[306,307] depressive mood,[308] enuresis,[309] and increased health-related costs,[310,311] further buttress the extensive and multifactorial impact of this condition.

In summary, it is becoming increasingly clear that OSA in children can have adverse effects on somatic growth, induce cardiovascular alterations such as pulmonary hypertension and systemic hypertension, and lead to substantial neurobehavioral deficits, some of which may not be reversible if treatment is delayed. Based on our current understanding of the morbidity affecting pediatric OSA, it is imperative to direct future efforts toward an improved definition of the spectrum of OSA-induced syndrome, such as to provide more accurate guidelines for treatment.

Treatment of Obstructive Sleep Apnea

Tonsillectomy and adenoidectomy is usually the first line of treatment for pediatric OSA, and a recent meta-analysis on the efficacy of T&A suggested a relatively high immediate curative rate of surgery for OSA in children.[312] Since OSA is the conglomerate result of the relative size and structure of the upper airway components, rather than the absolute size of the adenotonsillar tissue, both tonsils and adenoids should be removed, even when one or the other seems to be the primary culprit. Although the majority of children will have improvement in the severity of OSA, cure may actually occur in a smaller proportion than previously estimated, particularly in children with more severe OSA, in those who are obese, and in those with a positive family history of OSA.[70,313,314]

Children with OSA are at risk for respiratory compromise postoperatively, as a result of upper airway edema, increased secretions, respiratory depression secondary to analgesic and anesthetic agents, and postobstructive pulmonary edema. A high risk for such complications is particularly encountered among children younger than 3 years of age, those with severe OSA, and those with additional medical conditions such as craniofacial syndromes; these patients should not undergo outpatient surgery, and cardiorespiratory monitoring should be performed for at least 24 hours postoperatively to ensure their stability.[315–319] Postoperative polysomnographic evaluation 10 to 12 weeks after surgery is probably needed in most patients. However, it should definitely be recommended for those patients with additional risk factors and thus ensure that additional interventions are not required.

Additional treatment options are available for the management of OSA in children either before T&A, for those children who do not respond to T&A, or for the small minority in whom T&A is contraindicated. NCPAP has been reported to be both effective and well tolerated in hundreds of infants and older children, with only minor side effects (similar to those seen in adults), such as nasal symptoms and skin breakdown.[320–328] Younger children may develop central apneas or alveolar hypoventilation at higher pressure levels, presumably due to activation of the Hering-Breuer reflex by stimulating pulmonary stretch receptors. However, this can be remedied by the use of bilevel positive airway pressure ventilation with a backup rate. Supplemental O_2 results in improved arterial O_2 saturation in children with OSA without worsening of the degree of obstruction. However, since O_2 does not address many of the pathophysiologic features associated with the symptoms of OSA, it should be reserved as a temporary palliative measure preceding T&A, and it clearly should not be used as a first-line treatment. Furthermore, supplemental O_2 should never be used without monitoring the potential resultant changes in P_{CO_2}, since some patients with OSA can develop unpredictable and potentially life-threatening hypercapnia when breathing supplemental O_2.[329,330]

Uvulopharyngopalatoplasty has not been systematically evaluated in children. It has been found to be useful in patients with upper airway hypotonia, in other words, those with Down syndrome or cerebral palsy. Craniofacial reconstructive procedures are reserved for some children with craniofacial anomalies. Other procedures such as tongue wedge resection, epiglottoplasty, and mandibular advancement may occasionally be indicated. With the advent of CPAP, tracheostomy is now rarely required. Although pharmacologic agents are not usually useful in frank OSA, recent work has demonstrated that intranasal steroids[331,332] and oral leukotriene receptor modifiers may have a role in the clinical management of symptomatic children with either primary or secondary (after T&A) upper airway resistance syndrome.[333–335]

REFERENCES

1. Contreras D, Timofeev I, Steriade M: Mechanisms of long-lasting hyperpolarizations underlying slow sleep oscillations in cat corticothalamic networks. J Physiol 1996;494:251–264.
2. Hill SL, Tononi G: Modeling sleep and wakefulness in the thalamocortical system. J Neurophysiol 2005;93:1671–1698.
3. Anders T, Emde R, Parmelee AH: A Manual of Standardized Terminology, Techniques, and Criteria for Scoring of States of Sleep and Wakefulness in Newborn Infants. Los Angeles: UCLA Brain Information Services, NINDS Neurological Information Network, 1971.
4. Parmelee AH, Jr, Schulz HR, Disbrow MA: Sleep patterns of the newborn. J Pediatr 1961;58:241–250.
5. Parmelee AH Jr, Wenner WH, Schulz HR: Infant sleep patterns. From birth to 16 weeks of age. J Pediatr 1964;65:576–582.
6. Parmelee AH Jr, Wenner WH, Akiyama Y, Schultz M, Stern E: Sleep states in premature infants. Dev Med Child Neurol 1967;9:70–77.
7. Scher MS, Steppe DA, Banks DL, Guthrie RD, Sclabassi RJ: Maturational trends of EEG-sleep measures in the healthy preterm neonate. Pediatr Neurol 1995;12:314–322.
8. Curzi-Dascalova L, Peirano P, Morel-Kahn F: Development of sleep states in normal premature and fullterm newborns. Dev Psychobiol 1988;21:431–444.
9. Kohyama J, Iwakawa Y: Developmental changes in phasic sleep parameters as reflections of the brain-stem maturation. Polysomnographical examinations of infants, including premature neonates. Electroencephalogr Clin Neurophysiol 1990;76:325–330.
10. Gaultier C, Amiel J, Dauger S, Trang H, Lyonnet S, Gallego J, Simonneau M: Genetics and early disturbances of breathing control. Pediatr Res 2004;55: 729–733.

11. Smith JC, Ellenberger HH, Ballanyi K, Richter DW, Feldman JL: Pre-Botzinger complex. A brainstem region that may generate respiratory rhythm in mammals. Science 1991;254:726–729.
12. Gray PA, Rekling JC, Bocchiaro CM, Feldman JL: Modulation of respiratory frequency by peptidergic input to rhythmogenic neurons in the pre-Botzinger complex. Science 1999;286:1566–1568.
13. Del Negro CA, Morgado-Valle C, Feldman JL: Respiratory rhythm. An emergent network property? Neuron 2002;34:821–830.
14. Feldman JL, Mitchell GS, Nattie EE: Breathing. Rhythmicity, plasticity, chemosensitivity. Ann Rev Neurosci 2003;26:239–266.
15. Lieske SP, Thoby-Brisson M, Telgkamp P, Ramirez JM: Reconfiguration of the neural network controlling multiple breathing patterns. Eupnea, sighs and gasps. Nat Neurosci 2000;3:600–607.
16. Viemari JC, Bevengut M, Burnet H, Coulon P, Pequignot JM, Tiveron MC, Hilaire G: Phox2a gene, A6 neurons, and noradrenaline are essential for development of normal respiratory rhythm in mice. J Neurosci 2004;24: 928–937.
17. Chatonnet F, Dominguez del Toro E, Thoby-Brisson M, Champagnat J, Fortin G, Rijli FM, Thaeron-Antono C: From hindbrain segmentation to breathing after birth. Developmental patterning in rhombomeres 3 and 4. Mol Neurobiol 2003;28:277–294.
18. Fisher JT, Sant'Ambrogio G: Airway and lung receptors and their reflex effects in the newborn. Pediatr Pulmonol 1985;1:112–126.
19. Gaultier C, Praud JP, Canet E, Delaperche MF, D'Allest AM: Paradoxical inward rib cage motion during rapid eye movement sleep in infants and young children. J Dev Physiol 1987;9:391–397.
20. Kelly DH, Stellwagen LM, Kaitz E, Shannon DC: Apnea and periodic breathing in normal full term infants during the first twelve months. Pediatr Pulmonol 1985,1:215–219.
21. Gaultier C: Sleep apnea in infants. Sleep Med Rev 1999;3:303–312.
22. Harper RM, Schechtman VL, Kluge KA: Machine classification of infant sleep state using cardiorespiratory measures. Electroencephalogr Clin Neurophysiol 1987;67:379–387.
23. Gozal D, Hathout GM, Kirlew KA, Tang H, Woo MS, Zhang J, Lufkin RB, Harper RM: Localization of putative neural respiratory regions in the human by functional magnetic resonance imaging. J Appl Physiol 1994;76: 2076–2083.
24. Putnam RW: Intracellular pH regulation of neurons in chemosensitive and nonchemosensitive areas of brain slices. Respir Physiol 2001;129:37–56.
25. Nattie EE, Prabhakar NR: Peripheral and central chemosensitivity. Multiple mechanisms, multiple sites? A workshop summary. Adv Exp Med Biol 2001;499:73–80.
26. Kahn A, Groswasser J, Franco P, Scaillet S, Sawaguchi T, Kelmanson I, Dan B: Sudden infant deaths. Stress, arousal and SIDS. Early Hum Dev 2003;75 (Suppl):S147–S166.
27. Kato I, Franco P, Groswasser J, Scaillet S, Kelmanson I, Togari H, Kahn A: Incomplete arousal processes in infants who were victims of sudden death. Am J Respir Crit Care Med 2003;168:1298–1303.
28. Marcus CL, Glomb WB, Basinski DJ, Davidson SL, Keens TG: Developmental pattern of hypercapnic and hypoxic ventilatory responses from childhood to adulthood. J Appl Physiol 1994;76:314–320.
29. Gozal D, Arens R, Omlin KJ, Marcus CL, Keens TG: Maturational differences in step vs. ramp hypoxic and hypercapnic ventilatory responses. J Appl Physiol 1994;76:1968–1975.
30. Rebuck, AS, Campbell JM: A clinical method for assessing the ventilatory response to hypoxia. Am Rev Respir Dis 1974;109:345–350.
31. Shaw RA, Shonfeld SA, Whitcomb ME: Progressive and transient hypoxic ventilatory drive tests in healthy subjects. Am Rev Respir Dis 1982;126: 37–40.
32. Gabel RA, Kronenborg RS, Severinghaus JW: Vital capacity breaths of 5% or 15% CO_2 in N_2 or O_2 to test carotid chemosensitivity. Respir Physiol 1973;17:195–208.
33. Dejours P: Chemoreflexes in breathing. Physiol Rev 1962;42:335–352.
34. Calder NA, Williams BA, Kumar P, Hanson MA: The respiratory response of healthy term infants to breath-by-breath alternations in inspired oxygen at two postnatal ages. Pediatr Res 1994;35:321–324.
35. Calder NA, Williams BA, Smyth J, Boon AW, Kumar P, Hanson MA: Absence of ventilatory responses to alternating breaths of mild hypoxia and air in infants who have had bronchopulmonary dysplasia. Implications for the risk of sudden infant death. Pediatr Res 1994;35:677–681.
36. Bouferrache B, Krim G, Marbaix-Li Q, Freville M, Gaultier C: Reproducibility of the alternating breath test of fractional inspired O_2 in infants. Pediatr Res 1998;44:239–246.
37. Chardon K, Bach V, Telliez F, Tourneux P, Elabbassi EB, Cardot V, Gaultier C, Libert JP: Peripheral chemoreceptor activity in sleeping neonates exposed to warm environments. Neurophysiol Clin 2003;33:196–202.
38. Martin RJ, DiFiore JM, Jana L, Davis RL, Miller MJ, Coles SK, Dick TE: Persistence of the biphasic ventilatory response to hypoxia in preterm infants. J Pediatr 1998;132:960–964.
39. Arens R, Marcus CL: Pathophysiology of upper airway obstruction. A developmental perspective. Sleep 2004;27:997–1019.
40. Smith PL, Wise RA, Gold AR, Schwartz AR, Permutt S: Upper airway pressure-flow relationships in obstructive sleep apnea. J Appl Physiol 1988; 64:789–795.
41. Schwartz AR, Smith PL, Wise RA, Gold AR, Permutt S: Induction of upper airway occlusion in sleeping individuals with subatmospheric nasal pressure. J Appl Physiol 1988;64:535–542.
42. Marcus CL, McColley SA, Carroll JL, Loughlin GM, Smith PL, Schwartz AR: Upper airway collapsibility in children with obstructive sleep apnea syndrome. J Appl Physiol 1994;77:918–924.
43. Brouillette RT, Thach BT: A neuromuscular mechanism maintaining extrathoracic airway patency. J Appl Physiol 1979;46:772–729.
44. Hudgel DW, Hendricks C, Dadley A: Alteration in obstructive apnea pattern induced by changes in oxygen- and carbon-dioxide-inspired concentrations. Am Rev Respir Dis 1988;138:16–19.
45. Schwartz AR, Thut DC, Brower RG, Gauda EB, Roach D, Permutt S, Smith PL: Modulation of maximal inspiratory airflow by neuromuscular activity. Effect of CO_2. J Appl Physiol 1993;74:1597–1605.
46. Schwartz AR, Thut DC, Russ B, Seelagy M, Yuan X, Brower RG, Permutt S, Wise RA, Smith PL: Effect of electrical stimulation of the hypoglossal nerve on airflow mechanics in the isolated upper airway. Am Rev Respir Dis 1993;147:1144–1150.
47. Mezzanotte WS, Tangel DJ, White DP: Waking genioglossal electromyogram in sleep apnea patients versus normal controls (a neuromuscular compensatory mechanism). J Clin Invest 1992;89:1571–1579.
48. Mezzanotte WS, Tangel DJ, White DP: Influence of sleep onset on upper-airway muscle activity in apnea patients versus normal controls. Am J Respir Crit Care Med 1996;153:1880–1887.
49. Katz ES, White DP: Genioglossus activity during sleep in normal control subjects and children with obstructive sleep apnea. Am J Respir Crit Care Med. 2004;170:553–560.
50. Marcus CL, Katz ES, Lutz J, Black CA, Galster P, Carson KA: Upper airway dynamic responses in children with the obstructive sleep apnea syndrome. Pediatr Res 2005;57:99–107.
51. Marcus CL, Fernandes Do Prado LB, Lutz J, Katz ES, Black CA, Galster P, Carson KA: Developmental changes in upper airway dynamics. J Appl Physiol 2004;97:98–108.
52. Gozal D, Burnside MM: Increased upper airway collapsibility in children with obstructive sleep apnea during wakefulness. Am J Respir Crit Care Med 2004;169:163–167.
53. Longobardo GS, Gothe B, Goldman MD, Cherniack NS: Sleep apnea considered as a control system instability. Respir Physiol 1982;50:311–333.
54. Marcus CL, Lutz J, Carroll JL, Bamford O: Arousal and ventilatory responses during sleep in children with obstructive sleep apnea. J Appl Physiol 1998; 84:1926–1936.
55. Marcus CL, Gozal D, Arens R, Basinski DJ, Omlin KJ, Keens TG, Ward SL: Ventilatory responses during wakefulness in children with obstructive sleep apnea. Am J Respir Crit Care Med 1994;149:715–721.
56. Strauss SG, Lynn AM, Bratton SL, Nespeca MK: Ventilatory response to CO_2 in children with obstructive sleep apnea from adenotonsillar hypertrophy. Anesth Analg 1999;89:328–332.
57. Fregosi RF, Quan SF, Jackson AC, Kaemingk KL, Morgan WJ, Goodwin JL, Reeder JC, Cabrera RK, Antonio E: Ventilatory drive and the apnea-hypopnea index in six-to-twelve year old children. BMC Pulm Med 2004;4:4.
58. Gozal D, Ben-Ari JH, Harper RM, Keens TG: Ventilatory responses to repeated, short hypercapnic challenges. J Appl Physiol 1995;78:1374–1381.
59. Gozal D, Arens R, Omlin KJ, Ben-Ari JH, Aljadeff G, Harper RM, Keens TG: Ventilatory response to consecutive short hypercapnic challenges in children with obstructive sleep apnea. J Appl Physiol 1995;79:1608–1614.
60. Marcus CL, Moreira GA, Bamford O, Lutz J: Response to inspiratory resistive loading during sleep in normal children and children with obstructive apnea. J Appl Physiol 1999;87:1448–1454.
61. Onal E, Lopata M: Periodic breathing and the pathogenesis of occlusive sleep apneas. Am Rev Respir Dis 1982;126:676–680.
62. Schiffman PH, Rubin NK, Dominguez T, Mahboubi S, Udupa JK, O'Donnell AR, McDonough JM, Maislin G, Schwab RJ, Arens R: Mandibular dimensions in children with obstructive sleep apnea syndrome. Sleep 2004;27:959–965.
63. Arens R, McDonough JM, Costarino AT, Mahboubi S, Tayag-Kier CE, Maislin G, Schwab RJ, Pack AI: Magnetic resonance imaging of the upper airway structure of children with obstructive sleep apnea syndrome. Am J Respir Crit Care Med 2001;164:698–703.

64. Arens R, McDonough JM, Corbin AM, Rubin NK, Carroll ME, Pack AI, Liu J, Udupa JK: Upper airway size analysis by magnetic resonance imaging of children with obstructive sleep apnea syndrome. Am J Respir Crit Care Med 2003;167:65–70.
65. Jeans WD, Fernando DC, Maw AR, Leighton BC: A longitudinal study of the growth of the nasopharynx and its contents in normal children. Br J Radiol 1981;54:117–121.
66. Jeans WD, Fernando DC, Maw AR: How should adenoidal enlargement be measured? A radiological study based on interobserver agreement. Clin Radiol 1981;32:337–340.
67. Arens R, McDonough JM, Corbin AM, Hernandez ME, Maislin G, Schwab RJ, Pack AI: Linear dimensions of the upper airway structure during development. Assessment by magnetic resonance imaging. Am J Respir Crit Care Med 2002;165:117–122.
68. Goldbart AD, Goldman JL, Li RC, Brittian KR, Tauman R, Gozal D: Differential expression of cysteinyl leukotriene receptors 1 and 2 in tonsils of children with obstructive sleep apnea syndrome or recurrent infection. Chest 2004;126:13–18.
69. Brouillette RT, Fernbach SK, Hunt CE: Obstructive sleep apnea in infants and children. J Pediatr 1982;100:31–40.
70. Greenfeld M, Tauman R, DeRowe A, Sivan Y: Obstructive sleep apnea syndrome due to adenotonsillar hypertrophy in infants. Int J Pediatr Otorhinolaryngol 2003;67:1055–1060.
71. Suto Y, Inoue Y: Sleep apnea syndrome. Examination of pharyngeal obstruction with high-speed MR and polysomnography. Acta Radiol 1996; 37:315–320.
72. Don GW, Kirjavainen T, Broome C, Seton C, Waters KA: Site and mechanics of spontaneous, sleep-associated obstructive apnea in infants. J Appl Physiol 2000;89:2453–2462.
73. Pickens DL, Schefft GL, Storch GA, Thach BT: Characterization of prolonged apneic episodes associated with respiratory syncytial virus infection. Pediatr Pulmonol 1989;6:195–201.
74. Kahn A, Groswasser J, Sottiaux M, Kelmanson I, Rebuffat E, Franco P, Dramaix M, Wayenberg JL: Prenatal exposure to cigarettes in infants with obstructive sleep apneas. Pediatrics 1994;93:778–783.
75. Sawnani H, Jackson T, Murphy T, Beckerman R, Simakajornboon N: The effect of maternal smoking on respiratory and arousal patterns in preterm infants during sleep. Am J Respir Crit Care Med 2004;169:733–738.
76. Isono S, Shimada A, Utsugi M, Konno A, Nishino T: Comparison of static mechanical properties of the passive pharynx between normal children and children with sleep-disordered breathing. Am J Respir Crit Care Med 1998;157:1204–1212.
77. Ishikawa T, Isono S, Aiba J, Tanaka A, Nishino T: Prone position increases collapsibility of the passive pharynx in infants and small children. Am J Respir Crit Care Med 2002;166:760–764.
78. Shintani T, Asakura K, Kataura A: Adenotonsillar hypertrophy and skeletal morphology of children with obstructive sleep apnea syndrome. Acta Otolaryngol Suppl 1996;523:222–224.
79. Shintani T, Asakura K, Kataura A: Evaluation of the role of adenotonsillar hypertrophy and facial morphology in children with obstructive sleep apnea. ORL J Otorhinolaryngol Relat Spec 1997;59:286–291.
80. Fregosi RF, Quan SF, Kaemingk KL, Morgan WJ, Goodwin JL, Cabrera R, Gmitro A: Sleep-disordered breathing, pharyngeal size and soft tissue anatomy in children. J Appl Physiol 2003;95:2030–2038.
81. Mellins RB, Balfour HH Jr, Turino GM, Winters RW: Failure of automatic control of ventilation (Ondine's curse). Medicine 1970;49:487–504.
82. Deonna T, Arczynska W, Torrado A: Congenital failure of automatic ventilation (Ondine's curse). J Pediatr 1974;84:710–714.
83. Gozal D: Congenital central hypoventilation syndrome. An update. Pediatr Pulmonol 1998;26:273–282.
84. Vanderlaan M, Holbrook CR, Wang M, Tuell A, Gozal D: Epidemiologic survey of 196 patients with congenital central hypoventilation syndrome. Pediatr Pulmonol 2004;37:217–229.
85. Minutillo C, Pemberton PJ, Goldblatt J: Hirschsprung's disease and Ondine's curse. Further evidence for a distinct syndrome. Clin Genet 1989;36: 200–203.
86. Nakahara S, Yokomori K, Tamura K, Oku K, Tsuchida Y: Hirschsprung's disease associated with Ondine's curse. A special subgroup? J Pediatr Surg 1995;10:1481–1484.
87. Swaminathan S, Gilsanz V, Atkinson J, Keens TG: Congenital central hypoventilation syndrome associated with multiple ganglioneuromas. Chest 1989;96:423–424.
88. Rohrer T, Trachsel D, Engelcke G, Hammer J: Congenital central hypoventilation syndrome associated with Hirschsprung's disease and neuroblastoma. Case of multiple neurocristopathies. Pediatr Pulmonol 2002;33: 71–76.
89. Khalifa MM, Flavin MA, Wherrett BA: Congenital central hypoventilation syndrome in monozygotic twins. J Pediatr 1988;113:853–855.
90. Haddad GG, Mazza NM, Defendini R, Blanc WA, Driscoll JM, Epstein AF, Epstein RA, Mellins RB: Congenital failure of automatic control of ventilation, gastrointestinal motility and heart rate. Medicine 1978;57: 517–526.
91. Weese-Mayer DE, Silvestri JM, Marazita ML, Hoo JJ: Congenital central hypoventilation syndrome. Inheritance and relation to sudden infant death syndrome. Am J Med Genet 1993;47:360–367.
92. Weese-Mayer DE, Silvestri JM, Huffman AD, Smok-Pearsall SM, Kowal MH, Maher BS, Cooper ME, Marazita ML: Case/control family study of autonomic nervous system dysfunction in idiopathic congenital central hypoventilation syndrome. Am J Med Genet 2001;100:237–245.
93. Sritippayawan S, Hamutcu R, Kun SS, Ner Z, Ponce M, Keens TG: Mother-daughter transmission of congenital central hypoventilation syndrome. Am J Respir Crit Care Med 2002;166:367–369.
94. Silvestri JM, Chen ML, Weese-Mayer DE, McQuitty JM, Carveth HJ, Nielson DW, Borowitz D, Cerny F: Idiopathic congenital central hypoventilation syndrome. The next generation. Am J Med Genet 2002;112:46–50.
95. Attie T, Pelet A, Edery P, Eng C, Mulligan LM, Amiel J, Boutrand L, Beldjord C, Nihoul-Fekete C, Munnich A, Lyonnet S: Diversity of RET proto-oncogene mutations in familial and sporadic Hirschsprung disease. Hum Mol Genet 1995;4:1381–1386.
96. Edery P, Lyonnet S, Mulligan LM, Pelet A, Dow E, Abel L, Holder S, Nihoul-Fekete C, Ponder BA, Munnich A: Mutations of the RET protooncogene in Hirschsprung's disease. Nature 1994;367:378–380.
97. Romeo G, Ronchetto P, Luo Y, Barone V, Seri M, Ceccherini I, Pasini B, Bocciardi R, Lerone M, Kaariainen H: Point mutations affecting the tyrosine kinase domain of the RET proto-oncogene in Hirschsprung's disease. Nature 1994;367:377–378.
98. Amiel J, Laudier B, Attie-Bitach T, Trang H, de Pontual L, Gener B, Trochet D, Etchevers H, Ray P, Simonneau M, Vekemans M, Munnich A, Gaultier C, Lyonnet S: Polyalanine expansion and frameshift mutations of the paired-like homeobox gene *PHOX2B* in congenital central hypoventilation syndrome. Nat Genet 2003;33:459–461.
99. Pattyn A, Morin X, Cremer H, Goridis C, Brunet JF: The homeobox gene *Phox2b* is essential for the development of autonomic neural crest derivatives. Nature 1999;399:366–370.
100. Brunet JF, Pattyn A: *Phox2* genes—from patterning to connectivity. Curr Opin Genet Dev 2002;12:435–440.
101. Cross SH, Morgan JE, Pattyn A, West K, McKie L, Hart A, Thaung C, Brunet JF, Jackson IJ: Haploinsufficiency for *Phox2b* in mice causes dilated pupils and atrophy of the ciliary ganglion. Mechanistic insights into human congenital central hypoventilation syndrome. Hum Mol Genet 2004;13: 1433–1439.
102. Tsarovina K, Pattyn A, Stubbusch J, Muller F, van der Wees J, Schneider C, Brunet JF, Rohrer H: Essential role of Gata transcription factors in sympathetic neuron development. Development 2004;131:4775–4786.
103. Trang H, Laudier B, Trochet D, Munnich A, Lyonnet S, Gaultier C, Amiel J: *PHOX2B* gene mutation in a patient with late-onset central hypoventilation. Pediatr Pulmonol 2004;38:349–351.
104. Garcia-Barcelo M, Sham MH, Lui VC, Chen BL, Ott J, Tam PK: Association study of *PHOX2B* as a candidate gene for Hirschsprung's disease. Gut 2003;52:563–567.
105. Trochet D, O'Brien LM, Gozal D, Trang H, Nordenskjöld A, Laudier B, Uhrig S, Cole T, Munnich A, Gaultier C, Lyonnet S, Amiel J: *PHOX2B* genotype allows for prediction of tumour risk in congenital central hypoventilation syndrome. Am J Med Genet 2005;76:421–426.
106. Weese-Mayer DE, Berry-Kravis EM, Zhou L, Maher BS, Curran ME, Silvestri JM, Marazita ML: Sudden infant death syndrome. Case-control frequency differences at genes pertinent to early autonomic nervous system embryologic development. Pediatr Res 2004;56:391–395.
107. Macey PM, Woo MA, Macey KE, Keens TG, Saeed MM, Alger JR, Harper RM: Hypoxia reveals posterior thalamic, cerebellar, midbrain and limbic deficits in congenital central hypoventilation syndrome. J Appl Physiol 2005;98:958–969.
108. Harper RM, Macey PM, Woo MA, Macey KE, Keens TG, Gozal D, Alger JR: Hypercapnic exposure in congenital central hypoventilation syndrome reveals central nervous system respiratory control mechanisms. J Neurophysiol 2005;93:1647–1658.
109. Macey KE, Macey PM, Woo MA, Harper RK, Alger JR, Keens TG, Harper RM: fMRI signal changes in response to forced expiratory loading in congenital central hypoventilation syndrome. J Appl Physiol 2004;97: 1897–1907.
110. Hedner J, Hedner T, Breese GR, Lundell KH, Lundberg D, Lundstro NR, Ostergaar E, McCown TJ, Mueller RA: Changes in cerebrospinal fluid

homovanillic acid in children with Ondine's curse. Pediatr Pulmonol 1987;3:131–135.

111. Woo MS, Woo MA, Gozal D, Jansen MT, Keens TG, Harper RM: Heart rate variability in congenital central hypoventilation syndrome. Pediatr Res 1992;31:291–296.
112. O'Sullivan J, Cottrell AJ, Wren C: Ondine's curse and neurally mediated syncope—a new and important association. Eur Heart J 1993;14:1289–1291.
113. O'Brien LM, Holbrook CR, Vanderclaan M, Amiel J, Gozal D: Autonomic function in children with congenital central hypoventilation syndrome and their families. Chest 2005;128:2478–2484.
114. Trang H, Boureghda S, Denjoy I, Alia M, Kabaker M: 24-hour BP in children with congenital central hypoventilation syndrome. Chest 2003; 124:1393–1399.
115. Trang H, Girard A, Laude D, Elghozi JL: Short-term blood pressure and heart rate variability in congenital central hypoventilation syndrome (Ondine's curse). Clin Sci (Lond) 2005;108:225–230.
116. Macey PM, Valderama C, Kim AH, Woo MA, Gozal D, Keens TG, Harper RK, Harper RM: Temporal trends of cardiac and respiratory responses to ventilatory challenges in congenital central hypoventilation syndrome. Pediatr Res 2004;55:953–959.
117. Goldberg DS, Ludwig IH: Congenital central hypoventilation syndrome. Ocular findings in 37 children. J Pediatr Ophthalmol Strabismus 1996; 33:176–181.
118. Cutz E, Ma TK, Perrin DG, Moore AM, Becker LE: Peripheral chemoreceptors in congenital central hypoventilation syndrome. Am J Respir Crit Care Med 1997;155:358–363.
119. Spengler CM, Gozal D, Shea SA: Chemoreceptive mechanisms elucidated by studies of congenital central hypoventilation syndrome. Respir Physiol 2001;129:247–255.
120. Paton JY, Swaminathan S, Sargent CW, Keens TG: Hypoxic and hypercapnic ventilatory responses in awake children with congenital central hypoventilation syndrome. Am Rev Respir Dis 1989;140:368–372.
121. American Thoracic Society: Idiopathic congenital central hypoventilation syndrome. Diagnosis and management. Am J Respir Crit Care Med 1999; 160:368–373.
122. Weese-Mayer DE, Berry-Kravis EM: Genetics of congenital central hypoventilation syndrome. Lessons from a seemingly orphan disease. Am J Respir Crit Care Med 2004;170:16–21.
123. Weese-Mayer DE, Berry-Kravis EM, Zhou L, Maher BS, Silvestri JM, Curran ME, Marazita ML: Idiopathic congenital central hypoventilation syndrome. Analysis of genes pertinent to early autonomic nervous system embryologic development and identification of mutations in *PHOX2b*. Am J Med Genet 2003;123A:267–278.
124. Nielson DW, Black PG: Mask ventilation in congenital central alveolar hypoventilation syndrome. Pediatr Pulmonol 1990;9:44–45.
125. Pieters T, Amy JJ, Burrini D, Aubert G, Rodenstein DO, Collard P: Normal pregnancy in primary alveolar hypoventilation treated with nocturnal nasal intermittent positive pressure ventilation. Eur Resp J 1995;8:1424–1427.
126. Kerbl R, Litscher H, Grubbauer HM, Reiterer F, Zobel G, Trop M, Urlesberger B, Eber E, Kurz R: Congenital central hypoventilation syndrome (Ondine's curse syndrome) in two siblings. Delayed diagnosis and successful noninvasive treatment. Eur J Pediatr 1996;155:977–980.
127. Juhl B, Norregaard FO: Congenital central hypoventilation treated with nocturnal biphasic intermittent respiration via nasal mask. Ugeskr Laeger 1995;157:1683–1684.
128. Villa MPP, Dotta A, Castello D, Piro S, Pagani J, Palamides S, Ronchetti R: Bi-level positive airway pressure (biPAP) ventilation in an infant with central hypoventilation syndrome. Pediatr Pulmonol 1997;24:66–69.
129. Migliori C, Cavazza A, Motta M, Bottino R, Chirico G: Early use of nasal-BiPAP in two infants with congenital central hypoventilation syndrome. Acta Paediatr 2003;92:823–826.
130. Weese-Mayer DE, Morrow AS, Brouillette RT, Ilbawi MN, Hunt CE: Diaphragm pacing in infants and children. A life-table analysis of implanted components. Am Rev Respir Dis 1989;139:974–979.
131. Fitzgerald D, Davis GM, Gottesman R, Fecteau A, Guttman F: Diaphragmatic pacemaker failure in congenital central hypoventilation syndrome. A tale of two twiddlers. Pediatr Pulmonol 1996;22:319–321.
132. Silvestri JM, Weese-Mayer DE, Flanagan EA: Congenital central hypoventilation syndrome. Cardiorespiratory responses to moderate exercise, simulating daily activity. Pediatr Pulmonol 1995;20:89–93.
133. Weese-Mayer DE, Silvestri JM, Kenny AS, Ilbawi MN, Hauptman SA, Lipton JW, Talonen PP, Garcia HG, Watt JW, Exner G, Baer GA, Elefteriades JA, Peruzzi WT, Alex CG, Harlid R, Vincken W, Davis GM, Decramer M, Kuenzle C, Saeterhaug A, Schober JG: Diaphragm pacing with a quadripolar phrenic nerve electrode. An international study. Pacing Clin Electrophysiol 1996;19:1311–1319.
134. Waters KA, Forbes P, Morielli A, Hum C, O'Gorman AM, Vernet O, Davis GM, Tewfik TL, Ducharme FM, Brouillette RT: Sleep-disordered breathing in children with myelomeningocele. J Pediatr 1998;132: 672–681.
135. Kirk VG, Morielli A, Brouillette RT: Sleep-disordered breathing in patients with myelomeningocele. The missed diagnosis. Dev Med Child Neurol 1999;41:40–43.
136. Kirk VG, Morielli A, Gozal D, Marcus CL, Waters KA, D'Andrea LA, Rosen CL, Deray MJ, Brouillette RT: Treatment of sleep-disordered breathing in children with myelomeningocele. Pediatr Pulmonol 2000;30: 445–452.
137. Arens R, Gozal D, Omlin KJ, Livingston FR, Liu J, Keens TG, Ward SL: Hypoxic and hypercapnic ventilatory responses in Prader-Willi syndrome. J Appl Physiol 1994;77:2224–2230.
138. Gozal D, Arens R, Omlin KJ, Ward SL, Keens TG: Absent peripheral chemosensitivity in Prader-Willi syndrome. J Appl Physiol 1994;77: 2231–2236.
139. Arens R, Gozal D, Burrell BC, Bailey SL, Bautista DB, Keens TG, Ward SL: Arousal and cardiorespiratory responses to hypoxia in Prader-Willi syndrome. Am J Respir Crit Care Med 1996;153:283–287.
140. Gozal D, Torres JE, Menendez AA: Longitudinal assessment of hypercapnic ventilatory drive after tracheotomy in a patient with the Prader-Willi syndrome. Eur Respir J 1996;9:1565–1568.
141. Lindgren AC, Hellstrom LG, Ritzen EM, Milerad J: Growth hormone treatment increases CO_2 response, ventilation and central inspiratory drive in children with Prader-Willi syndrome. Eur J Pediatr 1999;158:936–940.
142. Nixon GM, Brouillette RT: Sleep and breathing in Prader-Willi syndrome. Pediatr Pulmonol 2002;34:209–217.
143. Katz ES, McGrath S, Marcus CL: Late-onset central hypoventilation with hypothalamic dysfunction. aA distinct clinical syndrome. Pediatr Pulmonol 2000;29:62–68.
144. Di Fiore JM, Arko MK, Miller MJ, Krauss A, Betkerur A, Zadell A, Kenney SR, Martin RJ: Cardiorespiratory events in preterm infants referred for apnea monitoring studies. Pediatrics 2001;108:1304–1308.
145. Ruggins NR, Milner AD: Site of upper airway obstruction in preterm infants with problematical apnoea. Arch Dis Child 1991;66:787–792.
146. Upton CJ, Milner AD, Stokes GM: Upper airway patency during apnoea of prematurity. Arch Dis Child 1992;67:419–424.
147. Lemke RP, Idiong N, Al-Saedi S, Kwiatkowski K, Cates DB, Rigatto H: Evidence of a critical period of airway instability during central apneas in preterm infants. Am J Respir Crit Care Med 1998;157:470–474.
148. Idiong N, Lemke RP, Lin YJ, Kwiatkowski K, Cates DB, Rigatto H: Airway closure during mixed apneas in preterm infants. Is respiratory effort necessary? J Pediatr 1998;133:509–512.
149. Ramanathan R, Corwin MJ, Hunt CE, Lister G, Tinsley LR, Baird T, Silvestri JM, Crowell DH, Hufford D, Martin RJ, Neuman MR, Weese-Mayer DE, Cupples LA, Peucker M, Willinger M, Keens TG; Collaborative Home Infant Monitoring Evaluation (CHIME) Study Group: Cardiorespiratory events recorded on home monitors. Comparison of healthy infants with those at increased risk for SIDS. JAMA 2001;285: 2199–2207.
150. Eichenwald EC, Aina A, Stark AR: Apnea frequently persists beyond term gestation in infants delivered at 24–28 weeks. Pediatrics 1997;100:354–359.
151. Krauss AN, Solomon GE, Auld PA: Sleep state, apnea and bradycardia in pre-term infants. Dev Med Child Neurol 1977;19:160–168.
152. Rehan VK, Fajardo CA, Haider AZ, Alvaro RE, Cates DB, Kwiatkowski K, Nowaczyk B, Rigatto H: Influence of sleep state and respiratory pattern on cyclical fluctuations of cerebral blood flow velocity in healthy preterm infants. Biol Neonate 1996;69:357–367.
153. al-Saedi SA, Lemke RP, Haider ZA, Cates DB, Kwiatkowski K, Rigatto H: Prolonged apnea in the preterm infant is not a random event. Am J Perinatol 1997;14:195–200.
154. Henslee JA, Schechtman VL, Lee MY, Harper RM: Developmental patterns of heart rate and variability in prematurely-born infants with apnea of prematurity. Early Hum Dev 1997;47:35–50.
155. Rigatto H, Brady JP, de la Torre Verduzco R: Chemoreceptor reflexes in preterm infants. II. The effect of gestational and postnatal age on the ventilatory response to inhaled carbon dioxide. Pediatrics. 1975;55(5): 614–620.
156. Gerhardt T, Bancalari E: Apnea of prematurity. II. Respiratory reflexes. Pediatrics 1984;74:63–66.
157. Oliven A, Deal EC Jr, Kelsen SG, Cherniack NS: Effects of hypercapnia on inspiratory and expiratory muscle activity during expiration. J Appl Physiol 1985;59:1560–1565.
158. Eichenwald EC, Ungarelli RA, Stark AR: Hypercapnia increases expiratory braking in preterm infants. J Appl Physiol 1993;75:2665–2670.

159. Abu-Shaweesh JM, Dreshaj IA, Thomas AJ, Haxhiu MA, Strohl KP, Martin RJ: Changes in respiratory timing induced by hypercapnia in maturing rats. J Appl Physiol 1999;87:484–490.
160. Dreshaj IA, Haxhiu MA, Abu-Shaweesh J, Carey RE, Martin RJ: CO_2-induced prolongation of expiratory time during early development. Respir Physiol 1999;116:125–132.
161. Martin RJ, Wilson CG, Abu-Shaweesh JM, Haxhiu MA: Role of inhibitory neurotransmitter interactions in the pathogenesis of neonatal apnea. Implications for management. Semin Perinatol 2004;28:273–278.
162. Rigatto H, Brady JP, de la Torre Verduzco R: Chemoreceptor reflexes in preterm infants. I. The effect of gestational and postnatal age on the ventilatory response to inhalation of 100% and 15% oxygen. Pediatrics 1975; 55:604–613.
163. Martin RJ, DiFiore JM, Jana L, Davis RL, Miller MJ, Coles SK, Dick TE: Persistence of the biphasic ventilatory response to hypoxia in preterm infants. J Pediatr 1998;132:960–964.
164. Burton MD, Kazemi H: Neurotransmitters in central respiratory control. Respir Physiol 2000;122:111–121.
165. Elnazir B, Marshall JM, Kumar P: Postnatal development of the pattern of respiratory and cardiovascular response to systemic hypoxia in the piglet: the roles of adenosine. J Physiol 1996;492:573–585.
166. Vlasic V, Simakajornboon N, Gozal E, Gozal D: PDGF β receptor expression in the dorsocaudal brainstem parallels hypoxic ventilatory depression in the developing rat. Pediatr Res 2001;50:236–241.
167. Nock ML, Difiore JM, Arko MK, Martin RJ: Relationship of the ventilatory response to hypoxia with neonatal apnea in preterm infants. J Pediatr 2004;144:291–295.
168. Gozal E, Gozal D: Respiratory plasticity following intermittent hypoxia. Developmental interactions. J Appl Physiol 2001;90:1995–1999.
169. Milner AD, Greenough A: The role of the upper airway in neonatal apnoea. Semin Neonatol 2004;9:213–219.
170. Kianicka I, Leroux JF, Praud JP: Thyroarytenoid muscle activity during hypocapnic central apneas in awake nonsedated lambs. J Appl Physiol 1994;76:1262–1268.
171. Renolleau S, Letourneau P, Niyonsenga T, Praud JP, Gagne B: Thyroarytenoid muscle electrical activity during spontaneous apneas in preterm lambs. Am J Respir Crit Care Med 1999;159:1396–1404.
172. Dorion D, Praud JP: The larynx and neonatal apneas. Otolaryngol Head Neck Surg 2003;128:463–469.
173. Hannam S, Ingram DM, Milner AD: A possible role for the Hering-Breuer deflation reflex in apnea of prematurity. J Pediatr 1998;132:35–39.
174. Davies AM, Koenig JS, Thach BT: Upper airway chemoreflex responses to saline and water in preterm infants. J Appl Physiol 1988;64:1412–1420.
175. Kneyber MC, Brandenburg AH, de Groot R, Joosten KF, Rothbarth PH, Ott A, Moll HA: Risk factors for respiratory syncytial virus associated apnoea. Eur J Pediatr 1998;157:331–335.
176. Lindgren C, Grogaard J.: Reflex apnoea response and inflammatory mediators in infants with respiratory tract infection. Acta Paediatr 1996;85: 798–803.
177. Lindgren C, Lin J, Graham BS, Gray ME, Parker RA, Sundell HW: Respiratory syncytial virus infection enhances the response to laryngeal chemostimulation and inhibits arousal from sleep in young lambs. Acta Paediatr 1996;85:789–797.
178. Martin RJ, Abu-Shaweesh JM, Baird TM: Apnea of prematurity. Pediatr Respir Rev 2004;4:s375–s380.
179. Kimball AL, Carlton DP: Gastroesophageal reflux medications in the treatment of apnea in premature infants. J Pediatr 2001;138:355–360.
180. Miller MJ, Kiatchoosakun P: Relationship between respiratory control and feeding in the developing infant. Semin Neonatol 2004;9:221–227.
181. Poets CF: Gastroesophageal reflux. A critical review of its role in preterm infants. Pediatrics 2004;113:e128–e132.
182. Kahn A, Rebuffat E, Sottiaux M, Dufour D, Cadrenal M, Reiterer F: Lack of temporal relation between acid reflux in the proximal esophagus and cardiorespiratory events in sleeping infants. Eur J Pediatr 1992;151:108–112.
183. Arad-Cohen N, Cohen A, Tirosh E: The relationship between gastroesophageal reflux and apnea in infants. J Pediatr 2000;137:321–326.
184. Mandich MB, Ritchie SK, Mullett M: Transition times to oral feeding in premature infants with and without apnea. J Obstet Gynecol Neonatal Nurs 1996;25:771–776.
185. Bhatt-Mehta V, Schumacher RE: Treatment of apnea of prematurity. Paediatr Drugs 2003;5:195–210.
186. Vandenplas Y, De Wolf D, Sacre L: Influence of xanthines on gastroesophageal reflux in infants at risk for sudden infant death syndrome. Pediatrics 1986;77:807–810.
187. Curzi-Dascalova L, Aujard Y, Gaultier C, Rajguru M: Sleep organization is unaffected by caffeine in premature infants. J Pediatr 2002;140:766–771.
188. Henderson-Smart DJ, Steer P: Methylxanthine treatment for apnea in preterm infants [review]. Cochrane Database Syst Rev 2001;3:CD000140.
189. Millar D, Schmidt B: Controversies surrounding xanthine therapy. Semin Neonatol 2004;9:239–244.
190. Kattwinkel J, Nearman HS, Fanaroff AA, Katona PG, Klaus MH: Apnea of prematurity. Comparative therapeutic effects of cutaneous stimulation and nasal continuous positive airway pressure. J Pediatr 1975;86:588–592.
191. Goldbart AD, Gozal D: Non-invasive ventilation in preterm infants. Pediatr Pulmonol Suppl 2004;26:158–161.
192. Davis PG, Henderson-Smart DJ: Nasal continuous positive airways pressure immediately after extubation for preventing morbidity in preterm infants [review]. Cochrane Database Syst Rev 2003;2:CD000143.
193. Lemyre B, Davis PG, de Paoli AG: Nasal intermittent positive pressure ventilation (NIPPV) versus nasal continuous positive airway pressure (NCPAP) for apnea of prematurity. Cochrane Database Syst Rev 2002; 1:CD002272.
194. Sreenan C, Lemke RP, Hudson-Mason A, Osiovich H: High-flow nasal cannulae in the management of apnea of prematurity. A comparison with conventional nasal continuous positive airway pressure. Pediatrics 2001;107:1081–1083.
195. Lemyre B, Davis PG, de Paoli AG: Nasal intermittent positive pressure ventilation (NIPPV) versus nasal continuous positive airway pressure (NCPAP) for apnea of prematurity [review]. Cochrane Database Syst Rev 2002;1:CD002272.
196. Fenner A, Schalk U, Hoenicke H, Wendenburg A, Roehling T: Periodic breathing in premature and neonatal babies. Incidence, breathing pattern, respiratory gas tensions, response to changes in the composition of ambient air. Pediatr Res 1973;7:174–183.
197. Rigatto H: Apnea and periodic breathing. Semin Perinatol 1977;1: 375–381.
198. Rigatto H, Brady JP: Periodic breathing and apnea in preterm infants. I. Evidence for hypoventilation possibly due to central respiratory depression. Pediatrics 1972;50:202–218.
199. Weintraub Z, Alvaro R, Kwiatkowski K, Cates D, Rigatto H: Effects of inhaled oxygen (up to 40%) on periodic breathing and apnea in preterm infants. J Appl Physiol 1992;72:116–120.
200. Simakajornboon N, Beckerman RC, Mack C, Sharon D, Gozal D: Effect of supplemental oxygen on sleep architecture and cardiorespiratory events in pre-term infants. Pediatrics 2002;110:884–888.
201. Tauman R, Sivan Y: Duration of home monitoring for infants discharged with apnea of prematurity. Biol Neonate 2000;78:168–173.
202. Darnall RA, Kattwinkel J, Nattie C, Robinson M: Margin of safety for discharge after apnea in preterm infants. Pediatrics 1997;100:795–801.
203. Poets CF, Stebbens VA, Alexander JR, Arrowsmith WA, Salfield SA, Southall DP: Oxygen saturation and breathing patterns in infancy. 2: Preterm infants at discharge from special care. Arch Dis Child 1991;66:574–578.
204. Poets CF, Samuels MP, Southall DP: Epidemiology and pathophysiology of apnoea of prematurity. Biol Neonate 1994;65:211–219.
205. Watkin SL, Spencer SA, Pryce A, Southall DP: Temporal relationship between pauses in nasal airflow and desaturation in preterm infants. Pediatr Pulmonol 1996;21:171–175.
206. Taylor HG, Klein N, Schatschneider C, Hack M: Predictors of early school age outcomes in very low birth weight children. J Dev Behav Pediatr 1998; 19:235–243.
207. Baird TM: Clinical correlates, natural history and outcome of neonatal apnoea. Semin Neonatol 2004;9:205–211.
208. American Thoracic Society: Standards and indications for cardiopulmonary sleep studies in children. Am J Respir Crit Care Med 1996;153:866–878.
209. McKenzie M: A Manual of Diseases of the Throat and Nose, including the Pharynx, Larynx, Trachea, Oesophagus, Nasal Cavities, and Neck. London: Churchill, 1880.
210. Guilleminault C, Eldridge F, Simmons FB, Dement WC: Sleep apnea in eight children. Pediatrics 1976;58:28–31.
211. Rosen CL, D'Andrea L, Haddad GG: Adult criteria for obstructive sleep apnea do not identify children with serious obstruction. Am Rev Respir Dis 1992;146:1231–1234.
212. Carroll JL, Loughlin GM: Diagnostic criteria for obstructive sleep apnea syndrome in children. Pediatr Pulmonol 1992;14:71–74.
213. Corbo GM, Forastiere F, Agabiti N, Pistelli R, Dell'Orco V, Perucci CA, Valente S: Snoring in 9- to 15-year-old children. Risk factors and clinical relevance. Pediatrics 2001;108:1149–1154.
214. Griffin MR, Walker FJ, Iwane MK, Weinberg GA, Staat MA, Erdman DD; New Vaccine Surveillance Network Study Group: Epidemiology of respiratory infections in young children. Insights from the New Vaccine Surveillance Network. Pediatr Infect Dis J 2004;23:S188–S192.

215. Ostlund MR, Wirgart BZ, Linde A, Grillner L: Respiratory virus infections in Stockholm during seven seasons. A retrospective study of laboratory diagnosis. Scand J Infect Dis 2004;36:460–465.
216. Hulcrantz E, Lofstarnd TB, Ahlquist RJ: The epidemiology of sleep related breathing disorders in children. Int J Pediatr Otorhinolaryngol 1995;6 (Suppl):S63–S66.
217. Ferreira AM, Clemente V, Gozal D, Gomes A, Pissarra C, César H, Coelho I, Silva CF, Azevedo MHP: Snoring in Portuguese primary school children. Pediatrics 2000;106(5):E64. Available at http://www.pediatrics.org/cgi/content/full/106/5/e64.
218. O'Brien LM, Holbrook CR, Mervis CB, Klaus CJ, Bruner J, Raffield TJ, Rutherford J, Mehl RC, Wang M, Tuell A, Hume BC, Gozal D: Sleep and neurobehavioral characteristics in 5–7-year-old hyperactive children. Pediatrics 2003;111:554–563.
219. Urschitz MS, Guenther A, Eitner S, Urschitz-Duprat PM, Schlaud M, Ipsiroglu OS, Poets CF: Risk factors and natural history of habitual snoring. Chest 2004;126:790–800.
220. Ersu R, Arman AR, Save D, Karadag B, Karakoc F, Berkem M, Dagli E: Prevalence of snoring and symptoms of sleep-disordered breathing in primary school children in Istanbul. Chest 2004;126:19–24.
221. Kaditis AG, Finder J, Alexopoulos EI, Starantzis K, Tanou K, Gampeta S, Agorogiannis E, Christodoulou S, Pantazidou A, Gourgoulianis K, Molyvdas PA: Sleep-disordered breathing in 3,680 Greek children. Pediatr Pulmonol 2004;37:499–509.
222. Rosen CL, Larkin EK, Kirchner HL, Emancipator JL, Bivins SF, Surovec SA, Martin RJ, Redline S: Prevalence and risk factors for sleep-disordered breathing in 8- to 11-year-old children. Association with race and prematurity. J Pediatr 2003;142:383–389.
223. Montgomery-Downs HE, O'Brien LM, Holbrook CR, Gozal D: Snoring and sleep-disordered breathing in young children. Subjective and objective correlates. Sleep 2004;27:87–94.
224. Schechter MS; Section on Pediatric Pulmonology, Subcommittee on Obstructive Sleep Apnea Syndrome: Technical report. Diagnosis and management of childhood obstructive sleep apnea syndrome. Pediatrics 2002;109:e69.
225. Tang JP, Rosen CL, Larkin EK, DiFiore JM, Arnold JL, Surovec SA, Youngblut JM, Redline S: Identification of sleep-disordered breathing in children. Variation with event definition. Sleep 2002;25:72–79.
226. Carroll JL, McColley SA, Marcus CL, Curtis S, Loughlin GM: Inability of clinical history to distinguish primary snoring from obstructive sleep apnea syndrome in children. Chest 1995;108:610–618.
227. Corbo GM, Fuciarelli F, Foresi A, De Benedetto F: Snoring in children. Association with respiratory symptoms and passive smoking. BMJ 1989; 299:1491–1494. Erratum in: BMJ 1990;300(6719):226.
228. McColley SA, Carroll JL, Curtis S, Loughlin GM, Sampson HA: High prevalence of allergic sensitization in children with habitual snoring and obstructive sleep apnea. Chest 1997;111:170–173.
229. Chng SY, Goh DY, Wang XS, Tan TN, Ong NB: Snoring and atopic disease. A strong association. Pediatr Pulmonol 2004;38:210–216.
230. Lu LR, Peat JK, Sullivan CE: Snoring in preschool children. Prevalence and association with nocturnal cough and asthma. Chest 2003;124:587–593.
231. Guilleminault C, Li KK, Khramtsov A, Pelayo R, Martinez S: Sleep disordered breathing. Surgical outcomes in prepubertal children. Laryngoscope 2004;114:132–137.
232. Guilleminault C, Li K, Quo S, Inouye RN: A prospective study on the surgical outcomes of children with sleep-disordered breathing. Sleep 2004; 27:95–100.
233. Redline S, Tishler PV, Schluchter M, Aylor J, Clark K, Graham G: Risk factors for sleep-disordered breathing in children. Associations with obesity, race, and respiratory problems. Am J Respir Crit Care Med 1999;159: 1527–1532.
234. Palmer LJ, Buxbaum SG, Larkin EK, Patel SR, Elston RC, Tishler PV, Redline S: Whole genome scan for obstructive sleep apnea and obesity in African-American families. Am J Respir Crit Care Med 2004;169: 1314–1321.
235. Erdamar B, Suoglu Y, Cuhadaroglu C, Katircioglu S, Guven M: Evaluation of clinical parameters in patients with obstructive sleep apnea and possible correlation with the severity of the disease. Eur Arch Otorhinolaryngol 2001;258:492–495.
236. Li AM, Wong E, Kew J, Hui S, Fok TF: Use of tonsil size in the evaluation of obstructive sleep apnoea. Arch Dis Child 2002;87:156–159.
237. D'Andrea LA: Diagnostic studies in the assessment of pediatric sleep-disordered breathing. Techniques and indications. Pediatr Clin North Am 2004;51:169–186.
238. Whiteford L, Fleming P, Henderson AJ: Who should have a sleep study for sleep related breathing disorders? Arch Dis Child 2004;89:851–855.
239. Marcus CL, Omlin KJ, Basinki DJ, Bailey SL, Rachal AB, Von Pechmann WS, Keens TG, Ward SL: Normal polysomnographic values for children and adolescents. Am Rev Respir Dis 1992;146:1235–1239.
240. American Thoracic Society: Cardiorespiratory sleep studies in children. Establishment of normative data and polysomnographic predictors of morbidity. Am J Respir Crit Care Med 1999;160:1381–1387.
241. Kahn A, Dan B, Groswasser J, Franco P, Sottiaux M: Normal sleep architecture in infants and children. J Clin Neurophysiol 1996;13:184–197.
242. Uliel S, Tauman R, Greenfeld M, Sivan Y: Normal polysomnographic respiratory values in children and adolescents. Chest 2004;125:872–878.
243. Crowell DH, Kulp TD, Kapuniai LE, Hunt CE, Brooks LJ, Weese-Mayer DE, Silvestri J, Ward SD, Corwin M, Tinsley L, Peucker M; CHIME Study Group: Infant polysomnography. Reliability and validity of infant arousal assessment. J Clin Neurophysiol 2002;19:469–483.
244. Morielli A, Desjardins D, Brouillette RT: Transcutaneous and end-tidal carbon dioxide pressures should be measured during pediatric polysomnography. Am Rev Respir Dis 1993;148:1599–1604.
245. Quan SF, Goodwin JL, Babar SI, Kaemingk KL, Enright PL, Rosen GM, Fregosi RF, Morgan WJ: Sleep architecture in normal Caucasian and Hispanic children aged 6–11 years recorded during unattended home polysomnography. Experience from the Tucson Children's Assessment of Sleep Apnea Study (TuCASA). Sleep Med 2003;4:13–19.
246. Stores G, Crawford C: Arousal norms for children age 5–16 years based on home polysomnography. Technol Health Care 2000;8:285–290.
247. Rosen CL: Clinical features of obstructive sleep apnea hypoventilation syndrome in otherwise healthy children. Pediatr Pulmonol 1999;27: 403–409.
248. McNamara F, Sullivan CE: Effects of nasal CPAP therapy on respiratory and spontaneous arousals in infants with OSA. J Appl Physiol 1999;87: 889–896.
249. McNamara F, Lijowska AS, Thach BT: Spontaneous arousal activity in infants during NREM and REM sleep. J Physiol 2002;538:263–269.
250. Goh DY, Galster P, Marcus CL: Sleep architecture and respiratory disturbances in children with obstructive sleep apnea. Am J Respir Crit Care Med 2000;162:682–686.
251. Gozal D, Wang M, Pope DW: Objective sleepiness measures in pediatric obstructive sleep apnea. Pediatrics 2001;108:693–697.
252. Tauman R, O'Brien LM, Holbrook CR, Gozal D: Sleep Pressure Score: A new index of sleep disruption in snoring children. Sleep 2004;27:274–278.
253. O'Brien LM, Tauman R, Gozal D: Sleep pressure correlates of cognitive and behavioral morbidity in snoring children. Sleep 2004;27:279–282.
254. Tauman R, O'Brien LM, Holbrook CR, Gozal D: Peripheral arterial tonometry events and EEG arousals in children. Sleep 2004;27:502–506.
255. Katz ES, Lutz J, Black C, Marcus CL: Pulse transit time as a measure of arousal and respiratory effort in children with sleep-disordered breathing. Pediatr Res 2003;53:580–588.
256. Bandla HPR, Gozal D: Dynamic changes in EEG spectra during obstructive apnea in children. Pediatr Pulmonol 2000;29:359–365.
257. Sivan Y, Kornecki A, Schonfeld T: Screening obstructive sleep apnoea syndrome by home videotape recording in children. Eur Respir J 1996;9: 2127–2131.
258. Brouillette RT, Morielli A, Leimanis A, Waters KA, Luciano R, Ducharme FM: Nocturnal pulse oximetry as an abbreviated testing modality for pediatric obstructive sleep apnea. Pediatrics 2000;105:405–412.
259. Nixon GM, Brouillette RT: Diagnostic techniques for obstructive sleep apnoea. Is polysomnography necessary? Paediatr Respir Rev 2002;3: 18–24.
260. Kirk VG, Bohn SG, Flemons WW, Remmers JE: Comparison of home oximetry monitoring with laboratory polysomnography in children. Chest 2003;124:1702–1708.
261. Nixon GM, Kermack AS, Davis GM, Manoukian JJ, Brown KA, Brouillette RT: Planning adenotonsillectomy in children with obstructive sleep apnea. The role of overnight oximetry. Pediatrics 2004;113:e19–e25.
262. Shouldice R, O'Brien LM, O'Brien C, de Chazal P, Gozal D, Heneghan C: Detection of obstructive sleep apnea in pediatric subjects using surface lead electrocardiogram features. Sleep 2004;27:784–792.
263. Marcus CL, Carroll JL, Koerner CB, Hamer A, Lutz J, Loughlin GM: Determinants of growth in children with the obstructive sleep apnea syndrome. J Pediatr 1994;125:556–562.
264. Bland RM, Bulgarelli S, Ventham JC, Jackson D, Reilly JJ, Paton JY: Total energy expenditure in children with obstructive sleep apnoea syndrome. Eur Resp J 2001;18:164–169.
265. Waters KA, Kirjavainen T, Jimenez M, Cowell CT, Sillence DO, Sullivan CE: Overnight growth hormone secretion in achondroplasia. Deconvolution analysis, correlation with sleep state, and changes after treatment of obstructive sleep apnea. Pediatr Res 1996;39:547–553.

266. Bar A, Tarasiuk A, Segev Y, Phillip M, Tal A: The effect of adenotonsillectomy on serum insulin-like growth factor-I and growth in children with obstructive sleep apnea syndrome. J Pediatr 1999;135:76–80.
267. Soultan Z, Wadowski S, Rao M, Kravath RE: Effect of treating obstructive sleep apnea by tonsillectomy and/or adeniodectomy on obesity in children. Arch Pediatr Adolesc Med 1999;153:33–37.
268. Shiomi T, Guilleminault C, Stoohs R, Schnittger I: Obstructed breathing in children during sleep monitored by echocardiography. Acta Paediatr 1993;82:863–871.
269. Amin RS, Daniels S, Kimball T, Willging P, Cotton R: Echocardiographic changes in children with obstructive sleep apnea. Sleep 2000;23:A99.
270. Tal A, Leiberman A, Margulis G, Sofer S: Ventricular dysfunction in children with obstructive sleep apnea. Radionuclide assessment. Pediatr Pulmonol 1988;4:139–143.
271. Amin RS, Kimball TR, Bean JA, Jeffries JL, Willging JP, Cotton RT, Witt SA, Glascock BJ, Daniels SR: Left ventricular hypertrophy and abnormal ventricular geometry in children and adolescents with obstructive sleep apnea. Am J Respir Crit Care Med 2002;165:1395–1399.
272. Fletcher EC, Bao G: Effect of episodic eucapnic and hypocapnic hypoxia on systemic blood pressure in hypertension-prone rats. J Appl Physiol 1996;81:2088–2094.
273. Aljadeff G, Gozal D, Schechtman VL, Burrell B, Harper RM, Ward SL: Heart rate variability in children with obstructive sleep apnea. Sleep 1997; 20:151–157.
274. Baharav A, Kotagal S, Rubin BK, Pratt J, Akselrod S: Autonomic cardiovascular control in children with obstructive sleep apnea. Clin Auton Res 1999;9:345–351.
275. Marcus CL, Greene MG, Carroll JL: Blood pressure in children with obstructive sleep apnea. Am J Respir Crit Care Med 1998;157:1098–1103.
276. Amin RS, Carroll JL, Jeffries JL, Grone C, Bean JA, Chini B, Bokulic R, Daniels SR: Twenty-four-hour ambulatory blood pressure in children with sleep-disordered breathing. Am J Respir Crit Care Med 2004;169:950–956.
277. Enright PL, Goodwin JL, Sherrill DL, Quan JR, Quan SF; Tucson Children's Assessment of Sleep Apnea study: Blood pressure elevation associated with sleep-related breathing disorder in a community sample of white and Hispanic children. The Tucson Children's Assessment of Sleep Apnea study. Arch Pediatr Adolesc Med 2003;157:901–904.
278. Tahawi Z, Orolinova N, Joshua IG, Bader M, Fletcher EC: Altered vascular reactivity in arterioles of chronic intermittent hypoxic rats. J Appl Physiol 2001;90:2007–2013.
279. Kraiczi H, Caidahl K, Samuelsson A, Peker Y, Hedner J: Impairment of vascular endothelial function and left ventricular filling. Association with the severity of apnea-induced hypoxemia during sleep. Chest 2001;119: 1085–1091.
280. Soukhova GK, Roberts AM, Lipton AJ, Gozal E, Gozal D: Early postnatal exposure to intermittent hypoxia attenuates baroreflex sensitivity in adult rats. Sleep 2002;25:A335.
281. Hill W: On some causes of backwardness and stupidity in children. And the relief of the symptoms in some instances by nasopharyngeal scarifications. BMJ 1889;II:711–712.
282. Weissbluth M, Davis A, Poncher J, Reiff J: Signs of airway obstruction during sleep and behavioral, developmental and academic problems. Dev Behav Pediatr 1983;4:119–121.
283. Gozal D: Sleep-disordered breathing and school performance in children. Pediatrics 1998;102:616–620.
284. Ali NJ, Pitson D, Stradling JR: Sleep disordered breathing. Effects of adenotonsillectomy on behaviour and psychological functioning. Eur J Pediatr 1996;155:56–62.
285. Urschitz MS, Eitner S, Guenther A, Eggebrecht E, Wolff J, Urschitz-Duprat PM, Schlaud M, Poets CF: Habitual snoring, intermittent hypoxia, and impaired behavior in primary school children. Pediatrics 2004;114:1041–1048.
286. Chervin R, Dillon J, Bassetti C, Ganoczy D, Pituch K: Symptoms of sleep disorders, inattention, and hyperactivity in children. Sleep 1997;20:1185–1192.
287. Rosen CL, Storfer-Isser A, Taylor HG, Kirchner HL, Emancipator JL, Redline S: Increased behavioral morbidity in school-aged children with sleep-disordered breathing. Pediatrics 2004;114:1640–1648.
288. Guilleminault C, Winkle R, Korobkin R, Simmons B: Children and nocturnal snoring—evaluation of the effects of sleep related respiratory resistive load and daytime functioning. Eur J Pediatr 1982;139:165–171.
289. Owens J, Opipari L, Nobile C, Spirito A: Sleep and daytime behavior in children with obstructive sleep apnea and behavioral sleep disorders. Pediatrics 1998;102:1178–1174.
290. LeBourgeois MK, Avis K, Mixon M, Olmi J, Harsh J: Snoring, sleep quality, and sleepiness across attention-deficit/hyperactivity disorder subtypes. Sleep 2004;27:520–525.
291. Melendres MC, Lutz JM, Rubin ED, Marcus CL: Daytime sleepiness and hyperactivity in children with suspected sleep-disordered breathing. Pediatrics 2004;114:768–775.
292. Montgomery-Downs HE, Jones VF, Molfese V, Gozal D: Snoring in preschoolers. Potential associations with sleepiness, ethnicity, and learning. Clin Pediatr 2003;42:719–726.
293. Kaemingk KL, Pasvogel AE, Goodwin JL, Mulvaney SA, Martinez F, Enright PL, Rosen GM, Morgan WJ, Fregosi RF, Quan SF: Learning in children and sleep disordered breathing. Findings of the Tucson Children's Assessment of Sleep Apnea (TuCASA) prospective cohort study. J Int Neuropsychol Soc 2003;9:1016–1026.
294. Gottlieb DJ, Vezina RM, Chase C, Lesko SM, Heeren TC, Weese-Mayer DE, Auerbach SH, Corwin MJ: Symptoms of sleep-disordered breathing in 5-year-old children are associated with sleepiness and problem behaviors. Pediatrics 2003;112:870–877.
295. O'Brien LM, Mervis CB, Holbrook CR, Bruner JL, Smith NH, McNally N, McClimment MC, Gozal D: Neurobehavioral correlates of sleep disordered breathing in children. J Sleep Res 2004;13:165–172.
296. O'Brien LM, Mervis CB, Holbrook CR, Bruner JL, Klaus CJ, Rutherford J, Raffield TJ, Gozal D: Neurobehavioral implications of habitual snoring in children. Pediatrics 2004;114:44–49.
297. Beebe DW, Gozal D: Obstructive sleep apnea and the prefrontal cortex. Towards a comprehensive model linking nocturnal upper airway dysfunction to daytime cognitive and behavioral deficits. J Sleep Res 2002;11:1–16.
298. Bass JL, Corwin M, Gozal D, Moore C, Nishida H, Parker S, Schonwald A, Wilker RE, Stehle S, Kinane TB: The effect of chronic or intermittent hypoxia on cognition in childhood. A review of the evidence. Pediatrics 2004;114:805–816.
299. Friedman BC, Hendeles-Amitai A, Kozminsky E, Leiberman A, Friger M, Tarasiuk A, Tal A: Adenotonsillectomy improves neurocognitive function in children with obstructive sleep apnea syndrome. Sleep 2003;26:999–1005.
300. Avior G, Fishman G, Leor A, Sivan Y, Kaysar N, Derowe A: The effect of tonsillectomy and adenoidectomy on inattention and impulsivity as measured by the Test of Variables of Attention (TOVA) in children with obstructive sleep apnea syndrome. Otolaryngol Head Neck Surg 2004; 131:367–371.
301. Montgomery-Downs HE, Crabtree VM, Gozal D: Changes in cognitive functions, sleep, and breathing characteristics following adenotonsillectomy in at-risk preschool children with obstructive sleep apnea. Eur J Resp Dis 2005;25:336–342.
302. Gozal D, Pope DW Jr: Snoring during early childhood and academic performance at ages 13–14 years. Pediatrics 2001;107:1394–1399.
303. Gozal D, Daniel JM, Dohanich GP: Behavioral and anatomical correlates of chronic episodic hypoxia during sleep in the rat. J Neurosci 2001;21: 2442–2450.
304. Gozal E, Row BW, Schurr A, Gozal D: Developmental differences in cortical and hippocampal vulnerability to intermittent hypoxia in the rat. Neurosci Lett 2001;305:197–201.
305. Row BW, Kheirandish L, Neville JJ, Gozal D: Impaired spatial learning and hyperactivity in developing rats exposed to intermittent hypoxia. Pediatr Res 2002;52:449–453.
306. Friedlander SL, Larkin EK, Rosen CL, Palermo TM, Redline S: Decreased quality of life associated with obesity in school-aged children. Arch Pediatr Adolesc Med 2003;157:1206–1211.
307. Rosen CL, Palermo TM, Larkin EK, Redline S: Health-related quality of life and sleep-disordered breathing in children. Sleep 2002;25:657–666.
308. Crabtree V, Varni JW, Gozal D: Quality of life and depressive symptoms in children with suspected sleep-disordered breathing. Sleep 2004;27: 1131–1138.
309. Brooks LJ, Topol HI: Enuresis in children with sleep apnea. J Pediatr 2003;142:515–518.
310. Reuveni H, Simon T, Tal A, Elhayany A, Tarasiuk A: Health care services utilization in children with obstructive sleep apnea syndrome. Pediatrics 2002;110:68–72.
311. Tarasiuk A, Simon T, Tal A, Reuveni H: Adenotonsillectomy in children with obstructive sleep apnea syndrome reduces health care utilization. Pediatrics 2004;113:351–356.
312. Lipton AJ, Gozal D: Treatment of obstructive sleep apnea in children. Do we really know how? Sleep Med Rev 2003;7:61–80.
313. Guilleminault C, Li K, Quo S, Inouye RN: A prospective study on the surgical outcomes of children with sleep-disordered breathing. Sleep 2004; 27:95–100.
314. Tauman R, Montgomery-Downs HE, Ivanenko A, O'Brien LM, Krishna J, Barnes ME, Gozal D: Changes in sleep architecture and respiratory function following adenotonsillectomy in children with obstructive sleep apnea syndrome [abstract]. Sleep 2004:A176.

315. McColley SA, April MM, Carroll JL, Naclerio RM, Loughlin GM: Respiratory compromise after adenotonsillectomy in children with obstructive sleep apnea. Arch Otolaryngol Head Neck Surg 1992;118: 940–943.
316. Rosen GM, Muckle RP, Mahowald MW, Goding GS, Ullevig C: Postoperative respiratory compromise in children with obstructive sleep apnea syndrome. Can it be anticipated? Pediatrics 1994;93:784–788.
317. Gerber ME, O'Connor DM, Adler E, Myer CM III: Selected risk factors in pediatric adenotonsillectomy. Arch Otolaryngol Head Neck Surg 1996;122:811–814.
318. Lalakea ML, Marquez-Biggs I, Messner AH: Safety of pediatric short-stay tonsillectomy. Arch Otolaryngol Head Neck Surg 1999;125:749–752.
319. Brown KA, Morin I, Hickey C, Manoukian JJ, Nixon GM, Brouillette RT: Urgent adenotonsillectomy. An analysis of risk factors associated with postoperative respiratory morbidity. Anesthesiology 2003;99:586–695.
320. Marcus CL, Ward SL, Mallory GB, Rosen CL, Beckerman RC, Weese-Mayer DE, Brouillette RT, Trang HT, Brooks LJ: Use of nasal continuous positive airway pressure as treatment of childhood obstructive sleep apnea. J Pediatr 1995;127:88–94.
321. Tirosh E, Tal Y, Jaffe M: CPAP treatment of obstructive sleep apnoea and neurodevelopmental deficits. Acta Paediatr 1995;84:791–794.
322. Waters KA, Everett FM, Bruderer JW, Sullivan CE: Obstructive sleep apnea. The use of nasal CPAP in 80 children. Am J Respir Crit Care Med 1995;152:780–785.
323. Rains JC: Treatment of obstructive sleep apnea in pediatric patients. Behavioral intervention for compliance with nasal continuous positive airway pressure. Clin Pediatr (Phila) 1995;34:535–541.
324. Massa F, Gonsalez S, Laverty A, Wallis C, Lane R: The use of nasal continuous positive airway pressure to treat obstructive sleep apnoea. Arch Dis Child 2002;87:438–443.
325. McNamara F, Sullivan CE: Obstructive sleep apnea in infants and its management with nasal continuous positive airway pressure. Chest 1999; 116:10–16.
326. Downey R III, Perkin RM, MacQuarrie J: Nasal continuous positive airway pressure use in children with obstructive sleep apnea younger than 2 years of age. Chest 2000;117:1608–1612.
327. Palombini L, Pelayo R, Guilleminault C: Efficacy of automated continuous positive airway pressure in children with sleep-related breathing disorders in an attended setting. Pediatrics 2004;113:e412–e417.
328. Koontz KL, Slifer KJ, Cataldo MD, Marcus CL: Improving pediatric compliance with positive airway pressure therapy. The impact of behavioral intervention. Sleep 2003;26:1010–1015.
329. Marcus CL, Carroll JL, Bamford O, Pyzik P, Loughlin GM: Supplemental oxygen during sleep in children with sleep-disordered breathing. Am J Respir Crit Care Med 1995;152:1297–1301.
330. Aljadeff G, Gozal D, Bailey-Wahl SL, Burrell B, Keens TG, Davidson Ward SL: Effect of overnight supplemental oxygen in obstructive sleep apnea in children. Am J Respir Crit Care Med 1996;153:51–55.
331. Brouillette RT, Manoukian JJ, Ducharme FM, Oudjhane K, Earle LG, Ladan S, Morielli A: Efficacy of fluticasone nasal spray for pediatric obstructive sleep apnea. J Pediatr 2001;138:838–844.
332. Alexopoulos EI, Kaditis AG, Kalampouka E, Kostadima E, Angelopoulos NV, Mikraki V, Skenteris N, Gourgoulianis K: Nasal corticosteroids for children with snoring. Pediatr Pulmonol 2004;38:161–167.
333. Goldbart AD, Goldman JL, Li RC, Tauman R, Brittian KR, Gozal D: Leukotriene receptors and inflammatory markers in tonsils of children with sleep apnea and recurrent infection [abstract]. Am J Respir Crit Care Med 2004;.
334. Goldbart AD, Goldman JL, Veling MC, Gozal D: Leukotriene modifier therapy for adenotonsillar hypertrophy and sleep disordered breathing in children. Am J Resp Crit Care Med 2005;172:364–370.
335. Kheirandish L, Goldbart AD, Gozal D: Intranasal steroids and oral leukotriene modifier therapy in residual sleep-disordered breathing following tonsillectomy and adenoidectomy in children. Pediatrics 2005 (in press).

Index

Note: Page numbers followed by f indicate figures; t, tables; b, boxes.

B

C

D

E

F

G

H

I

J

K

L

M

N

O

P

Q

R

S

T

U

V

W

X

Y

Z